Principles and Practice of

Echocardiography

PRINCIPLES AND PRACTICE OF

ECHOCARDIOGRAPHY

ARTHUR E. WEYMAN, M.D.

Associate Professor of Medicine
Harvard Medical School
Director, Cardiac Ultrasound Laboratories
Massachusetts General Hospital
Boston, Massachusetts

SECOND EDITION

Lea & Febiger

PHILADELPHIA • BALTIMORE • HONG KONG
LONDON • MUNICH • SYDNEY • TOKYO

A WAVERLY COMPANY
1994

Lea & Febiger
Box 3024
200 Chester Field Parkway
Malvern, Pennsylvania 19355-9725
U.S.A.
(215) 251-2230

Executive Editor—R. Kenneth Bussy
Development Editor—Tanya Lazar
Project Editor—Fran Klass
Production Manager—Thomas J. Colaiezzi

NOTE: Although the author(s) and the publisher have taken reasonable steps to ensure the accuracy of the drug information included in this text before publication, drug information may change without notice and readers are advised to consult the manufacturer's packaging inserts before prescribing medications.

First Edition, 1982
Reprinted, 1982, 1983
Second Edition, 1994

Library of Congress Cataloging-in-Publication Data

Weyman, Arthur E.
Principles and practice of echocardiography / Arthur E. Weyman. — 2nd ed.
p. cm.
Rev. ed. of: Cross-sectional echocardiography. 1982.
Includes bibliographical references and index.
ISBN 0-8121-1207-5
1. Echocardiography. I. Weyman, Arthur E. Cross-sectional echocardiography. II. Title.
[DNLM: 1. Echocardiography. WG 141.5.E2 W549p]
RC683.5.U5W49 1991
616.1'207543—dc20
DNLM/DLC
for Library of Congress 90-13578
CIP

Reprints of chapters may be purchased from Lea & Febiger in quantities of 100 or more. Contact Sally Grande in the Sales Department.

PRINTED IN THE UNITED STATES OF AMERICA

Print Number: 5 4 3 2 1

For Jean

Preface

In the years following publication of CROSS-SECTIONAL ECHOCARDIOGRAPHY, the field of cardiac ultrasound has undergone numerous and dramatic changes, with the growing importance and application of spectral Doppler and Doppler color flow mapping, as well as the new techniques of transesophageal and intravascular imaging. The need to integrate these new techniques in a way that would provide a unified and organized approach to any cardiovascular ultrasound study induced me to undertake the task of producing a second edition.

Although the vast majority of the text is new, the underlying principle remains unchanged: *echocardiography if fully understood can go far beyond simple clinical observation and provide unique quantitative information for clinical and research applications*. The first half of the text stresses the basic principles of image acquisition, Doppler sampling, and blood flow. I continue to feel that this is the most important section in the book, particularly those chapters that deal with the principles of image acquisition (4 and 5), Doppler flow recording (13), M-mode echocardiography (14), and transesophageal echocardiography (16). Although many people can be taught to interpret a high-quality echocardiographic study, far fewer can consistently record high-quality cross-sectional images and Doppler tracings in the heterogeneous patient population encountered routinely in the clinical laboratory. Without this ability, however, one will always be limited by the talents of those with whom one works and may fail to appreciate the effort often involved in acquiring a technically difficult study, or the superb achievement of the true artist. Obviously it is impossible to convey or teach a technical skill in a book. This section, therefore, approaches the examination from a conceptual viewpoint and, will, I hope, allow the reader to appreciate, at least in theory, the steps necessary to produce consistent images of optimal quality. The extensive consideration of basic principles in the remaining chapters of this section is based on my firm conviction that one needs to understand the operation of his tools thoroughly in order to use them wisely and to greatest effect.

The second half of this book deals with the clinical applications of imaging and Doppler echocardiography. I have organized and written this section from the perspective that cross-sectional echocardiography displays "functional anatomy." The individual chapters generally follow the path of blood flow through the left and right sides of the heart. The relative echocardiographic importance of individual structures further influences the order in which they are considered in each chapter. I have attempted in these chapters to describe both the functional and pathological anatomy of different structures and lesions in sufficient detail that the examiner can anticipate the principal anatomic variations that may be encountered. This is done in the hope that the greater the level of understanding, the less the reliance on pattern recognition.

Since over 25,000 references dealing with various applications of echo-Doppler methods are now available it was neither practical nor necessary to include all. Although I tried to recognize as many original contributions and major amplifications as possible, undoubtedly some important citations have been overlooked or underappreciated, for which I apologize. My goal is to be complete but not necessarily exhaustive. In areas of controversy I have tried to include all sides, explain differences, or offer some alternatives. In areas where present capabilities are less than ideal, I have described promising but not always proven alternatives. In reviewing the page proofs, I wished I had included more topics, but I feel that the sheer volume of the book precludes their incorporation.

The maturity of the field of echocardiography is reflected in the need to integrate clinical information with the principles of cardiovascular physiology, basic fluid mechanics, physical acoustics, materials science, digital data processing, and computer science. This maturity and increasing scope are also reflected in the fact that this book, although written primarily by one author, now includes additional contributors. I am indeed grateful for the support and input of many individuals who helped make this book possible. In particular I am indebted to my colleagues Robert Levine, James Thomas, Michael Picard, and Mary Etta King. The 6-year period during which this group was together was the most exciting of my career thus far. One learns most from his trainees and associates, and I can honestly say that I have never learned more than during this time. The imprint of these physicians is apparent throughout this book. Bob Levine's creativity and insight are particularly evident in the sections on the myopathies, mitral valve prolapse, and flow quantitation. The expertise in mathematics and computer modeling of Jim Thomas and his unique ability to apply these tools to illuminate questions of clinical relevance are found throughout the text, but particularly in the sections on fluid dynamics, digital image processing, and diastolic function. Mary Etta King's clarity of thought and skill as a teacher provide much of the foundation for the section on congenital heart disease. Mike Picard's work on the natural history of myocardial infarction and the quantitative effects of tamponade on Doppler indices provided important insights in writing these chapters. Although each played his or her own role, it was the complementarity of talent, creativity, drive, sense of competition, and personality that made this group unique.

Many others must also be recognized for their contributions, including: Chris Choong, who began our interest in diastolic function and who initially described the effects of loading on the Doppler mitral inflow profile; Bill Stewart and Kathy Ascah, whose work on the quantitation of volumetric flow by Doppler laid the foundation for the chapter on that subject; John O'Shea, who initiated our transesophageal echo program, and Brian Griffin, who continued this work; Sanjiv Kaul, who began his work on contrast echocardiography here and has gone on to become a leader in the field; David Guyer, who began our work on infarct mapping; Linda Gillam, who was at the head of the line and helped refine many of our methods of wall motion analysis; and the many other research fellows and staff whose creativity and effort are evident throughout the text. I would also like to thank Drs. Leng Jiang and Vivian Abascal for their numerous contributions of well-selected illustrations that have considerably enhanced the impact and teaching value of the text material; John Newell for the invaluable computational and statistical guidance he has provided for years; Luis Guerrero for his expertise in creating the experimental models from which much of our data is derived; my assistant Melissa Fox for her invaluable efforts in typing, compiling and editing this text; and the outstanding technical staff—Jane Marshall, Licia Mueller, Mark Adams, Kathy Fleming, Pamela Harrington, Jian Kang, Barbara Jones, Talbot Joziatis, Carlene McClanahan, Barbara McDade, Eleanor Morris, Susie Novick, Marc Roy, Claire Reilly, and MC Clark—with whom I have had the pleasure to work over the past decade and whose diligence and commitment to excellence are the foundation of this effort. Many others not specifically named contributed by proofreading, discussing ideas, providing data and illustrations or just being generally supportive. I am especially grateful to my family, Jean, Jenny, Shannon, Robert and Elizabeth, for their patience and continued encouragement throughout the writing of this book. Virtually all of the time spent on this effort was taken away from family activities, and despite this, they were always fully supportive, or at least tolerant. Apologies for time lost are a bit hollow—no one spends five years on something he really doesn't want to do. Perhaps a college education will help. I would also like to thank Mrs. Tina Rice, who has kept us all going for a long time.

I also express my appreciation to Dr. Edgar Haber for his support of our early efforts in establishing a group of bright and committed young echocardiographers in an environment of scientific excellence; to Dr. Roman DeSanctis for his friendship, counsel, and example; and to Dr. Valentin Fuster, for giving me the invaluable gift of time to finish this project when the last hurdle seemed insurmountable.

Finally, I trust that the effort of writing this book, which has occupied the majority of my time over the past years, will be rewarded by the increased understanding of its readers and their ability to apply the techniques of echocardiography for maximal patient benefit and generation of new knowledge.

Boston, Massachusetts Arthur E. Weyman

Contributors

Vivian M. Abascal, M.D.
Fellow in Cardiology
University Hospital and Boston City Hospital
Boston University School of Medicine
Boston, Massachusetts

Jayashri R. Aragam, M.D.
Staff Cardiologist
Fallon Clinic
Assistant Professor of Medicine
University of Massachusetts Medical School
Worcester, Massachusetts

Edward G. Cape, Ph.D.
Assistant Professor
Schools of Medicine and Engineering
University of Pittsburgh
Children's Hospital of Pittsburgh
Pittsburgh, Pennsylvania

Christopher Y.P. Choong, M.A.(Cantab.), M.B.B.Chir.(Cantab.), Ph.D., F.R.A.C.P., F.A.C.C., D.D.U.
Senior Staff Cardiologist
Director of Echocardiography Laboratory
Royal North Shore Hospital
Sydney, Australia

Ravin Davidoff, M.B., B.Ch.
Director, Echocardiography Laboratory
Boston University Medical Center/The University Hospital
Assistant Professor of Medicine
Boston University School of Medicine
Boston, Massachusetts

Annmarie Errichetti, M.D.
Assistant Professor of Medicine
University of Massachusetts Medical School
Director, Noninvasive Cardiology Laboratory
Medical Center of Central Massachusetts
Worcester, Massachusetts

Frank A. Flachskampf, M.D.
Med. Klinik I, RWTH Aachen
Aachen, Germany

Thomas L. Force, M.D.
Assistant Professor of Medicine
Harvard University
Cardiac Unit, Massachusetts General Hospital
Boston, Massachusetts

Brian P. Griffin, M.D.
Associate Staff Cardiologist
The Cleveland Clinic Foundation
Cleveland, Ohio

Mark D. Handschumacher
Senior Applications Program Analyst
Cardiac Unit
Massachusetts General Hospital
Boston, Massachusetts

Pamela Harrigan, R.D.C.S.
Director, Programs in Cardiac Ultrasound
School of Echocardiography
Hanson, Massachusetts

Leng Jiang, M.D.
Professor of Medicine
Shanghai Institute of Cardiovascular Diseases
Zhong-Shan Hospital
Shanghai Medical University
Senior Research Fellow in Medicine
Massachusetts General Hospital
Harvard University
Boston, Massachusetts

Sanjiv Kaul, M.D.
Professor of Medicine
Director, Cardiac Imaging Center
University of Virginia
Charlottesville, Virginia

Mary Etta E. King, M.D.
Associate Pediatrician, Children's Service
Director, Pediatric Echocardiography
Massachusetts General Hospital
Assistant Professor of Pediatrics
Harvard Medical School
Boston, Massachusetts

Robert A. Levine, M.D.
Assistant Professor of Medicine
Harvard Medical School
Staff Physician
Cardiac Ultrasound Laboratory
Massachusetts General Hospital
Boston, Massachusetts

Jane E. Marshall, B.S., R.D.C.S.
Technical Director
Cardiac Ultrasound Laboratory
Massachusetts General Hospital
Boston, Massachusetts

Shane A. Marshall, M.D., F.R.C.P.
Director, Cardiac Ultrasound Laboratory
King Edward VII Hospital
Paget, Bermuda

Stefan Mark Nidorf, M.D., M.B.B.S., F.R.A.C.P.
Instructor in Medicine
Harvard Medical School
Boston, Massachusetts

Justin Pearlman, M.D., Ph.D.
Assistant Professor
Harvard Medical School
Boston, Massachusetts
Assistant Professor
Department of Health Sciences and Technology
Massachusetts Institute of Technology
Cambridge, Massachusetts

Michael H. Picard, M.D.
Assistant Professor of Medicine
Harvard Medical School
Assistant in Medicine
Massachusetts General Hospital
Boston, Massachusetts

Anthony J. Sanfilippo, M.D.
Assistant Professor of Medicine
Queen's University
Attending Cardiologist and Director of Echocardiography
Hotel Dieu Hospital
Kingston, Ontario, Canada

Samuel C. Siu, M.D.
Staff Cardiologist
The Toronto Hospital
Assistant Professor of Medicine
University of Toronto
Toronto, Ontario, Canada

James D. Thomas, M.D., F.A.C.C.
Director of Cardiovascular Imaging
Department of Cardiology
Cleveland Clinic Foundation
Cleveland, Ohio

Wendy A. Thoreau, M.D., M.B., B.S., F.R.A.C.P.
Consultant Cardiologist
Mater Hospital
Pimlico, Australia
Townsville General Hospital
Townsville, Australia

Pieter M. Vandervoort
Clinical and Research Fellow in Medicine
Massachusetts General Hospital
Research Fellow in Medicine
Harvard Medical School
Boston, Massachusetts

Cedric Vuille, M.D.
Clinical and Research Fellow
Cardiac Ultrasound Laboratories
Massachusetts General Hospital
Research Fellow in Medicine
Harvard Medical School
Boston, Massachusetts

Arthur E. Weyman, M.D.
Associate Professor of Medicine
Harvard Medical School
Director, Cardiac Ultrasound Laboratories
Massachusetts General Hospital
Boston, Massachusetts

Susan E. Wiegers, M.D.
Assistant Professor of Medicine
University of Pennsylvania
Acting Director, Echocardiography Laboratory
Hospital of the University of Pennsylvania
Philadelphia, Pennsylvania

Gerard Thomas Wilkins, M.B., Ch.B., F.R.A.C.P.
Senior Lecturer in Medicine
Consultant Cardiologist
Dunedin Hospital
Otago Medical School
Dunedin, New Zealand

Contents

Part 2 CLINICAL APPLICATIONS

PART I

Physical Principles, Instrumentation, and Routine Examination

CHAPTER

1

PHYSICAL PRINCIPLES OF ULTRASOUND

Sound is a mechanical vibration in a physical medium, such as air or water; when it stimulates the auditory apparatus, it produces the sensation of hearing.[1] Sound is classified as infrasound, audible sound, and ultrasound, based on its rapidity of vibration or frequency. Ultrasound is sound with a frequency higher than the audible range for humans or greater than 20,000 cycles per second. The acoustic laws that govern the behavior of low frequency sound (audible sound) also apply to ultrasound. Ultrasound, however, can capitalize on properties that are not so apparent at lower frequencies (because of the relatively large wavelength-to-object-size relationship). These properties make ultrasound particularly useful in clinical medicine. Most significantly, ultrasound can be beamed in a particular direction and is reflected by relatively small objects (in the millimeter and submillimeter range).[2] The use of ultrasound in cardiac diagnosis is termed *echocardiography*.[3]

Historically, echocardiography can be traced to the demonstration by the Curie brothers in 1880 that a suitably cut plate of quartz, when subjected to a mechanical stress, develops electrical charges on its surface (Fig. 1–1).[4] This production of electrical energy, or voltage, by the application of a mechanical stress to a crystal is known as the *piezoelectric* or *pressure electric effect*.

The following year (1881), the same observers noted the converse of this principle; specifically, when a piezoelectric crystal is appropriately placed in an alternating electric field, it rapidly changes shape or is thrown into vibration in a characteristic fashion (Fig. 1–1). These basic principles of piezoelectricity—the transformation of electrical energy into mechanical energy and the subsequent transformation of mechanical energy into electrical energy—form the basis for all ultrasonic cardiac studies.

Figure 1–2 illustrates, in simplified form, the application of these principles in clinical echocardiography. Initially, a piezoelectric crystal or transducer is briefly subjected to a rapidly alternating electrical voltage. This alternating pulse shock excites the crystal, thereby causing it to change shape rapidly or to vibrate (Fig. 1–2A). As the crystal vibrates, it produces alternating areas of rarefaction and condensation of the molecules in the surrounding medium, which are, in effect, sound waves.[5] Once produced, these vibrations, or sound waves, are

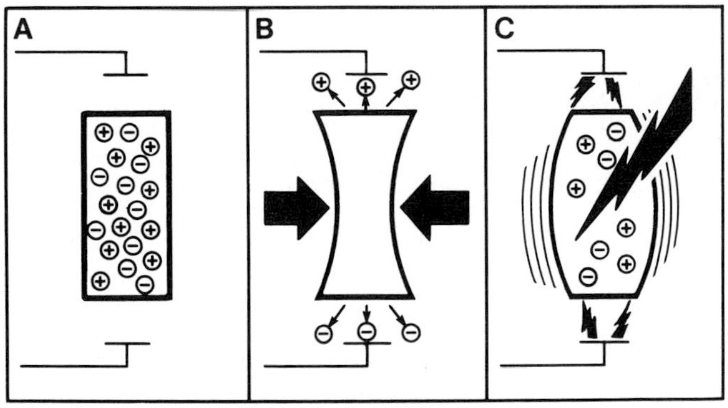

Fig. 1–1. The principles of piezoelectricity. **A.** A quiescent rectangular polar crystal is positioned between two electrodes. **B.** An external stress is applied, thereby deforming the crystal. This mechanical stress causes electrical charges bound within the crystal to shift to the surface, where they can be measured as a voltage. **C.** An electrical current is applied to the crystal. The interaction of this external electrical field with the charges in the ionic lattice of the crystal alters the crystal's shape. When the electric field is rapidly alternated, the crystal is thrown into a correspondingly rapid vibration, which produces a sound wave of like frequency.

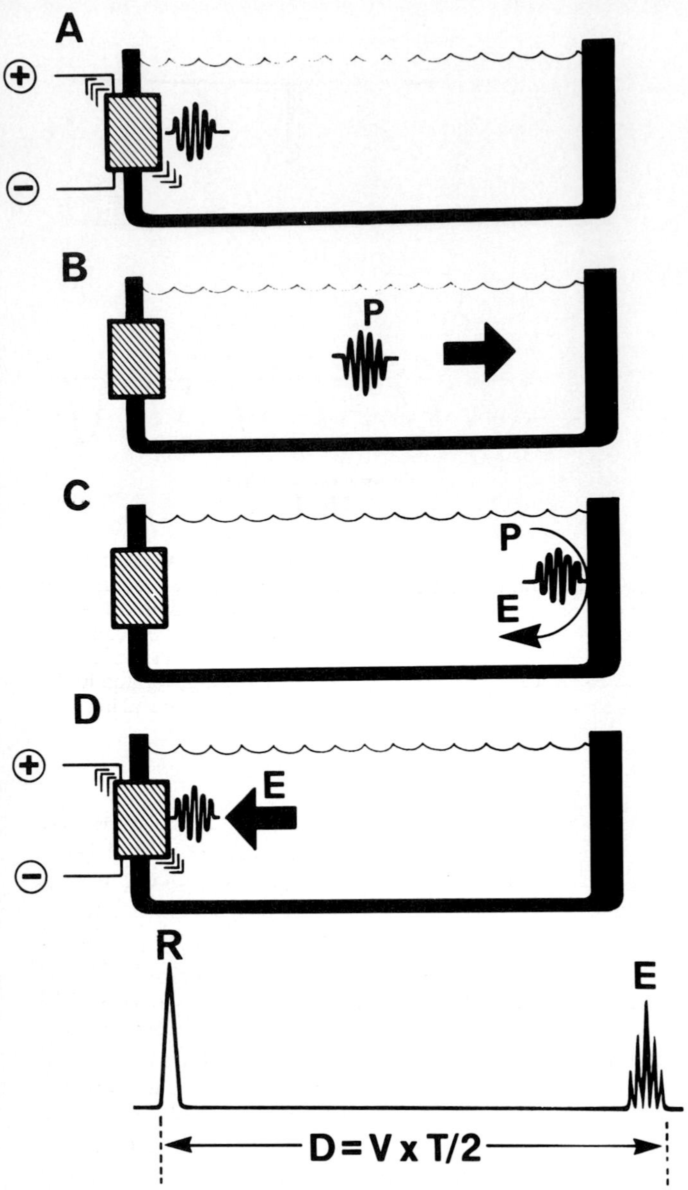

Fig. 1–2. A to D. The basic principles of echocardiographic imaging. R = reference spike indicating transducer position; P = transmitted pulse; E = echo; D = distance from transducer to reflector; V = velocity or speed of sound in that particular medium; T = time from pulse transmission to echo return. Because the distance of the target from the transducer is only one half of the total distance that the sound pulse must travel, the equation is divided by 2. (See text for details.)

propagated into the surrounding medium at a rate proportional to the speed of sound in that particular medium (Fig. 1–2B), until a reflecting interface is encountered (Fig. 1–2C). At this point, a portion of the sound energy is reflected back toward the transducer.[6] When the returning sound energy, or echo, strikes the now quiescent transducer element, the sound energy produces stresses within the crystal that cause electrical charges to form on its surface (Fig. 1–2D). By measuring the strength of the electrical charge reflected as a voltage, one can determine the amount of stress applied to the crystal and, hence, the amount of returning acoustic energy or echo strength. In addition, if one knows the speed of sound in that particular medium, by measuring the time taken for the sound pulse to travel from the transducer to the structure in question and return, one can calculate the total distance traveled by the pulse using the simple relationship:

$$D = V \times T \qquad [1.1]$$

where D is the distance traveled, V is the speed of sound, and T is the time of flight. Because the distance from the transducer to the reflecting interface is only one-half the total distance traversed by the sound wave (which must travel from the transducer to the reflecting target and back), one can divide the distance by two or use half the speed of sound in the equation (as is done in most commercial echographs), thereby making possible the direct determination and appropriate display of the distance of the reflector or target from the transducer.[6]

Multiple factors may contribute to the character of the transmitted and returning ultrasonic pulse and, as a result, to the derived echocardiographic data. These factors include (1) the properties of sound itself that govern its formation and transmission; (2) the specific characteristics of ultrasound that distinguish it from low frequency sound and facilitate its use in cardiac diagnosis; (3) the spatial configuration of the ultrasonic beam, which defines the area of the heart through which the ultrasonic energy passes and, hence, the area that can be illuminated and visualized; (4) the properties of the medium through which the sound passes and the interfaces or targets encountered that affect the intensity of the sound energy and the amplitude of the returning echoes; (5) the piezoelectric element or transducer, which determines the character of the generated ultrasonic pulse as well as the shape of the ultrasonic beam; and finally (6), the types of echo amplification and display that govern the properties of the final recording. Each of these elements contributes to the final ultrasonic output and, hence, is worthy of consideration.[6]

PROPERTIES OF SOUND

Sound travels through a medium in the form of a propagating wave. During the passage of a sound wave, the particles of the medium are thrown into vibrations that are either parallel to the line of propagation (longitudinal waves) or perpendicular to the line of propagation (transverse waves). Although both types of waves occur in solids, only longitudinal waves can be supported in fluids and air. A typical sound wave consists of areas in which the particles of the medium are tightly packed or compressed, alternating with areas in which the particles are spaced relatively farther apart (areas of rarefaction). These areas of particle compression and rarefaction correspond to changes in microscopic pressure within the tissue. Although the passage of a sound wave throws the particles of a medium into oscillation, no net particle motion occurs.[6]

Propagating ultrasonic waves contain energy, E, which is the capacity to perform work (e.g., to raise the temperature of a tissue) and is measured in joules.* In ultrasound the energy associated with the propagating pressure wave is the sum of the kinetic energy of the particle velocity of the tissue as well as the potential energy stored in the compressed or rarefied regions of the propagating wave. As a result, although the components of energy (kinetic and potential) vary, the total energy at any point along the beam path is constant.

Figure 1–3A is an example of a simple sound wave. The characteristics of a sound wave can be expressed graphically as a sine wave (Fig. 1–3B). When depicted in this manner, the height of the sine wave above and below the baseline represents the degree of particle compression and rarefaction, respectively, or the magnitude of the local change in microscopic tissue pressure. The distance between two similar areas along the wave path (e.g., two areas of maximum compression) is termed a *wavelength* (λ). The number of wavelengths per unit time is the frequency of the sound wave. Wavelength and frequency are, therefore, inversely related. Frequency may be expressed either in cycles per second (cps) or in hertz (Hz) (after the German physicist, Heinrich Hertz): 1 cps = 1 Hz; 1000 cps = 1 kilohertz (kHz); and 1,000,000 cps = 1 megahertz (MHz). The number of wavelengths passing a given point in space per unit time (the frequency) multiplied by the wavelength equals the velocity of sound in that medium.

A consideration of our auditory environment provides further understanding of the chief properties of sound waves that are important in echocardiography (i.e., intensity, frequency, and velocity). All sounds have intensity or loudness. A bell or piano key struck lightly produces a soft or low intensity sound. The same sound source struck more forcefully produces a higher intensity or stronger sound (i.e., a greater fluctuation in local pressure). Similarly, in echocardiography, the force or voltage applied to the piezoelectric element determines the amplitude of vibration of the crystal, which in turn, governs the sound pressure and, hence, the intensity of the transmitted pulse.**

The intensity of the transmitted pulse is important for two reasons. First, the amount of reflected energy or echo strength produced at any interface is a percentage of the strength of the ultrasonic wave striking that surface. Thus, if all other elements of a system are constant, the intensity of the transmitted pulse determines the strength of the returning echo. Second, high intensity sound may damage or destroy biologic systems.[7] Although the energy levels used in clinical echocardiography have not, to date, been associated with any recognized toxicity, the effect of sound on biologic tissues is an important consideration and is one of the factors limiting the intensities that may be used clinically.[7] The biologic effects of ultrasound are discussed in more detail later in this chapter.

Again, a consideration of our environment suggests several important characteristics of sound frequency. First, sounds of different frequencies travel at the same speed in the same medium. If one listens to an orchestra, the sounds produced by the high frequency instruments arrive at the ear simultaneously with those produced by the low frequency instruments. If sounds of varying frequencies traveled at different rates, harmony would be impossible. Second, high frequency sounds have a much lower penetration than low frequency sounds. If one stands close to a jet engine, one hears a high frequency, ear piercing whine. Conversely, at a distance from the same engine, only a low roar is audible. The high frequency components in this example are more intense and predominant when one is close to the source of sound, whereas at a greater distance, only the low frequency components are transmitted. In addition, as is considered later in the discussion of resolution, the higher the frequency of the sound wave, the smaller the structures that reflect it without entering the range in which scattering is apparent. Because small, closely spaced structures are examined in echocardiography, this characteristic of frequency is of paramount importance.

Finally, echocardiographic determination of interface location requires knowledge of the velocity or speed of sound. The velocity of sound in any medium depends on the density and elasticity of that medium.[5,6] The elastic constants of a medium are temperature-dependent, and as a result, velocity varies with temperature.[5,6] Because the temperature of the body is maintained within well-defined limits, the effects of temperature on velocity are generally disregarded in clinical echocardiography. In some media, velocity partially depends on the frequency of the sound wave, a phenomenon known as *velocity*

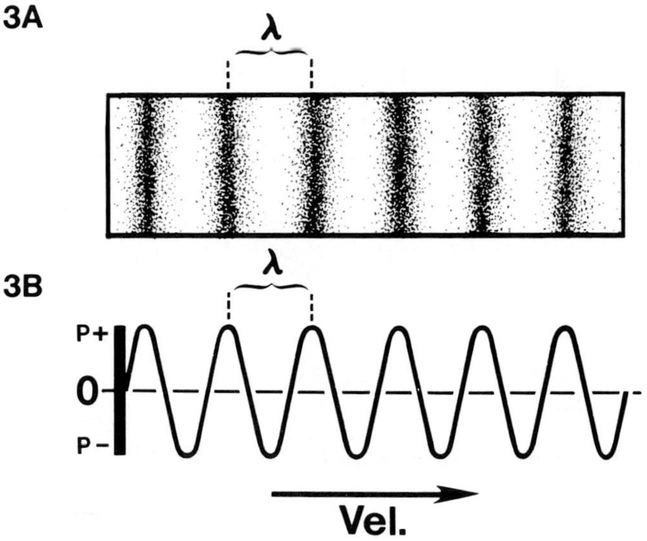

Fig. 1–3. Characteristics of a sound wave. **A.** The alternating compression and dispersion of the particles in any medium that occur during the passage of a sound wave. **B.** The amplitude and frequency of particle displacement are expressed graphically as a sine wave. P = the microscopic variation in local tissue pressure that occurs during passage of a sound wave and is related to the degree of particle displacement. Vel. = velocity of sound in a particular medium. λ = wavelength.

* The amount of acoustic energy produced by a sound-emitting device per unit time is the acoustic power of that device and is measured in watts (1 watt equals 1 joule/sec).

** The concentration of power within a specific area is the intensity (I). Intensity is commonly expressed as either watts per square meter or milliwatts per square centimeter.

dispersion. Velocity dispersion, when it does occur, is usually small and, hence, is likewise disregarded.

In general, as the density of a medium increases, the velocity of sound through the medium also increases. Thus, sound travels faster through such solids as bone than through either liquids or air. The velocity of sound in fluids is generally between 1000 and 1600 m/sec. In human tissue, the mean value for the velocity of sound is 1540 m/sec, or 1.54 mm/μsec.[6] For simplicity, 1.5 mm/μsec is used for the speed of sound in the examples throughout this book.

PROPERTIES OF ULTRASOUND

All the properties of low frequency sound apply also to ultrasound. Ultrasound, however, has specific characteristics that are particularly useful in cardiac diagnosis. Ultrasound can be beamed in a particular direction, obeys the laws of geometric optics regarding reflection, transmission, and refraction, and can be reflected by relatively small, closely spaced objects.

The Ultrasonic Beam

The sound energy produced by an ultrasonic generator (transducer) is propagated into an adjacent medium in the form of a beam. In the immediate vicinity of a typical disc-shaped transducer, the beam is cylindric with a diameter comparable to that of the disc. Farther from the transducer, the margins of the beam diverge, and the beam widens into a cone.[8] The well-columnated portion of the beam in close proximity to the transducer is called *the near field*, or the *Fresnel zone*, whereas the diverging conical portion of the beam is referred to as *the far field*, or the *Fraunhofer zone*. The junction of the near and far fields is the transition zone (Fig. 1–4).

The length of the near field can be calculated from the formula:

$$L_n = r^2/\lambda \qquad [1.2]$$

where r is the radius of the sound-generating surface and λ is the wavelength of the transmitted pulse. This

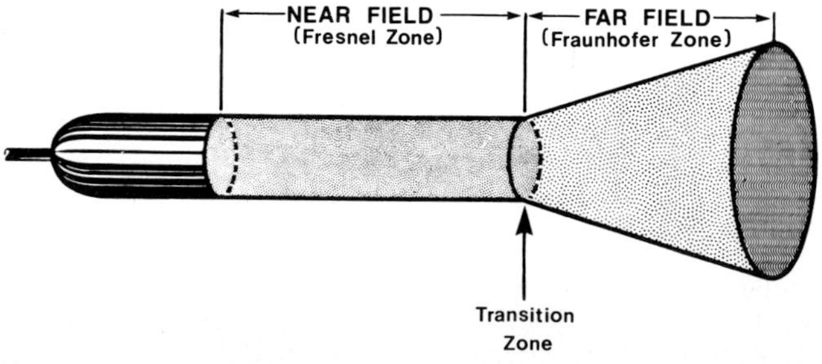

Fig. 1–4. The configuration of a sound beam as it progresses from the transducer. The near field is the region closest to the transducer face. The beam is relatively well columnated in this zone. In the transition zone, the beam begins to diverge. The far field is the conical diverging portion of the beam. The sound energy in an actual sound beam is not as uniformly distributed, and the beam margins are not as sharply demarcated as indicated in this diagram.

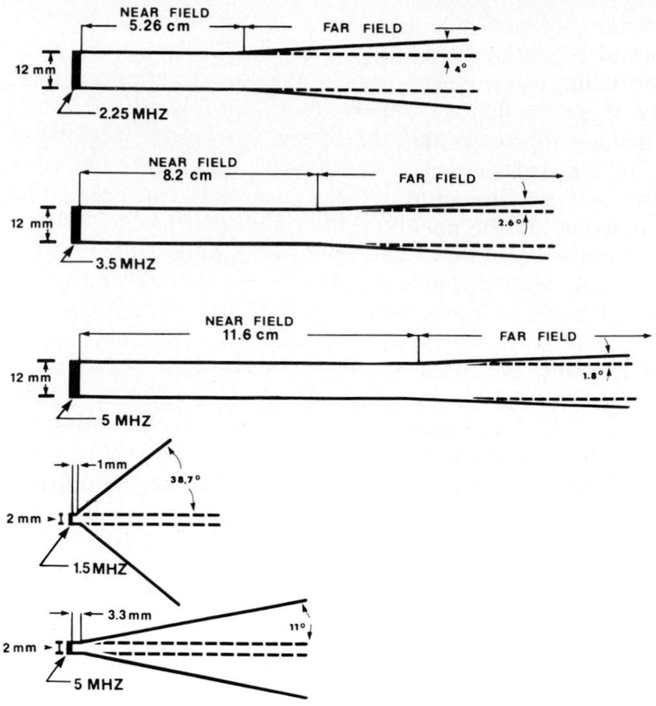

Fig. 1–5. The effects of transducer size and frequency on ultrasonic beam configuration. For transducers of similar size, an increase in frequency results in a longer near field and less beam dispersion in the far field. A decrease in transducer size, however, decreases near-field length and increases beam dispersion, even at higher frequencies.

formula shows that the length of the near zone increases when either the surface area of the transducer increases or the wavelength decreases. Because wavelength and frequency are inversely related, a decrease in wavelength is the same as an increase in frequency. The value of L_n provides two additional pieces of information. First, the peak acoustic amplitude of a nonfocused transducer occurs at this point and, second, a transducer can be focused only at a distance less than or equal to L_n and not at any arbitrary distance.

In the far field, the angle of the divergence of the beam (θ) can be derived from the formula:

$$\sin\theta = 0.61/r \qquad [1.3]$$

where r is the radius of the beam at the transition point. Here again, an increase in either frequency or transducer size decreases the spread of sound energy, thereby producing a narrower, more intense beam. Larger high frequency transducers, therefore, produce beams with longer near fields and less divergence in the far field, whereas smaller lower frequency transducers have shorter near fields and greater beam divergence. The beam configurations for a series of transducer elements of various sizes and frequencies are illustrated in Figure 1–5.

The shape of the ultrasonic beam is important because it determines the areas of the heart from which echoes may be recorded, affects intensity at any point along the beam path, and governs the lateral resolution of the system. In general, narrower beams are preferable to broad beams because they (1) produce echoes from a more limited area of the heart, thereby reducing ambiguity of echo origin; (2) are more intense and thus generate stronger echoes; and (3) have superior lateral resolution.

In addition to varying transducer size and frequency, one also can change the shape of the beam by focusing. Focusing can be accomplished in two ways; internally and externally (Fig. 1–6). Internal focusing is achieved by applying an appropriate radius of curvature to the piezoelectric ceramic. The radius of curvature in combination with the transducer frequency and element diameter then determines the focal point. In external focusing, a flat piezoelectric element is used and a concave acoustic lens is bonded to the front surface of the element.[8] By varying the concavity of the lens, one can focus the beam at a predetermined distance from the transducer. Decreasing the cross-sectional area of the beam within the focal zone increases its intensity, assuming constant transducer power output. Because the strength of the returning echoes is related to beam intensity, focusing increases the intensity of the echoes from all structures within the focal zone, both absolutely and in relation to targets elsewhere in the beam path. Beyond the focal zone, the beam again diverges. Because focusing decreases the radius (r) of the beam in the focal zone, the angle of divergence in the far field is greater for a focused beam than for an unfocused beam. Because beam divergence begins from a smaller cross-sectional area, however, the overall beam area within the working range of the transducer is generally smaller for a focused than for a nonfocused beam. Similarly, although beam width at the focal point decreases linearly with aperture size, depth of field decreases with the square of the aperture. This relationship forces a compromise between resolution at the focal point and depth of field whenever a fixed focus is used. The effects of focusing on beam pattern are illustrated in Figure 1–7.

When operating in the pulsed mode, the output of the transducer is not a continuous emission of energy as the beam concept implies. However, because each pulse of sound follows the same path and has the same shape and radius, the system behaves as if a beam were produced and the concept is valid.

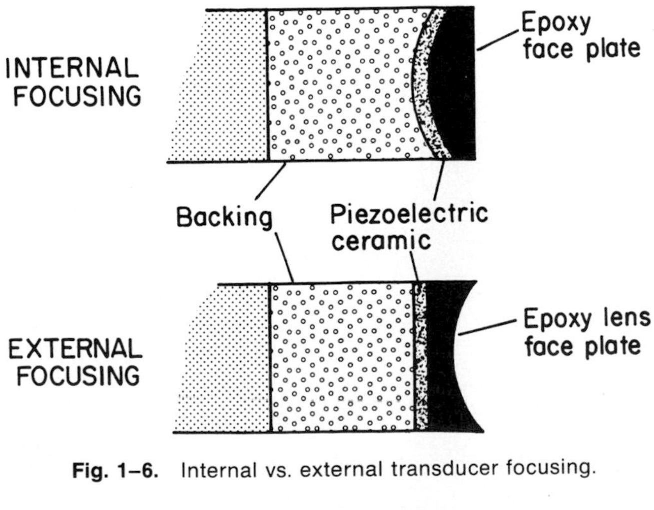

Fig. 1–6. Internal vs. external transducer focusing.

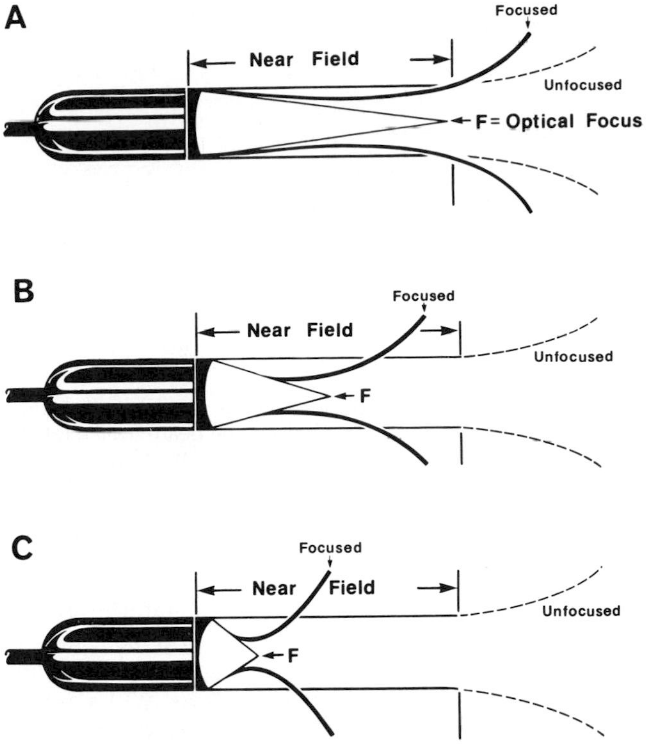

Fig. 1–7. The effects of focusing on beam patterns for a series of acoustic lenses with increasing radii of curvature. In each example, the beam pattern for an unfocused transducer of comparable size and frequency is indicated by the outer interrupted lines. The inner solid lines illustrate the beam pattern produced by the acoustic lens, and the innermost conical area is the focal pattern for a corresponding optical lens. Point F is the optical focus. **A.** The radius of curvature of the lens is such that the optical focus occurs at the transition zone for the unfocused beam. At this optical focus, the point of maximal acoustic focusing occurs slightly beyond the midpoint of the near field. Beyond the region of the acoustic focus, the beam diverges to a width that corresponds to the width of the unfocused transducer at the transition point. Beyond the transition point, the focused beam diverges more rapidly than the unfocused beam. **B** and **C.** As the radius of the curvature of the acoustic lens increases, the optical focus is brought closer to the transducer face, and the acoustic focus more closely approximates the optical focus. The degree of beam narrowing at the acoustic focus increases; however, the beam width at the transition point is greater than that for an unfocused transducer and increases as focusing is increased. As indicated by this figure, focusing always occurs in the near field of the corresponding unfocused transducer, and the acoustic focus always occurs closer to the transducer face than does the optical focus. As the focal point is brought closer to the transducer face, the acoustic focus more closely approximates the optical focus. When focusing is desired at a specific point in space, therefore, one must select a transducer with a sufficiently long near field so that the point of desired focusing lies within this range.

Distribution of Energy Within the Sound Beam

The preceding discussion suggests that the energy within the main beam of a simple disc-shaped transducer is homogenous. Although this simplification is useful conceptually, the actual distribution of energy within the cylindric and conical portions of the beam is not uniform and varies with both distance along the central beam axis and lateral offset from this axis. In the near field, the axial energy distribution is quite complex and results

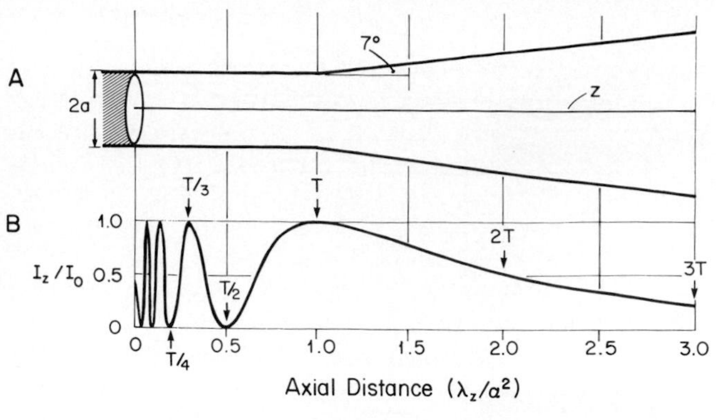

Fig. 1–8. The variation in axial intensity as a function of distance for a flat circular transducer. **A.** The general beam profile relative to the main axis (z). **B.** The variation in z axis intensity normalized to the intensity at the transducer face (I_z/I_0). λ = the wavelength of the transducer; α = the transducer radius; T = the transition distance.

from the constructive and destructive interference of three rays, one perpendicular to the piston face, and one from each of its extreme edges.[9] Figure 1–8 illustrates the varying near field intensity pattern, with maxima occurring at positions where the contributions of the three rays are most nearly in phase. Starting at the transition distance T (which is the same as the length of the near field L_n) and moving toward the transducer, the axial intensity begins to fall until, at a distance of T/2, the axial intensity is zero. The intensity then starts to increase and again reaches a maximum value of unity at T/3. As one continues to approach the transducer, the intensity continues to oscillate between a minimum value of zero at even distances, i.e., T/4, T/6, and a maximum value at odd distances, i.e., T/5, T/7. In the far field, the maximum axial intensity decreases with distance such that at a distance of 2T it is equal to half the value at the transition distance.

Figure 1–9 illustrates the off-axis intensity distribution within the receiver beam generated by a flat disc-shaped transducer. In the far field, the intensity drops off with lateral offset in the form of a bell-shaped curve until a zero value is reached. The position of the lateral offset where the zero value is reached is given by the divergence angle θ that confines the main beam, and mathematical analysis shows that 84% of the total energy is contained within this main beam.[10] As the lateral offset is increased further, the intensity again starts to increase corresponding to the energy associated with the first side lobe (see the following section). Continuing further laterally, the intensity again returns to zero and then through decreasing subsidiary maxima and minima as other side lobes are encountered.

The offset intensity distribution in the near field is more complex. As the distance T/2 is approached, the bell-shaped lateral distribution curve becomes humped and the off-axis maxima become more prominent, reaching 70 to 80% of the value of the maximum axial intensity. At T/3, where the axial intensity is again at a maximum, one off-axis minimum is found.

Side Lobes

Although the majority of the sound energy produced by a simple disc-shaped transducer propagates directly away from the transducer face to form the main beam, a small portion of the transmitted energy will concentrate in regions outside the main, or central, beam. These secondary, or side, lobes arise because at the lateral margins of the sound source a portion of the sound energy is transmitted radially away from the main beam axis. Radial transmission of sound energy occurs with all transducers and is referred to as the *edge effect*. Spatial variation in side lobe intensity occurs because the net energy arising from opposite "edges" arrives at varying points in space, either in phase or out of phase. When the sound energy from two opposite edges arrives in phase, the energy summates, and a region of high intensity occurs. Conversely, when the sound energy arrives out of phase, phase cancellation occurs, and a low intensity sound field results. The most common method for diagramming transducer side lobes is a polar two-dimensional coordinate representation such as that in Figure 1–10.[6] As indicated, the intensity of the side lobes decreases as one moves radially away from the main beam (0°). It should be understood, however, that side lobes are three-dimensional entities and for a disc-shaped

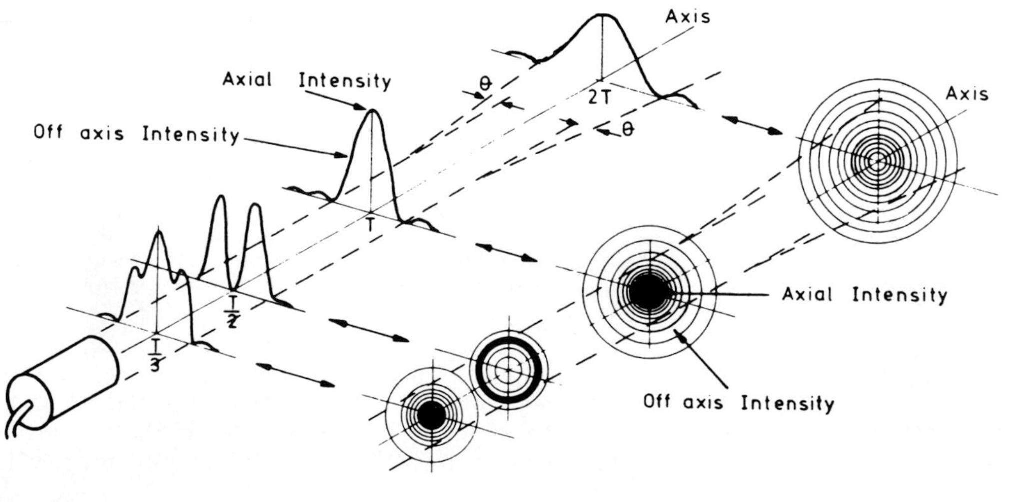

Fig. 1–9. The lateral, or off-axis, intensity distribution of a flat circular transducer. The top portion illustrates the off-axis intensity distribution along a line perpendicular to and passing through the central axis of the beam. The lower portion shows the two-dimensional intensity distribution in the plane at distances T/3, T/2, T, and 2T and illustrates the ring structure of the intensity distribution. θ = The angle of divergence of the beam in the far field.

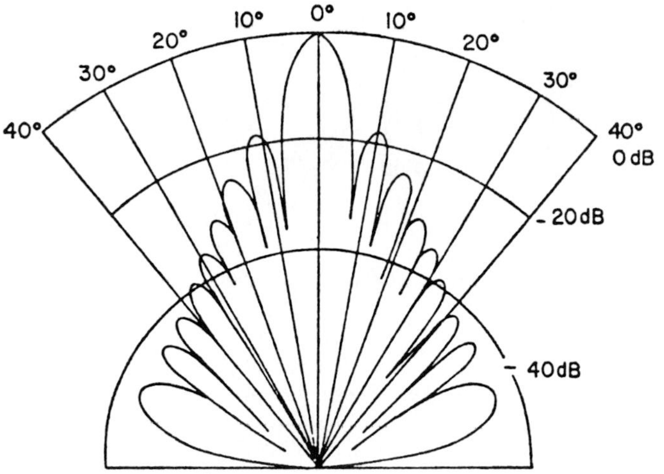

Fig. 1–10. Side lobe distribution and intensity as a function of degree of offset from the main lobe. Values given in decibels down from the intensity of the main lobe.

transducer have the same intensity at all points with an equal radial offset from the main beam axis. Side lobes are a potential source of artifact, because all echoes received by the transducer are displayed as if they arose from targets along the central axis of the main beam. Strong reflectors illuminated by side lobes, therefore, may be shifted on the display to a position that differs from their true location in space (Fig. 1–11).

Normally, side lobes are of relatively low amplitude and do not create serious imaging artifacts. In the more complex transducer arrays discussed in the next chapter, however, secondary lobes may be more intense, and their suppression becomes an important consideration.

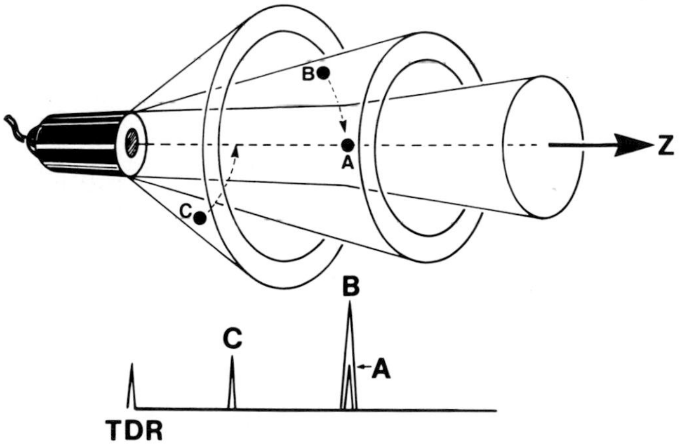

Fig. 1–11. The deleterious effects of side lobes on the displayed data. In this example, a disc-shaped transducer with a main beam and two side lobes is illustrated. Target A, a weak reflector, is located along the main axis of the sound beam. Target B, which is more highly reflective than target A, lies in the path of the inner side lobe. Target B is the same distance from the transducer as target A. On the display, target A produces a much weaker echo than does target B and hence is completely overshadowed by the stronger reflection arising from the side lobe. Target C is encountered by the outer side lobe. This target is also displayed as though positioned along the central axis of the beam, and hence its position on the display does not correspond to its true position in space.

Reflection, Refraction, and Transmission

When an ultrasonic beam meets the boundary between two different media, part of the acoustic energy is reflected and part continues into the second medium. When the linear dimensions of the boundary are large with respect to the wavelength, the amount of energy reflected is proportional to the difference in acoustic impedance, or the acoustic mismatch, of the two media.[11] Acoustic impedance is defined by the expression:

$$Z = \rho v \qquad [1.4]$$

where Z is the acoustic impedance in rayls, ρ is the density of the tissue in kilograms per cubic meter, and v is

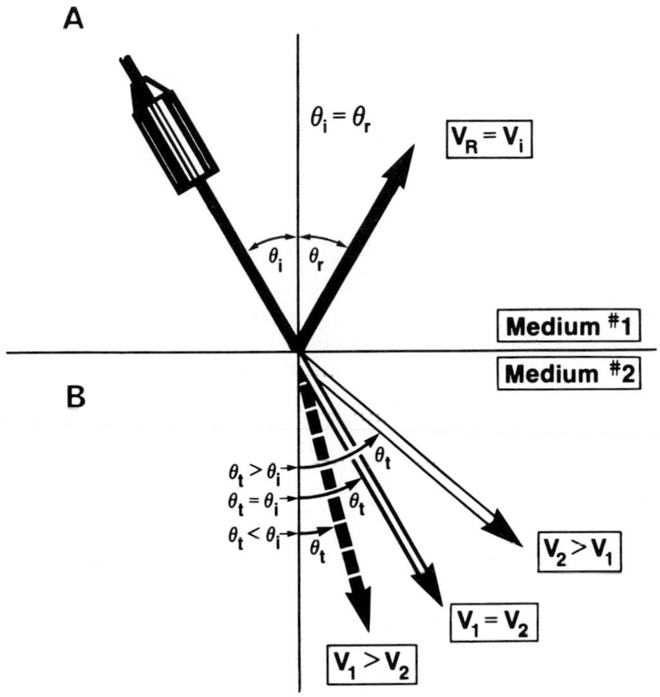

Fig. 1–12. Reflective and refractive characteristics of ultrasound. **A.** When a sound beam strikes an interface between two media of differing acoustic impedance, a portion of the sound energy is reflected into the incident medium. Because the velocity of the reflected wave (V_r) equals the velocity of the incident wave (V_i), the angle of reflection (θ_r) equals the angle of incidence (θ_i) in the same plane. **B.** The portion of the sound energy that continues into the second medium is propagated at an angle relative to the incident beam (θ_t), which is determined by the relative speed of sound in the two media. When the speed of sound in the second medium (V_2) is greater than that in the first (V_1), the sound energy in the left-hand portion of the incident beam begins to accelerate before the sound energy in the right-hand portion of the beam reaches the interface. This situation causes the sound wave to bend to the right and to be propagated at an angle that is greater than the angle of incidence. Conversely, when the speed of sound in the second medium (V_2) is slower than that in the first medium (V_1), the left-hand margin of the beam, which reaches the interface first, begins to decelerate as it enters the second medium. The right-hand margin of the beam continues at is original speed. This situation deflects the beam to the left, and the angle of transmission (θ_t) is less than the angle of incidence (θ_i). When the speed of sound in both media is the same ($V_1 = V_2$), there is no refraction, and the angle of transmission (θ_t) equals the angle of incidence (θ_i).

the velocity of sound in the medium in meters per second. For example, when a pulse crosses the boundary between muscle tissue ($Z = 1.7 \times 10^6$ rayls) and blood ($Z = 1.6 \times 10^6$ rayls), about 0.1% of the acoustic energy is reflected.[12] Reflectors that are large relative to the wavelength of the ultrasonic pulse and have a smooth surface (i.e., are mirror-like) are called *specular reflectors*.

When reflection occurs, the reflected wave is returned in a negative direction through the incident medium at the same velocity with which the boundary is approached. As in optics, the angle of reflection equals the angle of incidence in the same plane (Fig. 1–12A).[6]

The energy returning to the transducer from any reflective interface is referred to as the *backscattered energy* and is related not only to the acoustic mismatch at the interface but also to the angle of the incident beam relative to the plane of the reflector. As indicated in Figure 1–13, when the transducer is perpendicular to the plane of the reflector, a large percentage of the reflected energy returns directly to the transducer. As the angle between the transducer and the reflecting interface increases, however, the amount of reflected energy returning to the transducer rapidly diminishes. The strength of the recorded echo, therefore, is a function of both the acoustic mismatch at an individual interface and the angle of the transducer relative to the plane of that interface.

The portion of the ultrasonic energy that is transmitted beyond the interface is propagated into the second medium at a speed proportional to the speed of sound in that medium. When sound travels through both media at the same speed, the angle of incidence equals the angle of transmission (see Fig. 1–12B). When the speed of sound in the two media differs, the sound wave is refracted. The difference between the angle of incidence and the angle of transmission is proportional to the difference between the sound velocities in the two media. Because the velocity of sound in human tissue is fairly constant, little refraction occurs and the beam path is considered to remain straight.

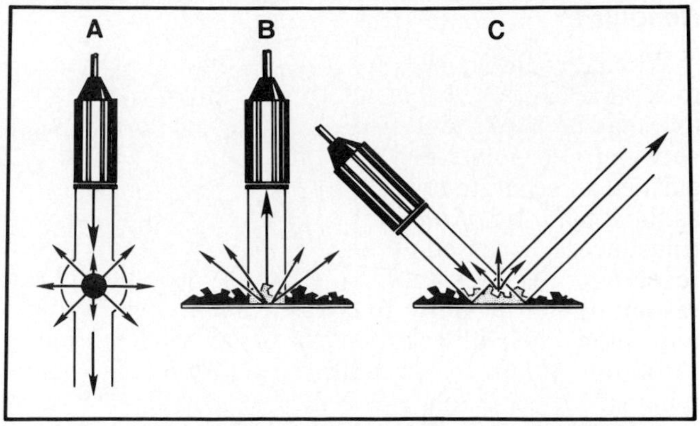

Fig. 1–14. **A.** Interaction of a sound wave with a target that is smaller than the wavelength of the ultrasonic pulse. **B.** Interaction of a sound wave with a rough or irregular but perpendicular surface. **C.** Interaction of a sound wave with a rough surface, which it strikes obliquely. The irregularity of the interface causes a portion of the sound energy to reflect back to the transducer. This reflective pattern can be contrasted to that depicted in Figure 1–13C, where no sound energy was reflected toward the transducer when the beam intersected a smooth surface at a similar angle.

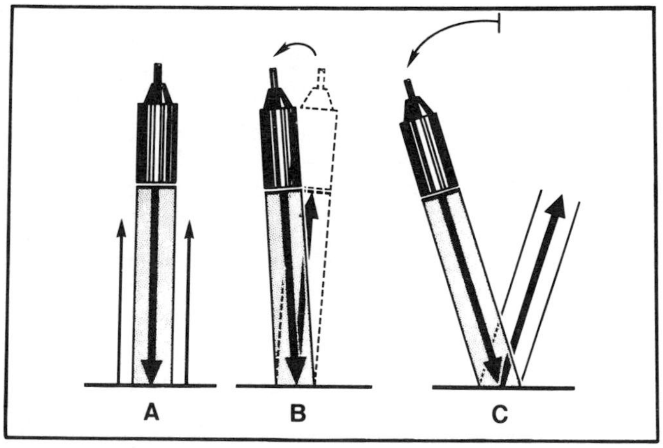

Fig. 1–13. The effects of transducer angle on the amount of reflected acoustic energy that returns to the transducer and is recorded as an echo. **A.** The transducer is perpendicular to the reflective interface. In this situation, the majority of the returning energy is transmitted directly toward the transducer and, hence, can be recorded. **B.** The transducer is at a slight angle to the reflecting interface. In this orientation, only a portion of the reflected energy strikes the transducer face and is recorded. **C.** The transducer lies at a relatively acute angle to the reflective interface and most, if not all, of the reflected energy is directed away from the transducer face. In this case, although the amount of energy reflected into the incident medium may be great, little if any of the reflected energy strikes the transducer face and is recorded.

In addition to specular reflectors, sound waves may encounter structures that are smaller than the wavelength of the ultrasonic pulse as well as structures that are larger with rough or uneven surfaces. When the sound waves strike an obstacle that is comparable to or smaller than the wavelength, diffraction occurs, and a portion of the sound energy changes direction and bends around the obstacle. The remainder is scattered in all directions (Fig. 1–14A). A sound wave that strikes a relatively large but rough surface produces a specular reflection with an additional scattered field (Fig. 1–14B). The presence of scattering is of clinical importance because, although the amount of energy returned to the transducer from a scatterer is significantly less than that from a specular reflector, scattered energy is propagated in all directions and, hence, is less angle-dependent, than are specular reflections (Fig. 1–14C). The echoes from the normal mitral valve, although relatively stronger when the transducer is directly perpendicular to the valve, diminish rapidly as the angle between the transducer and the reflecting surface decreases.[13] In contrast, although the peak amplitude of echo production from a deformed thickened mitral valve may be less, the echo strength remains fairly constant through a wide range of incident angles, reflecting the omnidirectional nature of the scattered field. Scattering from blood is critical to the generation of Doppler-shifted echoes and is discussed in greater detail in Chapter 9.

Resolution

When examining the heart, the examiner is attempting to separate and record small, rapidly moving structures that may be only 1 or 2 mm apart. The smallest distance between two points at which the points can be distinguished as separate by an imaging system is referred to as the *resolution of the system*. The simple disc-shaped transducers discussed to this point provide two types of resolution, axial resolution and lateral resolution. Axial resolution is the ability to differentiate between points lying along the path or axis of the beam, whereas lateral resolution refers to the ability to differentiate points lying side by side relative to the beam path.

Axial Resolution. The axial resolution of an ultrasonic beam is related to its wavelength or frequency and to the duration of the transmitted pulse. To illustrate the effects of wavelength and pulse duration on resolution, let us first calculate the wavelengths of two pulses of ultrasound: one of 300 kHz and a second of 3 MHz. Both of these sound frequencies are within the ultrasonic range; however, the difference in resolving power is significant. The wavelength of an ultrasonic pulse is calculated by using the formula wavelength equals velocity divided by frequency, or

$$\lambda = V/F \qquad [1.5]$$

therefore for the first case,

$$F = 300{,}000 \text{ Hz}$$

$$\lambda = \frac{1.5 \text{ mm/sec or } 1500 \text{ m/sec}}{300{,}000 \text{ cps}}$$

$$\lambda = .005 \text{ m or } 5 \text{ mm}$$

for the second case,

$$F = 3{,}000{,}000 \text{ Hz}$$

$$\lambda = \frac{1.5 \text{ m/sec or } 1500 \text{ m/sec}}{3{,}000{,}000}$$

$$\lambda = .0005 \text{ m or } 0.5 \text{ mm}$$

The wavelength of the 300-kHz pulse, therefore, is 5 mm, whereas that of the 3-MHz pulse is 0.5 mm.

Assume that a sound pulse of 4 cycles is transmitted into a test medium (such as that illustrated in Fig. 1–15) in which two targets (T_1 and T_2) are located at 10 and 11 cm from the transducer. At the lower frequency (300 kHz), the total length of the sound pulse is 20 mm (λ = 5 mm × 4 cycles = 20 mm). With a pulse train of this length, the echo from the closer of the two targets (T_1) is still striking the transducer when the echo from the second target (T_2) returns. The echocardiograph, therefore, senses and displays one long echo rather than two discrete echoes representing each of the reflecting surfaces. If a third reflector is placed between T_1 and T_2, it would be undetected. In contrast, when a frequency of 3 MHz is used, the wavelength is only 0.5 mm. With the same 4-cycle pulse train, the total pulse length is only 2 mm. At this pulse duration, there is a relatively long interval between the return of the echo from the first target and that from the second target. Thus, two separate echoes are displayed by the echocardiograph, and the presence of two distinct reflecting interfaces is "resolved." In addition, at 3 MHz, a third structure placed between T_1 and T_2 could still be resolved. This example shows that the higher the frequency of the transmitted pulse, the better the resolution along the path or axis of the beam. It also shows that resolution is a function not only of the wavelength or frequency, but also of pulse duration. Because the shortest pulse duration is a single half cycle, the wavelength sets the limit of resolution of the system. In practice, however, resolution is roughly twice the wavelength. Table 1–1 lists the frequencies and wavelengths for a series of commonly used transducers. The determinants of frequency and pulse duration are discussed in the section on transducers.

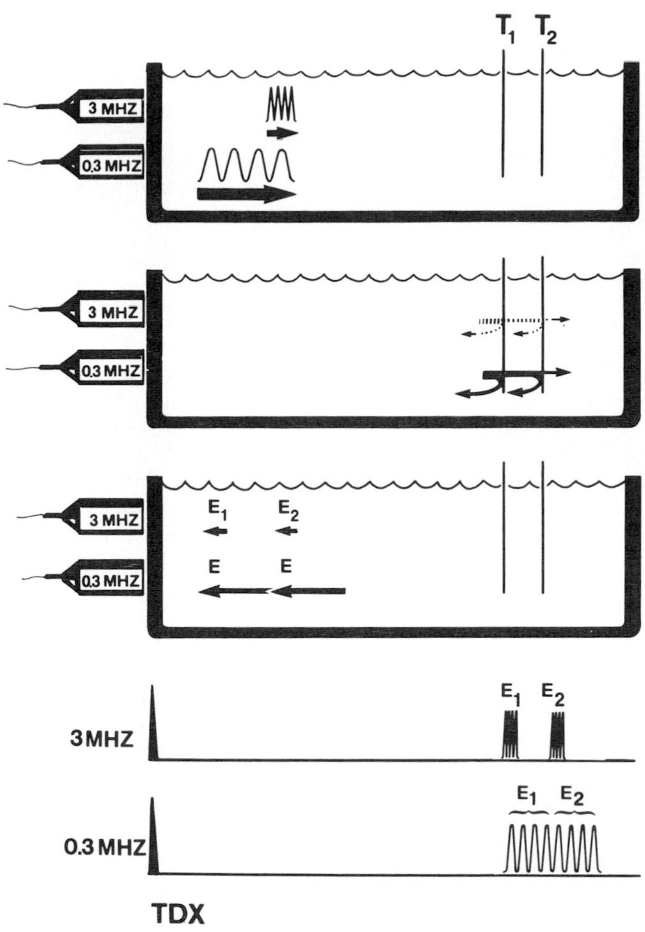

Fig. 1–15. The effects of frequency on axial resolution. In the upper panel, 2 pulses of 4 cycles each, one from a 3-MHz transducer and one from a 0.3-MHz transducer, are emitted into a test medium. Because of the higher frequency, the pulse from the 3-MHz transducer is much shorter than the corresponding pulse from the lower-frequency transducer. When these pulses strike two targets, T_1 and T_2, echoes are reflected at both interfaces. Because of the shorter pulse duration at the higher frequency (3 MHz), separate reflections (E_1 and E_2) arise from each target and are recorded as distinct. At the lower frequency (0.3 MHz), the pulse length is such that the echoes from T_1 and T_2 are continuous, and hence, these targets cannot be "resolved" as separate.

Table 1–1. Relationship of Transducer Frequency to Wavelength

Frequency (MHz)	Wavelength (mm)
1.0	1.50
1.6	0.94
2.2	0.68
3.5	0.43
5.0	0.30
7.5	0.20
10.0	0.15

Lateral Resolution. Although the ability to differentiate between points along the axis of the beam depends on frequency and pulse duration, the differentiation of points laterally oriented relative to the beam path is a function of beam width. Beam width, as indicated in Figures 1–5 and 1–7, is a function of transducer size, shape, frequency, and focusing. Beam width can be defined as the beam diameter measured at any consistent point; however, a standard reference is the width at −6 dB* or at the one-half amplitude point.[14]

To understand lateral resolution, one must first remember that the echocardiograph displays all structures within the beam path along a single line representing the axis of the beam. Figure 1–16 illustrates the types of distortion this display characteristic can produce. In Figure 1–16A, three pairs of reflectors, separated by 1 cm, are placed along the path of an ultrasonic beam. Reflectors A1 and A2 are oriented parallel to the path of the beam and, hence, the degree of separation is appropriately displayed. Reflectors B1 and B2 are separated by the same distance but lie at an angle to the beam axis. In this example, the true lateral separation is not evident, and hence, only the axial distance is displayed. In the final example, reflectors C1 and C2 are beside each other in the ultrasonic beam. In this example, not only is the true distance between the two reflectors not apparent, but the echoes from each source are superimposed on one another. The presence of two distinct reflecting sources cannot be detected. For this reason, parallel structures must be separated by more than the width of the ultrasonic beam to be "resolved" as laterally distinct.

Because of its effect on beam width, the overall gain or sensitivity of the system may also affect the apparent lateral resolution. This situation occurs because the sound energy is not evenly distributed across the beam and tends to be most intense in the center and to decrease toward the margins. Thus, similar reflectors in the center of the beam produce stronger echoes than those at the beam margin. When the sensitivity of the system is low, the weaker echoes from the beam margins are not recorded, and the beam appears narrower (Fig. 1–16B). When the gain is high, the echoes at the beam margins are recorded and the effective beam width appears greater.

Finally, as Figure 1–16C illustrates, the limitations encountered in displaying laterally positioned objects also apply to lateral motion. Thus, when the beam is held stationary, only the components of motion oriented parallel to the axis of the beam are appropriately displayed. Because both frequency and beam shape are determined by transducer design, transducer selection sets the theoretic limitations of resolution for any system.

* The decibel (dB) is the unit of measure of sound pressure and is defined as 20 times the logarithm to the base 10 of the ratio of the measured pressure (P) of sound to the reference sound pressure P_0, where $P_0 = 2 \times 10^{-4}$ dyn cm^{-2}.

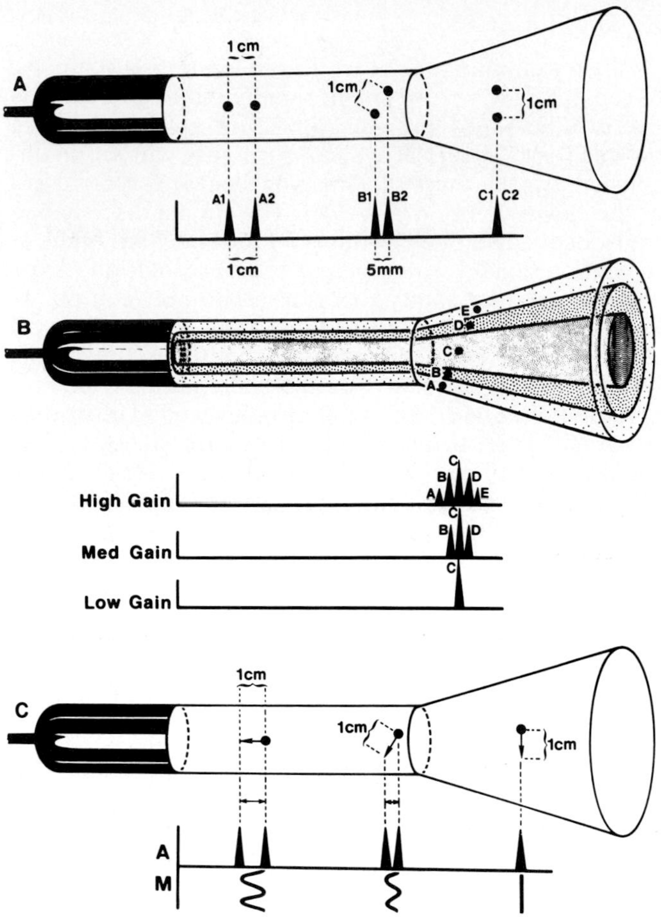

Fig. 1–16. **A** to **C**. The effects of beam width and gain on lateral resolution and the recording of off-axis motion. (See text for further details.)

Attenuation and Absorption

As a sound wave passes through the body, progressive loss of the sound energy, or attenuation, occurs. In homogeneous tissue, attenuation occurs as a result of both absorption and scatter. Absorption implies that the amplitude of sound is weakened primarily by inner friction or viscosity, which transforms sound energy into other forms of energy (heat).[5] Scattering occurs at the many small interfaces or elastic discontinuities encountered as the beam passes through even the most homogeneous medium.[5] The scattering of the sound energy at each of these interfaces decreases the amount of energy available to penetrate more deeply into the body. Atten-

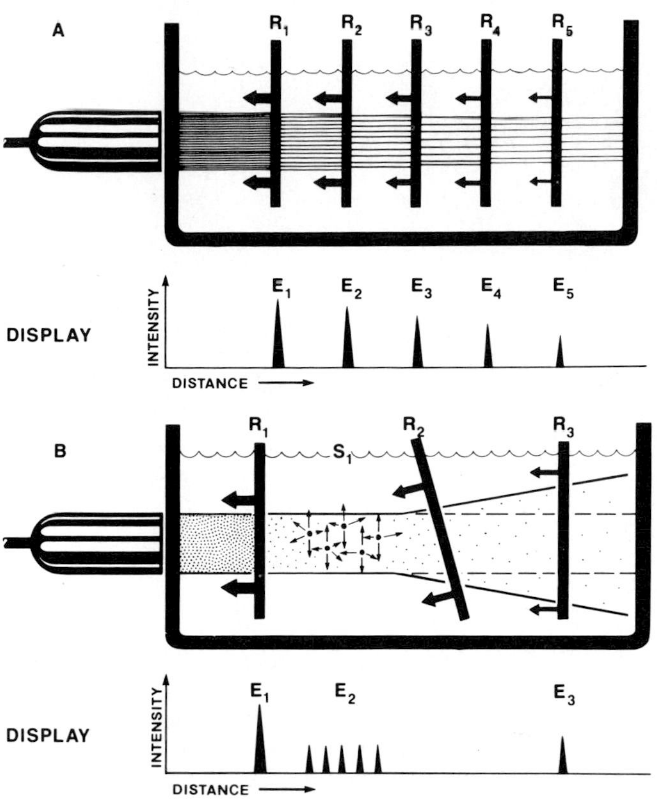

Fig. 1–17. Factors contributing to the attenuation of an ultrasonic pulse. **A.** The sound beam is transmitted into a homogeneous medium containing a series of equally spaced reflectors (R_1 to R_5). As the sound beam propagates into the medium, its intensity gradually decreases because of absorption and scattering. In addition, a portion of the sound energy at each interface is reflected toward the transducer as an echo (E). This further attenuates the sound beam, thereby decreasing the energy available to propagate beyond that reflector. When both the medium and reflector spacings are constant, the echo strength on the resultant display gradually and predictably decreases (E_1 to E_5). **B.** A more complex situation that is more comparable to the situation encountered in cardiac imaging. In this example, the beam is initially transmitted into a relatively homogeneous medium, resulting in some sound energy loss as a result of absorption and scattering. At reflector R_1, a larger amount of energy is directed toward the transducer as an echo (E_1). This action weakens the beam. The beam then encounters a series of larger scatterers (S_1), each of which further decreases the intensity of the beam. Beyond the scattering field, the beam begins to diverge, which further decreases its intensity. The beam then encounters a reflector at an angle to the transducer fact that produces echoes. These echoes are reflected into the incident medium but are propagated at an angle that prevents them from being recorded. The weakened beam then continues in a diverging pattern until reflector R_3 is encountered. The reflectivity of target R_3 is similar to that of R_1; however, the recorded echo (E_3) is much less, which is due to the loss in beam intensity that occurred because of the attenuation before this point. Because the in vivo system is complex and because many reflectors and scatterers significantly attenuate the ultrasonic beam without being detected, direct correction for this energy loss is virtually impossible.

uation may also be produced by deviation from a parallel beam. Any increase in beam diameter increases the cross-sectional area over which the sound energy is spread and, hence, decreases intensity per unit area.

In nonhomogeneous media, a portion of the sound energy is reflected at each interface encountered by the beam, thereby further attenuating beam strength. Figure 1–17 illustrates the effects of reflection, scattering, and beam dispersion on the intensity of the sound beam and the resulting display characteristic of sequentially encountered targets. The attenuation of the sound beam increases as its frequency increases. This is reasonable because each shift of the particles in a medium requires energy and high frequency waves cause more such shifts per unit distance traveled than lower frequency waves. The term *half-value layer* is frequently used to compare the attenuation of sound in different media. The half-value layer is the distance a sound wave travels in a given tissue before its energy is attenuated to half its original value. Some representative half-value layers include plasma, 100 cm; whole blood, 35 mm; and muscle, 3.6 cm. As a rule of thumb, the attenuation of sound in tissue is said to be approximately 1 dB/cm/MHz. For example, when imaging a structure that is 10 cm deep in the body at 2.5 MHz, the round-trip attenuation is 50 dB, resulting in an echo that should be detectable using acceptable transmission power. At 10 MHz, however, the round-trip attenuation would be 200 dB, resulting in a signal that would be too weak to detect.

THE TRANSDUCER

In echocardiography, the term *transducer* is generally used to refer to the small hand-held probe that transmits the acoustic energy into the heart and receives the returning echoes. The complete echocardiographic probe, or transducer, (Fig. 1–18) consists of (1) the piezoelectric element, which both generates and receives the acoustic impulse; (2) electrodes, which transmit the current required to shock-excite the crystal and record the

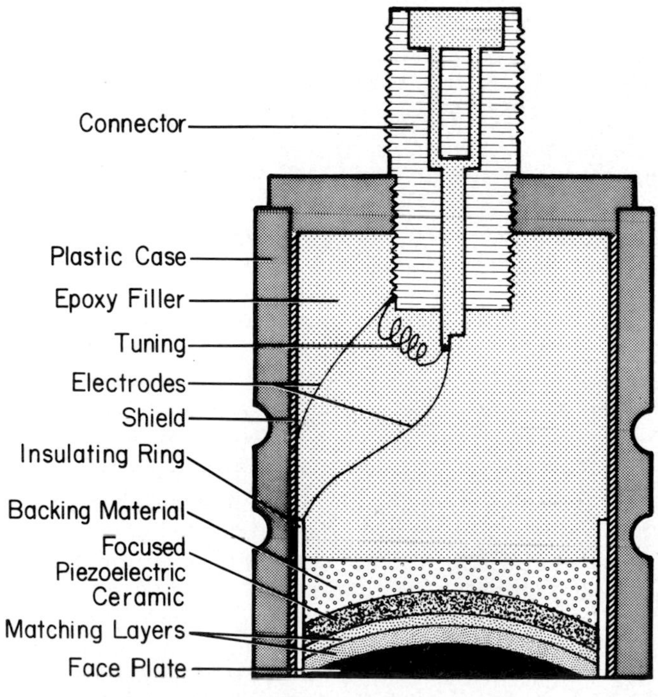

Fig. 1–18. Simple disc-shaped ultrasonic transducer. (See text for details.)

voltage produced by the returning echoes; (3) backing material, which helps to control the length of time the transducer vibrates following an electrical excitation and absorbs acoustic energy transmitted backward into the transducer (the backwave); (4) acoustic insulation, which prevents transmission of vibrations to the housing of the transducer, which otherwise cause interference with the returning signal; (5) a case, which provides a means of holding and directing the piezoelectric element; (6) matching layers, which reduce insertion losses caused by the large acoustic mismatch between the transducer and the patient; and finally, (7) a face plate, which permits contact of the piezoelectric element with the chest wall and focusing of the transducer when a lens is placed in this position.

The Piezoelectric Element

Transducers, more precisely, are devices capable of converting one form of energy into another. The piezoelectric materials, which convert electrical energy into sound energy, fall within this larger group of devices known as *transducers* and are commonly referred to as such. All piezoelectric materials are anisotropic, or lack a center of symmetry.[15] The electric charges bound within the ionic lattice of a piezoelectric crystal, therefore, can interact with an applied electrical field, thereby changing the shape of the crystal and producing a mechanical effect. This alteration in the shape of the crystal following the application of an electric charge is known as the *direct piezoelectric effect*. The amount of deformity is directly proportional to the applied voltage within the elastic limits of the crystal. Similarly, the voltage that appears across a piezoelectric material following a mechanical stress (the inverse piezoelectric effect) is directly proportional to the applied stress. A number of naturally occurring crystals, such as quartz, lithium sulfate, and potassium sodium tartrate (Rochelle salts), exhibit this piezoelectric property.

At present, however, a group of artificial ceramic materials, known as *ferroelectrics* (e.g., barium titanate and lead zirconate titanate), which show strong piezoelectric properties, are used as the active element in most ultrasonic transducers. The piezoelectric behavior of these ceramics is the result of either the zirconium or titanium ion locating in a stable, off-center position inside the otherwise symmetric lead and oxygen unit crystal cell (Fig. 1–19). Because the ion has a large charge, noncoincident centers of negative and positive charge are created in the unit cell, forming an electric dipole. Polarizing the material orients a majority of these dipoles in the same direction. This is achieved by heating the crystal above its Curie temperature at which the unit cell is body-centered, applying an external electric field, and then cooling the crystal (a process called *poling*). As the crystal cools, the ion in the center of the structure moves off center in a direction influenced by the applied electric field. After the crystal is cooled to room temperature and the electric field removed, the zirconium or titanium ions stay in their off-center locations to form the polarized crystal. If a voltage is applied to the opposite faces of such a polarized crystal, a field is produced in the crystal that acts on the dipoles to cause expansion and contraction.[16]

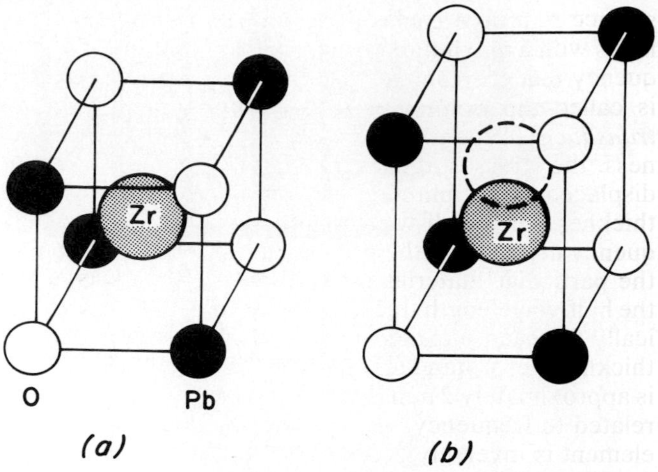

Fig. 1–19. The lead zirconate titanate crystal unit cell is a body-centered cubic structure above the Curie temperature (a). Below the Curie temperature, the zirconium ion moves off center to form a tetragonal structure (b).

Piezoelectric materials differ in their relative ability to convert electrical signals into mechanical vibrations (d_{33} value) and mechanical strain back into electrical signals (g_{33} value). For transducers operating in the pulsed echo mode, the piezoelectric material must both transmit and receive. Therefore, it is desirable for both the d_{33} and g_{33} constants to be large. Table 1–2 lists the transmitting and receiving constants of some of the more common piezoelectric materials.[17]

Transducer Frequency

The characteristic frequency of a transducer is determined by the thickness of the piezoelectric element. This occurs because shock-excitation of a piezoelectrical crystal results in the transmission of sound energy from both the front and back faces of the crystal. Unless the acoustic impedance of the surrounding medium is identical to that of the crystal, a portion of the sound energy is reflected at each interface back into the crystal. The sound energy then traverses the crystal at a speed proportional to the speed of sound in that material. The time it takes the sound wave to reach the opposite face is proportional to the width of the crystal. When the thickness of the element is exactly one half the wavelength, the reflected and transmitted stresses at each

Table 1–2. Transmitting and Receiving Characteristics of Common Piezoelectric Materials

Material	$d_{33}(10^{-12}$ m/V)	$g_{33}(10^{-3}$ Vm/N)
Quartz	2.3	57
Lead metaniobate	85	32
Barium titanate	~150	17
Lead zirconate titanate	150–600	20–40
PVF_2	20	190

surface reinforce each other, and the transducer resonates with a maximum displacement amplitude. The frequency that corresponds to a half-wavelength thickness is called the *fundamental resonant frequency of the transducer*. When the element is of wavelength thickness, the stresses at each surface are opposite, and the displacement amplitude is at a minimum. Because the thickness of a half-wavelength transducer at any frequency depends on the propagation velocity of sound in the particular material used in making the transducer, the half-wavelength thickness must be calculated specifically for each piezoelectric material. A representative thickness for a standard commercial, 1-MHz transducer is approximately 2 mm. Because wavelength is inversely related to frequency, the thickness of the piezoelectric element is inversely proportional to the frequency generated.

Transducer Damping

Because the resolution of an ultrasonic system depends on the total pulse duration (not just on the individual wavelength) and because the shortest pulse duration theoretically achievable is one-half cycle, the theoretic limit of resolution can be set at any frequency. Piezoelectric materials used in ultrasonic transducers, however, have a relatively long response to excitation. These ringing responses produce a long ultrasonic pulse, which, if undamped, results in poor range resolution. The length of this ringing response, or the "ringdown," of the transducer is measured in cycles and is calculated by counting the number of half-cycles required for the oscillations of the piezoelectric ceramic to decay to 10% (−20 dB) of the maximum peak to peak amplitude (Fig. 1–20).

The placement of a specially composed backing material behind the piezoelectric element shortens this ringing response by decreasing the length of time the crystal "rings," thus shortening the pulse length. In addition, this damping material absorbs sound energy emitted from the back face of the transducer. Such energy would otherwise reflect within the housing of the transducer and interfere with echoes returning from the examined medium. A high degree of transducer damping decreases pulse duration but also decreases transducer sensitivity, whereas poorly damped crystals have high sensitivity but have degraded range resolution. Thus, the backing

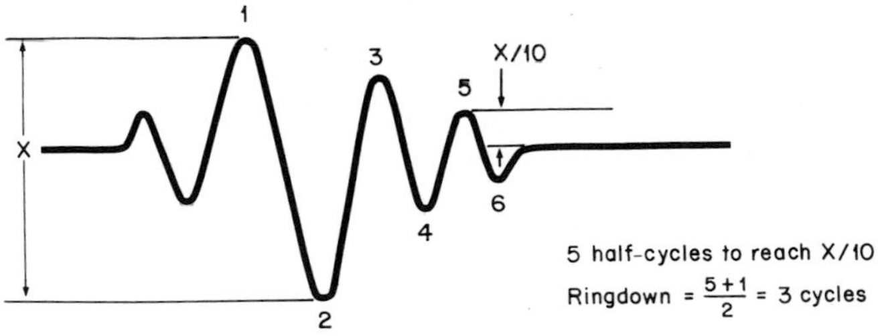

Fig. 1–20. Measurement of transducer ringdown. The ringdown is measured in cycles and is calculated by counting the number of half-cycles required for the pulse amplitude to decay to 10% of the maximum peak to peak amplitude. One half-cycle is added to the count, and the result is divided by 2.

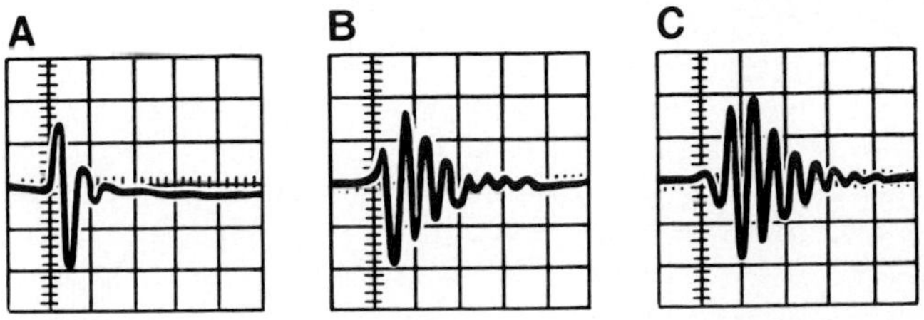

Fig. 1–21. The effects of damping on pulse configuration. **A.** A highly damped transducer with a short "ringing" response, which emits a pulse composed of a small number of cycles. **B** and **C.** The "ringing" response is increased by decreasing the damping of the transducer, and the pulse duration is correspondingly longer.

is required to match the piezoelectric acoustically and to have sufficiently high acoustic losses to damp any backwave to a level below the system noise. Typically, a 50- to 60-dB round-trip loss at any signal frequency above 1 MHz is required. If the loss is not large enough, multiple echoes will return and cause bright lines, or "range markers," in the image. The backing material chosen is usually composed of tungsten powder for high impedance and polyvinyl chloride (PVC) plastic as a binder and dissipative medium. Attenuation on the order of 20 dB/cm at 1 MHz is typically achieved and increases relative to frequency squared so that at 2 MHz the loss is 80 dB. Figure 1–21 illustrates the effect of varying degrees of damping on pulse configuration.

Impedance Matching

Another important component of the transducer is the impedance matching layer(s). The acoustic impedance of the transducer element (33×10^6 rayls) is about 25 times greater than that of the human body (1.5×10^6 rayls). This can potentially cause large reflective losses at the skin surface (i.e., 96%) unless some form of impedance matching is employed. By placing an impedance matching layer between the transducer element and the body, however, a sevenfold increase in the magnitude of the acoustic power input can be achieved. To prevent reverberations inside the layer and maximize the magnitude of the acoustic wave, the matching layer is made one-quarter wavelength thick at the transducer center frequency.* The one-quarter wavelength thickness results in constructive interference in the layer, as illustrated in Figure 1–22.[16–19] In this example, the initial acoustic pulse is represented by a ray, P, which strikes the layer at a normal incidence (here shown at a slight angle to allow the reflection from within the layer to be visualized). The reflected pulse, R, undergoes a 180° phase change as it travels the extra distance of one-half wavelength within the matching layer. This 180° phase

* One-quarter wavelength matching was first used by early astronomers who discovered that faint stars were brighter when viewed with telescopes that had old tarnished lenses rather than new untarnished ones. The tarnish layer turned out to be about one-quarter wavelength thick and have an intermediate index of refraction between that of the glass and the air. In modern times, coating optical components with one-quarter wavelength layers has become commonplace, and interest in one-quarter wavelength impedance matching of electrical transmissions lines has resulted in an extensive development of the theory.[16]

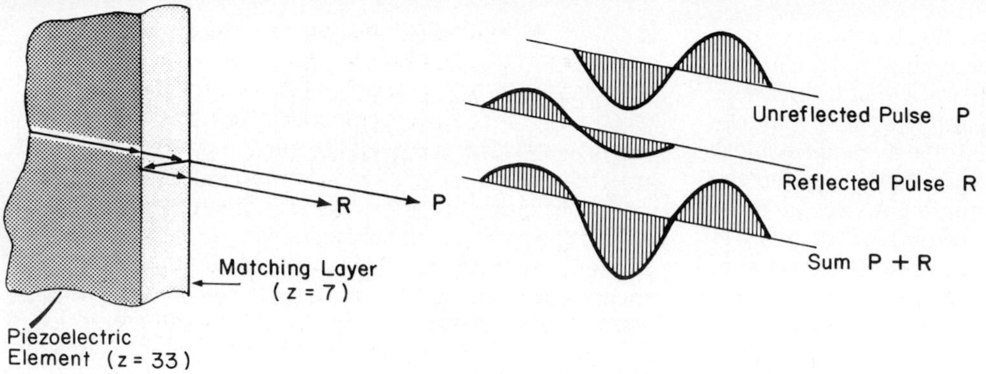

Fig. 1–22. Constructive interference in a matching layer one-quarter wave length thick. The normal rays P and R are drawn at a slight angle to their true direction so they both can be seen.

change aligns R to be in phase with P so that the original and reflected pulse amplitudes add as shown in the right panel of Figure 1–22.[16,18] Multiple matching layers have the additional advantage of further increasing power input, and therefore sensitivity, as well as increasing bandwidth and, hence, axial resolution.[19]

Electrical Matching

Electrical matching is another important determinant of transducer sensitivity. Electrical matching means selecting the material and tuning the transducer so that electrical compatability between the transducer and the diagnostic instrument is good. This is generally done by matching the impedance of the transducer to that of the pulser/receiver of the instrument, such that the transducer does not appear as a large perturbation to the overall electrical circuit. The electrical matching networks used in transducers range from a single inductor to more complex resistor-inductor-capacitor circuits and transformers. This tuning must be designed into the transducer based on a good understanding of the instrument's pulser/receiver characteristics and is not a user-variable function. One consequence of poor pulser-transducer matching is electrical ringing, which occurs when there is a large impedance mismatch between the instrument pulser and the transducer, such that a portion of the excitation pulse is reflected back into the pulser. Depending on the degree of mismatch this can significantly degrade the performance of the transducer in the diagnostic system. Electrical matching can often be the reason why a particular transducer performs well on one instrument and not another.[17]

Transducer Size

Finally, transducer size must be considered because it contributes to the shape of the ultrasonic field. In general, large transducers yield better circumscribed beams (longer near fields) and are easier to focus. When the area through which the ultrasonic beam can be directed to deeper structures (the acoustic window) is limited, use of a smaller transducer may be necessary.

Choice of Appropriate Transducer Frequency

From the foregoing discussion, it should be evident that increasing transducer frequency improves axial resolution as well as improving beam characteristics by both elongating the near field and diminishing beam divergence in the far field. Unfortunately, an increase in frequency also increases attenuation, thereby diminishing the ability of the beam to penetrate to deeper cardiac structures. In this trade-off between penetration and resolution, penetration is of primary importance because resolution becomes irrelevant when the echo beam cannot reach the structures of interest. As a general rule, therefore, one seeks to use the highest frequency that can still penetrate to the structures one wishes to examine. In adults, a 2.25-MHz transducer ordinarily provides sufficient penetration to reach the back wall of the heart and still provide satisfactory resolution. In younger children, a 3.5-MHz transducer frequently can be used, whereas in infants and neonates, a 5-MHz transducer provides excellent resolution and still has sufficient penetrating power to examine the entire cardiac area in these smaller subjects. In unusual circumstances, lower frequency transducers in the range of 1 MHz may be required to provide adequate penetration in thick-chested subjects or in older patients with emphysema or pulmonary obstructive changes.

System Sensitivity

Sensitivity is a widely used term to describe ultrasound system performance. Sensitivity describes the ability of the system to image small targets located at specific depths in an attenuative medium. The determinants of the sensitivity of an ultrasound system are difficult to define because sensitivity depends on the interaction of a host of system components including the transducer, pulser/receiver, and the signal processing and display circuitry. Because the transducer plays such an integral, if not independent, role in system sensitivity, it is important to understand its influence in more quantitative terms. Three basic transducer variables contribute to system sensitivity. These are beam geometry, frequency spectrum, and energy conversion efficiency. The effects of frequency and beam geometry have been described earlier, and this section, therefore, discusses the variables that affect energy conversion.

The conversion efficiency of a transducer describes how well the transducer converts both the electrical stimuli supplied by the instrument pulser into ultrasonic energy and the received echoes into electrical impulses. Sensitivity then can be related to conversion efficiency.[17] In fact, a simple definition would describe

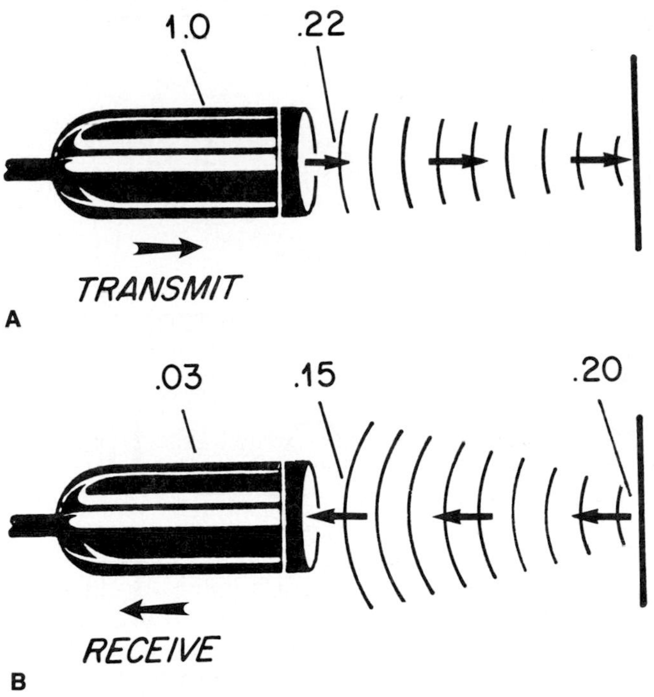

Fig. 1–23. Energy conversion efficiency of a typical ultrasonic system. (See text for details.)

transducer sensitivity as the product of the transmit and receive efficiencies.[17] Figure 1–23 represents a hypothetical transducer in pulse echo operation. In Figure 1–23A, the transducer is supplied with an excitation pulse that is equal to 1 "energy unit." The transducer, by means of the piezoelectric effect, converts this energy unit into a converging ultrasonic wavefront. The energy content of this input pulse is 0.22 energy units, indicating that only a portion of the energy in the excitation pulse was converted to ultrasound. The transmit efficiency, therefore, is 22% with the energy loss caused by imperfect electrical matching to the transducer and energy dissipation in the ceramic as heat. The ultrasonic pulse then travels through some intervening medium and strikes an acoustic interface, which directs the pulse back toward the transducer (Fig. 1–23B). The energy content of the reflected pulse is 0.20 energy units. A loss is indicated here because the pulse was not totally reflected (and in clinical practice never is). Next, because of the diverging nature of the reflected pulse, the assumption is made that the energy content of the pulse that strikes the transducer is 0.15 energy units. The transducer converts the received echoes back into an electrical signal, which in this example is 0.03 energy units, resulting in a receive efficiency of 20%. Based on this measure, the sensitivity of this transducer is the product of the transmit and receive efficiencies, or $0.22 \times 0.20 = 0.044$, or 4.4%. This value is typical of transducers in clinical use today.[17]

THE ECHOGRAPH

In the preceding section, the factors that determine the source, characteristics, and intensity of the echoes returning to the transducer from within the heart were examined. This section considers the methods of acoustic pulse generation and the different formats by which the returning echoes can be recorded and displayed to produce cardiac images. Doppler recording, analysis, and display are discussed in Chapters 7 through 13.

The circuitry necessary to transmit, receive, amplify, and display the acoustic pulse is contained in the basic echograph.[6] Figure 1–24 is a simplified block diagram of such an instrument. The main control component of the echograph is the master clock or oscillator (Fig. 1–24.1). The master clock is preset to transmit pulses at a designated frequency. Initially, the master clock signals the pulser to discharge stored electrical current to the transducer (TDR) (Fig. 1–24.2). This shock excites the transducer, thus generating the acoustic pulse. Simultaneously, the master clock activates the vertical or Y-sweep generator (Fig. 1–24.3), initiating the fast or downward deflection of the electron beam of the cathode ray tube (CRT) (Fig. 1–24.4). The CRT consists of an electron gun that produces a focused beam of high velocity electrons, a set of vertical and horizontal deflection plates that position the electron beam, and a display surface coated with a phosphor that glows where the electrons impinge on its surface. The CRT is ideally suited to display echocardiographic data because the electron beam has a low mass and, hence can be deflected rapidly. In addition, the position of this beam can be determined accurately by the voltage applied to the deflection plates.

Once activated, the Y-sweep generator rapidly displaces the electron beam vertically at a rate equal to one-half the speed of sound in tissue. Sweeping the beam at this fixed rate makes possible the conversion of time to distance and, hence, the display of echoes on the CRT at a distance from a reference point that is proportional to the physical distance of the echo-producing structures from the transducer face. Using half the speed of sound corrects for the round-trip passage of the acoustic pulse, thereby permitting the display of echoes from axially related structures at an appropriate depth and in correct spatial relationship to each other.

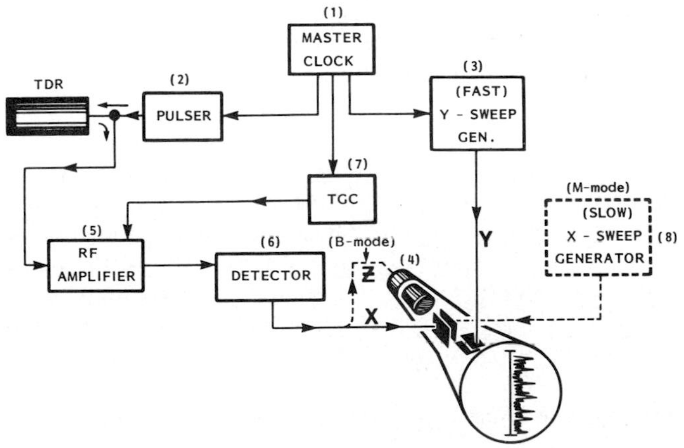

Fig. 1–24. Block diagram of a basic echograph. The primary components are labeled. (See text for further details.) RF = radio frequency; TDR = transducer; TGC = time-dependent gain.

Methods of Amplification

As the transmitted pulse passes through tissue, echoes from succeedingly deeper interfaces are received by the transducer. Each packet of ultrasonic energy or echo that strikes the transducer produces a transient vibrational stress within the crystal. This stress is converted by the piezoelectrical element to oscillatory electrical signals. The intensity of the electrical energy produced by these echoes is generally weak (in the low microvolt range). Because much higher voltages are needed to drive the display apparatus, some form of amplification is required. In addition, enormous variation (many 1000-fold) in intensity may exist between the weakest and strongest echoes. Because of the difficulty in displaying variations in signal strength of this magnitude on a linear scale, some form of nonlinear amplification or dynamic compression must also be introduced during the amplification process.

In its raw state, the oscillatory electrical signal is called a radio frequency (RF) signal. This RF signal is initially received and amplified by the RF amplifier (Fig. 1–24.5). The basic RF signal contains both amplitude and phase information. The amplified RF signals may be further processed to improve the resolving characteristics of the echo system. Commonly, the RF signal is first transformed to a video signal by displaying only the envelope of its positive components (Fig. 1–25). This signal processing occurs in the second component of the amplifier train, the detector (see Fig. 1–24.6).

In the video format, the signal reflects both the amplitude and the duration of the pulse train. Because the entire pulse train is displayed, a relatively long signal is produced. This prolonged signal makes differentiation of closely spaced structures difficult. In addition, because the leading edge of the pulse most appropriately reflects the position of the echo-producing interface, it is desirable to shorten the duration of the displayed echo while emphasizing the leading edge of the signal. This combination of features can be achieved by differentiating the signal and displaying only its positive components (see Fig. 1–25). Differentiation has the added advantage of making the width of the echo less gain-sensitive. In the RF or video format, an increasing system gain causes amplification of all signals. As a result, more of the lower intensity echoes at the onset and the termination of the pulse are displayed. Both signal amplitude and duration increase as gain increases. The differentiated signal also increases in amplitude with increasing gain; however, as illustrated in Figure 1–25B, the duration or width of the displayed echoes does not change significantly. This characteristic is important because if one is attempting to measure the distance between two echoes that are constantly changing in width as gain is varied, the measurements also vary and, hence, are unreliable. With a differentiated signal, the echo intensity may be increased without significantly changing the distance between echoes, thereby making measurements more reproducible.

Another component of the amplifier chain is the time-gain compensation (TGC), or gain as a function of depth (see Fig. 1–24.7). The TGC compensates for the relative decrease in the amplitude of echoes from more distant structures. This decrease occurs as a result of the attenuation of the sound beam as it progresses deeper into the body. When this attenuation is constant, it can be corrected for directly. Because, clinically, attenuation varies from patient to patient, this correction must be individualized, and hence, the depth-dependent increase in gain must be adjustable. Amplification circuitry in the TGC selectively increases the strength of far-field echoes to achieve this adjustability. In addition, it permits individual control of the rate at which this amplification is brought into play. In this manner, one can compensate for some of the normal depth-related decrease in echo intensity, and the relative intensities of both near- and far-field echoes can be displayed more appro-

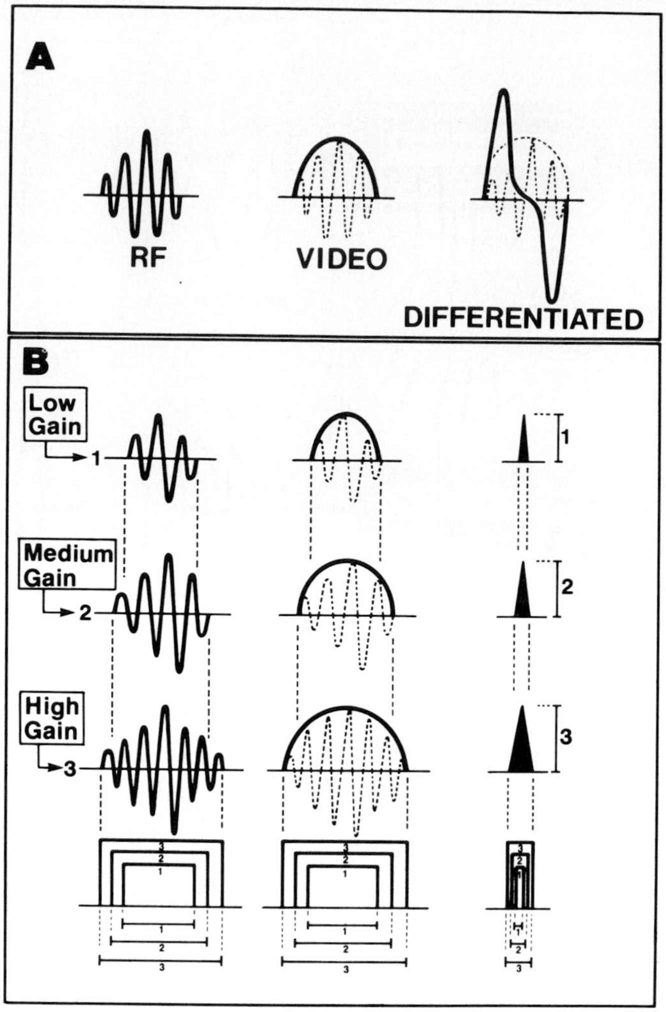

Fig. 1–25. The effects of amplification on the radio frequency (RF), video, and differentiated signal. The RF signal is the oscillatory electrical output of the transducer. In the video format only, the envelope of the positive components of this signal is displayed. Differentiating the signal accentuates the leading edge and effectively shortens the signal duration. **B.** The effects of increasing gain on these signals. When the gain is increased, both the amplitude and duration of the RF signal are increased because the lower intensity components of the RF signal are displayed at higher gains. This characteristic is also true of the video signal. With a differentiated signal, in contrast, signal width increases minimally with increasing amplitude.

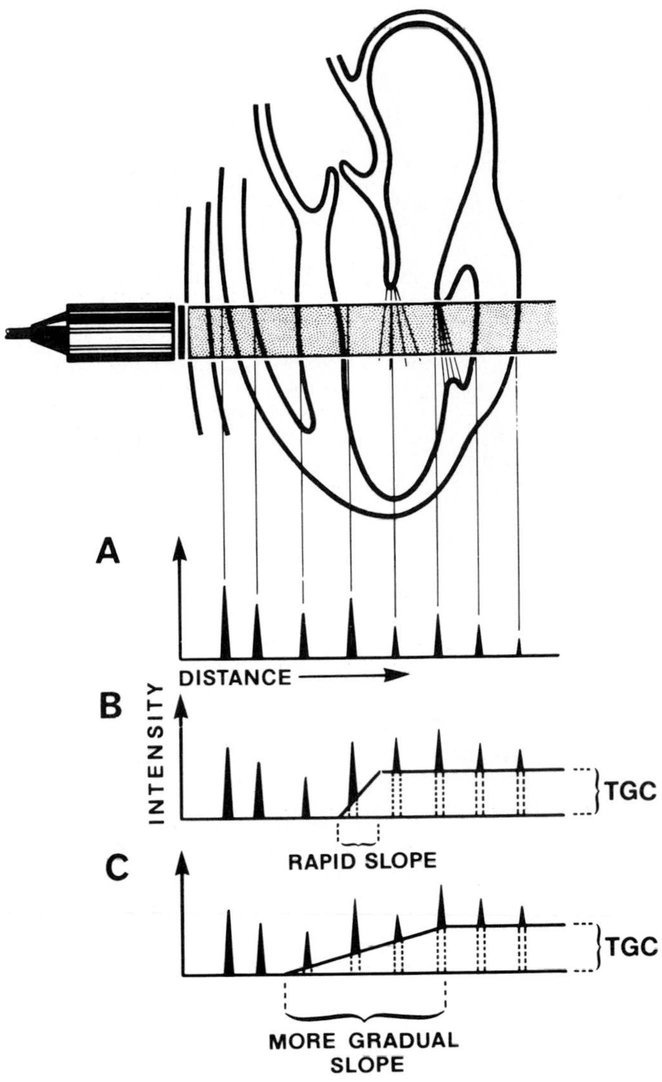

Fig. 1–26. The effect of the time-dependent gain (TGC) on the echoes from more distant structures. **A.** The normal loss in echo strength that is due to the decreasing intensity of the beam as it propagates through the heart. **B.** The effect of the TGC in boosting the intensity of far-field signals. Intensity is selectively increased to display far-field signals at an appropriate height relative to the near-field echoes. **C.** The position of this gain function and its rate of employment can be individualized to suit the needs of the operator.

priately (Fig. 1–26). After passing through the amplifier train, the amplified processed echo is transmitted to the CRT for final display.

Display Formats

There are two basic formats for displaying echocardiographic data: the A-mode and the B-mode. In each of these formats, individual echoes are displayed along a line that represents the beam axis. The difference between the two formats lies in the method of depicting echo amplitude.[6] In both the A- and the B-modes, the horizontal deflection plates of the CRT are attached to the fast or Y-sweep generator. When signaled by the time-base circuit (the master clock or oscillator), the Y-sweep generator sweeps the electron beam vertically at a rate corresponding to the speed of penetration into the heart of the interrogating sound beam. In the A-mode system, amplification circuitry is connected to the vertical deflection plates of the CRT, thereby producing horizontal deflections of the vertically sweeping electron beam each time a change in voltage is recorded (see Fig. 1–24, solid lines).

The amplitude of these horizontal deflections is proportional to the voltage transmitted to the CRT from the amplifier chain and, hence, reflects the relative strength of the recorded echoes. The A-mode format, therefore, displays individual echoes as spikes along a vertical line that represents the beam axis. The distance of these echoes from the start of the sweep is proportional to the distance of the echo-producing structure from the transducer. The amplitude of these spikes is proportional to the strength of the returning echo (Fig. 1–27). When moving structures are recorded, these spikes also move along the vertical axis in a pattern corresponding to the motion pattern of the structure from which they are reflected. The A-mode technique makes possible the detection of highly reflective structures that produce dominant spikes and of structures with characteristic motion patterns, such as the mitral valve or aortic root. Unfortunately, less highly reflective structures or those spaced closely together with similar motion patterns are difficult to differentiate and thus restrict the diagnostic value of A-mode echocardiography. Because of these inherent limitations, the A-mode method is not currently used as a primary clinical display format.

The second major display format, the B-mode or brightness-modulated mode, differs from the A-mode in that the amplified echoes are transmitted to the electron gun of the CRT as the z axis input rather than to the vertical deflection plates (see Fig. 1–24, interrupted

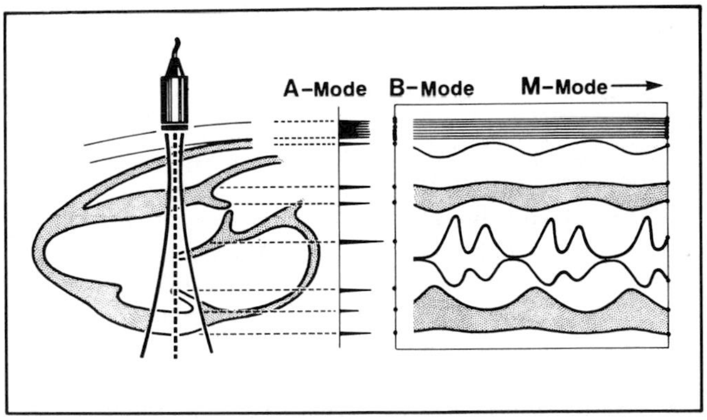

Fig. 1–27. Types of echocardiographic displays currently used. To the left, an ultrasonic beam is directed through the heart at the level of the mitral valve. In the A-mode format, the distance of the echo-producing interfaces from the transducer is depicted by a series of spikes along the vertical axis of the display. The strength of the echoes from each interface is indicated by the length of the horizontal spikes. In the B-mode format, distance is again depicted along the vertical axis by a series of dots. The intensity or brightness of the dots corresponds to the strength of the reflected echoes. In the M-mode format, the B-mode line sweeps across the face of a cathode ray tube. Because of the persistence of the phosphor of the tube, the B-mode dots leave a trail as they move. This trail depicts the motion of intracardiac structures relative to time.

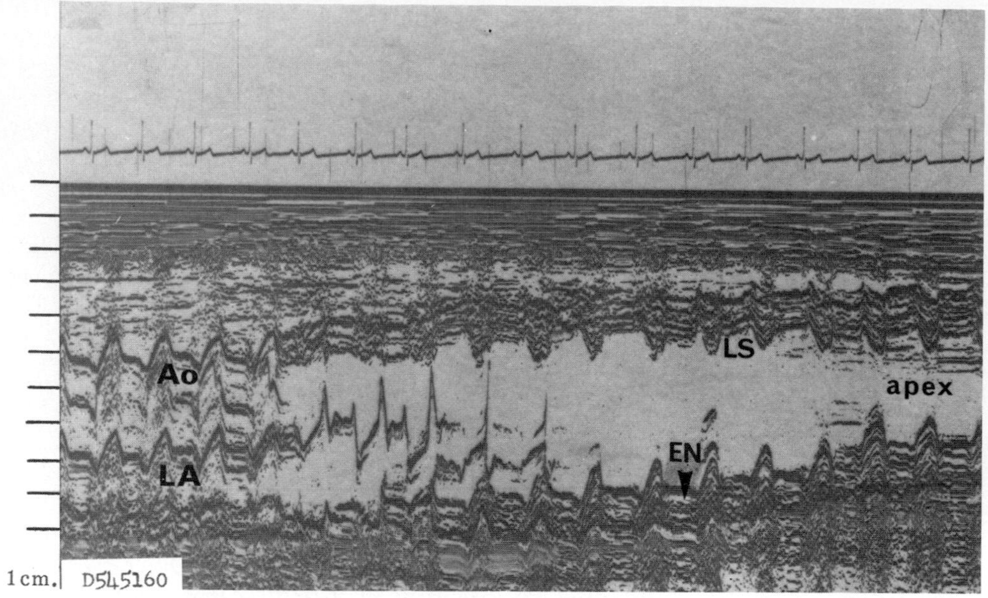

Fig. 1–28. Representative M-mode scan. This scan is obtained by sweeping the transducer from the aorta (Ao) and left atrium (LA) on the left through the left ventricle to the cardiac apex to the right. The overall configuration of the left ventricle, as well as the motion of patterns of specific areas, can be appreciated. The distance from the aortic root to the apex, however, is a function of the speed with which the transducer is angled and does not represent a true anatomic distance. EN = endocardium; LS = left septum.

line). Variations in the voltage from the amplifier train through the z axis input intermittently intensify the electron beam during its vertical sweep, producing points of increased brightness. The distance of these points along the vertical axis represents the depth of sequentially encountered, echo-producing structures, whereas the brightness of the points indicates the intensity of these reflectors (Fig. 1–27). In this basic format, the B-mode line contains little useful information. Conversion to the B-mode format, however, frees the vertical deflection plates, which can then be used to vary the pattern in which the B-mode lines are assembled and displayed. The individual B-mode lines form the basic building blocks for all subsequent echocardiographic imaging formats. The manner of display is varied to achieve particular clinical goals.

The first modification of the B-mode format, the M-mode—or time-motion display[20]—uses a slow sweep or x axis generator to sweep sequential B-mode lines across the face of a CRT (see Fig. 1–24 interrupted line). With an appropriate amount of persistence in the phosphor of the CRT, the B-mode lines leave a trail of echoes as they move. Sweeping the lines at a fixed rate permits the recording of the position and motion pattern of the echoes from intercardiac structures relative to time (see Fig. 1–27). The high resolution, rapid sampling rate, and convenient graphic format of M-mode echocardiography are ideal for imaging localized areas of the heart and analyzing time-related events. As a result, before the late 1970s, M-mode echocardiography was the primary clinical method for displaying echocardiographic data.

Unfortunately, the M-mode format provides only axial information concerning structure, motion, and depth. It is therefore limited because it fails to convey any appreciation of the true lateral distances between structures or to accurately reflect off-axis motion. Initial attempts to provide more spatial information led to the development of M-mode scanning (Fig. 1–28). An M-mode scan is obtained by manually sweeping the transducer from one area of the heart to another while continuously recording the resultant echocardiographic data on a strip-chart recorder.[21] This technical development provided some qualitative information concerning lateral structure relationships. Unfortunately, these scans vary with the speed and path of transducer movement, and because each of these variables changes from sweep to sweep and from examination to examination, the reproducibility of these data is limited.

The desire to add quantitative spatial information to the echocardiographic examination led to the development of the second modification of the B-mode format, which in the clinical context is termed two-dimensional or cross-sectional echocardiography. Cross-sectional echocardiography is an imaging format in which the ultrasonic reflections from a predetermined cross-sec-

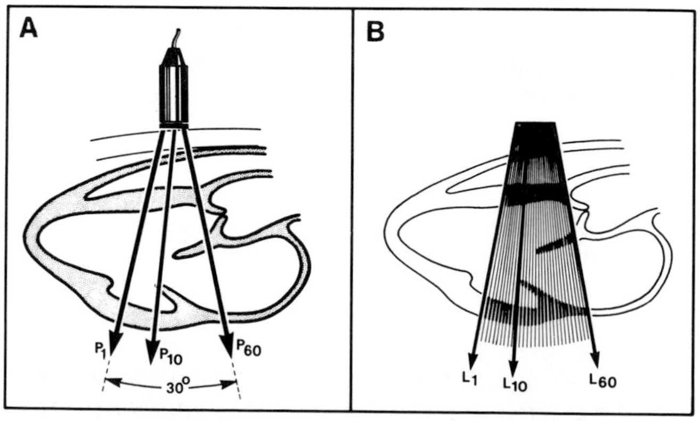

Fig. 1–29. Pulse transmission and image recording and display in the cross-sectional format. **A.** Pulses are continuously transmitted as the transducer is moved in a fixed plane through a 30° arc from the papillary muscles to the left atrium. **B.** B-mode lines, which correspond to each of these pulses, are recorded, assembled, and displayed in a pattern that corresponds to the pattern of pulse transmission. The first data line (L_1), therefore, corresponds to the position of the first pulse (P_1), the tenth data line (L_{10}) to the tenth pulse (P_{10}), and so on.

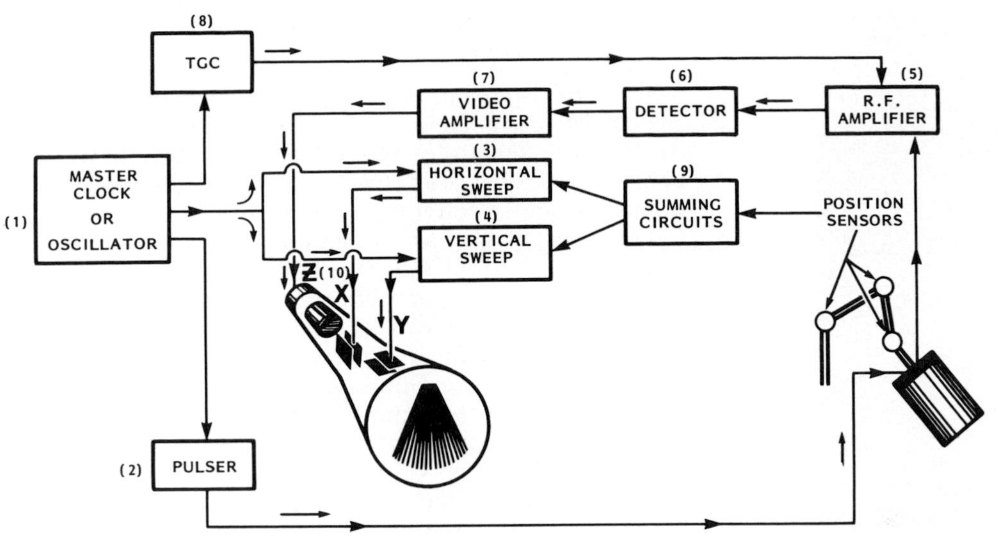

Fig. 1–30. Block diagram of a simple B-mode scanning system. RF = radio frequency; TGC = time-dependent gain.

tional or tomographic plane through the heart are recorded and displayed. To assemble a cross-sectional image, one moves the sound beam from one area of the heart to another through a fixed plane while continuously transmitting sound pulses and recording the resulting echoes. To display the acquired data in a coherent fashion, one continuously senses and transmits to the CRT the transducer position so that the resultant B-mode lines can be displayed in a position that corresponds to the spatial position of the ultrasonic beam at the time the data are recorded. Figure 1–29 illustrates how these B-mode lines can be assembled into a cross-sectional image of a fixed area of the heart.

The simplest example of this type of cross-sectional imaging is a static manual B-mode scanning system. Figure 1–30 is a block diagram of such a system. In this format, methods of pulse generation and echo amplification are similar to those previously described for the basic echograph. The chief differences in the scanning format are (1) the transducer is attached to an articulated arm, which limits the transducer's motion to a single plane, and (2) position-sensing devices in the arm continuously relay the transducer coordinates via the summing circuitry to the vertical and horizontal deflection plates of the CRT; the CRT then positions the path of the fast or Y-sweep on the oscilloscope to conform to the relative position of the ultrasonic beam in space. Because each B-mode line is recorded and can be stored in its appropriate spatial position, one can gradually assemble an image that depicts a two-dimensional or tomographic plane of the heart by manually moving the transducer across the precordium while continuously sampling.

Because cardiac structures are in constant motion, if data are randomly recorded at a slow rate during unselected portions of the cardiac cycle, the interfaces from which the data arise constantly vary in position, resulting in a blurred image. To overcome the effects of cardiac motion, slow manual or mechanical scanners are commonly modified, using a gating circuit triggered by the R-wave of the electrocardiogram. The gating circuit allows the recording oscilloscope to accept pulses only during specific portions of the cardiac cycle and, thus, effectively stops cardiac motion. Delay and duration controls within the gating circuitry vary the elapsed time between the R-wave and the onset and duration of the unblanking signal of the gate. Echoes received when the unblanking signal is active are recorded, whereas those received during the remainder of the cardiac cycle are eliminated. Multiple independent gates can be incorporated to permit the assembly of multiple images from varying points in the cardiac cycle.

During actual performance of a manual cross-sectional study, the transducer is slowly moved along the chest wall by the operator. With each cardiac cycle, a line representing the path of the sound beam during that cycle is written on a storage oscilloscope. Between the writing of individual lines, the direction of the sound beam is adjusted slightly to record additional anatomic information, and in this fashion, an image is gradually accumulated. Figure 1–31 is an example of such a scan. In this figure, the path of the transducer motion is parallel to the long axis of the left ventricle in a plane extending from the left ventricular apex to the aortic root. This type of image displays the spatial geometry of the heart, the interrelationship of various structures, and the lateral as well as axial distance between areas of interest.

If the B-mode scanning system is further modified to permit more rapid electronic or mechanical beam scanning, images can be accumulated at a sufficiently high rate to display dynamic cardiac motion in "real time." These "real time" or dynamic B-mode instruments are discussed in detail in Chapter 2. The data derived from them form the basis for much of the clinical material presented in this book.

System Controls

The types of signal processing and variations in display that occur in an echocardiograph are characteristic of the individual instrument and are not under operator control. Certain features of the display, however, can be controlled by the operator; these variable controls are discussed in the next section.

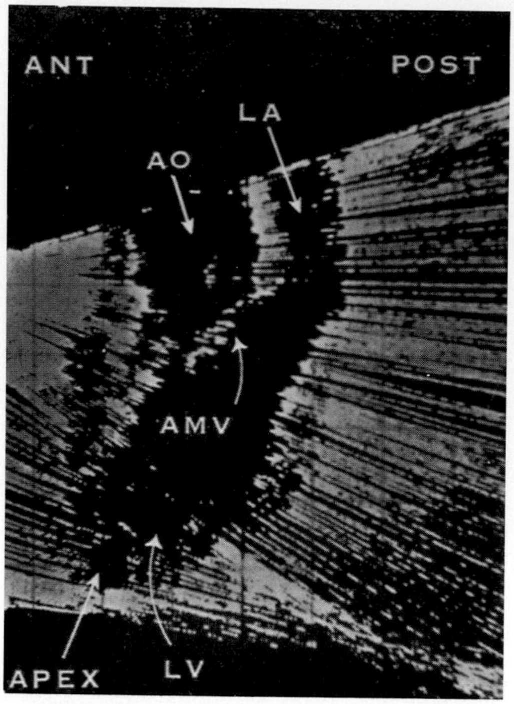

Fig. 1–31. Cross-sectional scan of the heart. This scan is assembled by recording sequential gated B-mode lines. These lines are displayed in a spatially oriented fashion to gradually build a two-dimensional image of the heart at a selected point in the cardiac cycle. LA = left atrium; AO = aorta; AMV = anterior mitral valve; LV = left ventricle. (From King DL: Cardiac ultrasonography: cross-sectional ultrasonic imaging of the heart. Circulation 47: 843, 1972. Reproduced by permission of the American Heart Association, Inc.)

All echocardiographs provide certain operator controls that, regardless of the kind of display, permit (1) the absolute amplitude of all echoes within the field of examination to be varied, (2) the selective amplification of echoes within specific portions of the field, or (3) echoes of only specified amplitudes to be included in the final display. The primary system controls that perform these functions and are common to most echocardiographic instruments include the system gain or coarse gain; the TGC, or gain as a function of time or depth; the near-field gain; the damping circuit; and the reject circuit.

System Gain or Coarse Gain

The system gain uniformly increases the amplitude of all echoes within the display. Depending on the degree of differentiation of the displayed signal, an increase in the overall gain may increase not only the amplitude of the displayed echo but also its duration or width. In addition, as previously noted, an increase in the overall gain permits display of weaker echoes and effectively increases beam width. Higher coarse gain settings, therefore, increase the ability to display weak or less distinct echoes; however, this ability always occurs at the expense of lateral resolution and, depending on display configuration, may also decrease axial resolution.

Time-Gain Compensation, or Gain as a Function of Depth

The TGC is an amplifier circuit that compensates for the natural loss in echo intensity or strength that occurs as the beam penetrates more deeply into the chest. To achieve these ends, the TGC consists of an amplification circuit, which selectively increases the strength of far-field echoes, as well as a ramp function, which permits individual control of the level and of the rate at which this depth-dependent amplification is brought into play. By varying the slope of this ramp, one can rapidly employ full amplification at a particular level or can gradually increase amplification as a function of time or depth (Fig. 1–26). In both M-mode and cross-sectional echocardiography, delineation of the interventricular septum is a difficult problem. Conventional practice, therefore, places the leading edge of the ramp at the right ventricular border of the septum, thereby abruptly boosting the level of all echoes in the septal region and onward to the posterior wall of the heart. This placement separates the septum from the less intensely amplified right ventricular cavity and highlights this region of the heart.[22] Many newer instruments have replaced the conventional TGC control with a series of slide pots, which permit gain to be varied independently at predetermined depths. This approach is simpler than the TGC but limits gain control to fixed increments of depth (e.g., 2-cm intervals) and a change in gain at one level usually affects the gain at adjacent levels.

Near-Field Gain

Because the strength of the echocardiographic beam is greatest in the near field, the echoes from structures most closely apposed to the transducer are the strongest and, if kept in their raw form, tend to dominate the display. To permit more detailed analysis of structure, configuration, and motion in the near field, one must frequently decrease the strength of the near-field echoes to a greater degree than that of those returning from more distal structures. This situation is, in effect, the reverse of the TGC function. For this reason, a selective near-field gain control is conventionally supplied to control the amplitude of these strong near-field echoes. This control determines the amplitude of all echoes in the portion of the display from the transducer to the ramp of the TGC. This near-field gain control, therefore, affects a variable portion of the display, depending on the position of the ramp, and must be distinguished from the near field of the ultrasonic beam, which depends on transducer properties and not on gain.

Damping Circuit

The damping circuit controls both the amplitude and the time constant of the transmitted pulse. This effectively decreases the power output of the transducer and shortens the pulse duration. The damping circuit decreases effective beam width and improves resolution. It does so, however, at the expense of signal strength. Although the coarse gain and the damping controls affect different portions of the signal, their net effects on the overall image are similar.

Reject Circuit

The echoes returning from within the heart vary widely in amplitude. Numerically, the low intensity signals from weak or off-axis reflectors and from scattering sources exceed the higher amplitude echoes from the more prominent structures of primary interest. When displayed in an unaltered state, these weak echoes dominate the display and obscure the higher amplitude signals. A reject circuit is incorporated into most echographs to eliminate the weak echoes. This circuit filters out all signals below a fixed amplitude, thereby removing weaker echoes and background noise from the final display and permitting the higher amplitude signals to be displayed in greater contrast.

BIOLOGIC EFFECTS OF ULTRASOUND

Ultrasound at relatively low intensities has been used for many years as a noninvasive imaging tool in clinical medicine without reported ill effects. One must recognize, however, that sound waves that contain sufficient mechanical energy to damage or to destroy biologic tissue can be produced.[23,24] The original Langevin underwater detection apparatus could generate intensities in the sound field sufficient to kill small fish or to induce severe pain in the human hands.[25] Subsequent reports have noted a variety of functional and structural changes in a wide range of biologic systems, including human beings, following ultrasonic radiation. Because the goal of any medical diagnostic technique is to obtain as much information as possible concerning the state of the human organism without adversely affecting that organism, the properties of ultrasound that determine its safe application and the mechanisms by which ultrasound produces tissue damage must be understood.

Properties of Ultrasound That Determine Its Biologic Effects (Pressure, Power, Energy, and Intensity)

The biologic effects of ultrasound depend on the total energy flux across a particular area, the spatial distribution of energy within the sound beam, the time duration and pattern over which a biologic system is exposed to the sound energy, the frequencies contained within the sound wave, and the sensitivity of the exposed tissue system. Acoustic pressure, p, is the fundamental physical quantity describing the propagation of an ultrasonic wave. Pressure is force, in newtons (N)* per unit area, in square meters (m^2).[26] Pressure can also be expressed in pascals (Pa), where 1 Pa is equal to 1 N/m^2, or in atmospheres (atm) with 1 atm being equal to approximately 10^5 Pa. Acoustic pressure varies with time, as indicated in Figure 1–32. The maximum pressure at any point is denoted by $p+$ and the minimum by $p-$. The maximum and minimum ultrasonic pressures (denoted $p+/p-$ in Fig. 1–32) are typically up to 50 atm.[26]

The amount of acoustic energy produced by a sound-emitting device per unit time (i.e., the rate at which energy is introduced into a tissue) is the acoustic power of the device and determines its ability to create a biologic effect. Power is usually measured in watts (joules/sec). Maximum values of ultrasonic power from diagnostic equipment are typically in the tens of milliwatts.

* 1 Newton = kg $msec^{-2}$

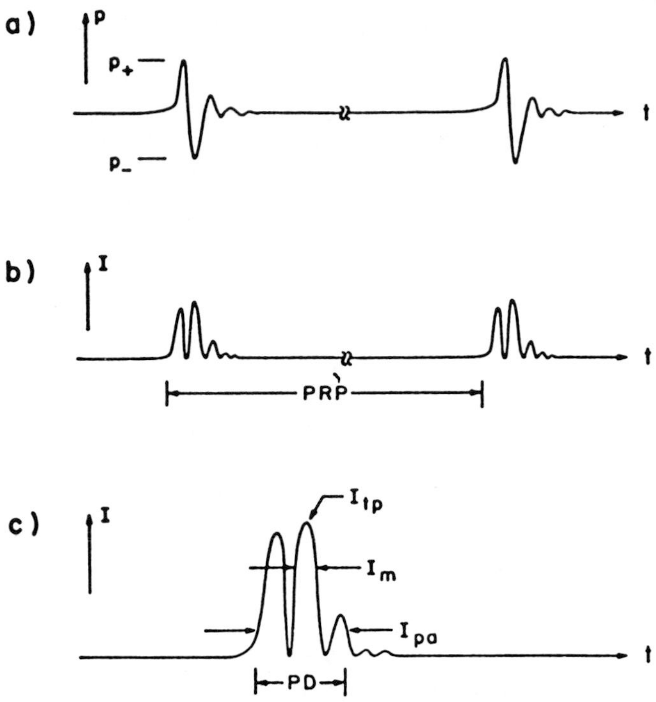

Fig. 1–32. Temporal representation of the pressure (a) and intensity (b) of an ultrasonic signal. The maximum positive (p_+) and negative (p_-) pressure are indicated in panel (a). The pulse repetition period (PRP) is the time between the same position on two adjacent pulses. The details of a single ultrasonic intensity pulse (c) show the pulse duration (PD), the temporal peak intensity (I_{tp}). The maximum intensity (I_m), and the pulse average intensity (I_{pa}). (From O'Brien WD: Biological effects of ultrasound: rationale for measurement of selected ultrasonic output quantities. Echocardiography 3:165, 1986.)

When actually transmitted into a tissue system, the acoustic power is largely concentrated within the margins of the sound beam. The concentration of power within a specific area is the intensity (I) (expressed as either watts per square meter or milliwatts per square centimeter). Measurement of the intensity of a sound beam is not simple, because intensity varies depending on the location within the sound beam at which it is measured.

Because the intensity can vary, depending on the point within the sound beam at which it is measured, a number of terms are used to describe spatial intensity. These include (1) the spatial peak intensity (I_{sp}), which typically occurs at the transition point along the beam axis for a nonfocused transducer and at the focal point along the beam axis for a focused transducer; (2) the spatial average intensity (I_{sa}), which can be calculated relative to the cross-sectional area of the sound beam or some other representative area such as the transducer face; or (3) the recorded intensity at a specific point in space ($I_{z,y}$).

Although relatively easy to determine, the spatial average intensity has the disadvantage of depending somewhat arbitrarily on the area selected to calculate this average (e.g., the area of the transducer face) and generally does not reflect the actual energy levels to which local tissue areas within the sound beam are exposed. For many purposes, therefore, intensity levels are referred to in terms of the peak intensity encountered by any tissue area within the path of the sound beam.

In addition to the total amount of acoustic energy produced by a sound-emitting device and the spatial distribution of that energy as it passes through a tissue system, the effects on that biologic system also depend on the time of exposure. The exposure time depends on whether the sound-emitting device transmits a continuous or an intermittent sound wave. A sound-emitting device that produces a constant sound wave is said to operate in a continuous wave (CW) mode, whereas a device that transmits a series of identical pulses, each consisting of only a few cycles, is said to operate in a pulsed mode. Most imaging systems operate in a pulsed mode; therefore, the tissue system imaged is subjected to sound energy intermittently, as illustrated in Figure 1–32A. In a pulsed system, the exposure time is a function of both the length of each pulse, or the pulse duration (PD), and the number of pulses transmitted per unit time, the pulse repetition frequency (PRF). The time between the onset or other corresponding points of successive pulses is the pulse repetition period (PRP). The PRP therefore, equals the reciprocal of a PRF. Thus, if pulses are transmitted at a frequency of 1000/sec, the PRP is 1/1000 of a second, or 1 msec. The fraction of the total time the instrument is operating (the time the sound is actually "on") is termed the *duty factor* (*D*) and is expressed by the ratio of the PD to the PRP (D = PD/PRP). Therefore, if the pulse duration is 1 μsec and the PRP is 1000 μsec, or 1 msec, the D is 1/1000, or 0.001 (0.10%). Duty factors for diagnostic ultrasonic instruments are typically in the range of 0.0005 to 0.002.

The power output of an ultrasonic device operating in the pulsed mode is the same when the device is "on" as that of a CW device operating at the same frequency.* Likewise, the spatial distribution of intensities is similar. Because tissue is subjected to these energy levels only intermittently in the pulsed mode, such energy levels can be described (1) in terms of the peak intensity to which tissue is subjected when the instrument is "on," the temporal peak intensity (I_{tp}); (2) in terms of the intensity averaged over the time the pulse is "on," the pulse average intensity (I_{pa}); or (3) in terms of the average intensity received by the tissue over the entire time period the instrument is in operation, the temporal average intensity (I_{ta}). When actually reported, therefore, intensities have both a spatial and a temporal value such as I_{sppa}, the spatial peak pulse average intensity, or I_{sptp}, the spatial peak temporal peak intensity.

* The output power for a CW device may actually be higher than that of a pulsed device for the same input voltage. This occurs because the CW element has time to achieve resonance and therefore may be more efficient in its energy conversion than a comparable element operating in pulsed mode.

From a measurement standpoint, it is difficult to determine high values of the I_{sptp} and significant measurement errors can occur.[26] A temporal definition of intensity that closely approximates the greatest temporal intensity is denoted by I_m. This intensity quantity, I_m, is defined at the spatial peak location to be the temporal average of the intensity over the largest half-cycle of the transmitted pulse (Fig. 1–32). The various values for intensity are listed in Table 1–3. The highest intensity value is the I_{sptp}, followed by the I_m, and the lowest value is the I_{sata}. The relative values of other parameters may vary depending on the pulse duration and the measured area.

The spatial peak, temporal average (SPTA) is apparently the most meaningful of these measurements because it describes the peak energy level to which any of the tissue areas lying within the sound beam are exposed, averaged over the total time of exposure. The total time of exposure reflects not only the actual exposure time but also the period available for potential recovery between pulses. In general terms, SPTA intensity levels in the low milliwatt per square centimeter range are used in diagnostic instruments. Therapeutic techniques, which rely on tissue heating, generally use CW devices with intensities in the range of 1 to 5 W/cm^2 and intensities of greater than 10 W/cm^2 are found in lesioning devices. The frequency of a sound wave also influences its biologic effects. Table 1–4 lists the inten-

Table 1–3. Various Measures of Intensity for Ultrasonic Beams

1. *Spatial peak, temporal peak intensity* (I_{sptp})—The peak intensity at the point in space where the intensity is highest and that occurs when the ultrasonic emitting device is "on." It is the highest of the measured intensities.
2. *Spatial average, temporal average intensity* (I_{sata})—The average power output of the device over the pulse repetition period divided by a reference area, usually that of the transducer face. This measurement of intensity is the most quickly determined and most frequently quoted by manufacturers. It also yields the lowest values of the more commonly used measures of intensity.
3. *Spatial average, temporal peak intensity* (I_{satp})—The peak intensity over a selected area, such as the transducer face, that occurs when the ultrasonic emitting device is "on."
4. *Spatial peak, temporal average intensity* (I_{spta})—The maximum spatial intensity occurring when the sound beam is "on," averaged over the pulse repetition period.
5. *Spatial peak pulse average intensity* (I_{sppa})—The pulse-averaged intensity measured at the point in space where this value is maximal.
6. *Spatial average pulse average* (I_{sapa})—The pulse average intensity averaged over the beam cross-sectional area.
7. *Temporal average intensity of the largest half cycle* (I_m)—This intensity measure is defined at the spatial peak location and, therefore, has only one value.

Table 1–4. Ultrasonic Power UM8

Mode	Scanhead	Absolute (mW)	(mW/cm²) Spatial Average Temporal Average (SATA)	Spatial Peak Temporal Average (SPTA)
Two-dimensional	Access, 3 MHz Medium focus	32.4	9.66	19.5
Two-dimensional	Access, 5 MHz Medium focus	18.3	9.18	17.4
Two-dimensional	Annular array 3.5 MHz	64.6	14.8	46.0
Two-dimensional	Annular array 5 MHz	18.2	5.8	21.2
Pulsed Doppler	Access, 2.25 MHz Medium focus	90.1	543	1021
Pulsed Doppler	Access, 3 MHz Medium focus	41.3	530	874

sity levels for a representative cardiac diagnostic system.

Mechanisms of Tissue Damage

The biologic effects of sound energy appear primarily related to the local heating properties of ultrasound, cavitation, and mechanical stresses induced in tissue during the passage of sound waves.[27–29]

Thermal Effects

By far the most common and best understood mechanism by which ultrasound can produce unwanted effects on tissue is through local heating. Heat is produced whenever ultrasonic energy is absorbed by any biologic material. The amount of heat produced is directly related to the intensity of the sound wave at any point in space. For a plane wave, this can be described by the equation

$$I = I_0 e^{-2\alpha x} \quad [1.6]$$

where I is the local intensity, x is the depth in the tissue, I_0 is the intensity at x equals zero, and α is the attenuation coefficient. For a focused wave, propagation is more complex, and intensity may actually increase with depth if focusing predominates over attenuation.

The relationship between local intensity and changes in temperature can be described as follows:

$$dT/dt = 2\alpha I/\rho C_m. \quad [1.7]$$

where dT/dt is the rate of increase in temperature, α is the absorption coefficient, t is time, ρ is the mass density of the tissue, I is local intensity, and C_m is the specific heat of the tissue.* Thus, temperature increases at a rate proportional to the local sound intensity and degree of absorption and is inversely proportional to tissue density and specific heat. The fundamental mechanisms of absorption in biologic tissues are not well understood, except that, in general, absorption is primarily related to the concentration of proteins and other large molecules and secondarily to the secondary and tertiary structures of these proteins.[30] The effects of density and specific heat are such that relatively dense tissue such as muscle (although absorbing energy at four times the rate)[31] will not heat as quickly as less dense tissue such as fat.†

Selective heating may occur at tissue interfaces because at such boundaries mode conversion takes place and part of the propagating longitudinal ultrasonic wave is converted to a shear wave. Shear waves have absorption coefficients orders of magnitude greater than those of longitudinal waves. Consequently, the wave energy quickly dissipates as heat within the immediate neighborhood of the interface. Scattering and reflection can also contribute to local heating by concentrating sound energy.

Perfusion of tissue by blood has a cooling effect and tends to offset temperature increases caused by exposure to ultrasound. The physical transport of heat from a tissue region by blood or fluid flow is called *convection*. Direct diffusion of heat through tissue also occurs, decreasing local temperature. This mechanism is called *conduction*.

Cavitation

Cavitation is the general term used to describe the formation, growth, and subsequent dynamic behavior of gas bubbles in an ultrasonically irradiated medium.[33,34] In a pure liquid, cavitation occurs when the local pressure falls below the vapor pressure of a fluid and gas "boils" from the liquid. In body tissues, pressures as low as the vapor pressure of water (47 mm at 37°C) are not reached with clinical ultrasound equipment, so bubble formation in tissue must occur primarily from dissolved gas (O_2 or CO_2). Bubbles of these dissolved gases are felt to form and grow from pre-existing microscopic gas nuclei trapped in cracks or corners of small tissue particles.

* Specific heat is the amount of heat, in calories, required to raise 1 g of tissue 1°C and is expressed relative to water.

† To illustrate how rapidly temperature would increase in a biologic material, given typical parameters, let us assume that density is 1 g/ml (the density of water) and that c_m is 1 calorie/g/°C (about the same as for water). Assuming α = 0.05 nepers (1 neper = 8.686 dB)/cm (which is approximately correct for liver at 3 MHz) and assuming intensity is 1 W/cm², we obtain a value of dT/dt of 0.024°C/sec or 1.44°C/min. Of course, most diagnostic systems do not expose tissues to such high energy continuously; however, during the short time of exposure, the temperature would rise at about this rate.[32]

Sound-induced oscillation of these small bubbles causes gas to diffuse inward and outward during each cycle because of the changing pressure within the bubble. If the diffusion inward and outward is asymmetric so that the sonically produced inward flow exceeds the outward diffusion flow, the bubble grows. This phenomenon, called *rectified diffusion*, is an important aspect of sonic cavitation. Limiting the process of rectified diffusion is bubble resonance. At each stage of growth, a bubble has a frequency at which it naturally vibrates. This resonant frequency is inversely related to bubble size and the density of the fluid surrounding it. The most efficient coupling of ultrasonic energy to the bubble occurs when the resonant frequency of the bubble is equal to the incident ultrasonic frequency. Thus, the microscopic gas nuclei, whose resonant frequencies are initially well above that of the ultrasound, will grow until their resonant frequency falls to that of the incident ultrasonic wave. At this point, diffusion in and out of the bubble is balanced so the mass of gas inside the bubble remains constant. However, because the bubble is "tuned" to the incoming ultrasound, significant energy continues to be absorbed, and this leads to an increase in the amplitude of bubble vibration.

Any vibrating bubble has associated with it a total energy reflecting the sum of the potential energy (alternate compression and rarefaction of the gas in the bubble) and kinetic energy (concentric motion of the fluid displaced by the bubble). When driven by incident ultrasonic waves at its resonant frequency, this total energy gradually increases. If there were no other counterbalancing forces, bubble vibration amplitude would grow without bound. In the real situation, however, fluid viscosity eventually limits the vibration amplitude as some of the kinetic energy of fluid motion is lost from the bubble by heat formation caused by viscosity. Additionally, some of the energy of vibration is radiated away by spherical waves from the bubble. For example, in water, a bubble resonating at 1 MHz in a sound field with an intensity of 100 mW/cm^2 can take 60 μW from the field, about 90% of which is converted to heat.[32] Therefore, tissues in a region containing distributions of such bubbles might reabsorb sound readily, causing increased local heating. In tissues that have distributions of bubbles of a size near the resonance frequency of the propagating sound field, heating can be expected to occur exponentially.[35] Thus, the growth in bubble amplitude stops when the amount of energy absorbed from the ultrasonic field is balanced by the loss of energy through viscous effects and radiation, and the bubble is said to be in equilibrium with its surroundings.

For all diagnostic ultrasound systems, this vibrational equilibrium is achieved at relatively low amplitudes (not enough to cause bubble collapse during the compressional phase of each vibratory cycle). Such cavitation is thus stable and will persist as long as there is incident ultrasonic energy to power it. Note that the fluid motion in the immediate vicinity of even stably resonating bubbles is much larger than would be seen with the bubbles alone. This increased motion leads to microstreaming or eddying of liquid near the bubbles, which can produce shear stresses that are high enough to break cell membranes and macromolecules. Depending on local conditions, the oscillations may be symmetric and predictable or asymmetric and unpredictable. Continuous wave ultrasound more likely causes stable cavitation because the bubbles need time to grow to resonance.

At extremely high intensities, unstable, "collapse," or transient cavitation occurs and bubbles collapse during the positive part of the pressure cycle. Because the cavity that has already absorbed energy from the ultrasonic field becomes smaller, the energy density increases, so that with complete collapse enormous local energy is produced, leading to shock waves and high local pressures.[36] It is estimated that a cavity of 10^{-3} mm in diameter collapsing in solid incompressable surroundings can create a local pressure of 1000 atm. Such pressures can open up other cavities, leading to a chain reaction known as "interaction cavitation." It is unlikely that interaction or collapse cavitation is a hazard in diagnostic ultrasound, because the threshold level in water is 300 W cm^{-2} at 1 MHz.[37]

Viscosity plays a critical role in limiting the vibrational amplitude of the bubbles. For example, typical diagnostic systems can produce powers of the order of 10 to 100 W for a few cycles. This represents peaks of 5 to 15 atm of pressure. It has been shown that the so-called viscous startup time for a bubble in water (with low viscosity) is small compared to an acoustic period and that bubbles with initial radii less than about 3 μm are not inertially limited, implying that significant growth could occur in water to a size maximum about 7 to 7.5 μm. The pressure of a bubble that starts at 3 μm and goes to 7 μm and collapses to a minimum size of less than 1 μm can be greater than 200 atm. The internal temperature could reach approximately 1000°C. This would give an energy density of about 100 joules/ml.[38] Although these are crude estimates, they demonstrate the order of magnitude of energy concentration that can be caused by cavitation *in water*. In tissues, however, the effective viscosity is 100 times greater than water, and therefore, bubble motion is greatly limited. In addition, little attenuation is required to decrease greatly the intensities of diagnostic units.

Mechanical Effects

Direct mechanical effects are caused by the large forces and accelerations to which particles in tissue can be exposed when they are in the path of an ultrasonic beam. Mechanical effects are usually grouped under the heading of "other" effects or "direct" mechanisms of action. Many such mechanisms of possible importance in ultrasound bioeffects are not based on thermal or acoustic cavitation processes. These mechanisms include acoustic microscopic streaming, effects of viscous stresses, radiation forces, and radiation torques.[39,40]

Stresses occur when velocity gradients are found resulting from either microstreaming or alterations in acoustic characteristics of the tissue within which the field is propagating. Micromolecules caught in a stream, either flowing or oscillating, in which the velocities vary strongly as a function of space can be subjected to a great deal of shear stress and perhaps be altered. However, the relationship of these phenomena to actual biologic effects at the diagnostic power levels output by echocardiographic equipment is unclear.

Summary of Bioeffects. Although all of the effects described here have been observed in in vitro and experimental in vivo studies, they are far less likely to occur in biologic tissues. Thermal effects are the most likely to occur clinically but should be most obvious close to the skin surface. Cavitation effects are far more complex and, though occurring with lower probability in biologic tissues, can be more serious than thermal effects. Even if the required bubbles or nucleation occur in tissues, the effects of absorption and viscosity will greatly moderate the possibility of cavitation effects. The other mechanisms, such as radiation pressure and radiation streaming, have an even lower probability of occurring in tissue.

Relationship of Ultrasonic Field Parameters to Patient Safety

Relating ultrasonic field parameters to patient safety, the committee on bioeffects of the American Institute of Ultrasound in Medicine (AIUM) has stated that, as of October 1982, no independently confirmed significant biologic effects had been observed in mammalian tissues exposed to intensities (SPTA as measured in a free field of water) below 100 mW/cm^2. Furthermore, such effects had not been demonstrated for ultrasonic exposure times (Total time, which includes "off" time as well as "on" time for repeated pulse regimen) of less than 500 seconds and more than 1 second, even at higher intensities when the product of intensity and exposure time is less than 50 joules/cm^2.[18] As noted in Table 1–4, current diagnostic levels often exceed these values. The AIUM statement, therefore, should not be interpreted as indicating that these higher intensities are associated with a definite risk of biologically adverse effects, but simply that no such effects have been documented at levels below 100 mW/cm^2. The committee further notes that

> diagnostic ultrasound has been in use for over 25 years. During that time no confirmed biological effects on patients or instrument operators caused by exposure at intensities typical of present diagnostic ultrasound instruments have ever been reported. Although the possibility exists that such biological effects may be identified in the future, current data indicate that the benefits to patients of the prudent use of diagnostic ultrasound outweigh the risks, if any, that may be present.[41]

Despite this optimistic clinical experience, large gaps exist in the knowledge base concerning the effects of ultrasound in humans. A threshold level below which sound can be used for an unlimited period without any ill effect has not been defined. Likewise, the cumulative effects of multiple, repeated ultrasonic pulses are poorly characterized. One must also remember that effects that occur on a gross scale are easily identified and, hence, appreciated. More subtle effects, which are not readily evident, may be retained within the system and may accumulate or may be passed to subsequent generations. Thus, despite the apparent safety of the low intensity sound levels used in diagnostic imaging, these instruments should be used judiciously and with sufficient medical justification.

In cross-sectional cardiac imaging, the actual exposure at any point within the heart is further affected by the variation in the pulse transmittal pattern and by the attenuating properties of the tissues that the sound energies must pass through to reach the heart. In the cross-sectional format, pulses are directed in a variable scan pattern. Consequently, a particular tissue area may actually receive sound energy from only a small fraction of the total number of transmitted pulses. Likewise, in the sector format, the amount of energy concentrated near the apex of the sector (where pulses tend to overlap) is greater than that encountered in the far field (where the individual waves are more widely separated). In addition, the sound energy emitted by the transducer face is attenuated as it passes through the superficial skin and muscle layers that overlie the heart. As a result, the sound intensity levels experienced by specific areas within the heart vary not only with the temporal and spatial field characteristics of the sound beam but also with the frequency at which a particular region is interrogated by the sound energy and with the characteristics of the tissue layers lying between the transducer and that area. Actual cardiac exposure, therefore, may represent a small fraction of the total energy level produced by the ultrasonic instrument. In Doppler studies, however, power is generally increased and the area of interest is insonated for a longer period. Good judgment suggests that Doppler studies be limited to the time required to obtain the desired clinical information and that in the fetus there be reasonable medical justification for such examinations.

REFERENCES

1. Lord Rayleigh: Theory of Sound. New York, Dover Publications, 1945.
2. Rschevkin SN: The Theory of Sound (translated by OM Blunn, PE Doak). New York, Pergamon Press, 1963.
3. Segal BL: Symposium on echocardiography (diagnostic ultrasound). Am J Cardiol 19:1, 1967.
4. Curie J, Curie P: Development par prission de l'electricite polaire dans les cristaux heimiedras a faces inclinees. CR Acad Sci 91:S294, 1880.
5. Kinsker LE, Frey AR: Fundamentals of Acoustics. New York, John Wiley & Sons, 1962.
6. Wells PNT: Biomedical Ultrasonics. New York, Academic Press, 1977.
7. Fry FJ (ed.): Intense focused ultrasound. *In* Ultrasound: Its Applications in Medicine and Biology. Amsterdam, Elsevier Science Publishing, 1978.
8. Kikuchi Y: Transducers for ultrasonic systems. *In* Fry FJ (ed.): Ultrasound: Its Applications in Medicine and Biology. Amsterdam, Elsevier Science Publishing, 1978.
9. Dehn JT: Interference patterns in the near field of a circular piston. J Acoust Soc Am 32:1692, 1960.
10. Kossoff G: The transducer. *In* DeVlieger M, et al.: Handbook of Clinical Ultrasound. New York, John Wiley & Sons, 1978.
11. Fry WJ, Dunn F: Ultrasound: analysis and experimental methods in biologic research. *In* Mastuk WL (ed.): Physical Techniques in Biological Research. Vol. 4. New York, Academic Press, 1962.
12. Karrer HE, Dickey AM: Ultrasound imaging: an overview. Hewlett-Packard J 34:3, 1983.
13. Reid J: A review of some basic limitations in ultrasonic diagnosis. *In* Grossman CC (ed.): Diagnostic Ultrasound. New York, Plenum Press, 1966.
14. Lateral resolution. *In* Aero-tech Reports. Vol. 1. Lewiston, PA, Krautkramer-Branson, 1979.
15. Meitzel AH: Piezoelectric transducer materials and techniques for ultrasonic devices operating above 100 MHz. *In* Mattist OE (ed.): Ultrasonic Transducer Materials. New York, Plenum Press, 1971.
16. Miller DG: An acoustic transducer array for medical imaging—part 11. Hewlett-Packard J 34:22, 1983.
17. Sensitivity 1. *In* Aero-tech Reports. Vol. 1. Lewiston, PA, Krautkramer-Branson, 1979.

18. One-quarter wavelength theory and application. *In* Aero-tech Reports. Vol. 1. Lewiston, PA, Krautkramer-Branson, 1979.
19. Multiple matching layer theory and application. *In* Aero-tech Reports. Vol. 1. Lewiston, PA, Krautkramer-Branson, 1980.
20. Edler I: Diagnostic use of ultrasound in heart disease. Acta Med Scand 308: 32, 1955.
21. Feigenbaum H: Use of echocardiography in evaluating left ventricular function. Second World Congress on Ultrasonics in Medicine. Excerpta Medica. June 1973.
22. Chang S: M-mode Echocardiographic Techniques and Pattern Recognition. 2nd Ed. Philadelphia, Lea & Febiger, 1981.
23. Langevin P: French patent. 505:703, 1918; British Patent. 145:691, 1921.
24. Fry FJ: Biological effects of ultrasound: a review. IEEE Trans Biomed Eng 67:604, 1979.
25. O'Brien WD Jr: Safety of ultrasound. In DeVleiger M (ed.): Handbook of Clinical Ultrasound. New York, John Wiley & Sons, 1978.
26. O'Brien WD: Biological effects of ultrasound: rationale for measurement of selected ultrasonic output quantities. Echocardiography 3:165, 1986.
27. Nyborg WL: Physical mechanisms for biological effects of ultrasound. *In* HEW Publications (FDA) 78-8062. Rockville, MD, US Department of Health Education, and Welfare, 1977.
28. National Institutes of Health Consensus Development Conference: Diagnostic ultrasound imaging in pregnancy. *In* HHS Publication 84-667. Bethesda, MD, US Department of Health and Human Services, 1984.
29. Proceedings of the workshop on interaction of ultrasound with biological tissues. *In* DHEW Publication (FDA) 73-8008. Seattle, WA, Battelle Seattle Research Center, 1971.
30. Haney MJ, O'Brien WD Jr: Temperature dependence of ultrasonic propagation properties in biological materials. *In* Greenleaf JF (ed.): Tissue Characterization with Ultrasound. Vol. 1. Boca Raton, FL, CRC Press, p. 15, 1986.
31. Goldman DE, Hueter TF: Tabular data of the velocity and absorption of high-frequency sound in mammalian tissue. J Acoust Soc Am 28:35, 1956.
32. Hellman LM, et al: Safety of diagnostic ultrasound in obstetrics. Lancet 1: 1133, 1970.
33. Flynn HG: Cavitation dynamics—part I. A mathematical formulation. J Acoust Soc Am 57:1379, 1975.
34. Flynn HG: Cavitation dynamics—part II: Free pulsations and models for cavitation bubbles. J Acoust Soc Am 58:1160, 1975.
35. Skorton DJ, et al.: Ultrasound bioeffects: an introduction for the echocardiographer—part I: acoustic output definitions and bioeffects mechanisms. Report of the ASE Committee of Physics and Instrumentation. JASE 1:240, 1988.
36. Taylor KJW, Pond JB: A study of the production of haemorrhagic injury and paraplegia in rat spinal cord by pulsed ultrasound of low megahertz frequencies in the context of the safety for clinical useage. Br J Radiol 45: 343, 1972.
37. Hueter TF, Bold RH: Sonics. New York, John Wiley & Sons, p. 237, 1955.
38. Apfel RE: Cavitation. *In* Edmonds PE (ed.): Methods of Experimental Physics: Ultrasonics. New York, Academic Press, p. 356, 1981.
39. Nyborg WL: Acoustic streaming. *In* Mason WP: Physical Acoustics. New York, Academic Press, 1965.
40. Williams AR, Hughes DE, Nyborg WL: Hemolysis near a transversely oscillating wire. Science 169:871, 1970.
41. Bioeffects Committee of the American Institute of Ultrasound in Medicine: Safety Considerations for Diagnostic Ultrasound. Bethesda, MD, American Institute of Ultrasound in Medicine, 1984.

CHAPTER

2

CROSS-SECTIONAL SCANNING: TECHNICAL PRINCIPLES AND INSTRUMENTATION

HISTORY OF CROSS-SECTIONAL IMAGING

The first two-dimensional ultrasonic imaging system was developed by Wild and Reid in 1952.[1] This "two-dimensional echoscope" consisted of a single, pivot-mounted crystal enclosed in a water-filled chamber (Fig. 2–1). The crystal was arced synchronously through a 45° sector by an oscillating cam. The cam also was mechanically attached to an electronic position-sensing unit, which synchronized the position of the sweep on a cathode ray tube (CRT) with the path of the sound beam in space (Fig. 2–2).

The same year, Howry and Bliss developed a conceptually similar instrument called a "sonoscope," which used a large, mechanically driven transducer submerged in a water tank to generate cross-sectional images of the extremities (Fig. 2–3).[2] Not until 1957, however, did Wild, et al., using a mechanically driven linear scanning instrument, first examine the freshly excised human heart and produce cross-sectional images of the poste-

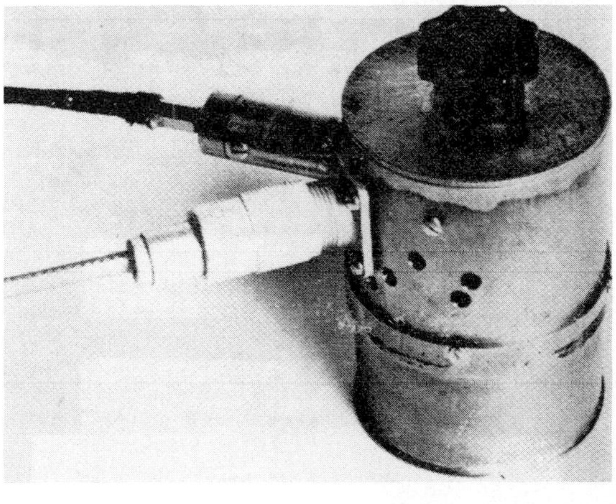

Fig. 2–1. The original two-dimensional transducer developed by Wild and Reid. (From Wild JJ, Reid JM: Application of echo ranging techniques to the determination of structure of biologic tissue. Science 115:226, 1952.)

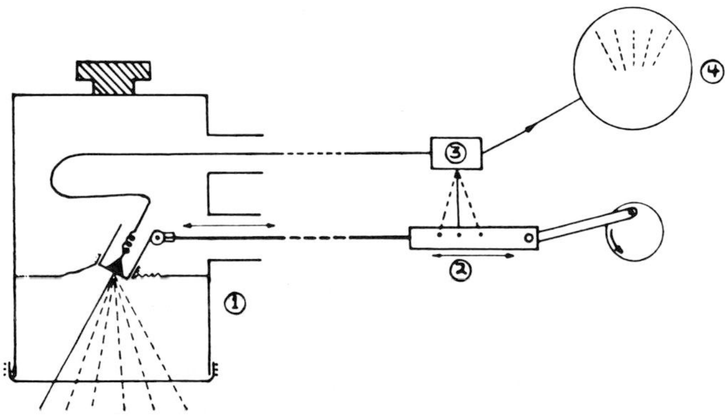

Fig. 2–2. Principles of operation of the echoscope. A pivot-mounted crystal (1) was driven by an oscillating cam (2), which was mechanically connected to an electronic position sensing device (3). This device, in turn, synchronized the position of the transducer with the orientation of the displayed data lines on the oscilloscope (4). (From Wild JJ, Reid JM: Application of echo ranging techniques to the determination of structure of biologic tissue. Science 115:226, 1952.)

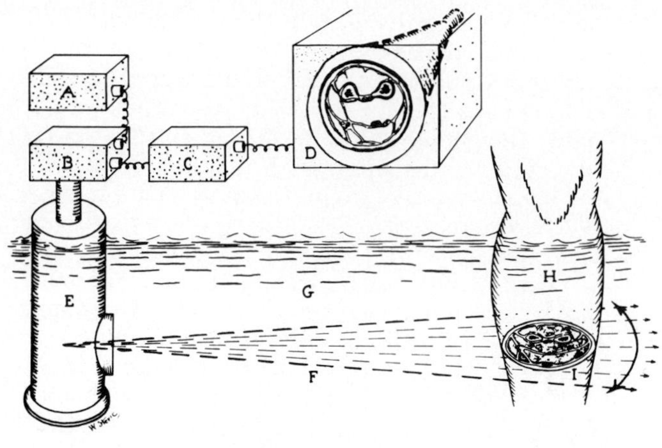

Fig. 2–3. Components and principles of operation of the sonoscope developed by Howry and Bliss. The pulser (A) activated the ultrasonic crystal, which was contained in a large submerged housing. The horizontal beam scanning and synchronization system (B) moved the transducer and housing (E) directed sequential ultrasonic pulses (F) in a controlled scan through a submerged (G) extremity, such as that indicated to the right (H). The received echoes were then amplified in the amplifier chain (C) and displayed in a spatially correct format on the oscilloscope (D). (From Howry D, Bliss W: Ultrasonic visualization of soft tissue structure of the body. J Lab Clin Med 40:579, 1952.)

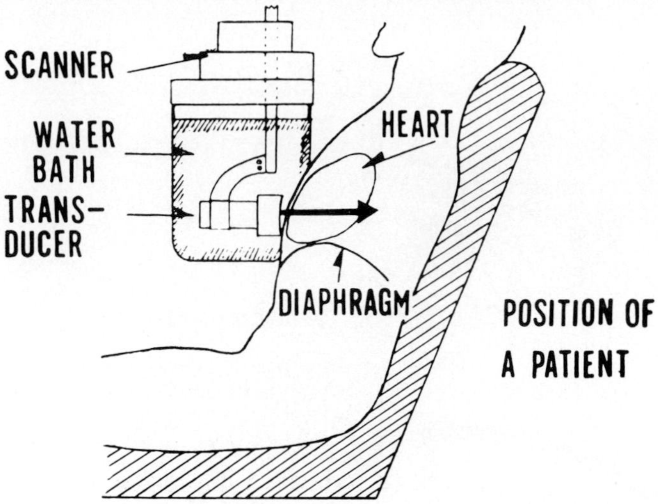

Fig. 2–4. The mechanically driven water path scanner developed by Ebina et al. During the examination, the patient was seated and the scanning instrument was applied directly to the anterior chest wall. (From Ebina T, et al.: The ultrasono-tomography of the heart and great vessels in living human subjects by means of the ultrasonic reflection technique. Jpn Heart J 8:331, 1967.)

rior wall, aorta, and a segment of the left coronary system.[3]

For the greater part of the next decade, advances in two-dimensional imaging were largely limited to studies of the abdomen and other areas that provided ready access to the exploring ultrasonic beam. Although preliminary attempts were made to generate two-dimensional cardiac images, the failure to appropriately display dynamic cardiac motion and the difficulties in gaining access to the heart limited progress.

In 1967, a group of Japanese investigators, led by Ebina, obtained the first large clinical series of static cross-sectional images of the cardiac chambers and great vessels using a compound, mechanically driven, water path scanner (Fig. 2–4). In addition, by synchronizing their ultrasonic sampling with the R-wave of an electrocardiogram, they were able to generate cardiac "ultrasono-tomograms" during both systole and diastole (Fig. 2–5).[4]

During the same period, Ashberg, using a scanning transducer and parabolic mirror system (Fig. 2–6), introduced dynamic motion to the cross-sectional format.[5]

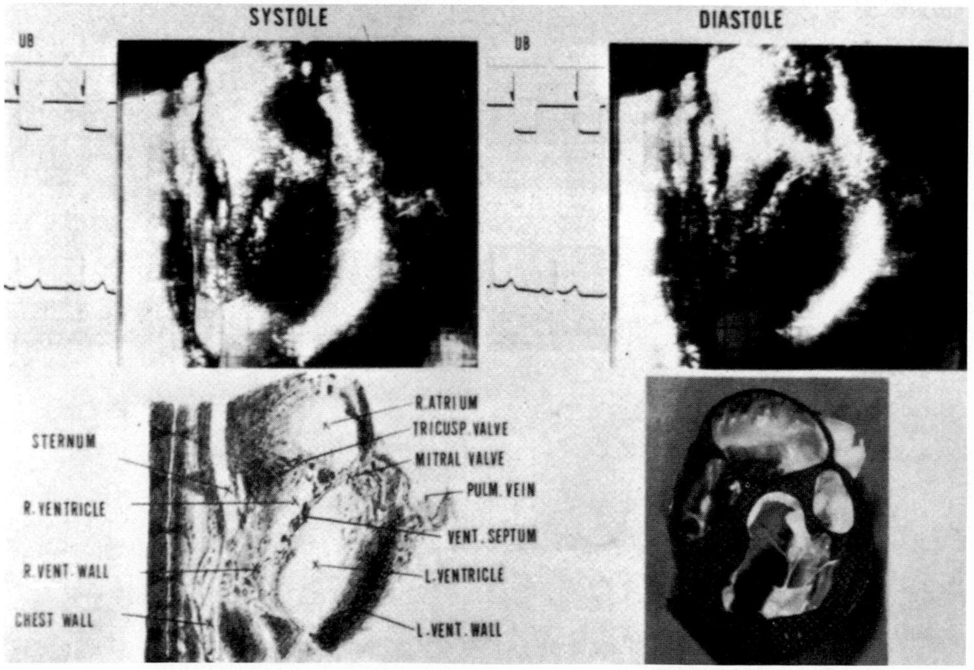

Fig. 2–5. Ultrasono-tomograms of the human heart recorded during diastole and systole. The path of the scan transects the right atrium, the left ventricle, and a portion of the interventricular septum. Changes in left ventricular and right atrial cavity sizes from systole to diastole are apparent. An anatomic section corresponding to the path of the imaging plane used to record these sections appears in the lower right of the figure. (From Ebina T, et al.: The ultrasono-tomography of the heart and great vessels in living human subjects by means of the ultrasonic reflection technique. Jpn Heart J 8:331, 1967.)

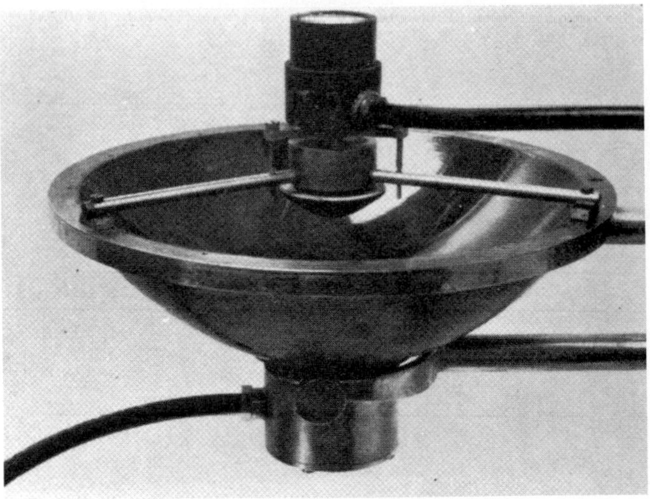

Fig. 2–6. Rotating transducer and parabolic mirror system used to create the first dynamic images of the heart. (From Hertz CH: Ultrasonic engineering in heart diagnosis. *In* Segal BL (ed.): Symposium on diagnostic ultrasound. Am J Cardiol 19:6, 1967.

This technique, which he called "ultrasonic cinematography," produced cardiac images at a rate of seven frames per second (Fig. 2–7). Although all the early scanning systems involved either mechanical or manual scanning of the transducer, Somer demonstrated in 1968 that, using existing electronic scanning techniques, a medical instrument could be developed in which beam scanning and position sensing could be achieved electronically.[6]

Despite steady improvement in cross-sectional instrumentation and increasing interest in cross-sectional cardiac scanning, these techniques were not applied clinically in a routine fashion until the appearance of the "real-time" imaging systems in the early 1970s.

The development by Bom, et al., of an electronically activated linear array system was the first practical method for deriving spatially correct, dynamic images of the moving heart.[7,8] This linear array consisted of a series of small transducers, aligned in a row, that could be activated in rapid sequence either individually or in groups (Fig. 2–8). The linear arrangement permitted the transmitted pulse to shift rapidly down the line of transducers, thereby achieving the same type of beam movement that had previously been attained by manual or mechanical motion of an individual transducer. Figure 2–9 is an example of how the resulting parallel data lines were recorded and assembled into a composite image.

Rapid electronic switching between transducers permitted image assembly at a sufficiently high frame rate to record dynamic cardiac motion. In addition, individual transducers could be used to generate M-mode recordings from preselected areas of the heart, thus adding spatial orientation to the derived M-mode data and improving understanding of the M-mode record. The linear array format, however, failed to achieve general acceptance because of (1) the almost compulsory use of small crystals, which had poor inherent beam characteristics and limited lateral resolution,[9] (2) the large composite transducer size, which was poorly suited to the available echocardiographic windows, and (3) the limited line density of the final image. This concept, however, represented a major advance because it proved that dynamic

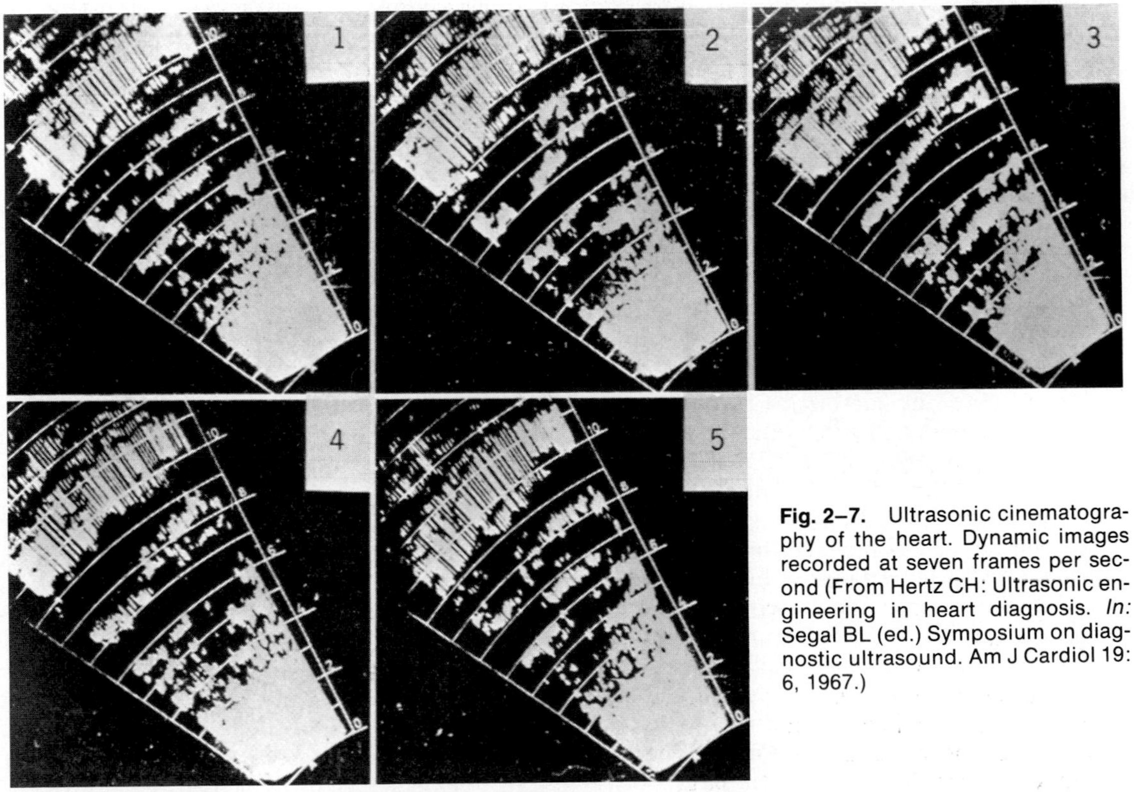

Fig. 2–7. Ultrasonic cinematography of the heart. Dynamic images recorded at seven frames per second (From Hertz CH: Ultrasonic engineering in heart diagnosis. *In:* Segal BL (ed.) Symposium on diagnostic ultrasound. Am J Cardiol 19: 6, 1967.)

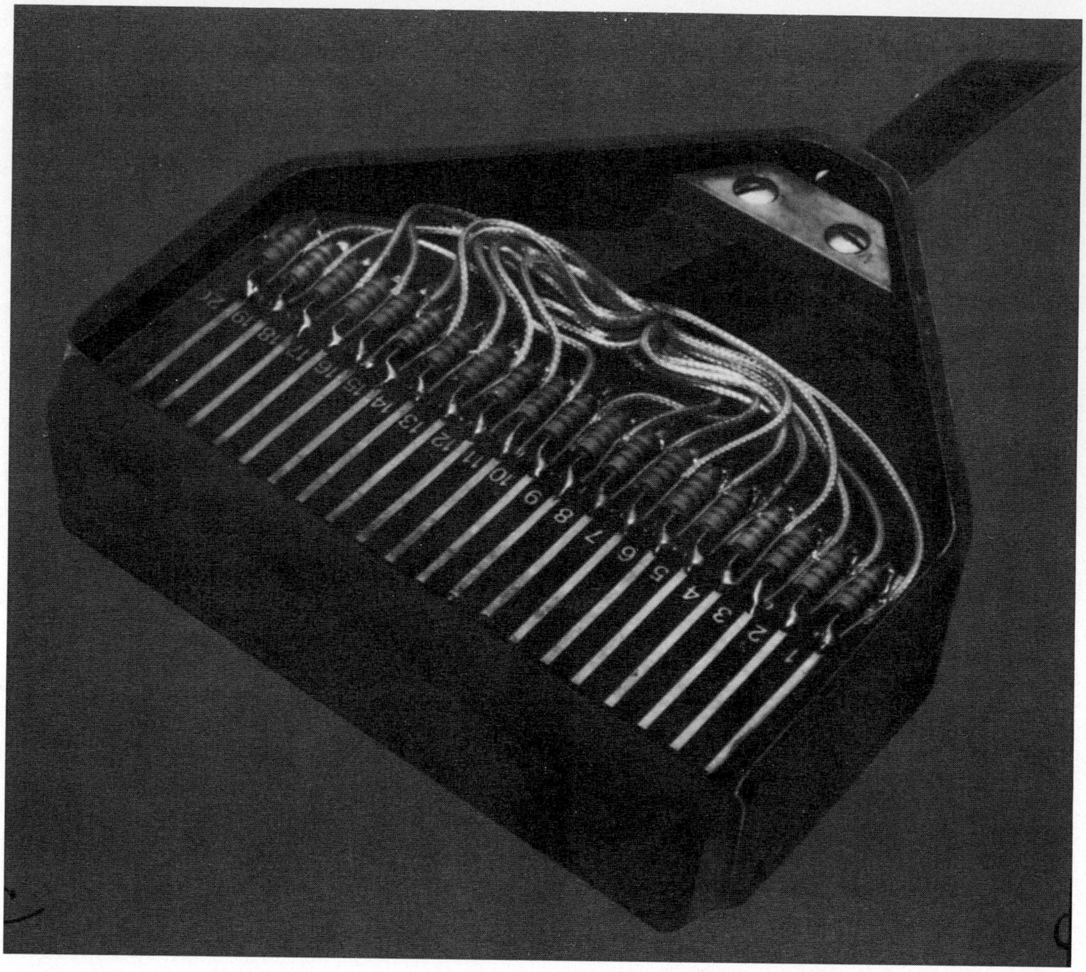

Fig. 2–8. Linear array transducer similar to that developed by Bom et al. (From Bom N, et al.: Multiscan echocardiography. 1: a technical description. Circulation 48:1066, 1973. Reproduced by permission of the American Heart Association, Inc.)

cardiac imaging not only was possible but could be applied to large groups of patients and could provide useful clinical information.[10,11]

The demonstration of the feasibility of dynamic cardiac imaging was followed by rapid advances in cross-sectional echocardiography from both the engineering and clinical standpoint. In 1973 and 1974, Griffith and Henry at the National Institutes of Health,[12] Eggleton and Johnston at Indiana University,[13–15] and McDicken in Scotland[16] developed prototype instruments for rapid mechanical sector scanning. These instruments provided both the high frame rate and line density required for high resolution cardiac imaging in a relatively simple and flexible format. During the same period, Thurstone and VonRamm, at Duke University,[17–19] using the principles suggested by Somer, developed a phased array system, which permitted electronic steering of the ultrasonic beam in a sector format. This sophisticated system, in addition to providing dynamic two-dimensional images of the heart, also incorporated transmit and receive focusing of the ultrasonic pulse. Subsequently, a number of other phased array systems have been developed with proven clinical application and reliability. In the intervening years, these basic systems have been improved and modified significantly, and a large body of clinical data has been assembled through their use. Although two-dimensional imaging is only one of the available echocardiographic techniques discussed in this book, all evidence to date indicates that it is and will remain the foundation of the echocardiographic examination.

Scan Formats

In all two-dimensional ultrasonic scanning systems, the sound beam is moved or scanned in a fixed plane across the precordium. As the beam moves, the echoes returning from structures along its path are continuously recorded. Each time a pulse is transmitted, the beam coordinates are simultaneously sensed and relayed to the CRT so that each new line of echocardiographic data can be oriented and displayed in a pattern that corresponds to the relative path of the sound beam in space. If the beam is swept rapidly enough, images can be assembled at a sufficiently high frame rate to depict dynamic cardiac motion.

Three predominant scan formats have been employed, either alone or in combination, to generate and record these images. These formats include the linear scan, the sector scan, and the arc scan (Fig. 2–10). In

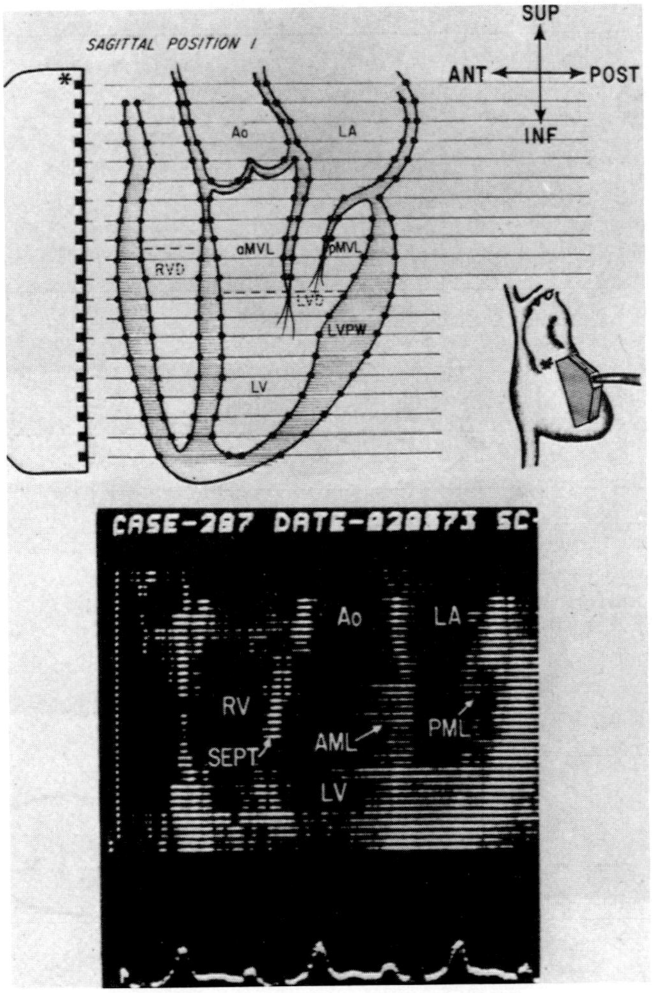

Fig. 2–9. A linear array transducer oriented parallel to the long axis of the left ventricle (LV) and aortic root (Ao). The path along which the sound pulses generated by the individual transducers transect the heart in this orientation is indicated. Also shown is the type of image obtained by assembling the resultant echoes. (From Sahn DJ, et al.: Multiple crystal cross-sectional echocardiography in the diagnosis of cyanotic congenital heart disease. Circulation 50:230, 1974. Reproduced by permission of the American Heart Association, Inc.)

the linear format, the point of origin of the ultrasonic pulse is moved in a straight line across the precordium so that the resulting sound waves propagate parallel to one another. This type of scan can be accomplished (1) by manually or mechanically moving a single transducer from one point to another (Fig. 2–10A); (2) by aligning a number of transducers next to one another and activating them in sequence (Fig. 2–10B); or (3) by using a rotating transducer(s) to reflect sequential pulses off the face of a parabolic mirror so that the pulses enter the chest in a parallel fashion (Fig. 2–10C). In the linear format, the scan area is of equal width in both the near and far field. The line density, or the number of individual B-mode lines contained in each image, depends on the method of scanning. When a single transducer is moved across the precordium (Fig. 2–10A), beam movement can be as slow as desired, and the resultant line density, therefore, may be high. Unless the scan rate is uniform, however, the image may be degraded by uneven line density. When numerous transducers are combined in a linear array (Fig. 2–10B), each transducer generates a single data line. The number of lines in the image, therefore, equals the number of transducers in the array and is, of necessity, limited. The regular spacing of the transducers in this format results in an even line distribution and a more visually acceptable image.

In the sector format (Fig. 2–10D), the transducer is held in a stationary position on the precordium, and from this fixed point, the sound beam is swept through a predetermined arc. A sector scan, therefore, is narrow in the region close to the transducer face and becomes wider as the imaging plane progresses farther from the transducer.

In the arc scan (Fig. 2–10E), the transducer is moved in an arcuate fashion while the ultrasonic beam is directed at a constant point in space. The arc scan permits examination of an individual point from multiple directions, thereby optimizing target description. A compound scan consists of a combination of two or more of the previously described scanning formats.

From the display standpoint, the linear scan has obvious advantages because it encompasses a large cross-sectional area that is the same in both the near and the far field. From a visualization standpoint, the compound scan, which permits individual points to be examined from multiple aspects, optimizes the chances for recording a given target. In clinical practice, however, the sector format, which is most readily adapted to the limited echocardiographic window and thus permits the greatest

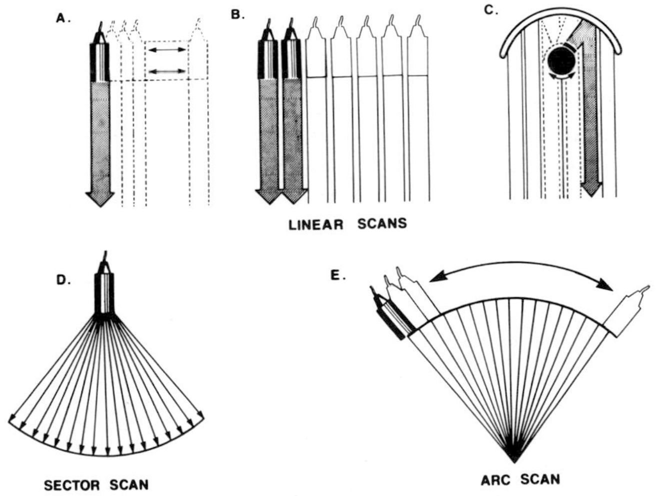

Fig. 2–10. Different scan formats that have been used to produce cross-sectional images. **A, B,** and **C** indicate the various methods used to generate linear scans. **A.** A single transducer is rapidly moved from one point to another while maintaining a constant orientation relative to the heart. **B.** A series of transducers is aligned in a row and activated in sequence to produce a series of parallel pulses. **C.** A rotating transducer is used to reflect pulses off a parabolic mirror such that they enter the tissue in a parallel orientation. **D.** A sector scan. In this format, the transducer is held in a fixed location while the sound beam is gradually swept through an arc of varying width. **E.** An arc scan in which the transducer is moved along an arcuate path while the beam is directed at a fixed point in space.

amount of information to be obtained in the largest number of patients, has become the scan pattern of choice. Instruments using this format have gained the widest acceptance.

Instrumentation

The various types of instruments that have been employed to obtain cross-sectional cardiac images are summarized in Table 2–1. These cross-sectional systems can be broadly classified as either static or dynamic, based on the rate at which individual frames are assembled. The static systems include both manual and mechanical scanning devices, which generate single composite images. When applied to the heart, these instruments are usually time-gated so that data are acquired only during specific points in the cardiac cycle. Each static image is assembled, therefore, from data derived from several cardiac cycles.

Dynamic systems involve fast movement of the ultrasonic beam across a predetermined area of the precordium at sufficiently high data acquisition rates to permit image assembly at a rapid frame rate. These instruments also can be conveniently subclassified, based on the method of the beam movement, into mechanical scanning systems and transducer arrays. Annular arrays combine mechanical transducer motion with electronic beam focusing and, therefore, represent a third class of dynamic system. More complex, two-dimensional block or orthogonal arrays also are listed because they provide dynamic images. At present, however, these intricate devices are of more theoretic and engineering interest than practical utility.

From a diagnostic standpoint, the dynamic nature of the heart makes assessment of cardiac motion at least as important as visualization of cardiac structure. Imaging systems that display dynamic cardiac motion in real time are therefore essential to an adequate assessment of cardiac performance. Therefore, only dynamic systems are currently in use and will be discussed further.

Table 2–1. Two-Dimensional Echo Instrumentation

1. Static
   - A. Manual
   - B. Mechanical
2. Dynamic
   - A. Mechanical sector scanners
     - i. Oscillatory
     - ii. Rotary
   - B. Transducer arrays
     - i. Linear arrays
     - ii. Phased arrays
     - iii. Two-dimensional arrays
       - a. Block arrays
       - b. Orthogonal arrays
   - C. Combined
     - i. Annular arrays

DYNAMIC CROSS-SECTIONAL IMAGING SYSTEMS

Mechanical Sector Scanning

In the mechanical sector scanning format, the ultrasonic beam is swept through a fixed plane by rapid mechanical oscillation of a single transducer or by rotation of multiple transducers. The transducer is housed in a small, hand-held scanning probe that permits flexible angulation and rotation of the scan plane. In addition to the transducer, the probe normally contains a position-sensing device and a small motor to drive the crystals. The transducer is similar to those used in conventional one-dimensional imaging systems. In oscillating systems, the transducer is generally constrained with a pivot bearing about which it is driven through a selected arc at a predetermined rate. The transducer drive also is connected to a position-sensing apparatus so that the position of the ultrasonic beam is continuously recorded as it sweeps through its arc. Various methods for position sensing have been used, including variable differential transformers, resistance pads, potentiometers, and photo-optical sensing devices. Figure 2–11 is an example of one of the early mechanical scanners that was developed at Indiana University.[14,15]

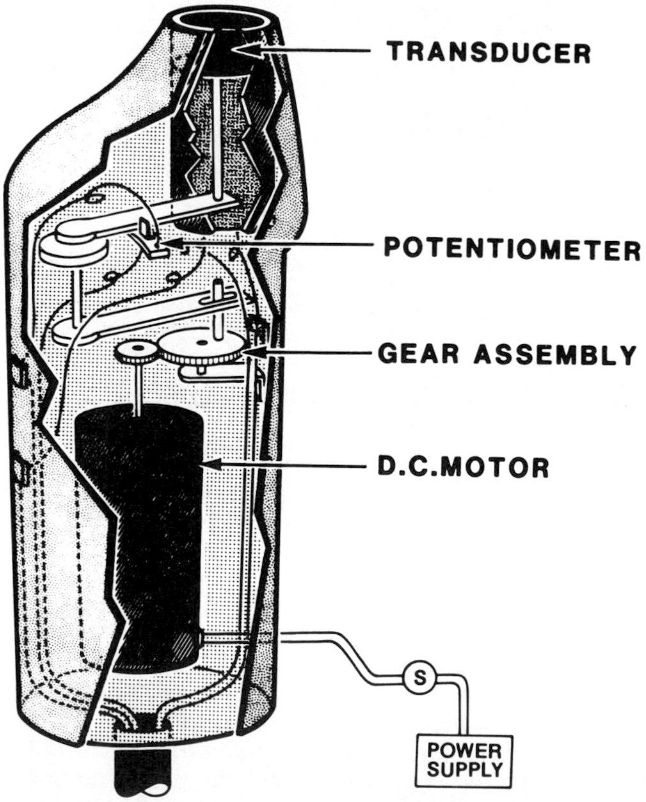

Fig. 2–11. The components of one of the early probes used for mechanical sector scanning. In this model, a small DC motor was attached to a gear assembly, which drove an oscillating transducer through a 30° arc. The probe position was sensed by a low-noise potentiometer, which recorded changes in the position of the drive shaft and, hence, of the transducer. The actual area of transducer contact with the skin was small, and the probe could be easily maneuvered to fit into any intercostal space.

Historically, the mechanical sector scanning concept proved advantageous when compared to the earlier dynamic systems (i.e., the linear array of parabolic mirror and rotary transducer) for several reasons. First, the mechanical scanners used single, relatively large, focused transducers that had comparatively well-collimated beam patterns. This construction improved lateral resolution as well as system sensitivity. Second, the smaller, more flexible probe could be placed in a variety of interspaces or echocardiographic windows, thereby permitting the examiner to adapt freely to the configuration of the patient's chest. In addition, the high pulse repetition frequency and relatively small scan angle of the mechanical scanners provided a high line density and resulted in a more pleasing and recognizable cross-sectional picture. The mechanical scanning concept also was relatively simple, and the amount of hardware required to drive the transducer and sense its position was limited. Figure 2–12 illustrates the original prototype mechanical scanner developed by Eggleton and Johnston. This scanner was assembled largely from existing components and was designed so that the scan module could be inexpensively retrofitted in an available M-mode system.

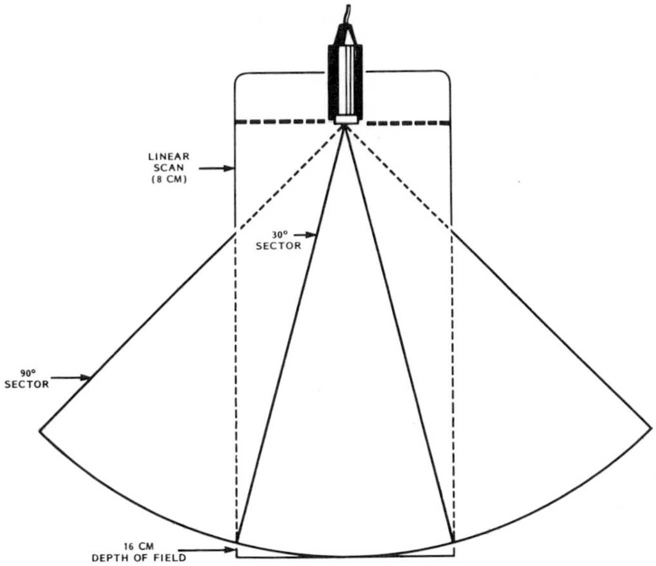

Fig. 2–13. The relative areas encompassed by a linear array with an 8-cm transducer face, a 16-cm depth of field, and 30 and 90° sector scans with comparable depths of field.

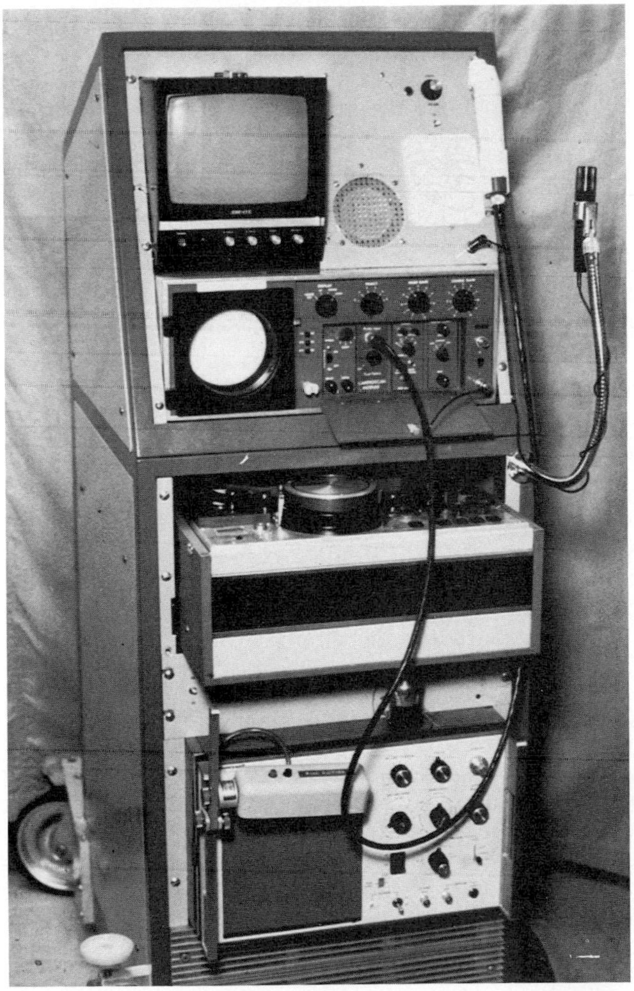

Fig. 2–12. The original prototype mechanical scanner developed by Eggleton and Johnston. This instrument, known as "the blue goose," provided much of the early cross-sectional data on which the first edition of the book was based.

Initial limitations of the mechanical scanning format included the small scan area of the first instruments, limited width at the apex of the sector, uneven line distribution with early oscillating probes, and mechanical vibration, which could be felt by the patient. Figure 2–13 compares the scan areas encompassed by a linear array with those encompassed by the 30° and 90° sector formats. The diagram shows that the sector format causes significant loss of near-field information at the apex of the sector. However, in the trade-off between the rectangular display and the ability to use a small echocardiographic window, the latter has proved more important in clinical practice. In the far field, the scan area depends on the size of the sector.

Second-generation recently oscillating mechanical probes generally have varying scan angles from 30 to 90°. Contact between the oscillating transducer and the patient's chest is now avoided by enclosing the transducer in a plastic housing. Unfortunately, because the apex of the sector lies back within the scanner housing, the area of acoustic contact must be larger than the element aperture. Transducer motion also has been made smoother through the use of magnetic, as opposed to mechanical, drives.

Uneven line distribution is a problem in all oscillating systems because the transducer is required to slow down, stop, reverse direction, and accelerate again at each border of the sector. When the activation rate of the transducer is constant, the line density at the margins of the sector (where the transducer is moving more slowly) is greater than the line density in the midportion of the sweep (where the transducer is moving at its most rapid rate). This uneven line density can be overcome by making the pulse frequency a function of scan speed. Stepper motors also can be used, which move the transducer in fixed increments between each pulse, thereby maintaining constant line density.

Rotary transducer systems that provide a wider scan angle also have become increasingly popular. Figure 2–14 is an example of a rotary transducer system. In this system, four single transducers are oriented at 90° to one another. Each transducer is then rotated through a full 360° arc. The individual transducers are activated only as they pass through an aperture in the probe head. The result in this example is an 82° sector. Transducer rotation occurs within a fixed plastic case. The rotary system produces an even line distribution without the need to vary the pulse repetition frequency and produces more even temporal sampling than does an oscillating transducer. In addition, the rotary format brings the active element closer to the surface of the housing, increasing the effective window/aperture ratio.

Transducer Arrays

Transducer arrays are composed of a group of individual transducers or transducer elements. Transducers have dimensions of several wavelengths and, thus, can transmit a highly directional beam. Transducer elements, in contrast, are small in comparison to the transmitted wavelength and are practically nondirectional. Transducers function independently, whereas transducer elements are effective only in groups.[20] A group of transducers or transducer elements, which are aligned next to one another in a straight row, is referred to as a *linear array*.

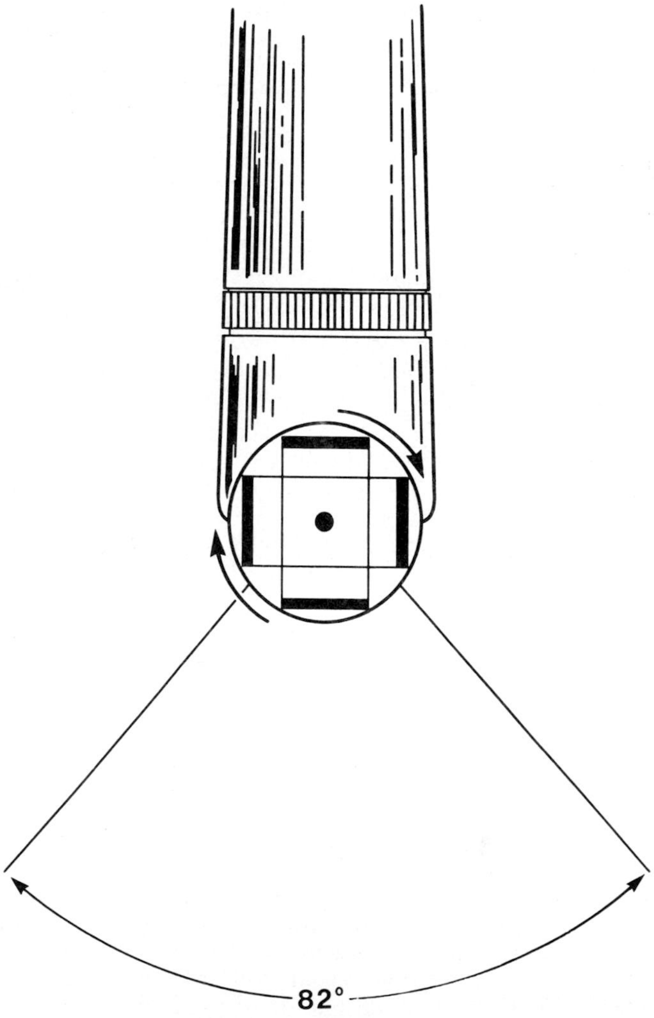

Fig. 2–14. Example of a rotary transducer system used in cross-sectional imaging.

Linear Arrays

Linear arrays may be composed of a group of transducers or transducer elements. A linear array that is composed of a row of equidistant transducers that are activated individually by switching the activation pulse from one transducer to another is termed a *simple switched array*. An array that is composed of a large series of transducer elements that are activated in groups such that each group forms a composite transducer is referred to as a *grouped switched array*.

The original linear array system developed by Bom et al. was a simple switched array.[7,8] In this system, 20 individual transducers, each 4 × 10 mm were aligned to yield a composite array with a transmitting surface of 1 × 8 cm. By briefly pulsing each transducer and leaving it on as a receiver for approximately 200 msec, one could record 20 individual B-mode data lines from a scan area (disregarding beam dispersion) of 1 × 8 × 16 cm with a line density of 1 line/4 mm. By pulsing each transducer twice and displaying the second line at half the distance between two adjacent transducers or by electronically doubling each line, one could increase the line density to 1 line/2 mm at a frame rate of either 80 or 160/sec. This line density still failed to produce a visually pleasing image. Increasing line density by decreasing transducer size would result in unacceptable lateral resolution. To overcome the problem of low line density in a linear array, grouped switched arrays were developed. Figure 2–15 compares a simple switched linear array with a grouped switched array. In the grouped format, multiple small transducer elements are arranged in a linear array. Groups of elements are then activated together and collectively form a large effective transducer face. This grouping results in an improved beam profile and, at the same time, increases the image line density. The large composite transducer, however, still lacks flexibility and requires a large "window" to obtain access to the heart. Such characteristics limit its value in adult cardiac imaging.

Phased Arrays

Phased arrays are multiple-element transducers that sweep the sound beam through a predetermined arc electronically rather than manually or mechanically. Each element in the array is narrow so that the divergence angle of the beam is wide and the element can be considered to emit a spheric wave front. Electronic beam steering is achieved using the principle of summation of time-sequenced wavelets first described by Huygens in the seventeenth century. Simply stated, when each of a series of linearly oriented transducers in an array is excited simultaneously, the resulting wavelets emanating from the individual transducers summate to

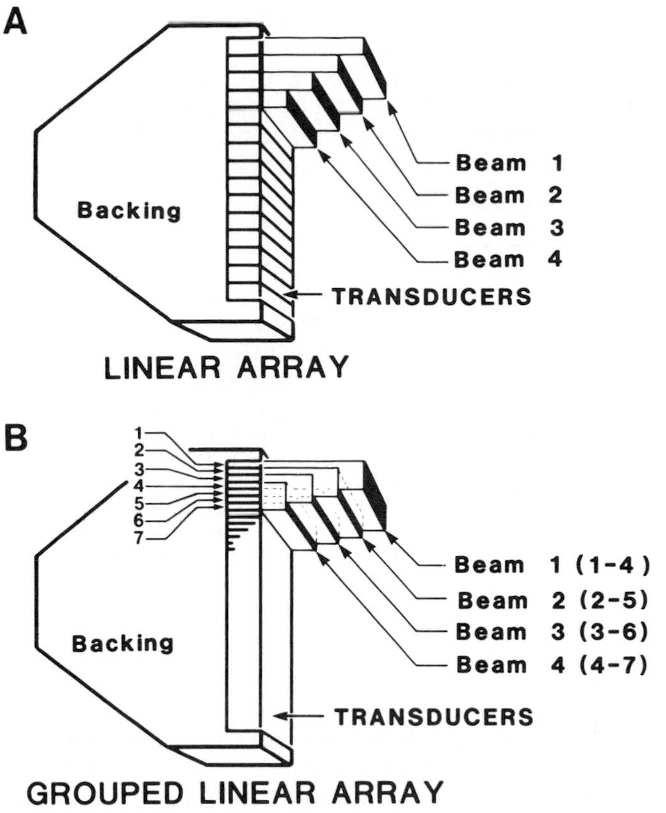

Fig. 2–15. Comparison of a simple switched linear array **(A)** with a grouped switched linear array **(B).** In the simple switched array, each transducer produces a separate ultrasonic beam. In the grouped array, groups of transducer elements are simultaneously activated, thereby producing a larger effective transducer face and increasing the image line density. **B.** Beam No. 1 is produced by a composite waveform resulting from the activation of transducer elements 1 through 4. Beam No. 2 is produced by the simultaneous activation of elements 2 through 5, beam No. 3 is produced by the activation of elements 3 through 6, and beam 4 is produced by the activation of elements 4 through 7.

form a single wave that propagates in a direction normal to or directly away from the transducer face. Conversely, when the transducers are excited in rapid sequence rather than simultaneously, the wavelets emanating from each transducer are propagated at an angle to the transducer face. This resultant angle is proportional to the time interval or delay between activation of the transducers. By rapidly varying the time sequence in which the transducers are excited, one can electronically direct or steer the wave front at correspondingly variable angles from the transducer face. Because the position of the array is fixed and the beam is swept from side to side, the resultant image is in a sector format. The first clinically useful phased array system was designed by Thurstone and VonRamm and can serve as an example of this type of imaging.[17,18]

In descriptions of the physical principles of any phased array system, the transmit and receive operations are customarily considered separately. In the transmit mode, ultrasonic energy is formed into a beam and propagates along a predetermined path by the constructive and destructive interference of sequentially created acoustic wave fronts. In the receive mode, ultra-

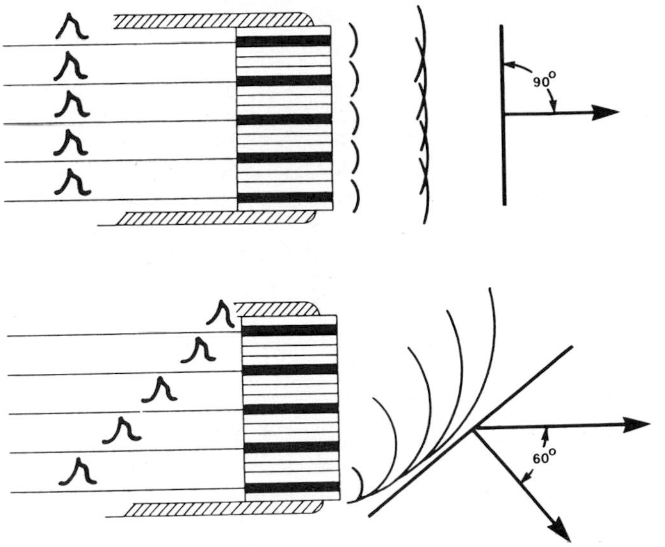

Fig. 2–16. The method of beam transmission and steering in the phased array format. **A.** A series of electrical pulses is depicted moving from left to right toward the transducer elements in the array. The pulses activate the elements, simultaneously producing a series of small wavelets. As these wavelets move from the transducer face, they summate to form a beam that propagates away from the transducer. **B.** The transducer elements are activated slightly out-of-phase. In this example, the upper transducer is activated first, producing an acoustic wavelet that propagates to the right and away from the array. Rapidly thereafter, the second element is excited, producing a second wavelet slightly behind the first. The sequence continues until the bottom element in the array is activated. In tissue, these five individual wavefronts summate to produce an acoustic beam that approximates in shape and direction the beam that would be produced by a transducer aimed in that direction.

sonic energy is sensed from a predetermined direction by the addition and subtraction of incoming ultrasonic energy of varying phases.

The method by which the ultrasonic beam is generated and steered in a phased array system is illustrated graphically in Figure 2–16. In these examples, 19 elements are depicted in each array; however, for simplicity, only the wavelets produced by five of these transducer elements are indicated.

During the beam transmission, a cylindric Gaussian focus can be produced at a specified range by imposing a spherical timing relationship on the excitation pulses (Fig. 2–17). The focusing produced by such a spherical

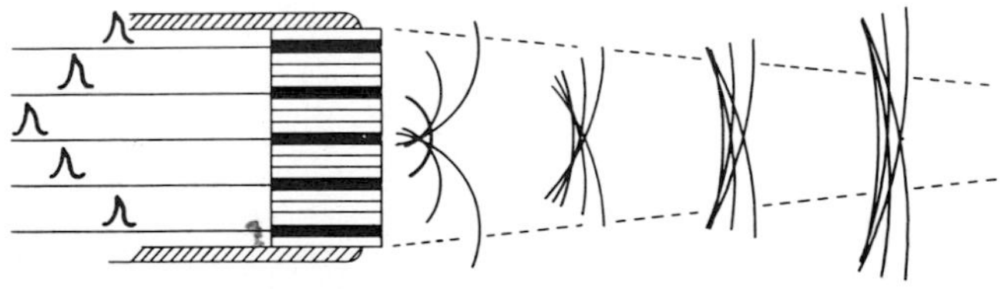

Fig. 2–17. The method of transmit focusing in the phased array format. In this diagram, the electrical pulses that activate the transducer elements have a spherical timing relationship. This relationship causes the elements at the margins of the array to be activated slightly before those in the center. This activation sequence causes the consolidation of the sound energy in the central portion of the beam and effectively focuses the array at a fixed point within the near field of the transducer.

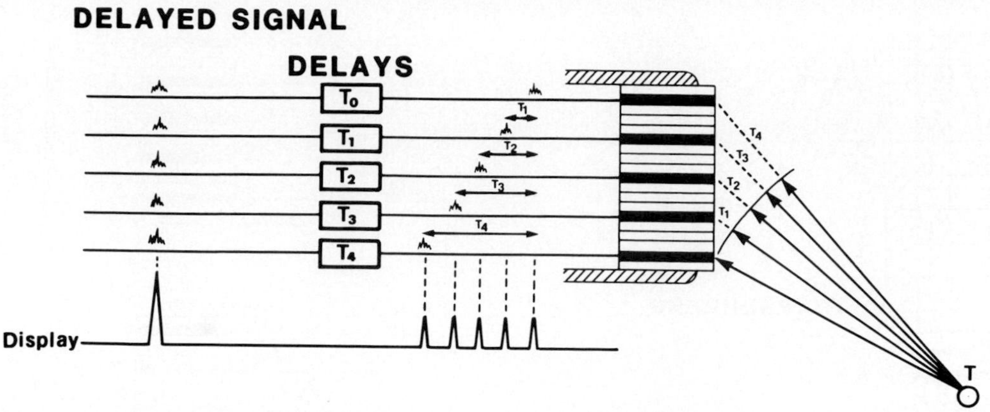

Fig. 2–18. The method by which the orientation of the array during reception corresponds to the path of the transmitted acoustic pulse. In this example, the time required for the echoes returning from the target (T) to strike the various elements of the transducer array increases from the bottom of the array to the top. If the electrical signals arising from these echoes are transmitted unaltered to the amplifier chain, the resulting signal from the target would be blurred and would fail to appropriately reflect the nature of the point target. By delaying the arrival of the first signal (and all subsequent signals) at the array until the final transducer element is activated, the echoes from the target can be brought into phase and thus can be appropriately displayed on the imaging scope. In this example, the electrical signal from the echo striking the bottom element would be delayed (T_4). The electrical pulse from the next lowest element (T_3) would then be delayed, and so on until each of the electrical signals is appropriately aligned with the signal activating the uppermost transducer. Hence, the array is effectively directed to look at signals returning from the path of the transmitted beam.

wave front, however, allows the focusing of each sound transmission in only a single area along the beam axis. As with fixed focusing, a single transmit focus improves the resolution of the system in the focal region; however, outside this region, the resolution may be degraded because of increased beam dispersion. In addition, although some beam focusing can be produced by this manner, theoretic considerations and beam pattern photographs indicate that the amount of sound energy along the axis of the beam outside the focal range is variable. Because each pulse must write one entire image line, blanks in the beam pattern result in gaps in the data line, thereby seriously degrading the resulting image. To produce a more uniform depth of focus throughout the scan area, the developers of the prototype system used five different focal points. Combining adjacent image lines recorded at different focal depths in an interlaced fashion was believed to improve the effective focal characteristics of the entire system.

In the receive mode, the array must appropriately record echoes from targets lying along the path of the transmit pulse. The width of the array, however, prohibits the echoes returning from an angle (with respect to the plane of the transducer face) from simultaneously striking each element on the array's surface. For the effective orientation of the array during reception to correspond to its orientation during transmission, delays in the processing of the echoes received by each element must be introduced. These delays are varied as necessary so that the echoes returning from a particular direc-

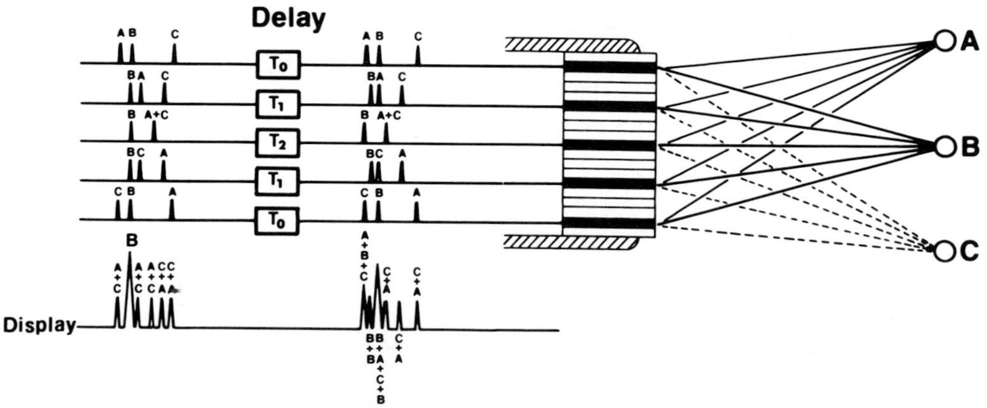

Fig. 2–19. The method by which the array can be focused to preferentially receive echoes from a particular point along the path of the transmitted beam. The echoes arising from a specific point target (B) arrive at the individual transducer elements in the array at different times. This variation in timing is reflected by the relationship of the electrical pulses to the left of the array. Echoes from other reflectors at the same depth (A and C) strike the transducer elements in timing sequences that differ slightly from one another as well as from those arising from reflector B. If all the pulses are delayed by the time required to appropriately summate and display echoes from target B, the echoes from this point will be in phase and, hence, will summate. Those from targets A and C will be further out of phase and, with appropriate filtering, can be eliminated.

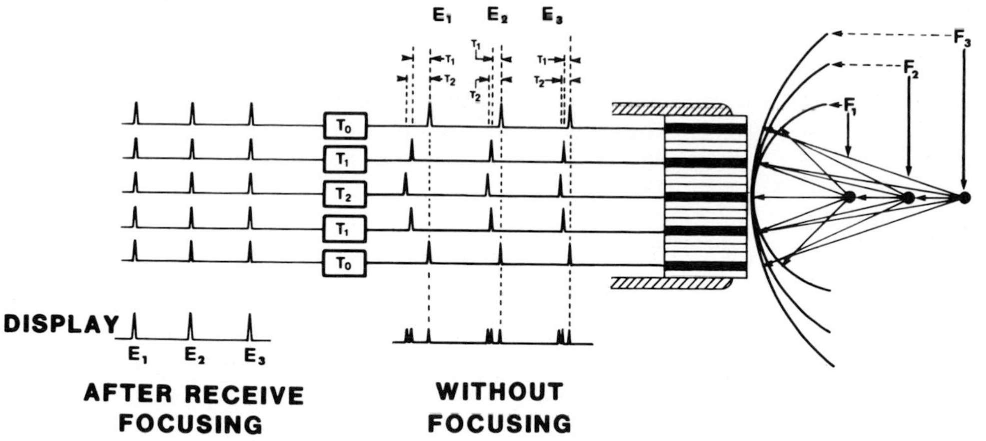

Fig. 2–20. The method by which the receive focus can be shifted to follow the progress of the transmitted pulse. The array is initially focused in the near field at F_1 by assigning the appropriate spherical timing relationship to the delays to place echoes from this point in phase. Then, by changing the spherical arrangement of the delays, the array can be sequentially refocused at increasingly deeper tissue depths, F_2 and F_3, thereby tracking the path of the transmitted pulse through the tissue.

tion will be in phase and, hence, will summate (Fig. 2–18). Echoes received from all other directions will not be in phase and, therefore, will partially cancel out.

In the prototype system, accurate phasing was accomplished using delay lines, which passed the acoustic information with different delay times from each element. In this fashion, echoes from a desired azimuthal orientation tend to be favored at the summing preamplifier. In addition to maintaining the effective orientation of the array during reception, the delay circuitry also permits the focusing of the receiver at any desired range and allows tracking of this focus in sync with the range of the returning echoes.

Figure 2–19 illustrates the method for obtaining this type of receive focusing. Echoes arising from a specific source at the center of the sound wave (reflector B) arrive at the individual transducer elements in the array at different times. This variation in timing also is indicated by the electrical pulses to the left of the array. Echoes from other reflectors at the same depth (A and C) strike the transducers in timing sequences that are slightly different from one another, as well as from reflector B. The controlling computer delays all the signals by the amount of time required to appropriately summate and display echoes from the particular area of interest (reflector B). This effectively places echoes from reflectors A an C out of phase in relation to those from reflector B, thereby producing a type of focusing. Because the returning echo information results from a known interrogating pulse, the time of the returning echoes is directly related to the depth of the echo-producing source. In practice, therefore, as illustrated in Figure 2–20, the receive system is focused initially in the near field (target F_1) for the period immediately after interrogation. The system is then refocused at successively deeper levels (targets F_2 and F_3) as the pulse continues to propagate to the maximum focal distance allowed by the near-field characteristics of the transducer array.

The near field of the array, like that of a simple disc-shaped transducer, is the distance from the array in which the ultrasonic energy is mainly confined within the dimensions of the transducer face. As discussed in Chapter 1, when the transducer is a single-element disc, the beam near the transducer is cylindric, propagating away from the transducer's face at a radius that approximates the radius of the disc. In a phased array, the transducer is rectangular (Fig. 2–21), and the beam has an elliptic shape. The shape of the ellipse is determined by the length and width of the array, the pattern of focusing, and the transmitted wavelength. Because lateral resolution is a function of beam width, for a rectangular array, "lateral resolution" has two components: azimuthal, also termed *lateral* (perpendicular to a scan line within the scanning plane), and elevation (the thickness of the scan plane at any depth). This spatial variation in beam width results in a complex scan plane (Fig. 2–22) where the near field for the lateral or azimuthal dimension of a nonfocus beam is greater than the near field for the elevation or thickness dimension because the total array width is greater than the height of the array elements. For a focused transducer, the opposite relationship may exist.

Because the phased array has separate transducer elements only in the lateral dimension, the ability to create an electronically positioned moving focus on receive is confined to the lateral dimension of the beam. Two types

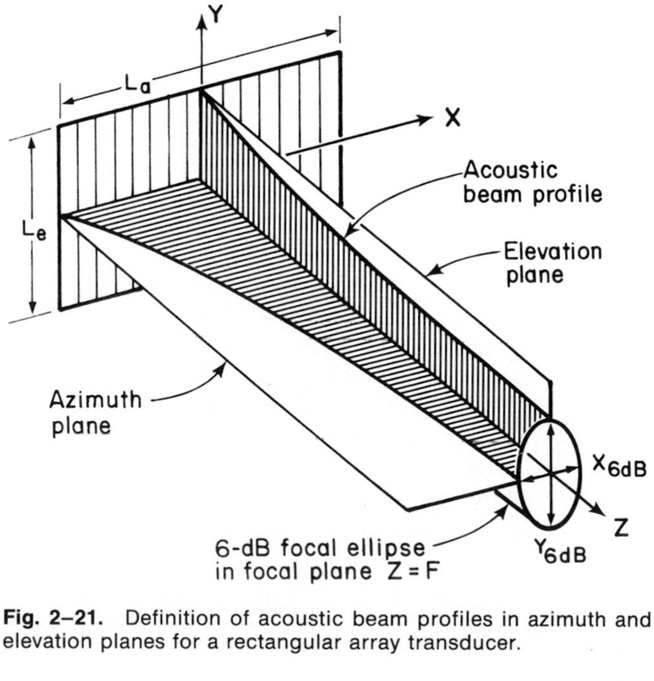

Fig. 2–21. Definition of acoustic beam profiles in azimuth and elevation planes for a rectangular array transducer.

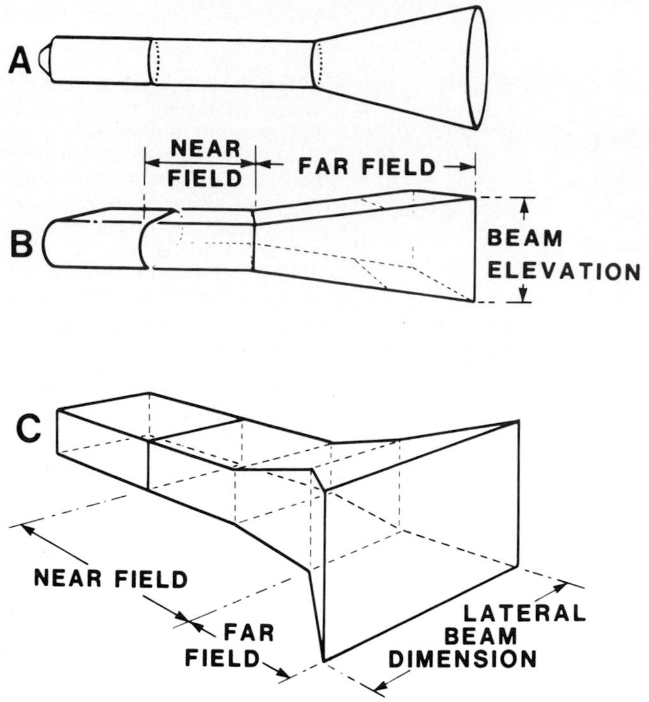

Fig. 2–22. The configuration of the sound beam arising from a simple disc-shaped transducer is compared with that generated by a rectangular transducer array. **A.** The beam is cylindric in the near field, paralleling the margins of the transducer face. In the far field, beyond the transition zone, the beam gradually diverges, thereby assuming a conical shape. The beam configuration of a rectangular array is more complicated. **B.** In the X or thickness dimension, the transducer width is relatively small, and hence, the near field is short and beam divergence begins relatively close to the transducer face. **C.** In the lateral, or Y, dimension, the near field is longer and beam divergence begins farther from the transducer because of the relatively greater length of the array.

of focusing can be used to improve the elevation characteristics of the array's beam. First, an acoustic lens can be used to focus the beam in the thickness dimension (Fig. 2–23).[21] Second, the technique of "shading" can be used. This technique involves widening the array by adding additional lines of transducers or varying the power output at the margins of the transducer elements when compared to the center of the element (Fig. 2–24). Each of these approaches decreases the power output at the edges, thereby minimizing the abrupt discontinuity found with a single element and reducing the side lobe amplitudes. These techniques for focusing the beam in the thickness dimension can be combined with the moving receive focus in the lateral dimension to optimize beam configuration.

In operation, the controlling computer of the phased array first provides the x-y deflection information to the CRT in the form of the sine and cosine of the deflection angle to be examined. The computer then sets the transmit timing circuits to produce a focused beam at the desired azimuthal direction. The transmit and deflection operations are then initiated, and the individual transmit pulses are triggered at appropriate times to produce the desired beam direction and focal point.

The returning echo data, which are received by the individual elements, are first amplified by a low noise preamplifier and are then amplified with logarithmic compression before beam delay. The echo data are then delayed for an appropriate length of time to permit the synchronization of the signals from the individual transducers. Appropriately delayed acoustic information from all receiving channels is then summed, and the resulting signal after detection is used to modulate the brightness of the CRT (z axis input). Immediately after the initiation of the transmit pulse, the computer sets the receiver delay lines to focus in the immediate proximity of the transducer. As the pulse progresses and as echoes are received from sources deeper in the tissue, the controller changes the receiver delays to maintain the focus of the receiving system at the appropriate point along the beam path. In this fashion, an electronically steered beam, which is focused in both its transmit and receive modes, is produced.

As with mechanical sector scanning, the phased array approach has inherent advantages and limitations. Advantages of these systems include (1) flexibility of beam angulation, depth of field examined, and line density, (2) ability to record Doppler and M-mode data from any azimuthal direction, (3) ability to focus in both the transmit and the receive mode. Limitations include the large size and the complexity of the required hardware, which limit portability and increase cost; limited transducer frequency, and increased side lobe intensity.

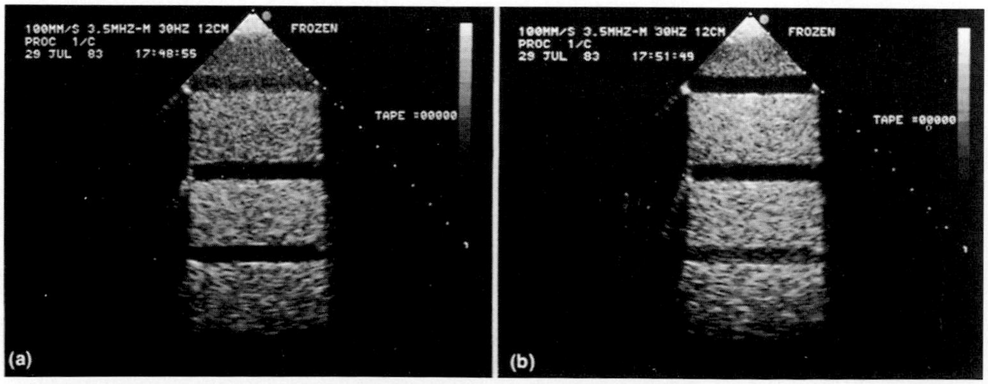

Fig. 2–23. Effect of transducer's elevation focal point on image quality. **A.** image with an elevation focal point at 8 cm. **B.** image with an elevation focal point at 4 cm. (From Snyder RA, Conrad RJ. Ultrasound image quality. Hewlett-Packard Journal 34:36, 1983. © Copyright 1983 Hewlett-Packard Company. Reproduced with permission.)

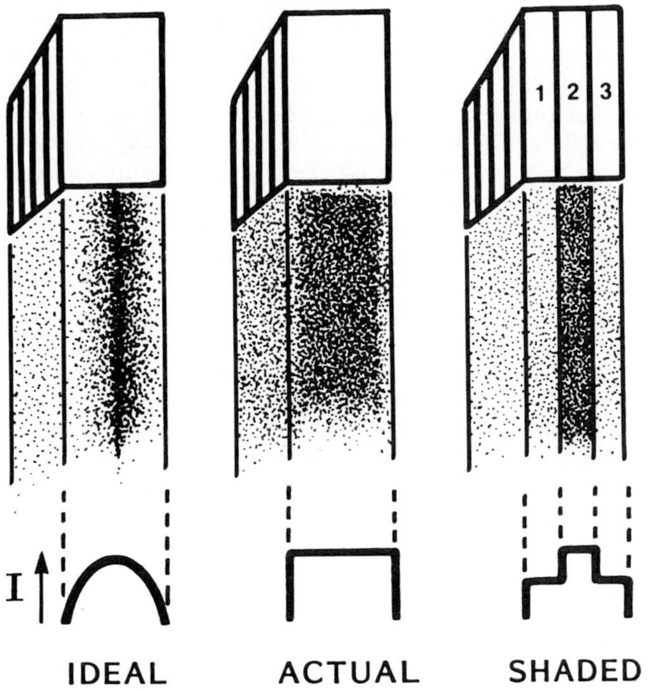

Fig. 2–24. The effects of shading on a series of representative beam intensity profiles. In the ideal beam, peak energy is concentrated in the center of the beam and gradually decays as the beam margins are approached. In practice, the drop in intensity at the beam margins is relatively abrupt. This change in intensity contributes to side lobe formation. This abrupt discontinuity at the beam margins can be decreased by placing one or more transducers beside the center transducer and by activating them less intensely.

ARRAY TRANSDUCERS

Array transducers are conceptually similar but practically far more complex than the basic transducer described in Chapter 1. The array transducers in current use contain from 32 to 128 individual elements that require all of the electrical connections and insulating layers of a single disc-shaped transducer but must fit into an aperture roughly 1.5 to 2.5 cm in length. Despite their close apposition, each element should ideally function identically and independently, isolated from the vibrations of its neighbors and of the array as a whole. To maintain consistency between elements, a single rectangular piezoelectric crystal is typically used, which is cut to appropriate dimensions and then ground and polished to a final thickness of 600 to 700 μm (Fig. 2–25). Appropriate matching and backing layers and electrical circuits are then bonded to the piezoelectric element using special epoxies, and the array is cut (diced) with microscopic precision into the desired number of elements (Fig. 2–25B and C). High voltage electrodes then are soldered to the external contacts bonded to the base of each element, and a thin metal foil is attached to the surface of the array to complete the ground connection and isolate the array elements from infiltration by grease, coupling gel, or water (Fig. 2–25D). An acoustic lens is then fitted to the front surface of the array to provide focusing in the elevation dimension. A convex single element lens, made of synthetic rubber, usually is chosen for this purpose. In order for focusing to occur with a convex lens, the velocity of sound in the lens must be less than that in human tissue.

Interelement Isolation

Because array transducers are composed of several closely spaced individual transducer elements in a single, compact housing, there is the potential for significant interelement interaction, which can degrade the resulting image. Ideally, when an electrical impulse is applied to an element to cause it to resonate, the elements on either side of the pulsed element should not be activated. In practice, this is difficult to achieve, and both electrical and mechanical coupling between array elements can occur. The elements can be isolated electrically by completely segmenting them and having a separate ground and high voltage electrode for each element. This electrical isolation is not total, however, because the individual array elements can behave like the plates in a parallel capacitor with the space, or kerf, between the elements acting as the dielectric. Although this capacitative coupling effect is not a critical problem, it does prevent the achievement of complete electrical isolation.[22]

A more significant problem is posed by mechanical coupling between array elements. Mechanical coupling occurs as a result of secondary or spurious modes of vibration of the array elements. Through the piezoelectric effect, an array element emits an ultrasonic beam by rapid oscillations in the thickness dimension, with the "resting" thickness of the element determining the frequency of the transmitted ultrasound. As the element changes shape, however, it also oscillates in the transverse or width dimension. This transverse vibration (also known as the dilational, or breathing, mode) is transmitted directly through the material between the elements and sets up a vibration in the adjacent elements. Because air is a poor carrier of ultrasound, an effective method of combatting this problem would be to allow only air to fill the spaces between elements.

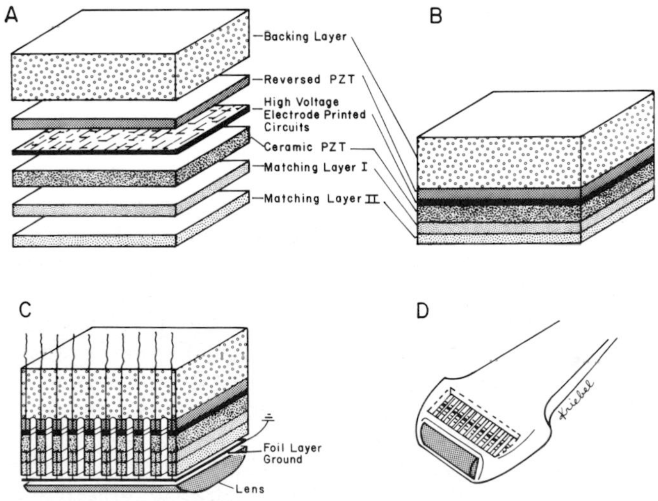

Fig. 2–25. **A** to **D.** Construction of a phased array transducer. (See text for details.)

Given the small spaces involved, however, this is difficult to accomplish. An alternative approach is to control the frequency of the transverse vibrations. As mentioned earlier, the thickness of the element determines the resonant frequency. Therefore, the transverse resonant frequency is determined by the width of the element. Transverse or lateral resonance coupling is most severe when the array element is as wide as it is thick. This aspect ratio of 1 : 1 means that the lateral resonance is at the same frequency as the operating frequency of the array, causing image degradation. The approach usually taken, therefore, is to reduce the width of the element and thereby increase the frequency of the lateral mode resonance. If the array element is made sufficiently thin, the lateral mode resonant frequency can be increased to a point where it lies outside the range of frequencies for which the signal processing electronics are designed. Typically, an aspect ratio of 2 : 1 (an element twice as thick as it is wide) achieves the desired reduction of lateral mode coupling.[22,23]

Array elements also are coupled to each other through the foil and lens attached to the front of the transducer, backing material, and the array housing. When an array element is pulsed or excited by a returning echo, the ultrasonic vibrations it produces will travel to a greater or lesser degree through all of these layers to the adjacent elements and induce them to resonate. The most common additional aberrant modes of vibration include mass-spring oscillation waves, Lamb waves, and Rayleigh surface waves. The mass-spring mode is the most troublesome of the aberrant modes to supress. Mass-spring waves are low frequency vibrations that result from harmonic oscillations of the element moving against the backing material. These waves are highly excited by the drive pulse, occur at frequencies of around 0.8 to 1 MHz, require 40 to 50 msec to decay below the system noise level following transducer discharge, and are difficult to filter because of their similarity to the fundamental frequency of the transducer. The main effect of the mass-spring mode on transducer performance is to add clutter to the images in the range from 0 to 7 cm.[24,25]

The mass-spring mode can be suppressed by using two oppositely poled pieces of lead zirconate titanate (PZT) to cause a zero net center of mass motion. This results in an order of magnitude reduction of the mode. Shorter ring-down times, less cross-coupling, and more uniform acoustic radiation patterns result.[25]

The metal foil bonded to the top of the array to seal the element interstices, and the lens, also can support a vibrational wave known as the *Lamb wave*.[26] There are two types of Lamb waves: symmetric and asymmetric. In the symmetric form, both sides of the layer move toward or away from each other, whereas in the asymmetric form the vibration is caused by flexural propagation. The Lamb wave is supressed by choosing a thin foil. Because the symmetric mode is largely responsible for Lamb-wave propagation, making the foil thin reduces the group velocity and prevents effective coupling from the array elements to the foil. Propagation in other layers remains a potential source of noise.

The last major mode that exists on the array is the Rayleigh surface wave.[27] This propagates on the backing as a retrograde ellipse with components along the surface and perpendicular to it. The vibrations decay exponentially with depth from the surface. This mode is driven by the motion of an element and is another cause of cross-coupling between elements. Because the Rayleigh wave is bound to within a few wavelengths of the backing surface, deep cuts extending well into the backing effectively suppress it.

The design and manufacturing of phased array transducers are obviously highly complex, and perfection of these processes has taken many years. Thus, despite the ever present theoretic advantages of dynamic focusing and flexibility of display, only in the last few years have the images from these complex systems become equal or, in some cases superior, to those produced by the simpler mechanical scanners.

ANNULAR PHASED ARRAYS

Annular phased arrays are constructed using piezoelectric elements that are concentrically, rather than linearly, oriented. Because of this arrangement, the typical annular array transducer is cylindric rather than rectangular (Fig. 2–26), containing a central disc-shaped element surrounded by a series of concentrically arranged ring-shaped elements. This arrangement allows both transmit and receive focusing at any desired range along the central axis. In the annular array format, both the transmit aperture and transmit focus are variable functions according to the tissue depth of interest. The transmit aperture can be varied by increasing or decreasing the number of rings used to produce the broadcast signal, whereas the range at which the output signal is focused can be controlled by varying the sequence in which the rings are activated. As with linear phased arrays, some improvement in system performance can be obtained by weakly focusing the transmitted beam. Likewise, although focal distance and depth of field can be varied for sequential pulses, each pulse can be focused at only one depth.[28–32]

For signal reception, the operative philosophy of the annular array is also similar to that of the linear phased array (i.e., the delays are set such that all echoes from a specific spatial location at the depth of interest are summed and those from all other locations cancel). The delays also can be varied to track the outgoing pulse as it travels through tissue, maintaining the focus at the depth from which the reflected signal is arising (Fig. 2–26).

The annular array design prevents electronic beam steering, and the array transducer therefore must be moved mechanically. The ideal drive mechanism is the conventional electrical stepper motor, which sectors the assembly through a rapid series of steps (starts and stops) corresponding to each scan line. Therefore, during sound propagation, the crystal is motionless and no correction is required for motion of the crystal as the echoes return from sequentially deeper tissue levels. Use of stepper motors does not affect the overall scan

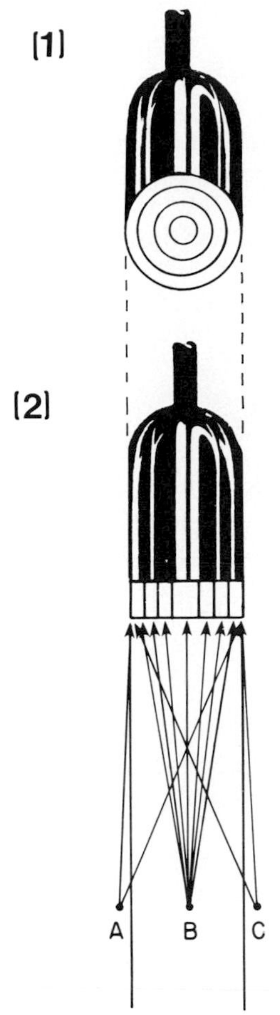

Fig. 2–26. Configuration of an annular array transducer (1) with a central circular element surrounded by a series of concentric ring-shaped elements. The array can be focused by applying a spherical receive pattern to the array elements (2) so that echoes from targets directly in front of the array (B) arrive in phase at all points on the rings while those from laterally positioned targets (A and C) arrive at different point on the ring out of phase and therefore cancel. By varying the delays of the receive circuitry, one can track the focus along the entire path of the sound pulse and maintain a relatively constant focus in all dimensions.

rate relative to traditional mechanical systems, and deriving each scan line only when the crystal is perpendicular to its path allows the same set of focusing algorithms to be used for all comparable depths in the display.

There are two main advantages of the annular format. First, because of the circular arrangement of the elements, focusing is not limited to the azimuthal and elevation planes. Rather, a spherical focus can be imposed, which constricts the beam equally in all dimensions. Changing the pattern of activation allows the focal distance and depth of field to be varied to include all ranges within the near field. Second, because the annular ring assembly is sectored mechanically, the computer algorithms required for beam control are much simpler than for a phased linear array because computer control is required only for beam focusing rather than simultaneous focusing and steering.

Array transducers are similar in size and method of use to those found in any conventional mechanical sector scanner. To permit appropriate phasing, the elements must be electronically and acoustically isolated because they are subject to the same undesirable vibrational modes found with linear arrays. It is important that the width of the outer annulus not be less than its thickness to avoid troublesome resonances. Moreover, each element should make an equal contribution to the signal power at the summing point, with the proviso that side lobe amplitudes may be reduced by tapering off the sensitivity toward the periphery of the array.

The mechanical sectoring requirements for the annular array create significant engineering and design problems because, as with all array transducers, each element must have its own electrical connections. When the crystal rings are moving within the stationary transducer body, significant degradation or loss of signal may occur if these potentially tenuous connections become disrupted.

Annular arrays are not a new concept[33] and are widely used in radar applications and in abdominal ultrasound. Their application in cardiology, however, has been relatively late. This is because the focal characteristics of the annular array relate directly to the number of rings in the array and aperture size. In echocardiography, where the aperture is almost always limited by the acoustic window, the number of rings in the array is also limited, reducing its theoretic effectiveness. Likewise, when portions of the array fall outside the area of available access to the heart, noise and reverberation will distort the summing process, further limiting effectiveness. To this point, therefore, annular array technology has not been as useful in cardiac imaging as elsewhere. The concepts are sound, however, and it is likely that with further improvements in technology, more of the inherent potential will be realized.

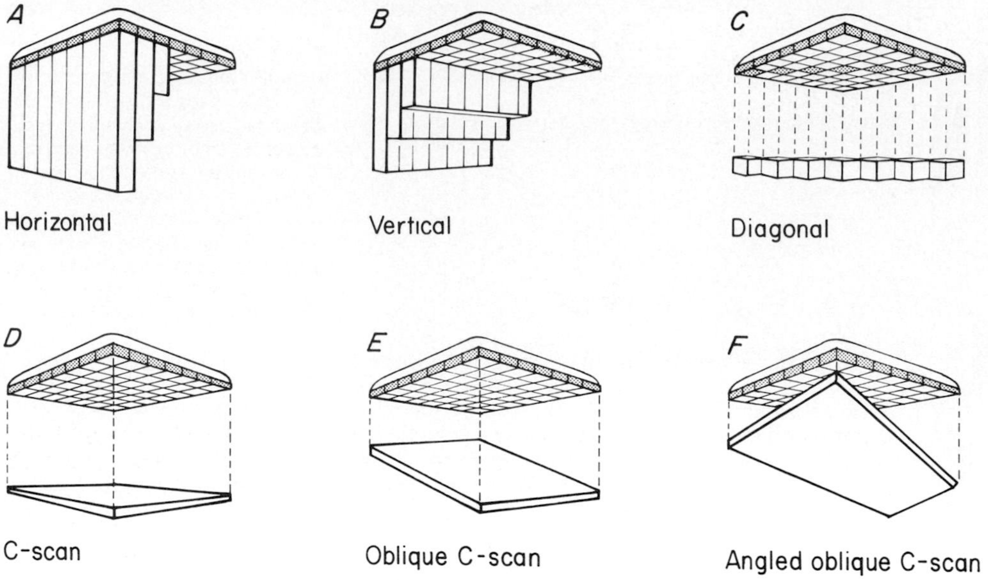

Fig. 2–27. **A** to **F.** A two-dimensional (block) array. (See text for details.)

TWO-DIMENSIONAL ARRAYS

The typical linear phased array provides a two-dimensional dynamic image of the heart in a single tomographic plane. Although this plane can be positioned to record different areas of the heart by moving the transducer, it would be ideal if a three-dimensional volume of the heart could be interrogated in any plane from the same transducer location. Two types of two-dimensional arrays have been developed: the rectangular, or block, phased array and the orthogonal, or O-mode, system. The block phased array design consists of a single large rectangular or square crystal that is cut in a grid pattern into numerous independent elements (Fig. 2–27). The result is a group of linear or linear-phased arrays operating at various levels of efficiency through all imaging planes. Theoretically, the block two-dimensional array of elements can generate two-dimensional images using elements aligned vertically, horizontally, or obliquely across the array (Fig. 2–27). Image planes oblique or parallel (C-scans) to the face of the array also can be obtained by electrocardiogram (ECG) gating and computer reassembly of multiple cross-sectional planes taken over many cardiac cycles from a single transducer location (Fig. 2–27D to F). Highly complex computer algorithms are obviously required to drive such a device. Further, the technologic difficulties in constructing piezoelectric arrays become much greater on moving from one to two dimensions. The major problems to be solved include electrical interconnections or access to the elements of the array using low-cost batch fabrication techniques, elimination of acoustic and electrical cross-talk, aliasing creating side lobes, the achievement of adequate bandwidth and sensitivity, and a high degree of uniformity in both amplitude and phase characteristics.[34]

Integrated circuit techniques have been used to construct several elegant two-dimensional arrays with various degrees of complexity up to 32×32 elements on 1-mm centers, operating typically at 3.5 MHz. The multiplexing switches used with these arrays are constructed as an integral part of the array and consist of field effect transducers arranged so that access to any element may be obtained by the application of two address signals.[35]

The major limitation of these devices for cardiac imaging is the obligate size of the array, which is much larger than any available portal of access to the heart. Again, however, the concepts are fascinating and undoubtedly will find application in some other format.

The second type of two-dimensional array uses two linear arrays aligned orthogonally or in a cross-like configuration (Fig. 2–28). By alternating the activation of each of the arrays, one can acquire orthogonal images

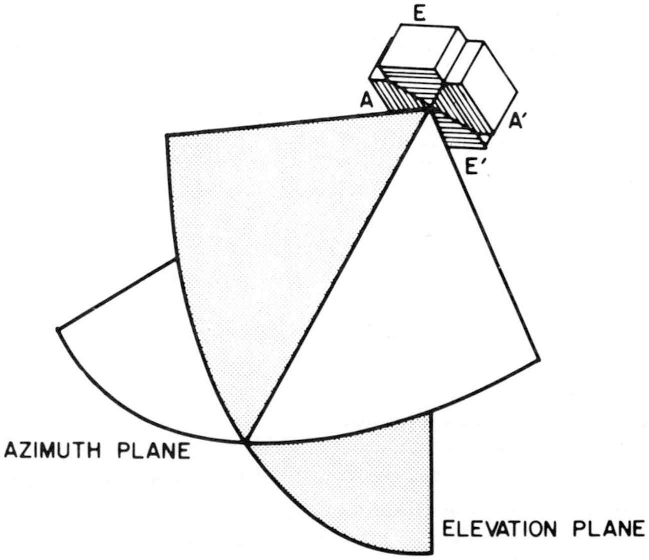

Fig. 2–28. An orthogonal or O-mode transducer and orientation of the orthogonal sector arcs from separate nearby triangular sections (A, A′, E, and E′) comprise the O-mode array. (From Snyder JE, Kisslo J, von Ramm OT: Real-time orthogonal mode scanning of the heart 1: system design. J Am Coll Cardiol 7:1279, 1986.)

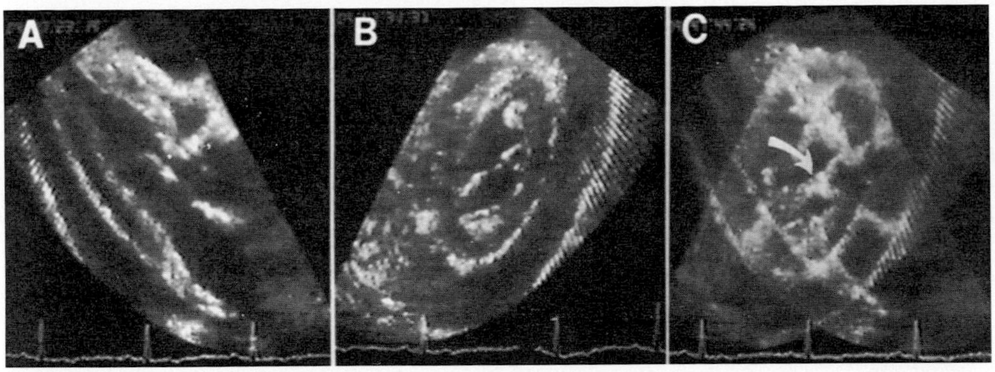

Fig. 2–29. Long **(A)** and short axis **(B)** projections of the left ventricle recorded using an orthogonal array. **C.** Simultaneous projections of the two sectors show the anterior mitral leaflet at the Z axis intersection of the two planes. (From Snyder JE, Kisslo J, von Ramm OT: Real-time orthogonal mode scanning of the heart 1: system design. J Am Coll Cardiol 7:1279, 1986.)

of the heart (Fig. 2–29). Although this approach has enormous potential as a foundation for three-dimensional cardiac imaging, application is limited by currently available display formats.[36]

PRINCIPLES OF DYNAMIC CARDIAC IMAGING COMMON TO ALL SYSTEMS

In dynamic, or "real time," two-dimensional cardiac imaging, ultrasonic data are displayed in a spatially oriented format relative to time. The introduction of time into the two-dimensional image creates several obligatory constraints. Instead of leisurely assembling a single picture of the heart, one must now create images at a rapid predetermined or fixed rate. Because one begins with a limitation in the amount of ultrasonic data that can be collected in a given time period (limited by the speed of sound in tissue), the number of image frames to be assembled determines the amount of data that can be included in each frame. If the image frames are assembled at a fixed rate, the size of the scan area then determines how thinly the data must be spread over the final ultrasonic image. As a result, several additional terms are required to describe dynamic imaging. These include pulse, or line, repetition frequency, frame rate, line density, depth of field, scan angle, and dead time. Each of these variables is interdependent; an alteration in one necessarily alters the others. Although different methods have been designed for generating ultrasonic images, the same basic physical constraints apply to all systems.

The Pulse, or Line, Repetition Frequency

The rate at which individual sound pulses are transmitted, resulting in lines of returning ultrasonic data, is referred to as the *pulse, or line, repetition frequency*. The maximum line repetition frequency that can be employed is governed by the speed of sound in tissue and by the depth of tissue one wishes to examine.

Figure 2–30 illustrates these relationships. In this example, we have assumed that the distance from the anterior chest wall to the posterior wall of the heart is 15 cm. Assuming that sound travels through the heart at 1.5 mm/μsec, 100 μsec are required for a sound pulse to travel from the anterior chest wall to the posterior wall of the heart. Because the returning echoes must transverse the same distance back to the transducer, the entire transit time for the burst of ultrasonic energy from the transducer to the posterior wall of the heart and back is 200 μsec. Each burst or pulse of acoustic energy results in the reception of a line of ultrasonic data. The maximum number of pulses that can be transmitted each second, and consequently the resultant line repetition frequency at a 15-cm tissue depth, therefore, is 1 pulse/0.0002 sec or 5000 pulses/sec.

If one were examining an infant or small child and thus needed to penetrate only 7.5 cm of tissue, the total transmit time of the pulse would be only 100 μsec, and

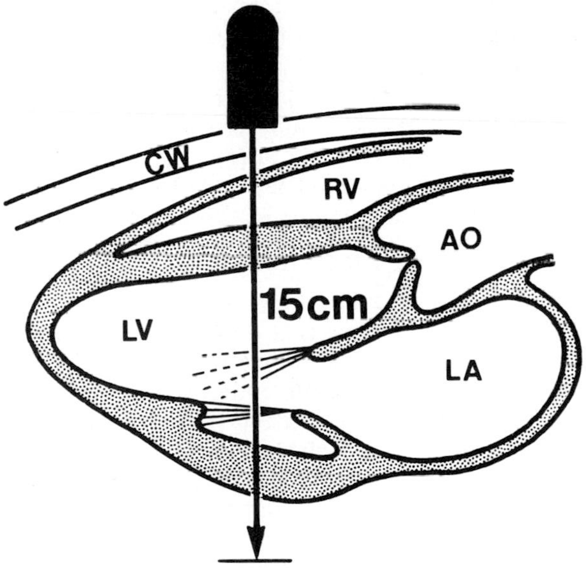

$$\text{P.D.} = \frac{D}{C'} = \frac{15\text{cm}}{1.5\text{mm}/\mu\text{sec}} = 100\mu\text{sec}\,(200)$$

$$\text{PRF} = \underline{.0002\ \text{sec}}/\text{pulse or } 5000\ \text{pulses/sec}$$

Fig. 2–30. The effects of the examined tissue depth on the pulse duration (P.D.) and, hence, on the number of pulses that can be transmitted in a given time period (the pulse repetition frequency, PRF). In this example, the tissue depth is 15 cm. If the speed of sound in tissue is 1.5 mm/μsec, the sound wave will require 100 μsec to reach this depth and an additional 100 μsec to return to the transducer. Because each pulse requires 200 μsec, a maximum of 5000 pulses can be transmitted per second. AO = aorta; LA = left atrium; LV = left ventricle; CW = chest wall; RV = right ventricle.

10,000 pulses could be transmitted per second. In the alternative case, if one were examining a large subject or were examining the heart from a relatively long distance, such as from the subcostal window, a depth of field greater than 15 cm might be necessary. At a field depth of 21.5 cm, the transit time of the pulse increases to 300 μsec, and the maximum pulse repetition frequency is 3333 pulses/sec. The depth of field one must examine, therefore, determines the pulse repetition frequency and, hence, the number of ultrasonic data lines available per second.

The optimum depth of field required in cardiac imaging depends on the size of the patient and on the position from which the examination is attempted. In the standard adult population, a field depth of between 16.5 and 17 cm normally allows the recording of the posterior surface of the heart from the anterior chest wall. Examination from the apex and subcostal region requires a greater field depth in the range of 20 to 21.5 cm.

In addition to the time the pulse has to travel, additional time is lost between pulses because the echograph cannot be converted from a transmitter to a receiver instantaneously. This retrace time, or dead time, further limits the number of pulses that can be transmitted and the amount of data that can be collected and displayed per unit time.

Frame Rate

After the line repetition frequency of the system is established, the frame rate should be determined next. Frame rate is important when one is attempting to resolve the motion of rapidly moving structures. For example, if we assume that the aortic valve opens at a speed of 300 mm/sec and that each leaflet moves approximately 1 cm from the open to the closed position, full excursion of the leaflet will occur in one thirtieth of a second. If the imaging system has a frame rate of 30 frames/sec, the valve will be closed in one frame and open in the next. When one is attempting to analyze the pattern of valvular motion, a frame rate of more than 30 frames/sec is required to examine intermediate positions along the leaflet's path. Increasing frame rate again allows more detailed motion analysis, although at a significant price. Because one begins with a fixed number of lines of information, an increase in frame rate decreases the lines available for individual frames. If we assume a pulse repetition frequency of 4500 pulses/sec at a frame rate of 10 frames/sec, we have 450 lines/frame. At 30 frames/sec, we have only 150 lines/frame, whereas at 100 frames/sec, we will have only 45 lines/frame. As the available ultrasonic data per frame are reduced, high quality images become increasingly difficult to produce. Higher frame rates, therefore, result in a trade-off between frame rate and image quality.

Scan Angle

The next important consideration is the size of the scan or the scan angle. Remember, the depth of field determines the line repetition rate, the line repetition rate determines the number of lines of information available, the frame rate determines the number of lines per individual frame, and the scan angle or picture size determines the density of these lines over the image field (Fig. 2–31). Line density, to a large degree, determines the quality of the image. When the lines are widely spread, reconstruction of the image is difficult because of a deficiency of information. As a general rule, a line density of about 2 lines/degree with a range of approximately 1.5 to 2.2 lines/degree provides sufficient data to create a clinically acceptable image.

Field Versus Frame

In addition to the general operating characteristics of two-dimensional systems, several other concepts in cross-sectional imaging must be defined and understood. The first is the difference between a field and a frame. A field is composed of the data recorded during one complete passage of the beam of ultrasound across the surface of an object. A frame is the sum of all data recorded until the beam returns to its original starting point, and new information is superimposed in an identical pattern on previously recorded data. Thus, when the received ultrasonic data lines are recorded in the same position, direction, and pattern each time the ultrasound beam sweeps across the patient, each field is equal to a frame. However, when data lines are accumulated from different directions or in a different pattern during each of multiple sweeps, several fields are required to compose a single frame.

To illustrate this more fully, consider two different types of mechanical scanning systems. In an oscillating

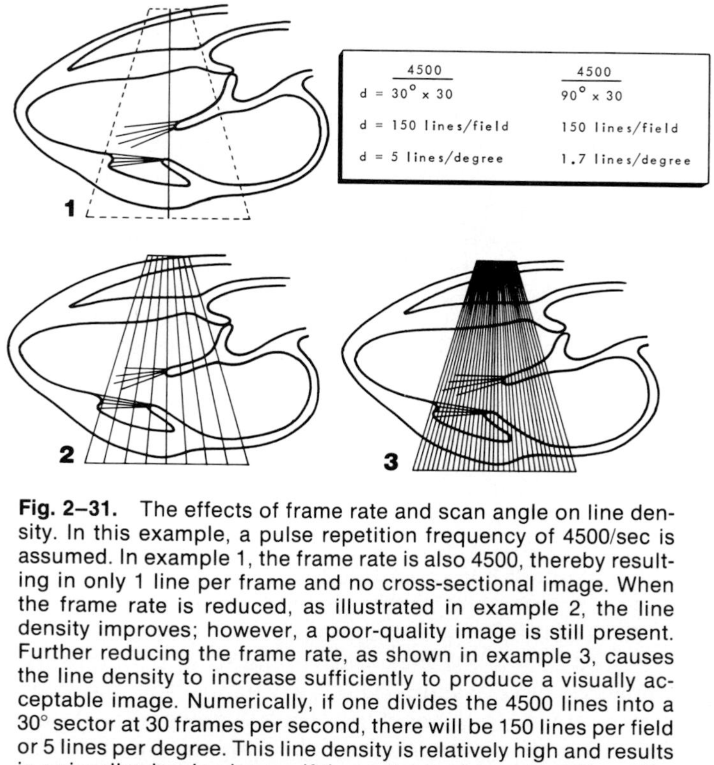

Fig. 2–31. The effects of frame rate and scan angle on line density. In this example, a pulse repetition frequency of 4500/sec is assumed. In example 1, the frame rate is also 4500, thereby resulting in only 1 line per frame and no cross-sectional image. When the frame rate is reduced, as illustrated in example 2, the line density improves; however, a poor-quality image is still present. Further reducing the frame rate, as shown in example 3, causes the line density to increase sufficiently to produce a visually acceptable image. Numerically, if one divides the 4500 lines into a 30° sector at 30 frames per second, there will be 150 lines per field or 5 lines per degree. This line density is relatively high and results in a visually pleasing image. If the sector is widened to 90° and the frame rate is held constant, the line density drops to 1.7 lines per degree. At this line density, the image is barely acceptable; below this density, the image quality becomes unacceptable to the average viewer.

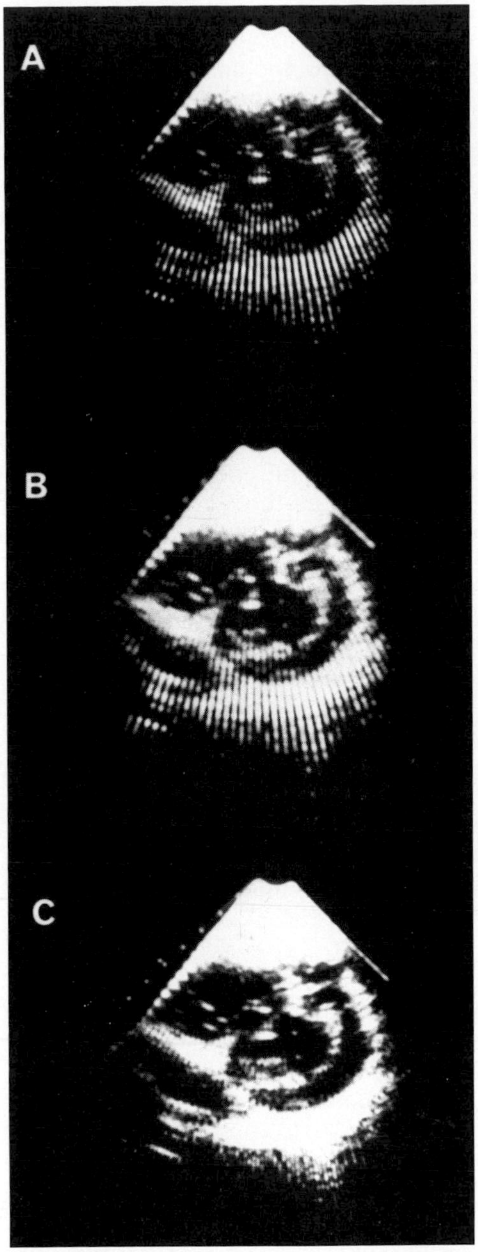

Fig. 2–32. Two methods of increasing the apparent line density. **A.** A single field of data is displayed. At the line density of this image, there is a clear separation between the individual data lines, producing a "spoking" effect. **B.** The system gain has been increased, causing the individual data points to bloom. The data lines widen, and the separation between lines decreases. **C.** The technique of interlacing has been used. In this example, a second field has been laid down such that the data lines are placed between the lines of the field illustrated in A. Interlacing further smooths the image; however, some blurring results because the data in the second field are recorded slightly later.

sector scanning system, the transducer and beam of ultrasound are initially swept from left to right across the surface of the chest. After reaching the opposite margin of its sector, the beam then returns from right to left before beginning the cycle again. Because each sweep and corresponding data display occurs in opposite directions, each constitutes an individual field. The combination of the two fields, which are displayed before the transducer begins in its original direction, constitutes a single frame.

In a rotary transducer system, the motion of the transducers is always in the same direction. As illustrated in Figure 2–32A, when the data lines that are recorded during each transducer sweep are displayed in the same position or on top of the lines from the preceding sweep, each field equals a frame. If, in contrast, lines from two or more consecutive transducer sweeps are displayed in the interspaces between the lines from preceding sweeps (interlacing), the number of fields required to complete a single frame depends on the number of lines that are interlaced (see Fig. 2–32).

Secondary Energy Lobes

One of the more serious problems encountered in array transducers is caused by image-degrading secondary lobes of ultrasonic energy. There are two basic types of secondary lobes: side lobes and grating lobes. Both are regions of ultrasonic energy occurring outside the main or central beam; however, they are caused by different mechanisms.

Side lobes (introduced in Chapter 1) are found with all types of ultrasonic transducers and are caused by the laterally directed energy arising from the transducer edges. Their intensity is determined by the diffraction pattern of this laterally directed energy and varies with the frequency and active area of the transducer. The active area contribution to the side lobes generated by an array is a function of element size and the number of elements pulsed simultaneously to form the beam. Generally, the greater the number and the smaller the size of the elements for a given active area, the lower the side lobe amplitudes.

Side lobes are three-dimensional entities and have an appearance similar to that in Figure 1–11. For a given frequency and active area, the side lobe pattern is similar for square and circular geometries. For a rectangular geometry, the side lobes tend to have a more elliptic configuration, similar to the overall beam pattern (see Fig. 2–21).

Grating lobes are a more significant problem for linear array transducers. Grating lobes are caused by the constructive interference pattern of the laterally directed energy from the edges of the individual array elements. Their intensity and angle from the main beam (which is itself a grating lobe) depend on the regular periodic spacing of array elements and their degree of separation. Plotting the sound field amplitude of a group of array elements as a function of angle from the central acoustic axis of the group gives a measurement of the sound field similar to the representation in Figure 2–33. The amplitudes of the first- and second-order grating lobes, expressed as a percentage of the main beam amplitude, are approximately 70 and 10%, respectively. As opposed to side lobes, grating lobes lie in the same plane as the main lobe, and their angular location relative to the main beam is given by the following expression:

$$\sin \theta = n\lambda/\Delta\chi \qquad [2.1]$$

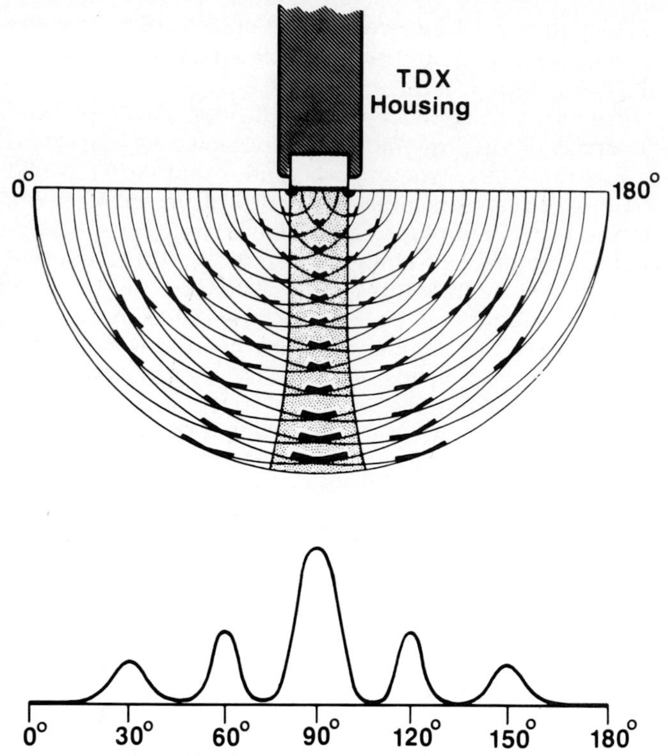

Fig. 2–33. The method of side lobe generation and the variations in sound intensity encountered at sequential sampling points through a 180° arc around the transducer face. In the upper panel, laterally directed echoes arise from the edges of the transducer. These echoes are alternately in and out of phase as they propagate radially away from the transducer face. Areas of increasing sound intensity can be detected at points where the echoes are in phase, whereas the sound intensity is relatively low in regions where the echoes are out of phase. In the lower panel, the relative sound intensities measured at various points in a 180° arc around the transducer are illustrated. The area of peak intensity represents the main beam. On either side of the main beam, regions of increasing intensity (corresponding to points where the radially directed sound energy is in phase) alternate with areas of lower intensity (where this energy arrives out of phase). TDX = transducer.

where θ is the angle in degrees from the beam's central axis, n is an integer denoting the order of grating lobe, λ is wavelength determined by the frequency of the array, and $\Delta\chi$ is the center-to-center spacing (pitch) of the array elements. For example, consider the case of an array with a center frequency of 3.5 MHz and an element pitch of 1.5 mm. The values are

$$\lambda = 0.44 \text{ mm}$$
$$\Delta\chi = 1.5 \text{ mm}$$

Substituting these values in Equation 2.1 yields:

$$\sin\theta = (1)\ 0.44/1.5$$
$$\theta = \text{arc sin } (.293)$$
$$\theta = 17°$$

The first-order grating lobe is located 17° from the acoustic axis. For the same array, the second-order grating lobes are located at approximately 35°. To eliminate or minimize the artifacts caused by grating lobes, it is necessary to make the location angle θ for all grating lobes greater than 90° from the main beam. Examining Equation 2.1 further demonstrates that for a given frequency array, the only design variable is the center-to-center spacing of the elements, $\Delta\chi$. When $\Delta\chi$ is made less than 1.0 λ, θ > 90°, and the grating lobes have been essentially eliminated. For a 3.5-MHz array, $\Delta\chi = 0.5\lambda = 0.2$ mm. Grating lobe intensity increases as the main beam is deflected from normal and is greatest when the main beam approaches the margins of the sector. Figure 2–34, for example, illustrates a grating lobe, which although displaced by almost 90° from the main beam, becomes apparent when the beam is fully deflected to the left.

Secondary lobes, both side lobes and grating lobes, are significant from the standpoint of artifact production, because all sound energy returning to the transducer is displayed as though it had originated along a line corresponding to the main beam axis. Although the intensity of the side lobes is usually considerably less than the intensity of the main beam, variability in reflector strength may cause an echo from a target within the secondary lobe to be displayed as strongly as a corresponding weaker source along the beam path. This problem is greater when logarithmic amplifiers are used because they tend to increase the intensity of these weak off-axis signals. As a result, side lobes can cause the image to become cluttered with meaningless echoes that reduce its interpretability. Figure 2–35 illustrates an ideal array beam profile with a high signal/noise ratio and strong side lobe suppression.

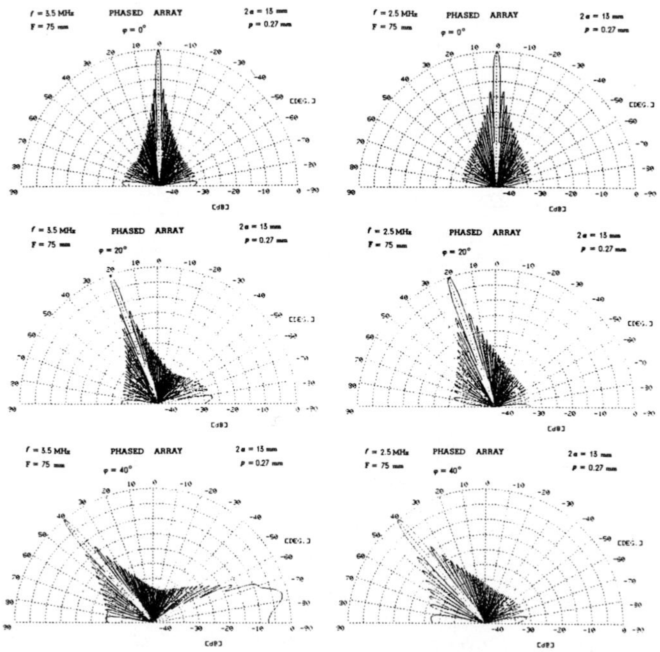

Fig. 2–34. Example of the effects of angle and frequency on grating lobe supression. On the right, a large grating lobe becomes apparent as the main beam is angled 40° to the left of center. By decreasing transducer frequency (increasing wavelength), one can supress the lobe. (From Omoto R: Color Atlas of Real-Time Two Dimensional Doppler Echocardiography. Tokyo, Shindan-To-Chiryo C. Ltd., 1984.)

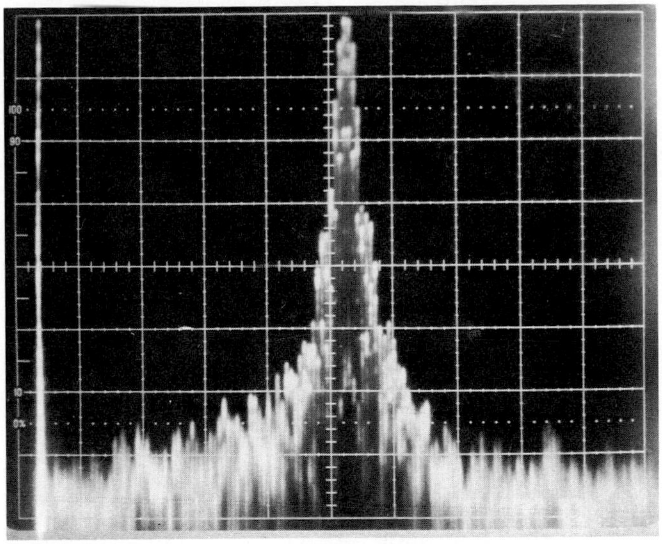

Fig. 2–35. Recording of an ideal ultrasonic beam with excellent signal/noise characteristics and low side lobe intensity.

Dynamic Range—Gray Scale

The acoustic transducers used in diagnostic echocardiography can record echoes over a range of pressures in excess of 100,000 to 1 (100 dB). Display devices, such as television monitors, oscilloscopes, and black and white video strip-chart recorders, used for the presentation of the ultrasonic information display an intensity range of only approximately 32 to 1 (30 dB). To ensure that the image presented to the diagnostician contains all the information present in the original echocardiographic signal, one must electronically manipulate the incoming ultrasonic data so that they can be faithfully displayed on the limited-range output device. To fully understand this important area, one must first define what is meant by the term "dynamic range."

Figure 2–36 schematically depicts the "dynamic range" of a representative system. This illustration, in the form of an A-mode display, indicates that all processed ultrasonic signals start at a zero signal level and can increase in amplitude until they reach the system's signal saturation level. A portion of the ultrasonic information falls in the same amplitude range as that of background noise and, therefore, is obscured. Noise, which is present in all electronic systems, is a combination of acoustic signals that reach the transducer from structures that do not lie on the central axis of the ultrasonic beam and random electronic fluctuations that are produced in the amplifiers of the system. When amplified signals are converted from ultrasonic energy to voltage by the transducer and are processed by a linear system, the dynamic range is defined as the ratio of the largest signal that can be faithfully depicted before signal saturation to the smallest signal amplitude that can be detected above the system noise. For a 100-dB range (100,000 to 1), this situation can include signal amplitudes ranging from 20 mV to 2 volts. This range is too broad for any linear system to handle.

Because all systems have a built-in reject function (i.e., they disallow the display of some small signal amplitudes), dynamic range is more practically defined as the ratio of the largest signal amplitude that can be faithfully depicted before signal saturation to the smallest signal amplitude that can just be perceived above the reject level. This latter interpretation applies equally well to the display devices used in echocardiographic image acquisition and processing systems because they all possess built-in reject functions and signal saturation levels.

Because an imaging system cannot display simultaneously the entire range of echo amplitudes despite the use of the entire dynamic range of its acquisition, processing, and display subsystems, most echographs use some form of dynamic range compression. The resulting image depicts varying echo amplitudes as varying shades of gray.

The first dynamic range compression method used by commercially available echocardiographs is schematically depicted in Figure 2–37. This approach, called *clipping*, simply clipped off all echoes above the amplitude at which the input signal exceeded the linear range of the amplifiers. Clipping thus restricted the range of output signals to one that the display devices could accept. This method produced an image that appeared to possess little gray scale (bistable). This loss of gray scale occurred because the gain controls were normally set to receive weak signals; consequently, the majority of signals exceeded the linear range of the amplifiers and were displayed only as maximum signals (white). These bright dots then tended to obscure the small gray scale, presenting echoes from the weaker reflectors that were adjacent to them. This resulted in a black and white image with no intermediate shades of gray.

A variety of more recent devices has been developed that permits the selection of variable relationships be-

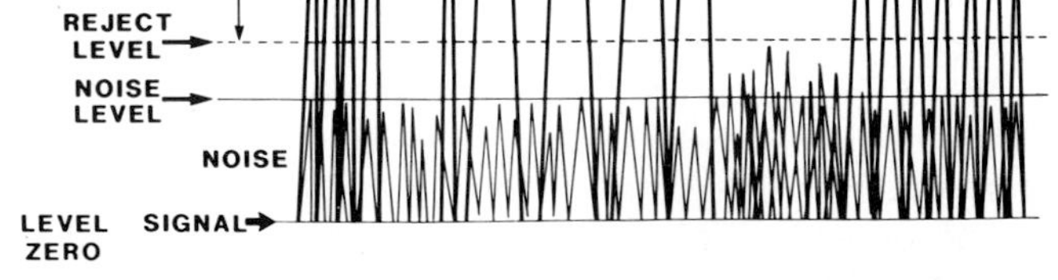

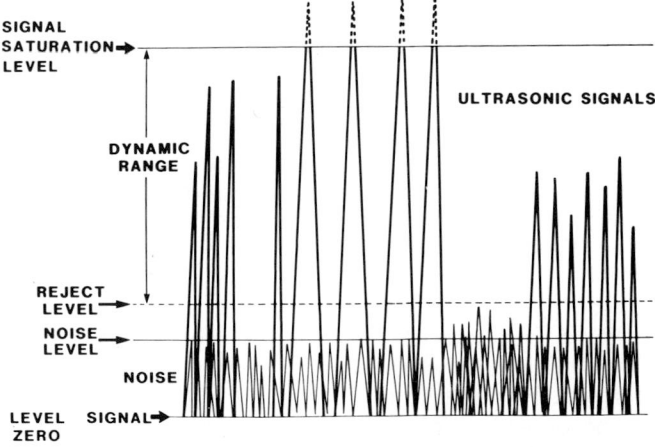

Fig. 2–36. The dynamic range of a representative echocardiographic display system. As indicated, all ultrasonic signals begin at a zero signal level and can increase in amplitude until they reach the system "signal saturation" level. Many of the low-intensity signals fall within the range of the background noise and are therefore obscured. All systems have a built-in system reject, which eliminates both the system noise and the low-intensity echoes that lie just above the noise level. The dynamic range of the system, therefore, is between the system reject level and the signal saturation level and represents the echoes that actually appear on the display scope.

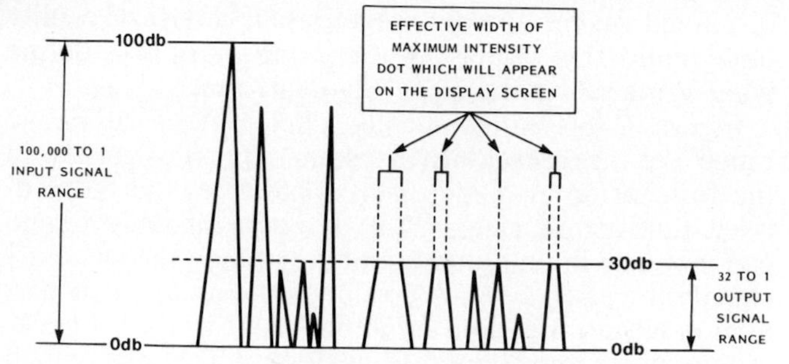

Fig. 2–37. The use of "clipping" to produce dynamic range compression. In this format, all echoes above the output capacity of the amplification and display apparatus are simply clipped when they reach a threshold level. Such action effectively restricts the range of the output signal to a level that the display devices can accept. The relative intensity of the signals above the clipping level is indicated by the width of the base of the remaining echo and, hence, by the intensity of the display dot on the imaging scope.

tween the input and output signals. In some instances, the operator can select the specific type of signal processing that is most appropriate to the study being performed. Figure 2–38 is an example of one type of signal processing that has been used to highlight higher intensity echoes when looking for increases in reflectivity arising from diseased vascular walls. This format is only one of an almost limitless series of relationships that can be established between the input and output signals. More complex algorithms are discussed in the next chapter.

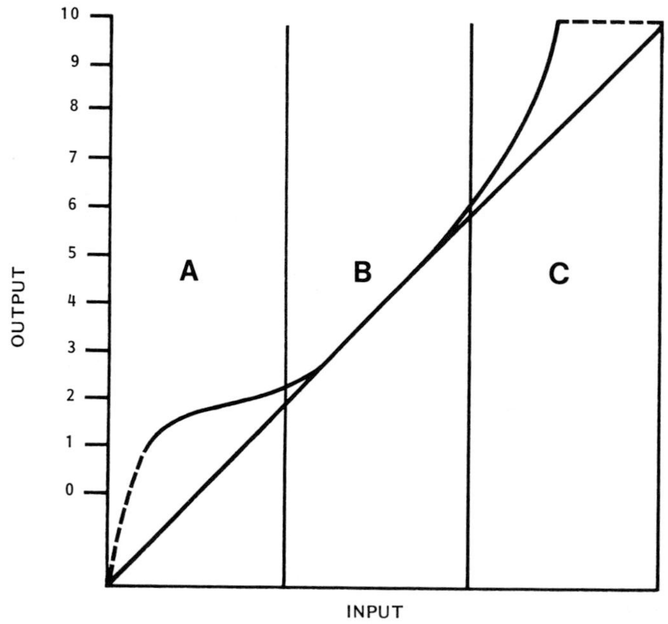

Fig. 2–38. A method of varying the relationship between the input and the output signals. In this format, the low-intensity signals (A) are logarithmically amplified and displayed over the lower two shades of gray on the output grade scale. The midrange signals (B) are then displayed in a linear fashion over the next four shades of gray. The high-intensity input signals (C) are exponentially amplified and displayed over the final four shades of the gray scale. This format compresses the lower-intensity signals into a relatively homogeneous field of gray while amplifying the higher-intensity signals, causing them to stand out in contrast to the homogeneous background.

The usefulness of various forms of gray scale imaging is well established in obstetric and abdominal ultrasonic imaging. In cardiac imaging, because structure location and motion have received more attention than has echo quality, this methodology has been less completely studied. It is anticipated, however, that gray scale, as well as other forms of signal processing, will become increasingly more important as more and more echocardiographic imaging systems with the ability to display the full range of diagnostic information in levels of gray become available.

Persistence

When the electron beam of a CRT strikes the front surface of the tube, the phosphor coating surface is illuminated and begins to glow. The length of time the phosphor glows after initial illumination is an inherent property of the phosphor and is termed *persistence*. Persistence is the basis of all image formation because, without some degree of persistence, the data would disappear immediately from the screen, and no image would result. The use of the persistence of the eye alone would require an impractically high frame rate. Thus, an aircraft propeller appears to the eye as a disc; however, the revolutions per minute (rpms) of the propeller are of a different order of magnitude than are those of standard imaging frame rates.

Persistence is seen and used daily in cardiology. The tracing on the standard bedside electrocardiographic monitor represents the persistent trail of the electron beam as it sweeps across the surface of the monitor, displaying voltage change relative to time. Similarly, the standard M-mode echocardiographic sweep represents information that is left behind or persists as the ultrasonic data line that displays echo amplitude and depth is swept across the face of the oscilloscope.

The same oscilloscopes (CRT) are used for repeated data visualization in most of these display formats; thus, the afterglow of the phosphor should gradually fade away, making that scope available for the next image. If further images are not displayed, the time required for the initial images to fade can be appreciated. If, however, a second image is written before the first image has completely disappeared, one must rely on the increased intensity of the new information to dominate the display, and the decaying data from the previous sweep become relatively less dominant. Because cross-sectional images are written rapidly, one on top of the other, four or more fields may be displayed before the recorded data from the first field totally fades.

The choice of phosphor determines the amount of "history" to be dealt with by the examiner. As a rule, the variation in intensity permits the eye to exclude data that are less intense or persistent and to concentrate on newly written or current information. In certain circumstances, however, the persistence may create significant artifacts. Thus, if a particularly strong echo source is displayed, the echo data from the first frame may be sufficiently bright to appear for three or four additional frames. These dominant, persistent echoes may then be confused with more recently written, but less intense, echo information, creating a "persistence artifact" (Fig. 2–39). In addition, the position of an interface may change from frame to frame during real-time dynamic imaging and, as a result, persistent data may lie next to, rather than beneath, previously recorded data. Such positioning blurs the display.

The effect of writing one image on top of another is particularly apparent in oscillating transducer systems. As the oscillating transducer sweeps in one direction (left to right), it continuously writes information on the oscilloscope. When it reaches the full extent of its arc

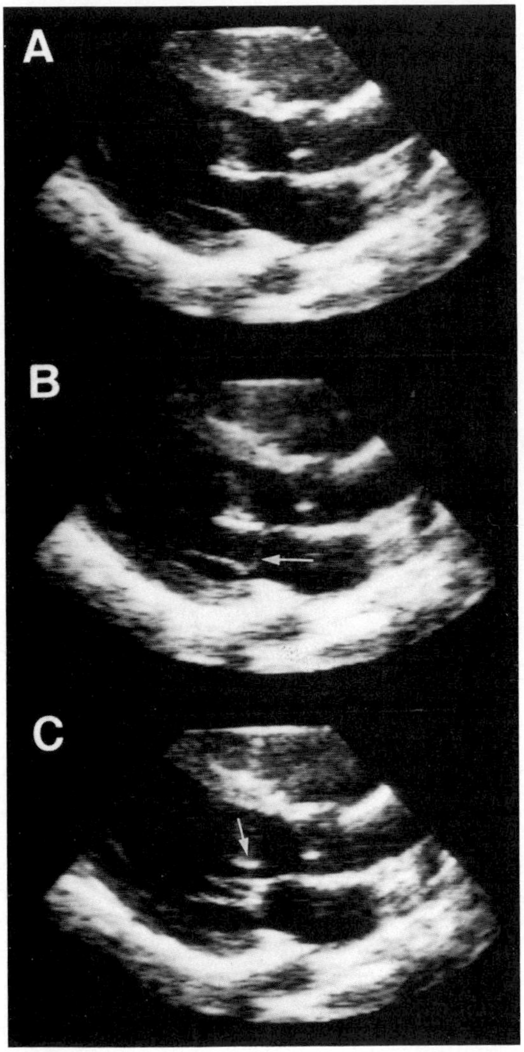

Fig. 2–39. Series of parasternal long axis recordings of the mitral valve during valve closure illustrates the effects of persistence of the resulting image. **A.** Recorded just before initial leaflet closure. The anterior mitral leaflet is in an open position and lies perpendicular to the path of the scan plane. In this position, it is highly reflective and produces a bright echo. **B.** The anterior leaflet has closed, as indicated by the horizontal arrow. The bright echo from the open leaflet recorded in the previous frame still persists and is more obvious than the true echo from the closed leaflet, which now lies parallel to the path of the scan plane. **C.** A later frame. The closed leaflets are now more prominent, but the echo from the previously open leaflet still persists (oblique arrow). If the effects of persistence were not recognized, the abnormal echo in B might have been interpreted as an abnormality of the mitral leaflet itself.

and reverses its course (right to left), it initially writes new data on top of the information from the end of the last sweep, which still persists brightly. Conversely, the data at the far end of the sweep have now been on the scope for a longer period of time and are beginning to fade. In this situation, on one half of the sector, recent data are inscribed twice, whereas on the other half, nothing has been written for a relatively long time. As a result, half of the screen is bright, and the other half is relatively less intense.

Although the inherent persistence in a single display tube may produce artifacts, many early echocardiographic instruments contained multiple CRTs in series leading to the final display. Each of these tubes had its individual persistence, and the sum of the persistent artifacts from each tube could be considerable. For example, in the standard display format used in many commercial instruments, the initial image was recorded directly on a CRT, which introduced persistence. The image on this CRT was then recorded using a television camera, which introduced a second persistence. The video information was then redisplayed on a television monitor, which introduced a third persistence. In addition to the variation in persistence of the individual components, the persistence of each tube tended to change in a dyssynchronous fashion over time as the phosphor aged. When one looked at an individual field, therefore, the resultant data represented the sum of current data plus persistent data. However, the amount and complexity of the persistent data were determined by the relative persistences of the multiple components in the display chain.

With the advent of digital scan converters, most of the intermediate analog steps in this image processing chain have been removed, and the only phosphor-related persistence occurs in the display monitor. However, the same types of artifact can be introduced by frame averaging in the digital scan converter (see Chapter 3), and recognition of the potential dyssynchrony between data acquisition and display remains important.

Complex Signal Processing

Because of the difficulties in appropriately displaying raw echo data, new approaches to signal processing have been developed. Many of the more sophisticated approaches to signal processing involve digitizing the returning echoes. Once in this form, the acoustic data can be mathematically manipulated with ease.[37]

Digital signal processing can be used to simulate different amplifier transfer functions. As a result, log, linear, exponential, and various other transfer functions can be obtained. Another signal processing approach is similar to the picture enhancement done for the space program. Echoes are selectively printed or deleted based on amplitude and density information of the surrounding echoes. These schemes can improve lateral and longitudinal resolution within their design limits. Fast Fourier transformation, autocorrelation, and convolution are some of the many other techniques available to process acoustic data. Usually, the signal is returned to analog form for display after processing is completed. This topic is discussed in greater detail in Chapter 3.

Image Recording Techniques

For maximum clinical utility, cross-sectional images must be displayed and recorded simultaneously. In addition, they should be available for instant playback and analysis. Detailed analysis further requires their availability for viewing in real-time, slow-motion, and stop-frame formats. In addition, the volume of data acquired in a single study makes a rapid scanning capability in both forward and reverse modes desirable. This flexibility is generally found only in a video recording format; consequently, cross-sectional images are primarily recorded on magnetic videotape.

For most clinical purposes, it is not necessary to be familiar with the steps involved in recording and transmitting video data. However, for quantitative analysis of echo images, a more detailed understanding of video signal processing and data storage are important because video images differ in both form and data acquisition rate from two-dimensional echo images.

At present, there are three worldwide television system standards: the National Television System Committee (NTSC), the Phase Alternating Line (PAL), and the Sequential Couleur a Memoire (SECAM).[38] North America and Japan employ the NTSC system; SECAM is used in France, Eastern Europe, and Russia; and PAL is the standard for the remainder of Europe, South America, and Africa.[37]

In the monochrome version of the NTSC television system, a television camera performs electro-optical line-by-line scanning of a scene. Each complete image scan, called a frame, is divided into even and odd fields composed of even and odd scan lines. A frame contains 525 horizontal scan lines; the frame is 1/30 second, and each field scan period is 1/60 second. The choice of a 60-Hz frame rate is motivated by the 60-Hz alternating current power lines employed in the United States. At the end of each scan line, a horizontal synchronization (sync) pulse is transmitted, and a vertical sync signal is transmitted at the end of each field.[38]

The composite analog video signal is passed through a low-pass electrical filter with a half-power bandwidth of about 4.0 MHz before amplitude modulation of a transmission carrier. At the receiver, after carrier demodulation, the sync signals are extracted from the composite video to drive the horizontal and vertical deflection circuits of the television display.[38]

The two-dimensional echo images, in contrast, are acquired in a polar or rectangular coordinate system and, as a result, some form of scan conversion is necessary to convert the echo image to a video image. This can be achieved using either a video camera, as discussed, or in a digital scan converter; however, in neither case is the frame or field rate of the two imaging systems typically synchronous. Likewise, the monochrome TV bandwidth of 4 MHz may undersample higher frequency echo data, losing potential resolution, and may be too low for processes such as tissue characterization, where most of the significant information lies in the higher frequency ranges. For such applications, direct analysis of the raw radio frequency (RF) data may be necessary.

In a color television system, the camera provides simultaneous red, green, and blue line scans of a scene; these are combined to form the scene luminance according to the following relationship:

$$Y = 0.299R + 0.587G + 0.114B \qquad [2.2]$$

The luminance signal is then transmitted along with two chrominance signals, I and Q, which are linear functions of the color difference signal R-Y and B-Y. The G-Y color difference signal can be generated from:

$$G\text{-}Y = -0.581(R\text{-}Y) - 0.394(B\text{-}Y) \qquad [2.3]$$

and the R, G, and B signals can then be reconstructed by adding Y to each color difference. The color differences are normalized to form the signals

$$U = R\text{-}Y/1.14 = 0.877(R\text{-}Y) \qquad [2.4]$$

$$V = B\text{-}Y/2.03 = 0.493(B\text{-}Y) \qquad [2.5]$$

This normalization, which is a standard for the NTSC, PAL, and SECAM systems, was chosen to limit the maximum excursion of the composite color television signal to the arbitrary value of 1.33 times the excursion of the monochrome television signal. In the NTSC system, the I and Q chrominance signals are formed by

$$I = U \cos(33°) - V \sin(33°) \qquad [2.6]$$

$$Q = U \sin(33°) + V \cos(33°) \qquad [2.7]$$

Alternately, the Y, I, and Q signals can be directly related to the R, G, and B camera signals by

$$Y = 0.299R + 0.587G + 0.114B \qquad [2.8]$$

$$I = 0.596R - 0.274G - 0.322B \qquad [2.9]$$

$$Q = 0.211R + 0.523G + 0.312B \qquad [2.10]$$

Figure 2–40 describes the NTSC video signal coding process. For transmission, the luminance signal is filtered to a bandwidth of about 4.0 MHz, whereas the I and Q signals are bandlimited to about 1.3 and 0.5 MHz, respectively.[37] This rather severe bandwidth limiting of I and Q at the transmitter affects the frequency spectrum of the reconstructed R, G, and B signals at the receiver; however, the degradation to a human viewer has proved minimal because of the poor spatial frequency response of the human visual system to colored light.[39] In the next stage of transmitter processing, the I and Q signals amplitude modulate subcarrier signals that are 90° but of phase with respect to each other. The modulated subcarrier signals are then summed together with the luminance signal. Because the frequency spectrum of a raster-scanned video signal has a line structure with a rather sparse energy distribution between lines, by frequency-shifting the combined chrominance signal by a frequency deviation of one-half the line frequency, one can sum the luminance and chrominance signals in a non-

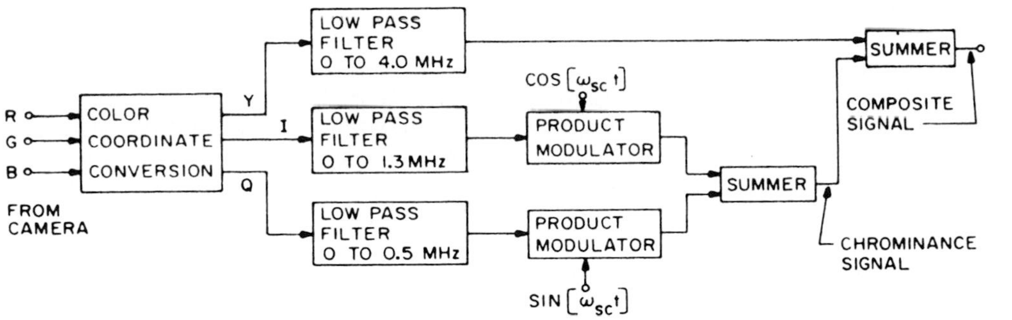

Fig. 2–40. National Television System Committee video signal coding process. For transmission, the luminance signal is filtered to a bandwidth of about 4.0 MHz. The I and Q chrominance signals are limited to a bandwidth of about 1.3 and 0.5 MHz, respectively. (From Pratt WK: Digital Image Processing. New York: John Wiley & Sons, 1978.)

overlapping comb-like fashion. In this manner, the chrominance signals can be combined with the luminance signal to form a color video signal with bandwidth the same as a conventional monochrome television signal. Horizontal and vertical sync signals are then combined with the color video signal during the horizontal and vertical retrace intervals to produce a composite color video signal. At the receiver, the color video signal is reconstructed by stripping its sync components. A color signal demodulation circuit separates the Y, I, and Q, signals which are converted to R, G, and B drive signals for display according to the relationships.[37]

$$R = 1.000Y + 0.956I + 0.621Q \quad [2.11]$$

$$G = 1.000Y - 0.272I - 0.647Q \quad [2.12]$$

$$B = 1.000Y - 1.106I + 1.703Q \quad [2.13]$$

This may all seem rather esoteric but has importance in the analysis of color flow images. For example, if the output of data by a color flow mapping system is a 512 × 512 matrix of color pixels/frame, at 30 frames/second, total output is 7,732,320 potential flow-related information samples. Unfortunately, the sampling rate of the lower frequency chrominance channel is only 0.5 MHz. The original color data therefore will be significantly undersampled when transformed to color video. When the data are recombined, the color output may represent the sum of the velocities in several originally discrete pixels.

Computer analysis of such data then yields pixel values that contain components of red, blue, and green, which for purposes of flow velocity analysis, are meaningless. These concepts are discussed further in the chapters on color flow mapping, wall motion analysis, and tissue characterization.

FACTORS AFFECTING THE CROSS-SECTIONAL DISPLAY CHARACTERISTICS OF A POINT TARGET

Many factors affect the manner in which a point target, swept by a cross-sectional beam, appears on the final display. These factors are summarized in Figure 2–41. Figure 2–41A illustrates a single circular point target. In Figure 2–41B, an ultrasonic beam is swept across the point target from left to right. As the right margin of the beam encounters the target, an echo is produced by the target. This echo, however, is displayed as though the point target were lying along the beam axis. Assuming the beam has a width of 1 cm at the level of the point target, the target is displaced 5 mm to the left on the display. As the beam continues across the point target for an additional 5 mm, the target is intersected by the true beam axis and, hence, is appropriately displayed. Further motion of the beam aligns the target at the left margin. In this position, the target again is displayed as though it were positioned along the beam axis, and, hence, is displaced 5 mm to the right.

Figure 2–41C illustrates the final display configuration of this single-point target. Because an echo is continuously produced by this target while it lies within the sound beam, the point is effectively spread in a lateral dimension equal to the diameter of the beam. This point-spread function, therefore, corresponds to the beam diameter. Targets positioned in the far field of the beam, where the lateral extent is greater, tend to undergo more spreading, whereas those in the narrower portion of the beam tend to be displayed more appropriately.

Figure 2–41D illustrates the effect of increasing gain on the displayed target. As the gain of the system is increased, the effective beam width also tends to increase, resulting in a grater point-spread function and image width. In the axial dimension, an increase in gain

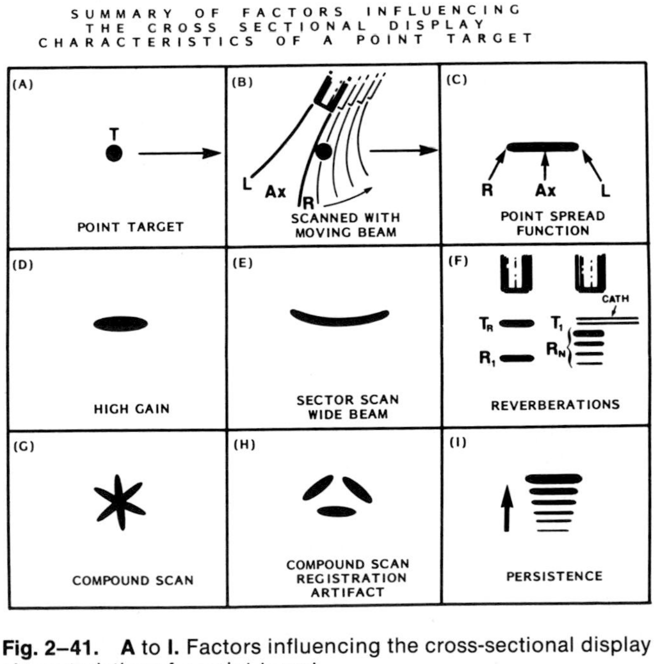

Fig. 2–41. **A** to **I.** Factors influencing the cross-sectional display characteristics of a point target.

tends to increase the width of the echo, particularly in the video format, as indicated in Chapter 1. Therefore, the point target is displayed as an elongated oval.

Figure 2–41E illustrates the effect of excessive beam width in a sector scanning format on the target echo. Because the beam sweeps in an arc, a target that is a constant distance from the transducer face is displayed in an arcuate fashion when scanned by a relatively wide beam. This phenomenon also affects targets that are scanned by narrower beams; however, when the beam width is limited, this effect is not as apparent and is generally undetected.

Figure 2–41F depicts two of the more characteristic patterns that can be seen as a result of internal reverberations of echoes. On the left, a single image (T_R), produced by the actual target, is followed by a second image, R_1, which represents a reverberation. This phenomenon occurs because the sound energy is reflected back to the transducer from the target and strikes the transducer face. It can then be reflected back to the target and then to the transducer a second time. This motion produces a second echo that is twice the distance of the first echo from the transducer.

The right side of Figure 2–41F illustrates the type of reverberation frequently seen when a pulse strikes a target composed of several highly reflected interfaces. In this example, an angiographic catheter has been used. The sound energy that strikes the catheter can be reflected back and forth several times by the interfaces that compose the catheter walls before returning to the transducer. When this occurs, a series of echoes is produced behind the catheter. The distance of the catheter from the transducers is a reflection of the number of internal reflections that occur before the echo's exit from the catheter. This type of reverberation frequently is seen in patients with Swan-Ganz or other hemodynamic catheters in place during the echocardiographic study.

Figure 2–41G illustrates the appearance of a target that is scanned from several different directions. The point-spread function, which occurs perpendicular to the axis of beams originating from a variety of directions, results in a rosette-like display of the point target. Thus, although compound scanning enhances the operator's chances of recording an individual target, it also may distort the final display characteristics of that target.

The combined effects of compound scanning and registration artifacts are indicated in Figure 2–41H. Registration artifacts arise because of variations in the speed of the sound wave as it approaches a target from different directions. The echograph assumes the speed of sound to be constant and, hence, displays all targets at a distance calculated from this assumed speed. The speed of sound through muscle, blood, and other tissues, however, varies slightly. As a result, a sound beam approaching a target along several different paths encounters each of these media in differing proportions. The actual time taken by the sound beam to reach the target, therefore, may vary slightly depending on the path taken. When this time variance occurs, the target appears on the display as a series of linear echoes that do not intersect at a common point.

The final artifact is produced by the persistence of the image frames themselves. Figure 2–41I illustrates the appearance of the persistence artifact during imaging of a point target that is moving anteriorly toward the transducer. The upper linear echo is the reflection from the point target. Each of the linear echoes beneath the dominant echo has a sequentially diminished intensity and represents the echoes from that target recorded in earlier frames. These earlier echoes are gradually fading with time. Because the echo is rapidly moving, any residual data from earlier frames are exposed and become evident. When the point target is a strong reflector, the residual data may persist for many frames and, hence, may blur the image.

REFERENCES

1. Wild JJ, Reid JM: Application of echoranging techniques to the determination of structure of biological tissues. Science 115:226, 1952.
2. Howry D, Bliss W: Ultrasonic visualization of soft tissue structure of the body. J Lab Clin Med 40:579, 1952.
3. Wild JJ, Crawford HD, Reid JM: Visualization of the excised human heart by means of reflected ultrasound or echocardiography. Am Heart J 54:903, 1957.
4. Ebina T, et al.: The ultrasono-tomography of the heart and great vessels in living human subjects by means of the ultrasonic reflection technique. Jpn Heart J 8:331, 1967.
5. Ashberg A: Cinematography of the living heart. Ultrasonics 5:143, 1967.
6. Somer FC: Electronic sector-scanning for ultrasonic diagnosis. Ultrasonics 6:153, 1968.
7. Bom N, Lancee CT, HonKoop J: Ultrasonic viewer for cross-sectional analysis of moving cardiac structures. Biomed Eng 6:500, 1971.
8. Bom N, et al.: Multiscan echocardiography I. Circulation 48:1066, 1973.
9. Roelandt J, et al.: Resolution problems in echocardiology: a source of interpretation errors. Am J Cardiol 37(2):256, 1976.
10. Kloster FE, et al.: Multiscan echocardiography II: technique and initial clinical results. Circulation 48:1075, 1973.
11. Bom N, et al.: Evaluation of structure recognition with the multiscan echograph: a cooperative study in 580 patients. Ultrasound Med Biol 1:243, 1974.
12. Griffith JM, Henry WL: A sector scanner for real time two-dimensional echocardiography. Circulation 49:1147, 1974.
13. Eggleton RC, et al.: Visualization of cardiac dynamics with real time B-mode ultrasonic scanner (abstr). Circulation (Suppl 3), 49, 50:26, 1974.
14. Eggleton RC, Johnston KW: Real time mechanical scanning system compared with array techniques. IEEE Proc Sonics Ultrasonics 1974.
15. Eggleton RC, et al.: Visualization of cardiac dynamics with real time B-mode ultrasonic scanners. *In* White D (ed.): Ultrasound in Medicine. New York, Plenum, 1975.
16. McDicken WM, Bruff K, Paton J: An ultrasonic instrument for rapid B-scanning of the heart. Ultrasonics 13:269, 1974.
17. VonRamm OT, Thurstone FL: Cardiac imaging using a phased array ultrasound system I: system design. Circulation 53(2):258, 1976.
18. Kisslo J, VonRamm OT, Thurstone FL: Cardiac imaging using a phased array ultrasound system II: clinical technique and application. Circulation 53(2):262, 1976.
19. Kisslo JA, VonRamm OT, Thurstone FL: Dynamic cardiac imaging using a focused, phased-array ultrasound system. Am J Med 63(1):61, 1977.
20. Somer JC: Transducer arrays. *In* deVlieger M, et al. (eds.): Handbook of Clinical Ultrasound. New York, John Wiley & Sons, 1978.
21. Jarnoczy J: Sound focusing lenses and waveguides. Ultrasonics, July–September p. 115, 1965.
22. Linear arrays: theory of operation and performance. In Aero-tech reports. Vol. 2. Lewiston, PA, Krautkramer-Branson, 1981.
23. Onoe M, Tiersten HF: Resonant frequencies of finite piezoelectric ceramic vibrators with high electromechanical coupling. IEEE Trans Sonics and Ultrasonics July, 32: 1963.
24. Larson JD: A new vibration mode in tall, narrow piezoelectric elements. IEEE Ultrasonics Symp Proc p. 108, 1979.
25. Larson JD: An acoustic transducer array for medical imaging: part 1. Hewlett-Packard Journal 34:17, 1983.
26. Grigsby TN, Tajchman EJ: Properties of lamb waves relevant to the ultrasonic inspection of thin plates. IRE Trans Ultrasonics Eng UE.8:1, 1961.
27. Viktorov IA: Rayleigh and Lamb waves. New York, Plenum, 1967.
28. Parks SI, Linzer M, Shawker TH: Further developments and clinical evalua-

tion of the expanding aperture annular array system. Ultrason Imaging 1: 378, 1979.

29. Arditi M, et al.: An annular array system for high resolution breast echography. Ultrason Imaging 4:1, 1982.
30. Patterson MS, Foster FS: The improvements and quantitative assessment of B-mode images produced by a annular array/cone hybrid. Ultrason Imaging 1:56, 1979.
31. Dietz DR, Parks SI, Linzer M: Expanding-aperture annular arrays. Ultrason Imaging 1:56, 1979.
32. Melton HE Jr, Thurstone FL: Annular array design and logarithmic processing for ultrasonic imaging. Ultrasound Med Biol 4:1, 1978.
33. Reid JM, Wild JJ: Current developments in ultrasonic equipment for mechanical diagnosis. Proc Natl Electron Council 12:44, 1956.
34. Wells PTN: Biomedical Ultrasonics. New York, Academic Press, p. 240, 1977.
35. Maginness MG, Plummer JD, Meindl JD: An acoustic image sensor using a transmit-receive array. In Green PS (ed.): *Acoustic Holography*. New York, Plenum Press, p. 619, 1974.
36. Snyder JE, Kisslo J, vonRamm OT: Real-time orthogonal mode scanning of the heart I: system design. J Am Coll Cardiol 7:1279, 1986.
37. Pratt WK: Digital Image Processing. New York, John Wiley & Sons, 593, 1978.
38. McLean FC: Worldwide color television standards. IEEE Spectrum 3:59, 1966.
39. McIlwain K: Requisite color bandwidth for simultaneous color television systems. IRE Proc 40:909, 1952.

CHAPTER

3

DIGITAL IMAGE PROCESSING

JAMES D. THOMAS

The description of ultrasound has thus far treated sound waves as continuously variable physical quantities (pressure and time) that are converted into a continuously variable voltage by the piezoelectric crystal. Such continuously variable quantities are said to be analog quantities. It is possible to perform all echocardiographic signal processing and video display in an analog fashion, as was done on the original M-mode and two-dimension imaging machines. Unfortunately, in the analog format, it is difficult to use this information for detailed analysis of the image or for integration with other data such as Doppler recordings, in particular color flow mapping. Also, it is difficult to design and build equipment to analyze and transform analog data properly. Arrays of precise capacitors, resistors, and inductors are needed to average, differentiate, and integrate signals, for example, and these are sensitive to changes in environmental conditions such as temperature and humidity. To change the analysis, even slightly, requires replacement of much of the analog circuitry.

Therefore, more and more of this processing and display is being done with digitized signals, which are sampled at discrete points in time and space and can take on only certain discrete values. Digital circuitry is much less exacting to design than its analog counterpart. Digital circuitry need only distinguish whether a voltage is "on" (i.e., above a certain level) or "off" (i.e below this voltage threshold). Precise linear amplifiers are not needed. Furthermore, digital analysis is much more flexible than analog. To change the analysis in a digital system requires only a modification of the computer program, not a change in the physical components of the system. This flexibility allows the testing and implementation of processing algorithms, which is not possible on an analog system.

Digitization can be done at almost any stage of echo processing. All contemporary cardiac ultrasound machines use a digital scan converter to change the image from the polar acquisition format of the sector scan to a rectangular grid that is compatible (after first converting back to an analog signal) with standard video output. Some machines digitize the signal earlier, while it is still raw radio frequency ultrasound. Digitization at this stage allows greater flexibility of the delay lines for better dynamic focusing and is critical for tissue characterization. Finally, digitization of the output video signal opens up the rapidly developing field of digital image processing, which may allow better quantification of cardiac features and eventually lead to automated systems of echo interpretation.

This chapter first reviews the differences between analog and digital representations of signals and the techniques for digitizing a signal. Next are descriptions of how digital processing is used in current echo machines. Finally, we describe an overall scheme for image processing with some of the mathematical techniques for noise reduction, edge detection, and feature interpretation.

DIGITAL SIGNAL PROCESSING

Analog vs. Digital Representation of Signals

Figure 3–1A displays a sine wave in analog format. This curve is a continuous function of time, which varies smoothly between +5 volts and −5 volts over a period of 1 minute (described mathematically as $V = 5 \sin \pi t/30$, where t is time in seconds). Because this is a continuous function, for every point in time (x axis), there is a corresponding voltage (y axis). Furthermore, there is

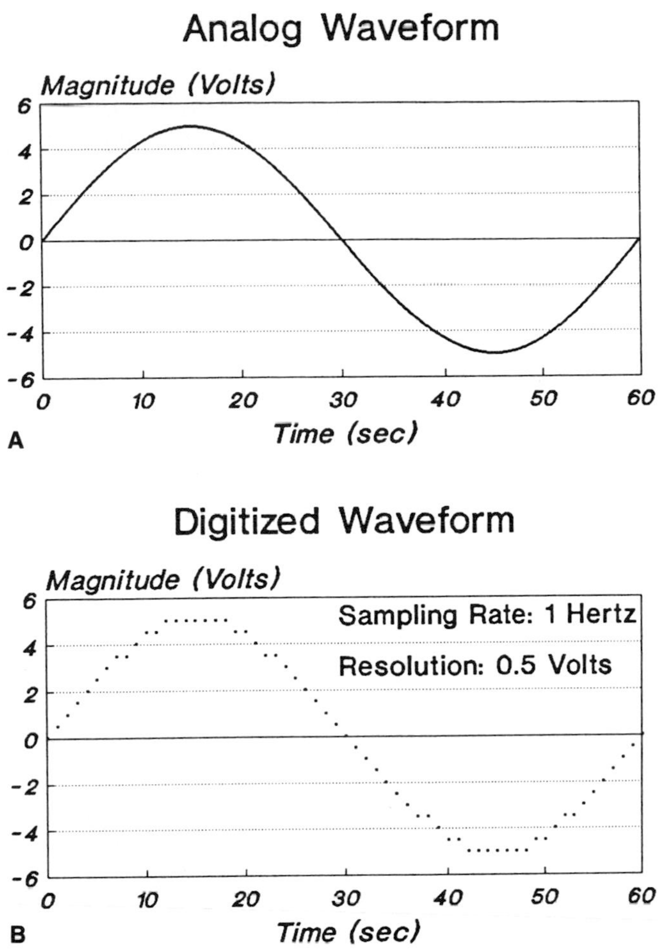

Fig. 3–1. Analog vs. digital representation of data. The same physical signal (a slowly varying voltage ranging between −5 and 5 volts and described mathematically as $5 \sin \pi t/30$) is represented in analog fashion in **A** and digital format in **B**. **A.** Both time and voltage are continuous quantities, the quality of the data determined by the intrinsic accuracy of the measuring equipment. **B.** The data are sampled only once per second (1 Hz), and no information is available between these points. Furthermore, the magnitude of the voltage is stored in 0.5-volt increments, leading to a less accurate representation than the analog signal.

no theoretical limitation to the accuracy of the voltage. Thus, we might read from Figure 3–1A that the voltage at 5 seconds is 2.5 volts and likewise at 5.0001 seconds is 2.500037 volts. The only limitation to this resolution is the accuracy of the "magnifying glass" used to examine the signal. In practice, however, analog equipment seldom has this accuracy, but there is no intrinsic limitation to the resolution of an analog signal.

In contrast, a digital representation of the same voltage wave is shown in Figure 3–1B. It differs in two important respects from Figure 3–1A. First, the signal is measured and displayed only at discrete time intervals, here every second. We know nothing about the signal between these points. Second, the measured voltage at these points in time can take on only certain values, here in half-volt intervals. Thus a voltage might be represented digitally as 4.5 or 5.0 volts, but there is no representation for 4.75 volts. Indeed, any analog voltage between 4.25 and 4.75 will be represented in this digital format as 4.5 volts. Figure 3–2, however, shows that it is possible to make digital signals as accurate as needed (certainly as accurate as the practical limitations of analog signals) by measuring the signal more frequently and storing the voltage more precisely.

Analog signals are stored as continuous variables such as the degree of magnetization on a video tape or the wavy excursion of a track on an audio record. Digital signals are stored as a series of binary bits, which can be in only one of two states: on or off, yes or no, 1 or 0. It is the proper interpretation of millions of these bits, taken sequentially, that allows digital signals to be represented and computer programs to operate.

Binary Representation of Numbers

The ability to represent numbers as either 0 or 1 is not useful by itself. We must combine a series of bits to represent a value with the desired degree of precision. This is done by using the binary or base two number system to build up larger numbers from individual bits. Consider a number formed from 8 bits (termed a byte), for example, 10011101. Just as in the decimal system, each digit in a number is multiplied by a power of 10, in the binary system, each digit is multiplied by a power of two. We can thus break down 10011101 as $1*2^7 + 0*2^6 + 0*2^5 + 1*2^4 + 1*2^3 + 1*2^2 + 0*2^1 + 1*2^0 = 1*128 + 0*64 + 0*32 + 1*16 + 1*8 + 1*4 + 0*2 + 1*1 =$ 157 (decimal). Thus an 8-bit number can represent an integer between 0 and 255, a 12-bit number is between 0 and 4095, and a 16-bit number is between 0 and 65,535.

Fractional Numbers

Fractional numbers can be created by using some of the bits in a number to represent a quantity between 0.5 and 1 and the other bits to define the power of two by which to multiply this fraction with a single bit used to specify if the number is positive or negative. Thus, a number may be made arbitrarily precise by simply using more bits to represent it. To return to our previous example, if it were important to represent 4.75 volts dis-

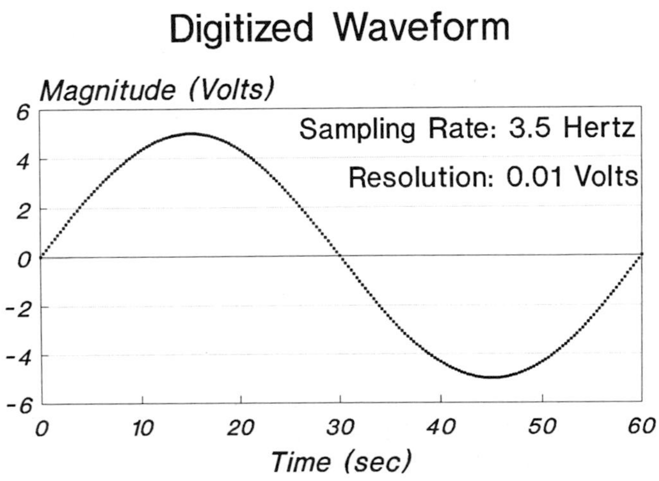

Fig. 3–2. Improved digital representation of the signal in Figure 3–1. Here the sampling rate has been increased to 3.5 Hz and the resolution of the data decreased to 0.01 volts, leading to a much more faithful rendering of the data.

tinct from 4.5 or 5.0 volts, we could use a binary representation containing one extra bit. Thus, in Figure 3–1B, a signal is digitized at a sampling rate of 1 Hz (sample per second) with a precision of 0.5 volts, whereas Figure 3–2 shows the same signal digitized at a sampling rate of 3.5 Hz and a resolution of 0.01 volts leading to a more faithful rendering of the signal. The price of this added precision is the increased storage need and processing time for the signal in Figure 3–2. Not only are there 3.5 times as many numbers to store (because of the more frequent sampling), but to obtain the 50-fold finer resolution, each number must have about 6 more bits of data than the data from Figure 3–1B. Thus, in general it pays to use a digital representation of a signal with a precision roughly equivalent to the accuracy of the original analog signal from which it was derived.

INTRODUCTION TO COMPUTER TECHNOLOGY

The principle components of any computing system are shown in Figure 3–3. The "brain" of the computer is the central processing unit (CPU). It is here that the instructions from a program come together with some data to produce a meaningful analysis. What form do these instructions take? As with any representation inside the computer, they are nothing but a series of 0s and 1s, which the CPU interprets as specific instructions. For example, on an Intel 8088 microprocessor (the CPU of the IBM PC), the code 0000001111011000 tells the CPU to add two numbers together. The CPU has dozens of such codes to perform numeric and logic tasks. A series of such codes makes up a computer program. Both the program and the data on which it operates must be stored in the computer's memory.

Computer Memory

Several complementary forms of memory exist within the computer. The most immediately accessible storage is termed *random access memory* (RAM) and is composed of semiconductor chips with thousands of electric cells that can be set either to 0 or 1 to store a bit of data. It is here that computer instructions and data are held during the actual processing of the program. The computer industry has seen an almost yearly doubling of the density of data storage so that now it is commonly possible to store over 4,000,000 bits (4 megabits) of information on a 12 × 6-mm chip with 16 megabit chips emerging and 64 megabit chips in development. A key characteristic of RAM is that it is "volatile," i.e., it exists only while power is supplied to the chip. If this power is cut off, the data are irretrievably lost. Clearly, a more permanent form of *long-term storage* is also needed, and currently this usually is either a thin magnetic disc or magnetic tape. The magnetic medium is divided into tiny domains, each of which are magnetized in one of two ways, corresponding to the 0 and 1 of the binary bit. The storage capacity can range from 360,000 bytes (360 kilobytes, KB) for a floppy drive on a personal computer to several billion bytes (gigabytes) on a large mainframe computer. Recently, there has been a revolution in storage technology: the read/write optical disc, capable of storing over a gigabyte of data (over 250,000 typewritten pages) on a disc smaller than a phonograph record.

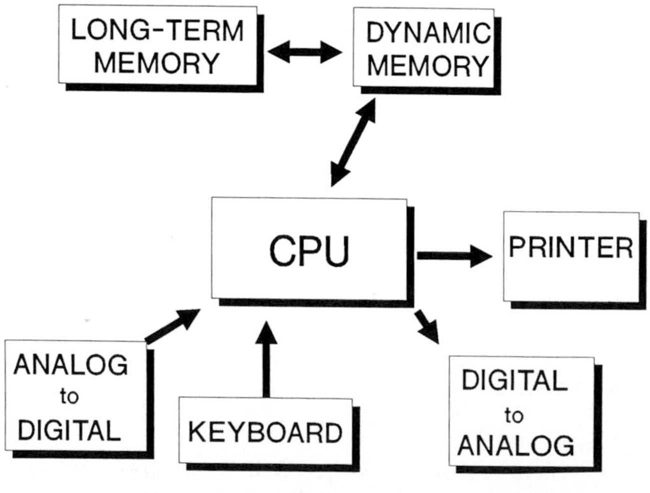

Fig. 3–3. Schematic of computer architecture. The central processing unit (CPU) is served by dynamic and long-term memory (top), input devices (lower left), and output devices (lower right). (See text for discussion.)

Communication

Finally, a computer must be able to communicate with the outside world: a keyboard and monitor to interact with the operator; a printer or plotter for hard copy; or a modem through a telephone line to another computer. These are generalized under the heading input/output (I/O). This communication may take place one bit at a time, in which case it is termed *serial*; or it may involve several (typically 8 to 32) bits transmitted at once, termed *parallel communication*. The presence of several industry standards for these interfaces, such as RS-232 for serial ports and IEEE-488 for parallel, allow computers of radically different internal architecture to communicate with each other. High-speed data links include Ethernet, at 10,000,000 bits/sec (10 megabauds), and FDDI (fiber distributed data interface) at 100 megabauds.

Analog-to-Digital Conversion

An especially important interface to the outside world is the analog-to-digital (A-to-D) converter, which takes the analog value of a signal (e.g., the magnitude of a reflected echo) and transforms it into a binary representation of the number. Two characteristics affect the performance of A-to-D converters: resolution and throughput, concepts demonstrated in Figures 3–1 and 3–2. Resolution is the precision with which a given signal can be represented and is stated in bits for the number of binary bits used to quantify each value. Six-bit resolution corresponds to a precision of 1 part in 2^6 or 64; 8 bit is 1 in 256; and 12 bit is 1 in 4096. The resolution should be carefully matched to the intrinsic accuracy of the signal being digitized. Resolution that is too low may discard valuable data, whereas resolution that is too high will waste storage space and processing time on meaningless data. Because the human observer can distinguish only about 50 different levels of grey in a black-and-white image, it is reasonable to use 6 bits in the video display of an echo. To perform quantitative analysis on this image, however, higher precision is needed, and typically 8 bits are used for manipulation of video signals. For representation of physiologic signals such as blood pressure or flow, 8-bit precision is too coarse, so 12-bit digitization is commonly used.

The second key characteristic of an analog-to-digital converter is throughput or sampling rate. This quantity is measured in Hertz (number of conversions per second) or seconds (interval between conversions). Like resolution, throughput must be carefully matched to the characteristics of the analog signal being digitized to achieved maximal efficiency and accuracy. In this case, however, we are most concerned with the component frequencies of the analog signal. The Nyquist sampling theorem states that for a waveform to be properly represented in digital form, it must be sampled at twice its maximal component frequency (see discussion on the Fourier transformation in Chapter 10 and Appendix B for more detail). Thus, raw ultrasonic data from a 5-MHz transducer must be sampled over 10,000,000 times/sec to be accurate. Physiologic data such as pressure of the electrocardiogram need be sampled only at 1 KHz or slower to maintain full fidelity to the analog signal.

Digital-to-Analog Converters

Digitizing an analog signal for computer analysis is only half of the I/O requirement for the system. To be appreciated by a human observer, the processed, digitized signal must be converted back to analog format for displaying on a monitor or plotting on a graph. This digital-to-analog conversion is characterized by the same resolution and throughput concerns of the A-to-D converter.

Analog and Digital Representation of Video

Because most echocardiographic images are ultimately displayed in video format, it is important to understand some of the technical features of the analog and digital representation of the video signal. The video image as it is displayed from either an echocardiographic instrument, video tape, or television broadcast is in analog format. That is, the intensity of any spot on the image is of continuously variable magnitude from a minimum level (black on the screen) to a maximum (bright white). As noted in Chapter 2, this spot is swept across and down the screen 30 times/sec to form a video frame. In actuality, each frame is composed of two fields, one containing the even-numbered scan lines (called raster lines), the other with the odd raster lines, so that there are 60 video fields/sec. This splitting of a frame into two fields is done to reduce the flicker that would be present if an area of the screen were illuminated only 30 times/sec. The video standard in the United States (NTSC) has 525 raster lines/frame.[1]

To digitize this image, we must convert each point in the image to a binary intensity. Some fundamental decisions to make about this process are (1) the number of raster lines in each digitized frame (Through interpolation it is possible to retain most of the information in an image while storing less than the original number of raster lines.), (2) the number of picture elements (termed pixels) to be digitized along each raster line (reflecting the intrinsic resolution of the analog video signal); and finally, (3) the resolution to be used to digitize each pixel. For a coarse representation, one might use $256 \times 256 \times 6$ digitization (256 pixels/raster; 256 raster lines/frame; and 6 bits/pixel). For more precise digitization, one might use $512 \times 512 \times 8$.

Simple arithmetic will demonstrate the tremendous storage and processing needs of video digitization. Digitization at $256 \times 256 \times 8$ requires, for 30 frames/sec, over 15 megabits (2 megabytes) of storage per second of video signal. A simple PC with only 640 KB of RAM can store only about one-third second of video in RAM. A standard high-density floppy drive holds less than 1 second of data at this rate. It is thus clear that very sophisticated data processing, compression, and storage techniques are needed to handle this volume of data.

CURRENT ECHOCARDIOGRAPHIC DIGITAL PROCESSING

Digital Processing of the Radio Frequency Ultrasound Signal

Digitization of the raw ultrasound signal is a demanding process requiring high resolution of at least 10-MHz throughput. To date, digital analysis of these data has been used in attempts at tissue characterization, discussed in Chapter 41. Recently, several companies have begun digitizing the ultrasonic signal directly and maintaining digital processing throughout the machine. In addition, digital techniques are being implemented to control the timing and aim of the multiple elements of the phased array transducer. This yields more accurate directing and dynamic focusing of the ultrasound beam.

Digital Scan Conversion

Perhaps the most ubiquitous use of digital processing in echocardiography is the digital scan converter (DSC), used to change the ultrasound image from the polar format of its acquisition to the rectangular format necessary to output the image in the NTSC standard (Fig. 3–4). It should be remembered that digital technology is not necessary to perform such a conversion. In the early days of sector scanning, a form of analog "scan conversion" was used in which the individual B-lines were drawn in a polar array on a long persistence oscilloscope, and this image was recorded by a separate video camera, in effect, reformatting the data, although with considerable degradation of the image quality. The DSC does the same thing, converting analog polar input into analog rectangular output, but the intermediate stages are digitized.[2]

A typical sector scan sweep consists of about 100 scan lines radiating out from a single point and equally spaced over a 60–90° wedge. These individual lines are processed in analog format by time-gain compensation; logarithmic amplification to compress the dynamic range;

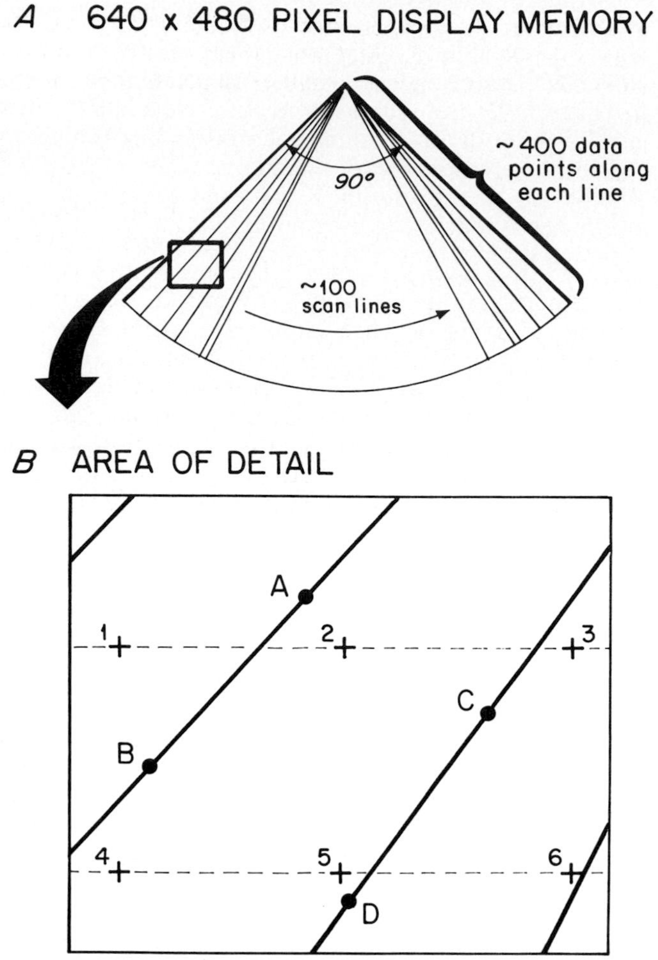

Fig. 3–4. Digital scan converter. **A.** The data from each sector sweep consist of approximately 100 scan lines, each of which is digitized at several hundred points. These data form a fan radiating out from the scan head. The digital scan converter maps these data, which are in a polar geometry, on a rectangular array of memory pixels. This output buffer is then scanned 60 times per second to generate the analog video output signal. **B.** In this close-up of a region of A, it is evident that the rectangular grid points do not generally line up with the polar data points. Simple algorithms assign the value of the nearest polar point to a given rectangular point, while more sophisticated techniques interpolate among the four nearest neighbors to yield a smoother video output.

rectification; and low-pass filtering to yield a B-mode scan line. The scan lines may have tissue interfaces highlighted by differentiating the signal (to detect changes in intensity) and adding this to the B-line. Each B-line is then digitized at about 4 MHz to yield several hundred equally spaced sampling points. Thus, several tens of thousands of digitized points form a complete scan, all arrayed in a polar coordinate system. The DSC maps the video intensity at each of these sampled points onto video memory, which is arranged in rectangular format. This video memory consists of a block of RAM organized into, say, a 640 × 480 rectangular array; such a memory storage area is termed a buffer. The polar scan lines radiate from a point at the top of this buffer and spread out to the bottom. Near the top, many scan lines overlap each pixel in the rectangular array and the DSC assigns the value of that pixel to the polar point falling closest to the center of the pixel. Toward the outer perimeter of the scan, many of the pixels in the rectangular video memory are not crossed by a scan line and so must be assigned values by the DSC by interpolating from adjacent pixels. This may be simple linear interpolation along a given horizontal raster line or, for a smoother display, by using data from the four nearest polar sampling points, termed R,θ interpolation,[3] as shown in Figure 3–4.

Once all of the data points in the polar rays are assigned, there is still considerable blank space in the rectangular raster video memory, outside of the sector scan. Into this section of the screen memory may be written the patient's name, the calibration line for the sector scan, a real-time clock, etc. It is also possible to assign the sector image into a much smaller portion of video memory and use the rest of the screen for an M-mode or Doppler display. Because all of the data are in digital format, it is simple to shift images about on the screen.

Of course, the digital video memory must be converted back to analog format before it can be displayed. Every 16.7 msec, the memory buffer is scanned and analog signals are calculated corresponding to the horizontal raster lines, first the odd lines, then the even ones. Because the number of raster lines (525/frame, 262 or 263/field) is different from the number of rows in the video memory buffer (e.g., 480), each raster line is formed by interpolating between adjacent rows in the buffer. Thus, the output buffer is written into continuously by the digital scan converter and the alphanumeric text editor and read from by the digital-to-analog converter 60 times/sec. Note that these writing and reading tasks need not be synchronized. Thus, there may be no relation between the rate at which the imaging transducer acquires data and the rate at which the image is displayed on the screen, and adjacent points on the screen may actually have been acquired on different sweeps of the transducer.

On-Screen Data Analysis

The presence of a digital memory buffer makes possible a great variety of on-screen analyses of echocardiograms. Placing a cursor on the screen is nothing more than writing the value for bright white (usually 255) to a group of bytes in RAM to form a cross in video memory. On the next sweep of the D-to-A converter, the cursor is displayed on the screen. Knowing the location in video memory and the calibration for the screen, the computer may compute dimensions, circumferences, and areas for various structures identified by the operator on the screen.

One is not limited to the use of a single video buffer for display. For example, the video content from 30 consecutive frames (1 second) could be stored (at 512 × 512 × 8) resolution in about 8 MB of RAM. These 30 buffers could be read in sequence by the D-to-A converter to display that second of the echocardiogram as a continuous loop. Such "frame-grabbing" hardware is becoming more common and less expensive yearly and forms the core for many of the off-line analysis systems as well as those built into contemporary echocardiographs.

IMAGE PROCESSING

The remainder of this chapter examines automated image processing and the elusive goal of automated image understanding. A number of the video algorithms discussed here are well established theoretically and practically, many are actively under investigation, and a few of them remain to be fully developed over the next several years. Although described specifically for echocardiography, this framework is applicable to many types of medical imaging (computed tomography, nuclear magnetic resonance, digital angiography, radionuclide imaging) and to the general field of machine vision. A more detailed description of the mathematics of image processing may be found in standard texts.[1,4,5]

Overview

The process of image understanding can be loosely divided into low level processing and high level processing (Fig. 3–5). Low level processing deals with the individual points or pixels that make up an image (termed icons in machine vision parlance). High level processing deals with the collection of features that make up objects in an image (also termed symbols). The task of low level processing is to extract from the myriad pixels streaming from an image a much smaller and more manageable list of features; high level processing takes these features and returns anatomic diagnoses and quantitative measurements about the objects being imaged. In many ways the retina and optic nerve act like a low level processor, responding to the billions of photons per second impinging on the rods and cones and passing to the occipital cortex a smaller list of edges, corners, movement, and texture. The cortex, then, is a high level processor taking these features, integrating them with prior knowledge and experience to yield an interpretation of the image.

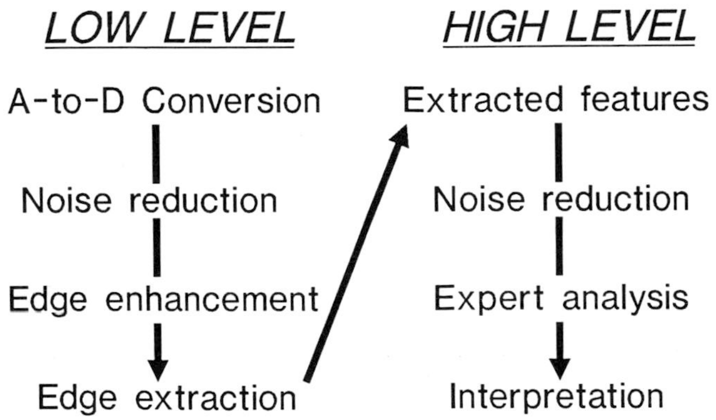

Fig. 3–5. Elements of image processing. The low level operations are performed on individual pixels and must occur several million times per second. High level operations, on the other hand, use features of the image, such as the location of edges or corners. High level interpretation requires a priori knowledge of the object being examined to tell normal from abnormal. High level processing can also guide the optimization of the low level algorithms, for instance, by ignoring regions with a great deal of artifact.

Low Level Processing

Low level processing may be subdivided into four steps. The first is analog-to-digital conversion, which has been discussed previously. The second step is noise reduction. This is especially crucial in echocardiographic analysis because ultrasonic images contain a great deal of noise caused by the stochastic (random) interaction of sound waves with matter. This noise is manifest as a high level of brightness variance between adjacent pixels in a given field (spatial noise) and between the same pixel in successive video fields (temporal noise). Because most edge-detection schemes use spatial gradient algorithms (see following discussion) that amplify noise, it is critical that effective noise reduction is used before edge enhancement.

The third step of low level processing is broadly called feature enhancement, whereby pixels corresponding to some feature of interest in describing the scene are made to stand out from the background of the image. For echocardiograms, this usually means myocardial border enhancement, though algorithms responding to corners, colors, and texture exist in the general image processing field. This step is the one in which most of the work in automated echo processing has been done and algorithms for enhancing (brightening) both static and moving edges have been described.

The final step in low level processing, feature extraction, is unfortunately both the most difficult and the most important one and also the step in which much progress remains to be made. Feature extraction is the bridge between low level and high level processing. One should recall that even after edge-enhancement, the video data still are in the form of individual pixels, typically about 8,000,000/second, streaming through the low level processor. High level processing, on the other hand, deals with much shorter lists of features, i.e., the actual coordinates over time of the left ventricle (LV) endocardial border, along with attributes such as speed and direction of motion of that border. Feature extraction, for example, must be able to extend enhanced borders through gaps of echocardiographic dropout and to reject extraneous edge points arising because of noise and so pass on to the high level processor the best possible description of the scene.

High Level Processing

High level processing is by definition an intelligent process that requires a priori knowledge of the object being analyzed. For example, it may receive the coordinates of the left ventricular endocardium at end-diastole and end-systole (either from an automated low level processor or by hand digitization) and from this determine the area and extent of abnormal wall motion. This implies that the high level processor has a knowledge base of what constitutes normal wall motion. It applies these rules to the observed features to arrive at an anatomic interpretation of the scene.

Techniques of Low Level Processing

Once a sequence of images has been digitized, four basic types of processing can be performed on it. These four types of processing differ in the extent of spatiotemporal impact on the image.

In the first approach, point processing, the output value for a pixel is based on the input value of only that pixel. Examples of this include contrast stretching, gray level equalization, and image inversion. The second type of processing yields an output value for a pixel that is based on the input value for that pixel and surrounding pixels in the same frame. Termed spatial convolution, examples include spatial noise reduction and edge enhancement. In the third approach, temporal convolution, a pixel output value is based on the input value of that pixel and on adjacent pixels in preceding and succeeding frames. Such processing is useful both for temporal noise reduction and for motion detection. The final major category of low level algorithms is termed Boolean processing. It differs fundamentally from the preceding types of processing in that it does not deal with numeric values, but rather with logical ones, items that can be only yes or no. Boolean processing is typically the final step in feature extraction; it is the step in which a decision is actually made regarding whether or not a pixel represents part of a border (or some other feature).

Computer Methods: Point Processing and Convolution

Point Processing. Point processing is the simplest low level operation. For each frame of video data, this operation alters the value of each pixel by a user-defined formula. For example, when an image is inverted, black features become white and vice versa. With 8-bit digitization, a total of 2^8 or 256 gray levels are available to represent the brightness of a pixel. These may be considered to run from 0 (for pure black) to 255 (for pure white), but frequently, to simplify the mathematics of the image processing algorithms, they are considered to be distributed symmetrically about 0, from -128 to $+127$ (the actual appearance is unaffected by this convention). Thus, inversion may be defined by the formula

$$I' = -I,$$

where I is the input pixel intensity, and I′ is the output.

Consider the computational load of this process: at the video frame rate of 30/sec and with 256 × 256 pixels/frame, this implies almost 2,000,000 negating operations per second. Though technically feasible, this task is greatly reduced by use of a look-up table (LUT). Notice that although there are almost 2,000,000 operations per second, only 256 possible answers can be obtained because there are only 256 different input values. It is much more efficient to evaluate the point processing formula just once for each of the possible input values and store the results in computer memory. Thereafter, the input value for each pixel is used only to reference the proper entry in the LUT where the output value can be read.

By using an LUT, point processing algorithms may be complex without increasing the computational burden of the array processor. In fact, a separate computer may be used to perform the calculations and then store the results in the array processor LUT. In this way a forbidding operation such as

$$I' = 256*(\sqrt{|\cos[\pi(I + 32)/192]|} - 0.5) \qquad [3.1]$$

may easily be performed (Fig. 3–6).

Some of the more common point-processing algorithms (illustrated in Figs. 3–7 and 3–8) include the following:

1. Stretching the contrast about an intensity I_0 (Figs. 3–7B and 3–8B):

$$I' = \alpha(I - I_0) + I_0 \qquad [3.2]$$

where α is the contrast ratio, values > 1 representing an increase in the image contrast, values < 1 signifying a contrast reduction. Because the output

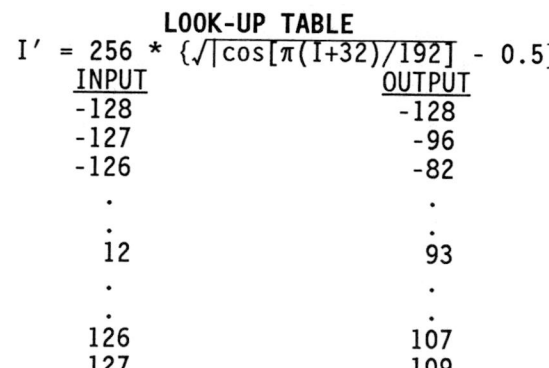

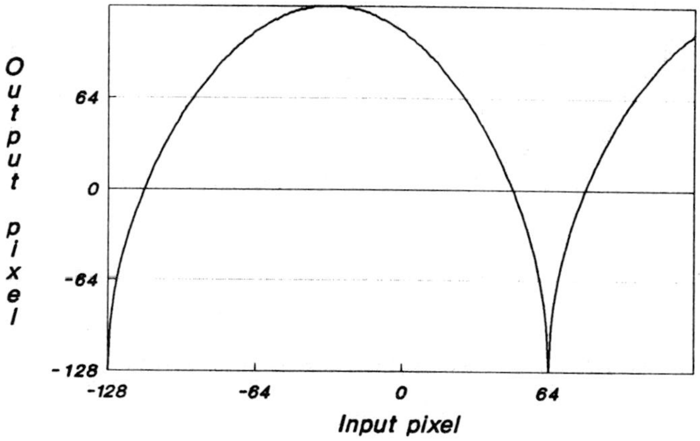

LOOK-UP TABLE

$$I' = 256 * \{\sqrt{|\cos[\pi(I+32)/192]|} - 0.5\}$$

INPUT	OUTPUT
-128	-128
-127	-96
-126	-82
.	.
.	.
12	93
.	.
.	.
126	107
127	109

Fig. 3–6. A look-up table is used to implement a complex point-processing algorithm. This transformation, $I' = 256*(\sqrt{|\cos[\pi(I + 32)/192]|} - 0.5)$ is far too complex to be calculated on each pixel as it streams by. However, because (for an image digitized with 8 bits of intensity resolution) there are only 256 possible input values, it is much simpler to calculate this expression once for each of these 256 numbers and store the results in a computer table, where they may be referred to. Note that this particular algorithm is unlikely to find utility in any image-processing scheme; it is shown for demonstration only.

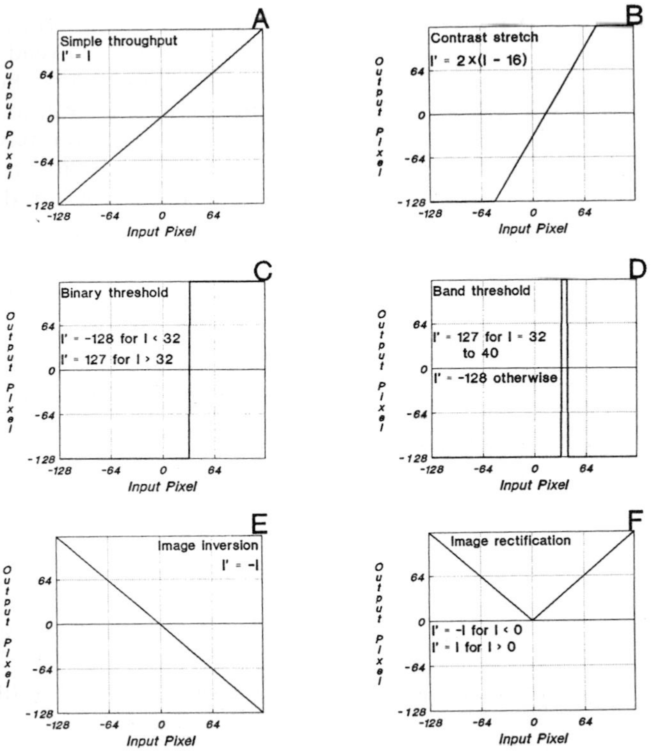

Fig. 3–7. Transfer graphs for several common point-processing algorithms. These graphs function the same way as look-up tables. The input pixel value corresponds to the x axis; the output pixel value is given by the y axis coordinate on the graph. **A.** Simple throughput; the output is identical to the input. **B.** Contrast stretch highlights differences in intensity among pixels near a brightness of 16. **C.** Binary threshold highlights all pixels with an input intensity above 32. **D.** Band threshold highlights only those pixels with an intensity between 32 and 40. **E.** Image inversion reverses black and white but keeps the level of contrast the same. **F.** Image rectification eliminates negative intensity values.

value I′ can have only 8 bits of data, output intensities < -128 are converted to -128 and those >127 are clipped at 127.

2. Thresholding on an intensity I_0 (Figs. 3–7C and 3–8C):

$$I' = -128 \text{ when } I < I_0;\ I' = 127 \text{ when } I \geq I_0. \quad [3.3]$$

This creates a binary image of just pure black and pure white. Although not particularly useful on the raw echo image, this algorithm is commonly applied to images after edge enhancement, to select out only edge pixels.

3. Highlighting a band between I_1 and I_2 (Figs. 3–7D and 3–8D):

$$I' = 127 \text{ when } I_1 \leq I \leq I_2 \text{ and } 0 \text{ elsewhere.} \quad [3.4]$$

4. Shifting the intensity by I_0:

$$I' = I + I_0. \quad [3.5]$$

$I_0 > 0$ brighten the image, and $I_0 < 0$ darken it.

Figure 3–7 displays the mapping curves corresponding to these and several other common point processing algorithms; Figure 3–8 demonstrates the effect that each of these algorithms has on an input echo image.

Spatial Convolution. Spatial convolution is the process whereby the output value of a pixel is determined by its input value and those of its neighbors. Critical to its application is the convolution kernel, a numeric mask with a center moved over each pixel in an image in turn. The numbers in the mask, which might be a 3 × 3, 5 × 5, or larger array overlap the pixels surrounding the center pixel. At once, each of these numbers is multiplied by the pixel that it overlies; these products are then added together to yield the output value for the central pixel. The kernel is then shifted 1 pixel, and the process is repeated until every pixel has been acted on as the central pixel.

As an initial example, consider simple averaging in which each pixel is replaced by the mean of itself and the 8 surrounding pixels (Fig. 3–9). The convolution kernel is a 3 × 3 matrix with one ninth in each cell, indicating that the 9 pixels are each multiplied by one ninth and summed. The mask is then shifted 1 pixel to the right and the process repeated. Clearly, this is an even more computationally expensive process than point processing with each convolution requiring 9 multiplications and 1 addition or about 20,000,000 operations per second. Again, the use of an LUT greatly reduces this burden (though its construction is more complicated than for

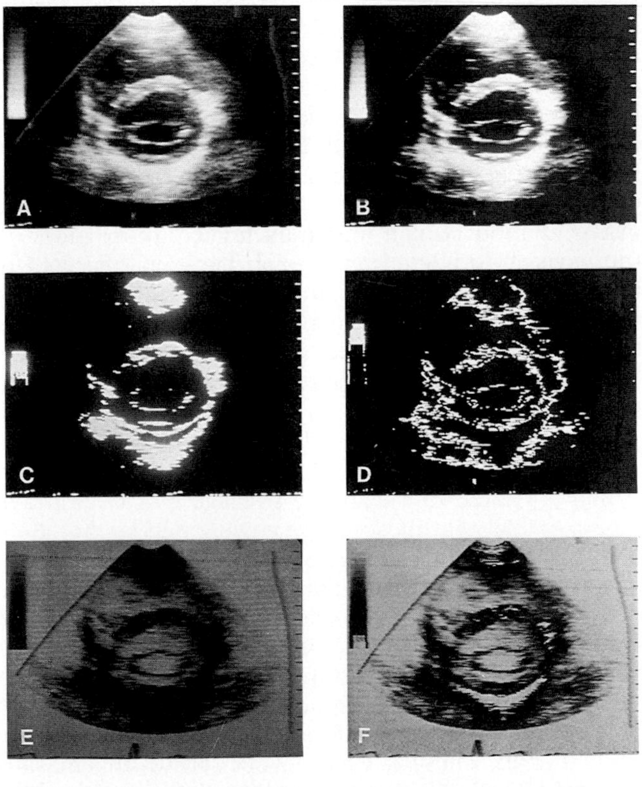

Fig. 3–8. **A** to **F.** Effect of point processing on an echocardiographic image. Each of the examples corresponds to the transfer graphs in Figure 3–7. Thus, **A,** which is a simple throughput, corresponds to the original image, digitized on a 256 × 256 grid.

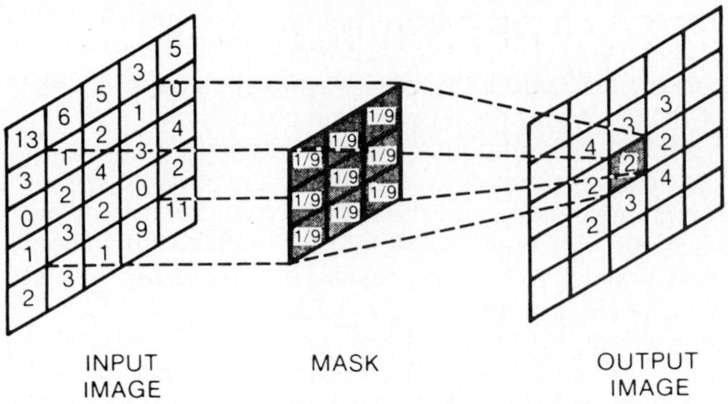

Fig. 3–9. Spatial convolution. The input image is on the left with the output image on the right. The convolution kernel, in this case a simple 3 × 3 average (all nine cells identical in value), lies between them. In turn, the kernel is moved so that its center cell overlies each pixel in the input image. Each time, the 9 pixels currently covered by the convolution mask are multiplied by the corresponding value from the kernel and added together. This sum is the value for the center pixel in the output image. The effect in this example is to replace each point in the input image with the average intensity of the nine surrounding points. (From Collins SM, Skorton DJ (eds.): Digital Image Processing. New York, McGraw-Hill, p. 143, 1986.

point processing). It is only in recent years that computer hardware has become available to perform convolution on video images at the real-time field rate.

Implementation of Low Level Algorithms

Noise Reduction vs. Feature Enhancement. Spatial convolution is used for many of the noise reduction and edge enhancement algorithms in echocardiographic image processing. Unfortunately, these two broad goals are fundamentally at odds with each other. Noise reduction tends to blur out sharp features such as endocardial borders along with random noise. Conversely, the edge enhancement algorithms described later all use spatial differentiation, which amplifies noise. Thus, much of the work in low level processing has been directed to minimizing these contradictory effects: apply too much noise reduction before edge enhancement and there may be no features left to detect; apply too little noise reduction and edge enhancement may produce predominantly spurious edge pixels.

Spatial Noise Reduction. The most commonly used spatial noise reduction algorithm is Gaussian smoothing, which is related to the simple average discussed previously, except that the average is weighted so that more centrally located parts of the mask have a greater effect on the convolution than distant pixels. It is derived from the Gaussian function, e^{-x^2/σ^2} (familiar as the bell shaped curve in statistics), which is maximal at $x = 0$ and falls smoothly to 0 with positive and negative x. For a two-dimensional convolution, as would be used on a video field, the Gaussian function is rotated around the central pixel. Thus, as Figure 3–10 shows, this mask is maximal at the center pixel, falling off smoothly and symmetrically on all four sides. The value of σ determines the width of the Gaussian function: the smaller σ is, the more quickly the curve falls to zero. This broadness of the kernel determines the degree of smoothing. A 3 × 3 kernel (Fig. 3–10A–C) thus provides much less noise reduction than does a 5 × 5 kernel (Fig. 3–10D to F). There is a trade-off in this, however: Gaussian smoothing reduces random noise but also smears out edges and other significant sharp features, making them harder to detect with subsequent edge enhancement schemes. Most reports of spatial noise reduction have used Gaussian convolution applied to single frames,[6,7] one used an asymmetric convolution kernels (9 pixels horizontally, 3 vertically) to exploit the difference between lateral and axial resolution in the echocardiogram.[8] Although good anatomic correlation has been reported with edges extracted following such linear filtering,[9] others have reported the detected edges to be displaced.[10]

Because simple Gaussian convolution indiscriminantly smooths both random noise and sharp features, it would be useful to devise techniques of edge-preserving smoothing, i.e., noise reduction schemes that maintain linear features such as edges. One approach (Fig. 3–11) is to examine the image for location and direction of edges (see Sobel operator, described later) and then apply selectively one of five convolution kernels to smooth along the edges but not across them.

The use of nonlinear filters allows noise reduction

1	2	1
2	4	2
1	2	1

A

1	2	4	2	1
2	5	7	5	2
4	7	9	7	4
2	5	7	5	2
1	2	4	2	1

D

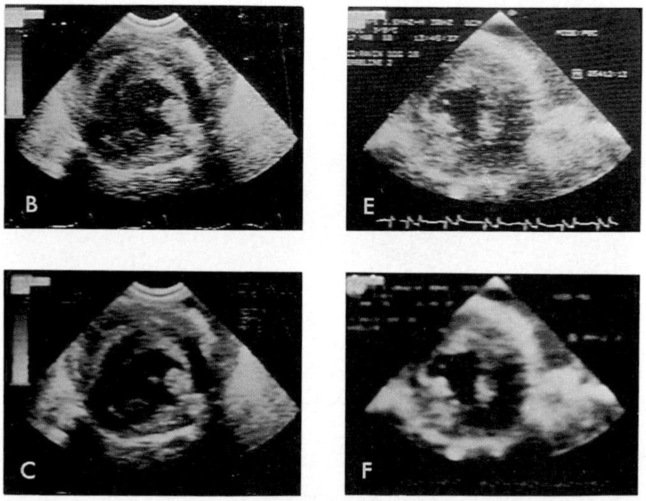

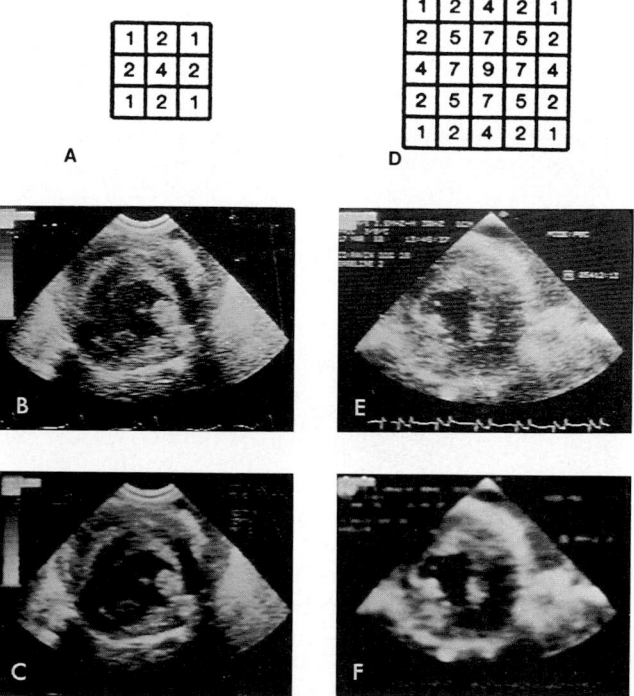

Fig. 3–10. Gaussian convolution. **A.** A 3 × 3 convolution kernel for noise reduction. For readability, the kernel values are whole numbers. In actual implementation, these numbers would be scaled down by a factor of 16, so that the sum of their absolute values would be 1. In this way, the values in the output image will remain within the −128 to 127 range of 8-bit digitization. **B.** Original input image. **C.** Output image following 3 × 3 smoothing. **D.** A 5 × 5 Gaussian convolution kernel (divide each cell by 93 to get actual values). **E.** Original input image. **F.** Output image following 5 × 5 Gaussian smoothing.

with relative edge preservation but at the cost of more complex calculations. For example, good smoothing has been reported with an algorithm that averaged only the 4 pixels closest in intensity to the center pixel within a 3 × 3 kernel.[11] Recently, a more sophisticated median filter, the symmetric nearest neighbor operator, has been applied to echocardiograms (Figs. 3–12 and 3–22B). This algorithm explicitly forces all pixels near an edge to lie on one side or the other, without averaging across it. Recent breakthroughs in processing hardware allows these complex operators to be performed in real-time at 60 fields/sec.[12] Such algorithms remain in the development stage.

Temporal Noise Reduction. Spatial noise reduction techniques help to reduce the "speckle" in individual frames caused by the random scattering of ultrasound from homogeneous tissue. There is also considerable randomness in the scattering from a single point over time. This temporal noise must be minimized for subsequent edge and motion analysis to be accurate.

Two general approaches to temporal noise reduction have been described. The first method is, in essence, a one-dimensional convolution in which the pixel under consideration is averaged with spatially corresponding pixels from the previous and subsequent frames. For instance, one group has used a 1:2:1 weighting for temporal smoothing before applying a 3 × 3 Gaussian spatial filter.[13] A fairly simple approach is to average in a portion of the output from each frame with the input from the succeeding frame.[12] Such a recursive filter behaves like a convolution with an exponential decay curve and significantly reduces the temporal variance in pixel intensity. Each of these filters tends to blur out rapidly moving structures, such as mitral valve opening, but appear acceptable for slower events, such as endocardial motion.

It is also possible to combine such spatial and temporal smoothing into a single 3 × 3 × 3 convolution encompassing three video fields. With faster hardware, it should be possible to use a nonlinear filter, such as the symmetric nearest neighbor operator on a 3 × 3 × 3 spatiotemporal kernel to preserve moving as well as static edges.

The second general approach to temporal noise reduction is gated averaging of corresponding video fields from successive cardiac cycles, taking advantage of the natural periodicity of cardiac movement, as is commonly done in nuclear cardiology.[14,15] The assumption is that true cardiac features will appear in the same location in each cycle, whereas the noise occurring randomly will average itself out. Averaging N images to-

EDGE-PRESERVING SMOOTHING

Symmetric Nearest Neighbor Operator

3X3 Convolution Kernal

B	C	D
E	A	F
G	H	I

Compare opposite pairs:

B ⟷ I
C ⟷ H
D ⟷ G
E ⟷ F

Select the one closest to 'A' (e.g., B, C, D, and F).

Average these 'nearest neighbors' with A:

$A_{NEW} = (A + B + C + D + F)/5$

Surpresses noise without blurring edges.

Fig. 3–12. Symmetric nearest neighbor operator. A nonlinear operator that segregates pixels on one side of an edge or the other. For the 3 × 3 kernel above, the four pairs of pixels arranged symmetrically around the center pixel (A and I, B and H, C and G, and D and F) are examined. From each of these four pairs, the pixel closest in magnitude to the center pixel is chosen, and then these four pixels and the center pixel are averaged together. If applied repeatedly to an image, the output ultimately will show several sharply divided smooth regions. In contrast, if Gaussian convolution is applied repeatedly, the output becomes a featureless gray. An example of this algorithm is depicted in Figure 3–22B.

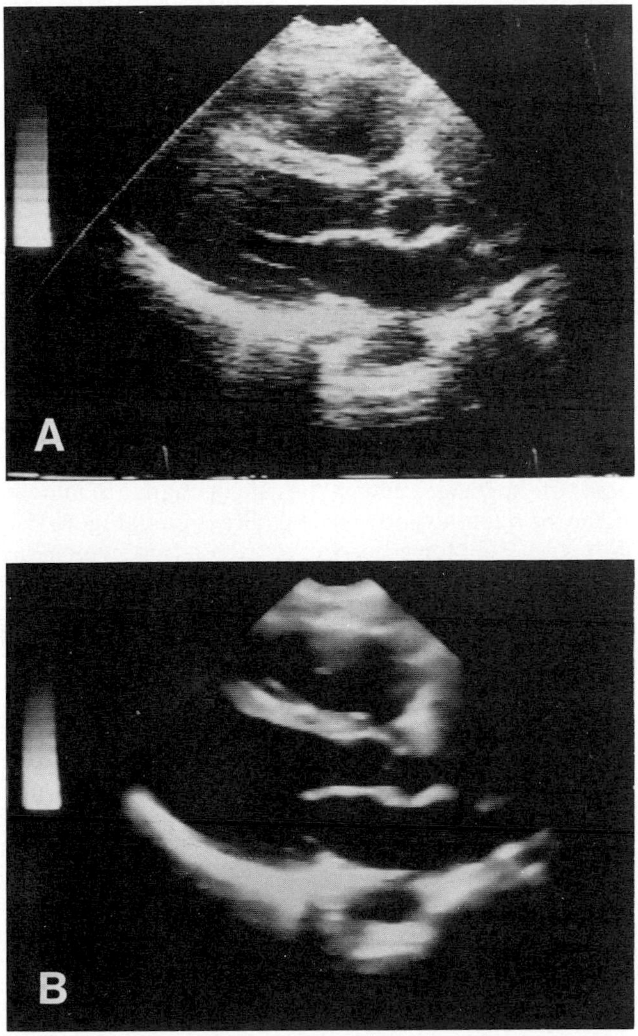

Fig. 3–11. Edge-preserving smoothing. **A.** For each pixel in the input image an edge detector is applied (Sobel operator), and if a significant edge is present, its angle is determined. **B.** Then one of five smoothing kernels is convolved with that pixel to smooth along but not across edges to yield the output image.

X-Derivative

-1	0	1
-2	0	2
-1	0	1

A

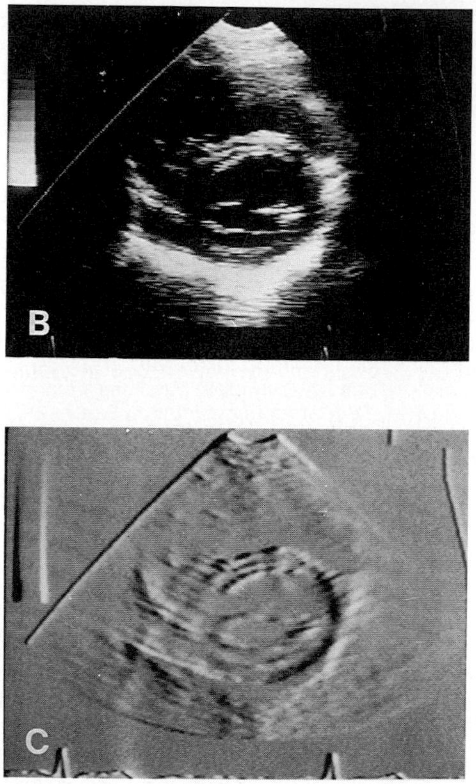

Fig. 3–13. X-derivative operator. **A.** A 3 × 3 convolution kernel to calculate the intensity gradient in the horizontal direction, ∂I/∂x, which will highlight vertical edges. **B.** Input image to x-derivative operator. **C.** Output image. Note that as one proceeds left to right along a horizontal raster line, where the input intensity rises (e.g., left side of gray bar), the output is black, whereas when the intensity falls (e.g., the right side of the gray bar), the output is white. In regions of constant intensity (e.g., within the gray bar), the output is neutral gray. Horizontal edges (e.g., the top and bottom of the gray bar) are not highlighted.

gether should decrease the random noise by a factor of $\sqrt{N}$. Unfortunately, two factors limit the utility of gated averaging in echocardiography: (1) The combination of high spatial resolution of the echo image and patient and transducer movement makes it difficult to align the images precisely before averaging, and (2) the type of noise resulting from ultrasonic "speckle" differs from the random variations about a mean value that gated averaging reduces effectively. For small features, such as valves, this misregistration leads to significant image degradation when averaged. In general, until the problem of misregistration of images is solved, temporal noise reduction is likely to be better handled within individual cardiac cycles rather than gated over several cycles.

Y-Derivative

1	2	1
0	0	0
-1	-2	-1

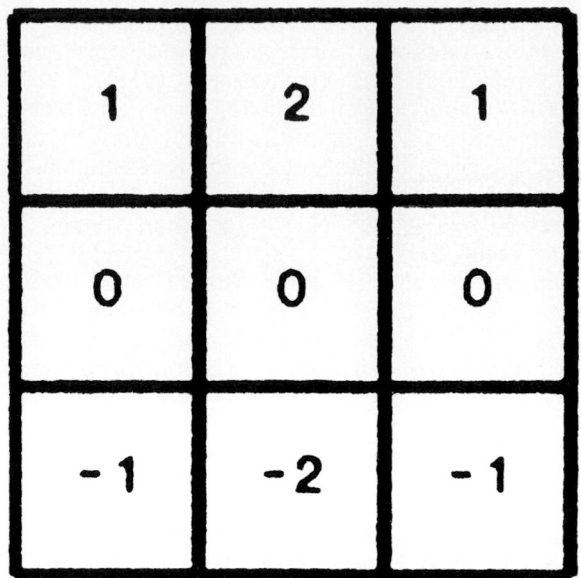

Fig. 3–14. Y-derivative operator. A 3 × 3 convolution kernel entirely analogous to the x-derivative operator (see Fig. 3–13), except that this one calculates the intensity gradient in the vertical direction, ∂I/∂y, and so highlights horizontal edges.

Spatial Edge Enhancement Algorithms. Once an adequate degree of spatial and temporal noise reduction has been achieved, several edge enhancement algorithms may be applied to the echocardiographic image. The simplest of these algorithms calculate the x and y gradients of the image, that is, the rate of change of intensity in the horizontal and vertical directions. Figure 3–13 shows a kernel for x-derivative calculation, which highlights vertical edges. Mathematically, this is equivalent to the operation $\partial I/\partial x$.* Note that in regions of constant brightness (e.g., within the gray scale bar), the two sides of the kernel cancel out, leaving no gradient. A vertical edge with the brighter part to the left is defined as having a large positive gradient and is marked by white, whereas if the brighter part is on the right, the gradient is negative and the pixel is marked black. This kernel is insensitive to horizontal edges: to highlight these, one would use the y-derivative convolution, $\partial I/\partial y$, in Figure 3–14.

Sobel Operator. To get a measure of overall edge intensity independent of orientation, one may combine the x and y derivative operators to yield the gradient, ∇I:

$$\nabla I = [(\partial I/\partial x)^2 + (\partial I/\partial y)^2]^{1/2}. \qquad [3.6]$$

* The partial derivative $\partial/\partial x$ is used instead of the simple derivative d/dx because the image intensity is a function of two variables, x and y (three variables if time is included). $\partial I/\partial x$ thus is the rate of change in intensity as x changes with y held constant, i.e., moving along a horizontal raster line.

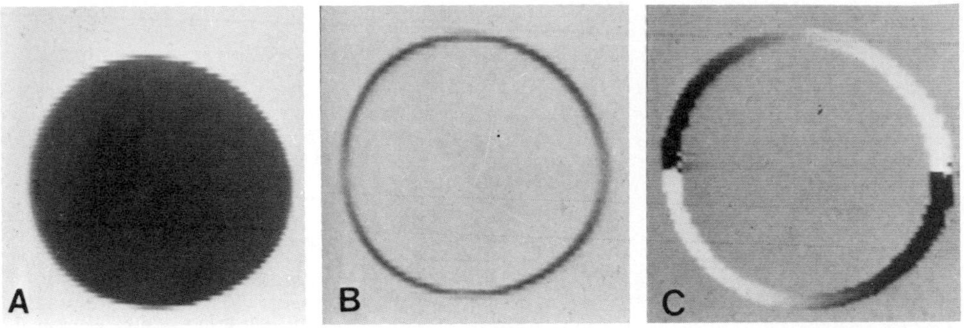

Fig. 3–15. Sobel operator. The Sobel operator uses the x- and y-derivative of an image to obtain the direction and magnitude of edges within the image. **A.** Circular input image. **B.** Sobel magnitude operator, $\nabla I = [(\partial I/\partial x)^2 + (\partial I/\partial y)^2]^{1/2}$, applied to circle. Edges are highlighted (in this case darkened) regardless of direction. **C.** Sobel angle operator, $\arctan[(\partial I/\partial x)/(\partial I/\partial y)]$, applied to circle. When edge is horizontal, output is neutral gray. As the line rotates through vertical the output changes abruptly from white to black, as $(\partial I/\partial y)/(\partial I/\partial x)$ suddenly changes from $+\infty$ to $-\infty$ and the arctangent changes from $+\pi$ to $-\pi$.

Using this expression, vertical and horizontal edges are enhanced identically, and thus this may be used as part of a general border detector. Figure 3–15A shows a circle that is input to this Sobel magnitude operator. The output shown in Figure 3–15B shows the edge to be highlighted equally, independent of direction.

Combining the x and y derivative in a different way yields the Sobel angle operator, which provides insight into the direction of the edge. Trigonometry suggests that this angle may be obtained by dividing the y derivative by the x derivative and taking the arctangent† of this ratio:

$$\arctan[(\partial I/\partial x)/(\partial I/\partial y)]. \qquad [3.7]$$

Horizontal edges (where $\partial I/\partial y \gg \partial I/\partial x$) will show up as neutral gray, becoming brighter as the edge is rotated counterclockwise to be pure white when the edge is vertical. As it is rotated further, the edge suddenly becomes black (the ratio of the derivatives shifts from $+\infty$ to $-\infty$), returning to neutral grey as the edge rotates back to the horizontal orientation. Figure 3–15C shows the application of this operator to the circle. The Sobel operator thus may be used to pick out pixels where the gradient is steep enough to favor their being edges and the orientation information may be used to connect these edge pixels into meaningful borders. Figure 3–16 shows the effect of the Sobel magnitude operator on an echocardiographic image.

Laplacian Operator. A different sort of edge enhancement can be obtained by calculating the Laplacian or second spatial derivative of the image:

$$\nabla^2 I = \partial^2 I/\partial x^2 + \partial^2 I/\partial y^2. \qquad [3.8]$$

Figure 3–17 shows a convolution kernel for the Laplacian operator, a high central pixel value surrounded by eight equal negative values, thus making it extremely sensitive to changes in pixel intensity. Although this operator effectively highlights edges, it is sensitive to noise: an isolated noise pixel will have its magnitude multiplied eightfold. Therefore, one would more commonly use an operator with some simultaneous noise reduction qualities, e.g., the difference of Gaussian operators.

Difference of Gaussian Convolution. As described previously, the Gaussian operator was used simply for noise reduction. Another way of saying this is that it is a *spatial low-pass filter*. It filters out features in the image with high spatial frequency (i.e., that greatly change intensity over a short distance, e.g., noise, and to a lesser extent, edges) while permitting low frequency features (gradual changes in intensity) to pass. The broader the Gaussian operator, the lower this high frequency cutoff becomes and the smoother the output. It is possible to use the difference of two Gaussian operators (one smaller than the other) to selectively highlight a band of spatial frequencies corresponding to edges while surpressing both the high frequencies associated with random noise and the lower frequencies resulting from gradual shifts in intensity. Figure 3–18A shows schematically a $3 \times 3 - 5 \times 5$ difference of Gaussians; Figures 3–18B and 3–18C show the effect of such an operation on an echocardiographic image. Note that each edge now is replaced by a white and black parallel stripe.

Edge Extraction Techniques. It is important to recognize that the edge enhancement methods just described are not edge detection techniques. That is, they may make edges stand out from the background, but they do not specify whether a pixel does or does not lie on an edge. Another way of looking at this is to recall that low level processing begins with an input of approximately 2,000,000 pixels/sec, and following edge enhancement, we still have 2,000,000 pixels/sec as output, far too many to perform anatomic analysis. Thus, the final stage of low level processing, edge extraction, seeks to define precisely those pixels that are edges while greatly distilling the volume of data, so that only the coordinates of these edge points are passed on for high level anatomic interpretation. This sort of decision making, which leads

† The tangent of an angle θ is 0 for $\theta = 0°$, 1 for $\theta = 45°$, rising to ∞ at $\theta = 90°$. The inverse tangent or arctangent reverses this process, taking as its input a number between $-\infty$ and $+\infty$ and returning a value between $-180°$ and $+180°$ (the angle whose tangent is the input number). This output value may then be scaled to fit within the 8-bit pixel range.

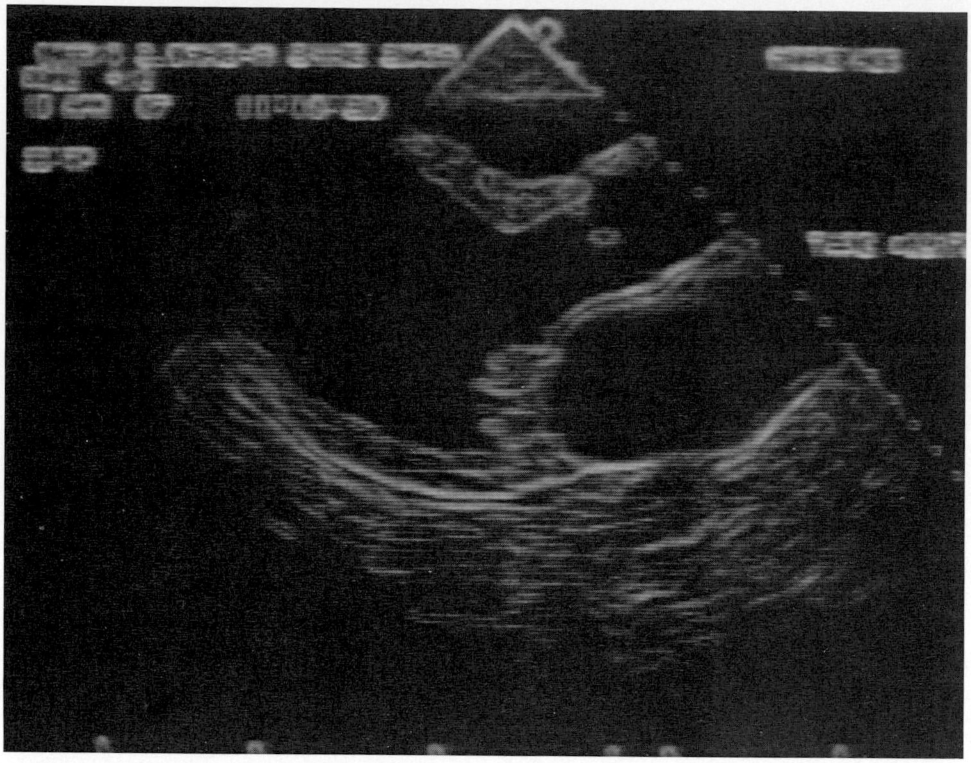

Fig. 3–16. Sobel magnitude operator applied to parasternal long axis echocardiogram. Edges are highlighted equally in all orientations.

to yes or no answers, is handled best by logical or Boolean processing.

Boolean Processing. All of the operators previously described have treated the 8 bits of pixel intensity information as combined into a single number with 256 possible values. Boolean processing, however, treats these 8 bits as separate entities, each of which can take on only two values as true or false or yes or no dichotomies. Treating these bits as separate binary variables permits the application of logical operations to keep track of features in the image. These Boolean operations help to provide the bridge between low level and high level analysis.

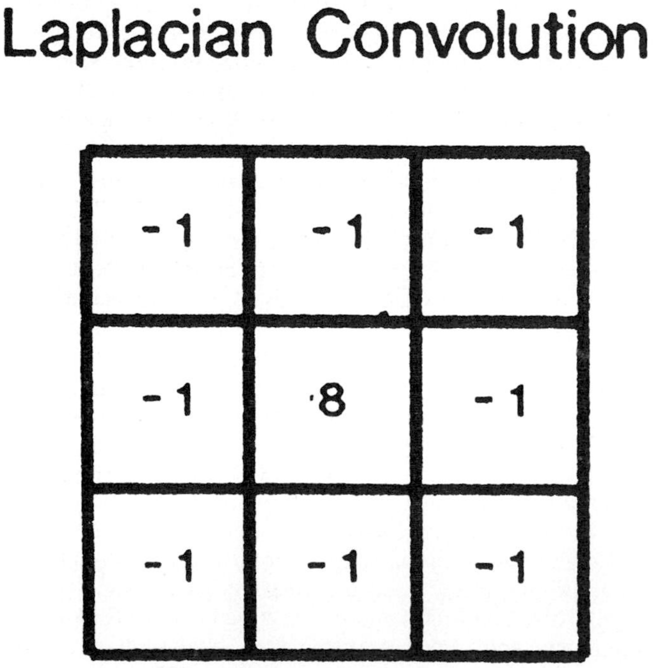

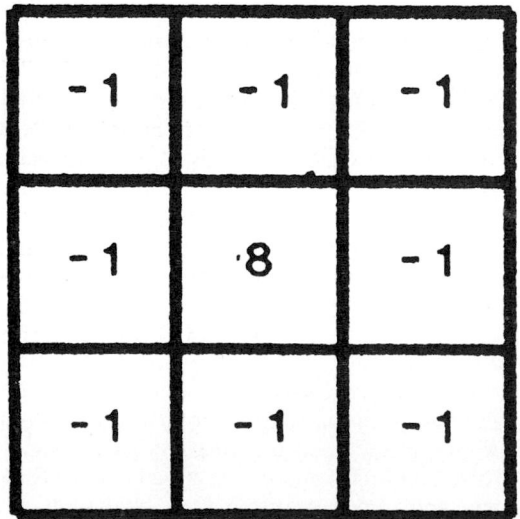

Fig. 3–17. Laplacian operator. A 3 × 3 convolution kernel that yields the Laplacian, or second derivative, of an image: $\nabla^2 I = \partial^2 I/\partial x^2 + \partial^2 I/\partial y^2$. Although effective at highlighting changes in image intensity (e.g., edges), it does so at the expense of 8-fold noise magnification.

A simple but common Boolean operation is binary thresholding, shown in Figures 3–7C and 3–8C. It is used, for example, to specify as "true" all pixels in an image with a Sobel magnitude above a certain value, thus dividing the pixels into two classes, those likely to lie on an edge (with high gradients) and those unlikely to lie on an edge (with low gradients). A thresholding point processing algorithm can be used to identify all pixels with a gradient above a certain intensity, and these data can be stored in a single bit of the output image.

A more complex Boolean operation is edge thinning. Commonly, simple thresholding of a Sobel magnitude image yields edges that are several pixels thick, leading to ambiguity of the true edge position. Boolean logic can be applied to such thresholded edges to thin them down to a single pixel wide. Similarly, it may be used to eliminate spurious edge points that are far removed from other edge pixels and, by a combination of thickening and thinning, to bridge small gaps between true edge pixels. In the latter case, knowing the orientation of the proposed edge pixels from the Sobel angle information permits grouping of these pixels into lines.

A final Boolean algorithm is zero crossing. It was noted previously that the difference of Gaussian convolutions converted edges into parallel white and black

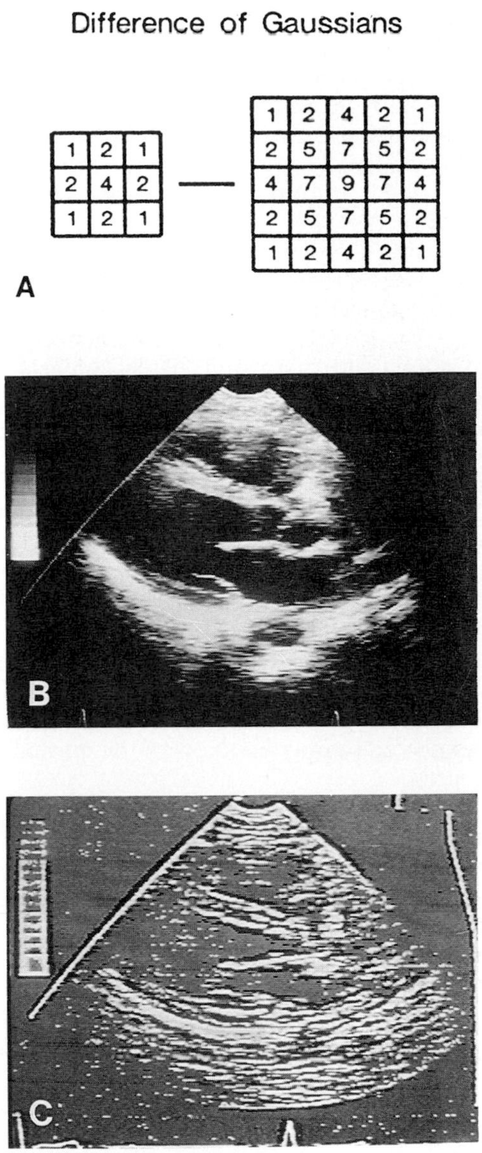

Fig. 3–18. Difference of Gaussian convolutions (DOG). Mathematically, this is approximately like the Laplacian operator, except that it provides a certain amount of noise suppression. **A.** Schematic of 3 × 3 − 5 × 5 DOG. Again, the actual numbers in the kernel would be scaled much lower so that their sum is 1. **B.** Input image. **C.** Output image from 5 × 5 − 9 × 9 DOG. Edges are characterized by parallel white and black stripes.

stripes. Zero crossing identifies those pixels that lie at the boundary between the two stripes, which closely approximates the true edge position.

Accurate edge detection is critically important to echocardiographic image processing. So, before discussing higher level algorithms and motion analysis, I will describe some of the reported methods for endocardial border detection.

Practical Experience With Edge Detection in Echocardiography

Many reports have described edge detection techniques for echocardiographic endocardial borders. These may be classified generally by the degree to which they depend on parallel versus serial computing methods.

Until now, all of the algorithms described have used parallel computing methods; that is, the algorithms act on all of the pixels in an image at once and largely independently. All of the processing goes on in small neighborhoods; no global information is available about the whole image to aid in making judgments about how individual edges connect together. By applying a sequence of these algorithms, one hopes to reduce the image to its key outlines without any a priori knowledge of the structure being visualized. Serial or sequential methods, on the other hand, in general require an understanding of the shape of the feature being searched for as well as some operator input to guide the algorithm. For instance, one might trace a single endocardial contour from a cardiac cycle; the computer would then identify subsequent borders within this neighborhood. Or, one might identify the center of the ventricular cavity, then select borders by searching radially from this point, using the computers knowledge of the endocardium as a closed smooth curve to bridge gaps in the border and exclude extraneous edge points. In practice, most edge detection schemes require at least some input from both local and global processing techniques.

An early report of predominantly parallel approaches to edge extraction used either the Sobel or Laplacian operators applied to an entire ventricular image.[9] In this study, the major user input was to adjust the threshold for declaring a pixel to be an edge. Others have described methods for automating this threshold selection.[16] An issue not fully resolved is the best technique to exclude extraneous edge points and fill in regions of echo drop-out. The most robust method is simply to allow the user to fill in gaps and override erroneous pixels. To do so in an automated fashion requires some a priori assumptions about the shape being scanned.

A fundamentally different edge detection algorithm has been reported, which exploits such an a priori fact, that the left ventricular endocardium in the short axis projection is a closed, nearly circular, curve.[17] After the user specifies a point within the ventricular cavity, a two-step algorithm is applied, first to define the ventricular centroid and then to search radially from this centroid for points where the derivative changes sign, which are defined as the endocardium and epicardium. Edge points are rejected if they cause too sharp a discontinuity in the border. Another difference between this method and those previously described is its use of the radio frequency envelopes from the original ultrasound scan lines (still in polar format) rather than the video image following digital scan conversion.

Efforts have also been directed at using the position of the endocardium in one field to guide the search for borders in subsequent frames.[18] The user must outline epicardial and endocardial borders in the first video field; these are then used to search, in an iterative fashion, for the borders in subsequent fields. Like the earlier serial methods,[17] these search radially from the ventricular centroid, but use pixel intensity, spatial gradient, and local variance in combination to assign a probability that a pixel is on an edge. Some recent methods have also allowed the user to correct computer errors on a single frame (e.g., to include or exclude the papillary muscles) and then extrapolate this correction throughout the cardiac cycle.[19]

It is possible to devise parallel algorithms that give global information about the image and so may help to refine the raw borders. The Hough transform, for instance, converts line segments into individual points and maps collinear line segments to the same point.[20,21] To understand this, recall that a line segment on a plane may be characterized by its slope and intercept. The Hough transform in effect charts the slope and intercept of all the line segments in an image on a separate graph. A long line, with gaps interrupting it, will have all of its fragments mapped to the same point by the transform and so provide a rationale for connecting the segments together. It is possible to devise transforms to search specifically for fragments of circles or ellipses, which might be useful for uniting endocardial surfaces.

Temporal Image Processing

Because much of the most useful information in an echocardiogram is contained in the motion of the heart, it is important to have effective algorithms that operate in the temporal domain, that is, on video frames from different points in time rather than just individual frames. This may be done either to reduce the noise inherent in raw echocardiograms (discussed previously) or to selectively highlight moving edges and calculate their velocity.

Temporal Feature Extraction. To conceptualize how temporal processing may enhance and extract moving features, consider the images from an echocardiogram as forming a three-dimensional array of pixels, with each video field forming a two-dimensional (spatial) plane in this structure, and successive frames stacked up to form the third dimension (time). Each pixel is surrounded by a spatiotemporal neighborhood of pixels consisting of those on adjacent rows and columns in the same video field as well as adjacent video fields. Simple edge detection operates as a two-dimensional convolution on a single frame. To gain information about the motion of these edges requires a full three-dimensional convolution, for instance using a $3 \times 3 \times 3$ kernel about each pixel. By use of a specific kernel, it might be possible to selectively highlight, for instance, a line with a slope of 30° moving vertically at a certain speed. Such edge and motion processing is thought to occur in the retinal ganglion cells.

In practice, the process of motion analysis is usually divided into edge enhancement and motion quantification. One common algorithm provides the normal optic flow of an edge;[22] that is, it yields the component of motion that is perpendicular (or "normal") to an edge. To calculate this flow requires two pieces of information: (1) the temporal derivative ($\partial I/\partial t$), the rate at which the intensity at a given pixel changes from one frame to the next, and (2) the spatial gradient (∇I), the rate at which pixel intensity changes as one moves around the given pixel in the same frame, given by the Sobel magnitude operator. Normal velocity, then, is given by their ratio, $(\partial I/\partial t)/\nabla I$. For example, suppose that at a given pixel, the intensity increases by 10 units in 1 second; also suppose that the intensity in the neighborhood of that point is increasing at 2 units/pixel traversed. Here, $\partial I/\partial t$ is 10, and ∇I is 2, and the ratio is 5 pixels/second, the speed at which motion is occurring perpendicular to the local edge.

One group has reported experience using this technique with echocardiographic images.[23,24] They hope to use such information to divide myocardial motion into normal convergence (contraction), divergence (dyskinesis), translation, and distortion. Such analysis is thus far untested, and there are two principle difficulties in applying it to ultrasonic images. First, this method returns normal flow (the component of motion that occurs perpendicular to a local edge). Any motion that occurs parallel to an edge (e.g., rotation of the ventricle in a parasternal short axis projection) will not be detected. Second, this algorithm explicitly assumes that the only change in the image occurring between successive frames is motion of the object being viewed. The object itself must be identical. Unfortunately, ultrasonic images are constantly changing because of the random interaction of sound with matter. Thus, ultrasonic speckle might be expected to play havoc with the normal optical flow algorithm.

One possible way around the problem of ultrasonic speckle is to perform motion analysis only on fully detected, binary border maps; that is, where a pixel is one if it is an edge, zero if it is not an edge. Convected activation is an algorithm that yields the normal motion of edges and is possible to implement at the video frame rate.[25,26] When input consists of a smooth accurate sequence of boundaries, the algorithm yields an accurate measure of the horizontal and vertical components (Fig. 3–19). However, it is critically dependent on the continuity and accuracy of the input edge maps.

Techniques of High Level Image Processing

We now turn briefly to a discussion of some of the issues involved in high level image processing, that portion of image analysis that yields an anatomic interpretation to a scene. Until this point the algorithms presented have acted on individual pixels within the original image. High level operations require for input specific features abstracted from the original echo. Commonly, these features are a sequence of endocardial borders from throughout the cardiac cycle. These borders might be obtained by the low level operations described previously, or they might be obtained by hand tracing the echocardiogram (letting the human eye and hand serve as the low level processor). Much of the experience with such analysis will be described in Chapters 20 and 21 on left ventricular function. Here we will only outline a few of the general approaches that might be applied.

Refinement of Endocardial Borders

As has been noted before in the discussions on edge and motion detection, it is critically important that the input to any algorithm be as "clean" as possible with

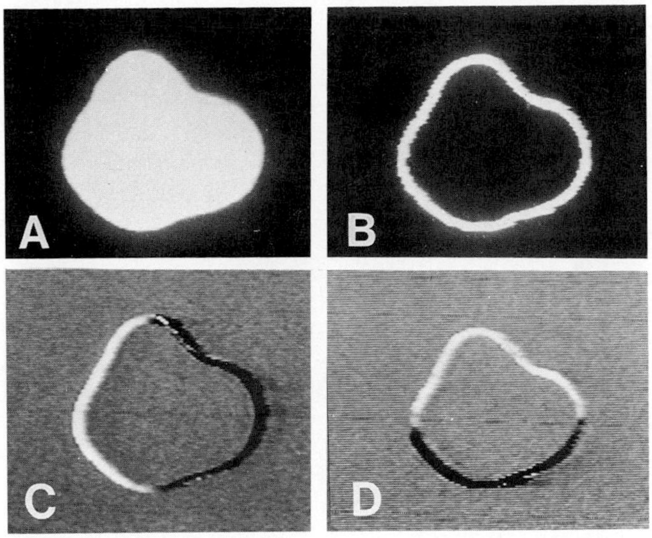

Fig. 3–19. Convected activation algorithm. This technique calculates the velocity at every point along a boundary throughout the cardiac cycle. It yields the velocity occurring perpendicular to the local edge, divided into horizontal **(C)** and vertical **(D)** components. This particular cross section **(A)** is traced from a short axis echocardiogram with the Sobel-enhanced edges shown **(B).** This frame is from midsystole, so all walls are moving inward. Thus, in **C,** leftward movement is coded whiter than background, rightward movement darker than background. Similarly in **D,** downward movement is white, upward is black.

accurate borders. Even after the endocardial borders have been extracted throughout the cardiac cycle, either by hand or automated method, some error on localization likely remains (Fig. 3–20). This error is in part random, which causes the extracted border to fluctuate around the true position. This is a common problem in signal analysis, and in general it is found that the "true" data consists primarily of low frequency information, whereas the "noise" is of higher frequency. Fourier analysis is a mathematical technique to extract the frequency information of any signal. We may consider the sequence of endocardial borders to be a "signal" on which higher frequency noise is superimposed. It is possible to remove the high frequency components from a Fourier transform (by setting their value to 0) and then to reconstruct a smoother version of the original sequence of borders by performing an inverse Fourier transform (Fig. 3–21). When applied to full cycle endocardial borders, this technique of Fourier filtration has been shown to reduce the number of "extraneous" endocardial motion reversals by over 90% and to yield a much truer representation of normal cardiac motion.[27] Optimal filtration was achieved by excluding temporal frequencies above six events per cardiac cycle and spatial frequencies above nine events per endocardial circumference.

Analysis of Endocardial Borders

Several high level analytical approaches have been used to quantify echocardiographic endocardial wall motion. These methods, which require knowledge of normal and pathologic echocardiographic anatomy, are discussed in greater detail in Chapter 21.

Artificial Intelligence Techniques. Many analytic methods are specific in their application: They require data from specific echocardiographic views in a particular format. The long-term (and so far elusive) goal of high level processing is a much more robust system that could accept data from the low level processor from a variety of views (perhaps nonstandard) and fit this information into a three-dimensional model of how a normal heart should appear and judge abnormality as a discrepancy from this normal model. Ideally, such a system should interact with the low level processing algorithms to optimize the features extracted and perhaps cue the echocardiographic examiner for additional views. Al-

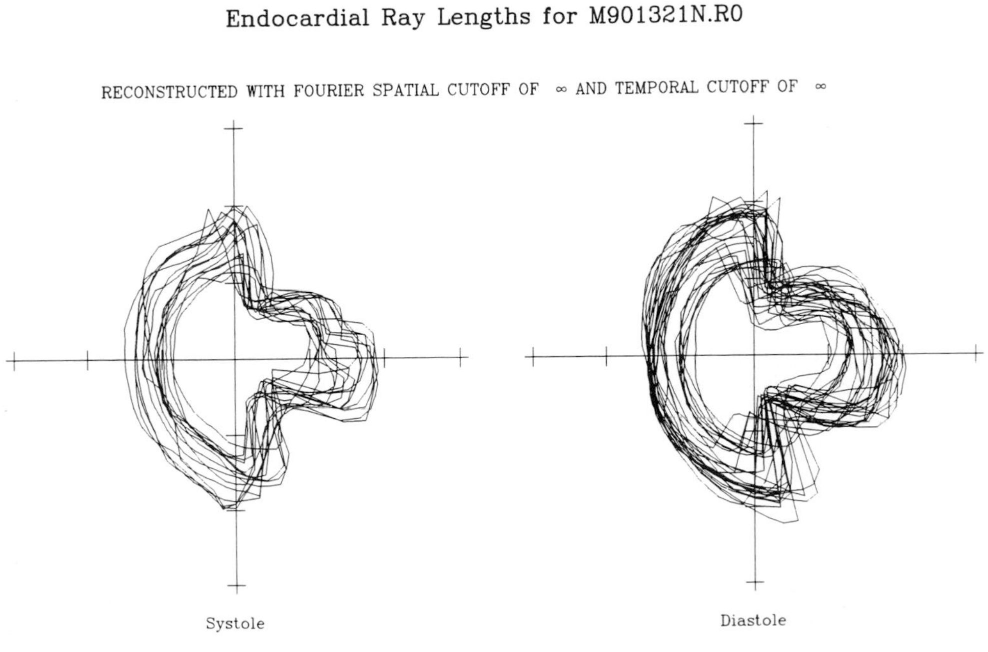

Fig. 3–20. Hand-traced endocardial borders. Endocardial borders from a parasternal short axis echocardiogram were traced for a complete cardiac cycle with systolic frames on the left, diastolic frames on the right. Although the general ventricular shape is discernible (including the papillary muscles at 2 and 4 o'clock) as well as the overall contraction sequence, there is a great deal of nonphysiologic "jitter" in the tracings.

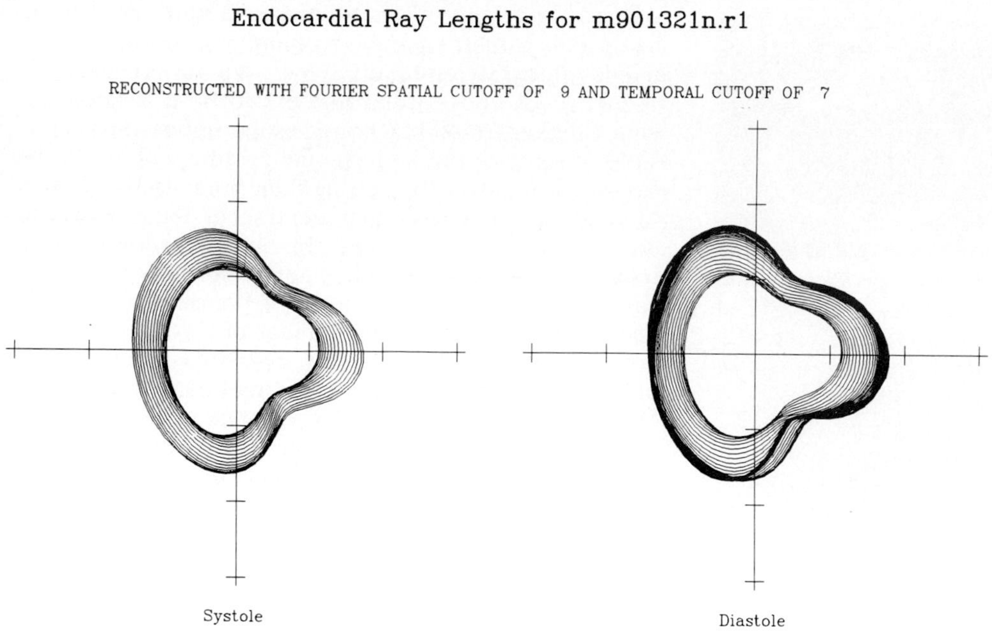

Fig. 3–21. Endocardial borders following Fourier filtration. These data are the same as Figure 3–20, reconstructed after eliminating all Fourier components above the sixth temporal and ninth spatial harmonics. The result is a more accurate representation of ventricular shape and motion than the input.

though such a system is far in the future, the use of artificial intelligence modeling has been described to guide ultrasonic data acquisition.[28] In this preliminary work, the size and shape of a balloon was reconstructed by sequential input of border information (hand tracing providing the feature extraction in this case) together with three-dimensional positioning data (provided by spark gaps mounted on the transducer; see Chapter 6 for more details). The computer used previously provided information concerning the typical appearance of a balloon to build a three-dimensional model of the object being imaged and request additional views as needed.

Current Status and Future Directions

There has been tremendous progress in echocardiographic image processing, but significant gaps remain to be bridged before true automated image analysis is achieved. With currently available hardware, it is possible to perform multiple sequential low level processing algorithms at the real-time video field rate (Fig. 3–22), with the raw image in Figure 3–22A, edge-preserving spatial smoothing in Figure 3–22B, Sobel edge enhancement in Figure 3–22C, edge extraction by thresholding the Sobel image in Figure 3–22D, and calculating velocity from this edge map by the convected activation algorithm Figure 3–22E. While this is a computational tour de force (requiring over a billion arithmetic operations per second), it is evident that the inherent noisiness of ultrasound leads to many extraneous edge pixels and regions of endocardial dropout. Indeed, when provided with a sequence of noiseless endocardial cavities, these algorithms work well (Fig. 3–19). Clearly, interaction with a "knowledgeable" serial computer is necessary to optimize these endocardial borders. Several such sys-

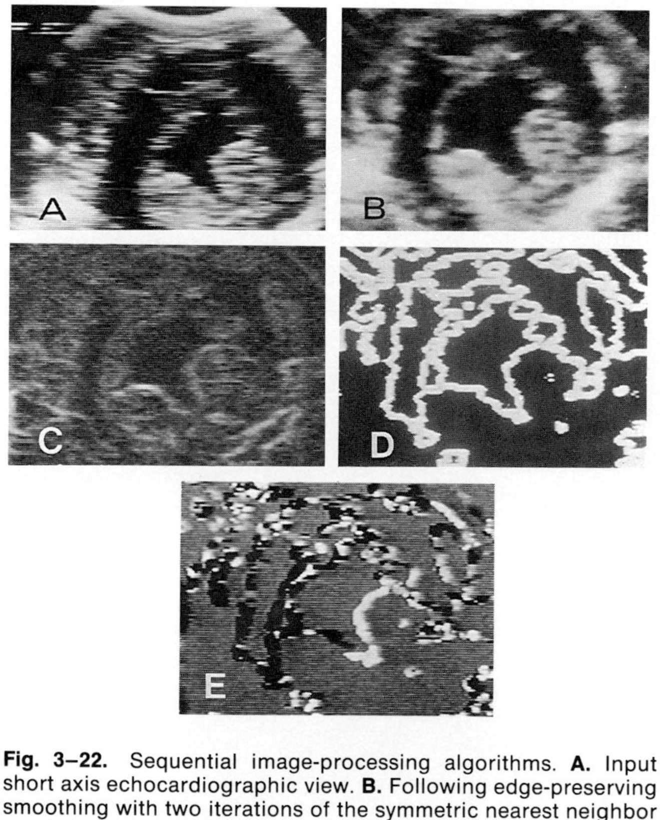

Fig. 3–22. Sequential image-processing algorithms. **A.** Input short axis echocardiographic view. **B.** Following edge-preserving smoothing with two iterations of the symmetric nearest neighbor operator. **C.** Sobel magnitude operator. **D.** Thresholding of Sobel magnitude image to yield binary edge map. **E.** Motion extraction (horizontal component) with convected activation algorithm. This frame is from mid-diastole, so the lateral wall is moving rightward and is marked whiter than the background, whereas the medial wall is darker (moving leftward). The failure to exclude extraneous edge pixels leads to the scattered artifactual motion seen around the heart.

tems have been developed, but none approach real-time speed and all can be fooled by a poor quality echocardiogram.

An encouraging trend is the increasing use of all-digital technology within echocardiographic machines. This will allow the use of signal enhancing techniques before digital scan conversion, which should aid subsequent border extraction. Furthermore, the use of digital beam formation in the phased array transducers might permit additional interrogation of regions with poorly visualized endocardium. If progress in computer technology over the next decade rivals that seen in the last decade, we may look forward to achievement of the elusive goal of automated image analysis.

Echocardiographic Border Detection. Recently, it has become possible to use processing algorithms built into the echocardiographic instrument to identify and track endocardial borders.[29] This general approach grows out of previous work in tissue characterization in which the backscattered ultrasound signal was integrated to yield an estimate of absolute tissue reflectivity.[30,31]

This general approach to edge detection analyzes individual scan lines separately. The returning radio frequency ultrasound signal is split into two components, which are processed in parallel within the echo machine. One is processed in the normal fashion to yield the standard two-dimensional image of the heart. The other component is analyzed by integrating the strength of the signal across its full frequency spectrum to yield absolute ultrasonic reflectivity. This signal is then thresholded by a binary operator to yield two families of pixels, one presumed to originate in the blood pool (those with backscattered strength below a specified threshold), the other presumed to originate from the myocardium. Endocardial borders then are assumed to occur at the boundary between these two regions and thus are identified on a real-time, frame-by-frame basis. Considerable user interaction is required to optimize the gain of this system so that machine-derived boundaries match as closely as possible those identified by the operator's visual assessment. Real-time assessment of ventricular cavity area can be obtained by plotting the count of blood pool pixels within a user-specified region of interest (Fig. 3–23). Care must be taken that the region of interest encircles the ventricular cavity throughout the cardiac cycle, while avoiding other blood pool regions (e.g., left atrium or right ventricle) that may translate into the region of interest. By choosing an apical view and assuming ventricular symmetry, it is possible to use a single plane area-length method to calculate ventricular volume on line as well.

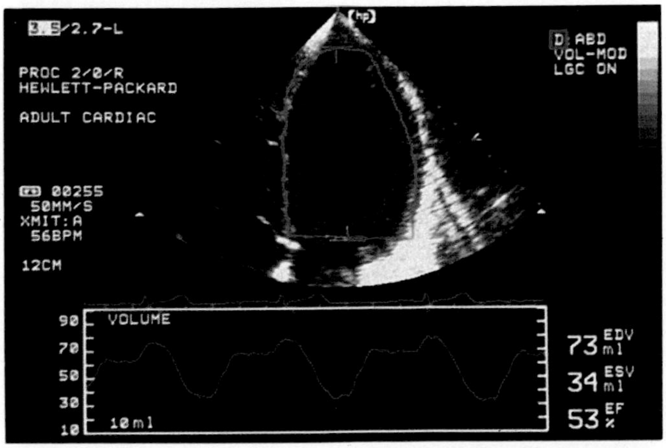

Fig. 3–23. Apical four-chamber recording with the left ventricle outlined by an operator-defined region of interest indicated in blue in the endocardium of the chamber automatically defined as an abrupt change in threshold between the blood pool and left ventricular myocardium. The lower panel indicates the instantaneous change in left ventricular volume for 3 cycles calculated using a modified single-plane Simpson's rule algorithm. In addition to the change in volume, the ejection fraction is automatically calculated for each cycle. (Illustration courtesy of Hewlett-Packard Company.)

REFERENCES

1. Pratt WK: Digital Imaging Processing. New York, John Wiley & Sons, p. 593, 1978.
2. Ophir J, Maklad NF: Digital scan converters in diagnostic ultrasound imaging. Proc IEEE 67:1979.
3. Leavitt SC, Hunt BF, Larsen HG: A scan conversion algorithm for displaying ultrasound images. Hewlett-Packard J 34:30, 1983.
4. Rosenfield A, Kak AC: Digital Picture Processing. 2nd Ed. New York, Academic Press, 1982.
5. Gonzalez RC, Wentz P: Digital Imaging Processing. Reading, MA, Addison-Wesley, 1987.
6. Skorton DJ, et al.: Digital imaging processing of two-dimensional echocardiograms: identification of the endocardium. Am J Cardiol 48:479, 1981.
7. Zwehl W, et al.: Validation of a computerized edge detection algorithm for quantitative two-dimensional echocardiography. Circulation 68:1127, 1983.
8. Parker DL, Pryor TA, Ridges JD: Enhancement of two-dimensional echocardiographic images by lateral filtering. Comput Biomed Res 12:265, 1979.
9. Collins SM, et al.: Computer-assisted edge detection in two-dimensional echocardiography: comparison with anatomic data. Am J Cardiol 53:1980, 1984.
10. Delp EJ, et al.: The analysis of two-dimensional echocardiograms using a time varying image approach. *In* Computers in Cardiology. Long Beach, CA, IEEE Computer Society, p. 391, 1982.
11. Linker DT, et al.: Automatic endocardial definition of 2-D echocardiograms: a comparison of four standard edge detectors and improved thresholding techniques. *In* Computers in Cardiology. Long Beach, CA, IEEE Computer Society, p. 395, 1982.
12. Thomas JD, et al.: Real-time echocardiographic noise reduction, edge enhancement, and motion detection: experience with a new programmable computerized array processor. Circulation 76:4, 1987.
13. Garcia E, et al.: Real-time computerization of two-dimensional echocardiography. Am Heart J 783, 1981.
14. Jenkins JM, et al.: Computer processing of echocardiographic images for automated edge detection of left ventricular boundaries. *In* Computers in Cardiology. Long Beach, CA, IEEE Computer Society, p. 391, 1981.
15. Brennecke R, et al.: Computerized enhancement techniques for echocardiographic sector scans. *In* Computers in Cardiology. Long Beach, CA, IEEE Computer Society, p. 7, 1981.
16. Zhang L, Geiser EL: An approach to optimal threshold selection on a sequence of two-dimensional echocardiographic images. IEEE Trans Biomed Eng 29:577, 1982.
17. Buda AJ, et al.: Automatic computer processing of 2-dimensional echocardiograms. Am J Cardiol 52:384, 1983.
18. Adam D, Hareuveni O, Sideman S: Semiautomated border tracking of cine echocardiographic ventricular images. IEEE Trans Med Imaging 6:266, 1987.
19. Angermann CE, et al.: Computerized quantitative evaluation of the endocardium in serial two-dimensional echocardiograms of the left ventricular short axis. *In* Computers in Cardiology. Long Beach, CA, IEEE Computer Society, 1987.
20. Hough PVC: Method and means for recognizing complex patterns. US Patent 3069654, December 18, 1962.
21. O'Gorman F, Clowes MB: Finding picture edges through collinearity of feature points. IEEE Trans Computers 25:449, 1976.
22. Horn BKP, Schunck BG: Determining optical flow. Artif Intel 17:185, 1981.
23. Mailloux GE, Bleau A, Bertrand M, Petticlerc R: Measurement of heart motion from two-dimensional echocardiograms. *In* Computers in Cardiology. Long Beach, CA, IEEE Computer Society, p. 397, 1986.
24. Mailloux GE, Langlois F, Bertrand M, Petticlerc R: Analysis of heart motions from two-dimensional echocardiograms by velocity field decomposi-

tion. *In* Computers in Cardiology. Long Beach, CA, IEEE Computer Society, p. 441, 1987.
25. Thomas JD, Waxman AM, Higginbotham R Jr, Weyman AE: Real-time detection of moving echocardiographic endocardial borders with automated velocity deprivation: description of a new algorithm. J Am Coll Cardiol 11: 5A, 1988.
26. Thomas JD, et al.: Real-time echocardiographic noise reduction, border extraction, and velocity derivation. *In* Computers in Cardiology 1988. Long Beach, CA, IEEE Computer Society p. 129, 1989.
27. Thomas JD, et al.: Improved accuracy of echocardiographic endocardial borders by spatiotemporal filtered Fourier reconstruction: description of the method and optimization of filter cutoffs. Circulation 77:415, 1988.
28. Brinkley JF: Knowledge driven ultrasonic three-dimensional organ modeling. IEEE Trans Pattern Anal Machine Intell 431, 1985.
29. Vandenberg BF, et al.: Estimation of left ventricular cavity area with an on-line, semiautomated echocardiographic edge detection system. Circulation 86:159, 1992.
30. Vered Z, et al.: Quantitative ultrasonic tissue characterization with real-time integrated backscatter imaging in normal human subjects and in patients with dilated cardiomyopathy. Circulation 76:1067, 1987.
31. Vered Z, et al.: Ultrasound integrated backscatter tissue characterization of remote myocardial infarction in human subjects. J Am Coll Cardiol 13:84, 1989.

CHAPTER

4

CROSS-SECTIONAL ECHOCARDIOGRAPHIC EXAMINATION

The goal of the cross-sectional examination is to optimally record the anatomic and functional characteristics of a particular area or areas of the heart in several tomographic imaging planes. If this goal can be achieved, the size, shape, relative position, and absolute and relative motion patterns of multiple cardiac structures can be assessed.[1–5]

To help the examiner achieve this goal, all cross-sectional echocardiographic instruments provide a small, flexible, hand-held probe that can be easily manipulated.[6–10] Figure 4–1 illustrates a typical probe and the fan-shaped imaging plane it generates. Three dimensions or axes characterize this imaging plane: (1) depth of field or distance from the transducer face (the Z axis), (2) width from one margin of the plane to the other (azimuthal dimension or X axis), and (3) thickness (the elevation dimension or Y axis). Although represented as a plane, the scan area is actually composed of a series of individual sound pulses or beams. The beam that propagates directly away from the transducer face and, as such, is an extension of the long axis of the probe is referred to as the *central ray*.

The flexibility of the probe permits almost limitless variation in the direction in which the imaging plane can be oriented to transect the heart. Despite this flexibility, aligning the probe and, hence, the examining plane to optimally record a particular structure may prove to be a formidable task for several reasons.

First, the examiner is attempting to visualize a specific area within an organ (the heart), which itself cannot be seen. External reference points on the chest wall may help to locate the heart; however, the position and orientation of individual cardiac structures within the chest are so variable that final plane orientation must be related to, and determined by, the particular area one wishes to visualize. This, in turn, requires that the examiner be able to (1) identify intracardiac structures from the images they produce, (2) define the plane in which they are visualized, (3) understand how to realign the imaging plane to achieve optimal visualization, and (4) recognize when such visualization is achieved. All these functions must occur almost simultaneously as the examination progresses to obtain the best final image.

Second, the flexibility of the transducer allows the imaging plane to be directed toward the heart from a number of different vantage points. From any of these transducer positions, the imaging plane can be rotated 360°, and at any degree of rotation, the plane can be angled through a wide arc. This enormous degree of flexibility presents the examiner with an equally enormous variety of potential image formats that must be recognized and interpreted.

Finally, the broad imaging plane encompasses a large area of the heart. Although the imaging plane configuration is fixed, the relationships of cardiac structures that fall within the plane are variable. Consequently, the plane may be appropriately aligned to optimally record a particular aspect of one structure while other areas within the same scan plane are poorly visualized. These nongeometric relationships of anatomic structures relative to the fixed planar area create further imaging artifacts, which must be recognized and their cause appreciated.

Despite these difficulties, one can perform a cross-

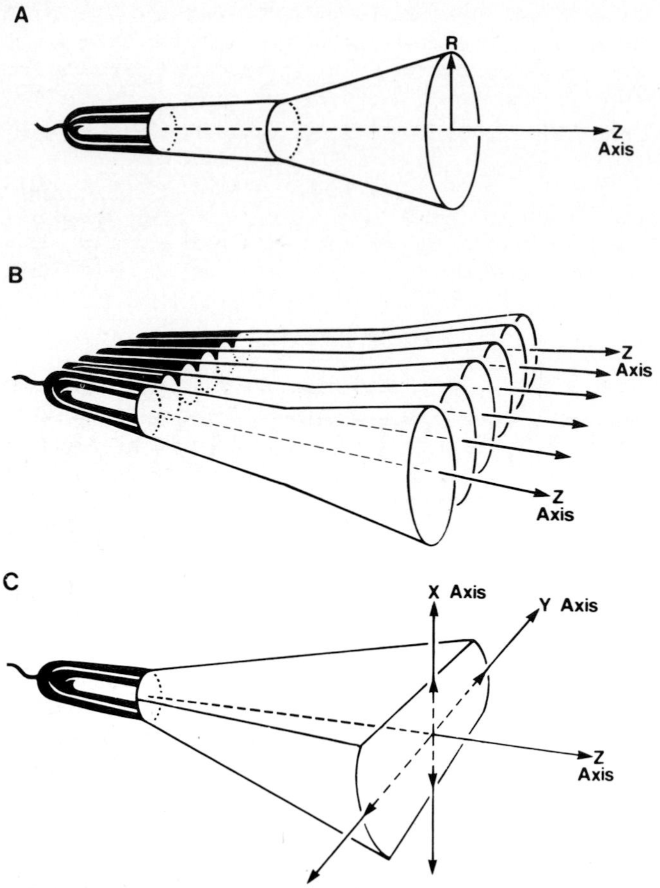

Fig. 4–1. The formation of a cross-sectional imaging plane from a series of individual ultrasonic beams or pulses. **A.** A single ultrasonic beam. The z axis corresponds to a long axis down the center of the beam. It propagates away from the transducer face and can be considered an extension of the long axis of the transducer. R = the radius of the sound beam at any point along the z axis for a disc-shaped transducer. **B.** How the series of sound beams can be aligned next to one another to form a scan plane. **C.** The resultant imaging plane. This plane can be described by three axes. The z axis, which corresponds to the path of the scan plane as it propagates away from the transducer, is an extension of the long axis of the transducer. The y axis is perpendicular to the z axis and extends from one lateral margin of the scan plane to the other. The x axis is orthogonal to both the y and z axes and represents the thickness of the scan plane. These axes obviously vary in length, depending on where in the scan plane they are measured. Therefore, these axes have no absolute values.

sectional study that records high quality images that appropriately depict the structural configuration and motion of numerous areas of the heart. Appropriate performance of the cross-sectional examination, however, requires that the examiner (1) appreciate the three-dimensional anatomy of the heart, (2) conceptualize how the same structure might appear when viewed in a number of different projections, (3) understand the patterns produced when a plane transects a variety of geometric figures along several paths, (4) know and understand the standardized imaging planes and recognize when these images are optimally recorded, and (5) recognize and allow for the effects of pathologic conditions on the appearance and orientation of a structure. The flexibility of the cross-sectional technique and the large variety of data that can be recorded, therefore, require a high degree of technical expertise to produce consistently useful clinical information.

The purpose of this and the following chapter is (1) to describe the steps necessary to record optimal cross-sectional images and (2) to review the most commonly used imaging planes and the method for standardizing image orientation.

The cross-sectional echocardiographic examination proceeds in a series of steps. These steps can be divided into those that are preliminary to the examination and those encompassed in the examination itself. Preliminary steps include (1) the initial approach to the patient, (2) considerations in dealing with uncooperative patients, (3) transducer selection, and (4) initial instrument control setting. The examination itself proceeds in a stepwise, albeit more integrated, fashion. The sequence of the examination is (1) location of the heart, (2) initial structure identification, (3) initial determination of plane orientation, and (4) fine plane positioning.

PRELIMINARY STEPS

Initial Approach to the Patient

The echocardiographic examination is appropriately performed on cardiac patients of all ages, from the premature infant to the elderly person.[11–14] The basic approach is similar for all patients regardless of age or sex. In preparation for the examination, the patient should be placed in the supine position on a comfortable examining surface. The room should be darkened slightly to permit maximal visualization of the display scope and also to provide a relaxed environment. The patient should be undressed to the waist. Exposure of a large area of the chest is necessary to make adequate use of all the probe positions from which the examining plane can be directed toward the heart. For female patients, this exposure occasionally results in some embarrassment. Such embarrassment should be overcome before beginning the study so that it does not become a recurrent problem as increasingly larger areas of the chest must be explored to record an adequate examination. An examining gown, open in the front, allows the patient to be covered and yet permits broad access to the chest wall.

Some form of timing information should be recorded so that the events occurring during the echocardiographic examination can be temporally related. For this purpose, an electrocardiogram is customarily recorded with the cross-sectional study.[11–14] The electrocardiographic data then can be redisplayed with the individual image frames within the cardiac cycle. When recording the electrocardiogram, only the limb leads are used because the exploring chest electrode would interfere with transducer placement. Additional timing information can be obtained from other graphic recording devices, such as the phonocardiogram and arterial and venous pulse tracings. Unfortunately, the cross-sectional images are recorded at a relatively slow frame rate, which limits the timing value of many of these graphic recordings. When an M-mode or Doppler study is recorded in conjunction with the cross-sectional examination, these recordings retain their inherent usefulness. When several studies are recorded simultaneously, all recording electrodes, microphones, or other sensing devices must be attached before the echocardiographic examination.

Before beginning the examination, both the patient and the examiner must be as comfortable as possible. If the patient is in an uncomfortable position, he will move about, thereby necessitating continual readjustment of the examining plane. If the examiner is uncomfortable, he will rapidly become fatigued, thereby shortening the time that can be devoted to the examination and limiting the quality of the data collected.

The examiner should be seated at the patient's side at the same level as the patient and should be able to reposition the patient (e.g., by using an electric bed) or to adjust the controls on the echocardiographic equipment without moving. This environment is most aptly achieved in a well-designed echocardiographic laboratory. Whenever possible, the echocardiographic examination should be performed in such a controlled setting (Fig. 4–2). When dealing with critically ill patients, however, one must frequently perform studies on a portable basis. The examiner is rarely as comfortable, and the patient is rarely as cooperative in such a setting. This is frequently reflected in the quality of the data.

The operator generally approaches the patient from the right side. The probe is then held in the right hand, and the instrument controls are adjusted with the left. The right-sided approach is preferable because (1) the majority of examiners are right-handed; therefore, the fine probe positioning, rotation, and angulation that are required during the examination can be performed more readily with the probe in the right hand rather than the left; (2) the right hand is generally stronger and does not fatigue as quickly as does the left; (3) many cross-sectional studies must be recorded with the patient on the left side or with the probe positioned at the cardiac apex. With the examiner on the patient's right side, the right arm naturally falls across the chest to the cardiac apex, thereby allowing easy probe manipulation in this area. Conversely, from the left side, the probe must be held in an awkward, backhanded fashion when attempting to examine a patient in the left lateral position or to record apical images. Such positioning limits probe control and flexibility.

Difficult or Uncooperative Patients

On occasion, the echocardiographic examination may be more difficult because of lack of patient cooperation, limited patient mobility, or restricted access to the precordium. In these circumstances, the approach to the patient may need modification.

Lack of patient cooperation is most frequently encountered in the pediatric age group and is most commonly caused by fright on initial exposure to a strange procedure or by fatigue in the latter stages of the examination.

As a rule, once a child's cooperation has been lost, the examination is effectively over. Attempts to re-establish rapport using distractions, such as cookies, rattles, or lollipops, may occasionally regain cooperation, but the cooperation usually is short-lived. Although useful data occasionally are obtained from a "moving target," such a situation is less than optimal. The examiner is then faced with the options of accepting an incomplete study, repeating the examination at a later date, or sedating the child. It is best, therefore, to make every effort to establish good rapport at the onset and to be assured that the child is comfortable during the study.

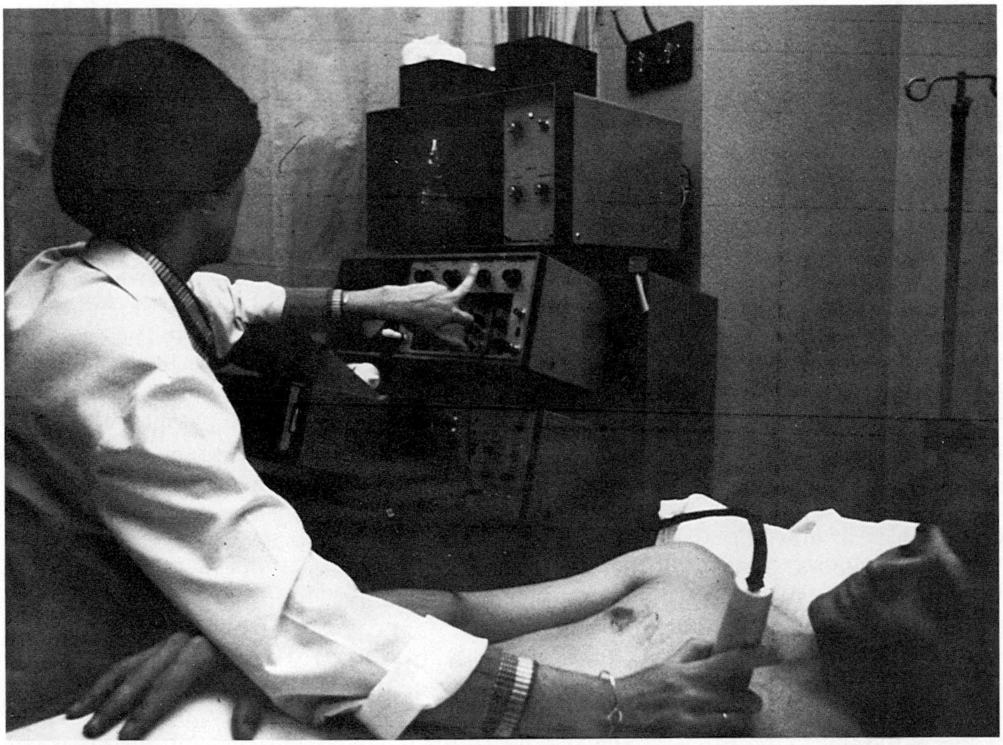

Fig. 4–2. Proper position of the echocardiographic technician relative to the patient and cross-sectional instrument.

Several steps may help to allay initial fear of the examination. If the child is old enough to understand, he should be introduced to the instrumentation and told how he will be able to "see his heart on television." He should be given a chance to hold the examining probe and to assure himself that the probe will not hurt. Such assurances are particularly helpful when using a mechanical probe because its noise and vibration sometimes cause even adults to expect that the examination will be painful. The probe should be initially applied to the hand or to the forearm as often as necessary to make the child comfortable. When actually applied to the chest, the probe can be supported by the examiner's little finger, thereby limiting actual skin contact. If the child still indicates discomfort, a sufficient amount of coupling gel can be used so that the probe never actually touches the chest during the examination. If parents are present, the examiner should inform them about the nature of the examination and may explain in general terms what is being recorded during the examination. This information puts them at ease, and their sense of calm is transmitted to the child. Once the examination has begun, the child should remain involved in the process and should be kept comfortable.

Another frightening aspect of the examination, particularly for small children, is the attachment of the electrocardiogram (ECG) electrodes. Experience suggests that this procedure may be more frightening than the examination itself. For examination of patients with congenital heart disease, structure orientation and identification are far more important than timing motion. If the electrocardiographic leads, therefore, prove disquieting, they can be easily omitted. Adequate timing information to establish the sequence of cardiac events generally can be derived from the cross-sectional echogram itself. But, if all else fails, sedation may be required. The decision to sedate a child is made after considering the importance of the information to be derived from the study and after consulting with the responsible physician.

Adult patients also may be uncooperative and even openly combative. This reaction is usually a reflection of their underlying disease process. Again, a decision must be made in conjunction with the responsible physician about whether the clinical question to be answered by the echocardiogram warrants sedating or restraining the patient.

Other situations related to the patient's clinical condition may prevent the positioning required to obtain an optimal study. Such difficulties arise most commonly in patients on ventilators, with arterial or venous pressure-monitoring catheters in place, or in traction. In these situations, the operators should attempt to record as much information as possible, recognizing that the quality of the examination may not be optimal. These studies should be interpreted in this light, and if circumstances permit, the patient may need to be restudied at a later date in the more controlled environment of the echocardiographic laboratory.

Finally, in many other situations, access to the chest may be limited. This occurs following cardiac surgery when the midportion of the patient's chest is commonly covered with bandages; in patients with acute myocardial infarction when monitoring electrodes may cover the principal echocardiographic windows; and in patients with chest wounds, burns, or extensive abrasions. Frequently, examinations in these situations are requested by physicians who are unfamiliar with the technical requirements of the echocardiographic study. When such requests are made, the primary physician should be contacted, and the requirements of the examination should be explained. Bandages or electrodes should never be removed by the operator independently, and the transducer should never be placed in an area of the chest in which the skin surface is not intact. In these cases, the esophageal approach (Chapter 16) is a particularly useful option.

Selection of a Transducer

Transducers vary in size, frequency, and focal characteristics. Selection of the appropriate transducer for a particular clinical study is determined by the physical characteristics of the patient and by the requirements of the examination.

Transducer size refers to the area or diameter of the transducer face. The area of the transducer face in a single-element system is a function of the size of the individual transducer. In an array of transducers, the area of the transducer face is the sum of the areas of all the transducers in the array. Both the size and shape of the transducer face are important from an imaging standpoint because they determine the area encompassed by the sound beam, the length of the near field in each dimension, the angle of divergence in the far field, and the depth at which the beam can be acoustically focused. As a rule, larger transducers have better beam characteristics and can be brought to a sharper, more intense focus at a deeper tissue depth (see Chapter 1).[15,16]

Transducer size also determines the size of the acoustic window required to transmit the examining plane into the chest. Because the window size for any patient is relatively fixed, transducer size must be appropriate to the clinical environment. The size of the transducer should correspond as closely as possible to the size of the echocardiographic window through which the imaging plane is directed. This relationship in size is important because the area of the raster (the raster is the area in the cathode ray tube [CRT] in which the image is reproduced) of the display corresponds to the physical area of the imaging plane. When transducer size is larger than window size, the portion of the imaging plane arising from the segment of the transducer face that lies outside the window is not transmitted, and the margins of the display raster are blank. When an interruption in the window lies beneath the transducer, information is missing in a more central portion of the raster, thereby producing an "acoustic shadow." Transducers that are small enough to fit cleanly within the clinical echocardiographic window provide uninterrupted images, whereas those that are too large for a single window or that overlie several separate windows produce truncated or interrupted images.

The second factor to be considered in transducer selection is frequency. When determining the appropriate transducer frequency, one must consider the relationship of resolution and penetration. *Resolution* is the ability to distinguish structures that are closely related in space as separate. *Penetration* is the ability of the sound beam to penetrate the heart and to reach the individual structures the examiner seeks to record. Resolution is directly related to frequency. As frequency increases, resolution also increases. Table 4–1 illustrates the wavelengths and, therefore, the relative resolving powers of a series of transducers of increasing frequencies. Increasing frequency, however, also increases attenuation. An increase in attenuation restricts the ability of the sound waves to penetrate the heart; consequently, frequency and penetration are inversely related. Without penetration, resolution is meaningless. Penetration, therefore, is of primary importance when considering these two variables.

In adults, the sound beam must often penetrate to tissue depths of 20 cm or more. This requirement is particularly true when using the apical or subcostal windows. When an intensity loss of 1 dB/cm/MHz is assumed, a pulse transmitted from a 2-MHz transducer loses 40 dB in reaching this 20-cm depth. Because another 40 dB are lost during the return trip to the transducer by the pulsed echo method, a total 80-dB, or a 10,000-fold, loss in signal strength is encountered at this transducer frequency. At the same tissue depth, a comparable pulse from a 4-MHz transducer undergoes a 160-dB intensity loss. By way of comparison, the dynamic range of the amplifiers of most echographs is only 80 to 100 dB. Therefore, although the intensity of any echo is a function of the intensity of the input pulse, a signal loss of 80 dB at conventional input intensities still permits the returning echoes to be recorded and amplified. A loss of 160 dB places the returning echo beyond the recording and amplification capabilities of most commercial instruments. An increase in the intensity of the input signal can compensate for the loss in signal strength encountered during tissue passage; however, at high input intensities, attenuation becomes nonlinear and increases as input power increases.

In the adult population, therefore, transducers with a frequency range of 2 to 3.5 MHz provide the penetration necessary to record the back wall of the heart and to still maintain an axial resolution in the range of 1 mm. Several recently developed instruments use 5.0-MHz transducers. Surprisingly good penetration has been achieved

Table 4–1. Relationship of Transducer Frequency to Wavelength

Frequency (MHz)	Wavelength (mm)	Wavelength (micron)
1	1.500	1,500
2.5	0.600	600
5	0.300	300
7.5	0.200	200
10	0.150	150
100	0.015	15

with these instruments in some patients while providing the increased resolution inherent in a higher frequency element. When evaluating such an instrument for routine use, however, one must examine typical rather than optimal patients to be sure that the penetration of the transducer is adequate for the routine clinical population of the laboratory.

Penetration may prove to be a particular problem in certain circumstances—most commonly in the barrel-chested or obese patient. Theoretically, a lower frequency transducer (in the 1-MHz range) would be most useful. In practice, however, the number of times this situation actually occurs rarely justifies the additional expense of such a low frequency probe. In addition, the increased field of vision and spatial orientation provided by the cross-sectional technique permit the examiner to approach the heart from many different vantage points, thereby increasing the opportunity to obtain useful data in all types of patients.

In infants and small children, the back wall of the heart is closer to the exploring probe, and penetration is less of a problem. For these situations, higher frequency transducers can more easily be used. Thus, when the back wall of the heart is 10 cm from the transducer, a 2-MHz probe encounters only a 40-dB loss in signal strength, whereas at 5 cm, this loss is only 20 dB. Thus, in a small infant, one can theoretically use a frequency as high as 10 MHz and still generate echoes with intensities within the recording and amplification capabilities of the instrument.

The choice of transducer frequency may also be limited by the operating characteristics of a particular system. In mechanical scanning systems, transducer frequency is not limited by instrument design, and hence, almost any frequency can be selected. In the phased array format, the choice of frequency is limited by the system itself. To date, the highest frequency obtained by using a phased array system has been 7.5 MHz.

In addition to defining the limits of frequency (as discussed in Chapter 2), the depth of field also determines the line or pulse repetition frequency. Thus, the closer the examined structures are to the transducer, the shorter the transit time of the ultrasonic pulse and the more rapidly pulses can be transmitted. Therefore, when one examines structures that are relatively close to the transducer, both the transducer frequency and the line repetition frequency can be increased, thereby producing an image in the infant and the young child that is of higher overall quality than that generally obtainable in the adult.

The final consideration in transducer selection is focusing characteristics. In the single-element mechanical or rotary systems, focusing is achieved by placing an acoustic lens over the front face of the transducer. This acoustic lens brings the beam to a focus within the near field of the transducer at a point determined by the radius of curvature of the lens. Increasing the size of the transducer increases the length of the near field and, hence, increases the depth at which the focus can be achieved. Once the radius of curvature of the lens is assigned, however, the focal length becomes fixed.

The possibility of achieving a variable focal length in

a mechanical system by the use of an annular array of transducers has been discussed earlier (see Chapter 2). In the annular array format, a series of concentrically oriented elements are used to transmit the interrogating pulse. As the pulse traverses the tissue, echoes arising from reflectors along the midportion of the beam strike each of the concentric rings in phase and, therefore, summate. Those arising from outside the central ray of the beam strike the concentric rings out-of-phase and, hence, tend to cancel each other. Optimizing the recording of reflectors along the central axis of the beam effectively focuses in both the azimuthal and the elevation dimensions of the imaging plane.

In the phased array format, as discussed in Chapter 2, focusing can be achieved by three different methods: (1) an acoustic lens, (2) dynamic transmit and receive focusing, and (3) shading.

Initial Control Settings

Before beginning the cross-sectional examination, the instrument settings under operator control must be adjusted to permit initial image recording. These controls were discussed in Chapter 1 and include the system gain or coarse gain, which controls the amplitude of all echoes within the examining plane; the time-again compensation (TGC), which selectively amplifies far-field echoes to correct for the normal loss of strength of the echo beam as it traverses the heart; the near gain, which controls the amplitude of echoes in close proximity to the transducer; the reject circuit, which selectively filters out all echoes below a certain predetermined amplitude; and the damping control, which adjusts the strength of the transmitted signal.

Specific control settings vary with different types of instrumentation and, as a result, must be individualized depending on the type of instrument used. Ideal gain settings are determined by examining several representative patients with a particular instrument and recording the control settings at which optimal studies are recorded. A clinical range of gain requirements can be determined from these settings. The gain controls should be set initially in the higher portion of this clinical range and then adjusted downward if necessary. When the initial settings are too low, even though the sound beam traverses the heart along an appropriate path, no recognizable signals may be recorded, and the operator never achieves the initial structure recognition required to pursue the examination. In contrast, when the gain settings are too high, even though the display scope may be cluttered with many extraneous signals, primary structures still can be discerned. It is best, therefore, to err by setting the gain too high.

Relating these principles to specific control settings suggests that a strong or weakly damped signal should be transmitted initially. Thus, the damping control is set at only 10 to 20% of maximum to initiate the examination. Similarly, with the coarse gain function, one is attempting to amplify any signals returning from the heart at a reasonably high level in hopes of recording some recognizable echoes. Therefore, in addition to transmitting a strong pulse initially, the operator seeks to amplify the reflected signals highly. As a result, the coarse gain is initially set at 80 to 90% of maximum. When too many signals are recorded, one can easily decrease either the amplification or the strength of the interrogating beam. When few or no signals are recorded, the operator never knows whether the control settings are inappropriate or whether the heart has not been located.

The TGC amplifies the echoes from structures that lie at increasingly greater distances from the transducer. The structures of greatest interest in clinical echocardiography lie at the level of the left ventricle. It has become customary, therefore, to amplify maximally all echoes from the proximal boundary of the left ventricle (the interventricular septum) distally. This amplification is achieved by initially placing the distal portion of the ramp of the TGC circuit at a depth that corresponds to the average distance of the interventricular septum from the chest wall. In the adult, the septum is usually between 5 and 8 cm from the anterior chest wall, most typically at approximately 6.5 cm. Any cross-sectional instruments have an additional display that can be used to view signals in an A-mode format. The A-mode best displays the effects of the TGC and, thus, permits a precise definition of its location.

The echoes that originate from structures close to the transducer generally have high amplitude and, therefore, require less amplification than those returning from deeper in the heart. The near gain controls the amplitude of all echoes from structures proximal to the ramp of the TGC. Because these echoes require less amplification, the setting of the near gain control is normally 20 to 40% of maximum.

Many newer instruments have replaced the conventional TGC control and near gain with a series of "slide pots" that permit gain to be varied independently at preselected ranges from the transducer. This approach has the same effects as the TGC, but is simple to teach and operate.

Finally, the reject circuitry must be adjusted. The objectives here are similar to those for the other control settings. Again, removing echoes that clutter an image is easier than trying to imagine what the image might look like if additional echoes were present. Therefore, the reject control is normally set at a relatively low level to allow the display of a wide range of signal amplitudes. When multiple low intensity signals obscure the image or prevent clear definition of more important structures, the amount of reject can be increased. A reject setting of 20 to 40% of maximum is therefore usually appropriate for an initial setting.

The control settings that are used to begin the examination are rarely those that are required to record the optimal final image. They are merely a starting point and should provide the examiner with enough data for initial structure identification and plane orientation.

EXAMINATION SEQUENCE

Locating the Heart

The first step in the actual cross-sectional examination is locating the heart. To locate the heart, the examiner must be familiar with (1) the principle echocardiographic windows; (2) three-dimensional cardiac anatomy, particularly the relationship of individual structures within the heart to each of the standard echocardiographic windows; and (3) the general imaging plane orientations that best record areas of initial interest.

In its normal position, the heart is enclosed within the bony skeleton of the thorax and is covered over most of its external surface by lung. Because ultrasound is poorly transmitted through bone and is reflected almost entirely by air-filled lung, the examiner must find a continuous soft tissue path, or window, through which the sound beam can travel to and from the heart. Unimpeded access can usually be obtained through four primary paths, or windows. These windows are located to the immediate left of the sternum in the interspaces between the third, fourth, fifth, and sixth ribs (parasternal); in the region of the cardiac apex (apical); over the anterior abdominal wall immediately beneath the lowest ribs (subcostal); and in the suprasternal notch (suprasternal). When the transducer is positioned over one of these windows, it is in a parasternal, apical, subcostal, or suprasternal location.[17]

Figure 4–3 illustrates the usual position of these windows in relation to the anterior chest wall and cardiac silhouette. The window positions indicated in this diagram apply to the normally positioned heart. When the heart is malpositioned or transposed, window position must shift accordingly. The suprasternal and subcostal windows that lie in the midline of the body usually do not change despite changes in cardiac position. The apical and parasternal windows, however, shift in parallel with the heart. When the heart is normally oriented in the left chest, the terms *apical* and *parasternal* are used alone to designate these window positions. In unusual situations when the apex is palpated on the right chest, however, the terms *right apical* and *right parasternal* should be substituted.[17] Likewise, if the transducer must be shifted far from the midline in the subcostal location, the designation *right subcostal* or *left subcostal* should be used. The suprasternal notch is so small that variation in transducer position is impossible. When the transducer is shifted to the right or left of the corresponding sternocleidomastoid muscle, it is referred to as in a *right supraclavicular* or *left supraclavicular* location.

The parasternal window is a series of small apertues that lie to the immediate left of the sternum at the level of the third, fourth, and fifth intercostal spaces. These windows are bordered medially by the left border of the sternum, superiorly and inferiorly by the contiguous ribs, and laterally by the lingula of the left lung. They directly overlie the base of the left ventricle and the mitral and aortic valves. The pulmonary and tricuspid valves are, as a rule, just beyond the margins of this composite window. All these important structures are closest to the transducer when it is in a parasternal location. In addition, their motion is largely perpendicular to the path of an imaging plane arising from the anterior chest wall, and hence, this motion is most appropriately assessed from this transducer location. The cross-sectional examination, therefore, is usually initiated and the majority of the study performed from a parasternal transducer location. Figure 4–4 illustrates the position of the cross-sectional probe when placed in a parasternal location.

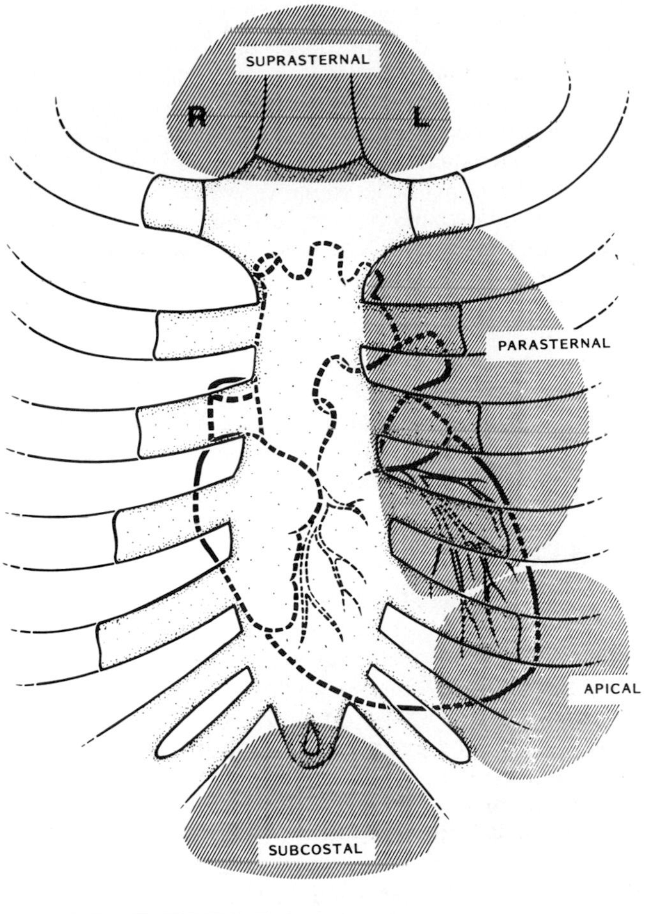

Fig. 4–3. The position of the four primary echocardiographic windows in relation to the thoracic cage and underlying regions of the heart.

The next most commonly used window is the cardiac apex. Apical position varies from patient to patient; consequently, the actual position of the cardiac apex must be located by palpation. Once the apex has been palpated, the transducer is placed directly over the apical impulse (Fig. 4–5). The apical impulse usually overlies a portion of the anterior left ventricular wall just proximal to the tip of the anatomic apex. From this position, one can direct the exploring plane either posteriorly (to record the apical region of the left ventricle) or superiorly and medially toward the right shoulder (to record structures at the base of the heart). The apical window has proved particularly useful because it is available in almost every case. In addition, the apical window is the only location from which all four cardiac chambers can be consistently recorded simultaneously in the adult.

The subcostal window[18] is located in the midline of the body immediately beneath the lowest ribs. When recording the heart from this location, the transducer is placed on the anterior abdominal wall and is pushed downward, depressing the skin until the transducer face lies beneath the plane of the anterior rib cage. The probe

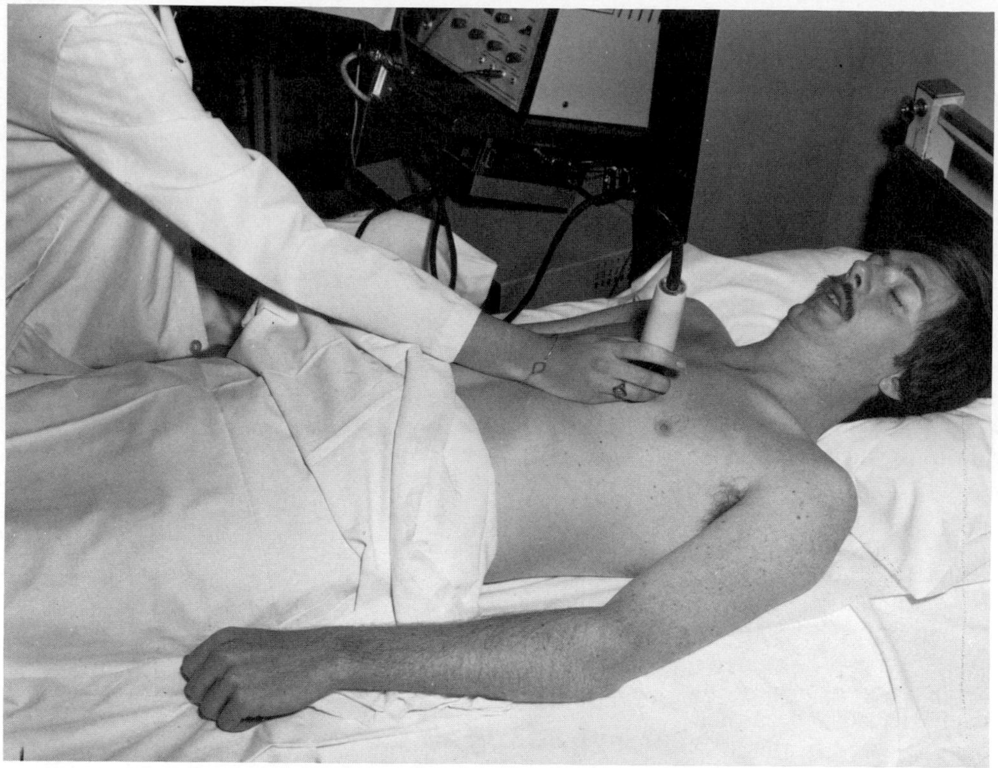

Fig. 4–4. Position of the cross-sectional probe on the anterior chest wall in the parasternal transducer location.

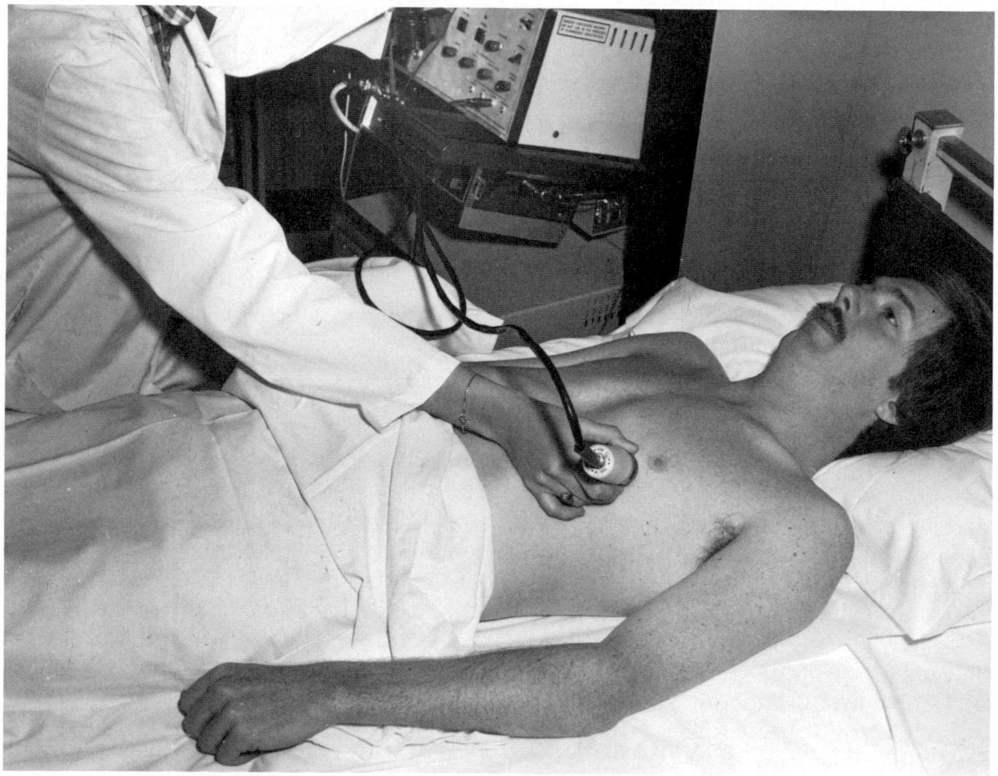

Fig. 4–5. Position of the cross-sectional probe at the cardiac apex. Although the patient in this illustration is supine, the apical window is frequently more accessible when the patient is in varying degrees of left lateral rotation.

is then angled superiorly and leftward (toward the left shoulder) to direct the central ray of the examining plane toward the heart (Fig. 4–6). This window is particularly useful in patients with chronic obstructive lung disease and chest deformities in whom access to the heart through the anterior parasternal or apical windows may be restricted. The subcostal window also is useful in small children and neonates because (as will be discussed later) it places the plane of the interventricular and interatrial septa perpendicular to the exploring sound beam and, hence, is optimally oriented to record these structures.

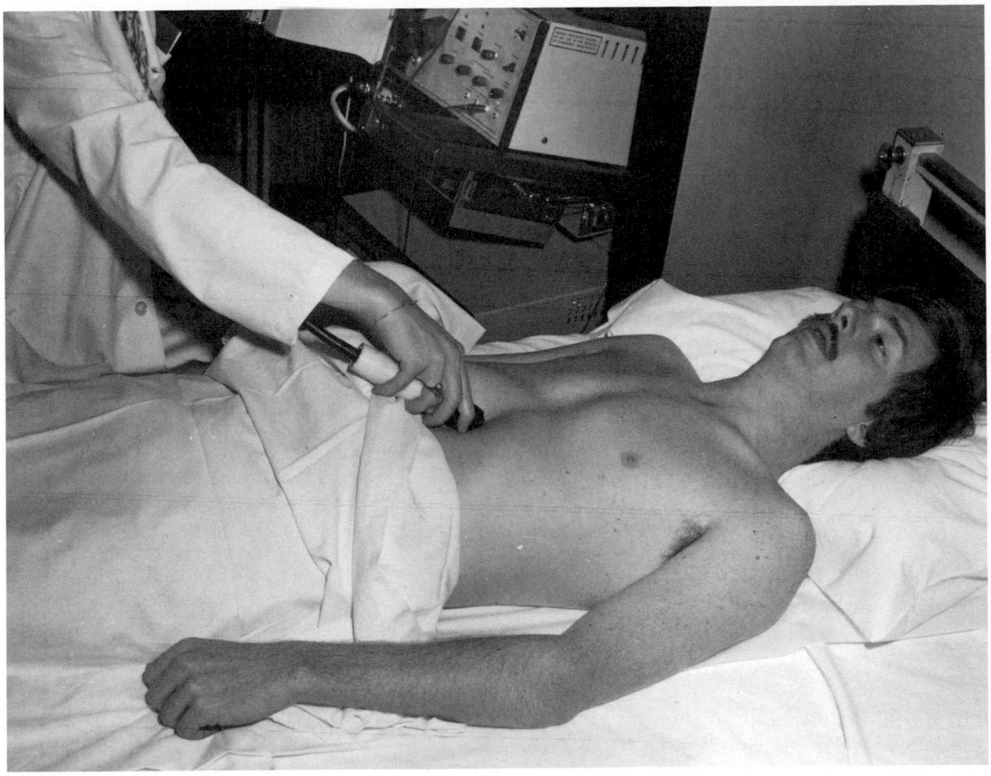

Fig. 4–6. Position of the cross-sectional probe in a subcostal location.

The suprasternal window is the last commonly employed transducer location. When this window is used, the exploring probe is placed directly in the suprasternal notch, and the sound beam is directed caudad, toward the left atrium (Fig. 4–7). From this location, the examining plane transects the aorta, the right pulmonary artery, and the left atrium in sequence as it penetrates into the chest. The aorta lies immediately beneath the suprasternal window. Little intervening tissue lies between the transducer face and the vessel. Thus, the sound beam readily passes into the aortic arch, thereby allowing this region to be recorded in almost every patient.

Although these areas represent the most common transducer locations, the transducer can and should be placed at any point on the chest wall or elsewhere from which useful information can be obtained. One helpful method for locating other such potential windows is quickly palpating the chest wall over a region of interest. If an impulse from any underlying cardiac structure is palpated, the structure itself should lie immediately beneath the chest wall at that point. If the transducer is placed directly over this impulse, the sound beam should pass unimpeded into the structures below. A common example is the pulmonary artery, which characteristically dilates in several disease states. Pulmonary artery dilation displaces the lung leftward and permits the transmission of the arterial impulse directly to the external surface of the chest. When this pulmonary artery pulsation is palpated and the exploring probe is placed directly over it, the pulmonary artery and pulmonary valves can be easily recorded.

A second technique that is helpful in locating alternative windows is simply to sweep the cross-sectional probe rapidly across the chest in a linear scan pattern. The large field of vision provided by this imaging format causes an image to flash on the display scope each time the sound beam finds access to the heart. Frequently, unexpected windows are uncovered in this fashion. The procedure can be carried out rapidly with broad strokes and does not require the "hunt and peck" that was characteristic of the M-mode method. As soon as the heart is located, the scanning probe can be more carefully oriented. This type of searching process is especially useful when the cardiac silhouette is grossly distorted (e.g., by a large anterolateral aneurysm) and a portion of the heart underlies an unusual area of the chest (e.g., the midaxillary line). If the examiner does not scan outside the normal echocardiographic windows in such cases, significant disorders can be missed.

Several factors influence the size of both the conventional and atypical echocardiographic windows and, as such, can facilitate or adversely affect the operator's initial search for the heart. Factors that increase window size are chamber dilation, change in patient position, and decreased lung volume. Expanded lung volume or bone area generally decrease window size.

Increased window size resulting from chamber dilation is most frequently noted in pathologic alterations of the right heart. In their normal orientations, the tricuspid valve and right ventricle lie beneath the sternum and, thus, may be difficult to record. As the right ventricle dilates, however, it expands leftward, shifting its position beneath and functionally enlarging the parasternal window. When right ventricular dilation is combined with pulmonary artery dilation, the area of the right

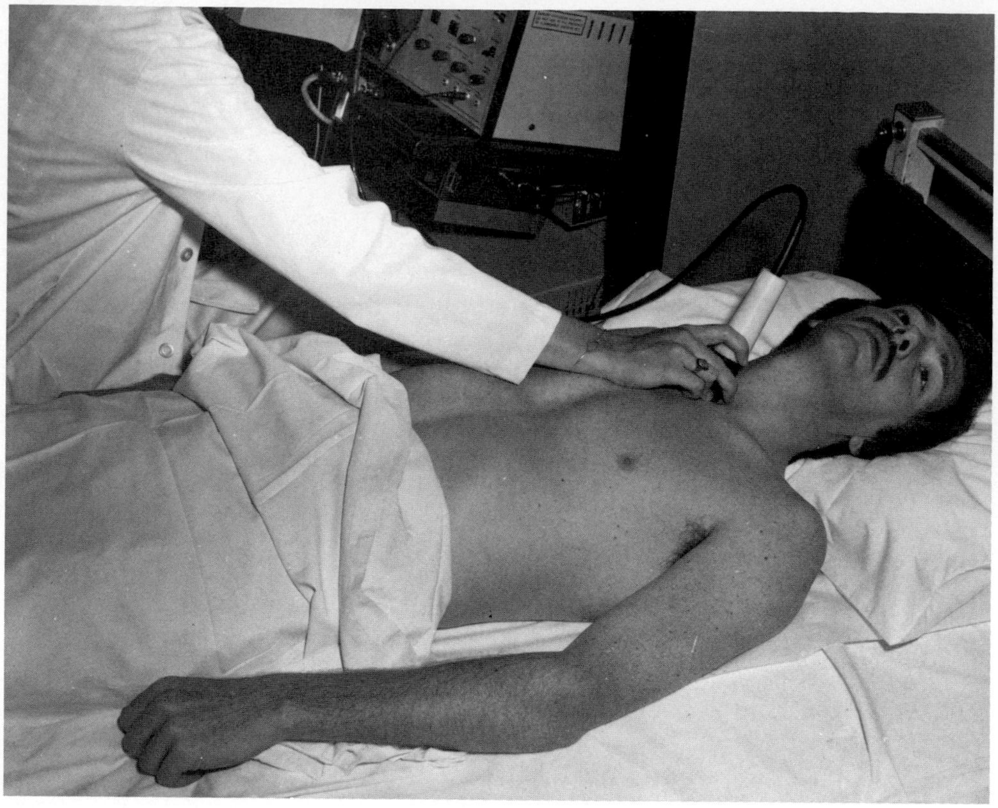

Fig. 4–7. Cross-sectional probe in suprasternal transducer location. Patient's neck is slightly extended, and the head is rotated slightly to the left.

heart that falls within the field of vision of the parasternal window may be vastly expanded.

Change in patient position may likewise increase window size or may shift structures into a position that facilitates viewing from a particular window. Rotating the patient from the supine to the left lateral position, for example, tends to shift the heart to the left. This change frequently moves the interventricular septum from beneath the sternum and permits its visualization from a parasternal transducer location. Positioning the patient on his left side also frequently increases the area of contact of the cardiac apex with the chest wall, thereby effectively expanding the apical window. Elevating the patient's head also may produce slight descent of mediastinal structures. Descent of the mitral or aortic valves may bring them out from under a rib and into a position where they can be recorded. Likewise, elevation of the head generally brings the heart closer to the subcostal window and decreases the penetration necessary to record structures from this location.

Increased bone density and lung volume occur most commonly in the elderly and combine to restrict access of the sound beam to the heart. In this population, calcification of the ribs narrows the intercostal spaces, whereas the expansion of the lungs commonly seen with chronic obstructive lung disease may totally obliterate the parasternal and apical windows. Other transient causes of pulmonary hyperexpansion, such as Valsalva's maneuver or hyperventilation, also can restrict access of the exploring beam to the heart.

A decrease in lung volume can be achieved by asking the patient to hold his breath after deep expiration. This temporary maneuver is difficult but occasionally useful. An important exception to the rule that inspiration makes the echocardiographic study more difficult is found in the subcostal views. Here, deeply held inspiration frequently improves visualization by shifting the heart closer to the transducer face.

Three-Dimensional Cardiac Anatomy

The examiner must next consider the position of the principal cardiac structures within the chest and their relationship to the primary echocardiographic windows. Figure 4–8 diagrammatically illustrates the normal orientation of the primary structures sought by the examiner for initial recording and identification. The importance of these structures lies in (1) their characteristic positions and motion patterns, which facilitate recognition, (2) their role as reference points for plane definition and fine plane positioning, and (3) their involvement in the more common cardiac disorders. The primary structures include the four cardiac valves, the apex, the papillary muscles, and the interventricular septum. When describing the relative positions of these structures within the chest, one should refer to those structures located toward the head or cranially as "superiorly oriented." Conversely, those positioned closer to the feet or caudally are referred to as "inferior." Structures located on the patient's right are designated as having a rightward orientation, whereas those on the patient's left are leftward. Structures near the anterior chest wall are anterior, whereas those closer to the posterior wall of the chest are posterior. Rotation of structures is described

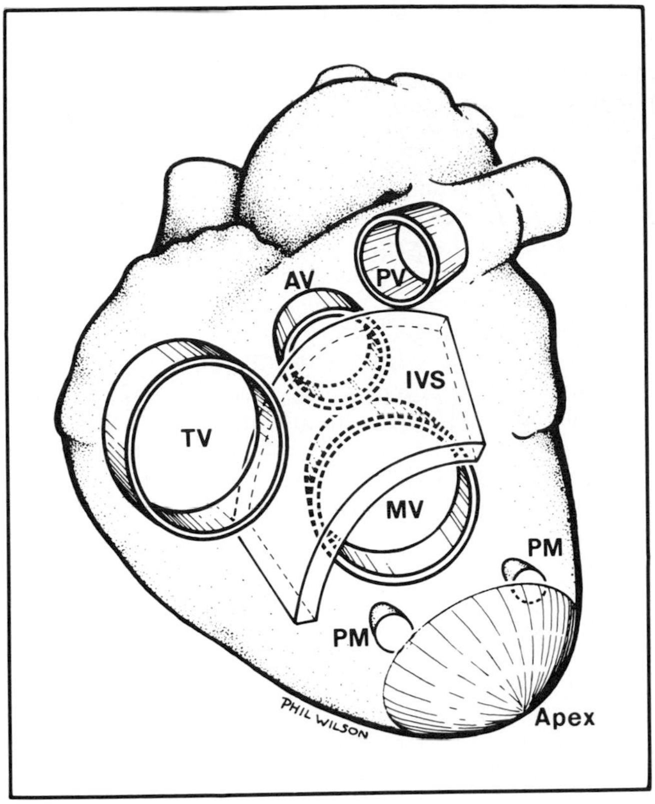

Fig. 4–8. The normal orientation and relationship of the major cardiac structures within the chest. PV = pulmonary valve; AV = aortic valve; TV = tricuspid valve; MV = mitral valve; IVS = interventricular septum; PM = papillary muscle. (See text for further details.)

as though the heart is viewed from below, looking upward toward the head.

The mitral valve, because of its central position within the heart, has historically formed the primary reference to which the position of other structures is related. As illustrated in Figure 4–8, the mitral valve is the most posteriorly positioned of the primary cardiac structures. It lies slightly to the left of the midline at the level of the fourth or fifth intercostal spaces. The tricuspid valve lies to the right of the mitral valve and is anterior and slightly inferior to the mitral valve. The aortic valve is superior to the mitral valve and also is anterior and slightly rightward in orientation. The pulmonary valve is the most superiorly positioned and is the most anterior of the structures at the base of the heart. It lies to the left of the aortic valve and almost directly superior to the mitral valve. The cardiac apex is the most inferior and leftward, as well as the most anterior, of the principal cardiac structures. The papillary muscles lie in the posterior hemisphere of the ventricle, parallel to the closure line of the mitral valve.

The examiner must be familiar not only with the position of these structures in the chest but also with their relationship to the primary echocardiographic windows. Figure 4–9 illustrates their positions in relation to the large parasternal window. The pulmonary valve lies at the left superior margin of this window and is the structure located most immediately beneath the window and, hence, closest to the transducer. The aortic valve is slightly more posterior and inferior and underlies the right margin of the window along its right superior border. The tricuspid valve lies beneath the sternum just beyond the right margin of the window, and at the annulus, its center is slightly inferior to that of the aortic valve. When the right heart dilates, its position within the chest rotates clockwise, and the anteroposterior relationships of the tricuspid and aortic valves may reverse. The mitral valve lies beneath the center of the window and is the most posteriorly positioned of the four cardiac valves. The interventricular septum curves posterior from left to right in an arcuate fashion beneath this window. Its left margin lies anteriorly almost immediately beneath the chest wall, whereas its right boundary is posteriorly positioned at approximately the level of the coaptation line of the mitral leaflets. The anterior one-third of the septum is almost perpendicular to the path of a sound beam emanating from the parasternal window and, hence, can be well recorded, whereas the posterior one-third of the septum is more parallel to the sound beam and is poorly visualized. The papillary muscles generally lie just beyond the left inferior border of the window and may be recorded by angling the imaging

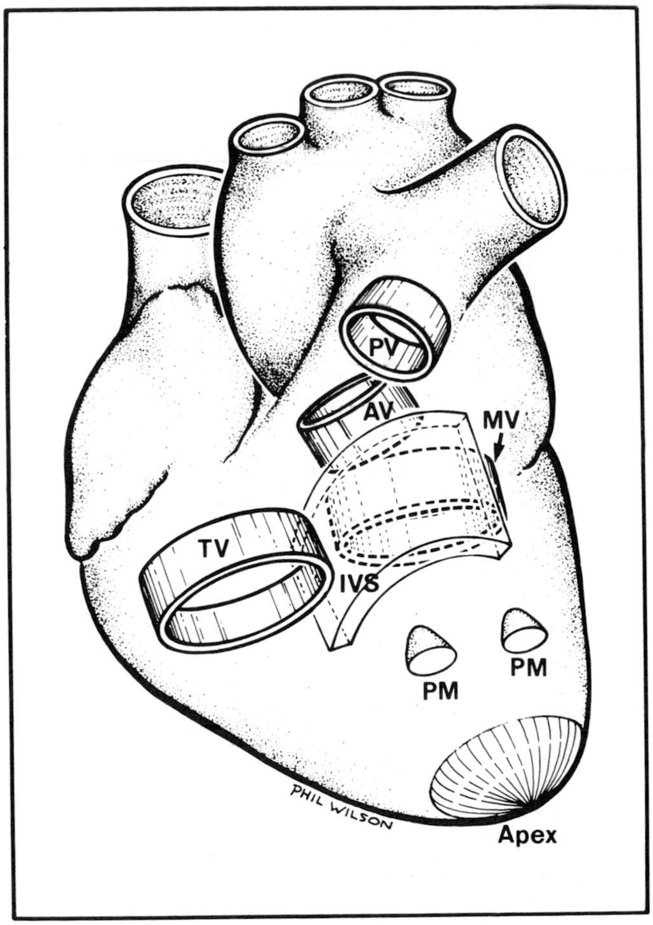

Fig. 4–9. Orientation and relative position of the primary echocardiographic structures when viewed from the parasternal transducer location. The center of this window normally overlies the medial third of the mitral valve. The abbreviations are the same as those in Figure 4–8. (See text for further details.)

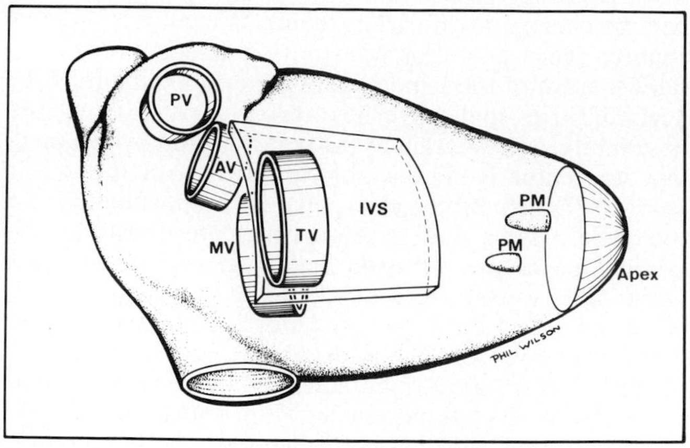

Fig. 4–10. The relative locations of the primary cardiac structures when viewed from the subcostal transducer location. Abbreviations are the same as those in Figure 4–8. (See text for further details.)

plane inferiorly and leftward. The cardiac apex, however, almost universally lies outside the parasternal window and cannot be visualized from this position.

Figure 4–10 illustrates the relative positions of these structures when viewed from a subcostal transducer location. From this vantage point, the tricuspid valve is positioned closest to the transducer. It is followed by the interventricular septum, the posteromedial surface of which is closest to the transducer and is oriented almost perpendicular to its face. The septum then curves superiorly and leftward away from the transducer such that the anterior portion of the septum lies parallel to the transducer. The mitral valve is slightly posterior and superior to the tricuspid valve. The papillary muscles and cardiac apex appear to the examiner's right and are situated farther from the transducer than the mitral valve. The aortic valve lies at the same depth as the mitral valve and is slightly anterior, whereas the pulmonary valve is the farthest structure from this transducer location and, after the apex, is the most anteriorly situated.

Figure 4–11 illustrates the positions of these structures relative to the cardiac apex. From this viewpoint, the apex itself is most closely related to the transducer face. As the plane passes away from the transducer, it first encounters the papillary muscles, followed sequentially by the tricuspid and mitral valves. The tricuspid valve lies slightly closer to the transducer than does the mitral and is positioned anteriorly in the chest. The next structure encountered is the aortic valve, which is still farther anterior. The pulmonary valve follows and, from this orientation, is the structure deepest to the transducer.

Finally, Figure 4–12 illustrates the orientation of the same structures viewed from the suprasternal notch. From this transducer location, the imaging plane must first pass through the aorta and right pulmonary artery before reaching the heart. Beneath the right pulmonary artery, the pulmonary valve lies closest to the transducer. This structure is followed sequentially by the aortic valve, the mitral valve, and the tricuspid valve. The papillary muscles and cardiac apex are too far from the transducer to be recorded in the normal situation.

The choice of a transducer location is ultimately determined by the orientation of the particular structure to be recorded relative to the available echocardiographic windows. As a rule, the transducer should be located in the position that places that structure as close as possible to the transducer face and in an orientation that is as perpendicular as possible to the path of the sound beam. After determining the appropriate transducer location, one must orient the imaging plane in the appropriate manner to best depict the specific features of the structures to be evaluated. As will be discussed later, differ-

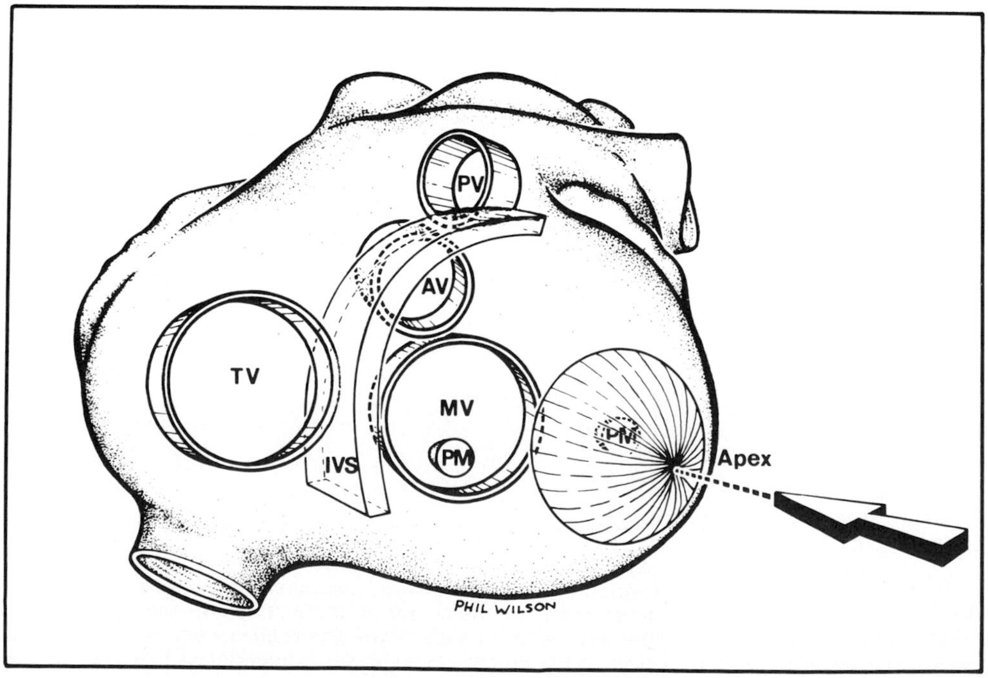

Fig. 4–11. The relative positions of the primary cardiac structures from the apical transducer location. Abbreviations are the same as those in Figure 4–8.

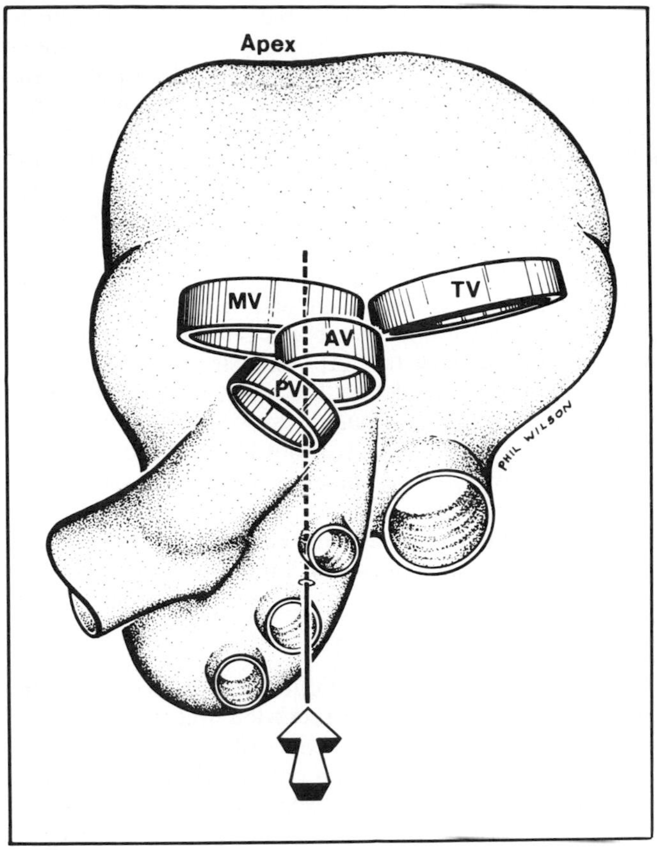

Fig. 4–12. Orientation of the primary cardiac structures from the suprasternal window. The arrow indicates the path along which the structures at the base of the heart are viewed from this location. Normally, the papillary muscles and apex cannot be recorded from this window. MV = mitral valve; TV = tricuspid valve; AV = aortic valve; PV = pulmonary valve.

ent considerations apply for Doppler flow recordings and as a result, optimal Doppler and imaging studies of the same region are rarely recorded from the same echocardiographic window.

General Plane Orientation

General plane orientation is an attempt by the examiner to correctly align the imaging plane (based on external references or the expected position of intracardiac structures in the chest) such that it passes through the heart in a manner that records a desired structure, dimension, or axis. The orientation of any plane in space can be described by three noncolinear points. When the transducer's position can be defined, it can be used as one point. The examiner must then determine two other points to orient the imaging plane. Because two points describe a line, the plane can be oriented using the transducer location and either a real or imaginary line in space. The line that is most commonly used is one of the axes of the structure to be examined.

An axis, by definition, is a straight line about which a body or geometric figure may be supposed to rotate and with respect to which the body or figure is symmetric.[19] The long axis of any structure, therefore, is the longest linear dimension about which that structure is symmetric, whereas the short axis is normally perpendicular to the long axis and is the shortest linear dimension about which that body would rotate in an orthogonal direction. Figure 4–13 illustrates the long and short axes of a series of simple geometric figures. Figure 4–14 depicts the long and short axes of the left ventricle. Because the borders of the left ventricle within any plane that includes the long axis are asymmetric, there is only one long axis of this chamber. Multiple planes, however, can pass through the ventricle parallel to and intersecting this long axis. In contrast, the borders of the ventricle are symmetric in a plane that intersects the short axis and is perpendicular to the long axis. A short axis, therefore, can be drawn between any two points along this 360° arc that can be connected by a line passing through the center of the ventricle. Thus, there are multiple short axes but only one plane that can contain more than one of these axes simultaneously.

The long axis of the ventricle is also easier to define. It runs from the tip of the cardiac apex to the midpoint of the base of the ventricle. Any plane through this long axis should, therefore, bisect the ventricle into two equal halves. The true short axis lies in a plane that also bisects the ventricle into two halves with equal masses. The halves of the ventricle on either side of this plane, however, are not geometrically similar; consequently, the position of this plane cannot be determined visually and must be calculated. Because of the inherent difficulties in attempting to calculate the true short axis from the cross-sectional image, the short axis views are generally considered as a family of planes oriented parallel to the true short axis plane, rather than as a single plane passing through the short axis itself.

When recording most structures, the examiner seeks

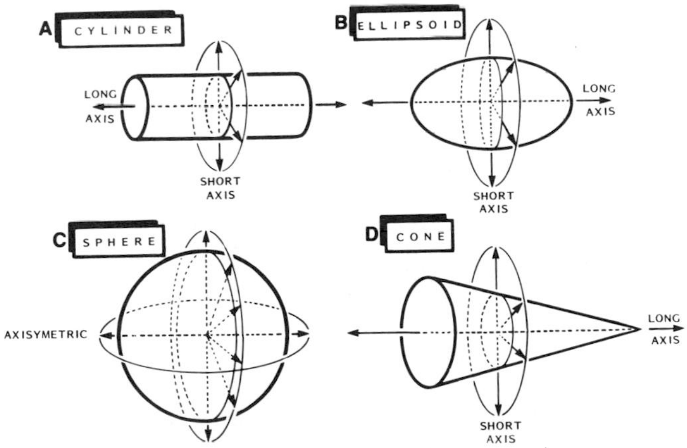

Fig. 4–13. The long and short axes of a series of simple geometric figures. The cylinder (A) ellipsoid (B) and cone (D) have only one long axis. There are, however, multiple short axes that can be drawn through the center of these figures and about which the figure is symmetric. Two or more of these short axes lie in a plane that is perpendicular to the long axis. In symmetric figures, such as the cylinder and the ellipsoid, the short axis can be measured directly. In more complicated figures, the short axis must generally be calculated. The sphere, in contrast to the other geometric figures, has no natural long or short axes and rotates about any line passing through its midpoint. Thus, the arbitrary long and short axes of a sphere must be assigned relative to some internal or external reference.

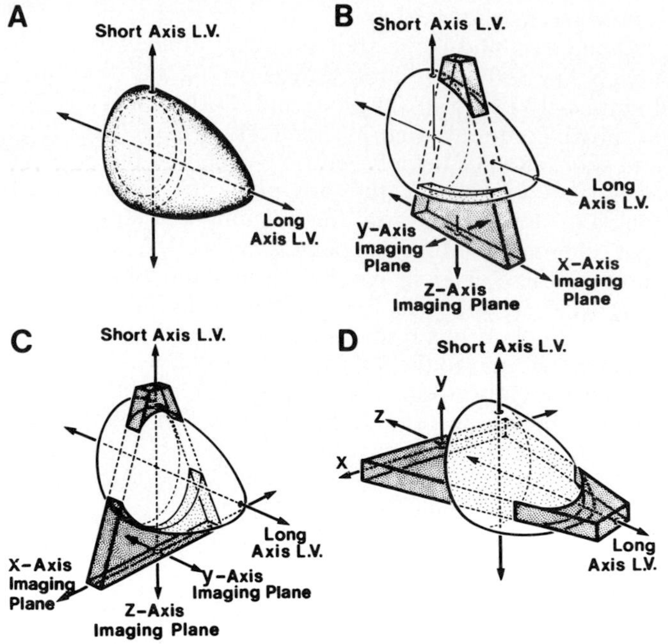

Fig. 4–14. **A.** The long and short axes of a figure similar in shape to the left ventricle (L.V.). As with the ellipse, the cylinder and the cone, the left ventricle has only one true long axis. Multiple planes rotated through a 360° arc, however, can pass through and can be parallel to this long axis. In addition, as with the cylinder, ellipse, and cone, multiple short axes of the left ventricle can be defined. However, only one plane can encompass more than one of these short axes. **B.** The relationship of the axes of a standard imaging plane to the axes of the left ventricle when the imaging plane is aligned parallel to the ventricular long axis and passes through it in an anteroposterior direction. **C.** The relationship of the axes of the imaging plane to those of the left ventricle when the imaging plane is aligned parallel to the ventricular short axis and is oriented in an anteroposterior direction. **D.** The relationship that would result if the imaging plane were directed from the left ventricular apex toward the base and if the plane included the ventricular long axis.

to align the x or z axis of the imaging plane (the y axis, which measures thickness or dimension, cannot be appreciated on the display and, hence, is not a useful reference) parallel to either the long or the short axis of the structure to be recorded. A long axis view of the left ventricle, e.g., is recorded by aligning the x axis of the imaging plane parallel to the long axis of the ventricular chamber (Fig. 4–14B). Both the y and z axis of the imaging plane are thereby aligned perpendicular to the long axis. Because numerous planes may intersect the long axis of the left ventricle, the third point required to define the position of the particular plane in space must be provided either by the transducer location or by another reference that is either internal or external to the left ventricle. Ideally, a combination of both transducer location and additional reference points is used to permit the most definitive determination of plane orientation. Thus, for example, a plane that passes through the long axis of the left ventricle from the anterior to the posterior surfaces of the heart (transducer in a parasternal location), and also passes between the papillary muscles without recording the echoes from either of these structures, is defined within narrow limits.

Orienting the imaging plane relative to the short axis plane of the left ventricle is achieved by aligning both the x and z axes of the imaging plane parallel to perpendicular short axes of the ventricle and orthogonal to the long axis (Fig. 4–14C). The y axis in this format is parallel to the long axis. Internal references are then used to define the point at which a plane oriented parallel to the short axes of the ventricle transects the chamber. These references include the mitral valve and supporting apparatus, the papillary muscles, and the apical segment of the ventricle distal to the papillary muscles.

When viewing the ventricle from the cardiac apex, the examiner seeks to align the z axis of the imaging plane along the long axis of the left ventricle. Both the x and y axes are then parallel to the short axis plane (Fig. 4–14D). From this particular transducer position, the plane can be rotated 360° without altering the relationships of the axes of the imaging plane to those of the ventricle. The precise angle in which the imaging plane transects the ventricle, therefore, must be again determined by use of an external or internal reference.

Initiating the Examination

After the examiner and patient are appropriately positioned, the structures to be recorded and their orientation relative to the available echocardiographic windows are defined and the ideal plane orientation to optimally view these structures is determined, the examiner is ready to begin the actual examination. The examination is initiated by placing the transducer in the selected location. The transducer face must then be coupled to the skin using an appropriate acoustic coupling gel. Coupling is important because it prevents air from entering between the transducer face and skin surface. Air in this location can produce a highly reflective interface and can cause significant loss in the acoustic energy available to penetrate the heart. When previously well-recorded structures begin to fade during the course of the examination, one can generally assume a loss of adequate coupling. This situation can be corrected by adding more gel.

When the transducer is appropriately positioned and coupled to the skin, the central ray of the imaging plane should be directed toward the structure of interest. This is achieved by angling the transducer in such a manner that an imaginary extension of the long axis of the probe passes through the desired area. The imaging plane is then rotated to align its x axis parallel to the appropriate axis of the structure to be recorded. When the imaging plane is properly oriented and gains access to the heart, an image should immediately appear on the display scope. When an image appears, the examiner must first identify the recorded structures to define the path of the imaging plane through the heart. When these structures are identified, they then form a reference for more precise alignment of the imaging plane or from which the plane position can be readjusted to record other structures of interest. If recognizable echoes do not appear, the imaging plane should be swept through the area where the heart is expected to lie until an identifiable image appears on the display scope.

The routine clinical examination is most frequently

initiated by placing the transducer in a parasternal location at the level of the fourth or fifth intercostal spaces. From this transducer location, the examiner normally seeks to record echoes from structures at the base of the heart (most particularly the mitral valve echo). The mitral valve is selected as a starting point because it lies most immediately beneath this window, is highly reflective, and has a characteristic motion pattern. Also, because of its central position within the heart, the mitral valve is a useful reference from which to locate other structures.

To record the mitral valve, the examiner directs the central ray of the imaging plane posteriorly and slightly leftward. The imaging plane is then rotated to align the x axis parallel to the long axis of the left ventricle and, hence, parallel to the path of the blood flow through the mitral leaflets. The long axis of the left ventricle runs roughly on a line from the cardiac apex to the right shoulder or 30 to 45° counterclockwise to the long axis of the body. In the majority of patients, when the transducer is oriented in this fashion, the imaging plane should pass directly into the heart and should record echoes from the mitral valve, the left ventricular myocardium at the base of the heart, and a portion of the left atrium and proximal aortic root (Fig. 4–15). When any echoes from underlying structures appear on the display scope, the examiner is ready to advance to more precise structure identification and fine plane positioning.

If echoes are not recorded from this initial transducer location and image plane orientation, the examiner should then explore other portions of the parasternal window to find access to the heart. If this step is unsuccessful, the patient can be rotated into the left lateral position in an attempt to shift the heart slightly to the left and to expand the parasternal window. If this maneuver is also unsuccessful, the examiner may have to explore other transducer locations from which access to the heart may be obtained.

Structure Identification

Intracardiac structures are identified on the basis of one or more characteristics of their ultrasonic reflections. These characteristics include (1) positions within the chest, (2) general appearance, (3) motion patterns, (4) associations with other known structures, and (5) unique anatomic characteristics.

The most common and perhaps easiest approach to structure identification is based on the expected position of the larger cardiac structures within the chest. Figure 4–16 illustrates how this method can be used. In this example, a transducer is placed on the anterior chest wall along the left sternal border, and the imaging plane is directed posteriorly into the chest parallel to the left ventricular short axis. If the heart is normally positioned, the first large echo-free space encountered by the sound beam should be the right ventricle. Moving echoes anterior to this space should then be reflected from the right ventricular free wall, whereas those beneath this space should arise from the interventricular septum. Assuming that this first group of structures is correctly identified, a second, large, echo-free space, lying beneath the septum, should represent the left ventricular cavity, whereas moving echoes bordering this space posteriorly may presumably arise from the left ventricular posterior wall. Echoes within the left ventricular cavity should arise from the mitral valve. When the heart is normally positioned in the chest and the cardiac chambers are appropriately related, this approach usually leads to correct structure identification. When the heart is malpositioned or when chamber relationships are distorted, reliance on this approach has resulted in a surprising amount of confusion and has led to incorrect structure identification.

The second approach to structure identification is based on an analysis of the geometric configuration of the structure(s) being imaged. The chamber that has a circular configuration when viewed from the anterior chest wall in a plane parallel to its short axis and also is

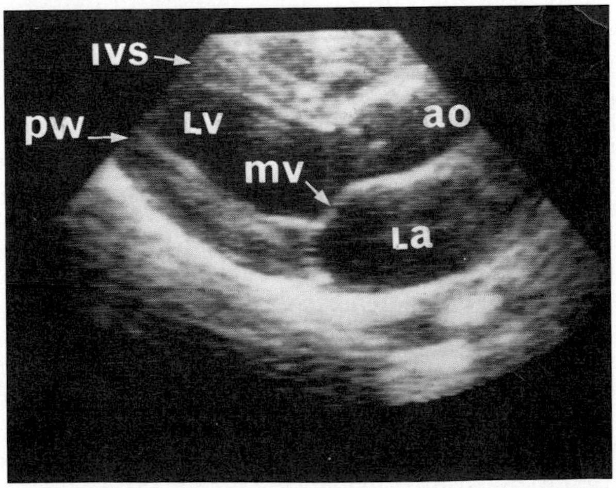

Fig. 4–15. Parasternal long axis view of the left ventricle similar to that usually sought as a starting point for the cross-sectional examination. LV = left ventricle; La = left atrium, mv = mitral valve; ao = aorta, ivs = interventricular septum, pw = posterior wall. The apex in this orientation is to the viewer's left, and the aorta is to the viewer's right.

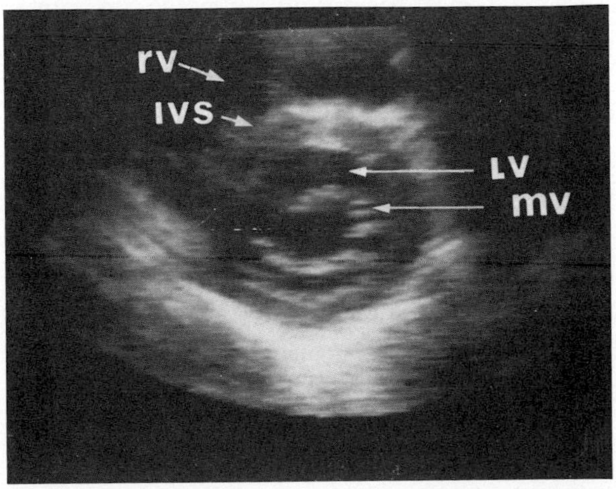

Fig. 4–16. Parasternal short axis view of the left ventricle illustrates the expected relative positions of the right ventricle (rv), interventricular septum (ivs), left ventricular cavity (LV), and mitral valve (mv) in this image orientation.

surrounded by a thick muscular wall is normally the left ventricle (see Fig. 4–16).

Exceptions to this kind of analysis also occur. In severe pulmonary hypertension and right ventricular volume overload, the right ventricle may become more circular than the left. Likewise, hypertrophy of a transposed right ventricle may prevent chamber identification on the basis of wall thickness.

Assessment of the motion patterns of intracardiac structures can be of particular value in structure identification. The broad amplitude and rapid motion of the cardiac valves serve to distinguish them from nonvalvular structures. Additionally, the opening or closing of these valves in relation to the cardiac cycle allows separation of the atrioventricular (AV) from the semilunar valves. Although separation of valves into those regulating ventricular inflow and outflow may be relatively easy, specific identification of the individual AV and semilunar valves is frequently more complicated. Such complication occurs because valve motion is not an inherent feature of the valve leaflets but is a passive function reflecting the pattern of blood flow through the valve and the relative pressure exerted on the opposing leaflet surfaces. Therefore, although the pattern and timing of valve motion may permit the identification of an AV valve, valve motion defines neither the number of leaflets the valve contains nor whether it lies in the mitral or tricuspid position. More precise valve identification must be gained through other means, such as comparing the relative position of these partially identified structures to one another or determining the number of leaflets the valve contains. The mitral valve inserts into the interventricular septum at a slightly more basal position than does the tricuspid valve when viewed from either the apical or subxiphoid window. Determination of the relative position of the valve leaflets as they insert into the septum, therefore, can permit differentiation of the AV valves. More simply, the mitral valve normally has two leaflets, and the tricuspid has three leaflets. Simply counting the number of leaflets in the AV valve may permit their separation.

Association with other structures of known identity is another method of identifying unknown areas of echo production. This method obviously requires the identification of the contiguous structures first, but it has proven particularly useful in recognizing structures that are known to be present anatomically but that may not have previously been appreciated by the examiner or described by others. An example of this approach was the original identification of the linear band of echoes arising from the interatrial septum. Taken by themselves, these echoes would have had little meaning. When placed between the posteromedial border of the aorta and the posterior left atrial wall, however, their origin and significance became apparent.

Finally, a few structures have unique anatomic characteristics that can be used for definitive identification. For example, when the great vessels are malaligned, differentiation of the aorta and pulmonary artery at their origins may prove difficult. Determination of the paths and distribution of these vessels, however, permits positive identification based on their branching patterns. Thus, the artery that courses into the neck and gives off numerous large branches to the head and upper extremities is always the aorta. Conversely, the vessel that bifurcates into two branches of relatively equal size is always the pulmonary artery. Likewise, the valve at the origin of the pulmonary artery is always the pulmonary valve, and the valve at the base of the aorta is always the aortic valve. Although such unique structural configurations are rare, they are valuable in structure identification.

Ideally, a combination of all the available methods should be used when attempting to identify any structure because the more characteristics of a particular structure that one can recognize, the more likely that the identification of the structure will be correct. For example, the determination that a structure with all of the following characteristics is the aorta is far more positive than an identification made on the basis of any one of these features alone: (1) It lies approximately 6 cm beneath the anterior chest wall; (2) is is characterized by two horizontal linear echoes when viewed with the scan plane parallel to its long axis and as a circle when viewed with the scan plane parallel to its short axis; (3) it moves anteriorly during systole and posteriorly during diastole; (4) it courses into the neck and gives off numerous large branches; (5) it has an anterior border that is continuous with the interventricular septum and a posterior border that is continuous with the mitral valve; and (6) it lies anterior to the left atrium and posterior to the right ventricular outflow tract. Although all structures are not as clearly defined as the aorta, an identification of a source of echoes is almost always possible if one carefully considers the location of a structure and its general configuration, motion patterns, and relationships to other known structures. Also, the identification of many structures independently is not necessary. If one or two structures can be identified, the other pieces of the puzzle can, as a rule, be easily fitted into place either by association or by exclusion.

In special cases, contrast echocardiography may aid in the identification of unusually positioned pathologic structures (see Chapter 15).

Fine Plane Positioning

The final step in recording any cross-sectional image involves positioning the imaging plane as precisely as possible to appropriately display the desired features of a structure of interest. Precise plane positioning is determined from the recorded image itself and is independent of the position of the heart in the chest or of the relative positions of other cardiac structures. Precise plane positioning is essential because it determines the reliability of dimensions, appreciation of motion, and reproducibility of derived data.

A typical long axis recording of the left ventricle can be used to illustrate how improper plane positioning adversely affects the data derived from the cross-sectional image. Figure 4–17 illustrates that when the imaging plane passes through the long axis of the ventricle (plane A), the distance between contralateral points on the ventricular wall represents a true ventricular diameter. Ad-

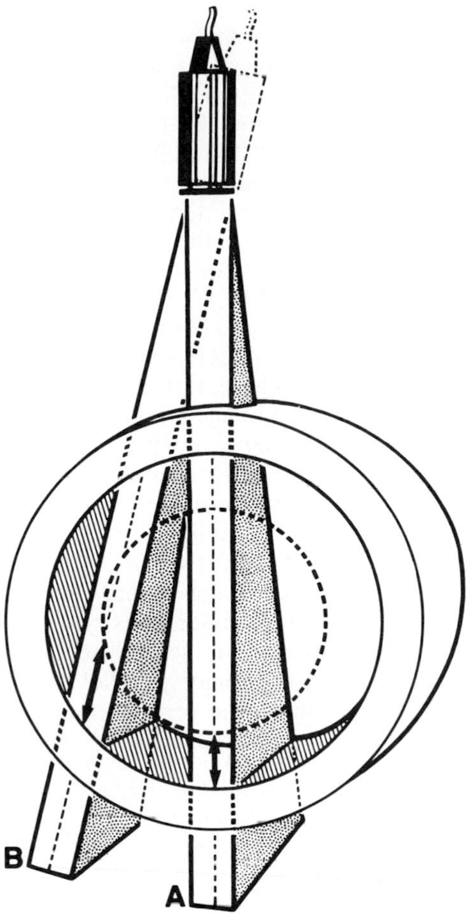

Fig. 4–17. The relative end-diastolic and end-systolic ventricular diameters and amplitudes of endocardial motion recorded in two different planes. Both planes are parallel to the ventricular long axis. Plane A passes through the center of the ventricle (long axis), recording a true ventricular diameter and appropriately depicting the amplitude of endocardial excursion. Plane B is eccentrically positioned and records a decreased ventricular diameter and an artifactually increased wall motion.

ditionally, motion of these points appropriately reflects actual left ventricular endocardial excursion. Conversely, as also indicated in Figure 4–17, when the plane is angled so that it is parallel to, but passes to one side of the long axis (plane B), the distance between points on the contralateral ventricular walls is less than a true diameter and motion is artifactually exaggerated.

If the examiner could see the structure to be recorded and the imaging plane simultaneously, it would be relatively simple to align the imaging plane parallel to any axis of the structure. Unfortunately, the examiner cannot directly visualize the structure to be recorded and must determine its shape, orientation, and position relative to the imaging plane from the image on the display scope. The probe must then be moved and the plane angled or rotated in an appropriate pattern to produce an optimal image based solely on the changes these movements produce in the image recorded. Fine plane positioning, therefore, requires the examiner's full understanding of the variations in the image that are produced by changes in plane positioning, the effects of improper plane orientation on image configuration, and the optimal structure configuration that can be recorded when the imaging plane is properly positioned.

To understand these concepts, one should consider the relationships of an imaging plane to a series of simple geometric figures. The simplest figure to consider is the cylinder. The cylinder has both a long axis and a short axis. Figure 4–18A illustrates that when an ultrasonic imaging plane transects the cylinder parallel to its long axis, two linear echoes, equally distant from each other at all points in the plane, are recorded. The effects of the improper transducer and, hence, plane positioning can be appreciated in Figure 4–18B and C. When the plane is angled to the right or left of the long axis (Fig. 4–18B), the distance between the two echoes decreases. Thus, the plane passes through the long axis of the cylinder only where the separation of the two imaged echoes is the greatest. Likewise, when the transducer is rotated such that the plane is no longer parallel to, but crosses, the long axis at an angle, it cuts through the cylinder obliquely (Fig. 4–18C). When this occurs, the echoes at the two margins of the imaging plane begin to curve inward toward one another and continue to decrease as the imaging plane is rotated further from the true long axis. The diameter in the center of the scan remains

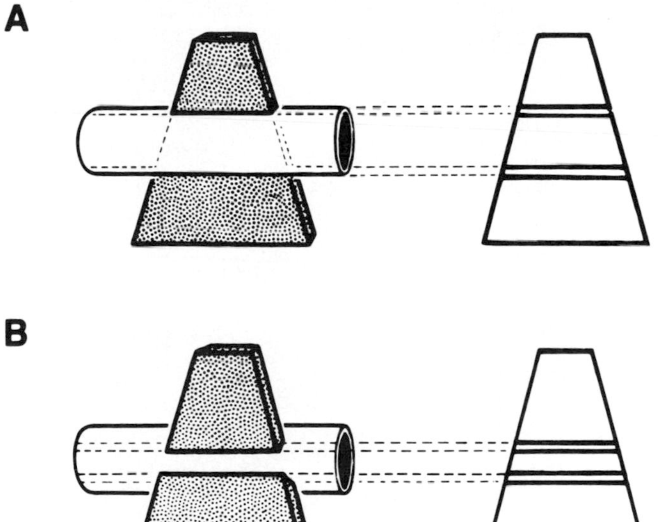

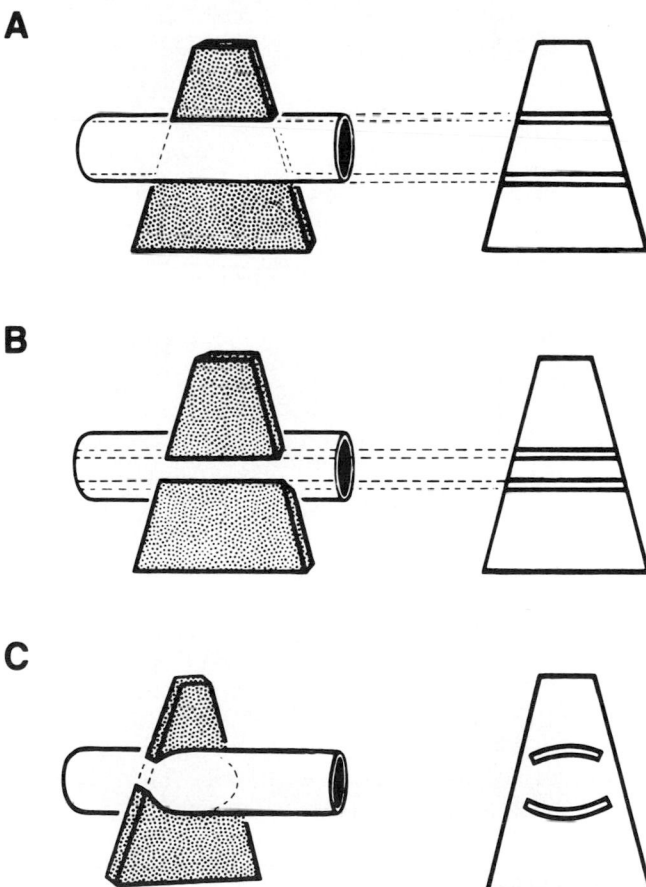

Fig. 4–18. **A.** Image recorded when a plane transects a cylinder along a path parallel to and intersecting its long axis. **B.** Image recorded when a plane transects a cylinder parallel to, but to the left or right of, its long axis. **C.** Image recorded when a plane transects the cylinder at an angle to its long axis.

maximal because the imaging plane passes through the long axis at this point. The plane is rotated parallel to the long axis of the cylinder then only when the diameter of the cylinder is equal at the center and both margins of the scan.

In Figure 4–18, the transducer is located over the middle of the cylinder. The transducer could obviously be moved either to the right or left without changing the recorded image. To determine the area of the cylinder transected by the plane, therefore, some external reference, such as the ends of the cylinder, is necessary.

Figure 4–19 contains three long axis, cross-sectional scans of the cylindric aorta, which demonstrate these principles. In Figure 4–19A, the scan is aligned parallel to the long axis of the vessel, and the vessel walls are parallel and widely separated. Figure 4–19B, the transducer is angled improperly, and the vessel diameter decreases; in Figure 4–19C, the plane is rotated such that it cuts through the external margin of the vessel. When attempting to align the imaging plane parallel to the long axis of a cylindric structure, the examiner should rotate the transducer clockwise and then counterclockwise until the distance between the linear echoes at the margins of the scan plane are at their maximum. Then, by angling the plane back and forth across the cylinder until the separation of the echoes in the midportion and the margins of the recorded image is equidistant, the examiner can plane the imaging plane not only parallel to but through the true long axis. Determination of transducer location depends on an external or internal reference.

Figure 4–20 illustrates the image produced when the imaging plane passes through the short axis of the cylinder. In this example, the image appears circular, and its diameters are equal in all dimensions. When the examiner angles the transducer in either direction such that the imaging plane is no longer parallel to the vertical short axis of the cylinder, the vertical dimensions of the

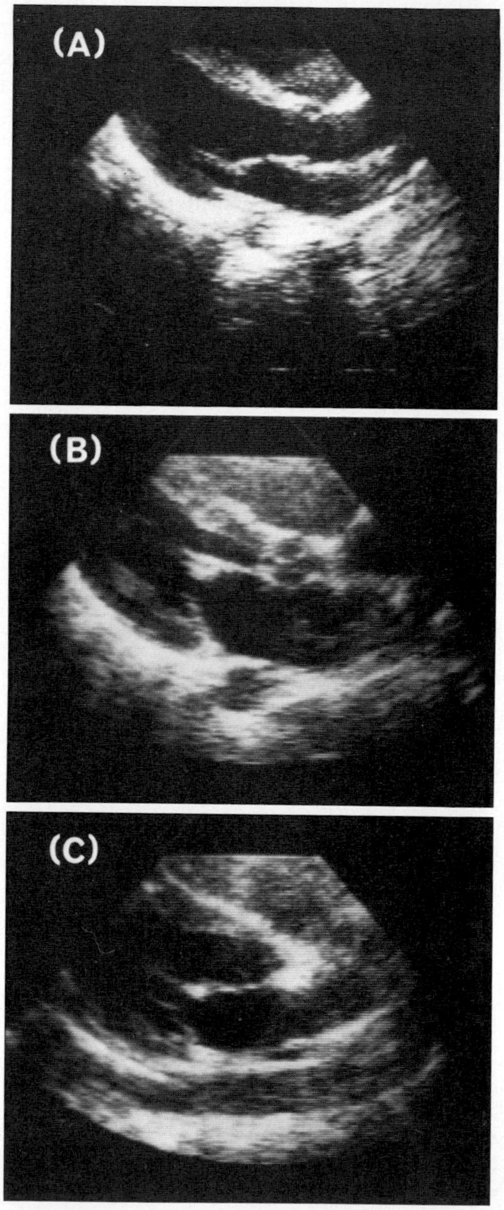

Fig. 4–19. Cross-sectional recordings illustrate the effects depicted diagrammatically in Figure 4–18. **A.** The scan plane passes through the aorta in an orientation that is parallel to and transects its long axis. **B.** The scan plane is angled to pass through the aorta parallel to but not through its long axis. The vessel, therefore, appears narrowed. **C.** The scan plane is rotated incorrectly and passes obliquely across the long axis of the aorta, thus transecting the lateral aortic wall.

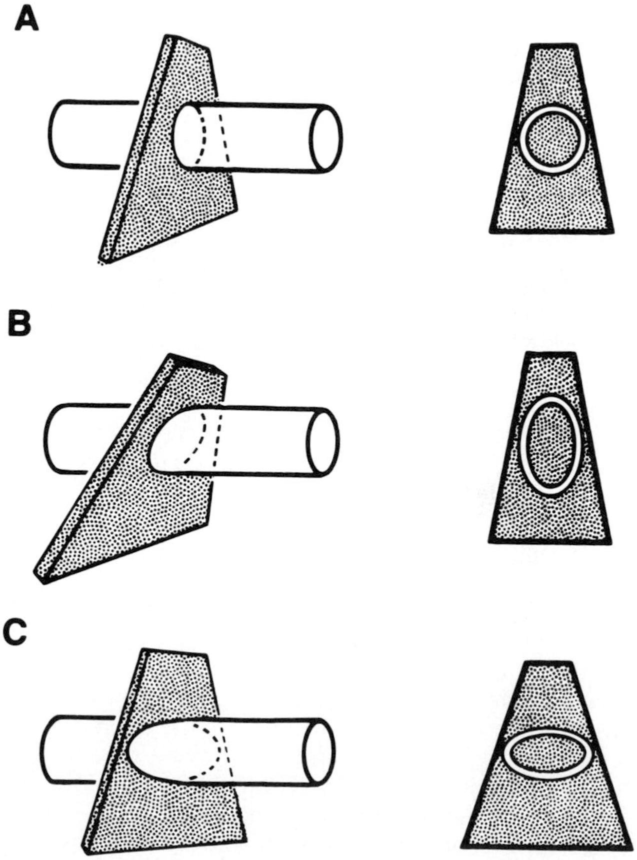

Fig. 4–20. A. Circular image recorded when a plane transects a cylinder parallel to its short axis. **B.** Vertically elongated image recorded when a plane passes through a cylinder at an angle to its short axis. **C.** Horizontally elongated image recorded when a plane is abnormally rotated relative to the short axis of the cylinder.

image gradually increase (Fig. 4–20B). The horizontal dimension, however, remains constant. Thus, improper angulation relative to the short axis results in an increase in vertical obliquity of the image. Conversely, when the imaging plane is rotated either clockwise or counterclockwise from the true short axis plane, the horizontal diameter of the image increases, and the vertical diameter remains the same (Fig. 4–20C). Thus, improper angulation of the transducer relative to a true short axis plane results in gradually increasing vertical obliquity, whereas improper rotation results in horizontal obliquity. To determine transducer position, one must again resort to some external reference. Figure 4–21 illustrates the type of distortion that can be produced in a normal ventricle, when the plane is inappropriately angled and rotated. In this example, the appearance of an aneurysm in the medial wall of the ventricle is created simply by improper plane alignment.

Finally, Figure 4–22 illustrates the image recorded when the examining plane is directed through the cylinder from its left base. When the imaging plane is aligned along the long axis of the cylinder, the echoes from its margins are parallel to one another. Rotating the imaging plane does not alter the image, and, hence, the degree of rotation of the plane must be determined from some external reference. Angling the plane, however, causes the echoes at the distal end of the image to curve inward toward one another, thereby indicating that the plane is no longer parallel to the long axis of the cylinder. Transducer position can be defined in this orientation by moving the transducer in an inferior-superior and medial-lateral direction until the distance between the echoes at the apex of the sector is as large as possible. When the distance between these echoes is the greatest,

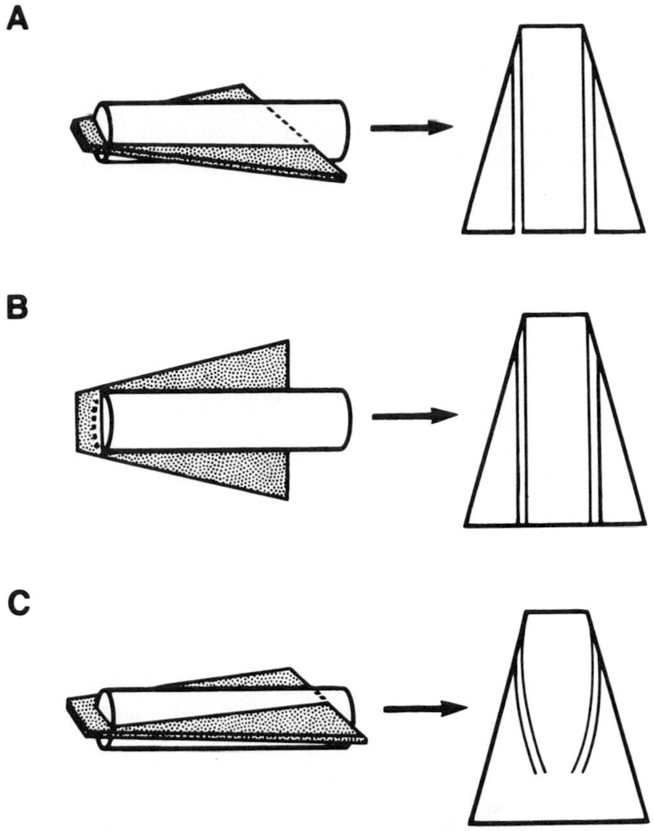

Fig. 4–22. **A.** Image recorded when a plane passes through a cylinder from apex to base through its long axis. **B.** The plane has been rotated; however, it remains parallel to the long axis and therefore, the image is unchanged. **C.** The plane has been angled above the long axis, and the image from the margins of the cylinder at the base of the scan plane begins to taper inward.

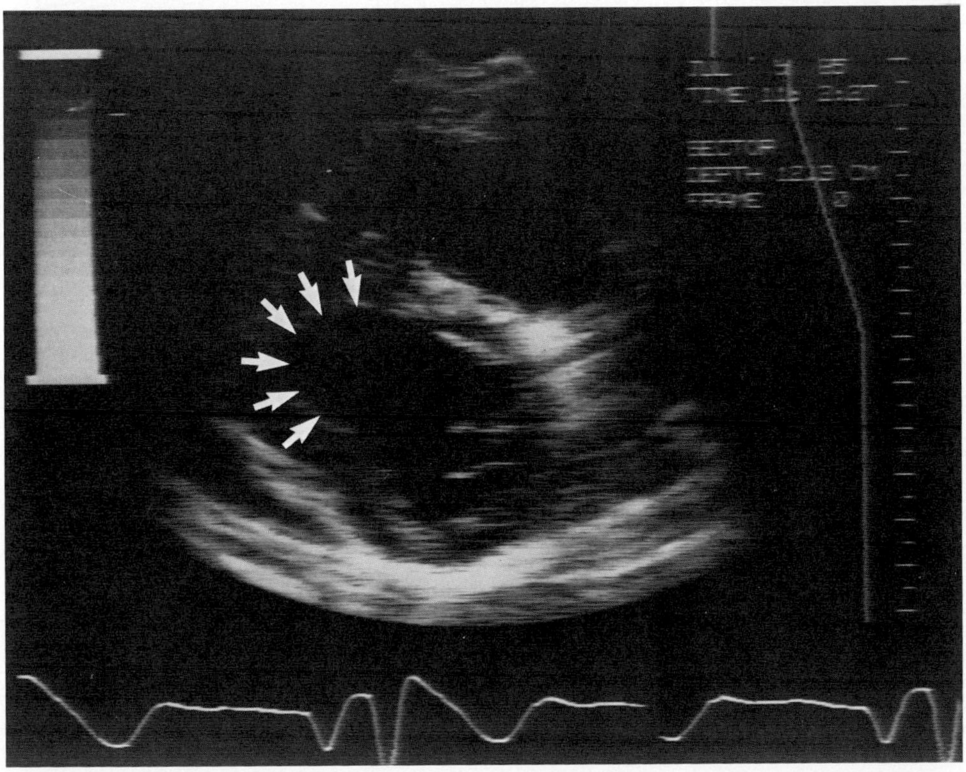

Fig. 4–21. The types of extreme artifact that can be created as a result of inferior transducer rotation and angulation. In this case, the plane passes obliquely through a normal left ventricle, creating the appearance of a ventricular aneurysm.

the transducer is lying over the true center of the base of the cylinder.

To record an appropriate image in this transducer orientation, the examiner must initially define the transducer location and then must angle the plane in an inferior-superior orientation until the maximal diameter of the image at the base of the sector is recorded. The degree of rotation of the plane can be determined only from an external reference. In each of these examples, two of the three variables in image plane orientation can be determined directly from the image itself. In the first two examples (the long and the short axes), transducer location could not be defined from the image alone. In the apical view, the degree of plane rotation could not be determined.

When recording a cross-sectional study, one can determine transducer location in several ways: (1) from the echocardiographic window over which the transducer is located and (2) from the image itself, by defining the orientation of recorded structures within the image or the position of the imaging plane relative to such anatomic references as the papillary muscles or mitral valve.

Figure 4–23 illustrates the images recorded when the scan plane transects a second simple geometric figure, the sphere. Because the sphere has neither true long nor short axes, the image produced is similar despite transducer location or degree of plane rotation. The only variable that can be directly determined from the image is that the plane passes through the center of the sphere. If the plane is angled either to the left or the right of center, the diameters of the sphere gradually shrink. To determine that the plane is passing through the center of the sphere, therefore, the examiner should sweep the plane from one side of the sphere to the other until the maximal diameter of the sphere is recorded. Both degree of plane rotation and transducer location must be defined by resorting to external references. Relating this illustration to the heart, the atria are relatively spherical structures without natural long or short axes. The long and short axes of the atria, therefore, are derived by relating them to the long and short axes of contiguous structures. Thus, the long axis of the left atrium is in a plane roughly parallel to the long axis of the left ventricle and the aorta. The same is true of the right atrium.

As structures become more complex, the orientation of the imaging plane becomes more difficult to define directly from the structure itself. In such cases, the examiner should seek to determine reproducible image orientation as an alternative to one that might be theoretically optimal. Figure 4–24 illustrates the relationship of an imaging plane to a pyramid with a triangular base. In

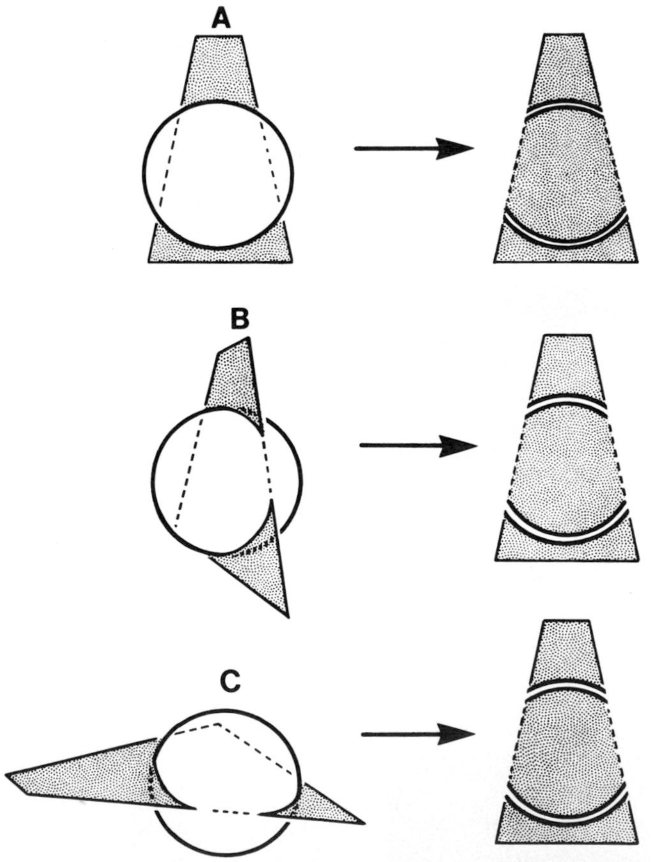

Fig. 4–23. A to **C.** Images obtained when a sphere is transected by a plane passing through its center. Because the spheres axes are symmetric, variation in the direction, rotation, or angulation of the plane does not affect the recorded image as long as the plane passes through the center of the sphere. The only variable that can be determined directly from the image is whether the plane has intersected the true center.

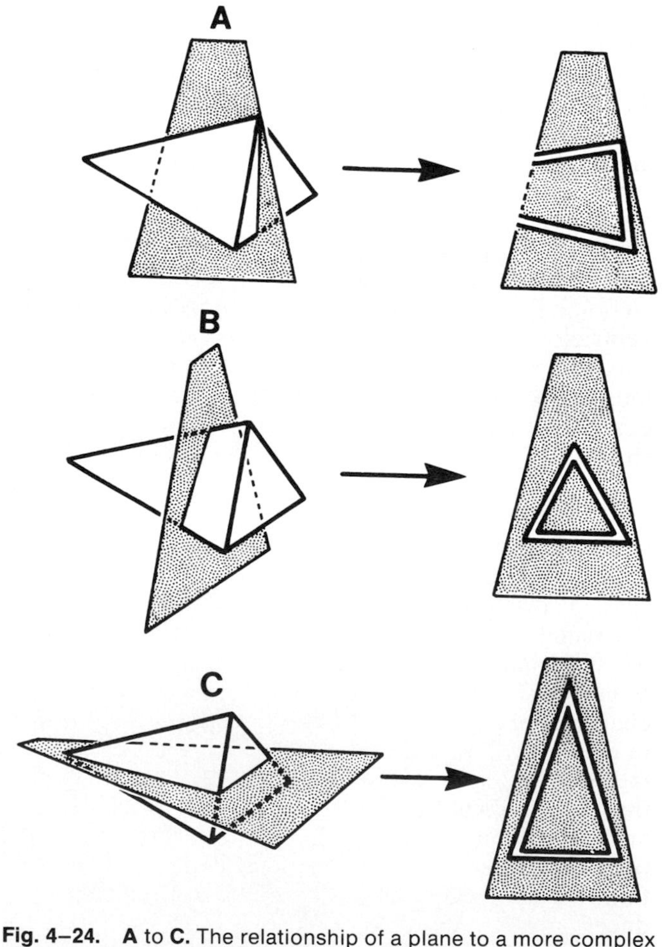

Fig. 4–24. A to **C.** The relationship of a plane to a more complex figure, the pyramid with a triangular base. The difficulties in aligning the plane relative to such a figure are discussed in the text.

Figure 4–24A, the plane is aligned parallel to the long axis of the pyramid. The plane passes through the base parallel to the long axis at the point where the superior angle is most acute and the height of the base is shortest. Using this reference axis, when the plane is then swung back and forth across the more apical segment of the pyramid, it crosses the long axis at a point where the length at the left margin of the sector is greatest. This type of orientation is difficult to achieve from the image itself, particularly when the structure is not perfectly symmetric.

Figure 4–24B illustrates a short axis recording of the same structure. By assuming that the three sides of the figure form an equilateral triangle, appropriate angulation can be achieved by sweeping the plane from apex to base of the pyramid until the shortest length of the arms of the triangle is recorded. An appropriate degree of rotation can be defined by rotating the plane until the base of the triangle is at its shortest length and is equal to the two arms. Here again, imaging plane position can be relatively assigned by moving the plane up and down the triangle and observing the changes in size.

Finally, in Figure 4–24C, the imaging plane is directed from the apex of the triangle toward the base and parallel to the long axis. In this example, transducer position relative to the apex can be determined by moving the transducer location until the point where the angle between the two limbs of the triangle at the apex is most acute. Aligning the plane parallel to the long axis from this point, however, is more difficult.

The standardized recording of complex structures can therefore be achieved more easily by relating the orientation of the imaging plane to the axes of contiguous, more easily defined structures or by using internal or external references. For example, the right ventricle is a complicated structure. Aligning the transducer over the apex of the right ventricle is a relatively simple maneuver if one uses the principles previously indicated. Defining plane orientation as it passes through the right ventricle, however, is far easier if one uses the point of maximal tricuspid excursion to define the base of the long axis rather than attempting to determine plane orientation based on observed changes in right ventricular shape.

The use of internal or external references can be invaluable in fine plane positioning. Figure 4–25 illustrates how these references can be used to examine an irregularly shaped structure. The example used here is a pear-shaped structure with a seed pod in the center. Aligning the plane parallel to the long axis of the pear, based on the distance between contralateral walls, is helpful. Because of the irregularity of the structure, however, change in angle may not be reflected by large variations in dimension, and, hence, lack of precision in position is possible. By aligning the plane such that it passes through both walls at a roughly maximal dimension and, at the same time, passes through the seed pod, one can obtain a precise, reproducible plane orientation. In addition, the irregularity of the figure helps to define transducer location because the area of the pear through which the imaging plane passes can be defined relative to the position of the seed pod.

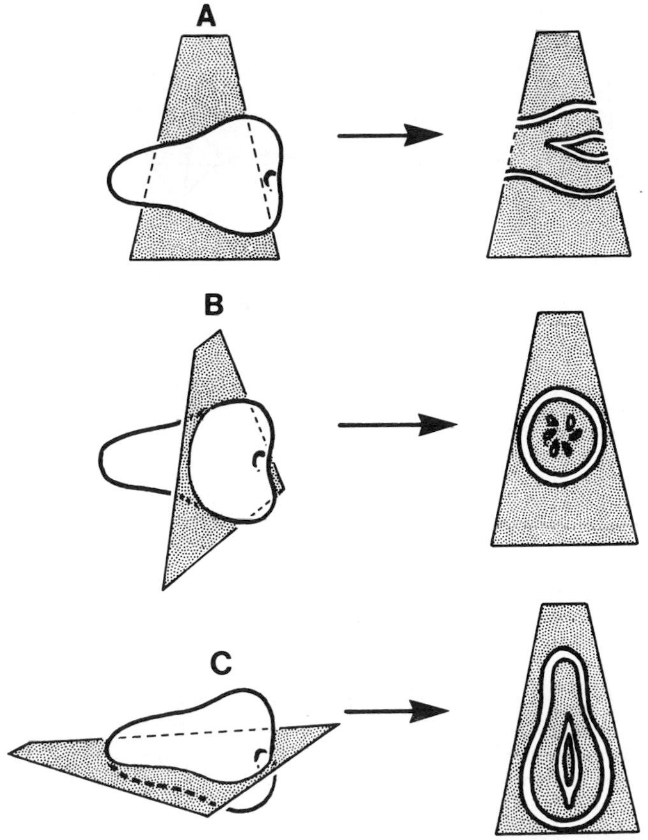

Fig. 4–25. Diagrams depict the images obtained when a plane passes through a structure with an internal reference—in this case, a pear with an internal seed pod. The single internal reference is invaluable because it permits one to define the position of the plane along the long axis (A), the orientation of the plane relative to the short axis (B), and the elevation of the plane (C). When the position of the transducer is known and two internal or external references can be defined, the plane can be positioned precisely in space.

Figure 4–25B illustrates a similar relationship for the short axis. Here the short axis orientation of the plane can be defined by angulation and rotation until the point of least horizontal and vertical obliquity is determined. Again, resorting to the position of the seed pod, the imaging plane can be easily determined to pass through the pear in a short axis orientation at the level of, or above or below, the seed pod and, hence, can be more precisely defined. Finally, relating this illustration to the apical view, the position of the seed pod presents a simple reference that is helpful in determining the degree of imaging plane angulation required to transect the long axis. Here again, the degree of plane rotation cannot be assigned even using this centrally located transducer reference. If a second pear were placed next to the first and the imaging plane adjusted so that it passed through the seed pods of both pears, the position of the plane would be precisely defined. Although plane positioning can usually be achieved without resorting to internal or external references, such references make this process easier.

Figure 4–26 illustrates how these simple figures can be related to the individual cardiac structures. The pul-

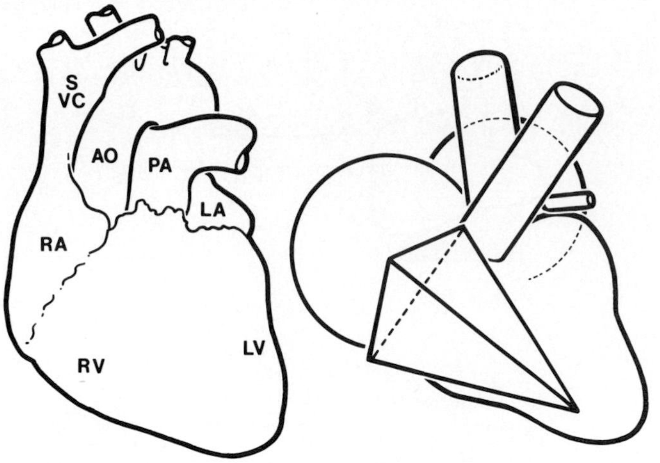

Fig. 4–26. Combination of simple figures represents the primary chambers and vessels of the heart. The principles used in recording the simple figures apply to the recording of each of the major areas of the heart. SVC = superior vena cava; AO = aorta; PA = pulmonary artery; LA = left atrium; RA = right atrium; RV = right ventricle; LV = left ventricle.

monary artery, aorta, and left main coronary artery are all cylindric in configuration. When examining these structures, a long axis view is customarily recorded first. This recording is achieved by (1) directing the central ray of the imaging plane toward the structure to be examined; (2) rotating the imaging plane until the echoes from the anterior and posterior margins of the vessel are as parallel to one another as possible; and (3) sweeping the plane back and forth across the vessel, parallel to the long axis, until the distances separating the linear echoes at the margins of the scan are as large as possible. In this manner, the plane is initially directed toward the arterial vessel, aligned parallel to its long axis, and then angled so that it passes directly through the long axis. Transducer location can then be varied, and these steps can be repeated to orient the imaging plane relative to the particular area of the vessel desired. These principles are applicable whether the vessel is oriented directly perpendicular to the path of the imaging plane or placed at an angle to this plane.

The same principles apply when recording a short axis view. The central ray is initially directed toward the structure. The imaging plane is then angled inferiorly to superiorly until the least vertical obliquity is recorded. It is then rotated in a clockwise to counterclockwise fashion until the least horizontal obliquity is achieved. The relationship of the plane to the short axis of the vessel is then defined by the use of internal or external references.

Similar principles can be applied to the examination of the left ventricle. The parasternal long axis is recorded when the ventricular dimensions at the left and right margins of the scan plane are the greatest and the plane has been angled back and forth across the ventricle to ensure that it passes parallel to, and through, the long axis. The plane position can be confirmed by ensuring that it passes between but does not record echoes from the papillary muscles and by optimizing it such that it passes through the mitral valve at the point of maximal mitral leaflet excursion, which should correspond to the midportion of the mitral valve. Short axis views are again optimized by defining the plane position with the least horizontal or vertical obliquity and by orienting the position at which the plane passes through the ventricle by the use of internal references, such as the mitral valve apparatus, the papillary muscles, or the apical segment distal to the papillary muscles.

The apical view can be recorded using the same principles. The transducer location is first defined either by moving the probe about the apex until the point of most acute angulation of the myocardium is observed or by stepping the transducer down the short axis to a point where the circular ventricle disappears, which should represent the true anatomic apex, and then angling the central ray toward the base of the heart. Orientation of the plane parallel to the long axis can be confirmed by angling the beam in a superior-inferior direction until the diameter at the base of the ventricle is greatest. The rotation of the plane is defined using internal or external references, such as the combined mitral and tricuspid valves, which, in addition to the cardiac apex, form the three points necessary to orient the plane in space.

Using these principles, one can reliably and reproducibly position the imaging plane such that chamber dimensions, wall motion, and structure abnormalities can be precisely recorded and their validity ensured. The imaging plane can only be related to a specific structure of interest. Recording multiple structures optimally from the same plane position is difficult, if not impossible.

The foregoing discussion has been directed primarily to the steps involved in initiating the cross-sectional examination and recording the first imaging plane. The total examination is nothing more than a collection of images recorded from a family of imaging planes. The steps involved in recording each of these planes, from the first to the last, are identical, and the processes involved in recording each subsequent plane are similar to those involved in recording the initial image.

REFERENCES

1. Weyman AE: Clinical application of cross-sectional echocardiography. *In* M deVlieger, et al. (eds.): Handbook of Clinical Ultrasound. New York, John Wiley & Sons, 1978.
2. Kisslo J, Von Ramm OT, Thurstone FL: Cardiac imaging using a phased array ultrasound system. Part II: Clinical technique and application. Circulation 53:262, 1976.
3. Sahn DJ, et al.: The validity of structure identification for cross-sectional echocardiography. J Clin Ultrasound 2:201, 1974.
4. Kotler MN, Mintz GS, Segal BL, Parry WR: Clinical uses of two-dimensional echocardiography. Am J Cardiol 45:1061, 1980.
5. Kloster FE, et al.: Multiscan echocardiography. Part II: Technique and initial clinical results. Circulation 48:1075, 1973.
6. Von Ramm OT, Thurstone FL: Cardiac imaging using a phased array ultrasound system. Part I: System design. Circulation 53:258, 1976.
7. Eggleton RC, et al.: Visualization of cardiac dynamics with real-time, B-mode ultrasonic scanner. *In* White D (ed.): Ultrasound in Medicine I. New York, Plenum, 1975.
8. Edler I: Ultrasound cardiogram in mitral valvular diseases. Acta Chir Scand 111:230, 1956.
9. McDicken WN, Bruff K, Paton J: An ultrasonic instrument for rapid B-scanning of the heart. Ultrasonics 13:269, 1974.
10. Bom N, et al.: Ultrasonic viewer for cross-sectional analysis of moving cardiac structures. Biomed Eng 6:500, 1971.
11. Meyer RA: Pediatric Echocardiography. Philadelphia, Lea & Febiger, 1977.

12. Goldberg SJ, Allen HD, Shan DJ: Pediatric and Adolescent Echocardiography. Chicago, Year Book Medical Publishers, 1975.
13. Reigenbaum H: Echocardiography, 4th Ed. Philadelphia, Lea & Febiger, 1976.
14. Chang S: M-mode Echocardiographic Techniques and Pattern Recognition. Philadelphia, Lea & Febiger, 1976.
15. Kossoff G: The transducer. *In* M deVlieger (ed.): Handbook of Clinical Ultrasound. New York, John Wiley & Sons, 1978.
16. Somer JC: Transducer arrays. *In* deVlieger M (ed.): Handbook of Clinical Ultrasound. New York, John Wiley & Sons, 1978.
17. Henry WL, et al.: Report of the American Society of Echocardiography Committee on nomenclature and standards in two-dimensional echocardiography. Circulation 62:212, 1980.
18. Chang S, Feigenbaum H: Subxyphoid echocardiography. J Clin Ultrasound 1:14, 1973.
19. Webster's New Collegiate Dictionary. Springfield, MA, Merriam Co., 1977.

CHAPTER

5

STANDARD PLANE POSITIONS—STANDARD IMAGING PLANES

A small group from the almost limitless number of possible cross-sectional imaging planes and display formats has been used so commonly in clinical studies that is has become recognized as a standard.[1–10] The recognition and use of these standardized image formats have many advantages because they (1) facilitate communication along individual users and laboratories, (2) permit reproducible data recording for serial comparison of individual patients or groups of patients, (3) aid in structure recognition, and (4) provide a format that can be consistently and easily taught to experienced and inexperienced users. In addition, they contain the vast majority of data required in any echocardiographic examination and permit most important structures to be viewed from several different vantage points.

The standard imaging planes are designated on the basis of (1) transducer location; (2) spatial orientation of the imaging plane, which is a combination of both the angle and degree of rotation of the plane, and (3) structure(s) recorded.[11] Thus, a plane recorded with the transducer in a parasternal location and the imaging plane orientation parallel to the long axis of the left ventricle would be termed a parasternal long axis of the left ventricle.

When applied to individual planes, these descriptors may be fairly general. As a result, a family of planes, rather than a specific plane, can be included within one standard plane designation. For example, when the transducer is described as in a parasternal location, it may be positioned anywhere from the second to the sixth intercostal spaces and from the immediate left sternal border to the anterior axillary line. Even when the angle and degree of rotation of the plane are constant, movement of the probe within these broad boundaries can generate a large series of parallel planes that would fall within this category. The same latitude is present in the apical and subcostal locations. Because of the anatomic limitations of this window, only the suprasternal designation defines probe position more precisely.

The description of general plane orientation relative to a particular set of reference axes likewise contains considerable latitude. Plane orientation can first be described in relation to several references including (1) the anatomic planes of the body, (2) the heart as a whole, or (3) the individual structures within the heart. Each of these methods has advantages and disadvantages, and the relationships of the standard imaging planes to each of these references are considered in this chapter. However, because final precise plane position must be related to the particular structure of interest, I prefer to describe and name the standard planes in a similar fashion. In most instances, the axes of the individual cardiac structures are similar to those of the entire heart, and a description based on either standard would be the same. There are several exceptions to this rule (e.g., the right ventricular outflow tract and left main coronary artery) in which these axes are not the same. In these circumstances, plane orientation is related to the axes of the individual structure.

Planes that pass through any axis of a structure may intersect that axis from any direction through a full 360° arc. The addition of the transducer location defines this intersection more narrowly, but it can be positioned precisely only by relating plane position to specific internal references. As a result, a plane that passes through the left ventricular long axis from a parasternal transducer location is probably defined within only a 90° arc, whereas a parasternal plane that passes through the long axis of the left ventricle and splits the papillary muscles is defined within narrow limits. Finally, even the designation of the structure to be examined may be fairly general. Thus, a plane parallel to the short axis of the left ventricle may transect that chamber at any level from the apex to the base and, as in the aforementioned examples, must also be more specifically defined by resorting to internal references. In this chapter, a method is described for precisely and reproducibly positioning each standard plane discussed.

The standard imaging planes described in this section are listed in Table 5–1. These planes are grouped initially by the transducer location from which they are recorded. They are then subgrouped on the basis of plane orientation and, finally, are related to the structure in question.

This listing of standard planes is not intended to be exhaustive. Other more inclusive systems have been devised, and additional planes have been described by individual authors.[1,2] This list does include, however, the planes that are most commonly used in routine clinical cross-sectional echocardiography and that contain the majority of the data required in any examination.

The concept used to describe each of these planes can be compared to photographing a ship on the horizon. When the ship is properly framed, the sea and sky are present in their proper proportions. Similarly, when the primary structures in each plane are correctly recorded, the other areas are naturally present and viewed in their proper perspective. In each series of figures, a reference mark (R) is included so that comparable points on the plane and the display can be related.

Table 5–1. Standard Cross-Sectional Imaging Planes

Parasternal
- A. Long axis
  - 1. Left heart
    - a. Optimized for the aortic valve
    - b. Optimized for the mitral valve and left ventricle
  - 2. Right ventricular inflow tract
  - 3. Right ventricular outflow tract
  - 4. Main pulmonary artery
  - 5. Cardiac apex
- B. Short axis
  - 6. Aortic valve and left atrium
  - 7. Left ventricle (mitral valve level)
  - 8. Left ventricle (papillary muscle level)
  - 9. Left ventricle (apex)

Apical
- 10. Four chamber
- 11. Five chamber
- 12. Two chamber
- 13. Long axis (left ventricle)

Subcostal
- 14. Long axis of the heart
- 15. Long axis of the right ventricular outflow tract

Suprasternal
- 16. Long axis of the aortic arch
- 17. Short axis of the aortic arch

PARASTERNAL LONG AXIS PLANES

Five long axis planes are conventionally recorded from the parasternal transducer location. These planes include the long axis of the left heart, the right ventricular inflow tract, the right ventricular outflow tract, the main pulmonary artery, and the cardiac apex. Because of the large number of structures contained in the parasternal long axis of the left heart, it must frequently be specifically aligned to optimally record certain areas. The two most common subplanes are the parasternal long axis of the aortic root (left ventricular outflow tract) and the parasternal long axis of the mitral valve and left ventricle (left ventricular inflow tract).

The inclusion of the long axis of the cardiac apex in the parasternal group of planes might appear surprising because it is recorded with the transducer close to the cardiac apex. This is done for several reasons. First, the cardiac apex does not generally lie in the same plane as does the left ventricular outflow tract and, hence, is rarely recorded in a parasternal long axis view of the left ventricle, which does include a well-recorded aortic root. When an apparent apex appears, it generally has a rounded configuration and has been termed a "foreshortened apex." This configuration represents the passage of the imaging plane through the diaphragmatic surface of the left ventricle and does not convey information concerning either the structure or the function of the actual cardiac apex, which must be recorded separately.

Second, the parasternal long axis of the apex is recorded by placing the transducer over the anterior wall of the left ventricle slightly above the apical tip. Thus, the transducer is not positioned appropriately to use the apex as a window. In addition, the central ray of the imaging plane is directed in an anteroposterior orientation, similar to that of the parasternal group, rather than upward toward the base of the heart, as occurs in the apical imaging planes. Finally, the apical plane is included as a separate entity to emphasize the importance of this region in patients with ischemic heart disease and to highlight the fact that apical structure and function are best recorded in an anteroposterior plane perpendicular to the long axis of this structure rather than in one of the apical views.

Parasternal Long Axis of the Left Side of the Heart

The parasternal long axis of the left heart is the most important and most frequently recorded of the standard cross-sectional imaging planes. It encompasses most of the primary echocardiographic structures on the left side of the heart (the aortic valve, mitral valve, and interventricular septum) and is oriented such that these structures lie perpendicular to the path of the imaging planes, are optimally reflective, and are recorded using the axial resolution of the imaging system.

This imaging plane is recorded with the transducer placed in a parasternal location, usually in either the third, fourth, or fifth intercostal spaces to the immediate left of the sternum. The best initial point to position the transducer can usually be determined by running the fingertips along the lower left sternal edge until the widest and deepest interspace in this region is defined. The transducer is then placed in this interspace with the central ray of the imaging plane (which is an extension of the long axis of the transducer) directed posteriorly toward the dorsal surface of the thorax. The examining plane is then rotated to align its x axis parallel to an imaginary line running from the right shoulder to the left flank. If the left ventricle is normally positioned, this plane orientation should align the imaging plane parallel to its long axis. Because the left ventricle is generally situated to the left of the sternum, a slight degree of leftward angulation (up to 30°) of the plane (toward the left shoulder) commonly is necessary to direct it through the true long axis of the ventricular cavity. Figure 5–1A illustrates the characteristic spatial orientation of this imaging plane and the path along which it transects the left heart. When displayed, the tip of the sector, indicated by the reference mark (R), is positioned to the lower left on the viewing scope. The left heart therefore appears sectioned from apex to base and viewed from the left shoulder. In this orientation, the right ventricle, which is closest to the transducer, is displayed anteriorly, whereas the left ventricle and left atrium are poste-

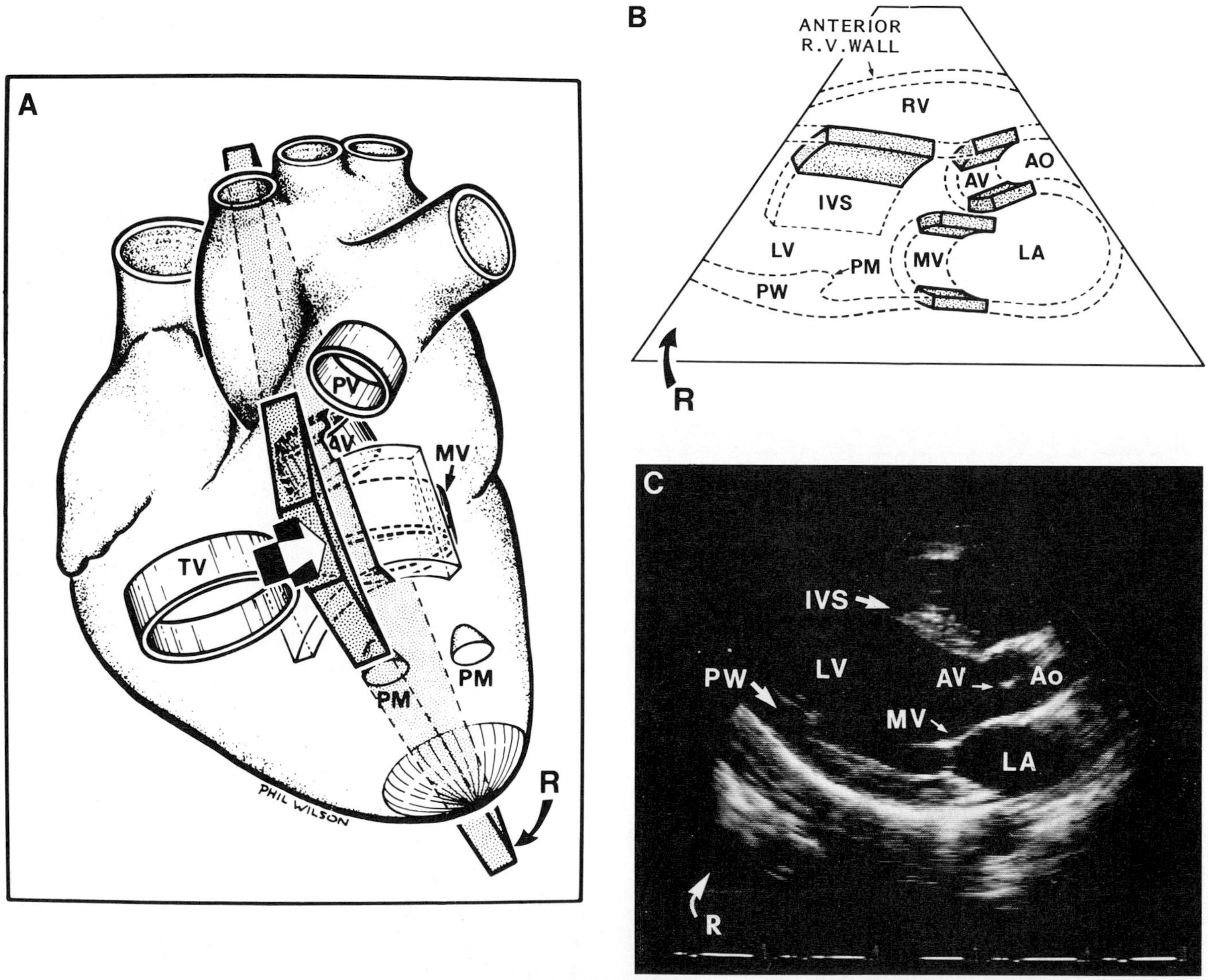

Fig. 5–1. A. The spatial orientation of the imaging plane in the parasternal long axis view of the left heart and the path along which this plane intersects the principal echocardiographic structures in this area. The reference mark (R) indicates the side of the plane that is positioned in the lower left corner of the display scope. PV = pulmonary valve; AV = aortic valve; MV = mitral valve; TV = tricuspid valve; PM = papillary muscles. **B.** The relative positions in which primary and adjacent structures recorded in the parasternal long axis view of the left heart appear on the display scope. The reference mark (R) in this diagram corresponds to the point indicated by the corresponding reference mark in A. AO = aorta; RV = right ventricle; PW = posterior wall of the left ventricle; IVS = interventricular septum; LA = left atrium; AV = aortic valve; MV = mitral valve; LV = left ventricle; PM = papillary muscle. **C.** Parasternal long axis recording of the base of the left heart. The labeling is the same as the preceding figures. (See text for further details.)

riorly positioned. The apex is to the left, and the aorta is to the right.

Figure 5–1B diagrammatically depicts the relative positions of the primary and associated cardiac structures that are recorded in this view. Figure 5–1C is an actual parasternal long axis recording. Beginning anteriorly at the apex of the sector, the chest wall echoes, followed by the moving echoes from the anterior right ventricular wall, are initially recorded. Beneath the anterior right ventricular wall lies a portion of the right ventricular cavity, which continues to the right as the infundibular portion of the right ventricular outflow tract. Continuing clockwise along the right margin of the image, the aortic root and aortic leaflets can be seen. Moving leftward, the anterior margin of the aortic root becomes continuous with the membranous portion of the intraventricular septum, whereas its posterior margin joins the anterior mitral leaflet at the anterior extreme of the left-sided atrioventricular ring. The left atrium lies behind the aortic root, and the posterior left atrial wall is the most posterior cardiac structure normally recorded in this view. Behind the left atrium, an oval, echo-free space is frequently noted. This space is produced by the descending aorta as it courses through the posterior thorax (see Chapter 19). The vessel typically appears oblong because this plane orientation is normally oblique to both its long and short axes. Continuing leftward, the left atrial posterior wall joins the left ventricular posterior wall at the posterior margin of the left-sided atrioventricular ring. In the groove between the atrial and ventricular walls, a circular echo-free space, representing the coronary sinus, occasionally is recorded (see Chapter 18). When the coronary sinus dilates, it may be confused with the larger descending aorta. They can be differentiated, however, by their motion patterns. The descending aorta is extracardiac and, therefore, does not move in concert with the heart, whereas the coronary sinus follows the motion pattern of the atrioventricular ring.

The left ventricular posterior wall extends leftward from the atrioventricular junction to the left margin of the image and can generally be visualized to the level of the papillary muscles. By angling the plane toward the cardiac apex, the examiner may slightly increase the extent of the posterior wall that can be recorded; however, the left ventricular apex normally lies directly beneath the anterior chest wall, one or more interspaces below the transducer level commonly used to record the base of the heart. Thus, except in small hearts, the plane cannot be angled sharply enough to record the cardiac apex. The apex, therefore, must be visualized using a separate view (to be discussed later). Anterior to the posterior left ventricular wall is the large, echo-free left ventricular cavity, which is the largest single structure recorded. Within the left ventricular cavity, the full extent of the anterior and posterior mitral leaflets can be visualized with their chordal attachments to the papillary muscles. Anterior to the left ventricular cavity is the muscular interventricular septum. This structure can be recorded from its junction with the membranous septum directly inferior to the anterior aortic root to a point directly proximal to the cardiac apex.

The number and variety of structures contained within this imaging plane present several problems from both a recording and an interpretive standpoint. First, the examiner's eye cannot simultaneously look at all the moving structures in a 90° image critically. Therefore, in both recording and analysis, the images must be optimized to specific areas.

Second, the long axes of all the structures contained within this view do not normally lie in the same anatomic plane. The long axis of the aorta, for example, is normally oriented at approximately a 30° angle to the long axis of the left ventricle, and hence, plane positioning must be individualized to the particular area of interest to record precisely a true long axis of either of these structures.

Failure to recognize this fact has led to one of the most common errors encountered in cross-sectional imaging. This error arises because most examiners instinctively attempt to align the imaging plane to optimally record the valvular structures at the base of the heart, particularly the aortic valve and the aortic root. The plane must be parallel to the long axis of the aorta to achieve such a recording. Such placement displaces the plane to the right of the long axis of the left ventricle. Consequently, the left margin of the plane passes through the diaphragmatic surface of the left ventricle in the region of the posteromedial papillary muscle. The resulting image depicts the anterior and posterior walls of the ventricle curving toward each other and meeting at the left margin of the scan. This pattern has been referred to as a *foreshortened apex,* or a *truncated apex,* but it clearly does not represent the true cardiac apex and may be displaced from it by several centimeters. Attempts to evaluate apical structure or wall motion or to derive a left ventricular long axis from this record are invalid.

Figure 5–1C, which has been optimized to record the aortic valve, would probably result in such a foreshortened apex if continued to the left. Precise positioning of this plane, therefore, requires that the plane be individually optimized to record the most important structures it contains. Those of major interest include (1) the aortic valve and aortic root, (2) the mitral valve, and (3) the left ventricular chamber.

Precise positioning of the scan plane to record the aortic valve and aortic root is achieved by using the principles described in Chapter 4. First, the plane is rotated until the diameters of the vessel at the annulus and right margin are maximal. This rotation aligns the plane parallel to the true long axis of the aorta. It is then swept across the vessel from the medial to lateral walls to ensure maximal diameters at all points. As a result, the plane passes through the true long axis. This movement permits a quantitative determination of aortic root diameter at all levels and a comparison of diameters at individual levels. It also permits the recording of the maximal excursion of the aortic leaflets.

The long axis of the mitral valve is optimally recorded by angling the scan plane back and forth across the mitral leaflets to define the point of maximal leaflet opening amplitude. Because the valve, when fully opened, parallels the circumferential margin of the left ventricle, the peak amplitude of opening occurs in the midportion of the valve. The point of maximal leaflet opening also should correspond to the maximal left ventricular internal diameter at the base of the heart because the valve orifice is concentrically positioned within the left ventricular cavity.

Alignment of the plane parallel to the long axis of both the left ventricle and mitral valve requires that the internal diameters of the left ventricle be maximal at the mitral valve level and at the left margin of the scan plane. To define the anteroposterior orientation more precisely, the examiner should align the left margin of the plane so that it passes between the two papillary muscles without recording echoes from either muscle. In this fashion, the plane passes through the true long axis of the left ventricle, and its anteroposterior position is defined within narrow limits. It should thus provide information that is both quantitative and reproducible.

The parasternal long axis of the left heart or one of its variations is ideally suited to evaluate the specific anatomic and functional characteristics of a number of structures, including the following:

1. The anterior right ventricular free wall and right ventricular cavity: Right ventricular free wall thickness, thickening, and excursion can be assessed. A right ventricular cavity dimension that correlates roughly with right ventricular size also can be obtained. This measurement, however, cannot be standardized, nor does it correspond to any natural right ventricular dimension. Although this measurement is comparable to the right ventricular dimension commonly recorded in M-mode studies, more representative right ventricular chamber measurements should be sought in other views (see Chapter 28).

2. The aortic root: Aortic root dimensions at multiple levels, from the aortic annulus to the proximal ascending aorta, can be visualized, and changes in aortic configuration characteristic of dilation, aneurysms, or supravalvular stenotic lesions can be appreciated. This view is not particularly useful for detecting sinus of Valsalva aneurysms because each of the sinuses lies outside the scan plane. When sinus of Valsalva aneurysms are large, they may be evident in this view, but, in general, they are better recorded by using a short axis plane at the aortic root level (plane 6).

3. The aortic valve: Aortic leaflet thickening, calcification, reduced leaflet excursion caused by anatomic restriction or disturbed transvalvular flow, doming of the congenitally stenotic valve, valvular vegetations, valvular motion relative to the aorta and left ventricular outflow tract, leaflet disruption, and prolapse can be recorded (see Chapter 19).

4. The left atrium: Left atrial anteroposterior and cranial-caudal dimensions, chamber area, phasic changes in chamber size, atrioventricular ring motion, and intracavitary masses, such as left atrial tumors and occasionally thrombi, can be appreciated (see Chapter 18).

5. The mitral valve: The systolic and diastolic configuration and motion patterns of the mitral leaflets, leaflet thickening, abnormalities of leaflet or chordal attachment, doming of the anterior mitral leaflet in mitral stenosis, the abnormal relationship of leaflet motion to the left ventricular and atrial chambers in anatomic mitral valve prolapse, mitral leaflet vegetations (see Chapter 17), and systolic anterior motion of the mitral valve such as occurs in idiopathic hypertrophic subaortic stenosis (IHSS) (see Chapter 25), can be visualized.

6. The anterobasal portion of the interventricular septum: Septal motion, thickness, systolic thickening, continuity with the anterior root of the aorta, location of the normal hinge point between systolic anterior motion of the basal septum in parallel with the aortic root and the posterior contractile movement of the body of the septum, and ventricular septal defects involving the membranous septum, particularly those associated with aortic overriding, can be appreciated. The ventricular septal defects that occur following acute myocardial infarction usually involve a more posterior portion of the apical septum and, hence, are not seen well in this view (see Chapter 29).

7. The left ventricle: This plane is optimally suited to record the anteroposterior or minor dimension of the left ventricle. This dimension can be optimized at the free edges of the mitral leaflets, or a maximal dimension can be obtained. On occasion, the abnormal intracavitary echoes associated with left ventricular thrombi or tumors can be detected. The majority of thrombi, however, lie in the apical region and are best seen in the long axis of the cardiac apex or one of the apical views (see Chapter 22).

8. The posterior left ventricular wall: Posterior wall motion, thickness, and thickening can be determined (see Chapter 22).

9. The pericardium: The region immediately beneath the left ventricular posterior wall at the base of the (AV) ring represents the most common area for pericardial fluid accumulation. This region is also a common area for tumor infiltration of the pericardium. This view, therefore, is the most important initial imaging plane for evaluating pericardial integrity (see Chapter 35).

10. Mitral-aortic continuity: Abnormal mitral-aortic continuity, which occurs in double-outlet right ventricle (see Chapter 32), or the increase in mitral-aortic separation seen in various forms of fixed discrete subaortic stenosis can be appreciated (see Chapter 19).

11. Coronary sinus size and differentiation of many of the causes of coronary sinus enlargement (see Chapter 18).

Chamber measurements ideally recorded in this view follow:

1. The anteroposterior left ventricular internal dimension or short axis (see Chapter 20).

2. Aortic dimensions at any point from the aortic annulus to the farthest recordable extent of the ascending aorta: The diameter measured at the level of the sinuses of Valsalva, however, depends on the angle at which the plane intersects the sinuses and, hence, is neither as reproducible nor as standardizable as are the other aortic dimensions (see Chapter 19). The aortic annular dimension serves as a reference for outflow tract and in Doppler measurements of cardiac output.

3. Maximal aortic cusp separation: This dimension is recorded in both normal and stenotic aortic valves. Because the orifice may be eccentrically positioned in a stenotic valve, the maximal dimension may not corre-

spond to the true long axis of the vessel and must be sought by scanning the imaging plane from the medial to the lateral walls of the aorta across the area of the stenotic valve (see Chapter 19).

4. The left atrial anteroposterior dimension: The left atrial superior-inferior dimension also can be obtained in this view. Recording this dimension may be easier, however, in an apical four-chamber view because the plane of the AV ring is more easily identified in that projection (see Chapter 18).

5. The atrioventricular ring diameter: This dimension is preferably recorded in this plane rather than in a short axis view because the short axis recording of the annulus is more difficult to standardize.

Measurements that generally cannot be recorded from this view are (1) a long axis of the left ventricle, (2) a short axis of the right ventricle, and (3) a right ventricular outflow tract dimension.

Parasternal Long Axis of the Right Ventricular Inflow Tract

The parasternal long axis view of the right ventricular inflow tract is intended to record the inferior portion of the right atrium, the tricuspid valve, and the basal two thirds of the right ventricle.

This view is recorded with the transducer in the parasternal location in either the third or the fourth intercostal spaces. As a rule, the transducer is moved laterally as far as possible from the sternum while still remaining within the parasternal window. The central ray is angled back beneath the sternum in the direction of the tricuspid valve. The transducer is then rotated approximately 15 to 30° clockwise from the long axis of the left ventricle. This rotation aligns the x axis of the imaging plane parallel to a line running from the right supraclavicular fossa to the left inguinal region. Figure 5–2A illustrates

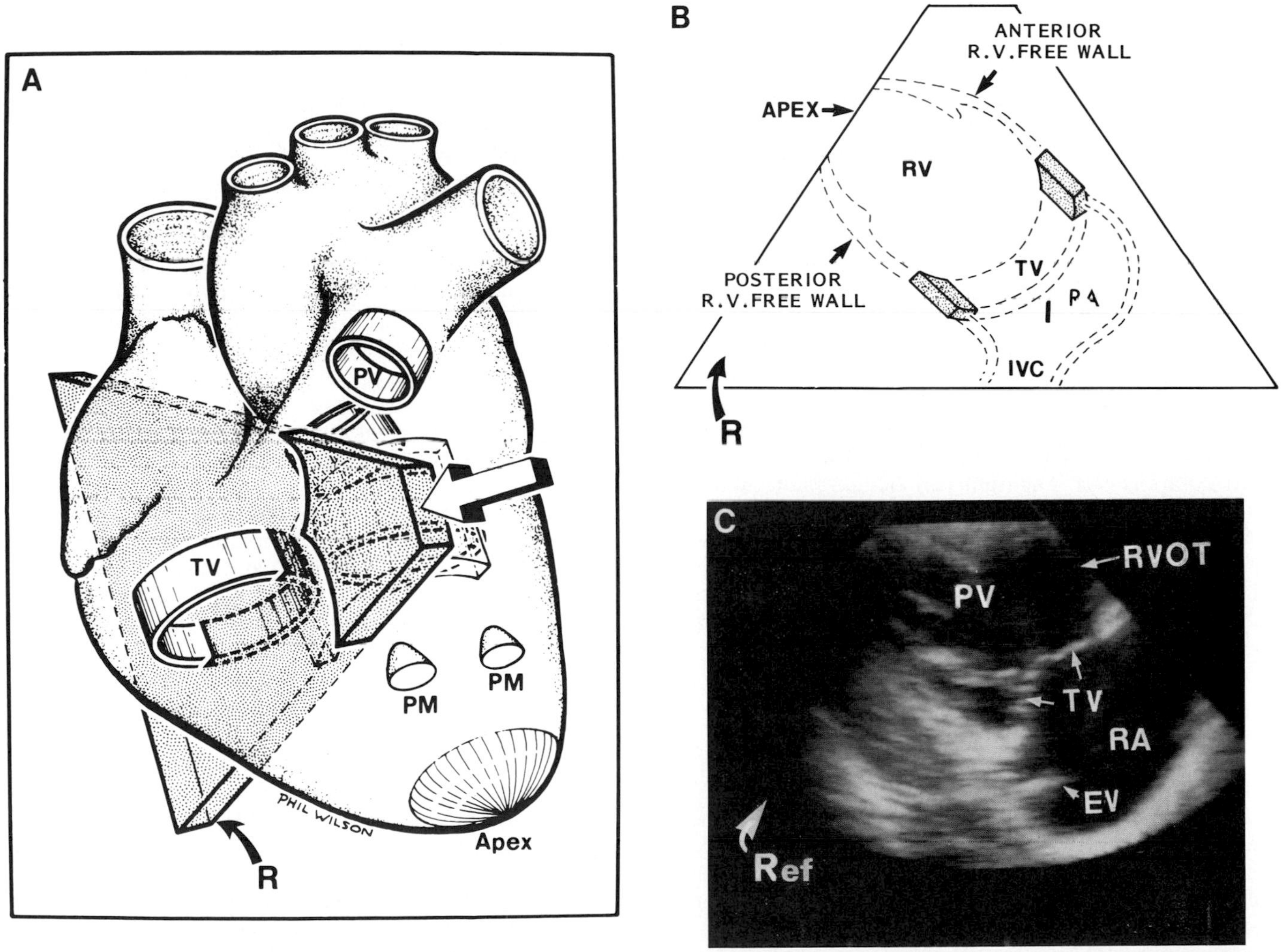

Fig. 5–2. A. The spatial orientation of the imaging plane in the parasternal long axis view of the right ventricular inflow tract. The only primary structure transected by this plane is the tricuspid valve (TV), and the plane is oriented to pass through the center of the tricuspid orifice. R = reference mark; PV = pulmonary valve; PM = papillary muscle. **B.** The relative positions on the display scope of the structures recorded in the parasternal long axis view of the right ventricular inflow tract. R = reference mark; IVS = interventricular septum; RV = right ventricle; TV = tricuspid valve. **C.** Cross-sectional recording of the right ventricular inflow tract including the basal two-thirds of the right ventricle (RV), two of the right ventricular papillary muscles, the anterior and posterior tricuspid valve (TV) leaflets, and the right atrium (RA). In addition, the eustachian valve (EV) and the proximal portion of the right ventricular outflow tract (RVOT), which bulges out from the anterior wall of the right ventricular cavity, also can be visualized. Ref = reference mark.

the spatial orientation of this plane. The only primary structure in this view is the tricuspid valve, and the scan plane is typically positioned such that the tricuspid valve is in its center. Figure 5–2B diagrammatically depicts the path along which this plane transects the right ventricular inflow tract, and Figure 5–2C is an actual long axis recording. In addition to the structures already mentioned, the proximal portion of the right ventricular outflow tract, bulging out from the anterior wall of the right ventricle above the anterior tricuspid leaflet, and the eustachian valve at the entrance of the inferior vena cava also are commonly recorded.

This plane is intended to record only the right ventricular inflow region, and the inclusion of any left-sided structures is inappropriate. The plane is optimized to record the right ventricle and tricuspid valve and is precisely positioned when both the anterior and posterior tricuspid leaflets are visualized at their point of maximal excursion and the right ventricular diameter at the left margin of the scan is maximal. When possible, following the tricuspid leaflets down to their insertion into the anterior and posterior right ventricular papillary muscles can be helpful because this should approximate the right ventricular long axis. Use of standard geometric reference figures to help to define precise positioning of this plane parallel to the right ventricular long axis is difficult because of the unusual shape of this chamber and the changes in its configuration that occur with dilation. As a result, this plane is the most difficult to position precisely.

The parasternal long axis of the right ventricular inflow tract is the best view for evaluating tricuspid leaflet structure and function, particularly doming of the tricuspid valve in tricuspid stenosis and tricuspid vegetations. Prolapse of the anterior and posterior tricuspid leaflets also can be appreciated. This view is useful for detecting right atrial thrombi or tumors and intracavitary right ventricular masses. The right ventricular and right atrial dimensions recorded in this view are difficult to standardize, and hence, right ventricular chamber size is better evaluated in the apical or subcostal views. This view yields neither a true right ventricular long nor short axis dimension. The disorders recorded using this view are discussed in more detail in Chapter 28.

Parasternal Long Axis of the Right Ventricular Outflow Tract

The parasternal long axis view of the right ventricular outflow tract is intended to record the infundibular portion of the right ventricle as it sweeps across the top of the aortic root, the pulmonary valve, and the proximal pulmonary artery. This view is recorded with the transducer placed in the parasternal window in the third or fourth intercostal spaces. It is best obtained with the transducer slightly below the true anatomic position of the right ventricular outflow tract and with the central ray of the imaging plane angled superiorly toward the right shoulder. The imaging plane is rotated approximately 30 to 45° clockwise from the sagittal plane of the body. This rotation places the y axis of the imaging plane parallel to a line running from the inner aspect of the left shoulder to the right flank.

Figure 5–3A illustrates the spatial orientation of this plane and the primary structures through which it passes. Figure 5–3B depicts diagrammatically the region of the heart transected by this plane, whereas Figure 5–3C is a representative recording of this region. When appropriately positioned, the right ventricular outflow tract should appear on the display immediately beneath the chest wall. The pulmonary artery and pulmonary valve should be to the right, and the right ventricle should appear to the left. The aorta is transected obliquely and lies in the center of the scan, whereas the left atrium is posteriorly positioned. The plane is optimally recorded when the diameters of the right ventricular outflow tract are maximal at its proximal and distal extremes, the pulmonary valve is visible, and its motion is appreciated.

This plane is primarily used for assessing right ventricular outflow dimensions and is particularly useful in assessing infundibular diameter in patients with infundibular pulmonary stenosis and tetralogy of Fallot. It is also useful for recording pulmonary valve motion and configuration in patients with valvular pulmonary stenosis and pulmonary vegetations.

Parasternal Long Axis of the Main Pulmonary Artery

The parasternal long axis of the main pulmonary artery is recorded with the transducer in the third intercostal space and the central ray of the scan plane angled superiorly and rotated slightly clockwise relative to the parasternal long axis of the right ventricular outflow tract. This plane is used to evaluate the distal segment of the pulmonary infundibulum, the pulmonary valve, and the main pulmonary artery to its bifurcation. Figure 5–4A illustrates the spatial orientation of this plane relative to the pulmonary artery and valve. Figure 5–4B diagrammatically depicts the path along which this scan plane transects the distal right ventricular outflow tract and main pulmonary artery. Figure 5–4C is a representative recording of these structures. This plane orientation places the proximal portion of the pulmonary artery and the region of the pulmonary valve at the apex of the sector. The pulmonary artery then courses posteriorly along the right margin of the display to its point of bifurcation into the right and left main pulmonary arteries. The pulmonary artery thus appears as if viewed from the cardiac apex. The aorta, which is transected obliquely, lies behind the proximal portion of this vessel and to its immediate left.

This imaging plane is appropriately recorded when the bifurcation of the main pulmonary artery into its two branches is well visualized, the diameter of the main pulmonary artery from the pulmonary valve to the point of bifurcation, is maximal, and the walls of the vessel are parallel. This plane is particularly useful for recording abnormalities of the main pulmonary artery and, in certain cases, is helpful for confirming the diagnosis of valvular pulmonary stenosis.

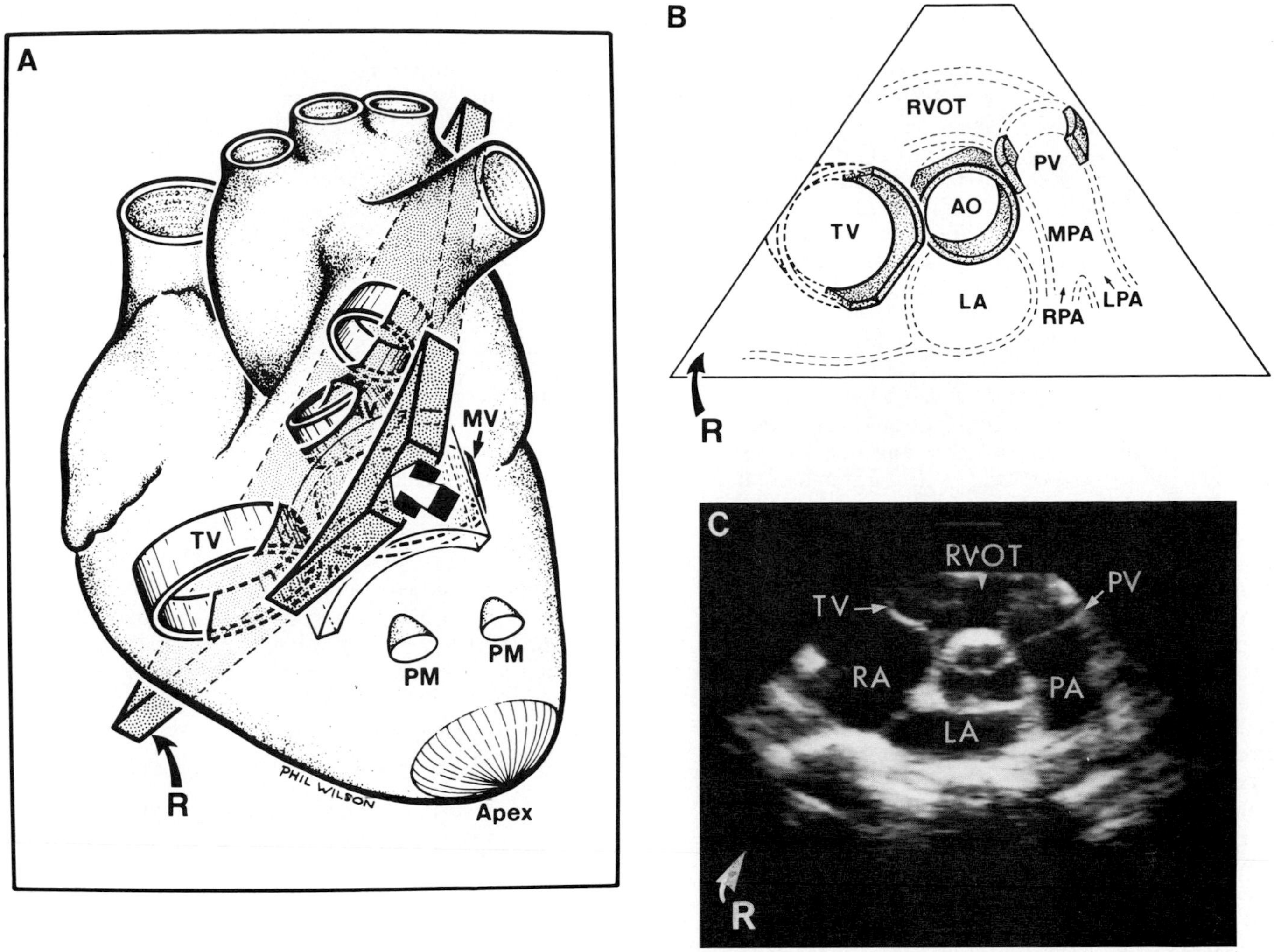

Fig. 5–3. A. The orientation of the imaging plane in the parasternal long axis view of the right ventricular outflow tract. This plane transects the midportion of the pulmonary valve and passes obliquely through the aortic valve (AV) and anterior margin of the tricuspid valve (TV). MV = mitral valve; PM = papillary muscle; R = reference mark. **B.** The relative positions on the display scope of the primary and adjacent structures recorded in the parasternal long axis view of the right ventricular outflow tract (RVOT). The stippled areas indicate the portions of the primary echocardiographic structures through which the imaging plane passes. Because the great vessels cross at their origins, the pulmonary valve (PV) is viewed in a plane that is oblique to their short axes. R = reference mark; LA = left atrium; RPA = right pulmonary artery; LPA = left pulmonary artery; MPA = main pulmonary artery. **C.** Parasternal long axis recording of the right ventricular outflow tract (RVOT). PV = pulmonary valve; PA = pulmonary artery; RA = right atrium; TV = tricuspid valve; LA = left atrium; R = reference mark. (See text for further details.)

Parasternal Long Axis of the Left Ventricular Apex

The parasternal long axis of the left ventricular apex is intended to record specifically the structural and functional characteristics of the apex. It is recorded with the transducer placed on the anterior chest wall above the apical impulse and the central ray directed toward the posterior thoracic wall. The imaging plane is then rotated to align its x axis parallel to the long axis of the left ventricle.

Figure 5–5A illustrates the spatial orientation of this plane. The apical long axis can be located by (1) aligning the imaging plane parallel to the short axis of the left ventricle at the apex (see plane 9, the parasternal short axis of the left ventricular apex); (2) placing the central ray of the imaging plane in the center of the ventricle; and then (3) rotating the plane 90° about its z axis. These steps should align the plane so that it is precisely parallel to the long axis of the ventricle and passes through the tip of the apex. Figure 5–5B diagrammatically depicts the path along which this plane transects the apex, whereas Figure 5–5C is a representative apical recording. The anatomic tip of the apex is displayed anteriorly and to the left. In addition to the apex, the anterior and posterior walls of the left ventricle to the level of the papillary muscles are recorded. This plane is precisely positioned by recording the most acute apical tip (the largest ventricular diameter at the right margin of the scan) and positioning the plane such that it passes between the papillary muscles. Its position relative to the circumference of the ventricle can be cross-checked by

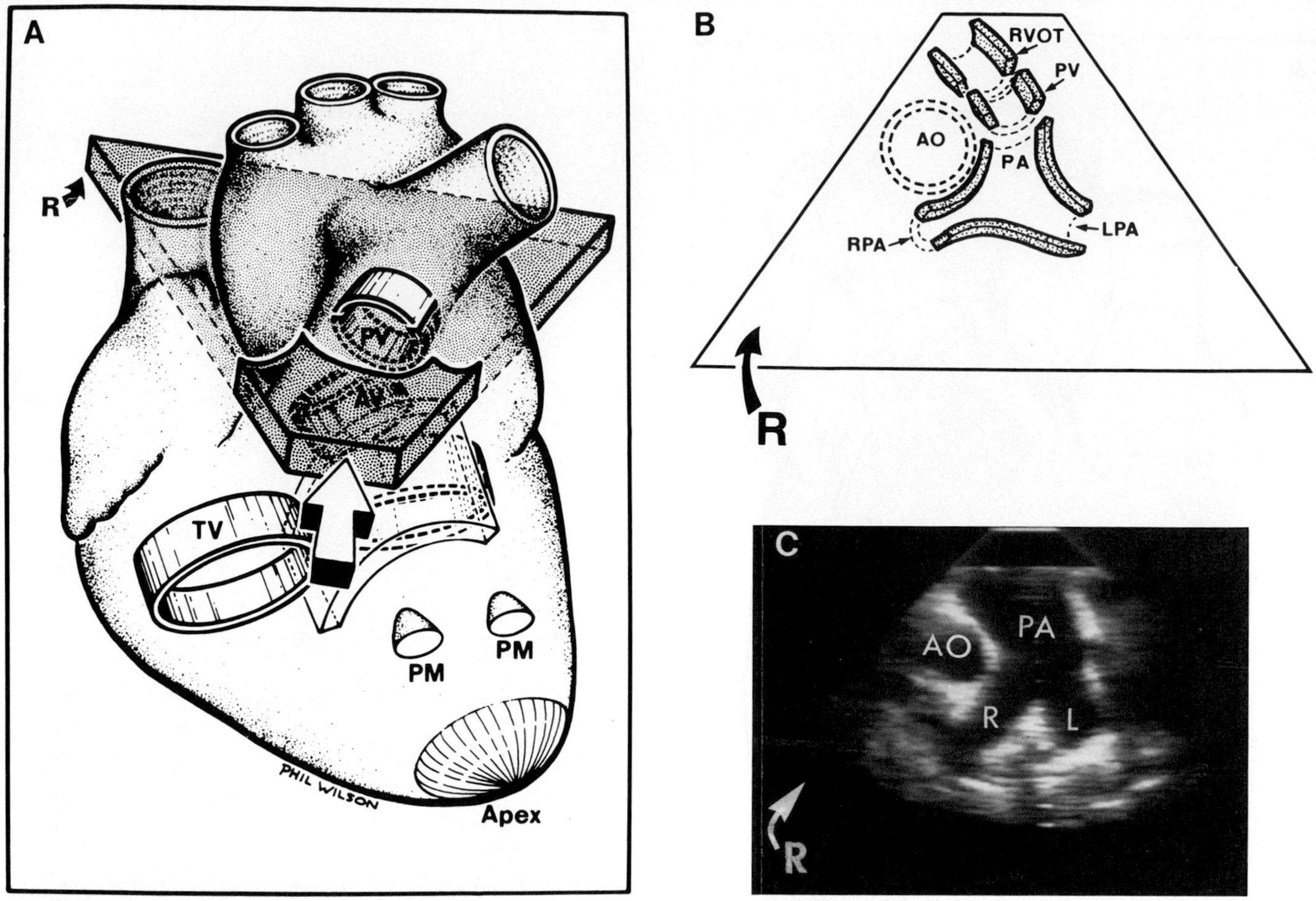

Fig. 5–4. **A.** The orientation of the imaging plane in the parasternal long axis view of the main pulmonary artery. This plane transects the midportion of the pulmonary valve (PV) and continues through the pulmonary artery to its bifurcation. AV = aortic valve; TV = tricuspid valve; PM = papillary muscle. **B.** The relative positions of the pulmonary valve (PV) and adjacent structures as they appear on the display scope in the parasternal long axis view of the main pulmonary artery (PA). The stippled areas indicate the portions of the vessels that are intersected by the imaging plane and, hence, are recorded on the final image. RVOT = right ventricular outflow tract; AO = aorta; LPA = left pulmonary artery; RPA = right pulmonary artery. **C.** Long axis cross-sectional recording of the main pulmonary artery illustrates the proximal right ventricular outflow tract, the region of the pulmonary valve, the main pulmonary artery (PA), and its bifurcation into the right (R) and left (L) pulmonary arteries. The aorta, which is viewed in a plane oblique to its short axis, lies beneath the right ventricular outflow tract and to the left of the main pulmonary artery. R = reference point; AO = aorta.

rotating to the short axis without shifting the position of the z axis or central ray.

This view is optimal for recording apical shape and wall motion. It is useful for detecting apical thrombi and intracavitary tumors involving the apex. However, its primary role is in the detection of apical dyskinesis[12] and aneurysms.[13]

PARASTERNAL SHORT AXIS PLANES

Four standard planes are recorded from the parasternal location with the imaging plane aligned parallel to the short axes of the left ventricle or aorta. These planes are the parasternal short axis of the aorta and left atrium, the left ventricle at the mitral valve level, the left ventricle at the papillary muscle level, and the left ventricular apex. Each of the ventricular planes is oriented parallel to, rather than through, the true short axis of the left ventricle. Their specific point of intersection is designated on the basis of the structures the plane transects. Again, one might argue that the apical short axis view is not truly a parasternal view, but rather an apical view. For reasons similar to those considered in the discussion of the apical long axis view (standard plane 5), this apical short axis is considered a parasternal plane.

The four short axis views are intended primarily to record the left heart. Although portions of right-sided structures are included in each of these views, the planes are not specifically oriented to record these structures optimally.

When the examiner wants to record any of the right-sided structures in their short axis configuration, the transducer can be angled toward the right ventricle and the plane realigned (based on the principles described in Chapter 4) to optimally record the features of the area desired. To date, short axis planes of right-sided structures have not been used frequently enough to be considered standard and, therefore, must be described individually.

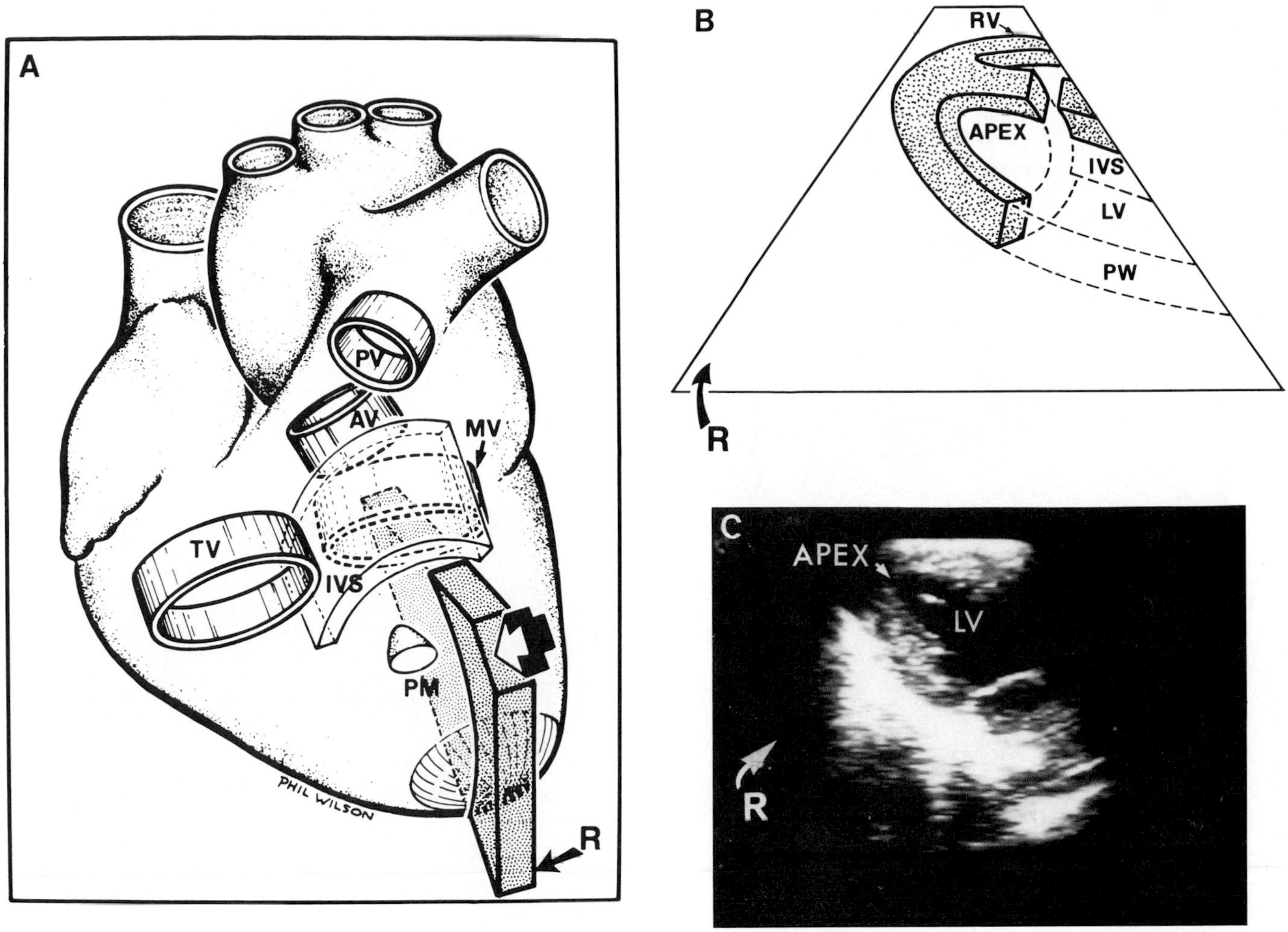

Fig. 5–5. **A.** Diagram illustrates the orientation of the imaging plane in the parasternal long axis view of the cardiac apex. This plane passes through the tip of the left ventricular apex, intersects the long axis of the left ventricle, and passes between the two papillary muscles (PM). PV = pulmonary valve; AV = aortic valve; MV = mitral valve; TV = tricuspid valve; IVS = interventricular septum; R = reference mark. **B.** The relative positions of the structures recorded in the parasternal long axis of the cardiac apex on the display scope. The tip of the apex is displayed to the left. The apical portion of the interventricular septum (IVS) and posterior left ventricular walls (PW) courses to the right from the apical tip. RV = right ventricle; LV = left ventricle; R = reference mark. **C.** Long axis parasternal recording of the left ventricular (LV) apex illustrates the normal apical configuration. R = reference mark.

Parasternal Short Axis of the Aortic Valve and Left Atrium

The parasternal short axis of the aortic valve and left atrium is recorded with the transducer in the third or fourth intercostal spaces to the immediate left of the sternum. The central ray of the imaging plane is directed either posteriorly toward the dorsal surface of the body or angled slightly rightward and superiorly toward the right shoulder. The plane is then rotated 90° clockwise from a parasternal long axis orientation at the aortic root level. This rotation places the x axis of the imaging plane parallel to a line extending from slightly beneath the left shoulder to the right subcostal region. The spatial orientation of this plane and the path along which it intersects the primary structures at the base of the heart are illustrated in Figure 5–6A. Figure 5–6B depicts diagrammatically the portion of these structures intersected by the plane and their relative positions on the display scope. The right ventricular outflow tract is transected first and, thus, appears at the apex of the sector with the pulmonary valve to the right and the right ventricle to the left. The aorta appears circular and is positioned in the center of the scan with the left atrium posteriorly behind the aorta. The heart is thus displayed as if viewed from the apex. Figure 5–6C is an actual short axis recording of the aortic root and surrounding structures. This imaging plane, although similar to that used in recording the long axis of the right ventricular outflow tract and the long axis of the left main coronary artery, lies midway between the two.

Recording of this plane is optimized to the short axis of the aortic root at the aortic valve level. Optimal alignment of this plane as with other short axis planes is achieved by angling and rotating the transducer until the aortic root shows the least degree of vertical and horizontal obliquity and the aortic leaflets are recorded in as much detail as possible.

This imaging plane is best for recording specific features of (1) the aortic valve, including the aortic valve

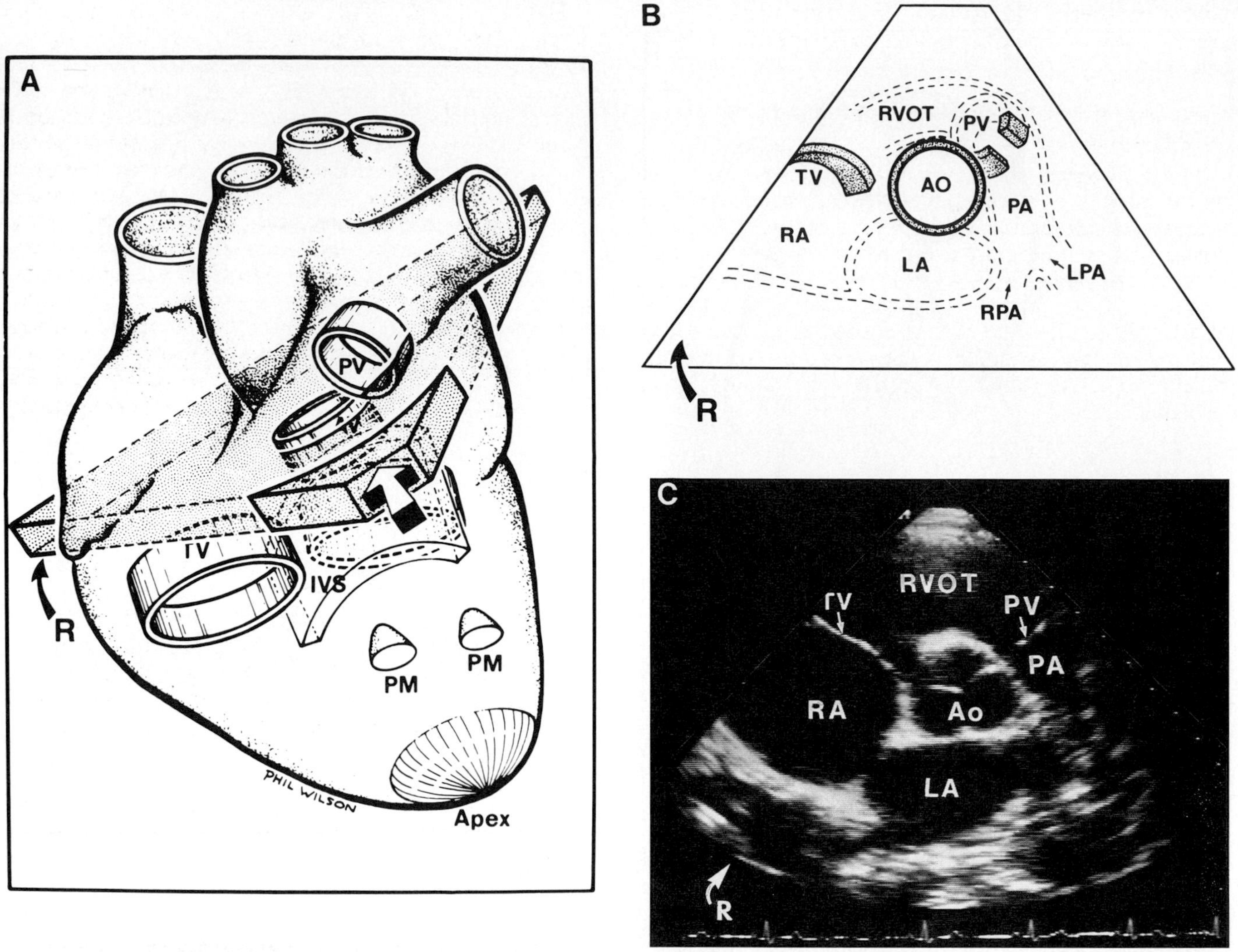

Fig. 5–6. **A.** The spatial orientation of the imaging plane in the parasternal short axis view of the aortic root and the left atrium. This plane passes through the aortic valve (AV) parallel to its short axis and passes obliquely through the inferior margin of the pulmonary valve (PV). The point of the sector indicated by the reference mark (R) is displayed at the lower left margin of the display scope. Structures recorded in this plane are therefore displayed as though viewed from the cardiac apex. TV = tricuspid valve; IVS = interventricular septum; PM = papillary muscle. **B.** The primary and adjacent cardiac structures that are recorded in the parasternal short axis view of the aortic root (AO) and left atrium (LA). Their relative positions on the final display are also evident. R = reference mark; RA = right atrium; TV = tricuspid valve; RVOT = right ventricular outflow tract; PV = pulmonary valve; PA = main pulmonary artery; LPA = left pulmonary artery; RPA = right pulmonary artery. **C.** Parasternal short axis recording of the aorta (Ao) and LA. The aorta, which is transected parallel to its short axis, appears as a circular structure in the center of the scan. The left atrium (LA) lies directly behind the aorta, and the RVOT crosses above the aorta from left to right. A portion of the tricuspid annulus is recorded separating the right ventricle and atrium, whereas the interatrial septum, stretching posteriorly and to the left from the posteromedial border of the aorta, separates the left (LA) and right atria (RA). PV = pulmonary valve; R = reference mark.

orifice, the number and orientation of the aortic leaflets, the position of the aortic commissures, the definition of aortic leaflet movement, and the degree of leaflet involvement with bacterial vegetations; (2) the aortic root, specifically the determination of the size of the sinuses of Valsalva and the presence or absence of aneurysms (it also may be helpful in detecting aortic dissection); (3) the left atrium, including atrial tumors or thrombi; an anteroposterior atrial diameter, which can be correlated with the anteroposterior dimension recorded in the long axis view; a medial-lateral dimension, and a long axis of the coronary sinus; and (4) the interatrial septum. Although the interatrial septum was first recorded and described using this view,[13,14] better visualization of the septum is obtained using either the apical four-chamber[9] or the subcostal planes.[7,8] The parasternal short axis is useful, however, for recording changes in anteroposterior atrial septal position and orientation in both left and right atrial enlargement. It also can be used to detect ostium primum and ostium secundum atrial septal defects and to observe contrast flow along the septum; however, it is not optimal for either of these tasks.

The parasternal short axis is also the primary view for assessing the relative position of the great vessels at the base of the heart and the number and orientation of the great vessels in the transposition complexes and truncus arteriosus.

Parasternal Short Axis of the Left Ventricle (Mitral Valve Level)

The parasternal short axis of the left ventricle at the mitral valve level is recorded with the transducer placed in a parasternal location in the third, fourth, or fifth intercostal spaces. The central ray of the scan plane is directed posteriorly or posteriorly and slightly leftward, and the imaging plane is rotated 90° from the long axis of the left ventricle so that it is aligned parallel to the ventricular short axis. This plane orientation is roughly parallel to a line running from the left shoulder to the right flank.

Figure 5–7A illustrates the typical spatial orientation of this plane. It encompasses the entire left ventricle, the mitral valve, and the medial portion of the tricuspid valve. Figure 5–7B diagrammatically depicts the path along which the plane intersects the primary structures at the base of the heart. The relative orientation of the primary structures on the display scope also is shown. The anterior portion of the right ventricle is recorded first and is displayed anteriorly and to the left. Fragments of the tricuspid valve are commonly visible and are recorded along the left margin of the scan. The interventricular septum separating the right and left ventricles lies beneath the right ventricle, is normally concave toward the left ventricle, and anatomically forms a portion of the left ventricular wall. The left ventricle, which appears circular when viewed in short axis is posterior

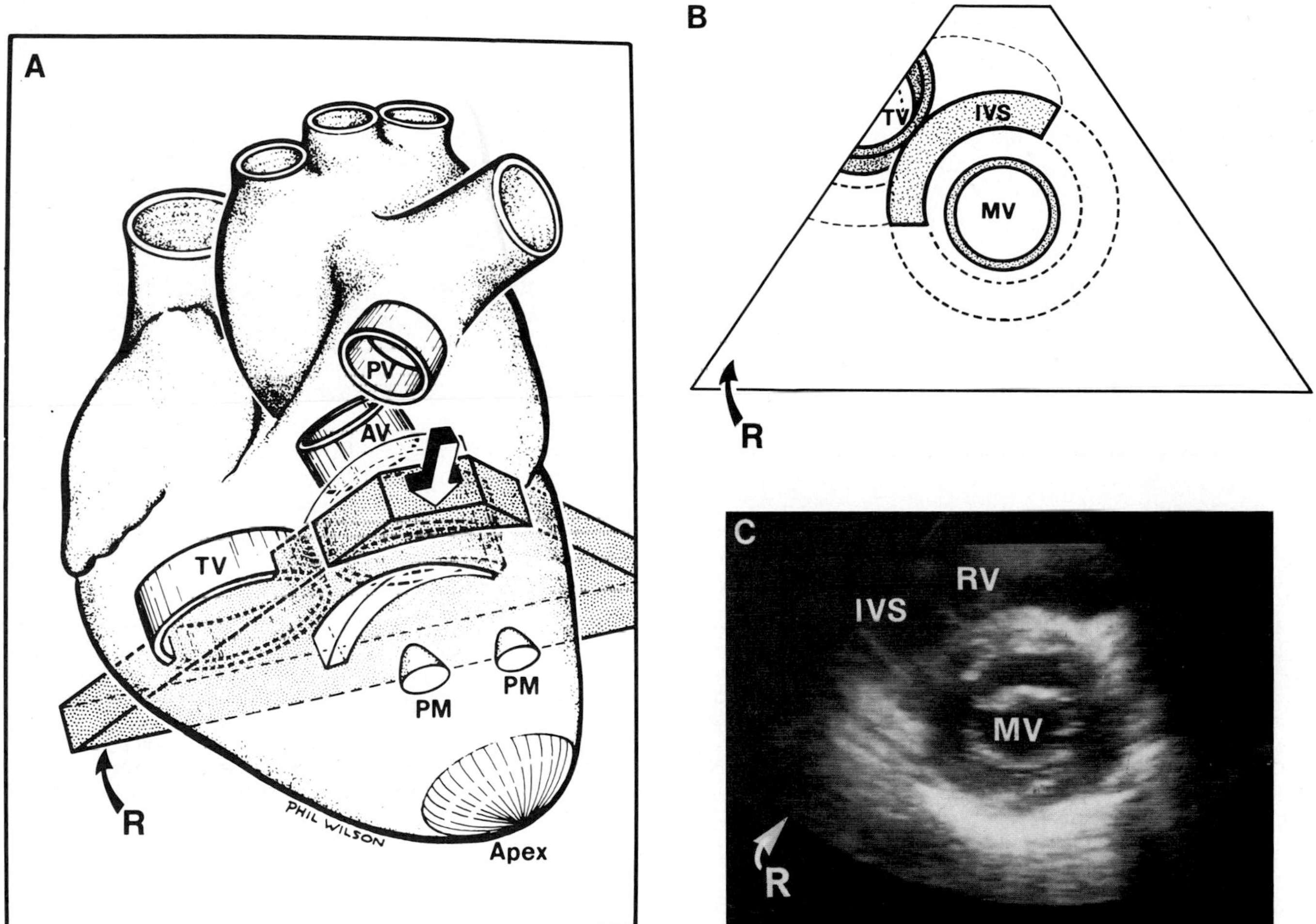

Fig. 5–7. A. The orientation of the imaging plane in the parasternal short axis view of the left ventricle at the mitral valve level. This plane transects the mitral valve in a path parallel to its short axis, the base of the interventricular septum, and the medial portion of the tricuspid valve (TV). R = reference mark; PM = papillary muscle; AV = aortic valve; PV = pulmonary valve. **B.** The relative positions on the display scope of the primary and adjacent structures recorded in the parasternal short axis view of the left ventricle at the mitral valve (MV) level. The medial portion of the tricuspid valve (TV) appears anterior and to the left immediately above the interventricular septum (IVS). The septum is to the left of center; the mitral valve is in the central portion of the scan. The medial anterior and posterior right ventricular walls and the entire circumference of the left ventricle at the base of the heart are also recorded in this view. R = reference mark. **C.** Parasternal short axis recording of the left ventricle at the mitral valve (MV) level. This frame is recorded during diastole, and the mitral valve orifice surrounded by the curvilinear anterior and posterior mitral leaflets can be appreciated. The mitral valve lies within the left ventricular cavity, which appears circular in this orientation. The medial portion of the right ventricle (RV) and the interventricular septum (IVS) are also evident. R = reference mark.

and to the left. The mitral leaflets are recorded in the center of the left ventricle. The left ventricle, therefore, is displayed as if viewed from the cardiac apex. Figure 5–7C is a representative short axis recording that illustrates the normal appearance and relative positions of these structures.

This plane is optimally recorded when both the anterior and posterior mitral leaflets are well visualized and when the left ventricular cavity shows the least vertical or horizontal obliquity. It is ideal for directly recording the mitral valve orifice and is used clinically to determine mitral valve area in mitral stenosis (see Chapter 17). This view is also useful for examining mitral leaflet redundancy in mitral valve prolapse, detecting the circumferential location of mitral vegetations, visualizing leaflet motion patterns in aortic insufficiency, and viewing incomplete leaflet closure in rheumatic mitral regurgitation.

The total circumference of the left ventricle also can be well recorded, and the absolute and relative patterns and amplitudes of left ventricular wall motion and thickening can be assessed. This plane is also used to detect distortions in left ventricular shape, specifically, anterolateral aneurysms and abnormalities of interventricular septal position and motion. It is the primary plane used for assessing abnormalities in septal configuration in patients with right ventricular volume and pressure overload because the greatest degree of septal deformity and, thus, of left ventricular eccentricity is apparent in this view (see Chapters 20 and 29).

Difficulties arise in attempting to visualize the anteromedial and anterolateral walls of the left ventricle. These two regions lie parallel to the ultrasonic beam, and the endocardial and epicardial targets in these areas are difficult to record. Both ventricular hypertrophy and increased endocardial infolding during systole make these targets easier to visualize. In many instances, however, the high lateral wall of the left ventricle cannot be recorded in this view, thereby making assessment of wall motion in this region impossible.

Parasternal Short Axis of the Left Ventricle (Papillary Muscle Level)

The parasternal short axis of the left ventricle at the papillary muscle level is recorded with the transducer in the fourth or fifth intercostal spaces to the immediate left of the sternum. Transducer position is generally similar to that used to record the short axis of the left ventricle at the mitral valve level. The papillary muscles can be recorded from this location by either angling the scan plane toward the cardiac apex or moving the transducer down one interspace. Plane rotation is identical to that used in recording the short axis of the left ventricle at the mitral valve level.

Figure 5–8A illustrates the orientation of this plane in space. Figure 5–8B diagrammatically depicts the path along which this plane intersects the papillary muscles and adjacent left ventricle. It typically encompasses the entire left ventricular cavity as well as the apical segment of the right ventricle. In this orientation, the right ventricle is displayed anteriorly and to the left. The interventricular septum is beneath the right ventricle, and the left ventricle is posterior. The papillary muscles are recorded along the medial and lateral walls of the left ventricular cavity. The posteromedial papillary muscle is displayed to the left, and the anterolateral papillary muscle is to the right. This plane, like all other short axis planes, is displayed as if viewed from the apex. Again, as with other short axis planes, fine plane positioning is achieved by alternately angling and rotating the plane until the least degree of horizontal and vertical obliquity is achieved. Both papillary muscles must be recorded because they are the internal reference that defines the final position of the plane. Figure 5–8C is an example of a parasternal short axis recording of the left ventricle.

This imaging plane is optimally suited for recording left ventricular cavity size and myocardial function at the level of the papillary muscles. Assessment of the contractile pattern of the left ventricle at this level is of major importance in patients with ischemic heart disease. In addition, an association has been demonstrated between left ventricular dyskinesis at the base of the papillary muscle and the clinical syndrome of papillary muscle dysfunction resulting from incomplete mitral valve closure. This relationship is discussed in detail in Chapter 17.

Parasternal Short Axis of the Left Ventricle (Apical Level)

The parasternal short axis of the left ventricle at the cardiac apex is recorded with the transducer located on the anterior chest wall above or just proximal to the apical impulse. This location is usually at least one interspace lower than that used to record the papillary muscles. The central ray of the examining plane is directed posteriorly, and the plane is rotated parallel to the orientation used to record the short axis views at the mitral valve and papillary muscle levels.

The spatial orientation of this plane is illustrated in Figure 5–9A. The plane normally transects the left ventricle just proximal to the apex and encompasses the entire circumference of the ventricle at a point midway between the papillary muscles and the apical tip. The only structures recorded at this level are the left ventricular cavity and the surrounding myocardium. A small segment of right ventricle is occasionally observed anteriorly. The position of this plane is defined by the absence of papillary muscles or apical endocardium. As depicted in Figure 5–9B, only the left ventricular wall is typically recorded. Figure 5–9C is a normal apical short axis. As with the other short axis views, precise plane position is achieved by angling and rotating the transducer until the least degree of horizontal or vertical obliquity of the left ventricle is obtained.

This imaging plane is primarily used in conjunction with the long axis and apical views to assess the magnitude and extent of regional dyssynergy. It can also be helpful in detecting apical thrombi and in assessing the degree of circumferential involvement of the apex when an apical aneurysm is present.

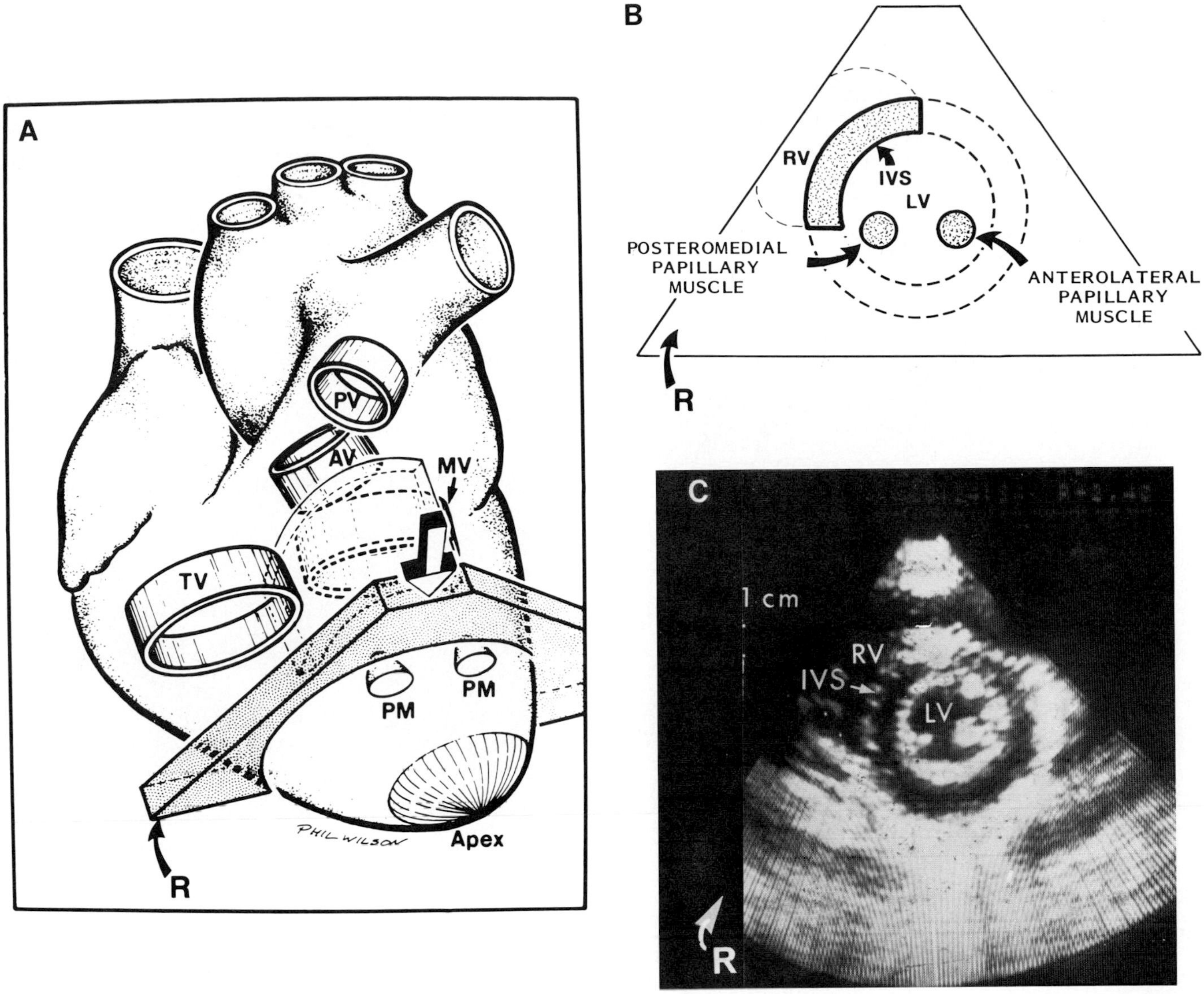

Fig. 5–8. **A.** The imaging plane orientation in the parasternal short axis view of the left ventricle at the papillary muscle (PM) level. This plane transects the entire circumference of the left ventricle, the apical portion of the right ventricle, and by definition, includes both the anterolateral and posteromedial papillary muscles. R = reference mark; TV = tricuspid valve; MV = mitral valve; AV = aortic valve; PV = pulmonary valve. **B.** The relative positions of the primary and adjacent echocardiographic structures recorded in the parasternal long axis view of the left ventricle (LV) as they appear on the display scope. The apical portion of the right ventricle (RV) is anterior and to the left, whereas the circular left ventricular cavity is in the center of the scan plane. The interventricular septum (IVS), which is concave toward the left ventricle, separates the right and left ventricular chambers. The posteromedial papillary muscle is displayed to the left, and the anterolateral papillary muscle is shown to the right. R = reference mark. **C.** Parasternal short axis recording of the left ventricle (LV) at the papillary muscle level. The circular left ventricle is apparent in the center of the scan plane. The right ventricle (RV) is anterior and to the left. The anterolateral and posteromedial papillary muscles can be visualized arising from the endocardial surface of the left ventricular cavity. R = reference mark; IVS = interventricular septum.

APICAL VIEWS

There are four primary apical views: the apical four-chamber, the apical five-chamber, the apical two-chamber, and the apical long-axis views of the left ventricle. Each of these views is recorded with the transducer located directly over the anatomic tip of the cardiac apex and the central ray of the imaging plane directed toward the base of the heart. The apex can be located in two ways. The first method is by palpating the apical impulse and placing the transducer directly over the region of apical activity. Unfortunately, the apical impulse frequently does not overlie the true anatomic apex but is produced by an adjacent area of the anterior left ventricular wall. In other cases, the apex may be distorted or its normal position occupied by structures other than the left ventricle. In these situations, the anatomic apex can be located by sequentially stepping the transducer down the short axis of the left ventricle. As the scan plane approaches the apex, the left ventricular cavity area

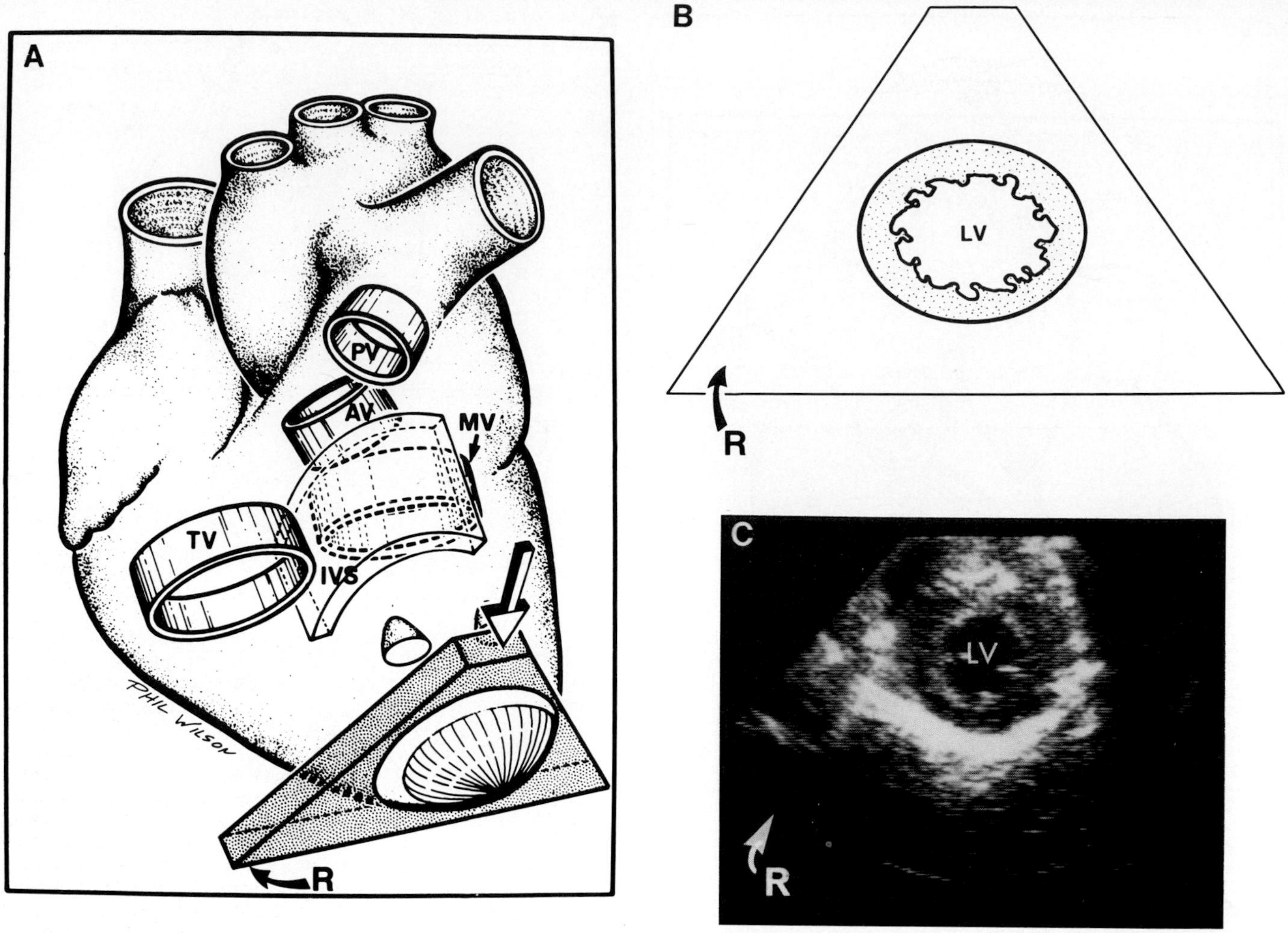

Fig. 5–9. A. The orientation of the imaging plane in the parasternal short axis view of the cardiac apex. This plane transects the ventricle midway between the papillary muscles and the tip of the anatomic apex. On occasion, a small portion of the apical segment of the right ventricle and the apical extreme of the interventricular septum (IVS) also are included. R = reference mark; PV = pulmonary valve; AV = aortic valve; MV = mitral valve; TV = tricuspid valve. **B.** Diagram illustrates the circular short axis appearance of the left ventricle (LV) at the apical level. This plane is defined by an absence of recognizable landmarks, and neither papillary muscles nor apical endocardium should be included. R = reference mark. **C.** Parasternal short axis recording of the left ventricular apex. The circular left ventricle (LV) is recorded in the center of the sector, and a small portion of the right ventricle is evident anteriorly and to the left. There is some irregularity of the ventricular wall, but no clearly defined papillary muscles are evident. R = reference mark.

gradually decreases, and the cavity is finally obliterated at the apical tip. This maneuver localizes the tip of the apex, and the apical views can then be recorded by angling the scan plane back toward the base of the heart. When the apical transducer position has been identified, all the apical views can be recorded from the same transducer location.

The Apical Four-Chamber View

The apical four-chamber view is recorded with the transducer located directly over the anatomic cardiac apex and the central ray of the scan plane directed superiorly and rightward toward the tip of the right scapula. The central ray is then angled to pass through the crux of the heart, and the plane is rotated until the full excursion of both the mitral and tricuspid valve leaflets are recorded. The spatial orientation of this plane is depicted in Figure 5–10A. The position of the plane in space is fixed by three specific points: the cardiac apex, the mitral valve, and the tricuspid valve. When positioned in this fashion, the plane encompasses the left ventricle and atrium, right ventricle and atrium, the two atrioventricular valves, and the interventricular and interatrial septa. Motion of the right ventricular free wall and septum relative to the right and left ventricular cavities also can be visualized.

The resultant image is displayed such that the left ventricular apex is positioned at the apex of the sector (Fig. 5–10B). The left ventricular cavity is anterior and to the right, and the left atrium is posterior and to the right behind the left ventricle. The right ventricle is anterior and to the left, and the right atrium is posterior along the left margin of the display. The septa course vertically down the midline, and the apical extreme of the interventricular septum is closest to the apex of the sector.

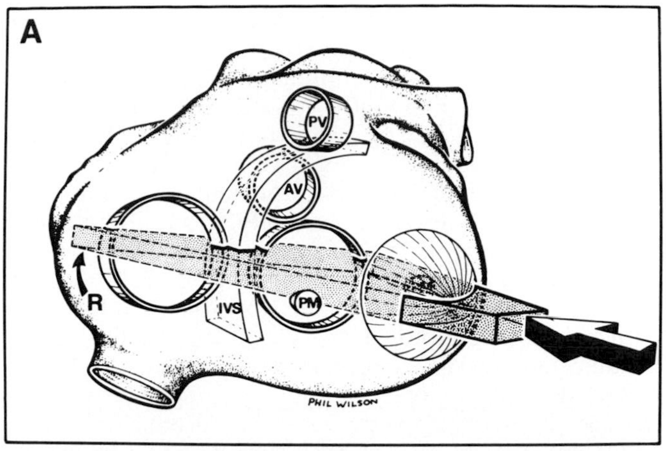

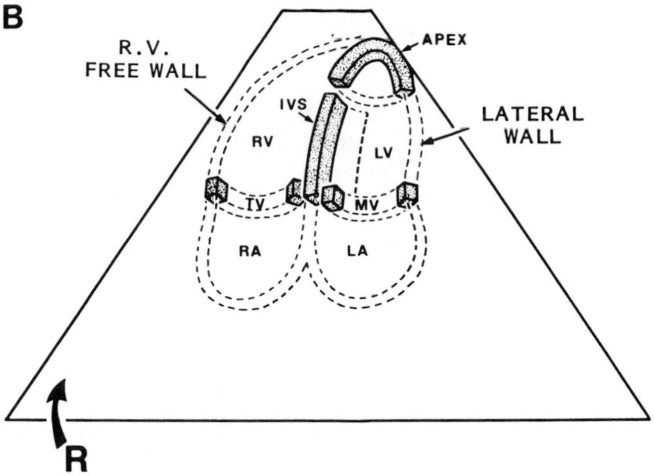

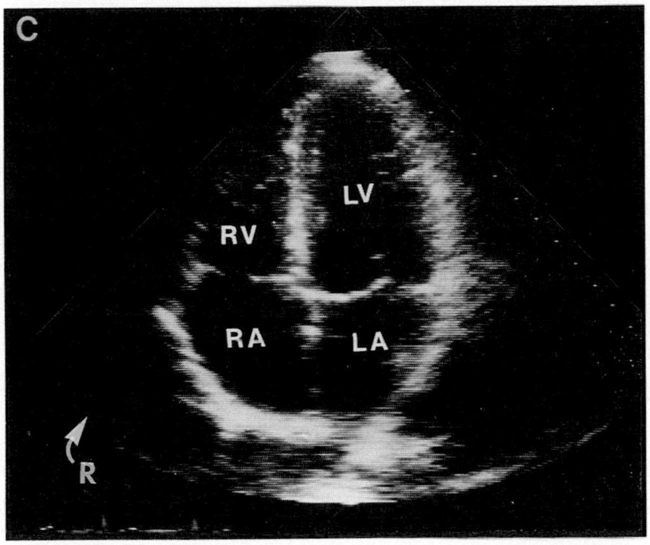

Fig. 5–10. **A.** Orientation of the imaging plane in the apical four-chamber view. This plane transects the heart from the tip of the cardiac apex to its superior border and passes through the center of both the mitral and tricuspid orifices. The point of the sector indicated by the reference mark (R) is displayed at the lower left of the display scope or as though viewed from beneath the heart. This plane transects the cardiac apex, the mitral and tricuspid valves, and the interventricular septum (IVS). It also encompasses both atria and ventricles and the interatrial septum. PM = papillary muscle; AV = aortic valve, PV = pulmonary valve. **B.** Orientation of the primary and adjacent cardiac structures as they appear on the display scope in the apical four-chamber view. IVS = interventricular septum; RV = right ventricle; LV = left ventricle; RA = right atrium; LA = left atrium; R = reference mark. **C.** Cross-sectional recording of the heart using the apical four-chamber view. The cardiac apex appears at the apex of the sector; the left ventricle (LV) is to the right, and the right ventricle (RV) is to the left. The interventricular septum dividing these two chambers courses posteriorly through the midportion of the scan. The mitral and tricuspid valves are in their systolic position and thus are oriented perpendicular to the scan plane. Behind the AV valves, the left atrium (LA), positioned to the right, and the right atrium (RA), positioned to the left, are evident. Portions of the interatrial septum separating these two chambers can be visualized. R = reference mark.

The atrioventricular valves are positioned horizontally and swing toward the apex of the sector during diastolic opening. Figure 5–10C is a representative recording of these structures.

Ideal positioning of this plane is achieved by placing the transducer over the precise anatomic cardiac apex and recording the maximal opening amplitude of both the mitral and tricuspid leaflets. Because the midpoint of the fully opened AV valves normally approximates the center of the corresponding ventricle, the valve orifices in the region of maximal leaflet opening should be intersected by the ventricular long axes. Because the long axis also passes through the apex, this plane alignment, when correctly positioned, should include the long axes of both ventricular chambers. Variations in plane angle may be used to record particular structures, such as the superior portion of the interatrial septum and the right and left inferior pulmonary veins. These variations are displaced from the ventricular long axis and are difficult to standardize and, thus, are useful only for imaging the particular area of interest.

The apical four-chamber view is one of the most important standard planes because it encompasses both ventricles and atria simultaneously, thereby permitting the evaluation of their relative sizes, orientation, and structural integrity.

The left ventricle is transected from apex to base in a plane extending from the medial portion of the interventricular septum to the free lateral wall (or roughly from the 10 to the 4 o'clock positions of the corresponding short axis planes). A ventricular area, long axis from the apical tip to the mitral annulus and short axis or minor dimension at any point along the long axis, can be measured (see Chapter 20). Endocardial targets along the medial and lateral walls unfortunately are recorded using the lateral resolution of the system and, therefore, are widened by the point-spread function of the beam at that level. This situation results in circumferential encroachment on the actual cavity area and in an underestimation of ventricular volumes and dimensions when the inner margins of the echoes are used to represent endocardial position. Motion of the septum and lateral wall can likewise be visualized but is recorded as movement across data lines rather than along the beam axis and, thus, is not optimally displayed. This view, therefore, is more useful for assessing differences in motion at individual points along the ventricular walls than for measuring absolute excursion at any point.

The left ventricular apex must, by definition, be recorded in this and all the apical views. The tip of the apical endocardium unfortunately lies close to the transducer face, and the proximal ventricular walls curve away from the transducer in an arc that roughly parallels the path of the sound beam. Therefore, the apical endocardium and ventricular wall motion in the apical region frequently are not well recorded. Apparent apical motion also can be varied greatly by small changes in transducer position. For example, slight transducer displacement up the anterior ventricular wall causes the apex to appear rounded, dilated, and artifactually hypokinetic. Apical function, therefore, is better recorded in the parasternal long axis view of the apex. The apical four-chamber view, however, is more useful for defining the apical intercept of the left ventricular long axis, detecting apical masses and thrombi, and recording gross distortions in apical geometry.

The right ventricle is likewise transected from apex to base in a plane extending from the midportion of the free lateral wall to the middle third of the interventricular septum. A right ventricular long axis, minor dimension at any point along the long axis, and right ventricular area can be determined (see Chapter 28). Motion of the right ventricular free wall and septum relative to the right and left ventricular cavities also can be visualized. The same limitations noted in attempting to record left ventricular medial and lateral wall endocardium also are encountered in the right ventricle. In addition, the right ventricular lateral wall is more difficult to record than the left. Because the standard plane is optimized to record the left ventricular apex, slight adjustment of plane position may be required when attempting to record the right ventricular long axis to ensure that the right ventricular apex is also included.

The left atrium is visualized in a plane extending from the AV ring to the superior atrial wall and from the interatrial septum to the free lateral border. Cranial-caudal and medial-lateral left atrial dimension, as well as an atrial area, can be obtained. Masses in the left atrium are well visualized, and their point of attachment to the atrial walls frequently can be assessed (see Chapter 18).

The pulmonary veins can often be visualized entering the superolateral and medial walls of the left atrium. Anomalies of pulmonary venous insertion also can be detected. The right atrium is recorded in a plane similar to that in which the left atrium is recorded, and comparable atrial dimensions and area measurements can be obtained (see Chapter 26). Intracavitary right atrial masses frequently can be visualized in this view, which forms an excellent complement to the parasternal long axis of the right ventricular inflow tract and subcostal long axis for demonstrating these lesions.

The entire extent of the midportion of the interventricular septum from the cardiac apex to the crux of the heart is displayed. Both acquired and congenital ventricular septal defects, particularly those of the ostium primum and AV canal varieties, are well visualized in this view. This apical view is particularly useful for recording the acquired ventricular septal defects that develop as a complication of acute myocardial infarction. These lesions are most commonly noted in the apical portion of the septum posteriorly, which is a well-visualized area (see Chapter 22).

The relationship of the interventricular and interatrial septa can also be defined. Normally, the ventricular and atrial septa do not lie along a straight line from apex to base, and the atrial septum is displaced slightly to the left of the ventricular septum[1] (toward the left atrium rather than toward the viewer's left). Right and left atrial volume and pressure overloads may alter these relationships, and their presence can be inferred from the changes in atrial septal position they produce.

Finally, the relative systolic and diastolic positions, motion and structural integrity of the mitral and tricuspid valves can be readily appreciated. The anterior mitral leaflet arises medially from the interventricular septum; the posterior leaflet arises from the lateral margin of the left-sided AV ring. The septal leaflet of the tricuspid valve likewise, inserts medially, whereas the large anterior tricuspid leaflet arises from the lateral ring margin. The posterior tricuspid leaflet is not recorded in this plane. The anterior leaflet of the mitral valve normally inserts into the left atrioventricular ring at the superior end of the membranous septum. The septal leaflet of the tricuspid valve, in contrast, inserts into the midportion of the membranous septum and, therefore, is displaced toward the cardiac apex approximately 5 to 10 mm relative to the anterior mitral leaflet.[1] This anatomic distinction is important because it permits identification of the AV valves and accompanying ventricular chamber.

During systole, the leaflets of both AV valves are positioned so that they are parallel to the plane of their respective atrioventricular rings and perpendicular to the path of the scan plane. This orientation permits optimal leaflet visualization, and hence, this view is ideal for detecting abnormalities characterized by abnormal systolic position of the leaflets relative to the AV ring such as mitral and tricuspid valve prolapse, flail leaflets, and incomplete leaflet closure, which typically occurs with papillary muscle dysfunction. During diastole, the open leaflets point toward the apex, are oriented parallel to the path of the ultrasonic beam, and, as a result, are less well visualized. Some diastolic abnormalities, such as valve doming with stenotic lesions, can be recorded, but in general, less useful information is available during this portion of the cardiac cycle.

The Apical Five-Chamber View

The apical five-chamber view is recorded using a transducer position and plane orientation similar to those used to obtain the four-chamber view. From this position, the plane is angled slightly anteriorly toward the anterior chest wall. As the plane is shifted, the area occupied by the crux of the heart in the four-chamber view is replaced by the left ventricular outflow tract and proximal aorta. Figure 5–11A illustrates the spatial position of this plane. Using this plane orientation, in addition to the original four chambers, the examiner can vis-

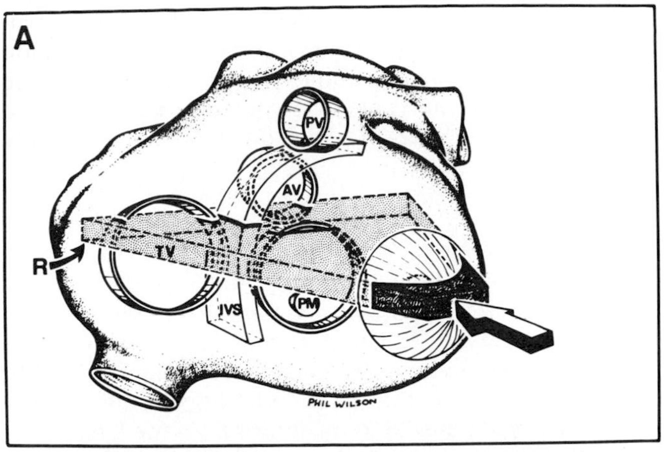

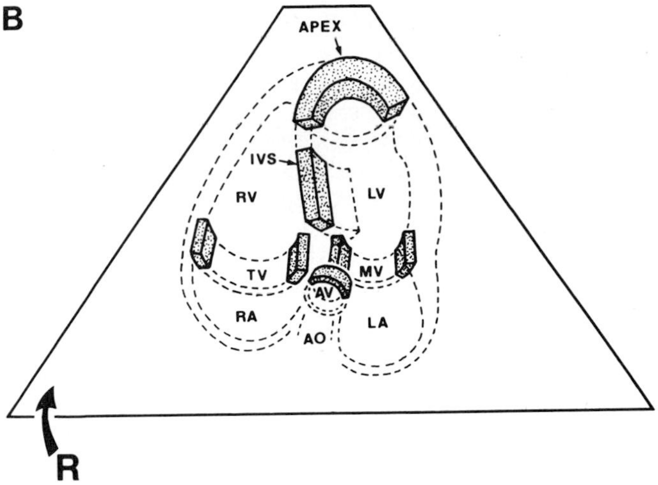

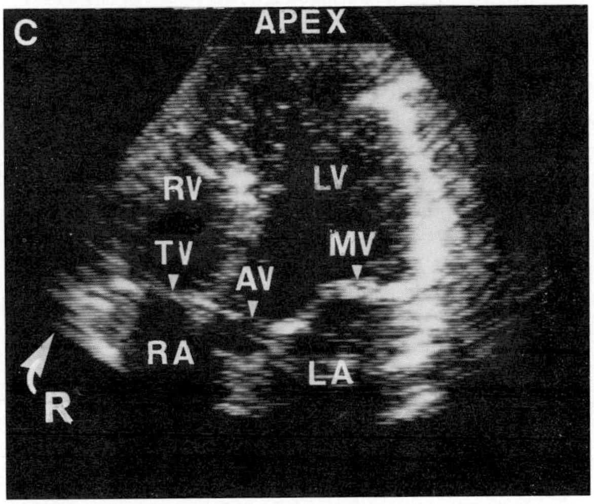

Fig. 5–11. **A.** Orientation of the imaging plane in the apical five-chamber view. This plane passes through the anatomic tip of the cardiac apex and is oriented to transect the superior margin of the mitral valve, the tricuspid valve (TV), and the inferior border of the aortic valve (AV). R = reference mark; PM = papillary muscle; IVS = interventricular septum; PV = pulmonary valve. **B.** The relative position of the major and adjacent cardiac structures recorded in the apical five-chamber view as they appear on the display scope. IVS = interventricular septum; RV = right ventricle; LV = left ventricle; TV = tricuspid valve; MV = mitral valve; AV = aortic valve; RA = right atrium; LA = left atrium; AO = aorta; R = reference mark. **C.** Cross-sectional recording of the heart obtained using the apical five-chamber view. As in the apical four-chamber view, the cardiac apex appears at the tip of the sector. The left ventricle (LV) and left atrium (LA) are displayed to the right, and the corresponding right-sided chambers are to the left. Portions of the mitral (MV) and tricuspid valves (TV) are evident. The left ventricular outflow tract appears posteriorly in the midportion of the scan. Aortic leaflets are apparent in the outflow tract. RV = right ventricle; AV = aortic valve; RA = right atrium; R = reference mark.

ualize the aortic valve and the aortic root or a fifth chamber.

The image orientation is similar to that for the four-chamber view with the apex positioned at the peak of the sector, the two ventricular chambers located anteriorly, and the two atrial chambers located posteriorly (Fig. 5–11B). The left ventricle and left atrium are located to the right, and the right ventricle and right atrium are to the left. The fifth or aortic chamber lies posteriorly between the two atria. Figure 5–11C is an example of the five-chamber view. In this figure, the proximal portion of the outflow tract originates from the medial portion of the left ventricle at the base of the heart. The ventricular portion of the outflow tract is bound medially by the interventricular septum, which continues distally as the medial border of the aortic root, and laterally by the anterior mitral leaflet and the base of the left ventricle, which are continuous with the lateral aortic root. The aortic leaflets can be seen in the proximal aorta.

This plane has limited utility beyond the assessment of the proximal portion of the left ventricular outflow tract and, as such, is optimally oriented when this region can be clearly visualized. Its major role is to assess left ventricular outflow disorders, specifically subvalvular membranous obstruction, subvalvular tunnels, and the relationship of interventricular septal hypertrophy to the left ventricular outflow tract.

The Apical Two-Chamber View

The apical two-chamber view is intended to record only the left ventricle and atrium with the interposed mitral valve. In contrast to other standard imaging planes with orientations defined by the structures they include, the apical two-chamber view is positioned on the basis of structures (specifically, the right side of the heart) that are not included. In recording this plane, the examiner again positions the transducer directly over the cardiac apex. The central ray of the scan plane is directed parallel to the long axis of the left ventricle. This position shifts the central ray slightly to the left of its position in the four-chamber view. The scan plane is then rotated until right-sided cardiac structures cannot be visualized. Because the right ventricle overlies between one third and two fifths of the circumference of the left ventricle at the base (see the section entitled Parasternal Short Axis of the Left Ventricle [Mitral Valve Level]), the area of the left ventricular free wall through which a plane can pass, which includes the long axis of the left ventricle and excludes the right ventricle, is limited. When one includes the thickness of the scan plane, this area becomes more limited.

Figure 5–12A diagrammatically illustrates the orientation of this plane and its relationship to the interventricular septum and other right-sided structures. When displayed (Fig. 5–12B), the image shows the left ventricular apex slightly to the left of the apex of the sector with the anterior left ventricular wall to the right and the posterior left ventricular wall to the left. The mitral valve is posterior, slightly to the right of center, with the anterior leaflet to the right and the posterior to the left. The left atrium is positioned posteriorly and to the right. Figure 5–12C is an example of a two-chamber view of the heart.

The apical two-chamber view is optimally recorded when the transducer is located over the true anatomic apex of the ventricle and the left ventricular diameter at the base of the ventricle is at its maximum. This indicates that the plane is positioned perpendicular to the maximal short axis and parallel to the true long axis of the ventricle. Right ventricular structures are completely excluded.

This imaging plane is orthogonal to the four-chamber view, and as such, should be useful for biplane cross-sectional imaging of the left ventricle. The plane provides a long axis to the left ventricle, which can be correlated with the long axis obtained in the four-chamber view, and a short axis in an orthogonal plane to the four-chamber short axis. The two-chamber view records the anterior and posterior wall endocardium in an orientation that is parallel to the beam axis and, hence, does not provide optimal visualization. This particular imaging plane has no unique value and is used primarily in conjunction with the apical four-chamber view to generate biplane data.

The Apical Long Axis of the Left Ventricle

The apical long axis view of the left ventricle is similar in orientation to the parasternal long axis of the left ventricle. The only difference is transducer location. To record the apical view, the transducer is placed directly over the cardiac apex, and the central ray of the imaging plane is aligned parallel to the long axis of the left ventricle. The path of the central ray is similar to that used in the apical two-chamber view. The transducer is then rotated to position the y axis of the scan plane such that it passes through the midportion of the aortic and mitral valves and includes the ventricular long axis (Fig. 5–13A). This position generally requires a 30° counterclockwise rotation from a true anteroposterior orientation. In addition to the apex and the mitral and aortic valves, the transducer encompasses the anterior portion of the interventricular septum, the posterior ventricular wall from apex to mitral annulus, the left atrium, and the proximal aortic root.

When displayed (Fig. 5–13B), the cardiac apex ap-

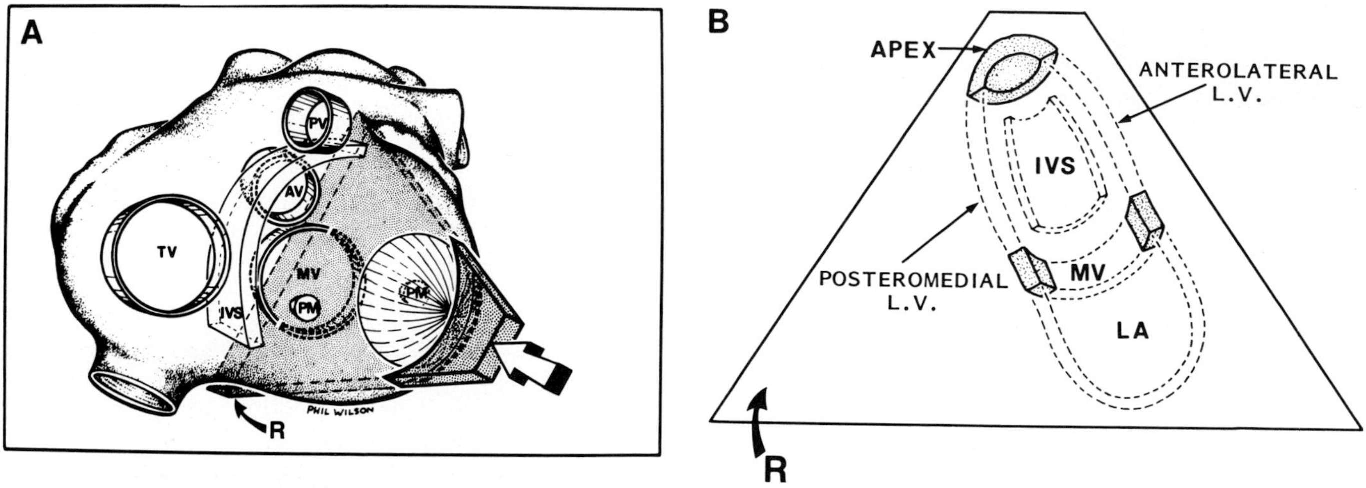

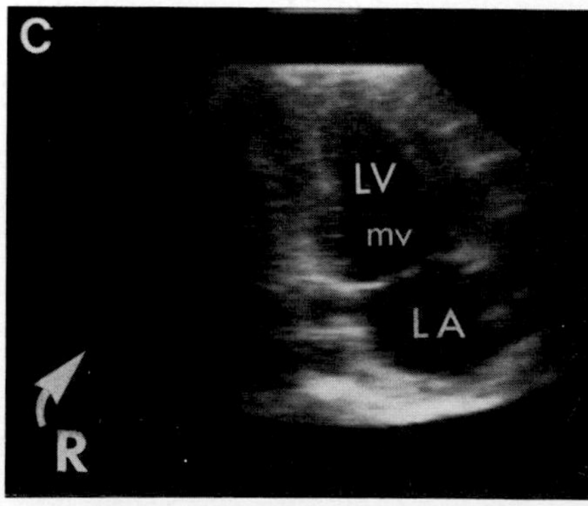

Fig. 5–12. **A.** Orientation of the imaging plane in the apical two-chamber view of the left heart. This plane transects the cardiac apex and passes through the midportion of the mitral valve (MV). The orientation of this plane is defined by the fact that no interventricular septum (IVS) or right ventricle is recorded. PV = pulmonary valve; AV = aortic valve; TV = tricuspid valve; PM = papillary muscle; R = reference mark. **B.** The relative positions of the primary and adjacent cardiac structures when displayed in the apical two-chamber view of the left ventricle (LV). IVS = interventricular septum; MV = mitral valve; LA = left atrium; R = reference mark. **C.** Cross-sectional recording of the left ventricle using the apical two-chamber view. The apex of the ventricle appears to the left and anteriorly in the sector. The anterior wall of the left ventricle is to the right, and the posteromedial wall is to the left. The mitral leaflets separating the left ventricle (LV) and left atrium (LA) are apparent posteriorly and to the right. The left atrium is behind the mitral valve (mv). R = reference mark.

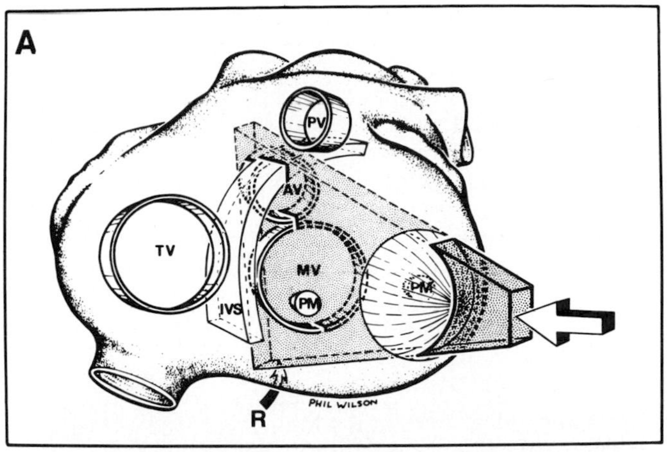

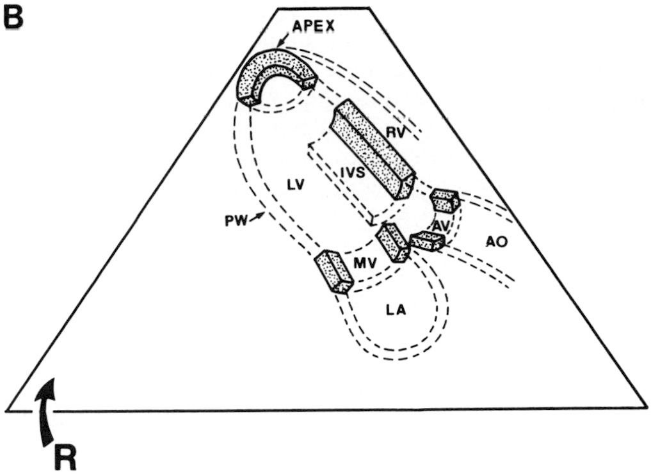

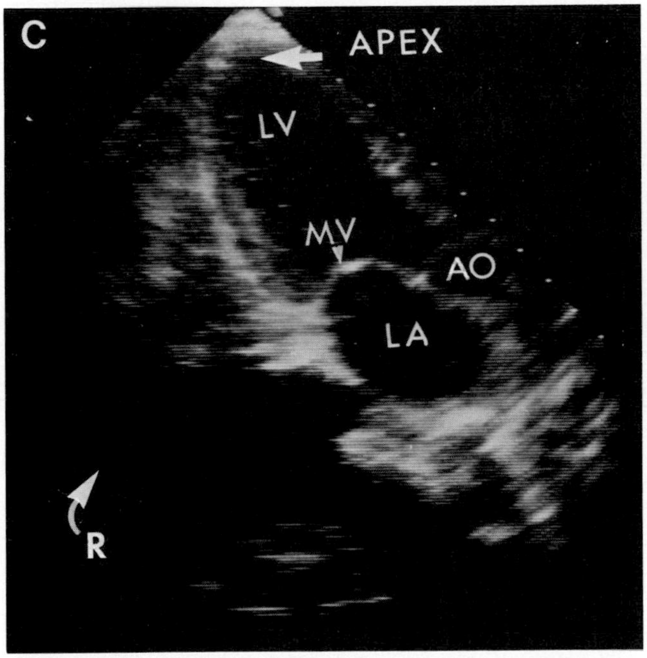

Fig. 5–13. **A.** Orientation of the imaging plane in the apical long axis view of the left ventricle. This plane passes through the tip of the cardiac apex, the center of the mitral valve (MV), and the midportion of the aortic valve (AV). It also transects the anterior portion of the interventricular septum (IVS) along a line stretching from the cardiac apex to the junction of the interventricular septum with the anterior aortic root. PV = pulmonary valve; TV = tricuspid valve; PM = papillary muscle; R = reference mark. **B.** The relative positions of the primary and adjacent cardiac structures as they appear on the display scope in the apical long axis view. RV = right ventricle; LV = left ventricle; IVS = interventricular septum; PW = posterior wall; AV = aortic valve; MV = mitral valve; AO = aorta; LA = left atrium; R = reference mark. **C.** Apical long axis recording of the left ventricle (LV), aortic valve, and mitral valve (MV). These structures are displayed in a fashion similar to their appearance in the parasternal long axis view of the left heart or as though viewed from the left shoulder. AO = aorta; LA = left atrium; R = reference mark.

pears at the tip of the sector with the right ventricle to the right and the left ventricular posterior wall to the left. The aorta is posterior and to the right, and the left atrium is posterior and to the left. Figure 5–13C is a representative recording of the apical long axis view of the left ventricle.

Fine plane positioning is defined by recording the cardiac apex and the maximal excursion of the mitral valve and aortic leaflets. In addition to recording these three points, the plane should be aligned such that the maximum short axis diameter of the ventricle at the base is recorded. This diameter should correspond to the point of peak mitral excursion and should fix the plane in a standardized and reproducible fashion.

This particular imaging plane provides little additional information when all the other examining planes are available. It is a reasonable alternative, however, to the parasternal long axis view and is used primarily to record the aortic valve and ventricular walls in a plane that corresponds to the parasternal long axis when the parasternal window is unavailable. Each of these areas, unfortunately, is less than optimally recorded. The aortic valve lies in the far field of the scan and is difficult to record in detail. The anterior septum courses directly under the chest wall. Often, the lateral extent of the imaging plane cannot be directed underneath the rib cage to record the distal one third to one half of this region. In addition, the anterior and posterior walls of the ventricle are oriented parallel to the beam axis. Endocardial resolution, therefore, is poor, and any assessment of the amplitude of wall motion is limited. Importantly, this transducer location places the path of the sound beam directly parallel to the flow vector in the aorta, and hence, this is an ideal orientation for recording aortic outflow velocity for Doppler measurement of cardiac output and aortic valve gradients.

SUBCOSTAL EXAMINATION

Echocardiographic recording of the heart from the subxiphoid or subcostal region developed initially as an alternative to parasternal recording in patients with chronic obstructive lung disease.[15] In these patients, the parasternal window was frequently obliterated by the hyperinflated lung, and the heart shifted medially and inferiorly toward the subxiphoid region. The frequency with which the cardiac impulse could be palpated in this region suggested that intracardiac structures might be recorded by directly placing the transducer in the subxiphoid area. Further experience with the cross-sectional technique has demonstrated that cardiac structures can be recorded in the majority of adult and virtually all pediatric patients from this transducer position and that a number of cardiac structures are optimally visualized in this particular orientation.[7,8,15] The two primary subcostal views are the subcostal long axis (four-chamber) view of the heart and the subcostal long axis view of the right ventricular outflow tract.

Subcostal Long Axis View of the Heart

The subcostal long axis view is recorded with the transducer placed in the subcostal window and the central ray directed superiorly and leftward toward the left clavicle. The transducer is then rotated to align the x axis of the imaging plane parallel to the long axis of the left ventricle. This view is comparable to the apical four-chamber view in that it permits visualization of the right and left ventricles, the right and left atria, and both atrioventricular valves. The z axis of the imaging plane, however, is orthogonal to that of the apical view and, hence, permits enhanced visualization of structures that are aligned parallel to the central ray of the scan plane in the apical position. Figure 5–14A illustrates the relative orientation of this plane.

The resulting image shows the right-sided cardiac structures, which are closest to the transducer, positioned anteriorly in the sector and the left-sided structures positioned posteriorly (Fig. 5–14B). The left and right ventricles are displayed to the viewer's right, and the left and right atria to the viewer's left. The heart is therefore displayed as if viewed from beneath the plane. Figure 5–14C, is a cross-sectional recording of a subcostal long axis and illustrates the typical appearance of these structures.

Fine plane positioning is achieved by angling the scan plane along a dorsal-to-ventral path to record the maximal amplitude of mitral and tricuspid valve motion combined with a maximal minor diameter of the left ventricle and left and right atria. When all these criteria cannot be achieved in one orientation, the examiner may have to align the plane to best record the individual area of inter-

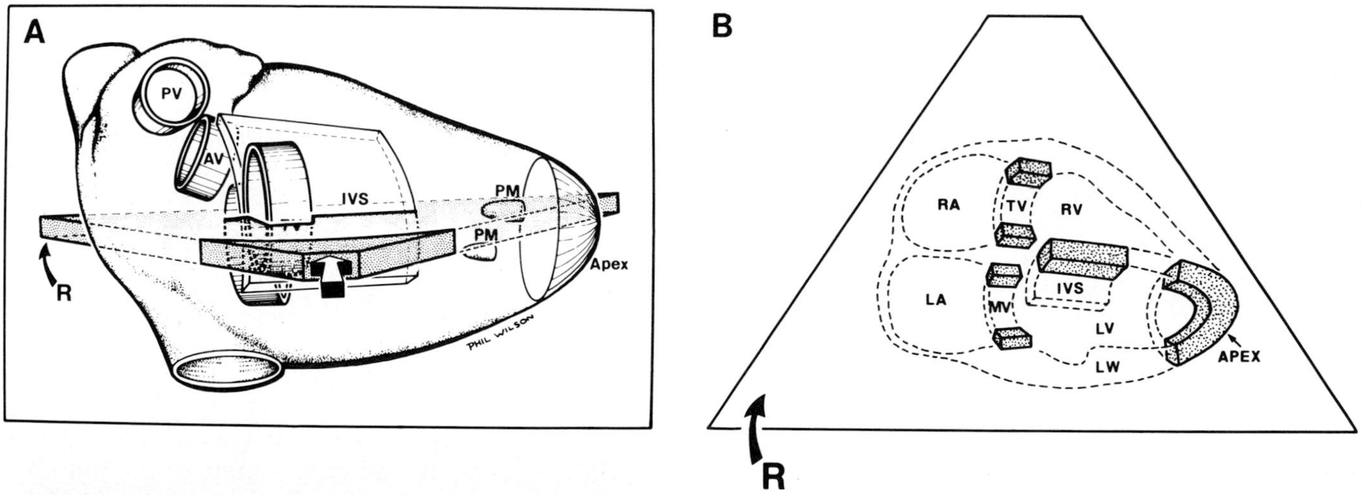

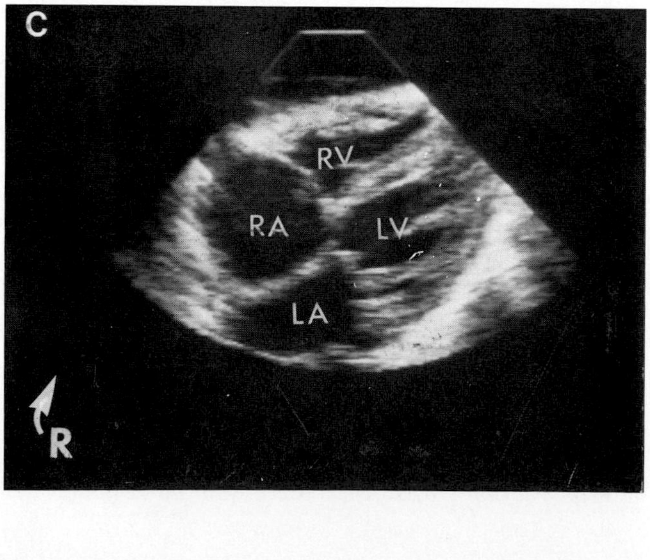

Fig. 5–14. **A.** Orientation of the imaging plane in the subcostal long axis view of the heart. This plane initially transects the lateral wall of the right ventricle; consequently, the tricuspid valve (TV) is recorded first, followed by the interventricular septum (IVS) and mitral valve. When displayed, the point of the sector indicated by the reference mark (R) is positioned at the lower left corner of the display scope. The resultant image, therefore, is displayed as though the structures were viewed from beneath the heart. PV = pulmonary valve; AV = aortic valve; PM = papillary muscle. **B.** The relative positions of the primary and adjacent structures recorded in the subcostal long axis view on the display scope. The apex in this orientation is positioned to the right and posteriorly. The right ventricle (RV), tricuspid valve (TV), and right atrium (RA) are closest to the apex of the sector. LW = lateral wall of the left ventricle; LA = left atrium; MV = mitral valve; IVS = interventricular septum; LV = left ventricle; R = reference mark. **C.** Subcostal long axis recording of the heart. RA = right atrium; RV = right ventricle; LA = left atrium; LV = left ventricle.

est. The right ventricular minor dimension varies greatly with plane angulation and hence, does not aid in plane alignment.

This image orientation permits a long axis view of both the left and right ventricles. Also, a short axis of both ventricular chambers drawn from the medial to lateral walls can be seen. Left ventricular free wall motion should be well visualized, as should motion of the posterolateral free wall of the right ventricle. The entire sweep of the interventricular and interatrial septa can be recorded in a plane that is perpendicular to the path of the sound beam. The left and right atria can be visualized, as can the insertion of the inferior vena cava into the right atrium.

This plane position best records the interventricular and interatrial septa, permits analysis of the relative positions of insertion of the septal leaflet of the tricuspid valve and the anterior leaflet of the mitral valve, and should theoretically be the best view for recording the character and amplitude of motion of the free right ventricular wall and free lateral left ventricular wall. It is the optimal view for assessing the integrity of the interatrial septum and for analyzing atrial septum motion.

Difficulties in recording this view relate to problems in defining transducer position and the initial orientation of the central ray. Because the subcostal window is broad and has no specific landmarks, the operator may sometimes have difficulty in precisely defining where the transducer should initially be placed. Further, the degree of transducer angulation in this particular view is greater than that of any of the other views, and hence, there is a tendency not to angle the beam deeply enough and, as a result, not to transect the heart. In addition, in many cases, the heart may lie deep to the transducer and may thus fall in an area of diminished lateral resolution. This situation may make the recording of laterally oriented structures more difficult. Despite these problems, the subcostal long axis view is useful in all patients, and in infants may be the best view for evaluating relative chamber size, septal integrity, and AV valve position and integrity.

Subcostal Long Axis of the Right Ventricular Outflow Tract

The subcostal long axis of the right ventricular outflow tract is recorded from the same transducer location used to record the subcostal long axis view of the heart. The central ray is initially oriented to pass through the base of the mitral leaflets. From this position, the central ray is directed cephalad toward the left clavicle, and the scan plane is rotated clockwise approximately 90° to

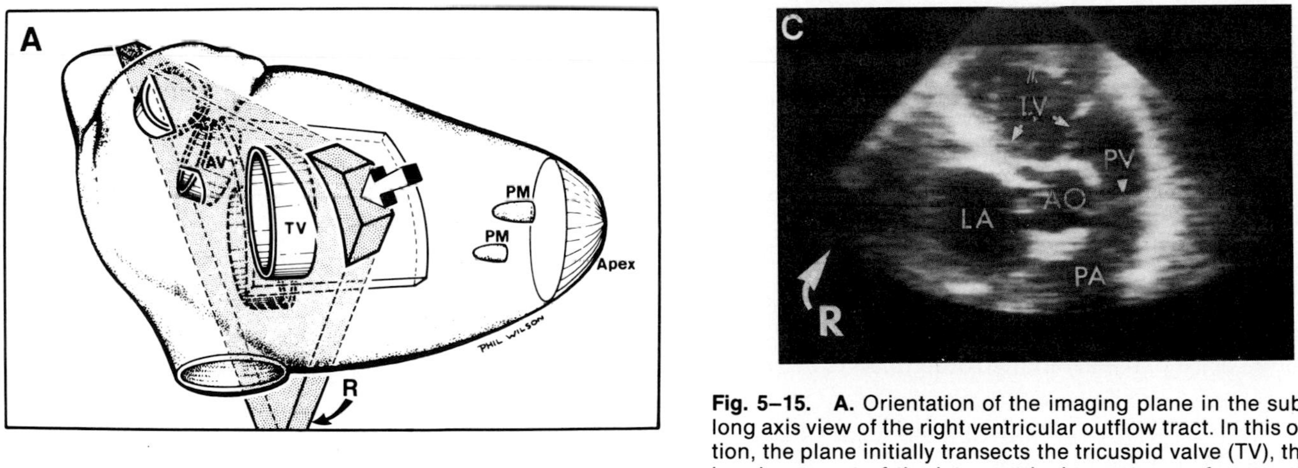

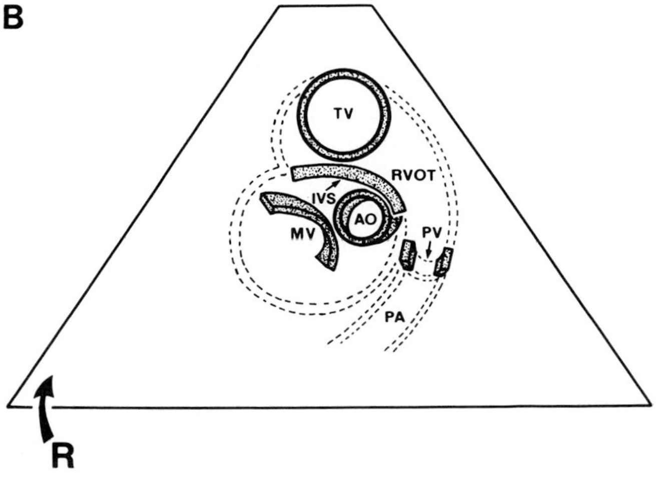

Fig. 5–15. **A.** Orientation of the imaging plane in the subcostal long axis view of the right ventricular outflow tract. In this orientation, the plane initially transects the tricuspid valve (TV), then the basal segment of the interventricular septum, a fragment of the mitral valve, the aortic valve (AV), and finally the pulmonary valve. R = reference mark; PM = papillary muscle. **B.** Relative positions of the primary and adjacent structures recorded in the subcostal long axis view of the right ventricular outflow tract on the display scope. The tricuspid valve (TV) is positioned anteriorly at the apex of the sector. The right ventricular outflow tract courses posteriorly along the right border of the sector. The pulmonary valve (PV) is the most posterior of the primary structures and, likewise, the farthest to the right on the display. RVOT = right ventricular outflow tract; IVS = interventricular septum; MV = mitral valve; AO = aorta; PA = pulmonary artery; R = reference mark. **C.** Cross-sectional recording of the right ventricular outflow tract from the subcostal transducer location. The entire sweep of the right ventricular outflow tract from the tricuspid valve (TV) level, through the pulmonary infundibulum and the pulmonary valve (PV) to the main pulmonary artery is evident. The aorta (AO), which is transected somewhat obliquely to its short axis, appears relatively circular and lies in the center of the scan. The structures are displayed as though viewed from the cardiac apex. LA = left atrium; PA = pulmonary artery; R = reference mark.

align it parallel to the long axis of the right ventricular outflow tract. In this orientation, the imaging plane transects the right ventricular outflow tract parallel to its long axis from the tricuspid valve orifice to the main pulmonary artery. Figure 5–15A illustrates this plane orientation.

On the display scope, the heart appears inverted with the right ventricular inflow region at the apex of the sector, the outflow tract along the right margin of the screen, and the left ventricle viewed in short axis along the left margin. Figure 5–15B diagrammatically depicts the structures recorded in this imaging plane; Figure 5–15C is an example of a subcostal long axis recording of the right ventricular outflow tract.

This view is primarily intended to record the full sweep of the right ventricular outflow tract and, as such, is optimally recorded when the maximal transverse diameters of the inflow and outflow areas are simultaneously visualized with the pulmonary leaflets. The subcostal view offers an alternative to the parasternal short axis view for recording the tricuspid valve orifice and may prove useful in tricuspid stenosis. It might also be anticipated that, in valvular pulmonary stenosis, systolic doming of the pulmonary leaflets could be best appreciated in this view because the domed leaflets should be oriented perpendicular to the imaging plane. The parasternal long axis of the right ventricular outflow tract, however, remains the view of choice for detecting valvular pulmonary stenosis because of the greater ease of the pulmonary valve recording and the favorable position of the valve in the near field of the scan plane.

This image orientation can be used as a starting point from which the transducer can be angled either superiorly toward the cranial margins of the atria or inferiorly toward the cardiac apex. This flexibility offers the potential to record multiple short axes of these chambers in an orientation that is orthogonal to the parasternal views. To date, these views are not sufficiently popular to be considered routine or standard. They may be of immense value, however, in patients with segmental wall motion abnormalities in whom the parasternal short axis views are technically limited or difficult to interpret.

Noncardiac Structures That Can Be Examined From the Subcostal Location

Many extracardiac vascular structures can be easily recorded from the subcostal region. These structures include the hepatic veins and their connection with the inferior vena cava, the inferior vena cava itself and its junction with the right atrium, and the abdominal aorta. There is potential for recording inferior vena caval obstruction and dilation, detecting backflow of contrast from the right atrium into the inferior vena cava and hepatic veins in instances of tricuspid regurgitation, and viewing tumor migration up the inferior vena cava in patients with metastatic abdominal malignancies. The abdominal aorta also can be traced from its origin beneath the diaphragm to its bifurcation into the iliac arteries. The anterior abdominal wall provides an uninterrupted window for the exploring transducer, and hence, multiple long or short axis recordings of these vessels are available.

SUPRASTERNAL VIEWS

The suprasternal views are used to examine the great vessels as they course cephalad from the heart. Structures that can be recorded from this transducer location include the aortic arch and its primary branches to the head and upper extremities, the proximal descending thoracic aorta, the primary branches of the pulmonary artery, and the major veins draining into the right atrium. The examination of this region is performed with the transducer placed directly in the suprasternal notch. To facilitate transducer placement, the patient should be positioned in a manner that makes the suprasternal notch as accessible as possible. The head should be in a neutral position and the chin angled either to the left or right at about 45°. When performing these maneuvers, the examiner tries to relax the sternocleidomastoid muscles as well as the skin in the suprasternal region to permit the transducer head to be positioned beneath the sternum. When this position is achieved, the aorta lies almost immediately beneath the transducer face, and access to the arch vessels can be achieved in almost every case. Two primary views have been described using the suprasternal transducer position—the suprasternal long and short axes of the aortic arch.

Suprasternal Long Axis of the Aortic Arch

The suprasternal long axis of the aortic arch is recorded with the transducer directly in the suprasternal notch and the central ray of the scan plane directed inferiorly and posteriorly. The transducer is then rotated until the scan plane is oriented approximately midway between the coronal and sagittal planes of the body. When oriented in this manner, the imaging plane should pass directly into the aortic arch allowing the arch, the arterial branches to the upper extremities and the distal portions of the ascending aorta, and the proximal descending aorta to be visualized. Figure 5–16A illustrates this plane position.

When displayed on the viewing scope (Fig. 5–16B), the aortic arch should be anterior at the apex of the sector with the descending aorta along the right margin and the ascending aorta along the left margin of the screen. The left atrium lies posteriorly. In some patients, the 90° scan is not wide enough in the near field to encompass the ascending and descending portions of the aorta in the same scan plane. In such patients, the transducer must be angled leftward to record specifically the descending thoracic aorta or rightward to record the ascending aorta. As a rule, the degree of transducer rotation is constant. Figure 5–16C is an example of a suprasternal long axis recording of the aortic arch that illustrates the typical appearance of the structures in this area.

This view is intended to record the aortic arch with as much of the ascending and descending aorta included as

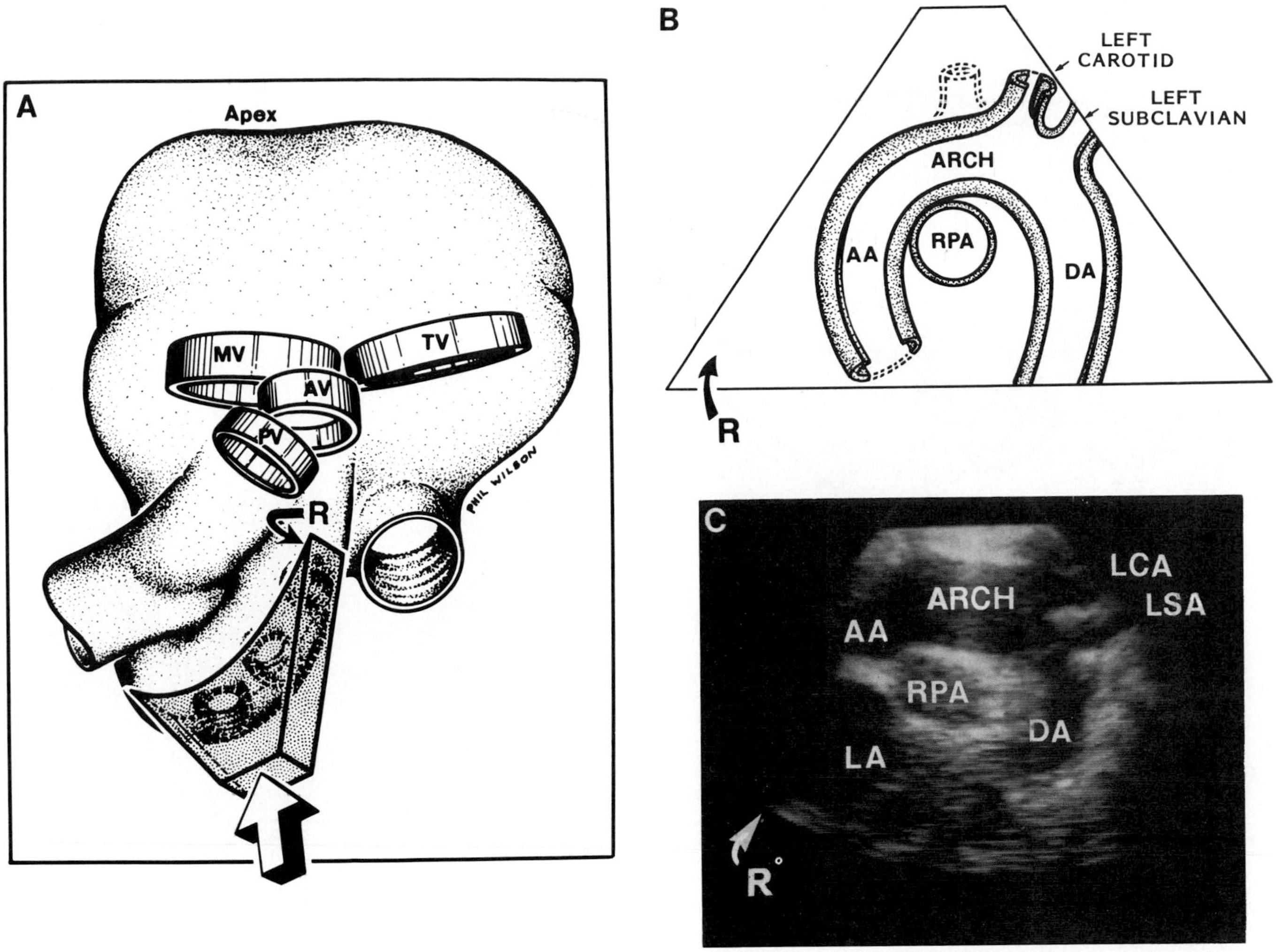

Fig. 5–16. A. Orientation of the imaging plane in the suprasternal long axis view of the aortic arch. As illustrated by the reference mark (R), the plane is displayed as though viewed from the anterior chest wall with the ascending aorta to the left and the descending aorta to the right. MV = mitral valve; TV = tricuspid valve; AV = aortic valve; PV = pulmonary valve. **B.** The relative positions of the structures recorded in the suprasternal long axis view of the aorta on the display scope. The ascending aorta (AA) is positioned to the left, the aortic arch is at the apex of the sector, and the descending aorta (DA) is to the right. The right pulmonary artery (RPA) is transected in a plane oblique to its short axis and appears relatively circular beneath the aortic arch. The left carotid artery is the first arterial vessel branching from the arch to the left of the apex of the sector and is used as a reference mark for identifying the other arterial branches. R = reference mark. **C.** Suprasternal long axis recording of the aortic arch with the ascending portion of the aorta (AA), the arch, and the descending aorta (DA) demonstrated. The left carotid (LCA) and left subclavian (LSA) branches of the aortic arch are also visible. The left atrium (LA) is behind the right pulmonary artery (RPA) and appears as the most posterior structure in the scan. The right pulmonary artery is oblong because it is transected in a plane oblique to its short axis. R = reference mark.

possible. The aortic arch is optimally recorded when the diameter of the aorta is at its maximum throughout the scan plane. Identification of the branches of the aorta is determined relative to the left carotid artery. This artery is readily recorded, and its identity can be determined by following its course into the neck. When this vessel is identified, the innominate and subclavian branches can be identified by their proximal and distal relationships. The suprasternal long axis view is optimally suited for recording dilation or aneurysm formation in the aortic arch, coarctation of the aorta, patent ductus arteriosus in infants, and evaluation of the size of the right pulmonary artery, and potentially for assessing ascending aorta to right pulmonary artery anastomoses.

Suprasternal Short Axis of the Aortic Arch

The suprasternal short axis of the aortic arch is obtained with the transducer in the suprasternal notch and the central ray directed inferiorly and slightly posteriorly. The short axis is recorded by rotating the transducer 90° from the long axis. In this orientation, the scan plane passes through the aorta in short axis, through a portion of the superior vena cava, through the right pulmonary artery parallel to its long axis, and through the left atrium. Figure 5–17A illustrates the orientation of this imaging plane.

On the display scope, the ascending aorta is positioned superiorly and slightly to the right (with the long

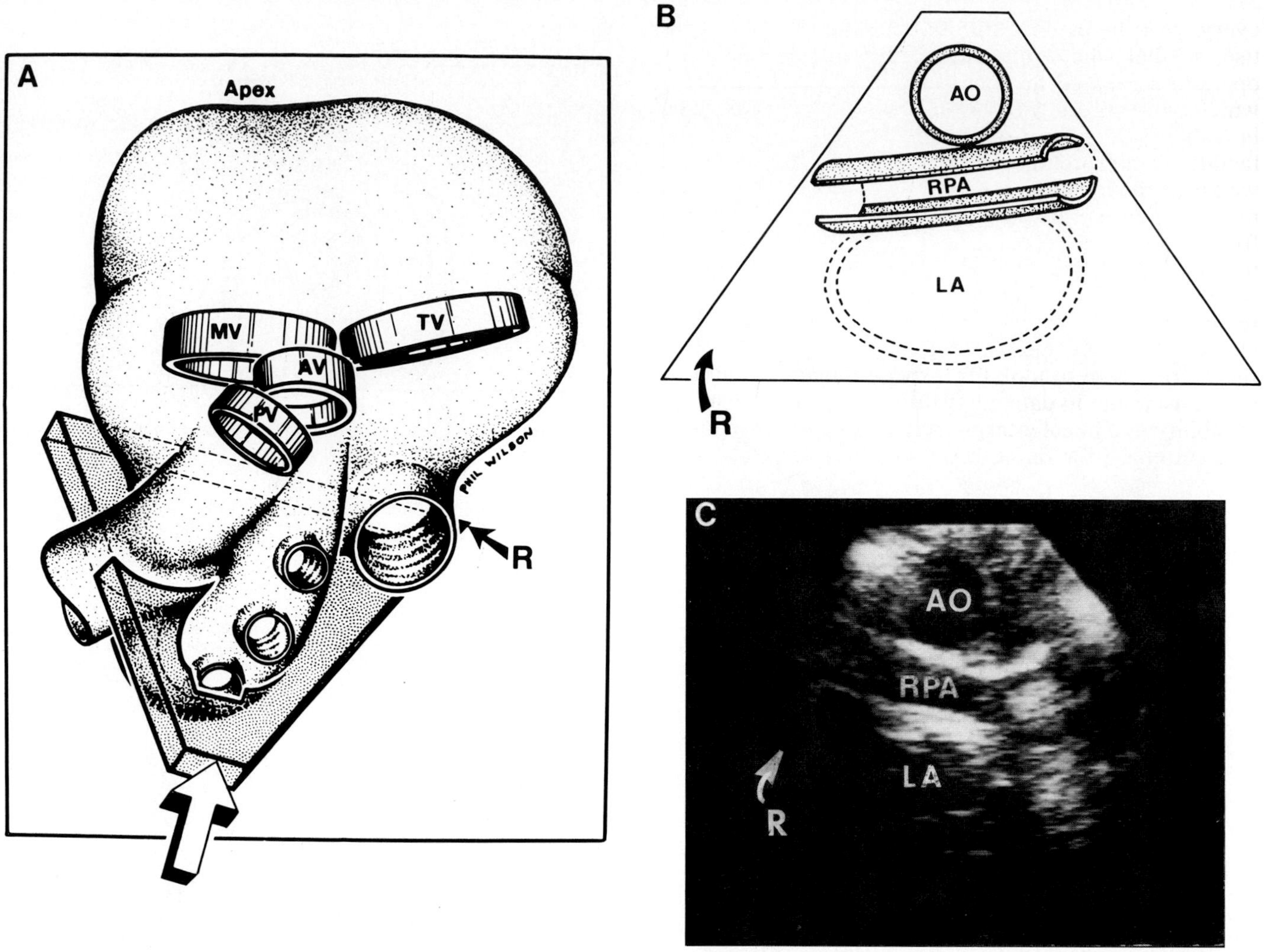

Fig. 5–17. **A.** Orientation of the imaging plane in the suprasternal short axis view of the aortic arch. MV = mitral valve; TV = tricuspid valve; AV = aortic valve; PV = pulmonary valve; R = reference mark. **B.** The relative positions of the structures recorded in the suprasternal short axis view of the aortic arch on the display scope. The aorta (AO), which is recorded in a plane parallel to its short axis, appears circular. The right pulmonary artery (RPA), which is transected in a plane that is roughly parallel to its long axis and thus appears as a cylindric structure, is beneath the aorta. The left atrium (LA), which is imaged in a superior-inferior orientation, is behind the right pulmonary artery. R = reference mark. **C.** Suprasternal short axis recording of the aortic arch illustrates the circular configuration of the aorta (AO), the linear echoes from the margins of the right pulmonary artery (RPA) and the left atrial (LA) superior segment behind the right pulmonary artery. R = reference mark.

axis of the pulmonary artery coursing from right to left in the midportion of the screen), and the left atrium is positioned posteriorly (Fig. 5–17B). Occasionally, the bifurcation of the right pulmonary artery is visualized to the left of the image. The superior vena cava is recorded to the left and anteriorly. Figure 5–17C is an example of a short axis view of the aorta from the suprasternal transducer location.

Optimal orientation of this view must be individualized depending on the structure the examiner wishes to visualize primarily. When one is interested in the short axis of the aorta, the image is optimally recorded when the least horizontal or vertical obliquity of the vessel is noted. When the right pulmonary artery is the structure of interest, the maximal diameter at the proximal and distal ends of the artery should be recorded. When one is interested in the superior vena cava, the plane must be angled toward the maximal expanse of this structure. Recording the entire long axis of the superior vena cava requires counterclockwise rotation and anterior angulation of the transducer. This plane orientation might be refined to a point where the superior vena cava can be visualized to join the right atrium.[1] The overall clinical role of this plane, however, remains to be defined.

SUMMARY

In our laboratory, we routinely record all the standard planes described in this chapter. We feel that this approach provides the opportunity to look at most areas of the heart from several vantage points and to confirm abnormalities, exclude artifacts, and detect subtleties that may be inapparent in only one view. Routine recording of subcostal views, although not necessary in every case, helps develop the requisite level of expertise, so that when only these views are available, the operator is skilled in their performance. The order in which we record these planes is the same as that listed in Table 5–1. This provides maximum efficiency and facilitates interpretation. Also, when a question arises, we know the location in the study of a plane image that may provide the answer. As a result, the interpreter is free to concentrate on successive images without remaining fixed on a single diagnostic question. Finally, when data are always recorded in the same order, the reviewer knows at any point in the study what data have already been presented and what are yet to come and therefore where to look for a specific piece of information. Discipline in data acquisition, therefore, results in reliability in clinical interpretation and ensures a consistent data base for future research studies.

REFERENCES

1. Tajik AJ, et al.: Two-dimensional real-time ultrasonic imaging of the heart and great vessels. Mayo Clin Proc 53:271, 1978.
2. Bansal RC, et al.: Feasibility of detailed two-dimensional echocardiographic examination in adults. Prospective study of 200 patients. Mayo Clin Proc 55:291, 1980.
3. Kloster FE, et al.: Multiscan echocardiography II: technique and initial clinical results. Circulation 48:1975, 1973.
4. Kisslo J, VonRamm OT, Thurstone FL: Cardiac imaging using a phased array ultrasound system: clinical technique and application. Circulation 53: 262, 1976.
5. Griffith JM, Henry WL: A sector scanner for real-time two-dimensional echocardiography. Circulation 49:1147, 1974.
6. Henry WL, et al.: Measurement of mitral valve orifice area in patients with mitral valve disease by real-time two-dimensional echocardiography. Circulation 51:827, 1975.
7. Lange LW, Sahn DJ, Allen HD, Goldberg SJ: Subxyphoid echocardiography in infants and children with congenital heart disease. Circulation 59: 513, 1979.
8. Bierman FZ, Williams RG: Subxyphoid two-dimensional imaging of the interatrial septum in infants and neonates with congenital heart disease. Circulation 60:80, 1979.
9. Silverman NH, Schiller NB: Apex echocardiography: a two-dimensional technique for evaluating congenital heart disease. Circulation 57:503, 1978.
10. Eggleton RC, et al.: Visualization of cardiac dynamics with real-time B-mode ultrasonic scanners. *In* White D (ed.): Ultasound Medicine. New York, Plenum, 1975.
11. Report of the American Society of Echocardiography Committee on Nomenclature and Standards in Two-Dimensional Imaging. Circulation 62:212, 1980.
12. Hickman HO, et al.: Cross-sectional echocardiography of the cardiac apex. Circulation 56:589, 1977.
13. Weyman AE, et al.: Detection of left ventricular aneurysms by cross-sectional echocardiography. Circulation 54:936, 1976.
14. Dillon JC, et al.: Cross-sectional echocardiographic examination of the interatrial septum. Circulation 55:115, 1977.
15. Schapira JN, Martin RP, Fowles RE, Popp RL: Single and two-dimensional echocardiographic features of the interatrial septum in normal subjects and patients with an atrial septal defect. Am J Cardiol 43:816, 1979.
16. Chang S, Feigenbaum H, Dillon J: Subxyphoid echocardiography. Chest 68:233, 1975.

CHAPTER

6

THREE-DIMENSIONAL RECONSTRUCTION OF ECHOCARDIOGRAPHIC IMAGES

MARK D. HANDSCHUMACHER and ANTHONY J. SANFILIPPO

In the preceding chapters we have discussed the methods for the formation and recording of dynamic two-dimensional cardiac images. Although these tomographic images provide an enormous amount of structural and functional information, their proper analysis requires that the observer be able to mentally integrate this planar data into a three-dimensional construct of the heart by interrelating information from one view with that from another. Thus, some form of cognitive three-dimensional reconstruction is implicit in every echocardiographic interpretation. Because the precise relationships of images to each other are not defined, the use of two-dimensional techniques to quantify three-dimensional measures of cardiac performance, such as ejection fraction and stroke volume, require the use of geometric assumptions. Although these methods may be satisfactory to analyze structures of known and regular shape, they become flawed when attempting to analyze or quantitatively describe structures of unknown or irregular shape. Three-dimensional reconstruction could eliminate the need for geometric assumptions and thereby facilitate more accurate evaluation of such structures. It would also allow quantitative description of structures whose surfaces do not form enclosed volumes (e.g., valve leaflets), structures for which simple geometric models are less applicable (e.g., the right ventricle and ischemic left ventricle), and intracardiac flow fields from color Doppler images. To achieve these goals, however, requires a method for registering the spatial location of multiple two-dimensional images and combining them in three dimensions at one or more points in the cardiac cycle.

As early as 1974, when two-dimensional scanning was being developed and refined, transducer locating systems had been designed to allow three-dimensional reconstruction of the planar data.[1,2] In the 1970s and 1980s, several groups demonstrated the feasibility of three-dimensional reconstruction in the research environment, but extension to larger populations was limited by the labor-intensive processes of acquiring and integrating the image and locating data to produce three-dimensional representations. As more sophisticated computer hardware and software and mechanisms for acquiring and displaying three-dimensional echo data have become available, many of these complex and labor-intensive tasks have been reduced or fully automated. Consequently, interest in and applications for this technology have expanded. The purpose of this chapter is to review the development and present status of the three-dimensional echocardiographic reconstruction and to describe its current and potential clinical applications.

BASIC CONCEPTS

Limitation of Two-Dimensional Techniques

When a standard two-dimensional echocardiographic study is performed or reviewed, the interpreter mentally

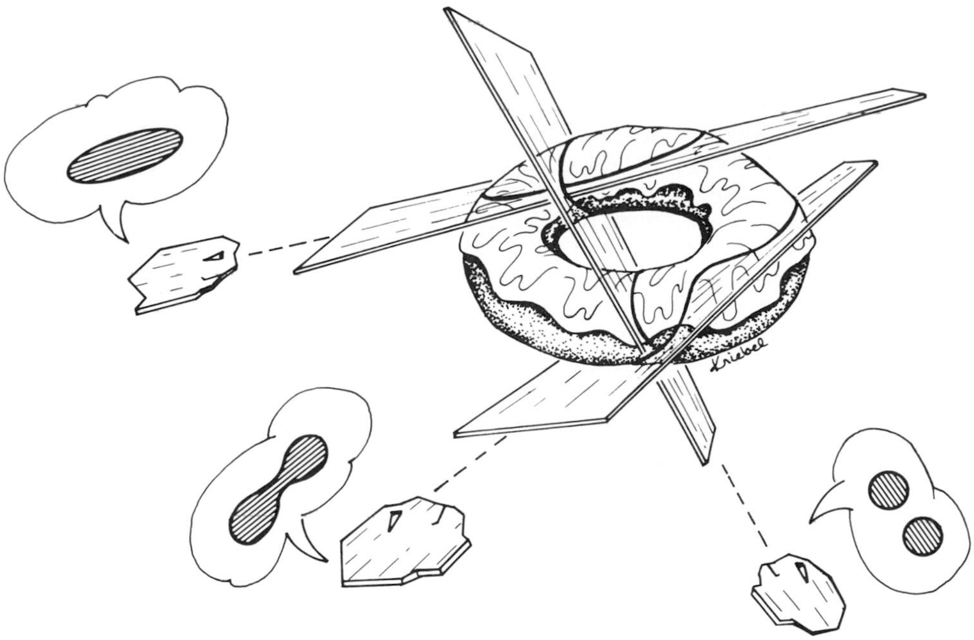

Fig. 6–1. Two-dimensional images produced by scanning of a simple geometric shape such as a "doughnut" are relatively simple and easy to understand in their three-dimensional context.

reconstructs a three-dimensional image of the heart from the visual images received. This requires intimate knowledge of the three-dimensional structure of the heart and great vessels and certain necessary assumptions about their internal structure and relationships to each other. As illustrated in Figure 6–1, determining the three-dimensional shape of an object from a series of two-dimensional images is valid and relatively easy when the structure is simple and symmetric, and the general shape is already known to the observer, as is the "doughnut" in this example. Similarly, the left ventricle, which has a relatively simple and symmetric shape in its normal state, yields images that are not difficult to appreciate in their three-dimensional context or to mentally reconstruct. However, interpretation becomes considerably more difficult and less reliable as the complexity of the object increases or when its underlying shape is poorly understood. The effect of increasing complexity is illustrated by the "pretzel" in Figure 6–2, where the basic shape is more variable and the relationship of spatially undefined slices to the original figure is less clear. In routine two-dimensional scanning, such spatial complexity is encountered when imaging irregular structures such as the right ventricle and mitral valve, or when the shape of the structure is unknown, as occurs with a variety of congenital or acquired malformations. In such cases, three-dimensional reconstruction could offer a more realistic, self-explanatory description of these features, thus decreasing or eliminating the need for assumptions on the part of the observer.

Need to Combine Images From Multiple Cardiac Cycles

Importantly, the imaging data necessary for three-dimensional reconstruction are already present in routine

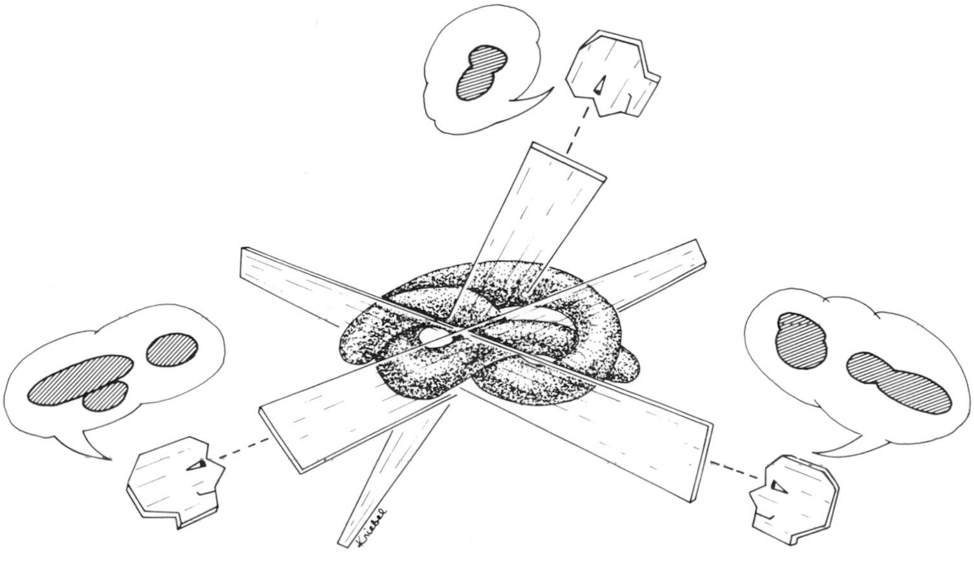

Fig. 6–2. In contrast to Figure 6–1, a more complex "pretzel" yields two-dimensional images that are complicated and not easily integrated into a three-dimensional shape. (See text for details.)

two-dimensional scans. By combining two-dimensional images from different tomographic views, three-dimensional information can be generated. At first glance it would seem reasonable that just as a single ultrasound beam can be scanned through a plane to produce a two-dimensional sector, such a sector could, in turn, be scanned through space to produce a three-dimensional acquisition. With existing technology, however, it would take too long to image a three-dimensional region the heart in real time. For example, scanning 30 sectors, each requiring 33 msec, would require close to a second, or about the duration of one full cardiac cycle. Because of the significant cardiac motion within this time, serious temporal artifacts would be introduced in the imaging data set. Therefore, until advances in transducer design and parallel processing permit real-time three-dimensional acquisition with sufficient imaging quality (see Chapter 2), two-dimensional images must be acquired over several cardiac cycles from different tomographic views, and information about their spatial and temporal relationships to each other must be determined.

Because many of the concepts and methods currently under development in the research environment are likely to appear in future clinical echocardiographic systems, the requisite components of such systems and the advantages and disadvantages of the different approaches taken bear some discussion.

System Requirements

Three-dimensional reconstruction requires the ability to collect the necessary raw data and then integrate these data into representations for analysis. The first step requires methods to collect and store (1) two-dimensional image data generated by the ultrasound machine; (2) data to locate these images in three-dimensional space, or more specifically, to localize the individual points that together constitute the image; and (3) data to define the time in the cardiac cycle that the two-dimensional images are recorded. Then the appropriate computer hardware and software must be available to process and integrate this information to produce three-dimensional representations that can be displayed to allow visual appreciation of the three-dimensionality of scanned structures. Furthermore, methods should be available for quantifying three-dimensional spatial and temporal relationships. Ideally, each of these steps could be integrated into one system that would allow rapid acquisition and processing of the data for three-dimensional analysis.

METHODS FOR ACQUIRING TWO-DIMENSIONAL IMAGE DATA

The two-dimensional echocardiographic images are the primary data on which the three-dimensional reconstruction depends and normally are stored on videotape by recording the analog video signal that is output by the ultrasound machine during the scan. The images can be reviewed during video playback by displaying the recorded data on a video monitor, and by placing the recorder in pause mode, it is possible to "freeze" on different images of interest at specific points in the cardiac cycle. Though videotape is a convenient and inexpensive storage media, the image data in this analog form are not easily manipulated for reconstruction. In some of the first attempts at three-dimensional reconstruction, these video images were photographed or printed with a hard-copy device, and the outlines of features for reconstruction were derived from the prints by hand or with the aid of a digital pointing device. Fortunately, this time-consuming process has been superseded by the advent of video frame grabbers that digitize the analog video signal, either directly from the ultrasound machine or from video playback. The images are then represented as a two-dimensional array of numeric values (commonly referred to as *pixels*) that correspond to the image intensity or color at a regularly spaced positions. These devices are usually directly interfaced to a computer so the image data can be easily stored and later recalled for display and processing as necessary. Ideally, image data could be acquired directly in a digital format from the ultrasound machine because it is represented in this form before conversion to the video signal by the scan converter. Although some of the more advanced systems currently provide access to the digital data for a limited number of images, the computer storage requirements, and data transfer rates have been prohibitively large to allow practical incorporation of this feature for real-time acquisition.

METHODS FOR LOCATING IMAGE DATA IN THREE-DIMENSIONAL SPACE

The position of any point or pixel on a two-dimensional echocardiographic image can be calculated with respect to the apex of the scan sector. This, in effect, localizes that point with respect to the imaging transducer. If, in turn, a method can be devised to define accurately the position and orientation of the transducer in space, the three-dimensional location of any point within the tomographic image can be determined. The methods for transducer or image plane localization can be grouped into three basic categories: (1) methods of best fit, which rely on assumed image orientation or visual cues to fit images from different views; (2) fixed acquisition formats that restrict the scan to a predetermined and regular geometric format, e.g., a series of equidistant parallel planes or equiangular rotations about a fixed axis; and (3) techniques that allow unrestricted scanning, with three-dimensional information provided by spatial locators (acoustic, electromagnetic, and articulated mechanical arms).

Best Fit Method

In the methods of best fit, anatomic landmarks are used to define a series of two-dimensional image orientations from which images are selected, traced, and realigned in space. The traces are first positioned in their assumed angular relationship to each other and then adjusted or translated until the intersecting traces align by visual or other criteria. In an example of this technique to measure ventricular volume,[3] a single apical long axis view served as the template to align a series of images selected from a short axis scan. The long axis view was assumed to intersect the central axis of the left ventricle in an anterior-posterior orientation. Each short axis trace was positioned in its assumed orientation perpendicular to the long axis view and then was adjusted from base to apex and translated within the plane until the anterior-posterior points of intersection of the two contours best fit each other. Combination of several of these fitted planes produced a "wire-and-frame" outline of the left ventricle was produced.

The best fit approach has been applied to the left ventricle because of its relatively simple and symmetric shape. It has the advantage of simplicity because scanning is unencumbered by additional hardware attached to the transducer and equipment requirements are modest. For asymmetric ventricles and other less simple structures, however, true three-dimensional registration is required. Even for simple structures, multiple solution often exist for the placement of the imaging planes and the selection of a particular orientation is highly subjective. Though a reconstruction may look coherent, it may not accurately reflect the shape of the original structure.

Techniques Based on Restricted Acquisition Format

The Method of Multiple Parallel Planes

One of the first approaches, and perhaps the simplest, to three-dimensional image reconstruction is through the acquisition of multiple parallel planes separated by fixed intervals. This method models any three-dimensional object as a series of two-dimensional images stacked on top of one another (Fig. 6–3). Because the two-dimensional images are derived from planes that have a known relative spatial orientation and separation, a three-dimensional representation of the original structure can be reconstructed if the space between these planes is filled in by connecting equivalent points on adjacent images. The accuracy of such a method will increase with the number of parallel slices that intersect the object of interest, and only objects larger than the distance between the slices can be faithfully reconstructed.

During image acquisition, the scanning transducer is generally held by some form of mechanical arm so that only movement in one direction, parallel to the surface of the chest (heart), is possible. By manually or mechanically shifting the transducer in measured increments, one can obtain images parallel to each other and can determine structure, volume, and mass using Simpson's rule. Ideally, structures of interest should be oriented perpendicular to the scan planes, or they may be poorly represented in the primary recordings. This method has been applied to reconstructions of the left ventricle, both in vitro and in vivo,[4–6] but may prove more applicable in the evolving fields of three-dimensional intravascular and transesophageal imaging.

The advantages of such a system are (1) ease of design and construction, (2) requirement that only relative plane separation be recorded, and (3) simplicity of the algorithms required to reconstruct structures of interest. Disadvantages are the constrained movement of the transducer, which severely limits image quality at some levels, and the fact that recording is generally limited to structures that underlie the anterior chest wall. Clinically, interference by ribs and lung makes the acquisition of multiple parallel planes extremely difficult, and this approach is best suited to open chest imaging, i.e., during surgery or in experimental animal preparations.

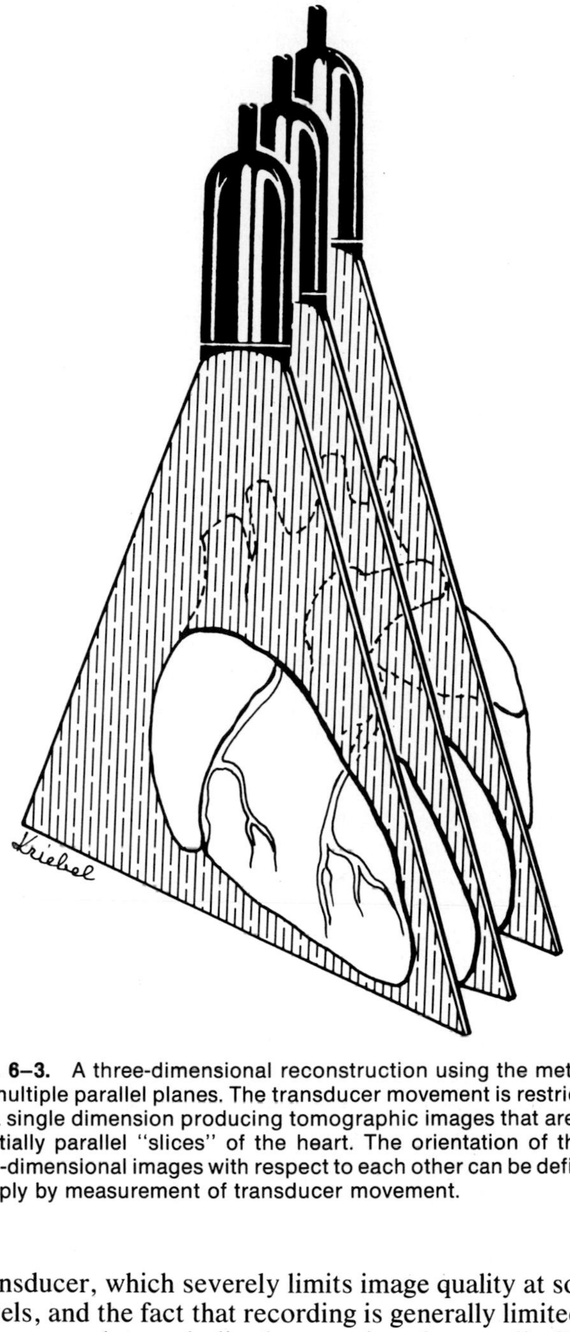

Fig. 6–3. A three-dimensional reconstruction using the method of multiple parallel planes. The transducer movement is restricted to a single dimension producing tomographic images that are essentially parallel "slices" of the heart. The orientation of these two-dimensional images with respect to each other can be defined simply by measurement of transducer movement.

The Pivot Point and Axial Rotation Methods

In the pivot point approach, the problem of transducer localization is avoided by imaging exclusively from a single, fixed recording point. Although angulation and rotation are allowed, the point of transducer contact with the chest wall is not altered. If the degree of transducer angulation or rotation is known, then the position of the images with respect to each other is defined, and three-dimensional relationships can be inferred.

In one application of this principle,[7] the transducer is

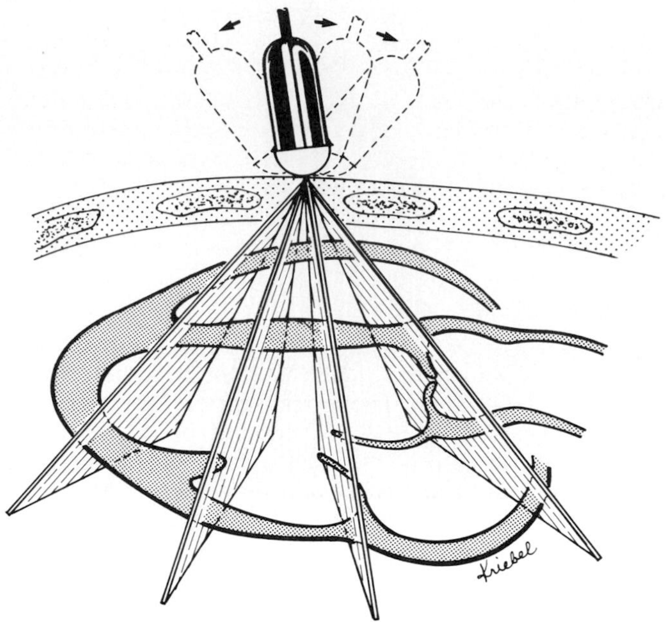

Fig. 6–4. The pivot point method for three-dimensional reconstruction. The acquisition of locating data is simplified by confining the transducer to a single point on the chest wall, and the position of recorded images can be defined by measuring transducer angulation.

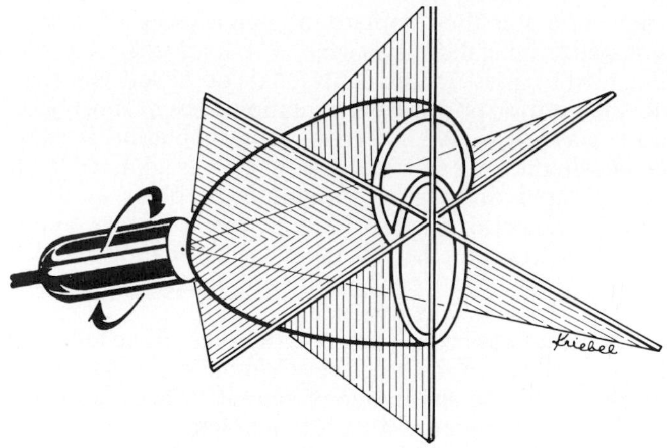

Fig. 6–6. An alternate form of the pivot point method. The transducer is placed at the cardiac apex and rotated through a full 360°. Recording the relative degree of rotation at which each image is recorded makes three-dimensional reconstruction possible.

initially positioned to record an optimal parasternal long axis view of the left ventricle. Then, without moving the transducer from this position on the chest, the examiner rotates it 90° and records serial short axis images by angling the scan plane from base to apex (Figs. 6–4 and 6–5). By gating image acquisition with the electrocardiogram, a series of tomographs are obtained at either end-systole or end-diastole. Because the pivot point is common for all the images, if the degree of angulation of the short axis cuts with respect to the long axis can be determined, the chamber can be reconstructed. Alternatively, the distance between anterior and posterior endocardial borders on the long axis image can be used to fit the short axis views into their proper location (a combination of the pivot point and best fit approaches).

Another application of the pivot point method is to place the transducer at the left ventricular apex and to rotate it about the long axis of the ventricle without altering its point of contact with the chest wall (Fig. 6–6).[8–10] Because the images share a common apical imaging point and axis of intersection, if the degree of rotation is known, then the recorded images of the left ventricle can be oriented with respect to each other. This technique has been used to determine left ventricular volume with good correlation to angiographic measurements.[8] Similarly, an inclinometer has been used to measure the rotation angle in a three-dimensional analysis of the annulus of the mitral valve.[10]

More recently, a mechanical device has been developed to automatically rotate the transducer in fixed increments about an axis.[11] This also has been used to image the left ventricle from an apical window generating full volumetric data sets of the raw echo data at multiple points in the cardiac cycle. By applying volumetric rendering algorithms to these three-dimensional data sets, researchers have produced two-dimensional representations of the beating left ventricle for qualitative review on a graphics monitor. Experimental validation of this technique for volume validation has also been performed.[12]

Also conceptually simple, this approach has several practical limitations. Most important, only cardiac structures that can be viewed completely from a single window can be reconstructed. Therefore, the operator's freedom to seek ideal images from multiple vantage points is restricted. Also, for correct image registration, the apex of the sector scan must remain stationary as the transducer is rotated or angulated. This can be especially difficult for acquisitions involving manual positioning of the transducer and during long image acquisitions.

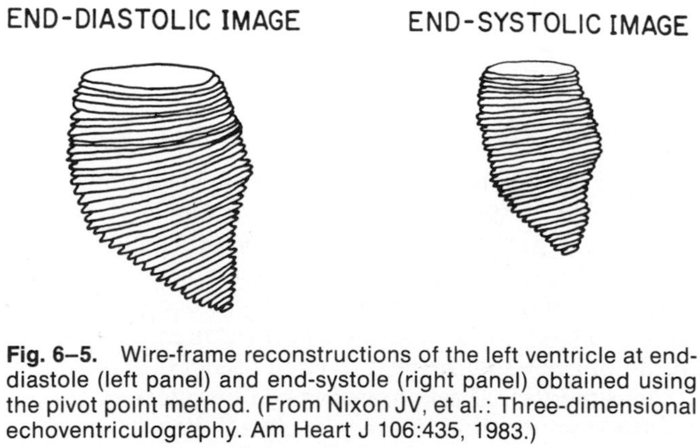

Fig. 6–5. Wire-frame reconstructions of the left ventricle at end-diastole (left panel) and end-systole (right panel) obtained using the pivot point method. (From Nixon JV, et al.: Three-dimensional echoventriculography. Am Heart J 106:435, 1983.)

Locating Systems That Allow Unrestricted Transducer Motion

Articulated Mechanical Arms

Several groups have attempted three-dimensional reconstruction of the heart using articulated mechanical

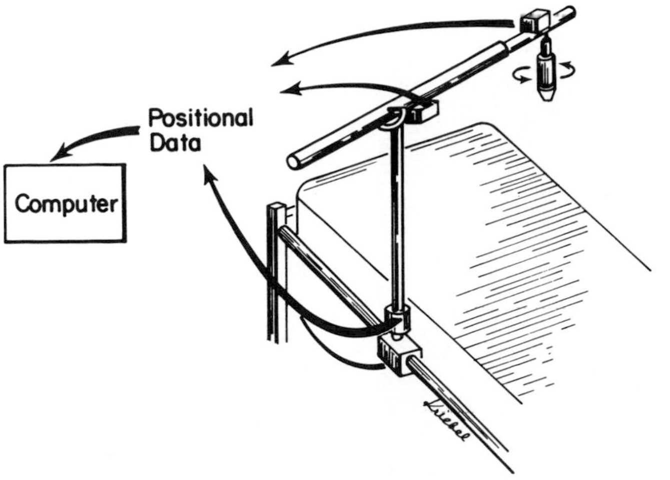

Fig. 6–7. An articulated mechanical arm for recording transducer location during an ultrasound scan.

arms, similar to those used in abdominal scanning, which accurately define transducer position in space, and yet allow considerable freedom of movement.[1,13–18] Devices of this type have been developed with up to six movable joints. If the lengths of the component arms (distance between the joints) are known, the three-dimensional position and orientation of the transducer can be calculated from the angular relationship of these arms to each other. Commonly, a potentiometer or optical encoder is positioned at each joint to automatically monitor angular changes during image acquisition. The output of these sensors is interfaced to a computer that can record the values and perform the necessary calculations to determine the three-dimensional position of the imaging data. In some systems, the entire apparatus is attached to a track that is secured to the bedside and along which the arm can slide (Fig. 6–7) for positioning with respect to the patient. Although articulated arms allows greater flexibility of transducer movement than systems that use a fixed acquisition format, the devices described thus far have generally been large and cumbersome and do not permit total freedom of motion.

Acoustic Locator Systems

Acoustic locator systems use three sound-emitting transmitters, which are rigidly attached to the transducer (Fig. 6–8).[19–21] These transmitters are fired in succession, and the sound is received by an array of fixed microphones. The time delay between sound generation from the transmitter and its detection by each microphone is then calculated and recorded by computer. Because the sound delay is proportional to the distance between transmitter and microphone, the position of each transmitter in space can be calculated by triangulation, and the position of the imaging plane of the transducer can be defined from its known location relative to the three transmitters. The positions of the microphones are assumed to be fixed in relation to the patient during scanning and their relative position to each other known.

This approach has the advantage of allowing considerable freedom of transducer movement within a wide range of transducer angles and positions relative to the microphone array, which allows the operator to acquire the imaging data like an ordinary two-dimensional scan (Fig. 6–9). The main limitation of this method is that

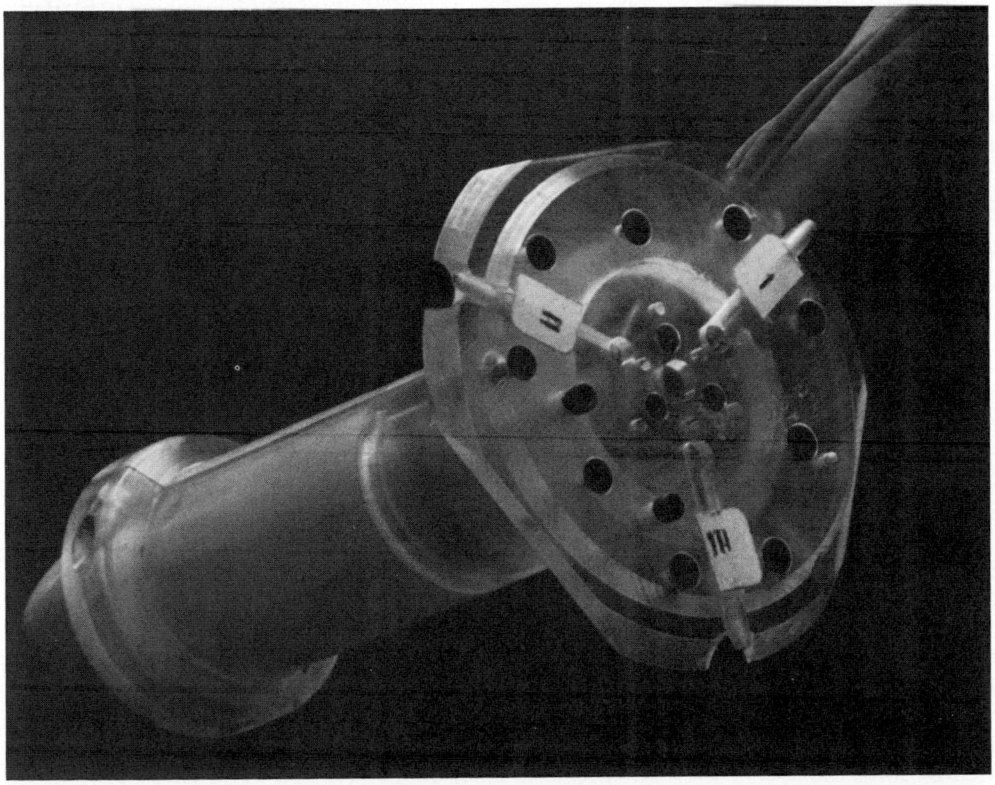

Fig. 6–8. A 3.5-MHz transducer with a specifically designed housing with three attached spark gaps that are sequentially fired during scanning for acoustic localization of image data.

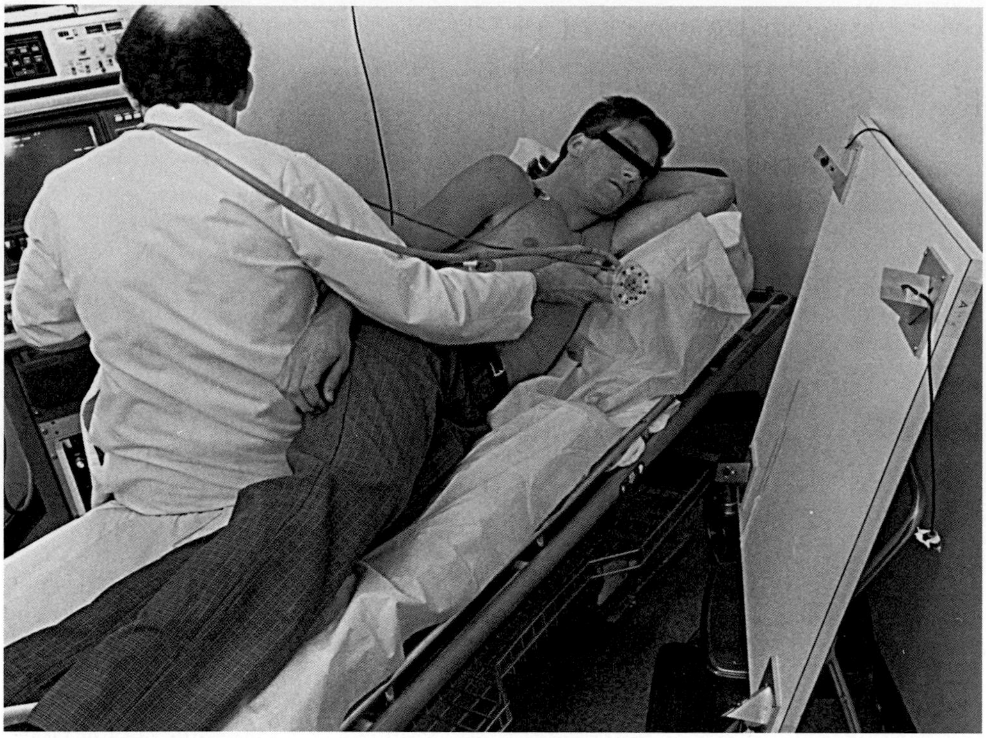

Fig. 6–9. Spark gap locating system in operation. The transducer with attached spark gaps is held in a parasternal location. Microphones attached to a board at the bedside record the sound emitted by the spark gaps. The time delay between sound production and its detection by the microphones is used to compute the position of the transducer in three-dimensional space continually throughout the examination.

there must be a direct, line-of-sight path between the sound transmitters and the microphones. This has prevented certain combinations of views, e.g., parasternal and apical orientations, from being obtained in a single acquisition: It is difficult to position the microphone array to accommodate both transducer orientations without occluding the sound path in one orientation or the other. This technique can also require some adjustment time to position of the microphone array for optimal data acquisition. Despite these restrictions, the acoustic locating technique has been an extremely useful method for routine research and clinical applications, as will be illustrated later in this chapter.

Electromagnetic Locator Systems

One of the more recent approaches to image localization has been the development of electromagnetic positional sensors (Polhemus Navigational Systems and Ascension Technologies). In these systems, a transmitter generates dipolar electromagnetic fields from three mutually orthogonal coils in rapid succession. The field strengths are measured by a three-coil (also mutually orthogonal) detector mounted on the transducer. The measured strengths of the three pulsed fields in each of the receiver coils are then used to define the receiver position (x, y, and z) and angular orientation (azimuth, elevation, and roll) in relation to the transmitter. Although similar in principle to the acoustic locating mechanism, the components of electromagnetic systems are considerably smaller and require minimal setup time. Furthermore, this method has the unique advantage that nonferromagnetic materials, such as body tissue or plastic mounting devices, can be placed between the transmitter and receiver without affecting the locating mechanism. This permits scanning from any angular orientation so that virtually any views, such as parasternal, apical or subcostal, can be combined from a single acquisition. In fact, it may be possible to make the receivers sufficiently small to fit on transesophageal probes with the transmitter placed adjacent to the patient's chest. An important limitation of this technique, however, is that ferromagnetic material in close proximity to the device will distort the magnetic fields and positional measurements. Therefore, care must be taken to ensure that such objects be removed from the scanning environment. Because of the components of electric motors, the technique may also be restricted to nonmechanical probes.

Summary of Locating Techniques

Reconstruction techniques that are completely objective in the acquisition of positional data, such as the fixed and unrestricted geometry techniques, offer a decided advantage over methods in which an operator or algorithm is required to fit planar images together (e.g., best fit methods), or where positional data depend on the nonvalidated assumption of a constant transducer position as in manual pivot point methods. The parallel plane and axial rotation methods are similar in concept to the mechanical arm or acoustic locator approaches but with restriction to 1° of freedom instead of 6°. Unfortunately, this restriction in flexibility of image acquisition often makes it impractical for transthoracic imaging of many structures: Obtaining images of sufficient quality throughout the scan and representing the entire structure of interest is difficult from restricted windows. The image quality for intravascular and transesophageal imaging, however, is generally more uniform and therefore better suited for fixed acquisition formats. One of the major advantages of unrestricted acquisitions is that images can be obtained from optimal imaging windows from multiple points on the chest wall. This allows regions that are better perceived from different views to be combined to produce a three-dimensional construct.

METHODS FOR TEMPORAL ALIGNMENT OF IMAGES TO THE CARDIAC CYCLE

Because the beating heart is not a stationary structure but rather is continually contracting and expanding, it is essential to locate images not only in space but also with respect to the time of their acquisition within the cardiac cycle. Therefore, a separate three-dimensional reconstruction must be performed for each temporal point of interest. This requires gathering images and their locating data over multiple cardiac cycles from a common temporal point within the cycle. The most widely used approach for temporal registration has been to use the electrocardiogram (ECG) signal that is simultaneously superimposed, in real-time, on the two-dimensional video images. During image selection, the most recent R wave of the QRS complex is identified and used as the reference from which the temporal offset of subsequent images can be measured. Commonly, the measurement unit is simply the number of video frames past the time of R-wave appearance. There is an assumption that the same temporal offset from different R waves correspond to the same point in the cardiac cycle. This technique has been incorporated in several on-line and off-line analysis systems to automatically allow acquisition of multiple, temporally registered sets of images and provides a convenient method to simplify the process of image selection for three-dimensional reconstruction. An alternative alignment technique is to use certain visual or auditory events, e.g., valve opening and closure, to identify common temporal points in the cardiac cycle. This method can be used independently or to assist in identifying the offsets from the R wave of specific temporal points of interest.

ALIGNMENT OF IMAGING DATA, POSITIONAL DATA, AND ECG DATA

Before the raw data produced by the techniques described previously can be integrated, the separate data sets must be correctly registered so that the individual elements correspond to the same point in acquisition time. Because the ECG signal can be directly recorded with the image data in real time, these data are inherently temporally registered with respect to each other. Locating data, however, is often acquired separately by a computer. Therefore, a method must be available for its synchronization to the image data.

In many image locating procedures, the position of the transducer is fixed over a period of one or more cardiac cycles for each tomographic view in the acquisition. This allows each set of positional data to correspond to a specific segment of image information on videotape. Some form of identification, e.g., entry of overlay characters or auditory flags, can be recorded on the videotape to identify the positional data that are associated with a particular segment of images. In some systems for multiplanar transesophageal imaging, this process has been fully automated and incorporated into the ultrasound system.[22] As the tip of the imaging transducer is rotated by manual adjustment of an external dial, the rotation angle is sensed and overlaid on a portion of the video image. The angle can then be read from the displayed image and manually entered into a computer.

Another simplified approach has been to digitize images directly from the ultrasound machine and simultaneously acquire the locating data at the time of the scan. The locating data can then be associated with the image data simply by the order of acquisition. Though this technique is straightforward, the number of tomographic views may be limited by the amount of high speed memory required for digital image storage.

For acquisitions that involve complete freedom of transducer movement, the position of the transducer can continuously change from one video frame to another. Therefore, the transducer location must be updated continuously throughout the scan, and a technique must be available to precisely register these data to the imaging data. In some systems, a visual or audio signal is generated by the computer and recorded on videotape to identify the onset of the three-dimensional scan. Each time data are received from the locating mechanism, the computer clock can be accessed and stored along with the locating data. The temporal offset of images from the initiation signal can then be used to select the appropriate locating data.

A more elegant approach for data alignment has been to rapidly acquire and overlay the positional data on an unused portion of the video signal for real-time recording on videotape.[23] Instead of representing the data in text format that must be read and manually entered into the computer, the data are encoded as a digital pattern. Because this pattern can be decoded from the image data, any image recorded during the scan can be digitized and positioned in space. Continuous data acquisition allows the operator to rapidly scan the patient to find the optimum imaging windows and to minimize the effects of patient motion and respiration. The ability to automatically decode positional information from the images saves considerable time and has the advantage that all the information necessary for reconstruction can be conveniently stored on videotape (the same storage requirement for two-dimensional scans).

Figure 6–10 illustrates the process of data alignment and selection for a scan with an acoustic locating system. Image data and ECG data are generated by the ultrasound system while, concurrently, data are recorded to locate the positions of the three sound emitters (spark gaps) on the transducer. If the imaging, ECG, and locating data are temporally aligned with respect to their time of acquisition, then images and their location in space can be selected from a particular point in the cardiac cycle using the ECG signal. In this example, the data for a single image in early diastole have been selected, and the location of the spark gaps has been used to calculate the three-dimensional orientation of

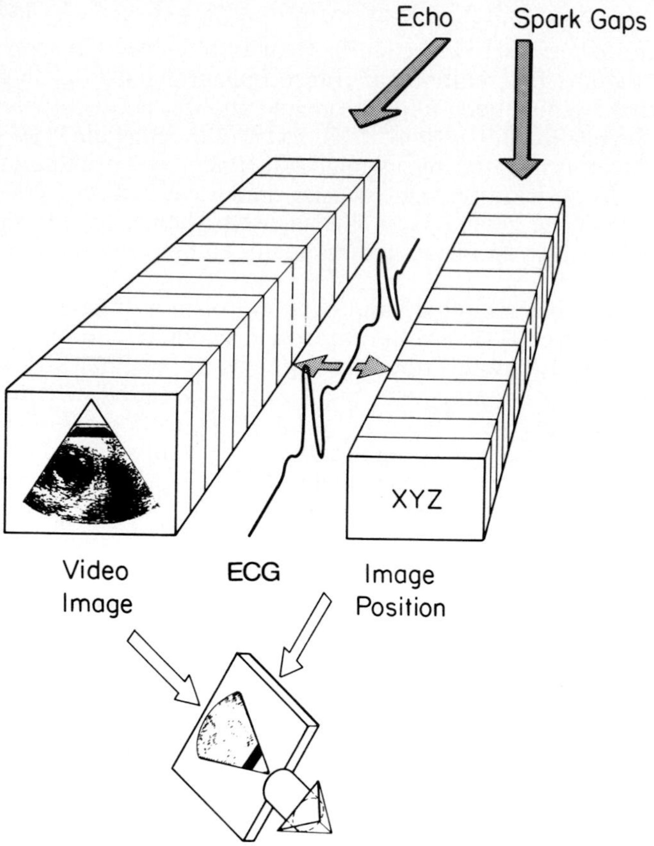

Fig. 6–10. Video images and positional data are acquired simultaneously and referenced to a common clock. The electrocardiogram can then be used to identify the position of each image of interest.

the transducer and image data. By adding other images from the same relative point in the cardiac cycle, the examiner can produce a three-dimensional representation.

PROCESSING, INTEGRATION, AND STORAGE OF IMAGING DATA

Because of the enormous quantity of data and number of calculations involved in three-dimensional reconstruction, the integration and processing of information for three-dimensional reconstruction must be performed on a computer. Therefore, the data, whether acquired directly or digitized from videotape, must be represented in a digital format. In essence, three characteristics need to be defined for each picture subunit or pixel of each two-dimensional image: intensity, spatial location, and time in cardiac cycle. A description of these components and their processing follows.

Intensity

Intensity is represented by a numeric value that corresponds to the particular gradation of shading from black to white, where black is usually assigned a value of zero and white is assigned a value of N, where N equals the number of gray levels. Digital frame grabbers can usually differentiate from 64 to 256 different pixel intensity levels from the video signal. The dimensions of the two-dimensional array of intensity values that describe an image commonly varies from 256 to 756 pixels in the horizontal direction and from 240 to 486 in the vertical direction. Therefore, depending on the dimensions, from 60,000 to 300,000 bytes could be required to store a single digitized video image.

Spatial Location

Spatial location of a pixel is ultimately defined as its reconstructed location in a three-dimensional Cartesian coordinate system and can be represented by three-numeric values (x, y, and z), each corresponding to a position along the separate orthogonal axes. The calculation of spatial location requires first defining the position of the pixel in two-dimensional space (x, y) (i.e., with respect to the sector scan) and then transforming the two-dimensional coordinates into three dimensions using the image locating data. The first step is accomplished by multiplying the particular column and row indices (ix, iy) that identify the location of the pixel in the two-dimensional image storage array by horizontal and vertical pixel scale factors (sx, sy):

$$x = ix * sx \qquad [6.1]$$

$$y = iy * sy \qquad [6.2]$$

The scale factors can vary for a particular acquisition depending on the number of pixels in each dimension of the digitized image array and the scan-depth setting on the ultrasound machine.

Once the locations are defined correctly in two dimensions, the appropriate three-dimensional transformation (derived from the transducer locating data) can be applied. The type of transformation will depend on the acquisition format. For instance, in parallel plane acquisitions, the orientation of the different images can remain in the x-y plane format with the position of each plane along the z axis varied to correspond to the acquired translation value. Therefore, the spatial location of all the pixels for a given image will have the same z coordinate.

Calculating spatial location from rotation about a fixed axis requires the location of the rotation axis to be known with respect to the two-dimensional image data and the rotation angle of each two-dimensional image relative to a reference plane. In most acquisitions, the rotation axis is the vertical axis, or y axis, of the image that passes through the origin or apex of the sector scan. The y coordinate therefore remains constant, while x and z can be computed from the distance of the pixel from the rotation axis in the x direction (dx) and the planar rotation angle of the image relative to the x-y plane (theta) as follows:

$$X = dx * \sin(theta) \qquad [6.3]$$

$$Z = dx * \cos(theta) \qquad [6.4]$$

When the imaging plane can be oriented and positioned arbitrarily in three-dimensional space, as occurs in unrestricted imaging scans, 6° of freedom can vary:

translation in the x, y and z direction (tx, ty, tz), and rotation angle about the x, y, and z axes (ax, ay, az) of the Cartesian coordinate system. With all the locating techniques used for such scans, computing the correct spatial location of a pixel requires the position and orientation of the locating device to be known with respect to the two-dimensional imaging data. This will allow the appropriate algorithms to compute (from the locating data generated by the device) the correct values for the 6° of freedom. Though the different locating mechanism provide different means of determining these values: the calculations to convert the two-dimensional position of a pixel (x, y) to its three-dimensional position (x, y, z) can be expressed ultimately in the form shown by the following formulas:

$$X = tx + x * \cos(ay) * \cos(az) + y * \cos(ay) * \sin(az) \qquad [6.5]$$

$$Y = ty + x * [-\cos(ax) * \sin(az) + \sin(ax) * \sin(ay) * \cos(az)] + y * [\cos(ax) * \cos(az) + \sin(ax) * \sin(ay) * \sin(az)] \qquad [6.6]$$

$$Z = tz + x * [\sin(ax) * \sin(az) + \cos(ax) * \sin(ay) * \cos(az)] + y * [-\sin(ax) * \cos(az) + \cos(ax) * \sin(ay) * \sin(az)] \qquad [6.7]$$

Temporal Location

Temporal location, or time, of image acquisition is usually defined by the number of video frames or milliseconds (33 per frame) past the onset of acquisition and also with respect to the most recent R wave. The latter can also be represented in a descriptive manner such as end-diastole or end-systole as long as common values correspond to common points in the cardiac cycle. Cardiac time is important for determining the selection of those images that can be combined to produce a reconstruction and to define the sequential order of a set of reconstructions for dynamic representations of the beating heart. The temporal location of data with respect to the start of a three-dimensional scan becomes important for aligning different data sets of interest that are collected independent of the image data.

Figure 6–11 shows a two-dimensional image using pixels and the subsequent positioning of these data in three dimensions with data from an acoustic locating system. The two-dimensional echo image is represented as a collection of individual rectangular tiles or pixels, each of which is assigned an intensity value that corresponds to the intensity of that region on the image. The position of a pixel on the two-dimensional image (a grid 256 × 240 pixels) is determined from its location in the storage array and the pixel scale factors that determine the horizontal and vertical dimensions of the image data. In turn, if the fixed relationship of the image data to the spark gaps on the transducer is known, then the coordinates of the spark gaps during acquisition (Fig. 6–11A, B, and C) will uniquely determine the location of the image data in three dimensions at a particular point in time. Combining multiple images from different tomographic views provides three-dimensional information about the region of interest. Each pixel of interest, then, can be assigned a set of numeric values that can be encoded into the computer memory to define its position in two-dimensional and three-dimensional space.

Digital Data Storage

With the availability of video frame grabbers, the acquisition of video images in a digital format for use by a computer is a relatively simple procedure. Saving digital image data, however, can require an enormous amount of computer disk space, especially for dynamic reconstructions. To illustrate this problem, let us consider storing an entire data set from a 60-second scan. As discussed in Chapter 3, the standard storage unit in computers is termed the *byte* which, as previously described is capable of representing 1 pixel. With a typical array size of 100,000 pixels per two-dimensional image and a standard video rate of 30 frames/sec, roughly 3 million bytes (megabytes) are required for the storage of each second of video recording. Sixty seconds of recording would therefore require about 180 megabytes of memory and is the equivalent of more than 100 standard high density floppy disks. Because the image locating data can be completely represented by 6 to 12 numeric values (3 for translation and 3 or 9 for rotation), each requiring 2 bytes, the storage requirement of 12 to 24 bytes per image is insignificant in relation to the image data.

Fortunately, many applications of three-dimensional imaging can be limited to reconstruction of one or two predetermined points in the cardiac cycle, e.g., end-systole and end-diastole. If combining 20 frames can adequately represent the structure of interest, then the data for an entire study could fit on one or two high density (1.2- to 1.4-megabyte) floppy disks.

Although the magnitude of data can be very large, advances in image compression technology and digital storage media are beginning to meet the challenges of providing a cost-effective solution to digital image storage. For instance, replaceable optical disk storage can hold 650 megabytes for under $200.00 (U.S.), and digital tape, though less convenient, can store up to 5 gigabytes for even less.

Border Identification

Once the images are retrieved from video tape and represented in a digital format, they can be displayed on a computer graphics monitor. They are then available for analysis in their current form or can be further refined to identify particular features of interest. The outlines of such structures can be traced from the image using a digital pointing device such as a light pen, digitizing tablet, or a mouse producing a series of two-dimensional points or connected line segments that can be superimposed on the ultrasound image. The coordinates and connectivity of the line drawing can then be digitally stored along with the image locating data for subsequent

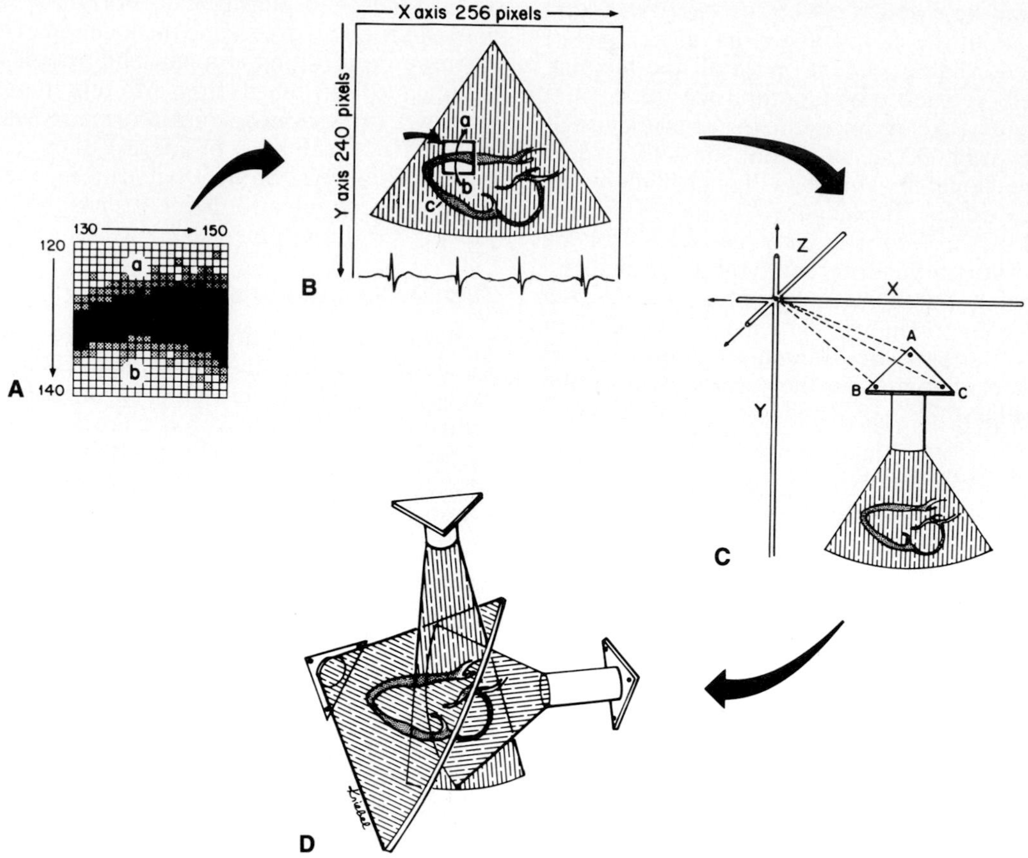

Fig. 6–11. Each video image obtained during a standard two-dimensional scan can be considered an array of picture elements or "pixels" (A) arranged in a 240 × 256 array (B). Each of these pixels can be characterized by its location in two dimensions (some combination of x and y values) and by its grey-scale intensity. Three-dimensional reconstruction further requires locating the pixel data in three-dimensional space using a three-axis coordinate system (i.e., X_i, Y_i and Z_i), as illustrated in C. This defines the position of each pixel in its orientation at the time the image was acquired (D).

integration in three dimensions. Because the line drawing is stored in the same coordinate framework as the image, and the spatial location of the image in three-dimensional space is known, the same geometric operations (described previously) can be used to reposition the trace data in three dimensions. Although certain techniques and algorithms have been available for automated border detection for other imaging modalities, such as magnetic resonance imaging (MRI) and computed tomography (CT), these techniques have been difficult to implement for echocardiographic images because of their lack of uniformity and variable quality. The development of more sophisticated algorithms for this purpose, however, is an area of ongoing interest and likely will be used to facilitate three-dimensional reconstruction in the future.

Examples of three-dimensional reconstruction of image data and their derived borders from a scan of a hemispherical object placed in a water bath are illustrated in Figures 6–12 and 6–13. The actual pixel data from two of the two-dimensional images are displayed in Figure 6–12. The pixels with intensity values below a given cutoff value have been eliminated to allow data normally obscured by the intersecting planes to be displayed. Figure 6–13 illustrates the reconstructed con-

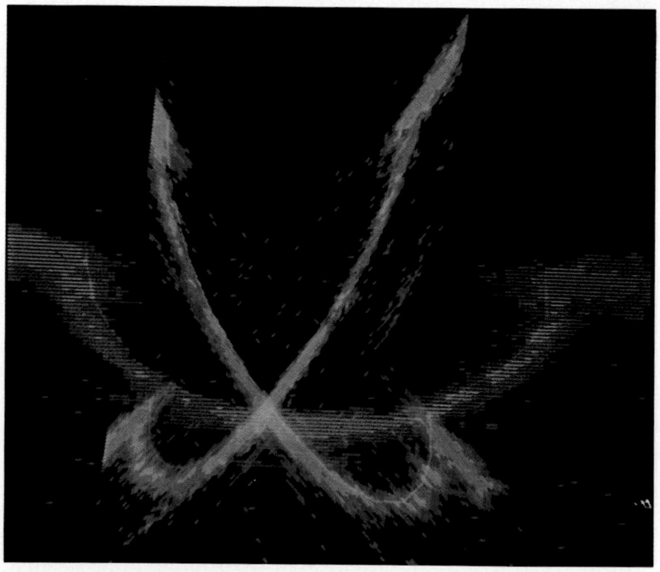

Fig. 6–12. Two-dimensional images of a hemispheric test object recorded with an acoustic locating system and realigned in space.

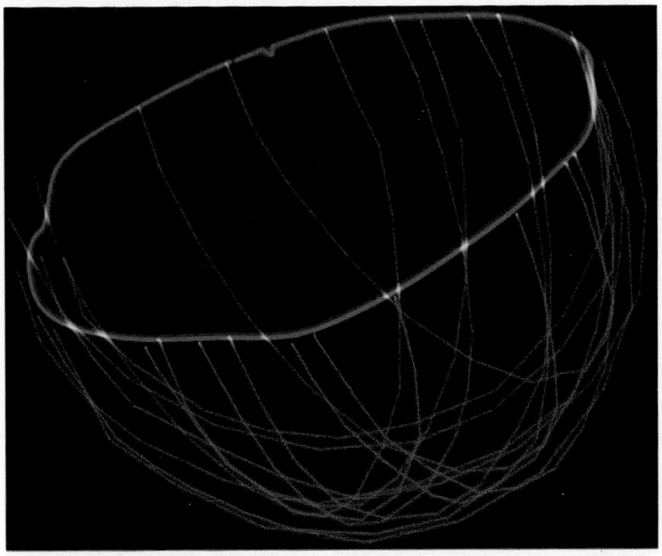

Fig. 6–13. Digitized contours from scans of the same hemispheric object illustrated in Figure 6–12. The contours are positioned in their correct three-dimensional orientation using locating data derived from the acoustic locator. Note that the connected end points of the traces accurately define the circular edge of the object.

tours of the inner surface of the hemisphere traced from a larger number of two-dimensional images. The endpoints of the traces have been connected to show the circular edge of the hemisphere, the shape of which can clearly be appreciated.

Similarly, traces derived from two-dimensional scans of the mitral valve leaflets are shown in Figure 6–14A in their three-dimensional orientation to each other. In Figure 6–14B, a grid surface has been calculated to conform to the traces that smooths the raw data and produces a more recognizable valve surface. The reconstruction is from a point in late systole so the leaflets are closed, and the traces, and surface, do not distinguish the commissure between the two leaflets.

METHODS FOR DISPLAYING THE RECONSTRUCTED DATA

To this point, methods have been described for acquiring the data required for three-dimensional reconstruction. The next step in the process is to display the accumulated data in a manner that allows the viewer to appreciate, as fully as possible, the three-dimensional nature of the structure under study.

Two-Dimensional Display of Three-Dimensional Data

Artists have recognized for centuries the value of perspective, shadowing, and image intensity for creating the impression of three-dimensionality on a flat surface. Computer hardware and software are now available that incorporate these techniques to automatically compute two-dimensional pictures from digital information that describes the three-dimensional shape of an object. Figure 6–15A through D illustrates several of the approaches used on a simplified representation of the left ventricle. Figure 6–15A is a simple line drawing of the ventricular chamber. These wire-frame diagrams are generated by mathematically transforming the coordinates of outlined borders, derived from two-dimensional images, to their three-dimensional positions, and then calculating the projection image of these data on a two-dimensional plane. The resulting image will depend on the particular perspective or vantage point from which the projection is made. Up to a certain limit, the representational power is proportional to the number of different slices available. Figure 6–15B illustrates the enhancement of the three-dimensionality of a wire-frame

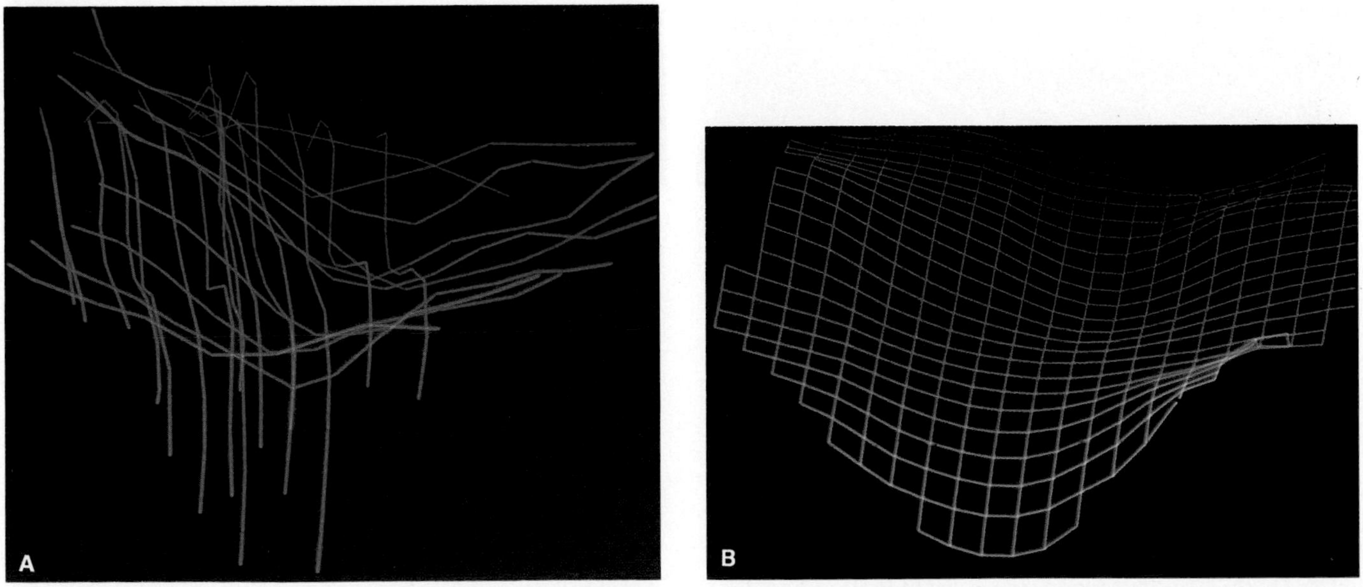

Fig. 6–14. **A.** Traces taken from two-dimensional scans of the mitral valve of a healthy volunteer in systole and oriented in three-dimensional space. **B.** A connected grid representation of the leaflet surface calculated from the reconstructed traces.

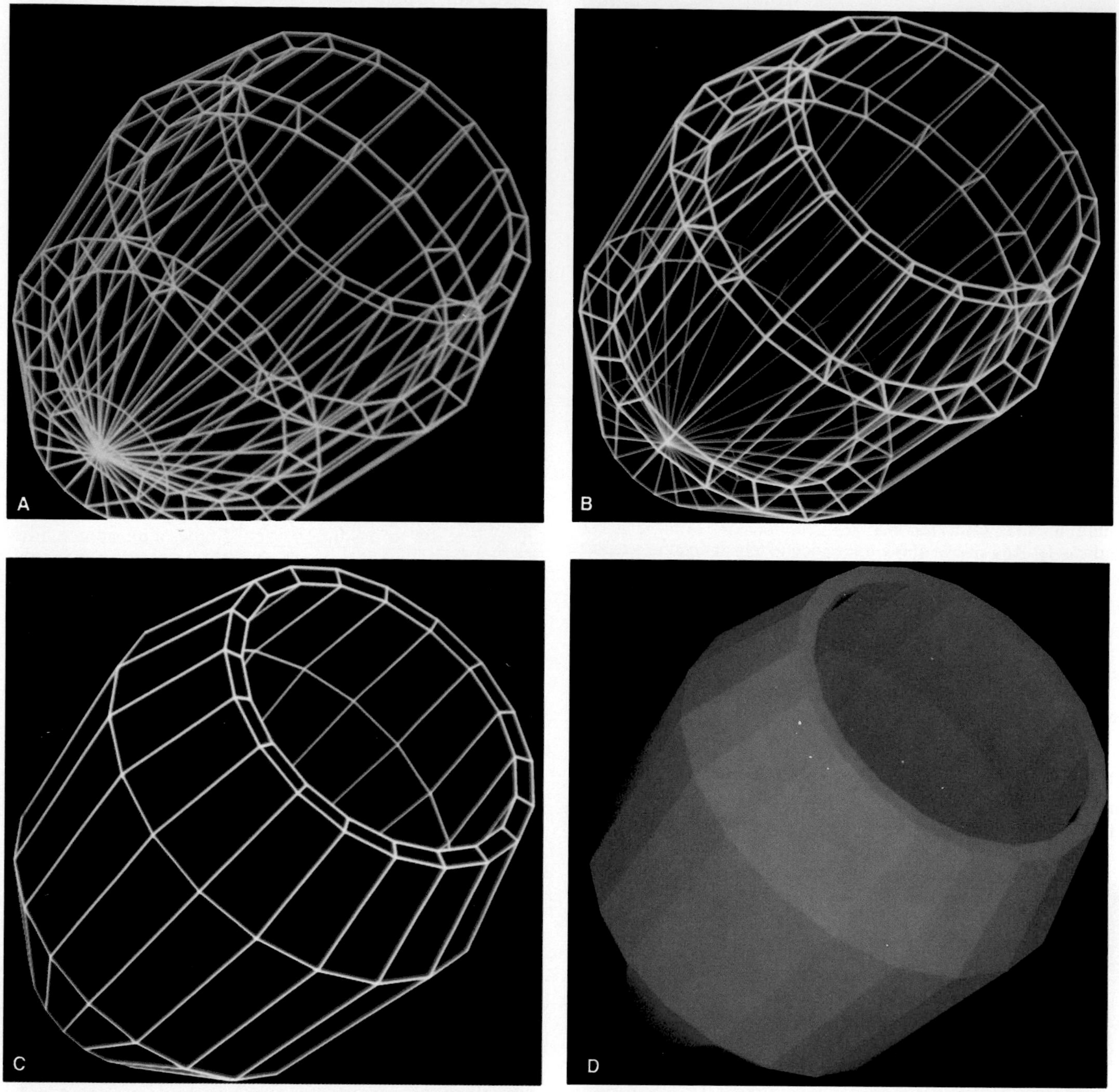

Fig. 6–15. A series of graphic representations of the left ventricle illustrating methods to enhance appreciation of three-dimensional structure. **A.** A simplified "wire frame" representation of the left ventricle. **B** to **D.** The same figure graphically rendered in various ways. **B.** Intensity depth cuing. **C.** Hidden line removal. **D.** Combination of hidden surface removal, surface shading, and intensity cuing.

image with intensity depth cuing. In this method, points that are closer to the viewer are displayed with greater intensity. The display algorithm simply converts the depth, or z coordinate, of line segments into an intensity level. Although useful for depicting simple structures, intensity cuing does not provide sufficient spatial resolution to enable the observer to appreciate small depth differences. If the digital representation of the object is in the form of a surface (usually defined as a series of connected polygonal patches), then techniques for hidden line and surface removal and surface shading can be implemented. In Figure 6–15C, the lines that would normally be obscured from view by closer portions of the structure have been removed and provide a more realistic sense of the object. Surface shading can further enhance the appearance of three-dimensionality and is performed by altering the intensity of the surface patches to correspond to the angle of their surfaces with respect to the direction of a light source (Fig. 6–15D). Hidden line and hidden surface representations, though able to provide more realistic representations of solid objects, are generated at the expense of some information about its internal structure. This problem can be partially overcome with a technique called polygon clipping and surface removal, an example of which is shown in Figure 6–16. In this example, an arbitrary plane is positioned with respect to the object and the portions of the polygonal surfaces that extend to one side of this surface have been removed. The remaining structure can then be rendered using the same algorithms described previously. In this example, the description of the polygonal surfaces has been extended to allow differentiation between solid and vacant regions of space that would reflect myocardial tissue versus empty ventricular chamber, respectively.

The surface rendering techniques described here can be particularly effective for illustrating three-dimensional anatomy in a static image, especially when views from multiple vantage points and processed with different clipping planes are presented together.

In the special case of image data that are acquired in a regular three-dimensional format, the use of voxel rendering techniques can be applied. Voxels are created by connecting the pixels from adjacent images to produce a three-dimensional volume element (usually a cube). In this form, the data represent a contiguous region of three-dimensional space and can be processed to produce cross-sectional images, projection images (like a radiograph), and shaded surfaces from any orientation. Surfaces can be derived by contouring the voxel data at specific intensity levels.

Stereoscopic Techniques

In normal human vision, a powerful sense of three-dimensionality occurs because the eyes are several inches apart and thus record slightly different images of an object. When these images are combined in the visual cortex of the brain, an impression of three-dimensionality results that is referred to as *stereopsis*. This same effect can be created by calculating two images (stereo pairs) of a scene from slightly different perspective angles, usually 5 to 7° apart) and then using any of several techniques to focus each eye on a separate image. This principle is certainly not new, having been used to produce the stereo viewers or stereopticons popular at the turn of the century. More recently, several types of devices have been developed to facilitate stereoscopic viewing of objects rendered from computer graphics systems. These include dual display monitors (one for each eye) mounted to a helmet[24] and stereo viewing glasses with special lenses that allow each eye to see one image of a stereo pair.[25] Although stereoscopic viewing has long been an integral part of areas such as molecular modeling and x-ray crystallography, it has not been widely used in the medical field. As techniques such as MRI and CT, in addition to ultrasound, generate more three-dimensional image data, the use of stereoscopic techniques will likely increase.

Dynamic Interactive Display Devices

Advanced graphics work stations are now available that can compute displays of objects with sufficient speed to provide real-time rotation, translation, and scaling of the three-dimensional image data. These systems often have input devices that allow the user to manually adjust the viewing perspective and other display parameters simply by the turning of a dial or touch of the keyboard. This interactive ability dramatically improves the ability to perceive the sense of three-dimensionality, particularly through kinetic depth cuing: the effect that is produced by the different motion of regions that are at different distances from the observers vantage point as they are smoothly rotated in space. Although this effect cannot be shown in print, Figure 6–17 illustrates

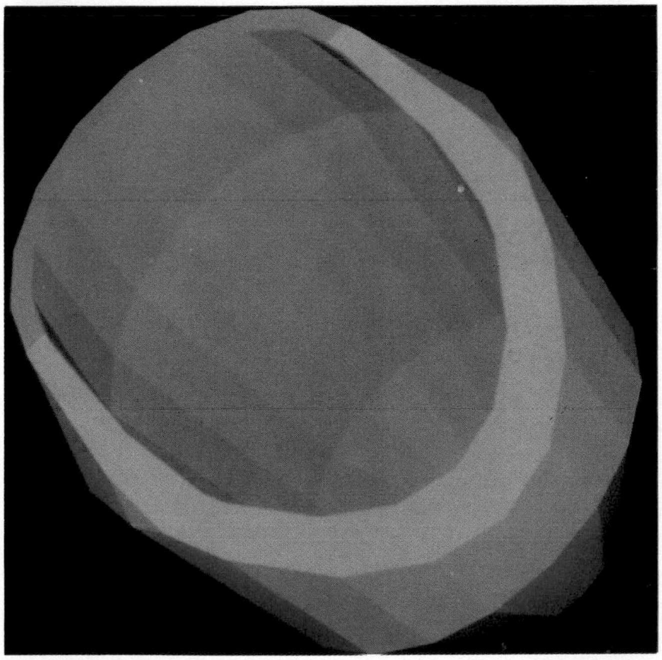

Fig. 6–16. Representation of the same ventricular model in Figure 6–15 illustrating the effect of surface clipping.

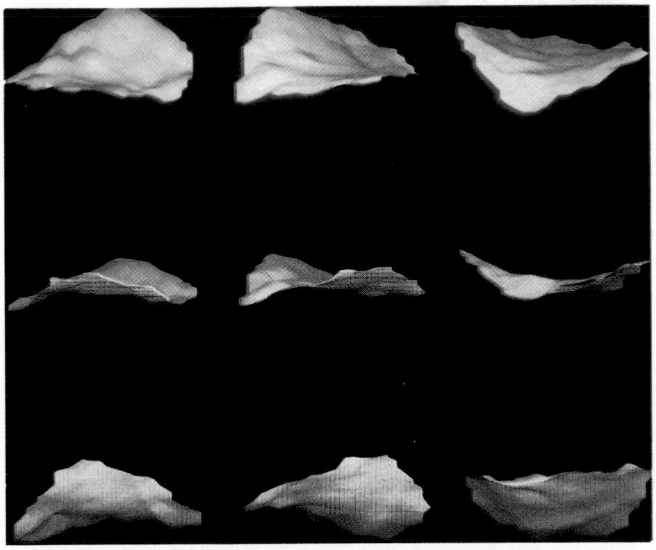

Fig. 6–17. Renderings of the surface of the closed mitral leaflets reconstructed in peak systole. The ventricular aspect is shown in yellow and the atrial in blue. Rotation and angulation of the valve reveal its appearance from different perspectives.

how rotation of the image allows more complete appreciation of its three-dimensional structure.

Surface Derivation

Many of the display techniques (described previously) and methods for quantifying volume (described later) require surface representations for their computation. Therefore, techniques must be available to interpolate the boundaries of structures from the regions between the reconstructed borders or contours (these are only samples of the original surface). The problem of best approximating a surface from a set of sample points has been a long-standing challenge to computer scientists and mathematical theorists, and the selection of an appropriate method may depend on the shape of the underlying surface and the sampling format of the contours. The simplest approach (and perhaps the most frequently used method) is to approximate the surface by a polyhedron of triangular faces that span the region between the traced borders. Several techniques have been developed for this purpose, many of which require that each of the traced borders form a closed planar contour and that separate contours must lie on separate parallel planes, or on nonintersecting regions of a plane. An example of one such triangulation method is illustrated in (Fig. 6–18).[26] Adjacent contours are selected and subdivided into multiple boundary points that are connected sequentially to form a series of contour segments. The end points of each segment are then connected to a single boundary point on the adjacent contour point by two lines (a left span and a right span) to create a triangular tile that spans the intervening space. This process is repeated until all the contour segments (from both contours) have been tiled.

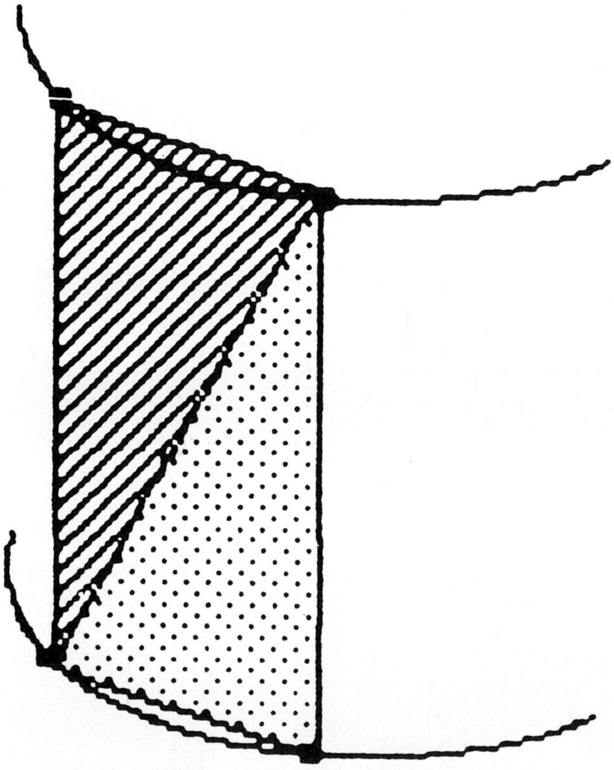

Fig. 6–18. Procedure for generating a polyhedral surface from nonintersection traces. (From Gopal AS, et al.: Three-dimensional echocardiographic volume computation by polyhedral surface reconstruction: in vitro validation and comparison to magnetic resonance imaging. J Am Soc Echocardiogr 5:115, 1992. With permission of Mosby Year-Book, Inc.)

Image acquisition from unrestricted scan formats, however, can result in intersecting image planes and the borders derived from them. Furthermore, in echocardiographic imaging in particular, it may be difficult to identify an entire closed border from the two-dimensional images. Ideally, it would be preferable to piece together partial traces of optimally imaged regions from multiple imaging windows without restriction of the acquisition format. However, applying the previously described surfacing methods to these data requires resampling the original contours with a set of predefined planes that conform to the required format, and then connecting the resulting points of intersection to produce a new set of contours. This method has been used by at least one group for right ventricular reconstruction.[27] Unfortunately, resampling reduces the amount of information provided by the original traces (the new contours are derived from a subset of the original data), and much of the information about the shape can be lost in the process.

To overcome this problem, a versatile algorithm has been developed for surfacing cardiac chambers that can take advantage of the full data set and also tolerates partial tracings.[23] An initially spherical template, positioned at the center of the cavity, is deformed to provide the best fit to the surrounding traces. The sphere is divided into evenly spaced lines of latitude and longitude to provide 800 grid points (intersection of 40 lines of longitude with 20 lines of latitude). Rays are then extended from the center of the sphere through these grid points toward the traced borders to calculate a corresponding grid point on the surface. The position of this point is obtained as a best fit to all traced line segments within a small conical sector (9.0°) around each ray, weighted by their proximity to the ray. Values for rays without adjacent traces are filled in by interpolating between nearest neighbors. Adjacent grid points are then connected to form an enclosed polyhedral surface.

METHODS FOR QUANTIFYING THREE-DIMENSIONAL RELATIONSHIPS

The attributes of structures represented by three-dimensional reconstruction can be quantified using measures of length, area, and volume. Techniques for determining length and area measurements in three-dimensional space are similar to those used to make similar measurements from two-dimensional images and simply represent the distance between two designated points or the area enclosed by a two-dimensional contour. Three-dimensional constructs are unique, however, because they offer the potential to directly quantify volume. The approaches for volume measurement depend, to some degree, on the format of the reconstructed information. For images that have been acquired in a fixed geometric format, such as parallel planes, volume can be quantified in terms of voxels or volume elements or as the region of space contained by an enclosed surface described by connected polygons. Voxels are three-dimensional picture elements, usually in the shape of an orthogonal box, with width and height, as in a two-dimensional image, and depth to define the third dimension. The voxel count can be used to compute the volume within a contour (i.e., ventricular volume), between contours (i.e., ventricular mass), or between a contour and a reference plane (i.e., the volume enclosed by the mitral leaflets relative to a least squares plane fit to the mitral annulus). Once data are acquired in a three-dimensional array, measurement of the array elements is one of the simplest tasks. The accuracy of these measurements in computer terms is related to the resolution of the pixels but in real terms is limited by the resolution of the raw data and the precision of the reconstruction.

When the data are described by a polyhedral surface, the volume can be computed by breaking up the region enclosed by a surface into a contiguous set of tetrahedra, for which the volume calculation is simple, and then summing the values. The formula for a tetrahedral volume with one vertex at the origin (x, y, z all equal 0) is described later (the coordinates of the other three vertices are identified by a numeric flag 1, 2, or 3):

$$v = [(y1 * z2 - z1 * y2) * x3 + (z1 * x2 - x1 * z2) * y3 + (x1 * y2 - y1 * x2) * z3]/6 \quad [6.8]$$

FUNDAMENTAL LIMITATIONS OF THREE-DIMENSIONAL RECONSTRUCTION

Accuracy of Image Locating Method. The different techniques for image localization each have some margin of error that will introduce positional noise in the image reconstruction. In general, however, this has not been a significant problem because most of the techniques, if properly implemented, can be made to accurately locate images at or beyond the resolution of the two-dimensional image data. An important factor that is often overlooked, and that can have a dramatic effect of the fidelity of a reconstruction, however, is the calibration of the position of the image data with respect to the locating mechanism. Particular attention must be paid to this process because small calibration errors in the angular relationships and image will be amplified the further the image data are from the locating mechanism.

Limits of Image Resolution. The quality of any three-dimensional reconstruction is inherently limited by the resolution and quality of the two-dimensional images on which it is based. This prevents meaningful reconstruction in patients whose basic images are technically limited. Also, when structures are too small to be resolved by two-dimensional imaging, they will not be resolved in three-dimensional reconstructions of these images.

Patient Motion and Respiration. Implicit in all of the three-dimensional imaging techniques is that the heart remain in the same location during the acquisition of the data for reconstruction. This requires the subject to remain motionless during data acquisition and, because the position of the heart may shift during breathing, requires that respiration either be suspended or somehow monitored to allow respiratory gating. In the former case, the procedure is limited to cooperative patients who can hold their breath long enough to acquire a representative sample of images from different transducer orientations.

Uniformity of Heart Beat. To combine images from different cardiac cycles, it is assumed that the heart is beating in a reproducible fashion. The beat-to-beat variation in the position of cardiac structures will limit the overall accuracy of their reconstruction. Although this may not be a significant problem in subjects with normal sinus rhythm, the technique may not be applicable to those presenting with atrial or ventricular arrhythmias.

Temporal Resolution. Another technical limitation, often overlooked, is the temporal resolution of image acquisition. In general, 30 two-dimensional images are generated per second of scan time. Therefore, consecutive image frames are separated by 33-msec intervals. If significant motion of a structure occurs within this time frame, such as the valve leaflets during opening and closing, then the ability to resolve the structure is limited. Furthermore, the temporal registration of images combined from other cardiac cycles may be subject to 33-msec alignment errors. Although this problem may be important for valvular structures at end-diastole and end-systole, it should not significantly effect reconstructions of the other slower moving structures and may be sufficient when leaflet motion is relatively smaller.

APPLICATIONS OF THREE-DIMENSIONAL ECHOCARDIOGRAPHIC RECONSTRUCTION

The major promise of the three-dimensional echocardiography must lie in elucidating specific features and abnormalities of cardiac structures that are not easily resolved by two-dimensional imaging and other competing technologies. Despite the long-standing clinical and research interest in three-dimensional reconstruction, practical applications have only recently been possible because of the significant improvements in techniques for acquiring and integrating the imaging and localizing data. There are, nevertheless, several examples that illustrate the advantages of this technology.

Mitral Valve

An example of the unique ability of three-dimensional echocardiographic reconstruction to answer complex questions can be found in the problem of mitral valve prolapse. To determine the exact relationship of the mitral leaflets to annulus, an acoustic locator system was used to reconstruct tracings of the leaflets in normal, healthy subjects with no auscultatory or echocardiographic markers of mitral valve prolapse. Using this approach, the mitral valve annulus was shown to have a saddle-like shape (Fig. 6–19) rather than a planar configuration, as was previously believed or inferred by certain diagnostic criteria. Once the configuration of the "normal" mitral valve was appreciated, its appearance

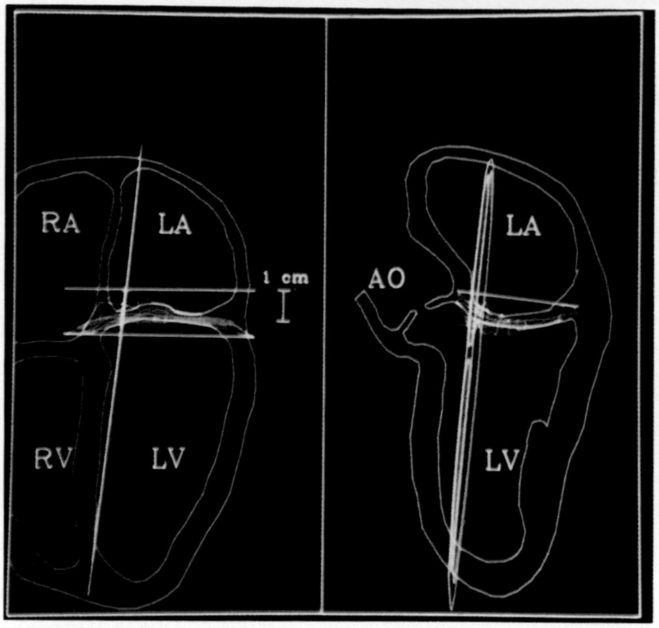

Fig. 6–19. Reconstruction of a mitral valve oriented with respect to two standard echocardiographic imaging planes. Left. The apical four-chamber perspective, or mediolateral imaging plane in which the high points of the mitral annulus can be seen to lie below (on the ventricular side of) the leaflets. Right. The long axis, or anterolateral, plane is shown, and the high points of the annulus are now consistently above (on the atrial side of) the leaflets. AO = aorta; LA = left atrium; LV = left ventricle; RA = right atrium; RV = right ventricle.

in various two-dimensional imaging planes could be better understood, and the erroneous diagnosis of prolapse avoided.[20]

Dynamic changes in annular morphology have also been reconstructed in three dimensions throughout the cardiac cycle.[22,27] This can provide information about the normal functioning of the mitral valve to aid the design of annuloplasty devices and may find applicability in surgical planning and intervention.

Ventricular Volume and Contractile Function

Although estimates of left ventricular volume and mass, stroke volume, and ejection fraction can be derived by extrapolation from one- and two-dimensional data, the underlying geometric assumptions often involved are least likely to be applicable when the ventricle is distorted by the effects of ischemic heart disease or right ventricular overload. To address this problem, several groups have demonstrated three-dimensional echocardiographic techniques for ventricular volume measurement that are independent of geometric assumptions.

The first reported clinical application of three-dimensional techniques appeared in 1978.[28] Using a pivot point method, Nixon and Saffer performed left ventricular volume determinations with good correlation to angiographically derived volumes. These preliminary data were subsequently confirmed for both end-systolic and end-diastolic left ventricular volumes.[3] Since then, three-dimensional ventricular reconstruction in humans has been carried out by a variety of techniques,[7,8,16,17] and the reliability of these measurements, when compared to angiography, has been consistently demonstrated (see Table 6–1).

Using another system, investigators accurately reconstructed a series of ventricular phantoms and excised ventricles over a wide range of shapes and sizes with excellent correlation of the computed volumes to actual measured values.[29] Localized features such as papillary muscle indentations and ventricular aneurysms were included in endocardial surface reconstruction and volume quantification. This same system was applied in patients for ventricular reconstruction at end-systole and end-diastole for computation of stroke volume and ejection fraction.[30] The ability to scan rapidly and continuously, with real-time integration of positional data with image data, greatly simplifies the reconstruction process for clinical applicability.

Studies are underway for in vivo validation of these methods in animal models and human patients.[30–32] Initial validation of three-dimensional techniques for measuring left-ventricular and right-ventricular volume have been carried out using both mechanical arm and acoustic locator systems in balloon models,[17] excised animal hearts,[5,6,15,19,33] excised human hearts,[7,8,12,13,16,17,28] and in open chest dogs.[28]

Intravascular Imaging

By placing the imaging catheter beyond a region of interest and then slowly withdrawing it at known rates or in fixed intervals, the examiner can establish the relation of successive two-dimensional images to one another and reconstruct them in three-dimensional space. Closely spaced images can provide a gray-scale representation of the vessel wall and lumen in three-dimensional voxel space, and thresholding programs can then produce a rendering of the intimal surface for convenient viewing.[34,35] These data can also be resected to provide longitudinal views of the vessel currently unavailable from the two-dimensional images and visualized with volume rendering techniques.[35] This method has been applied successfully to facilitate the recognition of extravascular lumens following angioplasty procedures[34] and

Table 6–1. Clinical studies of Three-Dimensional Left Ventricular Volume Determination in Multiple Patients In Vivo

Source	Year	Method	Patients	Correlation (r)
Ueda et al.[8]	1980	Pivot point	20	0.92
Nixon et al.[3]	1983	Pivot point	9	0.95 (ED) 0.94 (ES)
Sawada et al.[16]	1985	Mechanical arm	10	0.96 (ED) 0.97 (ES)
Sapoznikov et al.[7]	1987	Pivot point	15	NA

ED = end diastole; ES = end systole; NA = not available.

is being applied to integrate the thickness of vessel walls and their components.[36]

FUTURE DIRECTIONS IN TECHNOLOGY

Though significant advances have been made to streamline the process of data acquisition and reconstruction, the complexity of the overall process continues to limit the general utility of the method. The purpose of this section is to describe additional new technology that may further facilitate data acquisition and analysis.

Simultaneous Multiplanar Imaging. One of the current problems in three-dimensional reconstruction is that each plane must be recorded from a separate cardiac cycle and may, therefore, require long acquisition times for reconstructions requiring numerous tomographic views. Several approaches to simultaneous multidimensional image acquisition offer the possibility of simplifying the spatial registration of separately acquired planes and increasing the rate of data acquisition.[37,38] Orthogonal mode transducers (discussed and illustrated in Chapter 2), e.g., image in two orthogonal planes within the video refresh rate, so that the recorded two-dimensional scans are already defined with respect to each other in both time and space. This would increase the rate of data acquisition, reducing problems of patient motion, and would obviate the need for an external locating system for simpler applications. For example, the determination of ejection fraction could be made more precise by providing simultaneous orthogonal apical views of the ventricle with known geometric relationships. For more complete three-dimensional analysis requiring more than two imaging planes, a technique for transducer localization and reconstruction by combining images from several cardiac cycles would still be required. Simultaneous orthogonal image acquisition with position sensing would, nevertheless, cut the number of imaging frames required for reconstruction in half and would improve the accuracy of the reconstruction by guaranteeing that orthogonally recorded images were precisely aligned.

Color Doppler. Three-dimensional reconstruction of color Doppler data may be useful to improve the understanding of flow profiles in two-dimensional images and for deriving more accurate methods to quantify regurgitant volume. This could be accomplished by applying the technique to reconstruct flow through orifices of different shapes and sizes in a controlled environment with known flow profiles. In vivo applicability of three-dimensional reconstruction of proximal and regurgitant flow fields, however, may be limited by the small size and the beat-to-beat variability of these features. Further development of volumetric echocardiographic imaging could overcome some of the in vivo limitations by providing real-time three-dimensional reconstruction of flow fields.

Transesophageal Echocardiography. Transthoracic imaging does not always provide images of sufficient quality for uniform visualization of cardiac structures. The intervening chest wall in some patients may interfere with acquiring adequate images for feature recognition and three-dimensional reconstruction. Transesophageal imaging systems, however, provide excellent image quality, and systems for acquiring a series of parallel planes or rotations about an axis are being tested.[22,32,39] Though they are unlikely to be practical for routine examination, such systems could provide further information in applications where two-dimensional transesophageal imaging is indicated, such as surgical planning and intervention, and in the evaluation of a wide variety of pathologic conditions.

Direct Digital Data Storage. Direct access to the digital image information in the ultrasound machine can avoid the problem of image degradation and intensity clipping that occurs during data storage on videotape and subsequent retrieval with a frame grabber. Though this is currently impractical because of the massive storage requirements and the required speed of data transfer rates to recording media, advances will undoubtedly occur that will make these possible. It may ultimately be possible to store the digitized radio frequency signal for more sophisticated processing that cannot be performed in real time. Possible application could be to improve techniques for automated border detection and tissue characterization and to improved derivation of Doppler velocities for flow-field reconstruction.

System Integration. The success and practical utility of three-dimensional ultrasound techniques will ultimately depend on combining and streamlining the independent steps of data acquisition, processing, and display into a highly integrated environment such as a dedicated work station. Though this has been done in at least one system for transthoracic imaging, it is clear that the processes should be further simplified to minimize human intervention. The design of such a system will require further integration of several types of hardware devices as well as the development of more sophisticated computer software to control and manipulate the flow of imaging information.

On-Line Three-Dimensional Visualization. For qualitative assessment of the cardiac function, it should be possible to create three-dimensional representations in real time directly on an interactive computer graphics display and to gate the images so that only those corresponding to a given point in the cardiac cycle are displayed at one time. As each cycle is recorded, new information could be added to the display monitor and to be visualized with images from other cardiac cycles. With the interactive capabilities, and perhaps the incorporation of stereo viewing, certain regions could be inspected by manually adjusting scaling, rotation, translation, depth cuing, and depth clipping parameters. Such a system would need to rapidly calculate the spatial orientation of the imaging plane, extract the temporal location of images in the cardiac cycle from the electrocardiogram, and perform the geometric transformations to provide three-dimensional locations for each point on the image.

Border Identification. Manual tracing of cardiac morphology is often the most time-consuming and tedious step in the reconstruction procedure, especially in dynamic studies that involve a separate reconstruction for each point in time. Computer algorithms, such as those discussed in Chapter 3 and others under development may permit automated or semi-automated recognition of borders by following contiguous regions where the intensities in the image change rapidly. Techniques to guide the connection of separate disjointed edges on the image are also available and, with improvement, may allow digital recognition of features such as the endocardial border of the left ventricle, despite breaks in the ultrasound images. Manual intervention may be needed only to identify a few points on the image that lie on the border of the feature of interest. Then the computer algorithm could automatically follow and connect the edges in space as well as time. The results could be reviewed and revised by the operator.

SUMMARY

As was the case with two-dimensional imaging, the full impact of three-dimensional reconstruction will not likely be apparent until it has come into more widespread use. Many of the assumptions used in the routine interpretation of two-dimensional images, e.g., the assumption of planarity of the mitral annulus, may well be demonstrated to be erroneous and new insight into the relationship of structure and function will undoubtedly be gained.

Although currently a research tool, three-dimensional cardiac ultrasound holds great promise for widespread future applications in the diagnosis of cardiac disease. Recent advances in spatial monitoring devices, data storage and manipulation, and image display systems have greatly enhanced our ability to image cardiac anatomy in three dimensions. These and further developments expected in the future will bring three-dimensional imaging capability to a larger segment of the medical community and expand its clinical role.

REFERENCES

1. Dekker DL, Piziali RL, Deng E: A system for ultrasonically imaging the human heart in three dimensions. Comput Biomed Res 7:544, 1974.
2. Moritz WE, Shreve PL: A microprocessor-based spatial locating system for use with diagnostic ultrasound. Proc IEEE 64:966, 1974.
3. Nixon JV, Saffer SI, Lipscomb K, Blomqvist G: Three-dimensional echoventriculography. Am Heart J 106:435, 1983.
4. Matsumoto M, et al.: Three-dimensional echocardiography for spatial visualization and volume calculation of cardiac structures. J Clin Ultrasound 9: 157, 1981.
5. Eaton LW, Maughan WL, Shoukas AA, Weiss JL: Accurate volume determination in the isolated ejecting canine left ventricle by two-dimensional echocardiography. Circulation 60:320, 1979.
6. Weiss JL, Eaton LW, Kallman CH, Maughan WL: Accuracy of volume determination by two-dimensional echocardiography: defining requirements under controlled conditions in the ejecting canine left ventricle. Circulation 4:889, 1983.
7. Sapoznikov D, Fine DG, Mosseri M, Gotsman MS: Left ventricular shape, wall thickness and function based on three-dimensional reconstruction echocardiography. *In*: Computers in Cardiology 1986. IEEE Computer Society, p. 495, 1987.
8. Ueda K, Kuwaki K, Inoue K: Three-dimensional display and volume determination of the left ventricle by two-dimensional echocardiography (abstr). Am J Cardiol 45:471, 1980.
9. McCann HA, et al.: A method for three-dimensional ultrasonic imaging of the heart in vivo. Dynamic Cardiovasc Imaging 1:97, 1987.
10. Ormiston JA, Shah PM, Tei C, Wong M: Size and motion of the mitral annulus in man. I. A two-dimensional echocardiographic method and findings in normal subjects. Circulation 64:113, 1981.
11. Pini R, et al.: Computed tomography of the heart by ultrasound. Computers in Cardiology 1991. IEEE Computer Society, p. 17, 1992.
12. Mensah GA, et al.: Three-dimensional echocardiographic reconstruction: experimental validation of volume measurement (abstr). J Am Coll Cardiol 17:378A, 1991.
13. Geiser EA, et al.: Dynamic three-dimensional echocardiographic reconstruction of the intact human left ventricle: technique and initial observations in patients. Am Heart J 103:1056, 1982.
14. Geiser EA, et al.: A mechanical arm for spatial registration of two-dimensional echocardiographic sections. Cathet Cardiovasc Diagn 8:89, 1982.
15. Sawada H, et al.: Three-dimensional reconstruction of the left ventricle from multiple cross sectional echocardiograms. Br Heart J 50:438, 1983.
16. Sawada H, et al.: Three-dimensional reconstruction of the human left ventricle from multiple cross sectional echocardiograms: comparison with biplane cineventriculography using Simpson's rule. J Cardiogr 15:439, 1985.
17. Stickels KR, Wann LS: An analysis of three-dimensional reconstructive echocardiography. Ultrasound Med Biol 10:575, 1984.
18. Raichlen JS, et al.: Dynamic three-dimensional reconstruction of the left ventricle from two-dimensional echocardiograms. J Am Coll Cardiol 8:364, 1986.
19. Moritz WE, et al.: An ultrasonic technique for imaging the ventricle in three dimensions and calculating its volume. IEEE Trans Biomed Eng 30:482, 1983.
20. Levine RA, et al.: Three-dimensional echocardiographic reconstruction of the mitral valve, with implications for the diagnosis of mitral valve prolapse. Circulation 80:589, 1989.
21. King DL, King DL Jr., Shao MY: Three-dimensional spatial registration and interactive display of position and orientation of real-time ultrasound images. J Ultrasound Med 9:525, 1990.
22. Flachskampf FA, et al.: Dynamic, three-dimensional reconstruction of the mitral annulus using a multiplane transesophageal echo-transducer. Circulation 84(Suppl 2):II-686, 1991.
23. Handschumacher MD, et al.: A new integrated system for three-dimensional echocardiographic reconstruction and ventricular volume measurement. *In*: Computers in Cardiology 1991. IEEE Computer Society, p. 113, 1992.
24. Sutherland IE: A Head Mounted Three-Dimensional Display. Washington, DC, Thompson Books, p. 757, 1968.
25. Roese J, McCleary L: Stereoscopic computer graphics for simulation and modelling. Comput Graph 13(2):41, 1979.
26. Gopal AS, et al.: Three-dimensional echocardiographic volume computation by polyhedral surface reconstruction: in vitro validation and comparison to magnetic resonance imaging. J Am Soc Echocardiogr 5:115, 1992.
27. Handschumacher MD, Sanfilippo AJ, Weyman AE, Levine RA: Dynamic three-dimensional reconstruction of the normal human mitral valve from two-dimensional echocardiographic scans. *In*: Computers in Cardiology 1990. IEEE Computer Society, p. 385, 1991.
28. Nixon JV, Saffer SI: Three-dimensional echoventriculography (abstr). Circulation 57(Suppl 2):II-157, 1978.
29. Lethor JP, et al.: A new fully integrated system for three-dimensional echocardiographic reconstruction: validation for ventricular volume (abstr). Circulation 84(Suppl 2):II-684, 1991.
30. Lethor JP, et al.: Quantitative reconstruction of the left ventricle using a new fully integrated three-dimensional echocardiographic system: feasibility and validation in human subjects (abstr). J Am Coll Cardiol 19:381A, 1992.
31. Siu SC, et al.: Three-dimensional echocardiography: in vivo validation for left ventricular volume and function (abstr). J Am Coll Cardiol 19:18A, 1992.
32. Martin RW, Bashein G: Measurement of stroke volume with three-dimensional transesophageal ultrasonic scanning: comparison with thermodilution measurement. Anesthesiology 70:470, 1989.
33. Linker DT, Moritz WE, Pearlman AS: A new three-dimensional echocardiographic method of right ventricular volume measurement: in vitro validation. J Am Coll Cardiol 8:101, 1986.
34. Rosenfield K, et al.: Three-dimensional reconstruction of human coronary and peripheral arteries from images recorded during two-dimensional intravascular ultrasound examination. Circulation 84:1938, 1991.
35. Kitney RI, et al.: Ultrasonic imaging of arterial structures using three-dimensional solid modeling. *In*: Computers in Cardiology 1988. Vol. 15. IEEE Computer Society, p. 3, 1989.
36. Hibberd MG, et al.: Three-dimensional reconstruction of intravascular ultrasound images can measure intimal volume (abstr). J Am Soc Echocardiogr 5:319, 1992.
37. Snyder JE, Kisslo J, von Ramm OT: Real-time orthogonal mode scanning of the heart. I. System design. J Am Coll Cardiol 7:1279, 1986.
38. Sheikh KH, Smith SW, von Ramm OT, Kisslo J: Real-time, three-dimensional echocardiography: feasibility and initial use. Echocardiography 8: 119, 1991.
39. Wollschlager H, et al.: Transesophageal echo computer tomography: a new method for dynamic three-dimensional imaging of the heart (echo-CT). *In*: Computers in Cardiology 1989. IEEE Computer Society, p. 39, 1990.

CHAPTER

7

PRINCIPLES OF DOPPLER FLOW MEASUREMENT

The second major echocardiographic technique is Doppler echocardiography. Doppler echocardiography is based on the change in the frequency of a sound wave that occurs when it strikes a moving target.[1–4] From this frequency shift, the Doppler instrument can determine the presence, velocity, character, and timing of blood flow within the heart and great vessels. Although the Doppler technique has been used clinically for more than two decades, it is only in the last several years that it has become established as a major tool for cardiac investigation. This relatively slow development can be attributed to the conceptual difficulty in understanding the production of a Doppler shift frequency from moving structures, the complexity of the signal processing required before any meaningful data can be derived from a Doppler signal, and the problems inherent in measuring absolute blood velocity and volume flow.[1]

Two engineering advances, however, significantly enhanced the clinical utility and acceptance of Doppler technology. The first was the development of real-time spectrum analyzers, which can accurately and rapidly characterize the Doppler shift data and output it in a convenient graphic format.[1–7] The second was the combination of Doppler devices and cross-sectional imaging systems,[8,9] which permits visualization of the site and orientation of flow sampling.

These technical advances combined with the demonstration that flow velocity can be used to estimate transvalvular pressure gradients[10–12]—the first reliable quantitative clinical application of the Doppler technique and the first noninvasive measure of intracardiac pressure or pressure difference—have rapidly elevated the Doppler technique to a position of major diagnostic importance.

This importance lies not in the number of diagnoses that Doppler echocardiography makes possible, nor in the variety of lesions that can be detected using this technique, but rather because virtually all of the information it provides is unique. As such, it fills most of the major gaps in the data previously available from imaging echocardiography and contributes enormously to making the echocardiogram a definitive diagnostic test. Thus, although its general application is relatively new, the Doppler technique is presented after cross-sectional imaging but before M-mode echocardiography as a reflection of its relative importance.

HISTORY—CHRISTIAN JOHANN DOPPLER

The principle that the perceived frequency of a traveling wave is altered by motion of the source, the receiver, or both was first enunciated by the Austrian mathematician and physicist Christian Johann Doppler (1803 to 1853), and this effect has subsequently borne his name. As a professor of mathematics in Prague, Doppler (Fig. 7–1) became interested in the then well-recognized phenomenon that a moving source of sound seemed more highly pitched to an observer whom it was approaching and seemed lower in pitch to an observer from whom it was receding. He first explained this phenomenon qualitatively and then developed the mathematical formulas necessary to determine the exact change in pitch. The correct elementary formula for motion of source or observer along the line between them first appears in his classic article "Ueber das farbige Licht der Doppelsterne und einiger anderer Gestirne des Himmels" (Concerning the colored light of double stars and other stars of the heavens) published in 1842.[13] The initial experimental verification of Doppler's theory for acoustics

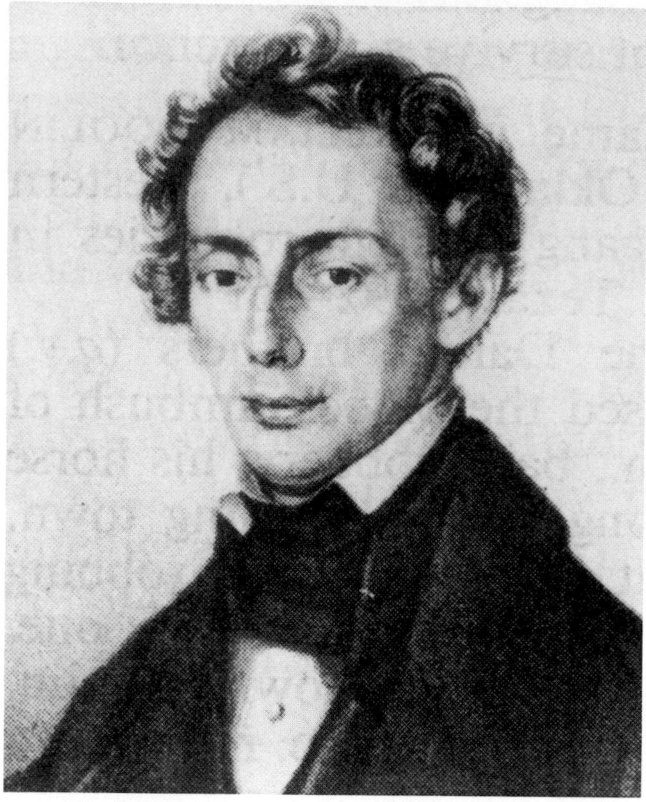

Fig. 7–1. Doppler, lithograph by Franz Sir (died 1865) after a drawing by Anton Machek (1771 to 1844). (Courtesy of the Bild-Archiv, Osterreichische Nationalbibliothek, Vienna.)

was obtained by Buys Ballot at Utrecht in 1845. To test the theory, several trumpeters were persuaded to ride in an open railroad carriage as it was pulled to and fro at different speeds and to play various notes on their instruments. Musicians with perfect pitch who could identify exact frequencies of musical notes sat at various points along the railroad track and recorded the notes they heard as the train approached or receded. This was continued for 2 days, and despite the rather crude experimental approach, Doppler's theory was confirmed.[14]

Doppler correctly suggested that his principle would apply to any wave motion including light. He believed that all stars emitted white light and that any differences in their colors observed on Earth occurred because the motion of the stars affected the observed frequency of the light and hence its color. This concept was not totally valid, because as we now know, stars vary in their basic color. In 1848, however, Armand Fizeau pointed out that shifts in the spectral lines of stars could be observed and ascribed to the Doppler effect, enabling their motion to be determined. Specifically, the frequency of light is shifted toward the red end of the spectrum if the light source is receding from the observer and toward the blue end if it is approaching. This idea was first applied by William Huggins (1824 to 1910), who found that the star Sirius is moving away from the solar system when he detected a small red shift in its spectrum (despite this celestial precedent, most manufacturers of color Doppler instruments have opted for the opposite convention, using red to indicate motion toward the transducer and blue motion away). With the linking of the velocity of a galaxy to its distance by Edwin Hubble (1889 to 1953) in 1929, it became possible to use the red shift to determine the distances of galaxies. The subsequent observation that the light from many stars and nebulae is red shifted, indicating high velocities of recession from the earth, led to the "big bang" theory, which holds that the cosmos was created when a single giant "molecule" or matter exploded, hurling its fragments apart to form the expanding universe.

Doppler Instrument Development

The first demonstrated use of Doppler ultrasound for the transcutaneous detection of blood flow was by Satomura in 1956.[15] His early vacuum tube instruments were sufficiently sensitive to detect signals that were felt to arise from areas of disturbed flow in superficial vessels and motion of the heart muscle and valves.[16–18] These early devices, however, recorded the intensity of the Doppler signal, rather than its frequency, and therefore could not indicate velocity. Following the demonstration that blood flow could be detected using ultrasound, the evolution of Doppler devices has progressed in an orderly and highly logical sequence. To understand the pattern of development, however, it must be recognized that from the beginning, the goal of most engineering groups working in this area has been the measurement of volumetric flow.[1] This measurement required the recording of blood velocity, the direction of flow, and the point within the vessel from which the flow signal arose. It was also necessary to measure the size of the vessel within which the blood was moving and to determine the orientation of the flow stream relative to the vessel walls. This focus on volumetric flow also explains why major applications, e.g., the relationship of flow velocity to transvalvular gradients, were not widely studied until long after instruments were available that could provide the necessary information.

The first true measurement of the Doppler shift frequency was by Franklin et al., in 1961, using an independently developed continuous wave device.[19] Their approach involved direct placement of transmitting and receiving transducers on opposite sides of the aorta in a canine model. The Doppler shift frequency was detected by mixing the transmitted and received signals in the receiving crystal and amplifier, with the "beat" frequency of the combined signals representing the Doppler difference frequency (see later discussion). Although these early instruments could measure flow velocity, they were not capable of measuring flow direction. McLeod, et al., started development of a flow direction sensing readout based on quadrature phase detection methods used in radio communication (see later discussion).[20,21] This approach permitted the separation of the forward and reverse components of the flow signal. With the advent of transistor technology, it became possible to develop miniaturized continuous wave Doppler equipment for transcutaneous use in man. The first such devices were developed by Baker et al.,[22] and Franklin et al.,[23] and formed the basis for several physiologic continuous wave flowmeter designs. The first commercial Doppler equipment, the SKI "doptone" and the Parks Doppler, were based on these models. These original devices were used predominantly to record the return of flow following peripheral vessel occlusion and to detect fetal and placental flow in pregnant women. Although there was early interest in Doppler techniques to detect flow signals from the heart and great vessels, this was difficult because continuous wave devices were sensitive to all motion in the path of the beam. Multiple attempts were made to eliminate interference from moving structures outside the region of interest by approaching the heart directly from the esophagus[1] or placing transducers at the tip of transvenous catheters,[24,25] which were introduced directly into the blood stream. Both of these approaches were complicated by difficulty in directly locating the tip of the catheter within the patient, maintaining the catheter in a stationary position from which blood flow could be sampled, and defining the exact location from which the flow signals were originating. Pulsed Doppler instruments designed to overcome limitations in the continuous wave approach were developed independently by Baker and Peronneau et al.[26–29] Although different in detail, the two approaches were able to detect flow signals from specific locations within the heart or great vessels and to exclude the masking effects of other nearby vessels or moving structures.

In terms of the ultimate objectives of flow quantification, however, these devices still contributed only velocity information. The flow angle and the dimensions of the vessel remained unknown. In 1971, Hokanson et al. demonstrated the use of the pulsed Doppler technique for producing flow images of the vessel lumen.[30] This approach used previously developed pulsed Doppler systems and mapped onto a storage oscilloscope the image of the vessel where flow exceeded a certain threshold velocity. This work demonstrated the possibility of using the display to determine the angle between the sound beam and the flow vector. The approach, however, required many cardiac cycles to generate a flow image and required the assumption that the flow vector is parallel to the vessel walls.

The first device that combined real-time two-dimensional imaging with simultaneous pulsed Doppler flow detection was developed by Barber et al. in 1974. His "duplex" scanning device allowed the relationship of the Doppler beam to the long axis of the vessel to be defined and the vessel diameter to be measured. In the original duplex systems, the Doppler and imaging transducers were separate and aligned to intersect at a selected depth within the scan plane. Although this configuration was impractical for cardiac work, the concept was rapidly extended to cardiac visualization and flow sampling by using the same transducer for both purposes.[31] This advance permitted the visualization of the great vessels and cardiac chambers and the recording of blood flow therein. It was still necessary, however, to assume that the flow vector was parallel to the long axis of the vessel being studied. In 1979, Brandestini et al. described a method for color encoding the velocity data and superimposing it on an M-mode image of the heart, making possible the display of flow and structural data simultaneously.[32] His initial observations were extended by Namekawa et al.[33] and Bommer and Miller[34] with the development of real-time two-dimensional color flow imaging, which in combination with pulsed Doppler, provided all of the requisite information for quantitation of volumetric flow. After 3 decades of development in Doppler engineering technology together with advances in electronic circuitry, communications theory and signal analysis, it has now become possible to achieve the initial goal of volumetric flow measurement. During the same period, other but no less important, uses of Doppler technology, e.g., the measurement of transvalvular gradients based on changes in velocity, have also been reported and refined, resulting in a methodology of major clinical import.

FREQUENCY DESCRIPTION AND ANALYSIS

Any meaningful discussion of Doppler principles requires an understanding of the various methods of waveform description, the basic mathematical operations that can be performed on waveforms, and sampling theory. These topics are, therefore, introduced before the discussion of Doppler-related frequency shifts and instrumentation because they are fundamental to these practical applications.

The basic features characterizing any wave are amplitude, frequency, and phase. Primary emphasis to this point has been on the time-varying changes in the amplitude of reflected ultrasonic waves, which are the basis for image generation. The concept of sound frequency was introduced in Chapter 1, however, to this point, only the relationship of frequency to axial resolution, beam pattern, and beam penetration have been discussed. Because all Doppler flow measurements are based on the detection and measurement of changes in ultrasonic frequencies, it is important to now review in more detail the methods by which the frequency or frequencies contained in a sound wave are typically represented and analyzed.

Time Domain Frequency Analysis and Display

Frequency is defined as the number of repetitions of a periodic process per unit time. Traveling sound waves produce the periodic compression and separation of the particles in the medium through which they pass and thus have an inherent frequency or frequencies. It is important to remember that any wave causes the propagation of not one but two physical properties. The areas of particle compression and separation produced by traveling sound waves are associated with microscopic troughs and peaks of pressure (see Fig. 1–2). In addition, the particles in the medium move back and forth to produce these pressure variations. We may consider the variations in pressure as representing potential energy, whereas the motion of the particles represents kinetic energy. A critical point is that these propagating properties (pressure and motion) are 90° out of phase with each other; i.e., when the pressure is highest or lowest, no particle motion is occurring. In contrast, when motion is greatest, pressure is at the ambient level. Most of our observations on waves are concerned with only one of these quantities. An ultrasound transducer, e.g., is sensitive to the microscopic pressure changes and not to the microscopic changes in kinetic energy. Thus, what we observe is the pressure "amplitude" of the wave, which has the usual up and down variation expected of a wave. It is important to remember, however, that there is always a second, "unseen" component to the wave and that the total energy (potential and kinetic) is always constant.

This periodicity of two quantities is not unique to sound but is a basic property of all propagating waves in nature, i.e., light and radio waves have electric fields (e.g., potential energy) and magnetic fields (e.g., kinetic energy) that are out of phase with each other; ocean waves have displacement of the surface above or below "sea level" (potential energy) and the motions of the surface between peaks and troughs (kinetic energy) that are out of phase with each other. With this unification in mind, let us turn to the mathematical representation of waves that is fundamental to so many branches of science.[39]

The most common method for graphically representing waves is to plot the periodic fluctuations in the amplitude of the wave as a function of time, f(t), as illustrated in Figure 7–2A. To store or manipulate these data, each point along the wave can be assigned a numeric value, recorded, and operated on individually (Fig. 7–2B), as is done using digital computers (see Chapter 3). For purposes of description and analysis, however, such an approach is quite tedious, and it is more convenient to represent the whole sound wave in a mathematically

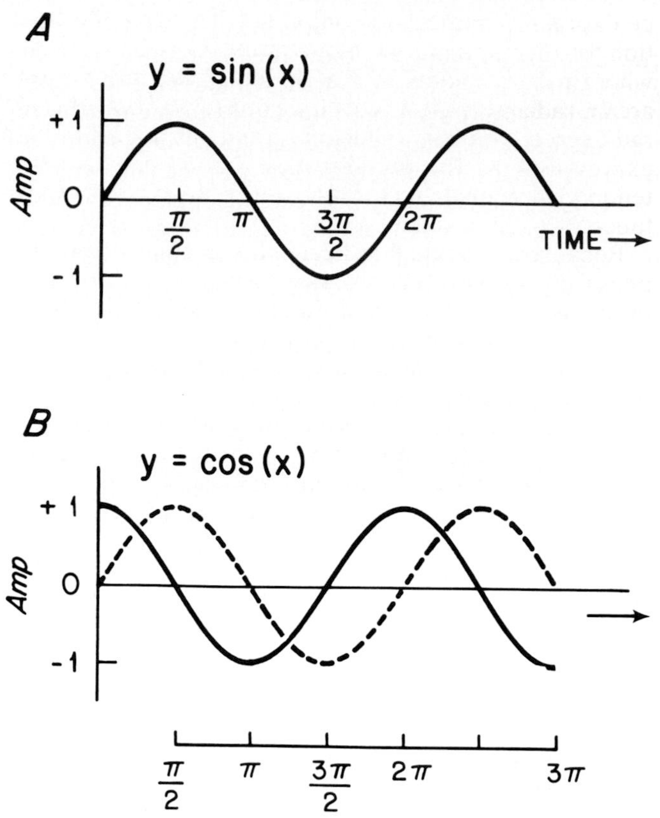

Fig. 7–3. Representation of sound waves by trigonometric functions (sines and cosines). **A.** Graph of expression y = sin(θ) is identical in form to the sound wave depicted in Figure 7–2A. **B.** Plot of the corresponding cosine function y = cos(θ), which is similar except for its starting point. The angle θ is conventionally expressed in radian measure. (See text for details.)

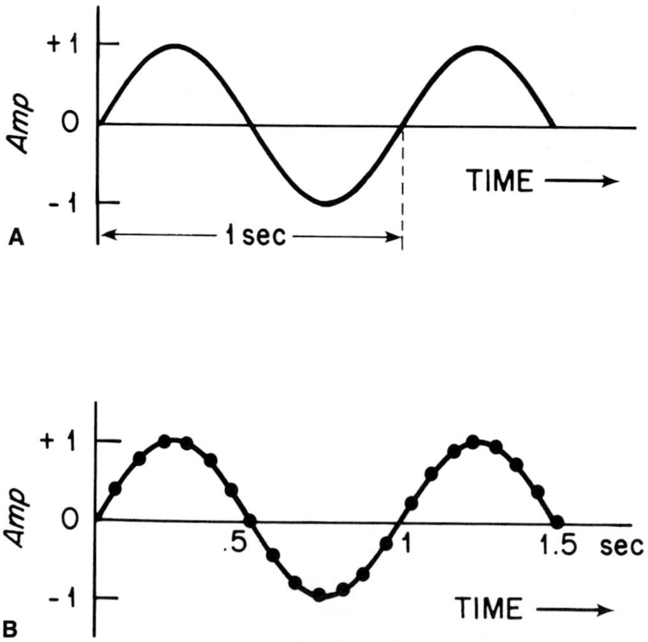

Fig. 7–2. **A.** Graphic representation of a wave as a periodic fluctuation in the amplitude of a quantity, such as pressure, as a function of time, f(t). **B.** To store or manipulate these data, each point along the wave can be assigned a numeric value, which is then recorded and operated on individually, as is done using digital computers.

compact form. A variety of forms has been devised for such representation, including trigonometric functions, rotating vectors, complex numbers and exponential functions, and Fourier (spectral) analysis. Some are better suited for illustrative purposes, some for compactness of expression and mathematical manipulation, and others for describing the electronic circuitry used in the practical processes of recording and analysis. It is important to remember that all of these forms describe the same waves and, thus, are identical in meaning.

The most familiar mathematical representation of sound waves is by trigonometric functions (sines and cosines), because all such functions are by nature periodic. For example, the expression $y = \sin \theta$ (theta is an angle whose sine is y), when plotted on a graph results in a curve such as that depicted in Figure 7–3A, which is identical in form to the sound wave depicted in Figure 7–2A. A plot of the corresponding cosine function $y = \cos \theta$ is similar except for its starting point (Fig. 7–3B). Because at $\theta = 0$, $\sin \theta = 0$, whereas $\cos \theta = 1$, the sine curve rises to its maximum (1) at $\theta = 90°$, whereas the cosine curve starts at 1 and falls to 0 at $\theta = 90°$. The cosine function, therefore, leads the sine function by 90°. When such curves are drawn, the angle θ is conventionally expressed in radian measure. The radian is a much more natural unit than degrees, because it allows both the amplitude and angular position of the wave to be expressed in the same units. It arises from the equation for the circumference of a circle, $C = 2\pi r$ or 6.28r, where r is the radius of the circle. By definition, there are 2π radians in a full 360° circle or 57.296°/rad or 0.1745 rad/degree. Use of radians greatly simplifies such expressions as the arc distance around a circle subtended by an angle θ at the center of the circle: arc distance = (θ [in radians])r.

Because the angle θ indicates the angular position or phase of the waveform at any point (i.e., the distance progressed through an oscillatory cycle) it is known as the *phase angle*. Sin θ and cos θ repeat themselves every 360° or 2π radians and vary between a maximum of +1 and a minimum of −1.

If we consider a wave propagating through space, the magnitude of the propagating quantity, e.g., pressure, at any point in space will vary cyclically with time, as illustrated in Figure 7–3. The phase angle, or point in the oscillatory cycle, will therefore also be a function of time: $\theta = \theta(t)$. Just as any linear distance, x, traversed by an object moving at velocity, v, equals $v \times t$, the phase angle achieved by a wave at any point in time equals the angular velocity, ω (expressed in radians per second) times t. In other words, $\theta(t) = \omega \times t$.

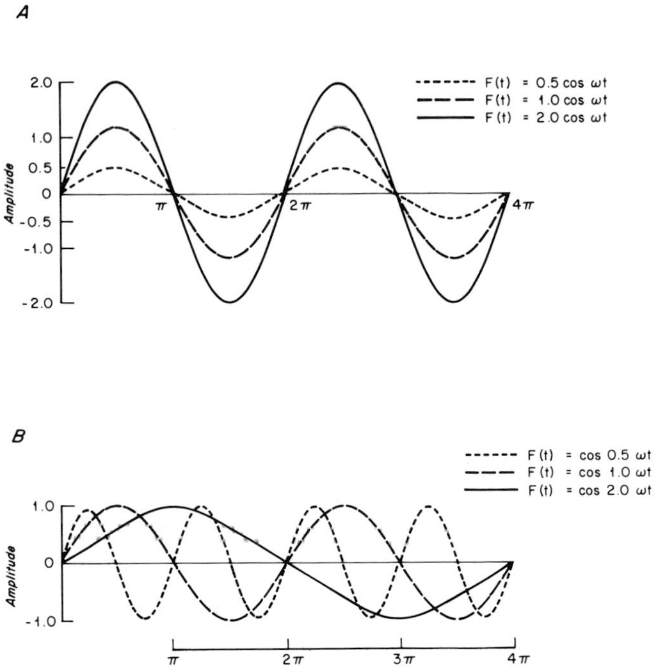

Fig. 7–4. Form of trigonometric functions used to represent differences in amplitude and frequency. **A.** Representation of changes in amplitude for a wave of constant frequency. **B.** Representation of changes in frequency for a wave of constant amplitude.

REPRESENTATION OF WAVEFORMS OF VARYING FREQUENCY AND AMPLITUDE

For sine and cosine functions to represent the wide range of naturally occurring periodic disturbances such as sound waves, it is necessary that they can be used to describe waves of varying amplitude, frequency, and phase. Variation in the amplitude of a sinusoid is specified by adding a coefficient M (the modulus or magnitude), giving the expressions $M\sin \omega t$ and $M\cos \omega t$. The peak-to-peak fluctuation in the sinusoid, therefore, equals 2M (Fig. 7–4A).

The angular frequency or velocity of the wave is given by the rate of change of the phase angle theta with time, or ω t, and measured in radians per second. Because the more familiar frequency, f, is measured in cycles per second or Hertz, these two are related by

$$\omega = 2\pi f \qquad [7.1]$$

A wave that completes a full cycle in 0.5 seconds therefore has f = 2 Hz and $\omega = 4\pi$ and could be expressed as $\cos(4\pi t)$ or $\sin(4\pi t)$. Figure 7–4B summarizes the effects of these operations.

Finally, to correlate an observed sinusoidal wave with other events in time, it is necessary to specify one other parameter, the phase of the waveform that defines the displacement along the horizontal axis of the wave at time t = 0. The final form of the function thus becomes $M\cos(\omega t - \phi)$, where ϕ is the phase shift in radians and expresses the amount by which the beginning of the wave lags behind the reference wave $M\cos(\omega t)$, which has a phase angle of 0 at time t = 0 (Fig. 7–5A). Because of the repetitive pattern of sinusoidal waves, an ambiguity of 2π radians always exists in computed phase relationships; i.e., a phase lag of $-\phi$ cannot be distinguished from a phase lag of $(2\pi - \phi)$ (Fig. 7–5B). The impor-

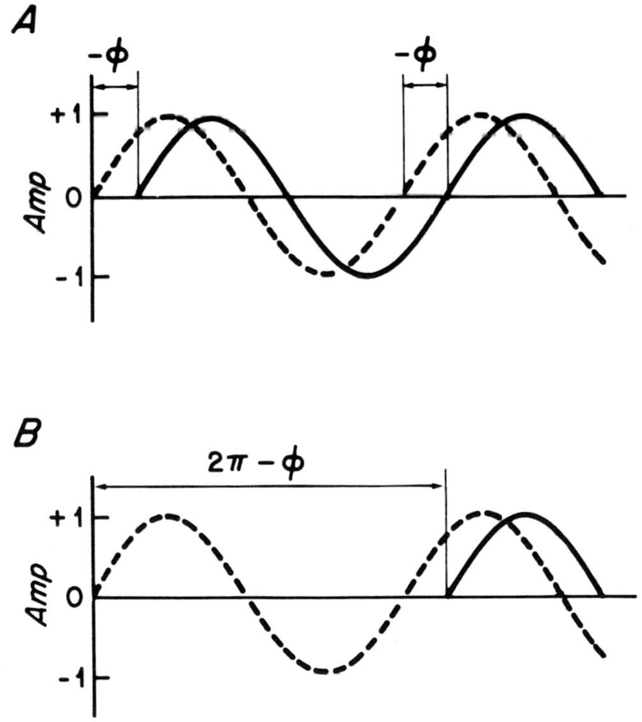

Fig. 7–5. **A.** The phase angle (ϕ) defines the displacement of the wave along the horizontal axis at time t = 0. **B.** Because of the repetitive pattern of sinusoidal waves, an ambiguity of 2π radians always exists in computed phase relationships; that is, a phase lag of $-\phi$ cannot be distinguished from a phase lag of $(2\pi - \phi)$. Amp = amplitude.

tance of this characteristic will become apparent later in the discussion of aliasing. Because both θ and ϕ are used to represent phase, it must be remembered that θ represents the instantaneous phase of the waveform at any point in time, t, whereas ϕ represents the phase difference between two such functions or a single function relative to a fixed reference; i.e., the phase θ at t = 0.

Thus far, this description of waves, both graphically and mathematically, has been in terms of amplitude as a function of time. This is referred to as analysis in the "time domain." As mentioned earlier, however, all waves have two propagating physical properties (though we are often only able to measure one). To display both pressure change and particle motion, e.g., in the time-amplitude plane, we must plot two curves, e.g., sin(ωt) and cos(ωt) (Fig. 7–3B), which are π/2 radians out of phase with each other (as are the sine and cosine functions). Fortunately, several other mathematical constructs for representing waves are more compact than this dual amplitude plot and, once initial unfamiliarity is overcome, prove much easier to analyze.

Description of Waveforms in Terms of Rotating Vectors

A conceptually useful way to represent waves is with rotating vectors. To develop this idea, consider a simple analogy, a runner on a circular track (Fig. 7–6). The track has a radius of M_0 meters, and the angular distance, θ, around the track is measured in radians, with the 0 direction taken to be east, π/2 being north, around to 2π at the east again. Thus, a runner's position at any point on the track is given by the pair of numbers (M_0,θ). If he is running around the track at an angular speed of ω rad/sec, his true speed in distance traversed per unit time is M_0 ω m/sec (Fig. 7–6A). If at time t = 0, he is located at −ϕ radians from the 0 ray, his position throughout time can be described as (M_0, ωt − ϕ) (Fig. 7–6B). The frequency/phase term ωt − ϕ has exactly the same meaning as it had in the amplitude-time plots of waves above. The magnitude term, M_0, need not be constrained to a single value. There might be multiple tracks around the center of the field, and a runner's distance from the center would be given by the variable M. A rotating vector is nothing more than an abstraction of this description of the runner's position (i.e., an arrow with its tail at the center of the track and its head on the runner as in Fig. 7–6C). This arrow has a length, M, and a direction, ωt − ϕ, and is termed a vector, (M, ωt − ϕ), the superscripted arrow traditionally identifying vectors. Because this vector follows the runner's position, it rotates about the center of the track with frequency ω rad/sec.

To turn this vector (M,θ) (said to be written in polar coordinates) into our familiar sines and cosines, we first superimpose the standard Cartesian coordinates (x-y grid) on our polar graph (track field) such that the origins coincide and the positive x axis is aligned along the θ = 0 ray (Fig. 7–7). Then the cosine component of the (M,θ) vector is given by its x value (the point where a vertical line from the vector crosses the x axis, also termed the *x projection*); the sine component is given by the projection of the vector onto the y axis.

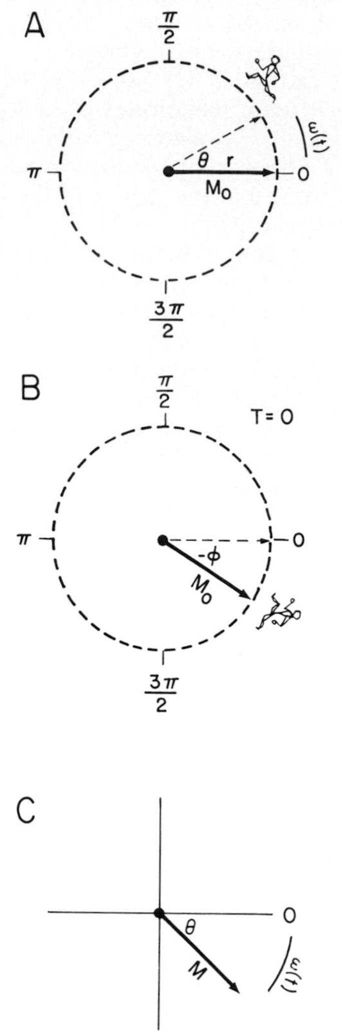

Fig. 7–6. The vector concept explained using the analogy of a runner on a circular track. **A.** The radius of the track corresponds to the magnitude of the vector and the runner's position at any point in time, relative to the start or zero reference is equal to the phase angle θ. **B.** The runner begins the race behind the starting line, and the angular distance between his starting position, and the zero reference is represented by the angle ϕ. **C.** Vectors are abstractions of this concept.

Thus, the vector, now written in terms of x and y coordinates, is

$$[M\cos(\theta),\ M\sin(\theta)] \quad [7.2]$$

Note that the vector itself is unchanged, only its representation in terms of coordinates. Thus, knowing the M and θ coordinates, we can translate into the x and y coordinates:

$$x = M\cos(\theta) \quad [7.3]$$

$$y = M\sin(\theta) \quad [7.4]$$

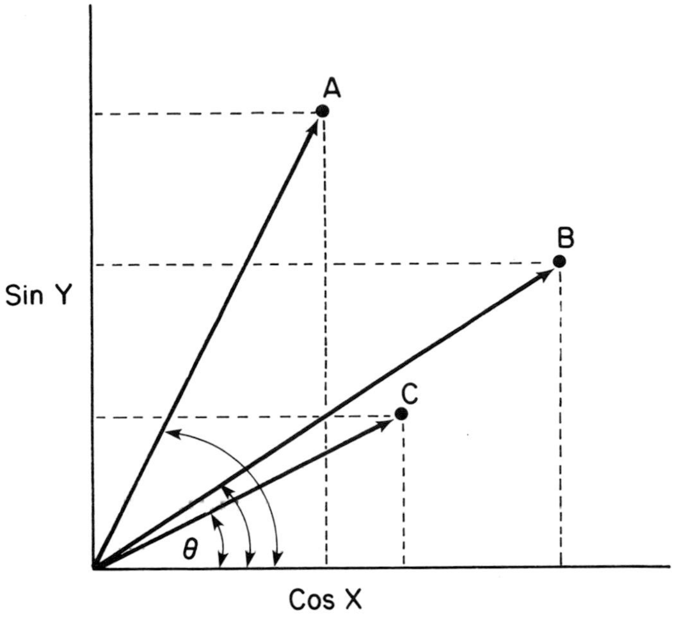

Fig. 7–7. The conversion of vectors to sines and cosines. Conversely, a wave (vector) of any magnitude and phase angle can be constructed from the combination of an appropriately weighted sine and cosine wave of the same frequency. (See text for details.)

and vice versa:

$$M = \sqrt{(x^2 + y^2)} \quad [7.5]$$

$$\theta = \text{arctangent}(y/x). \quad [7.6]$$

In these latter transformations: the first statement is nothing more than the Pythagorean theorem, because the vector and its x and y projections form a right triangle. The second statement uses the notion of the tangent, which is the ratio sine/cosine. Abbreviated tan(θ), it rises from 0 at $\theta = 0$ to ∞ at $\pi/2$ (where the cosine is zero). The arctangent, abbreviated arctan, or $\tan^{-1}$, is the inverse of this function; given a number, it yields the angle that has that number as its tangent.

Vectors can also be used to represent the instantaneous difference in phase between two waveforms as well as the combination of two waves. (Recall that vectors are added by placing the tail of vector 2 at the head of the vector 1.) The resultant sum is a vector extending from the tail of vector 1 to the head of vector 2. (Vector addition is commutative, so the choice of vector 1 and 2 is immaterial.) In the latter case, the vector sum represents the amplitude of the combined waves at any instant in time (Fig. 7–8).

It is important to recognize that this rotating vector describes the "whole" wave, i.e., both the microscopic pressure changes (the projection onto the y axis) and the microscopic particle motion changes (the projection onto the x axis). Graphically, therefore, the wave is fully represented by this single vector. However, performing any mathematical manipulation on this vector requires that it be written in terms of its coordinate parts, which differs little from the two-wave representation in the preceding time domain.

I therefore introduce the use of the complex number system to represent waves in a more mathematically malleable fashion. A word of explanation is in order here. Although I hope that the reader may gain an appreciation for this extremely useful technique of complex analysis, it is *not* a prerequisite for understanding the qualitative Doppler descriptions that follow. In particular, all of the basic notions of the Doppler shift, its detection, and display will be developed graphically using rotating vectors (and the track field analogy). For the interested reader, however, there will be short segments of more sophisticated mathematical exposition to explain these concepts. For the most part, I will use complex number theory to present these more advanced points, and this theory will be clearly delineated from the rest of the text. This first section on complex numbers should at least be skimmed by all so that complex notation will be recognizable, because it is used frequently in other forums.

The Complex Number System

A complex number has both real and imaginary components. This nomenclature is extremely unfortunate because it implies that imaginary numbers "do not really exist." In fact, they are no more "imaginary" than negative numbers. Just as the need for negative numbers arose quite naturally from equations such as

$$x + 5 = 3, \quad [7.7]$$

so imaginary numbers arose from commonly encoun-

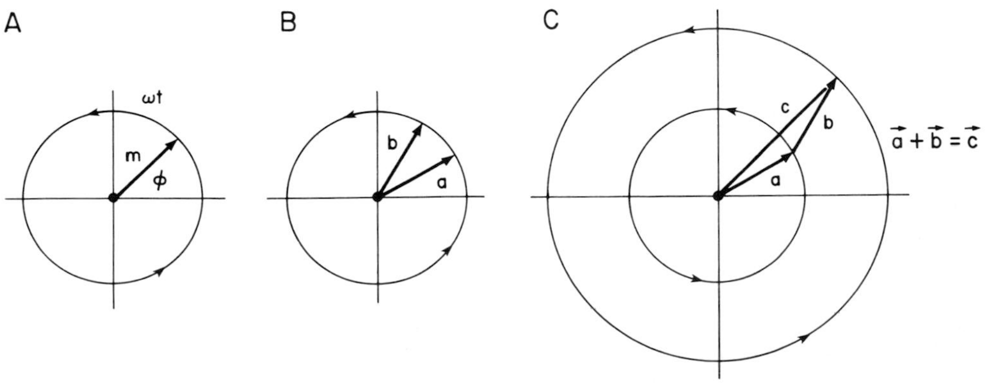

Fig. 7–8. Vector diagram illustrating a single waveform. **B.** Two waveforms of the same frequency and amplitude but different phase. **C.** The sum of the two waveforms in B. Note that as long as the vectors rotate with the same frequency the sum remains constant.

tered equations such as

$$x^2 + 1 = 0. \qquad [7.8]$$

The solution to this equation is $x = \sqrt{(-1)}$. But no real number has a square that is a negative number. Therefore, a new unit was introduced, the imaginary unit, i (sometimes called j), and defined as $i = \sqrt{(-1)}$. Thus, $\sqrt{(-4)} = 2i$, $\sqrt{(-25)} = 5i$, and so on. A complex number is just any real plus imaginary number: $2 + 3i$, $9 - 6i$, $4 + 0i$. (The last example shows that the real numbers are a subset of the complex numbers.)

Graphically, we represent complex numbers in the x-y plane, where the x axis corresponds to the pure real numbers (the real axis) and the y axis corresponds to the purely imaginary numbers (the imaginary axis) (see Fig. 7–8). The following arithmetic operations are defined for complex numbers:

Addition:

$$(A + iB) + (C + iD) = (A + C) + i(B + D) \qquad [7.9]$$

Subtraction:

$$(A + iB) - (C + iD) = (A - C) + i(B - D) \qquad [7.10]$$

Multiplication:

$$(A + iB) \times (C + iD) = (AC - BD) + i(AD + BC) \qquad [7.11]$$

Division:

$$(A + iB)/(C + iD) = [(AC + BD) + i(BC - AD)]/(C^2 + D^2) \qquad [7.12]$$

Complex conjugate:

$$(A + iB)^* = (A - iB) \qquad [7.13]$$

Magnitude:

$$\mathrm{MAG}(A + iB) = (A + iB) \times (A - iB)^* = (A^2 + B2) \qquad [7.14]$$

Real component:

$$\mathrm{Re}(A + iB) = A \qquad [7.15]$$

Imaginary component:

$$\mathrm{Im}(A + iB) = B \qquad [7.16]$$

Now comes one of the most profound (and perhaps mysterious) relationships in all of mathematics and from which all applications of complex analysis to wave theory derives. If θ is a real angle (as it has been in all discussions in this book), then

$$e^{i(\theta)} = \cos(\theta) + i\sin(\theta), \qquad [7.17]$$

where e is Euler's constant, 2.71828. What this means is that we are taking a real angle, θ, multiplying it by i (so that it becomes a purely imaginary number lying along the imaginary axis), and raising e to this power. What we end up with is a point on a circle of radius 1, centered on the complex origin, with the angular distance around that circle being θ radians, measured from the positive real axis. Although it is possible to prove this relation quite rigorously, we shall accept it simply as given.

Representing Waves With Complex Exponentials

If we substitute $(\omega t - \phi)$ for θ and multiply the whole expression by the magnitude M, we have the complex exponential form for the same wave described previously:

$$Me^{i(\omega t - \phi)} = M\cos(\omega t - \phi) + i\,M\sin(\omega t - \phi). \qquad [7.18]$$

Thus, as t advances, this describes a vector of length M rotating about the complex origin with an angular velocity of ω rad/sec, shown graphically in Figure 7–9. But this graph and this vector are exactly the same entities seen previously in Figures 7–6 and 7–7; only the coordinate system has been changed with the imaginary axis replacing the positive y axis. As before, at time $t = 0$, the vector is at $-\phi$ radians from the positive real axis.

As was noted in the discussion on rotating vectors, this notation also preserves both components of the propagating wave. In addition, complicated mathematical operations are easily performed using the notation $Me^{i(\omega t - \phi)}$. Once such operations are completed, one frequently needs only the real or the imaginary component of the final vector, and these are easily extracted from the expression

$$\mathrm{Re}\{Me^{i(\omega t - \phi)}\} = M\cos(\omega t - \phi), \qquad [7.19]$$

$$\mathrm{Im}\{Me^{i(\omega t - \phi)}\} = M\sin(\omega t - \phi). \qquad [7.20]$$

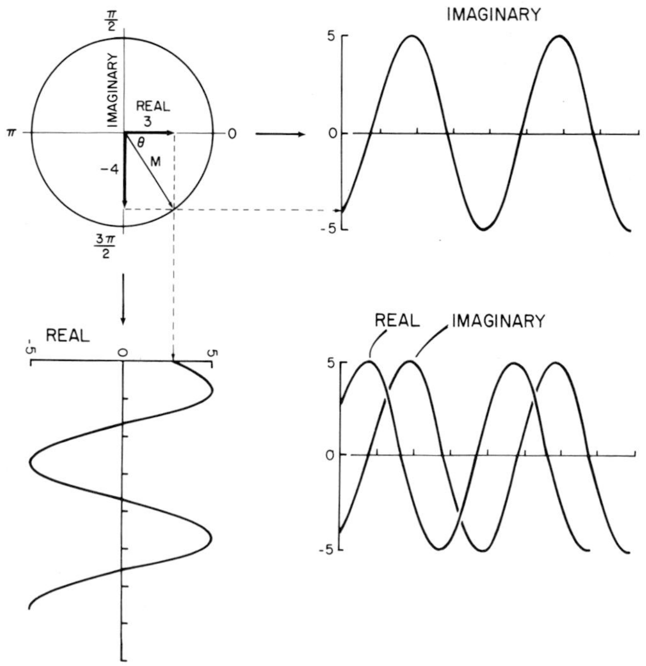

Fig. 7–9. **A.** Real and imaginary numbers. **B.** Real numbers are the projection of the rotating vector on the x axis. **C.** Imaginary numbers are its projection on the y axis. **D.** In this form the two components of a wave can be represented using a single number.

Following are the fundamental calculus operations on $f(t) = Me^{i(\omega t - \phi)}$:

Differentiation:

$$df/dt = i\omega Me^{i(\omega t - \phi)} = i\omega f(t); \quad [7.21]$$

Integration:

$$Me^{i(\omega t - \phi)}\,dt = Me^{i(\omega t - \phi)} = -i\,f(t)/\omega. \quad [7.22]$$

Note that multiplying a complex vector by i rotates it by $\pi/2$ rad (90° counterclockwise), whereas multiplying it by $-i$ rotates it by $-\pi/2$ rad (90° clockwise). Thus, integration and differentiation are simply vector rotations with the length scaled by the frequency, ω (multiplied for differentiation and divided for integration).

This mathematical framework allows the description of single waves in a variety of formats: trigonometric functions in the time-amplitude domain, rotating vectors in a phase plane, and complex exponential notation.*

COMBINATIONS OF WAVEFORMS

The foregoing expressions for the propagation of a single sinusoidal wave may be combined and manipulated to describe periodic waveforms of any shape. This is done by adding together waves with varying amplitude, frequency, and phase. Simple examples of such combinations are as follows:

Identical Frequency and Phase

One of the fundamental properties of sinusoidal waves is that a wave of any amplitude and phase angle can be produced by adding appropriately amplitude-weighted cosine and sine waves of the same frequency and zero phase angle. Thus,

$$M\cos(\omega t - \phi) = A\cos(\omega t) + B\sin(\omega t). \quad [7.23]$$

This could be considered nothing more than the separation of a rotating vector into its components. There is an engineering convention for this that breaks up the original vector into two vectors orthogonal to each other: the cosine vector oriented along the positive x (or real) axis and the sine vector oriented along the $-y$ (or imaginary) axis. The cosine and sine are then given by the x (real) component of the respective component vectors. These vectors are rigidly coupled and rotate around the origin at frequency ω. Some trigonometric manipulation will produce expressions for A and B:

$$A = M\cos(\phi) \quad [7.24]$$

$$B = M\sin(\phi). \quad [7.25]$$

Figure 7–9 illustrates this relationship and emphasizes again the correspondence between the real and imaginary numbers system and the sine and cosine functions.

Same Frequency-Varying Phase

In the previous example, we considered the addition or summation of two waves of the same frequency and phase. Now let us consider the interaction of two sound waves of the same frequency and amplitude but arising from different sources, the phases of which are initially adjusted so that the peaks arrive in phase at some point P. As we learned in Chapter 2, in the section on phased arrays, when two waves arrive at the same point "in phase," their amplitudes summate and the resulting signal intensity is maximal. Conversely, if the waves arrive 180° out of phase, they will cancel and their combined amplitude at that point will be at its minimum.

Now suppose that by turning a "phase knob" we can alter the phase of one wave relative to the other. If we begin with the waves arriving at point P in phase, the intensity of the signal heard by an observer will be maximal. If we then gradually turn the "phase knob" to shift the phase of one wave relative to the other, the signal will gradually decrease until it falls to zero at the point where they are 180° out of phase. If we continue beyond 180°, the signal will gradually increase again with alternating peaks and troughs occurring as long as we continue to turn the knob.[35]

Different Frequency

Because frequency is the change in phase over time, two waves of slightly different frequency will by definition gradually shift in phase relative to each other. Thus, if two waves of different frequency arrive at the same point, we should find a gradual rise and fall in the amplitude of the signal they produce. The amplitude of this pulsation will be maximum when they are in phase (phase difference equals 0) and minimum when they arrive totally out of phase (phase difference equals 180°). Mathematically, it can be shown that when two waves $\cos\omega_1 t$ and $\cos\omega_2 t$ are combined, the resultant wave

* Note that throughout this discussion, I have used the expression $\omega t - \phi$ to represent the instantaneous phase of the wave. Implicit in the use of this expression is the assumption that we are considering the wave properties as observed at a single point in space with time as the only variable. It is important to remember that propagating waves have both spatial and temporal variation: If one wishes to change the observed instantaneous phase (θ) of a wave, one may either wait a few milliseconds (temporal variation) or move (instantly!) a few millimeters (spatial variation). The fundamental spatial unit is the wavelength, $\lambda = c/f$, where c is velocity of wave propagation in space and f is the frequency. We can choose a different unit that is more closely analogous to our angular velocity, ω:

$$\nu = \omega/c,$$

where ν may be thought of as the spatial frequency of the wave and has units of rad/cm. For a wave propagating along the x direction, the space-time expression for the wave is

$$f(x, t) = Me^{i(\omega t - \nu x - \phi)} = Me^{i(\omega t - \omega x/c - \phi)}.$$

The real component of this is $M\cos(\omega t - \omega x/c - \phi)$. The spatial variation enters in a negative sense, $-\omega x/c$, because as we go along the x axis we reach waves emitted at an earlier point in time. We need not confine ourselves to one-dimensional propagation (and Doppler scattering produces spherical wavefronts). If r is the vector from the wave source to the observer, with distance given by $|r|$, then the wave equation becomes:

$$f(r, t) = Me^{i(\omega t - \nu|r| - \phi)} = Me^{i(\omega(t - |r|/c) - \phi)}.$$

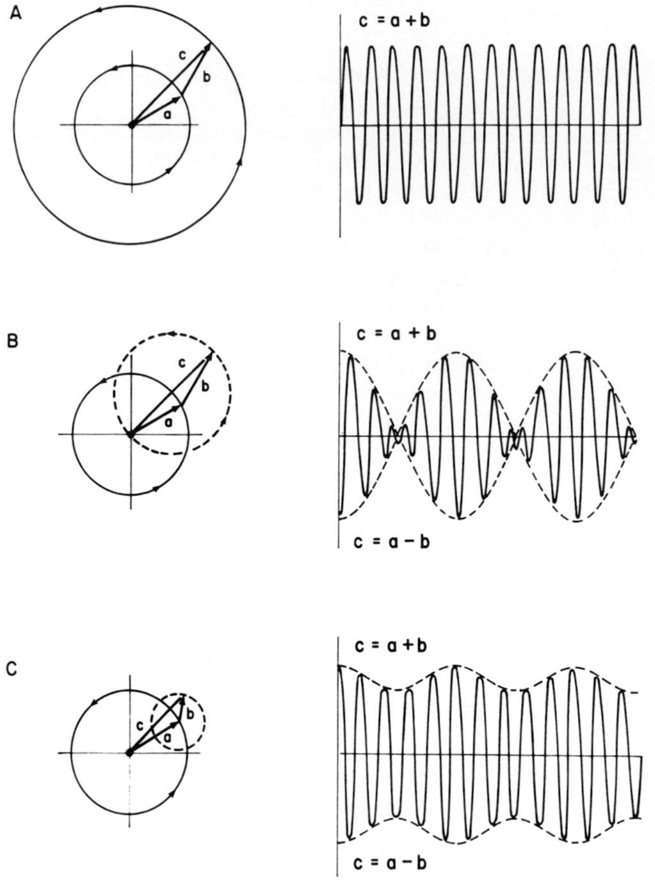

Fig. 7–10. **A.** The combination of waves (vectors) of the same amplitude and frequency. **B.** The same amplitude and different frequency. **C.** Different amplitude and frequency. Note that if the two vectors rotate at the same frequency (A), the sum is constant. If they rotate at different frequencies, the sum varies, being maximal when they point in the same direction (are in phase) and minimal when they point in opposite directions (are out of phase). The oscillation frequency of the output represents the frequency difference between the two vectors (waves).

will oscillate in amplitude at $\omega 1 - \omega 2$, which is the frequency difference between the two, termed the "beat frequency." This beat frequency will be shown later to be the same as the Doppler shift frequency, and its detection is the basis of the Doppler method.

We can use addition of rotating vectors to demonstrate graphically what occurs during this combination of waveforms. Figure 7–10 illustrates two rotating vectors, along with their sum at time (t) = 0. If they are rotating at the same frequency (i.e., represent waves of the same frequency), then they will maintain the same relative position to each other, and their sum will rotate with them (Fig. 7–10A). If instead they are rotating at different frequencies ω_1 and ω_2 (corresponding to waves of different frequencies), then they will not maintain the same relationship as they rotate. Sometimes the vectors will be in the same direction, and their sum will be of maximal amplitude and at other times they will be directed oppositely and their amplitudes will completely (Fig. 7–10B) or partially (Fig. 7–10C) cancel. Over time, the projection of the net vector onto either of the axes (i.e., its real or imaginary component), will vary, with the rate of fluctuation representing the difference in frequency of the two component vectors or waves. As the number of waves being added together rises, it becomes impractical to add rotating vectors. It is mathematically more tractable to treat each of the waves as a complex exponential, add them together, and then take the real or imaginary component (depending on the physical property being studied) for the time-amplitude plot.

METHODS FOR DETERMINING THE FREQUENCY OF UNKNOWN AND COMPLEX SINUSOIDAL WAVEFORMS

Frequency Description by Zero Crossings

The frequency of a simple sinusoid can be described most easily in terms of the number (N) of zero crossings of the wave per unit time (i.e., the number of times the sine wave crosses the zero reference line per second) or the zero crossing interval (time between zero crossings). The zero crossing interval is the most precise description of the frequency of a simple sine wave because for a constant zero crossing interval the frequency of the wave is independent of its amplitude. Because a sine wave crosses zero twice during each cycle, the frequency of the wave equals 2N or can be described by the zero crossing interval divided by 2 (Fig. 7–11A).

Two waves of similar frequency (Fig. 7–11B) but separated in time will have a constant time difference (Δt) between successive peaks or zero crossings, just as two

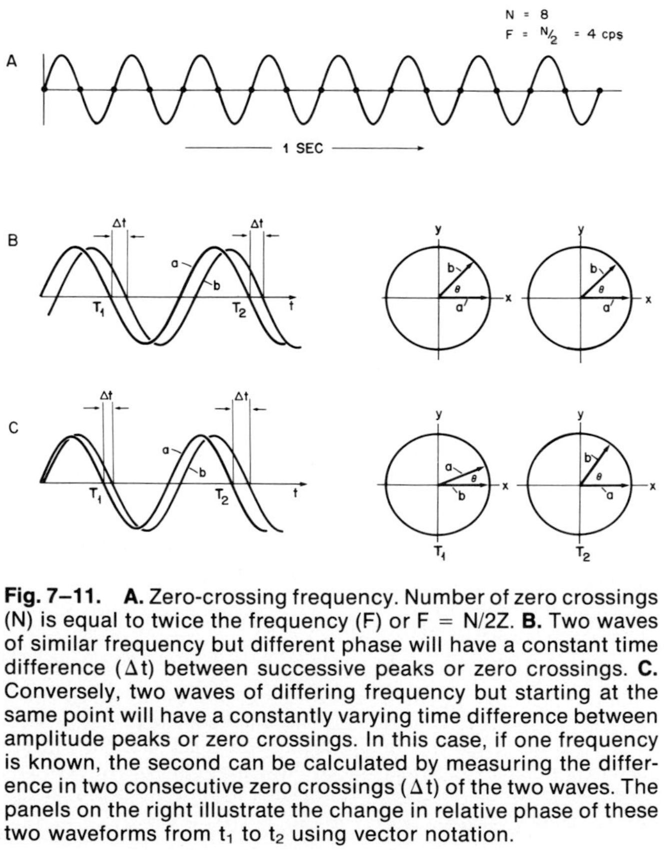

Fig. 7–11. **A.** Zero-crossing frequency. Number of zero crossings (N) is equal to twice the frequency (F) or F = N/2Z. **B.** Two waves of similar frequency but different phase will have a constant time difference (Δt) between successive peaks or zero crossings. **C.** Conversely, two waves of differing frequency but starting at the same point will have a constantly varying time difference between amplitude peaks or zero crossings. In this case, if one frequency is known, the second can be calculated by measuring the difference in two consecutive zero crossings (Δt) of the two waves. The panels on the right illustrate the change in relative phase of these two waveforms from t_1 to t_2 using vector notation.

runners starting at different points but moving at the same speed will maintain a constant separation between each other (i.e., a constant phase difference). Conversely, two waves of differing frequency but starting at the same point will have a constantly varying time difference between amplitude peaks or zero crossings (Fig. 7–11C). In the latter case, if one frequency is known, the second can be calculated by measuring the difference in two consecutive zero crossings (Δt) of the two waves. If ΔZC is the change in relative timing of zero crossings of the two waves observed between two successive crossings, then knowing f_1 yields the following for f_2:

$$f_2 = f_1/(1 - 2\Delta ZCf_1). \qquad [7.26]$$

This expression is accurate for a single Doppler-shifted wave being compared with the known output frequency. Unfortunately, a typical Doppler signal represents a complex combination of waves from millions of point scatterers within the heart and may contain many different frequencies. The frequency content of such a complex waveform cannot be completely described by changes in polarity or zero crossing intervals and, thus, a more detailed description of the frequency content of the wave is necessary.

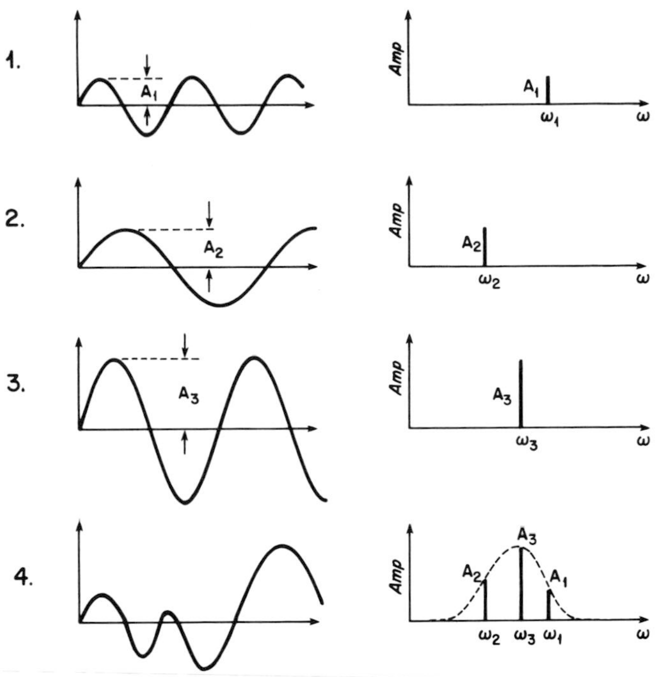

Fig. 7–12. Frequency domain analysis. In the left portion of this figure, three sinusoidal waves 1, 2, and 3, each with a different amplitude and frequency, are added together in the time domain to form the complex waveform 4. Alternatively, the amplitudes of each wave can be plotted as a function of frequency as illustrated on the right. In this format, the height and location of the spectral line correspond to the amplitude and frequency of the waveform, respectively. The complex waveform 4 can then be represented by its component frequencies. It is common practice to connect the tips of the frequency components to form a smooth curve known as the frequency power spectrum. It is important to remember, however, that this spectrum is composed of individual discrete frequency components. The width of the power spectrum is referred to as the frequency bandwidth.

Frequency Domain Analysis

As the frequency content of a wave becomes increasingly complex, it is often useful to display and operate on the component frequencies separately. This process, known as frequency domain analysis, is illustrated in Figure 7–12. In the left portion of this figure, three sinusoid waves 1, 2, and 3, each with a different amplitude and frequency, are added together in the time domain to form the resultant complicated waveform 4. Alternatively, the amplitudes of each wave can be plotted as a function of frequency as illustrated on the right. In this format, the height and location of the spectral line correspond to the amplitude and frequency of the waveform, respectively. The complex waveform 4 can then be represented by its component frequencies. It is common practice to connect the tips of the frequency components to form a smooth curve known as the *frequency power spectrum*. It is important to remember, however, that this spectrum is composed of individual discrete frequency components. The width of the power spectrum is also referred to as the *frequency bandwidth*. The frequency domain representation of waves is independent of time; however, the frequencies displayed must represent those present during some defined sampling period. This can extend from $+\infty$ to $-\infty$ or can be constrained to some discrete sampling period.

A fundamental property of frequency analysis is that a roughly inverse relationship exists between the length of the sampling period and the resulting frequency bandwidth (Fig. 7–13). Thus, a wave of constant frequency extending from infinity to minus infinity has a single infinitely narrow frequency peak in the spectral display (Fig. 7–13A). However, once beginning and end points to the wave are defined in time, then, in theory, some contribution of all frequencies is required to bring the wave from zero to its initial amplitude and permit its termination. For relatively long sampling periods, the contribution of these additional frequencies will be small (Fig. 7–13B). However, as the sampling time decreases, the contribution of the additional frequency components becomes relatively greater (Fig. 7–13C) such that a wave of infinitely short duration will contain an infinitely broad frequency bandwidth of uniform amplitude (Fig. 7–13D). Because any waveform that has a beginning and an end will contain some components of all frequencies, the bandwidth of all such waveforms would be infinity. Because such a description would be meaningless, it is conventional to take the bandwidth at the half-power level as the width of the frequency spectrum.

Fourier methods provide the link for converting complex waveforms between the time and frequency domains and therefore form the basis of Doppler signal processing. Using these methods, the component frequencies of any complex waveform can be defined. Fourier analysis is described in detail in Chapter 10 in the discussion on signal processing and in appendix B.

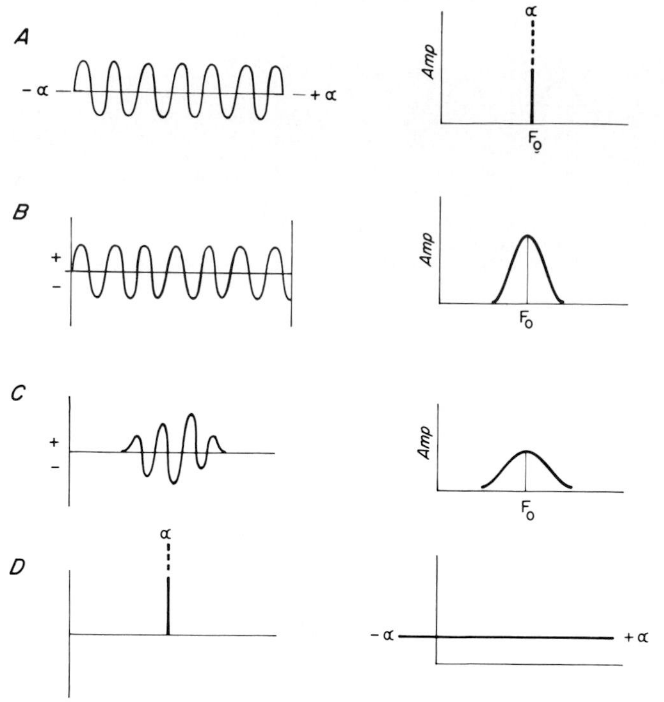

Fig. 7–13. The inverse relationship between the length of the sampling period and the frequency bandwidth. **A.** A wave of constant frequency extending from infinity to minus infinity has a single infinitely narrow frequency peak on the spectral display. **B.** Once the wave's beginning and end points are defined in time, some contribution of all frequencies is required to bring the wave from zero to its initial amplitude and permit its termination. For relatively long sampling periods, the contribution of these additional frequencies will be small and the frequency bandwidth will remain narrow. **C.** As the sampling time decreases, the contribution of the additional frequency components becomes relatively greater. **D.** Therefore, a wave of infinitely short duration will contain an infinitely broad frequency bandwidth of uniform amplitude.

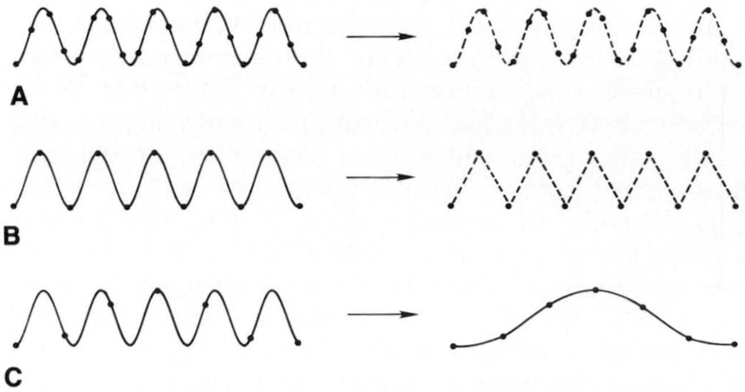

Fig. 7–14. The effects of sampling frequency on the reconstruction of a waveform. **A.** The waveform is sampled eight times per cycle and thus can be faithfully reconstructed. **B.** The waveform is sampled twice per cycle, and although the basic frequency is faithfully reconstructed, any information about the shape of the waveform is lost. **C.** The waveform is sampled less than twice per cycle (or below the Nyquist limit) and can no longer be accurately reproduced.

Differences Between Zero Crossing and Fourier Definition of Frequency

The zero crossing and Fourier definitions of frequency differ. The zero crossing definition considers only the time between shifts in polarity (+ to −) for each cycle and is, therefore, independent of amplitude and disregards any interruptions in the waveform. The Fourier definition includes all the frequencies required to reconstruct the waveform exactly and thus must include superimposed frequencies caused by variations in amplitude, interruptions, and the onset and termination of the waveform. When the term *frequency* is used in this discussion, it generally refers to the zero crossing frequency when simple sinusoids are considered and to the Fourier frequency when more complex waves are discussed. Frequency range or bandwidth (see following discussion) refers to the Fourier or spectral bandwidth. The differences in these two concepts of frequency are discussed in more detail later.

APPLICATION OF SAMPLING THEORY TO DOPPLER SIGNAL ANALYSIS

Many analyses of periodic functions are based on intermittent rather than continuous sampling. When sampling is intermittent, constraints in sampling rate may be imposed by the nature of the sampling process (i.e., pulsed Doppler), limitations in the available digitization rate, or the capacity for data storage. The effects of sampling frequency on waveform representation are illustrated in Figure 7–14. In Figure 7–14A, the wave is sampled eight times per cycle, and the frequency is accurately described. In Figure 7–14B, the wave is only sampled twice per wavelength. Again, the frequency is correctly represented but the waveform contour is lost. Below a sampling frequency of two per wavelength, the frequency of the waveform can no longer be accurately described. The requirement that a wave be sampled at least twice as fast as its maximal frequency to be correctly characterized is described by Shannon's theorem.[2] The numeric threshold for a given wave is known as the *Nyquist sampling limit*. Once this limit is exceeded, a phenomenon known as *frequency aliasing* occurs. Aliasing is the ambiguity in the representation of a wave that occurs when its inherent frequency exceeds one half the frequency at which it is sampled. This phenomenon is illustrated in Figure 7–14C.

FILTERS

A common method for separating or removing specific frequency components of a complex waveform is by filtering. Filters are electronic devices that permit a portion of the Doppler frequency spectrum to be transmitted while selectively blocking or eliminating the remainder of the spectrum. Because the full range is also referred to as the *frequency bandwidth*, the portion of this range that is allowed to pass through a filter is known as the *pass band* and that which is removed is termed the *stop band*. Various kinds of filters are encountered in Doppler instruments including high pass, low pass, and bandpass filters. High pass filters remove the frequency components below the filter cutoff while permitting frequencies above the level at which the filter is tuned to be transmitted. Low pass filters, in contrast, remove the higher frequency components; bandpass filters, in theory, transmit without attenuation frequencies

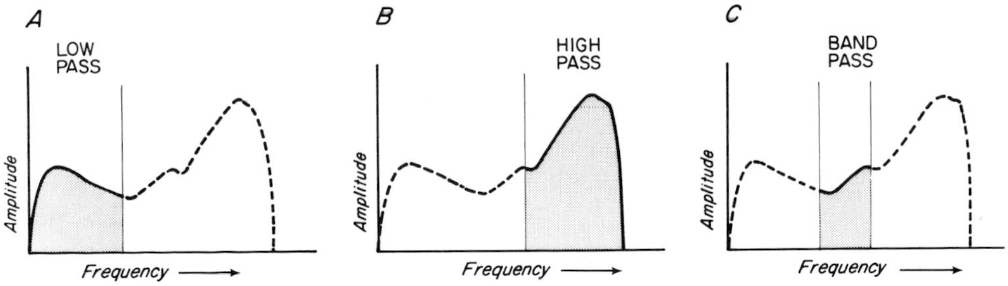

Fig. 7–15. The effect of low pass, high pass, and bandpass filters on the frequency spectrum. In each case, the portion of the spectrum that is allowed to pass through the filter is darkened.

lying within the pass band, while totally attenuating those lying outside. Figure 7–15 illustrates the effects of each of these types of filters. The concept of filters is introduced at this point because various types of filters are discussed in this chapter and in Chapter 8. In each of these cases, the filter is presumed to perform in an ideal fashion. Practical filters, unfortunately, differ from the ideal in several important respects, and the details of filter function are discussed in Chapter 10 under methods of spectral analysis.

THE DOPPLER EFFECT

The Doppler principle in its most basic form states that if a receiver is moving in relation to a stationary sound source, the frequency detected by the receiver will not be the same as that transmitted. Likewise, if the sound source is moving and the receiver stationary, a similar shift in frequency will be observed, with the magnitude of the frequency shift being directly related to the velocity of motion.[14] The reason for this frequency shift and the method by which it can be used to determine the velocity of relative transmitter-receiver motion are discussed in the following section.

Stationary Transmitter/Moving Receiver

The Doppler effect can be most simply illustrated using the case of the stationary transmitter and moving receiver (Fig. 7–16). To more clearly understand the effects of receiver motion, however, it is helpful first to review the characteristic reception pattern of a traveling wave passing from a stationary transmitter to a stationary receiver (Fig. 7–16A). In this example, a traveling wave is emitted at a frequency of 10 cycles/sec. Assuming that the transmission is continuous, 10 wavelengths or amplitude peaks will pass the stationary receiver during each 1-second interval, and the frequency received (F_r) will be the same as that transmitted (F_o). However, if the receiver moves toward the transmitter, as illustrated in Figure 7–16B, he will receive the same number of amplitude peaks (10) as if he had remained stationary, plus an additional number (3 in this example) proportional to the distance or number of wavelengths moved during the sampling period (1 second). The received frequency, therefore, will be 13 cycles/sec, with the difference between the transmitted and received frequency being the Doppler difference, or shift frequency. If the speed of sound (Fig. 7–16C) is known (in this example, 100 cm/sec), then the wavelength can be calculated as

$$\lambda = C/F_o \text{ or } 10 \text{ cm} \qquad [7.27]$$

The increase in frequency of three wavelengths, therefore, corresponds to a distance moved of 30 cm, and because this occurred in a 1-second sampling period, the velocity of motion of the receiver can be calculated as 30 cm/sec. It should also be apparent from this example that if the receiver moves faster or slower, then the number of wavelengths or the frequency received will correspondingly increase or decrease as will the Doppler difference frequency. The Doppler shift, therefore, varies directly with velocity, and by simply knowing the wavelength and frequency shift, one can calculate the velocity of motion.

$$Fd \alpha V \qquad [7.28]$$

Figure 7–16C illustrates the receiver moving away from the sound source. In this example, if the receiver moves away a distance of 3 wavelengths during a 1-second period, at the end of the second, only 7 of the transmitted amplitude peaks will have had time to reach the same position as that of the receiver. The received frequency (7 cycles/sec), therefore, will be 3 cycles/sec less than the transmitted frequency of 10 cycles/sec. Using the same calculations as in Figure 7–16B, it can

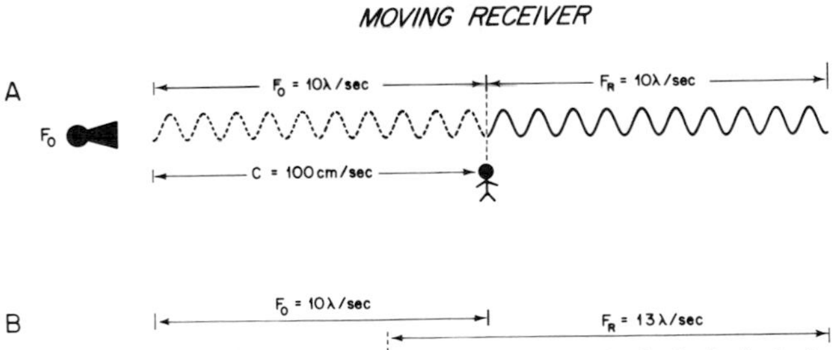

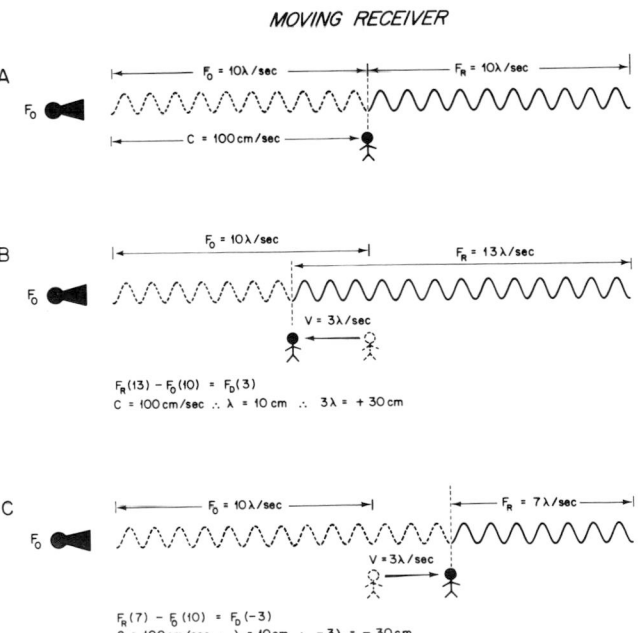

Fig. 7–16. Doppler effect caused by motion of a receiver relative to a stationary sound source. C = speed of sound. F_o = the original or transmitted frequency. F_r = the received frequency. λ = the wavelength.

be simply determined that F_d = negative 3 wavelengths and thus, the receiver has moved 30 cm away from the source. In this case (stationary transmitter moving receiver), the actual frequency of the traveling wave remains unchanged; it is simply perceived as being different because of the motion of the receiver.

Moving Transmitter/Stationary Receiver

The same general principles hold true if the transmitter is moving and the receiver is stationary. In this case, however, the explanation is different and it becomes necessary to understand how the movement of the transmitter affects the distance between peaks along a traveling wave. Again, it is helpful to begin with a consideration of a stationary transmitter and receiver (Fig. 7–17A). A stationary sound source can be imagined to be surrounded by successive spherical sound waves centered on itself and moving outward at a constant velocity. The frequency with which the wave peaks are transmitted determines their separation. In this example, the transmitted frequency is again considered to be 10 cycles/sec. Two observers, "a" and "b," positioned on opposite sides of the stationary source will both hear exactly the same frequency as that transmitted.

If, as in Fig. 7–17B, however, the transmitter moves and emits pulses at successive positions s_1, s_2, s_3 and s_4, each position becomes the center of a spherical wave that grows at the velocity of propagation of sound. At the instant depicted in this diagram, the pulse that started at s_1 has spread to a spherical wave front w_1, whereas that from position s_2 has spread to w_2, and so on. The distance between wavefronts, therefore, is reduced by the amount the transmitter is able to move toward receiver "a" between the transmission of two such peaks and is increased by the amount it moves away from receiver "b."

Stationary receiver "A," therefore detects a decreased peak separation and, hence, a higher frequency than that which originated from the transmitter, whereas stationary receiver "B" detects an increased spacing between peaks and the frequency appears to decrease. Mathematically, if VT is the velocity of the transmitter and $1/F_o$ is the time interval between peaks, then the distance moved by the transmitter between the transmission of successive peaks, ΔL, will be given by $\Delta L = VT \times 1/F_o$.

When the sound source is moving, therefore, the frequency of the traveling wave actually changes, with the degree of change varying depending on the position of the receiver in the surrounding sound field. Calculation of the Doppler shift in this situation assumes that the ratio of the velocity of motion to the speed of sound (V/C) is small and, hence, can be neglected. If this is not the case, the Doppler principle is no longer valid, and calculated velocities will be inaccurate (at the extreme, if V = C, the amplitude peaks will summate, causing energy accumulation but no detectable frequency change). In clinical Doppler studies, this ratio is normally in the range of 1:1000 and, hence, the calculated velocity for the moving transmitter will be similar to that of the moving receiver.

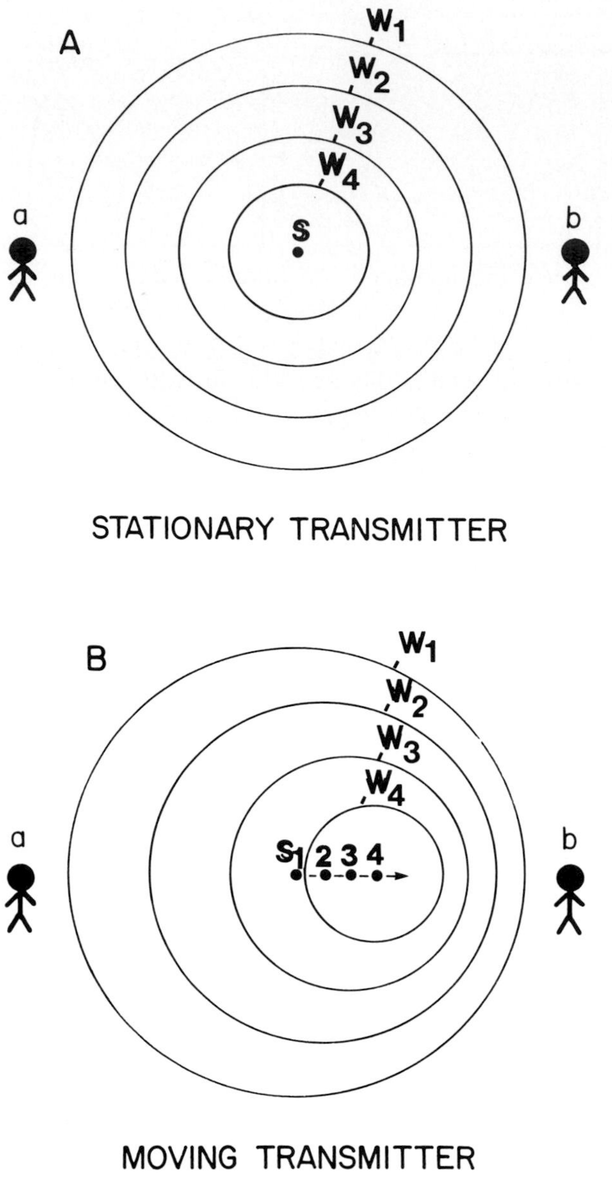

Fig. 7–17. The effect of motion of the sound source on the perceived frequency of sound by two receivers "a" and "b." **A.** The source is stationary, and both receivers hear the same frequency. **B.** The source moves to the right (toward receiver "b") and emits pulses at successive positions S_1 to S_4, each of which becomes the center of a spherical wave w_1 to w_4, which grows at the speed of sound. Motion of the source reduces the distance between these wavefronts in the direction toward which it is moving and increases it in the direction opposite to the path of motion. Because of this motion, receiver "b" hears a higher frequency, whereas receiver "a" hears a lower frequency. (See text for details.)

Effects of Transmit Frequency on the Recorded Doppler Shift

To this point, it has been demonstrated that the Doppler shift is a function of the velocity (distance per unit of time) of the source or receiver relative to the distance between amplitude peaks (wavelength) of the sound wave. Because for a constant speed of sound, a change in the transit frequency F_O will alter the wavelength, it can be expected to produce a corresponding change in the magnitude of the Doppler shift frequency. The effects of a change in frequency on the Doppler shift are illustrated in Figure 7–18, in which the frequency of the transmitted pulse is increased from 10 to 20 cycles/sec. For a stationary transmitter and receiver Fig. 7–18A), the frequency received (F_R) equals the frequency transmitted (in this case 20 cycles/sec). If the receiver moves toward the transmitter at the same velocity (30 cm/sec) used in the previous examples, however, he will encounter twice the number of amplitude peaks in the same distance because the separation between peaks is now only one half that present at a frequency of 10 cycles/sec. The Doppler shift will, therefore, be 6 wavelengths rather than 3. Because the increase in frequency decreases the wavelength by 50%, however, the calculated velocity will still be the same. Figure 7–18C illustrates the opposite case. Here the frequency is decreased by 50% to 5 cycles/sec, and the Doppler shift for the same distance of travel per unit time decreases. Thus, the Doppler shift varies directly with transmit frequency.

$$Fd \alpha V.\ F_o \qquad [7.29]$$

Varying the transmit frequency has many effects beyond those previously discussed for imaging. One important effect is that for a fixed sampling interval, a lower transmit frequency (F_o) will result in a lower Doppler shift frequency and, thus, if the sampling frequency is fixed, will permit a higher velocity to be detected before aliasing occurs. Transmit frequency also affects penetration, backscatter amplitude, signal bandwidth, and sample volume length. These effects of transmit and Doppler frequency on overall frequency resolution will, therefore, be discussed many times in different contexts.

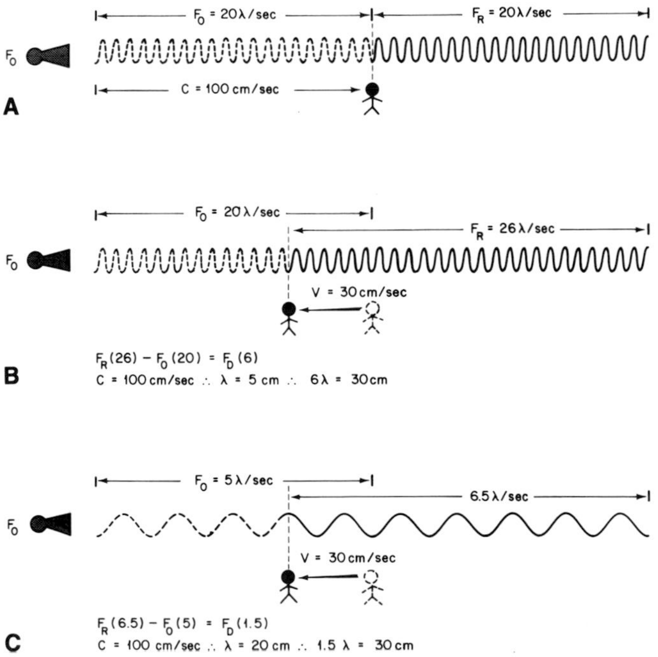

Fig. 7–18. The effect of changing carrier frequency on the Doppler shift frequency. (See text for details.)

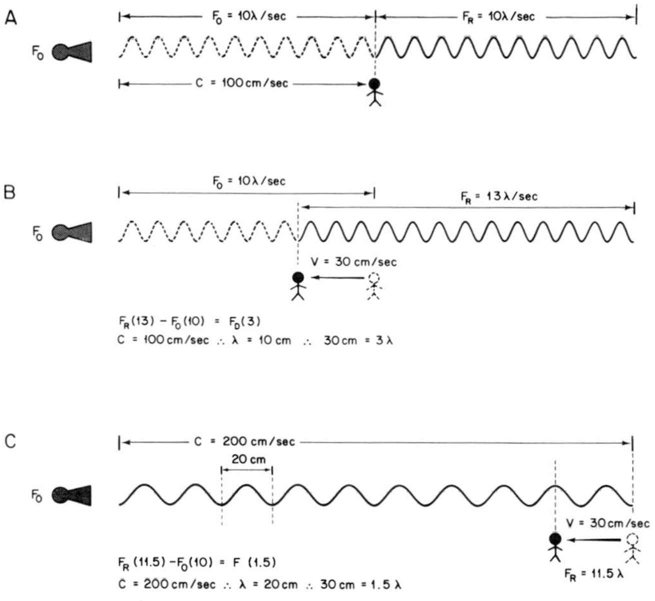

Fig. 7–19. The effect of changing the speed of sound on the Doppler shift frequency. (See text for details.)

Relationship of the Speed of Sound to the Recorded Doppler Shift

The speed of sound in the medium through which the source or receiver is moving also affects the recorded Doppler shift for any given velocity of motion. The effect of changes in the speed of sound on the detected Doppler shifts are illustrated in Figure 7–19. Figure 7–19A illustrates the frequency received by a stationary target at a transmit frequency of 10 cycles/sec and a speed of sound of 100 cm/sec. Figure 7–19B illustrates the frequency or Doppler shift encountered for the same transmit frequency and sound speed when the target moves at a velocity of 30 cm/sec. In Figure 7–19C, however, the speed of sound has doubled and is now 200 cm/sec. If the transmit frequency remains constant (10 cycles/sec), the increased sound speed has the effect of doubling the distance between amplitude peaks (wavelength). If the wavelength is now 20 cm, a receiver moving at 30 cm/sec will encounter only an additional 1.5 wavelengths, rather than the 3 wavelengths encountered at the slower sound speed in Figure 7–19B. Because increasing the speed of sound has the opposite effect as increasing the frequency, the Doppler shift, therefore, is inversely related to the speed of sound and hence,

$$Fd \alpha V \times F_o/C. \qquad [7.30]$$

The speed of sound in soft tissue is assumed to be constant and as a result, this term is typically disregarded. Even when sound speed does change, as during passage through a prosthetic valve, the associated change in wavelength is cancelled where the sound wave re-enters blood and, even though the reflected signals may appear to arise from a different location, no resulting Doppler shift occurs.

Effects of Angular Motion of the Receiver Relative to the Sound Source

In each of the examples to this point, it has been assumed that the receiver is moving in a direct line toward the sound source or vice versa. The effects of angular or radial motion of the receiver relative to the source are illustrated in Figure 7–20. Figure 7–20A illustrates the case for a stationary receiver. In this case, as in previous examples, the received frequency is equal to the transmitted frequency, and there is no Doppler shift. Figure 7–20B illustrates the case for motion of the receiver directly toward the sound source, where the receiver encounters the number of wavelengths that would have been received had he remained stationary plus the additional number caused by his movement. Figure 7–20C illustrates the case for a receiver moving at the same velocity (30 cm/sec) in a radial direction around the sound source. In this case, although movement is clearly present, because of the direction of movement, no additional amplitude peaks will be encountered and the recorded Doppler shift will be 0. Finally, Figure 7–20D illustrates the case in which the receiver moves toward, but at an angle to the point of origin of the ultrasonic wave. In this case, because of the angular motion, only one additional amplitude peak is encountered, rather than the three that would have been detected if the receiver was moving at the same velocity directly toward the source. If only the Doppler shift were recorded in this case, velocity would be significantly underestimated. However, if the angle between the actual direction of motion of the receiver and the direction of propagation of the sound waves is known, it is possible to determine true velocity by simple trigonometric relationship because true velocity is equal to the measured velocity divided by the cosine of this angle. In this example, the recorded Doppler shift would be 1 wavelength, the cosine of the angle .33, and the angle-corrected Doppler shift 3 wavelengths, which would correctly describe the velocity as 30 cm/sec. By rearranging the equation, it can be shown that the velocity times the cosine of the angle between the direction of motion and the source will equal the recorded Doppler shift. Therefore, when motion of source or receiver is not directly along a line connecting the two, F_d is equal not simply to the velocity but velocity times the cosine of the angle theta between the direction of ultrasonic propagation and the actual direction of motion.

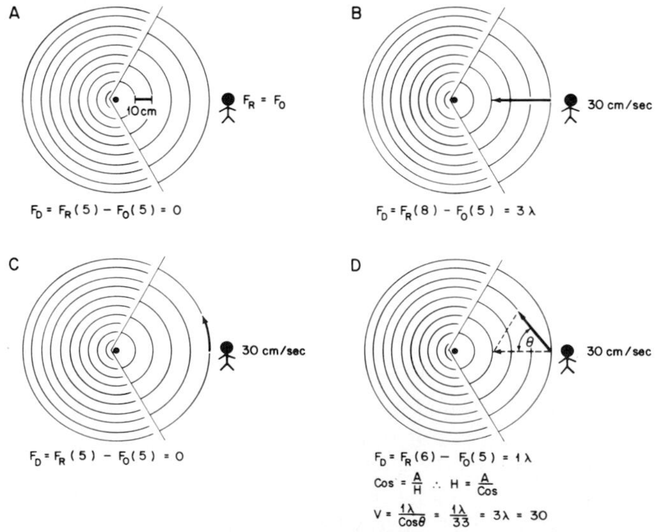

Fig. 7–20. The relationship of the direction of motion of the target relative to the path of the sound beam on the recorded Doppler shift frequency and velocity. (See text for details.)

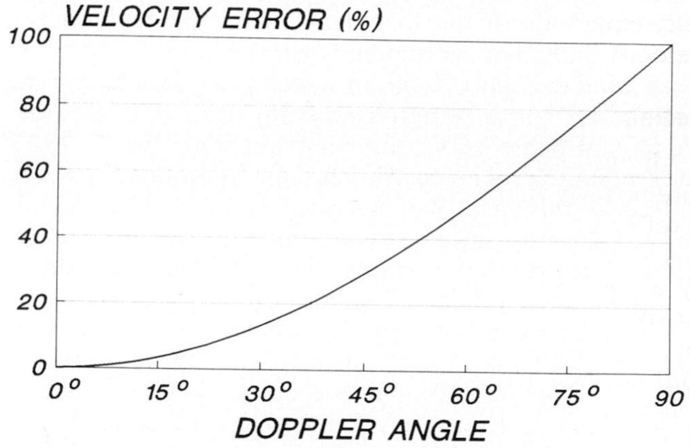

Fig. 7–21. Effects of the angle between the incident sound beam and the direction of motion on the recorded velocity for angles from 0 to 90°.

$$\text{Therefore, } F_d = F_o \times V \times \text{cosine } \theta/C. \quad [7.31]$$

This characteristic of Doppler sampling is similar to that illustrated in Figure 1–16 for motion of any target relative to an ultrasonic beam and occurs because only the component of motion along the beam axis is recorded.

Figure 7–21 illustrates the effects of angle on recorded velocity for a range of incident angles from 0 to 90°. When the beam angle is parallel to the direction of motion, the angular difference is 0°. Because the cosine of 0 is 1, multiplication by the cosine of 0 has no effect and, hence, this term can be disregarded. Angular deviations of less than 20° result in a change of less than 6% in recorded velocity, and it also is conventional to disregard the cosine function at these small angular differences. Beyond this point, however, the effects of beam angle relative to the direction of flow on the recorded Doppler shift become more important and must be taken into account.

When motion is perpendicular to the path of the ultrasonic beam, no Doppler shift should occur because the cosine of 1 is 0. This represents one of the fundamental differences between Doppler and imaging echocardiography. The specular reflectors of interest in imaging are best recorded when they are positioned at a right angle to the beam path whereas flow recording (velocity) is theoretically optimal when the sound beam is parallel to the flow vector.

In practice, however, even when the ultrasonic transducer is oriented perpendicular to a vessel, all the red cells within the vessel will not travel along exactly the same path, and hence, some of the scatterers will be moving toward and some away from the transducer. In this case positive and negative Doppler shifts are typically equal in amplitude, indicating that flow is present. Velocity, however, cannot be resolved.

Reflection

All clinical Doppler flow sampling is based on measurement of the frequency shifts that occur when sound is reflected from moving red blood cells (Fig. 7–22). In this situation, the ultrasonic waves are initially emitted by a stationary transducer and received by a moving receiver (the red cells). Because the red cells are moving, the received frequency is shifted by the Doppler shift frequency, and $F_r = F_o + F_d$. These targets then behave as moving sources radiating sound waves at an already Doppler-shifted frequency F_r. These sound waves are detected by a stationary receiver (the transducer), which receives a frequency of $F_r + F_d = F_{r'}$, which has thus been Doppler-shifted a second time. In an echo-dependent system, the Doppler shift frequency received, therefore, is doubled because both of the conditions of the Doppler equations are met. As a result, when using reflected sound, it is necessary to multiply the entire equation by 2 to determine the actual Doppler shift.

Thus, the final Doppler equation is

$$F_d = 2\ F_o \times V \times \text{cosine}\ \theta / C. \qquad [7.32]$$

Because it is the velocity of motion rather than the Doppler shift frequency that is usually of primary interest, the equation can be rearranged to solve for velocity such that

$$V = F_d \times C/2 \times F_o \times \text{cosine}\ \theta \qquad [7.33]$$

Ignoring the speed of sound and the cosine component, a direct relationship exists between the Doppler shift, the transmit frequency, and the target velocity, such that there is 1.3 KHz (of shift) per 1.0 MHz (of broadcast frequency) per 1.0 m/sec (of flow velocity). For example, using a 1.0-MHz transducer, a 1.3-KHz shift translates to 1.0 m/sec of blood flow; a 2.6-KHz shift to 2.0 m/sec of flow, a 5.2-KHz shift to 4 m/sec of flow, and so on. With a 2.0-MHz transducer, the same 5.2-KHz shift corresponds to a flow velocity of only 2.0 m/sec.

LIMITATIONS IN THE DIRECT APPLICATION OF THE DOPPLER EQUATION TO CLINICAL VELOCITY MEASUREMENT

The solution of the Doppler equation described previously yields a single frequency that can be directly related to target velocity. The precise interpretation of this equation in both the time and frequency domains is illustrated in Figure 7–23. Unfortunately, in its most basic form, the equation applies only when an infinitely wide planar target moves at a constant velocity through an ultrasonic field of uniform frequency and amplitude, and which is unlimited in any direction. If any of these conditions are not satisfied, the Doppler shift cannot be confined to a single frequency but will contain a whole spectrum of frequencies.[2]

In practice, none of the conditions of the basic Doppler equation are met: (1) The transmitted ultrasonic energy is not uniform in either frequency or amplitude. (2) The sound beam is limited laterally when the ultrasonic beam is transmitted continuously (continuous wave Doppler or CW) and is limited both axially and laterally when the beam is transmitted intermittently (pulsed wave Doppler, PD). (3) The targets with which the sound waves interact are neither planar nor infinite and do not move at a constant velocity. As a result, the Doppler shifts arising from flowing blood must comprise a spectrum of frequencies. As shown later, this characteristic complicates the detection, analysis, and description of the Doppler-shifted data.

Nonuniform Broadcast Frequency

As described previously, the basic Doppler equation in its most precise form assumes the transmission of an infinite sound field of uniform frequency and amplitude. In practice, this can never truly be achieved, because the wave duration must always be finite, and the response of the transducer crystal (piezoelectric element) to an input voltage is never perfectly uniform. Any interruption in sound wave transmission introduces additional fre-

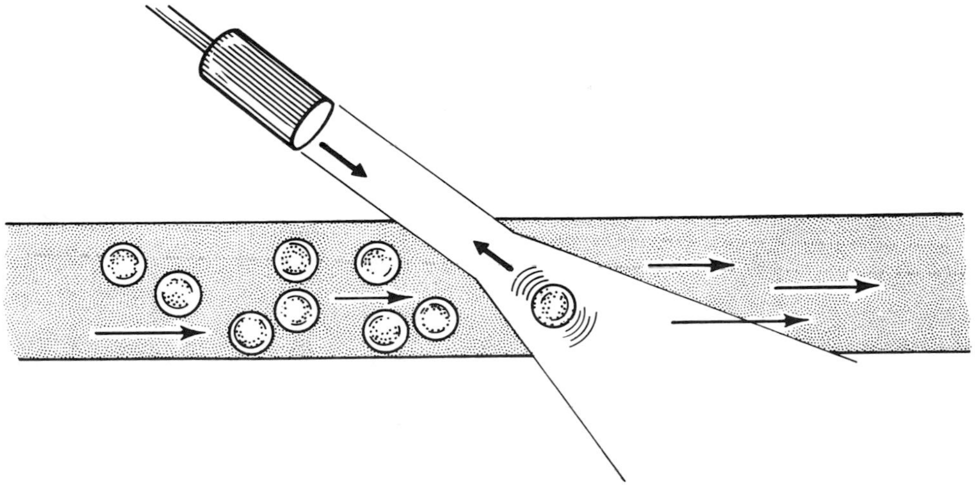

Fig. 7–22. The reflection of a sound wave from moving blood cells. The sound is initially emitted from a stationary transducer and received by the moving cells with the result that the received frequency is Doppler-shifted. The cells behave as moving sources radiating sound at the already Doppler-shifted frequency. When the reflected sound from the moving transmitters is received by the transducer, therefore, it has been Doppler-shifted twice.

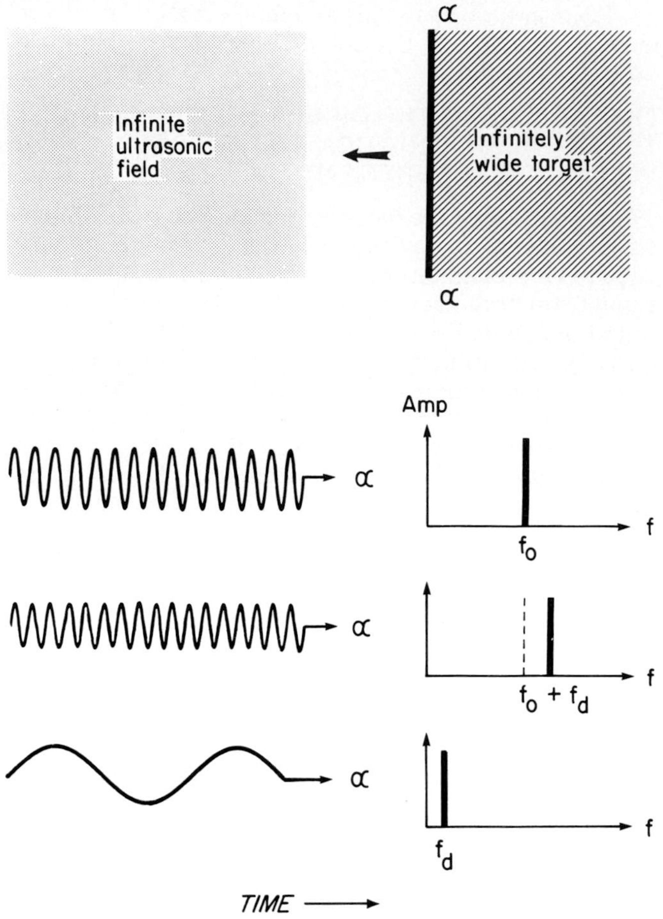

Fig. 7–23. Precise interpretation of the Doppler equation in both the time and frequency domains. In its most basic form, the equation relates only to the situation in which an infinitely wide planar target moves at a constant velocity through an ultrasonic field of uniform frequency and amplitude and that is unlimited in any direction. In this case a single Doppler-shift frequency will be recorded. If any of these conditions are not satisfied, then the Doppler shift cannot be confined to a single frequency but will contain a whole spectrum of frequencies. (After Atkinson and Woodcock, 1982.)

quency components during the period from initial transducer activation to the establishment of resonance and from the termination of activation to the cessation of oscillation. Because pulse duration and broadcast frequency spectrum (bandwidth) have an inverse relationship, more closely a Doppler device approaches continuous transmission, the narrower the transmitted bandwidth. Conversely, the shorter the pulse duration, the broader the transmitted frequency bandwidth (see Fig. 7–13).

Even if a pulse of infinite duration could be transmitted, it would still contain more than one frequency because of the finite nature of the sound-producing element and the variation in amplitude of the ultrasonic energy across the beam. It is the nature of transducers that an applied voltage will not affect all points on the crystal face equally. This is particularly true at the crystal borders, which generally do not respond in the same manner to the input energy as the center. This produces slight amplitude and frequency modulation even in a ''continuous'' signal, making the production of a single frequency broadcast beam virtually impossible.

Broadcast bandwidth has two important effects in Doppler studies: First, when a pulse containing multiple frequencies interacts with a moving object, each of the component frequencies will be Doppler-shifted, and the received signal will be a scaled-down version of the transmitted pulse with each frequency component shifted by the Doppler shift frequency.[36] If the signal bandwidth is small and the Doppler shift large, it is relatively easy to determine that a new frequency spectrum centered at $F_o + F_d$ is present, and to compare the difference in the two center frequencies (Fig. 7–24). As the broadcast bandwidth increases relative to the Doppler shift, however, it becomes more difficult to identify the new frequency or to define its spectral content. Second, the broadcast bandwidth determines the effects of frequency-dependent attenuation on the calculated center frequency of the received pulse.[37] Figure 7–25, for example, compares the transmitted and received characteristics of the power-frequency spectrum of a sound pulse typical of those used for cardiac imaging. When such a pulse returns from the body (dotted line), it is characteristically reduced in amplitude, and its center frequency is shifted downward because the higher frequency components of the spectrum are more highly attenuated than the lower frequencies. The range of frequencies present remains constant, and the change, therefore, occurs only in the relative amplitudes of the component frequencies.[38] In a Doppler instrument, every effort is made to transmit a pulse with as narrow a bandwidth as possible, and the returning signal contains new frequencies that were not present before.

In imaging studies, pulse duration is generally kept as short as possible to improve axial resolution, and the

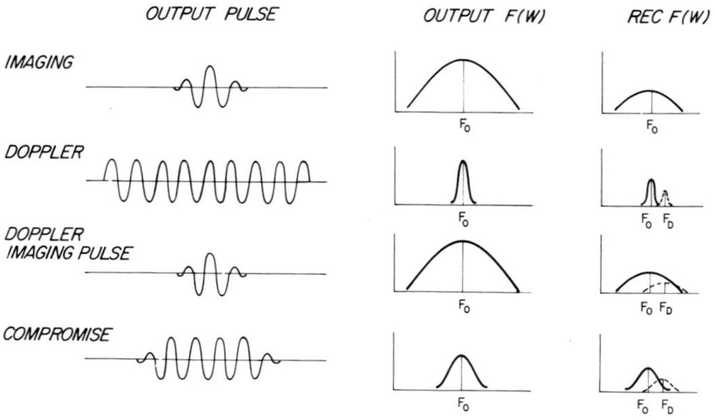

Fig. 7–24. Effects of broadcast bandwidth on the separation and detection of the Doppler-shift frequency. The first column illustrates a series of output pulses of varying lengths for different applications. The second column depicts the output bandwidth; the third column illustrates the received bandwidth. A typical imaging pulse has a short duration and broad bandwidth on both transmit and receive. A dedicated Doppler pulse, in contrast, would have a relatively longer duration and narrower bandwidth. This narrow bandwidth makes it relatively easy to separate a Doppler-shift frequency from the transmitted frequency spectrum. However, when an imaging pulse is used for Doppler recording, the transmit bandwidth is so broad that it is difficult to detect a Doppler shift. In the typical compromise, both Doppler and imaging resolution are sacrificed.

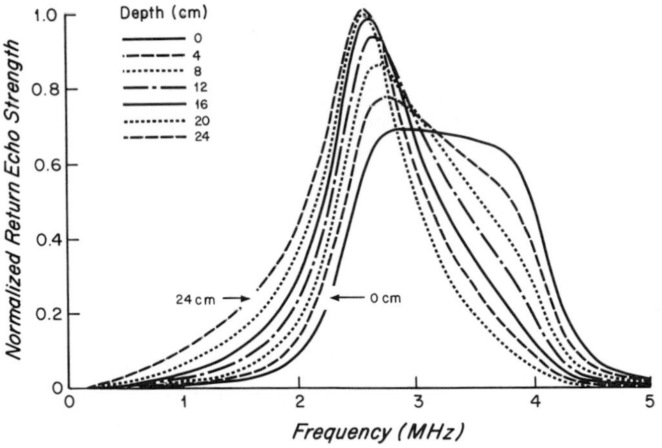

Fig. 7–25. Comparison of the transmitted and received power spectrum on a sound pulse typical of that used for cardiac imaging. The center frequency of the pulse is shifted downward as depth increases because of frequency-dependent attenuation.

broadcast bandwidth is ignored. In Doppler studies, when frequency resolution is paramount, it is desirable to transmit as narrow a bandwidth as possible. This can be achieved only by increasing pulse length, thereby degrading axial resolution. This basic conflict between spatial (axial) resolution and frequency resolution is a recurring theme of this discussion and will be dealt with in greater detail later.

The amplitude modulation within the beam also results in amplitude fluctuation in the individual components of the returning signal, because echo strength varies directly with the incident sound energy. Also, because any amplitude modulation in the returning signal is interpreted by Fourier methods as a new frequency or frequencies (see Chapter 10), this also increases, if only slightly, the apparent frequency bandwidth of the returning signal.

Finite Beam Dimensions—Transit Time Effect

The second assumption of the basic Doppler equation is that the sound field has no boundaries. In practice, this is not the case because one of the characteristics of ultrasound is that it can be transmitted as a well-circumscribed beam, and it is this property that allows it to be directed to intersect areas of flow. There are several important effects of this finite beam width on the resultant Doppler shift.

Continuous Wave Doppler

Figure 7–26 shows the ultrasonic wave form and spectral plots that result when a single point target (P) moves through a continuously transmitted ultrasonic beam. The motion of the target can be resolved into components directed parallel and perpendicular to the beam axis. The velocity component along the beam axis produces Doppler-shifted signals (Fig. 7–26A), whereas movement across the beam causes amplitude modulation of the reflected echoes. This variation in amplitude is interpreted by Fourier analysis as a new frequency that appears in the Doppler difference signal, broadening the Doppler shift spectrum (Fig. 7–26B). Amplitude modulation, therefore, introduces new frequency components that are not directly the result of target velocity. It can be shown that if the amplitude of a continuous sound wave varies with time, the modulating function (or the waveform envelope) determines the shape of the frequency spectrum, and the more rapid the modulation, the wider the frequency spread.[2]

If the sound beam is continuously transmitted, the amplitude modulation rate is determined by the transit time of the target across the beam ($\Delta F_d = 1/\Delta T$). For a target moving across the beam at a constant velocity, the frequency spread is in direct proportion to the beam width. For narrower beams, therefore, the transit time is relatively short, resulting in a more rapid amplitude modulation and broader frequency spectrum. Because the amplitude modulation is always finite in duration, even a single target traveling at a constant velocity through a continuously transmitted beam will produce a complete spectrum of Doppler shift frequencies. In addition to the rate of amplitude modulation, the transit time determines the length of the interaction between the target and the sound pulse and, hence, the relative dominance of the center frequency; following a briefer interaction, the center frequency will be represented to a lesser extent and the rest of the bandwidth to a greater one. Because the precision with which target velocity can be defined is determined by the width of the Doppler spectrum, which is inversely proportional to the beam width, the broader the beam the better the frequency resolution. Spatial resolution—i.e., the precision with which target position can be estimated—however, is di-

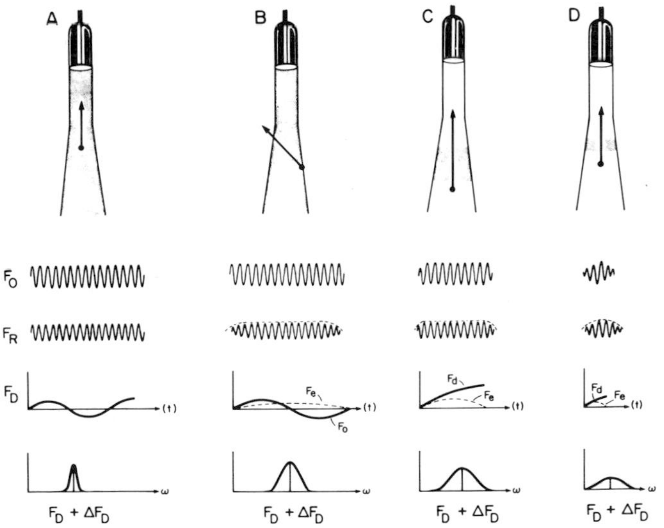

Fig. 7–26. Transit time effect. **A.** Continuous target motion parallel to a continuous wave beam produces a Doppler-shifted frequency F_D with slight spectral broadening ΔF_D because of the finite bandwidth of the transmit signal. **B.** Motion of the target across the beam introduces amplitude fluctuation and causes a further increase in the Doppler bandwidth. **C.** Pulse Doppler. The combination of a broader output bandwidth and shorter transit time further increases the Doppler bandwidth. **D.** Pulse Doppler with a small sample volume. This is the worst case situation and results in the lowest amplitude Doppler signal with the broadest bandwidth.

rectly proportional to beam width and, hence, improves as beam width narrows. Here again, we encounter the fundamental conflict between spatial and frequency resolution.

Pulsed Transmission. In the preceding example, the continuously transmitted sound beam was assumed to be constrained only at its lateral margins. If the sound energy is transmitted intermittently (pulsed Doppler), the finite pulse length also limits the axial length of the beam at any point in time. Blood moving through such an axially constrained pulse at a constant velocity (V) toward the transducer, will produce echoes that are both Doppler-shifted and amplitude-modulated, because of fluctuations in scattering power as different distributions of red cells pass through the sample volume. The resulting increase in Doppler shift bandwidth is again given by $\Delta F_D = 1/\Delta T$, where the bandwidth is inversely related to the transit time (Fig. 7–26). Basically, the longer the pulse-target interaction, the better the velocity of the target can be estimated (Fig. 7–26C). Conversely, the shorter the interaction, the less accurately target velocity can be estimated (Fig. 7–26D), a phenomenon known as transit time uncertainty. This uncertainty is a recurring theme in Doppler signal analysis and is discussed again in Chapter 10.

Finally, the basic Doppler equation assumes an infinitely wide planar target moving at a constant velocity. As described in detail in the next chapter, blood consists of multiple targets moving at different velocities that continually vary as a function of both space and time. Thus, the basic Doppler equation cannot be used to describe any of the practical situations encountered in the medical applications of flowmeters, and it is always necessary to consider the Doppler-shifted signals to contain a range of frequencies rather than a single discrete frequency shift. Many of the examples used throughout the remainder of the discussion describe operations on single frequencies; however, these should be recognized as simplifications for purposes of exposition.

REFERENCES

1. Baker DW: Principles of Doppler. *In* Fry (ed.): Ultrasound: Its Applications in Medicine and Biology. New York, Elsevier Science Publishing, 1978.
2. Atkinson P, Woodcock JP: Doppler Ultrasound and Its Use in Clinical Measurement. New York, Academic Press, 1982.
3. Wells PTN: Doppler methods. *In* Wells PTN (ed.): Biomedical Ultrasonics. New York, Academic Press, p. 354, 1977.
4. Hatle L, Angelsen B: Doppler Ultrasound in Cardiology: Physical Principles and Clinical Applications, 3rd Ed. Philadelphia, Lea & Febiger, 1985.
5. Cooley JW, Tukey JW: An algorithm for the machine calculation of complex Fourier series. Math Comp 19:297, 1965.
6. Bergland GD: A guided tour of the Fast Fourier Transform. IEEE Spectrum 6:41, 1969.
7. Bingham C, Godfrey MD, Tukey JW: Modern techniques of power spectrum estimation. IEEE Trans Audio Electroacoust 15:56, 1967.
8. Barber FE, et al.: Ultrasonic duplex echo Doppler scanner. IEEE Trans Biomed Eng 21:109, 1974.
9. Griffith JM, Henry WL: An ultrasound system for combined cardiac imaging and Doppler blood flow measurement in man. Circulation 57:925, 1978.
10. Holen J, et al.: Determination of pressure gradient in mitral stenosis with a non-invasive ultrasound Doppler technique. Acta Med Scand 199:455, 1976.
11. Hatle L, et al.: Non-invasive assessment of pressure drop in mitral stenosis by Doppler ultrasound. Br Heart J 40:131, 1978.
12. Hatle L, Angelsen BA, Tromsdal A: Non-invasive assessment of aortic stenosis by Doppler ultrasound. Br Heart J 43:284, 1980.
13. Doppler JC: Ueber das farbige Licht der Dopplesterne und einiger anderer Gestirne des Himmels. Abhandlungen der Konigl. Bohmischen Gesellschaft der Wissenschaften, 5th ser. 2:465, 1842.
14. Bullot's confirmation of Doppler's theory. *In* Gillespie EC (ed.): Dictionary of Scientific Biography. Vol. 4. New York, Charles Scribner's Sons, p. 167, 1971.
15. Satomura S: A study on examining the heart with ultrasonics. I: Principles. II: Instrumentation. Jpn Circ J 20:227, 1956.
16. Satomura S: Ultrasonic Doppler method for the inspection of cardiac functions. J Acoust Soc Am 29:1181, 1957.
17. Satomura S: Study of the flow patterns in peripheral arteries by ultrasounics. J Acoust Soc Jpn 15:151, 1959.
18. Yoshida T, et al.: Analysis of heart motion with ultrasonic Doppler method and its clinical application. Am Heart J 61:61, 1961.
19. Franklin DL, Schlegal W, Rushmer RF: Blood flow measured by Doppler frequency shift of backscattered ultrasound. Science 134:564, 1961.
20. McLeod FD: A Doppler ultrasonic physiologic flowmeter. Proc 17th Am Conf Eng Med Biol 6:81, 1964.
21. McLeod FD: A directional Doppler flowmeter. Digest, 7th Int Conf Med Biol Eng, p. 271, 1967.
22. Baker DW, Stegall HF, Schlegal WA: A sonic transuctaneous blood flow meter. Proc 17th Am Conf Eng Med Biol 6:76, 1964.
23. Franklin DL, Watson RL, VanCitters RL, Pierson KE: A miniature Doppler ultrasonic book flowmeter-calorimetry system. Proc 17th Am Conf Eng Med Biol 6:78, 1964.
24. Stone HL, et al.: Continuous measurement of blood flow velocity with an intravascular Doppler flowmeter. Digest, 7th Int Conf Med Biol Eng 13:6, 1967.
25. Reid JM, et al.: A new Doppler flowmeter system and its operation with catheter mounted transducers. *In* Reneman RS (ed.): Cardiovascular Applications of Ultrasound. Amsterdam, North Holland Publishing, p. 183, 1974.
26. Baker DW: Pulsed ultrasonic Doppler flow sensing. IEEE Trans Sonics Ultrasonics 17:170, 1970.
27. Peronneau P, et al.: Debitmetrie ultrasonore: developpements et applications experimentales. Eur Surg Res 1:147, 1969.
28. Baker DW: Pulsed ultrasonic Doppler blood flow sensing. IEEE Trans Sonics Ultrason 17:170, 1970.
29. Peronneau P, et al.: Velocimetre sanguin par effect Doppler a emission ultrasonore pulsee. L'Onde Electrique 59:369, 1970.
30. Hokanson DE, et al.: Ultrasonic arteriography: a new approach to arterial visulatization. J Biomed Eng 6:420, 1971.
31. Moritz WE, Shreve PL, Mace L: Analysis of an ultrasonic spatial locating system. IEEE Trans Inst Meas 25:43, 1976.
32. Brandestini MA, et al.: The synthesis of echo and Doppler in M-mode and sectorscan. Proc Annu Meet AIUM 125:704, 1979.
33. Namekawa K, et al.: Imaging of blood flow using autocorrelation. Ultrasound Med Biol 8:138, 1982.
34. Bommer W, Miller L: Real-time two-dimensional color flow Doppler-enchanced imaging in the diagnosis of cardiovascular disease. Am J Cardiol 49:944, 1982.
35. Feynman RP, Leighton RB, Sands M: The Feynman Lectures on Physics. Reading, MA, Addison-Wesley Publishing, 1963.
36. Newhouse VL, Bendick PJ, Varner LW: Analysis of transitime effects on Doppler flow measurement. IEEE Biomed Eng 23:381, 1976.
37. Snyder RA, Conrad RF: Ultrasound image quality. Hewlett Packard J 34: 34, 1983.
38. Harrigan P, Lee R: Principles of Interpretation in Echocardiography. New York, John Wiley & Sons, 1985.

CHAPTER

8

DOPPLER INSTRUMENTATION

The primary goal of any clinical Doppler instrument is to detect the velocity and direction of blood flow. To determine blood flow velocity, a Doppler instrument must (1) transmit a reference signal capable of penetrating to the depth at which flow occurs and returning to the transducer with sufficient remaining strength to be detected and (2) extract the Doppler-shifted frequencies from the other components of the complex reflected signal. The first requirement relates to the physical transmission, attenuation, and scattering characteristics of ultrasound. These physical characteristics can be considered to operate at the wavelength level and, hence, to pertain to Doppler instruments in general. More important, they describe the signal-to-noise characteristics of all Doppler devices and should be understood before specific instrument types are considered. The second requirement—Doppler signal extraction—occurs within the instrument. This is also a largely generic process and, therefore, is discussed before specific instrument types are considered. This chapter describes these processes for a simple sinusoidal waveform interacting with a uniform target of constant velocity. Later chapters examine the more complex interaction of sound waves with blood and the methods for analyzing and displaying the range of Doppler frequencies that arise from the complex blood target.

DOPPLER PULSE TRANSMISSION, ATTENUATION, AND SCATTERING: GENERAL CONCEPTS AND COMPARISON WITH IMAGING ECHOCARDIOGRAPHY

The ability of any flowmeter to detect and analyze an ultrasonic signal containing flow-related Doppler-shifted frequencies is governed by instrument design considerations and the physical characteristics of ultrasound in tissue. In general, these characteristics are similar to those previously discussed for imaging devices (see Chapter 1). However, several fundamental differences distinguish Doppler flow sampling from imaging echocardiography, and these should be kept in mind continually. First, Doppler devices are concerned solely with the analysis of frequencies and frequency differences. Because the frequency content of a waveform is far more difficult to define than its amplitude, factors that increase signal strength or limit noise by degrees, which are of little concern in imaging echocardiography, become critically important in flow studies. Second, the Doppler signals of interest arise from scatterers rather than specular reflectors. Scattered echoes tend to be weaker than specular reflections and are radiated in all directions, rather than along the relatively linear path that characterized the specular reflections from discrete interfaces. Third, imaging devices record and display all of the echoes returning to the transducer and, hence, the entire diffraction pattern of the transducer provides information that is of interest. A Doppler device, in contrast, is interested only in the signals that originate from a region of flow. All echoes that return from areas of the beam outside the region of flow are simply noise or clutter from which the Doppler signal must be separated.

Signal Transmission

Transducer Design

Imaging and Doppler devices both transmit ultrasound using transducers of similar overall design that operate within the same general frequency range. The major difference in the transducers used for Doppler studies lies in the degree of damping applied to the crystal. Imaging transducers typically have highly damped crystals so that the ringing response to an applied voltage (Q factor) is as short as possible to limit pulse duration and thereby increase axial resolution. As discussed in the preceding chapter, however, a short pulse duration increased frequency bandwidth, which limits frequency resolution. Therefore, dedicated Doppler transducers are less highly damped so that the response to a given input voltage results in a longer ringing response. This characteristic decreases the broadcast bandwidth, permits finer tuning of the oscillator and crystal frequencies, and increases transducer sensitivity in detecting low amplitude returning signals.[1]

Output Power

The power requirements in all diagnostic ultrasound examinations are critical because unless sufficient power is imparted to the transmitted wave to allow it to penetrate to the tissue depth of interest, no reflected signal will be generated.[2] Thus, reflected signal strength and output power are directly related, and it has been demonstrated that the performance of either a pulsed or continuous wave Doppler system is proportional to the average power transmitted into the vessel of interest.[1,2] There are three ways to increase the power in an outgoing sound pulse: increase pulse amplitude, extend the pulse length (number of cycles or wavelengths), or expand bandwidth.[2] The amplitude of the pulse can be increased by increasing the voltage applied to the transducer. This is probably the least desirable approach for diagnostic applications, however, because technical problems in rapid pulse generation are encountered and the tendency toward artifactual tissue reverberations is more pronounced at elevated excitation voltages.[2]

In imaging ultrasound, the third option—extended bandwidth—is used. Axial resolution preferences dictate that an imaging device broadcast a sound pulse of short duration, usually less than 5.0 wavelengths. When the excitation voltage is compressed into a short interval any crystal will be caused to emit a wide spectrum of simultaneous frequencies. The imaging device therefore transmits a broad range of frequencies, each of which contributes its component energy to the total pulse intensity. This combination of frequencies plus the energy contained in them is the power spectrum of the emitted sound pulse.

In Doppler studies, one is interested in what happens to a single frequency when it encounters a moving target. Accordingly, a wide spectrum of broadcast frequencies would be inappropriate because it would make it more difficult to monitor changes in any single frequency. Also, because excessive increases in amplitude or expansion in bandwidth would be self-defeating for Doppler studies, adequate penetration can be obtained only by increasing the length of the outgoing sound pulse or the number of cycles emitted by the crystal.[2] Since the average power for a pulsed device is the sum of the power contained in each wavelength, divided by the pulse repetition period, increasing pulse length increases average power. And because increasing pulse length also increases frequency resolution, this is the optimal approach for a Doppler device. However, this increased power and frequency resolution is attained at the expense of axial resolution.

Energy Attenuation

Dispersion

The strength of the signal that interacts with the target of interest is the difference between the energy output by the transducer and that lost from attenuation during transit from transducer to target. Attenuation, which is the product of absorption and scattering losses, is a function of the physical interaction of the ultrasonic wave with tissue and is the same for Doppler and imaging devices. The degree of attenuation varies with the tissue absorption coefficient, the range from the transducer to the target, and the frequency of the transmitted waveform. Increasing frequency increases signal attenuation because both absorbtion and scattering increase (see Chapter 1).

Energy concentration or dispersion is a function of beam pattern. The energy available at any depth may be concentrated into a narrow area if the beam is focused, or it may be dispersed over a broad front if the beam is defocused. Because force or intensity is equal to applied pressure per unit area, the beam pattern has a major effect on the energy impacting any point target in space. And because reflected energy is directly related to the incident energy, this also determines the strength of the reflected signal. Figure 8–1 illustrates the effect of beam profile on the energy impacting a point target.

Beam Pattern

The beam profile for a Doppler device, like that of an imaging system, is determined by transducer size, shape, frequency, and degree of focusing or defocusing. Beam pattern determines the diffusion or concentration of available power at any depth and the lateral resolution of the instrument (see preceding discussion). The effective beam width (see Chapter 1) is also modified by the output power and the receiver gain. The considerations that determine the ideal beam profile, however, differ

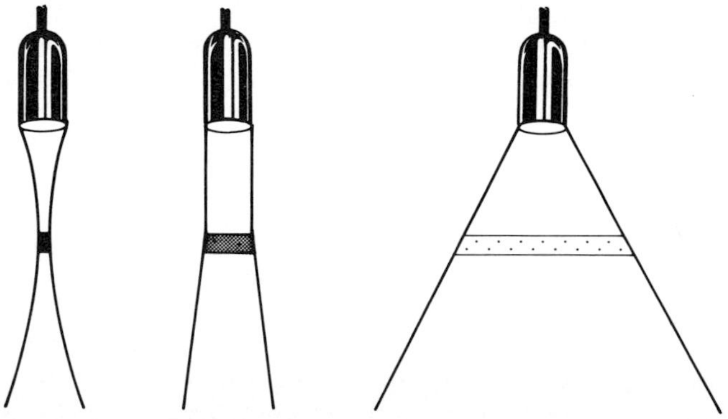

Fig. 8–1. Left. Effect of beam pattern on the sound energy available for interaction with a point target. Center. The beam is highly focused, and the energy is constrained into a narrow area. Right. The beam is nonfocused and the energy is spread over a broader area, thereby decreasing the intensity at any point in the beam path. The beam is defocused and spreads rapidly. This causes diffusion of the available energy over a wide area and a significant decrease in energy at any single point.

for imaging devices and flowmeters. For an imaging device, the narrowest beam profile possible appears desirable because this provides the best lateral resolution. For a Doppler device, the considerations are far more complex. A narrow beam, although increasing the spatial resolution of flow sampling and limiting power dissipation caused by diffusion, also increases reflected signal bandwidth caused by transit time effects (see Chapter 7), thereby decreasing frequency resolution. Likewise, if the beam profile is smaller than the flow area, it will fail to take advantage of all the available targets. A broad beam, in contrast, will decrease the spectral broadening related to nonaxially moving targets and will increase the potential scattering cross section that can be interrogated. Unfortunately, a broad beam has the potential to intersect areas outside the flow stream, which will result in reflections from non-flow-related targets (noise) returning simultaneously with those from the flow field, making the signal more difficult to detect. Because of these complex considerations, it is not possible to design a beam profile that will be optimal in all circumstances, and it is not uncommon to find an instrument or transducer that works better in one setting than in another. Doppler instruments, therefore, tend to be more application-specific than imaging devices.

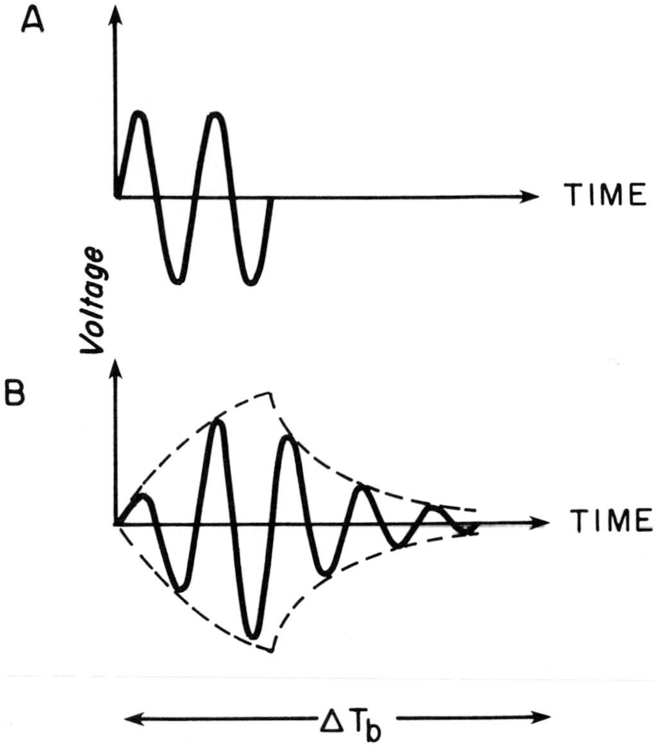

Fig. 8–2. The excitation pulse applied to the transducer (A) and the transducer response (B). To transmit a longer sound pulse, extend the length of the excitation pulse.

Sample Volume

The sample volume is that portion of the total beam diffraction pattern through which sound energy is traveling at any given point in time. Therefore, the Doppler sample volume is simply the envelope of the sound pulse described for imaging echocardiography and has the same meaning. Because echoes can arise only from targets that are in contact with sound energy, the sample volume or pulse volume defines the volume of tissue from which signals can originate at any instant. The lateral margins of this volume define the lateral beam margins and, hence, vary with range, degree of focusing, and output power (effective beam width). The axial length of the sample volume varies, depending on the pattern of pulse transmission. If the sound energy is transmitted continuously (continuous wave Doppler), the sample volume would occupy the entire diffraction pattern of the beam, and in fact, the concept of a beam implies continuous energy transmission. If, however, sound energy is transmitted intermittently (pulsed Doppler), the sample volume will be defined axially by the pulse length.

In theory, the shortest sample volume would be a single cycle. In practice, however, any crystal requires roughly three cycles to attain resonance after being shock-excited and requires two additional cycles for oscillations to decay. Figure 8–2 illustrates this relationship between the exciting pulse and the crystal output. The envelope of the signal is determined by the exponential rise in amplitude as the transducer is excited and the exponential decay as the crystal oscillates in free response.[1] Because the pulse amplitude begins at zero, rises to a peak at resonance, and decays more slowly to zero again, the sample volume has a teardrop shape. The smallest sample volume for pulsed systems is roughly 5 cycles or 2.5 mm at 3 MHz. In practice, longer pulses (8 to 14 cycles) are usually transmitted to increase frequency resolution; sample volume length increases proportionately. Figure 8–3 illustrates a representative sample volume configuration for a short duration pulse transmission. The sample volume determines many of the operating characteristics of a Doppler instrument because it defines the potential frequency resolution, the power within each pulse, and the spatial relationship of the sound energy to the area of blood flow.

Signal-Target Interaction

Scattering Cross Section

The volume of moving blood targets that interacts with the sample volume is termed the *scattering cross section*. The amplitude of the signal from this cross section is determined by the number and distribution of scatterers, which is in turn related to the hematocrit,

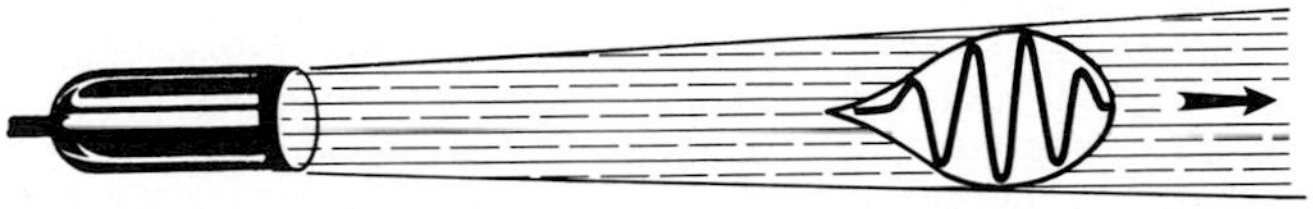
Fig. 8–3. Representative sample volume for a short output pulse. The sample volume is the envelope of the pulse and for short pulses has a teardrop shape. As the pulse length increases, so does the body of the pulse, and the sample volume assumes a more cylindric shape with a tapered head and tail.

degree of turbulence, and so on (see Chapter 9). For a comparable density and distribution of scatterers, however, the strength of the returning signal, for any input power, is directly related to the absolute size of the scattering volume or cross section.[1]

Spatially, the scattering cross section from which a Doppler device seeks to extract information generally occupies only a small portion of the entire diffraction pattern of the beam. Thus, while an imaging study uses all of the reflected data to create the final image, Doppler uses only the portion of the sound field that interacts with flowing blood. All echoes arising from outside this region represent clutter or noise, which tend to obscure the Doppler-shifted frequencies. Figure 8–4 illustrates the effects of the sample volume/scattering cross section relationship on the Doppler signal strength.

Target Motion

At the wavelength level, it is also important to remember that Doppler frequencies arise not only because the target moves during the time that the sound energy is being absorbed and rebroadcast but also because the target moves during the period between its interaction with each successive wave length. In imaging studies, the transmitted ultrasonic energy causes displacement of the particles in the medium as it passes. Between each peak, however, the particles return to their original position, and as a result, the distance each pulse must travel before it reaches the target is the same. In Doppler studies, the time each successive wavelength must travel to intersect a moving target constantly changes. If this were not the case, each intermittently transmitted wavelength would be shifted a constant amount and no new frequencies could be reconstructed using conventional pulsed Doppler methods (See Fig. 7–11B). The importance of this relationship will become apparent when pulsed Doppler systems are discussed.

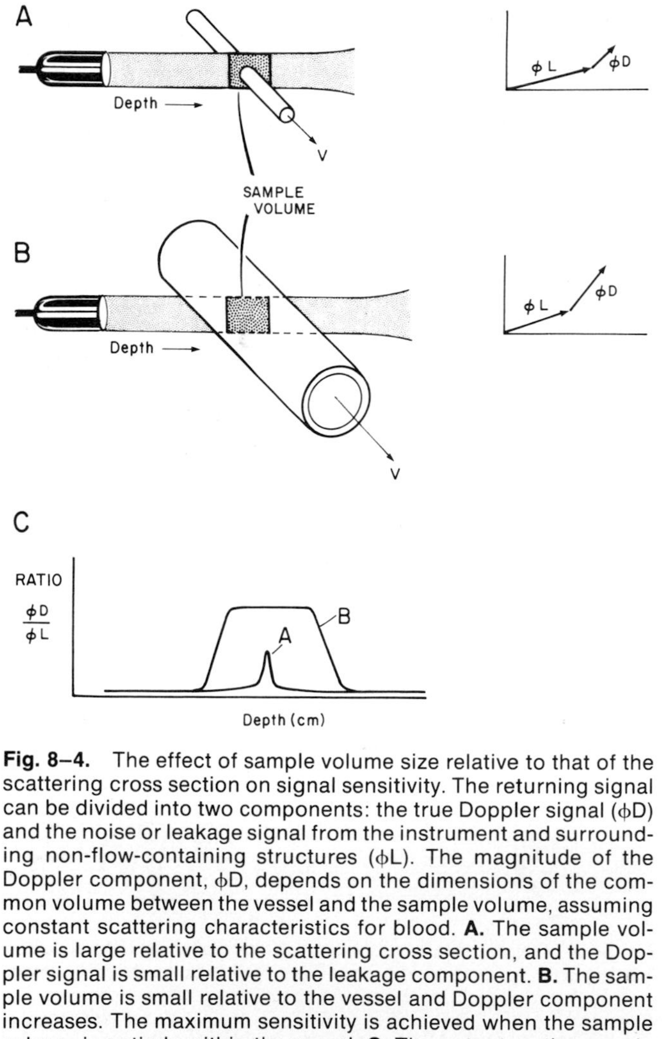

Fig. 8–4. The effect of sample volume size relative to that of the scattering cross section on signal sensitivity. The returning signal can be divided into two components: the true Doppler signal (ϕD) and the noise or leakage signal from the instrument and surrounding non-flow-containing structures (ϕL). The magnitude of the Doppler component, ϕD, depends on the dimensions of the common volume between the vessel and the sample volume, assuming constant scattering characteristics for blood. **A.** The sample volume is large relative to the scattering cross section, and the Doppler signal is small relative to the leakage component. **B.** The sample volume is small relative to the vessel and Doppler component increases. The maximum sensitivity is achieved when the sample volume is entirely within the vessel. **C.** The output as the sample volume is moved across the vessel in cases A and B.

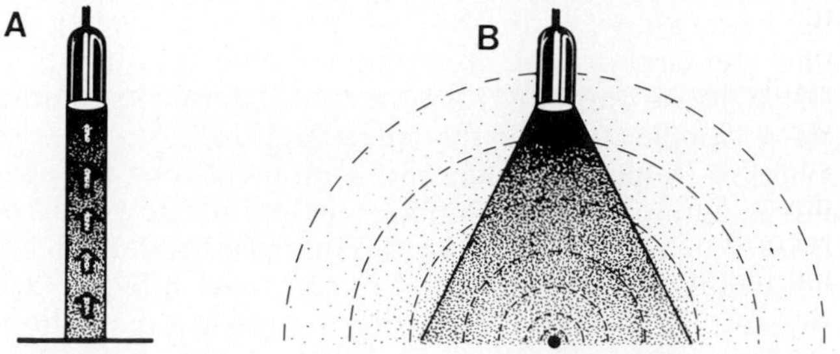

Fig. 8–5. Comparison of attenuation characteristics for specular reflectors (A) and scatterers (B). In both cases, energy is lost because of absorption and scattering during the round-trip passage from the transducer to the target and back. In the case of the scatterer, however, additional energy is dispersed because of the hemispheric pattern of reflection. **B.** A worst case example. Energy dispersion is depicted to occur on transmission because of beam defocusing and on reflection because of the hemispheric scattering pattern.

Attenuation of the Rebroadcast Signal

Scatterers, by definition, emit sound in all directions.[3] The reflected component therefore can be considered to propagate in a hemispheric pattern toward the transducer. This pattern of reflection causes the energy in the reflected wave to be spread over the entire hemispheric area of the returning wavefront. As a result, the strength of the reflect signal at any point along the wave front is diminished by the square of the radius (or range) between the scatterer and the transducer. In addition, the component of the reflected signal that propagates directly back to the transducer is also attenuated by the same factors that attenuate the input pulse. This linear component of attenuation is similar to that encountered in imaging systems; however, the hemispheric radiation of scattered energy is unique to Doppler devices and significantly reduces the strength of the Doppler signal for a given input power compared to that of an imaging device. Figure 8–5 illustrates these relationships.

SUMMARY OF FACTORS AFFECTING DOPPLER SENSITIVITY: SIGNAL/NOISE RATIO AND DYNAMIC RANGE

The discussion of echo intensity in Chapter 1 noted that the specular reflections that return to the transducer may be a factor of 10^3 below the intensity of the transmitted signal. Because the Doppler-shifted frequencies are only a small component of the total ultrasonic energy returning to the transducer and are generally much weaker than the specular reflections from adjacent tissue interfaces, a primary consideration in any Doppler device must be optimization of the factors necessary to record the strongest signal possible. Most of the individual factors that affect this ratio have been discussed in the preceding sections. A general equation also describes the interrelationship of the factors influencing this critical signal/noise ratio:[4]

$$s/n \propto \frac{V_v}{V_b} \frac{\theta e^{-2\alpha r}}{r^2 n} \frac{P_a}{bw} \qquad [8.1]$$

In this equation, V_v/V_b is the ratio of the volume of the vessel lumen (V_v) or flow stream falling within the sample volume to the total sample volume (V_b), θ is the scattering cross section of blood, e is Euler's constant of exponential growth or decay ($e = 2.71828$), α is the tissue absorption coefficient, r is the range from the target to the transducer, n is the electronic device noise, bw is the system bandwidth, and P_a is the average emission power.

Although seemingly complicated, when this equation is reduced from mathematical to conceptual terms it follows from the general principles previously discussed for ultrasound. Further, because it generally describes the performance of all Doppler systems, its understanding is extremely important for any intelligent clinical application of Doppler methodology.

Signal

The first term in the numerator and denominator is the ratio V_v/V_b or the ratio of the signal-producing volume to the beam sample volume. At the wavelength level, this ratio is directly proportional to the signal/noise ratio. As pulse duration increases, random noise tends to cancel over time, whereas nonrandom signal sums. Thus, this relationship becomes less critical as the pulse length increases. The second term in the numerator (θ) is the scattering cross section, which is directly related to the strength of the returning signal. The third term ($e^{-2\alpha r}$) is the signal attenuation term, which is expressed as a negative exponential. This term consists of the tissue absorption coefficient (α) and the range (r) and is doubled to reflect the round-trip, direct line passage of the sound wave from the transducer to the target. The final term that is directly related to signal strength is the average input power (P_a).

Noise

The noise terms in the denominator of the equation represent those factors that decrease the ability of the instrument to recognize the Doppler-shifted frequencies either by introducing extraneous frequencies or by decreasing the strength of the reflected signal that actually reaches the transducer. The first noise component V_b has already been discussed. The second is the range (r) squared. This term relates to the hemispheric reflective pattern of the scattered energy, which causes dispersion of the reflected signal. The enormous importance of range in determining Doppler signal strength should be readily apparent from the equation, because it appears in both the numerator and denominator and is doubled in one case and squared in the other. The third noise component (n), which has not been discussed to this point, is electronic noise, which is inherent in all high gain amplifiers. This type of noise can be recognized by simply turning up the volume on a home stereo without any input source (record or tape). This same phenomenon occurs whenever a weak signal must be highly amplified to make it audible or recordable. Added to the system noise is the ambient noise that arises from sources such as TV stations and FM radio channels, which are constantly emitting electronic noise into the atmosphere, and which any Doppler instruments will pick up to some extent. Likewise, every other piece of equipment in the laboratory contributes its own noise component. Hospitals are probably the worst environment for high gain amplifiers because of the thousands of miles of wiring within the walls, which act like a huge antenna. Although individually small, these components of noise may be significant in the aggregate, and in some environments (i.e., the operating room), isolation of the Doppler instrument may be both critical and extremely difficult. Even if all other sources of noise could be eliminated, there would still remain the thermal noise floor because the heat of the instruments causes some electron flow that is recorded as noise.

The last noise term is signal bandwidth (BW). Because frequency resolution is related to bandwidth, any increase in bandwidth is effectively an increase in noise. Signal/noise ratio is not the only factor influencing sensitivity; however, if both of these components (signal and noise) are small, their ratio may actually be relatively high and yet the signal too weak to be recorded. Hence, the dynamic range of the signal above the noise floor is also important (see Fig. 2–26), and it is the combination of these factors, signal/noise ratio, and dynamic range that determines overall system sensitivity.

Operator-Selectable Factors to Increase Signal Strength

The factors that can increase Doppler signal strength and are potentially operator selectable are transducer frequency and focal characteristics, output power, range, and sample volume length. Of these, the only truly useful approaches are to decrease transducer frequency and increase sample volume length. Decreasing frequency decreases absorption (attenuation) and increases penetration; however, it also decreases scattering, which varies with frequency to the fourth power. As previously discussed for imaging, unless the signal reaches the target, all other considerations become meaningless and, hence, penetration must be the primary consideration. Increasing sample volume length increases signal strength if the scattering cross section is larger than the original sample volume. Range can sometimes be modified by approaching the same target from a different window; however, this is the exception.

The output power of most instruments is already at the legally allowable level, and major increases are not possible.

Changes in Sound Frequency That Occur During Passage to and From the Transducer—Net Sum to Zero Motion

When an ultrasonic waveform encounters any scatterer, the sound energy is taken up by the target and then rebroadcast. If the target is moving, the signal will be rebroadcast at a Doppler-shifted frequency. Although the time of this interaction is extremely small, it is the basis of the Doppler shift formation. Given this fact, it should be apparent that every moving target encountered by both the transmitted and reflected sound wave affects the wavelength of the pulse and, hence, creates a frequency shift. Therefore, by the time the pulse reaches the final target from which it is reflected it has already been shifted numerous times. Because a single interrogation requires 1/1000 to 1/10,000 of a second to complete, it is assumed that any motion encountered by the emitted sound pulse is still present during the return flight and will create an equal but opposite frequency shift.[2] These oppositely directed frequency shifts, therefore, presumably sum to zero and the echo that returns to the transducer retains only the frequency shift imparted to it by the last encountered target. This concept holds for both pulsed and continuous wave (CW) systems because for each returning echo from within the sample volume only the last frequency shift will be retained. This net summing to zero of the frequency shifts imparted by intermediate targets is one of the basic assumptions of the Doppler method because, if this were not the case, the method could not produce meaningful data.

GENERAL APPROACHES TO SIGNAL DETECTION AND EXTRACTION

The echoes returning to the transducer after interacting with a moving target have a frequency equal to the broadcast frequency (the carrier) plus or minus the frequency shift imparted by the Doppler effect. This process by which information (i.e., the Doppler shift frequency) is impressed onto a carrying wave is known as modulation and the received waveform is the transmitted waveform modulated by the moving target that changes its frequency content. In any practical application of the Doppler method, the Doppler-shifted frequencies return in combination with the non-frequency-shifted echoes from surrounding structures, e.g., vessel walls and other tissue interfaces (clutter). For the motion-related signal to be identified, the Doppler-shifted frequencies must be separated from the complex returning echoes. In a Doppler device, this is achieved by a process known as *demodulation,* which is the detection and extraction of the signal from the carrier. Because the blood echoes are of low amplitude, relative to those from surrounding structures, the amplitude of the clutter component is usually much greater than that of the Doppler-shifted signals. In addition, because the relationship of target velocity, V, to the speed of sound, C, is usually small (less than 1/10,000 for physiologically encountered flows), successful Doppler demodulation demands the detection and extraction of Doppler-shifted signals that differ from the transmitted frequency by less than 1% and are buried in much larger amplitude clutter returns.

Because the Doppler frequency shifts are small relative to the broadcast frequency, it is difficult to separate them directly from the carrier and easier to compare the frequency of the returning echo with that transmitted.

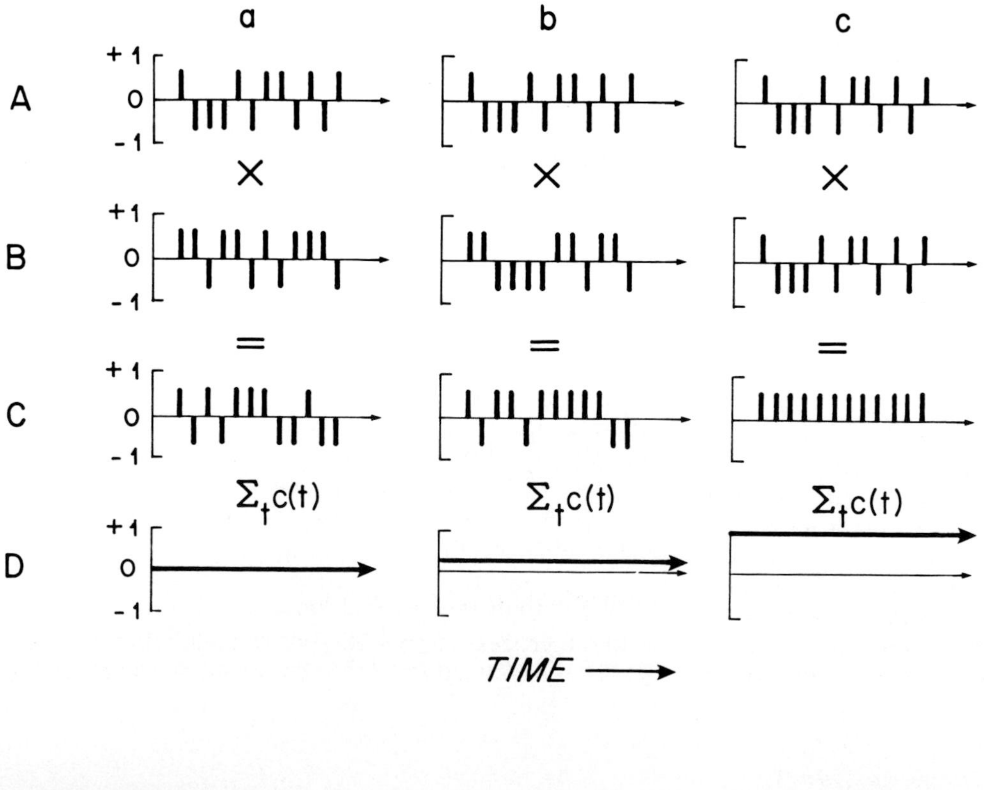

Fig. 8–6. The process of correlation. In column "a" two uncorrelated waveforms (A and B) are multiplied together (C), and the result summed over time (D) equals zero. For two partially correlated waveforms (column "b"), the output is proportional to the similarity or degree of correlation between the two waves (i.e., between zero and one). For two identical waves (column "c") the output will be unity. (After Atkinson and Woodcock, 1982.)

The process of comparing two waveforms is known as *correlation,* and the results of a correlation indicate to what extent the two waveforms are similar. One correlation method is to multiply two waveforms together and then average the results in a low pass filter. To illustrate this process, two noncorrelated random noise waveforms (A and B) are represented in Figure 8–6, column "a," by a random sequence of equally spaced impulses with an amplitude of +1 or −1. If A and B are multiplied together to give waveform C, the result is equally likely to be +1 as it is to be −1. When averaged in a low pass filter over a sufficiently long time, the contributions of each waveform will tend to cancel, giving zero output and indicating no correlation. However, if two waveforms show some degree of correlation (i.e., +1 in waveform A is more likely to coincide with +1 in waveform B than would be expected by chance; (Fig. 8–6, column b), the magnitude of the value of the filtered output will indicate the degree of correlation. Finally, if a waveform is correlated with an exact replica of itself, the result of each multiplication will be +1 as shown in Figure 8–6, column c, because $+1 \times +1 = +1$ and $-1 \times -1 = +1$. In this case, the correlator output will be at a maximum level and proportional to the power of the input waveform.[5]

When two waves of different frequency are similarly compared, they will alternately be in and out of phase. When they are multiplied together, the amplitudes will sum during the periods when they are in phase and the correlator output will be maximal. Conversely, when they are out of phase, their values will cancel when multiplied, and the correlator output will be minimal or zero. The frequency of periodic fluctuations in correlator output, in the form of a fluctuating voltage, can be shown to equal the difference in frequency between the two input waveforms.[1,2,5]

For a Doppler device to perform such a comparison, it is necessary for the instrument to have available some representation of the broadcast signal. This can be achieved by comparing the received waveform to the oscillator frequency (coherent demodulation) or to the clutter signal, which is higher in amplitude and should have the same frequency as the transmitted signal (noncoherent demodulation).[5]

Coherent Demodulation

In the process of coherent demodulation, the oscillator output is taken as the reference signal and is combined with the incoming received signal in a phase-sensitive detector. This approach is known as *coherent demodulation* because the oscillator maintains a constant phase and frequency reference against which all received waveforms are compared. The basic principles of phase-sensitive detection are illustrated in Figure 8–7. In this example, two sinusoidal waveforms (A and B) at frequencies Fo and Fo + Fd, representing the reference oscillation and the Doppler-shifted received waveform respectively, are multiplied together to give a product waveform. This produce waveform is then low pass filtered to remove components around 2Fo, and the result is Fd, the Doppler difference signal. It is important to note that the demodulation process destroys the directional information contained in the returning signal. The Doppler frequency that is output, therefore, is simply the difference, independent of sign, between the transmitted and received frequencies.[5]

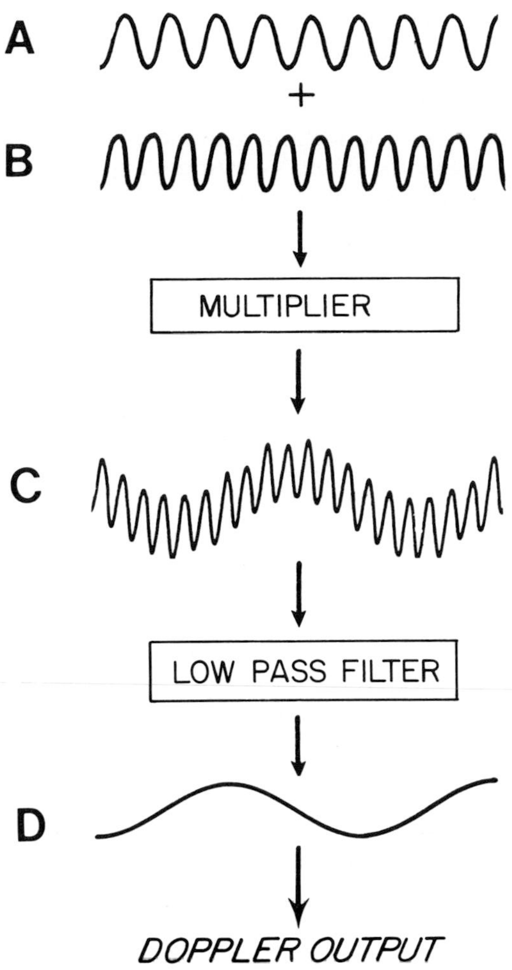

Fig. 8–7. The principles of coherent demodulation. The oscillator (A) and Doppler-shifted reflected waveforms (B) are multiplied together (C) and then low-pass filtered to discover the Doppler difference frequency (D).

This loss of directionality occurs because the carrier frequency demodulates to zero. Any frequency below the carrier, therefore, would have to be represented as a minus or negative frequency. Because negative frequencies have no meaning, the upper and lower Doppler sidebands demodulate to the same region above the baseband or above zero. More simply, using the analogy of runners on a track, the phase detector continuously determines the relative position of two runners, such that its output is maximum when they are abreast and minimum when they are on opposite sides of the track, but its output contains no information about which of the two is moving faster.

Noncoherent Demodulation

In the process of noncoherent demodulation, the clutter signal reflected from the stationary targets along the beam path, which can be regarded as an attenuated phase-shifted version of the transmitted waveform, is used as the reference against which to compare the Doppler-shifted echoes.

The principle of noncoherent demodulation for a continuous wave instrument is illustrated in Figure 8–8. The clutter signal (A) can originate not only from stationary targets but also from direct leakage of electrical and ultrasonic energy between the adjacent transmit and receiving transducer elements. Whatever its source, amplitude of the clutter signal is usually much greater than that of the echo (B) backscattered by blood. The two combine as ultrasonic echoes to produce the resultant (C) detected at the receiver. The Doppler-shifted components beat (i.e., interact to produce a difference or beat frequency) with the clutter-based reference, producing amplitude variations in the received signal. These modulations can be extracted by rectifying the signal (D) and smoothing the output to produce the Doppler difference waveform (E).

The simple amplitude detection system shown in Figure 8–8, which consists of half- or full-wave rectification followed by low pass filtering to remove the carrier, will extract the Doppler component B sin (Wd(t) + ϕ). More basic types of CW flowmeters still incorporate this rather straightforward method of noncoherent demodulation using transmitter-receiver breakthrough as the dominant source of the reference signal. Like coherent demodulation, noncoherent demodulation also destroys the directional information contained in the returning signal.

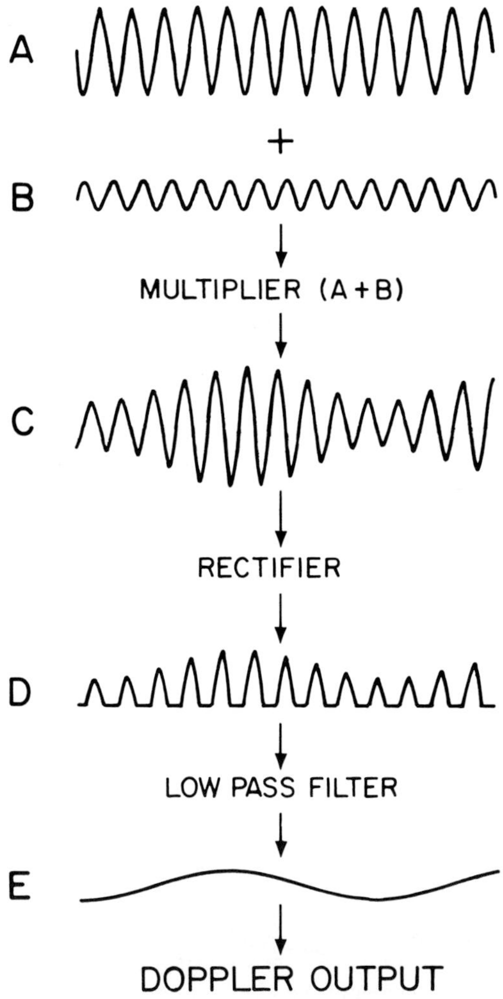

Fig. 8–8. The principles of noncoherent demodulation. The clutter signal (A) beats together with the Doppler signal (B) to form the combined echo (C). Following full- or half-wave rectification (D), the waveform is low-pass filtered to extract the Doppler difference frequency (E).

It might initially appear that noncoherent demodulation would have advantages over coherent demodulation because the reference signal is generated solely by clutter-producing targets within the beam diffraction pattern or sample volume. As a result, any cardiac motion caused by respiration, translation, or pulsation would impart a Doppler shift to the reference clutter signal, and the result would indicate the velocity of blood relative to its surroundings rather than the absolute velocity relative to the transducer. Further, the clutter signal is not subject to coherent demodulation, and so small movements, for example, of vessel walls, do not tend to produce the large amplitude, low frequency variations in the Doppler difference waveform that are found with coherent demodulation. Therefore, noncoherent demodulation, which is basically envelope detection should, in theory, result in a wider separation between clutter and blood Doppler flow signals. This, in turn, should allow more effective frequency filtering than would be possible with coherent demodulation. The problem with noncoherent demodulation, particularly in range discriminating flowmeters, is that the sample volume must contain sufficient targets to provide an adequate clutter signal to generate the reference waveform. Absence of sufficiently strong clutter returns results in Doppler signal dropout because of loss of reference, which is why the method is rarely incorporated into range discriminating systems.[5]

The same demodulation process can also be used for intermittently returning signals, as illustrated in Figure 8–9. In this case, the demodulator output is, likewise, intermittent but can still be used to reconstruct the Doppler shift frequency.

Practical Limitations Imposed on the Demodulation Process

The differences between the Doppler and carrier frequencies impose limitations on the demodulation process that should be recognized. If, e.g., the carrier frequency is 3 MHz, whereas the Doppler difference frequency is 3 KHz, then 1000 cycles of the broadcast and received waveform must be compared to extract a complete Doppler shift cycle. At 3 MHz, 1000 cycles would be equal to a wave 50 cm long, and the demodulator would require 333 μsec to extract a single cycle. In practice, an instrument that outputs data at 10-msec intervals, therefore, has at most 30 cycles of Doppler shift data from which to define the full frequency spectrum (Fig. 8–10). Hence, frequency determinations are generally estimates based on small fragments of the de-

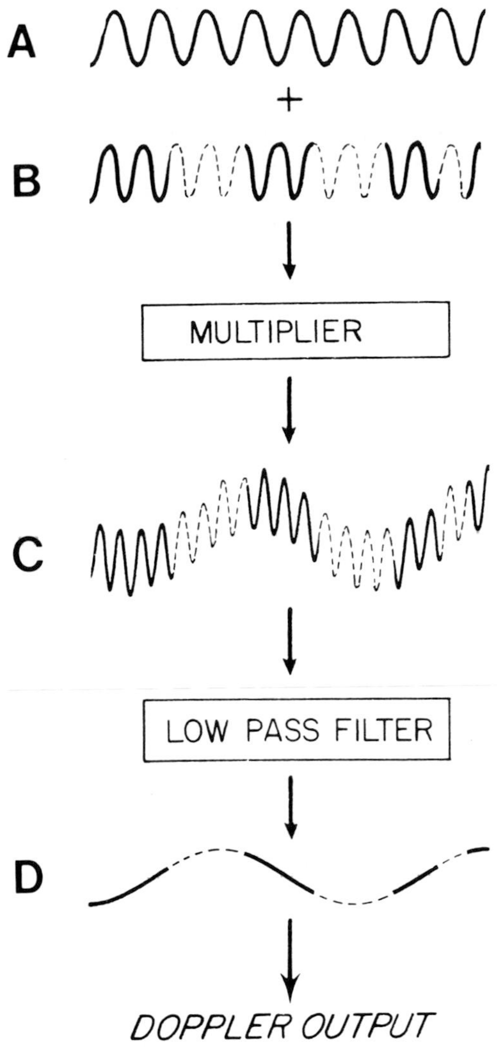

Fig. 8–9. The processes of coherent demodulation for an intermittently transmitted signal. Intermittent comparison still yields an approximation of the Doppler difference frequency. Note that the interpulse interval has been decreased relative to the wavelength for illustrative purposes. (After Atkinson and Woodcock, 1982.)

modulated Doppler shift frequency with the requisite imprecision in the frequency estimate.

Directional Doppler Demodulation

Clinically, it is usually important to determine the direction of flow as well as its velocity. However, straightforward demodulation techniques destroy the directional information contained in the Doppler-shifted echoes by shifting both the upper and lower Doppler sidebands (positive and negative Doppler shifts) into the same region of the baseband (generally taken to be zero frequency). Separation of upper and lower sidebands is a commonly encountered problem in communication theory, and several of the solutions that have been developed for communications application shave subsequently been adopted for directional Doppler demodulation. These include single sideband filtering, heterodyne demodulation, and quadrature phase demodulation.

Signal Sideband Filtering

The most direct method for directional demodulation is to separate the Doppler sidebands at the ultrasonic frequency using precisely tuned radio frequency filters.[6,7] In this process, the raw ultrasonic echo is fed to high and low pass filters, which are designed to pass only the signal in the upper and lower Doppler sidebands, respectively. These sidebands can then be coherently demodulated into separate channels to give independent forward and reverse Doppler difference signals. This frequency separation process is illustrated in Figure 8–11, which shows the filter characteristics and their effect on the echo spectrum. Although conceptually simple, this approach requires filters that are extremely precise and that remain highly stable. Likewise, it requires precise control of the master oscillator frequency to ensure that it does not drift into the passband of either filter. Although such stability can be achieved, it is enormously difficult and, at present, is not routinely used in clinical instrumentation.

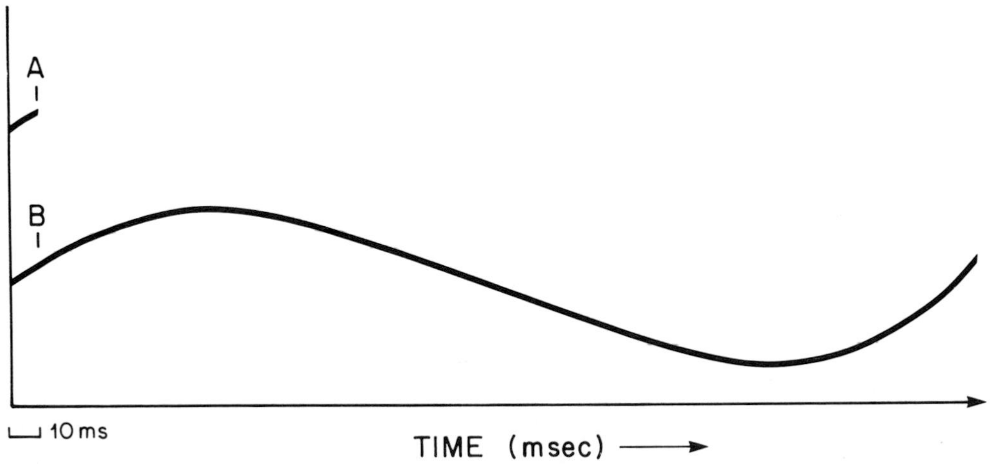

Fig. 8–10. Comparison of the time required to reconstruct one complete cycle of the Doppler difference frequency given a 3-MHz carrier and a 3-KHz Doppler shift (B) with the sampling time actually available to the typical analyzer (A). (After Atkinson and Woodcock, 1982.)

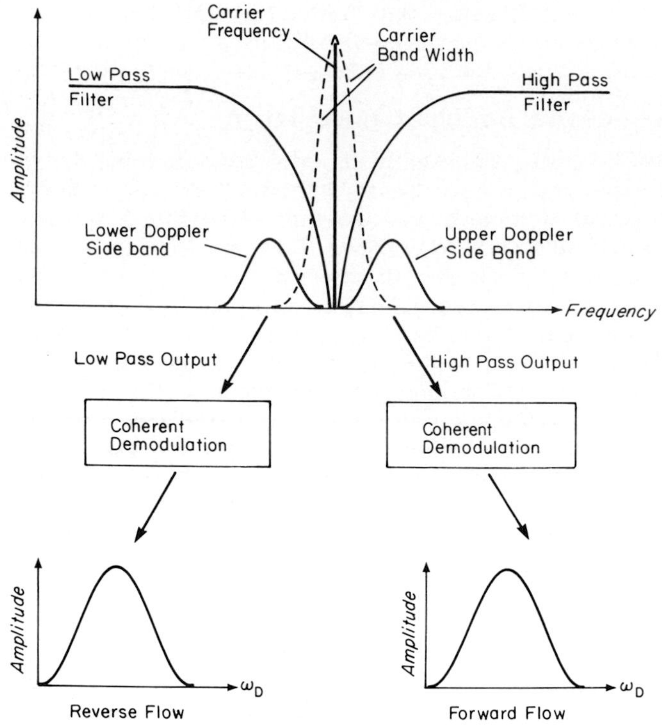

Fig. 8–11. Single sideband filtering. In this approach, high and low pass filters are used to separate the upper and lower Doppler sidebands from the carrier. The output of the filters is then coherently demodulated and processed to yield the upper and lower Doppler frequency components.

Heterodyne Demodulation

Coherent demodulation destroys directional information because both the upper and lower Doppler sidebands are shifted into the same region of the baseband. If, however, the carrier could be demodulated to a frequency that was offset from zero by more than the width of the lower sideband, then the directional separation could be maintained. Such an effect can be achieved by the process known as *heterodyne demodulation*.[5,8,9] The heterodyne process can be explained as follows. If instead of being stationary, the transducer is moved as illustrated in Figure 8–12, then the echo from a stationary target, A, is shifted by a positive frequency, proportional to the transducer velocity. Target movement toward the transducer increases the Doppler shift still further because the relative velocity has increased, whereas target movement away from the transducer reduces the Doppler shift frequency. Thus, by moving the transducer, the Doppler baseline corresponding to zero target velocity can, in effect, be offset to what is commonly known as *heterodyne frequency* (F_h). Directional information contained in the Doppler sidebands now lies on either side of this new "zero velocity" baseline. Coherent demodulation of the signal to the baseband retains this offset so that the Doppler difference signals lie on either side of the heterodyne frequency. For this method to work, however, the transducer velocity must be greater than any encountered target velocity to ensure that all targets are effectively closing toward the transducer. If a target were to move away at such a rate that it actually receded from the transducer, then the Doppler shift frequency would again become negative and the demodulated waveform would be ambiguous.[5]

In any practical situation, it is obviously not possible to move the transducer continuously toward the target. Fortunately, forward transducer movement can be simulated electronically by comparing the returning echo not with the transmitted frequency, but rather with a

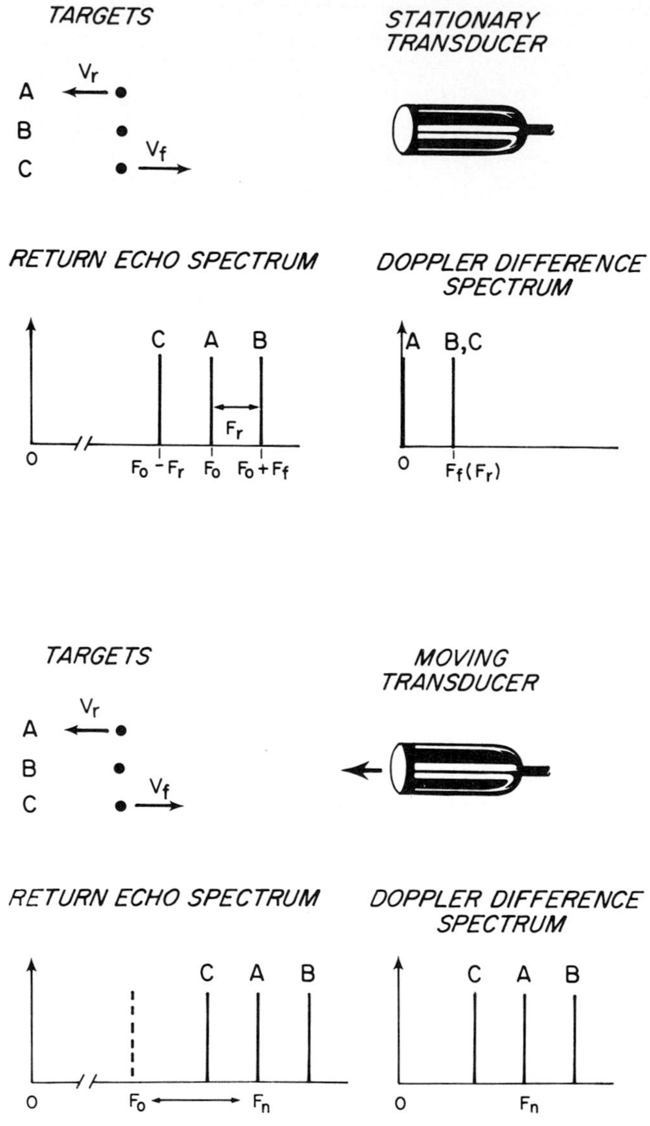

Fig. 8–12. Heterodyne demodulation. Top. Three targets, A, B, and C are recorded by a stationary transducer. A and C are advancing and receding from the transducer at the same speed, and hence their reflected signals differ from the carrier by the same amount. Following demodulation, the echoes from stationary target B with no Doppler shift will demodulate to the baseband (zero frequency difference); those from A and C will be offset from the baseband by the same amount but will be ambiguous in terms of direction. Bottom. The transducer moves toward the targets at a rate faster than that of the most rapidly receding target, A. Thus, the relative motion of all three targets is toward the transducer, and when demodulated, the frequencies of the moving targets are shifted to either side of the new or heterodyne frequency corresponding to transducer motion. By filtering at the heterodyne frequency, one can separate the upper and lower sidebands and restore directionality.

signal at the transmitted frequency minus a Doppler shift offset that is equivalent to transducer movement. The echoes from nonmoving targets beat with this heterodyned reference to give the offset frequency F_h, whereas moving targets produce higher or lower frequency beats depending on whether they are moving toward or away from the stationary transducer.[5] The advantage of heterodyne processing is that frequency analysis of the output waveform provides an immediate display of directional information. However, it is usually necessary to remove large amplitude clutter components using a notch filter precisely tuned to the heterodyne frequency.[1] The result is comparable to single sideband filtering at a lower frequency. The shift to a lower frequency, however, makes the requirements for such a filter much less demanding than for comparable filtering at the carrier because the heterodyning process has shifted all of the frequencies from the MHz to the KHz range. For example, at the carrier (frequency) a Doppler shift of ± 4 KHz would require the filter to discriminate between frequencies of 4,996,000 and 5,004,000. At a heterodyne frequency of 5 KHz, the same shift of 4 KHz results in sidebands at 1000 as 9000 Hz, resulting in an obvious difference in filter requirements.[5]

One problem with heterodyne demodulation is that, when output in an audible form, the heterodyne frequency sounds unfamiliar and is difficult to interpret. Thus, when an audio output is desired, it is often necessary to incorporate a nondirectional demodulator to provide an output frequency that is more recognizable to the ear.[5]

Quadrature Phase Demodulation

The two methods of directional demodulation described to this point operate in the frequency domain by directly filtering or shifting and then filtering the Doppler frequencies to separate their upper and lower sidebands. The final and most commonly used approach, quadrature phase demodulation, involves the detection of both the real and imaginary Doppler difference components and their manipulation to reveal the directional content of the signal.[10] In the process of quadrature demodulation, the received signal is first separated into two channels. The signal input into one channel, usually called the *direct channel,* is mixed with the direct oscillator frequency, whereas the signal in the second or quadrature channel is compared to a quadrature reference signal (the oscillator output shifted in phase by 90°). Figure 8–13 illustrates the effect of this process on the demodulated signals output from the two channels. Figure 8–13A illustrates the outputs from the direct and quadrature channels for the case of a frequency higher (positive Doppler shift) than the oscillator frequency. When the received signal is combined with the reference signal, the output from the direct channel leads that of the quadrature channel by 90°. Figure 8–13B illustrates the comparable situation for a reverse flow (negative Doppler shift). In this case, the output of the quadrature channel leads that of the direct channel by 90°. The result is to separate the positive and negative Doppler shift components by 180°. Once in this form, the upper and lower sidebands can be distinguished by their relative lead-lag relationship. This processer may be better understood by returning to our runner analogy, as illustrated in Figure 8–14. Suppose two runners, A and C, are going around the track at different speeds and are carrying transmitters designed such that each time they pass each other, a signal (beat signal) is transmitted. If we receive this signal intermittently, then we know that the runners are passing but not which one is going faster. This is analogous to the demodulated signal. If we wish to know whether runner C is faster or slower than runner A, we can introduce another runner B, traveling at the same speed as A, but leading him by 90° (quadrature phase shifted). We then start the Doppler race and set runners A (direct) and B (quadrature) off to a head start. When the received pulse (runner C) returns to enter the race,

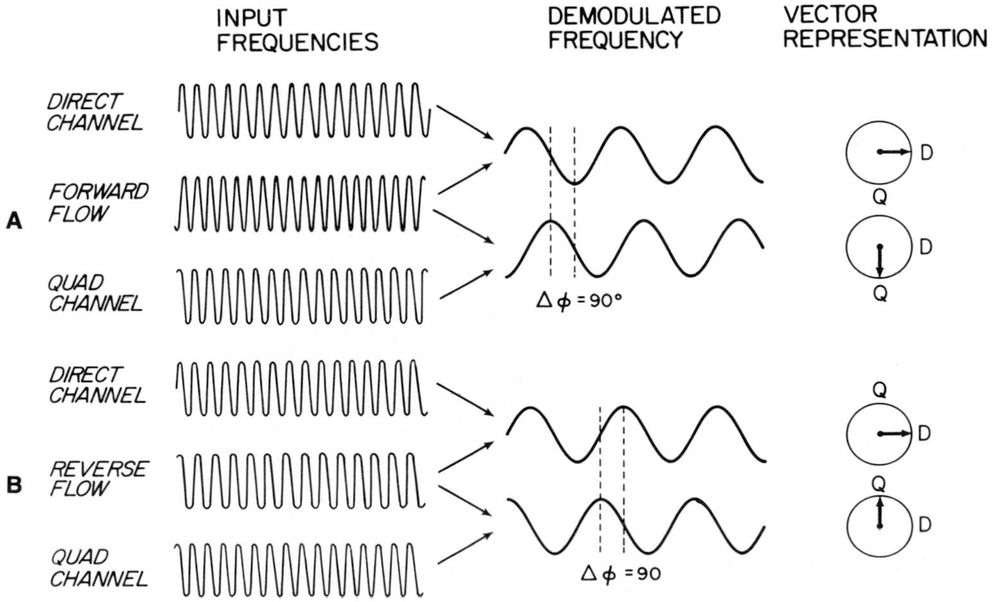

Fig. 8–13. Relative phase difference introduced in the quadrature demodulation process for a higher and lower frequency reflected waveform using both analogue and vector notation.

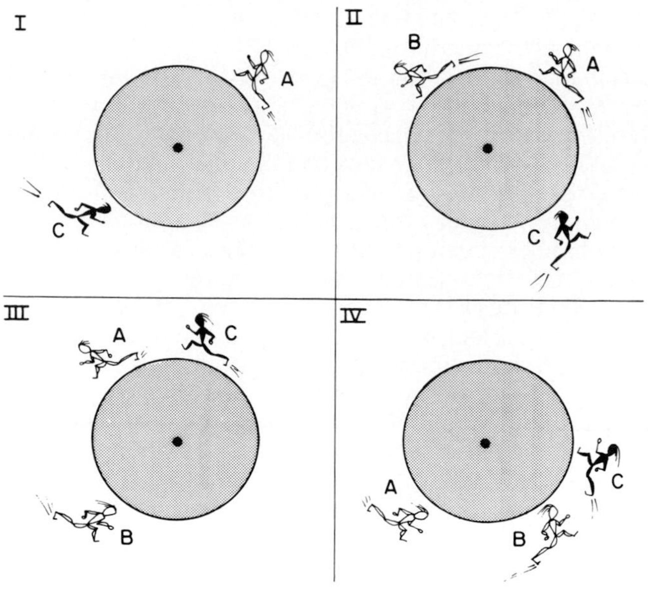

Fig. 8–14. The operation of the quadrature channels. (See Text for details.)

runner C is behind both A and B. If C is faster than A and B, he will catch up to A before B, and the beat signal from A will always precede the signal from B by 90° (i.e., the direct channel will lead the quadrature channel). If, on the other hand, the signal (runner C) is slower than runners A and B, runner B will eventually catch up to C first and, 90° later, runner A will do the same. In this case, the beat signal from B will precede that from (A) by 90°, and therefore, for a lower frequency reflected signal, the quadrature channel (B) will always precede the direct channel (A).

Having generated this differential lead-lag relationship, however, outputs from the direct and quadrature channels must be processed further to actually indicate flow direction. This processing can occur in the time domain, the phase domain, or the frequency domain.

Time Domain Processing

Because it has been shown that after quadrature demodulation, the forward and reverse flow waveforms can be distinguished by their relative lead-lag relationship, one approach to separating directional components has been to incorporate a logic system to monitor the phase angle between D(t) and Q(t), and then, depending on the lead-lag condition, to switch one of the demodulated Doppler channels through to the forward or reverse flow channel of the output device.[4] This is referred to as *time domain processing* because the directional information is retrieved directly from the demodulated quadrature channels.[11] This approach usually suffers from switching artifacts, and because of design principles, it can operate only under conditions of monodirectional flow. In addition, if simultaneous reverse and forward flow signals are received, then the lead-lag relationship is ambiguous and the flow direction cannot be resolved.

Phase Domain Processing

The direct and quadrature Doppler outputs can also be processed in the phase domain. This approach provides a more powerful method of separating forward and reverse flow. The process of phase domain processing is illustrated in Figure 8–15. Figure 8–15A depicts the relative phase of the outputs from the direct and quadrature channels when the input signal is a higher frequency (i.e., forward flow) than the reference waveform and the direct channel output leads the quadrature channel output by 90°. If the output from the quadrature channel is again shifted by $\pi/2$, the two channels will be in phase, and if the output from the quadrature channel is added to that from the direct channel, the forward flow signal will be doubled (i.e., +1). If the same process is performed for the reverse flow component (i.e., the quadrature channel is shifted 90° and multiplied by the direct channel output), the resultant waveforms will be 180° out of phase and they will cancel completely (Fig. 8–15C). As a result, only the upper Doppler sideband would be transmitted by the direct channel. Likewise,

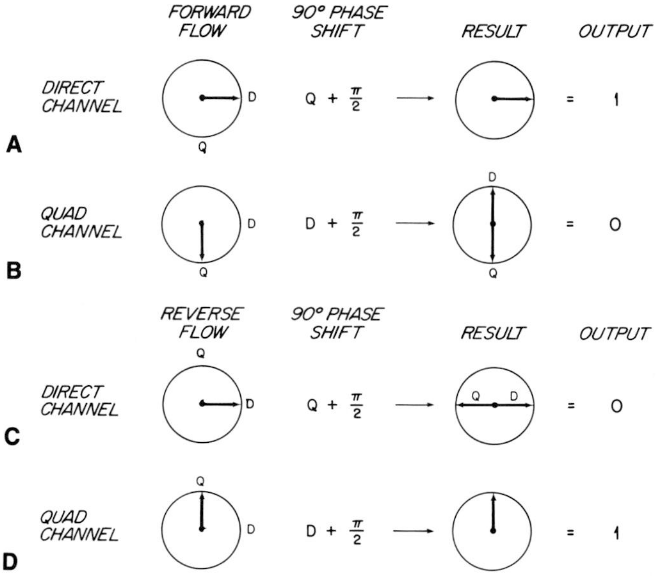

Fig. 8–15. The concept of phase domain processing of quadrature demodulated signals. **A** and **B.** For forward flow (top), the signal in the direct channel always leads that in the quadrature channel by 90°. Given this relationship, if the trailing signal in the quadrature channel is shifted forward 90° and added to the signal in the direct channel, they will sum and the output will be unity. Conversely, if the forward signal in the direct channel is shifted another 90° forward and added to the quadrature channel, it will be 180° out of phase with the forward signal already in this channel and they will cancel. By this process the forward components of the Doppler signal will be output completely by the direct channel and canceled in the quadrature channel. **C** and **D.** In contrast, the reverse flow component in the quadrature channel will lead that in the direct channel (bottom). **C.** In this case, if the signal in the quadrature channel is shifted forward an additional 90° and added to the signal in the direct channel, all reverse components will cancel. **D.** Alternatively, if the reverse flow signal in the direct channel is forward shifted 90° and added to the reverse flow signal in the quadrature channel, they will sum and the output will be unity. In this manner the entire forward component is output by the direct channel and the reverse component by the quadrature channel.

as illustrated in Figure 8–15D, if the input signal has a lower frequency (i.e., reverse flow), shifting the direct channel by $\pi/2$ and adding it to the quadrature channel Q(t) gives a double amplitude reverse flow component as the output of the quadrature channel and will completely eliminate the forward flow component (Fig. 8–15B).

Importantly, the unwanted Doppler sideband will cancel only if each Doppler component is shifted by precisely $\pi/2$ radians at the particular Doppler frequency. The $\pi/2$ phase shift is required to delay each component of the Doppler difference waveform by a time period that is inversely proportional to the Doppler difference frequency (the higher the frequency, the shorter the time delay required to produce a $\pi/2$ phase shift). Furthermore, separation of the sidebands requires precise equalization of gain in these channels, otherwise, the unwanted sideband will once again not cancel completely. Lack of complete cancellation because of amplitude difference will produce some output from the opposite channel, a phenomenon known as cross-talk. Some cross-talk between channels is inevitable; however, 1% matching in terms of phase and gain will reduce the cross-talk to approximately 40 dB.[5]

Frequency Domain Processing

The phase domain processors discussed previously separate the Doppler signal into distinct forward and reverse channels. This feature is essential if it is necessary to frequency-process the Doppler signals using devices such as zero-crossing counters or mean frequency followers (see Chapter 10). However, if the signal is to be frequency analyzed into discrete frequency bands (spectral analysis), it is sometimes advantageous to combine the forward and reverse components so that only one spectrum analyzer is required. Frequency domain processing of quadrature phase demodulated signals is a method that essentially shifts the Doppler signals to a pilot frequency (W_pt) while retaining directional information. Figure 8–16 contains a block diagram of a frequency domain processor. In this approach, the direct and quadrature demodulated channels enter twin multiplying networks fed, respectively, with sine and cosine waves at a pilot frequency (W_pt). When the two multiplier outputs are added together in a summing amplifier, the effect is to offset the Doppler difference frequency so that the Doppler sidebands lie on either side of the pilot frequency. This is comparable to heterodyne demodulation; however, because the forward and reverse channels are separated in phase by 90°, the signals in the respective channels are multiplied by the sine and cosine components of the pilot frequency (which are similar in phase to the signal already in the channels) to retain the 90° of phase separation of the two components. When the outputs of the two channels are multiplied together, the sine and cosine components combine to form the pilot frequency and the Doppler shifts assume their relative relationships above and below the pilot. In this method, the stationary clutter is offset to the pilot frequency, the forward and reverse flow signals have become sidebands lying on either side of the pilot frequency W_p, and frequency analysis in a single channel processor is now possible.

Thus, a variety of methods exist to restore the directional information lost in the demodulation process. Virtually all have found some application in Doppler devices; however, quadrature phase demodulation followed by frequency analysis is the approach most commonly used in current instruments.

SPECIFIC TYPES OF DOPPLER INSTRUMENTS

A variety of instruments has been developed to record the velocity of flow in the heart and great vessels using the Doppler principle. These include the CW Doppler, the pulsed wave Doppler (PD), the high pulse repetition frequency (HiPRF) Doppler, and the multigate Doppler. Other prototype devices such as the noise and FM Doppler are also of both historic and theoretic interest. This section discusses these classic approaches along with their specific applications and limitations. Color flow mapping, which combines imaging and Doppler technologies, is introduced in Chapter 11.

The Continuous Wave Flowmeter

The original, and by far the simplest, Doppler device is the CW flowmeter.[1] The basic components of a CW instrument are illustrated in Figure 8–17 and include the master oscillator, the transmitting amplifier, the transmitting and receiving transducers, the receiving amplifier, and the demodulator. During operation, the master oscillator produces a sinusoidal waveform, which is amplified and used to drive the transmitting transducer at its resonant frequency. The master oscillator is similar to those used in imaging devices, and in combined instruments provides the time reference for both operations. The transducers used in dedicated CW Doppler devices are composed of the same materials used in echo

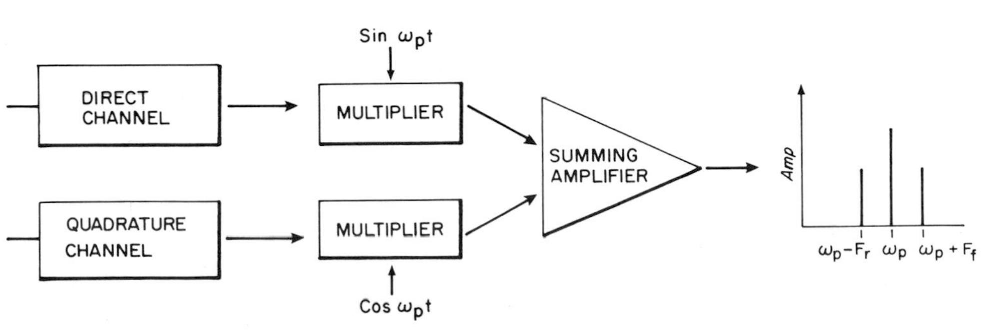

Fig. 8–16. Block diagram of a frequency domain processor. In this approach, the output of the forward and reverse channels is shifted to either side of a pilot or heterodyne frequency and in this form can be analyzed using a single transform analyzer. (See text for details.)

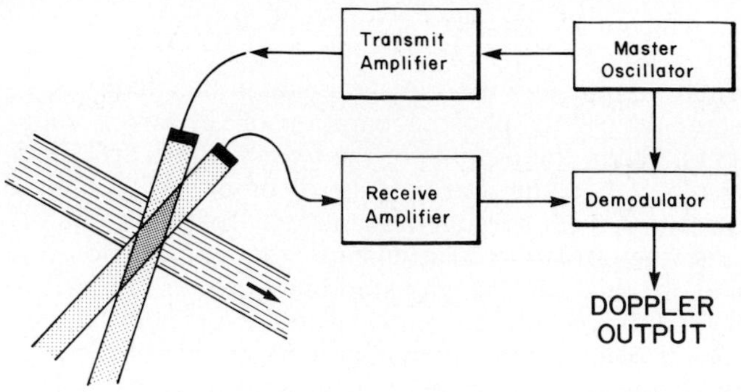

Fig. 8–17. Block diagram of a basic continuous wave Doppler instrument. (See text for details.)

instruments and function in the same frequency range (1 to 10 mHz). Continuous wave transducers typically have a high Q, air-backed construction to improve sensitivity. Because the CW Doppler is continuously transmitting ultrasound, echoes will be constantly returning to the transducer. Because it is difficult to receive and transmit simultaneously from the same transducer, CW instruments typically use separate transducers for transmission and reception. To limit transducer size (footprint) and match the frequency response of the two elements as closely as possible, a single circular crystal is usually cut in half to form the transmitting and receiving portions of the CW transducer (Fig. 8–18). The same effect can also be achieved using transducer arrays (linear and annular) by dedicating one group of elements to transmission and another to reception. The transmitting and receiving portion of the transducers are typically aligned such that their beam profiles overlap. In practice, only those targets moving within the beam area common to both transducers will contribute to the Doppler output.

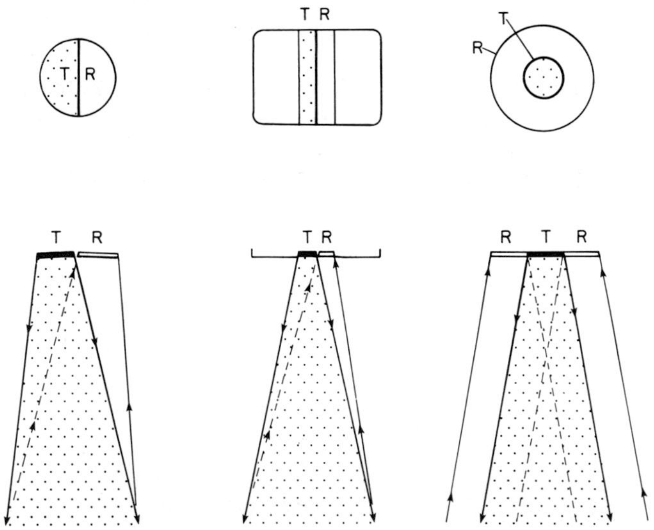

Fig. 8–18. Various types of continuous wave (CW) Doppler transducers. Left. Single circular transducer cut in half to form separate transmitting (T) and receiving (R) elements. Center. A linear array of elements with a segment dedicated to CW transmission and recording. Right. An annular array of elements with the central portion of the array used for transmission and the remainder for reception.

The beam broadcast by a dedicated CW transducer generally starts from a small semicircular area and disperses rapidly, resulting in a broad beam profile (Fig. 8–18, bottom). Because continuous excitation of the transducer produces an uninterrupted broadcast signal, sound energy is continuously present throughout the total diffraction field of the transmitting transducer. All targets within this beam reflect and backscatter echoes, some of which return to the receiving transducer. These weak received echoes are initially preamplified and then transmitted to the demodulator, where the frequency of the received waveform is compared with a replica of the transmitted waveform derived directly from the master oscillator (coherent demodulation) or from the transmitting transducer (noncoherent demodulation). The signal/noise ratio for the receiving amplifier is critical because the Doppler signal is generally 40 to 60 dB below that of the clutter signal. The output of the demodulator is the Doppler difference frequency. Note that the Doppler difference frequency first appears after the demodulation process and therefore exists only as an independent waveform in the instrument. Because the Doppler frequency is characteristically in the audible range, it can be output to an audio amplifier for auditory analysis. In addition, various signal processing readouts can be added to convert the raw Doppler signal to an analog or digital signal for flow velocity analysis (see Chapter 10).

The CW approach to Doppler flow sampling has many inherent advantages. First, the CW output contains the narrowest possible frequency bandwidth and hence provides optimal frequency resolution. Second, continuous wave systems provide optimal signal-to-noise discrimination because the signal, which is constant, sums over time, whereas noise, which is random, cancels. At the wavelength level, this property does not come into play, but for continuous pulse trains, it should reduce the random component of the noise signal. Third, the dedicated CW transducers have a small face area or footprint. As a result, they require a small acoustic window and, thus, provide optimal access for the ultrasonic energy to the heart. Fourth, the broad beam emitted by the CW device facilitates jet localization. Finally, and most important, the CW Doppler has no practical frequency limitation and thus can accurately describe any velocity encountered in clinical studies.

The major limitation of CW flowmeters is their inability to determine the range from which Doppler shifts originate because all targets moving within the beam diffraction pattern are continuously interrogated and contribute to the returning signal. Interest only in the highest velocities within the beam path creates no problem. When multiple vessels or jets lie within the CW beam, however, it is difficult if not impossible to define with certainty the origin of an individual signal. Further, to measure volumetric flow, the point at which the mean velocity of interest occurs must be measured, and this cannot be achieved using a CW flowmeter.

Because of the inability of CW devices to determine target range, a variety of instruments have been developed that attempt to record both range and velocity. The following sections describe the various methods of encoding the transmitted pulses and processing the received echo so that the range of moving targets can be defined.

Range Discriminating Flowmeters

Pulsed Dopplers

The first instrument designed to determine both range and velocity was the pulsed Doppler device.[12,13] As in any pulsed echo system, the principle of operation of the pulsed Doppler is to transmit a short burst of sound energy toward a target and then record the returning echoes. Because sound waves travel at a constant speed through soft tissue, the time delay between transmission of the pulse and detection of an echo (C/2) depends on the range of the target (see Fig. 1–2). As a result of this constant relationship between time and distance, these two parameters become interchangeable. In practice, if the instrument only analyzes and outputs signals received during a specific time window following pulse transmission, the resulting Doppler shifts can originate only from targets moving at a range from the transducer that corresponds to the selected time delay.

The Instrument. The basic elements of a pulsed Doppler system are illustrated in Figure 8–19. The master oscillator, like that of any echo system, generates a sinusoidal waveform at a selected clock frequency (e.g., 10 MHz). At specified intervals (determined by a PRF divider), a few cycles from the master oscillator are passed through a transmission gate and amplified to shock-excite the transducer. The shock produces a pulse that moves away from the transducer at the speed of sound (C). The frequency at which the transmission gate opens determines the number of pulses transmitted per unit time and, hence, defines the PRF of the instrument.

The Sample Volume. As noted earlier, the sound pulse transmitted by any pulsed Doppler instrument has dimensions of both length and width. The length of the pulse is determined by the wavelength and the number of cycles transmitted, and its width is determined by the transducer size, frequency, and degree of focusing. The pulse width defines the beam width at any depth. At any instant in time, echoes can arise only from structures that lie within the volume of tissue occupied by this pulse. Because roughly 3 cycles are required for an output burst to attain resonance and an additional 2 cycles for it to return to zero, the minimum sample volume at 3 MHz (λ = 0.5 mm) would be roughly 2.5 mm in length.

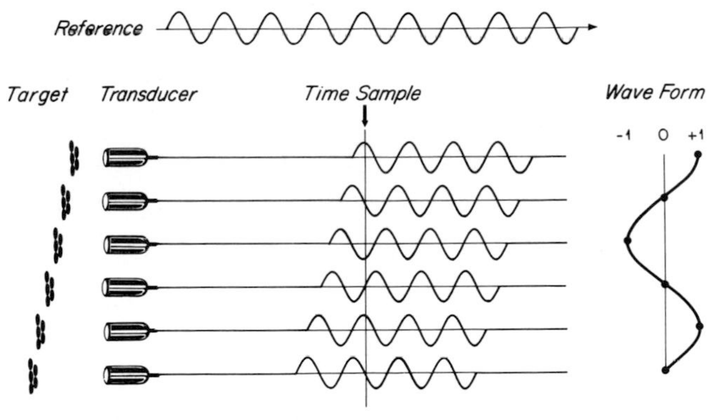

Fig. 8–20. Echo analysis for a pulsed Doppler system. (See text for details.)

Such a short sample volume, however, would result in poor frequency resolution because only one wavelength at the resonant frequency would be available to the demodulator. As a result, most pulsed Doppler instruments can transmit longer pulse trains (up to 14 cycles) so that at lower frequencies (i.e., 1 to 2 MHz), the length of the sample volume may reach 1 cm or more. These longer pulses provide better frequency resolution and an improved peak/average power ratio but at a loss of range resolution. Sample volume length is particularly important because it is one of the few operator selectable variables in most Doppler instruments and permits a choice between velocity and range resolution.

Frequency Analysis in a Pulsed Doppler System. Each of the echoes returning from the sample volume contain both phase and amplitude information. The phase component contains the Doppler shift data. This phase-shifted data can be extracted using the principles of coherent demodulation by comparing the received pulses to the oscillator frequency, which is taken as a continuous reference sine wave. This process is illustrated in Figure 8–20, in which short bursts of ultrasound are transmitted at regular intervals (T_p = interpulse interval = 1/PRF) toward a target moving away from the trans-

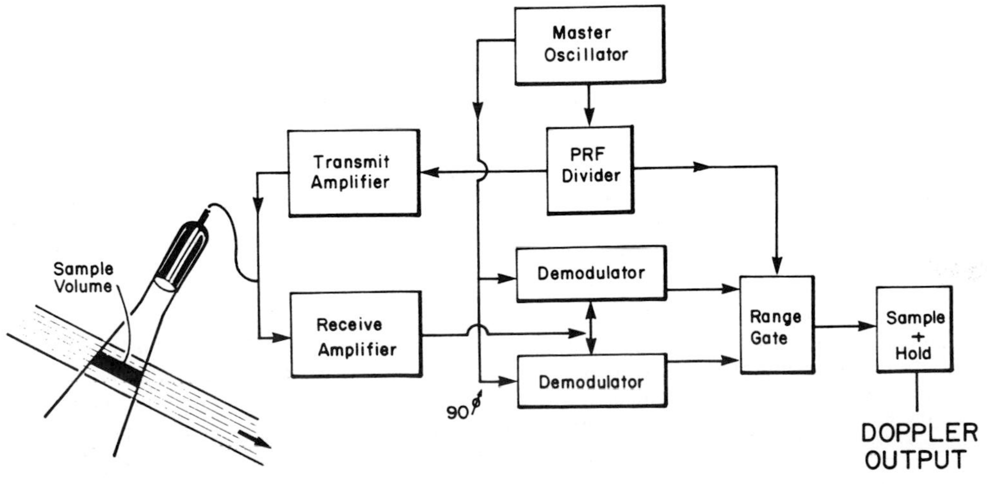

Fig. 8–19. Block diagram of a pulsed Doppler system. (See text for details.) PRF = pulse repetition frequency.

ducer. As the target recedes, the time of flight (T_f) of the pulse increases slightly with each successive transmission, causing the echo to gradually shift in phase relative to the reference wave. This gradual change in phase with time indicates that the frequency content of the returning pulse is different from that transmitted. When the Doppler component is revealed by the coherent demodulation process, the result is a series of pulses varying in amplitude at the Doppler shift frequency.[1] The output of the pulsed Doppler device is identical to that of the CW device but sampled at the PRF. The pulsed Doppler, therefore, interrogates the target only once every pulse repetition period, and this defines the rate at which data are collected and thus the maximum frequency at which the Doppler waveform can be updated.

Effects of Range Gate Position on the Frequency/Spatial Resolution of a Pulse Doppler. Several variations on this general approach to Doppler signal analysis have been described and implemented. To understand these different approaches, it is necessary first to recognize that the PRF determines the maximal range that can be unambiguously sampled but does not necessarily determine the range of interest, which may be less than the maximum distance set by the PRF. To sample only those echoes arising from the range of interest, a second time gate must be introduced into the receive circuitry, known as the range gate. The range gate can be positioned at any point within the interpulse interval and its length varied as desired. The location of the range gate in the analysis circuitry, however, changes the operating characteristics of the instrument. In the original instrument described by Peronneau,[13] the gate was placed before the demodulator. In this position, the duration of the gate determined range resolution because it could control the number of cycles that were passed on to the demodulator, irrespective of the sample volume length. This increase in range resolution, however, was achieved at the expense of frequency resolution and system sensitivity because some of the signals arising from the sample volume were discarded. In the device designed by Baker,[12] the range gate was positioned after the demodulator so that the entire signal from the sample volume interacted with the oscillator reference before the gate. The gate then sampled the output phase signal at range of interest and used the phase variation between pulses to reconstruct the Doppler signal. In this format range resolution was independent of gate duration because the entire echo from the sample volume interacted with the reference and contributed to the signal that was sampled. The latter approach proved more appropriate for cardiac studies because it made use of all the available signal power and frequency resolution.

Both of the reception formats produce short output pulses from the demodulator that form the sampled Doppler output from that device. If necessary, these samples can be stored before being updated by the return following the next transmission pulse. This so-called "sample and hold" technique tends to produce a smoother waveform, which can then be low pass filtered to remove any remaining components at the PRF and also high pass filtered to remove low frequency clutter.

Velocity Limitations in Pulse Doppler Recordings. During the brief interval when the ultrasonic pulse actually interacts with the target, the target moves only a fraction of a wavelength so that for practical purposes the frequency shift cannot be observed during a single echo. The period between pulses, in contrast, is much longer so the target can move much farther and produce a measurable change in pose between pulses.

In theory, no lower limit to the minimum Doppler shift can be coherently detected. However, because the Doppler waveform must be reconstructed from a series of samples taken at regular intervals (the PRF), the upper limit is constrained by the Nyquist sampling limit or one half of the sampling frequency. Because the sampling frequency of a pulse Doppler instrument is by definition the PRF:

$$F_{max} = PRF/2 \qquad [8.2]$$

If higher frequency signals are detected, then the waveform cannot be constructed correctly, and frequency aliasing occurs. Remember that aliasing is the ambiguity in the representation of a wave that occurs when its frequency exceeds one half the frequency at which it is sampled. Because the Doppler shift frequency is directly related to the velocity of target motion, this signal aliasing can be considered to occur because the Doppler shift frequency is undersampled or because the target moves faster than the ability of the instrument to record its velocity. It can be shown mathematically that the maximum velocity limit is equivalent to a $\lambda/4$ travel per pulse repetition period (Tp). Figure 8–20 shows how the phase of an echo from a moving target changes relative to the reference for six successive pulses. If the target moves less than one quarter of the ultrasonic wavelength between pulses, the reconstructed Doppler waveform on the right in Figure 8–20 is an accurate representation of the changing phase of the returning echoes. However if, as in Figure 8–21, the target is moving at such a high velocity that it can travel

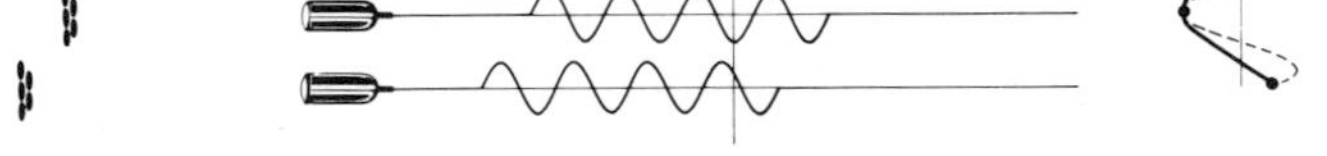

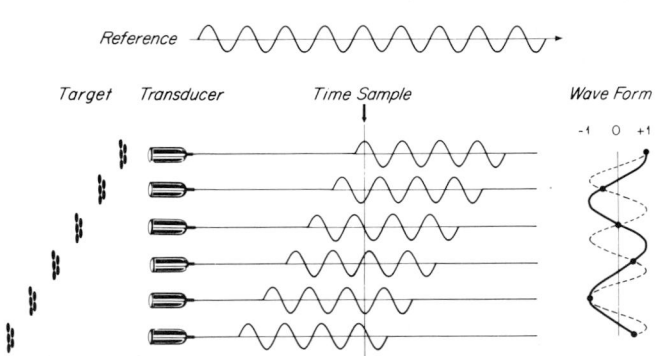

Fig. 8–21. Aliasing for a pulsed Doppler instrument that occurs when the target travels more than a quarter wavelength during the period between pulses. Interrupted waveform on the right would be the appropriate Doppler-shift frequency for the velocity of target motion. The solid waveform is the actual Doppler output, which is less than appropriate because of the aliasing produced by excessively rapid target motion.

more than one-quarter wavelength during the interpulse interval, the output of the coherent demodulator will not correspond unambiguously to the phase of the returning echo. Thus, the maximum velocity that can be detected is:

$$Vmax = \lambda/4/T_p \quad [8.3]$$

or since

$$\lambda = C/F \quad [8.4]$$

$$Vmax = C/4Fo/T_p \quad [8.5]$$

or since

$$T_p = 1/PRF \text{ or } 1/2R/C \quad [8.6]$$

$$Vmax = C^2/8F_oR \quad [8.7]$$

This is a fundamental limitation of all pulsed Doppler devices including color flow mappers and the concepts recur frequently throughout this text.

Range Velocity Limitations. In addition to the velocity limitation, pulsed Doppler systems are subject to maximum range restrictions, because it is necessary to wait for the echoes from the most distant target to reach the transducer before transmitting another burst. The maximum range, Zmax, which can unambiguously be determined is given by:

$$Zmax = T_p * C/2 \quad [8.8]$$

Combining Equations 2.23 and 2.24 gives the relationship for R = Rmax.

$$Vmax * Zmax = C2/8FoR * Rmax \quad [8.9]$$

or

$$Vmax * Zmax = C^2/8Fo \quad [8.10]$$

This relationship shows that the product of maximum observable velocity and range is limited for conventional pulsed Doppler systems. Figure 8–22 illustrates this maximum range velocity limitation for ultrasound propagating in human tissue for a range of ultrasonic frequencies. Typical range velocity products for various blood vessels are also indicated. These figures show that, in some cases, the pulsed Doppler flowmeter would have difficulty in determining flow in many critical parts of the cardiovascular system. If a vessel lies outside the range velocity limit, the blood within the vessel has moved more than one-quarter wavelength in the time it takes the ultrasound pulse to travel to and from the vessel, thus, making it impossible to track the changing phase of the Doppler-shifted echoes.

Doppler Systems Designed to Overcome Range Velocity Limitations

Because the CW Doppler fails to provide range resolution and the range velocity product limitation of the conventional pulsed Doppler is exceeded in many clinically important flow states, a variety of instruments have been developed that attempt to increase velocity resolution while maintaining range discrimination. These instruments fall into two general categories: (1) pulsed systems that operate at PRFs above the limitation specified by the range velocity product (HiPRF and noise Dopplers), and (2) CW systems into which the relative time of transmission of each output wavelength is encoded onto the carrier so that when an echo carrying a specific piece of code is detected, the time of flight of the pulse can be determined and the depth of the target defined (FM and pseudo-random binary sequencing Dopplers).

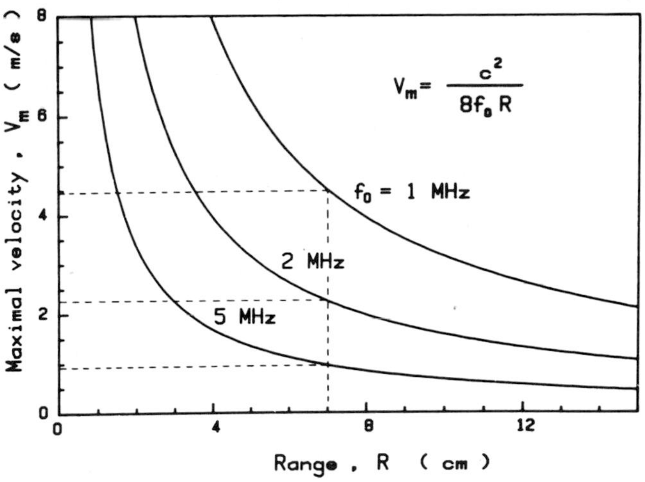

Fig. 8–22. Range velocity product for a pulsed Doppler instrument. (See text for details.) (Reproduced from Hatle L, Angelsen A: Doppler Ultrasound in Cardiology. 2nd ed. Philadelphia, Lea & Febiger, 1985.)

High Pulse Repetition Frequency Doppler

The HiPRF Doppler increases the frequency with which targets are interrogated by making use of the principle of range ambiguity. Range ambiguity is most easily understood by considering the range constraints imposed when creating a pulsed echo two-dimensional image. When these images are recorded, the instrument is initially set so that the scan encompasses the structures of interest that limits the depth of the sector. When the pulse that produces each B-mode line reaches the bottom of the sector, display of that line ceases, a new pulse is transmitted, and a new image line is initiated. Although no longer represented in the image, the first pulse (P) continues on, becoming weaker as it goes but retaining the capability of generating echoes if it encounters a strong reflector. Any echoes produced by this first pulse after it travels beyond the lower border of the sector return to the instrument after a time interval equal to the time between pulses (which was the time required for it to reach the bottom of the sector) plus the additional time required to reach the point from which the echoes originate. Because the second pulse (P2) is transmitted after T_p, the distance traveled from the transducer (t) is the same as the distance the first pulse traveled beyond the sector. Thus, echoes returning from Tp

+ t and t will arrive back at the transducer at the same time.

If the echoes from both ranges are of sufficient magnitude to create a signal, the site of origin of the two signals cannot be determined, and range becomes ambiguous. In pulsed echo studies, this range ambiguity is generally not a problem because the strength of the signal from t is much greater than those from Tp + t and it obscures the ambiguous signals. In Doppler studies, however, this may not be the case. For example, in Figure 8–23, if there is no active flow at sample site 1 (Fig. 8–23A), but high velocity flow at sample site 2 or 3 (Fig. 8–23B), there will be no signal from site 1 to obscure the signal from the more distal sites, and the instrument will detect and display the signal from site 2 or 3, as if it originated from site 1. If, as in Figure 8–23C, we decrease our primary sampling depth to 5 cm (T_p = 67 μsec), echoes from 4 cm will return along with echoes from 9 cm (T_p + t), 14 cm (2 T_p + t), and so on. The advantage of this change is that now the sample site at 14 cm is interrogated three times as often as in Figure 8–23A, but, because the signal must travel only 14 cm, it is theoretically as strong as the signal at site 1 in Figure 8–23A. Using this approach it is possible to increase the Nyquist limit

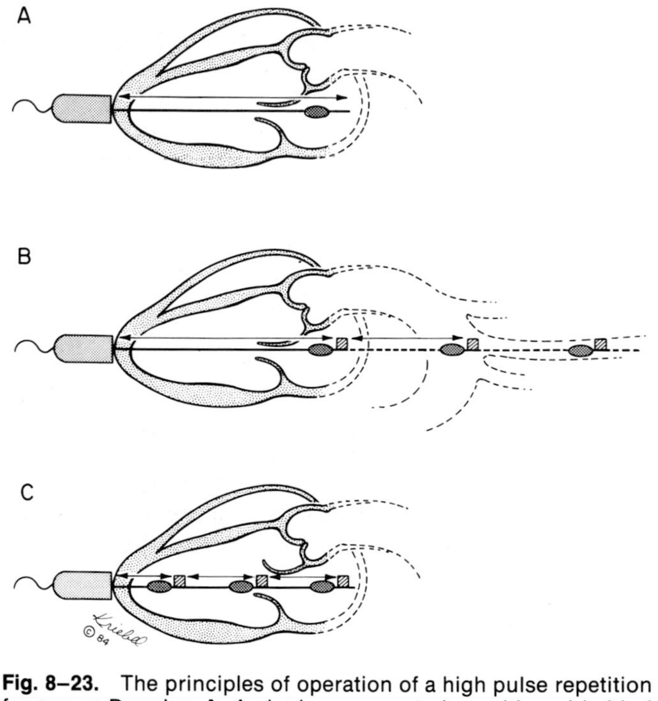

Fig. 8–23. The principles of operation of a high pulse repetition frequency Doppler. **A.** A single range gate is positioned behind the mitral valve. **B.** Although location of the primary range gate is behind the mitral valve, previously transmitted pulses continue to travel through tissue and are located at a distance equal to the time of flight of the most recent pulse (T) plus the number of interpulse intervals (T_p) that have elapsed between the earlier transmissions and that of the most recently transmitted pulse. If, in B, no flow is recorded behind the mitral valve, but high-velocity flow is present in the common carotid, this might be received by the transducer but will be displayed as if it occurred behind the mitral valve, an example of range ambiguity. **C.** If the depth of field is collapsed, the intensity of the signal at the third sample volume will be the same as at the first in A and B, but the range will be sampled three times as often. This increases the Nyquist limit, but introduces range ambiguity.

by a factor of 2 or more, depending on the number of pulses that are simultaneously traveling through the region of interest. Sampling frequency, therefore, has been increased but at the expense of range ambiguity.

This approach is attractive because it permits conventional pulsed Dopplers to increase their potential sampling frequency and, therefore, raise their velocity limit. The major limitation of the technique is the introduction of range ambiguity because signals from multiple sites arrive simultaneously and the site of origin of a specific velocity can only be presumed. Clinical results with these instruments have been variable: In pediatric and experimental studies, the maximal velocities have correlated closely with measured and predicted velocities.[14,15] In older patients, however, the results have been less reliable because examiners tend to underestimate peak velocity because of loss of signal strength.[16,17] This occurs because the power output of the instruments is usually held constant despite the fact that the pulse frequency is increased so that the average power per pulse decreases correspondingly. In most adult patients, it is not possible (because of loss of signal) to go beyond a threefold increase in PRF, which is insufficient to resolve the peak velocity in many stenotic and regurgitant lesions. For multiple high velocity lesions in series, however, the HiPRF approach is probably the only practical method for determining the velocity of each lesion.

Random Signal Coding—Noise Dopplers

From the previous sections, it should be apparent that conventional pulsed echo methods cannot completely overcome the problem of range/velocity ambiguity. The velocity limitation always recurs when the target of interest moves more than one-quarter wavelength between transmission sequences. Increasing the PRF above the Nyquist limit overcomes the velocity limitation, but introduces range ambiguity because each successive transmission sequence is indistinguishable. However, if successive transmissions could be made to retain their individuality in some way, additional pulses could be transmitted before previous signals had returned. This type of pulse encoding can be achieved either by transmitting random noise (unique signals)[18,19] or encoding each wavelength in such a way that it can be recognized as unique.[20,21]

The basic components of a random noise device are shown in Figure 8–24. The transducer is driven by a white noise generator, which results in the transmission of bursts of random noise limited only by the transducer bandwidth. The output of the noise generator can be thought of as a series of waves, all of which are different, and all of which are joined together to produce a continuous reference waveform of random amplitude and phase. The PRF of such a device must still be selected to satisfy the sampling theorum. By transmitting random noise, each pulse is unique, eliminating discrete range ambiguities at C/2*PRF.N for n = 1, 2, 3, etc. For the simple case, a random noise signal reflected from a single stationary point target will return to the receiving element after a delay equal to the time of flight to and

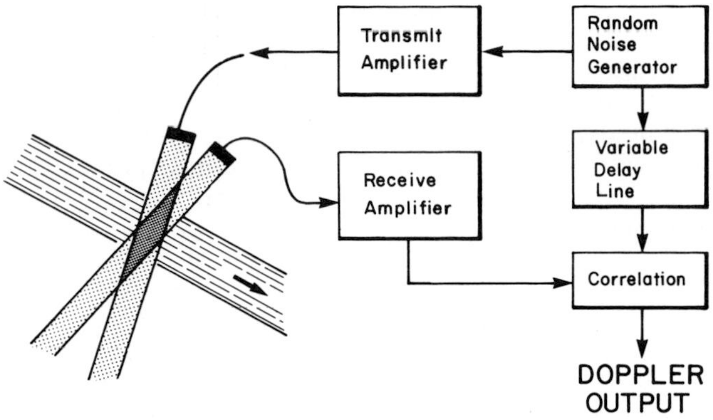

Fig. 8–24. Block diagram of a random noise Doppler device. (See text for details.)

from the target or Tf = R C/2. If the reference signal is routed through a variable delay line in which the delay is also T_f, then the reference and received signals should be uniquely related and, when compared in a correlator, the output should be at a maximum. If the target moves, however, all the returning echoes will gradually shift in phase relative to the "reference" provided by the delay line signal. After the target moves one-quarter wavelength, a situation of negative correlation will be reached, and each positive excursion of the echo will correspond to a negative excursion of the reference and vice versa. The correlator output will be a peak negative signal. Further, target movement will begin to increase the correlator output until another positive peak is reached (d). This second peak exists because the quasirandom signal is bandwidth-limited rather than pure white noise. This means that successive peaks of the transmitted waveform cannot be completely independent because the rate of change of the signal envelope is limited by the transducer bandwidth. However, the second peak will not be as large as the one produced by exact superimposition of two identical waveform. The output of the correlator will complete 1 cycle in the time that it takes for the target to move one-half wavelength because this movement increases the ultrasonic path in both directions by one wavelength.[1,5,18,19]

The random noise device is theoretically superior to a pulsed Doppler in two respects. First, because both range and velocity resolution depend on the transmitted noise bandwidth rather than the length of the transmitted pulse, the power in the noise Doppler can be spread over a much longer time than in the pulsed Doppler and the peak/mean power ratio, therefore, can be decreased. If peak power is limited by patient safety, the sensitivity of the random noise device can be considerably greater than pulsed systems. Second, and perhaps more important, a random signal flowmeter is not restricted by the range velocity limitations of the HiPRF Doppler. In the noise Doppler, range ambiguity has been removed because each interval or burst of signal differs from every other. Thus, echoes originating from any one burst will not correlate with any other burst, and so it is not necessary to wait for all echoes from one burst to return before transmitting the next. This also implies that there is no Nyquist limit on the maximum frequency that can be sampled and, therefore, no restriction on the maximum Doppler frequency that can be detected (in fact, a sampling limit is reached where the Doppler shift approaches the frequency corresponding to the averaging time of the correlator). As long as full use is made of the transducer bandwidth, however, this Doppler shift usually corresponds to velocities that are much higher than those encountered in clinical situations.[1,5,18,19]

A trade-off is made to achieve these advantages. As the number of pulses increases, uncorrelated clutter from ranges other than the range of interest results in an additional bandwidth limited noise component in the Doppler signal, which degrades the velocity resolution because the additional frequency components mask the true Doppler signal. The noise Doppler also requires a noise source different from the master oscillator and, therefore, complicates the design of dual purpose (imaging and Doppler) instruments. Thus, the random noise Doppler flowmeter represents an elegant solution to problems encountered using more simple transmission codes. Practical implementation of the technique is difficult, however, and at present, is not suitable for medical application.

Signal Encoded Continuous Wave Dopplers

Frequency Modulated Doppler. Several approaches to signal encoding the CW Doppler output have also been suggested to uniquely identify each transmitted wavelength so that the depth from which echoes that carry this code arise can be determined. The first type of signal encoding is frequency modulation (FM).[20] An FM device operates by transmitting a constantly changing ultrasonic frequency and then measuring the time it takes for the echo from a target to return at each particular (coded) frequency. The simplest method of coding the frequency is to increase or decrease it linearly with time. Figure 8–25 illustrates the effect of this frequency modulation in both the frequency and time domains when a single stationary target is in the ultrasonic beam.

In the frequency domain, ultrasound transmitted at frequency F_1 at time T_1 travels toward the target, is reflected, and arrives back at the source at T_2. By this time the transmitted frequency increases to F_2, and the difference in frequency ($F_2 - F_1$) between the received waveform and the currently transmitted waveform is related to the time of flight ($T_2 - T_1$) by the expression:

$$(F_2 - F_1) = q\,(T_2 - T_1) \qquad [8.11]$$

where q is the frequency vs. time gradient of the transmitted waveform.

As long as the transmission frequency increases linearly with time, the difference between the transmitted and received frequencies is constant and proportional to the range of the target. If the target is moving, the output frequency will vary at a rate proportional to target velocity.

In any practical situation, the transmission frequency cannot increase indefinitely, because it is limited by the bandwidth of the transducer. The modulated waveform,

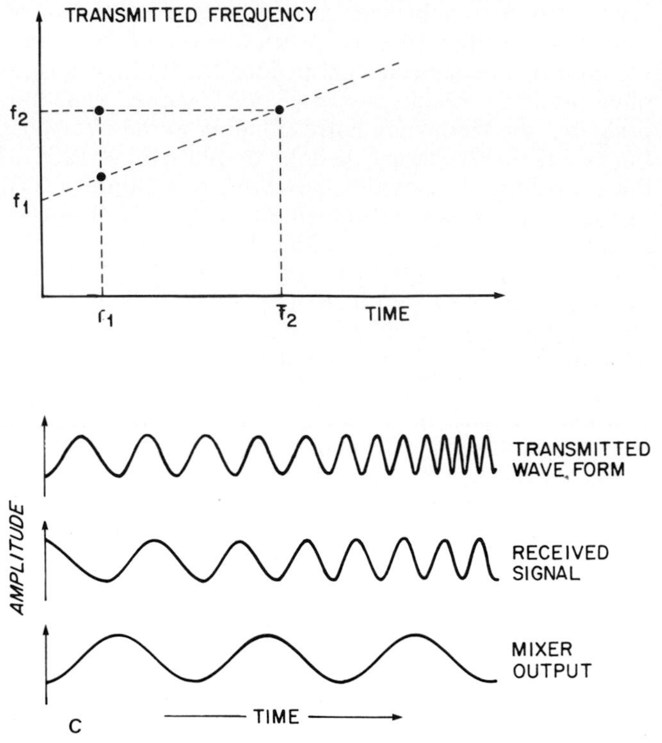

Fig. 8–25. Top. Principle of operation of a frequency modulation Doppler. The instrument transmits a constantly changing ultrasonic frequency. Ultrasound transmitted at frequency (f_1) at time (T_1) arrives back at the transducer at time (T_2). However, by this time the transmitted frequency has increased to (f_2). If the rate of change in frequency is known, the difference in frequency can be related to the time of flight or the range of the target. Bottom. These constantly varying frequencies can yield a constant Doppler difference frequency.

therefore, must either begin decreasing to produce a triangular modulation or be reset to produce a sawtooth modulation. In either case, the difference frequency is discontinuous and is no longer related unambiguously to target range. The rate at which these discontinuities occur is related to the transducer bandwidth, which defines the available range of frequency and the rate of change of frequency or the gradient (g).

In theory, it should be possible to resolve velocity using an FM system, but in practice, multiple targets confuse the analyzer. Using a simple sawtooth device, it is not possible to differentiate a stationary target at one range from moving targets with accompanying shift at a different range. In theory, one could devise a triangular sweep in which the apparent range of targets during an increase in frequency is compared to that during a decrease in transmission frequency. The range and Doppler shift component would then either add or subtract, depending on whether the transmission frequency sweep is increasing or decreasing. This complex type of system, however, has not been used to monitor flow.[1]

Pseudo-random Binary Sequencing. The final method is phase modulation of the output signal using a pseudo-random binary sequence (PRBS) of wavelengths.[21] For efficient phase modulation codes, ambiguities in range can be minimized to 1/N, where N is the total number of elements in the code. Neither the FM nor PRBS modifications have been implemented in clinical instruments. They are presented, however, because it appears useful for the reader to be familiar with the fact that other methods of signal coding do exist and may, in one form or another, play a role in future Doppler instruments.

Multigate Dopplers

The Doppler devices described to this point produce a signal that can be related to the peak velocity within the beam or to flow at specific points along the beam. When multiple targets are present, such as the red cells in flowing blood, their spatial location and distribution may also be of interest. This type of information can be obtained by Doppler flow mapping.

Doppler flow mapping uses the recorded presence of flow at a series of specific ranges to map the spatial distribution of flow within a specified sampling area. In its simplest form, flow mapping can be performed using a pulsed Doppler by varying the depth of the range gate along a specific line of site and recording the presence or absence of flow at each sampling point (Fig. 8–26). If

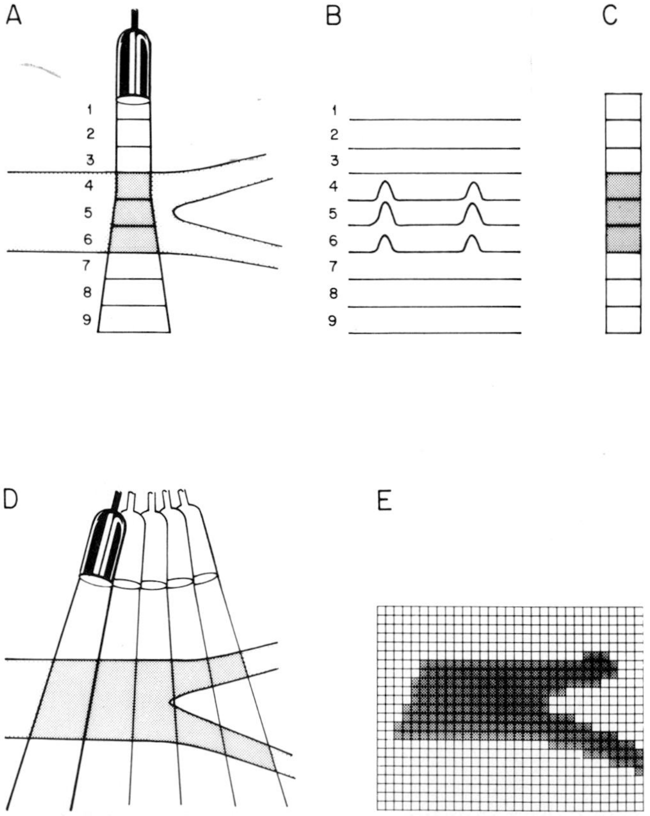

Fig. 8–26. Principles of operation of the multigate Doppler. **A.** Doppler sampling can be achieved at multiple locations along the beam (gates) either by advancing the sample volume in known increments or electronically gating at multiple points along the beam. **B.** Flow data from each gate can be output as a plot of velocity vs. time. **C.** Flow data output in a binary flow or nonflow format. **D.** By sweeping the beam while recording in a binary format, one can produce a two-dimensional map of the flow area. **E.** Two-dimensional map.

the process is repeated while shifting the orientation of the beam in an ordered progression, the spatial distribution of flow can be determined. This process, unfortunately, is time-consuming and subject to operator variability. As a result, flow mapping devices such as multichannel or multigate Dopplers and color flow mappers have been developed to increase speed and reduce variability.

Multigate Dopplers sample electronically from multiple range gates positioned at equal intervals along the beam path (Fig. 8–26A).[1,2] The velocity distribution is then determined by processing the signal received at each range. If the beam transects a large region of interest, the flow signal at each range can be defined and the velocity output continuously (Fig. 8–26B). However, two major problems arise with this type of display. First, many components are required because each channel requires a separate Doppler signal processor. Second, a large volume of data produced, which must be recorded and analyzed. Another approach is to output the data in a binary format indicating flow as the presence of a signal and no flow as its absence (Fig. 8–26C). In this format, the transducer can be swept across a two-dimensional region of a vessel (Fig. 8–26D) producing a map of the spatial distribution of flow (Fig. 8–26E). Although historically interesting, this approach presents flow in the absence of its structural references and fails to depict either velocity or direction. Because of these limitations, multigate Dopplers have been replaced by color flow mappers, which depict both the location of flow and an estimate of its direction and velocity in the context of associated structures. Color flow mapping is discussed in Chapter 11.

SUMMARY

In summary, although superficially, Doppler flow detection appears relatively simple, in any practical application it rapidly becomes more complicated. Useful modifications, e.g., range discrimination, inevitably introduce undesirable effects, e.g., range velocity ambiguities and transmit time fluctuations, which eventually limit Doppler performance. The operator, therefore, ought to be fully aware of all of these phenomenon because they can cause spurious output and can affect the interpretation of results.

REFERENCES

1. Baker DW, Foster FK, Daigle RE: Doppler Principles and techniques. *In* Fry FJ (ed): Ultrasound: Its Applications in Medicine and Biology. New York, Elsevier Scientific Publishing, 1978.
2. Lee R: Technology of Doppler echocardiography: Capabilities and Limitations. *In* Harrigan P, Lee R: Principles of Interpretation in Echocardiography. New York, John Wiley & Sons, 1985.
3. Rschevkin SN: A Course of Lectures on the Theory of Sound. Oxford, Pergamon Press, 1963.
4. McLeod FD: Multichannel pulsed Doppler techniques. In Reneman RS (ed.): Cardiovascular Applications of Ultrasound. Amsterdam, North Holland Publishing, p. 85, 1974.
5. Atkinson P, Woodcock JP: Doppler Ultrasound and its Use in Clinical Measurement. New York, Academic Press, 1982.
6. Dejong DA, et al.: A directional quantifying Doppler system for measurement of transport velocity of blood. Ultrasonics 13:138, 1975.
7. Sato, et al.: 13th Japanese Medical Electronics Society Convention, 2-C-54, 1974.
8. Kato K, Izumi T: On a method of indication of reverse flow in the ultrasonic Doppler flowmeter. Proc 10th Meet Jpn Soc Ultrasonics Med p. 78, 1966.
9. Cross G, Light LH: Direction resolving Doppler instrument with improved reflection of tissue artifacts. J Physiol 217:5, 1971.
10. McLeod FD: A directional Doppler flowmeter. Digest 7th Intl Conf Med Biol Eng p. 213, 1967.
11. Coghlan BA, Taylor MG: Directional Doppler techniques for detection of blood velocities. Ultrasound Med Biol 2:171, 1976.
12. Baker DW, Watkins D: A phase coherent pulse Doppler system for cardiovascular measurement. Proc 20th Annu Conf Eng Med Biol 27:2, 1967.
13. Peronneau PA, Leger F: Doppler ultrasonic pulsed blood flowmeter. Proc 8th Intl Conf Med Biol Eng p. 10, 1969.
14. Stevenson JG, Kawabori I: Noninvasive determination of pressure gradients in children: two methods employing pulsed Doppler echocardiography. J Am Coll Cardiol 3:179, 1984.
15. Valdez-Cruz LM, et al.: Studies in vitro of the relationship between ultrasound and laser Doppler velocimetry and applicability of the simplified Bernoulli relationship. Circulation 73:300, 1986.
16. Stewart WJ, et al.: Comparison of high pulse repetition frequency and continuous wave Doppler echocardiography in the assessment of high flow velocity in patients with valvular stenosis and regurgitation. J Am Coll Cardiol 6:565, 1985.
17. Rothbart RM, Gibson RS: Doppler quantitation of adult aortic valvular stenosis: comparison of continuous wave versus high pulse repetition frequency Doppler. J Am Coll Cardiol 5:484, 1985.
18. Jetwa GP, et al.: Blood flow measurement using ultrasonic pulsed random signal Doppler system. IEEE Trans Sonics Ultrasonics 22:1, 1975.
19. Bendick PJ, Newhouse VL: Ultrasonic random signal flow measurement system. J Acoust Soc Am 56:860, 1974.
20. McCarty K, Woodcock JP: Frequency modulated ultrasonic Doppler flowmeter. Med Biol Eng 13:59, 1975.
21. Waag RC, Rhoades WL, Gramiak R: Instrumentation for noninvasive cardiac chamber flow rate measurement. Proc IEEE Ultrasonics Symp p. 74, 1972.

CHAPTER

9

PRINCIPLES OF FLOW

Chapters 7 and 8 discussed the manner in which ultrasonic waves are shifted in frequency when they encounter moving targets and how the magnitude of this frequency shift can be used to determine target velocity. In each of the examples presented, it was assumed that the frequency-shifted signals arose from individual targets and that these targets moved at a constant velocity. It was also assumed that the Doppler difference frequency (i.e., the difference between the transmitted waveform and the Doppler-shifted waveform) could be analyzed in some way to compute target velocity using the simple Doppler equation.

The interaction of ultrasound with flowing blood in the heart and great vessels is more complicated than that described previously. In any practical application of the Doppler principle, the reflected signal arriving at the transducer is the sum of the reflected and scattered energy from multiple interactions with large numbers of stationary and moving targets. The moving target of primary interest, blood, is itself a complex of cells or groups of cells traveling at velocities that change with space and time and with individual and net characteristics that must be analyzed and interpreted.

The signal to be analyzed, therefore, is a complex of frequencies, some of which are similar to the transmitted waveform but vary widely in amplitude, whereas others are frequency-shifted by varying degrees from the carrier. To extract the Doppler shift frequencies of interest, each of these components must somehow be separated and displayed. It is the purpose of this chapter to describe the pattern of blood flow in various settings that form the physiologic basis of the returning signal. Chapter 10 discusses various methods by which individual components of the ultrasonic signal reflected from blood can be extracted and analyzed.

STRUCTURE OF BLOOD AND ITS RELATION TO ULTRASONIC SCATTERING

The Doppler shift frequencies of primary interest in clinical echocardiography arise from the interaction of sound waves with flowing blood. Human blood is a complex medium composed of a liquid (plasma), in which are suspended erythrocytes (red blood cells), leukocytes (white blood cells), and platelets. Available data suggest that the red cells are the primary source of the ultrasonic reflections from blood.[1] Because red cells are small (roughly 7×2 μm with a mean volume of 90 μm^3) relative to wavelength at clinically useful ultrasonic frequencies (0.3 mm at 5 MHz), they behave individually as point scatterers. The scattering coefficient, therefore, depends only on the volume of the red cell and the acoustic mismatch between it and the surrounding plasma and is independent of the shape of the cell.[2]

White cells, although much larger than red cells, are relatively few in number (7.5×10^3 vs. 5×10^3/ml). Platelets, although densely distributed, have a scattering cross section that is a factor of 10^3 lower than that of red cells and, in normal blood, platelet scattering can be considered to be negligible.[1]

The scattering and diffraction of sound at a single, small, flexible target, such as the red cell, has been described in detail, and its angular intensity can be calculated.[2] The scattering of waves in a dense distribution of small targets, such as the red cells in blood, however, is far more complex and varies with the density and distribution of the scatterers. At low densities (hematocrits of less than 10%), red cells behave as independent, randomly distributed scattering centers, and the reflected acoustic energy is a linear function of hematocrit.[3] Above this level, blood takes on an increasingly crystalline characteristic: interaction between particles becomes apparent, and constructive and destructive interference occurs between the defraction patterns arising from adjacent targets.[4] Figure 9–1 illustrates the relationship between scattering power and hematocrit. Experimental data suggest that scattering power increases with increasing target density up to a hematocrit of roughly 26%.[4] Beyond this density, destructive interference begins to predominate and the scattering power falls. At a hematocrit of 45%, the average separation between red cells is only 10% of the cell diameter, whereas above a hematocrit of 58%, blood has a nearly perfect crystalline character[3] and little scattering occurs.[3]

Because red cells are randomly distributed in blood, the number contained in different small volumes of the same size (V) will not simply be given by n × V, where n is the overall numeric density but rather will fluctuate about this mean value. This fluctuation in the number of cells contributing to the echo causes a continuing variation in the scattering power with the blood echo appearing to arise primarily from this "fluctuation" in local cell concentration (fluctuation scattering) rather than from individual cells as such. Because the scattering arises not from any particular structure, but from the random distribution of red cells, the dimensions of the ultrasonic pulse (which define the volume and distribution of scatterers sampled) determines the scale of fluctuations detected. Figure 9–2 illustrates the variation in scattering for a constant pulse volume when it is moved either axially or laterally within a larger volume of randomly distributed red cells. The same type of fluctuation about a statistical mean can be expected if random volumes of red cells pass through a stationary sample volume.[5,6]

Turbulence increases total scattering apparently because the eddy currents in regions of turbulent flow create a centrifugal force that separates plasma and red cells by their different mass densities. This separation in-

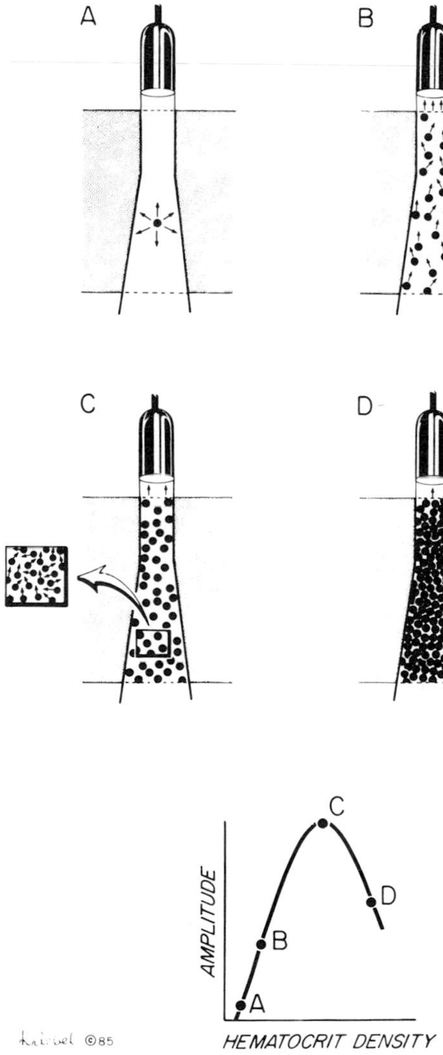

Fig. 9–1. Relationship between scatterer concentration and signal intensity. **A.** A single scatterer. **B.** A widely dispersed collection of scatterers. **C.** A denser concentration of scatterers with a maximal ratio of constructive to destructive interference. **D.** A dense concentration in which the scatterers take on a crystalline character.

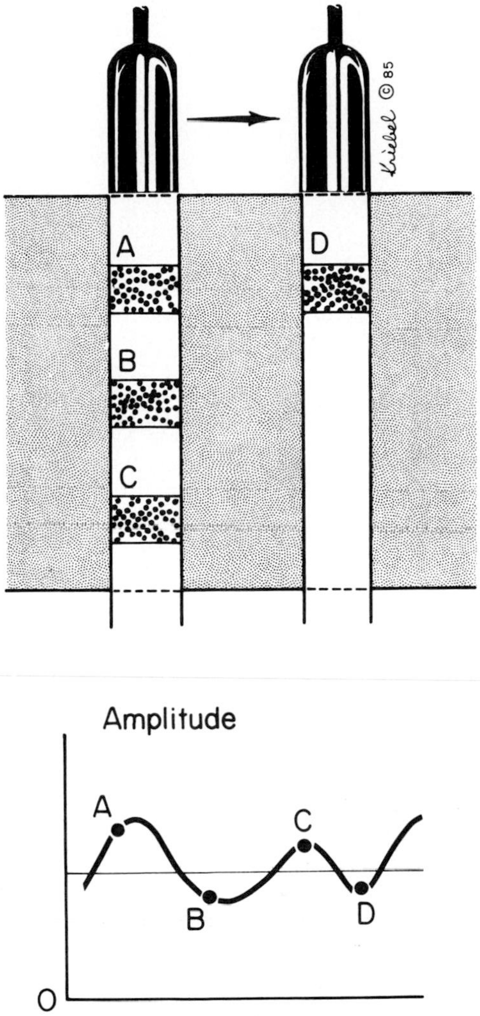

Fig. 9–2. Effect of fluctuation scattering on signal output. Because of the random distribution of scatterers in the sample volume, each spatially unique volume of blood cells produces a characteristic, independent echo amplitude. This occurs for both axially (A, B, and C) and laterally (D) separate samples.

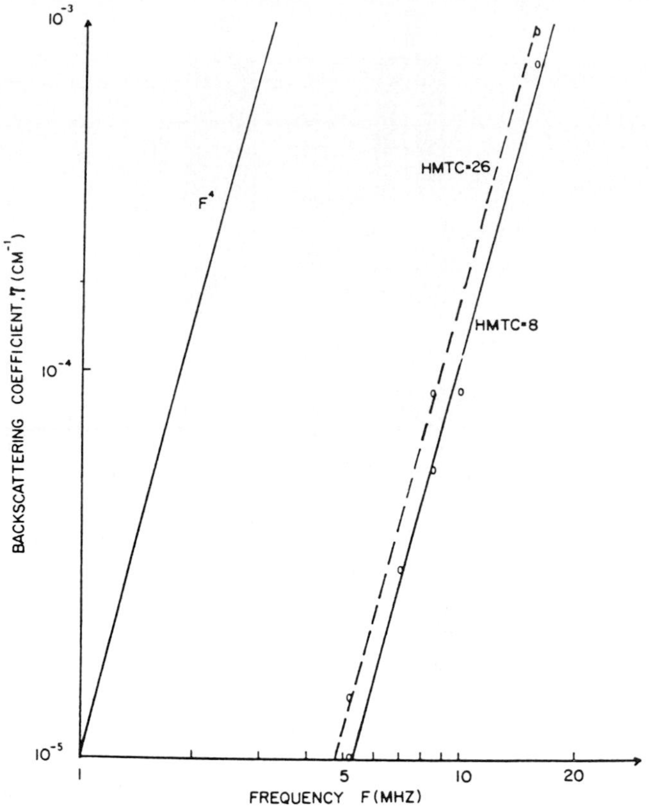

Fig. 9–3. Relationship of backscattered signal intensity to frequency. Backscattered signal intensity closely follows the fourth power of the frequency despite variation in hematocrit. (Reproduced from Shung KK, Sigelmann RA, Reid JM: Scattering of ultrasound by blood. IEEE Trans Biomed Eng BME 23:460, 1976.)

creases the fluctuation in the number and distribution of red cells within any volume, altering the relationship between constructive and destructive interference and augmenting scattering. This is probably the reason that areas of flow acceleration and turbulence cause stronger signals than ordinary flow.[6] This characteristic fluctuation in signal amplitude is important because amplitude modulation superimposes additional frequencies on the basic waveform when it is subject to Fourier analysis, and the intermittent "fading" associated with this type of signal complicates the tracking of specific frequency components (see following discussion).

The amplitude of the scattering from blood also varies with the frequency of the incident sound wave. Figure 9–3 illustrates the theoretic and observed fourth power relationship of scattering to frequency with the practical result that an increase in transducer frequency significantly increases both the scattered and Doppler signals.[4] Increasing frequency unfortunately also increases attenuation and, as discussed earlier, a frequency or range of frequencies must be defined that optimizes the relationship of penetration and frequency resolution.

BLOOD FLOW

Blood flow is a complex phenomenon, the characteristics of which vary with time, space, and location within the vascular system. Blood flow can be examined at many levels ranging from an average measurement of the forward movement of the entire blood column during periods of seconds or minutes to the instantaneous motion of individual blood cells or groups of cells at selected points in a single cardiac cycle. The precision of such flow measurements usually depends on the spatial and temporal resolution of the method used. Most clinical measures of flow report a mean flow averaged over many beats. The most common such measurement, e.g., the cardiac output, is an average of ventricular outflow, usually given in liters per minute. Such relatively gross measures of flow require little understanding of hemodynamics because the degree of averaging tends to obscure any spatial or temporal variation between the sampling points or within the sampling period. The Doppler method, in contrast, samples flow velocity several times during a single beat and allows its pattern to be studied at specific locations within larger vessels. Because the Doppler method looks at discrete spatial and temporal components of the total flow field, the resulting Doppler signals may vary greatly, and therefore, a detailed understanding of the patterns and principles of blood flow is required to interpret them intelligently.

Fortunately, blood flow is governed by basic hydraulic principles. An understanding of these principles makes the pattern of flow predictable in most clinically encountered situations. Once the common patterns of flow are understood, the Doppler shift signals from cells moving in these patterns should become interpretable, and unexpected or nonphysiological signals recognizable. Any serious student of the Doppler method, therefore, must be conversant with the principles of hydraulics and hemodynamics just as any imaging echocardiographer must understand normal and pathologic anatomy to interpret the data presented.

The variables most frequently measured in hemodynamics are pressure and flow. Pressure is defined as force per unit area and is most appropriately expressed in dyn/cm^2.* Alternatively, pressure can be expressed as the height of a column of mercury (mm Hg) or water (cm H_2O) that it will support. When measured at room temperature, 1 mm Hg is equivalent to 1329 dyn/cm^2 and 1 cm H_2O equals 980 dyn/cm^2. Thus, 1 cm H_2O is equivalent to 0.738 mm Hg. Blood flow refers to the volume moved per unit time in milliliters per second or liters per minute. The movement of fluid can also be described in terms of its velocity or distance moved per unit time, for example, in centimeters per second.

Steady Flow in a Rigid Cylindric Tube

The principles that govern the flow of blood can be most easily approached by first considering the simplest case: steady flow in a rigid cylindric tube. The dynamics of pulsatile flow can then be understood by extension of these principles, and the flow that results from the pumping action of the heart can be treated analytically as steady flow on which pulsations are superimposed.[7]

* The Dyne is the unit of force such that under its influence a body with a mass of 1 g would experience an acceleration of 1 cm/sec.

The relationship between steady flow and pressure in a rigid cylindric tube was first accurately described by the French physician, J.L.M. Pouiseuille (1799 to 1869). He observed that the relationship between volume flow (Q) and the drop in pressure (P) along a tube of length (L) and inner diameter (D) was equal to:

$$Q = K \times P \times D^4/L \qquad [9.1]$$

where K was a constant. Later investigators demonstrated that Poiseuille's Constant, K, was related to fluid viscosity and a subsequent form of this relationship, which includes a viscosity term (η), is known as Poiseuille's Law:

$$Q = \pi \times R^4 (P_1 - P_2)/8\eta L \qquad [9.2]$$

In this form, R is the radius of the tube, P_1 is the pressure at the beginning of the tube, P_2 is the pressure at the end of the tube, and the expression ($P_1 - P_2/L$) describes the pressure drop or energy expended in moving the fluid column one unit of length.* As described by this equation, the pressure drop along the tube is proportional to the fluid viscosity because any increase in viscosity must be matched by a proportional increase in expended pressure energy (manifest by a greater pressure drop per unit length) to maintain flow constant.[7]

To more fully understand the relationship between the force required to move a fluid a given distance and the viscosity opposing this motion, it is first necessary to understand the general patterns of fluid movement and the physical principles by which they are governed. Under steady state conditions, fluids move through a tube in a series of concentric layers, or lamina, as illustrated in Figure 9–4. The outermost layer, which is in contact with the tube wall, is fixed in place by the high degree of friction encountered at fluid-solid interfaces. Adjacent, axially positioned layers, however, slip past one another, with the velocity of motion of each layer increasing from the tube wall to the central axis. Particles in each layer move parallel to the vessel wall with no effective interaction occurring between the particles of individual layers. The parallel lines along which the fluid particles travel are termed *streamlines* and the overall pattern of flow is known as *laminar flow*.

Slippage of fluid lamina over one another is opposed by internal friction between fluid layers called *viscosity*,

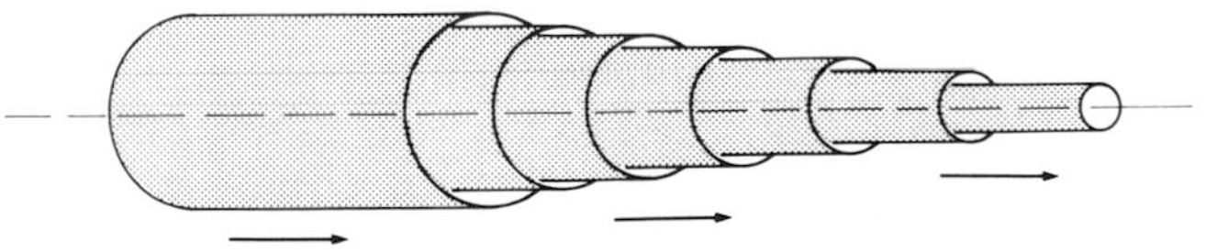

Fig. 9–4. Normal laminar flow, which is comparable to the slippage of a series of thin concentric cyclindric shells over one another. The outermost shell is stationary, and velocity increases to a maximum at the central axis of the tube. (After Milnor, 1982.)

* If radius and length are in centimeters, pressure in dynes per square centimeter, viscosity in dynes per second per square centimeter, then flow will be in milliliters per second.

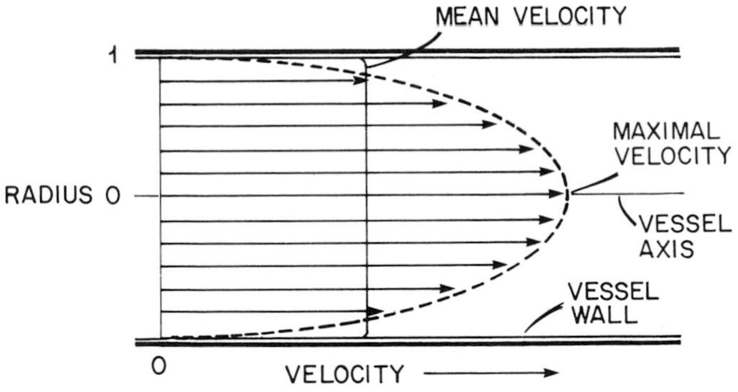

Fig. 9–5. Parabolic flow pattern that normally occurs during steady flow in a rigid cylindric tube.

a fundamental property of all fluids. The amount of force required to overcome the viscous resistance between layers is proportional to the area over which the layers are in contact and the velocity at which they are sliding past one another. The stress (S) or force per unit area required to slide the layers over one another is equal to the viscosity times the velocity gradient or:

$$S = \eta * dv/dx \qquad [9.3]$$

where dv/dx is the velocity gradient or the rate of shear across the tube. Viscosity, therefore, equals the ratio of stress to velocity gradient and is an inherent physical property of the fluid.* This relationship implies that within the limits of organized flow, the velocity gradient at any given viscosity is a function of the stress applied. Most liquids, including blood in larger vessels (greater than 0.5 mm diameter), behave in this fashion, and such fluids are called *ideal* or *Newtonian fluids*.[7–9]

The speed at which individual lamina move and the pattern or profile assumed by the blood column in different circumstances are the net result of the balance of the inertial forces promoting forward motion and the viscous (or shear) forces retarding that motion. For steady flow in a rigid tube, the profile is parabolic, as illustrated in Figure 9–5.[7,10] Such a parabolic profile assumes a velocity gradient that changes linearly across the tube (because the integral of a straight line is a parabola) and is the most energy-efficient form for fluid flow.

Volume flow, as described by Poiseuille's Law, thus represents the mean of the velocities within each lamina; this can be viewed as the average height of the solid of revolution of the parabola. This average velocity, which is volume flow divided by cross-sectional area ($\pi r2$), can be derived from the Poiseuille equation as

$$V_{mean} = R^2 \times (P_1 - P_2)/8\eta \times L. \qquad [9.4]$$

Based on the parabolic contour of the flowstream, the maximal velocity that occurs at the axis of the stream can be shown mathematically to be equal to approximately twice its mean velocity.

* The standard unit of viscosity, 1 dyn/sec/cm^2 is called the "Poise," and for water is approximately $\eta = 0.013$.

The pressure drop caused by viscous resistance can also be calculated for a tube of length L and radius r using Poiseuille's Law as

$$P_1 - P_2 = V_{mean} \times 8 \times \eta \times L/r^2 \qquad [9.5]$$

Vascular Resistance

Poiseuille's Law states, in effect, that the ratio of pressure gradient to flow is a function of the dimensions of the tube and the viscosity of the moving fluid. The physical properties of the system, in other words, determine how large a pressure gradient is required to produce a given flow. The ratio of mean pressure expenditure to mean flow is then a measure of the degree to which the system opposes flow, and this ratio is called the vascular resistance.[9]

$$R\ vasc. = (P_1 - P_2)/Q \qquad [9.6]$$

This relationship has been compared to the definition of electrical resistance in Ohm's law

$$R\ elect = E/I \qquad [9.7]$$

where I is the flow of current and E is the voltage drop across the circuit. Vascular and electrical resistances both express the dissipation of energy per unit flow within a system. In a cylindric tube under conditions that satisfy Poiseuille's Law (Equation 9.2), rearrangement of Equation 9.6 gives vascular resistance in terms of the properties of the system.[7]*

$$R = 8\eta L/\pi R^4 \qquad [9.8]$$

Relationship of Poiseuille's Law to In Vivo Blood Flow

Because Poiseuille's Law is based on observations of fluid flow in rigid tubes, it is reasonable to question the validity of its application to the study of pulsatile blood flow in the elastic, branching, tapering vessels of the human circulatory system. However, because Poiseuille's Law can be derived mathematically, the assumptions on which it is based are known, and it is thus possible to examine the degree to which deviation from these assumptions in the human circulation affects its accuracy. It is also possible to examine how these differences might be expected to affect Doppler flow measurements. The assumptions in the derivation of Poiseuille's Law include (1) a constant viscosity, defined as the ratio of stress to velocity gradient; (2) laminar flow; (3) no slip at blood-vessel wall interfaces; (4) steady flow; (5) tubes with parallel walls of circular cross section; and (6) inelastic tube or vessel walls.[7]

Blood behaves like a Newtonian fluid under most conditions, which is surprising because it is not a pure liquid but rather is a suspension of cells. Significant deviation from Newtonian behavior occurs only in narrow tubes (less than 1.0 to 0.5 mm in diameter),[8,9] which are far smaller than the vessels examined in most Doppler studies, and at low rates of shear.[11,12]

The increase in viscosity encountered at low shear rates is due to the formation of aggregates of red cells (rouleaux formation), which break down as velocity increases. Importantly, because blood is a suspension of cells, viscosity varies with hematocrit. Above a hematocrit of 10%, viscosity rises steadily as the proportion of cells increases, with an almost linear relationship existing between hematocrit and log viscosity.[13] Hence, conditions that significantly raise hematocrit (e.g., congenital heart disease and high altitude) or lower it (anemia) may affect blood viscosity significantly and thereby modify the pressure-flow relationship in the circulation.

The assumption that flow is laminar applies to almost all parts of the normal circulation; the only exceptions being the ascending aorta and main pulmonary artery just beyond the semilunar valves, where a brief period of turbulence may occur during peak systolic flow.[7,14,15] In pathologic situations, however, deformity of either artery can lead to turbulence, which would invalidate the Poiseuille relationship. Likewise, the concept of no slippage by the lamina in contact with the vessel wall is consistent with basic experimental hydrodynamic observation, where true slippage has not been demonstrated at any liquid-solid interface.[7]

The assumption of steady flow is obviously not met in the circulation, where flow is pulsatile in a major portion of the system. In such a pulsatile system, velocity profiles vary with time and are often nonparabolic. In addition, the inertial forces of acceleration are not taken into account in linear equations for steady flow. Nonetheless, pressures and flows in blood vessels can be treated as steady components on which pulsations are superimposed. The more important question is whether Poiseuille's Law accurately describes mean pressure and flow accurately. Theoretic data suggest that for a rigid tube, this should be the case. For an elastic tube, however, e.g., the arterial system, an error of roughly 10% or greater would be incurred with the direct use of the Poiseuille equation.[7] The effects of pulsatile flow are discussed in more detail later.

The assumptions of a circular tube and parallel walls are not uniformly met in the circulatory system. Most arteries of the systemic circulation are circular, but many veins and the pulmonary arteries[16] tend to be elliptic, rather than circular. Likewise, the requirement of parallel walls is probably never exactly met in blood vessels, because individual arteries tend to become narrower as they progress toward the periphery, whereas veins enlarge as they are followed centrally. Because Doppler measurements of volumetric flow are usually taken at specific points in the circulatory system, vascular tapering is not a problem. As will be discussed in Chapter 30, however, deviation from a circular shape can be an extremely difficult problem.

Finally, the assumption of a rigid tube is clearly not met because blood vessels are distensible, and their diameter is a function of transmural pressure. Here again, because Doppler studies are performed at a specific location with "simultaneous" imaging of the vessel, at

* If pressure is expressed in units of dyn per square centimeter and flow in milliliter per second, then resistance is in dyn per second per centimeter e+5.

least partial correction for pulsation-related changes in vessel size is possible.

The first three assumptions, therefore, are valid for blood vessels and the last three are not. The pulsatile nature of flow, tapering or elliptic cross sections of blood vessels, and blood vessel distensibility all seriously limit the application of Poiseuille's equation to the circulatory system. In general, the Poiseuille equation overestimates mean flow for a given pressure gradient, blood viscosity, and vascular dimension, particularly in smaller vessels, Nonetheless, the relationships are qualitatively correct, and their understanding is important to students of hemodynamics and the related Doppler flow measurements. Because the interaction of matter and motion encountered in the human circulation is so complex, no question of any real interest can be answered in closed mathematic terms. One's goal, therefore, should be an understanding of basic concepts and the clinical settings that alter these relationships rather than precise mathematic descriptions of phenomena. From this viewpoint, the Poiseuille relationship forms an ideal basis for understanding the factors that underlie Doppler velocity recordings. This is especially true because many of the limitations in applying Poiseuilles Law to the circulation relate to system properties that come into play only over relatively long distances and, hence, are not of concern in Doppler studies.

Flow at Vascular Inlets

All steady-state laminar flow does not invariably have a parabolic profile. The flow pattern at the entrance to a tube leading from the bottom of a reservoir, e.g., will initially have a relatively flat velocity profile, with a parabolic configuration developing only as flow progresses along the length of the tube (Fig. 9–6). This gradual evolution from a flat to a parabolic profile is seen because all lamina initially move at the same velocity at the entrance to the tube. Once in the tube, however, the layers nearest the wall are immediately slowed by the viscous friction at the boundary, whereas the inner core continues to advance with an almost flat profile. As the fluid moves farther along the tube, the blunt portion of the profile in the center becomes smaller and smaller, as velocity gradients produced by fluid viscosity are communicated to layers further and further from the wall until the profile assumes a completely parabolic shape.[17]

The distance required for the full development of a

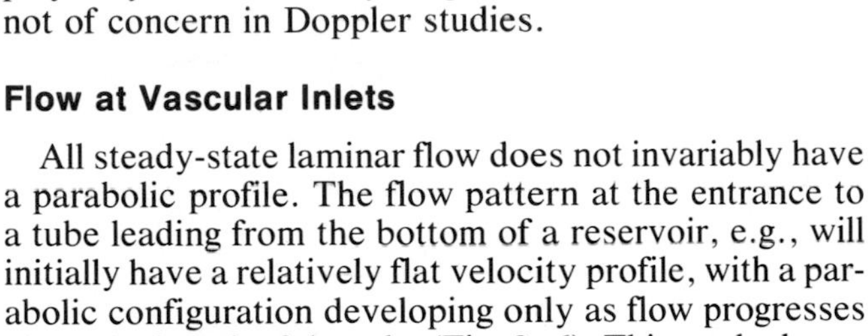

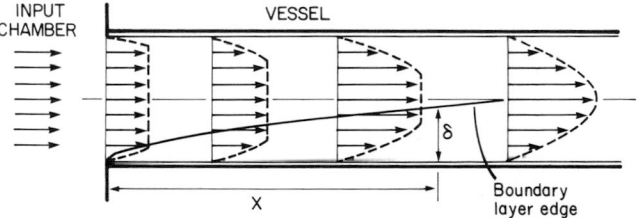

Fig. 9–6. Flow pattern at the entrance to a tube leading from the bottom of a reservoir. At the entrance to the tube, the profile is flat but progressively becomes more parabolic as flow progresses along the tube. This is accompanied by an increase in the width of the boundary layer (σ). X = the distance from the tube entrance. (After Caro et al., 1978.)

parabolic profile is referred to as the *entrance length*, and the progressive stages of development are called *entrance effects*. The outer portion of the fluid in which a radially directed gradient of velocity exists is called the *boundary layer*, in contrast to the *inner core* of uniform velocity. The boundary layer increases in width as the distance from the entrance increases until it constitutes the entire cross section of the tube at the point where the profile becomes parabolic.[7,17]

The thickness of the boundary layer T_b at any point is approximately

$$T_b \propto \frac{\eta}{\rho} \frac{x^{1/2}}{v} \qquad [9.9]$$

where η is the viscosity and ρ the density of blood, v the central core velocity, and x the distance from the tube entrance.[18,19] At the point where the parabolic profile first becomes fully developed, the boundary layer extends across the whole tube (R = r) and the distance x is the entrance length (L′). Rearrangement of the above equation shows that

$$L' \propto (R^2)v\rho/\eta \qquad [9.10]$$

Thus, for the vascular system, where the density and viscosity of blood are relatively constant, entrance length increases in direct relationship to vessel size and flow velocity. In large vessels, such as the aorta and pulmonary artery, entrance effects are nontrivial and may extend for the majority of the vessel length.

Flow Around Curves

Curves, branches, and projections all cause the streamlines of flow to change direction, which can lead to nonlaminar flow. Fluid moving through a curved pipe is affected by centrifugal forces, which tend to direct the lamina toward the outer wall of the curve. However, the net effect depends on the velocity profile at the entrance to the curve. If flow is laminar and the velocity profile at the beginning of the curve is parabolic, as in Figure 9–7, the axial lamina will be the most affected by the centrifugal force because it has the greatest velocity and inertia. As a result, the profile will be tilted toward the outer wall; the highest velocities will be found in the outer portion of the curve rather than at the stream axis. In addition, the shift of the central lamina toward the outer wall of the curve sets up secondary flow, which takes the form of helices rotating in two different directions, as shown in the cross section in Figure 9–7. If, on the other hand, flow at the entrance to the curve has a relatively flat profile, all of the lamina will have essentially the same inertia. Centrifugal force, then, does not displace the flow lines outward, but it does produce higher pressures at the outer wall relative to the inner wall. Assuming that the effects of viscosity and gravitation are the same at all lamina, the difference in pressure must be accompanied by a balancing difference in kinetic energy (as in Bernoulli's theorum, see following discussion). As a result, the highest velocities will be found near the inner wall of the curve. The velocity pro-

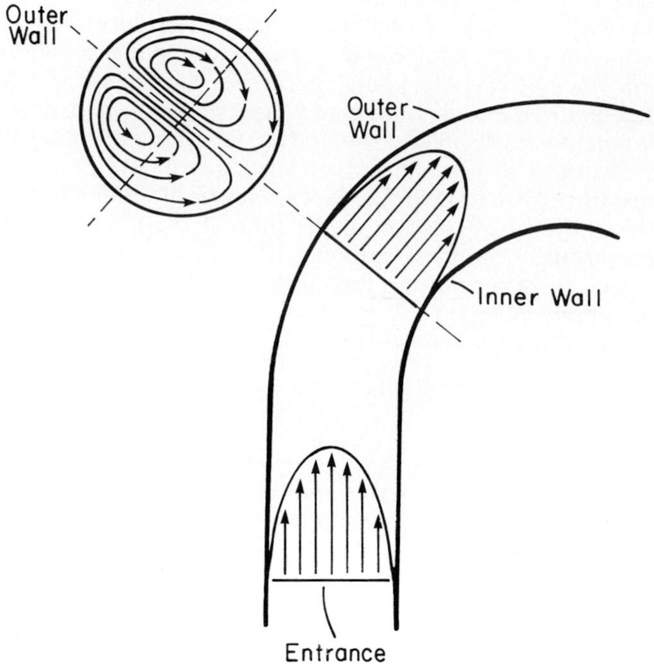

Fig. 9–7. Effect of a curve in a tube on the velocity profile when the profile at the entrance to the tube is parabolic. There is displacement of the profile toward the outer wall of the tube with secondary helical flow patterns arising because of the increased local pressure along the outer wall. (After Caro et al., 1978.)

file in the ascending aorta is relatively flat, and as a result, flow in the arch is similar to that described in Figure 9–8. Once the flat profile is disturbed, however, the lamina with the higher velocities become subject to greater centrifugal forces, and in a U-shaped curve, such as the aortic arch, they will shift toward the outer wall in the second half of the curve.[18]

Flow at Branch Points

Branching is a characteristic of the circulatory system. Branching generally takes place through the division of a main trunk into two daughter branches of roughly the same size or by a side branch that is smaller than the main vessel. In general, the cross section of each of the branches at the branch point is less than that of the parent vessel, but the sum of their areas is greater than that of the parent. Because total flow must remain constant while total area increases, the velocity of flow in the two branches must decrease relative to that in the parent vessel. The same relationship exists for uneven or multiple branches as long as the total area is greater than that of the parent vessel. Likewise, because both the area and velocity in each branch decrease, the Reynolds number (see following discussion) will be lower, and the stability of flow will increase. These conditions are exactly reversed in the converging channels of the venous system.

The flow pattern at branches is largely determined by the type of branching involved. When a parent vessel divides into two daughter vessels, as illustrated in Figure 9–9A, the streamlines of flow necessarily bend at the branch point, and the junction acts to some extent like an obstacle in the middle of the stream. At the bifurcation of the aorta, e.g., the axial stream of blood impinges on the wall joining the two vessels, creating eddies at the entrance of the branches. Near the outer wall, blood flows relatively smoothly into the outer portion of the daughter vessels. At side branches (Fig. 9–9B) blood flows smoothly into the side branch from the nearest lamina of the main vessel. Small eddies may form in the neighborhood of such junctions, but their effect on the overall flow profile is minimal. In addition, the increased stability of flow tends to prevent downstream propagation of any eddies that do form.[19]

Effects of Projections and Valves on Blood Flow

Projections or obstacles in any moving stream create eddies and turbulence. Whether or not the projection results in complete turbulence depends on the size and shape of the projection, creating the disturbance and the Reynolds number at that point, which is an indication of the stability of flow and, therefore, the tendency to return to a laminar condition downstream from a disturbance. For a sharp-edged projection in a pipe, laminar flow will be present only if

$$h/r < 4/\sqrt{N_r}$$

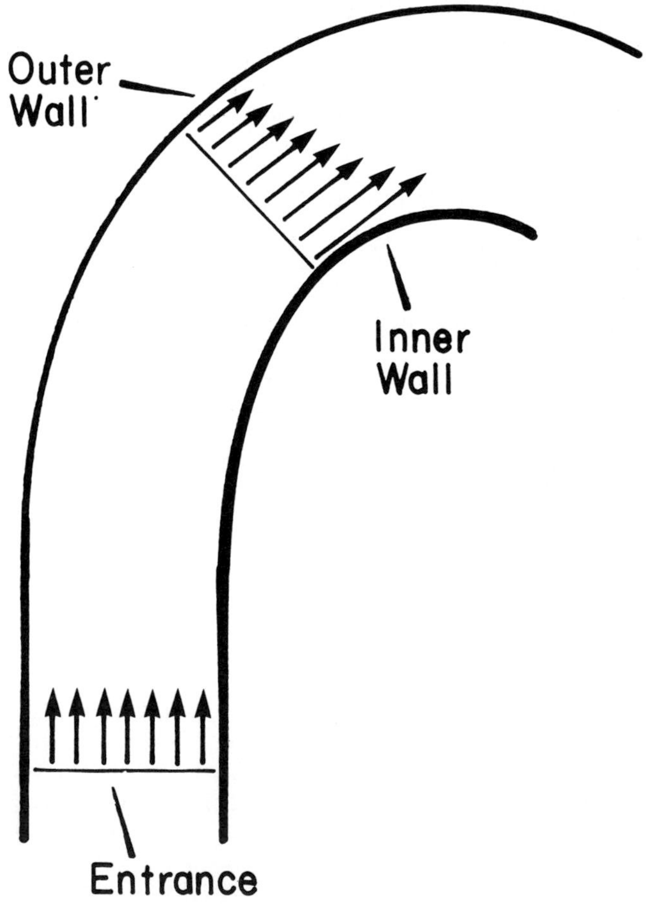

Fig. 9–8. Effects of a curve in a tube on the velocity profile when the profile at the entrance to the tube is flat, which is the normal situation in the ascending aorta. (See text for details.) (After Caro et al., 1978.)

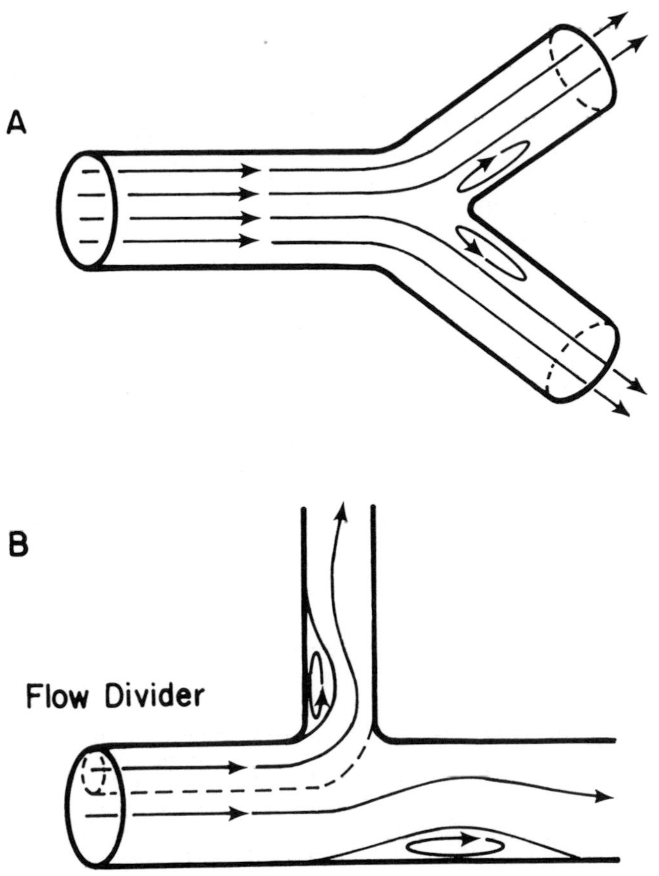

Fig. 9–9. Pattern of flow at branch points in vessels. **A.** Division of main trunk into two daughter vessels. **B.** Side branches.

where h/r is the ratio of the height of the obstruction to the radius of the pipe, and N_r is the Reynolds number, which is defined below. For a smooth obstacle of cylindric cross section, the critical condition is

$$h/r < 5/\sqrt{N_r}$$

The relatively small difference in the numeric coefficients of these equations (4 and 5), indicates that the shape is less important than the relative height of the obstruction.[7]

The only naturally occurring projections into the blood stream are valve cusps, which have the properties of sharp-edged projections. The application of the equation listed previously is only a rough approximation, but for a Reynolds number of 2300, turbulence would be expected if such a projection exceeded 8% of the vessel diameter.

Vortices do, in fact, develop as the aortic valve opens, but in its fully open position, these vortices lie behind the valve leaflets in the sinuses of Valsalva (Fig. 9–10) so that flow in the main stream is not obstructed.[20] Brief periods of turbulence that begin when velocity reaches a peak have been observed in the ascending aorta, but laminar flow is the rule in all other vessels, except for parts of the venae cavae nearest the right atrium.[21]

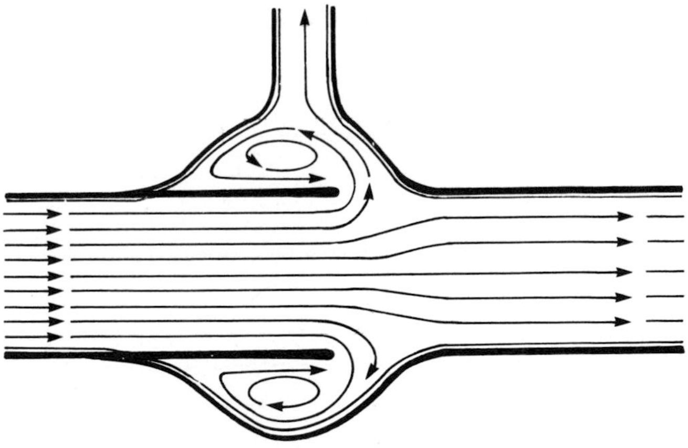

Fig. 9–10. Flow through and around the aortic leaflets in the fully opened position. Vortex formation occurs behind the valve leaflets.

Turbulent Flow

In the condition of laminar flow, the particles in the flow stream move in a constant direction, generally parallel to the wall of the vessel. This requires that sequential layers slip over each other at an increasingly rapid rate as velocity increases. At some critical threshold, this orderly flow pattern begins to break down and is replaced by an irregular, seemingly random, particle motion known as turbulence. The distinction between perfectly laminar and fully developed turbulent flow is clear-cut; however, in the progression from one state to the other, several intermediate but less well-defined stages typically occur (Fig. 9–11A). As velocity increases above some threshold, the parallel flow lines initially begin to exhibit wavy motion (Fig. 9–11B). As these oscillations become larger, vortices begin to appear, which, once established, are propagated downstream (Fig. 9–11C). At first, these vortices disappear, but if velocity is increased still further, they increase in number and duration, leading ultimately to the random particle motion that characterizes turbulent flow (Fig. 9–11D).[7,17]

The first person to describe in detail the factors that influence the transition from laminar to turbulent flow was Osbourne Reynolds in 1833. These variables were combined in a dimensionless term called the Reynolds number, which expresses the tendency of flow to become unstable. For a cylindric tube, the Reynolds number equals

$$N_r = 2r\ v\ p/\eta$$

where r is the radius of the tube, v is the mean velocity of flow, p is the mass density of blood, and η is the viscosity. The Reynolds number represents the ratio of the inertial to the viscous forces. The higher the Reynolds number, the greater the tendency toward turbulence. The critical threshold between laminar and turbulent flow is usually given as roughly 2300. However, as will be shown in the discussion of pulsatile flow, much higher Reynolds numbers have been recorded in the circulation without the occurrence of turbulence. Impor-

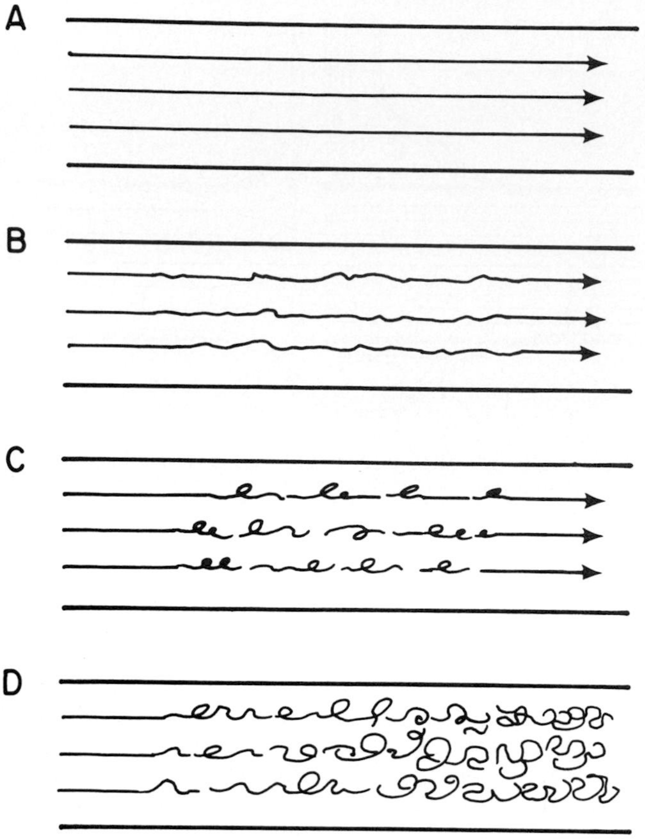

Fig. 9–11. Transition from laminar (A) to turbulent flow (D). (See text for details.)

tantly, when turbulence develops, the normal linear pressure-flow relationship changes abruptly (Fig. 9–12) and the pressure gradient per unit volume increases rapidly because of the dissipation of hydraulic energy in turbulent flow into friction and, therefore, heat energy.[22]

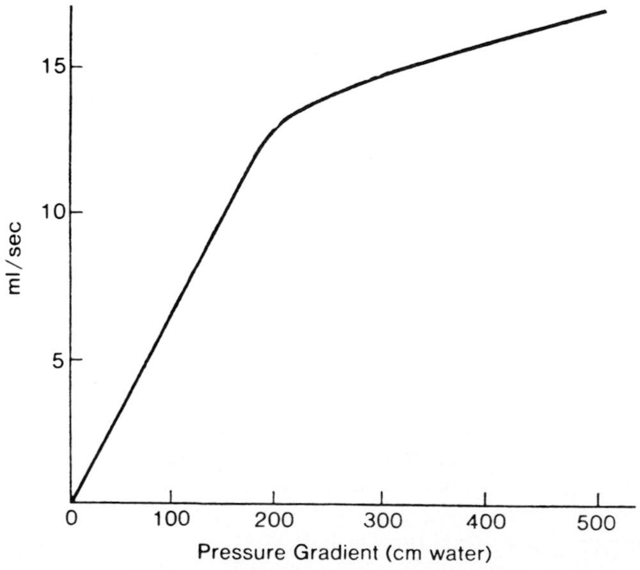

Fig. 9–12. Abrupt change in the relationship between pressure gradient and velocity, which occurs on transition from turbulent to laminar flow. (From Coulter NA Jr, Pappenheimer JR: Development of turbulence in flowing blood. Am J Physiol 159:401, 1949.)

HYDRAULIC ENERGIES

Doppler instruments measure the velocity of blood. However, it is often not the velocity itself but rather the energies or conversion of energy from one form to another to produce a given velocity that is of real interest. The Poiseuille equation describes pressure energy as the sole motive force for fluid flow. Under the special conditions of Poiseuille's experiments, this was correct. In the clinical setting, however, gravitational and kinetic energy also must be considered. Energy, which is the capacity to do work, is the produce of force and distance, and can be expressed in dyn cm. Pressure is defined as force per unit area (dyn cm^2), and it can also be considered as energy per unit volume or dyn cm/ml. The pressure energy (Wp) associated with a pressure P, in a volume of blood, v, is therefore

$$Wp = P \cdot V \qquad [9.11]$$

The second form of hydraulic energy is kinetic energy. Blood in motion possesses a kinetic energy (Wk) that depends on its mass and the square of its velocity. Mass, in turn, is the product of density (ρ, g (mass)/ml) and volume so that

$$Wk = 1/2\rho \cdot V \cdot v^2 \qquad [9.12]$$

For steady flow, v is the mean velocity. For pulsatile flow, take the integral of the time derivatives of the variables in equation 9.12.

The final form of energy is gravitational energy. This component (Wg) is the potential energy inherent in a volume of blood by virtue of its position relative to some arbitrary horizontal reference. It equals the product of the density of blood (ρ), the gravitational acceleration constant (g), which is roughly 981 cm/sec^2, the height of the blood above the reference level (h), and the volume of blood involved (V).

$$Wg = \rho g h V \qquad [9.13]$$

The total hydraulic energy, Wt, of the blood at any point in the circulation is the sum of these components or

$$Wt = pV + 1/2\rho\, V \cdot v^2 + \rho g h V \qquad [9.14]$$

Alternatively, each term can be expressed as energy per unit volume by dividing each term by V. All of the terms are then in dyn cm^2. The kinetic and gravitational energies per unit volume are referred to as *equivalent pressures*. The total equivalent pressure (P′) or the hydraulic energy per unit volume then equals

$$P' = P + 1/2\, \rho v^2 + \rho g h \qquad [9.15]$$

The energy gradient between any two points in the vascular system expressed as equivalent pressure is

$$P'_1 - P'_2 = (P_1 - P_2) + 1/2\rho\,(v_1^2 - v_2^2) + \rho g(h_1 - h_2) \qquad [9.16]$$

This is a more general expression of the energy available to move blood than the Poiseuille equation, which considers only the energy dissipated by viscous friction. Poiseuille could neglect the kinetic and gravitational terms because of the special conditions of his experiment; although the theoretic derivation of his equation specifically assumes that these terms remain constant. In the circulation, blood always moves toward regions of lower total hydraulic energy, and although pressure energy is typically much greater than the kinetic or gravitational energy, this is not always the case, as discussed later.[7]

Effects of Changes in Tube or Vessel Diameter on Hydraulic Energies

Conversion of Pressure to Kinetic Energy

The kinetic energy associated with blood flow normally is relatively small, but it can become significant when pressure energy is converted into kinetic energy and vice versa. Such conversions occur whenever the velocity of blood flow changes, as in a tube that narrows or widens abruptly. The law that describes this conversion of energy from one form to another is called Bernoulli's Law after the eighteenth century hydrodynamicist and mathematician Daniel Bernoulli. Bernoulli's law, which is based on the more fundamental law of conservation of mass and energy, states that the total energy at all points along a tube through which fluid is moving (providing that viscous frictional losses can be ignored) must be the same. Because kinetic energy is proportional to the product of density and the square of velocity, any change in velocity will alter the kinetic energy. Total energy must remain constant and, therefore, any increase in kinetic energy requires a corresponding change in one of the other energy components. For the purposes of this discussion, gravitational energy will be ignored and attention focused on the interconversion of kinetic and pressure energy. Figure 9–12 is an example of this law, in which kinetic energy is converted into pressure energy. This figure depicts a rigid tube that increases in cross-sectional area from A1 at point 1 to A2 at point 2. Small vertical tubes indicate the pressure at each site. The two points are assumed to be so close together that the viscous pressure gradient between them is negligible. Given a steady flow condition, the volume entering the tube must be the same as the volume leaving it, and the volume flow rate (Q) will be the same at every cross section of the tube. The average velocity at any cross section is then by definition

$$v\ (\text{average}) = Q/A \qquad [9.17]$$

so that;

$$A_1 v_1 = Q = A_2 v_2 \qquad [9.18]$$

Equation 9.18 is often called the *continuity equation* because it expresses the continuity of mass at sequential points along the flow stream. Because A_2 in Figure 9–13 is greater than A_1, it follows that v_2 must be less than v_1. The decrease in velocity as blood moves into the

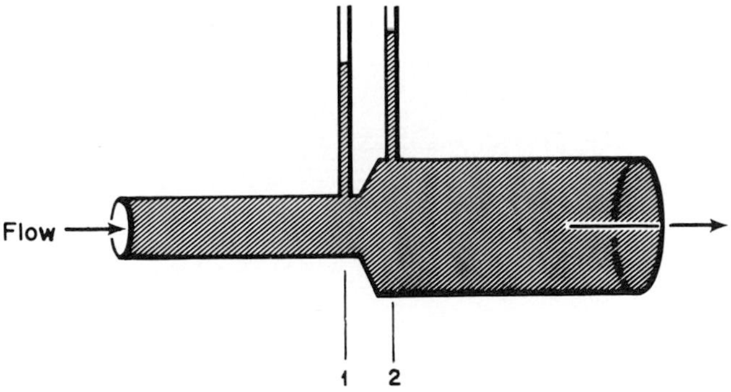

Fig. 9–13. Bernoulli's principle. Cross-sectional area of a tube increases from sampling point 1 to sampling point 2. Because area increases, velocity must decrease to keep flow constant. However, the loss of kinetic energy in the form of velocity must be balanced by an increase in pressure to maintain total energy constant. The pressure at site 2, therefore, is higher than at site 1. (See text for details.) (After Milnor, 1982.)

wider portion of the tube is accompanied by an associated decrease in kinetic energy, because by definition kinetic energy is proportional to the square of the velocity. Nevertheless, the total energy at point 2 must be the same as at point 1 in accordance with the laws of conservation of energy and mass. Therefore, from the equation for total hydraulic energy, omitting the gravitational term

$$P_1 + 1/2\ \rho v_1^2 = P_2 + 1/2\ \rho v_2^2 \qquad [9.19]$$

and the pressure at P_2 equals

$$P_2 = P_1 + 1/2\rho\ (v_1^2 - v_2^2) \qquad [9.20]$$

Because mean velocity, v, equals Q/A and Q is constant at both sites, the relationship of the change in pressure to the change in area can also be determined by substituting for velocity.

$$P_2 = P_1 + 1/2\rho\ (Q^2/A_1^2 - Q^2/A_2^2) \qquad [9.21]$$

or

$$P_2 = P_1 + \rho\ Q^2/2\ (1/A_1^2 - 1/A_2^2) \qquad [9.22]$$

The widening of the tube, in other words, increases the total pressure at site 2 by an amount that depends on the change in velocity and cross-sectional area. The right side of the equation represents the kinetic energy that is converted to pressure energy under these conditions. If the tube was to narrow rather than widen, velocity would increase and pressure energy would be converted to kinetic energy. This is the far more interesting situation from the Doppler viewpoint and is discussed in detail in the next section.

Effects of Stenotic Lesions. In accordance with the continuity equation, any abrupt narrowing of a tube or stenosis of a vessel causes the velocity of the fluid particles to increase (assuming that the fluid is incompressible) as they flow through the narrowed segment to maintain the flow volume constant at each cross section (see

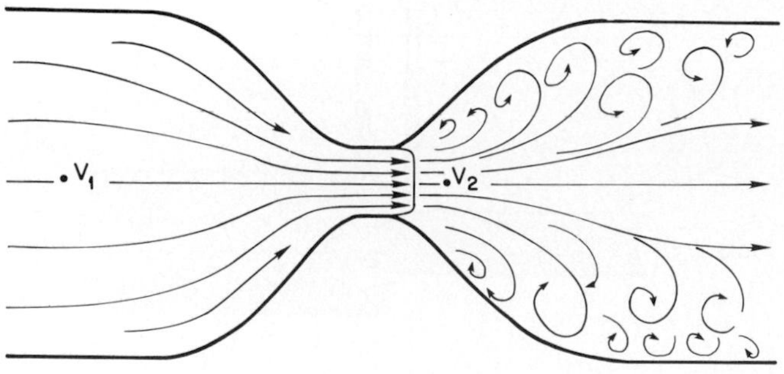

Fig. 9–14. The flow through a stenotic lesion.

equation 9.18). This increase in velocity is associated with convergence of the streamlines of flow and is, therefore, termed *convective acceleration*. Convective acceleration is associated with the conversion of pressure energy to kinetic energy and, therefore, a decrease in pressure within the narrowed area. The change in the pattern of flow and vascular area for a representative stenotic lesion is illustrated in Figure 9–14. In this diagram, point 1 is considered to be proximal to the narrowing and point 2 to lie along the same streamline of flow within the area of peak flow velocity. In addition to convective acceleration, this figure illustrates several other important concepts. First, the point of peak velocity (point 2) is not actually within the stenosis but slightly beyond. This placement is appropriate because the streamlines of flow continue to converge beyond the orifice, and the maximal velocity occurs at the point where the flow jet is narrowest (the vena contracta). Second, the flow profile in the stenosis is flat but retains its laminar character and associated pressure velocity relationship. Third, convective acceleration begins at the onset of narrowing, and the reference velocity, V_1, must be taken proximal to this point. Finally, distal to point 2 (the vena contracta), flow breaks down into a random pattern of eddies and turbulences, which dissipates the kinetic energy in the jet (Fig. 9–15). Because Bernoulli's

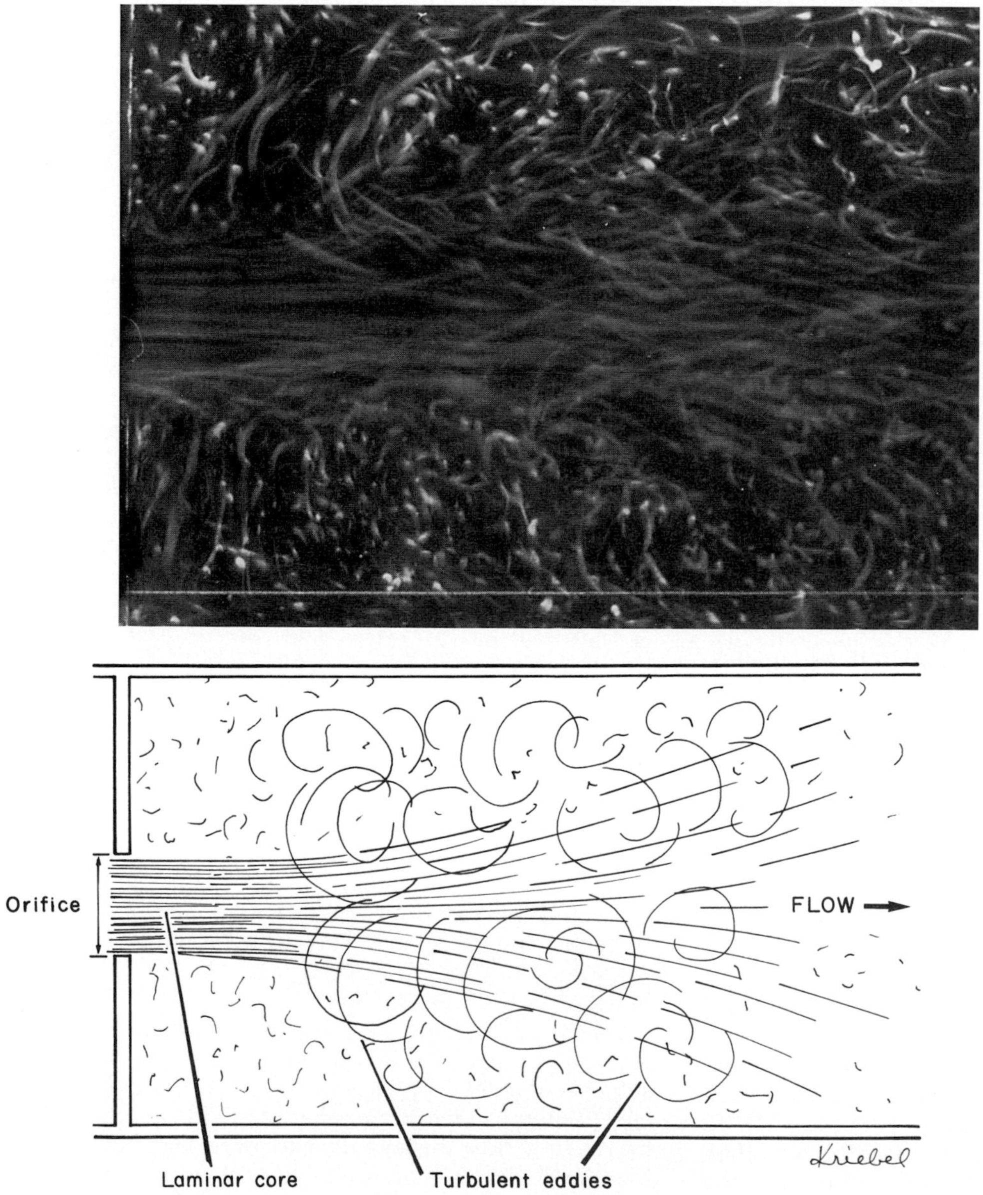

Fig. 9–15. Streamlines of flow breaking down into turbulence distal to a stenotic lesion. Because of the sudden expansion of the jet, the poststenotic jet interacts with adjacent stagnant regions creating turbulent eddies that invade the jet and limit pressure recovery. (From Levine RA, et al.: Pressure recovery distal to a stenosis: potential cause of gradient "overestimation" by Doppler echocardiography. J Am Coll Cardiol 13:706, 1989.)

Law requires that the energy at points 1 and 2 is equal, we again find that

$$P_1 + 1/2\ \rho v_1^2 = P_2 + 1/2\ p v_2^2$$

or

$$P_1 - P_2 = 1/2\ \rho(v_2^2 - v_1^2) \qquad [9.23]$$

Thus, using the Bernoulli relationship, we can calculate the difference in pressure between points 1 and 2 from the difference in velocity between the same two points. Further, because the kinetic energy at point 2 is dissipated downstream rather than being reconstituted to pressure energy, the pressure drop associated with convective acceleration is representative of the pressure gradient across the obstruction.* In clinical studies, this relationship can be further simplified as follows: First, because v_1 is usually much smaller than v_2 (roughly 0.2 m/sec for the mitral valve and 0.8 m/sec for the aortic valve), it can be ignored in most cases. Second, solving for p with appropriate correction for units of measure† yields a value of roughly 4 so the final equation becomes

$$P_1 - P_2 = 4v^2 \qquad [9.24]$$

This is the simplified Bernoulli equation. This equation, however, describes only the pressure drop that results from convective acceleration or the conversion of pressure energy to kinetic energy. It ignores viscous friction and the energy required to overcome inertial forces caused by changes in flow rate over time (flow acceleration) found in pulsatile systems such as the circulation. In the clinical setting where these factors must be considered, we obtain a more complete form of the Bernoulli equation with an added viscous friction term.[23]

$$P_1 - P_2 = 1/2\rho(v_2^2 - v_1^2) + \rho \int_1^2 \frac{d\vec{v}}{dt d\vec{s}} + R(\vec{v}) \qquad [9.25]$$

where v> is the velocity vector of the fluid element along its path and ds> is the path length. The flow acceleration term applies only during valve opening and closure, when flow acceleration is high. It causes a delay between the pressure drop curve and the velocity curve because during this period, pressure energy is being expended to overcome inertia rather than being converted to kinetic energy. The pressure drop calculated from the velocity, therefore, is delayed from the true curve, as indicated in Figure 9–16. Assuming that the acceleration is constant over the path length between points 1 and 2, the magnitude of this pressure loss can be calculated as follows:

$$P = \rho\ dv/dt\ L \qquad [9.26]$$

* This dissipation may be incomplete, leading to partial pressure recovery, particularly if the obstruction is stream lined.[36]

† $\rho = 1.06/981\ g\ s^2/cm^3 \times 1/1.36$ (to convert dyn cm to mm Hg) × 1/2, which after appropriate conversion of measurement units ($\cdot 10^4$) equals 3.972, or roughly 4.

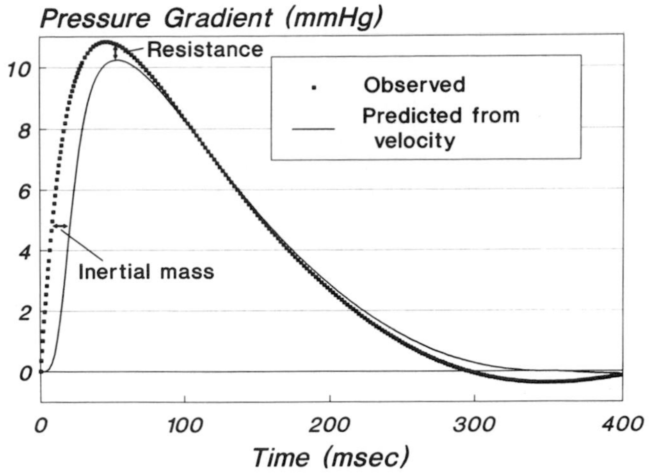

Fig. 9–16. Relationship of pressure gradient to velocity for flow through a valve orifice in an in vitro model. Squares indicate the recorded pressure gradient. The solid line represents the gradient that would be predicted from the instantaneous velocities. Separation of the two curves at the onset of flow is caused by the energy required to accelerate the inertial mass of blood. The difference in the observed and predicted gradients at peak flow reflects viscous losses. (Data courtesy of Thomas JD.)

Pressure loss caused by acceleration, therefore, increases in direct relation to the velocity gradient and the path length over which the acceleration occurs. For stenotic mitral valves, where the amount of acceleration is not great (e.g., 0 to 2 m/sec^2) and jet length relatively short (e.g., 3 cm), the calculated pressure drop caused by acceleration has been shown to be on the order of 5 mm Hg.[23] For aortic stenosis, where the peak velocity is typically greater (e.g., 5 m/sec) and the jet longer (e.g., 5 cm), the pressure drop caused by acceleration increases to roughly 20 mm Hg. Thus, during valve opening and closure, the flow acceleration term may be of the same order as the convective acceleration term. When the valve is open, however, flow acceleration decreases significantly, and the convective acceleration term becomes so dominant that any pressure loss caused by flow acceleration can be neglected. At the time of maximum velocity, flow acceleration is zero.

The magnitude of the pressure loss caused by viscous friction is more difficult to estimate. Viscous losses arise from friction between neighboring fluid elements and, therefore, will depend not only on v_2 but on the whole velocity profile. Provided that fluid remains laminar, these losses should be minimal over the short length of most stenoses. Deviation from a laminar profile, however, will greatly increase energy (pressure) loss. Most studies have examined the losses caused by viscous friction using steady flow conditions so that acceleration can be ignored. Given this experimental setting, any time the measured pressure drop deviates from that predicted by the convective acceleration term ($4v^2$), it can be related to viscous losses.

Experimental studies further suggest that the viscous friction term can be ignored until the size or length of the stenosis reaches a critical point at which normal laminar flow begins to break down.[24–26] At this point, the relation of measured pressure drop to that predicted from convective acceleration ($4v^2$) begins to fail (i.e., the pressure gradient will be greater than that predicted by convective acceleration alone). For orifices of 1 to 2 mm in length and ranging in area from 1.5 cm^2 to 0.1 cm^2, an excellent correlation has been noted between the measured gradient and that predicted using the simplified Bernoulli equation.[24–26] Below 0.1 cm^2, results differ, with some authors suggesting that the correlations remain excellent down to 0.01 cm^2,[26] whereas others report that at these levels the ratio of the directly measured to the Doppler-derived gradients falls below 1.[24,25] For orifices of this small size, however, high gradients become difficult to interpret because normal laminar flow is often converted to a fine spray that causes both dispersion of the Doppler signal and energy loss. Validity of the $4V^2$ relationship has also been verified for orifices of irregular shape and for orifices in parallel.[26] This is dictated by the Bernoulli equation because if the pressure gradient between two reservoirs is constant, the velocities through two parallel orifices connecting the reservoirs also must be the same, irrespective of size.

Finally, in vitro data[26] suggest that Doppler-measured gradients are also accurate for tunnel-like obstruction within certain anatomic limitations. Tunnels with cross-sectional areas of 0.5 cm^2 or greater yield accurate Doppler measurements for tunnel lengths up to 4 cm. At tunnel areas of 0.25 cm^2, however, it was found that Doppler examination underestimated pressure by 15% for a 4-cm tunnel length; for a 0.06-cm^2 tunnel area, this underestimation increased as tunnel length increased from 0.1 to 4 cm, with an underestimation of the manometric gradient of as much as 42% at the 4-cm length. These discrepancies result from viscous losses that become important as the length of the tunnels increase.

Thus, the modified Bernoulli equation accurately describes pressure gradient across most clinically encountered stenotic lesions. Although the relationships break down in experimental models of small orifices (less than 0.1 cm^2) and long tunnels (4 cm), lesions with these dimensions are of more concern to those involved in research applications of Doppler echocardiography (i.e, velocity measurements across a coronary stenosis) and are not relevant to typical stenosis of the cardiac valves or great vessels. The one simplification that may lead to error, however, is the assumption that $V_1 \ll V_2$. Although this is usually the case, in some situations, such as aortic insufficiency or coarctation of the aorta, failure to consider the proximal velocity may introduce significant error.

Valve Area Determination. Calculation of the cross-sectional area of the flow stream through a region of stenosis is also possible using Equations 9.19 and 9.20. In this case, however, the streamlines of flow in the jet issuing from the orifice will continue to converge for a short distance (the vena contracta). By the time the flow lines have again become parallel, the cross-sectional area of the jet (which in this case is A_2) will be smaller than the orifice area (A_o; Fig. 9–17). The ratio of A_2 to A_o, or the ratio of the area of the vena contracta to the orifice area, is called the *coefficient of contraction*. This ratio is affected by the original size of the tube (A1), the

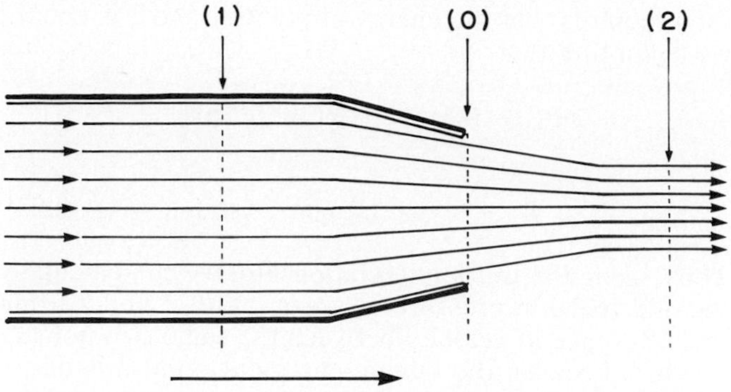

Figure 9–17. Flow pattern through a stenotic orifice. (1) Area proximal to the stenosis. (0) Anatomic orifice A_o. (2) Flow area at the vena contracta or the effective orifice A_e. (After Milnor, 1982.)

shape of the inlet, and the orifice size. To determine the anatomic orifice size, some correction must be introduced to account for this coefficient of contraction, which is unknown in most cases. Such calculations are facilitated by a term used in engineering called the *coefficient of discharge*. The coefficient of discharge can be defined such that the terms in the parentheses of equation 22 can be expressed as

$$(1/A_2^2 - 1/A_1^2) = 1/Ao^2\ Cd^2 \qquad [9.27]$$

with the result that equation becomes

$$P_1 - P_2 = \rho\ Q^2/2\ (1/AO^2\ Cd^2) \qquad [9.28]$$

and Ao is

$$Ao = Q/Cd\ \sqrt{(\rho/2(P_1 - P_2))} \qquad [9.29]$$

In other words, if Cd is known or has been determined experimentally for a given configuration (i.e., a stenosed valve), the orifice area can be calculated from measurement of pressure and flow.[7]

Gorlin and Gorlin were the first to apply this concept to the measurement of orifice size in patients with valvular stenosis.[27] Recognizing that blood viscosity, turbulence, pulsatile flow, and the inconstant shape of deformed valves made it almost impossible to predict the discharge coefficient analytically, they determined an empiric coefficient from direct measurement of mitral valves at surgery or autopsy. For the mitral valve, they concluded that valve area A_o is

$$A_o = Q/31\ \sqrt{(P_1 - P_2)} \qquad [9.30]$$

which corresponds to a discharge coefficient of roughly 0.7. It is important to remember that because ρ is a constant, the pressure gradient flow relationship in the orifice is entirely defined by the magnitude of A_e, the effective orifice at the vena contracta, which is the same as A2 in Figure 6–17. Thus, A_e is the measure of flow obstruction in the orifice so that the smaller the A_e, the greater the obstruction. The product Cd A_o is also a measure of obstruction, but A_o alone is not such a measure because Cd can be expected to vary from orifice to orifice. If velocity and area (flow proximal to the stenosis) are known and peak velocity at the stenosis can be measured, then area can be calculated using the continuity equation $A_1V_1 = Q = A_2V_2$ (Equation 9.18).

or $$A_1v_1/v_2 = A_2 \qquad [9.31]$$

This result, however, is A_e, not A_o, which is correct because A_e defines the pressure flow relationship across the orifice.

PULSATILE FLOW

The majority of the discussion of flow up to this point has dealt with steady-state flow. The concept of pulsatile flow has been introduced only in the analysis of the Bernoulli equation. This simplification has been deliberate because the analysis and mathematic description of pulsatile flow in the tapering, elastic vessels of the circulatory system is obviously more complex than that of constant flow in rigid tubes. As noted earlier, the concepts of flow in rigid tubes are qualitatively correct when applied to the circulation, and many of the effects of superimposed pulsations become apparent only over distance. Because of this latter property, most models of the circulatory system assume a tube of infinite length. Doppler studies, in contrast, deal with flow at specific locations or over short distances and are less affected by variables that relate to the cable properties of the circulation. The presence of pulsations, however, introduces four additional variables that are of interest in Doppler studies. First, pulsations introduce inertial forces associated with the acceleration and deceleration of the blood column. Second, they produce changes in the size and shape of the pressure and flow waves as they travel through the circulatory system. Third, they produce cyclic variations in the diameter of the elastic vessels through which they travel. Finally, and perhaps most importantly, they alter the velocity profile at various points in the vascular system.

The inertial forces required to accelerate the blood column with each pulsation are described by Newton's Second Law, which states that force equals mass times acceleration. It is a fundamental assumption of all models of pulsatile flow that the pressure or force per unit area required to move a particle of fluid is exactly balanced by the inertial forces associated with acceleration plus the viscous forces that must be overcome in moving the fluid. Because inertial forces are associated with acceleration and deceleration, they are strongest during the onset and termination of systole in the major arteries and at the onset and termination of diastole for flow across the atrioventricular valves. These inertial forces shift the velocity curves to the right, relative to the pressure curve but, as described previously, do not change velocity-pressure relationships during periods of established flow.

In the pulsatile flow state, intermittent cardiac contractions produce pulses of pressure and flow that propagate as sinusoidal waves along the receiving vessels. The mean pressure in the human ascending aorta is 85 mm Hg. Because of the relatively large vessel diameter, in the absence of pulsations the drop in mean pressure from the ascending to the terminal aorta would be small (less than 1 mm Hg). In a system free of reflections, the amplitude of the pressure pulse also would decrease gradually along the aorta because of the viscoelasticity of the vessels. Because of the pulsatile nature of the system, however, pressure waves are reflected back from the periphery and augment sequential incoming pulses in such a way that a given pressure wave actually increases in amplitude as it travels. A pulse pressure of 50 mm Hg in the ascending aorta increases to about 65 mm Hg at the terminal aorta and becomes even larger in the radial artery. The shape of the pressure wave also changes as it moves peripherally, the early portion rising more steeply and the secondary peak becoming more prominent. The amplification of the pressure pulse is a function of age; it is significant in children, diminishes with advancing years, and is usually absent after the age of 60.

Pressure and flow waves in the periphery are delayed by finite transit times that depend on the wave velocity and distance from the heart. Aortic wave velocities are 6 to 8 m/sec, and the transit time through the whole aorta is of the order of 50 msec.

The effects of reflections on flow and velocity waves are just the opposite of those on pressure waves (as transmission line theory predicts). Partial cancellation by reflections is added to the attenuating effects of viscosity, and the pulsations of the flow waves gradually decrease in amplitude as they travel down the aorta and out into the arterial tree. The ratio of pulse-to-mean flow falls from about 6.3 in the ascending aorta to 5.6 in the abdominal aorta, to 2 to 4 in the femoral artery, and to less than 2 in more distal arteries. Peak flow falls as the pulse amplitude diminishes, but diastolic flow rises, so that forward motion continues throughout the cardiac cycle.

The action of the arterial tree on the form of the pressure and flow waveforms is ultimately determined by three factors: vessel compliance, blood inertia, and peripheral conductance. The first two factors combine to produce the wave pulse transmission pattern that causes reflections. As discussed previously, this process changes the waveforms and can even cause oscillatory behavior of the flow pulse as one moves from the heart toward the periphery.

The effect of the conductive properties of the system on flow is proportional to pressure. An increase in peripheral conduction causes the flow waveform to more closely resemble the pressure waveform in the arteries of the organs and the brain and also in the arteries that feed muscles during work. The contractility of the heart therefore affects waveforms primarily in the arteries, closest to the ventricles (left and right), whereas the influence of transmission line effects on the pulse waveforms increases as one moves toward the periphery.[7]

VESSEL DIAMETER

Because blood vessels are distensible, their diameter is a function of transmural pressure. Given a fixed pressure gradient and external pressure, a distensible tube will naturally assume a slightly tapered shape because transmural pressure will fall along the length of the vessel. With pulsatile flow, the diameter of the vessel varies, becoming greatest as the pressure wave passes. This is a complex relationship because the elasticity of the wall will also affect the transmission and reflection characteristics of the pressure pulse as well as its shape. Because all Doppler measurements of flow require consideration of vessel diameter, some correction for the time varying changes in tube radius are obviously necessary. Methods of correction are discussed further in Chapter 30.

VELOCITY PROFILE

Finally, the superimposition of pulsations on steady-state flow influences the spatial as well as the temporal pattern of the velocity profile. Measurements in the ascending aorta show a significant blunting of the central portions of the velocity profile with nothing representing a true parabolic flow profile in any part of the cycle (Fig. 9–18).[17,28–30] In the lower thoracic and abdominal aorta, a more or less parabolic front, however, appears to develop.[14,28,29,31]

In the canine femoral artery (Fig. 9–19), in contrast, the profile is blunt at the onset of systole, becomes almost parabolic in midsystole, and then flattens again in diastole. In early diastole, a clear reversal of direction appears in the outer lamina, at a time when the central portion is still moving forward. Retrograde motion eventually occurs in all lamina, then dies away toward the end of the cycle.[30,31]

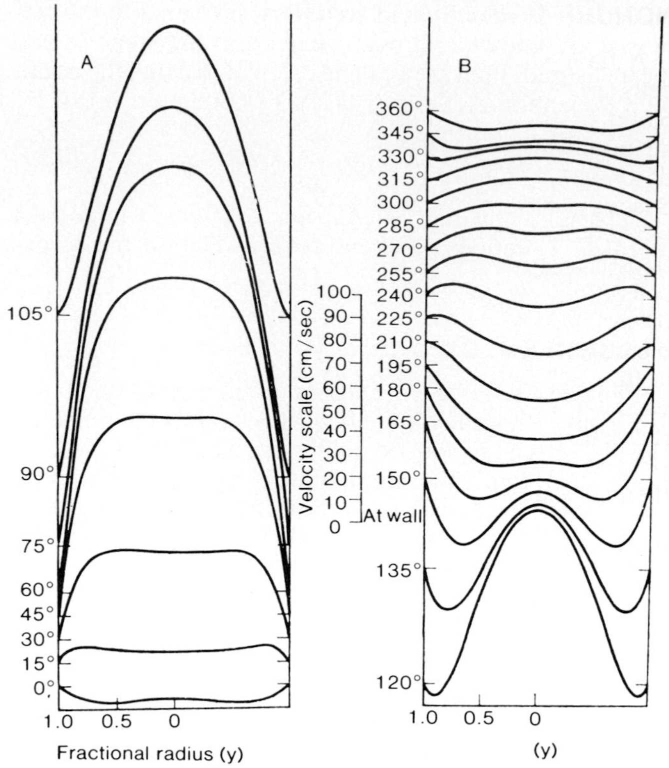

Fig. 9–19. Calculated velocity profiles in the femoral artery of the dog. The ordinate points are velocities at sequential points in the cardiac cycle from 0 to 360°. Abscissa: relative radial coordinates from the center of the vessel (0) to the outer wall (1). The amplitude of each curve from its baseline indicates the velocity of flow for each radial location at that point in the cardiac cycle. (From McDonald DA: Blood Flow in the Arteries. London, Edward Arnold, 1974.)

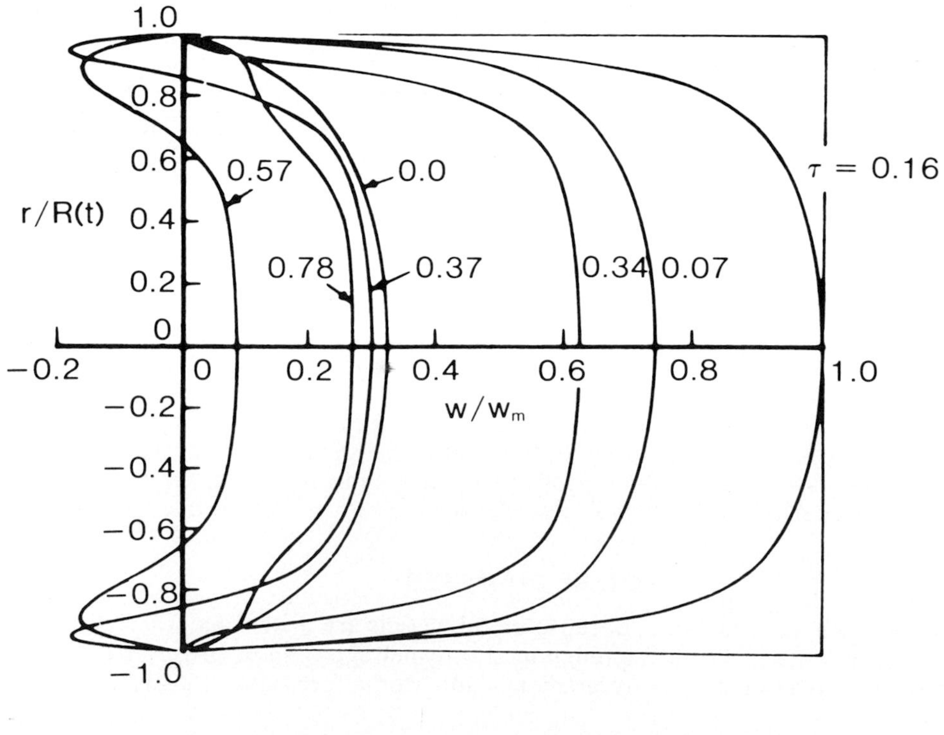

Fig. 9–18. Pattern of flow in the descending thoracic aorta of an anesthetized dog. Ordinate: radial position as a fraction of luminal radius; abscissa: ratio of measured velocity to maximal center line velocity (W/W_m). Profiles at seven different instants expressed as fractions of the cardiac cycle are shown. (From Ling SC, Atabek HB, Letzing WG, Patel DJ: Nonlinear analysis of aortic flow in living dogs. Circ Res 33:198, 1973.)

NONUNIFORM SUSPENSION OF CELLS

A final point of interest is the observation that red cells are not uniformly distributed in blood. The fact that blood is not a simple fluid but a suspension of cells has an influence on flow patterns quite apart from the factors described by the Reynolds number. Blood cells are not concentrated evenly across the lumen of blood vessels but tend to be fewer near the walls than in the rest of the stream. The cause of this preferential distribution of cells is not known with certainty, but the size and shape of the cell limits it proximity to the vessel wall. The major effect of the uneven radial distribution of cells is that the transit time of the erythrocyte through the vascular tree is shorter than that of plasma. Because red cells travel preferentially in the central parts of the stream, which has the highest velocity in laminar flow, their net velocity is higher than that of plasma.

Summary of Flow Patterns in Major Vessels

Because much of the data presented to this point are based on mathematical models and flow in rigid tubes, it is worthwhile to review the available experimental information concerning the normal flow patterns in the areas of greatest interest for Doppler studies, i.e., the proximal great vessels and the atrioventricular valves.

In the aorta, blood flow begins immediately after the opening of the aortic valve, rises rapidly to a peak, then falls continuously during the remainder of the ejection period. The contour of the flow wave is determined primarily by the contractile properties of ventricular muscle, but it is also influenced by the aortic input impedance. The area beneath the flow curve is proportional to the stroke volume. Peak aortic flow bears a fairly constant relationship to mean flow or cardiac output and is usually about six times as high as mean flow.[7] Acceleration of blood reaches a maximum during early ejection, amounting to 5000 to 8000 cm/sec^2 in the dog at rest. Relatively few direct measurements of this variable have been made in humans, but the published flow tracings suggest that it is somewhat lower than in the dog,[32–34] a difference that may be associated with heart rate. Peak acceleration is one of the many variables that have been proposed as an indication of myocardial contractility.[35]

The flow profile at the beginning of the ascending aorta, 1 or 2 cm beyond the aortic valve, is essentially flat.[17] There is a sleeve of relatively low velocity near the wall, but the rest of the blood moves like a cylindric "plug," just as it does at the entrance to a model tube supplied by a reservoir. As this flat profile moves into the aortic arch, it becomes skewed, with lamina moving more slowly near the outer wall of the curve.[9,18,31,36] This asymmetry is probably attributable in part to flow into the large branches of the arch as well as to the effects of curving on the initially blunt profile. It is sometimes much less significant than in Figure 9–8 and has not been observed in all experiments. The difference between inner and outer wall velocities is accentuated by relatively high cardiac outputs. At the beginning of the arch, secondary helical flow patterns similar to those demonstrated in curved pipes have been observed. Beyond the arch, the velocity profile again becomes symmetric, and in the lower thoracic aorta, the profile is typically parabolic.

Turbulence is occasionally recorded in the ascending aorta. In the upper thoracic aorta, at peak velocity and for a short time during deceleration, turbulence has also been suggested. Flow in the lower thoracic and abdominal aorta is essentially laminar.

Pulmonary Artery

Outflow from the right ventricle, like that from the left ventricle, rises rapidly in early systole. However, maximum acceleration in the pulmonary artery is only about half that in the ascending aorta, and the pulmonary arterial flow profile has a lower, more rounded peak. Normal respiration affects the volume, resistance, and compliance of the pulmonary bed. Right ventricular stroke volume and peak flow in the pulmonary artery normally increase in the beat immediately following the onset of inspiration. The velocity profile appears to be relatively flat under normal conditions.[7]

REFERENCES

1. Reid JM, et al.: The scattering of ultrasound by red blood cells. Proc 8th ICMBE 10:7, 1969.
2. Rschevkin SN: A Course of Lectures on the Theory of Sound. Oxford, Pergamon Press, 1963.
3. Shung KK, Sigelmann RA, Reid JM: Scattering of ultrasound by blood. IEEE Trans Biomed Eng BME 23:460, 1976.
4. Sigelmann RA, Reid JM: Analysis and measurement of ultrasound backscattering from an ensemble of scatterers excited by sine-wave bursts. J Acoust Soc Am 53:1351, 1973.
5. Atkinson P, Berry MV: Random noise in ultrasonic echoes diffracted by blood. J Physiol A 7:1293, 1974.
6. Angelsen BAJ: A theoretical study of the scattering of ultrasound from blood. IEEE Trans Biomed Eng BME 27:61, 1980.
7. Milnor WR: Hemodynamics. Baltimore, Williams & Wilkins, 1982.
8. Johnson PC: Hemodynamics. Annu Rev Physiol 31:331, 1969.
9. Whitmore RL: Rheology of the Circulation. Oxford, Pergamon Press, 1968.
10. McDonald DA: Blood Flow in Arteries. London, Edward Arnold, 1974.
11. Merrill EW: Rheology of Blood. Physiol Rev 49:863, 1969.
12. Cokelet GR, et al.: The rheology of human blood measurement near and at zero shear rate. Trans Soc Rheol 7:303, 1963.
13. Chien S, et al.: Effects of hematocrit and plasma proteins on human blood rheology at low shear rates. J Appl Physiol 21:81, 1966.
14. Nerem RM, et al.: Hot-film anemometer velocity measurements of arterial blood flow in horses. Circ Res 34:193, 1974.
15. Stein PD, Sabbah HN: Turbulent blood flow in the ascending aorta of humans with normal and diseased aortic valves. Circ Res 39:58, 1976.
16. Attinger EO: Pressure transmission in pulmonary arteries related to frequency and geometry. Circ Res 12:623, 1963.
17. Caro CG, et al.: The Mechanics of the Circulation. New York, Oxford University Press, 1978.
18. Lyne WH: Unsteady viscous flow in a curved pipe. J Fluid Mech 45:13, 1971.
19. McDonald DA: The occurrence of turbulent flow in the rabbit aorta. J Physiol 118:340, 1952.
20. Bellhouse BJ, Bellhouse FH: Mechanism of closure of the aortic valve. Nature 217:86, 1968.
21. Helps EPW, McDonald DA: Observations on laminar flow in veins. J Physiol 124:631, 1954.
22. Coulter NA Jr, Pappenheimer JR: Development of turbulence in flowing blood. Am J Physiol 159:401, 1949.
23. Hatle L, Angelsen B: Doppler Ultrasound in Cardiology. Philadelphia, Lea & Febiger, 1985.
24. Holen J, et al.: Determination of effective orifice area in mitral stenosis from non-invasive ultrasound Doppler data and mitral flow rate. Acta Med Scand 201:83, 1978.
25. Requarth JA, et al.: In vitro verification of Doppler prediction of transvalve pressure gradient and orifice area in stenosis. Am J Cardiol 53:1369, 1984.
26. Teirstein PS, Yock PG, Popp RL: The accuracy of Doppler ultrasound measurement of pressure gradients across irregular, dual, and tunnellike obstructions to blood flow. Circulation 72:577, 1985.
27. Gorlin R, Gorlin SG: Hydraulic formula for calculation of the area of the stenotic mitral valve, other cardiac valves, and central circulatory shunts. Am Heart J 41:1, 1951.

28. Schultz DL, et al.: Velocity distribution and transition in the arterial system. *In* Wolstenholme GEW, Knight J (eds.): Circulatory and Respiratory Mass Transport, Ciba Foundation Symposium. Boston, Little, Brown, p. 172, 1969.
29. Schultz DL: Pressure and flow in large arteries. *In* Bergel DH (ed.): Cardiovascular Fluid Dynamics. Vol. 1. London, Academic Press, p. 287, 1972.
30. Ling SC, et al.: Nonlinear analysis of aortic flow in living dogs. Circ Res 33:198, 1973.
31. Seed WA, Wood NB: Velocity patterns in the aorta. Cardiovasc Res 5:319, 1971.
32. Gabe IT, et al.: Measurement of instantaneous blood flow velocity and pressure in conscious man with a catheter-tip velocity probe. Circulation 40:603, 1969.
33. Mills CJ, et al.: Pressure-flow relationships and vascular impedance in man. Cardiovasc Res 4:405, 1970.
34. Nichols WW, et al.: Input impedance of the systemic circulation in man. Circ Res 40:451, 1977
35. Nobel MIM, Trenchard D, Guz A: Left ventricular ejection in conscious dogs: measurement and significance of the maximum acceleration of blood from the left ventricle. Circ Res 19:139, 1966.
36. Levine RA, et al.: Pressure recovery distal to a stenosis: potential cause of gradient "overestimation" by Doppler echocardiography. J Am Coll Cardiol 13:706, 1989.

CHAPTER

10

DOPPLER SIGNAL PROCESSING

To this point we have (1) shown how the frequency of a sound wave reflected from a moving target is shifted by an amount that is directly related to the velocity of target motion; (2) described the complex nature of the target of primary interest—flowing blood in the human circulatory system; and (3) examined the factors that determine the spatial and temporal pattern of the velocities at which the blood target moves. This chapter describes the various methods by which the complex signal produced by scattering from this blood target can be analyzed to identify its component Doppler frequencies and the relationship of these processed data to the original velocities.

Before discussing the various methods of signal analysis, however, it is first necessary to consider the information presented to the instrument to be analyzed, i.e., the complex signal arising from the interaction of the Doppler sample volume with the blood velocity profile. This relationship was discussed earlier in terms of its effect on signal/noise ratio. In this chapter, we view it from a different perspective; specifically, the velocity content or the portion of the spatial velocity profile falling within the scattering cross section. Remember that the scattering cross section is the common spatial volume within which the Doppler beam and the blood stream intersect. For a single target moving at a constant velocity through an infinite beam, we know that target velocity can be described as

$$V = c \cdot Fd / 2\ Fo \cdot \cos\theta \qquad [10.1]$$

and, hence, the Doppler shift and the target velocity can be viewed as being equivalent. The Doppler signal from blood, however, represents the sum of the contributions from the large number of scatterers, moving at different velocities, which pass through the ultrasonic beam during any analysis period (Fig. 10–1). It is important to note that this distribution of velocities is not necessarily the same as the velocity profile but represents only the component of the velocity profile that passes through the sample volume. Figure 10–2A illustrates the effect of this interaction for flow with a parabolic profile. Figure 10–2B illustrates the same relationship between the sample volume and velocity profile for flow with a more uniform velocity distribution. In each case, the frequency spectrum represents the velocity distribution within the sample volume, which often includes only a portion of the complete velocity profile.[1,2] In addition, because the sound intensity in the sample volume is not uniform, the amplitude of the reflected signal from similar targets may vary depending on their location in the sample volume. Therefore, when we analyze a Doppler signal for its component frequencies and velocities, we determine only those components of the velocity profile that fall within the sample volume and cannot tell the specific portion of the sample volume from which they arise.

SIGNAL PROCESSING

Remember that the Doppler difference frequency arises in the instrument only after it is detected by the demodulation process. Therefore, for the purpose of this discussion, the *Doppler signal* will be taken to mean the Doppler difference waveform output from the ultrasonic flowmeter, which contains the demodulated velocity information from the interrogated targets. The actual Doppler signal output is a time-varying voltage waveform that usually looks something like the tracing in Figure 10–3.[3] Because the underlying velocity information is related to the frequency content of this waveform, it is obviously of little value to view the raw Doppler signal by displaying it on an oscilloscope, as is done with the echoes used in image generation. Instead, the waveform

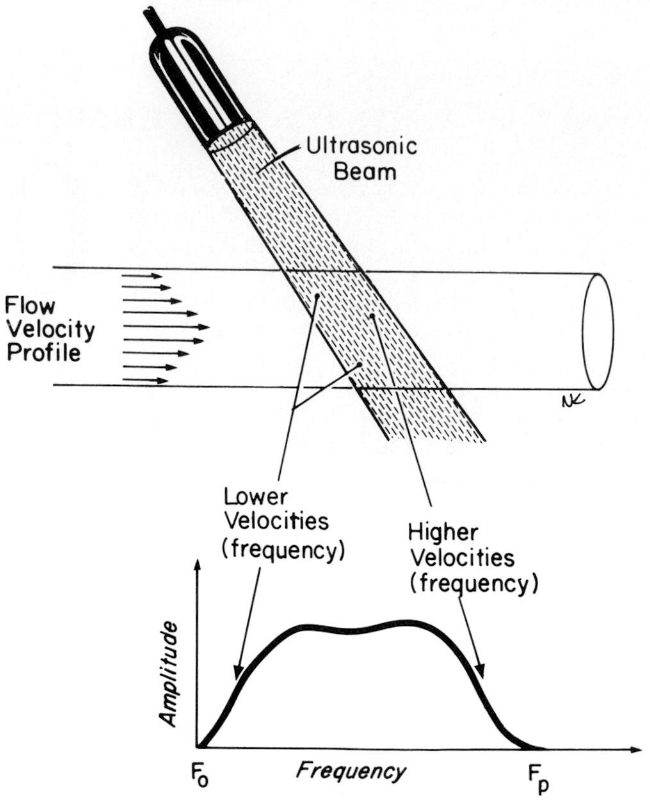

Fig. 10–1. Doppler recording of flow in a vessel produces a spectrum of frequencies of different amplitude corresponding to the number and velocities of the scatterers. (After Atkinson and Woodcock, 1982.)

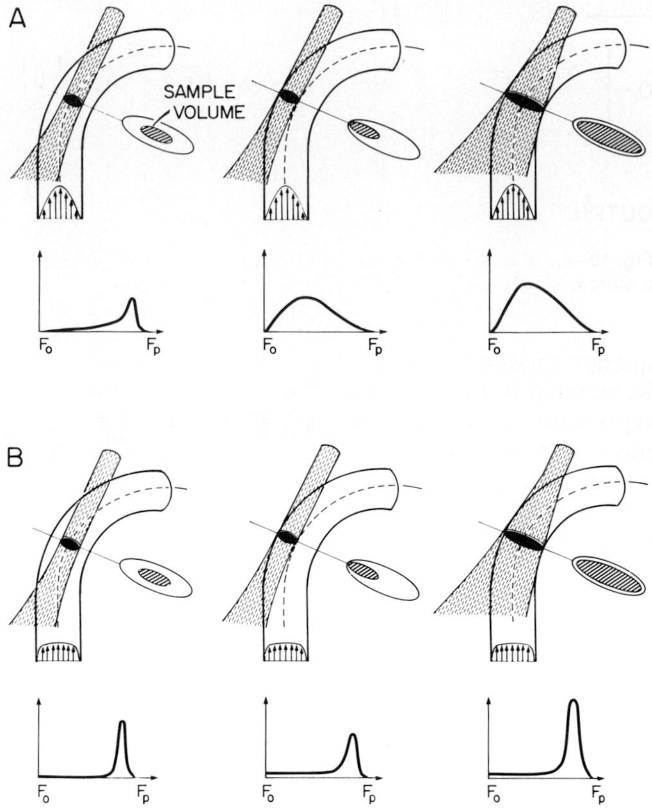

Fig. 10–2. Relationship of sample volume position within the flow stream to the recorded frequency spectrum for a parabolic (A) and flat flow profile (B). In each example, the left panel depicts a small centrally positioned sample volume; the middle panel, a small eccentrically placed sample volume; and the right panel, a large centrally placed sample volume.

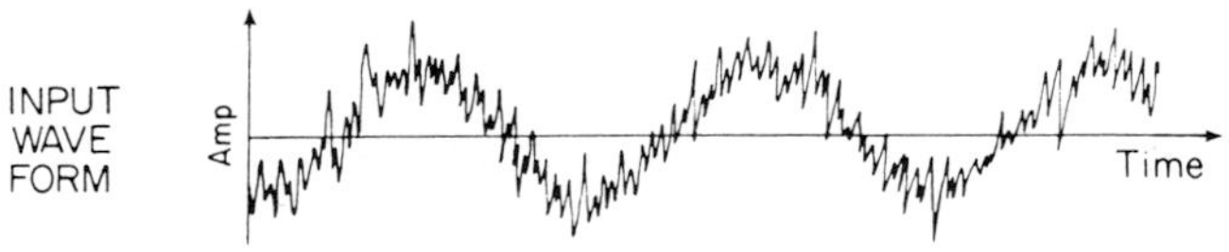

Fig. 10–3. Doppler signal output from the flowmeter.

requires some type of analysis to extract the frequency components to reveal the original velocities.

Ideally, we need a method for unambiguously determining and displaying all of the frequencies in the signal along with their relative amplitudes because this should tell us how many scatters are present and at what velocity they are moving. The result of such an analysis would give us the frequency spectrum of the signal, which is the average amount of power in the signal for each frequency. Several methods have been devised to provide this power spectrum. These include (1) auditory analysis, (2) zero-crossing detection, and (3) spectrum analysis. The latter group can be subdivided into the filter-based analyzers and the Fourier transform analyzers. In addition, specific components of this power spectrum can be identified and plotted over time. The most common of these components are the peak, mean, and modal frequency.

Auditory Analysis

One of the best and most widely used methods for Doppler spectral analysis is to simply listen to the Doppler signal with the human ear. Fortunately, using carrier frequencies in the 1- to 10-MHz range results in Doppler shifts from human blood that are in the audible range of from 250 to 20,000 cycles/sec. As a result, a subjective impression of frequency content can be gained simply by listening to the Doppler signal (using either earphones or, after amplification and broadcast, over a loudspeaker).

Virtually all Doppler instruments output an audible signal that is valuable in helping the operator direct the ultrasonic beam to intersect areas of peak velocity (based on signal frequency) and laminar flow (based on purity of tone). For subjective spectral analysis, the practiced human ear has a sensitivity with which no manmade instrument can compete, and most Doppler diagnoses can be made from the audible signal alone.[4] For more quantitative investigation, however, some objective form of frequency analysis is required.

Zero-Crossing Meters

Zero-crossing meters directly examine the time domain signal f(t) to determine its frequency content. The zero-crossing approach is relatively simple and easy to implement, and before 1980, it was the method of fre-

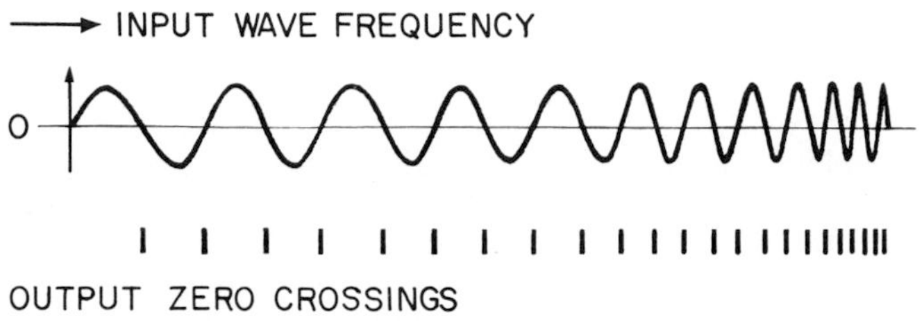

Fig. 10–4. Relationship of zero-crossing interval to frequency for a simple sinusoidal waveform of gradually increasing frequency.

quency analysis used in most Doppler instruments.[5,6] Remember that for a single scatterer, the Doppler signal represents a burst of oscillations with an internal frequency termed the *zero-crossing frequency*, which is inversely related to the time between zero-crossings (i.e., the points at which the waveform crosses the zero baseline). As the velocity of the scatterer increases, the Doppler frequency it produces likewise increases and the time between zero-crossings therefore decreases. Figure 10–4 illustrates the relationship between zero-crossing interval and frequency for a pure sinusoidal wave of increasing frequency. In this case, the frequency simply equals one half the number of times the wave crosses zero per unit time or the time interval between each zero-crossing pair. For the case of the Doppler waveform from flowing blood, however, the problem is far more complex. This signal is composed of many frequencies arising from the multiple scatterers passing through the sample volume during any sampling period. Each up and down motion or gyration of the wave is the product of these component frequencies each with a different zero-crossing interval and, hence, the gyration frequency of a complex wave does not have the same meaning as the zero-crossing frequency for a pure sinusoid. Fortunately, the expected number of zero-crossings can be predicted statistically for a given spectral content of a signal as the probability density of finding a zero-crossing event in a given time interval.[7–10] Thus, for a Doppler power spectrum, P(w), the zero-crossing rate, N, is given by:

$$N^2 = 2 \cdot \frac{\int_0^\infty \omega^2 P(\omega)\, d\omega}{\int_0^\infty P(\omega)\, d\omega} \qquad [10.2]$$

provided that there is no constant phase relationship between components at different frequencies (i.e., nonrandom associations). For a given sampling interval, therefore, the zero-crossing rate is proportional to the root mean square (RMS) frequency of the input signal.[11] This output is a statistical estimation of the mean frequency, which assumes a Gaussian distribution for the power spectrum and, hence, will show a varying correspondence to the actual spectral profile.

The principle of operation of the zero-crossing meter is illustrated in Figure 10–5. The instrument basically counts changes in polarity of the wave from positive to negative, or vice versa and plots changes in the derived zero-crossing interval as a representation of frequency vs. time. In operation, low frequency wall noise must be removed by high pass filtering. Also, because noise crosses zero, a set-reset system is introduced, as illustrated in Figure 10–5, to minimize any noise component. In this format, after a positive zero-crossing, the wave must cross a negative threshold before another positive crossing can be counted. Most commercial zero-crossing detectors use this set-reset system with an operator controllable threshold level. A practical limitation lies in the operator control of the set-reset system, because as the threshold of the set-reset system is varied, noise-related zero-crossings vary also, as does the displayed frequency or velocity. At high gain levels and a narrow set-reset window, a significant noise component may be misinterpreted as signal, resulting in reported velocity becoming a function of gain, rather than retaining its independent relationship to Doppler frequency.

Finally, zero-crossers, like spectral analyzers, assume that backscattered power relates directly to blood velocity distribution. If the vessel is not insonated uniformly, then this assumption is not valid. In addition, Equation 10.2 predicts the RMS frequency, which may

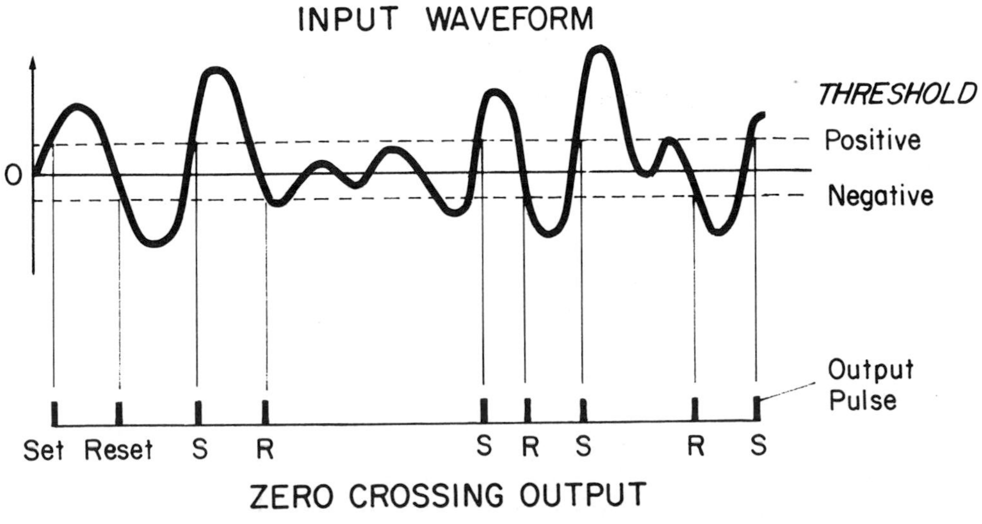

Fig. 10–5. Principles of operation of a set-reset zero-crossing meter. (See text for details.)

not be uniquely related to mean or peak flow. The ratio V mean to V rms varies with the flow profile, being unity for a flat profile and increasing to 1 to 16 for parabolic flow.[10]

Zero-crossing detectors suffer from several other theoretic and practical limitations. A major theoretic problem is that the broader the frequency bandwidth, the less clearly the mean and standard deviation will describe the envelope of the data. This problem can be overcome by shifting the data to a higher offset frequency (Fs), typically between 50 and 100 kHz. The Doppler spectrum then becomes extremely narrow relative to the offset frequency range, and zero-crossing detection more closely approximates the mean frequency of the Doppler shift.[2] The offset frequency corresponds to a DC level in the output that can be subtracted to yield a variation about zero volts, corresponding to velocities toward or away from the transducer. This is similar to the heterodyne process described earlier, except that in this case we are shifting to a higher frequency to narrow the relative signal bandwidth. The advantages of this step are (1) the output is more nearly proportional to the first moment of the Doppler shift spectrum; (2) the system becomes capable of a higher frequency response and can follow more rapid fluctuations in frequency (because the pulse train has a higher frequency and, therefore, less filtering is required to average the pulses to provide a voltage proportional to frequency); and (3) it provides a simple means of displaying the frequency content of the Doppler shift spectrum in a form similar to a continuous power spectral density plot (i.e., the time interval histogram, TIH). In contrast to the power spectrum, however, the TIH provides no amplitude information.[2]

Despite their significant limitation, zero-crossing meters should be capable of indicating component blood velocity to about 20% of their actual value and can detect changes in velocity of a few percent. The major problem with these instruments arise when the signal/noise ratio is poor. In these cases, the ability of the set-reset mechanism to separate signal from noise may be compromised and the output similarly misleading.

Because of their inherent limitations, zero-crossers were rapidly abandoned once more accurate real-time spectral analysis became available. They are discussed here in some detail, however, because most of the data in the literature before the early 1980s are based on the output of these devices. Because of their limitations, much of this information is either incorrect or severely limited, and it is important to understand why this is the case and the reasons for the confusion.

Spectral Analysis

Quantitative analysis of the Doppler frequency spectrum requires the use of instruments known as *spectrum analyzers*. These devices can detect the specific frequencies within a wave and measure the power level at each frequency. Before examining specific types of spectrum analyzers, however, it is useful to examine the characteristics of a typical Doppler shift spectrum to assess the performance requirements of such a frequency analysis system. Although the exact spectral characteristics will obviously vary with transducer frequency, angle of attack (Cos θ), site of examination, and so on, some general requirements can be defined. For example, at a 5-MHz carrier with the beam aligned parallel to flow, the Doppler spectrum for flow through a stenotic aortic valve or regurgitant mitral lesion could extend to 24 KHz, corresponding to a velocity of 6 m/sec. Furthermore, the blood might accelerate from zero to this peak velocity in 0.1 second. As a result, the Doppler spectrum analyzer must be capable of accommodating frequencies up to 25 to 30 KHz, and if it is to follow changes in velocity, it must be capable of updating the analysis at a rate of at least 100 spectra/sec. These are design specifications for high velocity arterial flow. If lower velocity flow was the subject of study, it might be preferable to use a lower range of analysis frequencies spaced closer together. The ideal analyzer, therefore, should have flexibility in both frequency range and frequency resolution. Given the limited sampling time available in clinical situations, there are restrictions on both of these parameters, as well as in the resolution of the raw data. These relationships are discussed in more detail as the specific types of analyses are discussed.

Filter-Based Spectrum Analyzers

The simplest form of spectrum analyzer is the filter-based analyzer. Although this form of analysis is no longer used in commercial instruments, filter-based analyzers are described here because their operation is relatively easy to understand. As such, they form a useful basis for the discussion of more complex Fourier methods.

Filter-based analyzers depend on bandpass filters used either independently or in groups to separate the component frequencies within a complex waveform. Bandpass filters, introduced briefly in Chapter 7, are electronic devices that permit a portion of the Doppler frequency spectrum to pass from one point to another (the passband) while selectively blocking or eliminating the remainder of the spectrum (the stopband). Bandpass filters, in theory, transmit without attenuation all frequencies lying within the bandpass region of the filter, and totally attenuate those lying outside the passband. Practical filters, unfortunately, differ from ideal filters in several respects.[3]

First, the power transmission generally is not uniform over the passband, and this effect is known as *passband ripple*. Second, signals in the stopband can never be completely eliminated, which is known as stopband ripple. Third, the point of filter cutoff will not be vertical but will fall away gradually with the rate of this slope, defined as the filter fall-off rate. These differences between an ideal and practical filter are illustrated in Figure 10–6.

It is also important to remember that the bandwidth associated with any particular analysis need not necessarily be determined by the filter bandwidth. The filter stopband only becomes limiting when the input signal has a wider bandwidth than that of the filter. As previously described, this varies with signal length, with the frequency spectrum being inversely proportional to sig-

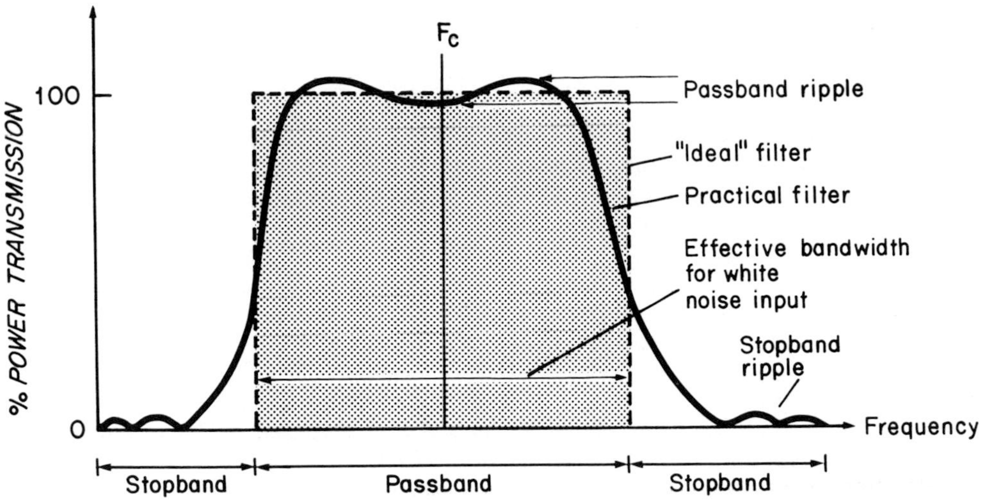

Fig. 10–6. Comparison of an ideal and a practical filter. (See text for details.) (After Atkinson and Woodcock, 1982.)

nal length or analysis time. An additional characteristic of filters is the filter response time. When a signal is suddenly applied to the input of a bandpass filter, it takes time for the output to respond. If, e.g., the input is a sine wave at a frequency within the passband, then the filter output will be a sine wave that gradually increases to its final amplitude, as shown in Figure 10–7. If the filter has a passband gain characteristic of unity, then the final output amplitude will be equal to the input amplitude. The time required for the output to approach this value is inversely proportional to the filter bandwidth. Thus, the narrower the filter, the longer the time required for the output amplitude of the signal to reach or equal the input amplitude. This limits precise separation of frequencies, as discussed later.[3]

There are two types of bandpass filters: the constant (absolute) bandpass filter, in which the filter bandwidth is constant at all frequencies, and the constant relative (or percentage) bandpass filter, in which the bandwidth is a fixed percentage of the tuned center frequency. The

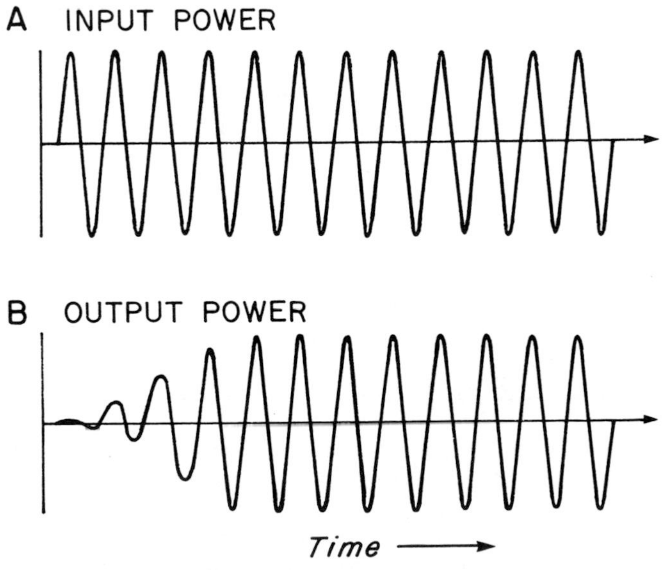

Fig. 10–7. Input signal (A) and output response (B) for a bandpass filter. (See text for details.)

constant bandwidth filter provides uniform resolution regardless of the center frequency because the bandwidth remains fixed and the response time of the filter is independent of its tuned center frequency. In contrast, the bandwidth of a constant percentage filter increases with tuned frequency. This means that the absolute bandwidth is narrow (slow response) at low frequencies and becomes wider (faster response) at higher frequencies.

Multichannel (Parallel) Filter Analyzers. There are two basic types of filter-based spectrum analyzers: the multichannel (or parallel processing) analyzers, and the swept filter analyzers. The multichannel analyzer is composed of a series of bandpass filters that can be either analog or digital construction. Whatever method is used, the output power of the bandpass unit is proportioned to that part of the input spectral power contained within the passband of each filter in the array, weighted by the bandpass characteristics of the filter. Thus, the output power spectrum G(W) from a bandpass filter can be estimated in the frequency domain simply by multiplying the input spectrum F(w) by the filter characteristic H(W). Figure 10–8 illustrates how a multichannel spectrum analyzer can be constructed from a bank of bandpass filters centered on a staggered range of consecutive frequencies, from F1 to Fn. Each filter output is fed to a full wave rectifier, which inverts the negative half-cycles, producing a unipolar waveform. This is then smoothed in an integrator to give a voltage A(F), which, as long as the filter bandwidth is kept constant and narrow, is a good estimate of the amplitude spectral density of the input waveform at the filter center frequency (Fi). The smoothed outputs from each channel are then sampled consecutively and displayed on an oscilloscope to a given histogram of A(F) against (F), which represent the amplitude frequency spectrum of the input signal.

The bandwidth of the filter and the smoothing time constant in the integrator determine the general performance characteristics of the spectrum analysis. The bandwidth of the filter not only defines the frequency (and hence velocity) resolution capability of the analyzer but also determines the maximum rate at which the output spectrum can follow input frequency changes. In

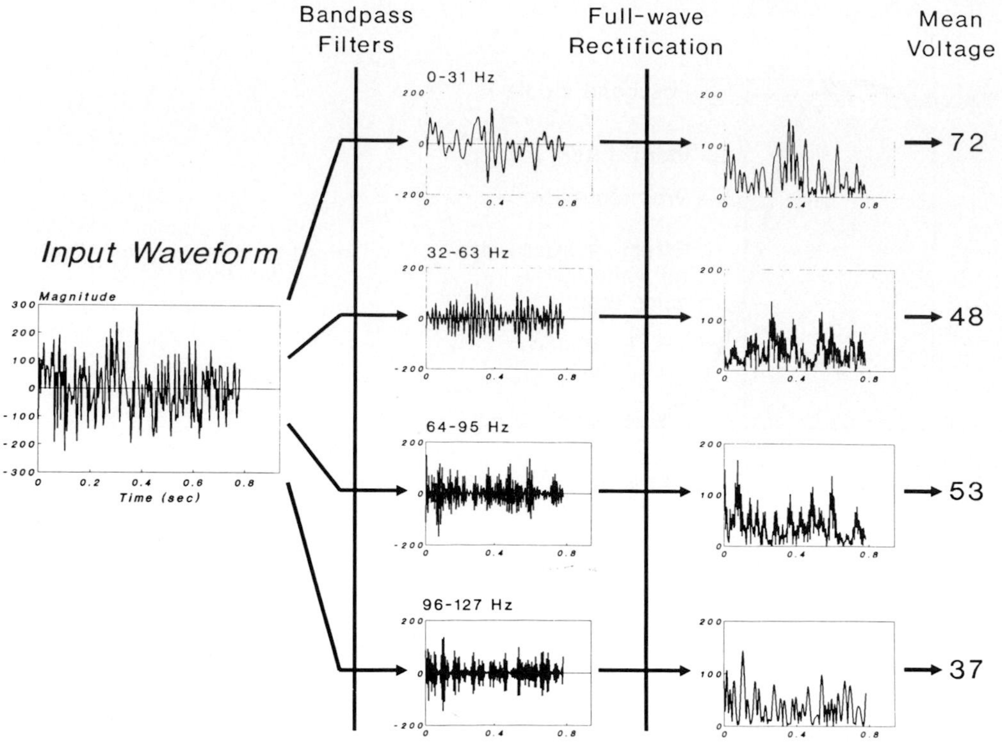

Fig. 10–8. Principles of operation of a filter-based spectrum analyzer. The input waveform is passed through a series of bandpass filters of increasing frequency. The output of each filter is then passed through a full-wave rectifier. The output of the rectifier is then smoothed in an integrator, and the output voltage of the integrator is a good estimate of the spectral power of the input waveform at the center frequency of the filter. (See text for details.)

general, as filter bandwidth is reduced, the frequency resolution of the filter improves, but the response and recovery time of the filter is increased. Slow response time followed by extended filter "ring down" can cause problems if the spectral content of the Doppler signal is changing rapidly with time, e.g., because of acceleration of the blood during systole. This can be overcome by increasing the filter bandwidth but at the expense of degrading the velocity resolution of the analysis. As a general rule, analysis time and frequency resolution are always inversely related.[3]

Multichannel analyzers are usually constructed from arrays of constant relative percentage filters. This means that the lower frequency filters respond slower but are capable of more precise absolute resolution than the higher frequency filters. The analyzed spectrum, therefore, is nonuniform in both its resolution and time response.

The multichannel spectrum analysis is probably the most straightforward method of Doppler signal processing. However, the analog filter bands suffer from two important disadvantages: (1) Analog filters are inflexible because each filter must be tuned to the preselected center frequency and, therefore, changing the frequency range of the analysis requires complete redesign of the filter components. (2) The instrument is usually complex and bulky because each processing network, including filter, rectifier, and integrator, must be duplicated for each frequency analysis channel. The inflexibility of the channels can be overcome using digital methods, but the large number of components in the instrument remains.

Swept Filter Analysis. Swept filter analysis reduces component number by using a single filter, which is swept over the frequency range of interest. This is achieved using a single bandpass filter with a center frequency that can be varied in a controlled manner. The Doppler spectrum is then analyzed, as illustrated in Figure 10–9, by slowly sweeping the bandpass region of the filter over the entire range of the Doppler frequency spectrum. The output of the ideal rectangular bandpass filter is detected (rectified and smoothed) in the same way as for the multichannel analyzer. The detector output is proportional to the shaded area (Fig. 10–9), which is common to both filter and spectrum. This represents the power of the input spectrum in the region of the filter. Thus, as the filter is swept in frequency from A to

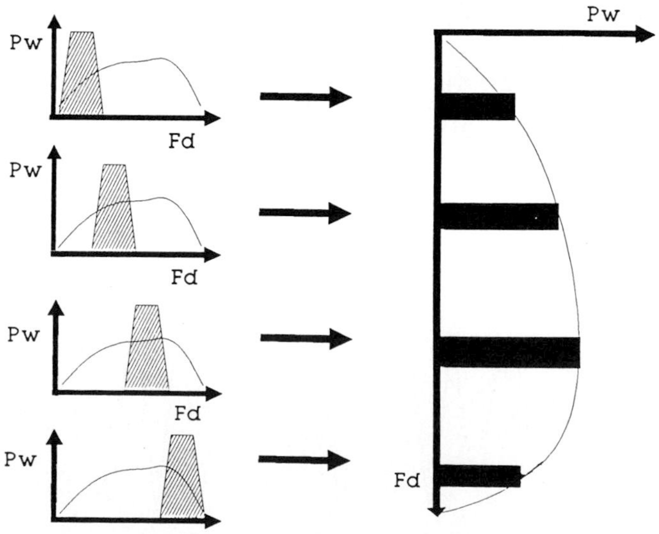

Fig. 10–9. Swept filter analysis of the Doppler frequency spectrum. (See text for details.) Fd = Doppler frequency; Pw = Power. (After Atkinson and Woodcock, 1982.)

D, the detected output sweeps out a profile of the input Doppler spectrum. The rate at which the bandpass filter can be swept depends on the filter settling time: The faster the output settles, the sooner the analysis can move onto the next frequency point.

The advantage of the swept filter concept is that only one signal processing channel is required. Unfortunately, direct application of the swept filter principle to Doppler analysis is impossible because this type of analysis requires a stable frequency spectrum through which to sweep the filter and the Doppler frequencies change rapidly during the cardiac cycle. This problem of the nonstationary Doppler signal can be solved, however, by recording the Doppler signal and playing the signal repeatedly through the filter, which is incremented in frequency after each complete replay. This procedure is time-consuming but can be accelerated by replaying the tape at a rate faster than the recording speed. For example, to analyze the Doppler signal into N channels, if the replay rate were the same as the record rate, it would take NT seconds to process a waveform that lasted T seconds. However, if the replay were to be sped up by N times, it would take only NT/N seconds to analyze the data. When N = N, the analysis time equals the recording time, and it becomes possible, in theory at least, to analyze one complete frame of data while the next one is being collected. An analysis working under these conditions is said to be operating in *real time*. Real-time analyzers can be recognized by their ability to process data without creating a backlog of data awaiting analysis. Note, however, that *real time* does not mean the same as *instantaneous*. In the swept filter analysis and the waveform analyzers that are described later, the analysis output always lags one frame behind the input signal.[3]

In practice, it is difficult to design and control a constant bandwidth bandpass filter that is able to sweep over a range of center frequencies. Thus, instead of sweeping the filter across the spectrum, it is easier to sweep the complete Doppler spectrum past a fixed frequency bandpass filter. However, the end result of the two approaches is similar.

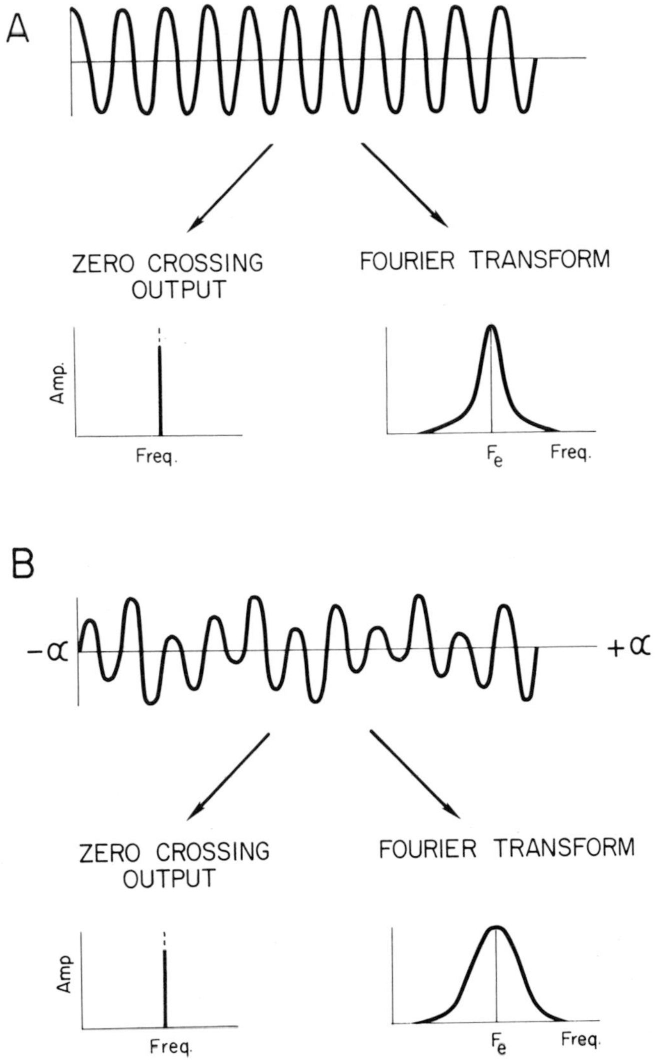

Fig. 10–10. Comparison of the zero-crossing and Fourier interpretations of frequency for the same waveforms. **A.** A wave of constant frequency and amplitude but finite duration. **B.** A wave of constant frequency and infinite duration but varying in amplitude. (See text for details.)

RELATIONSHIP OF THE ZERO-CROSSING DEFINITION OF FREQUENCY TO THE FOURIER DEFINITION OF FREQUENCY

In the preceding sections, we have discussed two different components of frequency: the zero-crossing frequency and the frequency distribution of the Fourier transform. It is important to understand the difference between these two representations of frequency and why they occur. To understand the difference, consider waveform A in Figure 10–10. This waveform is a simple sine wave with a constant zero-crossing interval, the zero-crossing representation of this wave is a single frequency, corresponding to the zero crossing interval. This representation, however, does not take into consideration the amplitude of the wave, its phase, the fact that it starts and stops, or its duration. The Fourier transform of the wave, in contrast, considers all of these factors. In transforming the wave from the time domain to the frequency domain, it must do so in such a way that the wave can be exactly reconstructed from the derived frequency components. The Fourier transform, therefore, must consider the frequency required to bring the wave from zero to its starting amplitude and the appropriate combinations of sine and cosine waves required to exactly reproduce this signal. Thus, because the Fourier transform must be able to operate in both directions, its representation of the waveform must be far more detailed and, hence, more complex than simply the frequency represented in terms of zero-crossings.

Figure 10–10B is a second example. In this case, the wave again has a constant frequency and extends from infinity to minus infinity. This wave, however, is amplitude-modulated. The zero-crossing representation will be identical to that in Figure 10–10A. However, the Fourier transform will differ because, in this case, it must include the secondary frequencies inherent in the amplitude modulation. Therefore, the zero-crossing frequency is the precise representation of the frequency of a simple sinusoid but contains no amplitude information. For a complex waveform, only Fourier analysis can describe the waveform in sufficient detail to reconstruct the wave from the descriptive information. When the Doppler frequency arises from a *single* target, it is identical to the zero-crossing frequency, and the use of the Fourier analysis introduces uncertainty into the detection of velocity because it introduces additional non-Doppler-related frequencies. For the composite Doppler signal, however, Fourier analysis retrieves all the information available and, therefore, is the most appropriate method of analysis.

Fourier Analysis

Fourier analysis provides the most direct link between the time and frequency domains and has become the standard method for Doppler signal analysis. In most treatments of this subject, the spectral analyzer that performs the Fourier analysis is described as simply a "black box" that resolves waveforms into their component frequencies. The concept behind Fourier analysis, however, is elegant and, yet simple enough that it warrants further discussion. To do so, let us return to the runner analogy. In the practical situation, we are faced with a track full of runners, all traveling at different, but unknown, speeds. The task is to determine the velocities or frequencies at which the runners are traveling and how many are moving at each frequency. To achieve this, suppose that we enter a new runner, A, into the race who is running at a known speed (velocity or frequency). As runner A moves around the track, each of the runners already on the track whom he passes (those moving slower), or who pass him (those moving faster), is eliminated. The faster or slower the other runners are moving relative to the speed of the reference runner (A), the more quickly they will be eliminated, and soon a situation will be reached when only the runners moving at approximately the same speed (frequency) as runner A are left. The word *approximately* is used deliberately because a runner may have a frequency that is so close to that of A that he will pass or be passed only after an hour. Another may require the race to continue for a week and another for a year to be eliminated. To be sure every runner moving at even the smallest difference in speed is eliminated, the process must continue for infinity because it is always possible that one runner is traveling at a frequency so close to that of runner A that he would pass or be passed at infinity minus a minute time difference.

Several relationships should be obvious from this analogy. First, a fundamental relationship between a known frequency and the components of that frequency in a larger group of frequencies should allow the frequency to be identified, and, second, the precision with which an individual frequency can be resolved is inversely related to sampling time.

$$\Delta F = 1/Ts \qquad [10.3]$$

The first time runner A goes around the track, he will eliminate the other runners whose frequencies differ the most from his own (i.e., all those greater than twice or less than one half the frequency of runner A). With each subsequent revolution, the speed (frequency range) of the remaining runners will be closer and closer to that of the known runner, until, at infinity, only those at precisely the same frequency will be left. Thus, the greater the degree of precision in frequency separation required, the longer the runners must continue. (Conversely, if the acceptable range of frequency estimation is fairly wide, the process can be completed quickly.)

The process described previously has identified only the velocity or frequency of the runners moving at (or close to) the known frequency of runner A. To identify all the runners in this race, we must continue to insert new runners B, C, D, and so on, and repeat the process. If we know nothing about the physical constraints of runners or racing, this process must continue to infinity because for an unknown system, an infinite number of possible frequencies exist. Fortunately, in racing and in Doppler frequency analysis, there are limits to the possible physiologically reasonable speeds or frequencies.

We can show the same relationship mathematically as we have in our runner analogy. Remember, we said earlier that any periodic function F(t) or cos $(\omega t + \phi)$ can be produced by summing sine and cosine waves of the same frequency and appropriate amplitude. Likewise, when dealing with unknown waveforms, it is necessary to use both the sine and cosine function of each frequency to determine its magnitude. Recall from basic algebra that $\cos(\omega t + \phi) = \cos\phi \cos\omega t - \sin\phi \sin\omega t$. Because ϕ is constant, any sinusoid oscillating at the frequency ω can be written as the sum of a term with $\cos \omega t$ and another term with $\sin \omega t$. Therefore, any function F(t) that is periodic with the period t can be written mathematically as:

$$\begin{aligned} F(t) = {} & Ao \\ & + A1 \cos \omega t + B1 \sin \omega t \\ & + A2 \cos 2\omega t + B2 \sin 2\omega t \qquad [10.4] \\ & + A3 \cos 3\omega t + B3 \sin 3\omega t \\ & + \ldots \qquad + \ldots \\ & \text{etc.} \end{aligned}$$

where $\omega = 2\pi/T$ and the As and Bs are numeric constants that tell us how much of each component oscillation is present in our periodic function F(t). The zero-frequency term (Ao) is included to represent any shift of the average above the zero level.[12]

If we can produce a periodic function by adding appropriately weighted sines and cosines, how, given the function, can we define its component parts? First look at Ao. We have already said that it is the average value of F(t) over one period (from $t = 0$ to $t = T$), but the average value of a sine or cosine function over one period is zero (i.e., half of the time the sinusoid is positive and half of the time it is negative and the sum is zero). Over 2, 3, or any whole number of periods, it is also zero, so that the average value of a term on the right side of the equation is zero, except Ao, which is a constant. Now suppose we multiply by some harmonic function (e.g., cos 5ωt). (This is similar to entering a runner at a known frequency.) We then have:

$$F(t) \cdot \cos 5\omega t = \qquad [10.5]$$

$$\begin{aligned}
&Ao \cdot \cos 5\omega t \\
&+ A1 \cos \omega T \cdot \cos 5\omega t \quad + B1 \sin \omega t \cdot \cos 5\omega t \\
&+ A2 \cos 2\omega t \cdot \cos 5\omega t \quad + B2 \sin 2\omega t \cdot \cos 5\omega t \\
&+ \ldots\ldots\ldots\ldots \quad + \ldots\ldots\ldots\ldots \\
&+ A5 \cos 5\omega t \cdot \cos 5\omega t \quad + B5 \sin 5\omega t \cdot \cos 5\omega t \\
&+ \ldots\ldots\ldots\ldots \quad + \ldots\ldots\ldots\ldots \\
&+ A9 \cos 9\omega t \cdot \cos 5\omega t \quad + B9 \sin 9\omega t \cdot \cos 5\omega t
\end{aligned}$$

Now let us average both sides. The average of cos 5ωt over time T is the average of a cosine over five whole periods, which is zero.

Looking at the A1 term, we known in general that

$$\cos A \cos B = 1/2 \cos(A + B) + 1/2 \cos(A - B) \qquad [10.6]$$

and the A1 term then becomes 1/2 A1 (cos 6ωt + cos 4ωt).

We thus have two cosine terms, one with six full periods and the other with four. They both average to zero. For the A2 term, we find 1/2 A2 (cos 7ωt + cos 3ωt), each of which also averages to zero. For the A9 term, we would find 1/2 A9 (cosine 14ωt and cos (−4ωt), but (−4ωt) is the same as cos 4ωt, so both of these average to zero. It is clear, then, that all terms average to zero except one and that one is the A5 term. For this term, we have 1/2 A5 (cos 10ωt + cos 0ωt), but, because cos 0 = 1, and 0 + 1 = 1, the average is one. As a result, the average of all the A terms of equation equals 1/2 A5. If that frequency is not present, then the entire sum will equal zero. Thus, when we multiply by a frequency (or enter a new runner), all terms except the components at that frequency cancel out. For the B terms, we can show that when we multiply by any cosine term such as cosine Nωt, all the B terms will average to zero. Thus, we have shown mathematically what we have reasoned from our runner analogy.

To be analyzed on a digital computer, a waveform must be sampled (digitized). Once sampling is introduced, there is no longer an infinite number of points available for analysis, and the finite discrete version of the Fourier transform (DFT) must be used. In practice, calculations usually are performed using a modification of the DFT known as the fast Fourier transform (FFT). The fast Fourier transform permits much more rapid computation of the frequency components of a signal, as illustrated in Figure 10–11.

The actual calculation of a Fourier series from a Doppler signal using the discrete transform can best be explained by example, as in Figure 10–12. In this example, one segment of a continuous wave is selected for analysis. This segment has a period, T, which is divided into N equally spaced samples. The period or time T defines the first harmonic of the Fourier series.

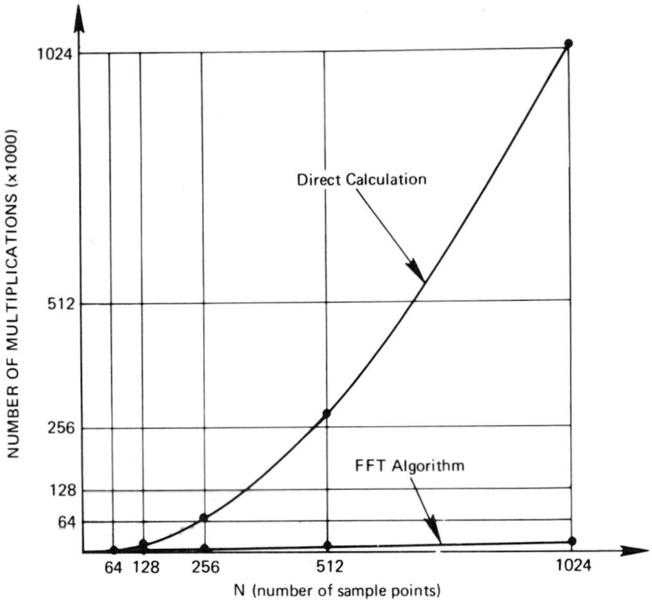

Fig. 10–11. Number of calculations required to compute a frequency spectrum using the discrete compared to the fast Fourier transform (FFT). (From Brigham EO: The Fast Fourier Transform. New York, Prentice-Hall, p. 152, 1974.)

The calibrated value of F(t) at each ordinate (Ys) is measured using an electronic analog-to-digital converter. The Fourier coefficients Ak and Bk, which represent the sine and cosine components at each frequency, can then be calculated from

$$A_K = \frac{2}{N} \sum_{s=0}^{N} y_s \cos K\omega t_s \text{ (for } K = 0, 1, 2, \cdots N/2) \qquad [10.7]$$

$$B_K = \frac{2}{N} \sum_{s=0}^{N} y_s \sin K\omega t_s \text{ (for } K = 1, 2, \cdots N/2). \qquad [10.8]$$

This operation for the first four cosine harmonics is illustrated in Figure 10–12B to E.

The results of such a discrete Fourier series analysis are usually displayed as a graphic spectrum of the real and imaginary components or sine and cosine coefficients as a function of frequency or harmonic number as illustrated in Figure 10–13. The modulus (M) and phase angle (ϕ) of any harmonic can easily be calculated from the Fourier coefficients (A + B) as

$$M = (A2 + B2)1/2 \qquad [10.9]$$

$$\phi = \text{Arctan } B/A \qquad [10.10]$$

The displays in Figure 10–13 are called *line spectra*, emphasizing that values can be computed only at specified frequencies. The same results are often plotted as connected points rather than lines (as is the case throughout this text), which is convenient if one remembers that this spectrum defined by a discrete Fourier series is not continuous.[13] (The Fourier transform is discussed in greater detail in Appendix B.)

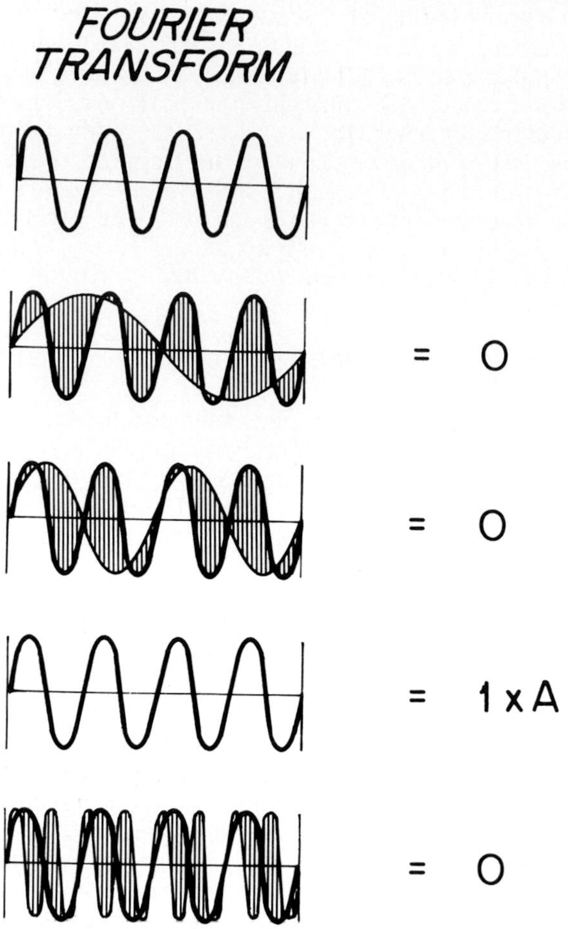

Fig. 10–12. The Fourier transform. Multiplication by the first harmonic at the sampling duration results in an equal number of positive and negative values, which when summed over the sampling period, result in zero output. The same is true for all other harmonics, except the fourth, which is exactly the same as the input waveform and hence the output sums to the maximum possible value.

Fast Fourier Transform Performance Characteristics

The performance characteristics of a generic FFT analyzer are determined by a variety of factors including (1) the sampling frequency, (2) the transform length, (3) the maximum frequency, (4) the frequency resolution, and (5) the time window. When dealing with physiologic data, such as Doppler signals, however, many of these variables are constrained by the nature of the raw data.

The sampling frequency, e.g., is defined by the upper limit of the Doppler bandwidth. To accurately characterize a sinusoidal wave at a given frequency, at least two points per wavelength must be known. The sampling frequency, therefore, must be at least twice the highest Doppler frequency of interest. In practice, this is in the range of 20 KHz, so that the sampling frequency must be at least 40 KHz.

The second factor is the time window. The power spectrum is strictly defined for velocities that do not change with time. In the clinical setting, however, velocities change greatly because of the pumping action of the heart. We, therefore, must examine a time window that is so short that, for practical purposes, the velocities can be considered constant during this period. We call this period the data acquisition time or Ta. For Doppler studies, the usual data acquisition time is in the range of 5 to 10 msec. Thus, in the ideal setting, if our sampling rate is 40-KHz and our data acquisition time is 10 msec, our sample number will be 400 equally spaced samples or 200 frequency points. Because these frequency points are equally spaced from DC to 20 KHz, we have a frequency resolution or maximal frequency separation of roughly 100 Hz. Note that this value of 100 is the reciprocal of the time window, and the frequency resolution is therefore the reciprocal of the input sample length in seconds. In theory, then, our spectrum analyzer will calculate frequencies at 100-Hz intervals from 0 to 20 KHz,

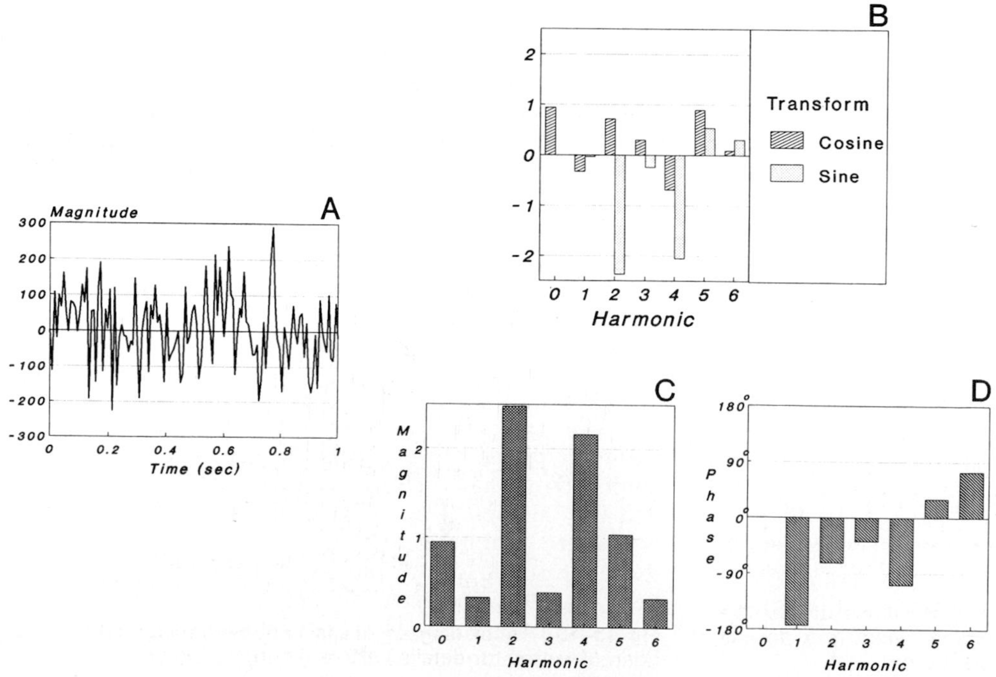

Fig. 10–13. A. Fourier transform of an input waveform. **B.** The sine and cosine magnitudes at the first six harmonics. **C.** The magnitude at each frequency. **D.** The phase at each frequency (harmonic). (See text for details.)

which at the usual carrier frequencies, corresponds to velocities of from 0 to 5 to 6 m/sec. If, at 10 msec, the frequency resolution is limited to 100 Hz at a 1-msec sampling interval, frequency resolution would be only 1000 Hz. In terms of velocity resolution, this is a difference in resolution of from roughly 3 to 4 cm/sec to roughly 30 to 40 cm/sec.

The finite sampling time Ta, therefore, introduces a variable degree of inaccuracy in the frequency estimate, when compared with an infinite analysis time, because all intermediate frequencies must be assigned a higher or lower value. As noted previously, the degree of inaccuracy varies with the frequency resolution and is inversely related to the acquisition time thus

$$\Delta FA = 1/TA. \qquad [10.11]$$

In addition, the limited data collection time also introduces a random inaccuracy in determining the amplitude of each frequency component. This is caused by the random fluctuation in scatterers passing through the sample volume. Figure 10–14 compares spectral estimates to infinite time analysis of the frequency spectrum.

Finally, it is reasonable to ask how the performance characteristics of a spectrum analyzer relate to the velocity resolution of the signal being analyzed (i.e., whether the analysis can characterize all the velocity information in the signal or whether its capability exceeds the resolution of the information to be analyzed). This is essentially a comparison of transit time uncertainty in the signal relative to the frequency resolution of the analyzer. As noted in Chapter 7, the accuracy with which the Doppler shift defines the target velocity is a function of the time available for the beam-target interaction. The finite nature of this interaction limits the frequency resolution of the signal.[1] A measure of the uncertainty introduced by the transit time effect is the width of the central lobe of the Fourier transform of the frequency spectrum from a single scatterer. Because this variable is inversely related to the transit time, the transit time uncertainty Ft equals

$$Ft = 1/Tt \qquad [10.12]$$

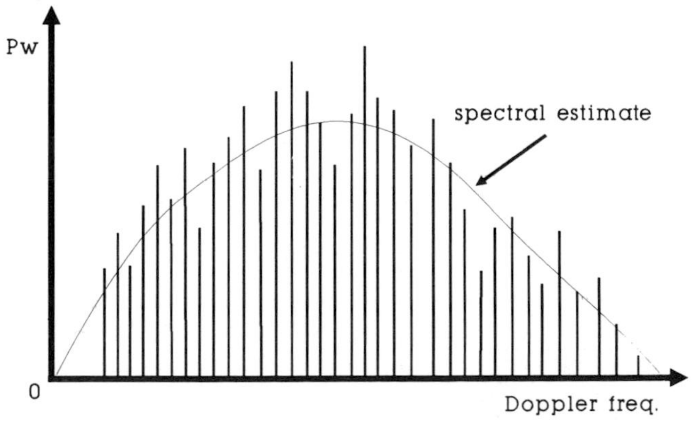

Fig. 10–14. Random inaccuracy in the amplitude at each frequency caused by limited sample collection compared to an "infinite time analysis" of the frequency spectrum.

The transit time of a scatterer is expressed by the relationship Tt = L/V, where L is the transit length of the scatterer through the region of interest and V is the scatterer velocity. Changes in either of these parameters change transit time. However, they affect it in different ways. If the velocity changes, the Doppler frequency Fd also changes so that the number of oscillations in a single scattered burst remains constant. The transit time broadening, therefore, is proportional to the Doppler shift and the relative degree of uncertainty remains constant.

$$Ft/Fd = 1/T \qquad [10.13]$$

If, on the other hand, the size of the region of observation increases, the number of oscillators in the received burst also increases and, therefore, the relative transit time uncertainty decreases. When Tt increases in this manner, the Fourier frequency distribution narrows and at the limit becomes a spike at the zero-crossing frequency. Remember in our analogy that the longer our runner of known frequency runs, the smaller the frequency range of the remaining runners. Infinite sampling obviously never occurs in practice, and some degree of uncertainty always exists. For a reference burst duration of 20 cycles, the uncertainty will be roughly 5%, at 14 cycles it will be 7%, and at 5 cycles 20%. Because the uncertainty is symmetrically distributed, a transit time uncertainty of 10% at a Doppler frequency of 5 KHz, will result in a variability in the signal of +250 Hz. Hence, any analyzer resolution higher than this is meaningless because its accuracy can be no better than that of the raw data. The analyzer resolution, therefore, need be no better than the frequency resolution contained in the Doppler signal.

To optimize performance, we can manipulate the length (time window) of the data string used for analysis (TA), the frequency resolution, and the variance in amplitude of the spectral estimate.

The Instrument

Figure 10–15 is a block diagram of an FFT analyzer, which is typical of the construction of most commercially available instruments. The processing sequence is under strict control of the internal timing unit (usually a microprocessor), which generates appropriate commands for sampling the input, performing the transform, and displaying the output. The input waveforms enter through an antialiasing filter that removes frequencies above the selected maximum of the processor and thereby removes artifacts. The synchronous analog-to-digital converter then samples the data at a suitable rate,

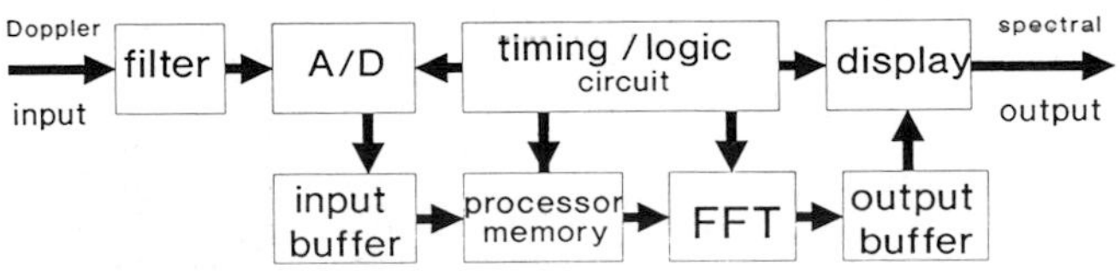

Fig. 10–15. Block diagram of a fast Fourier transform (FFT) analyzer. (See text for details.) A/D = Analog-to-Digital.

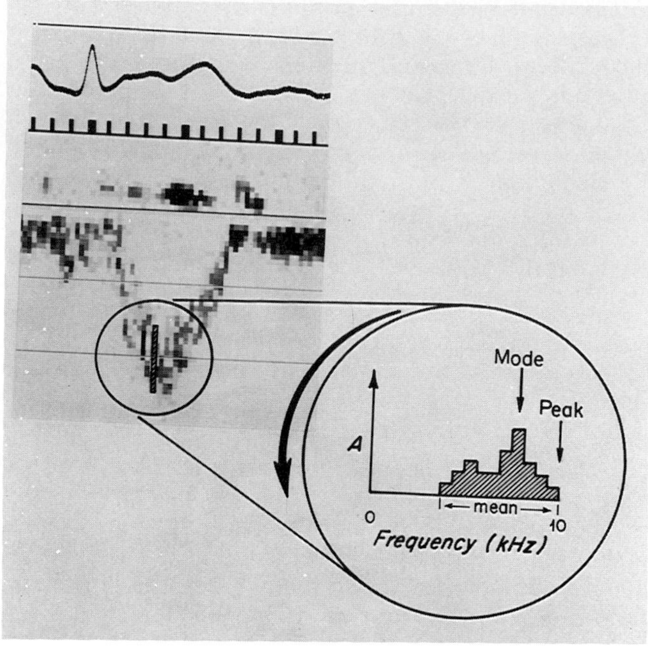

Fig. 10–16. Conventional method for displaying Doppler spectral data. (See text for details.)

converts it into digital form, and stores the results in the input buffer memory. When full, the contents of this memory are transferred to the processor memory. The time taken to fill the input buffer memory depends on the selected sampling rate (see following discussion). The processor thus computes an FFT from these data and stores the results in the output buffer memory. An output power P(F1) at each frequency point (Pi) can then be generated by repetitively scanning the output buffer, usually at a rate fast enough to provide a flicker-free trace on an oscilloscopic screen. By using the buffer in this way, the analyzer can continue recording new data and displaying the most recent transform while current signals are being processed so that real-time analysis is maintained. Note again that *real time* does not mean *instantaneous*.

Output of Frequency Spectra

Because velocity varies with time, the frequency spectra computed from the instantaneous velocities also vary with time. For clinical use, therefore, they must be output in some graphic format that depicts the frequency spectra for each acquisition period T2. Two such methods have been used. The most common approach is illustrated in Figure 10–16. In this gray scale display, time is plotted along the horizontal axis and frequency along the vertical axis. Each time increment corresponds to the processing time of the analyzer, in this case, 10 msec. For each interval of data collection (TA), a discrete set of frequency components is calculated with resolution ΔFa. The individual frequency cells ΔFa (e.g., 250-Hz increments) are plotted along the vertical axis on a scale from zero to Fmax. The intensity or power at each frequency is plotted in varying shades of gray with the time-frequency cell with the greatest signal power having the darkest intensity. The discreteness of the cells is a reflection of the velocity resolution limitations of the analyzer. They can be smoothed by interpolation, but this process does not improve the frequency resolution.

Another way to look at the same data is to display them in a three-dimensional plot, as illustrated in Figure 10–17. This format provides a better appreciation of the amplitude variations within the spectra than does the gray scale display. Connecting discrete frequency points also gives a sense of improved frequency resolution, but this is only a smoothing effect of the display and does not add further information. The major limitation of these plots is that they are time-consuming and generally can provide data for only 1 cycle. As a result, although artistically appealing, they provide little additional information.

METHODS OF EXTRACTING SPECIFIC COMPONENTS OF THE DOPPLER FREQUENCY SPECTRUM

Spectrum analyzers output the entire Doppler frequency spectrum. For clinical purposes, however, most of this information is discarded, and a single component

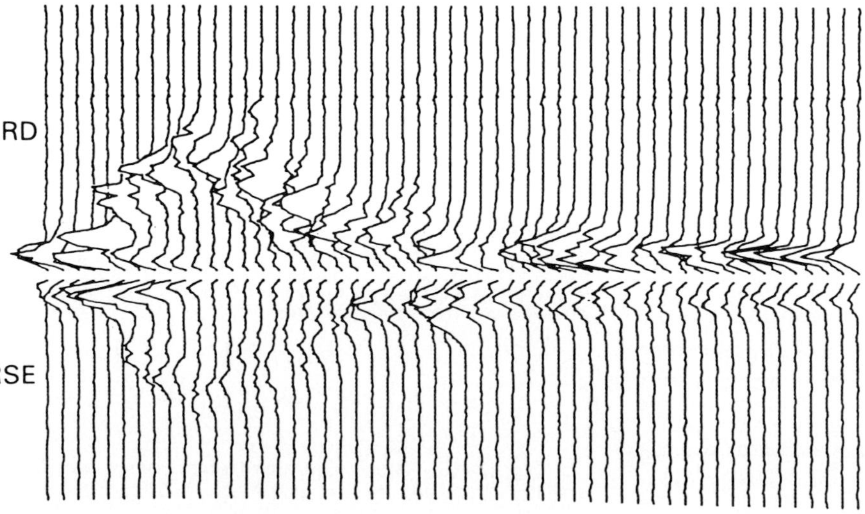

Fig. 10–17. Three-dimensional display of Doppler velocity data vs. time. (From Cannon SR, Richards KL, Rollwitz WT: Digital Fourier techniques in the diagnosis and quantification of aortic stenosis with pulsed-Doppler echocardiography. J Clin Ultrasound 10:101, 1982.)

of the Doppler frequency spectrum analyzed. This component is usually identified visually by the operator, and analysis is most often performed by manually tracing the components of interest.

Historically, the peak frequency has been used most often, simply because of the ease of tracing around the outside of the profile. Other components, e.g., the mean frequency and the modal frequency (i.e., the frequency with the highest amplitude corresponding to the velocity at which the greatest number of scatterers are moving), have also been used in various calculations, and their use in characterizing volumetric flow may be more appropriate. Drawing an outline of the peak or modal velocity by hand rapidly becomes time-consuming and introduces an additional source of variability into the data. Because these components of the spectrum form the data that are actually analyzed, various methods have been developed to output these parameters automatically by tracking the appropriate portion of the spectral profile or directly from the analog signal.

Peak Frequency Analyzers

Spectrum Samplers

Various methods have been described for detecting and outputing the peak Doppler frequency. The simplest approach is to sample automatically the output channels of a spectrum analyzer and determine the highest frequency channel registering a voltage. Figure 10–18 illustrates how such a peak frequency follower might work. In this diagram, the analysis channels are arranged in order from f1 to Fn, and each detected output is fed to a voltage comparator, which decides whether the signal is above a preset noise threshold. If the voltage exceeds this level, the comparator outputs a signal. A priority encoder then rapidly scans the comparator outputs, and the network produces a voltage proportional to the ranking of the highest channel that produces a signal. As the spectrum changes the output, voltage from the priority encoder follows the peak frequency content of the spectrum.[3] The main disadvantage of such an approach is that complete frequency analysis is still required and the complexity of the instrument is increased still further because each of the frequency channels now requires its own comparator circuitry.

Frequency Tracking Filters

Because it is inefficient to perform a complete spectral analysis to simply detect the peak frequency, several attempts have been made to derive the peak frequency directly from the time domain signal.[3] One such method is the use of a voltage-controlled high pass filter.[14] In this approach the Doppler signal is fed to a voltage-controlled high pass filter. The output of this filter is detected (rectified and smoothed) and applied to the control voltage input (Fig. 10–19). With no signal, the offset is adjusted so that the filter frequency rests at slightly above zero frequency. When a Doppler signal is fed into the system, the filter passes the signal and the control voltage increases, thereby raising the filter frequency and cutting off the Doppler input. The feedback loop settles to an equilibrium position, shown in Figure 10–20, in which the signal power passed by the filter is just sufficient to hold the filter in position. The control voltage is roughly proportional to the area in the figure that is common to both the Doppler spectrum and the filter bandpass. As the maximum Doppler frequency increases, the filter "rides" on the upper edge of the spectrum, maintaining the slight overlap necessary to produce the required control voltage. The feedback characteristics are controlled by the loop filter, which is designed to reduce overshoot.

Another approach is to position two filters such that their relative positions are fixed, but they can move together along the frequency axis (Fig. 10–21). The power output of the two filters are equated so that

$$P_2/P_1 = a \qquad [10.14]$$

where P_1 is the signal power in frequency window F_1, P_2 is the power in frequency window F_2, and a is a small number (roughly 0.1). Equation 10.14 can be satisfied

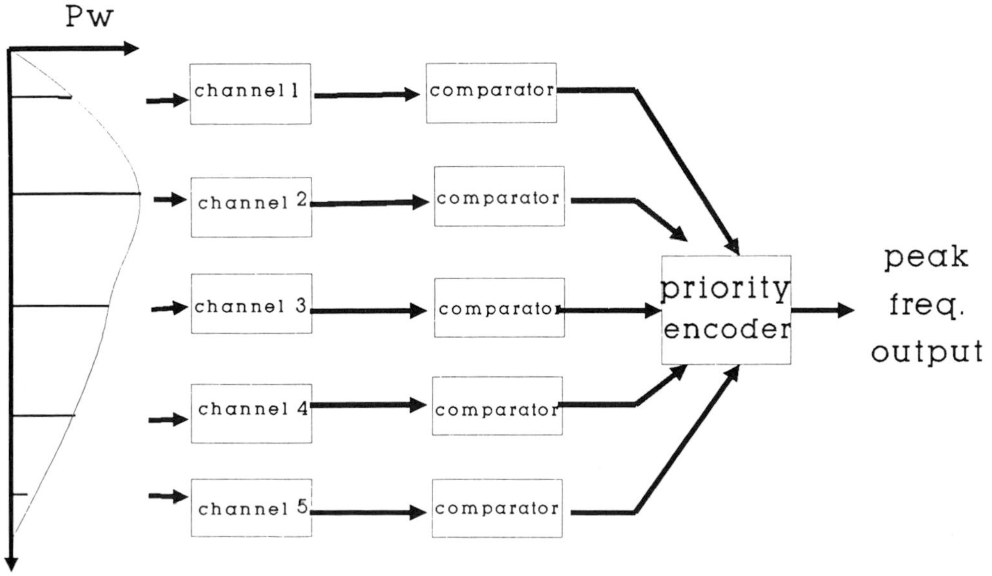

Fig. 10–18. Detection of peak frequency from an array of bandpass filters. (See text for details.) (After Atkinson and Woodcock, 1982.)

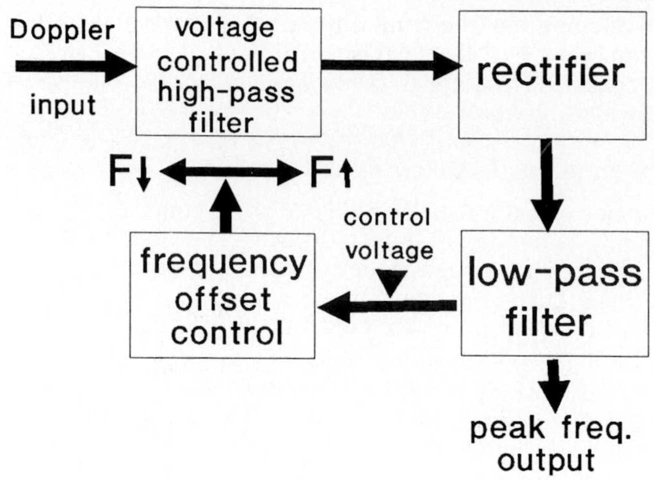

Fig. 10–19. Block diagram of a voltage-controlled high-pass filter in a feedback loop. When there is no signal, the filter rests just above the baseline. As input begins, it is smoothed, rectified, and passed through the low pass filter. This generates a control voltage that increases the frequency of the voltage-controlled high-pass filter, which decreases the input voltage. This process continues until the input voltage is eliminated and the filter thus rides along the top of the input spectrum. (See text for details.)

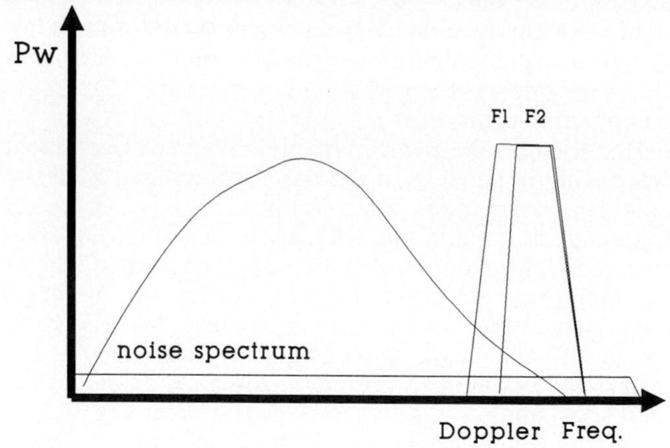

Fig. 10–21. Principle of operation of a dual filter maximum frequency estimator. (See text for details.) (After Hatle and Angelsen, 1985.)

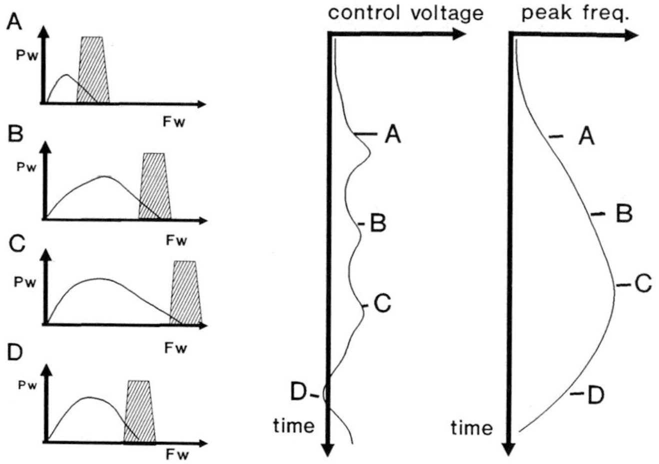

Fig. 10–20. Operation of a peak frequency tracking filter. **A.** Voltage increases resulting in an increase in filter and output frequency. **B** and **C.** As voltage continues to increase, the filter and output frequency, likewise, increase and the filter rides along the peak on the frequency spectrum. **D.** As the frequency falls, the control voltage decreases and the filter's positions correspondingly shift back toward the baseline. Outputs are smooth for illustrative purposes. Fw = frequency; Pw = power.

only when the lower slope of F_2 is located at a falling edge of the spectrum. If P_2/P_1 is less than a, the position of the windows is moved to the left, and if P_2/P_1 is greater than a, the position of the windows is moved to the right.[1]

Several major problems are encountered in all forms of peak frequency estimation. The first is the lack of any clear definition of the point at which the upper end of the frequency spectrum intersects the noise floor. By definition, the signal/noise ratio of the true peak frequency component must be close to unity because otherwise it would not be the maximum frequency present.

The second problem is the periodic fluctuation in the power level of the peak frequency over time. This occurs because the scattering from blood is a statistic process so that power fluctuates with time and periodically approaches zero. Finally, at its peak, the spectrum typically falls off slowly because of the combination of transit time effects and statistic variation in the peak velocity signal. The slope of the upper arm of the spectral envelope, therefore, is variable, and its intersection point is inconsistent. It is also affected by the height of the noise floor and the degree of high pass filtering.

Because the edge of the spectrum is so difficult to define at its upper extreme, an alternative approach has been suggested in which peak frequency is defined statistically as representing a percentile of the total power in the spectrum. In this format the peak frequency would be, e.g., the frequency below which 95% of the power in the spectrum falls. This method does not truly provide edge definition but is less sensitive to noise and is also simpler to implement on a microprocessor. It should be apparent that the ultimate lack of definition of peak frequency makes all of these approaches estimates rather than precise measures.

Mean Frequency Estimation

The mean frequency of the Doppler spectrum is the weighted average of the Doppler shifts for each instant in time. The mean frequency is of particular interest because it should be proportional to the space average velocity of flow if the artery is uniformly insonated. Because volume flow is equal to vessel area times mean velocity, this parameter should then be the appropriate Doppler measurement for volumetric flow calculations. The most direct method for calculating the mean frequency is to perform a spectral analysis and then (assuming the power spectrum is continuously distributed) compute the first moment of the Doppler power spectrum P(F) using the relationship

$$W(\text{mean}) = \frac{\int_0^\alpha F\, P(F)\, dF}{\int_0^\alpha P(F)\, d(F)} \qquad [10.15]$$

The mean frequency can then be related to V (mean) using the basic Doppler equation so that

$$F = 2V/C\ Fo \qquad [10.16]$$

This relationship assumes (1) that the blood vessel is uniformly insonated and (2) that blood is a homogenous scatterer of sound.

The preceding assumptions must be satisfied for the amount of backscattered power at each frequency to be directly and linearly related to the volume of blood moving at that frequency. If the blood were not uniformly insonated, then the echo from blood flowing in the more intensely insonated region would artifactually weight the integral. The same effect could also be caused if certain volumes of blood exhibited an increased backscattering power. In the clinical situation, both assumptions can generally be met. The main problem with defining the average frequency lies in the high pass or wall filters used by all instruments to remove low velocity signals from tissue. These filters also remove the signal from slowly moving blood and tend to lead to an overestimation of mean velocity. The degree of overestimation will tend to vary with the velocity profile. Because these filters are operator controlled, overestimation also varies with the selection of the filter threshold. The mean is also affected by the signal/noise ratio because noise above the high pass filter level will be included in the power spectrum, whereas signal below the threshold will be eliminated. Analog methods for computing the mean frequency have also been developed, but for the reasons stated are not widely used.[15–17]

Modal Velocity

Probably the component of the power spectrum that is simplest to determine is the modal velocity. The mode is simply the frequency with the highest amplitude that reflects the velocity at which the greatest number of scatterers are traveling. Given that noise is random, this parameter should be less affected by the noise level than either the mean or the peak frequency. Because it is by definition the highest amplitude signal, it is insensitive to high pass filtering. It is also easily identified by simply scanning the channel outputs and selecting the output with the highest voltage. Flow derived from the modal velocity has been shown to correlate better with independent measures of volumetric flow than with flow derived from the mean velocity which is very sensitive to noise. In addition, the ease of measurement and reproducibility of the modal velocity make it a particularly valuable parameter (see Chapter 30).

COMBINATION OF DOPPLER FLOW METERS WITH PULSED ECHO IMAGING SYSTEMS

Although Doppler devices were originally designed, and to this point in the discussion, have been considered as independent instruments in their current application, they are most often found in combination with some form of echo imaging system. This combination is highly advantageous from a diagnostic standpoint because it permits visualization of the location within the heart at which flow is being sampled (using pulsed Doppler systems), as well as the line of site along which continuous wave Doppler interrogation occurs. The combination of Doppler and imaging systems, however, requires tradeoffs in two areas. The first is the necessary compromise between frequency and spatial resolution, which has been alluded to repeatedly in the foregoing discussion. The second lies in the necessity of distributing data between the Doppler and imaging modes.

The first trade-off between frequency and spatial resolution is a function of the physical characteristics of the echo signal and arises because of fundamental differences in the physical requirements of the two modes of data acquisition. For the Doppler portion of the instrument, the primary concern is sensitivity because the amplitude of the Doppler signal is well below that of the specular echoes. Sensitivity is primarily determined by the signal/noise ratio, and this ratio is affected by many factors. The primary determinant of the signal/noise ratio that can be reasonably controlled is the volume of blood from which the Doppler signal is sampled. By increasing the size of the sample volume, we increase the signal strength and the sensitivity of the instrument, as well as the accuracy of our frequency estimate. An increase in sample volume length, however, implies an increase in pulse length and a corresponding loss of spatial resolution. In Doppler studies, spatial resolution is not as critical as in imaging studies, because velocities do not generally show abrupt spatial variation. The ability to use a long pulse train is also advantageous because it permits the use of narrow bandwidth, air-backed, low loss transducers which, likewise, improve sensitivity and, hence, signal/noise ratio.

In contrast, the primary consideration in the imaging component of the instrument is spatial resolution. High spatial resolution requires a short echo pulse that is generated by a highly damped, wide bandwidth transducer with relatively high losses. Because these two requirements—signal strength in the Doppler mode and spatial resolution in the imaging mode—cannot be reconciled, some compromise must be made, which results in loss of either Doppler sensitivity or image resolution. Because the image can be seen, and its quality immediately appreciated—whereas the sensitivity of Doppler is generally not apparent except to the highly trained observer, or by comparison with a more sensitive instrument—the compromise usually favors the imaging system. Much of this compromise occurs at the transducer level, therefore, it is possible to use separate transducers for imaging and Doppler studies. Use of a dedicated, stand alone Doppler transducer, however, sacrifices the advantage of the combination with the imaging device and requires that the flow signals themselves be used for appropriate positioning of the sound beam. However, despite the desirability of having some form of imaging guidance, the need for optimal sensitivity in a significant portion of the patients studied in a clinical laboratory has necessitated the inclusion of a stand alone Doppler transducer in most instruments.

Compromises Involved in Sharing Data Between the Imaging and Doppler Modes of a Combined Instrument

M-Mode and Doppler Combinations

By far, the simplest method for combining Doppler flow sampling and imaging is to combine a Doppler instrument with an M-mode echograph. In this combined format, the return pulse can simply be split and processed along twin paths to provide simultaneous M-mode and Doppler output. This is obviously possible only for pulsed Doppler systems because the M-mode, by definition, operates in a pulsed echo mode. In practice, however, the M-mode and Doppler are poorly suited for combination because the M-mode records interfaces optimally when they are aligned perpendicular to the path of the beam, whereas the Doppler records flow optimally when it is parallel to the beam path. Thus, in almost every application, the ideal orientation of the M-mode recordings is orthogonal to that of the Doppler recording. The major utility of this combination lies in use of the M-mode as a timing reference for the Doppler signals and the capability of continuously tracking the position of the Doppler sample volume, relative to specific structures of interest (Fig. 13–2).

Combination With Two-Dimensional Imaging Systems

Mechanical Sector Scanners

A more appropriate combination of modalities is the combination of Doppler flow sampling with two-dimensional echocardiographic imaging. This is particularly valuable in patients with complex lesions in whom the Doppler signal may be virtually uninterpretable without some spatial orientation. There are several problems in combining these modalities. First, the two-dimensional images are created by sweeping the beam of ultrasound across a predefined arc or sector, whereas the Doppler flow signal is recorded along a specific fixed line of site. In a mechanical system where the transducer is rotated or oscillated, it is necessary, therefore, to stop the transducer to record Doppler signals, so that imaging and Doppler cannot be performed simultaneously. Second, it is usually necessary to sample Doppler data for at least 5 msec to accurately characterize flow. To avoid rapid acceleration and deceleration with its associated wear and tear on mechanical parts, all existing mechanical systems stop the transducer for several seconds to record Doppler measurements and return to an imaging mode either on command or by storing and intermittently updating an image at fixed intervals. Because the transducer position required for optimal image generation usually differs from that required to record the best Doppler signal, one frequently moves the transducer while in the Doppler mode to optimize signal recording with resulting uncertainty as to precise sample location. The major limitation of these devices is the necessary compromise in transducer design to accommodate both imaging and flow studies. Although dedicated Doppler transducers can be used with mechanical systems just as they can be incorporated into phased arrays, this design feature is rarely implemented.

Phased Arrays

Using the phased array approach, it is possible to switch beam direction rapidly in any pattern desired. This makes it far easier to perform simultaneous Doppler and imaging studies. The initial concept for combination was to dedicate alternate pulses to imaging and Doppler, with the pulses allotted to imaging being swept through the usual scan plane and the Doppler pulses oriented along a specified line of sight. This, unfortunately, divided the total pulse repetition frequency (PRF) of the system in half. Therefore, because pulsed Doppler systems begin with an undesirably low PRF, this approach proved unacceptable. The second method was to fire several Doppler pulses in a row interrupted by a single imaging pulse. Although this approach did not result in a significant reduction in Doppler PRF, the resulting imaging had a slow sweeping appearance that was not visually pleasing.

An alternative method of time sharing between imaging and Doppler modes was developed that overcame many of the forgoing problems. In this format, Doppler sampling is interrupted for roughly 20 msec to record a full image scan. During this period, the missing Doppler signal can simply be left blank or can be filled in using a synthesized signal based on the directly measured signal in the period when the Doppler scanner is in use. This signal is obtained using a missing signal estimator (MSE). The Doppler "on" period must be long enough to collect sufficient data for the MSE to produce the synthesized signal in the Doppler "off" period, when the imaging is performed. This period can be roughly 10 msec, which makes the total imaging and pulsed Doppler cycle equal 30 msec. This technique gives an updated frame rate of 30 frames/sec. In the Doppler period, no reduction in pulse rate occurs, and mean velocity is not reduced. Thus, it is even possible to do continuous wave (CW) Doppler measurements in the Doppler "on" period, so that high velocities can be measured together with moving images. The relative length of the Doppler sampling period and the image update interval can be varied as desired by the operator. The last method gives practically no trade-offs between Doppler and imaging. Further, if the array can be designed so that specific elements are devoted to Doppler, the Doppler sensitivity increases. The transducer, however, remains large, and a separate, smaller, stand alone Doppler transducer is frequently required, to achieve better access and sensitivity. The optimal instrument should therefore, permit independent Doppler measurements along with the combined two-dimensional and Doppler measurement. In most patients, the combined instrument will perform both functions, but when sensitivity is critical the independent Doppler will provide better results.

REFERENCES

1. Hatle L, Anglesen B: Doppler Ultrasound in Cardiology. Philadelphia, Lea & Febiger, 1985.

2. Baker DW: Principles of Doppler. *In* Fry FJ (ed.): Ultrasound: Its Applications in Medicine and Biology. New York, Elsevier Science Publishing, 1978.
3. Atkinson P, Woodcock JP: Doppler Ultrasound and Its Use in Clinical Measurement. New York, Academic Press, 1982.
4. Johnson SL, Baker DW, Lute RA, Dodge HT: Doppler echocardiography: the localization of cardiac murmurs. Circulation 48:810, 1973.
5. Flax SW, Webster JG, Updyke SJ: Statistical evaluation of the ultrasonic blood flowmeter. *In* Biomedical Sciences Instrumentation. New York, Plenum, p. 201, 1970.
6. Peronneau P, Hinglais H, Pellet M, Leger F: Velocimetre sanguin par effect Doppler a emission ultra-sonore pulsee. L'Onde Electrique 59:369, 1970.
7. Rice SQ: Mathematical analysis of random noise. Bell Sys Tech J 23:282, 1944.
8. Rice SQ: Mathematical analysis of random noise. Bell Sys Tech J 24:1, 1945.
9. Bachman NM: Noise and its Effects on Communications. New York, McGraw-Hill, 1966.
10. Lunt MJ: Accuracy and limitations of the ultrasonic Doppler blood velcimeter and zero crossing detector. Ultrasound Med Biol 2:1, 1975.
11. Kato K, et al.: Linearity of readings on ultrasonic flowmeters. Dig 6th Intl Conf Med Elect Bio Eng p. 284, 1965.
12. Feynman RP, Leighton RB, Sands M: The Feynman Lectures in Physics. Reading, MA, Addison-Wesley, 1963.
13. Milnor WR: Hemodynamics. Baltimore, Williams & Wilkins, 1982.
14. Skidmore R, Follett DH: Maximum frequency follower for the processing of ultrasonic Doppler shift signals. Ultrasound Med Biol 14:145, 1978.
15. Arts MGJ, Roevros JMJG: On the instantaneous measurement of blood flow by ultrasonic means. Med Biol Eng 10:23, 1972.
16. Skidmore R, Woodcock JP: Physiological interpretation of arterial models derived using transcutaneous ultrasonic flowmeters. Proc Physiol Soc 277: 29, 1979.
17. Gill RW: Performance of the mean frequency Doppler modulator. Ultrasound Med Biol 5:237, 1979.

CHAPTER

11

PRINCIPLES OF COLOR FLOW MAPPING

Color flow mapping represents the synthesis of echo structure detection and Doppler flow recording to produce a composite two-dimensional images that depicts both anatomy and flow in a spatially correct, dynamic format. To construct these composite images, color flow mapping devices must be capable of sampling every point in the scan plane and determining the amplitude and phase of the returning signals at each of these locations. This is an enormous computational task because if each reflected waveform is divided, for example, into 256 points and the device has a pulse repetition frequency (PRF) of 5000/sec, then the instrument must analyze 1,180,000 points/sec. In addition, because the processes involved in amplitude detection and phase comparison differ, the returning signal must be processed separately and the resulting data recombined to form the final output. Finally, color flow mapping devices must also be capable of functioning as independent two-dimensional and M-mode imagers and pulsed and continuous wave Doppler flowmeters, making the final instrument highly complex from both an engineering and clinical viewpoint.[1–6]

The principles of two-dimensional image generation and conventional Doppler analysis and display have been discussed in detail in earlier chapters and will be described here only as they relate to the color flow mapping device. This chapter concentrates on the color flow mapping process and the integration of the multiple outputs to form the final display. In the next chapter we describe the interaction of color flow maps with complex flow fields.

GENERAL OVERVIEW AND SYSTEM DESIGN

Pulsed Echo Transmission and Reception

All color flow mapping devices operate in a pulsed echo mode to achieve range resolution. Color flow mappers are, therefore, subject to the same trade-offs in (1) axial vs. velocity resolution, and (2) depth of field vs. PRF and data line number that apply to conventional imaging and Doppler devices operating in the pulsed mode. The fundamental conflict between spatial (axial) and velocity resolution is always present because shorter pulses provide better axial resolution for both imaging and Doppler, whereas velocity resolution and sensitivity increase in direct relation to pulse length. This problem can be partially overcome in a dual function system by tightly linking the transducer output (burst length) to the length of the drive pulse. Then, if the imaging and Doppler functions are separated and long pulses are transmitted for Doppler sampling and short wide bandwidth pulses for imaging, differential axial (spatial and velocity) resolution can be achieved for the two separate operations. The spatial resolution of the Doppler sampling, however, will still be a function of pulse length and the inverse relationship between Doppler velocity and spatial resolution cannot be uncoupled. In addition, the receive characteristics of the transducer must be optimized for one of the two functions (i.e., Doppler or imaging, as discussed in Chapters 7 and 8). Thus, as with conventional dual or multipurpose devices, one of the operating modes must usually be compromised to achieve a desired level of performance in the other.

Determinants of Data Availability

The second important physical constraint encountered by any pulsed echo device is the inverse relationship between depth of field and PRF. As discussed earlier (Chapter 2), the PRF is determined by the depth of field (maximal sampling range R_{max}) because a pulse must travel to the furthest target of interest and the echoes return before a second pulse can be transmitted. Because the "time of flight" or the time per pulse (T_p) depends on the range (R) to the target, the time alotted to each pulse equals

$$T_p = R_{max} * c/2 \qquad [11.1]$$

and the maximal number of pulses transmitted per second or the PRF equals

$$PRF = 1/T_p \qquad [11.2]$$

Because each transmitted pulse generates one reflected waveform or data line, the number of data lines available to the color flow mapper for both imaging and Doppler is equal to the PRF. These data lines can be allocated to form color flow images based on the desired frame rate, scan angle, line density, and as will be shown later, velocity resolution. The absolute number, however, is always fixed by the depth of field. Because pulses of different burst length are used to obtain imaging and Doppler data, the same pulse is never used for both purposes. As a result, the available data lines must be further subdivided in a color flow mapping system into those used for Doppler and those available for imaging. This requires that an additional compromise be made in data allocation between the two processes.

Data Acquisition and Display Formats

In the most common acquisition and display format, the ultrasonic beam is swept through a predetermined spatial plane to produce a two-dimensional image. For most cardiac applications, a sector format is used; however, for epicardial and peripheral vascular studies, linear arrays with a rectangular scan format are more frequently used (Fig. 11–1). Beam movement during cardiac scanning is typically achieved using a phased array approach; however, mechanical beam scanning using stepper motors is possible.[7]

Imaging and Doppler data are acquired separately with different acquisition formats used in different instruments. Because images can be constructed from sequential data lines recorded along different lines of sight, whereas Doppler flow sampling requires at least two samples at each location to detect a phase shift, the Doppler component of the process requires more data, and therefore, a greater acquisition time. The two most common approaches for collecting the two data sets are (1) to perform a high speed imaging sweep and then a slower Doppler sweep recording multiple lines at each location or (2) to record an initial image data line at each transducer location (beam angle) and to then record multiple Doppler samples before moving the beam to a new interrogation angle (Fig. 11–2).

Color flow depiction in an M-mode format (Fig. 11–3) can also be achieved from a static beam position; however, as with imaging, this approach sacrifices the spatial information available in a two-dimensional display and is ordinarily used only for timing purposes. In the M-mode format, one data line is used to create the image, the next group of data lines is devoted to Doppler sampling and the process is repeated continuously for the duration of the recording.

THE COLOR FLOW MAPPER

Figure 11–4 is a block diagram of a representative color flow instrument. Pulse transmission and signal reception are similar to that of any other pulsed echo device. The signal processing and display portion of the instrument can be subdivided into six primary component areas: (1) the amplitude processing channel, (2)

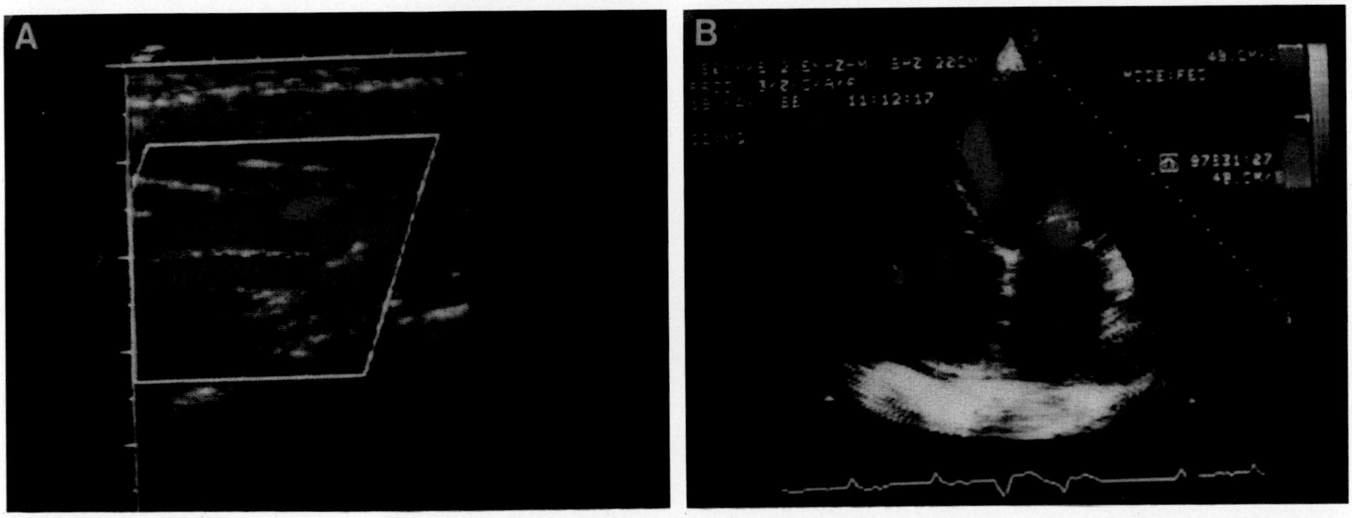

Fig. 11–1. **A.** Rectangular format for the display of color flow data. This format is more commonly used for peripheral vascular applications. **B.** Sector format. This format is preferred for cardiac imaging.

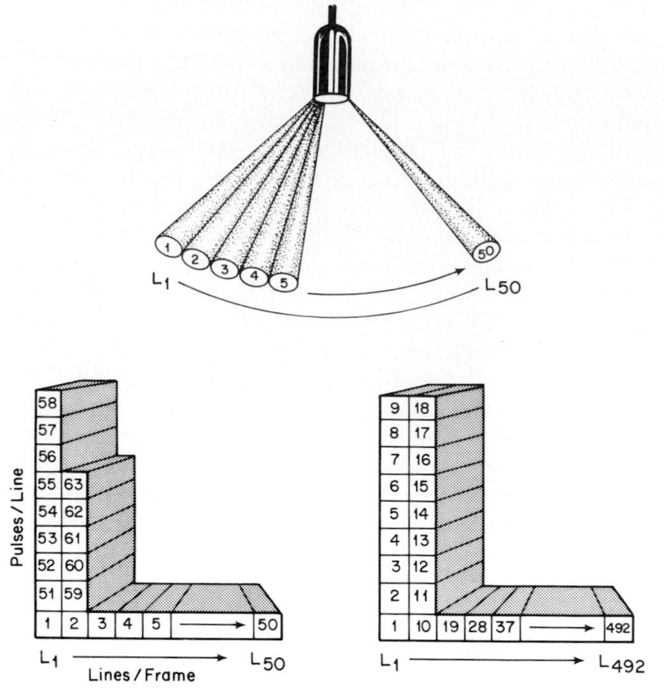

Fig. 11–2. Scan and image assembly formats used to construct color flow images. The upper panel illustrates the spatial beam locations. Lower left. A rapid imaging scan throughout the entire sector, followed by repeated pulsed data acquisition at each scan orientation to construct the Doppler image. Lower right. The first pulse is devoted to image construction; succeeding pulses along each line of site are devoted to Doppler flow mapping for the same line of site. (Numbers within boxes represent order in which data is collected).

quadrature phase demodulator, (3) the spectral Doppler analyzer, (4) the color flow processor, (5) the digital scan converter, and (6) the color processor and display components. Although each of these primary components is present in all color flow mappers, their mode of operations differs from instrument to instrument. Therefore, the following sections describe the generic function of these components rather than the specific operation of a particular instrument.

The Amplitude Channel

As noted previously, all color flow mappers acquire imaging and Doppler data separately with the result that the same pulse is never used to extract amplitude and frequency (phase) information. As the imaging data are acquired, they are transmitted to the amplitude channel that processes the signal using a detection format similar to that found in any pulsed echo imaging device to determine the location and amplitude of echoes arising from specific structures of interest. This process is discussed in detail in Chapters 1 and 2 and summarized in Figure 11–5. After appropriate amplification and processing, this channel produces a time varying digital output that corresponds in timing and magnitude to the range and amplitude of the reflected signals. This information is then passed on to the digital scan converter, which transforms the raw data acquired in polar coordinates into a rectangular array, as discussed in Chapter 3 and illustrated in Figure 11–6B to D. In the color flow mapping process, the large amount of data required for Doppler signal detection typically results in a low image line density and the imaging scan converter must compensate for gaps in the data using a variety of line-to-line and frame-to-frame interpolation algorithms to fill out the picture. Once the two data sets (amplitude and phase or

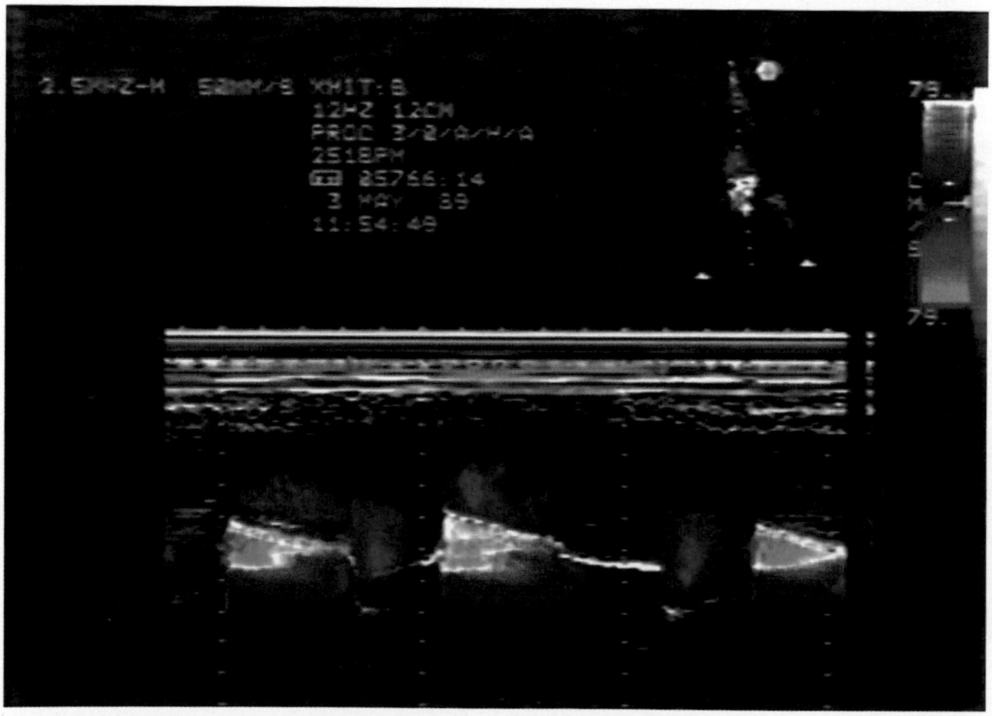

Fig. 11–3. Color flow M-mode. This format is ideal for defining the timing and location of the flow disturbance.

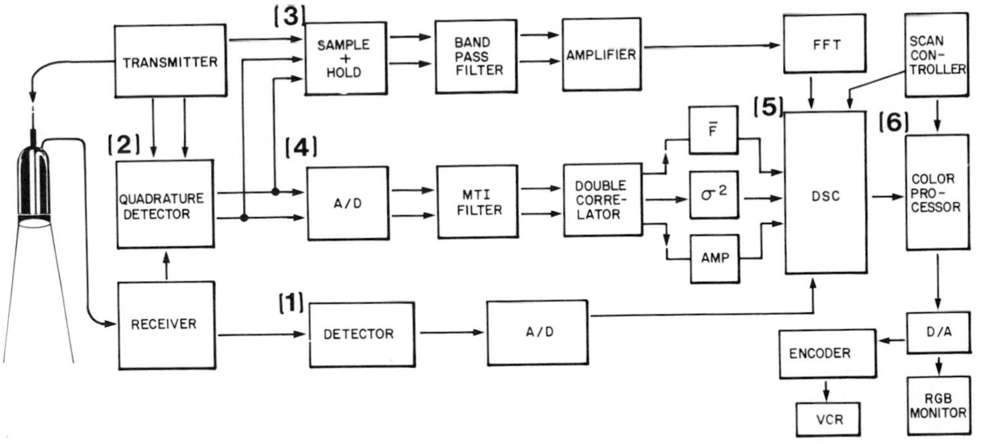

Fig. 11–4. Block diagram of a representative color flow mapping instrument. (1) Amplitude processing channel. (2) Quadrature phase demodulator. (3) Spectral Doppler analyzer. (4) Color flow processor. (5) Digital scan converter. (6) Color processor and display components. A/D = analogue to digital converter; DSC = digital scan converter; D/A = digital to analogue converter; RGB = red, green, blue; VCR = video cassette recorder; FFT = fast Fourier transform; MTI = moving target indicator; $\bar{F}$ = mean velocity; σ^2 = variance; AMP = amplitude (power).

structure and flow) are complete, a predefined algorithm (discussed later) determines those portions of the reflected signal that represent echoes arising from cardiac structures (Fig. 11–6D). These echoes are then displayed in a standard black and white format similar to that of any two-dimensional echo device.

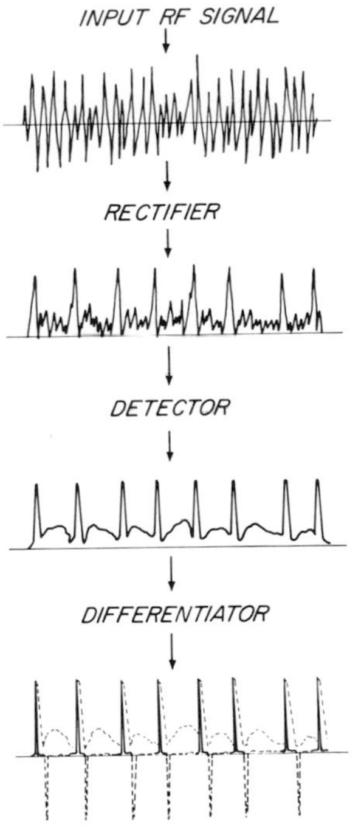

Fig. 11–5. Summary of the operations that occur in the amplitude processing channel. The input radio frequency (RF) signal is rectified, envelope detected, differentiated, digitized, and output in digital format to the digital scan converter. These operations are discussed in detail in Chapters 1 and 2.

If the instrument is operating as a dedicated imaging device, all the acquired data are devoted to image generation. Only the amplitude channel operates, and a standard two-dimensional image is output if the transducer is scanning or a conventional M-mode recording if the transducer or beam angle remains stationary.

The Quadrature Phase Demodulator

All signals not used for image generation are transmitted to the Doppler channel where they are processed to determine the presence, location, and velocity of flow. To identify or exclude the presence of flow at any point within the raster of the display, the instrument must essentially sample all points along each reflected wave. To understand this process, remember that echoes are returning from the transmitted pulse continuously during its passage through tissue. In the pulsed Doppler

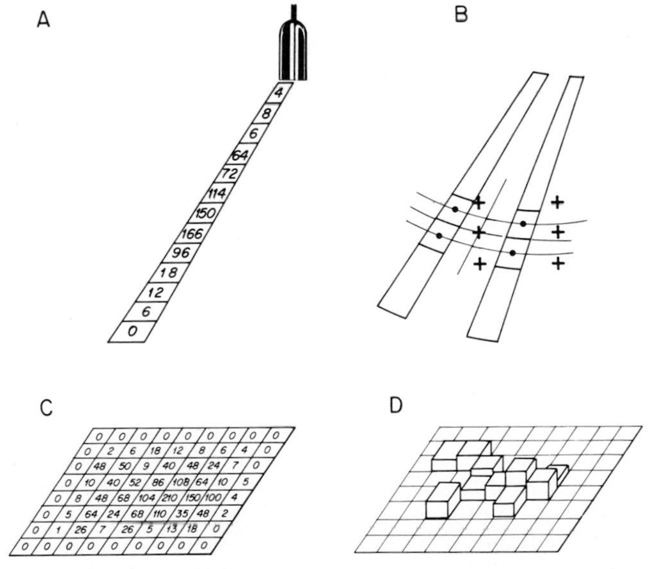

Fig. 11–6. The conversion of digital data in a polar format into a rectangular array in the digital scan converter. **A.** Polar digital data input. **B.** Interpolation of data during conversion from the polar to the rectangular format. (See Chapter 3 for details.) **C.** Rectangular array of digital data output by the scan converter. **D.** Digital data converted to a three-dimensional format with amplitude represented by the height of each pixel.

systems discussed in Chapter 8, this entire waveform (E_rt), which contains both the carrier (w_ot) and the Doppler-shifted frequencies (w_dt), is first split and then transmitted into two parallel processing channels: the direct and quadrature channels. In the direct channel, it is multiplied continuously by the oscillator frequency, whereas in the quadrature channel it is multiplied by a copy of the oscillator frequency shifted in phase by 90°. (The process of quadrature phase demodulation is discussed in detail in Chapter 8.) This initial multiplication or correlation produces waveforms with a primary frequency at roughly twice the carrier frequency ($2F_o$), modulated by low frequency components representing the Doppler phase shifts (w_dt) and clutter from high amplitude stationary or slow moving targets. The output of both channels is then low-pass-filtered to remove frequencies in the range of the carrier, and the result is a continuous output from both the direct and quadrature channels (Cos w_dt and Sin w_dt) plus any associated low frequency clutter. A *continuous* low frequency signal is produced from both channels because the returning waveform generally varies in amplitude, frequency, or both, relative to the reference oscillator waveform and, therefore, will never cancel completely. The output of the quadrature channels can then be directed into either a standard Doppler spectrum analyzer or a color flow processor for further analysis.

The Spectral Doppler Analyzer

In the Doppler processor, the signals from each of the quadrature channels are sampled at a point corresponding to the depth and duration of the range gate to reconstruct the Doppler waveforms. If the range gate is appropriately positioned and the signal is obtained from an area of blood flow, the returning signal will gradually vary in amplitude over time, and from this fluctuation in signal amplitude, the Doppler frequency can be reconstructed. The outputs of the sample and hold circuits are then bandpass filtered and multiplied by a pilot or offset frequency with a similar 90° phase shift (Cos w_pt and Sin w_pt) to that in the respective quadrature channels, and the output of the two channels is then summed. The sampled signal is then transmitted to a fast Fourier transform (FFT) analyzer and the component frequencies output. This process is summarized in Figure 11–7. Note that in this process all of the waveform outside the range gate has been discarded, and most of the signal that arises from non-flow-related fluctuations in amplitude between the reflected waveform and the oscillator frequency (clutter) is removed. To create a flow map it would be possible to position gates at preset intervals along the entire waveform and then process the output of each of these gates independently. This type of analysis is discussed in the section on multigate Dopplers in Chapter 8. Such a process is prohibitive, however, because each gate would require a separate sample and hold circuit and FFT processor, making the cost, complexity, and component count enormous.

The Color Flow Processor

To simplify the process of analysis while at the same time sampling the entire returning waveform for possible flow-related phase shifts, the color flow processor takes the entire waveform from the quadrature channels Cos w_dt and Sin w_dt and processes them using the concepts of moving target indication. The principles of operation of a moving target indicator (MTI) are illustrated in Figure 11–8. Basically, if a series of identical ultrasonic pulses interact with groups of targets, each target encountered by the pulse produces an echo (e), which returns to the transducer after a time delay proportional to its distance from the transducer. If successive pulses are compared, the echoes (waveform and interval) from stationary targets will be identical. The time interval be-

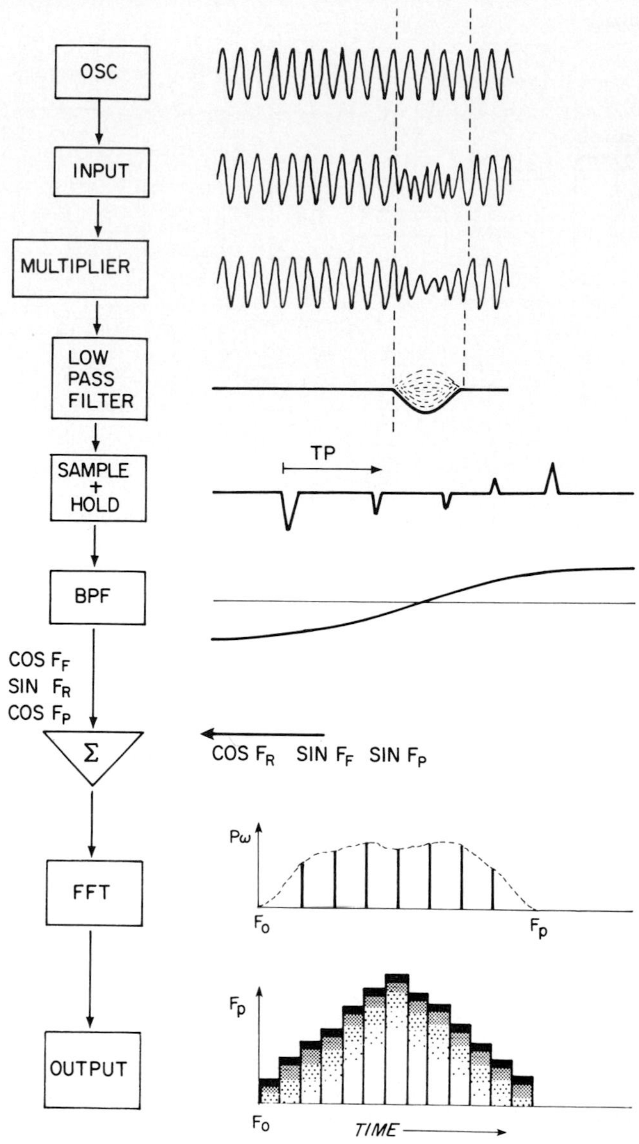

Fig. 11–7. Summary of the operations occurring in the pulsed Doppler channel. The input waveform is correlated with the oscillator frequency, low-pass-filtered to remove frequencies at the carrier, range-gated, and the output smoothed in a sample and hold circuit. Because these processes occur in both quadrature channels, the output is then summed in a summing amplifier, is processed in a fourier transform analyzer, and is output via the digital scan converter for display. Thee processes are discussed in detail in Chapters 7, 8, and 10. BPF = bandpass filter; FFT = fast Fourier transform; TP = interpulse interval; Pω = power; F_o = zero frequency; F_p = peak frequency.

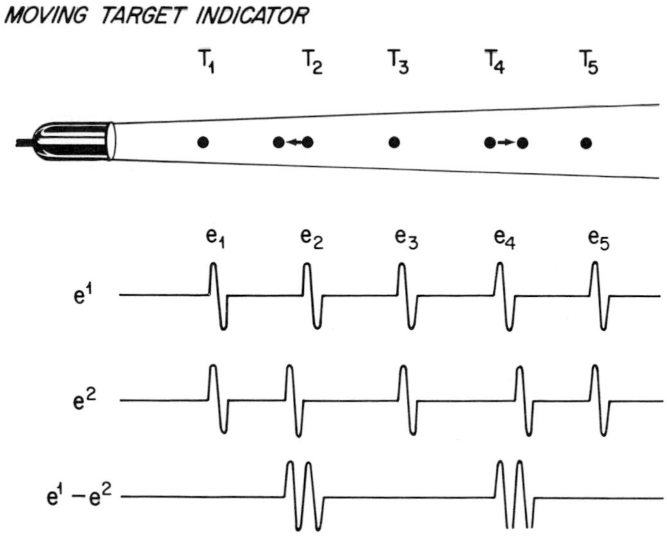

Fig. 11–8. Concept of moving target detection. T_{1-5} are the targets being interrogated by the sound beam. In this example, targets 1, 3, and 5 are stationary, whereas targets 2 and 4 are moving to the left and right, respectively; e^1 indicates the echo location from the first in a train of pulses; and e^2 illustrates the echo location from the second pulse in the train. As illustrated, the echoes from the stationary targets retain the same range, whereas those from moving targets have shifted in location. When the second pulse is subtracted from the first, the echoes from the stationary target will subtract out and those from the moving targets will not completely cancel. Likewise, the distance between these two echoes will indicate the speed of motion of the target.

tween echoes arising from moving targets, however, will change, producing a phase difference at points along successive returning waves, which corresponds to the velocity and range of the moving targets. If the second wavetrain is then subtracted from the first, the echoes from stationary targets will cancel and the difference will represent the phase shifts in signals from moving targets, which correspond in magnitude to the velocity of the target. Similarly, if the difference between successive pulses is determined using either an autocorrelator or a continuously running phase detector, differences in the waves will be apparent only at points where the returning echoes shift in time (phase).

Autocorrelation

To detect these changes in frequency or phase, commercial instruments take two approaches that are fundamentally different in concept but virtually identical in result. The first approach uses the autocorrelation principle to process the signals from the two quadrature channels. First, however, the signals are digitized and MTI filters are inserted along each line between the quadrature detector and the autocorrelator. This is essential because the output of the quadrature channels contains both amplitude- and phase-modulated data (i.e., echoes from either stationary or slowly moving organs as well as superimposed echoes from flowing blood) and the clutter echoes from stationary targets are much greater in amplitude than the signals from moving blood. These clutter echoes, therefore, would confound the subsequent analysis in the autocorrelator unless removed. The MTI filter selectively suppresses these high amplitude low frequency echoes and increases the amplitude of signals with higher frequency shifts, which presumably represent the Doppler shifted components.[8] Figure 11–9 shows a series of frequency response curves for an MTI filter. In practice the filter characteristic selected is determined by the diagnostic objective. Curve number 3, e.g., is a standard curve. Its input to output response is mathematically expressed as sin $[(\pi/2)(f/f_n)]$. In curves 1 and 2, the low frequency response is selectively boosted, and this serves to enhance low velocity blood flow in areas, e.g., the veins. Conversely, curve number 4 is used to reduce the lower frequencies and serves to suppress the intense artifact caused by wall motion.[8]

After clutter suppression in the MTI filters, the digitized signals are transmitted to the autocorrelator. The autocorrelator consists of delay lines, a complex multiplier, and integrators (Fig. 11–10). Upon entering the autocorrelator, each signal is again split into two, with one copy going directly to the complex multiplier and the second copy going to the complex multiplier via a delay line. The delay intervals are made equal to the pulse transmission interval of the instrument or 1/PRF. For an instrument operating at a PRF of 5000, this delay would be 200 msec. Thus, the analysis is performed by comparing the current reflected pulse with the preceding one (i.e., pulse 1 with pulse 2, 2 with 3, 3 with 4, and so on) (Fig. 11–11). In theory, the initial and delayed pulses should be identical except at points where one wave is out of phase with the other (as occurs when sequential reflections arise from a moving target). Thus, if the two waveforms are correlated (multiplied together), the result will differ from unity only at points along the waveform where the two waves are out of phase (i.e., where target motion has occurred) with the degree of phase

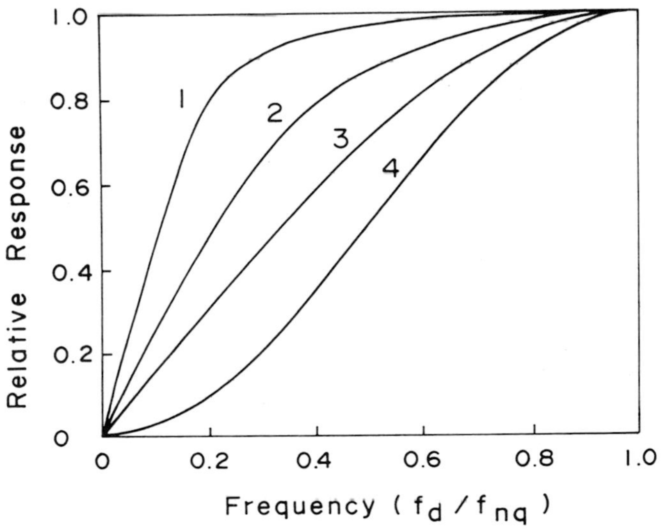

Fig. 11–9. Moving target indicator filter used to suppress clutter from stationary objects while amplifying signals from moving targets. Abscissa: ratio of the Doppler frequency to the Nyquist frequency. Ordinate: values equal the relative output response for each input ratio. (From Omoto R, et al.: Physics and instrumentation of Doppler color flow mapping. Echocardiography 4(6):467, 1987.)

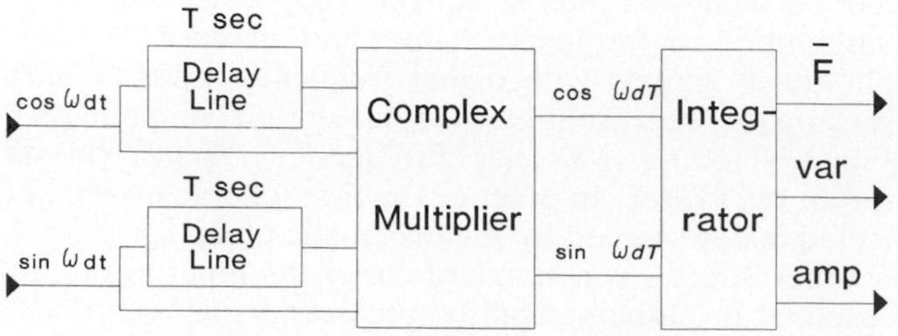

Fig. 11–10. Autocorrelator in the color processing channel. After passing through the analogue to digital (A/D) converter and moving target indicator filter, input pulses from the quadrature channels are delayed by a T second, which is equal to the interpulse interval. Delay and subsequent signal from each channel are then passed to the complex multiplier, which outputs the sine and cosine values for the interpulse phase difference, which are summed in the integrater to output the mean phase (frequency) difference for each packet for sequential spatial sampling intervals (range gates). Also output are the variance between individual pulses and the signal amplitude. (See text for further details.)

shift being equal to the velocity of target motion times the delay between pulses. Alternatively, an inverse correlation can be performed where the output reflects a lack of correlation and increases as the degree of correlation decreases. Mathematically, the complex multiplier carries out the following calculations and outputs a pair of results:

$$\cos \phi_1 * \cos \phi_2 + \sin \phi_1 * \sin \phi_2 = \cos(\phi_1 - \phi_2) \quad [11.3]$$

$$\sin \phi_1 * \cos \phi_2 - \cos \phi_1 * \sin \phi_2 * = \sin(\phi_1 - \phi_2) \quad [11.4]$$

where $\phi_1 = w_o t_1$ is the phase of the signal that has passed through the delay line, and $\phi_2 = w_d t_2$ is that of the undelayed signal (i.e., the signal that bypassed the delay lines). Considering that $T = t_2 - t_1$, $\Delta\phi$ therefore $= \phi_1 - \phi_2 = W_d T$. Thus, Equations 11.3 and 11.4 provide a pair of quadrature signals related to the phase shift between two signals, A sin $\Delta\phi$ and B cos $\Delta\phi$, where A and B are the amplitudes. These operations are illustrated in Figure 11–11. By calculating the quotient of the set of signals,

$$\sin \Delta\phi / \cos \Delta\phi = \tan \Delta\phi \quad [11.5]$$

the tangent of the phase angle is derived from its arctangent, and the phase shift angle $\Delta\phi = W_d T$ is obtained.[8] Direction is determined by the sign of the phase angle $+/- \Delta\phi$. Because these operations are performed continuously, the result describes the relative phase shift and signal amplitude for all points along the waveforms. To reduce computation time and decrease random noise, it is often more convenient to divide the digitized waveform into groups of bits corresponding to sequential spatial ranges or gates and to generate spatial average values for each of these gates. This has the same effect as increasing the range gate duration in a standard pulse Doppler system and should improve velocity resolution, albeit at the expense of spatial resolution.

Note that by using delay lines, each reflected waveform is compared to that preceding it rather than to the oscillator frequency, as in the process of coherent demodulation. As a result, for a constant phase shift, the output of the correlator should be a constant voltage rather than a time varying signal reflecting the Doppler frequency. The differences in these two processes are illustrated in Figure 11–12.

According to the principles described previously, the speed of any moving object may be determined simply by transmitting two ultrasonic pulses in the same direction and determining the phase shift between their echoes (Fig. 11–13A and B). In the case of flowing blood, however, the numerous cells (scatterers) that serve as the moving targets occur in a random and constantly fluctuating distribution. As a result, enormous errors may result if the blood flow velocity is derived from the phase shift between only two signals. Thus, to accurately measure the phase shift or velocity, many pulses are transmitted (Fig. 11–13C), and integrators beyond the complex multiplier average the signals to obtain a mean flow velocity (Fig. 11–13D). The final output, therefore, is the average of the velocities determined from a series of pulse-pairs, with the number of samples used to compute this average referred to as the *packet size*. Obviously, the more data that are integrated (or the larger the packet size), the more accurate the mean frequency.

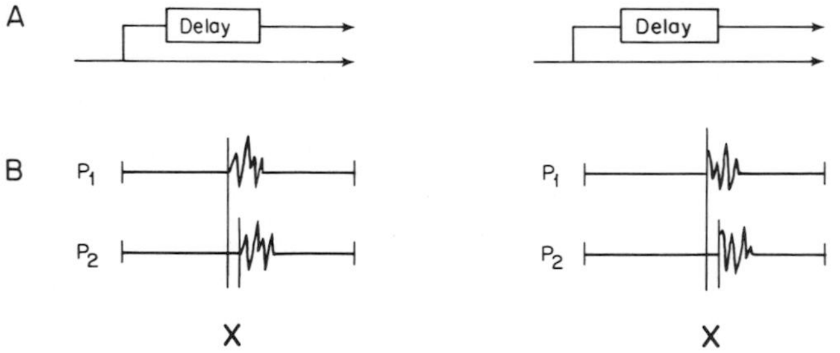

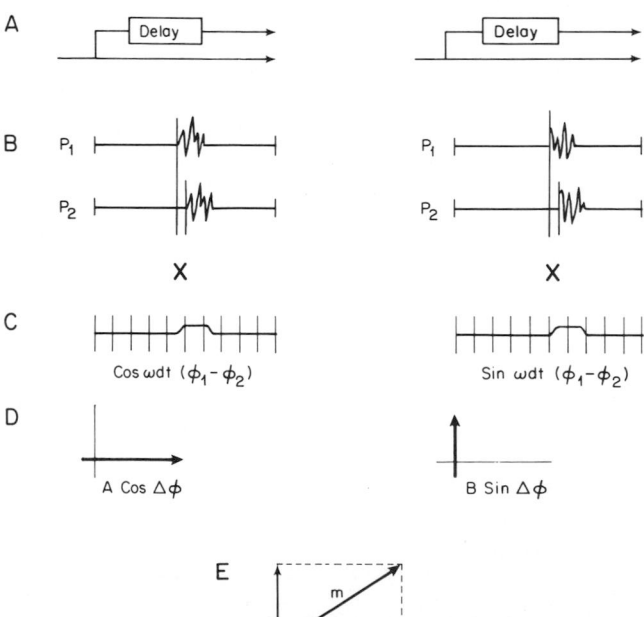

Fig. 11–11. Correlation of transmitted vs. delayed pulse in each of the processing channels (A, B) to yield a continuous output of the sine and cosine values (C, D) for the phase difference between the two signals (E). Also output is the modulus or amplitude of the signal.

Phase Detection

The second approach to flow mapping is based on the concept of phase detection and is illustrated diagramatically in Figure 11–14. In practice, this approach uses two delay lines in series and a phase detector in place of the quadrature channels and autocorrelator. The first delay line helps to cancel the echoes from stationary

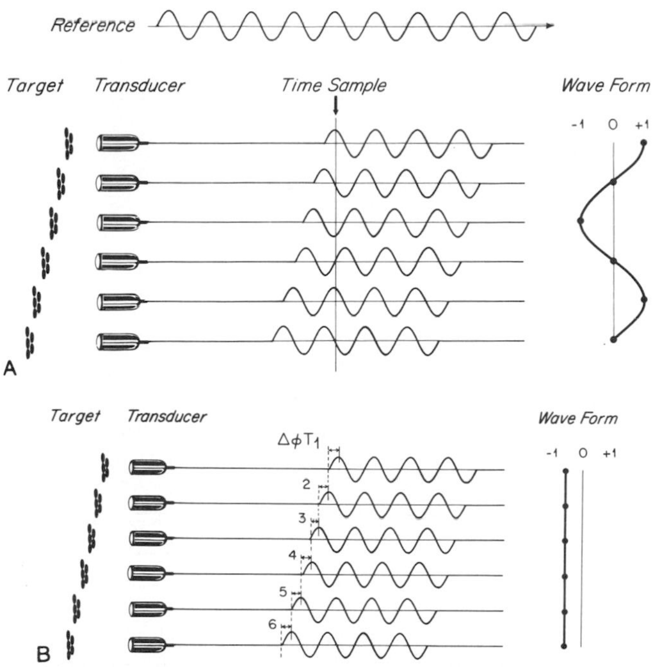

Fig. 11–12. **A.** Pulsed Doppler output. **B.** Moving target indicator output. For a constantly moving target, the pulsed Doppler compares the received signal with the oscillator frequency and outputs a waveform at the Doppler difference frequency. The moving target indicator, in contrast, compares each waveform with that preceding it, and for a constantly moving target will output a continuous voltage with amplitude reflecting target motion.

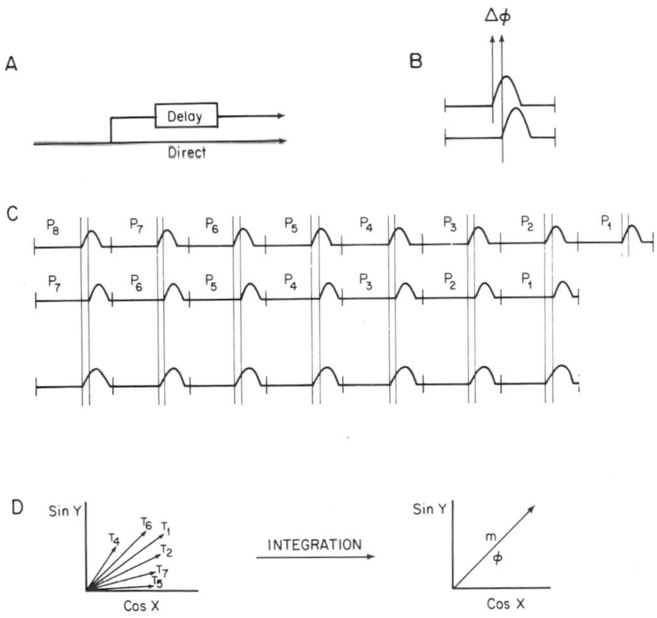

Fig. 11–13. Average output of a series of pulse pairs or a packet of pulses to achieve a more stable estimate of mean frequency. (See text for details.)

targets by subtracting successive wavetrains. This enhances the relative contributions of phase-shifted signals from moving targets ($P_1 - P_2 = \sigma_1$). The second delay line provides the delayed input or reference ($\sigma 1 - \sigma 2$) for the phase detector with output voltage equivalent to $\Delta\phi$.

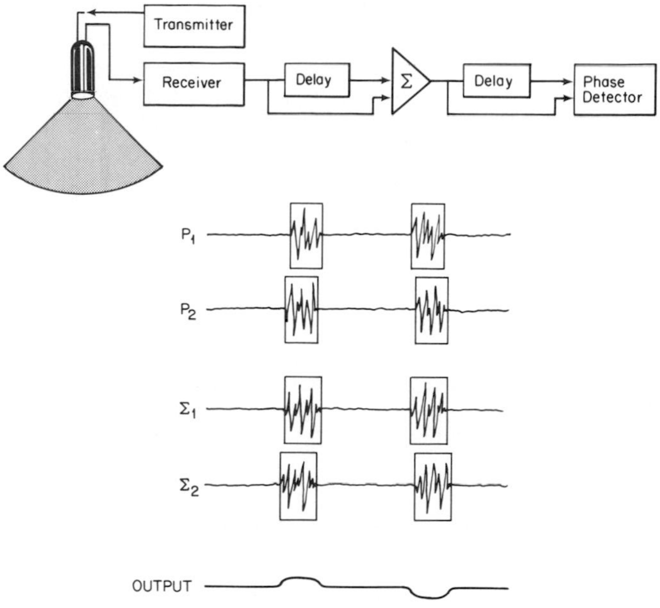

Fig. 11–14. Alternate approach to flow mapping based on the concept of phase detection. This approach employs two delay lines in series and a phase detector in place of the quadrature channels and autocorrelator. The first delay line helps to cancel the echoes from stationary targets by subtracting successive waves. This enhances the relative contributions of phase-shifted signals from moving targets ($P^1 - P_2 = \Sigma_1$). The second delay line provides the delayed input or reference ($\Sigma_1 - \Sigma_2$) for the phase detector with output voltage equivalent to $\Delta\phi$.

Essentially, the phase detector compares the instantaneous phases of the directly transmitted and delayed signals and outputs a voltage that indicates both the direction (positive or negative) and amplitude of the phase shift. Thus, both of these processes, phase detection and autocorrelation, use different methods of signal processing but result in the same final output. In the phase detection format, as in the autocorrelation process, the output of a number of pulses is averaged together to arrive at a relatively stable estimate of mean velocity.

Variance

In addition to achieving a more accurate assessment of mean velocity, the transmission of multiple pulses along the same line of sight also allows the instrument to calculate the variance of individual samples relative to the mean. Mathematically, the variance about the mean frequency for a noncontinuous sample is calculated as follows:

$$\sigma^2 = (F^1 - F_{mean})A_1^2 + (F_2 - F_{mean})A_2^2 + (F_3 - F_{mean})A_3^2/A_1^2 + A_2^2 + A_3^2, \text{ etc.} \quad [11.6]$$

In practice, this is achieved using a variance detector that determines the variability in the signals from which the mean is computed. Laminar flow, in theory, should show little variance; unstable or turbulent flow should have a variance that is directly related to the degree of flow disturbance.[8] It is important to note, however, that variance represents the variation about the mean frequency of the sample. Variance about the mean occurs not only when flow is turbulent but also when flow within the sample volume is accelerating or decelerating (Fig. 11–15A to C). In either case, even if the flow is basically laminar, the sampled information will contain a variety of velocities that result in the calculation of a variance even if no turbulence is present. Deceleration is a more disorganized process than acceleration, and deceleration instability, with its associated spectral broadening, is a characteristic of pulsed Doppler tracings of flows in great arteries as well as across atrioventricular valves. Thus, flow instability and deceleration may occur together, further complicating the physical correlate of the variance. Finally, variance can occur when the signal/noise ratio is poor, and samples containing a recordable Doppler shift are interspersed with those containing no recordable phase shift (Fig. 11–15D).

The color flow processor, therefore, outputs three sets of data: (1) the mean phase shift, which can be equated with velocity; (2) the variance about the mean, which can reflect either turbulence or acceleration; and (3) the amplitude, which reflects the degree of modulation of the carrier by the Doppler frequency and, by inference, the number of scatterers contributing to the Doppler frequency shift.

Digital Scan Converter and Color Processor

To produce a color flow image, the tissue data from the amplitude channel and the Doppler data from the color flow processor must be combined and output by the digital scan converter. Because tissue and Doppler data are not acquired simultaneously, but rather in series, they must be collected and initially processed separately before being combined. All of the data must first be converted from the polar format in which it is acquired to a rectangular format for analysis and processing. This process, illustrated in Figure 11–16 for amplitude data, is similar for the Doppler phase, variance and power input. Conceptually, this results in four stacked data planes (tissue amplitude, Doppler phase, Doppler variance, and Doppler amplitude) with each pixel having some value in each plane. To produce an appropriate output, the digital scan converter must compare the available data for each pixel ($P_{x,y}$) to decide whether to display the pixel as structural data (black and white) or flow data (color).

Although many algorithms exist for making this decision, the simplest is based on amplitude priority (tissue priority). In this format, the incoming signal from the tissue amplitude line, now formatted into a rectangular digital matrix, is initially interrogated to determine the tissue amplitude value at any pixel location. If the pixel value in the amplitude plane is sufficiently high, the pixel is assumed to represent structural data and is assigned a shade of gray determined by the input voltage. If the value for the pixel in the amplitude or tissue plane is below a predetermined threshold, the Doppler-velocity plane that contains a value equal to the magnitude of the phase angle (velocity) is next interrogated. If the value at the pixel location in this plane is above a preset threshold, it is assumed that the pixel contains data from a flow area, and it is assigned a color based on the direction and degree of the phase shift.

If the value in the Doppler plane is not above the preset threshold, the pixel can be left empty (black). Alternatively, the process of pixel location sampling can continue in an iterative fashion while the threshold is

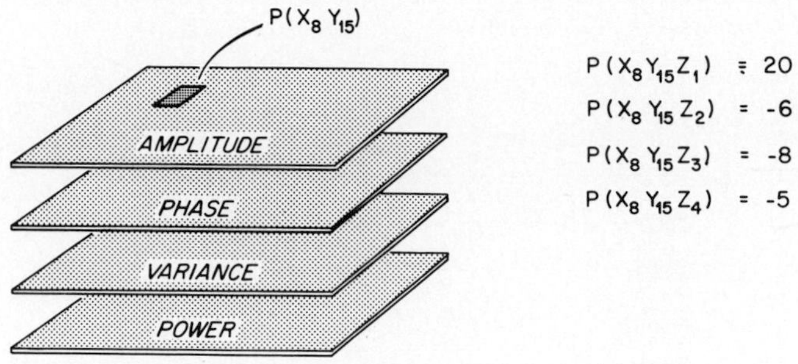

ALGORITHM	OUTPUT
Tissue Priority (T = 15, ± 5)	A20
Tissue Priority (T = 25, ± 5)	-6
Variance Display	V = -8
Power Mode	P = -5

Fig. 11–16. Stacked rectangular arrays of data representing, conceptually, the interaction of the four data sets—amplitude, phase, variance, and power—by assigning a value to each pixel in the color flow image. The numeric value of each parameter for an arbitrary pixel, e.g., X_8, Y_{15}, is given for each data plane (Z1 to Z4). The lower panel indicates the actual pixel value that will be output for a tissue priority algorithm with a threshold of 15, a threshold of 25, a variance display, and a power mode display.

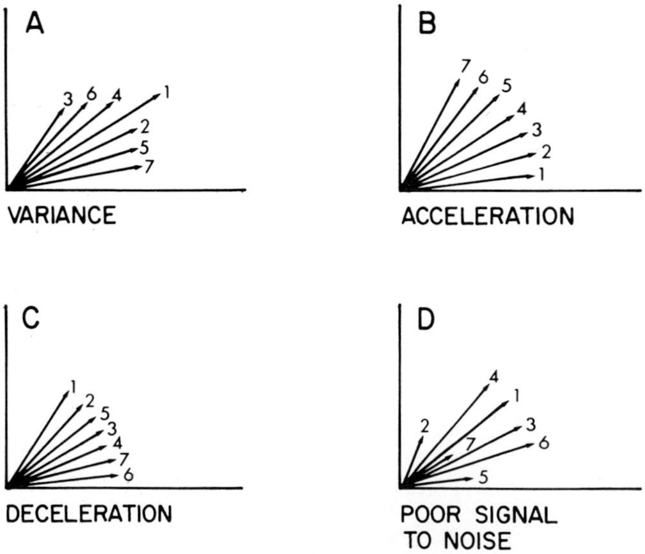

Fig. 11–15. The various phenomena that may produce variance about the mean phase shift for a series of sample pulses. **A.** Variance caused by random fluctuations in the input signal or turbulence. **B.** Variance caused by acceleration. **C.** Variance caused by deceleration. **D.** Variance caused by a poor signal/noise ratio.

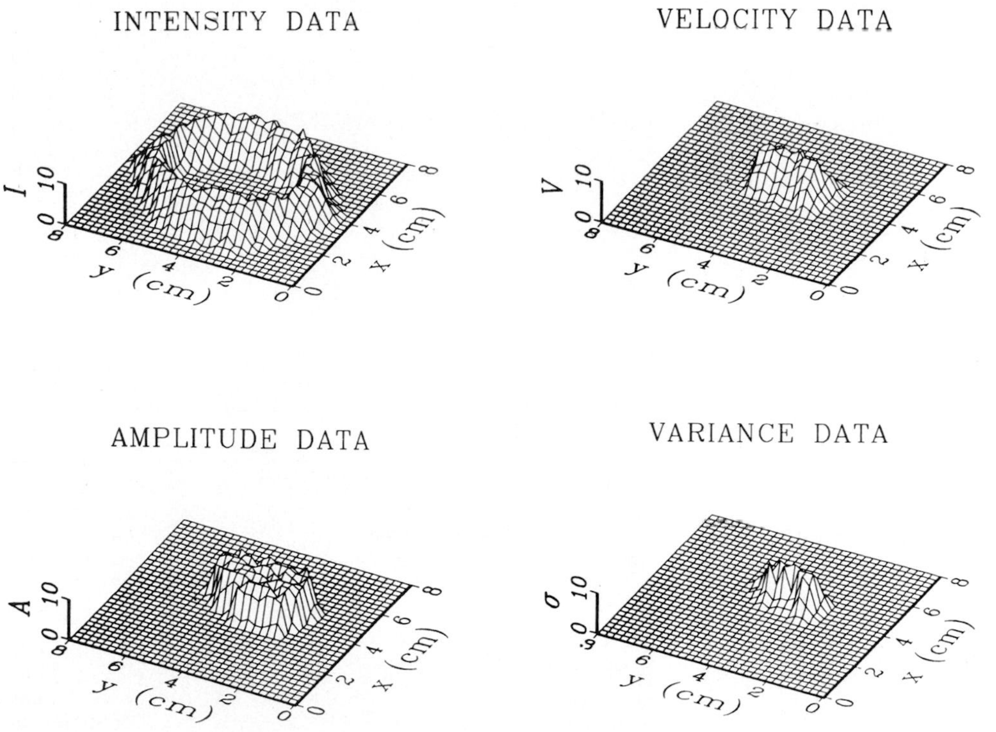

Fig. 11–17. Three-dimensional plots of digital values for each of the four data sets (intensity, velocity [phase], amplitude [power], and variance) for a short axis recording of the left ventricle. Increasing tissue or color gain has the effect of increasing the amplitude of all values for the affected plane. In the absence of some form of priority encoding, this will cause the parameter with the highest value (gain) to spill over into surrounding areas.

decreased incrementally for signal transmission until a value above the threshold is detected in one of the two planes. This process can continue until the signal from one of the planes is displayed or can stop after a preset number of iterations. Obviously, the longer the iterative process continues, the greater the chances for error in the data assignment. Figure 11–17 illustrates in a three-dimensional display examples of relative amplitudes for the data values in each of the four data planes in the scan converter. Altering the gain for any of the pixel values in any of the planes will obviously change its value relative to the other three and, if the magnitude of the change is sufficient, alter the output of the scan converter.

Choice of Color Assignment

The digital values for each pixel in the digital scan converter are transformed to color equivalent signals by the color processor. Most instruments use the primary colors red and blue to indicate flow toward and away from the transducer (Fig. 11–18). These provide the clearest contrast with the surrounding white tissue and

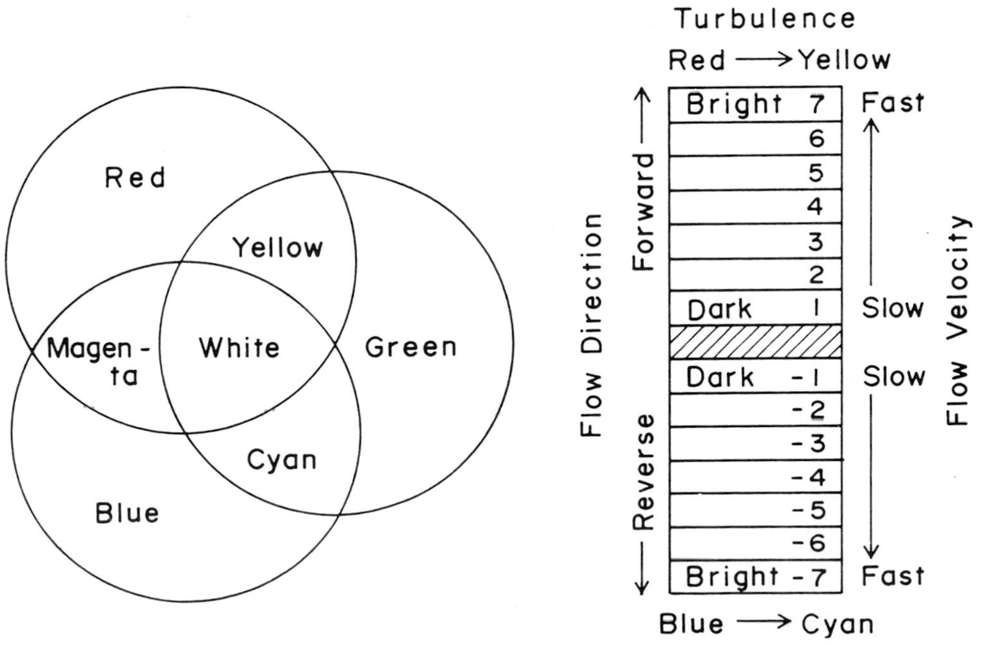

Fig. 11–18. Use of color encoding to depict the direction, velocity, and variance of a Doppler flow signal. Left. The primary colors red and blue are used to depict flow direction toward (red) and away (blue) from the transducer. Variance is depicted in the third primary color, green. Right. Velocity depiction by varying the hues of the primary color. (From Omoto R, et al.: Physics and instrumentation of Doppler color flow mapping. Echocardiography 4(6):467, 1987.)

black blood pool and are, therefore, the easiest for the eye to discriminate in real time. Given the choice of red for flow toward the transducer and blue for flow away, or vice versa, most manufacturers have opted for red indicating flow toward the transducer. This is the opposite of Doppler's original concept that stars moving away from the earth were shifted toward the red end of the spectrum. The "red-toward" convention appears to arise form carotid scanning, in which flow through the carotid artery toward the transducer was encoded in red because hues of red were more readily appreciated by the human eye. Venous flow in this convention was away from the transducer and, therefore, was encoded in blue.[9]

The concept of displaying arterial blood in red and venous blood in blue is intuitive and relatively easy for carotid imaging. Such a convention, however, is obviously impossible in the heart, where blood may flow in many directions within the same scan plane. Thus, the colors red and blue are indicators of flow direction relative to the transducer and are not indicative of oxygen content. Likewise, because color assignment is determined by the direction of flow relative to the transducer, flow in the same direction through the same anatomic region may be assigned different colors when viewed from different transducer locations.[9]

Velocity Depiction

In addition to simple direction, velocity information (based on the magnitude of the phase angle) is displayed by varying the hues of the primary direction colors red and blue. Figure 11–18 illustrates a typical color bar from a color flow mapping instrument that relates color intensity to velocity. The center of the standard color bar is black and represents zero flow. Preceding upward from this center bar, the intensity of the red color bar increases in evenly spaced increments representing increasing ranges of velocity from zero to the Nyquist limit for transducer frequency and PRF. In most current instruments, the frequency range assigned to each hue is similar (i.e., 0 to 10, 11 to 20, 21 to 30 cm/sec, etc.), however, this is not obligatory, and the lower or higher frequency or velocity range can be expanded or compressed using any output function desired. Figure 11–19 illustrates the complex output characteristics of the color processor. As noted earlier, altering the gain (magnitude) for any of the input values (amplitude, phase, variance or power) alters its output by the color processor. Figure 11–20 illustrates the effect of increasing color Doppler gain on the color flow image.

Color Aliasing

Because color flow mappers operate in a pulsed mode, they are subject to the same velocity-sampling rate limitations encountered by any pulsed Doppler device. Remember that for frequency or velocity to be appropriately recorded and displayed the sampling frequency must be at least twice the frequency of any Doppler shift encountered in the sample volume. If this is not the case and the Doppler shift frequency exceeds twice the sampling frequency (PRF/2 or the Nyquist limit), signal

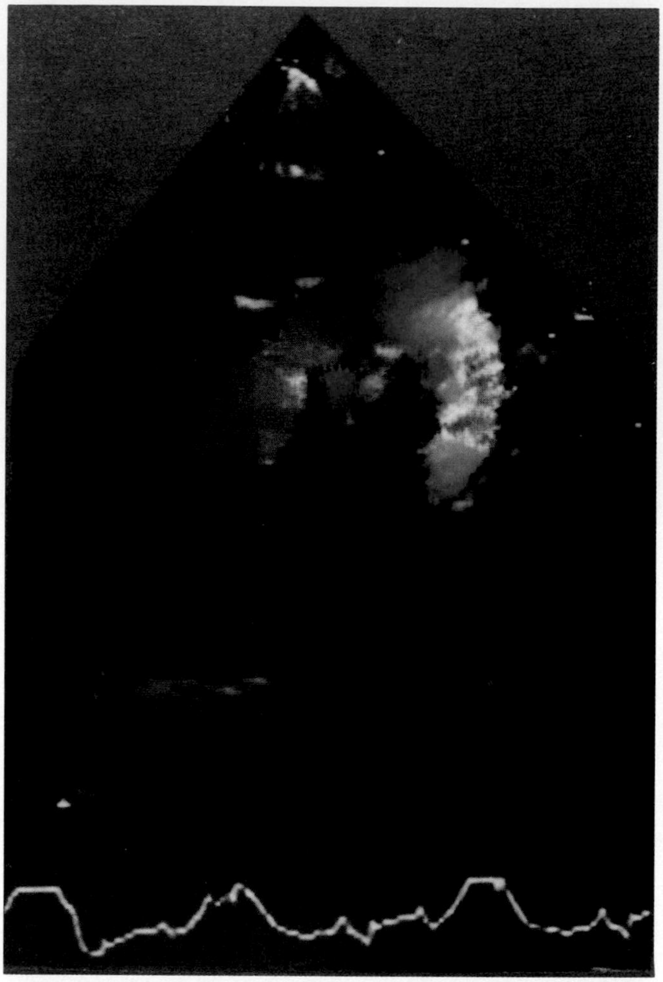

Fig. 11–19. The complex output of the color processor. In this recording, flow in the ascending aorta is depicted as red because it is directed toward the transducer. In the transverse arch, it transitions from red to dark blue, reflecting the shift in direction and effects of the large angle between the interrogating beam and the flow vector. In the descending arch, flow appears to accelerate as the angle between the beam and the flow vector increases. Highest velocities with color aliasing occur along the inner wall of the ascending aorta and the outer wall of the descending aorta. This pattern is consistent with the principles of flow in a curving tube, which are discussed in Chapter 9.

aliasing will occur. The effect can most easily be displayed using a color wheel (Fig. 11–21). In this example, if a target gradually accelerates toward the transducer, the recorded phase shift (output as increasingly brighter hues of red) will increase until it reaches 180°. If the velocity continues to increase beyond this point, the phase shift between pulses will exceed 180°, which will be recorded by the instrument as a decreasing negative value (hues of blue decreasing in brightness). If the velocity continues to increase, the phase vector will continue to rotate from red to blue and back to red until the maximum velocity is reached. Table 11–1 lists the maximal velocities that can be recorded before aliasing occurs for a series of typical transducer frequencies and PRFs or depths of field. Note that aliasing occurs sooner for a color flow mapper than for a conventional pulsed Doppler device because a portion of the PRF output by

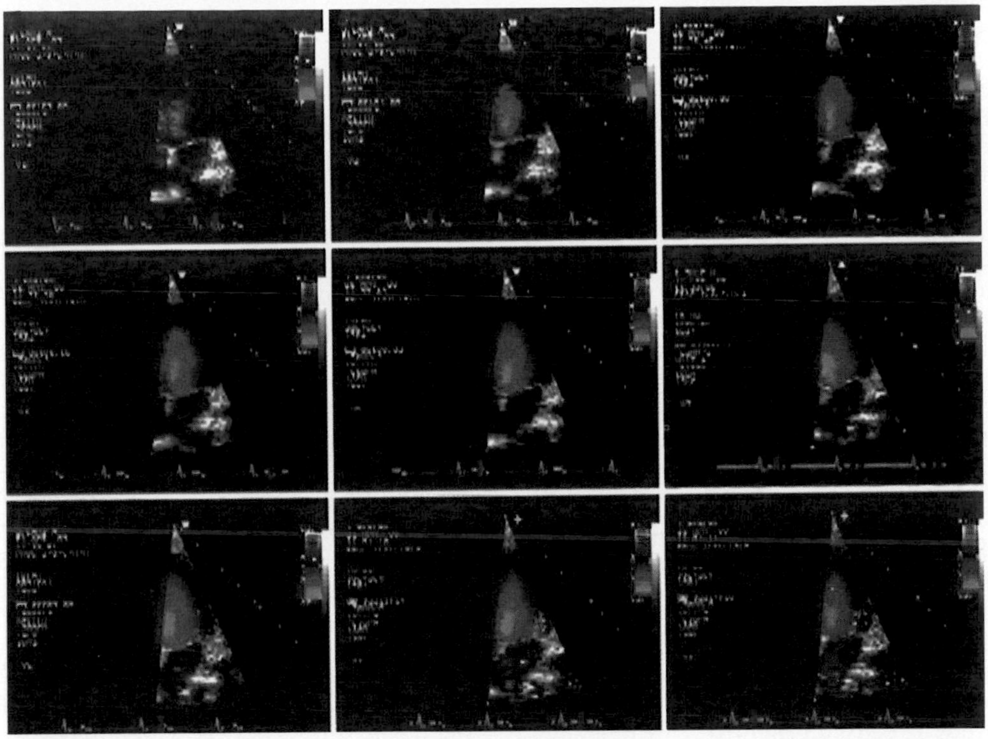

Fig. 11–20. Effect of increasing color gain on the output of a color flow mapper. Gain is gradually increased from upper left to lower right panels. Rows are read from left to right.

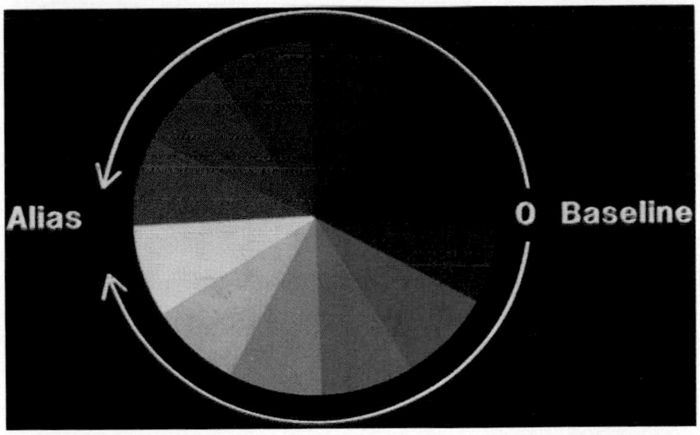

Fig. 11–21. Color wheel depicting color aliasing. As velocity increases through the alias point, color series shifts from red to blue or vice versa. (From Kisslo J, Adams DB, Belkin RN: Doppler Color Flow Imaging. New York, Churchill Livingstone, 1988.)

Table 11–1. Maximal Velocity Detectable Before Aliasing (m/sec)

	PRF (Depth)			
Transmit Frequency	4 KHz (18.8)	6 KHz (12.5)	8 KHz (9.2)	12 KHz (5.1)
2.5 MHz	0.64	0.93	1.23	1.91
3.5 MHz	0.48	0.70	0.93	1.43
5.0 MHz	0.32	0.47	0.62	0.96

the color instrument must be used for image generation, reducing the actual number of pulses available for Doppler sampling.

Variance Display. Flow variance, such as that seen in areas of turbulence or acceleration, can be displayed using the third primary color, green. The relationship of these color patterns and their combinations to depict velocity shifts are illustrated in Figure 11–18. The difference between acceleration and deceleration, which causes a continuous directional shift in the values used to compute the mean, and turbulence, which causes a random fluctuation about the mean, should be detectable by the instrument, but such discrimination is not presently available. Because some variance about the mean is virtually always present, it is again necessary to set some numeric threshold above which the additional color is added to the basic display. The variance data can also be displayed alone to generate a variance map. Such maps, however, have little practical value beyond assessing the performance characteristics of the instrument.

Power Mode

The final parameter output by the color processor is the amplitude of the Doppler signal, which presumably represents the strength of the backscattered echoes. In conventional Doppler processing, the signal amplitude is defined by the power spectrum, which is the amplitude at each frequency. Because the color flow processor does not perform a complete FFT, it can only approximate the power spectrum from the amplitudes of the frequencies (phase shifts) that are used to calculate the mean. If this mean amplitude or power value is output instead of the pause angle value, it gives an approximation of the strength of the backscattered signal at a spatial location.

Before outputting the power value, the instrument must first decide that a given pixel location represents a flow area. This can be determined from the magnitude of the phase angle or by assuming that any signal that passes through the MTI filter represents flow. Once this decision is made, the amplitude value rather than the phase data is output for that location. The amplitude data can be represented using any desired color assignments for flow toward or away from the transducer (based on the direction of the phase angle). The intensity of the color is used to represent differences in power. Note that because the direction of flow is still determined by the phase angle, the output will be subject to aliasing and color reversal will occur when the phase angle exceeds 180°, even though velocities are not being displayed.

This type of display is commonly called the *power mode*, and it should approximate the number of cells moving within a particular area. This may be helpful in determining the volume of a regurgitant lesion or in detecting large numbers of cells moving at low velocity as in venous flow. However, as indicated earlier (Chapter 9), because scattering amplitude is caused primarily by fluctuation in the density of the scatterers in a specific region rather than by scatterer number per se, this is an imprecise measure.

Output and Display of Color Flow Maps

Both the color information and the black and white information contained in a completed color flow image can be displayed directly as output from the scan converter using an RGB monitor (because white is the sum of the primary colors and black is the absence of color) or, after conversion to an analog video format, on a color TV monitor. The data can also be stored on videotape and replayed at a later time. Video display limits the spatial resolution of the image because the sampling rates of the upper and lower color side band of the video signal are much lower than the actual pixel output of the instrument (see Chapter 3). This causes image degradation and complicates color flow analysis because it has the effect of smearing together data from groups of adjacent pixels that cannot later be separated to calculate the velocity for each pixel.

INTERRELATIONSHIP OF VELOCITY RESOLUTION, DEPTH OF FIELD, LINE DENSITY, AND FRAME RATE

Because color flow devices must average many pulses together to arrive at a mean velocity, sequential pulses must be transmitted along the same line of sight, with the result that less unique data are available for image assembly. For example, if we assume a PRF of 5000 pulses/sec, these pulses or data lines can be divided into individual frames based on considerations of line density, frame rate, and in color flow Doppler scanning, mean velocity resolution (packet size). The ideal is to maintain a frame rate above the flicker vision frequency of the eye (15/sec), a wide scan angle (90°), accurate velocity resolution (e.g., 10 lines per sample), and an adequate line density (2 lines/degree). Unfortunately, to satisfy all of these requirements, using the preceding examples, would require 27,000 data lies (2 × 90 × 10 × 15), but only 5000 lines at most are available. Therefore, some compromises must be made, resulting in either a decrease in scan angle, image resolution, packet size, frame rate, or a combination of parameters. Empiric data suggest that a packet size of eight provides the best compromise between velocity resolution and data requirements (Fig. 11–22). At a PRF of 5000, this leaves 625 lines to be distributed among the total number of frames created. If we take 15 frames/sec as a threshold, 42 lines/frame are available. Assuming adequate image resolution requires roughly 1.5 lines/degree, the resulting sector size would be just under 30°. These relationships can be expressed using the equation

$$nT_pNF = 1 \qquad [11.7]$$

where n represents the number of pulses radiated along the same line of sight or the packet size, T_p is the pulse repetition period (1/PRF), N is the number of lines per frame, and F is the frame rate. These calculations disregard the fact that separate pulses must be used for imaging and Doppler, which further constrains the available data. They also ignore the electronic reset time required for conversion of the electronic data from transmission to reception and vice versa, which further decreases the actual PRF. As a result, color flow mappers must resort to various forms of data interpolation and cannot achieve the same performance parameters (sector angle, frame rate, and line density) that are found in conven-

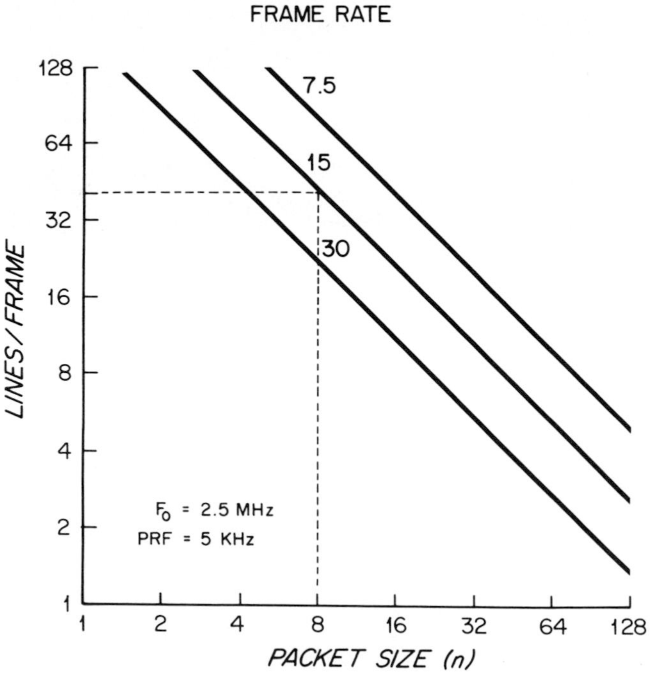

Fig. 11–22. Interrelationship between packet size, frame rate, and line density. Values for a carrier frequency (F_o) of 2.5 MHz and a PRF of 5 KHz.

Table 11–2. Typical Combinations of Depth of Field, Packet Size, Lines per Frame, and Frame Rate for Color Flow Images

Depth of Field (cm)	Packet Size	Lines per Frame	Frames per Second
6	4	30	30
8	8	45	20
10	8	30	30
12	4	45	30
14	8	30	20
16	8	45	15
18	4	30	30
18	4	45	20
18	8	45	12

tional two-dimensional images while simultaneously providing useful velocity information.

Table 11–2 lists some typical combinations for depth of field, packet size, lines per frame, and frame rate for color flow images. Obviously, the pattern in which these variables can be combined is almost infinite. However, given the fixed number of samples available at any depth, an increase in one parameter (image resolution, scan angle, velocity resolution, or frame rate) must result in a decrease in one or more of the others. Because depth of field and velocity resolution are the least flexible parameters, the compromises are usually made in sector angle, frame rate, or line density.

COLOR DOPPLER SPATIAL, TEMPORAL, AND VELOCITY RESOLUTION

Spatial Resolution

The spatial and velocity resolution of Doppler instruments are important considerations in clinical applications, particularly those that attempt to quantitate various portions of the flow signal. Doppler data, in general, have poorer axial resolution than tissue reflections in the same area. This is because the imaging pulse is shorter, and the signal processing in the amplitude channel is designed to detect only the leading edge of the reflected echo. The Doppler pulse, in contrast, is far longer, and the signal arises from the whole sample volume. For example, a Doppler pulse of 15 cycles at a transmit frequency of 2.5 MHz will be roughly 12 mm long. Thus, if the depth of field is 12 cm and the transmit pulse 12 mm, only 10 unique sample volumes exist between the transducer and the limit of sampling. If the resulting data line is sampled 256 times, these samples do not represent unique data, but rather a sliding average. As a result, a portion of the Doppler sample volume may be interacting with an area of flow while another portion is interacting with tissue. Therefore, a frequency or phase shift may be recorded even though the majority of the sample volume is within tissue. If only flow is displayed, it may appear to arise from locations beyond the confines of the blood pool. In early flow mapping systems, it was common to see flow (color) extending far into the tissue echoes.

To limit this effect and to tuck the Doppler resolution into the tissue resolution, most current instruments use a tissue priority algorithm (see preceding discussion) that samples the amplitude channel first to determine whether amplitude is sufficiently high to designate the pixel as a *tissue pixel*. Once the tissue pixel is assigned, the algorithm excludes all Doppler information (color) from the same location so that the two data sets cannot overlap. This has the effect of confining the Doppler signals within the structural echoes and thereby compensates for the lower Doppler resolution.

The lateral resolution of the imaging and Doppler components of the composite image should be the same because the beam profile in both modes of operation should be comparable. Remember, however, that the display width of a point target is expanded to the effective beam width. This point spread function tends to expand echoes from structural targets, causing them to encroach on the blood pool. It will similarly spread the spatial distribution of velocity data, a phenomenon that might be termed *the velocity spread function*. Because the magnitude of both of these functions is determined by the system gain, the relative lateral display of the imaging and Doppler signal depends on the relative gains in the two channels and the algorithm used to output the data.

Many in vitro studies have been performed to test the spatial accuracy of color Doppler velocity mapping using flow through tubes of known diameter as the reference. Although it is difficult to generalize because the studies used different models and instruments, they did provide some useful insights. In general, commercially available scanners maintain flow diameter within about 10% of known values for tube diameters in experimental studies. When poor lateral resolution defocuses the Doppler image, the tissue priority algorithm tends to improve the actual delineation of flow by tucking the flow echoes into the tube echoes. As might be anticipated, however, if echo gain for the amplitude channel (tissue signal) is too high, the point spread function of the system will cause the echoes arising from the tube walls to spread out and the area of flow to be underestimated. These effects are probably most important in imaging flow through stenotic lesions or at the base of regurgitant jets. In these cases, gain-related encroachment of the tissue portion of the echo on the orifice will limit the mapping of flow to pixels not assigned as tissue, and the actual diameter of the flow orifice may be underestimated.

The minimal diameter of flow visible in tube models has been on the order of 1 to 2 mm, which corresponds to the reported ability to see flow through ventricular septal defects (VSDs) on the order of 1 to 2 mm in diameter and on occasion in the coronary arteries.[10]

Similarly, animal studies of experimental mitral regurgitation at different gain settings, PRFs, and transducer frequencies have shown that for the same degree of mitral insufficiency, the area of the visualized "turbulent" jet increased as a function of the Doppler gain and transducer frequency and decreased with increasing PRF.

The jet width visualized immediately behind the valve in these studies exceeded the known size of the orifice in the animals, again relating to lateral resolution.[11] The variance imaged area also increases with increasing gain and transducer frequency and decreases with increasing PRF.[12] The observed relationship to PRF occurs because the same degree of statistic variation in velocity occupies a larger portion of the potentially available velocity scale at lower PRFs and, therefore, is proportionately assigned as more variance weighting. In summary, the spatial resolution of the Doppler image is much poorer than that of the tissue image, and "flow" will often appear to spread out into areas where it does not belong because of this differential resolution of the system. Flow can be confined to a cavity or orifice using a tissue priority algorithm, but the effects of this algorithm vary depending on relative strength of the Doppler and tissue signals and the gains in the two channels.

Temporal Resolution

The temporal resolution of a color flow mapping device is defined by the frame rate at which the color flow images are produced. Typically, color flow devices operate at between 10 to 30 frames/sec so that the image update rate is between 33 and 100 msec. This is relatively slow compared to the update time of 10 msec or less for the transform analyzers used in conventional pulsed and continuous wave instruments. The slow image assembly time has different effects depending on the method of data acquisition and frame assembly. If the frame is assembled by combining an image acquired by an initial fast sweep and a flow map assembled more slowly from multiple Doppler samples, the time in the cardiac cycle at which the two data sets are acquired can be different. For example, if the data are acquired at end systole, it is possible for the image portion of the frame to be recorded with the mitral valve closed and the subsequent flow data to be obtained 50 to 90 msec later during rapid ventricular filling. The combined image will then show flow through a closed mitral valve. Conversely if the first pulse along each line of sight is used to form the image and subsequent pulses for Doppler, temporal dyssynchrony can occur in both imaging and flow within the same frame (e.g., a frame in which both the mitral and aortic valves are open at the same time). Color M-mode does not suffer from these problems, because when sampling is confined to a single line of sight, the sampling rate is still extremely high, despite allocation of a significant portion of the data to color flow mapping.

Velocity Resolution

Velocity resolution is also decreased for a color flow mapping device when compared to a conventional pulsed Doppler. This occurs for several reasons. First, because a portion of the available pulses must be used for image generation, the actual Doppler sampling frequency for a given PRF is lower than for a comparable pulsed Doppler instrument. This reduces the Nyquist limit, causes aliasing to occur at a lower velocity, and decreases the range of frequencies that can be unambiguously displayed. Second, the accuracy of the velocity estimate is far less for a color flow system because the number of times a location is sampled is significantly reduced. For example, at a frame rate of 20, the color mapper will sample a specific location 7 or 8 times in 50 msec, whereas a pulsed Doppler operating at a PRF of 5000 will sample the same location 250 times. Because the accuracy of velocity discrimination increases with the sampling frequency, the pulsed Doppler signal will record and output a much better estimate of velocity. Third, the color flow imager outputs a single color that represents a velocity range, whereas the pulsed Doppler system outputs a range of velocities. Thus, for the color flow imager, the velocity resolution is defined by the velocity range, and component frequencies are not displayed. Finally, because the output velocity is a mean value, it can be affected greatly by outliers and loses resolution near the Nyquist limit because values above the Nyquist limit are interpreted as negative values and are, therefore, subtracted from the mean. Thus, as the velocity approaches the Nyquist limit, the mean may appear to fall rather than rise as the percentage of negative values being used to compute the mean increases.

The detection of low velocities is difficult in any Doppler system because these velocities, by definition, produce small phase shifts that are difficult to record. In addition, they lie near the threshold of the wall filter and, therefore, even when detected tend to be easily suppressed. Finally, because they begin close to the threshold for detection, they become particularly angle-dependent because any additional decrease in their recorded velocity may place them below the display threshold. In color flow systems this is further complicated by the use of darker colors to display lower velocities, which makes them particularly difficult to appreciate even when recorded. When the visualization of low velocities is important, reallocation of the color dynamic range toward a brighter color for lower velocity will make the detected low velocities more apparent. Although this type of processing will make the recorded velocities more obvious, it is important to remember that there will be a low velocity threshold at the margin of most flow fields beyond which low velocity flow occurs but is not detected or displayed.[9] The minimal flow velocity recordable is about 4 cm/sec.

SUMMARY

The color flow mapper represents an elegant combination of all of the functions of stand-alone imaging and Doppler devices into a single instrument. Its major advantage is that it allows the spatial distribution of velocities to be recorded and displayed along with the surrounding structures. Although providing unique diagnostic information, this gain in spatial information is achieved at a loss in velocity and temporal resolution and some compromise in spatial resolution between the imaging and Doppler display. Despite these trade-offs, these combined instruments have become and undoubtedly will remain the standard of practice.

REFERENCES

1. Brandistini MA, et al.: The synthesis of echo and Doppler in M-mode and sectorscan. Proc Annu Meet AIUM 125:704, 1979.
2. Namekawa K, Kasai C, Tsukamoto M, Koyano A: Imaging of blood flow using autocorrelation. Ultrasound Med Biol 8:138, 1982.
3. Bommer W, Miller L: Real time two-dimensional color flow Doppler-enhanced imaging in the diagnosis of cardiovascular disease. Am J Cardiol 49: 944, 1982.
4. Omoto R (ed.): Color Atlas of Real-Time Two-Dimensional Doppler Echocardiography. Tokyo, Shindan-To-Chiryosha, 1987.
5. Omoto R, Kasai C: Physics and instrumentation of Doppler color flow mapping. Echocardiography 4:467, 1987.
6. Gessert JM, Moore W: Color flow imaging display modes and data acquisition parameters. Echocardiography 4:375, 1987.
7. Angelsen BAJ: On the design of two-dimensional flow imaging system. Presented at the meeting of the University of Trondheim Biomedical Research Group, Trondheim, Norway, 1986.
8. Omoto R, Kasai C: Physics and instrumentation of Doppler color flow mapping. Echocardiography 6:467, 1987.
9. Kisslo J, Adams DB, Belkin RN: Doppler Color Flow Imaging. New York, Churchill Livingstone, 1988.
10. Sahn DJ: Instrumentation and physical factors related to visualization of stenotic and regurgitant jets by Doppler color flow mapping. J Am Coll Cardiol 12:1354, 1988.
11. Jones M, et al.: Variability of color flow mapping Doppler imaging of regurgitant jets in an animal model of mitral insufficiency. J Am Coll Cardiol 9:64, 1987.
12. Tamura T, et al.: In vitro studies of variance (turbulence) indicators in color flow mapping Doppler systems. Quantitative computer analysis of RGB digitized flow map images. Circulation 76(Suppl 4):IV-141, 1987.

CHAPTER

12

FLUID DYNAMICS OF REGURGITANT JETS AND THEIR IMAGING BY COLOR DOPPLER

JAMES D. THOMAS, RAVIN DAVIDOFF, and EDWARD G. CAPE

The development of color Doppler flow mapping allows one to visualize the spatial distribution of blood flow within the heart. Three primary types of flow can be discerned—normal forward flow, regurgitant jets, and flow through shunt lesions. The principles of normal forward flow were discussed in Chapter 9 and apply also to its color Doppler representation. Regurgitant jets, however, are more complex, and a discussion of the physical characteristics of these flow disturbances and their color flow display forms the basis of this chapter. Shunt lesions are dealt with later in the text.

The ability to visualize regurgitant jets has resulted in attempts to estimate regurgitant volume from the spatial distribution of the color jet. Numerous clinical studies have shown a correlation between the color flow representation of the regurgitant jet and the angiographic assessment of regurgitation[1–5] as well as a correlation between the color jet and the clinical severity of regurgitation.[6–8] It is tempting to extrapolate from these studies that the volume of the color jet reflects the volume of regurgitation. However, such simple attempts to correlate color jet appearance with the regurgitant flow's causing the jet bypasses a critical step: We must know how the true velocity distribution within the receiving chamber relates to the flow and driving pressure at the origin of the jet. Only after understanding the determinants of the physical jet can we hope to unravel the meaning of its color flow appearance. Fortunately the general field of fluid dynamics and the specific topic of turbulent jet flow have received intense theoretic and experimental study over the past two centuries because of their importance in hydraulics, jet propulsion, and pollution control.[9–11] By drawing on these lessons, we as cardiologists can hope to avoid "rediscovering the wheel" and maximize the quantitative data extractable using the remarkable tool of color flow Doppler echocardiography.

In this chapter, we first discuss the velocity distribution of a steady jet discharging through a round orifice into an infinitely large reservoir. We also derive expressions for the color flow Doppler appearance of such a free jet as if it were imaged with a "perfect" Doppler machine. Following this section of an idealized jet imaged with an idealized machine, we discuss some of the many ways in which intracardiac geometry and flow distort a regurgitant jet from its free form. Finally, we outline some of the ways in which current color Doppler imagers fall short of an ideal machine and how these shortcomings affect attempts at quantitation of regurgitant jets. To conclude the chapter, we discuss some of the algorithms that have been proposed for jet quantitation as well as future approaches that may give a more robust estimation of regurgitant volume, especially with the advent of more sophisticated Doppler equipment.

DEFINITIONS

Regurgitant volume may be defined as the volume of blood lost through an incompetent valve during one cardiac cycle. *Jet volume*, in contrast, describes the volume enclosed by the boundary of the regurgitant jet as imaged by color Doppler. On first glance, it may seem that these two similar terms describe the same physical volume. However, they are significantly different and extensive work has been done on jet flow, particularly under steady-state conditions, to evaluate this issue.[12–14] *Turbulence*, as previously described (Chapter 9), refers to the chaotic mixing of fluid flow in which the velocity at a given point varies erratically in magnitude and direction. These instantaneous variations cannot be predicted in detail by mathematic descriptions of the fluid flow; only average values can be predicted. *Laminar flow*, which describes flow along distinct and traceable stream lines, is less complex and can be described completely using fluid dynamics principles. Figure 12–1 demonstrates the striking difference between laminar and turbulent flow.

The transition from laminar to turbulent flow occurs over a wide range of flow rates rather than at a sharp, distinct rate. Definition of the zone beyond which turbulence occurs may be estimated by the *Reynolds number*, a dimensionless number used to characterize flow. It represents, in a general sense, the ratio between inertial forces within a fluid system (which tend to induce instability in the flow) and viscous forces (which tend to stabilize the flow). One representation of the Reynolds number is the equation

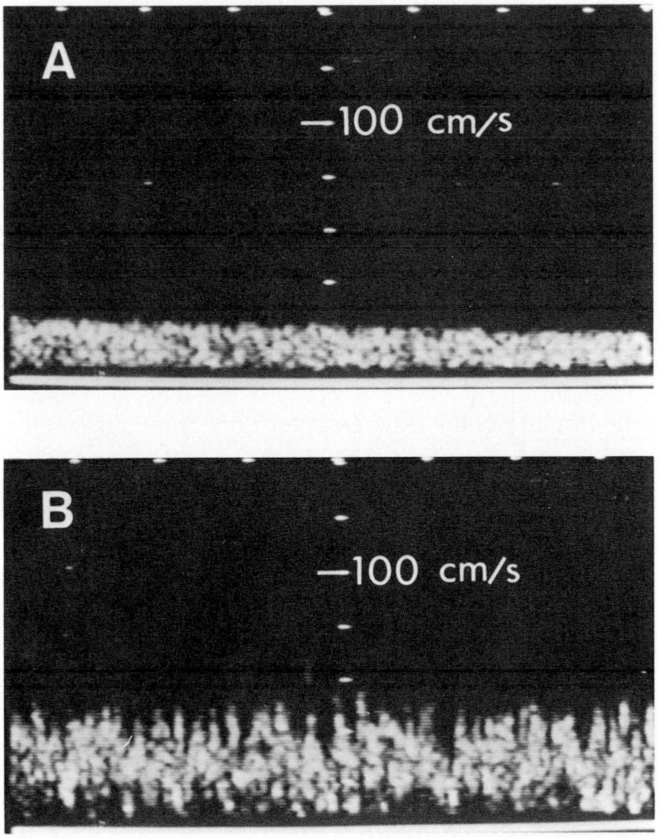

Fig. 12–1. Laminar vs. turbulent flow. Pulsed Doppler recordings obtained in an in vitro flow model. **A.** With a small orifice driving pressure (0.3 mm Hg), flow is laminar, without random fluctuation about the mean velocity. **B.** With an increase in driving pressure to 1.0 (9.1) mm Hg, flow is turbulent, characterized by chaotic fluctuations in velocity.

Table 12–1. Mathematic Symbols

a	Acceleration of an object (dv/dt) ($cm–sec^{-2}$)
A_o	Effective area of regurgitant orifice (cm^2)
F	Force acting on a body ($g–cm–sec^{-2}$)
m	Mass of an object (gram)
M	Momentum flux of a jet ($g–cm–sec^{-2}$) or momentum of a rigid object (g–cm/sec), both vector quantities
M	Kinematic momentum flux ($cm^4–sec^{-2}$): momentum divided by fluid density, M/ρ.
p	Pressure (mm Hg or $g–cm^{-1}–sec^{-2}$: 1 mm Hg = 1333 $g–cm^{-1}–cm^{-2}$
Δp	Driving pressure of jet (mm Hg or $g–cm^{-1}–sec^{-2}$)
Q	Jet flow (cm^3/sec)
Q_o	Flow at origin of jet (cm^3/sec)
r	Radial coordinate of the jet, distance from the centerline (cm)
r_o	Effective radius of regurgitant orifice (cm)
Re	Reynolds number (dimensionless): ratio of inertial and viscous forces within flow; represented (equivalently) by $2\rho rv/\mu$, $2rv/\nu$, $0.623/M_o/\nu$ (circular jet).
t	Time coordinate (sec)
T	Duration of the jet (sec)
u	Axial component of jet velocity (cm/sec)
u_o	Axial jet velocity at orifice (cm/sec)
u_c	Low velocity cutoff for color flow mapping; below this velocity no color is displayed (cm/sec)
v	Radial component of jet velocity (away from jet axis; used when velocity is treated as a vector quantity) or simple velocity magnitude when velocity is used as a scalar (cm/sec)
V	Regurgitant volume (cm^3)
$\vec{v}$	Vector representation of velocity (cm/sec)
x	Axial coordinate of jet, measured from jet virtual origin (cm)
μ	Fluid viscosity ($g–cm^{-1}–sec^{-1}$)
ν	Kinematic viscosity ($cm^2–sec^{-1}$): viscosity divided by density
ϵ_o	Turbulent viscosity
ρ	Density of fluid (1.05 $g–cm^{-3}$ for blood)
e	Base of natural logarithm (2.71828)
ln	Natural logarithm
∂	Partial derivative operator
∇	Gradient operator, $\vec{i}(\partial/\partial x) + \vec{j}(\partial/\partial y) + \vec{k}(\partial/\partial z)$ in Cartesian coordinates

$$Re = \text{inertia force/viscous force} = 2\rho vr/\mu, \quad [12.1]$$

where Re is the Reynolds number, v is the mean velocity of flow, r is the radius of the structure through which flow is occurring, ρ is the mass density of blood (1.05 g/cm^3), and μ is viscosity (0.03 $g–cm^{-1}–sec^{-1}$). (All mathematic symbols are defined in Table 12–1). As the Reynolds number increases, the tendency toward turbulent flow increases, and within pipes this threshold is approximately 2300. For flow through a small orifice into a large chamber (analogous to valvular regurgitation), this transition to turbulence occurs at a lower Re, approximately 200 to 500.[15,16] Thus, most regurgitant jets are turbulent because of their large driving pressure (which increases Re) and also because of the disparity between the size of the orifice and the relatively large receiving chamber (which lowers the turbulent threshold). Flow through a pinhole orifice (tiny r) may have a low enough Re to be laminar, but these jets are rarely of clinical significance.

MATHEMATIC DESCRIPTION OF JETS AND THEIR COLOR FLOW APPEARANCE

In this section, we shall discuss some of the physical principles that relate the physical jet to the driving pressure and flow rate at its orifice. This will initially be for a free jet discharging through a small round orifice into an infinitely large chamber of still fluid and imaged with a "perfect" color Doppler machine. We will provide equations that describe how color area should vary with these jet parameters, fluid viscosity, and the low velocity cutoff of the Doppler machine. Next, we will consider, in a more qualitative sense, the effects of jet constraint within a chamber, coflowing and swirling chamber fluid, and finally limitations of current color Doppler imagers.

Idealized Color Doppler Appearance of a Free Jet

Schematic Representation of a Free Jet. The jet to be studied theoretically is shown schematically in Figure 12–2. It is formed by the constant discharge of blood with velocity u_0 through an effective orifice area A_0 with radius r_0 ($A_0 = \pi r_0^2$). (The actual anatomic orifice area is somewhat larger than this because of vena contracta effects.) The flow rate (Q_0) is given by $A_0 u_0$. The distance along the jet axis is given by the variable x, whereas the radial distance from the jet axis is given by r. Velocity along the x axis is given by u, and the radial component of velocity given by v. We seek a description of axial velocity as a function of x and r: u(x,r). Knowing

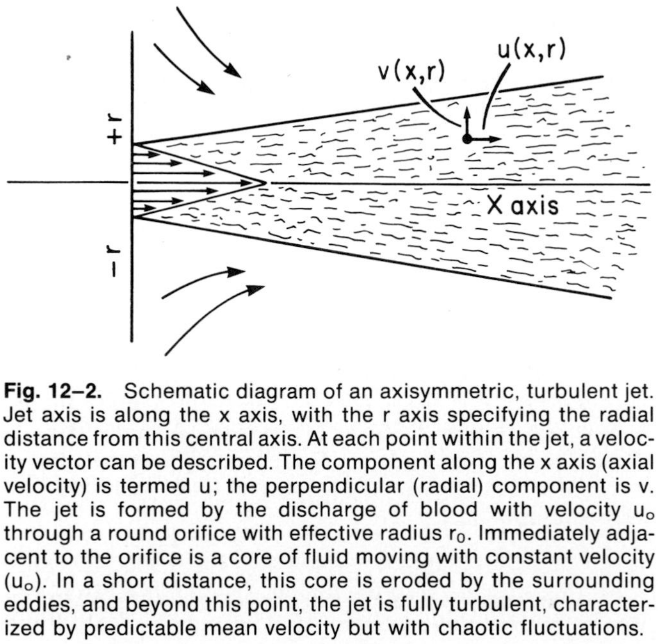

Fig. 12–2. Schematic diagram of an axisymmetric, turbulent jet. Jet axis is along the x axis, with the r axis specifying the radial distance from this central axis. At each point within the jet, a velocity vector can be described. The component along the x axis (axial velocity) is termed u; the perpendicular (radial) component is v. The jet is formed by the discharge of blood with velocity u_o through a round orifice with effective radius r_0. Immediately adjacent to the orifice is a core of fluid moving with constant velocity (u_o). In a short distance, this core is eroded by the surrounding eddies, and beyond this point, the jet is fully turbulent, characterized by predictable mean velocity but with chaotic fluctuations.

this, we should be able to predict the appearance of the jet by color flow Doppler mapping.

Turbulent Velocity is Chaotic. Because this jet is likely to be turbulent, the instantaneous velocity u(x,r,t) at any point in space and time will vary chaotically around a mean value, which we represent as a sum: u(x,r,t) = u(x,r) + u'(x,r,t), where u(x,r) is the mean velocity (does not vary with time) and u'(x,r,t) are random positive and negative velocities [about 20 to 30% of the magnitude of u(x,r)] the average of which is zero. It is impossible to describe u'(x,r,t) precisely (Fig. 12–1), only the mean value, u(x,r). Therefore, we seek to predict this mean value but must always bear in mind that the instantaneous velocity profile is likely to deviate significantly from this.

Conservation Law Applied to Jets

The jet may be thought of as a source of mass, energy, and momentum into the receiving chamber. Much of the behavior of the jet (and any physical system) is dictated by the conservation of these entities. For instance, the conservation of mass dictates that matter can be neither created nor destroyed, and so the amount of fluid within a chamber must precisely reflect flow into and out of that chamber. This principle is most widely used in application of the continuity equation, where flow through one part of a vessel (e.g., the left ventricular outflow tract) must be the same as flow elsewhere in the same vessel (e.g., aortic valve). We will later show that this does not imply that the flow within a free turbulent jet is constant at every point along the x axis, because stationary fluid within the receiving chamber is entrained into the jet and so the flow rate within the jet actually increases with distance from the orifice.

Conservation of Total Energy

The second physical parameter that must remain constant is total energy. Thus, the kinetic energy (KE) that a jet adds to a chamber must be reflected in the energy within that chamber. However, energy comes in many forms (e.g., kinetic energy, heat, and pressure), and only total energy is conserved. In stenotic valve flow, it is widely recognized that the pressure energy in the proximal chamber is converted into kinetic energy within the valve by the Bernoulli principle ($\Delta p = \frac{1}{2}\rho v^2$, where Δp is transvalvar driving pressure, v is blood velocity, and ρ is density) and that this kinetic energy is dissipated as heat in turbulent eddies downstream. Kinetic energy, however, is the only energy form readily quantifiable by Doppler scanning, because it is caused by fluid motion. Unfortunately, jet kinetic energy is not conserved within the receiving chamber, only total energy, which is not quantifiable by Doppler scanning.

Conservation of Momentum

The final conserved quantity is momentum (M), the "inertia" of the jet, and understanding this entity is critical to jet flow analysis. In rigid body mechanics (e.g., the flight of a baseball), momentum is defined as mass × velocity, and its change must precisely reflect applied forces (such as gravity), as specified by Newton's second law of motion:

Force = Mass
× Acceleration ≡ dM/dt (rate of change of momentum).

In fluid dynamics, we typically speak of momentum flux, the amount of momentum passing through a region per unit time. (In this discussion, we use *momentum* and *momentum flux* synonymously unless stated otherwise.) For the jet in Figure 12–2, its momentum is given by density × flow × velocity, or $\rho Q_0 u_0$. Conservation of momentum dictates that the total momentum flux crossing any vertical plane orthogonal to the jet axis must be constant throughout the full extent of the jet.

Advantages of Momentum Analysis in Doppler Jet Analysis. Momentum flux is especially attractive for describing jets as analyzed by color flow Doppler for three reasons. First, momentum exists only in one form, unlike energy, which is convertable from kinetic energy (measurable by Doppler) to heat (unmeasurable by Doppler). Second, momentum is a vector quantity. That is, it has components along each of the three coordinate directions, and each of these component momenta must be conserved. This is important because Doppler measures only the component of velocity that is parallel to the ultrasound beam. Thus, the momentum flux measured with this component must remain constant throughout the jet. Finally, momentum at the jet origin is expressible in many different ways. For instance, we have stated that the momentum flux is $\rho Q_0 u_0$, but flow (Q_0) is simply effective orifice area × velocity or $A_0 u_0$ (assuming plug flow). Thus, we could substitute this for Q_0 and write $M = \rho A_0 u_0^2$. Similarly, the Bernoulli equation relates velocity and driving pressure: $\Delta p = \frac{1}{2}\rho u_0^2$. Substituting this yields $M = 2A_0 \Delta p_0$ (Δp will need to be expressed in dyne–cm^{-2} or g–cm^{-1}–sec^{-2} where 1 mm Hg = 1333 dyne–cm^{-2}). In all, there are five expressions for M using the jet variables of flow, velocity, orifice area, and driving pressure:

$$M_0 = \rho Q_0 u_0 \qquad [12.1A]$$
$$= \rho A_0 u_0^2 \qquad [12.1B]$$
$$= \rho Q_0^2 / A_0 \qquad [12.1C]$$
$$= 2A_0 \Delta p \qquad [12.1D]$$
$$= Q_0 \sqrt{2\rho \Delta p}. \qquad [12.1E]$$

Examples of Jet Momentum. Because the concept of momentum flux may be unfamiliar, the following examples show how each of these formulas might be used to calculate the momentum of an intracardiac jet in a clinical situation. Equation 12.1A: A tricuspid regurgitant jet of 20 cm^3/sec moving at 300 cm/sec would have a momentum of 1.05 × 20 × 300 = 6300 g–cm–sec^{-2}. Equation 12.1B: A pulmonic regurgitant jet passing through a 0.1 cm^2 orifice at a speed of 200 cm/sec would have a momentum of 1.05 × 0.1 × 200^2 = 4200 g–cm–sec^{-2}. Equation 12.1C: An aortic stenotic jet of 200 cm^3/sec passing though an effective orifice area of 0.5 cm^2 would have a momentum of 1.05 × 200^2/0.5 = 84,000 g–cm–sec^{-2}. Equation 12.1D: A mitral regurgitant jet with a driving pressure of 150 mm Hg passing through a 0.2-cm^2 effective orifice would have a momentum of 2 × 0.2 × 150 × 1333 = 79,980 g–cm–sec^{-2}. Equation 12.1E: An aortic regurgitant jet of 50 cm^3/sec and a driving pressure of 100 mm Hg would have a momentum of 50 × (2 × 1.05 × 100 × 1333)$^{1/2}$ = 26,454 g–cm–sec^{-2}.

Equations 12.1A and 12.1B are especially interesting. They imply that, knowing the momentum of the jet and its velocity at the origin (readily obtainable by continuous wave Doppler), we should be able to derive the jet flow rate (Equation 12.1A) or regurgitant orifice area (Equation 12.1B).

Because density is constant for incompressible fluids (e.g., water or blood, not air), an equivalent kinematic momentum, M_0 with units cm^4–s^{-2}, is frequently used, which differs from Equations 12.1A to E by having density (ρ) divided out.

Calculating Momentum Elsewhere in the Jet. Farther down the x axis from the orifice, we know that the momentum passing through a vertical plane orthogonal to the jet axis must be the same as that entering the chamber. However, because velocity is no longer constant, we cannot use the simple Equations 12.1A to E (which assume plug flow through the orifice) for this but must integrate the momentum through each part of the plane to obtain a total momentum. This is analogous to Equation 12.1B, and for an axisymmetric jet becomes:

$$M = \int_A \rho u^2\, dA = 2\pi\rho \int_0^\infty u^2 r\, dr.^* \qquad [12.2]$$

Conservation of momentum requires that this x component of momentum always equal M_0 throughout the jet.

Jet Velocity Distribution

Overall Jet Appearance

We now attempt to describe the actual distribution of axial jet velocity as a function of x and r: u(x,r). In general, an axisymmetric turbulent jet expanding from a circular orifice can be divided into two regions (Fig. 12–2). The proximal part of the jet is termed the *potential core*; the zone beyond this is the *fully developed region*. The fluid leaves the hole as a core, which is practically free of shear (viscous friction between adjacent fluid). However, the velocity immediately begins to decrease on the fringes of the flow as it shears against the adjacent fluid. This shear or mixing layer, which forms the boundary between the core flow and reservoir fluid, consumes the core until it no longer exists. Beyond a transition zone is the fully developed region of the jet, which is turbulent throughout. As stated previously, the decrease in jet velocity must precisely balance its lateral spread so that total axial momentum flux (Equation 12.2) remains constant.

* We have used the relationship that in axisymmetric geometry, the rim of area dA between r and r + dr is $2\pi r\, dr$.

Mathematic Description

Unfortunately, a general description of the fully developed jet requires the solution of the Navier-Stokes equations, a set of four coupled partial differential equations with complex boundary conditions that must hold at every point in space and every instant in time. At best, this solution is prohibitively complex, requiring the services of a supercomputer; for turbulent flow, it can be shown that no unique solution exists. There are more unknowns in the system than there are equations to specify them. In fact this unpredictability is characteristic of turbulent flow.

Fortunately, several authors have suggested reasonable simplifications to these equations to obtain acceptably accurate descriptions of axisymmetric jet flow. One such simplification that agrees well with empiric observation[13,14] replaces the usual fluid viscosity of laminar flow with a much larger turbulent viscosity (ϵ_0), which relates to the mixing effect of turbulent eddies. This turbulent viscosity must be determined empirically. With this approximation, the following equation for mean axial velocity in an axisymmetric turbulent jet is obtained:

$$u(x,r) = 13.8(r_0/x)u_0\, e^{-94(r/x)^2} \quad [12.3]$$

What does Equation 12.3 mean? Consider first the velocity along the center axis of the jet (termed u_m for midline velocity). Along the x axis, r is 0, and so the exponential term in Equation 12.3, $e^{-94(r/x)^2}$, reduces to e^0, which is 1, and thus $u(x,0) = 13.8(r_0u_0)/x$; thus, the centerline velocity decreases inversely with distance from the jet origin (Fig. 12–3). Similarly, at any given distance, x, from the origin the velocity profile as a function of r is a Gaussian (bell-shaped) curve familiar from its use in statistics:

$$u(r) = u_m\, e^{-94(r/x)^2}$$

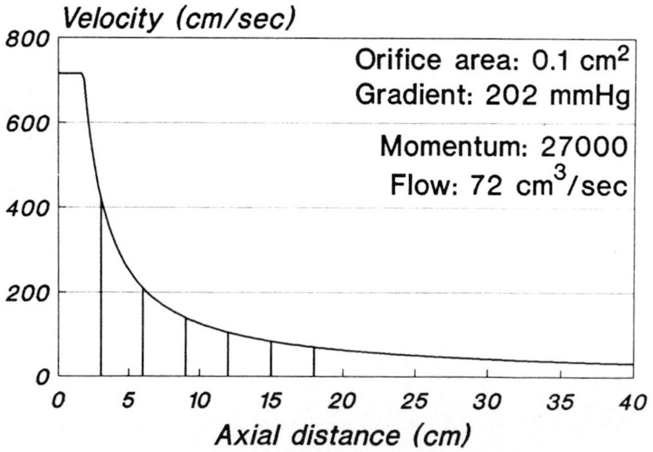

Fig. 12–3. Mean axial velocity measured along the center line of an axisymmetric jet with the parameters listed (similar to conditions encountered in moderate to severe mitral or aortic regurgitation). The center line velocity is proportional to (axial distance)$^{-1}$ but has a constant maximum velocity of 716 cm/sec within 2 cm of the orifice, where the potential core of plug flow still exists. The vertical lines mark the location of the radial profiles in Figure 12–4.

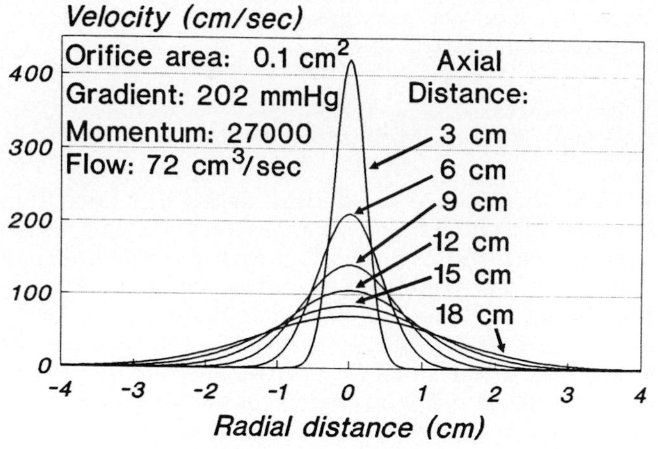

Fig. 12–4. Axial velocity profiles (as a function of radial distance from the jet centerline) for the indicated distances from the orifice. The physical jet is the same as for Figure 12–3, and the locations of these profiles are marked with vertical lines in that figure.

which falls to half of its centerline velocity ($u_m/2$) when $r = 0.086x$ (Fig. 12–4).

Equation 12.3 and Figure 12–4 demonstrate an important principle of jet flow: dynamic similarity. That is, all of the velocity profiles in Figure 12–4 have the same shape. If each curve is plotted so that u_m has the same height and the half-velocity has the same r value, then the curves are identical. This dynamic similarity is critical to the self-preserving nature of the jet. Far from the jet, there is no influence of the specific orifice shape, only the influence of fluid properties and total jet momentum.

Inspection of Equation 12.3 will demonstrate that this formula cannot be valid in the potential core region of the jet: When x approaches 0, u becomes infinite, whereas in the physical jet, u can never exceed u_0. In fact, Equation 12.3 is valid only beyond about $x = 10r_0$, where the potential core is completely eroded and the jet is said to be fully developed. Close to the orifice, the plug of constant velocity, u_m, is shown by the flat portion of the velocity curve in Figure 12–3, which is eroded into by the turbulent eddies induced by the jet shear. In this discussion, we ignore the specific details of this core flow, although computer solutions can be obtained for it.

Relationship of Jet Momentum to Equation 12.3. Note that the only parameter of the actual jet that enters Equation 12.3 is the product r_0u_0. We may relate this to jet momentum by noting that by Equation 12.1C, $M_0 = \rho A_0 u_0^2 = \rho(\pi r_0^2)u_0^2$ and so we may write $r_0u_0 = (M_0/\rho\pi)^{1/2} = .56\sqrt{M_0}$. Substituting this expression for r_0u_0, Equation 12.3 becomes

$$u(x,r) = 7.8\sqrt{M_0}/x\; e^{-94(r/x)^2}. \quad [12.4]$$

Thus, the kinematic momentum, M_0, is the only jet feature that determines its velocity profile.

This is an important prediction. It means that the color flow appearance of a regurgitant jet is not determined by the orifice flow rate, driving pressure, or orifice size alone, but rather by a combination of these parameters, which yields jet momentum flux (Equations 12.1A to 12.1E).

Calculation of Jet Flow Rate

We know that the flow rate at the jet orifice is Q_0. What is the flow rate downstream from the orifice? We can expect this flow rate to increase with distance from the orifice because of the entrainment of stationary fluid within the receiving chamber into the jet. In laminar flow, viscous effects slowly incorporate surrounding fluid while preserving axial streamlines. With turbulence, eddies within the jet draw in fluid and lead to more rapid jet expansion. To calculate the flow passing through a vertical plane, orthogonal to the jet axis, at a distance x cm from the orifice of a turbulent jet, we integrate the velocity profile (Equation 12.3) across this plane:

$$Q = \int_A u\, dA = 2\pi \int_0^\infty u\, r\, dr.$$

Expressing this in terms of the orifice flow (Q_0), this solution is approximately:

$$Q = 0.16 \times Q_0/r_0.$$

Thus, beyond about 6 orifice radii from the origin, the flow rate within the jet increases linearly so that at a distance of 100 radii downstream, the jet has 16 times the original flow rate (but its momentum remains the same).

Calculation of Jet Kinetic Energy

A similar approach can be used to estimate the kinetic energy within the jet. At the orifice, the kinetic energy flux (KE_0) is given by $\frac{1}{2}\rho u_0^2 Q_0$ or $\frac{1}{2}\rho u_0^3 A_0$. (This differs from the kinetic energy of rigid body mechanics, $\frac{1}{2}mu_0^2$, by the factor u_0, the same factor by which momentum flux differs from classic mechanical momentum.) Downstream from the orifice, we again calculate total kinetic energy flux by integrating across a plane orthogonal to the jet axis:

$$KE = \int_A \tfrac{1}{2}\rho u^3\, dA = \pi\rho \int_0^\infty u^3\, r\, dr.$$

Integrating this yields:

$$KE = 8.2\, r_0 KE_0/x.$$

Thus, jet kinetic energy decreases in inverse proportion to the distance from the orifice as it is converted into heat by viscosity and turbulent eddies.

Predicting Color Doppler Appearance

What is the relationship of Equations 12.3 and 12.4 to the appearance of the jet by color flow Doppler imaging? Current Doppler instruments will color a pixel if the velocity within that pixel rises above some threshold, typically 5 to 10 cm/sec. Thus, the color area should correspond to that velocity contour within the physical jet. We assume for the time being that we have a "perfect" Doppler machine that can display flow at any depth in the jet with equal sensitivity.

Graphic Display of Jet Profiles

To describe the jet profile at a given velocity contour (called u_c for color cutoff velocity), we must invert Equation 12.4 to express the jet radius (r) as a function of axial distance from the jet origin (x) and u_c. After some algebraic manipulation, we obtain:

$$r(x,u_c) = x\left(\frac{1}{94}\ln\frac{7.8\sqrt{M_0}}{u_c x}\right)^{1/2} = \frac{x}{9.7}\left(\ln\frac{7.8\sqrt{M_0}}{u_c x}\right)^{1/2} \quad [12.5]$$

Equation 12.5 looks rather unwieldy, but in fact, graphic display shows it to be a smooth, well-behaved function, as shown in Figures 12–5 to 12–10, and discussed in the sections to follow.

Jet Profile Versus Momentum. Figure 12–5 displays the expected color areas for jets of various momenta with a low velocity cutoff of 20 cm/sec. Inspection of these curves shows that both the length and width of the jet increase with increasing momentum, each roughly proportional to the square root of the increase in momentum. In fact, if the area of each of these jets is calculated, it is found to increase almost perfectly linearly with momentum (Fig. 12–6). Knowing the response of the jet to momentum changes allows us to predict the independent effects of changes in flow, velocity, driving pressure, or orifice area.

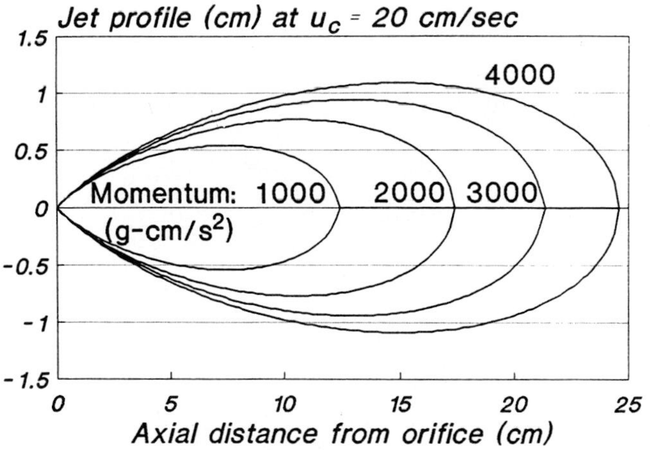

Fig. 12–5. Expected color flow Doppler appearance for turbulent jets of various momenta. In this figure and in Figures 12–6 to 12–8, and 12–10, the jet orifice is located at the graph origin (far left, center) and is directed toward the right. The Doppler probe is assumed to be imaging down the x axis and to display in color only those velocities above the color cutoff (u_c) of 20 cm/sec (located inside the indicated contours). These contours are for a jet discharging into an infinite reservoir and so are much longer than those observed inside the heart. It is further assumed that this is a "perfect" Doppler machine, without attenuation or aliasing problems.

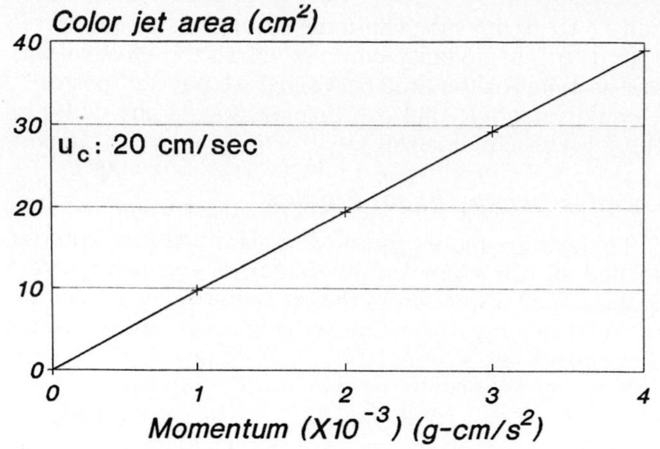

Fig. 12–6. Predicted color area as a function of jet momentum. The areas are derived from the contours in Figure 12–5 and are for an unconstrained jet. u_c = color cutoff.

Jet Profile Versus Flow. Figure 12–7 shows several jet profiles in which driving pressure is constant but flow is increased by enlarging the effective orifice area. By Equation 12.1B, this means that M_0 increases linearly with A_0 with the expected change in jet size.

Jet Profile Versus Pressure Gradient. In Figure 12–8 jet velocity increases while orifice area decreases so that flow (A_0u_0) remains constant; however, by Equation 12.1C, momentum increases inversely with the decrease in orifice area. Thus, high velocity (high pressure) jets produce a much larger color map than low velocity (pressure) jets of the same flow rate. Thus, we would expect left heart jets to be larger than right heart jets for a given flow rate.

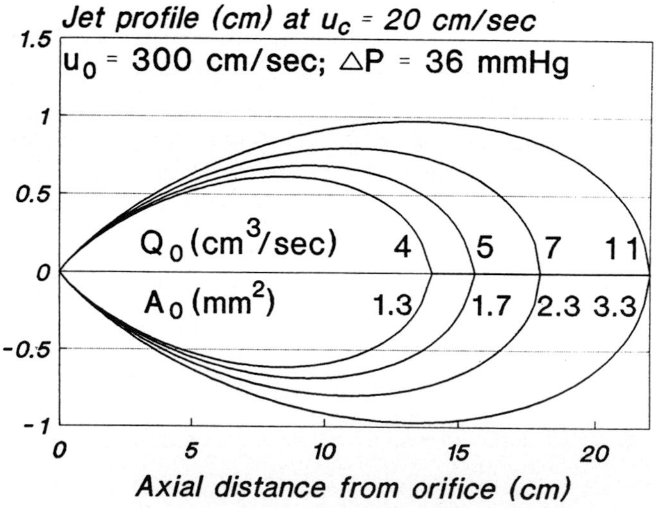

Fig. 12–7. Expected color flow profiles for jets with identical driving pressure (ΔP = 36 mm Hg) but with flow rate adjusted by changing the orifice size. For constant driving pressure, jet momentum is proportional to flow rate (or orifice area) and ranges from 624 g – cm/sec^2 for the smallest contour to 1584 g – cm/sec^2 for the largest. u_c = color cutoff; u_o = constant velocity; Q_o = orifice flow rate; A_o = orifice area.

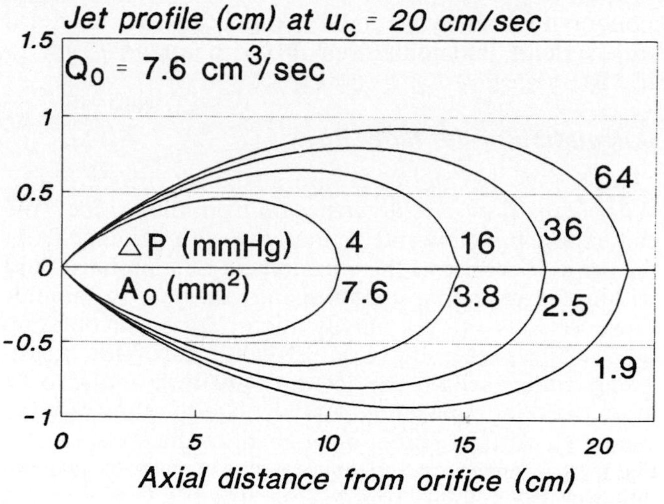

Fig. 12–8. Expected color flow profiles for jets with identical flow rates (Q_0 = 7.6 cm^3/sec) but with driving pressure (ΔP) and orifice area (A_o) adjusted in inverse proportion. For jets of constant flow, momentum is inversely proportional to orifice area (Equation 12.1C), ranging from 798 g – cm/sec^2 for the 7.6-mm^2 orifice to 3192 for the 1.9-mm^2 orifice. Thus, the higher pressure jets have the larger color Doppler profiles.

Jet Profile Versus Viscosity (Laminar and Turbulent). Fluid viscosity and the turbulent nature of the jet also have important effects on jet size and shape. In laminar flow, much less mixing occurs between the periphery of the jet and the stationary fluid surrounding it and, thus, for identical jet momentum, laminar flow leads to a much longer jet than does turbulent flow, although maximal jet width is little effected (Fig. 12–9). The length of laminar jets is inversely proportional to fluid viscosity; the more viscous fluids cause jets to spread more rapidly. As noted, however, there are few laminar intracardiac jets because of their high Reynolds numbers. Expressed in terms of momentum, the Reynolds number for a circular jet is approximately $0.6\sqrt{M}/\nu$, where ν is fluid kinematic viscosity, 0.01 cm^2–sec^{-1} for water, 0.03 for blood. For sharp-edged orifices, conversion to turbulent flow occurs at a kinematic momentum of about 100 cm^4/sec^2, which is a miniscule jet (e.g., 7-mm Hg pressure gradient across a 0.01-cm^2 orifice). It might be expected that the turbulent viscosity (ϵ_0) of blood would be higher than that of water, but this has not yet been examined. Figure 12–9 shows the effect on jet profile if ϵ_0 for blood was three times ϵ_0 for water. For the other graphs, no adjustment has been made for turbulent viscosity.

Jet Profile Versus Low Velocity Cutoff. Finally, a further variable is introduced by the echo machine into the color flow appearance of the jet: the low velocity cutoff. In fact, the current generation of color flow mappers do not have a sharp low velocity cutoff analogous to the wall filter of pulsed Doppler. However, the gain setting will vary the sensitivity of the instrument to low velocity signals and has much the same effect. As Figure 12–10 demonstrates, adjustments in u_c have profound effects on the color area. In fact, for the unconstrained jet, both

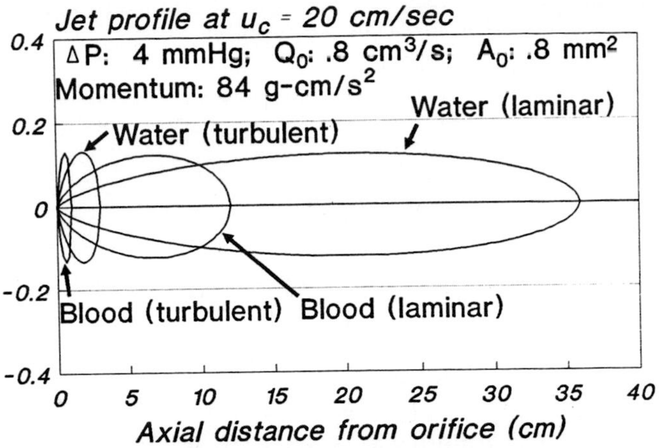

Fig. 12–9. Dependence of jet appearance on fluid viscosity and turbulent nature of flow. The four contours represent the same physical jet with the parameters listed (corresponding to a miniscule pulmonic regurgitant jet). The Reynolds number for this jet is about 600, approximately the transition point between laminar and turbulent flow for circular jets emerging from a sharp orifice. The two largest contours show the profoundly slow drop-off in velocity for laminar flow. With transition to turbulent flow, the jet spreads and dissipates much faster, and, consequently, the color profile is much shorter. Maximal width is little effected. These curves also demonstrate that laminar jet length is inversely proportional to fluid viscosity (here assumed to be 1 cP for water and 3 cP for blood). The two turbulent curves assume that a similar 3:1 ratio between blood and water turbulent viscosity exists, but this has not been verified empirically. u_c = color cutoff; ΔP = driving pressure; Q_0 = orifice flow rate; A_0 = orifice area.

length and width vary inversely with u_c and jet area varies inversely with the square of u_c. Decreasing the low velocity cutoff from 20 to 10 cm/sec quadruples the color area potentially visible.

Summary of Effects on Color Jet Area. To summarize, we would expect the total color area of an unconstrained jet to vary with other parameters as follows:

Color Area ∝ Momentum Flux
∝ Driving Pressure [Orifice Area Constant]
∝ (Velocity)^2 [Orifice Area Constant]
∝ (Flow)^2 [Orifice Area Constant]
∝ Effective Orifice Area [Driving Pressure Constant]
∝ Velocity [Flow Constant]
∝ (Orifice Area)$^{-1}$ [Flow Constant]
∝ (Color Cutoff)$^{-2}$
∝ (Turbulent Viscosity)$^{-1}$

In fact, it is possible to derive a numeric estimate for the color jet area based on M_0, u_0, and ϵ_{eff}, the effective turbulent viscosity (relative to that of water):

$$\text{Color Area} \approx \frac{3.8M_0}{u_c^2\ \epsilon_{eff}} \qquad [12.6]$$

Thus, the color flow area of an unconstrained jet can be expected to depend predominantly on machine-dependent factors (u_c^{-2}) and on turbulent viscosity, a quantity as yet undefined for blood and one that might be expected to vary with hematocrit. In the next section, we discuss how real regurgitant jets are greatly distorted by the effects of intracardiac geometry and flow and the limitations of current color flow Doppler technology. Because these factors make observed jet area an even more unpredictable property, we see that the observed color area is an imperfect way to characterize a jet by color flow Doppler analysis.

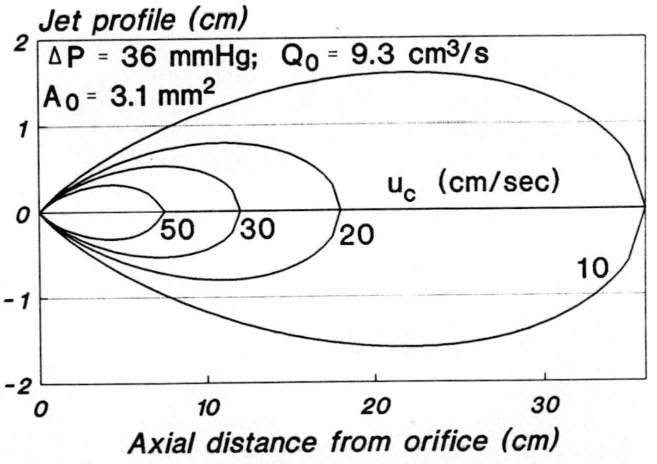

Fig. 12–10. "Gain" dependence of color flow profiles. All contours in this example are for the same physical jet with the parameters listed (momentum = 2930 g − cm/sec²) but with the low velocity cutoff varied from 10 to 50 cm/sec as shown. Decreasing the color cutoff (u_c) from 20 to 10 cm/sec quadruples the expected color area. ΔP = driving pressure; Q_0 = orifice flow rate; A_0 = orifice area.

Relationship of Jet Appearance to Regurgitant Volume

A critical point to recognize is that the color flow appearance of the jet depends on instantaneous, not cumulative, jet parameters. For example, the color flow area of a jet depends on the instantaneous flow rate, not on the cumulative regurgitant volume (V) that has flowed through the orifice. Consider the largest contour in Figure 12–9 (corresponding to a flow rate of 11 cm³/sec). If such a jet persisted for 1 second, a regurgitant volume of 11 cm³ would have flowed through the orifice. If the jet persisted for 10 seconds, a volume of 110 cm³ would have flowed through the orifice, but the jet itself would look the same. Thus, if one were able to estimate the orifice flow rate (Q_0) from the appearance of the jet, one could calculate the total volume injected by multiplying Q_0 by the duration of flow (T): $V = Q_0T$. Any algorithms that attempt to relate jet appearance to regurgitant volume directly contain the implicit assumption that the duration of regurgitation (T) is the same for all lesions.

Unfortunately, the situation is somewhat more complex. First, regurgitant flow is not constant but rises and falls during the regurgitant interval. Furthermore, the relation between jet momentum and color appearance is not quite instantaneous but delayed slightly. Thus, if flow started suddenly, it would take a few milliseconds for the jet to fully form. Also, if the flow is stopped abruptly, the jet remains visible for a period of time as the jet energy is dissipated. These warm-up and cool-down phenomena have been observed experimentally,[17] but their precise nature has not been worked out fully.

Restrictions to Jet Flow in the Heart

Thus far, discussion has focused on a nonphysiologic jet: one discharging at a constant rate through a round orifice into an infinitely large reservoir filled with stationary fluid. Inside the heart, all of these assumptions are violated. The receiving chamber is frequently constraining, with the jet striking either the end or side of the chamber; regurgitant orifices are irregular; the receiving fluid is usually in motion; and regurgitant flow is distinctly pulsatile, not steady. We shall examine the qualitative effects of each of these violations on the analysis already presented.

Constraining Effect of Cardiac Chambers

Inspection of the color profiles in Figures 12–5 to 12–10 demonstrates that the predicted lengths of free jets are much longer than those observed inside the heart. The primary reason for this (in addition to machine-dependent factors that are discussed later) is the constraining effect of the receiving cardiac chamber. It is self-evident that a mitral regurgitant jet entering a 5-cm long left atrium cannot be longer than 5 cm (Fig. 12–11). This limitation to axial penetration is termed *impingement*. Limits to jet flow may also result from restriction to lateral expansion.

Impingement may be approached theoretically by noting that linear momentum within a constrained jet is not

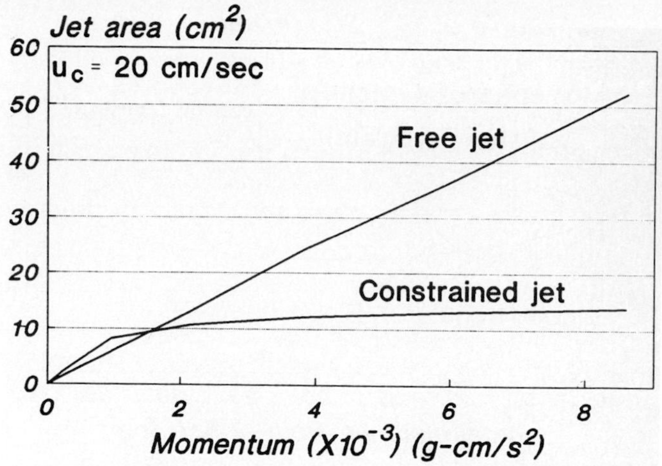

Fig. 12–12. Effect of jet constraint on expected color area. For the lower curve, the jets are assumed to be truncated 10 cm from the orifice by the chamber wall. For all but the smallest jets, the color area is significantly decreased by the chamber constraint. u_c = color cutoff.

constant (as it is in a free jet) but decreases along the axis of the jet as momentum is transferred to the walls of the chamber until, at the end of the chamber, momentum, flow rate, and jet velocity all fall to zero. It is not known precisely how momentum is transferred to the chamber walls, whether it falls linearly along the jet axis or is primarily lost from the distal part of the jet next to the wall. In any case, it greatly distorts the earlier predictions of color jet area vs. momentum, flow rate, and driving pressure. Let us apply a simple assumption: that momentum is constant until the end of the chamber, then is lost abruptly to the chamber. The effect of this is to truncate the profiles in Figure 12–5 at x = 10 cm. Figure 12–12 shows the color area vs. jet momentum for a free jet and one truncated at 10-cm length. The constrained jet shows a flat increase in area with momentum, a jet of 8000 g–cm/sec² having an area only

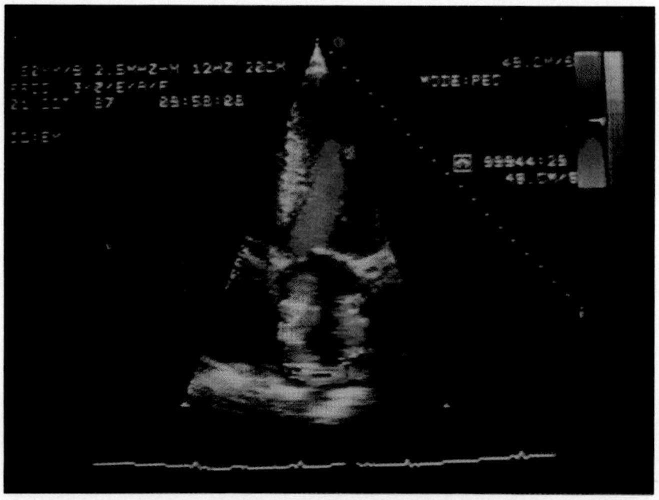

Fig. 12–11. Apical four-chamber view demonstrating impingement. The aliased mitral regurgitant jet is seen in orange as it passes through the mitral orifice and then impinges on the superior wall of the left atrium. In this instance, the jet retains enough momentum to turn back on itself with a velocity that still exceeds the Nyquist limit.

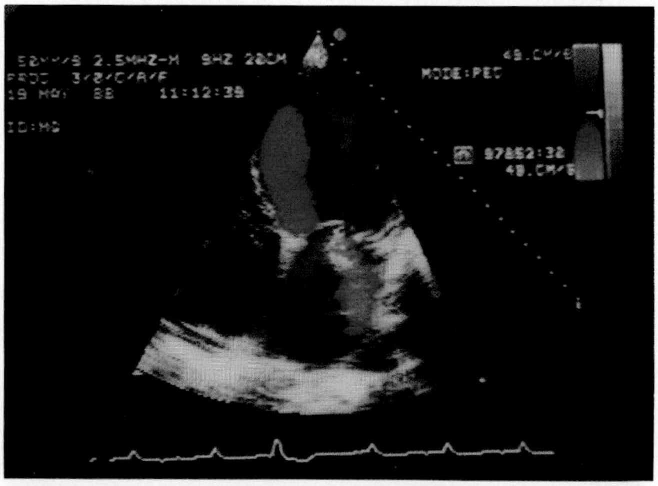

Fig. 12–13. Apical four-chamber view illustrating the Coanda effect. The mitral regurgitant jet (in blue) is seen to pass through the mitral orifice, hug the lateral wall of the left atrium, and then deviate from its long axis by maintaining its relationship to the wall of the atrium.

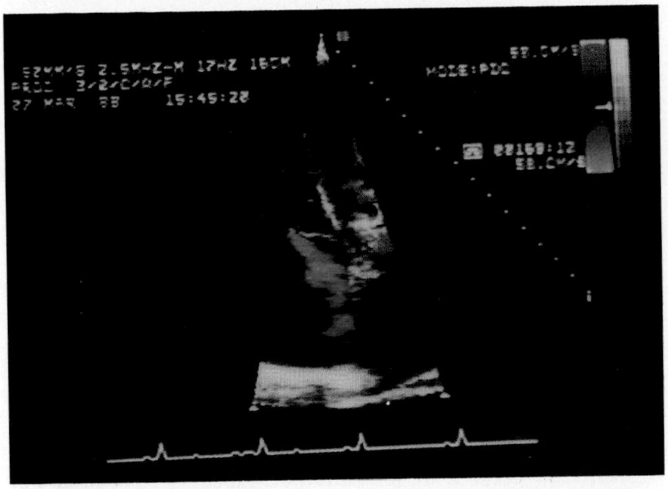

Fig. 12–14. The Coanda effect is further illustrated by this tricuspid regurgitant jet (in blue), which tracks along the interatrial septum.

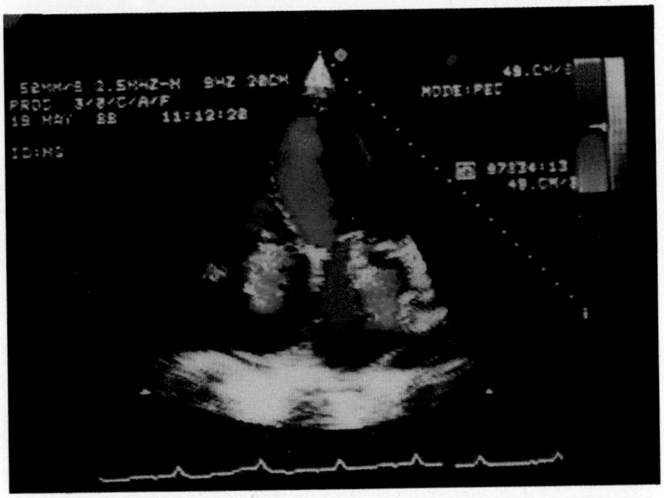

Fig. 12–16. Apical four-chamber view demonstrating both mitral and tricuspid regurgitation. On the left atrial side, pulmonary venous inflow (in orange) is seen to coflow in an opposite direction to the mitral regurgitant jet (in blue).

10% larger than one of 4000 g–cm/sec^2. As discussed below in the section on coflow, the backflow from the jet hitting the far wall of the chamber tends to broaden the jet and, thus, may increase the observed area somewhat more than this figure.

There is another distorting effect on jet flow caused by cardiac chamber geometry. The Coanda effect, described by Henri Coanda,[18] relates to the fact that jets often adhere to and flow around nearby solid boundaries. This is observed if a stream is allowed to run down one's finger, the stream attaches to and deflects around the finger to a new path. Clinically, this is apparent when mitral regurgitant jets are observed to hug the atrial wall (Fig. 12–13) and when tricuspid regurgitant jets track along the interatrial septum (Fig. 12–14), resulting in asymmetric jets. In addition, the arm pulse discrepancy observed in patients with supravalvular aortic stenosis is thought to result from the adherence of the jet to the vessel wall with selective streaming of blood into the innominate artery. The Coanda effect disturbs flow in a largely unpredictable manner, but axial momentum should be little affected beyond the impingement effect noted previously.

Coflow

Other flows are present within the receiving chamber that influence the velocity development of the regurgitant jet. This is termed *coflow*[9] and may create a compound or coaxial jet. Coflow situations may be divided into those resulting from flow extrinsic to the jet and those intrinsic to the jet. Extrinsic coflow may flow in the direction of the regurgitant jet (e.g., when mitral inflow absorbs aortic regurgitant flow) (Fig. 12–15), in a direction opposing the jet (e.g., pulmonary venous flow interrupts mitral regurgitant jets) (Fig. 12–16), or in a direction transverse to the jet (e.g., caval flow deflects tricuspid regurgitation or ventricular septal defect shunt flow intercepts pulmonic regurgitant flow (Figs. 12–17

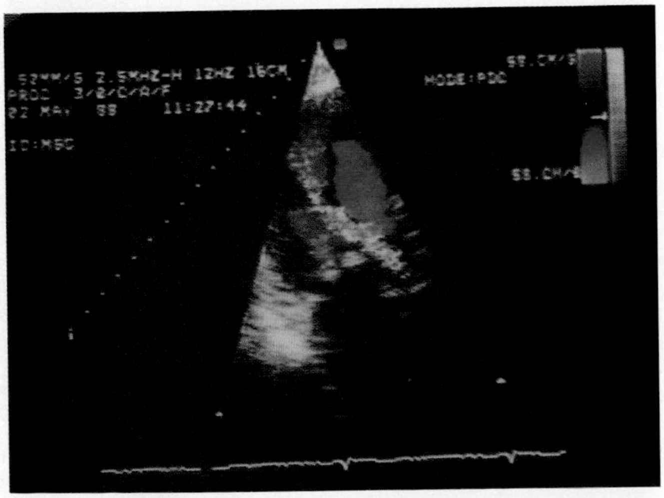

Fig. 12–15. Apical long axis view demonstrating extrinsic coflow in which mitral inflow coflows with and partly absorbs aortic regurgitant flow. This illustration also demonstrates impingement of the aortic regurgitant jet at the apex of the left ventricle.

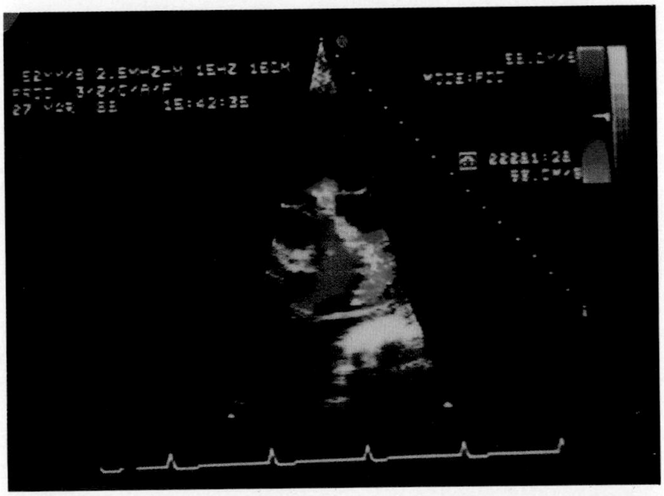

Fig. 12–17. Parasternal long axis view of the right ventricular inflow tract demonstrating extrinsic coflow of vena caval flow (in orange) in a transverse direction to the tricuspid regurgitant (in blue).

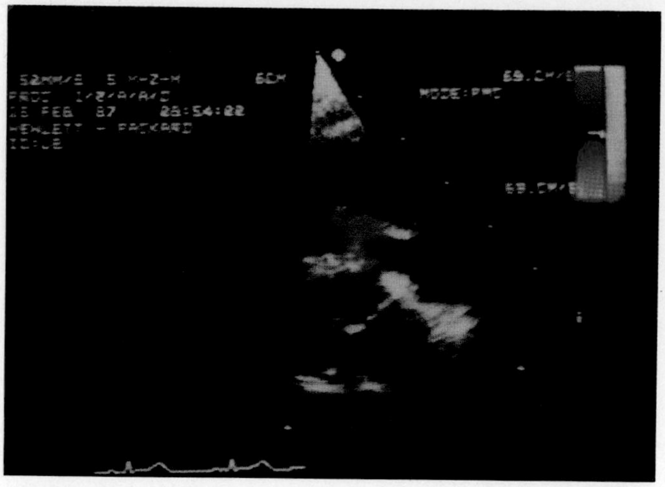

Fig. 12–18. Parasternal long axis view of the right ventricular outflow tract demonstrating a jet of pulmonary regurgitation coflowing with left to right shunt flow through a supracristal ventricular septal defect.

and 12–18). The two flow streams interact, and the jet may either be augmented or diminished depending on their relative velocities.

Intrinsic coflow is caused by the jet itself, typically by reflection of flow as the jet impinges on the wall of the chamber. As such, it usually flows opposite to the jet, increasing the shear rates at the periphery of the jet and causing it to spread more rapidly. Thus, constrained jets might be expected to be wider than free ones. In fact, this backflow is a likely mechanism for the transfer of jet momentum to the chamber walls.

Irregular Orifices

Regurgitant jet orifices are typically irregular in shape, and this irregularity can be expected to distort the jet from the axial symmetry assumed in the preceding analysis. This distortion, however, is predominantly confined to the proximal portion of the jet in the region of the potential core. It can be shown theoretically that jets with long and narrow cross sections tend to expand more rapidly in the narrow dimension than in the long dimension and eventually become round. In vitro experiments have shown that jets resulting from orifices with length to width ratios of 5:1 and areas between 0.1 and 0.5 cm^2 become axisymmetric within 3 cm of the orifice.[19] Thus, although irregular orifices can be expected to affect jet appearance, this alteration is likely to be less important than that resulting from impingement and coflow.

Unsteady Flow

Physiologic flow is unsteady. This greatly complicates analysis of jet flow because unsteady flow never yields a stable regurgitant jet. At the start of flow, it takes a certain amount of time for the regurgitant jet to develop and with cessation of flow, it takes a finite time for the regurgitant jet to dissipate. Thus, the jet may continue to appear even though no further flow is occurring across the orifice. It, therefore, is apparent that different parts of the jet reflect flow that is not occurring concurrently with the area being analyzed and that actually occurred at an earlier time.

Summary of Intracardiac Effects

Thus, we have seen that the single best characteristic to describe regurgitant jets is momentum. For an unconstrained jet, it is possible to predict with some confidence the velocity distribution throughout the jet. Inside the heart, however, jet flow is affected by multiple factors: irregular orifice shapes, impingement and backflow, the Coanda effect, external coflow, and the unsteady nature of flow. It may be possible to account for some of these variables and make a reasonable correlation of color jet appearance with the true jet parameters. Before discussing current and possible future methods of doing this, however, it is important to review some of the limitations of current color Doppler technology because these limitations further complicate the task of jet analysis.

Technical Limitations of Color Doppler Flow Displays

Thus far we have assumed a perfect measuring instrument with fine spatial and temporal resolution that can quantitate velocities of any magnitude. In fact, color flow mapping has several significant limitations.[20,21]

Limited Temporal Resolution. A single ultrasound pulse is sufficient to reconstruct the imaging information from one M-line of a two-dimensional sector scan. In contrast, to reconstruct the velocity information along the same M-line requires 3 to 7 ultrasound pulses (Chapter 11). This is the principal reason why color Doppler instruments typically generate only 10 to 20 images per second. Thus it is possible for one side of a sector scan to be as much as 100 msec removed from the other side and to miss completely flow events that persist for less than 50 to 100 msec.

Limited Spatial Resolution. Lateral and azimuthal spatial resolution are determined primarily by the focusing of the ultrasound beam. Axial resolution, on the other hand, depends primarily on the duration of the ultrasound packet used to interrogate the tissue: the shorter the packet, the finer the resolution. Unfortunately, a shorter packet requires more pulses to achieve the same signal/noise ratio, and so there is a trade-off between temporal and spatial resolution. Overall, typical resolutions are 10 to 20 Hz and 3 to 5 mm, respectively.

Limited Velocity Resolution. In an effort to maximize spatial and temporal resolution, current color flow mappers provide relatively coarse velocity resolution, typically only 8 to 16 gradations forward and reverse. In the usual algorithm, forward velocity is mapped into increasing saturation of red; reverse (or aliased) flow is output as blue. Unfortunately, the relatively poor intrinsic spatial and velocity resolution is further worsened by the limitations of standard color video. By the National Television System Committee (NTSC) television standard used in the United States, the intensity signal (monochrome image) is carried in a 4-MHz frequency band and the color information is carried in two signals of 0.5 and 1.3 MHz.[22] This means that sharp variations in intensity can be faithfully reproduced (the 4-MHz band allows black to white changes in the space of a single pixel). The color information, however, cannot be changed as rapidly; in fact, as many as 8 pixels within a horizontal scan line are smeared together into each output pixel, with consequent distortion of the apparent velocity and loss of spatial resolution.

Velocity Aliasing. Because the color flow image is generated by a pulsed wave modality, aliasing is a frequently encountered problem. The pulse repetition frequency (PRF) must be low enough to avoid range ambiguity throughout the full depth (R) of the image:

$$PRF = c/2R, \qquad [12.7]$$

where c is the velocity of sound in tissue. The Nyquist frequency is half of this, so the maximal forward and reverse velocity (v_m) is given by:

$$v_m = c^2/8Rf_0, \qquad [12.8]$$

where f_0 is the ultrasound frequency. In the adult, the color flow Nyquist limit is typically between 0.6 and 0.9 m/sec but can be raised by decreasing the sector depth or using a lower frequency transducer.

Mean Versus Maximal Velocity. With the correlation method of velocity decoding currently in use, most instruments estimate the mean Doppler shift, the bandwidth, and the intensity of the Doppler signal. These machines do not allow calculation of the maximum blood velocity in each pixel, which might help to factor out the multiple contributions to jet volume outlined previously.

Doppler Scanning Detects Only One Component of Velocity. It is commonly recognized that Doppler scanning detects only the component of velocity parallel to the ultrasound beam. To recover the absolute velocity, one must divide this detected component by cos Θ, where Θ is the angle between the jet flow and the ultrasound beam. Unfortunately, when the flow is turbulent, this angle correction is error prone. Because the random fluctuations in jet velocity can occur both in the axial and radial directions, it is possible for the actual instantaneous velocity direction to swing as much as 20° away from its mean direction. When mean flow is parallel to the ultrasound, this direction shift adds only about 6% to the observed turbulent velocity variations. However, if the mean flow stream is directed 70° from the ultrasound beam, then the calculated turbulent variation would exceed the corrected mean velocity, making estimation of the true mean velocity error prone.

Low Velocity Cutoff. Figures 12–7 to 12–12 were based on the color Doppler machine having a well defined low velocity cutoff that would define a velocity contour of the jet. Unfortunately, on current color flow mappers there is no sharp wall filter, as there is on standard pulsed Doppler units. In fact, the cutoff is quite soft, with little more than a linear fall-off in gain between the Nyquist velocity limit and zero velocity. Furthermore, this gain varies at different depth settings and at different locations within a given sector scan. Thus, it is difficult to standardize the gain so that the color areas of identical jets will be the same even if they lie at different depths in the chest.

CURRENT AND FUTURE APPROACHES TO COLOR JET QUANTIFICATION

Despite the previously mentioned limitations of cardiac geometry and Doppler technology, color flow maps provide a compelling spatiotemporal display of the intracardiac regurgitant jets. Numerous in vitro and clinical studies have demonstrated significant correlation between the color jet appearance and severity of regurgitation, but such assessments have generally been only semiquantitative and have been correlated with other semiquantitative measures of severity of regurgitation (e.g., angiography). The goal of true quantitation remains elusive.

Analyzing Color as a Binary or Continuous Quantity

There are two broad ways that the information in a color display may be used in analysis. The method used almost exclusively at present is to treat the color image as a dichotomy: color is either present or it is not. Thus, when the area or length of a color jet is measured, no discrimination is made between high velocity and low velocity flow. They are simply recorded as "flow." Clearly, a great deal of information is being discarded in such an analysis.

The alternative approach to color analysis is to use the actual velocity information present within the color image and to treat the color as a continuum ranging from low velocity to high velocity. Thus, high velocity regions of a jet would be weighted more heavily than low velocity regions in assessing the severity of regurgitation. Such an approach intuitively makes more sense in that it makes use of more of the data gathered by the echocardiograph than does simply measuring the area of the jet. There are two principal reasons why this more detailed approach to analysis has not been widely used. The first is the difficulty in recovering actual velocity data from the video output of the echo machine. Although each echo manufacturer provides a color bar that should map the output colors onto a velocity (and often variance) scale, until recently there was no way to use these data on a pixel-by-pixel basis to reconstruct the velocity map. Currently, off-line analyzers extract the red, green, and blue values from the video and use the color bar to derive velocity.[23] Experience with these analyzers is limited, however, and they remain dependent on the relatively unproven fidelity of the echo color bar to measure true intracardiac velocity. The distortions noted previously, caused by the limited bandwidth of the NTSC standard color video signal, alter velocity reconstructions, especially in regions of aliasing, in ways that cannot be completely corrected. The developing trend in direct digital storage by several manufacturers is a significant advance in velocity integrity. Figure 12–19 shows a digitally output color map of a mitral regurgitant jet. Because these velocity data are maintained in machine-

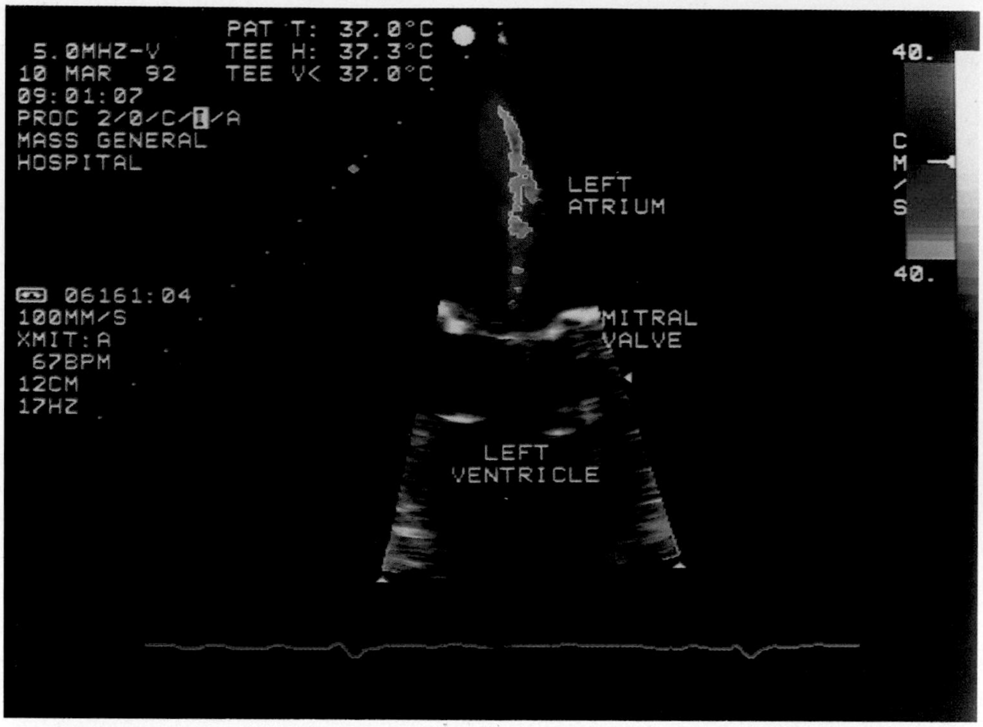

Fig. 12–19. Digital color Doppler velocity map of a mitral regurgitant jet.

readable format, they are available for further quantitative analysis.

However, even if true velocities can be reliably reconstructed, a second set of problems must be overcome to use velocity as a continuous variable in jet analysis: computational complexity. Analysis of a large jet might involve 30,000 pixels. To calculate, e.g., momentum flux throughout this region (see details later), would require coordinate transformation with velocity angle correction on each of the points with integration and averaging across the region. To perform this analysis on multiple frames from a cardiac cycle might be lengthy. Nevertheless, the extremely rapid progress in computer processing power over the past 20 years indicates that such algorithms soon will be feasible.

Prior Studies

Numerous in vitro and clinical studies have correlated color as a binary variable with severity of regurgitation. An in vitro study of aortic regurgitation[24] found that jet length increased in a curvilinear fashion with increasing driving pressure and orifice area (i.e., regurgitant flow rate). It also found that the proximal cross section of the jet correlated well with the orifice area. Another in vitro experiment designed to compare the effects of jet flow rate, driving pressure, and orifice area on jet area[25] found that for any given orifice area, jet area increased approximately linearly with flow rate and that larger orifices required higher flow rates to achieve the same jet area. Such an inverse relationship between flow rate and orifice area is consistent with the proposition that momentum is a key parameter in determining jet appearance because, by Equation 12.1C, momentum varies directly with flow rate and inversely with orifice area. Similarly, we found that the volume of a color jet varies directly with the flow rate.[26] When orifice area was also varied, the single jet parameter that best predicted the appearance of the jet was momentum flux. Indeed, it was found that color jet area increased in proportion to the square root of the momentum. This observation differs from the prediction of Equation 12.6 (that color area should be directly proportional to momentum) primarily because of the constraining effect of the in vitro model on the jet.

The ultimate goal in this analysis is to relate color jet appearance to orifice area or flow rate in a quantitative sense. For instance, if some combination of jet length, width, or area reliably predicted jet momentum flux (M_0), one could use continuous wave Doppler echocardiography to measure the orifice velocity (u_0) and calculate (by Equation 12.1A) orifice flow,

$$Q_0 = M_0/u_0$$

and (by Equation 12.1B) regurgitant orifice area,

$$A_0 = M_0/u_0^2$$

Unfortunately, such calculations have been unreliable because jet appearance depends so strongly on cardiac geometry and machine parameters, perhaps even more than on the magnitude of the jet itself. Furthermore, regurgitant flow is difficult to measure accurately by other modalities (angiography, conventional Doppler). Thus, most clinical color Doppler studies of regurgitation have made only semiquantitative correlations with other measurements. For instance, it was found that the ratio of jet cross-sectional area to left ventricular outflow tract area correlated well with angiographic grade of aortic regurgitation severity.[4] Interestingly, neither jet length nor area reliably distinguished between angiographic grades. Similarly, in evaluating mitral regurgitation, it was found that absolute color jet length and area failed to fully separate three angiographic grades of severity. Dividing the regurgitant area by the total left atrial area afforded better separation; however, no attempt was made to calculate actual regurgitant volume.[3]

Thus, there appear to be significant theoretic and practical barriers to calculating regurgitant flow when color Doppler scanning is treated simply as a binary quantity (i.e., present or not present). Therefore, to obtain better quantitation requires analyzing the actual velocities in a color Doppler map.

Quantitative Color Flow Analysis

We have thus far shown that momentum flux is probably the best single descriptor of the physical jet but that simple color area varies too much with machine gain and chamber constraint to provide a reliable measure of jet momentum. Thus we seek to calculate jet momentum directly from the observed jet velocities and then derive regurgitant flow rate and orifice area. Consider the jet in Figure 12–2. Color flow mapping should provide the spatial distribution of axial velocity, u(x,r), throughout the jet. We seek to calculate the momentum flux passing through a plane orthogonal to the jet axis at a distance x from the orifice. By the conservation principle, this momentum flux should be a constant throughout the jet (except for the effects of chamber constraint and impingement). If we assume that the jet is axisymmetric, each pixel represents a rim of blood moving at a radius, r, from the jet axis (Fig. 12–20). Thus, we may use Equation 12.2 to calculate the total kinematic momentum flux crossing the plane:

$$M = 2\pi \int_0^\infty r\, u(r)^2\, dr.$$

Again, by using continuous wave Doppler to provide the jet velocity at the orifice, we can calculate orifice area ($A_0 = M/u_0^2$) and flow rate ($Q_0 = M/u_0$).

As with our discussion of color jet area, we must be concerned about the effect of machine-dependent factors on the calculated jet momentum. In this regard, however, our calculations should be insensitive to variation in the low velocity cutoff for color display. This is because these low velocities contribute relatively little to the total momentum and their inclusion or exclusion matters little. Figure 12–21 compares the percentage of total jet momentum that would be expected to be measured and the predicted color jet area, each as a function of the low velocity cutoff u_c. Reducing u_c from 10 to 5 cm/sec only increases measured M from 97 to 99% of the actual total. Contrast this with the color area, which increases 400% when u_c is cut in half.

Practical experience in such calculations is extremely limited, however, largely because of the difficulty in recovering reliable velocity data from the color flow video. In an in vitro model, jets with momentum flux up to 19,000 g–cm/sec^2 were analyzed, and momentum flux was calculated using the preceding algorithm. To minimize the effect of turbulent variability in velocity, momentum flux was calculated across 60 to 100 planes for each jet. When averaged together, this observed momentum flux agreed with the known value with r = 0.99[27] (Fig. 12–22). Factoring in the orifice velocity provided an accurate estimate of instantaneous flow rate (Fig. 12–23). In this early work, the need for the color map to be nonaliased throughout its region of analysis

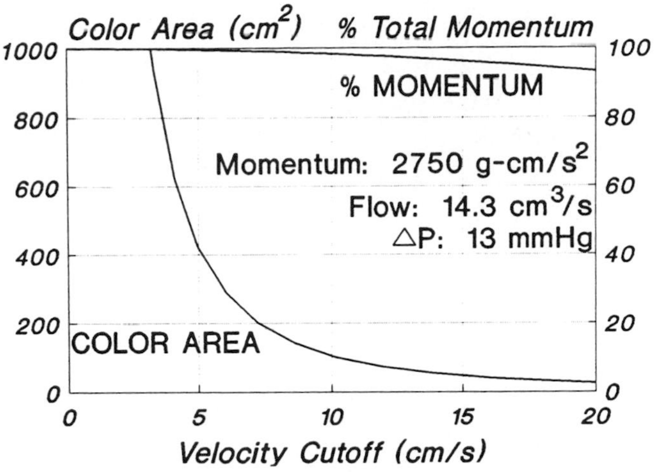

Fig. 12–21. Comparison of the changes in jet area and apparent jet momentum, each as a function of low velocity cutoff (u_o). Decreasing the cutoff from 20 to 5 cm/sec causes the color area of the unconstrained jet to increase 16-fold, whereas the measured jet momentum, because it weights high velocity flow much more than low velocity flow, only increases by 3%. ΔP = driving pressure.

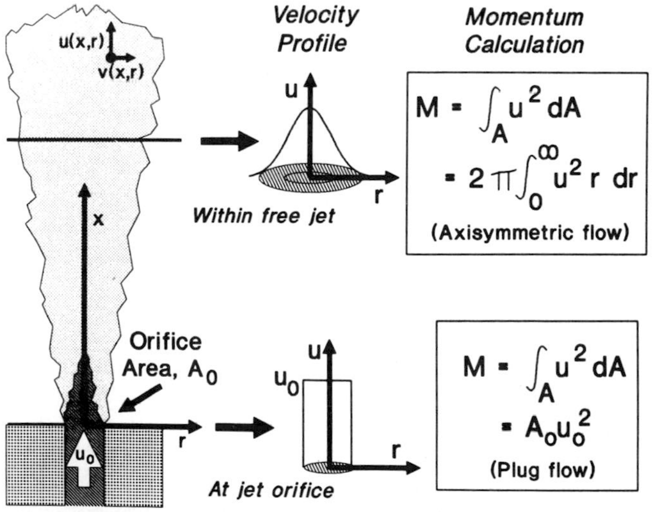

Fig. 12–20. Calculation of jet momentum assuming axial symmetry. At the round jet orifice, the velocity profile is flat and momentum is given by $A_o u_o^2$. As the jet spreads out in the chamber, it forms a Gaussian (bell-shaped) velocity profile. Because axial symmetry is maintained, momentum can be calculated by integrating $2\pi r u^2$ across a single profile, as shown. (From Thomas JD, O'Shea JP, Weyman AE: Quantification of jet flow by momentum analysis: An in vitro color Doppler study. Circulation 81:247, 1990. Reproduced by permission of the American Heart Association, Inc.)

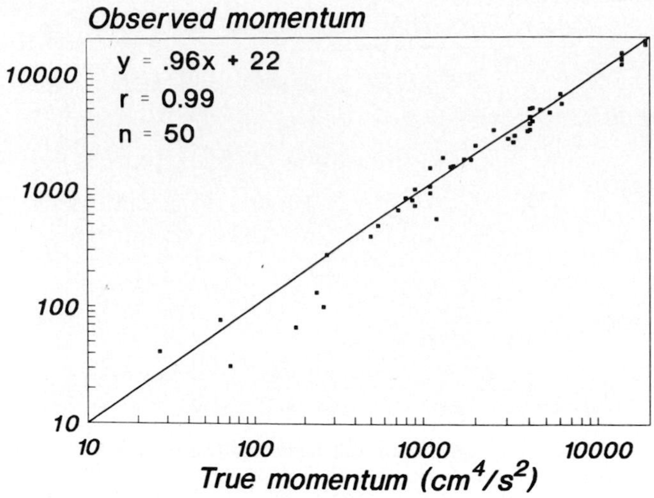

Fig. 12–22. Calculation of jet momentum in in vitro jets. Using velocities below the Nyquist limit, it is possible to obtain accurate estimates of jet momentum from color Doppler images. (From Thomas JD, O'Shea JP, Weyman AE: Quantification of jet flow by momentum analysis: An in vitro color Doppler study. Circulation 81:247, 1990. Reproduced by permission of the American Heart Association, Inc.)

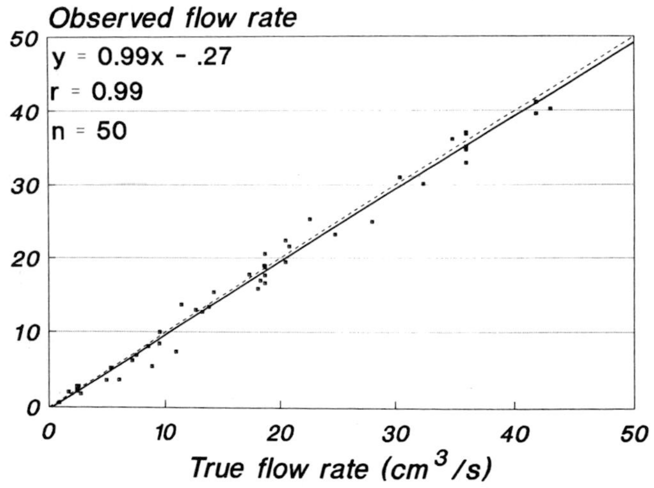

Fig. 12–23. Calculation of jet flow rate. Data from Figure 12–22 were divided by orifice velocity to obtain an estimate of orifice flow rate. (From Thomas JD, O'Shea JP, Weyman AE: Quantification of jet flow by momentum analysis: An in vitro color Doppler study. Circulation 81:247, 1990. Reproduced by permission of the American Heart Association, Inc.)

limited the magnitude of jets that could be quantified.

To obtain actual regurgitant volume (V), it is necessary to calculate flow rate for each video frame in which the jet is visible and to integrate the flow over time:

$$V = \int Q \, dt \qquad [12.9]$$

Even this relationship, however, is not as simple as one would hope. For example, at low flow rates, the color appears to take some time to be initiated, whereas at higher flow rates, the color jet persists beyond the end of the regurgitant interval, related to a cool-down time for the dissipation of jet momentum. Thus, duration of the visualized color jet may exceed the duration of physiologic jet. Because regurgitant volume is integrated over time, this cool-down time also tends to exaggerate the actual volume.

SUMMARY

The behavior of regurgitant jets is governed primarily by conservation of mass, momentum, and energy, of which momentum is most critical to color Doppler analysis. Momentum flux, which combines jet flow rate, orifice area, and driving pressure into a single parameter, best predicts the appearance of a jet by color flow mapping. Unfortunately, machine gain and intracardiac flow and geometry also have profound independent effects on the color flow appearance of the regurgitant jet.

Most current color flow analysis algorithms treat observed color as a binary quantity, which is either present or not, without considering actual blood velocity. Using such algorithms, it has been possible to obtain good semiquantitative correlations between jet appearance and severity of regurgitation but not to quantify actual regurgitant flow. With improvements in color Doppler technology and computer processing algorithms, it may be possible to use the actual velocities to calculate directly jet momentum and from this to derive the actual regurgitant flow rate, volume, and orifice area.

Quantification of Valvular Regurgitation by Analysis of the Proximal Convergence Zone

In recent years, a new quantitative method has emerged for evaluation of valvular regurgitation. In contrast to methods described previously, which analyze either the appearance or velocity distribution within the downstream regurgitant jet, this method analyzes velocities upstream from the regurgitant orifice.[28,29] In this zone, velocity must increase steadily in a series of roughly symmetric isovelocity shells. By the principle of conservation of mass, all flow that passes through any one of these shells is destined, ultimately, to pass through the regurgitant orifice (Fig. 12–24). The utility of this method depends critically on the predictable acceleration of flow toward the regurgitant orifice and the predictable shape of the isovelocity shells.

Physical Principles of the Proximal Acceleration Method

It was noted previously that one of the difficulties with analysis of the downstream jet is that flow is completely turbulent in this region, leading to significant difficulties in the accurate Doppler estimation of the mean velocity. In contrast, flow within the convergent zone proximal to a regurgitant orifice is better behaved and generally retains laminar character even to very high Reynolds numbers. The reason for this relative stability can be seen by analysis of the pressure gradients within this zone. As blood approaches the orifice, its velocity and kinetic energy increase, balanced (via conservation of energy) by a fall in local pressure. This favorable pressure gradient has the effect of suppressing the development of boundary layers within the flow. Because it is

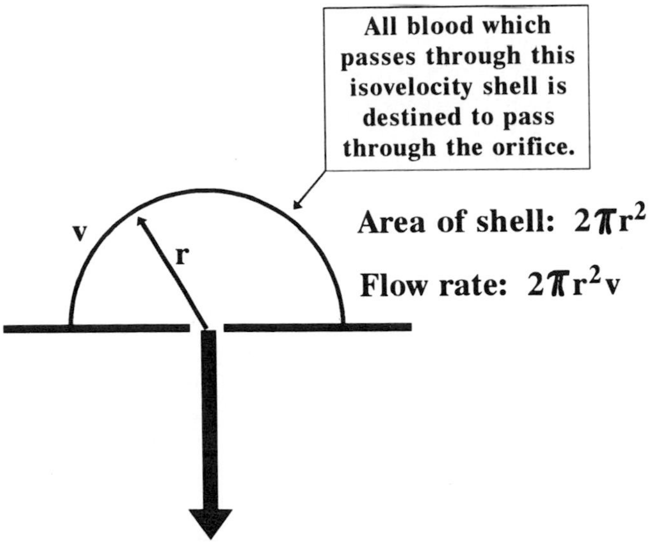

Fig. 12–24. Schematic representation of the proximal acceleration method. By the conservation of mass, all blood that passes through the isovelocity shell shown at a distance r from the orifice is destined ultimately to pass through the orifice (represented by large arrow).

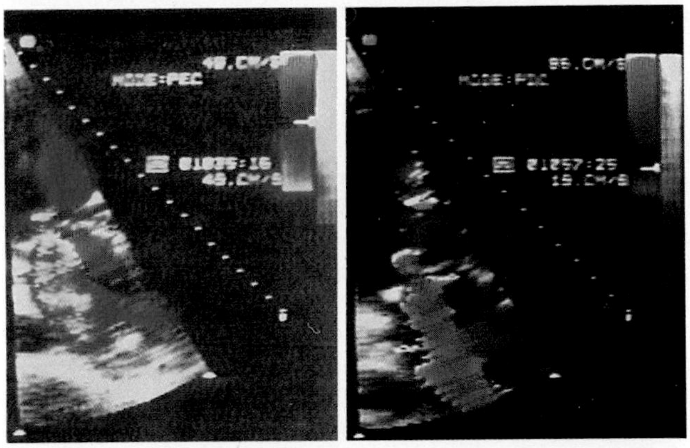

Fig. 12–26. An example of a proximal converging flow field at the ventricular surface of the mitral leaflets in a patient with mitral regurgitation. The blue-to-orange interface represents the isovelocity contour with a corresponding velocity of 19 cm/sec obtained after shifting the color baseline.

growth of boundary layers that leads to separation of the flow from walls and the development of turbulence, in the proximal convergence zone, flow separation does not occur and the effects of viscosity are essentially negligible.[30] In the absence of viscous effects, velocity increases symmetrically as flow approaches the orifice. If the orifice were a very small point within a flat plane, one would therefore expect the isovelocity shells to have a hemispheric shape. Figure 12–25 displays a finite difference solution of the Navier-Stokes equations of axisymmetric flow approaching a round orifice.[31] It can be seen in the zone far from the regurgitant orifice that the isovelocity contours are indeed hemispheric in shape. The distortion that occurs close to the orifice will be discussed later. It is the assumption of hemispheric symmetry that forms the basis for the clinical application of the proximal acceleration method.

Practical Quantification of Proximal Acceleration by Doppler Echocardiography

Figure 12–26 shows a color Doppler display of the proximal convergence zone in mitral regurgitation. Although the velocities are encoded in the colors, it is difficult to relate any given point to a particular velocity from the color display alone. At the aliasing bounding, however, there is a very sharp transition as blood changes from bright blue to bright yellow. At this point, blood is moving at 49 cm/sec; thus, this aliasing point defines the radius of the isovelocity contour of velocity of 49 cm/sec. Assuming that this isovelocity contour is actually hemispheric in shape, its area can be calculated at $2\pi r^2$, where r is the radius from the regurgitant orifice to this aliasing boundary. The instantaneous flow rate is

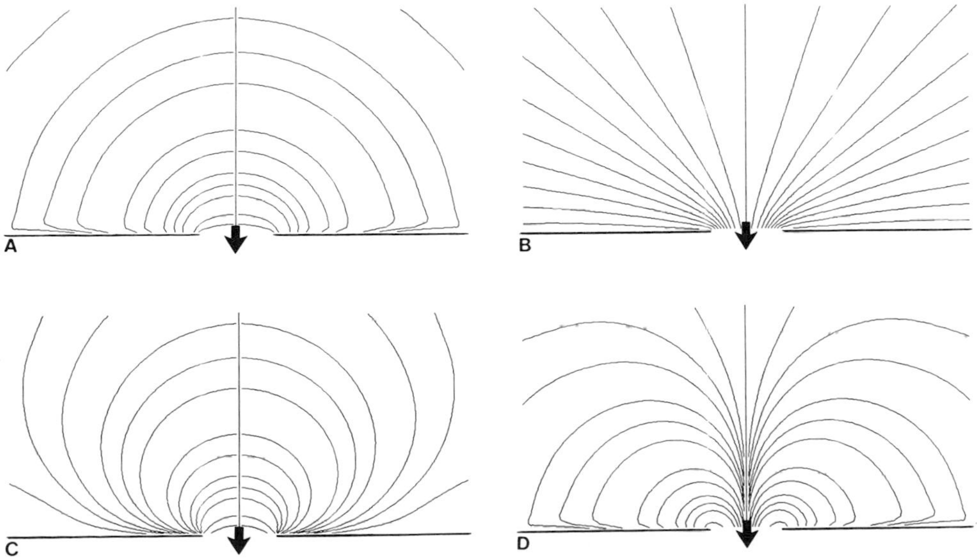

Fig. 12–25. Flow convergence toward a round orifice as modeled by finite difference solution to the Navier-Stokes equations. The domain shown here has a radius and axial length of 2.5 cm with 176 cm^3/sec flowing through an 8-mm diameter orifice. Fluid density and viscosity are physiologic. The panels show contours of velocity magnitude (A), streamlines of flow (B), and the axial (C) and radial (D) components of velocity. **A, C, and D.** Contours correspond (from distal to proximal) to velocities of 1, 2, 3, 5, 7, 10, 20, 30, 50, 70, 100, 200, and 300 cm/sec. Panel A has no 1 or 2 cm/sec contours and panel D has no 300 cm/sec contour. (From Rodriguez et al.: Circ Res 70:923, 1992. Reproduced by permission of the American Heart Association.)

then calculated by multiplying the area of this hemisphere by the aliasing velocity, $Q = 2\pi r^2 v$.

In practice, as shown in the left panel of Figure 12–26, this aliasing boundary often is very close to the regurgitant orifice, and the measurement of its radius can be imprecise. Accordingly, a common solution to this problem is to shift the baseline of the color Doppler display to allow the transition from blue to yellow to occur at lower velocities. As shown in the right panel of Figure 12–26, the Doppler display has been shifted so that aliasing occurs at a velocity of 19 cm/sec, with a corresponding increase in the aliasing radius. This larger radius is easier to measure, leading to more precise flow calculations.

In early in vitro studies of the proximal convergence method, it was shown that the assumption of hemispheric contour shape was valid.[28] However, further work demonstrated a slight flattening of the contours, suggesting that flow would be more accurately calculated if the isovelocity contours were hemielliptic, rather than hemispheric.[29] More detailed experiments have better defined the nature of this distortion and indicate that two broad types of geometric distortion can occur in the proximal convergence field, which render the hemispheric assumption inaccurate.

Impact of Local Geometry

The first of these geometric factors has to do with the flattening of the isovelocity contours as flow approaches the orifice. This is demonstrated in the numeric simulation in Figure 12–25 and leads to contours of hemielliptic shape.[29] Detailed analytic and in vitro study has demonstrated that this flattening of the isovelocity contours occurs in a predictable manner as flow approaches the orifice.

Analysis of finite difference simulations of proximal convergence flow has shown that this contour flattening near the orifice leads to progressive underestimation of the true flow rate when flow is calculated by the simple $2\pi r^2 v$ formula. The flow underestimation occurs because the velocity near a finite orifice falls predictably below that expected from the $1/r^2$ assumption (Fig. 12–27). Unfortunately, this observation would not help to correct this flow calculation, because in the clinical situation, the radius of the orifice cannot be directly determined echocardiographically. Alternatively, however, it was also found that the degree of flow underestimation could be predicted from the aliasing velocity of interest divided by the peak orifice velocity v_O. Indeed, the proportion of flow underestimation ($\Delta q/q$) when the simple formula $2\pi r^2 v$ was applied was found to be linearly related to v_N/v_O, as shown in Figure 12–28. This finding has important practical implications because it leads to a simple correction formula to account for the flattening of isovelocity contours. If flow rate is calculated in the usual manner as $2\pi r^2 v$, then the corrected flow rate can be obtained by multiplying this value by the ratio $v_O/(v_O - v_N)$. An in vitro experiment to test this hypothesis confirmed that the amount of flow underestimation can be almost completely corrected by this factor (Fig. 12–29).[32]

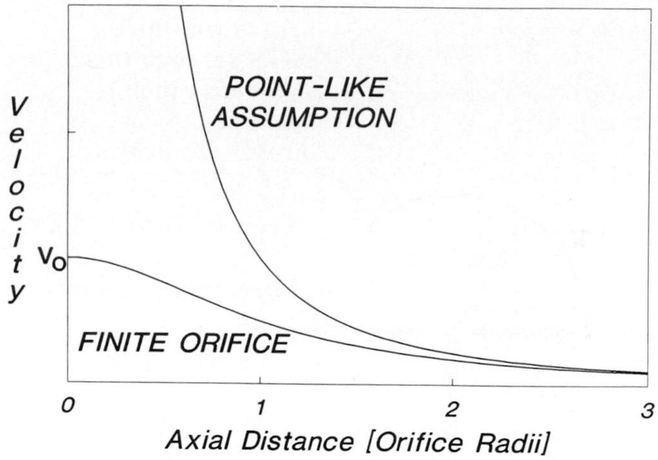

Fig. 12–27. Close to a finite orifice, the velocity falls below the $1/r^2$ relationship assumed for a pointlike orifice leading to progressive underestimation of flow in the immediate vicinity of the orifice. Beyond approximately three orifice radii, however, the two curves are virtually identical, indicating that the assumption of hemispheric isovelocity contour shape is appropriate in this region.

The impact of this error is minimal for the evaluation of left-sided regurgitant jets. In mitral regurgitation, for instance, the peak orifice velocity typically is 5 to 6 m/sec, whereas the aliasing velocity chosen to define the isovelocity contour is typically around 20 cm/sec. Therefore, the degree of flow underestimation that is due to flattening of the isovelocity contours is less than 5% in this circumstance, and correction by this factor is generally unnecessary. However, for right-sided regurgitant jets and other low velocity jets such as atrial septal defect (ASD) flow, the aliasing velocity of interest may be

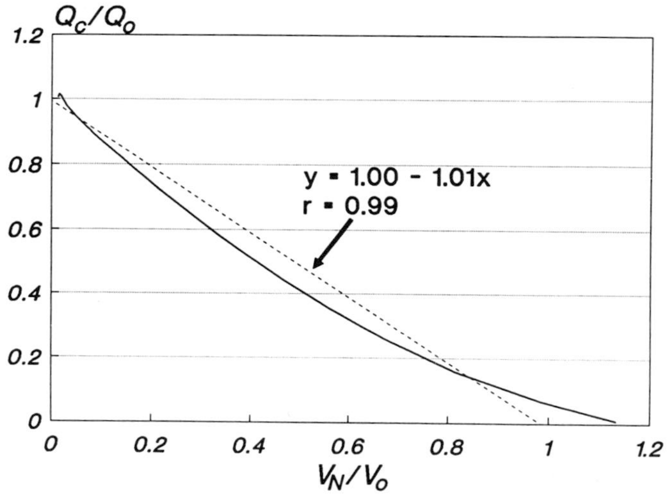

Fig. 12–28. Predictable underestimation of flow is seen when the aliasing velocity of interest approaches the orifice velocity. The solid line shows data from the finite difference simulations, and the dashed line shows the best linear approximation of this. As shown, the proportional underestimation of the flow rate by the hemispheric assumption is almost precisely equivalent to the ratio of the aliasing velocity of interest to orifice velocity. V_N = contour isovelocity of interest; V_o = orifice velocity; Q_c = flow rate calculated assuming hemispheric shape; Q_o = true flow rate. (From Rodriguez et al.: Circ Res 70:923, 1992. Reproduced by permission of the American Heart Association.)

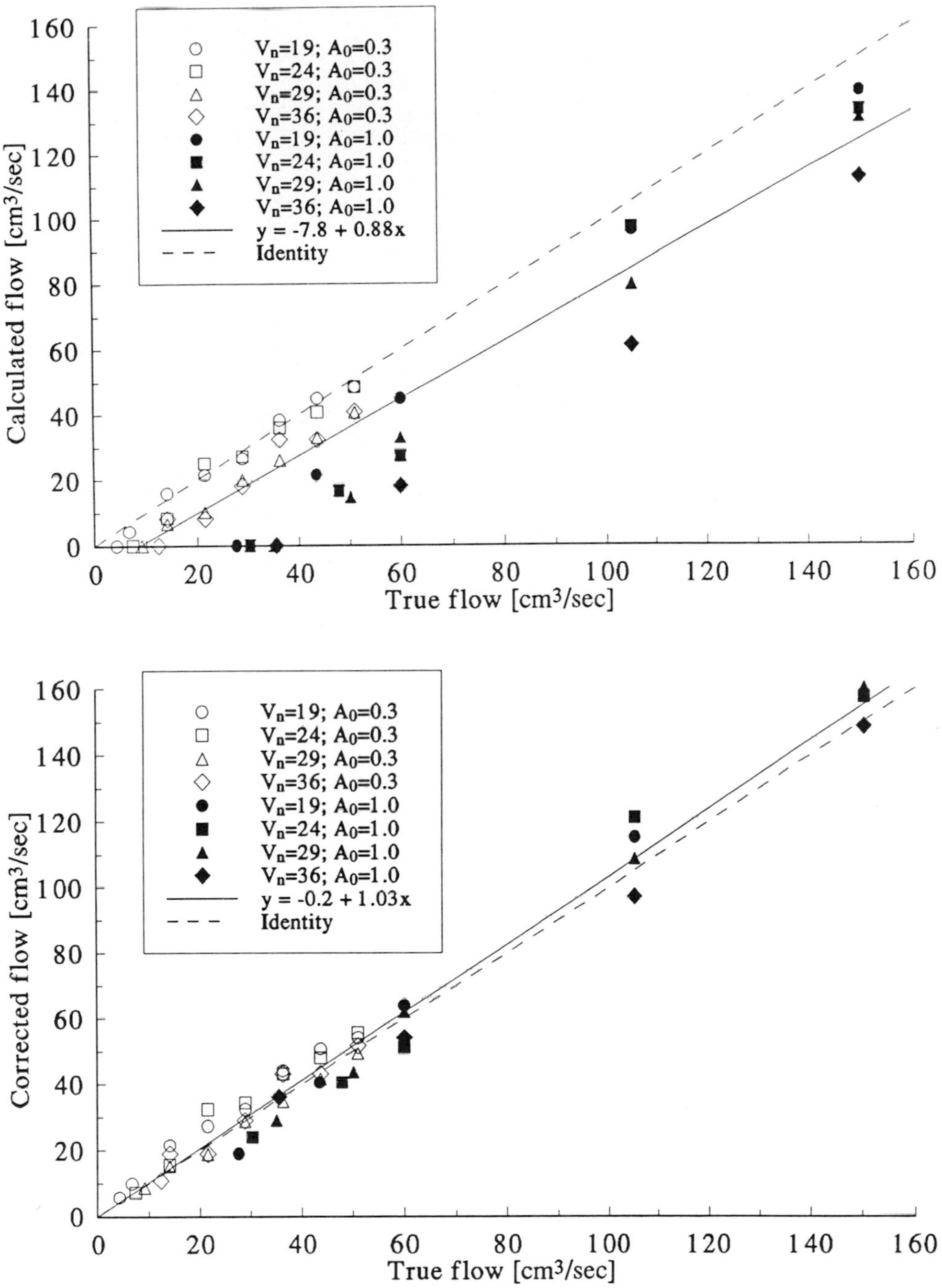

Fig. 12–29. Calculated flow vs. true flow using the proximal acceleration method with assumption of simple hemispheric symmetry (top) and correcting for the flattening of isovelocity contours near the orifice (bottom). Flow is progressively underestimated when larger aliasing velocities are used, which are a significant proportion of the orifice velocity. This flow underestimation can largely be corrected by recognizing the predictable underestimation as shown in Figure 12–28. V_N = contour isovelocity of interest; A_o = orifice area. (From Rodriguez et al.: Circ Res 70:723, 1992. Reproduced by permission of the American Heart Association.)

a significant proportion of the peak orifice velocity, and therefore, correction would be recommended. Application of this correction factor has been shown to be necessary in tricuspid regurgitation to achieve optimal accuracy.[33]

Effect of Global Geometry on Proximal Acceleration

The second broad cause of distortion of the proximal acceleration field is due to the global geometry within which the regurgitant orifice lies. It was noted previously that when the orifice lies in a plane, then flow converges in concentric hemispheric shells. However, it is obvious that an orifice that lies in a funnel could not have hemispherically shaped isovelocity shells because the full hemisphere is not available to the flow. Because the overall principles of flow convergence still hold in this situation, one would again expect viscosity to play a relatively minor role and the isovelocity shells to be roughly concentric; thus, one would expect the contours to appear as hemispheres that are truncated by the funnel-shaped geometry.

Numeric simulation of this situation lends support to this hypothesis. It was found that the constant of 2π used to calculate flow rate for orifices in a flat geometry had to be reduced when the orifices lay in a funnel-shaped geometry, and this degree of reduction reflected the solid angle subtended by the global geometry. For orifices that lie in axisymmetric funnel-shaped geometry, the appropriate constant for calculating flow is $2\pi \cdot (1 - \cos\theta)$ where θ is the angle from the central axis to the wall of the funnel (Fig. 12–30). For an orifice in a flat plain, θ is 90° with a cosine of 0; thus the constant reduces to 2π, the usual value used. For orifices that lie in a funnel that is much more pronounced in one dimension than the other, the appropriate reduction is simply $2\pi\alpha/180$, where α is the angular separation of the two funnel walls in the narrowest projection. Empiric evidence for this correction factor has been obtained in a model of mitral stenosis. In that study, flow rate was estimated from the proximal convergence radii of forward flow through the stenotic mitral valve with the empiric constant reduced by $\alpha/180$. The effective regurgitant orifice area was obtained by dividing this peak flow rate by peak orifice velocity and was compared with the mitral valve area obtained by mitral valve planimetry. As shown in Figure 12–31, there was an excellent correlation between valve area from planimetry and valve area from proximal acceleration supporting the overall approach to flow reduction in proportion to the solid angle subtended by the global geometry.

Clinical Studies

There have been relatively few clinical studies published on the use of proximal acceleration to quantify valvular regurgitation. One study used cardiac catheterization to obtain a semiquantitative assessment of regurgitant severity that correlated well with the estimates obtained from proximal acceleration.[34] A more detailed study quantified valvular regurgitation by measuring the forward stroke volume through the mitral valve and aortic valve by pulsed Doppler methods.[35] The difference (mitral regurgitant volume) was compared with the regurgitant stroke volume estimated by proximal acceleration. As shown in Figure 12–32, there was excellent correlation throughout a very wide range of regurgitant severity, and this relationship held both for patients in normal sinus rhythm and atrial fibrillation. Extension of this concept to tricuspid regurgitation also appears promising.[33] Thus far, there has been relatively little work on this subject in aortic regurgitation, although the overall principle should hold. One difficulty with this approach is that from the usual transthoracic windows used in aortic regurgitation (the apical views), the proxi-

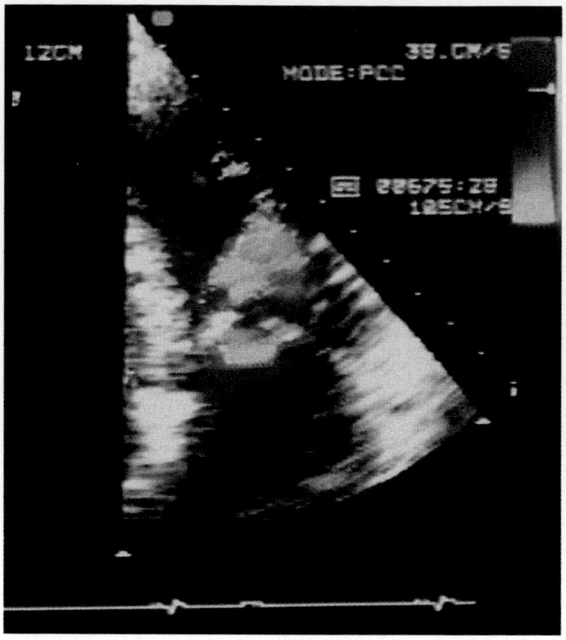

A

R = 1.06 cm

Aliasing velocity = 38 cm/sec

Angle α = 115°

Peak inflow velocity = 210 cm/sec

Peak flow rate $= 2\pi * (1.02\text{cm})^2 * 38\ \text{cm/sec} * (115/180)$

$= 171\ \text{cm}^3/\text{sec}$

$$\text{MVA} = \frac{171\ \text{cm}^3/\text{sec}}{210\ \text{cm/sec}} = 0.8\ \text{cm}^2$$

B

Fig. 12–31. Estimation of mitral valve area in mitral stenosis using the proximal acceleration concept. **A.** The region of acceleration (from low velocity red to high velocity blue) on the atrial side of the stenotic mitral orifice in an apical four-chamber view. This image, obtained when the proximal flow convergence region was largest, provides the radius R of that region, measured from the orifice to the red-blue interface, and the angle α subtended by the leaflets, which determines the fraction of a hemisphere ($\alpha/180$) over which flow can converge. **B.** Forward flow through the mitral valve was then calculated as shown in the equations using the proximal acceleration method, with the constant of 2π adjusted for the angle subtended by the stenotic leaflets. Regurgitant orifice area was then calculated as peak flow rate divided by peak forward velocity from the continuous-wave Doppler trace. Excellent agreement was observed with planimetered valve area. MVA = mitral valve area. (Courtesy of Drs. Leonardo Rodriguez and Robert Levine.)

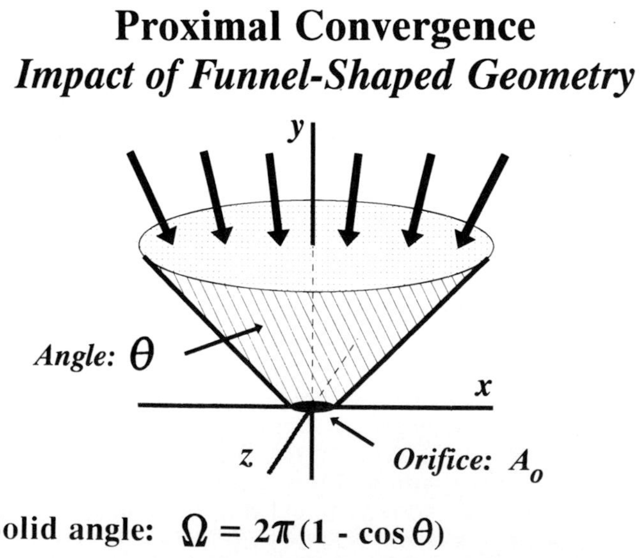

Fig. 12–30. Schematic representation of the impact of nonplanar geometry on the proximal acceleration field. For a funnel-shaped geometry with a central half angle of Θ, the usual constant of 2π must be reduced by $1 - \cos\Theta$.

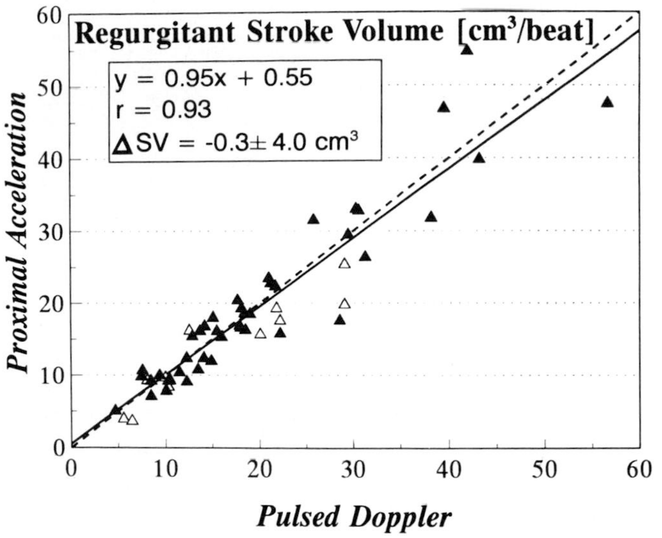

Fig. 12–32. Calculation of regurgitant stroke volume by proximal acceleration. In 53 patients with mitral regurgitation, regurgitant stroke volume (ΔSV) was calculated by the proximal acceleration method and showed excellent agreement with pulse Doppler methods. (From Rivera JM, et al.: Am Heart J 124:1289, 1992, with permission of Mosby Yearbook Publishers.)

mal convergence zone is obscured by an often calcific aortic valve. Recently, it has been reported that ventricular septal defect flow can be quantified by analysis of the proximal convergence zone on the ventricular side of the septum.[36]

It should also be recognized that there may be alternative regurgitant parameters obtainable by analysis of the proximal acceleration field that may be more clinically useful than peak flow rate or regurgitant volume. One such parameter is the effective regurgitant orifice area, a fundamental measure of valvular incompetence analogous in importance to the orifice area in the clinical follow-up of patients with valvular stenosis. Although previous methods have been described for obtaining regurgitant orifice area,[37] it is particularly easy with the proximal acceleration method. From a single color frame, peak regurgitant flow rate (Q_0) can be calculated. The peak orifice velocity (v_0) can then be measured by continuous wave Doppler, and the effective regurgitant orifice area (ROA) calculated as ROA $= Q_0/v_0$. If the assumption is made that the ROA is roughly constant throughout the regurgitant period, then regurgitant stroke volume may be obtained simply by multiplying ROA by the time velocity integral of the continuous wave Doppler signal. Calculation of the ROA in this way has recently been validated in vitro[38] and clinically.[39] In a group with mitral regurgitation, those with mild regurgitation by other criteria generally had an ROA less than 0.1 cm^2, while those with severe regurgitation had an ROA greater than 0.5 cm^2.

Future Developments in Proximal Convergence

Although the proximal convergence method has been validated theoretically and in clinical studies, its use would be more widespread if an automated method were available for calculating it.

One of the most difficult aspects of applying this method is determining the precise location of the regurgitant orifice. This is obviously of critical importance because it is the distance from this orifice to the isovelocity contour that generates the flow rate, and this value itself is squared, making any error in its measurement magnified when the flow rate is calculated. A recent approach to this problem has been described that uses the full velocity map from the proximal convergence zone.[40] In this approach, a small region is specified as likely to contain the regurgitant orifice. For each pixel within this zone, the velocity field surrounding it is analyzed to see how closely it correlates to the expected inverse squared decline in velocity magnitude from the orifice center. Because the velocity displayed is actually the velocity *component* parallel to the ultrasound beam, the anticipated velocity within the proximal convergence zone is

$$v \propto \frac{\cos \phi}{r^2} \qquad [12.10]$$

where r is the distance of a given pixel from the test orifice center and ϕ is the angle between the ultrasound beam and the anticipated blood flow convergence toward the orifice (Fig. 12–33).

The optimal orifice center is designated as the pixel that gives the highest correlation to the anticipated velocity dependence. Flow rate then is calculated as the slope of the line relating the observed velocity components to the cos ϕ/r^2 relationship:

$$Q = \frac{\sum_i v_i}{\sum_i \cos \phi / 2\pi r^2} \qquad [12.11]$$

As the orifice center is identified and the flow rate estimated, it is important to recognize that certain re-

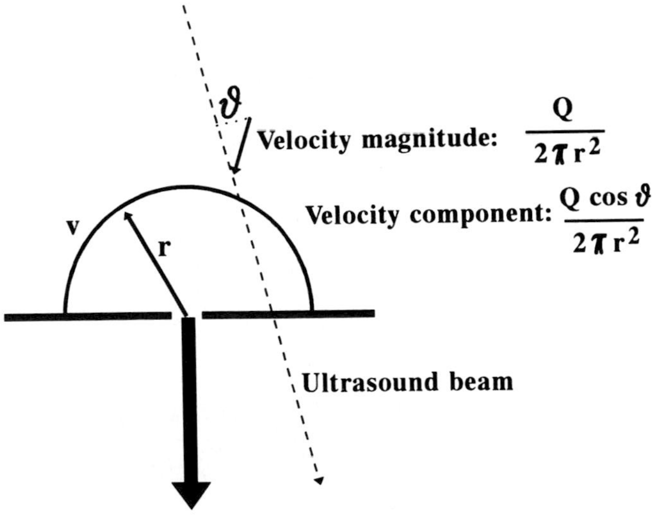

Fig. 12–33. Automated analysis of the proximal convergence zone. For flow converging toward a small orifice (large arrow), velocity magnitude (small arrow) is given by $Q/2\pi r^2$. The velocity component shown by color Doppler is given by the velocity magnitude multiplied by the cosine of the angle between the local velocity vector and the ultrasound beam (dashed line).

gions surrounding the orifice must be excluded in these calculations (Fig. 12–34). Points that are too close to the orifice would be expected to have a velocity high enough to be doubly (or more) aliased and thus would be unquantifiable. In addition, points that are too far away from the orifice will have very low velocities, which will be affected by the discretization error inherent in the color mapper with only 32 velocity bins. Finally, points that are located at too great an angle from the central axis of the ultrasound beam should be rejected because the velocity component parallel to the ultrasound beam will be too small to allow adequate quantification. When this method was applied to an in vitro study set, excellent determination of the regurgitant orifice was obtained, together with good estimation of the flow rate through the orifice (Fig. 12–35).[40]

A second automated approach to analysis of the proximal acceleration field also addresses the issue of integrating flow rate throughout the regurgitant period. This method uses the color M-mode from a single ultrasound vector directed through the regurgitant orifice.[41] With this approach, the isovelocity contour can be mapped throughout the regurgitant period and the regurgitant volume obtained from direct integration of these data. One potential problem with this method is that if the regurgitant orifice moves in and out of the plane of the ultrasound beam, there will be an artifactually low color M-mode estimation of the flow rate.

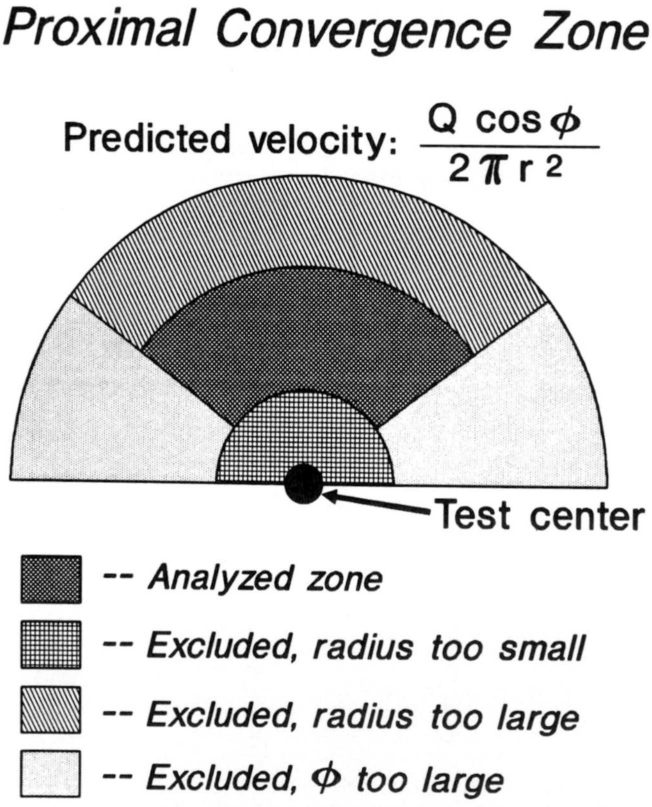

Fig. 12–34. Excluded zones from the proximal convergence analysis. (See text for details.) (From Thomas et al.: Computers in Cardiology. IEEE Computer Society Press, p. 14, 1991. With permission.)

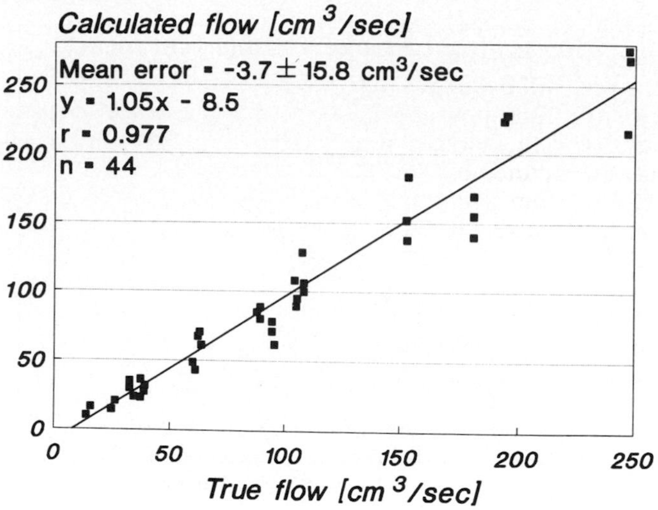

Fig. 12–35. Orifice flow rate calculated by automated analysis of proximal convergence zone. (From Thomas et al.: Computers in Cardiology. IEEE Computer Society Press, p. 15, 1991. With permission.)

Comparison of Quantitative Color Flow Methods for Assessing Valvular Regurgitation

Thus, there are two very different approaches to the quantification of valvular regurgitation using quantitative interpretation of color Doppler maps: application of conservation of mass within the proximal convergence zone and the use of conservation of momentum in the distal jet. These methods are not mutually exclusive, and in fact, complement each other in their application and limitations. Figure 12–36 demonstrates schematically how these methods are related. The momentum conservation method assumes that the momentum that is injected at the orifice level remains constant through-

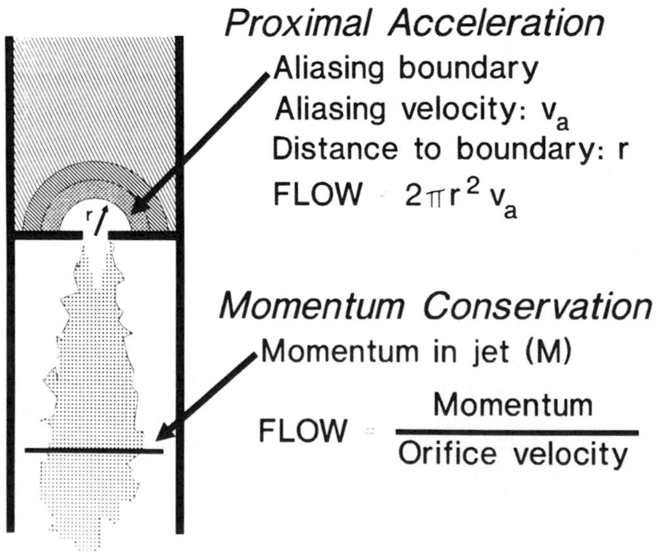

Fig. 12–36. Schematic comparison of proximal acceleration analysis with momentum analysis. Momentum quantification is best suited for low velocity or low flow jets, while quantification of flow by proximal acceleration is best suited for high flow jets.

out the free jet. Thus, if momentum can be quantified at any point within the regurgitant jet, then the regurgitant flow rate will be given by dividing momentum by orifice velocity. This method obviously depends critically on the ability to quantify momentum within the free jet. To do this, unambiguous velocities must be obtainable. Because from usual imaging depths, aliasing occurs at less than 1 m/sec, this method would appear to be limited to either very small left-sided regurgitant lesions or relatively low pressure right-sided regurgitant lesions. There are relatively new color Doppler processing algorithms (Quasar technology) that attempt to extend the Nyquist limit of color Doppler displays by effectively interrogating the jet with two ultrasonic frequencies simultaneously and analyzing the difference of their phase shift. Although this method is theoretically sound and appears to work in laminar flow fields,[42] there are great difficulties in applying it to the sort of turbulent velocity fields obtained in regurgitant jets.

In contrast, proximal acceleration method appears to work best in situations of relatively high flow. This is because accuracy is improved when calculations are based on isovelocity contours at a distance far enough from the orifice to allow proper measurement of the radius. Thus, momentum analysis may be most applicable to right-sided regurgitation and low flow, left-sided regurgitation, whereas proximal convergence may be most applicable to high flow regurgitation. This complementarity means that both methods may have important application in diagnosis.

REFERENCES

1. Omoto R, et al.: The development of real-time two-dimensional Doppler echocardiography and its clinical significance in acquired valvular diseases: with special references to the evaluation of valvular regurgitation. Jpn Heart J 25:325, 1984.
2. Miyatake K, et al.: Semiquantitative grading of severity of mitral regurgitation by real-time two-dimensional Doppler flow imaging technique. J Am Coll Cardiol 7:82, 1986.
3. Helmcke F, et al.: Color Doppler assessment of mitral regurgitation with orthogonal planes. Circulation 75:175, 1987.
4. Perry GJ, et al.: Evaluation of aortic insufficiency by Doppler color flow mapping. J Am Coll Cardiol 9:952, 1987.
5. Suzuki Y, et al.: The detection and evaluation of tricuspid regurgitation using a real-time two-dimensional color-coded, Doppler flow imaging system: comparison with contrast two-dimensional echocardiography and right ventriculography. Am J Cardiol 57:811, 1986.
6. Czer SCL, et al.: Intraoperative evaluation of mitral regurgitation by Doppler color flow mapping. Circulation 76:108, 1987.
7. Otsuji Y, et al.: Color Doppler echocardiographic assessment of the change in the mitral regurgitant volume. Am Heart J 114:349, 1987.
8. Maurer G, et al.: Intraoperative Doppler color flow mapping for assessment of valve repair for mitral regurgitation. Am J Cardiol 60:333, 1987.
9. Abramovich GN: The Theory of Turbulent Jets. Cambridge, MA, MIT Press, 1963.
10. Schlichting H: Boundary Layer Theory. 7th Ed. New York, McGraw-Hill, 1979.
11. Belvins RD: Applied Fluid Dynamics Handbook. New York, Van Nostrand Reinhold, p. 229, 1984.
12. Pai S-I: Fluid Dynamics of Jets. New York, McGraw-Hill, 1979.
13. Howarth L: Concerning the velocity and temperature distributions in plane and axially symmetrical jets. Proc Cambr Phil Soc 34:185, 1938.
14. Wygnanski I, Fiedler H: Some measurements in the self-preserving jet. J Fluid Mech 38:577, 1969.
15. Krabill KA, et al.: The shape of regurgitant jets: in vitro flow visualization and color flow Doppler studies. J Am Coll Cardiol 9:110A, 1987.
16. Thomas JD, Popovic AD, McGlew S: How turbulent is a turbulent jet? An in vitro color flow Doppler study. J Am Coll Cardiol 13:22A, 1989.
17. Thomas JD, et al.: The volume of a color flow jet varies directly with flow rate and inversely with orifice size: a hydrodynamic in vitro assessment. J Am Coll Cardiol 11:19A, 1988.
18. Newman BG: The deflection of plane jets by adjacent boundaries—Coanda effect. *In* Lachmann GV (ed.): Boundary Layer Control Principles and Application. New York, Pergamon Press, 1961.
19. Thomas JD, O'Shea JP, Rodriguez L: The impact of orifice geometry on the shape of jets: An in vitro color Doppler flow study. J Am Coll Cardiol 17:901, 1991.
20. Goldman ME: Real-time two-dimensional Doppler flow imaging: a word of caution. J Am Coll Cardiol 7:89, 1986.
21. Wong M, Matsumura M, Suzuki K, Omoto R: Technical and biologic sources of variability in the mapping of aortic, mitral and tricuspid color flow jets. Am J Cardiol 60:847, 1987.
22. Pratt WK: Digital Image Processing. New York, John Wiley & Sons, p. 591, 1978.
23. Lobadzinski SM, Ginzton LE, Laus MM: Quantitation of color Doppler images with the color image processor. J Am Coll Cardiol 11:99A, 1988.
24. Switzer DF, et al.: Calibration of color Doppler flow mapping during extreme hemodynamic conditions in vitro: a foundation for a reliable quantitative grading system for aortic incompetence. Circulation 75:837, 1987.
25. Simpson IA, et al.: Color Doppler flow mapping of simulated in vitro regurgitant jets: evaluation of the effects of orifice size and hemodynamic variables. J Am Coll Cardiol 13:1195, 1989.
26. Davidoff R, et al.: Regurgitant volumes by color flow over estimate injected volumes in an in vitro model. J Am Coll Cardiol 9:110A, 1987.
27. Thomas JD, O'Shea JP, Weyman AE: Quantification of jet flow by momentum analysis: an in vitro color Doppler study. Circulation 81:247, 1990.
28. Recusani F, et al.: A new method for quantification of regurgitant flow rate using color Doppler flow imaging of the flow convergence region proximal to a discrete orifice: an in vitro study. Circulation 83:594, 1991.
29. Utsonomiya T, et al.: Doppler color flow "proximal isovelocity surface area" method for estimating volume flow rate: effect of orifice shape and machine factors. J Am Coll Cardiol 17:1103, 1991.
30. Tritton DJ: Physical Fluid Dynamics. Clarendon Press, Oxford, 1988, p. 48.
31. Anderson DA, Tannehill JC, Pletcher RH: Computational Fluid Mechanics and Heat Transfer. New York, Hemisphere Publishing Corporation, p. 329, 1984.
32. Rodriguez L, et al.: Impact of finite orifice size on proximal flow convergence: Implications for Doppler quantification of valvular regurgitation. Circ Res 70:923, 1992.
33. Rivera JM, et al.: Quantification of tricuspid regurgitation using proximal flow convergence method: Clinical validation (abstr). J Am Soc Echocardiogr 5:318, 1992.
34. Bargiggia GS, et al.: A new method for quantitation of mitral regurgitation based on color flow Doppler imaging of flow convergence proximal to regurgitant orifice. Circulation 84:1481, 1991.
35. Rivera JM, et al.: Quantification of mitral regurgitation using the proximal flow convergence method: a clinical study. Am Heart J 124:1289, 1992.
36. Moises VA, et al.: A new method for non-invasive estimation of ventricular septal defect shunt flow by Doppler color flow mapping: imaging of the laminar convergence region on the left septal surface. J Am Coll Cardiol 18:824, 1991.
37. Reimold SC, et al.: Effective aortic regurgitant orifice area: description of a method based on the conservation of mass. J Am Coll Cardiol 18:761, 1991.
38. Vandervoort PM, et al.: Application of color Doppler flow imaging to calculate effective regurgitant orifice area: an assessment of valvular incompetence independent of hemodynamics (abstr). J Am Coll Cardiol 19:297A, 1992.
39. Rivera JM, et al.: Regurgitant orifice area, a fundamental measure of mitral incompetence: calculation by proximal acceleration (abstr). J Am Coll Cardiol 19:379A, 1992.
40. Thomas JD, et al.: Automated analysis of flow convergence proximal to regurgitant orifices: flow rate calculation using digital Doppler velocity maps. *In*: Computers in Cardiology 1991. Long Beach, CA, IEEE Computer Society, p. 13, 1991.
41. Zhang J, et al.: Flow convergence estimates of mitral regurgitation obtained by using the first, second, and third alias zones observed on color Doppler MQ traces in sheep with surgically produced mitral regurgitation (abstr). Circulation (Suppl)84:II-104, 1991.
42. Vandervoort P, et al.: High-velocity color Doppler flow mapping: validation in a stenotic model (abstr). J Am Soc Echocardiogr 4:296, 1991.

CHAPTER

13

THE ROUTINE DOPPLER EXAMINATION

The Doppler examination differs both conceptually and technically from an imaging study. In imaging echocardiography, the operator seeks to direct the sound beam in such a manner that the specular reflectors of interest lie perpendicular to its path. This orientation causes the reflected signals to have the highest amplitude and selected targets to be most clearly recorded. These reflective characteristics occur because sound waves striking specular reflectors obey the laws of geometric optics and the greatest amplitude of reflection occurs when the reflector is perpendicular to the path of the sound beam.[1,2]

In Doppler studies, different factors must be considered. First, the Doppler signals arise from groups of red blood cells that scatter rather than reflect the incident sound energy. Because scattering is omnidirectional, scatterer shape and orientation have little effect on the amplitude of the reflected signal, and the direction at which the sound beam intersects a volume of red cells, therefore, is of lesser importance in terms of signal amplitude.[3–5] Second, Doppler frequency shifts are maximal when the sound beam is parallel to the flow vector (i.e., aligned parallel to the path of blood flow in the vessel of interest), and cos Θ in the Doppler equation equals zero. The Doppler beam, therefore, is ideally aligned parallel, rather than perpendicular, to flow because larger frequency shifts are easier to detect and the output is less subject to random fluctuation. Third, detection of the Doppler frequency shift is critically dependent on the signal/noise ratio, and every effort must be made to maximize this relationship. This can often be achieved by decreasing range and avoiding passage of the sound beam through highly attenuating structures, such as prosthetic valves. Finally, it is desirable for the sample volume to encompass as much of the region of blood flow as possible, while avoiding surrounding nonmoving structures.[6–8]

Because blood flow through vessels and valves is typically parallel to the vessel walls or valve leaflets, flow, as a rule, will be best recorded using a beam direction that is orthogonal to that required to image the structure through which it is traveling. For example, flow through the aorta is best recorded from an apical or suprasternal transducer location, and the walls of the artery are best visualized from a parasternal window. This conflict between the optimal beam direction for flow recording and structure visualization, like that previously discussed between axial and velocity resolution, is a fundamental physical characteristic that must always be kept in mind. It is particularly important to remember the Doppler aspect of these obligate trade-offs because flow cannot be seen but becomes manifest only after it has been recorded and output by the instrument. The operator, therefore, must be continually aware of the expected direction of the blood flow he is seeking to record in order to obtain the best possible data.

In color flow studies, where both structure and flow are recorded together, it becomes even more important to remember these basic principles as there is a natural tendency to optimize structural recording first and then add flow data. This frequently gives a false sense of the adequacy of flow recording, because the ideal view for recording a structure will frequently not display the flow in that structure optimally. Thus, despite the fact that structure and flow are always present simultaneously in color flow studies, it is still often necessary to analyze structure in one projection and flow in another.[9]

INSTRUMENT CONTROLS

Most instruments provide several controls and visual aids to facilitate the performance of the Doppler examination. These controls allow selection of the direction and location of Doppler sampling and optimization of the reflected signal. Although the specific form and operation of individual controls varies from instrument to instrument, they are sufficiently generic to permit their function to be extrapolated from one instrument to another.

The Doppler Cursor

Most combined Doppler/imaging instruments provide a cursor line, which can be superimposed on the image to indicate the "line of sight" along which Doppler signals are being recorded (Fig. 13–1). The position of the cursor line is generally under operator control; changes in its position result in corresponding changes in the path along which Doppler sampling occurs.[10] In mechanical systems, the cursor indicates the direction in which the transducer will be pointed when it is stopped to record Doppler data, whereas in phased array systems, the cursor indicates the direction from which the echoes that are used to derive the Doppler data are obtained.

The Sample Volume Locator

The position of the sample volume is usually indicated on the monitor by a small marker on the cursor line at a point corresponding to the sample volume depth (Fig. 13–1). In pulsed mode, the position of the sample volume can be shifted axially along the cursor by altering the time delay between pulse transmission and signal sampling. In combined M-mode and Doppler studies, the sample volume depth is indicated by a line superimposed on the M-mode recording (Fig. 13–2).

Sample Volume Length

In addition to varying sample volume position, it is also generally possible to vary sample volume length.

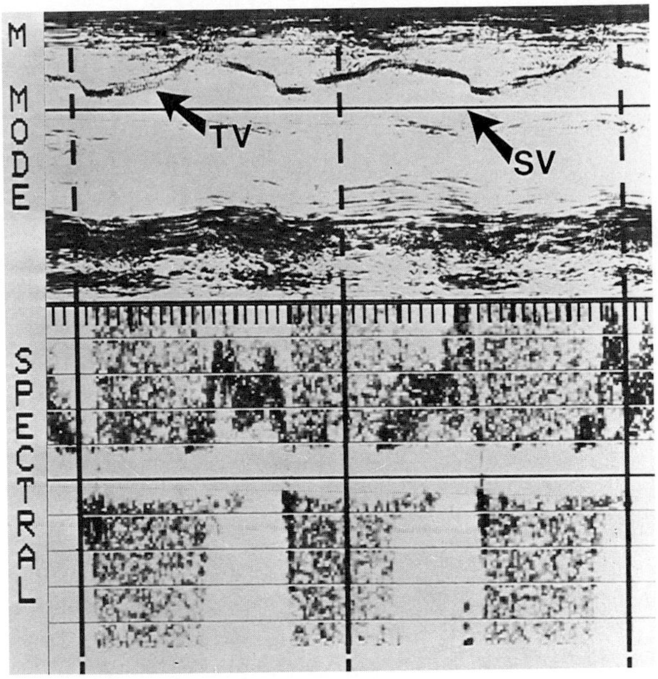

Fig. 13–2. Combined pulsed Doppler and M-mode recording. Top. The Doppler sample volume (SV) represented by the horizontal black line is positioned behind the tricuspid valve (TV). Bottom. Doppler spectral output depicts a normal m-shaped tricuspid inflow velocity profile during diastole, with turbulent, retrograde flow during systole indicative of tricuspid regurgitation.

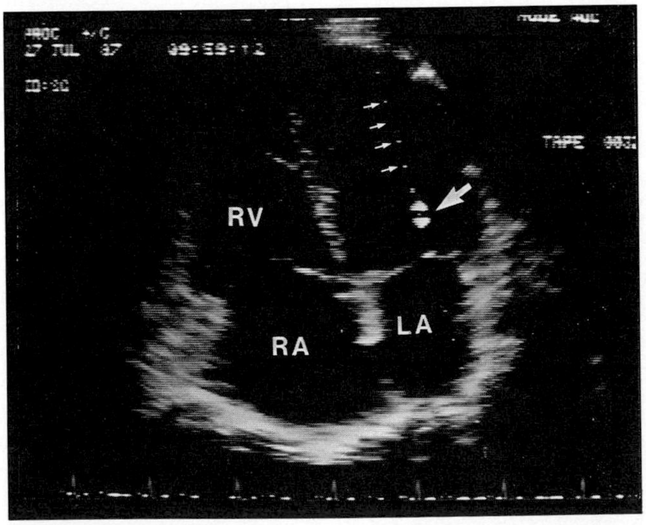

Fig. 13–1. Doppler cursor (small, right-pointing arrows) and sample volume locator (large, left-pointing arrow).

This is achieved by increasing pulse duration and is indicated on the monitor by expansion or contraction of the sample volume marker on the Doppler cursor.

Angle Correction

Many instruments also provide a second smaller cursor that originates from the primary Doppler cursor line at the level of the sample volume and can be rotated to place it parallel to the expected path of flow through an area of interest (Fig. 13–3). When activated, the instrument automatically calculates the angle between the two cursors and corrects the recorded velocity for the angular difference. Angle correction may be useful when technical constraints prevent the Doppler signals from being recorded in an orientation parallel to the flow vector. Unfortunately, the position of the second cursor is based on the expected path of flow though a particular area as assessed from the image. Because the actual direction of flow may not conform to that suggested by the image, particularly when dealing with stenotic lesions, angle correction introduces a major potential source of error, which increases as the angle between the direction of Doppler sampling and the presumed direction of flow increases. As a result, angle correction has become less popular and instead every effort is made to align the beam as parallel to the flow vector as possible.

Doppler Gain

The Doppler gain is similar to the gain control of any other echo instrument and determines the degree of am-

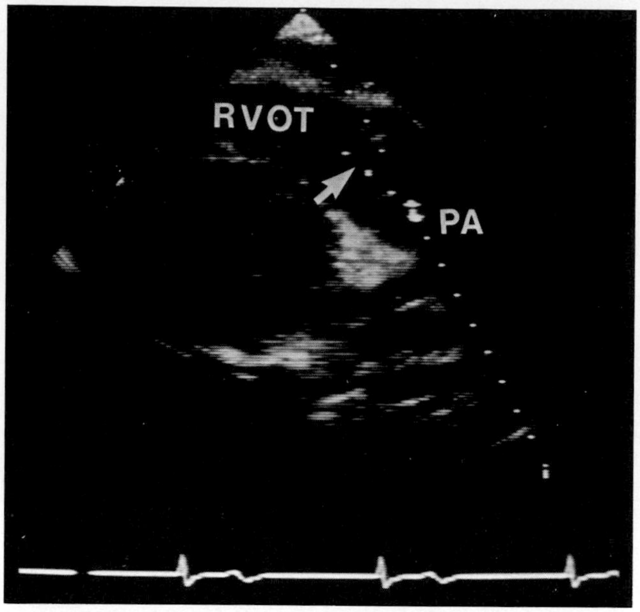

Fig. 13–3. Angle correction. A second cursor (arrow) arising from the sample volume indicator is positioned parallel to the presumed direction of flow in the pulmonary artery (PA). The instrument automatically corrects the recorded flow velocity for the cosine of the measured angle between the cursors. RVOT = right ventricular outflow tract.

plification of the returning signal before its entrance into the demodulator. Ideally, as in imaging studies, one begins with a high gain setting to be sure that all of the signal present is appreciated. The gain is then gradually decreased to a point where the signal is optimally displayed and the associated noise and mirroring artifacts (see following discussion) are at a minimum. Figure 13–4 illustrates the effect of increasing gain on the Doppler display. The effects of gain on a color flow image were discussed in Chapters 11 and 12.

Wall Filter

The wall filter is a high pass filter found on all Doppler instruments and is designed to eliminate low frequency signals from slowly moving structures, such as vessel walls and myocardium. Wall filters generally have selectable settings in the 200- to 800-Hz frequency range, with a setting of 400 Hz being most commonly used in our laboratory. Some degree of high pass filtering is usually necessary in all Doppler studies; however, the process also removes the signal from slowly moving blood and affects mean and peak frequency estimations. Likewise, when the wall filter is set too high, it will remove all signals on both sides of the baseline and thereby prevent display of the onset and termination of the flow signal. Figure 13–5 illustrates the effect of varying degrees of high pass filtering on the Doppler output.

Spectral Averaging

Many instruments have controls that permit two or more consecutive spectra to be averaged before output. The averaging process is based on the assumption that noise is random and, therefore, will cancel over time, whereas signal is constant and will sum. Averaging also is felt to eliminate some of the statistic variability in signal strength caused by random fluctuation scattering. The problem with averaging in physiologic systems is that the signal is not constant, and often significant variability is appropriate. Averaging also tends to blur the output signal and makes recognition of the individual spectral components more difficult. As a result, we prefer not to use signal averaging even when it is available.

Logarithmic Compression of Doppler Signals

Another form of postprocessing available in some Doppler instruments is logarithmic signal compression. Such compression schemes permit expansion of selected portions of the dynamic range of the signal while compressing others. This makes it possible, e.g., to emphasize high frequency, low amplitude signals while suppressing lower frequency signals of lesser interest. Figure 13–6 is an example of one such logarithmic compression scheme. Almost an infinite number of possible variations on this general theme are possible; however, as with most postprocessing algorithms, their theo-

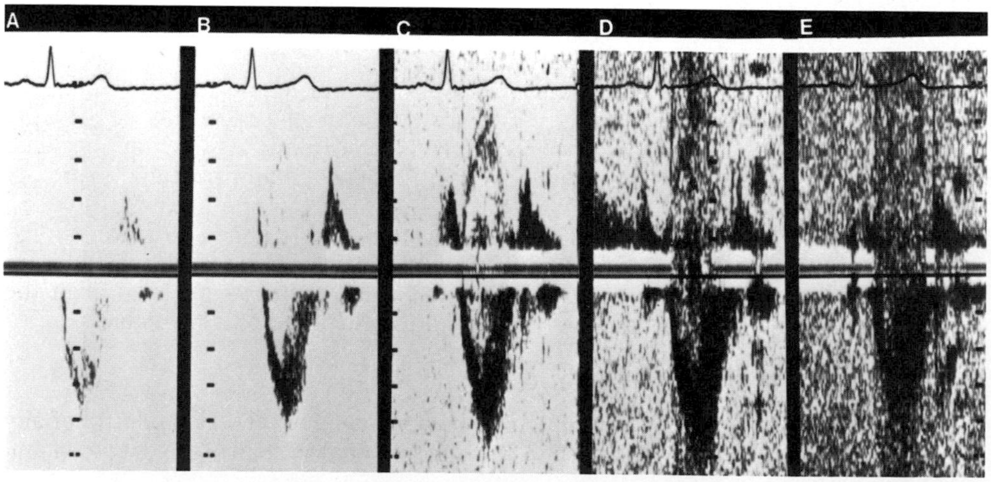

Fig. 13–4. Effects of increasing gain on the Doppler display. **A.** Low gain with loss of signal. **B.** Appropriate gain level. **C.** Slight oversaturation of the amplifiers with mirroring present. **D** and **E.** Excessive gain with inappropriate background noise and mirroring artifacts.

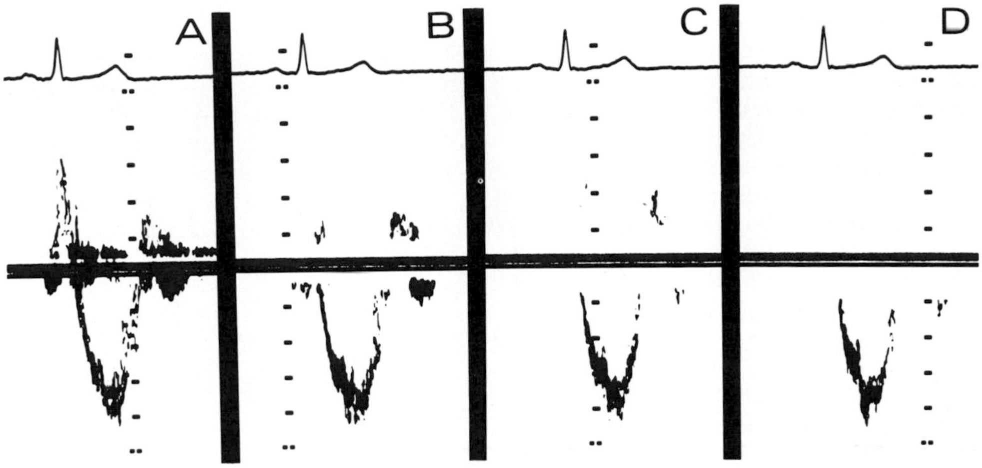

Fig. 13–5. Effects of increasing wall filter settings on the Doppler output. **A.** 200 Hz. **B.** 400 Hz. **C.** 600 Hz. **D.** 800 Hz. In this example the 200-Hz filter passes the most signal; the 400-Hz filter eliminates baseline noise while retaining the majority of the flow signal. Above 400 Hz, portions of the flow signals are lost along with the noise component.

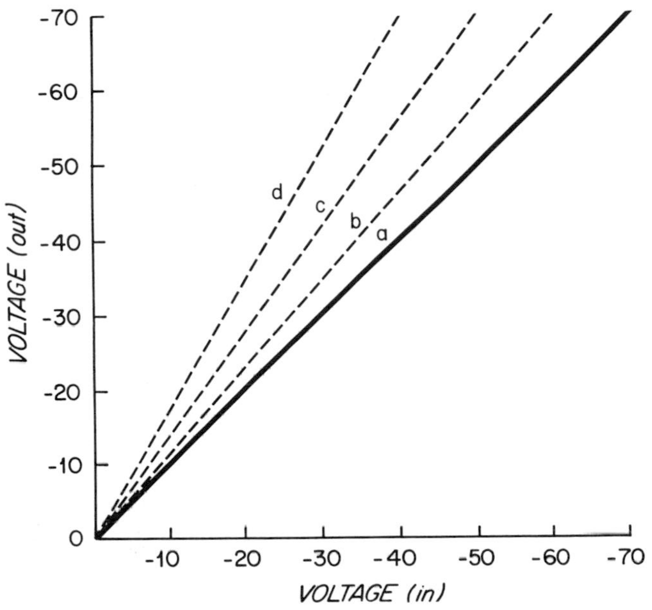

Fig. 13–6. Varying postprocessing curves for Doppler input signals. Voltage (in decibels) is output in a linear fashion in curve a. Curves b to d selectively eliminate low amplitude input signals. Higher amplitude signals are displayed with the full dynamic range.

retic potential is typically more exciting than any real data enhancement.

CHOICE OF ECHOCARDIOGRAPHIC WINDOWS FOR DOPPLER STUDIES

Doppler studies must make use of the same echocardiographic windows available for imaging studies because these areas of access to the heart are anatomically defined. The requirement that beam alignment be as parallel to flow as possible, however, suggests that the majority of the Doppler information will not come from the same windows that provide the major portion of the imaging data. The primary requirements for optimal Doppler signal recording are probably best achieved by recording from the apical window: alignment of the beam parallel to the flow stream, avoidance of intervening structures likely to cause a high degree of signal attenuation, and placement of the sample volume such that it includes as much of the flow stream as possible while avoiding surrounding non-flow-containing structures. The apical window is particularly useful because aortic, mitral, and tricuspid inflow and regurgitation are ideally recorded from this location. The apical window also permits the sample volume to be scanned along the interatrial and interventricular septae to detect or exclude most atrial and ventricular septal defects.

The parasternal window, from which the majority of imaging data is obtained, in contrast, places the ultrasonic beam perpendicular to flow through the aortic, mitral, and tricuspid orifices, and as a result, is less well suited for Doppler studies. It is, however, an appropriate location for studying the pulmonary artery, which courses almost directly away from the anterior chest wall with the result that flow in this vessel is directly away from a transducer positioned in a parasternal location. The parasternal window is also useful for confirming the presence of tricuspid, mitral, and aortic regurgitation. Although the primary flow vector in these lesions is perpendicular to the path of a sound beam originating from the parasternal window, there is typically sufficient turbulence in these regurgitant jets to direct components of the vector anteriorly and posteriorly, i.e., parallel to the orientation of the sound beam.

The same constraints also apply to color flow studies in which many of the imaging components are ideally recorded from the parasternal windows, but the major components of flow are perpendicular to the direction of propagation of the scan plane from this location. Only when turbulence is present to highlight specific flow areas are they generally well recorded from the parasternal window. The need in this format to combine imaging and flow data, therefore, often results in some compromise, e.g., the use of a low parasternal window in an attempt to obtain flow data while retaining image quality.

The suprasternal notch was originally believed to be the ideal Doppler window because it placed the transducer in direct contact with the anterior aortic wall in the midportion of the arch and permitted alignment of the beam parallel to flow in both the ascending and descending thoracic aorta. As applications have progressed, however, this transducer location has gradually receded in importance. Although a high degree of sensitivity (signal-to-noise) should be achieved from this location, other factors, e.g., the variation in the flow profile in the arch and difficulty in measuring vessel diameter at this location, have limited the applicability of the suprasternal window in volumetric flow studies. The flow jets of aortic stenosis, likewise, are rarely directed toward the suprasternal notch, and here again it provides the opportunity for confirmation rather than primary data. The areas where the suprasternal window is of unique value are the examination of the descending aorta in patients with suspected coarctation and in patent ductus arteriosus where aortic backflow into the ductus may be observed. Other studies have suggested that the ratio of forward to reverse flow in the descending thoracic aorta may provide quantitative information concerning the severity of aortic regurgitation; however, the true quantitative value of such measurements remains in question. (See Chapter 19.) Finally, this is the best window to record the abnormal flow patterns associated with arch dissection and, with the addition of color flow mapping, this application is gaining increasing importance.

The right parasternal window, which is of minimal use in imaging studies, is of particular value in the Doppler examination. This transducer location permits the operator to direct the sound beam parallel to most aortic jets from close range. When there is a difference in velocity noted between the apex, suprasternal notch, and right parasternal window, the latter generally gives the highest value and, in case of discrepancy, it is this peak velocity that should be the number of greatest interest.

Subcostal windows are of lesser importance in Doppler studies than in imaging, but in specific cases, such as atrial septal defect and the evaluation of caval flow, they often are valuable. In some cases, the subcostal location also permits better recording of the signal in the right ventricular outflow tract and pulmonary artery than does the parasternal window. But again, this is the exception and is primarily noted in small children in whom the outflow tract, pulmonary valve, and pulmonary artery are relatively close to the transducer.

USE OF THE FLOW SIGNALS AS THE PRIMARY METHOD FOR DIRECTING THE DOPPLER BEAM

Because most Doppler studies are performed in conjunction with imaging studies, there is a natural tendency to align the Doppler beam parallel to the path one would assume flow would take based on the image. Experience suggests, however, that the best flow signal frequently does not arise from the location suggested by the image. Because the pattern of flow cannot be seen, except by color flow mapping techniques, in the absence of such technology, it must be determined from the quality and amplitude of the Doppler signal itself. In laminar flow states, the appropriate signal has a narrow bandwidth with the peak and mean frequency components lying close together and the greatest signal power (modal velocity) indicated by the peak intensity of the spectral display (Fig. 13–7). Nonlaminar flow through regurgitant and stenotic lesions will virtually always contain some degree of turbulence and, hence, the velocity profile will be broader. Despite the presence of turbulence, organized flow elements virtually always remain and their Doppler shifts can be recorded. The location and orientation of these high velocity components, however, are not uniformly predictable from the image and, in the absence of direct flow mapping, can be defined only by patiently searching the area of interest until the strongest, highest velocity signal is recorded. In the study of stenotic lesions, however, the imaging data are helpful because the appearance of the valve often indicates the degree of severity one might expect and provides some indication of the amount of time that should be spent trying to document a high velocity jet.

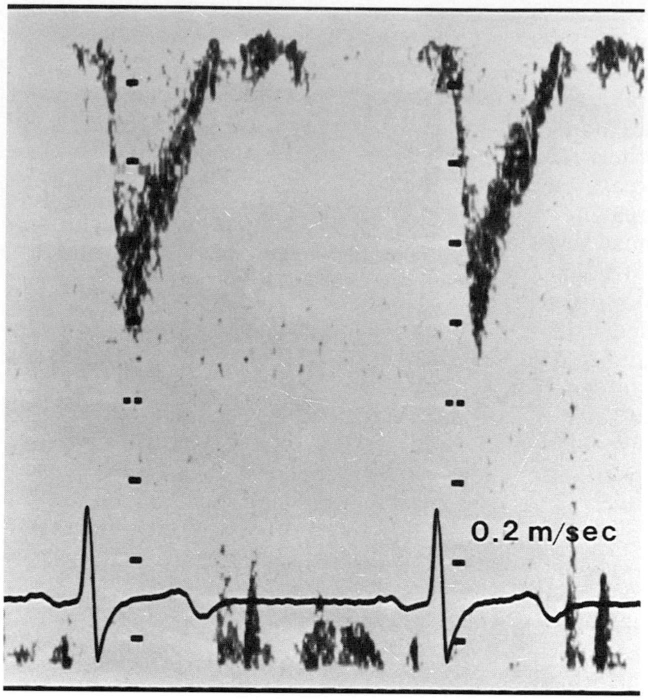

Fig. 13–7. Laminar flow characterized by a narrow bandwidth signal in which the peak and mean frequency components lie close together.

THE ROUTINE EXAMINATION

Although the Doppler examination differs in concept from the imaging examination, both should be performed with the same attention to order and consistency. In this section, we review the most efficient and complete approach to the routine Doppler study. This approach assumes that the Doppler examination is performed together with, but following, a two-dimensional imaging study. It is also possible to integrate these studies, and such an integrated approach is outlined at the end of this chapter. Integration does save some time. Unfortunately, the most efficient pattern of integration from a technical standpoint does not always result in data being presented in the most logical sequence for assimilation and interpretation. Therefore, although the imaging study builds logically from one view to the next, an integrated imaging/Doppler study requires that the operator assemble bits of information gathered at separate points in time and frequently not in the most logical order. As the length of all echocardiographic studies increases, however, the constraints of time become of increasing importance, and the interpretative process must adapt.

In discussing a routine examination, it is important to remember that *routine* does not equate with *normal*. Because flow lesions are not visible, they generally cannot be detected without actually performing the Doppler study and hence normality can be determined only after the fact. Likewise, the tendency to focus on areas of suspected high yield or to direct the study to answer specific questions, will result in lesions being missed, which are unsuspected by the observer or the requesting physician. Finally, only by routinely performing a complete examination will the operator gain sufficient experience with the multiple variations of normal to recognize unexpected patterns when they are encountered. It is therefore important that the routine examination be performed in all patients in whom the Doppler study is undertaken.

When Is a Routine Doppler Study Warranted?

Before discussing the routine Doppler examination itself, it is reasonable to ask in whom such an examination should be performed. Experience in our laboratory suggests that roughly 65% of patients referred for a routine echocardiographic examination will have new diagnostic information provided by the addition of a Doppler study. *New information* in this case is defined as detection of a previously unsuspected lesion, exclusion of a lesion thought to be present, or the determination of a transvalvular gradient. In patients with structurally normal hearts on their imaging studies, however, only 16% will have new diagnostic information provided by the addition of a Doppler study.[11] The yield in such patients, therefore, is low. As a result, a reasonable approach would be to perform a routine Doppler examination in all patients with obvious structural abnormality by imaging, while studying only patients with structurally normal hearts when a specific question has been asked that requires a Doppler examination for confirmation or exclusion.

DOPPLER EXAMINATION—APICAL WINDOW

Mitral Valve

A routine Doppler examination begins at the cardiac apex. The apical window generally provides excellent access to the heart, and from this location, the sound beam is parallel to most of the primary flow streams within the heart and great vessels. The study is normally begun by directing the sound beam superiorly toward the right clavicle with gradual angulation and rotation until the typical M-shaped pattern of mitral inflow is recorded. If a combined two-dimensional echo Doppler system is used, the scan plane is positioned to record an apical four-chamber view, and the Doppler cursor is directed through the center of the mitral valve orifice. The initial portion of the study is generally performed in the pulsed Doppler mode, with the sample volume placed on the left ventricular side of the mitral annulus to record mitral inflow velocity. Because some narrowing of the flow stream occurs at the mitral orifice, a

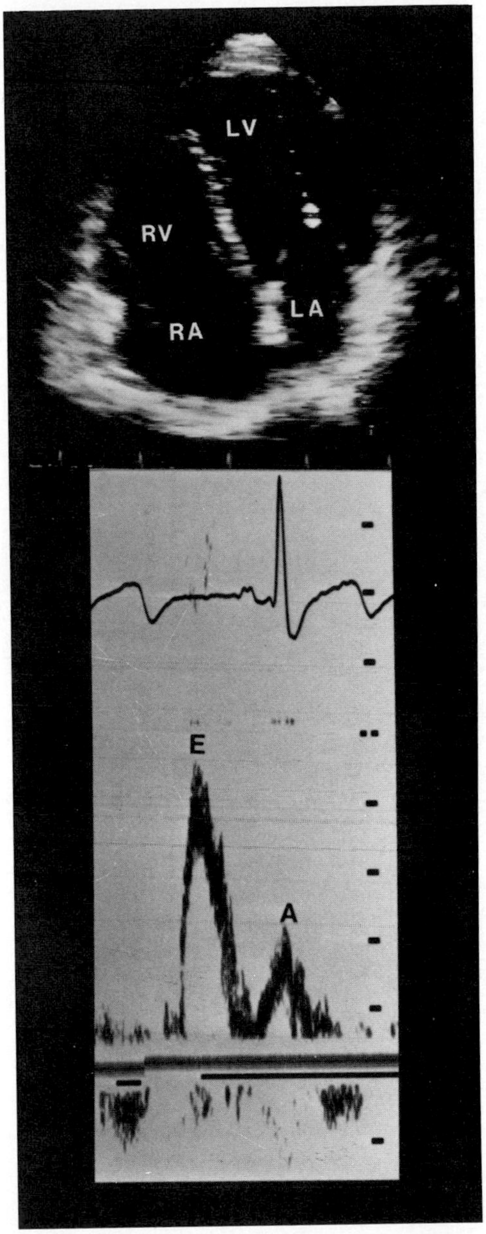

Fig. 13–8. Example of normal mitral inflow pattern recorded from the cardiac apex. Top. The sample volume positioned within the left ventricle near the free edges of the mitral leaflets. LA = left atrium; LV = left ventricle; RA = right atrium; RV = right ventricle. Bottom. Shows the normal pattern of mitral inflow velocities. Mitral flow begins with mitral valve opening at the onset of diastole and rapidly accelerates to a peak velocity at point E. Flow then decelerates as the transvalvular pressure gradient falls off during the period of diastasis. This is followed by a second increase in velocity following atrial contraction, which peaks at the A wave and then decreases in parallel with the atrioventricular gradient, terminating at the onset of ventricular systole with mitral valve closure.

slight degree of flow contraction is present, and the peak velocity normally will be found on the ventricular side of the valve, just beyond the annulus. Because, as noted previously, peak velocity does not always occur where one might predict from the image, it is useful to scan the inflow region by initially placing the sample volume in the center of the mitral annulus and gradually moving it outward in an expanding radial sweep. The sample volume can then be advanced in fixed increments toward the apex and the same process continued until the highest flow velocity with the narrowest spectral distribution is identified. If color flow mapping is available, this process can be simplified by locating the region of maximal inflow velocity on the color image and then using this information to direct the Doppler cursor. Figure 13–8 is an example of the normal M-shaped mitral flow pattern

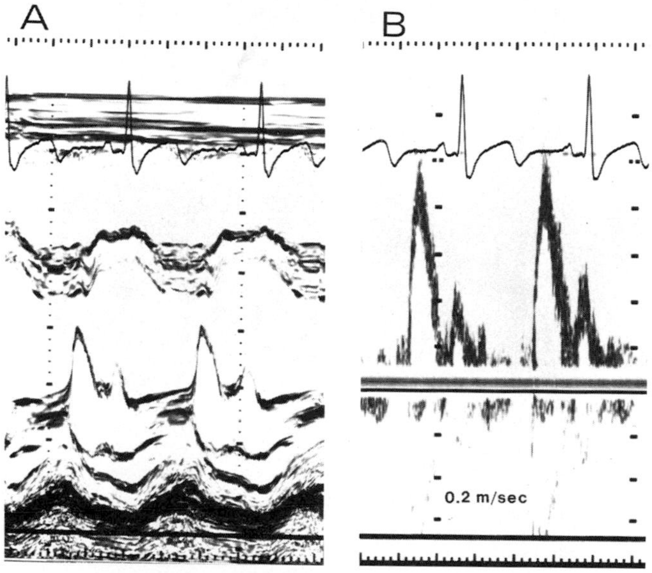

Fig. 13–9. Comparison of M-mode mitral leaflet motion with Doppler transvalvular flow patterns. **A.** Normal M-mode recording of mitral leaflet motion during systole and diastole. **B.** The corresponding Doppler velocity profile. Although in this case, the two profiles appear similar, this is often not the case, and important differences in leaflet motion and transvalvular velocity may frequently be noted.

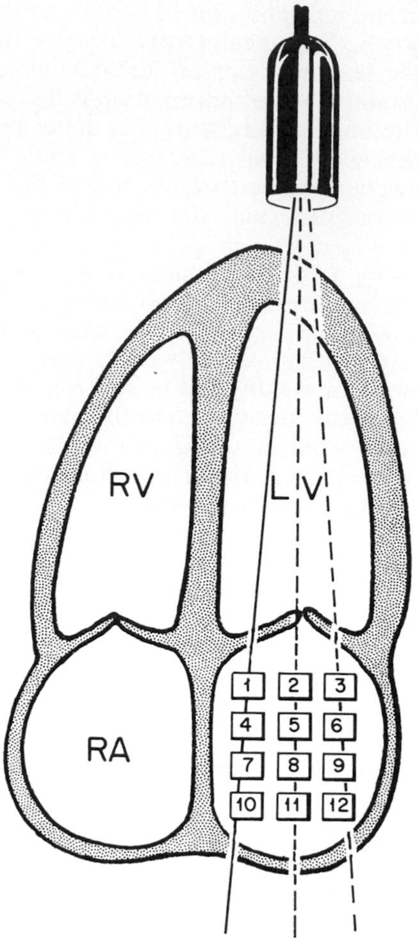

Fig. 13–11. A mapping sequence that may be used to define both the location and distribution of regurgitant flow in the left atrium using a pulsed Doppler system. LV = left ventricle; RA = right atrium; RV = right ventricle.

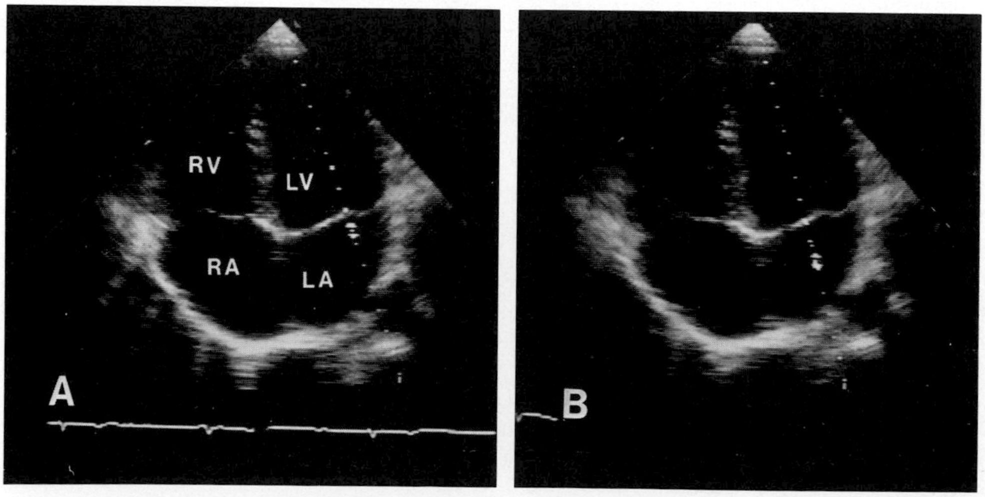

Fig. 13–10. **A.** Pulsed Doppler mapping of regurgitant flow in the left atrium (LA). The sample volume is positioned immediately behind the mitral leaflets to search for evidence of mitral regurgitation. LV = left ventricle; RA = right atrium; RV = right ventricle. **B.** If regurgitation is present, its spatial distribution can be mapped by tracking the abnormal flow pattern in the left atrium.

recorded from the cardiac apex. In this example, mitral flow begins immediately following valve opening, accelerates to a maximum (E point) during the rapid, passive phase of diastolic filling, decelerates following the nadir of the left ventricular pressure curve as the left atrial to left ventricular pressure gradient falls and stabilizes at a low flow rate in most patients during diastasis. With atrial contraction, a pressure gradient is reestablished between the left atrium and left ventricle and the flow velocity increases in response to this gradient, reaching its peak coincident with the peak of the transvalvular gradient and then decelerates before ventricular systole. The mitral flow pattern shows typical abnormalities in mitral stenosis, as will be discussed in Chapter 17 and bears a complex relationship to left ventricular diastolic function (see Chapter 24). Because the velocity profile bears a similarity to the pattern of leaflet motion on the M-mode echocardiogram, it is often questioned whether or not these two values are interchangeable. The two patterns, however, provide significantly different information because the M-mode study relates leaflet motion to the anterior chest wall, while the Doppler study examines the pattern of flow velocities across the valve throughout diastole. Thus, despite their apparent similarities, comparison of these two measurements in a large number of patients often reveals significant differences (Fig. 13–9).

Once the mitral inflow pattern is recorded, the sample volume is next positioned behind the valve, looking for mitral regurgitation. In most cases, regurgitant jets will be found near the center of the coaptation line; however, because important regurgitation can occur at any point along the line of valve closure, it is necessary to scan along the entire coaptation line, particularly when there is primary disease of the valve. When a regurgitant jet is located (Fig. 13–10), its distribution within the atrium can be mapped, using the pulsed Doppler technique (Fig. 13–11) or visualized directly with a color flow mapper (Fig. 13–12). When color flow mapping is available, this approach is clearly preferable because it is less time-consuming and provides a better appreciation of the spatial distribution of the velocity information.

In diagnosing regurgitation, it is important to remember that some backflow may occur behind any valve as the leaflets close (the closing volume), which should not be interpreted as abnormal. It is also important to remember that when sampling is conducted from the apex, the echo beam at the depth of the mitral valve may be fairly wide, particularly at high gain settings. In these cases, the lateral margin of the beam may overlap the posterior aorta, and high systolic velocities can be recorded that will inappropriately be displayed as if arising from along the beam axis (i.e., behind the mitral valve). This can artifactually suggest regurgitation that

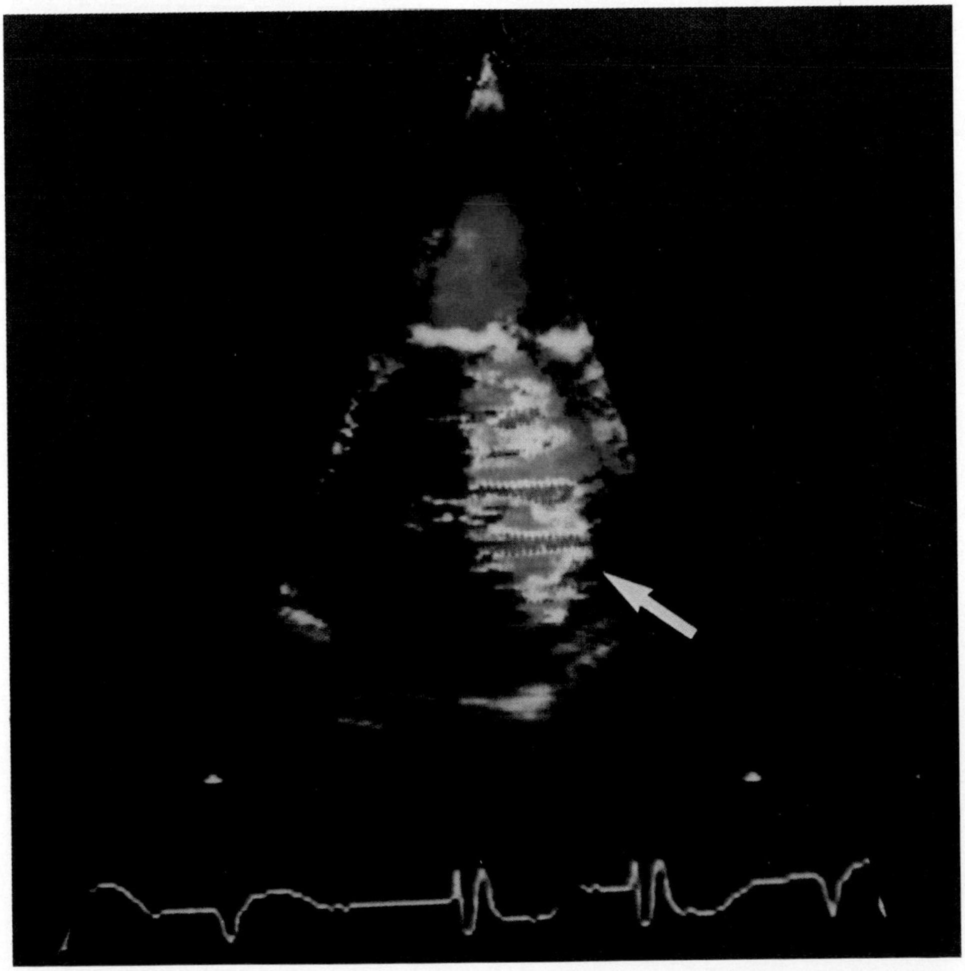

Fig. 13–12. Color flow map of a mitral regurgitant jet. In this example, regurgitant flow colored in blue (arrow) begins at the coaptation point of the mitral leaflets and extends for roughly 80% of the depth of the left atrium to approach the superior atrial wall. Multiple aliasing points are noted within the jet (orange–blue reversals) as it decelerates from its peak velocity at the orifice to zero velocity at the atrial wall.

is not truly present. This is discussed in more detail in the section on artifacts.

In studies of patients with prosthetic valves, regurgitation is often paravalvular, and in these cases, the annular attachment of the sewing ring must be sampled around the entire circumference of the valve. When the apical window is used, such sampling requires that the sound pass through the prosthetic material at the margins of the valve during both transmission and return. This frequently results in loss of signal and, hence, markedly reduced Doppler sensitivity. Prosthetic valves in the mitral position, therefore, should be studied from multiple transducer locations, particularly those that do not result in the beam passing through the prosthetic material, before regurgitation can be excluded.

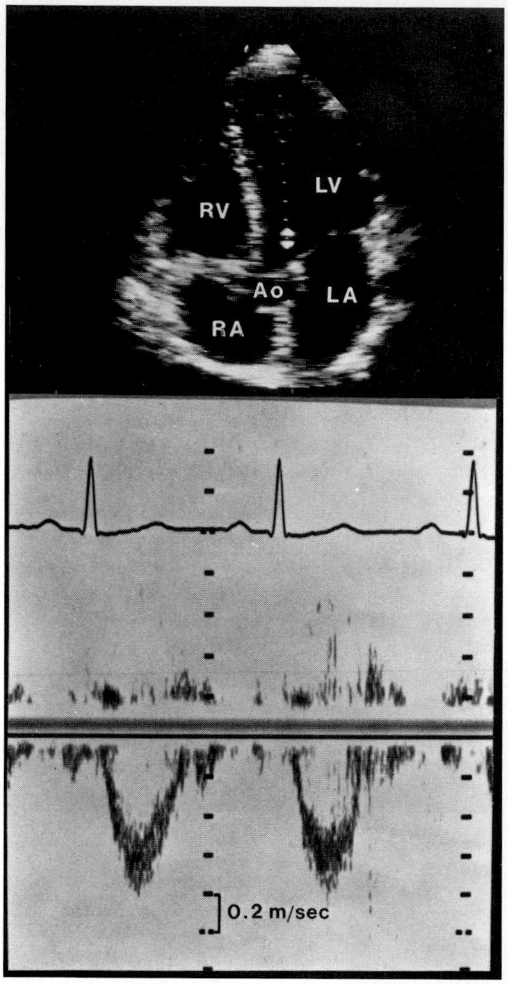

Fig. 13–13. Pulsed Doppler recording of flow in the left ventricular outflow tract proximal to the aortic valve (Ao). This sample volume location is also useful for detecting aortic insufficiency when present. LA = left atrium; LV = left ventricle; RA = right atrium; RV = right ventricle.

Aortic Valve

When the mitral examination is completed, the beam is then angled anteriorly toward the patients right shoulder to record aortic outflow. In combined imaging/Doppler studies, the scan plan is elevated to an apical five-chamber view, and the Doppler cursor is directed through the center of the aortic annulus. If this view does not expose the aorta adequately, rotation of the scan plane to an apical long axis view may be helpful, because this should facilitate alignment of the Doppler cursor parallel to the ascending aorta. The sample volume is positioned below the valve initially to record the outflow tract velocity (Fig. 13–13) for comparison with velocities encountered at the valvular level and to search for aortic insufficiency (Fig. 13–14). When subvalvular obstruction is suspected, the sample volume can initially be positioned apical to the mitral valve leaflets and gradually advanced to the level of the aortic annulus to look for a sudden increase in velocity (Fig. 13–15A and B). Once subvalvular flow has been adequately recorded, the sample volume is then advanced to a position at or slightly above the aortic annulus where the normal peak outflow velocity should be recorded (Fig. 13–16). Again, the level of maximal flow velocity cannot be defined from the image, although it will usually be found in the center of the aorta, several millimeters beyond the valve leaflet insertions points. Because this may vary, however, a radially expanding scan of the sample volume beginning at the annulus and advancing in increments of sample volume lengths should be performed until a clear laminar flow pattern showing the highest flow velocity is obtained. As with mitral inflow, initial color flow mapping of the area may facilitate this process.

In patients with aortic stenosis, the velocity of flow will increase as the sample volume is advanced through the valve orifice (Fig. 13–17). When the obstruction is

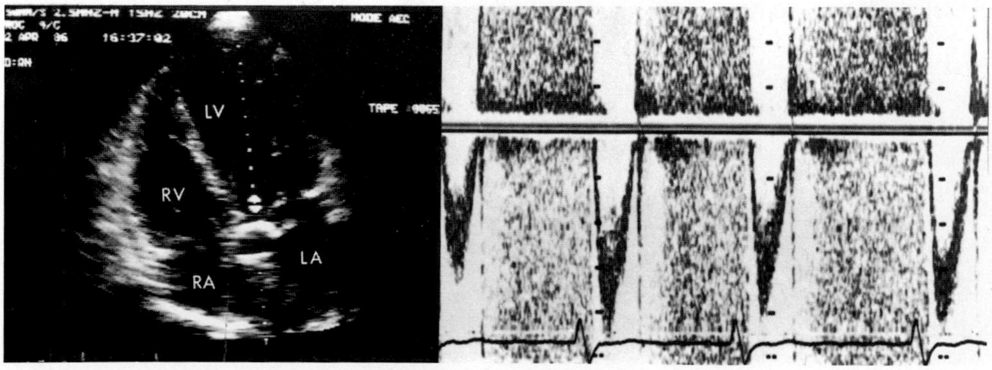

Fig. 13–14. Pulsed Doppler recording immediately beneath the aortic valve, illustrating normal systolic laminar flow and high velocity turbulent diastolic flow indicative of aortic regurgitation. LA = left atrium; LV = left ventricle; RA = right atrium; RV = right ventricle.

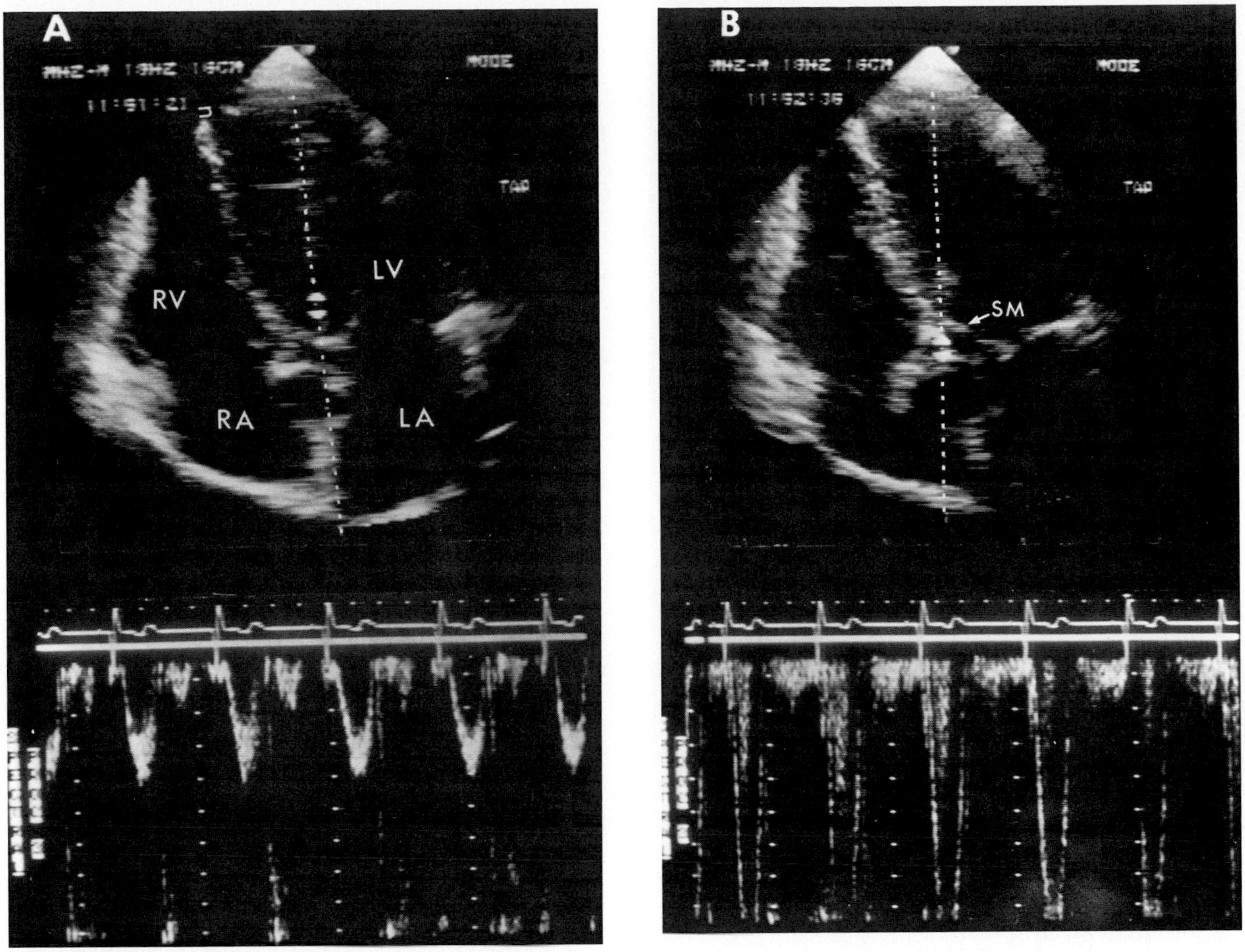

Fig. 13–15. The increase in velocity in the subvalvular region found when a fixed subvalvular obstruction (subvalvular membrane or tunnel) is present. **A.** A velocity of roughly 80 cm/sec, proximal to a subvalvular membrane. **B.** The velocity increases to roughly 2.6 m/sec as the sample volume is advanced across the subvalvular membrane (SM). LA = left atrium; LV = left ventricle; RA = right atrium; RV = right ventricle.

severe, the associated velocity increase that is due to convective acceleration may exceed the aliasing limit of the pulsed Doppler system. Likewise, the direction of flow through the diseased valve may differ from the direction of flow in the outflow tract, and the orientation of the jet exiting the valve may not correspond to the expected direction of flow in the aorta. The examination of the aortic valve in these cases, therefore, becomes more complex, and because this is the single most important component of the Doppler study and is an area where precision is critical, it is our policy to continue with the routine examination and return to study the aortic valve in detail at its conclusion, rather than to persist with the aortic valve at this point. If the assessment of aortic stenosis is left to the end, the aortic valve can then be studied using an appropriate combination of techniques i.e., pulsed Doppler to determine the proximal velocity, continuous wave (CW) to determine a maximal jet velocity, and color flow to determine jet orientation. The aortic jet can also be examined from several windows including the apex, the suprasternal notch, and the right parasternal border, which will almost invariably permit not only the highest velocity to be recorded (Fig. 13–18) but will increase the operator's confidence in the accuracy of individual measurements by confirmation from several locations.

Tricuspid Valve

When the aortic valve examination has been completed, the transducer is then angled further rightward (toward the patient's right shoulder) to direct the beam to intersect tricuspid inflow. The scan plane must typically be depressed slightly to return to an apical four-chamber view, and the sample volume is placed just proximal (apical) to the tricuspid valve annulus (Fig. 13–19). The tricuspid flow profile typically has a lower velocity and is more difficult to record that that of the mitral valve (Fig. 13–20). The lower velocity of flow is expected, because the tricuspid valve annulus is larger

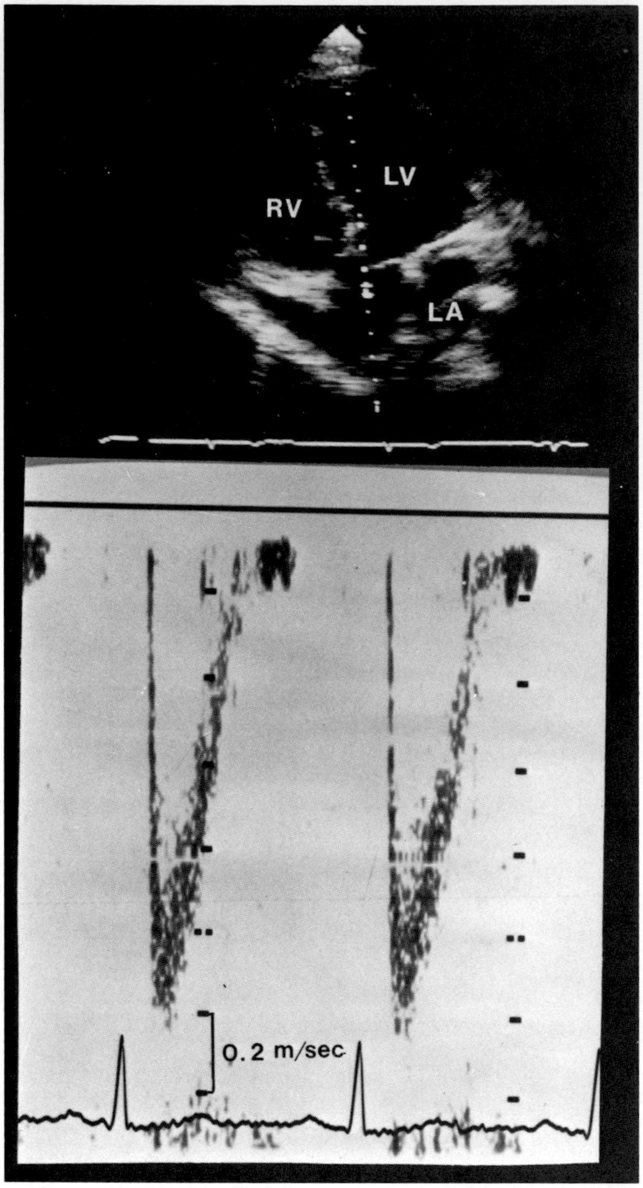

Fig. 13–16. Normal laminar aortic velocity profile recorded immediately distal to the aortic valve leaflets. LA = left atrium; LV = left ventricle; RA = right atrium.

than that of the mitral valve and in the absence of left-to-right shunting, flow velocity, by the continuity equation, must be lower. In addition, a typical apical window places the direction of the beam at a slight angle relative to the direction of flow through the tricuspid valve which decreases the recorded velocity (Fig. 13–19). This orientation further accentuates the recorded difference between mitral and tricuspid inflow velocities because from the apex the Doppler beam is generally parallel to mitral inflow. Finally, from the apex, the sound beam is generally directed obliquely through a large portion of the interventricular septum to reach the tricuspid valve, which slightly increases signal attenuation and decreases amplitude. To overcome these problems, it may be necessary to shift transducer position to the right of the left ventricular apex to more closely approach the apex of the right ventricle. This will align the path of the beam parallel to the direction of inflow through the tricuspid valve and should improve signal intensity (Fig. 13–19). In most normal patients, this window is not available because lung is interposed between the right ventricular apex and the anterior chest wall. Fortunately, tricuspid flow is rarely abnormal, and in those cases in which abnormal flow is expected, the right ventricle is generally dilated, enlarging the apical window and facilitating tricuspid recording.

When analyzing tricuspid flow patterns, it is also necessary to remember that all right-sided flows are aug-

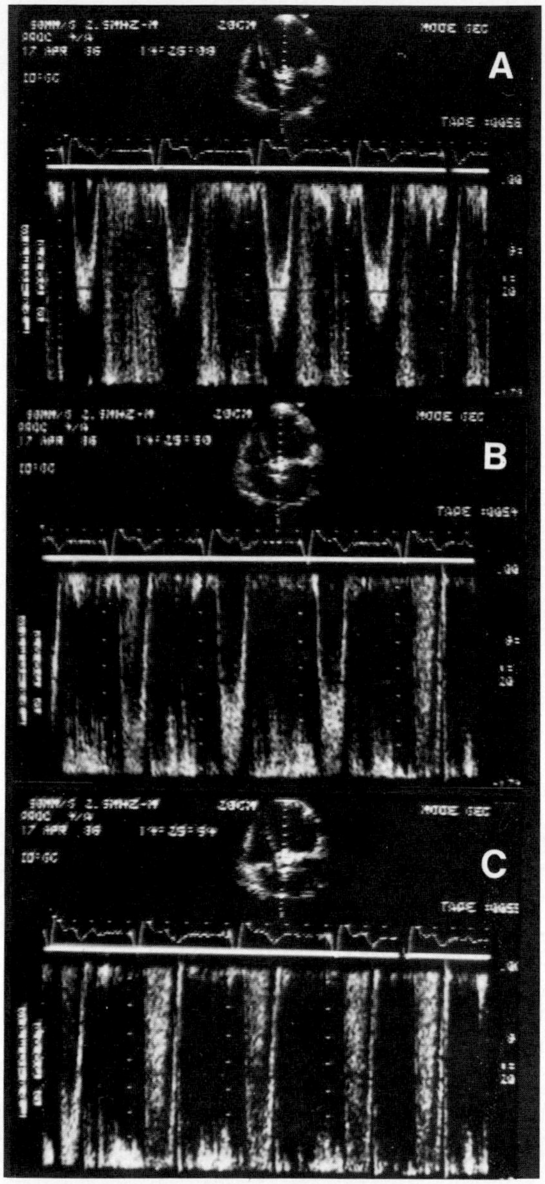

Fig. 13–17. The acceleration in velocity that occurs as the sample volume is advanced across a stenotic aortic valve. **A.** Normal velocity in the outflow tract proximal to the stenotic valve. A faint diastolic flow pattern indicative of aortic regurgitation also is present. **B.** The flow increase seen in the outflow tract immediately beneath the valve caused by convective acceleration. **C.** As the valve is crossed, the velocity increases abruptly and signal aliasing is noted.

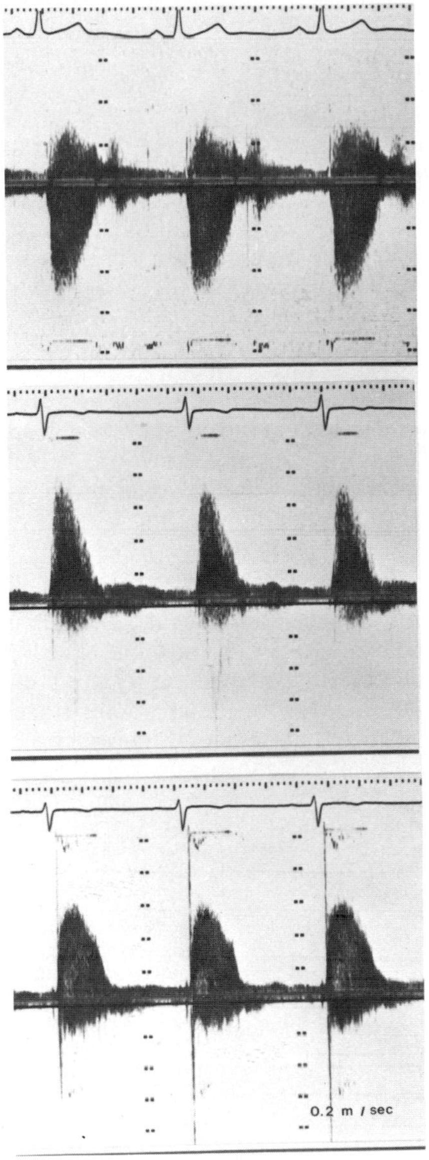

Fig. 13–18. Continuous wave Doppler recordings of an aortic stenotic jet obtained from the apical window (top), the right parasternal window (middle), and the suprasternal notch (bottom). Note that in this example, the highest velocity is recorded from the right parasternal location. Recording from multiple locations confirms the presence of a high velocity jet and offers the opportunity to interrogate the lesion from the vantage point that provides the greatest signal sensitivity.

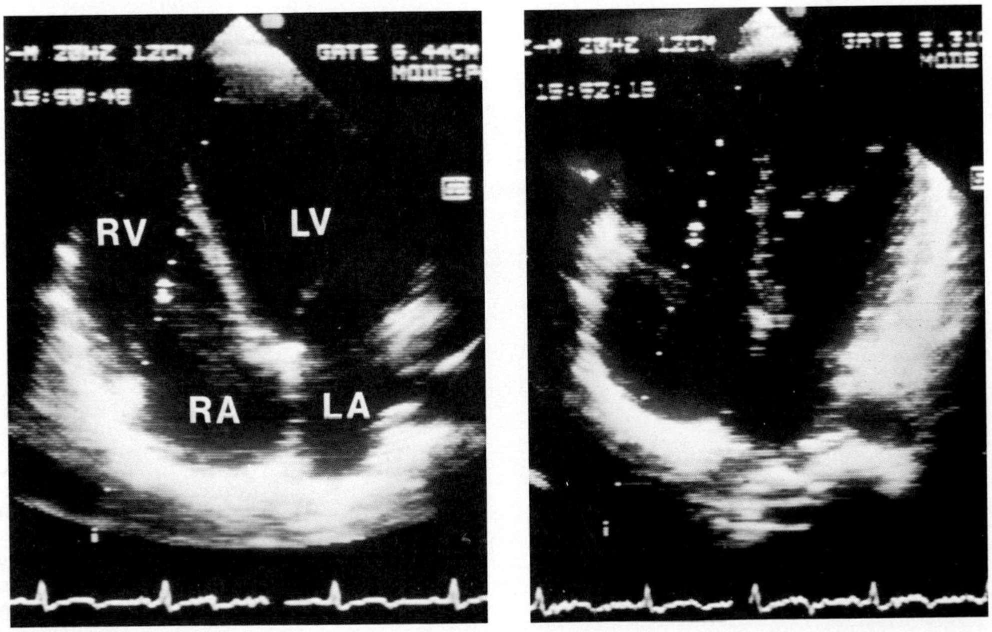

Fig. 13–19. Sample volume location in the right ventricle (RV) used to record RV inflow velocities. Left. The cursor originates from the cardiac apex and is oblique to the inflow velocities passing through the tricuspid orifice. Right. The transducer has been shifted medially, and the cursor lies more parallel to the true direction of tricuspid flow. This increases signal sensitivity and enhances velocity recording. LA = left atrium; LV = left ventricle; RA = right atrium.

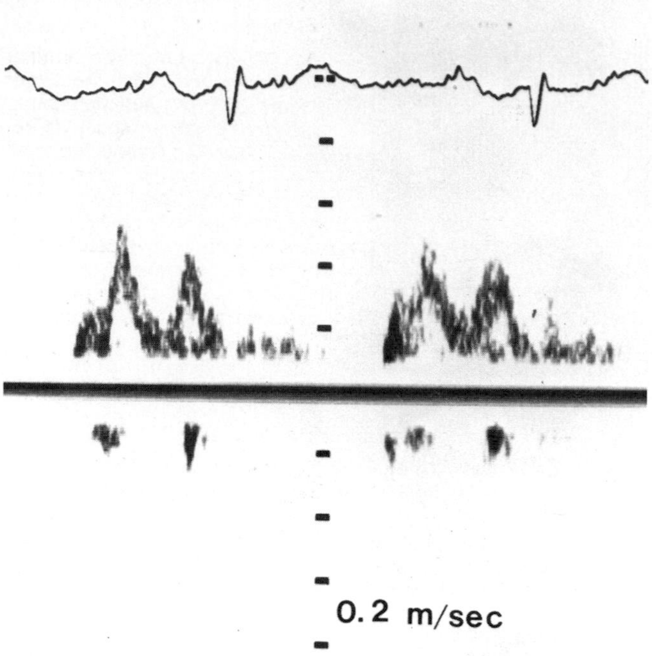

Fig. 13–20. Normal tricuspid flow velocity profile. The tricuspid velocity pattern is similar to that of the mitral valve; however, the absolute velocity is of slightly lower amplitude because the tricuspid annulus is typically larger.

mented by inspiration and tricuspid flow therefore may show marked inspiratory variation (Fig. 13–21).

Once tricuspid inflow is recorded, the sample volume can then be advanced through the valve orifice and positioned immediately behind the valve cusps to sample for tricuspid regurgitation (Fig. 13–22). Because the tricuspid valve has three commissures, the area along which leakage can occur is correspondingly increased. In most cases, however, the regurgitation will be centravalvular. This may well represent the fact that most pathologic tricuspid regurgitation is the result of right ventricular dilation secondary to either right ventricular volume or pressure overload rather than a primary leaflet abnormality. As the orifice expands, the leaflets are drawn apart and tend to leak at the point farthest from the annular margin or at the center of the valve. When regurgitation is due to a primary leaflet abnormality, it can occur at any point along the closure lines.

Atrial and Ventricular Septa

In addition to recording mitral, aortic, and tricuspid flows from the apex, it is also possible to scan the sample volume along both sides of the interatrial and interventricular septa, looking for the characteristic flow signals of atrial or ventricular defects. Figures 13–23 and 13–24 illustrate the typical flow signals recorded from each of

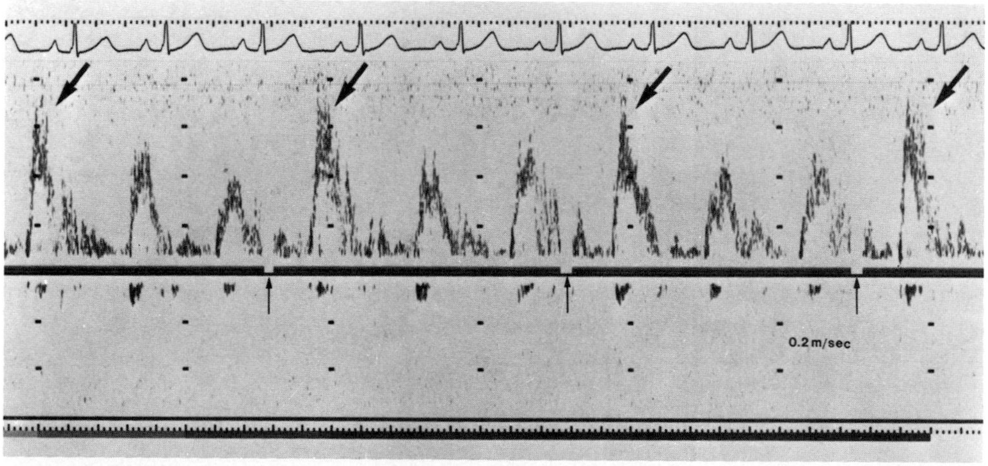

Fig. 13–21. Normal respiratory variation in tricuspid inflow velocities. The oblique downward pointing arrows indicate the augmentation of the peak inflow velocity, which is normally seen during inspiration. Upward pointing vertical arrows indicate points at which the data are transferred to update the "simultaneously" recorded image and, as a result, no Doppler signal is output.

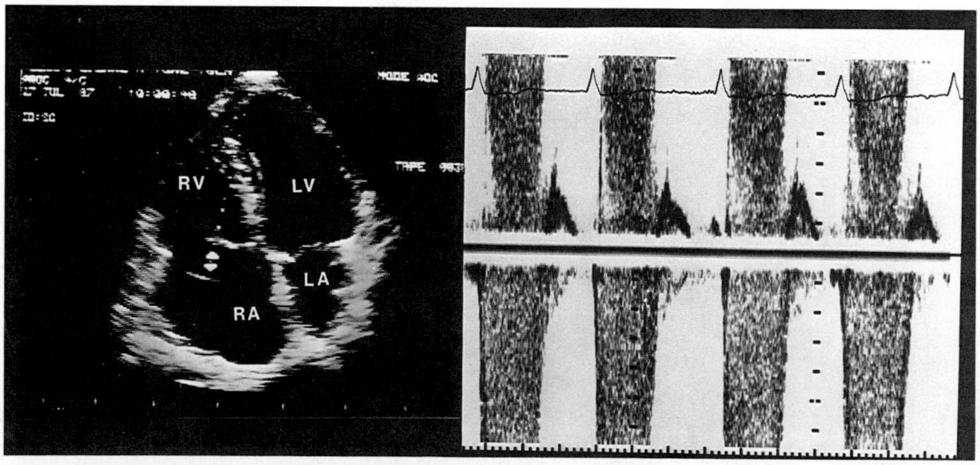

Fig. 13–22. The sample volume location behind the tricuspid leaflets used to record tricuspid regurgitation. Right. The high velocity turbulent systolic flow characteristic of a tricuspid regurgitant lesion. LA = left atrium; LV = left ventricle; RA = right atrium; RV = right ventricle.

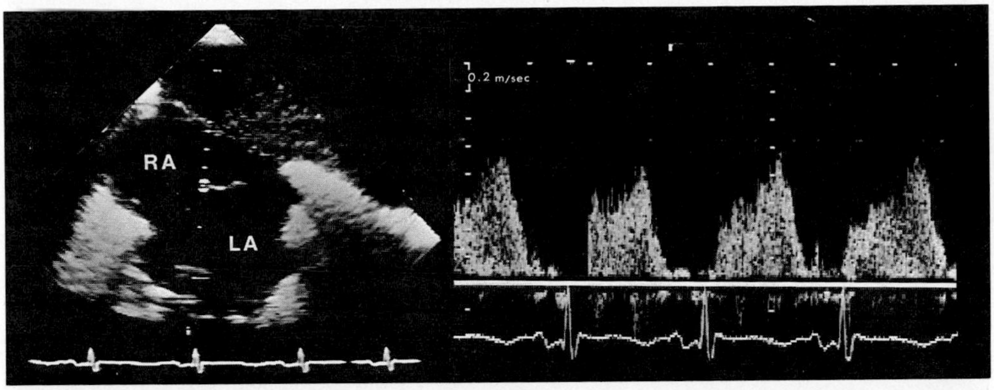

Fig. 13–23. Left. The sample volume placed in the right atrium (RA), immediately adjacent to a small atrial septal defect. Right. The typical flow pattern seen with a left-to-right shunt at the atrial level. Note that flow velocity peaks at end-systole and early-diastole at a point that corresponds to the maximal transatrial pressure gradient. LA = left atrium.

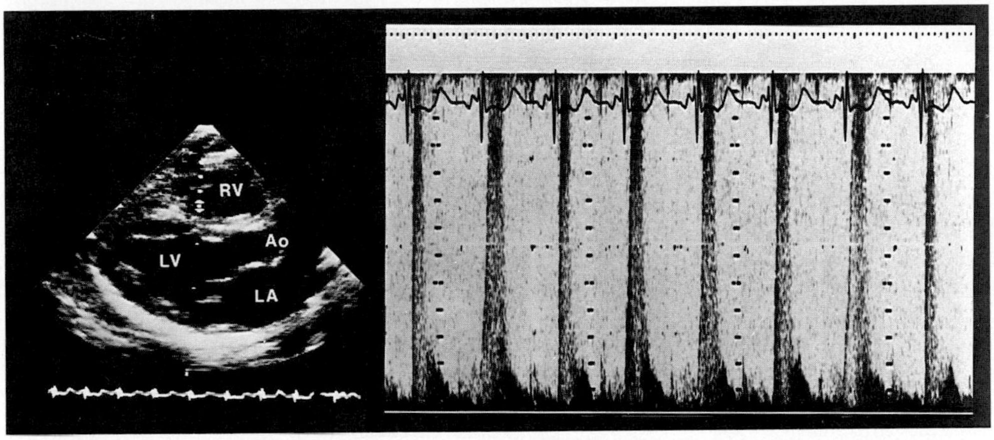

Fig. 13–24. Pulsed Doppler recording of ventricular septal defect (VSD) flow. Left. Sample volume is placed along the right side of the interventricular septum. Right. The high velocity left-to-right shunt flow indicative of a VSD with a large left-to-right pressure gradient. Ao = aorta; LA = left atrium; LV = left ventricle; RV = right ventricle.

these lesions. In the absence of some evidence of a ventricular septal defect, routine interrogation of the interventricular septum is probably a nonprofitable expenditure of time. Routine recording along the interatrial septum, however, is useful because the foramen ovale is patent in roughly 20% of the normal population, and it is worthwhile to document interatrial flow when present. Routine recording of flow along the right side of the interatrial septum also permits the sonographer to gain familiarity with the complex flow pattern in the right atrium, which originates from both vena cava, and the coronary sinus and may be complicated by flow through the atrial septum and tricuspid regurgitation when present. Familiarity with the normal variations in flow in the atrium is therefore extremely valuable because in the absence of such understanding the separation of normal flow from single or multiple abnormal jets may be extremely difficult.

DOPPLER EXAMINATION—PARASTERNAL WINDOW

Pulmonary Artery

Once the examination from the apex is completed, the transducer is then shifted to the parasternal window to record flow in the pulmonary artery. Typically, the sample volume is initially placed just proximal to the pulmonary valve leaflets in the right ventricular outflow tract to sample for pulmonary insufficiency (Fig. 13–25). This can be achieved in the pulsed Doppler mode, and the extent of regurgitant jet can be mapped either by repositioning the sample volume within the outflow tract or by using the color flow mapping technique (Fig. 13–26). Once the area behind the valve has been satisfactorily examined, the sample volume is then advanced through the valve leaflets to record forward flow in the pulmonary artery. Because the pulmonary artery follows an almost directly posterior course from the parasternal window, this is the ideal location for recording pulmonary flow. Care must be exercised, however, because the pulmonary artery curves roughly 90° from the superior margin of the aorta to the medial aortic wall, and hence, the pulmonary flow profile may be correspondingly shifted.

The normal pattern of pulmonary flow is a gradually accelerating and then decelerating laminar profile that peaks in midsystole. Such a profile can generally be found immediately distal to the pulmonary valve in the center of the pulmonary artery and will extend for several centimeters beyond the valve (Fig. 13–27). Inappropriate positioning of the sample volume medial or lateral to this central stream, however, can create alternations in the acceleration/deceleration phase, which may simulate pulmonary hypertension and alter both the form and the area of the systolic velocity interval. Figure 13–28 illustrates the patterns of pulmonary flow recorded at nine locations distal to the pulmonary valve, emphasiz-

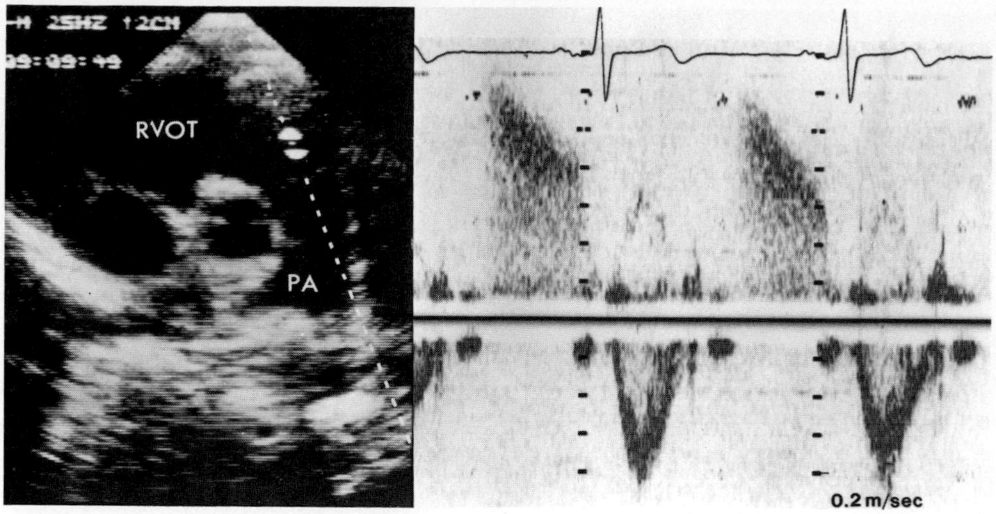

Fig. 13–25. Sample volume location and characteristic flow pattern noted in pulmonary regurgitation. Left. The sample volume position immediately behind the pulmonary leaflets in the right ventricular outflow tract (RVOT). Right. The diastolic regurgitant jet of pulmonary regurgitation, which is directed upward or toward the transducer. In this example, the early component of the regurgitant jet is not recorded because the jet volume is small and only becomes manifest as the position on the heart shifts downward during diastole, bringing the jet within the sample volume. PA = pulmonary artery.

ing the effect of sample volume location on the recorded peak velocity and the acceleration and deceleration times.

Sampling proximal and distal to the four cardiac valves and along the interatrial septum constitutes a routine study in our laboratory. If mitral, aortic, or tricuspid regurgitation is suspected from the apical study, it is our custom to confirm it from the parasternal window, which is frequently closer to the lesion and, hence, provides a stronger signal. Although these regurgitant jets are generally perpendicular or at an oblique angle to the beam path, they contain sufficient turbulence so that portions of the flow vector will be directed toward and away from the beam axis. Recording regurgitant lesions from several locations is a useful cross check, particularly when the signal from the apex is weak or when the character of the regurgitant lesion is atypical. It is also important to examine prosthetic valves from more than one location, particularly those in the mitral and tricuspid position, where the signal strength may be severely attenuated during apical sampling. Approaching the prosthesis from the parasternal window permits sampling behind the sewing ring without the beam's traversing any of the prosthetic material. This is particularly important because major degrees of insufficiency can be missed from the apical window as a result of loss of signal strength.

DOPPLER EXAMINATION—SUPRASTERNAL WINDOW

Once the parasternal study is finished, the routine examination is generally completed. If the aorta is inaccessible from the apex, flow in the ascending aorta can alter-

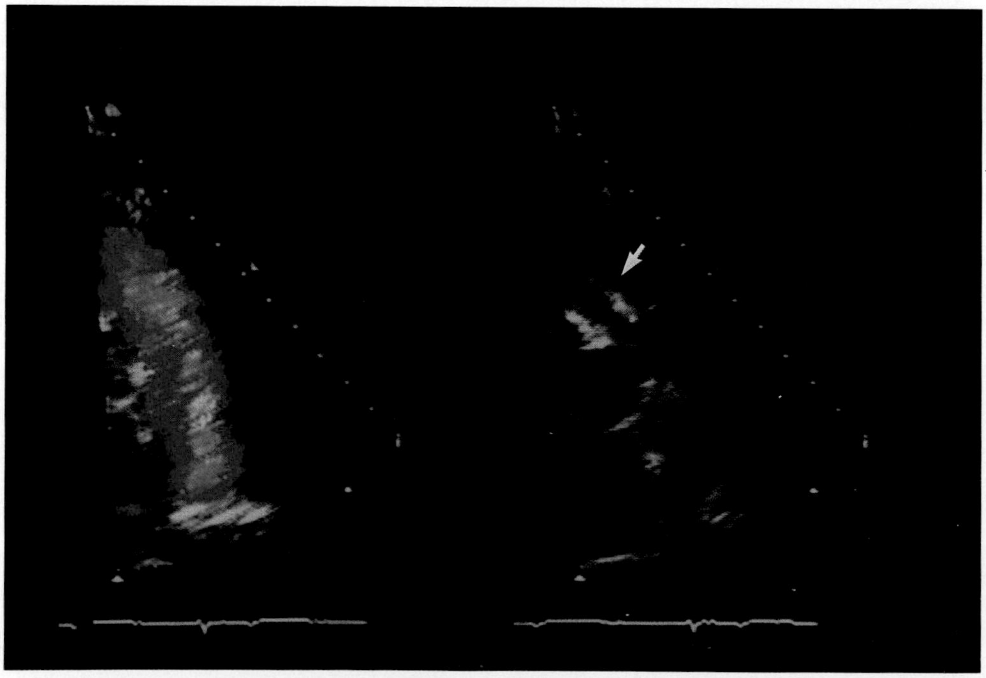

Fig. 13–26. Color flow map of the right ventricular outflow tract and pulmonary artery during systole (left) and diastole (right). In systole, the normal flow pattern in the pulmonary artery is apparent, with the highest velocities noted toward the center of the vessel. In diastole, there is a small regurgitant jet (arrow) similar to those frequently noted in normal patients.

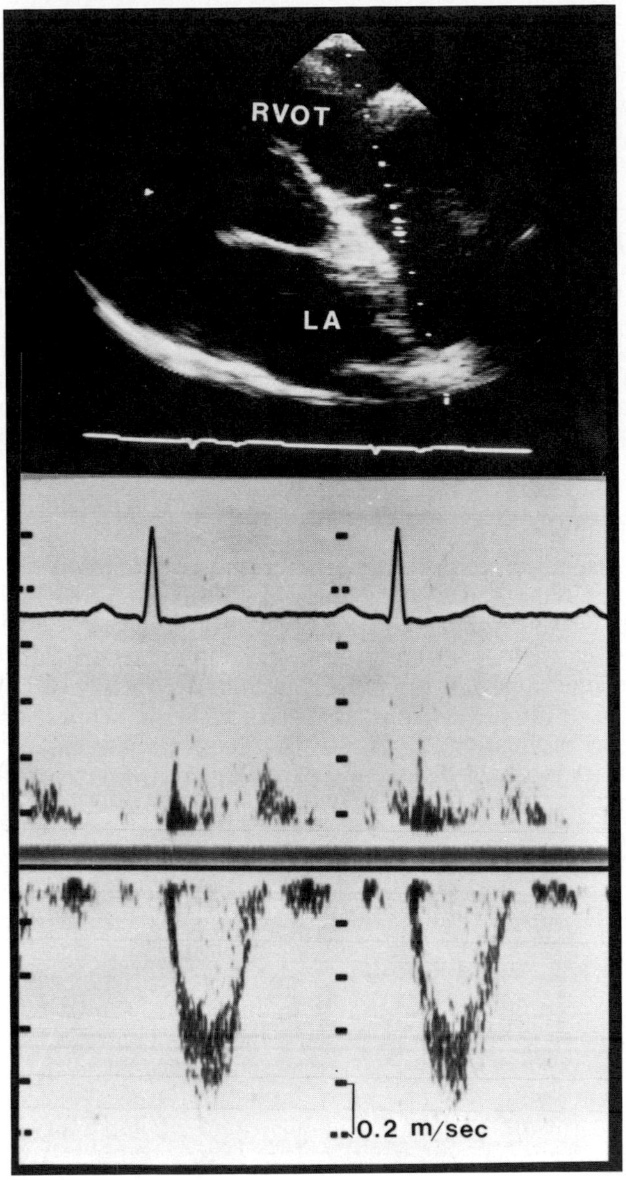

Fig. 13–27. Normal pulmonary artery flow recorded by pulsed Doppler. Top. The sample volume position within the pulmonary artery distal to the pulmonic valve. LA = left atrium; RVOT = right ventricular outflow tract. Bottom. The normal gradually accelerating and decelerating pattern of pulmonary artery flow with the peak velocity occurring in midsystole.

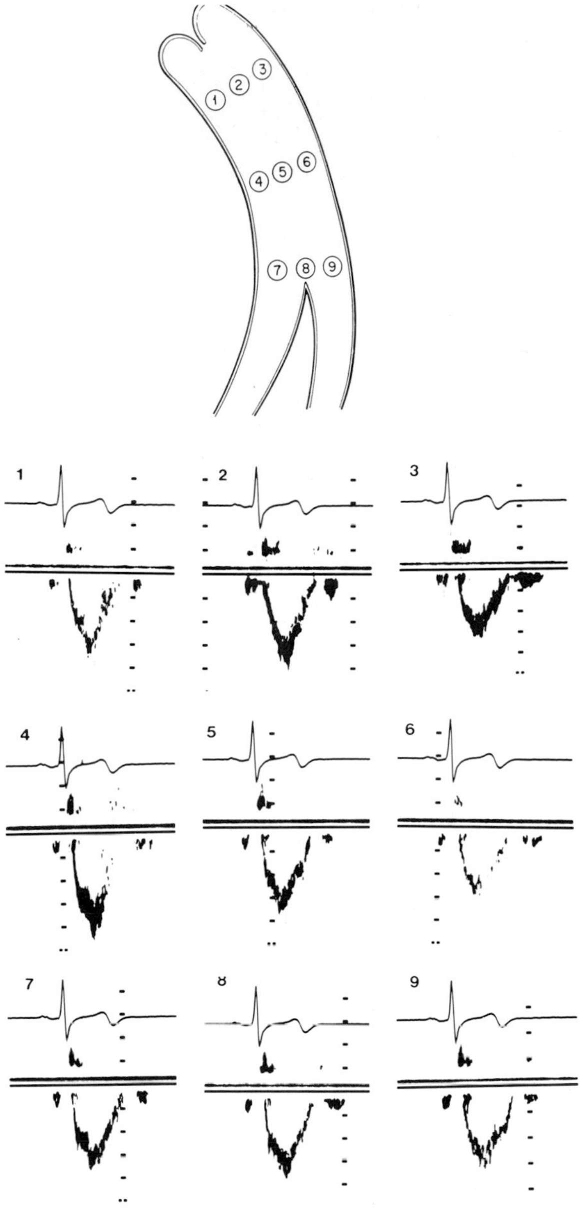

Fig. 13–28. Patterns of pulmonic flow recorded at nine different locations, distal to the pulmonic valve. This figure emphasizes the effect of sample location on the timing of peak velocity and the acceleration and deceleration times in the normal pulmonary artery.

natively be recorded from the suprasternal notch. When the suprasternal approach is used, the scan plane is initially aligned to record the long axis of the aortic arch, and the cursor is directed to record either ascending or descending aortic blood flow (Fig. 13–29). The suprasternal window can be used to verify the velocities recorded from the apex in aortic stenosis, to sample the descending thoracic aorta in patients with suspected coarctation, and to record aortic flow in the region of a suspected patent ductus arteriosus looking for backward flow through the duct. Despite the initial importance placed on this window, however, the suprasternal notch is less useful in the adult than either the apical or parasternal window and now finds its major utility in the assessment of the great vessels in children.

Once the routine examination is completed, it is our policy to return to study the aortic valve in more detail in patients with suspected aortic stenosis. This requires sampling from the apex, right parasternal window, and the suprasternal notch and can be a long (30 to 45 minutes) and tedious examination in itself. If this comes at the end of a two-dimensional echo, M-mode and routine Doppler study, both the patient and operator may be tired. Given the importance of the data, it is preferable

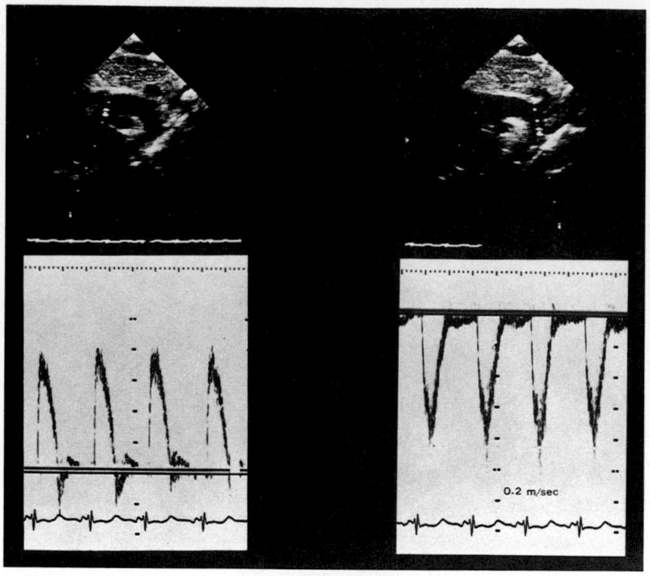

Fig. 13–29. Normal aortic flow recorded from the suprasternal notch. Left. The sample volume is positioned in the ascending aorta, and flow is directed positively or toward the transducer. Right. The sample volume is positioned in the descending aorta, and flow is away from the transducer or negatively directed on the recording.

to bring the patient back at another time, rather than to settle for suboptimal data resulting from operator fatigue or loss of patient cooperation.

USING COLOR FLOW MAPPING FOR ROUTINE DATA ACQUISITION

When color flow mapping capabilities are available, the general practice is to record the color flow pattern in each of the available imaging planes immediately following image acquisition. The color flow study therefore follows the same pattern as an imaging study, as discussed in Chapter 5. Because these planes are, by definition, oriented for optimal image acquisition, many are not ideal for Doppler flow recording. Thus, although some useful data may be derived from these additional views, the majority of the Doppler data will still be obtained from the transducer locations previously described for the routine pulsed and CW Doppler examination.

Integration of all three modalities provides the most information and represents an ideal study. In this approach, color flow mapping is used to define the spatial distribution of normal and abnormal flow, pulsed Doppler to define flow velocity at specific locations more accurately (i.e., with a higher temporal and velocity resolution than is available using color flow mapping), and CW Doppler to record peak velocities when aliasing confounds accurate velocity description by the color flow or pulsed techniques. The routine addition of this complex Doppler sampling to the imaging study markedly prolongs the examination. Although this is not inappropriate, it is important to remember that the majority of the significant diagnostic information still comes from the imaging study and that the images cannot be accurately interpreted while color flow mapping is occurring. Therefore, the operator should be sure to record sufficient imaging data before turning on the color flow Doppler.

COMMONLY ENCOUNTERED ARTIFACTS IN PULSED AND CONTINUOUS WAVE DOPPLER

Just as in imaging studies, a variety of phenomena produce artifacts in the output Doppler signal. The most common of these are aliasing, mirroring, data loss that is due to intermittent diversion for image formation, and reception by the transducer of extraneous sounds at the Doppler frequency, e.g., the crying of infants and talking in the area of the examination.

Aliasing

Aliasing is one of the artifacts most commonly encountered when a pulsed echo system is used for Doppler flow sampling. The use of any pulsed wave system implies that flow can be sampled only once per pulse transmission or at the pulse repetition frequency (PRF) of the system. As discussed earlier in the section on signal processing, aliasing is the inappropriate characterization of the frequency of a waveform that occurs when it is sampled at less than one half of its fundamental frequency. Because for a pulsed system the sampling frequency is the PRF, aliasing will occur whenever the frequency of the Doppler shift exceeds one half the PRF: the Nyquist frequency. Once this point is exceeded, a new or "aliased" signal is output, which although not describing the original signal, correctly bears a predictable relationship to it. It has also been shown that aliasing can occur either because the sampling frequency is low relative to the signal to be sampled or because the velocity of the target is so high that it produces a signal that is beyond the unambiguous sampling capability of the instrument.

The purpose of this section is to explain the effects of aliasing on the output of the Doppler device and the reasons that the pattern of aliasing appears as it does. Before discussing aliasing per se, several other basic facts should be remembered. First, aliasing is the result of effective undersampling of target velocity. As a result, CW Doppler instruments that interrogate targets continuously are not subject to aliasing at physiologically encountered frequencies/velocities. Second, the Nyquist limit is a function of the PRF, which in turn varies with the sampling depth with the result that the greater the depth to be examined the lower the velocity at which aliasing will be encountered. Third, in physiologic systems where velocity is constantly changing, it can be presumed that low frequency returns will, in general, be correctly displayed, while aliasing will occur at higher velocities, and situations in which aliasing is likely to be encountered can therefore be predicted. Finally, because aliasing is characterized as the inappropriate assignment and display of velocity data, its characteristics will vary depending on manner in which the instrument outputs this information (e.g., aliasing in a

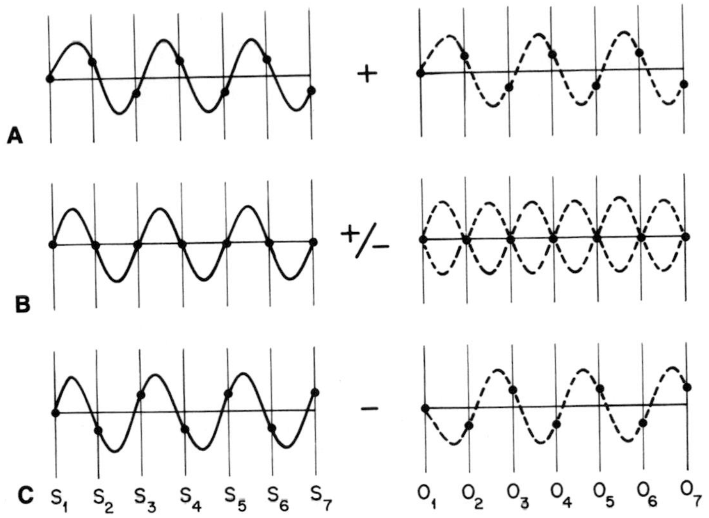

Fig. 13–30. The phenomenon of aliasing. This diagram emphasizes the transformation in the characterization of a sampled waveform that occurs as it approaches, equals, and just exceeds the Nyquist limit. Top. The frequency of the wave is slightly less than twice the sampling frequency, and hence the wave is output ($O_{1\text{-}N}$) in the appropriate direction and at the appropriate frequency. Middle. The frequency of the wave has increased slightly and is now at the aliasing frequency. In this case, the frequency of the wave is again appropriately represented, but the instrument cannot unambiguously determine its direction. Bottom. The frequency of the wave has increased to slightly above the Nyquist limit. In this case, the wave is undersampled and the output corresponds in frequency to that of the slower wave in the upper panel; however, it is now inverted in direction. (See text for further details.)

pulsed Doppler system will be manifest differently from aliasing in a color flow mapper), and hence different instruments will be dealt with separately.

To understand how aliasing occurs, let us first examine what happens as the frequency of a given wave approaches and then exceeds the Nyquist sampling limit. Figure 13–30 depicts three waves, which are sampled at a fixed interval Ts. For wave A, the sampling frequency is slightly greater than twice the frequency of the wave. For wave B, it is exactly twice the frequency of the wave, and for wave C, the sampling frequency is slightly less than twice the wave frequency. In each case, the value of the wave is sampled ($S_{1\text{-}N}$) only at the specified points. The amplitude of wave A will be recorded as first positive (S_2) then negative (S_3), and if the instrument assigns direction to the wave based on the polarity of the first sample, the wave will be depicted as positive going at the appropriate frequency. Wave B will reach π radians or 180° at S_2 and have returned to 0° at S_3. In this case, the frequency of the wave will again be correctly described, however, the direction of the wave becomes ambiguous and the instrument cannot tell if the wave is positive or negative. Wave C will have passed through 180° at S_2 and the instrument will read the first recorded phase angle as −179°. Because the value at the end of the first sampling interval is negative, the instrument will interpret this as a negative-going wave which has taken time (S_1 to S_2) to reach its current position at −179°. In fact, the wave will have passed through 180° to reach this point, but because the instrument samples intermittently, it knows only the position of the wave at S_2 and the time elapsed to reach that point and must assume that it took the shortest route. As a result, it will depict the wave as having a lower frequency than is the true case, because it will assume that the time required for a negative-going wave (wave C) to reach 179° (S_2) is the same as that required for a positive-going wave (wave A) to travel the same distance in a positive direction. Thus, it will output (wave C) as a negative-going wave, with the same frequency as wave A. As the frequency of the wave increases beyond wave C, the machine will continue to read it as being negatively directed but at an increasingly lower frequency until it reaches zero at twice the Nyquist limit. At this point, the polarity of the first sample again will become positive, and the process will continue as long as the frequency continues to increase.

This can be thought of as a clock, as illustrated in Figure 13–31. As the frequency of the signal (velocity of flow) increases, it will gradually move the hand (vector) counterclockwise until it reaches +179°. If the velocity

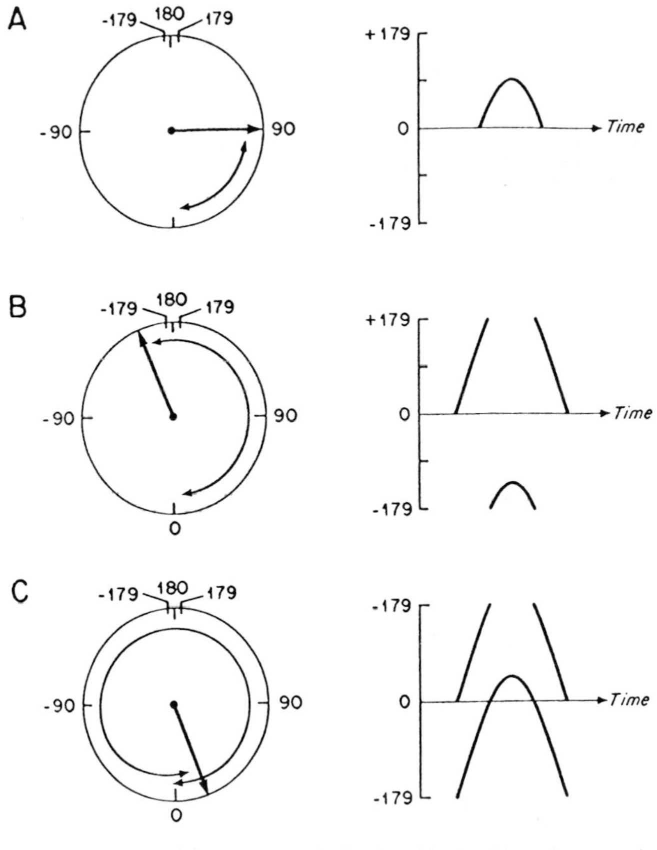

Fig. 13–31. Vector diagram of aliasing. Vector in each example represents the instantaneous phase shift in the Doppler signal and is considered to begin at 0°, rotate to its peak location indicated on the phase clock, and return to 0°. Right. The resulting phase-velocity output in the time domain. **A.** 90° peak positive phase shift in input signal is appropriately represented in the output display. **B.** Phase shift greater than 180° increases in value to 180°, becomes negative at −179°, and then decreases in value. Output shows the corresponding vector path over time. **C.** Positive phase shift-velocity increases to pass through both 180° and 0° before returning to baseline. Output signal correspondingly increases to 179°, then shifts to −179°, and then decreases in negative value to 0, where it again becomes positive.

increases further, the hand (vector) will pass through 180° (the Nyquist sampling limit), and it will then take on a decreasing minus value until it returns back to 0. If the frequency (velocity) continues to increase, the clock hand (vector) will continue to rotate up the positive side and down the negative side until the peak velocity is reached. Once this has happened and the flow velocity begins to decelerate, the Doppler frequency will begin to fall, and the clock hand can then be considered to reverse its direction and to unwind until it returns to its starting point.

On the Doppler display, the deflection of the output signal from the baseline will increase, corresponding to an increase in frequency/velocity until the Nyquist sampling limit is reached. At this point the output will shift to a negative value at the same frequency, which for the reasons cited previously, will then decrease toward zero as the frequency increases (Fig. 13–31). Once the baseline is reached, if velocity continues to increase, the output will continue in a positive direction until the sampling limit is reached again at twice the Nyquist frequency. The output will then invert again, and the process will continue until the peak frequency is reached. Once flow begins to decelerate, the process will reverse itself until it has reached its original starting point.

Approaches to Overcoming or Eliminating Signal Aliasing

Several approaches have been suggested for overcoming or eliminating the ambiguity introduced by signal aliasing. The simplest is to identify frequency shifts above the Nyquist limit by "unwrapping" the aliasing (i.e., for a signal that is initially positive and then negative to take the negative component and place it on top of the positive component) (Fig. 13–31B). The same result can be achieved by altering the display of the data by shifting the baseline. Baseline shifting is performed as follows. Because we know that the Nyquist range extends from +Fs/2 to −Fs/2, it is possible to displace the point of transition between positive and negative signals to any point within this range. This causes frequencies with one sign to alias sooner and those with another to alias later. The process is illustrated in Figure 13–32. Returning to our vector analogy, if instead of assuming that all samples shift from positive to negative at 180° (Fig. 13–32A), we instead shift the demarcation line between positive and negative by an additional 90°, then as illustrated in Figure 13–32B, the instrument will plot a larger shift in the phase angle as positive and for negatively shifted signals the aliasing point will occur sooner. If the instrument is instructed to assume that all signals are positive or the baseline is shifted to Fs (Fig. 13–32C), then we have effectively doubled the Nyquist limit and Fs is now equal to Fd. Figure 13–32D diagrammatically illustrates the effect of this process on a negative going signal while Figure 13–33 illustrates the same process for a negative-going signal on a Doppler recording. Thus, by zero-shifting the baseline, we can expand the apparent frequency range before aliasing by a factor of two. Once the vector rotates beyond zero, however, it

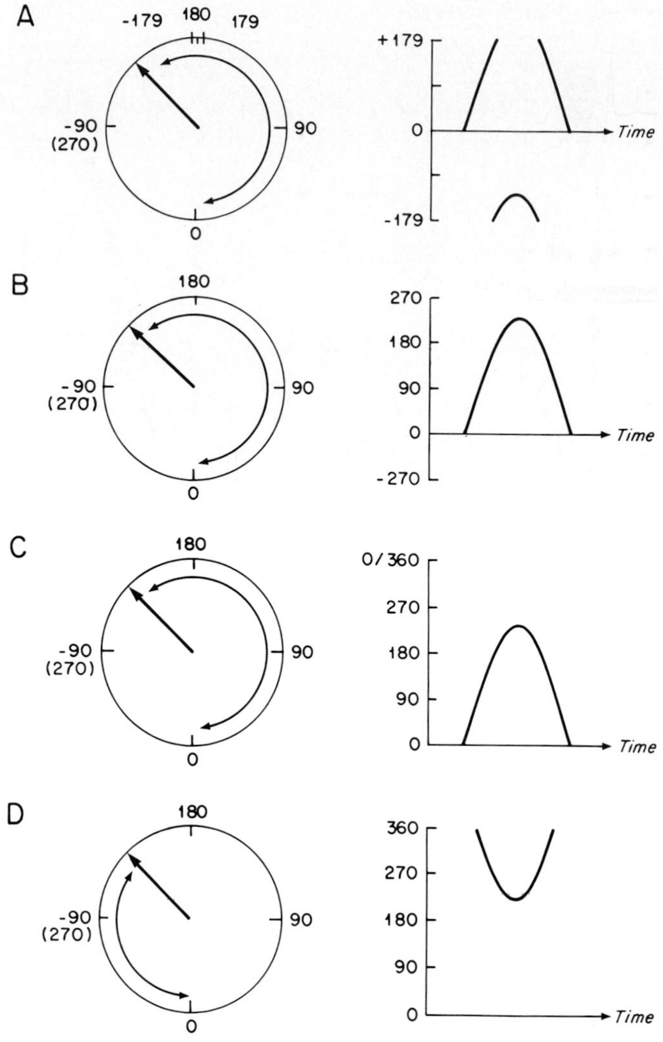

Fig. 13–32. Baseline shifting and its effect on the output signal. **A.** Baseline or aliasing point at 180°. **B.** Baseline or alias point shifted to +270 or −90°. **C.** Aliasing point shift to 0 or 359°. **D.** Output of a negative signal with a baseline of 360° and all signals considered positive. (See text for details.)

is again interpreted as a low value of the same sign, and aliasing occurs.

Another approach to overcoming aliasing is to use a lower carrier frequency. The use of a lower frequency carrier will result in a corresponding decrease in the Doppler shift frequency, which in turn increases the maximal velocity that can be recorded before the Nyquist limit is encountered. This method has all the additional effects inherent in decreasing transducer frequency discussed previously. It is most applicable in pediatrics, where the initial frequency employed is often high (5 to 7 mHz) but may also prove valuable in studies of adults. Figure 13–34 illustrates the effect of decreasing transducer frequency for both pulsed Doppler and color flow mapping. An alternative method for decreasing the Doppler shift frequency relative to the sampling frequency is to increase the angle between the direction of propagation of the beam and the flow vector. This decreases the recorded frequency shift by the cos of angle between the direction of the Doppler beam and the

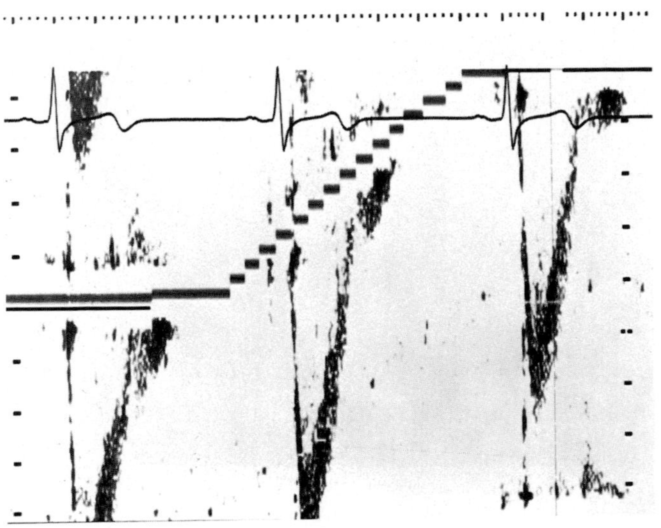

Fig. 13–33. Effects of baseline shifting on the Doppler spectral output. Left. The baseline is in the center of the display, and a negatively directed flow signal is depicted as accelerating until it reaches the aliasing frequency of −f/2 (180°), at which point it aliases and is initially displayed as a positive signal at the aliasing frequency or +f/2. As the velocity continues to increase, an incrementally decreasing positive velocity is recorded until the peak velocity is reached. After reaching its peak as the velocity decreases and the process is reversed, i.e., the signal becomes increasingly more positive until reaching the +/− crossover point, where it reverts to a maximal negative value before decelerating back out to the baseline. Middle. The baseline has been shifted to roughly +90 or −270°. In this case, the negative-going wave can accelerate through a phase shift of 270° before aliasing and reaches its peak velocity just beyond the aliasing point. In the final panel, all flow velocities are considered as negative; therefore, the velocity can accelerate a full 360° before aliasing. In this case, the entire negative-going velocity profile is displayed below the baseline, and no aliasing is apparent.

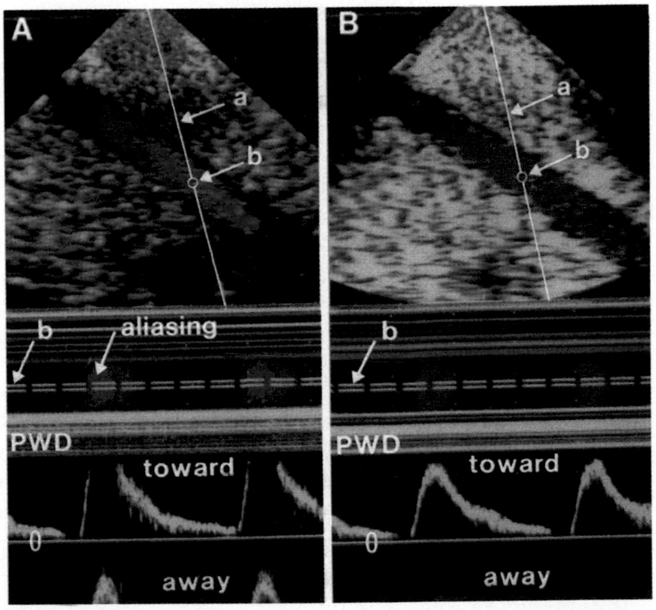

Fig. 13–34. The effect of lowering transducer frequency on the aliasing velocity for pulsed Doppler and color flow recordings. PWD = pulsed wave Doppler; a = high frequency; b = low frequency. (From Omoto R: Color Atlas of Real Time Two-Dimensional Doppler Echocardiography. Tokyo, Shindan-to-Chiryo, 1984.)

flow vector (cos Θ) and can often bring the recorded frequency below the Nyquist limit. The approach has several theoretic and practical limitations. First, it assumes that the direction of the flow vector is known. In pulsed Doppler studies, this is usually not the case, and the angle must be estimated from the image. At relatively small angular differences between the beam and flow vector, the error in this assumption is acceptable; however, as the angle between the flow vector and the interrogating beam increases, the error introduced by angle correction likewise increases. Even when the flow vector can be estimated using color flow mapping techniques, angle correction requires unnecessary assumptions and should be used only as a last resort. Finally, aliasing can be avoided by increasing the sampling frequency. This can be achieved first by decreasing the depth of sampling to include only the maximum range of interest and hence attaining the highest PRF possible. If this is unsuccessful, one can shift to high PRF (HiPRF) mode. Unfortunately, this approach, as noted earlier (see Chapter 8) decreases the power per pulse and introduces range ambiguity. Given adequate signal strength, however, HiPRF Doppler is generally felt to be accurate in adults for velocities below about 3 m/sec and to even higher levels in children.

Mirroring

Mirroring is a phenomenon that occurs when the amplitude of the Doppler shift spectrum is increased to a level where the incompletely canceled signal in the opposite quadrature channel exceeds the output threshold and a portion of the signal is output. The result is a second output signal of equal frequency (velocity) but decreased amplitude and opposite direction to the primary positive or negative signal. Figure 13–35 illustrates this phenomenon in the frequency domain. In Figure 13–35A, the positive and negative frequency bands are both present; however, only the amplitude of the positive component is above the threshold for output. As the gain is increased, however, (Fig. 13–35B), the +/− frequency amplitudes both increase, and at some point (Fig. 13–35C), the frequency band from the contralateral channel (in this example, negative) will exceed the output threshold and will be displayed as a signal of equal frequency but in the opposite direction. Figure 13–36 is an example of mirroring. In this recording, the gain has been increased until negative frequencies begin to appear in the output of the negative channel, which mirror the primary forward or positively directed velocities. This negative output increases in intensity as the gain increases.

Crying and Other External Input at the Doppler Shift Frequency

As noted earlier, physiologically encountered Doppler shift frequencies are in the range of normal human speech and hearing. Because the transducer acts as a microphone, it will pick up spoken words or the crying of an infant and transmit them to the system amplifiers. These sounds will obviously have an amplitude that is far greater than that of any returning Doppler-shifted echoes. They will therefore typically exceed the high

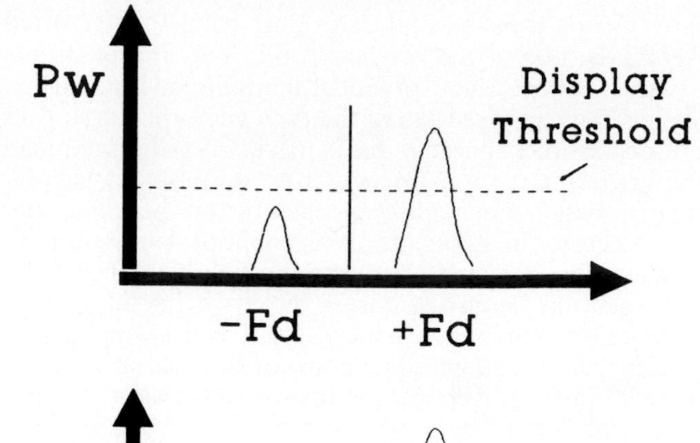

Fig. 13–35. Mirroring in the frequency domain. Top. The amplitude of the signal in the positive or forward channel is significantly higher than that of the negative channel and is plotted as a forward Doppler signal. Middle. The Doppler gain is increased, and the amplitude of the signals in both positive and negative channels increases. In this case, the amplitude in the negative channel just reaches the threshold for output and is displayed as a weak signal at the same frequency as that in the positive channel but in the opposite direction and at a significantly decreased amplitude. Bottom. The gain has been increased still further, and now a clear signal is output by both channels and is plotted as the same frequency but in opposite directions. Fd = Doppler shift frequency; Pw = amplitude.

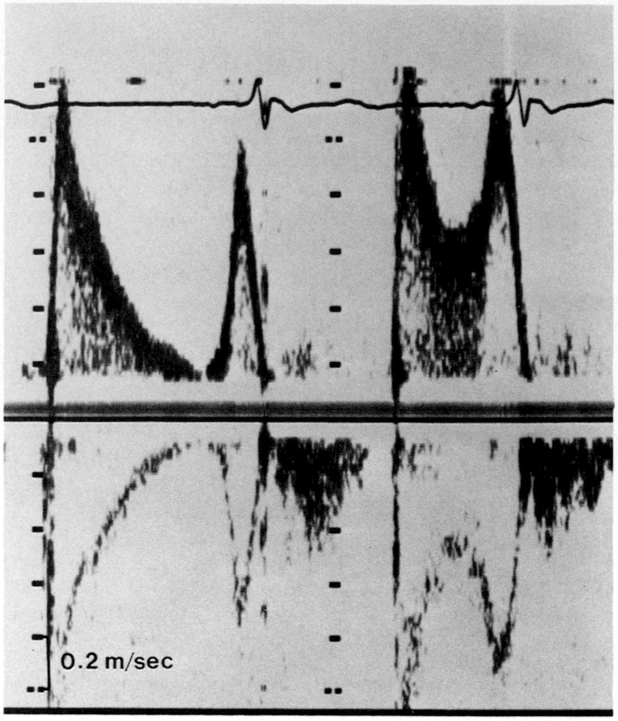

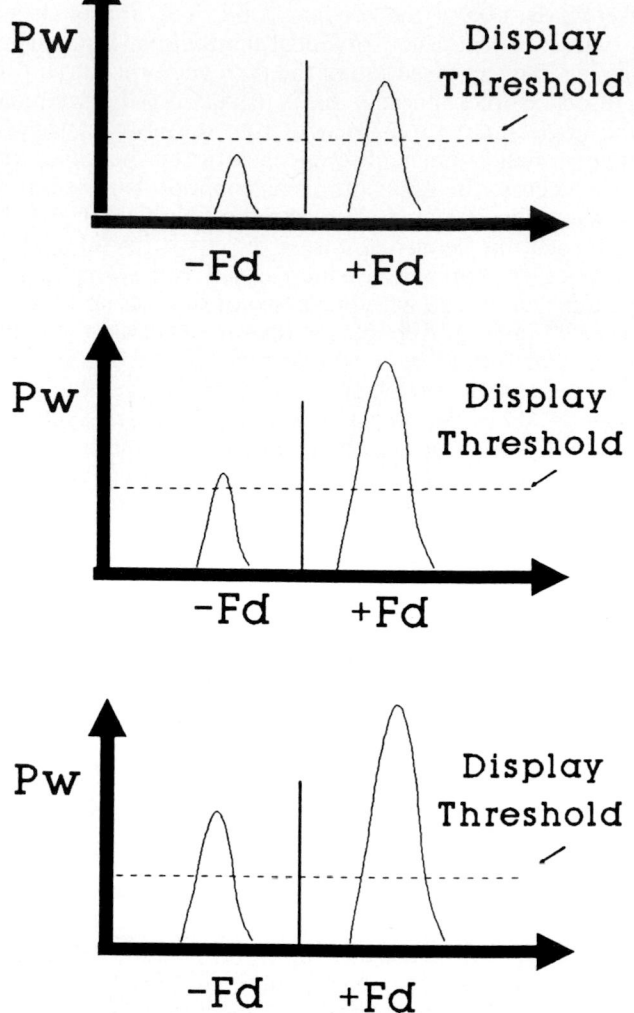

Fig. 13–36. An example of the mirroring phenomenon diagrammed in Figure 13–34. This represents cross-talk between positive and negative Doppler channels, which occurs at high gain settings.

amplitude cutoff of the amplifiers, will spill over into both quadrature channels, and will be output by the spectrum analyzer at the appropriate frequency, along with its upper and lower harmonics. Figure 13–37 is an example of the type of artifact produced in such a case.

When a child cries or a patient talks while the study is being performed, the source of these artifacts is obvious. Likewise, when such extraneous sounds are recorded on tape and replayed, they are usually recognizable although in a distorted form. However, when only a hardcopy record is available, these speech-related artifacts may create some confusion, and therefore their appearance should be recognized. Because the transducer is directly coupled to the chest and is insulated from sounds approaching it from other directions, the only speech typically recorded is that which comes from the patient. If room noise becomes loud enough, however, it may also be detected in the output.

Signal Loss Caused by Data Sharing

In Chapter 10, the concept of data sharing between the Doppler and imaging modes in combined imaging and Doppler instruments was discussed. In most such instruments, the majority of data is committed to Doppler sampling to maintain the PRF at as high a level as possible, and data are shifted to the imaging mode only intermittently to update the image. When this occurs, there is typically a gap in the Doppler output such as that indicated in Figure 13–21 and 13–38. Although these gaps can be filled in using some form of missing signal estimator, this is not usually necessary because the eye can fill in the information as accurately as the instrument, and it is sufficient to understand why these gaps in the Doppler data occur.

Beam Width Artifacts

Beam width can create spatial resolution problems in Doppler just as in imaging. In imaging studies, beam width degrades lateral resolution because it causes individual laterally positioned points to be spread to the effective width of the beam at any depth. In Doppler studies, beam width can cause inappropriate spatial localization, because all flow signals encountered at any

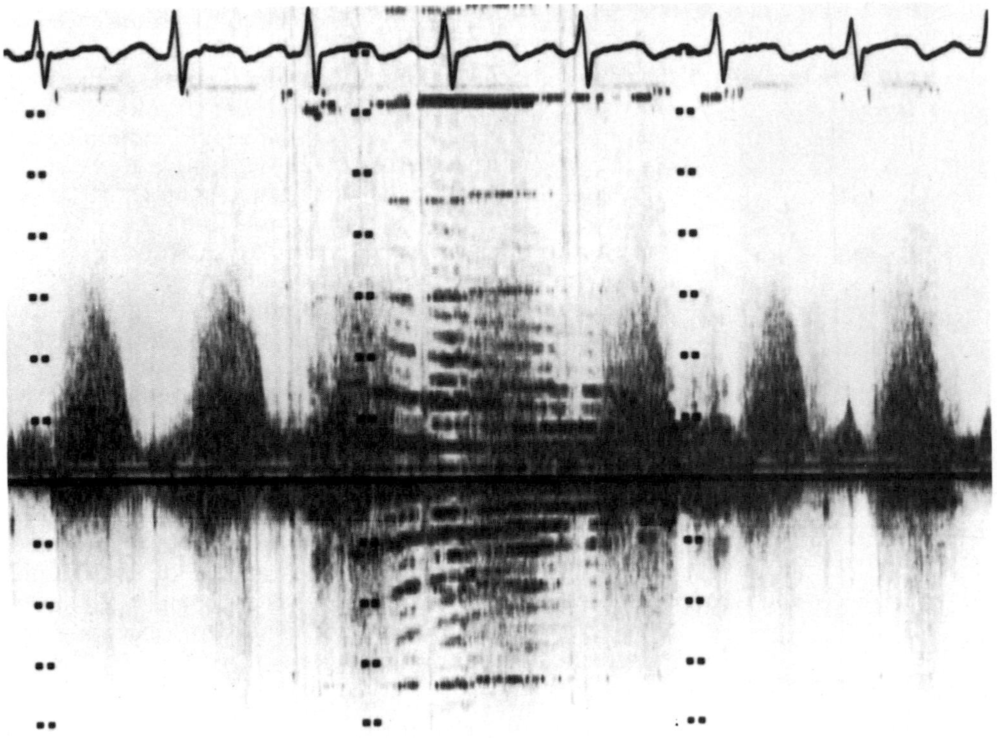

Fig. 13–37. An example of the artifact produced by a high amplitude sound in the Doppler frequency range. In this case a baby crying oversaturates the amplifiers and spills over into both quadrature channels to be output by the spectrum analyzer at the appropriate frequency with its upper and lower harmonics.

point across the beam are displayed as if they originate along the beam axis. As a result, strong flow signals at the margins of the beam may appear to arise from a point along the central axis rather than from their true location. This is particularly confusing when the flow signal arises from a chamber or a vessel other than the one in which the Doppler cursor and sample volume are positioned. This is a common problem when sampling from the cardiac apex because the areas of interest are frequently in the far field of the transducer, where the width of the beam is greatest and the boundaries between structures are parallel to the imaging beam and hence poorly recorded. Two commonly encountered Doppler beam width artifacts are illustrated in Figures 13–38 and 13–39. In Figure 13–39, aortic flow is recorded in early systole at the margin of the beam. However, because the cursor is directed through the mitral valve and the sample volume positioned behind the mitral orifice, it is displayed as if arising from behind the mitral valve. This occurs because the aortic signal is strong and even though the power at the margins of the beam is low, there is no other flow occurring to obscure the aortic signal. The apparent regurgitation is seen only during early systole because atrial filling moves the aorta anteriorly out of the beam path as systole progresses. A second common problem, illustrated in Figure 13–38, is encountered during tricuspid valve recording in patients with mitral regurgitation, left atrial volume overload, and a shift in interatrial septal position toward the right atrium. In these cases, the margins of the beam may actually cross the septum, despite the fact that the cursor is directed through the tricuspid valve orifice. When this occurs and the mitral regurgitant jet is directed to the right, it may inappropriately be interpreted as tricuspid regurgitation. Thus, beam width artifacts are probably

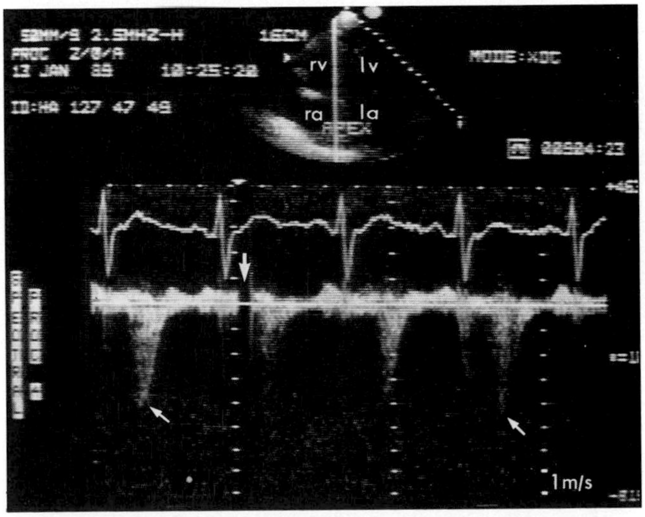

Fig. 13–38. A beamwidth artifact during continuous wave recording. In this example, the left atrium (la) is dilated and the interatrial septum is displaced toward the right atrium (ra). Although the continuous wave Doppler cursor clearly passes through the right atrium, the beamwidth at this level causes a mitral regurgitant jet, which is displaced along the left margin of the interatrial septum to be recorded and displayed as if arising from the right atrium. The oblique arrows indicate the peak velocity, which, in this case, could be inappropriately attributed to tricuspid regurgitation. The vertical arrow indicates an area where the Doppler data have been transferred to the imaging channel to update the "simultaneously recorded image." lv = left ventricle; rv = right ventricle.

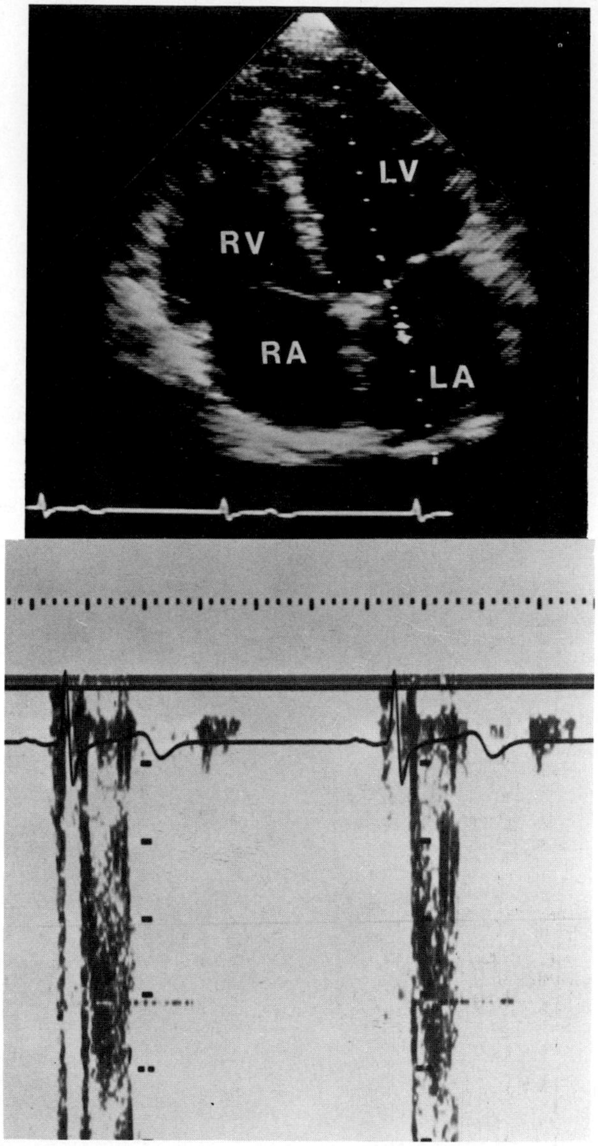

Fig. 13–39. Artifact caused by beamwidth in which aortic outflow velocity is recorded from a left atrial sample volume location. In this example, the beam extending from the apex to the left atrium (LA) has diverged considerably, and its width is well in excess of a centimeter. During systole, there is little flow in the left atrium; however, the margins of the beam encounter the intense outflow signal in the aorta (lower panel), which is displayed as if it arose from the left atrium. The aortic outflow signal is truncated because the aorta moves anteriorly with atrial filling and the flow stream therefore moves out of the beam path in the later part of the systole. LV = left ventricle; RA = right atrium; RV = right ventricle.

more important in Doppler than in imaging because they can lead to misdiagnosis and generally are inapparent unless anticipated and understood. In color flow mapping, these artifacts should be less of a problem and the effects of beam width should be more analogous to those encountered in imaging, i.e., velocity spreading rather than displacement.

Range Ambiguity

Range ambiguity was discussed in Chapter 8 in the section on HiPRF Doppler. In the HiPRF mode, range ambiguity is deliberately introduced to increase the frequency with which a specific target is sampled. The same phenomenon, however, may cause troublesome artifacts when encountered unexpectedly. Range ambiguity can occur whenever multiple pulses containing sufficient energy to generate a recordable echo are traveling through the heart at the same time. Figure 13–40 illustrates this situation. In this example, the sample volume is positioned close to the cardiac apex. However, at the time the most recently transmitted pulse reaches the sample volume location, the pulse from the previous transmission has traveled to the depth of the left atrium. If both of the pulses contain sufficient energy to generate an echo, then the output will be the sum of the two signals and the origin of an individual component will be ambiguous. If there is mitral regurgitation, it will generate the dominant signal; however, because the sample volume locator is set at the level of the apex, the origin of this flow signal would be inappropriately indicated. Although, in this example, the cause of the signal ambiguity should be obvious, other more complex examples are occasionally encountered. Failure to recognize this artifact can lead to misdiagnosis.

DISPLAY PHENOMENA AND ARTIFACTS UNIQUE TO COLOR FLOW MAPPING

Transducer Position and Blood Flow Imaging

Color flow images are by definition a composite of structural and flow data. As discussed earlier, these two parameters are typically not both optimally recorded from the same transducer position or beam direction. It may be less obvious, however, that the same conflicts can occur when imaging flow in different portions of the same scan plane (i.e., that flow in one chamber or area of a chamber may be best recorded from one transducer location, while that in a second region will require a different transducer position to be optimally detected). Thus, the transducer should be placed at the most appropriate position on the chest wall for obtaining blood flow images of optimal quality in the area of interest in the cardiac chamber being imaged, and flow in an entire scan area may require interrogation from multiple locations to be completely revealed. Remember that during life, blood is always moving within the heart, and failure to image flow does not mean that it is not present, but rather reflects inappropriate technique or lack of instrument sensitivity.

Effects of Flow Angle Within the Scan Plane on Color Output

In color flow mapping, the direction of flow is depicted by a certain color series with flow toward the transducer appearing in one color, usually red, and flow away in a second, usually blue. Because the scan plane is formed from a series of radially directed lines, however, flow through a horizontally positioned vessel will be toward the transducer on one side of the scan plane and away from the transducer on the other. Figure 13–41 illustrates this phenomenon. In this example, flow in the inferior vena cava is directed from left to right. At the

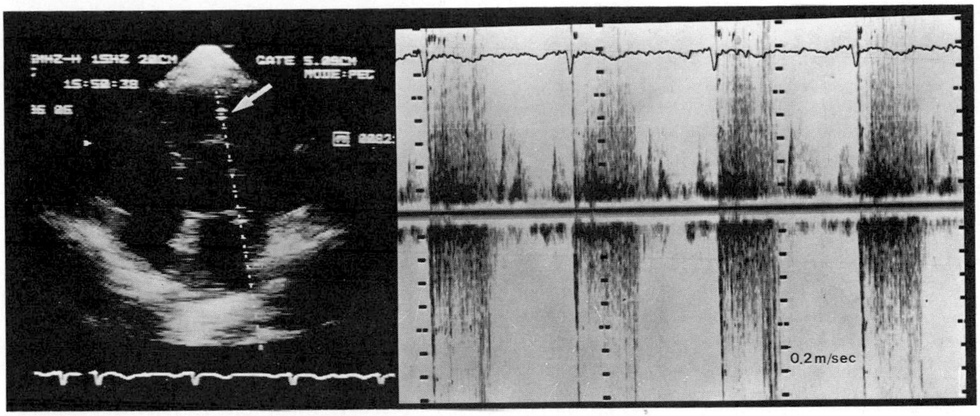

Fig. 13–40. The phenomenon of range ambiguity. In this recording from a patient with mitral regurgitation, the sample volume (white arrow) is placed at the cardiac apex, where no flow is occurring. At twice the range from the transducer to the sample volume or behind the mitral valve, however, there is high velocity flow resulting from mitral regurgitation. The pulse proceeding that indicated by the sample volume will have traveled far enough to place it behind the mitral valve, and the reflected signals from this pulse will be of higher intensity than those from the primary sample volume. As a result, the regurgitant jet will be displayed as if arising from the apex.

right margin of the raster, flow is depicted as red, or toward the transducer. Moving across the raster, flow continues in the same color but with gradually decreasing intensity as a result of an increase in cos Θ as it approaches the center of the scan plane; and once it passes the midpoint, it shifts to blue because the direction of flow is now away from the transducer. If the vessel were aligned at an angle to the scan plane, the point of cross-over would shift correspondingly. Thus, because the direction of flow is related solely to transducer position, the color of a flow stream may change within the image, despite the fact that the direction of flow remains the same.

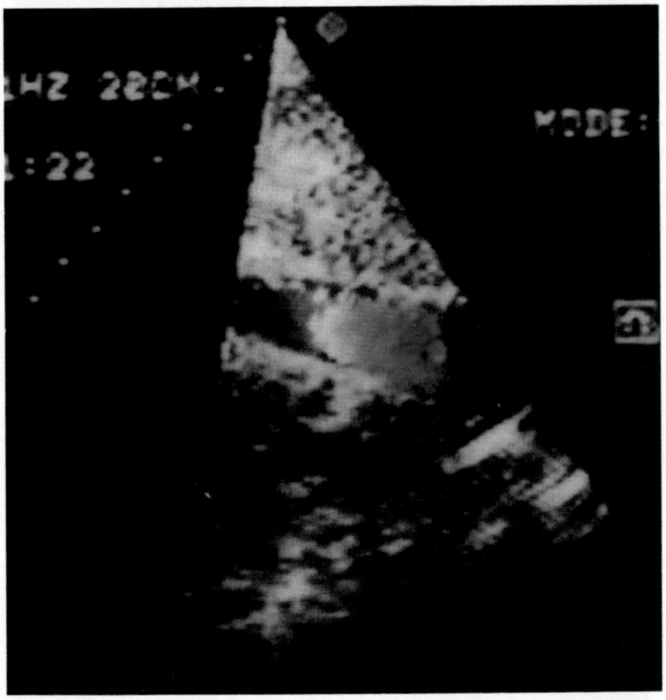

Fig. 13–41. The effects of changes in the orientation of the Doppler beam relative to the flow vector on the color output for flow through a tubular vessel passing obliquely through the scan plane. In this example, flow in the inferior vena cava is directed continuously from left to right. On the left, the flow is depicted as red, indicating flow toward the transducer. It then gradually transitions to blue or flow away from the transducer in the right portion of the scan. This occurs because the angle between the flow vector and the direction of sampling gradually changes as the flow stream proceeds through the scan plane, and hence the instrument output likewise indicates a shift in the direction of flow, despite the fact that none truly occurs.

Color Aliasing

Color flow mappers operate in a pulsed echo mode and hence are subject to the same sampling constraints of any pulsed Doppler system. Therefore, once the Doppler shift frequency exceeds the Nyquist limit, signal aliasing occurs. In a pulsed Doppler system, this is manifest by an apparent shift in the direction of flow, as illustrated in Figure 13–31. Because color flow mappers indicate direction by color series when aliasing occurs in a color flow system, it is represented by a shift from one color series to another. Once the color series changes, if velocity continues to increase, the intensity of the color will initially decrease then invert, increase, shift, etc. Figure 13–42 is a phase diagram for color similar to that for velocity depicted in Figure 13–31. As illustrated, once the phase vector reaches the peak of the red scale, any increase in the phase shift will move it into the blue series, where it will gradually decrease in intensity as velocity increases until eventually it again shifts to red. Velocities often vary spatially within a jet so that the slower moving boundary layers may appear in one color with aliasing occurring and the color reversing in the more rapidly moving central flow stream. For a high velocity lesion, this pattern may repeat several times from the margin of the jet to the central flow core, and an estimate of jet velocity can be obtained from the number of times the signal aliases. Figure 13–43 illustrates the phenomenon for a mitral inflow jet. Within the left atrium, flow toward the mitral orifice and transducer is red. As flow accelerates through the mitral orifice, the red color becomes brighter and then shifts to blue in the center of the jet as a result of aliasing. This shift in color occurs despite the fact that flow continues toward the

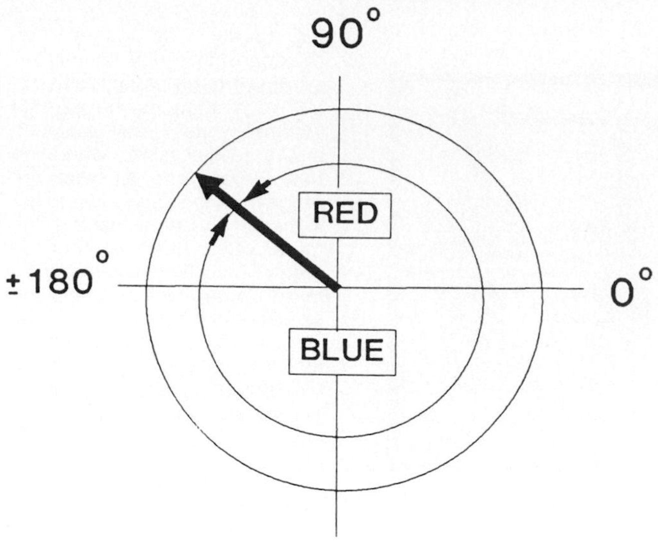

Fig. 13–42. The concept of aliasing for a color flow instrument. In this instance, a shift in color series occurs at the aliasing point, corresponding to the change in direction seen on conventional Doppler recordings. (See text for details.)

transducer. Within the left ventricle, the flow area increases, and velocity decreases. This decrease in flow is accompanied by a reversal of the aliasing pattern and a return to the red color series depicting forward flow.

Reverberations

The concept of reverberations was introduced in Chapter 2, and their effects on images are illustrated in Figure 2–30. Reverberations are secondary reflections that occur along the path of a sound pulse, delaying the return of the signal to the transducer and resulting in targets being displayed multiple times at successively greater depths. Reverberations may occur between a target and the transducer face when the signal strikes the target, is reflected back to the transducer, strikes the transducer face, and is reflected back to the target, etc. In this situation, the reverberations, or "ghost," are typically displayed at twice the distance of the primary target from the transducer, and if the target is moving, the amplitude of motion of the "ghost" will be twice that of the original target. Alternatively, the signal may reverberate between two targets along the beam path, in which case the "ghosts" will be displayed at even multiples of the distance between targets. If these targets are moving, then the apparent amplitude of motion

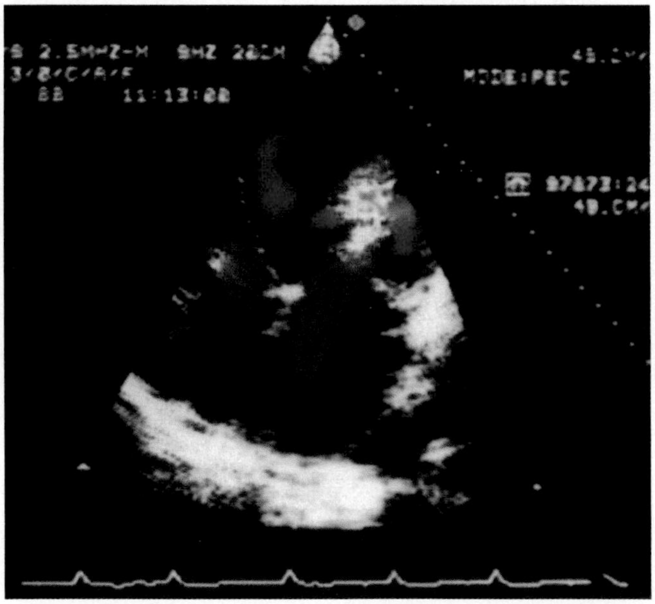

Fig. 13–43. Color flow recording of a mitral inflow jet from a patient with mitral stenosis illustrating the phenomenon of color aliasing. Within the left atrium, flow is toward the mitral orifice and transducer and is output as red. As the flow stream passes through the mitral valve, flow accelerates to reach the peak of the red scale and then aliases to become blue-white, as it enters the left ventricle. Further acceleration occurs at the vena contracta, decreasing the intensity of the blue color. In the body of the left ventricle, flow again decelerates as the area expands, and this process reverses itself with the color initially progressing up the blue spectrum until a cross-over occurs at the red-white interface and then gradually down the red spectrum as flow decelerates.

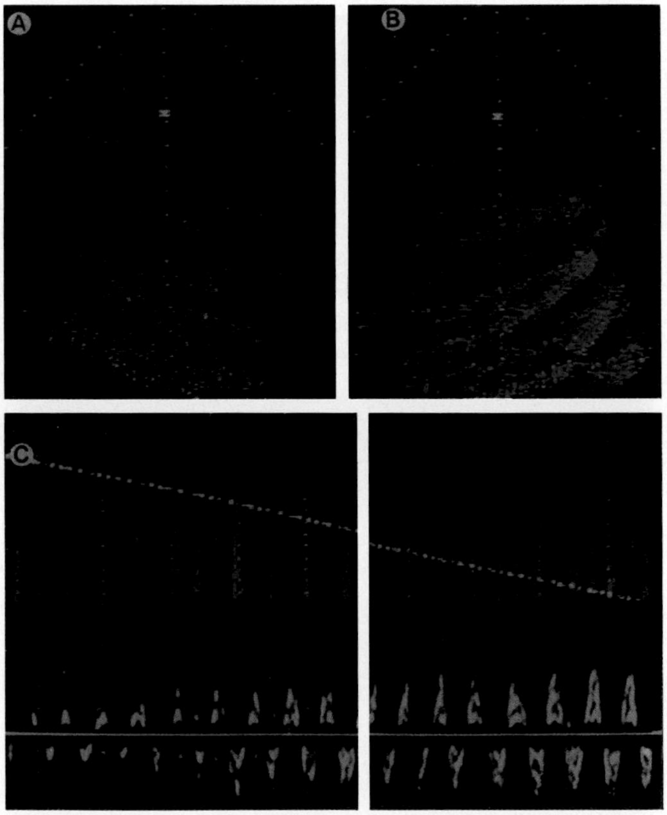

Fig. 13–44. A to **C.** A series of reverberations produced in the experimental model by moving a reflective plate between the transducer and a flow-containing tube. Because of the reverberations, the flow stream is depicted at several levels, which are even multiples of the distance between the tube and the plate. (From Omoto R: Color Atlas of Real-Time Two-Dimensional Doppler Echocardiography. Tokyo, Shindan-to-Chiryo, 1984.)

and velocity of the "ghosts" will also be increased by even multiples of the velocity of the primary target. Reverberations also affect the output of Doppler devices and are most obvious in the color flow format. Figure 13–44 illustrates a series of reverberations produced in an experimental model by moving a reflective plate between the transducer and a flow containing tube. Because of the reverberations, the flow stream is depicted at several levels, which are even multiples of the distance between the tube and the plate, and the apparent velocity of flow also increases (as manifest by an increase in color intensity) with each successive reverberation.

Effects of Wall Shadowing on the Color Display

Finally, in all imaging systems the amplifiers have a high amplitude cutoff, which limits the output of the amplifier to a predetermined peak. When a signal above the amplifier cutoff is followed by a weak signal, the amplifier suppression (high amplitude cutoff) must cease, and the amplifier must be reset to output the weaker signal. This process requires a minute time period, during which the weaker signal is suppressed, resulting in a phenomenon known as *acoustic shadowing*. In color flow mapping, a strong structural signal may result in transient suppression of immediately following but weaker Doppler signals with the result that there is insufficient voltage to produce any output from the digital scan converter and the image will be left blank for that pixel or series of pixels.

REFERENCES

1. Edler I: Diagnostic use of ultrasound in heart disease. Acta Med Scand 308: 32, 1955.
2. Wells PNT: Biomedical Ultrasonics. New York, Academic Press, 1977.
3. Sigelmann RA, Reid JM: Analysis and measurement of ultrasound backscatterers excited by sine wave bursts. J Acoust Soc Am 53:1351, 1973.
4. Shung KK, Sigelmann RA, Reid JM: The scattering of ultrasound by red blood cells. NBS Special Publication 453, October 1976.
5. Angelsen B: A theoretical study of the scattering of ultrasound from blood. IEEE Trans Biomed Eng 27:61, 1980.
6. Johnson SL, Baker DW, Lute RA, Dodge HT: Doppler echocardiography: the localization of cardiac murmurs. Circulation 48:810, 1973.
7. Baker DW, Rubenstein SA, Lorch GS: Pulsed Doppler echocardiography principles and application. Am J Med 63:69, 1977.
8. Hatle L, Angelsen B: Doppler Ultrasound in Cardiology: Physical Principles and Clinical Applications. Philadelphia, Lea & Febiger, 1985.
9. Omoto R: Color Atlas of Real Time Two-Dimensional Doppler Echocardiography. Tokyo, Shindan-to-Chiryo, 1984.
10. Griffith JM, Henry WL: An ultrasound system for combined cardiac imaging and Doppler blood flow measurement in man. Circulation 57:925, 1978.
11. Levine RA, et al.: How often does Doppler echocardiography provide information otherwise unavailable by imaging studies: experience in 100 patients. J Am Coll Cardiol 5:388, 1985.

CHAPTER

14

M-MODE ECHOCARDIOGRAPHY: PRINCIPLES AND EXAMINATION TECHNIQUES

MICHAEL H. PICARD

The last of the major echocardiographic techniques to be discussed is M-mode echocardiography. M-mode echocardiography was initially described in the early 1950s and for nearly two decades was the only clinically useful format for ultrasonic study of the heart. Therefore, during this period, virtually all the advances in ultrasonic cardiac imaging and diagnosis were based on M-mode recordings. Although the development of two-dimensional and Doppler echocardiography has diminished the importance of the M-mode approach, it is still an integral part of a complete cardiac ultrasound examination. Its role, however, has changed from that of a primary, independent procedure to a more limited adjunct to two-dimensional echocardiography.

HISTORY

M-mode echocardiography was first described by Edler and Hertz, working at the University of Lund, Sweden, in 1954.[1] Dr. Edler (Fig. 14–1) was motivated to explore the use of ultrasound as a means of studying the heart by the introduction of closed mitral commissurotomy for mitral stenosis. Appropriate referral for this procedure required separation of those patients with pure mitral stenosis from those with mixed mitral stenosis and regurgitation. Contrast ventriculography had yet to be invented, and there was a need to assess the severity of regurgitation because commissurotomy was contraindicated in patients with regurgitation as the primary lesion. To test the potential of ultrasound, Drs. Edler and Hertz borrowed a commercial echograph designed for metal flaw detection from the shipyards at Malmo, Sweden, With the transducer applied directly on the precordium and the sound pulse directed toward the heart, an echo was observed moving back and forth along the x axis of the oscilloscope screen at a depth of 8 to 9 cm from the chest wall (Fig. 14–2). Using a commercial ultrasonic reflectoscope, they continued their work and demonstrated that the blood-heart interface reflected sound to a sufficient degree that it could be detected and recorded. They confirmed their observations using water-filled, transected, isolated human heart preparations in which they validated the recorded thicknesses of the ventricular walls and detected echoes from a thrombus placed in the left ventricular cavity (Fig. 14–3).

To record continuously the changing depth of the echoes from the moving cardiac structures observed in clinical studies, Edler and colleagues devised the recording system now known as the *time-motion,* or *M-mode presentation*. In their original system, the output of the oscilloscope was photographed by film that was exposed as it passed in front of the oscilloscope at a constant speed (Figs. 14–4 and 14–5). The echoes from nonmoving structures appeared on the film as straight lines, while those from moving structures changed position in parallel with the motion of the structure from which they were reflected. With this technique, the posterior wall

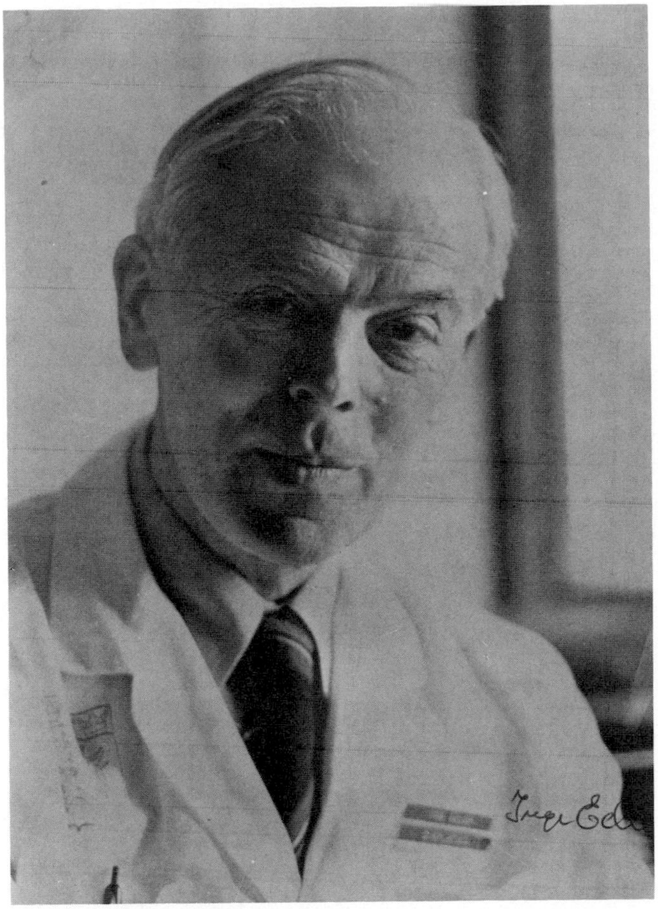

Fig. 14–1. Dr. Inge Edler, the first cardiologist to demonstrate the potential of ultrasound for cardiac diagnosis. For his pioneering work, he is generally recognized as "the father of echocardiography."

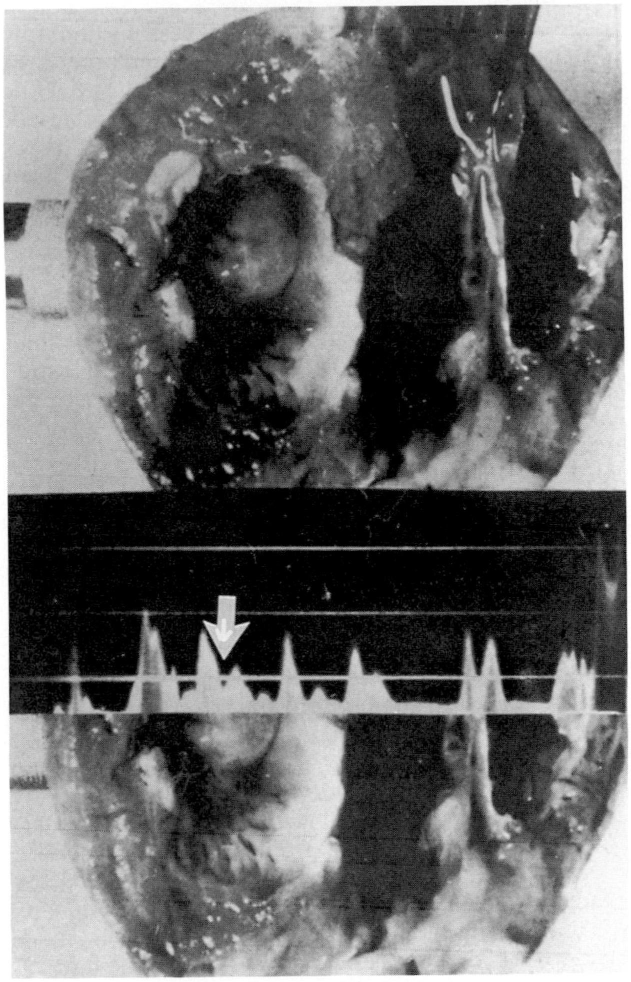

Fig. 14–3. The in vitro model of Edler and Hertz from which they measured the thickness of ventricular walls and recorded echoes from a left ventricular thrombus (arrow). (From Edler I, Hertz CH: The use of ultrasonic reflectoscope for the continuous recording of movements of heart walls. Kung Fysiogr Sallsk i Lund forhandl 24:5, 1954.)

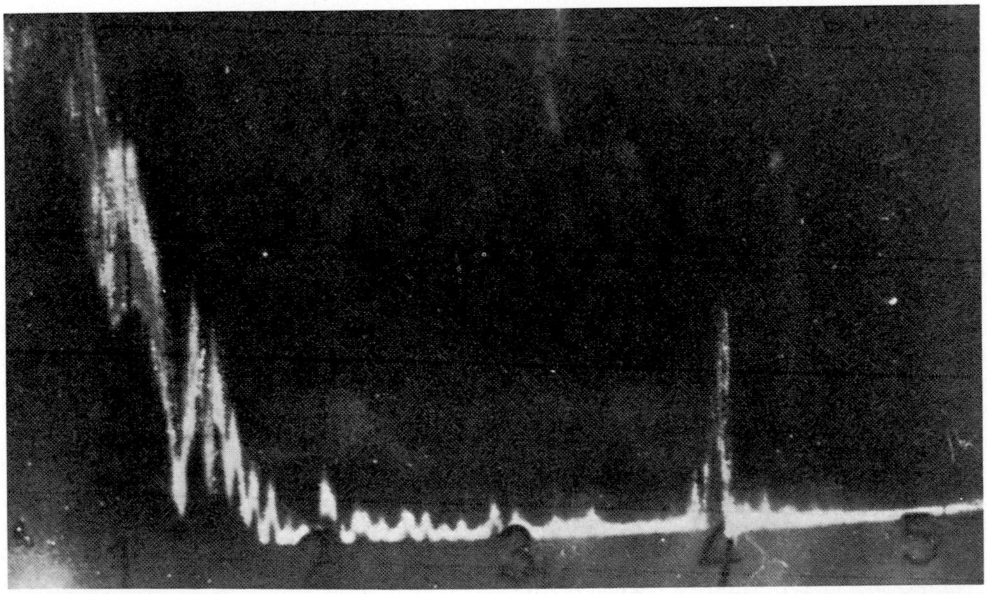

Fig. 14–2. Oscilloscopic recording of the first A-mode experiment by Edler and Hertz showing a clearly defined echo that moved back and forth along the X-axis. (From Edler I: *In* I. Donald and S. Levi (eds.): Diagnostic Ultrasound. Kooyker Scientific Publications, Rotterdam, Netherlands. 1976.)

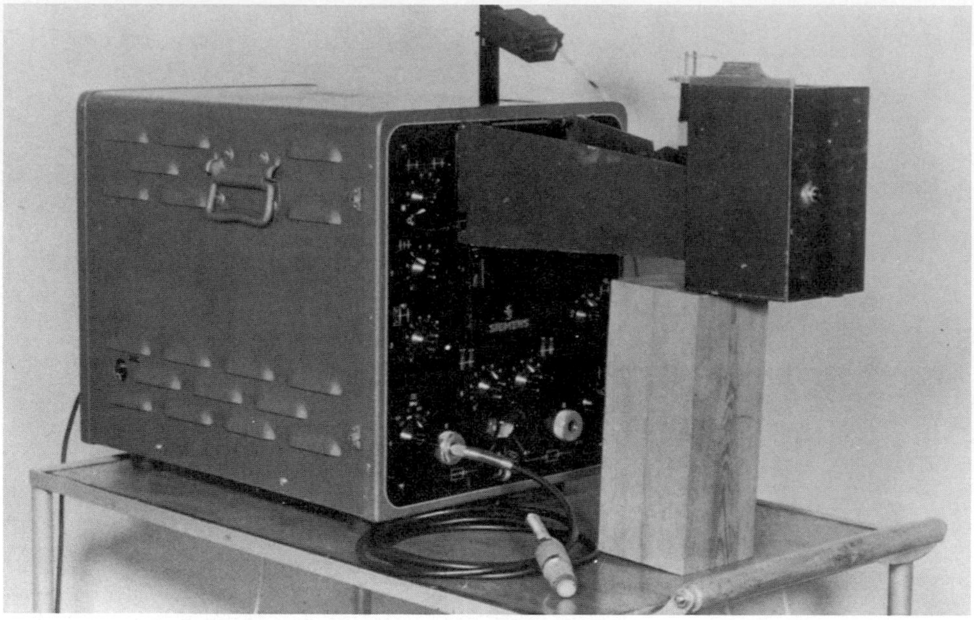

Fig. 14–4. The echograph used by Edler and Hertz. Originally designed for detection of flaws in metal structures, it was adapted for echocardiography. (From Edler I: The use of ultrasound as a diagnostic aid and its effects on biologic tissues. Acta Med Scand Suppl 370:39, 1961.)

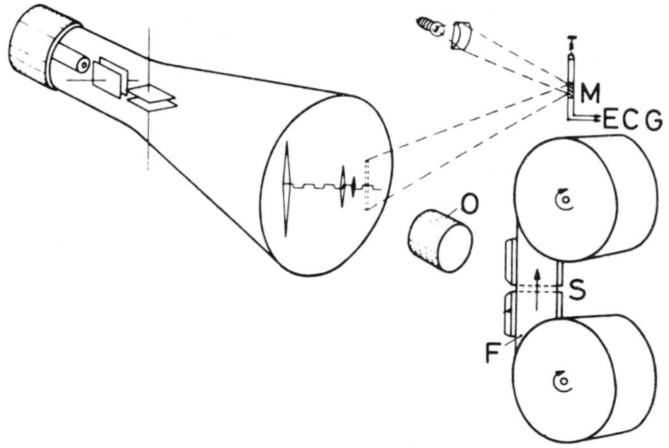

Fig. 14–5. The system for recording the first simultaneous M-mode echocardiogram and electrocardiogram on film. The film (F) passes a slot (S) at a constant speed. An oscilloscope mirror (M) reflects light from the electrocardiographic signal (ECG) as a vertical line on the oscilloscope screen at the same level as the echo signals, and both are projected to the film through a lens (O). (From Edler I: The use of ultrasound as a diagnostic aid and its effects on biologic tissues. Acta Med Scand Suppl 370:39, 1961.)

echoes of the left ventricle were recorded in adult patients and correlated with the location of the posterior wall on chest x-ray (Fig. 14–6).

The anterior leaflet of the mitral valve was also identified during these early investigations (Fig. 14–7). In 1955 Dr. Edler reported the difference in the mitral valve motion patterns of patients with pure mitral stenosis and those with mixed mitral valve disease.[2] This observation was extended to show the changes in the pattern of the stenotic mitral valve following commissurotomy.

Other early applications of M-mode echocardiography included the demonstration of atrial wall motion during atrial flutter and the diagnosis and follow-up of pericardial effusion (Fig. 14–8).[2–4] Edler and Hertz recorded

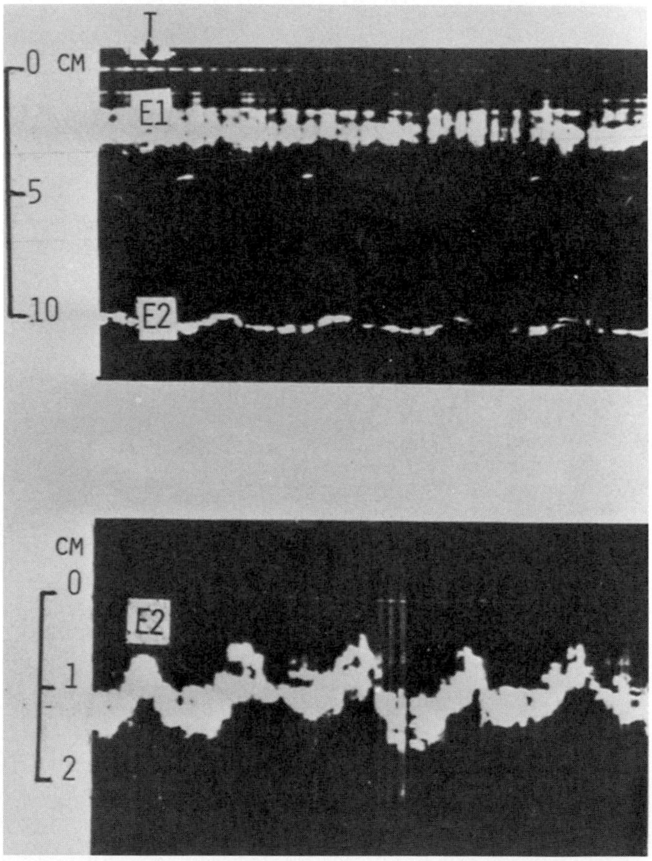

Fig. 14–6. The first recorded M-mode echocardiogram. Top. Low magnification photograph. E1 depicts echoes from the anterior chest wall, and E2 represents echoes from the posterior wall of the left ventricle at a depth of 10 cm from the transducer. Bottom. A higher magnification of the motion of the posterior wall of the left ventricle. (From Edler I: *In* I. Donald and S. Levi (eds.): Diagnostic Ultrasound. Rotterdam, Netherlands. Kooyker Scientific Publications, 1976.)

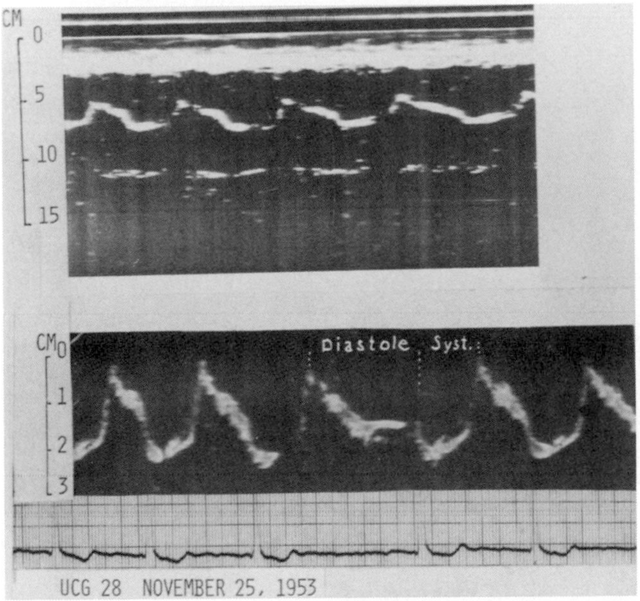

Fig. 14–7. The first M-mode echocardiographic recordings of the mitral valve. (From Edler I: The diagnostic use of ultrasound in heart disease. Acta Med Scand Suppl 308:32, 1955.)

the left atrial myxoma pattern in 1956 (Fig. 14–9), but the first published case was by Effert and Domanig in 1959.[5] Following the introduction of the more sensitive barium titanate crystal, the location, amplitude, and motion patterns of all the valves were recorded.

For his pioneering studies, Dr. Edler was awarded the Lasker Prize and is recognized as the Father of Echocardiography.

In 1959, Effert, Hertz, and Böhme described a method to simultaneously record the echocardiogram with other measurements such as the electrocardiogram, phonocardiogram, and intracardiac pressure. This sparked investigations into the significance of the motion patterns of various intracardiac echoes and their relationship to recognized physiologic events.[6]

In the early 1960s, Joyner, Reid, and Bond introduced echocardiography in the United States and confirmed the original work of Edler and Hertz in diagnosing mitral valve disease.[7–9] In 1965 Feigenbaum demonstrated the M-mode diagnosis of pericardial effusion in a canine model. Anterior pericardial effusions were soon demonstrated in humans.[10] These studies stimulated interest in echocardiography in this country, and soon similar results were reported by other investigators.[11–16] Feigenbaum and co-workers developed techniques for visualizing and measuring the posterior left ventricular wall thickness,[17] the left ventricular internal dimension,[18,19] and left ventricular stroke volume.[20–22] Further refinements in the M-mode technique were motivated by the hope that it could provide an accurate assessment of left ventricular function and obviate the need for invasive measurements.

Further identification of cardiac structures on M-mode was assisted by the use of contrast echocardiography by Gramiak and colleagues.[23] The use of contrast validated the location and motion of the aortic and pulmonic valves, the interatrial septum, the left ventricular endocardium, and a variety of other important cardiac structures (contrast echocardiography is discussed in greater detail in Chapter 15).

By 1970, the identities of most of the normal cardiac structures seen on the M-mode were established. The

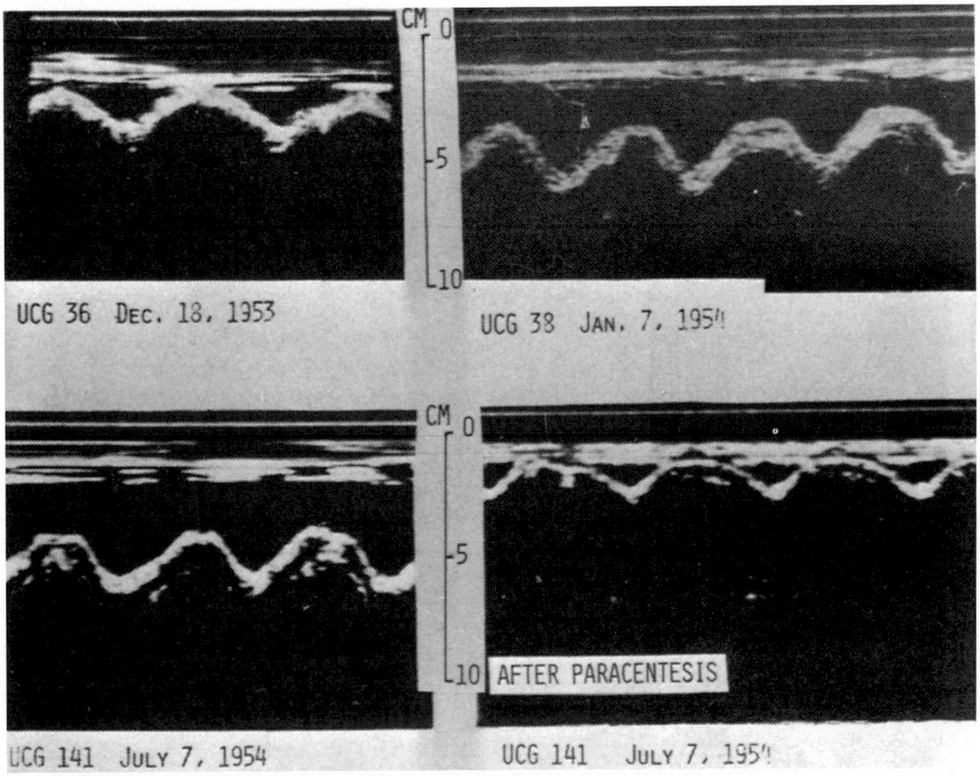

Fig. 14–8. Top. Serial echocardiograms from a patient with pericardial effusion. Bottom. The same patient after pericardiocentesis. (From Edler I: The history of cardiac ultrasound. *In* Giuliani ER (ed.): Two-Dimensional Real-Time Ultrasonic Imaging of the Heart. Boston, Martinus Nijhoff Publishing, 1985.)

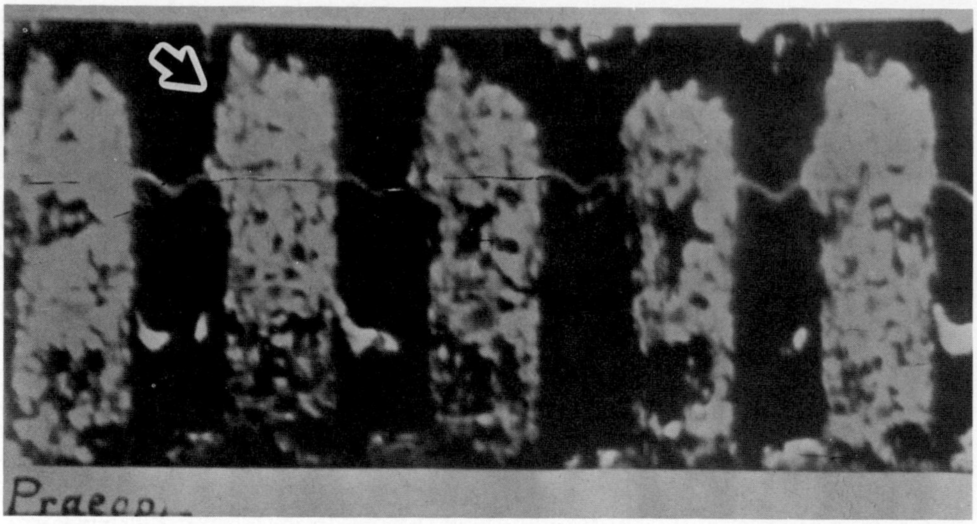

Fig. 14–9. An M-mode echocardiogram recorded by Edler in a patient with suspected mitral stenosis that was subsequently diagnosed as a left atrial myxoma. The echoes from the myxoma were best recorded in diastole as the tumor moved across the valve (arrow). (From Edler I: The history of cardiac ultrasound. *In* Giuliani ER (ed.): Two-Dimensional Real-Time Ultrasonic Imaging of the Heart. Boston, Martinus Nijhoff Publishing, 1985.)

next advance was the establishment of criteria for and use of M-mode echocardiography in the diagnosis and assessment of cardiac disease states. Abnormalities such as left atrial myxoma, idiopathic hypertrophic subaortic stenosis, pulmonic stenosis, mitral valve prolapse, and diseases associated with paradoxic ventricular septal motion such as atrial septal defect were reported in the late 1960s and early 1970s. As equipment improved and an increasing number of skilled investigators entered the field, there was rapid expansion of the role of the M-mode technique in cardiac diagnosis and functional assessment. This growth, however, was short-lived, peaking in the mid- to late 70s and then falling off rapidly as two-dimensional instrumentation became increasingly available. Today, M-mode echocardiography has virtually ceased to exist as a stand-alone modality. Despite this decline, M-mode clearly laid the foundation for modern echocardiography and continues to provide unique physiologic insights because of its high temporal resolution and convenient graphic display.

TECHNICAL ASPECTS

The M-Mode Display

The basic concepts of M-mode echocardiography have changed little from the original approach used by Edler. As discussed in Chapter 1, the M-mode, or time motion, display uses the basic B-mode data line as the source of image generation. In the M-mode format, sequentially recorded B-mode data lines from the same line of sight are swept across the face of the display screen from left to right at a constant, adjustable sweep rate. The rapid sampling of the same region, a result of the relatively fixed transducer location, places sequential parallel data lines so close together that individual points of brightness appear as continuous horizontal lines as they are swept across the screen. Sweeping the lines at a fixed rate permits the precise recording of the position and motion pattern of echoes from intracardiac structures relative to time.

The M-Mode Recording

Although, historically, most M-mode studies were performed using dedicated, stand-alone M-mode instruments, today, M-mode studies are almost universally acquired using instruments designed primarily for two-dimensional imaging. Most cross-sectional echographs permit M-mode recordings to be obtained with the same transducer and basic instrumentation used for two-dimensional studies. The location of M-mode sampling is determined by the position of a cursor superimposed on the cross-sectional display. This cursor appears as a line whose origin is fixed at the apex of the sector and thus is displayed as if it originated at the center of the transducer. The cursor can typically be directed through an arc of 90° or more, and an M-mode can be obtained at any location in this arc or along any ''line of sight'' within the two-dimensional image (Fig. 14–10).

The acquisition of data is a function of the basic type of instrument used (i.e., a mechanical sector or phased array scanner). To record and display M-mode data, mechanical scanners require the transducer to stop at a specific point and display all data lines in M-mode format. Phased array systems, in contrast, exhibit considerably more flexibility because they permit the direction of each data line to be individually determined. For example, (1) they can display all of the data acquired from any azimuthal angle in an M-mode format; (2) they can display a portion of the data lines in an M-mode format and use the remaining data to form a simultaneous cross-sectional image; (3) they can record simultaneous M-modes from two or more locations in the scan plane by alternately sampling from different directions and using the data from each angular direction to form a separate M-mode; and (4) finally, with a phased array system, they permit recording of two or more separate B-mode lines as simultaneous M-modes while still preserving a high enough line density to record a recognizable cross-sectional image (Fig. 14–11). Because the cross-sectional image is simultaneously recorded with the M-mode, the position of the M-mode can be more precisely maintained. Both mechanical and phased array systems can also record an M-mode sweep at a fixed rate through the full 90° sector. This is analogous to the manual M-mode sweep illustrated in Fig. 1–28. In the former case, however, the sweep speed is rigidly controlled. In the phased array format where data can be shared, both the M-mode sweep and the underlying two-dimensional image can be recorded simultaneously.

The depth of M-mode sampling, like that of two-dimensional echocardiographic display, is adjusted by changes in the depth of field. By varying the time of onset and the duration of sampling relative to the time of pulse transmission, one can create a variable window for localized M-mode sampling. This M-mode "window" can then be enlarged to the full area of the display

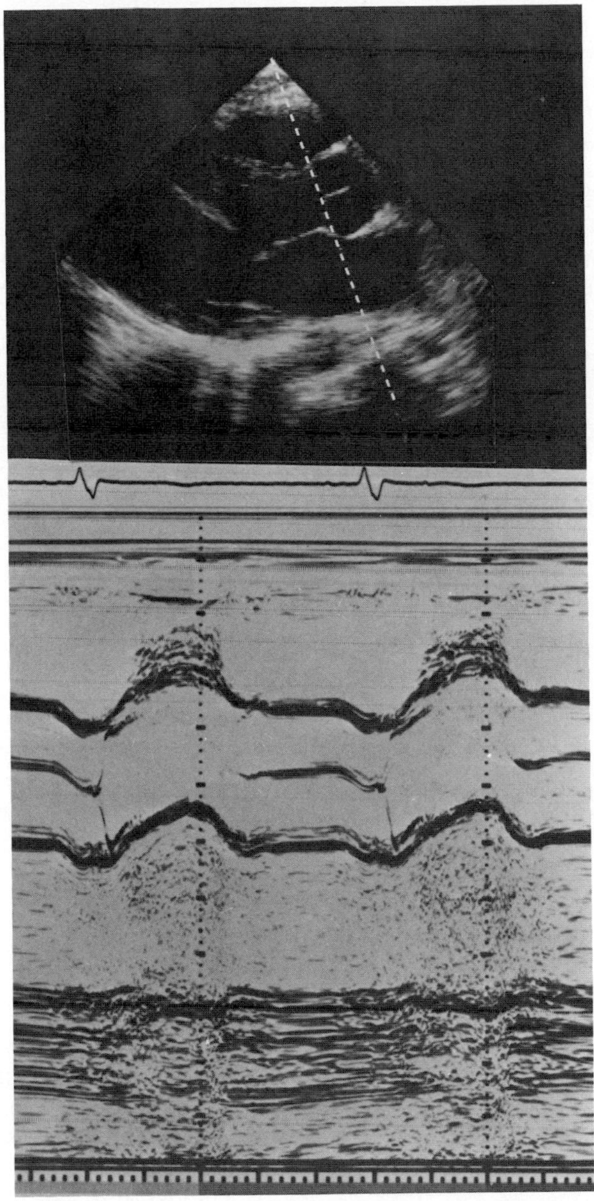

Fig. 14–10. M-mode cursor superimposed over a two-dimensional echocardiogram representing the location of M-mode sampling. The cursor can be directed across the sector, and the corresponding M-mode echocardiogram can be recorded at any of these locations.

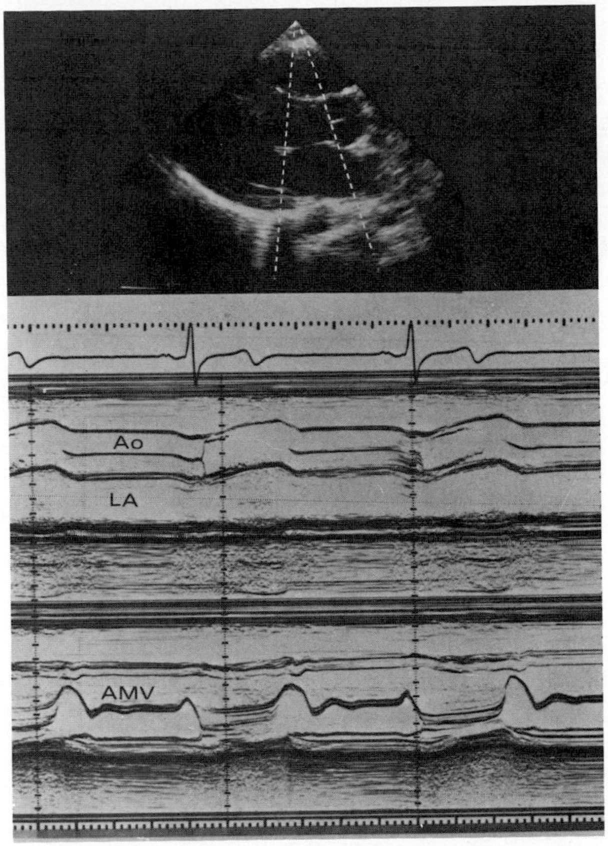

Fig. 14–11. With a phased array scanner, two separate M-mode echocardiograms can be simultaneously recorded while preserving a high enough line density to record a cross-sectional image. Ao = aorta; LA = left atrium; AMV = anterior mitral valve.

screen, thereby expanding the image with or without loss of resolution.

The M-Mode Examination

The routine M-mode echocardiographic examination includes recordings of the four cardiac valves, the left atrium, the aorta, and the left ventricle. The right ventricle is also transected, but the path along which the M-mode beam traverses the right ventricle is inconsistent and unpredictable. Hence, the derived measurements are only an approximation of right ventricular size. The majority of the M-mode data can be derived from the two-dimensional parasternal long axis view of the left ventricle because this view includes five of the seven M-mode structures of primary interest (aortic valve, aorta, left atrium, mitral valve, and left ventricle) (see Chapter 5). The remaining structures, the tricuspid and pulmonic valves, are generally recorded using the parasternal long axis views of the right ventricular inflow tract and pulmonary artery, respectively.

M-mode recordings can be obtained from several interspaces in the parasternal window. However, the optimum interspace is that from which the ultrasound beam will be perpendicular to the structure or structures of interest. Because the parasternal long axis plane includes an extensive area of the left heart, it is often not

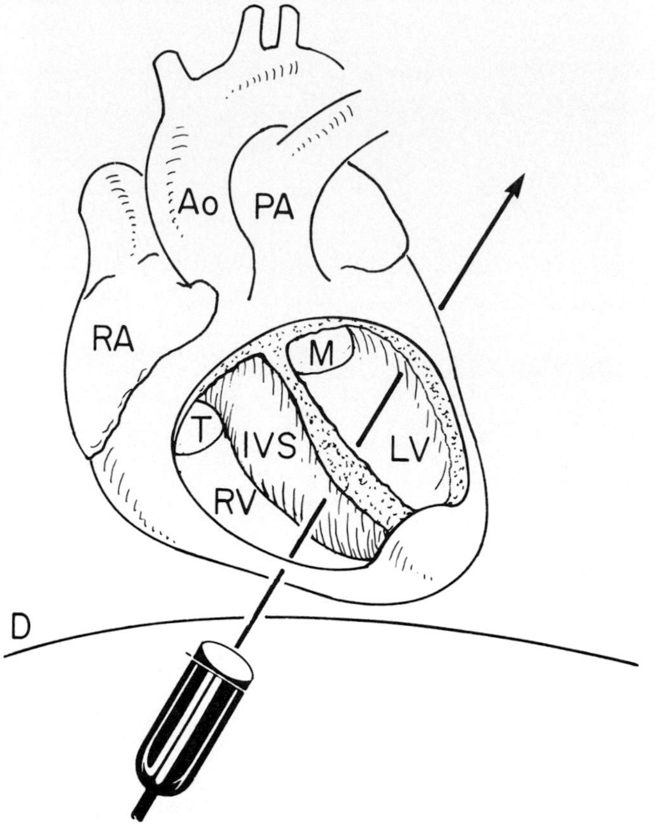

Fig. 14–12. The heart from the subcostal position. The M-mode transects the free wall of the right ventricle, the right ventricular cavity (RV), the interventricular septum (IVS), the left ventricular cavity (LV), and the lateral wall of the left ventricle. RA = right atrium; Ao = aorta; PA = pulmonary artery; T = tricuspid valve; M = mitral valve.

possible to align the cursor appropriately to record each of the structures of interest within the region from the same transducer location. In these cases, the transducer must be shifted up or down one or more interspaces or the scan plane angled or rotated slightly to direct the cursor to optimally transect the desired structure.

Although M-mode images are most often obtained from parasternal long axis planes, cardiac structures can be recorded from the parasternal short axis view. As with recordings from the parasternal long axis, the scan plane and the cursor must be properly angled to transect structures along a path that is perpendicular to the long axis of the structure of interest.

When images from the parasternal window are inadequate for analysis, M-mode recordings from the subcostal or suprasternal windows may provide the necessary information.[24,25] Figure 14–12 shows the path of the ultrasound beam from the subcostal transducer position. Although the beam transects the left ventricle from a different projection, the M-mode recordings of the ventricular cavity are similar to those from the parasternal window. In the symmetrically contracting left ventricle, measurements of subcostal M-mode images correlate highly with companion parasternal dimensions.[26] Measurements from the subcostal window, however, are subject to greater variation, presumably as a result of the difficulties in obtaining recordings that are perpendicular to the true long axis of the left ventricle.

Suprasternal M-mode echocardiography can provide recordings of the aortic arch, right pulmonary artery, and left atrium.[25,27] Although the ability to demonstrate the relationship of the aorta and pulmonary arteries was suggested to be of importance in differentiating subtypes of congenital heart disease, this application of suprasternal M-mode echocardiography has been superseded by two-dimensional imaging.[28–30]

MOTION PATTERNS AND MEASUREMENTS OF MAJOR STRUCTURES BY M-MODE

Mitral Valve

The mitral valve M-mode, as previously noted, is usually derived from the two-dimensional parasternal long axis view. To record the mitral valve M-mode from this cross-sectional view, the operator should position the cursor perpendicular to the ventricular long axis and pass through the mitral leaflet tips. This path will result in the beam passing through the anterior chest wall, the right ventricle, the interventricular septum, the anterior and posterior leaflets of the mitral valve, and the posterior left ventricular wall (Fig. 14–13C). By medial or lateral angulation of the scan plane or realignment of the

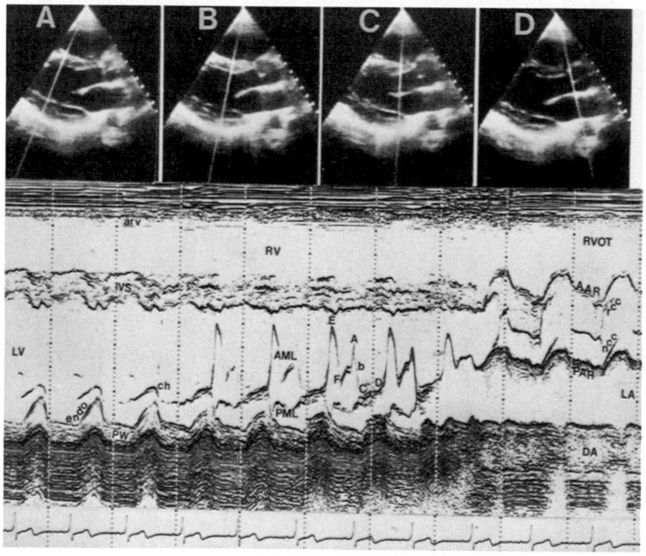

Fig. 14–13. Changes in M-mode cursor positions during a standard sweep from the left ventricular apex to the aortic valve. **A.** M-mode recorded through the mid left ventricle. **B.** M-mode recorded at the tips of the mitral leaflets, the standard path for recording the left ventricular internal dimension. **C.** The M-mode line represents the cursor position when optimally recording the mitral valve. **D.** The M-mode line illustrates the optimal path for recording the aortic valve and left atrium. arv = anterior wall of the right ventricle; RV = right ventricular cavity; RVOT = right ventricular outflow tract; IVS = interventricular septum; LV = left ventricular cavity; endo-posterior wall endocardium; PW = posterior wall of the left ventricle; ch = chordae tendinae; AML = anterior leaflet of the mitral valve; PML = posterior leaflet of the mitral valve; AAR = anterior wall of the aortic root; rcc = right coronary cusp; ncc = noncoronary cusp; PAR = posterior wall of the aortic root; LA = left atrium; DA = descending aorta. (From Harrigan P, Lee R: Principles of Interpretation in Echocardiography. New York, John Wiley & Sons, 1985.)

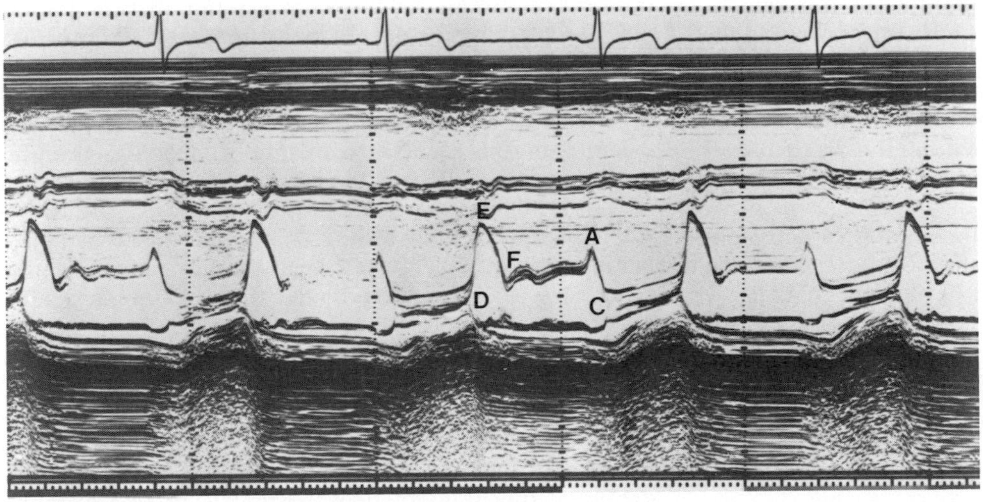

Fig. 14–14. A typical M-mode recording of the mitral valve including letter designations of the motion pattern. (See text for explanation.)

cursor, the image should be optimized to record echoes from both mitral valve leaflets. Figure 14–14 is an example of an M-mode recording of a normal mitral valve. The motion pattern of the anterior mitral leaflet has an M-shaped configuration, while the posterior leaflet appears as a blunted W. Various key points on the mitral valve echo have been designated by letters.[31] Taken sequentially, the A point corresponds to the point of peak leaflet separation following atrial contraction. With atrial relaxation, valve closure begins and the leaflets approach each other. The B point, although not apparent in this recording, corresponds to the position of the leaflets at the onset of ventricular systole, while the point at which they coapt is designated as the C point. The coapted leaflets then move gradually anteriorly in parallel with the normal anterior systolic motion of the base of the heart during systole. At the onset of diastole (point D), leaflet separation occurs with the leaflets moving rapidly apart to their point of maximal diastolic excursion in response to passive filling at the E point. As initial diastolic inflow diminishes, the leaflets drift toward each other, reaching their most closely apposed mid-diastolic position (F point) at the end of the rapid filling phase. The overall rate of this motion is described by the E-F slope. This is followed by a variable period (diastasis) leading up to the next A wave. The same points of posterior leaflet motion are noted by the same letter designations along with an apostrophe.

A variety of measurements can be made from the mitral valve M-mode recording and are shown in Figure 14–15. The diastolic opening velocity is measured as the slope from the D point to the E point. The maximum excursion of the anterior leaflet of the mitral valve is measured from the E point to the extension of the D point, and the maximum leaflet separation is measured from point E to point E′. Although the early diastolic closing velocity is composed of a deceleration phase (E-F_0) and an acceleration phase (F_0-F), the closing velocity is commonly measured as the E to F slope.

The Aortic Valve, Left Atrium, and Aorta

To record the aortic valve, left atrium, and aorta, the operator directs the cursor through the aorta at the level of the aortic valve cusps and as perpendicular as possible to the aortic long axis. The goal is to image two cusps simultaneously and record their full excursion pattern.

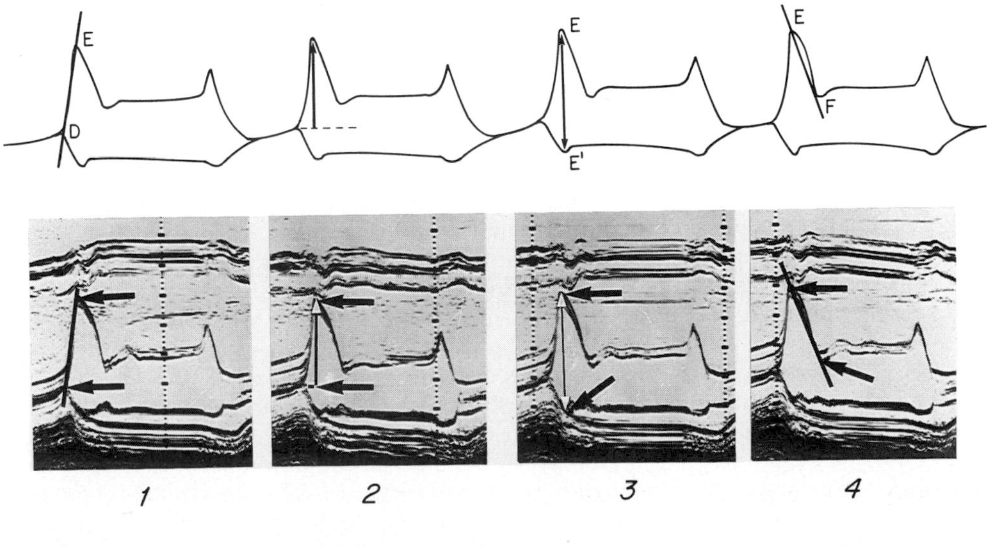

Fig. 14–15. Measurements from the mitral valve M-mode. (1) Diastolic opening velocity. (2) Maximum excursion of the anterior leaflet. (3) Maximum leaflet separation. (4) Early diastolic closing velocity. (See text for explanation.)

At the aortic valve level, the beam passes through the anterior chest wall, the right ventricle, the aorta, and the left atrium (Fig. 14–13D).

The two leaflets seen within the aortic root are typically the right coronary cusp anteriorly and the noncoronary cusp posteriorly. During diastole, the coapted leaflets appear as a single dark linear echo in the center of the aortic root. With the onset of ventricular ejection, the echoes from the two leaflets separate rapidly and, during systolic ejection, lie parallel to the anterior and posterior walls of the aortic root. At the onset of diastole (when left ventricular pressure falls below aortic pressure), the echoes rapidly return to the midline and continue in this coapted position until the next ejection. The single diastolic echo, rapid opening, systolic separation and rapid closure give a rectangular appearance to the aortic valve echo. Letter designations of the points of this pattern are not routinely used.

The left atrium is recorded from the same transducer position as the aortic valve recordings. Although the posterior wall of the aorta and the anterior wall of the left atrium are separate structures, they produce a single thick echo on the M-mode recording. The filling and emptying of the left atrium account for the motion pattern of this wall.[32] During ventricular systole, the left atrium fills and the wall is displaced anteriorly. With the onset of diastole, the wall moves rapidly posteriorly as the left atrium empties. This is followed by a variable period without significant wall motion, during which the left atrium acts as a conduit for blood flowing from the pulmonary veins to the left ventricle. With atrial contraction there is further posterior displacement of the anterior wall. The posterior wall of the left atrium is represented by a continuous echo posterior to the left atrial cavity. The posterior left atrial wall often appears flat without anteroposterior amplitude, although it can exhibit motion reflecting the filling and emptying of the chamber as well as atrial contraction.

With proper positioning of the transducer, M-mode recordings of the ascending aorta can be made at three different levels. At the level at which the aortic valve leaflets are recorded, the surrounding aortic root echoes, above and below the valve leaflets, originate from the sinuses of Valsalva. By moving the cursor caudad, the operator can record the aortic annulus at the point where the aortic valve leaflets are attached to the aortic walls. More cephalad, the aortic root is recorded at the junction of the sinuses of Valsalva and the tubular portion of the aorta (the sinotubular junction). The motion of the aorta at all three levels is similar. The motion of the posterior wall of the aorta is the same as described previously for the anterior wall of the left atrium. The anterior aortic wall motion is roughly parallel to this posterior wall. The amplitude of anterior motion of the anterior wall in systole is greater than that of the posterior wall, and this reflects the expansion of the aorta during ventricular ejection.[33]

The aorta is measured in the same fashion at all levels. The diameter of the vessel is measured at end-diastole from the inner edge of the echo of the anterior wall of the aorta to the leading edge of the echo of the posterior wall of the aorta. The importance of this measurement convention will be demonstrated in the chapter discussing Doppler cardiac output measurements (Chapter 30).

The recordings of the leaflets of the aortic valve reflect flow across the valve and can be used to calculate systolic time intervals (see Fig. 14–22). When calculating systolic time intervals, the examiner measures the preejection period (PEP) of the left ventricle from the onset of ventricular systole as noted by the onset of the Q wave on the electrocardiogram to the onset of aortic leaflet opening. The left ventricular ejection time (LVET) is the period from the onset of aortic leaflet opening to their closure. The ratio of these two values, PEP/LVET, provides an index of left ventricular performance.

The left atrium is measured from the same beat as that used for aortic measurements but at end-systole, as defined by the end of the T wave of the electrocardiogram or the point of peak anterior movement of the aorta. The goal is to measure the anteroposterior diameter of the left atrium at the point of its maximal distension. The diameter is measured from the trailing edge of the posterior aortic/anterior left atrial wall to the leading edge of the left atrial posterior wall.

The Tricuspid Valve

The tricuspid valve M-mode is recorded using the parasternal long axis right ventricular inflow view. As with the mitral valve, the cursor is positioned to pass through the bodies of the anterior and posterior tricuspid valve leaflets and to be roughly orthogonal to the right ventricular long axis. Note that in this orientation the posterior rather than septal tricuspid leaflet is recorded. The motion of the tricuspid valve is similar on M-mode recordings to mitral motion, although the timing differs slightly. The tricuspid valve usually closes within 40 msec after mitral valve closure.[34] In many cases, only the anterior leaflet is recorded, although two leaflets can be imaged when right ventricular enlargement is present. The same letter designations used in describing mitral valve motion are applied to the tricuspid valve motion pattern (Fig. 14–16).

Along with the timing of tricuspid valve opening and closure, the velocity of leaflet opening (D-E slope) and the rate of early diastolic closure (E-F slope) can be measured.

The Pulmonic Valve and Pulmonary Artery

The long and short axis parasternal right ventricular outflow views are used to record the pulmonic valve and pulmonary artery. Pulmonic valve M-mode motion is more difficult to record from the parasternal transducer location than that of the other cardiac valves, even though the anterior and posterior leaflets are visualized by the two-dimensional echocardiogram. This difficulty arises because the plane of the valve is situated such that when the transducer and M-mode cursor are positioned to record the pulmonic valve, the cursor commonly passes beneath the anterior leaflet and only intersects the posterior leaflet of the valve. Although both the anterior and a posterior pulmonary cusp are occasionally visualized (Fig. 14–17), an isolated posterior

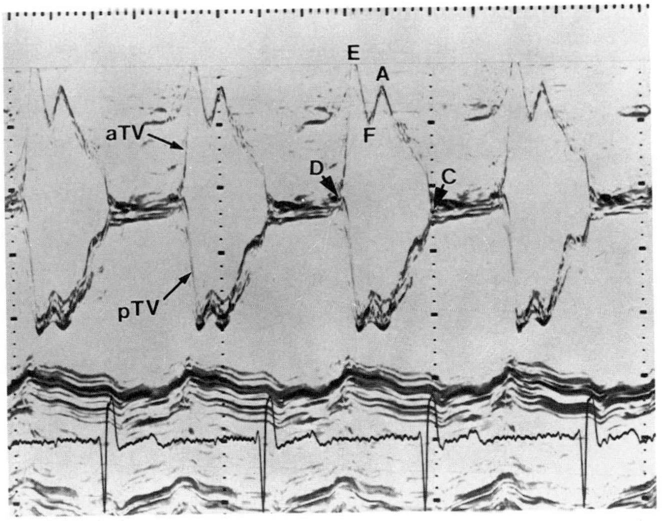

Fig. 14–16. An M-mode recording of the anterior and posterior leaflets of the tricuspid valve with letter designations of the motion pattern. aTV = anterior leaflet of the tricuspid valve; pTV = posterior leaflet of the tricuspid valve.

cusp is most commonly recorded. The motion of the posterior leaflet is recorded throughout the cardiac cycle because it opens and closes in an anteroposterior plane. The pulmonic valve tends to be obscured by hyperinflated lungs in patients with pulmonary disease and by expanding lung during normal inspiration. Recordings of the pulmonic valve are enhanced by right ventricular and pulmonary artery enlargement that displaces intervening lung from the field of interest.

On the M-mode tracing, the posterior pulmonic valve leaflet moves posteriorly to open during systole and anteriorly to close in diastole (Figs. 14–17 and 14–18). Often, the valve is recorded only during portions of the cardiac cycle. The major components of the pulmonic valve echo motion pattern have been designated by lowercase letters. The ''a'' wave follows the P wave of the electrocardiogram and reflects the effect of atrial contraction on valvular motion. From the ''b'' point, which is the onset of right ventricular ejection, the valve leaflets move to a maximally open position (point ''c''). The leaflets remain open until end ejection (point ''d''), which is followed by rapid movement to a closed position (point ''e''). During diastole, the leaflets move posteriorly to a point ''f,'' which precedes the onset of atrial contraction. The e-f slope is occasionally interrupted by anterior motion (e′), which represents transmitted motion. These lowercase letter designations are similar in timing to the corresponding labels of atrioventricular valve motion (Fig. 14–18).[35–37]

An accurate recording of the diameter of the pulmonary artery by M-mode is difficult to obtain from the parasternal window. From this transducer position, the vessel curves posteriorly, and the ultrasound beam generally transects the artery at an oblique angle. A similar problem exists with subcostal recordings of the pulmonary artery. The suprasternal window allows accurate recordings of the diameter of the right pulmonary artery. In general, all pulmonary artery measurements are better derived from the two-dimensional image of the structure.

A series of measurements are obtained from the pulmonic valve motion pattern. The ''a'' wave depth is measured from an extension of the ''f'' point perpendicular to the maximum posterior extent of the ''a'' wave

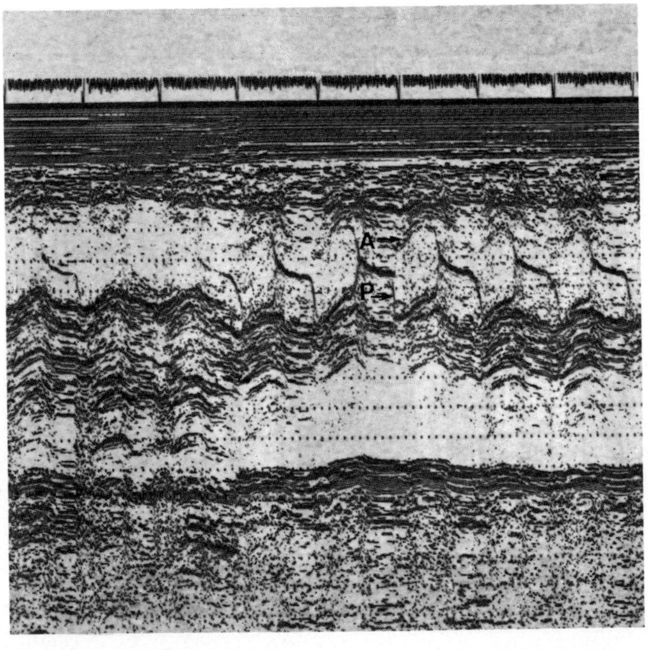

Fig. 14–17. M-mode recording of the pulmonic valve. The posterior leaflet (P) motion is completely recorded, and there is partial recording of the anterior leaflet (A) motion.

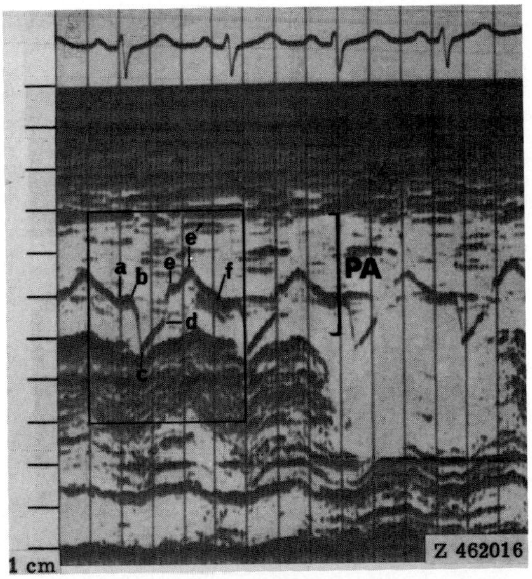

Fig. 14–18. M-mode echocardiogram illustrating the normal pattern of posterior pulmonic valve leaflet motion. The letter designations correspond to those discussed in the text. (From Weyman AE, et al.: Echocardiographic patterns of pulmonic valve motion with pulmonary hypertension. Circulation 50:905, 1974. Reproduced by permission of the American Heart Association, Inc.)

during inspiration. The maximum systolic opening of the posterior leaflet is taken as the amplitude of motion from points b to c. The e-f slope is obtained from the maximum anterior point of the leaflet after closure to the point before the onset of the "a" wave. Right ventricular systolic time intervals can be calculated from the pulmonic valve tracing in a similar fashion to that described for left ventricular systolic time intervals. The right ventricular pre-ejection period (RVPEP) is measured as the time from the onset of ventricular depolarization (Q wave of the electrocardiogram) to the onset of valve opening. The right ventricular ejection time (RVET) is the period during which the valve is open (b-e), and the RVPEP/RVET ratio is derived from these measures. The use of right ventricular systolic time intervals to estimate pulmonary artery pressure has been eclipsed by the more accurate Doppler derived measurements.

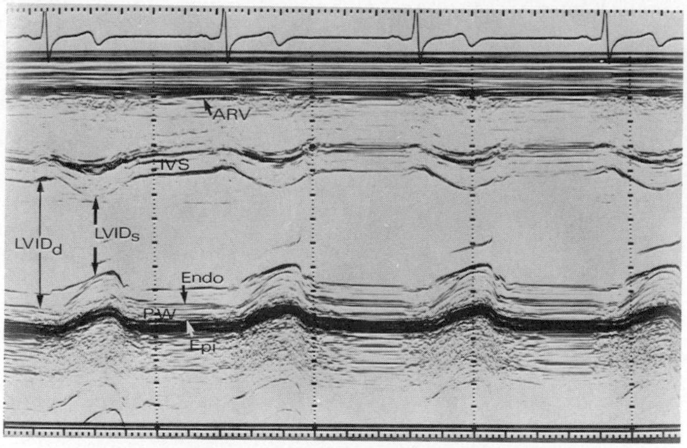

Fig. 14–19. M-mode recording of left ventricle illustrating structures and measurements. The left ventricular internal dimensions at end diastole and end systole (LVID$_d$, LVID$_s$) are taken from the trailing edge of the interventricular septum to the leading edge of the endocardium of the posterior left ventricular wall. ARV = anterior wall of the right ventricle; IVS = interventricular septum; PW = posterior wall of the left ventricle; Endo = endocardium of the posterior wall; Epi = epicardial-pericardial interface.

The Left Ventricle

Correct recording of left ventricular dimensions is one of the most important elements in echocardiography because numerous quantitative values are obtained from its measurement. The optimum left ventricular recording is obtained by positioning the cursor at the tips of the mitral valve leaflets so that it is perpendicular to the left ventricular long axis and passes through the center of the cavity (i.e., bisects the short axis area). Studies in our laboratory have shown that when the entire basal portion of the normal left ventricle is visualized on the accompanying two-dimensional recording, it is not critical to record the M-mode of the left ventricle at the chordal level.[38] Measurements of the left ventricle from the free edge of the mitral leaflet to the base of the left ventricle do not differ significantly from the chordal diameter, as long as the orientation of the M-mode cursor is correct. In children and infants, the M-mode echocardiogram of the left ventricle is recorded at the tips of the mitral valve because the chamber tapers more acutely. In the abnormal ventricle, standardization of the measurement at the leaflet tips is also appropriate.

After the left ventricular walls and cavity are recorded, the posterior pericardium is displayed by decreasing the intensity of the posterior wall echoes. Because the echoes from the posterior pericardium are usually bright, they will remain visible as the echoes of the posterior endocardium are damped. The controls of the echograph, discussed in Chapter 1, may need readjustments with each cursor movement to optimize the recording of specific structures.

Figure 14–19 is an example of a typical M-mode recording of the left ventricular walls and cavity obtained at the mitral chordal level. The anterior right ventricular wall is the most anterior moving echo recorded. This echo moves posteriorly during systole and anteriorly during diastole. Posterior to the anterior right ventricular wall is the right ventricular cavity, which is bordered posteriorly by the echoes of the right ventricular endocardial surface of the interventricular septum. This wall moves parallel to the echoes produced by the left ventricular endocardial surface of the interventricular septum. Contraction of the septum occurs at a mean of 90 msec after the onset of the QRS complex of the electrocardiogram[39] and is recorded as a rapid posterior motion of the echoes of the left ventricular septal endocardium. The maximum downward motion of this endocardium is often followed by a small notch before the onset of left ventricular relaxation. This notch reflects the earlier onset of filling of the right ventricle and development of a brief transseptal pressure gradient favoring the right side.[40–42] During the initial phase of ventricular relaxation, the septal echoes rapidly course anteriorly. During diastasis, the septal echoes continue anteriorly as passive filling progresses. At end-diastole, there is again an abrupt anterior motion, which reflects the change in left ventricular geometry that results from filling by atrial contraction.

The left ventricular cavity is bordered posteriorly by echoes from the endocardium of the posterior wall. Compared to septal motion, the systolic motion of the posterior wall is delayed and occurs at a mean of 159 msec after the onset of the QRS complex of the electrocardiogram.[39] This delay reflects the timing of the posterior wall depolarization during the normal activation sequence of the ventricles. The posterior wall endocardial echo on the M-mode echocardiogram moves anteriorly as the wall contracts and reaches a peak after the nadir of septal motion. Following peak contraction, the wall rapidly moves posterior. This is followed by a more gradual posterior motion during the diastolic filling of the left ventricle. An abrupt posterior dip of the wall may occur with atrial contraction.

The external border of the posterior left ventricular wall appears as a bright echo, which represents the epicardial-visceral pericardial interface. In the absence of a pericardial effusion or pericardial thickening, the epicardium and pericardium will produce a single thick linear echo. The direction of motion of the epicardial-pericardial echo is similar to the endocardial echo of the posterior wall. The amplitude of excursion of the epicardial-pericardial echo is much less than that of the endocardial echo. The difference in amplitude of these two echoes reflects the degree of myocardial thickening.

Because the M-mode is taken from the imaging planes of the two-dimensional echocardiogram, and the two-dimensional echocardiographic image is now the primary diagnostic imaging format, it is reasonable that measurements derived from the M-mode recordings should be the same as those taken from the two-dimensional image of the same structure.

The left ventricular internal dimension (LVID) is measured at both end-diastole and end-systole from the same beat ($LVID_d$ and $LVID_s$, respectively). To obtain dimensions that are equivalent to those from the two-dimensional echocardiographic structure, the LVID is measured from the trailing edge of the endocardial echoes of the interventricular septum to the leading edge of the posterior left ventricular endocardial echoes (Fig. 14–19).

Companion wall thickness of the interventricular septum (IVS) and the posterior wall (PW) should be obtained from the same beat as the LVID measurement. They are measured using the same inner edge technique described previously for measurement of two-dimensional echocardiographic structures. When applied to the M-mode, however, this measurement convention results in a trailing edge-to-trailing edge measurement for the septum and a leading edge-to-leading edge measurement for the posterior wall.

The right ventricular internal dimension (RVID) is conventionally measured along the same line of sight as that used to measure the LVID. It is measured in end-diastole and at end-expiration to avoid the effects of alterations in filling by respiration. The RVID extends from the anterior right ventricular echoes to the leading edge of the endocardial echoes of the IVS. As previously discussed, this measurement is variable because the position of the right ventricle varies from patient to patient and the orientation of the M-mode line through the right ventricle may not be consistent from study to study.

Derived Left Ventricular Measurements

From the dimensions discussed previously, a variety of derived measurements can be obtained. Such measurements include calculations of left ventricular volume, left ventricular mass, and left ventricular wall stress.

Left ventricular volume is calculated from M-mode measurements by assuming that the left ventricular cavity can be represented as a prolate ellipsoid, that the two minor axes of the ellipsoid are equal and represented by the LVID, and that the major axis of the ellipsoid is approximately double the minor axis.[21,43] With abnormal increases in heart size and in the setting of ventricular asynergy, this volume calculation is inaccurate because the relationship between the major and minor axes changes. Regression equations have been developed to describe the relation between the major and minor axes, which can be substituted into the volume calculation when cardiac enlargement or asynergy is present.[44] The calculation of ventricular volume is discussed in detail in Chapter 20.

Left ventricular mass is derived by multiplying the volume of the left ventricular walls by the specific gravity of cardiac muscle. The volume of the left ventricular walls is the difference between the combined left ventricular cavity and muscle volume, and the volume of the left ventricular cavity.[45] This calculation is also discussed in Chapter 20.

Left ventricular wall stress is derived by modifications of LaPlace's relationship that wall stress is directly related to cavity pressure and size and is inversely related to wall thickness. The wall stress can be derived from the M-mode measurements of wall thickness and LVID and the systemic blood pressure. This relation is discussed in detail in Chapter 20.

NORMAL M-MODE ECHOCARDIOGRAPHIC MEASUREMENTS

Tables of normal values for standard measurements are presented in Appendix A. Cardiac M-mode dimensions are independent of gender.[38,46] Although aortic root diameter has been shown to vary with age in previous M-mode studies,[47] standard left ventricular dimensions are independent of age.[38] Cardiac dimensions are related to body surface area,[48] and the correction of M-mode measurements for body surface area is of use for children. However, for adult patients with body surface area in the range from 1.4 to 2.1 m^2, there is minimal variation in size of structures, and thus there is little clinical utility for corrections (see Appendix A).

Historical Development and Basis of M-Mode Measurement Conventions

Over the 30 years of M-mode echocardiography, numerous criteria have been used to measure the cardiac structures represented on the M-mode echocardiograms. The methods differ primarily in the manner in which the thick echoes, representing the borders of structures, are included within the measurements. Figure 14–20 displays the measurement conventions commonly appearing in the literature.

In 1968, the first guidelines for M-mode measurements were published and have been referred to as the *standard convention*. These measurement criteria were developed during refinement of the M-mode recording of the posterior wall of the left ventricle and the interventricular septum.[17,19,45] This method includes the thickness of the endocardial echoes in the measurements of the interventricular septum and posterior wall. The thick pericardial echoes are excluded from the measurement of the posterior wall. Measurements of posterior wall thickness by this method correlate well with posterior wall measurements by surgical inspection and autopsy.[17] Measurement of the internal diameter of the left ventricular cavity by this convention showed a significant correlation with left ventricular end-diastolic diameters obtained by angiography. There was no validation of the septal measurement. Unfortunately, because the line of measurement of the epicardium must cross the

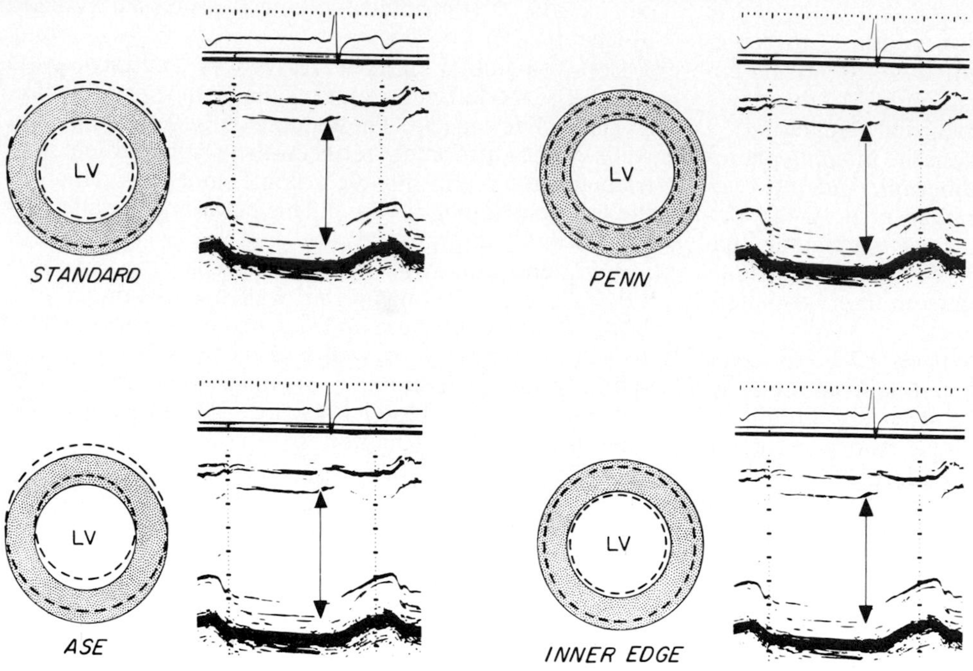

Fig. 14–20. Diagrams of the short axis, two-dimensional image of the left ventricle and corresponding M-modes illustrating the four major conventions for defining the edges from which to take M-mode and two-dimensional echocardiographic measurements. The shaded areas correspond to the myocardium; the interrupted lines follow the path of the line of measurement using each convention. See text for complete discussion of each convention. LV = left ventricle.

borders of the structure itself at some point around the ventricular circumference, this convention is difficult to apply to two-dimensional echocardiograms and results in a different convention for the measurement of septal thickness and posterior wall thickness.

In 1977 the Penn convention was derived to provide the best fit between anatomic mass and echocardiographically derived mass calculations.[49] This method includes the thickness of the endocardial echoes for the measurement of the LV internal diameter but not for wall thickness. It is not clear if the discrepancy between anatomic mass and echocardiographically derived mass measured by the standard convention is due to underestimation of mass by the model and formulas or to overestimation of mass by the standard M-mode measurements.

The most widely discussed convention was recommended by the American Society of Echocardiography (ASE) in 1978.[50] Using a survey, this organization attempted to define the M-mode measurement criteria used by individuals and to identify the criteria that led to the most consistently reproducible results. The committee recommended the leading edge-leading edge convention stating that it was least dependent on instrument gain or signal processing.

The strength of this study is based on its original premise that the convention would represent a consensus from echocardiographers. However, the recommendations were based on a low number (19%) of questionnaires returned, and these questionnaires revealed significant interobserver variability in measurement technique. The committee did not attempt to examine the accuracy or reproducibility of the measurements. Most important, this group made no attempt to integrate the measurements from the M-mode with those from the two-dimensional technique.

Our method of measurement (see preceding discussion) is essentially an inner edge method. The use of this method for M-mode echocardiographic recordings provides consistency between the structures measured on companion M-mode and two-dimensional echocardiographic studies and avoids the need for two sets of normative values for all structures. It also allows the measurement of structures where only the inner edge may be available, such as the left ventricular apex and superior wall of the left atrium. This measurement technique is also appropriate for Doppler-derived indices where the inner vessel or chamber area is of interest.

Timing of Measurements

The timing of measurements in the cardiac cycle must remain constant to ensure reproducibility. The definition of specific temporal points in the cardiac cycle is more critical with M-mode echocardiography than the cross-sectional technique, because the higher sampling rate allows for more precise timing of events by M-mode. Diversity exists in the M-mode literature for the notation of end-diastole. The peak of the R wave, the onset of the QRS complex, and the largest left ventricular diameter, regardless of timing, have been used to mark end-diastole. End-diastole or the start of mechanical systole occurs about 35 msec after the onset of the QRS complex.[51] Measurements at such a point require an additional measurement that will add to errors in reproducibility. The largest diameter of the left ventricle is a poor indicator of end-diastole because the ventricle may change shape during early phases of systole before emptying, and the largest diameter may occur at such a time. The onset of the R wave will vary depending on the electrocardiographic lead that is monitored or the existence of conduction delay. Thus, the onset of the QRS offers the most reproducible point for timing end-diastole.

End-systole is more difficult to define on the M-mode and electrocardiogram. Definitions for end-systole have included the end of the T wave on the electrocardiogram, the smallest left ventricular diameter on the M-mode, the occurrence of the aortic second sound, and the maximum excursion of the anterior or posterior left ventricular wall (Fig. 14–21).[50,52,53] The T wave as reference point is inaccurate. The use of the aortic second sound requires a simultaneous phonocardiogram. Because the septum is activated before the posterior left ventricular wall, it will reach its nadir before the peak anterior excursion of the posterior wall. One acceptable measure, if septal motion is normal, is to define the nadir of septal motion as the point to measure as end-systole. When abnormal septal motion is present, the timing of the peak anterior movement of the posterior wall can be used. This method also has the advantage that it can be reproduced in two-dimensional echocardiography. Another method that has been proposed is to measure end-systole by extrapolating the minimum distance between septum and posterior wall regardless of the timing of the wall excursions.[53] Although this has shown good correlation with angiography, it theoretically is not an acceptable method because it measures two points occurring at two separate instances in time and thus has no anatomic correlate.

Reproducibility of Measurements

Studies investigating the reproducibility of M-mode measurements have shown consistent results. Interobserver variability of standard measurements of the same study are less than 5%, while intraobserver variability ranges from 4% for left ventricular cavity dimensions to 12% for wall thickness measurements.[54,55] The intraobserver variability for measurements of wall thickness are large, because for these small structures, even a small absolute difference of 1 mm represents a large relative change.

Measurements from normal patients and those with stable heart disease exhibit no significant week-to-week variability when studies are performed by a single sonographer.[54] The variability increases when separate studies are recorded by two separate individuals.[43] This operator dependency represents variability in location and spatial orientation of the transducer.[55–58]

In the past, when the M-mode was recorded without the assistance of a two-dimensional image, an enlarged heart affected the reproducibility of left ventricular measurements.[58] This reflected the increased number of off-axis cuts through the left ventricle, which simulated the true perpendicular plane in patients with dilated left ventricles. However, with the current methods of deriving M-mode recordings from the two-dimensional image, such problems with reproducibility of measurement, even in abnormal hearts, should not exist.

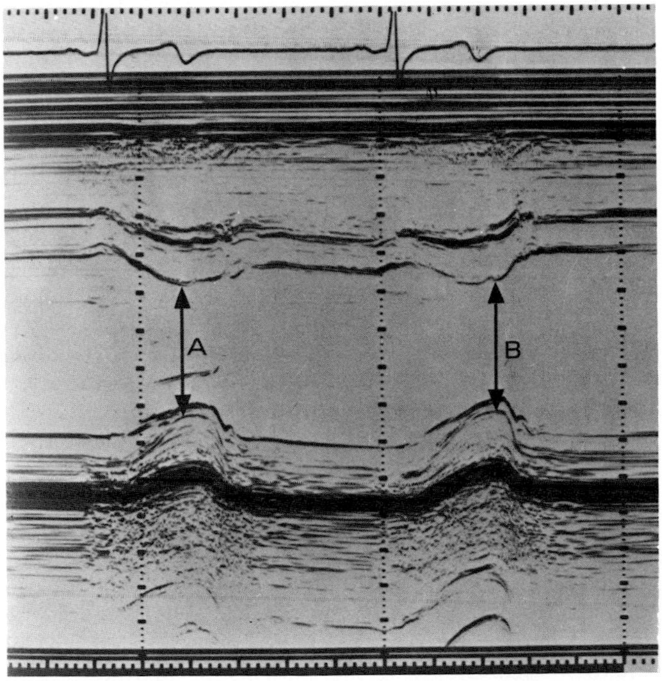

Fig. 14–21. The two conventions for measuring the left ventricular internal dimension at end systole. A = end systole as defined by the nadir of normal septal motion; B = end systole as defined by the peak movement of the posterior wall. (See text for complete discussion.)

Computer Analysis of the M-Mode Recording

The M-mode recording can be manually digitized to obtain further information on left ventricular function, such as peak rates of cavity and wall thickness changes. From such measurements, the peak filling rates of the ventricles can be determined.[59] Excellent correlations exist for comparisons of both multiple digitizations of the same image by a single observer and by different observers. As would be expected, more significant variability in the digitized image is observed between patients and within the same patient over time.[60] Controversy exists over the clinical utility of the information derived from the time-consuming process of digitization of the M-mode echocardiogram.

EXAMPLES OF CURRENT APPLICATIONS OF M-MODE ECHOCARDIOGRAPHY

The M-mode image remains an important part of the complete ultrasonic examination of the heart because of inherent features that differ in several important aspects from cross-sectional techniques. These features include the enhanced recording of individual targets, the higher sampling rate, and the concise graphic display.

M-mode permits enhanced recording of individual targets because the number of sound pulses directed toward a point target are increased up to 100-fold. This enormously enhances the potential for recording useful data from the target. Echocardiographic imaging of the left ventricular endocardium provides an illustration of the superior recording of targets by the M-mode technique. When attempting to record the endocardium, the M-mode beam must be optimized to record only two points, one from the interventricular septum, and the other from the endocardial surface of the posterior wall. At standard recording speeds, the M-mode lines are so densely packed together that if only 50% of the individual pulses actually generated echoes from both endocardial interfaces, the endocardium would still appear continuous. In contrast, in each cross-sectional image, more than 100 data lines must be positioned such that they intersect the left ventricular endocardium at appropriate angles to generate a continuous echo. The inability to achieve appropriate positioning frequently causes one or more segments of the ventricular endocardium to be well visualized, while other segments are poorly visualized on the two-dimensional image. In this latter case, if only 50% of the cross-sectional lines actually contained endocardial reflections, a poor-quality image would result. This will vary further with spatial heterogeneity of the reflected signal.

It is commonly stated that the resolution of M-mode echocardiography is superior to that of two-dimensional echocardiography. Actually, the resolving power of the two modalities along the beam axis is a function of the transducer frequency and is the same for both types of instruments. The lateral resolution of two-dimensional imaging is inferior to the axial resolution of the M-mode, but because the M-mode has no lateral resolution, a real comparison must favor the two-dimensional technique. It is the sampling frequency that differs between the two techniques and, for the reasons discussed previously, may result in an apparent increase in sensitivity, which is misinterpreted as "resolution." This feature of enhanced sensitivity allows for the detection by the M-mode technique of small pericardial effusions and subtle degrees of pericardial thickening that may escape detection by two-dimensional echocardiography.

In addition to superior local target sensitivity, the higher effective sampling rate of the M-mode format (1000 to 5000 pulses/sec) compared to the two-dimensional echocardiographic frame rates (15 to 60 frames/sec or fields/sec) improves the timing of cardiac events by M-mode echocardiography, and it allows for the precise recording of rapidly occurring movements.

Many cases illustrate the use of M-mode recordings to time cardiac events. One example is the precise timing of valve opening and closure. This allows for the calculations of systolic time intervals. In addition to the PEP and ejection time calculation previously discussed, the isovolumic relaxation time can be measured as the period from aortic valve closure to mitral valve opening (Fig. 14–22).[61,62]

Other values of the M-mode display for timing events include its use in contrast echocardiography (Chapter 15) and color flow mapping (Chapter 11).

The rapid sampling frequency of the M-mode technique enables detection and timing of movements of short duration, and visualization of the individual components of sets of high frequency repetitive motions that are missed at the slower frame rates of the two-dimensional images. This feature allows for the recording of subtle abnormalities of wall motion. Septal wall motion abnormalities detected by the M-mode technique have been associated with a variety of conditions including altered electrical activation of the left ventricle,[63] right ventricular volume overload,[64–66] cardiac surgery,[67,68] anterior myocardial infarction, large pericardial effusions, and congenital absence of the pericardium.[69] The motion patterns of the septum and their mechanisms are discussed in Chapter 29.

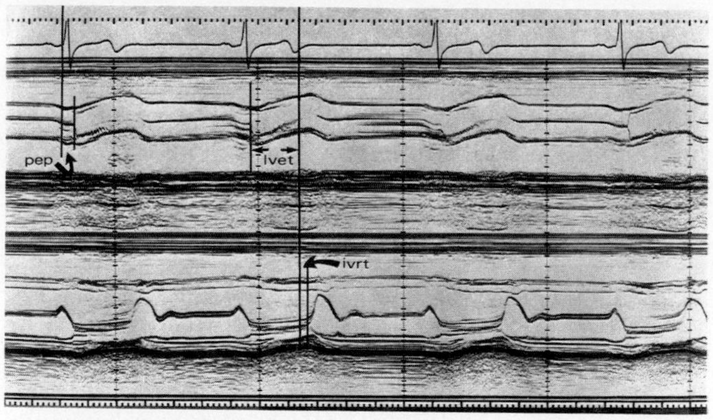

Fig. 14–22. Systolic time intervals by M-mode echocardiogram. Pre-ejection period (pep) corresponds to the onset of QRS to aortic valve opening. Left ventricular ejection time (lvet) corresponds to the duration of aortic valve opening. Isovolumic relaxation time (ivrt) corresponds to closure of aortic valve to opening of the mitral valve.

The M-mode recordings of the left ventricle in patients with Wolff-Parkinson-White syndrome provide another example of the discriminating power of the technique for displaying subtle alterations in wall motion. In the setting of pre-excitation, brief alterations in normal wall motion are a specific but not a sensitive finding.

In patients with type A Wolff-Parkinson-White syndrome, an early anterior motion of the posterior wall can be recorded within 100 msec of the onset of the electrocardiographic QRS complex (Fig. 14–23).[39] This early activation of the posterior wall is a variable finding and represents conduction through a posterior lateral accessory bypass tract to the left ventricle. With type B Wolff-Parkinson-White syndrome, a brief pre-ejection posterior motion of the interventricular septum is recorded within 56 msec of the QRS onset, and there is a delay in the normal septal posterior motion to approximately 160 msec after the QRS onset.[39] The abnormal interventricular septal motion has been shown to correlate with the presence of anterior right ventricular bypass tract conduction.[70] Both abnormal and normal posterior wall motion have been reported in association with this abnormal septal motion.[39,71,72]

M-mode echocardiography can also detect the high frequency diastolic flutterings of the anterior leaflet of the mitral valve and interventricular septum that are due to the regurgitant jet of aortic insufficiency (Fig. 14–24).[73–75]

This technique also is of value to detect the high velocity vibrations that are due to small fenestrations of the cardiac valves (Fig. 14–25). These fenestrations can be due to endocarditis or to other forms of valve degeneration,[76,77] and the associated fluttering is caused by the stream of regurgitant blood flowing past the freely mobile piece of leaflet tissue.

The linear display of variations in valvular motion by M-mode can assist in the diagnosis of pulmonary hyper-

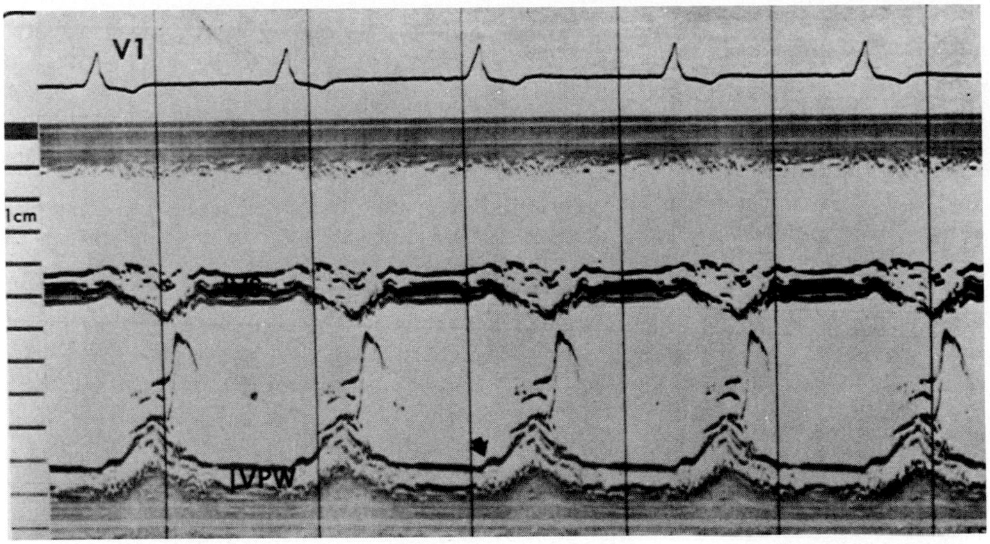

Fig. 14–23. M-mode recording from a patient with type A Wolff-Parkinson-White syndrome during normal sinus rhythm. The arrow indicates the premature contraction of the posterior wall of the left ventricle (LVPW). (From DeMaria AN, et al.: Alterations in ventricular contraction pattern in Wolff-Parkinson-White syndrome: detection by echocardiography. Circulation 53:249, 1976. Reproduced by permission of the American Heart Association, Inc.)

tension, idiopathic hypertrophic subaortic stenosis, and discrete subvalvular aortic stenosis.

Figure 14–26 displays the pulmonic valve recording associated with pulmonary hypertension. The characteristic alterations in the normal pulmonic valve motion include (1) diminution or absence of the "a" wave, (2) flattening or negative "e-f" slope, and (3) midsystolic notching between the c and d points (see Chapter 27).[36,37]

Although cross-sectional echocardiography provides a better assessment of the extent of septal thickening in idiopathic hypertrophic subaortic stenosis, a more accurate timing of the dynamic obstruction of left ventricular outflow is represented on the M-mode recording as a midsystolic closure of the aortic valve (Fig. 14–27), which may be inapparent on the two-dimensional recording. The M-mode recording also provides accurate graphic display and timing of the systolic anterior motion of the mitral valve (Fig. 14–28).[78,79]

Early systolic closure of the aortic valve is also recorded on the M-mode of discrete subvalvular aortic stenosis (Fig. 14–29).[80,81] Although the finding of aortic valve preclosure is most often associated with dynamic or fixed subvalvular aortic stenosis, it can also be found in mitral regurgitation and ventricular septal defects.

Another advantage of the M-mode echocardiogram is its concise and easily analyzed graphic format that depicts continuous motion vs. time. These records can be examined quickly, and measurements can be obtained from the graphic record. This technique allows for easy comparison within the same study or between studies. The M-mode echocardiogram in Figure 14–30 shows the variations in the timing of mitral valve A-wave motion in a patient with atrial flutter and variable atrioventricular block in which multiple cardiac cycles can be compared simultaneously. An M-mode study lasting 1 minute and recorded at 25 mm/sec would yield a tracing 150 cm long, which can be easily scanned, and the data from several

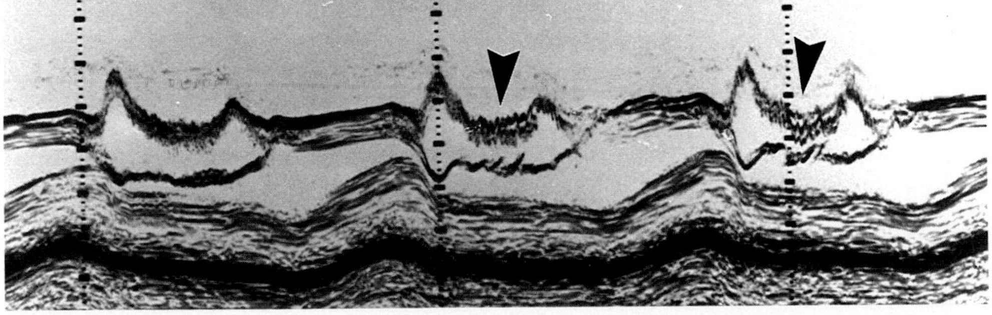

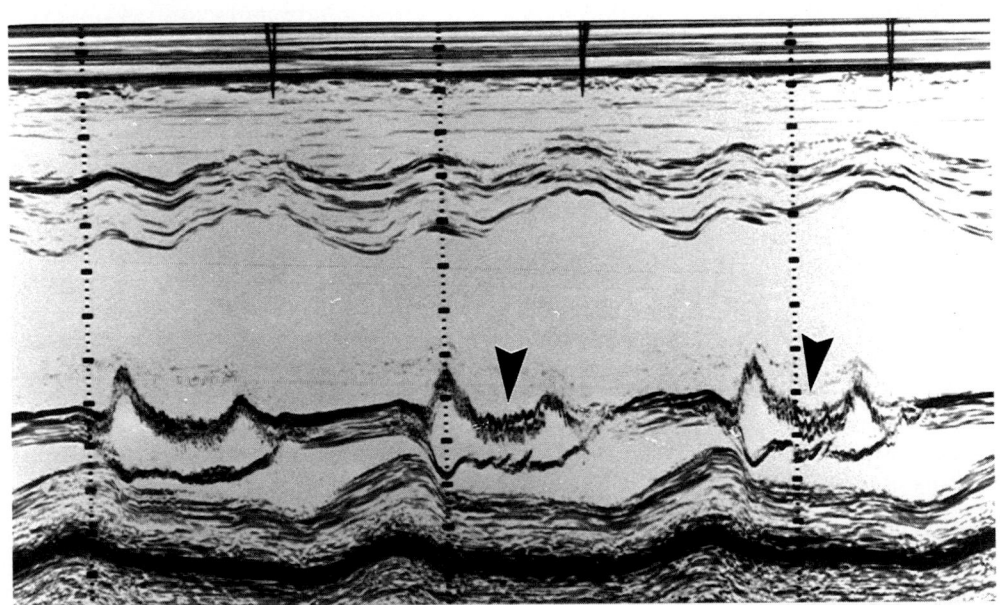

Fig. 14–24. High frequency flutterings (arrowheads) of the anterior leaflet of the mitral valve during diastole that are due to the regurgitant jet of aortic insufficiency.

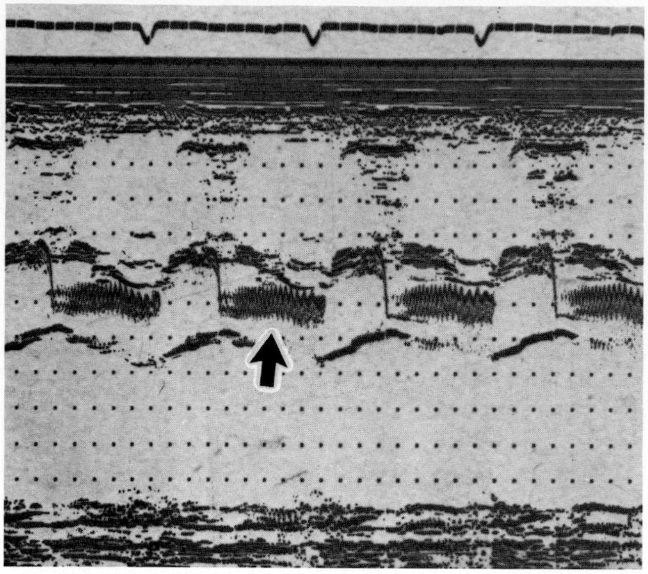

Fig. 14–25. High frequency flutterings (arrow) of an aortic valve leaflet during diastole caused by regurgitant flow through a partially torn leaflet. (From King ME, Weyman AE: Echocardiographic findings in ineffective endocarditis. Cardiovasc Clin 13:147, 1983.)

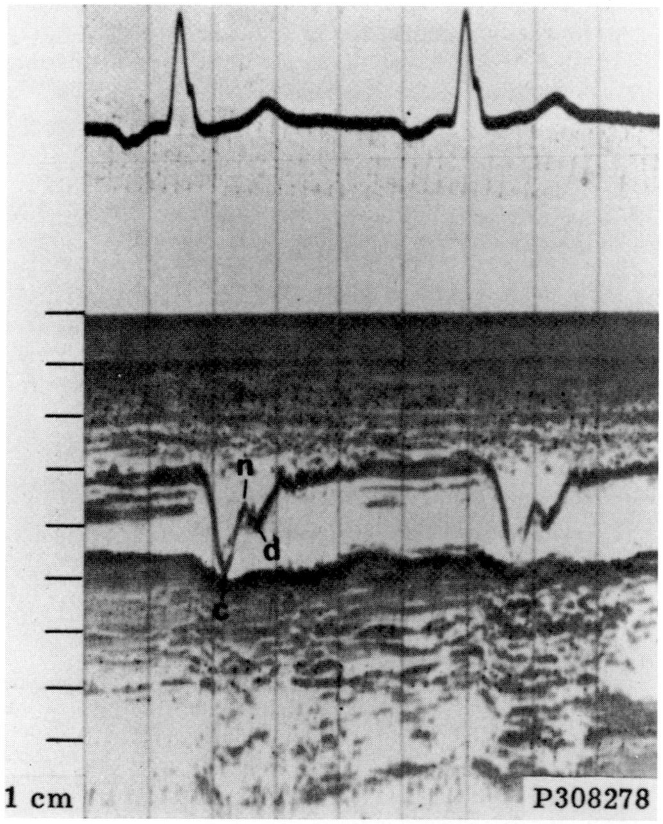

Fig. 14–26. Posterior leaflet pulmonic valve motion with pulmonary hypertension. The major findings include the decreased or absent "a" wave, flattened "e-f" slope, and midsystolic notching of the leaflet. c = fully opened leaflet; d = position of leaflet at onset of valve closure; n = midsystolic closure or notching of the leaflet. (From Weyman AE, et al.: Echocardiographic patterns of pulmonic valve motion with pulmonary hypertension. Circulation 50:905, 1974. Reproduced by permission of the American Heart Association, Inc.)

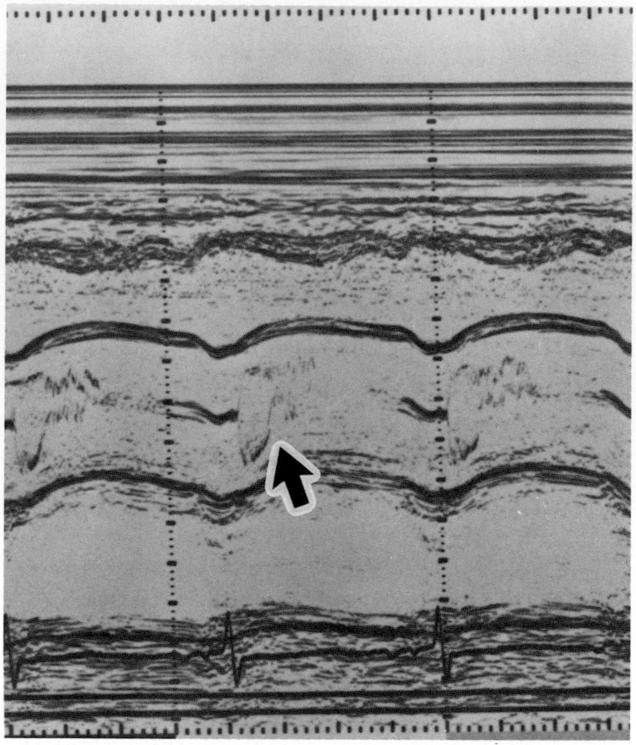

Fig. 14–27. Closure or notching of the aortic valve in midsystole (arrow) in a patient with idiopathic hypertrophic subaortic stenosis (IHSS). This notching represents the effects of the dynamic left ventricular outflow tract obstruction and provides a method to time the onset of the obstruction.

cycles can be compared. By contrast, a cross-sectional echocardiographic examination lasting 1 minute yields 3600 individual fields of data. Analyzing these fields individually represents an enormous task, and comparing images in one area of the video record with those in another area can be difficult.

Finally, the M-mode format allows for easy correlation with other graphic presentations of physiologic data. Simultaneously recorded phonocardiograms, respirations, cardiac chamber pressures, or Doppler signals can be displayed with the M-mode echocardiogram as a single record.

LIMITATIONS OF THE M-MODE TECHNIQUE

When M-mode echocardiography was performed without the aid of two-dimensional guidance, the blindly directed "ice pick view" led to imprecision in measurement, and the lack of spatial orientation required many assumptions about chamber shape and structure location, which were often incorrect. As a result, when two-dimensional imaging became available, it replaced the M-mode as the procedure of choice in many diagnostic areas. When guided by the two-dimensional image, however, most of the limitations of the technique as a measurement tool, including the errors that were due to obliquity of view, are resolved. Off-axis recordings are still produced if M-mode recordings are obtained from a two-dimensional image in which the cursor cannot be posi-

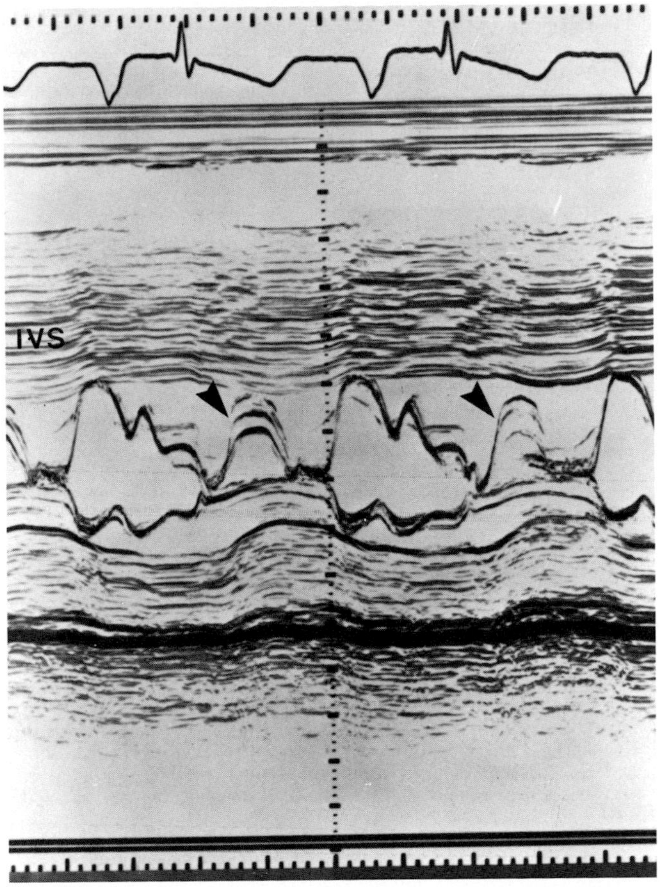

Fig. 14–28. Systolic anterior motion of the mitral valve (arrow) in idiopathic hypertrophic subaortic stenosis. IVS = interventricular septum.

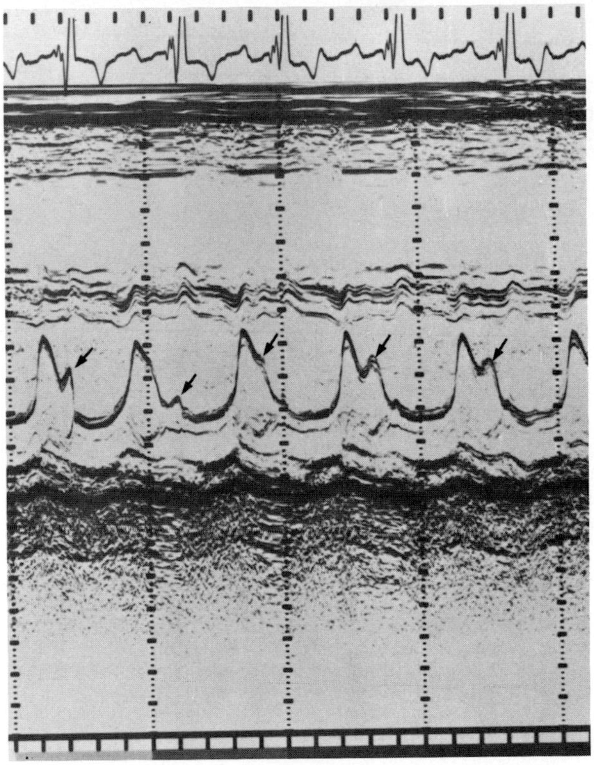

Fig. 14–30. An illustration of the ease of visualization and presentation by the M-mode format of the beat-to-beat variation in mitral valve A-wave timing (arrows) resulting from atrial flutter with variable atrioventricular block. (See text for explanation.)

tioned at right angles to the structure of interest. If the two-dimensional plane is poorly positioned, however, this is the fault of the operator and not the technique. Because the M-mode is derived from the two-dimensional image, the M-mode recording will only be as good as the corresponding two-dimensional recording, and M-mode derived measurements will be subject to the same limitations as those derived from the two-dimensional image.

SUMMARY

Although many of the former uses for M-mode echocardiography are now replaced by cross-sectional echocardiography, the technique remains an important ad-

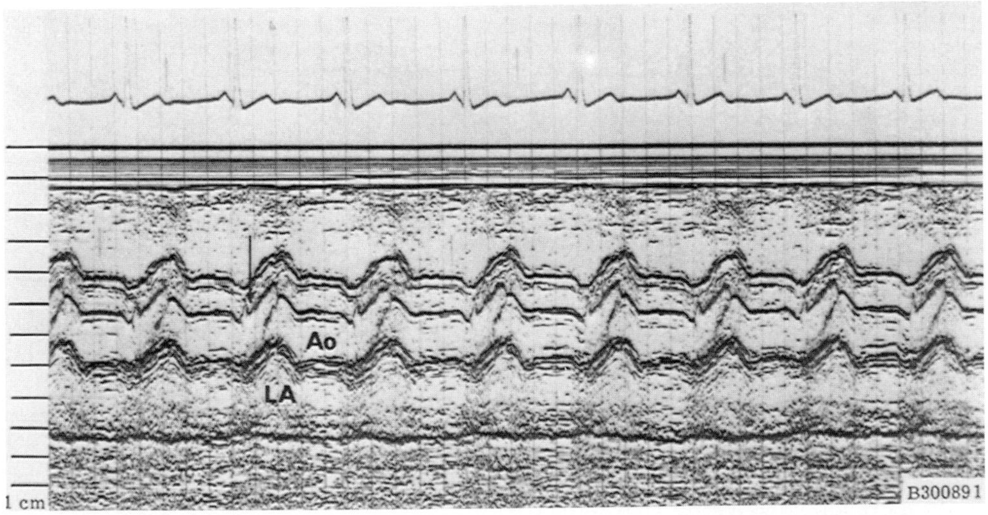

Fig. 14–29. Closure of the aortic valve in early systole (arrow) in a patient with discrete subvalvular aortic stenosis. Ao = aorta; LA = left atrium. (From Weyman AE, et al.: Cross-sectional echocardiography in evaluating patients with discrete subaortic stenosis. Am J Cardiol 37:358, 1976.)

junct to the complete echocardiographic examination. Its superior temporal resolution and convenient graphic display make the M-mode echocardiogram an accurate and reproducible method for the measurement of cardiac structures and for the analysis of time-related events.

REFERENCES

1. Edler I, Hertz CH: The use of ultrasonic reflectoscope for the continuous recording of movements of heart walls. Kungl Fysiogr Sallsk i Lund Forhandl 24:5, 1954.
2. Edler I: The diagnostic use of ultrasound in heart disease. Acta Med Scand Suppl 308:32, 1955.
3. Edler I: Ultrasound cardiogram in mitral valve diseases. Acta Chir Scand 111:230, 1956.
4. Edler I: Ultrasoundcardiogram in pericardial effusion. Follow up of six cases. Scientific Session, Swedish Society of Internal Medicine, Lund, Sweden, June 4, 1955.
5. Effert S, Domanig E: The diagnosis of intraatrial tumour and thrombi by the ultrasonic echo method. Germ Med Mth 4:1, 1959.
6. Effert S, Hertz CH, Böhme W: Direkte Regfistrierung des Ultraschall—Kardiogramms mit dem Electrokardiographen. Z Kreislaufforsch 48:230, 1959.
7. Joyner CR, Reid JM, Bond JP: Reflected ultrasound in the assessment of mitral valve disease. Circulation 27:506, 1963.
8. Joyner CR, Reid JM: Application of ultrasound in cardiology and cardiovascular physiology. Prog Cardiovasc Dis 5:482, 1963.
9. Joyner CR, Reid JM: Ultrasound cardiogram in the selection of patients for mtiral valve surgery. Ann NY Acad Sci 118:512, 1965.
10. Feigenbaum H, Waldhausen JA, Hyde LP: Ultrasound diagnosis of pericardial effusion. JAMA 191:107, 1965.
11. Feigenbaum H, Zaky A, Waldhausen JA: Use of ultrasound in the diagnosis of pericardial effusion. Ann Intern Med 65:443, 1966.
12. Feigenbaum H, Zaky A, Waldhausen JA: Use of reflected ultrasound in detecting pericardial effusion. Am J Cardiol 19:84, 1967.
13. Rothman J, et al.: Ultrasonic diagnosis of pericardial effusion. Circulation 35:358, 1967.
14. Pate JW, Gardner HC, Norman RS: Diagnosis of pericardial effusion by echocardiography. Ann Surg 165:826, 1967.
15. Goldberg BB, Ostrum BJ, Isard JJ: Ultrasonic determination of pericardial effusion. JAMA 202:103, 1967.
16. Klein JJ, Segal BL: Pericardial effusion diagnosed by reflected ultrasound. Am J Cardiol 22:57, 1968.
17. Feigenbaum H, Popp RL, Chip JN, Haine CL: Left ventricular wall thickness measured by ultrasound. Arch Intern Med 121:391, 1968.
18. Feigenbaum H, et al.: Correlation of ultrasound with angiocardiography in measuring left ventricular diastolic volume (abstr.) Am J Cardiol 23:111, 1969.
19. Popp RL, Wolfe SB, Hirata T, Feigenbaum H: Estimation of right and left ventricular size by ultrasound. A study of echoes from the interventricular septum. Am J Cardiol 24:523, 1969.
20. Feigenbaum H, Zaky A, Nasser WK: Use of ultrasound to measure left ventricular stroke volume. Circulation 35:1092, 1967.
21. Popp RL, Harrison DC: Ultrasonic cardiac echocardiography for determining stroke volume and valvular regurgitation. Circulation 41:493, 1970.
22. Feigenbaum H, et al.: Ultrasound measurements of the left ventricle: a correlative study with angiocardiography. Arch Intern Med 129:461, 1972.
23. Gramiak R, Shah PM, Kramer DH: Ultrasound cardiography: contrast studies in anatomy and function. Radiol 92:939, 1969.
24. Chang S, Feigenbaum H: Subxyphoid echocardiography. Chest 68:233, 1975.
25. Goldberg BB: Suprasternal ultrasonography. JAMA 215:245, 1971.
26. Starling MR, et al.: Accuracy of subxyphoid echocardiography for assessing left ventricular size and performance. Circulation 61:367, 1980.
27. Allen HD, et al.: Suprasternal notch echocardiography: assessment of its clinical utility in pediatric cardiology. Circulation 55:605, 1977.
28. Sahn DJ, Allen HD, McDonald G, Goldberg SJ: Real-time cross-sectional echocardiographic diagnosis of coarctation of the aorta. Circulation 56:762, 1977.
29. Weyman AE, et al.: Cross-sectional echocardiographic characterization of aortic obstruction 1. Supravalvular aortic stenosis and aortic hypoplasia. Circulation 57:491, 1978.
30. Snider AR, Silverman NH: Suprasternal notch echocardiography: a two-dimensional technique for evaluating congenital heart disease. Circulation 63:165, 1981.
31. Edler I: Atrioventricular valve motility in the living human heart recorded by ultrasound. Acta Med Scand Suppl 370:85, 1961.
32. Strunk BL, et al.: The posterior aortic wall echogram—Its relationship to left atrial volume change. Circulation 54:744, 1976.
33. Brewer RJ, Deck JD, Capati B, Nolan SP: The dynamic aortic root: its role in aortic valve function. J Thorac Cardiovasc Surg 72:413, 1976.
34. Tavel ME: Clinical Phonocardiography and External Pulse Recordings. 3rd Ed. Chicago, Year Book Medical Publishers, 1978.
35. Weyman AE, Dillon JC, Feigenbaum H, Chang S: Echocardiographic patterns of pulmonary valve motion in valvular pulmonic stenosis. Am J Cardiol 34:644, 1974.
36. Weyman AE, Dillon JC, Feigenbaum H, Chang S: Echocardiographic patterns of pulmonic valve motion with pulmonary hypertension. Circulation 50:905, 1974.
37. Weyman AE: Pulmonary valve echo motion in clinical practice. Am J Med 62:843, 1977.
38. Triulzi M, et al.: Normal cross-sectional echocardiographic values: linear dimensions and chamber areas. Echocardiography 1:403, 1984.
39. DeMaria AN, Vera Z, Neumann A, Mason DT: Alterations in ventricular contraction pattern in the Wolff-Parkinson-White syndrome: detection by echocardiography. Circulation 53:249, 1976.
40. Weyman AE: *Cross-Sectional Echocardiography*. Philadelphia, Lea & Febiger, 1982.
41. Kingma I, Tyberg JV, Smith ER: Effects of diastolic transseptal pressure gradient on ventricular septal position and motion. Circulation 68:1304, 1983.
42. Thompson CR, et al.: Trasseptal pressure gradient and diastolic ventricular septal motion in patients with mitral stenosis. Circulation 76:974, 1987.
43. Pombo JF, Troy BL, Russell RO: Left ventricular volumes and ejection fractions by echocardiography. Circulation 43:480, 1971.
44. Teichholz LE, Kreulen T, Herman MV, Gorlin R: Problems in echocardiographic volume determinations: echocardiographic-angiographic correlations in the presence or absence of asynergy. Am J Cardiol 37:7, 1976.
45. Troy BL, Pombo J, Rackley CE: Measurements of left ventricular wall thickness and mass by echocardiography. Circulation 45:602, 1972.
46. Henry WL, Gardin JM, Ware JH: Echocardiographic measurements in normal subjects from infancy to old age. Circulation 62:1054, 1980.
47. Gerstenblith G, et al.: Echocardiographic assessment of a normal adult aging population. Circulation 56:273, 1977.
48. Henry WL, et al.: Echocardiographic measurements in normal subjects. Circulation 57:278, 1978.
49. Devereux RB, Reichek N: Echocardiographic determination of left ventricular mass in man: anatomic validation of the method. Circulation 55:613, 1977.
50. Sahn DJ, DeMaria AN, Kisslo J, Weyman AE: Recommendations regarding quantitation in M-mode echocardiography: results of a survey of echocardiographic measurements. Circulation 58:1072, 1978.
51. Martin CE, et al.: Direct correlation of external systolic time intervals with internal indices of left ventricular function in man. Circulation 44:419, 1971.
52. Roelandt J, Gibson DG: Recommendations for standardization of measurements from M-mode echocardiograms. Eur Heart J 1:375, 1980.
53. Crawford MH, et al.: Accuracy and reproducibility of new M-mode echocardiographic recommendations for measuring left ventricular dimensions. Circulation 61:137, 1980.
54. Lapido GOA, et al.: Serial measurements of left ventricular dimensions by echocardiography. Assessment of week-to-week, inter- and intraobserver variability in normal subjects and patients with valvular heart disease. Br Heart J 44:284, 1980.
55. DeLeonardis V, Cinelli P: Evidence of no interobserver variability in M-mode echocardiography. Clin Cardiol 9:324, 1986.
56. Popp RL, Filly K, Brown O, Harrison DC: Effect of transducer placement on echocardiographic measurements of left ventricular dimensions. Am J Cardiol 35:537, 1975.
57. Stefadouros MA, Canedo MI: Reproducibility of echocardiographic estimates of left ventricular dimensions. Br Heart J 39:390, 1977.
58. Wong M, Shah PM, Taylor RD: Reproducibility of left ventricular internal dimensions with M-mode echocardiography: effects of heart size, body position, and transducer angulation. Am J Cardiol 47:1068, 1981.
59. Gibson DG, Brown D: Measurement of instantaneous left ventricular dimension and filling rate in man using echocardiography. Br Heart J 35:1141, 1973.
60. Pollock C, Fitzgerald PJ, Popp RL: Variability of digitized echocardiography: size, source and means of reduction. Am J Cardiol 51:576, 1983.
61. Hirschfeld S, et al.: Measurement of right and left ventricular systolic time intervals by echocardiography. Circulation 51:304, 1975.
62. Hirschfeld S, et al.: The isovolumic contraction time of the left ventricle: an echographic study. Circulation 54:751, 1976.
63. McDonald IG: Echocardiographic demonstration of abnormal motion of the interventricular septum in left bundle branch block. Circulation 48:272, 1973.
64. Diamond MA, et al.: Echocardiographic features of atrial septal defect. Circulation 43:129, 1971.
65. Meyer RA, Schwartz DC, Benzing III G, Kaplan S: Ventricular septum in right ventricular volume overload. Am J Cardiol 30:349, 1972.
66. Kerber RE, Dippel WF, Abboud FM: Abnormal motion of the interventricular septum in right ventricular volume overload: experimental and clinical echocardiographic studies. Circulation 48:86, 1973.
67. Righetti A, et al.: Interventricular septal motion and left ventricular function after coronary bypass surgery. Am J Cardiol 39:372, 1977.

68. Kerber RE, Litchfield R: Postoperative abnormalities of interventricular septal motion: Two-dimensional and M-mode echocardiographic correlations. Am Heart J 104:263, 1982.
69. Payvandi MN, Kerber RE: Echocardiography in congenital and acquired absence of the pericardium: an echocardiographic mimic of right ventricular volume overload. Circulation 53:86, 1976.
70. Ticzon AR, et al.: Interventricular septal motion during preexcitation and normal conduction in Wolff-Parkinson-White syndrome. Am J Cardiol 37: 840, 1976.
71. Francis GS, et al.: An echocardiographic study of interventricular septal motion in the Wolff-Parkinson-White syndrome. Circulation 54:174, 1976.
72. Hishida H, et al.: Echocardiographic patterns of ventricular contraction in the Wolff-Parkinson-White syndrome. Circulation 54:567, 1976.
73. Joyner CR, Dydra I, Reid JM: Behavior of the anterior leaflet of the mitral valve in patients with the Austin Flint murmur. Clin Res 14:251, 1966.
74. Winsberg F, Gabor GE, Hernberg JG, Weiss B: Fluttering of the mitral valve in aortic insufficiency. Circulation 41:225, 1971.
75. Cope GD, Kisslo JA, Johnson ML, Myers S: Diastolic fluttering of the interventricular septum in aortic insufficiency. Circulation 51:589, 1975.
76. Wray TM: Echocardiographic manifestations of flail aortic valve leaflets in bacterial endocarditis. Circulation 51:832, 1975.
77. Mintz GS, Kotler MN, Segal BL, Parry WR: Comparison of two-dimensional and M-mode echocardiography in the evaluation of patients with infective endocarditis. Am J Cardiol 43:738, 1979.
78. Shah PM, Gramiak R, Kramer DH: Ultrasound localization of left ventricular outflow obstruction in hypertrophic obstructive cardiomyopathy. Circulation 40:3, 1969.
79. O'Shea JP, Castellani S, Harrigan P, Levine RA: Anterior motion of the mitral valve—onset before systolic ejection: a Doppler-echocardiographic study. Circulation 78 (Suppl 2):II-548, 1988.
80. Davies RH, et al.: Echocardiographic manifestations of discrete subaortic stenosis. Am J Cardiol 33:277, 1974.
81. Kruger SK, et al.: Echocardiography in discrete subaortic stenosis. Circulation 59:506, 1979.

CHAPTER

15

MISCELLANEOUS ECHOCARDIOGRAPHIC TECHNIQUES I: CONTRAST ECHOCARDIOGRAPHY

The major echocardiographic techniques are often used in conjunction with agents that facilitate some aspect of the study (contrast echocardiography); adapted to examine the heart from some unique location (esophageal echocardiography and intracardiac echocardiography); employed in a specialized setting (intraoperative echocardiography and exercise echocardiography); or applied to a unique population (fetal echocardiography). Because of the specialized nature of these applications or approaches, they have received specific designations and are therefore considered separately in this and the next chapter. Two areas, exercise echocardiography and fetal echocardiography, however, are discussed later in the text. Exercise echocardiography, in its current application, is most often employed to assess the response of the left ventricle to stress. Because of this chamber-related application, "exercise echo" is included in the evaluation of the left ventricle. Likewise, because the diagnoses of cardiac defects in utero are based on the same criteria used in the neonate and infant, fetal echocardiography is discussed in a separate chapter following the section on the diagnosis of congenital heart disease.

In considering specific subcategories of echocardiography, it is important to remember that the use of ultrasound in conjunction with image-enhancing agents or in special settings in no way changes the basic principles or physical limitations of the imaging or flow-sensing components of the examination. New limitations or potential for complications or toxicity may be introduced because of the agents used, the more invasive nature of the study, or the sensitivity of the population. However, the basic operations of the systems and the properties of the ultrasound employed remain the same.

HISTORY

One of the major advantages of echocardiography for studying the heart is its inherent natural separation of solid cardiac structures from blood-filled cavities without the need for exogenous contrast materials. During early M-mode studies, however, it became apparent that some form of exogenous contrast agent would be useful because the M-mode display often did not provide sufficiently recognizable anatomic information for structure identity to be deduced. In 1967, Joyner reported the appearance of "clouds of dense echoes" within the heart following intracardiac injections of saline solution or indocyanine green.[1] Gramiak and Shah subsequently used this "contrast effect" to identify echocardiographic anatomy in vivo by injecting through catheters positioned in selected cardiac chambers and recording the location and sequence of contrast appearance on the echocardiogram (Fig. 15–1).[2] Using this approach, they confirmed and extended the observations of Edler and Hertz concerning the anatomic origin of the predominant echoes from within the heart; they described the chambers, vessels and valves recorded from various transducer locations; and they identified previously unrecorded structures such as the interatrial septum. They further demonstrated the potential of this technique for recording physiologic changes in structure motion such

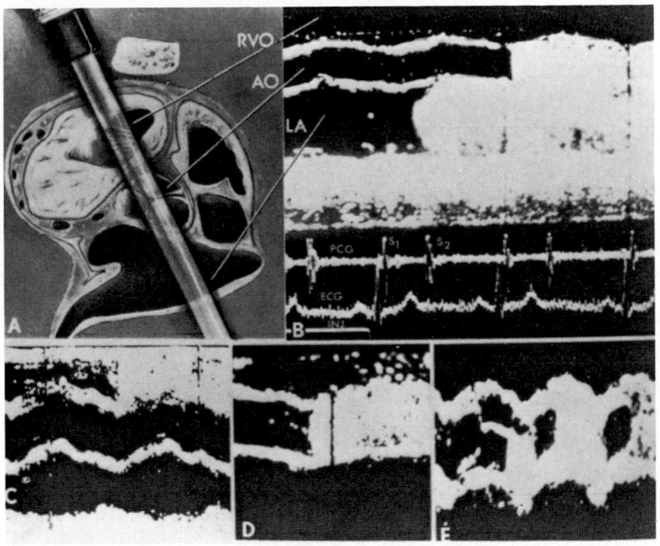

Fig. 15–1. Early contrast echo study for structure identification. **A.** M-mode beam transecting the right ventricular outflow tract (RVO) aortic root (AO) and left atrium (LA). **B.** Contrast injection in the left atrium, which opacifies the atrium and appears in the aorta during the following systolic ejection. ECG = electrocardiogram; PCG = phonocardiogram; **C.** Contrast in the right ventricular outflow tract following right-sided injection. **D.** Contrast in the aortic orifice and proximal ascending aorta following left ventricular injection. **E.** Aortic root injection shows negative contrast in the valve orifice as noncontrast-containing blood is ejected for the left ventricle. (From: Gramiak R, Shah PM: Echocardiography of the aortic root. Invest Radiol 3:356, 1968.)

as the midsystolic closure of the aortic valve in idiopathic hypertrophic subaortic stenosis (IHSS), the detection of regurgitant flow, and the determination of wall thickness.[3] It was also noted that the contrast effect was lost during passage through the lungs or systemic capillaries, and its appearance across cardiac septa was taken as evidence of an intracardiac shunt.[2] Subsequent studies by Bommer et al. showed that echo-contrast agents injected into the coronary arteries during echocardiographic recording produced myocardial opacification.[4] This property has subsequently been used to outline the perfusion territory of selected coronary vessels, while the absence of opacification of a region following intracoronary contrast injection has been shown to indicate lack of perfusion.[5–8] (See also Chapter 23).

SOURCE OF ECHO-CONTRAST

The likelihood that microbubbles* represented the echo source for the contrast effect was first suggested when small amounts of foam were noted in syringes of indocyanin green that were allowed to stand before use.[9] Additional support for microbubbles as the source of the contrast effect came from the observation that injections of degassed water, sucrose, or saline solution at atmospheric pressure produced echoes only when the injection velocity exceeded the threshold for transient cavitation.†[10] When the injections were repeated at similar cavitation velocities but with ambient pressure increased by 20 to 25 psi, no echoes, visible light scattering, or cavitation hiss were noted. It was concluded that the pressure-sensitive, light-scattering particles present exclusively during conditions of transient cavitation could only be microbubbles and that these represented the source of the contrast effect. Other possible causes of ultrasonic reflection, e.g., turbulence, temperature differential between the injectate and blood, and fluid acoustic impedance differences, were all examined and found to produce echo sources that would be insignificant in the clinical setting.[10] Subsequent studies demonstrating (1) microbubbles in the injectate by direct visualization, (2) a close correlation between the microbubble content of a liquid with its ultrasound contrast effect, and (3) the rate of rise of the contrast echoes in fluid to be the same as that of microbubbles firmly established that microbubbles are the "targets" that cause ultrasound contrast effects during peripheral or central injections of physiologic fluids into blood.[11] As a result, when the term *contrast* is used, microbubbles are usually understood.

MICROBUBBLES AS ECHO-CONTRAST AGENTS

Microbubbles are particularly strong reflectors because the gas within these bubbles has a markedly different acoustic impedance relative to that of blood. Studies of scattering from spheres at varying excitation frequencies[12] show that a 40-μm diameter microbubble excited by a 2-MHz frequency reflects 2×10^5 more signal than an equivalent size glass or steel sphere and nearly 4×10^5 as much as an equivalent diameter red cell aggregate.[12] This relative reflection ratio is even more pronounced for smaller bubbles.

The amplitude of the signal reflected from a bubble in a sound field of given frequency decreases approximately linearly with decreasing bubble diameter until the bubble resonant diameter is reached (Fig. 15–2) and then decreases as the cube of the diameter. This general trend is interrupted in two regions by perturbations in the response. The first causes fluctuations in response when bubble size is comparable to the wavelength of sound. The second causes a peak in response when the size corresponds to the bubble resonant frequency, which in water at 1 ata is approximated by;

$$d = 6.4/f \qquad [15.1]$$

where d is the diameter in microns and f the frequency

* Microbubbles are defined as gas bubbles smaller than 100 μm in diameter.

† Cavitation occurs at the tip of a catheter when the exhaust pressure decreases (because of the Bernoulli relationship $p + \rho v^2 = k$, where p, ρ, and v are the local stream pressure, fluid density, and velocity, respectively, and sum to equal a constant k) sufficiently that water vapor bubbles form. This characteristic is not a Reynolds number effect but rather a Thoma cavitation number effect. The Thoma cavitation number Th is defined as $Th = 2(p - p_v)/\rho v^2$, where p is the local catheter tip pressure (in dyne/cm², 1 mm Hg = 1333 dyne/cm²) and Pv is the fluid vapor pressure (47.035 mm Hg for H_2O at 37° C. Cavitation occurs whenever the Thoma cavitation number falls below a value of 0.35. When this occurs, microbubbles of water vapor are formed, and these bubbles are detected sonically as echo-contrast.

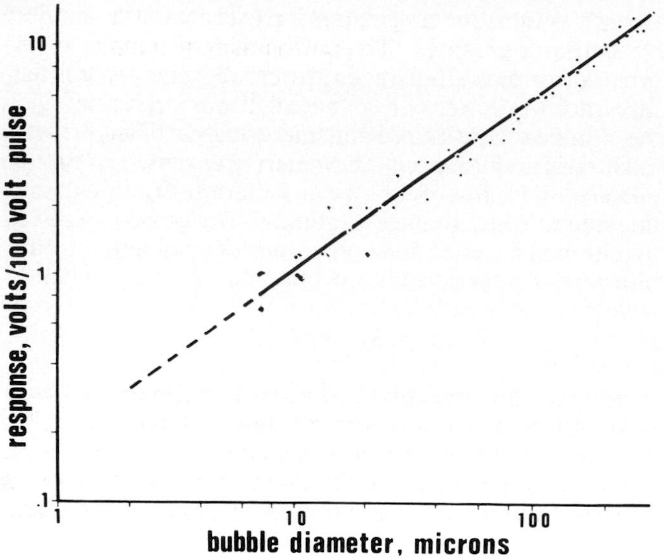

Fig. 15–2. Relationship of reflected signal intensity to bubble diameter. (From Rubissow GJ, Mackay RS: Ultrasonic studies during experimental decompression. *In* Meltzer RS, Roelandt J (eds.): Contrast Echocardiography. The Hague, Martinus Nijhoff, 1982.)

in MHz. The resonant frequency of a given diameter bubble further varies directly with the square root of the pressure inside the bubble.[13]

The minimum bubble size detectable by ultrasound depends on frequency, background noise surrounding the bubble, and scan depth, assuming optimum transducer and electronics design. An approximate limit to detectable size is probably set by the bubble resonant diameter. Based on an extrapolation of the curve in Figure 15–2, the smallest bubble detectable in water with a 7.5-MHz pulsed system is about 0.5 μm in diameter, or just below the resonant diameter. In practice, however, such measurements are difficult because bubbles of this size collapse almost instantly. The minimum size bubble detectable by Doppler is considerably larger than that using imaging because of the increased background noise that is due to blood flow.

In addition to their reflective properties, bubbles are also ideal targets because their spherical shape makes the intensity of their reflections independent of the direction of the sound source.

The reflective properties of a large group of microbubbles with diameters in the scattering range are far more complex. In theory, the reflective characteristics of such a suspension are determined by the individual microbubble properties (i.e., the type of gas they contain and their diameters), as well as their concentration and geometric distribution. In vivo recording of granular reflections from large numbers of microbubbles in the 4-μm range has clearly been demonstrated; however, the signal from reflectors of this size is generally weak relative to that from surrounding structures.[14]

Mathematic description of the relationship between contrast intensity and bubble concentration for a large ensemble of microbubbles would require injection of a standard amount of agent and be influenced by the range of scatterer sizes, because large scatterers reflect more energy and would interfere with those more deeply placed. In addition, because the geometric distribution in vivo would be unique for each case, precise definition of bubble concentration from contrast intensity appears intractable.

MICROBUBBLE CLEARANCE, COALESCENCE, AND DISSOLUTION

The observation that echo-contrast fails to pass the lungs and systemic capillaries implies that the microbubbles are somehow cleared from solution within these vascular networks. Clearly, if such bubbles are larger than the pulmonary capillary diameter of about 8 μm,[15] they will be held up by the pulmonary capillary "sieve." However, bubbles that are originally smaller than 10 μm, that are broken into fragments of this size or smaller within the pulmonary capillary bed, or that have their gas partly resorbed and "shrink" until they are smaller than 10 μm in diameter should be able to traverse the capillaries and emerge in the pulmonary or systemic veins. What then happens to these small bubbles? Studies of bubble dissolution dynamics[16,17] suggest that bubbles will shrink and disappear by diffusion in unsaturated solutions. In saturated solutions, bubble shrinkage and dissolution will also occur as a result of surface tension effects but at a slower rate. The additional incremental internal pressure within a bubble due to surface tension (P_i) is given as

$$P_i = 4\sigma/d \qquad [15.2]$$

where σ is the surface tension, and d is the bubble diameter. Thus, the small bubbles necessary to traverse the capillaries would have a high internal pressure as a result of their small diameters (for a 5-μm bubble, this excess pressure is about 420 mm Hg). The increased internal pressure would increase the gas concentration within the bubble. Gas inside the bubble would rapidly diffuse down the concentration gradient into the surrounding fluid, decreasing the bubble size further and increasing the internal pressure until total dissolution occurred. The time for total dissolution, taking into account the effects of surface tension, is presented in Figure 15–3 for both unsaturated and saturated solutions. An 8-μm bubble will completely dissolve in between 190 and 550 msec depending on the degree of saturation of the surrounding fluids. Nitrogen bubbles in this range, e.g., dissolve in blood plasma as if in an unsaturated solution, and their expected time for complete dissolution will be close to 190 msec.[18,19] Carbon dioxide bubbles, being more soluble in blood and body tissue, will dissolve even faster. Other effects, e.g., wiping away the diffusion boundary layer, can decrease this time dramatically and, as a result, this figure should be considered conservative. In humans, transit time from the pulmonary capillaries to the left atrium is 2 seconds or more, while the normal systemic circulation time is roughly 12 seconds. Hence, if bubbles smaller than 8 μm dissolve completely

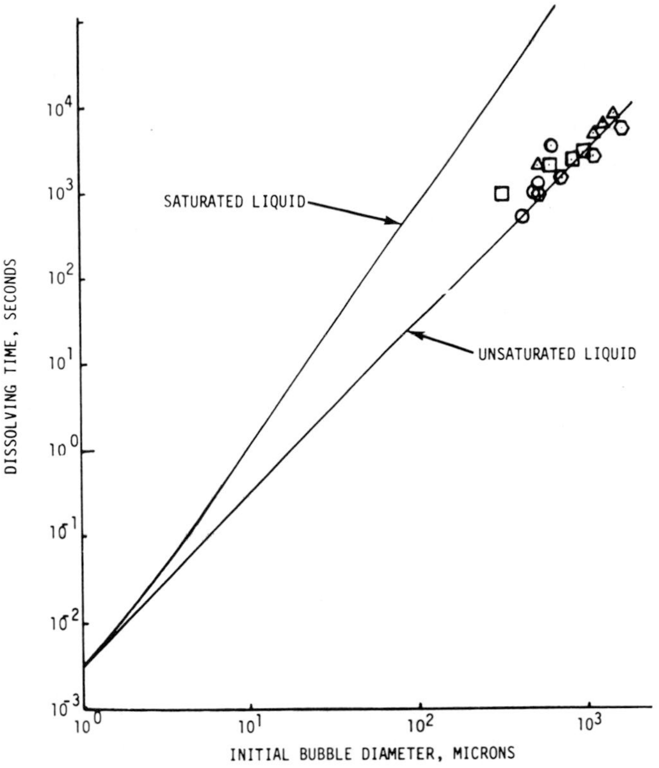

Fig. 15–3. Relationship between initial bubble diameter and time of total dissolution. Circles = oxygen bubbles in human blood; squares = oxygen bubbles in canine blood; triangles = nitrogen bubbles in human plasma; hexagons = oxygen bubbles in human plasma. (From Tickner EG, Meltzer RS: Why capillary beds remove ultrasonic contrast. *In* Meltzer RS, Roelandt J (eds.): Contrast Echocardiography. The Hague, Martinus Nijhoff, 1982.)

in less than 190 msec, they cannot survive for the time required to travel from the pulmonary capillaries to the left atrium or to transit the systemic circulation. Thus, microbubbles fail to pass from one side of the circulation to the other because those larger than capillary size are held up by the sieve action of the pulmonary and systemic capillary networks, and those that become small enough to get through the capillaries dissolve rapidly.

SPONTANEOUS BUBBLE FORMATION AND GROWTH IN SUPERSATURATED SOLUTIONS

Small bubbles in solution are inherently unstable and will grow or decay depending on the differences in gas tension inside and outside the bubble. In most clinical settings, the concentration of gas in the echo-contrast producing microbubbles is much higher than in blood, and the gas will diffuse down this gradient, causing the bubble to shrink. In certain cases, however, blood may be supersaturated with a gas (i.e., nitrogen) after ascent from a deep sea dive or following ether injection in experimental studies. In these cases, bubbles will arise spontaneously from solution and grow rather than shrink. Spontaneous bubble formation in tissue depends on the degree of supersaturation in that tissue, commonly measured by the supersaturation ratio.

$$\gamma = P_i/P_a \qquad [15.3]$$

where P_i is the inert gas tension and P_a is the ambient hydrostatic pressure. The mechanism of bubble formation is not clear, but recent research seems to confirm the traditional theory that bubble formation is related, at least in part, to pre-existing micronuclei.[14] Recent work also suggests that not only inert gas tension, but the tension of all dissolved gasses including O_2 plays a role in bubble formation and evolution. The growth of a bubble of initial radius R_o μm in a liquid of supersaturation ratio γ, in a time t (in seconds) is

$$R^2 = R_0^2 + 80t(\gamma - 1) \qquad [15.4]$$

where surface tension is neglected. Bubbles that arise spontaneously from supersaturated solutions are as easily detected by reflected ultrasound, as are those that are introduced from without. Such studies are frequently used to detect early signs of decompression sickness.[14]

SOURCE OF MICROBUBBLES IN INJECTED SOLUTIONS

Several theories have been advanced to explain the appearance of microbubbles during seemingly routine catheter injections. Those most commonly proposed are that (1) the bubbles are caused by cavitation as a result of the high velocity and low pressure at the catheter tip during injection, or (2) the bubbles represent air that is trapped in the injectate or the injecting apparatus. Although the early studies cited previously suggested that cavitation played a major role in microbubble formation, more recent data indicate that cavitation occurs only at catheter tip velocities that are well above those encountered clinically (about 24 m/sec). Conversely, the observations that the contrast effect directly relates to the bubble content in solution and that serial injections lead to decreasing gas content in the injectate (unless the injection apparatus is exposed to gases between studies) suggest that bubbles in the injectate and injecting apparatus are the source of the contrast effect. These observations further imply that the amount of contrast can be increased by maneuvers that increase the number of bubbles in solution, e.g., aeration or sonication, but not by forceful injection.

FACTORS AFFECTING MICROBUBBLE SURVIVAL

Because the contrast effect is related to the number of microbubbles in the solution, contrast can be enhanced by prolonging the life of the injected bubbles. Bubble survival can be prolonged by a variety of means including the use of physiologic solution with surfactant properties as the vehicle for injection, increasing gas content in the surrounding medium, interaction between bubbles in concentrated solution, and encapsulation or stabilization using substances such as gelatin or saccharides. Surfactants decrease the surface tension of bubbles in solution. Decreasing surface tension decreases the pressure within the bubble and as a result the decreases diffusion rate of gases out of the bubble core. This decreases the rate of shrinkage and prolongs survival. The most commonly used vehicles with good surfactant properties are meglumine diatrizoate (Renografin) and indocyanin green, both of which produce small noncoalescing bubbles with relatively long survival times.

Theoretically, if large concentrations of noncoalescing microbubbles are brought together, dissolution may also be reduced. This occurs because the outermost bubbles tend to protect the inner ones because they have the same gas concentration. Because bubble dissolution is caused by a concentration gradient, if such a gradient does not exist, dissolution will not occur. Eventually, the outer bubbles dissolve because they are only partially protected by the inner bubbles, but the net result is that a large group of closely spaced bubbles dissolves more slowly than an individual bubble. Precision bubbles encapsulated in gelatin can be produced and stabilized by freezing for prolonged periods of time. Although ideal for many applications, such precision bubbles are difficult to produce and hence have been employed only for selected research applications. The mechanism by which other agents, e.g., saccharide and albumin, stabilize bubbles in solution is less clear.

RELATIONSHIP OF BUBBLE SIZE TO RESONANT FREQUENCY

Bubble size determination based on variation in bubble resonant frequency with diameter has been discussed at length, and some promising results have been obtained. The importance of this line of investigation lies in the fact that changes in bubble size, which are recordable as changes in their resonant frequencies, in theory, reflect changes in the pressure of the surrounding fluid or intracardiac pressure (Fig. 15–4).

Bubbles in their purest form exhibit a simple one-degree-of-freedom, damped oscillatory behavior.[20,21] Their dynamic characteristics are comparable to a simple spring/mass system and for small excursions in radius may be described by an underdamped second-order linear differential equation. The spring constant is represented by the compression of the bubble gas, and the mass is equivalent to some effective mass of the liquid surrounding the bubble. Damping is caused by thermal and viscous effects of the gas and the surrounding liquid.

The free ringing frequency, f_r, of a bubble that oscillates as a sphere is given by

$$f_r = (3\gamma p/\rho)^{1/2}/\pi d, \qquad [15.5]$$

where p is the absolute pressure of gas in the bubble, γ is the specific heat ratio of the gas, ρ is the density of the liquid, and d is the bubble diameter. Thus, oscillatory frequency for a given gas bubble depends solely on the bubble diameter and its absolute pressure. Hence, if the physical properties and diameter are known, then the free ringing oscillation uniquely indicates the absolute local blood pressure.[22]

Because the bubble diameter $d = (6V/\pi)^{1/3}$ depends on the volume V, and the pressure and volume are related by the compressibility equation pV = constant,

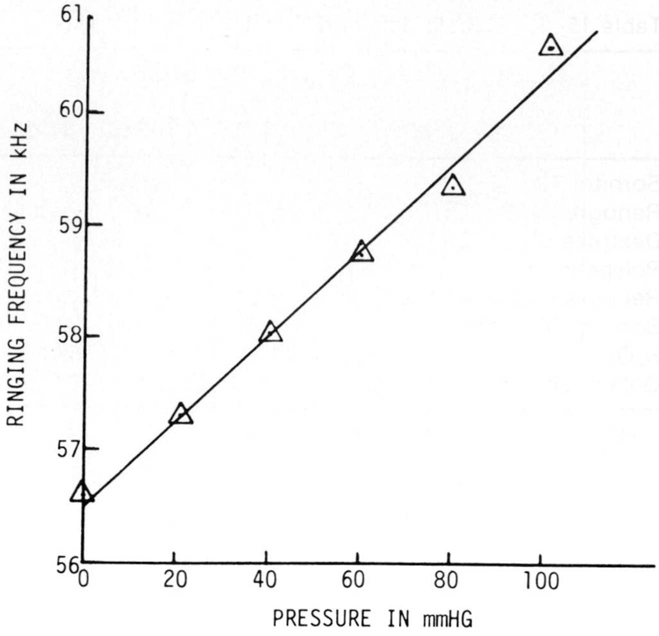

Fig. 15–4. Variation of free ringing bubble frequency with pressure. (From Tickner EG: Precision microbubbles for right side intracardiac pressure and flow measurements. *In* Meltzer RS, Roelandt J (eds.): Contrast Echocardiography. The Hague, Martinus Nijhoff, 1982.)

Equation 15.5 yields

$$p = p_0(f_r/f_0)^c \qquad [15.6]$$

where the zero subscript refers to the reference condition (e.g., atmospheric pressure), and c is a gas constant that depends solely on the polytropic coefficient at the excitation frequency.[22] The constant c is determined experimentally. Differentiating Equation 15.6 gives

$$dp/df_r = cp_0/f_0 \cdot (f_r/f_0)^{c-1} \qquad [15.7]$$

For oscillations near the reference pressure p_0 (atmospheric pressure), the factor $(f_r/f_0)^{c-1}$ is effectively 1, and Equation 15.7 may be approximated by

$$\Delta p/p_0 \approx c\,\Delta f_r/f_0. \qquad [15.8]$$

Thus, local changes in blood pressure can be directly determined by measurement of the change in ringing frequency Δf_r of bubbles in the blood stream. Two fundamental requirements exist however: The bubbles must ring in the blood stream, and they must be extremely precise to obtain accurate measurements. At atmospheric pressure, the resonant peak is sufficiently damped in blood to make this technique difficult, and results to date have been confined to in vitro experimental models.[23]

CONTRAST SOLUTIONS

Various physiologic solutions have been used as vehicles to carry microbubbles into solution. The simplest

Table 15–1. Bubble Size and Stability in a Representative Group of Contrast Solutions

Solution	Bubble Size (microns)	Source	Percent Remaining at 5 min
Sorbitol 70% (SON)	06 ± 2	Feinstein et al.[31]	80
Renografin-76 (SON)	10 ± 4	Feinstein et al.[31]	58
Dextrose 50% (SON)	11 ± 5	Feinstein et al.[31]	63
Polygelin col	12 ± 10	Santoso et al.[26]	78
Renografin/saline (HA)	16 ± 13	Feinstein et al.[31]	50
Sorbitol 70% (HA)	23 ± 26	Feinstein et al.[31]	92
H_2O_2	52 (10–100)	Kemper et al.[8]	—
Gelatin-encapsulated microbubbles	76 ± 1	Armstrong et al.[7]	—

HA = hand agitated; SON = sonicated.

and least expensive of these agents include sterile water, sterile saline solution, Ringer's lactate, and 5% dextrose in water. Microbubbles can be produced in these solutions either by hand agitation or sonication.* None of these solutions has good surfactant properties, and the bubbles formed by agitation tend to vary widely in size and to coalesce rapidly. Therefore, rapid injection after agitation is essential. If contrast is unsatisfactory, repeated agitation with 1 to 3 ml of CO_2 will generally improve the result. However, CO_2 solutions are also relatively unstable with rapidly changing bubble sizes and eventual coalescence into macrobubbles.[24] Therefore, rapid injection following agitation is again necessary. In addition to mixing CO_2 with other solutions, it has been reported that the gas can be injected directly in a dose of 0.25 ml/kg up to a maximum of 15 ml per injection with excellent contrast production.[25] Another simple approach is to withdraw and inject the patient's own blood. However, this appears less satisfactory than the other methods mentioned.

The second group of contrast agents are those with inherent surfactant properties. The two most commonly used agents in this group are indocyanine green (Cardiogreen) and meglumine diatrizoate (Renografin). Solutions of these substances tend to contain smaller bubbles, which are more stable, remain in solution longer, and do not tend to coalesce as rapidly. The normal injection of indocyanin green for adults is 1 ml (5 mg/ml) injected into a catheter and manually flushed with 5 to 10 ml of sterile saline solution or D_5W. Another agent used to stabilize bubbles because of its surfactant properties is 3.5% polygelin colloid solution, which is widely used for plasma substitution outside the United States. This solution contains degraded gelatin polypeptides cross-linked by urea bridges whose molecular weight is roughly 35,000.[26] The major disadvantages of these agents are the cost and time required to prepare the injectate.

The third group of agents are the "precision" microbubbles. The best characterized of these agents are the gelatin-encapsulated microbubbles, which contain CO_2 as the gaseous agent. These gelatin-encapsulated bubbles can be manufactured to fairly rigid size specifications, and bubbles ranging from 10 to 150 μm have been produced. Saccharide solutions have also been reported to yield "precision" microbubbles. These solutions appear to rely on the size and configuration of the saccharide particles to form selective attachments to bubbles of relatively uniform size rather than actual encapsulation of the gas.[27] Although such a process would tend to favor selection of bubbles of a particular size range, the percentage of the total population that falls within this range and the uniformity of this subpopulation remain unclear. Solutions of protein particles appear to act on the same principle. Note however, that these solutions also have separate surfactant properties so that their precise mechanism of bubble selection and stabilization is highly complex.

Other agents that have been used include hydrogen peroxide, perflurocarbons, and viscous solutions such as sorbitol (70%) and dextrose (50% and 70%). Hydrogen peroxide interacts with peroxidase in the blood to form water and free oxygen. Some of the oxygen combines with hemoglobin, while the remainder forms microbubbles of oxygen that disperse into the blood stream.[28–30] The mixture of dilute hydrogen peroxide and autologous blood results in the generation of a heterogeneous population of oxygen bubbles ranging in size from 10 to 100 μm (mean, 52 μm). The usual dosage of hydrogen peroxide is 2 to 10 ml of a 0.2 to 0.3% solution. Although reported safe in several large clinical series, the large bubbles that tend to form with this agent and potential for air embolism make us reluctant to use it clinically when other equally good agents are available. Perflurocarbons carry oxygen and have been used experimentally to preclude any ischemic effects resulting

* Sonication is an ultrasonic method for agitating a fluid that produces small, relatively uniform, stable microbubbles. The device used to perform this process, the sonicator, contains a piezoelectic element, which is capable of producing sound at sufficient energy levels to cavitate tissue and fluids. The process occurs in several stages. During the initial stage, nuclei of gas or particulate matter within the liquid are brought into the intense sound field transmitted from the horn tip of the sonicator unit. The sound field causes powerful cyclic compression and rarifaction of these preformed cavities, causing them to grow until they reach their resonant diameter. At this point, known as the *catastrophic phase*, the cavity begins to oscillate violently, radiating periodic shock waves, which open new microcavities that are extremely small but so plentiful that the solution becomes cloudy. These small, secondary, noncollapsing, bubbles outside the core of the energy beam can then act as highly effective echo-contrast targets.

from the replacement of oxygen-carrying blood by the contrast injectate. However, there seems to be little additional value to using such agents, because the ischemia has been shown to be due to mechanical obstruction by bubbles rather than blood replacement. Sonication of viscous solutions has been shown to produce microbubbles less than 10 μm in diameter, while more dilute, less viscous solutions typically result in microbubbles ranging in size from 10 to 23 μm.[31] Such considerations are important in experimental studies (see following discussion) but, to date, have not been demonstrated to be of clinical relevance. Table 15–1 lists the bubble size and stability found in a representative group of solutions.

INJECTION TECHNIQUE

To achieve the contrast effect, one can inject microbubble-containing solutions into either a peripheral vein or through a more centrally positioned catheter. The antecubital vein is typically used for peripheral venous injections; however, any of the smaller veins of the hand or arm will generally suffice. The choice of contrast agents for clinical studies is based on the reliability of a particular agent in producing opacification, expense, simplicity of preparation of the injectate, and potential for toxicity. The contrast solutions most commonly used clinically are sterile saline, D_5W, and indocyanine green. Because of their ready availability, sterile saline or D_5W are usually our agents of first choice for both peripheral venous and central injections. Five to ten ml of the solution is typically injected. To increase microbubble concentration, it is customary to draw up the solution to be injected along with a small amount of free air. The syringe is then shaken vigorously to aerate the injectate, the remaining free air is expelled, and the solution is injected rapidly. The solution can also be aerated by rapid injection into and out of the vial or by repeat injection from one syringe to another via a three-way stopcock. When adequately aerated, the saline solution will take on a cloudy gray appearance. If adequate contrast is not achieved with saline or D_5W, we then try indocyanine green (1 ml) followed by a 5 to 10 ml saline flush. Although larger bore needles (No. 14 to 18) or intravenous catheters are often recommended, adequate injections can be obtained with a No. 19 scalp vein.

High flow rates are probably important to flush the bolus of contrast along peripheral veins into the central circulation without margination but seem unnecessary in central catheter injections.

The use of a three-way stopcock contributes to the success of the contrast injection by enabling rapid access because agitated saline solution retains the suspended air for only a brief period. The transit time from the peripheral vein to the right atrium is usually between 5 and 7 seconds. Some of the microbubbles will typically stick to the vessel walls or be held in the periphery by their buoyancy. As a result, massage of the arm will often produce a second contrast flow without additional injection.

It is often recommended that contrast be injected into the left arm when possible, because this will disclose a persistent left superior vena cava if present. Likewise, it is customary to have all patients perform a Valsalva maneuver during at least one contrast injection. The Valsalva maneuver interrupts venous return during the strain phase as a result of the increased intrathoracic pressure. With release, the peripheral veins rapidly empty into the right atrium, while the left atrium receives little blood from the lungs. This alters the right-to-left atrial pressure gradient and will frequently result in small amounts of shunting when the foramen ovale is patent. This is important to document in all cases but particularly when paradoxic embolus is suspected.

Although contrast studies may be useful in patients of all ages, they are particularly easy to obtain in the sick newborn because of the large number of central lines that are typically in place, the short distances involved, and the small volume of the circulation.

LEFT-SIDED CONTRAST FOLLOWING RIGHT-SIDED INJECTION

Because microbubbles are entirely cleared by the lungs, left-sided contrast can normally be obtained only by direct catheterization of left-sided structures. This is obviously highly invasive and is typically done only as an adjunct to routine cardiac catheterization, significantly limiting the utility of the technique. Several authors have reported, however, that left-sided contrast can be produced by injecting D_5W, CO_2, or saccharide microbubbles through catheters wedged in the distal pulmonary artery.[32,33,45] Success rates for obtaining left heart contrast following pulmonary capillary wedge (PCW) injections approaching 95% have been reported. The reason for this level of success is not totally clear, because even if microbubbles do pass through the capillaries, they must still survive to reach the left heart. Several possible mechanisms have been suggested: (1) Direct intrapulmonary injection of contrast increases the concentration reaching the pulmonary bed, increasing local gas tension. (2) By introducing the agent closer to the pulmonary capillaries, there is less time for dissolution. (3) The injecting pressure may both expand the capillaries and deform the bubbles, permitting larger bubbles to cross the capillaries than would be possible with peripheral injections. The increased concentration of bubbles may have the additional effect of permitting the bubbles to enter the capillaries in a "packed train" so that those that dissolve will increase the local gas concentration and protect or even feed the survivors. The bubbles in the train will still dissolve but at a slower rate so that some of the bubbles in the train emerge from the pulmonary bed. Another approach to obtain left-sided contrast from right-sided injection relies on small, stabilized microbubbles. Sonication of albumin solution produces bubbles small enough (3 to 8 μ in diameter) to cross pulmonary capillary circulation and stable enough to survive more than the 10 seconds required to reach the left heart. Other contrast agents such as galactose solution are under development. Currently, optimal doses of these agents, their reproducibility, and their potential for clinical applications are under investigation.

EXAMINATION TECHNIQUE

Contrast material can be visualized using either the two-dimensional or M-mode methods or can be recorded as an increase in signal amplitude using the Doppler technique. The selection of imaging plane or sampling location, in general, is based on the specific lesion to be diagnosed or excluded and the clarity of a particular view in a given patient. The plane most frequently used for two-dimensional imaging is the apical four-chamber view, which displays the full extent of the atrial and ventricular septa followed by the parasternal long axis view. M-mode imaging is usually performed from the parasternal window using the transducer directed through the tips of the mitral valve leaflets (Fig. 15–5A), followed by a slightly higher view through the right ventricular outflow tract, aortic root, and left atrium (Fig. 15–5B). The suprasternal notch has also been reported to be of value in M-mode studies, because from this projection the aorta, right pulmonary artery, and left atrium bear a fixed relationship to one another and the

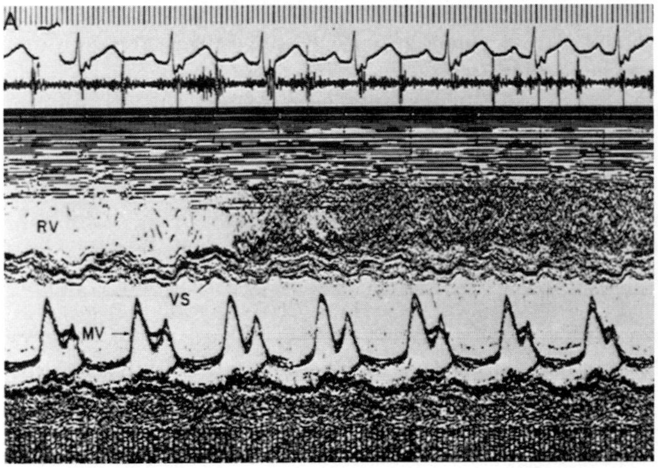

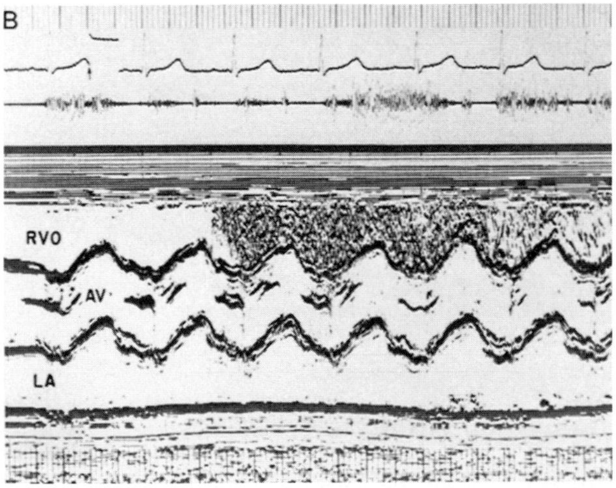

Fig. 15–5. **A.** Normal pattern of contrast appearance following peripheral venous injection on an M-mode recording of the left ventricle at the mitral valve (MV) level. RV = right ventricle; VS = ventricular septum. **B.** Normal pattern of contrast appearance following peripheral venous injection on an M-mode recording of the left heart at the aortic valve (AV) level. RVO = right ventricular outflow; LA = left atrium. (From Seward JB, Tajik AJ, Hagler DJ, Ritter DG: Peripheral venous contrast echocardiography. Am J Cardiol 39:202, 1977.)

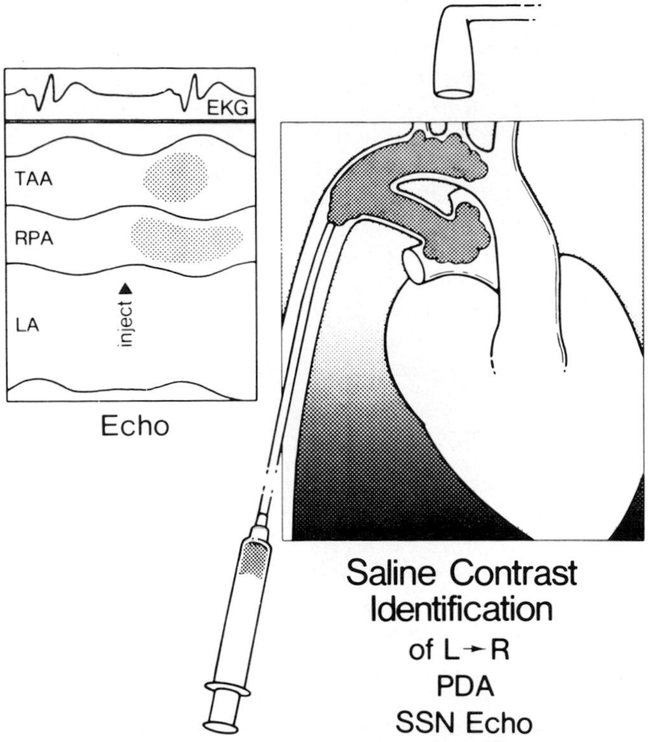

Fig. 15–6. A catheter positioned in the descending aorta via the umbilical artery in the neonate and the resulting suprasternal contrast echo pattern that would appear as a result of the left-to-right shunting through a patent ductus. EKG = electrocardiogram; TAA = transverse aotic arch; RPA = right pulmonary artery; LA = left atrium; PDA = patent ductus arteriovenous; SSN = suprasternal notch. (From Sahn, et al.: The utility of contrast echocardiographic techniques in the care of critically ill infants with cardiac and pulmonary disease. Circulation 56:959, 1977. Reproduced by permission of the American Heart Association, Inc.)

pattern of contrast flow into the great vessels can be of particular diagnostic value in complex congenital heart disease (Fig. 15–6).

In general, the two-dimensional examination with its spatial resolution and dynamic tomographic presentation is superior to the M-mode contrast study; however, for the purposes of accurate timing of the arrival of the contrast material and of correlating the contrast effect with other cardiac events, M-mode is superior.

EFFECTS OF INJECTED CONTRAST ON IMAGE RESOLUTION

As noted previously, the reflections that occur at the interface between the gas-containing microbubbles and the surrounding fluid are intense. This has the positive result of permitting small microbubbles to be visualized. However, when injected as a bolus, these strong reflectors have important effects on the contrast-enhanced image and on the ability of the imaging system to resolve the spatial distribution of the contrast pool. The most important of these effects is on spatial resolution. The intense contrast reflectors characteristically increase both the axial length of the reflected signal and the apparent lateral expanse of the contrast pool as a result of the point spread function of the system. Thus, when the area of a contrast-filled chamber is measured, it will be

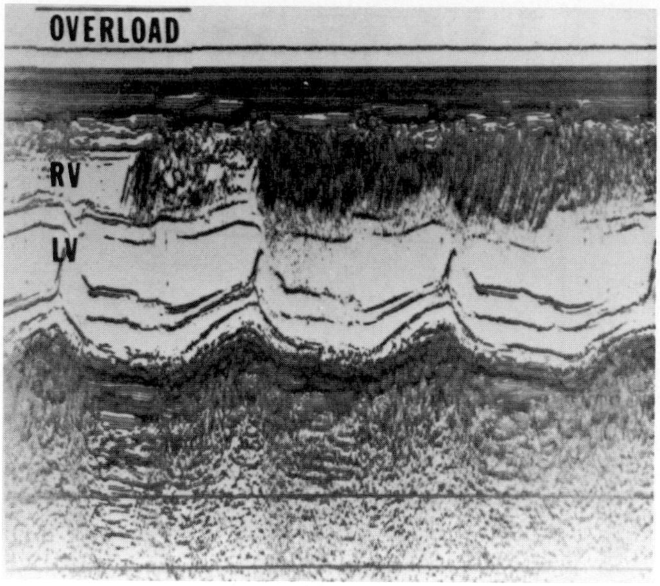

Fig. 15–7. Contrast overload. The contrast echoes recorded in the interventricular septum and left ventricle (LV) represent reverberations caused by the dense concentration of contrast in the right ventricle (RV). (From Valdez-Cruz, et al.: Recognition of residual post-operative shunts by contrast echocardiographic techniques. Circulation 55:148, 1977. Reproduced by permission of the American Heart Association, Inc.)

artifactually increased for the same reason that imaging the normal endocardial targets tends to constrict the chamber area. The degree of apparent expansion will be a function of gain and should be greater for a given gain setting than the normal constriction produced by imaging the endocardial targets because the contrast pool is a stronger reflector than the endocardium.

Other effects of contrast on the image include internal reverberations within the pool with apparent "spill over" of the contrast into subjacent chambers (Fig. 15–7); almost total absorption of the sound energy by the intense contrast-related reflections, which obscures more distal structures (shadowing); and the displacement of individual reflectors into adjacent chambers resulting from beam width. When this beam width displacement is in an axial or lateral direction, the target in question can usually be related to the primary contrast pool. However, when the beam width artifact relates to displacement in the thickness dimension, the origin of the artifact may be more difficult to appreciate.

ANALYSIS OF CONTRAST ECHOGRAMS

The analysis of any echo-contrast study requires consideration of several factors. These are listed in Table 15–2 and include the pattern and timing of contrast appearance; contrast intensity; cyclic changes in contrast intensity; the duration of opacification, or the clearance time; the effect of inflow of non-contrast-containing blood on the contrast pool, or the negative contrast effect; and the rate of microbubble motion as manifest by the slope of bubble trajectories.

Table 15–2. Factors To Be Considered in the Analysis of Contrast Echocardiograms

Pattern of contrast appearance
Timing of contrast appearance
Intensity
Cyclic opacification
Duration of opacification (clearance time)
Negative contrast effect
Slope of trajectories

Pattern of Contrast Appearance

Microbubbles injected into the circulation characteristically follow the path of blood flow through the heart and great vessels until they reach a point at which the size of the vessel becomes smaller than the bubble diameter (e.g., a capillary bed), where they become trapped, dissolve, and disappear from solution. The expected pattern of contrast appearance therefore parallels the path of blood flow, and changes in this pattern can be diagnostic of many flow-related lesions. Figures 15–8 and 15–9, e.g., illustrate the different patterns of contrast appearance that are recorded in patients with atrial and ventricular septal defects. In atrial septal defect (Fig. 15–8), peripherally injected contrast traverses the interatrial septum during systole and flows into both ventricles simultaneously during the peak filling phase of diastole. In the left ventricle, contrast initially appears in the mitral valve funnel, indicating that it originated from the left atrium, with subsequent opacification of the ventricular cavity. In ventricular septal defect (Fig. 15–9), flow is directed from the right-to-the left ventricles. The right ventricle is initially opacified during the rapid filling phase of diastole; however, contrast does not appear in the mitral funnel but rather becomes visible in the left ventricular cavity during the isovolumic

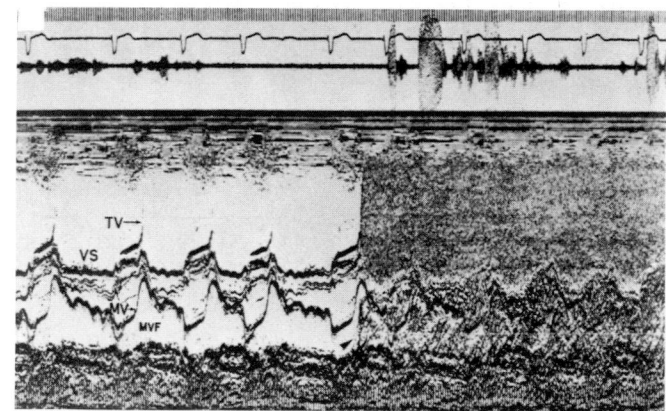

Fig. 15–8. Pattern of contrast appearance, following peripheral venous injection in a patient with an atrial septal defect. After peripheral venous injection of dye, echoes appear during diastole in the left ventricle through the mitral valve funnel (MVF) nearly simultaneously with the appearance of echoes in the right ventricle. MV = mitral valve; TV = tricuspid valve; VS = ventricular septum. (From Seward JB, Tajik AJ, Hagler DJ, Ritter DG: Peripheral venous contrast echocardiography. Am J Cardiol 39:202, 1977.)

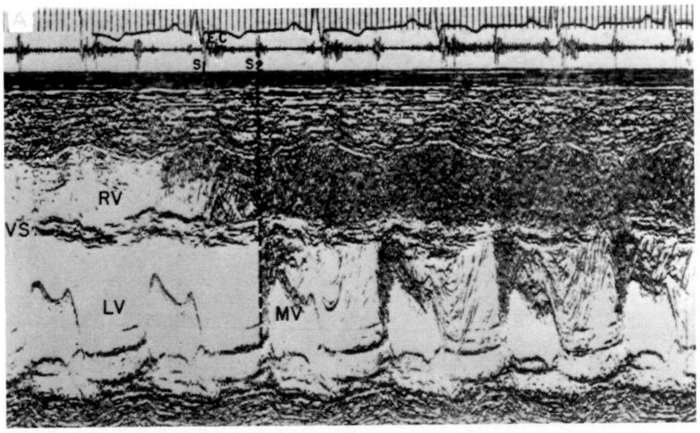

Fig. 15–9. Pattern of contrast appearance following peripheral venous injection in a patient with a ventricular septal defect and a right to left shunt. After diastolic opacification of the right ventricle (RV), no dye appears in the left ventricle (LV) for one complete cardiac cycle. During the next cycle, contrast appears anterior to the mitral valve (MV) during isovolumic relaxation (i.e., after aortic valve closure and before mitral valve opening). This pattern of right to left shunting is repeated in each subsequent cardiac cycle. EC = echo contrast, not visible on art; VS = interventricular septum, S_1 = first heart sound; S_2 = second heart sound. (From Assad-Morell JL et al.: Echophonocardiographic and contrast studies in conditions associated with systemic arterial trunk overriding the ventricular septum, truncus arteriosus, tetralogy of Fallot, and pulmonary atresia with ventricular septal defect. Circulation 53:663, 1976. Reproduced by permission of the American Heart Association, Inc.)

period of the next diastole. Figure 15–10 illustrates the more complex pattern of tricuspid atresia. In this case, following peripheral injection, flow is obstructed at the tricuspid valve and initially crosses the atrial septum from left to right. Therefore, contrast initially appears in the mitral funnel as a result of the right-to-left atrial shunt. Contrast is then visible in the left ventricle and finally is recorded in the right ventricle. Thus, although contrast appears in the right and left ventricles, in each case, the pattern of appearance results in three different diagnoses.

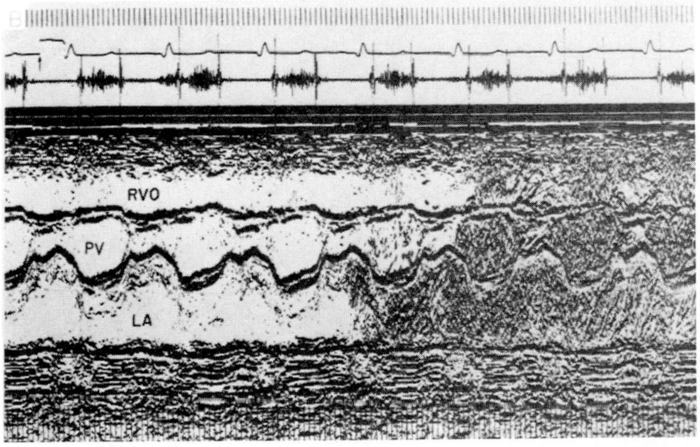

Fig. 15–10. Pattern of contrast appearance following peripheral venous injection in a patient with tricuspid atresia and transposed great arteries. The left atrium is initially opacified, and only with subsequent systoles are the pulmonary valve (PV) and finally the right ventricular outflow tract (RVO) opacified. LA = left atrium. (From Seward JB, Tajik AJ, Hagler DJ, Ritter DG: Peripheral venous contrast echocardiography. Am J Cardiol 39:202, 1977.)

Timing of Contrast Appearance

Although the pattern and timing of contrast appearance in most cases are inseparable, in certain instances the timing of appearance contains independent information. For example, in pulmonary A-V fistula, there is abnormal appearance of contrast in the left atrium following right-sided injection similar to that seen with an atrial septal defect (ASD). To pass through the fistula, however, the contrast must traverse the entire pulmonary circuit rather than just crossing the atrial septum. The arrival of contrast in the left atrium, therefore, is delayed 4 to 8 cycles after its arrival in the right ventricle, and it is this difference in timing rather than the pattern of appearance that distinguishes the two lesions (Fig. 15–11).

Cyclic Opacification

The pattern of contrast motion within individual cardiac cycles may also provide important diagnostic information. In ASD with left to right shunt, e.g., the flow of non-contrast-containing blood from left to right (negative contrast effect; see following discussion) is greatest at end-systole and early-diastole when the left-to-right gradient is maximal. Likewise, in D-transposition of the great vessels, peripherally injected contrast will be most apparent in the pulmonary artery during diastole when ductal flow is greatest and almost absent during systole when flow into the pulmonary artery is from the left-sided ventricle (Fig. 15–12). Ventricular septal defect with subsystemic pressures will typically show shunting only during the isovolumic phase of diastolic relaxation. In tricuspid regurgitation, contrast flow into the inferior vena cava following peripheral injection is only diagnostic when it occurs with the right atrial "v," wave and reflux of contrast at this point must be differentiated from that occurring during other points in the cycle. There are numerous other examples where the timing of

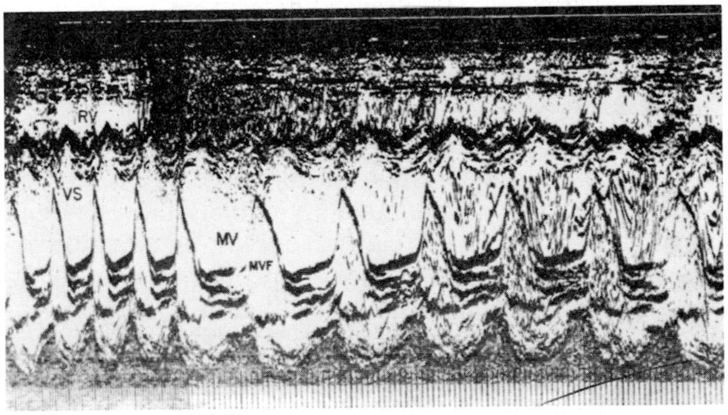

Fig. 15–11. Pattern of contrast appearance in a patient with pulmonary arteriovenous fistula. Contrast initially appears in the right ventricle (RV) and is then noted in the mitral valve funnel a number of cycles later. This delayed passage from right to left reflects the time required for the contrast to transit the pulmonary circulation. VS = ventricular septum; MV = mitral valve; MVF = mitral valve funnel. (From Shub C, Tajik AJ, Seward JB, Dines DE: Detecting intrapulmonary right-to-left shunt with contrast echocardiography: observations in a patient with diffuse pulmonary arteriovenous fistulas. Mayo Clin Proc 51:81, 1976.)

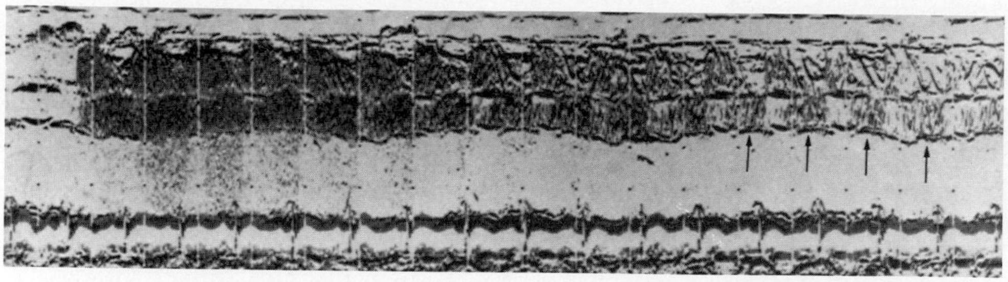

Fig. 15–12. Suprasternal notch M-mode recording illustrating predominant diastolic shunting (arrows) from the descending aorta into the pulmonary artery in a patient with transposition of the great vessels and a patent ductus arteriosus. (From Hunter S, Sutherland GR: Contrast M-mode echocardiography, the suprasternal notch approach. *In* Meltzer RS, Roelandt J (eds.): Contrast Echocardiography. The Hague, Martinus Nijhoff, 1982.)

contrast motion within the cardiac cycle is important, and these are discussed with the specific disease entity.

Intensity

The absolute intensity of contrast is variable from injection to injection and therefore is of little value. The relative contrast intensity, however, appears to contain more useful information. For example, in the presence of right-to-left shunt at the atrial or ventricular level, the great artery that opacifies more intensely and persistently can reasonably be assumed to receive most of the systemic venous return. This concept of relative intensity may be of practical value in conditions such as transposition of the great arteries. D-transposition differs from other forms of cyanotic congenital heart disease in that the greater the right-to-left shunt at the atrial or ventricular level, the higher the effective pulmonary blood flow will be and the higher the systemic arterial oxygen saturation. By comparing the percentage of aortic oxygen saturation to relative opacification of both great arteries, some idea can be derived about effective pulmonary blood flow. For example, when the aortic saturation is less than 40%, the amount of contrast appearing in the left atrium is minimal and the aorta opacifies for more than twice as many cycles as the pulmonary artery. When the aortic saturation is between 40 and 60%, the pulmonary artery opacifies for more than half as many cycles as the aorta, although there is usually still sufficient differential opacification to make the diagnosis of ventriculoarterial discordance (Fig. 15–13). When both great arteries opacify equally intensely and for the same number of cardiac cycles, an accurate assessment of ventriculoarterial connections becomes impossible. Under these conditions at cardiac catheterization, there is usually less than 10% difference between the aortic and pulmonary artery oxygen saturation.[34]

Duration

The rate of appearance and disappearance of contrast in the individual patient has been shown to bear a rough correlation to absolute flow at the time of study. When flow is high, contrast washes out quickly, while in low flow states, the converse is true. This effect can be quantitated and is discussed in more detail later in the section on cardiac output.

Negative Contrast Effect

The negative contrast effect occurs when non-contrast-containing blood enters a contrast-filled chamber or vessel, displacing the contrast already present and creating an echo-free area in a region where contrast would ordinarily be expected. This negative contrast effect can be seen in patients with ASD and left-to-right shunting, ventricular septal defect with left-to-right shunting, D-transposition in the region of left-to-right ductal flow, and at virtually any point where a significant non-contrast-containing stream enters a contrast-containing chamber. In patients with ASD and a left-to-right shunt, the area of negative contrast varies throughout the cardiac cycle, being greatest at the point of peak anterior motion of the aortic root, which corresponds to end-systole or initial diastole (Fig. 15–14). This is consistent with catheterization data, which show that the maximum gradient across an ASD and peak shunt flow occur during end-systole and initial diastole.[35] When making any diagnosis on the basis of the negative contrast effect, it is important to consider all of the possible sources of non-contrast-containing blood entering the chamber. Following initial contrast opacification, chambers such as the right atrium receive non-contrast-con-

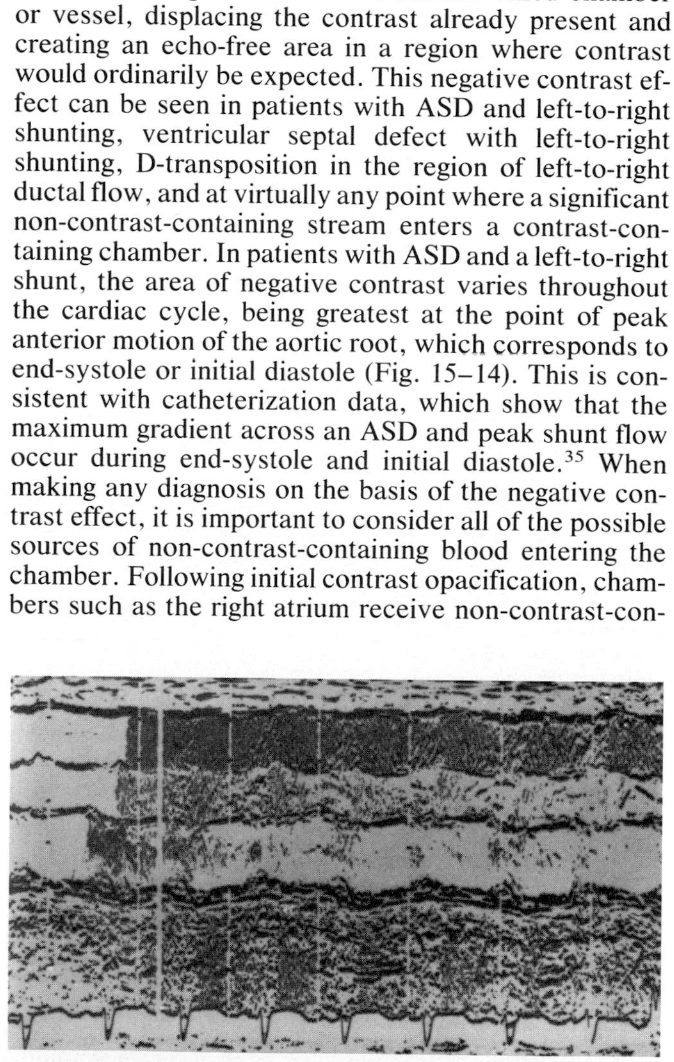

Fig. 15–13. Suprasternal notch echogram from a patient with transposition of the great arteries. The left atrium opacifies followed by both great arteries. The aorta is more persistently and intensely opacified, suggesting that it receives most of the systemic venous return. (From Hunter S, Sutherland GR: Contrast M-mode echocardiography: the suprasternal notch approach. *In* Meltzer RS, Roelandt J (eds.): Contrast Echocardiography, The Hague, Martinus Nijhoff, 1982.)

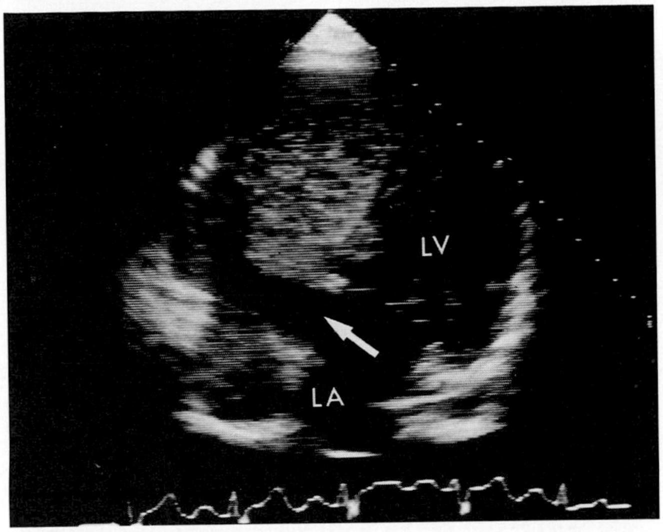

Fig. 15–14. Negative contrast effect in atrial septal defect. LA = left atrium; LV = left ventricle.

taining blood from sources other than an ASD. In normal patients, inflow from the inferior vena cana and coronary sinus will also be non-contrast-containing, while various types of heart disease, such as tricuspid regurgitation, may also contribute non-contrast-containing blood to the right atrial blood pool.

Slope of Trajectories

Theoretically, microbubbles in blood should travel at the same speed as that of the red blood cells. This being the case then, the speed of an individual bubble traveling parallel to the sound beam should be reflected by the slope of the trajectory of the bubble on an M-mode tracing. The rational for velocity calculation is that the distance traveled by the bubble is depicted by its movement toward or away from the transducer, while time is represented by the sweep speed of the M-mode trace. Thus, distance per unit time or velocity is represented by the slope of the trajectory of the bubble.[36] Figures 15–15 and 15–16 illustrate the method for calculating bubble velocities. Studies comparing velocities measured in this fashion with electromagnetic flow probe recordings and Doppler flow sampling have, in general, yielded good correlation[37] (Fig. 15–17), although some authors have found the approach less reliable than Doppler.[38] Accuracy requires that the target move parallel to the beam and that an individual target be recordable for at least 1.5 cm and preferably longer. Likewise, when echo and Doppler recordings are compared, correction must be introduced for the delay in signal output introduced by the Fourier analyzer.

Contrast trajectories can also be useful in documenting changes in flow direction and timing. In patients with normal pulmonary valve flow, e.g., forward contrast flow (negative trajectories) is noted throughout systole. In pulmonary hypertension (peak pulmonary artery pressure greater than 50 mm Hg, however, the contrast trajectories stop in midsystole with slight reversal in direction in some cases and complete reversal in others. Contrast echo lines reversing in early-diastole and crossing the pulmonary valve echogram during diastole have been reported in patients with pulmonary regurgitation.[39] In general, contrast trajectories suffer the same limitations as Doppler in that they reflect only flow velocity at the sampling site, which may not truly reflect either mean or peak velocity. Likewise, in routine practice, they can be studied only after peripheral venous injection and therefore only provide information concerning right-sided velocities. Doppler, therefore, is the obvious method of choice for measuring velocity. Contrast trajectories, however, do have several advantages that should be kept in mind. First, they have no depth or

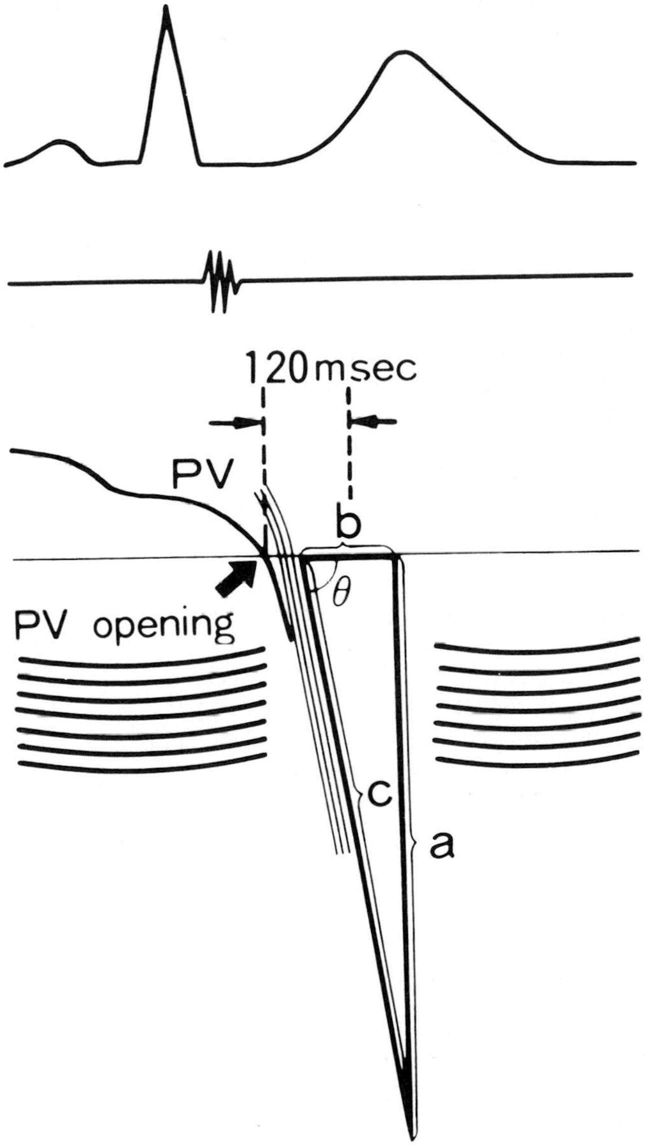

Fig. 15–15. Method for measurement of the flow velocity based on the linear contrast echo angle at the pulmonic valve (PV) orifice. A horizontal line is drawn at the position of pulmonic valve opening. Within 120 msec after pulmonic valve opening, the peak flow velocity is calculated as a/b mm/sec. (From Shiina A, et al.: Contrast echocardiographic evaluation of changes in flow velocity in the right side of the heart. Circulation 63:1408, 1981. Reproduced by permission of the American Heart Association, Inc.)

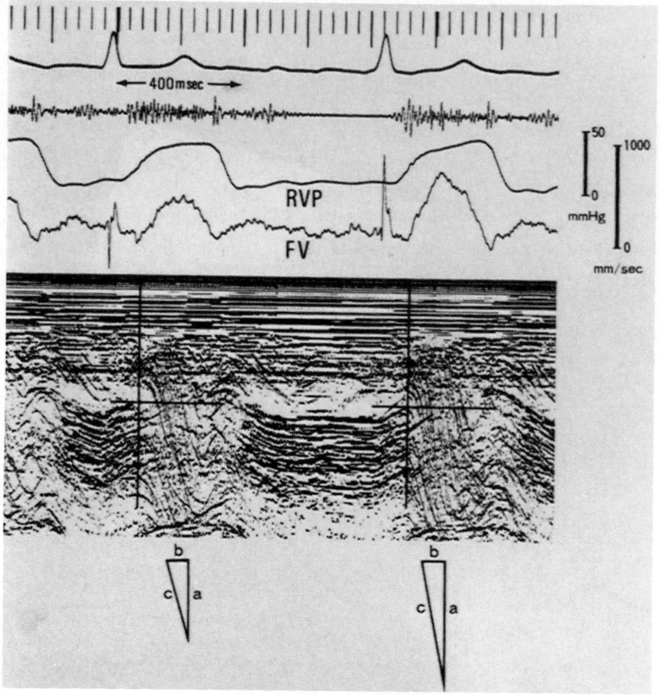

Fig. 15–16. Simultaneous recordings of contrast echoes at the pulmonic valve orifice, right ventricular pressure (RVP) and flow velocity (FV) obtained from a probe positioned at the valve orifice in a patient with atrial fibrillation. (Vertical and horizontal lines are drawn through the point of pulmonary valve opening.) Flow velocity changes according to the preceding R-R interval. When the flow velocity curve is higher, the ratio of a to b is greater (right), whereas when the flow velocity curve is lower, the ratio of a to b is smaller. (Shiina A, et al.: Contrast echocardiographic evaluation of changes in flow velocity in the right side of the heart. Circulation 63:1408, 1981. Reproduced by permission of the American Heart Association, Inc.)

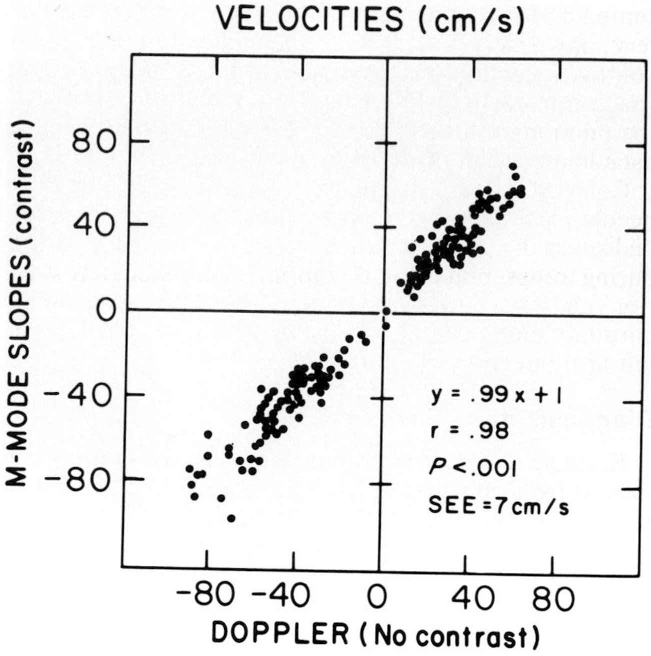

Fig. 15–17. Correlation between microbubble velocity derived from M-mode slopes (y axis) and red blood cell velocity (x axis) by Doppler for flows across the tricuspid and pulmonary valves. (From Levine RA, Telcholz LE, Goldman ME, et al.: Microbubbles have intracardiac velocities similar to those of red blood cells. J Am Coll Cardiol 3:28, 1984.)

velocity limitation, and second, they can sample several depths simultaneously. Despite these features, their practical application is limited. The concept, however, remains important because several authors have suggested using contrast to enhance faint Doppler signals, e.g., the tricuspid regurgitant jet, when measurement of right-sided pressures is important. Applications of this sort obviously would be valid only if contrast moved at the same velocity as red blood cells.

CLINICAL AND RESEARCH APPLICATIONS

Structure Identification

The first practical use of contrast echocardiography was to identify structures recorded on the M-mode echocardiogram. Peripheral or direct intracavitary injection of contrast aided in the correct M-mode identification of the aortic root and valve cusps,[3] the endocardium of the left ventricle, the interventricular septum, and the baffle after the Mustard procedure. In early two-dimensional studies, contrast played a similar role, permitting the identification of structures such as the interatrial septum,[40] left main coronary artery,[41] and coronary sinus. Although the identity of most major cardiac structures is now well established, contrast remains useful in determining structure identity of atypical or pathologic conditions. Figure 15–18 is an example of this application. In this case, a large echo-free space was recorded between the pulmonary artery and aorta in an infant following coarctation repair. It was unclear whether this repre-

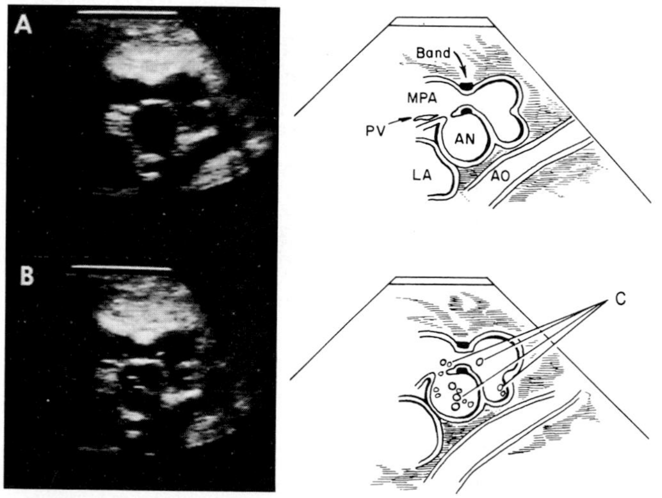

Fig. 15–18. Identification of pulmonary artery pseudoaneurysm. **A.** Parasternal long axis view oriented along the long axis of the main pulmonary artery (MPA). Note the echo-free aneurysmal (AN) cavity lying behind the pulmonary artery and the defect in the posterior artery wall. **B.** Similar long axis view with the appearance of contrast echoes in the pseudoaneurysm that stream across the tear in the posterior pulmonary artery wall proximal to the band. C = contrast echoes; PV = pulmonary valve; LA = left atrium; AO = aorta. (From Foale RA, et al.: Pseudoaneurysm of the pulmonary artery after the banding procedure: two-dimensional echocardiographic description. J Am Coll Cardiol 3:371, 1984.)

sented a pseudoaneurysm of the aorta or pulmonary artery, or was an extravascular fluid collection. Peripheral contrast injection caused opacification of the echo-free space immediately following the arrival of contrast in the pulmonary artery, confirming the fact that it was a pseudoaneurysm of the pulmonary artery.[42]

Contrast is also useful for confirming catheter or needle placement within structures such as the pericardial space during pericardiocentesis[43] and the left atrium during transseptal catheterization.[44] Persistent left superior vena cava entering the right atrium through a dilated coronary sinus can also be readily diagnosed following left arm injection of contrast.[45]

Diagnosis or Exclusion of Shunts

Because echocardiographic contrast is entirely removed from the circulation by the pulmonary and systemic capillary beds,[3,46] its appearance in the left heart after a peripheral venous injection is diagnostic of a right-to-left shunt. Similarly, its appearance in the right heart following direct left-sided, pulmonary venous, or capillary wedge injection is diagnostic of a left-to-right shunt. When injected proximal to the shunt, contrast is a highly sensitive indicator of the anomalous flow, having been demonstrated capable of detecting shunts as small as 3 to 5% or less, and when properly performed, it appears more sensitive than indocyanine green dye curves or oxymetry for shunt detection. If only one bubble is recorded in the left heart following right-sided injection, the presence of a defect is confirmed.

Because direct detection of left-to-right shunts requires catheter placement in the left heart or pulmonary wedge position, most clinical contrast studies in patients with left-to-right, right-to-left, or mixed shunts rely on information derived from peripheral venous injections. Using the peripheral venous approach, one can typically define three major levels of shunting, based on the pattern and appearance time of the echo-contrast on the right-and-left sides of the heart: ASD, ventricular septal defect, and pulmonary A-V fistula.

Atrial Septal Defect

To record contrast flow through an ASD using the M-mode technique, the operator usually directs the echo beam to pass through the left ventricle at the tips of the mitral leaflets, while for two-dimensional recording, we prefer the apical four-chamber view. If an ASD with right-to-left shunting is present, contrast can typically be recorded in the left atrium within one or two cardiac cycles following its appearance in the right atrium. Importantly, the passage of contrast from the right-to-left sides of the heart does not necessarily reflect a predominant right-to-left shunt. Transient reversal of the normal left-to-right pressure gradient at any point in the cardiac cycle will typically result in some reversal of flow direction and passage of contrast from right to left. Even if the pressures only equilibrate, the normal motion of the contrast-producing microbubbles within the right heart may lead to mixing between the right and left sides of the heart. Figure 15–19 illustrates the passage of contrast from the right-to-left atrium in a patient with an atrial septal defect and predominant left-to-right shunting.

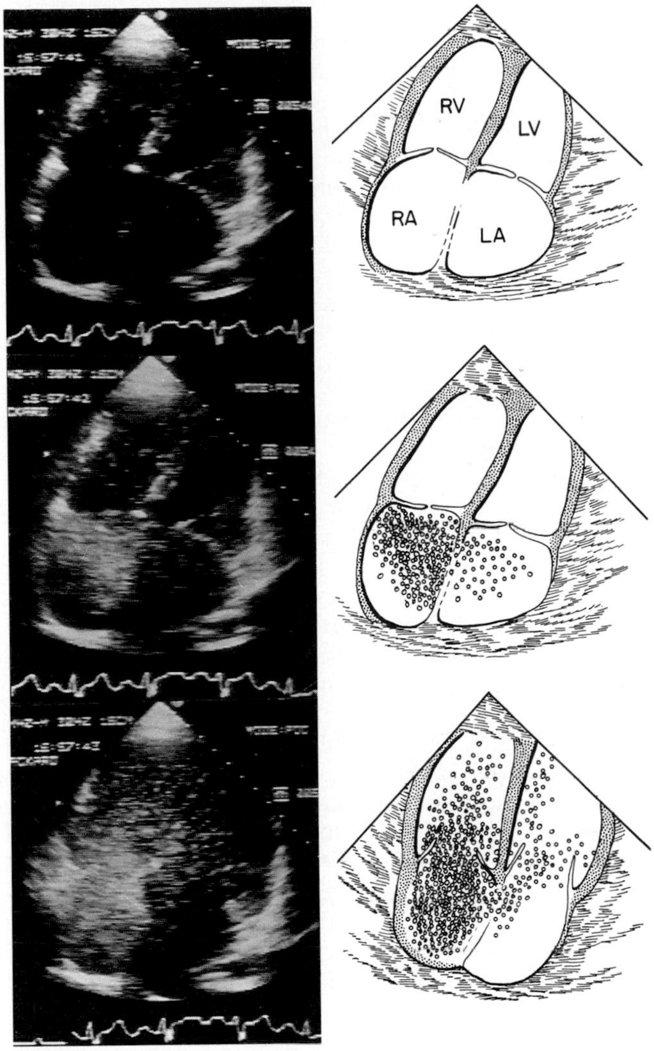

Fig. 15–19. Apical four-chamber recording of a patient with an atrial septal defect. Top. Before contrast injection. Middle. Following peripheral contrast injection. Initial contrast opacification of the right atrium with a small number of bubbles passing from right-to-left. Bottom. Diastolic flow of contrast into both the right and left ventricles. RV = right ventricle; LV = left ventricle; RA = right atrium; LA = left atrium.

Performance of the Valsalva maneuver may produce right-to-left shunting that is not present at rest. In some patients with large left-to-right shunts at the atrial level, no right-to-left component may be present and the contrast-containing blood will then be confined to the right heart. In these cases the flow of non-contrast-containing blood from left-to-right will often displace the contrast-containing blood from the right side of the defect, creating a contrast-free region or area of negative contrast (i.e., the absence of contrast in an area where it would be expected), which can be used to confirm the presence of the defect (see Fig. 15–14). The sensitivity of the contrast method in detecting ASD has varied from 96 to 100%, and these figures do appear appropriate.[47,48]

Note that persistent left superior vena cava appears more common in patients with ASD (3 to 10%) than in the general population (0.5%), and when unsuspected may complicate cardiac catheterization and the establishment of cardiopulmonary bypass during open heart surgery.[49,50]

Often, the demonstration of a patent foramen ovale (PFO) is important in the absence of an anatomic ASD, particularly in patients with unexplained cyanosis or paradoxic embolus. Contrast studies with associated Valsalva maneuver should allow demonstration of shunting through a PFO in at least two thirds of such cases, and with improved methods, the yield should currently be even higher. Another area where contrast may be of value is in the assessment of patch integrity immediately post-ASD repair. When present, such shunting requires re-evaluation because it may persist and require additional surgery.[51]

Contrast may also be useful in supporting the diagnosis of persistent pulmonary fetal circulation, because these patients virtually all have evidence of right-to-left shunting at the atrial level. This shunt may persist for as long as the pulmonary artery pressures are elevated and may be of significant magnitude. Contrast is, likewise, helpful in assessing the efficacy of mixing at the atrial level in infants with transposition of the great vessels (TGV) following balloon septostomy.[52]

A cautionary note regarding the neonatal circulation in the transition period is appropriate. The inferior vena caval return, which previously carried umbilical venous blood, is typically directed toward the left atrium, whereas superior vena caval blood is directed toward the tricuspid valve. As such, if a right-to-left shunt exists at the atrial level, it is often significantly overestimated on inferior vena caval injections and may be underestimated or even missed on superior vena caval injections.[53]

Ventricular Septal Defect

Demonstration of an uncomplicated ventricular septal defect usually requires the injection of contrast directly into the left heart. Although there may be some bidirectional flow across an uncomplicated defect, peripheral venous contrast studies generally fail to show right-to-left shunting in the absence of pulmonary hypertension. Occasional right-to-left contrast flow may be observed in the uncomplicated defect during the Valsalva maneuver or following premature beats, but this is unpredictable. Consistent right-to-left shunting of contrast typically begins when the right ventricular systolic pressure approaches 50% of the systemic systolic pressure. The shunting initially is noted during isovolumic relaxation when a transient right-to-left gradient occurs as a result of delayed right ventricular relaxation. With increasing right-sided pressures, specific changes in the pattern of right-to-left blood flow can be observed. At right ventricular peak pressures of 60 to 80% of left ventricle pressure, the transient right-to-left pressure gradient during isovolumic relaxation increases, and contrast flow from right to left occurs. During diastole, the left-to-right gradient is re-established, and the small volume of blood and its associated contrast, which was shunted into the left ventricle, rapidly returns to the right side, so that there is no evidence of a net systemic shunt. With larger defects,* the right and left ventricular peak systolic pressures equalize. Right-to-left shunting still occurs during isovolumic relaxation; however, contrast remains in the left ventricle during diastole and is ejected into the aorta during ventricular systole. This pattern may be seen in the face of a large left-to-right shunt and normal pulmonary vascular resistance.[54–56] In addition to its diagnostic implications, this observation also points out the potential for paradoxic emboli in patients in whom the predominant intracardiac shunt is left to right. Negative contrast jets are also commonly seen in the right ventricle in patients with pulmonary to systemic flow ratios greater than 2.0.[57] In patients with pulmonic stenosis or elevated pulmonary vascular resistance (greater than 15 units/m^2) and net right-to-left shunting Q_p/Q_s from 0.40 to 0.80 the right-to-left shunting appears increasingly earlier in the cycle, and the amount of the diastolic shunt likewise increases in parallel with the rise in right ventricular pressure.

Finally, in children with tetralogy of Fallot with significant pulmonary stenosis, there is a related, but distinctly different pattern of contrast flow.[58] During isovolumic contraction, the left ventricular pressure rises more rapidly than the right, resulting in a left-to-right pressure gradient, which rapidly reverses during early ventricular ejection. However, even though a small right-to-left gradient is established, flow from the right-to-left ventricles does not occur, because both ventricles eject into the aorta. With the commencement of isovolumic relaxation, the right-to-left pressure gradient is again established, which results in significant right-to-left shunting. The establishment of the right-to-left gradient appears earlier in the cardiac cycle than in an isolated ventricular septal defect with equal right and left ventricular pressures, and initial flow of contrast flow from the right-to-left ventricle, likewise, occurs earlier than is found in isolated ventricular septal defects. Thus, in tetralogy of Fallot, right-to-left shunting occurs during two phases of the cardiac cycle and in two different sites. During ventricular ejection, the shunt occurs directly into the aorta, while during isovolumic relaxation, it occurs across the ventricular septal defect into the left ventricle.

The injection of contrast material is particularly useful in D-transposition patients, because the right ventricle is the systemic ventricle and therefore at higher pressures than the left. If a ventricular septal defect is present, contrast echoes immediately traverse the ventricular septum and pass into the lower pressure "pulmonary" ventricle.

Minimal right-to-left contrast passage across ventricular septal defects is quite frequent in the newborn period when pulmonary pressure is high.

Despite the diagnostic information available, there are several important limitations in the contrast assessment of ventricular septal defects. First, adequate visualization is required so that shunt flow can be appreciated;

* Defects of less than 1 cm^2/m^2 have generally been felt to offer significant resistance to flow, whereas larger defects offer essentially no resistance.

second, studies are difficult to interpret in the face of an associated ASD,[36] and third, patterns of contrast flow depend on a normal activation sequence and are altered by right and left bundle branch block, Wolf-Parkinson-White complete heart block, and certain ventricular and atrial arrhythmias.

Pulmonary Arteriovenous Fistula

Late arrival of contrast in the left atrium after peripheral contrast injection (i.e., after 4 to 8 cycles after right atrial appearance) suggests the presence of pulmonary A-V fistula. The delayed left atrial appearance in this setting reflects the time required for passage through the pulmonary circulation. Figures 15–11 and 15–20 are examples of the relative delay in right vs. left atrial appearance that characterizes this lesion. Such A-V fistulas may be seen in patients with liver disease, with Osler-Weber-Rendu syndrome, or as isolated lesions. When a localized lesion is suspected, selective pulmonary arterial injection of contrast can be useful.

Diagnosis of Valvular Insufficiency

Direct intracardiac injection of contrast can be used to confirm or exclude the presence of regurgitation of

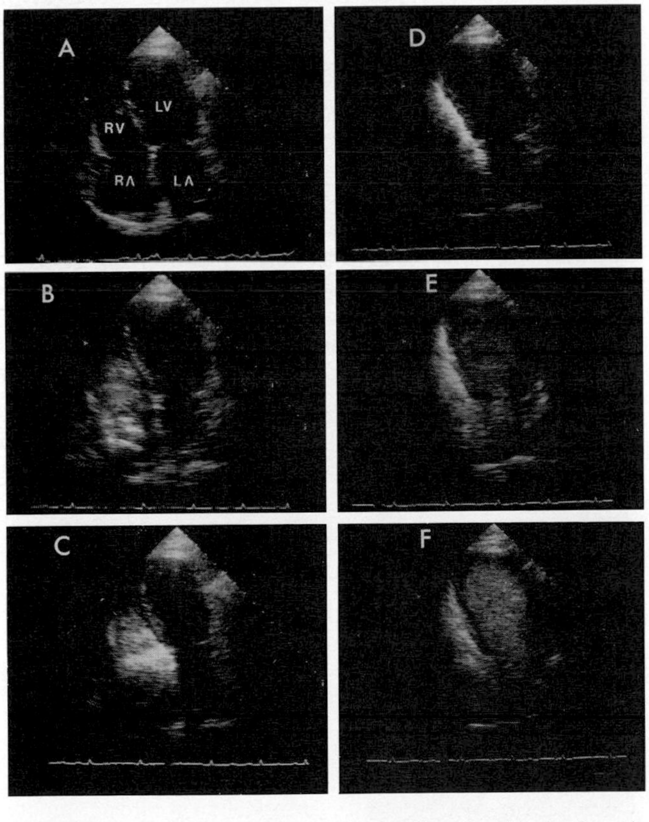

Fig. 15–20. Two-dimensional echocardiogram illustrating the delayed right-to-left passage of contrast in a patient with pulmonary arteriovenous fistula. **A.** Apical four-chamber view recorded before contrast injection. **B.** Peripherally injected contrast appears in the right atrium and ventricle. **C** and **D.** The right atrium and ventricle are densely opacified for a number of frames. **E.** Contrast initially appears in the left atrium and ventricle. **F.** The left ventricular contrast intensity increases as more of the contrast completes the pulmonary circuit. LA = left atrium; LV = left ventricle; RA = right atrium; RV = right ventricle.

the valve immediately proximal (upstream) to the site of injection.[59] This application can be useful in the operating room to assess the efficacy of valvuloplasty or the competence of a prosthetic valve and in the catheterization laboratory to assess valvular competence in patients who are allergic to angiographic contrast agents or in the study of patients during pregnancy.[60,61] Echo-contrast has the advantage over routine angiographic contrast agents in that it has less myocardial depressant effect and is without renal toxicity. Thus, it can be used without risk in most patients in whom angiographic contrast is contraindicated or the dose limited.

Contrast is most valuable in detecting valvular regurgitation when it can be injected directly into the chamber distal (downstream) to the valve suspected of leaking. The exception is the reported use of peripherally injected contrast to diagnose tricuspid insufficiency based on contrast appearance in the inferior vena cava during ventricular systole or v wave synchronous.[60,62]

Complex Congenital Heart Disease

In addition to enabling detection of simple shunt lesions, e.g., those described previously, echo-contrast can be a useful adjunct to the diagnosis of more complex congenital lesions such as tetralogy of Fallot, pulmonary atresia with ventricular septal defect, truncus arteriosus, Ebstein's anomaly, tricuspid atresia and hypoplastic right heart, univentricular heart, transposition of the great vessels, straddling and overriding atrioventricular valve, and crisscross heart. Many of these congenital anomalies have specific blood flow patterns that are pathognomic for the entity in question. In general, the more complex the cardiac lesion, the more likely one is to find a diagnostic echocardiographic blood flow pattern. The contrast pattern in each of these disorders is discussed later in this text under the discussion of the specific entity.

Echo-Contrast Ventriculography (Echoangiography)

One of the major problems in performing quantitative two-dimensional echocardiographic studies of the left ventricle has been the precise definition of the endocardium around the entire perimeter of the ventricle. Early M-mode studies suggested that the injection of contrast agents into the left ventricle outlined the cavity permitting better delineation of the margins of the blood pool and hence permitting endocardial definition.[62] Based on this concept, it has seemed reasonable that injection of contrast into the right and/or left ventricles during two-dimensional study would opacify the cavity, allowing the cavity area to be taken as the contrast area and obviating the need to visualize the endocardium. The contrast ventriculogram should be more easily recorded because contrast is a stronger reflector than the endocardium, and visualization of the spherical bubbles is independent of their location within the ventricular cavity. In addition, using digital subtraction methods, it should be possible to subtract the contrast-containing image from an earlier non-contrast-containing mask, further enhancing the blood pool definition and offering the potential for automated quantitation. In theory, the point spread function of the ultrasonic imaging system should enlarge the area of the echo-contrast ventriculogram as opposed to the area contraction, which results when the endocardium is used as the border reference (see Chapters 2 and 20). Not surprisingly, therefore, both long axis length and cavity area have been reported to be larger when the contrast ventriculogram is used as the reference.[63]

Separation of Flow From Non-flow Containing Areas

Contrast occasionally can be useful in separating flow-containing regions from non-flow-related structures. This is particularly useful in areas of low flow where the slowly moving blood may fail to produce a signal of sufficient strength to be recorded by Doppler. Examples are the separation of thrombus from stagnant blood in the left or right ventricular apex and the differentiation of atrial chamber blood from weakly reflective intracavitary masses. Differentiation of pseudoaneurysms from extracardiac echo-free spaces that are not in contact with a cardiac chamber (see preceding discussion) is another potential application.

Use as an Adjunct or Alternative to Fluoroscopy During Cardiac Catheterization

Although not yet fully appreciated, two-dimensional echocardiography may be a useful adjunct to cardiac catheterization, or in many cases, may provide an alternative.[64,65] The technique can aid in guiding catheter introduction and placement, reducing fluoroscopic control to a minimum. Selective echo-contrast injection can also determine proper catheter location before selective angiography, especially when the amount of radiographic contrast material that can be used is limited. Further, because entirely nontoxic echo-contrast agents are used, (1) multiple injections can be performed, (2) many different cardiac views can be obtained for analysis, and the hand injections of small amounts of fluid do not cause the premature beats frequently seen during standard cardiac angiography.

Videodensitometric Estimation of Shunt Flow and Cardiac Output

The intensity of the recorded two-dimensional echo signal arising from a bolus of echo-contrast is presented as brightness or luminance on a video monitor or cathode ray tube. This luminescence can readily be recorded by a photometer (light meter), or the image can be digitized and the video output can be recorded numerically. Both approaches permit the determination of instantaneous signal intensity and its pattern of change over time. In early videodensitometric studies, a photometer was directed at a fixed point on the video screen, and the luminance emitted by the video monitor continuously recorded and output as an analog signal (Fig. 15–21).[66] The result of the photometric analysis of two-dimensional contrast studies was to yield an indicator dilution-type curve whose upstroke was related to the luminance creator by the appearance of contrast on the video screen and whose downslope reflected the disappearance or washout of the contrast agent (Fig. 15–22). The variability of these early recordings was ±15%. Two parameters were defined for each contrast curve: the time from peak contrast effect (peak of the curve) to the point of 50% decrease in amplitude (DT/50), and the time from the peak of the curve to a 90% reduction in amplitude (DT/90). Marked differences were revealed using both of these measures between normal subjects and patients with ASD and those with a marked reduction in cardiac output or tricuspid regurgitation. In addition, both measures yielded a good correlation with thermodilution cardiac output. Direct calculation of cardiac output, unfortunately, has not been possible from such recording.

The calculation of cardiac output (CO) from any indicator dilution curve is usually computed by means of the Hamilton equation as $CO = i/(\bar{c}*t)$ where i is the mass of the injectate, $\bar{c}$ is the mean concentration of the indicator during its initial pass through the sampling area,

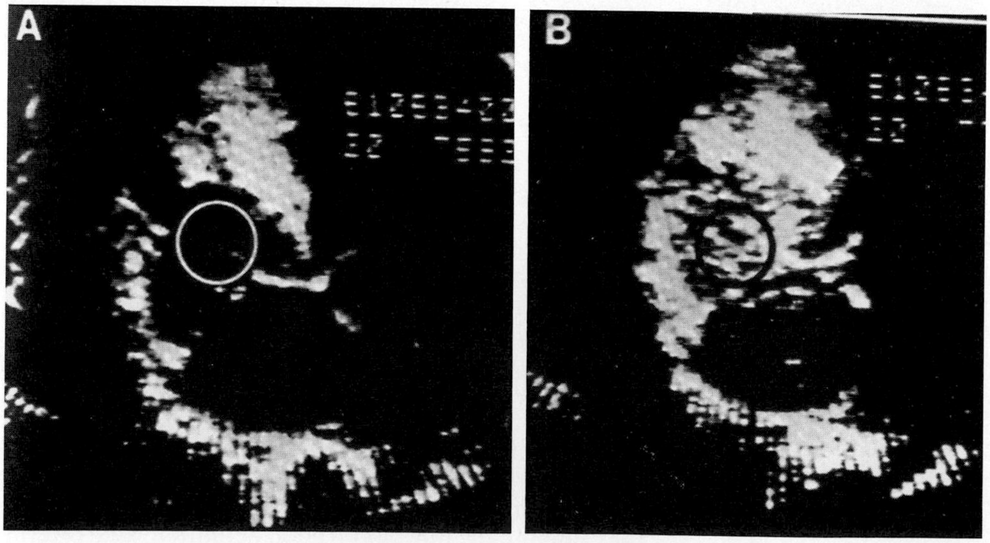

Fig. 15–21. Illustration of targeted area for photometric sampling in the right ventricular cavity. **A.** Recorded before contrast injection. **B.** Recorded during contrast flow into the right ventricle. (From DeMaria, et al.: Determination of cardiac output by two-dimensional contrast echocardiography. *In* Meltzer RS, Roelandt J (eds.): Contrast Echocardiography. The Hague, Martinus Nijhoff, 1982.)

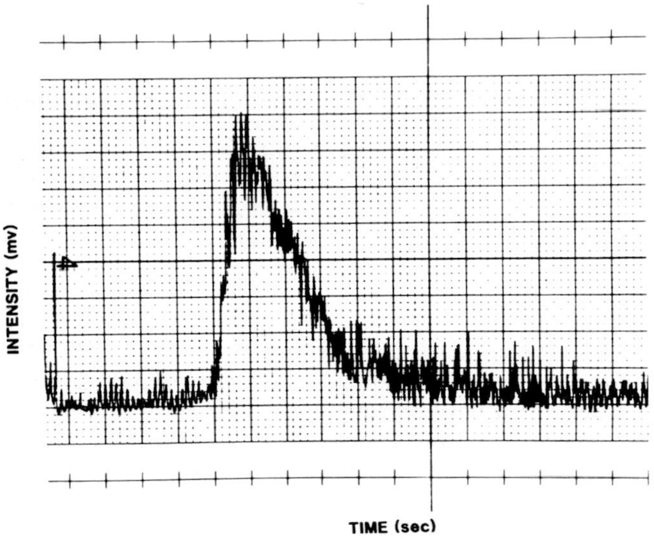

Fig. 15–22. Photometric indicator dilution-type curve. The upstroke is related to the appearance of contrast on the video screen, and the downslope is created by the disappearance or washout of the contrast agent. Ordinate: brightness (intensity), measured in microvolts appearing in the midright ventricle. Abscissa: time in seconds. (From Smith MD, et al.: Superior intensity and reproducibility of SHU-454, a new right heart contrast agent. J Am Coll Cardiol 3:992, 1984.)

and t is the total duration of the curve obtained. Accordingly, it is necessary to determine the mass of the contrast agent injected as well as to develop a method for computating the mean concentration of the agent during transit through the heart to calculate actual cardiac output from two-dimensional contrast echoes.

To determine the mass of the injectate, it is necessary to use an agent that yields a constant and predictable contrast effect. Two such agents have been studied. Plastic microballoons whose size varies in a bell-shape distribution about a mean of 30 μm, and gelatin-encapsulated microbubbles precisely 10 μm in size.[67] Agents such as these permit the mass of the injected contrast to be predicted. The next step is to determine the mean concentration of contrast at the recording site. This requires that a function $c = f(i)$ be known, relating contrast concentration to observed intensity. A linear relationship has been demonstrated for microballoons suspended in viscous medium for concentrations between 1.7 and 6.3×10^{-5}, implying that a simple constant, κ, would relate concentration to intensity, $c = \kappa i$. Unfortunately, this constant is likely to vary with gain and with the attenuation characteristic of the chest wall. Thus, at present, only directional curves, rather than absolute values, can be obtained. In addition to the lack of a calibration function, it is generally not possible to completely eliminate the extraneous introduction of microbubbles, and the contrast concentration must be controlled so as not to oversaturate the videodensitometric equipment.[68]

One circumstance, where ignorance of the absolute calibration function is acceptable, is in comparing contrast between chambers. For instance, shunt flow through a ventral septal defect can be estimated by injecting contrast into the left ventricle and measuring contrast intensity (a time-intensity histogram) in the aorta and pulmonary artery. In this case, the only assumption about f(i) is that it is linear over the range of contrast concentrations of interest. Such calculations have correlated well with similar measurements by Fick and green dye curves.[69]

Assessment of Myocardial Perfusion

Another area of current interest is the direct injection of contrast into the coronary arteries to define the perfusion territory of individual vessels, to detect areas of nonperfused myocardium, and to assess regional blood flow. This topic is discussed separately in Chapter 23.

UNIQUE APPLICATIONS OF CONTRAST ECHOCARDIOGRAPHY

Orthodeoxia (Platypnea and Orthostatic Cyanosis)

Orthodeoxia is a rare phenomenon in which the blood is predominantly desaturated only when the patient is in the upright position.[70] Platypnea, the accompanying symptom, is dyspnea in the upright position relieved in the supine position. This postural cyanosis has been reported most commonly in adults with various types of chronic lung disease or after pneumonectomy and is not associated with measurable pulmonary hypertension. The mechanism for this interesting and often dramatic postural cyanosis is not known. Nevertheless, in the upright position, these patients experience impressive right-to-left shunting at the atrial level, usually across a PFO or an ASD.[70–73] It has been reported that recumbent and upright peripheral venous contrast provides the most diagnostic and easily obtainable examination. With the use of a tilt table at the time of a contrast echocardiogram, minimal or no right-to-left shunt is observed in the recumbent position, whereas with a similar injection in the sitting or standing position, a pronounced increase in the amount of right-to-left shunt is visualized. Closure of a PFO or ASD has been shown to eliminate this unusual form of heart disease. We have also noted an orthostatic decrease in pO_2 in a patient with multiple pulmonary A-V fistulas, presumably that are due to redistribution of flow through the lungs while in the upright position.

Persistent Left Superior Vena Cava

A persistent left superior vena cava will typically drain into the coronary sinus and then into the right atrium. More rarely, however, the left superior vena cava will enter the left-or-right atrium directly. Persistence of the left superior vena cava is estimated to occur in roughly 3 to 4% of patients with congenital heart disease and in 7% of these to terminate in the left atrium.

To Coronary Sinus

When the left superior vena cava enters the coronary sinus, an injection of contrast into the left arm will initially opacify the coronary sinus and then fill the right atrium and other right heart structures in sequence (see

Chapter 18, Fig. 18–36). If an atrial septal defect is present, the dye may cross into the left atrium, and in this case, the pattern of contrast appearance is critical to correct diagnosis.

To Left Atrium

Anomalous systemic venous drainage into the left atrium is uncommon and most often is related to persistence of the left superior vena cava.[74] When the left superior vena cava connects directly to the left atrium, left upper extremity injection will cause the left atrium to opacify initially followed by the left ventricle and aorta. The coronary sinus in this case will not be dilated and will not opacify. When an ASD is present, there will usually be flow from the left atrium to the right, and again the sequence of contrast appearance is critical to appropriate diagnosis. Figure 15–23 illustrates the opacification of the left atrium following left arm injection in a patient with persistent left superior vena caval draining in the left atrium.

Right Superior Vena Caval Drainage to the Left Atrium

Rarer still are cases in which a persistent right superior vena cava empties into the left atrium.[75,76] Right superior vena caval drainage into the left atrium may occur with or without persistence of the left superior vena cava.[77] The condition is usually associated with obvious cyanosis, but this may be absent. Despite the absence of cyanosis patients with direct continuity between the systemic venous and arterial circuits are at risk for the complications of brain abscess or paradoxic embolization and surgical correction is necessary.[78] The anomaly can be identified by injection of contrast into the right arm with subsequent opacification of the left atrium (Fig. 15–24). An associated persistent left superior vena cava draining into the right atrium can be identified by left arm injection followed by right atrial opacification (Fig. 15–24). In either case, injection into a foot vein should opacify the right heart normally. Connection of the inferior vena cava to the left atrium[79–81] and total

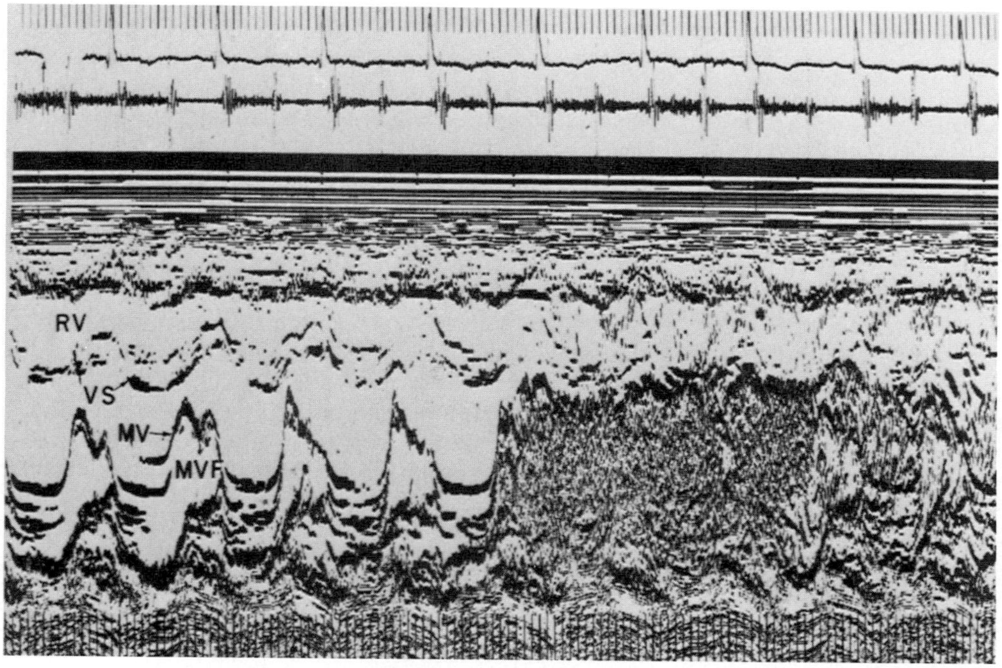

Fig. 15–23. Persistent left superior vena cava draining to left atrium. After a left upper extremity injection, contrast material initially appears in the left atrium and mitral valve. RV = right ventricle; VS = ventricular septum; MV = mitral valve; MVF = mitral valve funnel. (From Tajik AJ, Seward JB: Contrast echocardiography. Cardiovasc Clin 9:317, 1978.)

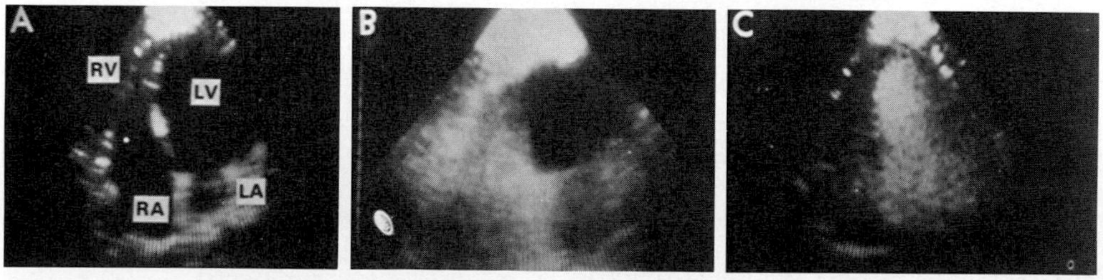

Fig. 15–24. Persistent right superior vena cava (SVC) draining into the left atrium (LA) along with a persistent left superior vena cava draining into the coronary sinus. **A.** Baseline recording. **B.** Opacification of the right heart by contrast after left antecubital venous injection. Flow in this instance is through the persistent left SVC and coronary sinus to the right atrium (RA) and ventricle (RV). **C.** Echocontrast completely fills the left heart chambers after right antecubital venous injection. Flow in this case is through the right SVC to the left atrium. LV = left ventricle. (From Schick EC, Lekakis J, Rothendler JA, Ryan TJ: Persistent left superior vena cava and right superior vena cava drainage into the left atrium without arterial hypoxemia. J Am Coll Cardiol 5:374, 1985.)

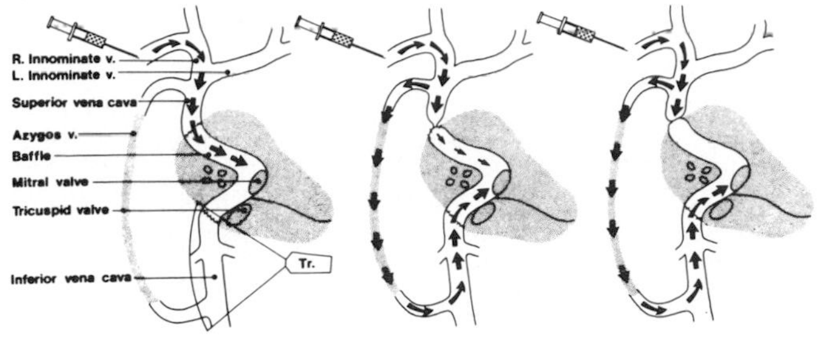

Fig. 15–25. The pattern of contrast flow in patients with and without superior vena cava obstruction after the Mustard operation. Left. In the absence of obstruction, peripherally injected contrast (arrows) fills the systemic venous atrium from above. No contrast echoes are seen in the lower inferior vena cava. Middle. With partial superior vena cava obstruction, contrast echoes fill the systemic venous atrium primarily from above. However, there is late contrast appearance in the lower inferior vena cava, flowing toward the systemic venous atrium. These contrast echoes arrive in the inferior vena cava by way of azygos-inferior vena cava collateral vessels. Right. With total superior vena cava obstruction, the contrast echoes fill the systemic venous atrium entirely from below by way of the azygos-inferior vena cava collateral vessels. (From Silverman NH, et al.: Superior vena caval obstruction after Mustard operation: detection by two-dimensional echocardiography. Circulation 64:392, 1981. Reproduced by permission of the American Heart Association, Inc.)

anomalous systemic venous drainage to the left atrium[82] have also been reported. In the former case, left-sided contrast opacification would be expected after lower but not upper extremity contrast injection. While in the latter, the left heart should opacify following contrast injection into any of the four extremities.

Glenn Anastomosis With Acquired Pulmonary Arteriovenous Fistula

A high percentage of patients with Glenn anastomosis will develop increasing numbers of pulmonary arteriovenous fistulas in the lower lobes of the shunted lung.[83] As a result, increasing cyanosis may be due to A-V fistula formation rather than to deterioration of the complex anomaly for which the shunt was performed. The presence of these fistulas can be detected by the appearance of contrast material in the left atrium following right upper extremity injection. In contrast, if shunt obstruction and acquired venous collaterals are present, the contrast material will initially appear in the inferior vena cava and right atrium, as opposed to the left atrium.

Superior Vena Cava Syndrome

Obstruction of the superior vena cava is associated with the development of collateral channels to the inferior vena cava.[84] Examples would be total or partial occlusion of the superior vena cava after the Mustard procedure or superior vena caval obstruction by tumor. In these situations, upper extremity contrast injection produces variable opacification of the inferior vena cava via the venous collaterals. The more marked the superior vena caval occlusion and the more extensive the collateral circulation, the more contrast will arrive in the right atrium from the inferior vena cava. Figure 15–25 diagramatically illustrates the pattern of flow that develops in response to partial and complete obstruction of the superior vena cava.

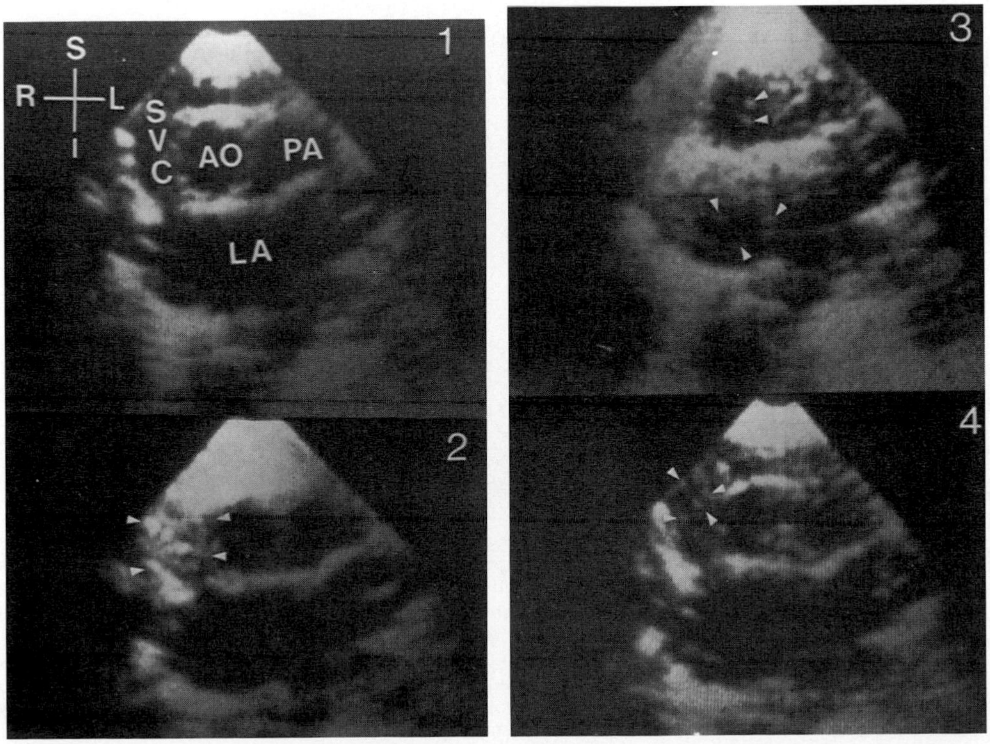

Fig. 15–26. Contrast echocardiograms from a patient with a large intercranial arteriovenous malformation of the vein of Galen. (1) Suprasternal short axis view of the superior vena cava (SVC), left atrium (LA), aorta (AO), and pulmonary artery (PA) before contrast injection. (2) Following left arm injection, contrast is seen in the SVC. (3) Contrast completely opacifies the SVC and PA and has passed into the LA and AO (arrows) via a right-to-left shunt. (4) The AO, PA, and LA are relatively free of echoes from the contrast injection; however, microcavitations (arrows) have reappeared in the SVC. The SVC recirculation in this case, is caused by contrast passing from left to right through the vein of Galen aneurysm. (From Snider, et al.: Detection of intracranial arteriovenous fistula by two-dimensional ultrasonography. Circulation 63:1179, 1981. Reproduced by permission of the American Heart Association, Inc.)

Detection of Intracranial Arteriovenous Fistula

Intracranial arteriovenous malformation is a rare cause of severe congestive heart failure in infancy.[85–88] Initial physical findings may include cranial bruits, hyperdynamic cardiac impulses, heart murmur, cyanosis, and bounding pulses. Although such infants are critically ill, the intracranial bruit may be of low intensity and the exact diagnosis difficult to establish. Pathophysiologically, the A-V malformation causes increased ductal shunting during the transition period as a result of the low systemic resistance caused by the malformation at a time when the pulmonary resistance is still high. The large right-to-left ductal shunt decreases pulmonary venous return and left atrial volume. In addition, the large flow volume passing through the fistula increases the return to the right atrium. This elevates right atrial volume and pressure in the face of low left atrial volume and pressure, holding the flap of the foramen ovale open and promoting right-to-left atrial shunting.[89] Persistence of the fetal circulatory pattern allows peripherally injected echo-contrast to pass directly through the atrial septum and thereby gain entrance to the systemic circulation.[90] The passage of echo-contrast from the systemic circulation into the low-resistance fistula can be imaged by two-dimensional echo of the brain. Further contrast passing through the fistula will not be removed from the circulation and will reappear rapidly in the carotid veins and superior vena cava (Fig. 15–26). The recognition of the lesion is also facilitated by the morphologic changes that correspond to the increased flow pattern, specifically, dilation of the superior vena cava, right atrium, right ventricle, pulmonary artery, ascending aorta, and carotid arteries.

LIMITATIONS

Despite its relative simplicity and lack of toxicity, contrast echocardiography has several important limitations. First, it requires venous or arterial cannulation and, hence, adds an invasive component to an otherwise noninvasive procedure. Second, the contrast response following apparently similar peripheral injections is not consistent and may vary from nonvisualization to intense opacification of the right heart. Third variation in injection rate, number, and volume of bubbles and their transit time through the system all influence the intensity of the contrast effect. Finally, echo-contrast can be an intense reflector that may artifactually be spread into neighboring chambers or obscure more distal structures.

POTENTIAL COMPLICATIONS

Reported side effects of echo-contrast injection are both rare and transient occurring in 0.062% of cases in one survey and lasting, at most, a few minutes with no reported residual complications.[91] The complications that are noted appear to relate to transient mechanical obstruction of small vessels by the injected microbubbles. When viewed microscopically, microbubbles flow downstream through successive branch points until they reach a point where the diameter of the vessel is smaller than that of the bubble where they then lodge, obstructing further flow (Fig. 15–27).[92,93] Over time, the gas in the bubble diffuses out, reducing its size. The fluid pressure behind the shrinking bubble then gradually deforms it until it can progress further or it breaks down into two smaller daughters, each of which can then continue downstream. These processes will continue until the original, or daughter bubbles, are small enough to clear the vascular bed or dissolve completely. In the process, however, there is transient occlusion of small portions of the vascular bed that may produce associated symptoms. The duration of occlusions varies with initial bub-

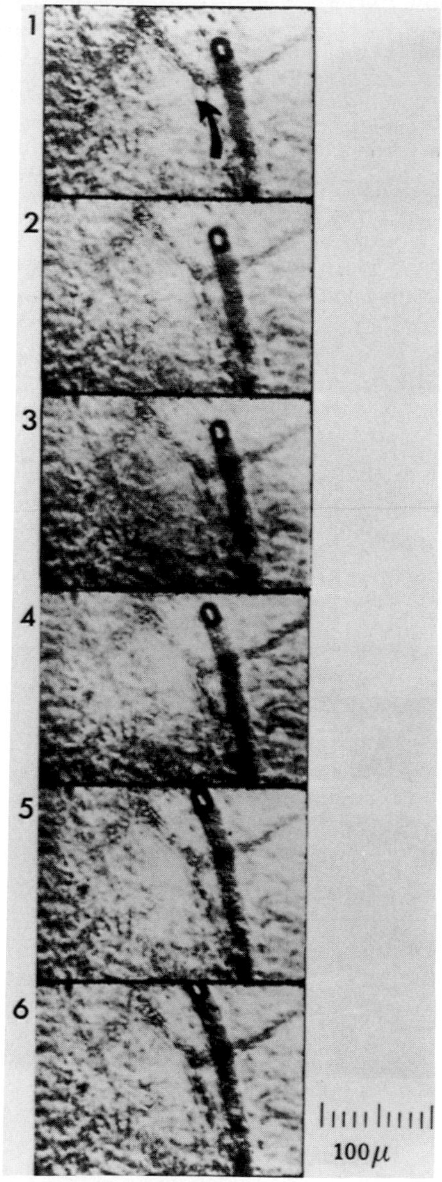

Fig. 15–27. Sequence of movie frames showing microbubble passage through a cat mesentery preparation. The bubble in this case is larger than the capillary diameter. Note the loss of the normal spherical shape of the bubble and the "backup" of red blood cells in the blood vessel, suggestive of vascular occlusion. Slow migration of the bubble is apparent, presumably caused by a gradual decrease in bubble diameter over time. (From Feinstein SB, et al.: Microbubble dynamics visualized in the intact capillary circulation. J Am Coll Cardiol 4:597, 1984.)

ble size and may last from a few seconds for small bubbles (10 to 15 μm) to several minutes for larger bubbles.[92,93]

Reported signs and symptoms include anxiety, slight increase in respiratory rate, wheezing, transient lightheadedness, cough, transient dyspnea, headache, transient bradycardia, occasional premature atrial contraction (PACs), tachycardia, T-wave changes following direct intracoronary injection, dysphasia and hemiparesis, and transient numbness and weakness of the arm, leg, and/or tongue. In one case, hallucinations, paresthesias, and abdominal and pelvic pain were noted for several minutes following the injection of bacteriostatic saline solution but were felt to be related to Paraben toxicity. Symptoms are usually related to the intensity of the contrast effect, implying that the more microbubbles injected, the greater the likelihood of side effects. Experimental studies in which a variety of contrast-producing agents were injected into the myocardium—including saline solution alone, Renografin and saline, perfluorocarbon, and oxygenated perfluorocarbon—revealed a transient depression in wall motion that was directly related to the contrast intensity but was independent of the injectate (Fig. 15–28). This confirms that the transient decrease in function is due to microbubble blockage of the myocardial capillaries rather than to replacement of oxygen-carrying blood by non-oxygen-carrying media or to a direct depressant effect of the vehicle (Renografin). Despite this transient loss of function, large amounts of contrast material repeatedly injected into the heart, brains, and kidneys of experimental animals with pathologic sectioning at 24 hours postinjection failed to reveal any lesions that could be directly attributed to the contrast media.[94] Thus, clinical and experimental data suggest that the echo-contrast microbubbles transiently occlude vessels and during the period of occlusion can cause transient symptoms of ischemia. The occlusion, however, lasts only seconds, and even repeat injections of large amounts of contrast into small vascular beds are not associated with any evidence of permanent pathologic change.

Clinically, intracavitary left ventricular microbubbles are often detected during cardiac operations, particularly during valve replacement, but are not predictive of obvious postoperative neurologic complications. This is true even if microbubbles are densely concentrated. Attempts to eradicate these microbubbles appear generally unsuccessful, and given the lack of associated complications, may be unnecessary.[95,96] However, this is an area that requires further study with long-term neurologic follow-up and specific psychological and cognitive testing before subclinical damage can be totally excluded.

CURRENT ROLE RELATIVE TO DOPPLER

Because both contrast echocardiography and Doppler imaging are methods for recording intracardiac blood flow, it is reasonable to examine the relative role of the two techniques in specific clinical situations. The relative merits of the two techniques in a series of common disorders are outlined in Table 15–3. In general, the Doppler method is preferable in any situation in which

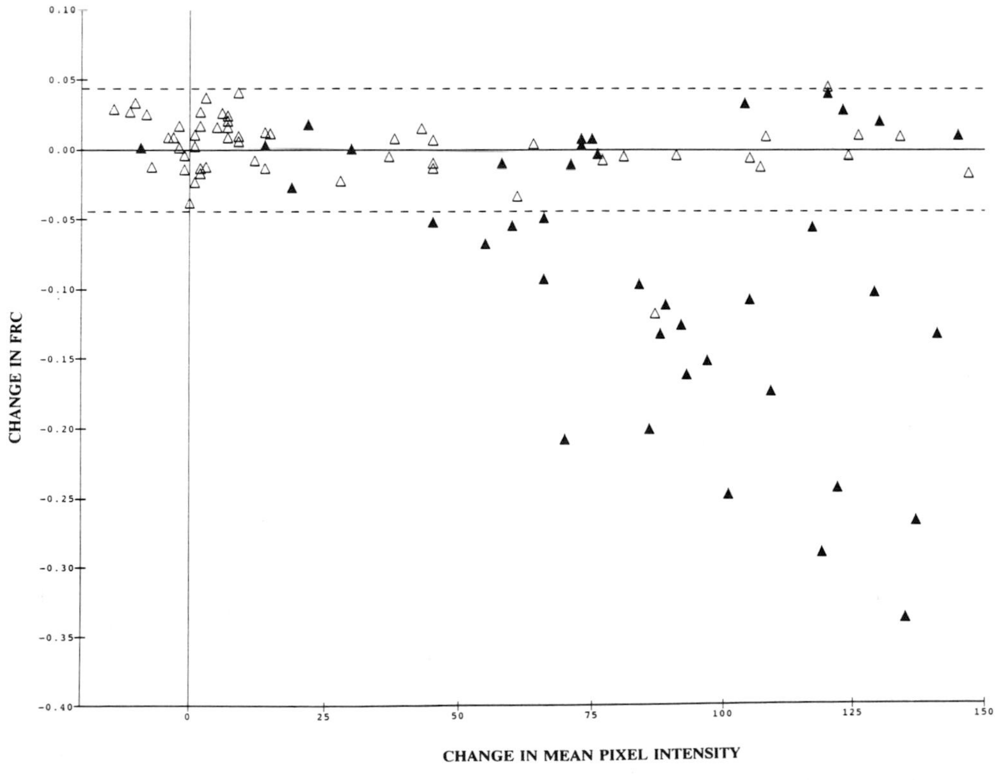

Fig. 15–28. Relationship of contrast intensity to myocardial depression for injections of unagitated and agitated solutions of normal saline solution, Renografin saline, perfluorocarbon, and oxygenated perfluorocarbon. Baseline indicates mean ±2 SD for the pooled data from the unagitated solutions (open triangles). Although varying contrast intensity is achieved, virtually no wall motion abnormalities are noted using unagitated solutions, presumably because of the predominance of small bubbles. The closed triangles represent data from agitated solutions, showing a clear relationship between contrast intensity and depression of function. This presumably reflects larger bubble sizes, producing both greater contrast intensity and more extensive capillary blockade. The effect was independent of the agent injected, suggesting a mechanical cause for the observed myocardial depression. FRC = fractional radical contraction. (From Levine RA, et al.: Wall motion abnormalities following myocardial echo contrast injection area caused by microbubbles. J Am Coll Cardiol 5:474, 1988.

Table 15–3. Relative Merits of Doppler Imaging and Contrast Echocardiography

	Doppler	Contrast
Noninvasive	+ +	−
Nontoxic	+ +	−
Aortic regurgitation	+ + + +	+ (DI)
Mitral regurgitation	+ + + +	+ (DI)
Pulmonic regurgitation	+ + + +	+ (DI)
Tricuspid regurgitation	+ + + +	+ (DI)
Flow velocity	+ + + +	+
Intracardiac shunts	+ + + +	+
Pulmonary and systemic Arteriovenous fistulas	−	+ + +
Myocardial perfusion	−	+ + +
Persistent left SVC	+	+ + +
SVC obstruction	+	+ + +

DI = direct injection; SVC = superior vena cava.

the same information can be obtained using either technique because it is totally noninvasive and without toxicity. Thus, for most routine clinical diagnoses, such as shunts and valvular regurgitation, the Doppler approach would be considered preferable. In certain instances (e.g., exclusion of a PFO), where a small flow volume or the need for an additional physiologic stress (i.e., a Valsalva maneuver) may make Doppler recording difficult, contrast can serve as a useful adjunct or provide confirmatory information; however, it is rarely the procedure of first choice.

In several specific instances, however, contrast provides unique information about abnormal flow occurring outside the recording area of the Doppler. These include pulmonary A-V fistula, superior vena cava syndrome, persistent left superior vena cava, anomalous left and right superior vena caval insertion into the left atrium, and the assessment of myocardial perfusion. In certain complex lesions, the portion of the aortic outflow that arises from the left ventricle may be separated in the aorta from that which arises from the right ventricle. Contrast will reveal this laminarization, which is inapparent in a Doppler study. Thus, despite the increasingly dominant role of Doppler in assessing blood flow, there remain important but more limited applications for the use of echo-contrast.

SPONTANEOUS CONTRAST

To this point we have discussed only echo-contrast that is due to microbubbles in the injectate or to bubbles arising from obviously supersaturated solutions of gas. Several authors, however, have reported the appearance of spontaneous contrast in patients without venous or arterial invasion or obvious decompression. The first and most widely studied form of spontaneous contrast is the small, discrete, mobile targets occasionally seen in the left and right ventricles in patients with prosthetic valves.[97] Several potential causes have been suggested including spontaneous cavitation or particulate matter, e.g., platelet aggregates or fibrin or fine pieces of the cloth sewing ring. Although the exact cause of these echoes is unknown, their similarity to the echoes arising from microbubbles, rapid movement, and short survival time suggest that they are small gas bubbles caused by spontaneous cavitation or hemolysis. Although the velocities of flow in regions where these echoes arise are much lower than those required to produce cavitation in water, cavitation characteristically occurs at much lower flow rates in gas-rich media, e.g., blood. Likewise, the bubbles that are formed persist considerably longer and do not collapse suddenly.* The possibility that hemolysis either causes or contributes to these echoes is supported by studies showing the formation of small gas bubbles in blood following the injection of hemolysins[98] and the clinical observation that the valves most prone to hemolysis have a particularly high incidence of spontaneous contrast.[99]

The second common cause of spontaneous contrast is the almost ubiquitous granular echoes seen in the proximal venous system (i.e., the inferior and superior vena cavae, innominate and subclavian veins) at high recording frequencies. These echoes are extremely small, large in number, continuously present, follow the path of blood flow precisely, and vary in velocity with respiration, suggesting that their origin is probably blood components rather than gas.[100] While commonly noted on the venous side of the circulation, similar mobile granular echoes are not normally seen in the arterial circulation. The difference in the reflective characteristics of venous and arterial blood may be explained by the difference in their physiochemical and rheologic characteristics, which in turn, is related to their varying CO_2 contents. Increasing CO_2 increases the density and viscosity of blood and may alter its reflective properties.

Finally, granular echoes are seen in areas of stagnant blood e.g., in the left atrium in patients with initial stenosis ("smoke") and arise to fill the ventricle following cardiac arrest. Here again, their formation most likely is related to aggregates of blood products (rouleaux formation, fibrin aggregation, etc.) rather than microbubbles.

INCIDENTAL CONTRAST

Finally, one should remember that in addition to the deliberate injection of microbubble-containing solutions, microbubbles can enter the circulation along with any solution that is injected or infused. In these cases, the bubbles may be trapped in the solution or the injecting apparatus and gradually or continuously released into the circulation. Likewise, whenever a catheter or indwelling line is flushed, contrast may appear. Contrast can also be seen during intracardiac procedures, e.g., ablation of the bundle of His, in which case it probably results from the destruction of blood elements and release of entrapped gases, as a consequence of the high local temperature and pressure associated with the electrical discharge.[101]

* This form of cavitation, therefore, is termed *stable cavitation* as opposed to the transient cavitation seen in water.

REFERENCES

1. Joyner CR: Cardiovascular Conference. Ultrasound in Cardiovascular Diagnosis. Am Heart Association Scientific Session, San Francisco, Oct 21, 1967.
2. Gramiak R, Shah PM: Echocardiography of the aortic root. Invest Radiol 3:356, 1968.
3. Gramiak R, Shah PM, Kramer DH: Ultrasound cardiography: contrast studies in anatomy and function. Radiology 92:939, 1969.
4. Bommer WJ, et al.: Quantitative regional myocardial perfusion scanning with contrast echocardiography. Am J Cardiol 47:403, 1981.
5. Armstrong WF, et al.: Assessment of myocardial perfusion abnormalities with contrast-enhanced two-dimensional echocardiography. Circulation 66:166, 1982.
6. Tei C, et al.: Myocardial contrast echocardiography. A reproducible technique of myocardial opacification for identifying regional perfusion deficits. Circulation 67:585, 1983.
7. Armstrong WF, et al.: Assessment of location and size of myocardial infarction with contrast enhanced echocardiography. J Am Coll Cardiol 2: 63, 1983.
8. Kemper AJ, et al.: Hydrogen peroxide contrast-enhanced two-dimensional echocardiography: real time in vivo delineation of regional myocardial perfusion. Circulation 68:603, 1983.
9. Gramiak R: Contrast agents for diagnostic ultrasound. *In* Meltzer RS, Roelandt J (eds.): Contrast Echocardiography. The Hague, Martinus Nijhoff Publishers, p. 17, 1982.
10. Kremkau FW, et al.: Ultrasonic cavitation at catheter tips. Am J Roentgenology 110:177, 1970.
11. Meltzer RS, Tickner EG, Sahines TP, Popp RL: The source of ultrasound contrast effect. J Clin Ultrasound 8:121, 1980.
12. Lubbers J, Van den Berg J: An ultrasonic detector for microgas emboli in a blood line. Ultrasound Med Biol 2:301, 1976.
13. Rubissow GJ, Mackay RS: Ultrasonic studies during experimental decompression. *In* Meltzer RS, Roelandt J (eds.): Contrast Echocardiography. The Hague, Martinus Nijhoff: p. 30, 1982.
14. Ten Cate FJ, et al.: Transpulmonary visualization of left ventricular structures using contrast 2D-echocardiography. Circulation 68(Suppl 3):III-329, 1983.
15. Weibel ER. Morphometry of the Human Lung. New York, Academic Press, p. 78, 1975.
16. Epstein P, Plesset M: On the stability of gas bubbles in liquid-gas solutions. J Chem Phys 18:1505, 1950.
17. Ward CA, Tucker AS: Thermodynamics theory of diffusion-controlled bubble growth or dissolution and experimental examination of the predictions. J Appl Physiol 46:233, 1975.
18. Yang WR, Echigo C, Molten D, Hwang J. Experimental studies of the dissolution of gas bubbles in whole blood and plasma: I. Stationary bubbles. J Biomech 3:275, 1971.
19. Yang WR, Echigo R, Molten D, Hwang J. Experimental studies of the dissolution of bubbles in whole blood and plasma: II. Moving bubbles. J Biomech 4:283, 1971.
20. Devin C: Survey of thermal, radiation and viscous damping of pulsating air bubbles in water. J Acoust Soc Am 31:1654, 1959.
21. Plesset M, Prosperetti A: Bubble dynamics and cavitation. Am Rev Fluid Mech 9:145, 1977.
22. Tickner EG: Precision microbubbles for right-side intracardiac pressure and flow measurements. *In* Meltzer RS, Roelandt J (eds.): Contrast Echocardiography. The Hague, Martinus Nijhoff, p. 313, 1982.
23. Tickner EG, Rasor N: Noninvasive assessment of pulmonary hypertension using the bubble ultrasonic resonance pressure (BURP) method. Annual Report #HR-62917-1A, NHLBI, 1977.
24. Meltzer RS, Serruys PW, Hugenholtz PG, Roelandt J: Intravenous carbon dioxide as an echocardiographic contrast agent. J Clin Ultrasound 9:127, 1981.
25. Munoz S, Berti C, Pulido C, Blanco P: Two-dimensional contrast echocardiography with carbon dioxide in the detection of congenital cardiac shunts. Am J Cardiol 53:206, 1984.
26. Santoso T, et al.: Myocardial Perfusion imaging in humans by contrast echocardiography using polygelin colloid solution. J Am Coll Cardiol 6: 612, 1985.
27. Smith MD, Kwan OL, Reiser J, DeMaria AN: Superior intensity and reproducibility of SHU-454, a new right heart contrast agent. J Am Coll Cardiol 3:992, 1984.
28. Gaffney FA, et al.: Hydrogen peroxide contrast echocardiography. Am J Cardiol 52:607, 1983.
29. Wang X, Jiaen W, Youzhen H, Chongde C: Contrast echocardiography with hydrogen peroxide: I experimental study. Chinese Med J 92:595, 1979.
30. Wang A, Wang J, Chen H, Lu C: Contrast echocardiography with hydrogen peroxide: II. Clinical application. Chinese Med J 92:693, 1979.
31. Feinstein SB, et al.: Two-dimensional contrast echocardiography: 1. In vitro development and quantitative analysis of echo contrast agents. J Am Coll Cardiol 3:14, 1984.
32. Bommer WJ, Mason DT, DeMaria AN: Studies in contrast echocardiography: development of new agents with superior reproducibility and transmission through lungs. Circulation 59, 60(Suppl 2):II-17, 1979.
33. Meltzer RS, et al.: Pulmonary wedge injections yielding left-sided echocardiographic contrast. Br Heart J 44:390, 1980.
34. Hunter S, Sutherland GR: Contrast M-mode echocardiography, the suprasternal notch approach. *In* Meltzer RS, Roeland J (eds.): Contrast Echocardiography. The Hague, Martinus Nijhoff, p. 1278, 1982.
35. Levin AR, et al.: Atrial pressure flow dynamics in atrial septal defects. Circulation 37:476, 1968.
36. Shiina A, et al.: Contrast echocardiographic evaluation of changes in flow velocity in the right side of the heart. Circulation 63:1408, 1981.
37. Meltzer RS, et al.: Correlation between velocity measurements from Doppler echocardiography and from M-mode contrast echocardiography. Br Heart J 49:244, 1983.
38. Valdes-Cruz L, et al.: Can tracking of contrast echocardiographic targets be used to measure intracardiac flow velocities? Am J Cardiol 51:215, 1983.
39. Gullace G, et al.: Contrast echocardiographic features of pulmonary hypertension and regurgitation. Br Heart J 46:369, 1981.
40. Dillon JC, et al.: Cross-sectional echocardiographic examination of the interatrial septum. Circulation 55:115, 1977.
41. Weyman AE, et al.: Non-invasive visualization of the left main coronary artery by cross-sectional echocardiography. Circulation 54:169, 1976.
42. Foale RA, et al.: Pseudoaneurysm of the pulmonary artery after the banding procedure: two-dimensional echocardiographic description. J Am Coll Cardiol 3:371, 1984.
43. Chandraratna PAN, Langevin E, O'Dell R: Echocardiographic contrast studies during pericardiocentesis. Ann Intern Med 87:199, 1977.
44. Kronzon I, et al.: The use of two-dimensional echocardiography during transeptal cardiac catheterization. J Am Coll Cardiol 4:425, 1984.
45. Reale A, et al.: Contrast echocardiography: transmission of echoes to the left heart across the pulmonary vascular bed. Eur Heart J 1:101, 1980.
46. Meltzer RS, Tickner EG, Popp RL: Why do the lungs clear ultrasonic contrast? Ultrasound Med Biol 6:263, 1980.
47. Fraker TD, Harris PJ, Behar VS, Kisslo JA: Detection and exclusion of interatrial shunts by two-dimensional echocardiography and peripheral venous injections. Circulation 59:379, 1979.
48. Kisslo J: Echo contrast for the detection of atrial septal defects. *In* Meltzer RS, Roelandt J (eds.): Contrast Echocardiography. The Hague, Martinus Nijhoff, p. 115, 1982.
49. Steinberg I, Deibilier W, Lukas I: Persistance of left superior vena cava. Dis Chest 24:479, 1953.
50. Campbell M, Deukar D: The left sided superior vena cava. Br Heart J 16: 423, 1954.
51. Valdes-Cruz LM, Pieroni DR, Rowland JM, Shematek JP: Recognition of residual post-operative shunts by contrast echocardiographic techniques. Circulation 55:148, 1977.
52. Sahn DJ, Friedman WF: Difficulties in distinguishing cardiac from pulmonary disease in the neonate. Pediatr Clin North Am 20:293, 1973.
53. Sahn DJ, Goldberg SJ, Allen HD, Valdez Cruz LM: Applications of contrast echocardiography in the newborn. *In* Meltzer RS, Roelandt J (eds.): Contrast Echocardiography. The Hague, Martinus Nijhoff, p. 215, 1982.
54. Savard M, Swan HJC, Kirklin JW, Wood EH: Hemodynamics alterations associated with ventricular septal defect. *In* Bass AD, Moe GK (eds.): Symposium on Congenital Heart Disease, Washington, DC, American Association for the Advancement of Science, p. 141, 1960.
55. Levin AR, et al.: Intracardiac pressure-flow dynamics in isolated ventricular septal defects. Circulation 35:430, 1967.
56. Serwer GA, et al.: Use of contrast echocardiography for evaluation of right ventricular hemodynamics in the presence of ventricular septal defects. Circulation 58:327, 1978.
57. Funabashi T, et al.: Echocardiographic visualization of ventricular septal defect in infants and assessment of hemodynamic status using a contrast technique: comparison of M-mode and two-dimensional Imaging. Circulation 64:1025, 1981.
58. Levin AR, et al.: Ventricular pressure-flow dynamics in Tetralogy of Fallot. Circulation 34:1, 1966.
59. Kerber RE, Kioschos JM, Lauer RM: Use of an ultrasonic contrast method in the diagnosis of valvular regurgitation and intracardiac shunts. Am J Cardiol 34:722, 1974.
60. Meltzer RS, et al.: The diagnosis of tricuspid regurgitation by contrast echocardiography. Circulation 63:1093, 1981.
61. Feigenbaum H, et al.: Identification of ultrasound echoes from the left ventricle by use of intracardiac injections of indocyanine green. Circulation 41:614, 1970.
62. Trippe W, Behar VS, Scallion R, Kisslo JA: Detection of tricuspid regurgitation with two-dimensional echocardiography and peripheral vein injection. Circulation 57:128, 1978.
63. Roelandt J, Meltzer RS, Serruys PW: Contrast echocardiography of the left ventricle. *In* Meltzer RS, Roelandt J (eds.): Contrast Echocardiography. The Hague, Martinus Nijhoff, p. 72, 1982.
64. Meltzer RS, et al.: Cardiac catheterization under echocardiographic control in a pregnant woman. Am J Med 71:481, 1981.
65. Elkayam U, et al.: Contrast echocardiography to reduce ionizing radiation during pregnancy. Am J Cardiol 52:213, 1983.
66. Bommer WJ, et al.: Indicator dilution dye curves obtained by photometric analysis of two-dimensional echo contrast studies (abstr). Am J Cardiol 41: 370, 1978.

67. Bommer WJ, et al.: Development of a new echocardiographic contrast agent capable of pulmonary transmission and left heart opacification following peripheral venous injection (abstr). Circulation 62(Suppl 3):III-111, 1980.
68. Zwehl W, et al.: Physical factors influencing quantitation of two-dimensional contrast echo amplitudes. J Am Coll Cardiol 4:157, 1984.
69. Hagler DJ, Tajik AJ, Seward JB, Ritman EL: Videodensitometric quantitation of left-to-right shunts with contrast echocardiography. *In* Meltzer RS, Roelandt J (eds.): Contrast Echocardiography. The Hague, Martinus Nijhoff, p. 298, 1982.
70. Schnabel TG, et al.: Postural cyanosis and angina pectoris following pneumonectomy: relief by closure of an interatrial septal defect. J Thorac Surg 32:246, 1956.
71. Begin R: Platypnea after pneumonectomy. N Engl J Med 293:342, 1975.
72. LaBresh KA, et al.: Platypnea syndrome after left pneumonectomy. Chest 79:605, 1981.
73. Winters WL, et al.: Venoarterial shunting from inferior vena cava to left atrium in atrial septal defects with normal right heart pressures. Am J Cardiol 19:293, 1967.
74. DeLeval MR, Ritter DG, McGoon DC, Danielson GK. Anomalous systemic venous connection. Mayo Clin Proc 50:599, 1975.
75. Wood P: Congenital Heart Disease. Diseases of the Heart and Circulation. Philadelphia, JB Lippincott, p. 554, 1975.
76. Kirsch WM, Carlson E, Hartmann AF: A case of anomalous drainage of the superior vena cava into the left atrium. J Thorac Cardiovasc Surg 41: 550, 1961.
77. Truman AT, Roa PS, Kulangara RJ: Use of contrast echocardiography in diagnosis of anomalous connection of right superior vena cava to left atrium. Br Heart J 44:718, 1980.
78. Schick EC, Lekakis J, Rothendler JA, Ryan TJ: Persistent left superior vena cava and right superior vena cava drainage into the left atrium without arterial hypoxemia. J Am Coll Cardiol 5:374, 1985.
79. Gardner DL, Cole L: Long survival with inferior vena cava draining into left atrium. Br Heart J 17:93, 1955.
80. Gautam HP: Left atrial inferior vena cava with atrial septal defect. J Thorac Cardiovasc Surg 55:827, 1968.
81. Kim YS, Serratto M, Long DM, Hastreiter AR: Left atrial inferior vena cava with atrial septal defect. Ann Thorac Surg 11:165, 1971.
82. Viart P, LeClerc JL, Primo G, Polis O: Total anomalous systemic venous drainage. Am J Dis Child 131:195, 1977.
83. McFaul RC, et al.: Development of pulmonary arteriovenous shunt after superior vena cava—right pulmonary artery (Glenn) anastomosis. Report of four cases. Circulation 55:212, 1977.
84. Levine RA, Gillam LD, Guerrero JL, Weyman AE: Wall motion abnormalities following myocardial echocardiographic contrast injection area caused by microbubbles. J Am Coll Cardiol 5:474, 1985.
85. Glatt BS, Rowe RD: Cerebral arteriovenous fistula associated with congestive heart failure in the newborn. Pediatrics 26:596, 1960.
86. Sunderland CO, Morgan CL, Lees HM: Cerebral arteriovenous fistula producing temporary heart failure in infancy. Clin Pediatr 10:309, 1971.
87. Holden AM, Fyler DC, Shillito J, Nadas AS: Congestive heart failure from intracranial arteriovenous fistula in infancy. Pediatrics 49:30, 1972.
88. Watson DG, Smith RR, Brann AW: Arteriovenous malformation of the vein of Galen. Am J Dis Child 130:520, 1976.
89. Cumming GR: Circulation in neonates with intracranial arteriovenous fistula and cardiac failure. Am J Cardiol 45:1019, 1980.
90. Snider AR, Soifer SJ, Silverman NH: Detection of intracranial arteriovenous fistula by two-dimensional ultrasonography. Circulation 63:1179, 1981.
91. Bommer WJ, et al.: The safety of contrast echocardiography: report of the Committee on Contrast Echocardiography for the American Society of Echocardiography 3:6, 1984.
92. Kort A, Kronzon I: Microbubble formation: in vitro and in vivo observations. JCU 10:117, 1982.
93. Feinstein SB, et al.: Microbubble dynamics visualized in the intact capillary circulation. J Am Coll Cardiol 4:595, 1984.
94. Gillam LD, et al.: Functional and pathologic effects of multiple echocardiographic contrast injections on the myocardium, brain and kidney. J Am Coll Cardiol 6:687, 1985.
95. Topol EJ, et al.: Value of intraoperative left ventricular microbubbles detected by transesophageal two-dimensional echocardiography in predicting neurologic outcome after cardiac operations. Am J Cardiol 56:773, 1985.
96. Rodigas PC, et al.: Intraoperative two-dimensional echocardiography: ejection of microbubbles from the left ventricle after cardiac surgery. Am J Cardiol 50:1130, 1982.
97. Schuchman H, Feigenbaum H, Dillon JC, Chang S: Intracavitary echoes in patients with mitral prosthetic valves. J Clin Ultra 3:107, 1975.
98. Gramiak R, Wang R (eds.): Cardiac Ultrasound. St. Louis, CV Mosby, p. 30, 1975.
99. Martin RD, Preis LK Jr: Spontaneous left ventricular microbubbles in patients with metallic mitral prosthetic valves. *In* Meltzer RS, Roelandt J (eds.): Contrast Echocardiography. The Hague, Martinus Nijhoff, p. 59, 1982.
100. Feinberg HJ: Ultrasonic visualization of in vivo flow phenomenon without introduced contrast material. Proc 25th Ann Convention Am Inst Ultra Med p. 17, 1980.
101. Rowland E, et al.: Intracardiac contrast echoes during transvenous HIS bundle ablation. Br Heart J 53:240, 1985.

CHAPTER

16

Miscellaneous Echocardiographic Techniques II: Transesophageal Echocardiography, Epicardial Echocardiography, Intraoperative Echocardiography, Catheter-Based (Intravascular and Intracardiac) Echocardiography, and Sonomicrometry

TRANSESOPHAGEAL ECHOCARDIOGRAPHY

Transesophageal echocardiography (*TEE*) is the term used to describe the study of the heart from the esophagus using two-dimensional, M-mode, or Doppler echocardiography. The esophagus is a muscular canal with an average diameter of 2 cm extending roughly 25 cm from the pharynx to the stomach. The general direction of the esophagus is vertical, with slight leftward deviation from the midline in the neck and at its junction with the stomach. The esophagus also curves anteroposteriorly in parallel with the curvature of the cervical and thoracic vertebrae. At it descends inferiorly in the thorax, the esophagus passes behind the trachea, left mainstem bronchus, left atrium, and left ventricle before it passes through the diaphragm (Fig. 16–1).[1] The esophageal introitus is the narrowest region of the esophagus, and the cricopharyngeus muscle contributes to this decrease in diameter. This constricted region has been referred to as the "pass of Bab-el Mandeb" or the "gate of tears."[2]

Because of its close apposition to the posterior surface of the heart, the esophagus is an ideal window for echocardiographic examination. The sound beam must pass through only the muscular esophageal wall before reaching the pericardium, with the result that there is little attenuation of the sound beam and virtually unlimited access. This close apposition to the heart overcomes many of the access problems encountered during transthoracic imaging, permits the use of high frequency transducers, which provide superb image quality, and improves the sensitivity of Doppler recordings.

Side and Gosling, in 1971, first reported use of the esophagus to record thoracic aortic flow in humans using continuous wave Doppler.[3] Two experimental studies using this approach to assess the blood flow dynamics and wall motion of the thoracic aorta in dogs followed in 1972 and 1975.[4,5] In 1976, Frazin et al. described a method for obtaining M-mode recordings of the heart from the esophagus using a single-element transducer.[6] The transducer was connected to the ultrasound machine by a thin (3 mm), flexible, shielded coax-

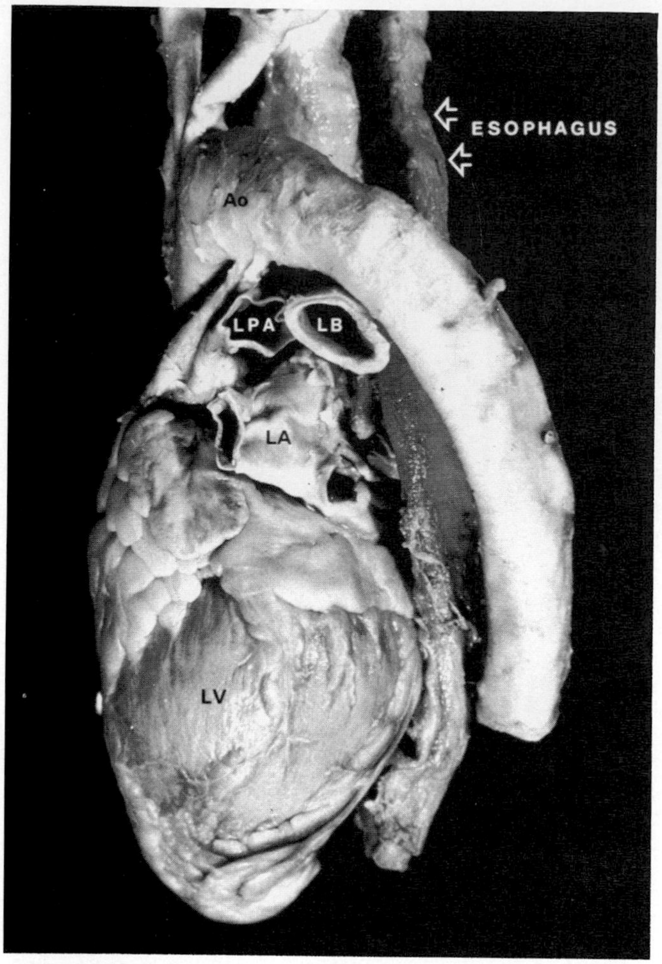

Fig. 16–1. Anatomic specimen illustrating the relationship of the esophagus to the heart, great vessels, and tracheobronchial system. Ao = aorta; LPA = left pulmonary artery; LB = left mainstream; LA = left atrium; LV = left ventricle.

ial cable, and the ability of the operator to control the transducer and direct the ultrasonic beam was severely limited. In 1977, Hisanaga et al. introduced the first two-dimensional echo device for recording images from the esophagus. Their instrument consisted of a high speed rotating ultrasound scanner fixed to the tip of a rigid gastroscope-like shaft.[7,8] The rotating transducer was enclosed in an inflatable oil bag to separate the moving elements from the surrounding tissues and to maintain contact with the esophageal wall.

Further clinical motivation for the development of esophageal echocardiography was provided by Matsumoto et al., who, in 1980, used the technique to monitor left ventricular performance during cardiothoracic surgery. They demonstrated that the esophagus offered a stable location for continuous cardiac examination that did not interfere with the surgical procedure and could be performed before the chest was opened and after it was closed.[9]

In 1982 Schluter et al. incorporated a phased array system into the tip of a flexible gastroscope, permitting greater flexibility and patient comfort and this probe design has become the standard for image acquisition.[10]

During the next decade, pulsed, continuous wave, and color flow Doppler were added to the basic two-dimensional imaging format, and the initial monoplane design was largely replaced by biplane imaging probes. To provide greater imaging flexibility, Souquet[11] and Hanrath et al.[12] suggested a rotating phased array transducer, in 1982, and such a device was designed by Harui and Souquet in 1985.[13]

Improved probe design and flexibility, together with the enhanced access and image resolution provided by TEE have led to expanded clinical application. At present, between 2.5 and 5% or more of all echocardiograms are being performed from the esophagus in major institutions,[14] and clinical applications continue to increase.

Instrumentation

Transesophageal studies are performed using the same basic echocardiographic instruments used for routine transthoracic studies with two-dimensional imaging and pulsed, continuous wave and color Doppler capabilities. The transesophageal probe is a modification of a standard gastroscope, with the optics removed and one or more phased array transducers inserted at its tip. A cable for establishing electrical connection between the echograph and transducer extends from the base of the probe. Mechanical oscillation of a single transducer is also possible and provides comparable results.

The original transducer constructed by Schluter et al. contained a single array of 32 elements, which operated at 3.5 MHz, was focused at 10 cm, and was aligned perpendicular to the long axis of the probe. The transducer was embedded in soft plastic material with carefully rounded edges to avoid damage to the esophagus and was fitted to the distal end of a standard flexible gastroscope. The outer diameter of the gastroscope was roughly 9 mm with a length of 100 cm. The only rigid part of the apparatus was the array transducer at the tip, which, in the earlier models, was 35 mm long, 15 mm wide, and 16 mm thick[10] (Fig. 16–2). As the technique has evolved, transducers with greater variety in design, frequency, focusing, and size have been developed. Transducers that image at multiple frequencies (3.5, 5.0, and 7.5 MHz) have also been devised with the higher frequencies, providing higher resolution and better anatomic detail, while Doppler studies are often best performed at lower frequencies. The wide array of transducer designs and sizes is shown in Figure 16–3.[15] Both single (monoplane) and biplane transducer are now in general use but will undoubtedly be replaced by multiplane devices in the near future.

Monoplane Transducers

Current monoplane transducers contain 64 elements in the array to improve image quality; most commonly operate at 5 MHz and have a distal tip that is 14 mm wide, 11 mm thick, and 27 mm long. The typical endoscope shaft diameter is 9.8 mm, although smaller devices (in the 6-mm range) are available for pediatric use.

Probe length is generally 100 cm, although probes with lengths ranging from 60 to 110 cm are also available. For intraoperative studies, a longer probe is desirable to

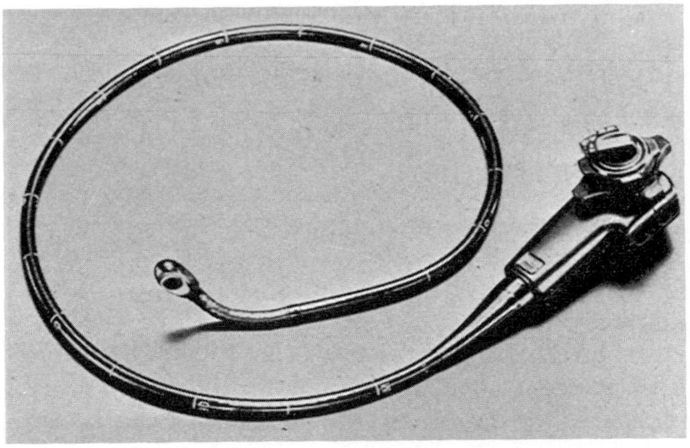

Fig. 16–2. Transducer for esophageal echocardiographic imaging. The probe consists of a flexible gastroscope with the optics removed and a phased array transducer placed at the tip of the probe.

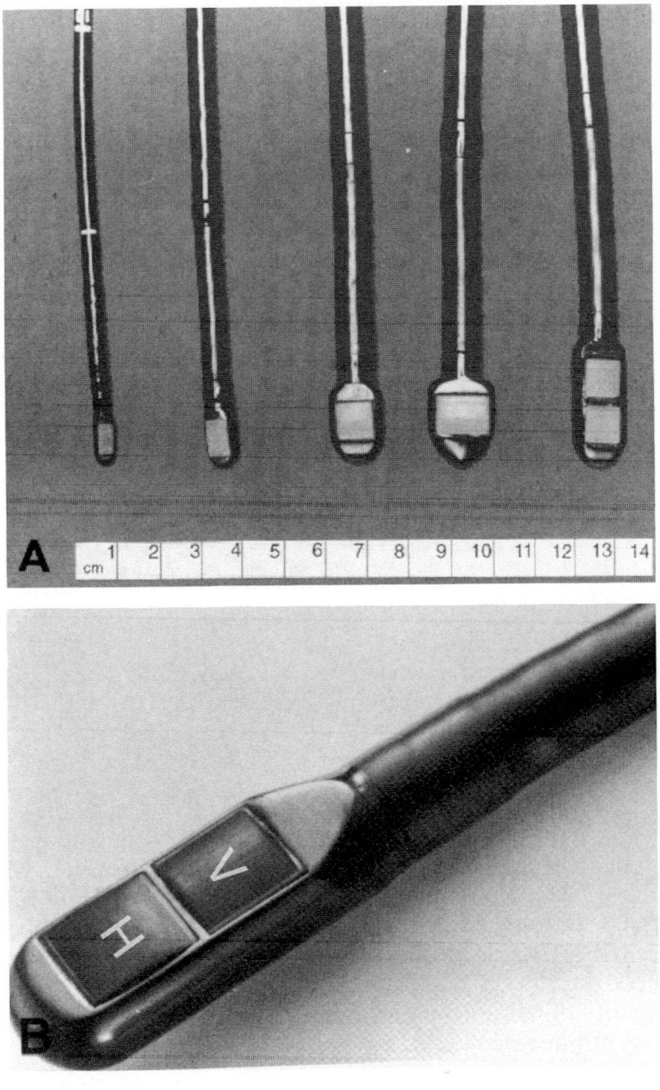

Fig. 16–3. A. The different sizes of transducers that are commercially available for use in transesophageal echocardiography. (From Khandheria BK, Oh J: Transesophageal echocardiography: state of the art and future directions. Am J Cardiol 69:61H, 1992.) **B.** Close-up of a transesophageal echocardiographic biplane endoscope tip with two separate phased array transducer elements. H = horizontal plane; V = vertical plane. (Courtesy of Advanced Technology Laboratories.)

permit access to the patient without interfering with the surgical or anesthesia environment.[16] Outpatient instruments can be shorter for ease of handling and control.

All transesophageal probes have a conventional endoscope handle with rotary controls and a locking mechanism for operation of the flexible tip.[16] Transducer position can be changed by (1) advancing or withdrawing the probe; (2) rotation of the gastroscope and (3) angulation of the probe tip (anteroposteriorly and mediolaterally). This combination of actions provides a high degree of freedom in transducer positioning (Fig. 16–4). The rotary controls in the endoscope handle consist of an inner (large) and outer (small) dial (Fig. 16–5). The inner dial generally controls anterior and posterior flexion, while the outer dial provides right and left lateral movement. Rotation of the dials toward the operator produces anteflexion and rightward angulation of the tip, while rotation in the opposite direction causes retroflexion and leftward tip displacement. The tip is capable of 120° of anterior motion and 90° of motion in the posterior and lateral directions.

Biplane Transducers

Biplane probes, which have now become standard, contain a second, proximal, array transducer aligned parallel to the long axis of the probe and thus orthogonal to the distal horizontal array. The centers of these two transducers are usually 1 cm apart (Fig. 16–6). By switching from one transducer to the other, one can display transverse and longitudinal planes in a sequential manner.[17] In early versions, each of the biplane transducers contained only 32 elements; however, later designs increased the element number to 48 × 48,[18] and current probes contain 64 elements in each array. The shaft size of the currently available biplane probes ranges in thickness from 6 to 14 mm, with the most common being 10.8 mm. Tip diameters (14.3 mm) and length (41.3 mm) are larger than those of monoplane probes to allow for the second transducer. Smaller size transducers provide less room for coaxial cables (transducer elements), and hence, there is compromise in image quality.

Because biplane probes have two separate imaging

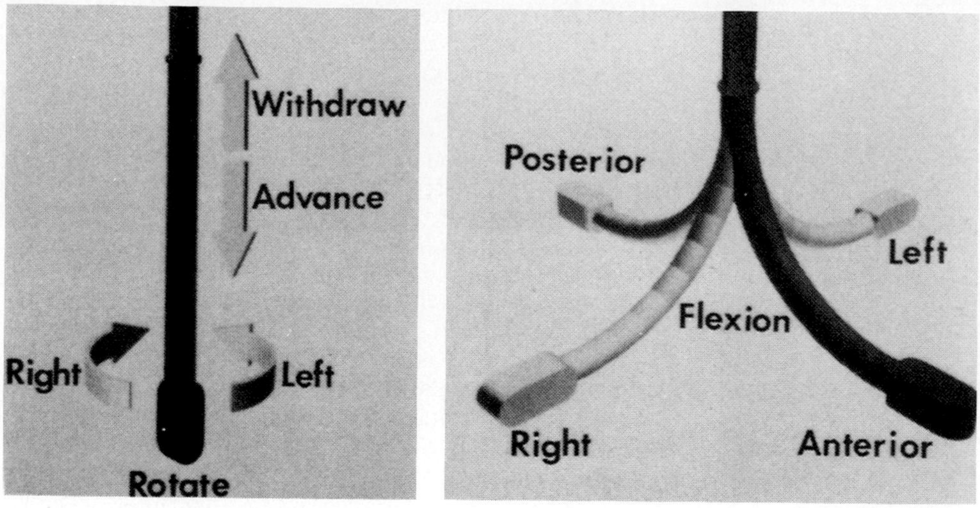

Fig. 16–4. Depiction of possible manipulations of biplanar transesophageal echocardiographic endoscope. Tip of scope can be advanced, withdrawn, rotated leftward or rightward, and flexed in four directions (anterior, posterior, left, and right). (From Seward JB, et al.: Biplanar transesophageal echocardiography: anatomic correlations, image orientation, and clinical applications. Mayo Clin Proc 65:1193, 1990. Reproduced with permission of the Mayo Foundation.)

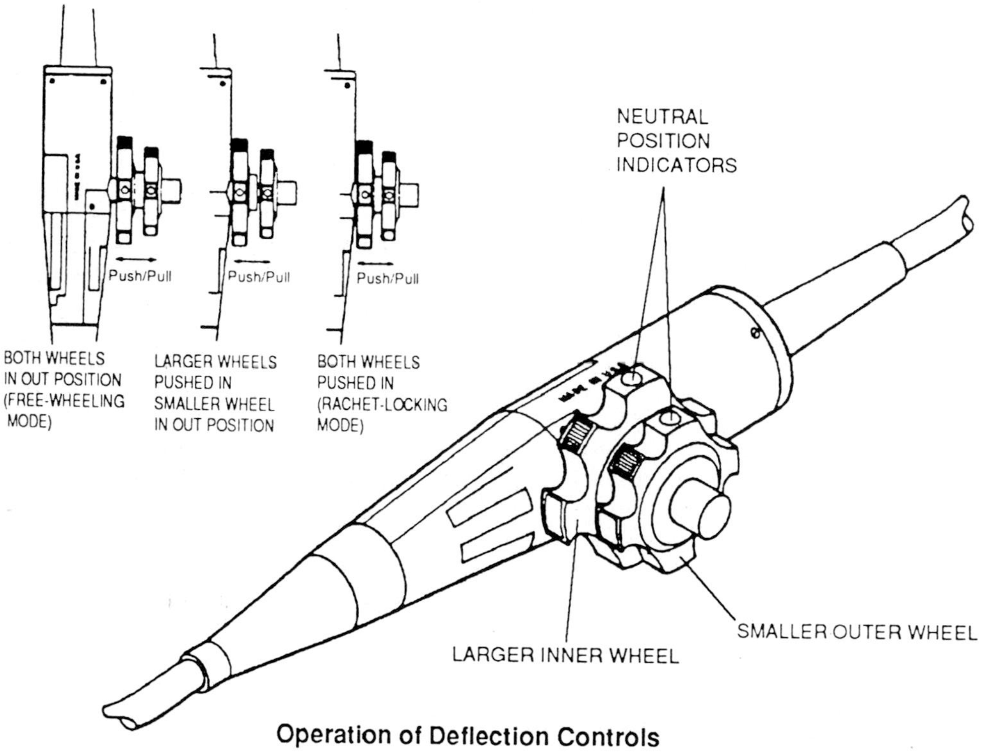

Fig. 16–5. The control device for movement and locking of the endoscope tip. (Courtesy of Hewlett-Packard Company.)

surfaces, repositioning is required to generate images orthogonal about the same central axis. Because of the relatively long imaging surface of the biplane probe, it is occasionally difficult to obtain the same degree of contact with both transducers, and image quality may vary importantly between planes.

Biplane imaging systems with cine-loop and split screen capabilities are available. These permit stored images or cycles from one plane to be displayed while data from the second plane are being acquired in real time. Biplane transducers capable of displaying horizontal and vertical images in rapid sequence or simultaneously are also available. Rapid sequence imaging can be achieved by alternately exciting each array, constructing a full image, and then switching to the orthogonal plane. Simultaneous imaging is achieved by alternately acquiring data lines from each plane and forming images in orthogonal sections simultaneously. Because both of these formats rely on perpendicular but spatially separated transducers, the planes do not arise from the same center. Biplane phased array matrix transducers have been developed to overcome this problem; however, the quality of the images produced by these devices to date has not been good.[19]

Multiplane Probes

Multiplane TEE probes with mechanical and phased array transducers are now available that permit rotation of a single plane around a central axis. The transducer can be rotated mechanically or by an electrically driven motor to provide continuous recording through an arc

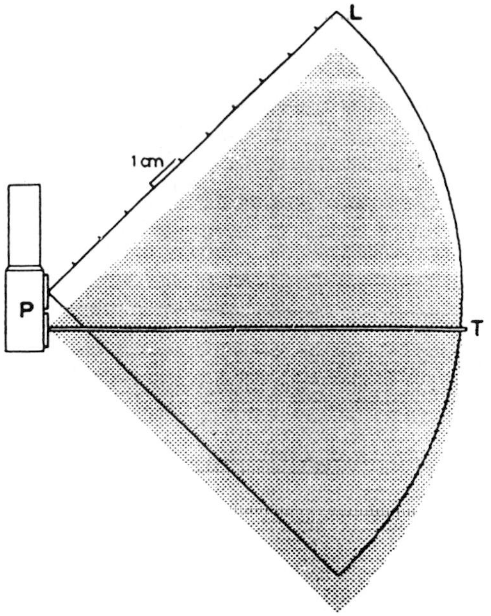

Fig. 16–6. Schematic drawing of the biplane probe tip (P) illustrating the effect of the distance between the two transducers. Observe that the transverse plane (T) intersects the longitudinal plane (L) approximately 1 cm from the probe, resulting in a lack of overlay in the proximal field. The shaded area represents the hypothetical situation of the longitudinal plane originating from the same transducer as the transverse plane. It is generally not necessary to advance the probe tip minimally to obtain exact correspondence between the two planes unless one is examining proximal structures such as the descending thoracic aorta. (From Nanda NC, Pinheiro L, Sanyal RS, Storey O: Transesophageal Biplane Echocardiographic Imaging: Technique, Planes, and Clinical Usefulness. Echocardiography 7:771, 1990.)

of 180° (Fig. 16–7). The standard horizontal and longitudinal planes are orthogonal to each other at 0 and 90°, respectively, with intermediate planes between 0 and 180°. Graphic display of the angle of rotation is available on the screen.[20,21]

The major problem with rotating array probes has been the size of the scan head. A standard 5-MHz, 64-element array transducer, e.g., is a rectangle 9 × 10 mm (diagonal, 13.5 mm). When the transducer housing is added, the outer diameter of the probe would be approximately 17 mm. Cutting the corners of the rectangle produces an octagonal array with a diameter of 15 mm; however, this is still relatively large. First-generation commercial probes image at 5.0/3.7 MHz, have a tip of 16.7 mm, thickness of 11.2 mm, and length of 45 mm. The gastroscope shaft diameter is 10.25 mm.

Multiplane transducers should facilitate fine plane positioning by allowing planes to be defined relative to cardiac anatomy, as is the custom with transthoracic recording. Precise plane positioning should provide more meaningful quantitation and hopefully permit three-dimensional reconstruction of structures of interest.

Temperature Sensing. Most transesophageal probes have self-contained thermal sensors to monitor probe temperature and to shut down the instrument when the external temperature exceeds the programmed threshold. The cutoff temperature varies between manufacturers. A common value is 42.25°C; however, this has been increased to 45 in some versions. When this temperature is exceeded, a warning message such as "probe auto cool" will appear, power will be cut off, and the system will stop scanning. This occurs most often in the operating room during active rewarming but can also be encountered in febrile patients. In patients with high fevers in whom an examination is essential, this function can be transiently overridden by cooling the probe before insertion. Activation of the warning in an afebrile patient suggests equipment malfunction.

Probe Care and Cleaning. The endoscope should be inspected before and after each case for perforations or tears in the outer case, which might prevent proper cleaning or pose an electrical risk. Following use, the probe should be cleaned with soap and water or an enzymatic solution (Protozyme) to remove saliva and then immersed in a glutaraldehyde solution (Cidex, Surgikos Inc.) for roughly 20 minutes to eradicate bacteria and

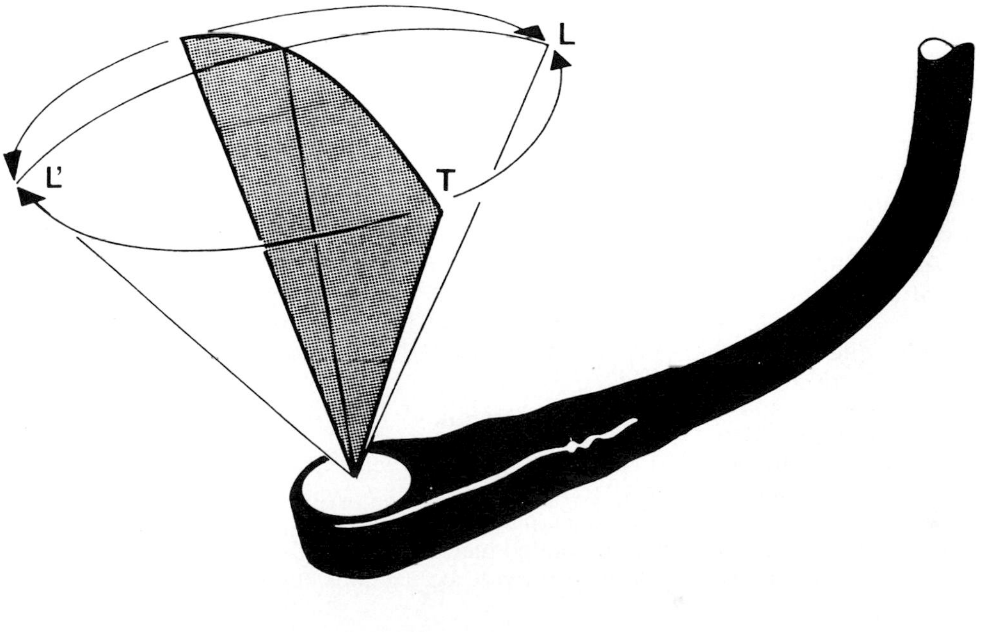

Fig. 16–7. Schema of the multiplane probe showing how the transducer and imaging plane can be rotated from an intermediate transverse position (T) in opposite directions over 90° to obtain longitudinal planes (L and L′). All intermediate oblique planes are sequentially visualized. (From Roelandt JRTC, et al.: Multiplane transesophageal echocardiography: latest evolution in an imaging revolution. J Am Soc Echocardiogr 5:361, 1992.)

viruses. The endoscope is then rinsed with tap water and allowed to air dry. Alternatively, the probe can be covered by a disposable sheath during use and then simply cleaned between studies. Most investigators, however, have found these sheaths to be cumbersome to use and irritating to the patient.

Examination Technique

Patient Preparation

Patients must fast for 4 to 6 hours before undergoing a TEE study. It is important to carefully explain the procedure to the patient and to obtain a detailed history of any gastroesophageal-related symptoms and prior endoscopy. Drug allergy and medication history are also important. In those suspected of esophageal disease, a barium swallow or endoscopic evaluation of the esophagus is recommended to rule out diverticula, strictures, or other disorders that might weaken the esophageal wall or obstruct passage of the endoscope. As with any other form of endoscopy, informed patient consent is obtained.

Dentures and oral prostheses must be removed before the examination, intravenous access established, and an oxygen delivery system (nasal prongs), airway, bite guard, suction, standard crash cart and sphygmomanometer must be immediately available. Cardiac rhythm should be continuously monitored and cuff blood pressure recorded periodically, especially during drug administration and initial intubation. Pulse oximetry can be used to monitor oxygen saturation in unstable patients. In patient with decreased respiratory function, supplemental oxygen is delivered via nasal cannula. A 12-lead electrocardiograph (ECG) should be immediately available for emergencies.

Medications used in conjunction with TEE in awake patients include (1) topical anesthesia of the oropharynx (and esophagus) to diminish pharyngeal sensation and resulting gagging, retching, and laryngospasm; (2) drying agents to reduce salivary and gastrointestinal secretions; (3) tranquilization to decrease fear and anxiety and provide amnesia for subsequent events (antegrade amnesia); and (4) antibiotics for endocarditis prophylaxis in selected cases.

Topical anesthesia is generally applied to the hypopharynx by 4% xylocaine spray, 10% cetacaine spray, and/or by having the patient gargle and swallow 2% viscous xylocaine. Peak anesthetic effect occurs in 2 to 5 minutes, and the effects persist for 30 to 45 minutes. Topical anesthesia of the pharynx may impair swallowing and increase risk of aspiration. As a result, nothing should be taken by mouth for at least 30 minutes after the procedure.[16]

Some authors advocate the use of drying agents to reduce secretions and obviate the need for oral suction. An anticholinergic (atropine, 0.5 mg subcutaneously or glycopyrrolate [Robinul] 0.1 to 0.2 mg) can be administered before the procedure to prevent bradycardia and hypersalivation. Glycopyrrolate has its peak effect 5 minutes after intravenous bolus administration. A mild increase in heart rate may be noted in patients with increased resting vagal tone.[16] Because of the potential for blurred vision or drowsiness, patients should be cautioned against operating a motor vehicle immediately after the procedure. We have not generally found it necessary to use these agents.

Sedation and analgesia are used for their calming effect, to prevent discomfort, and to produce antegrade or retrograde amnesia. Diazepam (Valium), 5 to 10 mg intravenously or midazolam (Versed), 0.5 to 5.0 mg, may be given immediately before the procedure to induce mild sedation. Midazolam can cause severe respiratory depression and hypotension, although this rarely occurs with a dose of less than 5 mg. An initial dose of 2 mg or less is usually administered slowly intravenously over 1 to 2 minutes, with several minutes elapsing before any additional drug is given. The dose should be reduced in elderly or debilitated patients. The goal is a calm, sedated, but cooperative patient. Cooperation of the awake patient is crucial, because an attempt by the patient to swallow greatly facilitates passage of the probe tip into the upper esophagus. Heavy sedation may make intubation more difficult as a result of lack of active patient cooperative. Associated discomfort can be relieved using meperidine with acetaminophen (Demerol) or morphine. In critically ill patients, where blood pressure and respiration are tenuous, short acting agents are preferred.

The clinical indications for TEE naturally select a patient population with a high prevalence of hemodynamically significant valvular lesions. As a result, the need for antimicrobial prophylaxis for the prevention of infective endocarditis in patients undergoing TEE is often questioned. The American Heart Association has categorized endoscopy as a low risk procedure not necessitating subacute bacterial endocarditis (SBE) prophylaxis. In studies of bacteremia associated with TEE, the frequency of positive blood cultures was no higher than the background contamination rate observed in the same patient population before the procedure. Further, no clinically significant bacteremias that were due to oral microbes susceptible to standard endocarditis prophylaxis regimens were detected.[22–24] Despite this, one case report appears to temporally link the occurrence of clinical, bacteriologic endocarditis with the TEE procedure.[25] We have also observed one case in which endocarditis appeared temporally related to a TEE procedure; however, this patient had received antibiotic prophylaxis.

Despite these background data, it is the practice in many laboratories to give antibiotic prophylaxis to patients at particular risk, e.g., those with artificial heart valves or intracardiac prostheses, poor dentition, or prior history of endocarditis.[26] In these cases, standard antibiotic prophylaxis is administered before the introduction of the gastroscope using currently recommended dosage.

Contraindications

TEE is contraindicated in patients with esophageal pathologies such as stricture, varices, tumors, diverticula, and scleroderma; severe atlantoaxial joint disease that prohibits flexing of the neck; prior radiation to the chest; and perforated viscus.

Probe Insertion

The operator who seeks to perform esophageal echocardiographic studies must become skilled in the insertion of the endoscope. This is particularly important in esophageal echocardiography, because the transducer replaces the optics of the gastroscope, and the insertion must be done blindly. The probe is typically introduced with the patient in a left lateral decubitus position, with gentle flexion of the neck to facilitate entry into the esophagus. In special circumstances the examination can be conducted in the sitting, supine, or prone positions; however, the left lateral decubitus position is preferred to prevent aspiration. When the probe is inserted, the index or index and middle fingers of the left (nondominant) hand are inserted into the patient's mouth and advanced to the base of the tongue. The tip of the partially flexed transducer is advanced into the mouth with the right (dominant) hand. The endoscope is always inserted with the transducer facing anteriorly. The probe tip is then passed beneath the left index finger and guided, using gentle downward pressure, toward the mouth of the esophagus until resistance is encountered.[16] Locking the lateral control knob will often aid in directing the probe. Adequate topical anesthesia will diminish the gag reflex; however, some transient gagging is usually encountered during introduction of the probe into the esophagus. With the tip of the probe at the esophageal inlet, the patient is requested to swallow. Swallowing will direct the probe into the upper part of the esophagus. Once the patient begins to swallow, the probe should be advanced firmly but without force. If resistance is encountered, the probe should be readjusted or redirected centrally. Many patients will continue to gag until the probe is advanced beyond the carina of the trachea or more than 25 cm from the incisors. Thus, rapid initial advancement to this point is essential. Once the probe is in the esophagus, most patients become more comfortable and will accept the remainder of the examination, and the probe can be advanced until cardiac structures appear on the viewing scope (Fig. 16–8). In large series, the rate of unsuccessful introduction has varied from 1.5%[15] to 1.9%.[27] In a large multicenter trial 201 (1.9%) of 10,419 transesophageal studies had to be aborted: 198 (98.5%) of these because of poor patient compliance or operator inexperience. In the remaining 3 cases, esophageal diverticula (2) or tracheostomy (1) prevented insertion. With difficult intubations, a laryngoscope may be used to assist in passing the endoscope.

When the patient cannot tolerate passage of the scope, the gag reflex can be completely abolished by blocking the internal branch of the superior laryngeal nerve (SLN), which blocks sensation to the epiglottis, the piriform fossa, the base of the tongue, and the mucous membranes of the larynx superior to the true cords. The internal branch of the SLN has only sensory fibers, and hence its blockade results in no laryngeal motor weakness.[28] When there is hypersalivation, excessive fluid accumulation can be removed by external suction. Forceful entry into the esophagus should always be avoided. If the probe cannot be passed easily, assistance from a gastroenterologist should be sought.

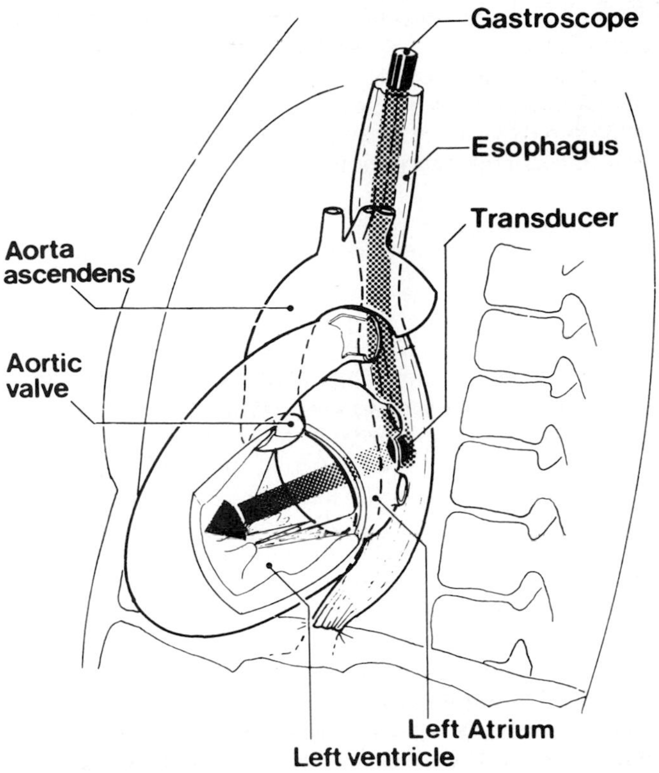

Fig. 16–8. Anatomic relationship of the esophagus and heart. The ultrasonic transducer is located in the esophagus, immediately behind the left atrium. From this location, and scan plane is aligned to pass through the mitral orifice parallel to the direction of transmitral flow. (From Schluter M, et al.: Assessment of transesophageal pulsed Doppler echocardiography in the detection of mitral regurgitation. Circulation 66:784, 1982. Reproduced by permission of the American Heart Association, Inc.)

During insertion, both the probe and the operator's fingers are at risk for being inadvertently or deliberately bitten. Greater risk is encountered in patients with behavior disorders, mental retardation, neurologic deficits, and those in an obtunded but restless state. In such patients, a mouth gag can be used to hold the teeth apart during probe insertion until the bite guard can be inserted or maintained in place throughout the procedure.[29]

When transesophageal studies are performed in the operating room, the transducer is usually not introduced until after general anesthesia is obtained. Introduction of the probe in the anesthetized is easier than in the conscious patient because there is no gagging, retching, or coughing.[16] Supine intubation is no problem because the trachea is protected. The head should be in the midline position and the neck slightly flexed. The endotracheal tube is shifted to one side to provide room for the transesophageal probe. Catheters within the esophagus such as nasogastric tubes, feeding tubes, or temperature probes are typically removed to prevent kinking, knotting, or intertwining of the devices. A second catheter in the esophagus can also become interposed between the transducer tip and the wall of the esophagus, obscuring vision. The transducer generally can be passed blindly by simply directing it toward the center of the posterior oropharynx and allowing the probe to flex passively. Occasionally, it is necessary to guide the probe digitally, to temporarily deflate the cuff of the endotracheal tube, or to introduce the probe under direct laryngoscopic vision. In this setting, success should approach 100%. When all of these maneuvers fail, however, esophageal pathology should be suspected and the procedure terminated.

Esophageal Imaging: Routine Imaging Planes

Esophageal studies tend to be more goal- or question-oriented than routine transthoracic echocardiograms. In addition, the views that can be routinely obtained from the esophagus cannot, in most cases, be considered standard (i.e., they cannot be precisely fixed in space (see Chapter 5) and therefore do not contain reproducible dimensional and area data that can be used for quantitative purposes. Fortunately, the esophageal views that can be recorded (see following discussion) are similar enough to standard transthoracic images to permit structure recognition and plane location. However, because they are recorded from the posterior surface of the heart, structure orientation differs considerably, and the identification and recording of specific features are often more complex than might be expected.

The esophagus also imposes constraints on the free movement of the endoscope, which makes precise alignment of individual planes with the axes of the heart difficult and in some cases impossible. As a result, the operator must often deal with images that are not only inverted but are oblique or rotated relative to their usual appearance. Thus, while the esophageal window improves access and resolution enormously when compared to the transthoracic approach, the technical and interpretative aspects of the study are often more difficult, and less quantitative data are available.

Despite these difficulties, it is important in all cases to attempt to record an ordered and comprehensive examination. Such an examination consists of a series of horizontal and vertically oriented planes that record as precisely as possible the four cardiac valves, the great vessels, the cardiac chambers, and the interventricular and interatrial septa. Probe position is initially determined by the distance the transducer has traveled down the esophagus. Most studies begin when the transducer reaches the most superior border of the left atrium and cardiac structures are first visualized. Alternatively, it has been suggested that the transducer be advanced into the stomach and that images be acquired as the probe is withdrawn up the esophagus. As with transthoracic imaging, the precise order in which images are acquired is less important than the fact that some order be determined for each laboratory and that the same order be maintained for every study. Likewise, the pattern in which images are acquired at each level varies, with some laboratories acquiring all horizontal images first and then all transverse images, while others alternate from one orientation to the other. Here again, it is not the pattern but the consistency that is important.

The next section describes the "standard" horizontal and the vertical views commonly obtained with a standard biplane imaging probe. In the future, multiplanar imaging will undoubtedly improve plane optimization with the result that a more standard long and short axis scheme can be used. Such devices, however, are not generally available, and thus, the following section describes what currently can be achieved rather than what might be considered optimal.

Transesophageal Horizontal and Transverse Views

Initial Probe Orientation. Although the probe is inserted with the transducer facing forward, it can often rotate inadvertently during passage. The primary landmarks for initial probe orientation are the descending thoracic aorta, which is leftward and posterior, and the left atrium, which is anterior to the esophagus. Because the heart and descending aorta are on roughly opposite sides of the esophagus, they are usually examined separately, with the cardiac examination performed first.

Once the probe is directly anteriorly toward the heart, the examination can begin. Horizontal views are recorded with the distal or transverse array of the biplane transducer. With the probe parallel to the long axis of the esophagus, the transverse array is roughly parallel to the short axis of the body. The transducer must therefore be angled to the left to more closely align the long axis of the probe tip with that of the heart and the transverse scan plane with the cardiac short axes. With the probe behind the superior border of the left atrium and retroflexed slightly, an inverted four-chamber view can be recorded. Continued advancement and anteroflexion will permit recording of sequential oblique and then true short axis views of the aortic valve, mitral valve, left ventricle at the base, papillary muscles, and finally, transgastric views of the distal ventricle and apex.

The Esophageal Four-Chamber View. As the probe is advanced down the esophagus, the first images of the heart are usually recorded when the transducer reaches the superior border of the left atrium (25 to 30 cm from the incisors) and have the appearance of an inverted transthoracic apical four-chamber view. This view usually includes portions of both atria and ventricles along with corresponding segments of the interatrial and interventricular septa and atrioventricular (AV) valves (Fig. 16–9). Unfortunately, from this transducer location, it is difficult to align the scan plane through the true long axis of either ventricle or atrium, and as a result, little unique quantitative information can be obtained. However, like the transthoracic apical four-chamber view, it encompasses a broad expanse of the heart and is extremely valuable for assessing qualitative abnormalities such as chamber enlargement, structural and functional disorders of the AV valves, and tumors or thrombi of the atria or ventricles. It is uniquely valuable for recording the superior wall of the left atrium and detecting thrombi at the origins of the pulmonary veins. Because the septa are only incompletely recorded in this view, imaging in multiple planes is required to record septal defects.

Esophageal Long Axis: Mitral Valve, Left Ventricular Outflow Tract, Aortic Valve View. Slight counterclockwise rotation of the transducer (elevation when the

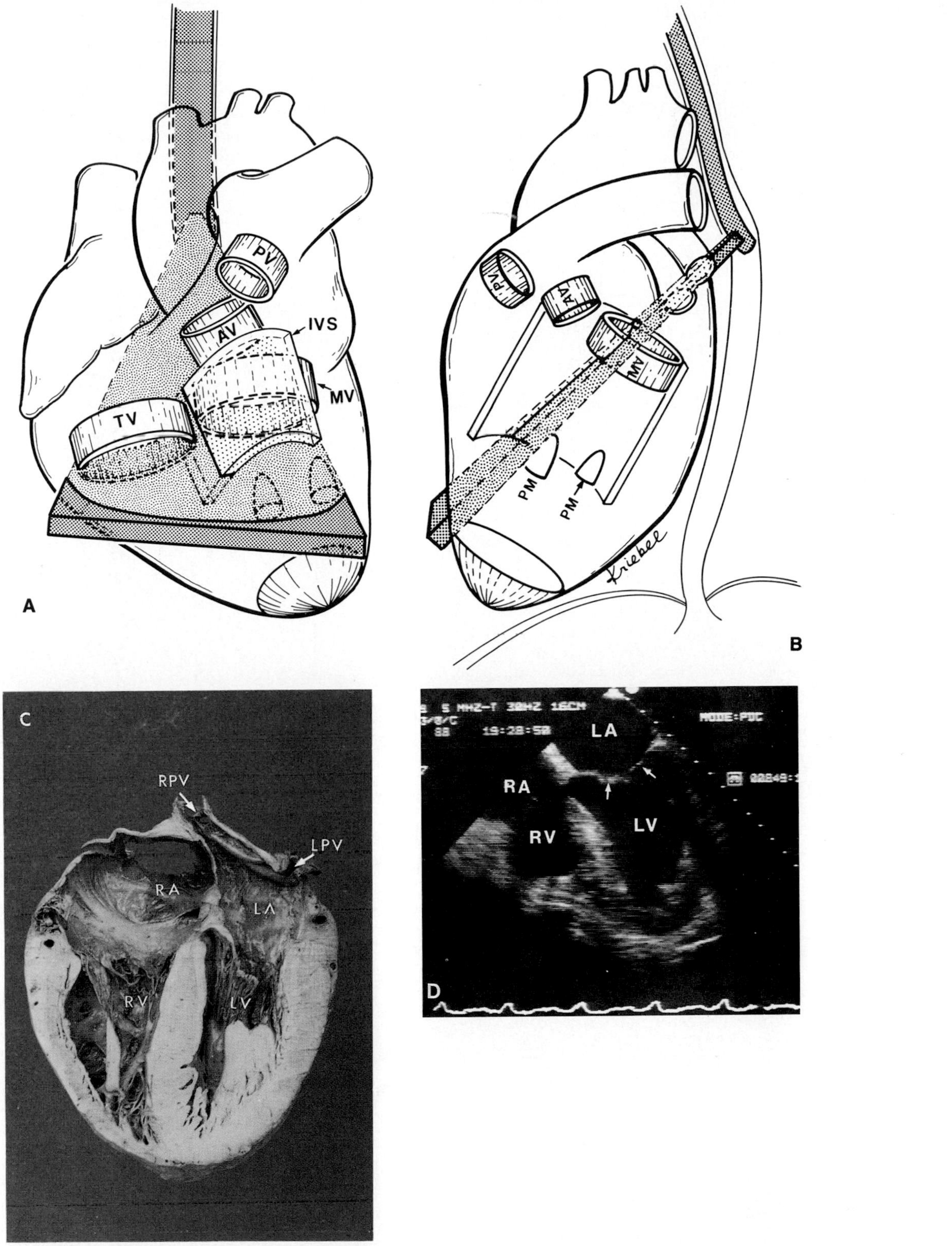

Fig. 16–9. **A.** The orientation of the imaging plane in the esophageal four-chamber view. This plane originates from the superior portion of the left atrium (LA) and transects the midportions of the mitral and tricuspid valves (MV and TV). It is ideally aligned to include the long axis of the right and left ventricles (RV and LV). Unfortunately, the esophagus usually prevents the degree of transducer angulation required to align the plane to include the ventricular long axis with the result that the plane often passes obliquely through the right and left ventricular cavities, exiting through the anterior wall near the apex. **B.** The orientation of the transducer and imaging plane, relative to the major cardiac structures when viewed in a lateral projection. **C.** Anatomic section corresponding to the echocardiographic plane. (Courtesy of Dr. Leng Jiang.) **D.** Apical four-chamber recording obtained with the transducer behind the LA and including the LA, a portion of the basal interatrial septum, the basal right atrium (RA), the anterior and posterior mitral leaflets (oblique arrows), the LV and RV, and the interventricular septum. AV = aortic valve; PV = pulmonic valve; RPV = right pulmonary vein; LPV = left pulmonary vein; IVS = interventricular septum; PM = papillary muscle.

probe is behind the posterior wall of the atrium) from the esophageal four-chamber view will elevate the right side of the scan plane, swinging it above the tricuspid valve and directing it through the left ventricular outflow tract, aortic valve, and proximal ascending aorta (Fig. 16–10). This view includes the mitral valve in an oblique long axis and often the chordae to the anterolateral papillary muscle. It also permits detailed assessment of the left ventricular outflow tract and aortic valve in an orientation approximating its long axis configuration. In patients with a more vertical heart, superior quality images of this region are generally obtained using the vertical transducer aligned parallel to the long axis of the outflow tract (see following discussion).

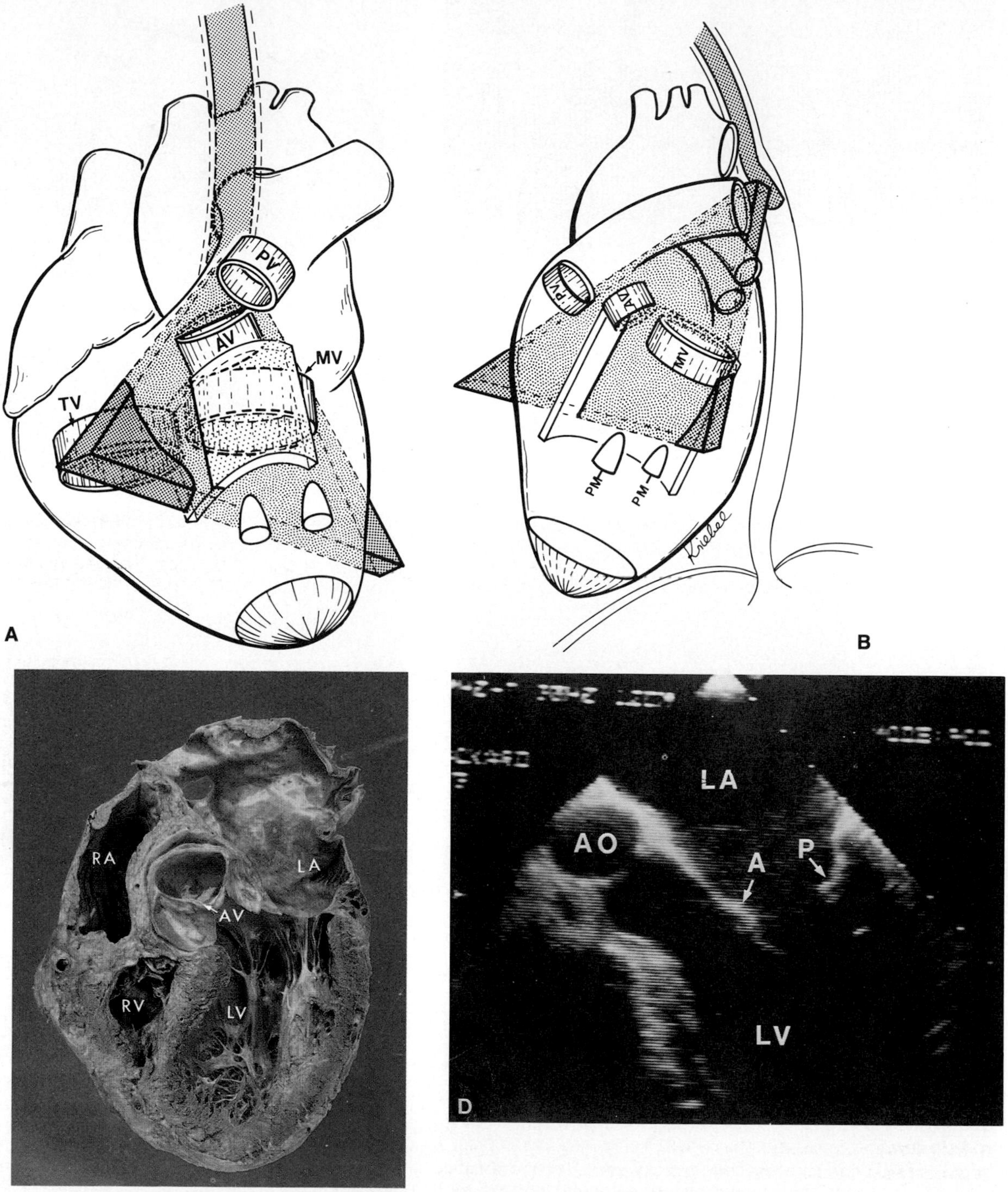

Fig. 16–10. **A.** The orientation of the imaging plane in the esophageal long axis view. This view includes the mitral valve (MV), the left ventricular outflow tract, the aortic valve (AV), and the proximal portion of the left ventricle (LV). **B.** The orientation of this imaging plane from a lateral perspective. The plane orientation is achieved by dorsiflection of the probe with leftward rotation, which elevates it from the four-chamber view to include the AV and outflow tract. The plane exits through the upper interventricular septum and lateral wall of the LV. **C.** Anatomic section corresponding to the echocardiographic plane. (Courtesy of Dr. Leng Jiang.) **D.** Esophageal long axis recording of the AV, left ventricular outflow tract, and MV. LA = left atrium; AO = aorta; A = anterior mitral leaflet; P = posterior mitral leaflet; TV = tricuspid valve; RA = right atrium; RV = right ventricle; PV = pulmonary valve; PM = papillary muscle.

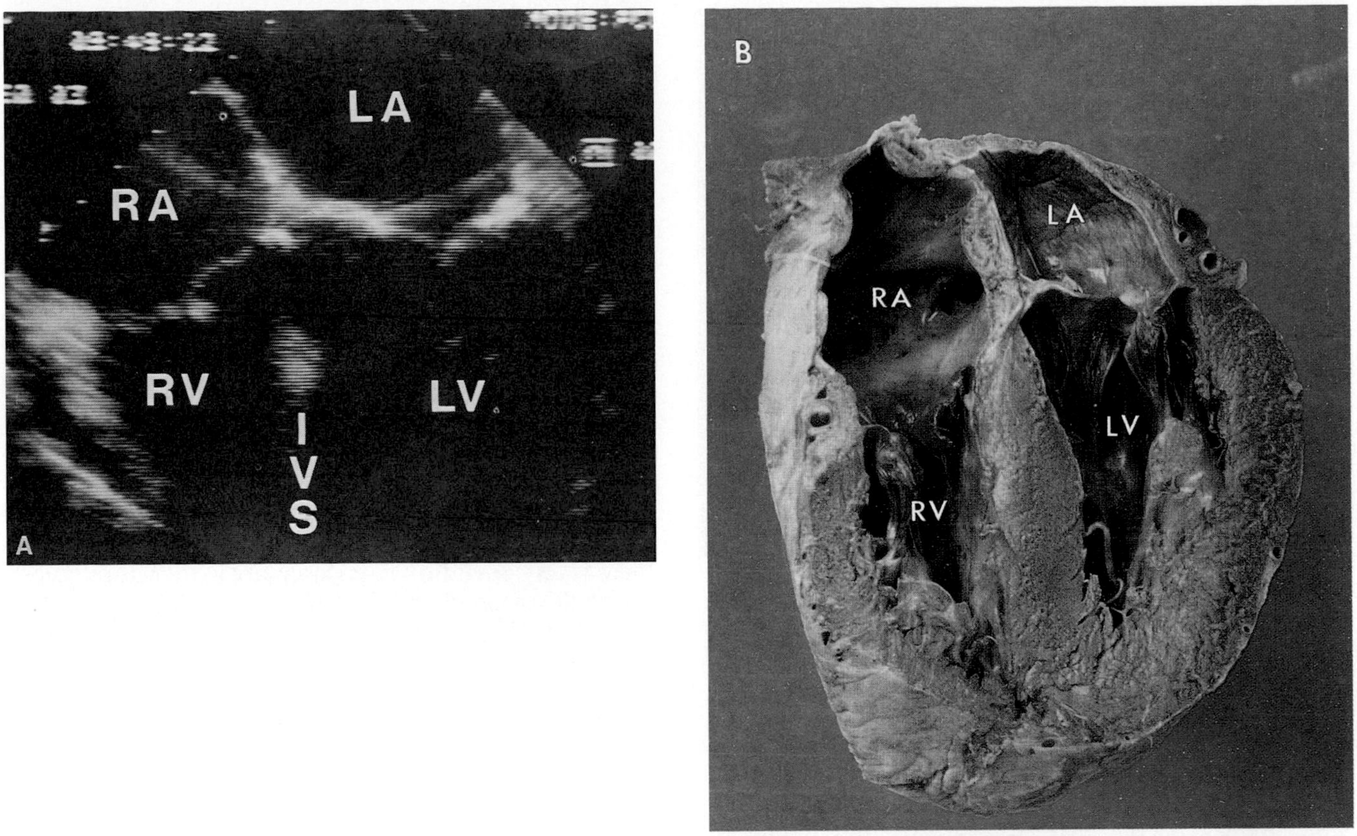

Fig. 16–11. **A.** Oblique recording of the mitral valve. This view is similar to the esophageal four-chamber view but is typically obtained with the transducer positioned further down the esophagus, behind the posterior wall of the left atrium (LA) with the plane transecting the mitral and tricuspid valves at a more oblique angle relative to the ventricular long axis than that of the true apical four-chamber view. **B.** Anatomic section corresponding to the echocardiographic plane. (Courtesy of Dr. Leng Jiang.) RA = right atrium; RV = right ventricle; IVS = interventricular septum; LV = left ventricle.

Mitral Valve View (Oblique). With continued advancement of the probe (1 to 2 cm), slight anterior angulation, and leftward rotation, the transducer faces leftward and laterally, and the scan plane traverses the inferior left atrium, mitral valve, and left ventricular cavity (Fig. 16–11). Because of the anterior orientation of the long axis of the left ventricle, this plane passes obliquely through the base of the left atrium (anterior in the sector), the mitral valve and the anterior wall of the left ventricle (posteriorly in the sector). This view provides the closest look at the mitral valve and is used primarily for detecting valvular disorders such as vegetations, torn chordae, fenestrations, and abnormalities of closure. Because of its oblique orientation, this view has no quantitative imaging value but is often useful for Doppler recordings of both forward mitral flow and regurgitant jets (Fig. 16–12). It is often the only view in which displacement of mitral structures into the left atrium can be clearly appreciated. It is the most commonly used esophageal view for evaluating the success of mitral valve reconstructive procedures. Occasionally, when the right atrium is dilated, the probe can be angled to the right from this position and placed directly behind the right atrium. One can then visualize the right atrium and tricuspid valve more directly without passing through the left atrium (Fig. 16–13).

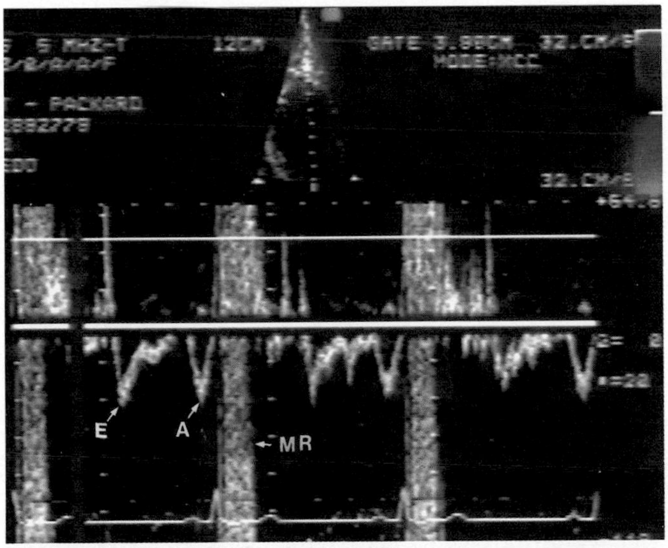

Fig. 16–12. Transesophageal Doppler recording of normal forward diastolic flow through the mitral valve with retrograde regurgitant systolic flow. Note that because the transducer is positioned in the esophagus behind the left atrium, flow through the mitral valve is normally away from the transducer reference and, therefore, is inverted on the recording. Regurgitant flow, likewise, is directed toward the transducer and, therefore, initially appears upright in contrast to the usual presentation from the cardiac apex. E = the E-point or peak of the rapid filling wave of the mitral valve; A = peak velocity following atrial contraction; MR = the mitral regurgitant jet.

Short Axis: Aortic Valve View. If the transducer is advanced further and tipped anteriorly, the aortic valve

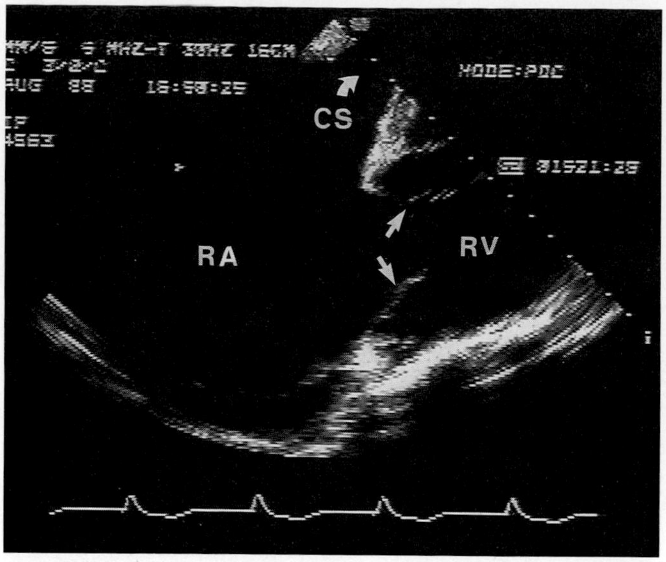

Fig. 16–13. Image recorded in a patient with marked dilation of the right atrium (RA) from the same transducer location as that used for an oblique mitral valve view. In this case, the dilated RA displaces the left atrium to the left, with the result that the esophagus lies behind the RA and the scan plane enters the heart through the right atrial posterior wall and passes directly through the tricuspid valve. Oblique arrows indicate the tricuspid leaflets. RV = right ventricle; CS = entrance of the coronary sinus into the RA.

echo appears on the viewing scope. At this point, the transducer is situated behind the posterior surface of the left atrium, and the scan plane traverses the heart from the posterior to the anterior surface. The result is an image in which the left atrium is closest to the transducer, with the aortic valve and root appearing beneath the left atrium and the right ventricular outflow tract below the aorta (Fig. 16–14). The three aortic leaflets are recorded in short axis along with their associated sinuses of Valsalva. Left atrial diameters recorded in this plane have correlated well with those obtained by standard transthoracic echocardiography[4] and cyclic changes in atrial diameter with angiographic volume changes.[30] Aortic root diameters have correlated less well in early studies,[4] however, this appears to be a question of technique rather than an inherent limitation of the method.

Leftward rotation and slight superior angulation in this plane permits visualization of the left atrial appendage and the left superior pulmonary vein. Muscular ridges (pectinate muscles) are easily visualized within the appendage and should not be confused with small thrombi. The orifice of the appendage is anterior to that of the left superior pulmonary vein, and the two are separated by a distinct infolding of the wall. Rightward rotation of the probe permits the superior vena cava to be recorded in short axis appearing as an ovoid or rounded triangular structure adjacent to the ascending aorta. Superiorly, the right upper pulmonary vein courses posteriorly and is orthogonal to the superior vena cava.

Mitral Valve View (Short Axis). As the probe is advanced further, it curves anteriorly with the esophagus, and the ultrasonic plane, likewise, tips anteriorly, more closely approximating a true short axis view of the left ventricle at the mitral valve level. The relative orientation of the probe and left ventricle varies depending on the position of the heart relative to the esophagus. Normally, the long axis of the heart, which is oblique in the chest, passes above the vertical esophagus at this level, and the scan plane must be directed leftward to transect the left ventricular-short axis. This alignment permits the anterior and posterior mitral leaflets, valve orifice, proximal chordae, and surrounding left ventricular myocardium to be readily appreciated (Fig. 16–15). This view can often be aligned parallel to the true short axis of the ventricle and thus can be considered a standard view for purposes of quantitation. Such an assumption, unfortunately, can be made only when the short axis image appears round because the limited mobility of the transducer in the esophagus prevents the requisite rotation and angulation required to ensure that the smallest major and minor dimensions are being recorded. When there is any deviation from circularity, therefore, it cannot be determined whether this is due to improper plane positioning or structural deformity (see Chapter 4). With minimal repositioning of the probe, the coronary sinus can be recorded from the lateral margin of the AV groove to its insertion into the right atrium.

Short Axis: Papillary Muscle View. Slight further advancement of the scope will bring the scan plane parallel to the short axis of the left ventricle at the level of the papillary muscles. At this level, the left ventricle is generally well to the left of the esophagus, and the plane must be directed leftward to transect the left ventricular cavity. In many patients, the left ventricle is positioned such that it is necessary to advance the probe into the stomach and approach the chamber from below. This is the primary view for assessing wall motion and left ventricular function and hence is used for monitoring left ventricular function intraoperatively (Fig. 16–16). Like the mitral valve view, it can also be aligned parallel to the short axis plane of the left ventricle and hence potentially contains quantitative area and dimensional data. Unfortunately, it is also subject to the same limitations outlined previously for quantitation at the mitral valve level.

Apical Short Axis View. Further advancement of the gastroscope will result in a cross-sectional view of the left ventricular apex (Fig. 16–17). This view is useful for recording isolated apical hypertrophy or apical segmental dysfunction. In dilated hearts where the apex is displaced to the left and laterally, a true transesophageal apical recording cannot be obtained, and the view is usually recorded from the fundus of the stomach. Thus, this view, along with the papillary muscle short axis view of the left ventricle, is more appropriately termed a *transgastric view* rather than a transesophageal view.

Biatrial View. If the gastroscope is withdrawn to the left atrial level and rotated clockwise until the transducer faces rightward and anteriorly, both atria can be viewed simultaneously (Fig. 16–18). In this orientation, the left atrial cavity is recorded in the left upper portion of the scan plane, and the right atrial cavity in the mid- to lower portion. The atrial chambers are separated by an oblique echo, which represents the interatrial sep-

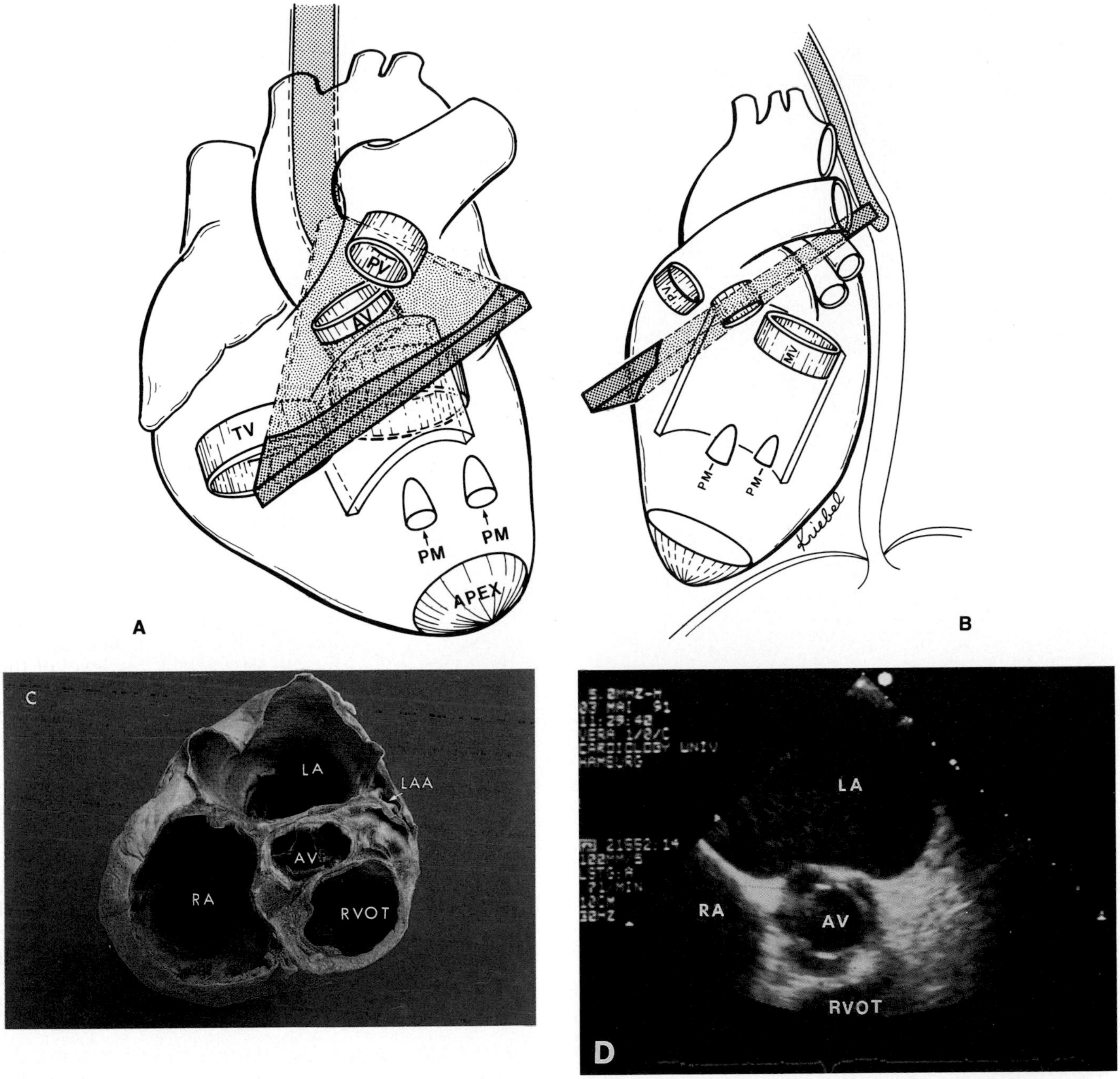

Fig. 16–14. **A.** The orientation of the scan plane in the esophageal short axis, aortic valve (AV) view. This plane transects the left atrium (LA) and AV in short axis and right ventricular outflow tract (RVOT) proximal to the pulmonary valve (PV). **B.** The orientation of the esophageal short axis AV view in a lateral projection. The plane is recorded by advancing the probe until it intersects the short axis plane, which includes the AV, and then angling and rotating the transducer until the three aortic leaflets are recorded in short axis. **C.** Anatomic section. (Illustration courtesy of Dr. Leng Jiang.) **D.** Short axis aortic valve recording. In this image orientation, the LA is superiorly positioned in the sector, the AV is in the midportion of the sector, and the RVOT is deep to the AV. In this image orientation, the left coronary cusp of the AV is to the viewer's right, in the sector closest to the pulmonary artery. The right coronary cusp is posterior in the sector, immediately above the RVOT, and the noncoronary cusp is anterior and to the viewer's left. LAA = left atrial appendage; RA = right atrium; TV = tricuspid valve; PM = papillary muscles; MV = mitral valve.

tum. By advancing and withdrawing the probe, the entire interatrial septum, including the fossa ovalis, can be viewed. This view is particularly important for investigating left and right atrial masses and abnormal intraatrial structures. Because it places the interatrial septum relatively perpendicular to the path of the scan plane, it is ideal for visualizing atrial septal defects (see following discussion) and defining their type, size, and the direction of shunt flow. Patency of the foramen ovale usually can be demonstrated using color Doppler; however, echo-contrast is generally more sensitive.

With small degrees of rotation and angulation, the superior vena cava, inferior vena cava, and eustachian valve also can be imaged. Medial and lateral rotation also permit imaging of both the left and right atrial appendages and their contents (Fig. 16–19).

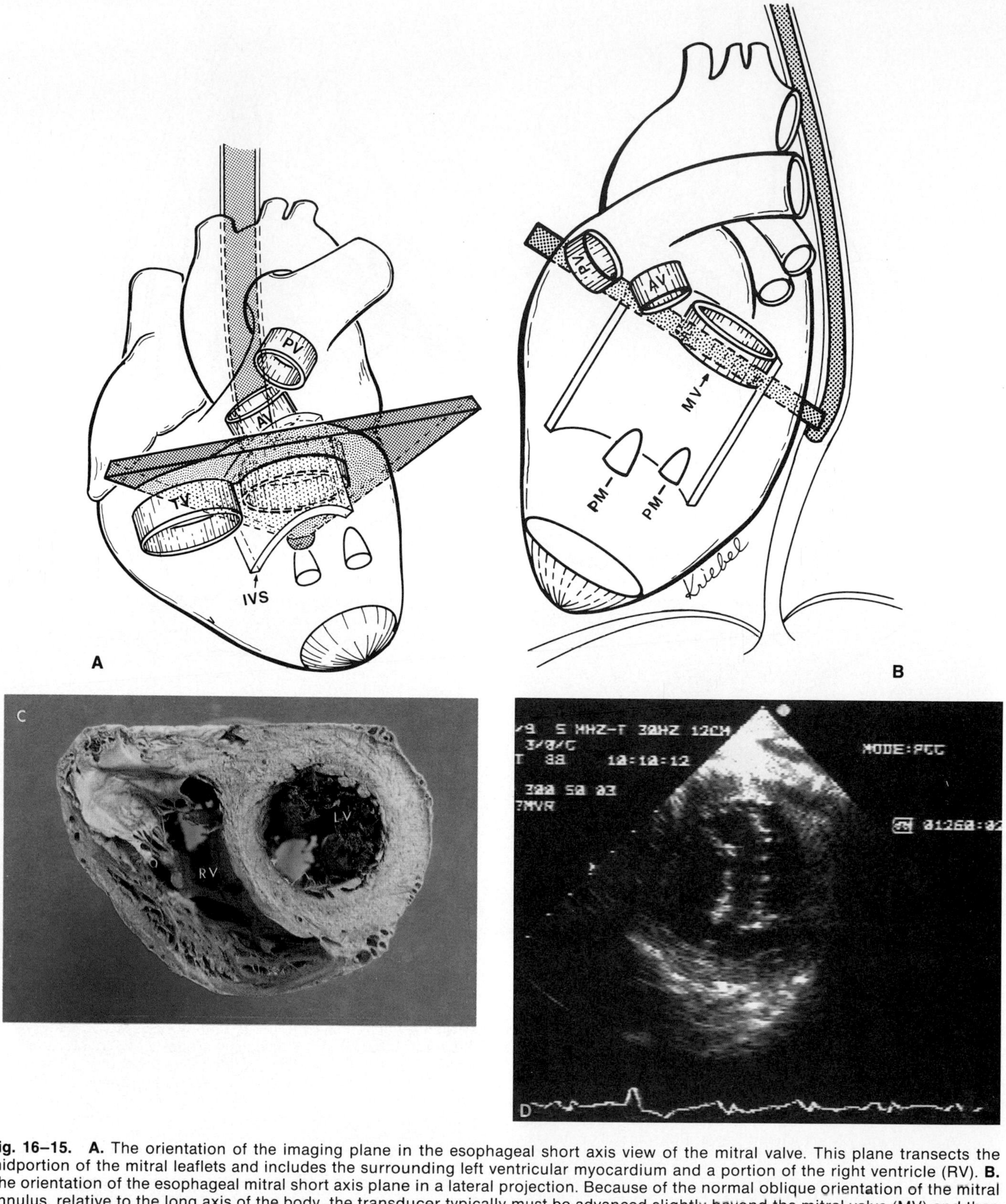

Fig. 16–15. **A.** The orientation of the imaging plane in the esophageal short axis view of the mitral valve. This plane transects the midportion of the mitral leaflets and includes the surrounding left ventricular myocardium and a portion of the right ventricle (RV). **B.** The orientation of the esophageal mitral short axis plane in a lateral projection. Because of the normal oblique orientation of the mitral annulus, relative to the long axis of the body, the transducer typically must be advanced slightly beyond the mitral valve (MV) and then angled anteriorly to bring the plane back through the short axis of the mitral orifice. Depending on the position of the left ventricle (LV), relative to the esophagus, a varying degree of leftward rotation may also be necessary for the plane to pass through the true MV orifice. **C.** Anatomic section corresponding to the echocardiographic plane. (Illustration courtesy of Dr. Leng Jiang.) **D.** Esophageal short axis recording of the MV. The leaflets are partially opened within the circular left ventricular cavity and appear vertically oriented within the scan plane. In this example, the LV was positioned to the left of the esophagus and the transducer was rotated leftward to record the mitral leaflets. The medial commissure of the MV, therefore, appears anterior in the scan plane, and the lateral commissure appears posterior. PV = pulmonary valve; AV = aortic valve; TV = tricuspid valve; IVS = interventricular septum; PM = papillary muscle.

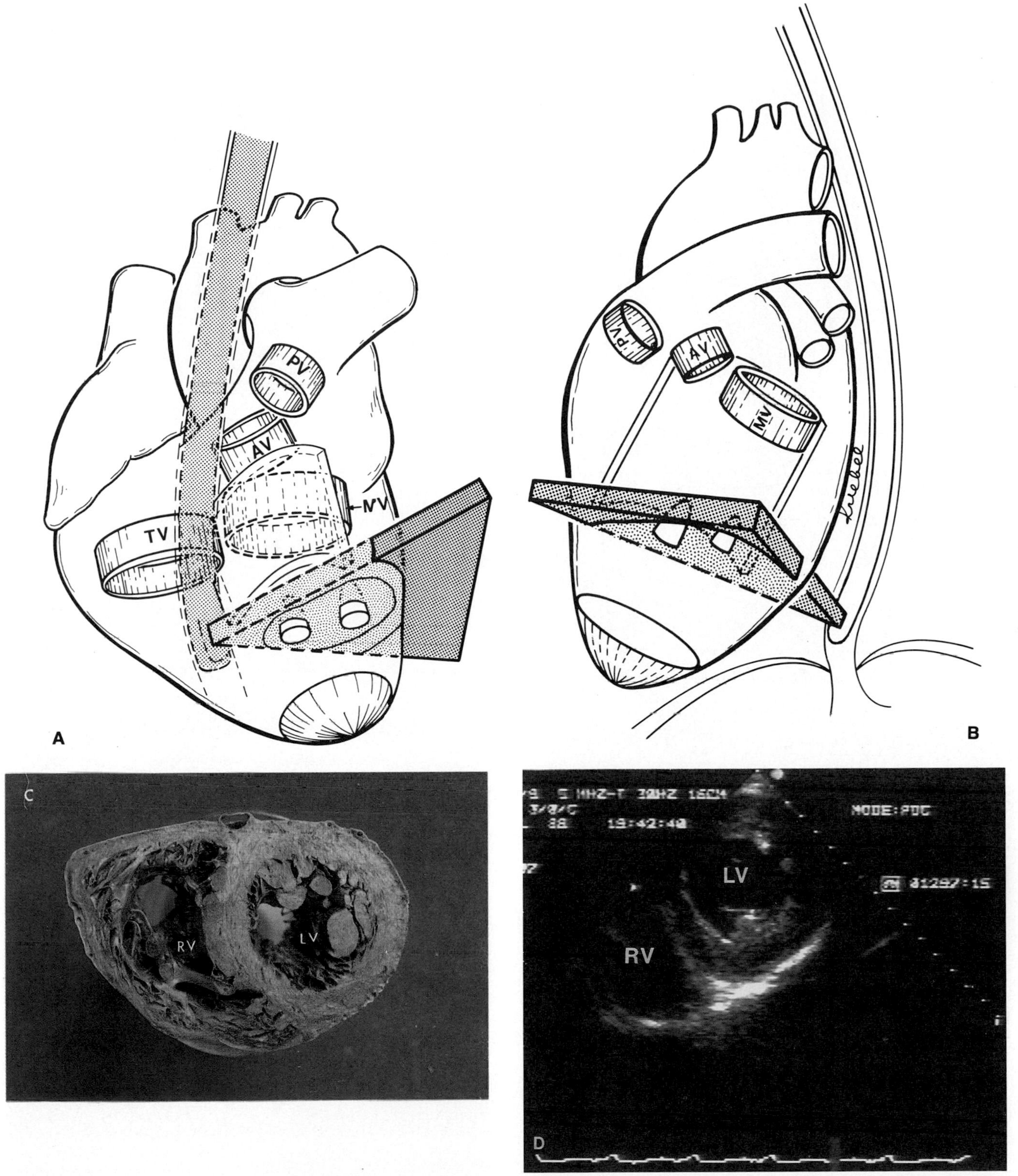

Fig. 16–16. A. The orientation of the imaging plane in the esophageal short axis view of the left ventricle (LV) at the papillary muscle level. This plane transects the LV parallel to its short axis plane. It includes the anterolateral and posteromedial papillary muscles. Because the esophagus generally has shifted to the right, relative to the LV, by this level, the plane must typically be recorded by directing the central axis of the imaging plane anteriorly and leftward, which positions the papillary muscles vertically, as opposed to horizontally in the image. **B.** The position of the transducer lateral to the LV and papillary muscles in the esophageal short axis plane of the LV at the papillary muscle level. The plane enters the LV from the right side and passes leftward and anteriorly before exiting through the free lateral wall of the LV. **C.** Anatomic secretion corresponding to the echocardiographic plane. (Illustration courtesy of Dr. Leng Jiang.) **D.** Esophageal short axis recording of the LV at the papillary muscle level. The posteromedial papillary muscle appears anteriorly in the imaging plane, and the anterolateral papillary muscle appears posteriorly. The papillary muscles are surrounded by the circular left ventricular myocardium. The right ventricle (RV) is positioned to the left in this image orientation. PV = pulmonary valve; AV = aortic valve; MV = mitral valve; TV = tricuspid valve.

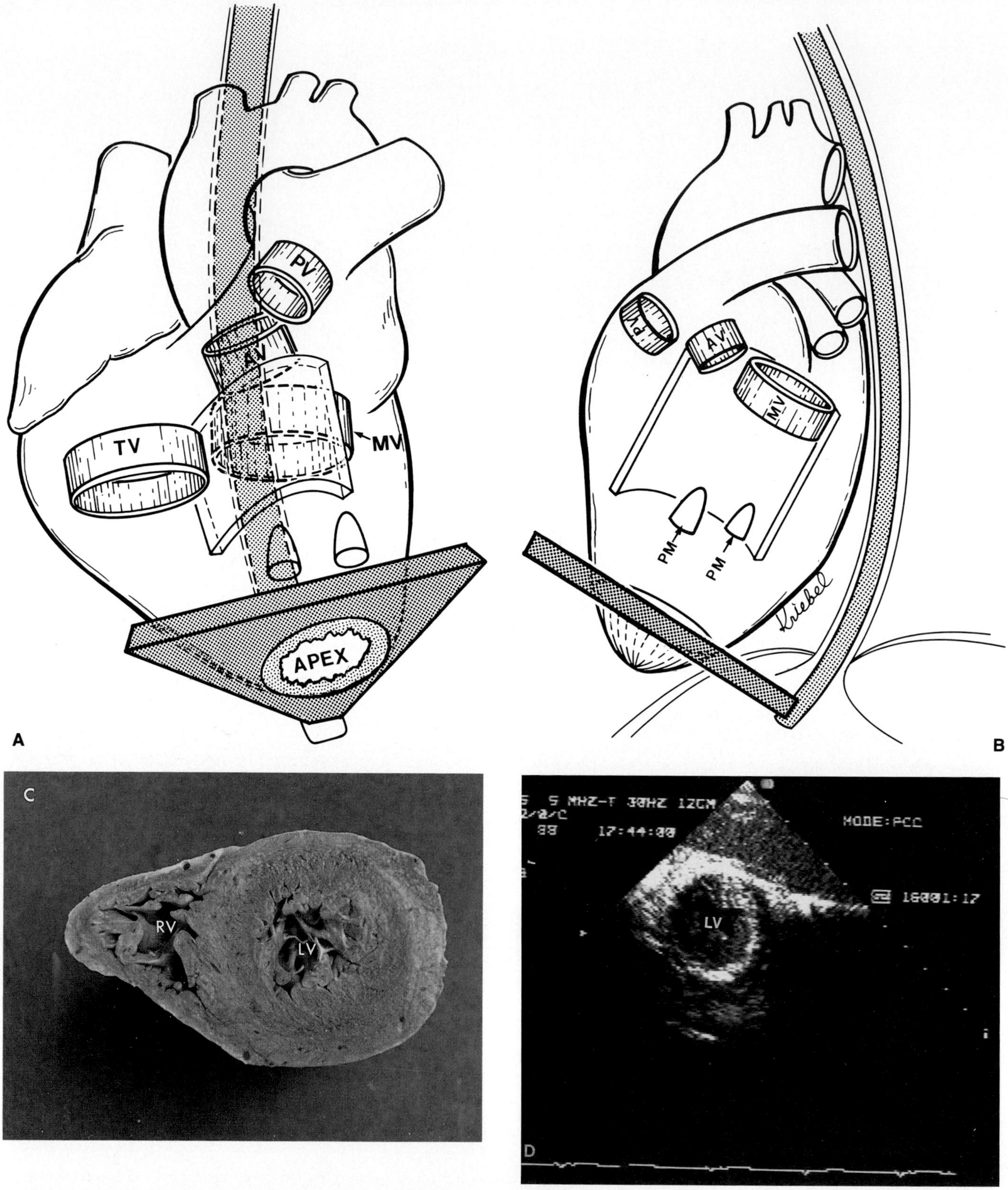

Fig. 16–17. **A.** The orientation of the imaging plane to the primary cardiac structure in the esophageal short axis view of the cardiac apex. Although nominally an esophageal plane, the transducer is typically positioned in the stomach to record this view and, hence, it might more appropriately be termed a *transgastric* view. **B.** The orientation of the scan plane relative to the cardiac apex in a lateral projection. As with the other short axis views, the orientation of the long axis of the heart relative to that of the transducer typically necessitates that the transducer be advanced beyond the structure or area of interest and angled anteriorly to align the imaging plane parallel to the short axis of the ventricular chamber. **C.** Anatomic section corresponding to the echocardiographic plane. (Courtesy of Dr. Leng Jiang.) **D.** Esophageal short axis recording of the cardiac apex. This image displays the apex in its normal circular configuration and permits both thickness and contractile function to be assessed. LV = left ventricle; PV = pulmonic valve; AV = aortic valve; TV = tricuspid valve; MV = mitral valve; PM = papillary muscles; RV = right ventricle.

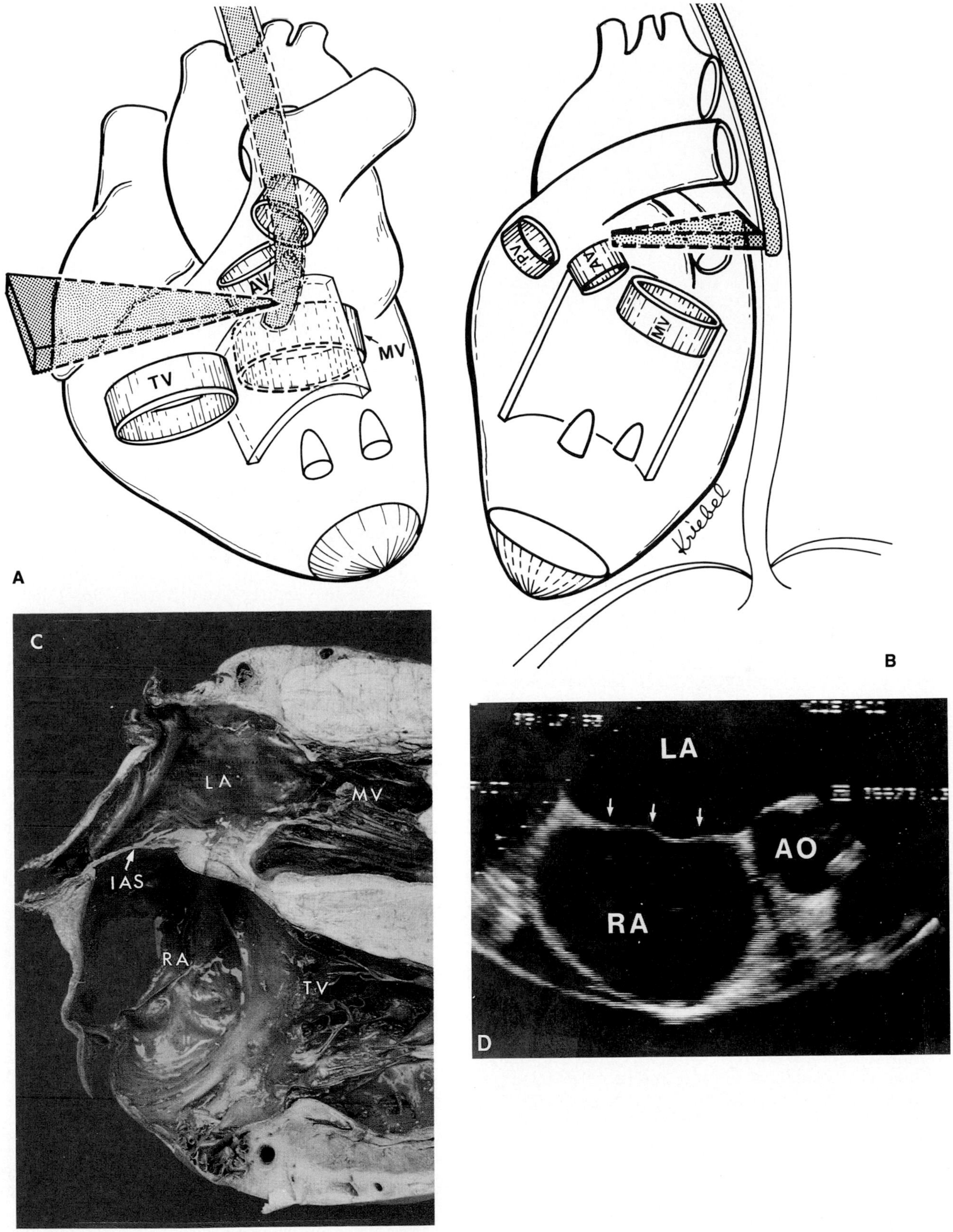

Fig. 16–18. **A.** The orientation of the imaging plane in the esophageal biatrial view. The plane transects the interatrial septum (IAS) obliquely along the line that extends from the aortic valve (AV) to the superior wall of the atrium. This plane displays the entire extent of the IAS in an oblique orientation. **B.** The position of the esophageal probe and orientation of the scan plane used to record the biatrial view. The plane is directed rightward and anteriorly. The atrial septum is transected in an orientation oblique to the long axis of the heart. **C.** Anatomic section corresponding to the echocardiographic plane. (Courtesy of Dr. Leng Jiang.) **D.** Because the esophageal biatrial view is recorded from behind the left atrium (LA), the LA is anterior in the scan plane; the IAS is displayed horizontally (arrows), and the right atrium (RA) appears in the posterior portion of the scan plane. The aorta (AO) is recorded obliquely and is displayed at the right margin of the image. MV = mitral valve; PV = pulmonic valve; TV = tricuspid valve.

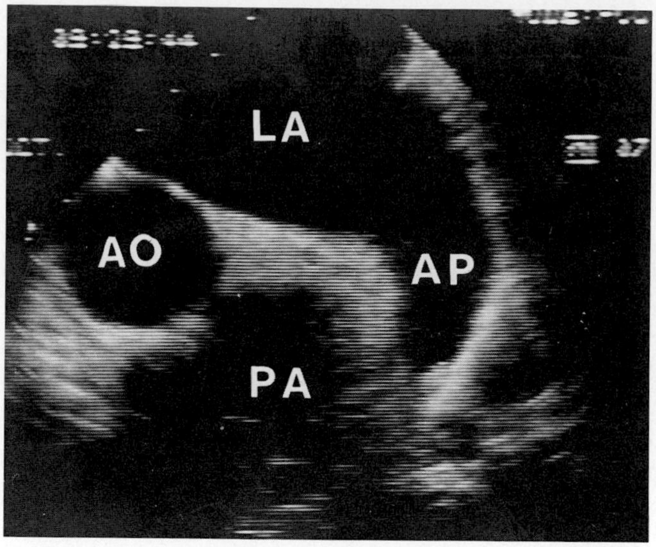

Fig. 16–19. Esophageal short axis image of the left atrial appendage. The atrial appendage can be imaged by slight leftward rotation of the probe from the normal biatrial view. LA = left atrium; AO = aorta; PA = pulmonary artery; AP = left atrial appendage.

Pulmonary Artery View. The last routine horizontal transesophageal view is obtained by rotating the gastroscope counterclockwise to again face anteriorly and withdrawing it another 1 to 2 cm. From this position, the great cardiac vessels are imaged, with the ascending aorta in a short axis orientation and the main and right pulmonary arteries in an oblique section (Fig. 16–20). This view is ideal for Doppler flow studies of the pulmonary artery, because it places the central ray of the scan plane parallel to the direction of pulmonary flow.

Although the transverse views described previously represent the "routine" views obtainable from the esophagus, a variety of other structures and regions of the heart can also be recorded. For example, the proximal coronary arteries can be recorded just above the short axis aortic valve by rotating the gastroscope slightly to the left or right. The origin of the left coronary artery from the left aortic sinus, the course of the left main branch, and its bifurcation into the anterior descending and circumflex branches can all be appreciated in most cases. Figure 16–21 is an example of the bifurcation of the left main coronary artery and the proximal segments of the left anterior and circumflex branches. Because of the high resolution and close proximity of the probe, it is often possible to record coronary flow. This is discussed in more detail in Chapter 34.

Vertical or Longitudinal Views

In addition to the horizontal views described previously, four additional tomographic planes are commonly acquired using the proximal, vertical transducer of the biplane pair. Initial longitudinal plane alignment is generally achieved by rotating the probe clockwise or counterclockwise from a midsagittal position. A different portion of the heart can then be recorded in the same plane by advancing or retracting the transducer. Once the central axis of the scan plane passes through the structure of interest, the transducer tip is angled to the left or right to align the plane parallel to the long or short axes of the structure of interest. Although commonly described based on the position of the transducer in the chest, these views are more appropriately defined by the structures recorded in each tomographic plane (i.e., more comparable to transthoracic imaging). Longitudinal views are described in sequence from the furthest degree of rightward rotation to the furthest degree of leftward rotation (Fig. 16–22).

Esophageal Long Axis of the Superior Vena Cava, Right Atrium, and Inferior Vena Cava. Rotating the probe approximately 20° to the right of the midsagittal plane of the body causes the right atrium and superior vena cava to appear in long axis. The continuity of the right atrium and interatrial septum with the superior venae cavae is clearly visualized (Fig. 16–23).[31] A longer segment of the atrial septum is recorded with longitudinal than with transverse imaging; especially when aortic root dilation is present.[32] The atrial septum can be thoroughly assessed for atrial septal defects, particularly sinus venosus defects, as well as for patency of the foramen ovale.[32] The right atrial appendage, cut obliquely near its base, is often seen anteriorly.[33] This view is useful for detecting masses in the venae cavae, right atrium and appendage, and other atrial septal pathology.[14] Minimal additional counterclockwise rotation of the transducer brings the anterior portion of the tricuspid valve into view.

The junction of the inferior vena cava with the right atrium lies slightly to the right of its junction with the superior vena cava. The right atrial, inferior vena caval, connection can be displayed by advancing the probe and rotating it slightly to the right. Apparent thickening of the atrial septum at its superior margin is caused by fat in Waterston's groove between the free walls of the atria.

Long Axis of the Aorta. Continued anterior rotation of the probe to a point roughly parallel to the midsagittal plane of the body positions the central ray of the scan plane through the aortic valve (Fig. 16–24). Leftward angulation of the probe is necessary to align the scan

Fig. 16–20. A. The orientation of the imaging plane in the esophageal short axis view of the pulmonary artery. With the probe in the esophagus, the plane enters the pulmonary arterial system through the right pulmonary artery and then continues upward through the main pulmonary artery and includes the pulmonary valve (PV) and a small portion of the right ventricular outflow tract. The aorta is also typically visualized obliquely. **B.** The position of the probe within the esophagus, and orientation of the scan plane when viewed from a lateral perspective. **C.** Anatomic section corresponding to the echocardiographic plane. (Courtesy of Dr. Leng Jiang.) **D.** Image of the right pulmonary artery (R), left pulmonary artery (L), and main pulmonary artery (PA). The pulmonary artery courses from the right ventricular outflow tract at the bottom of the image along the right border as the main pulmonary artery bifurcating into the right and left pulmonary arteries (top). The aorta (AO) is transected obliquely and displayed in the left midportion of the image. AAO = ascending aorta; RPA = right pulmonary artery; LPA = left pulmonary artery; SVC = superior vena cava; RB = right bronchus; LB = left bronchus; DAO = descending aorta; MV = mitral valve; PM = papillary muscle; AV = aortic valve.

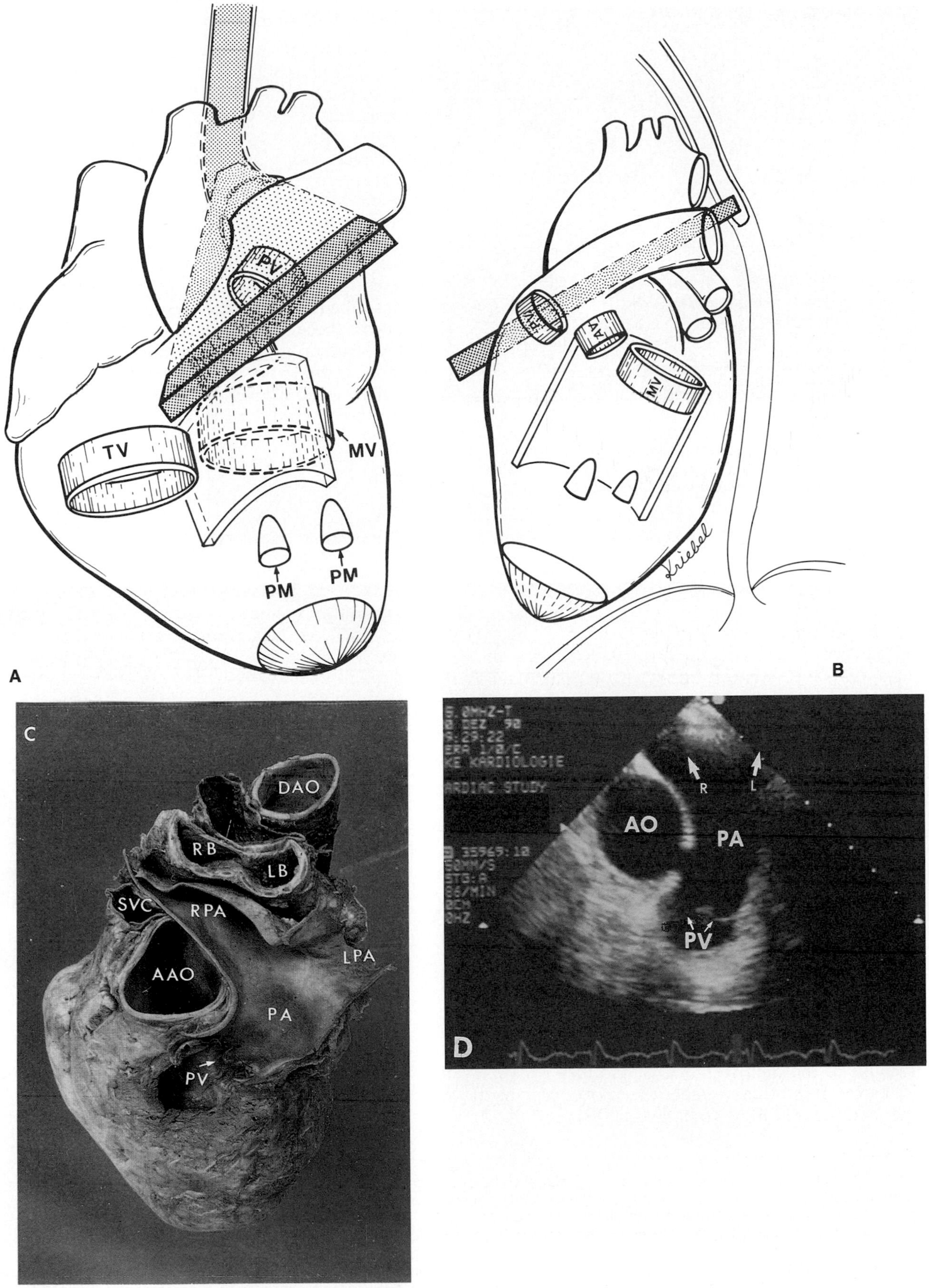
A
PV
TV
MV
PM
PM
B
AV
MV
Kriebel
C
DAO
RB
LB
SVC
RPA
AAO
PA
LPA
PV
AO
PA
R
L
PV
CARDIAC STUDY
D

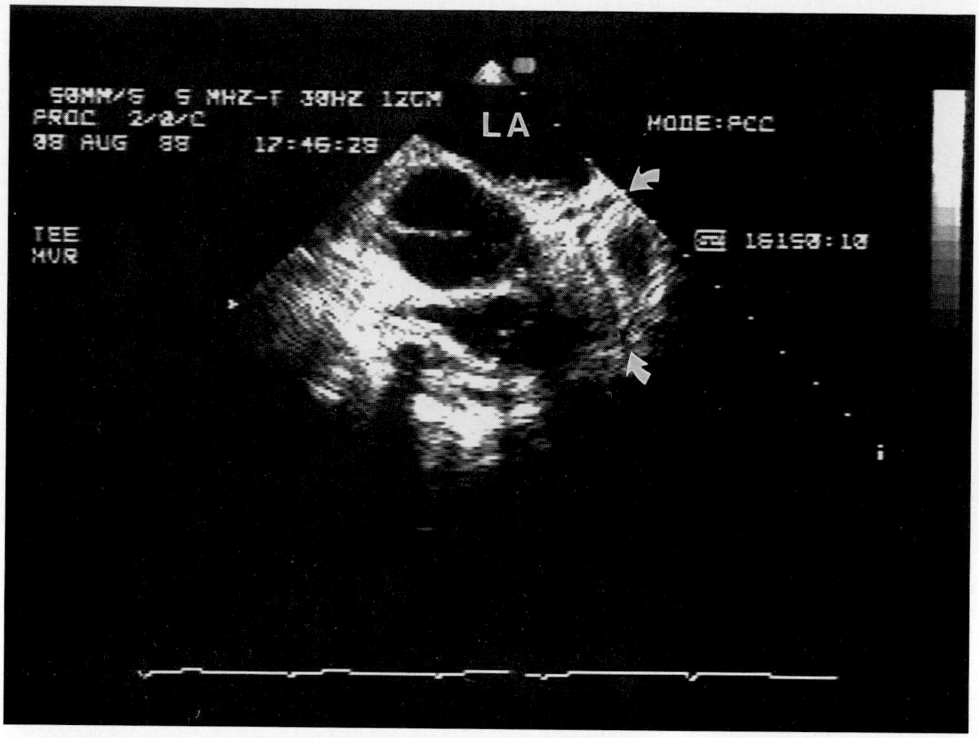

Fig. 16–21. Esophageal short axis recording of the coronary bifurcation and the proximal left anterior descending (LAD) (upward-pointing arrow) and circumflex vessels (downward-pointing arrows). The circumflex courses anteriorly toward the transducer, while the LAD courses posteriorly in the sector or away from the esophageal transducer. The aortic valve is recorded in a slightly oblique orientation to the viewer's left, with the left atrium (LA) at the apex of the sector.

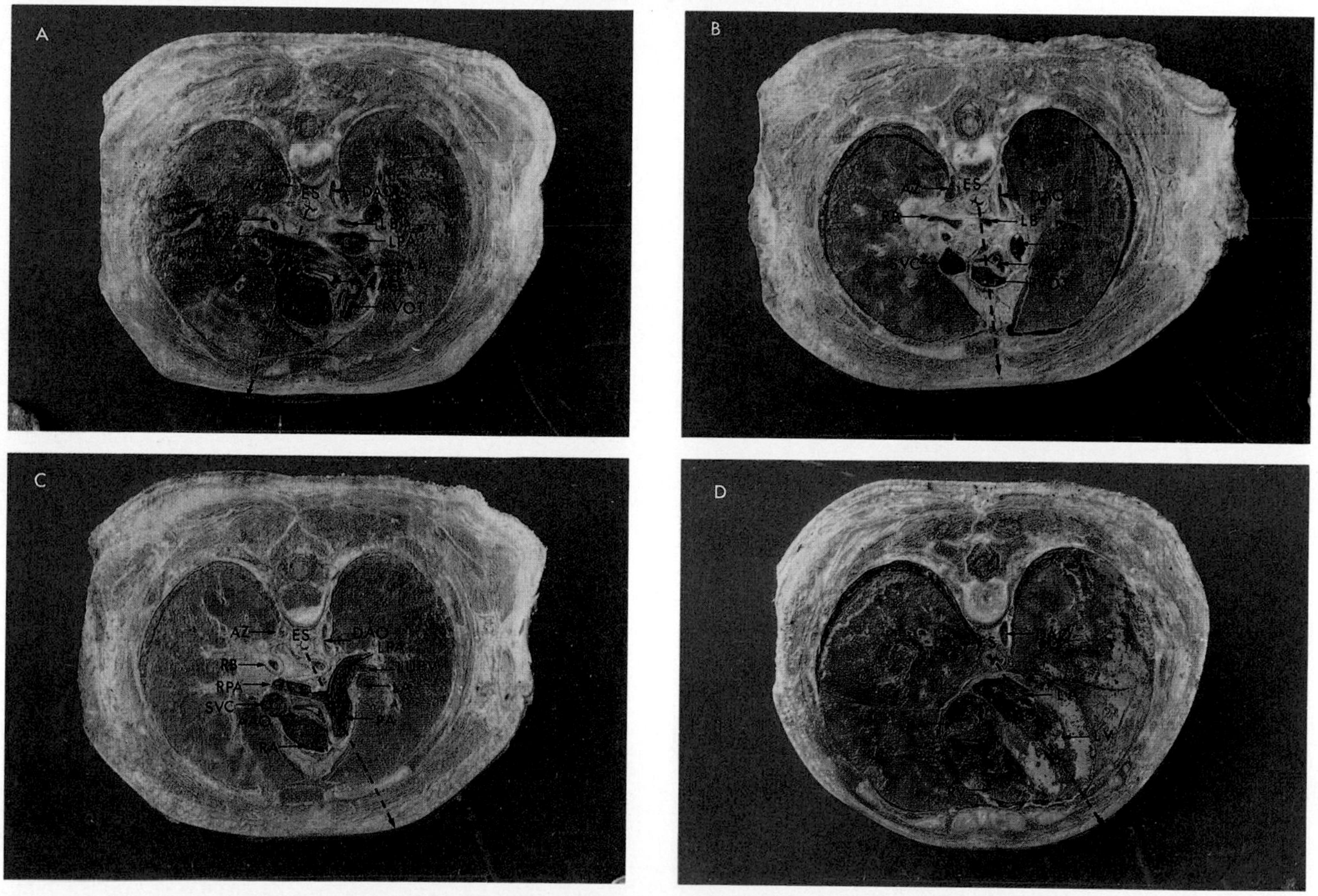

Fig. 16–22. Transverse sections of the body illustrating the relationship of the longitudinal planes to the primary cardiac structures. **A.** Line of section of the longitudinal view through the superior vena cava (SVC) and right atrium (RA). **B.** Aorta. **C.** Pulmonary artery. **D.** Left ventricle, mitral valve, and left atrium. ES = esophagus; AAO = ascending aorta; DAO = descending aorta; RV = right ventricle; RVOT = right ventricular outflow tract; LA = left atrium; LAA = left atrial appendage; LV = left ventricle; PA = pulmonary artery; LPA = left pulmonary artery; RPA = right pulmonary artery; RUPV = right upper pulmonary vein; LUPV = left upper pulmonary vein; AZ = azygos vein; RB = right bronchus; LB = left bronchus.

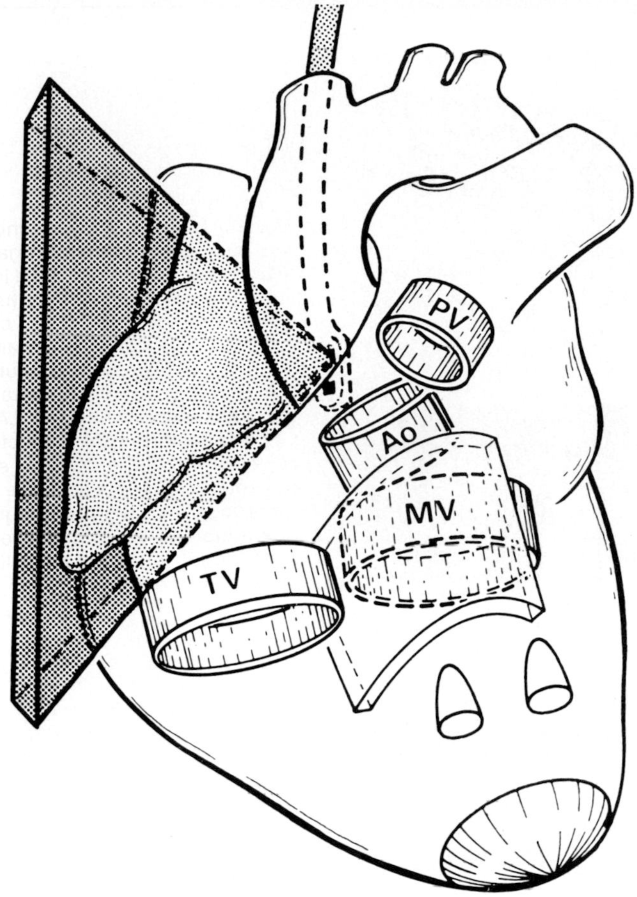

A

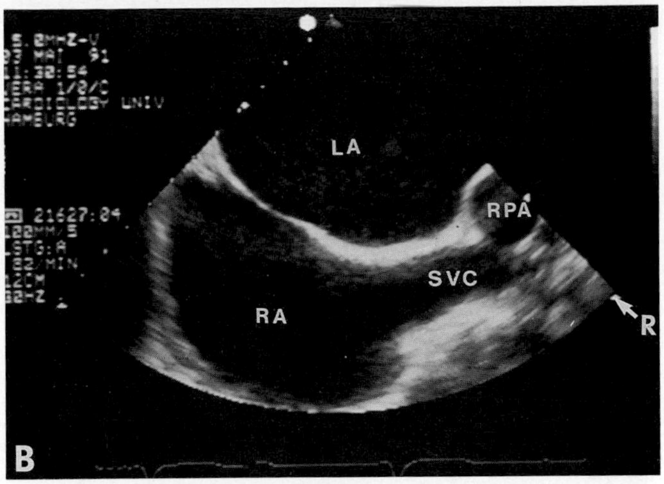

Fig. 16–23. A. The relationship of the longitudinal section of the right atrium (RA) and superior vena cava (SVC) to the primary cardiac structures. The scan plane originates from behind the left atrium (LA) and courses anteriorly and rightward, passing through the posterior interatrial septum, superior right atrium, and long axis of the SVC. The plane is positioned to specifically record the long axis of the SVC. **B.** Transesophageal recording of this view. TV = tricuspid valve; AV = aortic valve; MV = mitral valve; PV = pulmonary valve; RPA = right pulmonary artery.

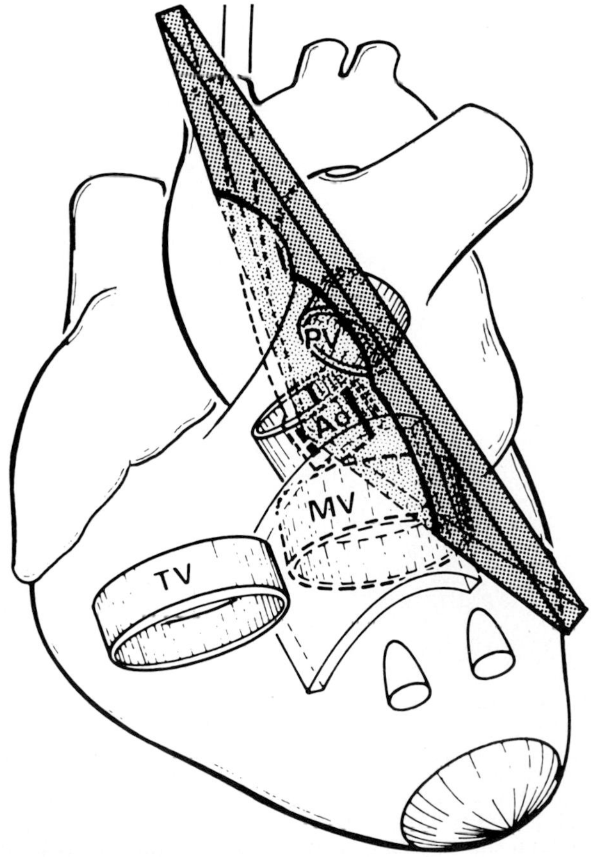

A

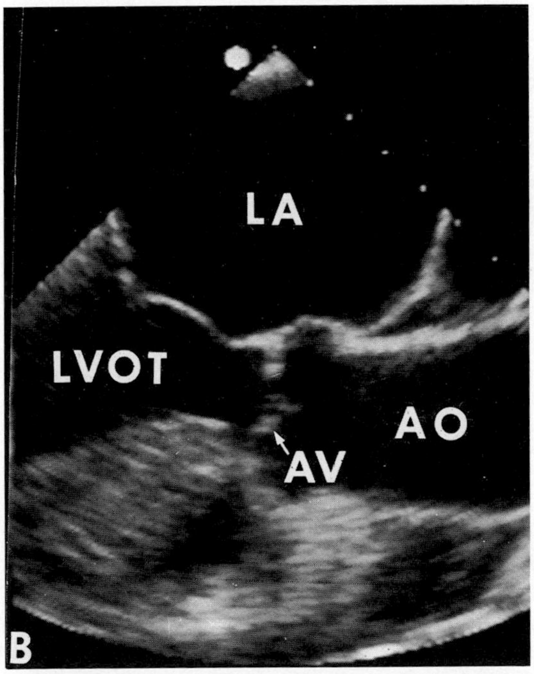

Fig. 16–24. A. The relationship of the esophageal longitudinal view of the aortic valve (AV) and long axis of the aorta to the other primary cardiac structures. The plane is positioned to pass through the aortic valve parallel to the aortic long axis. No other primary cardiac structures are necessarily included. **B.** Transesophageal recording of this view. TV = tricuspld valve; PV = pulmonary valve; MV = mitral valve. LVOT = left ventricular outflow tract; LA = left atrium; AO = aorta.

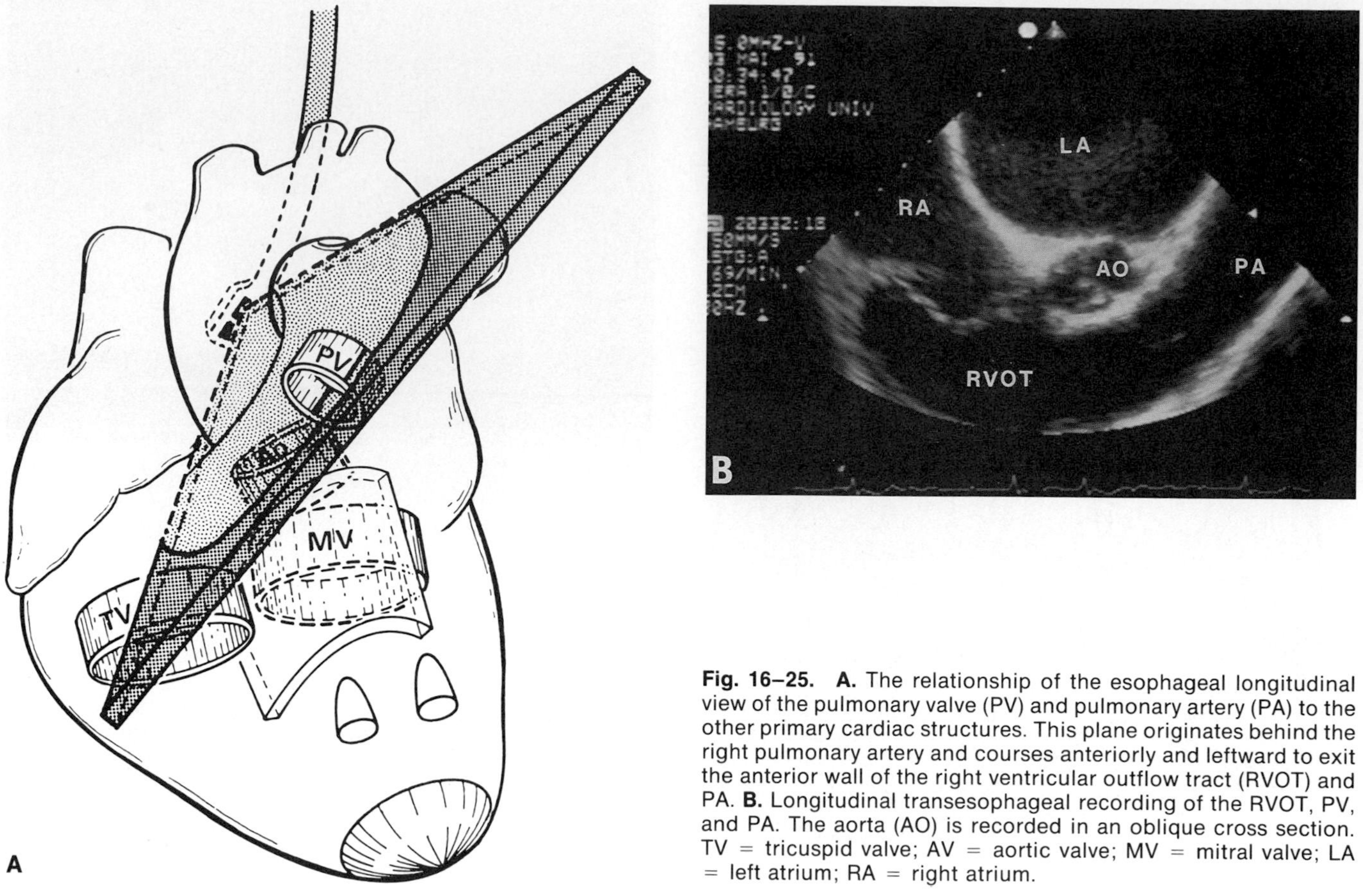

A

Fig. 16–25. **A.** The relationship of the esophageal longitudinal view of the pulmonary valve (PV) and pulmonary artery (PA) to the other primary cardiac structures. This plane originates behind the right pulmonary artery and courses anteriorly and leftward to exit the anterior wall of the right ventricular outflow tract (RVOT) and PA. **B.** Longitudinal transesophageal recording of the RVOT, PV, and PA. The aorta (AO) is recorded in an oblique cross section. TV = tricuspid valve; AV = aortic valve; MV = mitral valve; LA = left atrium; RA = right atrium.

plane parallel to the long axis of the aortic valve and ascending aorta.

Rightward flexion of the probe while maintaining the central ray of the scan plane through the aortic valve often allows the valve to be viewed in short axis. The best short axis view of the aorta (i.e., horizontal or vertical transducer) will depend on the relationship of the aortic root to the esophagus. In patients with aortic root dilation, it may be possible to record a true long axis only by using longitudinal imaging. This view is complementary and often preferred to the horizontal long axis view of the left ventricular outflow tract. It is useful in the assessment of valvular aortic stenosis; aortic valve calcification and vegetations; subvalvular and supravalvular aortic stenosis; and aortic dilation, aneurysm, and dissection.[34]

Long Axis: Right Ventricular Outflow Tract and Main Pulmonary Artery. Continued counterclockwise rotation of the probe with rightward flexion aligns the scan plane parallel to the long axis of the pulmonary artery, valve, and proximal outflow tract[32] (Fig. 16–25). This plane permits recognition of stenoses at various levels of the outflow tract and is particularly useful in patients with congenital heart disease. Visualization of the distal portion of both right and left pulmonary arteries is enhanced with longitudinal imaging. The right pulmonary artery in the longitudinal plane is visualized in the short axis as it courses superior to the left atrium and posterior to the ascending aorta and superior vena cava. The left pulmonary artery, which is poorly visualized in the horizontal plane, is better recorded using the longitudinal plane.[14]

Long Axis: Left Ventricle. Continued leftward and posterior rotation of the probe causes the scan plane to transsect the left atrium and left ventricle along a path similar to that of the transthoracic apical two-chamber view. When the probe is behind the left atrium, the left ventricular inflow tract is parallel to the path of the ultrasonic beam and the left ventricle is vertically oriented on the video screen (Fig. 16–26). The mitral valve and both papillary muscles are also recorded. When the probe is advanced below the gastroesophageal junction, the left ventricle is horizontally oriented on the video image, and the left ventricular inflow tract is perpendicular to the ultrasound beam. The apex, which is not visualized using the horizontal transducer, can usually be recorded using the vertical plane.

The Pulmonary Veins

Because the esophagus is close to the pulmonary veins, it is generally possible to clearly record the proximal portions of all four pulmonary veins using TEE when this is difficult or impossible from the transthoracic approach. Pulmonary venous imaging is important in patients with congenital heart disease, while Doppler assessment of venous inflow velocities is useful in assessing the severity of regurgitation and may play a role

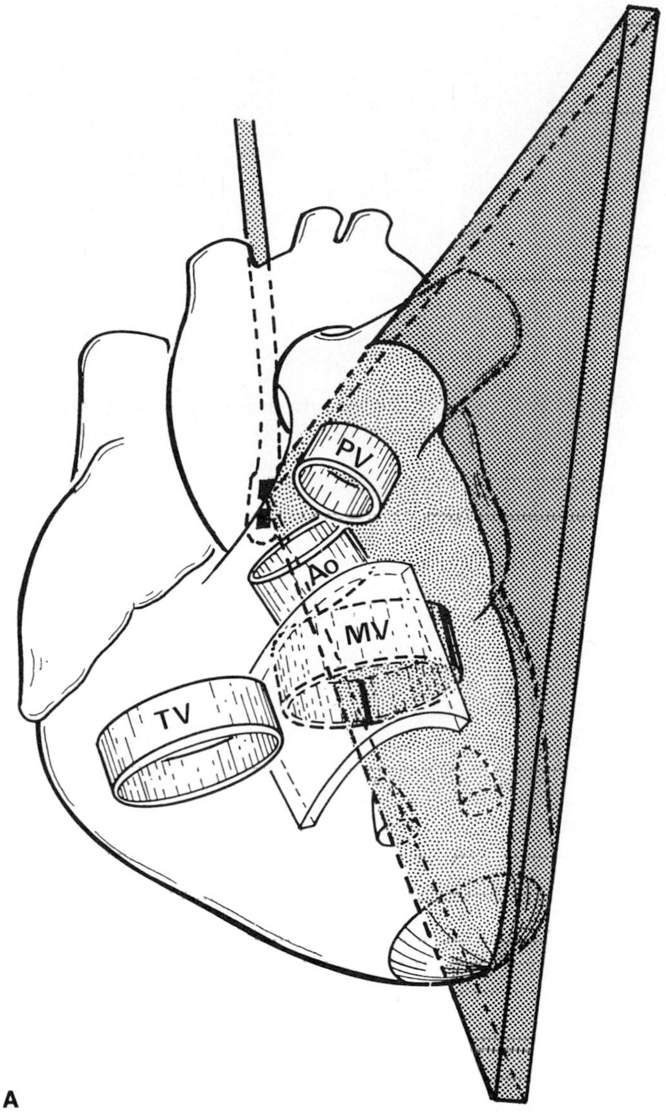

A

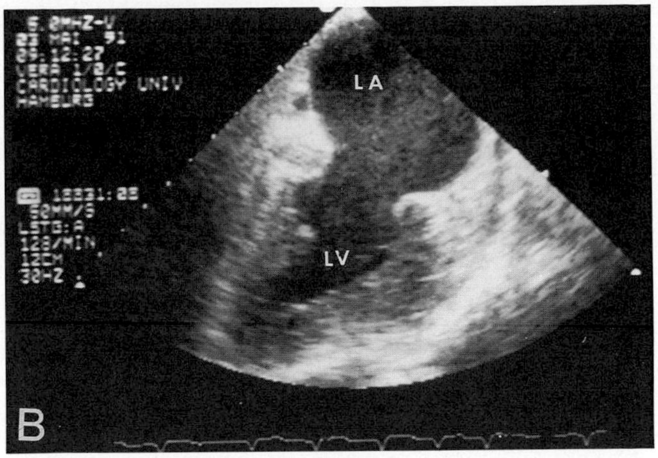

Fig. 16–26. A. The relationship of the esophageal longitudinal view of the left atrium (LA), mitral valve (MV), and left ventricle (LV) to the other primary cardiac structures. **B.** Transesophageal recording of the LA, MV, and LV. The same structures in roughly the same plane of section can be recorded with the transducer behind the superior LA (as illustrated here), the lower LA, the MV, or the base, mid- or apical sections of the LV. TV = tricuspid valve; PV = pulmonary valve; AV = aortic valve.

in the evaluation of atrial function. The right upper pulmonary vein is seen adjacent to the right pulmonary artery,[14] while the right lower vein inserts more inferiorly. Both right veins can often be recorded using one plane of the biplane pair (Fig. 16–27A). The left superior pulmonary vein is easily recorded using either the transverse or vertical plane immediately beneath the atrial appendage. With the vertical plane, it is often possible to record both the left inferior and superior vein in the same plane (Fig. 16–27B). An increase in chamber pressure with subsequent venous dilation facilitates recording (Fig. 16–28).

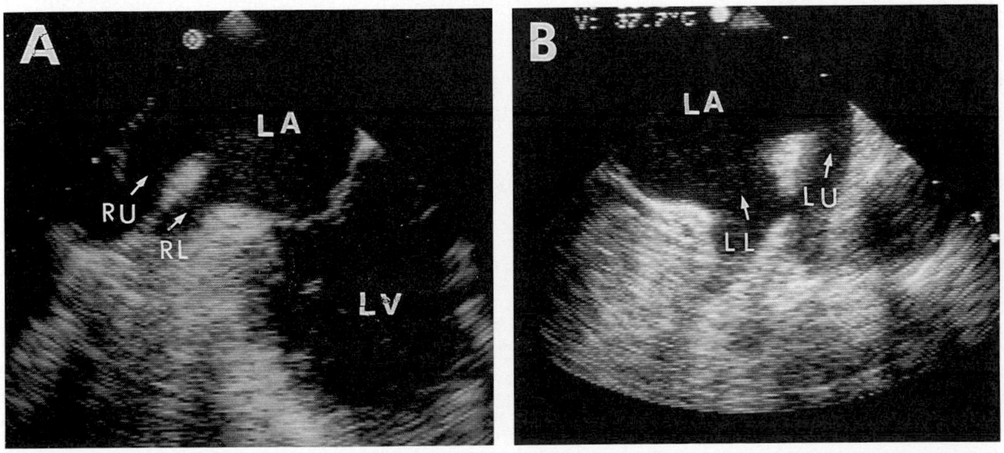

Fig. 16–27. Longitudinal views of the right **(A)** and left **(B)** pulmonary veins. RU = right upper pulmonary vein; RL = right lower pulmonary vein; LU = left upper pulmonary vein; LL = left lower pulmonary vein; LA = left atrium; LV = left ventricle.

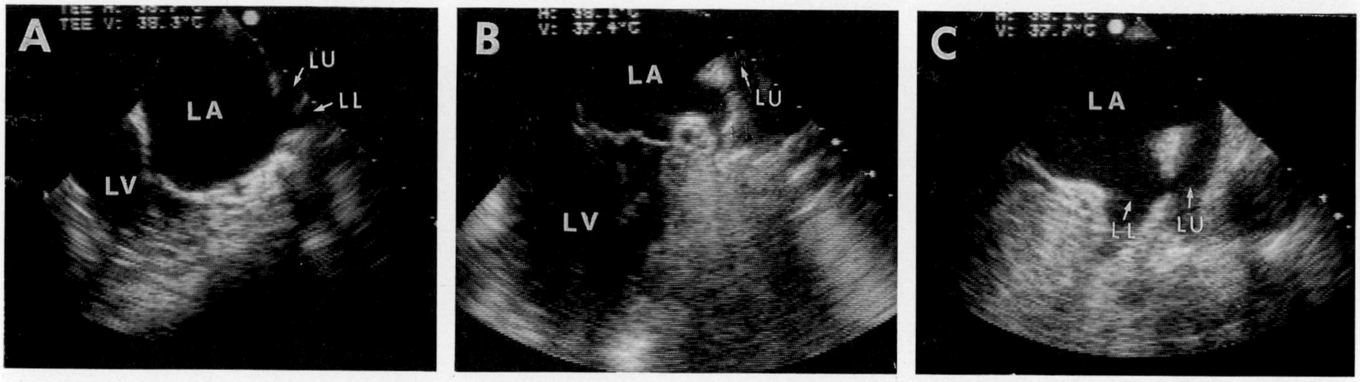

Fig. 16–28. Transesophageal recordings from patients with normal **(A)** and mildly **(B)**, and moderately **(C)** dilated left pulmonary veins. LA = left atrium; LV = left ventricle; LU = left upper pulmonary vein; LL = left lower pulmonary vein.

Thoracic Aortic Imaging

The examination of the thoracic aorta is one of the most important applications of TEE. Virtually the entire thoracic aorta can be recorded in both long and short axis using combined longitudinal and transverse imaging. The descending aorta, from the diaphragm to the aortic arch, is generally imaged by advancing the probe beyond the diaphragm and then gradually withdrawing while continuously recording. Using the horizontal array, the descending aorta presents as a pulsating circular structure (Fig. 16–29), with typical aortic flow characteristics evident on Doppler recordings.

Because there are no anatomic landmarks to define the level of the aorta being recorded, probe depth relative to the incisors is used as reference. Long axis images of the descending aorta can be obtained at selected intervals using the vertical array of the biplane probe.

Between the upper abdomen and the aortic arch, the intertwined aorta and esophagus gradually reverse their anteroposterior relationship. At the diaphragm, the esophagus is anterior to the aorta; at the midthorax, the esophagus is medial to the aorta, and at the arch, it is posterior to the aorta (Fig. 16–30). Thus, the probe must be rotated leftward and anteriorly as it is withdrawn to follow the aorta superiorly.

As the probe is withdrawn beyond the isthmus, the aorta begins to change direction and curve from left to right in front of the esophagus. The change in direction results in the horizontal plane being more closely aligned with the long axis of the vessel, which, because it is curving, appears as a sausage-shaped structure. The ver-

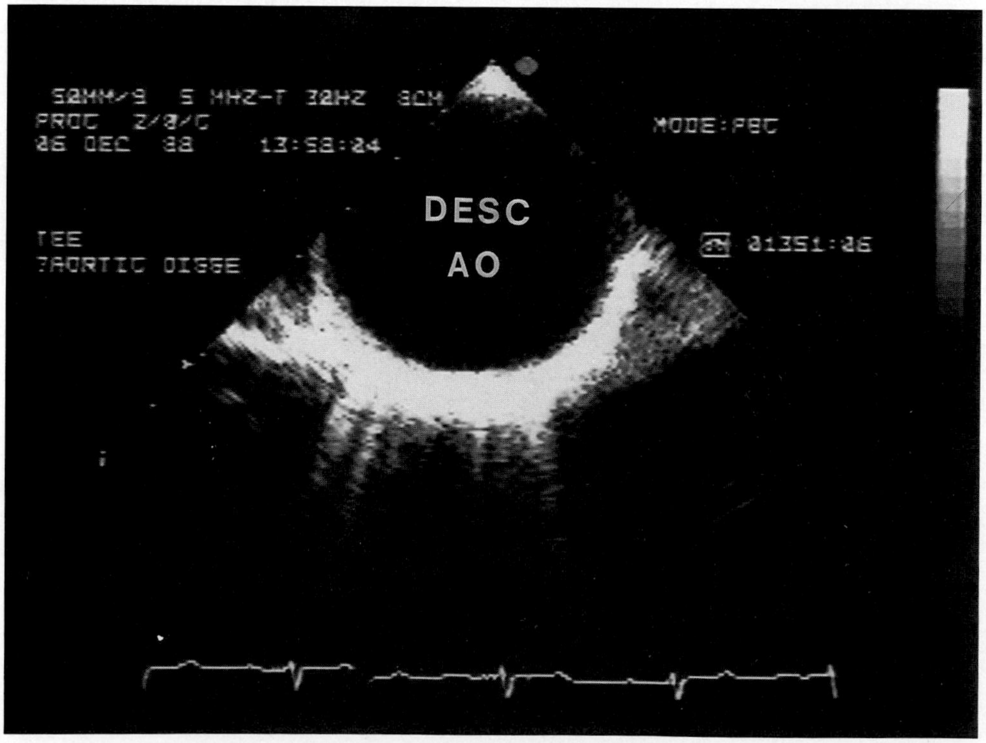

Fig. 16–29. Esophageal short axis view of the descending thoracic aorta (DESC AO). This image is obtained by rotating the plane roughly 180° from its normal orientation and aligning it to produce the most circular aortic configuration possible. The transducer can then be advanced along the esophagus from the level of the aortic isthmus to its penetration through the diaphragm to record the full extent of the descending thoracic aorta in short axis.

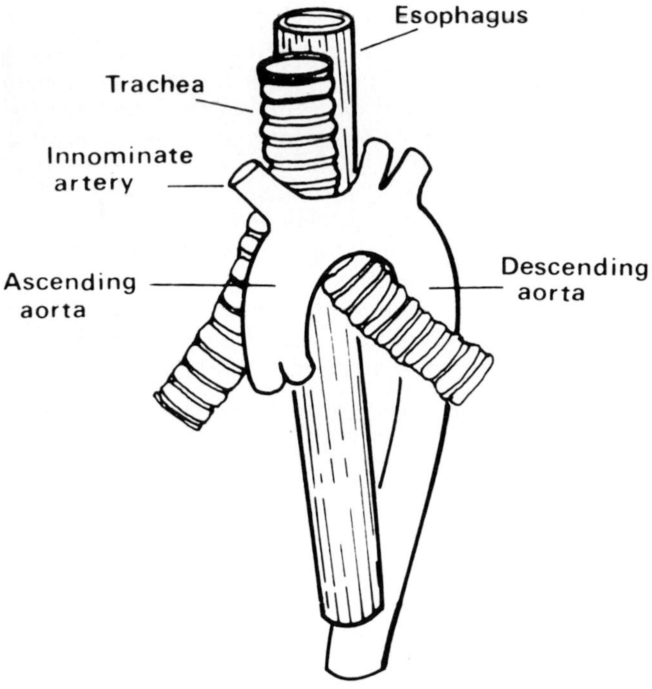

Fig. 16–30. Intertwining of aorta and esophagus from the diaphragm to the arch.

tical plane, in contrast, now records the arch in short axis as it passes in front of the esophagus. Using the vertical plane, it is also possible to record the origin of the left subclavian artery and occasionally one or more arch vessels.

The ascending aorta can be recorded in a true or slightly oblique short axis using the horizontal plane and in long axis using the vertical plane of the transducer. There is a blind spot in the upper ascending aorta where the air-filled trachea is directly interposed between esophagus and ascending aorta. This region is virtually impossible to examine in short axis using the horizontal plane; however, anteflexion of the vertical plane from a point just below the carina permits most of the region above the trachea to be imaged.

Both longitudinal and transverse imaging are important for detecting aortic aneurysms and dissection. Diagnosis is based on visualization of changes in vessel size, abnormal flow patterns, and/or an intimal flap with or without thrombus formation (Fig. 16–31).[35–37] Longitudinal scanning has been reported to be superior in detecting type I and type III entry sites.[38]

Applications

TEE studies are of value in (1) the study of hospitalized or ambulatory patients in whom a routine transthoracic examination fails to answer the clinical question or does so with an insufficient degree of certainty to permit appropriate decisions to be made concerning management; (2) the operating room where transthoracic studies are generally not possible; (3) the intensive care unit to study patients who are being artificially ventilated or have extensive surgical or traumatic chest wounds; (4) the catheterization laboratory to assess catheter location during transseptal puncture, balloon valvuloplasty, and electrical ablation; and (5) in the exercising patient to permit continuous image recording and to improve quality.

The distribution of patients studied in these various locations will vary depending on the nature of the institution. The majority of studies, however, are generally performed in ambulatory patients.

General Diagnostic Applications in Ambulatory or Hospitalized Patients

Esophageal echocardiography has been suggested to be useful as an alternative diagnostic procedure in cases in which transthoracic echocardiography is technically inadequate and the clinical question is important to re-

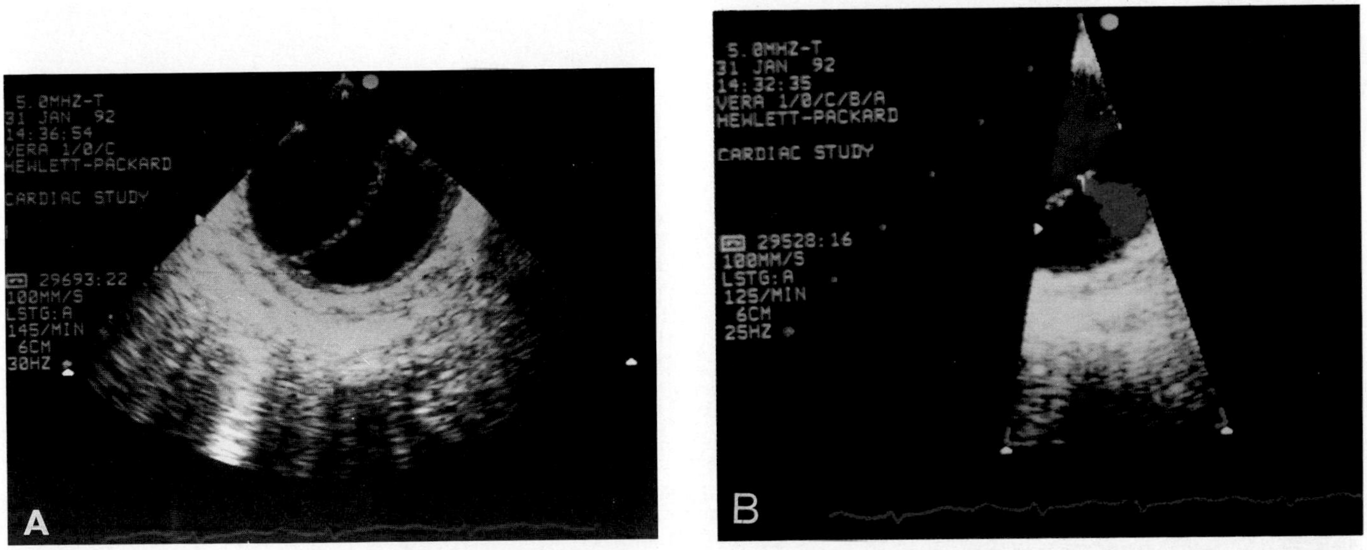

Fig. 16–31. Transesophageal short axis recording to an aortic dissection. **A.** The intimal flap runs from roughly the one-o'clock to seven-o'clock positions. **B.** Color Doppler recording illustrating a small communication between the true and false lumen of the dissection.

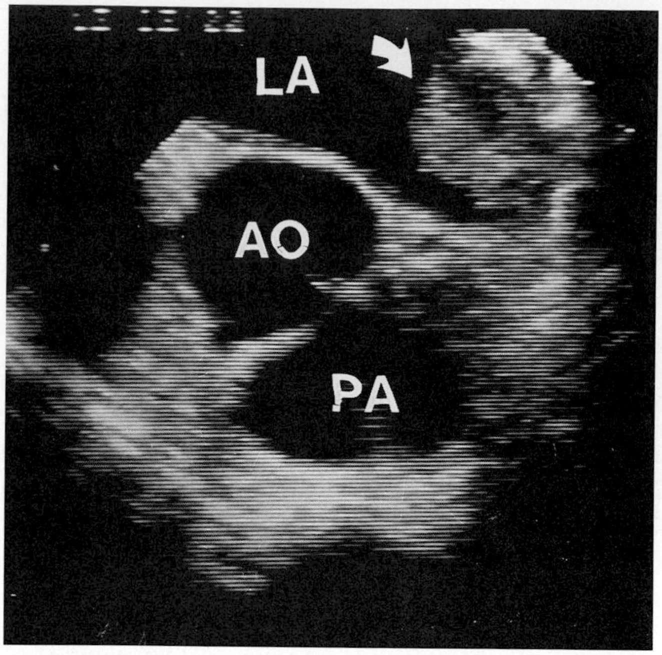

Fig. 16–32. Esophageal short axis recording of the aortic valve and left atrial appendage illustrating a large thrombus within the appendage (arrow). LA = left atrium; AO = aorta; PA = pulmonary artery.

solve. Thus, TEE is more commonly employed in obese patients, those with lung disease, or those with recent sternal or epigastric surgical wounds. Diagnostic questions for which this technique has been reported to be of particular value include the detection of intracardiac thrombi, particularly in the left atrial appendage; the evaluation of patients with a suspected cardiac source of embolic stroke;[39,40] the visualization of small bacterial vegetations[41–43] and endocarditis associated abscesses;[44] and the diagnosis of aortic dissection.[36,45–47] The technique has also been reported to be useful in detecting septal and papillary muscle rupture following acute myocardial infarction,[48] prosthetic valve dysfunction,[49–51] and specific features of native and postoperative congenital heart disease.[52–57]

The primary reported reason for performing a TEE (roughly one third of all diagnostic studies) has been as a preprocedure screen for atrial thrombi in patients undergoing a percutaneous mitral valvuloplasty and to rule out a cardiac source of embolus in patients with suspected embolic stroke. The diagnosis of left atrial thrombi is one of the areas in which two-dimensional echocardiography has been notably limited, particularly when the thrombus is localized to the atrial appendage.[58,59] The incidence of atrial thrombi is known to be particularly high in patients with mitral stenosis,[60,61] and the widespread use of percutaneous mitral balloon valvuloplasty as a primary form of treatment in these patients has made the accurate diagnosis of atrial thrombus increasingly important.[62–64] Likewise, in patients with recurrent systemic emboli, with or without mitral valve disease, detection or exclusion of atrial thrombus may play a role in appropriate therapeutic decision making. Studies of the left atrium from the esophageal approach have been shown to be particularly useful in visualizing thrombi, both fixed and mobile, in the atrial appendage that were not apparent during routine transthoracic studies[65] (Fig. 16–32). Although most attention has focused on the atrial appendage, thrombi can also be detected in other areas of the atrium that are difficult to visualize from the anterior chest wall. Figure 16–33, e.g., compares transthoracic (Fig. 16–33A) and TEE (Fig. 16–33B) recordings of the left atrium in a patient with a stenotic mitral valve. In this example, the atrium was reasonably well visualized in the standard apical four-chamber view, and no thrombus was apparent. When

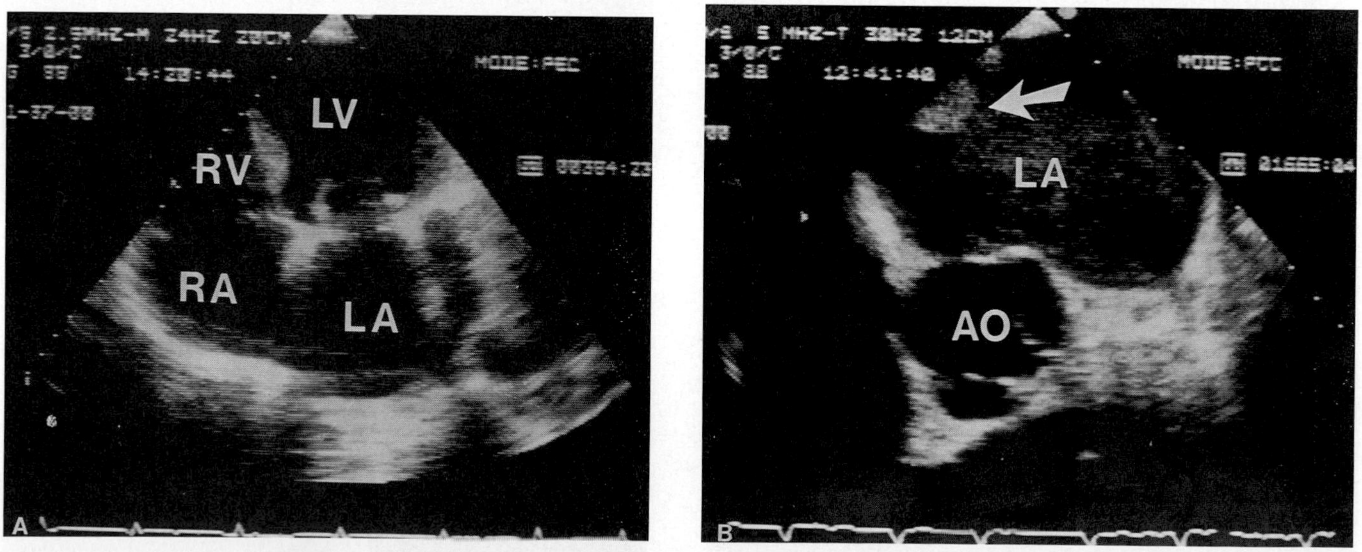

Fig. 16–33. Comparison of the transthoracic and transesophageal approaches for recording atrial thrombi. **A.** Apical four-chamber recording from a patient with mitral stenosis and a dilated left atrium (LA). Although the LA is well visualized in this and other planes, no obvious thrombus was noted. **B.** Transesophageal recording from the same patient illustrating spontaneous contrast in the LA and an obvious thrombus at the superior border of the atrium, near the entrance of the pulmonary veins. LV = left ventricle; RV = right ventricle; RA = right atrium; AO = aorta.

the atrium was examined from the esophagus, however, stasis of blood and a clearly defined thrombus along the superior atrial wall at the entrance to the pulmonary veins were recorded. It is also important to remember that despite reported amputation of the atrial appendage during a prior surgical procedure, a small stump can remain as a continued site for thrombus formation. Figure 16–34 is an example of such a case. In this longitudinal recording, thrombus is clearly evident in the atrial appendage despite reported prior surgical amputation. Atrial thrombi, when present, are virtually always found in patients recognized to be at high risk for embolic events, e.g., those with mitral stenosis, prosthetic valves, myopathy with marked decrease in cardiac output, and atrial fibrillation. In these cases, detection generally has little impact on management except in those undergoing a valvuloplasty because anticoagulation is recommended in any case. The use of TEE to exclude atrial thrombi before cardioversion has also been suggested and may prove useful in individual cases. TEE has proven valuable in at least one case in assessing the efficacy of thrombolytic therapy in a patient with a thrombosed prosthetic valve.[66]

TEE has also been reported to have a significantly higher yield in detecting other potential cardiac sources of embolism.[67–69] These studies, however, assume that abnormalities such as mitral valve prolapse, spontaneous echo-contrast, patent foramen ovale, or atrial septal aneurysm are all a direct cause of the embolic event in the population under investigation. Therefore, one must observe caution in the interpretation of these data, because not all of the entities can be clearly ascribed to be the cause of the unexplained embolic events, and their presence does not necessarily influence therapy.[15] Interatrial septal aneurysm, e.g., has been found more commonly in patients without evidence of stroke than in those with strokes.[70] Left atrial spontaneous echocontrast is an epiphenomenon occurring in patients with stasis of blood in the left atrium such as those with prosthetic mitral valves, mitral stenosis, and severe left ventricular failure—conditions that usually warrant anticoagulation, particularly in patients with atrial fibrillation. Intra-aortic debris, which is commonly detected by TEE, can also be a cause of an embolic event[71] and has been shown to be an independent risk factor for systemic embolization in a case-control study with an odds ratio of 3.2.[72] Thus, while TEE may permit detection of real or putative causes of embolic stroke, the impact on management, except in patients undergoing a mitral valvuloplasty, is likely to be small and should be considered before the procedure is performed.

In patients with endocarditis, TEE improves the sensitivity of detection of small vegetations and vegetations on prosthetic valves. The increase in sensitivity in detecting small vegetations on native valves clearly involves some loss of specificity, and patients have undergone surgery inappropriately because of misinterpreted degenerative changes on otherwise normal valves. In patients with prosthetic mitral valves, the improved resolution and ability to avoid the shadowing that obscures the atrial surface of the valve during transthoracic imaging appears to be a significant advantage of the transesophageal approach. Figure 16–35 compares the transthoracic and esophageal recordings from a patient with

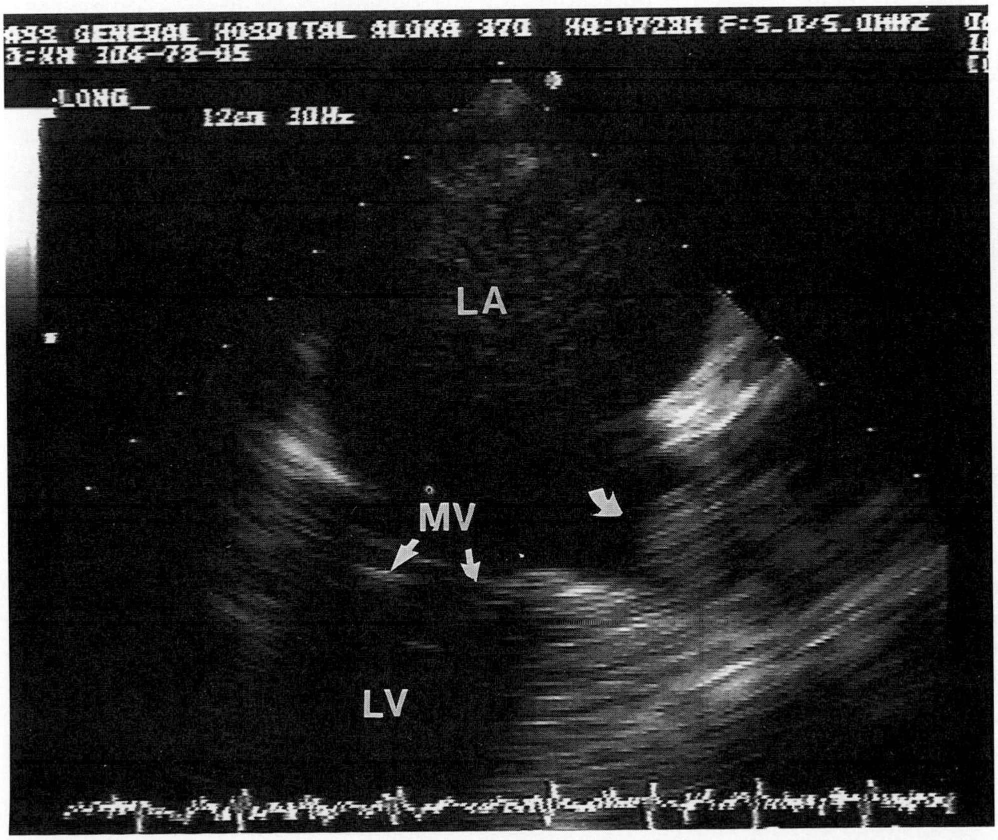

Fig. 16–34. Transesophageal echocardiogram recorded with the longitudinal array of a biplane probe. In this example, stasis of blood is clearly evident in the left atrium (LA), and there is a well-defined thrombus (curved arrow) in the atrial appendage. The residual appendage and thrombus were present, despite a prior surgical procedure during which the appendage had reportedly been amputated. MV = mitral valve; LV = left ventricle.

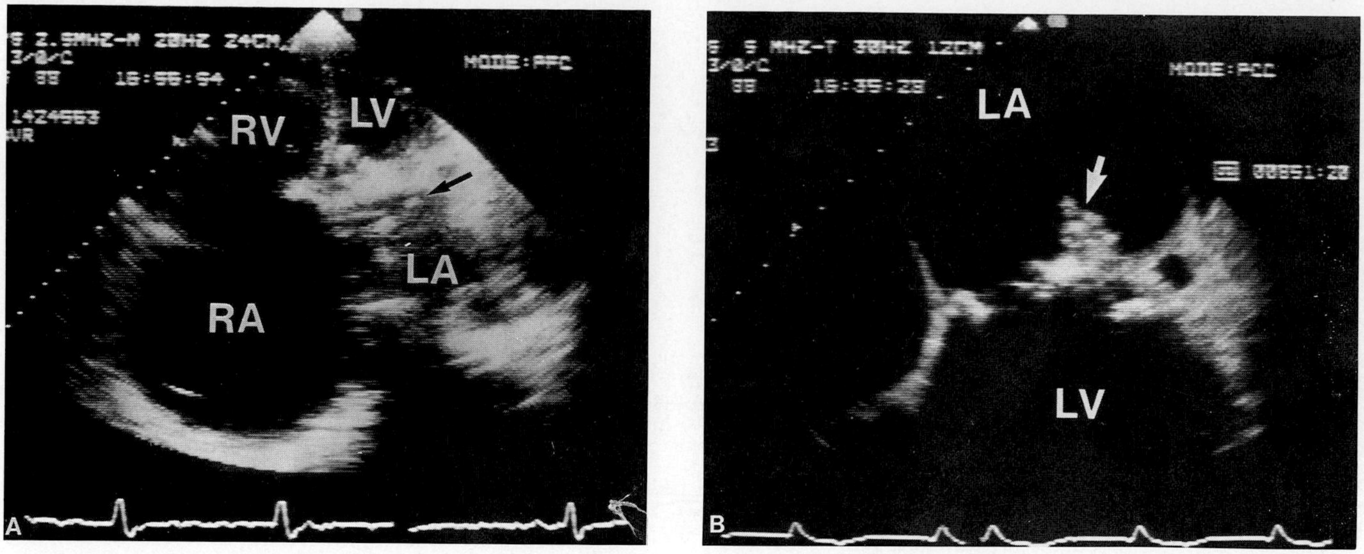

Fig. 16–35. Comparative recordings from the standard apical four-chamber and esophageal views from a patient with a prosthetic mitral valve and superimposed bacterial vegetation. **A.** A small mobile echo-producing mass (arrow) was apparent on the transthoracic recording and was correctly interpreted as a vegetation. **B.** The improved resolution obtainable from the esophageal window permitted the diagnosis of a bacterial vegetation (arrow) to be established with far greater certainty. LA = left atrium; LV = left ventricle; RV = right ventricle; RA = right atrium.

a mitral prosthesis and a superimposed valvular vegetation. Although a small mobile mass was detected on the transthoracic study, the size, nature, and morphology of the vegetative mass were far more clearly delineated on the transesophageal recording. TEE is particularly useful in defining the complications of endocarditis, including paravalvular leak, abnormal shunt, abscess and thrombus.[44]

Aortic dissection is another condition in which the improved image resolution and Doppler sensitivity of TEE may be particularly useful.[16] Esophageal imaging provides better visualization of the intimal flap, while pulsed and color flow Doppler can help define the asynchronous flow in the false lumen and exclude dissection in other cases in which an anomalous echo in a dilated aorta is misinterpreted as an intimal flap. The entry and exit site of the dissection can often be detected (see Fig. 16–31) when inadequately demonstrated by other techniques.[16] Figure 16–36 illustrates a large saccular aneurysm of the ascending aorta. On standard transthoracic imaging, a linear echo of unclear origin was present, raising the question of a dissection. TEE, however, clearly demonstrated the absence of dissection and confirmed the diagnosis of saccular aneurysms.

Papillary muscle rupture is an infrequent, but catastrophic, complication of acute myocardial infarction. Figure 16–37 compares transthoracic and esophageal recordings from a patient with papillary muscle rupture. Although a mobile mass, reflective of the papillary muscle head, was clearly apparent on the transthoracic study, the identity of the mass and its chordal attachments to the mitral valve were far more clearly defined from the esophagus.

TEE is of value in patients with congenital heart disease to more clearly delineate posterior structures, such as the pulmonary veins, main and branch pulmonary arteries, and the atrial appendages. Other lesions, e.g., coarctation and cor triatriatum, can also be clearly visualized. In older patients with congenital heart disease, thoracoskeletal deformity may limit transthoracic imaging, and in these cases TEE may be invaluable.

Other conditions for which TEE has been suggested to be of importance are right atrial thrombus and thromboembolism in the pulmonary artery, complications of myocardial infarction such as ventricular septal defect, and pseudoaneurysm, right atrial infarction, localized right atrial compression and tamponade, cardiac tumors and thrombi, and a host of other pathologies. Most of these lesions are routinely diagnosed using transthoracic imaging and Doppler, and examples appear throughout this text. In exceptional cases, it may be necessary to resort to an esophageal study to improve image resolution and hence, diagnostic accuracy; however, this is clearly the exception. In all cases, it is important to exert caution so that a procedure associated with obvious patient discomfort and potential risk not be used as a substitute for operator competence in performing routine studies.

The esophageal approach also has been suggested to be of value in the recording of unimpeded Doppler flow signals to close range and therefore increased sensitivity. A classic example is the obligate regurgitation, which is a design feature of the St. Jude valve and which can be recorded routinely from the esophagus while typically being inapparent during transthoracic studies (Fig. 16–38). Note that this improved sensitivity uniformly increases the size of all jets recorded from the esophagus when compared to their transthoracic appearance. As a result, gradation of severity based on standards established for jet size from transthoracic imaging must be correspondingly corrected.

Unfortunately, although Doppler recording is gener-

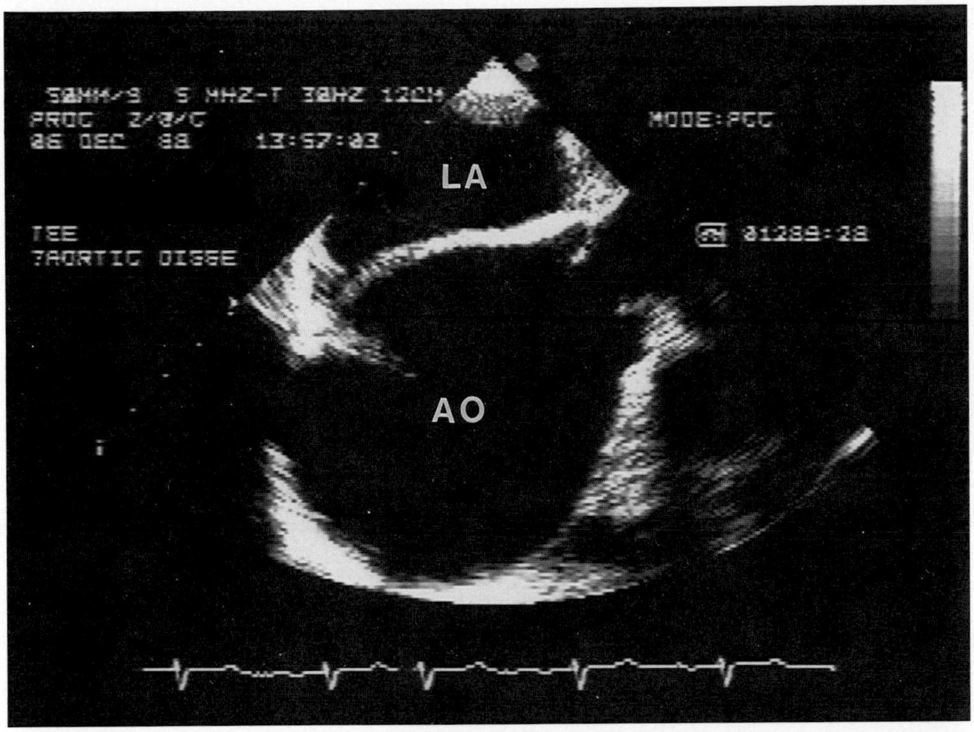

Fig. 16–36. A large saccular aneurysm of the ascending aorta (AO). On transthoracic imaging, aneurysmal dilation was appreciated; however, a linear echo suggestive of possible dissection was also noted. By transesophageal imaging and color flow, however, the presence of dissection could be confidently excluded, and the extent of the aneurysm was clearly defined. LA = left atrium.

ally improved from the esophagus, portions of the Doppler examination are more difficult to obtain as a result of the inability to align the ultrasonic beam parallel to the direction of flow or to avoid interfering flow fields. For example, the recording of accurate left ventricular outflow gradients is extremely difficult although sometimes feasible from the transgastric approach. Likewise, the continuous wave Doppler interrogation of tricuspid regurgitant jets tends to become contaminated by concomitant mitral regurgitation.

Intraoperative Transesophageal Echocardiography

With the transducer positioned behind the heart in the esophagus, it is possible to continuously record the left ventricle or other structures of interest during the induction of anesthesia, perfusion of the myocardium with cardioplegic solutions, performance of the surgical procedure, closure of the thorax, and postoperative recovery. The stability of the transducer in the esophagus per-

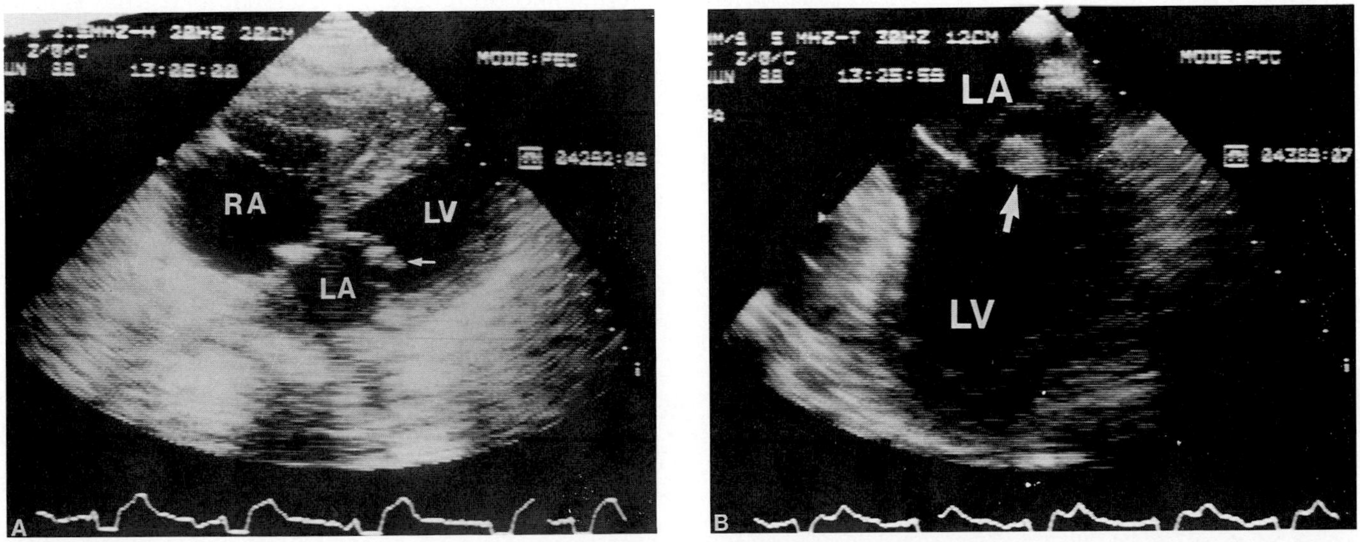

Fig. 16–37. Comparison of the diagnosis of ruptured papillary muscle using the transthoracic **(A)** and transesophageal **(B)** windows. **A.** From the transthoracic approach, a mobile, echo-producing mass attached to the posterior mitral leaflet is evident (arrow). **B.** On transesophageal imaging, however, the clear separation of this mass from the leaflets (arrow) and its attachment via chordae tendineae are more clearly delineated. LV = left ventricle; LA = left atrium; RA = right atrium.

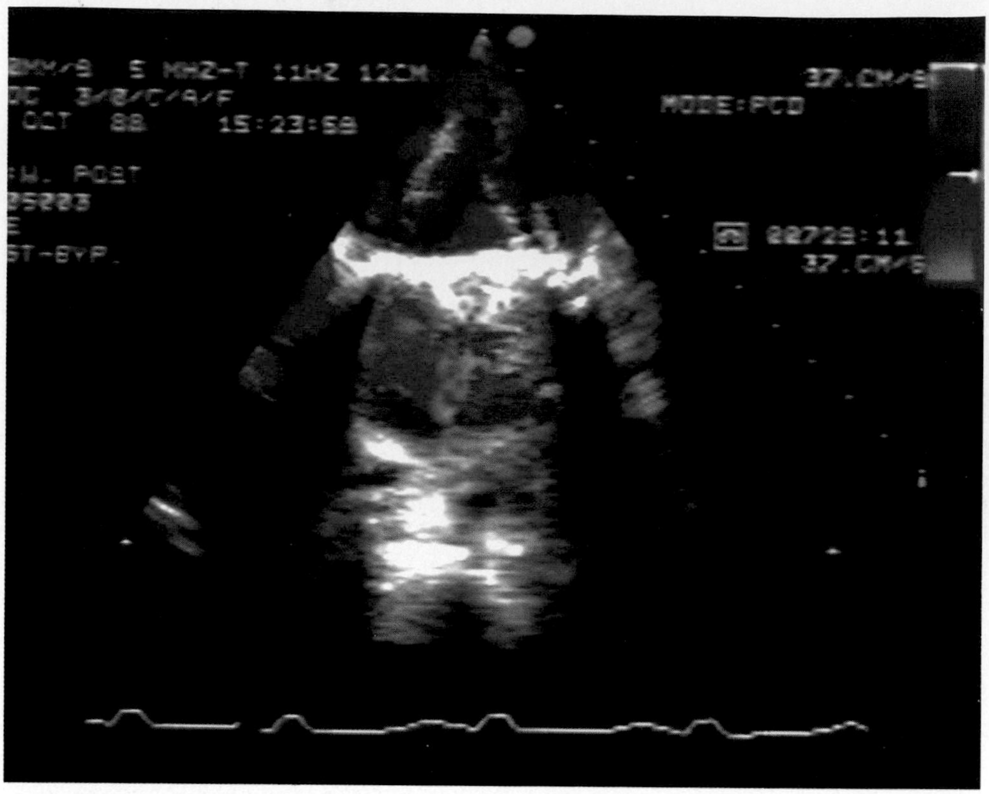

Fig. 16–38. Color flow Doppler recording of the multiple regurgitant jets normally visualized behind a St. Jude valve. These tiny areas of regurgitation are design features of the valve that are uniformly present but usually are recordable only from the esophagus.

mits continuous recording of the same region for monitoring purposes, while its flexibility is ideal for examining different structures as the procedure progresses. Because the heart lies directly on the esophagus, such recording is possible even though the chest is open and the anterior pericardium exposed to air. It has the added advantage of not interfering with the surgical field or sterility.

TEE has many applications in the operating room including the monitoring of left ventricular function and recording new segmental wall motion abnormalities;[73–75] continuous recording of cardiac output;[76] assessment of myocardial perfusion;[77] detection of valvular regurgitation;[78,79] assessment of valvular function following valvuloplasty, valvotomy, or valve replacement;[80] detection of intravascular air bubbles introduced during the surgical procedure;[81,82] confirmation of the integrity of shunt repairs; and localization of the site of origin and termination of dissection.[36,83–85] Specific intraoperative applications of esophageal echocardiography are discussed in greater detail in the section on intraoperative echocardiography later in this chapter.

The Intensive Care Unit

The intensive care unit is another area where transesophageal studies play a major role. These patients are traditionally difficult to study from the transthoracic approach because many are being artificially ventilated and/or have had major thoracic or abdominal surgery or extensive trauma. Any or all of these factors limit the available windows and prevent patient positioning to optimize the transthoracic study. In addition, the questions asked generally bear directly on patient management, making technically limited studies less acceptable. Fortunately, many of the same factors that limit routine studies often facilitate a transesophageal echo because these patients generally are sedated and the airway is controlled.

The diagnostic applications are similar to those of a routine examination in the critically ill patient and include the diagnosis of pericardial effusion or tamponade, the assessment of left ventricular function, the detection of valvular dysfunction and vegetations, and the diagnosis of dissection. The ability to answer these questions with confidence in the critically ill patient represents a major extension of echocardiography into an area where it was previously of limited value. In this type of patient, the examination is generally more question specific and may need to be halted abruptly. As a result, it is important to answer the diagnostic question first and then proceed with the full examination rather than run the risk of having to discontinue the study in the middle of a routine examination before the diagnostic question is answered.

The Catheterization Laboratory

TEE has been found useful during a variety of invasive procedures to aid in catheter placement, in the immediate assessment of results, and in the detection of complications. During balloon mitral valvuloplasty, TEE has been found to be useful in (1) guiding the transeptal catheterization; (2) positioning the balloon across the mitral valve; (3) immediately assessing the results of the valvuloplasty; (4) detecting the size of the iatrogenic atrial septal defect; and (5) identifying complications such as pericardial effusion and torn chordae.[86–88] TEE has also been found to be useful in positioning the clamshell devices used in percutaneous closure of atrial septal defects and in assessing residual shunting after the device is in place. Other applications include assisting catheter placement for radio frequency (RF) ablation of bypass tracts and assisting in the placement of the forceps during the intracardiac biopsy procedures.

The Exercising Patient

Two-dimensional and M-mode echocardiography have been shown to be accurate and reproducible methods for assessing left ventricular size and performance at rest. Both techniques are limited, however, in obtaining high quality, quantifiable left ventricular recordings during exercise. As a result, it has been suggested that these limitations might be overcome by recording the left ventricle from the esophagus during dynamic exercise or other non-exercise-induced stress. Early M-mode studies showed a reasonable correlation between left ventricular internal diameters recorded from the esophagus and those recorded transthoracically and also showed satisfactory reproducibility of the measurements.[89] Further validation of the technique to this point, however, has been based largely on recording the expected responses to exercise induced stress. Dynamic exercise, e.g., was shown to cause a progressive decrease in end-systolic dimension and an increase in fractional shortening and peak shortening rate. The end-diastolic diameter also decreased, which is probably related to a decrease in filling time with increasing heart rate and an increase in sympathetic tone. Studies in symptomatic patients with aortic regurgitation, in contrast, showed no change in end-diastolic dimension and a fall in shortening fraction.[90]

The added potential offered by orthogonal TEE imaging to record dynamic left ventricle function during various forms of exercise and non-exercise-induced stress is enormous given the improved resolution and enhanced spatial orientation inherent in this approach. Figure 16–39, e.g., illustrates orthogonal long and short axis views of the left ventricle recorded from the two transducers of an orthogonal array. The acquisition of the images about a "common" minor axis vastly simplifies the problem of chamber reconstruction and functional assessment. Despite this interesting preliminary data, the use of TEE during exercise remains a research tool.

Limitations and Potential Complications

The major limitation of esophageal echocardiography is obviously the need for the patient to swallow the gastroscopic probe. When the patient is already anesthetized for surgery, insertion of the transducer is a quick and relatively benign process. In the conscious patient, such procedures are always associated with some discomfort including retropharyngeal pressure, tearing, hypersalivation, gagging, and occasionally retching.

Major and minor complications have been reported to occur in 2.9% of patients. Complications leading to an aborted procedure occur in 0.88% of patients.[27] Figure 16–40 illustrates the number and type of complications noted in a group of 3827 patients studied at the Mayo Clinic over a 3-year period. Major complications, although rare, include death, aspiration, important arrhythmias, bleeding, bronchospasm, and esophageal injury. Two deaths have been reported; one that was due to bleeding in a patient with infiltration of the esophagus by lung cancer and the other presumably to arrhythmia in the immediate postprocedure period.[15]

The reported incidence of perforation associated with flexible esophagoscopy alone ranges from 0.02 to 0.03%,[91,92] with perforation occurring most commonly in the region of the cricopharyngeus muscle. Fortu-

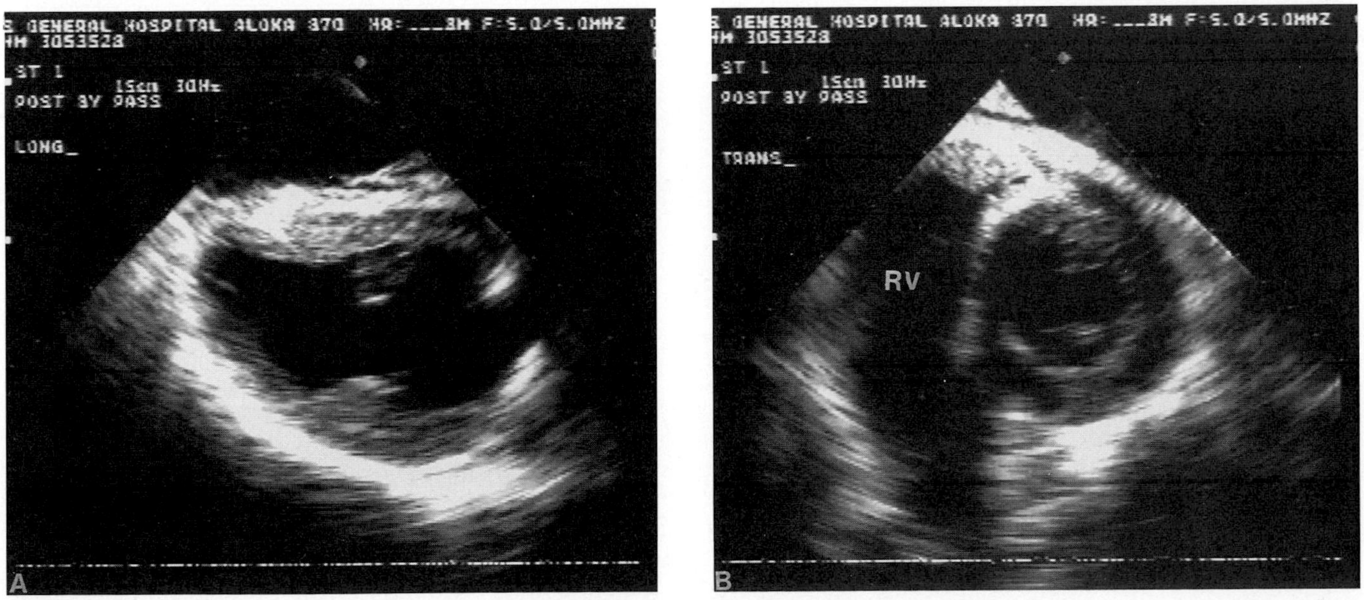

Fig. 16–39. Long **(A)** and short **(B)** axis images of the left ventricle recorded using the orthogonal arrays of a dual array esophageal probe. The resolution, fixed frame of reference, and potential for orthogonal image acquisition offer the potential for the assessment of left ventricular dynamic function at baseline and during various forms of induced stress. RV = right ventricle.

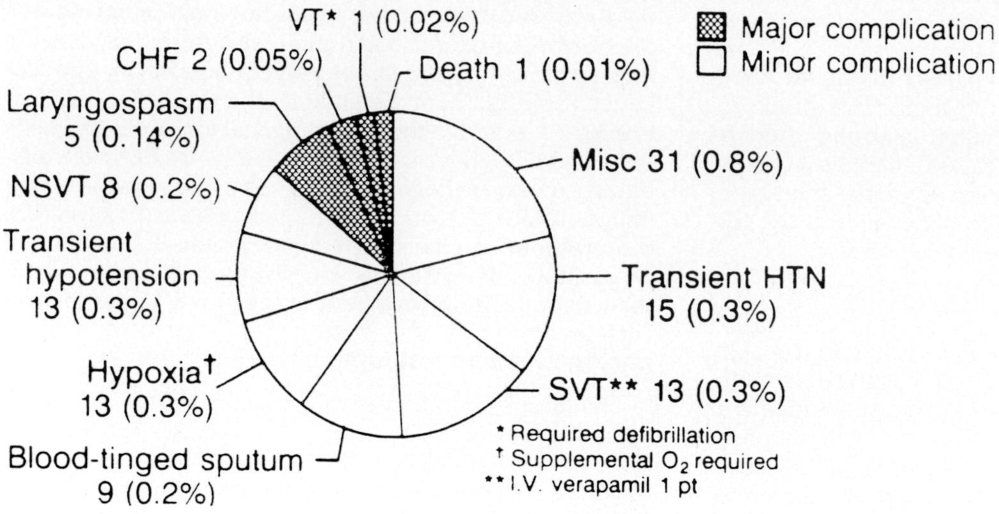

Fig. 16–40. The relative incidence of complications from transesophageal echocardiography in 3827 cases reported from the Mayo Clinic. CHF = congestive heart failure; NSVT = nonsustained ventricular tachycardia; SVT = supraventricular tachycardia; VT = ventricular tachycardia; HTN = hypertension. (From Seward JB, et al.: Critical appraisal of transesophageal echocardiography: limitations pitfalls and complications. J Am Soc Echocardiogr 5:228, 1992.)

nately, there have been few instances of esophageal trauma resulting from TEE, presumably because most centers routinely exclude patients with known or suspected esophageal disease.[93] Most trauma appears to occur during initial passage of the probe with little additional mechanical or thermal effect from prolonged intubation. Studies to date have failed to demonstrate pathologic evidence of esophageal trauma or thermal injury in animal models subjected to cardiopulmonary bypass and systemic heparinization when the probe was left in place and continuous imaging was conducted for several hours.[94]

Although major complications are relatively rare, minor complications occur more commonly. Minor complications include transient A-V block, nonsustained ventricular tachycardia,[95] acute bronchospasm,[45,96] vomiting, and laryngeal nerve paralysis in patients studied for prolonged periods in the sitting position during neurosurgical procedures.[97] A mild sore throat may be noted after the procedure and may continue for up to 24 hours. No specific treatment is necessary. Several authors have reported ischemic episodes requiring termination of the procedure.[98,99] One case of bronchial obstruction by the TEE probe, which resolved immediately after probe removal, in a pediatric patient during surgery has been reported. Transient hypoxia and allergic reactions to the sedatives or other drugs used during the procedure also occur.

Reactions have been reported to several of the medications used in preparing patients for TEE studies. These include toxic methemoglobinemia and a diffuse erythematous reaction or "red man syndrome." Toxic methemoglobinemia, reported in one case following lidocaine and benzocaine spray, is a rare complication of treatment with a variety of medications, including topical anesthetics.[100] Symptoms range from mild cyanosis to dyspnea, frank coma, and death. Acute toxic methemoglobinemia as a complication of treatment with topical benzocaine, lidocaine, or prilocaine has been reported most frequently in adults with congenital deficiency of methemoglobin reductase and in children after dental procedures. Methemoglobin is formed when ferrous iron (Fe^{2+}), chelated to the porphyrin ring in heme, is converted to ferric iron (Fe^{3+}) by endogenous or exogenous oxidizing agents. The methemoglobin molecule is unable to bind oxygen for transport, and there is a left shift in the hemoglobin/oxygen dissociation curve. Hence, while oxygen tension in blood (P_{O_2}) is normal, its total content (measured as saturation) for tissue delivery is markedly decreased. Treatment is methylene blue, 1 to 2 mg/kg given intravenously over 5 to 15 minutes. The diagnosis of methemoglobinemia can be confusing when pulse oximetry is used to monitor oxygen saturation, because spectroscopic methods cannot distinguish between methemoglobin and reduced hemoglobin. The oxygen saturation by pulse oximeter may continue to read 80 to 90%, despite lower actual levels of saturated oxyhemoglobin.

Technical Problems

A commonly encountered problem is air in the esophagus. Entrapped air consistently interferes with imaging during certain transducer maneuvers, particularly retroflexion of the scope tip in the midesophagus and imaging from the fundus of the stomach. As a rule, there is more air in the esophagus at the beginning of the examination than at the end because of continual clearing of air by esophageal and transducer action during the study. Passing the scope tip into the stomach also tends to clear air from the esophagus.[101]

Another problem is buckling of the tip of the probe in the esophagus. Buckling of the probe tip usually occurs with probes that are more flexible than normal. Buckling of the probe should be suspected if one or more of the following signs exist: difficulty obtaining an image, resistance to advancing or removing the probe, and fixation of the inner control knob in the fully clockwise position (maximal flexion). In general, the probe can be straightened by advancing it into the stomach, where the wider lumen permits unfolding of the buckled tip. The probe is then carefully withdrawn (Fig. 16–41).

Finally, the use of electrocautery in the operating room causes almost total disruption of the image and

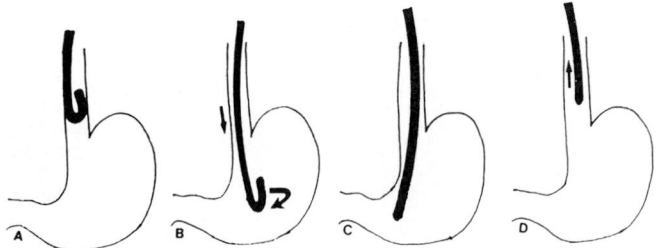

Fig. 16–41. **A.** Buckling of the tip of the transesophageal probe in the esophagus. When resistance was met on attempt to withdraw the probe, it was further advanced to the stomach **(B)**, where the wide lumen permitted straightening of the buckling **(C)**. The straight probe was then withdrawn without difficulty **(D)**. (From Kronzon I, et al.: Buckling of the tip of the transesophageal echocardiography probe: a potentially dangerous technical malfunction. J Am Soc Echocardiogr 5:176, 1992.)

loss of all useful information while it is in operation (Fig. 16–42).

Miscellaneous Considerations

Concern is occasionally voiced by the surgical staff concerning the possibility of damage to their eyes from the sound waves that are continuously directed toward them from behind the heart. TEE, when used in the operating room, has no appreciable risks to the surgeon or other medical/nursing staff present during cardiac or noncardiac procedures. This occurs for several reasons: First, when recommended procedures are followed, scanning is performed only as needed, thus minimizing the output of ultrasound energy. Second, ultrasound energy attenuates rapidly as it travels through esophageal, pericardial, and myocardial tissue and blood, because of energy absorption and beam scattering. After 5 cm, the ultrasound energy is reduced by 82% and after 7 cm by 91%. Furthermore, beyond 5 cm, the beam is past the focal point and begins to disperse, with intensities decreasing rapidly as energy is spread over a wider beam area. Third, the transmission of ultrasound through air is negligible as the tissue-air interface has poor acoustic coupling with low energy transfer and high beam scattering. Airborne attenuation from energy absorption and dispersion is much higher than in tissue and is virtually total at a distance of 6 inches. Thus, during an open-heart procedure, e.g., the ultrasound intensity at the upper surface of the heart (assuming that the transducer is emitting maximum intensity levels allowed for cardiac imaging) is reduced to levels allowed for ophthalmic scanning, and only infinitesimal amounts of ultrasound energy (too small to be measurable) reach as far as the surgeon's eyes.

EPICARDIAL ECHOCARDIOGRAPHY

Epicardial echocardiography is the term used to describe the acquisition of echocardiographic data from transducers placed directly on the surface of the heart or great vessels. The first such recordings were obtained by Edler and Hertz in cadaver hearts for the purpose of validating the source of intracardiac echoes (see Chapter 14). Kerber et al. demonstrated that high resolution echoes could be obtained, in vivo, by placing an M-mode transducer directly on the anterior epicardial surface of the beating canine heart and that these recordings could provide useful functional data.[102] In 1981, Marcus et al.[102a] developed and validated the use of an epicardial Doppler crystal, which could be transiently affixed to a coronary artery at the time of cardiac surgery to evaluate the physiologic significance of coronary stenoses in humans. At present, virtually all experimental animal studies using echocardiography are performed with the transducer applied to the anterior surface of the heart either directly or using a water bath standoff. Human studies can be obtained only at surgery because the chest must be open; however, important physiologic data have been generated in this environment.

Epicardial echocardiography offers several major ad-

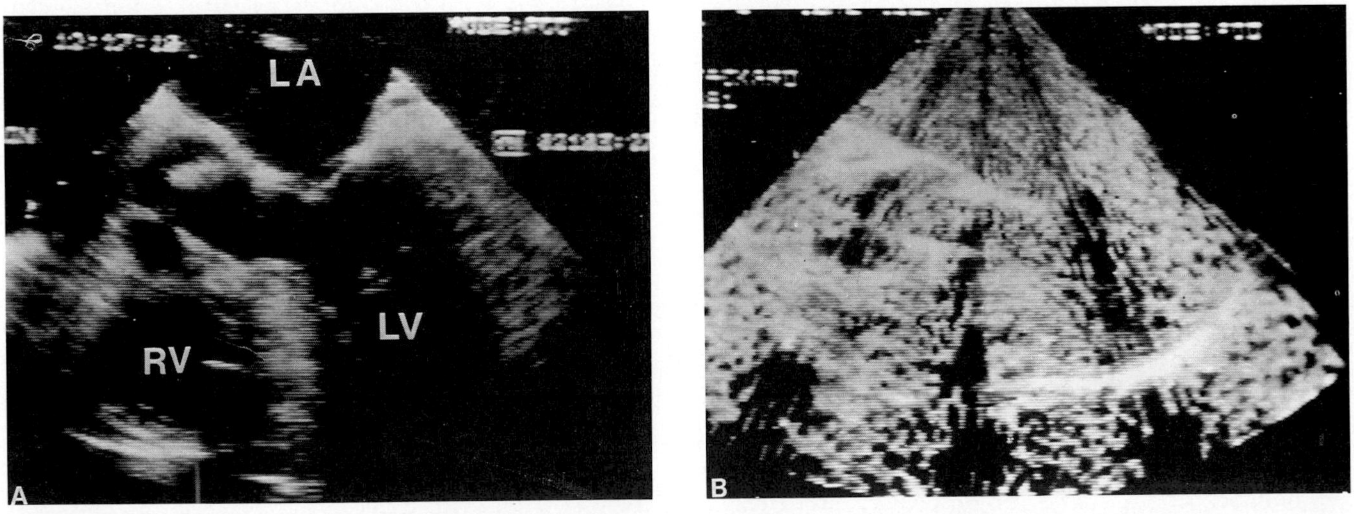

Fig. 16–42. Esophageal recordings before **(A)** and during **(B)** activation of electrocautery during a surgical procedure. The electrical interference produced by this instrument causes virtual total disruption of the image and loss of any useful information while it is in operation. LA = left atrium; LV = left ventricle; RV = right ventricle.

vantages over transthoracic imaging. First, by placing the transducer directly on the surface of the heart, one bypasses all of the intervening tissues encountered during normal transthoracic imaging. This permits the use of much higher frequency transducers than might otherwise be possible and can improve resolution considerably. Second, the ability to directly visualize the point on the chest where the transducer is being placed permits precise selection of the area to be examined (e.g., a specific coronary artery or a specific area of myocardium). Third, fixation of a transducer at a desired point on the epicardium permits chronic monitoring of local function over time and in response to interventions. Fourth, the ability to directly record the entire heart with visual external anatomic references provides even the unskilled operator with the entire diagnostic capabilities of an echocardiographic laboratory in an environment that does not require the technical expertise necessary to perform transthoracic studies.

Clinical Applications

The primary clinical applications of epicardial echocardiography include the intraoperative assessment of left ventricular function and the determination of the feasibility and results of valvular repair. Several investigators have also demonstrated the potential of high frequency epicardial echocardiography for the measurement of coronary arterial wall and luminal dimensions (Fig. 16–43).[103–106] In addition, it has been shown that coronary arterial bypass graft anastomoses can be accurately visualized using high frequency (12-MHz) epicardial echocardiography, and this offers the surgeon the potential for intraoperative correction of technical errors (Fig. 16–44).[107] When the precise location of a major epicardial coronary is obscured as a result of fat, myocardial bridging, or epicardial scarring, high frequency epicardial echocardiography can be used to quickly image and locate such arteries and to eliminate the need for time-consuming exploration.[108] Doppler sampling from a transducer directly affixed to the external surface of the epicardial coronaries or bypass grafts, likewise, permits monitoring of steady state flow as well

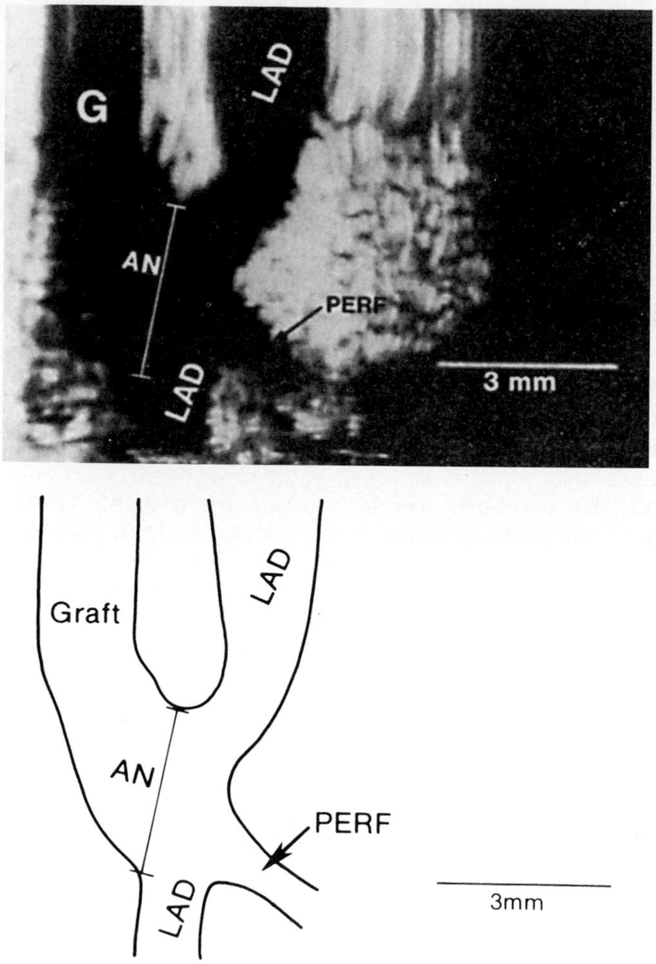

Fig. 16–44. Intraoperative epicardial recording of a vein bypass graft to the left anterior descending coronary artery (LAD) anastomotic site. AN = anastomosis; PERF = septal perforator; G = graft. (From Hiratzka LF, et al.: Intraoperative evaluation of coronary artery bypass graft anastomoses using high frequency epicardial echocardiography: experimental validation and initial patient studies. Circulation 73:1199, 1986. Reproduced by permission of the American Heart Association, Inc.)

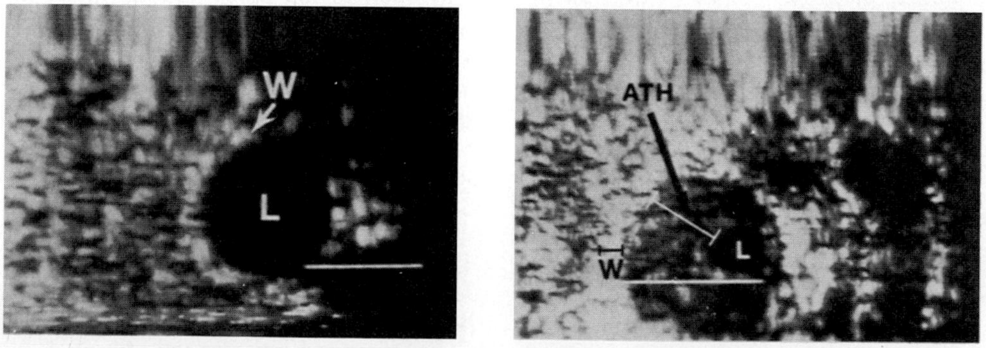

Fig. 16–43. Left. Epicardial short axis image of a coronary artery from a patient with no angiographic evidence of coronary disease. Right. Short axis epicardial image from a patient with severe coronary artery disease. The image is taken from an area of maximal angiographic stenosis. The reference for both studies is 3.0 mm in length. W = arterial wall; L = lumen; ATH = atherosclerosis. (From McPherson DD, Kerber RE: High frequency epicardial echocardiography for the intraoperative demonstration and evaluation of coronary atherosclerosis. Echocardiography 3:371, 1986. Reproduced with permission of Futura Publishing Company.)

as the response to interventions.[109] Assessment of segmental ventricular function is also possible with the same degree of resolution achieved in experimental studies. Such studies make possible extensive topographic sampling or long-term local monitoring of segmental myocardial function over the entire right and left ventricles.[110] Other applications such as the intraoperative assessment of ventricular and valvular morphology and function are discussed in the next section.

INTRAOPERATIVE ECHOCARDIOGRAPHY

Intraoperative echocardiography is the use of any of the standard echocardiographic techniques for cardiac diagnosis or monitoring in the operating room. Echocardiography is particularly valuable in this setting because it provides immediate information about ventricular and valvular function, which is often unobtainable using standard hemodynamic or electrocardiographic monitoring. Intraoperative echocardiographic studies can be of value during all phases of cardiac surgery as well as in the assessment of cardiac function during noncardiac surgery. In the cardiac surgical patient, studies can be performed from either the surface of the heart or esophagus, while in the noncardiac surgical patient, TEE is the primary form of examination. Intraoperative echocardiography represents a natural progression in which a well-accepted clinical tool is adapted to the operating room to gain further insight into cardiac pathophysiology and to provide immediate information to guide surgical therapeutic interventions.

Methods of Examination

Epicardial

Intraoperative epicardial two-dimensional and Doppler echocardiography can be performed during cardiac surgery using standard clinical echocardiographic equipment. The transducers can either be gas sterilized or covered with a sterile sheath and appropriately draped. To ensure patient safety, the cord of the transducer should be long enough to allow the machine to remain out of the operative field. To expedite the procedure, it is the surgeon who should perform the echocardiographic examination. Initially, an echocardiographer (preferably, a technically proficient cardiologist) should be in attendance in the operative suite to orient and guide the surgeon in obtaining optimal images. A team approach is absolutely necessary; all operating room personnel, including nurses, perfusionists, and technologists, should be familiar with the technique and the potential value of the study.[77]

Because the entire anterior surface of the heart is exposed after the chest is opened, most parasternal long and short axis planes can be easily obtained. Apical views are more difficult to record, but customized right angle phased array transducers have been developed for this purpose. Most information of interest, however, should be available from the anterior surface of the heart. Because the echocardiographic images are immediately available, they can be used to help guide therapeutic interventions and to select sites for aortic cannulation.[111] The echocardiographic examination also can be performed immediately after the operative procedure while the patient is being weaned from cardiopulmonary bypass. This permits evaluation of ventricular function, determination of appropriate interventions for smooth separation from bypass, and early recognition of myocardial or valvular dysfunction.[77]

Intraoperative Transesophageal Echocardiography

Intraoperative TEE probe insertion is generally performed by the anesthesiologist in collaboration with a cardiologist, because the anesthesiologist controls the mouth and airway. Manipulation of the probe and echocardiographic imaging is performed by the cardiologist in most cases, because the anesthesiology personnel lack specific echocardiographic training.[112] This practice, undoubtedly, will evolve as more anesthesiologists become trained in echocardiography. TEE imaging can be performed continuously and, therefore, is of particular value in monitoring ventricular function[13–15,113] during both cardiac and noncardiac surgery. (The technique of TEE is discussed earlier in this chapter.)

Comparison of Approaches

In the cardiac surgical patient, TEE is far more limited diagnostically than epicardial imaging because the intraesophageal probe is more difficult to maneuver and specific planes often cannot be recorded.[20] However, TEE is preferred for monitoring ventricular function during cardiac surgery and recovery because it can be performed continuously, does not interrupt the procedure, and does not require the attention of the surgeon. Because epicardial echocardiography can be performed only when the chest is opened, TEE is the procedure of choice for intraoperative monitoring of cardiac function in high risk cardiac patients undergoing noncardiac surgery or in the immediate postoperative period when transthoracic echocardiography is difficult.

Applications

Intraoperative Assessment of Valvular Heart Disease

Intraoperative echocardiography can be of value in the surgical management of all forms of valvular disease. It permits the surgeon (1) to directly assess the anatomy and function of the valves and their supporting apparatus;[17,18] (2) to visualize the extent of fibrous/calcific involvement, which may determine whether a conservative repair is feasible;[22] and (3) to determine the degree and location of regurgitation using echocontrast or one of the Doppler mapping techniques.[114,115] After prosthetic valve replacement, it permits the detection of valvular regurgitation or paravalvular leak and the recording of baseline gradients. Following valvuloplasty, it allows detailed assessment of valvular function including precise localization and grading of residual or de novo incompetence (Fig. 16–45), the measurement of residual transvalvular gradients, and the direct recording of valve area. The presence of significant regurgita-

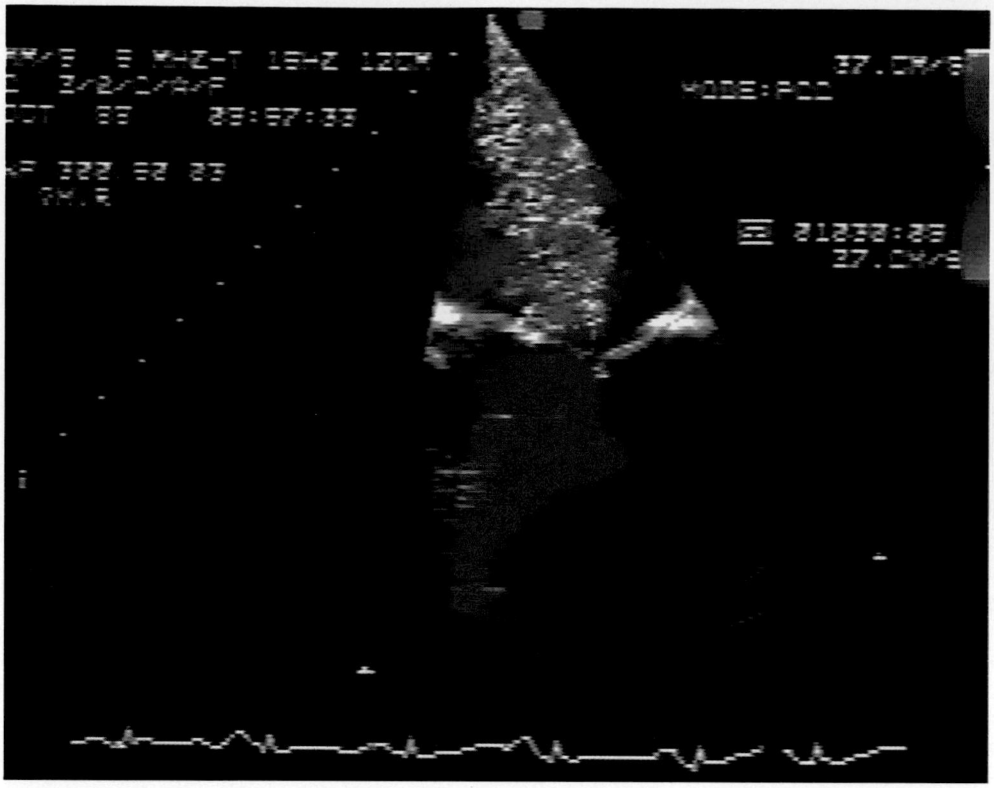

Fig. 16–45. Transesophageal color flow image illustrating residual mitral regurgitation following mitral valvuloplasty. The regurgitant jet depicted in the mosaic pattern is directed toward the transducer in the esophagus.

tion after removal from cardiopulmonary bypass permits additional valve repair or correction of prosthesis placement to be performed immediately.

Intraoperative echocardiography is particularly valuable in patients with combined aortic stenosis and moderate mitral regurgitation, because in some of these patients, the mitral regurgitation spontaneously improves after aortic valve replacement. Direct appreciation of this improvement may eliminate the need for mitral valve surgery.[22] Note that when either Doppler or contrast methods are used to assess intraoperative changes in the amount of regurgitation, studies must be performed at comparable intracavity pressures and, if possible, heart rates, because both of these factors can alter the degree of regurgitation independent of structural abnormalities of the valve or its supporting apparatus.

The significance of functional tricuspid regurgitation secondary to mitral stenosis or regurgitation is also often difficult to assess, and failure to appreciate its severity increases morbidity after mitral valve surgery.[116] Lesser degrees of tricuspid regurgitation are likely to diminish after the mitral lesion is corrected, while more severe regurgitation may persist and lead to progressive postoperative right ventricular dysfunction. Intraoperative evaluation of the degree of tricuspid regurgitation immediately after mitral valve repair allows the surgeon to determine whether tricuspid valve repair is necessary (Fig. 16–46). If the tricuspid valve is repaired, the efficacy of the repair can also be assessed before the patient leaves the operating room.

The use of intraoperative contrast to detect regurgitation may be complicated by the spontaneous bubbles that are frequently generated in the left atrium after open heart surgery[117] and must be differentiated from truly regurgitant bubbles (see following discussion). As a result, color flow mapping is generally preferred.

Assessment of Ventricular Structure and Function

One of the most important applications of intraoperative echocardiography is on-line assessment of myocardial function.[13–15,113] During the induction of anesthesia,

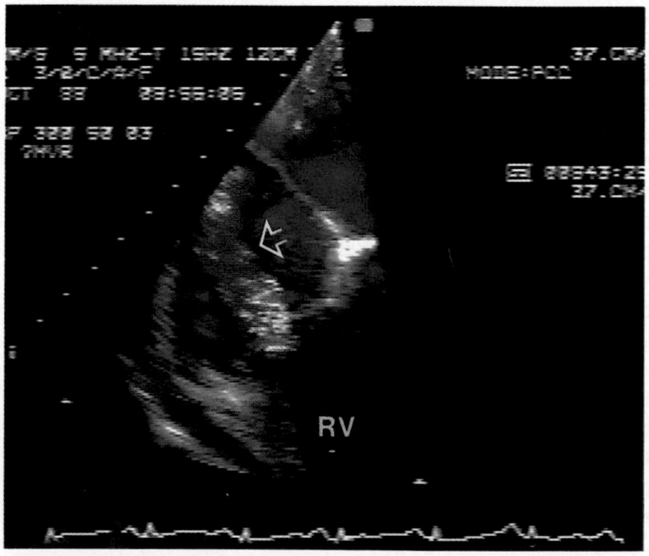

Fig. 16–46. Transesophageal color flow recording of residual tricuspid regurgitation (arrow) following mitral valve repair. The severity of the regurgitation in this case prompted repair of the tricuspid valve.

continuous monitoring of left ventricle function permits the anesthetist to detect the earliest signs of ischemia, manifest by the development of abnormal wall motion and/or thickening, and to take appropriate countermeasures. When ischemic dysfunction cannot be reversed, it suggests the need to move ahead rapidly to restore blood flow to the jeopardized region and thereby hopefully avoid intraoperative infarction.

With the chest open, normally, only the right ventricle and parts of the left ventricle are visible to the surgeon. Routine monitoring of the ECG and pulmonary and aortic hemodynamics are often insensitive to early ischemia. In experimental preparations, electrophysiologic changes rapidly follow the imposition of myocardial ischemia. However, the transthoracic ECG is relatively insensitive to subendocardial ischemia[118] and does not reflect abnormalities until minutes after changes in wall motion and lactate metabolism. Another major limitation of electrocardiography is the difficulty of detecting ischemia in the presence of conduction defects or ventricularly paced rhythms. The new occurrence of such conduction system defects is relatively common after cardiopulmonary bypass and does not accurately predict perioperative ischemia.[119,120] Studies, to date, suggest that the detection of ischemia during anesthesia and surgery, based on intraoperative wall motion abnormalities, is three to four times as sensitive as single or multiple lead intraoperative ECG monitoring.[121] Therefore, continuous monitoring of the left ventricle from the esophagus or periodic epicardial imaging may detect signs of ischemia (segmental wall motion abnormalities), which would otherwise be missed and can be immediately treated.[122]

Transesophageal echocardiography also permits detection of global or segmental changes in left ventricle function during aortic cross-clamping and the monitoring of left ventricle function in cardiac patients undergoing noncardiac procedures. Comparisons of TEE measurements of standard parameters such as left ventricular end-diastolic area, end-systolic area, and fractional area change have shown excellent correspondence to similar recordings made from the anterior cardiac surface immediately before and after pericardiotomy.[123] Continuous monitoring also provides clear evidence of improvement in wall motion or thickening when this occurs following bypass grafting. Transesophageal recordings are of particular value in the immediate postoperative period because they are free of the limited visualization and confounding translation that are found during transthoracic studies performed immediately after closure of the chest.

The echocardiogram can also fully evaluate left ventricular size and contractility intraoperatively and localize ventricular aneurysms. In patients with coronary artery disease, the response of the ventricle to various pharmacologic interventions can be evaluated both pre- and postoperatively and the decision to support ventricular function, pharmacologically or mechanically with intra-aortic balloon pumping or other assist devices, can be made more judiciously.[124]

Several studies have examined the effects of operative procedures on ventricular function using intraoperative echocardiography. Left ventricular ejection fraction has been shown to fall[124,125] in patients undergoing valve replacement for both mitral and aortic regurgitation, while ejection fraction increases after valve replacement for mitral and aortic stenosis.[124,125] After coronary bypass, reported changes in ventricular function have been variable, with improvement, no change, and depression of function all being recorded.[124–126] Early assessment of ventricular function has correlated well with results of other studies performed weeks to months after surgery, suggesting that hemodynamic alterations and underlying ventricular dysfunction are apparent immediately after the surgical procedure.[124,126]

In patients with hypertrophic cardiomyopathy, intraoperative epicardial echocardiography can guide the surgeon in determining the extent of myomectomy and evaluating the degree of baseline mitral regurgitation.[127] After surgery, echocardiographic imaging can permit exclusion of a ventricular septal defect and evaluation of ventricular function and residual mitral regurgitation. The degree of obstruction can also be assessed pre- and postmyectomy. Occasionally, obstructive hemodynamics similar to those of idiopathic hypertrophic subaortic stenosis (IHSS) are seen after routine operations in normal ventricles because of volume depletion and can cause elevated capillary wedge pressures and decreased cardiac output. The characteristic appearance of the ventricle and motion of the mitral valve in these cases can easily be observed.

Because of the interplay of multiple factors during and immediately after surgery, the operating room may not be the ideal physiology laboratory. Myocardial depressants (specifically, anesthetic agents, effect of aortic cross clamping, and different methods of myocardial preservation), pericardiotomy, hemolysis, anemia and subsequent volume loading, vasodilatory and inotropic agents, alterations in preload and afterload, and atrial pacing may all influence ventricular contractility and may affect the ejection fraction. Direct visualization of ventricular function, however, regardless of which influencing factors are predominant, is invaluable in guiding the surgeon's and anesthesiologist's therapeutic response.[77]

Continuous Monitoring of Cardiac Output

Cardiac output can also be monitored continuously using either the aortic flow velocity profile and vessel diameter or the corresponding pulmonary flow profile and area measurements. Such measurements have been shown to correlate closely with thermodilution measurements of cardiac output.[15] When serial changes in ventricular output are of interest, it is often simpler and more accurate to simply record changes in the velocity integral or stroke distance and assume that the vessel diameter remains constant.

Assessment of Myocardial Perfusion

Cold potassium cardioplegic solution is routinely infused into the aortic root to reduce myocardial metabolic requirements during aortic cross-clamping.[16] Significant coronary stenoses may impede cardioplegic flow, however, thereby leaving myocardial regions potentially ischemic. In patients with multivessel coronary disease, it is frequently difficult to determine the myocardial region at greatest ischemic jeopardy. Use of the echo-contrast effect permits imaging of cardioplegic flow as it perfuses the myocardium. This can be achieved by agitating or sonicating the cardioplegic solution before injection to induce microbubble formation and then following its distribution based on the echo-contrast effect. Areas not perfused do not show an increase in reflectance (whiteness), continue to finely fibrillate, and can be easily detected by TEE or epicardial echocardiography. This method appears most beneficial in detecting septal perfusion, which cannot be assessed by visual inspection or epicardial temperature probes. When an underperfused region is identified, the surgeon can provide selective cardioplegia distal to a proximal stenosis or can first perform proximal and distal coronary anastomosis to the ischemic region. When epicardial imaging is available, it appears preferred for this application because of its greater speed and flexibility.

Detection of Intracardiac Shunts

Intraoperative epicardial and/or esophageal echocardiography (Doppler or contrast) can permit assessment of the presence and severity of congenital, traumatic, or ischemic heart disease complicated by interventricular, interatrial, or extracardiac shunts.[128,129] Saline solution injected on the right side of the heart can permit detection of right-to-left shunts (Fig. 16–47), and injections on the left side of the heart can permit assessment of left-to-right shunts. Color flow Doppler imaging can provide similar information (Fig. 16–48). A minimal residual shunt may persist postoperatively at the margin of the patch material used for repair of interventricular and intra-atrial shunts.[67] Therefore, possible significant residual shunt after an operative procedure should be evaluated by intraoperative contrast or Doppler echocardiography to detect potential suture dehiscence or inadequate repair.

Congenital Heart Disease

Intraoperative echocardiography with contrast injections or flow mapping can permit localization of intracardiac shunts and definition of complex anatomy that may be difficult to fully appreciate by preoperative catheterization or closed chest imaging. The echocardiogram can also permit rapid assessment of the adequacy of shunt repairs and conduits before the patient leaves the operating room. This technique should allow a more aggressive approach to complex cardiac reconstructions, because the surgeon would be able to image the heart and evaluate the adequacy of the surgical repair during and immediately after the operative procedure. Given the complexity of the anatomy being studied, epicardial imaging appears preferred for this application.

Cardiac Tumors and Masses

Most cardiac tumors and masses are adequately diagnosed preoperatively. The extent of malignant tumors involving the heart, however, is often inadequately assessed by preoperative echocardiography or even computed tomography. Intraoperative imaging is effective in outlining the extent of disease and multichamber involvement unsuspected preoperatively. When an operation has entailed extensive reconstruction of cardiac chambers after removal of intracardiac tumors, the

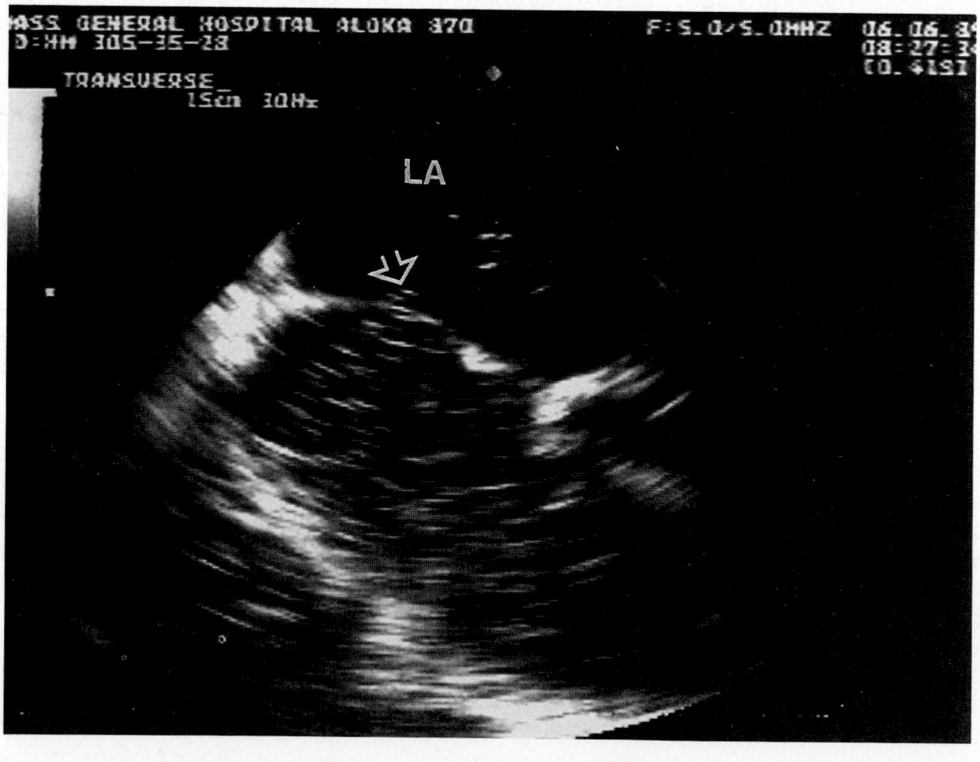

Fig. 16–47. Transesophageal recording of right-to-left shunting at the atrial level following direct right atrial injection of agitated saline. The arrow points to several bubbles passing through the septum via a patent foramen ovale. Five additional bubbles can be seen floating free in the left atrium (LA).

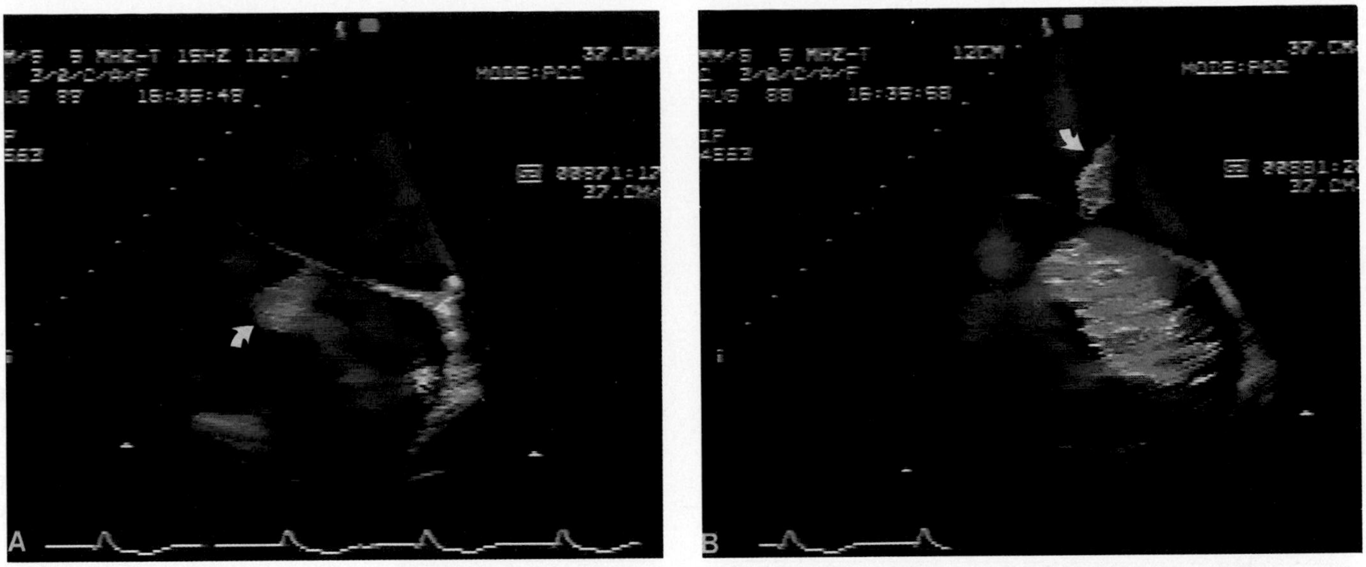

Fig. 16–48. Transesophageal color flow recordings of an alternating left-to-right **(A)** and right-to-left shunt **(B)** through an atrial septal defect created by a prior balloon valvuloplasty. The shunt in each case is indicated by the arrow.

echocardiogram is extremely helpful in assessing the adequacy of the procedure.[22]

Localization of the Longitudinal and Circumferential Extent of Aortic Dissection

Ascending aortic dissection (type 1) carries a high morbidity and mortality. Intraoperative imaging of the aorta should permit proper identification of the proximal origin of the dissection and detection of concomitant aortic valve involvement. This should facilitate surgical repair, which may improve survival. TEE also permits imaging of the descending aorta and arch, and the combination of procedures should allow complete visualization of aortic integrity and flow.[10–12]

Evaluation of the Epicardial Coronary Arteries and Bypass Grafts

Several research studies have suggested that high frequency epicardial echocardiography may permit visualization of the epicardial coronary arteries, location of atherosclerotic lesions, and assessment of bypass graft anastomoses. This exciting area, still in the early stages of investigation, is discussed in the preceding section on epicardial echocardiography.

Detection of Intracavitary Bubble Formation and Their Relationship to Air Emboli

Major central nervous system complications occur in approximately 5% of patients undergoing cardiac surgical procedures.[130,131] Although the specific origin of central nervous system complications is unknown, air embolism is certainly one of the many potential causes and is believed to be responsible for at least some postoperative strokes. Air embolism during cardiac surgery is particularly dreaded because this complication is potentially avoidable.

Using TEE, it is possible to continuously monitor the left ventricle, atrium, and aorta for the presence of microbubbles introduced during surgery (Fig. 16–49). Importantly, in comparative studies, TEE and precordial Doppler ultrasound were shown to be more sensitive methods for detecting intravascular air than alternative approaches such as recording pulmonary artery pressure, end-tidal CO_2, arterial oxygen tension, and transcutaneous oxygen tension. Not surprisingly, given its broader field of view and superior ability to record the signal from small numbers of bubbles, TEE imaging has proven more sensitive than Doppler.

TEE intraoperative monitoring has shown evidence of intracardiac microbubbles in a high percentage of patients (up to 62%) after cardiopulmonary bypass is discontinued.[56,132,133] Although the number of bubbles appearing in any given patient is variable, large numbers of bubbles have been found in roughly 26% of these cases.[71] Microbubbles are found far more often following valve replacement than coronary bypass surgery (roughly 80 vs. 10%).[56,71,72] Although microbubbles can be detected easily with ultrasound techniques, their clinical significance is not known. In one study,[56] no gross neurologic deficits developed, despite the presence of bubbles in 62% of patients. In a second study, transient central nervous system disturbances occurred in 3 of 14 patients with microbubbles evident, while in a third, prolonged encephalopathy occurred in 7 patients but was present in 4 patients without observable bubbles in addition to the 3 in whom bubbles were present.[71] Manual attempts to eradicate bubbles have also met with varying success.[71,72] At present, therefore, although TEE is clearly the most sensitive tool for identifying patients who develop intracavitary micro- or macrobubbles following cardiopulmonary bypass, their significance and the approach to be taken when they are found is unclear.

In addition to its applications in cardiac surgery, TEE may be a more sensitive and accurate method for detect-

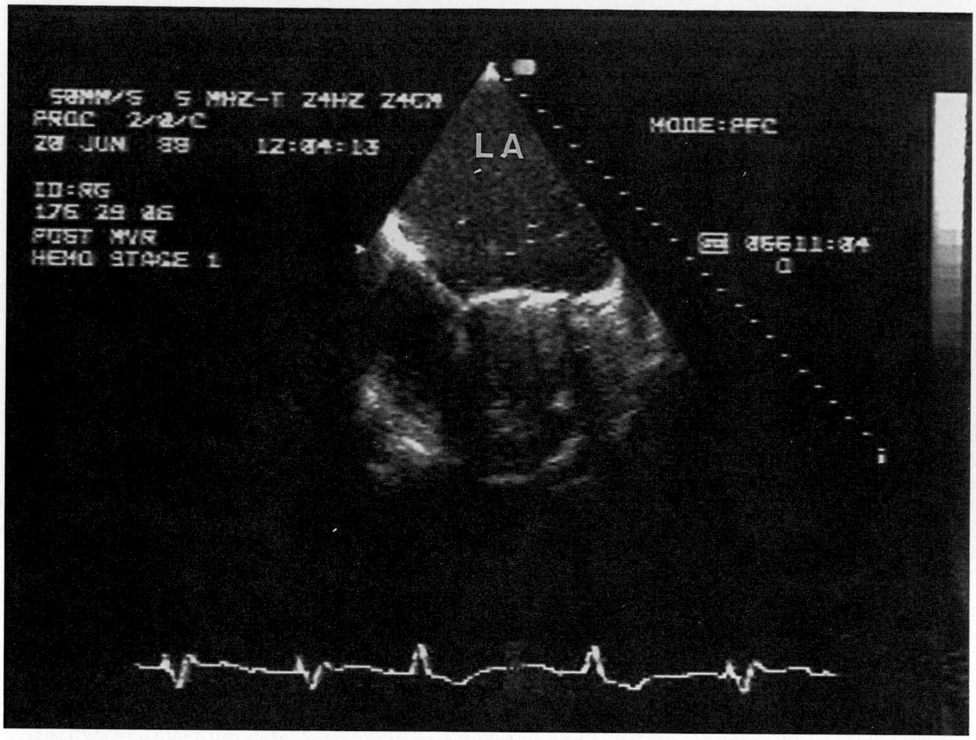

Fig. 16–49. Microbubbles in the left atrium detected during reperfusion following cardiac bypass and mitral valve replacement with a St. Jude valve. LA = left atrium.

ing venous air and fat embolism than other commonly used monitors in patients undergoing neurosurgical and orthopedic procedures.[20] This approach may also permit detection of air in the aorta in patients experiencing paradoxic air embolism during surgery resulting from intracardiac or pulmonary shunts.[21]

Summary

Intraoperative epicardial echocardiography is a relatively simple technique to learn and teach. The procedure is expedited when it is performed by the surgeon. Intraoperative echocardiograms allow precise definitions of both myocardial and valvular function. The technique allows immediate pre- and postoperative imaging, facilitating the earliest detection of valvular and ventricular dysfunction, which can significantly reduce therapeutic response time. The entire procedure, in experienced hands, should take no more than 1 to 2 minutes per imaging period. The apparatus can remain in the surgical suite and can be used as often as required by the surgeon without concern for adverse effects to the patient. At this juncture, there are no known risks or complications of the procedure, and none should be expected, as long as sterile technique is maintained.[22] Use of the transesophageal approach provides more limited information but permits continuous monitoring and does not interfere with the operative field or require the surgeon to take the time to perform an additional task.

CATHETER-BASED IMAGING AND FLOW RECORDING: INTRAVASCULAR AND INTRACARDIAC IMAGING AND FLOW VELOCITY RECORDINGS

The first catheter-based imaging system was described by Cieszynski in 1960.[134] During the next 25 years, a variety of catheter-based ultrasonic devices were developed and applied. These included two-dimensional imaging catheters that could record the dynamic motion of the internal circumference of the left ventricle,[135] high-frequency M-mode catheters capable of defining subtle functional changes (e.g., right atrial wall thickening) inapparent from the chest wall,[136,137] and Doppler catheters for recording intracoronary flow both at baseline and following a variety of interventions.[138,139] Despite this clearly demonstrated capability for catheter-based ultrasonic recording of intracardiac structure and function and intravascular flow, the method attracted little attention. This lack of enthusiasm was primarily due to the absence of a clearly defined, unique application that would justify the necessary development of instrumentation and catheters necessary to extend this previously noninvasive imaging technique broadly into the interventional arena.

More recently, the recent rapid advance in interventional catheter techniques for the treatment of atherosclerotic lesions and the more aggressive pharmacologic strategies for lowering serum lipids made clear the need for more specific diagnostic information about vessel wall morphology and response to therapy. Currently available techniques such as angiography and more recently angioscopy are limited in that they cannot look beneath the surface of the vessel, where the atherosclerotic process begins and develops. They also cannot fully assess the effects of interventions on vessel wall and plaque morphology. Newer methods to assess coronary arteries, e.g., computerized tomography or magnetic resonance imaging, have yet to achieve a resolution sufficient to distinguish the different wall layers of medium-sized vessels.

Catheter-based ultrasonic imaging, in contrast, has the ability to look beneath the luminal surface and provide high resolution dynamic images of the vessel. Using this technique, the physician can determine lumen size and wall thickness, define vessel layers, identify the presence of atherosclerotic plaque, and reasonably estimate plaque composition. In addition, it permits assessment of the alterations in vessel wall morphology produced by various interventions and, it is hoped, will permit both definition of lesions most suitable for specific types of interventional devices and, in some cases, tailoring of therapy. This combination of need and capability has accelerated progress in catheter development and directed the current focus toward the coronary arteries, aorta, and peripheral vessels, where atherosclerosis is most prevalent. The following section therefore begins with a discussion of intravascular imaging, followed by intracardiac imaging and intravascular Doppler.

Intravascular Imaging

Instrumentation

General Principles. Routine ultrasonic interrogation of vascular walls from an intraluminal location has been made possible by the development of low profile (1.1 to 3 mm in diameter), flexible catheters that can be passed over conventional arterial guide wires (0.014 inches) and directed safely into the more distal arteries of most vascular beds, including the coronary arteries. Intraluminal imaging catheters can use high frequency ultrasound (up to 40 MHz) because of the close apposition of the catheter tip and transducer to the vessel wall, the low attenuation of the intervening fluid medium, and the small vessel diameters that must be penetrated. These frequencies permit structures on the order of 150 μm to be resolved and many of the components of the vascular wall to be distinguished.[140,141]

To construct two-dimensional ultrasound images in real time, the ultrasound beam must be rapidly directed to different areas of the target. As in other areas of ultrasonography, two approaches to real-time intraluminal scanning have been developed—electronic and mechanical.[142]

Mechanical Intraluminal Imaging Catheters. The simplest method for obtaining rapid tomographic images of vessels is to mechanically direct the ultrasound beam through a 360° arc around the catheter. This is most commonly achieved by (1) mechanical rotation of a single crystal within the tip of an intraluminal catheter (direct view design) (Fig. 16–50A) or (2) use of a fixed transducer with a mechanically rotated mirror that deflects the ultrasonic beam at a right angle to the catheter (rotating mirror design) (Fig. 16–50B).

The direct view design, in which the piezoelectric element is mounted roughly parallel to the long axis of the catheter, allows the sound beam to proceed directly away from the catheter. This design provides the largest possible aperture in a plane perpendicular to the catheter long axis and produces the shortest sound path from the transducer to the vessel wall. As a result, relatively little of the near-field focal zone is wasted within the catheter, and the best lateral resolution at the vessel wall is achieved. This design also minimizes the amount of machinery or electronics at the catheter tip, giving more

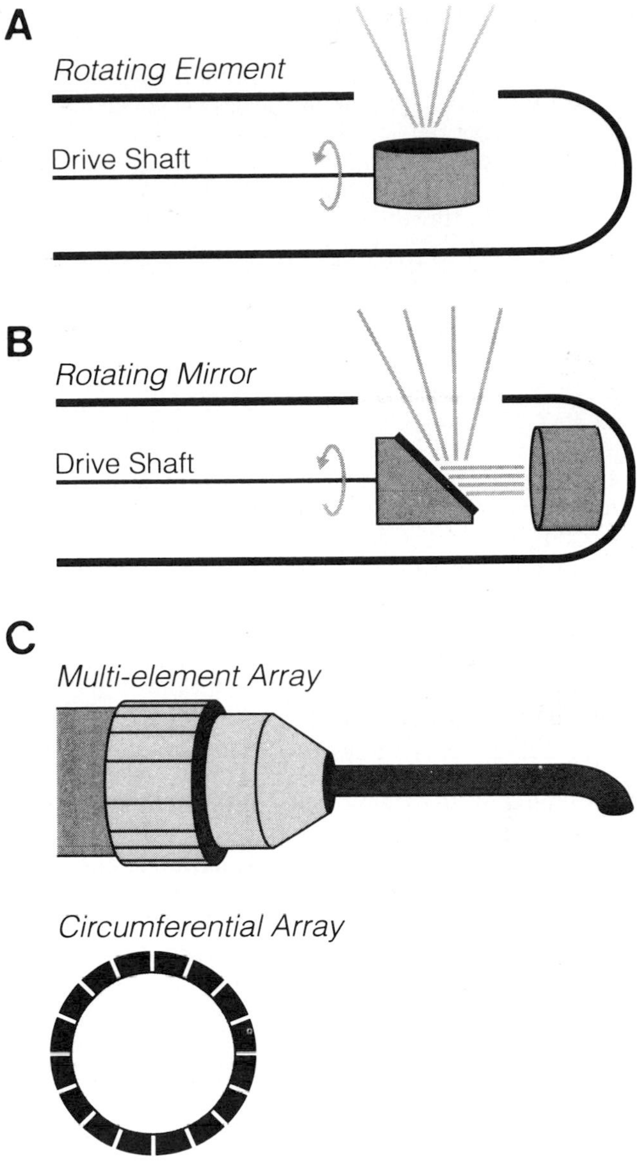

Fig. 16–50. Intravascular ultrasound transducer designs. **A.** Mechanical device with rotatory crystal. **B.** Mechanical device with rotating mirror. **C.** Electronic device with a multiple element array. (From Nissen SE, Gurley JC: Application of intravascular ultrasound for detection and quantification of coronary atherosclerosis. Int J Cardiac Imaging 6:165, 1991. Reproduced with permission from Kluwer Academic Publishers.)

flexibility to the assembly, which aids in catheter positioning within the arterial bed.[143]

Unfortunately, direct view catheters are subject to ring-down artifacts, which appear as a bright circle or halo around the outer surface of the catheter. Because imaging is often done within tenths of millimeters from the transducer face, the system electronics damp the transmit pulse quickly to eliminate halo artifacts near the catheter surface, which can obscure objects close to the transducer. Similar artifacts can be caused by reverberations between the transducer and catheter sheath. The transducer can be positioned at a slight angle to the sheath to suppress these acoustic vibrations; however, the result is imperfect, and new problems are introduced.

The rotating mirror design tends to increase the sound path within the catheter thereby and to suppress the reverberations and halo artifacts common with the direct view design. The disadvantages of this design are (1) part of the near field focal zone is lost during passage along the extended sound path within the catheter; (2) strong echoes from the wires to the element can appear in the image in those catheters in which the mirror rotates proximal to a stationary element; and (3) the mirror assembly, wires, and need to maintain precise alignment between the transducer and mirror tend to increase the stiffness of the end of the catheter, which can impede placement within tortuous anatomy.[143]

In all mechanical designs, the transducer or mirror is rotated by a flexible drive cable within the catheter assembly, which is connected to a motor at the proximal end. The transducer/mirror can be rotated at variable speeds, typically ranging from 600 to 1800 rpm, yielding 10 to 30 frames/sec. Catheters with transducer frequencies ranging from 10 to 40 MHz have been developed, with lower frequencies generally being used for intracardiac applications and higher frequencies for intravascular imaging. For a representative 30-MHz mechanical transducer, the reported axial resolution at the focal point is 150 μm. The lateral resolution depends on transducer aperture size, frequency, focusing, and catheter design. In the near field of the transducer (roughly 5 to 7 mm including the sound path in the catheter), lateral resolution may be as fine as 200 μm; however, beyond the focal zone, the beam diverges rapidly, and in the far field, lateral resolution is generally poor.

Advantages and Disadvantages of Single-Crystal Mechanical Designs. The mechanical systems are simple to design, provide high resolution images, and require no complicated acoustic or electronic technology. Single-crystal transducers also have the advantage of greater output power and signal-to-noise characteristics than multielement arrays.

The disadvantages of mechanical systems include (1) the need for a central drive shaft to rotate the transducer or mirror, which precludes the use of a central guide wire and makes it more difficult to combine mechanical imaging systems with other types of catheters; (2) lack of flexibility of a small (5- to 8-mm) region at the tip of the catheter containing the transducer element, making it more difficult to image the more tortuous segments of the coronary tree; (3) occasional distortion of the ultrasound image, which can be caused by variable rotational velocity of the drive shaft, resulting in a "rubber sheet" deformation of the image; and (4) the fact that all mechanical transducers ride on an external guide wire that adds at least 1 French (Fr) to the catheter diameter and can often be seen in the ultrasonic image.

Electronic Multiple-Element Arrays

Phased Arrays. The first real-time intraluminal scanner was developed in 1972 by Bom et al.[142] The array included 16 transducer elements embedded around the circumference of a 3-mm catheter (Fig. 16–51). Because each element in the array was small compared to the ultrasound wavelength, a directed ultrasound beam could not be generated from any single element. Hence, directional ultrasound scanning was produced by combining the responses of several elements, as shown in Figure 16–52. The beam shown in position 1 is formed by summing the incoming signals from each of the active elements (blackened in the figure), after introduction of a phase delay, which compensates for the acoustic path difference from each of the elements. The next acoustic beam is formed by rotating the active group of elements

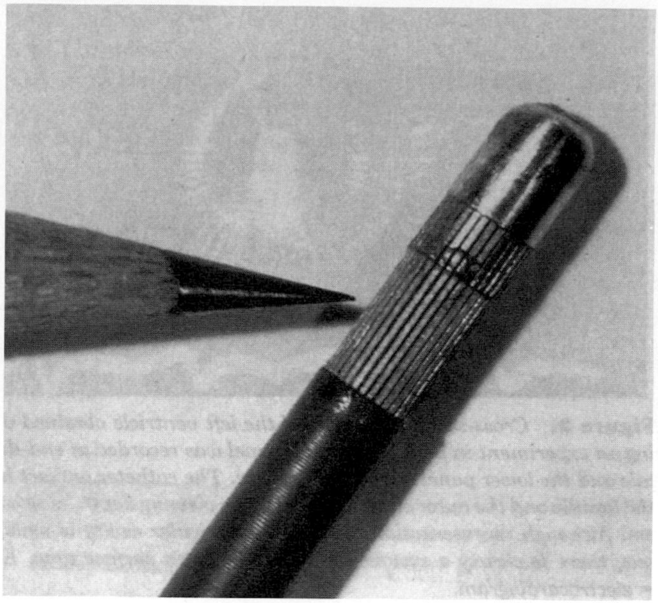

Fig. 16–51. Comparison of the size of the original intracardiac catheter tip array transducer to the head of a pencil. (From Bom N, Lancee CT, Van Egmond FC: An ultrasonic intracardiac scanner. Ultrasonics 10(2):72, 1972.)

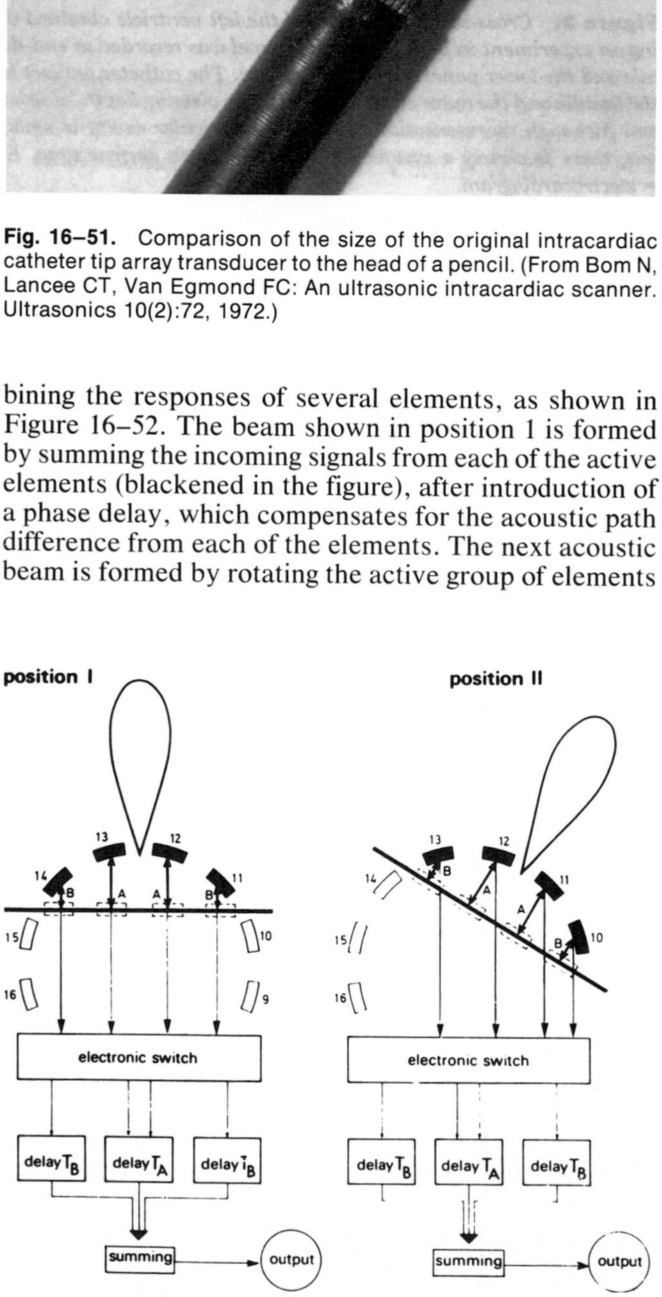

Fig. 16–52. Directional ultrasound scanning produced with multiple-element arrays (see text for details). (From Bom N, Lancee CT, Van Egmond FC: An ultrasonic intracardiac scanner. Ultrasonics 10(2):72, 1972.)

as illustrated. The total number of beams created in this way is equal to the number of elements in the complete array. The acoustic aperture is fixed, so that the acoustic power and degree of focusing (which affects lateral resolution) at any point in the image plane is predetermined.

Synthetic Aperture Arrays. Although Bom's system was capable of real-time intracardiac scanning, recent technological advances have allowed the refinements necessary for imaging small to medium-sized arteries. Hodgson et al. described the operation of a catheter-based array of 64 elements, in which the effective acoustic aperture is varied according to the distance from the array surface to the target.[144] Each element is activated alone, and its response recorded in a digital memory bank. After all the elements around the circumference have been sequentially activated, digital processing creates a "synthetic" aperture, by combining the signals from groups of elements. The computer refers to a preset focus map, which contains delay and amplitude weighting factors for the response of each element. The delay and weighting factors vary for each element, depending on the distance to the target and whether or not the target is central or peripheral in the acoustic field of that particular element. For the near field, the responses from a small number of elements are combined, to keep the effective near-field aperture small and hence improve the lateral resolution in close proximity to the catheter. For more distant points in the acoustic field, more elements are grouped together. The larger the synthetic aperture created, the longer the length of the near-field where focusing and lateral resolution are optimized.

Because of the tight radius of curvature of the catheter, however, the effective aperture is smaller for an array-tipped catheter than for a mechanical catheter of the same diameter. Grating lobes have also been a problem when groups of elements are fired in sequence.[145]

Advantages and Disadvantages of Array Designs. Electronic scanning by an array eliminates the need for moving parts. This allows flexibility in catheter design, because there is no need to accommodate a long mechanical drive shaft. As a result, catheters can be made smaller, are more flexible, and the nonuniform rotational distortion that occurs in mechanical systems is eliminated.

However, because array crystal elements are mounted on the catheter surface, the ring-down artifact caused by crystal oscillations fills the zone immediately adjacent to the crystals. While the ring-down artifact can be electronically eliminated, nothing can be imaged within this space. Additionally, the peak power generated by array crystals is less than that of a comparably sized single-crystal transducer, with the result that ultrasound penetration and signal/noise ratio are poorer.[146]

Normal Arterial Structure and Imaging Characteristics

To interpret the images produced by intraluminal catheters, it is necessary to be familiar with the structure of arterial wall and the normally expected interactions between ultrasound with its varying components.

Histology. Arteries are three-layered structures comprising a thin inner layer, the intima; a muscular, or musculoelastic, middle layer, the media; and an outer connective tissue layer, the adventitia. Thin layers of concentrically arranged elastic fibers, the internal and external elastic lamina, separate the intima from the media and the media from the adventitia. Arteries are subclassified based on the structure of the media into muscular (coronaries, femoral, and more distal leg arteries), elastic (aorta, proximal coronaries), and transitional types (iliac). The media of muscular arteries is composed mainly of smooth muscle cells with very few elastic lamellae, resulting in a relatively homogeneous layer. The normal medial thickness in adult *coronary arteries* ranges from 125 to 350 μm (average, 200).[147] Elastic arteries differ from muscular arteries in that the medial is composed of densely packed, concentrically arranged elastin fibers with interspersed smooth muscle cells. The difference in elastic and muscular arteries is illustrated in Figure 16–53.

The intima is primarily involved in the evolution of coronary disease and has been studied most extensively. The intima is the region of the arterial wall extending from the endothelial surface at the lumen to the internal elastic lamina. The internal elastic lamina defines the border between the intima and media but is generally considered part of the media. An internal elastic lamina is absent in some parts of geometric transitions of arteries such as bifurcations, branches, and curvatures, and in these regions, recognition of the demarkation between the intima and media may be difficult.

The thickness of the arterial intima is not uniform. The range of normal thickness is broad and is conveniently expressed quantitatively as an intima/media ratio. This ratio may vary from 0.1 to 1.0 or more in normal arteries of humans.[148] Thick segments of intima exist in arteries obtained from healthy human subjects of all ages and from many other species. The thick segments may be focal (eccentric) or may be more extensive (diffuse). In human coronary arteries, eccentric thickening has been observed from the first week of life and thereafter, although considerable individual variation in degree is found. Adaptive intimal thickening is the result of a range of physiologic stimuli and is an attempt by the tissue to maintain normal conditions of flow, wall tension, or both in response to changes in pulse rate, blood pressure, arterial geometry, flow rate, and resistance to flow in distal vascular segments and in supplied organs.[149]

Atherosclerosis tends to develop first in areas of adaptive luminal thickening; however, thickening may exist for decades without any accumulation of atherogenic lipoproteins.[149]

Imaging Characteristics: Theoretic Considerations. Three factors primarily determine the ultrasonic image obtained from an arterial wall: (1) the reflective properties of the tissue components and their pattern of organization, (2) the dynamic range and resolution of the recording device, and (3) the pattern of interaction between the ultrasound beam and the arterial wall.

Reflective Properties of Arterial Wall. Ultrasound is reflected at interfaces between structures (tissues) of dif-

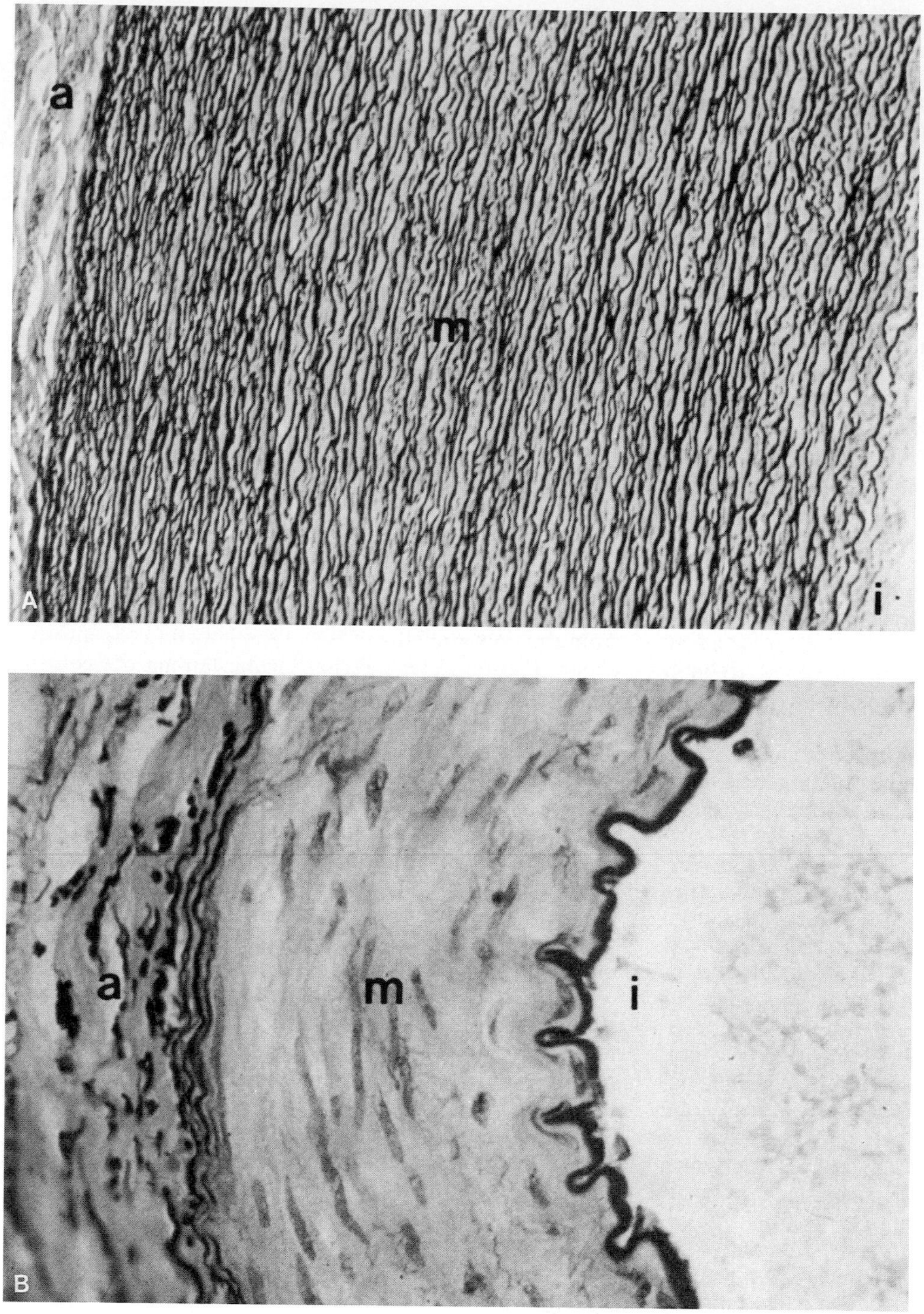

Fig. 16–53. Histologic pattern of elastic **(A)** and muscular **(B)** arteries. **A.** The media (m) of the elastic artery contains many elastic fibers, appearing dense and homogeneous. **B.** The media (m) of the muscular artery contains few elastic fibers and appears distinct from the intima (i) and adventitia (a). From Goss CM (ed.), Anatomy of the Human Body. Philadelphia, Lea & Febiger, p. 1251, 1962.

fering acoustic impedance. The acoustic impedance of the various tissues that make up arteries varies with their density, compressibility, and viscosity. Calcium salts are the most highly reflective substance followed by organized elastic tissue, fibrous tissue, smooth muscle, and other cellular elements. Layers of tissue composed of cellular elements of similar acoustic impedance (i.e., the muscular media) produce few internal reflections, whereas layers composed of organized tissue planes of varying density (i.e., the media of elastic arteries and the internal and external elastic lamina) may be highly reflective. Intensely reflective regions such as collections of calcium salts often return all of the ultrasonic energy that impacts on their surface, preventing any echo production by more distal structures.[141]

The Dynamic Range and Resolution of the Instrument. The dynamic range of an instrument, which is the range from the signal saturation level of the amplifiers to the noise floor, determines the weakest signals that can be perceived as distinct. This characteristic defines both the weakest reflectors that can be detected and displayed and the smallest difference in the signal amplitude reflected from different tissue elements that can be distinguished. Thus, an instrument with a low dynamic range may fail to detect interfaces at both the borders of layers and those between tissue components within layers, which are clearly defined by a more sensitive device (Fig. 16–54). The impact of the dynamic range is modified by intrinsic tissue reflectivity, and because diseased arteries generally contain more highly reflective elements such as collagen, elastin fibrils, and calcium, more components of the wall will be visualized by a lower dynamic range instrument when an artery is diseased than normal. Increasing output power also increases echo strength and thus the sensitivity of the instrument.

Resolution determines the separation between structures that is required for them to be displayed as distinct. For a transducer with an axial resolution of 150 μm, the lumen-intimal echo must be greater than 150 μm from the internal elastic lamina for it to be interpreted as separate. If these two layers are closer together, a single echo will be detected that is the sum of the two. Without discrete borders, the intima will be inapparent. If the width of the composite echo is taken as the width of the intima, intimal size will be overestimated, because the internal elastic lamina is part of the media and it will be broadened by the trail-edge effect of the signal. Because normal intima is frequently less than 0.1 mm in thickness, this occurrence is not infrequent.[140] Confusion quickly arises as the distinction between borders and layers becomes blurred. For example, when the echo from the lumen-intimal border fuses with that of the internal elastic lamina, the combined echo should roughly approximate intimal thickness. If, in contrast, the lumen-intima echo is not recorded as a result of a poor signal/noise ratio, then the echo from the internal elastic lamina will be the border echo and will bear a relationship to intimal thickness by chance only, because both are small.

Pattern of Interaction Between the Ultrasound Beam and the Arterial Wall. The amplitude of the echo reflected from an interface depends not only on the input power and difference in acoustic impedance of the tissue but also on the angle at which the beam strikes the interface. Maximal reflectance occurs when the beam strikes the target at a 90° angle but decreases rapidly as the angle of intersection increases. Thus, for an intraluminal catheter, the strongest signals from all targets should be obtained when the catheter is in the center of and coaxial with the vessel. As the catheter is moved from the center of the vessel, the echoes from targets toward and away from the vector of motion will remain roughly the same in amplitude, but all others will decrease because the beam no longer intersects these targets at a right angle. This is true not only for the intima but for all vessel layers. With the catheter in the center of the vessel, the same effect will be observed if the catheter is angled so the sound plane intersects the wall obliquely. In this case, the echoes from the intercepts of the minor dimension should be unaffected, while those closer to the intercept of the major dimension will be reduced because of the increasing angle at which the beam strikes the wall. Again, disease will generally increase tissue density and surface irregularity, diminishing but not negating these effects. In summary, because there are several types of artery, the internal components of these arteries differ in health and disease, and the manner in which the same components are displayed can differ depending on the type imaging system used and the angle at which the beam intersects the wall, extensive correlation is necessary to interpret the image data arising from this complex system.

Correlation With Histology: General Observations and Limitations

The origin of the echoes in intravascular images has been established primarily by comparing in vitro ultrasonic recordings with light micrographs obtained from the same arterial section. Although the state in which the vessel is studied (pressure perfused vs. immersed, fixed vs. fresh) creates some differences in both the ultrasonic and histologic appearance of the artery, general observations appear consistent. In normal muscular arteries, the intima is represented by a single circumferential echo, which represents the confluence of the echoes from the lumen-intimal interface and the internal elastic lamina (Fig. 16–55). As the intima thickens, these two interfaces can generally be separated, and the intervening space has a reticular pattern of faint echoes (Fig. 16–56).[150] The media lies beneath the internal elastic lamina and in muscular arteries appears anechoic or hypoechoic. This pattern is due to the homogenous nature

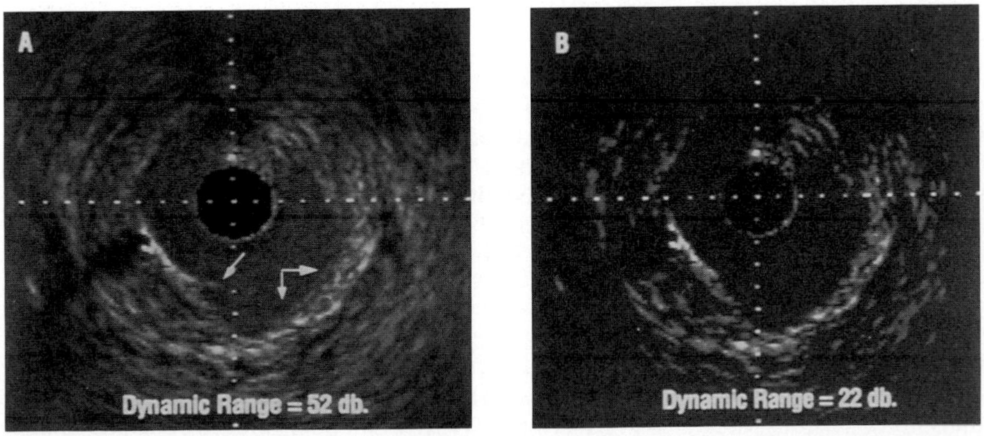

Fig. 16–54. Artery imaged with a high **(A)** and low **(B)** dynamic range. (Reproduced with permission from Dr. P.L. Fitzgerald. Unpublished data.)

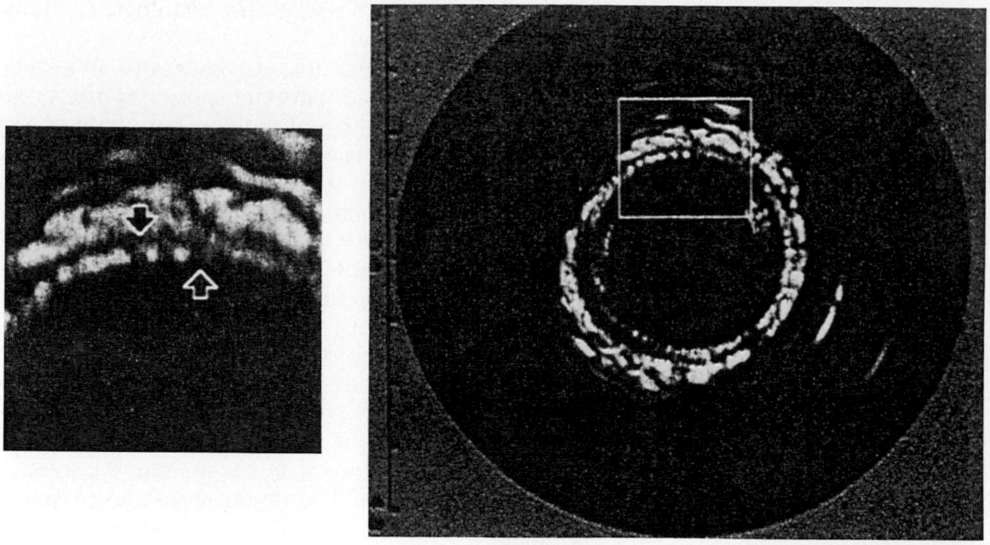

Fig. 16–55. Layers of a muscular artery imaged by intravascular echocardiography in vitro: intima (inner bright line), media (dark line), and adventitia (outer bright line). (From Nissen SE, Gurley JC: Application of intravascular ultrasound for detection and quantification of coronary atherosclerosis. Int J Cardiac Imaging 6:165, 1991. Reproduced with permission from Kluwer Academic Publishers.)

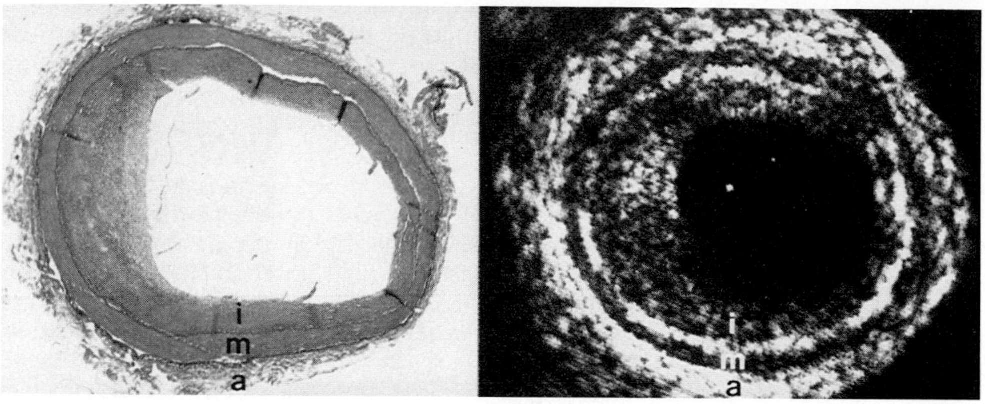

Fig. 16–56. Left. Histologic section from the right coronary artery showing an eccentric fibrous plaque. Right. Bright and fairly homogeneous echoes are reflected by the fibrous tissue in the corresponding ultrasound image. The internal elastic lamina is clearly seen between the intima and the media in both images. a = adventitia; m = media; i = intima. (From Potkin BN, et al.: Coronary artery imaging with intravascular high-frequency ultrasound. Circulation 81:1575, 1990. Reproduced by permission of the American Heart Association, Inc.)

of this muscle layer, which is composed of smooth muscle cells and is practically devoid of elastic components. The fact that this echo-free zone represents the media has been confirmed both by direct histologic comparison and by imaging the arterial wall after dissection of the adventitia from the media. The adventitia in contrast is generally highly reflective as a result of the presence of collagen bands within loose connective tissue. When smooth muscle is absent from the adventitia or occupies only its outer fringe, the interface between the media and adventitia is distinct on both macroscopic and ultrasound examination. When smooth muscle is diffusely intermixed with collagen, the adventitial smooth muscle blends with that of the media, and the ultrasound appearance is more diffusely homogeneous, blurring the boundary between the two layers.[151]

In vitro comparisons of ultrasonic images of elastic arteries with histologic sections reveals a similar, single reflective layer from the intima. The media of elastic arteries, however, such as the aorta, is composed of elastic lamellae, which are highly reflective and whose dense arrangement produces a bright homogeneous tissue layer, which is of similar intensity to intima. In arteries in which the adventitia contains dense collagen, the entire wall image is bright and homogeneous (Fig. 16–57). However, when the adventitia contains loose collagen with little or no smooth muscle, a media-adventitia interface is seen. Depending on the relative density of the two layers, either can appear brighter, or the pattern can be completely homogeneous without any distinct layers visible. This is also true for transitional arteries where the density and locations of tissue concentrations within layers varies. This can result in images in which the arterial wall appears homogeneous or in which either the media or adventitia is brighter, and hence the two layers are separable.

Ultrasonic images recorded in vitro may not be totally representative of those obtained in vivo. Fixation causes arteries to shrink and as a result, borders become irregular or wrinkled. This increases the reflectivity of interfaces such as the internal elastic lamina and often permits tissue layer discrimination, which cannot be obtained in clinical studies.

Although the classic three-layer appearance is generally observed in clinical images of coronary arteries, this has not been a universal finding.[152,153] Such variation is to be expected given the small space between individual arterial layers relative to the resolution of current imaging systems, the displayed echo width, and the changes in echo intensity that can be produced by small changes

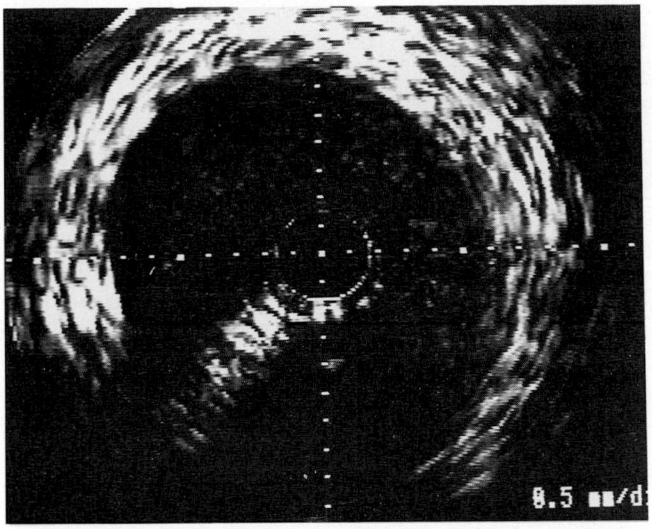

Fig. 16–57. In vitro ultrasound imaging of a canine aorta, showing a dense homogeneous wall. The probe, in the center of the picture, creates an artifact at the 7-o'clock position.

in catheter position. Often, images of arterial wall will change with millimeter movements of the catheter. Fortunately, information from adjacent sections can be extrapolated to fill in missing data. Note that the left main coronary artery changes from elastic to muscular in its first few millimeters. As a result, arterial images will likewise change from homogeneous to three-layered over this transition.

Accuracy of Intravascular Ultrasound in Measuring Arterial Lumen Diameter and Cross-Sectional Area

Many studies have been performed to validate ultrasonic measurements of lumen diameter and wall thickness by comparison with phantoms, histologic sections, and angiography.

Phantoms. The accuracy of distance and area measurements by ultrasonic catheter-based systems has been confirmed by several authors using phantoms of known size.[151,154] Extremely close correlations have been reported (r = .98) with differences on the order of 0.1 mm. For small phantoms, the results have been virtually identical; however, slight but increasing deviation from the line of identity is noted as phantom size increases. This trend appears to relate to difficulties in positioning the catheter precisely coaxial with the phantom and reflects the increase in absolute error that will occur for the same deviation from perpendicular as phantom size increases.

Dimensional measurements are identical whether the catheter is central or eccentric within the phantom as long as the long axis of the catheter is parallel to that of the phantom.[151]

Histology. Ultrasonic area measurements have correlated closely (r = .85 to .98) with those determined from pathologic sections.[150,151,154] The best correlation (r = .98) was achieved by comparing images recorded from pressure-perfused arteries with histologic measurements obtained following pressure perfusion fixation (Fig. 16–58).[151] Discrepancies observed in other studies have been systematic and attributed to geometric distortion and shrinkage of tissue during fixation. Geometric distortion produces a smaller area for the same circumference and thus caused the histologic area to underestimate the ultrasound value by 17%.[154] Radial shrinkage of the wall in contrast caused the histologic measurement to result in overestimation of the ultrasound value by 18%.[150]

Angiography. Because angiography has been the clinical gold standard for determining vessel size, comparison between angiographic and echocardiographic measures of lumen size and area have been particularly

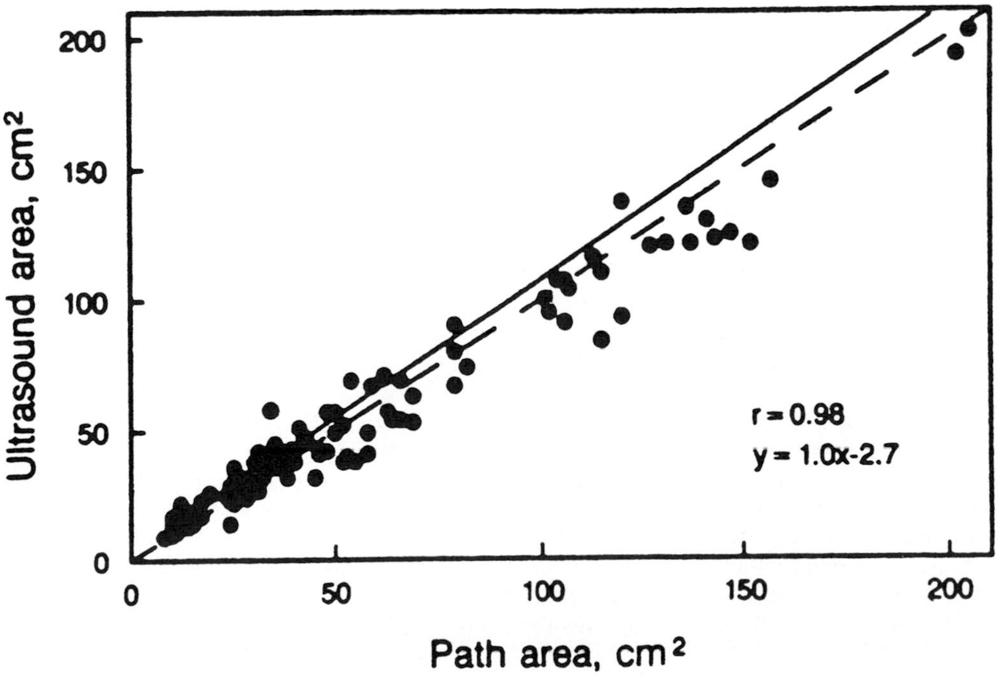

Fig. 16–58. Correlation of measurements of luminal areas of in vitro perfused arteries imaged by ultrasound (y axis) with histologic section areas (x axis). (From Nishimura RA, et al.: Intravascular ultrasound imaging: in vitro validation and pathologic correlation. J Am Coll Cardiol 16:145, 1990. Reprinted with permission from the American College of Cardiology. Journal of the American College of Cardiology. 1990, 16, 145.)

instructive. Correlations in normal peripheral and coronary arteries have in general been excellent (r = .86 to r = .95).[140,154] Intraluminal ultrasound data can result in overestimation of vessel diameter and area when the scan plane is not orthogonal to the long axis of the vessel, but such errors are generally small[151,140] and can be largely eliminated when care is taken to align the catheter with the arterial wall in orthogonal angiographic views.[140] Ultrasound data have also been observed to result in overestimation of lumen area when the dynamic range of the instrument is insufficient to detect weak intimal echoes.[155] This effect varied linearly, so that the measured lumen area increased by 26% as the dynamic range of an intravascular scanner was reduced from 52 to 22 dB (see Fig. 16–54).

In diseased vessels, the relationship between ultrasound and angiography has varied more widely. When the true lumen has a highly irregular or eccentric profile, such as after angioplasty,[156] multiple angiographic views are required for accurate assessment of the residual lumen area. In some cases (i.e., when the lumen is crescent shaped), it is impossible for a shadow image to correctly describe vessel area. Because ultrasound is better able to describe irregularly shaped vessels, it should be more accurate in assessing vessel area in those cases for which the measurement is most important.

Assessment of Degree of Stenosis

Ultrasound may also be used to assess the degree of luminal stenosis by comparing the area at the stenosis and that of unaffected regions of the same artery, in the same way that stenosis is assessed angiographically. Ultrasound, however, may be preferred in many cases because of its ability to frequently detect diseased segments that are taken as a "normal" reference. For example, diffuse concentric intimal thickening or post-transplant intimal proliferation cannot be accounted for by angiography (Fig. 16–59). If, however, such an abnormal but nonstenosed area is used as a "normal" angiographic reference, the degree of stenosis will be underestimated. The same situation can occur in studies of restenosis if changes in the degree of intimal thickening in regions neighboring the stenosis increase at the same rate as restenosis develops. In both situations, ultrasound can identify the abnormalities in the walls of presumably normal segments and more appropriately determine the degree of vessel narrowing produced by the lesion. In addition, serial ultrasound examination of the site of angioplasty might be able to separate the components of restenosis that were due to recoil or hyperplasia of the arterial wall.

Ultrasonic measurements of wall thickness in diseased arteries have correlated closely (r = .92) with those reported by histology.[150] Histologic measurements, however, are generally smaller for both wall (19 to 41%) and intima (33%), with the difference being attributed to tissue shrinkage that was due to processing after imaging.

Characterization of Atherosclerotic Lesions

Most atherosclerotic plaque is echogenic and thus can be imaged directly as a layer of variable thickness between the lumen and the media (both appearing darker than plaque). Quantitative studies[157,158] of plaque thickness have shown generally good correlation (r = .84 to r = .97) between measurements made from ultrasound images and corresponding histologic sections. Estimation of plaque size in muscular arteries, however, depends on the identification of the plaque-media interface, and this can be difficult for several reasons.[159] First, the media tends to decrease in thickness in areas underlying plaque, with reported diameters ranging from 16 to 190 μm (mean, 80 μm). Second, the acoustic mismatch between plaque and media may be large, resulting in a strong echo from the interface that encroaches on and may obliterate the thin media. Finally the hypoechoic medial layer may be totally obscured by atheroma eroding into and destroying the media or by shadow from intimal calcifications. When the media cannot be defined, it is difficult to detect the thickness of atheroma. In elastic arteries where there is often no interface between intima and media, atherosclerotic plaque can be particularly difficult to identify.

Plaque Distribution (Eccentric Versus Concentric). In addition to determining the presence and size of plaque,

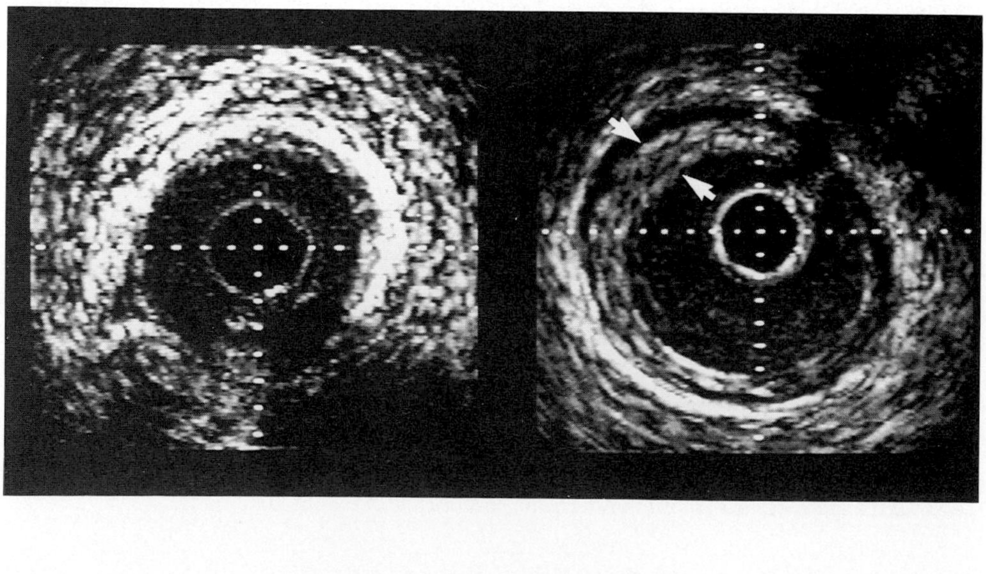

Fig. 16–59. In vivo images from human cardiac transplant recipients early (left) and several years post-transplantation (right). Diffuse concentric thickening of the intima (arrows) evolves during the post-transplant period. (Reproduced with permission from Drs. F. St. Goar and R. Popp. Unpublished data.)

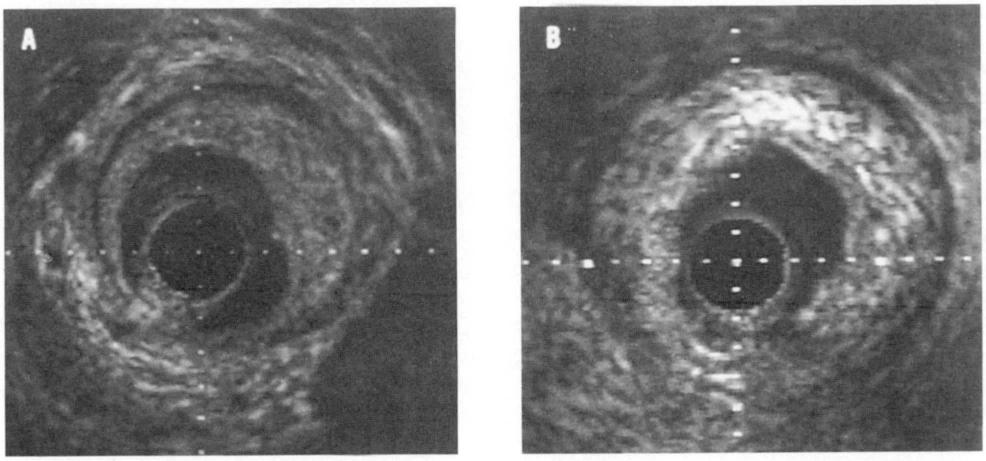

Fig. 16–60. Eccentric **(A)** vs. concentric **(B)** plaque distribution. (Reproduced with permission from Dr. P.L. Fitzgerald. Unpublished data.)

intravascular imaging can also be used to determine its spatial distribution (Fig. 16–60). Eccentric plaque is more obvious because it produces regional variation in layer thickness and reflective patterns within a single image. Symmetric plaque may be more difficult to identify, particularly when thin, because its presence must be determined with reference to values for normal intimal thickness, which as we have seen, are highly variable. Further, small atheroma do not cause luminal stenosis because reactive medial thinning and overall enlargement of the artery accommodate the early lesions.[160] In these cases, stenosis does not draw attention to the intimal lesion. Despite these difficulties, recent intravascular ultrasound studies have demonstrated small, diffuse lesions[152] in angiographically normal arteries. This observation is consistent with pathologic observations and suggests that the technique may make it possible to track the evolution of early, concentric, angiographically invisible lesions and to assess the effects of early intervention.

Plaque Composition (Fatty, Fibrous, Calcified). Atherosclerotic plaque is composed to varying degrees of lipid, smooth muscle, fibrous and elastic tissue, and calcium. Dense collection of lipid (lipid pools or lakes) are weakly reflective[158] and present as anechoic zones within plaque. Unfortunately, similar hypoechoic or anechoic regions can be caused by local shadowing resulting from neighboring or overlying calcium or dense fibrotic tissue reducing specificity.[150]

Fibromuscular plaque generally has a soft homogeneous appearance and is less intensely reflective than either fibrous or calcific plaques.[157] Calcium is characterized by intense reflections with distal shadowing (Fig. 16–61). This pattern is found in all types of arteries.[151] When the intima is calcified, the medial and adventitial layers generally cannot be seen.[151]

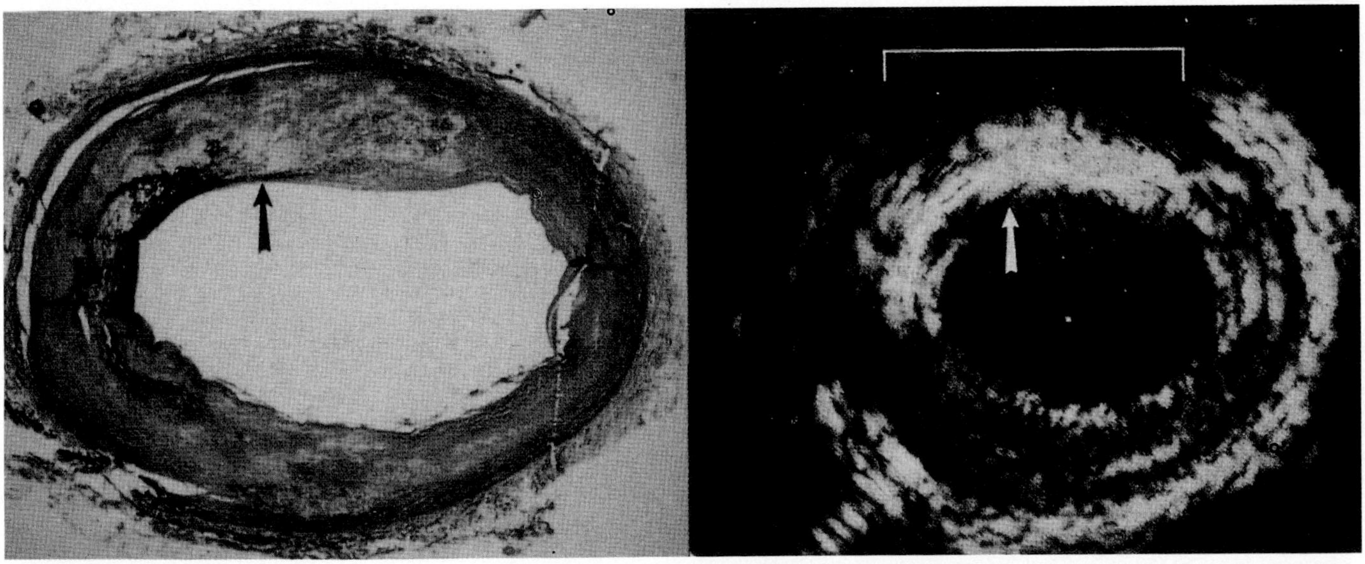

Fig. 16–61. Left. Histologic section from the left anterior descending coronary artery showing a calcified plaque (black arrow). Right. In the corresponding ultrasound image, the very bright echoes that are due to the calcium deposits (white arrow) and the acoustic shadow behind the calcium (bracket) are visible. Also shown in the ultrasound image are the echo reverberations from the needle marker inserted in the adventitia (seven o'clock). (From Potkin BN, et al.: Coronary artery imaging with intravascular high-frequency ultrasound. Circulation 81:1575, 1990. Reproduced by permission of the American Heart Association, Inc.)

In more severely diseased arteries, neither the internal nor the external elastic lamina are clearly visualized.[158]

Using the gray scale ultrasonic criteria described previously, fibrous and calcific lesions have been predicted with over 90% accuracy.[150] Predictive accuracy decreases to 78% for lipid-filled lesions.[150]

Although encouraging, these results suggest limitations in the prediction of tissue type from gray scale comparisons alone. Thus, a hypoechoic region could be due to a normal media, a lipid-filled region, acoustic shadowing, or simply failure to record local low intensity echoes as a result of limitations in the dynamic range of the instrument.

Thrombus. Loosely organized fresh thrombus has an acoustic impedance similar to both blood and soft atheroma and is therefore difficult to clearly identify. In several reports, however, thrombus was recorded both in vitro and in vivo.[151,161] While these studies demonstrate feasibility, true sensitivity and specificity remain to be established.

Also encouraging are recent data indicating that thrombus can be separated from hypoechoic plaque based on differences in the radio frequency backscatter,[162] although their gray scale appearance may often be similar. Figure 16–62 is an intraluminal recording taken following laser angioplasty with adjunctive balloon dilation, of a severely stenotic saphenous vein bypass graft. Although luminal patency was restored, there was a small angiographic filling defect in the lumen. Ultrasound imaging at the same location showed a structure protruding into the lumen with characteristics consistent with thrombus. Real-time observation of the rapidly moving echoes associated with blood flow can also help separate stagnant blood from thrombus because flow is only present in unobstructed areas of the lumen and is excluded for areas occupied by clot.

Role in Assessing the Effects of Interventions

Clearly, a major clinical application of catheter-based ultrasound should be improving the efficacy and control of vascular interventions.[163,164] Potential applications include (1) assessment of plaque morphology to determine the most appropriate type of intervention; (2) guiding the procedure to achieve maximal benefit at minimal risk (i.e., the degree of debulking with atherectomy); (3) measurement of the actual increase in cross-sectional area produced by the intervention; (4) assessment of the mechanism of luminal expansion (stretching of normal wall or plaque compression/disruption); (5) assessment of the complications of the procedures (fissures or dissection); and (6) evaluation of the effect of postintervention plaque morphology on the natural history of the lesion.

Angioplasty. The characteristics of plaque that determine its response to angioplasty are the presence and extent of calcium and the geometry of the plaque (eccentric or concentric). Pathologic data suggest that the amount and distribution of calcium within a lesion may influence the likelihood of success following balloon angioplasty.[147] Lesions with extensive calcific concretions often undergo excessive disruption with angioplasty, as

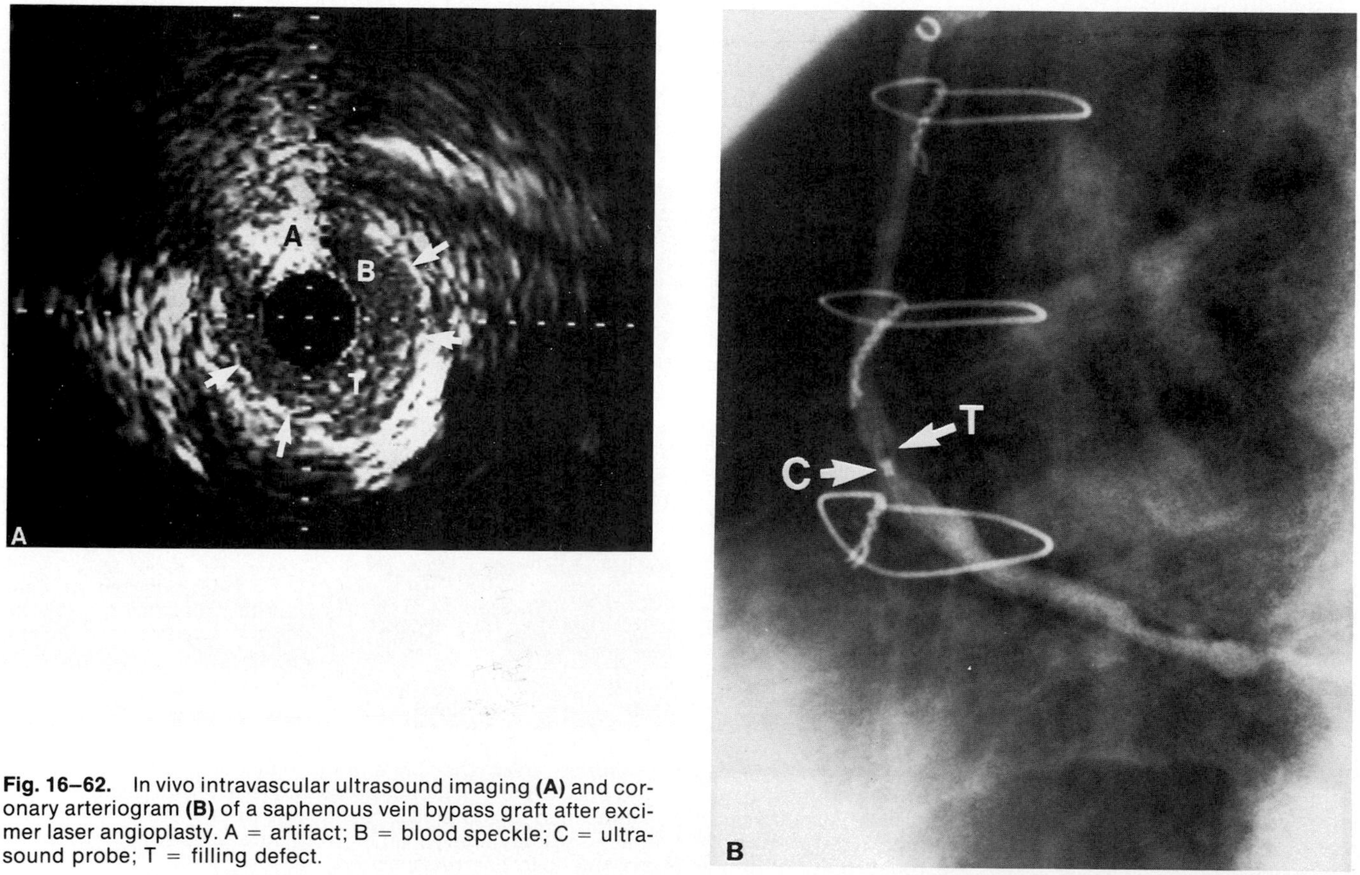

Fig. 16–62. In vivo intravascular ultrasound imaging **(A)** and coronary arteriogram **(B)** of a saphenous vein bypass graft after excimer laser angioplasty. A = artifact; B = blood speckle; C = ultrasound probe; T = filling defect.

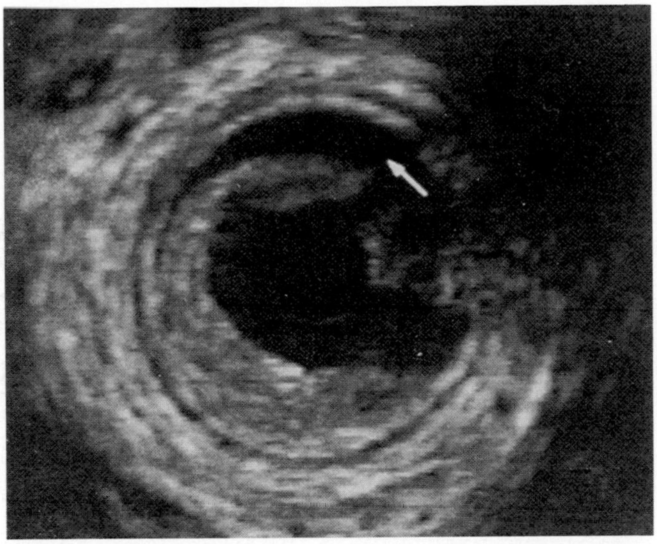

Fig. 16–63. Extensive intimal dissection (arrow) following angioplasty. (Reproduced with permission from Dr. P.L. Fitzgerald. Unpublished data.)

a result of the unequal distribution of forces within the vessel wall. In contrast, lesions with little or no calcification and/or fibrosis may be excessively elastic, stretching during dilation and later returning to their original size.

The ability of intravascular ultrasound to identify the location and extent of calcification in vivo has been established in both in vitro and clinical studies. Intravascular ultrasound is more sensitive than angiography in identifying calcium (54 vs. 25%)[165] and has demonstrated that extensive dissection is more common in calcified than in noncalcified plaque (62 vs. 27%). Angioplasty of softer, less echogenic plaque more often results in multiple superficial fissures or abrupt closure resulting from thrombosis.[166] Preliminary data also suggest that eccentric lesions by intravascular ultrasound (IVUS) are three times more likely to dissect or fracture than concentric lesions.[167]

Recently, dilating balloons and imaging elements have been combined in the same catheter in the hopes of fine tuning the procedure based on changes in the wall during inflation.[168] Unfortunately, this combination may be of limited value for several reasons. First, because the action of the balloon is symmetric and the length of the balloon is greater than that of the lesion in most cases, it is unlikely that balloon positioning will be greatly facilitated. Second, it is unlikely that effective control of inflation variables can be obtained by imaging during inflation because (1) individual sections provide only a two-dimensional representation of the complex three-dimensional process of plaque responding to pressure; (2) the relatively long delay in the response of the balloon to changes in inflation pressure means that it may be impossible to respond appropriately to the instantaneous information from the ultrasound images; and (3) pressure-volume studies[167] indicate that cracking of plaque often occurs abruptly over a period too short to allow the operator to react with a change in pressure. As clinical experience increases, the true value of the combined catheter will become more apparent.[169]

Postangioplasty intravascular ultrasound should prove valuable in depicting the degree and mechanism of luminal expansion and the presence of complication. The mechanism of expansion in eccentric lesions (vessel stretching vs. plaque compression or disruption) can be determined by comparing the changes in absolute extent of the circumference that overlies plaque and more normal vessel. Changes in plaque thickness, fissuring, and dissection can also be determined directly from the image. Intravascular ultrasound is particularly suited to assess plaque dissection because of its ability to see beyond the surface of the tear into the deeper layers of the vessel wall (Fig. 16–63). Animal data suggest that lesions with deep extension of a dissection and exposure of the media to the blood are more prone to initiate an aggressive platelet response and are potentially more likely to close abruptly.[170] Human pathologic studies and animal models of restenosis also suggest that myointimal proliferation appears to originate in areas of medial dissection and fracture of the internal elastic lamina, leading to restenosis.[170]

Atherectomy. The ability of intravascular ultrasound to define the location and depth of plaque within the vessel wall makes it potentially well suited for guiding atherectomy catheters and assessing the extent of plaque removal (Fig. 16–64). The success of atherec-

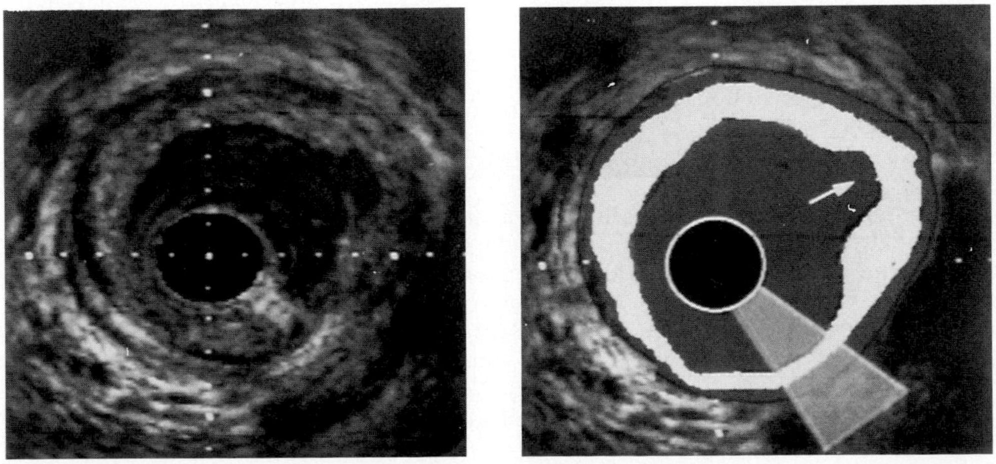

Fig. 16–64. Postatherectomy recording illustrating a cut extending deep into the intimal layer (arrow) but avoiding subintimal tissue.

tomy appears to relate to the removal of the maximum amount of plaque without disrupting the vascular media or adventitia. Restenosis rates have been shown to increase in relation to the presence of media or adventitia in the pathologic specimen.[171] During atherectomy procedures, ultrasound can be used to define the borders of eccentric plaque and appropriately orient the cutting tool. Reevaluation of the lesion between atherectomy cuts allows the operator to optimize intimal "debulking" and luminal enlargement, without causing perforation or medial injury.[172]

Ultrasound is clearly preferred to angiography for this purpose. In one study in which ultrasound imaging was performed after directional atherectomy was taken to angiographic completion (mean residual stenosis was 14% by angiography), ultrasound scans demonstrated that, on average, 43% of the available lumen was still occupied by plaque.[173]

Combined atherectomy and imaging devices make it possible to scan a portion of plaque before cutting to ensure that there is a sufficient margin of plaque to prevent trauma to normal components of vessel wall. Imaging guidance also appears to facilitate more efficient and complete removal of plaque. The images serve as a guide to optimal positioning of the cutter, so that an organized approach with progressive cuts can be taken in a manner that leads to the creation of a more regular lumen rather than an eccentric trough.

Intracoronary imaging may also be useful when using concentric atherectomy devices such as the transluminal extraction catheter and rotablator catheters to determine appropriate catheter size and to assess the amount of debulking achieved as the procedure progresses.

Lasers. Intravascular ultrasound may also prove to be an important adjunct of laser therapy because of its ability to look more than a centimeter into the vessel wall. This depth of penetration may aid in the development of systems to address complete occlusions by directing the catheter along an optimal route to stay centered in the vessel.[174] Although the discharge of an excimer laser causes "local spontaneous contrast," this phenomenon is transient and should not seriously effect the imaging process. The major limitation of combined laser-ultrasound catheters is the complexity of trying to mate two highly complex technologies in the same catheter while still retaining the low profile necessary for application in smaller vessels.

Stents. Stents, which are composed of a highly reflective metal lattice, are easily visualized by ultrasound. Because of the tomographic nature of the image, stents appear as a series of evenly spaced, highly reflective points around the circumference of the vessel (Fig. 16–65). Because stents are symmetric and extend beyond the margins of the lesion, angiography is adequate for positioning and deploying the stent. Ultrasound, however, has been suggested to be useful in sizing the vessel for stenting and assessing the apposition of the stent to the vessel wall.[175] Ultrasound may also be useful in the evaluation of intimal hyperplasia after stenting, because the metal wires of the stent can be imaged clearly within the mass of hyperplastic tissue.[169]

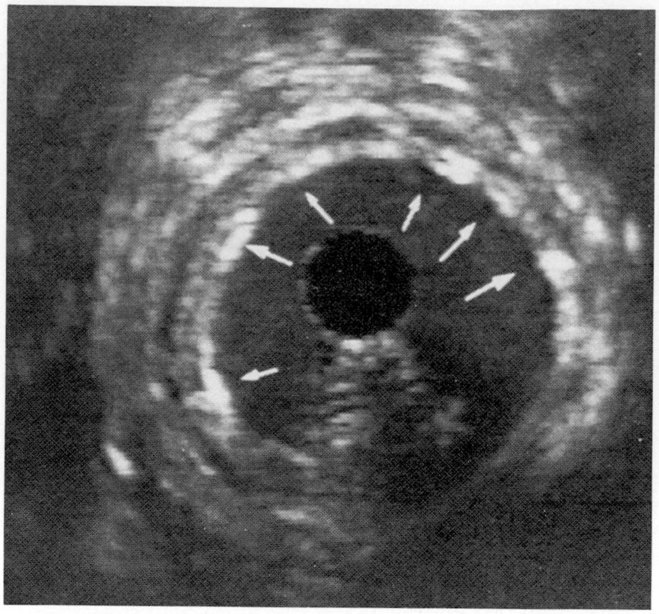

Fig. 16–65. Reflective points on the intima (arrows) corresponding to the mesh wire of a stent. (Reproduced with permission from Dr. P.L. Fitzgerald. Unpublished data.)

Assessing Vascular Reactivity

Intravascular ultrasound can assess physiologic changes in vascular tone and reactivity to pharmacologic agents based on changes in cross-sectional area during the intervention.[176]

It also has the potential to allow measurement of the motion of selected local regions within the arterial wall, and, if arterial pressure is simultaneously determined, the static and dynamic stiffness of regions of the artery should be calculable.

Initial ultrasound studies show a reduction in the systolic-diastolic change in cross-sectional area in patients with significant coronary disease compared with a cohort with minimal or no disease.[151]

Vascular reactivity has also been studied in transplant patients, both as a function of time after transplantation, and during rejection.[177] In patients with biopsy-proven rejection, the ability of the coronaries to dilate was significantly blunted (9 vs. 27% for cross-sectional area; and 4 vs. 12% for diameter). Patients studied less than 1 month after transplantation tend to have a lower vasodilator response compared to those studied greater than 1 year after transplantation.[177]

Other Diagnostic Imaging Applications

Many other diagnostic applications for intravascular ultrasound have been suggested. These include the evaluation of bypass graft anastomoses during surgery;[178] the assessment of angioplasty for aortic coarctation;[179] the diagnosis of aortic dissection;[180] the distinction of renal artery fibromuscular dysplasia from atherosclerotic stenosis;[181] the assessment of the extent of pulmonary artery thromboembolic disease before surgical thromboendarterectomy;[182] visualization of thrombi associated with acute pulmonary embolism;[183] and the diagnosis of post-transplant intimal hyperplasia.[184]

Future Directions

Improved Catheter Development. Although striking examples of normal arteries and specific lesion types have been published, these are clearly not reflective of the image quality produced by most instruments in the average clinical study. Although the presentation of unique examples of superb quality is important because it demonstrates capability, a great deal of work needs to be done to improve overall catheter performance and consistency. It is difficult to expect the same image quality from a transducer within a disposable catheter that costs several hundred dollars as from a clinical imaging transducer costing many thousands of dollars and designed to last the lifetime of the instrument. Despite this, the bottom line in all echocardiographic studies is image quality, and much work needs to be done to make today's ideal images tomorrow's norm.

In addition, catheter size needs to be reduced to allow tighter lesions to be crossed if the technique is to truly be of value in selecting therapeutic approach based on plaque morphology. It would also be desirable for the catheter tip to be controllable so the imaging plane could be aligned parallel with the short axis of the vessel, which would improve accuracy of measurement and should also improve image quality.

Three-Dimensional Reconstruction. Recent efforts at three-dimensional reconstruction of the serial ultrasound images along an arterial segment have been encouraging. The tomographic nature of the two-dimensional images facilitates the reconstruction process by either voxel modeling techniques[185] or the implementation of surfacing algorithms[186] (Fig. 16–66). Useful three-dimensional reconstructions that reveal the extent of dissection, stent location and degree of expansion, and details of the luminal surface can now be accomplished quickly enough to guide interventional procedures. If two-dimensional imaging can be improved, it should be possible to make rapid measurements of plaque volumes and follow changes in these volumes in response to interventions.

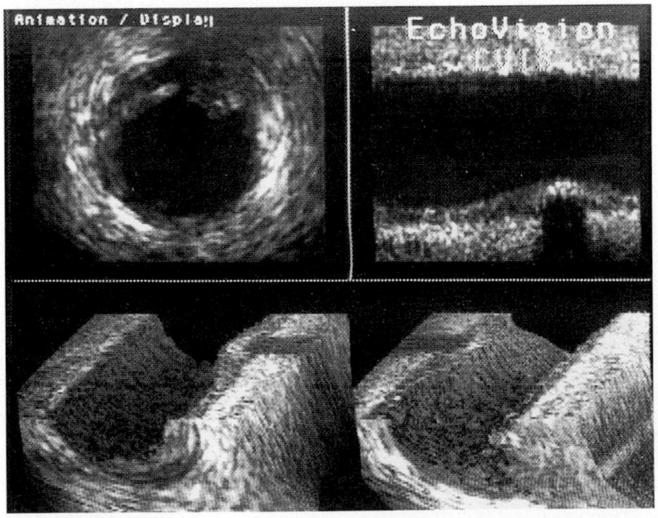

Fig. 16–66. Three-dimensional reconstruction of intravascular images. (Courtesy of Cardiovascular Imaging Systems.)

Tissue Characterization. The obvious differences in the gray scale images of different types of tissues noted in this and other areas of ultrasonic imaging have prompted numerous investigators to propose quantitative approaches to tissue characterization based on measurable changes in specific parameters of the reflected ultrasound signal. Unfortunately, these efforts, although often successful in controlled experimental studies, have not proven useful in the more complex clinical environment. However, many of the physical and biologic characteristics that facilitate intravascular imaging (i.e., use of high sampling frequencies, lack of attenuation between the transducer structure of interest, maintenance of a relatively normal beam interface relationship at all layers, and limited biologic variation in tissue types) should also enhance the potential for ultrasonic tissue characterization.

Preliminary data support the feasibility of quantitative tissue analysis. In one study, using 30-MHz ultrasound, soft plaque was discriminated from thrombus ex vivo based on the analysis of radio frequency backscattered signals.[162] In another study, angle-dependent backscatter—recorded in orthogonal planes, from unrolled, flattened arterial wall and integrated over a frequency range of 1 to 70 MHz—was shown to vary with tissue type.[187] The lowest values were obtained from loose collagenous intima, followed by muscular media, adventitia, dense collagenous intima, elastic media and external elastic lamina. There was considerable overlap between groups, however, with the result that peak power alone would not differentiate tissue types reliably.

A final approach, which has been suggested for this and other applications, is to analyze the frequency dependency of backscatter following the interrogation of tissue with a broad-banded input signal.[141] It has been observed that the returning signal from tissue will have local frequency-related amplitude spikes that correspond to dominant scatterer spacings. In theory, by associating these scatterer spacings with specific tissues, it should be possible to predict local tissue type from the amplitude and frequency distribution of depth-gated signals. Validation of these concepts is lacking to date.

Development of Catheters With Multiple Capabilities. Various combined-capability catheters have been developed as prototypes or suggested as theoretic possibilities. These include angioplasty, atherectomy, and laser catheters with combined imaging capabilities. In addition, combined imaging and Doppler catheters have been described in the hopes of measuring flow volume rather than just velocity. In concept, the multiple capabilities of such a catheter (e.g., sideways and forward imaging capabilities combined with lasers of some other interventional device) could be compared to a Swiss army knife. Unfortunately, like the Swiss army knife, the more it can do, the more difficult it is to get into one's pocket (i.e., coronary artery).

Intracardiac Echocardiography

Intracardiac echocardiography is a technique that uses transducer-tipped catheters to sample ultrasonic data directly from within the heart.[134,188–192] Intracardiac imaging generally uses larger catheters than intervascular imaging to maintain stability, and the transducers mated with these catheters operate at lower frequencies because the structures of interest are generally further from the transducer tip. Because of the ability to use larger catheters and lower frequencies, the capability for intracardiac imaging was demonstrated more than two decades before miniaturized transducers and catheters with two-dimensional imaging capabilities made it possible to record smaller vessels. The first intracardiac recordings were obtained by Cieszynski in 1960, using a miniature ultrasonic probe inserted via the jugular vein of an anesthetized dog.[134] Kimoto et al., in 1964, developed a method of transducer control and gating that allowed recording of C-scans of the atrial septum to and imaging of septal defects in humans.[193] Eggleton et al., in 1969, described a four-crystal catheter that, when rotated with gated sampling and computer reconstruction, produced a composite dynamic two-dimensional image of the left ventricular endocardium.[192] Bom et al. subsequently developed a circular 32-element catheter tip-phased array system (outer diameter, 3 mm) that permitted real-time study of intracardiac structures (see following discussion).[194] In the early 1980s, guide wires with a transducer imbedded in their tips became available, and M-mode recordings of right heart structures were demonstrated (Fig. 16–67).[75,76] Figure 16–68 illustrates one of these transducer-tipped guide wires in the cavity of the right atrium. The smaller horizontal arrows indicate the lateral atrial border, and the larger arrow points to the transducer as it emerges from the catheter tip. Figure 16–69 is an example of a recording of the right atrial free wall from within the right atrium. Both the endocardial and epicardial surfaces of the atrial myocardium can be clearly visualized, as can the excursion and thickening of the wall during atrial systole. During ventricular systole, passive thinning of the atrial wall is apparent as a result of the apical displacement of the AV groove (the accordion effect). Newer catheter-tip transducers have been fabricated, which permit recording of two-dimensional circumferential images from the heart and great vessels.[195]

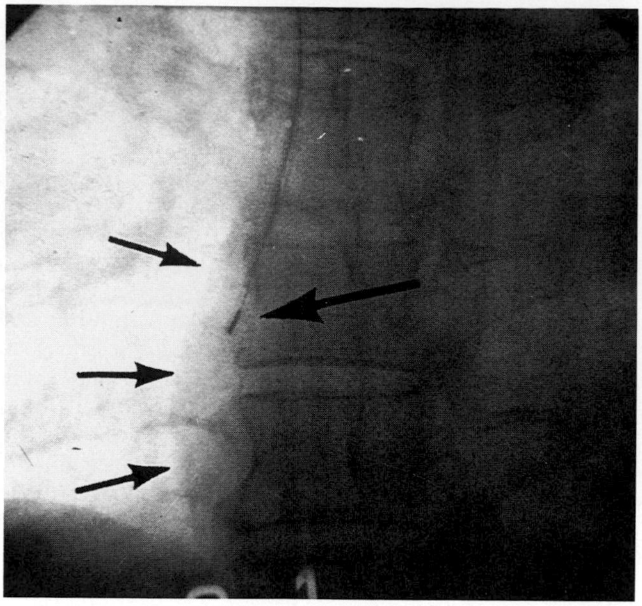

Fig. 16–68. Transducer-tipped guide wire in the right atrial cavity (large left-pointing arrow). The smaller right-pointing arrows indicate the lateral margin of the right atrium.

Applications. Although there are currently no established clinical applications for this technique, potential applications exist in many areas including on-line, high resolution assessment of ventricular function, tissue

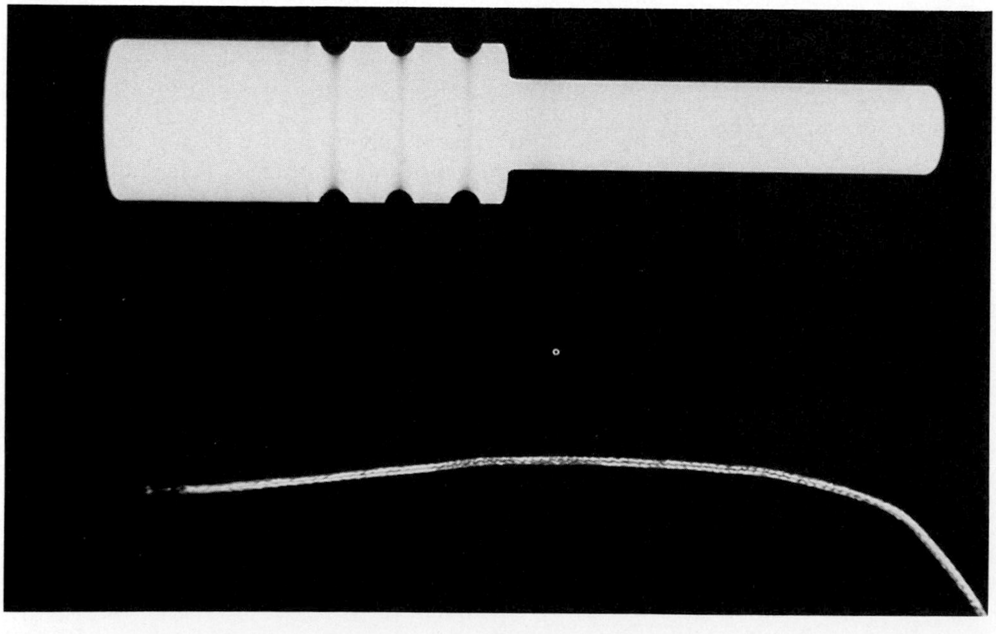

Fig. 16–67. M-mode transducer affixed to the tip of a guide wire small enough to pass through a 7F catheter compared to a standard M-mode transducer.

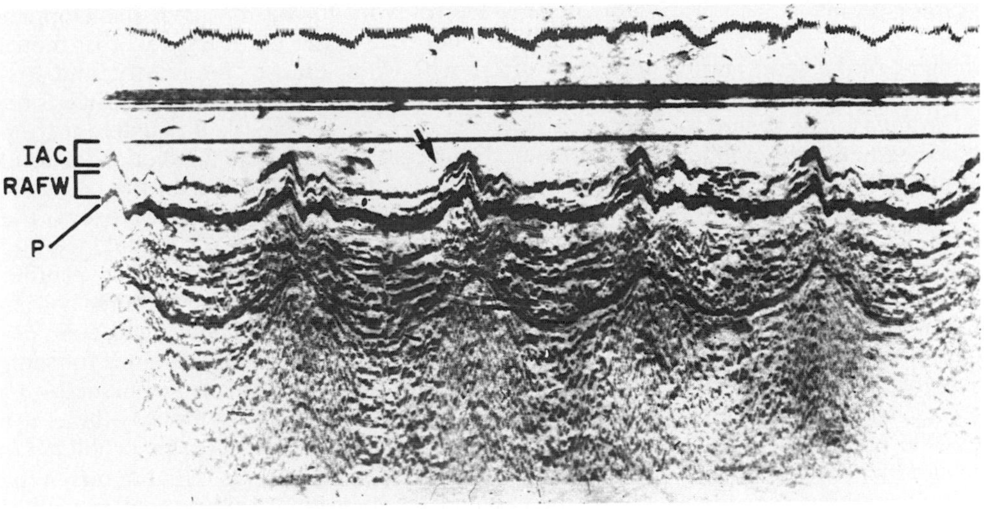

Fig. 16–69. Recording of the right atrial free wall (RAFW), epicardial pericardial interface (P), and atrial cavity (IAC) from a transducer-tipped guide wire in the right atrium. Note the contraction of the atrial wall following atrial systole (arrow).

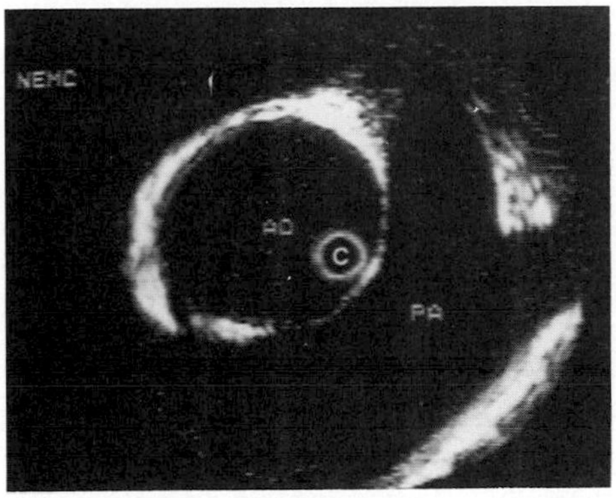

Fig. 16–70. Ultrasound image obtained from a catheter (C) in the anterior portion of the ascending aorta displaying the aorta (AO) in short axis and the adjoining main pulmonary artery (PA) and its major branches in long axis. (From Pandian NG, et al.: Real-time, intracardiac, two-dimensional echocardiography. Echocardiography 8:407, 1991. Reproduced with permission of Futura Publishing Company.)

characterization, facilitation of intracardiac catheter placement through direct "ahead" or "to-the-side" visualization from the catheter tip, and the mapping of myocardial contrast distribution, to name a few. To date, most studies have been limited to animal validation with excellent resolution demonstrated. Figure 16–70, e.g., is a recording of the aorta and pulmonary artery from a catheter in the aortic root. Figure 16–71 illustrates the canine left ventricle during diastole and systole.[196]

Potential Complications. The complications of intracardiac echocardiography are those of any catheterization procedure and vary with the size of the catheter, the site of insertion, and the receiving chamber. Small transducers affixed to the tips of guide wires, as illustrated in Figure 16–67, should add no additional risk to that associated with the insertion of the primary catheter. "Look-ahead" imaging may make procedures such as transeptal catheterization safer than with radiographic positioning.

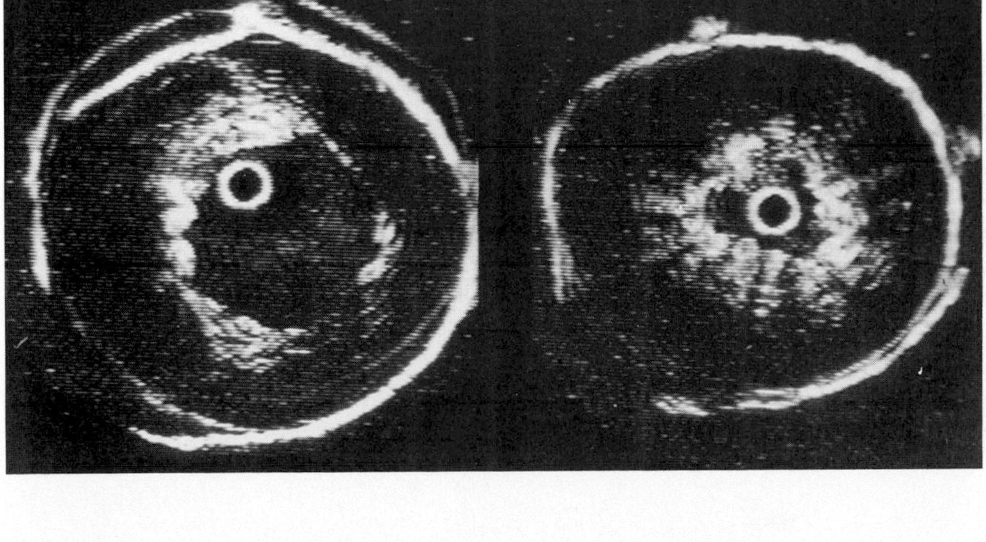

Fig. 16–71. Intracardiac echocardiographic images of the canine left ventricle obtained with the ultrasound catheter positioned within the left ventricular cavity. Resulting short axis images of the left ventricle during diastole (left) and systole (right) demonstrate normal ventricular function. (From Pandian NG, et al.: Real-time, intracardiac, two-dimensional echocardiography. Echocardiography 8:407, 1991. Reproduced with permission of Futura Publishing Company.)

Intravascular Doppler Flow Measurement

In addition to catheter-based imaging of the heart and blood vessels, it is also possible to record blood flow velocity at specific points in the cardiovascular system using Doppler transducers affixed to catheters or guide wires. Direct intravascular recording of intravascular and intracoronary flow offers several theoretic advantages over external methods. First, flexible catheters can be designed to follow the path of flow, and the detected frequency can be considered to parallel actual flow. Second, because intravascular catheters can be positioned close to lesions of interest, the pulse path from the catheter to the lesion is short. This improves signal sensitivity and decreases pulse duration, which result in an increase in the allowable pulse repetition frequency (PRF). Because of this high PRF, high velocities can be recorded at known locations without exceeding the Nyquist limit.

Intravascular Doppler flow recording was first attempted in 1967 by Stegall et al., who affixed two piezoelectric crystals to the tips of 7- to 9-Fr catheters to obtain continuous wave recordings of flow in the aorta, great veins, and cardiac chambers.[197] Benchimol et al., in 1969, first reported the use of a continuous wave Doppler catheter to measure intracoronary velocity signals.[198] In 1974, Hartley and Cole developed a catheter-based pulsed Doppler system to measure blood flow velocity in the ostia of native coronary arteries and bypass grafts.[199,200] Their system employed an 8-Fr catheter with a 20-MHz transducer at its tip and was capable of recording velocity at any point from 1 to 10 mm from the catheter tip. Although initial studies with these catheters showed excellent results, subsequent data were more variable. These differing and often disappointing results were primarily related to the relatively large size of early catheters but are relevant for all intravascular Doppler applications. Generally, larger catheters (5-Fr or more) tend to interfere with flow velocity, laminarity, and possibly even flow volume. These catheters produce a region of turbulence or "wake effect" downstream from the catheter; this region's length is a function of fluid viscosity and velocity and the diameter of the catheter. As a result, Doppler measurements taken close to the catheter may be contaminated by wake turbulence and become nonrepresentative of the native flow profile. Thus, the minimum useful range gate distance varies directly with catheter diameter, and larger catheters demand an extended minimum range gate distance for sampling to occur beyond the downstream turbulence.

Unfortunately, placement of the sample volume at a distance from the catheter tip often creates problems in the normal tortuous coronary vessels. Near bends in the vessel the catheter tip may point toward the far wall of the vessel and the range gate can lie off center in the parabolic coronary flow stream or even outside the lumen. Space-occupying lesions may further complicate range gate positioning and distort data derived from a distant sample volume.

Second-generation devices have used smaller catheters with side-looking transducers or very small Doppler probes incorporated into floppy guide-wire tips. Figure 16–72 is an example of a Doppler catheter developed at the University of Iowa. This "steerable" 4-Fr Doppler catheter has a 3-Fr distal tip containing an 0.018-inch lumen through which a movable guide wire can be inserted. A 20-MHz piezoelectric crystal is side mounted at a 45° angle to flow.[201] In validation experiments, the velocities recorded by this catheter have correlated closely with those obtained by an epicardial suction Doppler transducer and with timed volume collections of coronary sinus flow.[202]

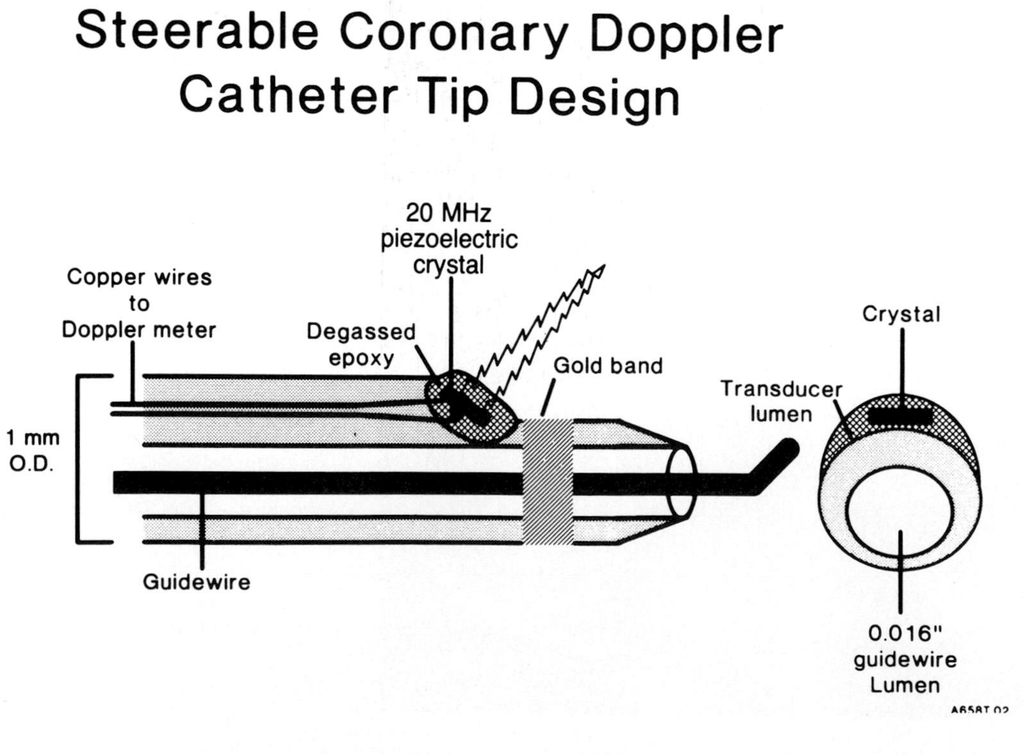

Fig. 16–72. Tip configuration of the second-generation steerable selective intracoronary Doppler catheter. The copper wires attached to the piezoelectric crystal exit from the proximal end of the catheter and are connected to a pulsed Doppler meter. (From White CW, Wilson RF, Marcus ML: Methods of measuring myocardial blood flow in humans. Prog Cardiovasc Dis 31:88, 1988.)

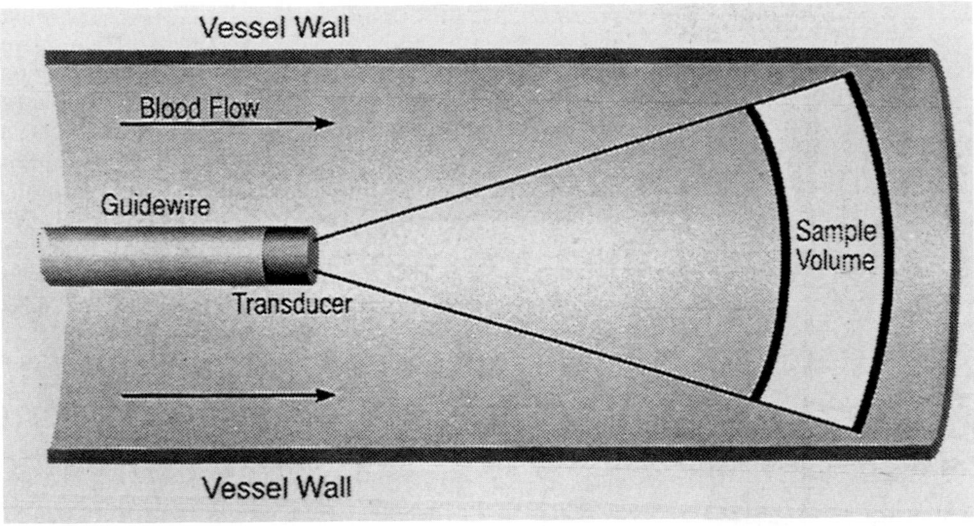

Fig. 16–73. A guidewire tip Doppler transducer (12 MHz) in a proximal coronary artery. A 15° diverging concentric beam is adequate to insonate the cross-sectional area of a 3.5-mm vessel within a distance of 5 mm from the catheter tip. The catheter diameter permits the range gate to be positioned 5 mm (more than 10 catheter diameters) from the transducer face and still avoid the wake effect. The sample volume in this example is 1 mm in axial length. (Reproduced with permission from Lee R, et al.: Intravascular ultrasound: technology and applications. *In* Nanda NC (eds.): Doppler Echocardiography. Philadelphia, Lea & Febiger, 1993.)

Very small Doppler probes have also been incorporated into floppy guide-wire tips (0.014 or 0.018 inches) for insertion into the proximal and distal coronary tree.[143] The piezoelectric element is positioned parallel to the long axis of catheter, producing a forward-looking sound beam. The small-diameter floppy guide wires tend to be flow seeking, which aids in placement within the flow stream, and the wire can be used to insert other catheters for therapeutic or imaging purposes.[143] The small diameter of the wire allows flow to relaminarize quickly, minimizing the length of the wake effect and allowing the sample volume to be positioned closer to the probe. Although the small crystal diameter leads to rapid beam spread, this is tolerable, because the distance to the range gate is small. Divergence of the sound path, however, creates increasing vector angles between the direction of sound propagation and the direction of blood flow. Use of lower frequencies (10 to 12.5 MHz) can constrain beam dispersion to within 15°, which introduces a relatively small error in the calculated velocities (less than 5%). Figure 16–73 illustrates the geometric consideration encountered when using a small Doppler device in the coronary arteries.

The absolute magnitude of the Doppler signal depends on the cross-sectional area of the vessel, the angle between the Doppler beam and the flow axis, the shape of the velocity profile, and the position of the sample volume within the velocity profile.

Applications

Intravascular and intracoronary catheter-based Doppler devices remain largely research tools. Their value has been studied in assessing coronary flow reserve, measurement of any increase in flow velocity across local stenoses, and measurement of coronary flow.

The normal coronary circulation can increase its flow by fourfold to fivefold during maximal vasodilation. The relationship between resting and peak flow after maximal vasodilation has been termed the *coronary flow reserve* or vasodilator reserve. In most cases Doppler-recorded velocities are used as a surrogate for flow and results expressed in terms of coronary blood flow velocity. In clinical studies, maximal coronary vasodilation has been produced using papaverine, dipyridamole, and adenosine with similar increases in flow demonstrated. Coronary flow reserve measurements can be used in the functional assessment of coronary stenoses of intermediate severity,[203,204] in assessing the functional significance of individual lesions in patients with multivessel disease,[205] in assessing bypass graft and graft vessel anastomotic lesions,[206] in assessing the coronary microcirculation, in evaluating post-transplant rejection,[207] and in assessing the results of coronary angioplasty[208,209] (Fig. 16–74). In each of these cases, a normal coronary flow reserve indicates the absence of functionally significant stenosis or microcirculatory disease. Following successful percutaneous transluminal coronary angioplasty (PTCA), coronary flow reserve increases in virtually every instance; however, in approximately 50% of patients, normalization does not occur for several days after the procedure.[208,209]

Stenosis severity can also be assessed by measuring the increase in velocity that occurs at the lesion. Either the proximal to peak velocity ratio or the pressure gradient determined from the modified Bernoulli equation ($\Delta P = 4V^2$) can be used as measures of stenosis severity. A translesion pressure gradient suggests functional significance, whereas successful intervention tends to eliminate the gradient. Absolute flow measurements using combined imaging and Doppler catheters have also been proposed, but their accuracy has yet to be established.

The degree of coronary stenosis has also been determined in the experimental model using the continuity equation by measuring the peak velocity proximal to and within the stenosis and the absolute area of the normal segment.[210] Further validation, however, in a more representative environment is clearly necessary.

Limitations and Technical Considerations

Although Doppler measurement of coronary flow dynamics have provided important physiologic insight, the

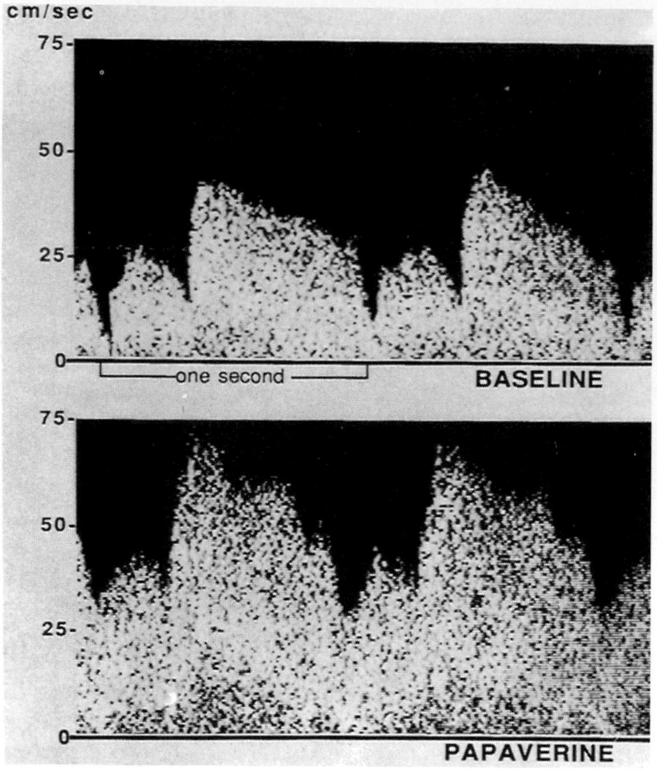

Fig. 16–74. Intravascular Doppler recordings from a patient following percutaneous transluminal coronary angioplasty (PTCA). Top. Baseline recording. Overall velocity is slightly increased with a distinct systolic/diastolic contour. The increase in velocity may be due to low-grade coronary hyperemia following multiple balloon inflations. Bottom. With papaverine, the hyperemic response is improved (2.8 times) but is still below normal for post-PTCA patients. (From Yock PG, Johnson EL, Linker DT: Intravascular ultrasound: development and clinical potential. Am J Cardiac Imaging 2:185, 1988.)

accuracy of individual recordings is difficult to establish because the location of the sample volume relative to the parabolic coronary flow profile and vessel wall cannot be determined. Reliable measurements depend on obtaining a normal biphasic stable flow profile, free of wall noise. The flow profile should be primarily diastolic and show zero velocity in part of systole (systolic zero touchdown). The sample volume should be advanced and withdrawn until the maximal flow velocity is determined. The position of the catheter must not change during interventions. Positioning the catheter at a bend in a vessel will increase the absolute velocities but not the relative change in velocity following interventions. Despite all attempts to align the Doppler beam parallel to the flow stream, the vagaries of exact catheter placement coaxially within the often curving coronary vessel often make calculation of absolute volume flow in patients using Doppler techniques unreliable.

SONOMICROMETRY

Miniature locally implanted piezoelectric crystals or sonomicrometers are often used to measure small distances with precision in experimental biologic systems. Using this technique, the transit time of a sound pulse between a transmitting and receiving transducer is recorded directly, and because the speed of sound in tissue is known, the time-varying distance between the transducers can be determined with a high degree of precision (Fig. 16–75). In the typical preparation, 1- to 2-mm piezoelectric disks with relatively high dominant frequencies (5 MHz or above) are sutured into the myocardium 1 to 2 cm apart. A crystal pair can be positioned: (1) along the endocardial or epicardial circumference of the left ventricle so that their separation reflects segment length; (2) perpendicular to the ventricular wall to measure its thickness; (3) at the extremes of a ventricular diameter or orthogonal diameters to assess ventricular function (Fig. 16–76); or (4) along the axis of a papillary muscle to describe its length as a function of time.[211–213]

This technique allows measurements of distances to within 0.05 mm and also provides high temporal resolution, because the small distances involve permit high PRFs.

Although superficially straightforward, the use of sonomicrometers entails several difficulties. First, the transducers are generally implanted blindly into the myocardium and subsequent adjustments must be made to ensure that their faces are parallel and that they are properly positioned (e.g., that they lie perpendicular and not oblique to the myocardium if they are to measure its thickness). Second, the movements recorded by this method can be confounded by nonaxial or shear components (e.g., transducers placed obliquely across a muscle wall will sense both wall thickening and changes in segment length). Third, the transducers may migrate after placement if not sutured in place. Finally, implantation of the crystals may cause tissue damage, which can independently effect the resulting measurements. Despite these technical problems, the spatial and temporal accuracy of this approach appear to be unparalleled for measuring instantaneous changes in wall and chamber dimensions.[85] Transmission methods can also be used to characterize myocardium in terms of the effects of tissue transit on beam characteristics.

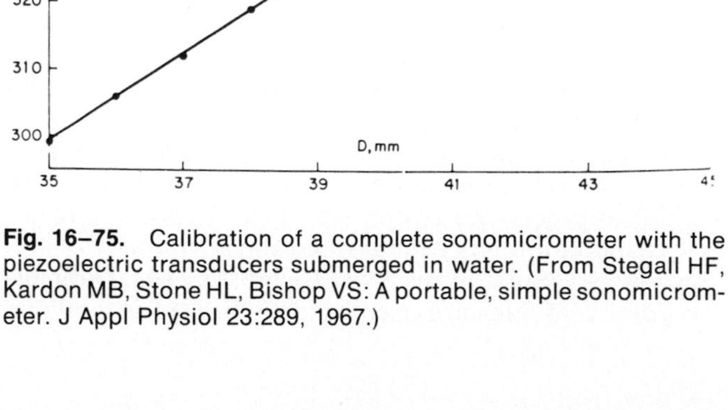

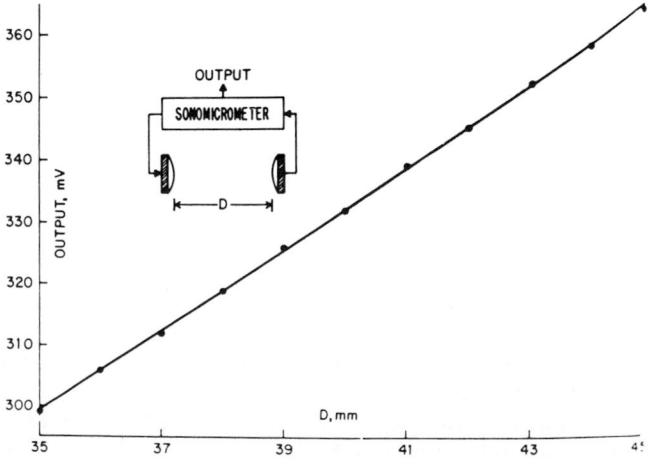

Fig. 16–75. Calibration of a complete sonomicrometer with the piezoelectric transducers submerged in water. (From Stegall HF, Kardon MB, Stone HL, Bishop VS: A portable, simple sonomicrometer. J Appl Physiol 23:289, 1967.)

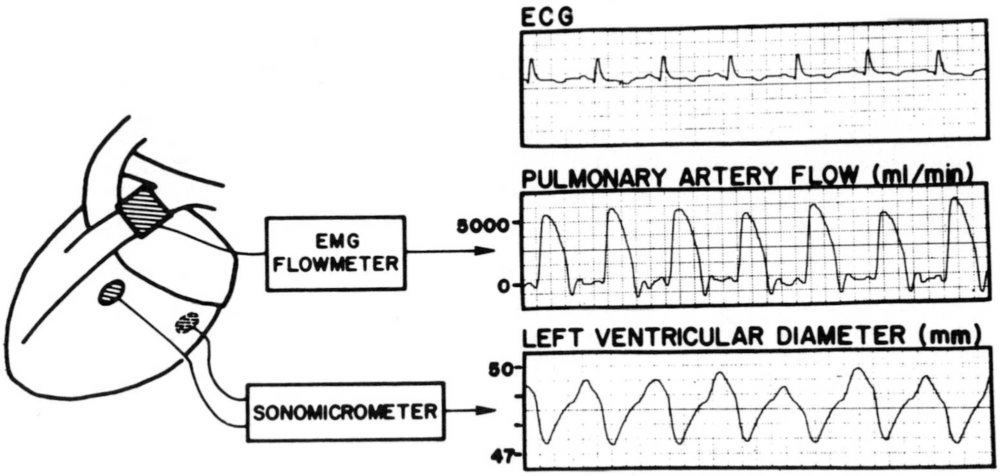

Fig. 16–76. Simultaneous recording of precordial electrocardiogram (ECG), pulmonary artery flow, and left ventricular diameter in a conscious dog. EMG = electromagnetic flowmeter. (From Stegall HF, Kardon MB, Stone H, Bishop VS: A portable, simple sonomicrometer. J Appl Physiol 23:289, 1967.)

Because of the need to use locally implanted transducers, however, these methods are poorly suited to the clinical environment. Likewise, because crystal implantation and alignment are time-consuming and cause some tissue trauma, sampling from more than a few sites in any one heart is difficult and often impractical.

REFERENCES

1. Williams PL, Warwick R (eds.): Gray's Anatomy (16th ed.), New York, Churchill Livingstone, 1980.
2. Jackson CL: Foreign bodies in the esophagus. Am J Surg 93:308, 1957.
3. Side CD, Gosling RG: Non-surgical assessment of cardiac function. Nature 232:335, 1971.
4. Olson RM, Shelton DK: A nondestructive technique to measure wall displacement in the thoracic aorta. J Appl Physiol 32:147, 1972.
5. Daigle RE, et al.: Non-traumatic aortic blood flow sensing by use of an ultrasonic esophageal probe. J Appl Physiol 38:1153, 1975.
6. Frazin L, et al.: Esophageal echocardiography. Circulation 54:102, 1976.
7. Hisanaga K, Hisanaga A, Nagata K, Ichie Y: Transesophageal cross-sectional echocardiography. Am Heart J 100:605, 1980.
8. Hisanaga K, et al.: High speed rotating scanner for transesophageal cross-sectional echocardiography. Am J Cardiol 47:412, 1981.
9. Matsumoto M, et al.: Application of transesophageal echocardiography to continuous monitoring of left ventricular performance. Am J Cardiol 46: 95, 1980.
10. Schluter M, et al.: Tranesophageal cross-sectional echocardiography with a phased array transducer system: technique and initial clinical results. Br Heart J 48:67, 1982.
11. Souquet J: Phased array transducer technology for transesophageal imaging of the heart: current status and future aspects. *In* Hanrath P, et al. (eds.): Cardiovascular Diagnosis by Ultrasound. The Hague, Martinus Nijhoff, p. 251, 1982.
12. Hanrath P, et al.: Transesophageal horizontal and sagittal imaging of the heart with a phased array system. Initial clinical results. *In* Hanrath P, et al. (eds.): Cardiovascular Diagnosis by ultrasound. The Hague, Martinus Nijhoff, p. 280, 1982.
13. Harui N, Souquet J: Transesophageal echocardiography scanhead. United States Patent No. 4.543.960, October 1, 1985.
14. Seward JB, et al.: Biplanar transesophageal echocardiography: anatomic correlations, image orientation, and clinical applications. Mayo Clin Proc 65:1193, 1990.
15. Khandheria BK, Oh J: Transesophageal echocardiography: state of the art and future directions. Am J Cardiol 69:61H, 1992.
16. Seward JB, et al.: Transesophageal echocardiography: technique, anatomic correlations, implementation, and clinical applications. Mayo Clin Proc 63:649, 1988.
17. Omoto R, et al.: Biplane color Doppler transesophageal echocardiography: its impact on cardiovascular surgery and further technological progress in the probe, a matrix phased-array biplane probe. Echocardiography 6:423, 1990.
18. Pearson AC, Pasierski T: Initial experience with a 48 by 48 element biplane transesophageal probe. Am Heart J 122:559, 1991.
19. Omoto R, et al.: New direction of biplane transesophageal echocardiography with special emphasis on real-time biplane imaging and matrix phase-array biplane transducer. Echocardiography 7:691, 1990.
20. Flachskampf FA, et al.: Initial experience with a multiplane transesophageal echotransducer: assessment of diagnostic potential. Euro Heart J 13: 1201, 1992.
21. Roelandt JRTC, et al.: Multiplane transesophageal echocardiography: latest evolution in an imaging revolution. J Am Soc Echocardiogr 5:361, 1992.
22. Steckelberg JM, et al.: Prospective evaluation of the risk of bacteremia associated with transesophageal echocardiography. Circulation 84:177, 1991.
23. Nikutta P, et al.: Risk of bacteremia induced by transesophageal echocardiography: analysis of 100 consecutive procedures. J Am Soc Echocardiogr 5:168, 1992.
24. Khandheria BK: Prophylaxis or no prophylaxis before transesophageal echocardiography? J Am Soc Echocardiogr 5:285, 1992.
25. Foster E, Kusumoro FM, Sobol SM, Schiller NB: Streptococcal endocarditis temporally related to transesophageal echocardiography. J Am Soc Echocardiogr 3:424, 1990.
26. Steckelberg JM, et al.: Prospective evaluation of the risks of bacteremia associated with transesophageal echocardiography. Circulation 84:177, 1991.
27. Daniel WG, et al.: Safety of transesophageal echocardiography. A multicenter survey of 10,419 examinations. Circulation 83:817, 1991.
28. Risk C, Fine R, D'Ambra MN, O'Shea JP: A new application for superior laryngeal nerve block: transesophageal echocardiography. Anesthesiology 72:746, 1990.
29. Lightly GW, Hare CL, Kaplan DS: Use of a mouth gag instrument to facilitate bite block insertion and prevent finger and probe bites during transesophageal echocardiography. Echocardiography 9:485, 1992.
30. Toma Y, et al.: Determination of atrial size by esophageal echocardiography. Am J Cardiol 52:878, 1983.
31. Cohen GI, Chan KL, Walley VM: Anatomic correlations of the long-axis views in biplane transesophageal echocardiography. Am J Cardiol 66:1007, 1990.
32. Cohen GI, Chan KL: Biplane transesophageal echocardiography: clinical applications of the long-axis plane. J Am Soc Echocardiogr 4:155, 1991.
33. Stumper O, et al.: Transesophageal echocardiography in the longitudinal axis: correlation between anatomy and images and its clinical implications. Br Heart J 64:282, 1990.
34. Wang X, et al.: Biplane transesophageal echocardiography: an anatomic-ultrasonic-clinical correlative study. Am Heart J 123:1027, 1992.
35. Borner N, et al.: Diagnosis of aortic dissection by transesophageal echocardiography. Am J Cardiol 54:1157, 1984.
36. Engberding R, et al.: Identification of dissection or aneurysm of the descending thoracic aorta by conventional and transesophageal two-dimensional echocardiography. Am J Cardiol 59:717, 1987.
37. Takamoto S, Omoto R: Visualization of thoracic dissecting aortic aneurysm by transesophageal Doppler color flow mapping. Herz 12:187, 1987.
38. Omoto R, et al.: Evaluation of biplane color Doppler transesophageal echocardiography in 200 consecutive patients. Circulation 85:1237, 1992.
39. Aschenberg W, et al.: Transesophageal two-dimensional echocardiography for the detection of left atrial appendage thrombus. J Am Coll Cardiol 7: 163, 1986.
40. Nellessen U, et al.: Impending paradoxical embolism from atrial thrombus: correct diagnosis by transesophageal echocardiography and prevention by surgery. J Am Coll Cardiol 5:1002, 1988.
41. Gussenhoven EJ, et al.: Detailed analysis of aortic valve endocarditis: comparison of precordial, esophageal and epicardial two-dimensional echocardiography with surgical findings. J Clin Ultrasound 14:209, 1986.
42. Erbel R, et al.: Improved diagnostic value of echocardiography in patients with infective endocarditis by transesophageal approach: a prospective study. Eur Heart J 9:43, 1988.

43. Mugge A, Daniel WG, Frank G, Lichtlen PR: Echocardiography in infective endocarditis: reassessment of prognostic implications of vegetation size determined by the transthoracic and the transesophageal approach. J Am Coll Cardiol 14:631, 1989.
44. Daniel WG, et al.: Improvement in the diagnosis of abscesses associated with endocarditis by transesophageal echocardiography. N Engl J Med 324: 795, 1991.
45. Erbel R, et al.: Detection of aortic dissection by transesophageal echocardiography. Br Heart J 58:45, 1987.
46. Erbel R, et al.: European Cooperative Study Group for Echocardiography: Echocardiography in diagnosis of aortic dissection. Lancet 1:457, 1989.
47. Mohr-Kahaly S, et al.: Ambulatory follow-up of aortic dissection by transesophageal two-dimensional and color-coded Doppler echocardiography. Circulation 80:24, 1989.
48. Koenig K, et al.: Transesophageal echocardiography for diagnosis of rupture of the ventricular septum or left ventricular papillary muscle during acute myocardial infarction. Am J Cardiol 59:362, 1987.
49. Currie PJ, et al.: Evaluation of mitral prosthetic dysfunction with transesophageal color flow Doppler in ambulatory patients (abstr). Circulation 76(Suppl. 4):IV-39, 1987.
50. Taams MA, et al.: Transesophageal Doppler color flow imaging in the detection on native and Bjork-Shiley mitral valve regurgitation. J Am Coll Cardiol 13:95, 1989.
51. Nellessen U, et al.: Transesophageal two-dimensional echocardiography and color Doppler flow velocity mapping in the evaluation of cardiac valve prostheses. Circulation 78:848, 1988.
52. Schluter M, et al.: Transesophageal two-dimensional echocardiography in the diagnosis of cor triatriatum in the adult. J Am Coll Cardiol 2:1011, 1983.
53. Hanrath P, et al.: Detection of ostium secundum atrial septal defects by transesophageal cross-sectional echocardiography. Br Heart J 49:350, 1983.
54. Kaulitz R, et al.: Comparative values of the precordial and transesophageal approaches in the echocardiographic evaluation of atrial baffle function after an atrial correction procedure. J Am Coll Cardiol 16:686, 1990.
55. Kronzon I, et al.: Transesophageal echocardiography is superior to transthoracic echocardiography in the diagnosis of sinus venous atrial septal defect. J Am Coll Cardiol 17:537, 1991.
56. Morimoto K, et al.: Diagnosis and quantitative evaluation of secundum-type atrial septal defect by transesophageal Doppler echocardiography. Am J Cardiol 66:85, 1990.
57. Stumper OFW, Sreeram N, Elzenga NF, Sutherland GR: Diagnosis of atrial situs by transesophageal echocardiography. J Am Coll Cardiol 16: 442, 1990.
58. DePace NL, Soulen RL, Kotler MN, Mintz GS: Two-dimensional echocardiographic detection of intra-atrial masses. Am J Cardiol 48:954, 1981.
59. Come PC, Riley MF, Markis JE, Malagold M: Limitations of echocardiographic techniques in evaluation of left atrial masses. Am J Cardiol 48:947, 1981.
60. Jordan NA, Scheifly CH, Edwards JE: Mural thrombus and arterial embolism in mitral stenosis. Circulation 3:363, 1951.
61. Wallach JB, Lukash L, Angrist AA: An interpretation of the incidence of mural thrombi in the left auricle and appendage with particular reference to mitral commissurotomy. Am Heart J 45:252, 1953.
62. Palacios I, et al.: Percutaneous balloon valvotomy for patients with severe mitral stenosis. Circulation 75:778, 1987.
63. McKay RG, et al.: Percutaneous mitral valvotomy in an adult patient with calcific rheumatic mitral stenosis. J Am Coll Cardiol 7:1410, 1986.
64. Palacios IF, Block PC, Wilkins GT, Weyman AE: Follow-up of patients undergoing percutaneous mitral balloon valvotomy: analysis of factors determining restenosis. Circulation 79:573, 1989.
65. Aschenberg W, et al.: Transesophageal two-dimensional echocardiography for the detection of left atrial appendage thrombus. J Am Coll Cardiol 7: 163, 1986.
66. Young E, Shapiro SM, French WJ, Ginzton LE: Use of transesophageal echocardiography during thrombolysis with tissue plasminogen activator of a thrombosed prosthetic mitral valve. J Am Soc Echocardiogr 5:153, 1992.
67. Pearson AC, Labovitz AJ, Tatineni S, Gomez CR: Superiority of transesophageal echocardiography in detecting cardiac source of embolism in patients with cerebral ischemia of uncertain etiology. J Am Coll Cardiol 17:66, 1991.
68. Hofman T, et al.: Echocardiographic evaluation of patients with clinically suspected arterial emboli. Lancet 336:1421, 1990.
69. Pearson AC, et al.: Atrial septal aneurysm and stroke—a transesophageal echocardiographic study. J Am Coll Cardiol 18:1223, 1991.
70. Fisher EA, Stahl JA, Budd JH, Goldman ME: Transesophageal echocardiography: procedures and clinical application. J Am Coll Cardiol 18:1333, 1991.
71. Karalis DG, et al.: Recognition and embolic potential of intra-aortic debris. J Am Coll Cardiol 17:73, 1991.
72. Tunick PA, Perez JL, Kronzon I: Protruding atheromas in the thoracic aorta and systemic embolization. Ann Intern Med 115:423, 1991.
73. Kremer P, et al.: Intraoperative monitoring by two-dimensional echocardiography. Anaesthetist 34:111, 1985.
74. Schiller NB: Evaluation of cardiac function during surgery by transesophageal 2-dimensional echocardiography. *In* Hanrath P, Bleifeld W, Souquet J (eds.): Cardiovascular Diagnosis by Ultrasound. The Hague, Martinus Nijhoff, p. 289, 1982.
75. Smith JS, et al. Intraoperative detection of myocardial ischemia in high risk patients. Electrocardiography versus two dimensional transesophageal echocardiography. Circulation 72:1015, 1985.
76. Mark JB, et al.: Continuous monitoring of cardiac output with esophageal Doppler ultrasound during cardiac surgery. Anesth Analg 65:1013, 1986.
77. Goldman ME, Mindich BP: Intraoperative cardioplegic contrast echocardiography for assessing myocardial perfusion during open heart surgery. J Am Coll Cardiol 4:1035, 1984.
78. Schluter M, et al.: Assessment of transesophageal pulsed Doppler echocardiography in the detection of mitral regurgitation. Circulation 66:784, 1982.
79. Schluter M, Kremer P, Hanrath P: Transesophageal 2-D echocardiographic feature of flail mitral leaflet due to ruptured chordae tendineae. Am Heart J 108:609, 1984.
80. Dahm M, et al.: Intraoperative evaluation of reconstruction of the atrioventricular valves by transesophageal echocardiography. Thorac Cardiovasc Surg 35(Special Issue 2):140, 1987.
81. Furuya H, et al.: Detection of air embolism by transesophageal echocardiography. Anesthesiology 58:124, 1983.
82. Cucchiara RF, Nugent M, Seward JB, Messick JM: Air embolism in upright neurosurgical patients: detection and localization by two-dimensional transesophageal echocardiography. Anesthesiology 60:353, 1984.
83. Borner N, et al.: Diagnosis of aortic dissection by transesophageal echocardiography. Am J Cardiol 54:1157, 1984.
84. Takamoto S, Omoto R: Visualization of thoracic dissecting aortic aneurysm by transesophageal Doppler color flow mapping. Herz 12:187, 1987.
85. Goldman ME, Mindich BP: Intraoperative two-dimensional echocardiography: new application of an old technique. J Am Coll Cardiol 7:374, 1986.
86. Ballal RS, Mahan EF, Nanda NC, Dean LS: Utility of transesophageal echocardiography in interatrial septal puncture during percutaneous mitral balloon commissurotomy. Am J Cardiol 66:230, 1990.
87. Chan KL, et al.: Role of transesophageal echocardiography in percutaneous balloon mitral valvuloplasty. Echocardiography 7:115, 1990.
88. Jaarsma W, et al.: Transesophageal echocardiography during percutaneous balloon mitral valvuloplasty. J Am Soc Echocardiogr 3:384, 1990.
89. Matsumoto M, et al.: Evaluation of left ventricular performance during supine exercise by transesophageal M-mode echocardiography in normal subjects. Br Heart J 48:61, 1982.
90. Matsumoto M, Hanrath P, Kremer P, Bleifeld W: Transesophageal echocardiographic evaluation of left ventricular function at rest and during dynamic exercise in aortic insufficiency. J Cardiogr 11:1147, 1981.
91. Dawson J, Cockel R: Oesophageal perforation at fibreoptic gastroscopy. Br Med J 283:583, 1981.
92. Silvis SE, et al.: Endoscopic complications: results of the 1974 American Society of Gastrointestinal Endoscopy Survey. JAMA 235:928, 1976.
93. Dewhirst WE, Stragand JJ, Fleming BM: Mallory-Weiss tear complicating intraoperative transesophageal echocardiography in a patient undergoing aortic valve replacement. Anesthesiology 73:777, 1990.
94. O'Shea JP, et al.: Effects of prolonged transesophageal echocardiographic imaging and probe manipulation on the esophagus—an echocardiographic-pathologic study. J Am Coll Cardiol 17:1426, 1991.
95. Geibel A, et al.: Risk of transesophageal echocardiography in awake patients with cardiac diseases. Am J Cardiol 62:337, 1988.
96. Chan K, Cohen G, Sochowski RA, Baird MG: Complications of transesophageal echocardiography in ambulatory adult patients: analysis of 1500 consecutive examinations. J Am Soc Echocardiogr 4:577, 1991.
97. Erbel R, et al.: Detection of spontaneous echocardiographic contrast within the left atrium by transesophageal echocardiography. Clinical Cardiology 9:245, 1986.
98. Geibel A, et al.: Risk of transesophageal echocardiography in awake patients with cardiac diseases. Am J Cardiol 62:337, 1988.
99. Matsuzaki M, Toma Y, Kusukawa R: Clinical applications of transesophageal echocardiography. Circulation 82:709, 1990.
100. Marcovitz PA, Williamson BD, Armstrong WF: Toxic Methemoglobinemia caused by topical anesthetic given before transesophageal echocardiography. J Am Soc Echocardiogr 4:615, 1991.
101. Seward JB, et al.: Critical appraisal of transesophageal echocardiography: limitations, pitfalls, and complications. J Am Soc Echocardiogr 5:288, 1992.
102. Kerber RE, et al.: Correlation between echocardiographically demonstrated segmental wall motion and regional myocardial perfusion. Circulation 59:662, 1975.
102a. Marcus M, et al.: Measurements of coronary velocity and reactive hyperemia in the coronary circulation of humans. Circ Res 49:877, 1981.
103. Sahn DJ, et al.: Ultrasonic imaging of the coronary arteries in open chest humans: evaluation of coronary arteriosclerotic lesions during cardiac surgery. Circulation 66:1034, 1982.
104. Sahn DJ, et al.: Anatomic ultrasound correlations for intraoperative, open-chest imaging of coronary artery atherosclerotic lesions in human beings. J Am Coll Cardiol 3:1169, 1984.
105. McPherson D, et al.: Evaluation of the coronary arterial wall and lumen

by high-frequency 2-dimensional epicardial echocardiography: comparison with histologic measurements. J Am Coll Cardiol 3:565, 1984.
106. McPherson DD, et al.: High-frequency epicardial echocardiographic assessment of coronary arteries: further validation. J Am Coll Cardiol 5:387, 1985.
107. Hiratzka LF, et al.: Intraoperative evaluation of coronary artery bypass graft anastomoses with high frequency epicardial echocardiography: experimental validation and initial patient studies. Circulation 73:1199, 1986.
108. Hiratzka LF, et al.: Intraoperative high frequency epicardial echocardiography in coronary revascularization: locating deeply embedded coronary arteries. Ann Thorac Surg 42:s9, 1986.
109. Payen D, et al.: Comparison of perioperative and postoperative phasic blood flow in aortocoronary venous bypass grafts by means of pulsed Doppler echocardiography with implantable microprobes. Circulation 74(Suppl. 3):III-61, 1986.
110. Likoff M, et al.: Epicardial mapping of segmental myocardial function: an echocardiographic method applicable in man. Circulation 66:1050, 1982.
111. Davila-Roman VG, et al.: Intraoperative ultrasonographic evaluation of the ascending aorta in 100 consecutive patients undergoing cardiac surgery. Circulation 84:(Suppl. 3):III-47, 1991.
112. Kaplan JA: Monitoring technology: Advances and restraints (editorial). J Cardiothoracic Anesthesia 3:257, 1989.
113. Beaupre PN, et al.: Intraoperative detection of changes in left ventricular segmental wall motion by transesophageal two-dimensional echocardiography. Am Heart J 107:1021, 1984.
114. Equaras MG, et al.: Interoperative contrast two-dimensional echocardiography: evaluation of the presence and severity of aortic and mitral regurgitation during cardiac operations. J Thorac Cardiovasc Surg 89:573, 1985.
115. Takamoto S, et al.: Intraoperative color flow mapping by real-time two-dimensional Doppler echocardiography for evaluation of valvular and congenital heart disease and vascular disease. J Thorac Cardiovasc Surg 90: 802, 1985.
116. King RM, et al.: Surgery for tricuspid regurgitation late after mitral valve replacement circulation 70(Suppl. 1):I-193, 1984.
117. Rodigas PC, et al.: Intraoperative two-dimensional echocardiography: ejection of microbubbles from the left ventricle after cardiac surgery. Am J Cardiol 50:1130, 1982.
118. Barnard RJ, Buckberg GD, Duncan HW: Limitations of the standard transthoracic electrocardiogram in detecting subendocardial ischemia. Am Heart J 99:476, 1980.
119. Zeldis SM, et al.: Fascicular conduction disturbances after coronary bypass surgery. Am J Cardiol 41:860, 1978.
120. O'Connell JB, et al.: Transient bundle branch block following use of hypothermic cardioplegia in coronary artery bypass surgery: high incidence without perioperative myocardial infarction. Am Heart J 103:85, 1982.
121. Battler A, et al.: Dissociation between regional myocardial dysfunction and ECG changes during ischemia in the conscious dog. Circulation 62: 735, 1980.
122. Braunwald E, Kloner RA: The stunned myocardium: prolonged, postischemic ventricular dysfunction. Circulation 66:1146, 1982.
123. Konstadt SN, et al.: Validation of quantitative intraoperative transesophageal echocardiography. Anesthesiology 65:418, 1986.
124. Ren J, et al.: Effect of coronary bypass surgery and valve replacement on left ventricular function: assessment by intraoperative two-dimensional echocardiography. Am Heart J 109:281, 1985.
125. Dubroff JM, et al.: Left ventricular ejection fraction during cardiac surgery: a two-dimensional echocardiographic study. Circulation 68:95, 1983.
126. Topol EJ, et al.: Immediate improvement of dysfunctional myocardial segments after coronary revascularization: detection by intraoperative transesophageal echocardiography. J Am Coll Cardiol 4(6):1123, 1984.
127. Syracuse DS, et al.: Intraoperative intracardiac echocardiography during left ventriculotomy and myectomy for IHSS (abstr.). Circulation 56(Suppl. 3):III-27, 1977.
128. Valdex-Cruz L, Pieroni D, Roland J, Shematek J: Recognition of residual postoperative shunts by contrast echocardiographic techniques. Circulation 55:148, 1977.
129. Fraker T, Harris P, Behar V, Kisslo J: Detection and exclusion of interatrial shunts by two-dimensional echocardiography and peripheral venous injection. Circulation 59:379, 1979.
130. Furlan AJ, Breuer AC: Central nervous system complications of open heart surgery. Cur Con Cerebro Dis 19:7, 1984.
131. Breuer AC, et al.: Central nervous system complications of coronary artery bypass graft surgery: prospective analysis of 421 patients. Stroke 14:682, 1983.
132. Topol EJ, et al.: Value of intraoperative left ventricular microbubbles detected by transesophageal two-dimensional echocardiography in predicting neurologic outcome after cardiac operations. Am J Cardiol 56:773, 1985.
133. Oka Y, et al.: Retained intracardiac air: transesophageal echocardiography for definition of incidence and monitoring removal by improved techniques. J Thorac Cardiovasc Surg 91:329, 1986.
134. Cieszynski T: Intracardiac method for the investigation of structure of the heart with the aid of ultrasonics. Arch Immun Ter Dosw 8:551, 1960.
135. Eggleton RC, et al.: Ultrasonic visualization of left ventricular dynamics. Ultrasonics 8:143, 1970.
136. Glassman E, Kronzon I: Transvenous intracardiac echocardiography. Am J Cardiol 47:1255, 1981.
137. Stephens DD, Palacios I, Block P, Weyman AE: Intracardiac echocardiographic evaluation of phasic right atrial free wall dynamics. Circulation 64: 128, 1981.
138. Hartley CJ, Cole JS: A single-crystal ultrasonic catheter-tip velocity probe. Med Instrum 8:241, 1974.
139. Cole JS, Hartley CJ: The pulsed Doppler coronary artery catheter: preliminary report of a new technique for measuring rapid changes in coronary artery flow velocity in man. Circulation 56:18, 1977.
140. St. Goar FG, et al.: Intravascular ultrasound imaging of angiographically normal coronary arteries: an in vivo comparison with quantitative angiography. J Am Coll Cardiol 18:952, 1991.
141. Linker DT, et al.: Analysis of backscattered ultrasound from normal and diseased arterial wall. Int J Card Imaging 4:177, 1989.
142. Bom N, et al.: Early and recent intraluminal ultrasound devices. Int J Cardiac Imaging 4:79, 1989.
143. Lee R, et al.: Intravascular ultrasound: technology and applications. *In* Nanda NC (ed.): Doppler Echocardiography. Philadelphia, Lea & Febiger, p. 383, 1993.
144. Hodgson JMcB, et al.: Clinical percutaneous imaging of coronary anatomy using an over-the-wire ultrasound catheter system. Int J Cardiac Imaging 4:187, 1989.
145. Roelandt JR, et al.: Intravascular high-resolution real-time cross-sectional echocardiography. Echocardiography 6:9, 1989.
146. Linker DT, et al.: Instantaneous arterial flow estimated with an ultrasound imaging and Doppler catheter (abstr.). Circulation 80:2302, 1989.
147. Waller BF: Anatomy, histology, and pathology of the major epicardial coronary arteries relevant to echocardiographic imaging techniques. J Am Soc Echo Cardiogr 2:232, 1989.
148. Stary HC: Macrophages, macrophage foam cells, and eccentric intimal thickening in the coronary arteries of young children. Atherosclerosis 64: 91, 1987.
149. Stary HC, et al.: A definition of the intima of human arteries and of its atherosclerosis-prone regions. Circulation 85:391, 1992.
150. Potkin BN, et al.: Coronary artery imaging with intravascular high-frequency ultrasound. Circulation 81:1575, 1990.
151. Nishimura RA, et al.: Intravascular ultrasound imaging: in vitro validation and pathologic correlation. J Am Coll Cardiol 16:145, 1990.
152. Nissen SE, Gurley JC: Application of intravascular ultrasound for detection and quantification of coronary atherosclerosis. Int J Cardiac Imaging 6:165, 1991.
153. Borst C, et al.: Imaging of post-mortem coronary arteries by 30 MHz intravascular ultrasound. Int J Cardiac Imaging 6:239, 1991.
154. Wenguang L, et al.: Validation of quantitative analysis of intravascular ultrasound images. Int J Cardiac Imaging 6:247, 1991.
155. Fitzgerald PJ, et al.: Errors in ultrasound image interpretation and measurement due to limited dynamic range (abstr.). Circulation 84(Suppl. 2): II-438, 1991.
156. Werner SG, et al.: Intravascular ultrasound imaging of human coronary arteries after percutaneous transluminal angioplasty: morphologic and quantitative assessment. Am Heart J 122:212, 1991.
157. Gussenhoven EJ, et al.: Arterial wall characteristics determined by intravascular ultrasound imaging: an in vitro study. J Am Coll Cardiol 14:947, 1989.
158. Mallery JA, et al.: Assessment of normal and atherosclerotic arterial wall thickness with an intravascular ultrasound imaging catheter. Am Heart J 119:1392, 1990.
159. Fitzgerald PJ, et al.: Intravascular ultrasound imaging of coronary arteries: is three layers the norm? (abstr.). J Am Coll Cardiol 17:217A, 1991.
160. Glagov S, et al.: Compensatory enlargement of human atherosclerotic coronary arteries. N Engl J Med 316:1371, 1987.
161. Pandian NG, Kreis A, Brockway B: Detection of intraarterial thrombus by intravascular high frequency two-dimensional ultrasound imaging in vitro and in vivo studies. Am J Cardiol 65:1280, 1990.
162. Fitzgerald PJ, et al.: Combined catheter ultrasound imaging with on-line tissue characterization: feasibility study (abstr.). Circulation 84(Suppl. 2): II-372, 1991.
163. Yock PG, et al.: Intravascular ultrasound imaging for guidance of atherectomy and other plaque removal techniques. Int J Cardiac Imaging 6:179, 1991.
164. Siegel RJ, et al.: Angiography, angioscopy, and ultrasound imaging before and after percutaneous balloon angioplasty. Am Heart J 120:1086, 1990.
165. Potkin BN, et al.: Ultrasound assessment of lesion composition predicts mechanisms of PTCA (abstr.). Circulation 84:(Suppl.)II-722, 1991.
166. Leon M, et al.: Intravascular ultrasound assessment of plaque responses to PTCA helps to explain angiographic findings (abstr.). J Am Coll Cardiol 17:47A, 1991.
167. Honye J, Jain A, Mahon DJ, Tobis JM: Atherosclerotic plaque eccentricity: a comparison of angiography and intravascular ultrasound imaging. Circulation 84(Suppl. 2):II-701, 1991.
168. Isner JM, et al.: Combination balloon-ultrasound imaging catheter for percutaneous transluminal angioplasty. Validation of imaging, analysis of recoil, and identification of plaque fracture. Circulation 84:739, 1991.

169. Yock PG, Fitzgerald PJ, Linker DT, Angelsen BJ: Intravascular ultrasound guidance for catheter-based coronary interventions. J Am Coll Cardiol 17: 39B, 1991.
170. Steele PM, et al.: Balloon angioplasty: natural history of the pathophysiological response to injury in a pig model. Circ Res 57:105, 1985.
171. Garratt KN, et al.: Restenosis after directional coronary atherectomy: differences between primary atheromatous and restenosis lesions and influence of subintimal tissue resection. J Am Coll Cardiol 16:1665, 1990.
172. Yock PG, et al.: Intravascular ultrasound as a guiding modality for mechanical atherectomy and laser ablation. Echocardiography 7:425, 1990.
173. White NW, et al.: Atherectomy guidance using intravascular ultrasound: quantitation of plaque burden (abstr.). J Am Coll Cardiol 80(Suppl. 2):II-374, 1989.
174. Aretz HT, et al.: Ultrasound guidance of laser atherectomy. Int J Cardiac Imaging 6:231, 1991.
175. Slepian MJ: Application of intraluminal ultrasound imaging to vascular stenting. Int J Cardiac Imaging 6:285, 1991.
176. Hodgsen J, et al.: Clinical percutaneous-imaging of coronary anatomy using an over the wire ultrasound catheter system. Int J Cardiac Imaging 4:187, 1989.
177. Pinto FG, et al.: Nitroglycerin-induced coronary vasodilation in cardiac transplant recipients: evaluation with in vivo intracoronary ultrasound. Circulation 85:69, 1991.
178. Yeon EB, et al.: Size and shape of the anastomotic junction as seen with intravascular ultrasound during coronary bypass surgery (abstr.). Circulation 84:(Suppl. 2):II-702, 1991.
179. Harrison JK, et al.: Balloon angioplasty of coarctation of the aorta evaluated with intravascular ultrasound imaging. J Am Coll Cardiol 15:906, 1990.
180. Weintraub AR, et al.: Evaluation of acute aortic dissection by intravascular ultrasonography. N Engl J Med 3323:1566, 1990.
181. Sheikh KH, et al.: Intravascular ultrasound assessment of the renal artery. Ann Intern Med 115:22, 1991.
182. Ricou F, et al.: Catheter-based intravascular ultrasound imaging of chronic thromboembolic pulmonary disease. Am J Cardiol 67:749, 1991.
183. Gorge G, et al.: Intravascular ultrasound in diagnosis of acute pulmonary embolism. Lancet 337:623, 1991.
184. St. Goar FG, et al.: Intimal disease in young coronary arteries: detection by intracoronary ultrasound (abstr.). Circulation 84(Suppl. 2):II-700, 1991.
185. Kitney RI, Moura L, Straughan K: 3-D visualization of arterial structures using ultrasound and voxel modelling. Int J Cardiac Imaging 4:135, 1989.
186. Rosenfield K, et al.: Three-dimensional reconstruction of human coronary and peripheral arteries from images recorded during two-dimensional intravascular ultrasound examination. Circulation 84:1938, 1991.
187. de Kroon MGM, et al.: Backscatter directivity and integrated backscatter power of arterial tissue. Int J Cardiac Imaging 6:265, 1991.
188. Omoto R, et al.: Ultrasonic tomography of the liver and detection of heart atrial septal defect with the aid of ultrasonic intravenous probes. Jap J Med Elect Biol Engin 1:90, 1963.
189. Glassman E, Kronzon I: Transvenous intracardiac echocardiography. Am J Cardiol 47:1255, 1981.
190. Stephens DD, et al.: Differentiation of constrictive pericarditis from restrictive cardiomyopathy by combined intracardiac echocardiography and transvenous endomyocardial biopsy. Circulation 64:25, 1981.
191. Carleton RA, Sessions RW, Graettinger JS: Diameter of heart measured by intracavitary ultrasound. Medical Res Engin p. 28, May–June 1969.
192. Eggleton RC, et al.: Computerized ultrasonic visualization of dynamic ventricular configurations. Presented at the Eighth ICEMB, Palmer House, Chicago, July 1969.
193. Kimoto S, et al.: Ultrasonic tomography of the liver and detection of heart atrial septal defect with the aid of ultrasonic intravenous probes. Ultrasonics 2:82, 1964.
194. Bom N, Lancee CT, Van Egmond FC: An ultrasonic intracardiac scanner. Ultrasonics 10(2):72, 1972.
195. Yock PG, Johnson EL, Linker DT: Intracavitary ultrasound: development and clinical potential. Am J Cardiac Imaging 2:185, 1988.
196. Pandian NG, et al.: Real-time, intracardiac, two-dimensional echocardiography. Echocardiography 8:407, 1991.
197. Stegall HF, Stone HL, Bishop VS: A catheter-tip pressure and velocity sensor. Proceedings of the 20th Conference on Engineering in Medicine and Biology. 27:4, 1967.
198. Benchimol A, et al.: Aortic flow velocity in man during cardiac arrhythmias measured with the Doppler catheter-flowmeter system. Am Heart J 78:649, 1969.
199. Hartley CJ, Cole JS: A single-crystal ultrasonic catheter-tip velocity probe. Med Instrum 8:241, 1974.
200. Cole JS, Hartley CJ: The pulsed Doppler coronary artery catheter: preliminary report of a new technique for measuring rapid changes in coronary flow velocity in man. Circulation 56:18, 1977.
201. White CW, Wilson RF, Marcus ML: Methods of measuring myocardial blood flow in humans. Prog Cardiovasc Dis 31:79, 1988.
202. Wilson RF, et al.: Transluminal, subselective measurement of coronary artery blood flow velocity and vasodilator reserve in man. Circulation 72: 82, 1985.
203. Wilson RF, Marcus ML, White CW: Prediction of the physiologic significance of coronary arterial lesions by quantitative lesion geometry in patients with limited coronary artery disease. Circulation 75:723, 1987.
204. Wilson RF, Marcus ML, White CW: Effects of coronary bypass surgery and angioplasty on coronary blood flow reserve. Prog Cardiovasc Dis 31: 95, 1988.
205. Lesser RF, Wilson RF, White CW: Physiologic assessment of coronary stenoses of intermediate severity can facilitate patient selection of coronary angioplasty. Coronary Artery Dis 1:697, 1990.
206. Wilson RF, White CW: Does coronary bypass surgery restore normal maximal coronary flow reserve: the effects of diffuse atherosclerosis and focal obstructive lesions. Circulation 76:563, 1987.
207. McGinn A, et al.: Coronary vasodilator reserve following human orthotopic cardiac transplantation. Circulation 78:1200, 1988.
208. Wilson RF, et al.: The effect of coronary angioplasty on coronary flow reserve. Circulation 77:873, 1988.
209. Vaterrodt D, Dirschinger J, Dacian S, Rudolph W: Normalization of coronary flow reserve with 24 hours post PTCA. Circulation 82(Suppl. 3):III-626, 1990.
210. Johnson EL, et al.: Assessment of severity of coronary stenoses using a Doppler catheter: validation of a method based on the continuity equation. Circulation 80:625, 1989.
211. Rushmer RF, Franklin DL, Ellis RM: Left ventricular dimensions recorded by sonocardiometry. Circ Res 4:684, 1956.
212. Hagl S, et al.: In-situ function of the papillary muscles in the intact canine left ventricle. *In* Duran C et al. (eds.): Recent Progress in Mitral Valve Disease. Butterworth, London, p. 397.
213. Theroux P, Franklin D, Ross J, Kemper WS: Regional myocardial function during acute coronary artery occlusion and its modification by pharmacologic agents in the dog. Circ Res 35:896, 1974.

PART 2

Clinical Applications

CHAPTER

17

LEFT VENTRICULAR INFLOW TRACT I: THE MITRAL VALVE

The left ventricular inflow tract has three major components: the mitral valve and supporting apparatus, the left atrium, and the pulmonary veins (Fig. 17–1). This portion of the heart collects oxygenated blood from the pulmonary vascular bed, stores the blood transiently, and then transports it to the left ventricle for subsequent ejection to the systemic circulation. The mitral valve, in addition to permitting unimpeded flow into the left ventricle during diastole, prevents systolic regurgitation into the left atrium and helps to funnel blood into the aorta.

The coronary sinus is also included in this section. This structure, although contributing to right ventricular inflow, lies immediately beneath and is consistently recorded with the left atrium. Consequently, the coronary sinus is discussed with this region.

THE NORMAL VALVE

The mitral valve has historically been a structure of principal echocardiographic interest. The pioneering studies of Edler and Hertz on the role of pulsed reflected ultrasound in cardiac diagnosis dealt primarily with the identification and analysis of the echoes returning from the mitral valve.[1,2] Likewise, the changes in the motion pattern of the mitral valve echo in mitral stenosis, which were observed by these investigators, represent the first clinical application of the echocardiographic technique and continue to remain the cornerstone of echocardiographic diagnosis.[2–4]

The early interest in the mitral valve occurred because of its high reflectivity, characteristic motion pattern, and position directly beneath the parasternal echocardiographic window, which combined to facilitate its location and recording. Additional features that have contributed to the continued echocardiographic importance of the mitral valve are its central position within the heart (which makes the mitral valve an ideal landmark from which to locate other structures) and its frequent involvement in a variety of disorders that affect the structure and function of the left side of the heart.

Anatomy

Anatomically, the mitral valve is a complex structure composed of the mitral leaflet tissue, chordae tendineae, papillary muscles, left ventricular myocardium subjacent to the papillary muscles, and fibromuscular mitral annulus.[5–9] Functional integrity of the valve requires that each of these components performs appropriately and acts in concert with its other members. The mitral leaflets actually represent a continuous veil of fibrous tissue whose base is attached around the entire circumference of the mitral orifice to the fibromuscular ring, the mitral annulus. The free edges of the leaflet veil show several indentations. Two of these indentations, the anterolateral and posteromedial mitral commissures, are regularly placed and permit the mitral valve's division into the anterior and posterior leaflets.[10] A line drawn between these two commissures runs parallel to the coaptation line of the mitral leaflets and likewise parallels a line drawn between the tips of the two papillary muscles. The anterior mitral leaflet is a relatively long, semicircular or triangular structure, whereas the posterior leaflet, although shorter, has a more extensive area of attachment to the mitral annulus. The distal third of both leaflets is roughened and opaque, whereas the proximal two thirds are smooth and clear.[8] The roughened area is important because it receives the insertions of the chordae

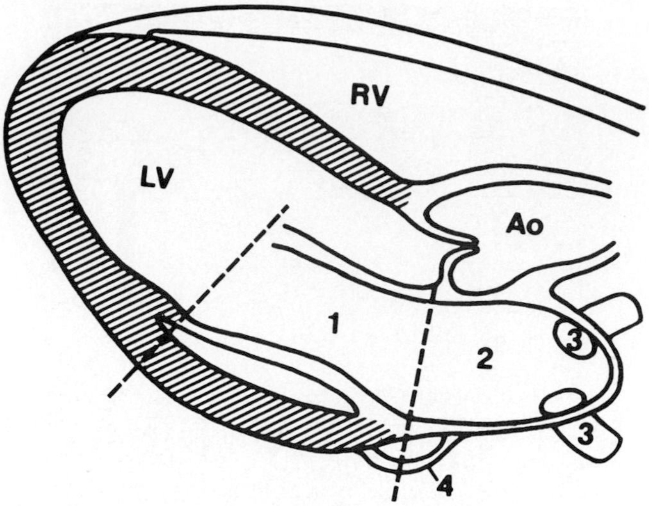

Fig. 17–1. Diagram of the left ventricular inflow tract. The mitral valve region (1) includes the area from the tips of the papillary muscles to the mitral annulus. The left atrial chamber (2) extends from the mitral annulus to the superior atrial wall. Two pairs of pulmonary veins, the right and left superior and inferior veins (3), insert into the corresponding superior medial and lateral walls of the left atrium. The coronary sinus (4) is anatomically incorporated into the posterior wall of the left atrium beneath the atrioventricular groove. The coronary sinus appears circular because it is transected parallel to its short axis. Ao = aorta; LV = left ventricle; RV = right ventricle.

tendineae on its ventricular surface. A ridge at the superior margin of this roughened area marks the line of coaptation of the anterior and posterior leaflets.[9]

The anterior mitral leaflet has a common point of attachment to the fibrous skeleton of the heart with the left coronary cusp and half of the noncoronary cusp of the aortic valve.[10]

The chordae tendineae arise from the tips of the anterolateral and posteromedial papillary muscles and course superiorly to insert into the mitral leaflets at both the free leaflet edges and superior margins of the roughened area. The chordae from the posteromedial papillary muscle supply the medial half of both the anterior and posterior mitral leaflets, whereas those from the anterolateral papillary muscles supply the lateral half of both leaflets.[10]

Although the left ventricular papillary muscles are anatomically termed *anterolateral* and *posteromedial*, both of these muscle groups, from an echocardiographic standpoint, lie in the posterior hemisphere of the ventricle with their tips oriented parallel to the closure line of the mitral leaflets. Therefore, the terms *anterior* and *posterior* appear unnecessary, and hence, they are referred to throughout this book as the *medial* and *lateral papillary muscles*. Either papillary muscle group may have one or more distinct "bellies of muscle." They may, likewise, arise as separate finger-like projections from the left ventricular myocardium or may be more intimately involved with the left ventricular trabeculae.[11] The papillary muscles move in concert with the subjacent left ventricular myocardium during systolic ventricular contraction. Dysfunction of the papillary muscles appears to be related to the concomitant dysfunction of the myocardium at their base.[12,13]

Methods of Cross-Sectional Examination

The mitral valve is examined using three primary imaging planes. These include (1) the parasternal long axis of the left ventricle, (2) the parasternal short axis of the left ventricle at the mitral valve level, and (3) the apical four-chamber view. The mitral valve can also be recorded, albeit less optimally, in a variety of other planes, including the apical long axis, two-chamber, and five-chamber views, and the subcostal long axis view of the left ventricle. A portion of the mitral valve is frequently recorded in the subcostal long axis of the right ventricular outflow tract, and a subcostal short axis of the left ventricle at the mitral valve level can be recorded if necessary. To determine the contractile function of the left ventricular myocardium at the base of the papillary muscles (which may affect normal mitral closure), one must also record a short axis view of the left ventricle at the papillary muscle level.

The primary view for recording the mitral valve is the parasternal long axis (Fig. 17–2A).[14] This imaging plane transects the midportion of the bodies of both the anterior and posterior mitral leaflets from their points of insertion into the mitral annulus to their free edges. It also includes the anterior and posterior extremes of the mitral annulus and some of the chordae tendineae. The precise point at which the free edge of the mitral leaflets joins the chordae is often difficult to define, and they frequently appear as one continuous structure.[15] When appropriately aligned parallel to the long axis of the left ventricle, this plane should pass between but fail to record the two papillary muscles. The plane, however, can be angled in a medial or lateral direction to record either of the papillary muscles if desired. This imaging plane records the motion of both mitral leaflets in an anteroposterior direction, their systolic and diastolic positions and spatial configurations (Fig. 17–2B and C), the anteroposterior mitral annular diameter, the motion pattern of the mitral annulus in both a superoinferior and anteroposterior direction, and the temporal and spatial positions of the mitral leaflets in relation to the left ventricular cavity, annulus, and atrium.

The parasternal short axis of the left ventricle at the mitral valve level is depicted in Figure 17–3. This view is important because it permits direct visualization of the mitral valve orifice.[16] It is the primary plane for recording mitral valve orifice area and for assessing the location and extent of involvement for the mitral valve orifice in focal disorders. It encompasses the entire circumferential area of both the anterior and posterior mitral valve leaflets and can be positioned to record these leaflets at any level from the free edges to the point of annular insertion.

The apical four-chamber view passes through the mitral leaflets obliquely at approximately a 30° angle to the line of leaflet coaptation (Fig. 17–4).[17] Because the coaptation line of the leaflets is ordinarily displaced toward the posterior portion of the ventricle, this oblique orientation causes the plane to transect more of the anterior mitral leaflet than of the posterior. The anterior leaflet is displayed medially and the posterior leaflet laterally. This plane orientation is ideal for determining the position of the atrioventricular ring and for defining the point of leaflet closure relative to this anatomic landmark. It is also useful for defining the point of mitral leaflet insertion into the interventricular septum and for relating it to the level of insertion of the tricuspid leaflet.

Normal Mitral Leaflet Motion: Long Axis View

The normal mitral leaflets are thin, pliable structures that move freely in response to the relative forces acting on their surfaces. The diastolic motion of these leaflets

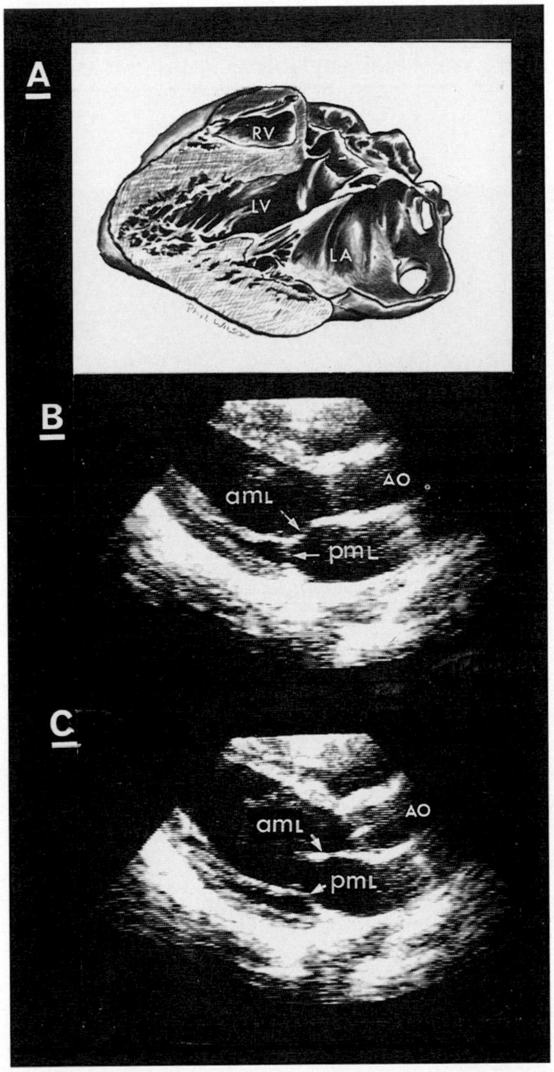

Fig. 17–2. An anatomic section through the left ventricle (LV), mitral valve, and left atrium (LA) corresponding to the path of the imaging plane in the parasternal long axis view of the left ventricular inflow tract. **B.** Systolic configuration of the mitral valve and adjacent structures in this long axis plane. The anterior (aml) and posterior mitral leaflets (pml), their coaptation point, and the chordae tendineae, stretching from the region of leaflet coaptation toward the papillary muscles, are recorded. **C.** Diastolic frame demonstrates the open mitral valve. The anterior mitral leaflet and the full extent of the posterior mitral leaflet and its chordal extension to the papillary muscles can be visualized. Ao = aorta; RV = right ventricle.

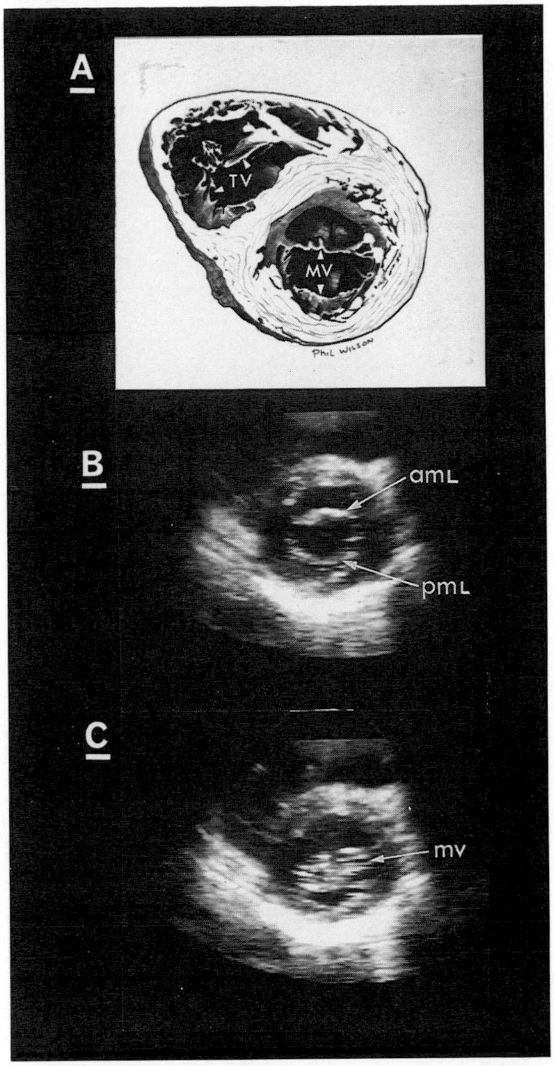

Fig. 17–3. A. An anatomic section through the right and left ventricles at the free edges of the mitral leaflets corresponding to the region recorded in the parasternal short axis view of the mitral valve (MV). **B.** Diastolic frame illustrates the separated anterior (aml) and posterior mitral leaflets (pml) surrounding the mitral valve orifice. The normal circular diastolic configuration of the left ventricle in short axis is evident. **C.** Systolic frame illustrates the coapted mitral leaflets. The left ventricular cavity area is decreased, and the circular left ventricular walls are thicker than those in the comparable diastolic recording. TV = tricuspid valve.

is a combination of both independent leaflet motion in response to blood flow through the valve orifice and motion of the mitral annulus to which the leaflets are attached. Systolic motion of the coapted leaflets, in contrast, passively follows that of the mitral annulus and papillary muscles.

The normal pattern of mitral leaflet motion recorded in the long axis, cross-sectional view is depicted and described in Figure 17–5A through H. At the onset of ventricular systole (Fig. 17–5A), the left ventricle is maximally dilated, and the coapted mitral leaflets and mitral annulus are in their most posterior and cephalad position. At this point, the leaflets appear as a horizontally placed, narrow-based funnel. The base of this fun-

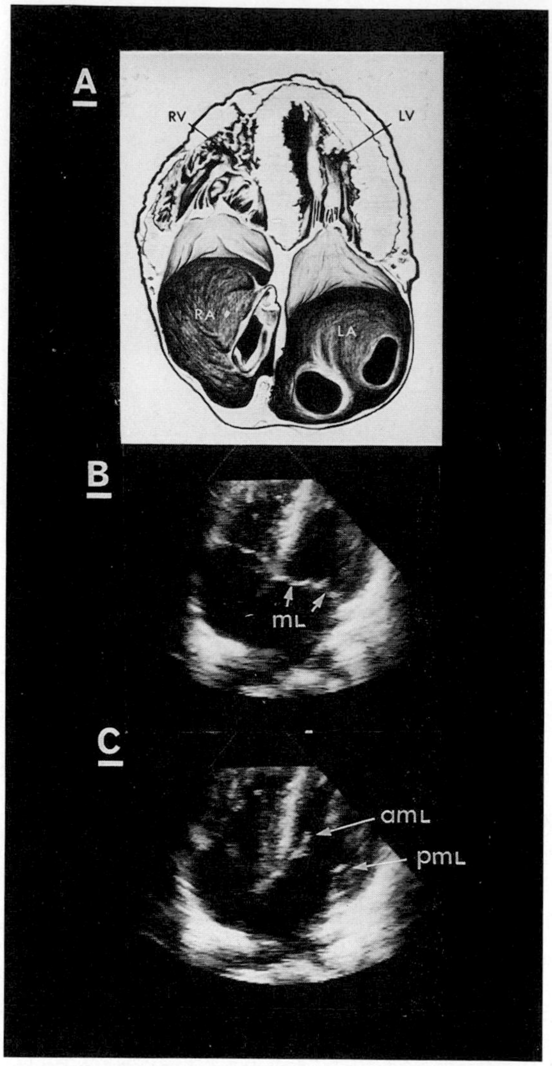

Fig. 17–4. Apical four-chamber view of the mitral valve. **A.** An anatomic section through the left (LV) and right (RV) ventricles and left (LA) and right (RA) atria. The diagram corresponds to the path of the imaging plane in this view. **B.** Systolic frame illustrates the coapted mitral leaflets (ml). The anterior mitral leaflet arises at the superior margin of the interventricular septum and extends laterally perpendicular to the septum. The posterior leaflet arises from the lateral margin of the atrioventricular ring and extends medially to join the anterior leaflet. **C.** Diastolic frame with the (medial) anterior (aml) and (lateral) posterior (pml) mitral leaflets widely separated and pointing toward the apex of the left ventricle.

nel is formed by the mitral annulus, the curvilinear sides by the basal two thirds of the mitral leaflets, and the spout by the distal third of the leaflets and the chordae tendineae. As systole progresses (Fig. 17–5B), the mitral valve and annulus are drawn anteriorly and toward the cardiac apex so that, by end-systole, the valve is in its most anterior and apical position. Left atrial filling during this period elevates the posterior aortic root and increases the diameter of the mitral annulus. This increase in annular diameter separates the basal attachment points of the mitral leaflets and causes them to become more vertically oriented in the ventricle. During isovolumic relaxation (Fig. 17–5C), the leaflets shift downward toward the left ventricular cavity.

At the onset of diastolic inflow, the leaflet tips fly rapidly apart (Fig. 17–5D) and continue this motion until they approach the endocardial surfaces of the ventricle. At the point of peak leaflet separation, the distance between the leaflets exceeds the mitral annular diameter, and the annulus thus represents the area of anatomic limitation to left ventricular inflow. Having reached the point of peak opening, the leaflets almost immediately begin to reclose (Fig. 17–5E). Downward or closing motion of the anterior leaflet is initiated by downward movement of the posterior aortic root in response to left atrial emptying. The leaflets then swing inward toward each other and, during the slow phase of ventricular filling, assume a neutral or floating position within the left ventricular cavity (Fig. 17–5F). Following atrial systole (Fig. 17–5G), the leaflets reopen. Final leaflet closure is initiated by atrial relaxation (Fig. 17–5H) and is completed by ventricular systole.

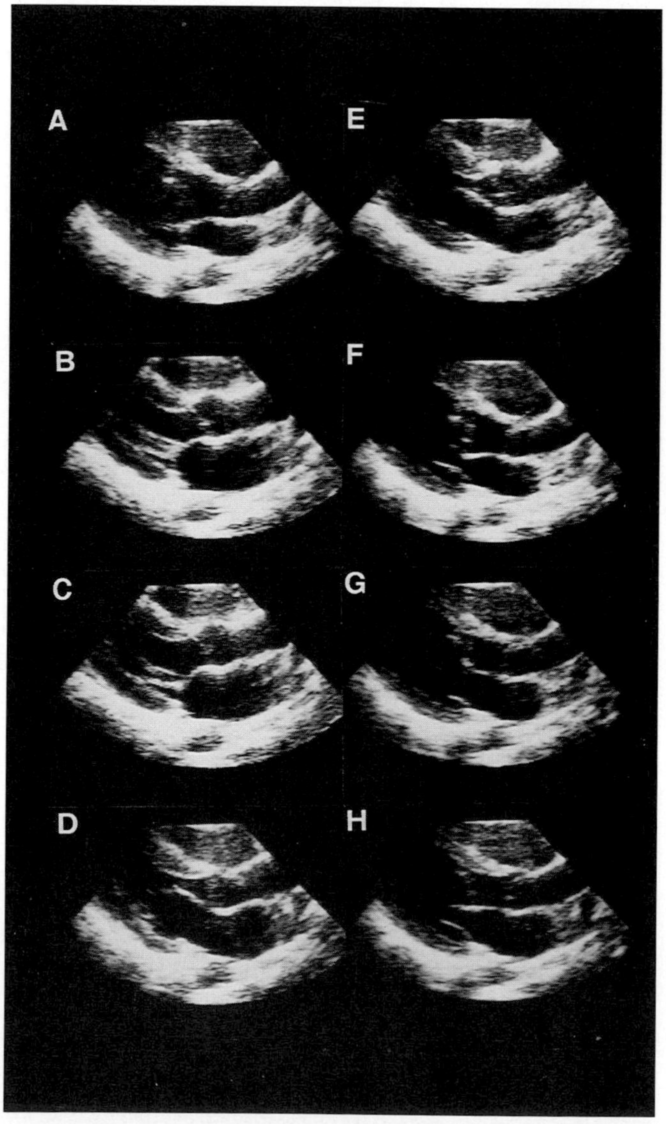

Fig. 17–5. The normal sequence of mitral leaflet motion in the parasternal long axis view. (See text for details.)

Normal Mitral Leaflet Motion: Short Axis View

The short axis projection is ideally suited to evaluate the changes that mitral leaflet motion produces on the configuration of the mitral orifice and on the relationship of the ventricular surface of the leaflets to the endocardial margins of the ventricle at sequential points during the diastolic filling period. The normal pattern of mitral leaflet motion in the short axis view is depicted in Figure 17–6A through H. Beginning at end-systole (Fig. 17–6A), the coapted mitral leaflets are positioned posteriorly in the ventricle in a line that roughly parallels the anterior chest wall. At the onset of diastole (Fig. 17–6B), an initial anterior movement of the coapted leaflets is followed almost immediately by the onset of rapid valve opening. During the rapid opening phase (Fig. 17–6C), the leaflets initially separate evenly along the entire width of the closure line. This separation causes the orifice to appear transiently more rectangular than circular. As motion of a central portion of the leaflets continues, however, they become more parallel to the circular endocardial margin of the ventricle, and the orifice assumes a circular configuration (Fig. 17–6D). Almost immediately after reaching the point of peak opening (Fig. 17–6E), the leaflets begin to move inward toward the center of the ventricle. Movement at the center of the leaflets is greater than at the margins, and the orifice, therefore, becomes more oval in configuration.

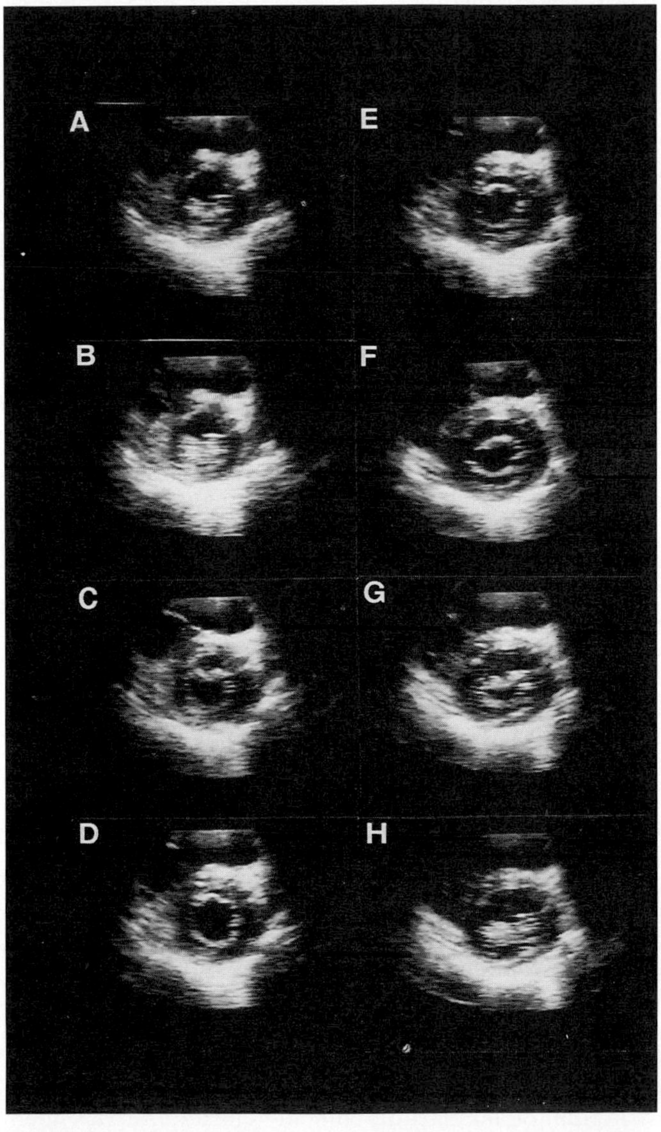

Fig. 17–6. Normal pattern of mitral leaflet motion in the parasternal short axis view. (See text for details.)

During the slow phase of ventricular filling, the leaflets assume a floating position within the ventricular chamber (Fig. 17–6F), and the orifice assumes a consistent oval appearance. At the onset of atrial systole, the leaflets separate again, the orifice becomes more circular, and the orifice area increases. With atrial relaxation, the leaflets move toward a closed position (Fig. 17–6G). This motion is primarily caused by downward movement of the anterior leaflet, which may actually assume an orientation that is convex anteriorly before final systolic closure. At the point of leaflet coaptation (Fig. 17–6H), the anterior and posterior leaflets with their chordal attachments appear as a linear band or mass of echoes horizontally positioned in the posterior portion of the ventricle. During systole, the coapted leaflets move anteriorly in concert with the anterior motion of the posterior wall of the ventricle, and as the ventricular area decreases, they become more closely associated with the posterior wall endocardial echoes.

Normal Mitral Leaflet Motion: Apical Four-Chamber View

Mitral leaflet motion is more difficult to analyze in the apical four-chamber view than in either the long or short axis views for two reasons. First, in the four-chamber orientation, the imaging plane transects the mitral valve along a line that passes just above the medial commissure and below the lateral commissure. As noted in the section on short axis motion, movement of the leaflets is lesser in these areas than in their midportions. As a result, more subtle changes in the pattern of leaflet motion may be more difficult to appreciate. Second, although the leaflets are oriented perpendicular to the path of the ultrasonic beam during systole and, hence, are well visualized, the opened leaflets during diastole point almost directly toward the transducer and thus become far more difficult to record. The apical four-chamber view, therefore, is better for analyzing the configuration and motion patterns of the mitral leaflets during systole than during diastole.

Figure 17–7A through H depicts the motion pattern of the mitral leaflets in this view. At end-systole (Fig. 17–7A), the mitral leaflets are coapted and lie in the plane of the mitral annulus. At the onset of diastole (Fig. 17–7B), the leaflets initially bow outward toward the cardiac apex. As the rapid phase of leaflet opening continues, the leaflet tips swing freely from about their insertion points into the anteromedial and posterolateral margins of the mitral annulus until they lie parallel to the septum and the lateral wall of the ventricle, respectively (Fig. 17–7C). When the leaflets are fully open, one can frequently record the entire sweep of the chordae, from the anterior leaflet to the lateral papillary muscle, as they

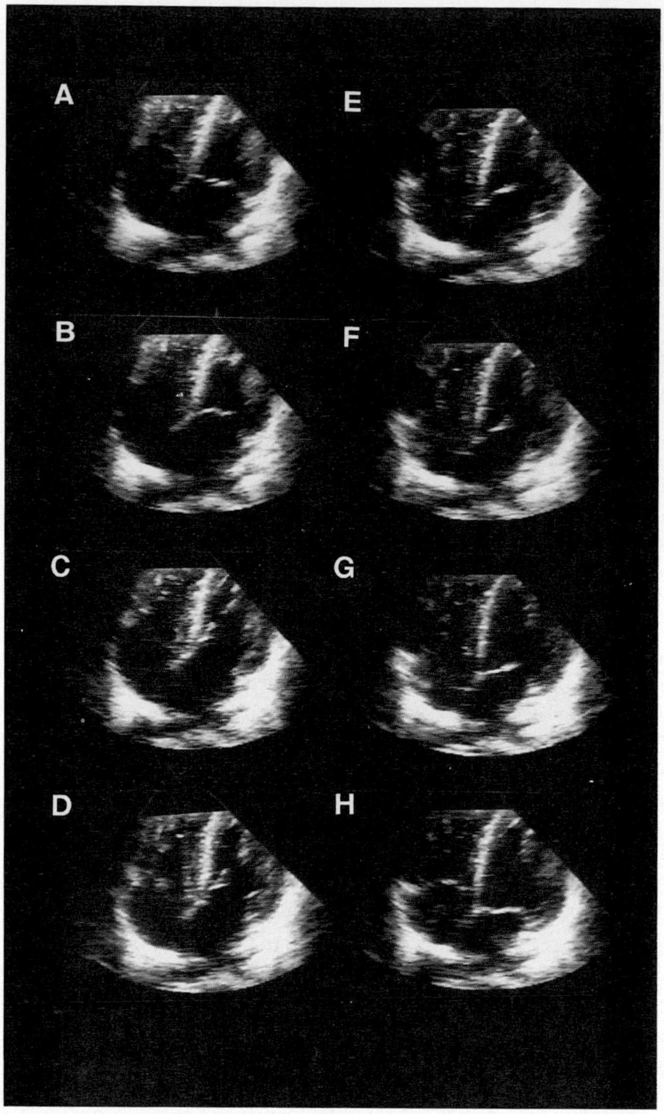

Fig. 17–7. Normal mitral leaflet motion in the apical four-chamber view. (See text for details.)

arc through the ventricular chamber. After reaching full excursion, the leaflets almost immediately separate from the ventricular walls (Fig. 17–7D) and move slightly inward toward the center of the ventricle. This inward motion continues until a mid-diastolic resting or floating position in the ventricular chamber is reached (Fig. 17–7E). Atrial contraction is accompanied by variable leaflet reopening (Fig. 17–7F). As the atrium relaxes, there is corresponding movement inward toward the mitral annulus (Fig. 17–7G), and a fully closed position. When closed, the leaflets are positioned parallel to the plane of the mitral annulus and perpendicular to the long axis of the left ventricle. During ventricular systole (Fig. 17–7H), the annulus moves upward toward the cardiac apex. As annular movement progresses, the coapted leaflets sink slightly posteriorly and appear to "set" within the annulus before reopening during the next diastolic period. The leaflet bodies may normally come to rest slightly superior to the plane of the mitral annulus at the point of peak systolic closure (see following discussion).

Factors Affecting Timing, Amplitude, and Rate of Mitral Leaflet Motion

Mitral leaflet motion is influenced by a variety of factors including (1) the relative pressures in the left atrium and left ventricle;[18–21] (2) the velocity and volume of blood flow through the mitral orifice;[18,20,22–24] (3) motion of the points of leaflet attachment at the mitral annulus[25] and papillary muscles; (4) left ventricular and atrial diastolic compliance;[26] and (5) the systolic performance of the left ventricle.[27] Figure 17–8 diagrammatically depicts the relationships of the left atrial and left ventricular pressures and mitral valve flow to mitral leaflet motion. Beginning at the point of aortic valve closure, left ventricular pressure falls rapidly. As ventricular pressure approaches left atrial pressure, the mitral leaflets shift downward into the ventricle (see Fig. 17–5B and C). This motion is associated with a low rate and volume of flow recorded at the mitral annulus but not with actual leaflet opening.[18] Following the intersection of the left ventricular and left atrial pressure curves, a positive left atrial-left ventricular gradient develops, the mitral leaflets fly open, and the flow through the valve rapidly accelerates.[18,23,28] The rate of leaflet opening (D-E slope) appears directly related to flow into the left ventricle[29] and like flow is inversely related to initial diastolic left ventricular pressure.[19] The degree of leaflet separation at peak diastolic opening can likewise be related to transmitral flow at low flow rates.[29] At higher flow rates, leaflet separation is limited by the endocardial surface of the ventricle, and this relationship can no longer exist.[23]

On reaching their full excursion, the leaflets immediately begin to reclose.[30] The point of peak leaflet excursion (E point) is reached before peak flow velocity is recorded, and the leaflets begin their initial closing motion (E-F slope) while flow is still accelerating.[18,23]

The factors that influence the pattern and rate of initial diastolic closure are complex. Several mechanisms have been proposed to explain this dissociation between transmitral flow and leaflet motion. It was initially felt that, as the leaflets opened, tension was produced because of chordal stretching with resultant recoil of the leaflets as they reached their point of peak opening.[31] In contrast, early echocardiographic data suggested that the initial downward motion of the leaflets occurred as a result of posterior motion of the mitral annulus.[21,23] More recently, it has been postulated that flow through the mitral orifice causes tip vortices to form at the leaflet edges, which initiate leaflet closure.[22,32] Analysis of leaflet motion in cross-sectional studies supports the early M-mode observations that the initial downward motion of the anterior mitral leaflet occurs in response to downward displacement of the mitral annulus and posterior wall of the aortic root (see Fig. 17–5E).

The greater portion of the leaflet closure (E-F slope), however, results from free motion of the leaflets about their point of annular attachment. This motion has been attributed to the formation of a ring vortex system within the ventricle.[22,30,32,33] These vortices begin immediately

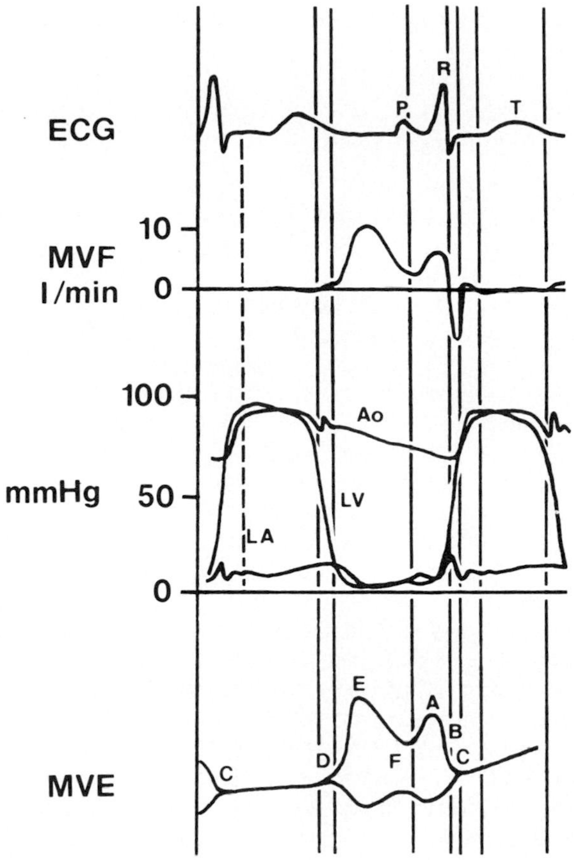

Fig. 17–8. Comparison of the temporal sequence and relative magnitudes of mitral valve flow (MVF) in liters per minute (l/min); the aortic (Ao), left ventricular (LV), and left atrial (LA) pressure curves in millimeters of mercury (mm Hg), and the motion pattern of the mitral valve echo (MVE). The MVE depicted here corresponds to a typical M-mode recording of mitral leaflet motion at the free edges of the valve leaflets. The D-point is the position of the leaflets at the onset of diastolic opening. The E-point represents the point of peak leaflet opening. The E-F slope represents the initial diastolic closing motion of the valve leaflets, and the A wave represents leaflet reopening in response to atrial systole. The A-C slope corresponds to end-diastolic leaflet closure, and the C-point reflects final leaflet coaptation. Point B is the position of the mitral leaflets at the onset of ventricular systole. Normally, leaflet closure is initiated by atrial relaxation and completed by the systolic rise in left ventricular pressure. Relating the points on the mitral valve echogram to the long axis cross-sectional recording in Figure 17–5, the C-point of the mitral valve echogram corresponds to the leaflet position in panel A. The D-point corresponds to panel B, whereas panel C occurs slightly after the D-point (just as the leaflets are beginning to open). The E-point of the mitral valve echogram corresponds to panel D. Downward motion following the E-point is reflected in panel E. The F-point of the mitral valve echogram corresponds to panel F, whereas the A wave corresponds to panel G. Panel H then corresponds to the B-point of the mitral valve echogram. (See text for further details.) ECG = electrocardiogram. (Adapted from Nolan SP: Patterns of instantaneous mitral valve flow and the atrial contribution to ventricular filling. *In* Kalmanson (ed.): The Mitral Valve: A Pluridisciplinary Approach. Littleton, MA, Publishing Sciences Group, 1976.)

after valve opening with the formation of small tip vortices at the free margins of the cusps and continue to expand as the in-rushing blood strikes the cardiac apex, spreads out, and flows back up along the walls of the ventricle. The vortices then turn back behind the leaflets toward the apex, thereby forming the ring vortex system. Because of the configuration of the ventricle, the main strength of this vortex system is concentrated behind the anterior leaflet. The strength of these vortices is related to flow into the ventricle, and the rate of leaflet closure should also be related to the rate and volume of diastolic inflow.

In support of these concepts, clinical studies have shown a direct correlation between the percentage of ventricular inflow during the first third of diastole and early diastolic mitral closing velocity [E-F slope, Fig. 17–8 mitral valve echo (MVE)].[24] In contrast, a decrease in initial diastolic closing rate has been observed in patients with increased left ventricular initial diastolic volume or decreased compliance, which are both associated with a shift in the percentage of ventricular filling toward the latter third of diastole.[24]

A mid-diastolic opening and closing motion of the mitral valve (L wave) is commonly seen at slow heart rates in normal subjects. This motion is due to reestablishment of a positive left atrial pressure > left ventricular pressure (LAP > LVP) gradient during mid-diastole and is associated with low velocity forward flow. The increase in atrial pressure during this period is due to increased pulmonary venous flow into the atrium during the period of early diastolic transmitral flow deceleration and pressure reversal. This increase in inflow from the pulmonary bed occurs because the atrial pressure is low and the gradient from the pulmonary bed to the atrium is relatively high. As venous inflow continues, left atrial pressure rises toward left ventricular pressure, eventually reestablishing a positive atrioventricular pressure gradient and reaccelerating mitral flow and reopening the mitral leaflets.[34]

Following atrial contraction, the left atrial-left ventricular pressure gradient increases as does the flow velocity through the mitral valve.[18] As the atrium relaxes, there is a decrease or even reversal in this gradient as well as in mitral valve flow. This change is accompanied by movement of the leaflets toward a closed position (A-C slope).[35] With ventricular systole, the left ventricular and left atrial pressure cross and valve closure is completed.[18] Note, however, that flow through the valve may continue after atrial and ventricular pressures have intersected, thereby reflecting the higher pressure required to stem the established flow through the valve leaflets.[18]

Several conditions may alter the normal pattern of late diastolic mitral leaflet closure (A-C slope, Fig. 17–8). The most noteworthy of these are (1) an increase in PR interval and (2) a rapid rise in left ventricular diastolic pressures (e.g., with aortic insufficiency). Prolongation of the PR interval causes atrial contraction to occur earlier in diastole. As the atrium relaxes, the atrioventricular pressure gradient reverses and the mitral valve flow decelerates rapidly.[23] These changes are followed by premature apposition of the valve cusp.

In patients with severe aortic insufficiency, the rapid rise in ventricular diastolic pressure may also reverse the atrioventricular pressure gradient and cause premature closure of the valve leaflets.[36–38] This early closure may be protective because it prevents the left atrium and pulmonary circuit from exposure to the inordinately high end-diastolic pressures in the left ventricle.

Effects of Abnormal Pressure and Flow on Mitral Valve Motion

Marked reduction in flow through the mitral valve reduces maximal leaflet opening amplitude and the rate of leaflet movement. The diminished mitral leaflet opening increases the separation between the ventricular surface of the leaflets at peak opening and the ventricular endocardium (E-point septal separation) (Fig. 17–9B and D). M-mode studies have demonstrated that an increased distance between the anterior leaflet and the septum (greater than 5 mm) at peak leaflet opening is associated with a reduced ejection fraction (less than 50%).[39] This relationship is based on the assumption that the volume of blood entering the ventricle during diastole is directly related to the percentage ejected during the preceding systole. These relationships are also noted in the cross-sectional format and form a useful basis for roughly estimating left ventricular performance in a manner that is independent of ventricular geometry.

In the short axis view, the reduced leaflet motion caused by diminished transmitral flow is reflected by a decrease in the mitral valve orifice area. Figure 17–9D illustrates this reduction in absolute orifice area at peak leaflet opening. The maximal orifice area that occurs in response to mitral valve flow is termed the functional mitral valve area. This area is in contrast to the anatomic orifice area, which is the maximal allowable anatomic separation of the leaflets. The relationship of these two areas becomes important when considering stenotic values because flow can be reduced to a point where an orifice that is anatomically reduced is no longer functionally restrictive. Likewise, at high flow rates, a deformed orifice, which is within the normal absolute range for valve areas, may be functionally restrictive because it is still smaller than the separation that would be achieved by the leaflets if anatomic restriction were not present. Absolute values for orifice area therefore must be treated with caution. An orifice that is restrictive in one flow setting may be more than adequate to accept the reduced flow volume in another setting.

In the apical four-chamber view, the decrease in rate and amplitude of leaflet motion is again noted. As illustrated in Figure 17–9F, this decrease is characterized by failure of the leaflet tips to approach the lateral margins of the ventricular wall at peak diastolic separation. Also, in this case there is displacement of the leaflets downward into the ventricular cavity during systole (Fig. 17–9E) (see the section entitled Papillary Muscle Dysfunction later in this chapter).

Although precise measurement of rate and timing of leaflet motion is better recorded in the M-mode format, decrease in amplitude of leaflet excursion, increase in separation between the leaflets and ventricular walls, and decrease in or distortion of the mitral orifice area are readily appreciated on the cross-sectional record.

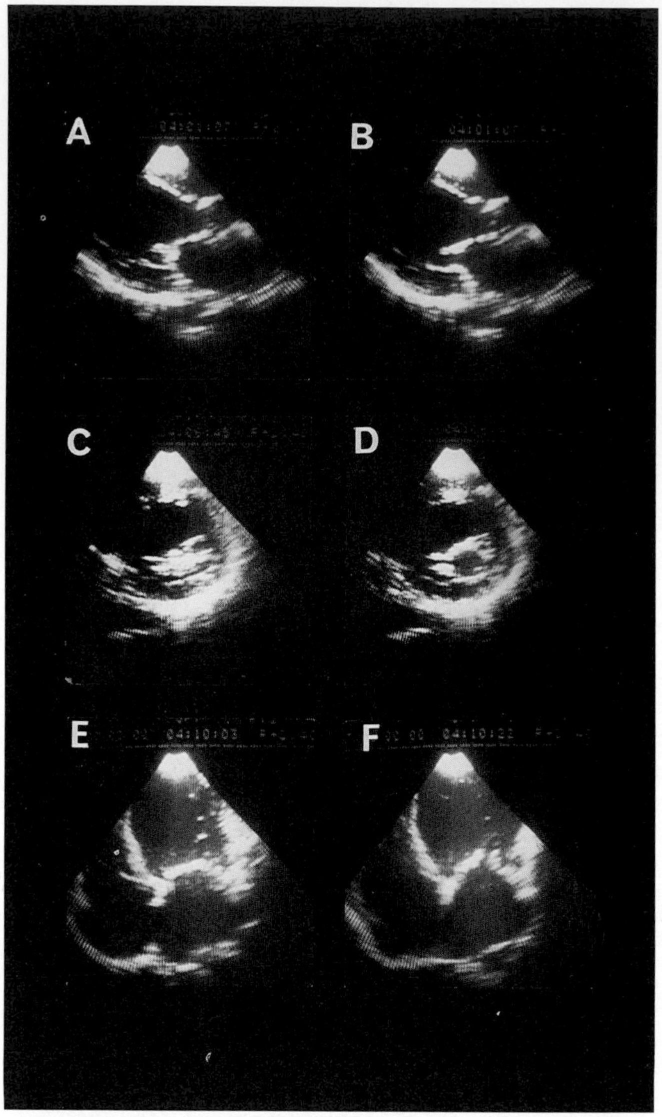

Fig. 17–9. Cross-sectional echogram from a patient with severe cardiomyopathy, left atrial and ventricular dilation, and a marked reduction in left ventricular stroke volume and ejection fraction. **A** and **B.** Systolic and diastolic long axis recordings of the mitral valve illustrate a decrease in diastolic mitral leaflet separation and an increase in distance between the ventricular surface of the anterior mitral leaflet and the endocardium of the interventricular septum at peak leaflet excursion (E-point, septal separation). **C** and **D.** Systolic and diastolic short axis recordings illustrate the reduction in mitral valve orifice area at peak diastolic opening in relation to the left ventricular cavity size. **E** and **F.** Systolic and diastolic frames recorded in the apical four-chamber view again illustrate the reduction in diastolic mitral leaflet separation. During systole **(E),** the coapted leaflets fail to reach the plane of the mitral annulus during peak systolic closure. This failure results in the displacement of the leaflets into the left ventricular cavity and has been associated with the clinical syndrome of papillary muscle dysfunction (see section on papillary muscle dysfunction).

Transmitral Flow

The pattern of the instantaneous velocities present in the left atrium and ventricle at any point in diastole is highly complex and varies both spatially and temporally in response to the locally varying pressure gradients in the flow field. This complex phenomenon can be considered in terms of (1) the mean spatial flow velocity crossing the valve (limiting orifice) at any point in time or integrated over the diastolic filling period; (2) the local velocities in the flow field passing through the orifice at any point in diastole; (3) the velocities along a streamline of flow extending from an arbitrary point in the left atrium to a comparable point in the left ventricle or (4) the entire two- or three-dimensional velocity distribution in the atrium and ventricle at one or multiple points in diastole.

The mean spatial velocity at sequential temporal points during the filling period is the most commonly used measure of the rate at which blood crosses the mitral valve. This value is usually derived from pulsed Doppler recordings obtained from the cardiac apex with the sample volume positioned to record the peak spatial inflow velocity that is typically found on the left ventricular side of the mitral annulus close to the leaflet tips. Because the impetus for blood to move through the mitral valve is the development of the diastolic atrioventricular pressure gradient, the velocity of flow generally follows the gradient throughout diastole.[40] Although the "gradient," like the velocity profile, varies at different points within the ventricle, it can be most simply considered as the pressure difference between the midatrium and midventricle.[40] Figure 17–10 illustrates the relationship between transmitral flow and mid-left atrial and mid-left ventricular pressure. At slow heart rates (Fig. 17–10A and B), early transmitral flow begins immediately after the pressure in the relaxing left ventricle falls below that in the left atrium. Flow then accelerates as the gradient increases, reaches its peak at or slightly before the second crossover of left atrial and left ventricular pressure, and then decelerates rapidly to zero at or near the third pressure crossover.[40] As the atrioventricular pressure gradient falls, mitral flow decelerates; however, inertia maintains forward flow even as the gradient becomes negative. Deceleration is completed by the reversed pressure gradient and dissipation of inertial energy. A period of diastasis then follows, during which atrial and ventricular pressure can remain essentially equal or a distinct mid-diastolic forward pressure gradient can occur (Fig. 17–10B), which is accompanied by a forward velocity on the Doppler recording (L wave). This gradient is caused by continued atrial filling from the pulmonary veins and is exaggerated when E wave deceleration is rapid. A small reversed gradient associated with deceleration of the L wave is also seen.

Atrial contraction produces another forward (LAP > LVP) pressure gradient and accelerates flow across the mitral valve as evidence by the A wave on the Doppler flow profile. At more rapid heart rates (Fig. 17–10C), diastole is shortened and atrial contraction (A wave in the Doppler flow profile) immediately follows ventricular relaxation and often shortens this phase of diastole.

The determinants of the various components of the early diastolic mitral velocity profile (Fig. 17–11) have been examined extensively in clinical studies,[41,42] animal experiments,[43–45] and by mathematic modeling.[46–48] These variables are discussed in detail in Chapter 24. Briefly, flow acceleration (a_m) during passive filling is primarily determined by the rate at which the atrioventricular pressure gradient increases following mitral valve opening. This in turn is governed by the initial left atrial pressure, the rate of left ventricular relaxation, and the resistance to flow offered by the mitral valve apparatus. Increasing left atrial pressure augments the atrioventricular gradient for any ventricular relaxation rate and increases both flow acceleration and peak velocity. An increase in ventricular relaxation rate shortens the time to peak gradient and likewise increases flow acceleration. Opposing acceleration is the mass of blood that must be set in motion. This can be considered as a column whose length has been shown experimentally to be equal to roughly twice the diameter of the mitral orifice.[49] Thus, as the orifice area decreases, acceleration increases (i.e., in mitral stenosis).[50,51]

The deceleration of early diastolic flow (d_m) is determined by the rate at which the atrial and ventricular pressures approach each other following the peak atrio-

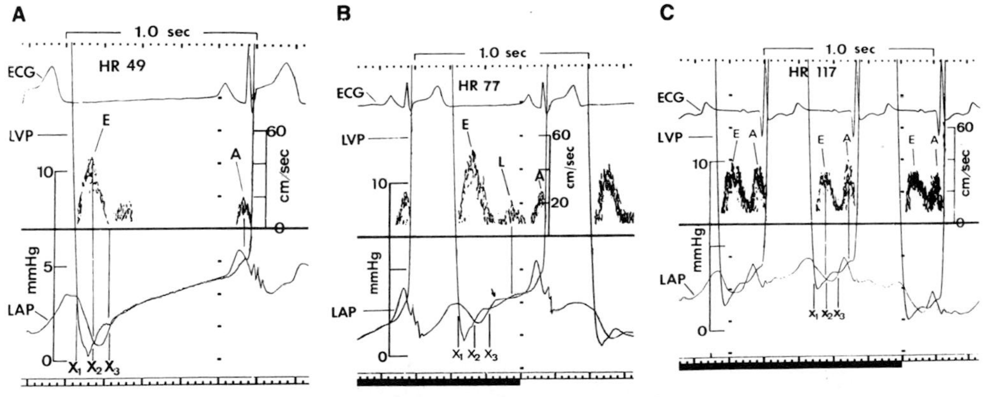

Fig. 17–10. Records of simultaneous transmitral pressures recorded at the midatrial and midventricular (4 cm from the apex) levels aligned with Doppler time-velocity plots recorded from an apical four-chamber view at heart rates of 49, 77, and 117 beats per minute in an experimental animal model. **A.** Heart rate of 49 beats per minute. Presence of a reversed (LVP > LAP) transmitral pressure gradient is temporally associated with the deceleration of the early filling wave (E) throughout a wide range of heart rates. **B.** Heart rate of 77 beats per minute. Same basic pressure-flow velocity relation is observed. In addition, in animals exhibiting heart rates of less than 90 beats per minute, a distinct mid-diastolic wave of flow (L) is recorded with an accompanying positive pressure gradient (arrow). **C.** Heart rate of 117 beats per minute. Same basic pressure-flow velocity relation is observed. However, flow during the early rapid-filling phase is accelerated again before it has completely decelerated, resulting in incomplete separation of the E and A waves. HR = heart rate; ECG = electrocardiogram; LVP = left ventricular pressure; LAP = left atrial pressure. (From Courtois M, Kovacs SJ Jr, Ludbrook PA: Transmitral pressure-flow velocity relation. Importance of regional pressure gradients in the left ventricle during diastole. Circulation 78:667, 1988. Reproduced by permission of the American Heart Association, Inc.)

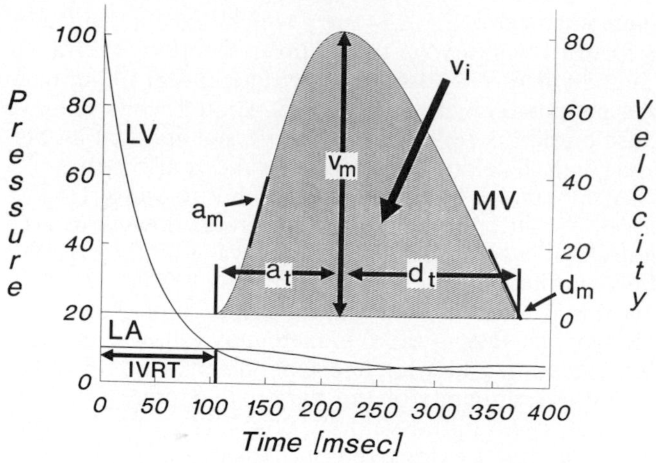

Fig. 17–11. Sample output from mitral flow simulation, showing derivable Doppler and other indices (dependent parameters) used in the analyses in Figures 17–12 and 17–13. LV = left ventricular pressure, LA = left atrial pressure; IVRT = isovolumic relaxation time; a_m = maximal acceleration rate (dv/dt) of mitral velocity, cm/sec^2; a_t = acceleration time of early mitral inflow, seconds or milliseconds; v_m = maximum mitral velocity, cm/sec; d_t = mitral deceleration time, time between peak and 0 velocity, seconds or milliseconds; d_m = maximal deceleration rate (−dv/dt) of mitral velocity following peak velocity, cm/sec^2; v_i = time velocity integral of mitral velocity from mitral valve opening until velocity returns to 0 cm. (From Thomas JD, Choong CYP, Flachskampf FA, Weyman AE: Analysis of early transmitral Doppler velocity curve: effect of primary physiologic changes and compensatory preload adjustment. J Am Coll Cardiol 16:644, 1990. Reprinted with permission from the American College of Cardiology.)

ventricular gradient. This in turn is governed by the relative stiffness of the two chambers (i.e., the fall in atrial and rise in ventricular pressure that occurs for each milliliter of blood that moves from atrium to ventricle) and the resistance of the mitral valve per se (i.e., the mitral valve area). In patients with nonobstructive valves, net atrial and ventricular stiffness is the primary determinant of deceleration because it is the pressure gradient not the absolute chamber pressure that governs flow. Thus, the effect on the gradient will be the same, whether 1 ml of blood passing from the atrium to the ventricle causes the atrial pressure to fall by 2 mm Hg and the ventricular pressure to rise by 1 mm Hg or the atrial pressure to fall by 1 mm Hg and the ventricular pressure to rise by 2 mm Hg. This same relationship applies to chamber compliance (Cn), which is the reciprocal of stiffness. Stiffness and compliance are altered by factors that either change the basic pressure volume relationship of the chamber (e.g., ischemia, intrinsic myocardial disease, or constriction) or alter the location on the pressure volume curve at which the chamber is operating (changes in end-systolic volume). Changes in the intrinsic properties of the atrium or ventricle that increase stiffness (or decrease compliance) will increase the rate of flow deceleration as will an increase in atrial pressure or ventricular end-systolic volume.[50,51]

The peak mitral velocity (V_m or E-wave height) is generally increased by factors that augment flow acceleration and diminished by factors the increase deceleration. Peak velocity has been shown to be most directly affected by initial left atrial pressure, with a mean increase in peak E-wave velocity of roughly 3.9 cm/sec being observed for each mm Hg atrial pressure increase. It is also lowered somewhat by prolonged relaxation, low atrial and ventricular compliance and systolic dysfunction. Figure 17–12 graphically illustrates the effects of left atrial pressure, ventricular relaxation, ventricular compliance, and end-systolic volume on the early filling wave of mitral inflow. Figure 17–13 summarizes the quantitative effects of changes in each of these parameters in a mathematic simulation in which a single measure is altered while the others are kept constant. Unfortunately, these relationships suggest that the mitral velocity curve can give no unique information about individual chamber pressures or compliances, only the pressure gradient and the net stiffness/compliance.

Mid-diastolic filling of the ventricle (L wave) also appears to be related to ventricular stiffness and the rate of initial diastolic flow deceleration. Specifically, as ventricular stiffness increases, the magnitude of the atrioventricular gradient reversal in early diastole increases, flow decelerates more rapidly, atrial filling from the pulmonary veins increases,[34] and the second gradient reversal becomes more marked. The degree of filling that occurs during diastasis is primarily determined by ventricular compliance because the forward pressure gradients that are present during this period are small.

The atrial filling wave has four primary physiologic determinants: (1) left atrial volume/pressure at the time of atrial contraction (Starling's law of the atrium); (2) the contractility of the atrium; (3) the compliance of the ventricle (the stiffer the ventricle, the more blood will be ejected retrograde into the pulmonary veins); and (4) the systolic function of the ventricle (which determines the point on the pressure volume curve at which the ventricle is operating when the atrium contracts).

Mean transmitral velocities have been used extensively in studies seeking to relate diastolic filling to diastolic function and in the quantitation of transmitral flow. These applications are discussed in detail in Chapters 24 and 30, respectively.

Spatial Distribution of Transmitral Velocities

More detailed mapping of the velocity profile across the limiting orifice as well as the local velocities within the three-dimensional flow field proximal and distal to the valve can be achieved by color flow mapping. Color M-mode recordings reveal the spatial pattern of velocities along a streamline of flow while preserving the temporal accuracy of sampling (Fig. 17–14). In general, the peak velocity at the E wave occurs more apically than that following atrial contraction; however, this is not an invariable finding, and the factors that determine these spatial relationships remain to be defined.

Color flow maps of the inflow stream reveal the relative velocities at all points in two-dimensional space. These flow maps are far more complex than measures of mean or axial velocities and the increase in spatial resolution is achieved at the expense of both velocity

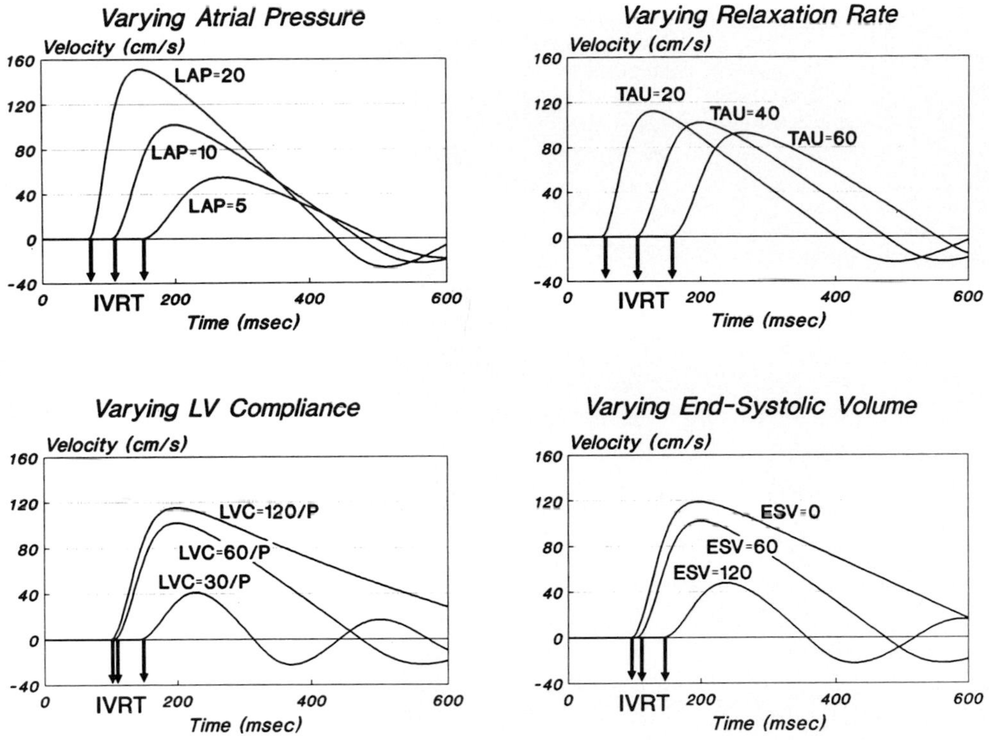

Fig. 17–12. The effects of varying left atrial pressure (mm Hg), ventricular relaxation rate (milliseconds), left ventricular compliance milliliters per milliliters of mercury, and end-systolic volume (ml) on early diastolic mitral inflow. LAP = left atrial pressure; LVC = left ventricular compliance; ESV = end systolic volume; TAU = time constant of ventricular relaxation (T_L); IVRT = isovolumic relaxation time. (Courtesy of Dr. James D. Thomas.)

and temporal resolution. At present, color velocity maps are used to visually assess the spatial distribution of velocities with quantitative analysis reserved for specific research applications. Figure 17–15 illustrates the spatial acceleration of velocities from the left atrium to the left ventricular side of the mitral orifice and their deceleration within the left ventricular cavity at peak passive filling. The maximal transmitral velocity occurs between the mitral annulus and the leaflet tips, and the axial profile appears relatively flattened at its peak. Although in this example the velocity profile at the orifice appears flat, quantitative analysis of the flow field crossing the valve has demonstrated that the profile can be variably skewed both at the leaflet tips and annulus.[52] Analysis of the complete three-dimensional flow field is beyond the capability of most clinical laboratories, and current understanding of these data even when available is incomplete at best.

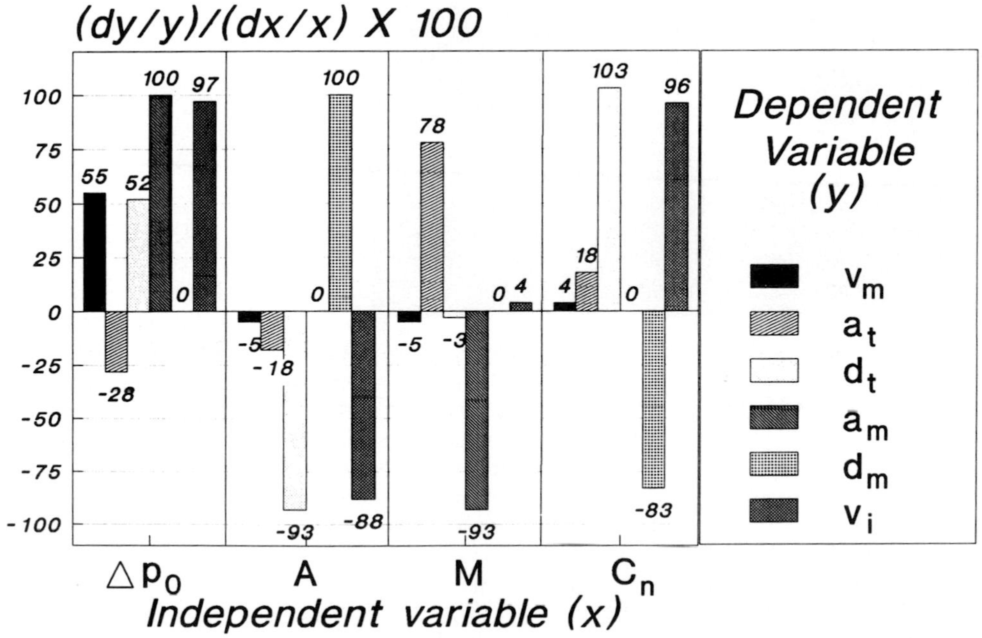

Fig. 17–13. Proportional change in noninvasive indices for small proportional changes in physiologic parameters. For example, a 10% increase in left atrial pressure would lead to a (55 × .10) 5.5% increase in V_m or E-wave velocity, a 2.8% decrease in acceleration time (a_m) a 5.2% increase in deceleration time (d_t), and a 9.7% increase in the velocity time integral of the E wave (V_i). V_m = maximum velocity; a_t = acceleration time; d_m = maximum deceleration; Δp_o = change in initial left atrial pressure; A = valve areas; M = mass; C_n = net compliance. (Adapted from Thomas JD, Newell JB, Choong CYP, Weyman AE: Physical and physiological determinants of transmitral velocity: numerical analysis. Am J Physiol 260:H1718, 1991.)

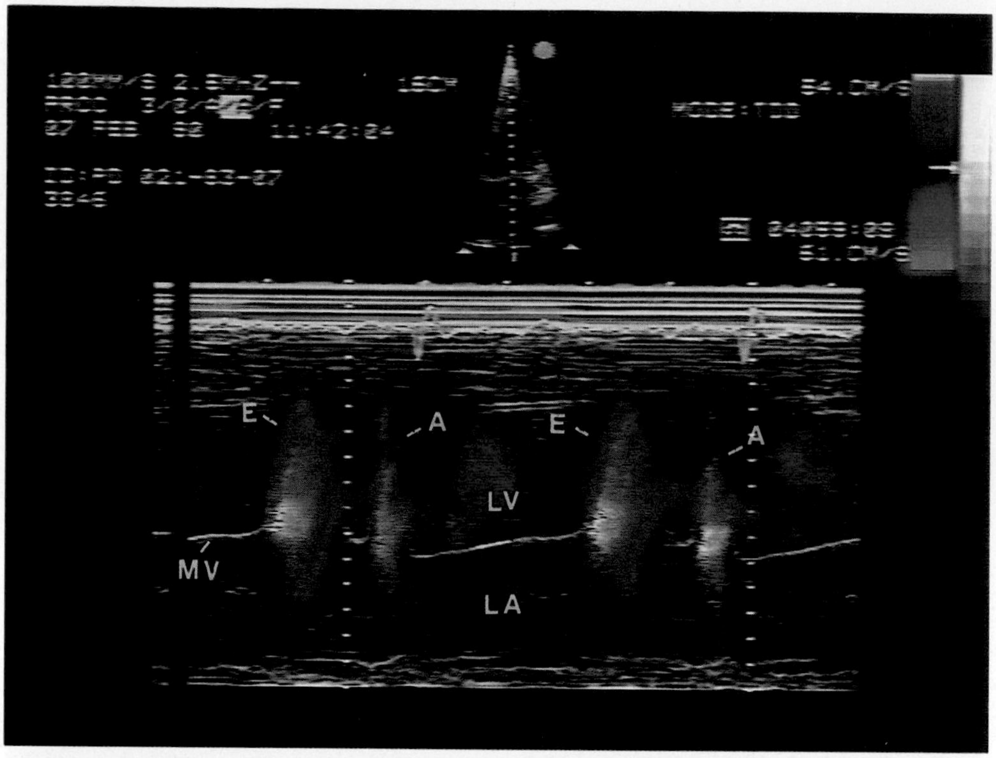

Fig. 17–14. Color M-mode recorded for the cardiac apex illustrating the spatial and temporal velocity pattern along a streamline of flow extending from the left atrium (LA) to the left ventricle (LV) through the center of the mitral valve (MV) during early rapid filling (E) and following atrial contraction (A).

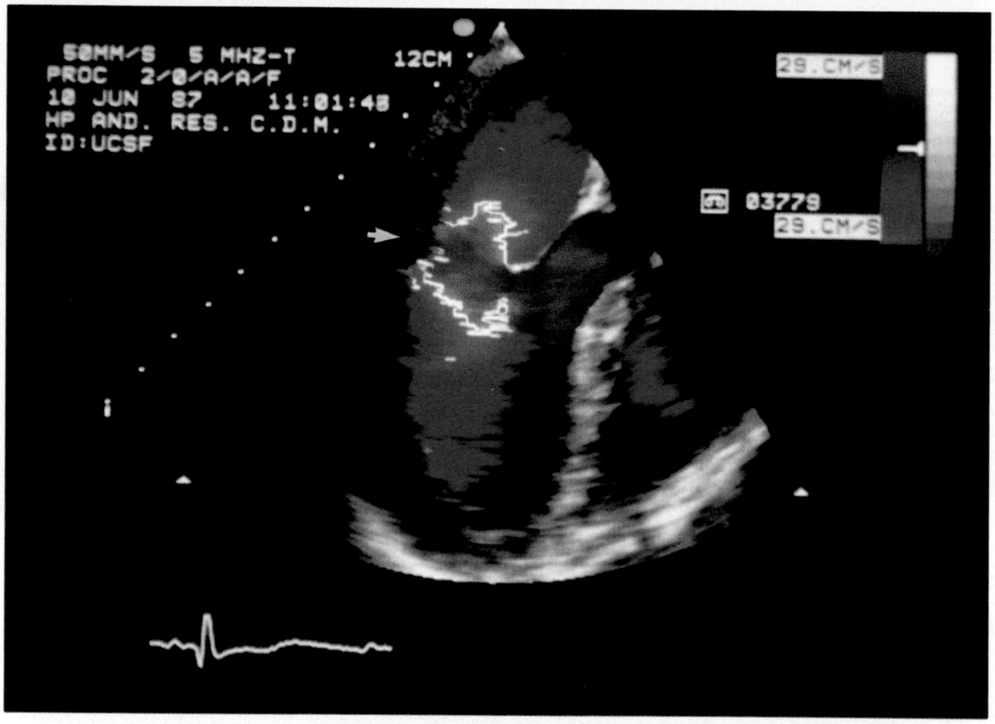

Fig. 17–15. Transesophageal color Doppler recording illustrating the spatial velocity pattern in the region of the mitral valve (arrow) immediately following atrial contraction.

THE ABNORMAL MITRAL VALVE ECHOGRAM

Proper function of the mitral valve requires unimpeded passage of blood from the left atrium into the left ventricle during diastole and the prevention of backflow into the left atrium during systole. On the basis of these functional requirements, mitral valve disorders can be divided into (1) those that restrict diastolic flow into the left ventricle and are characterized echocardiographically by a decrease in orifice size or distortion in orifice configuration; (2) those that primarily affect the systolic competence of the valve and are associated with abnormalities of leaflet closure; and (3) structural abnormalities of the valve leaflets or supporting structures, which may occur with or without disruption of valvular function.

Abnormalities Associated With Restricted Left Ventricular Inflow

Valvular lesions that primarily obstruct left ventricular inflow include rheumatic mitral stenosis, mitral stenosis and insufficiency, congenital mitral stenosis, parachute mitral valve, mitral arcade, and supravalvar mitral ring. A variety of other structural disorders of the mitral valve and left atrium (e.g., mitral annular calcification, mitral annular and leaflet tumors, and cor triatriatum) may secondarily impede left ventricular inflow; however, these abnormalities are discussed in the sections describing the primary lesions. The mitral valve orifice is also frequently distorted in aortic insufficiency, and inflow may be disturbed in this condition.

Rheumatic Mitral Stenosis

Rheumatic mitral stenosis is by far the most common lesion that produces obstruction to left ventricular inflow. This acquired form of chronic valvular heart disease is characterized pathologically by a diffuse thickening of the mitral leaflets, fusion of the commissures, and shortening and fusion of the chordae tendineae. These abnormalities combine to decrease the size of the mitral valve orifice, thereby restricting the flow of blood into the left ventricle.[53]

Diagnosis

Two-dimensional Echocardiography. Mitral stenosis is generally diagnosed by two-dimensional echocardiographic imaging and is characterized by (1) an increase in echo production from the thickened, deformed mitral leaflets; (2) abnormal diastolic leaflet motion; (3) fusion of the commissures; and (4) a reduction in mitral valve orifice area.[16,54–58]

Increased echo production from the deformed mitral leaflets can be observed in almost every instance of rheumatic mitral stenosis.[16,56] This increased reflectivity generally involves both the anterior and posterior leaflets and is most prominent at the margins of the valve orifice and along the line of commissural fusion (Fig. 17–16A and B).[56] As leaflet deformity becomes more severe, the area of increased reflectivity expands superiorly toward the mitral annulus (Fig. 17–16C and D). Calcification of the rheumatic valve also begins at the tips of the leaflets and spreads upward toward the annulus (Fig. 17–16D). This pattern is in contrast to the distribution of calcification and the corresponding area of increased echo production noted in mitral annular calcification, where initial involvement occurs at the annulus and subvalvular region and spreads downward toward the leaflet tips.[59]

Abnormal mitral leaflet motion may be evident throughout diastole or only during the initial phase. It is

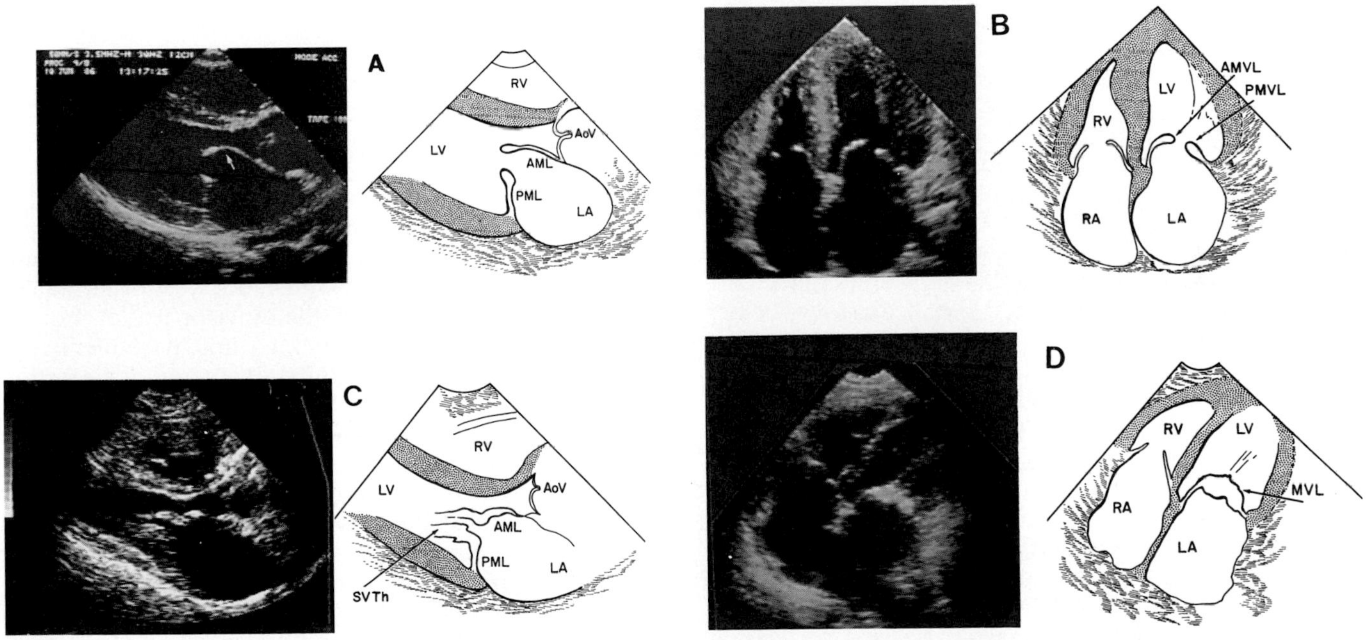

Fig. 17–16. **A.** A parasternal long axis recording illustrating a domed, stenotic, mitral valve at peak diastolic opening. There is minimal thickening of the leaflet tips, restriction of anterior leaflet excursion, and a reduction in orifice diameter. The posterior leaflet is fixed and erect. The arrow indicates the point of maximal leaflet flexion or doming. **B.** An apical four-chamber recording; the minimally deformed leaflets show slight thickening at the tips and marked doming. **C.** A parasternal long axis recording from a patient with more severe mitral stenosis showing right ventricular dilation, left atrial dilation, extensive thickening of both the anterior and posterior mitral leaflets, limited leaflet mobility, and diffuse chordal thickening. **D.** An apical four-chamber recording. There is extensive leaflet calcification, minimal doming, and moderate involvement of the subvalvular apparatus. **B** and **D.** There is associated stenosis of the tricuspid valve, with doming of both the septal and anterior tricuspid leaflets. RV = right ventricle; LV = left ventricle; AoV = aortic valve; AML = anterior mitral leaflet; PML = posterior mitral leaflet; RA = right atrium; LA = left atrium. SVTh = subvalvular thickening; MVL = mitral valve leaflet. (From Wilkins GT, et al.: Percutaneous balloon dilatation of the mitral valve: an analysis of echocardiographic variables related to outcome and the mechanism of dilatation. Br Heart J 60:299, 1988. Used with permission of the British Heart Journal.)

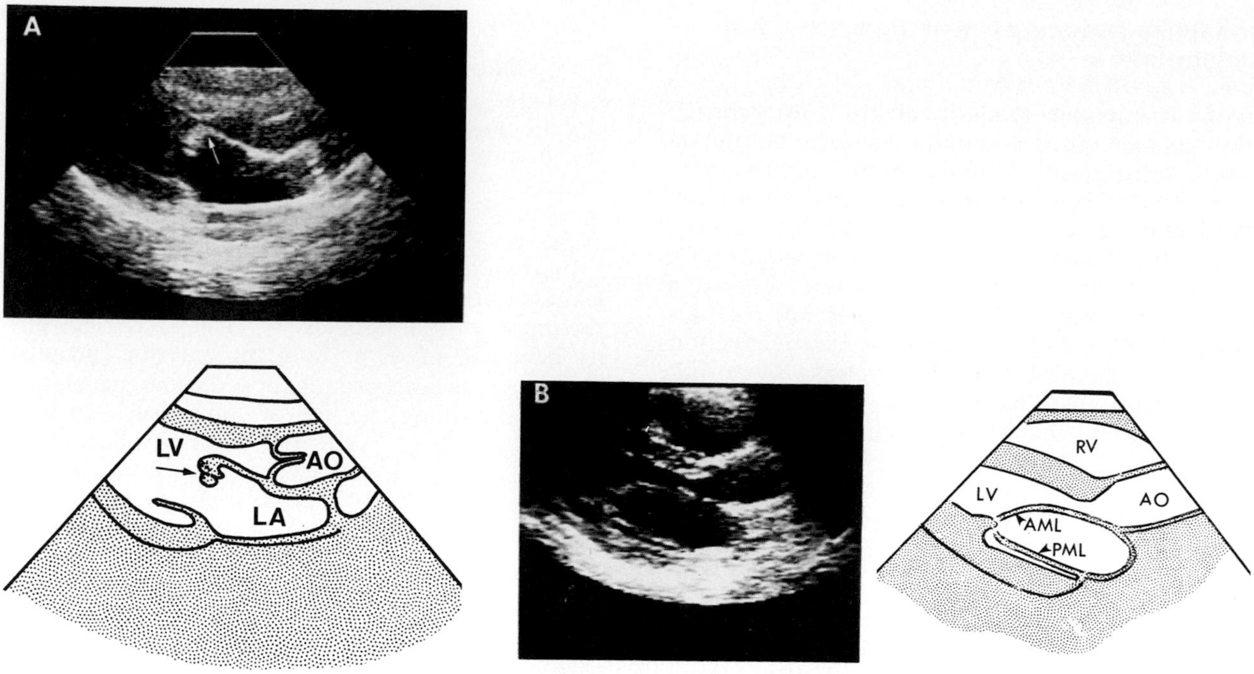

Fig. 17–17. **A.** Top. Diastolic recording from a patient with mitral valve prolapse and an apparent mass lesion involving the free edge of the anterior mitral leaflet. An abrupt, almost right-angle bend in the midportion of the anterior leaflet simulates the doming seen in mitral stenosis (arrow). Bottom. The increased echo density at the tip of the anterior leaflet is indicated by the horizontal arrow. LV = left ventricle; Ao = aorta; LA = left atrium. **B.** Parasternal long axis view of the mitral valve from a normal patient, in whom the full extent of the anterior mitral leaflet is recorded (from the anterior point of insertion into the mitral annulus to the papillary muscles). This gives the valve the appearance of an elongated dome and has been confused with mitral stenosis. This configuration is usually produced by either abnormal medial or lateral angulation of the transducer and can readily be differentiated from true mitral stenosis by the position of the tip of the arc at the level of the papillary muscles and by the smooth acceleration and deceleration of the anterior leaflet in real time. RV = right ventricle; LV = left ventricle; Ao = aorta; AML = anterior mitral leaflet; PML = posterior mitral leaflet.

best recorded in the parasternal long axis view but can also be appreciated in the apical views (Figs. 17–16A and B). Changes in anterior leaflet motion are most evident,[16,54] although restricted posterior leaflet motion is also present. The abnormal motion is characterized by (1) restricted excursion of the leaflet tips;[16,54–57] (2) prominent diastolic doming of the anterior leaflet into the left ventricular outflow tract;[16,54,56] and (3) decrease in, or total loss of, the normal initial diastolic closing motion of the anterior mitral leaflet (E-F slope, see Fig. 17–8).[54]

The initial diastolic motion abnormalities occur in the following sequence. At end-systole, the leaflets are coapted, the posterior leaflet is frequently more prominent and erect than normal, and its body is oriented in a convex arc toward the left atrium.[54] Immediately before valve opening, the leaflets shift downward toward the left ventricular cavity. The posterior leaflet reverses its position and becomes concave toward the left atrium, and the anterior leaflet bows inward toward the left ventricle.[54] Almost immediately, the leaflets initiate their rapid opening sequence, and the leaflet tips separate. Motion of the tip of the anterior leaflet, however, is quickly arrested because of the commissural fusion.[16,54,56] The body of the leaflet, in contrast, continues anteriorly and, in the absence of corresponding motion of the leaflet tip, produces an abrupt knee-like bend in the midportion of the anterior leaflet (convex toward the septum) (Figs. 17–16A and B). Continued distention of the body of the anterior leaflet pulls the anterior and posterior leaflet tips farther anteriorly. The leaflet tips, however, remain in close apposition, thereby resulting in an obvious decrease in orifice diameter.

The body of the anterior leaflet must be pliable for diastolic doming to occur. When the leaflet is extensively fibrosed or calcified, doming may not be evident (Fig. 17–16C and D). In these instances, real-time analysis of leaflet motion shows the anterior leaflet moving stiffly and stopping abruptly, as though suddenly restrained at its point of maximal excursion. This action is in contrast to the free motion and smooth acceleration and deceleration of normal valve leaflets and indicates that stenosis is present.

Although diastolic doming is a relatively specific characteristic of mitral stenosis, there are several situations in which apparent doming of the valve may occur in the absence of stenosis. The most common situations are the redundant floppy valves sometimes seen in mitral valve prolapse syndrome and mass lesions or vegetations involving the free edge of the anterior mitral leaflet.

Figure 17–17A is an example of a patient with both mitral valve prolapse and an apparent mass lesion on the free edge of the anterior mitral leaflet. The abrupt, nearly right-angle curve of the anterior leaflet in this example is similar to the type of doming seen in mitral stenosis. The free unrestricted motion of these leaflets and a normal mitral valve orifice diameter, however, differentiate the apparent stenotic valves from the truly stenotic valves. Finally, in normal persons, when the full extent of the mitral valve leaflets and chordae are recorded, a gradual arc is inscribed, extending from the aortic root to the papillary muscle tips (Fig. 17–17B). This arc has been confused with valvular doming and stenosis. It can be readily differentiated from true mitral stenosis, however, by the smooth deceleration of the normal anterior leaflet as it reaches complete excursion; by the position of the apical tip of the arc at the level of the papillary muscles rather than at the free edges of the mitral leaflets; and by the normal mitral valve orifice diameter.

After reaching full excursion, the domed anterior leaflet of mitral stenosis either may be held in this fully distended position throughout diastole or may gradually begin to reclose. The rate of diastolic leaflet closure (E-F slope) depends on the duration of the distending pressure against the atrial surface of the valve. With moderate or severe stenosis, the pressure gradient may persist throughout diastole, thereby maintaining the leaflets in their fully distended position and preventing diastolic closure. In this setting, the only independent leaflet motion occurs during initial diastolic valve opening and with systolic closure.[54] Any movement of the leaflets during this period therefore is caused by motion of the mitral annulus, which is displaced superiorly and posteriorly as the ventricle fills. The leaflets are displaced in the same manner. With less severe obstruction, the pressure gradient across the valve may dissipate during the latter portion of diastole, thereby allowing the anterior leaflet to gradually fall back toward a closed position. When sinus rhythm is present, reopening may occur in response to atrial systole.

Commissural fusion and the resultant changes in valve area are best recorded in the parasternal short axis view (Fig. 17–18). In cases in which mild stenosis is questioned and long axis valve motion is equivocal, the presence or lack of commissural fusion will usually establish or exclude the diagnosis.

Doppler. The pattern of flow through the stenotic mitral valve varies with the severity of the lesion. As the mitral orifice area decreases and the left atrial pressure increases, flow acceleration and peak velocity increase and the rate of deceleration decreases (Fig. 17–19). The increase in velocity is primarily related to the increase in left atrial pressure, which augments the atrioventricular pressure gradient (Fig. 17–20). Stenosis cannot be differentiated from normal based on peak velocity alone because velocities above the normal range (50 to 75 cm/sec) can be recorded in lesions associated with increased transmitral flow such as mitral regurgitation and ventricular septal defect. In these cases however, the deceleration rate is usually normal or increased. Figure 17–21A to C illustrates the patterns of transmitral flow in three patients with increasingly severe stenosis. When normal atrial contraction persists (Fig. 17–21A), flow velocity typically increases after atrial contraction, while in patients with atrial fibrillation (Fig. 17–21B), flow velocity decreases gradually until the gradient disappears or flow is terminated by ventricular contraction.

M-Mode. The assessment of mitral stenosis by the M-mode technique was the first clinical application of echocardiography and is mentioned largely for historical purposes.[3,4,60] The M-mode diagnosis of mitral stenosis is based on an increase in echo production from the thickened, deformed, often calcified leaflets; a decrease in the opening amplitude of the valve; anterior motion of the posterior leaflet; and a decrease in the diastolic or E-F slope. Figure 17–22 illustrates the characteristic M-mode features of mitral stenosis.

Many attempts have been made to relate the rate of diastolic leaflet closure (E-F slope) measured from M-mode recordings to severity of stenosis.[2,61–65] Although a rough correlation should exist between this closure rate and the duration of the pressure gradient across the valve, the E-F slope is affected by factors other than mitral valve orifice size, such as the severity of fibrosis or calcification of the leaflets, compliance of the left ventricle,[66] rate and volume of flow through the mitral orifice,[23,29,61,67] heart rate, and diastolic motion of the mitral annulus.[25,54] Consequently, in individual cases, attempts to estimate severity of stenosis from rate of leaflet closure alone may be misleading.[54,55,68] Anterior diastolic motion of the posterior leaflet, concordant with

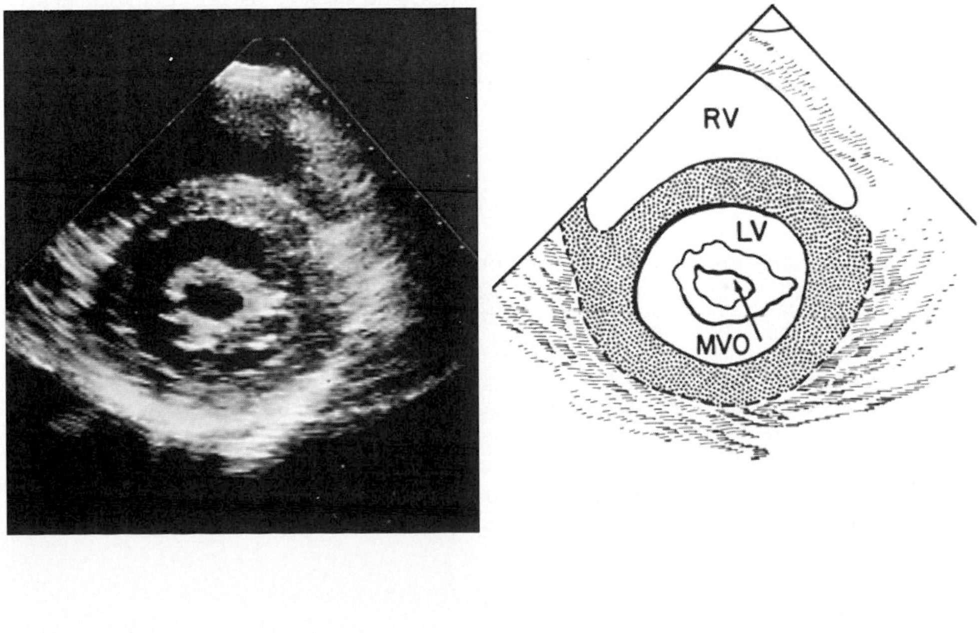

Fig. 17–18. A parasternal short axis recording of a patient with mitral stenosis, illustrating effusion of the mediolateral mitral commissures, diffuse thickening of the leaflet tips, and a marked reduction in mitral valve orifice (MVO) area. The arrow in the accompanying diagram indicates the stenotic valve orifice. LV = left ventricle; RV = right ventricle.

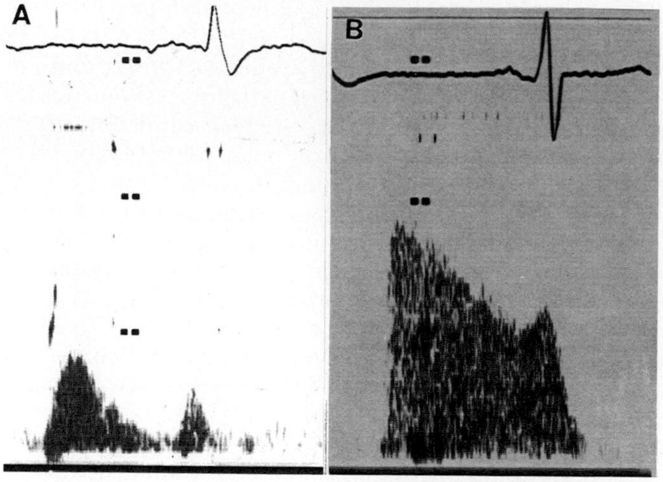

Fig. 17–19. A comparison of normal transmitral flow **(A)** recorded by continuous wave Doppler with that in a patient with mitral stenosis **(B).** In normal persons, there is relatively rapid acceleration and deceleration of the E wave and a clearly defined A wave on the mitral valve tracing. In contrast, in patients with mitral stenosis, there is an increase in the acceleration of flow through the stenotic valve and in the peak transvalvular velocity as well as a decrease in the deceleration rate that roughly corresponds to the severity of stenosis.

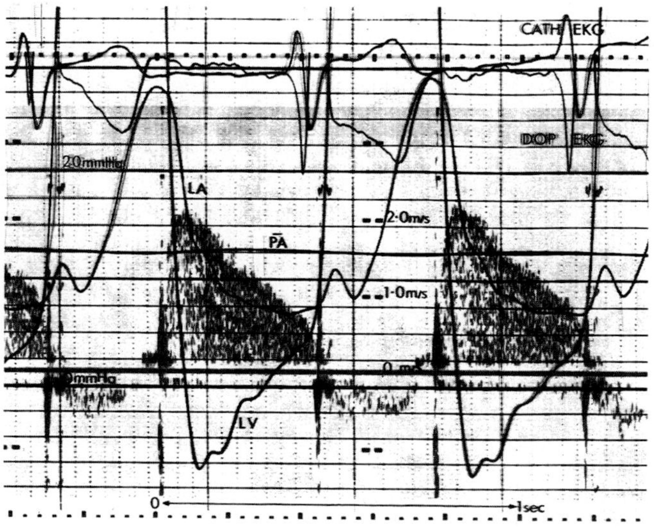

Fig. 17–20. Simultaneous transmitral velocity profiles and left atrial and left ventricular pressure recordings from a patient with a stenotic mitral valve. Note the similarity in timing and magnitude between the instantaneous transvalvular pressure gradient and the transvalvular velocity. The absolute pressures and velocities are as indicated by the accompanying scales. LA = direct left atrial pressure; LV = left ventricular pressure; PA = mean pulmonary arterial pressure. (From Wilkins G, et al.: Validation of continuous-wave Doppler echocardiographic measurements of mitral and tricuspid prosthetic valve gradients: a simultaneous Doppler-catheter study. Circulation 74:789, 1986. Reproduced by permission of the American Heart Association, Inc.)

the motion of the anterior leaflet, is absent in as many as 18% of patients with stenosis, in whom the body of the posterior leaflet is pliable and domes posteriorly.[69,70] Preservation of leaflet opening during atrial contraction, however, appears to be useful: in one study, this sign implied that valve area was greater than 1.2 cm^2.[71]

Estimation of Severity

The severity of stenosis is generally defined by the pressure gradient required to force blood across the stenotic valve and the anatomic reduction in valve area.

Transvalvular Gradient. Doppler offers an ideal noninvasive method for measuring the pressure gradient across the mitral valve.[72–74] The instantaneous pressure gradient can be calculated from the instantaneous velocity across the valve using the modified Bernoulli equation:

$$\Delta P = 4\,v^2 \qquad [17.1]$$

Where V is the instantaneous or peak transvalvular velocity usually measured by the continuous wave technique. The derivation of this equation and the assumptions inherent in its use are discussed in detail in Chapter 9. In vitro and in vivo data suggest that equation 17.1 is an accurate approximation of ΔP at clinically encountered mitral valve areas and flow velocities and thus provides a reliable measure of the transvalvular pressure gradient.[72] Although the gradient is affected by flow across the valve and therefore by heart rate, cardiac output, and valvular regurgitation, none of these factors alters the fundamental accuracy of the measurement.

Although the transvalvular gradient can be determined at any point in diastole, the values most commonly reported clinically are the peak initial diastolic gradient, the end-diastolic gradient—measured immediately before ventricular systole—and the mean gradient. The mathematically correct method for calculating the mean gradient is to measure velocity at fixed intervals (i.e., 10, 20, 40 msec) throughout diastole, to convert the velocities into pressures (using the $4v^2$ relationship), to sum the pressures, and then to divide this sum by the number of samples (Fig. 17–23). Thus, the mean gradient is appropriately calculated from the sum of the squares of the velocities rather than by squaring the mean velocity. Mean gradients by Doppler have been shown to have an excellent correlation with similar hemodynamic measurements in patients with both mitral stenosis and prosthetic mitral valves.

Pressure gradients can be underestimated by the Doppler method if the angle between the sampling beam and the flow vector is too large. When sampling from the apex, this is rarely a problem. With the combined use of color flow and continuous wave Doppler, the direction of the jet can be visualized and any necessary correction incorporated. Gradients can also potentially be overestimated in patients with aortic insufficiency that is due to contamination of the mitral flow stream with the higher velocity aortic flow. This problem can also be overcome with the help of color flow mapping

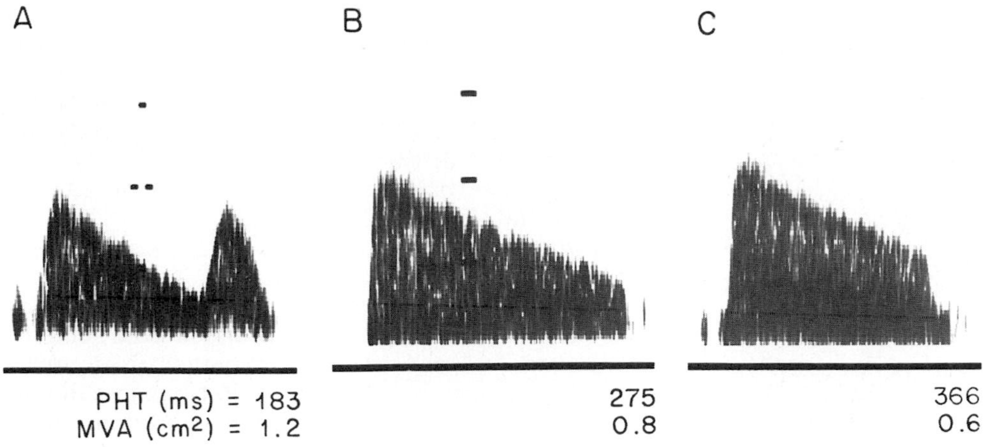

Fig. 17–21. Continuous wave Doppler recordings from three patients with mitral stenosis of increasingly greater severity. **A.** The patient is in sinus rhythm, and velocity increases following atrial contraction. **B.** The mitral area is smaller, and the peak and mean velocities are higher. **C.** Recorded from the patient with the smallest valve area; shows the highest peak velocity and the slowest deceleration slope. PHT = pressure half time; MVA = mitral valve area.

by separating the two streams and placing the sample volume at the mitral orifice.

Mitral Valve Area

Planimetry. Anatomic reduction in mitral orifice area is the hallmark of mitral stenosis, and the severity of stenosis can be assessed by direct visualization of the valve orifice and measurement of its area.[16,54–57] The mitral valve orifice is best visualized in the parasternal short axis view with the scan plane positioned such that it is parallel to and passes directly through the valve orifice.[16] This positioning is most easily achieved by first determining the location of the mitral valve orifice in the parasternal long axis view. If the orifice is then placed in the center of the scan plane, the rotation of the transducer 90° should align the scan plane directly across the valve orifice. The limiting orifice can also be recorded by angling the short axis scan plane in a superior-inferior arc until the smallest anatomic valve orifice recorded during maximal initial diastolic leaflet distention is visualized.

The characteristic features of the stenotic mitral valve in the short axis projection are illustrated in Figure 17–24. The stenotic valve shows a general increase in reflectivity from the orifice margins, limitation of leaflet separation at the commissures, and a marked decrease in orifice area. The orifice typically has a fish-mouthed shape, is longer in its horizontal than vertical dimension, and tapers smoothly at each lateral margin.

The true mitral valve orifice can be measured as soon as it has been properly imaged. Measurement can be accomplished by transferring the image to some form of hard copy for manual measurement or by use of one of

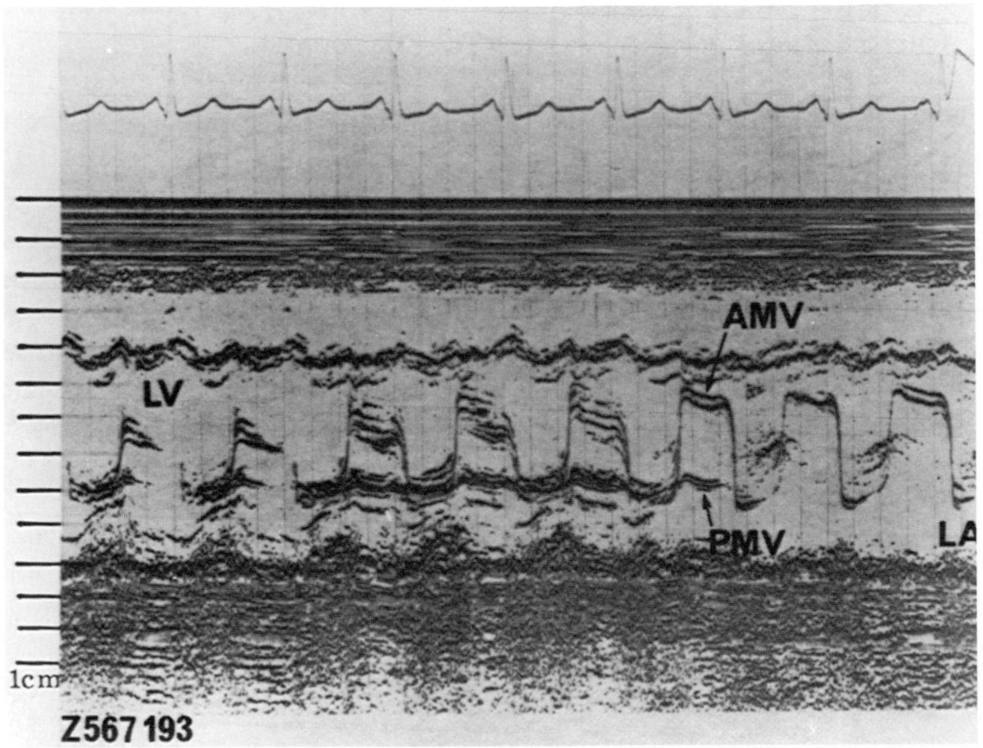

Fig. 17–22. M-mode recording of a patient with mitral stenosis. The initial excursion of the mitral valve is preserved because the M-mode beam passes through the area of maximal doming of the stenotic leaflet. The anterior leaflet is thickened, and the posterior leaflet moves anteriorly. LV = left ventricle; AMV = anterior mitral valve; PMV = posterior mitral valve; LA = left atrium. (From Chang S: M-Mode Echocardiographic Techniques and Pattern Recognition. Philadelphia, Lea & Febiger, p. 23, 1976.)

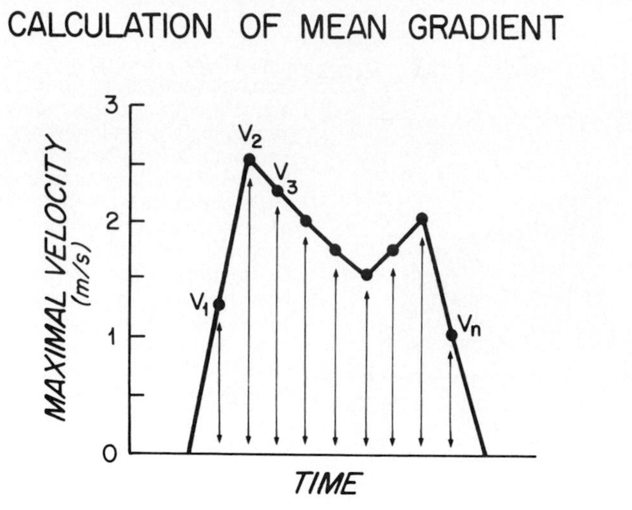

$$\text{MEAN GRADIENT (mm Hg)} = \frac{4\left[\Sigma (V_1)^2 + (V_2)^2 + (V_3)^2 + \cdots (V_n)^2\right]}{n}$$

Fig. 17–23. Calculating the mean transmitral pressure gradients. Gradients at fixed intervals in time are calculated, the values at each point of diastole are summed, and the total is divided by the number of samples.

the many computer devices now available for measuring areas directly from the video screen.

Reported success rates for recording a measurable mitral valve orifice vary from 83[54] to 100%.[56] Figure 17–25 illustrates the success rates for mitral valve orifice recording from the Indiana laboratory for the years 1974 to 1978 and the first quarter of 1979 for patients undergoing hemodynamic studies. Although the overall success rate for this group is only 87%, the results include studies performed during the earlier learning phase of the technique, and the success rate improved to 96% for the years 1977 to 1979. Although these data are now more than a decade old, they remain representative of our current practice both in terms of the initial learning curve and the ultimate success rate.

The accuracy of the echocardiographic measurement of the mitral valve orifice has been established by comparing this value to the mitral valve area measured directly at the time of surgery,[16] calculated from hemodynamic data,[54–58] and determined pathologically from excised specimens.[55,57] Figure 17–26 compares the mitral valve orifice measured by the cross-sectional echogram with that obtained at surgery in 14 patients. In 12 of these 14 instances, the two measurements were within 0.3 cm² of each other, and the echocardiogram tended to underestimate the surgical valve area. This underestimation can be attributed to areas of dense fibrosis or calcification along the orifice margin, which increase the intensity of the returning echoes and thereby encroach on the orifice area.[16] In addition, targets at the lateral margins of the orifice are imaged by using the lateral resolution of the system. The echoes from these points, therefore, are widened by the point-spread function of the scanning beam and also encroach on the lumen. Fortunately, the stenotic valve orifice has a consistent fish-mouthed shape. Its long dimension is oriented perpendicular to the direction of propagation of the scan plane. Because of this orientation, the majority of the orifice is recorded using the axial resolution of the system, and the effects of decreased lateral resolution on orifice size are minimized.

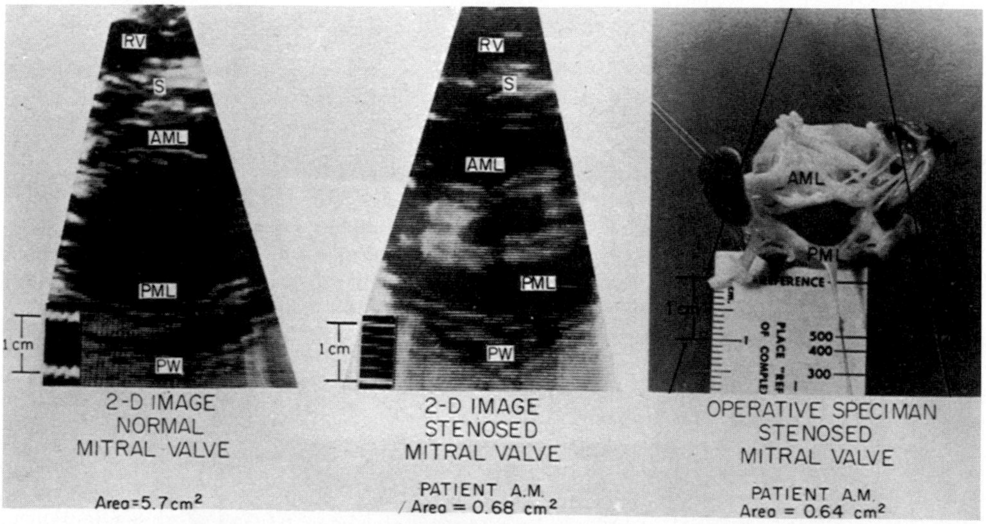

Fig. 17–24. Parasternal short axis recordings compare the normal mitral valve orifice with the mitral valve seen in rheumatic mitral stenosis. Left. The normal mitral valve. The leaflets are thin and, at peak diastolic opening, separate widely and lie parallel to the circumferential margin of the left ventricular endocardium. Center. A stenotic mitral valve. The margins of the orifice are thickened, the commissures are fused, and the orifice area is decreased. Right. An anatomic specimen from the same patient illustrating the similarity in both orifice configuration and size between the echocardiographic image and the pathologic anatomy. RV = right ventricle; S = septum; AML = anterior mitral leaflet; PML = posterior mitral leaflet; PW = posterior wall. (From Henry WL, et al.: Measurement of mitral orifice area in patients with mitral valve disease by real-time two-dimensional echocardiography. Circulation 51:827, 1975. Reproduced by permission of the American Heart Association, Inc.)

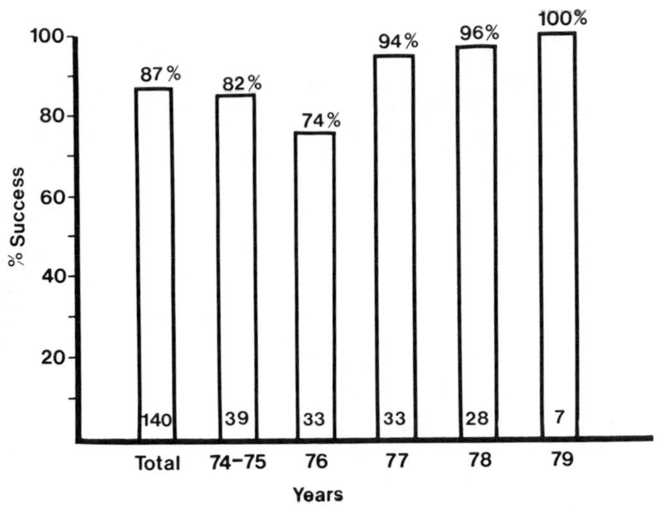

Fig. 17–25. Success rate for recording a measurable mitral valve orifice by cross-sectional echocardiography for the years 1974 to 1978 and the first quarter of 1979. (Data compiled from studies performed at the Indiana University Hospital laboratory.)

Studies examining the relationship of the echocardiographic mitral valve orifice size and the mitral valve area calculated from hemodynamic data have also shown a good correlation when both measurements could be obtained.[54–58] Figure 17–27 compares the success rates of the echocardiographic and hemodynamic methods of determining mitral valve orifice area in a group of 140 con-

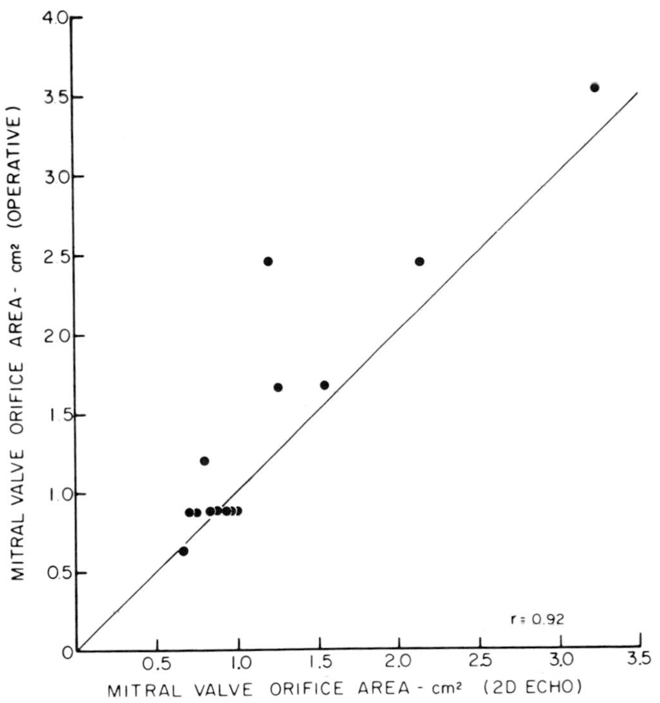

Fig. 17–26. Original comparison of the mitral valve orifice area measured by two-dimensional echocardiography with the area determined at surgery. (From Henry WL, et al.: Measurement of mitral orifice area in patients with mitral valve disease by real-time two-dimensional echocardiography. Circulation 51:827, 1975. Reproduced by permission of the American Heart Association, Inc.)

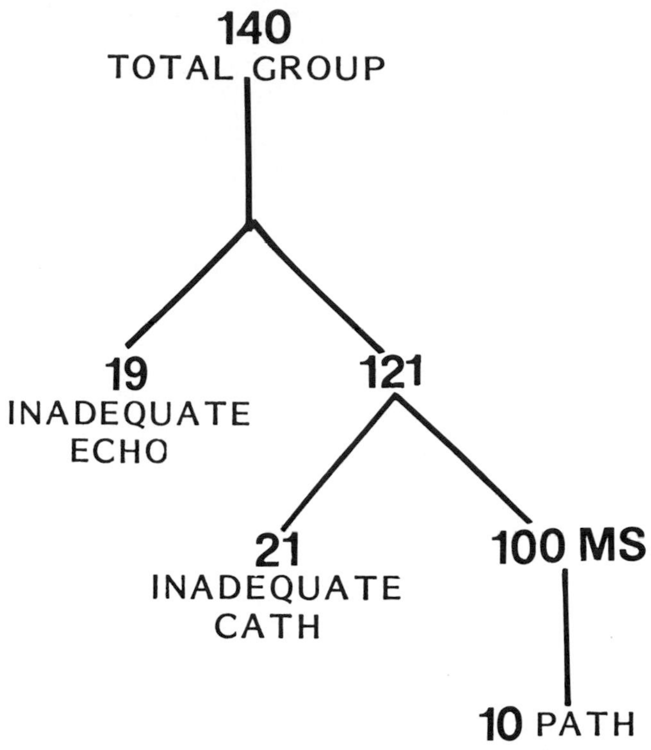

Fig. 17–27. Comparative success rates for echocardiographic and hemodynamic determinations of mitral valve orifice area in 140 consecutive patients examined by both techniques.

secutively examined patients.[57] In 19 of these 140 patients, the mitral valve orifice could not be recorded echocardiographically. In comparison, the mitral valve area could not be calculated from the available hemodynamic data in 21 of the 140 cases. This occurred primarily in patients with combined mitral stenosis and insufficiency and results from an inability to determine an angiographic cardiac output because of associated aortic insufficiency, arrhythmia, or incomplete opacification or visualization of the ventricle. Figure 17–28A illustrates the correlation between the echocardiographic and hemodynamic mitral valve areas in the 100 patients in whom both sets of data were available. Correlation is good through a wide range of orifice sizes in patients with both isolated mitral stenosis and mitral stenosis and insufficiency. The echocardiographic valve area in these cases tends to overestimate the hemodynamic area by approximately 0.3 cm^2. This overestimation presumably occurs because the cross-sectional echogram records only the limiting orifice, whereas the transvalvular gradient is composed of all the factors that contribute to inflow obstruction: the funnel shape of the valve, the decrease in orifice size, and the resistance to ventricular inflow offered by the thickened, fused chordae. Figure 17–28B illustrates virtually identical data from another group of 53 patients studied before balloon valvuloplasty, roughly 10 years later.

When patients with isolated mitral stenosis are considered separately (Fig. 17–29), the correlation between echocardiographic and hemodynamic valve areas is not as good. In an attempt to explain the difference, we com-

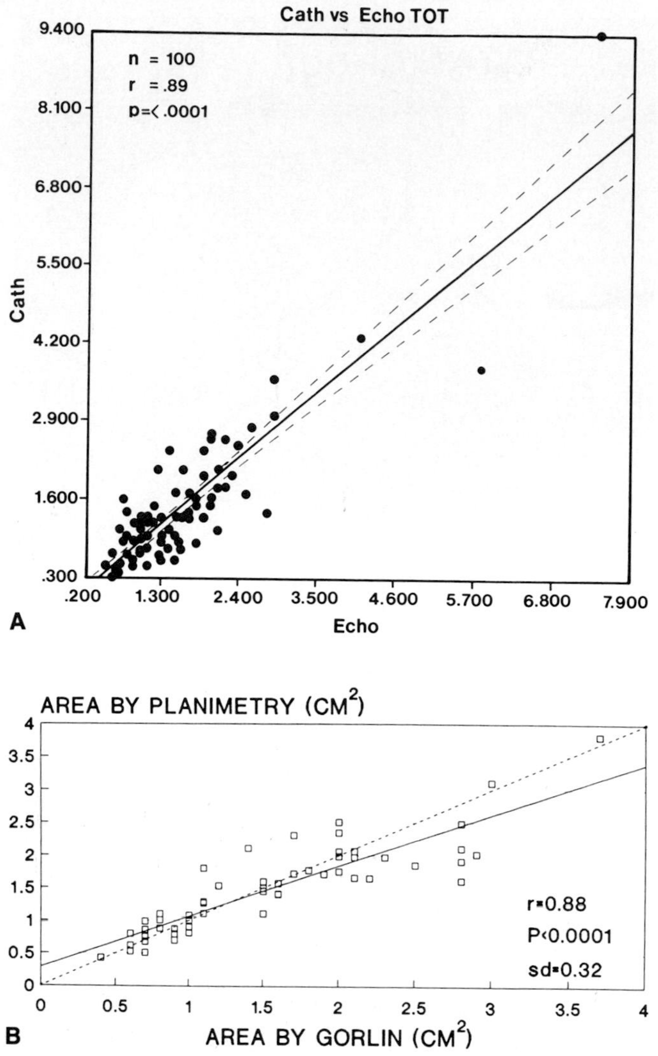

Fig. 17–28. **A.** Original correlation between echocardiographic and hemodynamic measurements of mitral valve area for a total group of 100 patients with valvular mitral stenosis. **B.** Virtually identical correlation obtained 10 years later in a second group of 53 patients with a narrower range of valve areas studied before valvuloplasty.

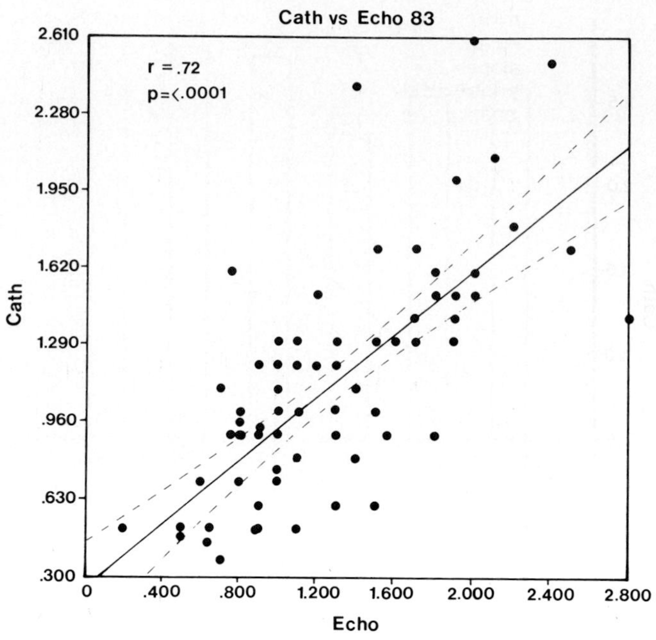

Fig. 17–29. Correlation between echocardiographic and hemodynamic estimates of mitral valve area only in patients with isolated mitral stenosis (N = 83). This correlation is not as good as that for the total group because of the narrowed range of valve areas included and the measurement errors inherent in both methods.

pared both of these parameters with direct pathologic measurement in 10 patients in whom the valves were excised en bloc at surgery. Figure 17–30 illustrates the correlation between the echocardiographic mitral valve area and the pathologic measurements, whereas Figure 17–31 illustrates the corresponding relationship for the hemodynamic valve areas with the same pathologic data. Although the correlation is good in both instances, the echocardiographic measurement of valve area correlates more closely with the pathologic measurement than does the hemodynamic estimate. The greatest variation in the echocardiographic data occurs at the smaller valve areas where the measurement error is greatest. The largest difference between the hemodynamic and pathologic data, in contrast, occurs at larger valve areas where a small change in measured transvalvular gradient results in a large variation in the calculated valve area. Unfortunately, this type of correlation tends to select in favor of the echocardiogram because densely calcified or deformed valves, which are recorded least accurately by the echocardiogram, can rarely be removed intact and, hence, are not available for comparison.

Several factors may distort the echocardiographic appearance of the mitral valve orifice and thus affect the

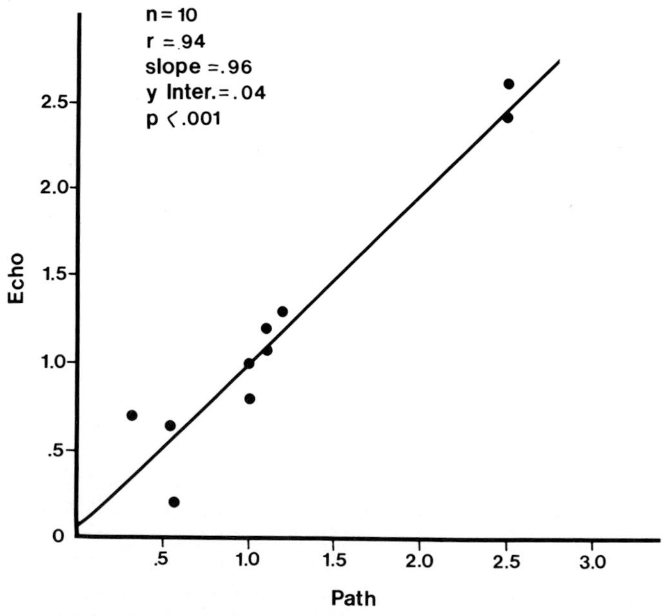

Fig. 17–30. Correlation between the echocardiographic measurement of mitral valve area and direct pathologic measurement of the excised valve. Correlation is excellent with a slight degree of scattering in the lower range.

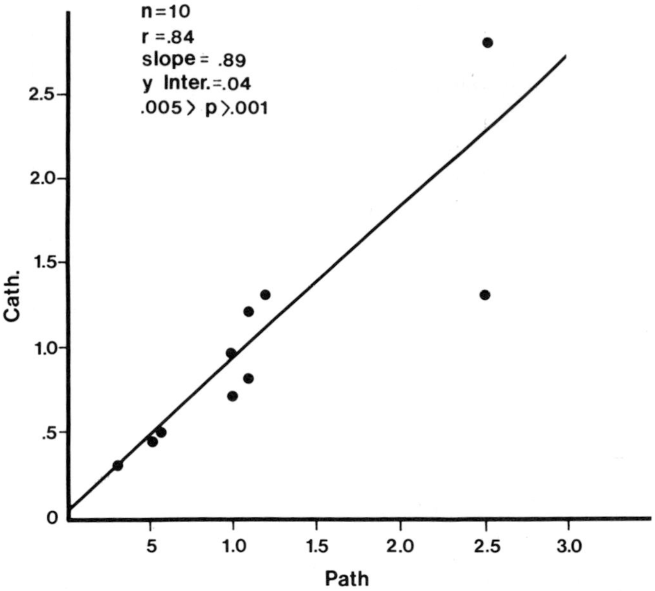

Fig. 17–31. Correlation between the hemodynamic estimate of mitral valve area and the directly measured mitral valve area for the 10 patients reviewed in Figure 17–30. Here, the correlation is not as good, and the scatter is greater at the larger valve areas.

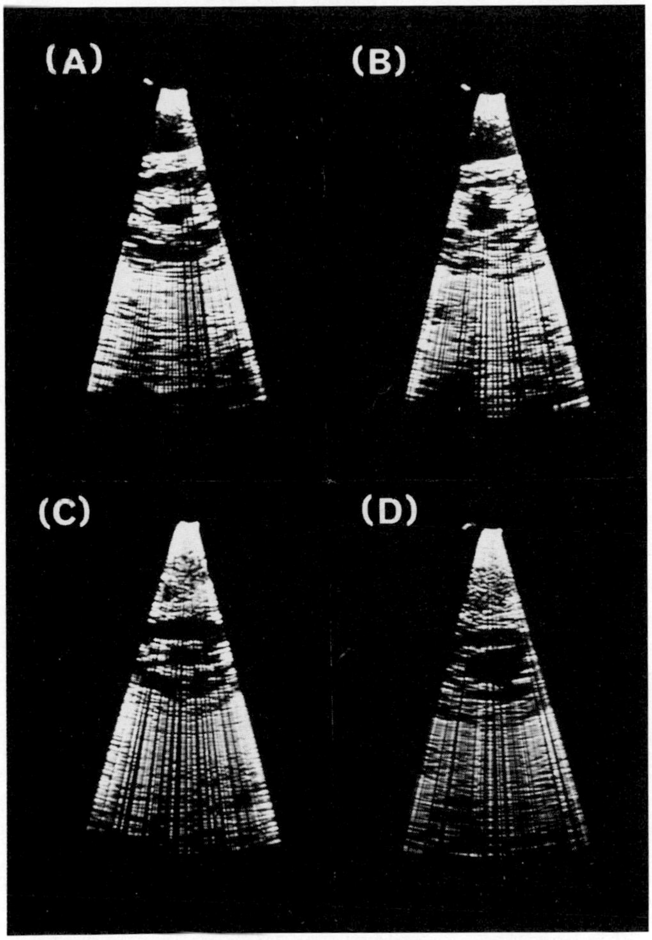

Fig. 17–32. Series of four mitral valve orifices recorded from the one patient with mitral stenosis. This figure illustrates the variations in orifice configuration that can be produced by improper plane angulation and/or rotation. **A.** The appropriately recorded valve orifice. **B.** The orifice is distorted vertically by improper angulation. **C.** The orifice is distorted horizontally by improper rotation. **D.** The orifice is enlarged in both dimensions by the improper placement of the imaging plane in relation to the valve orifice. (See text for further details.)

accuracy of orifice measurements. These include (1) improper imaging plane orientation relative to the valve orifice,[16] (2) inappropriate receiver gain settings,[54,56] (3) selecting an orifice for measurement that is recorded after valve closure has begun, and (4) confusing an extraneous echo-free area for the valve orifice.

Improper imaging plane orientation characteristically produces an orifice that appears larger than the true limiting orifice.[16] This enlargement can result from improper plane angulation, rotation, or placement relative to the tip of the dome. Each of these factors distorts the orifice in a different manner and can be recognized by the alterations they produce. Figure 17–32 contains a series of mitral valves recorded from the same patient that illustrate each of these distortions. Figure 17–32A contains the appropriately recorded, fish-mouth-shaped, stenotic orifice. In Figure 17–32B, the same orifice is distorted in a vertical dimension. This distortion occurs because the imaging plane is angled improperly and enters the dome of the valve anteriorly above the level of the orifice and then passes through the valve obliquely to exit through the posterior tip of the orifice. This angle increases the vertical dimension of the orifice disproportionately to the horizontal dimension and enlarges the apparent valve area. In Figure 17–32C, the orifice is elongated horizontally. This configuration is recorded when the plane is rotated improperly and passes through one of the lateral margins of the dome above the true orifice. In addition to increasing the horizontal dimension disproportionately to the vertical dimension, this pattern also causes the improperly recorded orifice margin to lose its normal tapered configuration and to become more rounded. Finally, in Figure 17–32D, the imaging plane passes through the dome parallel to but above the true orifice. This orientation increases both the vertical and horizontal dimensions and causes both orifice margins to appear more rounded than tapered.

Inappropriate receiver gain settings can either enlarge or constrict the orifice.[54,56] If the gain is too low, echo dropout often occurs at the margins of the orifice. The echo dropout increases the apparent orifice area.[54] Conversely, abnormally high gain settings increase both the axial and the lateral echo width, consequently encroaching on the orifice and reducing its apparent area (Fig. 17–33).[56] This effect is greater in densely fibrotic or calcified valves where the echoes are stronger initially.[16]

Whenever possible, the mitral valve orifice should be recorded and measured during initial diastole when the valve is always maximally distended. In patients with more severe lesions, the time of measurement is less important because pressure is exerted against the valve throughout diastole, and little change in orifice area occurs. With less severe lesions, however, partial closure

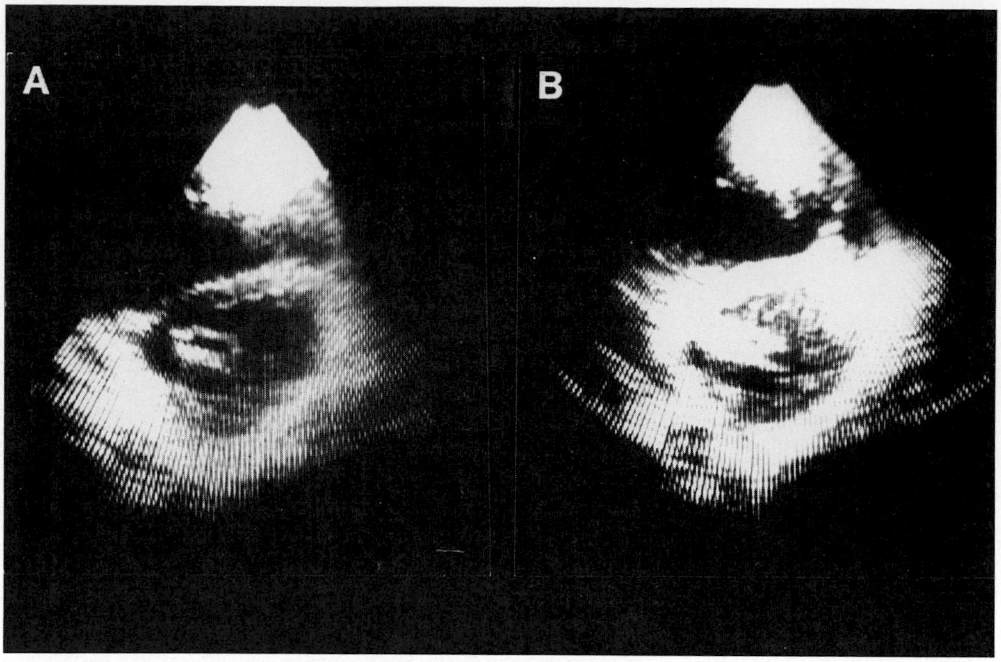

Fig. 17–33. The effects of gain setting on mitral valve orifice size. **A.** The gain is appropriately set, and the mitral valve orifice is clearly visualized. **B.** The gain is inappropriately high and almost completely obliterates the orifice.

may occur as diastole progresses, and orifice measurements made later in the diastolic filling period may underestimate the maximal valve area. This possibility is particularly true with atrial fibrillation during long diastolic filling periods.

Movement of the valve in a direction perpendicular to or into the short axis imaging plane may also affect the recorded size of the mitral valve orifice. This motion is due to the normal superior diastolic motion of the mitral annulus, which draws the distended mitral leaflets superiorly as the ventricle fills. Thus, when the imaging plane is positioned above the limiting orifice at initial diastole, the superior motion of the valve draws the dome through the imaging plane as diastole progresses, and the orifice decreases as it approaches the apex.

Occasionally, an echo-free area in the chordal-papillary muscle region or an apparent secondary orifice in the valve itself can be recorded. These areas generally have indistinct margins and do not demonstrate the normal fish-mouthed configuration. Confusion concerning the location of the actual orifice can be resolved by returning to the long-axis view and defining the point of leaflet separation at the tip of the valve. Also, because the maximal leaflet separation in long axis should equal the vertical dimension of the orifice in short axis, comparison of these dimensions can help the define the true limiting orifice.

Finally, some valvular orifices are so densely calcified that the area of leaflet opening cannot be identified.[16] Failure to record an orifice in a densely calcified valve usually indicates that severe stenosis is present, which can be confirmed by Doppler methods (see following discussion).

Flow Area. An alternative to visualizing the restrictive orifice by two-dimensional imaging is to visualize the margins of the flow stream passing through the orifice by color Doppler.[75,76] Conceptually, the two-dimen-

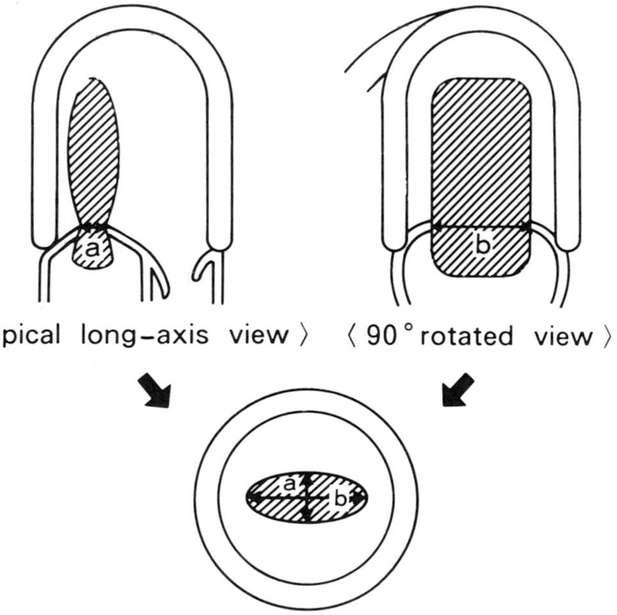

$$MVA = \frac{\pi}{4} ab$$

Fig. 17–34. The diameters of the color Doppler jet emanating from a stenotic mitral valve can be used to calculate valve area. Top, left. The diameter is measured in the apical long axis view. Top, right. The maximum diameter of the jet is measured in a view roughly orthogonal to the apical long axis. Bottom. Valve area is calculated from the product of these diameters using the formula for the area of an ellipse. MVA = mitral valve area. (From Kawahara T, et al.: Applications of Doppler color flow imaging to determine valve area in mitral stenosis. J Am Coll Cardiol 18:87, 1991. Reprinted with permission from the American College of Cardiology.)

sional approach might be compared to measuring the inner edge of the doughnut, while the margins of the flow stream define the outer edge of the hole. Direct short axis recording of the flow area is difficult because the direction of flow is parallel to the interrogating beam. As a result, orifice diameters are typically recorded from the apex, and the valve area is calculated as the area of an ellipse:

$$MVA = \frac{\pi}{4} ab \qquad [17.2]$$

where MVA is mitral valve area and the minor axis of the ellipse (a) is taken as the maximal diameter of the flow stream recorded in the apical long axis view and the major axis (b) as the maximal orifice diameter that can be recorded in a plane rotated roughly 90°[75] (Fig. 17–34). Care must be taken to measure the narrowest flow diameter of the central laminar core at the orifice because the flow jet will tend to widen as it progresses downstream. Experimental data indicate that this flow "waist" correlates closely with orifice diameter in orifices of known size.

Excellent correlations have been observed between the mitral valve area calculated from the diameters of the flow stream and the area determined at catheterization,[75,76] by direct planimetry,[76] and by the half-time method[76] (Fig. 17–35). This method is an excellent check on values obtained by planimetry in cases in which the orifice is not clearly defined. Further, it is

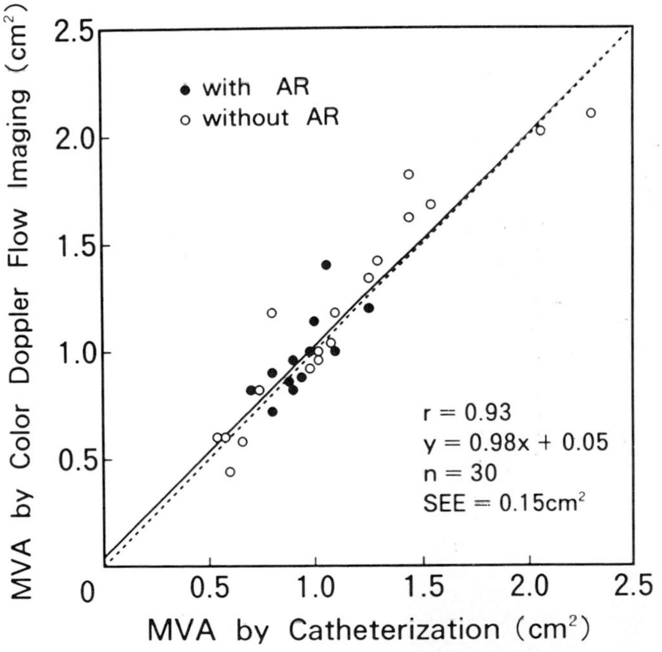

Fig. 17–35. Correlation of the mitral valve area (MVA) determined using the color Doppler jet diameters with that determined at catheterization. AR = aortic regurgitation; SEE = standard error of estimation. (From Kawahara T, et al.: Applications of Doppler color flow imaging to determine valve area in mitral stenosis. J Am Coll Cardiol 18:90, 1991. Reprinted with permission from the American College of Cardiology.)

unaffected by mitral or aortic regurgitation and should not be influenced by ventricular function or atrial pressure.

The method does, however, assume that the mitral orifice is elliptic, which may not be the case in patients with severely deformed valves. The measurements are also gain dependent, and both Doppler and tissue gains must be carefully set to optimize image quality.

Continuity-Based Methods

Continuity Equation. Mitral valve area can also be calculated using the continuity principle.[77,78] As discussed in detail in Chapter 9, the continuity equation is based on the law of conservation of mass and energy, which states that the flow at all points along a tube is constant and is equal to the product of the mean velocity and the cross-sectional area, hence,

$$Q = v_1 * A_1 = v_2 * A_2 \qquad [17.3]$$

where v_1 and A_1 are usually taken as a reference area and velocity and v_2 and A_2 are the area and velocity at the stenosis. To determine the area of a stenotic orifice (A_2), the equation is rearranged so that:

$$A_2 = A_1 * v_1/v_2 \qquad [17.4]$$

or for the mitral valve

$$MVA = A_1 \times \frac{TvI_1}{TvI_m} \qquad [17.5]$$

where MVA equals the mitral valve area, and TvI_m is the time velocity integral of transmitral flow. This equation requires that flow through both the mitral and reference valves is the same. When the continuity equation is used to determine mitral flow, the reference is usually the flow (stroke volume) passing through the aortic or pulmonic valves.[78] In clinical studies, mitral valve areas calculated using Doppler-derived aortic or pulmonic flow have correlated well with catheterization data (r = .91; standard error of estimate [SEE] = .26 cm²). The continuity-derived areas slightly underestimate those obtained at catheterization (y = 0.84x).[78]

When there is regurgitation of either the mitral or reference valve, the flow through both valves will not be equal (except by chance), and therefore the equation will be invalid. This is a significant limitation in mitral stenosis that is commonly associated with regurgitation. The continuity equation therefore is used more commonly to determine aortic than mitral valve area because the reference for flow through the aortic valve is flow in the left ventricular outflow tract, and hence the equation is not invalidated by aortic regurgitation. Note also that the continuity equation gives the effective valve area A_e and not the anatomic valve area A_0. As a result, the continuity-derived valve area should be smaller than that measured at cardiac catheterization because the Gorlin formula yields the anatomic area (see following discussion).

A simplified version of the continuity equation that relates mitral valve area to the ratio of the aortic or pulmonic time velocity integral to the mitral time velocity integral has been suggested.[78] Although reasonable correlations have been reported using this approach it is theoretically unsound (see Chapter 30), and thus its use cannot be advocated.

Proximal Acceleration. The second continuity-based method for determining mitral valve area uses the proximal convergence zone proximal to the valve to derive instantaneous flow rate. This approach is based on the observation that flow converges uniformly and radially toward an orifice that is small relative to the proximal chamber, forming concentric isovelocity layers (Fig. 17–36). When the orifice is circular or small relative to the region of acceleration, these isovelocity surfaces are hemispheric, and the flow through any isovelocity surface is the product of the area of the surface and its velocity. By conservation of mass, flow at each layer must equal orifice flow because it must all pass through the orifice. Once orifice flow is known, orifice area can be determined by dividing instantaneous flow by instantaneous velocity.

Color flow mapping displays both the isovelocity contour and its distance from the orifice, which is most easily identified by the first aliasing boundary encountered as flow begins to accelerate toward the orifice. Flow through this isovelocity surface can be calculated by multiplying the area of the surface ($2\pi r^2$ for a hemispheric surface) by the aliasing velocity. Flow through both elliptic and circular orifices of equal area can be described by the same $2\pi r^2$ formula because flow senses the same axial pressure gradient for a given restriction in area. Because the funnel shape of the stenotic mitral valve prevents blood from approaching the orifice hemispherically, it is necessary to correct for the inflow angle formed by the mitral leaflets in the flow convergence region.

In practice, color flow Doppler recordings of mitral inflow are obtained from the cardiac apex (apical four-chamber view), and the radius of the proximal convergence region is measured as the peak diastolic distance from the orifice to the first color alias along the axis of flow. Flow is recorded at a low aliasing velocity to place the initial aliasing boundary as far from the orifice as possible, thereby increasing the accuracy of measurement, diminishing any effect of imprecise orifice location, and limiting any inaccuracy that is due to finite orifice size. Peak flow rate is calculated assuming uniform radial flow convergence toward the orifice, modified by a factor that accounts for the inflow funnel angle formed by the mitral leaflets. This factor is the funnel angle α divided by 180°; the inflow angle without such restriction (Fig. 17–37). Mitral valve area is then calculated as peak flow rate/peak velocity:

$$\mathrm{MVA} = 2\pi r^2 \times \frac{\alpha}{180^\circ} \times \frac{v_n}{v_{peak}} \qquad [17.6]$$

with peak flow velocity recorded from the cardiac apex using continuous wave Doppler.[79]

Valve areas calculated in this manner have been shown to agree with planimetered values over a range of 0.5 to 2.2 cm^2 (r = .9, slope 1.08, SEE = .21). Agreement was similar in patients with and without mitral regurgitation as well as in those with atrial fibrillation.[79]

Doppler Half-Time. In addition to altering the morphology of the mitral valve, rheumatic mitral stenosis also obstructs flow from the left atrium to the left ventricle, increasing left atrial pressure and both the magnitude and duration of the diastolic transvalvular pressure gradient. In mild lesions, this increased gradient may persist for only a portion of diastole, while in more se-

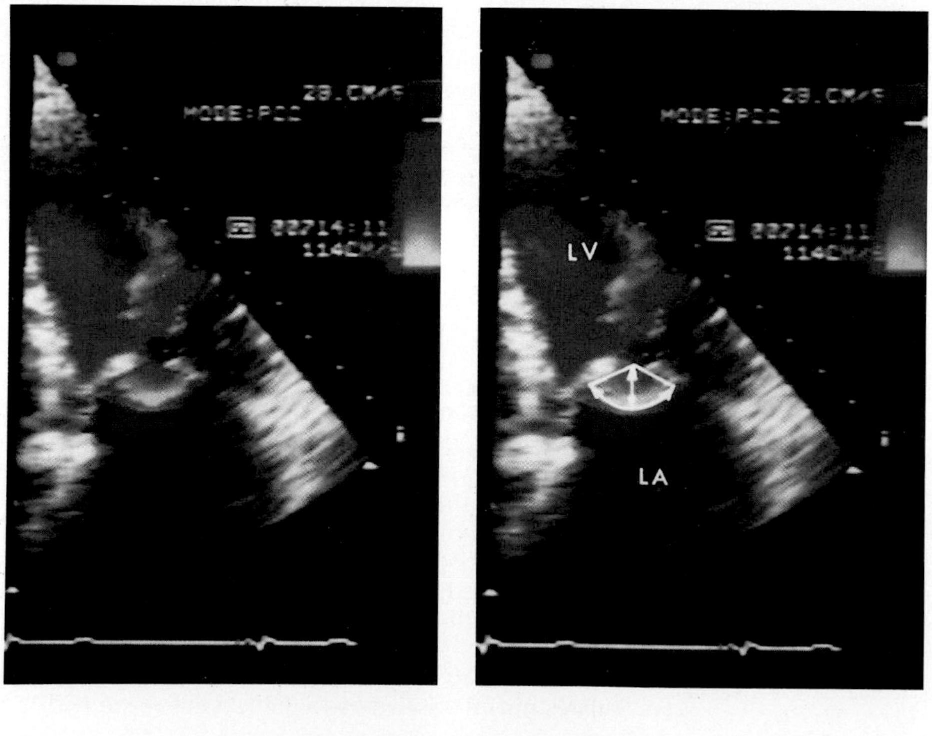

Fig. 17–36. Apical four-chamber color flow recording of the outflow acceleration field proximal to a stenotic mitral valve. LV = left ventricle; LA = left atrium.

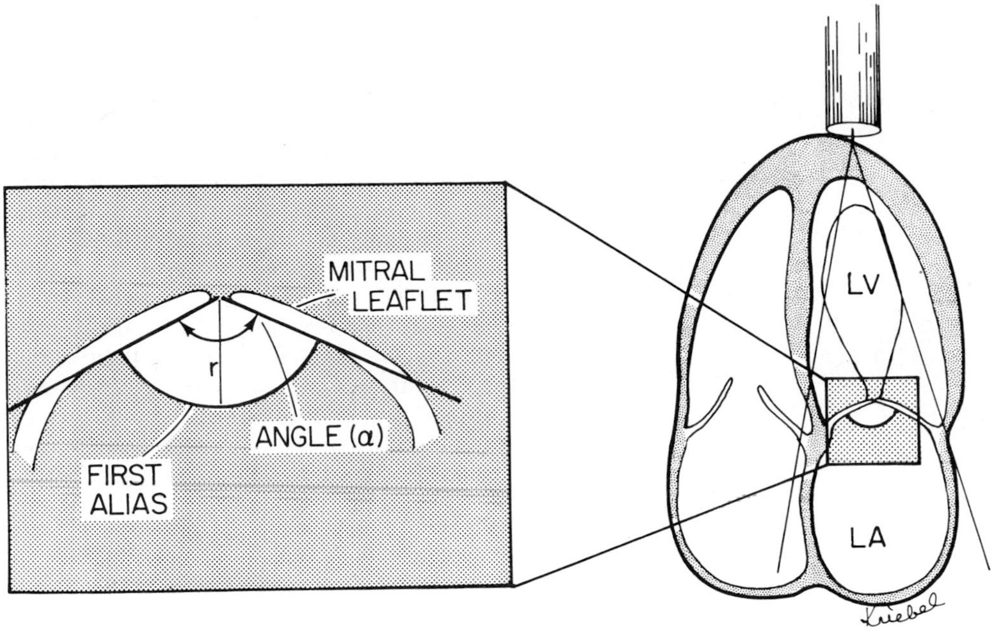

Fig. 17–37. Because of the funnel shape of the stenotic mitral orifice, flow cannot converge along hemispheric surfaces, and hence some correction must be introduced to allow for the constriction of the flow field by the mitral leaflets. This diagram illustrates the method for calculating the angle subtended by the stenotic valve, which is then used to correct for the actual deviation from the ideal hemispheric surface. LV = left ventricle; LA = left atrium.

vere obstruction, the gradient tends to be present throughout the diastolic filling period. A quantitative index of the rate of decay of this gradient, the mitral pressure half-time (i.e., the time required for the gradient to fall to half its maximal early diastolic value) was proposed in the late 1960s as a method for estimating mitral valve area from catheterization data that was relatively independent of changes in heart rate, cardiac output, or degree of regurgitation.[80,81]

In 1979, Hatle et al.[82]—recognizing from the Bernoulli equation that instantaneous transmitral blood velocity is proportional to the square root of the driving pressure gradient (i.e., $\Delta p = 4v^2$)—defined the Doppler half-time as the time required for the transmitral velocity to fall from its peak by a factor of the square root of 2. By definition, the pressure half-time (written as $t_{1/2}$) equals the time required for the pressure gradient to fall to one half its original value.

$$Pt_{1/2} = \frac{P_0}{2} \quad \text{The pressure gradient at pressure half-time equals one half the original peak value.} \qquad [17.7]$$

The relationship between the pressure gradient and the velocity at pressure half-time can be derived as follows:

$$P(t) = 4[v(t)]^2 \quad \text{The pressure gradient at any time (t) is equal to } 4v^2 \text{ by the modified Bernoulli equation.} \qquad [17.8]$$

Therefore, equation 17.7 can be written as

$$4[vt_{1/2}]^2 = \frac{4v_0^2}{2} \qquad [17.9]$$

Then one can extract the velocity at pressure half-time:

$$vt_{1/2} = \frac{v_0}{\sqrt{2}} \approx \frac{v_0}{1.4} \approx 0.71v_0 \qquad [17.10]$$

Figure 17–38 illustrates the method for measuring the half-time from a mitral velocity recording. The peak velocity is first identified, and a vertical line is drawn from the baseline through the peak. The velocity representing half the initial pressure gradient is then determined by dividing the peak velocity by 1.4 (or multiplying by 0.71). A horizontal line is then drawn from the velocity representing half-pressure to intercept the slope of maximal instantaneous velocities, and a vertical line is dropped from this intercept point to the baseline. The time between the vertical lines passing through the peak velocity and the velocity representing the half-pressure is then measured, and this is the pressure half-time. The pressure half-time for normal persons has been reported to range between 20 and 60 msec (mean, 49 msec), while in patients with mitral stenosis, it ranges from 90 to 383 msec.[82] Although the slope of the diastolic velocity decay is usually linear, as illustrated in Figure 17–38, in some cases there is an early diastolic velocity peak followed by a more linear slope, while in others the late diastolic velocity slope curves.[82] In both situations, it is the dominant slope that is measured; the early spike and late curvature are ignored. When sinus rhythm is present and the P-R interval is prolonged, there is often an increase in velocity that is due to atrial contraction in early diastole. In these cases, the half-time cannot be measured. Similarly, in patients with atrial flutter or atrial tachycardia, the frequent atrial contractions may prevent measurement of the pressure half-time.[82] Despite these difficulties, it is our experience that half-time measurements are easily obtained in most cases and are sub-

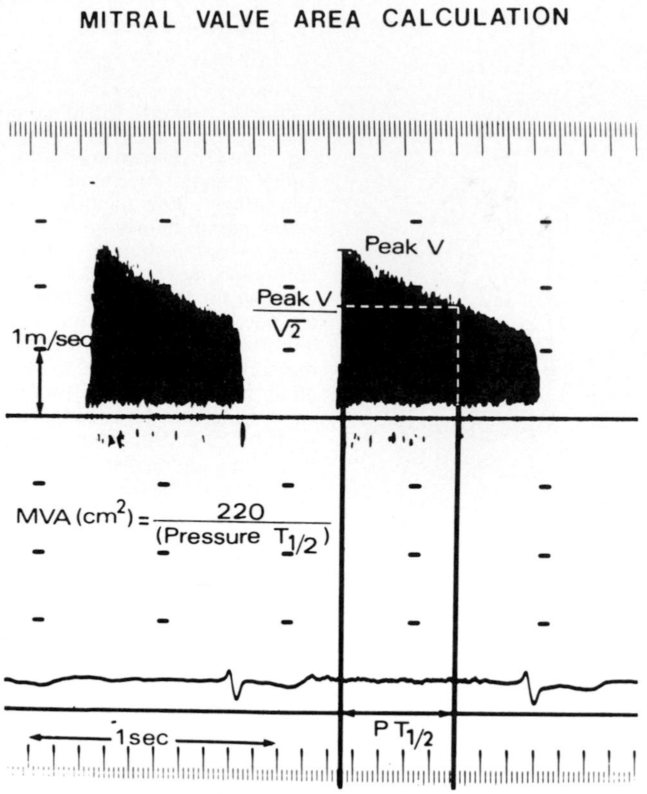

Fig. 17–38. Method for calculating the mitral valve half-time. (See text for details.) MVA = mitral valve area.

ject to less inter- and intraobserver variability than planimetry or other methods of Doppler analysis. An increase in the angle between the Doppler beam and the direction of flow through the valve will decrease all velocities proportionally and will not affect the half-time.

Hatle and Angelsen subsequently provided an empiric mathematic expression relating the Doppler half-time to mitral valve area:

$$\text{MVA (cm}^2) = 220/T_{1/2}\ \text{(msec)} \qquad [17.11]$$

They validated this against catheterization data in 20 patients.[83] Subsequent studies have shown a good correlation between the half-time calculated valve area and the valve area calculated using the Gorlin equation in patients with mitral stenosis and combined stenosis and insufficiency.[84–86] However, variations in this relationship with exercise, change in heart rate, and following commissurotomy, and the failure of the half-time following balloon valvotomy suggest that the half-time is not completely independent of other hemodynamic factors.[87,88]

Theoretic Background. The Doppler velocity half-time is a measure of the rate at which the atrioventricular pressure gradient decays during diastole. The rate at which the transvalvular gradient falls is, in turn, determined by the volume flow across the mitral valve and the effects of this transfer in volume from the atrium to the ventricle on the respective chamber pressures which, in turn, is determined by the respective chamber stiffnesses or compliances (compliance is the inverse of stiffness). As noted earlier in the discussion of normal E-wave deceleration, it is the net compliance of the two chambers that is the important variable because the transfer of 1 ml of blood from the atrium to the ventricle will result in a fall in atrial pressure that is determined by the compliance characteristics of the atrium and a rise in ventricular pressure that is determined by ventricular compliance; the sum of these two changes (C_{net}) will represent the net effect on the gradient.

To understand the relationship of the half-time to these hemodynamic variables, it is necessary to consider the primary determinants of instantaneous mitral valve flow. Because flow (Q) in milliliters per second through the orifice is simply the velocity (v) multiplied by the effective orifice area (assuming plug flow across the orifice):

$$Q = v \times \text{MVA} \qquad [17.12]$$

By the Bernoulli principle, the velocity (v) of the outgoing blood (ignoring the tiny terms representing viscous drag and bulk acceleration and assuming a negligible velocity proximal to the valve) is related to the driving pressure (p) by: $\Delta p = 1/2\,\rho\,v^2$ (ρ is the density of blood), for a variety of shapes and sizes of orifices. For pressure in millimeters of mercury and velocity in meters per second, this relation is approximated by: $\Delta p = 4v^2$ (the constant is actually 3.94). Solving for v yields: $v = (\sqrt{\Delta p})/2$ for v in meters per second or, multiplying by 100 to yield v (in centimeters per second); v roughly equals $50\sqrt{\Delta p}$ (using 3.94 instead of 4 gives $v = 50.4\sqrt{\Delta p}$).

$$Q = v \times \text{MVA} = 50.4\,\rho\sqrt{p}\ \text{MVA} \qquad [17.13]$$

Because the changes in velocity and flow over time are determined by the compliances (dV/dP) of the atrium and ventricle and because both volume and pressure are functions of time, left atrial compliance (LAC) (or net compliance)* can be expressed in terms of the time derivatives of these variables:

$$C_{net} = \frac{dV}{dp} = \frac{dV/dt}{dp/dt} = \frac{-Q}{dp/dt} \qquad [17.14]$$

where $dV/dt = -Q$ (negative because flow is out of the left atrium, causing V to decrease). Expressing dp/dt as function of p yields:

$$\frac{dp}{dt} = \frac{-Q}{C_{net}} = \frac{-v\ \text{MVA}}{C_{net}} = \frac{50.4\ \text{MVA}\ \sqrt{p}}{C_{net}} \qquad [17.15]$$

$$C_{net} = \frac{1}{1/\text{LAC} + 1/\text{LVC}} = \frac{\text{LAC} \times \text{LVC}}{\text{LAC} + \text{LVC}}$$

* Thus, net compliance is always lower than either atrial or ventricular compliance. LVC = left ventricular compliance.

From this differential equation, we can see that pressure falls more rapidly if the valve area is larger, if the pressure gradient is larger, or if the compliance is smaller. The only additional variable to specify is the initial pressure (P_0). As shown by Thomas,[87] when this is specified, the solution to equation 17.15 becomes:

$$p(t) = (\sqrt{Po} - 25.2 \text{ MVA } t/C_{net})^2 \qquad [17.16]$$

which is the overall time course of atrial depressurization. The pressure half-time then is the time (t) at which the pressure (p[t]) equals half the initial pressure ($p_0/2$), or:

$$T_{1/2} = \frac{11.6\, C_{net} \sqrt{P_0}}{\text{MVA}} \qquad [17.17]$$

Thus, while the half-time is inversely related to the mitral valve area, it also depends directly on left atrial compliance and the square root of peak transmitral pressure gradient.

Figure 17–39 displays computer-generated solutions of equation 17.15, showing the dependence of pressure decay on the mitral valve area, LAC, and initial pressure (P_0). The baseline curve in each figure (denoted by the arrow) is for an orifice area of 1.5 cm^2, initial pressure of 10 mm Hg, and compliance of 6 ml/mm Hg, with the respective variable altered as shown. Figure 17–39A demonstrates that the pressure fall-off becomes flatter in inverse proportion to the valve area, which prolongs the pressure half-time proportionally. In this example, the half-time increases from 110 msec for an orifice area of 2 cm^2 to 440 msec for an orifice area of 0.5 cm^2. Note that the proportionality constant in this case, 220 msec/cm^2, is the same as that generally used in the application of mitral pressure half-time in Doppler echocardiography: this, however, is only coincidental and depends on the fortuitous combination of initial left atrial pressure and compliance. Similarly, Figure 17–39B shows a prolongation of the pressure half-time from 73 msec for a compliance of 3 ml/mm Hg to 293 msec for a compliance of 12 ml/mm Hg, with mitral valve area and P_0 held constant. In Figure 17–39C, we see that the initial pressure fall-off does increase with increasing peak transmitral gradient; however, the pressure half-time still increases from 104 msec for a peak gradient of 5 mm Hg to 208 msec for a gradient of 20 mm Hg.

Clinically increasing left atrial pressure typically causes a corresponding decrease in left atrial compliance, leaving the half-time dependent more purely on mitral valve area. However, when anatomic distortion or physiologic derangement independently changes either pressure or compliance, one should expect 220/$T_{1/2}$ to be a poor predictor of mitral valve area. Thus, the pressure half-time fails to accurately predict changes in valve area[88] immediately following balloon mitral valvotomy, which causes dramatic changes in atrial volume and pressure, shifting the chamber to a different portion of its pressure volume curve. Similarly, in patients with aortic regurgitation, the pressure half-time is decreased, and mitral valve area is overestimated, which is due to

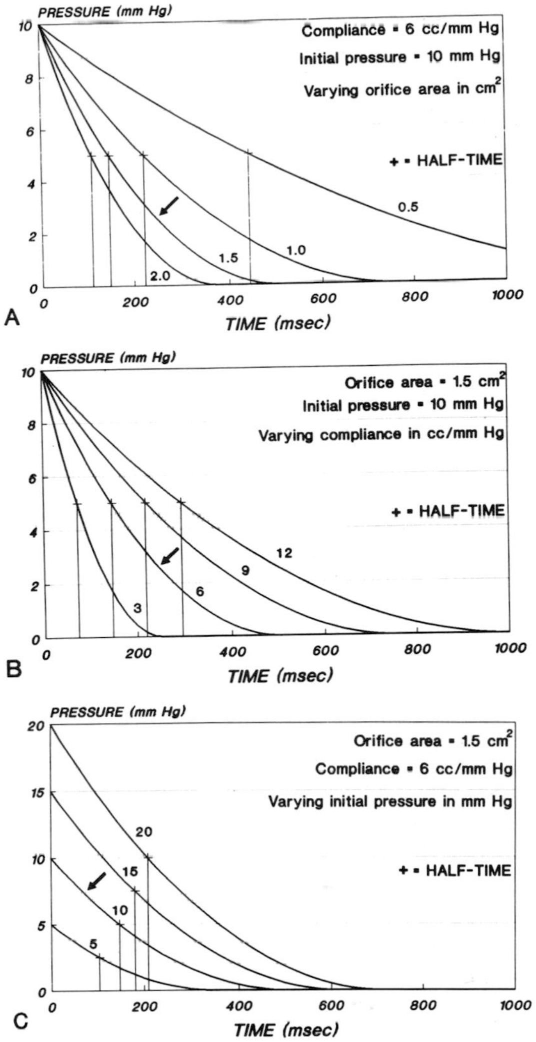

Fig. 17–39. Time course of the transmitral pressure gradient calculated using the relationship $p(t) = (\sqrt{P_0} - 25.2 \text{ MVA } t/\text{LAC})^2$ with **(A)** varying mitral valve area (MVA), **(B)** left atrial compliance, (LAC), and **(C)** initial transmitral gradient. The arrow denotes a curve with identical conditions in each figure: effective orifice area = 1.5 cm^2, compliance = 6 ml/mm Hg, and initial pressure = 10 mm Hg. The respective variables are then altered as shown and the resulting curves plotted. The vertical lines show the pressure half-time for the given condition. This mathematical model demonstrates that mitral pressure half-time varies inversely with valve area and directly with atrial compliance and the square root of the initial pressure gradient. (From Thomas JD, Weyman AE: Doppler mitral pressure half-time: a clinical tool in search of theoretical justification. J Am Coll Cardiol 10:923, 1987. Reprinted with permission from the American College of Cardiology. Journal of the American College of Cardiology, 1987, 10, 923.)

the second source of blood filling the left ventricle.[78,89,90] Figure 17–40 is a computer simulation that shows the effects of varying degrees of aortic insufficiency (expressed as regurgitant orifice area) on the time course of transmitral velocity. The augmented ventricular filling from the aorta raises ventricular pressure prematurely and shortens the mitral pressure half-time, even though the mitral valve area remains constant.[90] If ventricular compliance is sufficiently increased however, the pressure half-time may return to baseline be-

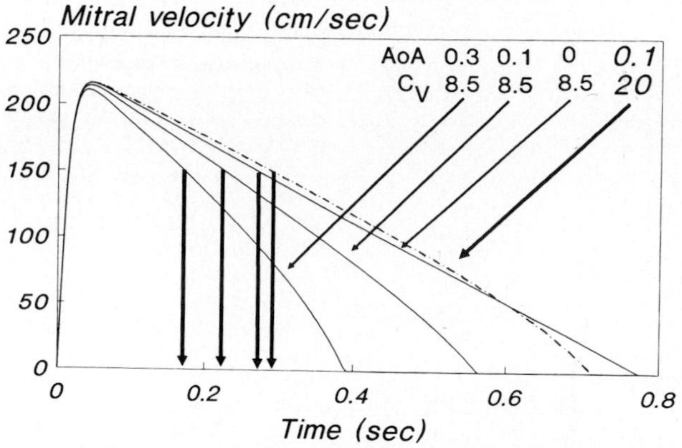

Fig. 17–40. Computer simulation showing the effects of increasing aortic regurgitation on the transmitral flow curve. Flow decays faster and pressure half-time shortens (vertical arrows) with increasing regurgitation (regurgitant orifice areas [AoA] 0, 0.1, and 0.3 cm^2). The other parameters are held constant: mitral valve area (MVA) 1 cm^2, atrial and ventricular compliance = 8.5 ml/mm Hg, aortic compliance = 5 ml/mm Hg, initial atrial pressure = 20 mm Hg, initial ventricular pressure 0 mm Hg, initial aortic pressure = 100 mm Hg. However, if in the presence of a 0.1-cm^2 aortic regurgitant orifice, ventricular compliance (C_V) is increased to 20 ml/mm Hg (dashed line), the flow curve and pressure half-time are similar to that calculated with a compliance of 8.5 ml/mm Hg and no aortic regurgitation. (From Flachskampf FA, et al.: Aortic regurgitation shortens Doppler pressure half-time in mitral stenosis: clinical evidence, in vitro simulation, and theoretic analysis. J Am Coll Cardiol 16:396: 1990. Reprinted with permission from the American College of Cardiology.)

cause the regurgitant volume may be accommodated without significant pressure rise. The combined effects of regurgitant volume and ventricular compliance on half-time are shown in Figure 17–41. At any level of compliance, regurgitation always shortens half-time.[90]

Because of the competing effects of regurgitant volume and ventricular compliance, acute and chronic regurgitation should have different effects on mitral pressure half-time. In acute aortic regurgitation, the abruptly imposed volume load both increases pressure and causes a shift to a steeper portion of the pressure volume curve; both of which should shorten the half-time. In chronic aortic regurgitation, the situation is more complex because ventricular dilation leads to an increase in ventricular compliance, which could partially offset the effect of aortic regurgitation on the pressure half-time.[90] In practice, while differences in chamber compliance may account for intersubject variation in the effects of chronic aortic regurgitation on the pressure half-time, they do not completely negate the effect of the added volume load.

When compliance is constant throughout the diastolic filling period, the velocity decay curve will be linear with a slope that is inversely related to the net chamber compliance. Temporal variation in net compliance during diastole alters the velocity decay curve. When net compliance decreases during diastole (i.e., when the ventricle moves to a steeper portion of its pressure-volume curve), the transorifice velocity profile will be concave downward, whereas when net compliance increases, the velocity profile will be concave upward. As a result, increasing net compliance shortens and decreasing net compliance lengthens the pressure half-time (Fig. 17–42). The linear velocity decay curve seen in most patients with mitral stenosis implies that the net atrioventricular compliance is relatively constant throughout diastole. Because neither the atrium nor the ventricle would be expected to have a linear pressure-volume relationship, it must be that the rise in atrial compliance as it empties is offset by a fall in ventricular compliance as it fills.[88,91] When the velocity decay slope is not linear, a concave upward curve implies that the increase in atrial compliance is greater than the fall in ventricular compliance, while a concave downward curve indicates that the fall in ventricular compliance is the predominant effect.[91]

The Mitral Depressurization Time. An alternative to the half-time method has been proposed that is based on the time taken for the pressure gradient to fall to zero as opposed to one-half its peak value. In this approach, the mitral valve area is calculated as follows:

$$MVA = 750/AC \qquad [17.18]$$

where AC is the time taken for a line drawn from the peak velocity of the mitral valve Doppler velocity profile along the slope of maximal velocities to reach the baseline or zero level.[92] Although the depressurization time may be simpler to measure than the half-time, its accuracy should be affected by the same hemodynamic variables.

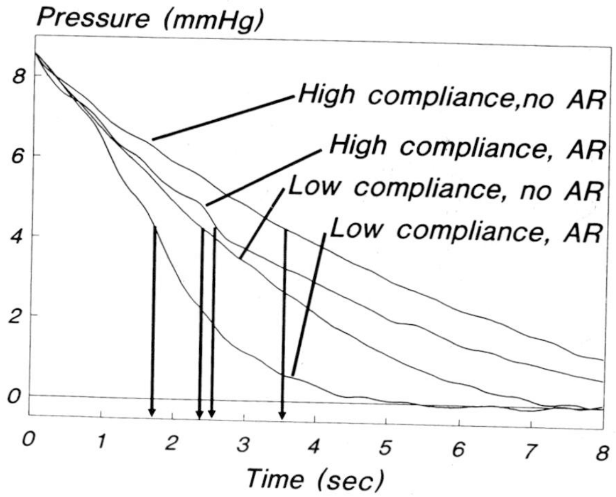

Fig. 17–41. Effect of aortic regurgitation and compliance on pressure half-time in an in vitro model. The top pair of curves are generated with high ventricular compliance, the bottom pair with low compliance (all with a 0.3-cm^2 mitral orifice. Addition of aortic regurgitation (60 ml, denoted as AR) shortens pressure half-time in each compliance setting. However, pressure half-time for high compliance with aortic regurgitation is the same as in the setting of low compliance with no regurgitation. Thus, the reduction of pressure half-time by aortic regurgitation can be counteracted by a concomitant increase in compliance. (From Flachskampf FA, et al.: Aortic regurgitation shortens Doppler pressure half-time in mitral stenosis: clinical evidence, in vitro simulation, and theoretic analysis. J Am Coll Cardiol 16:396, 1990. Reprinted with permission from the American College of Cardiology.)

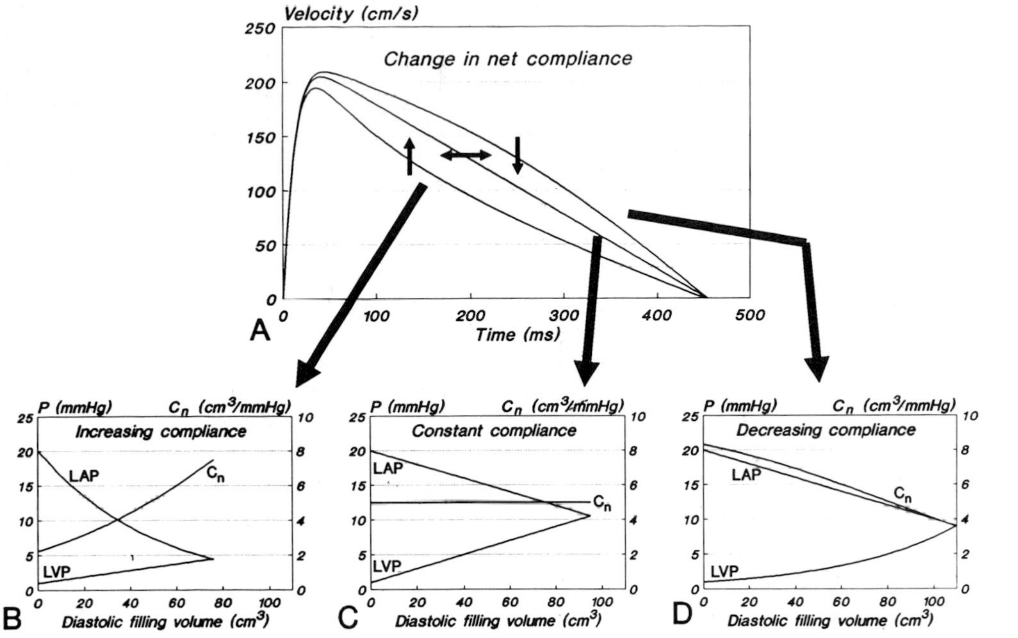

Fig. 17–42. A. Computer modeling of the effects of variable net compliance on the velocity downslope. During diastole, the emptying atrium shifts to a less steep portion of its pressure volume curve, and the filling ventricle shifts to a steeper portion. **B** to **D.** However, the result can be an increasing **(B)**, constant **(C)**, or decreasing **(D)** net compliance, depending on the individual chamber pressure volume curves. C_n = net compliance; LAP = left atrial pressure; LVP = left ventricular pressure. (From Flachskampf FA, Weyman AE, Guerrero JL, Thomas JD: Calculation of atrioventricular compliance from the mitral flow profile: analytical and in vitro study. J Am Coll Cardiol 19: 998, 1992. Reprinted with permission from the American College of Cardiology.)

Conceptual Integration of Invasive and Noninvasive Methods for Determining the Mitral Valve Area. In the preceding sections, four different methods were discussed for defining the mitral valve area: echocardiographic planimetry, the continuity equation, the Gorlin equation, and the Doppler pressure half-time. Although each of these methods yields a measure of mitral valve area, the reported valves are not necessarily the same, and it is important to understand the similarities and differences between these methods to correctly interpret the results they yield.

The most straightforward of these approaches is echocardiographic planimetry, which is equivalent to tracing around the edges of the mitral valve at autopsy or surgery. Planimetry therefore yields the in vivo anatomic area (A_0) free from the distortion encountered in fixation or during surgical measurement. Measurement of the flow area yields a similar result but requires the assumption that the valve orifice is elliptic.

The two echo-Doppler methods and the hemodynamic standard (the Gorlin equation) are often thought differ fundamentally from each other; however, they are all based on the same fundamental relationship:

$$\text{flow} = \text{velocity} * \text{area} \qquad [17.19]$$

or

$$\text{area} = \text{flow/velocity} \qquad [17.20]$$

The continuity equation is based on the principle that the flow passing through the mitral valve must be the same as that passing through all other parts of the heart (assuming no shunting or regurgitation). Flow can be measured hemodynamically as the cardiac output (determined by the Fick, thermodilution, or dye dilution methods) divided by the diastolic filling period or more commonly by Doppler methods. Velocity is the mean temporal velocity usually determined by the continuous wave Doppler method. Dividing mean flow by mean velocity will yield the narrowest area through which blood is flowing. This area, the vena contracta, is by definition the effective valve area (A_e) and is normally between 65 and 85% of the anatomic area. The ratio of the effective to the anatomic valve areas is the coefficient of contraction.

The Gorlin equation begins with the continuity equation $A_e = Q/v$. Flow in the hemodynamic laboratory is typically obtained from the cardiac output (determined by the thermodilution, Fick or dye dilution methods) divided by the diastolic filling period to give the mean flow rate. Because it is pressure rather than velocity that is measured at catheterization, pressure must be converted to velocity. This is achieved using the modified Bernoulli equation $\Delta p = 1/2\ \rho\ v^2$ or $\Delta p = 4\ v^2$ for pressure in millimeters of mercury and velocity in meters per second. Because flow is in milliliters per second, velocity must be expressed in centimeters per second. This is achieved by inverting the equation and multiplying by 100 (to convert meters to centimeters). Thus, velocity $= 100\ \sqrt{\Delta p/4}$ or $v = 50\ \sqrt{\Delta p}$. With this substitution, the continuity equation becomes $A_e = Q/50\ \sqrt{\Delta p}$. Because Gorlin's standard of comparison was a series of excised mitral valves, it was necessary to divide by the coefficient of discharge to correct the effective area to the anatomic area: $A_0 = A_e/C_D = A_e/.75$ or $Q/.75 \times 50\ \sqrt{\Delta p} = Q/37.5\ \sqrt{\Delta p}$, which is the familiar Gorlin equation.[93] Others have modified the Gorlin constant by using different values for the coefficient of discharge or solving for water rather than blood, but in all these modifications, the basic relationships remain the same.[94]

The half-time method, like the Gorlin formula, combines the continuity principles for mass and energy. It differs, however, in that it does not use mean values for pressure and flow to determine area but rather seeks to define the specific point in time at which the gradient falls to half of its initial valve. Thus, the half-time method begins with the same basic equation for flow through the mitral valve $Q = A_e * v =$ (by the modified Bernoulli equation) $50.4\ A_e \sqrt{\Delta p}$. Because the half-time is the time for Δp to fall from its initial value (Δp_0) to $\Delta p/2$, it is necessary to know how the pressure gradient changes with time. Because the net compliance (C_n) of the atrium and ventricle determines the rate at which flow through the valve diminishes the pressure gradient,

$$d\Delta p/dt = -Q/C_n \qquad [17.21]$$

Substituting for Q yields the differential equation

$$d\Delta p/dt = -\ 50.4\ A_e/C_n \qquad [17.22]$$

whose solution is a parabolic decay curve for pressure gradient versus time. Solving for the time ($T_{1/2}$) when pressure has fallen to half of its initial value yields the following expression:

$$T_{1/2} = \frac{11.6\ C_n \sqrt{\Delta p_0}}{C_D\ E_A} \qquad [17.23]$$

or

$$E_A = \frac{11.6\ C_n \sqrt{\Delta p_0}}{C_D\ T_{1/2}} \qquad [17.24]$$

If $11.6\ C_n$ square root p_0/C_D happens to equal 220 (which it approximates in a remarkable number of clinical circumstances) then this reduces to the familiar $MVA = 220/T_{1/2}$.

Note that all of the flow-based equations derived here initially yield the effective valve area (A_e) or the area at the vena contracta. The Gorlin equation corrects for the coefficient of contraction to approximate the anatomic orifice. Because the constant 220 in the half-time equation was derived by correlation with Gorlin-derived values, it implicitly includes a correction for the coefficient of discharge and should also yield anatomic valve areas. Continuity-derived values yield the effective orifice area and should underestimate Gorlin, planimetry, and half-time measures. Although the value of A_0 should be closer to that measured at surgery and by planimetry, the value A_e is more appropriate from a physiologic viewpoint because it is the area to which flow is actually constricted.

Summary. We prefer to measure the mitral valve area using echocardiographic planimetry when the orifice can be clearly recorded. This method contains no assumptions, and in skilled hands, the orifice can be accurately measured in the majority of cases. When the lateral orifice margins are indistinct, border identification can be confirmed from the margin of the flow stream. Our second choice is the half-time method. This approach is the simplest and has the least observer variability. Unfortunately, it is affected by atrial and ventricular compliance, and the initial transvalvular pressure gradient and the magnitude of the resulting error cannot be predicted in the individual case. Continuity-based methods are more difficult to apply but in appropriate cases should yield accurate results. Hemodynamic measurement of valve area based on the Gorlin equation is probably less accurate than any of the echo-Doppler methods because of the imprecision in both cardiac output and pressure measurements in most clinical studies. However, the differences in the results obtained by any of these methods are generally so small that absolute truth is difficult to establish in the clinical environment, and accuracy in most cases depends more on the quality of the raw data than on the method of calculation.

Mitral Stenosis and Insufficiency

The combination of mitral stenosis and insufficiency includes a broad spectrum of valvular deformities ranging from the predominantly stenotic lesion with minimal valve leakage to the severely insufficient valve that offers only limited obstruction to left ventricular inflow. As with pure mitral stenosis, the stenotic component of the combined lesions is indicated by diastolic doming of the anterior mitral leaflet.[16,55] This finding is even more important in the combined lesion because, in many patients with predominant insufficiency, the absolute valve area may be within the normal range. The stenosis then becomes a relative phenomenon because the deformed orifice, although not reduced below the normal range, is inadequate to handle the combined forward and regurgitant volumes that must pass through the valve during diastole. This situation is evidenced, however, only by diastolic doming and not through the measurement of valve area. Figure 17–43 is a recording of the mitral valve of a patient with mitral stenosis and insufficiency that illustrates diastolic doming of the valve in the setting of a relatively large leaflet separation.

When the stenotic component of the combined lesion predominates, leaflet separation in long axis and valve orifice in short axis are reduced. Likewise, left ventricular size and stroke volume are usually normal. As the regurgitant component becomes more dominant, the mitral valve orifice, as a rule, becomes larger, as do left ventricular chamber size and stroke volume.

The correlation between echocardiographic and hemodynamic mitral valve area is better with combined lesions than with isolated stenosis (Fig. 17–44). This fact reflects the wider range of valve areas seen with combined lesions and the greater accuracy in the echocardiographic measurement of large valve orifices.

Also note that the rate of diastolic mitral valve closure or E-F slope has correlated better with mitral valve area in patients with combined mitral stenosis and insufficiency than in those with mitral stenosis alone.[55] This improved correlation probably occurs because both the posterior motion of the annulus and the closure rate of the anterior leaflet bear a direct relationship to the rate of left ventricular inflow and an inverse relationship to mitral valve area. The high inflow rates of predominant mitral insufficiency, therefore, should increase both the annular and the leaflet components of the E-F slope and

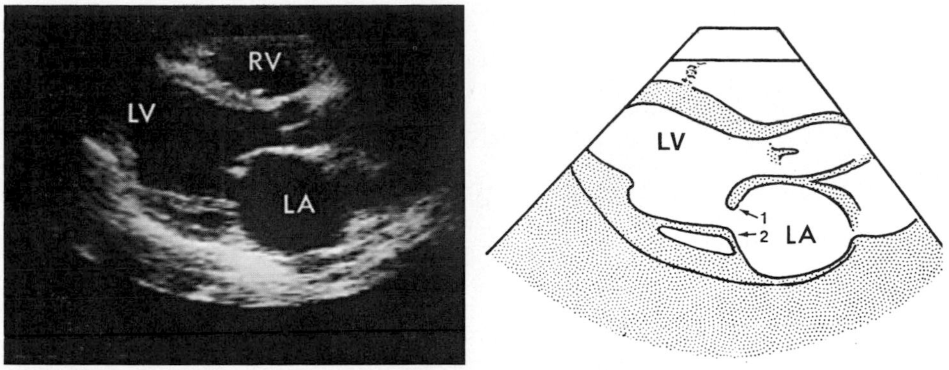

Fig. 17–43. Long axis recording of the mitral valve, left ventricle (LV), and left atrium (LA) in a patient with mitral stenosis and mitral insufficiency. Diastolic doming of the anterior mitral leaflet is prominent, indicating that the valve is stenotic despite the reasonably large separation between the anterior and posterior borders of the mitral valve orifice (arrows 1 and 2, respectively). The posterior leaflet is stiff and immobile and stands erect during diastole. RV = right ventricle.

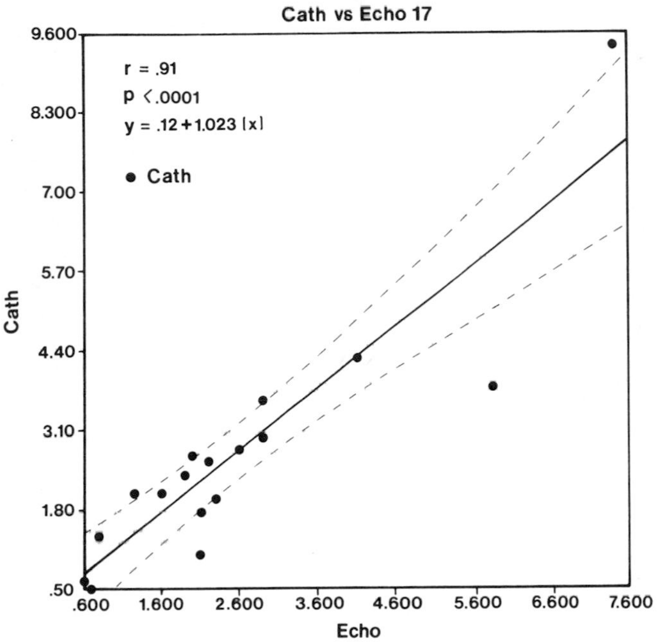

Fig. 17–44. Correlations between echocardiographic and hemodynamic estimates of mitral valve orifice area in patients with combined mitral stenosis and insufficiency. Hemodynamic values are derived using the Gorlin formula and angiographic cardiac output.

thus exaggerate the difference in initial diastolic leaflet closure rate when compared to the low inflow rates of predominant stenosis.

Most Doppler measures of transmitral gradients and valve area are similar and have the same degree of accuracy in patients with combined stenosis and insufficiency as in patients with isolated stenosis. The obvious exception is the determination of valve area using continuity-based methods, which use the cardiac output or flow across other valves as the reference flow. When mitral regurgitation is present, flow across the mitral valve is not the same as that across other valves or to the periphery, and thus the continuity principle is invalidated. The proximal convergence method measures all of the flow passing through the mitral orifice and hence remains valid for determining orifice area.

Mitral Stenosis and Prolapse

Prolapse of the mitral valve is frequently noted in patients with mitral stenosis. An incidence of between 10[95] and 40%[54] has been reported. When prolapse does occur in association with mitral stenosis, it almost invariably involves the anterior mitral leaflet and is associated with extreme leaflet pliability and prominent diastolic doming. Figure 17–45 is a recording from a patient with mitral stenosis and prolapse that demonstrates both the

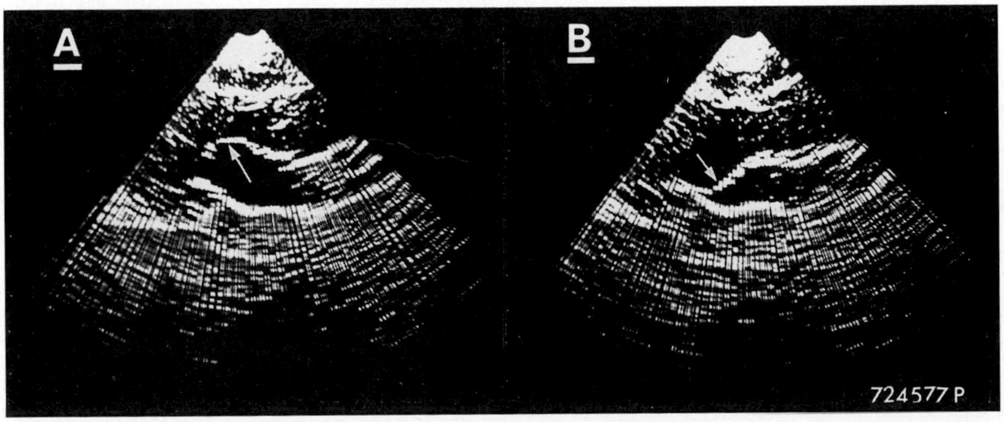

Fig. 17–45. Long axis recordings of the mitral valve demonstrate both mitral stenosis and mitral valve prolapse. **A.** During diastole, there is diastolic doming of the anterior leaflet (arrow) with a reduction in mitral orifice diameter. **B.** Systolic prolapse of the anterior leaflet (arrow).

marked diastolic doming and systolic prolapse of the anterior mitral leaflet.

The reason for this association is unclear. Both prolapse and mitral stenosis affect predominantly females and may therefore represent the chance association of the two relatively common disorders with the superimposition of the rheumatic process on a valve that is already predisposed to prolapse. Alternatively, the continued wear and tear on a pliable leaflet resulting from repeated diastolic distention might result in leaflet degeneration and/or stretching.

Posterior leaflet prolapse is much less common and usually occurs in association with bacterial endocarditis and/or chordal rupture. The almost exclusive involvement of the anterior leaflet and association with pronounced doming suggest that continued diastolic distention of the leaflet either is a direct cause or exaggerates an underlying predisposition.

Mitral Commissurotomy

When the decrease in the orifice area of the stenotic mitral valve reaches a critical level, surgical intervention is generally necessary. This procedure may involve either replacement of the diseased valve with a prosthesis or enlargement of the valve orifice by means of a mitral commissurotomy. Commissurotomy, when possible, appears to be the procedure of choice because of its lower incidence of mortality, morbidity, and postoperative complications in comparison to valve replacement.[96]

Several reports have indicated that cross-sectional echocardiography is a useful technique for defining the structure and area of the mitral valve orifice following commissurotomy,[96,98] determining the increase in orifice size resulting from the surgical procedure,[58] assessing the long-term effects of the commissurotomy on valve area,[96] and potentially identifying suitable patients for this surgical procedure.[64] Commissurotomy characteristically alters the appearance of the mitral valve orifice in short axis by elongating the horizontal dimension of the orifice disproportionately to the vertical dimension. Vertical leaflet excursion typically remains restricted and stiff. In some instances, the enlargement of one commissure may be greater than that of the other, further distorting the postoperative orifice configuration. Figure 17–46A and B shows recordings of the mitral valve orifice from the same patient taken before and after commissurotomy. On occasion, surgery can so deform the valve orifice that planimetry is impossible, and in these instances the Doppler half-time may provide a more accurate measure of orifice area.[86]

In a group of 10 patients studied by cross-sectional echocardiography and cardiac catheterization both before and 6 months after commissurotomy, a good correlation in the mitral valve area, determined by both techniques at both sampling periods, was demonstrated.[58] In the postoperative state, the echocardiogram again slightly overestimated the hemodynamic valve area (0.3 cm^2), and the overall correlation ($r = .84$) was similar to that noted in uninstrumented valves.[58]

In addition to aiding in determining the short-term effects of commissurotomy, the echocardiographic method has also proven useful in determining the long-term influence of mitral commissurotomy on mitral valve area.[96] In a study of 18 patients examined 10 to 14 years after a documented successful commissurotomy (Fig. 17–47), no change in valve area was noted in 13 patients, whereas in 5 patients (28%), restenosis was evident. This method further helped to separate the patients with increasing symptoms who had evidence of restenosis (3) from those with recurrent symptoms but no change in valve area (3).[96]

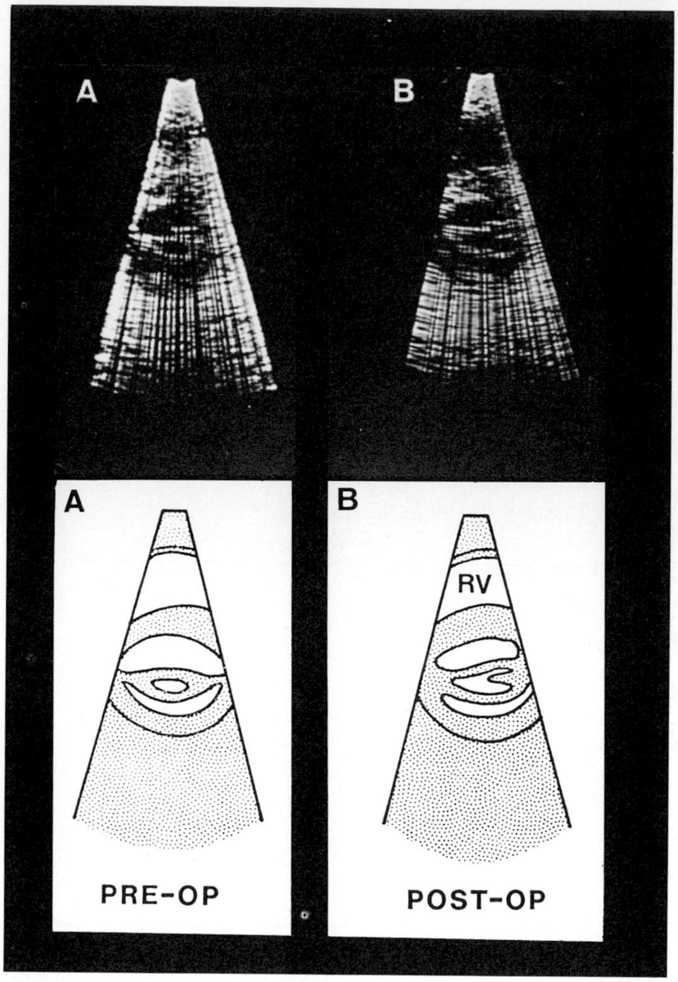

Fig. 17–46. Pre- and postcommissurotomy recordings of the mitral valve orifice from a patient with mitral stenosis. **A.** Before the operation, the orifice is markedly decreased and has a fish-mouthed appearance. **B.** After the operation, an increase in valve area is most prominent in the lateral or horizontal dimension. In addition, separation of the valve leaflets is greater at the lateral commissure, and there is a second lateral indentation in the anterior leaflet just above the native commissure. RV = right ventricle.

Although precise correlation of symptoms with echocardiographic valve areas is not possible, it has been suggested that symptoms are commonly noted in patients with valve areas of less than 1.1 cm^2/m^2 after commissurotomy and are less frequently observed in patients with larger postoperative valve areas.[58]

Finally, the echocardiographic method may be helpful in determining the suitability of a patient for commissur-

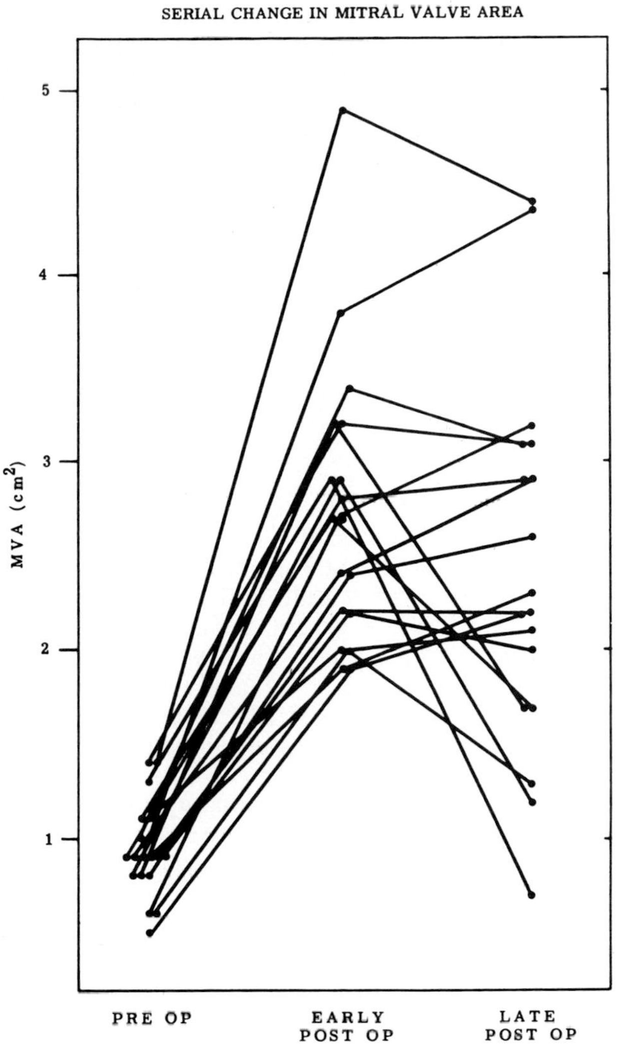

Fig. 17–47. Long-term changes in mitral valve area (MVA) following successful commissurotomy. Both preoperative and early postoperative values for mitral valve area were determined hemodynamically. The late postoperative values were cross-sectional studies recorded 10 to 14 years after the documentation of successful commissurotomy. (From Heger JJ, et al.: Long-term changes in mitral valve area after successful mitral commissurotomy. Circulation 59:443, 1979. Reproduced by permission of the American Heart Association, Inc.)

otomy.[58] Extensive fibrosis, calcification, and mitral insufficiency are considered at least as relative contraindications to commissurotomy. The echocardiographic method can clearly demonstrate significant calcification and distortion of the valve orifice and can evaluate leaflet pliability. Doppler techniques can identify mitral regurgitation and provide an estimate of its severity. Thus, although precise criteria have not yet been established for selecting a patient for commissurotomy, the presence of a thin, freely mobile leaflet in the absence of dense fibrosis or calcification should indicate a good candidate for prospective commissurotomy.

Percutaneous Mitral Balloon Valvotomy. Percutaneous mitral balloon valvotomy (PMV) is a new nonsurgical technique for the treatment of patients with mitral stenosis.[97–103] An increase in valve area is achieved by inflating a balloon catheter that has been passed antegrade through the interatrial septum and positioned across the stenotic mitral valve orifice. Inflation of the balloon(s) splits the valve along its commissures without traumatic evulsion or damage to the valve leaflets,[101,103–106] a process resembling the changes seen after surgical commissurotomy.[96] Figure 17–48 shows a mitral valve orifice pre- and postvalvotomy. The orifice in this example is increased by 1.7 cm^2 following the procedure. Figure 17–49 is a second example with an even better result obtained in a young patient with a less severely deformed valve. Percutaneous mitral valvotomy has gained rapid acceptance because it is less invasive than surgery, can be performed in patients who would not be considered surgical candidates, and can be repeated as necessary. Echo-Doppler techniques have proven highly valuable in (1) selecting patients for valvuloplasty, (2) detecting complications during the procedure, and (3) evaluating the short- and long-term results of the intervention.

Patient Selection. Echo-Doppler studies of potential candidates for PMV establish the diagnosis of rheumatic stenosis, provide information about the severity of the lesion (the transvalvular gradient and mitral valve area), identify important complications (i.e., mitral regurgitation, aortic stenosis and regurgitation, tricuspid stenosis and regurgitation, pulmonary hypertension, left atrial thrombi, and left and right ventricular dysfunction) and display the morphology of the valve. Morphologic features such as leaflet mobility, thickening, calcification, and the degree of subvalvular involvement have been shown to help identify patients most likely to profit from

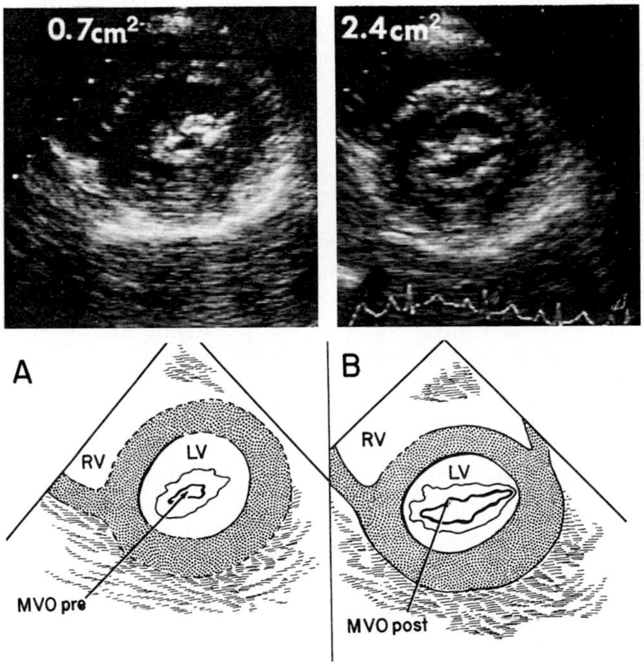

Fig. 17–48. Parasternal short axis recordings of a mitral valve orifice before **(A)** and after **(B)** balloon mitral valvotomy. Note that splitting of the valve occurs along the line of commissural fusion and that the valve area in this case increases from 0.7 cm^2 to 2.4 cm^2. RV = right ventricle; LV = left ventricle; MVO = mitral valve orifice.

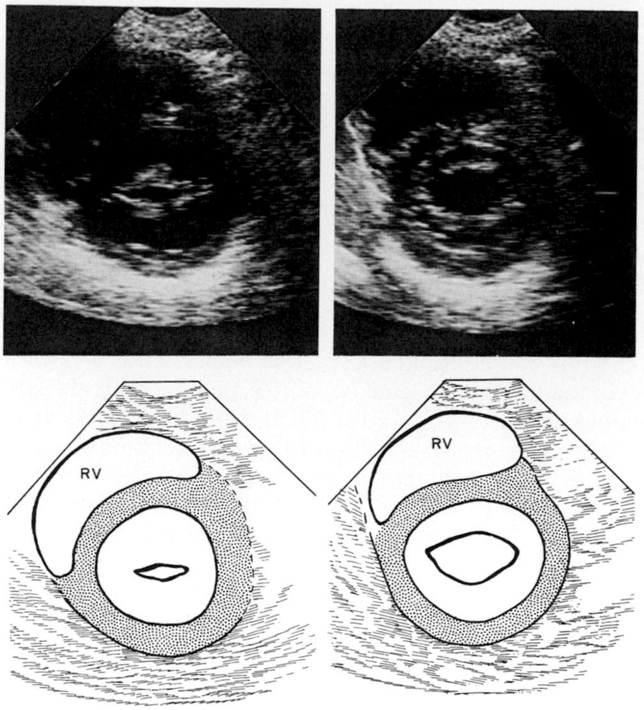

Fig. 17–49. Parasternal short axis recording of the mitral valve before and after balloon valvotomy. The valve area in this example increased from 1.1 cm^2 before the procedure to 4 cm^2 postvalvotomy. This unusually good result occurred in a patient with little morphologic deformity of the valve before valvotomy. RV = right ventricle.

the valvuloplasty procedure.[105,106] Table 17–1 lists a series of criteria developed by Wilkins to grade valvular involvement by each of these processes on a scale of 0 to 4. These individual values are then summed to yield a "score" that reflects the overall severity of morphologic derangement.[105] In this schema, higher scores indicated a greater degree of derangement.

Mobility, calcification, and fibrosis are assessed in standard parasternal long and short axis and apical views. To assess subvalvar thickening, one must angle the standard parasternal long axis view medially and laterally so that the long axis of each papillary muscle and its attached chordal apparatus can be recorded. From the apical window, the extent of subvalvar shortening and scar is best defined in a four-chamber view with the transducer angled posteriorly.[105]

Several studies have suggested that the echo score is a better predictor of outcome than any other clinical or hemodynamic variable.[105] In a series of 130 patients, the echo score was significantly lower (mean 7.3 ± 2.1) in patients with a "good" result (defined as a postvalvotomy mitral valve area ≥ 1.5 cm^2 and an increase in valve area of at least 25%) than in those who failed to meet these criteria (mean 10.0 ± 2.3) and who were considered to have a suboptimal result. Figure 17–50 shows the number of good and suboptimal results stratified according to total echocardiographic score. Note that all patients with a very low echocardiographic score (4 and 5) had a "good" outcome and that the proportion of patients with a "good" outcome decreased progressively as the score increased. The sensitivity and specificity of the echo score for predicting a "good" result are shown in Figure 17–51. Sensitivity increased, and specificity decreased as the echocardiographic score increased. The optimal combination of sensitivity and specificity, as defined by the cross-over point of the two

Table 17–1. Grading of Mitral Valve Characteristics From the Echocardiographic Examination

Grade	Mobility	Subvalvar Thickening	Thickening	Calcification
1	Highly mobile valve with only leaflet tips restricted	Minimal thickening just below the mitral leaflets	Leaflets near normal in thickness (4–5 mm)	A single area of increased echo brightness
2	Leaflet mild and base portions have normal mobility	Thickening of chordal structures extending up to one third of the chordal length	Mid-leaflets normal, considerable thickening of margins (5–8 mm)	Scattered areas of brightness confined to leaflet margins
3	Valve continues to move forward in diastole, mainly from the base	Thickening extending to the distal third of the chords	Thickening extending through the entire leaflet (5–8 mm)	Brightness extending into the mid-portion of the leaflets
4	No or minimal forward movement of the leaflets in diastole	Extensive thickening and shortening of all chordal structures extending down to the papillary muscles	Considerable thickening of all leaflet tissue (>8–10 mm)	Extensive brightness throughout much of the leaflet tissue

The total echocardiographic score was derived from an analysis of mitral leaflet mobility, valvar and subvalvar thickening, and calcification which were graded from 0 to 4 according to the above criteria. This gave a total score of 0 to 16.

(From Wilkins GT, et al.: Percutaneous balloon dilatation of the mitral valve: an analysis of echocardiographic variables related to outcome and the mechanism of dilatation. Br Heart J 60:299, 1988.

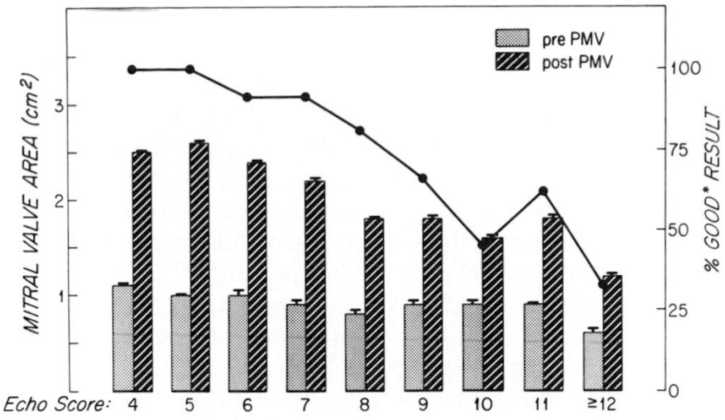

Fig. 17–50. Relationship of echo score on the abscissa to mitral valve area before and after balloon valvuloplasty on the ordinate. Abscissa values equal echo scores ranging from 4 to more than 12. The solid line indicates the percentage of patients with a "good" result (defined as an absolute valve area equal to or greater than 1.5 cm² and an increase in valve area of 25% or more) in relation to the preprocedure echoscore. (Courtesy of Dr. Igor Palacios.)

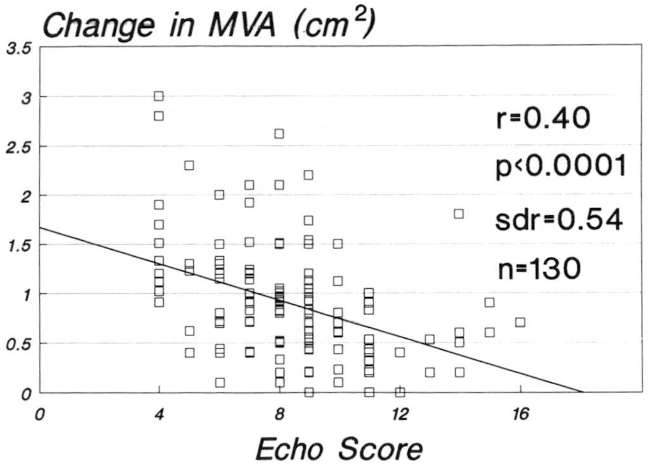

Fig. 17–52. Absolute change in mitral valve area (MVA) (cm²) produced by balloon mitral valvotomy in relation to the prevalvotomy echo score for 130 patients. Note that although there is a weak but highly significant correlation, it is impossible to predict an absolute change in valve area from the morphologic characteristics of the valve. sdr = standard deviation of the regress. (From Abascal VM, et al.: Prediction of successful outcome in 130 patients undergoing percutaneous balloon mitral valvotomy. Circulation 82:448, 1990. Reproduced by permission of the American Heart Association, Inc.)

curves, occurred at an echocardiographic score of 8. Eighty-four percent of patients with an echo score ≤8 had a good result, while 58% of those with scores greater than 8 had a suboptimal outcome. Figure 17–52 illustrates the relationship between the echocardiographic score and the absolute change in valve area. A fair (r = .40) but highly significant correlation is present, with substantial scatter in the data. When all relevant hemodynamic, demographic, and morphologic aspects of the mitral valve were considered, the echocardiographic score was the most significant univariate predictor of absolute change in valve area followed by the effective balloon-dilating area. No other parameter proved to be a statistically significant predictor. When the individual components of the score were cross correlated, significant relationships were uniformly found, indicating that these abnormalities tended to progress together in the

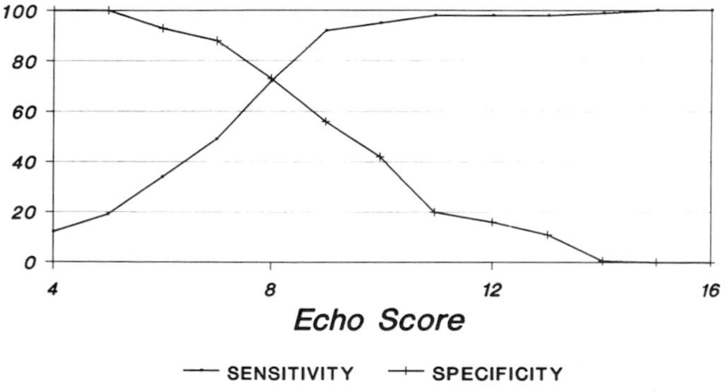

Fig. 17–51. Relationship of sensitivity and specificity of individual echo score values in the prediction of a good outcome following balloon valvuloplasty. Note that low scores are highly specific but insensitive (because many patients with higher scores will have good results). The optimum combination of sensitivity and specificity occurs at an echo score of 8. (From Abascal VM, et al.: Prediction of successful outcome in 130 patients undergoing percutaneous balloon mitral valvotomy. Circulation 82:448, 1990. Reproduced by permission of the American Heart Association, Inc.)

same patient. Of all the individual components of the score, thickening was the most highly correlated with absolute change in valve area, but the relationship was not significantly different from that for the total score. Thus, while the echo score appears of value in identifying patients most likely to benefit from percutaneous valvotomy, it cannot accurately predict the absolute change in area that will be achieved. Likewise, although patients with high scores are less likely to benefit from the procedure, a high score does not preclude a "good" result.

Asymmetric fibrosis or calcification of the mitral commissures does not appear to affect the results of the procedure or to lead to an increased incidence of complications.[107] In some patients with a high score, balloon dilation seems to produce extensive commissural splitting, yet the separation of the leaflets in diastole remains poor. As a result, the orifice area fails to increase in proportion to the increase in circumference.[105]

Guiding the Procedure and Detecting Acute Complications. During the percutaneous valvotomy procedure, echo-Doppler studies can be valuable in helping guide the transeptal puncture, assessing acute complications such as atrial or ventricular perforation with tamponade, and identifying acute mitral regurgitation and valvular disruption.

Assessment of Results and Follow-Up. Immediately following PMV, the mitral valve area increases, left atrial pressure and pulmonary artery pressure decrease, and the cardiac output increases. Figure 17–53 illustrates the observed magnitude of these changes for 357 patients studied at our institution from 1986 to 1991. Morphologically, splitting along the lines of commissural fusion is noted, and as a result, the transverse diameter of the orifice increases. In most cases, splitting is observed

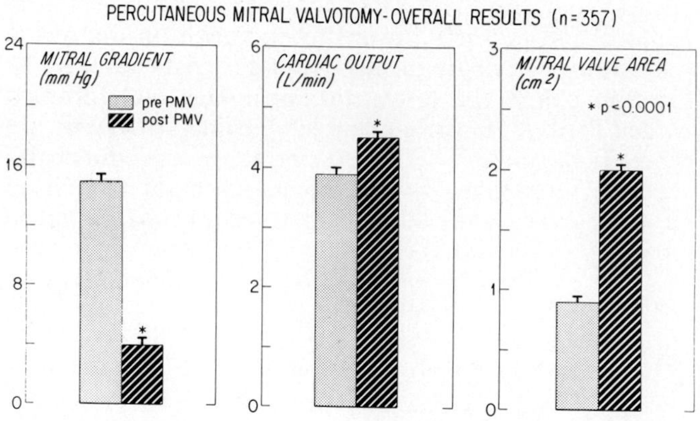

Fig. 17–53. Hemodynamic results of percutaneous mitral valvotomy (PMV) for a group of 357 patients studied at the Massachusetts General Hospital. The procedure results in a significant decrease in transmitral gradient, slight but significant increase in cardiac output, and a mean 1.1 cm^2 increase in mitral valve area. (Courtesy of Dr. Igor Palacios.)

along both commissures, although on occasion, only one commissure may appear to have torn.[106]

In immediate postprocedure studies, the severity of mitral regurgitation does not change in roughly 50% of patients studied; it increases in severity by 1 grade in another 33% and by 2 grades in the remainder.[108] No preprocedure clinical, hemodynamic, or morphologic characteristic is useful in predicting patients in whom regurgitation is likely to appear or increase.[108] Although balloon size has generally not been associated with an increase in regurgitation, a recent study suggested that large balloon diameters (>27.5 mm) did increase regurgitation significantly.[109] Left atrial volume decreases significantly in the majority of patients, including those with regurgitation, suggesting that despite the increase in regurgitation in some patients, the overall effect is positive. An atrial septal defect at the site of the transeptal catheterization has been reported in from 15 to 89% of patients.[110,111] The incidence reported in echocardiographic studies is generally higher than that in hemodynamic series, reflecting the greater sensitivity of the Doppler technique.[112]

Immediate postprocedure recordings of mitral valve area and transmitral gradients are important because these are the primary noninvasive parameters that will be used to follow patients. The Doppler half-time method for determining mitral valve area has been shown to be inaccurate for several days following the valvuloplasty procedure.[88,113] This transient inaccuracy relates to the rapid change in atrial pressure caused by the valvuloplasty that occurs without a commensurate change in atrial compliance. Over a period of days, atrial compliance appears to adapt to the acutely reduced pressure and to the accuracy of the half-time returns. In the immediate postvalvulotomy period, however, planimetry or continuity-based methods should be used. Once a reference is established, changes in valve area should be followed using the same standard, lest normal differences between methodologies be interpreted as evidence of restenosis.

Experience gained from patients after surgical commissurotomy indicates that a portion of the patients with good initial results develop restenosis at a variable period after surgery. In a group of 20 patients studied 6 to 11 months following PMV, mitral valve area decreased from a mean of 1.90 ± 0.59 cm^2 to a mean of 1.62 ± 0.55 cm^2 at follow-up. Valve area remained unchanged in 55% of patients, decreased by <25% in 5 (25%), and decreased by >25% in 4 (20%) patients. At follow-up, the transverse diameter of the orifice decreased slightly but significantly, while the anteroposterior diameter did not change, suggesting that valvular restenosis occurred primarily by refusion of the commissures. The morphologic characteristics of the valve did not change from pre- to postprocedure or at the >6-month follow-up. The degree of mitral regurgitation appears to decrease from immediate follow-up to the >6-month study. The only significant predictors of the percentage of decrease in valve area were the echocardiographic score described previously and the valve area following the procedure, with higher scores and smaller areas being associated with restenosis. Although this relationship was subsequently confirmed in a larger series,[114] it has not been a universal finding.[115]

Congenital Mitral Stenosis

Congenital mitral stenosis is a rare disorder of the mitral valve and is characterized by variable and often extensive deformity of the valve apparatus. Such deformity may include thickening, fibrosis, and nodularity of the mitral leaflets; fused, rudimentary, or absent commissures; thickened, shortened, and intra-adherent chordae; and fibrotic papillary muscles. These lesions may combine to transform the valve into a thickened, funnel-shaped, flat, or diaphragm-like structure that offers variable obstruction to left ventricular inflow.[116–120] Echocardiographically, the appearance of the valve depends on the degree of deformity. When the valve is more severely deformed, the leaflets appear highly reflective and thickened, leaflet motion is stiff and restricted, and diastolic leaflet excursion is reduced.[121,122] When the leaflets are more pliable, diastolic doming may be evident.

Figure 17–54 is a recording from a 6-month-old child with congenital mitral stenosis and illustrates diastolic mitral leaflet doming and systolic prolapse. In short axis, the mitral orifice was reduced in size, and two papillary muscles were recorded. Calcification of the valve is not typical. The left ventricle in such instances is normal in size, which serves to distinguish this lesion from mitral atresia. Diastolic vibration of the mitral leaflets was noted in one report;[121] however, the reason for its appearance is unclear because the area of turbulence should be distal to the valve. When obstruction is significant, the left atrium may dilate, and when long-standing pulmonary hypertension occurs, right-sided structures may also be enlarged. The reported accuracy of valve area measurement in the congenitally stenotic valve is similar to that in rheumatic mitral stenosis.[122]

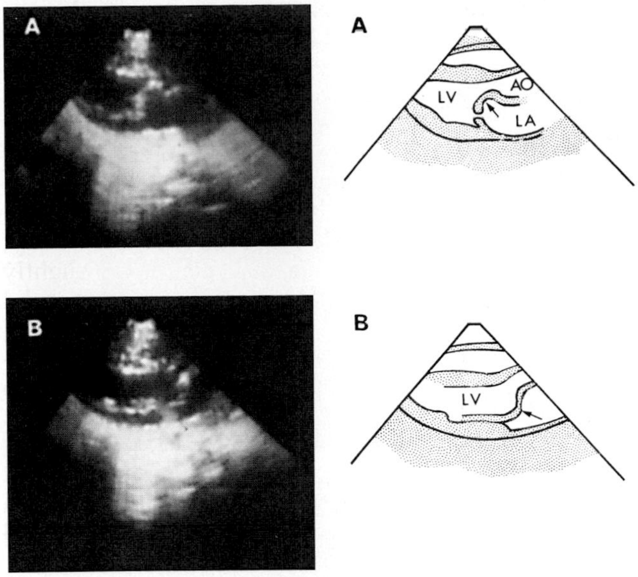

Fig. 17–54. Long axis recording of the mitral valve from a 6-month-old child with congenital mitral stenosis and systolic prolapse. **A.** The diastolic doming of the pliable stenotic anterior leaflet. The point of peak doming is indicated by the oblique arrow in the accompanying diagram. **B.** A systolic recording illustrates the pronounced systolic prolapse. The region of prolapse is indicated by the arrow in the accompanying diagram. Ao = aorta; LV = left ventricle; LA = left atrium.

Parachute Mitral Valve

Parachute mitral valve is a congenital form of mitral stenosis characterized by a single, large, papillary muscle—usually, the posteromedial—originating from the floor of the left ventricle. The leaflets and chordae are typically normal. The chordae, however, converge to insert into the single papillary muscle, restricting leaflet opening and causing blood to flow through the intrachordal spaces to reach the left ventricle. This can restrict mitral inflow at both the valvular and chordal level, particularly when the intrachordal spaces are narrowed.[123,124] In some patients, two papillary muscles are present; however, one is usually rudimentary and the chordae only insert into the larger of the pair.[122,125]

Echocardiographically, the long axis mitral valve configuration shows an increase in reflectivity and a reduction in leaflet motion.[121] The characteristic feature of this disorder, however, is the recording in short axis of a single (or dominant), large, papillary muscle that is positioned posteriorly in the center of the left ventricle.[121] Figure 17–55 illustrates a case of parachute mitral valve in which the posteromedial papillary muscle is dominant and receives all of the chordae tendineae. The mitral orifice is also restricted and directed toward the dominant papillary muscle.

Supravalvular Mitral Ring

Another form of congenital, left ventricular inflow obstruction is the supravalvular mitral ring. The supravalvular ring or membrane is composed of connective tissue, arises from the base of the atrial aspects of mitral leaflets, and extends inward to encroach on the mitral inlet. It can be distinguished from cor triatriatum by its location below the left atrial appendage and foramen ovale. The valve leaflets and supporting structures are typically normal.[126–128] These rings appear on the cross-sectional echogram as an anomalous band of echoes stretching across the left atrium at the level of the mitral annulus.[121] This band of echoes typically moves inward toward the mitral valve in diastole and superiorly away from the mitral valve in systole.[121]

Figure 17–56 illustrates a supravalvular ring recorded in the parasternal and apical long axis views. Although in this example the membrane is clearly recorded in the parasternal long axis view, apical recordings generally display these delicate structures more clearly because they are perpendicular to the path of a scan plane arising from this transducer location. The ring in this case appears as a band of linear echoes arising from the posterior margin of the mitral annulus and extending inward to partially obstruct the mitral inflow area. The mitral leaflets that lie in the region of the turbulence beyond the area of obstruction often vibrate during diastolic inflow.[121]

Figure 17–57 illustrates the combined occurrence of a supravalvar mitral ring and a subvalvar aortic membrane. These combined lesions are often associated with parachute mitral valve and coarctation of the aorta (Shone's syndrome).[123]

The Mitral Valve in Aortic Insufficiency

Mitral valve motion and diastolic orifice configuration may be altered in aortic insufficiency. These abnormalities involve primarily the anterior leaflet and are characterized by (1) a decrease in the opening amplitude of the anterior leaflet in long and short axis; (2) an abnormal short axis mitral orifice configuration; and (3) diastolic leaflet oscillation.[129] The reduced amplitude of anterior leaflet excursion is apparently caused by the regurgitant stream of blood from the aorta that strikes the leaflet and impedes its normal opening pattern. This reduction in leaflet opening is most prominent in mid- and late diastole; however, even the initial portions of diastolic opening may be impaired in more severe cases.

The valve orifice in short axis is deformed because the restriction in anterior leaflet excursion is most pronounced in the center of the leaflet, where peak vertical separation normally occurs. This restriction causes the anterior leaflet to appear flattened rather than convex anteriorly, and in severe cases, it may actually be concave toward the left ventricular outflow tract. As diastole progresses, the deformity generally becomes more pronounced. Figure 17–58A and B shows short-axis recordings of the mitral valve orifice from two patients with aortic insufficiency and illustrates this pattern.

In these instances, the curvature of the anterior leaflet parallels that of the posterior leaflet, and the mitral orifice assumes a curved slit-like appearance rather than the normal circular or oval pattern. Once this abnormal configuration is assumed, it is generally maintained

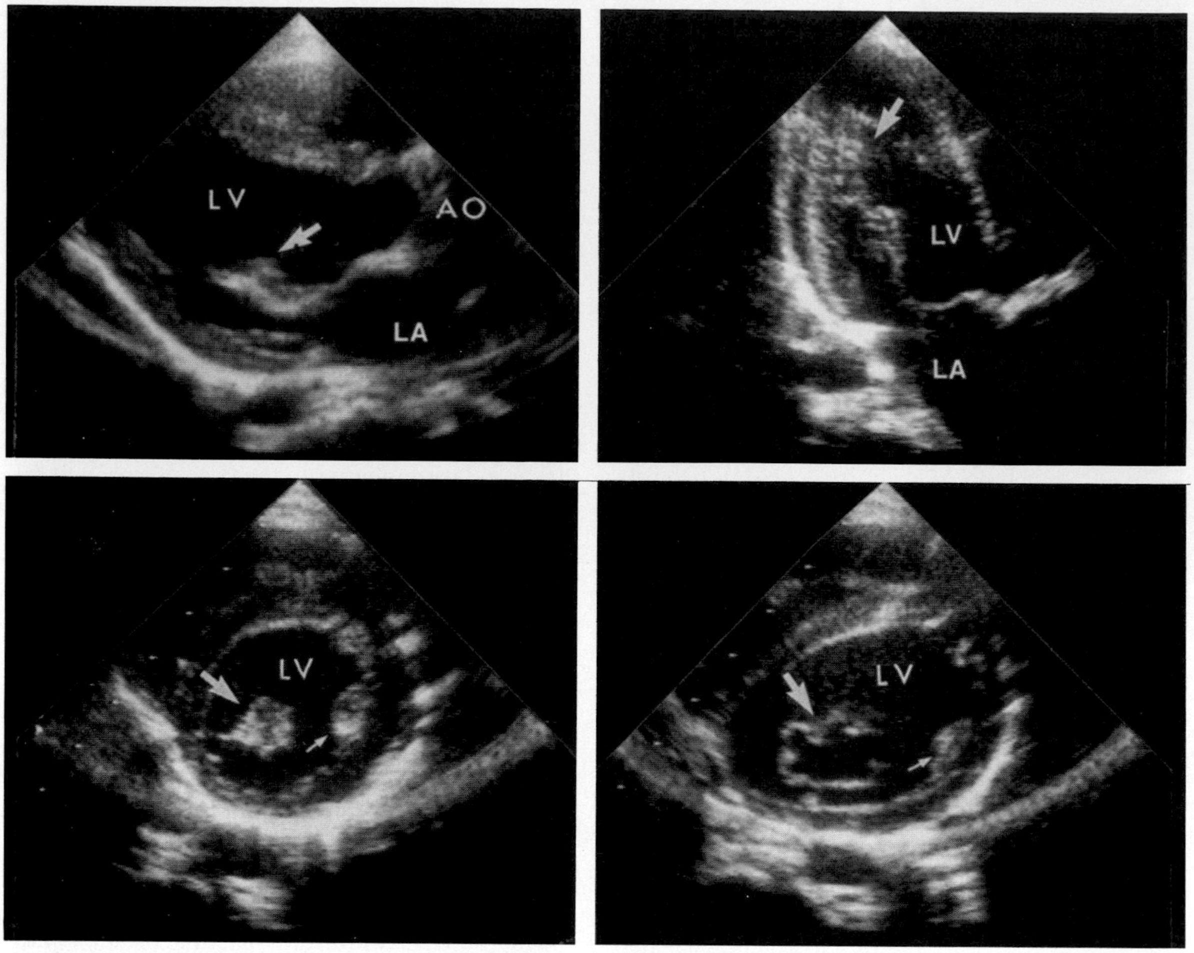

Fig. 17–55. Series of recordings from a patient with a variant of parachute mitral valve. Top, left. Parasternal long axis recording showing a large papillary muscle (arrow) that extends far into the ventricle and attaches by thick, short cords to the anterior mitral leaflet. Top, right. Apical long axis view illustrates the morphology of the enlarged papillary muscle in greater detail, along with its relationship to the mitral leaflet. Bottom, left. A parasternal short axis recording illustrating the large (large arrow) posterior medial papillary muscle that lies to the right of center in the left ventricular cavity and a small, rudimentary (small arrow) anterolateral papillary muscle. Bottom, right. Mitral valve orifice during valve opening (large oblique arrow). Note that the orifice appears serrated, which is due to the restricted motion by the abnormal cords, is small, and is committed to the posterolateral papillary muscle. Mild stenosis was present in this case. LV = left ventricle; LA = left atrium; Ao = aorta.

throughout the remainder of the diastolic filling period. Atrial systole may cause the anterior leaflet to move anteriorly; however, as a rule, the movement is not sufficient to restore the orifice to a normal configuration. Although this deformity of the mitral valve orifice has not been related to the Austin Flint murmur, it does occur most prominently during the phase of diastole in which this murmur is recorded.[130–132] It also is consistent with intracardiac phonocardiographic evidence suggesting that the murmur arises from the left ventricular inflow tract.[133]

The abnormal pattern of mitral leaflet diastolic motion and the orifice configuration, although characteristic of aortic insufficiency, are not seen in all cases and, therefore, are not sensitive indicators of this disorder. This atypical orifice configuration, however, has not been observed in other disorders and, hence, appears to be fairly specific. A similar pattern can be seen in normal patients in the frame or frames immediately preceding valve closure; however, this pattern occurs late in the diastolic cycle and is associated with otherwise normal leaflet motion. As such, it should offer no confusion.

Mitral Insufficiency

Normal systolic closure of the mitral valve depends on the integrated function of the mitral leaflets, chordae tendineae, papillary muscles, and subjacent left ventricular myocardium. Failure of any of these components to function normally can result in improper leaflet closure and valvular regurgitation.[8,134]

Diagnosis

Mitral regurgitation characteristically produces a high velocity, turbulent, systolic flow disturbance (jet) in the left atrium, which can be detected by pulsed (Fig. 17–59), continuous wave, or color flow Doppler. The high peak velocity of the jet (i.e., 5 to 6 m/sec) is due to

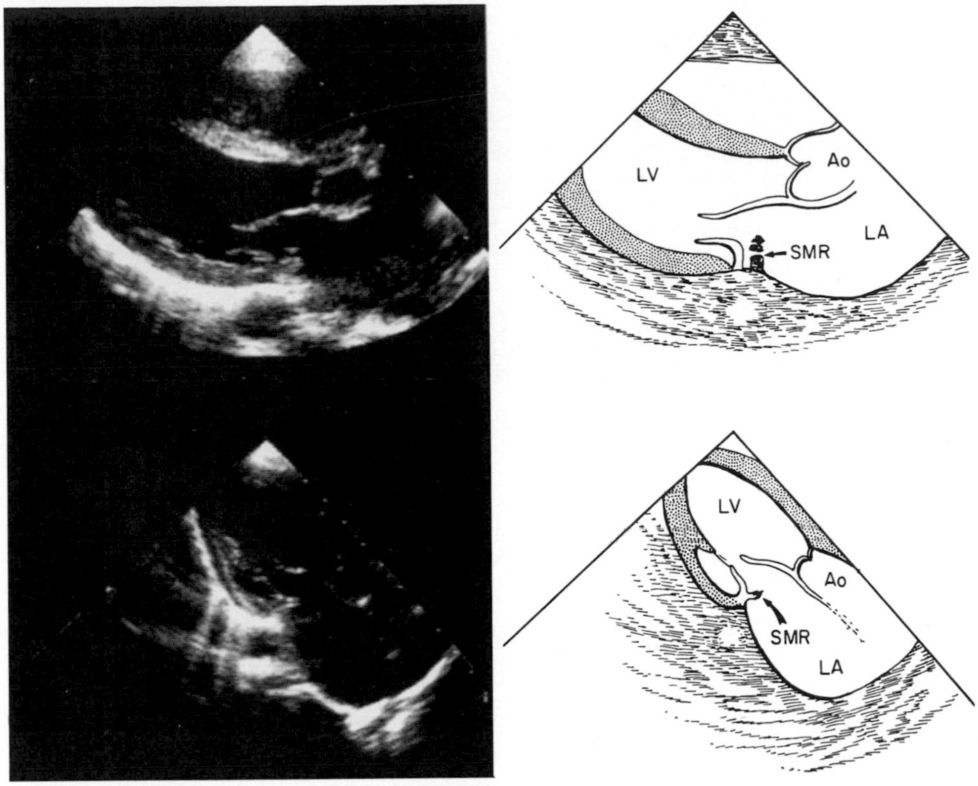

Fig. 17–56. Top. Parasternal long axis recording of a supravalvar mitral ring (SMR). The ring presents as a linear mass of echoes arising just superior to the atrioventricular groove and partially obstructing the mitral orifice. Bottom. Apical long axis recording from the same patient, illustrating the ring in a slightly different projection. In this view the encroachment of the ring on the orifice is more apparent. LV = left ventricle; Ao = aorta; LA = left atrium.

the large pressure difference between the left ventricle and left atrium during systole (Fig. 17–60). Jet turbulence produces a wide range of velocities, which broadens the frequency spectrum of the Doppler signal. Mitral regurgitant flow typically begins immediately after mitral closure and continues throughout most or all of systole. Regurgitation confined to late systole may also be seen in disorders such as mitral valve prolapse.

The pulsed Doppler technique has a sensitivity of at least 90% and a specificity of ≤95% for the detection of mitral regurgitation. This sensitivity is even greater when mild lesions are not considered.[135–142] Sensitivity is a function of the diligence with which the atrium is searched for systolic flow and the degree to which the regurgitant jet is eccentrically oriented or directed out of the scan plane and approaches 100% with careful search in multiple planes.[143] Color Doppler (Fig. 17–61) is slightly more sensitive than the pulsed or continuous wave technique because it is less likely to miss small or eccentrically positioned jets. In three series totaling 189 patients with angiographically documented regurgitation,[143–145] the color Doppler sensitivity averaged 94% (range, 86 to 100%), while the specificity in 97 patients with angiographically competent valves was 100%.[146] However, the obligatory regurgitation that is characteristic of the tilting disc-type mitral prosthesis can be routinely recorded from the esophagus when it is inapparent from the precordium, which indicates that even color Doppler is limited in its ability to detect discrete low volume jets.[147]

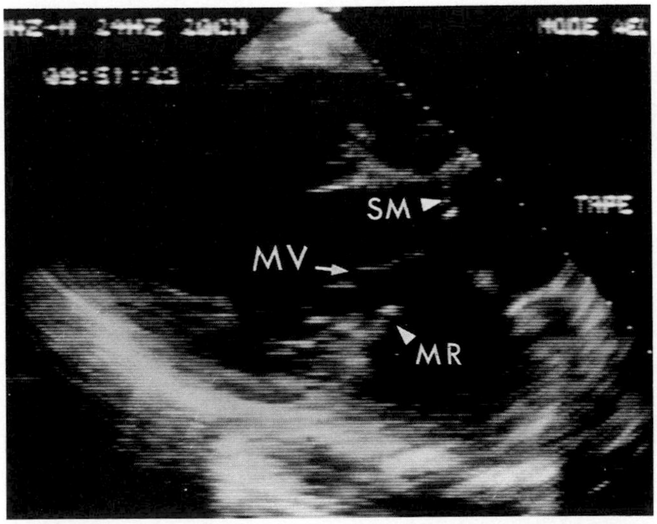

Fig. 17–57. A parasternal long axis recording from a patient with Shone's syndrome, illustrating a supravalvular mitral ring (MR) and a discrete subaortic membrane (SM). MV = mitral valve.

Regurgitation is more difficult to detect in patients with prosthetic mitral valves, which is due to the acoustic shadowing and reverberations produced by the prosthesis. This interference can be avoided by examining the valve from transducer locations that do not require the sound beam to pass through the valve to reach the jet (parasternal rather than apical). Because regurgitation can also occur between the sewing ring and the annulus (paravalvular), it is necessary to scan the entire circumference of the valve to diagnose or exclude a leak. Paravalvular leaks are identified by the left atrial origin of the jet outside the sewing ring or by recording an area

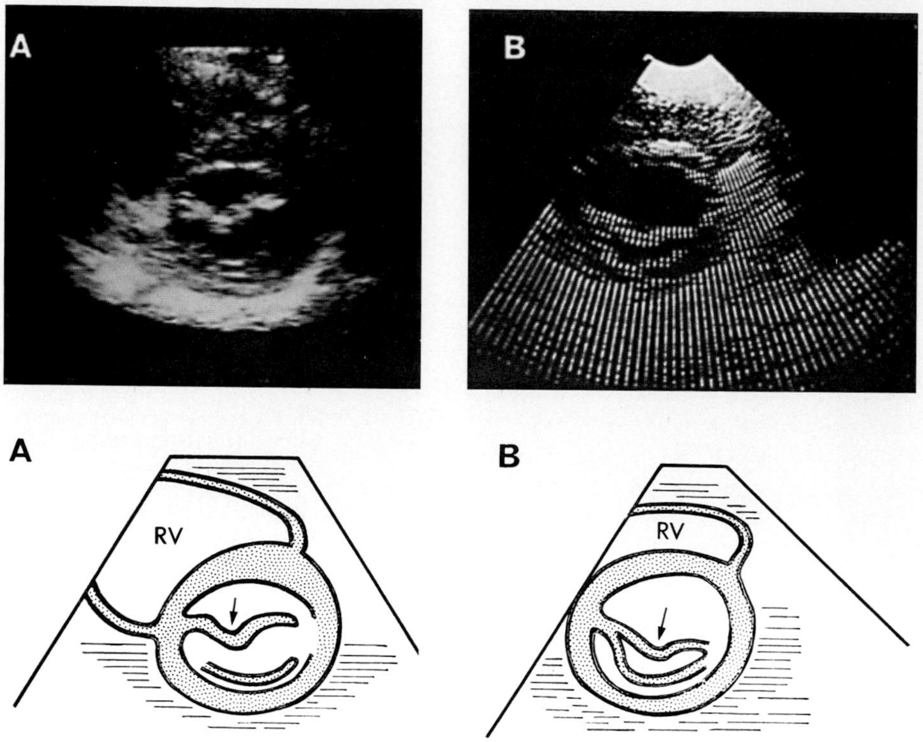

Fig. 17–58. Short-axis recordings of the mitral valve orifice in mid-diastole from two patients with aortic insufficiency. In each case, the midportion of the anterior mitral leaflet is inverted. The leaflet is, therefore, concave toward the left ventricular outflow tract in contrast to its normal convex orientation. The area of peak concavity is indicated in each case by the arrow in the accompanying diagram. RV = right ventricle.

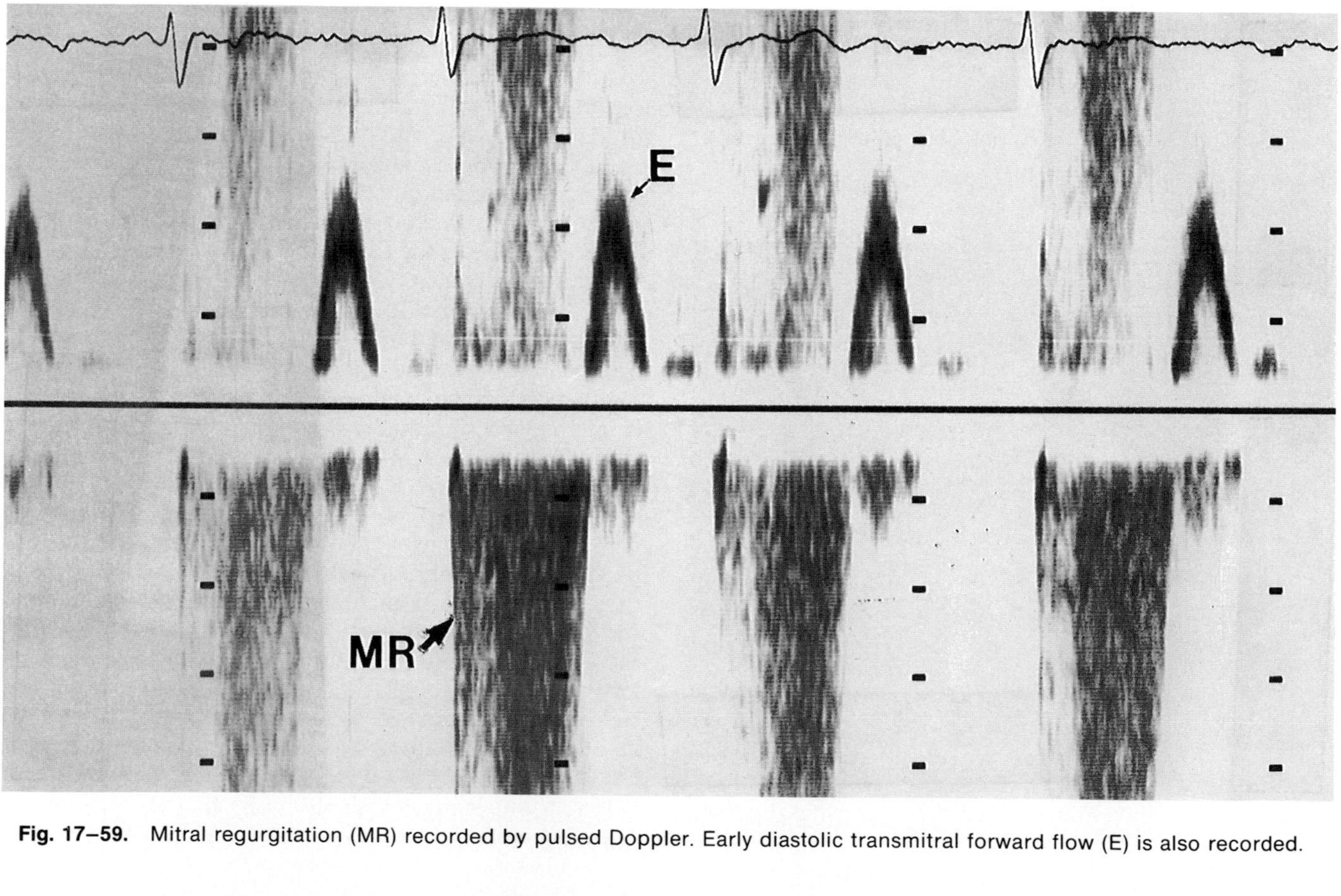

Fig. 17–59. Mitral regurgitation (MR) recorded by pulsed Doppler. Early diastolic transmitral forward flow (E) is also recorded.

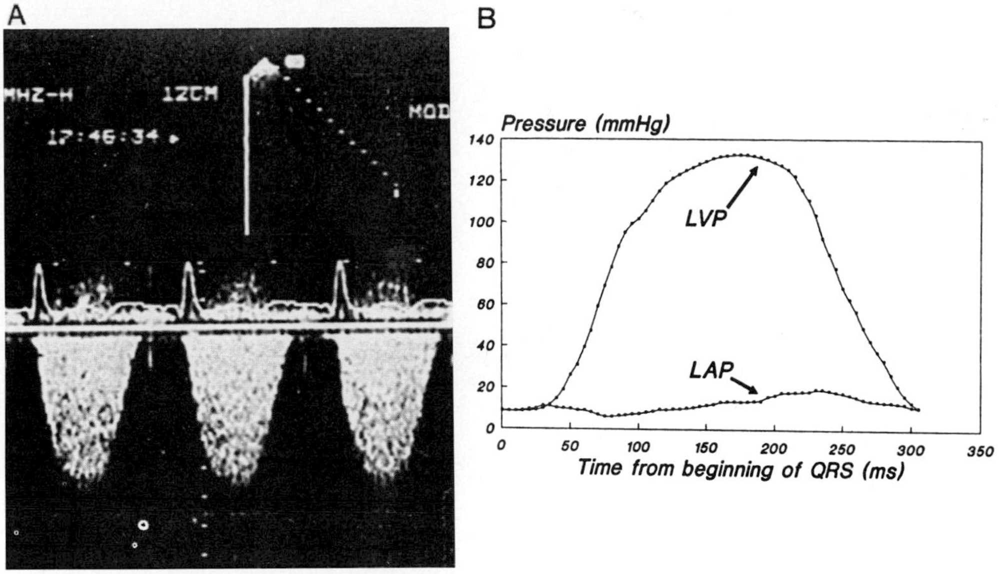

Fig. 17–60. A. Continuous wave Doppler recording of mitral regurgitation illustrating the typical high peak velocity. **B.** Simultaneous left atrial (LAP) and left ventricular (LVP) pressure recording illustrating the instantaneous transmitral pressure gradient.

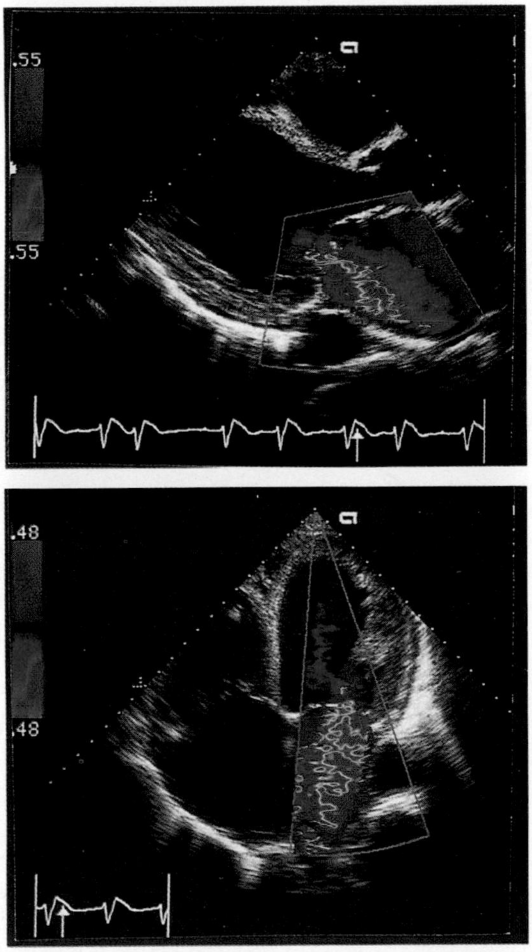

Fig. 17–61. Top. Parasternal long axis color Doppler recording of mitral regurgitant jet (blue-yellow mosaic color) in left atrium. Bottom. Apical four-chamber color Doppler recording of a large mitral regurgitant jet (blue-yellow mosaic color). (Reprinted with permission of Acuson, Inc.)

of flow acceleration in the left ventricle outside the valve struts. Prosthetic regurgitation is discussed in greater detail in Chapter 38.

It should be noted that trace or mild regurgitation detectable only in the immediate vicinity of the valve occurs frequently in otherwise normal individuals. In a review of 7000 patients in our laboratory, trace to mild regurgitation was observed in 19% of patients with otherwise normal hearts in this echocardiographic referral population, similar to findings of other groups for the atrioventricular and pulmonic valves.[148–150]

Backward displacement of blood into the left atrium that is due to closure of the valve leaflets can also be recorded. This motion of the blood pool immediately behind the valve is usually of short duration ($\leq$0.1 second) and does not reach velocities usually associated with regurgitant jets. Therefore, it is not considered to represent regurgitant flow.[151]

Estimation of Severity

The severity of regurgitation can be viewed in terms of both the regurgitant volume and the effects of that volume on the cardiovascular system. Methods for estimating regurgitant volume are discussed in this section. Assessment of the effects of regurgitation on left ventricular size and function (see Chapter 21), left atrial size (see Chapter 18), and pulmonary artery and right ventricular pressure (see Chapter 27) are discussed in the relevant chapters.

Regurgitant blood flow can be assessed qualitatively, semiquantitatively, or quantitatively. In assessing the accuracy of all of these methods, researchers have been hampered by the lack of an ideal gold standard and the limitations of angiographic semiquantitative grading systems as well as more quantitative approaches.[152–154]

Qualitative Assessment of Severity

Qualitative approaches for assessing the severity of mitral regurgitation generally derive from the older continuous wave Doppler literature and reflect the limited ability of this technique to estimate regurgitant volume more directly. Two such methods have been described. The first is based on the relationship of the regurgitant volume to signal strength. Because the amplitude of the reflected Doppler signal "generally" relates to the number of scatterers producing the signal, large regurgitant volumes will typically produce strong harsh signals, while small volumes (jets) will yield faint signals (Fig. 17–62). Because signal strength is also a function of attenuation, the regurgitant signal is usually compared to the forward flow signal, which arises from roughly the same depth and should represent all of the red cells passing through the valve. With this approach, mild lesions will produce weak reflections relative to the amplitude of the inflow signal; when the jet volume is larger, the signals should be more comparable.

The second qualitative approach is based on the pattern of the late systolic velocity profile. When the systolic left atrial pressure increase (V wave) is large, the left ventricle-left atrium gradient will fall rapidly, producing a "shoulder" on the downslope of the continuous wave velocity curve. Figure 17–63 illustrates this characteristic late systolic shoulder, which generally implies more severe regurgitation.

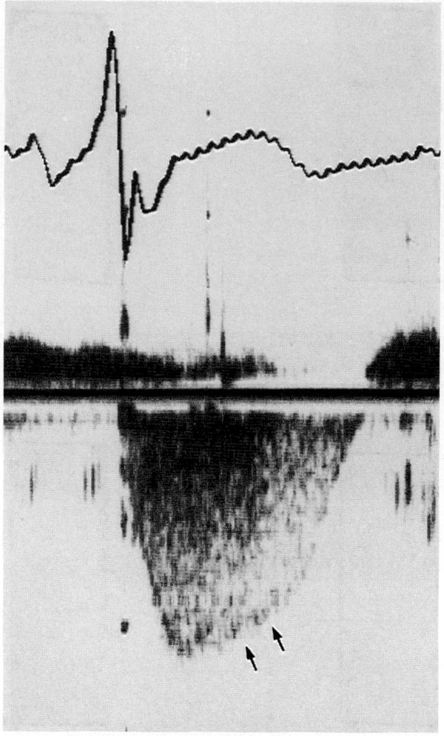

Fig. 17–63. Late systolic shoulder (arrows) seen on a continuous wave Doppler recording seen in patients with severe mitral regurgitation that is due to a rapid rise in left atrial pressure (V wave) and resulting decrease in the transvalvular gradient.

Semiquantitative Estimates of Severity Based on Regurgitant Jet Size

Jet Length and Area. The use of Doppler-derived measures of jet size to estimate severity of regurgitation is based on the assumption that the spatial distribution of regurgitant velocities reflects or at least is proportional to the regurgitant volume. To understand the relationship between Doppler measures of jet size and regurgitant volume, it is first necessary to appreciate the physical processes governing jet flow (this topic is discussed in detail in Chapter 12 but reviewed briefly here). Figure 17–64 illustrates the simple case of an axisymmetric jet discharging into an infinite reservoir. The regurgitant flow rate (Q_o) is the product of the orifice area (A_o) and the jet velocity at the orifice (u_o), so that $Q_o = A_o * u_o$. In the immediate vicinity of the orifice, flow is laminar, but the laminar core is rapidly eroded into by eddies with the result that flow becomes fully turbulent within 10 orifice diameters from the origin. As the jet progresses, fluid from the surrounding chamber is entrained into it, so that the jet volume increases with distance from the orifice. The total jet volume (regurgitant volume plus entrained volume) is determined both by the flow rate (Q_o) and the velocity at which the jet enters the receiving chamber (u_o): jet area and volume increase when either flow rate or driving pressure/velocity are increased, but the relationship is nonlinear.[155]

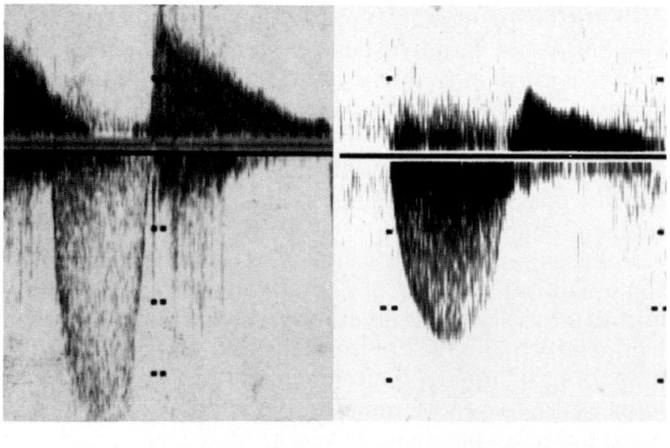

Fig. 17–62. Continuous wave Doppler recordings illustrating the difference between the weak signals arising from a small mitral regurgitant jet (left) compared to the stronger signals from a more important jet (right).

The behavior of any physical system is governed by the fact that mass, energy, and momentum either are constant or change in a predictable manner in response to an applied force. In a free jet, mass increases as fluid is entrained into the jet, and kinetic energy is dissipated as heat. Momentum, however, remains constant throughout the jet and is the best descriptor of its physical behavior. In fluid dynamics, the relevant quantity is momentum flux, which is the product of flow rate, velocity, and density (although the latter term is often omitted for incompressible flow). Conservation principles predict that the center-line velocity of the jet will decrease inversely with distance from the orifice (Fig. 17–64) and that the cross-sectional profiles will be Gaussian (bell-shaped) curves that become flatter and wider with distance (Fig. 17–65). For free jets, area is a direct function of momentum and, if driving pressure or orifice velocity remains constant, of flow rate. Jet volume is

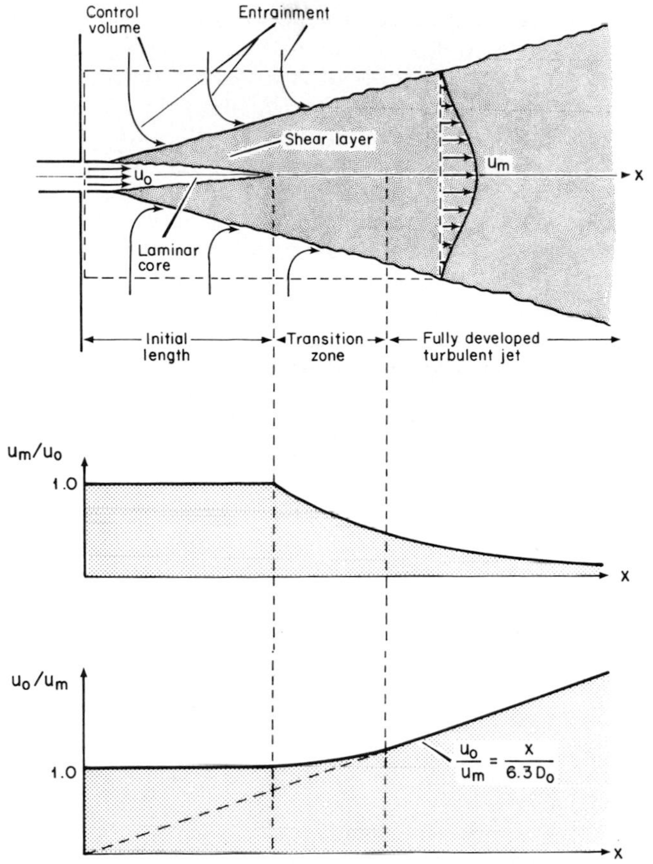

Fig. 17–64. Schematic of free turbulent jet. Top. Flow emerging from an orifice with an effectively uniform velocity u_o to form a core of laminar flow. Turbulent shear stresses caused by the interaction of moving and stagnant fluid generate eddies that propagate from the borders of the jet inward, thereby diminishing the laminar core and entraining fluid. Equations describing a fully developed turbulent jet apply five to eight orifice diameters or more beyond the origin. The *control volume,* indicated by the dashed lines, permits the equations for conservation of axial momentum to be formulated. The momentum of the jet at the orifice must equal that at any distance x along the axis in the absence of imposed pressure gradients. Therefore, as jet mass increases, its velocity must fall. Axial momentum relates to the component of jet velocity parallel to the jet axis. Entrainment, which occurs in a radial direction, does not alter axial momentum. u_o = centerline velocity at any axial distance x. Middle. Behavior of axial velocity u_m, normalized to orifice velocity u_m as a function of axial distance. Bottom. The reciprocal plot of u_o/u_m permits identification of the laminar core, transitional zones, and fully developed turbulent jet. D_o = orifice diameter. (From Cape E, et al.: A new method for noninvasive quantification of valvular regurgitation based on conservation of momentum. In vitro validation. Circulation 79: 1344, 1989. Reproduced by permission of the American Heart Association, Inc.)

affected by orifice size only in so far as this alters flow rate or driving pressure (e.g., for a constant flow rate, decreasing orifice size will increase driving pressure and hence jet size). Because all systems have a threshold below which velocity cannot be detected, free jets will appear to have a tear-drop shape, when sectioned in a plane including the long axis. Note that jet size is related to flow rate, not regurgitant volume, which is flow rate multiplied by the time during which flow occurs. Although these physical relationships hold for free axisymmetric jets, important mitral regurgitant jets are rarely free and are often nonsymmetric.

In practice, the limited size of the left atrium profoundly affects the jet area. Jets that reach the far wall of the atrium are truncated at that point and transfer their momentum to the wall (see Chapter 12). Thus, for constrained jets, an increase or decrease in chamber size will cause a directionally similar change in jet area. In addition, fully 30% of mitral regurgitant jets strike one of the walls of the atrium almost immediately after they exit from the regurgitant orifice.[156] Wall-impinging jets present a more complicated case because they can de-

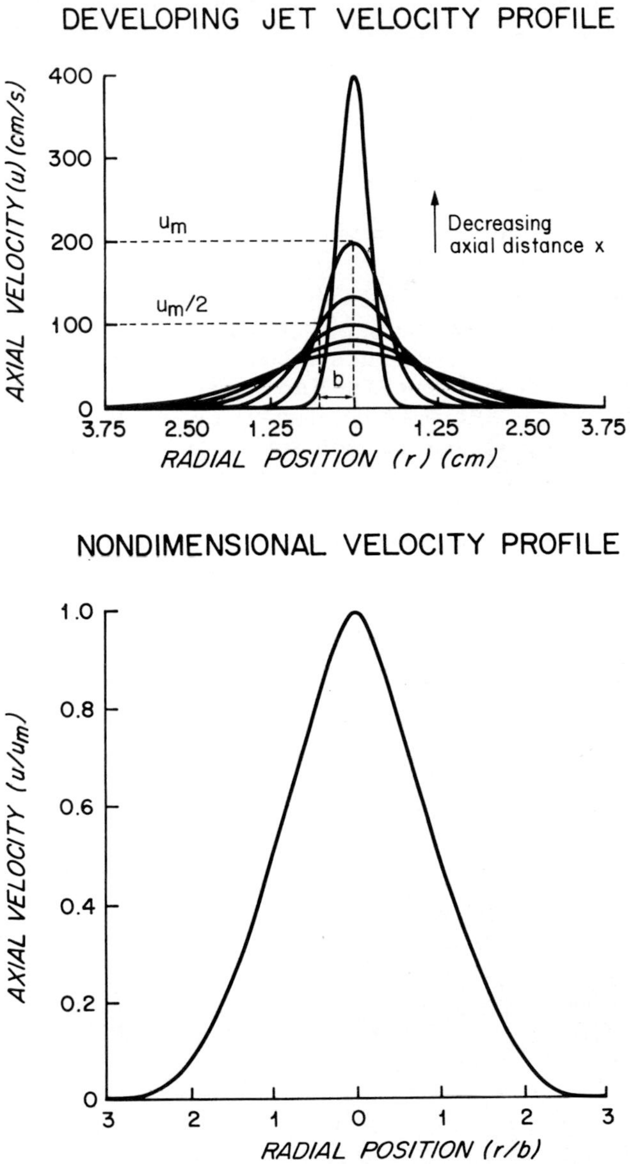

Fig. 17–65. Curves of dynamic similarity of the nondimensional (normalized) profiles of axial velocity across the face of a free turbulent jet. Curves at various axial levels coincide when velocity is expressed as a fraction of the centerline velocity u_m at that level and when radial distance r from the center of the jet is divided by b, the half-width of the jet, that is, the radius at which $u = u_m/2$. (From Cape E, et al.: A new method for noninvasive quantification of valvular regurgitation based on conservation of momentum. In vitro validation. Circulation 79:1344, 1989. Reproduced by permission of the American Heart Association, Inc.)

crease in size as a result of the transfer of momentum to the wall or simply can change shape as they spread out along the wall. Because these jets are not axisymmetric, they cannot be simply represented by their area in any one plane. In addition, their center-line velocity appears to increase relative to that of a free jet with the same momentum as a result of decreased entrainment and thus the transfer of momentum to a smaller mass.[157] As a result of this increase in center-line velocity, their displayed length will be greater than that of comparable free jets.

A variety of other factors can also influence the size and shape of both free and constrained mitral regurgitant jets. These include coflow, orifice shape, jet pulsatility, and turbulence. Flow into the left atrium from the pulmonary veins (coflow) can modify both jet size and shape independent of jet momentum. The effects of coflow will vary with its amount and the direction at which the opposing flow strikes the free jet—parameters that are virtually impossible to quantitate clinically. Orifice shape can also influence jet shape and symmetry. Although the orifices used to derive in vitro data are usually round or elliptic, many regurgitant orifices encountered clinically are irregular and, at least near the jet origin, may produce very irregular jets.[158] Far from the orifice, however, circular symmetry again prevails. Turbulent jets appear to lose approximately 90% of their eccentricity within 3 orifice diameters of the jet origin.[158]

Because regurgitant jets are pulsatile, they never reach a steady state. As a result, the rate of flow into the jet is constantly changing, and jet area at any point will have a varying relationship to regurgitant volume. Hence, any true measure of regurgitant volume must integrate flow rate over the duration of systole rather than assuming that flow rate at a particular point is reflective of regurgitant volume. Finally, regurgitant jets are almost always turbulent. As a result, their mean velocity can be predicted on the basis of fluid dynamics principles, but the instantaneous velocity may vary chaotically as much as 30% around this value, with consequent fluctuations in jet size and shape.

Given the many variables that influence jet size, simple binary measures such as jet length, jet area, or jet volume cannot be reasonably equated with regurgitant volume in vivo. Clinical studies that relate parameters of jet size to severity of regurgitation as assessed by semi-quantitative angiographic methods must therefore be considered as relationships based on empiric observation rather than clearly definable hydrodynamic principles.

Length

Pulsed Doppler Mapping. Jet length was first measured by pulsed Doppler and the spatial extent of the turbulent flow signal shown to coincide well with semiquantitative angiographic assessment of severity.[138] Pulsed Doppler determination of jet size—defined by the presence of abnormally directed systolic flow—requires systematic, point by point sampling of the entire area of the left atrium in multiple tomographic imaging planes (Fig. 17–66A).[135,141,159,160] In practice, the pulsed Doppler sample volume is initially positioned immediately behind the mitral leaflets and then is swept in gradually expanding radial arcs until the entire expanse of the atrium is mapped. Figure 17–66B illustrates one semiquantitative method for describing the extent of the jet. Flow limited to the region of leaflet apposition is designated *trace;* the atrium is then divided along its long axis into four equal segments so that flow that is

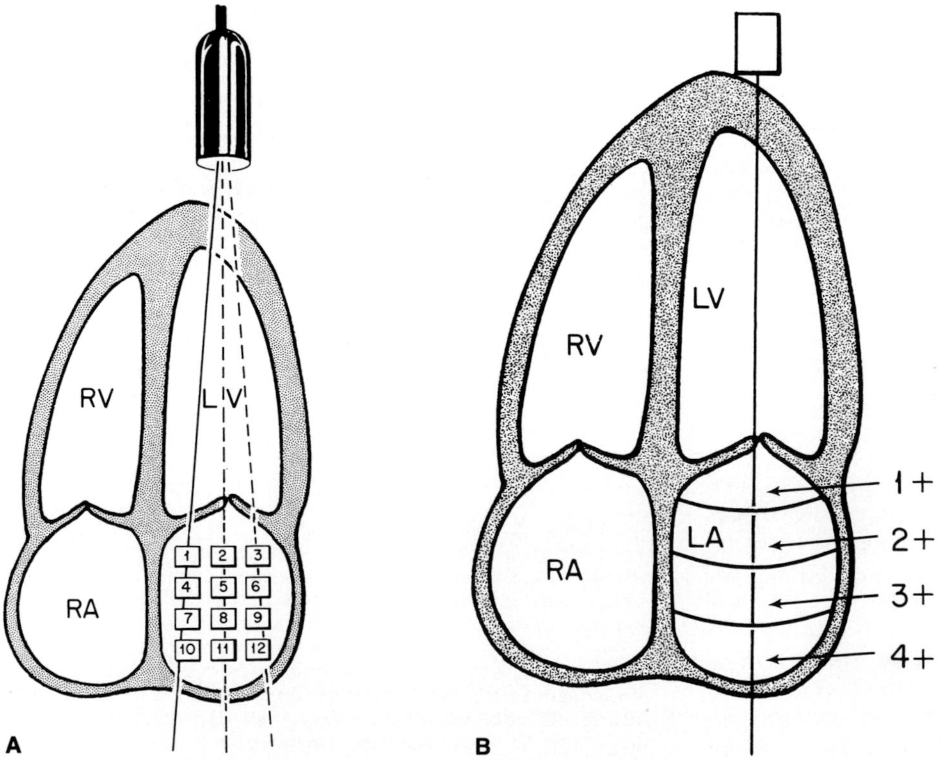

Fig. 17–66. A. The extensive mapping of the left atrium required to detect or exclude with confidence mitral regurgitant flow. **B.** One format for relating depth of jet penetration into the atrium to severity of regurgitation. RV = right ventricle; LV = left ventricle; RA = right atrium; LA = left atrium.

confined to the segment closest to the valve is designated 1+, and flow extending to the roof of the atrium, 4+. Results have been variable, with some authors reporting correlation coefficients of r = .87 to .88 when Doppler data are compared to the 1+ to 4+ angiographic grading system,[135,139] whereas others describe significant differences between only the mild and severe grades.[159]

This approach has several limitations: (1) Mapping the entire atrium is tedious and time-consuming and thus is poorly suited for routine clinical studies. (2) Because the grading system is indexed to atrial size, atrial dilation may result in a change in grade with no change in jet volume; this can result in a different grade for the same regurgitant volume between subjects or within the same subject if the atrial volume is changing rapidly (e.g., postballoon valvotomy). (3) Because the search for regurgitant flow is generally performed in an apical view, the returning Doppler signal may be weak as a result of tissue attentuation, causing severity to be underestimated—a deficiency that can be remedied by searching in a parasternal long axis view as well as using the maximum extent detected. Because of these inherent limitations of pulsed Doppler mapping, it has largely been replaced by color Doppler flow mapping.

Color Flow Mapping. Color flow mapping is a quicker and more accurate method for defining mitral regurgitant jet length. An early study suggested that absolute jet length (≤1.5 cm = 1+, mild; 1.5 to 2.9 cm, moderate; 3.0 to 4.4 cm, moderately severe; ≥4.5, severe) correlated reasonably well (r = .87) with the angiographically graded severity of regurgitation.[139] Subsequent data, however, indicate that jet area, or area corrected for left atrial size, yields an improved correlation with angiographic severity than simple length,[143] and as a result, length alone is not generally reported.

Area. The area of mitral regurgitant jets is usually determined from color Doppler flow images,[139] although pulsed Doppler mapping has been described.[151,161] Figure 17–67 is an example of a regurgitant jet displayed in blue-yellow, which originates from the center of the coapted mitral leaflets and spreads out in a tear-drop shape in the center of the atrial cavity. The color Doppler-defined jet area can be directly planimetered and reported in absolute terms or expressed as a percentage of the area of the atrium. To relate the color jet area to other measures of regurgitation, it is essential that the measured area accurately and consistently reflect the hydrodynamic area of the jet. To achieve this, it is necessary to understand the spatial, temporal, hydrodynamic, chamber, and instrument-related factors that can affect the measured area.

Spatial Considerations. The regurgitant jets encountered clinically are dynamic three-dimensional structures that can change size, shape, and direction during systole. Thus, some fixed parameter must be defined to represent the dynamic jet or jet area continuously recorded throughout systole and averaged or integrated over time. Generally, the maximum jet area occurring at any point during systole is taken as the representative value. Because the long axis of the jet will parallel the long axis of one of the standard imaging planes only by chance, it is necessary to scan the atrium in multiple views and to angle and rotate the scan plane until the long axis of the jet is located. Once the plane containing the greatest jet length/area is identified, the maximal jet area in any frame is planimetered. An alternative approach has been proposed in which jet area is averaged in two or three standard views (Fig. 17–68), but this method is more complicated and less theoretically accurate than simply locating and measuring the maximal jet area. Averaging in multiple planes is probably only necessary when jet direction changes during systole and the jet cannot be completely encompassed in any single plane.[162]

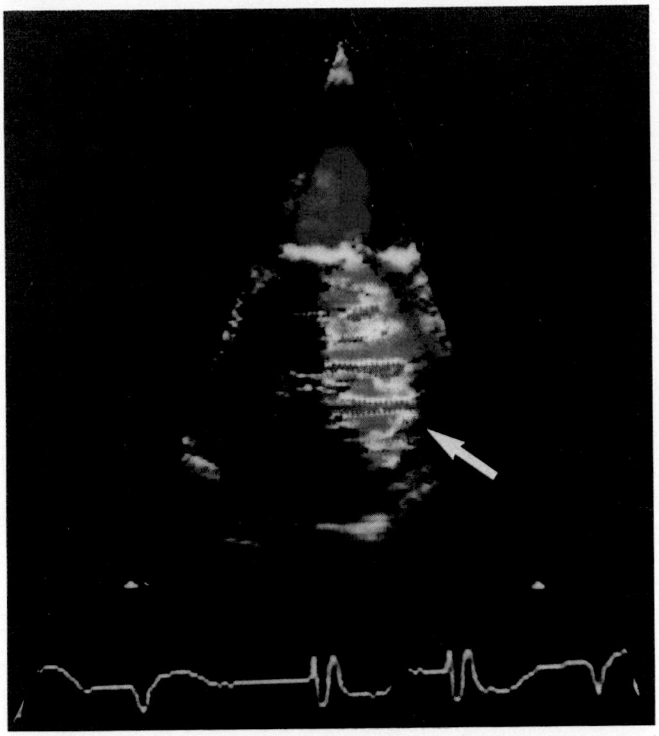

Fig. 17–67. Color Doppler flow recording of a moderately large mitral regurgitant jet obtained from the apical window. The jet (arrow) presents as a mosaic blue-yellow turbulent flow pattern that extends almost to the superior wall of the atrium.

Jet size often varies when recorded for different transducer locations (parasternal vs. apical) even when these recording planes pass through the long axis of the jet. These differences are a function of the varying interaction between sensitivity (apical > parasternal) and attenuation (apical > parasternal). Maximal jet area is recorded with roughly equal frequency in the apical and parasternal long axis views but much less frequently in the parasternal short axis view.[143,162] The largest recorded area should be used regardless of the plane in which it is recorded.

Jets that strike one of the lateral walls of the atrium spread out along the wall and lose their circular symmetry (Fig. 17–69). These jets are most commonly recorded at a plane parallel to their smaller minor dimension, and hence, jet area underestimates jet volume. When two or more jets are present, the area of each jet is recorded,

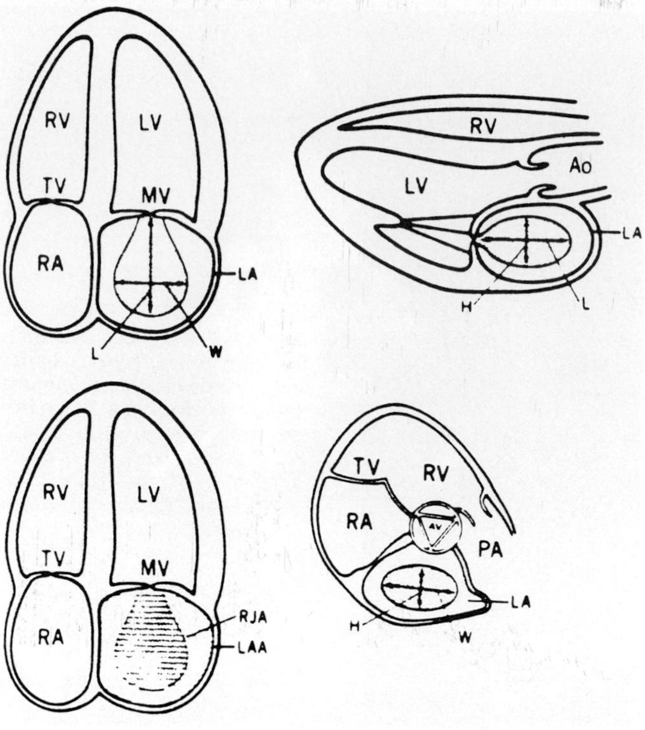

Fig. 17–68. The components of the regurgitant mitral jet conventionally measured from color Doppler recordings. Top, left. Apical four-chamber view. Top, right. Parasternal long-axis view. Bottom, left. Apical four-chamber view with measurements of regurgitant jet area (RJA) and left atrial area (LAA) indicated. Bottom, right. Parasternal short-axis view. RV = right ventricle; TV = tricuspid valve; RA = right atrium; LV = left ventricle; MV = mitral valve; L = maximum length of the regurgitant jet; W = maximum width of the regurgitant jet; H = maximum height of the regurgitant jet; LA = left atrium; Ao = aorta; AV = aortic valve. The shaded area represents the abnormal color Doppler signals produced by mitral regurgitation. (From Helmcke F, et al.: Color Doppler assessment of mitral regurgitation with orthogonal planes. Circulation 75:175, 1987. Reproduced by permission of the American Heart Association, Inc.)

and the total area of all jets is used in any calculation (Fig. 17–70).

It is common practice to average the maximal jet area from several cycles and to report a mean value.[162] This is appropriate if the maximal jet area is truly recorded in each frame to account for normal physiologic variability between cycles and to allow for variation in jet area resulting from turbulence. Averaging does not correct for frames in which the full extent of the jet is not imaged and will only reduce the appropriately recorded areas.

Temporal Considerations. Jet size (area and volume) varies with the instantaneously changing pressure gradient between the left ventricle and atrium during systole. The jet area usually reaches its peak in midsystole, when the gradient is maximal. For consistency, the maximal systolic (temporal) jet area is taken as the representative measure. Use of the maximal temporal jet area assumes that the peak flow rate has a fixed relationship to the regurgitant volume, which is the product of the instantaneous flow rate integrated over the time during which systole occurs. When the duration of systole changes (changing heart rate) or when regurgitant flow is confined to only a portion of systole (i.e., mitral valve prolapse), the relationship of the peak area to the regurgitant volume will vary. In patients with premature beats or atrial fibrillation, the color jet area may vary from cycle to cycle as the duration of systole and ventricular pressure change. In such cases, it is important to average the color jet area from a number of beats to attain a representative measure of regurgitant flow. Alternatively, jet area can be summed for the entire duration of systole, which is theoretically more correct but not routinely practical.

Hydrodynamic Effects. Changes in peak left ventricular pressure alter the maximal jet area, just as cyclic variation in driving pressure alters instantaneous systolic jet area. Changes in arterial blood pressure therefore can produce dramatic changes in jet area that are augmented if the change in pressure is associated with a corresponding increase in orifice area (i.e., flow rate).[163,164] Thus, comparative assessment of jet size must be performed under comparable hemodynamic conditions to be meaningful.

Chamber Effects. Jets that are large relative to atrial size are constrained by the superior atrial wall. Atrial enlargement will reduce the degree of constraint and increase jet area for a constant jet momentum. Thus, there is an interaction between the jet, which causes the chamber to enlarge, and the chamber, which constrains large jets. This raises the question whether jet area should be corrected for chamber area or presented as an absolute value. There are pros and cons to both approaches. Reporting absolute size fails to account for differences in patient size and the effects of chamber constraint. Con-

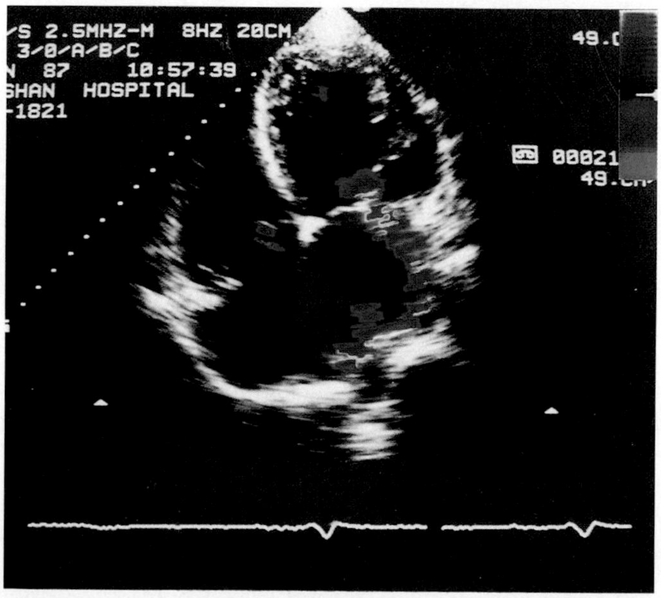

Fig. 17–69. Apical four-chamber view illustrating a mitral regurgitant jet in a blue-red mosaic color, which is directed toward and flows along the left atrial lateral wall. An area of proximal acceleration on the left atrial side of the regurgitant orifice is apparent. In this case the large jet flows completely along the atrial wall from the valve to the superior atrial margin and then curves backward in red toward the valve orifice. (Courtesy of Dr. Leng Jiang.)

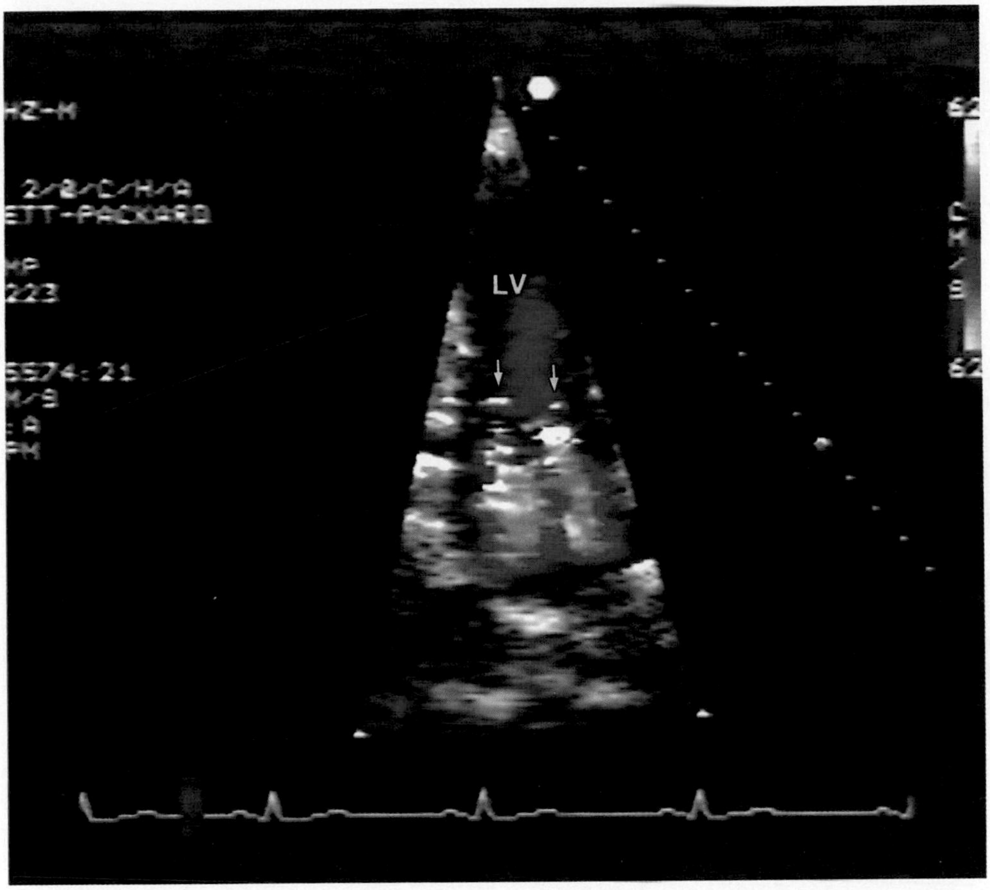

Fig. 17–70. Apical two-chamber recording from a patient with two distinct mitral regurgitant jets. Both jets arise from separate orifices, as indicated by discrete zones of proximal acceleration (arrows) on the left ventricular (LV) side of the mitral valve.

versely, while correction for atrial size is reasonable when patients of differing anatomic size are being compared (i.e., children and adults), it assumes a proportionality between jet size and chamber size that has no physiologic basis. For a receiving chamber that is large relative to jet size, absolute color flow area should relate to jet momentum, independent of chamber size. When the chamber is small relative to jet size, the jet will be constrained, but because jets are typically long and narrow, it is chamber length rather than area that determines the amount of constraint (i.e., a short, wide chamber will be more constraining than a long, narrow chamber of the same size). Further, for unconstrained jets, correction for chamber size can artifactually increase or decrease jet size despite the fact that momentum remains constant. Not surprisingly, conflicting data exist concerning the merits of correction for atrial size. In our experience, area-corrected values correlate slightly better with regurgitant volume and fraction than absolute values, but the difference is statistically insignificant.[156] Normalization by atrial size seems reasonable when patients of different size are compared and when constrained jets are analyzed. For unconstrained jets, absolute values are theoretically more appropriate.

Instrument Considerations. The displayed area of any jet is affected by several instrument variables including gain, pulse repetition frequency, transducer frequency, and beam pattern. Jet size varies directly with instrument gain, which determines the lowest velocities that are encoded in color and thus the margins of the jet at its periphery. To attain consistency, gain is usually increased until noise appears in the background and then reduced until the background noise just disappears.[143,162] In addition, the jet area is inversely related to the pulse repetition frequency and is directly related to the transducer frequency.[163] The display algorithm can also affect jet size. This limits comparisons of absolute data recorded on different instruments. Despite control and instrument variability, techniques have been derived to obtain reproducible data. When comparing patients, however, it is essential to use similar instrumentation and acquisition parameters.

Clinical Correlations. Several studies have shown that the maximal absolute jet area correlates reasonably well with angiographic grade of severity (r = .76 to .83) in adults.[143,162] In one study, a maximal jet area > 8 cm^2 predicted severe mitral regurgitation with a sensitivity of 82% and specificity of 94%, whereas a maximal jet area < 4 cm^2 predicted mild mitral regurgitation with a sensitivity and specificity of 85 and 75%, respectively. Patients with a maximal jet area between 4 and 8 cm^2 tended to have moderate mitral regurgitation by angiography, although these measures had little predictive value. In another study, roughly the same numeric values and relationship with angiographic severity were reported for maximal area.[143] Not surprisingly, neither jet dimensions nor area in any single plane correlate well with angiographic severity (presumably because the jet long axis does not fall consistently in any one plane).[143] Averaging values from multiple planes improves correlation, but this approach seems nothing more than an alternative method for converging on the largest area. Correction for atrial area has been reported to improve the correlation with semiquantitative angiographic severity; however, this is controversial,[162] and as discussed previously, the effects of such correction may differ with different populations. Figure 17–71 illustrates the relationship between maximal jet area corrected for left atrial area and angiographic severity. Jet areas less than 20% of left atrial area generally correspond to mild mitral regurgitation (predictive value 100%, sensitivity 94%, specificity 100%); areas between 20 and 40% with moderate regurgitation (predictive value 85%, sensitivity 94%, specificity 95%); and areas > 40% with severe regurgitation (predictive value 93%, sensitivity 93%, specificity 96%).

Jet area measurements have shown limited correlation with regurgitant volume (r = .55) and fraction (r = .62 to .78), respectively; however (as indicated later), this

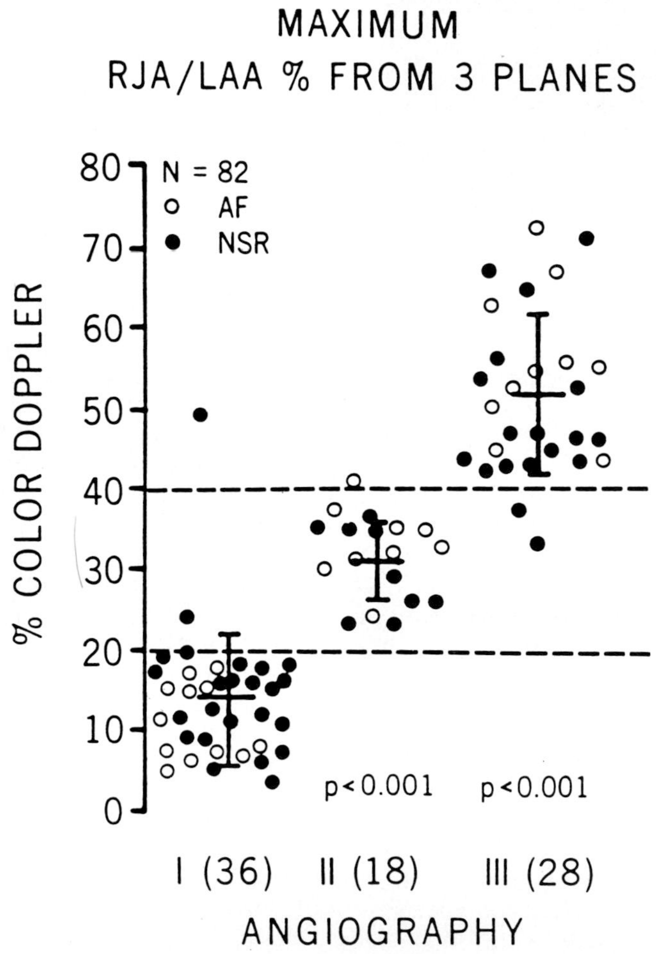

Fig. 17–71. Maximal color Doppler-defined mitral regurgitant jet area (RJA) normalized to left atrial area (LAA) in any plane compared with angiographic grade of severity. AF = atrial fibrillation; NSR = normal sinus rhythm. (From Helmcke F, et al.: Color Doppler assessment of mitral regurgitation with orthogonal planes. Circulation 75:175, 1987. Reproduced by permission of the American Heart Association, Inc.)

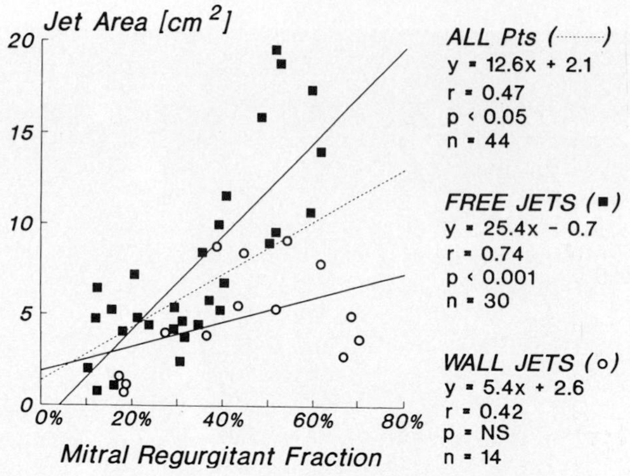

Fig. 17–72. Correlation between mitral regurgitant fraction and maximal jet area for all patients with free jets and those with wall jets. Dotted line shows linear regression relation for the combined group, whereas solid lines show regression lines for the two groups separately (with the more horizontal line reflecting wall jet data). (From Chen C, et al.: Impact of impinging wall jet on color Doppler quantification of mitral regurgitation. Circulation 84:712, 1991. Reproduced by permission of the American Heart Association, Inc.)

correlation improves when only free jets are considered. Jet area does not appear to be predictive of hemodynamic abnormalities including stroke volume or ventricular volumes, although a weak relationship with wedge pressure has been reported.[162]

On average, wall jets (see Fig. 17–69) are only 40% of the size of free jets with the same regurgitant fraction.[156] As indicated in Figure 17–72, there is a reasonable correlation between jet area and regurgitant fraction for free jets. For wall jets, however, the relationship is weak and, for the data presented in Figure 17–72, did not reach statistical significance. The smaller appearance of wall jets may simply be due to transfer of momentum to the wall very close to the valve, with the result that they become physically smaller jets. Distortion in the three-dimensional shape of the jet may also play an important role. In the vicinity of a solid boundary, jets preferentially spread laterally along the wall with their minor dimension perpendicular to the wall.[157,165,166] An imaging plane aligned perpendicular to the wall would therefore show only a very thin jet, whereas a plane that was parallel to the wall might show a broader-than-normal jet (Fig. 17–73). One of the difficulties in comparing data from available series is that the number of patients with wall jets in each study is unstated but will obviously influence the results.

Measurements of color Doppler jet areas are reproducible. In one study, measurements by two observers of jet area corrected for left atrial in the parasternal long axis view were highly correlative (r = .99).[143] In another, intraobserver and interobserver correlations for mitral jet area in the apical views were excellent (r = .97, SEE = .76 cm^2, and r = .93, SEE = 1.34 cm^2, respectively).[167]

Given the multiple factors that can affect the relationship of color jet size to regurgitant volume, these mea-

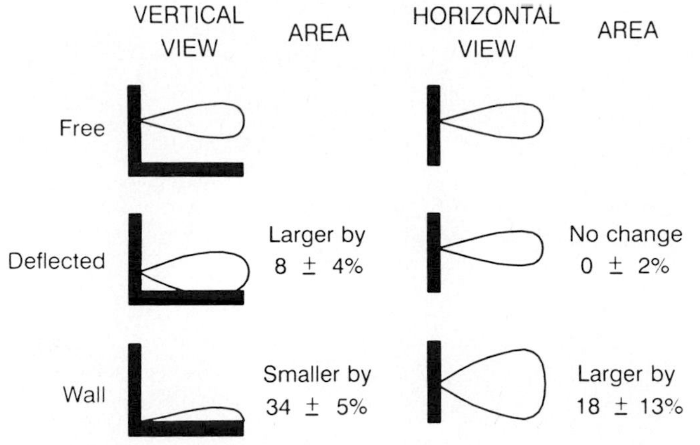

Fig. 17–73. Changes in the configuration of a free jet when it impinges against an adjacent wall. Data were obtained during an in vitro experiment in which the adjacent wall was gradually brought closer to the jet orifice. The vertical view corresponds to the usual color Doppler plane used to record the jet, while the horizontal view represents jet area in the orthogonal dimension. For free axisymmetric jets, the jet area viewed in any plane passing through the long axis of the jet is approximately equal. When the wall approaches the jet, a negative pressure zone develops between the jet and the wall, which attracts a portion of the flow, resulting in deflection of the jet toward the wall. When this occurs, the vertical jet area increases by a mean of 8%, although no change is evident in the horizontal view. When the jet actually flows completely along the wall, jet area is decreased by 34%, which is similar to the clinical observation of a 40% decrease in jet area relative to regurgitant volume. In contrast, the horizontal view increases by 18%; however, jet recording in this projection is very difficult to achieve in the clinical setting. (From Cape EG, Yoganathan AP, Weyman AE, Levine RA: Adjacent solid boundaries alter the size of regurgitant jets on Doppler color flow maps. J Am Coll Cardiol 17:1094, 1991. Reprinted with permission from the American College of Cardiology.)

sures are most useful in comparing the degree of regurgitation pre- and postintervention in the same patient. Figure 17–74 illustrates jet sizes in four patients following mitral valve repair, all of whom had severe regurgitation preoperatively. The assessment of jet size in such cases is extremely helpful in assessing the adequacy of repair.

Volume. Jet dimensions have been determined clinically by pulsed Doppler mapping of the atrium and volume calculated using the formula for the volume of a wedge (V = 0.5 × length × height × width).[168] Although good correlations were reported with semiquantitative angiographic grading, the complexity of the method is prohibitive. Calculation of the volume of free axisymmetric jets by color Doppler would appear to add complexity for little theoretic gain. Calculation of the volume of wall jets would be ideal but is practically limited by the inability of the technique to accurately record the short axis areas of jets whose predominant direction is perpendicular to the path of the scan plane.

In summary, color Doppler measurements of jet area and volume show a reasonable correlation with other clinical measures of regurgitant volume and fraction. These correlations are imperfect, as are the standards against which the Doppler measures are compared. Thus, the Doppler data, although ordered, can only be considered semiquantitative. However, it should yield results that are at least as good as other semiquantitative measures, particularly when patients with free jets are considered and physiologic and technical variables are controlled.

Difference in Flow Volume. The third, or quantitative approach calculates regurgitant volume as the difference between diastolic flow across the mitral valve (which is equal to forward plus regurgitant flow), and systolic flow across the aortic valve (which in the absence of aortic regurgitation is equal to forward flow). Forward flow across any valve can be measured by integrating the Doppler velocity over the period of antegrade flow and multiplying by the annular cross-sectional area. Such measurements have been validated in a variety of clinical and experimental settings.[169–176] In an experimental model, we have demonstrated that Doppler estimates of regurgitant volume correlate closely with electromagnetic flow probe measurements (r = .84), but more importantly, the standard error in these experiments was only 0.35 liter/min.[169] Clinical studies comparing Doppler with angiographic or scintigraphic measures of regurgitant volume or fraction have yielded comparable correlations (r = .82 to .91),[177,178] however, in these instances where there is no true gold standard and the meaning of such correlations is less clear. The limitations of this approach include (1) the requirement that aortic insufficiency be absent (although pulmonary flow can be substituted for aortic flow) and (2) the multiple steps involved in the calculations increasing the potential for error (e.g., regurgitant fractions of up to 20% can be calculated in the absence of any regurgitation).[178] Probably the greatest problem with this approach, however, lies not in the methodology but in the lack of familiarity with the results. Regurgitant volumes in milliliters per beat or liters per minute are simply not familiar terms, and in the current state of our knowledge they are difficult to relate to a particular severity of disease. Details of this method are discussed in Chapter 30.

Preliminary reports also indicate that severe regurgitation may also be differentiated from mild-to-moderate lesions by the presence of an increased left atrial emptying volume (maximum minus minimum volume exceeding 40 ml). However, this cumbersome technique, ideally requiring biplane cross-sectional area measurements, may not be routinely practical.[179,180]

Newer Approaches. Measurements of jet area or volume treat the jet velocities as a binary quantity (i.e., present or absent). Several approaches have been described that make use of all the velocity information in the jets and thus appropriately consider velocity as a continuous variable. Two general approaches to this type of analysis have been described. The first is based on conservation of momentum within the jet and the second on the conservation of mass in the acceleration zone proximal to the jet orifice.

Momentum Flux. Momentum is a conserved property within a free jet and hence should remain constant at all points along the jet until it strikes a wall. At the orifice, momentum is equal to flow times velocity ($Q_o \times u_o$ or $A_o \times v_o^2$). Thus, if momentum can be measured any-

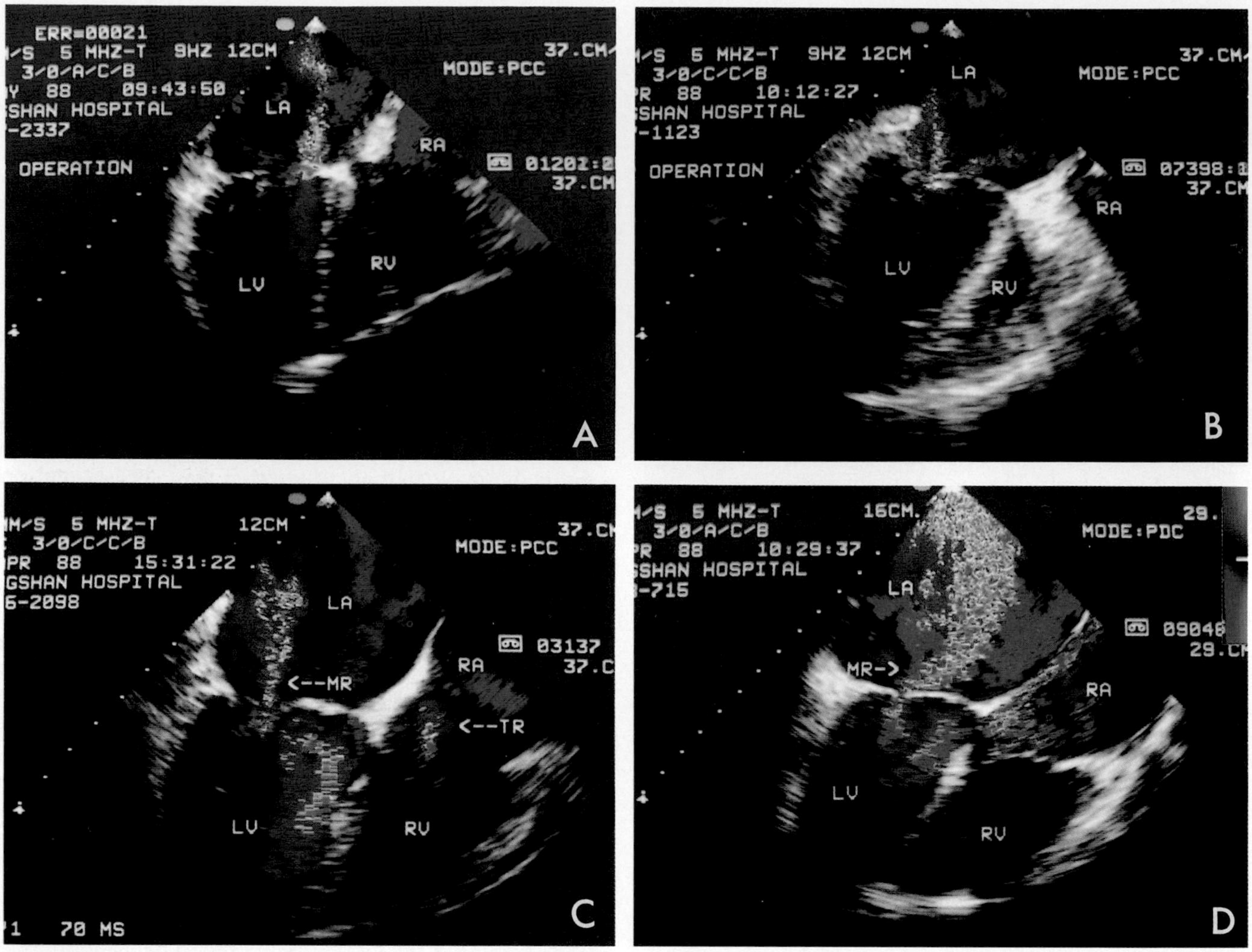

Fig. 17–74. Transesophageal echocardiographic recordings of the mitral regurgitant jet in four patients following mitral valve reconstruction. In each case, severe regurgitation was present before the valve repair. **A.** A small, slightly eccentric jet extends superiorly in the left atrial cavity. **B.** Three discrete but still small regurgitant jets are evident, indicating mild mitral regurgitation. **C.** A larger central jet, consistent with moderate regurgitation, is present. **D.** Severe regurgitation remains. LA = left atrium; RA = right atrium; LV = left ventricle; RV = right ventricle; MR = mitral regurgitation; TR = tricuspid regurgitation. (Courtesy of Dr. Leng Jiang.)

where within the jet from the color map and U_o obtained by continuous wave Doppler, then orifice flow rate can be calculated as M/U_o.

Momentum can be calculated directly from an axisymmetric color jet as

$$M = \int \pi r u^2 \, dr \qquad [17.25]$$

where r is the distance from the centerline of the jet, and the integration is carried from one side of the jet to the other at a given distance from the orifice. This principle can also be applied to the decay of the jet centerline velocity. Assuming a velocity decay inversely proportional to distance from the orifice, it can be shown that $Q_o = \pi \times u_m^2 \times x^2/K \times u_x$ where u is the centerline velocity at a distance x from the orifice, and K is an empirically derived constant (26.46).[181] Both of these approaches have been validated in vitro in steady flow models.[181,182] The centerline method has also been validated for pulsatile flow and in animal experiments. Two factors limit application for mitral regurgitant jets. First, to derive jet velocities from color flow maps, these velocities must be accurately reported. The Nyquist limit of color flow mapping devices is relatively low, and hence aliasing is routinely encountered in the center of mitral regurgitant jets. Although it may be possible to unwrap one alias, accuracy decreases beyond this point. Because momentum is related to velocity squared, the central velocities that contribute most to this calculation are least accurately represented. The second factor is chamber constraint. When using the centerline method, it is necessary to plot a velocity decay curve for the nonlaminar portion of the jet. This requires that the high core velocities be recorded at measurable distances from the orifice and that the jet expand free of chamber constraint. Although center line velocities might be measured using a high pulse repetition frequency Doppler, the distance over which velocities can decay in the atrium is so limited that measurement may be impractical. Thus, momentum principles will likely be applied to lower velocity, right-sided jets, until instrumentation advances to a point where nonaliased left-sided jet velocities can be accurately recorded.

For nonsymmetric or wall jets, the application of momentum principles is more complex. However, the distribution of velocities within these jets should be predictable, and hence, should the method prove reliable for free jets, extension to wall jets is not impossible.

Proximal Velocity Acceleration. Proximal to the regurgitant orifice, blood velocity increases in a predictable fashion, with the isovelocity contours forming concentric hemispheric shells. The flow passing through each of these shells is identical to the flow that finally passes through the orifice. Thus, knowing the velocity v at a distance r from the orifice, orifice flow rate can be calculated as $Q_o = 2\pi r^2 v$. The easiest method for determining velocity and radius is to use the first point where the color display aliases, generally, a sharp dividing line at which flow, by definition, is moving at the aliasing velocity.[183] In vitro studies further suggest that by aligning a color M-mode coaxial with the color jet it is possible to measure velocity and radius throughout the pulsatile flow cycle to provide an accurate estimate of the total regurgitant stroke volume.[184] Recent clinical studies also report good correlations between peak regurgitant flow rate measured by the proximal acceleration method and both semiquantitative angiographic measures of severity[184a] and Doppler derived regurgitant volumes.[184b]

In summary, techniques for quantitating the severity of mitral regurgitation are currently in flux. The semiquantitative Doppler flow-mapping technique has the advantage of simplicity but is affected by a variety of factors that demand further investigation. At present, we feel justified in using the flow map (color display or pulsed Doppler search) to describe regurgitation as trace, 1+ to 4+, as outlined previously, bearing in mind the need to search for the maximum jet extent in multiple planes. When wall jets are encountered, we increase assessed severity by one grade. When truly quantitative measures of regurgitant volume are necessary, we rely on the Doppler-derived difference between forward and regurgitant volumes. Newer methods based on conservation of mass and momentum are promising, but only the proximal acceleration method is currently ready for clinical application.

Diastolic Mitral Regurgitation

Although mitral regurgitation is generally thought of as occurring during systole, retrograde blood flow from the left ventricle to the left atrium can also be recorded during diastole.[185–188] Diastolic mitral regurgitation is due to a positive left ventricular-to-left atrial pressure gradient and is most commonly observed in patients with varying degrees of atrioventricular (AV) block.[185] It can also be recorded in atrial flutter, atrial fibrillation with effective mechanical contraction, severe aortic regurgitation, and disorders associated with reduced ventricular distensibility.[187] The positive gradient (left ventricular to left atrial) generally develops, because atrial relaxation is not followed by a properly timed ventricular contraction allowing left atrial pressure to fall below the left ventricular pressure, which has been increased by the preceding atrial contraction. In experimental studies of first- and second-degree heart block, these reverse gradients (3.7 ± 1.1 mm Hg in first-degree AV block and 3.2 ± 1.5 mm Hg in second-degree AV block) were found to be as large as the maximal forward transmitral gradients in early diastole and approximately 1.5 to 2.3 mm Hg larger than the maximal forward gradients associated with atrial contraction.[189] The delay between the onset of the P wave and the onset of diastolic regurgitation is reported to vary from 0.24 to 0.34 seconds. As illustrated in Figure 17–75, the diastolic velocity acceler-

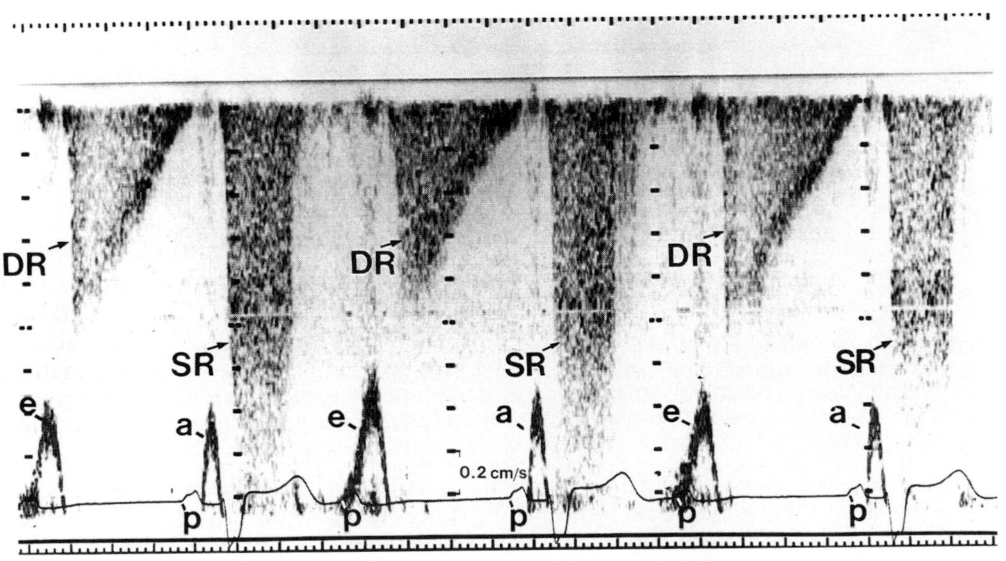

Fig. 17–75. Doppler recording from a patient with second-degree heart block and both systolic and diastolic mitral regurgitation. The systolic regurgitation (SR) begins immediately after the onset of the QRS complex of the electrocardiogram and terminates just before the end of the T wave. Following the T wave, there is a blocked atrial contraction (p) with associated antegrade flow through the mitral valve (e). Atrial relaxation is accompanied by a diastolic regurgitant jet (DR) with a peak velocity of roughly 1 cm/sec, which is higher than the velocity of forward flow wave (e). The diastolic regurgitant jet velocity then decays as the retrograde gradient diminishes. This is followed by a second, conducted P wave, which again restores antegrade transmitral flow (a).

ates rapidly as the atrium relaxes and then gradually diminishes as the atrial pressure rises as a result of continued inflow from the pulmonary veins. In second-degree AV block, the velocity and duration of diastolic regurgitation vary, with smaller reverse gradients and flow velocities being recorded in cycles with short Q-P intervals (Fig. 17–76). Ventricular systole abruptly interrupts diastolic regurgitation.

The fact that regurgitation occurs implies that the mitral valve is not fully closed by the developed gradient. This in turn implies either that the valve is intrinsically abnormal or that the chordal tension holding the valve open is greater than the small pressure gradient seeking to force it closed. Both mechanisms appear to be operative because diastolic regurgitation commonly occurs in patients with systolic regurgitation but may also be present when the valve is competent during systole. Because the developed gradient is small, the retrograde velocity is likewise low (≤ 1.5 m/sec). Although the velocity of retrograde flow can be greater than that of antegrade diastolic filling, the volume is much less because the mitral orifice is smaller and is of no apparent hemodynamic significance. Diastolic regurgitation is generally not observed in patients with prosthetic mitral valves.[186] On occasion, however, disc valves may be positioned such that the disc deflects an aortic regurgitant flow into the left atrium. Figure 17–77 is a recording from a patient with a disc valve in the mitral position in which the disc opens into the left ventricular outflow tract. During diastole (Fig. 17–77B), the open disc directs a regurgitant aortic jet into the left atrium, leading to high velocity pandiastolic mitral regurgitation.

Specific Abnormalities Associated With Mitral Regurgitation

Although Doppler echocardiography is a highly sensitive and specific method for detecting mitral regurgitation, by itself, it provides little insight into the cause of the leakage. Fortunately, two-dimensional imaging reveals many abnormal leaflet closure patterns that are highly associated with valvular insufficiency and is of unique value in determining the cause of the valvular abnormality in patients with recognized valvular leakage.[190] Patterns of abnormal systolic leaflet closure or motion have been described in patients with both congenital and acquired forms of valvular dysfunction.

Congenital

A variety of congenital anomalies of the mitral valve predispose to mitral regurgitation. These include cleft anterior or posterior mitral leaflet, deficiency of tissue of the anterior leaflet, double orifice mitral valve, mitral arcade, anomalous origin of the mitral chordae, and apical displacement of the left-sided valve with or without ventricular inversion (the latter situation representing Ebstein's anomaly of the mitral valve).[191]

Cleft Mitral Valve

Clefts in the anterior mitral leaflet occur in association with other defects in the endocardial cushions or as isolated lesions.[192] The anterior leaflet may be partially or completely cleft. Accessory chordae, not found in a normal heart, characteristically arise from the interventric-

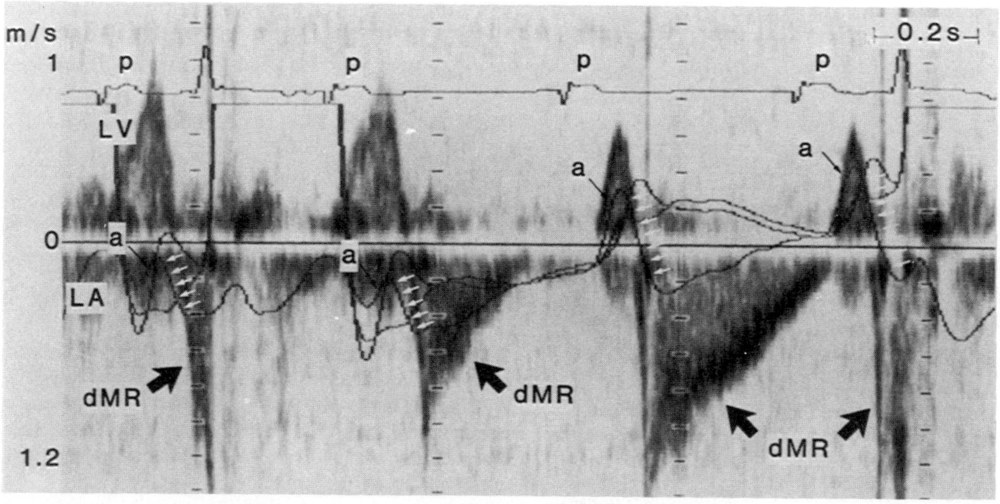

Fig. 17–76. Pulsed Doppler mitral flow velocity recording from the mitral annulus showing the relation of velocity and duration of diastolic mitral regurgitation to the reverse transmitral pressure gradient. Simultaneous left atrial and left ventricular pressures from both the apex and the base are recorded. First- and second-degree atrioventricular (A-V) block are present. The P waves are labeled; the first and fourth beats are conducted, and the second and third beats are blocked. Diastolic regurgitation is most apparent in the beats showing complete A-V block but can also be observed briefly during beats showing first-degree heart block. The left atrial pressure X-descent (small white arrows) shows that the larger reverse pressure gradients occur during the beats with the largest decrease in atrial pressure during atrial relaxation. The largest increase in atrial pressure with contraction (a, small black arrows) also occurs during these beats. dMR = diastolic mitral regurgitation; p = P wave of electrocardiogram; a = Doppler "a" wave. LA = left atrial pressure; LV = left ventricular pressure. (From Appleton CP, et al.: Diastolic mitral regurgitation with atrioventricular conduction abnormalities: relation of mitral flow velocity to transmitral pressure gradients in conscious dogs. J Am Coll Cardiol 18:843, 1991. Reprinted with permission from the American College of Cardiology.)

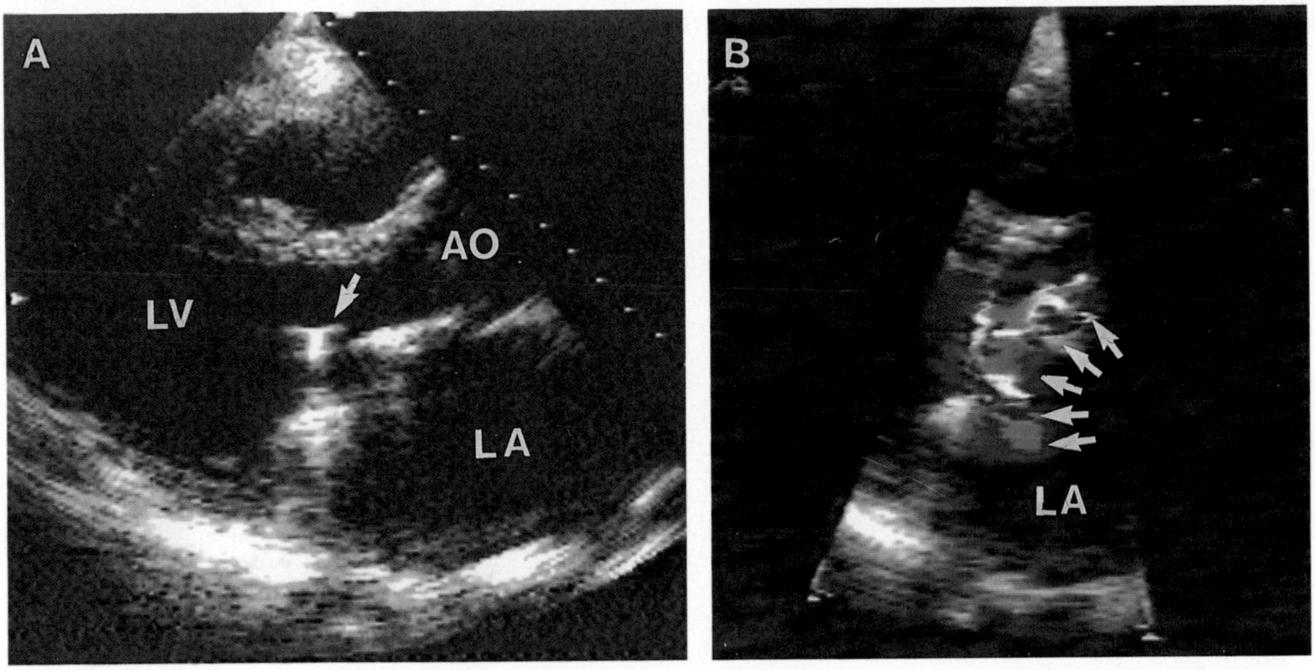

Fig. 17–77. A. Parasternal long axis recording of a disc valve in the mitral position in which the disc (arrow) opens at a right angle to the long axis of the left ventricular outflow tract. **B.** A color flow recording illustrating an aortic regurgitant jet (arrows), which strikes the open disc and is deflected directly into the left atrium. AO = aorta; LV = left ventricle; LA = left atrium; arrow points to the jet entering the left atrial cavity.

ular septum and attach to the margins of the cleft. These chordae tend to hold the leaflets anteriorly in the outflow tract during systole and frequently provide inadequate leaflet support. Valvular insufficiency results. Although the major functional abnormality occurs during systole, the cleft valves are most easily detected during diastole.

Figure 17–78 is an example of a cleft mitral valve. The cleft is best visualized in short axis at the free edges of the leaflet and is characterized by a separation between the medial and lateral leaflet halves, which move independently.[193] During diastole (Fig. 17–78B), disturbed flow through the cleft may also highlight the abnormality. Systolic regurgitant jets also originate from the cleft (Fig. 17–78C) and are generally directed posteriorly into the atrium. The cleft mitral valve may be confused with an anatomic tricuspid valve. They can be differentiated,

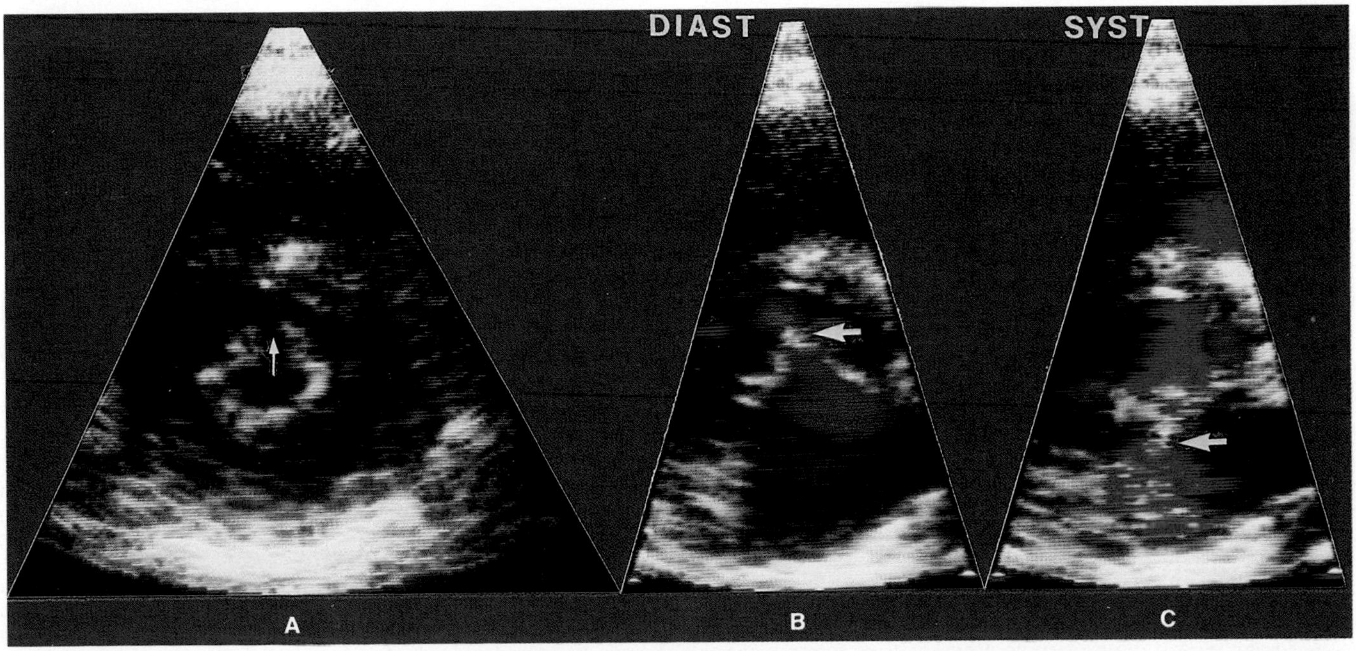

Fig. 17–78. A. Parasternal short axis recording illustrating a cleft (arrow) anterior mitral leaflet. **B.** Diastolic recording showing flow in red passing through the cleft (arrow) and the anterior mitral valve. **C.** Systolic recording illustrating a mitral regurgitant jet (arrow) passing through the cleft into the left atrium.

however, by the appearance of only two points of leaflet attachment in the cleft mitral valve.

At the base of the valve, anterior displacement of the medial insertion point may also be noted, and in the long axis, the leaflets are frequently thickened.

Double-Orifice Mitral Valve

Double-orifice mitral valve is a relatively rare congenital disorder of the mitral valve.[194–196] Three types of double-orifice valve have been described: (1) The *complete bridge* type in which two separate, complete, funnel-shaped orifices extend from the leaflet edges to the valve ring; (2) the *incomplete bridge* type in which there is a connection between the anterior and posterior leaflets only at the leaflet edge; and (3) the *hole* type in which a single orifice is present at the leaflet tips with a second smaller hole in a lateral commissure oriented at a roughly right angle to the main orifice.[197–199] The papillary muscles are usually normally oriented in this condition. The chordae from the lateral (anterior) orifice typically attach only to the anterolateral papillary, while the chordae of the medial (posterior) orifice attach to the posteromedial papillary muscle.

The double-orifice mitral valve is usually recognized echocardiographically during short axis scanning of the mitral valve orifice. Once the anomaly is recognized, sweeping the scan plane from the valve orifice to the annulus permits the extent of orifice separation to be defined.[199,200] Figures 17–79 and 17–80 are two examples of double-orifice mitral valves. In each case, the parasternal long axis appearance of the closed valve is normal, while in short axis, two orifices of different size are recorded. In Figure 17–80, the two discrete orifices along with the extent of separation can also be recognized in the apical two-chamber view. The four-chamber view may be particularly useful in patients with hole-type defects because in these cases the two orifices do not lie in the same plane and hence cannot be recorded in short axis. Note, however, that in patients with severe aortic regurgitation, the anterior mitral leaflet is frequently concave upward during diastole, and a plane originating at the apex can transect the medial and lateral portions of the orifice but not the center, giving the appearance of a double-orifice valve.

A double-orifice mitral valve can also be created iatrogenically during balloon valvuloplasty if the guide wire passes through a weak portion of the medial or lateral commissure, outside an area of more dense commissural adhesion. Balloon inflation can then create a secondary orifice while leaving the more dense central area of leaflet fusion intact. Figure 17–81 is an example of such a valve.

Congenital double-orifice mitral valve may be seen in association with AV canal defects, coarctation of the aorta, or hypoplastic left heart syndrome or may present as an isolated lesion. These valves may be stenotic or regurgitant or in some cases function normally. When

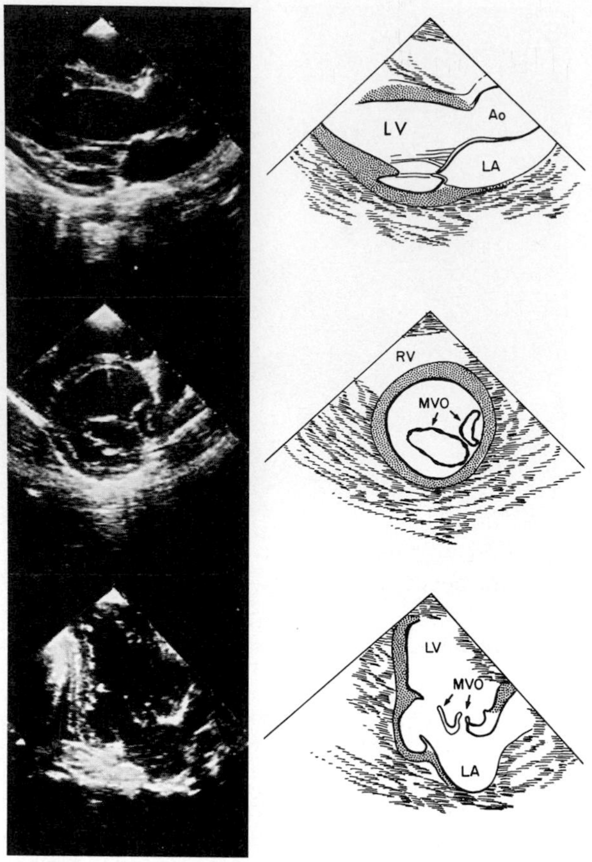

Fig. 17–80. Top. Parasternal long-axis systolic recording from a second patient with a double orifice mitral valve. Again, the valve appears normal in its closed position. Middle. Short-axis recording illustrating the two uneven sides of valve orifices. Bottom. Apical two-chamber view illustrating the two separate orifices as well as the separation extending from the annulus to the free edges of the valve. LA = left atrium; LV = left ventricle; Ao = aorta; RV = right ventricle; MVO = mitral valve orifice.

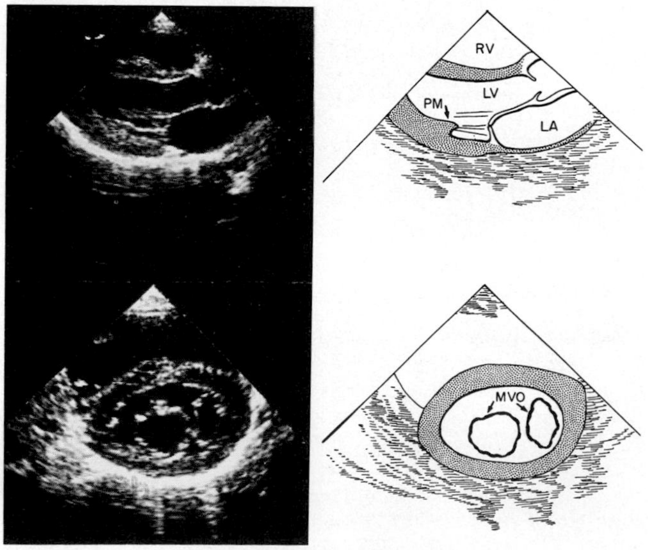

Fig. 17–79. Top. Parasternal long axis recording from a patient with a double orifice mitral valve. In this view the valve appears normal when closed during systole. Bottom. A parasternal short axis recording illustrating two separate mitral valve orifices (MVO). RV = right ventricle; LV = left ventricle; LA = left atrium; PM = papillary muscles.

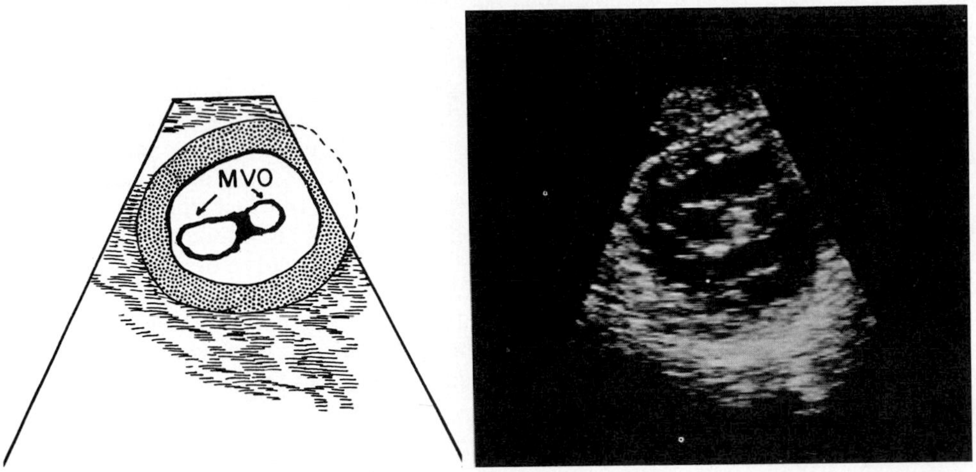

Fig. 17–81. Parasternal short axis recording from a patient with an iatrogenically created double orifice mitral valve during balloon mitral valvotomy. In this example, there is a dense area of calcified adhesion between the medial, native orifice and the lateral, iatrogenically created orifice. During a second procedure, a complete separation of the leaflets was achieved. MVO = mitral valve orifice.

associated with AV canal defects, their recognition is important because they may complicate surgical repair.

Mitral Arcade

Mitral arcade is a developmental abnormality of the mitral valve characterized by a bridge of fibrous tissue between the tips of the papillary muscles that directly attaches to the anterior mitral leaflet in some areas, while in others poorly differentiated chordae extend between the leaflet and the bridge. Somewhat more differentiated chordae generally extend between the papillary muscles and the posterior mitral leaflet. Development of the mitral commissures is rudimentary, and the commissures themselves may not be clearly identifiable.[201] The arcade typically prevents complete closure of the mitral valve and leads to valvular regurgitation. Incomplete separation at the commissures may partially obstruct mitral inflow.

Figure 17–82 is an example from a patient with a variant of mitral arcade. In the parasternal long axis view, there is a thick band of fibrous tissue incorporated into the anterior mitral leaflet. The leaflet itself is shortened, and the leaflet tip fails to reach that of the posterior leaflet. Medial angulation reveals an elongated, anteriorly displaced papillary muscle that is connected by short thickened chordae to the fibrous mass. Other short chordae attach to the free edge and body of the rudimentary leaflet. Longer chords extend to the posterior leaflet, which is larger than the anterior leaflet and domes slightly when fully opened. On short axis (Fig. 17–83), the fibrous mass can be seen to extend between the papillary muscle tips, and although the leaflet tips are mobile, the anterior and posterior portions of the valve appear continuous without evidence of commissural separation. Apical scanning demonstrates large elongated papillary muscles whose tips extend to almost directly insert into the mitral leaflets.

Acquired Lesions Associated With Mitral Regurgitation

Acquired lesions associated with mitral insufficiency include rheumatic mitral insufficiency, mitral valve prolapse, ruptured chordae tendineae and flail mitral leaflets, and papillary muscle dysfunction. Structural changes in the valve leaflets and supporting apparatus have also been noted in other disorders that may be associated with mitral insufficiency, such as bacterial endocarditis, mitral annular calcification, and left atrial myxoma.

Rheumatic Mitral Regurgitation

Rheumatic mitral regurgitation is characterized pathologically by loss of leaflet tissue from fibrosis and con-

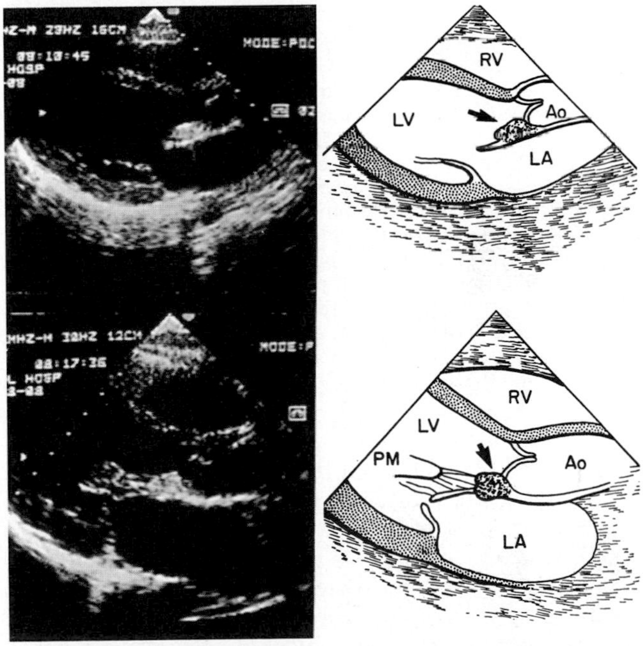

Fig. 17–82. Parasternal long axis recording from a patient with mitral arcade. Top. A dense band of fibrous tissue (arrow) is attached to a rudimentary anterior mitral leaflet. The more normal posterior leaflet is fixed, with restriction of diastolic opening motion. Bottom. This recording, after slight medial transducer angulation, illustrates the thickened chordae that bridge a short separation between the large elongated papillary muscle and the fibrous band (arrow), which is incorporated into the anterior mitral leaflet. RV = right ventricle; LV = left ventricle; Ao = aorta; LA = left atrium; PM = papillary muscle.

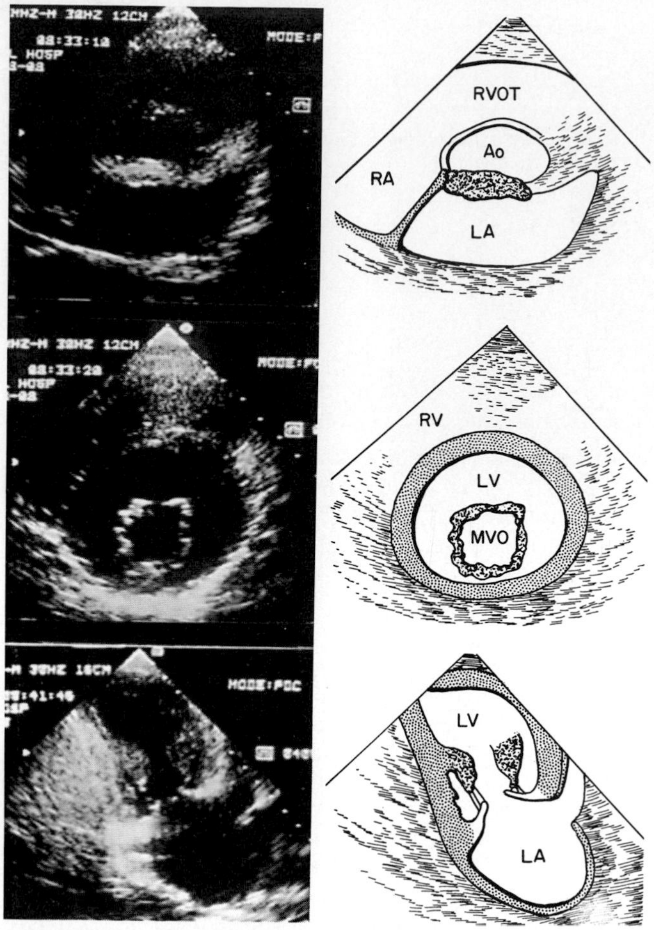

Fig. 17–83. Top. Parasternal short axis recording of the base of the mitral leaflet from the same patient illustrated in Figure 17–82. The dense fibrous band extends to involve the full width of the mitral leaflet. Middle. Parasternal short-axis recording of the mitral valve at the level of the valve orifice illustrating thickening of the free edges of the valve leaflets without separation of the leaflet commissures and slight restriction of orifice area. Bottom. Apical two-chamber recording illustrating the enlarged, elongated papillary muscles, which extend to and almost abut the mitral leaflets and are attached to the leaflets by very short, thickened chordae tendineae. RVOT = right ventricular outflow tract; RA = right atrium; LA = left atrium; Ao = aorta; MVO = mitral valve orifice; RV = right ventricle; LV = left ventricle.

traction and by thickening and fibrosis of the chordae tendineae.[202] Commissural fusion is not evident in pure mitral insufficiency, and this characteristic differentiates pure mitral insufficiency from combined lesions. In some instances, the fibrosis and chordal fusion may primarily affect the posterior leaflet with little or no anterior leaflet involvement.[203] Pure mitral regurgitation occurs in approximately 10% of patients with rheumatic mitral valve disease.[204]

Echocardiographically, rheumatic mitral insufficiency is characterized by an increase in echo production from the thickened deformed leaflets primarily in the region of the leaflet tips.[190,205] Long axis motion of the anterior leaflet is unrestricted, and in the absence of associated mitral stenosis, leaflet doming is not evident. The posterior leaflet is frequently more erect than normal and may be so deformed that motion is not evident. In one series, anterior leaflet prolapse was noted in 3 of 10 patients with pure rheumatic mitral insufficiency.[190]

In short axis, the orifice area is typically normal in size, and the leaflet edges are thickened. No commissural fusion is evident. Incomplete leaflet coaptation can be noted during early systole in some instances and can be related to the severity of the insufficiency.[205] This incomplete closure is usually seen at one of the commissural margins, but it may also involve the central portion of the coaptation line. When the area of incomplete closure involves only one leaflet margin, regurgitation is usually mild. When both margins or the entire closure line are involved, regurgitation tends to be more severe.[205]

Mitral Valve Prolapse

Mitral valve prolapse is the most common cause of pure isolated mitral regurgitation, often leading to valve repair or replacements.[206] The general term *prolapse* refers to the slipping or displacement of a bodily part from its usual position or relationships.[207] *Mitral valve prolapse* is the displacement of the mitral leaflets with respect to surrounding structures generally taken to be the mitral annulus. The sine qua non for prolapse, therefore, is the anatomic derangement as opposed to any associated clinical manifestations constituting a syndrome. The mitral annulus is generally selected as the structure to which leaflet motion and position are related because it identifies the boundary between the left ventricle and left atrium and is a clearly definable anatomic and echocardiographic reference.

The proper diagnosis of mitral valve prolapse requires both a technique that can display the fundamental anatomic leaflet-annular relationship and requires a knowledge of the normal range of leaflet motion. Two-dimensional echocardiographic imaging is ideally suited for recording the morphology, motion, and position of both mitral leaflets throughout the cardiac cycle in relation to each other, to external reference points, to surrounding cardiac structures (i.e., the mitral annulus), and to time.[208,209] The technique permits these relationships to be analyzed not only at rest but also during physiologic stress or pharmacologic intervention. Despite the availability of this tool for over 15 years, the definition of normal mitral leaflet motion and the clear separation of normal from abnormal have been continuing problems that are only now being resolved.[210]

Definition of Normal. To define normal leaflet annular relationships, it is essential to understand how normality is established. The normality of a given finding can be defined in either of two ways: (1) statistical normality—i.e., whether the finding occurs with sufficient frequency in the general population so that it may be considered normal—or (2) operational normality—i.e., whether the presence of the finding correlates with a state of health and confers a prognosis no worse than those pertaining in its absence. Statistical normality is generally considered to occur when a finding falls within two standard deviations of the mean of the normal population. Thus, a pattern found in 10 to 20% of the random population would be considered statistically normal. Because the establishment of normality by either of these criteria requires large population studies, the normality of a finding reported by a new technique is often established by comparison with an existing standard for which it has already been defined.

Both angiography and clinical signs have been used as gold standards for defining prolapse; however, neither is ideal. Angiography is fundamentally limited in the study of a generally benign disorder such as prolapse because angiographic studies of large populations, even on a research basis, are unjustified, and populations identified in angiographic series will be inherently biased. In addition, the technique itself is limited because the x-ray beam must be exactly parallel to the mitral annulus or else leaflet tissue will be overlaid by dye in the ventricle. The precise anatomic correlation of various angiographic patterns is poorly defined, as is the range of normal.[211] Marked intraobserver and interobserver variability also occur.[212] In one study, 13 left ventriculograms were reviewed by 20 observers, and in no case was there complete agreement regarding the presence or absence of prolapse, even in patients in whom clinical assessment was unequivocal.[213]

Clinical signs such as nonejection clicks and late systolic murmurs have also been used to identify patients with prolapse.[214–220] Clicks and murmurs, however, are found in a large percentage of the normal population, and no study has found a uniform association between clicks and murmurs and prolapse defined by any independent criteria.

Evolution of Echocardiographic Criteria for Prolapse

M-Mode Echocardiography. Early M-mode studies performed in small selected populations suggested that mitral prolapse was associated with a characteristic pattern of prominent midsystolic posterior displacement of the mitral leaflet echo.[221–225] This possibility raised the hope that M-mode echocardiography might offer a simple reliable, noninvasive method of objectively defining the presence of this abnormality. Unfortunately, with increased experience, questions concerning the appropriate diagnostic criteria and resulting sensitivity and specificity of this technique arose.[225,226] Commonly used M-mode criteria established in small groups of selected patients identified prolapse in up to 21% of normal persons, suggesting that statistically the criteria identify normality rather than a disease.[226] Likewise, these criteria defined operational normality because patients selected as normal are without an illness. Consequently, such basic questions as the incidence of prolapse and its relationship to other diseases were impossible to resolve.[226–228] Although M-mode echocardiography was the standard of diagnosis for mitral valve prolapse for less than a decade, it created enormous confusion about almost every aspect of the disorder and as a result diminished the general perception of echocardiography as a diagnostic tool.

Much of this confusion occurred because the M-mode method relates leaflet motion to the fixed transducer located on the anterior chest wall rather than to surrounding structures within the heart. As a result, if the transducer is relatively low and angled upward, the normal downward systolic motion of the base of the heart will produce an apparent upward systolic motion of the leaflets, potentially masking prolapse. Conversely, false-positives can be created by angling the transducer downward from a higher interspace.[229,230] The classically correct perpendicular transducer angulation has been defined only by statistical correlation of observed patterns with clicks and murmurs, the presence of which does not uniformly coincide with prolapse on the cross-sectional study.[230] Thus, because there are no M-mode criteria for prolapse with reasonable sensitivity and specificity, the method can produce false-positives and false-negatives, and it provides no unique information, it is no longer used for this purpose. Likewise, the validity of existing M-mode data based on criteria that classify up to 21% of normal persons as having a disease must be questioned.

Two-Dimensional Echocardiographic Criteria for Prolapse. The original two-dimensional echocardiographic studies showed that normal mitral leaflets coapted below (on the ventricular side of) a line connecting the annular hinge points in the parasternal long axis view of the ventricle and that leaflet displacement above this line correlated with angiographic prolapse.[208,209] Figure 17–84 compares the normal pattern of leaflet closure (Fig. 17–84A) with that seen with isolated prolapse of the leaflet (Fig. 17–84B) and bileaflet prolapse (Fig. 17–84C). In each instance, the prolapsing leaflets are displaced into the left atrium above the plane of the mitral annulus. The motion of the leaflets required to reach this point represents the combined effects of superior motion of the valve leaflets and apical motion of the mitral annulus. Because the maximum extent of these oppositely directed movements occurs at end-systole, the most pronounced degree of prolapse is also evident at this point of the cardiac cycle.

Subsequently, the criteria for prolapse were extended to include superior leaflet displacement in the apical four-chamber view as well; this view is oriented to intersect the medial and lateral margins of the annulus and is roughly orthogonal to the parasternal long axis view.[231,232] This extension was readily accepted because of the greater ease with which leaflet-annular relationships could be determined in the four-chamber view, which displays the leaflets and their hinge points in a horizontal orientation, and the apparently increased sensitivity attained when the valve was examined in this projection. Although unstated, extending the criteria to include both views implied the assumption that the mitral annulus must be a Euclidean plane, so that leaflet-annular relationships would be comparable in the two views.

The introduction of this assumption led to two observations that raised questions as to its validity. First, prolapse by these criteria was found in 11 to 13% or more of the general population, including individuals preselected to be normal, suggesting that the criteria were far too sensitive.[233,234] Second, when prolapse was present in the apical four-chamber view, it was frequently absent in the long axis view (Fig. 17–85), which would be unexpected if the mitral annulus is truly a plane.[233]

In vitro and in vivo studies have subsequently demon-

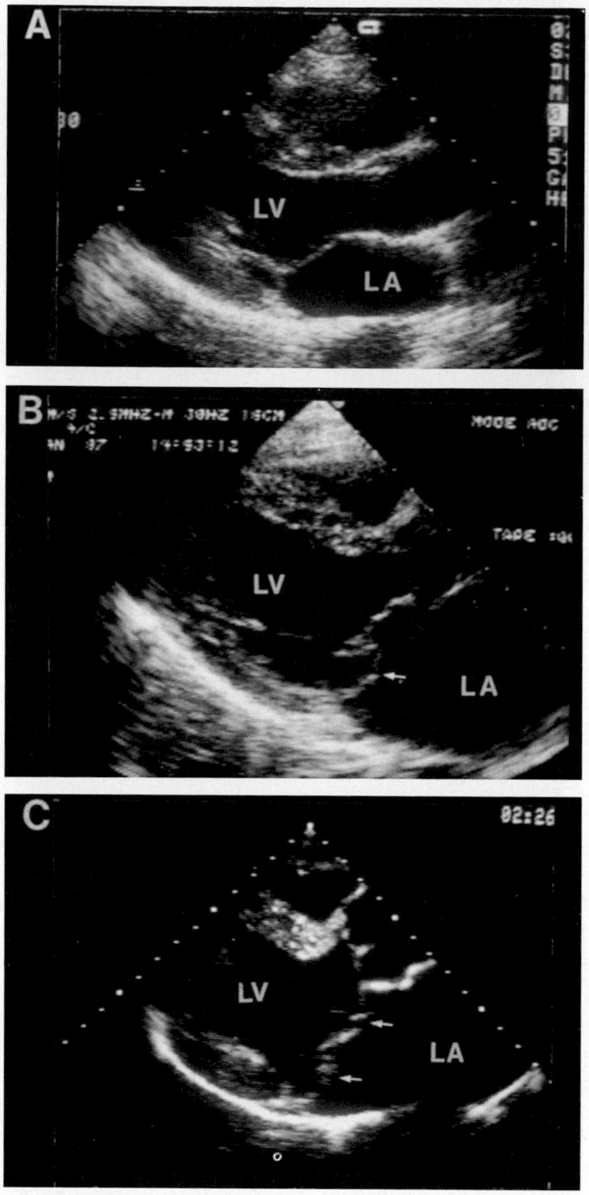

Fig. 17–84. Parasternal long axis recordings. **A.** A patient with a normal mitral valve. **B.** Mitral valve with isolated posterior leaflet prolapse. **C.** Bileaflet prolapse. LV = left ventricle; LA = left atrium; arrows point to the prolapsing leaflets.

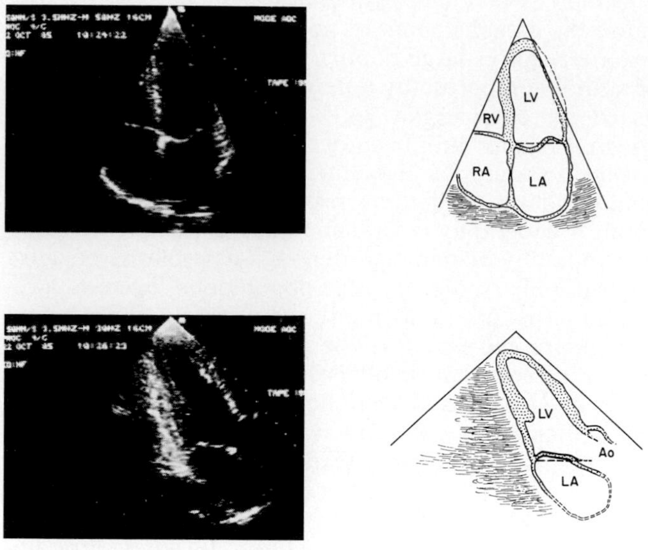

Fig. 17–85. Discrepancy of leaflet-annular relationships in a normal individual. Top. The anterior mitral leaflet extends *superior* to a line connecting the annular hinge joints (dashed line) in the apical four-chamber view. Bottom. In the roughly orthogonal apical long axis view, the leaflets appear to lie entirely on the ventricular side of the line connecting the hinge points. Note that the overall leaflet structure has opposite concavities in these two perpendicular views—a feature that defines a three-dimensional saddle surface. RV = right ventricle; LV = left ventricle; RA = right atrium; LA = left atrium; Ao = aorta. (Courtesy of Dr. Robert A. Levine.)

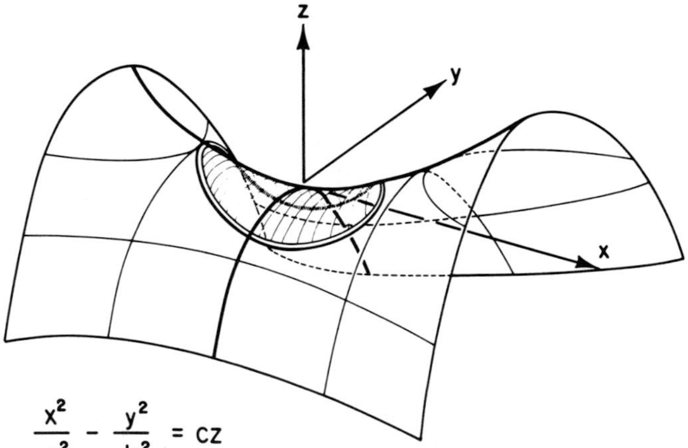

$$\frac{x^2}{a^2} - \frac{y^2}{b^2} = cz$$

Fig. 17–86. The saddle-shaped nature of the mitral annulus and its effect on the position of the mitral leaflets relative to the annular plane in different projections. The mitral annulus is depicted as the central elliptic portion of a hyperbolic paraboloid or saddle-shaped surface, which is concave downward in one direction (parallel to the yz plane) and upward in a perpendicular direction (parallel to the xz plane). In the equation, a, b, and c are constants and determine the shape of the structure. (From Levine RA, et al.: The relationship of mitral annular shape to the diagnosis of mitral valve prolapse. Circulation 75:756, 1987. Reproduced by permission of the American Heart Association, Inc.)

strated that the mitral annulus does not define a flat or Euclidian plane but rather has a saddle-like shape with high points positioned anteriorly and posteriorly and low points medially and laterally (Fig. 17–86).[235,236] Because of this shape, the mitral leaflets can appear to be displaced above the annulus when imaged in a plane that intersects the annulus through its medial and lateral low points (Fig. 17–87) but below the annulus in a plane that transects the annulus through its high points.[235,236] These observations explained the clinically observed discrepancy between leaflet-annular relationships in roughly orthogonal views without the need to postulate

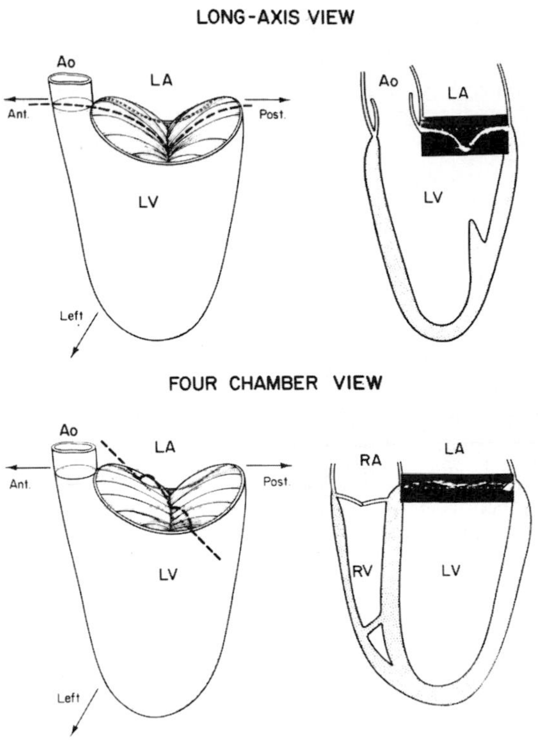

Fig. 17–87. Discrepancy of mitral leaflet relations in two-dimensional echocardiographic views (long axis and four chamber) of an in vitro model (left) with a saddle-shaped annulus and leaflets that are concave toward the left ventricle (LV), reflecting its distending pressure. The highest points of the saddle (farthest from the apex) are considered to be located anteriorly (Ant.) and posteriorly (Post.), with medial and lateral low points consistent with in vivo observations. The heavy interrupted lines on the left indicate the plane of view. On the right, echocardiographic images of the model are shown, along with diagrams of surrounding structures. The dotted lines in the echocardiographic images demarcate an apparent annular plane in each view; they are manually placed with the aid of the echocardiographic instrument. Of note, the leaflets lie below the annular plane in the long axis view, and above the plane in the four-chamber view. Ao = aorta; LA = left atrium; RA = right atrium; RV = right ventricle. (From Levine RA, Triulzi MO, Harrigan P, Weyman AE: The relationship of mitral annular shape to the diagnosis of mitral valve prolapse. Circulation 75: 761, 1987. Reproduced by permission of the American Heart Association, Inc.)

localized leaflet distortion and suggested that superior systolic leaflet displacement limited to the apical four-chamber view might well constitute a normal geometric finding without pathologic significance. This hypothesis was tested in a retrospective study of 312 patients, and it was shown that patients with superior systolic leaflet displacement limited to the apical four-chamber view are no more likely to have associated abnormalities connoting mitral valve pathology or dysfunction than patients with no displacement in any view and no other echocardiographic evidence of heart disease[237] (Table 17–2). Thus, abnormal displacement of the mitral leaflets (prolapse) occurs when the leaflets lie above the high points of the annulus, which are recorded in the parasternal long axis or apical long axis views; superior systolic displacement above the low points of the annulus is merely a normal anatomic variant.*

Relationship of Leaflet Morphology and Patterns of Closure to Valve Function. The observation that patients with prolapse tend to have leaflet displacement above the high points of the mitral annulus does not, by itself, imply that all patients with displacement above the annulus are abnormal or have prolapse. Four other characteristics of the valve appear to be important in defining patients whose leaflet displacement is associated with functional abnormalities: (1) location of leaflet displacement, (2) the degree of leaflet displacement, (3) leaflet thickening, and (4) symmetry of displacement (i.e., single- or double-leaflet prolapse). Use of the annular high points to diagnose leaflet prolapse implies that the maximal degree of leaflet displacement occurs in the same plane as the most superior portion of the annulus. In most cases, this assumption is correct; however, exceptions do exist. Specifically, isolated posterior leaflet displacement can involve only the medial or more commonly lateral scallop and can be evident in an apical view (lateral, apical four-chamber; medial, apical two-chamber) when it is not obvious in the parasternal long axis view. This focal posterior leaflet displacement is limited to the apical views and occurs infrequently enough to be considered statistically abnormal,[233] but when associated with significant functional abnormality, it is usually also apparent in the parasternal long axis view.

The degree of leaflet displacement can be defined as the peak linear distance of the leaflet body or (bodies) above a line connecting the anterior and posterior margins of the annulus in the parasternal long axis view (Fig. 17–88), the area between the leaflet bodies and this line,[238] or the three-dimensional volume enclosed between the leaflet body and a plane defining the annulus (Fig. 17–89). As illustrated in Figure 17–90, the degree of linear displacement above the annulus correlates with the degree of dysfunction and changes in leaflet morphology. Based on these data, we do not consider patients with leaflet displacement $\leq$ 2 mm to have prolapse, because the prevalence of associated abnormalities is no greater in these patients than in individuals without displacement.

Roughly 18% of patients with parasternal long axis displacement have a distinctive form of prolapse characterized by diffuse leaflet thickening ($\geq$ 5 mm) and obvious redundancy, which we have termed *classic mitral valve prolapse.*[239] Thickening is often most prominent near the tips of the leaflets and appears to represent the myxomatous degeneration noted pathologically in patients with mitral valve prolapse (Fig. 17–91). Associated tricuspid valve prolapse is more common in patients with classic prolapse than in those with displacement but without leaflet thickening.[239] Leaflet

*An exception to this rule is isolated posterior leaflet prolapse, which is seen very infrequently in the apical four-chamber view, thus meeting a statistical definition for abnormality. Until sufficient numbers are found to study its operational significance, it is our custom to consider it an abnormality and report it as such.

Table 17–2. Echocardiographic Findings in the Three Leaflet Displacement Groups

	Group 1 (No Displacement)	Group 2 (A4C Only)	Group 3 (PLA at Least)
No. of patients	135	57	120
Increased leaflet thickness	1 (0.7%)	0	29 (24%)
Increased LA dimensions	3 (2%)	0	19 (16%)
Increased LA volume	0	0	14 (12%)
Mitral regurgitation/No. of Doppler studies	7/90 (8%)	2/31 (6%)	35/87 (40%)
MR >1+/Doppler studies	0/90	0/31	14/87 (16%)

p > .5 (Group 1 vs. Group 2)
p < .005 (Group 2 vs. Group 3)
p < .005 (Group 1 vs. Group 3)

A4C = apical four chamber view; LA = left atrium; MR = mitral regurgitation; PLA = parasternal long-axis view. (From Levine RA, et al.: Reconsideration of echocardiographic standards for mitral valve prolapse: lack of association between leaflet displacement isolated to the apical four-chamber view and independent echocardiographic evidence of abnormality. J Am Coll Cardiol 11:1013, 1988. Reprinted with permission from the American College of Cardiology.)

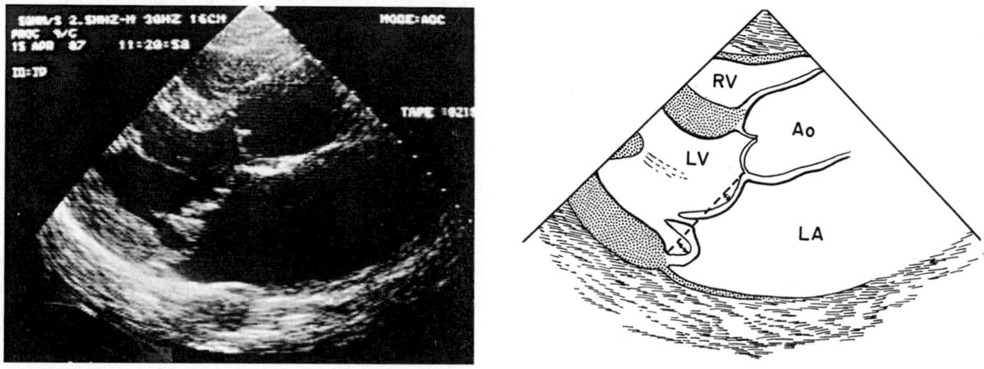

Fig. 17–88. Measurement of leaflet displacement above a line connecting the annular hinge points in the parasternal long axis view (left) and line drawing (right). RV = right ventricle; LV = left ventricle; Ao = aorta; LA = left atrium. (From Levine RA, et al.: Reconsideration of echocardiographic standards for mitral valve prolapse: lack of association between leaflet displacement isolated to the apical four-chamber view and independent echocardiographic evidence of abnormality. J Am Coll Cardiol 11:1010, 1988. Reprinted with permission from the American College of Cardiology.)

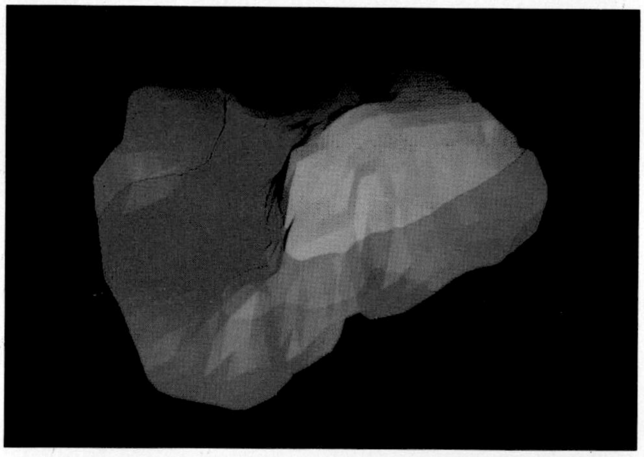

Fig. 17–89. Leaflet displacement can also be quantitated in three-dimensional space and expressed in terms of a volume. This figure illustrates a three-dimensional model of the coapted mitral leaflets with leaflet tissue below a least-squares plane fitted to the mitral annulus illustrated in blue, leaflet tissue between the least-squares plane and the high points of the annulus indicated in green, and displacement above the high points of the annulus illustrated in gray. (Courtesy of Dr. Robert A. Levine and Mark D. Handschumacher.)

thickening and redundancy appear to identify a subgroup of patients at risk for complications such as endocarditis, severe mitral regurgitation, and mitral valve replacement[239,240] (Table 17–3). However, the frequency of stroke is similar in patients with classic and nonclassic prolapse.[239] Note that increased leaflet thickness occurs in patients with greater displacement so that these two characteristics move in parallel.

Finally, when mitral prolapse is observed on two-dimensional echocardiography, it most frequently involves both leaflets. In four series involving a total of over 500 patients,[190,209,241,242] prolapse of both leaflets was noted in 75 to 90% of cases. Isolated prolapse of the posterior leaflet was the next most common occurrence (10 to 20%), whereas anterior leaflet prolapse was infrequently seen (3 to 5%). The pattern of displacement appears to relate to the degree of regurgitation. In a study of 329 patients, at least moderate mitral regurgitation was noted in a far higher percentage (73%) of patients with asymmetric prolapse (i.e., prolapse of only one leaflet—usually, the posterior, or prolapse of two leaflets in which one was dominant) than in patients with symmetric classic mitral valve prolapse (22%).[242] In this

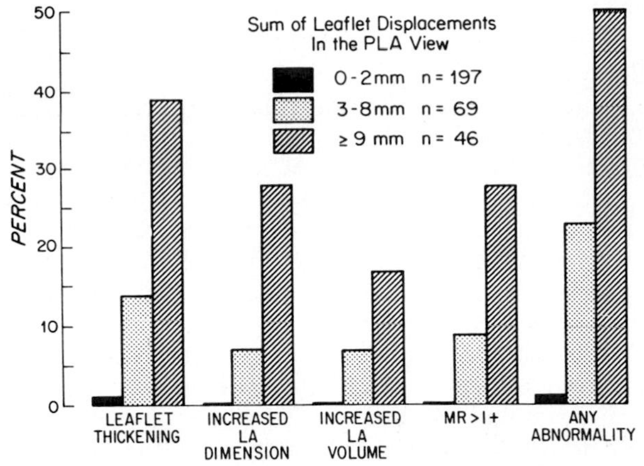

Fig. 17–90. Frequency of associated abnormalities as a function of the degree of leaflet displacement in the parasternal long axis (PLA) view. The 312 patients in this study are grouped according to the sum of leaflet displacements (anterior and posterior leaflets) in the long axis view. The height of the bars expresses the percentage of each group having a given abnormality. LA = left atrium; MR = mitral regurgitation. (From Levine RA, et al.: Reconsideration of echocardiographic standards for mitral valve prolapse: lack of association between leaflet displacement isolated to the apical four-chamber view and independent echocardiographic evidence of abnormality. J Am Coll Cardiol 11:1010, 1988. Reprinted with permission from the American College of Cardiology.)

study, important regurgitation was not found in patients with displacement ≤ 5 mm without associated leaflet thickening. Although the reason for this observation is as yet unclear, patients with predominant single-leaflet prolapse may represent those with early valvular disruption and chordal rupture, while those with bileaflet symmetric prolapse have redundant but intact leaflets.

Additional Echocardiographic Features Associated With Prolapse. Additional echocardiographic features reported in mitral valve prolapse include (1) exaggerated superior motion of the papillary muscles toward the mitral annulus during the later half of systole;[243] (2) an abnormal rocking motion of the posterior mitral annulus;[190,209,241,244] (3) an increase in mitral annular diameter;[244] and (4) displacement of the mitral coaptation point.[190,209] Exaggerated superior motion of the papillary muscles has been noted in patients with classic mitral valve prolapse. This exaggerated motion is characterized by a decrease in the distance between the papillary muscle tips and the annulus, which parallels the degree and time course of superior displacement of the leaflets above the annulus.[243] The exaggerated superior motion of the papillary muscles appears to result from traction by the prolapsing leaflets, which cannot

Table 17–3. Complications in Classic and Nonclassic Mitral Valve Prolapse

Complication	Mitral Valve Prolapse: Classic (N = 319) Percent (No. of Patients)	Mitral Valve Prolapse: Nonclassic (N = 137) Percent (No. of Patients)	p Value
Endocarditis	3.5 (11)*	0	<.02
Severe mitral regurgitation	11.9 (30)†	0	<.001
Mitral valve replacement	6.6 (21)	0.7 (1)	<.02
Stroke	7.5 (24)§	5.8 (8)¶	NS‖

* Endocarditis developed in two patients after index echocardiography; nine others underwent index echocardiography during an admission for endocarditis.

† Calculations for mitral regurgitation are based on the patients who had Doppler examinations (n = 252 and 99 for the classic and nonclassic groups, respectively).

‡ All mitral-valve replacements occurred after index echocardiography.

§ Three of the 24 patients had strokes after index echocardiography.

¶ One of the eight patients had a stroke after index echocardiography.

‖ NS denotes not significant.

(From Marks AR, et al.: Identification of high-risk and low-risk subgroups of patients with mitral valve prolapse. N Engl J Med 320:1031, 1989.)

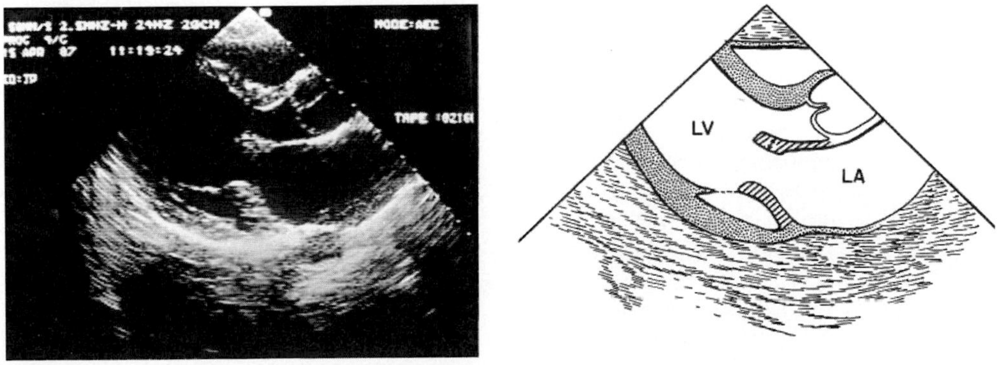

Fig. 17–91. Parasternal long axis recording of the mitral valve from a patient with classic mitral valve prolapse and thickened mitral leaflets, illustrating the measurement of leaflet thickness. LV = left ventricle; LA = left atrium; thickness measurement is indicated by the double-headed arrow in the accompanying diagram. (From Levine RA, et al.: Reconsideration of echocardiographic standards for mitral valve prolapse: lack of association between leaflet displacement isolated to the apical four-chamber view and independent echocardiographic evidence of abnormality. J Am Coll Cardiol 11:1013, 1988. Reprinted with permission from the American College of Cardiology.)

be counteracted by the normal force of contraction.[243] Experimentally, traction on the papillary muscles has been shown to cause electrical instability and may predispose to ventricular arrhythmia.[245] However, the clinical significance of this finding remains to be established.

Exaggerated apical motion of the posterior mitral annulus, without a corresponding increase in the normally associated apical motion of the anterior annulus, has also been reported in a large percentage of patients with prolapse.[209,244] However, actual measurements of annular displacement[243] and rotation[246] fail to demonstrate a quantitative difference in the motion of the posterior annulus in patients with mitral valve prolapse when compared to normals.[243] The visual perception of exaggerated motion may be due to the oppositely directed movement of the annulus and papillary muscles, which increases relative annular movement and attracts the eye. Alternatively, more specific methods of measurement may be needed to characterize this phenomenon.

An increase in mitral annular diameter has also been reported in patients with mitral valve prolapse.[247,248] This has not been a uniform finding,[246] however, and it is unclear whether annular dilation is a primary abnormality or occurs secondary to associated mitral regurgitation.

Both anterior and posterior displacement of the mitral leaflet coaptation point have also been described.[190,209] In our experience, anterior displacement is seen most often in patients with posterior leaflet prolapse. In contrast, posterior displacement is more common in patients with secondary prolapse (see following discussion), which is due to conditions such as atrial septal defect and pancake heart. In the majority of patients with bileaflet prolapse (classic and nonclassic), the point of leaflet coaptation within the ventricle is normal. Displacement of coaptation may also be seen in conditions other than prolapse and, by itself, adds little to the diagnosis.

Relationship of Prolapse to Clinical Signs and Symptoms. Clinical signs and symptoms have been widely used in an attempt to identify patients with mitral valve prolapse. The clinical signs classically associated with prolapse are the systolic click and apical systolic murmur. This association was initially based on the frequent occurrence of clicks and murmurs in small groups of patients sufficiently ill to be studied by angiography or surgery.[215,217,218,220,223–225] By extrapolation, investigators then assumed that clicks and murmurs imply mitral valve prolapse whenever they occur regardless of the population studied. In some cases this extrapolation was taken a step further, and these findings were used as a diagnostic gold standard, to substitute for the anatomic demonstration of leaflet displacement or regurgitation.[219,226,228,249,250] Unfortunately, although the original surgical and angiographic standard identified a small, symptomatic population as having prolapse, the assumption that clicks and murmurs *imply* prolapse led to its diagnosis in 5 to 15% of the general population, even in apparently healthy individuals.[226,228] These findings were variously interpreted as indicating widespread disease or potential disease or simply reflecting the lack of sensitivity and specificity of the diagnostic criteria.[210,226]

Because two-dimensional echocardiographic imaging can demonstrate the anatomic relationships fundamental to the diagnosis of prolapse, it forms a useful reference to define the true sensitivity and specificity of these clinical signs in identifying patients at risk. Unfortunately, as the echocardiographic criteria for prolapse have evolved over the past 20 years, these relations have also changed. Thus, while there are a great deal of data comparing signs and symptoms to M-mode criteria—which are no longer accepted as a primary reference—there is much less information relating the more appropriate two-dimensional imaging criteria to clinical findings. Available data (Table 17–4) suggest that clicks have a sensitivity of 59% and a specificity of roughly 90% for prolapse defined as superior systolic leaflet displacement in the parasternal long axis view.[251] Similar data have been obtained in probands of patients with mitral valve prolapse in whom M-mode findings have been largely corroborated in the long axis view.[252] The sensitivity of a systolic murmur, when patients with other recognized forms of heart disease are excluded, is approximately 54%, which increases slightly when the murmur is required to be late systolic. The specificity of an apical systolic murmur is roughly 64%, which likewise increases when the murmur is required to be late systolic. The combined specificity of both a click and murmur is good (97%), but the sensitivity of these combined findings is poor (32%). The combination of a click and *late* systolic murmur, although not present in patients without displacement, identified only 14% of patients (3 of 22) with displacement. The predictive value of a click (Table 17–5) has been calculated as roughly 24% and may in fact prove to be even lower as the criteria for prolapse become further refined. Figures 17–92 through 17–95 illustrate the varying relationship between leaflet morphology and physical findings. Figure 17–92 contains the two-dimensional echocardiogram, carotid pulse tracing, and phonocardiogram from a pa-

Table 17–4. Physical Findings by Auscultation or Phonocardiography

	No Displacement n = 72	Displacement n = 22
Click	7 (10%)*	13 (59%)
Murmur	26 (36%)†	12 (55%)
Both	2 (3%)*	7 (32%)

* $p < .005$.

† NS, $p > .05$.

Click = systolic click, with or without associated murmur: murmur = apical systolic murmur, with or without associated click.

(From Abascal VA, Hagege AA, Brady CL, Levine RA: Mitral valve prolapse: lack of sensitivity and specificity of clicks and murmurs for leaflet displacement by 2D echocardiography. Circulation 76[Suppl IV]:IV–316, 1987.)

Table 17–5. Predictive Value (Auscultation or Phonocardiography)

	Click n = 20	Murmur n = 38	Both n = 9
No displacement	7 (35%)	26 (68%)	2 (22%)
Displacement	13 (65%)	12 (32%)	7 (78%)

(Data from Abascal VA, Hagege AA, Brady CL, Levine RA: Mitral valve prolapse: lack of sensitivity and specificity of clicks and murmurs for leaflet displacement by 2D echocardiography. Circulation 76[Suppl IV]:IV-316, 1987.)

tient with a clearly defined midsystolic click and normal mitral leaflet morphologic and closure. Figures 17–93 and 17–94 illustrate similar midsystolic murmurs in two patients; one with classic mitral valve prolapse and the second with a morphologically normal mitral valve. Finally, Figure 17–95 illustrates classic mitral valve prolapse in a patient with no abnormal auscultatory or phonocardiographic findings.

Symptoms bear no clear association with anatomic and functional evidence of prolapse[251,252] (Table 17–6).

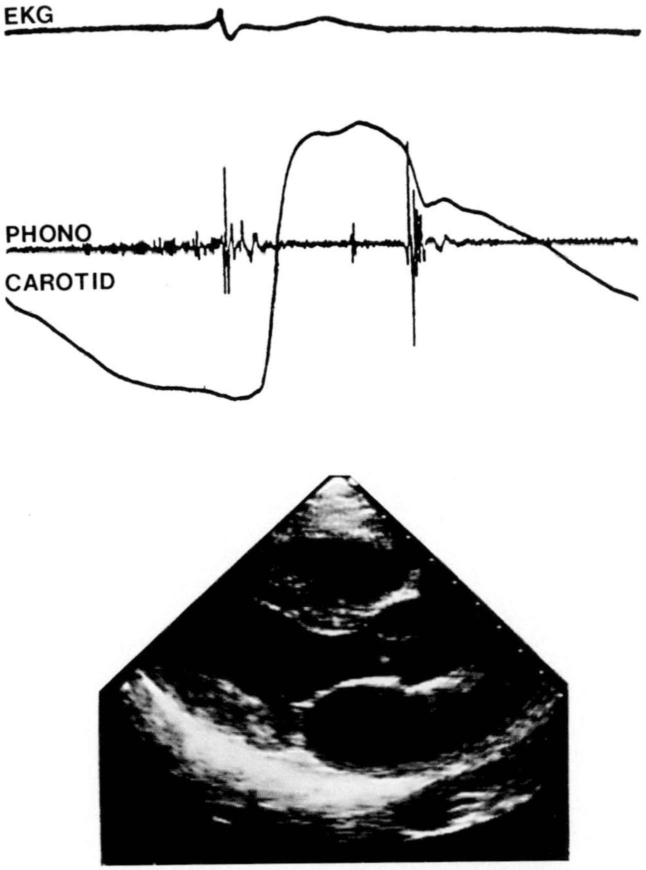

Fig. 17–92. Electrocardiogram, phonocardiogram, carotid pulse tracing, and parasternal long axis mitral valve recording from a patient with a clearly defined midsystolic click and normal mitral valve coaptation.

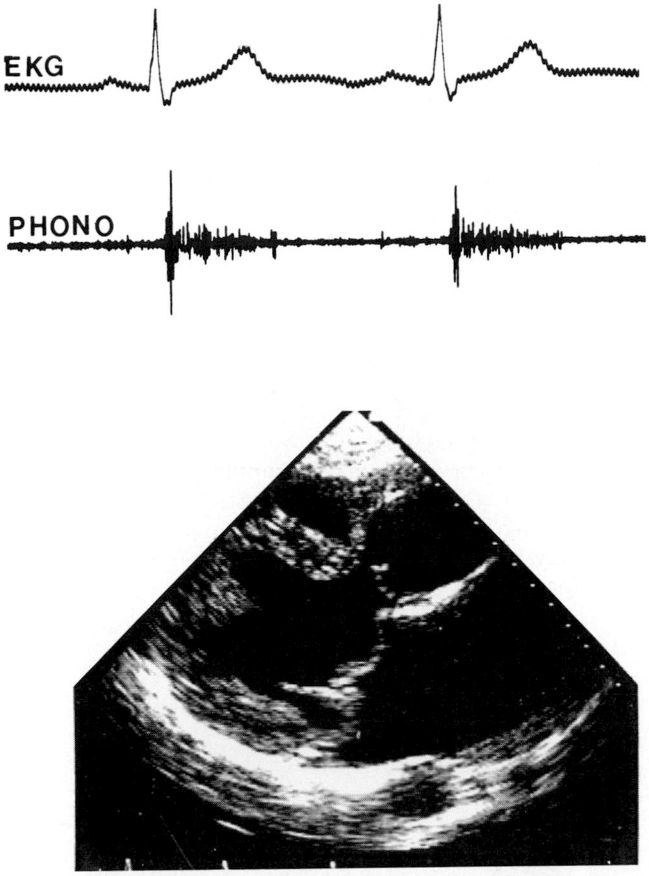

Fig. 17–93. Electrocardiogram, phonocardiogram, and parasternal long axis recording from a patient with classic bileaflet mitral valve prolapse and a midsystolic murmur.

Chest pain is equally common in patients with prolapse and in patients referred for evaluation who subsequently prove not to have prolapse; the same is true of nonspecific dyspnea. The only significant correlation we have noted is with palpitations, and in this case the correlation is negative; specifically, palpitations are 95% predictive of not having mitral valve prolapse.[251] This lack of positive association of symptoms with anatomic prolapse has consistently been reported by many groups using a variety of criteria for the diagnosis of prolapse[234,239,252–257] and suggest that the original associations largely reflected the ascertainment bias caused by studying symptomatic patients.[258]

Complications Associated With Mitral Valve Prolapse. Mitral valve prolapse is generally felt to be a benign condition with an overall mortality not significantly different from that of an age- and sex-matched control population.[240,259] It is now becoming increasingly clear, however, that there are subgroups within this larger population who are at increased risk for important complications such as bacterial endocarditis and progressive mitral regurgitation leading to valve replacement.

Infectious endocarditis is a clearly established complication of mitral valve prolapse with an incidence ranging from 1 to 10% in follow-up series.[240,259–261] Endocarditis

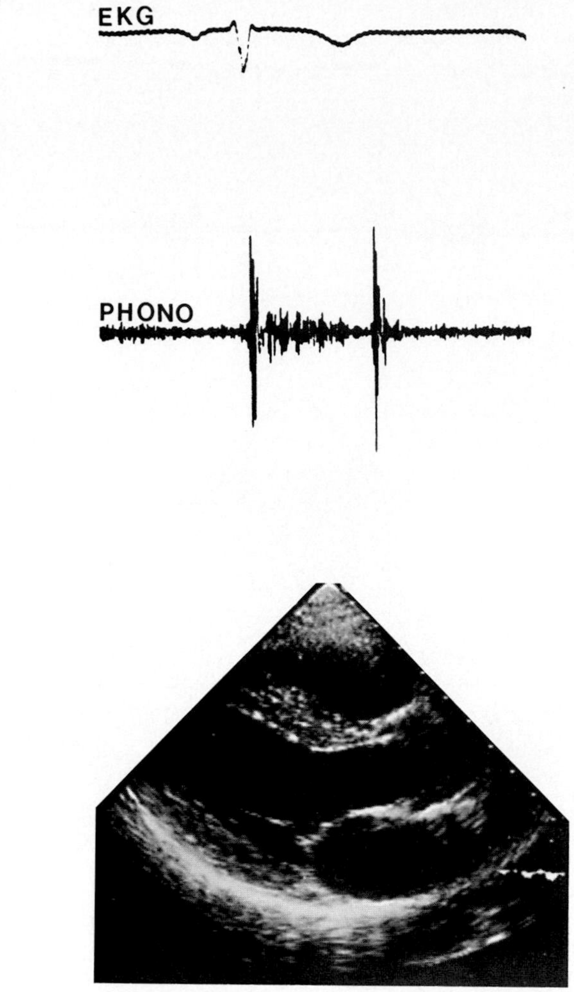

Fig. 17–94. Electrocardiogram, phonocardiogram, and parasternal long axis mitral valve recording illustrating a midsystolic murmur similar to that recorded in the patient illustrated in Figure 17–93. In this case, however, mitral leaflet motion and coaptation are normal.

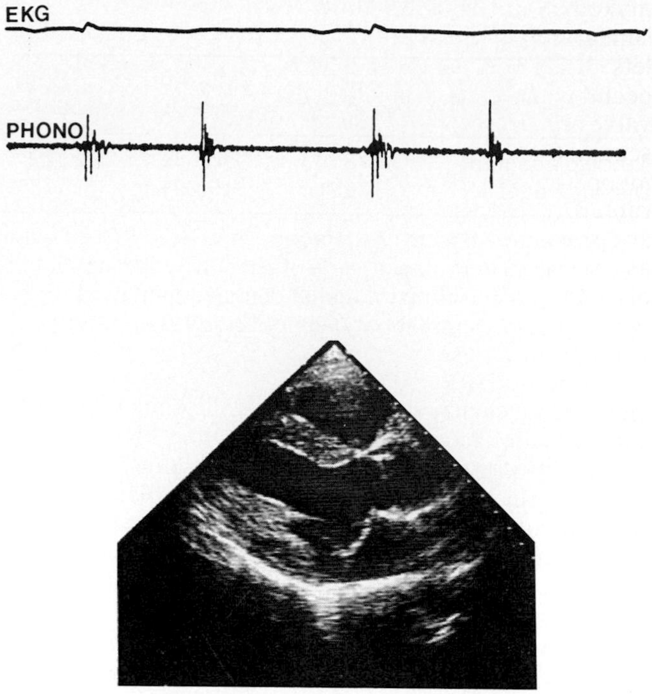

Fig. 17–95. Electrocardiogram, phonocardiogram, and parasternal long axis mitral valve recording from a patient with classic severe bileaflet mitral valve prolapse and no evidence of either a systolic click or a murmur.

appears to be associated with leaflet thickening[239,240] and can involve any affected valve in patients with polyvalvular prolapse. Most major studies have estimated the relative risk of endocarditis at 2.9 to 8.2%.[262–265] The reported risk of subacute bacterial endocarditis (SBE) increases in patients with mitral regurgitation manifested by a systolic murmur and is relatively low in patients without mitral regurgitation. Other independent risk factors appear to be the male sex and age over 45 years.

The cumulative risk of valve surgery in both men and women below the age of 50 with mitral valve prolapse is minimal. The risk of valve surgery rises steeply after the age of 50, particularly in men, approaching 4% by age 70.[266] Important regurgitation and valve replacement are far more common in patients with thickened leaflets, particularly in those with single posterior leaflet prolapse.

Sudden death has been reported in patients with mitral valve prolapse but appears to be rare. Sudden death, like other major complications, appears related to leaflet redundancy and has been attributed to ventricular tachycardia and fibrillation.[267] However, further study is required to clearly define risk and pathophysiology.

Primary Versus Secondary Prolapse. Prolapse as described to this point is due to an intrinsic or primary abnormality of the mitral leaflets and chordal apparatus. Such changes have been described in association with

Table 17–6. Association of Symptoms With Leaflet Displacement

	No Displacement n = 72	Displacement n = 22
Chest pain, exertional	3 (4%)*	0
Chest pain, atypical	14 (19%)*	2 (9%)
Dyspnea, exertional	6 (8%)*	2 (9%)
Dyspnea, nonexertional	2 (3%)*	0
Palpitations	19 (26%)†	1 (5%)
Syncope	0*	0
One or more symptoms	30 (42%)‡	4 (18%)

* NS, $p > .3$.
† $p < .035$.
‡ $p = .04$.
(Data from Abascal VA, Hagege AA, Brady CL, Levine RA: Mitral valve prolapse: lack of sensitivity and specificity of clicks and murmurs for leaflet displacement by 2D echocardiography. Circulation 76[Suppl IV]:IV-316, 1987.)

myxomatous degeneration, Marfan's syndrome, and similar conditions with thickened and redundant leaflets. It is important to remember that prolapse can also occur when disproportion develops between a normal valve and a small ventricle, as in mitral stenosis, ostium secundum atrial septal defect, and hypertrophic cardiomyopathy,[268] or when systolic chordal support is disrupted, as in the case of bacterial endocarditis (secondary prolapse). Ventriculovalvar disproportion may arise as a result of abnormalities of ventricular size, function, or geometry that distort or shorten the ventricular support base for the leaflets. Thus, a disproportion between ventricular and valve size may be sufficient to cause anatomic prolapse in the absence of pathologic changes inherent to the leaflets or chordal structures. Theoretically, because valve size is fixed whereas chamber size is variable, sufficient reduction in chamber size should be attainable in any heart so that the leaflets become relatively redundant and, if under pressure, prolapse into the left atrium.

Atrial septal defect is a natural example of this phenomenon. Anatomic mitral valve prolapse by two-dimensional echocardiography occurs in at least 50% of patients with secundum atrial septal defects who have been studied. Left ventricular geometry is prominently distorted in this condition, leading to the hypothesis that the observed prolapse is secondary to the ventricular abnormalities. This contention is supported by the observation that mitral valve abnormalities are infrequently noted at surgery despite preoperative angiographic prolapse[269] and that the degree of prolapse decreases or normalizes in parallel with postoperative normalization of ventricular geometry.[238] Prolapse occurs more frequently in older patients with atrial septal defects, leading to the speculation that secondary prolapse can ultimately lead to primary pathologic changes in an abnormally stressed valve.[270,271]

Prolapse that is due to loss of chordal support most commonly occurs in patients with bacterial endocarditis and ischemic heart disease. The relationship between bacterial endocarditis and prolapse is particularly difficult to assess because valvular thickening and prolapse can provide the anatomic substrate for infection or can be the result of the infectious process. When the leaflets are diffusely thickened and redundant, we generally consider prolapse to have been the primary process. This relationship is supported when other valves are similarly involved.[239] In patients with focal thickening and prolapse, the infection is considered causative. Precise definition of prolapse as cause or effect requires prior knowledge of valve morphology. As a general rule, prolapse occurring de novo in patients with ischemic heart disease is due to chordal rupture. Prolapse can also be seen in patients with congenital abnormalities of the mitral leaflets (Fig. 17–96) or papillary muscles (Fig. 17–97).

It is unclear whether secondary prolapse differs in functional effect from primary prolapse with a similar degree of displacement and morphologic change. Until similarity is proven, it seems appropriate to retain this distinction.

Doppler Studies. One of the major complications associated with mitral valve prolapse is mitral regurgitation. Significant mitral regurgitation is reported to increase the risk of sudden death and underlies the need for valve replacement in patients with mitral valve prolapse. Doppler provides a sensitive method for detecting both the presence and severity of regurgitation associated with mitral valve prolapse.[272,273] Color flow mapping has proven particularly valuable for the intraoperative evaluation of the changes in regurgitation produced by mitral valve repair. When the leaflets are difficult to visualize, the color Doppler jet can often help to define the border of the leaflet and hence aid in the primary diagnosis.

Summary. In summary, therefore, we consider prolapse to be present when there is greater than 2 mm displacement of one or both mitral leaflets in the parasternal long axis or apical long axis views. Focal prolapse of the medial or lateral scallop of the posterior leaflet recorded in the apical four- or two-chamber views is unusual and is also considered abnormal. The combination of leaflet displacement together with increased leaflet thickness (≥ 5 mm) and redundancy—termed *classic mitral valve prolapse*—identifies a subgroup most likely to have complications such as endocarditis, moderate-to-severe mitral regurgitation, and progressive disease leading to valve replacement. It is our prac-

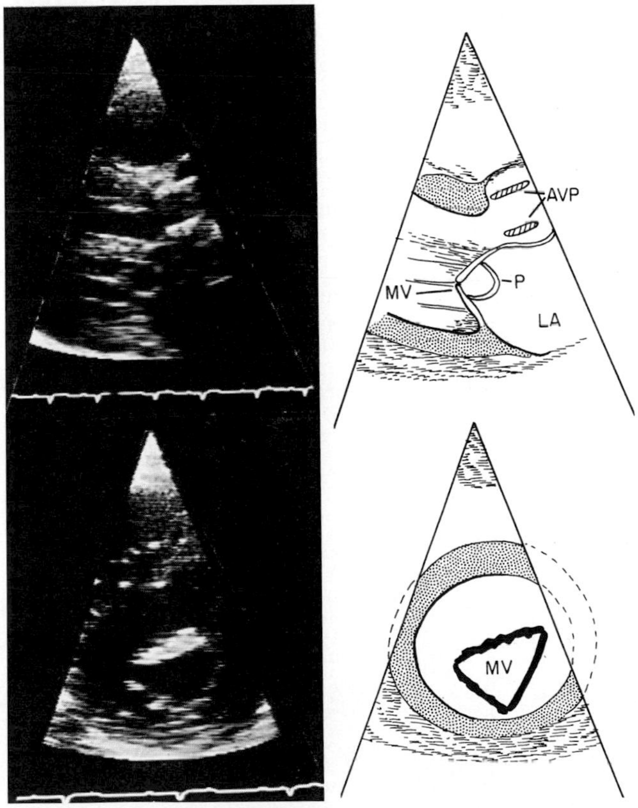

Fig. 17–96. Top. Parasternal long axis recording from a patient with a prosthetic aortic valve illustrating focal prolapse of a lateral segment of the mitral valve. Bottom. Parasternal short axis recording illustrating a trileaflet mitral valve with otherwise normal left ventricular morphology. AVP = aortic valve prosthesis; P = prolapse; LA = left atrium; MV = mitral valve.

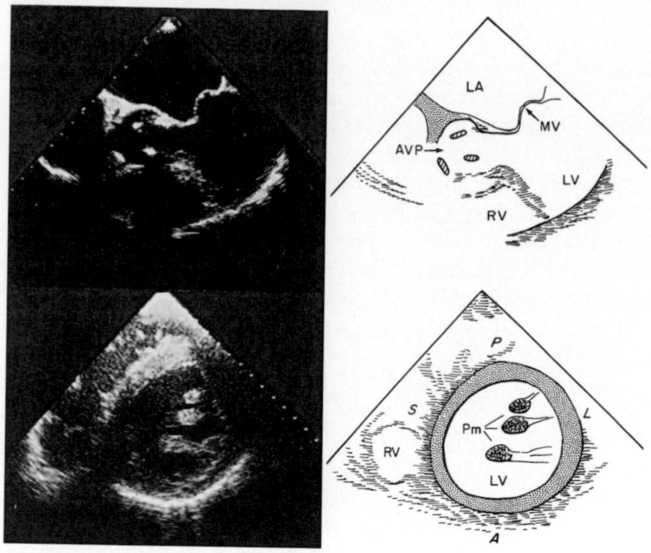

Fig. 17–97. Top. Transesophageal recording illustrating prolapse of the anterior mitral leaflet. Bottom. Transesophageal short axis recording of the left ventricle at the papillary muscle level showing enlargement and elongation of the anteromedial papillary muscle and reduplication of the posteromedial papillary muscle. Pm = papillary muscle; LV = left ventricle; AVP = aortic valve prosthesis; MV = mitral valve; RV = right ventricle; LA = left atrium.

tice not to diagnose prolapse on the basis of M-mode patterns or four-chamber view findings alone with the exception noted previously.

Papillary Muscle Dysfunction

The papillary muscles and subjacent left ventricular myocardium provide the foundation that supports the mitral leaflets during ventricular systole. Abnormal function of the papillary muscles has been associated with improper leaflet closure and resultant valvular insufficiency.[274–278]

Papillary muscle dysfunction is most commonly associated with ischemic heart disease; however, other causes—such as cardiomyopathy, left ventricular dilation, trauma, and a variety of disorders of the endocardium and myocardium that disturb function in the region of the papillary muscles—have been implicated.[190] The presence of this disorder has been most commonly established on clinical grounds by the occurrence of a new murmur of mitral insufficiency in a setting consistent with dysfunction of the papillary muscles.

Cross-sectional echocardiographic studies have demonstrated abnormalities of both leaflet motion and systolic leaflet position in patients with clinical evidence of papillary muscle dysfunction.[279,280] These leaflet abnormalities are almost invariably associated with left ventricular dysfunction, either dyskinesis at the base of one or both papillary muscles, and/or generalized ventricular dilation. Calcification or fibrosis of the papillary muscles themselves has also been reported. The most common pattern of abnormal leaflet motion is characterized by the apparent failure of one or both mitral leaflets to reach the normal peak systolic position relative to the mitral annulus.[279] This pattern is best recorded and has been most extensively studied in the apical four-chamber view.[279] The pattern has been referred to as *incomplete leaflet closure;* however, the leaflet tips actually coapt along most of their margins, and echocardiographic evidence of apical leaflet displacement can be present before regurgitation develops.[281] Thus, the leaflet pattern defines the cause but not always the presence of mitral regurgitation.

Figure 17–98 is an example of this phenomenon. In this figure, both the anterior and posterior mitral leaflets are restrained more deeply than normal in the left ventricular cavity. Characteristically, there is an abrupt bend in the midportion of the anterior mitral leaflet with the tip curving inward toward the center of the left ventricular cavity at approximately a 30° angle to the base of the leaflet. This pattern has been reported in a high percentage (91%) of patients with ischemic heart disease and clinical evidence of papillary muscle dysfunction.[279] It is rarely noted in patients with ischemic disease without clinical evidence of papillary muscle dysfunction

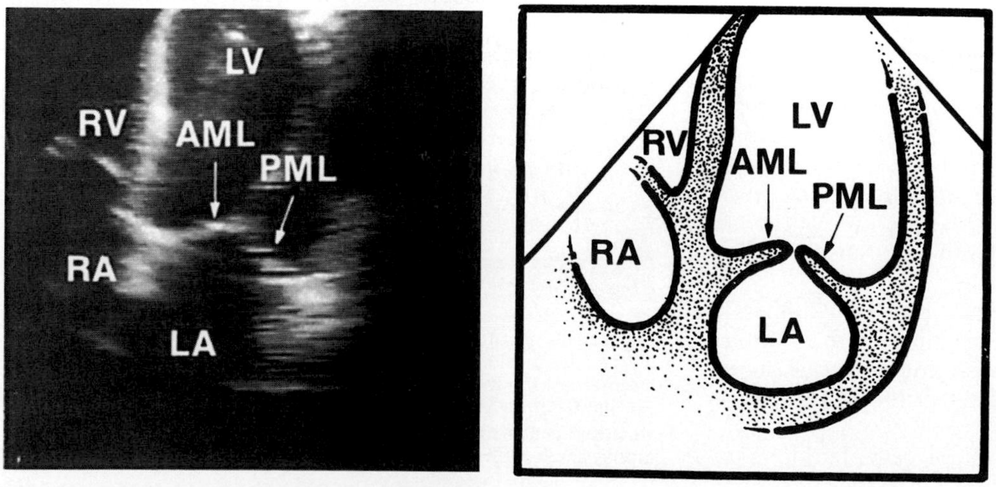

Fig. 17–98. Apical four-chamber view from a patient with cardiomyopathy and generalized left ventricular dilation. In this case, tension on both the anterior (AML) and posterior mitral leaflets (PML) is increased because of a generalized increase in chordal-leaflet separation. This generalized increase in tension on both leaflets results in failure of either leaflet to reach the plane of the mitral annulus during systole. LV = left ventricle; RV = right ventricle; RA = right atrium; LA = left atrium.

(8%) and is never seen in normal patients. The anterior leaflet is always involved, and apical displacement of the posterior leaflet, while present, is usually less pronounced (12%). This phenomenon may be seen in patients with a normal-size ventricle and dyskinesis at the base of one papillary muscle or with generalized ventricular dilation. When dyskinesis involves only one papillary muscle, the leaflet pattern is the same regardless of the papillary muscle involved.[279]

Long axis studies have likewise shown that the leaflets are tethered more deeply in the left ventricular cavity during systole.[280] This tethered configuration is characterized by apical displacement of the coaptation point in both early and late systole and by outward bowing of the lower third of the bodies of the leaflets with increased convexity toward the left ventricular cavity.

Figures 17–99 and 17–100 explain diagrammatically (1) the forces that produce the type of incomplete closure noted in Figure 17–98, (2) the reason for the universal involvement of the anterior mitral leaflet, and (3) the observation that the leaflet pattern is the same regardless of which papillary muscle is involved. As illustrated in these diagrams, each papillary muscle gives off chordal attachments to both the anterior and posterior mitral leaflets equally. These chordae attach to both the free edges and bodies of the leaflets. Presumably, the chordal length is such that tension is normally equally distributed during systole. Echocardiographically, both papillary muscles lie in the posterior half of the left ventricle. A line, which joins their tips, runs parallel to the coaptation line of the mitral leaflets. When dyskinesis occurs at the base of either papillary muscle, the papillary muscle is displaced posteriorly relative to the coaptation line of the mitral leaflets and medially or laterally relative to the midportion of the leaflet body. As illustrated in Figure 17–99, the posterior displacement increases the distance from the tip of the papillary muscle to the body of the anterior leaflet, thereby resulting in increased tension in this region. The corresponding distance from the papillary muscle tip to the body of the posterior leaflet should remain relatively unchanged until the dyskinesis becomes profound. Thus, the anterior leaflet should selectively be pulled toward the cardiac apex, and its complete systolic closure should be prevented. In contrast, little additional tension is exerted on the posterior leaflet, and its closure pattern should remain relatively normal.

Applying the same reasoning to the medial or lateral component of the dyskinetic process, Figure 17–100 suggests that the maximum tension should be exerted in the central portion of the mitral leaflet. When both of these components are combined, the maximum tension should occur in the midportion of the anterior leaflet. The degree of abnormal tension in the midportion of the anterior leaflet should depend on the presence and degree of dyskinesis and should be relatively independent of the papillary muscle involved. Because of the uneven tension exerted on the anterior and posterior leaflets, the anterior mitral leaflet should be involved uniformly, whereas posterior leaflet involvement is expected only with more severe degrees of dyskinesis. With generalized left ventricular dilation, symmetric and

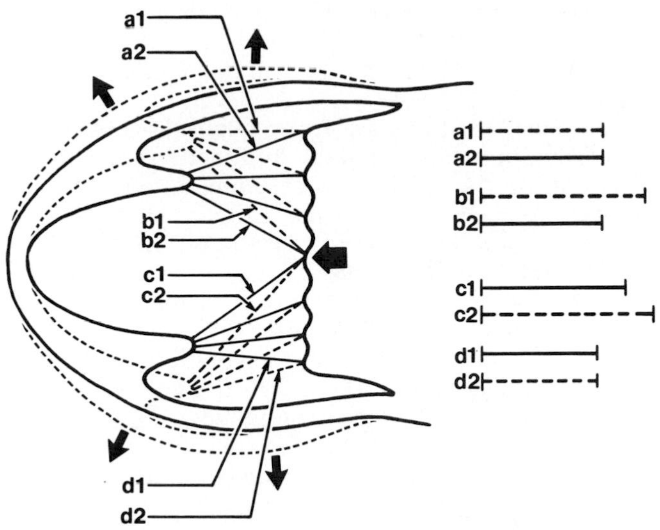

Fig. 17–100. The two papillary muscles and a mitral leaflet viewed from above. This diagram illustrates the effects of the medial or lateral component of dyskinesis at the base of either papillary muscle on the mitral leaflet. The solid lines illustrate the normal papillary muscle-chordal-leaflet orientation, whereas the interrupted lines illustrate the dyskinetic orientation. Dyskinesis of either papillary muscle results in the exertion of maximum tension in the midportion of the mitral leaflet (b1 vs. b2 and c1 vs. c2). The lateral margins of the leaflet, in contrast, are subjected to little increase in tension (a1 vs. a2 and d1 vs. d2). This medial lateral component, combined with the posterior component described in Figure 17–99, suggests that the increased tension produced by the dyskinetic process, irrespective of the papillary muscle involved, should always affect the midportion of the body of the anterior mitral leaflet.

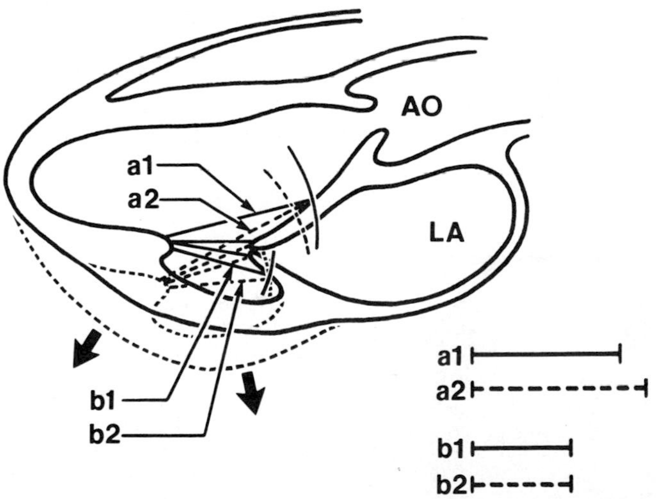

Fig. 17–99. The relative effects of the posterior component of the dyskinetic motion of the left ventricle at the base of the papillary muscles on the anterior and posterior mitral leaflets. The solid lines illustrate the normal relationship of the papillary muscles and chordae to the leaflets. The interrupted lines illustrate the relationship occurring with dyskinesis. The distance from the papillary muscle to the body of the anterior leaflet (a1 vs. a2) increases more than the distance to either the tip or body of the posterior leaflet (b1 vs. b2). AO = aorta; LA = left atrium.

additive tension on both leaflets may displace them into the left ventricular cavity; however, any disproportion in tension always affects the anterior leaflet preferentially.

Although these observations explain the leaflet position found in papillary muscle dysfunction, they do not fully explain the mechanism of regurgitation. Although the apical displacement of the leaflet(s) should reduce the leaflet area available for coaptation, this would be insufficient in itself to cause valvular regurgitation. Presumably, other factors such as ventricular, atrial, and annular dilatation further decrease the area available for coaptation and increase the tension on the chordae until failure of effective closure occurs at some point along the leaflet margin.[282] Once regurgitation is initiated, this can then begin a vicious cycle, with the increased volume load leading to increased chamber and annular size and chordal tension, which in turn leads to further regurgitation.

Although mitral valve prolapse has also been suggested as a mechanism underlying insufficiency in some patients with papillary muscle dysfunction,[279] in our experience, prolapse arising de novo in these patients is virtually always caused by rupture of one or more chordae tendineae.

Ruptured Chordae Tendineae

The most common cause of acute severe mitral insufficiency is ruptured chordae tendineae. Chordal rupture may occur in the absence of underlying disease or may be secondary to rheumatic heart disease, bacterial endocarditis, mitral valve prolapse, connective tissue disorders, myocardial infarction, idiopathic hypertrophic subaortic stenosis (IHSS), and trauma. Patients with spontaneous rupture most often have posterior leaflet involvement, whereas chordal rupture secondary to other disorders apparently involves the anterior and posterior leaflets equally.[283–285]

The echocardiographic pattern of chordal rupture varies depending on the degree of loss of leaflet support. In mild cases, this pattern may take the form of exaggerated mitral prolapse, whereas in more severe cases, flail mitral leaflet may be present.[190,286,287] In some instances, the chordae themselves can be seen flying wildly about the left ventricular cavity. When the disrupted chordae cannot be visualized directly, the diagnosis rests on the pattern of leaflet motion. Marked leaflet abnormalities, such as the flail leaflet (see following discussion), imply chordal or papillary muscle rupture. Less dramatic leaflet abnormalities, however, such as the development or extension of mitral prolapse, require that the presence of chordal rupture be inferred from the clinical situation. When chordal rupture is associated with marked insufficiency of the mitral valve, the associated increase in heart rate and left ventricular stroke volume also draw attention to the leaflet abnormality.

Papillary Muscle Rupture

Papillary muscle rupture is a rare complication of acute myocardial infarction, being found in 0.9% of fatal infarcts examined at necropsy.[288] Rupture of the posteromedial papillary muscle is 2.5 times more common than that of the anterolateral papillary muscle as a result of its single blood supply from the posterior descending coronary artery.[134] Rupture usually occurs during the second or third day after infarction but may occur later.

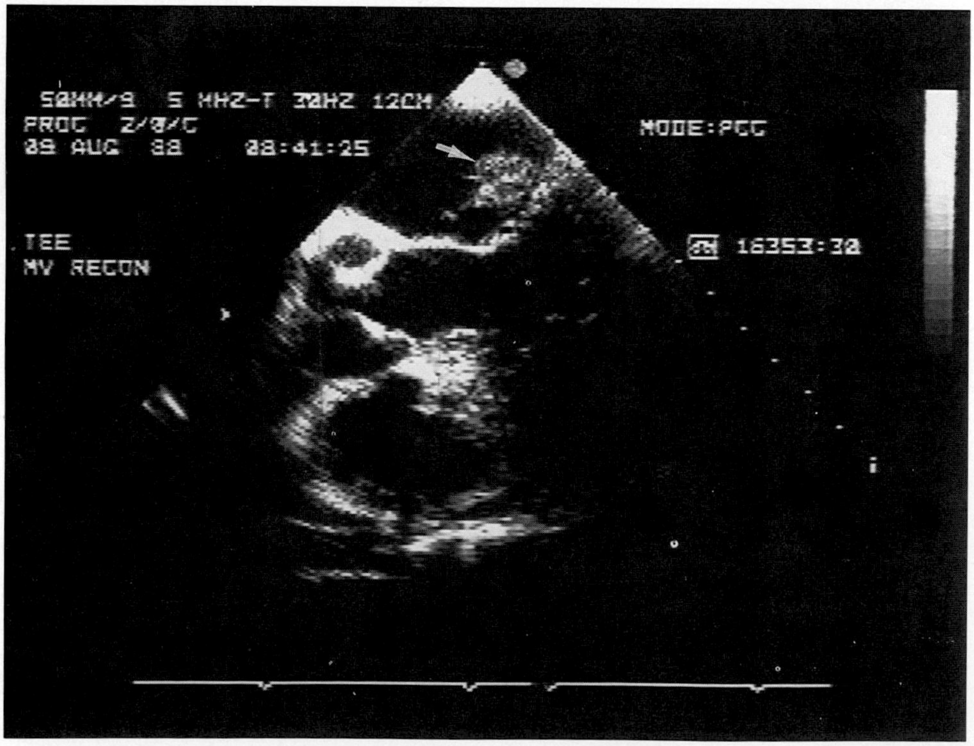

Fig. 17–101. Transesophageal echocardiogram from a patient with a ruptured head of the anterolateral papillary muscle. The papillary muscle head with attached chordae appears as a circular mass (arrow) in the left atrium behind the closed mitral leaflets during ventricular systole.

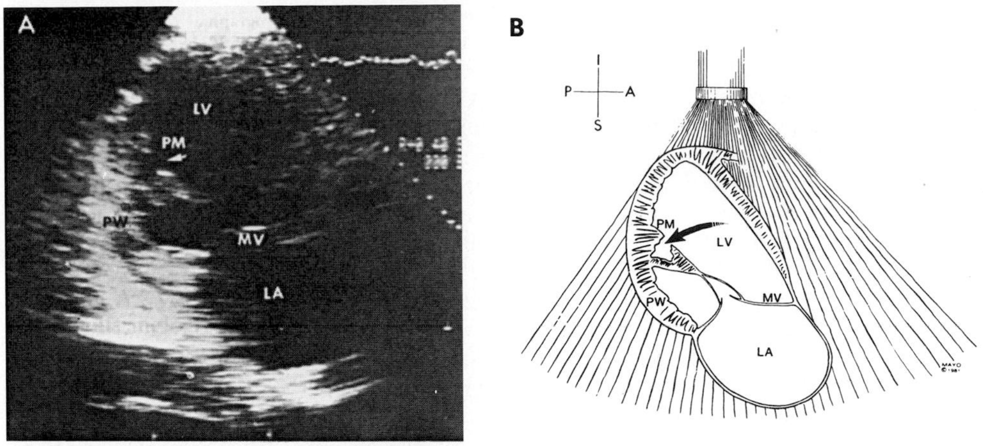

Fig. 17–102. **A.** Apical view showing partial rupture (arrow) of the posteromedial papillary muscle (PM). **B.** Schematic diagram of the same structures. PW, posterior wall; LV, left ventricle; LA, left atrium; MV, mitral valve. (From Nishimura RA, Shub C, Tajik AJ: Two dimensional echocardiographic diagnosis of partial papillary muscle rupture. Br Heart J 48:599, 1982.

Rupture is associated with acute severe mitral regurgitation with death occurring within 24 hours in 50% of patients.[288] Two-dimensional imaging can rapidly display the detached papillary muscle head swinging freely from its remaining chordae in parallel with the motion of blood from the atrium to the ventricle.[289,290] Often the papillary muscle head becomes knotted in the chordae, and its distance from the leaflet tips appears shorter than that observed in situ (Fig. 17–101). The portion of the mitral leaflet usually supported by the affected papillary muscle is typically flail. Severe mitral regurgitation can be demonstrated by Doppler techniques.

Partial papillary muscle rupture has also been observed.[291] Figure 17–102 demonstrates partial rupture of the trunk of the posteromedial papillary muscle with normal coaptation of the mitral leaflets. This partial rupture was followed by complete rupture several days later, suggesting that in some cases this process may occur in stages and that partial rupture is a harbinger of complete rupture.[291]

Flail Mitral Leaflet

Flail mitral leaflet is the most severe form of mitral leaflet motion disturbance that results from disruption of the supporting apparatus (chordae tendineae and/or papillary muscles). The flail motion of the mitral leaflets is most prominent in a plane parallel to the long axis of the left ventricle and left atrium and, thus, can be best visualized in the parasternal long axis, apical long axis, or apical four-chamber views. Because only a portion of the mitral leaflet may be flail, the scan plane must be swept from one margin of the mitral orifice to the other so that a localized area of distorted leaflet motion is not overlooked.

A flail valve is characterized by a whipping motion of the tip of the affected leaflet through a 180° or greater arc about its point of annular attachment.[286,287] This motion has been compared to that of a detached sail in the wind. During diastole, the leaflet tip points into the left ventricular cavity, and the leaflet body is concave toward the left ventricle. With the onset of systole, the leaflet is thrust upward into the left atrium. The leaflet tip completely reverses its direction and points toward the left atrium. The body of the leaflet, therefore, is concave toward the left atrium or superiorly. This pattern is in contrast to the prolapsing leaflet in which the leaflet body always remains concave toward the left ventricle. Normal systolic coaptation of the anterior and posterior leaflets is lost, and a clearly defined separation between these leaflets in both the parasternal long axis and apical four chamber views can usually be determined. Figure 17–103 is an example of a flail posterior mitral leaflet. When the loss of leaflet support is caused by bacterial endocarditis, an increase in echo production from the free edges of the ruptured chordae and leaflet tips is frequently noted (see Fig. 37–17).

Mitral Valve Vegetations

Valvular vegetations are the characteristic lesions of bacterial endocarditis. These vegetations are friable, verrucous masses composed of clumps of bacteria or fungi, platelets, fibrin, white blood cells, red blood cells,

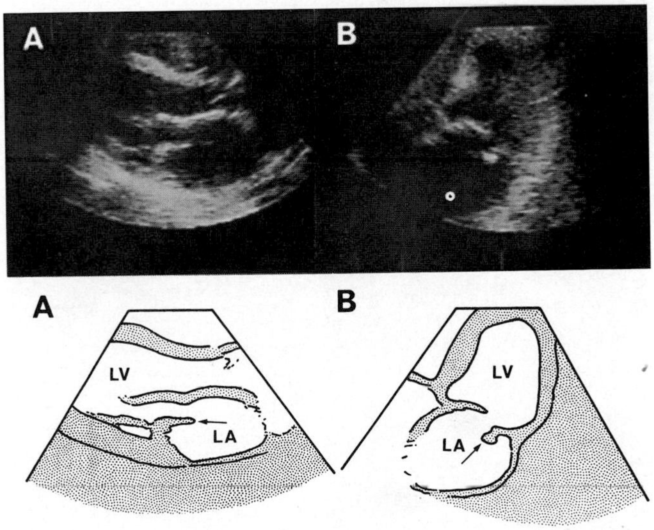

Fig. 17–103. Parasternal long axis and apical four-chamber systolic recordings from a patient with a flail posterior mitral leaflet. The free leaflet tip is directed toward the left atrium (LA), and the body of the leaflet is concave superiorly toward the atrium. The leaflet tip is indicated by the arrows in each diagram. LV = left ventricle.

and varying amounts of necrotic tissue. They are usually located in areas previously altered by rheumatic, congenital, or syphilitic cardiac lesions but may be found on apparently normal surfaces. The vegetative lesion is usually attached to a broad-based area of degenerated valvular tissue. Vegetations may assume a variety of sizes and shapes, varying from small, flat, granular lesions to large, fungating, friable masses. Vegetations may erode and disrupt the valve leaflets and adjacent structures or, when large, may obstruct flow through the valve. Pieces of the vegetation may dislodge, resulting in peripheral emboli. Healing is initiated by the invasion of polymorphonuclear leukocytes, and eventually, the infecting organisms disappear. Fibroblasts infiltrate the area, and the vegetations may become hyalinized and may even calcify. The remnant of the vegetation is then finally covered with a layer of endothelium.[292]

Vegetations appear on the echogram as an irregular mass of echoes that is usually attached to a valve leaflet and moves in concert with that leaflet.[293] When the vegetations are small, they may appear as no more than an irregular lump or bump in the leaflet, most commonly toward the tip. In other patients, the vegetations may be attached to the leaflet by a stalk, or a portion of the vegetation may be more loosely supported and more freely moving (Fig. 17–104). When such situations occur, the corresponding echoes are highly mobile and more easily identified because of this mobility. Vegetations are more prominent when they are large or associated with damage to the valvular structures. The classic features and implications of the vegetations that are the hallmark of bacterial endocarditis are discussed in Chapter 37. Nonbacterial vegetation may also be recorded. For example, Figure 17–105 is a long axis, cross-sectional recording of a patient with verrucous endocarditis with a rim of small vegetations along the ventricular margins of both the anterior and posterior mitral leaflets. These vegetations appear as a focal accumulation of echoes along the leaflet margins (vertical arrows). Figure 17–106 is a pathologic specimen from the same patient illustrating the gross appearance of these vegetations and the correspondence of their location to the increase in echo production in the clinical recording.

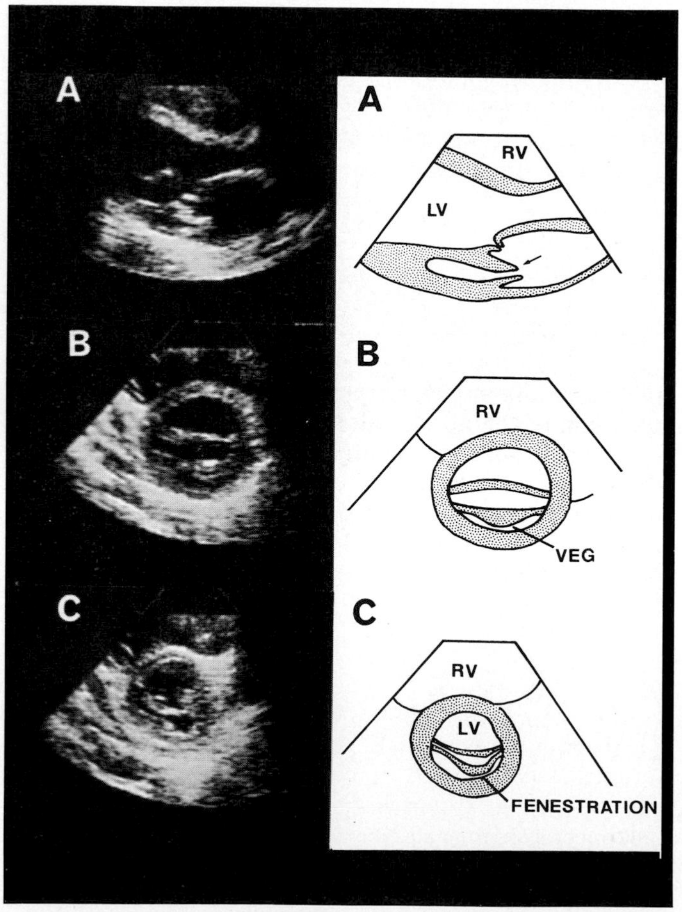

Fig. 17–104. **A.** Parasternal long axis recording of a vegetative lesion of the posterior mitral leaflet with a fenestration in the leaflet body (arrow in accompanying diagram). **B.** Short axis recording with the circumferential location of the vegetation (VEG) indicated at the tip of the arrow in the diagram. **C.** Short axis systolic recording illustrates the fenestration through the valve leaflet caused by the disruptive infectious process. RV = right ventricle; LV = left ventricle.

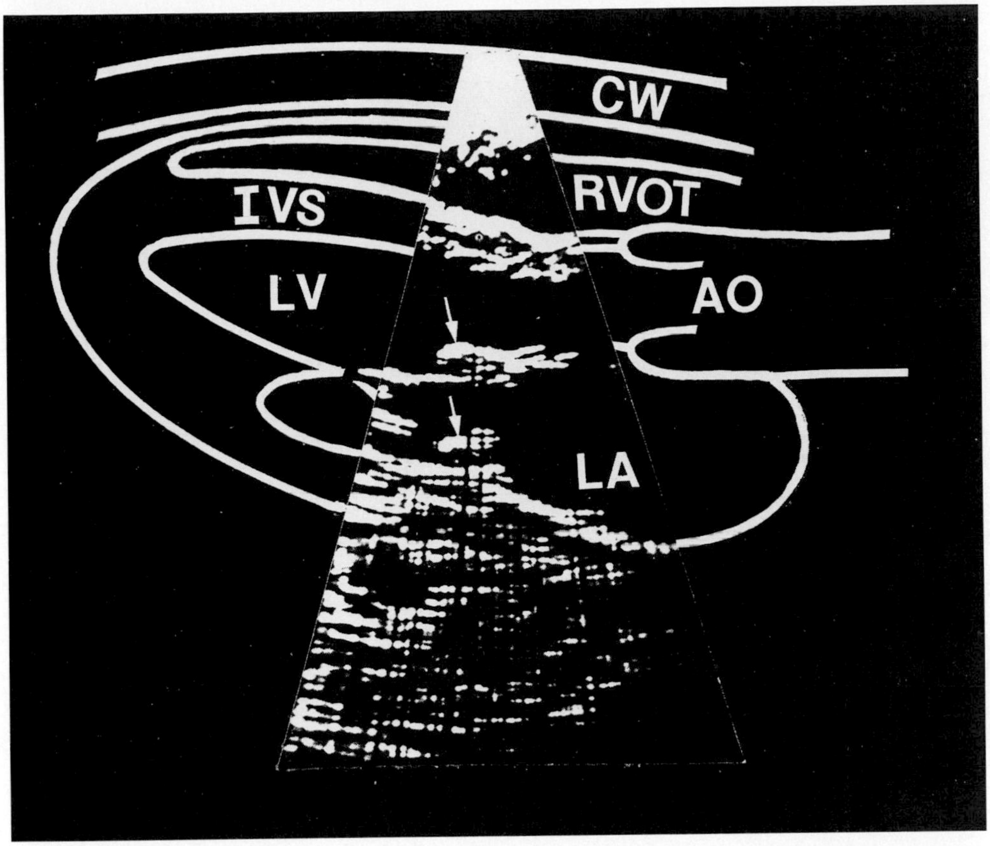

Fig. 17–105. Long axis parasternal recording of the mitral leaflets from a patient with verrucous endocarditis (Libman-Sacks endocarditis). The vegetations appear as focal accumulations of echoes on the ventricular surfaces of the anterior and posterior leaflets (arrows). CW = chest wall; RVOT = right ventricular outflow tract; IVS = interventricular septum; LV = left ventricle; AO = aorta; LA = left atrium.

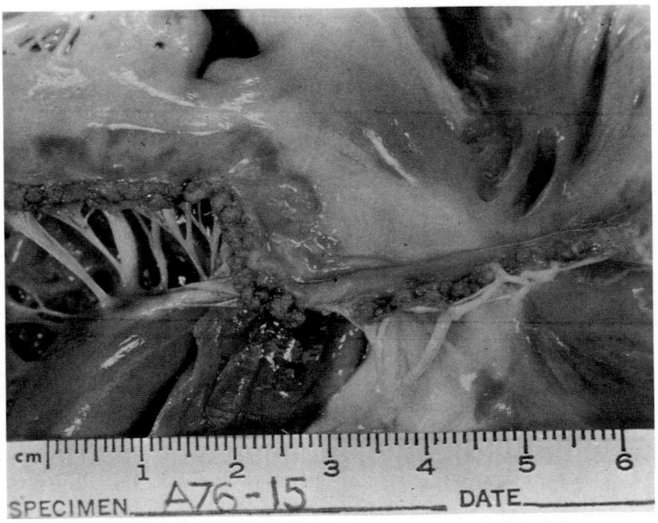

Fig. 17–106. Gross specimen from the same patient as in Figure 17–105 indicates the small, warty vegetations along the margins of the leaflets.

STRUCTURAL ABNORMALITIES OF LEAFLETS OR SUPPORTING STRUCTURES

Mitral Valve Aneurysms

Mitral valve aneurysms are uncommon lesions that occur in association with infective endocarditis of the aortic and mitral valves.[294–300] The aneurysm(s) may be single or multiple and although involving the anterior leaflet most commonly may also arise from the posterior leaflet. The primary site of infection in patients with mitral valve aneurysm is typically the aortic valve. Destruction of the aortic valve leaflets produces aortic insufficiency, and the regurgitant jet is thought to strike the anterior leaflet of the mitral valve producing a jet lesion and associated secondary infection. The mitral infection then leads to the development of the aneurysm. Mitral regurgitation in these patients can result from perforation of the aneurysm or valve leaflet, rupture of infected chordae tendineae, associated disease of the mitral valve such as mitral valve prolapse, or rheumatic mitral valve disease.

The aneurysm typically appears as a localized bulge arising from the mitral leaflet and extending for a variable distance (up to several centimeters) into the left atrium during ventricular systole (Fig. 17–107).[301,302] Such a bulge is typically larger in systole than diastole, but in contrast to prolapse or a flail leaflet, the bulge generally persists throughout the cardiac cycle. The an-

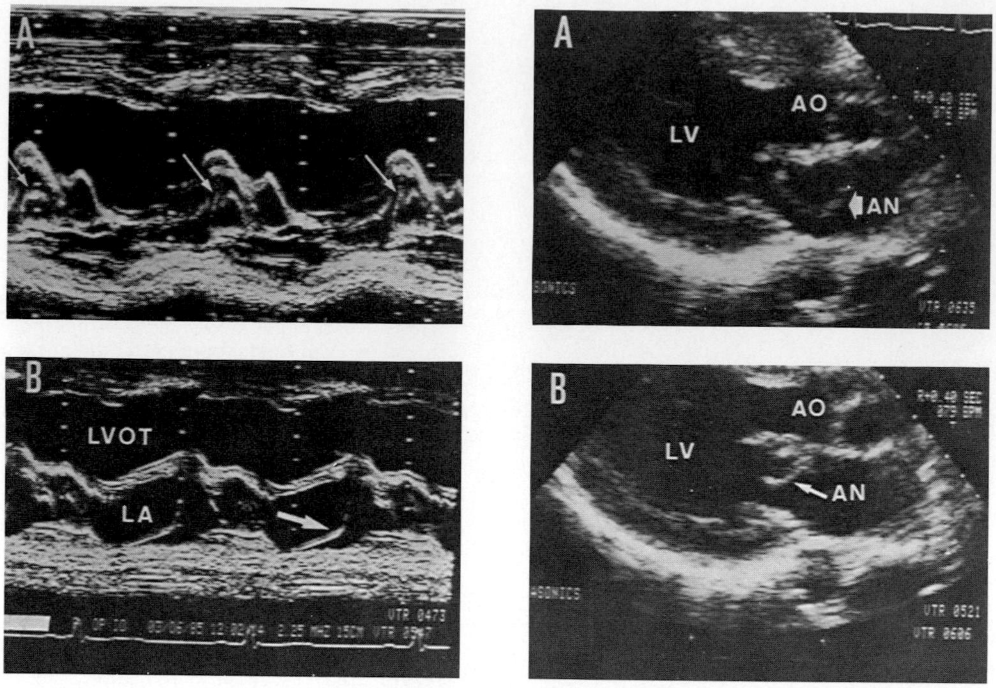

Fig. 17–107. M-mode and two dimensional echocardiographic recordings from a patient with a large mitral leaflet aneurysm. **A.** Left. M-mode recording at the level of the mitral valve illustrating the mobile aneurysm prolapsing through the mitral leaflets during diastole. Right. Parasternal long-axis recording illustrating the aneurysm displaced into the left atrial cavity during systole. **B.** Left. M-mode echocardiogram depicting the linear echo from the posterior margin of the aneurysm in the left atrial cavity during ventricular systole and its motion toward the ventricle during diastole. Right. Parasternal long axis recording of the mitral valve during diastole with the free edge of the aneurysm displaced into the mitral valve orifice. AO = aorta; LV = left ventricle; AN = aneurysm; LVOT = left ventricular outflow tract; the arrow in each illustration points to the aneurysm. (From Oquendo I, et al.: Mitral valve aneurysm: M-mode and 2-dimensional echocardiographic features. Texas Heart Inst J 14:312, 1987.)

eurysm typically moves with the affected leaflet; however, a portion of the aneurysm may become adherent to the atrial wall, limiting mobility.

In patients being considered for acute aortic valve replacement, early preoperative recognition of these aneurysms is important because (1) they may rupture acutely and produce catastrophic mitral regurgitation in an already seriously ill patient, or (2) they may be overlooked at the time of aortic valve replacement and lead to mitral regurgitation at a later time.

False Aneurysm of the Mitral-Aortic Intervalvular Fibrosa

False aneurysm of the mitral-aortic intervalvular fibrosa may also occur as a complication of aortic valve infective endocarditis.[303] The intervalvular fibrosa attaches to the aortic root and to the anterior leaflet of the mitral valve. Perforation from infection in this region can cause an aneurysm to develop in the epicardial tissue between the aorta and the left atrium, which is in direct communication with the pericardial space. As a result, these aneurysms can rupture, causing death, develop thrombi with secondary systemic embolization, and/or cause detachment of the aortic or mitral valve(s).[303,304] These aneurysms present echocardiographically as saccular echo-free spaces between the posterior aortic root and left atrium and can extend to the superior border of the left atrium. They are typically in contact with the left ventricle and therefore expand during systole and contract during diastole.[305] Figure 17–108 is an example of such an aneurysm.

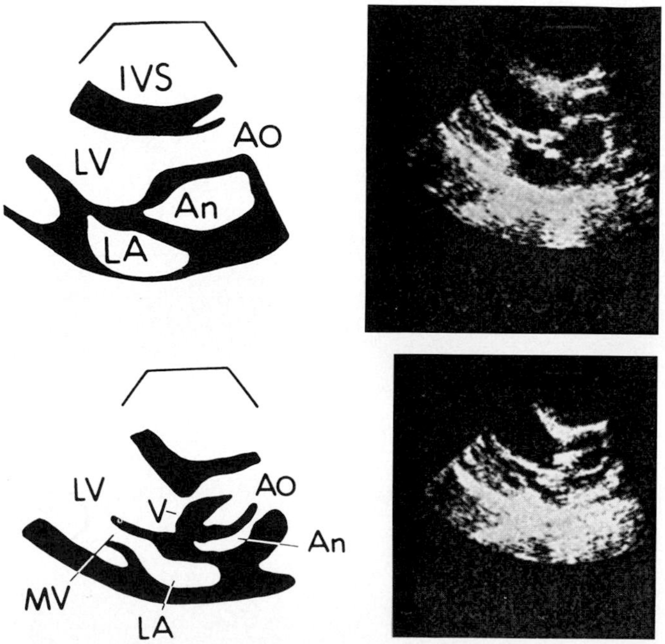

Fig. 17–108. False aneurysm of the intervalvular fibrosa. Top. A systolic recording showing systolic expansion of the aneurysm. Bottom. A diastolic recording in which the aneurysm is partially collapsed. IVS = interventricular septum; Ao = aorta; LV = left ventricle; An = aneurysm; LA = left atrium; V = aortic valve; MV = mitral valve. (From Reid CL, et al.: False aneurysm of mitral-aortic intervalvular fibrosa: diagnosis by 2-dimensional contrast echocardiography at cardiac catheterization. Am J Cardiol 51: 1801, 1983. Used with permission of Cahners Publishing Co.)

Mitral Annular Calcification

Mitral annular calcification is a degenerative disorder that occurs in elderly people and is characterized by calcium deposition in the mitral annular region or in the angular space between the posterior mitral leaflet and the subjacent left ventricular posterior wall. This disorder may be associated with mitral insufficiency, conduction abnormalities, congestive heart failure, endocarditis, and when extremely severe, obstruction to left ventricular inflow.[134,306–309]

Cross-sectional echocardiography appears to be a sensitive method for detecting the presence of calcium in the region of the mitral annulus and may be more specific than radiographic studies in differentiating this type of calcification from that involving the mitral leaflets.[310] Although the term *mitral annular calcification* is commonly used, one cannot differentiate true calcification from dense sclerosis by echocardiography.

The presence of mitral annular calcification is indicated on the echogram by a dense localized, highly reflective area at the base of the posterior mitral leaflet.[310] This echogenic area may be small and discrete or may extend to involve the entire annular region and posterior mitral leaflet, thereby making discrete leaflet visualization impossible. Calcification of the posterior mitral annulus occurs approximately five times as frequently as calcification of the anterior portion of the annulus.[310] Mitral annular calcification, when present, may be combined with aortic annular calcification. Isolated calcification of the anterior margin of the annulus is rarely observed, and involvement of the anterior annulus generally results from medial and/or lateral extension around the annular circumference in severely involved cases. Figure 17–109 is a recording of a patient with calcification of the posterior margin of the mitral annulus. This area of increased reflectivity can be observed in each of the standard views and is confined to the posterior margins of the annulus at approximately the six-o'clock position. Figure 17–110, in contrast, is a recording of a patient with massive calcification involving both the anterior and posterior margins of the mitral annulus and the aortic root. In this example, visualization of the mitral leaflets is difficult. Moderate-to-severe degrees of annular calcification located along the medial border of the annulus—near the conduction system—appear to be more commonly associated with conduction disturbances, especially intraventricular conduction delay, than calcification involving other regions of the annulus.[311] Bacterial vegetations may also be superimposed on regions of annular calcification. In these cases, identification of the vegetation is based on independent motion of a portion of the infected mass and a high degree of clinical suspicion.[312]

Nonrheumatic Fibrosis and Calcification of the Chordae and Papillary Muscles

Although far less common than annular calcification, nonrheumatic fibrosis and calcification of the chordae and papillary muscles may also be recorded echocardiographically. The fibrotic/calcified chordae appear as dense, generally mobile, echoes within the body of the left ventricle extending from the free leaflet tips to the insertion point of the papillary muscle base into the left ventricular wall (Fig. 17–110). The extent and density of the fibrosis/calcification is variable and may involve one or both papillary muscle-chordal complexes. These changes appear to be degenerative in nature, being associated with mitral annular calcification in more than 90% of cases and with aortic annular calcification in the majority.[313] No specific cause has been defined, however, and a variety of associated disorders have been reported, including myocardial infarction, chronic renal failure,[314] hypertension, endocarditis,[315] and mitral prolapse.

The majority of patients with papillary muscle/chordal fibrosis or calcification have mitral regurgitation and a history of congestive heart failure; associated left atrial enlargement is common.

Mitral Valve Abnormalities Associated With Coarctation of the Aorta

Coarctation of the aorta is frequently associated with other cardiac malformations, including ventricular and atrial septal defects, patent ductus arteriosus, and left ventricular inflow and outflow tract lesions. The reported incidence of mitral valve disease associated with coarctation varies from 26 to 58% in autopsy se-

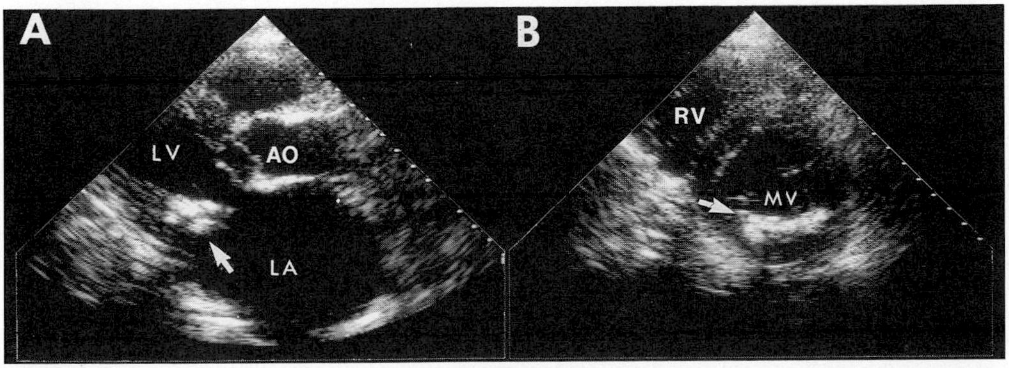

Fig. 17–109. Parasternal long **(A)** and short axis **(B)** recordings from a patient with posterior mitral annular calcification. The area of calcification (arrow) presents as a high-intensity globular collection of echoes in the region of the aortic annulus and myocardium immediately subjacent to the posterior mitral leaflet. In short axis, a 3-cm bar of calcium (arrow) can be appreciated extending from the medial to lateral posterior margins of the annulus. MV = mitral valve; AO = aorta; LV = left ventricle; LA = left atrium; RV = right ventricle.

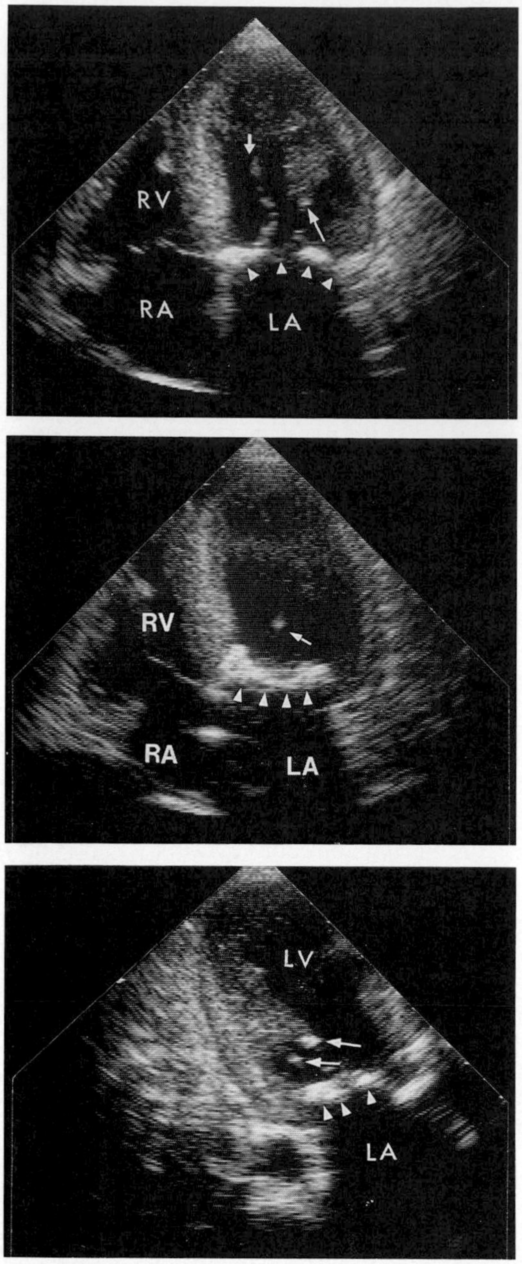

Fig. 17–110. Top. Apical four-chamber view from a patient with more extensive annular calcification involving both the medial and the lateral portions of the annulus (arrowheads). Fibrosis of the tip of the papillary muscle is also indicated by the long vertical arrow. Middle. Depressed apical four-chamber view illustrating the posterior extent of the calcification, which involves the full expanse of the annulus (arrowheads). Fibrotic/calcified papillary muscle tip is again evident (small arrow). Bottom. Apical long axis view indicating the interior extension of the annular calcification (arrowheads) with calcification of both tips (small arrows) of the anterolateral papillary muscle. LV = left ventricle; RV = right ventricle; LA = left atrium; RA = right atrium; arrowheads indicate areas of calcification; arrows with shafts point to calcified papillary muscle tips.

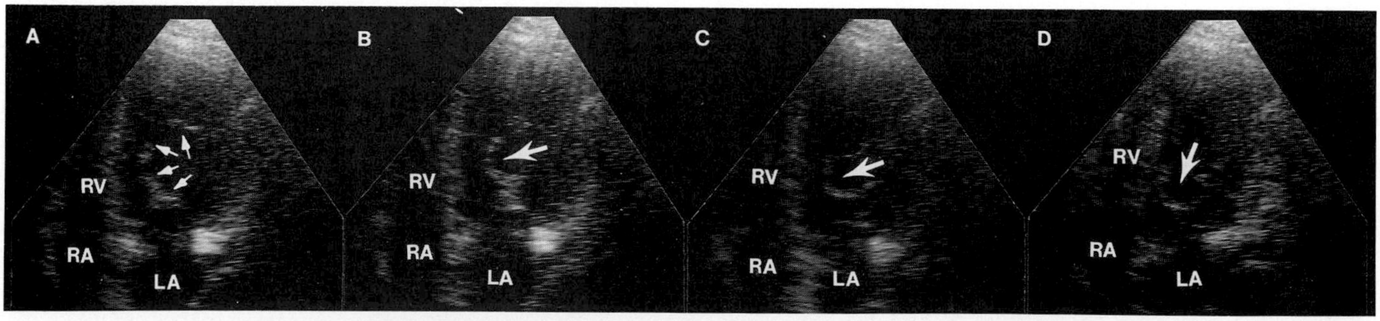

Fig. 17–111. **A** to **D.** Apical four-chamber recordings of the mitral valve in a patient with coarctation of the aorta. During late diastole (A and B), the chordae tendineae are elongated, thickened, and matted. During systole (C and D), (arrows) the chords (arrow) are displaced into the outflow tract (arrows) by the ejected blood, causing partial obstruction to left ventricular outflow. RV = right ventricle; RA = right atrium; LA = left atrium.

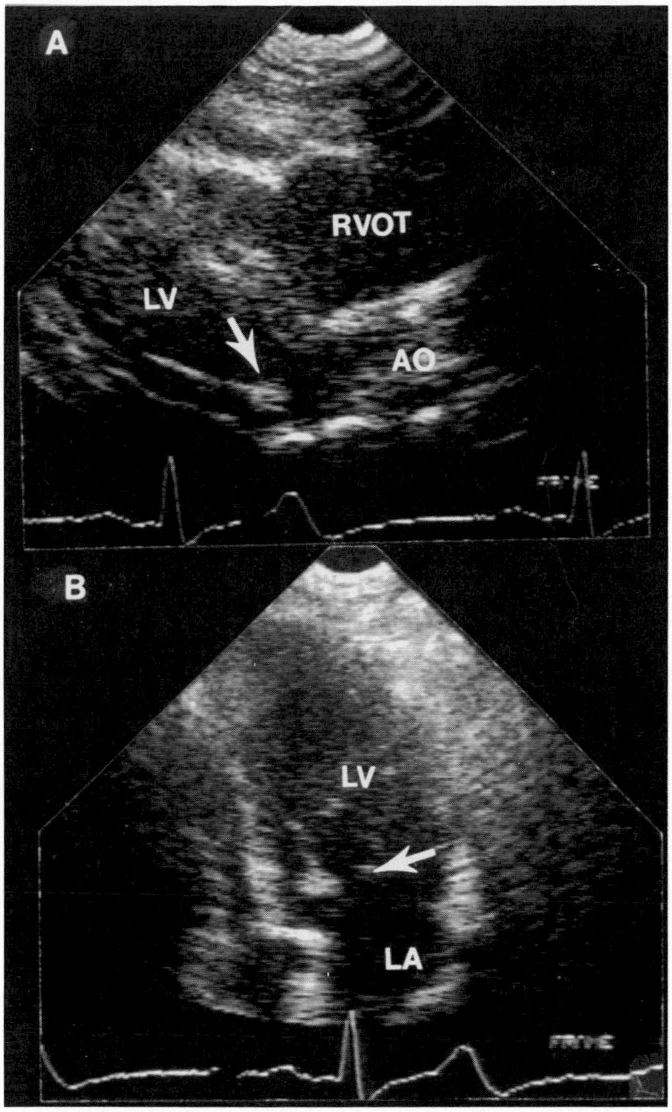

Fig. 17–112. **A.** Parasternal long axis recording illustrating a small mass (myxoma) arising from one of the chordae tendineae and prolapsing into the left ventricular outflow tract during ventricular systole. **B.** Apical five-chamber recording illustrating the myxoma (arrow) immediately beneath the aortic valve. RVOT = right ventricular outflow tract; LV = left ventricle; AO = aorta; LA = left atrium.

ries.[316–318] Anomalies of the mitral valve that are readily detectable echocardiographically include cleft mitral valve in association with endocardial cushion defects; congenital mitral stenosis that is due to supravalvar ring; congenital valvar mitral stenosis; anomalies of papillary muscle location, size, and number; parachute mitral valve; anomalous chordal attachments (e.g., from the anterior mitral leaflet to the septum); chordal redundancy; and mitral valve prolapse.

Figure 17–111 is an example of a patient with elongated thickened matted chordae tendineae detected a number of years after primary coarctation repair as a child. The redundant chords and mitral leaflet billow into the left ventricular outflow tract during systole, causing functional subvalvular obstruction. On the M-mode recording, the leaflet appearance was similar to that seen in IHSS; however, there was no septal hypertrophy.

Leaflet and Chordal Tumors

Tumors, usually benign, can arise from any of the cell types found in the mitral leaflet or supporting chordal structures. The most common are the myxoma, fibroma, and fibroelastoma. Figure 17–112 is an example of a primary chordal myxoma that presented as a harsh outflow murmur of varying intensity. The tumor in this case prolapsed into the outflow tract during systole and at catheterization was associated with intermittent outflow obstruction.

REFERENCES

1. Edler I, Hertz C: Use of ultrasonic reflectoscope for the continuous recording of movements of heart walls. Kung Fysiograf Sallsk Lund Fordhandl 24:40, 1954.
2. Edler I: The diagnostic use of ultrasound in heart disease. Acta Med Scand (Suppl) 308:32, 1955.
3. Edler I: Ultrasound cardiogram in mitral valve disease. Acta Chir Scand 3:230, 1956.
4. Edler I, Gustafson A: Ultrasonic cardiogram in mitral stenosis. Acta Med Scand 159:85, 1957.
5. Rusted IE, Schiefley CH, Edwards JE: Studies of the mitral valve: I. Anatomic features of the normal mitral valve and associated structures. Circulation 6:825, 1952.
6. Chiechi MA, Lees WM, Thompson R: Functional anatomy of the normal mitral valve. J Thorac Surg 32:378, 1956.
7. Silverman ME, Hurst JW: The mitral complex. Am Heart J 76:399, 1968.
8. Lam JHC, Ranganathan N, Wigle ED, Silver MD: Morphology of the human mitral valve: I. Chordae tendineae: a new classification. Circulation 41:449, 1970.
9. Ranganathan N, Lam JHC, Wigle ED, Silver MD: Morphology of the human mitral valve: II. The valve leaflets. Circulation 41:459, 1970.
10. Ranganathan N, Silver MD, Wigle ED: Recent knowledge of the anatomy of the mitral valve. *In* Kalmanson D (ed.): The Mitral Valve. Acton, MA: Publishing Sciences Group, 1976.
11. Ranganathan N, Burch GE: Gross morphology and arterial supply of the papillary muscles of the left ventricle of man. Am Heart J 77:506, 1969.
12. Rider CF, Taylor DEM, Wade JD: The effect of papillary muscle damage on atrioventricular valve function in the left heart. Q J Exp Physiol 50:15, 1965.
13. Tsakiris AG, Rastelli GC, Amorim D: Effects of experimental papillary muscle damage on mitral valve closure in intact anesthetized dogs. Mayo Clin Proc 45:275, 1970.
14. Griffith JM, Henry WL: A sector scanner for real-time two-dimensional echocardiography. Circulation 49:1147, 1974.
15. Roelandt J, et al.: Ultrasonic two-dimensional analysis of the mitral valve. *In* Kalmanson D (ed.): The Mitral Valve. Acton, MA, Publishing Sciences Group, 1976.
16. Henry WL, et al.: Measurement of mitral orifice area in patients with mitral valve disease by real-time two-dimensional echocardiography. Circulation 51:827, 1975.
17. Silverman NH, Schiller NB: Apex echocardiography: a two-dimensional technique for evaluating congenital heart disease. Circulation 57:503, 1978.
18. Nolan SP: The normal mitral valve. Patterns of instantaneous mitral valve flow and the atrial contribution to ventricular filling. *In* Kalmanson D (ed.): The Mitral Valve. Acton, MA: Publishing Sciences Group, 1976.
19. Konecke L, Feigenbaum H, Chang S: Abnormal mitral valve motion in patients with elevated left ventricular end diastolic pressure. Circulation 47:989, 1973.
20. Lewis JR, Parker JO, Burggraf GW: Mitral valve motion and changes in left ventricular end-diastolic pressure: a correlative study of the PR-AC Interval. Am J Cardiol 42:383, 1978.
21. Zaky A, Nasser WK, Feigenbaum H: A study of mitral action recorded by reflected ultrasound and its application in the diagnosis of mitral stenosis. Circulation 37:789, 1968.
22. Bellhouse BJ: Fluid mechanics of a model mitral valve and left ventricle. Cardiovasc Res 6:199, 1972.
23. Laniado S, et al.: A study of the dynamic relations between the mitral valve echogram and phasic mitral flow. Circulation 51:104, 1975.
24. DeMaria AN, et al.: Mitral valve early diastolic closing velocity in the echocardiogram: relation to sequential diastolic flow and ventricular compliance. Am J Cardiol 37:693, 1976.

25. Zaky A, Grabhorn L, Feigenbaum H: Movement of the mitral ring. A study of ultrasound cardiography. Cardiovasc Res 1:121, 1967.
26. Quinones MA, Gaasch WH, Waisser E, Alexander J: Reduction in the rate of diastolic descent of the mitral valve echogram in patients with altered left ventricular diastolic pressure-volume relations. Circulation 49:246, 1974.
27. Massie BM, Schiller NB, Ratshin RA, Parmley WW: Mitral-septal separation: new echocardiographic index of left ventricular function. Am J Cardiol 39:1008, 1977.
28. Pohost GM, et al.: The echocardiogram of the anterior leaflet of the mitral valve: correlation with hemodynamic and cineroentgenographic studies in dogs. Circulation 51:88, 1975.
29. Rasmussen S, et al.: Stroke volume calculated from the mitral valve echogram in patients with and without ventricular dyssynergy. Circulation 58: 125, 1978.
30. Tsakiris AG, Gordon DA, Mathieu Y, Lipton I: Motion of both mitral valve leaflets: a cineroentgenographic study in intact dogs. J Appl Physiol 39:359, 1975.
31. Rushmer RF, Finlayson BL, Nash AA: Movements of the mitral valve. Circ Res 4:337, 1956.
32. Taylor DE, Wade JE: The pattern of flow around the atrioventricular valves during diastolic ventricular filling. J Physiol 207:71, 1970.
33. Taylor DE, Wade JE: Patterns of blood flow within the heart: a stable system. Cardiovasc Res 7:14, 1973.
34. Keren G, et al.: Interrelationship of mid-diastolic mitral valve motion, pulmonary venous flow, and transmitral flow. Circulation 74:36, 1986.
35. Zaky A, Steinmetz E, Feigenbaum H: Role of the atrium in closure of mitral valve in man. Am J Physiol 217:1652, 1969.
36. Pridie RB, Beham R, Oakley CM: Echocardiography of the mitral valve in aortic valve disease. Br Heart J 33:296, 1971.
37. Mann T, McLaurin L, Grossman W, Craige E: Assessing the hemodynamic severity of acute aortic regurgitation due to infective endocarditis. N Engl J Med 293:108, 1975.
38. Botvinick EH, et al.: Echocardiographic demonstration of early mitral valve closure in severe aortic insufficiency. Its clinical implications. Circulation 51:836, 1975.
39. Massie BM, Schiller NB, Ratshin RA, Parmley WW: Mitral-septal separation: new echocardiographic index of left ventricular function. Am J Cardiol 39:1008, 1977.
40. Courtois M, Kovacs SJ, Ludbrook PA: Transmitral pressure-flow velocity relation: importance of regional pressure gradients in the left ventricle during diastole. Circulation 78:661, 1988.
41. Choong CYP, Herrmann HC, Weyman AE, Fifer MA: Preload dependence of Doppler-derived indices of left ventricular diastolic function in humans. J Am Coll Cardiol 10:800, 1987.
42. Stoddard MF, et al.: Influence of alteration in preload on the pattern of left ventricular diastolic filling as assessed by Doppler echocardiography in humans. Circulation 79:1226, 1989.
43. Choong CY, et al.: Combined influence of ventricular loading and relaxation on the transmitral flow velocity profile in dogs measured by Doppler echocardiography. Circulation 78:672, 1988.
44. Ishida Y, et al.: Left ventricular filling dynamics: influence of left ventricular relaxation and left atrial pressure. Circulation 74:187, 1986.
45. Rokey R, et al.: Determination of parameters of left ventricular diastolic filling with pulsed Doppler echocardiography: comparison with cineangiography. Circulation 71:543, 1985.
46. Thomas JD, Choong CYP, Flachskampf FA, Weyman AE: Analysis of the early transmitral Doppler velocity curve: effect of primary physiologic changes and compensatory preload adjustment. J Am Coll Cardiol 16:644, 1990.
47. Yellin EL, Nikolic S, Frater RW: Left ventricular filling dynamics and diastolic function. Prog Cardiovasc Dis 32:242, 1990.
48. Mirsky I, Pasipoularides A: Clinical assessment of diastolic function. Prog Cardiovasc Dis 32:291, 1990.
49. Flachskampf FA, Rodriguez L, Chen C, Thomas JD: Calculation of mitral inertial mass: a factor critical to extracting relaxation from Doppler filling profiles; an in vitro study (abstr). Circulation 80(Suppl 2):II-567, 1989.
50. Thomas JD, Newell JB, Choong CYP, Weyman AE: Physical and physiological determinants of transmitral velocity: numerical analysis. Am J Physiol 260 (Heart Circ Physiol 29):H1718, 1991.
51. Thomas JD: Flow in the descending aorta: a turn of the screw or a sideways glance? (Editorial comment). Circulation 82:2263, 1990.
52. Samstad A, et al.: Cross-sectional early mitral flow velocity profiles from colour Doppler. Br Heart J 62:177, 1989.
53. Pomerance A, Davies MJ: The Pathology of the Heart. London, Blackwell Scientific Publications, 1975.
54. Nichol PM, Gilbert BW, Kisslo JA: Two-dimensional echocardiographic assessment of mitral stenosis. Circulation 55:120, 1977.
55. Wann LS, et al.: Determination of mitral valve area by cross-sectional echocardiography. Ann Intern Med 88:337, 1978.
56. Martin RP, et al.: Reliability and reproducibility of two-dimensional echocardiographic measurement of the stenotic mitral valve orifice area. Am J Cardiol 43:560, 1979.
57. Weyman AE, et al.: Five-year experience in correlating cross-sectional echocardiographic assessment of the mitral valve area with hemodynamic valve area determinations (abstr). Am J Cardiol 43:386, 1979.
58. Henry WL, Kastl DG: Echocardiographic evaluation of patients with mitral stenosis. Am J Med 62:813, 1977.
59. D'Cruz I, Panetta F, Cohen H, Glick G: Submitral calcification or sclerosis in elderly patients: M-mode and two-dimensional echocardiography in "mitral anulus calcification." Am J Cardiol 44:31, 1979.
60. Segal BL, Likoff W, Kingsley B: Echocardiography: clinical application in combined mitral stenosis and mitral regurgitation. Am J Cardiol 19:42, 1967.
61. DeMaria AN, et al.: Mitral valve early diastolic closing velocity in the echocardiogram: relation to sequential diastolic flow and ventricular compliance. Am J Cardiol 37:693, 1976.
62. Segal B, Likoff W, Kingsley B: Echocardiography. Clinical application in mitral stenosis. J Am Med Assoc 195:99, 1966.
63. Gustafson A: The correlation between ultrasound cardiography, hemodynamics and surgical findings in mitral stenosis. Am J Cardiol 19:32, 1967.
64. Winters WL, et al.: Reflected ultrasound as a diagnostic instrument in study of mitral disease. Br Heart J 29:188, 1967.
65. Wharton CFP, Lopez-Bescos L: Mitral valve movement. A study using an ultrasound technique. Br Heart J 32:344, 1970.
66. Quinones MA, Gaasch WH, Waisser E, Alexander J: Reduction in the rate of diastolic descent of the mitral valve echogram in patients with altered left ventricular diastolic pressure-volume relations. Circulation 49:246, 1974.
67. Bellhouse BJ: Fluid mechanics of a model mitral valve and left ventricle. Cardiovasc Res 6:199, 1972.
68. Cope GD, Kisslo JA, Johnson ML, Behan VS: A reassessment of the echocardiogram in mitral stenosis. Circulation 52:664, 1975.
69. Levisman JA, Abbasi AS, Pierce ML: Posterior mitral leaflet motion in mitral stenosis. Circulation 51:511, 1975.
70. Shiu MF, Jenkins BS, Webb-Peploe MM: Echocardiographic analysis of posterior mitral leaflet movement in mitral stenosis. Br Heart J 40:372, 1978.
71. Dabestani A, et al.: Mitral valve A wave in mitral stenosis. J Clin Ultrasound 9:91, 1987.
72. Holen J, Aaslic R, Landmark K, Simonsen S: Determination of pressure gradients in mitral stenosis with a non-invasive ultrasound Doppler technique. Acta Med Scand 199:455, 1976.
73. Hatle L, Brubakk A, Tromsdal A, Angelsen B: Non-invasive assessment of pressure drop in mitral stenosis by Doppler ultrasound. Br Heart J 40: 131, 1978.
74. Holen J, Simonsen S: Determination of pressure gradient in mitral stenosis with Doppler echocardiography. Br Heart J 41:529, 1979.
75. Kawahara T, et al.: Application of Doppler color flow imaging to determine valve area in mitral stenosis. J Am Coll Cardiol 18:85, 1991.
76. Monterroso VH, et al.: Estimation of mitral valve area by color Doppler flow mapping. Circulation 80 (Suppl 2):II-167, 1989.
77. Robson DJ, Flaxman JC: Measurement of the end-diastolic pressure gradient and mitral valve area in mitral stenosis by Doppler ultrasound. Eur Heart J 5:660, 1984.
78. Nakatani S, et al.: Value and limitations of Doppler echocardiography in the quantification of stenotic mitral valve area: comparison of the pressure half-time and continuity equation methods. Circulation 77:78, 1988.
79. Rodriguez L, et al.: Validation of the proximal flow convergence method: calculation of orifice area in patients with mitral stenosis. Circulation, in press.
80. Libanoff AJ, Rodbard S: Evaluation of the severity of mitral stenosis and regurgitation. Circulation 33:218, 1966.
81. Libanoff AJ, Rodbard S: Atrioventricular pressure half-time: measure of mitral valve area. Circulation 38:144, 1968.
82. Hatle L, Angelsen B, Tromsdal A: Noninvasive assessment of atrioventricular pressure half-time by Doppler ultrasound. Circulation 60:1096, 1979.
83. Hatle L, Angelsen B: Doppler Ultrasound in cardiology: physical principles and clinical applications. Philadelphia, Lea & Febiger, p. 83, 1982.
84. Stamm RB, Martin RP: Quantification of pressure gradients across stenotic valves by Doppler ultrasound. J Am Coll Cardiol 2:707, 1983.
85. Byrg RJ, et al.: Effect of atrial fibrillation and mitral regurgitation on calculated mitral valve area in mitral stenosis. Am J Cardiol 57:634, 1986.
86. Smith MD, et al.: Comparative accuracy of two-dimensional echocardiography and Doppler pressure half-time methods in assessing severity of mitral stenosis in patients with and without prior commisurotomy. Circulation 73:100, 1986.
87. Thomas JD, Weyman AE: Doppler mitral pressure half-time: a clinical tool in search of theoretical justification. J Am Coll Cardiol 10:923, 1987.
88. Thomas JD, et al.: Inaccuracy of mitral pressure half-time immediately after percutaneous mitral valvotomy. Circulation 78:980, 1988.
89. Gillam LD, Choong CY, Wilkins GT, Marshall JE: The effect of aortic insufficiency on Doppler pressure half-time calculations of mitral valve area in mitral stenosis. Circulation 74 (suppl 2):II-217, 1986.
90. Flachskampf FA, et al.: Aortic regurgitation shortens Doppler pressure half-time in mitral stenosis: clinical evidence, *in vitro* simulation, and theoretical analysis. J Am Coll Cardiol 16:396, 1990.
91. Flachskampf FA, Weyman AE, Guerrero JL, Thomas JD: Calculation of atrioventricular compliance from the mitral flow profile: analytical and in vitro study. J Am Coll Cardiol 19:998, 1992.
92. Yang SS, Goldberg H: Simplified Doppler estimation of mitral valve area. Am J Cardiol 56:488, 1985.

93. Herman MV, Cohn PF, Gorlin R: Resistance to blood flow by stenotic valves: calculation of orifice area. *In* Grossman W (ed.): Cardiac Catheterization and Angiography. Philadelphia, Lea & Febiger, 1974.
94. Holen J, et al.: Determination of effective orifice area in mitral stenosis from non-invasive ultrasound Doppler data and mitral flow rate. Acta Med Scand 201:83, 1977.
95. Beasley B, Kerber R: Does mitral prolapse occur in mitral stenosis? Am J Cardiol 43:443, 1979.
96. Heger JJ, et al.: Long-term changes in mitral valve area after successful mitral commissurotomy. Circulation 59:443, 1979.
97. Lock JE, et al.: Percutaneous catheter commissurotomy in rheumatic mitral stenosis. N Engl J Med 313:1515, 1985.
98. Al-Zaibag M, Ribeiro PA, Al-Kasab S, Al Fagih MR: Percutaneous double balloon mitral valvotomy for rheumatic mitral valve stenosis. Lancet 20: 757, 1986.
99. Babic UU, et al.: Percutaneous transarterial balloon valvuloplasty for mitral valve stenosis. Am J Cardiol 57:1101, 1986.
100. Kveselis DA, et al.: Balloon angioplasty for congenital and rheumatic mitral stenosis. Am J Cardiol 57:348, 1986.
101. Palacios I, et al.: Percutaneous balloon valvotomy for patients with severe mitral stenosis, Circulation 75:778, 1987.
102. McKay RG, et al.: Balloon dilatation of mitral stenosis in adult patients: post-mortem and percutaneous mitral valvuloplasty studies. J Am Coll Cardiol 9:723, 1987.
103. Inoue K, et al.: Clinical application of transvenous mitral commissurotomy by a new balloon catheter. J Thorac Cardiovasc Surg 87:394, 1984.
104. Block PC, Palacios IF, Jacobs M, Fallon J: The mechanism of successful mitral valvotomy in humans. Am J Cardiol 59:178, 1987.
105. Wilkins GT, et al.: Percutaneous balloon dilatation of the mitral valve: an analysis of echocardiographic variables related to outcome and the mechanism of dilatation. Br Heart J 60:299, 1988.
106. Reid CL, et al.: Mechanisms of increase in mitral valve area and influence of anatomic features in double-balloon, catheter balloon valvuloplasty in adults with rheumatic mitral stenosis: a Doppler and two-dimensional echocardiographic study. Circulation 76:628, 1987.
107. Rodriguez L, et al.: Does asymmetric mitral valve disease predict an adverse outcome following percutaneous balloon mitral valvotomy? An echocardiographic study. Am Heart J, in press (June), 1992.
108. Abascal VM, et al.: Mitral regurgitation after percutaneous balloon valvuloplasty in adults: Evaluation by pulsed Doppler Echocardiography. J Am Coll Cardiol 11:257, 1988.
109. Chen C, et al.: Effects of technical selection on results of percutaneous mitral valvuloplasty: a comparative study of three different techniques. J Am Coll Cardiol [in press.] 1992.
110. Bernard Y, et al.: Assessment with color flow mapping of mitral regurgitation and left to right atrial shunting after percutaneous mitral valvuloplasty. (abstr) Circulation 78(II):1, 1988.
111. Yoshida K, et al.: Assessment of left-to-right atrial shunting after percutaneous mitral valvuloplasty by transesophageal color Doppler flow-mapping. Circulation 80:1521, 1989.
112. Chen C, et al.: Transesophageal color Doppler flow mapping of iatrogenic left-to-right interatrial shunting after percutaneous transluminal mitral valvotomy. Echocardiography 8:649, 1991.
113. Wilkins GT, et al.: Failure of the Doppler half-time to accurately demonstrate change in mitral valve area following percutaneous mitral valvotomy. J Am Coll Cardiol 9:218A, 1987.
114. Palacios IF, Block PC, Wilkins GT, Weyman AE: Follow-up of patients undergoing percutaneous mitral balloon valvotomy. Circulation 79:1, 1989.
115. Reid CL, et al.: Influence of mitral valve morphology on double-balloon catheter balloon valvuloplasty in patients with mitral stenosis: Analysis of factors predicting immediate and three-month results. Circulation 80: 515, 1989.
116. Bernstein A, Weiss F, Gilbert L: Uncomplicated congenital mitral stenosis. Am J Cardiol 2:102, 1958.
117. Daoud G, et al.: Congenital mitral stenosis. Circulation 27:185, 1963.
118. Ferencz C, Johnson AL, Wiglesworth FW: Congenital mitral stenosis. Circulation 9:161, 1954.
119. Singh SP, et al.: Congenital mitral stenosis. Br Heart J 29:83, 1967.
120. Van der Horst RL, Hastreiter AR: Congenital heart stenosis. Am J Cardiol 20:773, 1967.
121. Snider RA, Roge CL, Schiller NB, Silverman NH: Congenital left ventricular inflow obstruction evaluated by two-dimensional echocardiography. Circulation 61:848, 1980,
122. Vitarelli A, et al.: Echocardiographic assessment of congenital mitral stenosis. Am Heart J 108:523, 1984.
123. Shone JD, et al.: The development complex of "parachute mitral valve," supravalvular ring of left atrium, subaortic stenosis, and coarctation of aorta. Am J Cardiol 11:714, 1963.
124. Simon AL, Friedman WF, Roberts WC: The angiographic features of a case of parachute mitral valve. Am Heart J 77:809, 1969.
125. Grenadier E, et al.: Two-dimensional echo Doppler study of congenital disorders of the mitral valve. Am Heart J 107:319, 1984.
126. Perloff JK: Congenital mitral stenosis. In The Clinical Recognition of Congenital Heart Disease. Philadelphia, Saunders 1970.
127. Johnson MJ, Dodd K: Obstruction to left atrial outflow by a supravalvular stenosing ring. J Pediatr 51:190, 1957.
128. Rogers HM, Waldron BR, Murphey DFH, Edwards JE: Supravalvular stenosing ring of left atrium in association with endocardial sclerosis [endocardial fibroelastosis] and mitral insufficiency. Am Heart J 50:777, 1955.
129. Feigenbaum H: Echocardiography. 3rd Ed. Philadelphia, Lea and Febiger, 1981.
130. Flint A: On cardiac murmurs. Am J Med Sci 44:29, 1862.
131. White PD: A note on the differentiation of the diastolic murmur of aortic regurgitation and of mitral stenosis. Bostom Med Surg J 195:1146, 1926.
132. Segal JP, Harvey WP, Corrado MA: The Austin Flint murmur: its differentiation from the murmur of rheumatic mitral stenosis. Circulation 18:1205, 1958.
133. Reddy PS, et al.: Sound pressure correlates of the Austin-Flint murmur. An intracardiac sound study. Circulation 53:210, 1976.
134. Roberts WC, Perloff JK: Mitral valvular disease: a clinicopathologic survey of the conditions causing the mitral valve to function abnormally. Ann Intern Med 77:939, 1972.
135. Abbasi AS, Allen MW, DeCristofara D, Ungar T: Detection and estimation of the degree of mitral regurgitation by range-gated pulsed Doppler echocardiography. Circulation 61:143, 1980.
136. Blanchard D, et al.: Non-invasive diagnosis of mitral regurgitation by Doppler-echocardiography. Br Heart J 45:589, 1981.
137. Knutsen KM, Bae EA, Sivertssen E, Hiseth A: Detection of mitral regurgitation by Doppler ultrasound. Acta Med Scand. 210:349, 1981.
138. Matsuo H, et al.: Detection and visualization of regurgitant flow in valvular diseases by pulsed Doppler technique. Jpn Circ J 46:377, 1982.
139. Miyatake K, et al.: Semiquantitative grading of severity of mitral regurgitation by real-time two-dimensional Doppler flow imaging. J Am Coll Cardiol 7:82, 1986.
140. Patel AK, et al.: Detection and estimation of rheumatic mitral regurgitation in the presence of mitral stenosis by pulsed Doppler echocardiography. Am J Cardiol 51:986, 1983.
141. Pearlman AS, et al.: Echocardiographic detection of mitral regurgitation in mitral valve prolapse. In C. T. Lancee (ed.), Echocardiography. The Hague: Martinus Nijhoff, 1979.
142. Richards KL, Cannon SR, Crawford MH, Sorensen SG: Non-invasive diagnosis of aortic and mitral valve disease with pulsed-Doppler spectral analysis. Am J Cardiol 51:1122, 1983.
143. Helmcke R, et al.: Color Doppler assessment of mitral regurgitation with orthogonal planes. Circulation 75:175, 1987.
144. Miyatake K, et al.: Clinical applications of a new type of real-time two-dimensional Doppler flow imaging system. Am J Cardiol 54:857, 1984.
145. Omoto R, et al.: The development of real-time two-dimensional Doppler echocardiography and its clinical significance in acquired valvular diseases. Jpn Heart J 25:325, 1984.
146. Perry GJ, Nanda NC: Recent advances in color Doppler evaluation of valvular regurgitation. Echocardiography: a review of cardiovascular ultrasound 4:503, 1987.
147. Flachskampf FA, et al.: Patterns of normal transvalvular regurgitation in mechanical valve prostheses. J Am Coll Cardiol 18:1493, 1991.
148. Kostucki W, Vandenbossche JL, Friart A, Englert M: Pulsed Doppler regurgitant flow patterns of normal valves. Am J Cardiol 58:309, 1986.
149. Yock PG, Naasz C, Schnittger I, Popp RL: Doppler tricuspid and pulmonic regurgitation in normals: Is it real? (abstr). Circ 70 (II):II-240, 1984.
150. Choong CY, et al.: Prevalence of valvular regurgitation by Doppler echocardiography in patients with structurally normal hearts by two-dimensional echocardiography. Am Heart J 117:636, 1989.
151. Miyatake K, et al.: Intracardiac flow pattern in mitral regurgitation studied with combined use of the ultrasonic pulsed Doppler technique and cross-sectional echocardiography. Am J Cardiol 45:155, 1980.
152. Croft CH, et al.: Limitations of qualitative angiographic grading in aortic or mitral regurgitation. Am J Cardiol 53:1593, 1984.
153. Schuster AH, Nanda NC: Doppler echocardiographic measurement of cardiac output: comparison with a non-golden standard. Am J Cardiol 53:257, 1984.
154. Reddy PS, et al.: Determinants of variation between Fick and indicator dilution estimates of cardic output during diagnostic catheterization. J Lab Clin Med 87:568, 1976.
155. Bolger AF, et al.: Computer analysis of Doppler color flow mapping images for quantitative assessment of in vitro fluid jets. J Am Coll Cardiol 12:450, 1988.
156. Chen C, et al.: Impact of impinging wall jet on color Doppler quantification of mitral regurgitation. Circulation 84:712, 1991.
157. Cape EG, Yoganathan AP, Weyman AE, Levine RA: Adjacent solid boundaries alter the size of regurgitant jets on Doppler color flow maps. J Am Coll Cardiol 17:1094, 1991.
158. Thomas JD, et al.: The impact of orifice geometry on the shape of jets: an in vitro Doppler color flow study. J Am Coll Cardiol 17:901, 1991.
159. Quinones MA, et al.: Assessment of pulsed Doppler echocardiography in the detection and quantification of aortic and mitral regurgitation. Br Heart J 44:612, 1980.
160. Stevenson JG: Pulsed Doppler characterization of intracardiac flow patterns. In W. Berman, Jr. (ed.), Pulsed Doppler Ultrasound in Clinical Pediatrics. Mount Kisco, NY: Futura Publishing Co., 1983.

161. Miyatake K, et al.: Localisation and direction of mitral regurgitant flow in mitral orifice studied with combined use of ultrasonic pulsed Doppler technique and two dimensional echocardiography. Br Heart J 48:449, 1982.
162. Spain MG, et al.: Quantitative assessment of mitral regurgitation by Doppler color flow imaging: angiographic and hemodynamic correlations. J Am Coll Cardiol 13:585, 1989.
163. Hoit BD, et al.: Sources of variability for Doppler color flow mapping of regurgitant jets in an animal model of mitral regurgitation. J Am Coll Cardiol 13:1631, 1989.
164. Yellin EL, et al.: Dynamic changes in the canine mitral regurgitant orifice area during ventricular ejection. Circ Res 45:677, 1979.
165. Blevins RD: Applied Fluid Dynamics Handbook. New York, Van Nostrand Reinhold Co., 1984, pp. 229–241.
166. Launder BE, Rodi W: The turbulent wall jet—measurements and modeling. Ann Rev Fluid Mech 15:429, 1983.
167. Smith MC, et al.: Observer variability in the quantitation of Doppler color flow jet areas for mitral and aortic regurgitation. J Am Coll Cardiol 11:579, 1988.
168. Veyrat C, et al.: Pulsed Doppler echocardiographic indices for assessing mitral regurgitation. Br Heart J 51:130, 1984.
169. Ascah KJ, et al.: A Doppler-two-dimensional echocardiographic method for quantitation of mitral regurgitation. Circulation 72:377, 1985.
170. Colocousis JS, Huntsman LL, Carreri PW: Estimation of stroke volume changes by ultrasonic Doppler. Circulation 56:914, 1977.
171. Elkayam U, et al.: The use of Doppler flow velocity measurement to assess the hemodynamic response to vasodilators in patients with heart failure. Circulation 67:377, 1983.
172. Fisher DC, et al.: The mitral valve orifice method for noninvasive two-dimensional echo-Doppler determinations of cardiac output. Circulation 67:872, 1983.
173. Labovitz AJ, et al.: The effects of sampling site on the two-dimensional echo-Doppler determination of cardiac output. Am Heart J 109:327, 1985.
174. Lewis JF, et al.: Pulsed Doppler echocardiographic determination of stroke volume and cardiac output: Clinical validation of two new methods using the apical window. Circulation 70:425, 1984.
175. Steingart RM, et al.: Pulsed Doppler echocardiographic measurement of beat-to-beat changes in stroke volume in dogs. Circulation 62:542, 1980.
176. Stewart WJ, et al.: Variable effects of changes in flow rate through the aortic, pulmonary and mitral valves on valve area and flow velocity: Impact on quantitative Doppler flow calculations. J Am Coll Cardiol 6:653, 1985.
177. Blumlein S, et al.: Quantitation of mitral regurgitation by Doppler echocardiography. Circulation 74:306, 1986.
178. Rokey R, et al.; Determination of regurgitant fraction in isolated mitral or aortic regurgitation by pulsed Doppler two-dimensional echocardiography. J Am Coll Cardiol 7:1273, 1986.
179. Gehl L, et al.: Left atrial volume overload in mitral regurgitation. A two-dimensional echocardiographic study. Am J Cardiol 49:33, 1982.
180. Ren JF, et al.: Two-dimensional echocardiographic determination of left atrial emptying volume: A non-invasive index in quantifying the degree of non-rheumatic mitral regurgitation. J Am Coll Cardiol 2:729, 1983.
181. Cape EG, et al.: A new method for noninvasive quantification of valvular regurgitation based on conservation of momentum: In vitro validation. Circulation 79:1343, 1989.
182. Thomas JD, et al.: Quantification of jet flow by momentum analysis: an in vitro color Doppler flow study. Circulation 81:247, 1990.
183. Recusani F, et al.: A new method for quantification of regurgitant flow rate using color Doppler flow imaging of the flow convergence region proximal to a discrete orifice: An in vitro study. Circulation 83:594, 1991.
184. Cape EG, et al.: The proximal flow convergence method can be extended to calculate regurgitant stroke volume: in vitro application of the color Doppler M-mode. Abstract presented at National Scientific Sessions of the American College of Cardiology, 1990.
184a. Bargiggia GS, et al.: A new method for quantitation of mitral regurgitation based on color flow Doppler imaging of flow convergence proximal to regurgitant orifice. Circulation: 84:1481, 1991.
184b. Rivera JM, et al.: Regurgitant orifice area, a fundamental measure of mitral incompetence: Calculation by proximal acceleration. J Am Coll Cardiol 19:379A, 1992.
185. Panidis JP, et al.: Diastolic mitral regurgitation in patients with atrioventricular conduction abnormalities: A common finding by Doppler echocardiography. J Am Coll Cardiol 7:768, 1986.
186. Schnittger I, Appleton CP, Hatle LK, Popp RL: Diastolic mitral and tricuspid regurgitation by Doppler echocardiography in patients with atrioventricular block: New insight into the mechanism of atrioventricular valve closure. J Am Coll Cardiol 11:83, 1988.
187. Rokey R, et al.: Detection of diastolic atrioventricular valvular regurgitation by pulse Doppler echocardiography and its association with complete heart block. Am J Cardiol 57:692, 1986.
188. Clyne CA, Cuenoud HF, Pape LA: Diastolic mitral regurgitation occurring with complete atrioventricular block detected by Doppler color flow mapping. Echocardiography 6:543, 1989.
189. Appleton CP, Basnight MA, Gonzalez MS: Diastolic mitral regurgitation with atrioventricular conduction abnormalities: relation of mitral flow velocity to transmitral pressure gradients in conscious dogs. J Am Coll Cardiol 18:843, 1991.
190. Mintz GS, Kotler MN, Segal BL, Parry WR: Two-dimensional echocardiographic evaluation of patients with mitral insufficiency. Am J Cardiol 44: 670, 1979.
191. Levy TE, Edwards JE: Anatomy of mitral insufficiency. Prog Cardiovasc Dis 5:119, 1962.
192. Perloff JK: The clinical recognition of congenital heart disease. Philadelphia, Saunders 1970.
193. Beppu S, et al.: Mitral cleft in ostium primum atrial septal defect assessed by cross-sectional echocardiography. Circulation 62:1099, 1980.
194. Greenfield W: Double mitral valve. Trans Pathol Soc (London) 27:128, 1876.
195. Schraft WC, Lisa JR: Duplication of the mitral valve: case report and review of the literature. Am Heart J 39:136, 1950.
196. Edwards JE, Carey LS, Neufeld HN, Lester RG: Congenital heart disease: correlation of pathologic anatomy and angiocardiography. Philadelphia, WB Saunders, p. 785, 1965.
197. Hartmann B: Zur Lehre der Verdopplung des linken Atrioventrikularostiums. Arch Kreislaufforsch 1:286, 1937.
198. Cascos AS, Rabago P, Sokolowski M: Duplication of the tricuspid valve. Br Heart J 29:943, 1967.
199. Trowitzsch E, et al.: Two-dimensional echocardiographic findings in double orifice mitral valve. J Am Coll Cardiol 6:383, 1985.
200. Warmes C, Somerville J: Double mitral valve orifice in atrioventricular defects. Br Heart J 49:59, 1983.
201. Layman TE, Edwards JE: Anomalous mitral arcade. A type of congenital mitral insufficiency. Circulation 35:389, 1967.
202. Levy MJ, Edwards JE: Anatomy of mitral insufficiency. Prog Cardiovasc Dis 5:119, 1962.
203. Nixon PG, Woller GH, Radigan LR: Mitral incompetence caused by disease of the mural cusp. Circulation 19:839, 1959.
204. Seltzer A, Katayama F: Mitral regurgitation: clinical patterns pathophysiology and natural history. Medicine 51:337, 1972.
205. Wann LS, Feigenbaum H, Weyman AE, Dillon JC: Cross-sectional echocardiographic detection of rheumatic mitral regurgitation. Am J Cardiol 41:1258, 1978.
206. Waller BF, et al.: Etiology of clinically isolated, severe, chronic, pure mitral regurgitation: analysis of 97 patients over 30 years of age having mitral valve replacement. Am Heart J 104:276, 1982.
207. Webster's New Collegiate Dictionary. Springfield, MA, G. & C. Merriam, 1975.
208. Sahn DJ, Allen HD, Goldberg SJ, Friedman WF: Mitral valve prolapse in children: a problem defined by real-time cross-sectional echocardiography. Circulation 53:651, 1976.
209. Gilbert BW, et al.: Mitral valve prolapse: two-dimensional echocardiographic and angiographic correlation. Circulation 54:716, 1976.
210. Levine RA, Weyman AE: Mitral valve prolapse: a disease in search of, or created by, its definition. Echocardiography 1:3, 1984.
211. Cohen MV, Shah PM, Spindola-Franco H: Angiographic-echocardiographic correlation in mitral valve prolapse. Am Heart J 97:43, 1979.
212. Kennett JD, et al.: Observer variation in the angiocardiographic diagnosis of mitral valve prolapse. Chest 79:146, 1981.
213. DeMaria AN, et al.: Echocardiographic identification of the mitral valve prolapse syndrome. Am J Med 62:819, 1977.
214. Reid JVO: Mid-systolic clicks. S Afr Med J 35:353, 1961.
215. Barlow JB, Bosman CK: Aneurysmal protrusion of the posterior leaflet of the mitral valve. Am Heart J 71:166, 1966.
216. Kesteloot H, VanHoute O: On the origin of the telesystolic murmur preceded by a click. Acta Cardiologica 20:197, 1965.
217. Barlow JB, et al.: The significance of late systolic murmurs. Am Heart J 66:444, 1963.
218. Criley JM, et al.: Prolapse of the mitral valve. Clinical and cineangiographic findings. Br Heart J 28:488, 1966.
219. Hancock EW, Cohn K: The syndrome associated with midsystolic click and late systolic murmur. Am J Med 41:183, 1966.
220. Barlow JB, Bosman CK, Pocock WA, Marchand P: Late systolic murmurs and non-ejection ("mid-late") systolic clicks: an analysis of 90 patients. Br Heart J 30:203, 1968.
221. Shah PM, Gramiak R: Echocardiographic recognition of mitral valve prolapse. Circulation 42 (Suppl 3):III-45, 1970.
222. Kerber RE, Isaeff DM, Hancock EW: Echocardiographic patterns in patients with the syndrome of systolic click and late systolic murmur. N Engl J Med 284:691, 1971.
223. Dillon JC, Haine CL, Chang S, Feigenbaum H: Use of echocardiography in patients with prolapsed mitral valve. Circulation 43:503, 1971.
224. Popp RL, et al.: Echocardiographic abnormalities in the mitral valve prolapse syndrome. Circulation 49:428, 1974.
225. DeMaria AN, et al.: The variable spectrum of echocardiographic manifestations of the mitral valve prolapse syndrome. Circulation 50:33, 1974.
226. Markiewicz W: Mitral valve prolapse in one-hundred presumably healthy young females. Circulation 53:464, 1976.
227. Brown OR, Kloster FE, DeMots H: Incidence of mitral valve prolapse in the asymptomatic normal. Circulation 52(Suppl 2):II-27, 1975.
228. Procacci PM, Savran SV, Schreiter SL, Bryson AL: Prevalence of clinical mitral valve prolapse in 1169 young women. N Engl J Med 294:1086, 1976.
229. Weiss AN, et al.: Echocardiographic detection of mitral valve prolapse:

exclusion of false positive diagnosis and determination of inheritance. Circulation 52:1091, 1975.
230. Markiewicz W, London E, Popp RL: Effect of transducer placement on echocardiographic mitral valve motion. Am Heart J 96:555, 1978.
231. Morganroth J, Jones RH, Chen CC, Naito M: Two-dimensional echocardiography in mitral, aortic and tricuspid valve prolapse: the clinical problem, cardiac nuclear imaging considerations and a proposed standard for diagnosis. Am J Cardiol 46:1164, 1980.
232. Morganroth J, Mardelli TJ, Naito M, Chen CC: Apical cross-sectional echocardiography: standard for the diagnosis of idiopathic mitral valve prolapse syndrome. Chest 79:23, 1981.
233. Warth DC, et al.: Prevalence of mitral valve prolapse in normal children. J Am Coll Cardiol 5:1173, 1985.
234. Sasaki H, et al.: Two-dimensional echocardiographic diagnosis of mitral valve prolapse syndrome in presumably healthy young students. J Cardiogr 12:23, 1982.
235. Levine RA, Triulzi MO, Harrigan P, Weyman AE: The relationship of mitral annular shape to the diagnosis of mitral valve prolapse. Circulation 75:756, 1987.
236. Levine RA, et al.: Three-dimensional echocardiographic reconstruction of the mitral valve, with implications for the diagnosis of mitral valve prolapse. Circulation 80:589, 1989.
237. Levine RA, et al.: Reconsideration of echocardiographic standards for mitral valve prolapse: lack of association between leaflet displacement isolated to the apical four-chamber view and independent echocardiographic evidence of abnormality. J Am Coll Cardiol 11:1013, 1988.
238. Schreiber TL, Feigenbaum H, Weyman AE: Effect of atrial septal defect repair on left ventricular geometry and degree of mitral valve prolapse. Circulation 61:888, 1980.
239. Marks AR, et al.: Identification of high-risk and low-risk subgroups of patients with mitral valve prolapse. N Engl J Med 320:1031, 1989.
240. Nishimura RA, et al.: Echocardiographically documented mitral valve prolapse: long term follow-up of 232 patients. N Engl J Med 313:1305, 1985.
241. Mardelli TJ, Morganroth J, Chen CC, Naito M: Apical cross-sectional echocardiography: the standard for the diagnosis of mitral valve prolapse (abstr). Circulation 60:11, 1979.
242. Nidorf SM, Weyman AE, Levine RA: A new 2-dimensional echocardiographic classification of mitral valve prolapse which relates mitral valve morphology to mitral valve function. (in preparation)
242a. Nidorf SM, Weyman AE, Levine RA. A new 2-dimensional echocardiographic classification of mitral valve prolapse which relates mitral valve morphology to mitral valve function. J Am Coll Cardiol 19:157A, 1992.
243. Sanfilippo AJ, et al.: Papillary muscle traction by two-dimensional echocardiography. J Am Coll Cardiol 19(March):1992.
244. D'Cruz I, Shah S, Hirsch L, Goldberg A: Abnormal systolic motion of the posterolateral basal left ventricle in mitral valve prolapse: a new cross-sectional echocardiographic sign (abstr). Am J Cardiol 45:434, 1980.
245. Gornick CC, et al.: Electrophysiologic effects of papillary muscle traction in the intact heart. Circulation 73:1013, 1986.
246. Pini R, et al.: Mitral valve dimensions and motion and familial transmission of mitral valve prolapse with and without mitral leaflet billowing. J Am Coll Cardiol 12:1423, 1988.
247. Cohen IS: Two-dimensional echocardiographic mitral valve prolapse: evidence for a relationship of echocardiographic morphology to clinical findings and to mitral annular size. Am Heart J 113:859, 1987.
248. Roberts WC, McIntosh CL, Wallace RB: Mechanisms of severe mitral regurgitation in mitral valve prolapse determined from analysis of operatively excised valves. Am Heart J 113:1316, 1987.
249. Haikal M, et al.: Sensitivity and specificity of M-mode echocardiographic signs of mitral valve prolapse. Am J Cardiol 50:185, 1982.
250. Krivokapich J, Child JS, Dadourian BJ, Perloff JK: Reassessment of echocardiographic criteria for diagnosis of mitral valve prolapse. Am J Cardiol 61:131, 1988.
251. Abascal VA, Hagege AA, Brady CL, Levine RA: Mitral valve prolapse: lack of sensitivity and specificity of clicks and murmurs for leaflet displacement by 2D echocardiography. Circulation 76 (Suppl IV):IV-316, 1987.
252. Devereux RB, et al.: Relation between clinical features of the mitral prolapse syndrome and echocardiographically documented mitral valve prolapse. J Am Coll Cardiol 8:763, 1986.
253. Hickey AJ, Wolfers J, Wilcken DEL: Mitral valve prolapse: prevalence in an Australian population. Med J Australia 1:31, 1981.
254. Sbabaro JA, Mehlman DJ, Wu L, Brooks HL: A prospective study of mitral valvular prolapse in young men. Chest 75:555, 1979.
255. Savage DD, et al.: Mitral valve prolapse in the general population: 2. Clinical features: the Framingham study. Am Heart J 106:577, 1983.
256. Uretsky DF: Does mitral valve prolapse cause nonspecific symptoms? Int J Cardiol 1:435, 1982.
257. Retchin SM, et al.: Mitral valve prolapse. Disease or illness? Arch Intern Med 146:1081, 1986.
258. Motulsky AG: Biased ascertainment and the natural history of diseases. N Engl J Med 298:1196, 1978.
259. Allen H, Harris A, Leatham A: Significance and prognosis of an isolated late systolic murmur: a 9–22 year follow-up. Br Heart J 36:525, 1974.
260. Mills P, et al.: Long-term prognosis of mitral-valve prolapse. N Engl J Med 297:13, 1977.
261. Bisset GS III, et al.: Clinical spectrum and long term follow-up of isolated mitral valve prolapse in 119 children. Circulation 62:423, 1980.
262. Clemens JD, et al.: A controlled evaluation of the risk of bacterial endocarditis in persons with mitral valve prolapse. N Engl J Med 307:776, 1982.
263. Hickey AJ, MacMahon SW, Wilcken DEL: Mitral valve prolapse and bacterial endocarditis: When is antibiotic prophylaxis necessary? Am Heart J 109:431, 1985.
264. Devereux RB, et al.: Complications of mitral valve prolapse. Disproportionate occurrence in men and older patients. Am J Med 81:751, 1986.
265. McMahon SW, et al.: Mitral valve prolapse and infective endocarditis. Am Heart J 113:1291, 1987.
266. Wilcken DEL, Hickey AJ: Lifetime risk for patients with mitral valve prolapse of developing severe valve regurgitation requiring surgery. Circulation 78:10, 1988.
267. Campbell RWF, et al.: Ventricular arrhythmias in syndrome of balloon deformity of mitral valve: definition of possible high risk group. Br Heart J 38:1053, 1976.
268. Perloff JK, Roberts WC: The mitral apparatus. Functional anatomy of mitral regurgitation. Circulation 46:227, 1972.
269. Somerville J, Kaku S, Saravalli O: Prolapsed mitral cusps in atrial septal defect: An erroneous radiological interpretation. Br Heart J 40:58, 1978.
270. Nagata S, et al.: Mitral valve lesion associated with secundum atrial septal defect: analysis by real time two dimensional echocardiography. Br Heart J 49:51, 1983.
271. Liberthson RR, Boucher CA, Fallon JT, Buckley MJ: Severe mitral regurgitation: A common occurrence in the aging patient with secundum atrial septal defect. Clin Cardiol 4:229, 1981.
272. Abbasi AS, DeCristofara, Anabtawi J, Irwin L: Mitral valve prolapse: comparative value of M-mode, two-dimensional and Doppler echocardiography. J Am Coll Cardiol 2:1219, 1983.
273. Panidis JP, McAllister M, Ross J, Mintz GS: Prevalence and severity of mitral regurgitation in the mitral valve prolapse syndrome: a Doppler echocardiographic study of 80 patients. J Am Coll Cardiol 7:975, 1986.
274. Wiggers C, Feil H: The cardiodynamics of mitral insufficiency. Heart 1: 149, 1922.
275. Levy MJ, Edwards JE: Anatomy of mitral insufficiency. Prog Cardiovasc Dis 5:119, 1962.
276. Perloff JK, Roberts WC: The mitral apparatus. Functional anatomy of mitral regurgitation. Circulation 46:227, 1972.
277. Burch GE, DePasquale NP, Phillips JH: Clinical manifestation of papillary muscle dysfunction. Arch Intern Med 112:112, 1963.
278. Burch GE, DePasquale NP, Phillips JH: The syndrome of papillary muscle dysfunction. Am Heart J 75:399, 1968.
279. Godley RW, et al.: Incomplete mitral leaflet closure in patients with papillary muscle dysfunction. Circulation 63:565, 1981.
280. Ogawa S, Hubbard FE, Mardelli TJ, Dreifus LS: Cross-sectional echocardiographic spectrum of papillary muscle dysfunction. Am Heart J 97:312, 1979.
281. Kinney EL, Frangi MJ: Value of two-dimensional echocardiographic detection of incomplete mitral leaflet closure. Am Heart J 109:87, 1985.
282. Boltwood CM, Tei C, Wong M, Shah PM: Quantitative echocardiography of the mitral complex in dilated cardiomyopathy: the mechanism of functional mitral regurgitation. Circulation 68:498, 1983.
283. Sanders CA, et al.: Diagnosis and surgical treatment of mitral regurgitation secondary to ruptured chordae tendineae. N Engl J Med 276:943, 1967.
284. Luther RR, Meyers SN: Acute mitral insufficiency secondary to ruptured chordae tendineae. Arch Intern Med 134:568, 1974.
285. Sanders CA, Armstrong PW, Wilkerson JT, Dinsmore RE: Etiology and differential diagnosis of acute mitral regurgitation. Prog Cardiovasc Dis 14: 129, 1971.
286. Child JS, et al.: M-mode and cross-sectional echocardiographic features of flail posterior mitral leaflets. Am J Cardiol 44:1383, 1979.
287. Mintz GS, Kotler MN, Segal BL, Parry WR: Two-dimensional echocardiographic recognition of ruptured chordae tendineae. Circulation 57:244, 1978.
288. Sanders RJ, Neubuerger KT, Ravin A: Rupture of papillary muscles: occurrence of rupture of the posterior papillary muscle in posterior myocardial infarction. Dis Chest 31:316, 1957.
289. Mintz RF, et al.: Two-dimensional echocardiographic identification of surgically correctable complications of acute myocardial infarction. Circulation 64:91, 1981.
290. Erbel R, Schweizer P, Bardos P, Meyer J: Two-dimensional echocardiographic diagnosis of papillary muscle rupture. Chest 79:595, 1981.
291. Nishimura RA, Shub C, Tajik AJ: Two dimensional echocardiographic diagnosis of partial papillary muscle rupture. Br Heart J 48:598, 1982.
292. Friedberg CL: Diseases of the Heart. Philadelphia, WB Saunders, 1966.
293. Gilbert BW, et al.: Two-dimensional echocardiographic assessment of vegetative endocarditis. Circulation 55:346, 1977.
294. Maclean N, Macdonald MK: Aneurysm of the mitral valve in subacute bacterial endocarditis. Br Heart J 19:550, 1957.
295. Morgan WL, Bland EF: Bacterial endocarditis in the antibiotic era: with special reference to the later complications. Circulation 19:753, 1959.
296. Hoffman FG, Robinson JJ: Aneurysm of the mitral valve associated with bacterial endocarditis. Am Heart J 63:826, 1962.
297. Jarcho S: Aneurysm of heart valves. Am J Cardiol 22:273, 1968.

298. Edwards JE: Mitral insufficiency secondary to aortic valvular bacterial endocarditis. Circulation 46:623, 1972.
299. Pomerance A: Rarities and miscellaneous endocardial abnormalities. Aneurysms of valve cusps. *In* Pomerance A, Davies MJ (eds.): The Pathology of the Heart. Oxford, Blackwell Scientific Publications, p. 486, 1975.
300. Pocock WA, Lakier JB, Hitchcock JF, Barlow JB: Mitral valve aneurysm after infective endocarditis in the billowing mitral leaflet syndrome. Am J Cardiol 40:130, 1977.
301. Reid CL, et al.: Mitral valve aneurysm: clinical features, echocardiographic-pathologic correlations. J Am Coll Cardiol 2:460, 1983.
302. Lewis BS, et al.: An unusual case of mitral valve aneurysm: Two dimensional echocardiographic and cineangiographic features. Am J Cardiol 49: 1293, 1982.
303. Chesler E, et al.: False aneurysm of the left ventricle secondary to bacterial endocarditis with perforation of the mitral-aortic intervalvular fibrosa. Circulation 37:518, 1968.
304. Gonzalez-Lavin L, Scappatina E, Lise M, Ross DN: Mycotic aneurysms of the aortic root: a complication of aortic valve endocarditis. Ann Thorac Surg 9:551, 1970.
305. Reid CL, et al.: False aneurysm of mitral-aortic intervalvular fibrosa: diagnosis by 2-dimensional contrast echocardiography at cardiac catheterization. Am J Cardiol 52:1801, 1983.
306. Geill T: Calcification of the left annulus fibrosus [230] cases. Acta Med Scand Suppl 239:153, 1950.
307. Simon MA, Liu SF: Calcification of the mitral valve annulus and its relation to functional valvular disturbance. Am Heart J 48:497, 1954.
308. Kirk RS, Russell JGB: Subvalvular calcification of mitral valve. Br Heart J 31:684, 1969.
309. Pomerance A: Pathological and clinical study of calcification of the mitral valve ring. J Clin Pathol 23:354, 1970.
310. D'Cruz I, Panetta F, Cohen H, Glick G: Submitral calcification or sclerosis in elderly patients: M-mode and two-dimensional echocardiography in "mitral annulus calcification." Am J Cardiol 44:31, 1979.
311. Takamoto T, Popp RL: Conduction disturbances related to the site and severity of mitral annular calcification: a 2-dimensional echocardiographic and electrocardiographic correlative study. Am J Cardiol 51:1644, 1983.
312. D'Cruz IA, Collison HK, Gerrardo L, Hensel P: Two-dimensional echocardiographic detection of staphylococcal vegetation attached to calcified mitral annulus. Am Heart J 103:295, 1982.
313. Come PC, Riley MF: M-mode and cross-sectional echocardiographic recognition of fibrosis and calcification of the mitral valve chordae and left ventricular papillary muscles. Am J Cardiol 49:461, 1982.
314. Terman DS, et al.: Cardiac calcification in uremia: a clinical, biochemical and pathologic study. Am J Med 50:744, 1971.
315. Buchbinder NA, Roberts WC: Left-sided active infective endocarditis. Am J Med 53:20, 1972.
316. Ruckman RN, Van Praagh R: Anatomic types of congenital mitral stenosis: report of 49 autopsy cases with consideration of diagnosis and surgical implications. Am J Cardiol 42:592, 1978.
317. Becker AE, Becker MJ, Edwards JE: Anomalies associated with coarctation of aorta: particular reference to infancy. Circulation 41:1067, 1970.
318. Rosenquist GC: Congenital mitral valve disease associated with coarctation of the aorta: a spectrum that includes parachute deformity of the mitral valves. Circulation 49:985, 1974.

CHAPTER

18

LEFT VENTRICULAR INFLOW TRACT II: THE LEFT ATRIUM, PULMONARY VEINS, AND CORONARY SINUS

LEFT ATRIUM

Anatomy

The left atrium is a thin-walled, ovoid chamber that lies directly beneath the aorta and, with the right atrium, is the most posteriorly positioned cardiac structure.[1,2] The left atrium is bordered inferiorly by the mitral annulus and medially by the interatrial septum. The posterior, lateral, and superior walls are not typically in contact with other cardiac structures; however, the right pulmonary artery and pulmonary veins may frequently be recorded along the superior margin of the left atrium, and the descending aorta is seen commonly beneath its posterior wall. The endocardial surface of the left atrial wall is normally smooth and continuous and is interrupted only by the insertions of the right and left pulmonary veins superiorly, by the orifice of the atrial appendage anterolaterally, and by the mitral orifice inferiorly. An additional depression in the midportion of the interatrial septum represents the position of the foramen ovale.

Left Atrial Function

The left atrium functions as a reservoir for the collection and storage of blood during left ventricular systole, as a conduit for the passage of blood from the pulmonary veins to the left ventricle during early left ventricular diastole, and as a contractile chamber to augment end-diastolic left ventricular filling. An understanding of each of these functions in normal and diseased hearts is important to correctly interpret changes in chamber size and patterns of flow into and out of the left atrium.

The instantaneous changes in normal left atrial pressure and volume during a representative cardiac cycle are illustrated in Figure 18–1, top. Four phases characterize left ventricular filling and emptying. Phase 1 begins at mitral valve closure and extends to mitral opening. During this period (the reservoir phase), blood flows into the left atrium from the pulmonary veins, increasing atrial volume to a maximum just before mitral valve opening. The increase in volume is accompanied by a continuous rise in pressure (the "v" wave). Phase 2 begins with the opening of the mitral valve; atrial volume then decreases rapidly (passive atrial emptying), with an accompanying fall in left atrial pressure. During phase 3, atrial volume remains relatively constant (atrial diastasis), but atrial pressure increases sharply as the ventricle shifts to a steeper portion of its compliance curve. At the beginning of atrial contraction (phase 4), atrial volume starts to decrease (active atrial emptying) and reaches its minimum just before mitral valve closure. The peak atrial systolic pressure is also attained during this phase (the "a" wave).[3] Figure 18–1, bottom, depicts the atrial pressure-volume relationship. The left atrial volume before active atrial emptying corresponds to the preload for atrial contraction.

The change in left atrial volume from end-systole to end-diastole does not provide an accurate measure of the total volume of blood entering the left ventricle during ventricular diastole. During passive atrial emptying and diastasis, blood also flows directly from the pulmo-

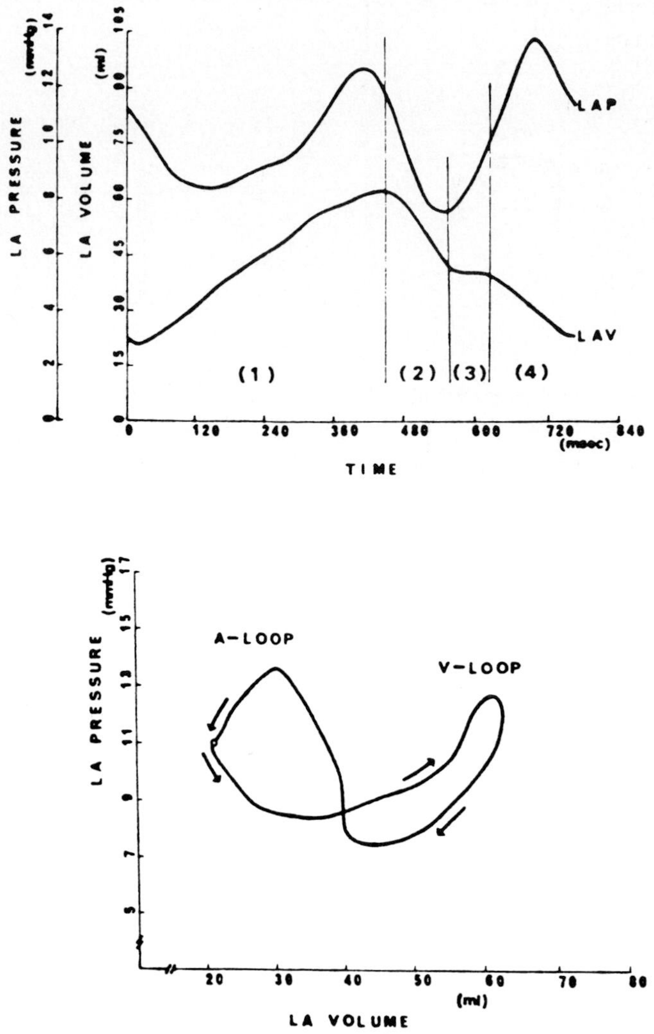

Fig. 18–1. Top. Instantaneous changes in left atrial pressure (LAP) and volume (LAV) for one cardiac cycle. Bottom. Atrial pressure-volume loop for the cycle in the upper panel. The pressure-volume curve forms a double loop, with the beginning of phase 1 situated at the left lower corner. During phase 1, the curve is directed upward and to the right. After maximal diastolic pressure and volume are reached, the curve turns clockwise and downward, corresponding to phase 2. The curve then proceeds almost parallel to the y axis (phase 3), as systolic atrial pressure increases while the volume does not change. After the rising curve has closed the first loop (v-loop) by crossing the segment corresponding to atrial filling, the curve turns counterclockwise and closes the second loop (A-loop). The left atrial volume before active atrial emptying corresponds to the preload for atrial contraction. (From Matsuda Y, et al.: Importance of left atrial function in patients with myocardial infarction. Circulation 67:566, 1983. Reproduced by permission of the American Heart Association, Inc.)

nary veins to the left ventricle, while during active atrial emptying, some blood may flow back to the pulmonary veins. The ratio of left atrial volumetric change to left ventricular stroke volume in normal subjects is roughly 50%. A direct relationship has been demonstrated between the cyclic left atrial volume change and left atrial maximal volume (i.e., patients with larger left atria tend to have a greater cyclic change in atrial volume).[4,5] Left atrial work (millimeters of mercury per milliliter) during active emptying also correlates significantly with left atrial volume at the onset of atrial contraction, suggesting that the Frank-Starling mechanism is also operative in the atrium.[3]

Examining Planes and Linear Dimensions

The left atrium is imaged using the parasternal long axis, short axis, and apical four-chamber views.[6,7] Because of its spherical or ovoid shape, the left atrium has no natural long or short axis. The axes of the left atrium, therefore, are defined echocardiographically relative to those of the major adjacent structures. Thus, the echocardiographic long axis of the left atrium lies in the same plane and is roughly parallel to the long axes of the aorta and left ventricle. Likewise, the short axis of this chamber corresponds to the short axes of these adjacent structures. The longest dimension of the atrium, however, may not always lie in the long axis plane.[6] Two additional planes, the subcostal long axis and right parasternal long axis, are particularly useful for recording the interatrial septum (see Chapter 29), because the septum is perpendicular to the path of the ultrasonic scan in both of these views. The subcostal long axis view is also particularly useful for detecting left atrial disorders in children.[7–9]

Figure 18–2 illustrates the parasternal long axis view of the left atrium. This plane passes through the atrium in an anteroposterior direction. The x axis of the imaging plane is oriented parallel to a line running from the midportion of the superior atrial border to the midportion of the mitral annulus. This plane should pass between but should not record the ostia of the pulmonary veins.

Two linear dimensions can be derived from the parasternal long axis view: an anteroposterior dimension (D_1) and a superior-inferior dimension (D_3). The anteroposterior dimension is taken as the distance between the posterior root of the aorta and the posterior left atrial wall at the level of the aortic valve. This line should pass through and be perpendicular to the superior-inferior axis and should approximate the longest anteroposterior dimension of the atrium at any level in this plane.

The superior-inferior dimension (D_3) is measured from the superior atrial wall to the plane of the mitral annulus through a point that roughly bisects the anteroposterior dimension. The plane of the mitral annulus (rather than the atrial surface of the mitral leaflets) is used as the inferior boundary of this dimension because it is a constant reference in both systole and diastole. Measurements are taken from the inner border of the endocardial echoes of the chamber walls. This procedure is in contrast to M-mode dimensions where the leading-edge method has been recommended.[10] In the cross-sectional format, however, the inner-edge method appears preferable because these points are also included in area measurements. In addition, these points permit consistency because the leading edge of the superior margin of the atrium is frequently not visualized.

The superior border of the atrium may be difficult to record in the parasternal long axis view because it lies parallel to the path of the imaging plane. This border should normally arise from the posterior aortic root at the level of the superior margin of the left coronary sinus

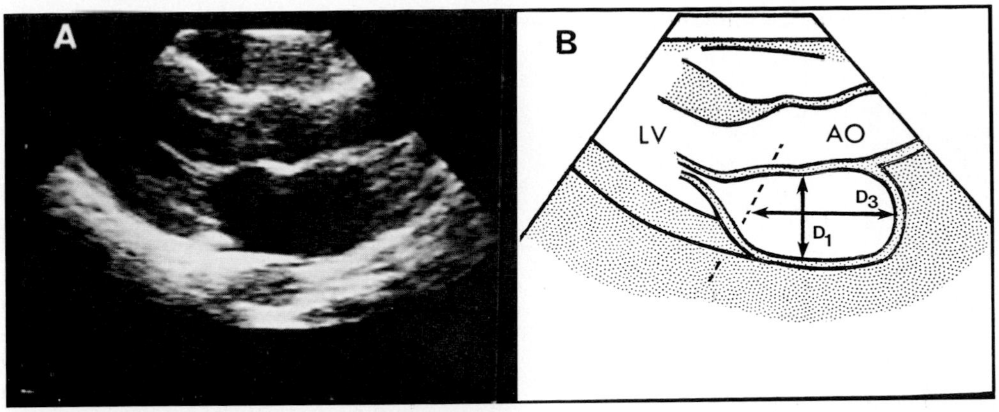

Fig. 18–2. **A.** Parasternal long axis recording of the left atrium. **B.** The anteroposterior dimension (D_1) and the superior-inferior dimension (D_3) are indicated. AO = aorta; LV = left ventricle.

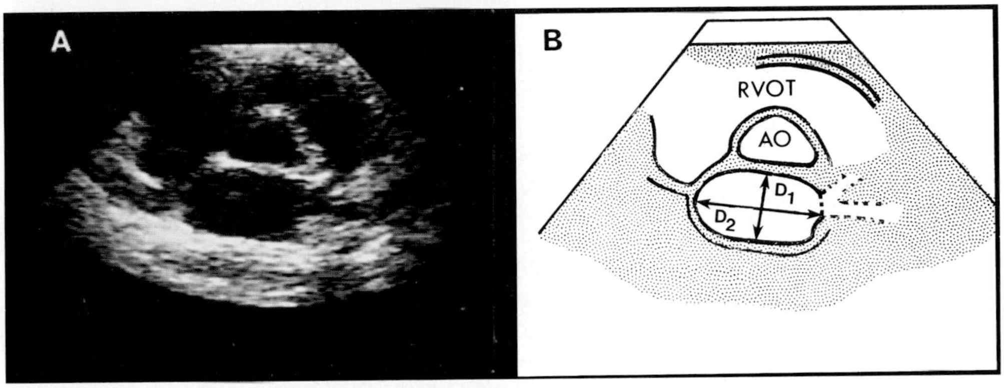

Fig. 18–3. **A.** Parasternal short axis view of the left atrium. **B.** The anteroposterior dimension recorded in this plane (D_1) and the medial lateral dimension (D_2) are indicated. AO = aorta; RVOT = right ventricular outflow tract.

of Valsalva. When the superior border is not visualized at this level, one can assume that it has not been adequately recorded and that D_3 is artifactually long. In addition, when the imaging plane is angled too far laterally or medially, it may pass through the orifice of one of the pulmonary veins, again causing loss of definition of the superior border of the atrium.

In the parasternal short axis view of the left atrium (Fig. 18–3), the imaging plane passes through this chamber from the anterior to the posterior borders. The x axis of the imaging plane is oriented parallel to a line running from its medial to lateral margins. This plane may transect the atrium at any point along its long axis from the annulus to the superior border; however, for purposes of measurement, the plane should be positioned at the level of the aortic leaflets. Two linear dimensions can also be derived from this plane: an anteroposterior dimension (D_{1s})* and a medial-lateral dimension (D_{2s}). The anteroposterior dimension is taken as the length of a line drawn from the midportion of the posterior aortic root anteriorly to the posterior atrial wall. If properly recorded, the length of this line should correspond to the anteroposterior dimension recorded in the long axis view (D_1). The medial-lateral dimension (D_{2s}) is the distance between the endocardial intercepts of a line that is perpendicular to and bisects the anteroposterior dimension. The medial and lateral borders of the atrium may be difficult to record in this view because they are oriented parallel to the imaging plane. In addition, targets along these walls are recorded using the lateral resolution of the system. These targets are consequently widened by the point-spread function of the beam, thus encroaching on the chamber lumen.

The apical four-chamber view transects the atrium from the mitral annulus to its superior wall (Fig. 18–4). In this orientation, the x axis of the imaging plane is slightly oblique to a true transverse plane of the atrium and, thus, is parallel to a line that is rotated between 15 and 30° clockwise from the true medial-lateral dimension of this chamber. The linear dimensions derived from this plane are a superior-inferior dimension (D_{3a}) and a medial-lateral dimension (D_{2a}). The superior-inferior dimension is taken from the midpoint of the mitral annular plane to the center of the superior atrial wall. The medial-lateral dimension is taken as the length of a line from the interatrial septum to the free lateral wall that bisects D_{3a}.

The optimal plane for recording each of the atrial dimensions is determined (1) by the orientation relative to the scan plane of the endocardial surfaces that define the limits of that measurement, (2) by the proximity of these surfaces to the transducer, and (3) by the ease of defining plane angulation and rotation. Although correlation between similar dimensions derived from each of the different views has been good, differences have been

* Because the same dimension may be recorded in two or more planes, the subscript (s) for short axis and (a) for apical four-chamber are used in the text to denote dimensions recorded in those planes. When a subscript is not present, the reader can presume that the dimension is recorded in a parasternal long axis. Subscripts are not included in the figures because the reference plane itself is always provided.

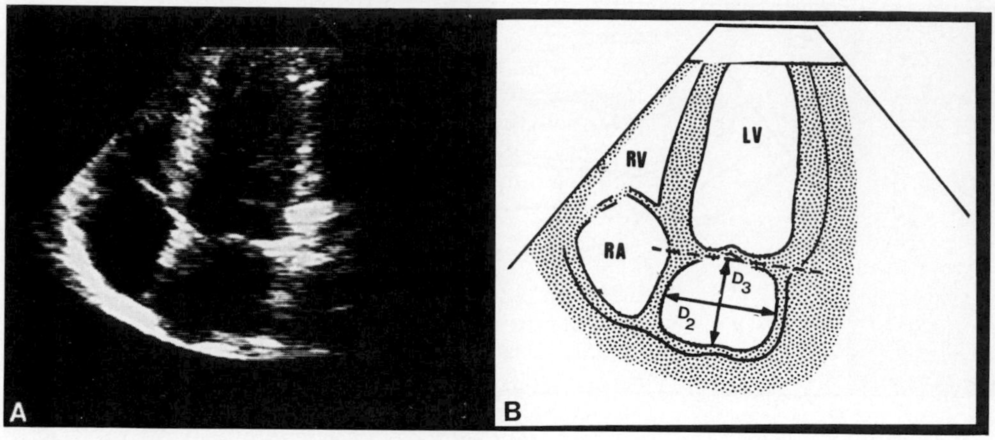

Fig. 18–4. A. Apical four-chamber view of left atrium. **B.** The linear dimensions obtainable from this view. A medial lateral dimension (D_2) and a superior inferior dimension (D_3) can be derived as indicated. LV = left ventricle; RV = right ventricle; RA = right atrium.

noted that can be related to the imaging difficulties inherent in each plane.[6] Analysis of these differences suggests the appropriate plane for recording each dimension. Thus, in a large group of patients with atria of varying sizes, the anteroposterior dimension (D_1) was noted as generally longer when recorded in the short axis than when recorded in the long axis view.[6] This discrepancy probably reflects the difficulties in defining plane angulation in the short axis because improper angulation elongates the vertical or anteroposterior dimension and suggests that the long axis plane is preferable for recording this measurement.

Likewise, the medial-lateral dimension (D_2) was noted as consistently shorter in the apical four-chamber view in both normal patients and patients with dilated atria when compared with the corresponding dimension in the short axis plane.[6] Here again, this discrepancy can be explained by the imaging characteristics of the system. In both views, the walls are parallel to the scan plane. In the apical view, however, the walls are farther from the focal zone, and hence, the point-spread function is greater, thereby leading to greater encroachment of the endocardial targets on the atrial lumen. Unfortunately, the variance in this dimension in normal persons when recorded in the short axis view is greater than when the same dimension is obtained from the apical four-chamber view. This presumably relates to the greater difficulty in defining its medial and lateral intercepts. Consequently, when the walls of the atrium are clearly defined, the short axis view should be preferable for recording the medial-lateral dimension; however, when border definition is difficult, apically derived data will be more reproducible.

The superior-inferior dimension, in contrast, appears comparable when recorded in both the four-chamber and long axis views.[6] The four-chamber view may prove to be preferable, however, because the plane of the mitral annulus is generally more easily defined in this orientation.

Normal Cyclic Variations in Left Atrial Dimensions

The size of the atrium normally changes throughout the cardiac cycle, as does the normal relationship of its dimensions. The major increase in atrial volume occurs during mechanical ventricle systole as the atrium fills from the pulmonary veins.[11]

Figures 18–5 and 18–6 illustrate this change in atrial size as well as the corresponding change in the linear dimensions. As these recordings demonstrate, the atrium expands primarily by elongating in anteroposterior and superoinferior directions. This expansion is accompanied by elevation of the aortic root and inferior motion of the mitral annulus. The medial-lateral dimension does not change markedly, because these walls are pulled in the same direction as the aortic root as it moves anteriorly. The atrium, therefore, is more spherical at end-systole than at end-diastole.

The atrial dimensions are most often measured at end-ventricular systole (just before mitral valve opening) because the atrial volume is greatest at this point.[10,12] Fortunately, as illustrated in Figures 18–5 and 18–6, the atrium is also most spherical at this point, and thus, a

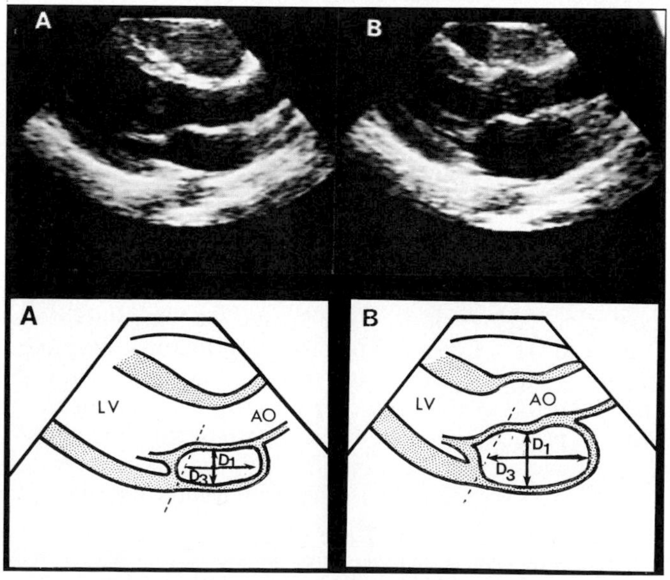

Fig. 18–5. Parasternal long axis recordings of the left atrium at end-diastole **(A)** and end-systole **(B).** In this plane, the atrium expands by both elevation of the aortic root with an increase in D_1 and expansion in a superior-inferior direction with an increase in D_3. AO = aorta; LV = left ventricle.

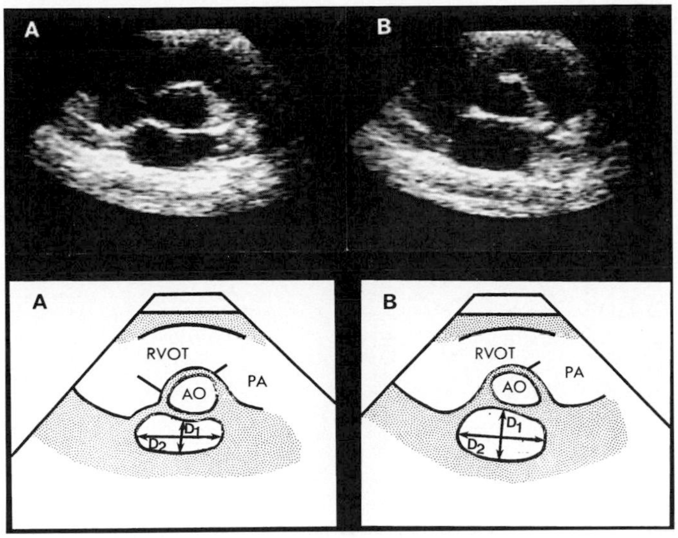

Fig. 18–6. Parasternal short axis recordings of the left atrium at end-diastole **(A)** and end-systole **(B).** The primary direction of atrial expansion in this plane is in the anteroposterior dimension. There is little change in the medial-lateral dimension (D_2). The atrium, therefore, shifts in configuration from a flattened oval shape at end-diastole to a more circular configuration at end-systole. RVOT = right ventricular outflow tract; AO = aorta; PA = pulmonary artery.

single dimension is most representative of chamber volume.

Normal Changes in Atrial Dimensions During Growth and Development

By birth, the measured dimensions of the left atrium have reached almost 50% of their adult value; this increases to almost 65% by 12 to 18 months of age. Subsequently, the growth rate slows so that by 5 years these dimensions have attained 75% of their adult value, and by the time of puberty (12 to 15 years of age), this has increased to 90%. Beyond this point, the rate of cardiac growth slows even further, and significant increases in dimension are not seen after 15 years of age. Univariate analysis predicts a strong correlation between the anteroposterior atrial dimension and height, weight, body surface area, and age. However, although the relationships between atrial dimensions and both weight and body surface area are nonlinear and predicted by a quadratic equation (Fig. 18–7A to D), the relationship between height and left atrial dimension is linear (left atrial anteroposterior dimensional = 0.014 × height + 0.69) (Fig. 18–8) and hence more easily determined and not affected by fluctuations in an individual's weight.[12A] Although multivariate analysis indicates that weight should be included with height in a model to predict left atrial dimension, the additional effect is minimal and beyond the resolution of the basic measurement.

Atrial Dilation and Compression

The left atrium dilates in a variety of pathologic states, including chronic mitral valve disease, left ventricular failure, and such left-to-right shunts as patent ductus arteriosus[13–15] and ventricular septal defect.[16] The left atrium also dilates in patients with atrial fibrillation in the absence of other cardiac disease.[17] When the left atrium dilates, all end-systolic dimensions tend to increase symmetrically,[6] the medial and lateral walls bow outward, and the atrium becomes more spherical. The configuration of the dilated left atrium is illustrated in Figure 18–9.

The left atrium may be smaller than normal in several situations. This typically occurs with (1) left-to-right shunting at the atrial level, which partially or completely bypasses the left atrium, as in total or partial anomalous pulmonary venous connection,[18] or (2) atrial septal defect with partial anomalous pulmonary venous drainage. On occasion, a large atrial septal defect may result in extreme right atrial dilation and clockwise rotation of the structures at the base of the heart. Such rotation shifts the aortic root to the left and posteriorly, thereby compressing the left atrium; (2) marked dilation of the aortic root (e.g., Marfan's syndrome, sinus of Valsalva aneurysms, and aortic dissection) may encroach on the left atrium; (3) extracardiac masses, which elevate the atrial floor; and (4) hypoplasia of the left heart. Atrial compression tends to be asymmetric, and in these cases, the normal relationship of the atrial dimensions is often lost, as is the relationship of a single dimension to atrial volume.

Methods for Quantitating Left Atrial Size

Atrial size can be determined using the anteroposterior linear dimension derived from the parasternal long axis view (or an equivalent view), or the atrial volume can be calculated using dimensions and areas derived from several orthogonal views.

The Anteroposterior Linear Dimension

The anteroposterior dimension (D_1) has been the traditional basis for estimating left atrial size in both M-mode and two-dimensional studies[19,20] and has been found to correlate well with the angiographic anteroposterior minor axis of the atrium,[12,21] with the angiographic area of the left atrium recorded in the right anterior oblique projection,[20,22] and with biplane angiographic volumes.[21]

Left atrial enlargement can usually be detected by simply relating the echocardiographic end-systolic, anteroposterior diameter of the atrium to the aortic root diameter at the same point in the cardiac cycle. In normal persons, the left atrial/aortic root ratio should be equal to or less than 1.1:1.[23] This relationship assumes that the aortic root is neither dilated nor hypoplastic. In the majority of cases, this assumption is valid, and an increase in this ratio can be used as a ready visual reference to indicate the presence of left atrial enlargement (see Figure 18–9 top and middle panels).

Despite the almost universal use of the standard anteroposterior left atrial dimension (D_1) to assess left atrial size, its accuracy is based on the assumption that the minor dimension bears a consistent relationship to atrial volume throughout the cardiac cycle and that this relationship is constant from patient to patient and in all

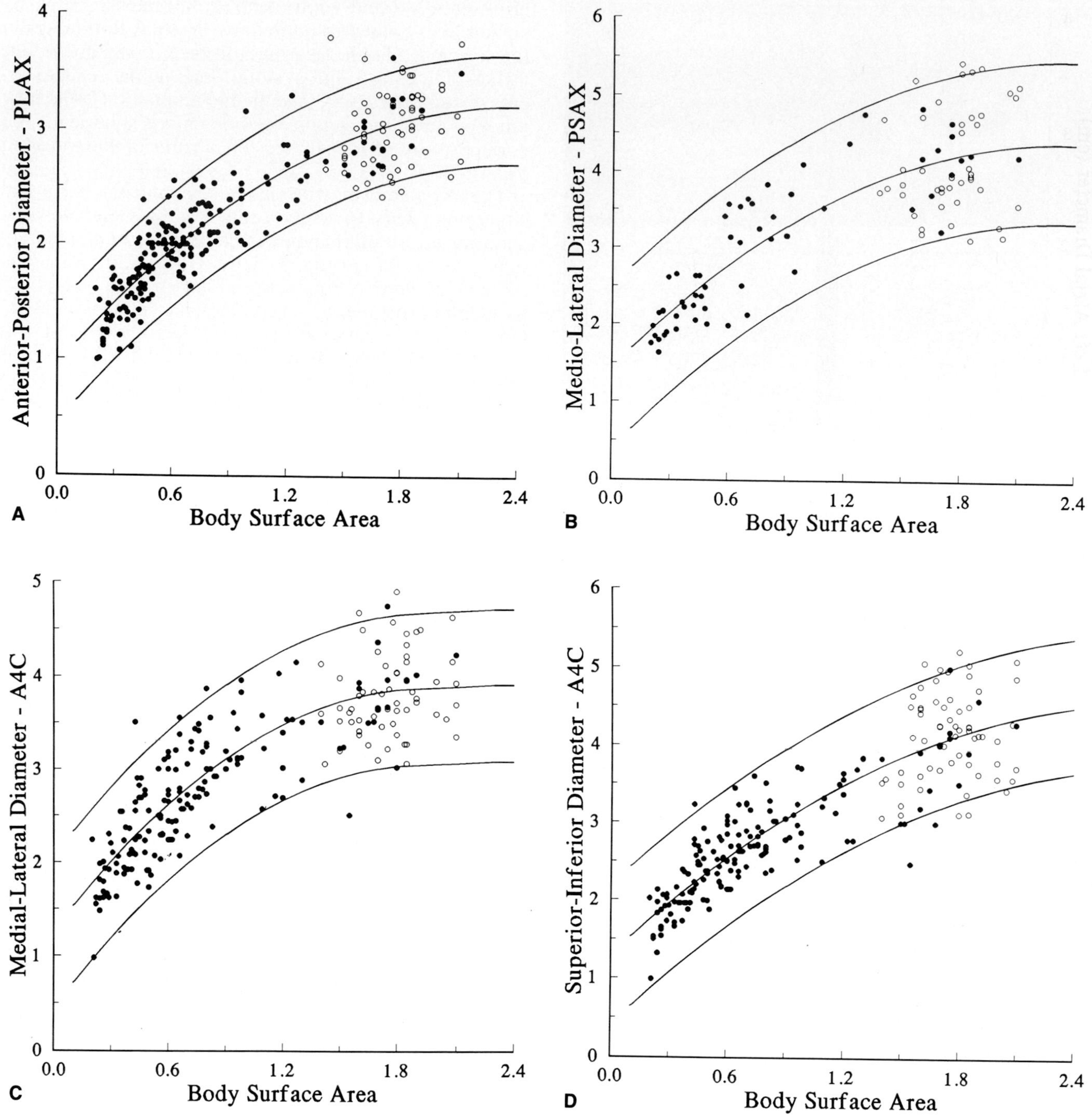

Fig. 18–7. Relationship of atrial dimensions to body surface area in normal from infancy to adulthood. **A.** Parasternal long axis antero posterior (PLAX) dimension (D_1). **B.** Parasternal short axis medial-lateral (PSAX) dimension (D_{2s}). **C.** Apical four-chamber medial-lateral dimension (D_{2a}). **D.** Apical four-chamber superior-inferior dimension (D_3). Note the decreased frequency with which the medial-lateral dimension could be measured in the parasternal view and the greater variance in the derived values. Solid circles = infants and children; open circles = adults. (From Nidorf SM, Picard MH, Triulzi MO, et al.: New perspectives in the assessment of cardiac chamber dimensions during development and adulthood. J Am Coll Cardiol 19:983, 1992.)

disease states. Normal atrial shape changes from end-ventricular-systole (maximal atrial volume) to end-ventricular-diastole (minimal atrial volume), and hence this relationship is not maintained. These assumptions are also invalid in clinical situations in which the atrium is asymmetric (i.e., atrial septal defect; distortion of the cardiothoracic architecture; cardiac tamponade; intracavitary, mural, and extramural tumors; and thoracic aortic aneurysm).

Use of the single atrial dimension to assess atrial dilation resulting from disease processes (i.e., mitral stenosis or regurgitation) or contraction following interventions (e.g., mitral valve surgery or balloon valvuloplasty) additionally assumes that the chamber di-

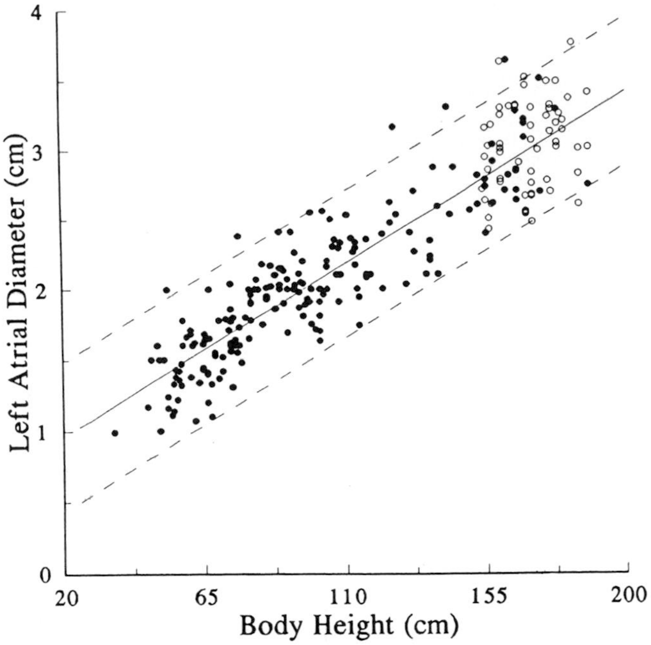

Fig. 18–8. Relationship of the left atrial anteroposterior dimension to body height in normal persons from infancy to adulthood. Solid circles = infants and children; open circles = adults. (From Nidorf SM, Picard MH, Triulzi MO, et al.: New perspectives in the assessment of cardiac chamber dimensions during development and adulthood. J Am Coll Cardiol 19:983, 1992.)

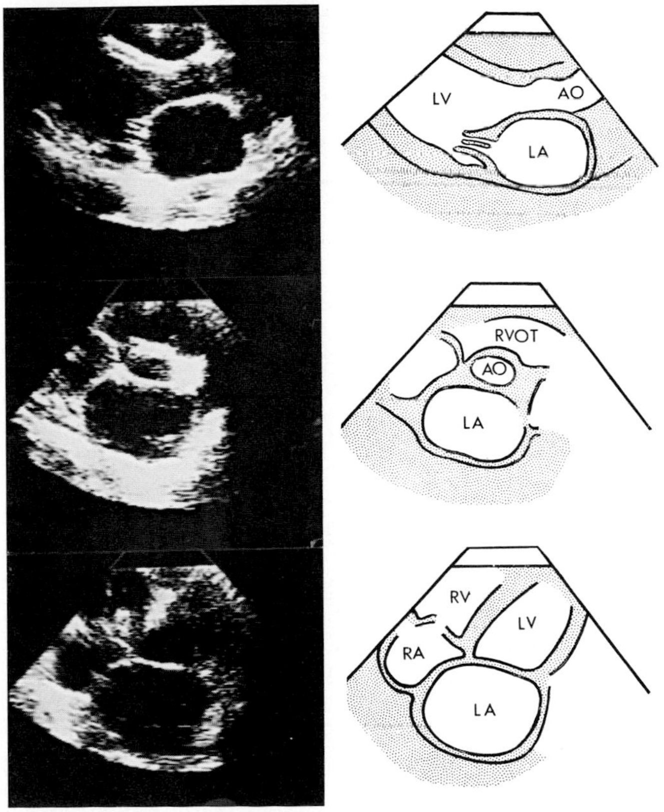

Fig. 18–9. Long axis, short axis, and apical four-chamber views from a patient with marked left atrial dilation. The atrium expands in all directions and becomes more spherical as it dilates. LV = left ventricle; AO = aorta; LA = left atrium; RVOT = right ventricular outflow tract; RV = right ventricle; RA = right atrium.

lates and contracts symmetrically, thereby maintaining a constant shape. Although this assumption is generally correct, the atrium may enlarge asymmetrically.[24] For example, in one study of 30 patients with mitral valve disease and left atrial enlargement, only 16 patients had all three atrial dimensions outside the normal range, and 5 had normal values for the anteroposterior dimension.[24] Thus, atrial volume should be determined in all clinical studies in which atrial distortion would make the information provided by the anteroposterior dimension misleading, and in follow-up studies where quantitative accuracy is important.

Left Atrial Volume

Left atrial volume can be calculated using either an ellipsoid model or a Simpson's rule algorithm.[24] The simplest approach is to use the length diameter ellipsoid method where the semiminor diameters are taken as the anteroposterior and medial-lateral dimensions (D_1, D_2) from the parasternal long and short axis views, and the long axis (L, or in this case D_{3a}) from the apical four-chamber view (Fig. 18–10). Volume is then calculated as follows:

$$\text{Volume} = \frac{4}{3}\pi\left(\frac{L}{2}\right)*\left(\frac{D_1}{2}\right)*\left(\frac{D_2}{2}\right) \qquad [18.1]$$

Alternatively, volume can be calculated using the biplane ellipsoid area length approach where:

$$\text{Volume} = \frac{8A_1 * A_2}{3\pi L} \qquad [18.2]$$

All ellipsoid volume determinations, however, assume that the atrium can be represented appropriately by an ellipsoid of revolution. When the atrium is deformed as a result of either external compression or generalized distortion of the heart, use of a Simpson's rule algorithm is more appropriate. Simpson's rule basically states that the volume of a large figure can be calculated from the sum of the volumes of a series of smaller figures of like shape. Thus, the volume of the atrium might be calculated from the sum of the volumes of a series of smaller elliptic cylinders of known height where

$$\text{Volume} = \frac{\pi}{4}\sum_{0}^{n} D_1 * D_2 \qquad [18.3]$$

Such calculations generally require the input of biplane chamber contours to derive the necessary diameters. These contours should be orthogonal about the long axis of the atrium and as such would be most appropriately derived from views such as the apical two- and four-chamber. Calculation of volumes using Simpson's rule also requires use of a computer analysis system, so that when appropriate the ellipsoid model is easier to apply.

The correlation of echocardiographic volume measurements with corresponding angiographic values has been excellent, with correlation coefficients consistently

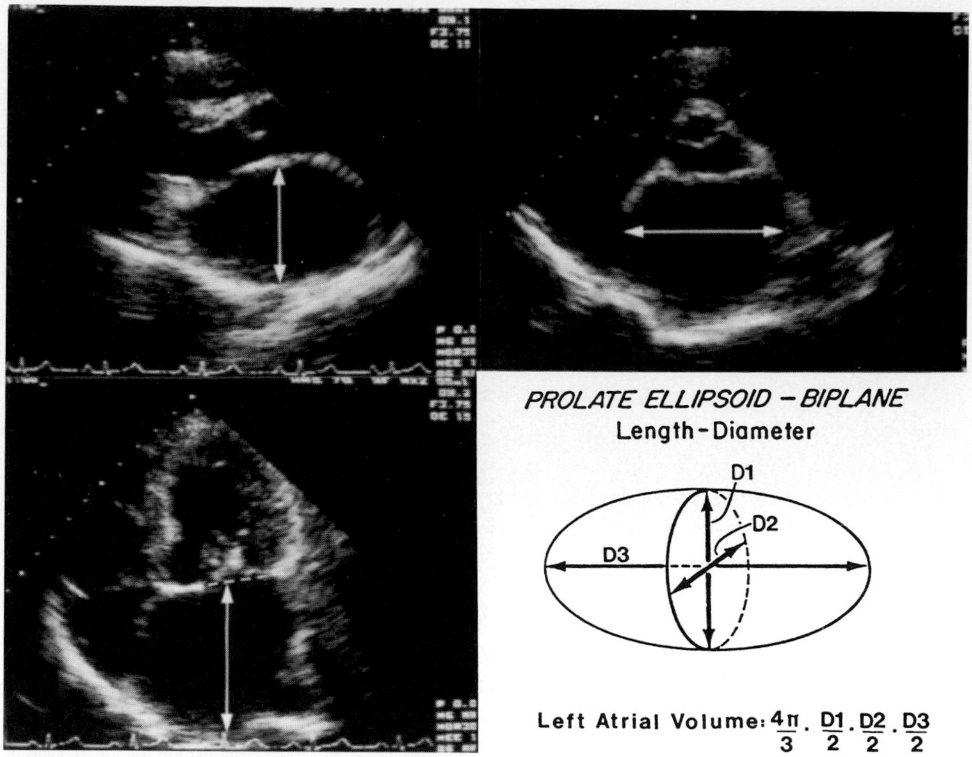

Fig. 18–10. Orthogonal atrial dimensions used to calculate volume using the prolate ellipsoid formula. This example is taken from a patient with mitral stenosis and a dilated left atrium.

above r = .9 and small standard errors. Figure 18–11 is an example of the results of one such study. Left atrial volume has also been calculated from a single plane area, assuming a spherical geometry.[25] This approach, however, appears less optimal because it fails to account for shape changes during expansion and contraction and may significantly over- or underestimate volume in the asymmetric ventricle.

Atrial Emptying Volumes

Atrial emptying volumes (the difference between end-systolic and end-diastolic volume) from two-dimensional echo studies have also been suggested as a means of determining the severity of mitral regurgitation, because a clear difference in emptying volume between normal persons and patients with mitral regurgitation can be demonstrated.[26] The emptying volume seems directly related to left atrial size and increases proportionally with severity of mitral regurgitation. Patients with moderate and severe regurgitation generally have emptying volumes greater than 40 ml.[26] In addition, the emptying volume has been shown to correlate remarkably well with the catheterization regurgitant fraction, given the imprecision of the latter measurement.[26]

Unfortunately, despite these positive correlations, no real separation between mild and moderate regurgitation and normal has been achieved, so that in individual patients, the measure can be considered at best a rough estimate of severity. Likewise, it fails to account for the blood entering the ventricle directly from the pulmonary veins and hence is not a measure of ventricular filling. Thus, left ventricular regurgitant volume and regurgitant fraction assessed by echo-Doppler methods (see Chapters 17 and 30) appear to be preferable.

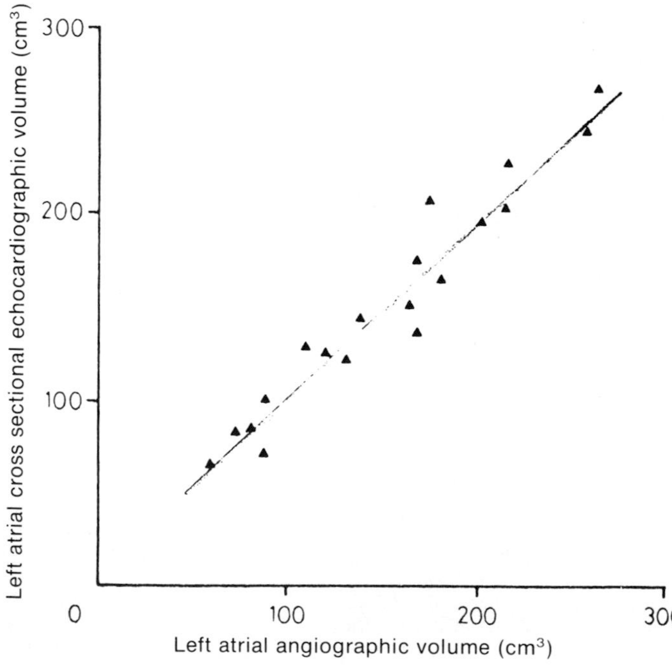

Fig. 18–11. Comparison of angiographic and echocardiographic measures of atrial volume. (From Loperfido F, et al.: Assessment of left atrial dimensions by cross-sectional echocardiography in patients with mitral valve disease. Br Heart J 50:570, 1983.)

Giant Left Atrium and Atrial Prolapse

In some patients with rheumatic mitral valve disease, the left atrium may undergo such extreme dilation that it compresses neighboring intrathoracic structures and expands behind the posterior wall of the left ventricle. Such extreme dilation is usually found in patients with predominant mitral regurgitation, and the term *giant left atrium* is often applied. Although there is no uniform agreement as to when an enlarged left atrium becomes a giant atrium, we arbitrarily set this threshold at 8 cm.

Profound atrial dilation and "prolapse" are generally evident in the parasternal long axis view (Fig. 18–12). Prolapse occurs when the dilating atrium meets external resistance and begins to expand inferiorly within the pericardial space between the posterior left ventricular wall and the epicardium. As the process progresses, the enlarging atrium undermines the posterior portion of the annulus and posterior left ventricular wall. During diastole, when the pressure in the atrium is higher than that in the ventricle (i.e., when there is mitral stenosis), the basal left ventricular segment overlying this atrial reflection will often be pushed forward or indented as a result of the positive atrial-ventricular pressure gradient (Fig. 18–12). This changes the shape of the ventricle at the base, causing it to become convex toward the short axis centroid. As the ventricle contracts during systole and left ventricular pressure increases, this area of the ventricle will return to its normal circular short axis configuration.[27] This is analogous to the change in septal shape that occurs from diastole to systole in patients with right ventricular volume overload. The change in shape results in a net outward or dyskinetic motion of the base of the ventricle. Although dyskinesis due to rearrangement in shape does not have the same pathologic significance as that seen in ischemic heart disease, it may have a similar functional consequence. The degree to which the atrium extends behind the left ventricle appears directly related to atrial size. Recognition of this phenomenon is important because the prolapsed portion of the left atrium appears as an echo-free space behind the left ventricle and can be misinterpreted as either a pericardial effusion or a pseudoaneurysm.[28] Likewise, the abnormal movement of the base might be felt to represent ischemic dysfunction or rheumatic involvement of the myocardium when in fact this is simply a rearrangement in ventricular shape.[29]

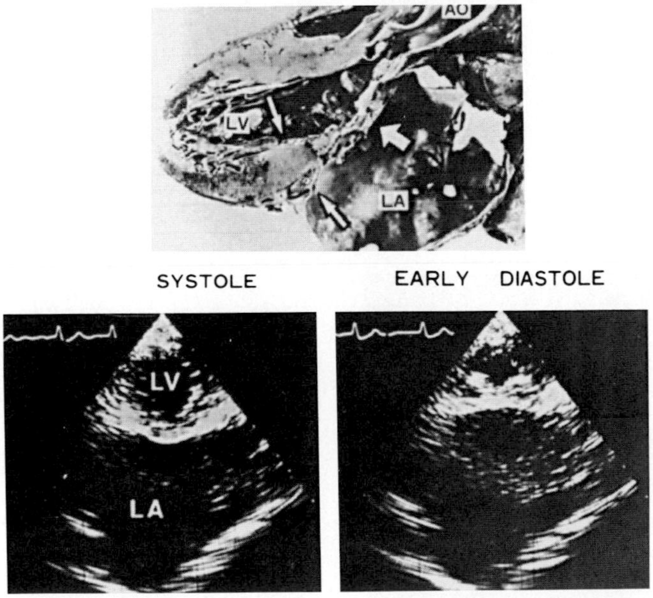

Fig. 18–12. Top. Postmortem specimen cut in a plane corresponding to the echocardiographic parasternal long axis view. The mitral valve has been replaced by a Hancock prosthesis (wide arrow). The left atrium (LA) is extremely dilated, extending to behind the left ventricle (LV). Note that the posterobasal wall of the LV (thin arrows) is entrapped between the LA and LV. Bottom. Parasternal short axis recording of the LV in early diastole (left) and early systole (right). Note that at end-diastole the base of the ventricle is pushed inward by the prolapsed atrium. With the onset of systole, the pressure in the LV increases, causing the cavity to return to a more normal circular configuration. AO = aorta. (From Beppu S, et al.: Echocardiographic study of abnormal position and motion of the posterobasal wall of the left ventricle in cases of giant left atrium. Am J Cardiol 49:467, 1982.)

Left Atrial Tumors

Tumors involving the left atrium may be intracavitary, mural, or extracardiac (see also Chapter 36). The most common intracavitary tumor is the left atrial myxoma. These myxomata are gelatinous, friable masses that commonly arise on a pedicle from the rim of the interatrial septum in the region of the fossa ovalis. Myxomata vary in size and may become large enough to fill the left atrium almost completely and to obstruct the mitral valve orifice. When obstructive, they may present clinically with signs and symptoms suggestive of mitral stenosis. Alternatively, the continual pounding of the tumor against the mitral valve may disrupt the valve apparatus, producing mitral insufficiency.[30] They may also produce constitutional symptoms that mimic bacterial endocarditis, and portions of the tumor may break off, releasing embolic material into the systemic circulation.[31] Because of the variable manifestations of these tumors, they are rarely detected clinically, and patients are usually referred for echocardiographic evaluation with a suspected diagnosis of rheumatic mitral valve disease.

Atrial myxomata appear echocardiographically as mobile, well-circumscribed masses of echoes within the cavity of the left atrium.[32–34] Because of the histologic composition of the tumors, there are multiple reflective interfaces within the interior, which result in an internal speckled pattern and make the body of the tumor as reflective as its edges. Myxomas may also contain a single or multiple internal cyst-like structures containing serous fluid or blood and may show varying degrees of calcification.[35–37] These tumors are typically mobile, prolapse through the mitral valve orifice during diastole, and are thrust back into the left atrial cavity during systolic ejection. On occasion, myxomas may be fixed or nonprolapsing. In these cases, diagnosis is more difficult and rests on location, site of origin, shape, and consistency.[38,39]

Figure 18–13 is an example of a large prolapsing myxoma recorded in long axis, and Figures 18–14 and 18–15 are examples of another myxoma in both the long axis

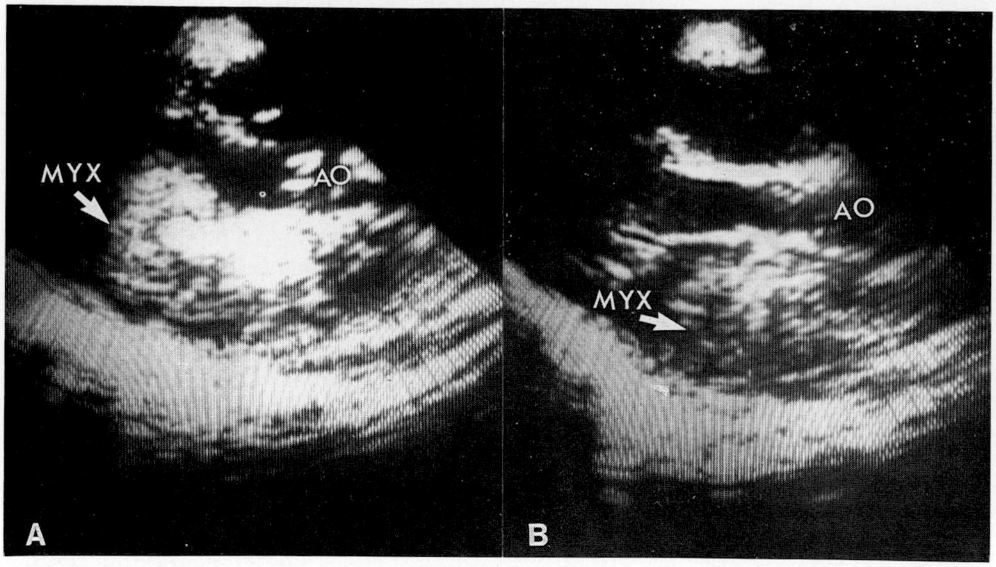

Fig. 18–13. Long axis recording of a large left atrial myxoma (MYX) during diastole **(A)** and systole **(B).** The tumor appears as a large, circular, echo-producing mass that can be visualized within the confines of the left atrial cavity during systole. During diastole, the tumor shifts toward the left ventricle almost totally filling the mitral valve orifice. AO = aorta.

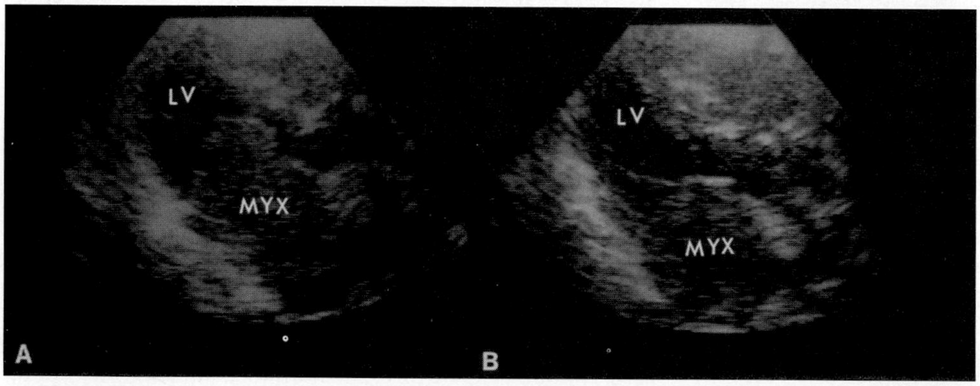

Fig. 18–14. Long axis recording illustrating another atrial myxoma (MYX). As in Figure 18–13, the tumor presents as a large circular mass of echoes within the confines of the left atrial cavity during systole **(B).** During diastole **(A),** the tumor prolapses through the mitral valve into the left ventricular (LV) cavity, completely filling the valve orifice.

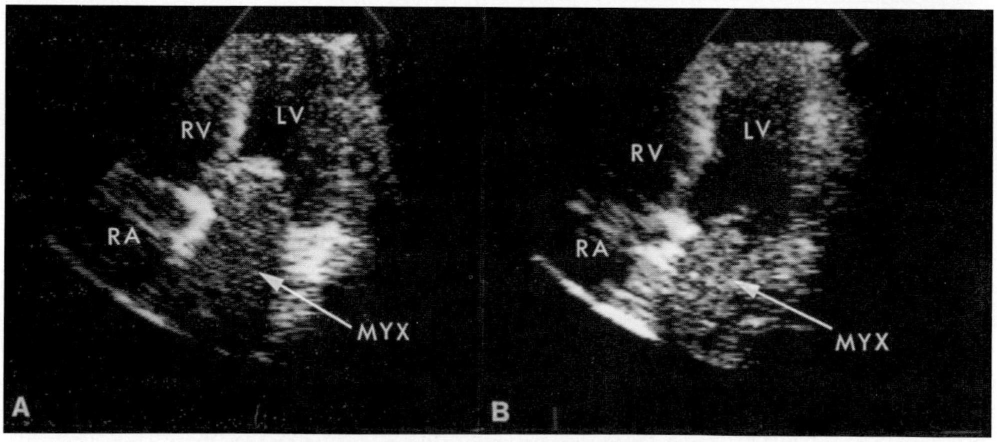

Fig. 18–15. Apical four-chamber view of the tumor demonstrated in Figure 18–12 during diastole **(A)** and systole **(B). B.** The anterior mitral leaflet can be visualized closing behind the tumor as it shifts back into the left atrium. RV = right ventricle; LV = left ventricle; RA = right atrium; MYX = myxoma.

and the apical four-chamber views. Motion of the tumor generally trails slightly behind that of the mitral valve. As a result, the valve usually opens fully before the tumor swings into the valve orifice. When the tumor obstructs the mitral orifice during diastole, the mitral valve is held open both by the tumor itself and by flow through the orifice around the tumor. No diastolic closing motion (E-F slope) is noted. Remember that multiple myxomas may be present in the same chamber and that myxomas may be found in multiple chambers at the same time. Therefore, the identification of a myxoma in the left atrium should stimulate a rigorous search for other accompanying tumors elsewhere in the heart.[40]

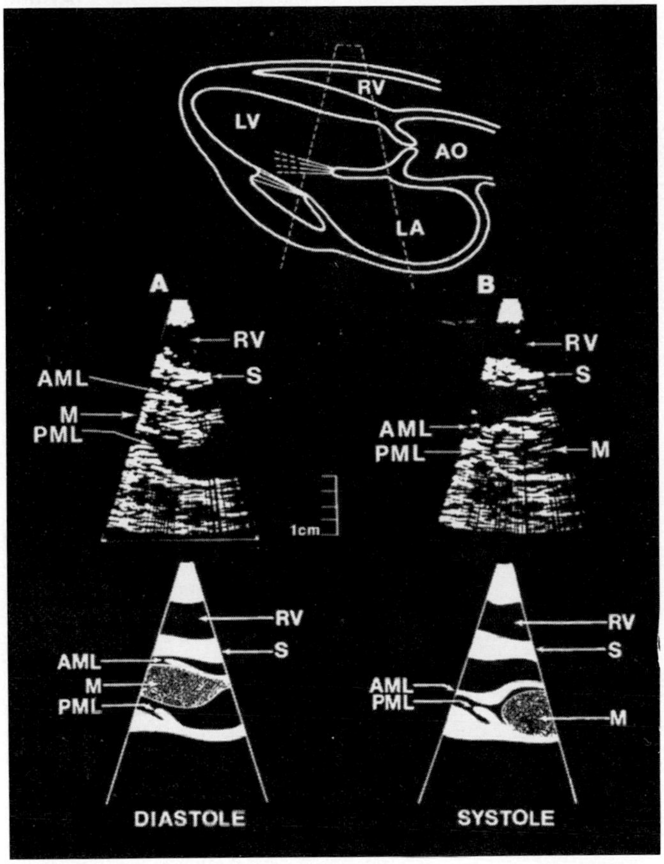

Fig. 18–16. Long axis recording from a patient with disseminated histoplasmosis and a secondarily infected left atrial myxoma. The diastolic frame illustrates the tumor prolapsing through the mitral orifice. During systole, the tumor lies within the left atrial cavity. RV = right ventricle; LV = left ventricle; AO = aorta; LA = left atrium; AML = anterior mitral leaflet; M = mass; PML = posterior mitral leaflet; S = septum. (From Rogers EW, et al.: Left atrial myxoma infected with histoplasma capsulatum. Am J Med 64:643, 1978.)

Atrial myxomata may become secondarily infected. If so, the patient's complaints may relate to the tumor itself or to the infectious process.[41,42] Figure 18–16 is an example of a large atrial mass discovered unexpectedly in a patient with disseminated histoplasmosis. Histologically, a small nidus of myxomatous tissue was present; however, the majority of the mass was composed of vegetative material and fungi. The similarity between this mass and those previously illustrated emphasizes again that, although the echogram can detect the presence of intracardiac masses, it cannot define their histologic composition.

Patients with left atrial myxomas obstructing the mitral valve orifice have transmitral flow patterns almost indistinguishable from those seen in patients with mitral stenosis. Absolute velocities are also in the range characteristic of mitral stenosis, and gradients can be determined using the modified Bernoulli equation. However, the mitral half-time should be less meaningful as a result of the independent effect of the tumor on left atrial compliance. In addition to the increased velocity, a lower frequency sound can be recorded at the beginning and end of diastole, reflecting movement of the tumor. This sound is simultaneous with, but of longer duration than, normal valve opening and closure and has a different quality from the short, sharp clicks that characterize valve movements.

Metastatic tumors may also extend into the left atrium and can simulate an atrial myxoma. Figure 18–17 is an example of a large intra-atrial tumor that was noted in a patient with metastatic osteogenic sarcoma.[43] This tumor mass can be distinguished from the typical myxoma because it arises from a broad base along the superoposterior atrial floor, rather than from the interatrial septum, and extends into one of the pulmonary veins. Although rare in general, the most common tumors growing into the left atrium from the pulmonary veins are the primary bronchogenic carcinomas and sar-

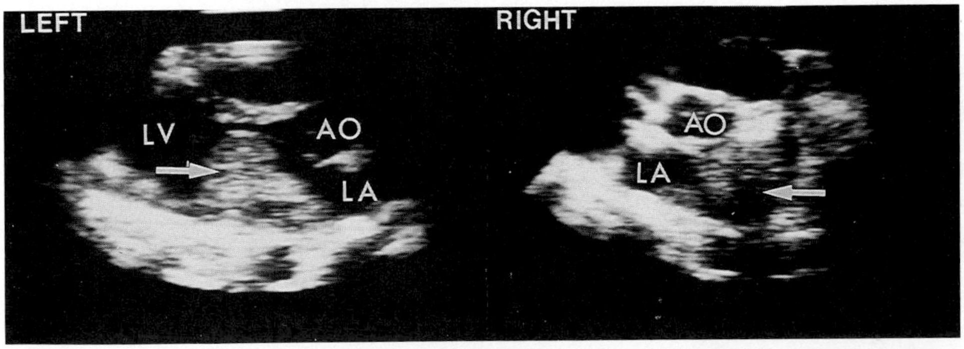

Fig. 18–17. Parasternal long and short axis recordings from a patient with metastatic osteogenic sarcoma and a large intra-atrial tumor mass. Left. During diastole, the tumor prolapses through the mitral valve orifice; however, its origin by a broad base from the atrial floor is still apparent. Right. The short axis recording demonstrates that the tumor is confined to the central and lateral portions of the atrium and appears to obstruct the pulmonary veins. The tumor is clearly separated from the interatrial septum, and its location serves to differentiate it from a typical myxoma. AO = aorta; LV = left ventricle; LA = left atrium.

comas.[44] Of this latter group, the primary or secondary osteogenic sarcoma and chondrosarcoma are the most common.[43–46] Sarcomas that are mobile like the myxoma can generally be differentiated from the solid carcinomas.

Mural tumors are detected by irregularities they produce in the atrial wall, by infringement on the cavity of the atrium, or by calcification of the tumor. In contrast to intracavitary masses, mural tumors are typically immobile. Figure 18–18 is an example of a calcified fibroma that produces an irregularity along the inferior-posterior border of the atrium. This tumor actually arises from the myocardium at the base of the left ventricle but has expanded into the cavity of the left atrium above the mitral annulus. This mass is highly reflective and suggests calcification within the tumor. During the pathologic examination, both fibrous encapsulation and calcification of the tumor were noted.

Tumors located in the posterior mediastinum may also enlarge to compress the left atrium from behind.[47] Figure 18–19 illustrates a large, small cell carcinoma originating from the posterior mediastinum and extending anteriorly to distort the posterior atrial wall and to compress the atrial cavity.

A large diaphragmatic hernia may also impinge on the left or right atrium, simulating an extracardiac tumor. This can be differentiated by its posterior location and the typical presence of stomach contents and air, which will cause changing echo density and a swirling appearance of the reflective targets. Having the patient drink a carbonated beverage during the examination can enhance this effect and aid in the diagnosis.[48]

Left Atrial Thrombi

Left atrial thrombi typically develop when blood stagnates within the atrium or when the integrity of the endocardial surface is interrupted. These situations may occur with left atrial dilation, atrial arrhythmias with resultant loss of normal coordinate atrial contraction, mitral valve disorders, or following mitral valve replacement. Very slow-moving or stagnant blood appears on two-dimensional echo as a cloud of echoes in the center of the atrium moving in a slow circular or spiral pattern.[49,50] This cloud of echoes constantly changes its configuration and reflective characteristics. The increased blood echogenicity has been attributed to both rouleaux formation and physical layering of blood components; however, the precise cause remains unclear.

Left atrial thrombi, in contrast, appear as well-demarcated masses of echoes that are generally attached to one of the atrial walls (most commonly, the posterior, lateral, or superior) and protrude into the atrial cavity. Although many thrombi are fixed, they may show some mobility, which, when present, is usually characterized by motion toward the mitral valve orifice during diastole. As with all masses, to be confident of the diagnosis of atrial thrombus, the mass should be visible in at least two different echocardiographic views.[51] Intracavitary

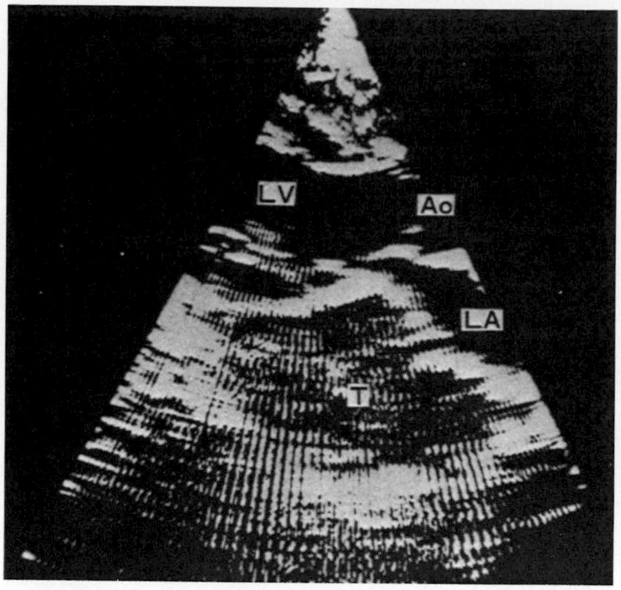

Fig. 18–19. Long axis recording of the left atrium demonstrates a small cell carcinoma of the posterior mediastinum that has expanded anteriorly, thereby displacing the left atrial wall and compressing the left atrial cavity from below. LA = left atrium; LV = left ventricle; T = tumor; Ao = aorta. (From Yoshikawa J, et al.: Cross-sectional echocardiographic diagnosis of large left atrial tumor and extracardiac tumor compressing the left atrium. Am J Cardiol 42:853, 1978. Reproduced with permission of Mosby Year-Book, Inc.)

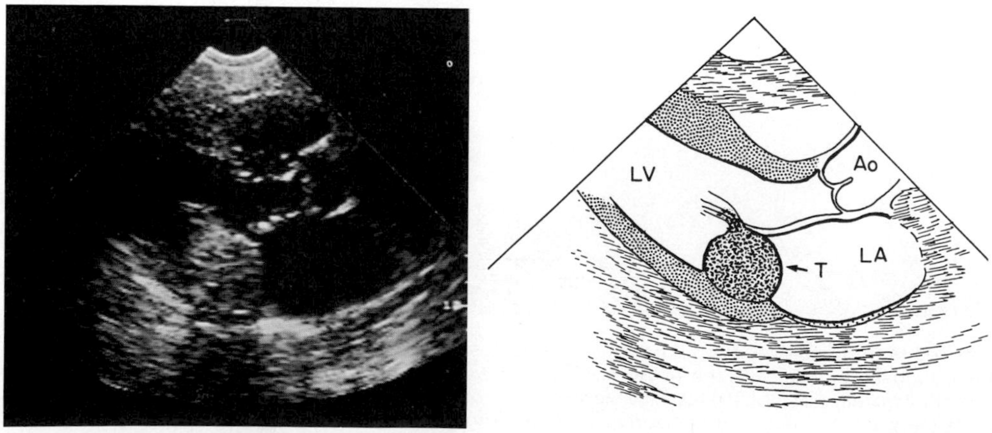

Fig. 18–18. Parasternal long axis recording of a calcified fibroma of the mitral annulus. The tumor partially obstructs mitral inflow, producing a transvalvular gradient. T = tumor, LA = left atrium; LV = left ventricle; Ao = aorta.

thrombi are detected most commonly in patients with predominant mitral stenosis, being reported in roughly 4% of such cases in large series.[52,53] Figure 18–20 is an example of a large and globular mass of echoes in the posterior region of the left atrium produced by one of these atrial thrombi.

The reported sensitivity of the cross-sectional echocardiogram in detecting intracavitary left atrial thrombi has been in the range of 75 to 80%.[53] This sensitivity varies with transducer frequency and has improved constantly as instrument sensitivity has improved. False-negatives occur principally in patients with small thrombi, mural thrombus without clear projection into the atrial cavity, and thrombi within the atrial appendage. The reported specificity for detection of intracavitary thrombi is roughly 98%.[53] Unfortunately, despite the good sensitivity in detecting intracavitary thrombi, clinicopathologic studies indicate that mural thrombi in mitral stenosis are restricted to the left atrial appendage in more than half of all cases,[54] and the echocardiographic sensitivity in detecting thrombi in the appendage using the transthoracic approach has been poor. Figure 18–21 illustrates a thrombus in the atrial appendages. Although in this case, the appendage and thrombus were clearly visualized, this is the exception, and failure to detect a thrombus in the appendage from the transthoracic approach does not absolutely exclude its presence. A transesophageal examination therefore may be indicated when the diagnosis or exclusion of a thrombus in the left atrial appendage is critical. Note that prior surgical amputation of the atrial appendage does not exclude thrombus formation in this region, and a small residual stump-like appendix with superimposed thrombus is not an uncommon finding.

Occasionally, free-floating ball thrombi will be detected in the left atrium.[55,56] These ball thrombi are generally associated with mitral stenosis, and the restricted mitral orifice retains the free-floating thrombus in the atrium. The unattached thrombus can intermittently be seen to drift into the mitral orifice during diastole, completely or partially obstructing flow for one cycle. During systole, they are typically ejected by the closing leaflets back into the atrium. Ball thrombi are generally prevented from lodging in the mitral valve orifice by the incomplete emptying of the atrium, the blood's tendency for rotary motion, and the smooth spherical surface of the thrombus itself.[56] Detection is important, however, because acute hemodynamic alterations and occasional sudden death may occur.

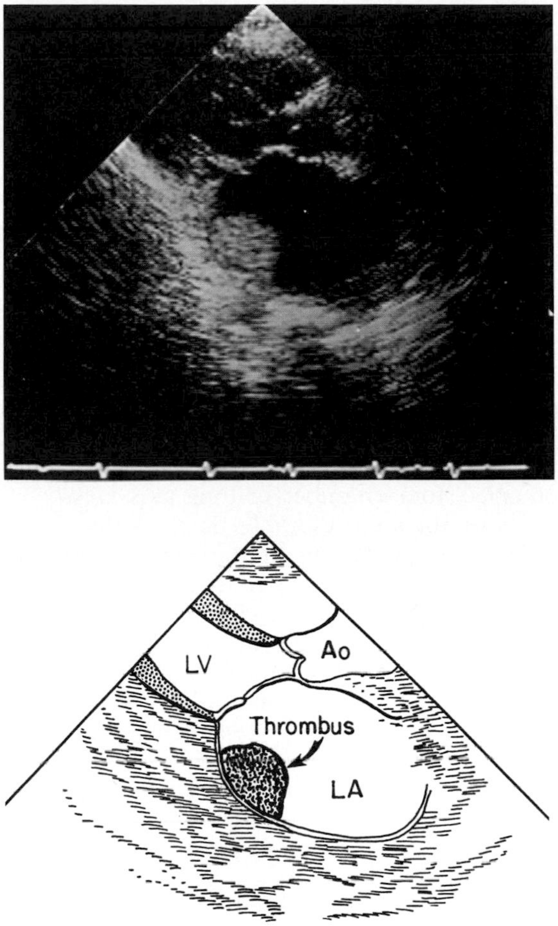

Fig. 18–20. A long axis recording of a large left atrial thrombus in a patient with mitral stenosis. The thrombus appears as a relatively homogenous, large echo-producing mass within the posterior left atrial cavity (arrow). LA = left atrium; Ao = aorta; LV = left ventricle.

Congenital Aneurysms of the Left Atrium

Isolated aneurysms of the left atrium in the absence of mitral valve or left ventricular disease are rare. These aneurysms, although considered to be congenital in ori-

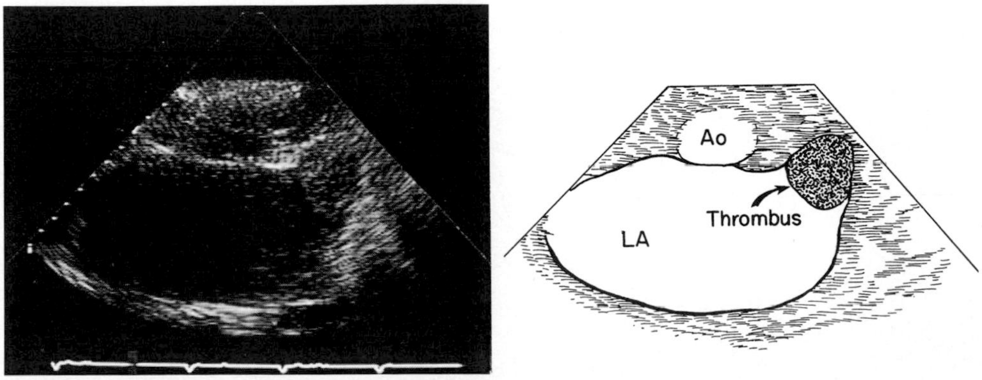

Fig. 18–21. Parasternal short axis recording from a patient with mitral stenosis and a dilated left atrium illustrating a thrombus in the atrial appendage. Ao = aorta; LA = left atrium.

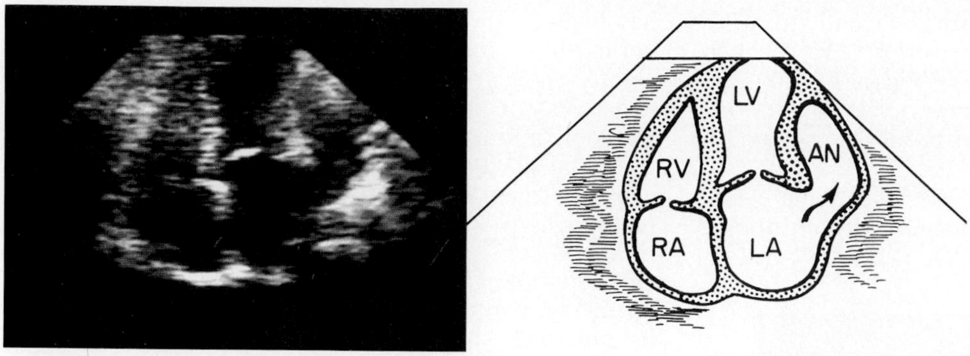

Fig. 18–22. Apical four-chamber recording illustrates a congenital aneurysm of the left atrial appendage. The aneurysm (AN) has dissected along the lateral wall of the left ventricle (LV) and distorts the shape of the base of the ventricle. It is connected to the left atrial cavity (LA) by a large neck. The entrance to the aneurysm is indicated by the arrow. RV = right ventricle; RA = right atrium.

gin, are usually clinically silent until the second to fourth decade. They may involve the wall of the body of the atrium; however, they are more frequently confined to the left atrial appendage. Congenital aneurysms are associated with systemic embolization and/or recurrent supraventricular tachyarrhythmias, and when present, aneurysectomy is usually recommended.[57]

Figure 18–22 is an example of a congenital aneurysm of the left atrial appendage. The aneurysm appears as an echo-free space along the lateral margins of the left atrium and the basal half of the left ventricle, which indents the wall of the left ventricular chamber. The aneurysm communicates with the left atrial cavity through a broad neck. This aneurysm was an unsuspected finding in a patient who was referred for echocardiographic study following a systemic embolic event.[58] These aneurysms are best appreciated in the apical four-chamber view, which typically depicts both the enlarged appendage and its site of origin from the left atrium.[59]

Cor Triatriatum

Cor triatriatum is an uncommon congenital cardiac disorder that can occur as an isolated lesion or can be associated with other congenital cardiac anomalies. The basic disorder is characterized by partition of the left atrium into two discrete chambers by a fibrous or fibromuscular diaphragm. This diaphragm typically divides the atria above the atrial appendage and fossa ovalis. Such a location serves to differentiate the membrane of cor triatriatum from the supravalvular mitral ring. One or more openings in the fibrous membrane permit the flow of blood from the pulmonary venous system into the true left atrium.[60,61] The size of these openings determines the degree of left atrial obstruction. Although the diagnosis is generally made in childhood, patients may occasionally experience their first symptoms as adults.

The obstructing membrane of cor triatriatum appears echocardiographically as an anomalous band of echoes stretching across the chamber at a level midway between the mitral ring and the superior atrial border.[62,63] This membrane shows phasic motion and is displaced inferiorly toward the mitral orifice during diastole and superiorly toward the superior left atrial border during systole.[62] Although these membranes can be viewed in either the parasternal long axis, the subcostal long axis, or the apical four-chamber or long axis views,[62,63] the latter views appear preferable because they place the membrane perpendicular to the path of the imaging plane. The peak instantaneous and mean gradients across the membrane can be calculated using the modified Bernoulli equation and the size of the orifice(s) by the continuity equation. Color flow mapping may demonstrate the number, location, and size of the orifice(s) in the membrane. When the turbulent jet produced by the midcavity obstruction strikes the mitral valve, it can produce mitral leaflet flutter, which is obvious on M-mode recordings.

Although all four pulmonary veins generally empty into the proximal chamber, a membrane obstructing only right pulmonary venous inflow has been reported.[64] In evaluating patients with cor triatriatum, it is important to record all four pulmonary veins because partial anomalous pulmonary venous drainage is an associated anomaly.

Figure 18–23 is a recording from a patient with cor

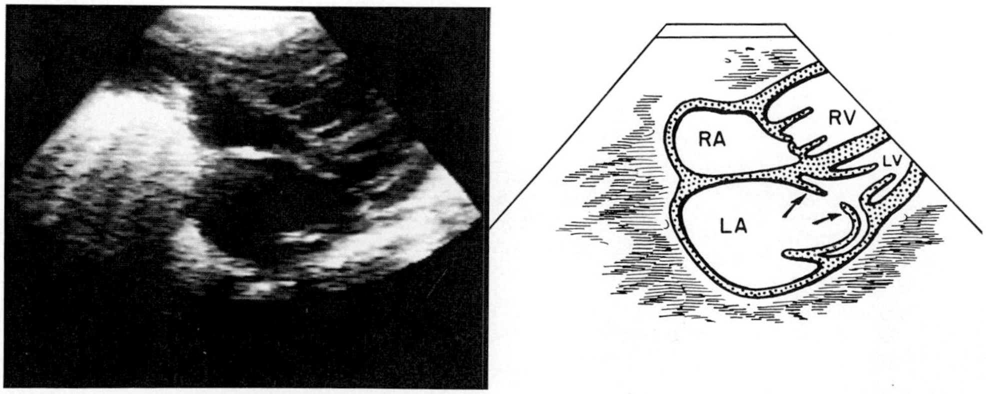

Fig. 18–23. Subcostal long axis recording from a patient with cor triatriatum. The transatrial membrane (arrowheads) is elongated and during diastole lies just above the mitral inlet. Its origin, however, is above the left atrial appendage. The atrium above the membrane is markedly dilated. RA = right atrium; RV = right ventricle; LV = left ventricle; LA = left atrium.

triatriatum. In this patient, the membrane appears as a pair of thin, elongated linear echoes originating from the medial and lateral margins of the atrium and stretching downward toward the mitral orifice. A central perforation is evident in the membrane, which permits blood flow into the small residual left atrial chamber and left ventricle. Figure 18–24 is a color Doppler recording illustrating pulmonary venous flow passing around a midatrial membrane in another patient with cor triatriatum. In this case there is no significant obstruction, and no increase in velocity is apparent.[65]

Left Juxtaposition of the Atrial Appendages

Left juxtaposition of the atrial appendages is a rare congenital malformation in which the right atrial appendage is displaced leftward beneath the great vessels such that it lies anterior to the left atrium and adjacent and slightly anterior to the left atrial appendage. The anomaly is usually associated with transposed great vessels. Hypoplasia of the right heart with inflow or outflow obstruction is also common. Recognition is important because the orifice of the appendage can be mistaken for an atrial septal defect at surgery, and the associated distortion in the alignment of the atrial septum complicates balloon septostomy, septectomy, and baffle placement in the Mustard and Senning procedures. The Fontan procedure can also be modified by anastomosis of the juxtaposed appendage to the pulmonary artery.

Echocardiographically, the malpositioned atrial appendage is first apparent in the parasternal long axis view,[66] presenting as an ovoid echo-free space immediately posterior to the aorta (Fig. 18–25A). The abnormally positioned appendage displaces the true left atrium posteriorly and creates a waist in its midportion. The malpositioned appendage can be differentiated from the right pulmonary artery by its location beneath the aortic sinuses; the inferior border of the right pulmonary

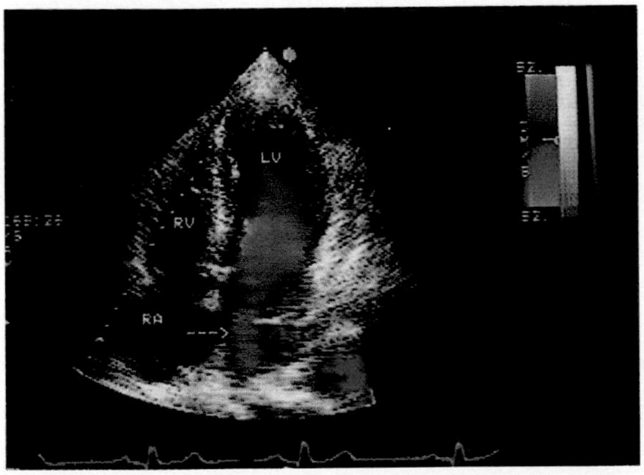

Fig. 18–24. Color Doppler recording of forward atrial flow (red) passing around a midatrial membrane characteristic of cor triatriatum. In this case, the membrane is nonobstructive, and although the flow stream appears constricted, there is no significant increase in velocity. LV = left ventricle; RV = right ventricle; RA = right atrium. (From Patt MV, Obeid AI: Cor triatriatum with isolated pulmonary venous stenosis in an adult: diagnosis with transesophageal two-dimensional echocardiography. J Am Soc Echocardiogr 4:185, 1991. Reproduced with permission from Mosby Year-Book, Inc.)

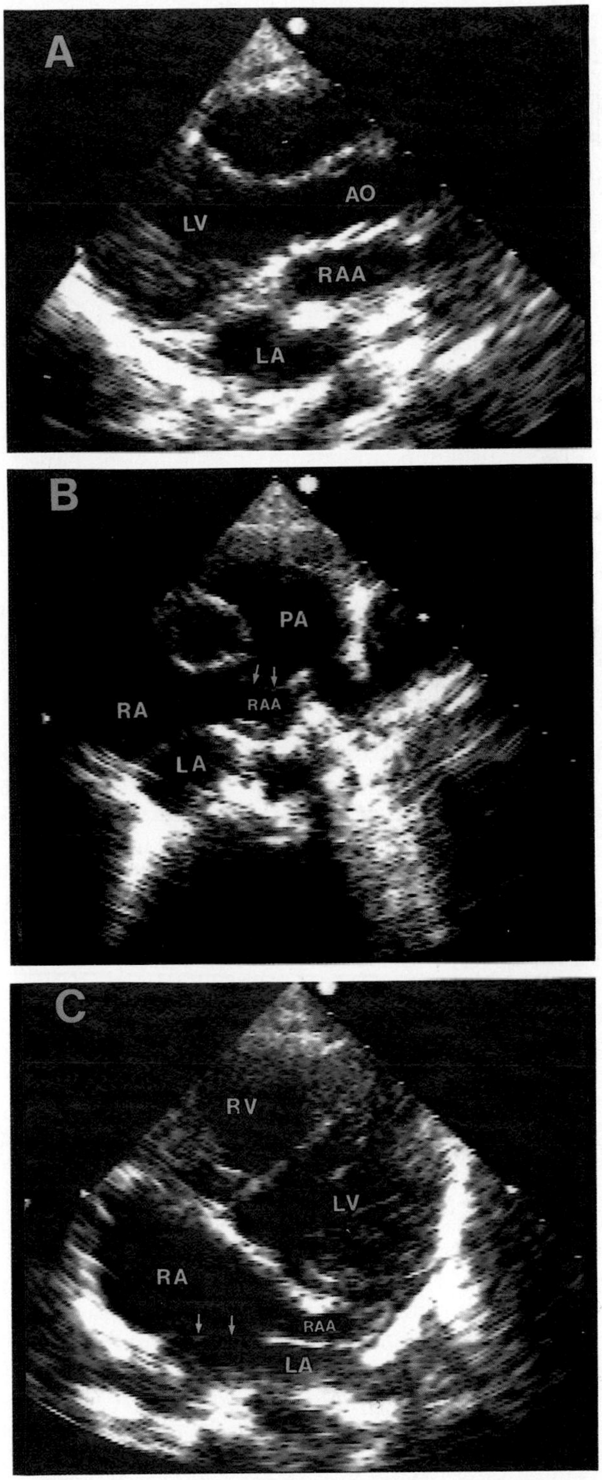

Fig. 18–25. Left juxtaposition of the atrial appendages. **A.** Long axis view. **B.** Short axis recording. **C.** Apical four-chamber recording. LV = left ventricle; AO = aorta; RAA = right atrial appendage; LA = left atrium; PA = pulmonary artery; RA = right atrium; RV = right ventricle.

artery typically lies at the sinotubular junction. The basic abnormality is most obvious in a parasternal short axis view recorded at or just above the semilunar valve level[66] (Fig. 18–25B). Normally in this view, the atrial septum courses vertically from the posterior atrial wall to the inferoposterior wall of the aorta. In patients with juxtaposition of the atrial appendages, the septum originates at the same point posteriorly and extends vertically about one third of the distance to the posterior great vessel. It then curves leftward, however, becoming horizontal relative to the anterior chest wall and crosses in front of the left atrium. At the left margin of the left atrium, it curves back to the right beneath the posterior great vessel and inserts normally into its posterior wall. This results in a finger-like projection (cavity) between the posterior great vessel and the left atrium: the leftwardly displaced right atrial appendage. At the extreme of its leftward extension, the walls of the left and right atrial appendages are in contact and hence are juxtaposed. The appearance is the same as would be expected if the right atrial appendage were pulled through the potential space between the posterior great vessel and the anterior atrial wall (Fig. 18–25B).

In the apical four-chamber view there is also a characteristic but nondiagnostic alteration in the superior atrial septal configuration in which the atrial septum appears to wrap around the superior aspect of the right atrium, making the right atrium appear slightly smaller than the left.[66] Anterior elevation of the atrial four-chamber plane (Fig. 18–25C) can also demonstrate the anteriorly located right atrial appendage coursing beneath the great arteries and leftward above the left atrial cavity.[66]

When the diagnosis is in question, peripherally injected contrast may be useful to outline the abnormally positioned appendage and to clarify its communication with the right atrium.

An associated secundum atrial septal defect is common and is located in either the normally oriented posterior portion of the septum or at the junction of the normal vertical and horizontal portions.[66]

PULMONARY VEINS

Normal Appearance

Normally, four separate veins connect the pulmonary vascular bed with the left atrium. The upper and lower veins from the right lung enter the superior-medial border of the left atrium, and the corresponding pair from the left lung insert into the superior-lateral border. *In roughly 2% of normal persons, three or more veins drain the right lung.*[67] The position and orientation of the pulmonary veins make them difficult to visualize transthoracically. Although segments of one or more pulmonary veins can be recorded in each of the standard atrial imaging planes, recording of all the venous connections in any single view is generally not possible. In some patients, all four veins can be recorded from the suprasternal notch using the so-called "crab view," which is a coronal section through the aorta, right pulmonary artery, and posterior left atrium angled to transect the orifices of the four pulmonary veins.

Figure 18–26A is a long axis recording that illustrates the right upper and lower pulmonary veins as they enter the superior-medial border of the left atrium. When viewed in this orientation, the veins lie next to one another. Their long axes are oriented parallel to that of the aorta. Figure 18–26B is a short axis recording that illustrates the left upper and left lower pulmonary veins as they enter the lateral border of the left atrium. In this view, the veins separate at a slight angle as they course leftward from the atrial wall. Figure 18–26C demonstrates the venous connection in the four-chamber view. From this vantage point, both the medial and lateral venous insertions of three (two lateral and one medial) of the pulmonary veins can be visualized. Figure 18–27 is an example of a "crab view" of the pulmonary veins recorded from the suprasternal notch in an adult. In this plane of section, each of the pulmonary veins is clearly recorded and their relative orientation is defined. The four pulmonary veins can also be routinely recorded from the esophagus and their flow patterns assessed.

Success rates for pulmonary venous visualization using the transthoracic approach have been reported pri-

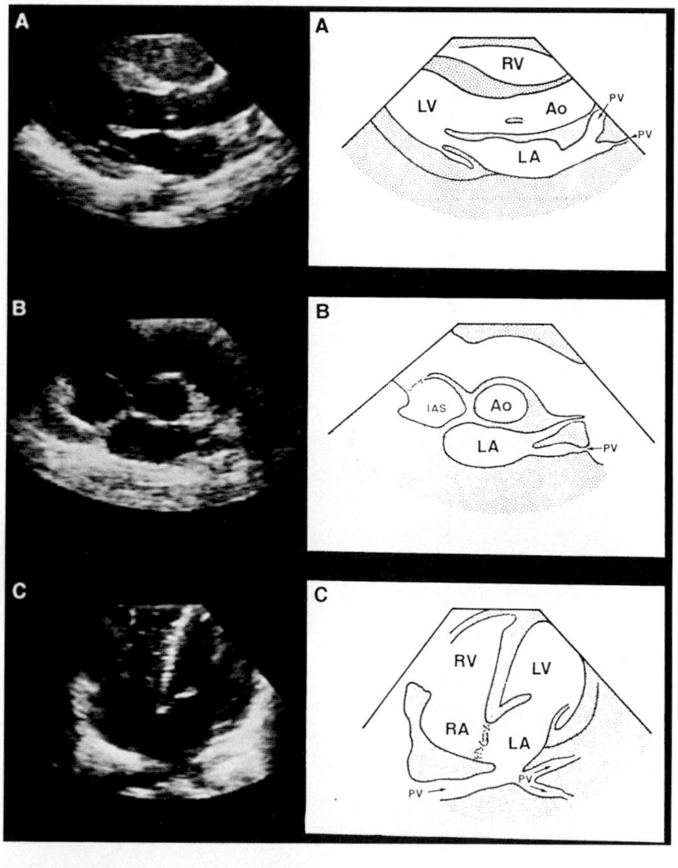

Fig. 18–26. **A.** Long axis recording of the left atrium (LA) with the transducer angled medially illustrates the right superior and inferior pulmonary veins (PV) inserting into the superior border of the left atrium. **B.** Short axis recording of the left atrium (LA) illustrates the superior and inferior left pulmonary veins (PV) inserting into the lateral walls of the atrial chamber. **C.** Apical four-chamber view illustrates the insertion of three of the four pulmonary veins (PV) (two lateral and one medial). Ao = aorta; IAS = interatrial septum; RV = right ventricle; LV = left ventricle; RA = right atrium; LA = left atrium.

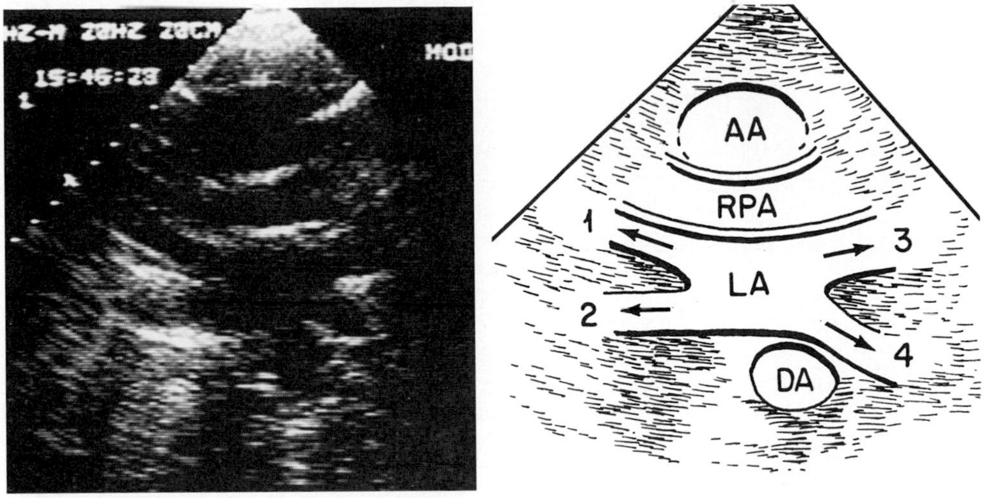

Fig. 18–27. Suprasternal recording illustrating the entry of the four pulmonary veins into the left atrium. In this so-called "crab view," (1) the right upper vein is superior and to the left; (2) the right lower is inferior and to the left; (3) the left upper is superior and to the right; and (4) the left lower is inferior and to the left. AA = aortic arch; DA = descending aorta; RPA = right pulmonary artery; LA = left atrium.

marily in infants.[68] In one study, at least one pulmonary vein was recorded in 94% of infants with a variety of congenital cardiac disorders. Two veins were visualized less frequently (77%). The best single view for recording the pulmonary veins proved to be the apical four-chamber view (86% of infants had at least one vein recorded in this view alone). The most consistently imaged vein was the left upper pulmonary vein, noted in 54% of cases. Although data are limited, in our experience, all four pulmonary veins can be routinely recorded from the esophagus.

Pulmonary Venous Flow

Pulmonary venous flow patterns have been studied using pulsed Doppler from both transthoracic and transesophageal approaches. Normal pulmonary venous flow can be divided into three phases: antegrade systolic, antegrade diastolic, and retrograde following atrial contraction (Fig. 18–28). Antegrade systolic flow is due to both the fall in atrial pressure that accompanies atrial muscular relaxation and the increase in atrial volume caused by apical systolic motion of the mitral annulus. Although atrial relaxation contributes to systolic forward flow, it does not appear to be the primary determinant because systolic forward flow persists, although at reduced velocity, in patients with atrial fibrillation (Fig. 18–29).[69,70] Annular displacement is an inherent component of ventricular contraction, and its amplitude relates to left ventricular output. Annular displacement causes an increase in atrial volume and fall in pressure with a corresponding increase in flow from the pulmonary veins into the left atrium. A direct linear relation has been reported between the cardiac output and the velocity of systolic forward flow[71] and an inverse relationship between the percentage of systolic filling (the percentage of total forward velocity occurring during systole) and the mean left atrial pressure.[72]

In patients with low filling pressures, systolic forward flow becomes biphasic, which appears to represent dissociation of the atrial and annular components of atrial filling. In these cases, the systolic filling from annular motion peaks later and continues longer than that due

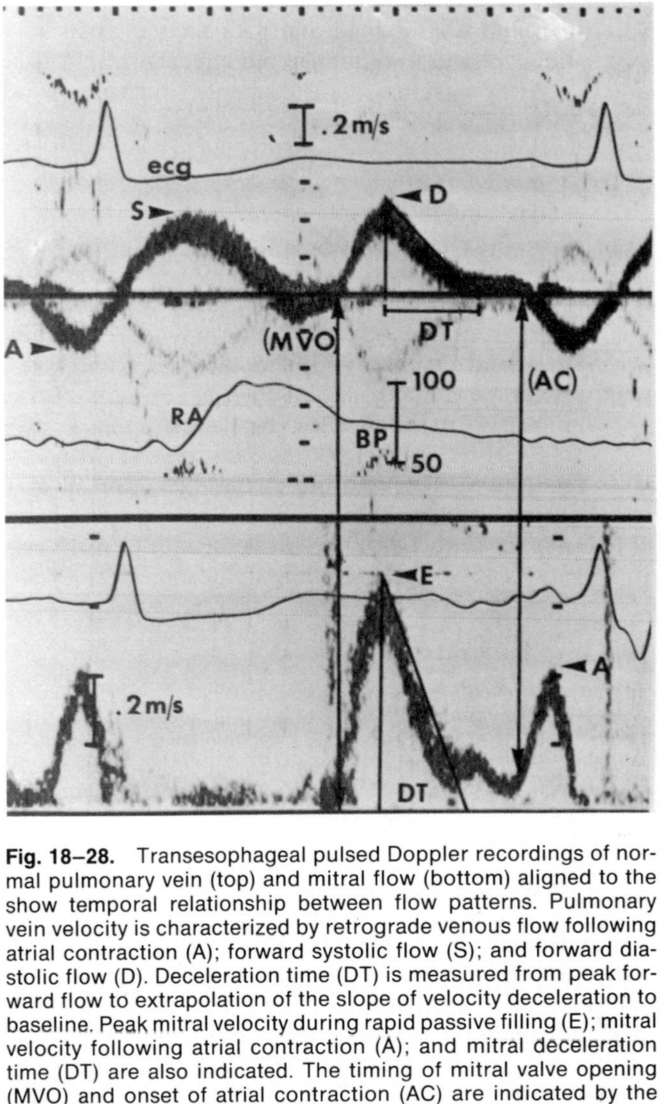

Fig. 18–28. Transesophageal pulsed Doppler recordings of normal pulmonary vein (top) and mitral flow (bottom) aligned to the show temporal relationship between flow patterns. Pulmonary vein velocity is characterized by retrograde venous flow following atrial contraction (A); forward systolic flow (S); and forward diastolic flow (D). Deceleration time (DT) is measured from peak forward flow to extrapolation of the slope of velocity deceleration to baseline. Peak mitral velocity during rapid passive filling (E); mitral velocity following atrial contraction (A); and mitral deceleration time (DT) are also indicated. The timing of mitral valve opening (MVO) and onset of atrial contraction (AC) are indicated by the vertical arrows. RA = radial artery pressure recording; ecg = electrocardiogram. (From Nishimura RA, Abel MF, Hatle LK, Tajik AJ: Relation of pulmonary vein to mitral flow velocities by transesophageal Doppler echocardiography: effect of different loading conditions. Circulation 81:1488, 1990. Reproduced by permission of the American Heart Association, Inc.)

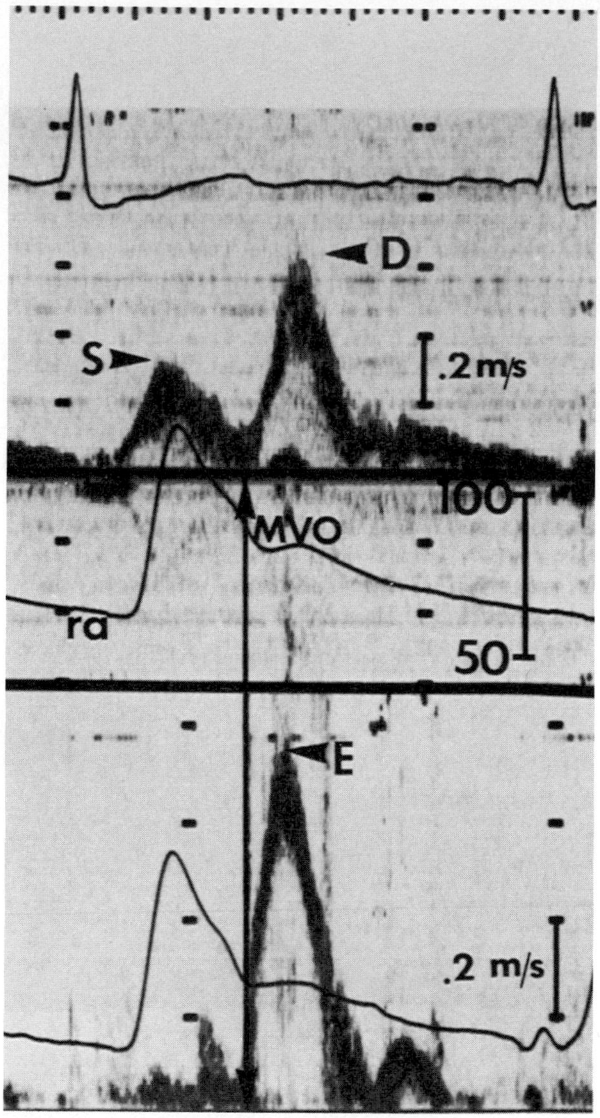

Fig. 18–29. Transesophageal pulsed Doppler recordings of pulmonary vein velocity curve (top) and mitral flow velocity curve (bottom) in a patient with atrial fibrillation. Forward velocities normally recorded following atrial contraction are absent. Systolic (S) forward velocity is lower than diastolic (D) velocity. Vertical arrow indicates timing of mitral valve opening (MVO). ra = radial artery pressure. E = peak velocity of E (passive filling) wave (From Nishimura RA, Abel MF, Hatle LK, Tajik AJ: Relation of pulmonary vein to mitral flow velocities by transesophageal Doppler echocardiography: effect of different loading conditions. Circulation 81:1488, 1990. Reproduced with permission of the American Heart Association, Inc.)

to atrial contraction. In patients with high degree AV block, the antegrade component of pulmonary flow that is due to atrial relaxation follows the P waves of the electrocardiogram including those not conducted to the ventricle.[69] Other variables that effect atrial pressure and pulmonary vein systolic flow are atrial compliance and mitral regurgitation. In clinical and experimental studies, increasing left atrial pressure resulting from mitral regurgitation has been shown to cause a decrease in forward flow in late systole with complete reversal of flow when regurgitation was severe (Fig. 18–30).[73,74]

Diastolic forward flow in the pulmonary veins reflects the pattern of transmitral flow. Initial mitral valve opening causes the pressure in the left atrium to drop, increasing the atrial-venous gradient and causing blood flow from the pulmonary veins to begin. Because the atrium is open to the ventricle during diastole, the pulmonary veins essentially "see" ventricular pressure, and flow is determined by the ventricular-venous gradient. Both the peak diastolic velocity and the deceleration time of pulmonary venous flow are similar to the peak E velocity and deceleration time of the mitral valve. However, the peak velocity of pulmonary diastolic flow occurs roughly 50 msec after the peak of the mitral E wave.[70] Because the diastolic pulmonary and mitral flow profiles are similar, they must be determined by the same forces (i.e., left atrial pressure, ventricular relaxation, and atrial and ventricular compliance; see Chapter 24).

In patients with high filling pressures and high afterload, mid-diastolic forward flow has been noted following rapid mitral E-wave deceleration. It has been postulated that this flow causes continued atrial filling, thereby restoring the positive pressure gradient between the atrium and ventricle and reopening the mitral valve.

Atrial contraction causes both forward flow through the mitral valve and reversed flow into the pulmonary veins.[75] The atrial systolic pressure and amount of forward flow are influenced by the ventricular pressure against which the atrium must contract with higher pres-

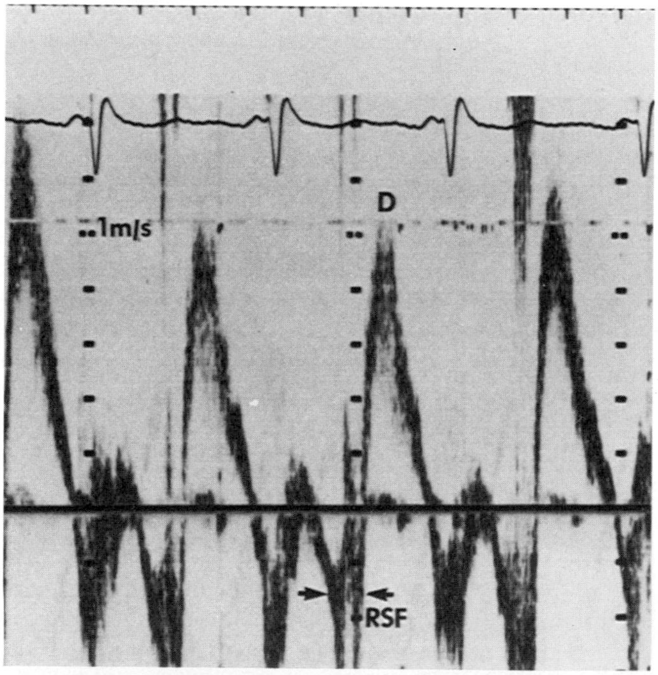

Fig. 18–30. Pulsed Doppler transesophageal recording from the left upper pulmonary vein in a 44-year-old man with 4+ mitral regurgitation secondary to a flail posterior leaflet. Note the reversed systolic flow (RSF) with increased peak diastolic (D) filling. (From Klein AL, et al.: Transesophageal Doppler echocardiography of pulmonary venous flow: A new marker of mitral regurgitation severity. J Am Coll Cardiol 18:518, 1991. Reprinted with permission from the American College of Cardiology.)

sures and less ventricular filling occurring in patients with higher ventricular pressures. For any given atrial systolic pressure, retrograde flow into the pulmonary veins will increase in proportion to the resistance to forward flow into the left ventricle because pulmonary venous compliance is greater than ventricular compliance. When atrial contraction increases independently as a result of an increase in atrial preload, both forward and reverse flow velocities increase.

In addition to its normal physiologic variability, the pattern of pulmonary venous flow is reportedly altered in several disease states including mitral stenosis,[76] cor triatriatum,[77] constrictive pericarditis,[78] and restrictive myopathy.[79] Figure 18–31, e.g., compares the difference in mean inspiratory and expiratory pulmonary flow velocities in small groups of normal persons and in patients with constrictive pericarditis and restrictive cardiomyopathy. Unfortunately, all available data to date are from small groups of selected patients, and the ultimate diagnostic value of these changes in pulmonary flow patterns remains to be defined.

Anomalous Pulmonary Venous Connection and Return

Abnormalities of the pulmonary venous system are many and varied. Two general terms are used to describe these abnormalities: (1) *anomalous pulmonary venous connection,* which indicates that all (total) or part (partial) of the pulmonary venous system is connected to the right atrium either directly or via one of its tributary veins, and (2) *anomalous pulmonary venous drainage,* which is a functional term and implies that one or more of the pulmonary veins is directed so that its flow passes preferentially into the right atrium, usually by way of an associated atrial septal defect.[80]

When anomalous pulmonary venous connection is total, the pulmonary veins may connect with the right atrium separately or, more often, may combine into a venous chamber behind the left atrium. A separate vascular channel then arises from this accessory chamber to connect with the right atrium or one of its tributaries. Common sites of connection include the coronary sinus, innominate vein, superior vena cava, and right atrium directly. Several echocardiographic findings, which although not specific for total anomalous pulmonary venous connection, are uniformly associated with this disorder. These nonspecific features, in general, are easily defined and must be present before the diagnosis can be entertained. They include (1) a right ventricular volume overload pattern and (2) an atrial septal defect with obligatory right-to-left shunting. The right ventricular volume overload pattern occurs because both systemic and pulmonary venous blood enters the right atrium, and the majority of this increased volume must be borne by the right ventricle. The volume overload pattern is characterized by an increase in right ventricular chamber size, displacement of the interventricular septum toward the left ventricle, and paradoxic septal motion. The atrial septal defect is necessary for survival because, without it, blood cannot reach the left side of the heart. The septal defect can be visualized directly in the short axis, four-chamber or subcostal long axis views and can be confirmed by peripheral contrast injection with the demonstration of a right-to-left shunt at the atrial level. In addition, the left atrium is usually smaller than normal because of the reduced inflow into the chamber; however, this finding by itself is not of diagnostic value.[8]

Specific echocardiographic characteristics of total anomalous pulmonary venous return relate to the direct demonstration of the venous chamber behind the left atrium and of additional changes that may be recorded in the tributary veins to which this chamber is connected.[18,63] The common venous chamber appears as an echo-free space that is best visualized on the apical and subxiphoid views, is separated from the atria by a linear band of echoes, and thus appears as a subdivision behind the true left atrium. The position of this chamber may vary, depending on the site of connection of the anomalous pulmonary venous inflow into the right heart.[68] These changes in position, however, appear subtle and may be difficult to appreciate.

It has also been reported that the level of entry of the anomalous venous connection into the systemic circulation can be detected based on the visualization of an accessory venous pattern and/or dilation of the tributary vein receiving the anomalous pulmonary venous flow.[18] The easiest abnormal tributary vein to record is the coronary sinus. When the anomalous pulmonary veins connect with the coronary sinus, the coronary sinus typically dilates. When coronary sinus dilation is combined with an anomalous chamber behind the left atrial wall, a right ventricular volume overload pattern, and an atrial septal defect with right-to-left shunting, total anomalous pulmonary venous return to the coronary sinus is strongly suggested. (Total anomalous pulmonary venous return is discussed in greater detail in Chapter 32.)

Partial anomalous pulmonary venous return is usually confined to the right pulmonary veins. The most common types of partial anomalous pulmonary venous con-

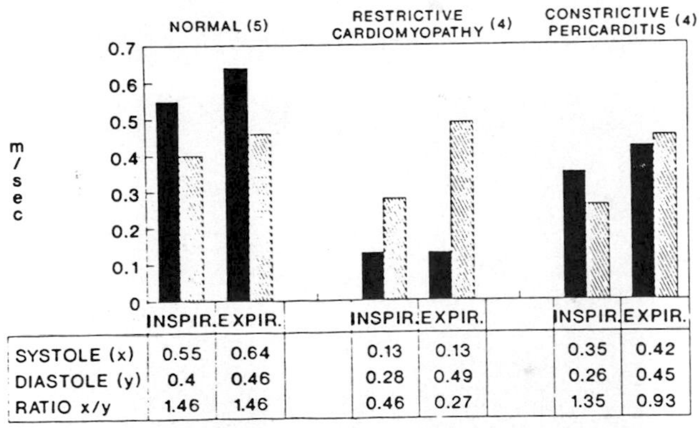

	NORMAL (5) INSPIR.	NORMAL (5) EXPIR.	RESTRICTIVE CARDIOMYOPATHY (4) INSPIR.	RESTRICTIVE CARDIOMYOPATHY (4) EXPIR.	CONSTRICTIVE PERICARDITIS (4) INSPIR.	CONSTRICTIVE PERICARDITIS (4) EXPIR.
SYSTOLE (x)	0.55	0.64	0.13	0.13	0.35	0.42
DIASTOLE (y)	0.4	0.46	0.28	0.49	0.26	0.45
RATIO x/y	1.46	1.46	0.46	0.27	1.35	0.93

Fig. 18–31. Comparison of difference in mean inspiratory and expiratory pulmonary flow velocities in small groups of normal persons and in patients with constrictive pericarditis and restrictive cardiomyopathy. (From Schiavone WA, Calafiore PA, Salcedo EE: Transesophageal Doppler echocardiographic demonstration of pulmonary venous flow velocity in restrictive cardiomyopathy and constrictive pericarditis. Am J Cardiol 63:1286, 1989.)

nection are drainage of the right upper pulmonary vein to the superior vena cava and drainage of all or part of the right pulmonary venous system to the right atrium. Echocardiographic findings will vary depending on the degree of shunt flow, with larger shunts producing a right ventricular volume overload pattern. Color Doppler will often permit the abnormal venous inflow to be identified, particularly when the vein(s) enter the right atrium. In one patient with three separate right pulmonary veins entering the right atrium (Fig. 18–32), the right upper vein entered the right atrium near the superior-vena caval-right atrial junction; the right middle vein near the junction of the atrial septum and the supero-posterior atrial wall, and the right lower vein just superior to the orifice of the inferior vena cava.[67]

Anomalous pulmonary venous drainage is difficult to diagnose echocardiographically. On occasion, an anomalous jet can be recorded by color flow Doppler entering the right atrium adjacent to the superior vena caval-right atrial junction, but this finding is neither sensitive nor specific. It has also been observed during cardiac catheterization that if a catheter is placed in the pulmonary veins and echocardiographic contrast is injected, the resulting pattern of venous blood flow can be defined from the distribution of contrast within the left and right sides of the heart.[81] This procedure may be adjunctive when color flow studies are inconclusive and the angiographic definition of venous flow patterns proves difficult.

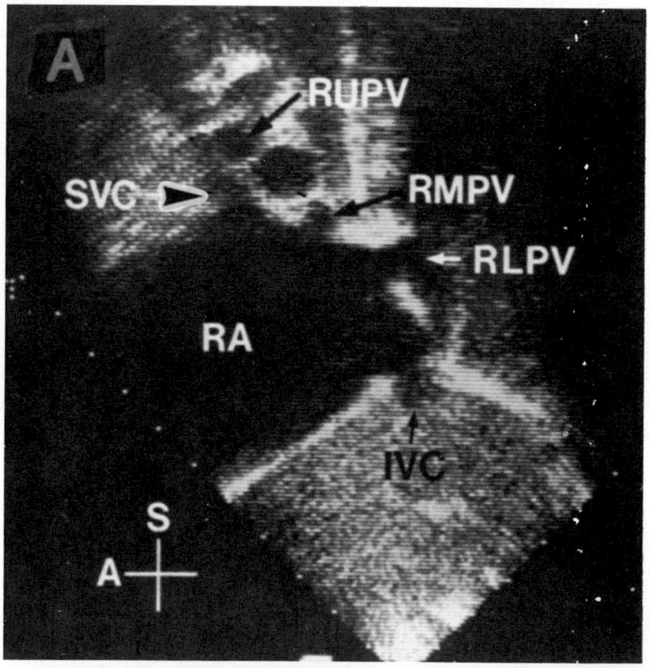

Fig. 18–32. Entrance of three separate pulmonary veins into the right atrium. SVC = superior vena cave; RA = right atrium; RUPV = right upper pulmonary vein; RMPV = right middle pulmonary vein; RLPV = right lower pulmonary vein; IVC = inferior vena cava. (From Vermilion RP, Snider R, Peters JA, Merida-Asmus LM: Two-dimensional echocardiographic and color flow Doppler detection of an unusual pulmonary venous anomaly: anomalous right pulmonary venous return to the right atrium by way of three separate orifices. J Am Soc Echocardiogr 3:135, 1990. Reproduced with permission from Mosby Year-Book, Inc.)

Pulmonary Venous Obstruction

Isolated pulmonary venous obstruction is a rare anomaly that may involve a single or multiple pulmonary veins. The obstruction may be due to a localized stenotic segment, a partially obstructing fibrous diaphragm, and on occasion, the entire extrapulmonary vessel may be atretic.[82] In most cases, the obstruction is congenital, although acquired lesions have been reported.[82]

Postoperative venous inflow obstruction can also be observed in patients who have undergone the Mustard

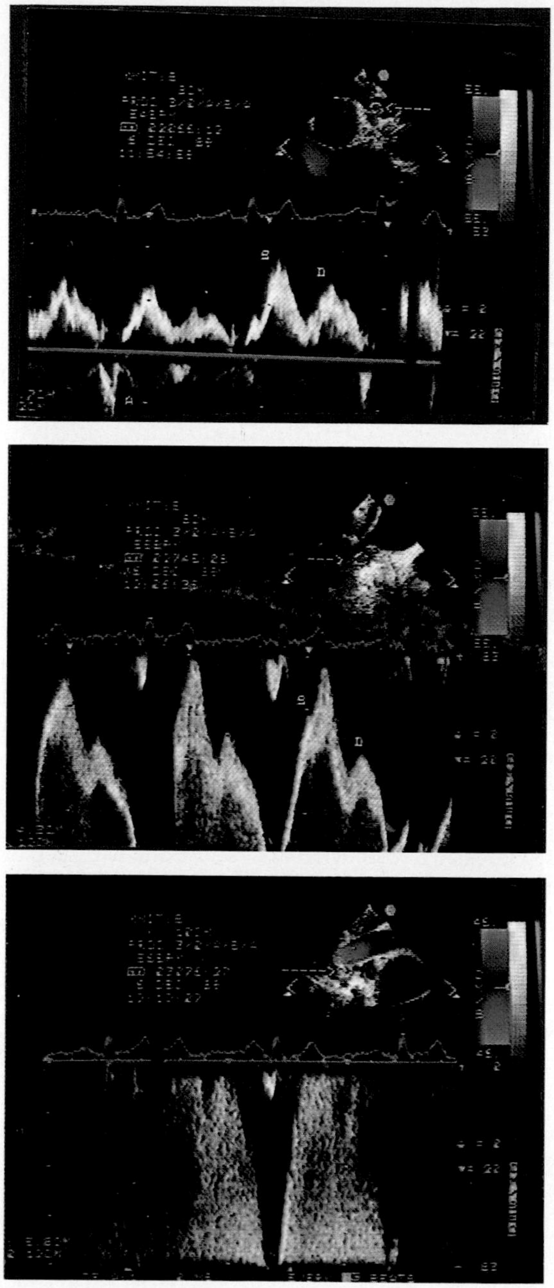

Fig. 18–33. Velocities in three pulmonary veins. (From Patt MV, Obeid AI: Cor triatriatum with isolated pulmonary venous stenosis in an adult: diagnosis with transesophageal two-dimensional echocardiography. J Am Soc Echocardiogr 4:185, 1991. Reproduced with permission from Mosby Year-Book, Inc.)

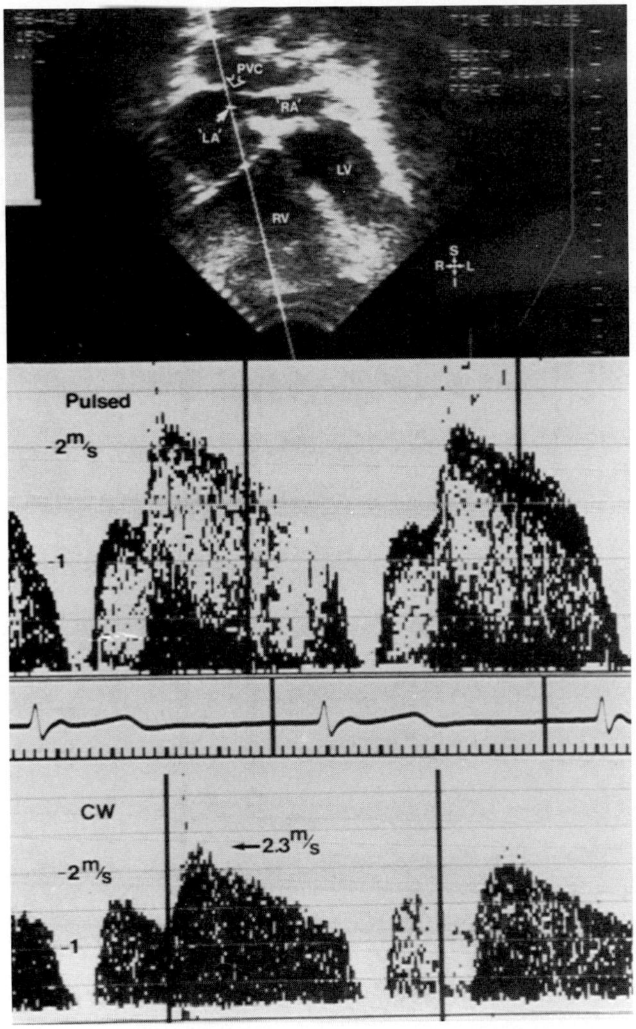

Fig. 18–34. Velocity pattern in a patient with pulmonary venous obstruction following a Mustard procedure. Top. Two-dimensional recording illustrating narrowing at the junction of the pulmonary venous confluence (PVC) and the main body of the pulmonary venous atrium ('LA'). The pulsed Doppler sample volume is positioned near the junction of the pulmonary venous confluence and the main body of the venous atrium. Middle. The pulsed Doppler study revealed a velocity of >2 m/sec., Bottom. By continuous wave (CW) Doppler, the velocity was measured at 2.3 m/sec. 'RA' = right atrium; LV = left ventricle; RV = right ventricle. (From Vick GW III, et al.: Pulmonary venous and systemic ventricular inflow obstruction in patients with congenital heart disease: detection by combined two-dimensional and Doppler echocardiography. J Am Coll Cardiol 9:580, 1987. Reprinted with permission from the American College of Cardiology.)

or Senning procedure for transposition of the great arteries.[83,84] Although uncommon, anastomotic stricture causing pulmonary venous obstruction is the most common mode of surgical failure following correction for total anomalous connection of the pulmonary veins.

Pulmonary venous obstruction alters the normal pattern of flow from the pulmonary veins producing a biphasic or continuous high velocity turbulent flow pattern at the site of obstruction, similar to that seen with ductus arteriosus.[85–88] Figure 18–33 illustrates flow velocities recorded from three different pulmonary veins with varying degrees of obstruction in the same patient. A similar increase in velocity is seen in patients with mid-baffle or pulmonary vein obstruction following the Mustard or Senning procedures[89] and with stricture of the inflow anastomosis following surgical correction of total anomalous pulmonary venous return.[87] In these cases, the highest velocities occur during initial diastole (Fig. 18–34) when atrial pressure falls most rapidly and the atrial-venous gradient therefore is greatest. In a heterogenous group of patients with various types of left ventricular inflow obstruction, severe stenosis was predicted by a diastolic inflow velocity of ≥ 2 m/sec at any level of the left ventricular inflow tract.[88] Milder degrees of obstruction may be more difficult to identify; however, a comparison of the velocities and flow patterns in the different pulmonary veins can be helpful. Recording of both absolute peak velocity and relative velocity is complicated by the different angles at which the pulmonary veins enter the atrium, but the presence of local turbulence and anatomic evidence of narrowing should aid in diagnosis. The degree of obstruction can also be underestimated by the gradient when there is low pulmonary venous return resulting from obstruction to pulmonary blood flow, low cardiac output, or pulmonary atelectasis.[88]

CORONARY SINUS

The coronary sinus is located in the atrioventricular groove along the posterior surface of the heart. It is covered by a layer of muscle fibers from the left atrial wall and by the pericardium and therefore is partially incorporated into the atrial wall.

Echocardiographically, the coronary sinus is best visualized in the parasternal long axis view. When recorded, it appears as a circular echo-free space lying posterior to the left atrial wall just superior to the atrioventricular junction. This echo-free space characteristically moves in concert with the atrioventricular ring. This motion pattern differentiates the coronary sinus, particularly when dilated, from the descending aorta, which may likewise appear circular and lie behind the left atrial wall. The aorta, however, is independent of the heart, and therefore, its motion pattern does not follow that of the atrioventricular ring. The normal coronary sinus is visualized relatively infrequently in adults and rarely, if at all, in children.[90]

Dilation

Dilation of the coronary sinus is frequently noted in patients with right ventricular dysfunction and right atrial hypertension (Fig. 18–35). Marked coronary sinus dilation also occurs owing to increased volume flow into this structure from anomalous venous communications.[91] Four patterns of anomalous venous drainage into the coronary sinus have been characterized echocardiographically.[90] These include (1) persistent left superior vena cava with drainage into the coronary sinus, (2) total anomalous pulmonary venous return with coronary sinus drainage, (3) coronary AV fistula with drainage into the coronary sinus, and (4) anomalous hepatic venous drainage to the coronary sinus. Persistent left

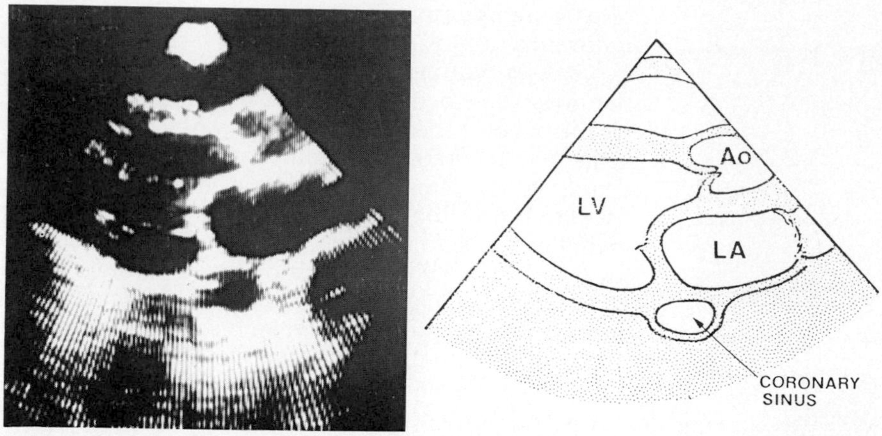

Fig. 18–35. Long axis recording of the left atrium (LA) and left ventricle (LV) illustrates a dilated coronary sinus lying posterior to the left atrium in the region of the atrioventricular groove. The dilated coronary sinus appears circular because this plane transects the vessel parallel to its short axis. This recording was obtained in a patient with severe biventricular failure and right atrial hypertension. The fact that this vessel represents the coronary sinus and not the descending aorta can be confirmed by its motion, which is parallel with that of the atrioventricular ring. Ao = aorta.

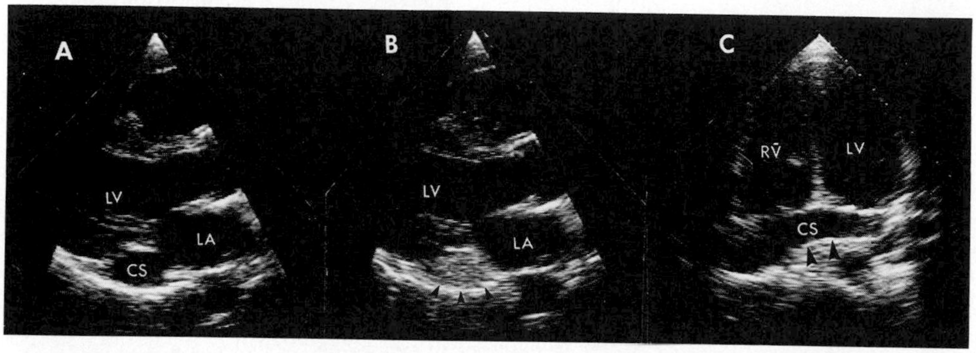

Fig. 18–36. A. parasternal long axis recording from a patient with a dilated coronary sinus (CS) that is due to a persistent left superior vena cava. **B.** Opacification of the CS following contrast injection into the left antecubital vein. **C.** Apical four-chamber view showing the dilated CS emptying into the right atrium. LV = left ventricle; LA = left atrium; RV = right ventricle.

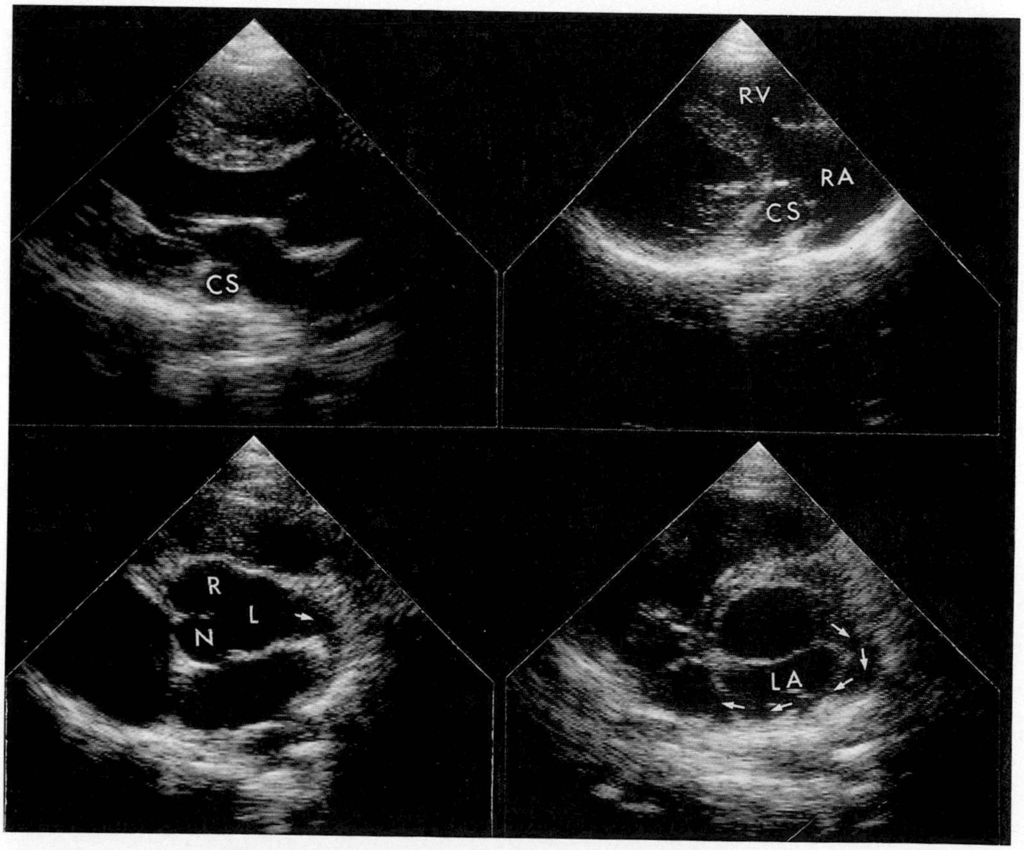

Fig. 18–37. Coronary arteriovenous fistula draining into the coronary sinus (CS). Top, right. Parasternal long axis recording illustrating a dilated CS in the posterior atrioventricular groove. Top, right. Right ventricular inflow view showing the dilated CS bulging into right atrium (RA). Bottom, left. Parasternal long axis recording to the left main coronary artery illustrating dilation of the left coronary ostium and left circumflex coronary artery. Bottom, right. Course (arrows) of flow from the left circumflex coronary artery to the coronary sinus. LA = left atrium; R = right coronary aortic cusp of aortic valve; N = noncoronary aortic valve cusp; L = left coronary aortic valve cusp; RV = right ventricle.

superior vena cava is a fairly common congenital anomaly that is found in 0.5%[92,93] of normal patients and in from 3 to 10% of patients with congenital heart disease.[91] This diagnosis is suspected whenever the coronary sinus is dilated and can be confirmed by injection of echocardiographic contrast into the left basilic vein. When injected into the left arm, contrast should flow through the persistent left superior vena cava into the coronary sinus, thereby opacifying this dilated chamber.

Figure 18–36 is an example of a patient with a persistent left superior vena cava recorded before and after contrast injection. In the left panel, the dilated echo-free coronary sinus is illustrated at the base of the atrioventricular ring. Following contrast injection into the left arm, this entire area is opacified, thereby confirming this diagnosis. Contrast injected into the right basilic vein conversely flows normally through the right superior vena cava into the right atrium. The coronary sinus remains echo free. Rarely, the right superior vena cava may be absent, and all upper extremity venous flow returns to the heart via the left superior vena cava and coronary sinus. In these cases, the coronary sinus will be much larger than with simple persistence of the left superior vena cava with a patent right superior cava, and contrast injected into either arm will enter the right atrium via the coronary sinus.[94] When the persistent left superior vena cava communicates with the left atrium rather than with the coronary sinus, this chamber is opacified following left-arm injection.[95]

Coronary sinus dilation that is due to total anomalous pulmonary venous connection is detected by the associated presence of a right ventricular volume overload pattern, an atrial septal defect with a mandatory right-to-left shunt, and the demonstration of a common venous chamber behind the left atrium. Contrast injection in either the right or the left basilic vein results in total opacification of both the left and right sides of the heart, and the contrast fails to enter the dilated coronary sinus.

A coronary AV fistula with drainage into the coronary sinus produces a high-pressure shunt and, in addition to coronary sinus dilation, should be associated with obvious dilation of the coronary artery involved (Fig. 18–37).

Anomalous hepatic venous connection to the coronary sinus is a rare congenital anomaly that can also cause coronary sinus dilation. Because the coronary sinus connects to the right atrium, this anomaly does not produce any hemodynamic disturbance, and its importance lies only in its similarity of appearance to that of subdiaphragmatic total anomalous pulmonary venous connection. Common features include a third vascular channel penetrating the diaphragm between the inferior vena cava and aorta, which could be mistaken for the vertical venous channel in subdiaphragmatic total anomalous pulmonary venous return (TAPVR). The direction of flow, however, should be opposite, with pulmonary venous flow coursing in a superior-inferior direction, while hepatic venous flow is directed superiorly through the diaphragm. In the infant, if an umbilical vein catheter is in place, contrast injection can also be used to outline the path of venous flow through the hepatic veins and coronary sinus.[96]

The coronary sinus may also become dilated as a result of postoperative obstruction, thrombosis, or ventricularization (see following discussion).

Unroofed Coronary Sinus

Unroofed coronary sinus is a rare congenital cardiac anomaly in which there is a defect in the tissue separating the coronary sinus and the left atrium. This defect permits communication between the venous blood in the great vein and the arterial (oxygenated) blood in the left atrium. The defect may be only a few millimeters in diameter, or the whole roof of the sinus may be absent. Figure 18–38 illustrates the anatomy of this defect. Physiologically, the defect typically causes a shunt from the left to the right atrium via the coronary sinus (see Chapter 29). When right atrial pressures are elevated, however, a right-to-left shunt may develop with systemic desaturation.

The optimal views for recording the defect depend on its size and location. Visualization has been reported in the parasternal long axis, parasternal short axis, and subxyphoid four-chamber views of the coronary sinus.[97] When unroofed coronary sinus is associated with anomalous left superior vena cava, contrast injected into the

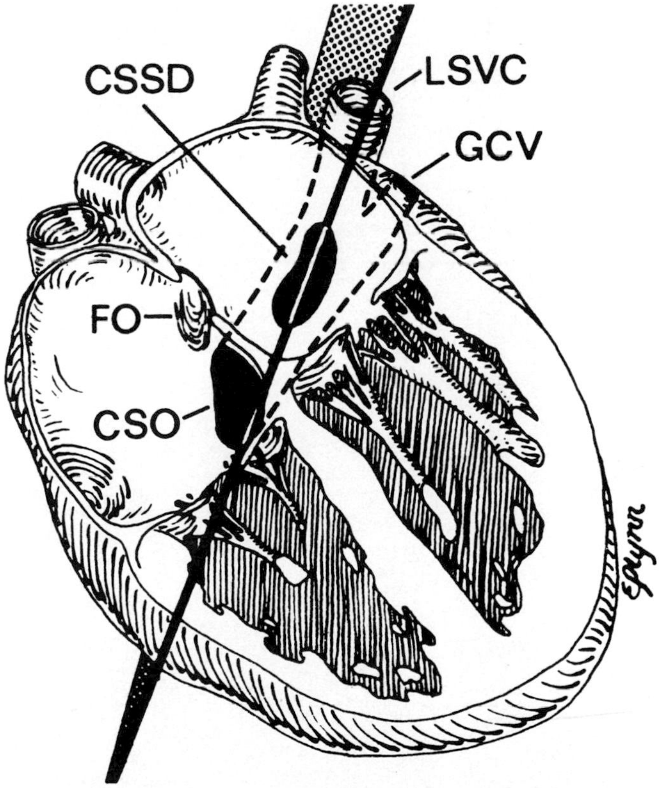

Fig. 18–38. Unroofed coronary sinus. Two-dimensional plane used for displaying coronary sinus defect is indicated. The ostium of the coronary sinus (CSO) is depicted as it enters the right atrium. An echo-free gap (CSSD) indicates the unroofed portion of the coronary sinus. Also indicated is a persistent left superior vena cava (LSVC), which can be recorded behind the left atrium. GCV = great cardiac vein. (From Yeager SB, Chin AJ, Sanders SP: Subxiphoid two-dimensional echocardiographic diagnosis of coronary sinus septal defects. Am J Cardiol 54:686, 1984.)

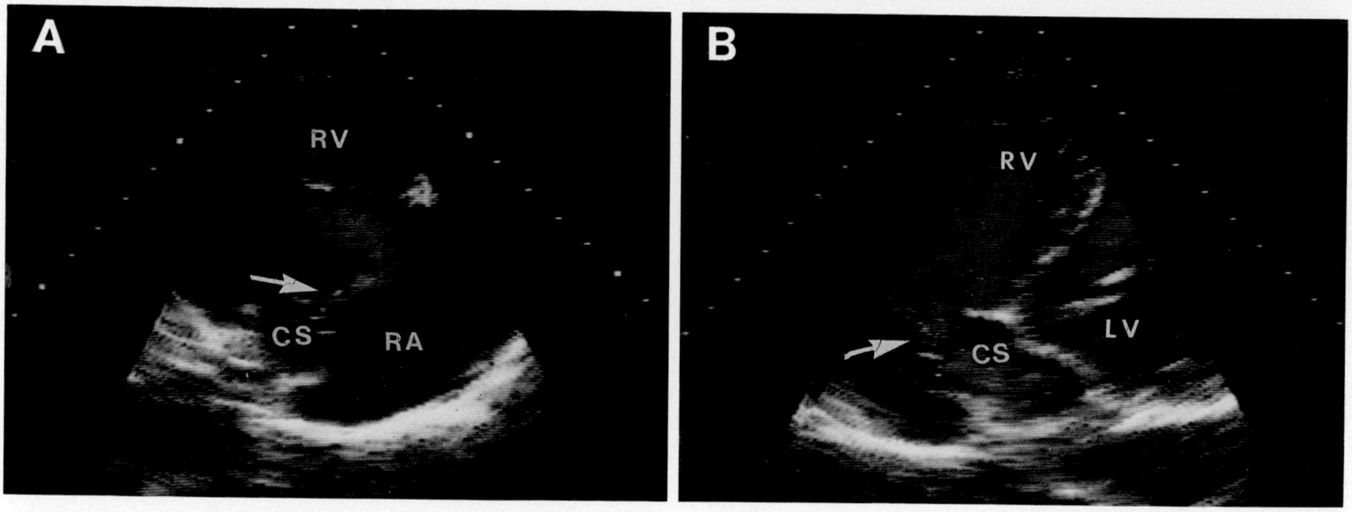

Fig. 18–39. High velocity flow from the coronary sinus (CS) that is due to partial obstruction to coronary sinus outflow. **A.** Right ventricular inflow view showing the high velocity jet (red) arising from the narrow outlet of the sinus and curving toward the tricuspid valve along with the diastolic flow stream. **B.** Depressed apical four-chamber view illustrating turbulent flow (arrow) arising from the coronary sinus. RV = right ventricle; LV = left ventricle.

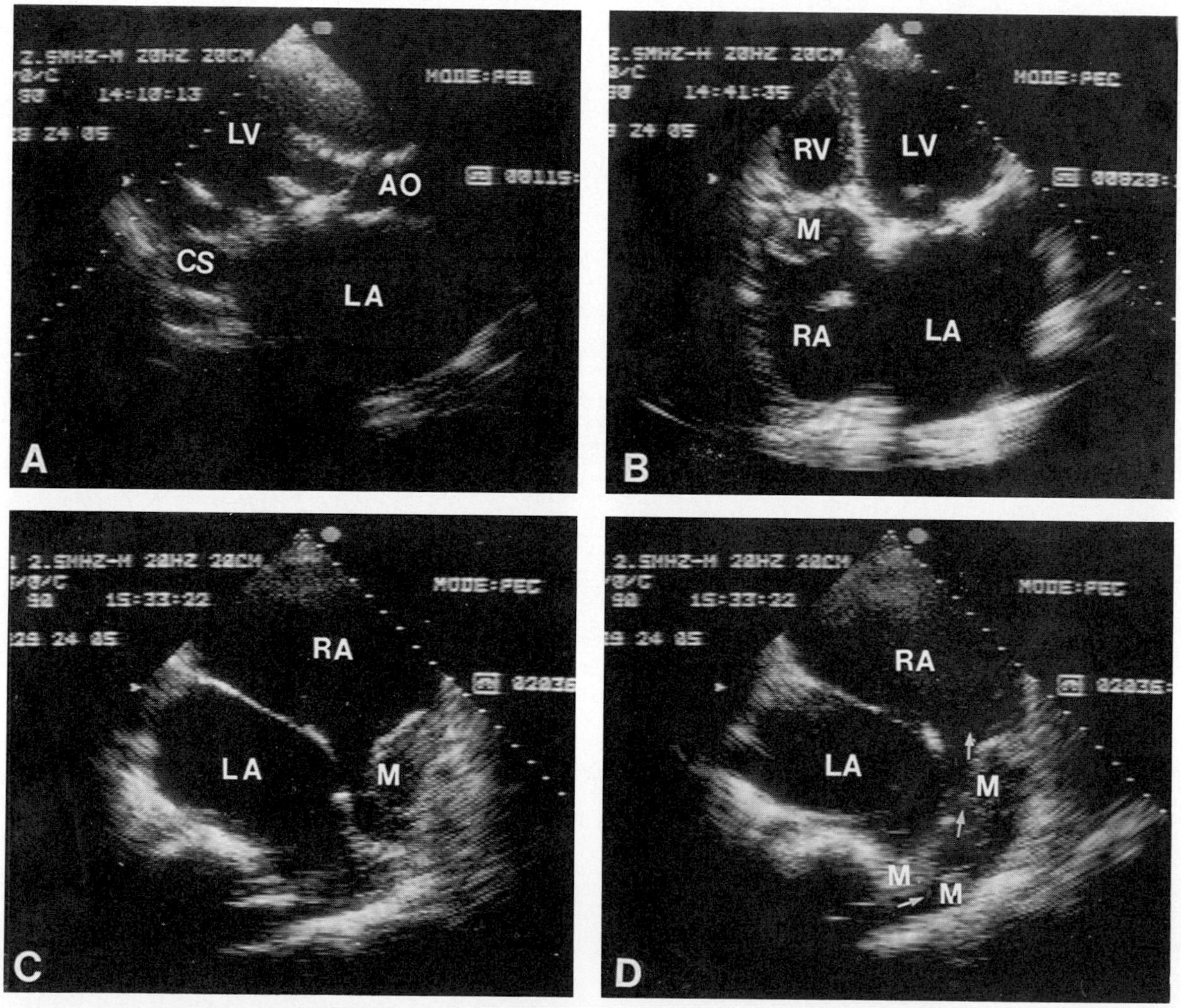

Fig. 18–40. Series of recordings from a patient following mitral and tricuspid valve replacement illustrating partial thrombosis of the coronary sinus (CS). **A.** Parasternal long axis view. The left atrium (LA) and CS are dilated, and there is a prosthetic valve in the mitral position. **B.** Apical four-chamber recording illustrating a mass (M) in the right atrium (RA) behind the prosthetic tricuspid valve near the orifice of the CS. **C.** Transesophageal recording from the same patient illustrating thrombus in the coronary sinus near its origin with the right ventricle. **D.** Transesophageal recording angled to display a longer segment of the CS and illustrating both sinus dilation and extension of the thrombus roughly 6 cm back from the orifice. The arrows indicate the path of flow around the thrombus. LV = left ventricle; AO = aorta; RV = right ventricle.

left arm will usually enter the left atrium through the defect and then continue on to opacify the right atrium. Note, however, that the anomalous left superior vena cava may connect directly to the left atrium, and the appearance of contrast in the left atrium following left arm injection does not, by itself, establish the diagnosis of unroofed coronary sinus.

Postoperative Abnormalities

A variety of abnormalities of the coronary sinus can be observed postoperatively. These include (1) partial coronary sinus obstruction, (2) coronary sinus thrombosis, (3) ventricularization of the coronary sinus, and (4) left atrial insertion of the coronary sinus. Coronary sinus obstruction usually complicates tricuspid valve repair but can also occur as a component of a complex congenital anomaly. Outlet obstruction leads to coronary sinus dilation and an increase in pressure within the great vein. The difference in pressure between the sinus and the atrium produces an increase in the velocity of the efflux into the atrium and can alter the normal phasic pattern of flow (Fig. 18–39). Coronary sinus thrombosis is also seen after tricuspid valve surgery, and like other thrombi, presents as an echogenic mass within the normally fluid-filled chamber (Fig. 18–40). The effects of ventricularization of the sinus depend on whether it is displaced below a prosthetic tricuspid or mitral valve. Displacement below the tricuspid valve subjects the sinus to right ventricular systolic pressure and can lead to massive dilation. Figure 18–41, e.g., is a recording from a patient with Ebstein's anomaly in whom a prosthetic valve was implanted on the atrial side of the sinus.

Placement of a prosthetic mitral valve superior to the sinus results in an echo-free space in the myocardium on the ventricular side of the sewing ring. This generally occupies the whole ventricular wall and may be quite large because in many cases the sinus was dilated—as a result of associated right heart disease—before the prosthetic mitral valve was implanted. Although not of functional significance, this echo-free space can easily be confused with a pseudoaneurysm at the base of the valve ring or a ring abscess. This becomes particularly difficult when the clinical situation suggests confounding

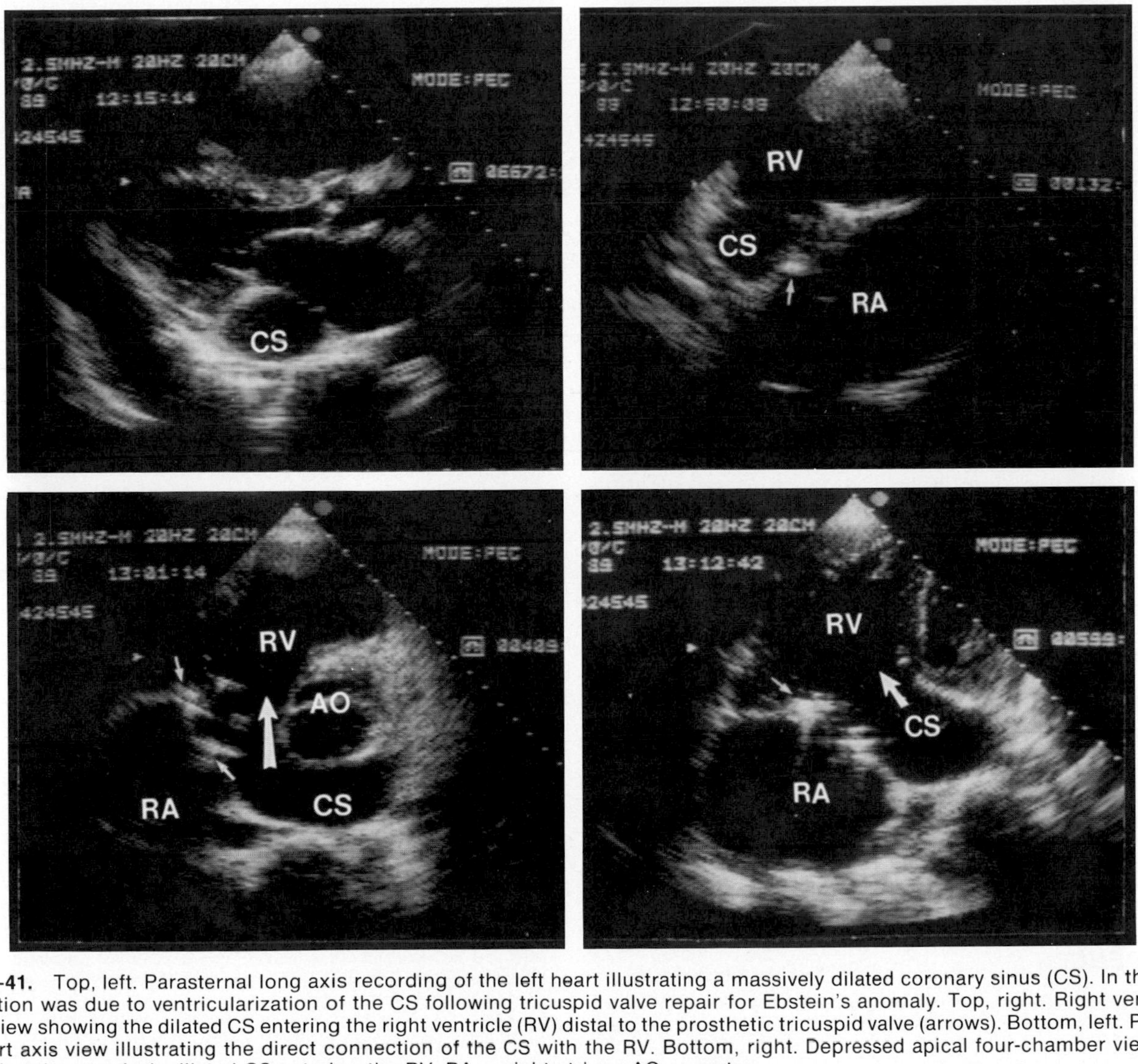

Fig. 18–41. Top, left. Parasternal long axis recording of the left heart illustrating a massively dilated coronary sinus (CS). In this case, CS dilation was due to ventricularization of the CS following tricuspid valve repair for Ebstein's anomaly. Top, right. Right ventricular inflow view showing the dilated CS entering the right ventricle (RV) distal to the prosthetic tricuspid valve (arrows). Bottom, left. Parasternal short axis view illustrating the direct connection of the CS with the RV. Bottom, right. Depressed apical four-chamber view again illustrating the massively dilated CS entering the RV. RA = right atrium; AO = aorta.

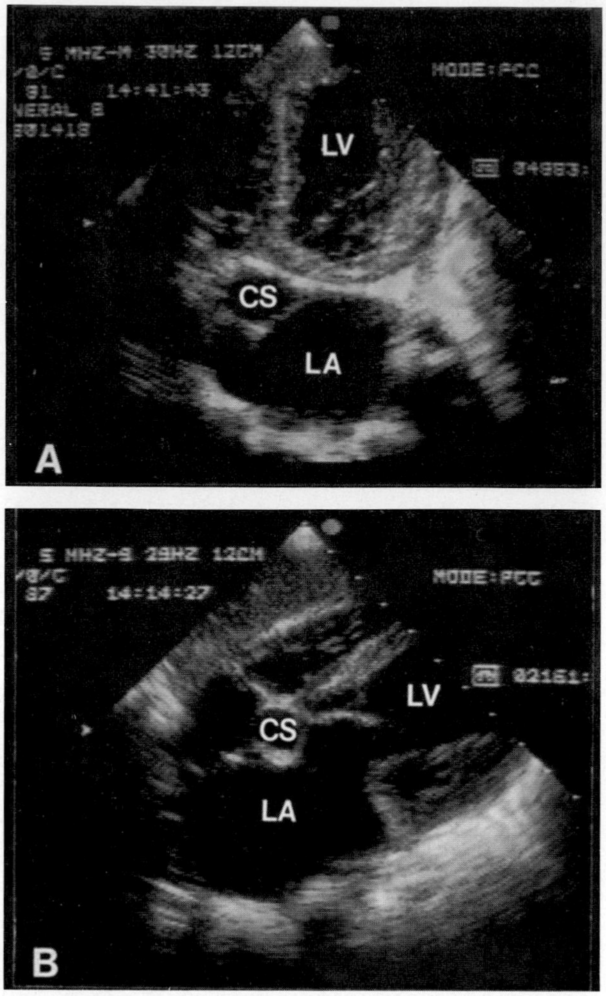

Fig. 18–42. A. Depressed apical four-chamber view illustrating the coronary sinus (CS) entering the left ventricle (LV) following surgical repair of an atrioventricular canal defect. **B.** Subcostal four-chamber view from the same patient, again illustrating the left-sided entry of the CS. LA = left atrium.

disease. Correct diagnosis is possible by following the path of the sinus and demonstrating its communication with the right atrium. Demonstration of flow in the sinus is also useful but tends to be difficult. Surgical ligation of the circumflex coronary artery during mitral valve replacement has also been reported to cause local necrosis and a left ventricular-coronary sinus fistula. The fistula was characterized by dilation of the coronary sinus, a large left-to-right shunt, and high velocity flow in the coronary sinus detectable by Doppler techniques.[98]

Finally, during surgical repair of an A-V canal, the atrial septal patch can be inserted such that the orifice of the coronary sinus is on the left side of the septum and the sinus drains into the left atrium. In these cases, the orifice of the sinus can be imaged on the left atrial side of the septal patch (Fig. 18–42), and coronary sinus flow will be recorded in the left atrium.

REFERENCES

1. Hurst JW: The Heart. New York, McGraw-Hill, 1974.
2. Gray H: Gray's Anatomy. Edited by CM Goss. Philadelphia, Lea & Febiger, 1959.
3. Matsuda Y, et al.: Importance of left atrial function in patients with myocardial infarction. Circulation 67:566, 1983.
4. Hawley RR, Dodge HT, Graham TP: Left atrial volume and its changes in heart disease. Circulation 34:989, 1966.
5. Murray JA, Kennedy JW, Figley MM: Quantitative angiocardiography: II. The normal left atrial volume in man. Circulation 37:800, 1968.
6. Schabelman SE, et al.: Comparison of four two-dimensional echocardiographic views for measuring left atrial size (abstr). Am J Cardiol 41:391, 1978.
7. Tajik A, et al.: Two-dimensional real-time ultrasonic imaging of the heart and great vessels. Technique, image orientation, structure identification and evaluation. Mayo Clin Proc 53:281, 1978.
8. Bierman FZ, Williams RG: Subxiphoid two-dimensional imaging of the atrial septum. Am J Cardiol 41:354, 1978.
9. Lange LW, Sahn DJ, Allen HD, Goldberg SJ: Subxiphoid cross-sectional echocardiography in infants and children with congenital heart disease. Circulation 59:513, 1979.
10. Sahn DJ, DeMaria A, Kisslo J, Weyman AE: Recommendations regarding quantitation in M-mode echocardiography: results of a survey of echocardiographic measurements. Circulation 58:1072, 1978.
11. Murray JA, Kennedy JW, Figley MM: Quantitative angiocardiography: II. The normal left atrial volume in man. Circulation 37:800, 1968.
12. Lundstrom NR, Mortensson W: Clinical applications of echocardiography in infants and children: II. Acta Paediatr Scand 63:33, 1974.

12A. Nidorf SM, Picard MH, Triulzi MO, et al: New perspectives in the assessment of cardiac chamber dimensions during development and adulthood. J Am Coll Cardiol 19:983, 1992.

13. Silverman NH, Lewis AB, Heymann MA, Rudolph AM: Echocardiographic assessment of ductus arteriosus in premature infants. Circulation 50:821, 1974.
14. Baylen B, Meyer RA, Kaplan S: Echocardiographic assessment of patent ductus arteriosus in prematures with respiratory distress. Circulation 50(Suppl 3):III-16, 1974.
15. Goldberg SJ, et al.: A prospective 2-½ year experience with echocardiographic evaluation of prematures with patent ductus arteriosus (PDA) and respiratory distress syndrome (RDS) (abstr). Am J Cardiol 35:139, 1975.
16. Carter WH, Bowman CR: Estimation of shunt flow in isolated ventricular septal defect by echocardiogram. Circulation (Suppl 4)48:IV-64, 1973.
17. Sanfilippo AJ, et al.: Atrial enlargement as a consequence of atrial fibrillation: a prospective echocardiographic study. Circulation 82:792, 1990.
18. Bierman FZ, Williams RG: Subxiphoid two-dimensional echocardiographic diagnosis of total anomalous pulmonary venous return in infants (abstr). Am J Cardiol 43:401, 1979.
19. Feigenbaum H: Echocardiography. 2nd Ed. Philadelphia, Lea & Febiger, 1976.
20. Hirata T, et al.: Estimation of left atrial size using ultrasound. Am Heart J 78:43, 1969.
21. Yabek SM, et al.: Echocardiographic determination of left atrial volumes in children with congenital heart disease. Circulation 53:268, 1976.
22. tenCate FJ, et al.: Dimensions and volumes of left atrium and ventricle determined by single beam echocardiography. Br Heart J 36:737, 1974.
23. Brown OR, Harrison DC, Popp RL: An improved method for echographic detection of left atrial enlargement. Circulation 50:58, 1974.
24. Loperfido F, et al.: Assessment of left atrial dimension by cross-sectional echocardiography in patients with mitral valve disease. Br Heart J 50:570, 1983.
25. Gehl LG, Mintz GS, Kotler MN, Segal BL: Left atrial volume overload in mitral regurgitation: a two dimensional echocardiographic study. Am J Cardiol 49:33, 1982.
26. Ren J-F, et al.: Two-dimensional echocardiographic determination of left atrial emptying volume: a noninvasive index in quantifying the degree of nonrheumatic mitral regurgitation. J Am Coll Cardiol 2:729, 1983.
27. Beppu S, et al.: Echocardiographic study of abnormal position and motion of the posterobasal wall of the left ventricle in cases of giant left atrium. Am J Cardiol 49:467, 1982.
28. Reeves WC, et al.: Prolapsed left atrium behind the left ventricular posterior wall: two dimensional echocardiographic and angiographic features. Am J Cardiol 47:708, 1981.
29. Beppu S, et al.: Echocardiographic study of abnormal position and motion of the posterobasal wall of the left ventricle in cases of giant left atrium. Am J Cardiol 49:467, 1982.
30. Nasser WK, et al.: Atrial myxoma: I. Clinical and pathologic features in nine cases. Am Heart J 83:694, 1972.
31. Greenwood WF: Profile of atrial myxoma. Am J Cardiol 21:367, 1968.
32. Lappe DL, Bulkley BH, Weiss JL: Two-dimensional echocardiographic diagnosis of left atrial myxoma. Chest 74:55, 1978.
33. Lewis BS, et al.: Diagnostic value of cross-sectional echocardiography in left atrial myxoma. Isr J Med Sci 15:426, 1979.
34. Perry LS, et al.: Two-dimensional echocardiography in the diagnosis of left atrial myxoma. Br Heart J 45:667, 1981.
35. Come PC, Kurland GS, Vine HS: Two dimensional echocardiography in differentiating right atrial and tricuspid valve mass lesions. Am J Cardiol 44:1207, 1979.
36. Rahilly GT, Nanda NC: Two dimensional echocardiographic identification of tumor hemorrhages in atrial myxomas. Am Heart J 101:237, 1981.

37. Thier W, et al.: Cysts in left atrial myxomas identified by transesophageal cross sectional echocardiography. Am J Cardiol 51:1793, 1983.
38. Lee YC, Magram MY: Nonprolapsing left atrial tumor. Chest 78:332, 1980.
39. Sung RJ, et al.: Hemodynamic features of prolapsing left atrial myxoma. Circulation 51:342, 1975.
40. Abramowitz R, Majdan JF, Plzak LF, Berger BC: Two-dimensional echocardiographic diagnosis of separate myxomas of both left atrium and left ventricle. Am J Cardiol 53:379, 1984.
41. Rogers EW, Weyman AE, Noble RJ, Bruins SG: Left atrial myxoma infected with histoplasma capsulatum. Am J Med 64:683, 1978.
42. Quinn TJ, Codini MA, Harris AA: Infected cardiac myxoma. Am J Cardiol 53:361, 1984.
43. Mich RJ, Gillam LD, Weyman AE: Osteogenic sarcoma mimicking left atrial myxomas: clinical and two-dimensional echocardiographic features. J Am Coll Cardiol 6:1422, 1985.
44. Schiller HM, Madge CE: Neoplasms within the pulmonary veins. Chest 58: 535, 1970.
45. Boland TW, Winga ER, Kalfayan B: Chondrosarcoma: a case report with left atrial involvement and systemic embolization. J Thorac Cardiovasc Surg 74:268, 1977.
46. Gardner MAH, Bett JHN, Stafford EG, Matar K: Pulmonary metastatic chondrosarcoma with intracardiac extension. Ann Thorac Surg 27:238, 1978.
47. Yoshikawa J, et al.: Cross-sectional echocardiographic diagnosis of large left atrial tumor and extracardiac tumor compressing the left atrium. Am J Cardiol 42:853, 1978.
48. Nishimura RA, Tajik J, Schattenberg TT, Seward JB: Diaphragmatic hernia mimicking an atrial mass: a two-dimensional echocardiographic pitfall. J Am Coll Cardiol 5:992, 1985.
49. Garcia-Fernandez MA, Moreno M, Banuelos F: Two-dimensional echocardiographic identification of blood stasis in the left atrium. Am Heart J 109: 600, 1985.
50. Iliceto S, et al.: Dynamic intracavitary left atrial echoes in mitral stenosis. Am J Cardiol 55:603, 1985.
51. Mikell FL, et al.: Two-dimensional echocardiographic demonstration of left atrial thrombi in patients with prosthetic mitral valves. Circulation 60:1183, 1979.
52. Shrestha NK, et al.: Two-dimensional echocardiographic diagnosis of left atrial thrombus in rheumatic heart disease: a clinicopathologic study. Circulation 67:341, 1983.
53. Schweizer P, et al.: Detection of left atrial thrombi by echocardiography. Br Heart J 45:148, 1981.
54. Jordan RA, Scheifley CH, Edwards JE: Mural thrombosis and arterial embolism in mitral stenosis: a clinicopathologic study of fifty one cases. Circulation 3:363, 1951.
55. Sunagawa K, et al.: Left atrial ball thrombus diagnosed by two-dimensional echocardiography. Am Heart J 100:89, 1980.
56. Warda M, et al.: Auscultatory and echocardiographic features of mobile left atrial thrombus. J Am Coll Cardiol 5:379, 1985.
57. Bramlet DA, Edwards JE: Congenital aneurysm of left atrial appendage. Br Heart J 45:97, 1980.
58. Foale RA, et al.: Congenital aneurysms of the left atrium: recognition by cross-sectional echocardiography. Circulation 66:1065, 1982.
59. Lipkin D, Colli A, Somerville J: Aneurysmal dilatation of the atrial appendage diagnosed by cross-sectional echocardiography and surgically removed. Br Heart J 53:69, 1985.
60. Lucas RV Jr, et al.: Congenital causes of pulmonary venous obstruction. Pediatr Clin North Am 10:781, 1963.
61. Niwayama G: Cor triatriatum. Am Heart J 59:291, 1960.
62. Snider AR, Roge CH, Schiller NB, Silverman NJ: Congenital left ventricular inflow obstruction evaluated by two-dimensional echocardiography. Circulation 61:848, 1980.
63. Breitweser JA, Meyer RA: Use of echocardiography to evaluate structure and function in congenital heart disease. *In* Yu PN, Goodwin NJ (eds.): Progress in Cardiology. Philadelphia, Lea & Febiger, 1979.
64. Porter BA, Bogren HG, DeMaria AN: Cor triatriatum in an adult with mitral regurgitation and massive left atrial enlargement. Cardiovasc Intervent Radiol 6:37, 1983.
65. Fagan LE, et al.: Two-dimensional, spectral Doppler, and color flow imaging in adults with acquired and congenital cor triatriatum. J Am Soc Echocardiogr 4:177, 1991.
66. Rice MJ, et al.: Left juxtaposed atrial appendages: diagnostic two-dimensional echocardiographic features. J Am Coll Cardiol 1:1330, 1983.
67. Vermilion RP, Snider AR, Peters JA, Merida-Asmus LM: Two-dimensional echocardiography and color flow Doppler detection of an unusual pulmonary venous anomaly: anomalous pulmonary venous return to the right atrium by way of three separate orifices. J Am Soc Echocardiogr 3:135, 1990.
68. Sahn DJ, Allen HD, Lange LW, Goldberg SJ: Cross-sectional echocardiographic diagnosis of the sites of total anomalous pulmonary venous drainage. Circulation 60:1317, 1979.
69. Keren G, et al.: Pulmonary venous flow pattern—its relationship to cardiac dynamics: a pulsed Doppler echocardiographic study. Circulation 71:1105, 1985.
70. Keren G, Sonnenblick EH, LeJemtel TH: Mitral annulus motion: relation to pulmonary venous and transmitral flows in normal subjects and in patients with dilated cardiomyopathy. Circulation 78:621, 1988.
71. Nishimura RA, Abel MD, Hatle LK, Tajik AJ: Relation of pulmonary vein to mitral flow velocities by transesophageal Doppler echocardiography: effect of different loading conditions. Circulation 81:1488, 1990.
72. Kuecherer H, et al.: Estimation of mean left atrial pressure form transesophageal pulsed Doppler echocardiography of pulmonary venous flow. Circulation 82:1127, 1990.
73. Dixon SH Jr, Nolan SP, Morrow AG: Pulmonary venous blood flow: the effects of alteration in left atrial pressure, pulmonary arterial occlusion, and mitral regurgitation in the dog. Ann Surg 174:944, 1971.
74. Klein AL, et al.: Transesophageal Doppler echocardiography of pulmonary venous flow: a new marker of mitral regurgitation severity. J Am Coll Cardiol 18:518, 1991.
75. Naito M, et al.: Reevaluation of the role of atrial systole to cardiac hemodynamics: evidence for pulmonary venous regurgitation during abnormal atrioventricular sequencing. Am Heart J 105:295, 1983.
76. Keren G, et al.: Pulmonary venous flow determined by Doppler echocardiography in mitral stenosis. Am J Cardiol 65:246, 1990.
77. Mori K, Dohi T: Mitral and pulmonary vein blood flow patterns in cor triatriatum. Am Heart J 117:1167, 1989.
78. Schiavone WA, Calafiore PA, Currie PJ, Lytle BW: Doppler echocardiographic demonstration of pulmonary venous flow velocity in three patients with constrictive pericarditis before and after pericardiectomy. Am J Cardiol 63:145, 1989.
79. Schiavone WA, Calafiore PA, Salcedo EE: Transesophageal Doppler echocardiographic demonstration of pulmonary venous flow velocity in restrictive cardiomyopathy and constrictive pericarditis. Am J Cardiol 63:1286, 1989.
80. Perloff JN: The Clinical Recognition of Congenital Heart Disease. Philadelphia, WB Saunders, 1970.
81. Denilowicz D, Kronzon I: Use of contrast echocardiography in the diagnosis of partial anomalous pulmonary venous connection. Am J Cardiol 43:248, 1979.
82. Sade RD, Freed MD, Matthews EC, Castaneda AR: Stenosis of individual pulmonary veins. Review of the literature and report of a surgical case. J Thorac Cardiovasc Surg 67:953, 1974.
83. Driscoll EJ, Nihill MR: Late development of pulmonary venous obstruction following Mustard's operation using a Dacron baffle. Circulation 55:484, 1977.
84. Graham TP, Jr: Hemodynamic residua and sequelae following intra-atrial repair of transposition of the great arteries: a review. Pediatr Cardiol 2:203, 1982.
85. Smallhorn JF, Freedom RM, Olley PM: Pulsed Doppler echocardiographic assessment of the intraparenchymal pulmonary vein flow. J Am Coll Cardiol 9:573, 1987.
86. Smallhorn JF, et al.: Pulsed Doppler assessment of pulmonary vein obstruction. Am Heart J 110:483, 1985.
87. Leung MP, Mok CK, Cheung DLC, Lau KC: Echocardiographic diagnosis of anastomotic stricture following surgical correction of supracardiac total anomalous pulmonary venous connection. Am Heart J 114:1518, 1987.
88. Vick GW III, et al.: Pulmonary venous and systemic ventricular inflow obstruction in patients with congenital heart disease: detection by combined two-dimensional and Doppler echocardiography. J Am Coll Cardiol 9:580, 1987.
89. Smallhorn JG, et al.: Pulsed Doppler echocardiographic assessment of the pulmonary venous pathway after the mustard or senning procedure for transposition of the great arteries. Circulation 73:765, 1986.
90. Snider AR, Ports TA, Silverman NJ: Venous anomalies of the coronary sinus: detection by M-mode, two-dimensional and contrast echocardiography. Circulation 60:721, 1979.
91. Mantini E, Grondin CM, Lillehei CW, Edwards JE: Congenital anomalies involving the coronary sinus. Circulation 33:317, 1966.
92. Fraser RS, Dvorkin J, Rossal RE, Eidem R: Left superior vena cava: a review of associated congenital heart lesions. Catheterization data and roentgenologic findings. Am J Med 31:711, 1961.
93. Cha EM, Khoury GH: Persistent left superior vena cava. Radiology 103: 375, 1972.
94. Oguni H, et al.: A case of absent right superior vena cava: cross-sectional echocardiographic diagnosis. Heart Vessels 1:239, 1985.
95. Foale RA, Bourdillon PD, Somerville J, Rickards AF: Cross-sectional echocardiographic features of anomalous systemic and coronary venous return (abstr.). Am J Cardiol 43:385, 1979.
96. Sanders S: Anomalous hepatic venous connection to the coronary sinus diagnosed by two-dimensional echocardiography. Am J Cardiol 54:458, 1984.
97. Hamada Y, et al.: Unroofed coronary sinus demonstrated by two-dimensional echocardiography. Am Heart J 108:1558, 1984.
98. Yee G, et al.: Doppler diagnosis of left ventricle to coronary sinus fistula: an unusual complication of mitral valve replacement. J Am Soc Echocardiogr 1: 458, 1988.

CHAPTER

19

LEFT VENTRICULAR OUTFLOW TRACT: THE AORTIC VALVE, AORTA, AND SUBVALVULAR OUTFLOW TRACT

ARTHUR E. WEYMAN and BRIAN P. GRIFFIN

The left ventricular outflow tract can be considered to extend from the free edges of the mitral leaflets to the aortic bifurcation. It can be conveniently divided at the aortic valve into three primary segments: (1) the aortic valve and supporting structures, (2) the cylindric aorta, and (3) the funnel-shaped subvalvular region. The outflow tract courses in a wide arc through the thorax and abdomen. It begins within the left ventricular cavity in the midportion of the left chest and sweeps cephalad toward the neck. It then arcs posteriorly and caudad, passing behind the posterior border of the left pulmonary artery and left ventricle before penetrating the diaphragm and continuing along the midline of the abdomen.[1] Such an extensive area obviously cannot be examined from a single transducer location, and as a result, the outflow tract must be imaged from several different vantage points to determine its overall integrity.

The precise methods for examining the individual segments of the outflow tract are discussed in the appropriate section. In general, however, the subvalvular portion, which lies within the left ventricular cavity, is examined from a low parasternal or apical transducer location; the valvular region and ascending aorta are recorded from a slightly higher precordial location; and the transverse aortic arch (with the contiguous portions of the ascending and descending aorta) are viewed from the suprasternal notch. The descending aorta can be visualized in standard and modified parasternal views as it passes behind the left atrium and ventricle. Higher resolution images of this area can also be obtained using the transesophageal approach. The abdominal aorta, from the diaphragm to the bifurcation can readily be recorded from the anterior abdominal wall.[2,3]

Because the left ventricular outflow tract is a cylindric or tubular structure, it is optimally recorded with the scan plane aligned parallel to its long axis (see Chapter 4). This alignment permits the diameter of the vessel within the entire scan area to be visualized and local areas of narrowing or dilation to be appreciated. Scans across the short axis of the outflow tract can also be obtained at multiple levels.

Doppler recordings of flow velocity in the left ventricular outflow tract and aorta are ideally obtained from transducer locations that align the ultrasonic beam parallel to the direction of flow. Thus, flow in the left ventricular outflow tract, through the aortic valve, and in the proximal aortic root are best recorded from the apex. Right parasternal and suprasternal views can also be used to assess transvalvular and supravalvular flow. The distal ascending aorta, arch, and proximal descending aorta are best interrogated from the suprasternal notch, while distal thoracic and abdominal aortic flow can be sampled from the subcostal location.

THE AORTIC VALVE

Normal Anatomy

The aortic valve is both clinically and echocardiographically the most important single component of the left ventricular outflow tract. Anatomically, the aortic valve is composed of three leaflets, their associated sinuses, and the fibrous interleaflet triangles between the sinuses (Fig. 19–1).[4] Each leaflet is crescent shaped, is attached at its curved edge to the aortic wall, and is separated from its neighbors by a commissure (Fig. 19–2A). There is a slight thickening at the tip of each leaflet called the *node of Arantius*, which becomes more prominent with age. Two ridges curve slightly downward from each node to the lateral cusp margins, marking the line along which the cusp abuts its two neighbors.

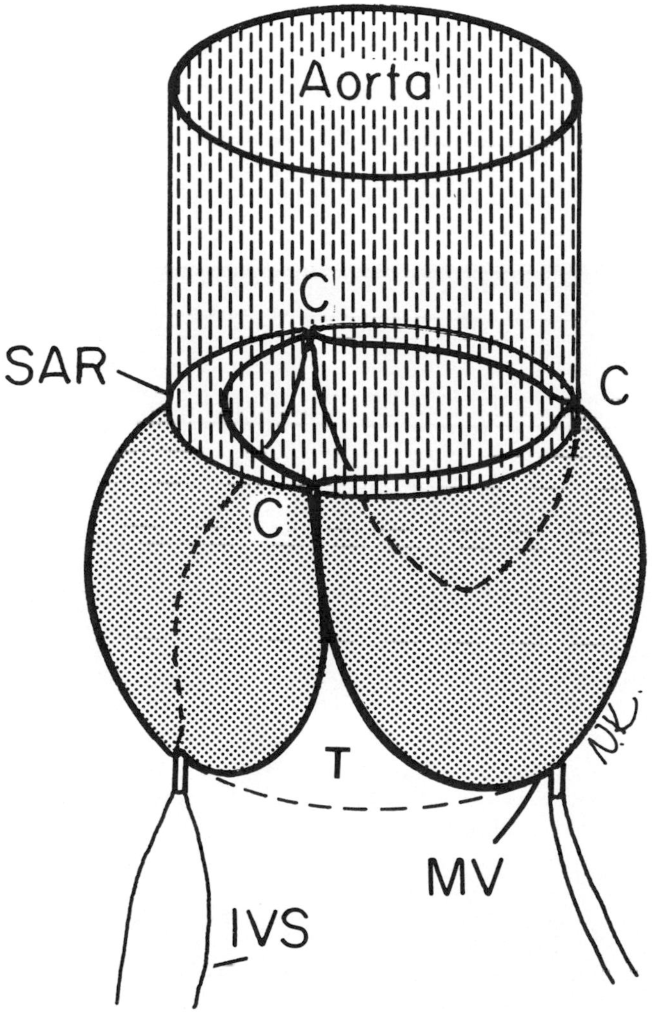

Fig. 19–1. Aortic valve and supporting structures. The three crescent-shaped aortic leaflets attach at their curved edges to the aortic wall and are separated at their superior margins by a commissure (C) and inferiorly by three interleaflet fibrous triangles (T). SAR = supra-aortic ridge; MV = mitral valve; IVS = interventricular septum. (Redrawn from Davies MJ: Pathology of Cardiac Valves. Butterworths, London, 1980.)

The portion of the valve above the closure line is known as the *lunula* and is often fenestrated (Fig. 19–2B). The total cusp area is about 40% greater than that of the aortic root.[5] When closed, each leaflet overlaps its neighbors by 2 or 3 mm, thus allowing a tight seal against backflow of blood despite substantial diastolic pressure in the aorta.

The normal tricuspid configuration is theoretically optimal because two cusps of equal size can close tightly but cannot open completely without considerable elastic stretch. Four or more cusps, in contrast, can open fully but lack sufficient basal support relative to the leaflet area to maintain diastolic competence. Three cusps can open to the full dimensions of the valve ring and still produce a perfect seal when closed.[6] Although normally functioning bicuspid and quadricuspid valves are encountered in young people, the natural history of these valve types is ultimately to develop either stenosis or incompetence.[7,8] Unicuspid valves are almost always congenitally stenotic.[9]

The sinuses of Valsalva are outpouchings of the fibrous aortic wall that are positioned behind the aortic cusps when the valve is open. The sinuses support the leaflets of the aortic valve at their superior or aortic surfaces. The right coronary artery arises from the sinus that is positioned to the right and anteriorly, whereas the left coronary artery arises from the left posterior sinus (Fig. 19–2A). The third sinus, positioned to the right and posteriorly, does not give rise to a coronary artery and is therefore termed the *noncoronary sinus*. The aortic leaflets take their names from the sinuses with which they are associated and, thus, are termed the *right, left,* and *noncoronary leaflets*. The sinuses are anatomically configured such that, in addition to giving rise to the coronary arteries, they also provide a reservoir for diastolic blood flow to the coronary vessels. During systole, the open aortic leaflets, which lie in front of the coronary ostia, shield the ostia from the main force of the ejected blood. The separation of the leaflets from the ostia provided by the sinuses also prevents coronary occlusion because if a leaflet were to come into direct contract with the coronary orifice, it would shut off flow from the aorta. The coronary pressure would then fall rapidly as blood left the distal coronary arterial system, and the leaflet would be held against the orifice by the high differential pressure. This catastrophe is presumably prevented by the presence of adequate space behind the open valve cusps.[6]

Transvalvular Flow Patterns

Normal flow through the aortic valve is systolic, beginning at aortic valve opening with initial acceleration, generally reaching a peak toward midsystole, and then decelerating with completion of flow occurring before valve closure (Fig. 19–3). Normal transvalvular flow is laminar, though a degree of turbulence may be recorded at peak systole and during initial deceleration. The normal spatial flow profile in the left ventricular outflow tract and across the valve is blunted, with the result that the spatial mean and peak velocities are similar (Fig. 19–4). Some spatial acceleration occurs in the outflow

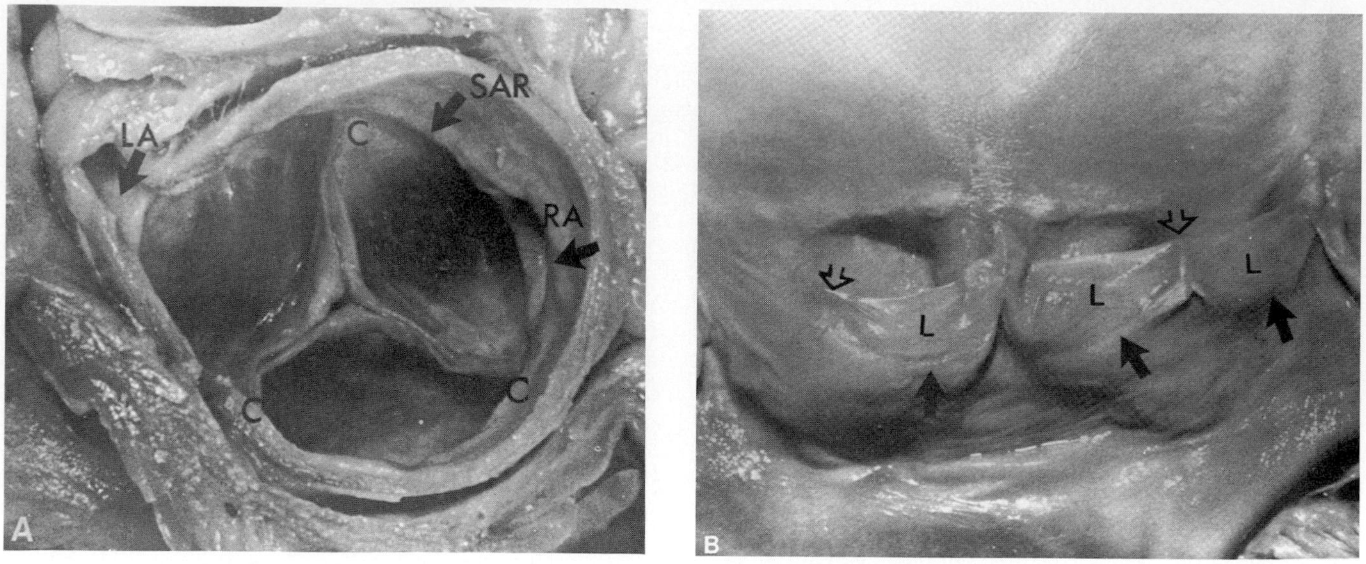

Fig. 19–2. **A.** Pathologic section of the aortic valve viewed from above illustrating the three aortic leaflets, the three commissures (C), the supra-aortic ring (SAR), and the ostia of the left (LA) and right coronary arteries (RA). **B.** Longitudinal view of two of the three aortic cusps illustrating their crescent shape, the area of thickening at the tip of each leaflet (open arrows), and the coaptation lines arising from each region of central thickening (solid arrows). The portion of the valve between the closure line and the free edge is the lunula (L). (From Davies MJ: Pathology of cardiac valves. Butterworths, London, 1980.)

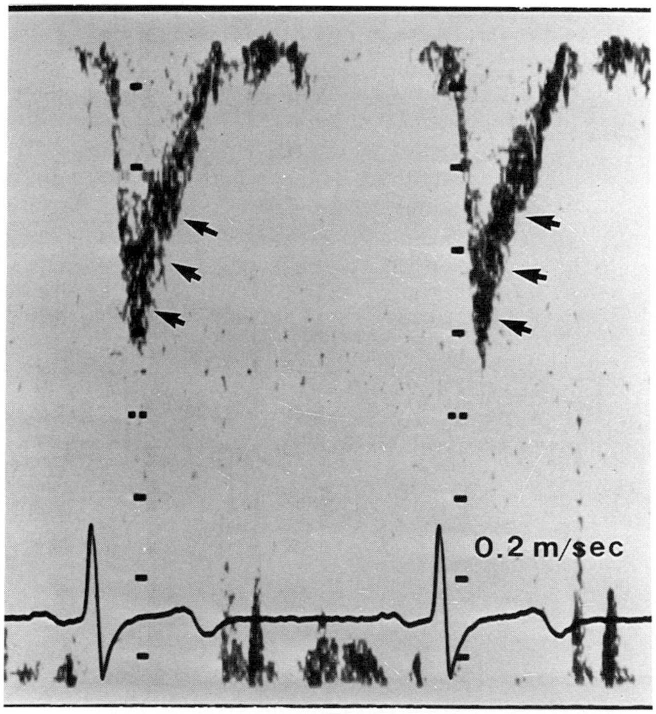

Fig. 19–3. Pulsed Doppler recording of normal aortic flow recorded at the aortic annulus. Flow accelerates rapidly to a relatively sharp peak and then decelerates more gradually. A period of flow instability manifest by slight spectral broadening (arrows) is typically evident during deceleration.

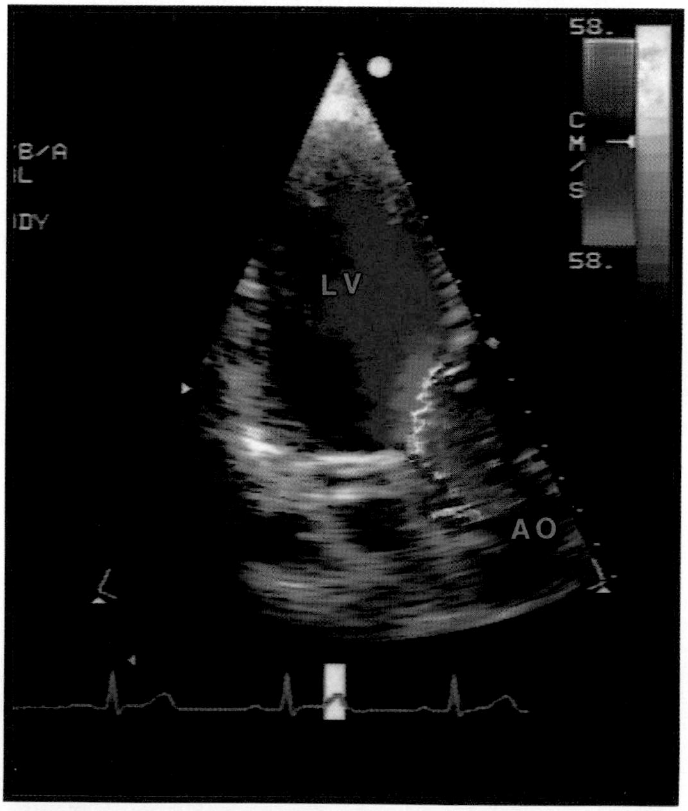

Fig. 19–4. Apical long axis color Doppler recording of normal aortic outflow illustrating the gradual acceleration of flow as the flow stream narrows to pass through the outflow tract and the relatively flat flow profiles at each level of the outflow tract. LV = left ventricle. AO = aorta.

tract because, as the flow stream narrows, velocity must increase to maintain volume flow constant (Fig. 19–5). Distal to the valve eddy, currents arise that form vortices in the sinuses of Valsalva; however, the primary flow stream retains its laminar character and flat profile. Little in the way of diastolic flow is normally present on the ventricular side of the valve, although transient retrograde flow may be recorded in the proximal aorta immediately after valve closure. Aortic flow velocity varies with cardiac output and systemic vascular resistance. Normal resting left ventricular outflow tract velocities in adults average 0.90 m/sec (range, 0.7 to 1.1) and velocities in the aorta average 1.35 m/sec (range, 1.0 to 1.7). In children, these values are slightly higher, with a mean velocity for the left ventricular outflow tract of 1.0 (range, 0.7 to 1.27) and for the aorta, 1.50 (range, 1.2 to 1.80).[10]

Pre-ejection flow toward the aortic valve can be recorded in the left ventricular outflow tract, beginning after atrial systole and continuing until the onset of ventricular ejection. It can be either monophasic or biphasic. In normal persons, pre-ejection flow is monophasic, peaking roughly 0.18 ± 0.05 seconds after the onset of the P wave of the electrocardiogram (ECG). In patients with atrial fibrillation, a monophasic pattern is also seen that peaks 0.06 ± 0.01 seconds after the Q wave. In patients with first-degree AV block, pre-ejection flow is biphasic. The first peak occurs roughly 0.2 seconds after the onset of the P wave, as in normal persons, and the second occurs 0.05 seconds after the Q wave, as in atrial fibrillation. In second-degree block of the Wenkebach type, the first peak occurs at a constant interval after the P wave, while the second peak is related to left ventricular contraction and disappears when atrial contraction fails to induce a ventricular response. Thus, it appears that pre-ejection flow consists of two components. The first is due to atrial contraction and is caused by atrial systolic flow curving around the apex and circling up toward the aortic valve. The second flow component corresponds to ventricular contraction and reflects basal movement of blood, which is presumably due to shortening of the ventricular long axis and mitral valve closure (Fig. 19–6). The velocity of pre-ejection flow is highest close to the tip of the anterior mitral leaflet and decreases higher up in the outflow tract (see Fig. 19–5).[11] In our experience, presystolic flow is more prominent in patients with noncompliant ventricles and may result in a presystolic anterior movement of the mitral valve in patients with idiopathic hypertrophic subaortic stenosis (IHSS).

Examining Planes

The aortic valve is examined echocardiographically in two primary imaging planes: (1) the parasternal long axis and (2) the parasternal short axis at the aortic valve level. The valve can also be recorded in the apical five-chamber view, which is orthogonal to the long and short axis planes, the apical long axis view and in both a long and short axis projection from the subcostal transducer location.[12–15]

In the parasternal long axis view, the imaging plane

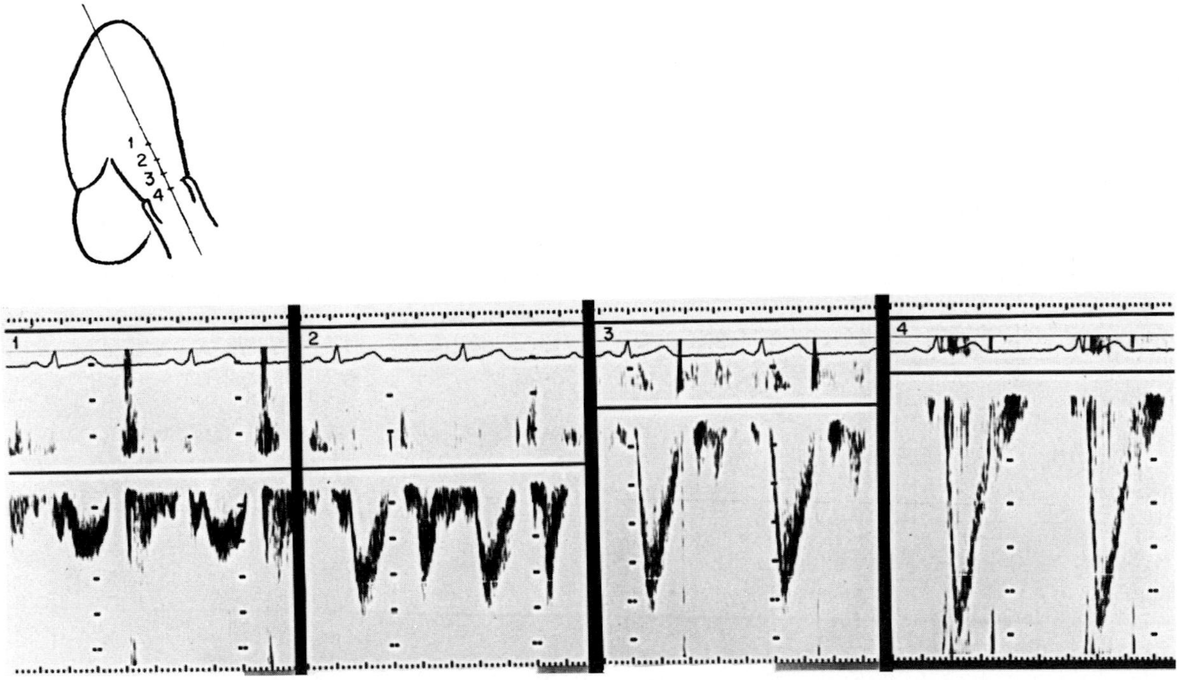

Fig. 19–5. Pulsed Doppler recording of aortic outflow velocity with the sample volume **(1)** at the tip of the anterior mitral leaflet; **(2)** at the midportion of the anterior mitral leaflet; **(3)** at the aortic annulus; and **(4)** just beyond the annulus. **1.** At the tip of the mitral leaflet, the velocity is relatively low; the contour is symmetric, and there is evidence of presystolic forward flow as a result of atrial inflow, which curves around the apex and into the outflow tract. **2.** At the midleaflet, acceleration is more rapid and the peak velocity is higher. **3.** At the annulus acceleration, even more rapid, peak velocity is higher and the atrial presystolic flow is no longer apparent. **4.** Just beyond the annulus, the rate of flow acceleration is greatest, as is the peak velocity.

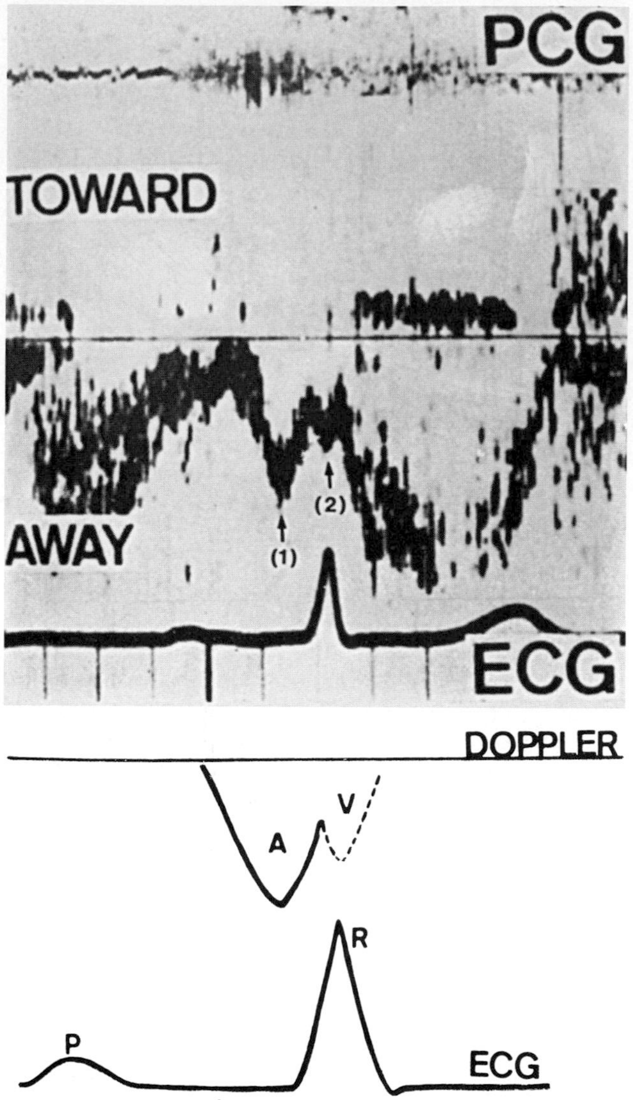

Fig. 19–6. Presystolic flow in the left ventricular outflow tract in a patient with first-degree heart block. Two peaks are evident before the onset of systolic ejection. The first peak (1) bears a constant relation to the p wave of the electrocardiogram as the degree of heart block varies. The second peak (2) occurs after the Q wave of the electrocardiogram (ECG) and is independent of atrial contraction. See text for further details. PCG = phone cardiogram. (From Mizushige K, et al.: Pre-ejection flow in the left ventricular outflow tract elucidated by pulsed Doppler technique. J Cardiography 14:507, 1984. Reproduced with permission of the Japanese College of Cardiology.)

transects the aortic valve in an anteroposterior direction, and its x axis is aligned parallel to the long axis of the aorta. Because the aorta is normally to the right of the transducer when it is in the parasternal location, the long axis plane is usually oriented such that it passes through the right and noncoronary aortic leaflets.

Figure 19–7 is an example of a normal aortic valve recorded in the parasternal long axis view. During diastole (Fig. 19–7A), a thin linear echo is recorded in the midportion of the aortic root. This echo is produced by the coapted free edges of the aortic cusps, which are oriented perpendicular to the path of the imaging plane. The bodies of the thin, smooth leaflets, in contrast, are oriented parallel to the imaging plane and, thus, are less well visualized. In Figure 19–7B, recorded during systole, the leaflet echoes are separated and lie in close apposition to the walls of the aorta. The right coronary leaflet is anterior, and the noncoronary leaflet is posterior. At peak systolic opening, the aortic cusps normally parallel the inner margins of the aortic annulus.

Because the parasternal long axis view is oriented such that the direction of aortic outflow is perpendicular to the path of the ultrasonic beam, Doppler data are poorly recorded in this plane. Although turbulent jets of aortic stenosis and regurgitation can be appreciated, more useful information concerning flow velocities is derived from apical views. An exception is the color flow recording of regurgitant jet diameter, which along with the outflow tract diameter, are imaged using the axial resolution of the system, and their ratio may have value in estimating the severity of aortic regurgitation (see following discussion).

The parasternal short axis view of the aortic valve is recorded with the imaging plane aligned parallel to the short axis of the aortic root at or just superior to the level of the aortic annulus. Ideally, the commissures separating the three aortic leaflets should be visualized during diastole, and the open aortic leaflets should be recorded during systole. In routine clinical studies, however, the aortic commissures can be clearly visualized in only about 73% of cases.[3]

Figure 19–8 illustrates the normal short axis appearance of a tricuspid aortic valve during diastole (Fig. 19–8A) and systole (Fig. 19–8B). In the diastolic recording, the three aortic commissures are evident and outline the position of the aortic leaflets. The right coronary leaflet (R) is positioned anterior and leftward, the left coronary leaflet (L) is to the right and posterior, and the

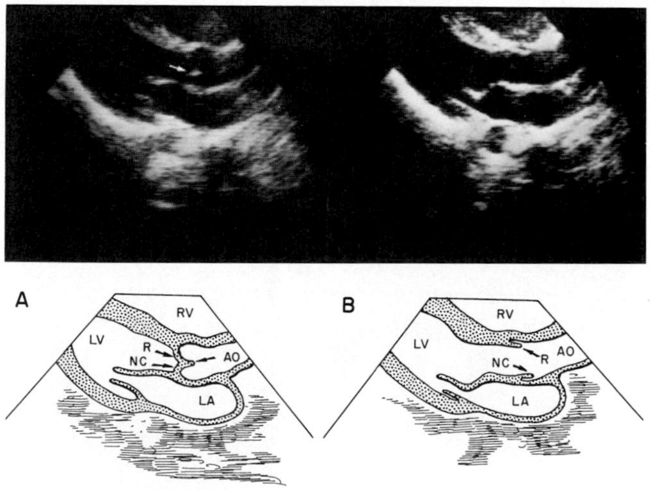

Fig. 19–7. Parasternal long axis recording of a normal aortic valve. The positions of the right (R) and noncoronary (NC) aortic leaflets during diastole **(A)** and systole **(B)** are illustrated. **A.** Top. The single linear echo arising from the coapted aortic leaflets is indicated by the horizontal arrow. RV = right ventricle; LV = left ventricle; AO = aorta; LA = left atrium.

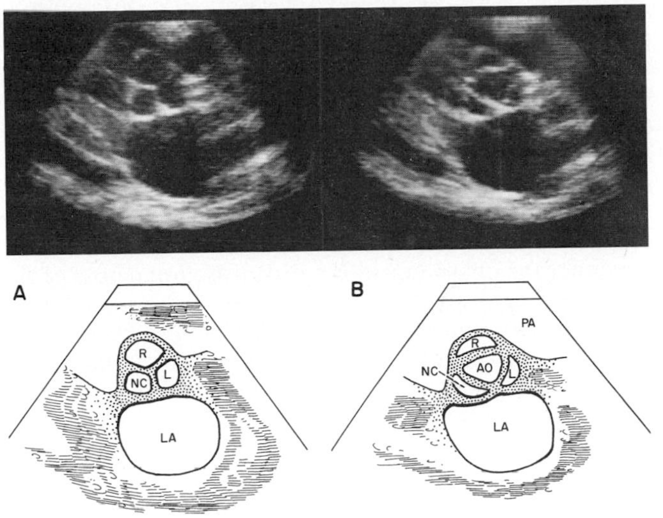

Fig. 19–8. Parasternal short axis recording of a normal aortic valve during diastole **(A)** and systole **(B).** During systole, the commissures of the trileaflet valve outline the positions of the right (R), noncoronary (NC), and left (L) coronary leaflets. During systole, the leaflets separate widely, producing an orifice that appears as a triangle with curved sides. LA = left atrium; PA = pulmonary artery; AO = aorta.

noncoronary leaflet is to the left and posterior.* This normal diastolic short axis configuration of the tricuspid aortic valve has been likened to the Mercedes-Benz emblem lying on its side. Figure 19–8B illustrates the systolic configuration of the aortic leaflets and their relationship to the semicircular sinuses of Valsalva. In this example, the aortic orifice appears as a triangle with curved sides.

The short axis view is ideal for recording the aortic orifice and for defining the location of focal aortic valve abnormalities. It is also useful for evaluating disorders of the aortic root, such as sinus of Valsalva aneurysms and aortic root dissection. When recording this view, remember that the aortic root normally moves in a superior-inferior direction with cardiac contraction and relaxation. At the onset of ventricular systole, the aortic root is in its most superior position. As the ventricle contracts, the aortic root and valve are drawn in an apical or inferior direction. Consequently, a stationary imaging plane records a more superior portion of the aortic valve at end-systole than at end-diastole. This motion of the valve through the imaging plane creates particular problems when trying to visualize the valve orifice in valvular aortic stenosis because the position of the orifice continuously shifts relative to the examining plane.

The short axis view is also useful for determining the location of aortic regurgitant jets using color Doppler flow mapping, measuring the area of these jets at their origin, and separating valvular from paravalvular leaks.

* Because the leaflets are displayed as if view from below, their right-left orientation in the image is the opposite of their anatomic orientation; i.e., the right coronary leaflet, which is positioned to the patient's right, appears on the left side of the recorded image and, thus, to the viewer's left.

Although the dominant flow vector in most cases is perpendicular to the path of the ultrasonic beam, there is usually sufficient turbulence in the regurgitant jets to permit their origin to be defined.

In the apical five-chamber view, the imaging plane is oriented such that it passes through the open aortic valve from the point of basal attachment to the leaflet tips. Although the five-chamber view may be more difficult to obtain than the parasternal views, it is often useful in demonstrating the domed, stenotic valve of congenital aortic stenosis or the presence of subvalvular membranes. In these instances, the lesions are placed perpendicular to the path of the imaging plane, and their visualization may be facilitated. The apical long axis view may also be useful in visualizing the subvalvular region and, in addition, offers an alternative to the parasternal long axis view for recording the aortic valve and proximal ascending aorta. Both the apical long axis and five-chamber views provide an ideal orientation (i.e., roughly parallel to blood flow) for Doppler interrogation of both subvalvular and transvalvular outflow velocities.

Aortic regurgitation is also best recorded from the apical window. Aortic regurgitant jets typically present as areas of high velocity turbulent flow originating at the valve and extending for a varying distance into the left ventricle (Fig. 19–9). Apical imaging permits their width, spatial distribution within the left ventricle, and interaction with mitral inflow to be appreciated.

Relationship of Aortic Leaflet Motion to Cardiac Output and Transvalvular Flow Patterns

Normal aortic leaflet motion depends on both the volume and the character of flow through the aortic valve. A marked reduction in forward cardiac output characteristically decreases both the rate and the amplitude of aortic leaflet opening and can result in valve closure beginning before the end of mechanical systole (Fig. 19–10).[16,17] A decrease in amplitude of aortic leaflet motion is associated with a corresponding decrease in systolic aortic valve area. When valve closure begins before the end of systole, a further decrease in instantaneous and mean systolic valve area can be noted. Figure 19–11 is a short axis aortic valve recording from a patient with

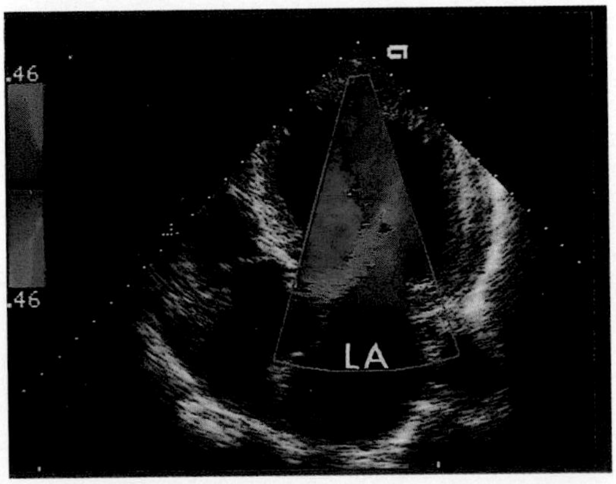

Fig. 19–9. Apical five-chamber color Doppler recording from a patient with aortic insufficiency (blue-yellow mosaic). LA = left atrium. (Courtesy of Acuson Corporation.)

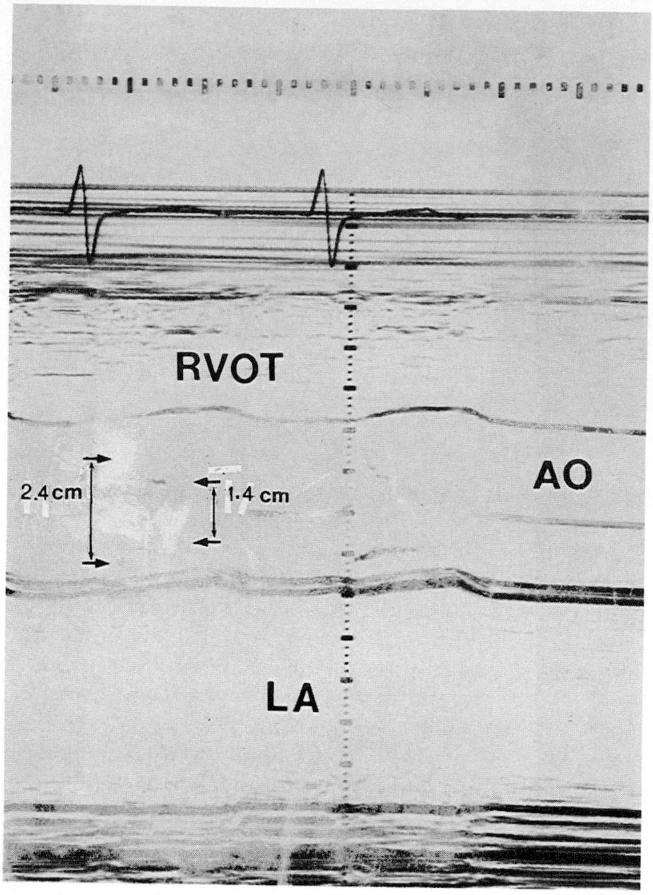

Fig. 19–10. M-mode recording of the aortic root, aortic valve, and left atrium (LA) from a patient with low cardiac output. In this example, the valve leaflets initially separate at a slower than normal rate and reach a diameter of 2.4 cm, which is considerably smaller than that of the aortic root. The leaflets then gradually drift together, with a separation of only 1.4 cm during midsystole, and then continue to close at a more rapid rate until end-systole. RVOT = right ventricular outflow tract; AO = aorta.

congestive cardiomyopathy and illustrates the reduced aortic valve opening that can occur in low flow states. In any measurement of aortic valve area, therefore, one must remember that reduced flow through the valve may reduce the valve area independent of any leaflet disorder or may exaggerate the anatomic decrease in valve area in patients with aortic stenosis.

Obstructive lesions located beneath the valve also characteristically affect aortic leaflet motion by changing either the character or the cross-sectional area of the flow stream passing through the valve orifice. Turbulent flow typically induces high-frequency vibrations of the freely mobile leaflets, whereas a transient reduction in systolic outflow or a decrease in the cross-sectional area of the flow jet may cause the leaflets to move toward a closed position before end-systole. Thus, in discrete subaortic stenosis, initial leaflet opening is typically normal, i.e., to the margins of the aortic annulus. Once flow is established, however, the leaflets fall back to parallel the margins of the narrowed flow stream caused by the subvalvular lesion[18,19] (see Fig. 14–29). In IHSS, the midsystolic decrease in forward cardiac output caused by the functional subvalvular obstruction produces a corresponding midsystolic closing movement of the aortic leaflets with subsequent reopening if forward flow is re-established at end-systole (see Fig. 14–27).[20,21] Although these abnormalities of aortic leaflet motion are best demonstrated with an M-mode recording, they can clearly be seen during the cross-sectional study, and their presence frequently draws attention to the subvalvular lesions.

An early abrupt closing motion of one or more aortic leaflets has also been noted in a variety of other conditions including aortic root dilation, ascending aortic aneurysm or dissection,[22–24] floppy aortic valve,[25] surgically corrected tetralogy of Fallot, truncus ateriosus,[26] double-outlet right ventricle,[22] ventricular septal defect,[22] left ventricular diverticulum,[22] mitral regurgitation, and dilated cardiomyopathy.[27] In general, this "notching" (Fig. 19–12) represents either transient overshoot of the leaflet(s) beyond the annulus resulting from dilation of the root with return of the leaflets to their normal systolic position parallel to the annulus

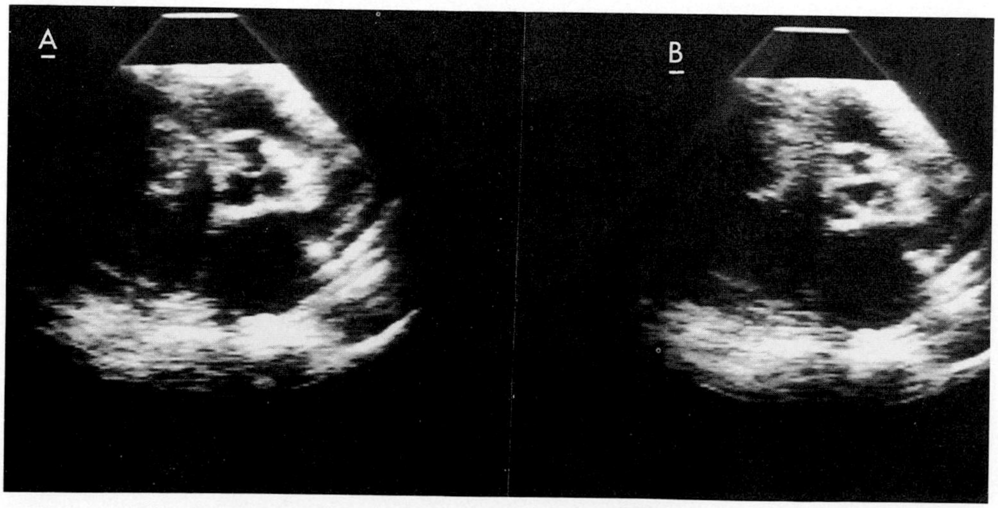

Fig. 19–11. Parasternal short axis recording of the aortic valve, illustrating the effects of reduced cardiac output on the systolic aortic valve orifice configuration. **A.** During diastole, the normal trileaflet aortic configuration is evident. **B.** During systole, there is a reduction in leaflet separation and a corresponding decrease in aortic valve orifice area at peak opening.

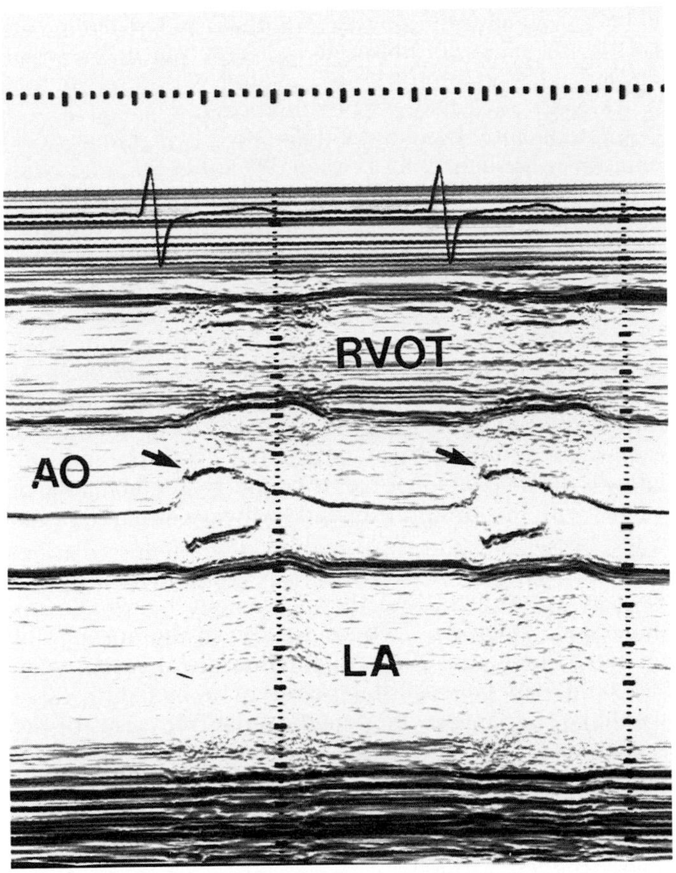

Fig. 19–12. M-mode recording illustrating aortic valve "notching" (arrow) that is due to aortic root dilation. LA = left atrium; AO = aorta; RVOT = right ventricular outflow tract.

once flow is established or failure of the leaflet to maintain its normal systolic position resulting from contraction of the flow stream. In either case, the "notching" pattern per se simply reflects the effects of pressure and flow on the ventricular and arterial leaflet surfaces, and its only diagnostic value lies in drawing attention to the fact that these relationships are abnormal.

Changes in volume flow through the aortic valve are also reflected in the Doppler velocity profile. Low cardiac output is typically associated with a reduced peak velocity and systolic velocity integral and a delay in the time to maximal velocity (Fig. 19–13A). In severe left ventricular dysfunction, flow volume may vary from beat to beat without obvious changes in heart rate.

Conversely, in high output states, peak velocity and systolic velocity integral are increased, and the time to peak velocity is reduced (Fig. 19–13C). Understanding these relationships is important because apparently normal velocities may be recorded through a stenotic valve in the presence of low cardiac output, whereas high velocities can be recorded across normal valves when cardiac output is increased (i.e., during pregnancy, exercise, conditions that increase sympathetic activity, and with augmented outflow resulting from shunt or regurgitant flow).

Arrhythmias can alter stroke volume and associated aortic valve motion. Diminished opening excursion or failure of opening can occur following premature ventricular contractions, whereas postextrasystolic ventricular potentiation can be recorded as an increase in both peak velocity and systolic velocity integral. Similar findings may be recorded during the irregular cycles of atrial fibrillation (see Chapter 40). Characteristic changes in the aortic flow profile in specific conditions such as hypertrophic cardiomyopathy and cardiac tamponade are described in Chapters 25 and 35, respectively.

THE ABNORMAL AORTIC VALVE ECHOGRAM

Congenital Abnormalities in Aortic Leaflet Number

Congenital anomalies in the number of aortic valve leaflets range from the extremely rare congenital absence of the valve to the hexacuspid valve occasionally seen in patients with truncus arteriosus.[28] Abnormalities of leaflet number are of clinical import because they can either be associated with functional impairment at birth or predispose the individual to stenosis or insufficiency later in life.

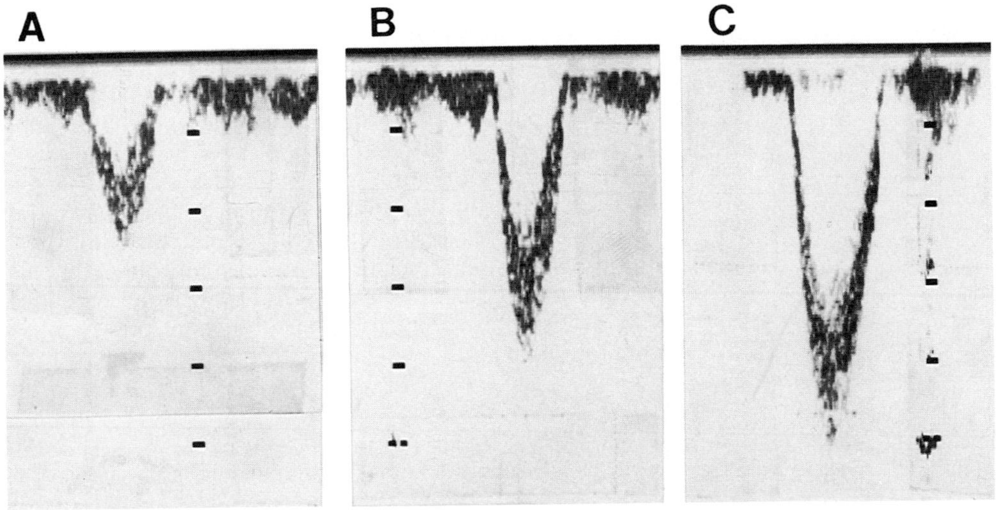

Fig. 19–13. Comparison of pulsed Doppler flow profiles from patients with low (A), normal (B), and high (C) cardiac output. See text for details.

Unicuspid Aortic Valves

Unicuspid aortic valves are separated pathologically into two types: acommissural and unicommissural. The acommissural valve is a rare anomaly and morphologically resembles that seen in congenital pulmonic stenosis. In this form of unicuspid valve, there is a single membrane-like leaflet with a central circular orifice (Fig. 19–14).[28]

Unicommissural unicuspid aortic valves occur more frequently and are the most common cause of symptomatic aortic stenosis in infants. Anatomically, unicommissural valves consist of a single leaflet that begins at the aortic wall, attaches around the aortic annulus, and folds back to its point of origin without touching the far wall of the aorta distal to its annular insertion (Fig. 19–15A and B). The orifice is typically eccentric and has an elliptic shape.[28,29] Both acommissural and unicommissural unicuspid valves are generally stenotic, although sufficient redundancy may be present to prevent stenosis during infancy or childhood. As a result, initial presentation can occur in adult life.[30] Unicuspid valves may close completely during diastole as a result of leaflet redundancy or regurgitation can occur.

Bicuspid Aortic Valve

The bicuspid aortic valve is the most common congenital cardiac anomaly and is found in 0.9 to 2.5% of patients in autopsy series.[7,31] Bicuspid valves are clinically important because they can be associated with hemodynamically significant aortic stenosis in the child or may undergo progressive thickening, fibrosis, and eventually, calcification, leading to critical obstruction in later life.[7,32,33] In addition, bicuspid valves are frequently insufficient, are a common site of infection in bacterial endocarditis, and may be associated with a variety of other congenital disorders of the heart.[7,34]

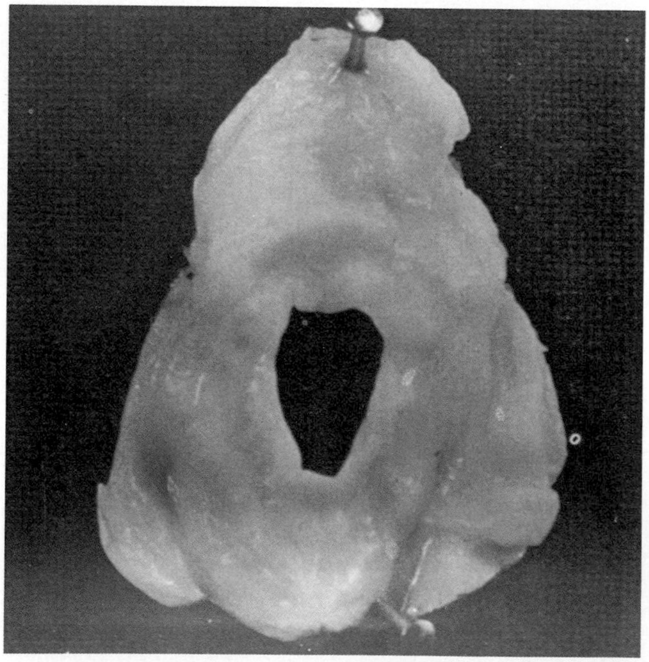

Fig. 19–14. Pathologic specimen of a unicuspid acommissural aortic valve. The valve is dome-like with a central perforation. No commissure is evident. (From Davies MJ: Pathology of Cardiac Valves. Butterworths, London, 1980.)

Anatomically, bicuspid valves have two primary orientations. In slightly more than 50% of cases, one cusp is positioned anteriorly, and the second is positioned posteriorly. The commissures are to the right and left, respectively. In this configuration, both coronary arteries arise in front of the anterior cusp. A raphe, present in roughly one half of these cases, is always located in the anterior cusp.* Alternatively, the cusps may be positioned to the right and left, and the two commissures may have an anteroposterior orientation. In this configuration, the right coronary artery arises from behind the right cusp and the left main coronary from behind the left. A raphe is also present in approximately 50% of valves with this orientation and is always situated in the right cusp.[7]

The percentage of bicuspid valves that becomes stenotic or insufficient and the mechanism by which this occurs are unknown.[7] Theoretically, in the absence of leaflet redundancy, the straight line distance between the points of lateral attachment of a bicuspid valve would be the same as the length of the free edges of the leaflets, and the valve should be inherently stenotic. It has been suggested pathologically, however, that although bicuspid valves are frequently stenotic, sufficient redundancy exists in many instances to permit the valve to open normally.[7,35]

Insufficiency of a bicuspid valve may develop for several reasons. The redundancy of the valve leaflets required to permit systolic opening may result in diastolic leaflet prolapse. Some degree of prolapse occurs in roughly 85% of patients with bicuspid valves, and the degree of prolapse is greater in those with aortic regurgitation than in those without.[36] Another cause of valvular insufficiency is leaflet damage that is due to bacterial endocarditis. The incidence of bicuspid valves in patients dying of acute aortic endocarditis ranges from 9 to 31%,[37–40] whereas in patients with bicuspid valves, and pure aortic regurgitation, the valvular incompetence in as many as 73% of the patients may be due to infective endocarditis.[7] In addition, valvular insufficiency may develop as a result of degeneration of the leaflets caused by the effects of aging and the continued stress of improper closure or superimposed rheumatic disease.[7] Bicuspid valves occur in association with coarctation of the aorta, patent ductus arteriosus, and ventricular septal defect.[7] They may also be familial.[41]

The echocardiographic diagnosis of a bicuspid aortic valve is based on the demonstration of two cusps and two commissures during direct short axis recording. Additional short axis features that support this diagnosis include leaflet redundancy and infolding and eccentric valve closure. In long axis, an abnormal or eccentric coaptation line may also be apparent along with systolic

* An exception to this rule is D-transposition of the great vessels with a bicuspid valve where the raphe is typically located in the posterior cusp.

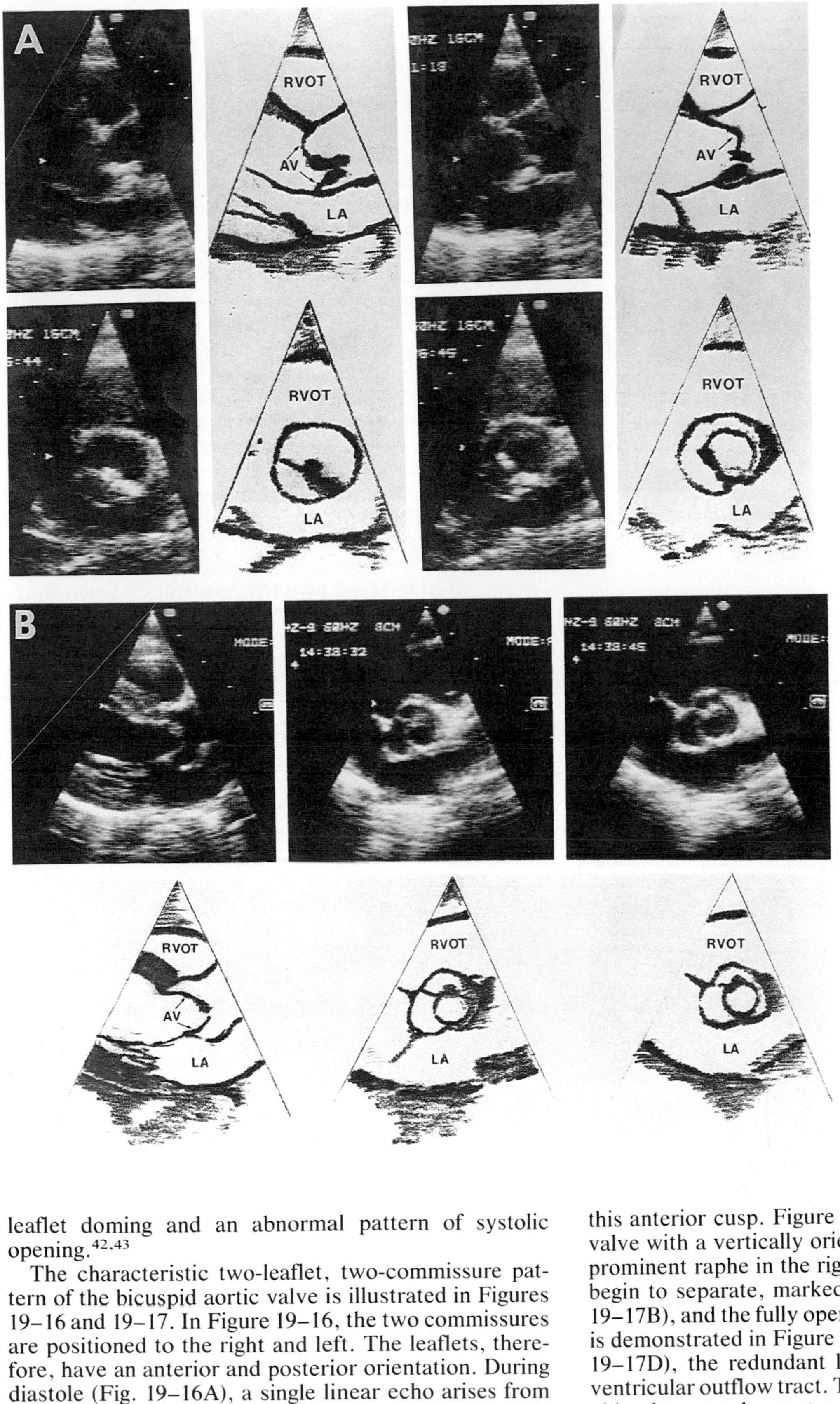

Fig. 19–15. Recordings from two patients with unicuspid unicommissural aortic valves. **A.** Top, left. Parasternal long axis recording illustrating leaflet thickening and an eccentric closure line. Top, right. Parasternal long axis systolic recording illustrating systolic doming (arrow) and a restricted orifice. Bottom, left. Parasternal short axis diastolic recording illustrating the single commissure. Bottom, right. Parasternal short axis systolic recording illustrates the restricted circular valve orifice. **B.** Example of a unicuspid unicommissural valve with more severe associated stenosis. Left. Parasternal long axis recording showing systolic doming of the stenotic valve. Middle and right. Parasternal short axis recordings showing the stenotic valve orifice. In both of these examples, the short axis panel transsects the domed valve above the limiting orifice, and hence the recorded orifice is not the limiting orifice. RVOT = right ventricular outflow tract; AV = aortic valve; LA = left atrium.

leaflet doming and an abnormal pattern of systolic opening.[42,43]

The characteristic two-leaflet, two-commissure pattern of the bicuspid aortic valve is illustrated in Figures 19–16 and 19–17. In Figure 19–16, the two commissures are positioned to the right and left. The leaflets, therefore, have an anterior and posterior orientation. During diastole (Fig. 19–16A), a single linear echo arises from the coaptation line between the two leaflets, which divides the aortic root horizontally. The anterior leaflet in this example is larger than the posterior leaflet, and both the left and the right coronary arteries arise from behind this anterior cusp. Figure 19–17A illustrates a bicuspid valve with a vertically oriented line of coaptation and a prominent raphe in the right-sided cusp. As the leaflets begin to separate, marked redundancy is evident (Fig. 19–17B), and the fully open systolic leaflet configuration is demonstrated in Figure 19–17C. During diastole (Fig. 19–17D), the redundant leaflets prolapse into the left ventricular outflow tract. The appearance of these bicuspid valves can be contrasted with the tricuspid valves illustrated in Figures 19–8, 19–11, and 19–20. When the leaflets are not ideally visualized, the opening pattern of the aortic valve can be particularly helpful in making

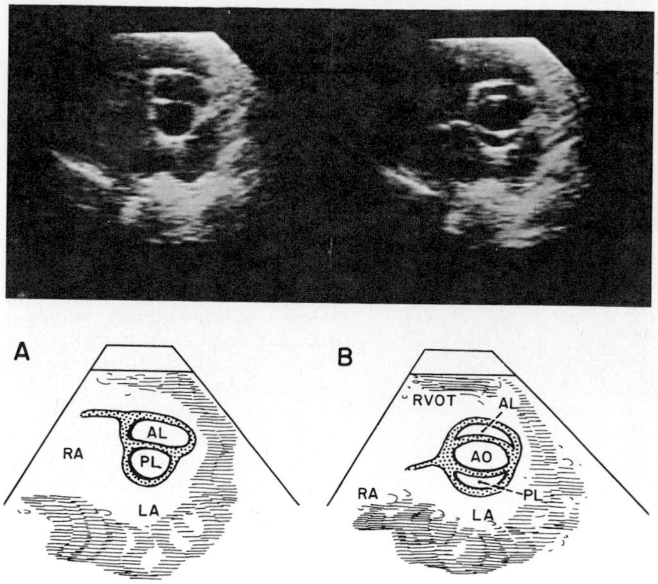

Fig. 19–16. Parasternal short axis recording of a bicuspid aortic valve. **A.** In the diastolic frame, a single horizontal coaptation line separates the anterior (AL) and posterior (PL) leaflets. The anterior leaflet in this example is the larger of the two leaflets, and both coronary arteries arise from behind this cusp. **B.** During systole, the open leaflets produce a circular orifice, which is apparent within the margins of the aortic root. AO = aorta; RVOT = right ventricular outflow tract; LA = left atrium; RA = right atrium.

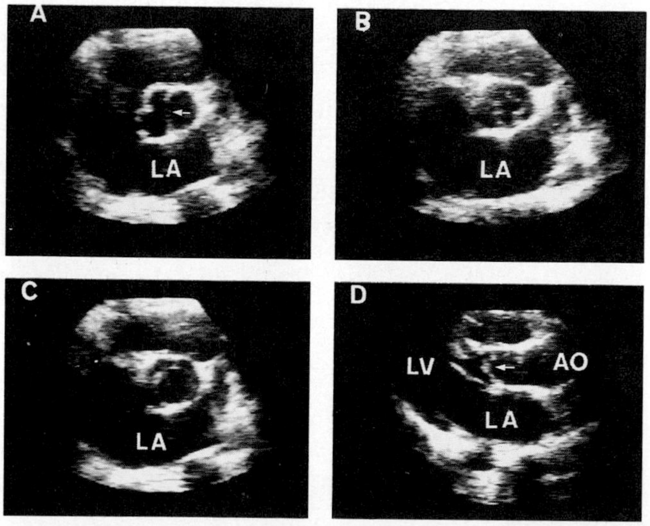

Fig. 19–17. Series of recordings of a bicuspid aortic valve. **A.** A vertically oriented coaptation line (arrow) and a prominent raphe in the right cusp are noted during diastole. **B.** During initial systolic opening, redundancy and infolding of the valve leaflets are obvious. **C.** At full systolic opening, the leaflets parallel the concentric margins of the aorta, producing a circular orifice. **D.** In the parasternal long axis view, diastolic prolapse of the bicuspid valve is evident (arrow). LA = left atrium; LV = left ventricle; AO = aorta.

the diagnosis. Bicuspid valves appear to open from the center and separate at the commissures in a curvilinear fashion much like a rope suddenly going slack in the center. Tricuspid valves, in contrast, maintain their straight diastolic shape and pivot from the point of annular insertion.

The sensitivity of the cross-sectional technique in detecting bicuspid aortic valve is unknown. In studies in which angiographic and surgical confirmation have been available, sensitivity has been excellent; however, these patients represent only a small percentage of the total population with bicuspid valves.[44] Both false-positives and false-negatives may be encountered. A false-negative diagnosis is most likely when a prominent raphe is evident, giving the appearance of a third coaptation line. This is compounded when leaflet redundancy obscures the typical opening pattern of a bicuspid valve. False-positives occur when one leaflet and coaptation line of a tricuspid valve are poorly visualized or when one of the three leaflets is significantly smaller than the other two. In the adult, when a bicuspid valve becomes fibrotic or calcified, the underlying disorder is frequently no longer apparent.

Figure 19–18 depicts a bicuspid valve in long axis. During systole (Fig. 19–18A), the fully opened aortic leaflets are parallel to the aortic root, suggesting that, in this example, leaflet redundancy was sufficient to permit full opening of the valve. Although normal leaflet opening may be observed, systolic doming is common and is reported in approximately 50% of patients.[42] The degree of doming becomes more prominent as leaflet separation decreases and stenosis increases. During diastole (Fig. 19–18B), the coaptation line between the two leaflets of the bicuspid aortic valve is often positioned eccentrically within the aortic root.[43] The degree of eccentricity can be expressed quantitatively by calculating an eccentricity index (EI) using the following formula:

$$EI = \frac{1}{2}\frac{A}{a} \qquad [19.1]$$

where "A" is the aortic root diameter at the onset of diastole and "a" is the distance from the line of aortic cusp coaptation to the nearest aortic wall at the same point in the cardiac cycle. It was originally suggested that all bicuspid valves had an eccentricity index of greater than 1.5, whereas all tricuspid valves had a degree of eccentricity of 1.25 or less.[45] Subsequently, approximately 25% of patients with bicuspid valves were shown to have normal eccentricity indexes, whereas on occasion, tricuspid valves appeared eccentric.[42,45] Despite these difficulties, eccentric valve closure in the long axis should always suggest the possibility of a bicuspid valve and should prompt a more detailed short axis examination in an attempt to demonstrate the leaflet structure.

Abnormalities of the Trileaflet (Tricuspid) Aortic Valve

Tricuspid aortic valves generally appear symmetric to the naked eye; however, detailed measurements can

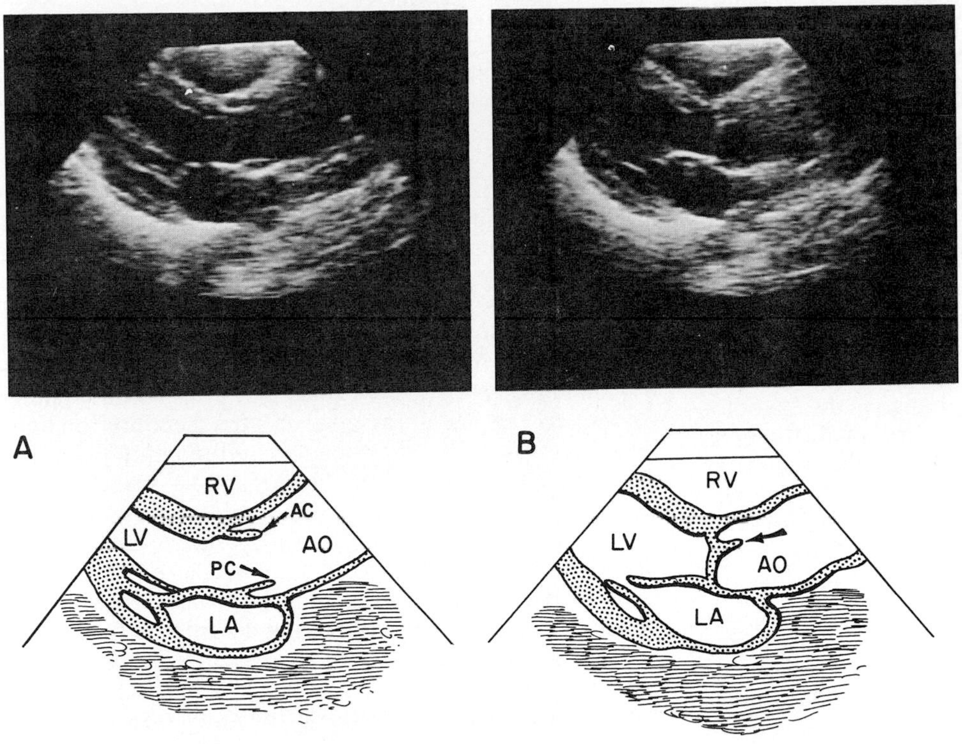

Fig. 19–18. Parasternal long axis recording of a bicuspid aortic valve. **A.** During systole, the aortic leaflets separate widely and lie parallel to the margins of the aortic root. **B.** During diastole, the coaptation line of the aortic leaflets is markedly eccentric and is displaced closer to the anterior margin of the aortic root. RV = right ventricle; LV = left ventricle; AO = aorta; LA = left atrium; AC = anterior cusp; PC = posterior cusp.

reveal marked asymmetry in leaflet size. Variation in cusp size leads to asymmetric closure, which is rarely of functional significance early in life but is felt to predispose individuals to premature senile calcification.[46] Other congenital anomalies of trileaflet aortic valves that have been reported to give rise to stenosis include dystrophic valve leaflets[47] and miniature aortic annulus.[48]

Quadricuspid Aortic Valve

Quadricuspid aortic valve is a rare anomaly with a reported incidence of between 1 in 2500 and 1 in 10,000 in autopsy studies.[49] The presence of four cusps is compatible with normal aortic valve function, although significant regurgitation has been reported in up to 50% of cases, and rarely stenosis can occur. This lesion is detected echocardiographically by the x-shaped short axis commissural pattern of the closed valve (Fig. 19–19).[50]

There may be inequality in the sizes of the four cusps, or all may be of equal size.[51] Quadricuspid valves are rarely associated with other congenital cardiac anomalies, with the exception of truncus arteriosus, in which four or more cusps are frequently noted.[28] Isolated examples of quinticuspid aortic valves have also been reported.[52–54]

Aortic Leaflet Thickening Without Stenosis

Focal or generalized thickening of one or more of the aortic leaflets without associated valvular stenosis is not infrequent. Focal thickening is commonly seen as part of the normal aging process, while generalized thickening may be seen in patients with cardiac amyloidosis and polyvalvular prolapse syndrome.

Aging characteristically accentuates the topographic features of the aortic valve.[5] The central nodules of Arantius enlarge, and the closure lines become more

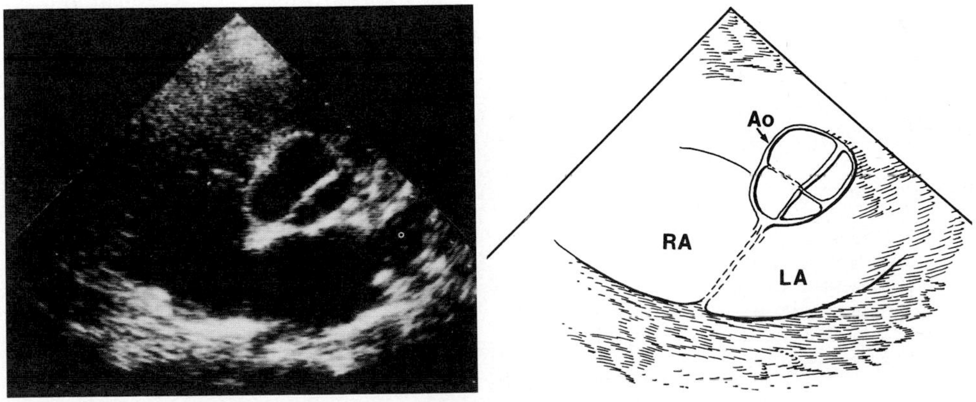

Fig. 19–19. Parasternal short axis recording of a quadricuspid aortic valve. Ao = aorta; RA = right atrium; LA = left atrium.

prominent. The bodies of the cusps tend to thicken, while the lunulae often thin and develop fenestrations. These changes reflect mechanical wear and tear and are characterized histologically by fibroelastic tissue developing on the ventricular surface of the cusps at their points of maximal impact. Calcification also occurs beginning deep within the fibrosa of the valve cusps at the points of maximal cusp flexion. This dystrophic calcification extends toward the center surface of the cusps, forming C-shaped nodular masses of calcium. This calcification ultimately leads to stiffening of the cusps, limitation of motion, and valvular stenosis. Up to 20% of valves from patients over the age of 70 years have been found to have macroscopic calcification.[55]

A specific form of degenerative change is the Lambl's excrescence. Lambl's excrescences are small filamentous or comb-shaped lesions that commonly arise from the free borders of the aortic leaflets or from the ventricular surface of the cusp.[56] These lesions consist of connective tissue with an elastin-like center and may serve as a nidus for thrombus formation or bacterial growth. The prevalence of these lesions increases with age, and like other degenerative lesions, they are generally attributed to normal wear and tear. In one large autopsy series, Lambl's excrescences were noted in all patients above 60 years of age.[57] The excrescences may be several centimeters long but are generally very thin and were rarely recorded with standard transthoracic imaging.[58] With the increased resolution obtainable from the esophagus, however, it is now possible to record these fine mobile threads with some regularity, and it is important to recognize their existence lest they be confused with small vegetations, leading to inappropriate therapy.

Diffuse thickening of the aortic leaflets may be seen with cardiac amyloidosis and appears to be useful in differentiating this disorder from other infiltrative myopathies. Figure 19–20 is an aortic valve recording from a patient with amyloidosis that illustrates this diffuse aortic leaflet thickening.

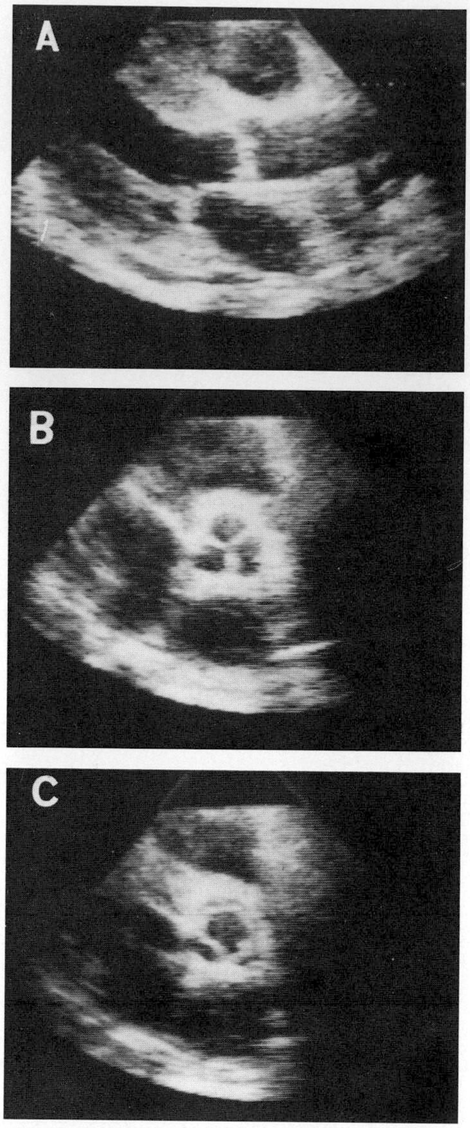

Fig. 19–20. Marked aortic leaflet thickening, which may be noted in patients with amyloidosis. **A.** Parasternal long axis recording. **B.** Parasternal short axis recording during diastole. **C.** Parasternal short axis systolic recording.

Valvular Aortic Stenosis

Morphologic Characteristics and Diagnostic Features

Valvular aortic stenosis is the most common cause of left ventricular outflow obstruction.[28] Aortic stenosis may be due to congenital malformation of the valve, rheumatic fusion of the commissures, secondary calcification of congenitally bicuspid valves, or primary degenerative calcification of otherwise normal aortic valves.[5,59] Echocardiographically, stenosis is defined as any abnormality of the aortic valve in which the leaflets physically encroach on the lumen of the outflow tract. Depending on its severity, such anatomic deformity may or may not produce hemodynamically significant obstruction, defined by the presence of an abnormal transvalvular pressure gradient.

Because valvular stenosis narrows the outflow tract, flow velocity through the restricted area must increase to maintain the flow volume constant. The increased flow velocity starts just proximal to the obstruction (flow acceleration) and reaches its maximum at a point distal to the obstruction where the flow jet is narrowest, termed the *vena contracta*. The exact location of the maximal jet velocity (vena contracta) is determined by the shape of the aortic inlet and the size of the orifice at its most narrow point. Distal to the vena contracta, the streamlines of flow break down into turbulent eddies that propagate upstream until relaminarization occurs.* Detection of this local increase in velocity is the basis for the Doppler diagnosis of valvular stenosis, and the degree to which the velocity increases is related to the severity of stenosis.

* Theoretic data suggest that relaminarization, with restoration of normal symmetric flow, has occurred by approximately five vessel diameters distal to the stenosis.

Congenital Aortic Stenosis

The term *congenital aortic stenosis* usually refers to valves that are stenotic at birth. Congenitally stenotic valves may be acommissural or unicommissural (see preceding discussion) or, more commonly, are bicuspid with two distinct leaflets and commissures. Congenital aortic stenosis can present as an isolated lesion or can be part of generalized hypoplasia of the aorta and/or left heart (Chapters 31 and 32). Congenital stenosis is characterized by an increase in echo production that is due to cusp thickening, systolic doming of the leaflets, and a decrease in leaflet number.[60] Leaflet thickening is apparent in long axis and can be appreciated during both diastole and systole. Doming, likewise, is best seen in long axis at peak systole when the leaflets lose their normal parallel orientation and swing inward toward the center of the aortic lumen (Fig. 19–21).

The specific valve type can be determined in short axis by the number of commissures and the shape of the valve orifice. Three patterns are encountered: complete absence of a clearly defined commissure and a circular orifice (acommissural unicuspid); a single commissure with a coaptation line extending from the vessel wall to an elliptic orifice (unicommissural unicuspid); or a single coaptation line extending between two commissures (bicuspid) (Fig. 19–22).

Congenitally stenotic aortic valves tend to calcify with advancing age. When calcification occurs, mobility of the valve is further limited, and severity of stenosis may increase. When calcification is severe, the differentiation of a congenitally deformed valve from acquired stenosis may be difficult without prior historical data.[61]

Rheumatic Aortic Stenosis

Rheumatic aortic stenosis is the result of an inflammatory endocarditis, which causes adhesion of the leaflet

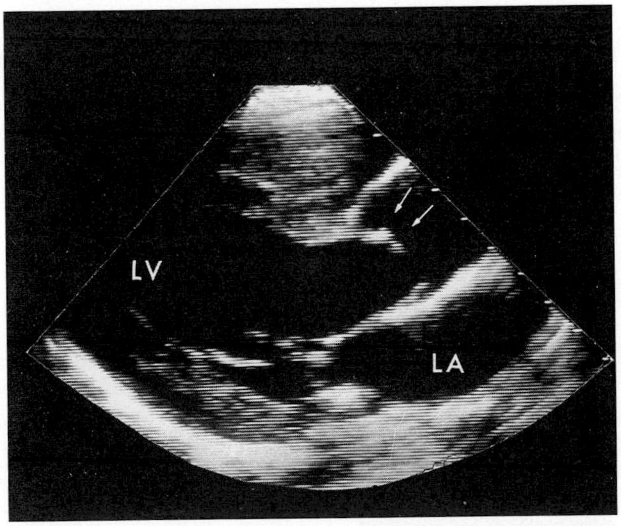

Fig. 19–21. Parasternal long axis recording illustrating systolic doming (arrows) of the aortic valve consistent with congenital aortic stenosis. In this example, both the anterior and posterior leaflet curve inward to encroach on the aortic lumen. However, doming of the anterior leaflet is more prominent. LV = left ventricle; LA = left atrium.

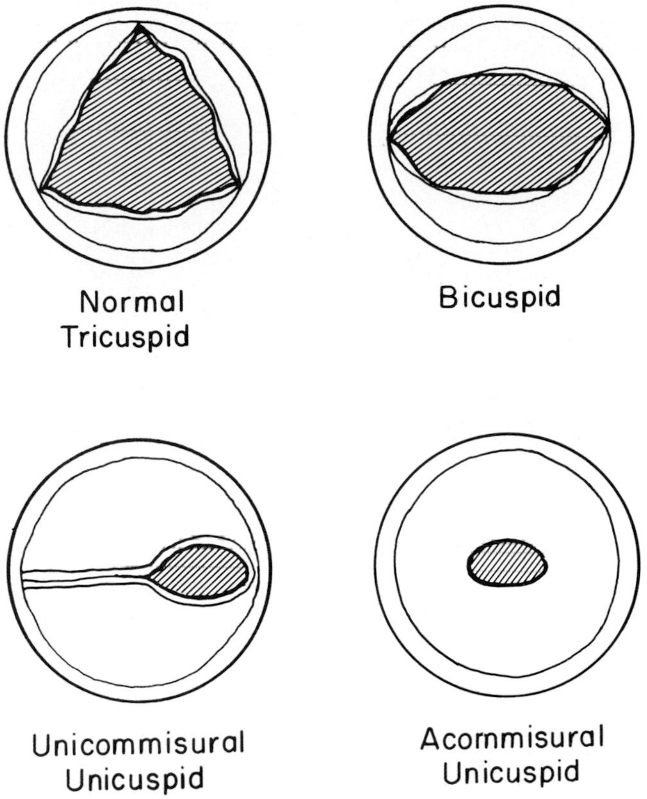

Fig. 19–22. Comparison of the short axis configuration of the normal trileaflet aortic valve with that of the bicuspid, unicommissural unicuspid, and acommissural unicuspid valves.

commissures and leaflet thickening and/or retraction. Fusion usually affects all commissures equally, producing a central triangular valve orifice, but may be limited to only a single commissure. The severity of the valvular stenosis depends on the number of commissures that are adherent and the extent of fusion. When only one commissure is involved, the normal tricuspid aortic valve is converted to a bicuspid valve with little resulting obstruction. When two or more commissures are fused, the degree of valve opening decreases progressively, and the leaflets likewise tend to be more deformed and thickened. Secondary calcification is common and further restricts leaflet motion and distorts the valve orifice.[5]

Rheumatic aortic stenosis presents echocardiographically as it does pathologically as thickening of the aortic leaflet edges with variable fusion of the aortic commissures (Fig. 19–23). The valve is normally tricuspid, although rheumatic fever can affect patients with congenitally bicuspid valves. Mitral stenosis is virtually always present and is typically the predominant lesion.

Rheumatic valvular disease generally presents initially in middle age when the leaflets are still pliable, and therefore doming is recorded in the parasternal long axis view. As a rule, there is obvious focal thickening limited to the free edges of both domed leaflets that is slightly globular and more intense than the reflections from the rest of the leaflet (Fig. 19–24).

In older patients, calcification is usually superimposed on the deformed valve, and leaflet motion be-

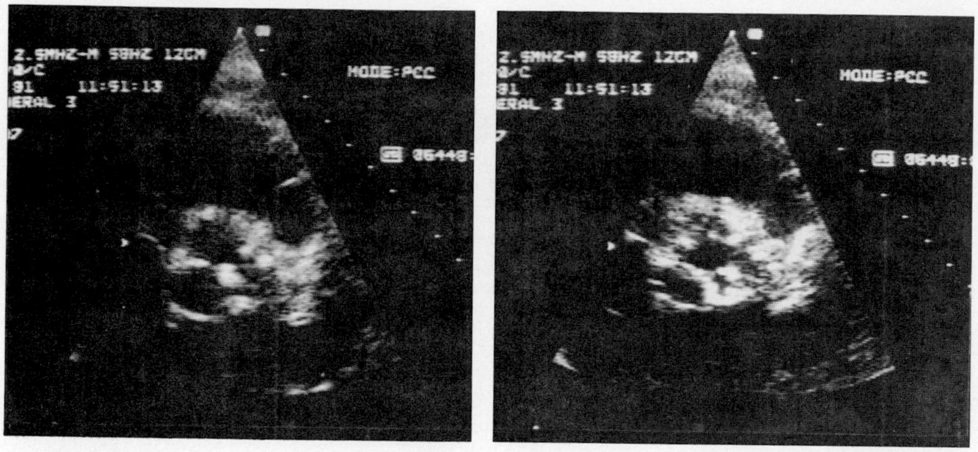

Fig. 19–23. Parasternal short axis recordings from a patient with rheumatic aortic stenosis. Left. During diastole, the leaflet margins are thickened and produce thick globular echoes. Right. During systole, increased echo production from the margins of the thickened valve are again evident, the valve orifice is reduced in size, and the commissures are fused.

comes further restricted. At the extreme, all topographic features of the valve can become obscured, and the diagnosis of rheumatic disease can be established by only history or the presence of associated mitral stenosis.

Adult Calcific Aortic Stenosis

The term *calcific aortic stenosis,* although applicable to all calcified valves in adults, is generally reserved for aortic stenosis in which calcium deposition is the principal process. This includes late calcification of congenitally bicuspid aortic valves and senile calcification of previously normal tricuspid valve.[33] The former occurs at an earlier age, most frequently in the sixth, seventh, or eighth decades of life. The calcification occurring in bicuspid valves is of the dystrophic type and is identical in nature to the process occurring in tricuspid aortic valves (Fig. 19–25).[5] Within bicuspid valves, calcification often involves the raphe first and initiates obstruction by holding one cusp across the outflow tract. Calcification later extends throughout both cusps as bars and nodular masses. Senile calcification of tricuspid valves is found in the late eighth and ninth decades and progresses from the base of the leaflets toward the free edges. Paget's disease of bone is recognized to potentiate early senile aortic valve calcification.[62]

The calcified, stenotic aortic valve of the adult is characterized echocardiographically by an increase in reflection from the thickened, deformed valve cusps, by decreased mobility of the leaflets, and by an absolute decrease in maximal leaflet separation and orifice size.[13,63,64]

The right coronary cusp appears by far the most commonly affected. Commissural fusion, likewise, is most frequently noted between the right and noncoronary leaflets. The left coronary cusp, in contrast, shows the least tendency for deformity and calcification. When fibrosis or calcification is severe, the leaflets may be more highly reflective than surrounding structures and may stand out in sharp contrast to the less dominant background.

Systolic leaflet motion is characteristically reduced. In contrast to the normal full excursion of the leaflets to the margins of the aortic annulus, all or a portion of the leaflet(s) become fixed, thereby limiting motion. This may involve only a portion of one leaflet or may progress to a point where the entire valve is fixed and immobile. The pattern of leaflet fixation follows that of calcification and fibrosis, beginning at the base of the involved leaflet and progressing toward the free edge. It is not uncommon to see a leaflet whose base is fixed and calcified, while the free edge remains thin and mobile. Commissural fusion can occur but is not a primary component of the disease process.

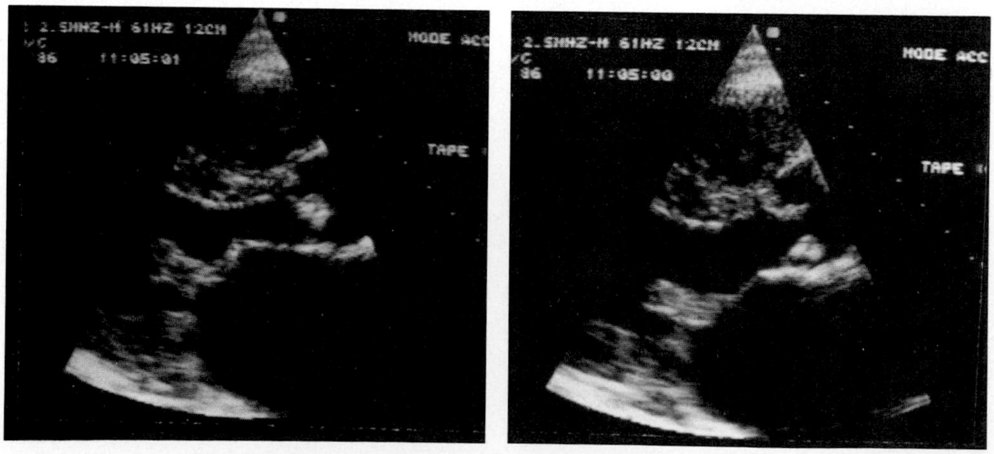

Fig. 19–24. Parasternal long axis recordings from a patient with rheumatic aortic stenosis. Left. During diastole, the leaflet tips are thickened and produce a globular appearing mass of echoes. Right. During systole there is restricted leaflet opening, thickening of the anterior leaflet, and a marked globular collection of echoes at the tip of the posterior leaflet.

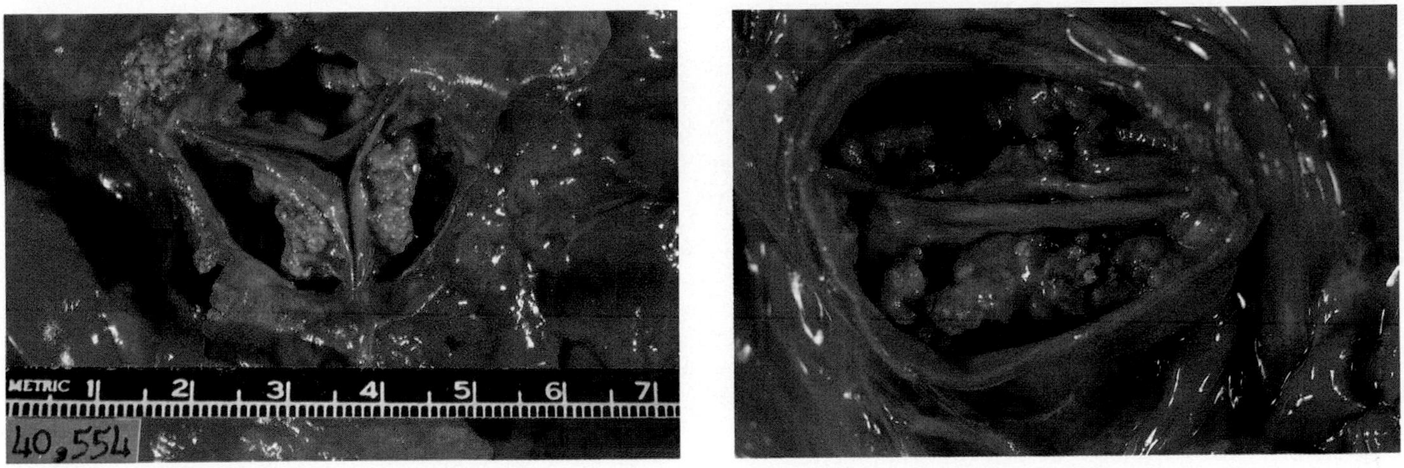

Fig. 19–25. Anatomic sections illustrating dystrophic calcification with stenosis of both a tricuspid (left panel) and a bicuspid (right panel) aortic valve. (Courtesy of Dr. John T. Fallon.)

The restricted motion reduces the absolute separation between the leaflets and thereby narrows the aortic orifice. Although the maximum leaflet separation may vary depending on the portion of the valve examined, peak separation has been shown to be roughly related to severity of stenosis.[13,63,64] Figure 19–26 illustrates the long and short axis appearance of a severely stenotic aortic valve.

Congenital, rather than acquired, abnormalities of leaflet structure appear to underlie the majority of cases of adult calcific aortic stenosis. In one series of 105 patients with isolated aortic stenosis, e.g., 51% had bicuspid, 31% tricuspid, and 12% unicuspid valves.[7] This combined predominance of bicuspid and unicuspid valves, which can be presumed to represent congenital deformities, underscores the significance of these lesions in the late development of clinically important aortic stenosis.

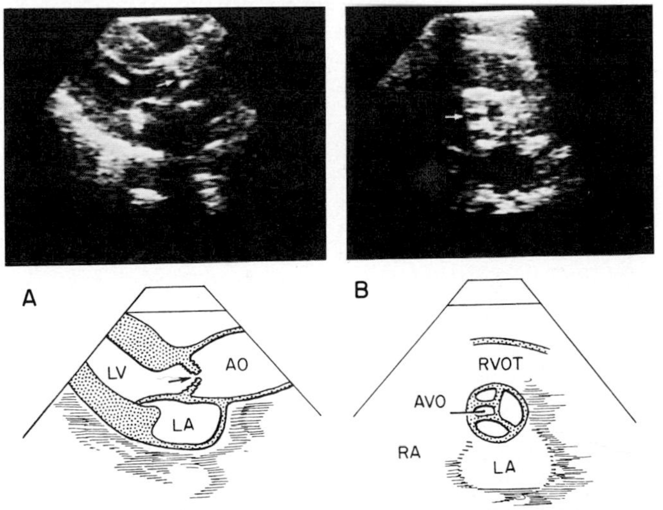

Fig. 19–26. A. Parasternal long axis recording illustrating severe valvular aortic stenosis. The valve leaflets are more highly reflective than normal and dome slightly during systolic opening. Leaflet separation at the valve orifice is reduced (arrow). There is concentric hypertrophy of the left ventricle (LV). **B.** Parasternal short axis recording illustrating the decreased aortic valve orifice area with cusp separation occurring only in the commissure between the right and noncoronary leaflets. The arrow points to the valve orifice (AVO). AO = aorta; RVOT = right ventricular outflow tract; RA = right atrium; LA = left atrium.

Sensitivity and Specificity of Diagnosis

The echocardiographic detection of valvular aortic stenosis has been excellent, with success rates of 100% being reported in two large series.[63,64] In each of these studies, however, normal persons were compared with patients with hemodynamically significant valvular aortic stenosis. Because the valve orifice must be decreased by roughly 75% before a significant gradient develops, major anatomic deformity must have been present in the majority of the aortic stenosis group, and this sensitivity is therefore not unexpected.[65] The overall sensitivity of two-dimensional imaging in detecting lesser degrees of anatomic deformity has not been determined. Many patients are examined in whom there is basal thickening and decreased motion of one or more leaflets but in whom the decrease in orifice area is noncritical.

Although a systolic ejection murmur typically prompts the clinical examination, these patients are generally not surgical candidates, and confirmation of the limitation in orifice area has not been obtained to date. Despite this lack of surgical or postmortem confirmation, the uniform association of leaflet thickening and decreased motion with significant valvular aortic stenosis and its absence in normal persons suggests that the echogram is a highly sensitive method for visualizing leaflet deformity of lesser degrees than can be detected hemodynamically. Although these valves may not impose a hemodynamic burden on the left ventricle, their detection is clinically important, because they place the patient at risk for the development of more severe stenosis as well as for other complications, such as bacterial endocarditis (see following discussion).

The sensitivity and specificity of Doppler methods in detecting aortic stenosis cannot be equated with the sensitivity and specificity of imaging studies, because they evaluate different characteristics of the lesion. As illustrated in Figure 19–27, valve area must decrease significantly before the transvalvular gradient/velocity shows an important increase. Thus, imaging echocardiography reveals the anatomic deformity of the valve, whereas Doppler data define its hemodynamic impact at any point in time.

Estimation of the Severity

Methods have been described for estimating the severity of aortic stenosis (1) directly from the anatomic features of the valve on the imaging study and (2) from Doppler estimates of transvalvular gradients and valve area. An indirect estimation of the peak systolic left ventricular pressure can also be derived from the left ventricular systolic wall thickness and cavity dimension using the constant wall-stress hypothesis. Since the advent of Doppler techniques, however, indirect measures such as those based on wall stress are rarely used.

Imaging

Anatomic characteristics of the valve used to estimate severity include (1) direct short axis measurement of the aortic valve area and (2) measurement of the maximum, long axis, aortic cusp separation (MACS). In addition, qualitative information is frequently available from the short axis evaluation of leaflet motion (even when the orifice itself cannot be fully recorded).

Direct Short Axis Measurement of Aortic Valve Area. The direct determination of mitral valve orifice size has proved to be one of the most accurate and reliable quantitative measurements in clinical cross-sectional echocardiography (see Chapter 17). Visualization and measurement of the aortic valve orifice, in contrast, have proven far more difficult for a variety of reasons.[13,63,64] First, in the adult with calcific aortic stenosis, the valve orifice tends to be smaller, more irregular, and more densely calcified than that of the stenotic mitral valve. Second, the aortic valve moves more rapidly through the scan plane than does the mitral valve, thereby making localization of the true orifice more difficult. Finally, the range in valve areas from a mildly to a severely stenotic aortic valve is small (0.25 cm^2), and as a result, variations between the echocardiographic and hemodynamic measurements that are acceptable in mitral stenosis have proved unacceptable with aortic lesions.

Reported success rates for direct recording of the aortic valve orifice have varied from 13%[64] to greater than 85%,[66] with the majority of clinical experience favoring the lower figure.[63,64] In patients in whom a well-defined orifice can be recorded, however, there does appear to be a reasonable correlation between the echocardiographic and hemodynamic estimate of orifice area. Figure 19–28 illustrates this relationship for a group of eight patients. Unfortunately, these eight patients represent the only instances from a total group of 81 consecutive patients referred for cardiac catheterization for suspected aortic stenosis in whom a measurable aortic orifice could be recorded. Thus, although the clinical value of direct aortic valve area measurement would be enormous, visualization of the aortic valve orifice cannot, at present, be achieved in a large enough percentage of patients to play a major clinical role.

Maximal Aortic Cusp Separation. During the routine echocardiographic examination, aortic stenosis is usually first recognized in the parasternal long axis view based on the typical increased reflectance of the valve and restricted leaflet motion. Several studies have suggested that the maximal aortic cusp separation recorded in this view during careful lateral sweeps of the scan plane across the valve bears a rough relationship to the severity of stenosis (Fig. 19–29). Given the wide varia-

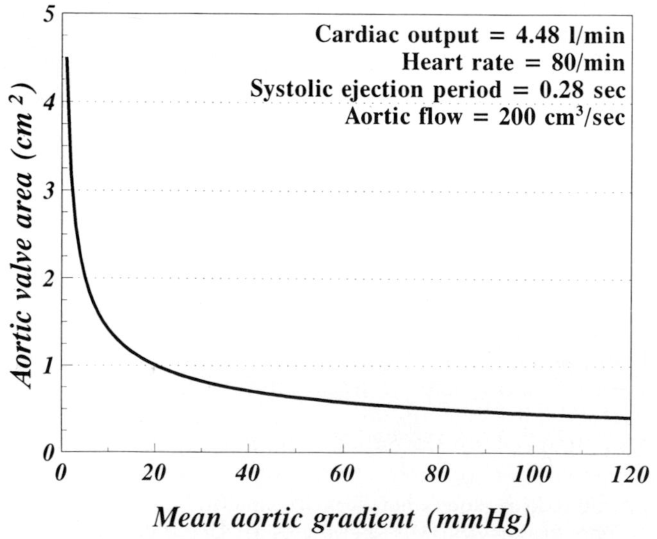

Fig. 19–27. Relationship of valve area to gradient.

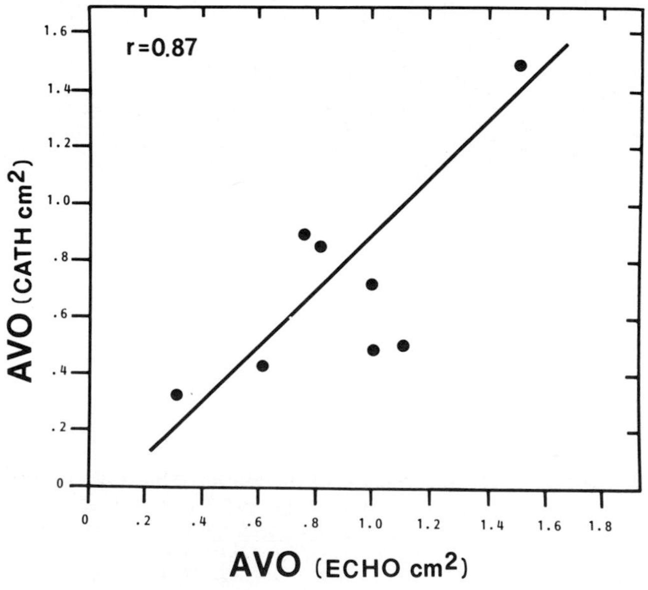

Fig. 19–28. Relationship of directly measured echocardiographic aortic valve orifice (AVO) to the aortic valve determined at cardiac catheterization.

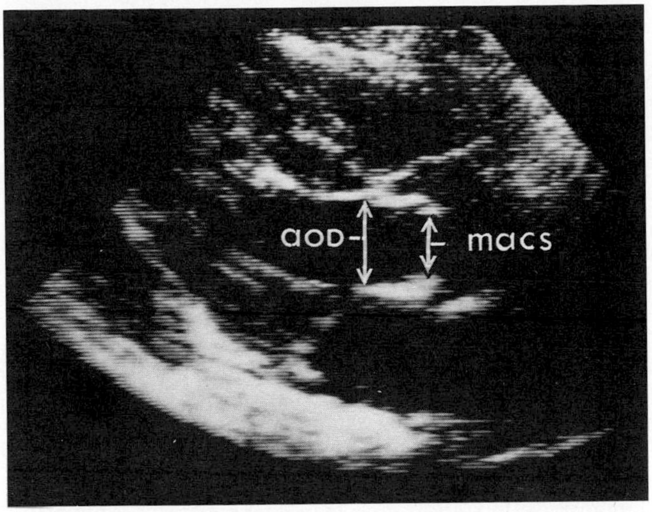

Fig. 19–29. Parasternal long axis recording of a congenitally stenotic aortic valve illustrates the method of measurement of the maximum aortic cusp separation (macs) and aortic diameter (aoD). The macs is taken from the inner margins of the echoes of the anterior and posterior borders of the aortic orifice, whereas the aoD is taken at the level of the aortic annulus.

tion in orifice geometry, such a unidimensional measure cannot be used to predict valve area precisely. It has been shown, however, that in the presence of critical aortic stenosis (aortic valve area <0.75 cm), the maximal separation is always <11 mm,[13,63,64] whereas if the maximal cusp separation is >13 cm, then mild stenosis is the rule, with a 96% predictive value for a valve area of >1 cm^2.[64] In children, the orifice is generally more symmetric, and the MACS normalized by the aortic root diameter is a better, but still less than ideal, discriminator of severity.[60]

Since the advent of more precise Doppler techniques, the MACS is no longer measured; however, the concept remains useful because analysis of leaflet motion consciously or unconsciously biases the operator concerning the severity of the lesion. This impression is then carried over to the Doppler study and appropriately influences the amount of time spent trying to record a high gradient in patients with severely deformed valves as well as one's readiness to accept a lower gradient when valve opening appears reasonable (i.e., an MACS ≥12 mm or a valve area ≥1.0 cm^2).

Qualitative Assessment of Leaflet Motion. Two qualitative patterns of aortic leaflet motion are sufficiently distinctive to permit rapid, visual assessment of severity. First, it can be presumed that if any leaflet in either short or long axis opens completely to the margin of the aortic wall, there can be no more than mild stenosis. This presumption applies because full opening of one leaflet of a three-leaflet valve means that the orifice can be reduced by no more than 66%, which is less than the degree of stenosis required for the development of a significant gradient. Second, if the valve is severely deformed and there is no observable leaflet motion, the lesion can be considered severe.

Doppler

Doppler methods permit direct noninvasive measurement of transvalvular pressure drop or gradient* and calculation of aortic valve area. Doppler ultrasound has the further advantage of providing this information on a beat-to-beat basis and without causing any hemodynamic alterations (as may occur with invasive pressure gradient measurements).

Pressure Gradients. Doppler measurement of the transvalvular pressure drop or gradient is based on the law of conservation of energy, which states that for flow in a closed system the total energy at all points must remain constant. In practice, for any given blood flow (milliliters per second), the linear velocity in centimeters per second through a valve must increase as the valve area decreases. Therefore, as blood crosses a stenotic valve, its kinetic energy, which is proportional to the square of the linear velocity, increases. As a result, its potential energy (lateral pressure) must decrease to maintain total energy constant. In pulsatile systems, additional energy may be required to overcome inertia and accelerate blood to its peak velocity. Energy can also be lost as heat as a result of viscous friction. These relationships can be expressed mathematically using the Bernoulli equation (see Chapter 9), as,

$$\Delta P = \frac{1}{2}\rho(v_2^2 - v_1^2) + \rho\int_1^2 \frac{dv}{dt}\,ds + R(\mu, v) \qquad [19.2]$$

where ΔP is the difference in the pressures proximal and distal to the stenosis, V_1 and V_2 are the velocities proximal to the stenosis and at the vena contracta, s is the distance over which flow accelerates, R is viscous resistance, ρ is the mass density of blood, and μ is the viscosity. In the clinical situation, viscous friction has been shown to be negligible for discrete orifices ≥0.25 cm^2, because blood velocity is approximately constant across the orifice, and as a result there is no frictional loss between adjacent fluid layers. In addition, although the need for flow to accelerate from zero delays the velocity waveform slightly relative to the pressure waveform, it does not significantly alter the calculation of the peak gradient (because at peak velocity dv/dt [acceleration] = 0). The mean gradient is also unaffected because the lag in velocity is roughly symmetric during acceleration and deceleration. At other points in the cardiac cycle, the acceleration term produces small discrepancies between pressure gradient and velocity, but these are not clinically important.[67] Because the viscous friction and flow acceleration terms are negligible,[68,69] they can be ignored, and Equation 19.2 simplifies to

$$\Delta P = \frac{1}{2}\rho(v_2^2 - v_1^2) \qquad [19.3]$$

In addition, in most stenotic lesions, $v_2^2 \gg v_1^2$, so that V_1

* Although in strict terms, *pressure gradient* refers to the loss of pressure as a function of distance, the terms *pressure gradient* and *pressure drop* are generally used interchangeably.

Doppler Calculation of Gradients
Components of Bernoulli Equation

$$p_1 - p_2 = \underbrace{\tfrac{1}{2}\rho(v_2^2 - v_1^2)}_{\text{Convective acceleration}} + \underbrace{\rho \int_1^2 \frac{dv}{dt}\, ds}_{\text{Flow acceleration}} + \underbrace{R(\mu, v)}_{\text{Viscous friction}}$$

$$\Delta p = \tfrac{1}{2}\rho(v_2^2 - v_1^2) \quad \text{[Short acceleration, brief contact with walls]}$$

$$\Delta p = 4(v_2^2 - v_1^2) \quad \text{[Pressure in mmHg velocity in m/sec]}$$

$$\Delta p = 4v^2 \quad [v_1 \ll v_2]$$

Fig. 19–30. Derivation of simplified Bernoulli equation.

can be ignored, and the pressure gradient (after correction for different units of measure) can be regarded as equal to approximately:

$$\Delta P = 4\, v_2^2 \qquad [19.4]$$

Derivation of the simplified Bernoulli equation (Equation 19.3) from the complete equation is summarized in Figure 19–30 and discussed in more detail in Chapter 9. Figure 19–31 illustrates the characteristic changes in both the aortic flow velocity and velocity profile that occur with increasing degrees of stenosis. In addition to the increase in instantaneous velocity, the velocity peak occurs later in systole as the severity of stenosis increases. Although this delay in the time to peak velocity is consistently observed, the time to peak velocity divided by the systolic ejection time has been shown to correlate poorly with aortic valve area (r = .30).[70]

Technical Considerations. To accurately determine transaortic pressure gradients, the peak instantaneous velocities within the stenotic jet must be recorded. To record these velocities, the jet must be sampled from a location that provides an adequate signal/noise ratio and permits the ultrasonic beam to be aligned as parallel as possible to the jet axis. In patients with significant stenosis, the peak velocities in the jet are above the Nyquist limit for pulsed Doppler devices, and continuous wave recordings are required.

Signal Sensitivity. The signal/noise ratio of Doppler devices, operating at a constant output power, depends on the range of the stenotic jet from the transducer, the jet size relative to the beam volume, and the sensitivity of the transducer. In adults, the signal/noise ratio may be poor, because the jet often lies in the far field of the transducer, the jet area is small relative to the beam volume, and the vena contracta typically lies within or just beyond a region of dense calcification that returns a high amplitude signal and blocks ultrasonic propagation when the jet is recorded from below the valve. These factors combine to diminish the contribution of the higher jet velocities to the total returning signal. When the overall signal is weak, the high velocity components may fall below the noise floor and thus fail to be displayed. Failure to record the peak jet velocity can result in significant underestimation of the derived gradient.

The signal/noise ratio can be optimized by precisely aligning the central beam axis (where intensity is highest) with the center of the jet (Fig. 19–32), recording the jet from the closest possible window (Fig. 19–33), and using a small dedicated continuous wave transducer. Because the spatial orientation of the jet will vary from individual to individual, alignment of the beam parallel to the jet axis usually requires recording from multiple windows. It is our custom to record all aortic jets from the apex first and then to confirm the accuracy of the recorded velocity from the right parasternal window. If a discrepancy exists in these values, suprasternal recording is also attempted. As a rule, when the peak velocities differ, the highest value will be obtained from the right parasternal window, which places the transducer

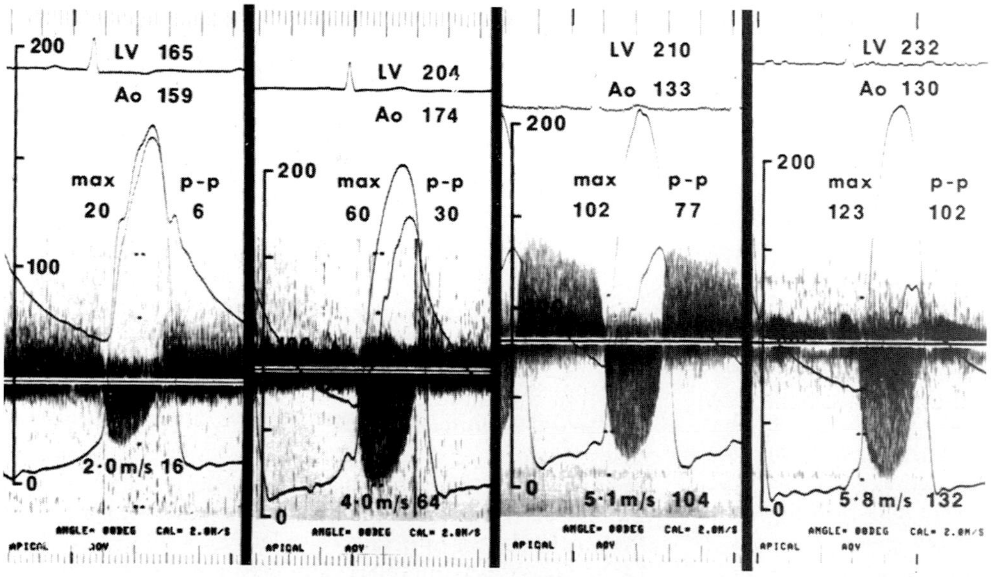

Fig. 19–31. Characteristic changes in velocity and velocity profile with increasing degrees of stenosis. LV = left ventricle; Ao = aorta; max = maximal instantaneous pressure; p-p = peak to peak pressure. (From Currie PJ, et al.: Continuous-wave Doppler echocardiographic assessment of severity of calcific aortic stenosis: a simultaneous Doppler-catheter correlative study in 100 adult patients. Circulation 71:1162, 1985. Reproduced by permission of the American Heart Association, Inc.)

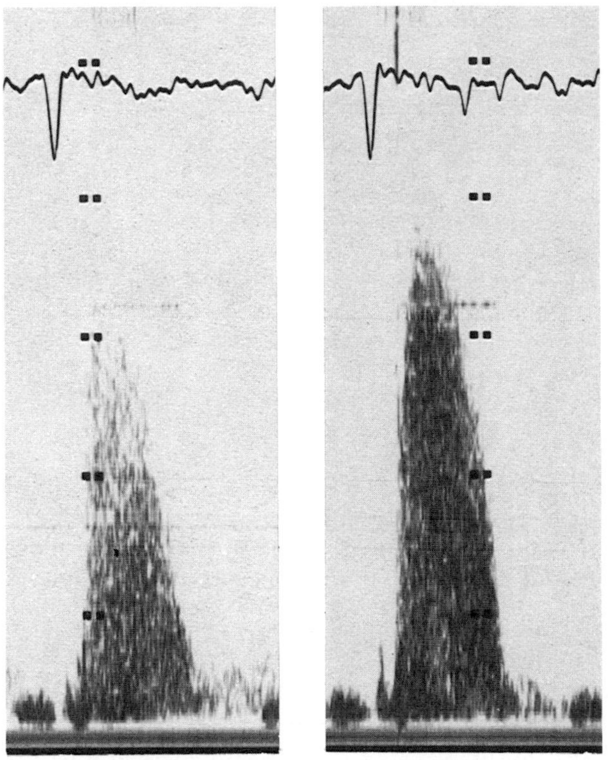

Fig. 19–32. Continuous wave Doppler recordings of aortic jet velocity recorded from the right parasternal window. Left. The beam is not coaxial with the stenotic jet; as a result, the recorded signal is weak and the peak velocity (Vmax) is only 3.0 m/sec. Right. Angling the transducer slightly causes the beam to align coaxial with the jet, which increases the signal intensity and the peak recorded velocity to 3.7 m/sec. PPG = peak pressure gradient.

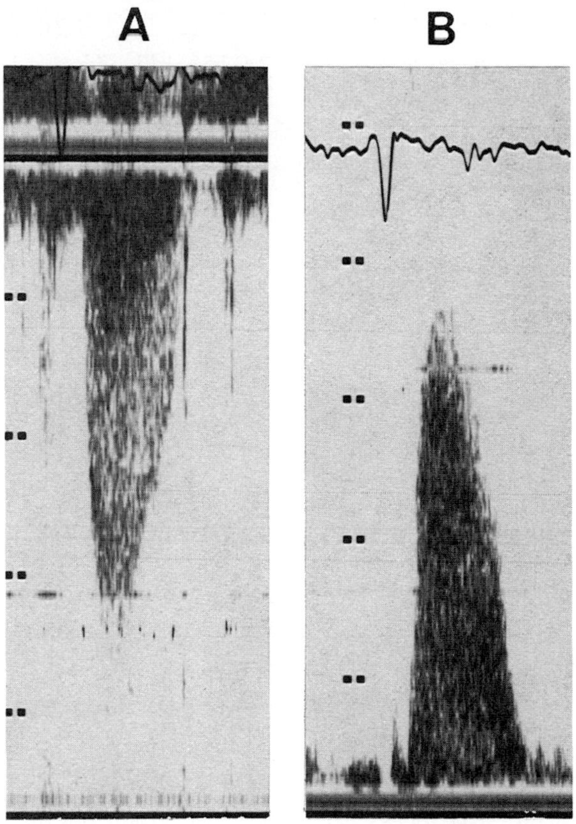

Fig. 19–33. Effects of recording proximity on Doppler velocity profiles. Continuous wave recordings from the cardiac apex **(A)** and right parasternal windows **(B)** in the same patient. In both cases the Doppler beam appeared to be parallel to the jet. The stronger signal and higher velocity recorded from the right parasternal window appear to be a function of decreased signal attenuation when the jet is recorded from a point closer to its origin. Vmax = peak velocity; PPG = peak pressure gradient.

closest to the jet and thus is associated with the least attenuation. Right parasternal velocities have also been shown to correlate most closely with catheterization data (Fig. 19–34).[71] Unfortunately, the overall success rate for jet velocity recording from this site is low.[71,72] In some cases, subcostal recordings will provide velocity information that is unobtainable from the three primary windows.[72] Importantly, the highest Doppler velocity, irrespective of the location from which it is recorded, is used for gradient determination.

In many cases, an adequate velocity signal can be recorded using a steerable continuous wave transducer that facilitates location of the stenotic valve and beam alignment. When necessary, the signal/noise ratio can be improved by using the more sensitive, air-backed, dedicated continuous wave transducer supplied with most instruments. The narrow aperture of these small transducers improves contact and energy transmission, while their lower frequencies increases penetration.

Respiratory variation in cardiac position can alter the spatial location of the jet relative to the beam axis, causing the highest jet velocities to be intermittently recorded (Fig. 19–35). In these cases, the velocity profile typically becomes ragged during the periods when the jet and beam are not coaxial, and this phenomenon must be differentiated from physiologic variation in gradient resulting from changes in output (see following discussion).

Interrogation Angle. Peak velocity will be underestimated if the Doppler beam intersects the jet at an angle because, in this case cos Θ in the Doppler equation will be less than 1. This error is magnified in the calculation of transvalvular gradients because the velocity is squared. For example, if the beam intersects the jet at an angle of 20°, the velocity will be underestimated by 6% and the gradient by roughly 12%. As the velocity increases, the percentage of underestimation will remain constant but the absolute underestimation will increase. This is a particular problem in patients with eccentric jets that are directed at an angle to one or more of the primary recording windows, which reinforces the need to interrogate the jet from multiple sites. Appropriate alignment of the beam parallel to the jet axis can be facilitated by using the audio output of the instrument. When the beam intersects the jet at an angle, both the high velocities from the jet and the lower velocities from

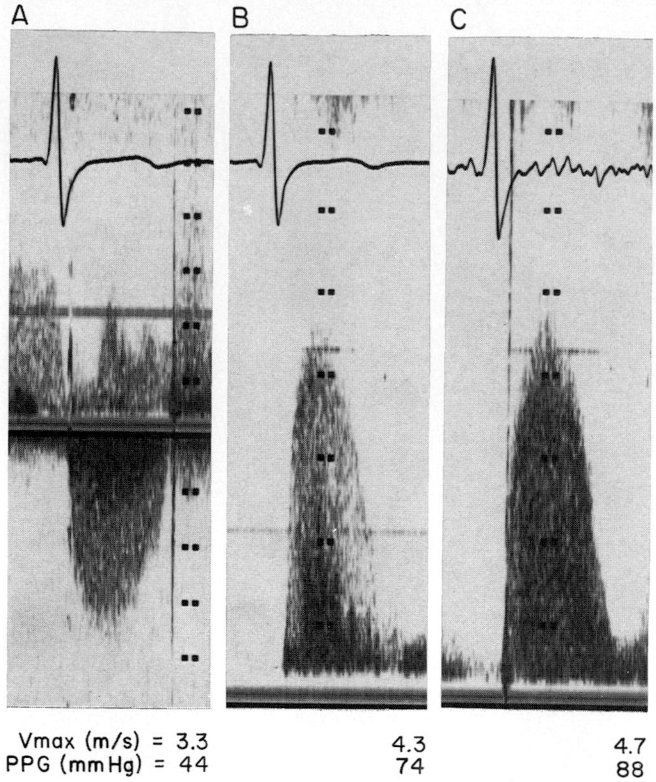

Fig. 19–34. Continuous wave Doppler velocity profiles recorded from the apex **(A)**, suprasternal notch **(B)**, and right parasternal window **(C)** in the same patient. The difference in recorded velocities despite seemingly adequate Doppler profiles emphasizes the need to record from multiple windows to ensure that the maximal velocity is reported. Vmax = peak velocities; PPG = peak pressure gradients.

alongside the jet are recorded. As the intercept angle decreases, the frequencies contributed by the jet will increase, and the low velocity components will decrease, yielding a purer high frequency tone.[73] Use of steerable continuous wave Doppler transducers and color flow mapping may also be helpful in determining the direction of the jet and locating the maximal jet velocity.[74] When the interrogating beam intersects the jet at an angle of >20°, angle correction should be introduced. Angle correction, however, requires some assumptions about the three-dimensional jet vector, and it is preferable to identify a window that aligns the beam parallel to the jet.

Technical Expertise. Experience and skill are required to consistently obtain the clearest recordable Doppler signal (highest signal/noise ratio) with the interrogating beam aligned parallel to the flow stream. Most investigators find that the correlation between catheter and Doppler gradients improves as the number of patients studied increases.[75,76] For example, in a study of 100 consecutive patients, correlation between Doppler and catheter mean gradients improved from r = .88 for the first 33 patients studied to r = .97 for the last 34 patients.[77]

Because the peak velocity remains unknown until it is recorded, it is important to approach the Doppler examination with some idea of severity from the imaging study. This is particularly important in difficult studies because the accuracy with which peak jet velocity is recorded is often directly related to the diligence with which it is pursued.

Doppler-Derived Gradients. Two measures of transvalvular pressure gradient are usually calculated from Doppler aortic velocity profiles; the peak gradient and the mean gradient. The peak gradient is determined from the peak velocity using the relationship $\Delta p = 4v^2$. The mean velocity is determined as the mean of the squared instantaneous velocities recorded during the systolic ejection period. Note that squaring the instantaneous velocities and then calculating the mean is the appropriate method and will yield a slightly higher result than calculating the mean velocity and squaring this value.[78]

Pressure gradients calculated from Doppler flow velocities using the simplified Bernoulli equation have been shown to accurately predict hydrodynamic gradients in in vitro studies of flow through stenotic orifices of variable shape and size (within the physiologic range) when pressures are precisely measured proximal to the stenotic orifice and at the vena contracta.[69,79] In several experimental and clinical studies, similar excellent correlations have been obtained when gradients (Doppler

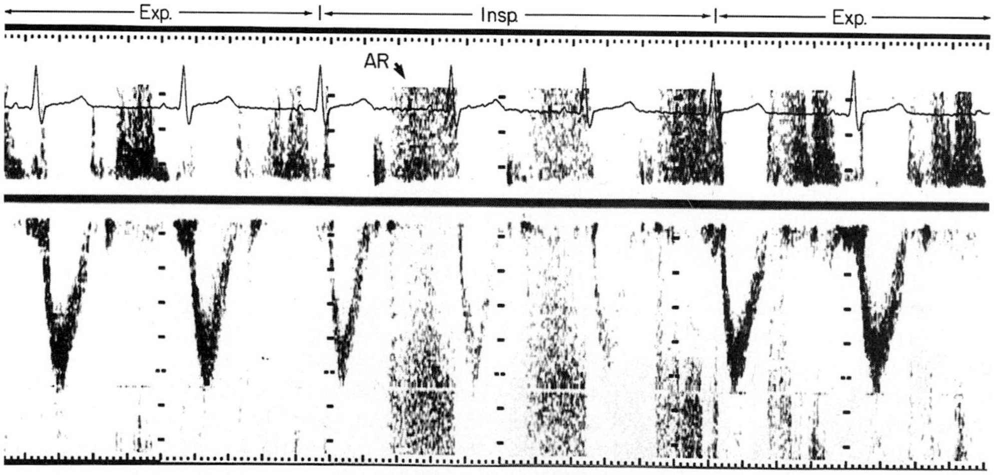

Fig. 19–35. Effects of respiration on the relative position of the flow vector and transducer axis in a patient with aortic stenosis and insufficiency. With the pulsed Doppler cursor placed beneath the valve, the outflow velocity is clearly recorded, and the regurgitant flow is apparent during only a portion of systole during expiration (Exp.). During inspiration (Insp.), the systolic velocity profile almost completely disappears while the retrograde flow from the regurgitant jet becomes more obvious. AR = aortic regurgitation.

and hemodynamic) are measured simultaneously, and both data sets are acquired appropriately.[77,80–82] Figure 19–36 compares maximal and mean Doppler and catheter gradients for a group of 100 patients in whom the majority of measurements were obtained simultaneously.[77]

When the instantaneous pressure and velocity are recorded simultaneously, the velocity curve trails the pressure curve slightly. This delay, which reflects the inertial resistance offered by the blood column, is roughly 60 msec in normal persons and decreases with exercise.[83]

It is important to remember that Doppler measures the change in velocity from a point proximal to the onset of convective acceleration toward the stenosis to the peak velocity at the vena contracta. A critical but unstated assumption in using this increase in velocity as a measure of the pressure gradient across the valve is that all of the pressure that is converted to kinetic energy (velocity) is lost as heat in the turbulent eddies downstream from the stenosis and that none of the kinetic energy is reconverted to pressure. It is this downstream loss of energy that is the important effect of the stenosis because, if velocity were simply reconverted to pressure, there would be no energy loss to the system and the stenosis would have no hemodynamic effect (Fig. 19–37). This lack of effect would occur despite the fact that Doppler would record an increase in velocity at the stenosis and pressure taps would register a corresponding fall in pressure. The assumption that no pressure is recovered is also implied when hemodynamic measures of transvalvular gradient are used to calculate valve area. Although approximately correct in most cases, as indicated by the good correlations between Doppler and hemodynamic studies listed previously, the pressure field distal to the stenosis is complex, and beyond the vena contracta, pressure can vary locally. In addition, the conversion of kinetic energy to heat is not always complete and some pressure can be recovered (see following discussion).

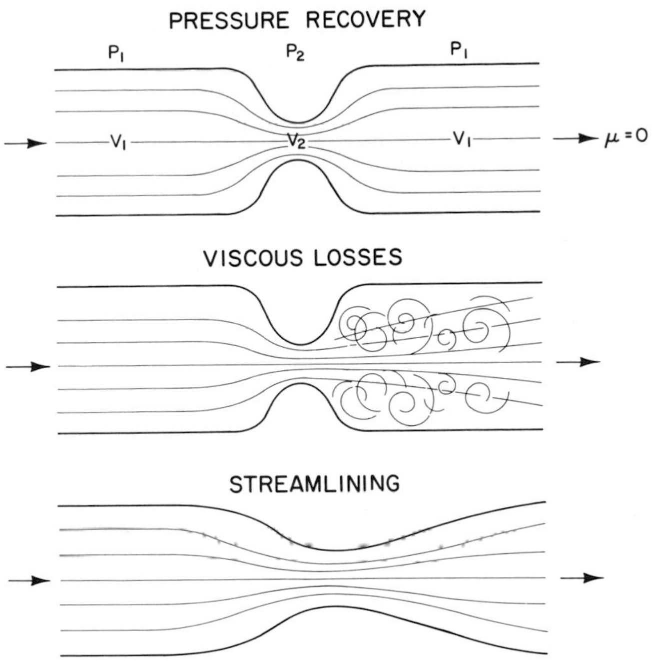

Fig. 19–37. Top. Complete recovery of pressure (P) for inviscid flow ($\mu = 0$), where velocity (V_1) increases (V_2) and then decreases to its original value (V_1) distal to the stenosis. Middle. In the more common clinical case, pressure recovery is limited by turbulence distal to the stenosis, created by flow separation from the chamber walls and viscous interactions between the jet and adjacent fluid. Bottom. Streamlining the stenosis to minimize flow separation increases pressure recovery. (From Levine RA, et al.: Pressure recovery distal to a stenosis: potential cause of gradient "overestimation" by Doppler echocardiography. J Am Coll Cardiol 13:706, 1989. Reprinted with permission from the American College of Cardiology.)

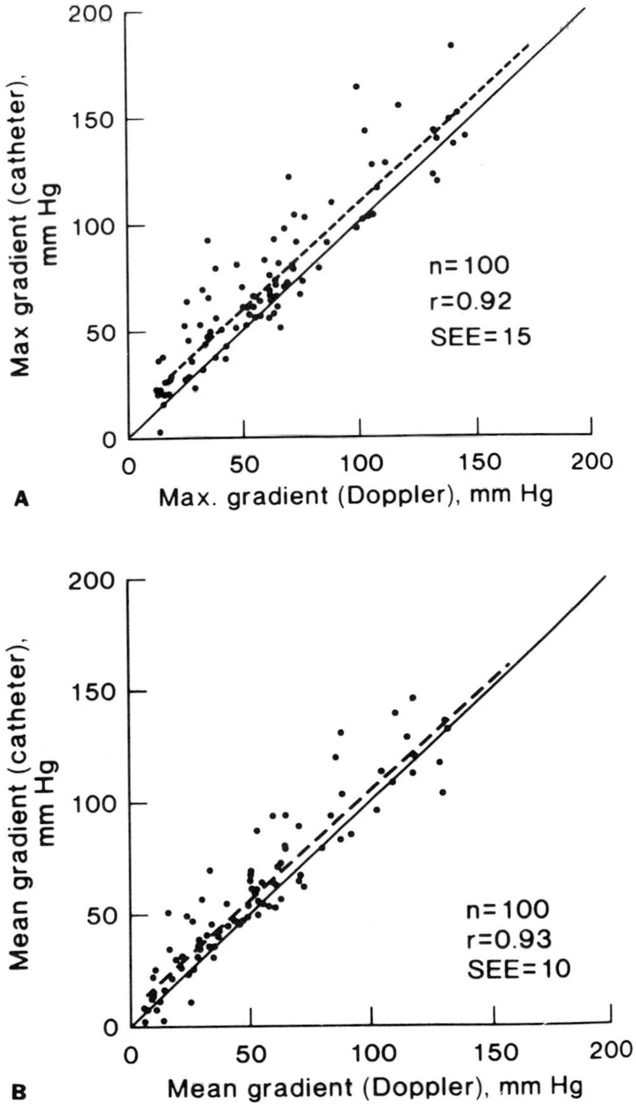

Fig. 19–36. Comparison of maximal **(A)** and mean **(B)** Doppler- and catheter-derived gradients in a group of 100 patients with valvular aortic stenosis. SEE = standard error of estimate. The solid line is the line of identity. (From Currie PJ, et al.: Continuous-wave Doppler echocardiographic assessment of severity of calcific aortic stenosis: a simultaneous Doppler-catheter correlative study in 100 adult patients. Circulation 71:1162, 1985. Reproduced by permission of the American Heart Association, Inc.)

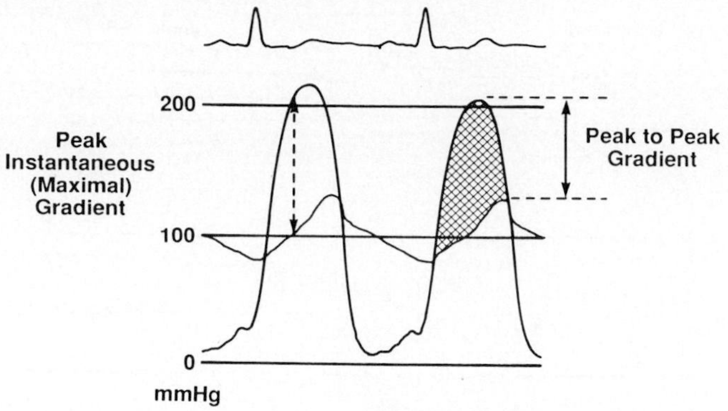

Fig. 19–38. Simultaneous left ventricular and ascending aortic pressure tracings in a patient with aortic stenosis. Measurements of peak instantaneous and peak-to-peak gradients are indicated. The sum of the instantaneous gradients within the shaded area divided by the number of samples is the mean gradient. (From Zoghbi WA, et al.: Echocardiographic and Doppler ultrasonic evaluation of valvular aortic stenosis. Echocardiography 5:28, 1988. Reproduced by permission of the American Heart Association, Inc.)

Difference Between the Doppler Peak and the Catheter-Derived Peak-to-Peak Gradients. Probably the most common reason for apparent differences between the Doppler and catheter measurements of pressure gradient results from confusion of the peak gradient measured by Doppler with the peak-to-peak gradient generally reported by the catheterization laboratory. The peak velocity recorded by Doppler corresponds to the peak transvalvular gradient, which is the maximal difference between the instantaneous left ventricular and aortic pressures at any point during the systolic ejection period (Fig. 19–38). This differs for the peak-to-peak gradient measured at catheterization, which is a nonsimultaneous measurement determined as the difference between the peak left ventricular systolic pressure and the peak aortic systolic pressure (Fig. 19–38). Because these two peaks occur at different points at the ejection period, the peak-to-peak gradient never actually exists and is thus a nonphysiologic measure. Despite this limitation, the peak-to-peak gradient is commonly reported by the catheterization laboratory and is used extensively in the literature as a measure of the severity of aortic stenosis.

The peak instantaneous gradient is always higher than the peak-to-peak gradient, although the difference in these values decreases as the absolute gradient increases. The peak gradient also tends to occur later during the ejection period as the stenosis becomes more severe.[73] The confusion that arises between the Doppler peak and the catheterization peak-to-peak gradients can be diminished by also reporting the mean gradient. The mean gradient, which is the average of the instantaneous gradients throughout systole, is required for the estimation of valve area by the Gorlin equation, and mean gradients obtained by both Doppler and cardiac catheterization should theoretically be equivalent and have correlated closely in comparative studies.[77]

Reproducibility of Doppler Data. To be useful as measures of aortic stenosis, Doppler velocities must be both accurate and reproducible. Intra- and interobserver variability for the same Doppler velocities measured repeatedly has been reported as 3.2 and 3.1% for maximal jet velocity and 3.0 and 3.9% for outflow tract velocity. The reported coefficient of variance for maximal aortic jet velocity recorded by two different observers independently on different occasions separated by a mean interval of 28 ± 36 days without intervening change in clinical status was 3.2%. This variance obviously includes some physiologic variability as well as measurement error. Outflow tract velocity recorded in 10 patients by two sonographers separated by 15 minutes showed a mean coefficient of variance was 4.6%. Reported intraobserver variability for the systolic velocity integral at the aortic valve level and the left ventricular outflow tract were 6.0 and 5.9%, respectively, while the interobserver variabilities for both these measures were 7.5%.[70]

Factors Leading to Differences Between Doppler- and Catheter-Recorded Gradients. Although in vitro and in vivo studies demonstrate that, when accurately and simultaneously recorded, Doppler and hemodynamic gradients correlate closely, in the complex clinical environment there are many physical, technical, and physiologic reasons why these values may differ. Reasons for these differences must be understood to appropriately interpret both data sets. The most common causes are listed in Table 19–1 and discussed in the following paragraphs. This discussion assumes that the catheter recordings are appropriately acquired and form a reference. There are numerous reasons why catheter measurements may be in error, but a discussion of this topic is beyond the scope of this text.

Reasons for the Doppler-Derived Pressure Drop to Exceed That Measured by Catheter Recording. Although it is not theoretically possible for a properly calibrated Doppler device to overestimate the peak velocity at the vena contracta, cases in which the Doppler pressure drop is higher than the gradient recorded by pressure measuring devices do occur, even when the data are

Table 19–1. Factors Responsible for Differences in the Doppler- and Catheter-Derived Pressure Gradients

1. Apparent overestimation of the catheter-derived gradient by Doppler
   - A. Comparison of peak gradient with peak-to-peak gradient
   - B. Failure to account for an increased subvalvular velocity
   - C. Pressure recovery
   - D. Recording the wrong jet
   - E. Nonrepresentative selection of velocity data
2. Apparent underestimation of the catheter-derived gradient by Doppler
   - A. Failure to record the peak velocities present
     - a. Inadequate signal
     - b. Inappropriate recording angle
     - c. Lack of technical expertise
   - B. Use of the proximal velocity in the Doppler equation
3. Unpredictable differences in Doppler and catheter gradients
   - A. Changing physiologic conditions

recorded simultaneously. The most common cause for apparent overestimation of the catheter gradient by Doppler is confusion of the Doppler peak with the catheter peak-to-peak gradient as discussed previously. Other causes for apparent overestimation include (1) failure to consider the proximal velocity in the gradient determination when transvalvular flow is increased, (2) pressure recovery, (3) inadvertently recording the wrong jet, and (4) nonrepresentative selection of velocity profiles to report.

Failure to Account for Increased Transvalvular Flow. Just as the hemodynamically measured pressure gradient is the difference in pressure between the left ventricle and aorta, the Doppler estimate of pressure drop is based on the difference between the peak velocity at the stenosis and the velocity proximal to the area of narrowing. In most cases, the proximal velocity is ≤1 m/sec, and thus v_1 is ≤4 mm Hg. Because failure to account for the proximal velocity in these cases results in overestimation of the gradient by ≤4 mm Hg, which is clinically insignificant, v_1 is customarily ignored. However, when the stroke volume is increased (i.e., in high output states or aortic insufficiency), the proximal velocity may be ≥2 m/sec. Once the proximal velocity exceeds 1.5 m/sec, the overestimation will exceed 10 mm Hg, which cannot be ignored. Thus, it is common practice to calculate the gradient using Equation 19.3, which includes the proximal velocity in all cases in which v_1 equal or exceeds 1.5 m/sec.

Pressure Recovery. The use of the Bernoulli equation to measure transvalvular gradients assumes that all of the pressure energy that is converted to kinetic energy is lost as turbulence (heat) distal to the vena contracta. In most cases, this assumption is approximately correct, and the Doppler gradient reflects the energy loss to the system. Occasionally, however, when the poststenotic jet expands, some of the streamlines reattach to the vessel wall. In these cases, the kinetic energy is not completely dissipated as turbulence, and a portion is reconverted to pressure energy distal to the stenosis.[84] As a result, the directly measured pressure rises and the gradient decreases downstream from the orifice. When pressure recovery occurs, the actual pressure loss to the system, termed the *head loss,* will be less than that reflected by the increase in kinetic energy at the vena contracta. Figure 19–39 illustrates flow through a Venturi tube, which permits almost complete pressure recovery. In this example, despite the fact that pressure energy is almost totally converted to kinetic energy at the point of maximal narrowing, most of the kinetic energy is reconverted to pressure energy downstream, and the head loss is only 15%. Figure 19–40 demonstrates flow through a nozzle, which more closely approximates the clinical situation. In this example, the degree of narrowing is the same as that in Figure 19–39, and the gradient at the vena contracta likewise is similar. In this case, however, most of the energy is lost as turbulence downstream from the nozzle, and only 35% of the pressure is recovered.[85] The fact that Doppler-derived gradients correlated so well with simultaneously recorded hemodynamic gradients in patients with native stenosis and prosthetic valves suggests that significant pressure

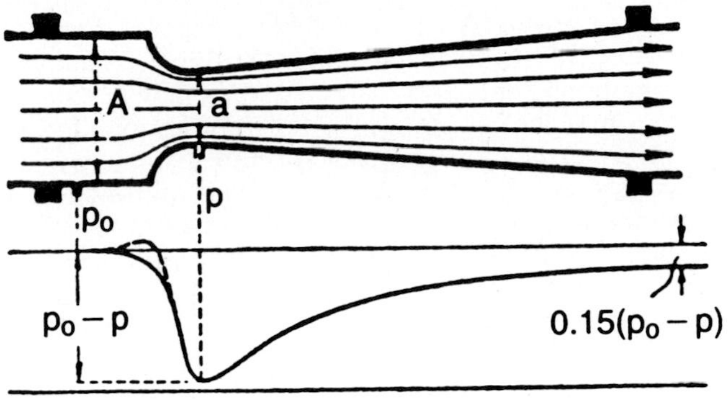

Fig. 19–39. Pressure recovery—flow through a Venturi tube. The solid line gives the pressure distribution along the center line; the dashed curve gives the pressure distribution along the wall. (From Prandtl L, Tietjens OJ: Applied Hydro- and Aeromechanics. New York, Dover, 1957.) A = tube area upstream from the stenosis; a = stenosis area at the vena contracta; Po = pressure proximal to the stenosis; P = pressure at the vena contracta.

recovery is rarely encountered in the clinical setting. In the rare cases in which pressure recovery does occur, the head loss (which is the loss of energy to the system) is the appropriate measure of pressure gradient. *However, the Doppler gradient—which measures the conversion of pressure to kinetic energy induced by the stenosis—is the appropriate gradient to use in any calculation of valve area.* For more tapering stenosis—such as those that often characterize subvalvular and supravalvular obstruction and coarctation—pressure recovery may cause a greater disparity between Doppler- and catheter-measured gradients. This phenomenon is discussed again when these lesions are described.

Recording the Wrong Jet. The peak transaortic velocity must often be differentiated from systolic jets across neighboring valves (i.e., mitral and tricuspid regurgitation and pulmonic stenosis), particularly when velocities are recorded using a blind continuous wave transducer. The most common source of confusion is the high velocity mitral regurgitant jet because both the

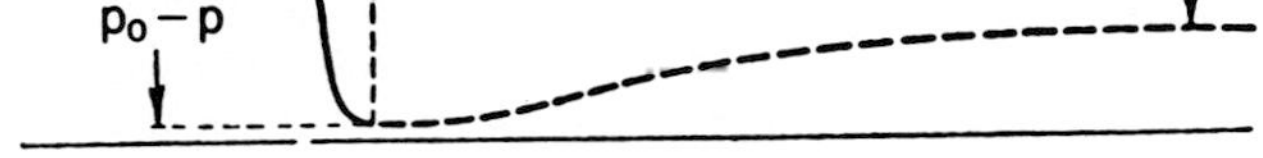

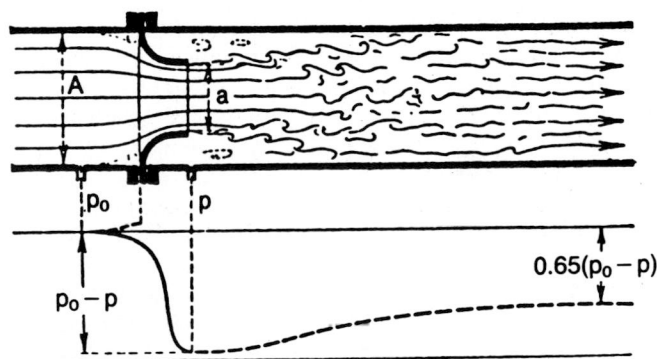

Fig. 19–40. Pressure recovery—flow through a nozzle. Solid and dashed lines as in Figure 19–39. (From Prandtl L, Tietjens OJ: Applied Hydro- and Aeromechanics. New York, Dover, 1957.) A = tube area upstream from the stenosis; a = stenosis area at the vena contracta; Po = pressure proximal to the stenosis; P = pressure at the vena contracta.

mitral and aortic jets have the same general direction relative to the transducer, and when the jet of mitral regurgitation is anteriorly directed, they may be closely related in space. Misinterpretation can be avoided by (1) ensuring that the Doppler spectral display has the typical characteristics of left ventricular outflow rather than that of atrioventricular valvular regurgitation (see Chapter 13); (2) obtaining a consistent Doppler velocity across the stenosis from several windows (e.g., suprasternal and right parasternal, in addition to the standard apical site); (3) examining the timing of the jet relative to the opening and closing clicks of the mitral and aortic valves (because aortic opening follows mitral closure and aortic closure precedes mitral opening, holosystolic mitral jets should always begin before and end after aortic stenotic jets); and (4) using ancillary information from the imaging study, to ensure internal consistency; e.g., if the aortic valve leaflets are thickened with relatively well-preserved excursion, suggesting mild aortic stenosis, but the peak velocity obtained is 6 m/sec (corresponding to a gradient of 144 mm Hg), lesions other than aortic stenosis such as mitral regurgitation should be considered as the cause of the Doppler recordings). Figure 19–41 compares the shape, timing, and velocity of aortic stenotic and mitral regurgitant jets in the same patient.

Nonrepresentative Selection of Velocity Data. Another cause of apparent overestimation is reporting a temporal peak gradient rather than a temporal mean gradient in patients with varying stroke volume (i.e., those with arrhythmia). When measuring Doppler velocities, there is a natural tendency to select the highest recorded velocity with the most prominent velocity profile as the value to report. Even when values are averaged, there is a tendency to select the highest velocities under the assumption that these represent the "best" recordings. Although this yields the most impressive value, it is often not representative of the average gradient, and multiple *consecutive* values should be measured and averaged. Figure 19–42 illustrates the physiologic variability in gradient as a function of cycle length and the importance of measuring several consecutive gradients to obtain a meaningful temporal average.

Causes for Doppler Gradients Appearing Lower Than Those Recorded by Catheter Measurement. Doppler underestimation of the catheter gradient is most often the result of failure to record the peak velocities present in the stenotic jets. This can be due to inadequate signal intensity or inappropriate recording angle and reflects a lack of technical expertise. Gradients can also be underestimated if an erroneous jet is recorded, which has a velocity lower than that across the aortic valve. Such a jet can originate only from the tricuspid or pulmonic valves because the jet of mitral regurgitation must have a higher velocity than that across the aortic valve.

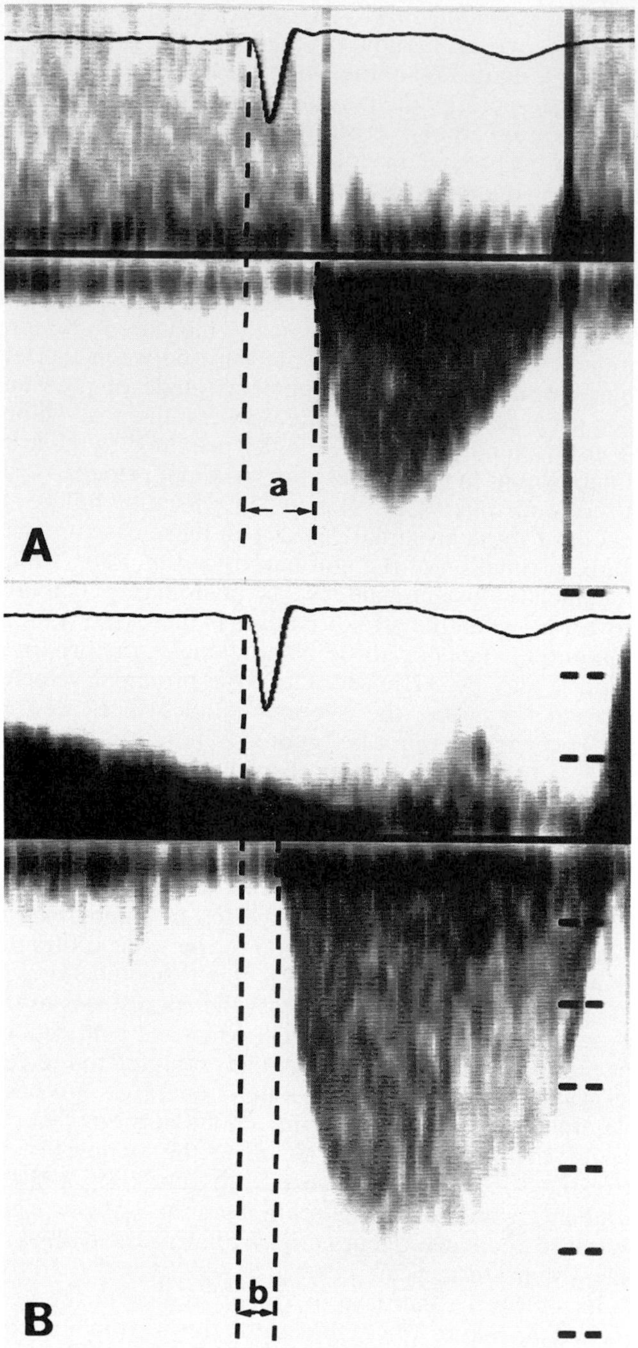

Fig. 19–41. Comparison of aortic stenotic **(A)** and mitral regurgitant **(B)** jets in the same patient. The aortic stenotic jet begins later (A vs. B) and ends earlier than that of mitral regurgitation. In addition, the peak velocity of the mitral regurgitant jet is always higher than that of the aortic stenotic jet. a = time from outset of Q-wave to start of aortic outflow; b = time from onset of Q-wave to start of mitral regurgitation.

Another cause of potential underestimation of catheter-derived gradients relates to the use of the proximal velocity term (V_1) in the Bernoulli equation. In this format, the calculated gradient represents the convective acceleration occurring from just below the valve to the peak at the vena contracta, which appropriately represents the increase in velocity induced by the valvular stenosis. However, because the reference velocity is that recorded immediately below the valve, any geometric acceleration occurring as the blood stream is constricted by the tapering outflow tract is ignored (Fig. 19–43). Geometric acceleration can cause a small gradient between the ventricular cavity and the region immediately beneath the valve, which can be measured

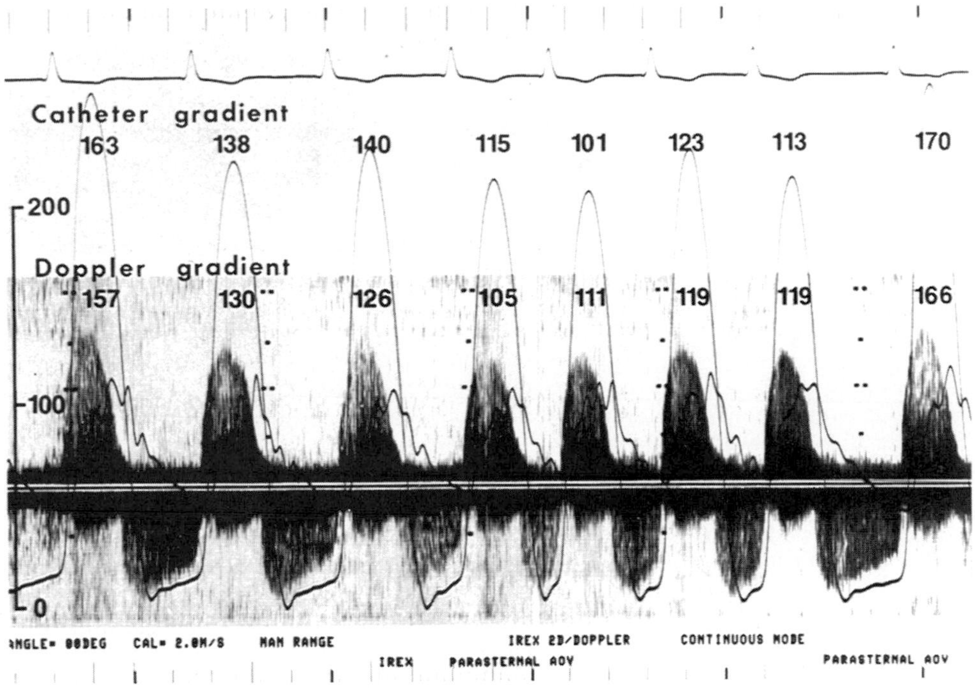

Fig. 19–42. Simultaneous Doppler-catheter pressure measurements with a dual catheter technique showing the beat-to-beat comparison in a patient with atrial fibrillation and severe aortic stenosis. The catheter and Doppler-derived gradients are maximum systolic gradients. Aortic regurgitation is also present. (From Currie PJ, et al.: Continuous-wave Doppler echocardiographic assessment of severity of calcific aortic stenosis: a simultaneous Doppler-catheter correlative study in 100 adult patients. Circulation 71: 1162, 1985. Reproduced by permission of the American Heart Association, Inc.)

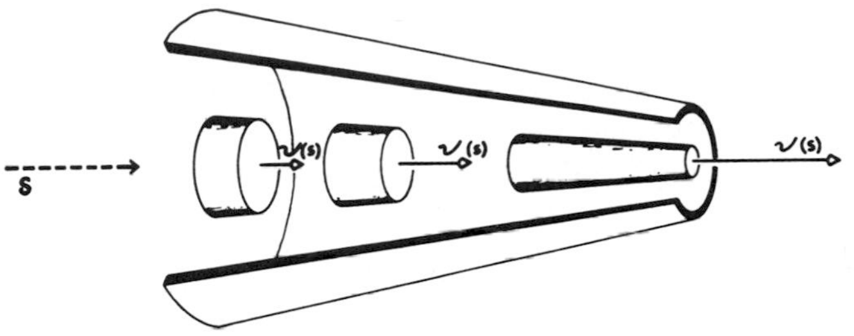

Fig. 19–43. Convective change in streamwise velocity in a tapering flow field. A fluid particle accelerates as it moves successively through axial positions of narrower cross-section and higher velocity [v(s)]. This convective acceleration depends on the velocity gradient $\delta \nu / \delta s$ and on the velocity ν, which determines how quickly the fluid moves through the spatial variations. (From Bird JJ, Murgo JP, Pasipoularides A: Fluid dynamics of aortic stenosis: subvalvular gradients without subvalvular obstruction. Circulation 66:835, 1982. Reproduced by permission of the American Heart Association, Inc.)

by micromanometer-tipped catheters (Fig. 19–44) and is included in catheter measurements of the gradient from the body of the left ventricle to the aorta. It is also included in the $4V^2$ approximation because in this form blood is assumed to accelerate from zero. Although of theoretic interest, this factor should affect the measured gradient by only a few mm Hg.

Unpredictable Differences in Doppler and Catheter Gradients Caused by Changing Physiologic Conditions. In addition to the physical, methodologic, and technical causes described previously for differences between hemodynamic and Doppler gradients observed during simultaneous recordings, physiologic changes in patient status can result in important but unpredictable differences in nonsimultaneous measurements. Several studies have indicated that, whereas Doppler-derived gradients are reproducible on different occasions and with different experienced operators,[70] gradients meas-

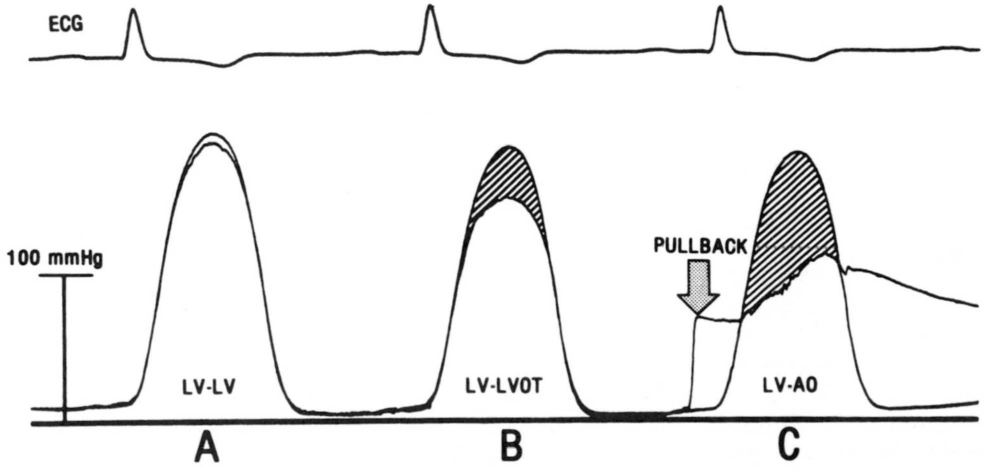

Fig. 19–44. Intraventricular deep (A), subvalvular (B), and transvalvular (C) ejection gradients in aortic stenosis. AO = aorta; LV = deep left ventricle; LVOT = left ventricular outflow tract at or immediately proximal to the aortic orifice. (From Pasipoularides A: Clinical assessment of ventricular ejection dynamics with and without outflow obstruction. J Am Coll Cardiol 15:859, 1990. Reprinted with permission from the American College of Cardiology.)

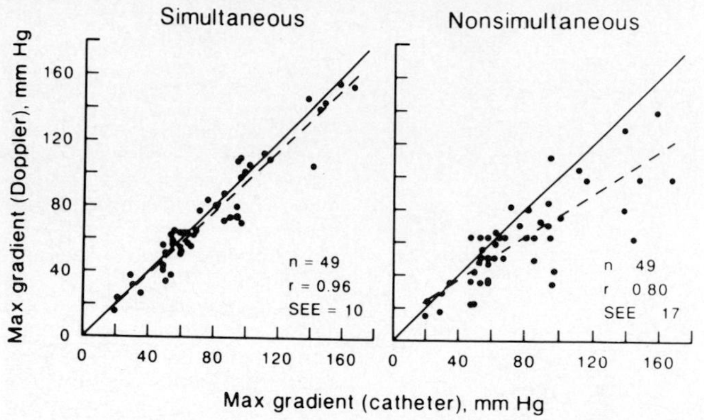

Fig. 19–45. Comparison of catheter- and Doppler-derived maximal gradients measured simultaneously (left) and nonsimultaneously (right). Note the decrease in correlation and increased scatter in the nonsimultaneous values. SEE = standard error of estimate. (From Currie, et al.: Instantaneous pressure gradient: simultaneous Doppler and dual catheter correlative study. J Am Coll Cardiol 7:800, 1986. Reprinted with permission from the American College of Cardiology.)

ured in the cardiac catheterization laboratory have only a fair correlation with those determined independently in the noninvasive laboratory. This appears to relate to dynamic changes in cardiac output, which is a primary determinant of gradient and which in turn is affected by circulatory volume status and autonomic tone. In one large study, the correlation between maximal gradients measured in the outpatient laboratory and at catheterization (r = .80; standard error of estimate [SEE] = 17 mm Hg) was significantly lower than simultaneously recorded Doppler and catheterization values (r = .96; SEE = 10 mm Hg) in 49 patients with two Doppler studies[77] (Fig. 19–45). In another study, the correlation between consecutively measured gradients in the catheterization laboratory and the noninvasive laboratory was modest (r = .66).[86] However, despite the short time interval between examinations (15 to 30 minutes), several patients had major hemodynamic changes between the catheter and Doppler studies. The mean percentage of difference for systolic ejection period was 5% (range, 0 to 33%); for heart rate, 10% (range, 0 to 41%); and for cardiac output, 13% (range 1 to 61%). Despite these changes, aortic valve areas calculated using independently measured cardiac output showed an excellent correlation (r = .99).[86] Given the wide variation in resting hemodynamics between the catheterization and noninvasive laboratories, identity in gradient measurements should be considered fortuitous and only simultaneously derived values should be considered appropriate for validation studies.

Significance of the Aortic Pressure Gradient. The aortic pressure gradient is a useful parameter in assessing the severity of aortic stenosis and following its progression over time. For the same degree of stenosis, however, the pressure drop varies with flow across the valve. Thus, high gradients can be found in patients with mild stenosis if the cardiac output is elevated (e.g., during exercise, pregnancy, or acute anxiety states). Similarly, in patients with mixed aortic stenosis and incompetence, the augmentation of the forward stroke volume by the regurgitant volume will result in a greater transvalvular gradient for the same valve area. In contrast, when the cardiac output is reduced, transvalvular gradient may be relatively low despite important stenosis. This is particularly common in patients with severe aortic stenosis who develop left ventricular failure and in whom reliance on the gradient alone can lead to underestimation of the severity of stenosis. Figure 19–46 illustrates the dependence of mean transvalvular gradient on cardiac output and heart rate.

Several studies have suggested that when the mean transvalvular gradient assessed by Doppler is >50 mm Hg, critical aortic stenosis defined as a valve area of <0.75 cm^2 is the rule,[87,88] whereas a mean gradient of <20 mm Hg is generally indicative of mild aortic stenosis. The severity of aortic stenosis when the mean valve gradient is between 20 and 50 mm Hg is more difficult to define, and under these circumstances, the valve area should be determined. An assessment of valve area should also be performed when ventricular function is

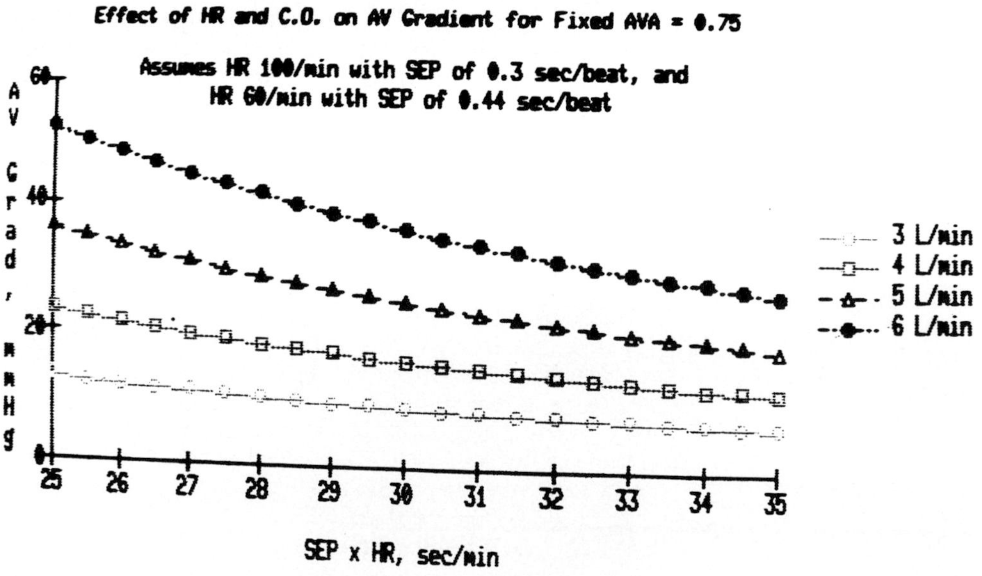

Fig. 19–46. Effects of heart rate (HR) and cardiac output (CO) on the mean aortic valve (AV) gradient for a fixed aortic valve area (AVA) of 0.75 cm^2. SEP = systolic ejection period.

poor or when cardiac output is low, which may be suggested by low velocities in the left ventricular outflow tract.

Assessment of Valve Area by Doppler-Continuity Equation. To determine the anatomic severity of valvular stenosis, it is necessary to calculate the valve area. The normal aortic valve has an effective orifice area of 2 to 4 cm^2, which decreases as stenosis progresses. Mild stenosis is considered to be present from the point of initial encroachment on the outflow tract to a valve area of 1 cm^2. Moderate stenosis is defined as a valve area of 0.75 to 1 cm^2, while severe stenosis is defined as a valve area of <0.75 cm.

Using Subvalvular Aortic Flow as a Reference. The calculation of the aortic valve area from Doppler recordings is based on the law of conservation of mass, which states that for an incompressible fluid in a closed system flow (Q) at all points must remain constant. Thus, for the example illustrated in Figure 19–47, the flow through the outflow tract must be the same as the flow through the valve ($Q_1 = Q_2$). In addition, because flow equals mean velocity times area at any point

$$Q_1 = Q_2 = v_1 \times A_1 = A_2 \times v_2 \qquad [19.5]$$

If flow through the valve is known or can be determined from the product of area and velocity at a reference level, and the velocity at the stenosis can be recorded, then the area at the point of stenosis can be calculated as follows:

$$A_2 = v_1 \times A_1/v_2 \qquad [19.6]$$

This is simply another way of saying that the ratio of the velocities is the inverse of the ratio of the areas, or

$$v_1/v_2 = A_2/A_1 \qquad [19.7]$$

For an incompressible fluid in a tube, the continuity equation is instantaneously valid (assuming that the flow profile does not change between the two points of measurement), and as a result, for pulsatile flow either the peak flow velocity or the mean velocity can be used in the equation. Obviously, the same measure of velocity,

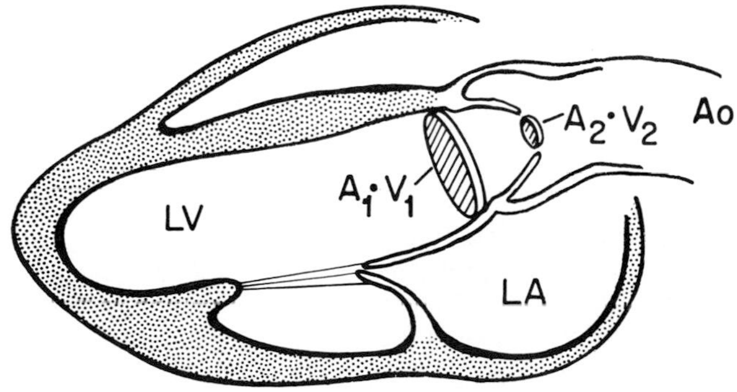

Fig. 19–47. Calculation of aortic valve area using the continuity principle. Aortic outflow is calculated as the product of the subvalvular area A_1 and velocity V_1. The stenotic valve area is then equal to $A_1 * V_1$ divided by the peak transvalvular velocity V_2. LA = left atrium; Ao = aorta; LV = left ventricle.

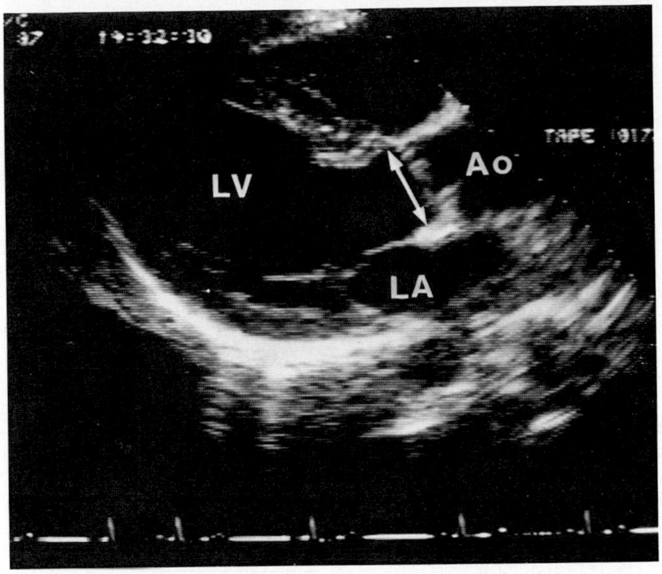

Fig. 19–48. Parasternal long axis recording illustrating the measurement of the subvalvular aortic diameter used to calculate the outflow tract area in the continuity equation. Ao = aorta; LA = left atrium; LV = left ventricle.

peak or mean, must be used for both v_1 and v_2. The most common method for calculating aortic valve area using the continuity equation is to measure flow proximal to the aortic valve by calculating area from the left ventricular outflow tract diameter immediately below the valve (Fig. 19–48) assuming a circular area ($A = \pi r^2$) and to record the velocity at the same level. To avoid inappropriately high velocities resulting from the acceleration of blood as it converges to enter the stenosis, the sample volume is typically advanced up the outflow tract until flow begins to accelerate rapidly (usually from 1.5 to 0.5 cm below the valve) and then withdrawn slightly. This reference flow is then divided by the velocity across the stenotic lesion recorded by continuous wave Doppler yield the area of the stenosis.

The continuity equation also assumes that the area of the valve A_2 is constant. If the orifice is elastic and varies because of changes in the gradient across the obstruction during pulsatile flow, the size of the valve area calculated by Equation 19.6 will depend on when v_1 and v_2 are determined. If peak v_1 and v_2 are used, it can be assumed that the maximal A_2 is calculated because the gradient is greatest at this point, forcing the valve to open maximally. Figure 19–49 compares valve areas calculated using the peak velocity and the velocity integral. Areas calculated using the peak velocity are equal to or slightly larger than those determined using the velocity integral.[89] This supports the concept that the peak velocity yields a maximal area while the velocity integral gives the mean or effective area. The differences are less meaningful at small areas, suggesting that these valves are more densely calcified and less elastic. In studies of patients postaortic balloon valvuloplasty, where the valve has presumably been maximally stretched, we have not noted any significant difference in valve areas calculated by the two methods or changes in valve area following dobutamine infusion.

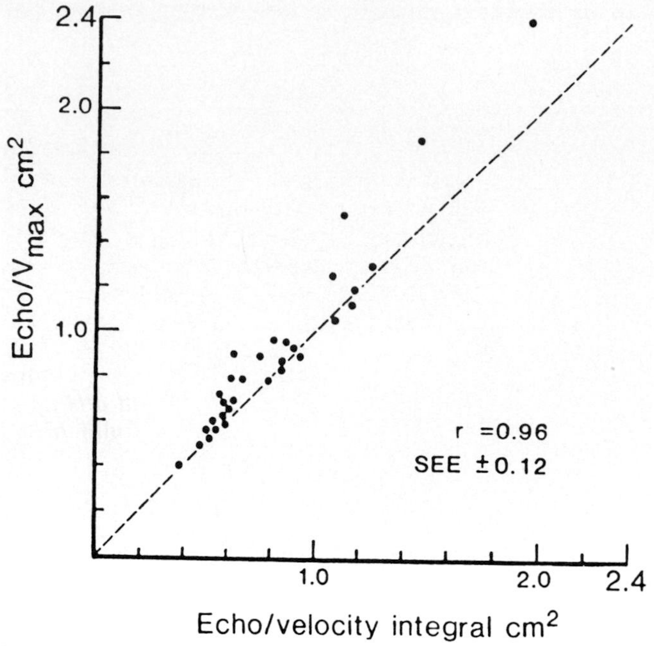

Fig. 19–49. Comparison of aortic valve areas calculated using the peak outflow tract and transaortic velocities (echo/V_{max}cm^2) and that calculated using the mean velocities (echo/velocity integral cm^2). In general, the peak velocities yield a slightly higher value for valve area, suggesting the possibility of some degree of orifice stretching, particularly for less severely stenotic valves. (From Skjaerpe T, Hegrenaes L, Hatle L: Noninvasive estimation of valve area in patients with aortic stenosis by Doppler ultrasound and two-dimensional echocardiography. Circulation 72:810, 1985. Reproduced by permission of the American Heart Association, Inc.)

Several points should be remembered in these calculations:

1. The continuity equation is instantaneously valid so that the velocities used in the equation can be either the stroke velocity integrals or the peak velocities (assuming that the valve area does not change).

2. Flow through the outflow tract includes both forward and aortic regurgitant flow so that the valve areas calculated using the continuity equation will be accurate whether aortic regurgitation is present or not. This is in contrast to hemodynamic measures based on cardiac output, which generally fail to account for regurgitant aortic flow and hence underestimate anatomic valve area.

3. Because the peak Doppler velocity is the velocity at the vena contracta, the calculated valve area will be the smallest area of the flow stream, which will be equal to that anatomic area reduced by the coefficient of discharge of the orifice (see Chapter 9). This is the appropriate hydrodynamic area but should be smaller than the area calculated at catheterization using the Gorlin formula, which includes a constant to account for the coefficient of discharge and thus convert hydrodynamic area to the anatomic area (the accuracy of this constant for the aortic valve has never been validated).[90]

4. When the cardiac output is used as a reference, it must be converted to the stroke volume (i.e., milliliters per beat) to reflect flow crossing the valve during each systole (see following discussion).

5. If echo-Doppler derived flow through other valves is used as the reference, one must be sure that flow through the aortic valve and the reference valve are identical. For example, mitral valve flow can be used as the reference if there is no mitral or aortic regurgitation. If regurgitation of either valve is present, flow through the two valves will not be equal (except by chance), and the continuity equation will be invalid.

6. Although the continuity equation is instantaneously valid, velocities are usually recorded using different techniques (i.e., the proximal velocity is recorded using pulsed Doppler and the peak transvalvular velocity using continuous wave Doppler) and thus cannot be recorded simultaneously. This is not a problem in patients with stable heart rates but can lead to considerable error in patients with widely varying cycle lengths. In the latter cases, care must be taken to use velocities recorded at comparable cycle lengths or, if this is not practical, to average values over several beats to obtain the representative velocities.

Using Doppler Velocities in Conjunction With Cardiac Output (Measured Either by Right Heart Catheterization or by Doppler Techniques). An alternative method for calculating valve area is to use the Doppler transvalvular velocity (v_2) or the derived gradient, together with an independently calculated cardiac output. This cardiac output can be determined by thermodilution,[86,70] Fick, or dye dilution methods, or a Doppler cardiac output measured at an intracardiac site other than the aortic valve can be used.[91] The principle underlying this approach is that volumetric flow (milliliters per second) through a valve is simply equal to the cross-sectional area of the valve (square centimeters), multiplied by the velocity of blood through the valve (centimeters per second) (see Chapter 9). Hence, valve area can be calculated if cardiac output and blood flow velocity are known as:

$$\text{aortic valve area} = \frac{\text{cardiac output}}{(\text{systolic ejection period}) \times (\text{mean post-stenotic flow velocity})} \quad [19.8]$$

or

$$\text{aortic valve area} = \frac{\text{stroke volume}}{\text{mean post-stenotic flow velocity}} \quad [19.9]$$

This approach has been shown to yield aortic valve areas that are closely correlated (r = .99) with those obtained at catheterization.[86] In this formula, it is necessary to divide by the systolic ejection period because the whole cardiac output crosses the valve during systole, and hence the relationship between flow and area is established only during seconds of systole. Also note that because the cardiac output is a mean value, the relationship with area must be based on the mean temporal post-stenotic flow velocity as expressed by the systolic velocity integral rather than the peak velocity.

Miscellaneous Approaches Based on the Continuity Principle. Other approaches based on the continuity principle have been described that reportedly separate degrees of stenosis with reasonable accuracy. These include (1) the ratio of the mitral mean linear velocity to the aortic mean linear velocity,[92] (2) a dimensionless index based on the ratio of the systolic velocity integral in the left ventricular outflow tract to the systolic velocity integral of flow across the valve,[70] and (3) the ratio of the left ventricular outflow velocity to the left ventricular fractional shortening.[93] None of these approaches is uniformly accurate in determining severity, and although the goal of simplification is commendable, reliance on such contrived indices seems inappropriate when direct calculation of valve area is possible.

Wall Stress Hypothesis

In children, if Doppler is unavailable, the transvalvular gradient can be estimated using the constant wall-stress hypothesis, which holds that the left ventricle hypertrophies in response to a pressure overload in such a way that peak systolic wall stress remains constant. Empirical correlations have yielded the following equation:

$$\text{peak LV systolic pressure} = \frac{225 \times \text{LV wall thickness}}{\text{LV internal diameter}_s} \quad [19.10]$$

where LV is left ventricle and s signifies end systole. The gradient is then obtained by subtracting systolic arterial pressure from ventricular pressure. Results in aortic valvular and discrete subvalvular obstructions in children correlate well with hemodynamic measurement.[94–97] In adults, however, the method has proven less reliable.[98] The disparity between the good results obtained in children and the limited utility of this approach in adults may relate to the effects of superimposed factors, such as hypertension and myocardial dysfunction, on wall thickness and stress.[99] Given the numerous factors that can affect wall thickness independent of chamber pressure in both populations, Doppler is the technique of choice for gradient estimation.

Natural History of Aortic Stenosis

Valvular aortic stenosis is recognized to be a progressive disease; however, the rate and nature (incremental or sporadic) of progression remain to be defined.[100] In children with congenital aortic stenosis, an absolute reduction of aortic valve area appears relatively uncommon, and changes in the transvalvular gradient appear to be due to the growth-related increase in stroke volume relative to the congenitally restricted valve orifice.[101] In the adult, progression is characterized by an absolute decrease in valve area, increase in transvalvular pressure gradient, and a decrease in cardiac output with the onset of left ventricular failure. In hemodynamic studies, progression has been reported in between 41[102] and roughly 90%[103] of patients.

The mean rate of progression of aortic valve gradient and area from hemodynamic and Doppler studies are listed in Table 19–2. Although these data provide a general sense of the rate of progression of stenosis, they are difficult to apply clinically as a result of enormous individual variability. For example, in one hemodynamic study, one patient showed an increase in peak systolic gradient of 90 mm Hg over a 2-year period (3.7 mm Hg/month), while another showed no change in gradient during a 10-year follow-up.[104] Several studies have divided patients into rapid and slow progressors in an attempt to identify factors predictive of accelerated progression. Progression appears unrelated to age, sex, symptoms at initial study, ventricular function, presence or absence of associated coronary disease,[106] or associated aortic insufficiency. In individual studies, cause (degenerative calcific stenosis), decreased cardiac output, and milder degree of stenosis at entry have been associated with increased progression, but these same features have not proven predictive in others. Progression does show a consistent but not uniform association with increasing symptoms during follow-up.[106] In one study in which three or more samples were obtained, the rate of progression appeared linear, but the duration

Table 19–2. Rate of Progress in Aortic Valve Gradient and Area

Study	N	d AVA/Year	%d AVA/Year	d MAVG/Year
Bogart et al.[103]	11	0.2 (0.02–0.6)		11.6 (1.2–24)
Cheitlin et al.[104]	29	NA		8.4 (−12–45)
Nestico et al.[102]	29	0.05 (0–0.5)		0.8 (−8–10.4)
Wagner and Selzer[100]	50			
Rapid	21	0.3 ± 0.2		
Slow	29	0.02 ± 0.08		
Otto et al.[105]	42	0.1 (0–0.5)		8.0 (−7–23)
Thoreau[105a]	84	0.07 ± 0.11	4.09 ± 6.14	4.12 ± 4.86
AVA_i				
<1.0	35	0.02 ± 0.06	1.99 ± 6.89	4.64 ± 5.60
1.0–2.0	38	0.07 ± 0.07	4.67 ± 4.87	3.79 ± 4.58
>2.0	11	0.24 ± 0.16	8.77 ± 4.70	3.63 ± 3.27

d AVA = change in aortic valve area; d MAVG = change in mean aortic valve gradient; NA = not available.

of follow-up was limited.[106] Further, this observed linearity was based on changes in velocity, which do not bear a linear relationship to gradient. Thus, although echo-Doppler methods appear ideal for defining the natural history of aortic stenosis, further studies are required to clarify the nature of this complex process.

Aortic Insufficiency

Structural Abnormalities Associated With Aortic Insufficiency

Aortic insufficiency may result from a primary disorder of either the aortic valve, the aortic root, or a combination of both. Aortic insufficiency on a valvular basis may be either acquired (occurring most often as a result of rheumatic fever or bacterial endocarditis) or congenital (in association with congenital valvular aortic stenosis, bicuspid aortic valve, or aortic valve prolapse.)[7,107–109] In pure rheumatic aortic regurgitation, commissural fusion is absent but fibrosis extending outward from the base retracts the cusps. This process ultimately leads to failure of cusp apposition in the center of the valve. Pure regurgitation is rare in patients with rheumatic aortic valve disease and is usually associated with some degree of commissural fusion and stenosis. Rare cases are reported in which one cusp is retracted and fibrotic without abnormality of the other two.[5] Bacterial endocarditis can cause valvular regurgitation that is due to leaflet perforation, cusp fibrosis, and retraction or loss of basal support with a portion of the valve cusp becoming flail (Fig. 19–50). Aortic endocarditis is discussed in detail in Chapter 37.

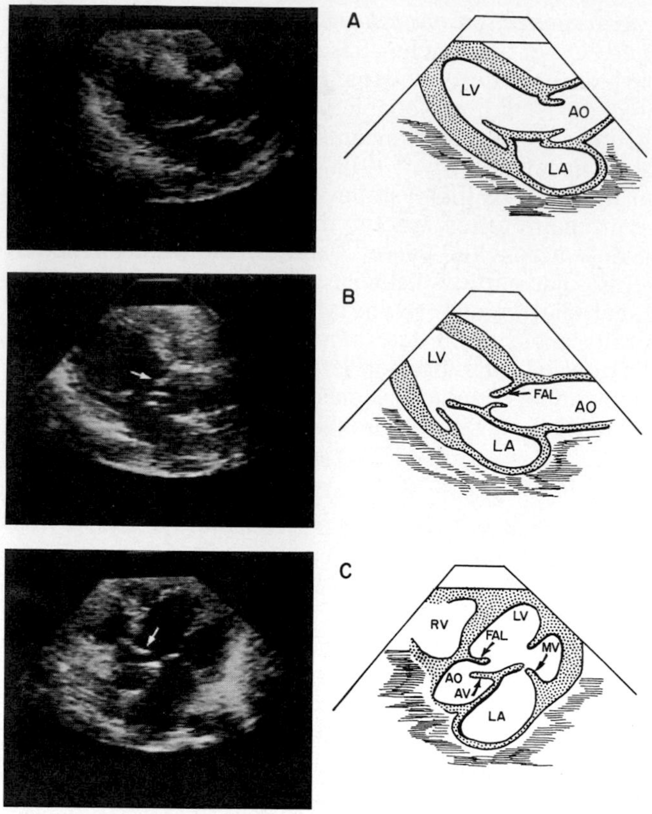

Fig. 19–50. Flail right coronary aortic leaflet. **A.** Parasternal long axis recording indicating the relatively normal systolic appearance of the flail valve. **B.** Diastolic recording demonstrating the reversal in direction of the freely moving leaflet. The leaflet tip (FAL) points down toward the left ventricle (LV). **C.** An obliquely recorded apical five-chamber view that again illustrates lack of coaptation of the flail leaflet and reversal of the normal diastolic orientation. RV = right ventricle; AO = aorta; AV = aortic valve; LA = left atrium; MV = mitral valve.

Congenital abnormalities of leaflet morphology and number frequently result in aortic regurgitation. These range from rare morphologic disorders such as congenital absence of the aortic valve[110] or dysmorphic aortic leaflets[111] to the more common unicuspid and bicuspid aortic valves (see preceding discussion). Aortic valve prolapse is generally an inherited disorder defined as the abnormal inferior or apical displacement of one or more aortic cusps below the plane of the aortic annulus (Fig. 19–51). Although a slight amount of apical displacement of the aortic leaflets may be recorded normally at peak diastole,[112] abnormal displacement or prolapse can occur in many conditions such as in bicuspid aortic valve, in myxomatous degeneration of the aortic valve, in connective tissue disorders such as Marfan's syndrome, in sinus of Valsalva aneurysm, following aortic valvotomy, and occasionally with a ventricular septal defect located immediately below the valve. Aortic valve prolapse can also be seen in up to 20% of patients with mitral valve prolapse (polyvalvular prolapse syndrome).[113] Aortic valve prolapse can progress to flail leaflet, particularly when the cause is primary myxomatous degeneration of the valve. Echocardiographic differentiation of a flail leaflet caused by bacterial infection from disruption of a myxomatous valve may not be possible on purely morphologic grounds, and both conditions can coexist.

Aortic root abnormalities (i.e., dilation, aneurysm, dissection) must involve the plane of commissural insertion (the supra-aortic ridge or sinotubular junction) to cause valvular insufficiency. Both generalized root dilation and focal dilation and distortion can lead to valvular insufficiency. Leakage occurs because the cusps are unable to expand as the root diameter increases, and the degree of cusp overlap decreases until the valve becomes incompetent. If the process is symmetric, a central leak will typically occur, whereas local dilation leads to eccentric malposition and regurgitation. In either case, regurgitant flow over the cusp edge(s) leads to thickening of the free edge with a normal leaflet body.[5] Aortic root dilation is most commonly idiopathic and is due to noninflammatory destruction of the elastic fibers and smooth muscle of the media.[114] Other less common causes include Marfan's syndrome, Ehlers-Danlos syndrome, and osteogenesis imperfecta. Inflammatory disorders involving the aorta such as ankylosing spondylitis, Reiter's syndrome, rheumatoid arthritis, syphilis, and giant cell aortitis are also associated with aortic dilation and regurgitation.

Infective or destructive processes in the aortic wall such as aortic root abscess or dissection cause root dilation and can also lead to inadequate leaflet support and flail leaflet (see Chapter 37).

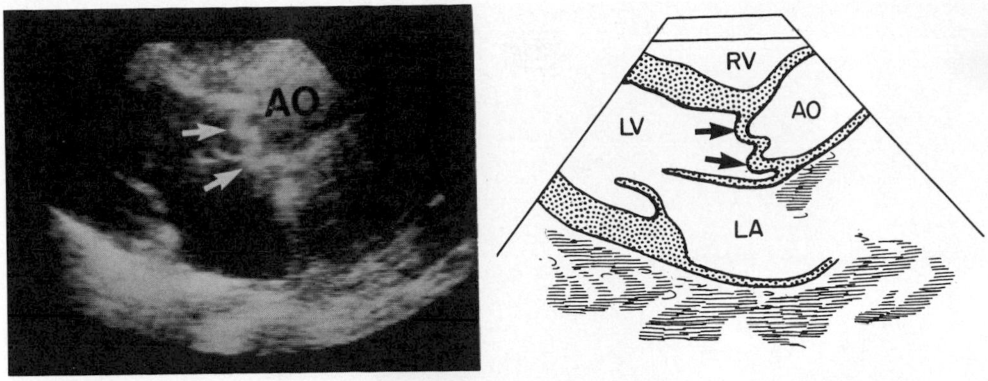

Fig. 19–51. Parasternal long axis recording of the aortic valve illustrating prolapse of both the right and noncoronary aortic leaflets (horizontal arrows). LV = left ventricle; RV = right ventricle; LA = left atrium; AO = aorta.

Detection of Aortic Insufficiency

Although the presence of aortic regurgitation may be suspected from the appearance of the valve (i.e., flail aortic valve) or root, demonstration of the abnormal regurgitant jet is achieved by Doppler methods. Aortic regurgitation is detected by Doppler as a high velocity, turbulent, diastolic flow originating just below the aortic valve (Fig. 19–52) immediately after valve closure and generally continuing throughout diastole. Although the jet can be recorded using any of the Doppler techniques, color flow mapping, which depicts jet origin, size, and spatial distribution (Fig. 19–53), and continuous wave Doppler (Fig. 19–54), which reports the maximum jet velocities and the timing of flow, provide the primary information.

Sensitivity and Specificity

Multiple studies have shown all Doppler modalities to have sensitivities and specificities for the detection of aortic regurgitation of greater than 90% when compared with angiography.[115–118] In a composite analysis of eight studies with a total of 388 patients studied by aortography, pulsed Doppler had an overall sensitivity of 95% and specificity of 96% for the detection of aortic regurgitation.[119] In a study of 42 patients, continuous wave Doppler was 94% sensitive and 100% specific when compared to aortography for the detection of aortic regurgitation.[120] Color flow mapping has been shown to have similar sensitivity and specificity.[121–123] When compared to auscultation, Doppler methods were proven to be more sensitive (96 vs. 73%) and specific (96 vs. 92%) in the recognition of aortic regurgitation.[124] In an in vitro study, two jets originating from defects placed only 3 mm apart in the same leaflet could be differentiated by color Doppler regardless of hemodynamic setting up to a mean aortic pressure of >150 mm Hg.

Given the high sensitivity and specificity of Doppler techniques in identifying aortic regurgitation, false-posi-

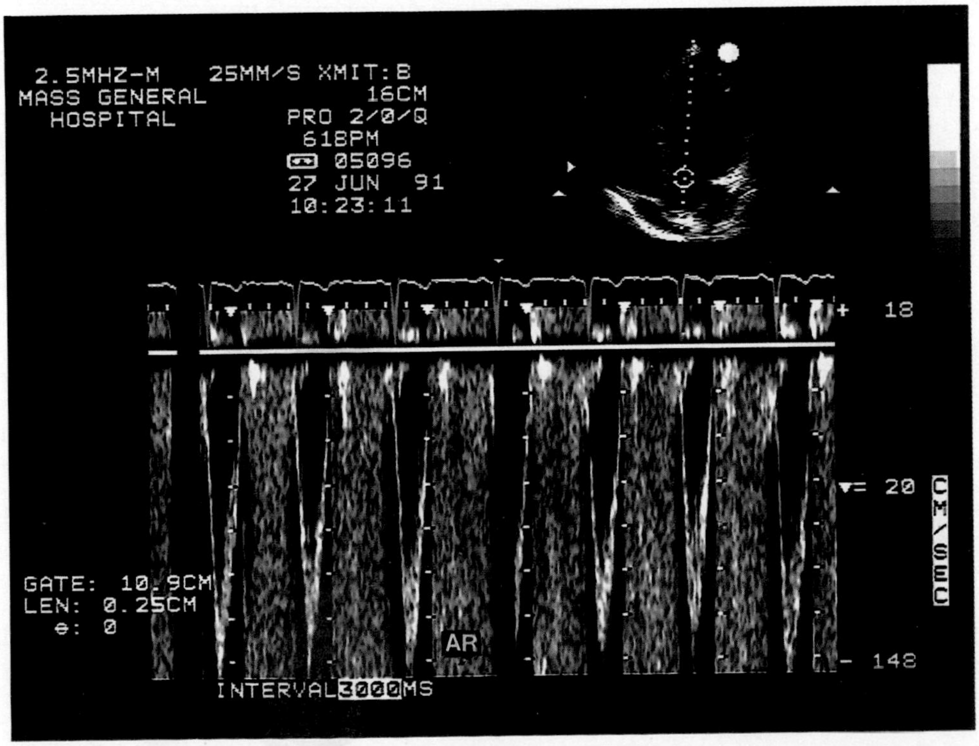

Fig. 19–52. Pulsed Doppler recording from a patient with aortic regurgitation (AR) illustrating high velocity turbulent diastolic flow in the left ventricular outflow tract immediately below the aortic valve.

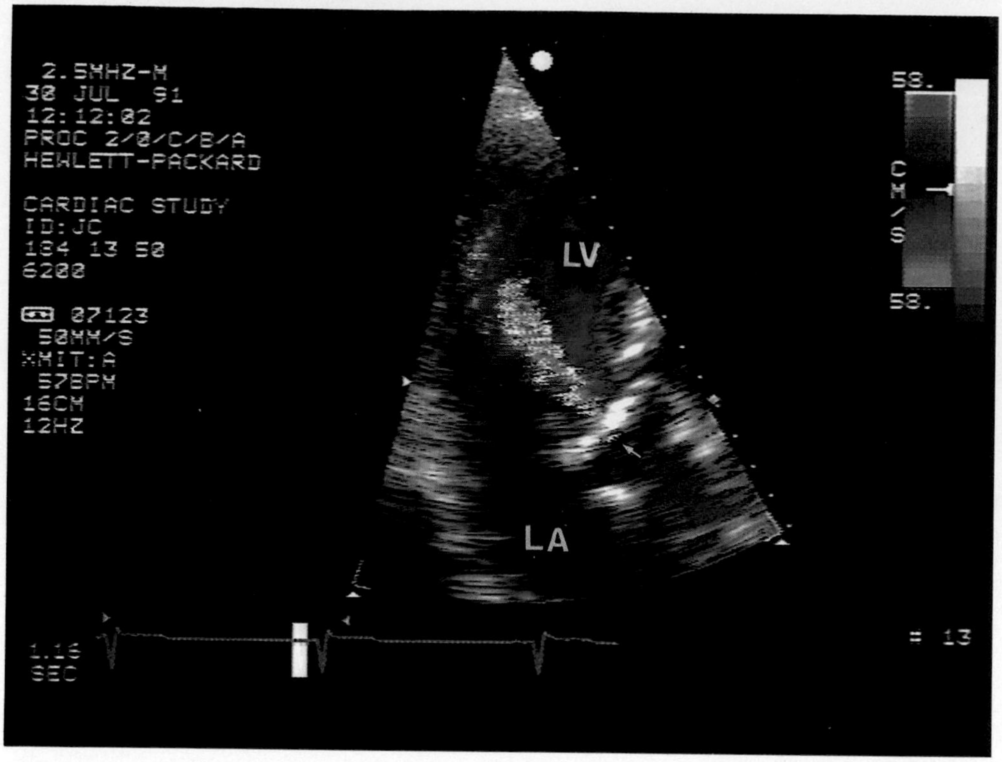

Fig. 19–53. Apical long axis color Doppler recording of an aortic regurgitant jet. The jet (blue-yellow mosaic color) originates from the center of the aortic valve and extends to the middle of the left ventricular cavity. A small area of proximal acceleration (arrow) is evident on the aortic side of the valve. LA = left atrium; LV = left ventricle.

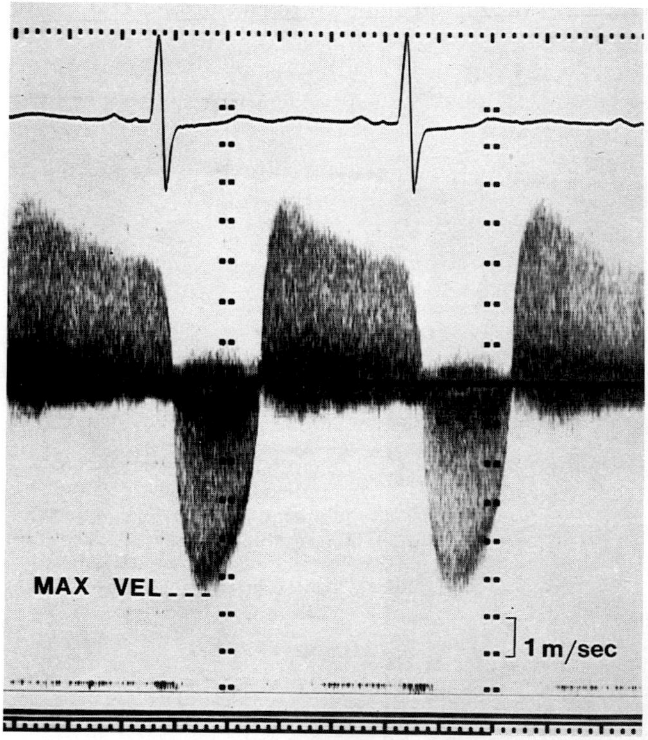

Fig. 19–54. Continuous wave Doppler recording from the cardiac apex from a patient with aortic stenosis and insufficiency. The peak systolic velocity is roughly 5.3 m/sec, which is equivalent to a transvalvular gradient of 116 mm Hg. The peak regurgitant velocity (flow toward the transducer) is roughly 4.5 m/sec and falls to 3 m/sec by end-diastole.

tives and false-negatives are uncommon and when present often relate to the specific type of Doppler device employed. False-positives are generally reported using pulsed Doppler in patients with prosthetic mitral valves oriented such that the flow stream is directed into the outflow tract immediately beneath the aortic valve. Both color flow and continuous wave Doppler are useful in differentiating this turbulent inflow from true aortic insufficiency. On color flow images, intact aortic valves can usually be seen to close and be competent for at least one frame before the mitral valve opens, and even when the anteriorly directed mitral inflow jet is established, a clear space is typically present between the ventricular side of the closed aortic valve and the mitral jet. Even when aortic regurgitation is present, the regurgitant jet can usually be clearly separated from anteriorly directed mitral inflow (Fig. 19–55). On continuous wave Doppler recordings, the peak velocity of the mitral inflow jet, which represents the left atrial-left ventricular gradient, never approaches the peak velocity of the aortic regurgitant jet, which corresponds to the aortic-to-left ventricular gradient (Fig. 19–56). In addition, a clear separation can be recorded between the aortic closure sound and the onset of the mitral inflow. During blind continuous wave recording, the inflow pattern of mitral stenosis has been confused with aortic regurgitation, but careful analysis of the peak jet velocity and timing of onset should permit appropriate diagnosis.

False-negatives generally occur when the regurgitant volume is small or the jet eccentric. Small paravalvular leaks around aortic prostheses may be particularly difficult to record. The limits of sensitivity are reflected in the examination of tilting disc valves in the aortic position. As discussed in Chapter 38, all disc valves leak as

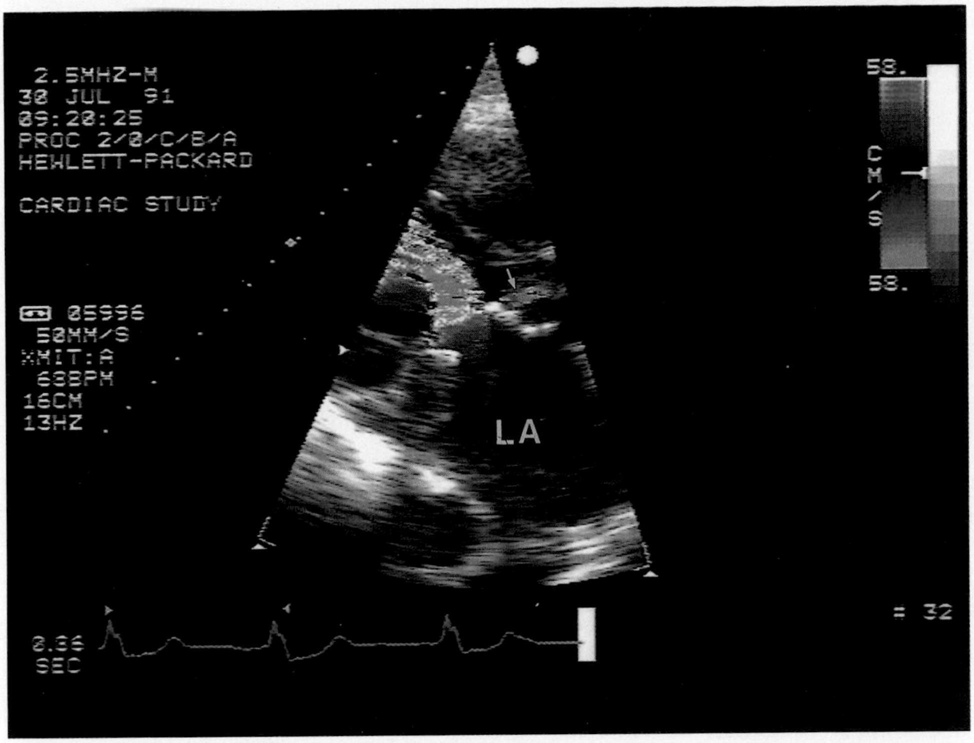

Fig. 19–55. Parasternal long axis color flow recording from a patient with a prosthetic valve in the mitral position and aortic regurgitation. Note that in this case mitral inflow is directed toward the interventricular septum and by pulsed Doppler might be confused with aortic regurgitant flow. By color Doppler, the small regurgitant jet (arrow) can be clearly differentiated from the mitral inflow. LA = left atrium.

a design feature, yet this obligate regurgitation is rarely recorded on any surface Doppler study. Fortunately, such leaks are trivial and without clinical significance.

Aortic Regurgitation With a Normal Valve and Root

A small amount of aortic regurgitation can occasionally be detected in the absence of structural abnormalities of the aortic valve and root.[125,126] The prevalence of regurgitation in patients with presumably normal valves increase with age. In patients with structurally normal hearts, we observed regurgitation in 0.3% of those under 19 years of age, increasing to 13% in those over 60[125] (Fig. 19–57). In a similar study of a normal population, the prevalence of trace aortic regurgitation increased from 0 at age 40 to 49 to 89% in those over the age of 80.[126] This age-related increase in regurgitation most likely reflects the effects of normal wear and tear on the valve apparatus, and hence we consider it to be abnormal, despite the lack of obvious change in valve morphology.

Assessment of the Severity of Aortic Regurgitation

Several echo-Doppler methods have been proposed to assess the severity of aortic regurgitation. These

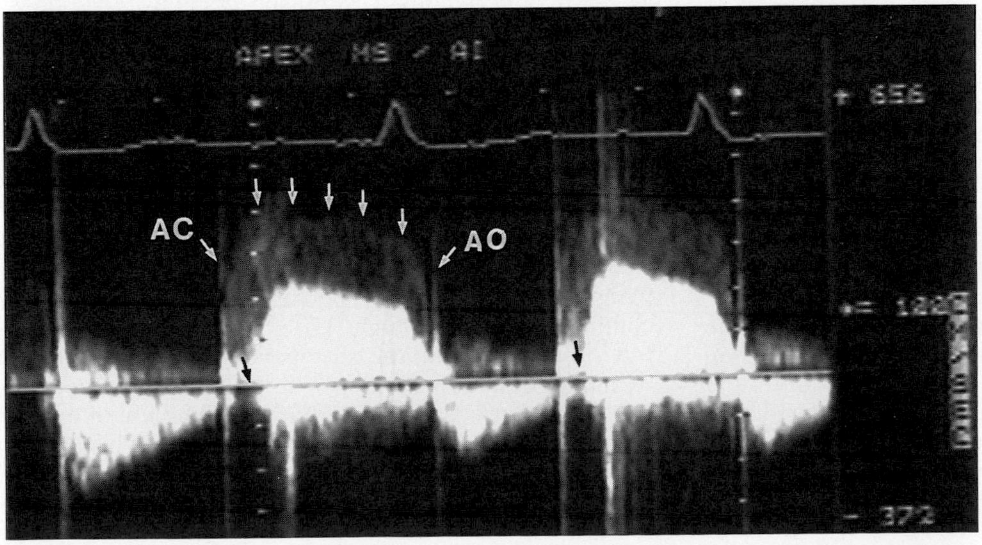

Fig. 19–56. Continuous wave Doppler recording from the cardiac apex in a patient with combined mitral stenosis and aortic regurgitation. The mitral inflow begins after the onset of the aortic regurgitation and ends before aortic valve opening. In contrast, the aortic regurgitant flow (arrows) begins immediately after aortic valve closure (AC), reaches a higher velocity (arrows), and ends at aortic valve opening (AO). The aortic outflow velocity is slightly elevated, consistent with mild aortic stenosis.

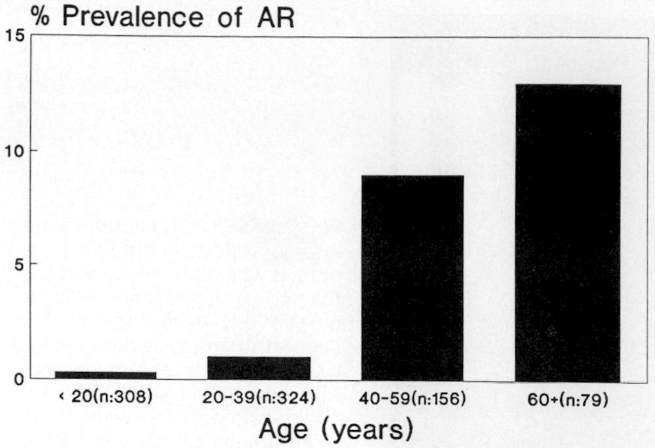

Fig. 19–57. Prevalence of aortic regurgitation (AR) as a function of age in patients without clinical evidence of heart disease and with normal imaging studies. Percent equals the percentage of the total number in each group with AR. (From Choong CY, et al.: Prevalence of valvular regurgitation by Doppler echocardiography in patients with structurally normal hearts by two-dimensional echocardiography. Am Heart J 117:636, 1989. Reproduced with permission of Mosby-Year Book, Inc.)

methods seek to assess severity based on (1) the size of the fully developed regurgitant jet, (2) the size of regurgitant orifice, or (3) the regurgitant volume or fraction.

The hemodynamic significance of aortic regurgitation has historically been determined using angiographic techniques.[127,128] Although of limited accuracy,[129] these techniques have been the standard by which newer clinical methods such as Doppler-echocardiography are validated. Both semiquantitative and quantitative angiographic methods are available. Semiquantitative assessment is based on the degree and time course of the opacification of the left ventricle following a contrast injection into the aortic root and reports severity as mild, moderate, or severe,[127] This method is subjective and is affected by factors such as the site and quantity of the contrast injection, the size of the receiving chamber, and contrast-induced ectopy. In the quantitative approach, the regurgitant volume is calculated as the difference between the total left ventricular stroke volume determined by cineangiography and forward stroke volume determined by the Fick or thermodilution method.[128] Regurgitant fraction is the ratio of regurgitant volume to total left ventricular stroke volume. This method is invalid in the presence of significant mitral regurgitation or of a ventricular septal defect.

Methods Based on Assessing the Size of the Fully Developed Regurgitant Jet

One of the simplest methods for quantitating the severity of aortic regurgitation is to map the extent of the flow disturbance produced by the regurgitant jet using pulsed Doppler or color flow mapping.[130] Both the length, maximal area, and "volume" of the fully developed regurgitant jet have been used for this purpose.

Length of the Jet. Jet length was first examined as a measure of the severity of regurgitation by mapping the extent of the turbulent flow stream in the left ventricular outflow tract using pulsed Doppler.[116,130,131] Severity was defined relative to anatomic landmarks. Because recorded jet length varies according to the window from which the turbulent flow is sampled (i.e., jets appear larger from the apex than from the parasternal window), different anatomic references have been employed. From the parasternal window, an aortic regurgitant jet was arbitrarily defined as mild if it was localized just below the aortic valve in the distal portion of the left ventricular outflow tract, as moderate if it extended from the proximal portion of the left ventricular outflow tract to the level of the anterior mitral leaflet, and severe if it was detected below the mitral valve within the left ventricular cavity.[116] From the apical window, jets have been considered mild if they extend <2 cm below the aortic valve, moderate from 2 cm below the valve to the papillary muscles, and severe if they extend beyond the papillary muscles.[132] In several reports, the pulsed Doppler assessment of severity correlated well with the angiographic grade ($r \geq .86$). Furthermore, when discordant the methods generally varied by only a single grade, such that mild and severe regurgitation were rarely mistaken.[116] Some of the observed overlap may relate to the use of fixed anatomic references because it is clear that a jet reaching the papillary muscle level has a different meaning in the dilated ventricle of chronic aortic regurgitation than it does in the small ventricle of mitral stenosis.

More recent studies using color flow mapping techniques have failed to confirm the correlation between aortic regurgitant jet length and severity of aortic regurgitation as assessed by angiography. Indeed, several studies have indicated that the length of a regurgitant jet more closely relates to the driving pressure across the regurgitant orifice than to the size of the regurgitant orifice or the regurgitant fraction (Fig. 19–58).[123,133] Despite these apparently conflicting data, it is the general experience that jet length bears a rough if imperfect relationship to severity.

Jet Area and Volume. Mapping the area and volume of the flow disturbance caused by the regurgitant jet has also been reported as a means of determining the severity of aortic regurgitation (Fig. 19–59). These methods are extremely tedious with pulsed Doppler techniques, but the advent of color flow mapping has facilitated measurement. Initial experience suggested that the area of the regurgitant jet in the long axis plane could predict the aortic regurgitant fraction under controlled conditions in animal experiments or in patients undergoing surgery. More recent reports indicate that the correlation between the maximal jet area and the severity of aortic regurgitation as determined by angiography is weak ($r = .63$) and that this correlation is not improved by correcting for the size of the left ventricle or by excluding patients with high velocity flow through the mitral valve.[123] Jet volume has also correlated reasonably with independent measures of severity but is more complex to measure and seems to add little to length or area alone.

The use of jet mapping to measure severity or regurgitation is limited by both physiologic and physical factors. In experimental models of regurgitation, the color

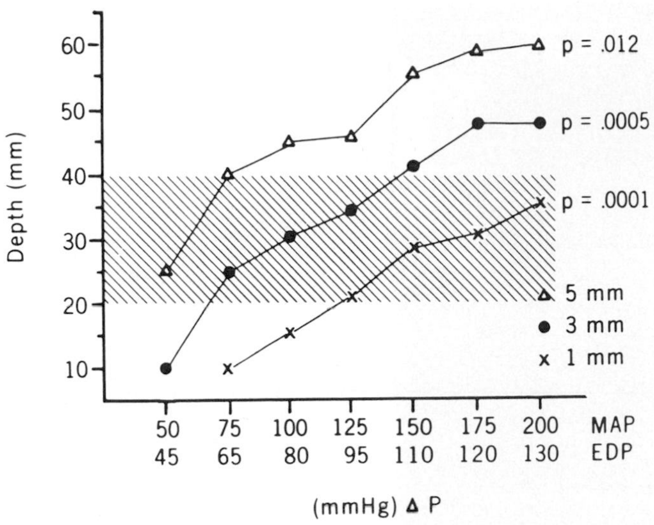

Fig. 19–58. Relationship of regurgitant jet "depth" to orifice size and driving pressure. Although the jet depth is proportional to regurgitant orifice size (5 > 3 > 1-mm diameter defects), there is also a very strong dependence of depth on the imposed instantaneous pressure gradient. The shaded area emphasizes that a jet of 20 to 40 mm in depth could originate for a 1-, 3-, or 5-mm defect, depending on the ΔP. ΔP = pressure gradient. (From Switzer DF, et al.: Calibration of color Doppler flow mapping during extreme hemodynamic conditions in vitro: a foundation for a reliable quantitative grading system for aortic incompetence. Circulation 75: 837, 1987. Reproduced by permission of the American Heart Association, Inc.)

flow jet size is best predicted by the momentum flux within the regurgitant stream, which accounts for both jet velocity (driving pressure) and volume, rather than simple binary measures of jet area.[134] Clinically, regurgitant jets tend to adhere to adjacent structures, such as the interventricular septum or the anterior mitral leaflet (the Coanda effect), which affects both their shape and area.[135–136] In addition, aortic regurgitant jets often join with the mitral inflow stream in the ventricular cavity (coflow), which can obscure or falsely magnify the regurgitant jet area as well as changing its course (Fig. 19–60). This is a particular problem when aortic regurgitation occurs in patients with mitral stenosis or prosthetic mitral valves where the transmitral velocities are high and the flow stream may be abnormally directed. Technical factors, such as gain, carrier frequency, pulse repetition frequency, and color display algorithm, may also alter jet size independent of any actual change in regurgitant volume.[138–140] Despite these limitations, the general truism holds that big things are big, small things are small, and everything else is in the middle. Thus, jet size must bear a general relationship with severity, although absolute values may be less meaningful than they might appear.

Measurement of Regurgitant Orifice Size

The second general approach to assessing the severity of aortic regurgitation is based on the measurement of

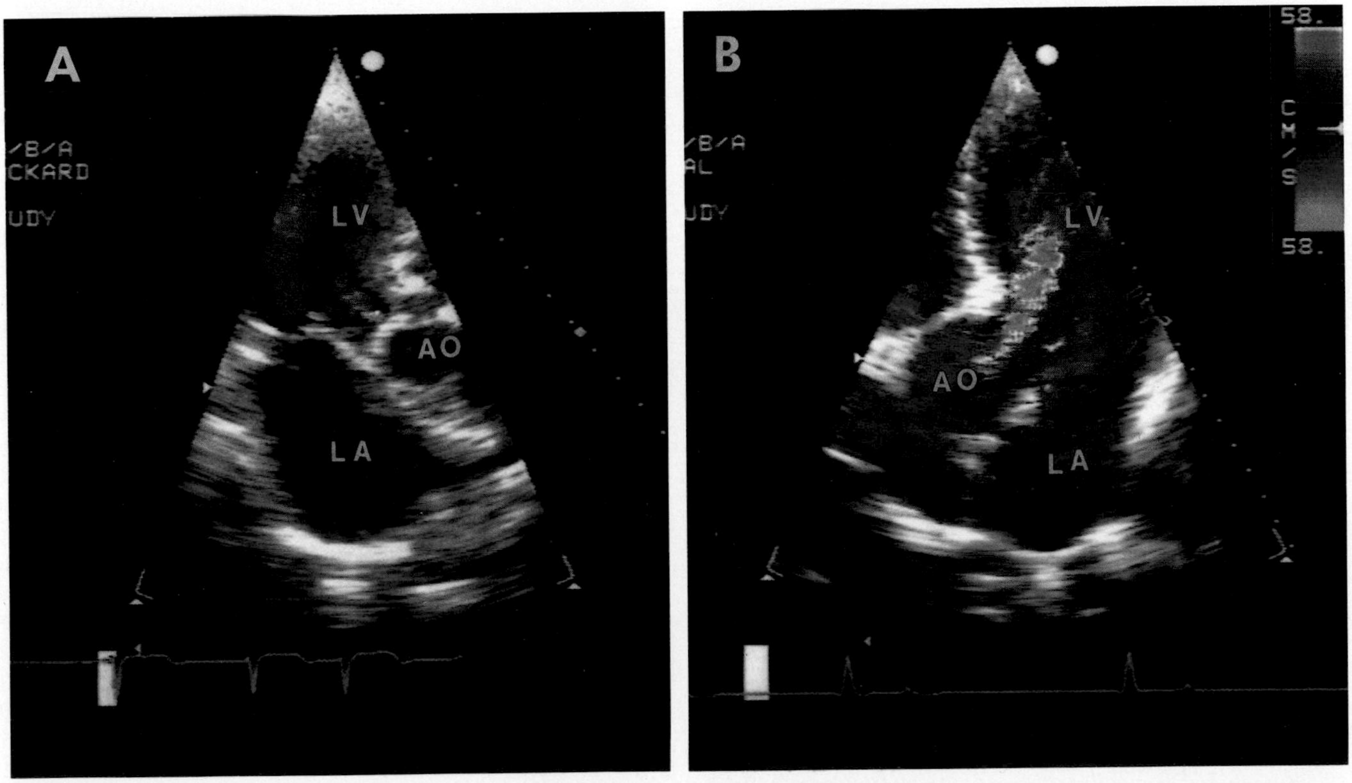

Fig. 19–59. Apical long axis color recordings illustrating the difference in the area encompassed by a small- **(A)** and moderate-sized **(B)** aortic regurgitant jet. **A.** The small-volume jet loses momentum quickly, and although aliasing is present at the orifice, the velocity quickly falls below the aliasing velocity and is displayed in red. **B.** In contrast, the higher momentum jet is displayed in a blue-yellow mosaic color for 6 cm beyond the orifice. LV = left ventricle; AO = aorta; LA = left atrium.

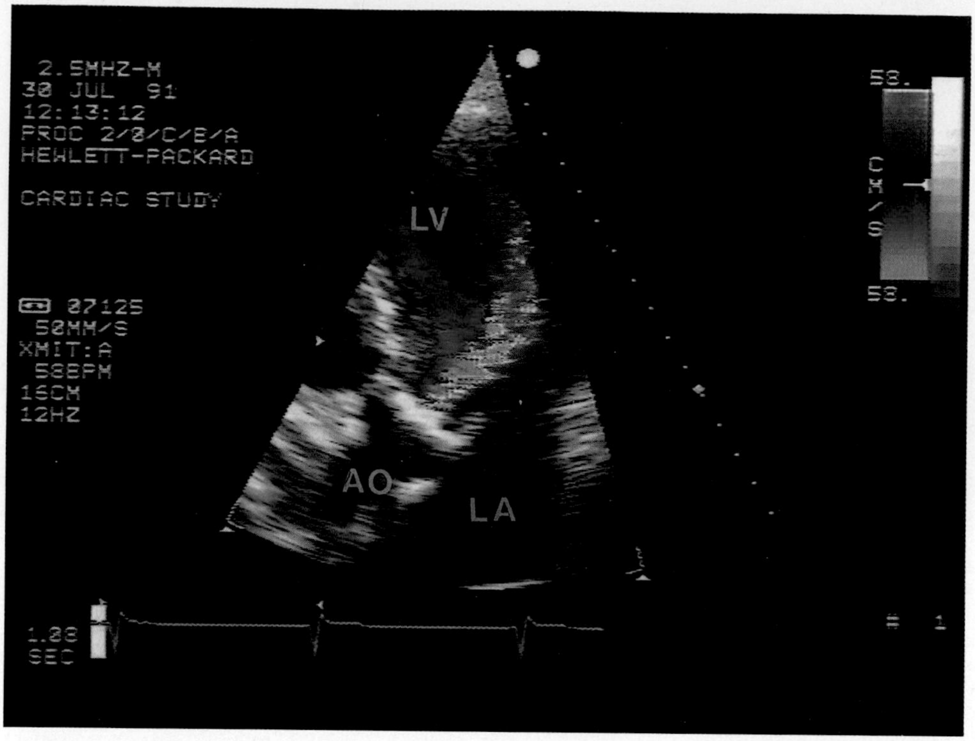

Fig. 19–60. Apical long axis recording of an aortic regurgitant jet that is directed inferiorly toward the mitral inflow stream, with which it becomes confluent. In this case, it would be impossible to define precisely the aortic component of the combined flow streams and hence to map its length or area. LA = left atrium; LV = left ventricle; AO = aorta.

the size of the regurgitant orifice. The size of the regurgitant orifice has been approximated based on (1) the proximal jet area and height assessed by color flow mapping and (2) the slope and half-time of the velocity decay curve.

Proximal Jet Area and Height. The size of the regurgitant orifice can be approximated from the cross-sectional area and/or height of the regurgitant jet at its origin just below the aortic valve, and this "orifice size" has been used as a measure of the severity of regurgitation (Fig. 19–61). Using pulsed Doppler, it was shown that

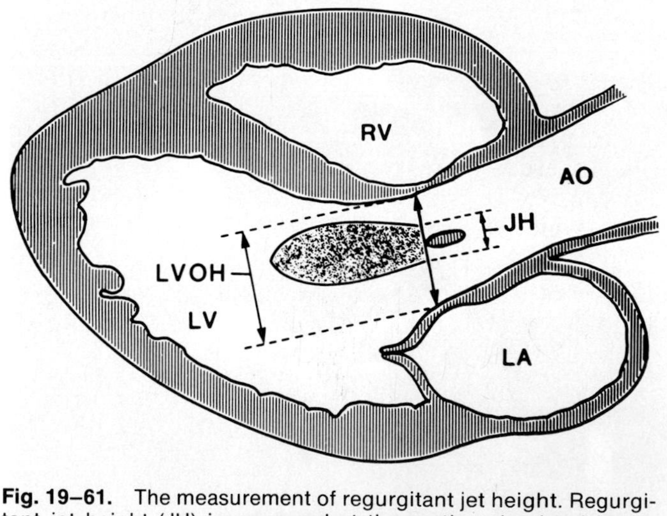

Fig. 19–61. The measurement of regurgitant jet height. Regurgitant jet height (JH) is measured at the aortic valve level in the parasternal long axis view. AO = aorta; LA = left atrium; LV = left ventricle; LVOH = left ventricular outflow tract height; RV = right ventricle. (From Perry GJ, et al.: Evaluation of aortic insufficiency by Doppler color flow mapping. J Am Coll Cardiol 9:952, 1987. Reprinted with permission from the American College of Cardiology.

the mapped area of a regurgitant jet recorded from a parasternal short axis window at the aortic valve level correlated well (r = .87) with the angiographic grade of regurgitation.[118] Color flow mapping has provided a simpler method to determine jet area and has been shown to correlate equally well with angiographic grade (r = .87). When absolute jet area was compared to angiographic grade, however, there was considerable overlap between groups. Expressing the color jet area as a percentage of the area of the outflow tract improved the overall correlation and decreased overlap (Fig. 19–62A). A ratio of color jet to left ventricular short axis area of >60% was reported to indicate severe regurgitation, a ratio of 25 to 59% was reported to indicate moderate regurgitation, while mild regurgitation was represented by a ratio of less than 25%.[123] To ensure that the jet is imaged at its origin, measurements should be made only in areas where valve components are also recorded.[123] Note that jet area/diameter are consistently larger than the actual defect and hence should be used to predict approximate rather than actual defect sizes.[133]

The height of the regurgitant jet as it enters the left ventricular outflow tract on long axis color flow images has also been used to assess the severity of regurgitation. Use of this single dimension is based on the assumption that the jet rapidly becomes symmetric after it exits the irregular regurgitant orifice, and thus the jet diameter is a reasonable representation of its area. Jet height has been reported to show a fair correlation with the angiographic grade (r = .78), which is improved by indexing for the diameter of the left ventricular outflow tract at the site of measurement (r = .91). A ratio of jet height to outflow tract diameter of >65% has been reported in severe aortic regurgitation, a ratio of 47 to 64% in moderate aortic regurgitation, and a ratio of less

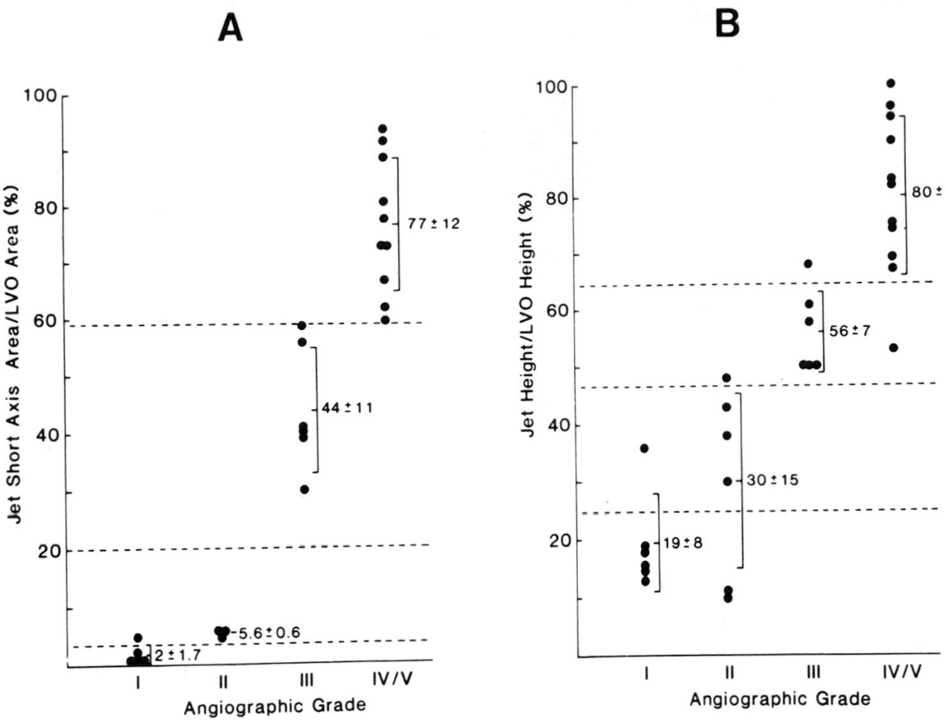

Fig. 19–62. **A.** Jet short axis area/left ventricular outflow tract (LVO) short axis area compared with angiographic grade. **B.** Relationship of jet height/left ventricular outflow tract (LVO) height, measured in the high LVO (see Fig. 19–61) compared with angiographic grade of aortic insufficiency. (From Perry GJ, et al.: Evaluation of aortic insufficiency by Doppler color flow mapping. J Am Coll Cardiol 9:952, 1987. Reprinted with permission from the American College of Cardiology.)

than 46% in mild cases (Fig. 19–62B).[123] Although jet area has been reported to predict angiographic grade slightly better than jet diameter, the latter is a simpler measurement and is unaffected by translation. Figure 19–63 illustrates a jet characteristic of severe aortic regurgitation imaged in both long and short axis views. When jets are eccentric, it is important to relate maximal jet diameter to maximal outflow tract diameter, which may not lie in the same plane.

In vitro studies confirm that the dimensions of a jet just distal to a restrictive orifice are closely related to the size of the orifice, which is an important independent determinant of regurgitant volume.[133] Orifice area, however, is only one measure of flow, and thus it must be assumed that driving pressure is similar across patients for these indices to be useful. In addition, jets expand as they progress downstream from an orifice, and translation of the aortic valve in an inferosuperior plane may lead to changes in the short axis area of the jet displayed at various points in diastole and at different points in the respiratory cycle. Further, the relationship between jet area/diameter and orifice size assumes that the jet

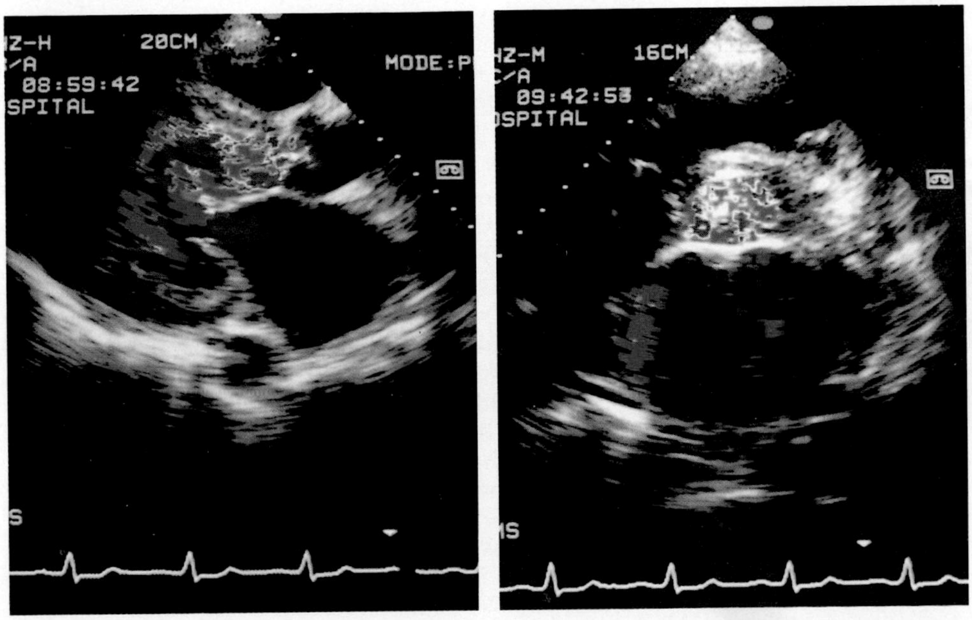

Fig. 19–63. Parasternal long and short axis recordings from a patient with severe aortic regurgitation. In this example, the jet height and area occupy virtually the whole diameter and area of the outflow tract. (Courtesy of Dr. Leng Jiang.)

courses directly away from the regurgitant orifice. When the jet splays out along the undersurface of the valve, the relationship of jet diameter/area to orifice size does not hold. Finally, the relationship between regurgitant orifice area and the size of the jet distal to it is affected both by machine factors[138,139] and orifice shape.[141] Despite these limitations, if aortic diastolic pressure is reasonably constant, and the jet remains free as it progresses away from the valve, flow area and diameter should reflect regurgitant orifice area and hence severity.

Decay Rate of the Aortic Regurgitant Velocities (Slope and Half-Time). The use of the aortic regurgitant velocity slope and half-time as measures of regurgitant orifice area is based on the assumption that the aortic valve is a restrictive orifice that controls the rate of diastolic flow from the high pressure aorta to the low pressure left ventricle. Flow between the two chambers therefore will vary directly with orifice size, as will the rate at which the diastolic pressure gradient falls. Because the aortic regurgitant jet velocity reflects the pressure difference between the aorta and left ventricle at any instant during diastole, its slope should reflect the rate of decline in the pressure gradient and hence the size of the restrictive orifice.

In practice, the highest velocity occurs shortly after aortic valve closure when the gradient between the left ventricle and aorta is at its maximum, which roughly corresponds to the nadir of the left ventricular pressure curve. The magnitude of the regurgitant velocity then declines throughout diastole as aortic pressure falls (which is due to both forward run-off and regurgitation back into the left ventricle), while left ventricular pressure rises (which is due to the combination of normal mitral inflow and aortic regurgitant volume). In mild aortic regurgitation, the aortic diastolic pressure falls slowly, and left ventricular pressure rises slowly, so that at end-diastole, there is still a significant pressure gradient between the aorta and left ventricle. This gradual convergence of the aortic and left ventricular pressure curves is reflected in a slow decline in the aortic regurgitant velocity (Fig. 19–64A). In contrast, in severe aortic regurgitation, diastolic aortic pressure falls rapidly and left ventricular pressure rises more quickly than normal, which is due to the increased filling volume. Rarely, equilibration occurs before end-diastole. The rapid convergence of aortic and left ventricular pressures is reflected by a rapid decline in the aortic regurgitant velocity (Fig. 19–64B). Because the velocity of the aortic regurgitant jet is generally >2 m/sec, continuous wave Doppler is required to obtain a complete velocity profile.

The rate of decline of the aortic regurgitant velocity has been quantitated using both the slope and the pressure half-time (Fig. 19–64). The slope is measured as the rate of decline on the aortic velocities from their initial peak. When this decline is linear, the slope is simply defined by drawing a straight line along the peak of the velocity profile. In some cases, however, the profile is curvilinear, with a rapid initial slope and a flatter terminal component. In these cases, the initial slope, the slope taken from the initial peak to the point at which the velocity profile falls to $1/\sqrt{2}$ of its initial peak, or an

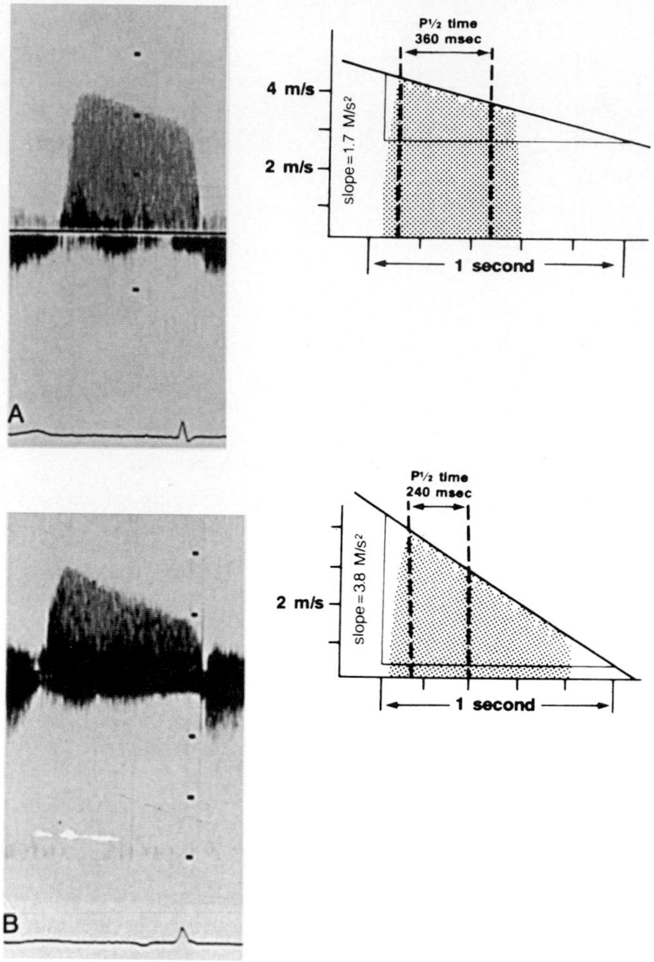

Fig. 19–64. Continuous wave Doppler recordings from a patient with mild **(A)** and severe **(B)** aortic insufficiency. Diagrams to the right illustrate the measurement of the slope and half-time in these cases. Note that the slope is greater and the pressure half-time (P½) is shorter in the patient with more severe aortic insufficiency, indicating a more rapid equilibration between left ventricular and aortic diastolic pressures. (From Labovitz AJ, et al.: Quantitative evaluation of aortic insufficiency by continuous-wave Doppler echocardiography. J Am Coll Cardiol 8:1341, 1986. Reprinted with permission from the American College of Cardiology.

average slope drawn between the peak and end-diastolic velocities can be taken. Each of these approaches will yield a different result, and no standard exists.[141a] The initial slope shows the least variation with heart rate but overestimates the mean velocity decay. The slope from the peak velocity to the point at which the velocity falls by $1/\sqrt{2}$ requires that the latter value first be calculated, which is time-consuming and may be complicated by the fact that this point may fall beyond the termination of the velocity contour (see following discussion). The mean slope varies with heart rate but appears most representative in normal sinus rhythm. It is also the easiest to derive using computer-assisted calculation packages and hence is the most commonly applied.

The pressure half-time of the aortic regurgitant velocity is analogous to that in mitral stenosis and represents the time taken for the pressure gradient to fall to half of its initial value. Because velocity is related to the square

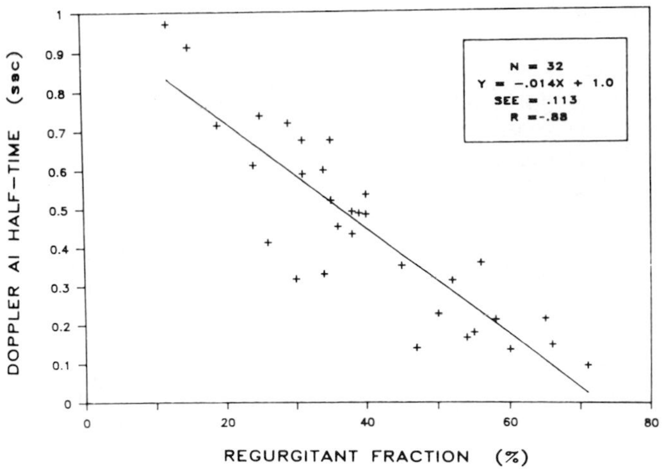

Fig. 19–65. Doppler velocity half-time plotted against regurgitant volume, expressed as a percentage of angiographic cardiac output in a group of 32 patients. AI = aortic insufficiency; SEE = standard error of estimate. (From Teague SM, et al.: Quantification of aortic regurgitation utilizing continuous-wave Doppler ultrasound. J Am Coll Cardiol 8:592, 1986. Reprinted with permission from the American College of Cardiology.

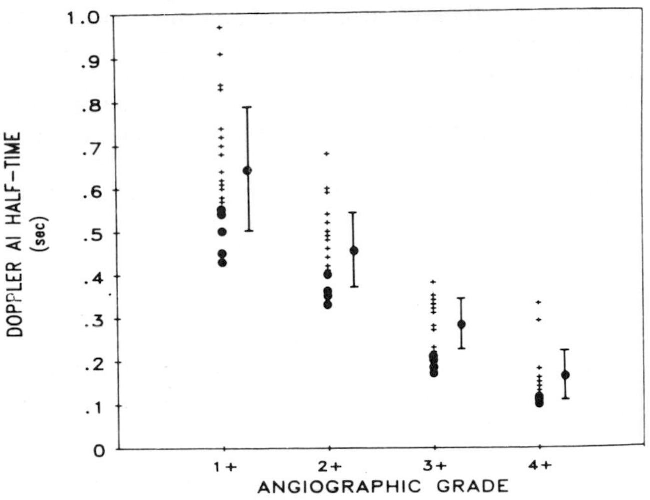

Fig. 19–66. Doppler aortic regurgitation (AI) velocity half-time plotted as a function of angiographic grade. Patients with left ventricular end-diastolic pressures greater than 26 mm Hg are represented by solid circles. Means and standard deviations of Doppler half-time are plotted for each angiographic range. (From Teague SM, et al.: Quantification of aortic regurgitation utilizing continuous-wave Doppler ultrasound. J Am Coll Cardiol 8:592, 1986. Reprinted with permission from the American College of Cardiology.

root of pressure, the velocity half-time is the time taken for the initial velocity to fall to $1/\sqrt{2}$ (0.71) of its initial peak value. When aortic regurgitation is mild, the half-time is frequently not reached before the end of diastole, and the line connecting the velocity peaks must be extended beyond the actual duration of flow, to measure the half-time.

Although reasonable correlations between these indices (Fig. 19–65) and invasively measured regurgitant volume have been reported, most studies have indicated significant overlap among groups classified on the basis of angiographic severity (Fig. 19–66).[120,132,141a,142–144] Table 19–3 lists the relationship of slope and half-time to severity of aortic regurgitation for the studies reported to date. Note that although each study reports reasonable separation of patients with differing degrees of severity, the absolute value of slope and half-time at which this separation occurs varies widely.

In general, a mean slope of >2 m/sec has been reported in groups of patients with mild regurgitation; a mean slope between 2 and 3 m/sec in groups with moderate regurgitation; and a mean slope of >3 m/sec in those with severe regurgitation. In individual studies, however, the specific slope values found to permit discrimination between groups have not been consistent. For example, in one study a slope of 2 m/sec was reported to separated patients with mild, from those with moderate or severe disease, whereas in another study, a slope of 3 m/sec was 100% specific but only 53% sensitive in the detection of significant (3 to 4+) regurgitation.[143]

A pressure half-time of 400 msec has also been reported to separate mild (1 to 2+) from significant (3 to 4+) regurgitation with a specificity of 92% and predictive value of 90%.[142] However, half-time results have also been inconsistent. Hence, the values 2, 3, and 4 (slopes of 2 m/sec and 3 m/sec and half-time of 400 msec), while useful as a mnemonic, cannot be considered as providing definitive group separation.

Much of the observed variation in slope and half-time values between studies and overlap between groups within studies can be explained by factors other than regurgitant volume that affect these variables. Technically, it is often difficult to record the upper envelope of the Doppler velocity profile, particularly, in patients

Table 19–3. Relationship of Slope and Half-Time to Severity of Aortic Regurgitation

	Slope (m/sec)			Half-Time (msec)		
Study	Mild	Moderate	Severe	Mild	Moderate	Severe
Masuyama[120]	1.5 ± 0.5	2.2 ± 0.4	4.0 ± 1.0	1220	890	520
Grayburn[143]	1.89 ± 0.54		3.12 ± 1.05	—	—	—
Labovitz[132]	1.6 ± 0.5	2.7 ± 0.5	4.7 ± 1.5	432 ± 118		284 ± 114
Beyer[144]	1.8 ± 0.7	2.5 ± 1.3	5.7 ± 2.4	820 ± 392	600 ± 200	283 ± 141
Teague[142]	—			650 ± 140	450 ± 90	280 ± 70 170 ± 70
Samstad[141a]			>3 m/sec	628 (500–702)	444 (353–600)	385 (205–670)

with mild aortic regurgitation. This is especially important in measuring the pressure half-time, because the accuracy of this parameter depends on recording the initial peak velocity. Failure to record adequate tracings has been reported in 14 to 31% of patients with aortic regurgitation.[142,143]

There are also conceptual limitations because both the pressure half-time and deceleration slope, in effect, treat the insufficient aortic valve as a "stenotic orifice" whose size determines the regurgitant flow rate and the rate of pressure change.[132] Use of the pressure half-time to quantitate this orifice depends on passage of flow from one chamber with a single outlet into another with a single inlet. This condition holds for mitral stenosis where the pressure half-time method has been applied successfully (provided that the relationship between initial atrial pressure and net compliance remains constant). In patients with aortic insufficiency, however, there is a double outlet (flow to the periphery and left ventricle), and the left ventricular receiving chamber has a double inlet (the mitral valve and regurgitant aortic valve). In this case, the relationship between the pressure half-time and the orifice area is far more complex because factors such as systemic vascular resistance and aortic and left ventricular compliance also affect the rate at which aortic and ventricular pressure tend to equilibrate. For example, in the presence of a stiff left ventricle, the aortic and left ventricular pressure will tend to equilibrate faster for any degree of aortic regurgitation, giving rise to a steeper slope and a shorter pressure half-time. In clinical studies, patients with higher left ventricular end-diastolic pressures tend to have the shortest pressure half-time and steepest slope in a given angiographic grade.[142,144] Finally, although these indices have been used to classify groups of patients, there is little information concerning their use in following individual patients over time. Experimental data suggest that the slope and pressure half-time vary opposite to conventional clinical expectation when the regurgitant orifice is fixed and the severity of the regurgitation is decreased by lowering the systemic vascular resistance.[145] The same effect has been observed clinically in individual patients receiving afterload reduction.[146] Clinically, the slope has also been found to correlate with the systemic vascular resistance in patients with severe aortic regurgitation.

Thus, although the slope and half-time are attractive in that they are simple to derive and represent ordered variables, they do not appear to perform better than measurement of jet size in assessing severity of regurgitation and appear less accurate than the direct measurement of jet area or diameter in determining orifice size.

Quantification of Regurgitant Volume and Regurgitant Fraction

Quantitation of regurgitant volume and fraction is the most direct method for assessing the severity of regurgitation and corresponds most closely to the quantitative angiographic "gold standard." Regurgitant volume and fraction can be calculated (1) as the difference between aortic flow, which represents forward and regurgitant flow and some reference that describes only forward flow; (2) as the difference between aortic forward and reverse flow; or (3) from the direct calculation of regurgitant volume using the continuity principle and its expression as a percentage of total aortic flow.

Direct Calculation as the Difference Between Transaortic Flow (Forward and Regurgitant) and Forward Flow. Aortic regurgitant volume can be directly calculated as the difference between the forward stroke volume across the aortic valve, which represents both forward and regurgitant flow, and the cardiac output, which represents only forward flow. Flow across the aortic valve can be calculated using Doppler echocardiography as the product of the systolic velocity integral and the aortic valve area. Alternatively, in the absence of mitral regurgitation, it can be determined from the difference in echocardiographic end diastolic and end-systolic volumes. Forward cardiac output can be determined from the cross-sectional area and Doppler-derived time velocity integral at any other competent cardiac valve. The details of these measurements are given in Chapters 20 and 30. The regurgitant fraction can then be calculated as the regurgitant volume over the forward stroke volume.

In one small series, aortic regurgitant volume determined as the difference between the total left ventricular stroke volume calculated by two-dimensional echocardiography and forward flow through the mitral valve, determined using Doppler echocardiographic methods correlated well with similar radionuclide measures and was most accurate in those patients without mitral regurgitation.[147] Similarly, when aortic regurgitant fraction was determined as the difference between Doppler-derived aortic and pulmonary flow in 20 patients with aortic regurgitation, an excellent correlation of .94 with the invasively determined regurgitant fraction was recorded. This correlation was further improved when patients with mitral regurgitation were excluded (Fig. 19–67).[148] Others have shown a good correlation between the invasively determined aortic regurgitant fraction and that determined as the difference between Doppler derived aortic and mitral flow. However, the correlation between Doppler derived regurgitant volume and that measured invasively was less good ($r = .62$).[149]

Like other approaches, quantitation of regurgitation based on differences in flow volumes has limitations. First, accurate measurements are time-consuming and tedious to perform. Second, these methods do not measure regurgitant volume directly but rather calculate the difference between total left ventricular stroke volume and forward stroke volume. Both of these calculations have inherent error, which can be presumed to propagate, and the values are not measured simultaneously. Despite these limitations, the approach provides quantitative, ordered data, which when measured accurately in appropriate patients should provide a reasonable measure of regurgitant volume.

Differences in Amplitude-Weighted Mean Flow Velocities. Another method that has been proposed for calculating regurgitant fraction based on relative differences in intracardiac flow is to compare the amplitude weighted mean flow velocities in the aorta and pulmo-

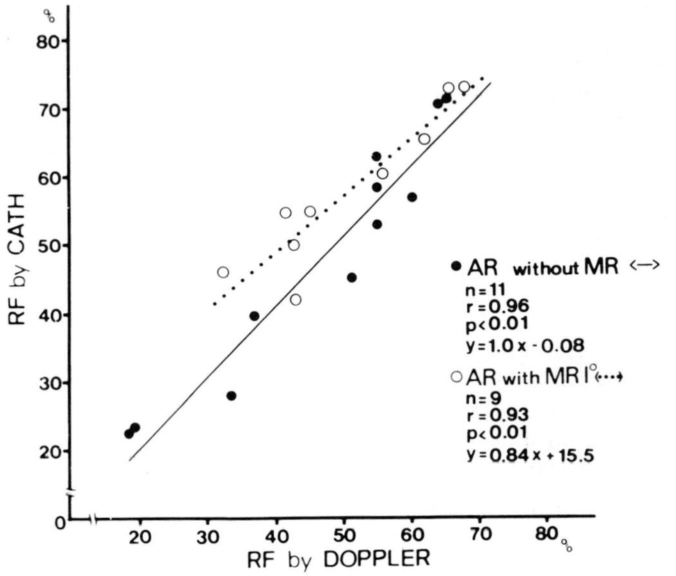

Fig. 19–67. Doppler estimates of regurgitant fraction (RF) (difference between aortic and pulmonary artery flow) plotted against those obtained by catheter technique (difference between angiographic and thermodilution cardiac output). In patients without mitral regurgitation (MR), there is a good correlation between Doppler and hemodynamic estimates (solid circles). In patients with MR, the catheterization values overestimate regurgitation compared with the Doppler measures. AR = aortic regurgitation. (From Kitabatake A, et al.: A new approach to noninvasive evaluation of aortic regurgitant fraction by two-dimensional Doppler echocardiography. Circulation 72:523, 1985. Reproduced by permission of the American Heart Association, Inc.)

nary artery.[150] This approach is based on the assumption that at physiologic hematocrits the amplitude of the reflected Doppler signal at each frequency/velocity is proportional to the number of scattering erythrocytes moving at that velocity. Given that this assumption is approximately correct, the individual velocities in the Doppler signal multiplied by their respective amplitudes should be proportional to the instantaneous blood flow. This can be expressed mathematically as:

$$Q \sim AWMV = \int_{F_o}^{F_x} A(f)\, f df \qquad [19.11]$$

where Q is flow, AWMV is the amplitude-weighted mean velocity, A(f) is the amplitude of the spectral density, f is the Doppler shift, F_x is the spectral range, and F_o is the frequency limit of the wall filter. In addition to the basic assumption that the backscattered energy is proportional to cell number, this approach also assumes that the flow stream is completely and uniformly sampled. Ideally, the amplitude-weighted mean velocity of a thin layer of cells within the orifice of interest should be used to assess blood volume flow rates. In practice, this condition is approximated by low pass filtering the continuous wave Doppler signal to confine the values of interest to the fastest moving scattering particles, which presumably are those passing through the annulus where the area is narrowest. It must also be assumed that the intensity of the beam reaching the scatterers is the same at both the reference and study location. Because the aorta and pulmonary artery generally lie at different depths relative to the transducer, this requirement is difficult to satisfy. Aortic or pulmonic annular dilation would also effect results because the flow area/beam volume ratio would be altered. The method also provides only a relative measure of stroke volume and does not allow calculation of absolute regurgitant volume. It can assess only the incompetence of one valve and requires laminar flow. Thus, it is invalid when either aortic or pulmonic stenosis are present because in these cases turbulence will increase scattering independent of cell number and will falsely increase signal amplitude.

In practice, regurgitant fraction (RF) is calculated as

$$RF_{ao} = \frac{AWMF_{ao} - AWMF_{pa}}{AWMF_{ao}} \qquad [19.12]$$

Preliminary clinical results using this method have been good. In normal persons, the differences between pulmonary and systemic flow averaged +4.3% with a range of −2.9 to 12%. In a group of 20 patients, correlation between the amplitude weighting method and catheterization-determined regurgitant fraction was excellent (r = .95). Although an interesting approach, it is unlikely, given the many assumptions that must be satisfied for accurate measurement that these initial results can be maintained in larger populations.[150]

Comparison of Antegrade and Retrograde Flow in the Thoracic Aorta. Normal flow in the proximal descending thoracic aorta is predominantly systolic, although a small amount of retrograde early diastolic flow can occasionally be recorded. When aortic regurgitation is present, the amount of retrograde diastolic flow increases as the volume of blood leaking back though the regurgitant aortic valve becomes greater (Fig. 19–68). Assuming that the cross-sectional area of the aorta remains constant throughout the cardiac cycle, and that the forward and reverse flows in the aorta represent a constant percentage of the volume ejected from and returning to the heart, then the ratio of diastolic to systolic flow should represent the regurgitant fraction. This method was first applied using continuous wave Doppler measurements of flow in the aortic arch.[115] Subsequent pulsed Doppler studies applied the same concept to the analysis of flow in the ascending aorta and proximal portion of the descending thoracic aorta.[151] The ratio of the diastolic to systolic flow integrals has correlated well with both the angiographic grade of aortic regurgitation (r = .81)[151] and with invasively determined regurgitant volume (r = .91).[115] Correlation with invasive methods have been less good in the presence of associated aortic stenosis and in patients with less severe degrees of regurgitation.[151] The latter may be explained by the fact that some retrograde aortic flow can be seen normally in early diastole, with the result that differentiation of normal flow from mild regurgitation may be difficult. Another factor that can affect the accuracy of this method is the variation in aortic cross-sectional area from systole to diastole. Systolic cross-sectional area is greater than that measured during diastole, and thus, the simple ratio of diastolic to systolic velocity time inte-

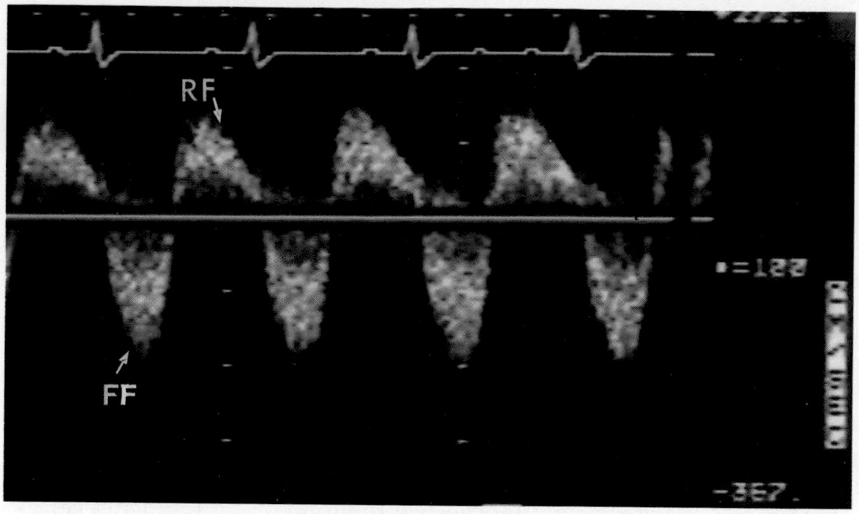

Fig. 19–68. Continuous wave Doppler recording of flow in the descending aorta demonstrating retrograde flow throughout diastole consistent with severe aortic regurgitation. FF = forward flow; RF = reversed flow.

grals can overestimate the regurgitant fraction. Correction for this change in vessel area can be introduced by using the ratio of aortic diastolic to systolic area derived as the diastolic diameter squared (D_d^2)/systolic diameter squared (D_s^1). The mean diastolic diameter is approximated as the average of mean and maximal diameters of the aortic arch obtained from M-mode recordings, whereas the maximal diameter recorded during systole is taken to approximate the systolic diameter (Fig. 19–69). Applying this correction slightly improved the correlation of Doppler-derived aortic regurgitant fraction and that determined at cardiac catheterization from r = .86 to r = .90[152] (Fig. 19–70).

Although theoretically attractive, this method is not widely used in practice as a result of technical difficulties in recording descending aortic flow in many patients and separating patients with mild lesions from normal persons. Localized flow disturbance in the aorta as may occur with coarctation or patent ductus arteriosus can also invalidate the method.

A conceptually similar but simpler approach, based on the pattern of flow in the abdominal aorta has also been used to determine the severity of aortic regurgitation. Using this method, the abdominal aorta below the diaphragm is interrogated by pulsed Doppler from a subcostal window. Under normal circumstances, only antegrade systolic flow is recorded in the abdominal aorta. In patients with severe aortic regurgitation, however,

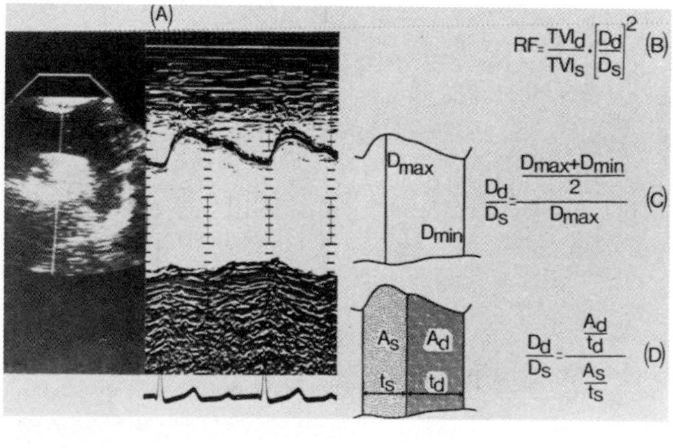

Fig. 19–69. Method for correcting for changes in aortic diameter from systole to diastole in the calculation of forward and reversed aortic flow. **A.** M-mode record of the aortic arch. **B.** The regurgitant fraction (RF) is equal to a diastolic (d)≠systolic (s) time-velocity integral (TVI) ratio, times a squared diastolic≠systolic diameter (D) ratio. **C.** Simplified determination of the diameter ratio; the systolic diameter is the maximal diameter (D_{max}), and the diastolic diameter is the mean of maximal and minimal (D_{min}) diameters. **D.** Determination of the ratio of the true mean diastolic diameter to the true mean systolic diameter. Mean diameters were obtained by dividing planimetered M-mode aortic systolic and diastolic areas (A) by the duration (t) of systole and diastole, respectively. This more complicated calculation of the diameter ratio has not proven to differ significantly from the diameter ratio obtained by the simplified determination. (From Touche T, et al.: Assessment and follow-up of patients with aortic regurgitation by an updated Doppler echocardiographic measurement of the regurgitant fraction in the aortic arch. Circulation 72:819, 1985. Reproduced by permission of the American Heart Association, Inc.)

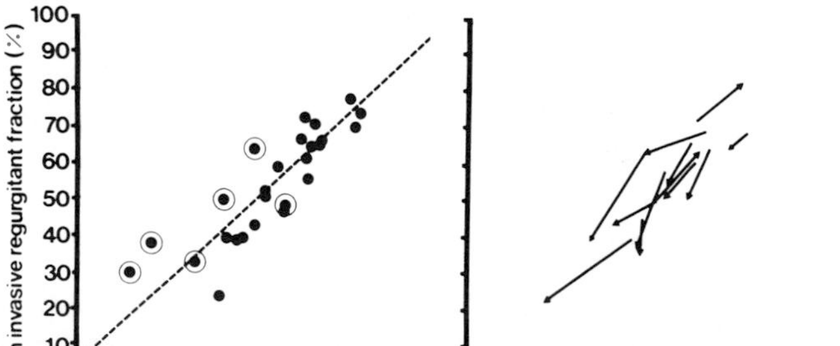

Fig. 19–70. Comparison between invasive and noninvasive measurements of the aortic regurgitant fraction. Left. Basal result in patient with (closed circles) and without (open circles) high velocity systolic flow. Right. Correlation between invasive and noninvasive measures during induced variations of the regurgitation fraction (simplified determination). (From Touche T, et al.: Assessment and follow-up of patients with aortic regurgitation by an updated Doppler echocardiographic measurement of the regurgitant fraction in the aortic arch. Circulation 72:819, 1985. Reproduced by permission of the American Heart Association, Inc.)

pandiastolic retrograde flow is usually present (see Figs. 19–68 and 19–82). When aortic regurgitation is less severe, flow reversal that does not extend throughout diastole may be seen. In a study in which angiographic validation was available, pandiastolic flow reversal was seen in all patients with 3 or 4+ aortic regurgitation, whereas this sign was absent in all 10 normal patients and in 21 of 22 patients with 1 to 2+ aortic regurgitation. The false-positive recording of pandiastolic flow in the abdominal aorta in a patient with mild aortic regurgitation was accounted for by the presence of a patent ductus arteriosus.[153]

Direct Calculation of the Regurgitant Volume Based on the Continuity Principle (Proximal Convergence). Hemodynamic theory suggests that flow velocity accelerates in a predictable manner toward a restrictive orifice in a flat plate such that the isovelocity contours form concentric hemispheric shells radiating out from the orifice. Because the flow passing through each of these shells is equivalent to that which eventually passes through the orifice, orifice flow (Q) can be derived as $Q = 2\pi r^2 u$ where u is the velocity at a distance r from the orifice. Clinically, this characteristic flow acceleration can be recorded by color Doppler proximal to a regurgitant or stenotic orifice. The most easily identified isovelocity contour is that at which the velocity first aliases on the color flow display as it begins to accelerate toward the orifice. Knowing the velocity at which flow first aliases and the distance from the point of aliasing to the orifice should permit the calculation of flow through the orifice or the instantaneous regurgitant flow. Likewise, integration of these data throughout diastole should provide a measure of regurgitant volume. In one study, a proximal acceleration zone in the aorta above the aortic valve was evident on the parasternal long axis view in all 18 patients with evidence of severe or moderate aortic regurgitation on aortography whereas it was seen in only 1 of 11 patients who had mild aortic regurgitation. The presence of a proximal acceleration area of greater than 45 mm^2 was 89% sensitive and 80% specific for the presence of severe aortic regurgitation.[53a]

Although these interesting preliminary observations suggest that proximal acceleration may be of value in assessing the amount of regurgitation there are many theoretical and practical limitations to the method as applied. The color display of the proximal acceleration region is affected by machine factors such as the color display algorithms used, gain settings and pulse repetition frequency, all of which can influence the absolute size of the proximal acceleration zone. Similarly, the parasternal long axis plane may not be the ideal plane in which to assess the presence or size of the proximal acceleration region because regurgitant flow is generally orthogonal to the transducer in this plane. Finally, use of absolute values to separate grades of severity fails to employ the quantitative potential of the method. Quantitative application will have to account for other variables such as valve morphology—because the aortic valve is not a flat plate—and orifice shape, with the result that the true potential of the method remains to be defined.

Associated Echocardiographic Findings in Aortic Regurgitation

Associated echocardiographic findings of aortic regurgitation may be due to (1) direct impingement of the regurgitant jet on other cardiac structures, (2) rapid increase in the left ventricular pressure in diastole, and (3) volume overload of the left ventricle.

Jet Effects

Vibratory Effects on Cardiac Structures. The aortic regurgitant jet can strike either the anterior mitral leaflet, or the interventricular septum giving rise to a high frequency diastolic flutter of the affected structure (Fig. 19–71).[154,155] These jet effects are best demonstrated with the high temporal resolution of an M-mode scan (Fig. 19–72) but are neither sensitive nor specific for the presence of aortic regurgitation.[130,155] In a large series, the sensitivity of anterior mitral leaflet flutter for aortic regurgitation was only 46%, while the specificity was 81%. Interventricular septal flutter was even less sensitive (9%) but had a specificity of 90%. The differential diagnosis of mitral leaflet flutter includes severe mitral regurgitation (even with intact chordae), atrial flutter, and rarely, high flow states such as anemia. The leaflet flutter seen in ruptured chordae tendineae tends to be coarser,[156] whereas that produced by atrial flutter tends to have a lower frequency.[157] Mitral valvular vegetations can also give rise to diastolic flutter of that valve, but the presence of the valvular mass usually indicates the true diagnosis.

The motion and configuration of the anterior mitral valve leaflet on two-dimensional images may also be affected by the regurgitant aortic jet.[158] The early diastolic opening of this leaflet may be blunted or absent. In the parasternal long axis or apical views, reverse doming of the anterior mitral leaflet may be recognized, such that this leaflet bows away from the septum. On the parasternal short axis view, diastolic indentation of the anterior mitral leaflet by the regurgitant jet may be detected (see Chapter 17).

Jet Lesions. Jet lesions present pathologically as white, opaque, roughened areas of endocardium caused by the force of the regurgitant jet hitting the interventricular septum or anterior mitral leaflet. On two-dimensional echo, these lesions are characterized by a focal increase in the intensity of the endocardial echoes at the point at where the jet impacts the ventricular wall.

Rapid Increase in the Diastolic Pressure in the Left Ventricle

Large, acutely developing regurgitant lesion can cause left ventricular pressure to exceed left atrial pressure during diastole. This reversal of the normal atrioventricular pressure gradient can lead to premature closure of the mitral valve,[159–161] (see Chapter 37), diastolic mitral regurgitation (Chapter 17),[162] and premature opening of the aortic valve if ventricular pressure transiently exceeds aortic pressure.[163,164] M-mode recordings in these cases demonstrate both the early mitral

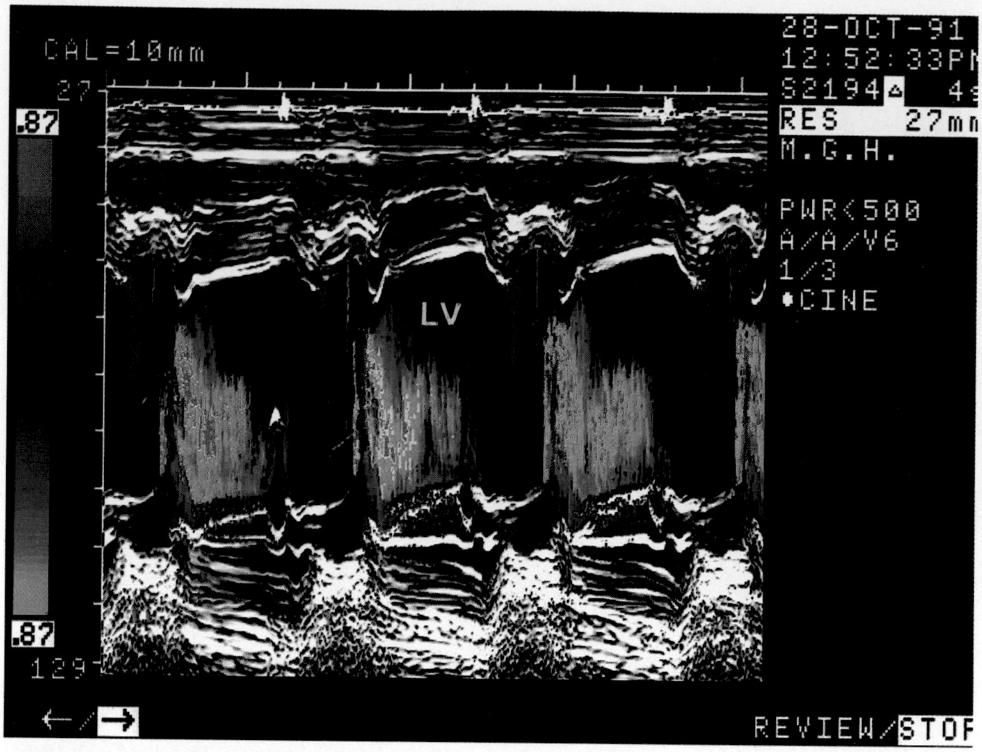

Fig. 19–71. Color M-mode recording of the high velocity turbulent aortic regurgitant jet (turquoise) immediately above the anterior mitral leaflet. LV = left ventricle.

closure and premature aortic opening. Doppler studies reveal a rapid decrease in the transaortic regurgitant velocities, diastolic mitral regurgitation, and rarely antegrade diastolic flow into the aorta. Diastolic reversal of the atrioventricular pressure gradient, premature mitral valve closure, and diastolic mitral regurgitation suggest overwhelming regurgitation and usually occur only in patients requiring urgent valve repair. Note, however, that mitral valve closure is normally initiated by atrial relaxation and completed by ventricular systole. Thus, mitral closure before ventricular systole and diastolic mitral regurgitation can occur in patients with varying degrees of heart block. As a result, to be of prognostic value in aortic regurgitation, these phenomena must occur before atrial contraction.

Left Ventricular Volume Overload

Chronic aortic regurgitation gives rise to left ventricular volume overload (Chapter 20), left ventricular hypertrophy, and a characteristic pattern of diastolic septal motion (Chapter 29).

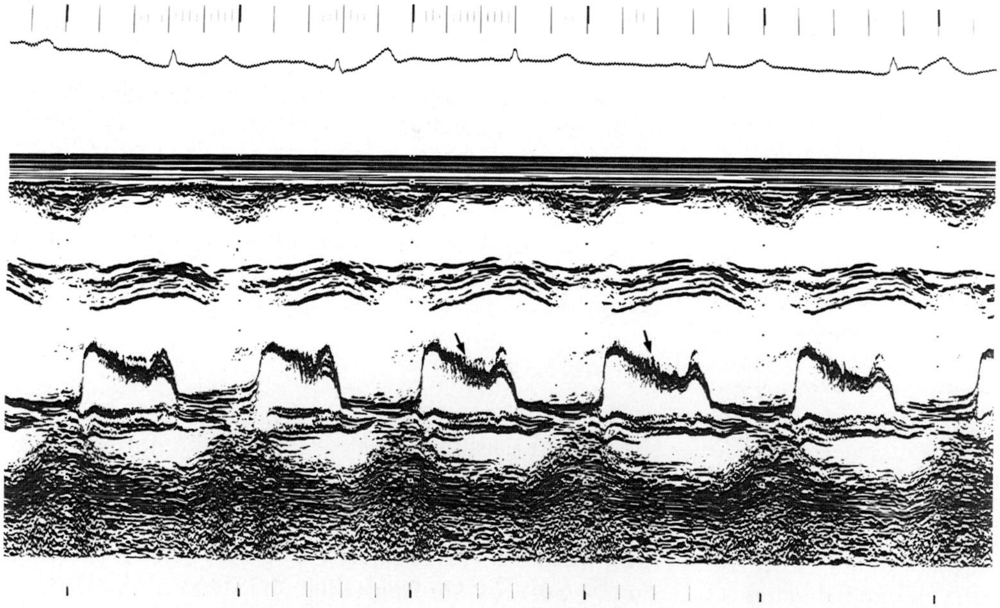

Fig. 19–72. M-mode recording of the mitral valve illustrating the high frequency fluttering (arrows) of the anterior leaflet characteristic of aortic regurgitation.

Overview of Doppler-Echocardiographic Assessment of Aortic Regurgitation

No single Doppler-echocardiographic method for assessing the severity of aortic regurgitation provides definitive information in all cases. All of the techniques described previously appear capable of permitting separation of mild from severe aortic regurgitation but are less satisfactory in classifying intermediate degrees of severity. The confidence with which the severity of aortic regurgitation is classified can be improved by using several methods when they agree. Unfortunately, different criteria yield different results all too frequently, and the final impression is often a compromise (moderately severe or mild to moderate).

Most observers assess severity clinically based on the jet appearance on color flow mapping from the apex, with the additional measurement of proximal jet area or diameter when separation is unclear. Measure of regurgitant velocity slope and half-time provide further confirmation of the initial impression or can modify it when they yield disparate results. Quantitation can be achieved using volumetric methods—either as the difference between aortic flow by two-dimensional echo or Doppler and a reference flow at some other site or the difference between forward and reverse flow in the aorta. Newer methods such as proximal acceleration appear to await further refinement.

The effect of the regurgitant volume on the ventricular size and function is important complementary information, which is discussed in Chapter 20.

THE AORTA

The aorta is the major arterial trunk connecting the left ventricle with the systemic arterial system. The aorta has a thick, tough musculoelastic wall that normally can withstand pressures of thousands of millimeters of mercury without rupturing.[6] The aortic wall is composed of three primary layers: a thin inner tunica intima, a thick tunica media, and a thin outer tunica adventitia. Structurally, the tunica media is the most important of these layers, composing more than 80% of the arterial wall. This layer comprises multiple, concentric, elastic sheets made of broad, interwoven, fenestrated bands. These sheets are connected by interposed smooth muscle, collagen, and ground substance. The inner portion of the media is nourished by diffusion from the vascular lumen, whereas its outer portion is supplied by small, diffusely branching intramural arteries, the vasa vasorum.[165,166]

In addition to its role as a conduit, the aortic wall, because of its elastic properties, serves to damp the surge of aortic pressure in systole, and after inflow has ceased, by use of the stored energy in its walls, is able to drive blood through the peripheral vessels. This dual function prevents wide swings in systemic arterial pressure and maintains a relatively constant perfusion pressure throughout the peripheral vascular system.[6]

Normal Echocardiographic Features

The aorta can be divided anatomically into three primary regions: the ascending aorta, the aortic arch, and the descending aorta. The descending aorta can be further divided at the diaphragm into thoracic and abdominal segments.[1] In neonates and infants, the entire aorta can often be recorded in a single image plane (Fig. 19–73), and local flow patterns assessed (Fig. 19–74). However, in the child and adult, each section of the aorta must be examined separately and the information often combined to acquire a complete picture of aortic morphology or disease involvement.

The Ascending Aorta

The ascending aorta begins at the aortic valve and extends roughly 5 cm to its junction with the aortic arch. Its origin typically lies beneath the third costal cartilage along the left sternal margin.[1] From this point, it courses anteriorly, superiorly, and rightward, joining the arch beneath the superior border of the second right costal cartilage.

Figure 19–75 diagrammatically illustrates the normal appearance of the ascending aorta from its origin at the aortic annulus to its disappearance beneath the sternum. The diameter of the vessel normally varies in this region, increasing from the aortic annulus to the sinuses by a mean of 5.4 mm (range, 2 to 10 mm).[167] At the sinotubular junction, the diameter decreases to equal or slightly exceed (mean, 3.1 mm) that recorded at the aortic annulus. The normal decrease in diameter from the sinuses to the beginning of the tubular portion of the ascending aorta averages 10% (range, 0 to 26%). Importantly, the diameter of the tubular portion of the ascending aorta in normal persons is never less than that recorded at the aortic annulus.[167]

Flow in the ascending aorta is predominantly systolic and has a flat velocity profile for its initial few centimeters (Chapter 9).[168] Curvature of the distal ascending aorta causes the velocity profile to be skewed so that the highest velocities are recorded along the inner wall.[169–171] During the early portion of systole, flow acceleration reduces the tendency toward turbulent transition. During deceleration, however, flow is less stable and turbulence is observed at normal flow rates.[172–174] The combination of flow deceleration and vessel curvature may lead to flow separation along the inner wall of the ascending aorta, and reversed flow may be detected in this region in late systole.[170,171] Along the outer wall, antegrade flow may persist into diastole.[169,171]

The Aortic Arch

The aortic arch begins beneath the superior border of the second right costal cartilage and curves superiorly, posteriorly, and to the left, passing in front of the trachea and then curving inferior to its left border. It joins the descending aorta at the inferior border of the fourth thoracic vertebra, posteriorly. At its most superior point, it is roughly 2.5 cm below the upper border of the ster-

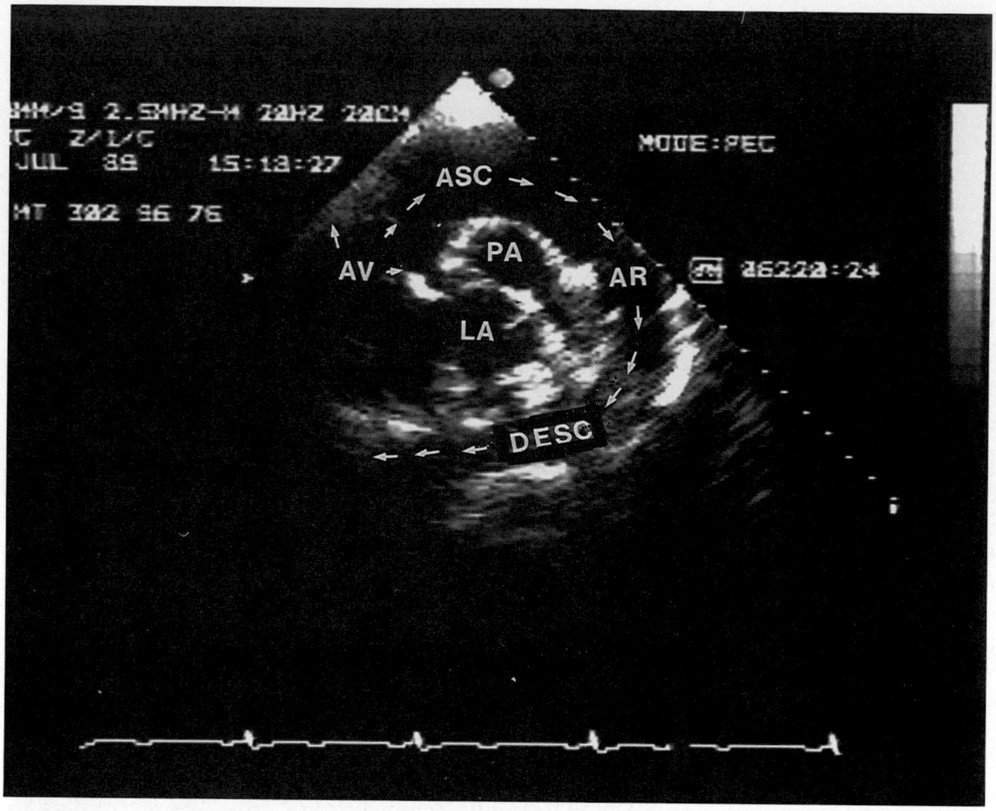

Fig. 19–73. High parasternal long axis recording illustrating the full sweep of the aorta from the aortic valve (AV) to the diaphragm in a child. Line of arrows indicates the path of blood flow in the aorta. ASC = ascending aorta; AR = aortic arch; DESC = descending aorta; PA = pulmonary artery; LA = left atrium.

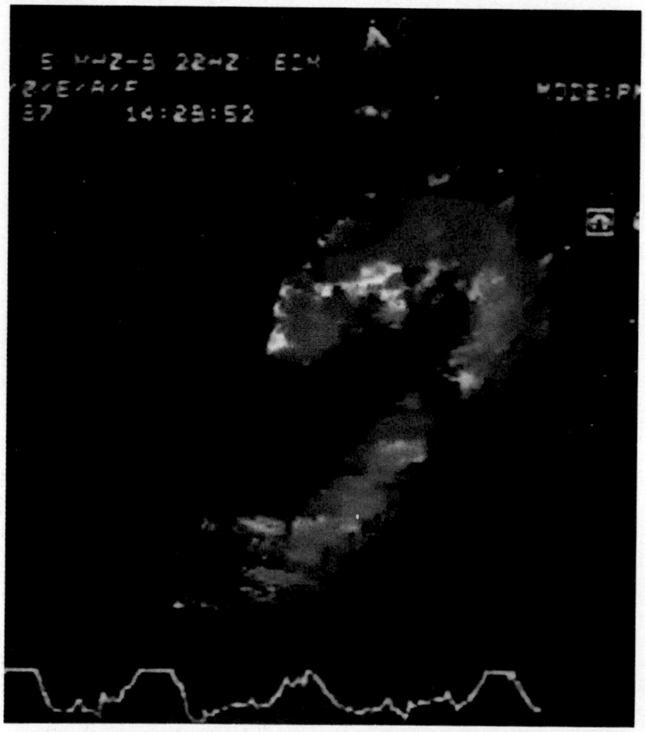

Fig. 19–74. Color flow recording of flow in the aorta from the aortic valve to the diaphragm. Flow in the ascending aorta is toward the transducer and therefore is displayed in orange, while flow in the aortic arch and descending aorta is away from the transducer and therefore is displayed in blue.

num. The aortic arch gives off three major arterial branches: the innominate, the left common carotid, and the left subclavian arteries.

The aortic arch is recorded with the transducer placed directly in the suprasternal notch and the scan plane directed posteriorly, inferiorly, and leftward to align it with the long axis of the aorta.[175,176] In this position, the transducer is between the innominate and left common carotid branches of the aortic arch. When displayed, the left common carotid is positioned to the right of the apex of the sector, and the innominate artery is to the left. The ascending aorta courses superiorly along the left margin of the scan, whereas the descending aorta sweeps posteriorly along the right margin. Figure 19–76 illustrates the probe position and scan plane orientation used to record the aortic arch.

The normal aortic arch appears as an arcuate echo-free structure. Its walls are parallel and roughly equidistant throughout the scan area. Figure 19–77 is a long axis recording of a normal aortic arch and proximal descending aorta. The origin of the major branches are also shown. The right pulmonary artery is commonly recorded beneath the aortic arch with the left atrium and pulmonary veins behind the pulmonary artery. The close proximity of the aortic arch to the suprasternal notch makes this portion of the aorta relatively easy to record, and it can be uniformly imaged in normal subjects.[175,176] Visualization of the branches of the arch is slightly more difficult from the suprasternal transducer location with

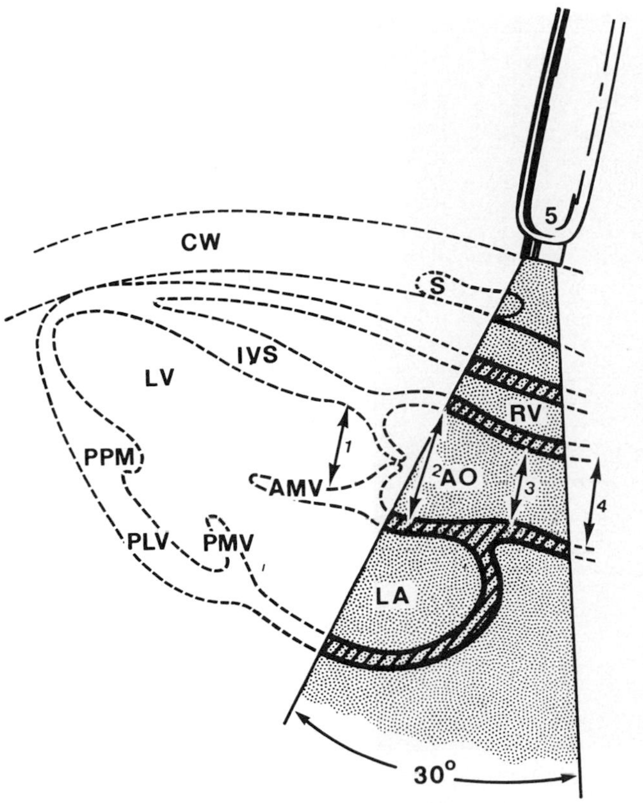

Fig. 19–75. The relationship of a 30° cross-sectional scan to the supravalvular portion of the ascending aorta. The aortic diameter is generally measured at the levels indicated by the arrows: (1) aortic annulus; (2) sinuses of Valsalva; (3) the junction of the superior margin of the sinuses of Valsalva and the tubular ascending aorta (the sinotubular junction); and (4) the ascending aorta at the most distal margin of the scan plane or at the first junction with the aortic arch. CW = chest wall; S = sternum; IVS = interventricular septum; LV = left ventricle; PPM = posterior papillary muscle; PLV = posterior left ventricular wall; PMV = posterior mitral valve leaflet: AMV = anterior mitral valve leaflet; LA = left atrium; AO = aorta; RV = right ventricle. (From Weyman AE, et al.: Cross-sectional echocardiographic characterization of aortic obstruction. I: Supravalvular aortic stenosis and aortic hypoplasia. Circulation 57:491, 1978. Reproduced by permission of the American Heart Association, Inc.)

the carotid and subclavian being recorded in 92% of cases compared to 60% for the innominate.[176] Beyond their origin, the carotid arteries can be directly imaged from the neck in the vast majority of patients.

Flow in the proximal portion of the aortic arch is similar to that in the ascending aorta, while flow in the distal arch is comparable to descending aortic flow. In the midportion of the arch, the flow vector is perpendicular to the transducer, and optimal interrogation of flow in this area is difficult. Figure 19–78 is a color Doppler recording of flow in the aortic arch illustrating the change in direction and apparent velocity (which is due to the changing relationship between the flow vector and the central axis of the interrogating beam) as blood courses around the arch. The effect of vessel curvature on the spatial velocity profile is also apparent.

The Descending Aorta

The descending aorta originates at the lower border of the fourth thoracic vertebra and extends inferiorly to its bifurcation into the common iliac arteries in front of the fourth lumbar vertebra. It can be divided at the diaphragm into the thoracic and abdominal segments. At its origin, the descending thoracic aorta normally lies to the left of the vertebra column. As it descends, it curves toward the midline and is positioned directly in front of the vertebral column at its termination.[1]

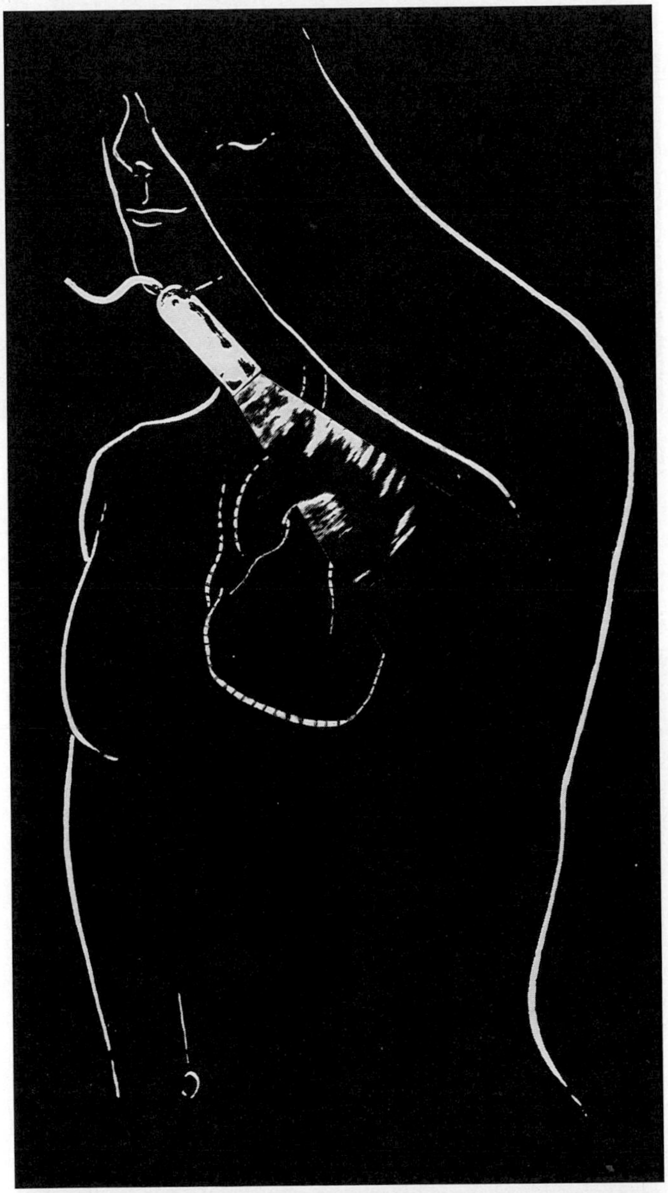

Fig. 19–76. The position and orientation of the cross-sectional probe in the suprasternal notch. This orientation is used to record the aortic arch and proximal descending aorta. The probe is normally directed inferiorly, posteriorly, and slightly to the left when recording this region. The scan plane is oriented approximately 45° to both the sagittal and coronal planes of the body. (From Weyman AE, et al.: Cross-sectional echocardiographic characterization of aortic obstruction. II: Coarctation of the aorta. Circulation 57:498. Reproduced by permission of the American Heart Association, Inc.)

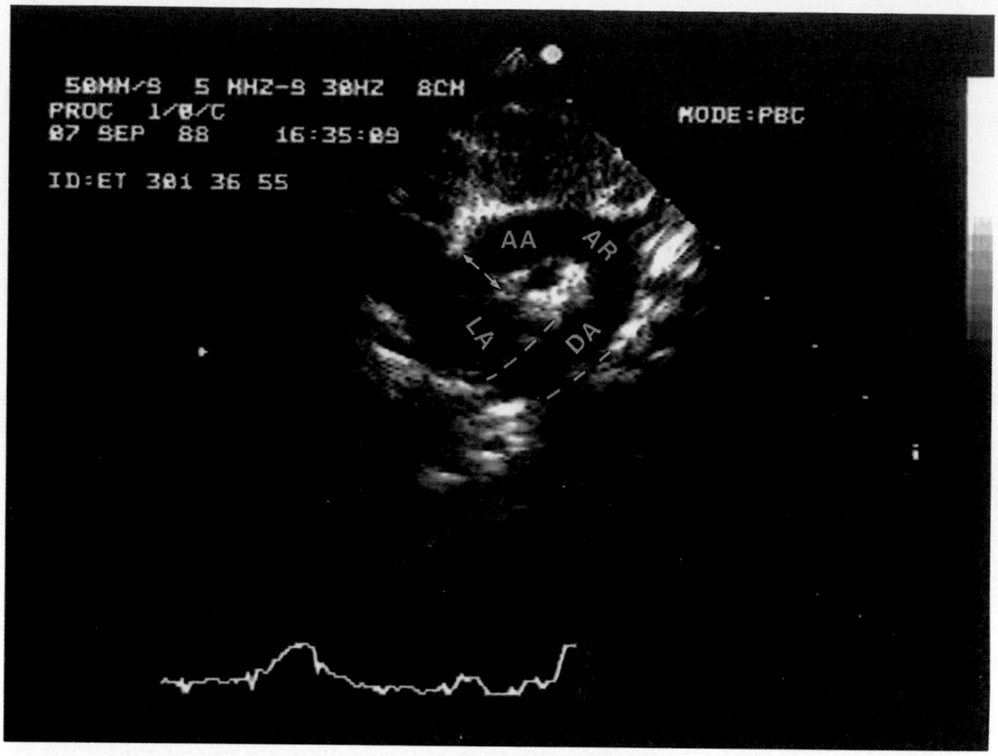

Fig. 19–77. Long axis recording of normal arch. AA = ascending aorta; AR = aortic arch; LA = left atrium; DA = descending aorta.

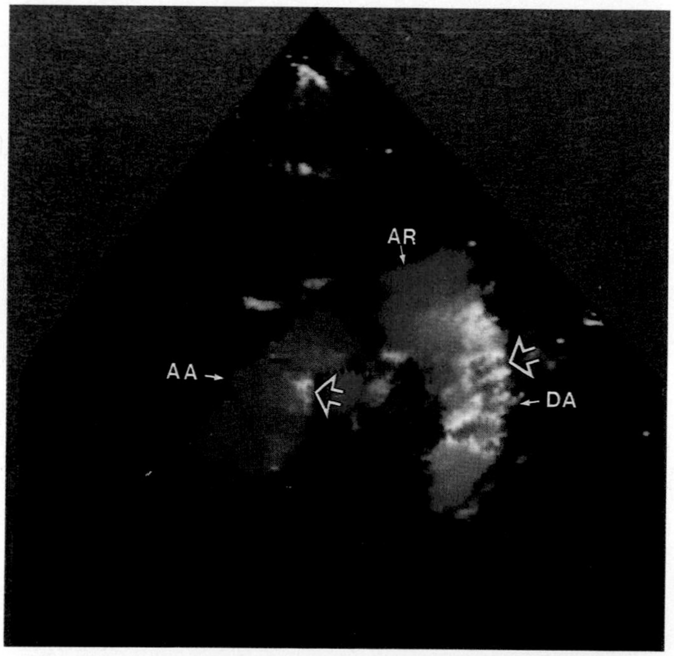

Fig. 19–78. Color Doppler recording of flow in the ascending aorta, arch (AR) and descending thoracic aorta. Flow in the ascending aorta (AA) is toward the transducer (orange), while flow in the descending aorta (DA) is away from the transducer (blue). Note that flow velocity in the ascending aorta is greatest along the inner wall (yellow, open arrow), while beyond the arch it is greatest along the outer vessel wall (yellow-orange, open arrow).

The Descending Thoracic Aorta

The descending thoracic aorta is best visualized transthoracically from a parasternal transducer location as it passes behind the left side of the heart.[2,177–179] In the typical long axis view of the left ventricle, the descending aorta appears as a pulsatile, circular or oval, echo-free space located beneath the posterior atrioventricular groove (see also Chapters 5 and 35). During short axis scans from the apex to the base of the left heart, the position of the aorta appears to shift relative to the center of the left ventricle because of the acute angle at which the long axis of these two structures intersect (Fig. 19–79). At the papillary muscle level, the descending aorta is generally medial to the center of the left ventricle; at the mitral valve level, it is more directly behind the left ventricle; at the left atrial level, it is slightly lateral or leftward in position; and at the pulmonary artery level, it lies beneath the arterial bifurcation.[177] The long axis position of the descending aorta is also reported to vary when there is left atrial or left ventricular dilation.[177] When the left atrium is enlarged, the descending aorta is typically displaced superiorly from its normal position behind the atrioventricular groove, whereas with left ventricular hypertrophy, the descending aorta is displaced inferiorly. These variations in relative positions do not represent movements of the aorta, but rather a shift in cardiac position relative to the aorta produced by the variation in chamber size. The normal descending thoracic aorta is smaller than the aortic root or ascending aorta. It has a reported mean diastolic diameter of $17 + 3$ mm in contrast to a mean diastolic diameter of $22 + 4$ mm for the ascending aorta. The descending aorta is reported to be larger than nor-

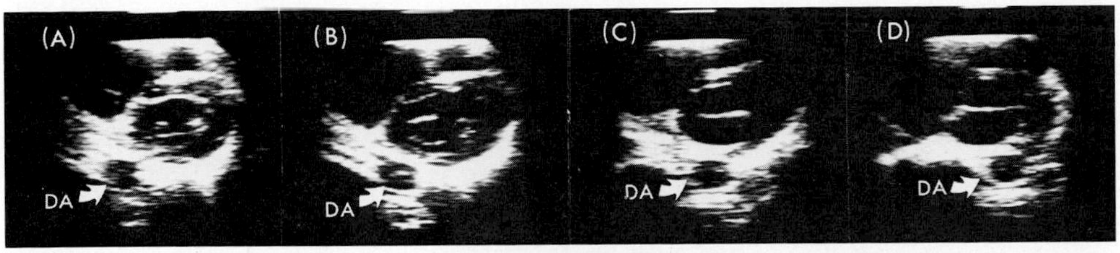

Fig. 19–79. Short axis scans recorded as the transducer is swept from the left ventricle **(A)** to the aortic root **(D)**. Because the aorta crosses obliquely beneath the left ventricle, its position shifts from left to right as the scan plane is moved superiorly. DA = descending aorta.

mal in patients with hypertension, aortic valve disease, and coronary atherosclerosis.[177] It is also enlarged in patients with thoracic aortic aneurysms.

An additional cause of dilation of the descending thoracic aorta in the newborn is cerebral or hepatic arteriovenous malformations.[178] These arteriovenous connections increase venous return to the right side of the heart during intrauterine life. This increased flow is transmitted to the descending aorta via the ductus arteriosus, thereby causing aortic dilation. The combination of features may suggest the diagnosis. An abnormally small thoracic aorta may be noted with aortic hypoplasia.[177]

The position of the descending thoracic aorta may be useful in differentiating pleural from pericardial effusion because pericardial effusion displaces the extra pericardial thoracic aorta posteriorly; whereas a pleural effusion should not change the position of the aorta relative to the left side of the heart (see Chapter 35).

Transesophageal echocardiography has markedly improved the quality of the images that can be obtained of the descending thoracic aorta because the proximity of the esophagus to the aorta improves access, decreases attenuation, and increases the transducer frequencies that can be employed. Using single-plane transesophageal probes, the aorta is usually imaged at multiple short axis levels, whereas with a biplane probe, it can be recorded in both long and short axis (Fig. 19–80). Because few anatomic landmarks are available, plane position is typically defined by the distance the probe has been advanced relative to the incisors.

Axial flow velocity in the descending aorta can be recorded from the suprasternal, subcostal, or transesophageal transducer positions. Rotational flow in the descending thoracic aorta has been described in short axis transesophageal color Doppler recording.[180] The perception of rotational flow about the long axis of the vessel was based on the recording of a red color on one side (indicating flow toward the transducer) and a blue color on the other (indicating flow away from the transducer). However, it has also been shown by computer simulation (Fig. 19–81) that this appearance can be produced in the absence of rotatory flow if the aorta is not imaged precisely across its short axis.[181]

The Abdominal Aorta

The abdominal aorta, which extends from the diaphragm to the iliac bifurcation, is readily examined throughout its course from the anterior abdominal wall. Areas of aneurysmal dilation, external compression, and abdominal coarctation can readily be appreciated. Flow in the abdominal aorta is similar to that recorded in the ascending aorta except that there is usually no flow reversal in early diastole (Fig. 19–82A). In aortic regurgitation, flow reversal typically extends to the abdominal aorta and may be pandiastolic when the lesion is severe (Fig. 19–82B).

Structural Abnormalities of the Aorta

From an echocardiographic viewpoint, disorders involving the tubular aorta can be grouped into (1) developmental anomalies associated with vascular ring symptoms, (2) lesions that produce aortic stenosis or obstruction, (3) lesions characterized by dilation of the vessel walls, and (4) miscellaneous disorders such as aorto-left ventricular tunnel.

Developmental Anomalies Associated With Vascular Rings

Developmental anomalies of the aortic arch and its branches often give rise to a pattern of symptoms known as the vascular ring complex.[182,183] The anomalous course of these vessels causes entrapment of either the esophagus, the trachea, or of both, giving rise to symptoms of dysphagia and/or stridor. The most common anomalies causing this complex are anomalous origin of the right subclavian artery, double aortic arch, right aortic arch, and cervical aorta (Fig. 19–83). Persistence of the ductus arteriosus may also contribute to the vascular entrapment of the esophagus and trachea.

Echocardiographically, the suprasternal and subcostal imaging windows have proved most useful in the delineation of the course of the aorta in this symptom complex and in imaging the origin of its branches.[184–189]

Anomalous Right Subclavian Artery

Anomalous origin of the right subclavian artery is the most common vascular ring anomaly occurring in patients with a normal left-sided aortic arch.[183] In this condition, the right subclavian artery arises from the aorta distal to the left subclavian artery and passes behind the esophagus to reach the right arm. Symptomatic compression of the trachea or esophagus is rare. The anomaly may be recognized echocardiographically by the absence of the normal branching of the first aortic branch vessel (the innominate).[190] The anomalous right subclavian artery should also be apparent using the transesophageal approach.

Double Aortic Arch

Double aortic arch is a congenital condition in which the ascending aorta divides into right and left aortic

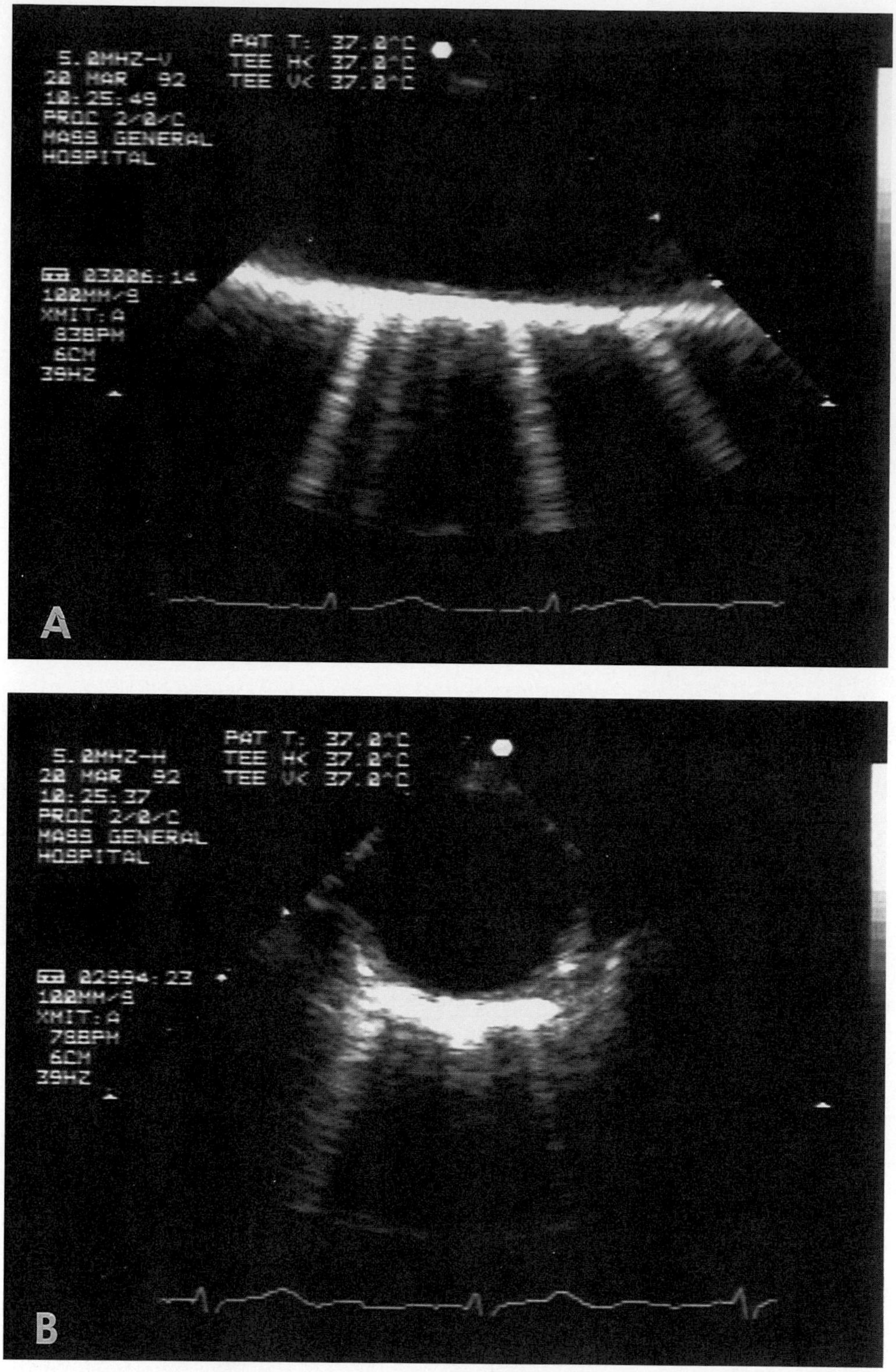

Fig. 19–80. Long- **(A)** and short **(B)** axis recordings of normal descending aorta, using biplane probe.

arches.[182,183] The double aortic arch is a remnant of the embryonic pattern in which the aorta and great vessels are paired structures. The right and left arches in this condition encircle the trachea and esophagus and subsequently fuse to form a single descending aorta. Double aortic arch is usually an isolated abnormality.[183] The right arch is generally larger than the left.[183] Separate common carotid and subclavian vessels arise from each arch. Both arches are generally functional, but atresia of the smaller arch is occasionally seen.[182] When present, the atretic segment is usually observed between the common carotid and subclavian arteries or just distal to the origin of the subclavian. The aorta may descend on either side. The ductus arteriosus, however, is generally left-sided.[183]

The presence of a double aortic arch may be detected echocardiographically from the suprasternal or subcostal imaging positions.[185,186,191] From the latter window,

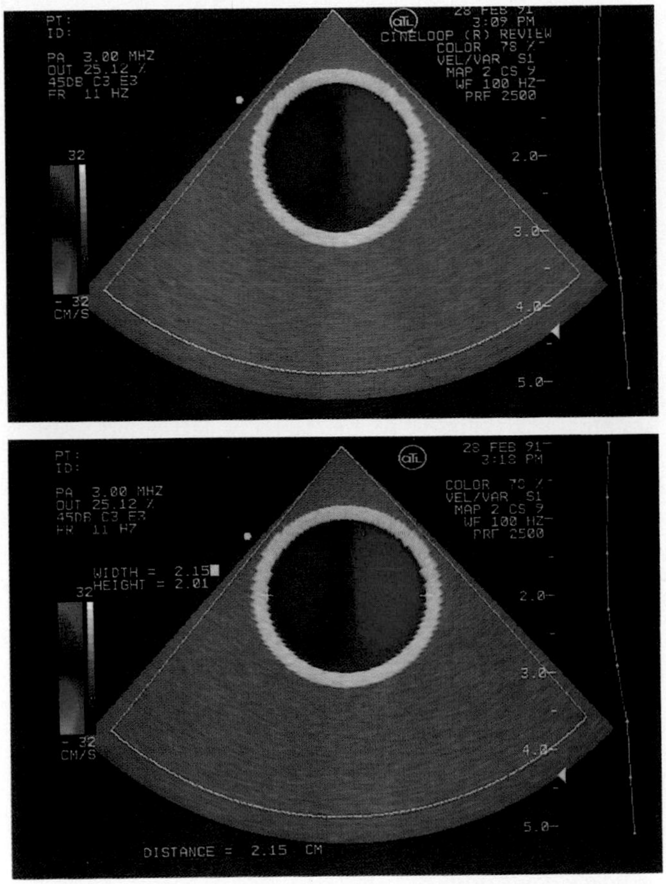

Fig. 19–81. Computer simulation of short axis color flow appearance in a circular vessel for rotary flow (top) and laminar flow (bottom) recorded with the transducer rotated 5° from the true short axis. (Courtesy of Advanced Technology Laboratories.)

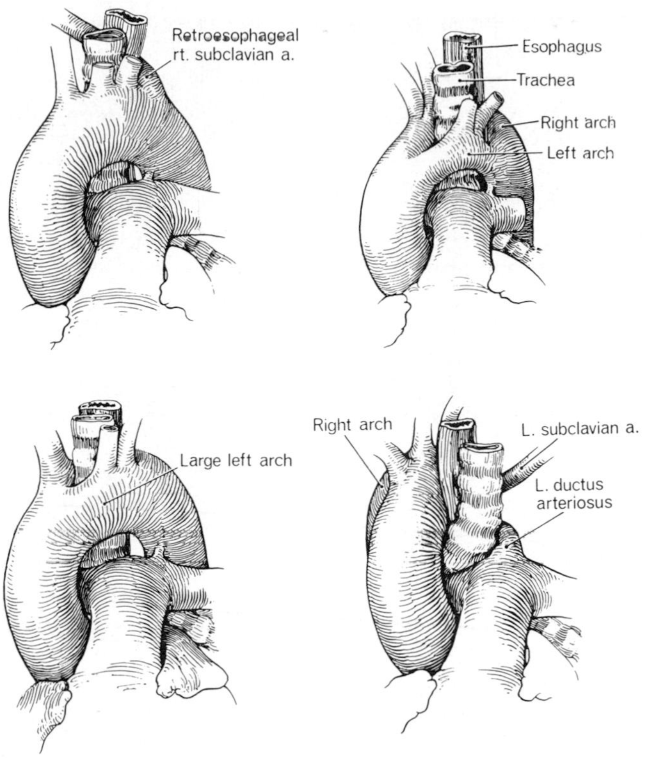

Fig. 19–83. Diagram of common developmental anomalies of the aortic arch associated with vascular ring anomalies. Top, left. Retroesophageal right subclavian artery. Top, right. Double aortic arch with dominant right arch. Bottom, left. Double aortic arch with dominant left arch. Bottom, right. Right aortic arch. (From Cooley DA, Wukasch DC: Techniques in Vascular Surgery. Philadelphia, Saunders, 1979.)

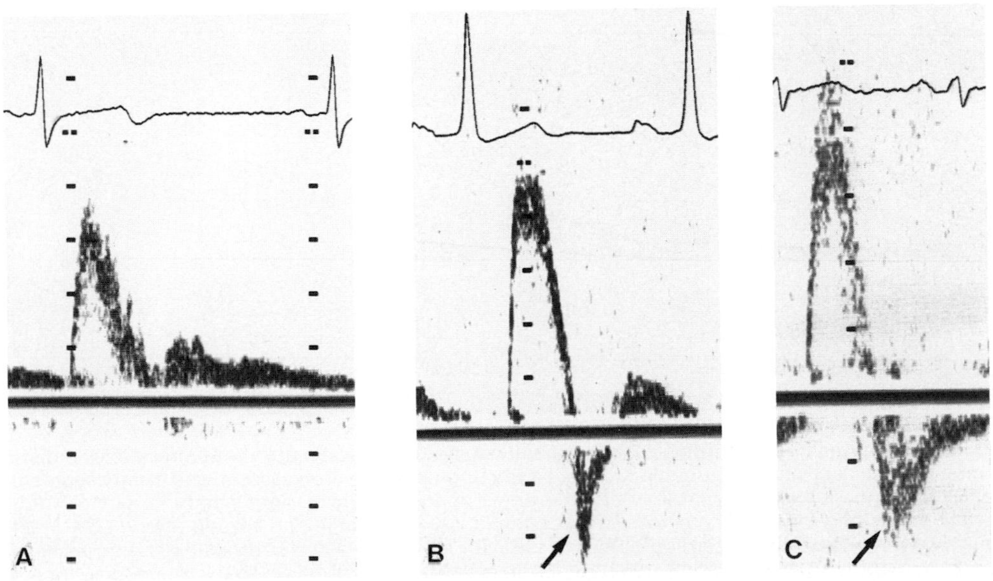

Fig. 19–82. **A.** Normal abdominal aortic flow pulsed Doppler. **B.** Brief area of flow reversal (arrow) in a patient with moderate aortic regurgitation. **C.** Pansystolic flow reversal (arrow) in severe aortic regurgitation.

the bifurcation of the aorta distal to the aortic valve has been recognized by tilting the transducer anteriorly from the five-chamber view (Fig. 19–84).[185] Doppler interrogation is helpful in demonstrating the presence of flow in both vascular lumens.

Right Aortic Arch

Right aortic arch is a congenital condition in which the ascending aorta arises normally, but the arch and proximal portion of the descending aorta remain to the right of the midline. The course of the descending thoracic aorta is variable. It may remain on the right side or cross the midline to enter the abdomen on the left. Right-sided arch is seen in approximately 0.1% of the population[192] and is classified into several types on the basis of the origin of the great vessels. The two major types of right-sided arch are characterized by (1) mirror-image branching of the brachycephalic arteries and (2) four major vessels (two subclavian and two common carotid arteries) arising independently from the aortic arch, usually anomalously.[182] The classification is of importance because mirror-image branching is associated with significant congenital heart disease in up to 98% of patients, whereas a right-sided arch with independently arising vessels to the head and neck is less frequently associated with other significant congenital cardiac abnormalities.[193,194] Vascular ring symptoms may occur with right-sided aortic arch that is due to (1) anomalous origin of an arch branch, (2) left-sided insertion of the ductus arteriosus or (3) retroesophageal passage of the arch. A combination of these anomalies can also occur.

Several imaging planes and maneuvers are useful in the detection of right-sided aortic arch Figure 19–85.[187,188,195] From a standard suprasternal long axis imaging plane, the ascending aorta alone is visualized in right-sided aortic arch (Fig. 19–85B). Rotating the transducer clockwise 15 to 20° from the standard suprasternal long axis view will bring the arch and rightward coursing descending thoracic aorta into view (Fig. 19–85C). It is important to label these maneuvers while recording the study on videotape, because knowledge of plane orientation during image acquisition is required for accurate diagnosis. Tilting the transducer rightward and superiorly to examine the first arch vessel provides additional information. Normally, the first vessel encountered is the brachiocephalic, which bifurcates shortly after its origin. Therefore, if the first branch bifurcates and courses to the right, a left-sided arch is present. However, if the first branch vessel bifurcates and courses to the left, then a mirror-image right-sided arch is probable. If the first vessel fails to bifurcate, then an aberrant right subclavian artery should be considered. Left and right parasternal long axis views are used to determine the sidedness of the descending thoracic aorta, while subcostal recordings help determine the location of the aorta as it enters the abdomen.

Cervical Arch

A cervical arch is a rare anomaly in which the aortic arch lies more superiorly than normal and may extend into the neck.[196,197] Vascular ring symptoms may occur with this condition, but the presence of a pulsatile mass in the neck is the usual presenting feature. The location of the vessel in this anomaly is easily visualized from the neck or from a suprasternal long axis plane.[198]

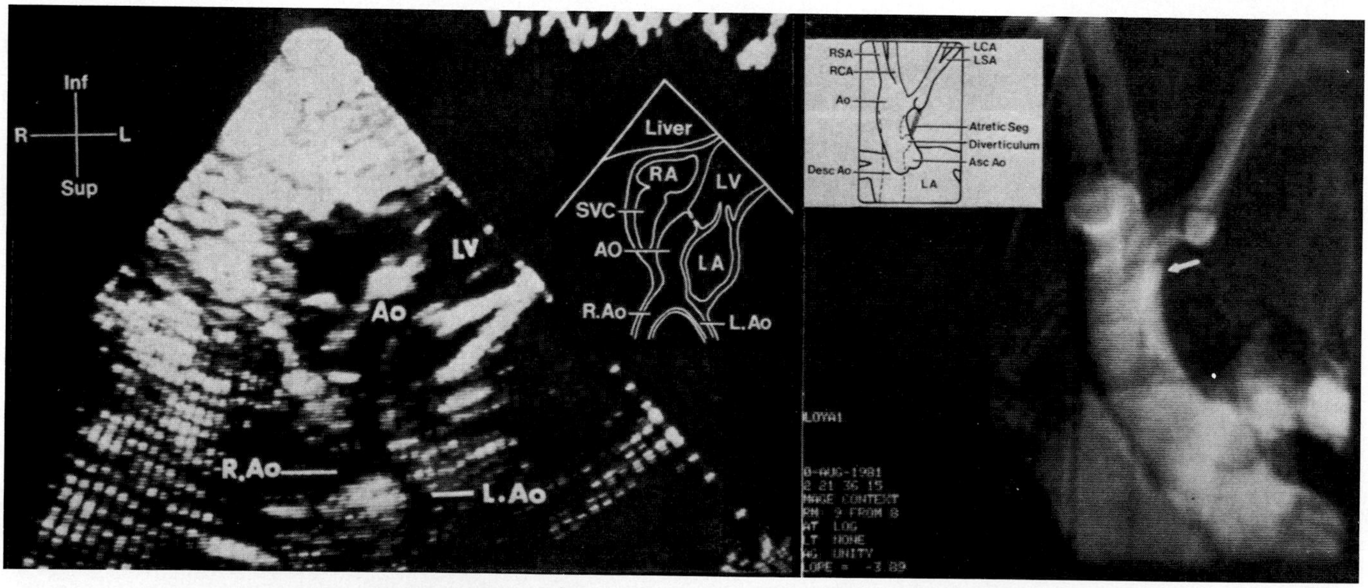

Fig. 19–84. Left. Anteriorly angled subcostal five-chamber recording from a patient with a double aortic arch with atresia of the distal left arch. Right. Angiogram from the same patient illustrating the double arch, separate origins of the arch vessels, and atretic segment. RA = right atrium; LV = left ventricle; SVC = superior vena cava; LA = left atrium; AO = aorta; R.Ao = right-sided arch; L.Ao = left-sided aortic arch; RSA = right subclavian artery; RCA = right common carotid artery; LCA = left common carotid artery; LSA = left subclavian artery. (From Sahn DJ, et al.: Two-dimensional echocardiography and intravenous digital video subtraction angiography for diagnosis and evaluation of Double aortic arch. Am J Cardiol 50:342, 1982. Reproduced with permission of Mosby Year-Book, Inc.)

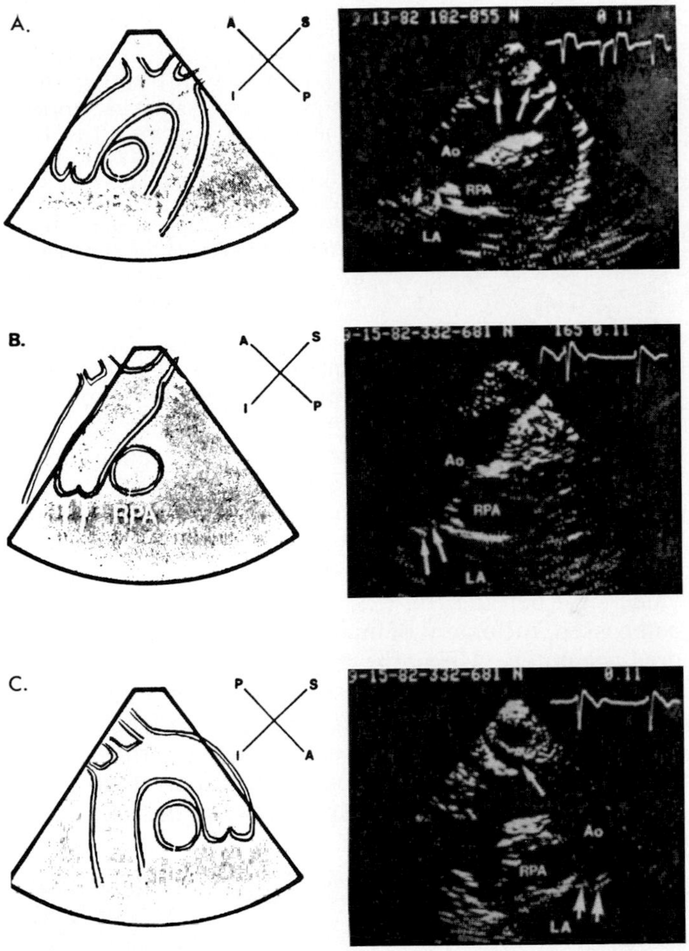

Fig. 19–85. **A.** Suprasternal notch recording of a normal aortic arch. **B.** A right-sided arch recorded with the transducer aligned in the standard position to record a normal arch. **C.** A right-sided arch recorded with the transducer rotated counter clockwise to a position roughly 20° to the right of the midline. Ao = aorta; RPA = right pulmonary artery; LA = left atrium. (From Celano V, Pieroni DR, Gingell RL, Roland JA: Two-dimensional echocardiographic recognition of the right aortic arch. Am J Cardiol 51:1507, 1983. Reproduced with permission of Mosby Year-Book, Inc.)

Lesions Associated With Stenosis or Obstruction of the Aorta

Supravalvular Aortic Stenosis

Supravalvular aortic stenosis is an obstructive, congenital deformity of the ascending aorta that originates just distal to the coronary arteries and produces either localized or diffuse narrowing of the vessel.[199] Although the designation *supravalvular aortic stenosis* encompasses a heterogeneous group of lesions, three specific anatomic types have been characterized. First is the so-called membranous type, which consists of a simple fibrous diaphragm containing a single perforation. At the opposite extreme is a uniform hypoplasia of the entire ascending aorta, designated the *hypoplastic type*. Between these two is the hourglass lesion. This type of obstruction is characterized by extreme thickening of the media of the ascending aorta with an hourglass-like narrowing of the external aspect of the affected segment and corresponding narrowing of the aortic lumen. Intimal fibrous thickening may appear over the narrowed segment, further accentuating the degree of obstruction.[199]

The hourglass deformity is clearly the most common, representing roughly 66% of cases, whereas diffuse narrowing of the vessel accounts for more than 20%. Membranous lesions are the least common, occurring in no more than 10% of patients with supravalvular obstruction.[200–202] Although supravalvular stenosis is not common (it accounts for only 0.6 to 6% of obstructive lesions[199,203,204] occurring in the region of the aortic valve), it does occur with sufficient frequency to warrant continued diagnostic consideration.

In addition to the different anatomic types of supravalvular aortic stenosis, three separate clinical presentations have also been described. The most common of these is the sporadic type in which the lesion occurs in otherwise normal individuals. In approximately a third of cases, the supravalvular stenosis is found in association with an extended syndrome, which includes an abnormal elfin facies, mental retardation, and idiopathic hypercalcemia.[205–208] Finally, there have been reports of familial aggregates of patients in which the disorder appears to be transmitted as an autosomal dominant disorder with variable expression.[209,210]

Echocardiographically, supravalvular aortic stenosis is characterized by an obvious decrease in aortic diameter originating at the superior border of the sinuses of Valsalva.[167] The area of obstruction may vary in both severity and extent, but the point of peak aortic narrowing usually is found just anterior to the junction of the superior border of the left atrium and the aortic root.[167]

The membranous lesion generally appears as a discrete, thin, linear echo extending inward from the walls of the aorta and encroaching on the vascular lumen. The membrane is typically located at the sinotubular junction just above the insertion of the superior left atrial wall into the posterior aortic root. The lesion is considered obstructive when the separation between the inner margins of the membrane is less than the diameter of the outflow tract at the annulus. Figure 19–86 is an example of a supravalvular membrane.

Figure 19–87 is an example of an hourglass lesion in which there is more marked luminal narrowing as well as a more extensive area of involvement of the ascending aorta, while Figure 19–88 illustrates a small membrane superimposed on an area of more extensive narrowing. Figure 19–89 illustrates aortic hypoplasia. In this example, the aorta appears small, thin, and strandlike. The area of hypoplasia involves the entire ascending aorta and aortic arch. The diminutive vessel is evident throughout the scan plane and, as indicated in the accompanying diagram, was associated with hypoplasia of the left ventricle and mitral valve. In the left portion of the scan, a small area of dilation reflects the rudimentary sinuses of Valsalva. Figure 19–90 is an angiogram from the same patient that confirms the extent and severity of the aortic hypoplasia.

Supravalvular aortic stenosis has also been described in familial homozygous hypercholesterolemia. In this condition, atheroma is preferentially deposited at the

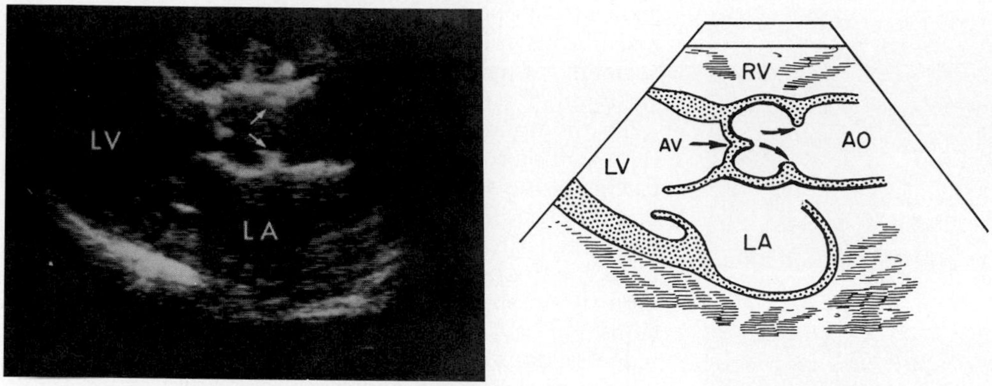

Fig. 19–86. Parasternal long axis recording of the ascending aorta illustrating a discrete supravalvular membrane. The membrane, indicated by the oblique arrows, appears as two discrete linear bands of echoes arising from the anterior and posterior margins of the aortic root at the level of the sinotubular junction and encroaching on the vessel lumen. AO = aorta; RV = right ventricle; AV = aortic valve; LA = left atrium; LV = left ventricle.

level of the sinuses of Valsalva and sinotubular junction, giving rise to localized stenosis. Echocardiography has proven sensitive and specific when compared with aortography in detecting these atheromatous deposits. Atheromatous involvement of the coronary ostia can also be visualized.[211]

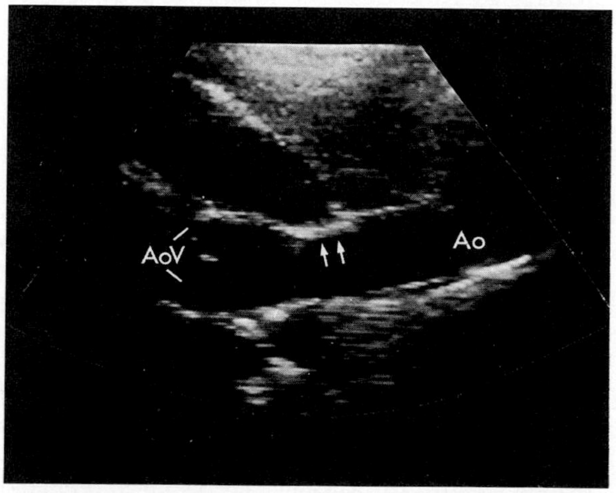

Fig. 19–87. Parasternal long axis recording illustrating a more diffuse hourglass type of supravalvular narrowing (arrows). AoV = aortic valve; Ao = aorta.

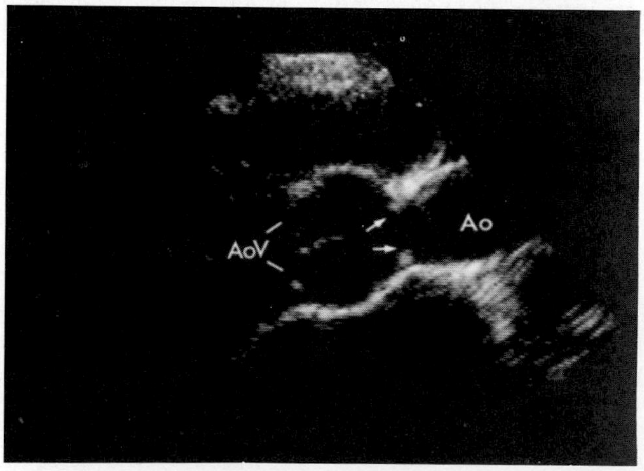

Fig. 19–88. Parasternal long axis recording illustrating a diffuse area of supravalvular narrowing (hourglass lesion) with a superimposed membrane (arrows). AoV = aortic valve; Ao = aorta.

Comparisons between cross-sectional echocardiographic and angiographic studies of the aortic root have revealed a good correlation in both morphologic appearance and estimates of severity, with a tendency for echocardiography to slightly underestimate the angiographic value.[167] When the full extent of the lesion can be encompassed, the extent of involvement can also be measured accurately. Using the diameter of the aorta at the annulus as a reference, investigators noted a mean decrease in diameter of 47% in four patients with hourglass lesions.[167] This finding is in contrast to the normal mean increase of 12.5%. In addition, a rough correlation existed in this small patient group between the small de-

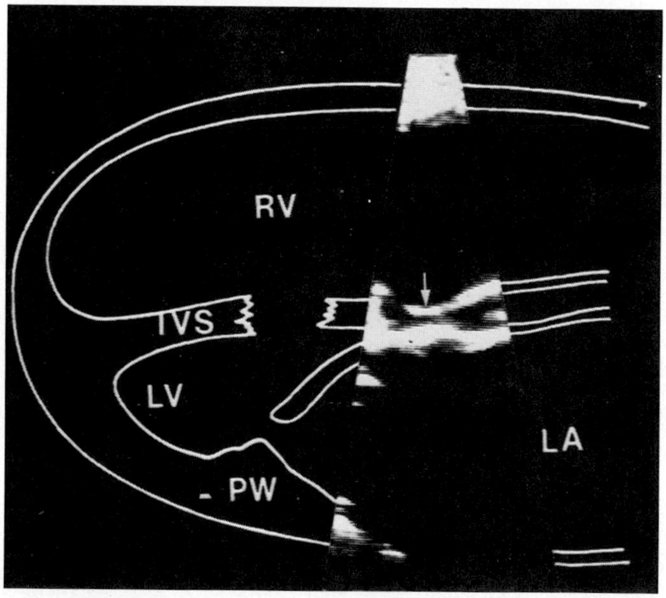

Fig. 19–89. Cross-sectional echogram of the supravalvular aorta from a patient with severe hypoplasia of the aortic annulus and ascending vessel. The area of greatest narrowing is indicated by the vertical arrow. Proximal to the obstruction, rudimentary sinuses of Valsalva are visible. Distally, hypoplasia of the entire ascending aorta continues. As indicated in the accompanying diagram, there was also hypoplasia of the left ventricle (LV) and mitral valve, a ventricular septal defect, and a dilated right ventricle (RV) and pulmonary artery. IVS = interventricular septum; PW = posterior wall; LA = left atrium. (From Weyman AE, et al.: Cross-sectional echocardiographic characterization of aortic obstruction. I: Supravalvular aortic stenosis and aortic hypoplasia. Circulation 57:491, 1978. Reproduced by permission of the American Heart Association, Inc.)

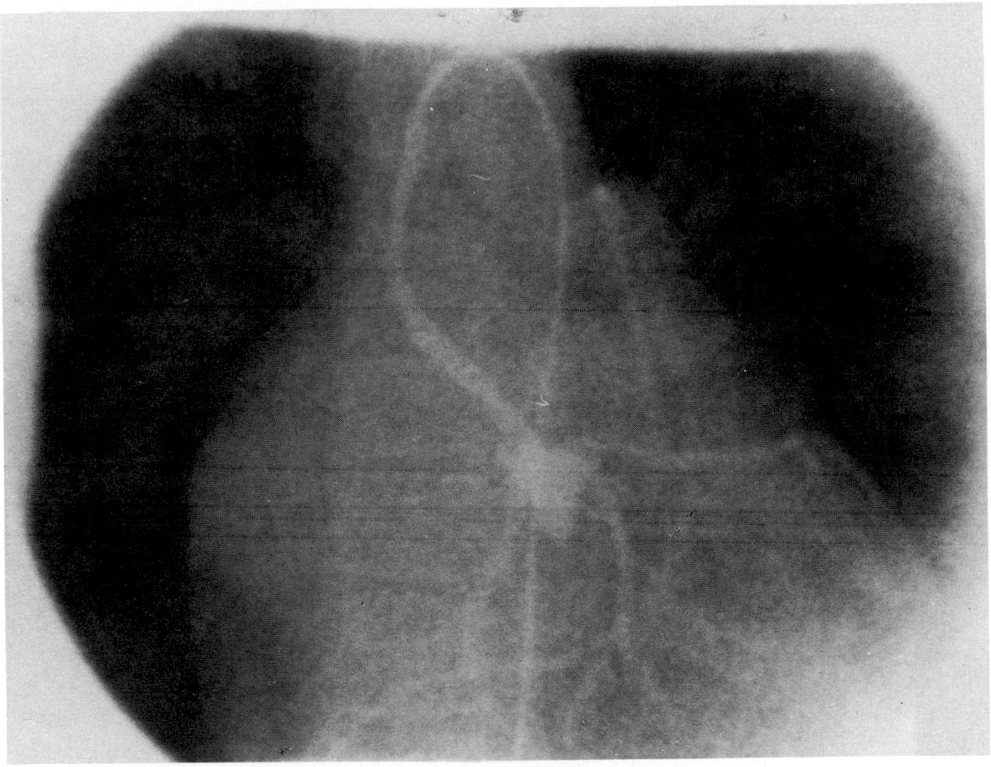

Fig. 19–90. Angiographic recording of the ascending aorta corresponds to the cross-sectional echogram in Figure 19–89. This recording again demonstrates severe hypoplasia of the entire ascending aortic arch. Diminutive sinuses of Valsalva, from which the coronary arterial system arises, are also evident. (From Weyman AE, et al.: Cross-sectional echocardiographic characterization of aortic obstruction. I: Supravalvular aortic stenosis and aortic hypoplasia. Circulation 57:491, 1978. Reproduced by permission of the American Heart Association, Inc.)

crease in diameter and the severity of obstruction. When the aorta is diffusely hypoplastic, the annulus is frequently also involved and can no longer be used as a reference for estimating severity.

Doppler interrogation of the aortic root can aid in confirming the diagnosis of supravalvular aortic stenosis and in assessing its severity. The site of the stenosis can be localized with both color flow or pulsed Doppler, while continuous wave Doppler is used to record the maximal velocity. The pressure gradient across the stenosis can be determined using the modified Bernoulli equation ($\Delta P = 4\ V^2$).[212] In hourglass lesions, however, gradual re-expansion of the aorta distal to the site of the stenosis may lead to pressure recovery.[84,213] Under these circumstances, the pressure gradient across the stenotic segment estimated by Doppler will exceed that measured at cardiac catheterization. In a 1989 study of five patients with this form of supravalvular aortic or pulmonary stenosis, Doppler was shown to overestimate the gradient measured at cardiac catheterization in each case (Fig. 19–91).[213]

Figures 19–92 illustrates the effects of the downstream shape of the vessel beyond a stenosis on the degree of pressure recovery and hence the difference between the actual head loss and the pressure drop at the stenosis. Note that the more gradually the vessel re-expands, the less the actual head loss. Figure 19–93 is an angiogram from a patient with supravalvular stenosis illustrating the similarity between the actual anatomy and the model contours in Figure 19–92.

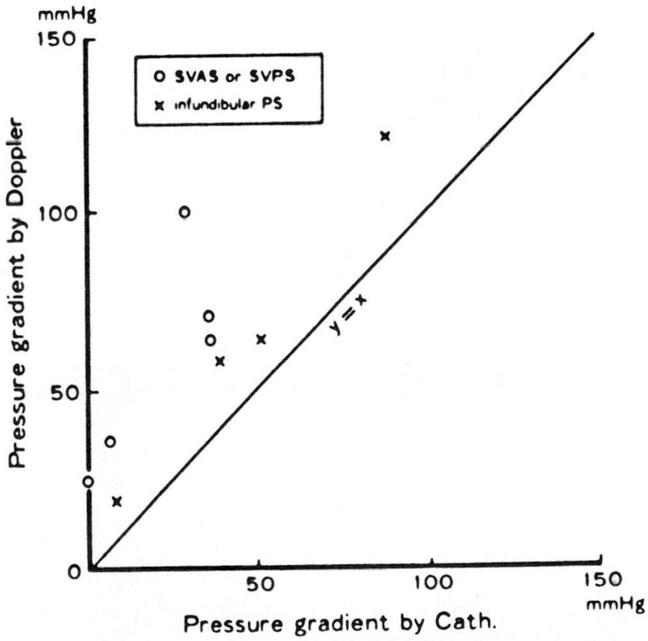

Fig. 19–91. The relationship between Doppler- and catheter-measured gradients in patients with supravalvular aortic stenosis (SVAS), supravalvular pulmonic stenosis (SVPS) and infundibular pulmonic stenosis (PS). Note that in each case the Doppler-derived gradient is greater than that measured at catheterization, indicating pressure recovery distal to the lesion. (From Nakajima T, et al.: Doppler echocardiographic estimates of pressure gradients in various types of stenoses: usefulness and limitations. J Cardiol 19:851, 1989. Reproduced by permission of the Japanese College of Cardiology.)

Coarctation of the Aorta

Coarctation of the aorta is characterized anatomically by a localized deformity of the media of the aortic wall

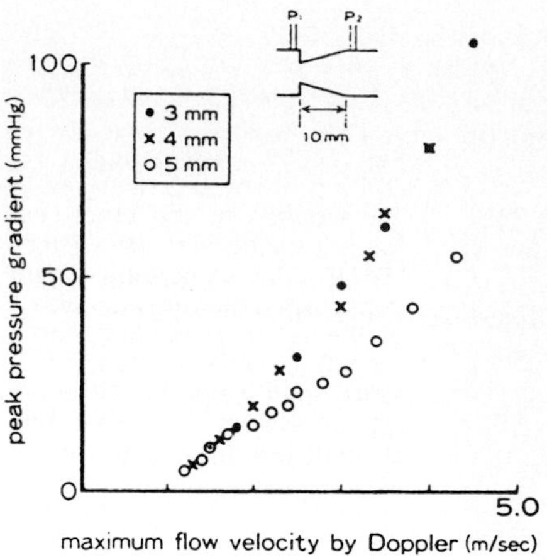

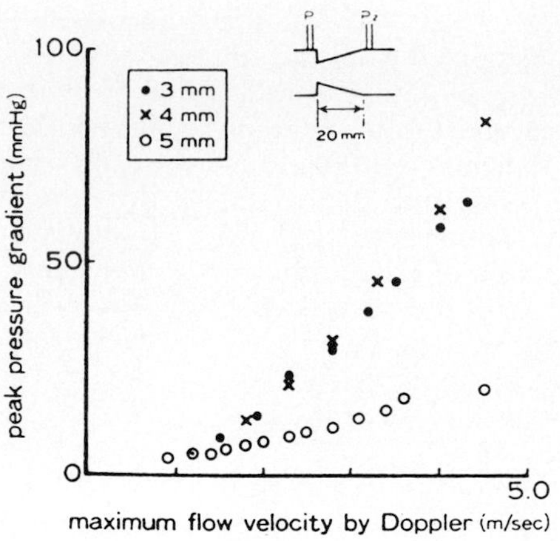

Fig. 19–92. In vitro studies demonstrating the relationship of stenotic orifice size and exit length to pressure gradient measured directly and by continuous wave Doppler. Left. 3-, 4-, and 5-mm-diameter orifices with a 10-mm-long tapering outlet. Right. Same as left but with a 20-mm-long tapering outlet. The larger orifices and longer tapering outlet permit overestimation of the head loss by the Doppler method. (From Nakajima T, et al.: Doppler echocardiographic estimates of pressure gradients in various types of stenoses: usefulness and limitations. J Cardiol 19:851, 1989. Reproduced by permission of the Japanese College of Cardiology.)

that produces a curtain-like infolding, which narrows the vascular lumen in an eccentric fashion. Externally, the aorta exhibits an indentation or localized concavity.[214] Coarctation may occur at any level of the thoracic aorta,[215] but it is most commonly located just beyond the origin of the left subclavian artery or distal to the

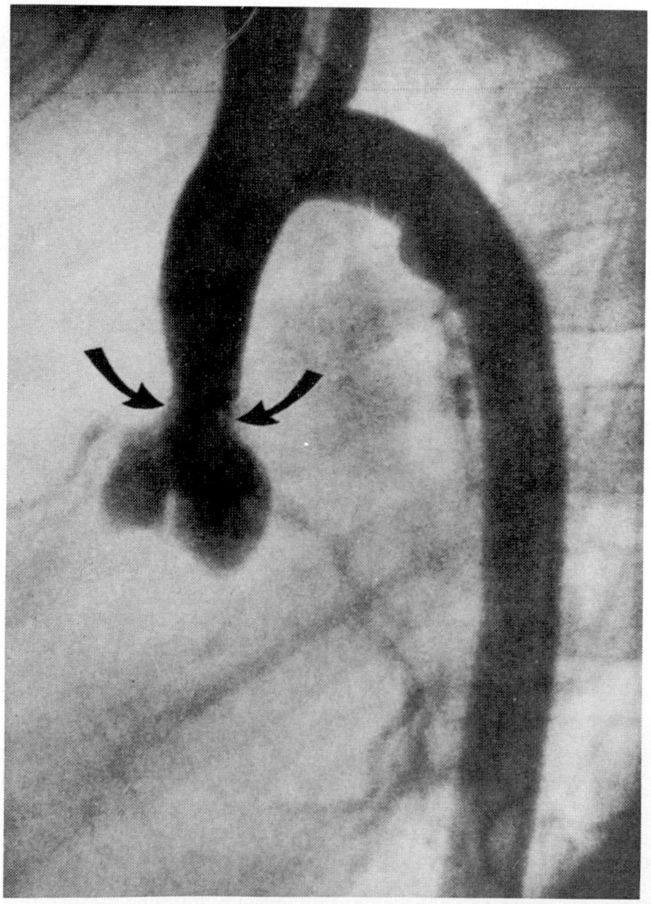

Fig. 19–93. Angiogram showing the similarity of the actual anatomic lesion of supravalvular aortic stenosis with the models depicted in Figure 19–92.

insertion of the ligamentum arteriosum.[216] The area of coarctation may be well defined and localized, or the aortic segment may be diffusely narrowed.

Coarctation is commonly divided at the ductus arteriosus into the postductal or adult type, and the preductal or infantile type. Postductal coarctation is usually localized and appears almost as a diaphragm with the aorta widening immediately below the area of constriction to a diameter greater than that above the obstruction.[202]

In the preductal or infantile type, the coarctation is proximal to the entrance of the ductus arteriosus. Preductal coarctation can be further divided into three general categories: (1) localized constriction just above the entrance to the ductus, (2) diffuse isthmic narrowing extending from the entrance of the ductus superiorly to the left subclavian artery, (3) constriction not only involving the isthmus but extending to include a variable portion of the aortic arch.[202] Isolated coarctations are usually postductal, whereas coarctations associated with other major congenital anomalies are more frequently preductal. In preductal lesions, there is a further association between the extent and location of the narrowing and the presence of other major defects. Thus, studies have shown that focal preductal constriction is associated in 16% of patients with other major abnormalities; isthmic hypoplasia in 28%; and more diffuse obstruction involving the isthmus and aortic arch in 80%.[202] A bicuspid aortic valve is found in between 40 and 80% of patients with isolated coarctation of the postductal type. Coarctation is also the most common cardiac anomaly associated with Turner's syndrome.[217]

Direct echocardiographic visualization of the area of coarctation has been reported in many series.[218–222] The degree of success has varied, however, depending on the size, age, and clinical condition of the patient. In neonates, excellent sensitivity and specificity in the diagnosis of coarctation have been reported;[220] however, direct visualization of the area of coarctation is not easy. Left ventricular failure in the newborn in the absence of other obvious pathology should suggest the diagnosis. On occasion, diagnostic confusion may occur in patients with an interrupted aortic arch distal to the left subclavian artery or in patients with a shelf simulating a coarctation (pseudocoarctation) at the site of entry of the normal ductus into the aorta.

The site of coarctation is best visualized from the suprasternal notch or a parasternal plane aligned parallel to the long axis of the aortic arch and the descending thoracic aorta. Coarctation presents echocardiographically as a localized decrease in the diameter of the aortic lumen, with the area of maximal narrowing distal to the left subclavian artery. The area of coarctation is characteristically more reflective than the surrounding vascular wall because of focal thickening in the affected region and the tendency for the obstructing shelf to be more perpendicular than the curvilinear wall of the normal descending aorta to the path of the scan plane.[175,176] Proximal to the obstruction, the left carotid and the left subclavian arteries may be enlarged, and the aortic pulsations are increased. Distal to the lesion, the aorta may again dilate, but in this region the normal aortic pulsations are damped.[175] The striking disparity between the markedly pulsatile proximal vessel and the quiescent distal vessel, highlights the presence of the obstructing lesion. In many cases, it is this discrepancy in pulsation that initially alerts the examiner to the possible presence of a coarctation.[175]

Figure 19–94 illustrates an area of discrete coarctation. In this example, a localized area of luminal narrowing is present distal to the left subclavian artery. The area of coarctation is small and well demarcated and almost obliterates the aortic lumen.

Color flow mapping usually reveals an increase in flow velocity at the site of the coarctation, which is helpful in identifying both the site and length of the stenosis. Excellent correlations have been reported between the diameter of the color flow jet at the site of the coarctation and that measured angiographically.[223] However, given the poor lateral resolution of color flow images of this area and their dependence on machine factors (gain, wall filter setting, pulse repetition frequency), caution should be exercised in the use of the dimensions of the color jet alone in determining the severity of stenosis. The flow disturbance at the site of the coarctation frequently extends into diastole as a result of the persistent gradient across the stenosis[224,225] (Fig. 19–94), and the finding of antegrade diastolic flow in the descending aorta has been used to diagnose coarctation. However, when a patent ductus arteriosus is also present, flow in the descending aorta is generally confined to systole.[224]

The increase in velocity through the coarctation recorded by continuous wave Doppler can be used to derive the pressure drop across the lesion. Good correlations have been reported between Doppler-derived pressure gradients and those obtained by sphygmomanometry of upper and lower limbs or measured invasively.[226,227] The modified Bernoulli equation ($\Delta P = 4v^2$) is generally used to derive these gradients. However, if the velocity proximal to the coarctation is greater than 1.5 m/sec, then the proximal velocity should be taken into account ($\Delta P = 4(v_{distal}^2 - v_{proximal}^2)$) in calculating the pressure gradient. In neonates with long tunnel-like obstructions, the increased importance of viscous forces may invalidate the use of the Bernoulli equations.[69,228,229] The relationship between velocity and mean pressure gradient may be further complicated by pressure recovery distal to the site of obstruction, which causes the Doppler-derived pressure gradient to overestimate that measured invasively.[84] Jet eccentricity can also make it difficult to obtain an adequate velocity profile.[227] When a patent ductus arteriosus is also present, there may be no velocity increase at the site of the obstruction. Under these circumstances, imaging alone should be used to establish the diagnosis of coarctation.

Interrupted Aortic Arch

Interrupted aortic arch is a rare anomaly in which a portion of the aorta distal to the right brachiocephalic artery is absent or atretic.[230–232] It is classified into three types on the basis of the anatomic site of the interrupted segment. Type A is an interruption distal to the left subclavian artery; type B occurs between the left subclavian and common carotid arteries; type C occurs between the right brachiocephalic and left common carotid and is the least common variety.[232,233] Subtypes have also been described based on the site of origin of the right subclavian artery, which is also frequently anomalous.[233,234]

Blood flow to the descending aorta is maintained early postpartum by the presence of a patent ductus arterio-

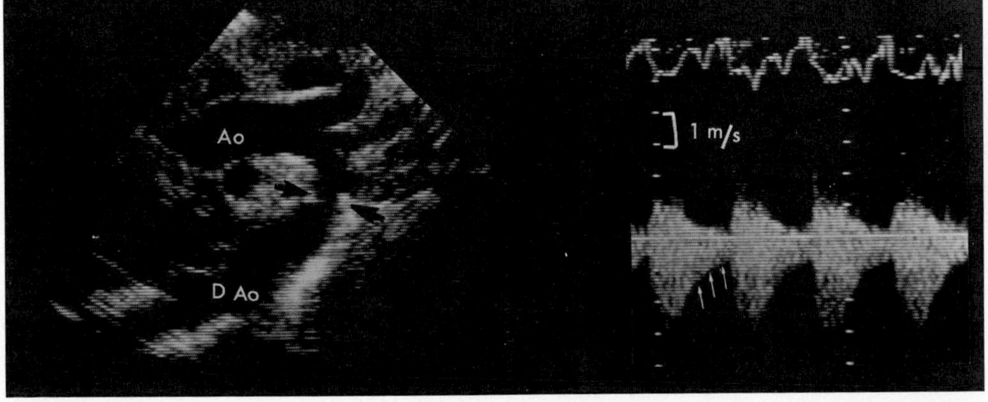

Fig. 19–94. Two-dimensional echocardiogram and continuous wave Doppler recording of the descending aorta from the aortic suprasternal notch in a child with a discrete postductal coarctation (black arrows). The peak gradient across the area of stenosis is 3 m/sec, consistent with a gradient of 36 mm Hg. Note the presence of persistent forward flow throughout diastole (white arrows). Ao = ascending aorta; D Ao = descending aorta.

sus.[235] Additionally, in a majority of cases (50% type A, almost 100% type B), a ventricular septal defect (VSD) is present.[230,231,233,236,237] In the absence of a VSD, an aortopulmonary window is generally found.[235] Pulmonary hypertension exaggerated by the VSD shunts blood from the pulmonary artery to the aorta, thus maintaining flow to the lower extremities. Interrupted arch becomes hemodynamically apparent once the ductus arteriosus closes and intractable heart failure develops as a result of the pressure and volume load on the pulmonary circulation. Death within the first few weeks of life was the rule before surgical intervention.

Interrupted aortic arch has been successfully diagnosed prospectively by echocardiography in several series.[220,221,238,239] The aorta should be scanned in multiple planes, with the suprasternal and right parasternal transducer positions often providing the most information. The diagnosis is suggested by prominence of the pulmonary artery relative to the aorta. This is in contradistinction to the usual finding in coarctation in which dilation and increased pulsation of the aorta proximal to the site of coarctation are seen. In type B, the most common form of interrupted arch, the left common carotid is particularly prominent and points cephalad in a manner analogous to a pointing index finger (Fig. 19–95). In many cases it may not be possible to image both ascending and descending aorta from the same viewing plane, but this should be attempted because identification of the extent of the interrupted segment is important in planning surgical reconstruction of the aorta (Fig. 19–96). Color flow imaging helps in identifying the site of interruption and with other Doppler modalities assists in the diagnosis of associated anomalies such as patent ductus arteriosus, VSD, or subaortic obstruction.

Aortic Aneurysms

Aneurysms are abnormal localized areas of dilation of the wall of a blood vessel, usually an artery.[61,240] Aneurysms may be saccular (involving only a portion of the vascular wall) or fusiform (encompassing all or almost all of the circumference of the vessel). True aneurysms involve all the layers of the vascular wall. False aneurysms, in contrast, result from the destruction of

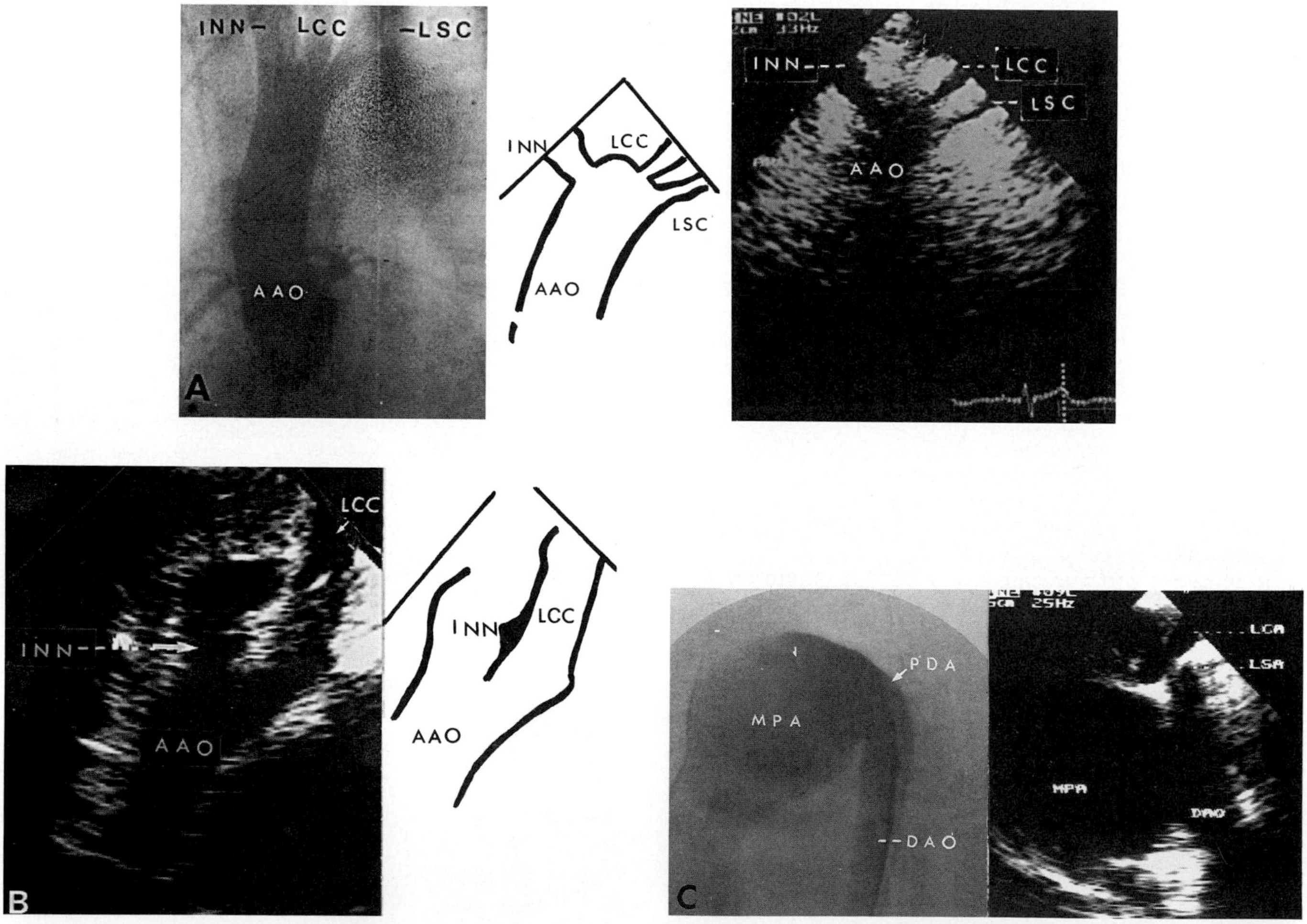

Fig. 19–95. **A.** Angiogram and cross-sectional echocardiographic suprasternal notch recording of the ascending aorta, innominate (INN), left common carotid arteries (LCC), and left subclavian arteries (LSC) from a patient with type A interruption of the aortic arch (AAO). **B.** Two-dimensional recording from a patient with type B interruption of the aortic arch. The LCC has the typical appearance of the pointing finger described in this anomaly. **C.** Angiogram and two-dimensional echocardiogram of the pulmonary artery and descending aorta from the patient in **B.** The pulmonary artery is markedly dilated, and flow into the descending aorta is through the ductus arteriosus. MPA = main pulmonary artery; DAO = descending aorta. (Courtesy of Dr. George Xie.)

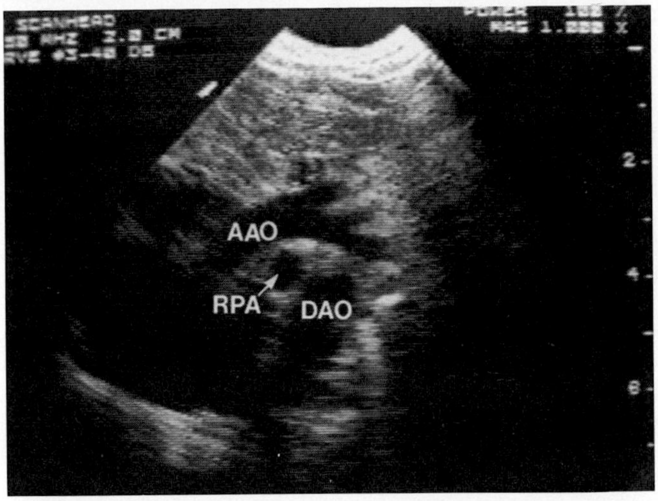

Fig. 19–96. Suprasternal long axis view from an infant with an interruption of the aortic arch beyond the origin of the left subclavian artery. The vessels to the head and neck arise from the ascending aorta (AAO). DAO = descending aorta; RPA = right pulmonary artery. (From Snider AR, Serwer GA: Echocardiography in Pediatric Heart Disease. Chicago, Year Book Medical Publishers, 1990.)

the vessel wall, usually by trauma. The external border of the false aneurysm is composed of perivascular clot and connective tissue. Dissecting aneurysms are characterized by separation of the layers of the aortic wall. The process of dissection is commonly initiated by rupture of a vasa vasorum with subsequent formation of an intramural hematoma. This intramural hematoma separates the medial layers and produces an intimal tear, which allows the hematoma to communicate with the vascular lumen. Once this connection is established, the force of aortic pressure continues the process of dissection.[61]

Aortic aneurysms may be congenital or acquired. The most common congenital aneurysms include those arising from a sinus of Valsalva and those associated with Marfan's syndrome and other connective tissue disorders. Acquired aneurysms may result from atherosclerosis, idiopathic cystic medial necrosis, syphilis, trauma, or infection (mycotic aneurysms).[61]

Regardless of their cause or location, aneurysms of the aorta result from disease of the musculoelastic media, which is the major barrier against aortic pressure. Deterioration of the media progressively weakens the aortic wall, resulting in dilation at the site of involvement. Dilation increases wall stress in the affected region, which may lead to continued local expansion and, finally, to rupture.

Congenital Aneurysms of the Aorta

Sinus of Valsalva Aneurysm. Congenital aneurysms of the sinuses of Valsalva appear to result from a lack of continuity between the media of the aortic root and the annulus of the aortic valve.[241] These aneurysms are reported to involve the right coronary sinus in approximately 69% of cases, the noncoronary sinus in 26%, and the left coronary sinus in 5%.[242] Aneurysmal involvement of more than one sinus has also been reported.[243] Because the sinuses are largely intracardiac, their relationship to adjacent structures determines the direction of aneurysmal expansion and the site of rupture.[244–246] Aneurysms of the right coronary sinus tend to project the right ventricle and, occasionally, the right atrium, whereas those of the noncoronary sinus almost invariably project into the right atrium.[247] More rarely, sinus of Valsalva aneurysms may protrude into the right ventricular outflow tract, causing outflow obstruction;[248,249] dissect into the interventricular septum and then rupture into the right or left ventricles;[250,251] or communicate directly with the left atrium, ventricle, or pericardial space. Occasionally, dilation of a sinus may cause prolapse of the associated aortic leaflet with resulting valvular insufficiency.[252–255]

Echocardiographically, sinus of Valsalva aneurysms are best identified in a parasternal short axis view of the aortic root. The aneurysmal sinus is typically larger and has a thinner wall than the adjacent nonaffected sinuses. Figure 19–97 is a short axis recording of a right coronary sinus aneurysm that illustrates these features. Transesophageal recordings may also aid in defining the presence and extent of sinus of Valsalva aneurysms. Figure 19–98 illustrates a large aneurysm of the right coronary sinus that almost completely fills the right ventricle, causing both restriction to inflow and an outflow gradient.

When a sinus ruptures, the resulting echocardiographic pattern is determined largely by the size of the

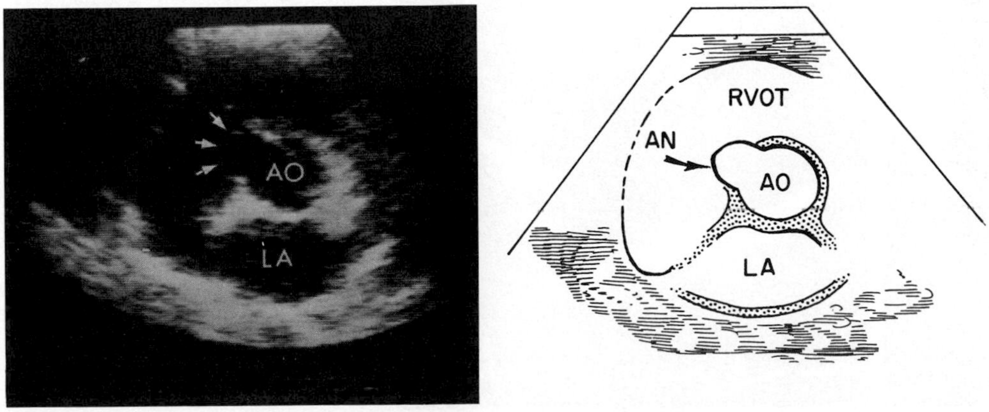

Fig. 19–97. Parasternal short axis recording illustrates aneurysmal dilation (AN) of the right coronary sinus of Valsalva. The aneurysm is thin-walled and, in this instance, projects into the right atrium. RVOT = right ventricular outflow tract; AO = aorta; LA = left atrium.

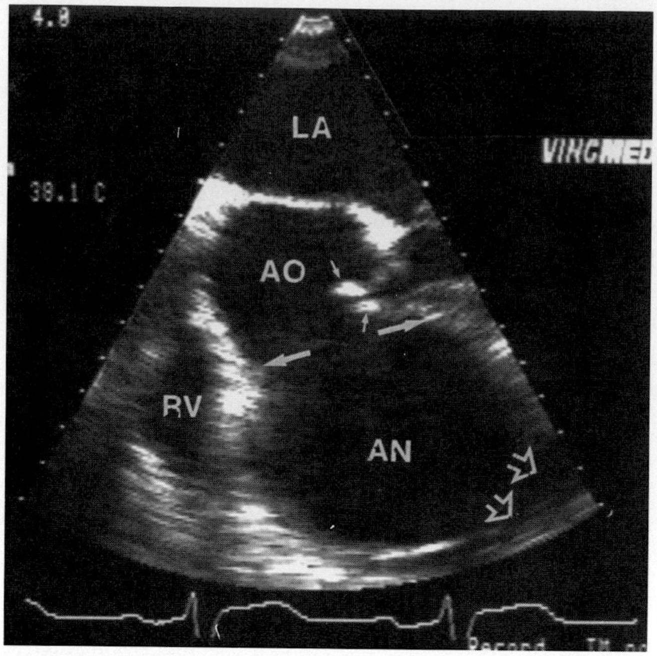

Fig. 19–98. Transesophageal recording of a massive sinus of Valsalva aneurysm that fills the right ventricle. The aneurysm (AN) obstructed right ventricular filling and produced an outflow gradient at catheterization. RV = right ventricle; LA = left atrium; AO = aorta. Small arrows point to aortic valve leaflets; larger horizontal arrows indicate expected position of aortic wall; open arrows indicate the inferior margins of the aneurysm. (Courtesy of Dr. Alan Weiss.)

leak, the rapidity with which the leak develops, and the chamber that receives the shunt flow. Color flow mapping allows rapid diagnosis and localization of the shunt flow associated with a ruptured sinus of Valsalva aneurysm (Fig. 19–99). Continuous wave Doppler is generally required to resolve the high velocities generated by the aortic to right heart pressure gradient. Because the aortic pressure is generally higher in both systole and diastole than that in the receiving chamber, high velocity turbulent flow is typically recorded throughout the cardiac cycle. Doppler is also useful in detecting the presence of associated abnormalities such as VSD or aortic regurgitation. When the shunt is into the right side of the heart, the increased flow must pass through the pulmonary artery, the left atrium, and the left ventricle before reaching the aorta again. Therefore, a left ventricular volume overload pattern can always be expected. When the aneurysm ruptures into the right ventricle, volume overload of this chamber is also present, whereas rupture into the right atrium causes volume overload of both the right atrium and ventricle. Despite the right ventricular volume overload, paradoxic septal motion should not be expected, because the right and left ventricular volume loads should balance each other. Rupture into the right side of the heart has also been associated with premature opening of the pulmonary valve caused by the rapid rise in right ventricular diastolic pressure.[256]

Differential diagnosis of sinus of Valsalva aneurysm includes coronary arteriovenous fistula and membranous aneurysm of the ventricular septum. In coronary arteriovenous fistula, a tubular structure is seen on the parasternal short axis view of the aorta reflecting the presence of the fistulous tract. This may mimic the presence of a sinus of Valsalva aneurysm, but dilation of the coronary artery feeding the fistula should suggest the true diagnosis. An aneurysm of the membranous ventricular septum may also be mistaken for a sinus of Valsalva aneurysm. Careful short axis scanning of the left ventricular outflow tract and aortic root in short axis allows the appropriate diagnosis to be established, because a membranous VSD arises below the aortic annulus, whereas a sinus of Valsalva aneurysm originates between the annulus and the supravalvular ridge. However, clear separation is occasionally difficult because a membranous VSD extending into the interleaflet tri-

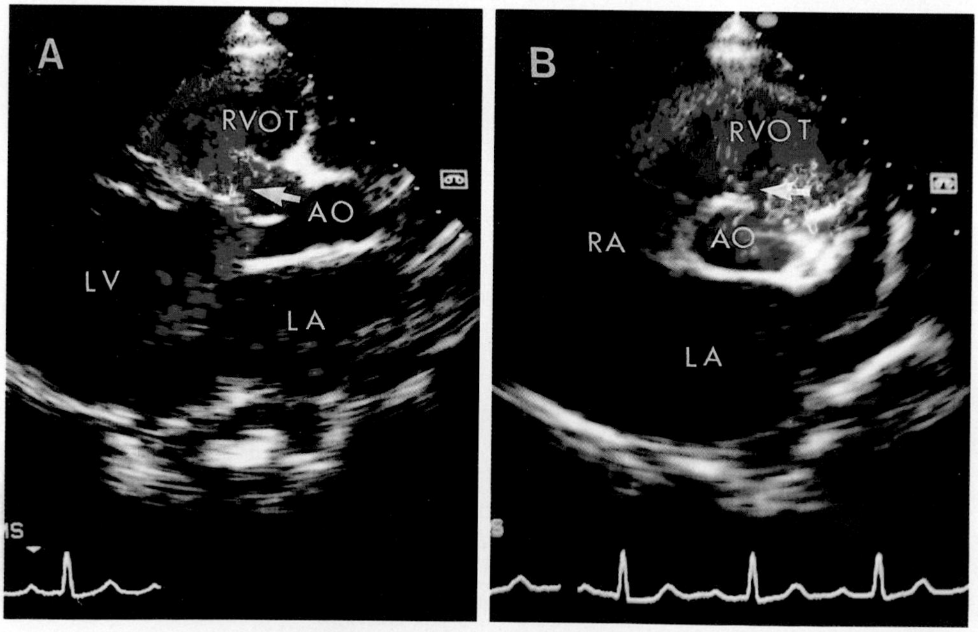

Fig. 19–99. Color Doppler recordings of a sinus of Valsalva aneurysm that has ruptured into the right ventricular outflow tract (RVOT). The aortoventricular shunt is depicted in red as it swirls in the outflow tract. (Courtesy of Dr. Leng Jiang.) AO = aorta; LA = left atrium; LV = left ventricle; RA = right atrium.

gones may arise at almost the same level as an aneurysm of the adjacent sinus. Differentiation must then be based on the timing of the shunt flow: systolic for the VSD and both systolic and diastolic for the ruptured sinus aneurysm. In cases of diagnostic uncertainty, higher resolution images of the aortic root and sinuses can be obtained from the esophagus. Acquired sinus of Valsalva aneurysm is seen in endocarditis and may mimic the congenital appearance.

Marfan's Syndrome. Marfan's syndrome is a generalized disorder of connective tissue inherited as an autosomal dominant trait. Marfan's syndrome is characterized by abnormalities of the eye (myopia and ectopia lentis); the skeletal system (excessive limb length, loose joints, kyphoscoliosis, arachnodactyly, pectus excavatum, and pectus carinatum); and the cardiovascular system.[257] Cardiovascular abnormalities include aortic aneurysm, which may be complicated by dissection; aortic insufficiency that is due to dilation of the aortic root and annulus; and myxomatous degeneration of the aortic leaflets.[257–259] Myxomatous degeneration of the mitral valve and chordal apparatus is also frequently noted.[257–259] Cardiovascular abnormalities are seen in a majority of patients with classic features of Marfan's syndrome, with both aortic root dilation and mitral valve prolapse reported in up to 70% of patients.[260,261] Obviously, the true prevalence of cardiovascular abnormalities depends on the age of the population studied and the diagnostic criteria used for mitral valve prolapse. Nevertheless, cardiovascular involvement is the most important cause of premature death in this condition, accounting for up to 95% of all mortality. Aortic dissection is the most common cardiac cause of death.[262]

Cardiac abnormalities tend to be progressive and are believed to represent the response of the defective connective tissue to hemodynamic stress.[257,263] This hypothesis is supported by the fact that such abnormalities are less pronounced and rarely involve the aortic root in children, whereas in adults, the abnormalities center about areas of greatest hemodynamic stress—the left-sided cardiac valves and the proximal aorta.[258] The primary defect underlying the aortic root abnormality of Marfan's syndrome is unknown. Histologically, there is a striking loss of medial elastic tissue in the affected segment, disorganization of smooth muscle bundles, and an increase in collagen with focal accumulation of mucopolysaccharide.[257–259,263]

Echocardiographically, the aortic root is typically dilated (often massively), and the aortic walls appear thin. The pattern of dilation is unique in that it involves the annulus, sinuses of Valsalva, and the distal ascending aorta, symmetrically.[264] Massive enlargement of sinuses of Valsalva is a characteristic feature of this condition. Aortic root enlargement may be so great that left atrial compression is seen.[260] The aortic leaflets are elongated and may prolapse. With increased dilation of the aortic root, failure of adequate coaptation of the aortic leaflets may occur with resultant aortic insufficiency and left ventricular volume overload. Aortic dissection is a common complication (see following discussion).

Figure 19–100 illustrates the characteristic aortic valve and root involvement in Marfan's syndrome. In long axis (Fig. 19–100A), the aortic root is markedly dilated, and the aortic leaflets are elongated. The pronounced dilation at the level of the sinuses of Valsalva compresses the left atrium from above, thereby reducing its anteroposterior expanse. In short axis (Fig. 19–100B), the marked dilation of the aortic root is again evident, as is the symmetric dilation of the three sinuses of Valsalva. The extended commissure of the coapted aortic leaflets can also be appreciated.

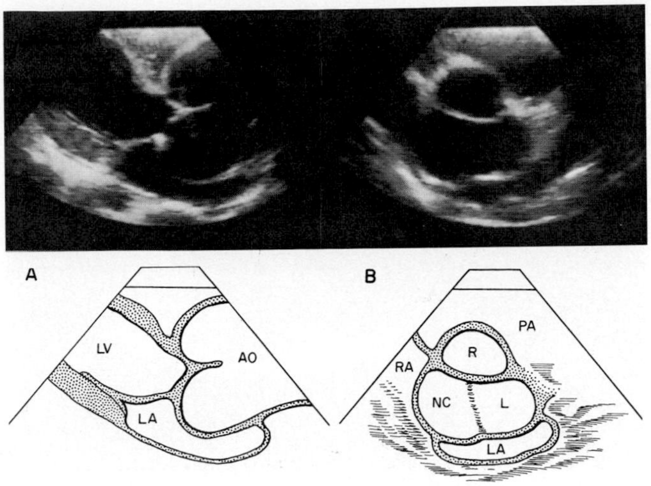

Fig. 19–100. Aneurysmal dilation of the aortic root in Marfan's syndrome. **A.** Parasternal long axis recording of the aortic root illustrates the dilation of the aortic root and the thinning of the vascular wall, which are characteristic of Marfan's syndrome. The prominent posterior sinus of Valsalva compresses the left atrium (LA) from above. The aortic leaflets appear thin and elongated. **B.** Short axis recording illustrates the symmetric dilation of the three sinuses of Valsalva. Although only one coaptation line is apparent in this recording, the valve was tricuspid. PA = pulmonary artery; R = right coronary aortic cusp; NC = noncoronary aortic cusp; L = left coronary aortic cusp; RA = right atrium; AO = aorta; LV = left ventricle.

Echo-Doppler studies are an important part of the routine follow-up of patients with Marfan's syndrome to detect changes in aortic root size and the development of complications. Because of the high premature mortality—survival beyond the fourth decade being rare in unoperated groups—the current practice is to perform prophylactic aortic valve and root replacement once the aortic root diameter exceeds 6 cm.[265,266] Once the aortic root diameter reaches 5 cm, more frequent echocardiographic evaluations of root size are required. Echocardiography has also been used to screen for the presence of cardiovascular abnormalities in first degree relatives of patients with Marfan's syndrome.[261,267] The appearance of the aorta in other connective tissue disorders is similar to that of Marfan's syndrome. Figure 19–101, for example, is a recording from a patient with Ehlers-Danlos syndrome in which diffuse aneurysmal dilation of the aorta is also present.

Acquired Aneurysms

Four types of acquired aortic aneurysms can be detected echocardiographically: dissecting aneurysms,

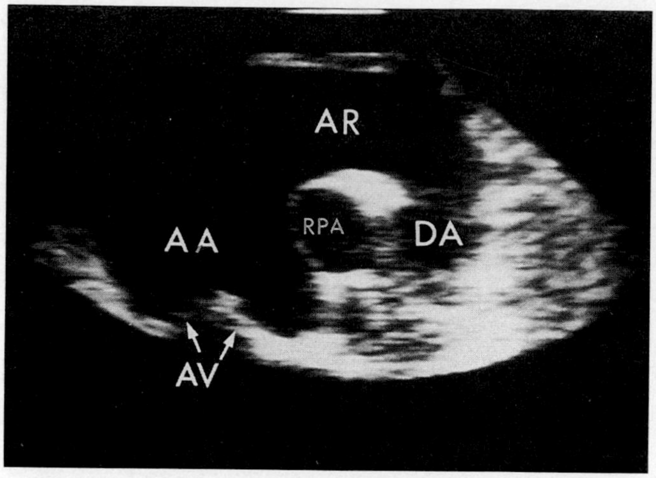

Fig. 19–101. Diffuse dilation of the ascending aorta (AA) and aortic arch (AR) in a patient with Ehlers-Danlos syndrome. AV = aortic valve; DA = descending aorta; RPA = right pulmonary artery.

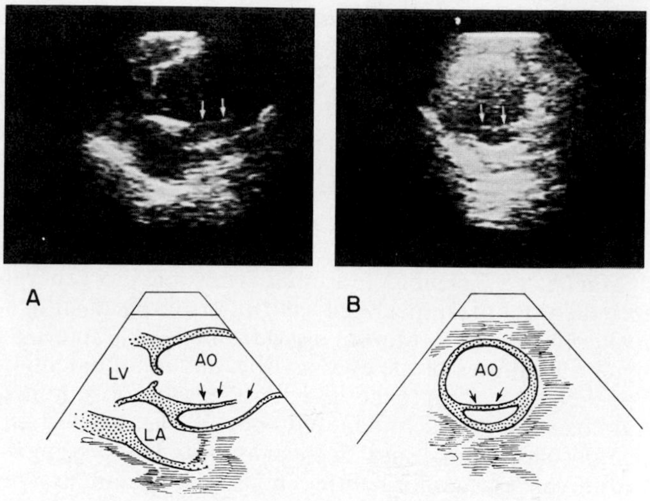

Fig. 19–102. Long and short axis recordings of the aortic root illustrate an isolated posterior dissection. The intimal flap is indicated by the vertical arrowheads. The aortic root is markedly dilated. LV = left ventricle; LA = left atrium; AO = aorta.

atherosclerotic aneurysms, traumatic aneurysms, and mycotic aneurysms (see Chapter 37).[264]

Dissecting Aneurysms. Dissecting aneurysms develop as a result of degenerative or destructive disease of the aortic media, usually in association with systemic hypertension.[268–270] The most common underlying cause is idiopathic cystic medial necrosis. Dissection may also occur in other conditions that are associated with weakening of the aortic media or that place an increased stress on the aortic wall, such as Marfan's syndrome, Ehlers-Danlos syndrome, idiopathic kyphoscoliosis, Turner's syndrome, and coarctation of the aorta. Dissection may also be seen in younger women in the third trimester of pregnancy and following cardiac surgery. Dissecting aneurysms are categorized into three types.[271] Both type 1 and type 2 dissections have their origin in the proximal ascending aorta; type 1 extends into the descending thoracic aorta, whereas type 2 is confined to the ascending aorta. Type 3 dissections originate in the descending thoracic aorta; occasionally, these may track back into the ascending aorta but most commonly they propagate antegradely.

Echocardiographically, dissecting aneurysms are characterized by local or generalized dilation of the aorta and by separation of the normal single dominant echo from the aortic wall in the region of the dissection into two discrete echoes that generally move in unison with one another (Figs. 19–102 and 19–103).[264,272,273] The inner echo arises from the tunica intima, whereas the outer echo arises from the medial and adventitial structures external to the tear. Because dissection may involve any portion of the aorta, the entire vessel must be examined in detail to exclude dissection. Absence of aortic dilation is strong evidence against dissection, but rare exceptions do occur. Additional imaging features that may aid in diagnosis include swirling echoes (spontaneous contrast) and thrombus in the false lumen resulting from reduced flow (Fig. 19–104).[274,275] Color flow mapping can document reduced or absent flow in the false lumen or flow directed opposite to that in the true lumen[275–277] (Fig. 19–105B). The site of communication between true and false lumen has also been demonstrated by color flow mapping[275,276] (Figs. 19–105C and 19–106).

Transthoracic echocardiographic imaging has been reported to be from 79 to 100% sensitive, and up to 90% specific in the detection of aortic root dissection.[278–280] Higher resolution images of the ascending and descending thoracic aorta can be obtained from the esophagus, and in a recent multicenter study,[281] the sensitivity and

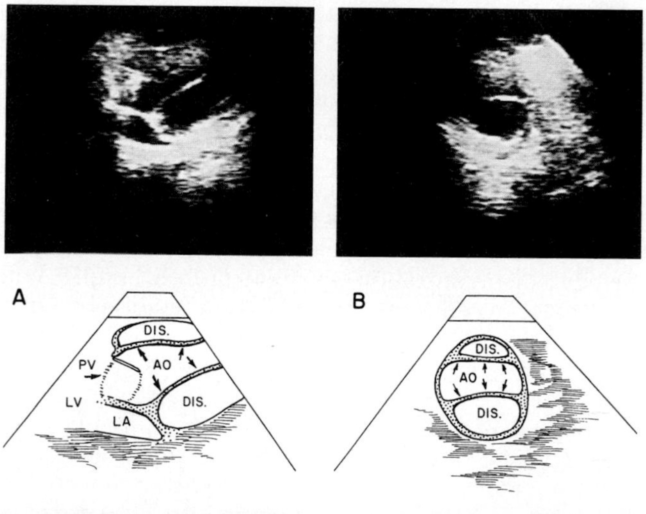

Fig. 19–103. Parasternal long and short axis recordings of the ascending aorta illustrate aortic dissection (DIS). **A.** In the long-axis recording, large echo-free space posterior to the aortic root and a smaller, anterior, echo-free space are produced by the dissection. The aortic intima is indicated by the vertical arrowheads. A Starr-Edwards valve is present in the aortic position. **B.** In the short-axis view, the posterior dissection elevates the intima from below. This pattern suggests that the pressure in the false channel is high enough to deform the aorta (AO) and thus excludes the left atrium as a possible cause of this echo-free area. PV = prosthetic valve; LV = left ventricle; LA = left atrium.

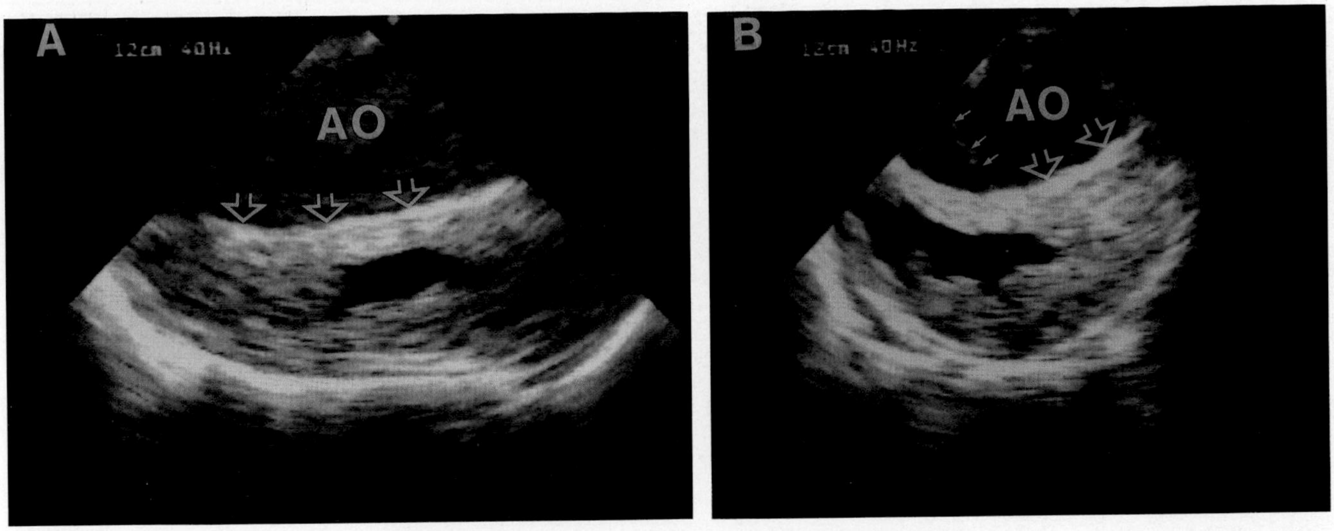

Fig. 19–104. Transesophageal long (A) and short (B) axis recordings illustrating a large dissecting aneurysm with the false lumen filled with thrombus (open arrows). The true lumen also shows evidence of thrombus (small closed arrows) and "smoke" indicative of stagnant flow.

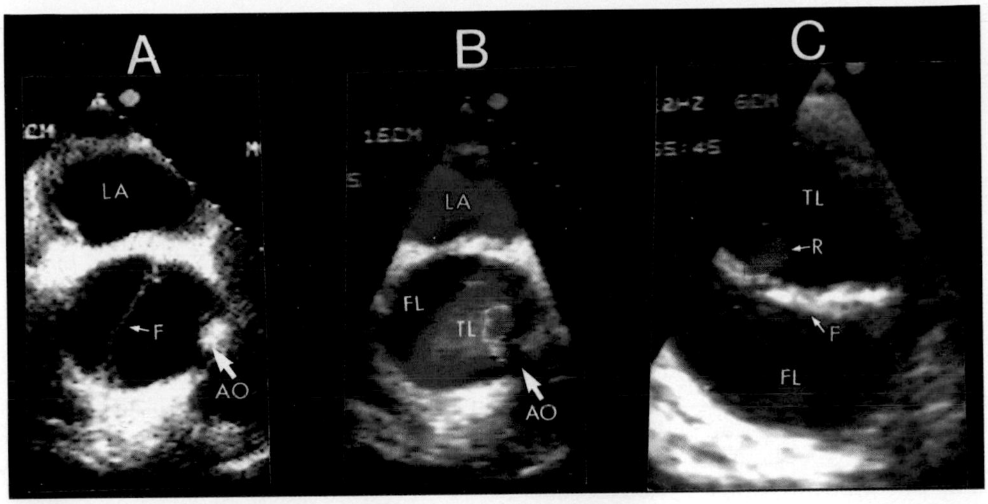

Fig. 19–105. Color flow Doppler recording from a patient with a dissection of the ascending aorta. **A.** Dissection flap is shown in the center of the aorta. **B.** Color recording in which flow (blue) is evident in the true channel but not in the false channel. **C.** Color Doppler recording of the descending aorta showing the distal site of communication between the true and false lumens. TL = true lumen; LA = left atrium; FL = false lumen; F = dissection flap; AO = aorta; R = site of flow reentry.

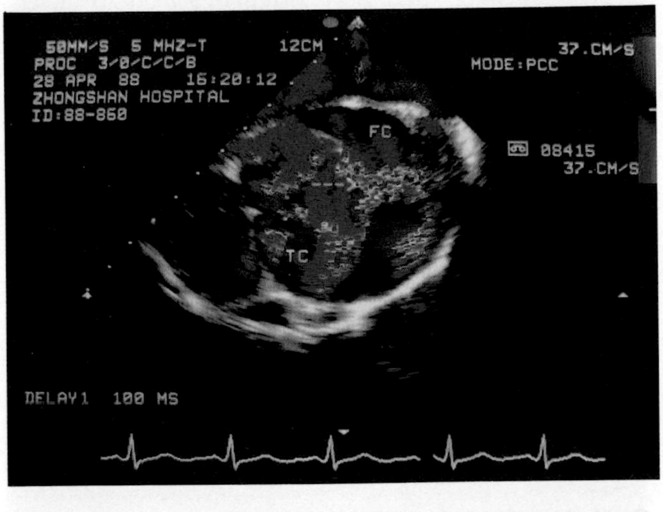

Fig. 19–106. Transesophageal color flow recording of the ascending aorta in a patient with acute dissection, illustrating flow (arrow) from the true channel (TC) or lumen into the false channel (FC). (Courtesy of Dr. Leng Jiang.)

specificity of transesophageal echocardiography in the detection of aortic dissection were 99 and 98%, respectively. These values were equivalent to or superior to those obtained using other invasive and noninvasive techniques.[281] The extent of dissection can be mapped by sequential examination of the ascending aorta, the arch, and the descending aorta using transthoracic imaging (Fig. 19–107), transesophageal imaging, or a combination of both. Although the esophagus provides clearer definition of the primary lesion and often permits involvement of the coronary ostia to be visualized, the interposition of the trachea between the esophagus and the distal portion of ascending aorta and the proximal arch may prevent adequate imaging of this portion of the aorta with a transversely mounted esophageal transducer. Similarly, imaging of the major branches of the aortic arch may not be possible from the esophagus, but these branches are generally accessible from the suprasternal notch. With biplane transesophageal imaging, the longitudinal transducer allows the aorta to be exam-

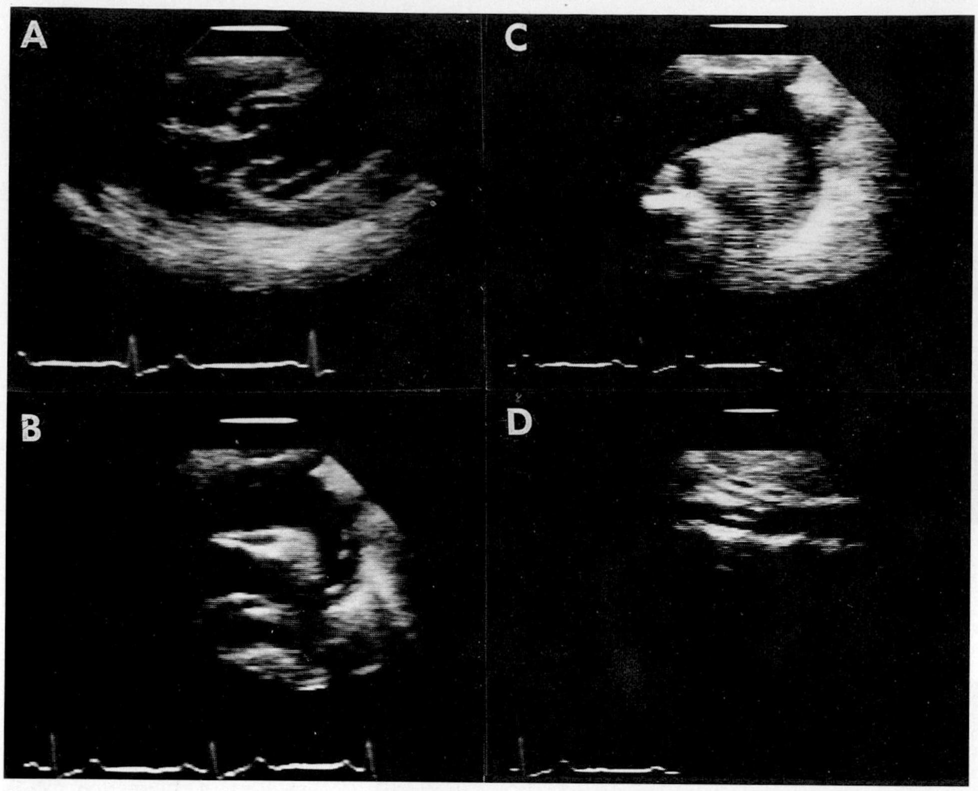

Fig. 19–107. Series of two-dimensional echocardiographic recordings that map the extent of a dissection from its origin as a spiral flap at the level of the aortic valve **(A)** into the ascending aorta **(B)**; around the arch and into the descending thoracic aorta **(C)**; and finally into the abdominal aorta **(D)**.

ined in long axis and generally increases the extent of the aorta that can be reliably imaged,[282] but external evaluation is still necessary to assess branch vessel involvement.

Although the diagnostic accuracy of transthoracic and particularly transesophageal echocardiography in the detection of aortic dissection is excellent, false-positives and false-negatives can occur. False-positives may be due to reverberations distal to atherosclerotic plaques or intravascular catheters as well as side lobe and other interference patterns in the sound field.[281] Flow separation on color flow mapping at the site of the presumed dissection improves the diagnostic specificity. False-negatives may be due to inadequate imaging of the aorta or thrombosis of the false lumen simulating a saccular atherosclerotic aortic aneurysm.[279] Echocardiography can also detect the sequelae of aortic dissection such as aortic regurgitation and pericardial effusion and assess their hemodynamic impact.

Atherosclerotic Aneurysms. Atherosclerosis is now the most common cause of aortic aneurysm formation. These aneurysms have a predilection for the abdominal aorta, particularly, the infrarenal segment. However, approximately 25% of atherosclerotic aneurysms affect the ascending or descending thoracic aorta.[283] Atherosclerotic aortic aneurysms confined to the proximal ascending aorta are readily imaged by transthoracic echocardiography using the parasternal long and short axis windows.[264,284] Transesophageal imaging facilitates diagnosis of both ascending and descending thoracic aortic aneurysms[285] and is particularly helpful in differentiating atherosclerotic from dissecting aneurysms.[286] Differentiation can be aided by the visualization of asymmetric thrombus and diffuse swirling echoes suggestive of low flow within thoracic aneurysms (Fig. 19–108).

Traumatic Aneurysms. Traumatic aneurysms arise most commonly in the isthmic region between the left subclavian artery and ligamentum arteriosum.[287] Although these aneurysms are of major clinical importance, no specific echocardiographic features that separate traumatic from other types of aneurysms. Thus, diagnosis is based on local or more generalized dilation of the vessel with or without dissection and an appropriate history. Diverticula at the origin of the ductus arteri-

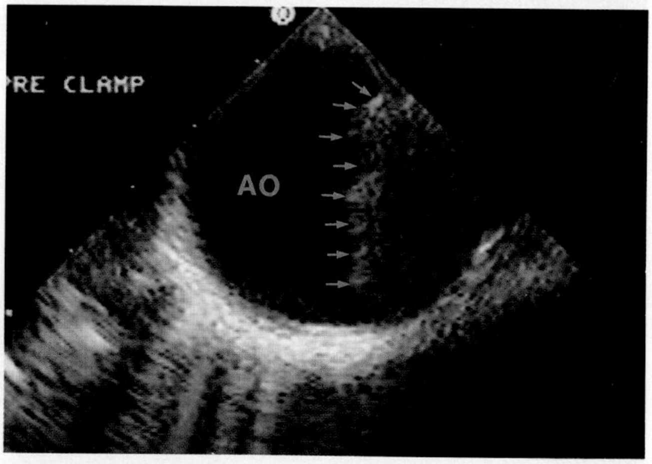

Fig. 19–108. Transesophageal short axis recording illustrating thrombus (arrows) within a dilated aorta (AO).

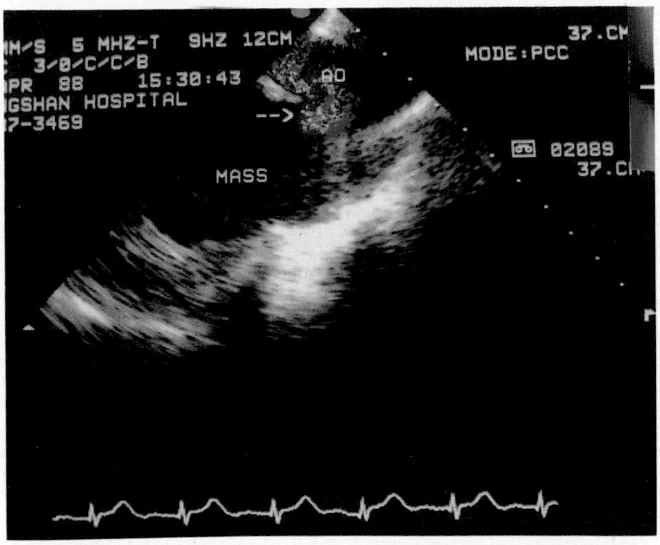

Fig. 19–109. Transesophageal short axis recording illustrating a pseudoaneurysm of the aorta with a large accumulation of thrombus (mass) outside the vessel wall. The arrow indicates the local area of flow within and extending slightly beyond the vessel wall. AO = aorta. (Courtesy of Dr. Leng Jiang.)

osus have also been described using transesophageal echocardiography.[286]

Pseudoaneurysm of the Aorta. Pseudoaneurysm or rupture of the aorta may occur as a result of trauma, penetration, of an ulcerative atherosclerotic plaque, infection, or following ductal ligation. Rupture of the ascending aorta into the pericardium usually leads to rapid cardiac compression and death. However, when the descending thoracic aorta ruptures, but the adventitia remains intact, bleeding into the adventitia is contained by the pleura and other mediastinal tissues, and a false aneurysm can develop, limiting the rupture. The continuity of flow is maintained by thrombus in the false aneurysm.[288–290]

Echocardiographically, the false aneurysm typically shows an area of flow within the wall of the aorta, extending a variable distance beyond the lumen. Figure 19–109 is an example of a false aneurysm recorded from the esophageal window. Flow is present within the aorta and extends slightly beyond the lumen in the area of rupture. The large mass posterior to the lumen was demonstrated at surgery to be a large extravascular thrombus.

Aortico-Left Ventricular Tunnel

Aortico-left ventricular tunnel is a rare congenital condition in which there is an abnormal tunnel-like communication between the ascending aorta and the left ventricle.[291] This communication bypasses the aortic valve and is considered to have an extracardiac and intracardiac segment. Typically, the tunnel originates from the upper portion of a dilated right sinus of Valsalva, passes between the aortic annulus and pulmonary trunk (the extracardiac segment), and continues through the interventricular septum to enter the left ventricle beneath the aortic commissure between the right and left cusps (intracardiac segment). Hemodynamically, this condition simulates severe aortic regurgitation, and patients with aortico-left ventricular tunnel present at birth or in the early neonatal period with severe congestive heart failure. Associated developmental abnormalities are

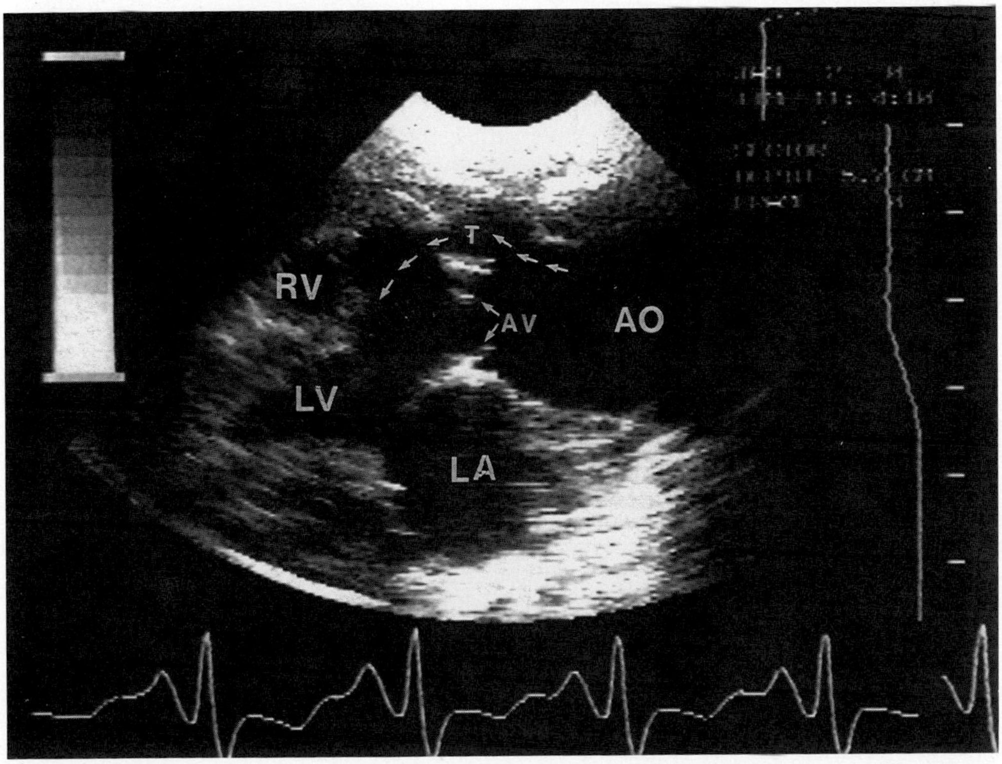

Fig. 19–110. Parasternal long axis recording of an aortoventricular tunnel. The tunnel (T) courses above the aortic valve (AV) to connect the aorta (AO) and left ventricle (LV) directly. The angled small arrows point to the aortic valve leaflets. The curvilinear small arrows indicate the path of retrograde flow through the tunnel. LA = left atrium; RV = right ventricle.

common and include bicuspid aortic valve, pulmonary stenosis, and VSD.[291]

Echocardiographically, two conduits for the passage of blood between the aorta and left ventricle are apparent.[292–294] The anterior conduit represents the aortico-left ventricular tunnel, whereas the posterior conduit represents the left ventricular outflow tract. On the parasternal and apical long axis views, the anterior conduit is seen to communicate with the right sinus of Valsalva at its aortic end (Fig. 19–110). Echo dropout is seen in the interventricular septum below the aortic valve representing the opening of the conduit into the left ventricle. On the parasternal short axis view, the aortico-left ventricular tunnel is seen as a crescent-shaped structure distinct from the aorta that passes anterior to the right coronary cusp. The ascending aorta is frequently dilated. Doppler interrogation of the tunnel demonstrates retrograde flow into the left ventricle during diastole and antegrade flow into the aorta in systole.[295] The echocardiographic appearances may simulate VSD, sinus of Valsalva aneurysm, or coronary arteriovenous fistula. The detection of two anatomically symmetric conduits for passage of blood between the left ventricle and aorta on the parasternal long axis view should suggest the true diagnosis.

THE SUBVALVULAR LEFT VENTRICULAR OUTFLOW TRACT

The subvalvular portion of the left ventricular outflow tract is a funnel-shaped area extending from the free edges of the mitral leaflets to the aortic annulus. It is bounded anteriorly by the interventricular septum and posteriorly by the anterior mitral leaflet. Disorders of primary interest in this region are those that obstruct left ventricular outflow. In this chapter, only fixed subvalvular obstructive lesions will be detailed. IHSS and functional subvalvular aortic stenosis are discussed in Chapter 25.

Discrete Subaortic Stenosis

Discrete subvalvular aortic stenosis is a relatively frequent cause of left ventricular outflow obstruction and accounts for approximately 10% of all cases of childhood aortic stenosis.[296,297] This obstruction is generally caused by either a thin discrete, fibrous membrane located immediately below the aortic valve and obstructing an otherwise normal outflow tract (type 1) or a thick, fibrous ring associated with muscular hypertrophy and located approximately 1 cm below the valve and extending downward 1 to 2 cm (type 2).[298] The type 2 lesions not only produce a more diffuse area of left ventricular outflow obstruction but also frequently encroach on the anterior mitral leaflet. A third variety, the fibromuscular tunnel, may narrow the outflow tract for several centimeters.[299,300] Subvalvular tunnels are relatively uncommon, representing only 6 to 20%[299] of fixed subvalvular obstructive lesions. The subvalvular tunnels, however, produce the greatest deformity of the subvalvular region.

Separation of the various types of subvalvular obstruction is important because, as a rule, simple surgical resection of the thin membrane relieves the obstruction in type 1 lesions, whereas fibromuscular rings and subvalvular tunnels require more extensive fibromuscular revision of the outflow tract with frequent, residual obstruction.[298] Associated defects are common in the discrete subvalvular stenoses and are present in from 10 to 57% of reported cases. The most common associated lesions are VSDs and areas of obstruction at other levels of the left ventricular outflow tract such as bicuspid aortic valve and coarctation.[299] The high velocity jet produced by the subaortic obstruction often leads to thickening of the aortic valve leaflets and aortic incompetence. Left ventricular outflow obstruction that is due to a discrete subvalvular membrane developing after aortic valve replacement has also been reported, but the exact pathogenesis remains unclear.[301]

Echocardiographically, discrete areas of subvalvular obstruction may be visualized in a parasternal long axis, apical long axis and apical five-chamber views. The diagnosis of subaortic obstruction should be entertained whenever the distance between the anterior mitral leaflet and interventricular septum is narrower than the diameter of the aortic annulus.[302] Short axis scanning of the outflow tract in an attempt to directly record the decrease in outflow area has proved less useful because precise alignment of the short axis scan plane across the area of maximal obstruction is difficult.

Early systolic closure of one or more of the aortic valve leaflets is also frequently associated with subaortic obstruction (Fig. 19–111). The aortic valve closure begins immediately after maximal excursion and the affected leaflets remain substantially closed for the remainder of systole. Coarse systolic fluttering of the valve leaflets is also typical. Early systolic closure of the aortic valve may occur in other conditions such as aortic root dilation but is rarely of the severity or duration of that recorded in subaortic stenoses.[303–306] In hypertrophic cardiomyopathy, systolic aortic valve closure is also seen, but this is usually recorded in midsystole rather than in early systole. Early systolic closure may be absent in subaortic stenosis if the aortic valve is thickened or bicuspid.[305]

Although several mechanisms have been postulated to account for early systolic closure of the aortic valve, the leaflets consistently assume a position parallel to the margins of the flow stream distal to the stenotic orifice. This position presumably reflects the balance of forces created by the low lateral pressure of the jet attracting the leaflets while the forward jet pressure prevents them from actually encroaching on the flow stream.

Discrete Membranous Subaortic Stenosis

Discrete subvalvular membranes appear echocardiographically as thin, linear bands of echoes protruding from both the anterior and posterior margins of the outflow tract immediately beneath the aortic valve.[307–309] The inner margins of the membrane are characteristically more highly reflective than the membrane itself. Figure 19–112 illustrates a thin subvalvular membrane lying immediately beneath the aortic valve. The mem-

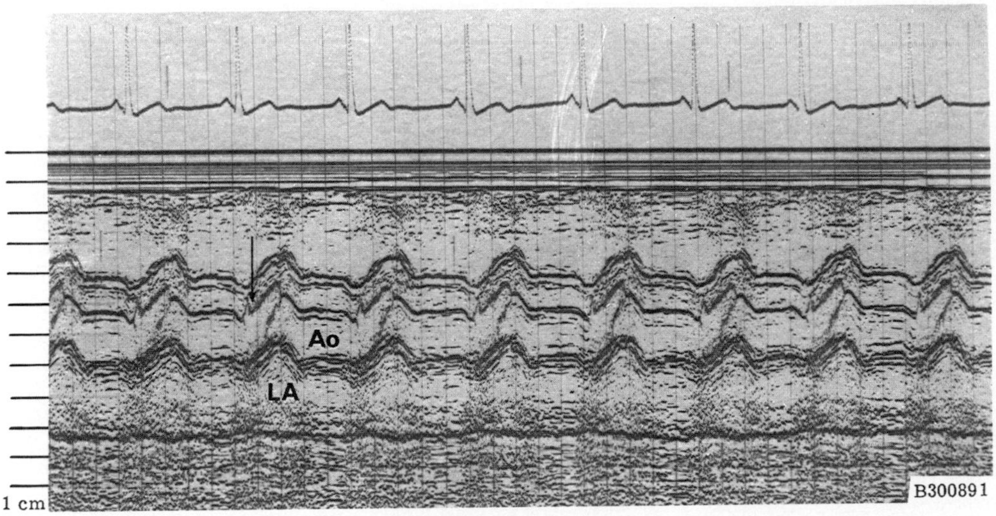

Fig. 19–111. M-mode recording from a patient with discrete subaortic stenosis illustrating the typical early systolic notch (arrow) followed by high frequency fluttering of the valve leaflet throughout the remainder of ejection. Ao = aorta; LA = left atrium. (From Weyman AE, et al.: Cross-sectional echocardiography in evaluating patients with discrete subaortic stenosis. Am J Cardiol 37:358, 1976. Reproduced with permission of Mosby Year-Book, Inc.)

brane extends downward into the outflow tract from the interventricular septum, partially obstructing the outflow area. In this systolic recording, the membrane domes or curves slightly toward the aortic valve. These membranes are generally mobile and move toward the aortic valve during systole and shift back into the left ventricle during diastole. When a membrane is present, the rest of the outflow tract is usually normal, and the subvalvular fibrous curtain, or separation between the insertion of the left and the noncoronary aortic leaflet and the anterior mitral leaflet, is not elongated. Associated disease of the aortic valve is common. In Figure 19–113 the aortic valve is bicuspid and domes slightly in this systolic frame, while in Figure 19–114 the aortic valve is calcified and stenotic. When discrete membranes are difficult to record, the apical views are particularly valuable because they place the membrane perpendicular to the path of the scan plane, thereby enhancing visualization (Fig. 19–115).

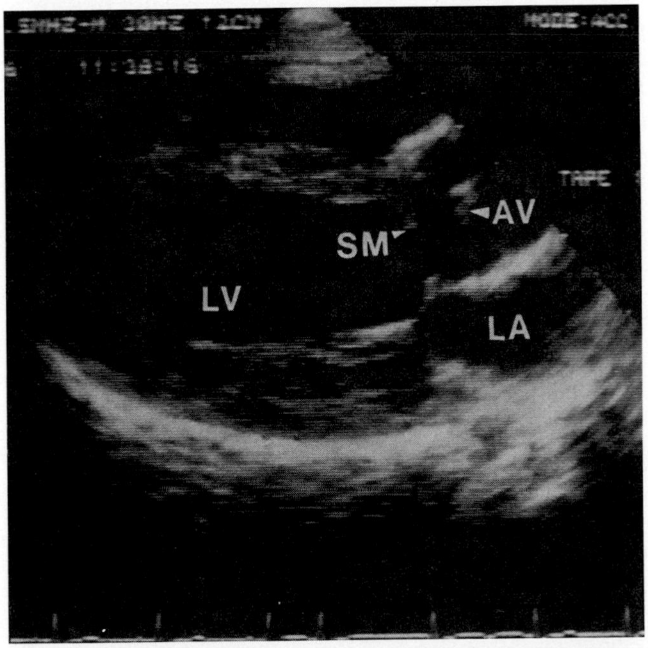

Fig. 19–112. Parasternal long axis recording from a patient with a discrete subvalvular membrane. The membrane (SM) presents as two thin linear bands of echoes arising from the anterior and posterior borders of the outflow tract. The membrane is slightly curved and concave toward the left ventricle. AV = aortic valve; LA = left atrium; LV = left ventricle.

Diffuse Fibromuscular Subvalvular Obstruction

Subvalvular fibromuscular collars or tunnels produce a more extensive area of obstruction, which is characterized by an inward bowing of the echoes from the anterior and posterior margins of the outflow tract immediately below the aortic valve.[300] Both the anterior and posterior borders of the outflow tract must be deformed before this diagnosis can be considered. Focal areas of upper septal hypertrophy, which encroach on the anterior margin of the outflow tract, are common but not as a rule obstructive. Obstructive lesions almost invariably involve the base of the anterior mitral leaflet as well as the upper septum. They elongate the subvalvular fibrous curtain and thereby increase the separation between the noncoronary and the left coronary aortic leaflets and the anterior mitral leaflet. The area of obstruction may extend for several centimeters, with increased narrowing of the outflow space being commonly noted as systole progresses. Figure 19–116 is an example of diffuse subvalvular obstruction. In this example, the area of obstruction is located approximately 1 cm below the aortic valve and extends downward approximately 1.5 cm.

An additional type of outflow obstruction has been noted echocardiographically in one patient. In this case, illustrated in Figure 19–117, a narrow shelf-like protrusion of the basal end of the muscular interventricular septum encroached on the outflow tract from above. A corresponding shelf-like bulge protruded anteriorly from the midportion of the anterior mitral leaflet. Although there was systolic anterior motion of this abnormal anterior leaflet echo, the leaflet abnormality was also present during diastole, suggesting a fixed deformity of the valve associated with an additional functional constrictive component.

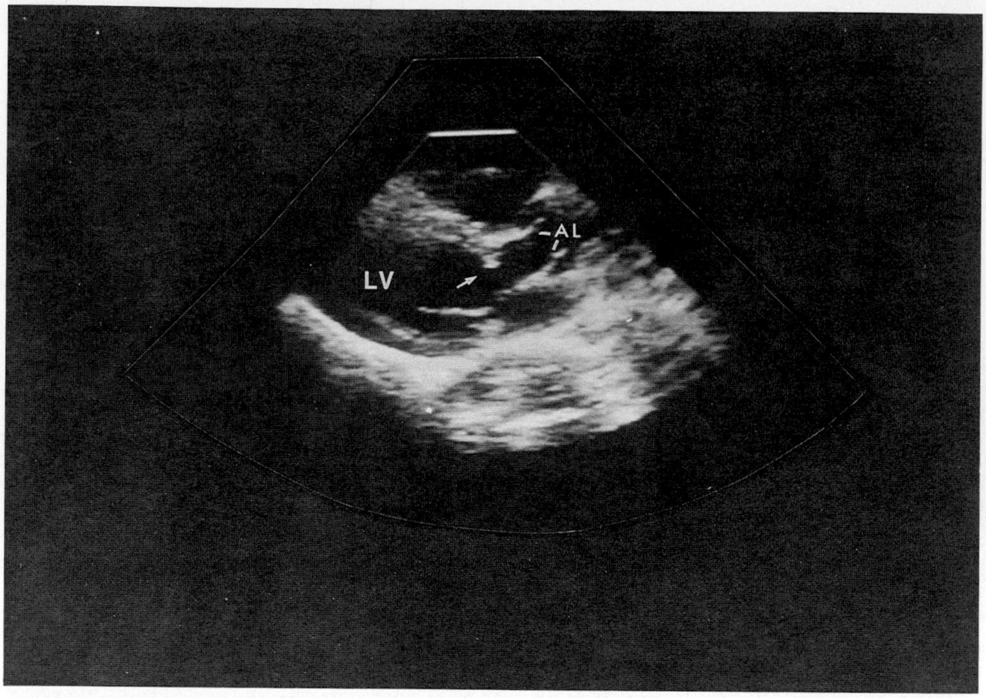

Fig. 19–113. Parasternal long axis recording from a patient with a discrete subvalvular membrane and a bicuspid aortic valve. The membrane (arrow) projects downward from the base of the interventricular septum and is associated with a slight elevation at the base of the anterior mitral leaflet. There is minimal systolic doming of the bicuspid aortic leaflets (AL). LV = left ventricle.

Postoperative Studies

After surgical intervention, the subvalvular left ventricular outflow tract generally remains abnormal. Residual fragments of the base of the membrane are often visible both anteriorly and posteriorly. These fragments may be isolated or superimposed on more diffuse areas of subvalvular narrowing and are commonly associated with a residual gradient. Figure 19–118 illustrates a recording obtained following surgical resection of a subvalvular membrane. Both basal remnants of the resected membrane and an associated area of more diffuse out-

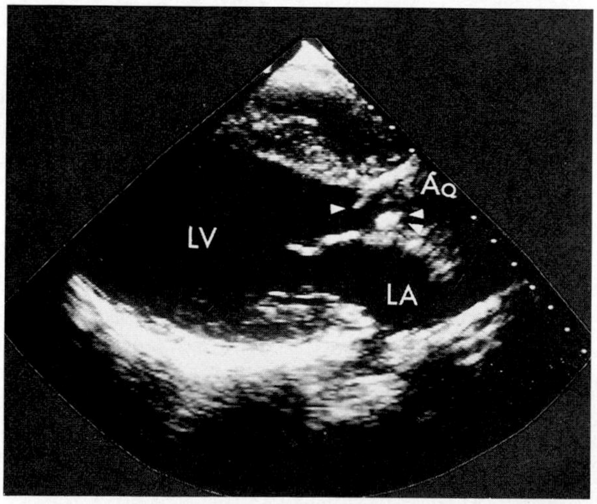

Fig. 19–114. Parasternal long axis recording of a discrete subvalvular membrane (arrowhead) with a stenotic calcified aortic valve (double arrowhead). The membrane in this case points downward toward the left ventricle, which is not an uncommon orientation. LV = left ventricle; Ao = aorta; LA = left atrium.

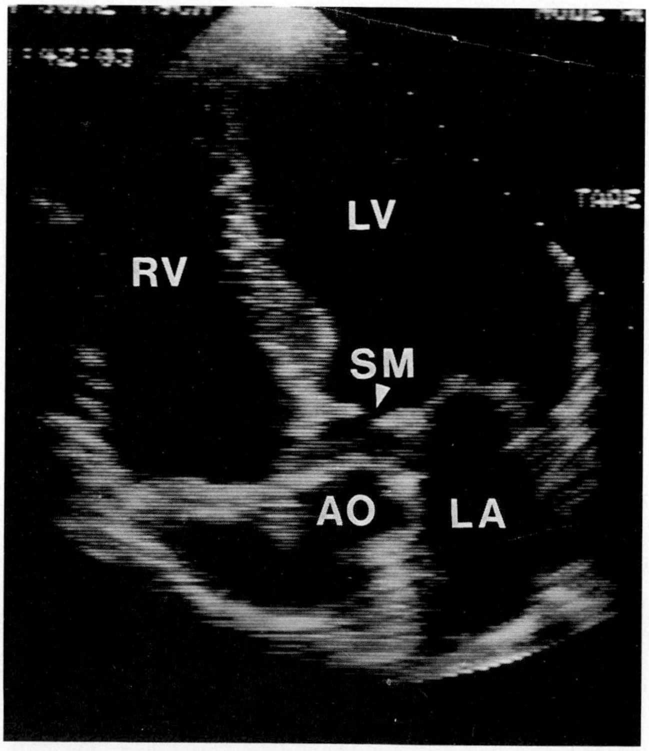

Fig. 19–115. Apical five-chamber recording of a subvalvular membrane (SM). In this view, the membrane is perpendicular to the path of the scan plane, which enhances its visibility. RV = right ventricle; LV = left ventricle; AO = aorta; LA = left atrium.

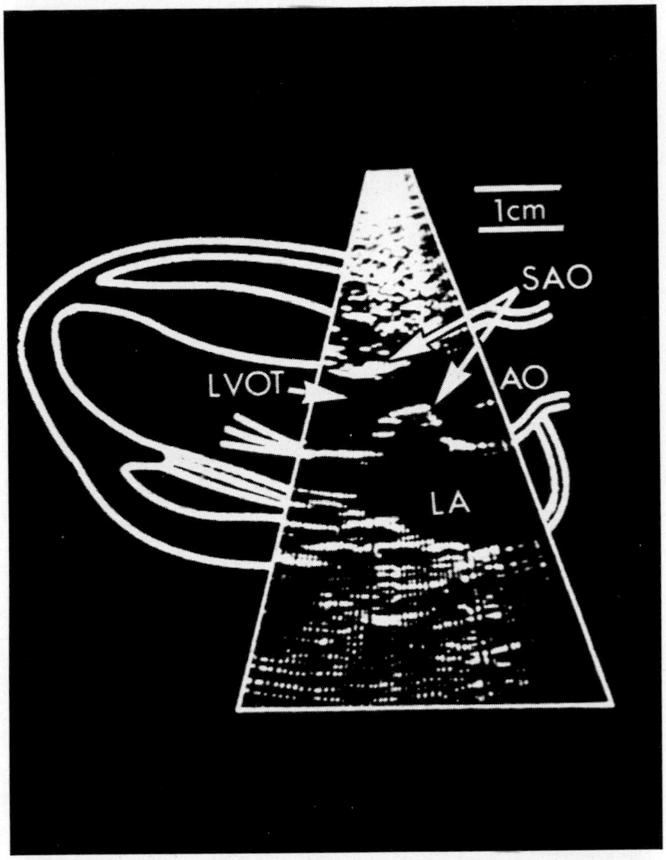

Fig. 19–116. Parasternal long axis recording of the left ventricular outflow tract (LVOT) illustrates diffuse subvalvular aortic obstruction (SAO). In this example, the echoes from the interventricular septum and anterior mitral leaflet bow inward from the anterior and posterior margins of the outflow tract, producing an elongated area of outflow obstruction. AO = aorta; LA = left atrium.

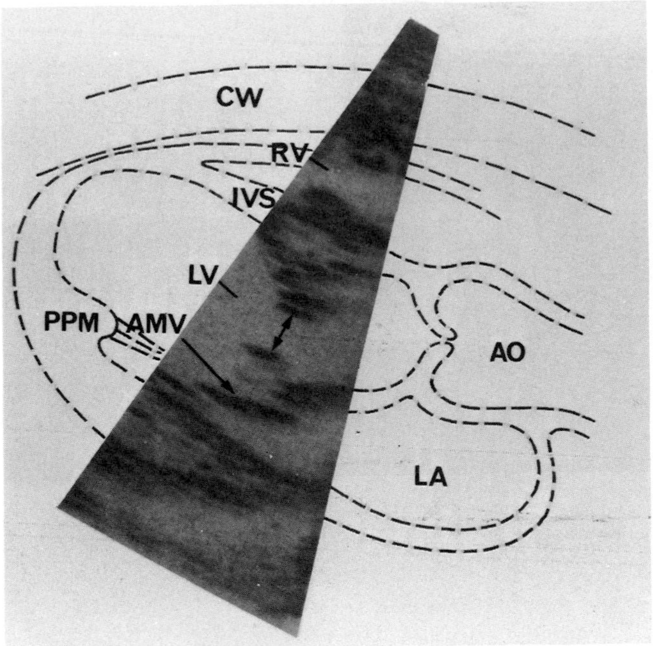

Fig. 19–117. Parasternal long axis scan of the subvalvular left ventricular outflow tract illustrates a third type of fixed subvalvular obstruction. In this example a prominent muscular shelf arises from the base of the interventricular septum (IVS) and is associated with a fixed deformity in the midportion of the anterior mitral leaflet. This type of obstruction can be distinguished from idiopathic hypertrophic subaortic stenosis (IHSS) because the anterior protrusion from the anterior mitral valve (AMV) is present during both systole and diastole, whereas the functional obstruction of IHSS is noted only during the systolic phase of the cardiac cycle. CW = chest wall; RV = right ventricle; LV = left ventricle; PPM = posterior papillary muscle; AO = aorta; LA = left atrium. (From Weyman AE, et al.: Cross-sectional echocardiography in evaluating patients with discrete subaortic stenosis. Am J Cardiol 37:358, 1976. Reproduced with permission of Mosby Year-Book, Inc.)

flow obstruction are present. With more extensive outflow obstruction, the residual postoperative deformity of the outflow tract is usually greater than that noted following simple membrane resection, and in some patients, little change may be seen from the preoperative study.

Doppler Assessment of Subaortic Obstruction

Doppler interrogation of the left ventricular outflow tract is useful in subaortic stenosis.[310] An area of local flow acceleration beneath the aortic valve in the left ventricular outflow tract may initially suggest the diagnosis. Continuous wave Doppler is usually required to fully resolve the high velocities produced by the subaortic obstruction and to determine the peak gradient across the left ventricular outflow tract. Excellent correlations have been reported between Doppler-derived pressure gradients in subaortic stenosis and those measured invasively both in animal models and in patients.[310,311]

Several pitfalls may be encountered when using Doppler in the assessment of the severity of subaortic obstruction. These relate to the shape of the stenosis and the pressure of associated lesions. Shape is more problematic in subvalvular tunnels than in discrete membranes. Flow velocity across discrete membranes generally reflects the local gradient, whereas elongated cylindric stenoses may predispose patients to pressure recovery.[84] In these cases, the Doppler-derived gradient will exceed that measured hemodynamically. The presence of substantive viscous forces may also invalidate the use of the Bernoulli equation in patients with subvalvular tunnels.[69] Associated lesions cause further difficulties in interpreting Doppler data. When there is an associated VSD, the gradient across the subvalvular obstruction may not reflect the severity of obstruction because flow is shunted preferentially across the interventricular septum. In these cases, the real severity of the subaortic obstruction may become evident only after repair of the septal defect.[299,312] When valvular and subvalvular stenosis coexist, a continuous wave Doppler recording of outflow velocities will reflect only the velocity across the lesion causing the greatest convective acceleration. This may not reflect the total pressure drop between the ventricle and aorta, which is the sum of the gradients at the two sites of obstruction. To accurately measure the

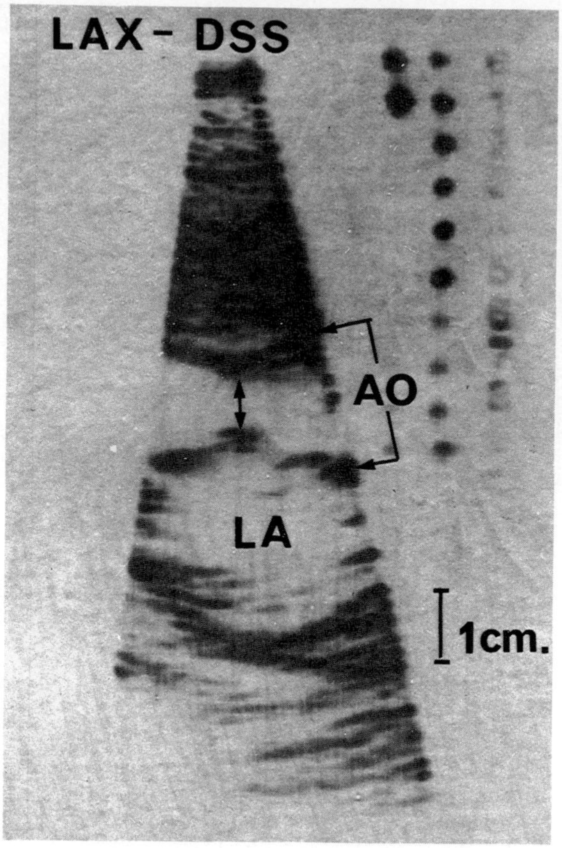

Fig. 19–118. Parasternal long axis recording of the left ventricular outflow tract obtained following surgical resection of a subvalvular membrane. The basal remnants of the resected membrane and a more diffuse generalized narrowing of the outflow space are apparent. The area of peak narrowing is indicated by the vertical arrows. AO = aorta; LA = left atrium; LAX-DSS = long axis-discrete subaortic stenosis. (From Weyman AE, et al.: Cross-sectional echocardiography in evaluating patients with discrete subaortic stenosis. Am J Cardiol 37:358, 1976. Reproduced with permission of Mosby Year-Book, Inc.)

total gradient, it is necessary to measure the velocity across each stenosis separately, which may be difficult when they are close to each other.[228,229]

In general, although it is important to understand the effects of pressure recovery and viscous losses on the hemodynamic measurements, they are of limited clinical significance. The presence of associated lesions, however, significantly complicates the clinical interpretation, and in these cases, the anatomy of the lesions takes on increasing importance in assessing severity.

Acquired Subvalvular Outflow Tract Obstruction

In addition to the congenital forms, subvalvular outflow obstruction may occur following valve repair with mitral annuloplasty and mitral valve replacement.[313–316] Subvalvular obstruction following mitral valve repair and annuloplasty has been reported in approximately 4.5 to 10% of cases. The obstruction in these cases is due to displacement of the redundant mitral leaflet tissue into the outflow tract during systole in a manner similar to that seen in patients with IHSS. This phenomenon is discussed in detail in Chapter 25. Outflow obstruction that is due to prosthetic mitral valves (Fig. 19–119) is described in Chapter 38. Finally, ventricular outflow obstruction can be caused by accessory mitral leaflet tissue in the outflow tract[317] (Fig. 19–120).

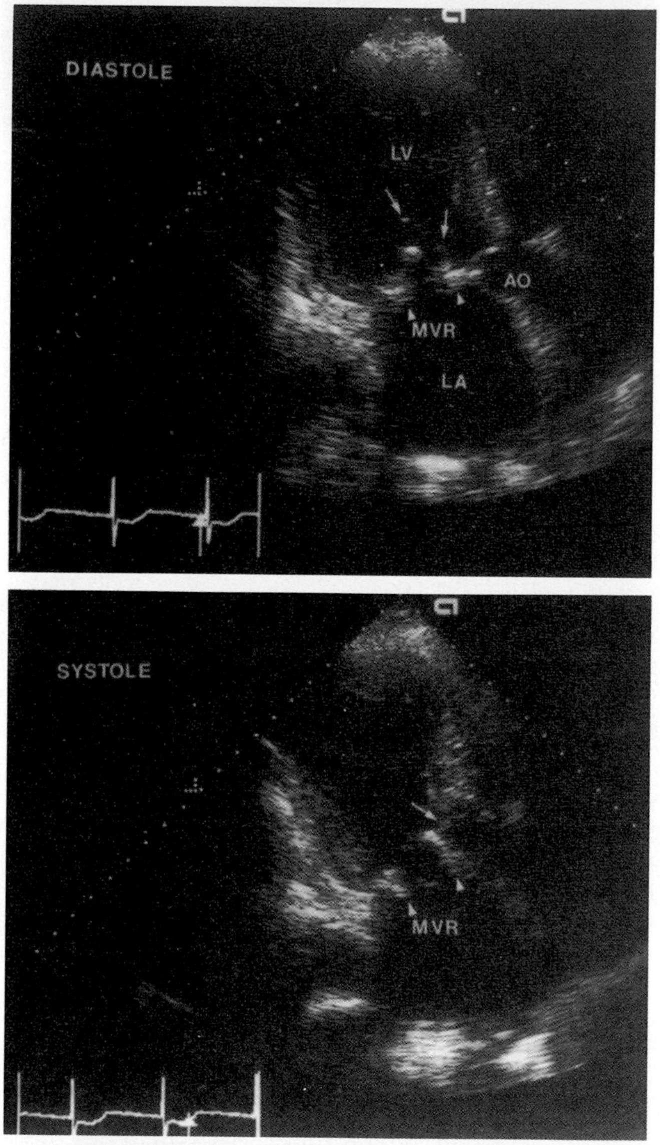

Fig. 19–119. Apical long axis recording from a patient with a Carpentier-Edwards mitral prosthesis in the mitral position. Although the mitral valve was left intact and pledgeted to the mitral annulus, a systolic murmur was noted postoperatively. Top. A flail native anterior leaflet was visualized along the mitral prosthesis. Bottom. During systole, the leaflet (arrow) wedged itself between the strut of the prosthetic valve (MVR) and the interventricular septum. LV = left ventricle; AO = aorta; LA = left atrium. (From Jacobs LE, Kotler MN, Ioli A: Left ventricular outflow tract obstruction following mitral valve replacement with Carpentier-Edwards prosthesis. Echocardiography 7:147, 1990.)

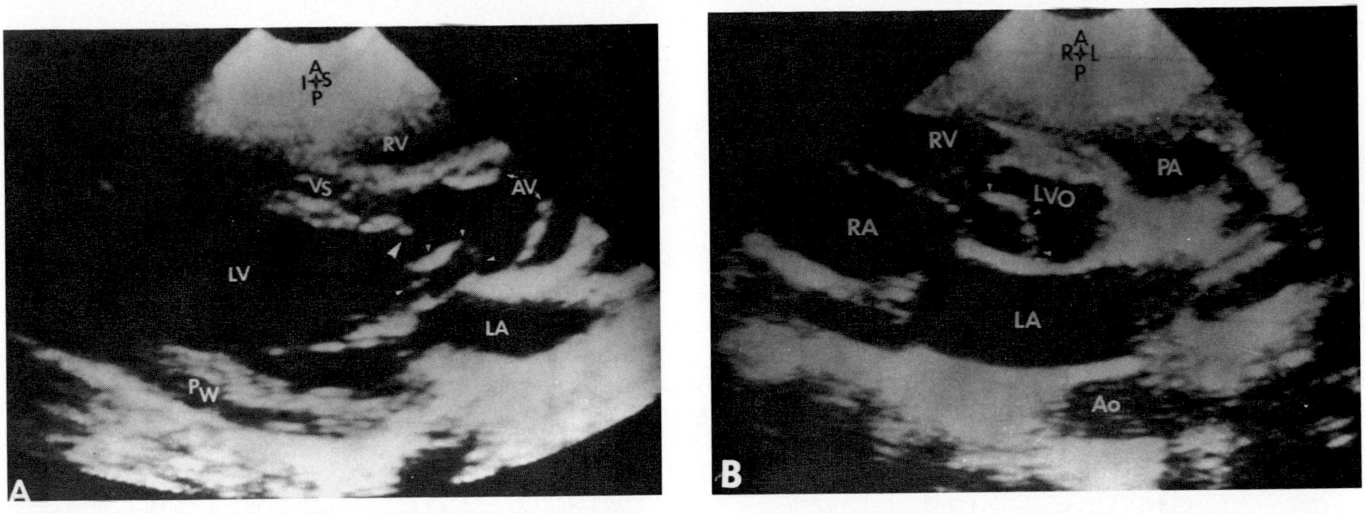

Fig. 19–120. **A.** Parasternal long axis recording illustrating the accessory leaflet tissue (arrowheads) in the outflow tract during systole. **B.** Short axis recording from the same patient illustrating the cowl-like appearance of the accessory leaflet tissue beneath the noncoronary aortic cusp, which partially obstructs left ventricular outflow (LVO). RV = right ventricle; AV = aortic valve; VS = ventricular septum; LV = left ventricle; LA = left atrium; PW = posterior wall; RA = right atrium; PA = pulmonary artery; Ao = aorta. (From Alboliras ET, et al.: Accessory mitral valve tissue in association with discrete subaortic stenosis: a two-dimensional echocardiographic diagnosis. Echocardiography 2:191, 1985.)

REFERENCES

1. Gray H: Gray's Anatomy. Goss CM (ed.) Philadelphia, Lea & Febiger, 1959.
2. Seward JB, Tajik AJ: Non-invasive visualization of the entire thoracic aorta: a new application of wide-angle two dimensional sector echocardiographic technique. Am J Cardiol 43:387, 1979.
3. Bansal RC, Tajik AJ, Seward JB, Offord RP: Feasibility of detailed two-dimensional echocardiographic examination in adults: prospective study of 200 patients. Mayo Clinic Proc 55:291, 1980.
4. Angelini A, et al.: The morphology of the normal aortic valve as compared with the aortic valve having two leaflets. J Thorac Cardiovasc Surg 98: 362, 1989.
5. Davies MJ: Pathology of Cardiac Valves. Butterworths, London, 1980.
6. Rushmer RF: Cardiovascular Dynamics. Philadelphia, WB Saunders, 1970.
7. Roberts WC: The congenitally bicuspid aortic valve. A study of 85 autopsy cases. Am J Cardiol 26:72, 1970.
8. Hurwitz LE, Roberts WC: Quadricuspid semilunar valve. Am J Cardiol 31:623, 1973.
9. Falcone MW, Roberts WC, Morrow AG, Perloff JK: Congenital aortic stenosis resulting from a unicommissural valve. Clinical and anatomical features in 21 adult patients. Circulation 44:272, 1971.
10. Hatle L, Anglesen B: Doppler Ultrasound in Cardiology. Physical Principles and Clinical Applications. 2nd Ed. Philadelphia, Lea & Febiger, 1985.
11. Mizushige K, et al.: Pre-ejection flow in the left ventricular outflow tract elucidated by pulsed Doppler technique. J Cardiography 14:507, 1984.
12. Tajik AJ, et al.: Two-dimensional real-time ultrasonic imaging of the heart and great vessels. Technique, image orientation, structures, identification, and validation. Mayo Clin Proc 53:271, 1978.
13. Weyman AE, Feigenbaum H, Dillon JC, Chang S: Cross-sectional echocardiography in assessing the severity of valvular aortic stenosis. Circulation 52:828, 1975.
14. Weyman AE, et al.: Localization of left ventricular outflow obstruction by cross-sectional echocardiography. Am J Med 60:33, 1976.
15. Lange LW, Sahn DJ, Allen HD, Goldberg SJ: Subxiphoid cross-sectional echocardiography in infants and children with congenital heart disease. Circulation 59:513, 1979.
16. Yeh HC, Winsberg F, Mercer EM: Echocardiographic aortic valve orifice dimension: its use in evaluating aortic stenosis and cardiac output. J Clin Ultrasound 1:182, 1973.
17. Rasmussen S, et al.: Forward stroke volume derived from aortic valve echograms. Clin Res 27:672A, 1979.
18. Davis HA, et al.: Echocardiographic manifestations of discrete subaortic stenosis. Am J Cardiol 33:277, 1974.
19. Laurenceau JL, Guay JM, Gagne S: Echocardiography in the diagnosis of subaortic membranous stenosis (abstr.). Circulation (Suppl 4)48:46, 1976.
20. Gramiak R, Shah PM, Kramer DH: Ultrasound cardiography: contrast studies in anatomy and function. Radiology 92:939, 1969.
21. Feigenbaum H: Clinical applications of echocardiography. Prog Cardiovasc Dis 14:531, 1972.
22. Wong P, Cotter L, Gibson DG: Early systolic closure of the aortic valve. Br Heart J 44:386, 1980.
23. Atsuchi Y, et al.: Echocardiographic manifestations of annuloaortic ectasia: its "paradoxical" motion of the aorta and premature systolic closure of the aortic valve. Am Heart J 93:428, 1977.
24. Candell-Riera J, del Castello HG, Rius J: Aortic root dissection. Another cause of early systolic closure of the aortic valve. Br Heart J 43:579, 1980.
25. Chandraratna PA, Samet P, Robinson MJ, Byrd C: Echocardiography of the "floppy" aortic valve. Report of a case. Circulation 52:959, 1975.
26. Hess PG, et al.: M-mode echocardiographic systolic motion patterns of the aortic valve: clinical-echocardiographic correlates. *In* White D, Lyons EA (eds.): Ultrasound in Medicine. Vol. 4. New York, Plenum Press, p. 37, 1978.
27. Gardin JM, Tommaso CL, Talano JV: Echographic early systolic partial closure (notching) of the aortic valve in congestive cardiomyopathy. Am Heart J 107:135, 1984.
28. Roberts WC: Valvular, subvalvular and supravalvular aortic stenosis. Cardiovasc Clin 5:104, 1973.
29. Roberts WC, Morrow AG: Congenital aortic stenosis produced by a unicommissural valve. Br Heart J 27:505, 1965.
30. Falcone MW, Roberts WC, Morrow AG, Perloff JK: Congenital aortic stenosis resulting from a unicommissural valve. Circulation 44:272, 1971.
31. Osler W: The bicuspid condition of the aortic valve. Trans Assoc Am Phys 2:185, 1886.
32. Campbell M: Calcific aortic stenosis and congenital bicuspid aortic valves. Br Heart J 30:606, 1968.
33. Pomerance A: Pathogenesis of aortic stenosis and its relation to age. Br Heart J 34:569, 1972.
34. Carter JB, Sethi S, Lee GB, Edwards JE: Prolapse of semilunar cusps as causes of aortic insufficiency. Circulation 43:922, 1971.
35. Edwards JE: The congenital bicuspid aortic valve. Circulation 23:485, 1961.
36. Stewart WJ, et al.: Prevalence of aortic valve prolapse with bicuspid aortic valve and its relation to aortic regurgitation: a cross-sectional echocardiographic study. Am J Cardiol 54:1277, 1984.
37. Lewis T, Grant RT: Observations relating to subacute infective endocarditis. Heart 10:21, 1923.
38. Grant RT, Wood JE, Jones TD: Heart valve irregularities in relation to subacute bacterial endocarditis. Heart 14:247, 1928.
39. Fulton MN, Levine SA: Subacute bacterial endocarditis with special reference to the valvular lesions and previous history. Am J Med Sci 183:60, 1932.
40. Bayles TB, Lewis WH: Subacute bacterial endocarditis in older people. Ann Intern Med 13:2154, 1940.
41. Emanuel R, et al.: Congenitally bicuspid aortic valves. Clinicogenetic study of 41 families. Br Heart J 40:1402, 1978.
42. Fowles RE, et al.: Two dimensional echocardiographic features of bicuspid aortic valve. Chest 75:434, 1979.

43. Nanda NC, Gramiak R: Evaluation of bi-cuspid valves by two-dimensional echocardiography. Am J Cardiol 11:372, 1978.
44. Brandenburg RO, et al.: Accuracy of two-dimensional echocardiographic diagnosis of congenitally bicuspid aortic valve. Am J Cardiol 51:1469, 1983.
45. Nanda NC, et al.: Echocardiographic recognition of the congenital bicuspid aortic valve. Circulation 49:870, 1974.
46. Vollebergh FE, Becker AE: Minor congenital variations of cusp size in aortic valves. Possible link with isolated aortic stenosis. Br Heart J 39: 1006, 1977.
47. Davis GL, McAlister WH, Friedenberg MM: Congenital aortic stenosis due to failure of histogenesis of the aortic valve (Myxoid dysplasia). Am J Roentgenol 95:621, 1965.
48. Reeve R Jr, Robinson SJ: Hypoplastic annulus—an unusual type of aortic stenosis: a report of three cases in children. Dis Chest 45:99, 1964.
49. Hurwitz LE, Roberts WC: Quadricuspid semilunar valves. Am J Cardiol 31:622, 1973.
50. Barbosa M, Motta M: Quadricuspid aortic valve and aortic regurgitation diagnosed by Doppler echocardiography: Report of two cases and review of the literature. J Am Soc Echocardiogr 4:69, 1991.
51. Davia JE, et al.: Quadricuspid semilunar valves. Chest 72:186, 1977.
52. Simonds JP: Congenital malformations of the aortic and pulmonic valves. Am J Med Sci 166:584, 1923.
53. Luisi VS, et al.: Quadricuspid aortic valves. J Cardiovasc Surg 25:252, 1984.
54. Rogers AJ, Zulfukar A, Hendriks F, Huysmans H: Quinticuspid aortic valve causing aortic valve incompetence and stenosis. Thorax 37:542, 1982.
55. Pomerance A: Aging changes in human heart valves. Br Heart J 29:222, 1967.
56. Lambl VA: Papillare Exkrescenzen an der Simulararklappe der Aorta. Wien Med Wochenschr 6:244, 1856.
57. Magarey FR: On the mode of formation of Lambl's excrescences and their relation to chronic thickening of the mitral valve. J Pathol Bacteriol 61: 203, 1949.
58. Cogswell T, Komorowski RA, Galbraith TA, Singh S: Giant Lambl's excrescences of the left ventricular outflow tract in rheumatic heart disease. Echocardiography 4:424, 1987.
59. Selzer A: Changing aspects of the natural history of valvular aortic stenosis. N Engl J Med 317:91, 1987.
60. Weyman AE, et al.: Cross-sectional echocardiographic assessment of the severity of aortic stenosis in children. Circulation 55:773, 1977.
61. Friedberg CW: Diseases of the Heart. Philadelphia, WB Saunders, 1966.
62. King M, Huang JM, Glassman E: Paget's disease with cardiac calcification and complete heart block. Am J Med 64:302, 1969.
63. DeMaria AN, et al.: Valve and limitations of cross-sectional echocardiography of the aortic valve in the diagnosis and quantification of valvular aortic stenosis. Circulation 62:304, 1980.
64. Godley RW, et al.: Reliability of two-dimensional echocardiography in assessing the severity of valvular aortic stenosis. Chest 79:657, 1981.
65. Grossman W (ed.): Cardiac Catheterization and Angiography. Philadelphia, Lea & Febiger, 1980.
66. Leo LP, et al.: Determination of aortic valve area by cross-sectional echocardiography. Circulation 60(Suppl. 2):II-203, 1979.
67. Borow KM, et al.: Can the modified Bernoulli equation be used to accurately determine intraventricular pressures throughout systole in patients with valvular aortic stenosis? (abstr.) J Am Coll Cardiol 9:236A, 1987.
68. Holen J, et al.: Doppler ultrasound in orifice flow: in vitro studies of the relationship between pressure difference and fluid velocity. Ultrasound Med Biol 11:261, 1985.
69. Teirstein P, Yock PG, Popp RL: The accuracy of Doppler ultrasound measurement of pressure gradients across irregular and tunnellike obstruction to blood flow. Circulation 72:577, 1985.
70. Otto CM, et al.: Determination of the stenotic aortic valve area in adults using Doppler echocardiography. J Am Coll Cardiol 7:509, 1986.
71. Williams GA, Labovitz AJ, Nelson JG, Kennedy HL: Value of multiple echocardiographic views in the evaluation of aortic stenosis in adults by continuous wave Doppler. Am J Cardiol 55:445, 1985.
72. Ramirez ML, Wong M, Shah PM: Subcostal window: a new portal for recording continuous-wave Doppler aortic flow velocities. Am J Cardiol 56:199, 1985.
73. Hatle L: Noninvasive assessment and differentiation of left ventricular outflow obstruction with Doppler ultrasound. Circulation 64:381, 1981.
74. Fan PH, Kapur KK, Nanda NC: Color-guided Doppler echocardiographic assessment of aortic valve stenosis. J Am Coll Cardiol 12:441, 1988.
75. Panidis IP, Mintz GS, Ross J: Value and limitations of Doppler ultrasound in the evaluation of aortic stenosis: a statistical analysis of 70 consecutive patients. Am Heart J 112:150, 1986.
76. Danielson R, Nordreburg JE, Strangeland L, Vik-Mo H: Limitations in assessing the severity of aortic stenosis by Doppler gradients. Br Heart J 59:551, 1988.
77. Currie PJ, et al.: Continuous wave Doppler echocardiographic assessment of severity of calcific aortic stenosis: a simultaneous Doppler-catheter correlative study in 100 adult patients. Circulation 71:1162, 1985.
78. Mich RJ, et al.: Mean pressure estimation: mean of the squares vs. square of the means? Circulation 74(Suppl. 2):II-229, 1986.
79. Holen J, et al.: Doppler ultrasound in orifice flow: in vitro studies of the relationship between pressure difference and fluid velocity. Ultrasound Med Biol 11:261, 1985.
80. Callahan MJ, Tajik AJ, Su-Fan Q, Bove AA: Validation of instantaneous pressure gradients measured by continuous wave Doppler in experimentally induced aortic stenosis. Am J Cardiol 56:989, 1985.
81. Smith MD, et al.: Correlation of continuous wave Doppler velocities with cardiac catheterization gradients: an experimental model of aortic stenosis. J Am Coll Cardiol 6:1306, 1985.
82. Currie PJ, et al.: Instantaneous pressure gradient: a simultaneous Doppler and dual catheter correlative study. J Am Coll Cardiol 7:509, 1986.
83. Murgo JP, et al.: Normal ventricular ejection dynamics in man during rest and exercise. *In* Leon SF, Shaver JA (eds.): Physiologic Principles of Heart Sounds and Murmurs. American Heart Association, Dallas, p. 92, 1975.
84. Levine RA, et al.: Pressure recovery distal to a stenosis: potential cause of gradient "overestimation" by Doppler echocardiography. J Am Coll Cardiol 13:706, 1989.
85. Sugawara M: Stenosis: theoretical background. *In* Sugawara M, Kajiya F, Kitabatake A, Matsuo H (eds.): Blood Flow in the Heart and Large Vessels. Tokyo, Springer-Verlag, 1989.
86. Warth DC, Stewart WJ, Block PC, Weyman AE: A new method to calculate aortic valve area without left heart catheterization. Circulation 70:978, 1984.
87. Oh JK, et al.: Prediction of the severity of aortic stenosis by Doppler aortic valve area determination: prospective Doppler-catheterization correlation in 100 patients. J Am Coll Cardiol 11:1227, 1988.
88. Yeager M, Yock PG, Popp PL: Comparison of Doppler derived pressure gradient to that determined at cardiac catheterization in adults with aortic valve stenosis: implications for management. Am J Cardiol 57:644, 1986.
89. Skjaerpe T, Hegrenaes L, Hatle L: Noninvasive estimation of valve area in patients with aortic stenosis by Doppler ultrasound and two-dimensional echocardiography. Circulation 72:810, 1985.
90. Gorlin R, Gorlin SG: Hydraulic formula for calculation of the area of the stenotic mitral valve, other cardiac valves and central circulatory shunts. Am Heart J 41:1, 1951.
91. Zoghbi WA, et al.: Accurate noninvasive quantitation of stenotic aortic valve area by Doppler echocardiography. Circulation 73:452, 1986.
92. Richards KL, Cannon SR, Miller JF, Crawford MH: Calculation of aortic valve area by Doppler echocardiography: a direct application of the continuity equation. Circulation 73;964, 1986.
93. Mann DL, et al.: The fractional shortening velocity ratio: validation of a new echocardiographic Doppler method for identifying patients with significant aortic stenosis. J Am Coll Cardiol 15:1578, 1990.
94. Glanz S, Hellenbrand WE, Berman MA, Talner NS: Echocardiographic assessment of the severity of aortic stenosis in children and adolescents. Am J Cardiol 38:620, 1976.
95. Johnson GL, et al.: Echocardiographic evaluation of fixed left ventricular outlet obstruction in children. Pre- and postoperative assessment of ventricular systolic pressures. Circulation 56:299, 1977.
96. Blackwood AR, Bloom KR, William CM: Aortic stenosis in children: experience with echocardiographic prediction of severity. Circulation 57:263, 1978.
97. Schwartz A, et al.: Echocardiographic estimation of aortic valve gradient in aortic stenosis. Ann Intern Med 89:329, 1978.
98. Gewitz HM, et al.: Role of echocardiography in aortic stenosis: Pre- and postoperative studies. Am J Cardiol 43:67, 1979.
99. DePace NL, et al.: Correlation of echocardiographic wall stress and left ventricular pressure and function in aortic stenosis. Circulation 67:854, 1983.
100. Wagner S, Selzer A: Patterns of progression of aortic stenosis: a longitudinal study. Circulation 65:709, 1982.
101. Wagner HR, Ellison RC, Keane JF, Humphries JO, Nadas AS. Clinical course of aortic stenosis. Circulation 36 (suppl I):1–47, 1977.
102. Nestico PF, et al.: Progression of isolated aortic stenosis: analysis of 29 patients having more than 1 cardiac catheterization. Am J Cardiol 52:1054, 1983.
103. Bogart DB, et al.: Progression of aortic stenosis. Chest 76:391, 1979.
104. Cheitlin MD, et al.: Rate of progression of severity of valvular aortic stenosis in the adult. Am Heart J 98:689, 1979.
105. Otto CM, Pearlman AS, Gardner CL: Hemodynamic progression of aortic stenosis in adults assessed by Doppler echocardiography. J Am Coll Cardiol 13:545, 1989.
105a. Thoreau EA, et al.: The rate and pattern of change of valve area in aortic stenosis: Long term Doppler follow-up. J Am Coll Cardiol 19:331A, 1992.
106. Roger VL, et al.: Progression of aortic stenosis in adults: new appraisal using Doppler echocardiography. Am Heart J 119:331, 1990.
107. Stapleton JF, Harvey WP: A clinical analysis of aortic incompetence. Postgrad Med 46:156, 1969.
108. Carter JB, Sethi S, Lee GB, Edwards JE: Prolapse of semilunar cusps as causes of aortic insufficiency. Circulation 43:922, 1971.

109. Frahm CJ, Braunwald E, Morrow AG: Congenital aortic regurgitation, clinical and hemodynamic findings in four patients. Am J Med 31:63, 1961.
110. Bierman FZ, et al.: Absence of the aortic valve: antenatal and postnatal two-dimensional and Doppler echocardiographic features. J Am Coll Cardiol 3:833, 1984.
111. Hashimoto R, Miyamura H, Eguchi S: Congenital aortic regurgitation in a child with trileaflet non-stenotic aortic valve. Br Heart J 51:358, 1984.
112. Stewart WJ, et al.: Prevalence of aortic valve prolapse with bicuspid aortic valve and its relation to aortic regurgitation: a cross-sectional echocardiographic study. Am J Cardiol 54:1277, 1984.
113. Ogawa S, Hayashi J, Sasaki H, et al.: Evaluation of combined valvular prolapse by two-dimensional echocardiography. Circulation 65:174, 1982.
114. Guiney TE, et al.: The aetiology and course of isolated severe aortic regurgitation: a clinical, pathological and echocardiographic study. Br Heart J 53:358, 1987.
115. Boughner DR: Assessment of aortic insufficiency by transcutaneous Doppler ultrasound. Circulation 52:874, 1975.
116. Ciobanu M, et al.: Pulsed Doppler echocardiography in the diagnosis and estimation of severity of aortic insufficiency. Am J Cardiol 49:339, 1982.
117. Esper RJ: Detection of mild aortic regurgitation by range-gated pulsed Doppler echocardiography. Am J Cardiol 50:1037, 1982.
118. Veyrat C, et al.: New indexes for assessing aortic regurgitation with two-dimensional Doppler echocardiographic measurements of the regurgitant aortic valve area. Circulation 68:998, 1983.
119. Pearlman AS, Otto CM: Quantification of valvular regurgitation. Echocardiography 4:271, 1987.
120. Masuyama T, Kodama K, Kitabatake A, et al.: Noninvasive evaluation of aortic regurgitation by continuous-wave Doppler echocardiography. Circulation 73:460, 1986.
121. Miyatake K, et al.: Clinical applications of a new type of real-time two-dimensional Doppler flow imaging system. Am J Cardiol 54:857, 1984.
122. Omoto R, et al.: The development of real-time two-dimensional Doppler echocardiography and its clinical significance in acquired valvular diseases. Jpn Heart J 25:325, 1984.
123. Perry GJ, et al.: Evaluation of aortic insufficiency by Doppler color flow mapping. J Am Coll Cardiol 9:952, 1987.
124. Grayburn PA, et al.: Detection of aortic insufficiency by standard echocardiography, pulsed Doppler echocardiography and auscultation. Ann Int Med 104:599, 1986.
125. Choong CY, et al.: Prevalence of valvular regurgitation by Doppler echocardiography in patients with structurally normal hearts by two-dimensional echocardiography. Am Heart J 117:636, 1989.
126. Akasaka T, et al.: Age-related valvular regurgitation: a study by pulsed Doppler echocardiography. Circulation 76:262, 1987.
127. Sellers RD, et al.: Left retrograde cardioangiography in acquired cardiac diseases—technique, indications, and interpretations in 700 cases. Am J Cardiol 14:437, 1964.
128. Sandler H, et al.: Quantitation of valvular insufficiency in man by angiocardiography. Am Heart J 65:501, 1963.
129. Croft CH, et al.: Limitations of qualitative angiographic grading in aortic or mitral regurgitation. Am J Cardiol 53:1393, 1984.
130. Matsuo H, et al.: Detection and visualization of regurgitant flow in valvular diseases by pulsed Doppler technique. Jpn Circ J 46:377, 1982.
131. Esper RJ: Detection of mild aortic regurgitation by range-gated pulsed Doppler echocardiography. Am J Cardiol 50:1037, 1982.
132. Labovitz AJ, et al.: Quantitative evaluation of aortic insufficiency by continuous-wave Doppler echocardiography. J Am Coll Cardiol 8:1341, 1986.
133. Switzer DF, et al.: Calibration of color Doppler flow mapping during extreme hemodynamic conditions in vitro: a foundation for a reliable quantitative grading for aortic incompetence. Circulation 75:837, 1987.
134. Thomas JD, et al.: Quantification of jet flow by momentum analysis: an in vitro color Doppler analysis. Circulation 81:247, 1990.
135. Stevenson JG: Lessons provided by color flow imagery: disturbed flow jets tend to adhere to adjacent walls (abstr.). J Am Coll Cardiol 9:3A, 1987.
136. Chen C, et al.: Impact of eccentrically directed impinging wall jets on quantitation of mitral regurgitation by color Doppler flow mapping (abstr.). Circulation 80(Suppl. 2):II-578, 1989.
137. Krabill KA, et al.: Factors influencing the structure and shape of stenotic and regurgitant jets: an in vitro investigation using Doppler color flow mapping and optical flow visualization. J Am Coll Cardiol 13:1672, 1989.
138. Stevenson JG: Critical importance of gain, pulse repetition frequency and carrier frequency on apparent 2D color Doppler jet size (abstr.). Circulation 78(Suppl. 2):II-12, 1988.
139. Utsonomiya T, et al.: Effect of machine parameters on variance image display in Doppler color flow mapping (abstr.). Circulation 78(Suppl. 2): II-12. 1988.
140. Holt BD, et al.: Sources of variability for Doppler color flow mapping of regurgitant jets in an animal model of mitral regurgitation. J Am Coll Cardiol 13:1361, 1989.
141. Thomas JD, et al.: Impact of orifice geometry on the shape of jets: an in vitro Doppler color flow study. J Am Coll Cardiol 17:901, 1991.
141a. Samstad SO, Hegrenaes L, Skjaerpe T, Hatle L. Half time of the diastolic aortoventricular pressure difference by continuous wave Doppler ultrasound: a measure of the severity of aortic regurgitation? Br Heart J 61: 336, 1989.
142. Teague SM, et al.: Quantification of aortic regurgitation utilizing continuous-wave Doppler ultrasound. J Am Coll Cardiol 8:592, 1986.
143. Grayburn PA, et al.: Quantitative assessment of the hemodynamic consequences of aortic regurgitation. J Am Coll Cardiol 10:135, 1987.
144. Beyer RW, Ramirez M, Josephson MA, Shah PM: Correlation of continuous wave Doppler assessment of chronic aortic regurgitation with hemodynamics and angiography. Am J Cardiol 60:852, 1987.
145. Griffin BP, et al.: The effects of regurgitant orifice size, chamber compliance, and systemic vascular resistance on aortic regurgitant velocity slope and pressure half-time. Am Heart J 122:1049, 1991.
146. Montemurro D, et al.: Spectral analysis and color code Doppler study of the changes in aortic regurgitation induced by vasodilators in asymptomatic patients affected by aortic incompetence. G Ital Cardiol 20:842, 1990.
147. Zhang Y, et al.: Measurement of aortic regurgitation by Doppler echocardiography. Br Heart J 55:32, 1986.
148. Kitabatake A, et al.: A new approach to noninvasive evaluation of aortic regurgitant fraction by two-dimensional Doppler echocardiography. Circulation 72:523, 1985.
149. Rokey R, et al.: Determination of regurgitant fraction in isolated mitral or aortic regurgitation by pulsed Doppler two-dimensional echocardiography. J Am Coll Cardiol 7:1273, 1986.
150. Hoppeler H, Jenni R, Ritter M, Krayenbuhl H: Quantification of aortic regurgitation with amplitude-weighted velocity from continuous wave Doppler spectra. J Am Coll Cardiol 15:1305, 1990.
151. Diebold B, et al.: Non-invasive quantification of aortic regurgitation by Doppler echocardiography. Br Heart J 49:167, 1983.
152. Touche T, et al.: Assessment and follow-up of patients with aortic regurgitation by an updated Doppler echocardiographic measurement of the regurgitant fraction in the aortic arch. Circulation 72:819, 1985.
153. Takenaka K, et al.: A simple Doppler echocardiographic method for estimating severity of aortic regurgitation. Am J Cardiol 57:1340, 1986.
153a. Okamoto M, et al.: Assessment of supra-valvular abnormal signal with color Doppler flow mapping in patients with aortic regurgitation. Am Heart J 119:339, 1990.
154. Nakao S, et al.: A regurgitant jet and echocardiographic abnormalities in aortic regurgitation: an experimental study. Circulation 77:78, 1988.
155. Winsberg F, Gabor GE, Hernberg JG: Fluttering of the mitral valve in aortic insufficiency. Circulation 41:225, 1970.
156. Mintz GS, et al.: Statistical comparison of M-mode and two-dimensional echocardiographic diagnosis of flail mitral leaflets. Am J Cardiol 45:253, 1980.
157. David D, et al.: Echocardiography in the diagnosis and quantification of valvular heart disease. Cardiovasc Clin 13:67, 1983.
158. Robertson WS, et al.: Reverse doming of the anterior mitral leaflet with severe aortic regurgitation. J Am Coll Cardiol 3:431, 1984.
159. Ambrose JA, et al.: Premature closure of the mitral valve: echocardiographic clue for the diagnosis of aortic dissection. Chest 73:121, 1978.
160. Botvinick EH, et al.: Echocardiographic demonstration of early mitral valve closure in severe aortic insufficiency: its clinical applications. Circulation 51:836, 1975.
161. Mann T, et al.: Assessing the hemodynamic severity of acute aortic regurgitation due to infective endocarditis. N Engl J Med 293:108, 1975.
162. Vandenbossche JL, Englert M: Doppler color flow mapping demonstration of diastolic mitral regurgitation in severe acute aortic regurgitation. Am Heart J 11:889, 1987.
163. Weaver WF, et al.: Mid-diastolic aortic valve opening in severe acute aortic regurgitation. Circulation 55:145, 1977.
164. Pietro DA, et al.: Premature opening of the aortic valve: an index of highly advanced aortic regurgitation. J Clin Ultrasound 6:170, 1978.
165. Weiss L, Greep R: Histology. New York, McGraw-Hill, 1977.
166. Quinquera L, Carneiro J, Contopoulos A: Basic Histology. Los Altos, CA, Lange Medical Publications, 1977.
167. Weyman AE, et al.: Cross-sectional echocardiographic characterization of aortic obstruction. I: Supravalvular aortic stenosis and aortic hypoplasia. Circulation 57:491, 1978.
168. Farthing S, Peronneau P: Flow in the thoracic aorta. Cardiovasc Res 13: 607, 1979.
169. Segadal L, Matre K: Blood velocity in the human ascending aorta. Circulation 76:90, 1987.
170. Louie EK, Maron BJ, Green KJ: Variations in flow velocity waveforms obtained by pulsed Doppler echocardiography in the normal human aorta. Am J Cardiol 58:821, 1986.
171. Klipstein RH, et al.: Blood flow patterns in the human aorta studied by magnetic resonance. Br Heart J 58:316, 1987.
172. Clark C, Schultz DL: Velocity distribution in aortic flow. Cardiovasc Res 7:601, 1973.
173. Yamaguchi T, Kikkawa S, Yoshikawa T: Measurement of turbulence intensity in the center of the canine ascending aorta with a hot-film anemometer. J Biomech Eng 105:107, 1983.

174. Stein PD, Sabbah HN: Turbulent blood flow in the ascending aorta of humans with normal and diseased aortic valves. Circ Res 39:58, 1976.
175. Weyman AE, et al.: Cross-sectional echocardiographic detection of aortic obstruction. II: Coarctation of the aorta. Circulation 57:498, 1978.
176. Sahn DJ, Allen HD, McDonald G, Goldberg SJ: Real-time cross-sectional echocardiographic diagnosis of coarctation of the aorta: a prospective study of echocardiographic angiographic correlations. Circulation 56:762, 1977.
177. Mintz GS, Kotler MN, Segal BL, Parry WR: Two-dimensional echocardiographic recognition of the descending thoracic aorta. Am J Cardiol 44:232, 1979.
178. Sapire DW, et al.: Dilatation of the descending aorta: a radiologic and echocardiographic diagnostic sign in arteriovenous malformations in neonates and young infants. Am J Cardiol 44:493, 1979.
179. Come PC: Improved cross-sectional echocardiographic technique for visualization of the retrocardiac descending aorta in its long axis. Am J Cardiol 51:1029, 1983.
180. Frazin LJ, et al.: Functional chiral asymmetry in descending thoracic aorta. Circulation 82:1985, 1990.
181. Thomas JD: Flow in the descending aorta. A turn of the screw or a sideways glance. Circulation 82:2263, 1990.
182. Stewart JR, Kincaid OW, Edwards JE: An Atlas of Vascular Rings and Related Malformations of the Aortic Arch System. Springfield, IL, Charles C Thomas, 1964.
183. Moes CAF: Vascular rings and anomalies of the aortic arch. *In* Keith JD, Rowe RR, Vlad P (eds.): Heart Disease in Infancy and Childhood. 3rd Ed. New York, MacMillan, 1978.
184. Gutgesell HP, et al.: Accuracy of two-dimensional echocardiography in the diagnosis of congenital heart disease. Am J Cardiol 55:514, 1985.
185. Sahn DJ, et al.: Two-dimensional echocardiography and intravenous digital subtraction angiography for diagnosis and evaluation of double aortic arch. Am J Cardiol 50:342, 1982.
186. Enderlein MA, et al.: Usefulness of suprasternal notch echocardiography for diagnosis of double aortic arch. Am J Cardiol 57:359, 1986.
187. Celano V, et al.: Two-dimensional echocardiographic recognition of the right aortic arch. Am J Cardiol 51:1507, 1983.
188. Kveselis DA, et al.: Echocardiographic diagnosis of right aortic arch with a retroesophageal segment and left descending aorta. Am J Cardiol 57: 1198, 1986.
189. Murdison KA, Andrews BA, Chin AJ: Ultrasonographic display of complex vascular rings. J Am Coll Cardiol 15:1645, 1990.
190. Snider AR, Serwer GA: Echocardiography in Pediatric Heart Disease. Chicago, Yearbook p. 289. 1990.
191. Kan MN, Nanda NC, Stopa AR: Diagnosis of double aorrtic arch by cross sectional echocardiography with Doppler colour flow mapping. Br Heart J 58:284, 1987.
192. Hastreiter AR, D'Cruz IA, Cantez T: Right sided aorta: 1. Occurrence of right sided aortic arch in various types of congenital heart disease. Br Heart J 28:722, 1966.
193. Felson B, Palayew MJ: The two types of right aortic arch. Radiology 81: 745, 1963.
194. Stewart JR, Kincaid OW, Titus JL: Right aortic arch: plain film diagnosis and significance. Am J Roentgenol Radium Ther Nucl Med 97:377, 1966.
195. Shrivastava S, et al.: Parasternal cross-sectional echocardiographic determination of aortic arch situs: a new approach. Am J Cardiol 55:1236, 1985.
196. McCue CM, Mavck P Jr, Tinglestead JB, Kellett GN: Cervical aortic arch. Am J Dis Child 125:738, 1973.
197. Mullins CE, Gillette PC, McNamara DG: The complex of cervical arch. Pediatrics 51:210, 1973.
198. Kronzon I, Mehta SS, Zelefsky M: Cervical aorta presenting as superior mediastinal mass: diagnosis by echography. Br J Radiol 47:900, 1974.
199. Peterson TA, Todd B, Edwards JE: Supravalvular aortic stenosis. J Thorac Cardiovasc Surg 50:734, 1968.
200. Denie JJ, Verleugt AP: Supravalvular aortic stenosis. Circulation 18:902, 1958.
201. Morrow AG, et al.: Supravalvular aortic stenosis. Circulation 20:1003, 1959.
202. Keith JD, Rowe RD, Vlad P: Heart Disease in Infancy and Childhood. New York, Macmillan, 1978.
203. Beuren AJ, Apitz J, Ronceg J: Die Diagnose und Beurteilung der Verschiedenen Formen der Supravalvularen Aortenstenose. Zeitschrift fuer Kreislaufforschung 51:829, 1962.
204. Hancock EW: Differentiation of valvar, subvalvar and supravalvar aortic stenosis. Guys Hosp Rep 110:1, 1961.
205. Williams JC, Barrat-Boyes BG, Lowe JB: Supravalvular aortic stenosis. Circulation 24:1311, 1961.
206. Beuren AJ, et al.: The syndrome of supravalvular aortic stenosis, peripheral pulmonary stenosis, mental retardation and similar facial appearance. Am J Cardiol 13:471, 1964.
207. Black JA, Bonham-Carter RE: Association between aortic stenosis and facies of severe infantile hypercalcemia. Lancet 2:745, 1963.
208. Garcia RE, Friedman WF, Kaback MM, Rowe RD: Idiopathic hypercalcemia in supravalvular aortic stenosis: documentation of a new syndrome. N Engl J Med 271:117, 1964.
209. McCue CM, Spicuzza TT, Robinson LW, Mauck HP: Familial supravalvular aortic stenosis. J Pediatr 73:889, 1968.
210. Wooley CF, et al.: Supravalvular aortic stenosis. Clinical experience with four patients including familial occurrence. Am J Med 31:717, 1961.
211. Beppu S, et al.: Supravalvular aortic stenosis and coronary ostial stenosis in familial hypercholesterolemia: two-dimensional echocardiographic assessment. Circulation 67:878, 1983.
212. Smith MD, et al.: Correlation of continuous wave Doppler velocities with cardiac catheterization gradients: an experimental model of aortic stenosis. J Am Coll Cardiol 6:1306, 1985.
213. Nakajima T, et al.: Doppler echocardiographic estimates of pressure gradients in various types of stenoses: usefulness and limitations. J Cardiol 19:851, 1989.
214. Edwards JE, Casey IS, Neufeld HN, Lester RG: Congenital Heart Disease. Philadelphia, WB Saunders, 1965.
215. Bahnson HT, Cooley RN, Sloan RD: Coarctation of the aorta at unusual sites. Am Heart J 38:905, 1949.
216. Elliot LP, Schiebler GL: X-ray Diagnosis of Congenital Cardiac Diseases. Springfield, IL, Charles C. Thomas, 1968.
217. Nora JJ, Torres FG, Sinhas AK, McNamara DG: Characteristic cardiovascular anomalies of XO Turner syndrome, XX and YY phenotype and XO/XX Turner mosaic. Am J Cardiol 25:639, 1970.
218. Snider AR, Silverman NH: Suprasternal notch echocardiography: a two-dimensional technique for evaluating congenital heart disease. Circulation 63:165, 1981.
219. Smallhorn JF, et al.: Cross-sectional echocardiographic assessment of coarctation of the aorta in the sick neonate and infant. Br Heart J 50:349, 1983.
220. Huhta JC, Gutgesell HP, Latson LA, Huffines FD: Two-dimensional echocardiographic assessment of the aorta in infants and children with congenital heart disease. Circulation 70:417, 1984.
221. Nihoyannopolous P, et al.: Accuracy of two-dimensional echocardiography in the diagnosis of aortic arch obstruction. J Am Coll Cardiol 10:1072, 1987.
222. Duncan WJ, Ninomiya K, Cook DH, Rowe RD: Noninvasive diagnosis of neonatal coarctation and associated anomalies using two-dimensional echocardiography. Am Heart J 106:63, 1983.
223. Simpson IA, et al.: Color Doppler flow mapping in patients with coarctation of the aorta: new observations and improved evaluation with color flow diameter and proximal acceleration as predictors of severity. Circulation 77:736, 1988.
224. Sanders SP, MacPherson D, Yeager SB: Temporal flow velocity profile in the descending aorta in coarctation. J Am Coll Cardiol 7:603, 1986.
225. Shaddy RE, et al.: Pulsed Doppler findings in patients with coarctation of the aorta. Circulation 73:82, 1986.
226. Wyse RKH, et al.: Use of continuous wave velocimetry to assess the severity of coarctation of the aorta by measurement of aortic flow velocities. Br Heart J 52:278, 1984.
227. Marx GR, Allen HD: Accuracy and pitfalls of Doppler evaluation of the pressure gradient in aortic coarctation. J Am Coll Cardiol 7:1379, 1986.
228. Yoganathan A, et al.: Continuous wave Doppler velocities and gradients across fixed tunnel stenoses in an in vitro flow model. Circulation 76:657, 1987.
229. Simpson IA, et al.: Spatial velocity distribution and acceleration in serial subvalve tunnel and valvular obstructions: an in vitro study using Doppler color flow mapping. J Am Coll Cardiol 13:241, 1989.
230. Moller JH, Edwards JE: Interruption of the aortic arch. Anatomic patterns and associated cardiac malformations. Am J Roentgenol 95:557, 1965.
231. Roberts WC, Morrow AC, Braunwald E: Complete interruption of the aortic arch. Circulation 26:39, 1962.
232. Celoria GC, Patton RB: Congenital absence of the aortic arch. Am Heart J 58:407, 1959.
233. Jaffe RB: Complete interruption of the aortic arch: characteristic radiographic findings in 21 patients. Circulation 52:714, 1975.
234. Subramanian AR: Coarctation or interruption of aorta proximal to origin of both subclavian arteries. Br Heart J 34:1225, 1972.
235. VanPraagh R, et al.: Interrupted aortic arch: surgical treatment. Am J Cardiol 27:200, 1971.
236. Freedom RM, et al.: Ventricular septal defect in interruption of the arch. Am J Cardiol 39:572, 1977.
237. Braulin E, et al.: Interruption of the aortic arch with aorticopulmonary septal defect. Pediatr Cardiol 3:329, 1982.
238. Riggs TW, Berry TE, Aziz KV, Paul MH: Two-dimensional echocardiographic features of interruption of the aortic arch. Am J Cardiol 50:1385, 1982.
239. Smallhorn JF, Anderson RH, Macartney FJ: Cross-sectional echocardiographic recognition of interruption of the aortic arch between left carotid and subclavian arteries. Br Heart J 48:229, 1982.
240. Hopps HC: Principles of Pathology. New York, Appleton-Century Crofts, 1959.

241. Edwards JE, Burchell HB: The pathologic anatomy of deficiencies between the aortic root and the heart including aortic sinus aneurysms. Thorax 12: 125, 1957.
242. Sawyers JL, Adams JE, Scott HW: Surgical treatment for aneurysms of the aortic sinuses with aorticoatrial fistula. Surgery 41:26, 1957.
243. Chamsi-Pasha H, Musgrove C, Morton R: Echocardiographic diagnosis of multiple congenital aneurysms of the sinus of valsalva. Br Heart J 59:724, 1988.
244. Bardy GH, et al.: Two-dimensional echocardiographic identification of sinus of valsalva-right heart fistula due to infective endocarditis. Am Heart J 103:1068, 1982.
245. Lewis BS, Agathangelou NE: Echocardiographic diagnosis of unruptured sinus of valsalve aneurysm. Am Heart J 107:1025, 1984.
246. Haaz WS, et al.: Ruptured sinus of Valsalva aneurysm: diagnosis by echocardiography. Chest 78:781, 1980.
247. Sakakibara S, Konno S: Congenital aneurysms of the sinus of Valsalva—anatomy and classification. Am Heart J 63:405, 1962.
248. Kerber RE, et al.: Unruptured aneurysm of the sinus of Valsalva producing right ventricular outflow obstruction. Am J Med 53:775, 1972.
249. Kiefaber RW, Tabakin BS, Coffin LH, Gibson TC: Unruptured sinus of Valsalva aneurysm with right ventricular outflow obstruction diagnosed by two-dimensional and Doppler echocardiography. J Am Coll Cardiol 7: 438, 1986.
250. Onat A, Ersanli O, Kanuni A, Aykan TB: Congenital aortic sinus aneurysms with particular reference to dissection of the interventricular septum. Am Heart J 72:158, 1966.
251. Chen WWC, Tai YT: Dissection of interventricular septum by aneurysm of sinus of Valsalva: a rare complication diagnosed by echocardiography. Br Heart J 50:293, 1983.
252. Davidson HG, Tabricium J, Husfeldt E: Five cases of congenital aneurysm of the aortic sinuses of Valsalva and notes of the prognosis. Acta Med Scand 160:455, 1968.
253. Falholt W, Thomson G: Congenital aneurysm of the right sinus of Valsalva diagnosed by aortography. Circulation 8:549, 1953.
254. London SB, London RE: Production of aortic regurgitation by unperforated aneurysm of the sinuses of Valsalva. Circulation 24:1403, 1961.
255. Rothbaum DA, Dillon JC, Chang S, Feigenbaum H: Echocardiographic manifestation of right sinus of Valsalva aneurysm. Circulation 49:768, 1974.
256. Weyman AE, Dillon JC, Feigenbaum H, Chang S: Premature pulmonic valve opening following sinus of Valsalva aneurysm rupture into the right atrium. Circulation 51:556, 1975.
257. McKusick VA: Heritable Disorders of Connective Tissue. 4th Ed. St. Louis, CV Mosby, 1972.
258. Hirst AE, Gore I: Marfan's syndrome: a review. Prog Cardiovasc Dis 16: 187, 1973.
259. Phorphutkul C, Rosenthal A, Nadas AS: Cardiac manifestations of Marfan's syndrome in infancy and childhood. Circulation 47:587, 1973.
260. Come PC, Fortuin NJ, White R Jr, McKusick VA: Echocardiographic assessment of cardiovascular abnormalities in the Marfan's syndrome. Am J Med 74:465, 1983.
261. Bruno L, et al.: Cardiac, skeletal and ocular abnormalities in patients with Marfan's syndrome and in their relatives. Br Heart J 51:220, 1984.
262. Murdoch JL, et al.: Life expectancy and causes of death in the Marfan syndrome. N Engl J Med 286:804, 1972.
263. Bowers D: Pathogenesis of primary abnormalities of the mitral valve in the Marfan's syndrome. Br Heart J 31:679, 1969.
264. De Maria AN, et al.: Identification and localization of aneurysms of the ascending aorta by cross-sectional echocardiography. Circulation 59:755, 1979.
265. McDonald GR, et al.: Surgical management of patients with the Marfan syndrome and dilatation of the ascending aorta. J Thorac Cardiovasc Surg 81:180, 1981.
266. Donaldson RM, et al.: Management of cardiovascular complications in Marfan's syndrome. Lancet 1:1178, 1980.
267. Pan CW, et al.: Echocardiographic study of cardiac abnormalities in families of patients with Marfan's syndrome. J Am Coll Cardiol 6:1016, 1985.
268. Hirst AE, Johns VJ, Kime SE: Dissecting aneurysm of the aorta: a review of 505 cases. Medicine 37:217, 1958.
269. Braunstein H: Pathogenesis of dissecting aneurysm. Circulation 28:1071, 1963.
270. Sethi GF, Hughes RK, Takaro T: Dissecting aortic aneurysms. Am J Thoracic Surgery 18:201, 1974.
271. DeBakey ME, et al.: Surgical management of dissecting aneurysms of the aorta. J Thorac Cardiovasc Surg 49:130, 1965.
272. Smuckler AL, Nomeir A, Watts E, Hackshaw BT: Echocardiographic diagnosis of aortic root dissection by M-mode and two-dimensional techniques. Am Heart J 103:897, 1982.
273. Granata JE, Dee P, Gibson RS: Utility of two-dimensional echocardiography in suspected ascending aortic dissection. Am J Cardiol 56:123, 1985.
274. Panidis JP, Kotler MN, Mintz GS, Ross J: Intracavitary echoes in the ascending aorta in type III aortic dissection. Am J Cardiol 54:1159, 1984.
275. Mohr-Kahaly S, et al.: Ambulatory follow-up of aortic dissection by transesophageal two-dimensional and color-coded echocardiography. Circulation 80:24, 1989.
276. Iliceto S, et al.: Color Doppler evaluation of aortic dissection. Circulation 75:748, 1987.
277. Dagli SV, et al.: Evaluation of aortic dissection by Doppler color flow mapping. Am J Cardiol 56:497, 1985.
278. Victor MF, et al.: Two-dimensional echocardiographic diagnosis of aortic dissection. Am J Cardiol 48:1155, 1981.
279. Khandheria BK, et al.: Aortic dissection: review of value and limitations of two-dimensional echocardiography in a six-year experience. J Am Soc Echocardiogr 2:17, 1989.
280. Granato JE, Dee P, Gibson RS: Utility of two-dimensional echocardiography in suspected ascending aortic dissection. Am J Cardiol 56:123, 1985.
281. Erbel R, et al.: Echocardiography in diagnosis of aortic dissection. Lancet 1:457, 1989.
282. Hashimoto S, et al.: Assessment of transesophageal Doppler echography in dissecting aortic aneurysm. J Am Coll Cardiol 14:1253, 1989.
283. Lindsay J Jr: Thoracic aneurysms. *In* Lindsay J Jr, Hurst JW (eds.): The Aorta. New York, Grune & Stratton, p. 121, 1979.
284. Mathew T, Nanda NC: Two-dimensional and Doppler echocardiographic evaluation of aortic aneurysm and dissection. Am J Cardiol 54:379, 1984.
285. Taams MA, Gussenhoven WJ, Bos E, Roelandt J: Saccular aneurysm of the transverse thoracic aorta detected by transesophageal echocardiography. Chest 93:436, 1988.
286. Taams MA, Gussenhoven WJ, Schippers LA: The value of transesophageal echocardiography for diagnosis of thoracic aorta pathology. Eur Heart J 9:1318, 1988.
287. Parmley LF, et al.: Non-penetrating traumatic injury of the aorta. Circulation 17:1086, 1958.
288. Turney SZ, et al.: Traumatic rupture of the aorta: a five year experience. J Thorasc Cardiovasc Surg 72:727, 1976.
289. Bochly K: Salvageability of patients with post-traumatic rupture of the descending thoracic aorta in a primary trauma center. J Trauma 17:754, 1977.
290. Cheitlin MD: Cardiovascular injury. *In* Parmley WW, Chatterjee K: Cardiology, San Francisco, JB Lippincott, 1982.
291. Levy MJ, Schachner A, Blieden LC: Aortico-left ventricular tunnel. J Thorac Cardiovasc Surg 84:102, 1982.
292. Turley K, et al.: Repair of aortico-left ventricular tunnel in the neonate: surgical, anatomic and echocardiographic considerations. Circulation 65: 1015, 1982.
293. Perry JC, Nanda NC, Hicks DG, Harris JP: Two-dimensional echocardiographic identification of aortico-left ventricular tunnel. Am J Cardiol 52: 913, 1983.
294. Fripp RR, et al.: Pulsed Doppler and two-dimensional echocardiographic findings in aortico-left ventricular tunnel. J Am Coll Cardiol 4:1012, 1984.
295. Bash SE, et al.: Aortico-left ventricular tunnel with ventricular septal defect: two-dimensional/Doppler echocardiographic diagnosis. J Am Coll Cardiol 5:757, 1985.
296. Braunwald E, et al.: Congenital aortic stenosis. I. Clinical and hemodynamic findings in 100 patients. Circulation 27:426, 1963.
297. Campbell M: The natural history of congenital aortic stenosis. Br Heart J 30:514, 1968.
298. Kelly DT, Wulfsberg E, Rowe RD: Discrete subaortic stenosis. Circulation 46:309, 1972.
299. Newfeld EA, et al.: Discrete subvalvular aortic stenosis in childhood. Study of 51 patients. Am J Cardiol 38:53, 1976.
300. Reis RL, et al.: Congenital fixed subvalvular aortic stenosis: an anatomic classification and correlations with operative results. Circulation (Suppl 1)43:1, 1971.
301. Wilkes HS, et al.: Left ventricular outflow obstruction after aortic valve replacement: detection with continuous wave Doppler ultrasound recording. J Am Coll Cardiol 1:550, 1983.
302. Motro M, et al.: Two-dimensional echocardiography in discrete subaortic stenosis. Am J Cardiol 53:897, 1984.
303. Eldar M, et al.: Systolic closure of aortic valve in patients with prosthetic mitral valves. Br Heart J 48:48, 1982.
304. Gardin JM, Tommaso CL, Talano JV: Echographic early systolic partial closure (notching) of the aortic valve in congestive cardiomyopathy. Am Heart J 107:135, 1984.
305. Khan MM, et al.: Discrete subaortic stenosis. Br Heart J 46:421, 1974.
306. Krajcer Z, et al.: Early systolic closure of the aortic valve in patients with hypertrophic subaortic stenosis and discrete subaortic stenosis. Am J Cardiol 41:823, 1978.
307. Weyman AE, et al.: Localization of left ventricular outflow obstruction by cross-sectional echocardiography. Am J Med 60:33, 1976.
308. Weyman AE, Feigenbaum H, Hurwitz RA, et al.: Cross-sectional echocardiography in evaluating patients with discrete subaortic stenosis. Am J Cardiol 37:358, 1976.
309. Williams DE, Sahn DJ, Friedman WF: Cross-sectional echocardiographic localization of sites of left ventricular outflow obstruction. Am J Cardiol 37:250, 1976.

310. Valdes-Cruz LM, et al.: Prediction of gradients in fibrous subaortic stenosis by continuous wave two-dimensional Doppler echocardiography: animal studies. J Am Coll Cardiol 5:1363, 1985.
311. Lima CL, et al.: Prediction of severity of left ventricular outflow tract obstruction by quantitative two-dimensional echocardiographic Doppler studies. Circulation 63:348, 1983.
312. Fisher DJ, et al.: Ventricular septal defect with silent discrete subaortic stenosis. Pediatr Cardiol 2:265, 1982.
313. Jacobs LE, Kotler MN, Ioli A: Left ventricular outflow obstruction following mitral valve replacement with Carpentier-Edwards prosthesis. Echocardiography 7:147, 1990.
314. Kreindel MS, et al.: Systolic anterior motion of the mitral valve after Carpentier ring valvuloplasty for mitral valve prolapse. Am J Cardiol 57:408, 1986.
315. Kronzon I, et al.: Left ventricular outflow obstruction: a complication of mitral valvuloplasty. J Am Coll Cardiol 4:825, 1984.
316. Come PC, et al.: Dynamic left ventricular outflow tract obstruction when the anterior leaflet is retained at prosthetic mitral valve replacement. Ann Thorac Surg 43:561, 1987.
317. Alboliras ET, et al.: Accessory mitral valve tissue in association with discrete subaortic stenosis: a two-dimensional echocardiographic diagnosis. Echocardiography 2:191, 1985.

CHAPTER

20

LEFT VENTRICLE I: GENERAL CONSIDERATIONS, ASSESSMENT OF CHAMBER SIZE AND FUNCTION

CEDRIC VUILLE and ARTHUR E. WEYMAN

"Everything should be as simple as can be, but not simpler."
A. Einstein

The primary function of the heart is to provide the energy necessary to propel blood through the vascular channels of the body to supply oxygen, nutrients, and other substances to tissues and to remove the waste products of cellular metabolism.[1] Rhythmic contraction of the muscular left ventricle creates the force needed to overcome systemic vascular resistance and to initiate and maintain this circulation of blood.[2] An assessment of left ventricular function is, therefore, of primary importance in the overall evaluation of any patient with cardiac disease. This functional assessment further represents one of the major challenges of cross-sectional echocardiography because it requires greater quantitative accuracy than does any other application of this imaging format.

Anatomically, the left ventricle is a thick-walled, bullet-shaped chamber with a large, roughly cylindric base and a smaller, cone-shaped apical cap.[2,3] In cross-section, the ventricle has a nearly circular configuration that increases in area from apex to base.[2,3]

The left ventricle is positioned obliquely in the chest such that its apex points to the left, inferiorly and anteriorly. It lies posterior and to the left of the right ventricle and inferior and anterior to the left atrium. The anteromedial portion of the left ventricle is formed by the triangular interventricular septum, which is shared with the right ventricle. The remainder of the ventricular wall is not in contract with any other cardiac chamber and is, therefore, termed the *free wall*.[3]

The left ventricle has several important internal and external anatomic features that serve as references for locating the scan plane during cross-sectional imaging and permit the division of the chamber into specific regions of interest. The major internal landmarks include the mitral valve, the aortic valve, the papillary muscles, and the apical tip.

The mitral valve divides the ventricle at its base into an anterior outflow and a posterior inflow region. It also forms a reference for determining the position of the ventricular long axis and the anteroposterior minor dimension. In short axis, the plane of the mitral commissures can be used to define the orientation of orthogonal minor diameters and to align radial coordinate systems.

The aortic valve provides a precise landmark for aligning the parasternal and apical long axis planes for comparison and measurement.

The two large papillary muscles arise from the anterolateral and posteromedial left ventricular free walls inferior to the medial and lateral mitral commissures. They are positioned such that a line joining their tips parallels a similar line connecting the mitral commissures. The mitral valve and papillary muscles, therefore, combine to provide a constant spatial reference at two separate levels within the ventricle.

The left ventricular apex is a particularly important landmark because it represents the most clearly defined intercept of the left ventricular long axis and forms the reference for transducer placement in each apical view.

The primary external landmarks are the anterior and posterior junctions of the right and left ventricular free walls. These points define the boundaries of the interventricular septum and the paths of the left anterior descending and posterior descending coronary arteries.[3]

The muscular walls that surround the left ventricle are between 9 and 12 mm thick or approximately three times as thick as those of the right ventricle.[2,3] These walls are composed of sheets of muscle fibers, which encircle the ventricular cavity like the windings of a turban.[4–6] Contraction of these muscular sheets decreases both the radius of the cylindric portion of the ventricle and the ventricular long axis. The major power and volume of ejection, however, are produced by contraction of the circumferentially oriented muscle bundles because the volume of a cylinder decreases with the square of its radius. Long axis shortening is less effective in ejecting blood because volume displacement is only in direct proportion to change in length.[2]

The inner surface of the ventricle is lined by multiple small muscular bands—the trabeculae carneae.[2,3] Although they do not contribute directly to tension development, the trabeculae represent preformed wrinkles in the ventricular wall that provide a template for further endocardial infolding during ventricular contraction. They also displace volume and permit more complete systolic emptying than would be possible if the inner walls of the ventricle were smooth.[2]

GENERAL PRINCIPLES OF ECHOCARDIOGRAPHIC IMAGING PERTINENT TO THE LEFT VENTRICULAR EXAMINATION

Several basic principles of ultrasonic imaging should be considered when attempting to record, interpret, or quantitate cross-sectional images of the left ventricle. First, remember that, in any evaluation of the left ventricle, the structures of primary interest are the endocardial and epicardial interfaces. The endocardial interface is the most important of the two because the area encompassed within the boundaries of the endocardium corresponds to the left ventricular blood pool and, hence, the chamber volume. Endocardial motion, likewise, is the primary determinant of volume change and, hence, overall ventricular function. Neither the structure nor the function of the ventricle can be evaluated unless the endocardium is well visualized.

The epicardial interface, in contrast, encompasses both the intracardiac blood pool and the ventricular musculature. By itself, the epicardial interface provides little information about the relative magnitude or the functional integrity of the muscle contained within its boundaries. From an echocardiographic standpoint, the epicardial interface serves primarily as a reference in determining wall thickness, systolic thickening, and ventricular muscle mass.

Ideally, both the endocardium and epicardium should be visualized in their entirety throughout the cardiac cycle, and point targets along their surfaces should be recorded accurately and uniformly. Unfortunately, the closed-loop configuration of these interfaces results in only a small portion being aligned perpendicular to the path of the scan plane in the majority of the standard views. The ability to record individual segments of these interfaces, therefore, varies with the difference in the acoustic impedance of the tissues that form the interface, their orientation in the scan plane, and their surface characteristics.[7] When the interfaces are perpendicular to the path of the scan plane, as occurs in the parasternal and subcostal long axis views, the primary determinant of reflectivity is the difference in acoustic density of the tissues that border the interface. Because the difference in acoustic impedance between lung and heart muscle is greater than that between heart muscle and intracavitary blood, the reflectivity of the posterior wall epicardium is greater than that of any of the internal borders of the ventricle.[7] The anterior right ventricular epicardium, in contrast, abuts the soft tissue of the anterior chest wall, which differs little from the right ventricular epicardium in acoustic impedance. As a result, the right ventricular epicardium is the most difficult surface to visualize.

When the interfaces are oblique or parallel to the path of the scan plane, their spatial orientation and surface characteristics play a more important role in determining their reflectivity. Figure 20–1 illustrates the relationship

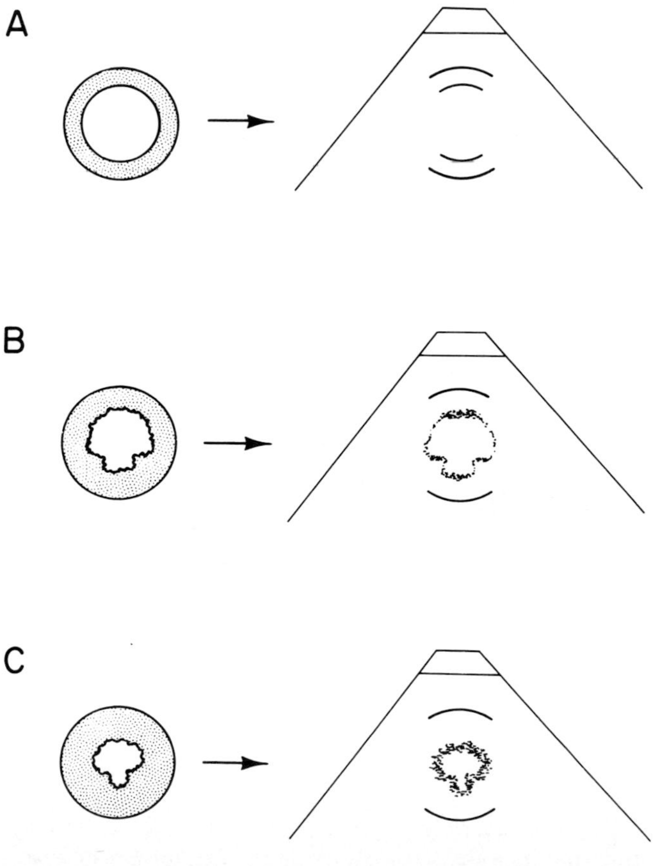

Fig. 20–1. The relationship of the left ventricular endocardial and epicardial interfaces to the path of the ultrasonic scan plane in the short axis projection. **A.** Reflections that would arise from a smooth-walled chamber. **B.** Change in the reflective pattern occurring when the interface is irregular. **C.** Increased reflectivity from the medial and lateral walls of the endocardium that is due to more marked systolic infolding. In each of these examples, the epicardial interface remains smooth; consequently, its medial and lateral borders are not clearly defined.

of the endocardial and epicardial interfaces of the left ventricle to the scan plane in a representative short axis view. If the chamber were smooth walled (Fig. 20–1A), only a small portion of the anterior segment of each surface and a slightly larger portion of the posterior segment would be visualized. This problem is even more marked in the apical views, where only the apical tip is perpendicular to the ultrasonic beam. Fortunately, the endocardial surface is irregular, and such rough surfaces scatter a portion of the incident sound energy in all directions. This scatter decreases the reflected energy recorded from surfaces that are perpendicular to the sound beam but permits some reflections to originate from areas that are oblique or parallel to the incidence sound energy. Figure 20–1B illustrates the effect of this surface irregularity on a representative diastolic image. Endocardial infolding increases during systolic contraction, further increasing the reflective characteristics of the walls that are parallel or oblique to the path of the scan plane (Fig. 20–1C). The epicardial interface, in contrast, remains smooth, and its reflective characteristics vary little from systole to diastole.

The resolution and display characteristics of individual targets along the endocardial and epicardial surfaces also vary depending on the position of the targets within the scan plane (Fig. 20–2). From a resolution standpoint, only targets that are perpendicular to the path of the ultrasonic beam are viewed with the axial resolution of the imaging system. Resolution in this dimension can be achieved at the millimeter or submillimeter level. Points that are oblique or parallel to the ultrasonic beam are resolved to varying degrees using the lateral resolution of the system. Only points separated laterally by more than the beam width can actually be resolved as being distinct. Likewise, individual targets are laterally broadened to the effective beam width (point spread function) at the target level. Again, using the short axis view as an example, the greatest point spreading occurs along the medial and lateral walls of the ventricle, which are oriented parallel to the path of the ultrasonic beam (Fig. 20–2B). Spreading of individual points along these interfaces causes the resulting echoes to encroach on contiguous chamber or muscle areas. Because the degree of point spreading varies, depending on the gain level and on the position of individual targets within the beam, direct correction for these errors is difficult and their recognition, therefore, becomes even more important. The length of the ultrasonic pulse also affects the perceived axial width of individual targets (Fig. 20–2C) but to a much lesser degree than the lateral beam width distortion.[8,9] The combined effects of beam width and pulse duration on a circular target are illustrated in Figure 20–2D.

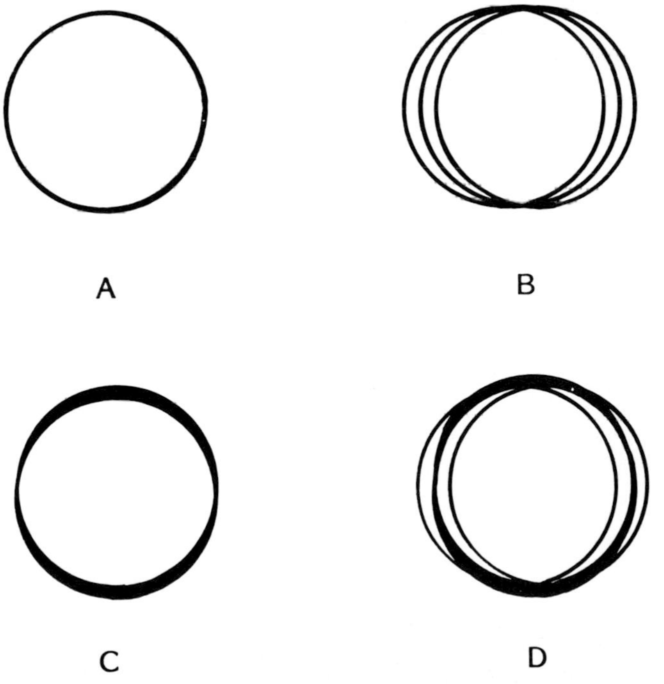

Fig. 20–2. The effects of beam width and pulse width on the image recorded from a circular target. It is assumed that the scan plane originates above the test object and that the beam is swept from left to right. **A.** Ideal image obtained if beam width and pulse width were infinitely small. **B.** Effect of beam width, which broadens the echoes from targets positioned around the medial and lateral surfaces of the circular test object. **C.** Effect of pulse width, which thickens the echoes arising from the anterior and posterior margins of the test object. **D.** Combined effects of beam width and pulse width, which thicken the echoes from targets that are anteriorly and posteriorly positioned and broaden those arising from targets that are oriented medially and laterally.

Finally, accurate description of the motion of targets along any interface is affected by the position of the target within the scan plane and its direction of motion. Motion of targets perpendicular to the path of the ultrasonic beam (axial motion) can be precisely recorded to the millimeter or submillimeter range. Motion across the scan plane, however, is recorded as movement of the target echo from one data line to the next and is, therefore, measured in degrees. The accuracy with which lateral motion can be determined depends on the separation between data lines and, therefore, is inversely related to the line density and varies from the apex to the base of the sector. In addition, the ability to perceive motion is related to the amount of movement and to the size of the moving object. For example, a fly may move only 1 or 2 mm, and yet, this small movement will be apparent, whereas a suspension bridge or skyscraper may sway many feet in the wind but will appear motionless. The motion of interfaces that are oriented parallel to the path of the sound beam and move laterally is therefore more difficult to appreciate and can be less accurately measured than that of perpendicularly oriented and axially moving regions. For this reason, wall motion is recorded less accurately in the apical than in the long axis views. Likewise, the excursion of the anterior and posterior walls of the ventricle is more easily defined in the short axis views than is the excursion of the medial and lateral walls.

Examining Planes and Linear Dimensions

Because random manipulation of the transducer can potentially provide an unlimited number of imaging planes of the left ventricle, standardization is necessary to measure reproducible and comparable dimensions and to quantitate the systolic function. The primary imaging planes used to record the left ventricle are listed in Table 20–1. The orientation of these planes is based on the assumed geometric symmetry of the ventricle and is fixed by specific internal and/or external references. Because these planes are positioned with reference to the left ventricular major or minor axes (see Chapters 4 and 5), the axes themselves, portions thereof, or dimensions that parallel these axes should be included in the recorded images. The short axis planes, for example, use the circular configuration of the ventricle when viewed in cross section to align the individual planes parallel to the true ventricular short axes. As a result, when appropriately positioned, these planes should inherently include orthogonal minor ventricular dimensions. The use of geometric assumptions to define these planes makes the areas and dimensions contained by the planes naturally suited to the reconstruction of the geometric figures on which these assumptions are based.

Unfortunately, no single view or simple combination of views provides all the data necessary for a complete evaluation of the left ventricle. This occurs primarily because access to the ventricular chamber is restricted by the available acoustic windows. As a result, with the exception of the short axis planes, some compromise must uniformly be made in terms of completeness of the image or appropriate orientation to achieve optimal interface definition. Thus, although linear and/or area measurements can be derived from the majority of these views, data must frequently be combined from multiple planes to assemble a complete picture of ventricular structure and function.

The Parasternal Long Axis Views

The parasternal long axis is the initial and most commonly used plane for recording the left ventricle. As illustrated in Figure 20–3, the parasternal long axis view transects the ventricle along a line extending from the anterior portion of the interventricular septum to the posterolateral free wall. It includes the basal two thirds of the septum and the posterolateral free wall from the atrioventricular groove to the base of the papillary muscles. This orientation places both the right and left septal surfaces and the endocardial and epicardial borders of the posterior wall perpendicular to the path of the ultrasonic beam. As a result, visualization of these interfaces is optimal and motion is along the beam axis. This combination of factors makes the parasternal long axis view ideal for defining the distances between contralateral points along the ventricular walls and for measuring endocardial excursion and myocardial thickness and thickening.

Because this plane fails to include the ventricular apex, no area measurement can be obtained. Likewise, only an anteroposterior linear dimension is available. This dimension, also referred to as the *left ventricular internal dimension* (*LVID*), however, has formed the basis for most of the M-mode determinations of left ventricular function[10–15] and, as such, is probably the most important single echocardiographic measurement. In M-mode studies, the LVID has conventionally been taken at the chordal level between the free edges of the mitral leaflets and the tips of the papillary muscles.[16] This point was chosen because it could be readily defined and, in the absence of spatial orientation, provided a means for standardization of data between patients, examinations, and laboratories. The inherent spatial orientation of the cross-sectional image makes the chordal reference less critical. Because of the established historical precedent, however, its use has persisted.

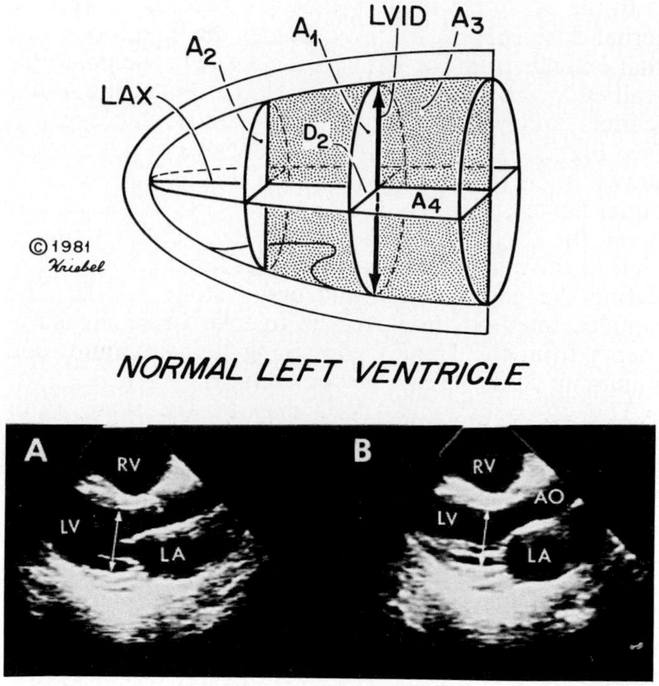

Fig. 20–3. Parasternal long axis (LAX) recording of the left ventricle (LV) during diastole (A) and systole (B) illustrating the method for obtaining the left ventricular internal dimension (LVID). The LVID is the distance between the tips of the vertically oriented arrowheads in each panel. RV = right ventricle; AO = aorta; LA = left atrium. The accompanying diagram illustrates the position of this dimension within an idealized left ventricular cavity and its relationship to areas and dimensions derived from the other ventricular views. The absence of shading at the apex is to emphasize that this plane does not include the apex and hence does not provide an area measurement.

Table 20–1. Left Ventricular Imaging Planes

- A. Parasternal long axis
  1. Left ventricle
  2. Left ventricular apex
- B. Parasternal short axis
  1. Mitral valve level
  2. Papillary muscle level
  3. Apical level
- C. Apical
  1. Four chamber
  2. Two chamber
  3. Long axis
- D. Subcostal
  1. Long axis (four chamber)
  2. Short axis

In the cross-sectional format, the anteroposterior internal dimension (LVID) is taken as the length of a line that extends from the left septal surface to the posterior wall endocardium, passes through the tips of the mitral leaflets, and is perpendicular to the ventricular long axis (see Fig. 20–3). The ventricular long axis in this view is drawn such that it divides the chamber into roughly equal halves. Because the ventricle is cylindric at this level, the LVID should approximate a maximal dimension in this plane. Various methods have been used to define the end-diastolic and end-systolic LVID. The simplest method, however, is to take these measurements from the frames containing the maximum and minimum cavity areas, respectively.

The cross-sectional LVID may be the same as or smaller than the corresponding M-mode measurement. The reason for this variation is illustrated in Figure 20–4. Specifically, when the M-mode transducer is positioned on the chest below the chordal level or when the left ventricle slopes posteriorly from apex to base, the M-mode beam transects the ventricle obliquely and the LVID is artifactually elongated. The ability in the cross-sectional format to orient this dimension perpendicular to the long axis should overcome this problem and should result in a more accurate and reproducible measurement.

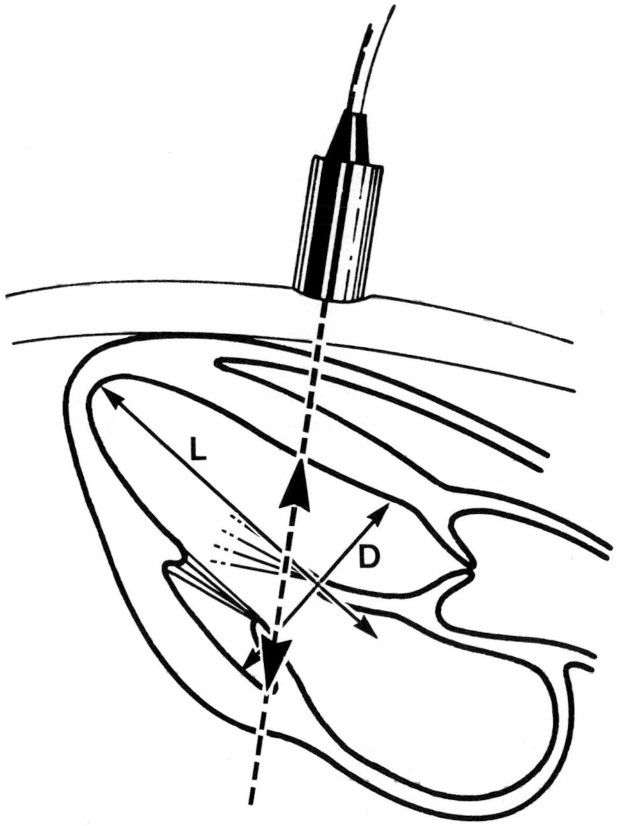

Fig. 20–4. The variation in the length of the M-mode left ventricular internal dimension that can arise as a result of apical displacement of the transducer or oblique orientation of the heart within the chest. L = length; D = diameter. (From Rodgers EW, et al.: Echocardiography for quantitation of cardiac chambers. *In* Yu PN, Goodwin JF (ed.): Progress in Cardiology. Vol. 8. Philadelphia, Lea & Febiger, 1979.)

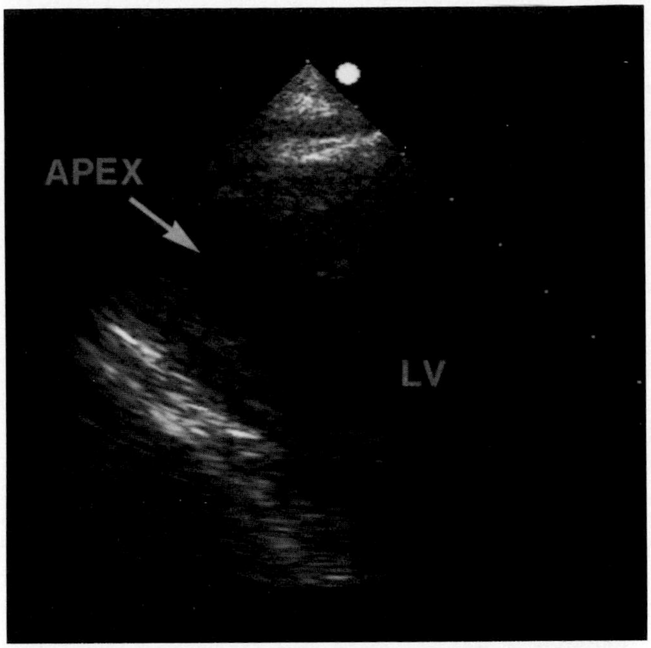

Fig. 20–5. Parasternal long axis recording of the cardiac apex. LV = left ventricle.

A similar anteroposterior dimension (D_1) can be obtained from a short axis view at the free edge of the mitral valve. As with the left atrial anteroposterior dimension (see Chapter 18), this measurement is better taken from the long axis plane because the true anteroposterior orientation and motion of the ventricle parallel to its long axis are more easily appreciated in long axis.

The parasternal long axis view of the cardiac apex is illustrated in Figure 20–5. In this view, the imaging plane transects the apex in an anteroposterior direction, and the scan plane is oriented parallel to and passes through the ventricular long axis and the apical tip. Because the parasternal long axis view of the cardiac apex contains no internal references but the apex itself, this view provides no standardizable linear dimensions. Likewise, because the basal side of the scan is not enclosed, area measurements cannot be recorded.

The long axis view of the apex is primarily used for evaluating apical configuration and wall motion. Apical wall motion is optimally recorded because the long axis view of the apex is the only view in which both the anterior and the posterior margins of the apex are perpendicular to the path of the scan, and thus, motion is along the beam axis.[17]

Short Axis Planes

Theoretically, an almost limitless number of planes might be oriented parallel to the true short axes of the left ventricle. The lack of internal references by which these planes can be standardized, however, has limited reproducible sampling to three levels. These levels include the parasternal short axis views through the mitral valve leaflets, through the bodies of the papillary muscles, and through the apex between the papillary muscles and the apical tip.

The *parasternal short axis view of the left ventricle at the mitral valve level* is illustrated in Figure 20–6A. This plane transects the ventricle from its anterior to its posterior surfaces, is parallel to the plane of its true short axes, and passes through the free edges of the mitral leaflets. The free edges of the mitral leaflets are normally defined as the point at which maximal leaflet excursion occurs. In low flow states or mitral stenosis, this may not pertain because maximal leaflet separation may be less than the annular diameter. In these instances, the free edges can be defined by sweeping the short axis scan plane down the mitral valve to a point just before the disappearance of the leaflet echoes.

Because this plane passes through the ventricle at its cylindric base, the image should appear roughly circular. The circular short axis configuration of the ventricle permits measurement of a chamber area and provides many options for obtaining ventricular diameters and chordal or radial measurements. The simplest method for drawing perpendicular short axis diameters relates these dimensions to the scan plane, thereby defining an anteroposterior diameter and a perpendicular, medial-to-lateral ventricular diameter. Though this method is attractive from the standpoint of simplicity, dimensions related to the transducer may vary considerably in their orientation relative to specific points around the ventricular circumference in different individuals, with examination from different transducer angles, or when ventricular rotation occurs from systole or diastole. This variance may affect the reproducibility of data, particularly when the radial excursions of individual points around the ventricular circumference are compared.[18] These differences are not trivial because the position of the papillary muscles and, hence, the orientation of the mitral commissures may vary considerably.[19] The ventricle may also rotate about its long axis by as much as 29°.[18]

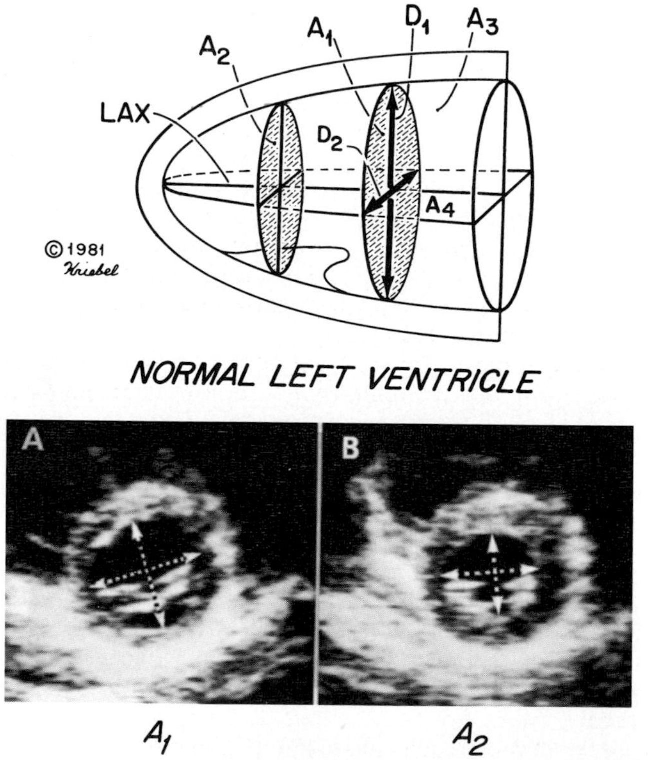

Fig. 20–6. Parasternal short axis view of the left ventricle at the mitral valve **(A)** and papillary muscle levels **(B)**. The method we prefer for aligning ventricular diameters is illustrated. Because these views encompass the circumference of the ventricular cavity, an area can be measured at both the mitral valve (A_1) and the papillary muscle levels (A_2). The accompanying diagram again illustrates the relative positions of these areas and dimensions to those obtained from the other standard ventricular views. LAX = long axis.

A second method relates the orientation of the minor axes to single or multiple fixed internal references. Different references have been used for this purpose. In one approach, an axis was constructed from the midpoint of the interventricular septum to the posterolateral wall such that it divided the diastolic ventricular cavity in half.[20] Once this orientation was established, a second perpendicular diameter or several diameters at varying angles could then be defined relative to the first. Unfortunately, this method is limited because the anterior and posterior margins of the interventricular septum are frequently difficult to define. An alternative method for orienting the short axis diameters of the ventricle uses the mitral valve commissures as the internal references. The initial diameter is then drawn through the midpoint of the ventricular cavity such that it parallels a line connecting these commissures. A second diameter can be constructed perpendicular to and can bisect the first diameter, which should pass through the midpoint of the mitral valve orifice. This method is illustrated in Figure 20–6.

The *parasternal short axis view of the left ventricle at the papillary muscle level* is depicted in Figure 20–6B. This view, like the short axis at the mitral valve level, provides a left ventricular area and orthogonal minor dimensions. In addition, multiple radial measurements can be obtained once the center of the cavity is defined. The minor ventricular dimensions obtained in the view can be aligned with reference to the scan plane, the interventricular septum, or the papillary muscles. Again, we prefer to relate these dimensions to the papillary muscles and to draw the initial diameter through the center of the left ventricular cavity from the medial to the lateral walls such that it parallels a line connecting the tips of the papillary muscles. A second dimension can then be obtained that is perpendicular to and bisects the first dimension and, thus, should pass vertically between the two papillary muscles. The left ventricular area obtained from this view is an integral part of several of the volume formulas discussed later in this chapter. Likewise, the radial excursion of individual points on the ventricular circumference is of major importance in the evaluation of patients with ischemic heart disease.

In symmetric or circular ventricles, almost any method for measuring minor ventricular diameters suffices as long as the linear dimensions are obtained from consistent points along the ventricular circumference.

When the ventricle is asymmetric, however, the lengths of individual minor dimensions may differ significantly. It has been suggested, in these instances, that the noncircular shape of the ventricle itself be used as a means of orientation.[21] In one format, which highlights the discrepancy between the major and minor ventricular short axes, an ellipse is constructed with the posterior wall of the left ventricular endocardium comprising the posterior arc of its circumference (Fig. 20–7).[18,21] The major axis (B) of the ellipse is taken as the longer

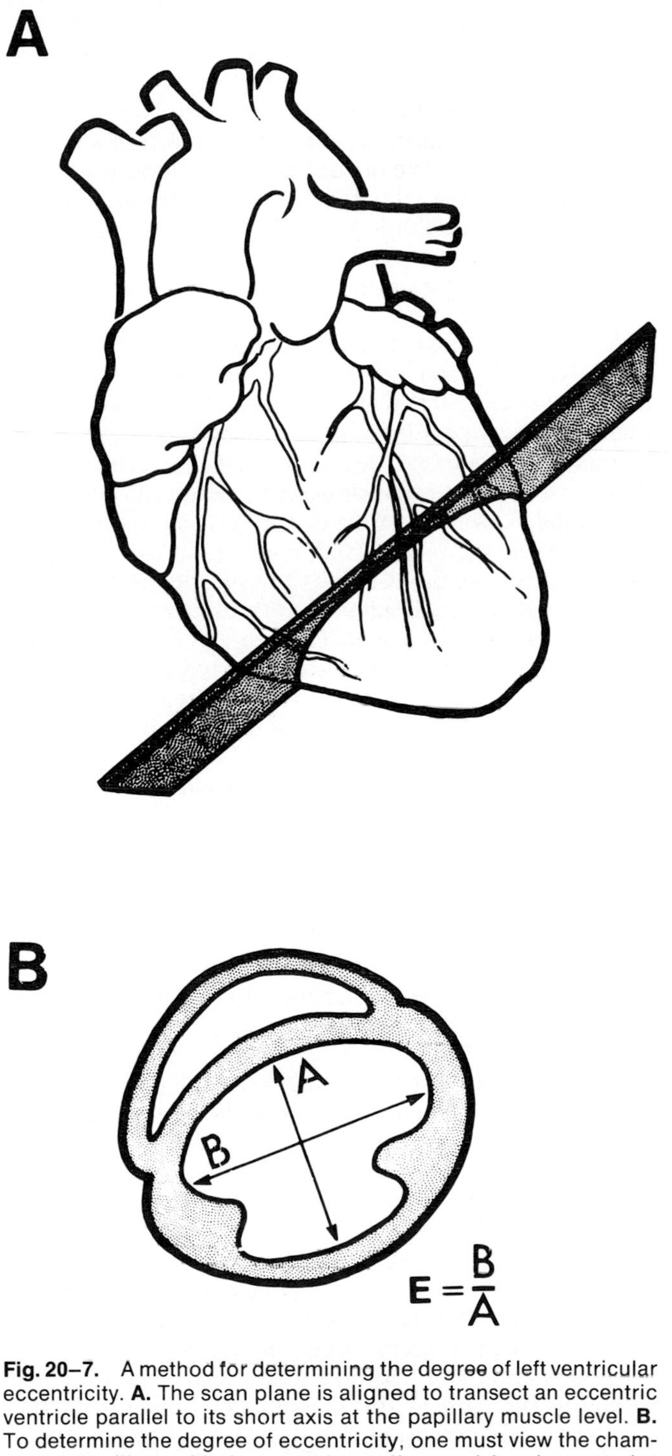

Fig. 20–7. A method for determining the degree of left ventricular eccentricity. **A.** The scan plane is aligned to transect an eccentric ventricle parallel to its short axis at the papillary muscle level. **B.** To determine the degree of eccentricity, one must view the chamber as an ellipse with the posterior wall comprising the posterior arc of its circumference. The major axis of the ellipse (B) is taken as the longer of the two minor axes of the ventricle. A second minor axis (A), which bisects and is perpendicular to the major axis, is then constructed. The eccentricity index (E) can then be defined as a ratio of B to A.

of the two minor axes of the left ventricle. The minor axis (A) is then defined as the length of a line that bisects and is perpendicular to the major axis. An eccentricity index can then be defined as the ratio of B to A. For circular ventricles, this ratio equals unity but increases as the degree of ventricular deformity becomes greater.[21]

The parasternal short axis view of the left ventricular apex is illustrated in Figure 5–9C. Although this plane encompasses a ventricular area, this measurement cannot be precisely fixed and therefore, has little quantitative value. Likewise, any linear dimension that might be obtained from this plane could not be considered reproducible. This view is used primarily to determine the degree of apical involvement in patients with ischemic heart disease, to visualize the circumferential extent of apical thrombus, and to define the position of the apical tip and ventricular long axis for the orientation of subsequent long axis and apical views.

Effects of Ventricular Motion on Short Axis Measurements. Because the short axis planes are fixed in space, whereas the ventricle moves about all its axes as it contracts, "misperception" of the true pattern of contraction can be introduced by ventricular rotation or translation. Three types of motion are important: (1) rotation of the ventricle about its long axis and short axes, (2) motion of the ventricle in space (translation), and (3) motion of the ventricle parallel to its long axis, i.e., base-to-apex shortening or through the scan plane.

The left ventricle normally rotates by as much as 7° in a counterclockwise direction about its long axis as it contracts.[18] This rotation may increase to 29° in patients with ostium secundum atrial septal defects[18] and may occur in a reverse or clockwise direction in patients with ostium primum defects and atrioventricular canals.[22] Rotation of the left ventricle about its short axes produces phasic changes in recorded images of the left ventricle, from a spherical end-diastolic shape to a more elliptical end-systolic shape, assuming a proper alignment in end-diastole.

Translation of the ventricle along its short axes has little effect on two-dimensional measurement of short axis views. M-mode measurements, however, can be significantly altered, as occurs during normal respiration:[22] As the diaphragm descends during inspiration, the heart shifts to a more medial position and the cursor intercepts a more lateral section of the ventricle. Inspiratory and expiratory dimensions thus may not be equal. In addition, translation of the ventricle may affect the assessment of wall motion. Figure 20–8 illustrates the effects of movement of the ventricle in space on the perceived excursion of individual points along the ventricular wall. Failure to appreciate or to correct for this type of motion results in an underestimation of the radial excursion of points toward which the centroid moves and in a corresponding artifactual augmentation of the excursion of points on the opposite surface of the ventricle. Centroid definition is described further in Chapter 21.

Motion of the ventricle parallel to its long axis is caused by long axis shortening, which draws the base of the ventricle inferiorly toward the apex and the apex

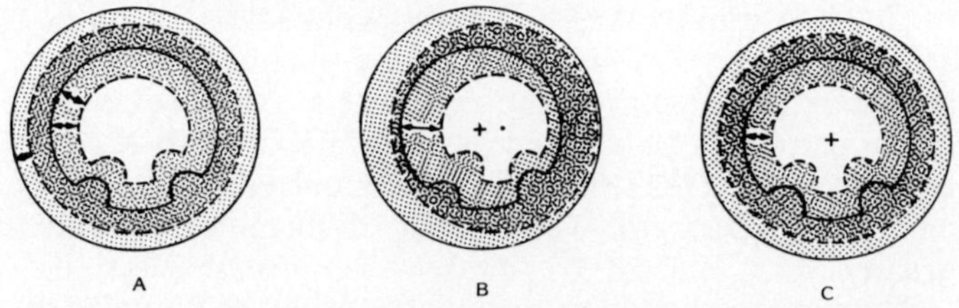

Fig. 20–8. The effects of spatial motion of the left ventricle during contraction on the perceived amplitude of wall motion. **A.** There is no spatial motion of the ventricle, and contraction around the circumference of the chamber is symmetric. **B.** The ventricular chamber shifts to the right as it contracts. This motion augments the perceived contraction of the left-sided endocardial surface (horizontal arrow) and diminishes the perceived contraction of the right margin of the chamber. The diastolic center of the ventricle is indicated by the cross and the systolic center by the point. The distance between the two centers is the motion of the centroid during contraction. **C.** Both the systolic and diastolic frames have been realigned about the centroid for each frame. Appropriate correction has been made for motion of the ventricle in space, and contraction again is correctly perceived.

superiorly toward the base. Consequently, a more basal portion of the ventricle is transected by the scan plane at end-systole than at end-diastole. Because the base of the ventricle is larger than the apex, this type of motion artifactually increases both the end-systolic cavity area and decreases the apparent endocardial excursion. The effects of this type of motion are illustrated diagrammatically in Figure 20–9. Long axis shortening also increases

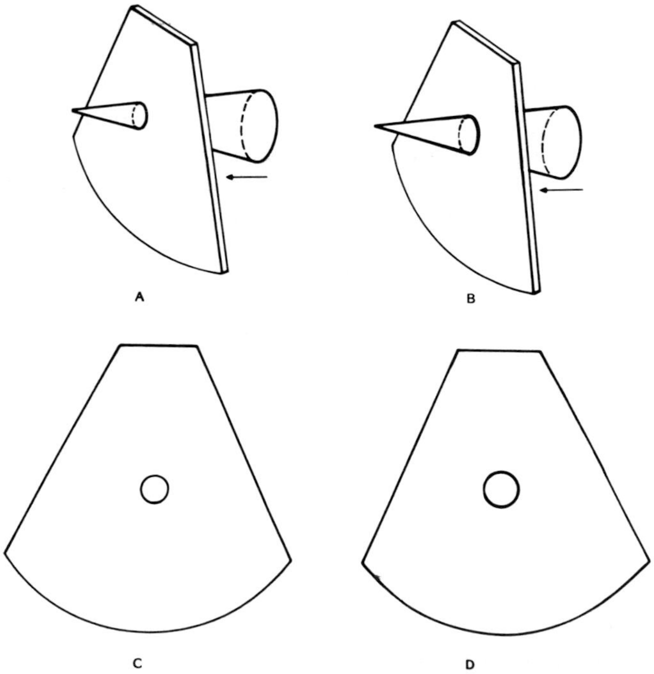

Fig. 20–9. The effects of apical motion of the ventricle during systolic contraction on the recorded short axis area. A representative imaging plane passes through the apical segment of a cone **(A)**, producing the cross-sectional area shown in **C.** When the cone advances through the plane, as indicated in **B,** the cross-sectional area on the display increases correspondingly **(D).** These variations in the cross-sectional area of the cone are analogous to the changes in the ventricular area that can be produced by motion of the left ventricle parallel to its long axis.

the muscle mass contained within the fixed area of the scan plane at end-systole when compared to the end-diastolic mass.

Ventricular rotation and spatial motion of the ventricle along any of its minor axes can be appreciated from the short axis image, and therefore, direct correction can be achieved. Motion of the ventricle parallel to its long axis cannot be appreciated from the short axis image alone, and direct correction for this type of motion is not possible. Although the motion of the ventricle from systole to diastole could be tracked by varying the angle of the scan plane to hold it on a fixed point within the chamber, this is clearly not practical. As a result, when excessive motion of the left ventricle along its long axis is noted, linear dimensions may preferably be obtained from one of the long axis or apical views.

The Apical Views

The apical views are recorded with the transducer positioned directly over the tip of the left ventricular apex and, therefore, at the distal extreme of the ventricular long axis. The scan plane is then angled until the maximal minor dimension at the ventricular base is recorded. The apical views are thus aligned by definition such that they include the full extent of the left ventricular long axis.

The difficulty of positioning the transducer exactly on the apex was demonstrated by filming the echo transducer position during ventriculography: in all but 2 of 46 patients, the transducer was found to be anterior and superior to the anatomic apex, thereby producing a tangential cut of the left ventricle and resulting in underestimation of the true size.[23]

Once positioned to include the long axis, a plane originating at the left ventricular apex theoretically could be rotated a full 360° about this axis. The lack of internal and external references available to fix such a plane in space, however, has limited apical sampling to three primary views. These views include the apical four-chamber, long axis, and two-chamber views.

The apical four-chamber view, illustrated in Figure 20–10A, is the most commonly used apical imaging plane. In this view, the plane is rotated such that it transects the midportion of the interventricular septum and the lateral left ventricular free wall in the region of the anterolateral papillary muscle. It includes a ventricular long axis that extends from the left ventricular apex to the midportion of the mitral annular plane, as illustrated in the diagram in Figure 20–10A. Minor dimensions can be drawn perpendicular to this long axis at any desired point(s) along the major axis. The area of the left ventricle within this plane can also be determined.

Unfortunately, targets along the septum and the left ventricular free wall are positioned such that they are parallel to the path of the scan plane. As a result, the echoes arising from point targets along these interfaces are widened by the point-spread function of the beam and encroach on the ventricular cavity. This artifactually reduces the measured cavity area and the length of linear distances between points along these walls. This phenomenon probably explains, in part, why volumes

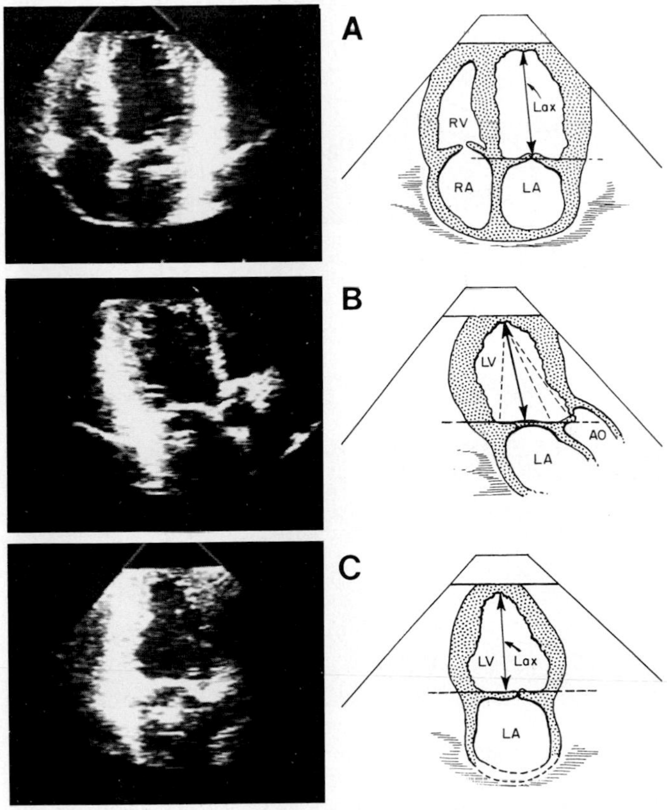

Fig. 20–10. Apical four-chamber **(A)**, long axis **(B)**, and two-chamber **(C)**, views of the left ventricle and accompanying diagrams illustrating the ventricular long axis (Lax). The interrupted lines in the apical long axis view **(B)** indicate alternative basal intercepts of the long axis (i.e., the aortic annulus, insertion point of the noncoronary aortic leaflet, or insertion point of the posterior mitral leaflet). For consistency, the basal intercept of the ventricular long axis in this view should be defined as the midpoint of the ventricular base. LA = left atrium; AO = aorta; RA = right atrium; LV = left ventricle.

calculated from the areas and dimensions obtained in this and other apical views tend to underestimate true ventricular volume. The motion of the ventricular walls in this and the other apical views is also laterally rather than axially directed and, thus, not optimally appreciated.

Assessment of apical wall motion using the apical four-chamber view may be misleading. A normal apex frequently appears hypokinetic because of the combined effects of poor near-field endocardial definition, motion of the apex into the scan plane, and positioning of the transducer above or below the true apical tip.

The major role of the apical four-chamber view is to provide a ventricular long axis and to permit the total extent of the ventricular borders that surround this long axis to be defined (albeit not optimally). This view is particularly useful for identifying ventricular thrombi, apical aneurysms, and in certain instances, pseudoaneurysms. It is also useful when assessing relative right and left ventricular chamber areas.

The apical long axis view of the left ventricle is illustrated in Figure 20–10B. In this view, the scan plane is rotated approximately 135° counterclockwise from the four-chamber view and is positioned such that it includes the aortic and mitral orifices. As illustrated in the diagram in Figure 20–10B, a ventricular long axis can theoretically be drawn from the apical tip to the junction of the mitral and aortic valves, the midportion of the mitral or the aortic annuli, or the insertion point of the posterior mitral leaflet. The midpoint of the ventricular base appears to be the most consistent basal intercept of this axis because it corresponds to the method used for defining this dimension in the parasternal long axis and other apical views. Once this long axis is defined, any number of orthogonal minor dimensions can be drawn perpendicular to the major axis at selected points within the ventricle. As with all other apical views, targets along the ventricular walls are resolved with the lateral resolution of the scan plane, and their motion is laterally directed.

The apical two-chamber view is illustrated in Figure 20–10C. In this view, the scan plane transects the anterior and inferior left ventricular free walls and is oriented by definition such that it fails to intersect any part of the right ventricle. This view, like the other apical views, contains a ventricular long axis extending from the tip of the left ventricle to a point that bisects the plane of the mitral annulus, multiple minor dimensions, and a ventricular area. Importantly, this plane is rotated approximately 90° to the apical four-chamber view. The apical two- and four-chamber views are the only two imaging planes that are orthogonally positioned about the ventricular long axis and include all the points around the circumference of the ventricle. They are, therefore, the ideal combination of planes for calculating ventricular volumes using either the ellipsoid area-length or the Simpson's rule method. Figure 20–11 illustrates how, in the idealized ventricular model, these orthogonal apical areas and the apically derived long axis relate to the areas and dimensions derived from the other standard views of the left ventricle.

Effects of Ventricular Motion on Apical Views and Measurements. As is the case with short axis views, apical views are affected by left ventricular translation and rotation. Only rotation about the minor axis perpendicular to the imaging plane and base-to-apex shortening can be appreciated directly from the image. Rotation about the minor axis included in the imaging plane and lateral translation might not be perceived as motion artifacts, hence leading to miscalculation of volumes and ejection fraction, and misperception of regional wall motion. Rotation about the long axis has no significant effect in quantitation of perfectly ellipsoid ventricles but creates artifacts in asymmetric ventricles.

Another source of motion artifact is breathing. As already noted, the translation of the heart to a medial position during inspiration may move the long axis of the left ventricle out of the imaging plane. Measurements should be made during suspended respiration at end-expiration.[24]

The Subcostal Views

The left ventricle can be visualized from the subcostal transducer location in either the long axis or the multiple short axis projections.

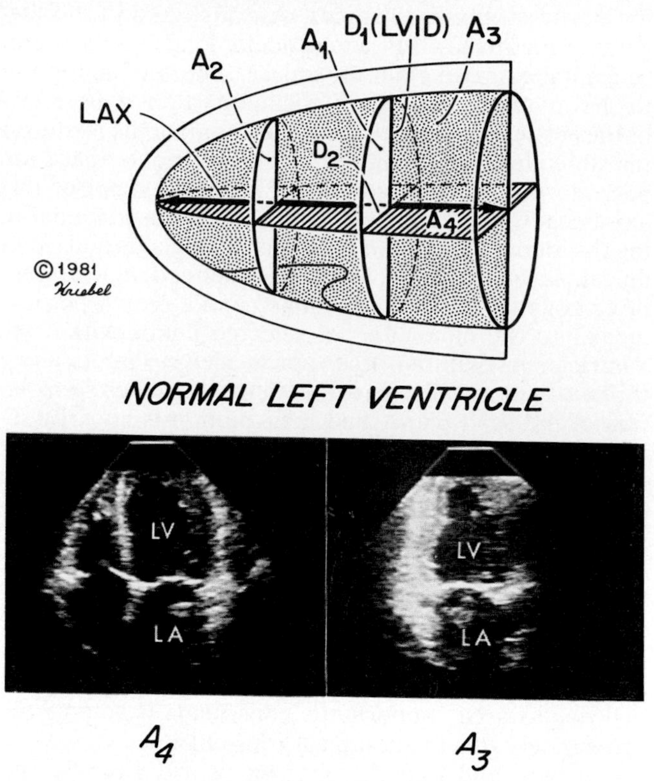

Fig. 20–11. The relationship of the orthogonal areas derived from the apical four-chamber (A_4) and two-chamber (A_3) views and the left ventricular long axis (LAX) to the areas and dimensions obtainable from the other left ventricular imaging planes. The position of these apical planes in space obviously varies with that of the internal landmarks about which they are fixed, and their positions in the diagram are intended to illustrate geometric and not necessarily anatomic relationships. LVID = left ventricular internal dimension; LV = left ventricle; LA = left atrium.

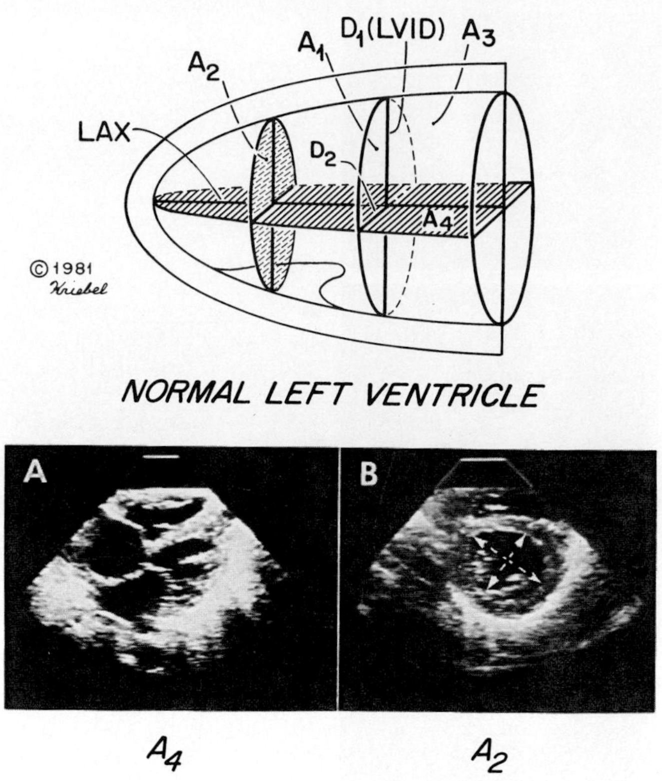

Fig. 20–12. A. Subcostal long axis (LAX) view of the left ventricle. **B.** Subcostal short axis view with the minor dimension aligned relative to the papillary muscles. The diagram illustrates how the planes fit into the idealized model of the left ventricle. LVID = left ventricular internal dimension.

The subcostal long axis (four-chamber) view of the left ventricle is illustrated in Figure 20–12A. In this projection, the imaging plane passes through the posterior third of the right ventricle, the posterior segment of the interventricular septum, the left ventricular long axis, and the anterolateral left ventricular free wall at or just above the anterolateral papillary muscle. This orientation places both the septum and the lateral left ventricular free wall perpendicular to the path of the scan plane and is theoretically optimal for recording targets along their surfaces. Left ventricular wall motion is also axially directed in this view and should be accurately recorded. In children, this view is extremely valuable for recording left ventricular structure and function. In the adult, the left ventricle is so deep to the transducer face that clear structure visualization is frequently difficult to obtain. When the ventricle can be clearly recorded, however, major and multiple minor dimensions can be obtained. A cavity area can also be outlined, and the excursion of points along the ventricular walls can be recorded.

Multiple short axis views of the left ventricle can theoretically be obtained from the subcostal transducer location. The landmarks available to orient these planes, however, are similar to those in the parasternal short-axis views and limit sampling to the levels of the mitral valve, papillary muscles, and cardiac apex. In the subcostal position, the transducer and hence the origin of the scan plane are rotated counterclockwise between 60 and 90° from the parasternal transducer location. This rotation causes the images to appear rotated in the opposite or clockwise direction. Figure 20–12B is a subcostal short axis view of the left ventricle taken at the papillary muscle level. This view contains the same dimensions and area that are available in the corresponding parasternal short axis view. Furthermore, when these dimensions are aligned relative to an internal reference, such as the papillary muscle tips, they should, as indicated, be identical to comparable parasternal measurements. The same relationships apply at the mitral valve and apical levels, and when available, the subcostal views should offer an alternative to the parasternal views. In addition, because of the shift in transducer orientation, the subcostal views may permit the recording of some areas of the ventricle that are less well visualized from the precordium.

LEFT VENTRICULAR VOLUME

The collection of imaging planes described in the preceding section contains a variety of dimensions and areas that can be used to calculate left ventricular volume. Before the volume of any chamber can be determined from a planar image or group of images, however,

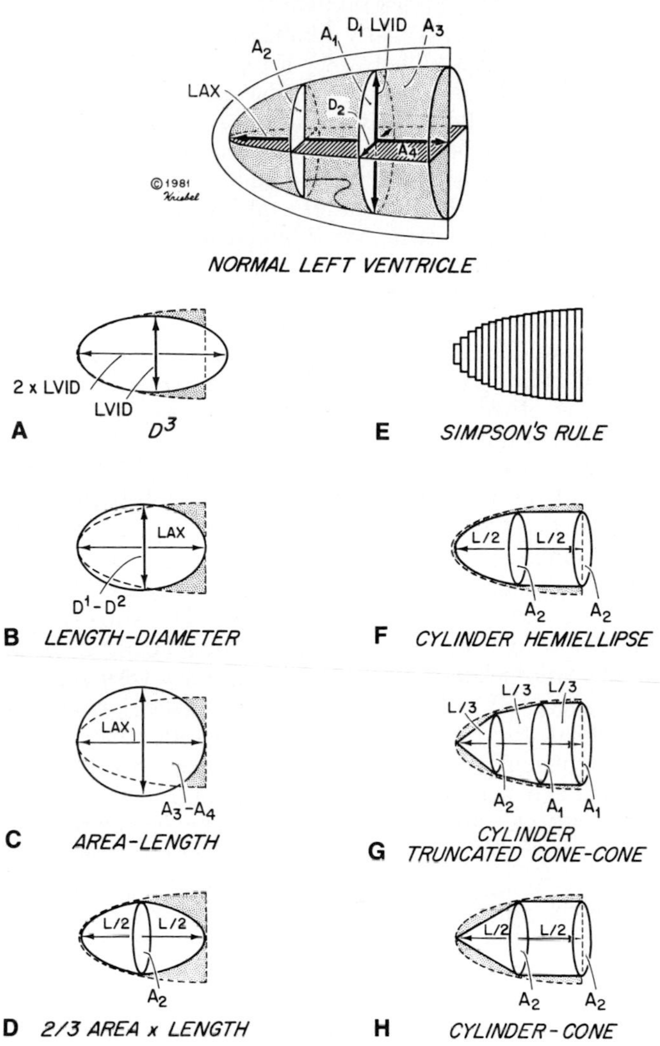

Fig. 20–13. The primary geometric figures that have been used to represent the left ventricle are shown, as well as the echocardiographic dimensions and areas used to construct these figures. **A.** Prolate ellipsoid, D^3 method. **B.** Prolate ellipsoid, length-diameter method. **C.** Prolate ellipsoid, area-length using the biapical areas and the ventricular length. **D.** Prolate ellipsoid using the short axis area and length. **E.** Simpson's rule. **F.** Cylinder-hemiellipse. **G.** Cylinder-truncated cone-cone. **H.** Cylinder-cone. The truncated cone-hemiellipsoid method is shown in Fig. 20–20. LVID = left ventricular internal dimension.

the chamber must first be represented by a mathematical model with dimensions that are directly available or can be calculated from the image(s). A variety of geometric figures or combinations of figures have been used to represent the left ventricle. The most common of these are illustrated in Figure 20–13. They represent three basic approaches to ventricular volume calculation (1) representation of ventricular volume as the volume of a single figure, e.g., the prolate ellipsoid; (2) the sum of the volumes of multiple smaller figures of like configuration (the Simpson's rule method); or (3) the volumes of a combination of different figures, e.g., a cylinder, and a cone. The first two methods have been extensively studied and validated angiographically.[25–32] The third uses the short axis area measurements that are easily provided by cross-sectional echocardiography and greatly increase the number and variety of geometric models that can be conveniently used to represent the ventricular chamber.

Ventricular Volume Calculations Using the Prolate Ellipsoid Model

The single figure that has been used most extensively to represent the left ventricle is the prolate ellipsoid. This figure forms the basis for most angiographic calculations of left ventricular volume, and its validity as a model of the left ventricle has been well documented.[25–30] The prolate ellipsoid is illustrated in Figure 20–14. This figure has two minor axes (D_1 and D_2) and a major axis (L). It can also be sectioned through its long axis to provide orthogonal areas (A_1 and A_2) or through its short axes to yield a third area (A_3). The volume of the ellipsoid can be calculated by using the following formula:

$$\text{Volume} = \frac{4}{3}\pi \frac{L}{2}\frac{D_1}{2}\frac{D_2}{2} \qquad [20.1]$$

The ellipsoid model can be applied to echocardiographic images by (1) extension of the M-mode D^3 method; (2) adaptation of angiographic ellipsoid volume formulas; and (3) use of the short axis area to derive a unique echocardiographic ellipsoid area-length formula.

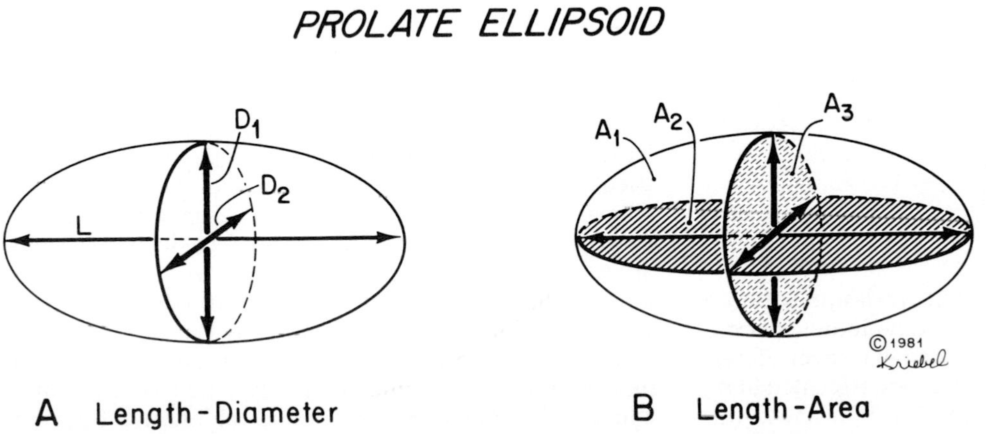

Fig. 20–14. The prolate ellipsoid figures. **A.** Minor diameters (D_1 and D_2) and long axis length (L). **B.** Three areas obtained either by projecting the figure or by sectioning it through its long or short axes. For reasons of convention, plane labeling in this figure does not correspond to the normal left ventricular illustration in Figures 20–8 to 20–13, and these should not be confused.

D^3 Method

The D^3 method is the simplest approach to left ventricular volume calculation because it permits volume to be estimated from a single linear dimension.[11] This method was originally developed specifically for M-mode echocardiographic studies where only one ventricular dimension was available. It is based on the following observations:

1. Left ventricular dilatation occurs primarily along the minor axis. Consequently, a linear relationship can be demonstrated between minor axis length[33] and chamber volume over a wide range of ventricular sizes.
2. A good correlation can be demonstrated between the M-mode LVID and the angiographic minor axis.
3. The LVID is directly related to left ventricular volume,[33–35] and this relationship improves when the linear dimension is cubed.[10,11]

The D^3 method for left ventricular volume can be derived from the ellipsoid volume formula if it is assumed that the LVID is equal to one of the minor axes of the ellipse (D_1), that both minor dimensions are equal ($D_1 = D_2$) and that the major axis (L) is equal to twice the minor axis ($L = 2D_1$). After substitution, the formula for the volume of the ellipsoid becomes:

$$\text{Volume} = \frac{4}{3}\pi \frac{2D_1}{2}\frac{D_1}{2}\frac{D_1}{2}$$

or

$$V = \frac{\pi}{3} \times D^3$$

or

$$V = 1.047 \times D^3$$

or

$$V \simeq D^3 \qquad [20.2]$$

Because the ventricle becomes more spherical as it dilates, the ratio of (L) to (D) decreases. As a result, the D^3 method may seriously overestimate the volume of larger ventricles.[13,36–44] Several regression formulas have been developed to correct for the effect of ventricle size on the relationship of L to D. The most widely used formula is that derived by Teichholz et al.,[45] in which:

$$\text{Volume} = \left(\frac{7.0}{2.4 + D}\right) \times D^3 \qquad [20.3]$$

This correction permits more direct correlation between echocardiographic and angiographic volumes over a wide range of ventricular sizes[45] and has been determined the most accurate M-mode method for calculating stroke volume.[46]

The D^3 method is easily adapted to the cross-sectional format.[20,47–50] As illustrated in Figure 20–3, the LVID can be directly obtained from the parasternal long axis view or an orthogonal short axis projection. Measurements taken from the cross-sectional image should be more reliable and, thereby, should increase the accuracy of the method. Unfortunately, although the simplicity of this method is attractive, it has major limitations. The most important limitation is that the method seeks to define left ventricular size and function from a single arbitrary dimension and consequently must assume that the recorded measurement actually corresponds to one of the minor axes of the ellipsoid model and that the function of the ventricle in the region in which the dimension is taken is representative of global ventricular function.

There are important exceptions to both of these assumptions. In ischemic heart disease, e.g., major local abnormalities in left ventricular structures and function may be present in areas of the ventricle that are removed from the region sampled by the LVID. Not surprisingly, several studies have demonstrated the inaccuracy of M-mode volume determinations in patients with regional dyssynergy.[38,42,46,48,51,52] In right ventricular volume overload, the LVID may also fail to reflect accurately left ventricular volume. This occurs because the interventricular septum is frequently displaced toward the left ventricle. Such displacement alters the relationship of the two minor dimensions, and because the LVID more closely approximates the smaller dimension, chamber volume is underestimated. Even with in vitro studies of symmetric formalin-fixed ventricles, the D^3 method correlated less well with measured ventricular volumes than did methods based on more extensive substitution into the ellipsoid formula or on combined geometric figures (Table 20–2).[47] Likewise, in clinical studies, the corrected D^3 method correlated less well with angiographic volumes than did the single or biplane angiographic formula or a modified Simpson's rule approach.[20] In addition, any error in the measurement of LVID will be roughly tripled in the calculation of volume. Thus, despite its historical import and the large body of data generated by the use of this method, the D^3 formula, with or without correction, appears to be the least accurate echocardiographic approach to volume calculation.

Angiographic Ellipsoid Volume Formulas: The Length-Diameter and Area-Length Methods

Many of the echocardiographic sections of the left ventricle contain dimensions and areas that appear similar to those found in angiographic projections of the ventricular chamber. As a result, several of the angiographic ellipsoid volume formulas have been applied to echocardiographic volume calculations. Two basic angiographic approaches to volume calculation use the ellipsoid model: the length-diameter method, in which the minor ventricular dimension is measured directly from the image,[26–28] and the area-length method, in which the minor dimension is calculated rather than directly measured.[25,29,30] The rationale for and the method by which each of these angiographic approaches can be applied to cross-sectional echocardiography are more easily understood if the angiographic derivations of the formulas are first considered.

Angiographic Derivations. Figure 20–15 illustrates how the ellipsoid model is applied angiographically. This figure contains two orthogonal angiographic images of the left ventricle recorded in the anteroposterior and left lateral projections. As indicated in the accompanying diagrams, each of these images contains a long axis drawn from the aortic valve to the ventricular apex, a minor axis that is perpendicular to the major dimension, and an elliptic area that is contained within the ventricular silhouette. Together, the two planar images provide the orthogonal minor dimensions and ventricular length required by the prolate ellipsoid formula. Application of this formula, however, requires two assumptions: (1) The ventricle must be oriented parallel to at least one of the angiographic planes so that a true long axis is projected, and (2) the ventricle must be a true ellipse. In practice, the true left ventricular long axis generally cannot be determined angiographically, and because L is not usually equal in the two projections, the larger length must be assumed to approximate more nearly the ventricular long axis.[25,29] Likewise, the ventricle is rarely a true ellipse, and as a result, correction for shape becomes necessary. This can be done by assuming that the projected area of the ventricle (A) represents a true ellipse. By knowing the ventricular length (L), the minor axis for that projection (D) can be calculated from the relationship:

$$\text{Area} = \pi \times \frac{L}{2} \times \frac{D}{2} \quad \text{or} \quad D = \frac{4A}{\pi L} \qquad [20.4]$$

This correction permits the irregular silhouette of the left ventricle in each projection to be represented by a true ellipse, and the volume formula then becomes:

$$\text{Volume} = \frac{4}{3}\pi\left(\frac{L_{max}}{2}\right)\left(\frac{4A_1}{2\pi L_1}\right)\left(\frac{4A_2}{2\pi L_2}\right) \qquad [20.5]$$

Ventricular volume can also be calculated from a single planar image (generally, the right anterior oblique (RAO) angiographic image) using the length-diameter method if the two minor diameters are assumed equal. If $D_1 = D_2$, then:

$$\text{Volume} = \frac{4}{3}\pi \frac{L}{2}\frac{D_1}{2}\frac{D_1}{2} \qquad [20.6]$$

or

$$V = \frac{\pi}{6} L \times D^2$$

The area-length method can also be used, by assuming the ventricular area and long axis in the two projections are the same, with the result that:

$$\text{Volume} = \frac{4}{3}\pi\left(\frac{L_1}{2}\right)\left(\frac{4A_1}{2\pi L_1}\right)\left(\frac{4A_1}{2\pi L_1}\right) \qquad [20.7]$$

or

$$V = \frac{8A^2}{3\pi L}$$

Either the single plane or the biplane ellipsoid formulas can be applied to any appropriately derived planar image of the ventricle.

For angiographic use, two additional corrections are required. The first correction is necessary to allow for the image magnification, which is caused by the divergence of the x-ray beam.[25,53] The second correction is necessary to compensate for the slight overestimation of ventricular volume that is due to the inclusion of the papillary muscles and mitral valve apparatus in the measured volume.[25,30] The biplane angiographic volume formula including both of these corrections can be expressed[54] as

$$V = \frac{0.788\ A_a \times A_L \times CF_m^2 \times CF_s}{L_{min}} - 3.8 \qquad [20.8]$$

where CF_m is the correction factor for the image with the larger major axis, CF_s is the correction factor for the second image, A_a is the area in the anteroposterior projection, A_L is the area in the lateral projection, and L_{min} is the smaller of the two uncorrected major axes.

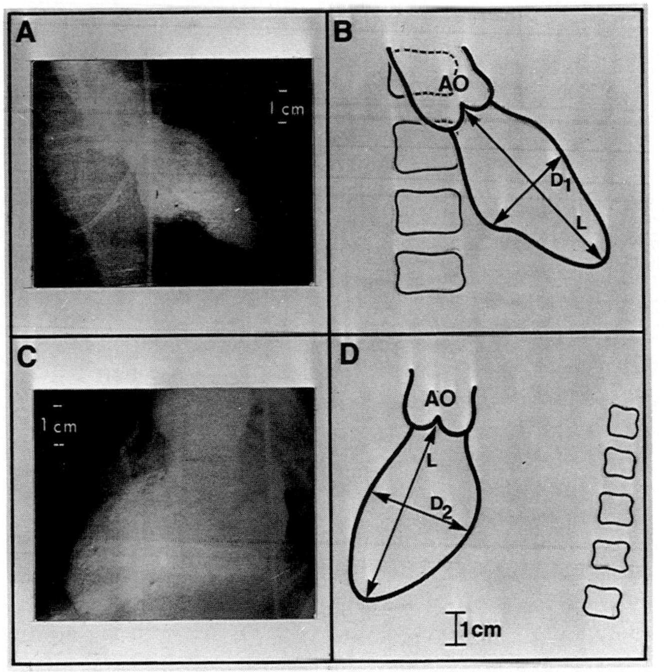

Fig. 20–15. Anteroposterior (**A** and **B**) and lateral angiographic (**C** and **D**) projections of the left ventricle and accompanying diagrams illustrating how the ellipsoid figure can be used to represent the angiographic silhouette of the ventricular chamber. AO = aorta; L = length; D_1, D_2 = diameter. (From Rogers EW, et al.: Echocardiography for quantitation of cardiac chambers. *In* Yu PN, Goodwin JF (eds.): Progress in Cardiology. Vol. 8. Philadelphia, Lea & Febiger, 1979.)

Table 20–2. Left Ventricular Volumes and Ejection Fraction

Geometric Model	Volume Formula	Reference	Subjects of Study	Segmental Diseases	Dilated Ventricles	Standard of Comparison	Cross-Sectional Views	Ejection Fraction		End-Systolic Volume		End-Diastolic Volume		In Vitro Volume		
								r	SEE	r	SEE (ml)	r	SEE (ml)	r	% Error	SEE (ml)
Prolate ellipsoid (length-diameter)	D^3	Wyatt et al.[47]	21 dogs, in vitro			Direct volume measurements	SAX-Pap; LAXp							.84	49.9	40.4
		Wyatt et al.[48]	10 dogs, in vitro	Symmetric ventricles		Direct volume measurements	SAX-Pap							.97	29.8	15.6
		Wyatt et al.[48]	9 dogs, in vitro	Asymmetric ventricles		Direct volume measurements	SAX-Pap							.87	53.5	34.2
	$\frac{7}{2.4 + D} D^3$	Folland et al.[20]	35 patients	20	8	Single-plane cineangiogram	4Ch; SAX-MV	.55	13.0%	.81	37	.72	46			
		Stamm et al.[49]	49 patients			Single-plane or biplane	SAX-MV	.70	11.3%							
		Stamm et al.[49]	23 patients			Single-plane or biplane	2CH; 4Ch	.69	10.5%							
		Mercier et al.[59]	25 children, CHD			Biplane cineangiogram	M-mode, MV, parasternal	.65	10.9%	.93	11	.79	30			
	$\frac{\pi}{6} L D_1 D_2$	Mercier et al.[59]	25 children, CHD			Biplane cineangiogram	SAX-MV; 4Ch	.89	7.0%	.95	6.6	.97	9.6			
		Mercier et al.[59]	25 children, CHD			Biplane cineangiogram	SAX-Pap; 4Ch	.91	6.7%	.93	6.3	.97	8.4			
		Chaudry et al.[50]	30 patients	20		Single-plane cineangiogram	SAX-MV; 2Ch	.73		.91		.86				
		Wyatt et al.[48]	10 dogs, in vitro	Symmetric ventricles		Direct volume measurements	SAX-Pap; LAXp							.98	26.6	6.8
		Wyatt et al.[48]	9 dogs, in vitro	Asymmetric ventricles		Direct volume measurements	SAX-Pap; LAXp							.96	35.4	7.5
		Wyatt et al.[47]	21 dogs, in vitro			Direct volume measurements	SAX-Pap; LAXp							.96	31.4	8.7
		Erbel et al.[58]	22 rubber casts of human aneurysmal ventricles	22		Direct volume measurements	2 orthogonal LAX planes							.97		22.0
		Smith et al.[69]	36 patients	4		Single-plane or biplane	TEE 4Ch, SAX-MV	.73	11.9%	.95	17	.88	30			
Prolate ellipsoid (length-area)	$\frac{\pi}{6} L \left(\frac{4A_1}{\pi D_2}\right)\left(\frac{4A_4}{\pi L}\right)$	Stamm et al.[49]	46 patients			Single-plane or biplane	4Ch; SAX-MV	.83	8.8%							
		Stamm et al.[49]	17 patients			Single-plane or biplane	2Ch; SAX-MV	.81	8.6%							
		Folland et al.[20]	35 patients	20	8	Single-plane cineangiogram	4Ch; SAX-MV	.78	9.8%	.72	44	.67	49			
	$\frac{8A_4^2}{3\pi L}$	Folland et al.[20]	35 patients	20	8	Single-plane cineangiogram	4Ch	.76	10.1%	.64	48	.61	52			
		Stamm et al.[49]	56 patients			Single-plane or biplane	4Ch	.80	9.1%							
		Stamm et al.[49]	23 patients			Single-plane or biplane	2Ch	.72	10.3%							
	$\frac{8A_3A_4}{3\pi L}$	Erbel et al.[58]	22 ventricular casts	22		Direct volume measurements	2 orthogonal LAX planes							.99		14.0
	$0.85 \frac{A^2}{L}$	Mercier et al.[59]	25 children, CHD			Biplane cineangiogram	4Ch	.68	10.7%	.83	10	.93	12			

(Continued)

		Mercier et al.[59]	25 children, CHD			Biplane cineangiogram	2Ch	.51	9.2%	.64	11	.73	20			
		Wyatt et al.[47]	21 dogs, in vitro			Direct volume measurements	LAXp							.90	42.8	9.5
		Wyatt et al.[48]	10 dogs, in vitro	Symmetric ventricles		Direct volume measurements	LAXp							.97	30.9	7.5
		Wyatt et al.[48]	9 dogs, in vitro	Asymmetric ventricles		Direct volume measurements	LAXp							.89	52.1	8.9
Simpson's rule	$\frac{\pi}{4} h \sum_{i=1}^{n} D1_i \times D2_i$ 100–250 slices	Erbel et al.[58]	22 ventricular casts	22		Direct volume measurements	2 orthogonal planes							.99		12.8
	Multiple slices by computer	Erbel et al.[23]	46 patients	23	9	Single-plane cineangiogram	LAXa	.80	9.1%	.94	19	.91	26			
	20 slices by computer	Starling et al.[66]	70 patients	30		70 single-plane cineangiogram	4Ch; 2Ch	.90	7%	.88	27	.80	34			
		Starling et al.[66]	30 patients			30 biplane cineangiogram	4Ch; 2Ch	.87	9%	.92	28	.81	37			
		Starling et al.[66]	60 patients			60 radionuclide angiography	4Ch; 2Ch	.81	10%							
	15–19 slices	Weiss et al.[64]	5 isolated ejecting canine hearts			Volumetric chamber measurement	Multiple SAX							.97	6.6	2.4
	8–10 slices	Weiss et al.[64]				Volumetric chamber measurement	Multiple SAX							.95	8.1	3.0
	5–9 slices	Weiss et al.[64]	52 volume measurements			Volumetric chamber measurement	Multiple SAX							.94	9.4	3.5
	4 slices	Weiss et al.[64]				Volumetric chamber measurement	Multiple SAX							.94	8.6	3.3
	3 slices	Weiss et al.[64]				Volumetric chamber measurement	Multiple SAX							.91	11.3	4.5
	2 slices	Weiss et al.[64]				Volumetric chamber measurement	Multiple SAX							.88	17.3	6.8
	1 slice	Weiss et al.[64]				Volumetric chamber measurement	Multiple SAX							.85	26.6	7.1
Modified Simpson's rule	$(A_1 + A_2)\frac{L}{3} + \frac{A_3}{2}\frac{L}{3} + \frac{\pi}{6}\left(\frac{L}{3}\right)^3$	Mercier et al.[59]	25 children, CHD			Biplane cineangiogram	SAX-MV, Pap1, Pap2; 4Ch	.91	4.9%	.93	8.6	.98	9.1			
		Smith et al.[69]	36 patients	4		Single-plane cineangiogram	TEE SAX-MV, Pap, apex; 4Ch	.85	8.0%	.94	22	.85	42			
	$(A_1 + A_2 + A_3)h + \frac{A_4 h}{2} + \frac{\pi h^3}{6}$	Wyatt et al.[47]	21 dogs, in vitro			Direct volume measurements	4 SAX; LAXp							.98	9.6	6.6
		Wyatt et al.[48]	10 dogs, in vitro	Symmetric ventricles		Direct volume measurements	Multiple SAX; LAXp							.996	5.9	3.4
		Wyatt et al.[48]	9 dogs, in vitro	Asymmetric ventricles		Direct volume measurements	Multiple SAX; LAXp							.98	9.8	5.8
	$(A + A_2 + A_3 + A_4)h + \frac{A_5 h}{2} + \frac{\pi h^3}{6}$	Guéret et al.[67]	30 dogs	0		Single-plane cineangiogram	5 SAX; 4Ch	.90	3.6%	.93	4.5	.92	7.1			
		Guéret et al.[67]	11 dogs	11		Single-plane cineangiogram	5 SAX; 4Ch	.92	5.1%	.86	8.7	.89	9.9			
		Guéret et al.[68]	25 dogs	6		Single-plane cineangiogram	5 SAX; LAXp	.89	4.3%	.97	3.8	.94	8.4			
Cylinder-cone = ellipsoid	$\frac{2}{3}AL$	Wyatt et al.[47]	21 dogs, in vitro			Direct volume measurements	SAX-Pap; LAXp							.97	22.4	8.6
		Stamm et al.[49]	47 patients			Single-plane or biplane	SAX-MV; 4Ch	.86	8.0%							
Cylinder-truncated cone-cone	$A_1\frac{L}{3} + \left(\frac{A_1 + A_2}{2}\right)\frac{L}{3} + \frac{1}{3}A_2\frac{L}{3}$	Folland et al.[20]	35 patients	20	8	Single-plane cineangiogram	SAX-MV, Pap; 4Ch	.78	9.7%	.86	32	.76	43			
		Stamm et al.[49]	34 patients			Single-plane or biplane	SAX-MV, Pap; 4Ch	.89	7.9%							

(Continued)

Table 20–2. Left Ventricular Volumes and Ejection Fraction—*Continued*

Geometric Model	Volume Formula	Reference	Subjects of Study	Segmental Diseases	Dilated Ventricles	Standard of Comparison	Cross-Sectional Views	Ejection Fraction		End-Systolic Volume		End-Diastolic Volume		In Vitro Volume		
								r	SEE	r	SEE (ml)	r	SEE (ml)	r	% Error	SEE (ml)
Cylinder-2 truncated cones-cone	$\frac{L}{4}\left[A_1 + \left(\frac{A_1 + A_2}{2}\right) + \left(\frac{A_2 + A_3}{2}\right) + \frac{A_3}{3}\right]$	Mercier et al.[59]	25 children, CHD			Biplane cineangiogram	SAX-MV, Pap1, Pap2; 4Ch	.90	4.9%	.93	7.0	.98	7.2			
Cylinder-hemiellipsoid	$\frac{5}{6}AL$	Folland et al.[20]	35 patients	20	8	Single-plane cineangiogram	SAX-MV; 4Ch	.66	11.6%	.75	42	.68	49			
		Guéret et al.[68]	12 patients	10		Single-plane cineangiogram	SAX-Pap; 4Ch	.97	3.7%	.91	25.3	.73	40			
		Mercier et al.[59]	25 children, CHD			Biplane cineangiogram	SAX-MV; 4Ch	.85	5.8%	.91	10.7	.98	10.9			
		Mercier et al.[59]	25 children, CHD			Biplane cineangiogram	SAX-Pap; 4Ch	.89	6.4%	.91	8.5	.96	11.7			
		Smith et al.[69]	36 patients	4		Single-plane cineangiogram	TEE SAX-MV; 4Ch	.80	8.7%	.93	25	.84	46			
		Wyatt et al.[47]	21 dogs, in vitro			Direct volume measurements	SAX-Pap: LAXp							.97	17.9	10.9
		Wyatt et al.[48]	10 dogs, in vitro	Symmetric ventricles		Direct volume measurements	LAXp; SAX-Pap							.99	10.1	6.1
		Wyatt et al.[48]	9 dogs, in vitro	Asymmetric ventricles		Direct volume measurements	LAXp; SAX-Pap							.97	20.3	9.1
		Guéret et al.[67]	30 dogs	0		Single-plane cineangiogram	SAX-MV; 4Ch	.70	5.8%	.85	6.3	.89	8.1			
		Guéret et al.[67]	11 dogs	11		Single-plane cineangiogram	SAX-MV; 4Ch	.60		.56		.90	9.4			
		Guéret et al.[67]	30 dogs	0		Single-plane cineangiogram	SAX-Pap; 4Ch	.82	4.7%	.92	4.7	.89	8.0			
		Guéret et al.[67]	11 dogs	11		Single-plane cineangiogram	SAX-Pap; 4Ch	.92	4.8%	.87	8.4	.82	12.4			

CHD = congenital heart disease; 2Ch = apical two-chamber view; 4Ch = apical four-chamber view; LAX = long axis; LAXa = apical long axis view; LAXp = parasternal long axis view; MV = mitral valve; SAX-MV = parasternal short axis view at the level of the mitral valve; SAX-Pap = parasternal short axis view at the level of the papillary muscles; SEE = standard error of the estimate; TEE = transesophageal echocardiography.

In clinical practice, this method has a standard error of approximately 5%.[30] To arrive at this formula, however, it has been necessary (1) to assume that the ventricle can be represented by a prolate ellipse; (2) to assume that the maximal angiographic long axis is representative of the true long axis; (3) to derive the minor axis to correct for deviation from a true ellipse; (4) to correct for magnification; and (5) to allow for the volume displaced by the trabeculae, papillary muscles, and mitral apparatus.

In the single-plane format, other elements of the formula may also be less accurately derived, because (1) only a single projection of the long axis is available and, thus, must be assumed to be the true long axis, and (2) only one correction factor for image magnification can be determined and must be cubed. This magnification correction factor is also less accurate because the true center of the ventricle cannot be determined from a single plane. Despite these additional assumptions, the single-plane method has an error of only approximately 9%.[30]

Echocardiographic Applications of the Length-Diameter and Area-Length Ellipsoid Volume Formulas

The role of the angiographic length-diameter and area-length methods in echocardiographic left ventricular volume calculation has been examined in a variety of clinical and experimental studies.[20,46–50,53,55–61]

The echocardiographic application of these formulas is slightly more complicated because most angiographic studies are limited to two orthogonal planes that include the ventricular long axis, whereas the echocardiogram provides several additional short axis planes. These additional planes increase both the available points for data sampling and the methods of substitution into the ellipsoid formula.[47] Despite these differences, the basic assumptions of the formulas are similar, and the data required for their use appear to be readily available. These similarities can be appreciated by comparing the echocardiographic areas and dimensions illustrated in the idealized ventricular model in Figure 20–13 with those of the ellipsoid figures illustrated in Figure. 20–14.

The Length-Diameter Method. The length-diameter method is easily adapted to the echocardiographic format. The ventricular length (L) can be obtained from any of the apical views,[50,59] whereas the minor diameters (D_1 and D_2) can be taken from lines drawn perpendicular to the long axis in orthogonal apical views or, more commonly, from a short axis plane.[46,47,54,59] All the dimensions are taken from the inner margins of the endocardial echoes.

The echocardiographic length-diameter method has been compared in experimental studies to direct in vitro volume measurements[47,58] and clinically to angiographically derived volume.[50,59] The results of these correlations and their relationship to other methods of volume calculation are illustrated in Table 20–2. Use of this ellipsoid equation results in better correlation with other methods of volume calculation than can be achieved using the cubed linear dimension with or without correction for ventricular shape.

Area-Length Method. It has been observed in angiographic studies that because of the irregular outline of the left ventricle, choice of the location and direction of the minor dimensions used in the length-diameter format may be somewhat arbitrary and inconsistent. Furthermore, these measurements can be more accurately derived from the ventricular area (A) and major axis length (L) (see Equation 20.4).[25,30]

Although the fixed internal references that are available in the cross-sectional images should permit more reproducible orientation of the minor dimensions, the variable nature of their placement is again apparent in the different short axis planes from which they have been obtained.[20,47,59] To avoid the inaccuracies that appear inherent in the arbitrary placement of ventricular dimensions and to better allow for irregularities in ventricular shape, it seems reasonable to make use of the angiographic experience and calculate the echocardiographic minor axis from the ventricular area and major dimension.

Both the biplane and single-plane area-length formulas have been employed echocardiographically.[20,47–49,55,58–61] In the biplane format, one left ventricular area (A_4) and length (L) are obtained from one of the apical planes, usually the four-chamber view. The second orthogonal plane is usually the short axis at the mitral valve level, where the area is equal to A_1 (see Fig. 20–13) and the length is equal to the larger of the minor dimensions (D_1) in this plane.[20,49,55,60,61] The ellipsoid volume formula then becomes:

$$\text{Volume} = \frac{\pi}{6} L_1 \left(\frac{4A_4}{\pi L}\right)\left(\frac{4A_1}{\pi D_1}\right) \qquad [20.9]$$

Use of any short axis view in this model appears inappropriate because, for a circular ventricle, the calculated dimension is the same as the measured dimension, D_1, and is prejudiced by the level at which the plane is taken. In addition, the calculated minor axes, in all likelihood, will not intersect the long axis at the same point and, therefore, will not be truly orthogonal.

Therefore, it appears that the minor dimensions are more appropriately calculated from two orthogonal planes that include the ventricular long axis, such as the apical two- and four-chamber views. Areas (A_3 and A_4, see Fig. 20–13) and ventricular length (L_1 and L_2) are measured in the apical views.[60,61]

Volume is then calculated as:

$$\text{Volume} = \frac{\pi}{6} L_1 \left(\frac{4A_3}{\pi L_1}\right)\left(\frac{4A_4}{\pi L_2}\right) \qquad [20.10]$$

Volume can also be determined using the area-length method from a single projection using the single-plane formula:[20,47–49,58,59]

$$\text{Volume} = \frac{8(A_4)^2}{3\pi L}$$

The single-plane formula is only valid for projections that include the true ventricular long axis, i.e., the apical view. The correlations that have been achieved using the area-length method are good in experimental studies[47,48,58] but only fair in clinical trials[20,49,59] (see Table 20–2). In practice, use of the apical 4-chamber view has yielded better results than use of the apical 2-chamber view.[49,59] In general, the biplane methods have proved superior to the single-plane methods, and the area-length methods are better than the length-diameter methods.[20,47,49,58] These data suggest that, in any application of the ellipsoid model, the greater the number of dimensions that are either directly measured or directly calculated, the greater the accuracy of the volume determinations.

Determining Ventricular Volume Using the Ellipsoid Model From the Short Axis Area and Ventricular Length. A third method for determining ventricular volume from the ellipsoid figure uses the short axis areas (A_2) (Fig. 20–13D) and the ventricular length (L).[47] Because the short axis area is equal to

$$\pi \times \left(\frac{D_1}{2}\right) \times \left(\frac{D_2}{2}\right)$$

the ellipsoid volume equation then becomes

$$\text{Volume} = \frac{4}{3} A \times \frac{L}{2} \qquad [20.11]$$

or

$$\frac{2}{3} A \times L$$

In formalin-fixed hearts, volumes calculated using this derivation have correlated extremely well with directly measured volume.[47] Use of the constant 2/3, however, results in a consistent, slight underestimation of true volume. Ejection fraction determined using this model has resulted in a slight overestimation when compared to angiography[49] but has shown a better correlation than other ellipsoid formulae (see Table 20–2).

The figures that are actually formed when the echocardiographic dimensions and areas are substituted into the ellipsoid volume formulas and their relationship to the idealized ventricle are illustrated in Figure 20–13 A to D.

Simpson's Rule Method

The second general method for calculating left ventricular volumes employs Simpson's rule. According to Simpson's rule, the volume of a large figure can be calculated from the sum of the volumes of a series of smaller, similar figures. Although sometimes called the "disc summation method," this method does not require that figures be circular discs. The volume of an evenly sliced stick of butter, for example, might be determined from the sum of the volumes of each rectangular slice.

Figure 20–16 illustrates how Simpson's rule can be applied to the left ventricle. In this example, the chamber is divided along its long axis into a series of cylinders or ellipsoid cylinders. The volume of each cylinder is determined from the following formula:

$$\text{Volume} = \left(\pi \frac{D_1}{2} \frac{D_2}{2}\right) \times H \qquad [20.12]$$

where H equals the height of the cylinder and D_1 and D_2 are the orthogonal diameters. This method can be applied echocardiographically in several ways. The first method, illustrated in Figure 20–17, records serial short axis cross-sectional scans of the ventricle at known increments from apex to base. The height of each cylindric section is then determined directly as the distance between short axis scans (in this example, 5 mm) and the area of the cylinder can be either planimetered from the short axis section or calculated from two measured minor diameters. The volume of the ventricle can then be determined by summing the volumes of the individual sections,[62] or

$$\text{Volume} = (A_1 + A_2 + A_3 \ldots) \times H \qquad [20.13]$$

In experimental studies, this method has yielded accurate volume measurements with correlation coefficients

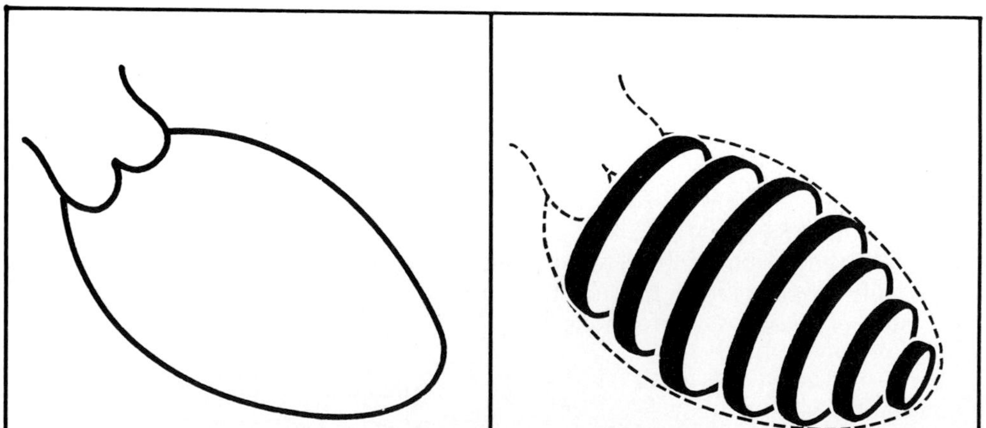

Fig. 20–16. The division of an ellipsoid ventricle into a series of cylinders using Simpson's rule. (From Rogers EW, et al.: Echocardiography for quantitation of cardiac chambers. *In* Yu PN, Goodwin JF (eds.): Progress in Cardiology. Vol. 8. Philadelphia, Lea & Febiger, 1979).

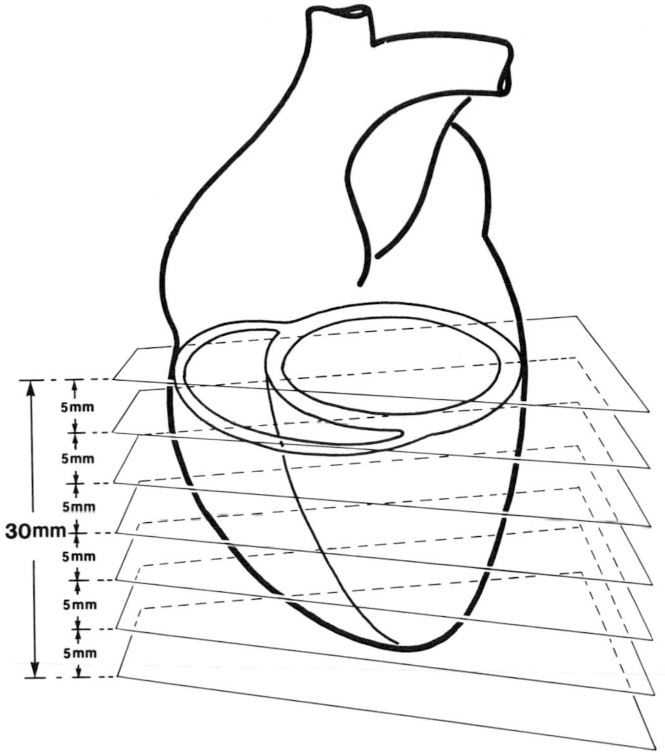

Fig. 20–17. Serial cross-sections of the ventricle can be obtained at fixed increments and then summed to determine the volume of the entire ventricle.

greater than .97 and low standard errors (see Table 20–2).[63,64] The accuracy of this method is influenced by the sampling intervals, and a clear relationship has been demonstrated between the number of sections recorded and both the correlation coefficient and standard error; at least four slices are needed to achieve acceptable accuracy (see Table 20–2).[64] Unfortunately, although accurate, this method is not applicable clinically because the limited acoustic windows do not permit the scan plane to be stepped down the ventricle in fixed increments from base to apex.

A second adaptation of Simpson's rule, which can be applied clinically, uses two cross-sectional views that are orthogonal about the long axis, i.e., four- and two-chamber apical views, to define the margins of the left ventricle and divides the chamber along this common axis into a series of even slices.[58,60,65,66] Each of these slices is then represented by an ellipsoid cylinder, and the height of each cylinder (H) is determined by dividing the ventricular long axis by the number of slices. The orthogonal diameters of each cylinder are then derived from the two planes by taking the distances between the endocardial intercepts of lines drawn perpendicular to the long axis at each interval and ventricular volume calculated as:

$$\text{Volume} = \frac{\pi}{4} H \sum_{0}^{N} D_1 \times D_2 \qquad [20.14]$$

A simplified method has been reported, which uses only one apical view.[23,58] In asymmetric ventricles, however, there was no significant correlation between direct measurement and single-plane echocardiographic calculations, whereas biplane Simpson's rule was accurate.[58]

The Simpson's rule method is attractive because it does not require that the ventricle correspond to any geometric figure and, as illustrated in Figure 20–18, readily adapts to gross distortions in ventricular shape.

The data accumulated using the Simpson's rule approach to ventricular volume calculation are listed in Table 20–2. In general, excellent correlations have been obtained with this method, provided that the sampling intervals are sufficiently narrow. Its major limitation lies in the complexity of the calculations, which are laborious by hand and generally require computer support.

A third method, illustrated in Figure 20–19, uses a modification of Simpson's rule.[47] In this model, the volume of the body of the ventricle is determined in the usual Simpson's rule format, whereas the apex is considered as a separate ellipsoid segment. The formula for an ellipsoid segment is:

$$V = \frac{Ah}{2} + \frac{a^2}{b^2}\frac{\pi h^3}{6}$$

where A and h are the area and the height of the segment, a and b are the radii of the total ellipsoid; i.e., in this case a is the semidiameter of the left ventricle at the base and b is the length of the ventricle. As a simplification, the factor a^2/b^2 is omitted, leading to overestimation of the segment volume. The volume of the overall figure is calculated from the formula:

$$\text{Volume} = (A_1 + A_2 + A_3)\,h + \frac{A_4 h}{2} + \frac{\pi h^3}{6} \qquad [20.15]$$

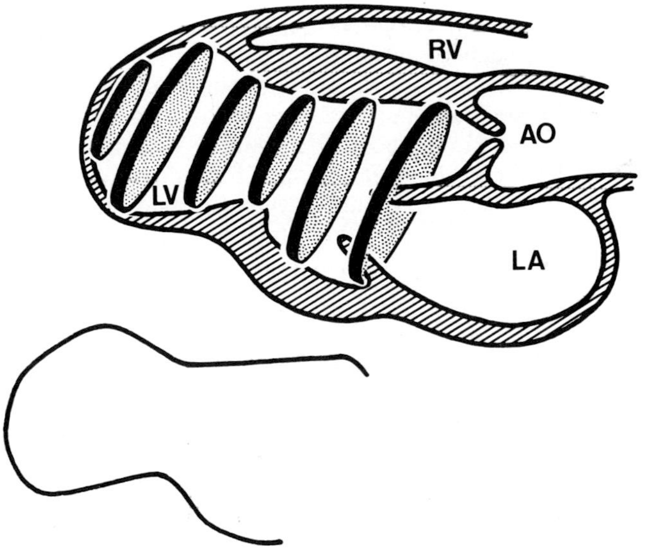

Fig. 20–18. Simpson's rule readily adapts to gross distortions in ventricular shape. RV = right ventricle; AO = aorta; LV = left ventricle; LA = left atrium. (From Rogers EW, et al.: Echocardiography for quantitation of cardiac chambers. *In* Yu PN, Goodwin JF (eds.): Progress in Cardiology. Vol 8. Philadelphia, Lea & Febiger, 1979).

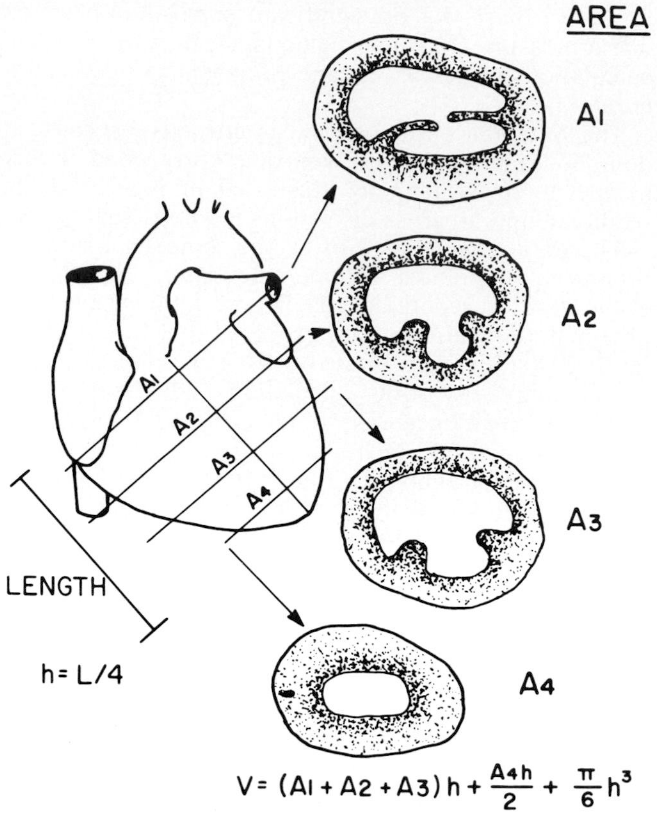

Fig. 20–19. A modified Simpson's rule approach to left ventricular volume calculation. The volume of the basal three quarters of the ventricle is determined using Simpson's rule, whereas the volume of the apex is determined as the volume of an ellipsoid volume segment. (From Wyatt H, et al.: Cross-sectional echocardiography. I. Analysis of mathematic models for quantifying mass of the left ventricle in dogs. Circulation 60:1104, 1979. Reproduced by permission of the American Heart Association, Inc.)

In spite of the inaccuracy of the last term, a better correlation has been demonstrated with measured volume both in experimental[47,48,67,68] and clinical studies[59] with use of this formula than with any of the ellipsoid formulas or the combined geometric figures. Although technically a combination of figures, this formula is included in this section because the majority of the data are derived using the Simpson's rule method.

Combined Geometric Figures

The final approach to left ventricular volume calculations uses the short axis planes to divide the ventricle into two or more sections that can be represented individually by different geometric figures.[20,47,48,67,68] The figures most commonly used to represent these ventricular sections are the cylinder (volume = area of the base × height), the hemiellipsoid (volume = 2/3 area of the base × height), the cone (volume = 1/3 area of the base × height), and the truncated cone

$$\text{Volume} = \pi \times \left(\frac{r_1^2 + r_2^2 + r_1 r_2}{3}\right) \times H \qquad [20.16]$$

where r_1 is the radius of the base, r_2 is the radius of the apex, and H is height. A simplified formula for the truncated cone is often used:

$$\text{Volume} = \left(\frac{A_1 + A_2}{2}\right) \times H$$

where A_1 and A_2 are the areas at the base and the apex. With this formula, the volume of the truncated cone is slightly overestimated, but this approximation is acceptable if A_1 and A_2 are similar in size. Once the volumes of each of these subfigures are known, they can be added to determine the volume of the whole ventricle. Four such combined figures are the cylinder-hemiellipsoid (illustrated in Fig. 20–13F), the cylinder truncated cone-cone (Fig. 20–13G), the cylinder-cone (Fig. 20–13H), and the truncated cone-hemiellipsoid (Fig. 20–20).

In each of these combined figures, the overall length is equal to the ventricular length taken from one of the apical views. The areas are short axis cavity areas recorded at the mitral valve level (A_1) or the papillary muscle level (A_2). In each instance, the short axis sections presumably divide the long axis into segments of equal length. As a result, the height of each subfigure is the same and can be determined by dividing the ventricular length (L) by the total number of subfigures.

The Cylinder-Cone

The simplest combined figure represents the base of the ventricle as a cylinder and the apex as a cone. The volume of this figure can be determined by using the formula:

$$V = A\frac{L}{2} + \frac{1}{3}A\frac{L}{2} \quad \text{or} \quad \frac{2}{3}A \times L \qquad [20.17]$$

where A is the short axis ventricular area, and L is the ventricular length. An excellent correlation has been re-

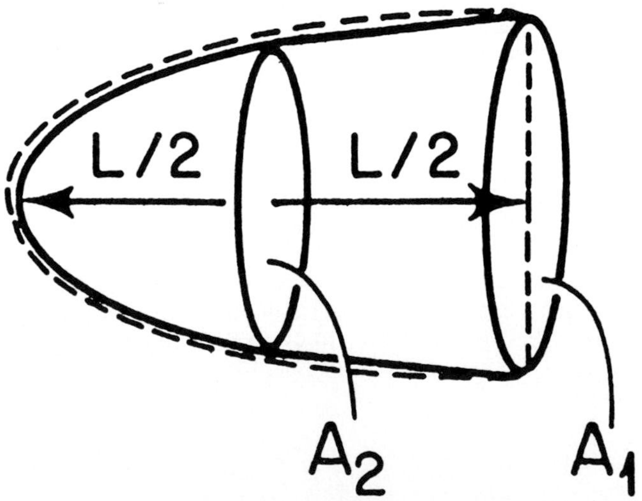

Fig. 20–20. The truncated cone-hemiellipsoid method. (From Triulzi MO, et al.: Normal adult cross-sectional echocardiographic values: left ventricular volumes. Echocardiography 2:153, 1985.)

ported between volumes calculated using this model and directly measured volumes from formalin-fixed hearts.[47] It has not, to date, been evaluated in either the in vivo experimental setting or in clinical studies, but normal values have been reported.[61] Consequently, its true value remains unclear. It is interesting to note that this figure has the same formula as that of the ellipsoid figure, where volume is calculated from the short axis area and ventricular length.[47] In the ellipsoid format, the formula has been more extensively tested in vitro[47] and again has been found to have an excellent correlation (r equals .97) with measured volume. The formula has a slight tendency to underestimate true ventricular volume. The underestimation appears related to the constant 2/3, because volumes calculated using the same basic formula but with the constant 5/6 show a similar correlation but more closely approximate true volume. It is assumed in this model that the short axis plane divides the ventricle in half so that the height of each subfigure is equal to L/2.

The Cylinder-Truncated Cone-Cone

The volume of the second combined figure, the cylinder-truncated cone-cone (Fig. 20–13G) can be calculated from the following formula:[20]

$$\text{Volume} = A_1 \frac{L}{3} + \pi \left(\frac{r_1^2 + r_2^2 + r_1 r_2}{3} \right) \frac{L}{3} + \frac{1}{3} A_2 \frac{L}{3} \qquad [20.18]$$

where A_1 is the short axis of the ventricle at the mitral valve level, and A_2 is the corresponding short axis area at the papillary muscle level. In practice, a simplified formula is used:[20,49,59]

$$\text{Volume} = A_1 \frac{L}{3} + \left(\frac{A_1 + A_2}{2} \right) \frac{L}{3} + \frac{1}{3} A_2 \frac{L}{3}$$

which yields a slightly larger end-diastolic volume.[61]

In the cylinder-truncated cone-cone model, it is assumed that the short-axis planes divide the ventricle into three equal parts such that the height of each figure is equal to one third of the overall ventricular length in the apical four-chamber view. A similar model divides the ventricle into four segments, represented by a cylinder, two truncated cones, and a cone.[59] Volumes calculated using these models have correlated well with angiographic volumes in clinical studies.[20,59] The overall correlation has proved superior to that observed with either the single or the biplane ellipsoid volume method, the cylinder hemiellipsoid model (see the following), or the corrected D^3 method.

The Cylinder Hemiellipsoid

Another combined figure that has been applied clinically is the cylinder-hemiellipsoid (Fig. 20–13F). The volume of this figure is calculated from the formula:

$$\text{Volume} = A \frac{L}{2} + \frac{2}{3} A \times \frac{L}{2} \qquad [20.19]$$

or

$$V = \frac{5}{6} A \times L$$

This model has been evaluated in both experimental[47,48,67] and clinical studies.[20,59,61,68] In experimental studies, a high correlation with direct volume measurements was obtained when the area was taken at the level of the papillary muscle,[47,48] which is assumed to divide the ventricle in half such that the height of each subfigure is equal to L/2. In asymmetric ventricles, the papillary muscle level provides better volume estimates than the mitral valve level.[67] In a clinical study of children with congenital heart disease, no significant difference was found using either the mitral valve or the papillary muscle level area.[59]

Among the combined figure models, the cylinder-hemiellipsoid formula, with the area taken at the papillary level, provides good estimates of left ventricular volumes, approaching those obtained using Simpson's rule.

The Truncated Cone-Hemiellipsoid

The final combined figure is the truncated cone-hemiellipsoid, illustrated in Figure 20–20. The volume of this figure is calculated as:[61]

$$V = L \left(\frac{7}{12} A_2 + \frac{1}{4} A_1 \right) \qquad [20.20]$$

It requires two short-axis areas, at the level of the mitral valve (A_1) and of the papillary muscle (A_2), and the left ventricular length (L) from a an apical view. Normal values for this model have been published,[61] but the model has, to date, not been validated, and their clinical value remains unknown.

Left Ventricular Volume Measurements With Transesophageal Echocardiography

Three different methods have been validated for estimation of left ventricular volume by transesophageal echocardiography: length-diameter, modified Simpson's rule, and the cylinder-hemiellipsoid model.[69] Although the correlation with angiographic measurements has been good, it has not been better than that achieved using transthoracic echocardiography (see Table 20–2). In addition, using transesophageal data all three methods result in significant and systematic underestimation of volume for both diastolic and systolic measurements. The reason may be foreshortening of the ventricular length in the esophageal four-chamber view.

Three-Dimensional Methods of Volume Measurements

Three-dimensional reconstruction of the left ventricle permits the spatial integration of a number of randomly acquired planes and the precise calculation of ventricular volume, without the need for geometric assumptions. This technique can combine as many target locations as necessary and does not require that images be acquired from any predetermined plane orientation. In contrast to geometry-based methods, appropriate three-dimensional systems should eliminate (1) ventricular foreshortening, (2) the need for assumptions concerning short-axis plane location relative to the ventricular long axis, and (3) the need for the complete endocardial contour to be recorded around the circumference of the ventricle. Further, they should adapt to various ventricular shapes and should perform equally well in nondistorted as in distorted left ventricles.

The accuracy of three-dimensional reconstruction of the left ventricle has recently been validated in a series of in vitro, in vivo, and clinical studies.[70–74] In vitro studies of excised left ventricles of normal shape and known volume (21 to 101 ml) revealed an excellent correlation ($r = 0.99$, $y = 1.00x + 0.17$) and a small difference (0.2 ± 3.6 ml) between echocardiographic and true volume.[72] Further, in these symmetric ventricles where two-dimensional methods should be most accurate, the correlation between three-dimensional and known volume was significantly better than that obtained for the same volumes calculated using the area-length ellipsoid, the cylinder hemiellipsoid (bullet), and the Simpson's rule methods. In deformed ventricles designed to simulate apical aneurysms and right ventricular volume overload, the difference in accuracy between three-dimensional and two-dimensional methods was even more apparent. In vivo studies in a beating heart model in which volume could be measured continuously, likewise, revealed an excellent correlation between directly measured and three-dimensionally reconstructed left ventricular volumes ($r = .97$), stroke volume ($r = .94$) and ejection fraction ($r = .94$).[73] Finally, in humans, three-dimensional reconstruction of the left ventricle at end-diastole and end-systole from data acquired during a single held expiration yielded stroke volumes that correlated closely with Doppler-derived stroke volume ($r = .94$, $y = .92x + 4.3$; standard error of estimate [SEE] = 3.1 ml).[74]

Technical Considerations

One of the main limitations in left ventricular volume quantitation is delineating the endocardial borders, especially in technically limited studies.

One approach to enhancing border delineation is to color encode the amplitude distribution of two-dimensional images. Based on the principle that the human eye can distinguish a greater number of colors than shades of gray, the method uses color scales instead of a gray scale to display the full dynamic range of the echo signals (see Fig. 20–21). Initial hopes that this technique might allow better cavity delineation and more accurate volume measurements have not been fulfilled. Echocardiographic left ventricular volumes have been calculated, using a modified Simpson's rule, from images with different color scales and compared with volumes derived from gray scale images. Color-encoded images provided similar but not significantly better correlation with single-plane angiographic measurements of end-systolic and end-diastolic volumes. A statistically significant but unimportant improvement was obtained in the estimation of the ejection fraction.[75]

Another method to improve quantitative accuracy may be automatic border detection. This method would help to simplify the time-consuming tracing of the borders and measurements of length and diameters. Although many such algorithms have been described, the only widely tested and commercially available approach uses the integrated backscatter of the ultrasonic signal to delineate the border between endocardium and blood, to provide an on-line real-time automatic measure of cavity area. Comparison of such a system with traditional, extensively validated off-line operator-dependent procedures has shown good correlation for cavity areas from parasternal short axis and apical views.[76] However, satisfactory studies were obtained in only 72% of patients studied.

Despite its potential (see Chapter 3), automatic border detection systems are still hindered by the relatively low signal-to-noise ratio of echocardiographic images, by areas of echo dropout, and by the need to define a stable region of interest. Once perfected, however, such systems should have widespread application in the assessment of left ventricular function, in quantitation of wall motion abnormalities, and in hemodynamic monitoring during surgery or of critically ill patients.

Reproducibility of Volume Measurements

In order to be reliable, quantification of left ventricular volumes requires not only accuracy but also reproducibility. Several studies have specifically addressed the problem of reproducibility.[77–79]

Ventricular volume calculations using the length-area method [$V = 8A^2/(3\pi L)$], with measurements taken in the apical four-chamber view, was repeated several days apart in 30 subjects.[77] The correlation between the first and the second study was very good for end-diastolic and end-systolic volumes ($r = .96$ and $.97$; SEE = 6.3 and 5.7 ml), and slightly lower for ejection fraction ($r = .84$; SEE = 5.3%). The 95% confidence limits of individual results were ±15% for the end-diastolic volume, ±25% for the end-systolic volume, and ±10% for the ejection fraction. The mean values of the whole group of 30 subjects were included in 95% confidence limits of, respectively, 2%, 5%, and 2%. Interobserver variability and beat-to-beat variability were higher than intraobserver variability, suggesting that serial measurements should be done by a single person, averaging several cycles.

Using Simpson's rule with apical four- and two-chamber views in three subjects studied five times, variability was lower for ejection fraction (±7%) than for end-diastolic and end-systolic volumes (±11% and ±15%).[78] In this study, tracing the borders was responsible for most of the variability, which suggests that an average of several measurements are needed to obtain a reliable result. Variability was higher in a subject whose study was technically difficult.

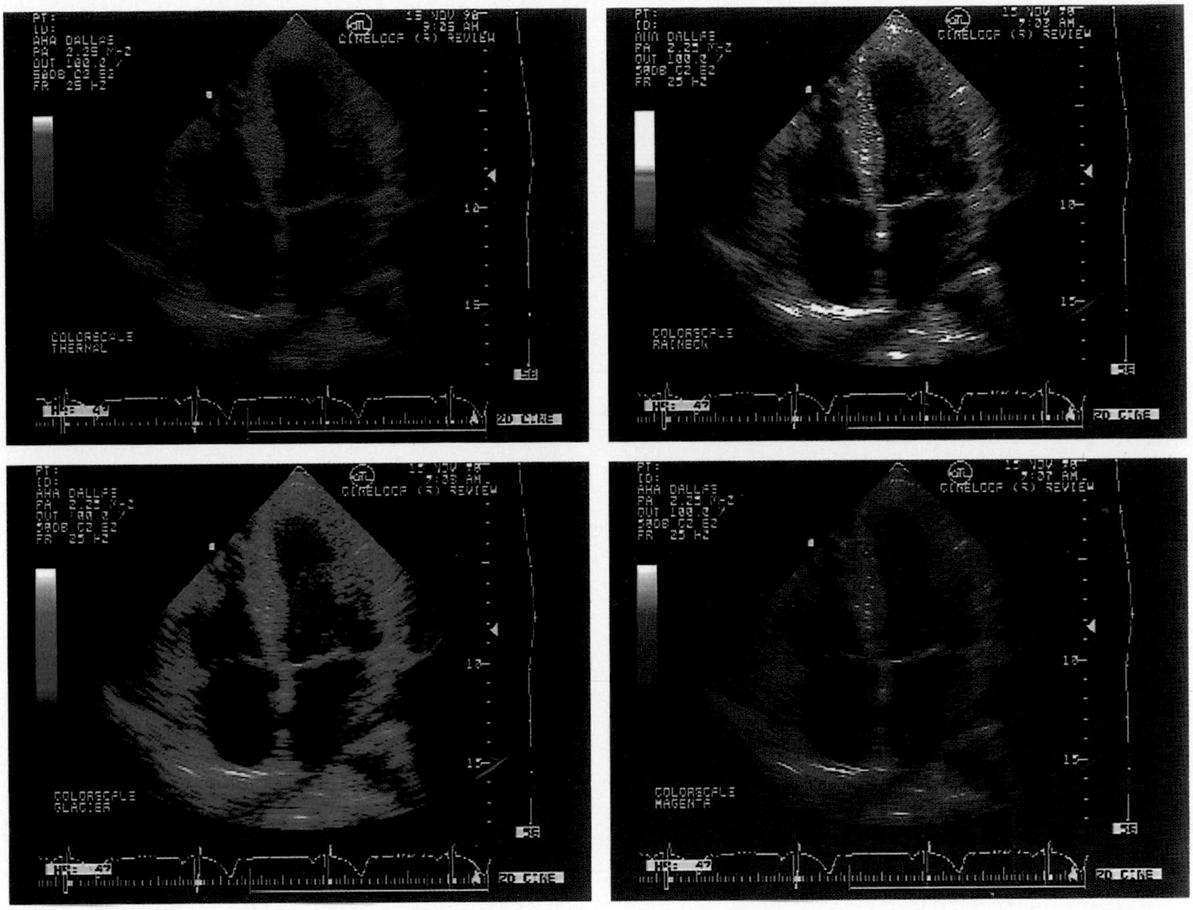

Fig. 20–21. Apical four-chamber views of the heart illustrating the effect of color-encoding on endocardial border definition. Top, left. "Thermal" scale. Top, right. "Rainbow" scale. Bottom, left. "Glacier" scale. Bottom, right. "Magenta" scale.

An objective method to delineate borders, such as a computer edge-detection algorithm, would be expected to increase the reproducibility of measurements. Among 10 subjects studied five times, volumes were determined according to the cylinder-hemiellipsoid formula ($V = 5/6$ AL); endocardial borders on the short-axis midpapillary plane were automatically detected and the area computed, whereas the ventricular length from the apical four-chamber view was manually measured.[79] The 95% confidence limits for end-diastolic volume were ±16.7%, for end-systolic volume ±17.0%, and for ejection fraction ±9.7%. Although different formulae were used, the computer edge-detection system did not seem to improve the reproducibility of volume measurements.

Normal Values of Left Ventricular Volume

When volumes are compared, the method must be taken into account; different formulae, or the same formula with different planes, yield different results for the same ventricle. Normal echocardiographic values[60,61] are provided in Table 20–3, together with angiographic and dye dilution values for comparison.[80–82] It should be noted that men have larger end-diastolic left ventricular volumes than women, even after normalization for body surface area (58 vs. 50 ml/m^2 using Simpson's rule, $p < .005$), and slightly higher ejection fraction (69% vs. 64%, p = not significant).[60]

Summary

Despite the large volume of data presented in Table 20–2, no optional method for the clinical determination of ventricular volume is apparent. No study compares the accuracy of all the available formulas, nor do studies using the same formulas employ similar methods. These data do, however, provide important insight into the accuracy and limitations of echocardiographic volume calculations.

First, they demonstrate that echocardiographic volumes consistently underestimate true ventricular cavity volume because of (1) the effects of pulse width and beam width, which broaden the echoes from the endocardial interface and thereby encroach on the ventricular chamber; (2) the use of the plane of the mitral valve annulus as the basal intercept of the ventricular long axis, which slightly foreshortens ventricular length measurements when compared with angiographic measurements taken from the aortic valve; (3) frequent failure to identify the true apical extreme of the ventricular cavity, resulting in an underestimation of ventricular length; (4) the exclusion of the portion of the cavity volume con-

Table 20–3. Normal Values of Left Ventricular Volumes and Ejection Fraction

Geometric Model	Method	Formula	Cross-Sectional Views	Reference	Subjects (N)	End-Diastolic Volume (ml/m²)	End-Systolic Volume (ml/m²)	Ejection Fraction (%)
Prolate ellipsoid	Area-length	$\frac{8A^2}{3\pi L}$	2Ch	Triulzi et al.[61]	43	69 +/− 26	23 +/− 11	67 +/− 9
				Wahr et al.[60]	52	63 +/− 13	20 +/− 7	68
			4Ch	Triulzi et al.[61]	62	70 +/− 26	25 +/− 13	64 +/− 10
				Wahr et al.[60]	52	57 +/− 13	19 +/− 8	67
		$\frac{8}{3\pi}\frac{A_1A_4}{D_1}$	4Ch; SAX-MV	Triulzi et al.[61]	55	73 +/− 21	28 +/− 11	62 +/− 8
				Wahr et al.[60]	52	60 +/− 12	19 +/− 6	68
		$\frac{8}{3\pi}\frac{A_3A_4}{L}$	4Ch; 2Ch	Triulzi et al.[61]	39	71 +/− 24	23 +/− 11	68 +/− 11
				Wahr et al.[60]	52	61 +/− 12	20 +/− 7	67
	Length-diameter	$\frac{\pi}{6} L D_1D_2$	2Ch; SAX-MV	Triulzi et al.[61]	53	59 +/− 13	25 +/− 7	58 +/− 7
Cylinder-cone		$\frac{2}{3}AL$	4Ch; SAX-MV	Triulzi et al.[61]	53	71 +/− 16	28 +/− 8	61 +/− 7
Cylinder-truncated cone-cone	Simplified formula	$A_1\frac{L}{3} + \left(\frac{A_1 + A_2}{2}\right)\frac{L}{3} + \frac{1}{3}A_2\frac{L}{3}$	4Ch; SAX-MV; SAX-Pap	Triulzi et al.[61]	52	81 +/− 17	30 +/− 9	63 +/− 6
	Exact formula	$A_1\frac{L}{3} + \pi\left(\frac{r_1^2 + r_2^2 + r_1r_2}{3}\right)\frac{L}{3} + \frac{1}{3}A_2\frac{L}{3}$		Triulzi et al.[61]	52	75 +/− 15	29 +/− 7	61 +/− 8
Cylinder-hemiellipsoid		$\frac{5}{6}AL$	4Ch; SAX-Pap	Triulzi et al.[61]	52	84 +/− 18	28 +/− 9	67 +/− 7
Truncated cone-hemiellipsoid		$L\left(\frac{7}{12}A_2 + \frac{1}{4}A_1\right)$	4Ch; SAX-MV; SAX-Pap	Triulzi et al.[61]	52	85 +/− 17	30 +/− 9	65 +/− 7
Simpson's rule		$F\frac{\pi}{4}\sum_{i=1}^{20} D_{1_i}D_{2_i}$	4Ch; 2Ch	Wahr et al.[60]	52	55 +/− 10	18 +/− 6	67
Prolate ellipsoid	Cineangiogram		AP; LAT	Kennedy et al.[80]	16	70 +/− 20	24 +/− 10	67 +/− 8
	Cineangiogram		RAO; LAO	Wynne et al.[81]	17	72 +/−15	20 +/− 8	72 +/− 8
	Dye dilution			Levinson et al.[82]	11	82 +/− 12	37 +/− 11	55 +/− 8

2Ch = apical two-chamber view; 4Ch = apical four-chamber view; SAX-MV = short-axis view at the level of the mitral valve; SAX-Pap = short-axis view at the level of the papillary muscles; AP = anteroposterior projection; LAT = lateral projection; RAO = right anterior oblique projection; LAO = left anterior oblique projection.

tained within the trabeculae; and (5) the systolic motion of the ventricle through the scan plane with artifactual reduction in either diastolic or systolic volume.[47,55]

These limitations of the echocardiographic method are in direct contrast to the angiographic silhouette image in which true volumes are consistently overestimated because of (1) inclusion of the papillary muscles and mitral valve apparatus in the calculated volume; (2) the effects of the silhouette format, which gives a maximal projected area; and (3) inclusion of the trabeculae in the ventricular volume because dye within the invaginations between the muscles extends to the edge of the projected silhouette.

Second, end-systolic echocardiographic volumes almost uniformly show a better correlation with angiographic volumes than do end-diastolic volumes. This difference apparently relates to the more reliable definition of the endocardial interface at end-systole than at end-diastole, and possibly to the more regular, ellipsoidal shape of the ventricle in systole.

Finally, the overall accuracy of the various formulas appears to relate to the frequency of sampling and the ease with which the model adapts to changes in ventricular contour. Thus, the Simpson's rule method, with sections taken at 3-mm intervals, is clearly the most accurate, whereas the D^3 method, which uses the least amount of available data and requires the greatest number of assumptions, is the least precise.

A theoretic "worst case" comparison of these formulas can be used to point out individual strengths and weaknesses. Figure 20–22 illustrates a cross-sectional image of a large ventricular aneurysm originating below the papillary muscles. The accompanying diagram shows the points at which the standard measurements of ventricular length (L), mitral valve short axis area (A_1), papillary muscle short axis area (A_2), and LVID would be taken. The figures that would be calculated from each of these measurements are then superimposed on the outline of the actual echo. The only figures that truly approximate the "worst case" ventricle are the Simpson's rule method and the area-length ellipsoid model. The Simpson's rule method provides the most accurate representation. The area-length method converts the irregular figure to an ellipse by deriving the

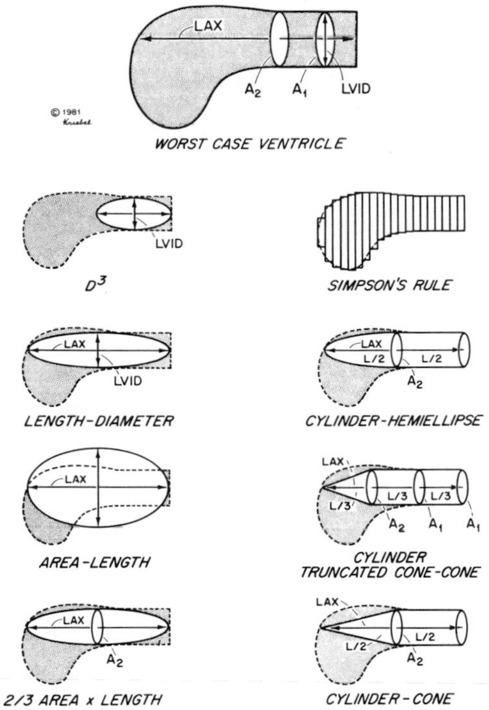

Fig. 20–22. The adaptive ability of each of the ventricular volume formulas to a theoretic worst-case ventricle. Only Simpson's rule and the area-length ellipsoid volume formulas accurately approximate the volume of this distorted figure. A_1 = short axis area at the mitral valve level; A_2 = short axis area at the papillary muscle level; LVID = left ventricular internal dimension; LAX = long axis.

minor dimension and thereby gives a reasonable representation of the area and volume of the ventricle. The D^3 method fails completely to approximate the ventricle, whereas the figures that rely on short axis areas significantly underestimate true ventricular volume. Data derived from symmetric ventricles may be misleading because any reproducible area or dimension should show a relationship to the volume of a symmetric figure. Methods that are valid in both the symmetric ventricle and the "worst case" model should have the greatest applicability to the general cardiac population.

LEFT VENTRICULAR MASS

One of the primary mechanisms by which the left ventricle adapts to an abnormal pressure or volume load is muscular hypertrophy. The degree of hypertrophy parallels the severity of the increased load,[83–87] and extreme hypertrophy may indicate a poor prognosis.[88–90] Left ventricular hypertrophy as defined by echocardiography is a predictor of cardiovascular risk and higher mortality.[91–94] Anatomically, left ventricular hypertrophy is characterized by an increase in muscle mass or weight. Left ventricular mass is determined by two factors: (1) chamber volume and (2) wall thickness. In chronic pressure loads, mass generally increases as a result of wall thickening without a marked increase in chamber volume (Fig. 20–23A and B), whereas with volume overloads, the increase in mass is predominantly due to chamber dilatation (Fig. 20–23C and D). The common association of the term *left ventricular hypertrophy* with wall thickening may lead to confusion because mass may increase without an increase in wall thickness.

All echocardiographic calculations of left ventricular mass are based on the assumption that the volume of the myocardium is equal to the total volume contained within the epicardial borders of the ventricle less the chamber volume[95–98] or

$$V_m = V_t\,(ep) - V_c\,(en)$$

where V_m is the muscle volume, V_t is the total left ventricular volume or the volume contained within the epicardial interface, and V_c is the chamber volume or volume contained within the endocardial interface. The muscle volume (V_m) can then be converted to mass (LVM) by multiplying by the specific gravity of the cardiac muscle (1.05) such that

$$LVM = [V_t\,(ep) - V_c\,(en)] \times 1.05 \qquad [20.21]$$

In all left ventricular mass calculations, the interventricular septum is assumed to be a part of the left ventricle. As a result, the right septal surface is considered to form the external border of the left ventricle in the septal region.

A variety of echocardiographic methods have been described to calculate ventricular mass. These differ principally in (1) the conventions used to measure wall thickness and chamber area and (2) the formula used to calculate volume.

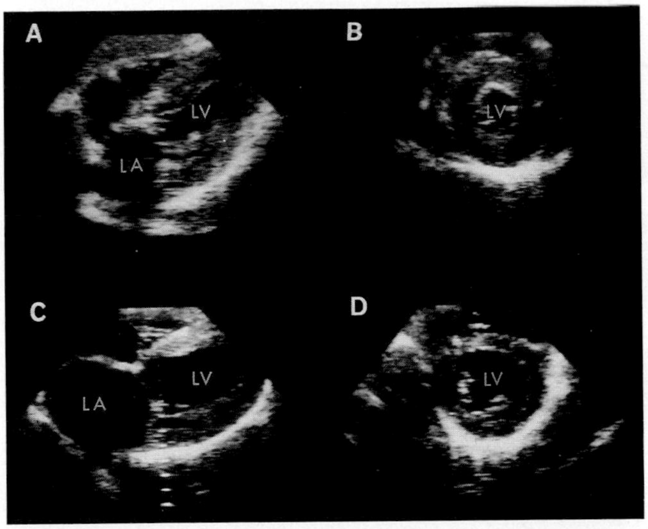

Fig. 20–23. Subcostal long axis **(A)** and parasternal short axis **(B)** recordings of the left ventricle (LV) illustrating concentric left ventricular hypertrophy. The ventricular walls are thickened, and the chamber size is decreased. **C** and **D.** Corresponding subcostal long and short axis views that illustrate eccentric hypertrophy. In these examples, there is a predominant increase in the chamber volume and a corresponding, although lesser, increase in wall thickness. LA = left atrium.

Conventions Used to Measure Wall Thickness and Chamber Area

The first major factor in any mass calculation is the definition of the endocardial and epicardial interfaces or, more specifically, whether the echoes from these interfaces are included in the wall thickness measurement, are considered part of the chamber volume, or, in the case of the epicardial echo, are excluded completely. At least four different conventions have been described for making these measurements: (1) standard,[95,99] (2) Penn,[97] (3) American Society of Echocardiography (ASE) M-mode,[100] and (4) Wyatt[98] or ASE for two-dimensional echocardiography.[24] These measurement formats are illustrated in Figure 20–24.

The first three formats were developed specifically for M-mode echocardiography, whereas the fourth has been applied solely to cross-sectional studies. When methods were compared in vitro, using different gain settings, measurements of wall thickness were most accurate with the leading edge to leading edge convention (M-mode ASE), while the leading edge to trailing edge method (standard) overestimated the true thickness and the trailing edge to leading edge method (Penn) underestimated it.[101] Both the standard and the ASE M-mode conventions, however, appear inappropriate for use in the cross-sectional format, because they require the line of measurement to cross the interface at two points around the circumference of the ventricle. In the Penn and Wyatt conventions, the line of measurement follows the same border of the interface around the ventricular circumference, and they appear better suited to the cross-sectional method. We prefer to use the Wyatt method because the internal margins of both the endocardial and epicardial interfaces are usually more easily defined than are the external margins and because this method is consistent with the other dimensional and area measurements described in this text. Although seemingly a trivial point, the inclusion of these echoes is important because a 1-mm variation represents approximately a 10% difference in wall thickness.[97] These differences become even more significant when determining mass because the calculated volumes vary with the cube of the linear measurement.

In addition to these theoretic considerations, measurement is further complicated by the basic structure of the left ventricular wall, which can vary in thickness from point to point with the result that a representative dimension can be difficult to establish (Fig. 20–25). Although echocardiography provides both point-to-point and circumferential images of the myocardial boundaries and the main trabeculations, no method of border tracing can take into account all anatomic details.

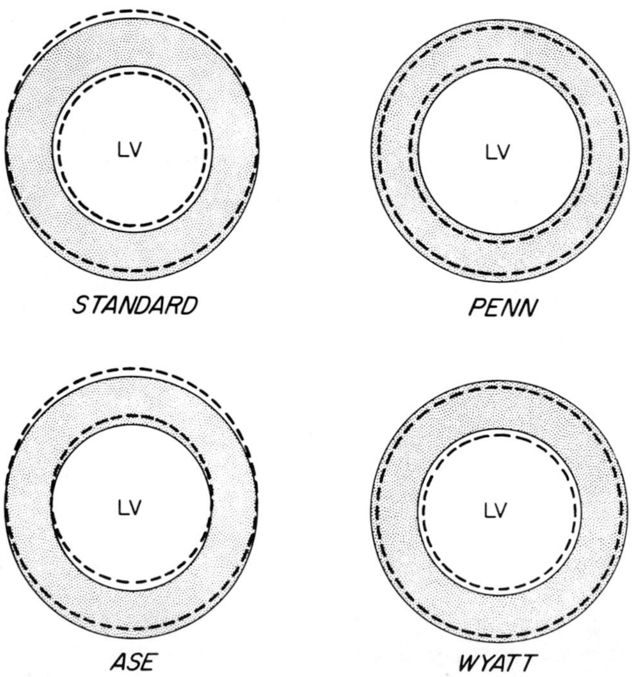

Fig. 20–24. The adaptation of the four major conventions for defining the endocardial and epicardial interfaces to the short axis, cross-sectional image of the left ventricle. The shaded areas correspond to the myocardium, while the interrupted lines follow the path of the line of measurement using each convention. ASE = American Society of Echocardiography, M-mode convention. The method proposed by Wyatt is similar to the ASE two-dimensional convention.

Approaches to Calculating Volume for the Mass Equation

The volume component of the mass formula can be derived using any of the methods described in the preceding section for ventricular volume calculation: (1) Simpson's rule, (2) the combined geometric figure, or (3) the single figure.

Simpson's Rule Method

The modified Simpson's rule formula has been applied to calculate the volume component of the mass formula. Using this approach, both epicardial and endocardial volumes are considered to be represented by a series of cylinders, to which are added ellipsoid segments to represent the apex.[98,102] The volume of each apical segment is calculated using a simplified formula (see Fig. 20–19), Simpson's rule is applied to separately calculate endocardial and epicardial volumes, and endocardial volume is subtracted from epicardial volume to yield muscle volume.

In pathologic studies, the echocardiographically derived area of individual short axis sections has correlated extremely well with the photographic section area ($r = .95$). Likewise, multiplying each echocardiographic section area by its thickness measured in vitro provided a close estimate of section volume ($r = .97$) and permitted calculation of section weight and total ventricular mass.[102]

In the experimental model,[98] the ventricle has been represented as the sum of three cylinders and one ellipsoid segment. The volume of the whole figure is expressed as:

$$V = (A_1 + A_2 + A_3)h + \frac{A_4 h}{2} + \frac{\pi h^3}{6} \qquad [20.22]$$

Areas A_1, A_2, A_3, and A_4 are obtained on short axis

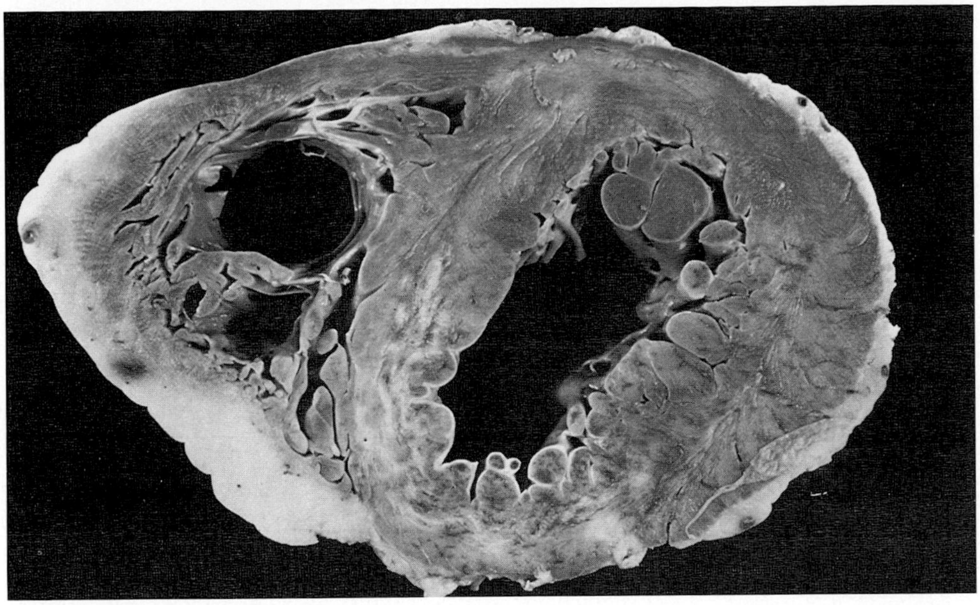

Fig. 20–25. Pathologic section of the heart corresponding to a short axis view illustrating the variation of wall thickness at different points around the ventricle, as well as the difficulty in measuring thickness at any point.

views at the mitral valve level, at the high and low papillary muscle level, and at the apex. The height h is calculated by dividing the ventricular length, measured in a long axis view, by four. In the calculation of the epicardial volume of the apical ellipsoid segment, 4 mm have been added to the height, to represent the apical thickness of a canine ventricle. This method has yielded a good correlation with actual mass (r = .95) and should be applicable clinically.

Combined Geometric Figures

Only one combined figure has been tested to date for determining the volume component of the mass formula.[98,102–104] This figure is the cylinder-hemiellipsoid (Fig. 20–14F) where

$$V = \frac{5}{6} A \times L \qquad [20.23]$$

The same formula is used to determine the volumes contained within both the endocardial and epicardial interfaces, and mass is calculated as

$$\text{LVM} = (\text{LVV of epicardium} - \text{LVV endocardium}) \times \text{muscle density} \qquad [20.24]$$

where LVV is left ventricular volume. The areas within each interface are measured directly from a short axis scan of the ventricle at the high papillary muscle level, and the length (L) is taken from the base to the endocardial interface at the apex; the epicardial length is obtained by adding a constant value representing the apical wall thickness: 4 mm in the canine model[98] and 10 mm in the human model.[103] In the experimental studies, this method has yielded an excellent correlation with ventricular weight with a small standard error and even scatter of individual points about the line of identity.[98]

The model has also been validated in 21 patients who had an echocardiographic examination 2 to 76 days before their death.[103] After "instrument-specific" corrections,* a good correlation was found (r = .93) with an SEE of 31 g. In a smaller series, left ventricular mass without such corrections had a lower correlation (r = .68).[104]

This model further allows for the absence of myocardium at the base of the ventricle because the length measurement is derived such that the bases of the concentric shells are the same. It also makes allowance for the contribution of the papillary muscles to overall mass. Although this model does not readily adapt to gross changes in ventricular shape (as noted in the "worst case" example in Fig. 20–22), clinically important changes in mass are most commonly sought when the ventricle is symmetric. This model, therefore, appears to represent a simple method for volume calculation for which the necessary data should be available in most patients.

Single-Figure Method

The single-figure method for calculating the volume component of the mass equation has been tested using both the prolate ellipsoid model,[97,98,103,104] the truncated ellipsoid,[105] and the simple cylinder.[98]

Although valuable in volume calculation, the ellipsoid model has major limitations in this setting because, when constructing concentric ellipsoid figures, it is necessary to assume that the ventricle is surrounded by a uniform shell of even thickness (D^3) or by a shell that tapers at both extremes of the long axis (area-length or length-diameter). In either case, the ellipsoid fails to

* Regression equations derived in vitro were used to correct left ventricular mass. LV mass = $1.055 \times k \times 5/6(A_tL_t - A_cL_c) + b$, where k is the instrument-specific regression slope and b is the instrument-specific intercept.

allow for the absence of myocardium over the mitral and aortic orifices. This limitation has been previously demonstrated in postmortem measurements, which indicate that, for mass calculation, the ventricle is better represented by a truncated ellipsoid.[106] Not surprisingly, therefore, comparative studies show that mass calculations using the basic ellipsoid figure have correlated less well with measured mass than have those using either the Simpson's rule or the combined figure methods. The D^3 derivation of the ellipsoid model in pathologic studies is least accurate.[106]

Subtracting a constant to correct for the absence of myocardium at the base partially overcomes one of the limitations of the M-mode-derived D^3 formula. This constant was determined from a group of 34 patients who had echocardiographic studies and later postmortem measurements.[97] Using the Penn convention, the modified D^3 formula that provided the best estimate of mass was

$$LVM = 1.04[(LVID + IVS + PW)^3 - (LVID)^3] - 13.6 \qquad [20.25]$$

where LVID is the left ventricle internal diameter at end diastole, IVS is the interventricular septum thickness, and PW is the posterior wall thickness. Other studies using the same method,[103,104,107] yielded similar results, but the SEE is fairly large (see Table 20–4). Left ventricular mass determined by this method has been shown to correlate with body surface area and to be significantly different in men and women.[108] Normal values in a healthy population sample of 78 men and 55 women were 93 ± 22 g/m^2 for men and 76 ± 18 g/m^2 for women (mean ± SD).

The truncated ellipsoid is another approach to left ventricular mass assessment. The center of the ellipsoid is included in a short axis plane at the level of the papillary muscle tip, as illustrated in Figure 20–26. A mean thickness of the ventricular wall is computed from the myocardial area in this short axis:

$$\text{Wall thickness } t = \sqrt{\frac{A_1}{\pi}} - \sqrt{\frac{A_2}{\pi}}$$

This mean thickness and the different radii illustrated in Figure 20–26 are included in a complex formula:[105]

$$V = \pi\left((b+t)^2 \int_0^{d+a+t} \left[1 - \frac{(x-d)^2}{(a+t)^2}\right] dx - b^2 \int_0^{d+a} \left[1 - \frac{(x-d)^2}{a^2}\right] dx\right)$$

$$= \pi\left((b+t)^2 \left[\frac{2}{3}(a+t) + d - \frac{d^3}{3(a+t)^2}\right] - b^2\left[\frac{2}{3}a + d - \frac{d^3}{3a^2}\right]\right)$$

The resulting volume, multiplied by 1.05, gave a very good estimate of left ventricular mass in an experimental canine model.[105] In contrast to most other models of mass calculation, which have only been validated at end-diastole, this formula has been reported to be valid in systole as well as in diastole. Unfortunately, in a small group of patients studied before death, this model predicted left ventricular mass at necropsy with a lower correlation (r = .82) and a constant underestimation (mean underestimation = 34%).[104] Normal values of human left ventricular mass with this method have been published: 130 ± 31 g (mean ± SD); mass is higher in men than in women, even after correction for body surface area (men 76 ± 13 g/m^2, women 66 ± 11 g/m^2).[109]

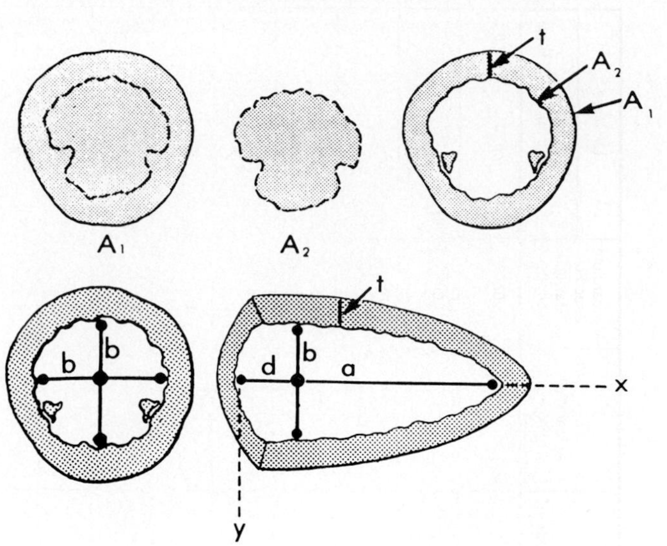

Fig. 20–26. The truncated ellipsoid model. Top. Wall thickness (t) is computed from planimetry of the epicardial area (A_1) and cavity area (A_2), measured on a short axis plane at the level of the papillary muscle tip. Bottom. The minor-axis radius (b) of the left ventricle is measured at the level of the papillary muscle tip. Its placement determines the division of the major axis of the left ventricle into a full major radius (a) and a truncated major radius (d). x and y are the Cartesian coordinates of the system. (Modified from Schiller NB, et al.: Canine left ventricular mass estimation by two-dimensional echocardiography. Circulation 68:210, 1983.)

The simple cylinder has also been used for mass calculation in several studies.[98,107] This figure consistently overestimates true mass. Even with corrections, it yielded a poor estimate of postmortem left ventricular mass (see Table 20–4), and this two-dimensional method has also proven inferior to the M-mode modified D^3 formula (Equation 20.25).[107]

There is no general agreement about the optimal method for mass calculation. The Simpson's rule method appears to be an accurate but complex approach to mass calculation. In the symmetric ventricle of the experimental model, the ellipsoid figure has been less accurate than the combined cylinder-hemiellipsoid or the cylinder alone.[98] In more irregular ventricles, such as the "worst case" example presented in Figure 20–22, the accuracy of the area-length ellipsoid model might prove superior; however, mass is rarely determined in this setting. Because of its simplicity and accuracy, the combined cylinder-hemiellipsoid appears to be a good clinical alternative. The truncated ellipsoid method con-

Table 20–4. Left Ventricular Mass

Geometric Model	Volume Formula	Reference	Subjects of Study	Method of Measurement	Cross-Sectional Views	Convention	Apical Wall Thickness	Myocardium Specific Gravity (g/ml)	LV Mass r	LV Mass SEE (g)	LV Mass % Error
Prolate ellipsoid	D^3	Wyatt et al.[98]	21 dogs	Direct	M-mode at the mitral valve tip	Wyatt	—	1.055	0.83	30.0	8.8
Length-diameter	D^3	Devereux et al.[104]	52 patients	Postmortem	M-mode at the mitral valve tip	ASE M-mode	—	1.040	0.90	47	
	$V = D^3$ $LVM = 1.04(V_{epi} - V_{endo}) - 13.6$	Devereux et al.[97]	34 patients	Postmortem	M-mode at the mitral valve tip	Penn	—	1.040	0.96	29.1	
		Reichek et al.[103]	18 patients	Postmortem	M-mode at the mitral valve tip	Penn	—	1.040	0.86	59	
		Devereux et al.[104]	52 patients	Postmortem	M-mode at the mitral valve tip	Penn	—	1.040	0.92	43	
		Woythaler et al.[107]	48 patients	Postmortem	M-mode at the mitral valve tip	ASE M-mode	—	1.040	0.81	51	
	$\frac{7}{2.4 + D} D^3$	Devereux et al.[104]	52 patients	Postmortem	M-mode at the mitral valve tip	ASE M-mode	—	1.040	0.84	60	
	$\frac{\pi}{6} L D_1 D_2$	Wyatt et al.[98]	21 dogs	Direct	SAX-Pap; LAXp	Wyatt	4 mm	1.055	0.89	9.8	8.6
Area-length	$0.85 \frac{A^2}{L}$	Wyatt et al.[98]	21 dogs	Direct	LAXp	Wyatt	4 mm	1.055	0.74	20.8	10.0
Modified Simpson's rule	$\sum_{i=1}^{n-1} A_i h + \frac{A_n h}{2} + \frac{\pi h^3}{3}$	Helak et al.[102]	13 human hearts in vitro	Direct	6–11 SAX†	Wyatt	†	0.964	0.93	59.5	
	$(A_1 + A_2 + A_3)h + \frac{A_4 h}{2} + \frac{\pi h^3}{6}$	Wyatt et al.[98]	21 dogs	Direct	SAX-MV, Pap1, Pap2, apex; LAXp	Wyatt	4 mm	1.055	0.95	9.0	6.3
Cylinder	A L	Wyatt et al.[98]	21 dogs	Direct	SAX-Pap; LAXp	Wyatt	4 mm	1.055	0.94	12.8	7.0
	A L $LVM = \frac{5}{6}(V_{epi} - V_{endo})$	Woythaler et al.[107]	19 patients	Postmortem	SAX-MV; 4Ch	Wyatt	0 mm	1.00	0.50		
Ellipsoid-cylinder cone	$\frac{2}{3} AL$	Wyatt et al.[98]	21 dogs	Direct	SAX-Pap; LAXp	Wyatt	4 mm	1.055	0.94	8.5	6.9
Cylinder-hemiellipsoid	$\frac{5}{6} AL$	Helak et al.[102]	13 human hearts in vitro	Direct	SAX-Pap†	Wyatt	†	0.964	0.92	74.7	
		Wyatt et al.[98]	21 dogs	Direct	SAX-Pap; LAXp	Wyatt	4 mm	1.055	0.94	11.4	6.9
		Devereux et al.[104]	9 patients	Postmortem	SAX-Pap; 4Ch	Standard	10 mm	1.055	0.68		
	$V = \frac{5}{6} AL$ $LVM = 1.055k(V_{epi} - V_{endo}) + b^*$	Reichek et al.[103]	21 patients	Postmortem	SAX-Pap; 4Ch	Standard	10 mm	1.055	0.93	31	
Truncated ellipsoid	See Fig. 20–26 and equations on p. 602.	Schiller et al.[105]	10 dogs	Direct	SAX-Pap; LAXa	Wyatt	Wall thickness in short axis	1.050	0.98	6.0	
		Devereux et al.[104]	9 patients	Postmortem	SAX-Pap; 4Ch	Standard	Wall thickness in short axis	1.055	0.82		

* k And b are instrument-specific correction factors.
† Nonechocardiographic direct measurement of slice thickness, ventricular length, and apical thickness.
4Ch = apical four-chamber view; LAXa = apical long axis view; LAXp = parasternal long axis view; LVM = left ventricular mass; SAX-MV = parasternal short-axis view at the level of the mitral valve; SAX-Pap = parasternal short-axis view at the level of the papillary muscles; SEE = standard error of the estimate; V = volume.

tains several assumptions, adds a great deal of complexity, and in clinical studies has not been proven more accurate than other simpler approaches. Because of its ease of use, the modified D^3 formula (Equation 20.25) has been the most widely applied model in clinical trials and epidemiologic studies,[93] but its limitations have been noted previously.

Definition of Left Ventricular Hypertrophy

To define left ventricular hypertrophy (LVH) by echocardiography, two approaches are possible: (1) criteria from other methods, such as necropsy, can be used or (2) a normal population can be sampled, all values within ± 2 SD of the population mean considered as "normal" and values out of this range as "abnormal." Abnormal values are thus below the 3rd percentile or above the 97th percentile.

At necropsy, LVH has been defined as a left ventricular mass of 220 g or more.[110] In echocardiographic studies, LVH has usually been defined as a left ventricular mass >215 g[111,104] or >225 g.[107] Because mass is significantly different in men and women and is correlated with height and body surface area, indexed limits have been established, for use with the modified D^3 formula (Equation 20.25). Upper limits indexed for height, from the Framingham Heart Study, are 143 g/m for men and 102 g/m for women.[112] Using the same D^3 formula, limits indexed for body surface area (based on a sample of 78 men and 55 women), set at 2 SD above the mean value, are 134 g/m² in men and 110 g/m² in women.[108]

The criteria used to define LVH are critical. If the upper limit of normal is set very high, specificity will be very good but sensitivity will decrease. Different echocardiographic criteria for mass and for wall thickness were applied in a group of normotensive subjects and in a population of urban workers with untreated hypertension or who had stopped treatment for at least 3 weeks, to determine the prevalence of LVH.[113] Mass was calculated using the modified D^3 formula (Equation 20.25) and the Penn convention; wall thickness was measured using the ASE M-mode convention. Results, shown in Table 20–5, illustrate how prevalence can vary, depending on the definition of LVH. Based on these data, use of the same criterion for both men and women seems inappropriate, and sex-specific criteria should be used.

In very small left ventricles (small patients; hypovolemia), concentric hypertrophy sometimes results in a mass within the normal range, even after correction for body surface area. In these cases, the ratio of left ventricular volume and mass can be used. Its normal value at end-diastole is 0.80 ± 15 ml/g, using the truncated ellipsoid model;[109] in concentric LVH, the ratio can be expected to be below 0.50 ml/g.

Left ventricular mass determined by echocardiography is significantly correlated not only with height[112] and body surface area[108] but also with obesity,[114] expressed as body mass index (i.e., weight/[height]²); lean body mass;[113] subscapular skinfold;[114] hypertension (see following discussion of left ventricle in hypertension); and blood viscosity.[115] Age is positively correlated with left ventricular mass;[114] however, the reason may be that hypertension and other diseases are also more frequent in old age. Indeed, increased left ventricular mass seems not to be an inevitable consequence of aging: echocardiographic examination of a group of healthy normotensive old people did not reveal any increase in mass.[116]

Sensitivity and Specificity of Echocardiographic Assessment of Left Ventricular Hypertrophy

In hypertensive patients, increase in left ventricular mass is known to occur before any change can be detected on the electrocardiogram or on the chest roentgenogram. Therefore, echocardiography should be more sensitive than other commonly used screening tech-

Table 20–5. Prevalence of Left Ventricular Hypertrophy in Three Populations, Based on Different Echocardiographic Criteria

Criteria	% Normal Blood Pressure (n = 160)	% Borderline Hypertension (n = 145)	% Sustained Hypertension (n = 316)
Left ventricular mass			
>134 g/m² for men and >110 g/m² for women	3.1%	12.4%	19.4%
>120 g/m² (for both sexes)	7.5%	17.4%	21.1%
>130 g/m² (for both sexes)	3.1%	11.6%	14.1%
>140 g/m² (for both sexes)	1.3%	8.0%	9.0%
>143 g/m for men and >102 g/m for women	9.4%	19.6%	30.1%
Interventricular septum thickness ≥1.28 cm	3.8%	12.3%	18.4%
Posterior wall thickness ≥1.13 cm	3.8%	14.5%	16.4%

Explanations: In the group of 160 patients with normal blood pressure, 7.5% are diagnosed as having LVH if the criterion is >120 g/m². In the same group, only 1.3% are diagnosed as having LVH if the criterion is >140 g/m².

(Adapted from Hammond IW, et al.: The prevalence and correlates of echocardiographic left ventricular hypertrophy among employed patients with uncomplicated hypertension. J Am Coll Cardiol 7:639, 1986.)

niques to detect hypertrophy. This hypothesis has been confirmed in postmortem studies. Commonly used electrocardiographic criteria for left ventricular hypertrophy, such as a Sokolow index (S in V_1 + R in V_5 or V_6) ≥ 35 mm, or a Romhilt-Estes score ≥5, have a specificity of 86 to 95% but a sensitivity of only 21 to 54%.[107,111] In the same groups, the modified D^3 formula (Equation 20.25) using >265 g[107] or >215 g[111] as the definition of hypertrophy achieves a similar specificity (84 to 95%) and a much higher sensitivity (88 to 93%).

Relationship of Mass to Volume

Left ventricular mass may be increased either because of thickened walls with a small or normal ventricular cavity, sometimes called *concentric hypertrophy*, or because of an increase in cavity size with near-normal wall thickness, sometimes called *eccentric hypertrophy*, and seen, e.g., in volume overloads. One way to quantify these patterns of hypertrophy is the index of relative wall thickness (RWT); it is expressed as the ratio of twice the posterior wall thickness (PWT) to LVID, measured at the end of diastole:

$$RWT = \frac{2\ PWT}{LVID} \qquad [20.26]$$

Echocardiographic values in a normal population were similar for men and women: 0.34 ± 0.07 and 0.35 ± 0.08.[108] In hypertrophy that is due to hypertension[117] and to aortic stenosis,[118] relative wall thickness is significantly increased.

DYNAMIC OR EJECTION PHASE INDICES OF LEFT VENTRICULAR PERFORMANCE

The principle dynamic- or ejection-phase indices that can be calculated echocardiographically are stroke volume, ejection fraction (EF), shortening fraction (%ΔD), and velocity of circumferential fiber shortening (Vcf).

Stroke Volume

Stroke volume (SV) can be determined as

$$SV = \text{end-diastolic volume} - \text{end-systolic volume}$$

Both volumes are calculated using one of the methods described earlier. As might be expected, the most accurate clinical correlations have been obtained using a modification of Simpson's rule (see Table 20–2). The echocardiographic stroke volume generally shows a better correlation with the comparable angiographic measurement than does the end-diastolic volume but a lower correlation than the end-systolic volume. In absolute terms, the echocardiographic stroke volume appears to be a more accurate estimate of the comparable angiographic volume than are either the end-diastolic or the end-systolic volumes taken by themselves. This increased accuracy occurs because the consistent errors in both volume calculations cancel out when the values are subtracted. Angiographically, the normal stroke volume has been reported to average 45 ± 13 ml/m^2.[119]

An indirect method of calculating stroke volume from the M-mode mitral valve echogram has been reported,[120] which is based on the maximum vertical separation of the leaflets, the EF slope, the PR interval on the electrocardiogram (ECG), and the heart rate. It has the advantage of being independent of ventricular geometry but is based on the assumption that the mitral valve is anatomically intact and that flow through the valve is unimpeded. Direct methods of measuring the stroke volume are now preferred.

In clinical correlations, stroke volume is frequently determined by dividing the cardiac output, obtained by thermodilution or the Fick method, by the heart rate. Remember that many techniques that measure cardiac output, such as the Fick method, reflect only the forward component of the stroke volume. In the presence of valvular regurgitation or ventricular septal defect, they may significantly underestimate the total volume ejected by the left ventricle and measured by the direct echocardiographic method.

In all methods, stroke volume should be determined at end-expiration, because it has been shown that stroke volume normally decreases during inspiration.[121,122]

Ejection Fraction

The ejection fraction is the ratio of the stroke volume to the end-diastolic volume,

$$EF = \frac{EDV - ESV}{EDV} \times 100 \qquad [20.27]$$

The ejection fraction is a global index of left ventricular fiber shortening and is generally considered as one of the most meaningful measures of left ventricular pump function. Angiographic studies have shown that the normal ejection fraction averages 72% ± 8% (SD),[81] and ranges from 56 to 78%.[80] Values below 50% in the resting supine individual are generally considered abnormal.

Two-dimensional echocardiographic assessment of ejection fractions is generally based on measuring end-diastolic and end-systolic volumes, as described earlier in this chapter. Correlation with angiographic studies and normal values of ejection fraction by echocardiography are reported in Tables 20–2 and 20–3.

Simplified Methods of Ejection Fraction Measurement

Simplified methods have been developed to measure ejection fraction, without the need for planimetry. One such method relies on eight left ventricular diameters.[123] These diameters are measured on two-dimensional images at different levels of the left ventricle in the parasternal long axis, apical four-chamber, and long axis views. These eight dimensions are averaged at end-diastole (D_d) and end-systole (D_s), and a fractional "area" shortening is calculated:

$$\%\Delta D^2 = \frac{(D_d)^2 - (D_s)^2}{(D_d)^2}$$

The fractional shortening of the long axis of the left ventricle, %ΔL, is then subjectively assessed and given a value of 15% when normal apical contraction is present, 5% when it appears hypokinetic, 0 when it appears akinetic and −5 or −10% when it appears slightly or frankly dyskinetic. The ejection fraction is expressed as:

$$EF = (\%\Delta D^2) + [(1 - \%\Delta D^2)(\%\Delta L)]$$

Averaging diameters at multiple locations takes into account regional contraction defects. Good correlation has been reported between this method and radionuclide or angiographic measurements of ejection fraction (r = .89 to .93), with an SEE close to 7%.[123,124] This method, however, was developed before computer analysis programs were widely available and is rarely used at this time.

Another simplified method, derived from the cylinder-hemiellipsoid formula and requiring less measurements, has been proposed:[125]

$$EF = \frac{(D_d)^2L_d - (D_s)^2L_s}{(D_d)^2L_d}$$

where D_d and D_s are the minor diameters at the midventricular cavity level measured at the end of diastole and systole in the apical four-chamber view and length (L_d and L_s) is measured in the same view from the ventricular apex to the base of the mitral valve. Correlation with angiographic measurements was fair in a group of 60 patients (r = .79) but poor in the subgroup of 24 patients with abnormal wall motion (r = .38). To overcome this limitation, diameters had to be measured at different levels, thus increasing the complexity of the method.

An even simpler adaptation of this method uses the commonly measured end-diastolic and end-systolic diameters of the left ventricle in the parasternal long axis view, with a correction for the apex:

$$EF = \frac{EDD^2 - ESD^2}{EDD^2} \times 100 + K$$

K is given a value of +10% for a normal apex, +5% for hypokinesis, 0 for akinesis, and −5% for dyskinesis. This formula appears reasonably accurate in symmetric ventricles, which represent the vast majority of patients. Although invalid in patients with important wall motion abnormalities and distorted ventricles, it provides acceptable results quickly and, when applied appropriately, has proven useful in our experience.

E-Point Septal Separation

A normal ejection fraction can be differentiated from an abnormal one based on the minimum separation between its anterior mitral leaflet at its E point (see Chapter 17) and the most posterior excursion of the interventricular septum.[126] An E-point septal separation ≤5 mm is considered normal, whereas an increased separation is consistent with a reduced ejection fraction. This index has the advantage of being independent of ventricular geometry, size, and abnormal wall motion. It has been shown to have a reasonable correlation (r = −.86) with angiographic ejection fraction.[126] An abnormal E-point septal separation of more than 7 mm has a sensitivity of 87% and a specificity of 75% in identifying reduced ejection fraction (less than 50% by angiography) in patients with coronary artery disease.[127] The index is limited, however, because it must assume normal mitral valve motion and unimpeded left ventricular inflow. Thus, it is inaccurate in patients with aortic insufficiency and mitral stenosis. This method provides a rapid approximation of function but is less accurate than two-dimensional methods.

Visual Assessment

In the clinical setting, visual estimation of left ventricular systolic function has become a common practice. It can be described as normal or mildly, moderately, or severely impaired. Alternatively, an ejection fraction can be estimated. In one study,[128] visual estimates were shown to have a good correlation with angiographic measurement (r = .89, SEE 7.3%), and to be as good as the best echocardiographic measurements using Simpson's rule (see Table 20–2). Another study[129] also reported a good correlation of visually estimated echocardiographic ejection fraction with that obtained by radionuclide angiography (r = .88, SEE 7.1%). Unfortunately, the correlation between observers was less good (r = .77), and the mean percentage difference was high (MPD = 22.9% ± 36.7%); it improved to r = .88 and MPD 9.2% ± 20.5 when only patients with adequate apical views were analyzed.

Visual estimation of ejection fraction allows the observer to take into account all possible views and real-time analysis aids in endocardial detection compared to stop-frame images. The method is rapid and widely applicable. However, it requires an observer with experience both in echocardiography and in assessment of ejection fraction derived from another source. Its subjective nature makes it prone to errors, and the method is clearly unacceptable for scientific studies where highly reproducible measures of ejection fraction are needed. In clinical practice, echocardiographic reports should mention when ejection fraction is based on a visual estimate and not on a measured value.

Effect of Respiration

A common source of error in ejection fraction assessment is respiration. Inspiration decreases the intrathoracic pressure, causing an increase in systemic venous return and in right ventricular volume, which itself reduces left ventricular end-diastolic volume via diastolic ventricular interdependence. In addition, inspiration increases the left ventricular afterload, thus reducing the left ventricular stroke volume.[130] These different mechanisms combine to produce a decrease in end-diastolic left ventricular dimensions, with no change in end-systolic dimensions and a decrease in stroke volume and ejection fraction.[121,122,131,132] Beat-to-beat variability at end-expiration in the measurement of ejection fraction is significantly less than during inspiration.[133] Therefore, as mentioned earlier, measurements should be taken during held expiration. Simultaneous recording of respiration facilitates analysis of echocardiographic images at end-expiration and provides a more reliable assessment of left ventricular function.

Fractional Shortening

The shortening fraction, %ΔD, and the velocity of circumferential fiber shortening, Vcf, have been mainly derived from M-mode recordings and rely on minor axis shortening as a representation of overall ventricular systolic function. They are based on the angiographic observation that the systolic decrease in ventricular volume is primarily due to minor axis shortening and that the percentage of change in the minor axis during systole shows a linear correlation with ejection fraction.[33] These assumptions are similar to those underlying the D^3 method of volume calculation, and their limitations have already been discussed. Fractional shortening (FS) represents a simple method for estimating ventricular function in the symmetrically contracting ventricle and can be calculated from the LVID using the following formula:[134,135]

$$\%\Delta D = \frac{LVID_d - LVID_s}{LVID_d} \times 100 \qquad [20.28]$$

In patients with normal left ventricular function, %ΔD is usually greater than 25%.

M-mode fractional shortening is a rapid and easy method to evaluate ventricular function but does not take into account asymmetric ventricles. To overcome this limitation, two-dimensional cavity area, A_c, can be planimetered to express an area change. Alternatively, the area can be converted into a mean ventricular diameter, and LVID can be expressed as:

$$LVID = 2 \times \sqrt{\frac{A_c}{\pi}}$$

Such a method, with A_c measured at the high papillary muscle level in the short axis view, provides smaller normal values for shortening than M-mode measurements (30 ± 5% vs. 34 ± 5%).[136]

Unfortunately, major changes in ventricular morphology often appear near the apex and remain unaccounted for by the fractional shortening approach.

Velocity of Circumferential Fiber Shortening

The velocity of circumferential fiber shortening (Vcf) may be a more meaningful estimate of left ventricular function than the more familiar ejection fraction because it reflects not only the normalized amplitude but also the rate of fiber shortening.[12,40,135,137–139] The Vcf, expressed in circumferences per second, is normally calculated by assuming that the LVID reliably represents the circumference of the ventricle at the base and is expressed as

$$Vcf = \frac{LVID_d - LVID_s}{LVID_d \times ET} \qquad [20.29]$$

where ET is the ejection time derived from the carotid pulse tracing, from the duration of aortic valve opening, or from the onset to the peak of posterior left ventricular wall movement. The lower limit of normal for Vcf is 1.1 circumferences per second.

M-mode-derived mean circumferential fiber shortening velocity is misnamed; in reality, Vcf represents the velocity of the shortening of the minor axis and not of the whole circumference. It does not reflect the change in geometry during contraction or regional wall motion abnormality. Correlation between M-mode Vcf and circumferential fiber shortening based on two-dimensional short axis echocardiographic measurements is only fair ($r = .68$).[140] This consideration does not minimize the usefulness of M-mode-derived mean Vcf but pinpoints one of its limitations.

The ejection-phase indices, although generally considered to reflect myocardial contractility, are also subject to changes of preload and afterload.[141] When either end-diastolic volume (preload) is reduced or aortic pressure (afterload) is elevated, the ejection phase indices decline. Conversely, the ejection phase indices may appear normal when afterload is reduced, as in acute mitral insufficiency or ventricular septal defect, even though contractility may be depressed. Afterload reduction with nifedipine results in a higher fractional shortening during maximal exercise, when ventricular function is at its peak.[141]

Helical Shortening

Based on studies suggesting that the great proportion of myocardial fibers are oriented helically around the left ventricular cavity, a mathematical model has been developed to express the length of the helical fibers, from base to apex, and their shortening during systole. Using M-mode echocardiographic measurements of diameter and wall thickness, and length from a two-dimensional apical view, helical shortening was calculated at endocardium and epicardium;[142] left ventricular volumes were calculated using a length-diameter formula, to estimate the ejection fraction. A curvilinear relationship was found between helical shortening and ejection fraction, ejection fraction increasing as the natural logarithm of helical shortening.

dP/dt: The Rate of Change of Left Ventricular Pressure

An important parameter in the assessment of myocardial systolic and diastolic function is the rate of change of left ventricular pressure during the cardiac cycle. The first derivative of pressure, dP/dt, is conventionally derived from the left ventricular pressure curve obtained at cardiac catheterization using micromanometer catheter recordings. Noninvasive evaluation of dP/dt is possible by Doppler echocardiography in patients with mitral regurgitation. The complete velocity profile of regurgitant flow through the mitral valve can be recorded by continuous wave Doppler echocardiography. Using the simplified Bernoulli equation, the velocity curve can be converted to a pressure gradient (ΔP) curve, the derivative of which gives instantaneous dΔP/dt (Fig. 20–27).

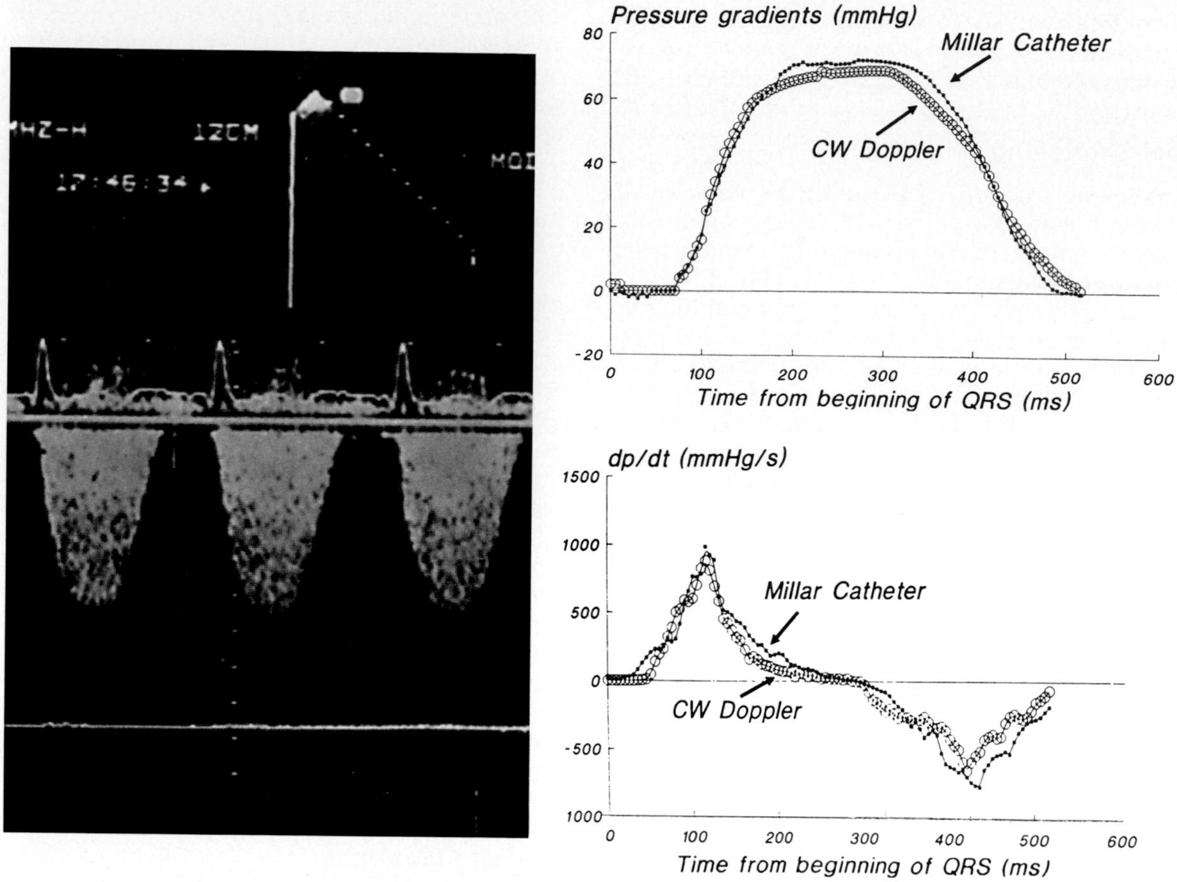

Fig. 20–27. dP/dt: Rate of change of left ventricular pressure. Left. Continuous wave (CW) Doppler recordings showing mitral regurgitant velocity spectrum. Horizontal white dots represent time scale (time period between two dots = 200 msec); vertical white dots represent velocity amplitude scale (amplitude between two dots = 1 m/sec). Top, right. Graph comparing Doppler-derived left ventriculoatrial pressure gradient curve (CW Doppler) with gradient curve derived from Millar catheter-recorded simultaneous left atrial and ventricular pressures. Bottom, right. Graph comparing dP/dt curve determined by Doppler mitral regurgitant velocity spectrum (CW Doppler) with dP/dt curve derived from Millar catheter-recorded left ventricular pressure curve. (Modified from Chen C, et al.: Noninvasive estimation of the instantaneous first derivative of left ventricular pressure using continuous-wave Doppler echocardiography. Circulation 83:2101, 1991.)

Continuous Doppler-derived pressure gradients and $d\Delta P/dt$ have been demonstrated to correlate closely to those obtained at catheterization in patients[143] and by direct measurements in experimental models.[144] The latter model allowed calculation of instantaneous $d\Delta P/dt$ from Doppler recording throughout systole (correlation factor with invasive measurements r = .92). Peak dP/dt has been obtained from continuous Doppler recordings using two different approaches.

The first method to estimate dP/dt is the mean rate of pressure rise measured from the steepest rising segment of the velocity curve, between 2 points arbitrarily selected at 1 m/sec and 3 m/sec, corresponding to 4 and 36 mm Hg. This method has correlated well with peak dP/dt obtained from pressure curves at catheterization (r = .87, SEE = 316 mm Hg/sec, slope = 1.05).[143] The mean rate of pressure rise, however, underestimates peak dP/dt, because the time point of dP/dt_{max} on the pressure curve depends in part on the peak systolic pressure attained. Peak dP/dt occurs at lower pressure when peak ventricular pressure is low and at a higher pressure when peak pressure is high. Thus, in patients with congestive cardiomyopathy, where peak dP/dt occurs early in the upstroke of the pressure curve, this method is less reliable (r = .84, slope of .55).[145]

From the measurements of *instantaneous* dP/dt by continuous Doppler, peak dP/dt can easily be obtained and has an excellent correlation with invasive measurements (r = .97).[144] This method is more accurate than the mean rate of pressure rise and is not subject to underestimation.[144]

The rate of left ventricular pressure decline in early isovolumic diastole, −dP/dt, can be obtained by the same method from the mitral regurgitation velocity. It reflects relaxation of the left ventricle and provides an index of diastolic function. Doppler-derived −dP/dt is slightly lower than catheter-derived measurements, by an average of 8.5%.[144] This may be due to the simultaneous decline of the atrial pressure, causing a prolongation of the gradient and therefore a blunted decrease in the velocity of the mitral regurgitation jet. Nevertheless, it represents a useful noninvasive approach to evaluate diastolic function.

The main limitations of the Doppler method are: (1)

mitral regurgitation must be present, which is not the case in all patients; (2) the maximal spectra of the regurgitant flow must be recorded, which may be impractical with eccentric jets or with minimal regurgitant flow; and (3) early systole is not truly isovolumic, because of mitral regurgitation. The latter concern, however, has not been a significant problem in the experimental settings.

Left Ventricular Wall Stress

The common noninvasive measures of left ventricular systolic function—such as stroke volume, ejection fraction, fractional shortening, Vcf, and also, to some extent, dP/dt—do not differentiate between abnormalities of myocardial contractility and alterations in afterload or preload. To truly characterize myocardial contractility, therefore, some measure of the force-length relationship of the myofibril is required. The end-systolic stress-length and the end-systolic pressure-volume relations, which incorporate afterload and are relatively independent of preload, are sensitive indicators of left ventricular contractility.[146] As a result, left ventricular wall stress, as the load opposing ejection, is commonly used to describe systolic function.

The use of wall stress as a measure of myocardial function is based on the principle that, for equilibrium to exist at any point in the cardiac cycle, the forces acting within the ventricular wall must exactly balance the forces acting on the wall. The force present in the wall per unit cross-sectional area is defined as stress and expressed as dynes/cm^2. Left ventricular wall stress is a function of chamber size, configuration, thickness of the ventricular wall, and intraventricular pressure. Figure 20–28 illustrates the circumferential, meridional, and radial stress acting on the ventricular wall. For an ellipsoid model, the average meridional stress, σ_m, can be defined as the force per unit area acting at the midplane of the heart toward the apex.[147] With the assumptions of uniform ventricular wall thickness and homogeneous elasticity, the wall stress is derived by equating the meridional wall forces ($\sigma_m \times \pi(R_o^2 - R_i^2)$) to the pressure loading forces ($P\pi R_i^2$), because these must be equal for the chamber to hold its shape.

$$\sigma_m \times \pi(R_o^2 - R_i^2) = P\pi R_i^2$$

where, P is the left ventricular pressure in g/cm^2, R_i is the left ventricular inner radius in centimeters, and R_o is the left ventricular outer radius in centimeters. Wall stress can thus be expressed as:

$$\sigma_m = \frac{PR_i^2}{R_o^2 - R_i^2} = \frac{PR_i^2}{(R_o - R_i)(R_o + R_i)}$$

and when wall thickness (h) is substituted for $(R_o - R_i)$ the expression becomes:

$$\sigma_m = \frac{PR_i^2}{h(R_o + R_i)} = \frac{PR_i}{2h\left(1 + \frac{h}{2R_i}\right)}$$

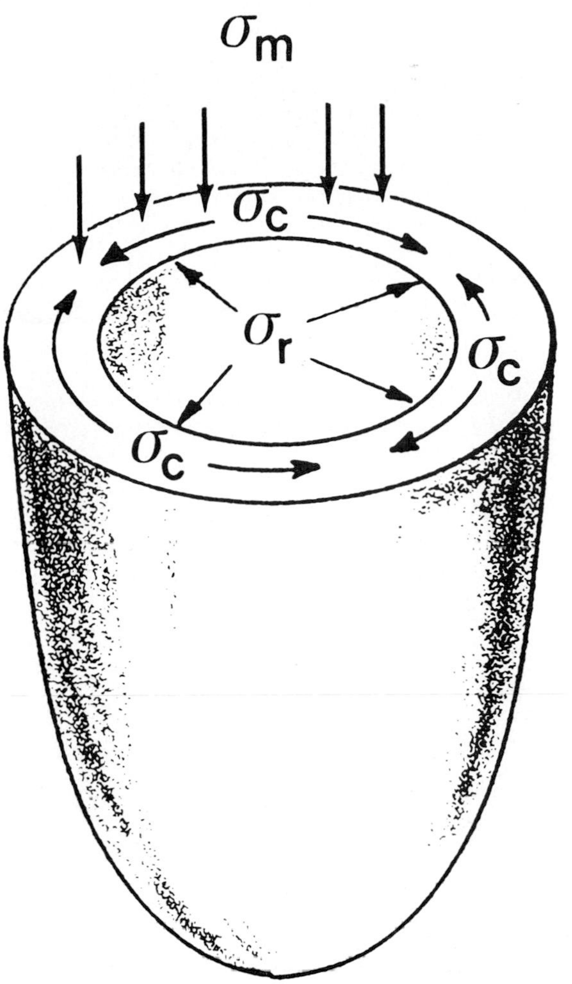

Fig. 20–28. Circumferential (σ_c), meridional (σ_m), and radial (σ_r) components of left ventricular wall stress for an ellipsoid model. The three components of wall stress are mutually perpendicular. (From Fifer MA, Grossman W: Measurement of ventricular volumes, ejection fraction, mass, and wall stress. *In* Grossman W (ed.): Cardiac Catheterization and Angiography. 3rd Ed. Philadelphia, Lea & Febiger, 1986.)

which can be simplified by substituting LVID for $2R_i$:

$$\sigma_m = \frac{P(LVID)}{4h\left(1 + \frac{h}{LVID}\right)}$$

Thus, the average meridional or longitudinal left ventricular wall stress may be calculated throughout the cardiac cycle from the simultaneous left ventricular pressure (P), wall thickness (h), and left ventricular diameter (LVID). Because instantaneous wall thickness and minor axis chamber dimensions are available from the M-mode echocardiogram, stress measurements are most often derived from M-mode recordings.[147]

Assessment of wall stress throughout the cardiac cycle requires continuous pressure recording, obtained by left ventricular catheterization or, in the absence of outflow obstruction, aortic catheterization. At end-systole, however, wall stress can be determined totally noninvasively. End-systolic wall stress, $\sigma_{m(es)}$, requires measurement of the $LVID_s$, the end-systolic left ventricular wall thickness (either posterior wall or mean of thickness of the IVS and posterior wall) and an estimate of left ventricular end-systolic pressure. Sphygmomanometric pressure provides peak systolic pressure, but in the absence of obstruction to left ventricular outflow and of severe mitral regurgitation, this value is close to the end-systolic pressure and can be used to calculate end-systolic wall stress. Some authors have suggested that a better estimate of the end-systolic pressure can be derived from calibrated carotid pulse tracing at the time of the dicrotic notch.[146]

To convert from millimeters of mercury to dynes/cm², multiply the systolic blood pressure (BP_{sys}) by 1.35 dynes/cm²/mm Hg.

$$\sigma_{m(es)} = \frac{1.35(BP_{sys})(LVID_s)}{4h\left(1 + \frac{h}{LVID_s}\right)} = \frac{0.334(BP_{sys})(LVID_s)}{h\left(1 + \frac{h}{LVID_s}\right)}$$

The noninvasive method to assess end-systolic meridional wall stress, using cuff pressure and M-mode measurements, has been shown to correlate very closely (r = .97, SEE 10 × 10³ dynes/cm²) with invasive measurements.[148] Normal values have varied from 64.8 ± 19.5 × 10³ dynes/cm² to 73 ± 21 × 10³ dynes/cm².[136,148]

Meridional stress can also be calculated from two-dimensional echo recordings using the formula

$$\sigma_{m(es)} = 1.33\, P \frac{A_m}{A_c} \times 10^3 \ \frac{\text{dynes}}{\text{cm}^2}$$

where P is the left ventricular pressure, A_m is the myocardial area, and A_c is the left ventricular cavity area in the short axis view. Normal two-dimensional values have been reported to be slightly higher than those for M-mode recordings because of averaging of ventricular wall thickness: 86 ± 16 × 10³ dynes/cm².[136]

A simplified index of meridional wall stress has been suggested:[149]

$$\frac{PR}{W} = \frac{P\frac{LVID}{2}}{W} \ \text{(mm Hg)}$$

where P is left ventricular pressure, R is minor radius of the left ventricle, W is wall thickness, and LVID is left ventricular diameter. Normal end-systolic values of this index have been reported to be 134 ± 23 mm Hg.[150]

Circumferential stress will act perpendicular to the long axis. For a sphere, the circumferential stress will equal the meridional stress; however, for an ellipse the circumferential stress is larger. Circumferential stress can be calculated only from the two-dimensional echocardiogram because it requires measurement of the ventricular long axis. Circumferential stress can be calculated as[151]

$$\sigma_c = \frac{1.33P\sqrt{A_c}}{\sqrt{A_m + A_c} - \sqrt{A_c}}\left[\frac{\frac{4(A_c)^{3/2}}{\pi L^2}}{\sqrt{A_m + A_c} + \sqrt{A_c}}\right]$$

where P is left ventricular pressure, L is left ventricular long axis length, A_m is myocardial area, and A_c is left ventricular cavity area. Normal end-systolic circumferential stress has been reported as 213 ± 29 × 10³ dynes/cm².[136]

Wall stress is directly related to the shape of the ventricle, which changes during the cardiac cycle and also in heart failure. Circumferential stress is higher at the end of diastole than during systole, which is due to the systolic thickening of the walls. At the end of systole, circumferential stress exceeds meridional stress, with their normal ratio being 2.57 ± 0.33.[136] In heart failure, however, as the ventricle becomes more spherical, meridional stress increases more than the circumferential stress, and their ratio decreases toward a value of 1. It has been reported to be 1.71 ± 0.21 in a group with congestive cardiomyopathy.[136]

The loss of the ventricular elliptic shape in systole can be an early indicator of impaired function. In experimental heart failure caused by adriamycin, the left ventricle became more spherical before any reduction in ejection fraction, stroke volume, or cardiac index could be noted.[152] In more advanced stages, two- and three-dimensional shape indices also correlated well with the decrease in ejection fraction (r = −.803 and −.855).

Calculating wall stress requires the assumption that the radius of curvature of the left ventricle is equal along the whole perimeter. This is clearly invalid in patients with regional ischemia. Regional wall stress can be calculated, based on a formula developed by Janz:[153]

$$\sigma = \frac{PrR\left(2 - \frac{r}{R}\sin\phi\right)}{2h\sin\phi\left(R + \frac{h}{2}\right)}$$

where P is left ventricular pressure, r is the circumferential radius of curvature at endocardial surface, R is the meridional radius of curvature at endocardial surface, h is wall thickness, and φ is the angle between R and the axis of symmetry (i.e., the ventricular long axis). Regional wall stress has been shown to be inversely related to the velocity of circumferential fiber shortening, with a linear relation independent of preload and sensitive to changes in contractility.[154] Analysis of regional systolic function of the left ventricle has thus been possible in experimental ischemia and reperfusion.

Wall stress can be useful in distinguishing different groups of patients (i.e., normal hearts and congestive cardiomyopathy[136,148] or aortic regurgitation[136]) or in studying individuals under different loading conditions.[148] However, because of considerable overlap of values from different groups, an isolated value cannot be used reliably to determine the cardiac status of a patient or to guide clinical decisions.

End-Systolic Stress-Dimension, Force-Length, and Pressure-Dimension Relations

A slightly different approach to describe contractility is also based on the following principle: At any given level of myocardial contractility, the length of a muscle at the end of contraction (the end-systolic length) depends on the tension at the end of contraction (the end-systolic tension) but is not influenced importantly by the initial length (i.e., the end-diastolic length) or the mode of contraction, i.e., whether it is isometric or isotonic.[155,156] In the heart, tension can be represented by left ventricular pressure, and length can be represented by ventricular diameter[146,157] or volume.[158] Thus, the end-systolic ratio of pressure/volume provides an index of contractility that is independent of load. Poorly contractile ventricles have lower values than normal ones.[158]

Clinically, end-systolic pressure can be obtained noninvasively from calibrated carotid pulse tracings at the time of the dicrotic notch.[146] End-systolic pressure measured by this method has been shown to be more reliable than peak-systolic pressure to express the pressure-dimension relation and to detect changes in contractility.[159]

Although the method has been validated in humans,[146] it has not been widely used in clinical practice, which is mainly due to its complexity: at least two dimension values, measured at different pressure, are needed to reconstruct the pressure-dimension slope, requiring afterload manipulation. Simplification of the method by measuring the pressure noninvasively from carotid tracings or by cuff pressure impairs its accuracy.

Attempts to express the force-length relation without the need for afterload manipulation have relied on the stress-dimension relation. This relation is linear during nonisovolumic systole, and its slope value constitutes another index of contractility. Unfortunately, this index is not independent of afterload, as shown in a study with pharmacologic manipulation of both contractility and loading.[160] The ratio of end-systolic wall stress/volume, also suggested as an index of contractility, is itself dependent on the end-diastolic ventricular size and on the underlying cardiac disease.[161] Because circumferential stress occurs in the same plane as minor axis dimension measurements and shortening, it is the appropriate load to consider in the stress-dimension relation.[136]

Sophisticated indices of left ventricular systolic function provide interesting insights into the mechanisms of cardiac function. They have been useful to assess different interventions in research. In clinical practice, assessment of cardiac function generally relies on simpler indices, mainly ejection fraction.

In population studies left ventricular end systolic dimension and fractional shortening may provide sufficient information on systolic function without the need to assess variables that are independent of load.[162]

LEFT VENTRICULAR RESPONSE TO EXERCISE

Various forms of controlled stress are frequently employed in conjunction with the echocardiographic examination to assess the ability of the left ventricle to respond to increased demand.[141,163–171] These challenges are directed primarily toward identifying early global abnormalities of left ventricular function that are not apparent at rest or toward inducing wall motion abnormalities in patients with ischemic heart disease (see Chapter 22).

Dynamic (treadmill, upright and supine bicycle)[141,163–168] and isometric (handgrip)[163,168–171] exercise are most commonly employed. In addition, the left ventricular response to dobutamine stimulation, to pharmacologic variation in afterload and preload, to cold exposure, and to a variety of physiologic maneuvers, such as the Valsalva and Muller maneuvers, and to the gravitational test (tilt-test), can also be assessed echocardiographically. The general cardiac response to all forms of exercise is an increase in heart rate, blood pressure, and cardiac output.[163] Dynamic exercise produces a greater increase in heart rate for a given change in blood pressure than does isometric exercise. Isometric exercise, in contrast, causes a predominant increase in blood pressure. The changes in left ventricular size and function that are noted during various forms of exercise are listed in Table 20–6.

Dynamic Exercise

Dynamic, or isotonic, exercise normally causes a progressive decrease in the left ventricular end-systolic dimension and end-systolic volume and an increase in

Table 20–6. Characteristic Responses to Dynamic Exercise, Handgrip, and Dobutamine

	HR	SBP	D_d	D_s	%ΔD	Vcf	End-Systolic Wall Stress
Bicycle exercise	↑↑	↑	— (↑)	↓	↑	↑	↓
Handgrip	↑	↑	— (↑)	↑	— (↓)	↓ (—)	↑
Dobutamine	↑	↑	—	↓	↑	↑	↓

HR = heart rate; SBP = systolic blood pressure; D_d = diastolic left ventricular dimension; D_s = Systolic left ventricular dimension; %ΔD = percentage left ventricular minor dimension shortening (fractional shortening); Vcf = normalized mean rate of left ventricular dimension shortening.

↑↑ = marked increase; ↑ = increase; — = no change; ↓ = decrease.

stroke volume.[163] An increase in ejection fraction from 59 to 72% has been reported during exercise in normal subjects.[165,166] Controversy exists concerning the response of the end-diastolic dimension and volume to dynamic exercise. In general, end-diastolic volume changes little during mild or moderate dynamic exercise. An increase in diastolic volume is generally noted during severe exercise,[172–175] although a report to the contrary has appeared.[141] The change in diastolic volume seems to be related to the level of physical training of the subjects. In a group of trained athletes, the increase in diastolic volume (+5.6 mm) reached significance, but the increase was only 4.1 mm (nonsignificant) in a group of healthy untrained men whose maximal exercise level was inferior to that of the athletes.[167]

In supine studies, diastolic volume changes little following the initiation of exercise. This is in contrast to upright exercise, where an initial increase in diastolic volume is noted and attributed to increased venous return following initial contraction of the leg muscles.[163]

The shortening fraction[141,167,168] (%ΔD) and the mean velocity of circumferential shortening[167,168] (Vcf) increase during dynamic exercise. In an isolated study, meridional and circumferential end-systolic wall stress decreased slightly.[169]

The changes in end-systolic volume and systolic indices during dynamic exercise are not only due to increased myocardial contractility. A decrease in afterload may also play a significant role, as demonstrated by the additional decrease in end-systolic dimension and the additional increase in fractional shortening when a vasodilator, nifedipine, is administered before maximal dynamic exercise.[141] The effect of tachycardia, distinct from the effect of increased contractility, can be assessed by pacing the heart. In one study, where heart rate was accelerated by atrial pacing from 80 to 140 beats per minute, end-diastolic left ventricular volume decreased slightly more than end-systolic volume. A significant decrease in stroke volume and in ejection fraction was observed in normal subjects (from 51 to 45%) and in a group of patients with coronary artery disease or dilated cardiomyopathy (from 31 to 21%).[176]

After prolonged and strenuous exercise in healthy young subjects, systolic blood pressure, left ventricular end-diastolic diameter, fractional shortening, and Vcf were shown to decrease.[177] This suggests that exhaustion may result in depressed left ventricular function.

Isometric Exercise: Handgrip and Deadlift

The normal response to handgrip exercise is complex. The diastolic volume is typically unchanged,[163] although a minimal increase has also been reported.[170] In contrast to changes seen during dynamic exercise, end-systolic volume increases during handgrip.[163,170] Conflicting changes have been reported in systolic indices: decrease[163,169] or no change[168,170,171] in fractional shortening; decrease,[163,168] or no change in mean Vcf,[171] and even an initial increase in Vcf during the first minute of handgrip with return to baseline values later in the test.[170] In contrast to dynamic exercise, meridional and circumferential end-systolic wall stress increase markedly during isometric exercise.[169] Given these inconsistent changes during handgrip, this test is not widely used to assess cardiac function.

Deadlift permits achievement of a higher level of isometric exercise. At 50 and 100% of maximum voluntary effort, an initial increase in heart rate, blood pressure, left ventricular end-systolic diameter and a decrease in ejection fraction have been noted.[178] Sustained effort produced an increase in end-diastolic diameter and tended to bring ejection fraction back to baseline value. Immediately after cessation of effort, blood pressure, end-diastolic and end-systolic diameters decreased sharply, with an increase in ejection fraction. This kind of maximal exercise, however, is not applicable to sick subjects.

Pharmacologic Testing

Intravenous infusion of inotropic agents produces an increase in heart rate and blood pressure. The most commonly used agent has been dobutamine, which produces a decrease in end-systolic diameter with no change in end-diastolic diameter;[179] peak meridional wall stress, which occurs in early-systole, increases, while end-systolic meridional wall stress decreases.[160] Dobutamine stress testing has been used primarily in assessing cardiac function in coronary artery disease (see Chapter 22).

VALVULAR DISEASES AND THE LEFT VENTRICLE

A critical issue in valvular disease is the timing of valve replacement. Early intervention may expose the patient to the complications of surgery and of a prosthetic valve years before necessary, whereas delayed intervention may fail to result in clinical improvement because the left ventricle may have already been irremediably damaged. Echocardiography permits repeated assessment of the progression of disease and provides important data for clinical decision making. In aortic insufficiency, aortic stenosis, and mitral regurgitation, volume or pressure overload directly affects the left ventricle. Cardiac chambers enlarge, wall thickness and ventricular mass increase, and myocardial function often deteriorates—all changes that can be detected by echocardiography.

Aortic Regurgitation

Aortic regurgitation imposes an increased volume on the left ventricle, which often produces important changes: end-diastolic and end-systolic volume increase, the left ventricle assumes a more spherical shape, ventricular mass increases,[150,180,181] and circumferential and meridional wall stress also increase.[182] In an experimental study,[183] increased end-diastolic wall stress appeared to stimulate left ventricular hypertrophy until wall thickness reduced stress to an acceptable level.

Ejection fraction is affected by two main parameters: myocardial function and systemic vascular resistance (afterload). As vascular resistance is low in chronic aortic insufficiency, the ejection fraction may remain normal for a long period, despite severe regurgitation, although it will eventually decrease.[181] Exercise-induced change in ejection fraction has been suggested as an early index of impaired systolic performance. The response to exercise is variable, however, and correlates mainly with changes in systemic vascular resistance.[184] In aortic regurgitation, isometric exercise causes an increase in end-systolic diameter, and a fall in fractional shortening, especially marked in severe regurgitation.[185]

Natural History

The natural history of asymptomatic aortic regurgitation is relatively good; among patients with a normal ejection fraction at rest and a normal fractional shortening, the risk of undergoing valve replacement was 10% at 3 years, 19% at 5 years, and 25% at 7 years, i.e., about 4% a year.[180] However, patients whose ventricular end-systolic dimension reaches ≥55 mm have an increased risk of becoming symptomatic and needing valve replacement.[186] The increase of end-systolic dimension rarely exceeds 7 mm/year.[186] Ejection fraction during exercise is not a useful predictor, particularly when the ventricular end-systolic dimension is already taken into consideration: Most patients whose ejection fraction decreased during exercise continued to be asymptomatic, had a stable normal ejection fraction at rest, and did not need valvular replacement in a 4-year follow-up period.[180]

Surgery

Following valve replacement for aortic regurgitation, the 5-year survival rate was 83% in the 1976 to 1983 period and showed a clear improvement over the previous years.[187] The main effect of valve replacement on the left ventricle is a decrease in preload, although afterload may also be altered.

Intraoperative studies with epicardial echocardiography have shown the immediate effects of valve replacement to be a decrease in end-diastolic volume,[188] cavity area,[189] and ejection fraction.[188,189] The decrease in end-diastolic dimension has been confirmed in the first postoperative days,[190] with some additional decrease after 3 weeks,[191] but little further reduction beyond this point.[191,192] Valve replacement causes temporary thickening of the ventricular walls (which is due to the decrease in chamber volume without a change in wall thickness), which produces concentric hypertrophy.[193] During the 6 months following valve replacement, left ventricular mass regresses, and the walls become thinner.[190,192,194] Ejection fraction and other systolic indices (fractional shortening and Vcf) continue to improve over several months to years after operation.[180,192,193]

When intraoperative mortality is included, valve replacement does not consistently improve survival for patients with isolated aortic insufficiency. For example, in a group for whom aortic valve replacement was recommended based on clinical and hemodynamic data, the 5-year survival rate was 86% in 127 patients who underwent surgery and 87% in 28 patients who did not.[195]

Preoperative Factors Predicting Postoperative Function

Despite generally positive results, some patients with chronic aortic regurgitation do not benefit clinically from surgery. Their symptoms persist, as does left ventricular dilatation, and on occasion, the ejection fraction may even decrease. The end-systolic dimension appears to be one of the primary predictive parameters of a poor outcome; high values are associated with persistence of symptoms, ventricular dilatation, congestive heart failure, and a higher mortality (Figs. 20–29 and 20–30 and Table 20–7).[150,191,196] An increased end-diastolic dimension, representing left ventricular dilatation, is also a sign of unfavorable prognosis, but its predictive value is less than that of the end-systolic dimension.[150,196]

Wall stress and relative wall thickness also have prognostic value. The ratio of left ventricular radius (LVID/2) to posterior wall thickness (or mean thickness of posterior wall and interventricular septum) can be calculated at the end of diastole[196] or as an average of diastolic and systolic measurements.[150] Increased values are predictive of unfavorable postoperative evolution (see Table 20–7). A simplified index of wall stress (pressure × radius/wall thickness) calculated at the end of systole[150] or diastole[196] has a similar significance.

Preoperative systolic dysfunction implies a poor postoperative prognosis, especially if present for a prolonged period.[197] It is associated with a higher mortality: The 5-year postoperative survival rate was 96% in patients with normal preoperative ejection fraction but was only 63% in patients with an ejection fraction of less than

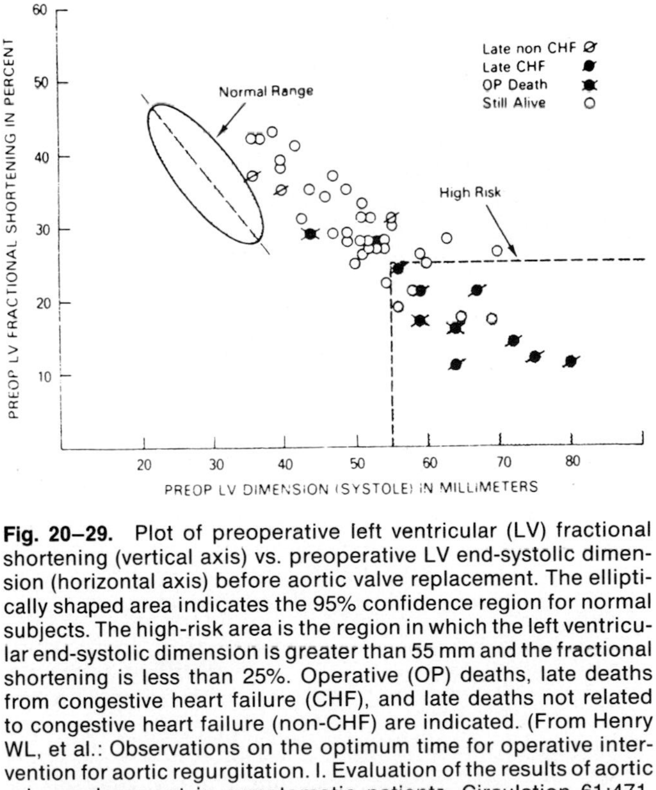

Fig. 20–29. Plot of preoperative left ventricular (LV) fractional shortening (vertical axis) vs. preoperative LV end-systolic dimension (horizontal axis) before aortic valve replacement. The elliptically shaped area indicates the 95% confidence region for normal subjects. The high-risk area is the region in which the left ventricular end-systolic dimension is greater than 55 mm and the fractional shortening is less than 25%. Operative (OP) deaths, late deaths from congestive heart failure (CHF), and late deaths not related to congestive heart failure (non-CHF) are indicated. (From Henry WL, et al.: Observations on the optimum time for operative intervention for aortic regurgitation. I. Evaluation of the results of aortic valve replacement in symptomatic patients. Circulation 61:471, 1980. Reproduced by permission of the American Heart Association, Inc.)

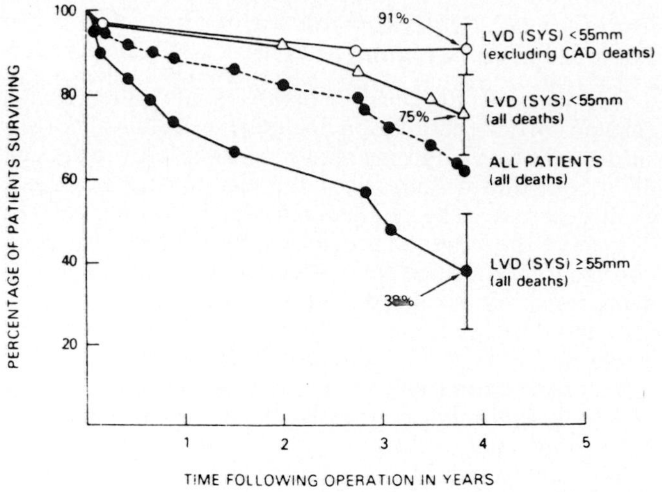

Fig. 20–30. Plot of the percentage of patients surviving after aortic valve replacement (vertical axis) vs. time after operation (horizontal axis) in a group of 49 patients. Survival curves calculated using the method of Kaplan and Meier are shown for patients with left ventricular end-systolic dimensions (LVD[SYS]) greater than or equal to 55 mm and those with LVD(SYS) less than 55 mm. These two curves differ from each other at a statistical significance of p = .006. Two patients died late from complications of coronary artery disease (CAD), and both had end-systolic dimensions less than 55 mm. A third survival curve is shown with these deaths excluded. This survival curve differs from the survival curve of patients with an end-systolic dimension greater than or equal to 55 mm (p = .0009). Vertical bars indicate the standard error of the estimate for the curves. The survival curve for the entire patient group is shown by the dashed line. (From Henry WL, et al.: Observations on the optimum time for operative intervention for aortic regurgitation. I. Evaluation of the results of aortic valve replacement in symptomatic patients. Circulation 61:471, 1980. Reproduced by permission of the American Heart Association, Inc.)

45%, as assessed by radionuclide angiography.[187] In patients with an ejection fraction less then 55%, calculated by the cylinder-hemiellipsoid method, no significant change was observed in left ventricular volume, mass, meridional wall stress, or systolic function at either 6 weeks or 6 months following surgery.[181] Patients without improvement in systolic function during the first 6 months after operation did not experience improvement in the subsequent 5 years.[192]

The duration of aortic insufficiency before valve replacement is also an important predictor of postoperative response. Patients with endocarditis or aortic root dissection causing acute aortic regurgitation, of less than 6 months duration, had normalization of left ventricular dimension in the 8 months after valve replacement, regardless of preoperative values.[150] Patients with preoperative left ventricular dysfunction, defined as fractional shortening less than 29%, had postoperative improvement of radionuclide angiographic ejection fraction only if the dysfunction has been present for no longer than 14 months; if fractional shortening had been "subnormal" for 18 months or longer, the dysfunction persisted, and regression of end-diastolic dimension was incomplete after valve replacement.[197] Preoperative ejection fraction during exercise or its change from baseline are not useful prognostic factors and have not shown any significant correlation with mortality after aortic valve replacement.[187]

Aortic Stenosis

Aortic stenosis creates an increase in afterload because the left ventricle has to generate higher pressures to maintain a normal cardiac output. In response to this increased pressure, the left ventricular mass increases,[181,198] the walls thicken (Fig. 20–31) while vol-

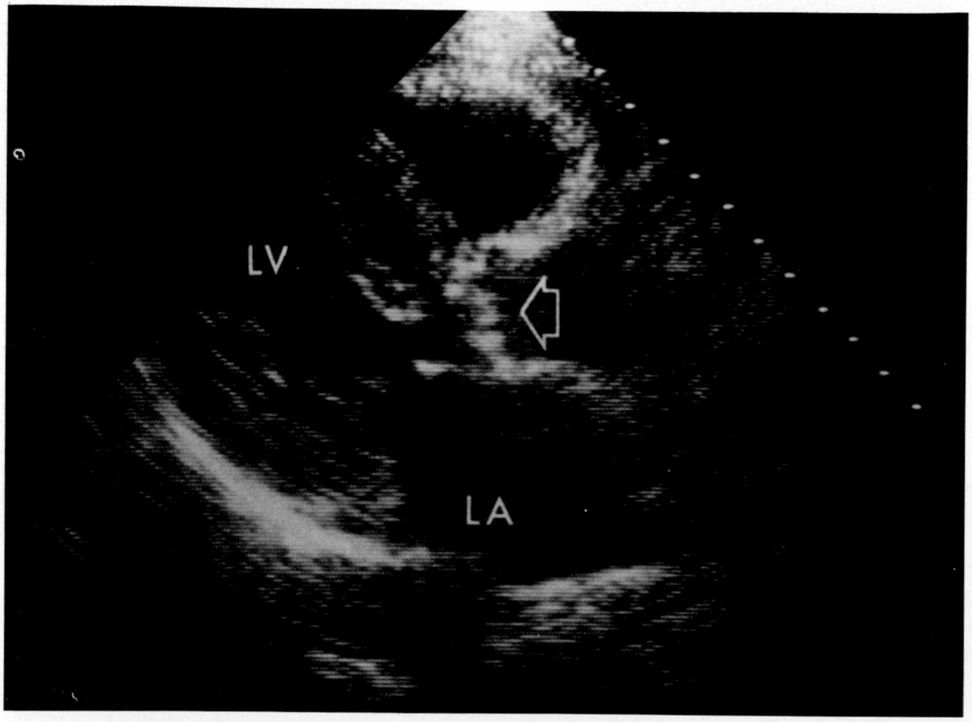

Fig. 20–31. Parasternal long axis view illustrating concentric hypertrophy and reduced cavity size in a patient with severe aortic stenosis. LA = left atrium; LV = left ventricle; Arrowhead = aortic valve.

Table 20–7. Echocardiographic Preoperative Factors Predictive of Evolution After Valve Replacement

Reference	Number of Patients	Postoperative Follow-up (Mean)	Preoperative Criteria	Postoperative Evolution	% Sensitivity	% Specificity
AORTIC INSUFFICIENCY						
Bonow et al.[196]	37	6 months	Fractional shortening < 29% for > 16 months	Persistent LV dilatation and dysfunction		
Bonow et al.[197]	80	45 months	Fractional shortening < 29%	Lower 5-year survival rate		
			Radionuclide angiography EF < 45%	Lower 5 year survival (63 vs. 96%)		
Gaasch et al.[195]	32	1–6 years	ES LV diameter > 2.6 cm/m^2	Persistent LV dilatation	100	85
			ES wall stress index P × R/Th > 600 mm Hg	Persistent LV dilatation	100	85
Henry et al.[190]	49	6 months	ES LV diameter > 55 mm	Higher mortality (53 vs. 6%)		
			Fractional shortening < 25%	Higher mortality (64 vs. 6%)		
Kumpuris et al.[150]	43	8 months	ES LV diameter > 50 mm	Persistent LV dilatation	92	86
			ED LV diameter > 72 mm	Persistent LV dilatation	82	67
			Fractional shortening < 28%	Persistent LV dilatation	80	56
			ED relative wall thickness R/Th > 3.2	Persistent LV dilatation	92	82
			Mean relative wall thickness R/Th > 2.5	Persistent LV dilatation	93	93
			ES wall stress index P × R/Th > 235 mm Hg	Persistent LV dilatation	88	100
MITRAL REGURGITATION						
Reed et al.[207]	176	3.8 years	LA index < 7.0 cm^2	RR of cardiac-related deaths: 2.42		
			ES ratio wall thickness/cavity dimension > 0.20	RR of cardiac-related deaths: 0.35		
Zile et al.[202]	20	1.7 years	ES LV diameter > 2.6 cm/m^2	Persistent LV dilatation	100	88
			Fractional shortening < 31%	Persistent LV dilatation	100	88
			ES wall stress index P × R/Th > 195 mm Hg	Persistent LV dilatation	100	63
Schuler et al.[203]	16	15 months	ED LV diameter > 70 mm	Persistent LV dilatation and hypertrophy; decreasing EF		
			ES LV diameter > 50 mm	Persistent LV dilatation and hypertrophy; decreasing EF		

Echocardiographic measurements: LV diameter in parasternal view. LA index = product of maximal longitudinal and transverse left atrial diameter in four-chamber view.

ED = end-diastolic; EF = ejection fraction; ES = end-systolic; LA = left atrium; LV = left ventricle; P = pressure; R = left ventricular radius (½ diameter); RR = relative risk; Th = average of septal and posterior wall thickness.

ume remains unchanged. This results in a low end-systolic wall stress, with increased values for systolic performance indices (Vcf and fractional shortening).[198] Sometimes, a pattern of asymmetric septal hypertrophy occurs, with septal/posterior wall ratio reaching 1.5, without coexistence of idiopathic hypertrophic cardiomyopathy, which regresses after valve replacement.[199] Late in the course of severe aortic stenosis, the ejection fraction may decrease, while end-diastolic and end-systolic volumes increase;[181,200] wall stress stays near normal[181] or may even increase.[200] In congenital valvular aortic stenosis, there is higher than normal shortening fraction and Vcf, higher wall mass, lower end-systolic wall stress, but no difference in left ventricular dimensions or peak wall stress.[198]

Valve replacement causes a sudden decrease in afterload. Improvement of ejection fraction has been reported during operation, with epicardial echocardiography.[188,189] As elevated intraventricular pressure suddenly decreases after valve replacement, meridional and circumferential wall stress fall to abnormally low levels.[181] Later, wall thickness decreases and wall stress tends to normalize. In a group of patients, most of whom had preoperative systolic dysfunction, there was a significant decrease in left ventricular mass, in end-diastolic and end-systolic volumes, and an improvement in ejection fraction noted 6 weeks after surgery.[181]

Aortic valve replacement is clearly superior to medical treatment in severe aortic stenosis and improves survival in symptomatic patients.[195,201] Among patients with predominant aortic stenosis, for whom operation was recommended, the reported 3-year survival rate was 87% in operated and 21% in unoperated patients.[195] Potentially all symptomatic patients will benefit from valve replacement in severe aortic stenosis and experience an improvement of systolic function. Even late in the course of the disease, surgery is warranted, in contrast to aortic regurgitation, where the left ventricle may have been irremedially damaged.

Mitral Regurgitation

Mitral regurgitation may be acute or chronic. In acute mitral insufficiency that is due to a torn or perforated leaflet, or to a ruptured chord, there is no significant change in left ventricular volume. In contrast, chronic mitral regurgitation causes an increase in volume of left atrium and ventricle.[202] Left ventricular end-diastolic and end-systolic dimensions increase, as does left ventricular muscle area, an index of mass.[203] As the regurgitant fraction is included in such parameters as ejection fraction or fractional shortening, systolic indices may appear preserved until late in the course of the disease.[202] In patients with congestive heart failure and mitral regurgitation, isometric exercise causes a decrease in forward cardiac output and an increase in mitral regurgitation.[204]

The ultimate treatment for patients with severe mitral regurgitation is valve replacement or repair. The immediate effect of mitral valve replacement has been studied intraoperatively, with epicardial echocardiography.[189,197] The ejection fraction usually decreases by about one third, following the correction of mitral regurgitation, which is due to a decrease in end-diastolic volume.[197] The afterload is increased, which is due to the removal of outflow into the left atrium, but it does not produce a significant increase in end-systolic volume. The fractional shortening decreases and wall stress increases, with the elimination of the low impedance left atrial pathway.[205]

In the following months, the left ventricle shrinks and symptoms are reduced or disappear;[202] muscle area decreases, and a small decrease in ejection fraction (70% preoperatively; 59% 15 months postoperatively) has been noted.[203]

In some patients, however, the ventricle has been damaged beyond the point of recovery, and the goal of echocardiography is therefore to define a threshold at which surgery should be strongly considered. Several preoperative echocardiographic criteria have been described, which identify patients who are not likely to improve following surgery.

In a study of patients with important preoperative left ventricular dilatation (end-systolic dimension >50 mm, end-diastolic dimension >70 mm), muscle area increased and ejection fraction fell from 57 to 26%.[203] An end-systolic left ventricular dimension index greater than 2.6 cm/m^2, a fractional shortening less than 31%, and an elevated index of wall stress[202] have also been shown to identify patients who experience persistent symptoms and no regression of left ventricular enlargement after valve replacement (Fig. 20–32). The specificity of these criteria was imperfect (88%), however, because some patients improved despite such preoperative values. Patients with persistent left ventricular dilatation after surgery have retrospectively been found to have an elevated mean preoperative value of end-systolic stress and a decreased mean preoperative value of fractional shortening.[206]

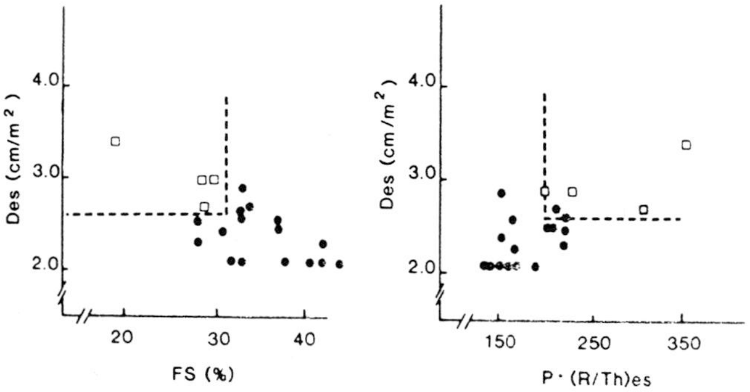

Fig. 20–32. Preoperative echocardiographic variables prognostic of evolution following mitral valve replacement. Des = left ventricular dimension at end-systole. FS (%) = fractional shortening. P·(R/Th)es = index of late systolic stress, which is the product of systolic arterial pressure (P) and the end-systolic radius/thickness ratio (R/Th)es; closed circles = 16 patients with postoperative normalization of left ventricular end-diastolic dimension; open squares = 4 patients with postoperative persistent left ventricular enlargement. (From Zile MR, Gaasch WH, Carroll JD, Levine HJ: Chronic mitral regurgitation: predictive value of preoperative echocardiographic indexes of left ventricular function and wall stress. J Am Coll Cardiol 3:235, 1984. Reprinted with permission from the American College of Cardiology.)

A large study found that echocardiographic assessment of left atrial size and left ventricular systolic function provide prognostic information that is significantly greater than those obtained from clinical and laboratory parameters alone; catheterization variables did not increase the prognostic value of the clinical and echocardiographic data.[207] Among 176 patients who underwent mitral valve replacement, 61 died. Predictors of cardiac death were the presence of pulmonary rales, increased left atrial index, and a decreased ratio of left ventricular free wall thickness divided by the left ventricular cavity dimension at end systole (see Table 20–7).

Left ventricular end-systolic size is affected by loading conditions, but despite this limitation, it has been shown to be a useful prognostic factor and has been widely used in clinical studies.

Mitral Stenosis

Mitral stenosis has little effect on left ventricular size and function. No significant abnormalities in end-diastolic and end-systolic dimensions or in muscle cross-sectional area are generally found before valve replacement.[203]

During valve replacement, there may be a transient but significant intraoperative increase in ejection fraction,[189] which may be due to increased preload. Fifteen months after operation, left ventricular volumes and ejection fraction are at the same levels as those found preoperatively.[203]

THE LEFT VENTRICLE IN HYPERTENSION

The responses of the left ventricle to hypertension have been intensively investigated and include (1) an increase in wall stress, (2) a change in left ventricular diastolic filling, and (3) thickening of the ventricular walls and an increase in mass (Fig. 20–33). Echocardiography is an extremely useful tool for detecting these changes and is widely used in clinical and epidemiologic studies to identify LVH and to assess its prevalence, its prognostic meaning, and the effects of antihypertensive therapy.

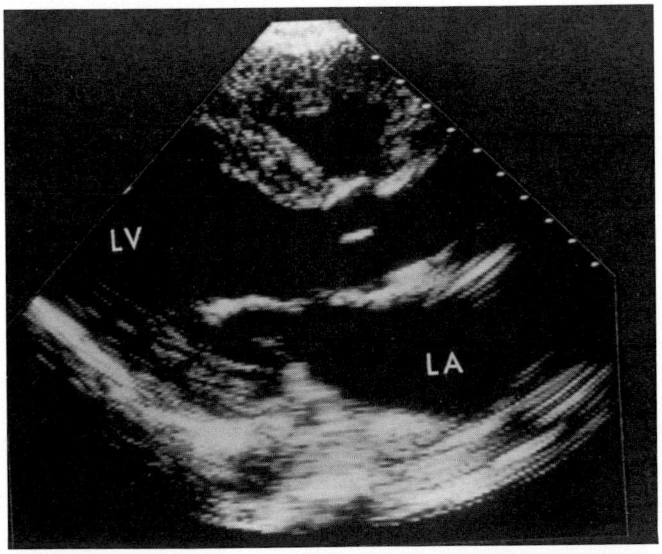

Fig. 20–33. Parasternal long axis view, recorded immediately before mitral valve closure, illustrating concentric left ventricular hypertrophy in a patient with long-standing arterial hypertension. LA = left atrium; LV = left ventricle.

Diastolic Function in Hypertension

In hypertension, diastolic function is altered first, before any significant increase in wall thickness or in systolic function is noticed.[208,209]

Isovolumic relaxation time is increased in hypertension, even before a significant increase in wall thickness can be detected;[208] the maximum rate of early left ventricular filling (assessed by radionuclide study) is lower and is inversely correlated to left ventricular mass and meridional wall stress.[209]

In more advanced stages, with wall thickening, other abnormalities are noted: a decrease in the peak rate of thinning (early relaxation) of the posterior wall,[208,210] an increase in the duration of thinning, and a slower peak rate of dimension increase.[208]

Elderly patients with marked concentric LVH, excessive left ventricular systolic emptying (increased ejection fraction), and congestive heart failure have a prolonged early diastolic filling period and a reduced peak increase in left ventricular diastolic dimension.[211] These patients are prone to severe hypotensive episodes if hypovolemia occurs. This is discussed in detail in Chapter 24.

Development of Left Ventricular Hypertrophy in Hypertension

A relationship between blood pressure and left ventricular mass seem obvious, but few studies have shown a good correlation. This is partially due to the fact that hypertrophy develops over several years whereas blood pressure generally is measured only at one point in time, which may not necessarily represent the pressure burden born by the ventricle in the past. In addition, other parameters such as heart rate, hormone levels, level of physical activity, myocardial ischemia, and coronary disease can influence the development of hypertrophy.

An experimental study[212] has shown that wall thickness may significantly increase even with a minimal increase in mean arterial pressure and that there is dissociation between the rate of development of hypertension and of hypertrophy, suggesting that other factors contribute to LVH.

In the Framingham Heart Study,[87] among normotensive or untreated hypertensive adults, left ventricular mass, indexed for height, correlated weakly with systolic blood pressure measured at the time of echocardiography ($r = .23$ in men, .24 in women), and no significant correlation with diastolic blood pressure was noted. When the average of blood pressure over the last 30 years (biennial examinations) was taken into consideration, the correlation improved slightly ($r = .27$ in men, .31 in women for systolic blood pressure, $p < .001$; $r = .18$ for diastolic pressure). Note that the relatively low correlation is partially due to the narrow range of pressure values recorded in that population sample, most of whom were normotensive.

Ambulatory 24-hour recordings of blood pressure provide a better assessment of hypertension than casual measurements, and they have shown a higher correlation with left ventricular mass determined by M-mode echocardiography.[213–215] The best correlation (r = .81) was noted between 24-hour systolic pressure and left ventricular mass in a small group of 12 hypertensive male patients, after 2 weeks without antihypertensive medication.[213]

Left ventricular mass has also been found to significantly correlate with systolic blood pressure during exercise[216] and with blood pressure measured at work.[214] No influence of "white coat" hypertension has been detected on left ventricular mass.[217] The effect of race on hypertrophy is debated, as LVH is more prevalent in blacks, but so is hypertension. After ventricular mass was matched for blood pressure, no racial difference has been detected by some authors,[218] whereas LVH seemed to be more frequent in blacks in other studies.[219,220]

In summary, there is a weak but significant correlation of left ventricular mass and systolic blood pressure. Average of blood pressure measurements over several years and ambulatory blood pressure recordings are better predictors of left ventricular mass than casual measure of blood pressure.

Systolic Performance and Wall Stress in Hypertension

Systolic performance indices, such as fractional shortening, Vcf, and ejection fraction, change little in hypertensive patients, except in the advanced stages preceding cardiac failure. An increase in end-systolic wall stress have been found in several groups of untreated hypertensive patients but is not related to the degree of hypertrophy. Elevated blood pressure causes an increase in wall stress, which leads to thickening of the walls, itself tending to normalize wall stress.

Although many studies[113,117,221–229] have described the effect of hypertension on left ventricular function, they used different methods and included dissimilar groups of hypertensive patients. As the presence of antihypertensive medication can significantly affect systolic performance, some results and comparisons must be assessed with caution.

In the early stages of hypertension, sometimes called *borderline hypertension,* before any increase in wall thickness can be detected, only few, isolated studies noted any significant changes in systolic function parameters. Two studies found that the end-diastolic and end-systolic dimensions of the left ventricle were slightly decreased, whereas FS and Vcf were normal.[221,222] No significant increase in meridional wall stress, FS, or Vcf was found in borderline hypertension.[223] In newly diagnosed marked hypertension, however, an increase in circumferential wall stress was found, before any change in wall thickness or FS.[224]

In the same study,[224] another group of patients with LVH had normal wall stress, whereas Vcf was increased. This "supranormal" systolic function has also been found in a group with mild hypertension, with an increase in the thickness of the septum (significant) and of the posterior wall (nonsignificant).[222] A group of untreated hypertensive patients with increased left ventricular performance has been identified with increased fractional shortening.[225] Compared to other hypertensive patients, they have a smaller relative wall thickness, increased left ventricular end-diastolic dimension, increased cardiac index, increased systemic pressure and pulse pressure, and lower total peripheral resistance. This group of patients has minimally increased wall stress, less hypertrophy, and a better contractility. The authors suggest that increased preload may be responsible for the increased systolic performance.[225] Similar observations were made in a subgroup of patients with moderate hypertension;[223] in addition, wall stress was higher but the increase in left ventricular dimension was not significant.

In treated patients with mild or moderate hypertension and electrocardiographic signs of LVH, M-mode echocardiography confirmed the increased wall thickness and found normal wall stress and no change in functional shortening, Vcf, or ejection fraction.[226] In untreated hypertension with LVH, however, left ventricular dimensions and wall stress were significantly increased, compared to a group of normotensive subjects, with no change in FS.[117] In untreated mild and moderate hypertension, there was an increase in wall stress and no change in FS.[223] Similarly, in a large series of 461 active subjects with untreated hypertension (or where treatment had been withdrawn for at least 3 weeks),[113] an increased wall stress and a normal FS were noted. These studies tend to show that an increased wall stress is common in untreated hypertension.

In more advanced stages of hypertension, impairment of systolic function has been described. Fractional shortening,[227] Vcf,[224,227,228] and ejection fraction[229] may decrease, while end-systolic wall stress increases. Ultimately, the left ventricle dilates, leading to further increase in wall stress in spite of the very high ventricular mass.[224,227]

During dynamic exercise in hypertensive patients, the increase in ejection fraction is inversely correlated to the left ventricular mass.[229]

In summary, wall stress, increased by hypertension, can be considered to trigger LVH in an attempt to compensate. Contractility is preserved, or even increased in the early stages of hypertension. In later stages, hypertrophy seem to be insufficient to compensate for the increased wall stress, and systolic function deteriorates.

Clinical Significance of Hypertensive Hypertrophy

Echocardiography is very useful for large-scale screening for LVH; it is the safest and most sensitive and specific tool for serial assessment of LVH. In the Framingham Heart Study, a general population over 40 years of age was studied. It included 1403 men, with a mean blood pressure of 131/82 mm Hg and 1817 women with a mean blood pressure of 130/77 mm Hg. The prevalence of LVH was 15.5% in men and 21.0% in women.[93]

LVH, as determined by echocardiography, represents a risk factor of cardiovascular disease, independent of systolic blood pressure, as well as of age, smoking, and cholesterol.[91–93] In a 4.8-year follow-up period, patients with LVH experienced three times more cardiovascular morbid events such as myocardial infarction, angina, congestive heart failure, stroke and cardiovascular death, than patients without LVH.[91] For each increment of 50 g/m in height-adjusted mass, the relative risk was between 1.5 and 2 over 4 years for the incidence of cardiovascular disease, for cardiovascular mortality, and for overall mortality.[92,93] Decreased survival has been related to LVH independent of ejection fraction and of the extent of coronary artery disease.[94] The presence of LVH has also been related to a higher frequency of ventricular arrhythmia,[112] ventricular fibrillation, and sudden cardiac death.[230] In addition, among hypertensive patients, an increased posterior wall thickness (>11 mm) is an indicator of a greater prevalence of disease in other target organs, especially hypertensive retinopathy and impairment of renal function.[231]

In malignant hypertension, an increase in wall thickness is found only in patients with a previous history of hypertension; in the absence of a history of elevated blood pressure, wall thickness has been normal, suggesting a rapid onset of hypertension.[232]

Regression of Left Ventricular Hypertrophy

As left ventricular mass has been shown to be related to blood pressure, treatment of hypertension can be expected to cause a decrease in left ventricular mass. Since the first positive clinical study,[233] many studies have been published, using different drugs, tested singly or in combination, in different groups of hypertensive patients, for different durations.

In a review of 66 studies published before 1990, where the effect of antihypertensive treatment on LVH was assessed by echocardiography, it was noted that left ventricular mass can regress and that the changes are sometimes measurable within the first 3 months of treatment.[234] Usually, a decrease in mass is associated with decrease in systemic pressure; these studies, analyzed together, showed a modest but significant correlation ($r = .33$; $p < .025$).[234] Other factors affect regression, however, as suggested by the observation that a decrease in left ventricular mass can occur without a significant change in blood pressure,[235] and conversely, a significant decrease in blood pressure sometimes produces no change in left ventricular mass.[236,237] Selection of hypertensive patients with very thick walls and normal ventricular diameter identified a group of patients with low meridional end-systolic wall stress.[238] During therapy these patients experienced a decrease in blood pressure with an increase in left ventricular mass. This finding strongly suggests the role of factors other than blood pressure in the development and regression of hypertrophy.

Most studies assessing reduction in left ventricular mass[234] have shown no change in systolic cardiac function, although a few have shown an improvement in systolic indices, and even fewer, a decrease in systolic function. Similarly, wall stress has generally been reported to remain unchanged or to decrease. Diastolic function may improve with left ventricular mass regression.

Among antihypertensive agents, angiotensin-converting enzyme inhibitors, calcium channel blockers, and sympatholytic agents, including β-blockers, have usually demonstrated a decrease in wall mass together with a decrease in blood pressure. Diuretics and peripheral vasodilators (non-calcium channel blockers) have produced little or no effect on wall mass.[234] A decrease in wall mass has also been reported with nonpharmacologic interventions: salt restriction,[239] and weight reduction in obese hypertensive patients.[240]

As additional evidence of the effect of antihypertensive medications, discontinuation of therapy has been reported to cause an increase in interventricular septum thickness in 4 weeks.[241]

Regression of LVH is possible, but it remains to be demonstrated that patient outcome improves. In trials such as the Multiple Risk Factor Intervention Trial and the Hypertension Detection and Followup Study, which involved 8,000 to 10,000 participants for 5 to 6 years, the significant decrease in the prevalence of electrocardiographic LVH was not associated with a significant effect on prognosis.[234]

Differential Diagnosis With Hypertrophic Cardiomyopathy

Asymmetric hypertrophy of the left ventricle has been found in many hypertensive patients, raising the problem of differential diagnosis with idiopathic subaortic stenosis. The frequency of disproportionate septal thickening, i.e., a septum/posterior wall ratio ≥1.3 has varied between 1 and 50% in hypertensive patients.[242] It has been found to be 12% in a normal population, 32% in LVH that is due to chronic renal failure, and 95% in idiopathic hypertrophic subaortic stenosis.[243] Hypertension may not be the only factor influencing the septal thickness: heredity, right ventricular overload, and coronary heart disease may also play a role.[244]

In borderline hypertension, a study demonstrated an increase in septal thickness but not of posterior wall thickness, leading to a septum/posterior wall ratio of 1.25 ± 0.09.[245] The ratio decreased to normal values in the group with sustained hypertension because of the increase in posterior wall thickness. In another group of hypertensive patients with increased posterior wall thickness, 8 of 37 patients had a disproportionate septal thickening (ratio, ≥1.3).[231]

The problem of asymmetric hypertrophy is not surprising, if one considers the relative accuracy of the measurements and the normal range of value. Measurement errors of 1 mm in the septum and as much in the posterior wall can be enough to produce a ratio of 1.3 in a normal heart. Therefore, one should measure wall thickness several times, in different cycles, to obtain a correct ratio. However, it may also be true that, either at a certain point in the course of hypertension-induced LVH or in a certain subset of patients, real asymmetric hypertrophy occurs. To distinguish this type of hypertrophy from idiopathic obstructive hypertrophy, the patient should be assessed for the presence of other echocardiographic features of obstructive cardiomyopathy.

Athletes' Left Ventricular Hypertrophy

Hypertrophy is known to occur in athletes, and its morphologic pattern is similar to hypertrophy induced by hypertension. However, a few differences have been noted.

No abnormality of diastolic function have been reported in athletes. There is no increase in isovolumic relaxation time,[208] no decrease in left ventricular filling rate,[246] and no decrease in peak rates of left ventricular cavity enlargement and wall thinning.[247]

In contrast to untreated hypertensive patients whose wall stress is increased, sportsmen have either normal or decreased wall stress.[247–250] Thus, the increase of wall thickness is, in some cases, "disproportionate" to the blood pressure at rest.

Detraining of athletes results in rapid decrease of left ventricular mass. In a group of 6 competitive runners who stopped training, posterior wall thickness decreased from 10.7 to 8 mm over 3 weeks.[251] The first changes in the group's mean were already significant on the fourth day. Left ventricular mass calculated with the modified cubed formula (Equation 20.25) underwent the same changes: 109 to 67 g/m^2. At the same time, left ventricular diameter decreased. A reduction of the left ventricular mass by 20% was noted after 3 weeks of deconditioning in endurance athletes.[252] Continuous training therefore seems necessary to maintain exercise-induced LVH, and the rate of regression is much more rapid than for hypertension-induced LVH.

Summary

Echocardiography is an extremely valuable tool for hypertensive patients. It permits assessment of left ventricular mass and of systolic and diastolic function, which not only provides an evaluation of the effect of hypertension on the heart at the time of the study but also has prognostic value. Further, serial echocardiographic studies generate unique information on the effect of antihypertensive therapy.

REFERENCES

1. Schlant RC, Sonneblick EH: Normal physioloy of the cardiovascular system. *In* Hurst JW (ed.): The Heart. 7th Ed. New York, McGraw-Hill, 1990.
2. Rushmer RF: Cardiovascular Dynamics. Philadelphia, Saunders, 1970.
3. Williams PL, Warwick R, Dyson M, Bannister LH: Gray's Anatomy. 37th Ed. Edinburgh, Churchill Livingstone, 1989.
4. Mall FP: On the muscular architecture of the ventricles of the human heart. Am J Anat 11:211, 1911.
5. Robb JS, Robb RC: The normal heart. Am Heart J 23:455, 1942.
6. Streeter DD: Gross morphology and fiber geometry of the heart. *In* Dow P (ed.): Handbook of Physiology. Vol 1. Baltimore, Williams & Wilkins, 1962.
7. Wells PNT: Biomedical Ultrasonics. New York, Academic Press, 1977.
8. Roelandt J, et al.: Resolution problems in echocardiography: a source of interpretation errors. Am J Cardiol 37:256, 1976.
9. Garrison JB, et al.: Quantifying regional wall motion and thickening in two-dimensional echocardiography with a computer-aided contouring system. *In* Ostrow H, Ripley K (eds.): Proceedings of Computers in Cardiology 1977. Long Beach, CA, Institute of Electrical and Electronics Engineers, 1977.
10. Feigenbaum H, et al.: Correlation of ultrasound with angiocardiography in measuring left ventricular diastolic volume. Am J Cardiol 23:111, 1969.
11. Feigenbaum H, Popp RL, Wolfe SB: Ultrasound measurements of the left ventricle: a correlative study with angiocardiography. Arch Intern Med 129:461, 1972.
12. Fortuin NH, Hood WP, Craige E: Evaluation of left ventricular function by echocardiography. Circulation 46:26, 1972.
13. Gibson DG: Estimation of left ventricular size by echocardiography. Br Heart J 35:128, 1973.
14. Pombo JF, Troy BL, Russell RO: Left ventricular volumes and ejection fraction by echocardiography. Circulation 43:480, 1971.
15. Popp RL, Harrison DC: Ultrasonic cardiac echocardiography for determining stroke volume and valvular regurgitation. Circulation 41:493, 1970.
16. Feigenbaum H: Echocardiography. Philadelphia, Lea & Febiger, 1976.
17. Hickman H, et al.: Cross-sectional echocardiography of the cardiac apex (abstr.). Circulation 56(Suppl. 3):III-153, 1977.
18. Mirro MJ, Rogers EW, Weyman AE, Feigenbaum H: Angular displacement of the papillary muscles during the cardiac cycle. Circulation 60:327, 1979.
19. Bansal RC, Tajik AJ, Seward JB, Offord KP: Feasibility of detailed two-dimensional echocardiographic examination in adults: prospective study of 200 patients. Mayo Clin Proc 55:291, 1980.
20. Folland ED, et al.: Assessment of left ventricular ejection fraction and volumes by real-time, two-dimensional echocardiography. Circulation 60: 760, 1979.
21. Schreiber FL, Weyman AE, Feigenbaum H, Stewart J: Effects of atrial septal defect repair on left ventricular geometry and degree of mitral valve prolapse. Circulation 61:888, 1980.
22. Brenner JI, Waugh RA: Effect of phasic respiration on left ventricular dimension and performance in a normal population: an echocardiographic study. Circulation 57:122, 1978.
23. Erbel R, et al.: Echoventriculography—a simultaneous analysis of two-dimensional echocardiography and cineventriculography. Circulation 67: 205, 1983.
24. Schiller NB, et al.: Recommendations for quantitation of the left ventricle by two-dimensional echocardiography. J Am Soc Echocardiogr 2:358, 1989.
25. Dodge HT, Sandler H, Ballen DW, Lord JDJ: The use of biplane angiocardiography for the measurement of left ventricular volume in man. Am Heart J 60:762, 1960.
26. Arvidsson H: Angiocardiographic determinations of left ventricular volume. Acta Radiol 56:321, 1961.
27. Bunnell IL, Grant C, Greene DG: Left ventricular function derived from the pressure volume diagram. Am J Med 39:881, 1965.
28. Herman HJ, Bartle SH: Left ventricular volumes by angiocardiography: comparison of models and simplification of techniques. Cardiovasc Res 4: 404, 1968.
29. Sandler H, Dodge HT: The use of single plane angiocardiograms for the calculation of left ventricular volume in man. Am Heart J 75:325, 1968.
30. Dodge HT, Sandler H, Bailey WA, Henley RR: Usefulness and limitations of radiographic methods for determining left ventricular volume. Am J Cardiol 18:10, 1966.
31. Davila JC, SanMarco ME: An analysis of the fit of mathematical models applicable to the measurement of the left ventricle. Am J Cardiol 18:31, 1966.
32. Chapman CB, Baker O, Reynolds J, Bonet FJ: Use of biplane cinefluorigraphy for measurement of ventricular volume. Circulation 18:1105, 1958.
33. Lewis RP, Sandler H: Relationship between changes in left ventricular dimension and the ejection fraction in man. Circulation 44:548, 1971.
34. Murray JA, Johnston W, Reid JM: Echocardiographic determination of left ventricular dimensions, volumes and performance. Am J Cardiol 30: 252, 1972.
35. Belenkie I, Nutter DO, Clark DW: Assessment of left ventricular dimensions and function by echocardiography. Am J Cardiol 31:755, 1973.
36. Ratshin RA, Rackley CE, Russell RO: Determination of left ventricular preload and afterload by quantitative echocardiography in man. Circ Res 34:711, 1974.
37. Rackley CE, Hood WP: Quantitative angiographic evaluation and pathophysiologic mechanisms in valvular heart disease. Prog Cardiovasc Dis 15: 427, 1973.
38. Fortuin NJ, Wood WP, Sherman ME, Craige E: Determination of left ventricular volume by ultrasound. Circulation 44:575, 1971.
39. Johnston ML: Echocardiographic evaluation of left ventricular size and function and its application to coronary artery disease. Adv Cardiol 17: 105, 1976.
40. Ludbrook P, et al.: Comparison of ultrasound and cineangiographic measurements in patients with and without wall motion abnormalities. Br Heart J 35:1026, 1973.
41. Machii K, Tamura T, Natsume T, Umeda T: Echocardiographic left ventricular volume determination by direct measurements of the major and minor axes. Jpn Circ J 41:501, 1977.
42. Mashiro I, et al.: Comparison of measurements of left ventricle by echography and cineangiography. Jpn Circ J 39:23, 1975.
43. Ratshin RA, Rackley CE, Russell RO: Quantitative echocardiography: accuracy of ventricular volume analysis by area length linear regression and quadratic regression formulae. Am J Cardiol 35:165, 1975.

44. Redwood DR, Henry WL, Epstein SE: Evaluation of the ability of echocardiography to measure acute alterations in left ventricular volume. Circulation 50:901, 1974.
45. Teichholz LE, Kreulen T, Herman MV, Gorlin R: Problems in echocardiographic volume determinations: echocardiographic-angiographic correlations in the presence or absence of asynergy. Am J Cardiol 37:7, 1976.
46. Kronik G, Slany J, Mosslacher H: Comparative value of eight M-mode echocardiographic formulas for determining left ventricular stroke volume. Circulation 60:1308, 1979.
47. Wyatt HL, et al.: Cross-sectional echocardiography: II. Analysis of mathematic models for quantifying volume of formalin fixed left ventricle. Circulation 61:1119, 1980.
48. Wyatt HL, et al.: Cross-sectional echocardiography: III. Analysis of mathematic models for quantifying volume of symmetric and asymmetric left ventricles. Am Heart J 100:821, 1980.
49. Stamm RB, Carabello BA, Mayers DL, Martin RP: Two-dimensional echocardiographic measurement of left ventricular ejection fraction: prospective analysis of what constitutes an adequate determination. Am Heart J 104:136, 1982.
50. Chaudry KR, et al.: Biplane measurements of left and right ventricular volumes using wide angle cross-sectional echocardiography (abstr.). Am J Cardiol 41:391, 1978.
51. Feigenbaum H: New aspects of echocardiography. Circulation 61:1119, 1973.
52. Popp RL, Alderman EL, Brown OR, Harrison DC: Sources of error in calculation of left ventricular volume by echocardiography. Am J Cardiol 31:152, 1973.
53. Rackley CE, Hood WP: Quantitative angiographic evaluation and pathophysiologic mechanisms in valvular heart disease. Prog Cardiovasc Dis 15: 427, 1969.
54. Yang SS, Bentivoglio LG, Maranhao V, Goldberg H: Cardiac volumes. *In:* From Cardiac Catheterization to Hemodynamic Parameters. Philadelphia, FA Davis, 1978.
55. Carr K, et al.: Measurement of left ventricular ejection fraction by mechanical cross-sectional echocardiography. Circulation 59:1196, 1979.
56. King DL, Jaffe CC, Schmidt DH, Ellis K: Left ventricular volume determination by cross-sectional cardiac ultrasonography. Radiology 104:201, 1972.
57. Teichholz LE, Cohen MV, Sonnenblick BM, Gorlin R: Study of left ventricular geometry and function by B-scan ultrasonography in patients with and without asynergy. N Engl J Med 291:1220, 1964.
58. Erbel R, et al.: Comparison of single-plane and biplane volume determination by two-dimensional echocardiography: 1. Asymmetric model hearts. Eur Heart J 3:469, 1982.
59. Mercier JC, et al.: Two-dimensional echocardiographic assessment of left ventricular volumes and ejection fraction in children. Circulation 65:962, 1982.
60. Wahr DW, Wang YS, Schiller NB: Left ventricular volumes determined by two-dimensional echocardiography in a normal adult population. J Am Coll Cardiol 1:863, 1983.
61. Triulzi MO, et al.: Normal adult cross-sectional echocardiographic values: left ventricular volumes. Echocardiography 2:153, 1985.
62. Georke RJ, Carlsson E: Calculation of right and left ventricular volumes: methods using standard computer equipment and biplane angiograms. Invest Radiol 2:360, 1967.
63. Eaton LW, Maughan WL, Shoukas AA, Weiss JL: Accurate volume determination in the isolated ejecting canine left ventricle by two-dimensional echocardiography. Circulation 60:320, 1979.
64. Weiss JL, Eaton LW, Kallman CH, Maughan WL: Accuracy of volume determination by two-dimensional echocardiography: defining requirements under controlled conditions in the ejecting canine left ventricle. Circulation 67:889, 1983.
65. Schiller N, et al.: Left ventricular volume from paired biplane two-dimensional echocardiography. Circulation 60:547, 1979.
66. Starling MR, et al.: Comparative accuracy of apical biplane cross-sectional echocardiography and gated equilibrium radionuclide angiography for estimating left ventricular size and performance. Circulation 63:1075, 1981.
67. Guéret P, et al.: Two-dimensional echocardiographic quantitation of left ventricular volumes and ejection fraction. Importance of accounting for dyssynergy in short-axis reconstruction models. Circulation 62:1308, 1980.
68. Guéret P, Corday E: Etude quantitative de la fonction ventriculaire gauche par l'échocardiographie bidimensionnelle. Arch Mal Coeur 74:329, 1981.
69. Smith MD, et al.: Value and limitations of transesophageal echocardiography in determination of left ventricular volumes and ejection fraction. J Am Coll Cardiol 19:1213, 1992.
70. Handschumacher MD, et al.: A new integrated system for three-dimensional echocardiographic reconstruction and ventricular volume measurement. Comput Cardiol 113, 1991.
71. Lethor JP, Handschumacher MD, Siu SC: A new fully integrated system for three-dimensional echocardiographic reconstruction: validation for ventricular volume (abstr.). Circulation 84(Suppl. 2):II-684, 1991.
72. Siu SC, et al.: Three-dimensional echocardiography improves noninvasive left ventricular volume quantitation (abstr.). J Am Coll Cardiol 19:18A, 1992.
73. Siu SC, et al.: Three-dimensional echocardiography: in vivo validation for left ventricular volume and function (abstr.). J Am Coll Cardiol 19:18A, 1992.
74. Lethor JP, et al.: Quantitative reconstruction of the left ventricle using a new fully integrated three-dimensional echocardiographic system: feasibility and validation in human subjects (abstr.). J Am Coll Cardiol 19:381A, 1992.
75. Huang ZH, et al.: Comparison of gray-scale and B-color ultrasound images in evaluating left ventricular systolic function in coronary artery disease. Am Heart J 123:395, 1992.
76. Pérez JE, et al.: On-line assessment of ventricular function by automatic boundary detection and ultrasonic backscatter imaging. J Am Coll Cardiol 19:313, 1992.
77. Gordon EP, et al.: Reproducibility of left ventricular volumes by two-dimensional echocardiography. J Am Coll Cardiol 2:506, 1983.
78. Himelman RB, Cassidy MM, Landzberg JS, Schiller NB: Reproducibility of quantitative two-dimensional echocardiography. Am Heart J 115:425, 1988.
79. Conetta DA, et al.: Reproducibility of left ventricular area and volume measurements using a computer endocardial edge-detection algorithm in normal subjects. Am J Cardiol 56:947, 1985.
80. Kennedy JW, et al.: Quantitative angiography: I. The normal left ventricle in man. Circulation 34:272, 1966.
81. Wynne J, et al.: Estimation of left ventricular volumes in man from biplane cineangiograms filmed in oblique position. Am J Cardiol 41:726, 1978.
82. Levinson GE, Frank MJ, Nadimi M, Braunstein M: Studies of cardiopulmonary blood volume. Measurements of left ventricular volume by dye dilution. Circulation 35:1038, 1967.
83. Badeer HS: Biologic significance of cardiac hypertrophy. Am J Cardiol 14:133, 1964.
84. Hood WB: Dynamics of hypertrophy of the left ventricular wall of man. *In* Alpert N (ed.): Cardiac Hypertrophy. New York, Grune & Stratton, 1971.
85. Sasayama S, et al.: Adaptations of the left ventricle to chronic pressure overload. Circ Res 38:172, 1976.
86. Ross J: Afterload mismatch and preload reserve: a conceptual framework for the analysis of ventricular function. Prog Cardiovasc Dis 18:255, 1976.
87. Lauer MS, Anderson KM, Levy D: Influence of contemporary versus 30-year blood pressure levels on left ventricular mass and geometry: the Framingham Heart Study. J Am Coll Cardiol 18:1287, 1991.
88. Sokolow M, Perloff D: The prognosis of essential hypertension treated conservatively. Circulation 23:697, 1961.
89. Spagnuolo M, et al.: Natural history of rheumatic aortic regurgitation. Circulation 44:368, 1971.
90. Tremouth RS, Phelps NC, Neill WA: Determinants of left ventricular hypertrophy and oxygen supply in chronic aortic valve disease. Circulation 53:644, 1976.
91. Casale PN, et al.: Value of echocardiographic measurement of left ventricular mass in predicting cardiovascular morbid events in hypertensive men. Ann Intern Med 105:173, 1986.
92. Levy D, et al.: Left ventricular mass and incidence of coronary heart disease in an elderly cohort. The Framingham Heart Study. Ann Intern Med 110:101, 1989.
93. Levy D, et al.: Prognostic implications of echocardiographically determined left ventricular mass in the Framingham Heart Study. N Engl J Med 322:1561, 1990.
94. Cooper RS, et al.: Left ventricular hypertrophy is associated with worse survival independent of ventricular function and number of coronary arteries severely narrowed. Am J Cardiol 65:441, 1990.
95. Troy BL, Pombo J, Rackley CE: Measurement of left ventricular wall thickness and mass by echocardiography. Circulation 40:602, 1972.
96. Murray JA, Johnson W, Reid JM: Echocardiographic determination of left ventricular dimension volumes and performance. Am J Cardiol 30:252, 1972.
97. Devereux R, Reichek N: Echocardiographic determination of left ventricular mass in man. Circulation 55:613, 1977.
98. Wyatt H, et al.: Cross-sectional echocardiography: I. Analysis of mathematic models for quantifying mass of the left ventricle in dogs. Circulation 60:1104, 1979.
99. Feigenbaum H, Popp RL, Chip JN, Haine CL: Left ventricular wall thickness measured by ultrasound. Arch Intern Med 121:391, 1968.
100. Sahn DJ, DeMaria A, Kisslo J, Weyman AE: Recommendations regarding quantitation in M-mode echocardiography: results of a survey of echocardiographic measurements. Circulation 58:1072, 1978.
101. Wyatt HL, Haendchen RV, Meerbaum S, Corday E: Assessment of quantitative methods for 2-dimensional echocardiography. Am J Cardiol 52:396, 1983.
102. Helak, JW, Reichert NP: Quantitation of human left ventricular mass and volume by two-dimensional echocardiography: in vitro anatomic validation. Circulation 63:1398, 1981.
103. Reichek N, et al.: Anatomic validation of left ventricular mass estimates from clinical two-dimensional echocardiography: initial results. Circulation 67:348, 1983.

104. Devereux RB, et al.: Echocardiographic assessment of left ventricular hypertrophy: comparison to necropsy findings. Am J Cardiol 57:450, 1986.
105. Schiller NB, et al.: Canine left ventricular mass estimation by two-dimensional echocardiography. Circulation 68:210, 1983.
106. Geiser E, Bove K: Calculation of left ventricular mass and relative wall thickness. Arch Pathol 97:13, 1974.
107. Woythaler JN, et al.: Accuracy of echocardiography versus electrocardiography in detecting left ventricular hypertrophy: comparison with postmortem mass measurement. J Am Coll Cardiol 2:305, 1983.
108. Devereux RB, et al.: Standardization of M-mode echocardiographic left ventricular anatomic measurements. J Am Coll Cardiol 4:1220, 1984.
109. Byrd BF, et al.: Left ventricular mass and volume/mass ratio determined by two-dimensional echocardiography in normal adults. J Am Coll Cardiol 6:1021, 1985.
110. Fulton RM, Hutchinson EC, Jones AM: Ventricular weight in cardiac hypertrophy. Br Heart J 14:413, 1952.
111. Reichek N, Devereux RB: Left ventricular hypertrophy: relationship of anatomic, echocardiographic and electrocardiographic findings. Circulation 63:1391, 1981.
112. Levy D, et al.: Echocardiographic criteria for left ventricular hypertrophy: the Framingham Heart Study. Am J Cardiol 59:956, 1987.
113. Hammond IW, et al.: The prevalence and correlates of echocardiographic left ventricular hypertrophy among employed patients with uncomplicated hypertension. J Am Coll Cardiol 7:639, 1986.
114. Savage DD, et al.: Association of echocardiographic left ventricular mass with body size, blood pressure and physical activity (The Framingham Study). Am J Cardiol 65:371, 1990.
115. Devereux RB, et al.: Whole blood viscosity as determinant of cardiac hypertrophy in systemic hypertension. Am J Cardiol 54:592, 1984.
116. Dannenberg AL, Levy D, Garrison RJ: Impact of age on echocardiographic left ventricular mass in a healthy population (The Framingham Study). Am J Cardiol 64:1066, 1989.
117. De Simone G, et al.: Hemodynamic hypertrophied left ventricular patterns in systemic hypertension. Am J Cardiol 60:1317, 1987.
118. Reichek N, Devereux RB: Reliable estimation of peak left ventricular systolic pressure by M-mode echocardiographic determined end-diastolic relative wall thickness: identification of severe valvular aortic stenosis in adult patients. Am Heart J 103:202, 1982.
119. Dodge H, Kennedy J, Peterson J: Quantitative angiocardiographic methods in the evaluation of valvular heart disease. Prog Cardiovasc Dis 16:1, 1973.
120. Rasmussen S, et al.: Stroke volume calculated from the mitral valve echogram in patients with and without ventricular dyssynergy. Circulation 58: 125, 1978.
121. Shuler RH, et al.: The differential effects of respiration on the left and right ventricles. Am J Physiol 137:620, 1942.
122. Ruskin J, Bache RJ, Rembert JC, Greenfield JC: Pressure-flow studies in man: effect of respiration of left ventricular stroke volume. Circulation 48: 79, 1973.
123. Quinones MA, et al.: A new, simplified and accurate method for determining ejection fraction with two-dimensional echocardiography. Circulation 64:744, 1981.
124. Tortoledo FA, et al.: Quantification of left ventricular volumes by two-dimensional echocardiography: a simplified and accurate approach. Circulation 67:579, 1983.
125. Baran AO, Rogal GJ, Nanda NC: Ejection fraction determination without planimetry by two-dimensional echocardiography: a new method. J Am Coll Cardiol 1:1471, 1983.
126. Massie BM, Schiller NB, Ratshin RD, Parmley WW: Mitral-septal separation: new echocardiographic index of left ventricular function. Am J Cardiol 39:1008, 1977.
127. Ahmadpour H, et al.: Mitral E point septal separation: a reliable index of left ventricular performance in coronary artery disease. Am Heart J 106: 21, 1983.
128. Stamm RB, et al.: Two-dimensional echocardiographic measurement of left ventricular ejection fraction: prospective analysis of what constitutes an adequate determination. Am Heart J 104:136, 1982.
129. Amico AF, et al.: Superiority of visual versus computerized echocardiographic estimation of radionuclide left ventricular ejection fraction. Am Heart J 118:1259, 1989.
130. Amoore JN, Santamore WP: Model studies of the contribution of ventricular interdependence to the transient changes in ventricular function with respiratory efforts. Cardiovasc Res 23:683, 1989.
131. Brenner JI, Waugh RA: Effect of phasic respiration on left ventricular dimension and performance in a normal population: an echocardiographic study. Circulation 57:122, 1978.
132. Andersen K, Vik-Mo H: Effects of spontaneous respiration on left ventricular function assessed by echocardiography. Circulation 69:874, 1984.
133. Assmann PE, et al.: Quantitative echocardiographic analysis of global and regional left ventricular function: a problem revisited. J Am Soc Echocardiogr 3:478, 1990.
134. Quinones MA, Gaasch WH, Alexander JK: Echocardiographic assessment of left ventricular function: with special reference to normalized velocities. Circulation 50:42, 1974.
135. Mason S, Fortuin N: The use of echocardiography for quantitative evaluation of left ventricular function. Prog Cardiovasc Dis 21:119, 1978.
136. Douglas PS, et al.: Comparison of echocardiographic methods for assessment of left ventricular shortening and wall stress. J Am Coll Cardiol 9: 945, 1987.
137. Cooper RH, et al.: Comparison of ultrasound and cineangiographic measurements of the mean rate of circumferential shortening in man. Circulation 46:914, 1972.
138. Quinones MA, Gaasch WH, Alexander JK: Influences of acute changes in preload, afterload, contractile state, and heart rate on ejection and isovolumic indices of myocardial contractility in man. Circulation 53:293, 1976.
139. Rosenblatt A, Clark R, Burgess JE, Cohn K: Echocardiographic assessment of the level of cardiac compensation in valvular heart disease. Circulation 54:509, 1976.
140. Ruschhaupt D, et al.: Estimation of circumferential fiber shortening velocity by echocardiography. J Am Coll Cardiol 2:77, 1983.
141. Andersen K, Vik-Mo H: Increased left ventricular emptying at maximal exercise after reduction in afterload. Circulation 69:492, 1984.
142. Jobin J, et al.: Clinical evaluation of left ventricular function using the helical fiber model: an echocardiographic study. Am Heart J 110:1226, 1985.
143. Bargiggia GS, et al.: A new method for estimating left ventricular dP/dt by continuous wave Doppler-echocardiography: validation studies at catheterization. Circulation 80:1287, 1989.
144. Chen C, et al.: Noninvasive estimation of the instantaneous first derivative of left ventricular pressure using continuous-wave Doppler echocardiography. Circulation 83:2101, 1991.
145. Neumann A, et al.: Comparison of Doppler vs catheterization derived dP/dt in dilated cardiomyopathy (abstr.). Circulation 80(Suppl.):II-170, 1989.
146. Marsh JD, et al.: Left ventricular end-systolic pressure-dimension and stress-length relations in normal human subjects. Am J Cardiol 44:1311, 1979.
147. Grossman W, Jones D, McLaurin LP: Wall stress and patterns of hypertrophy in the human left ventricle. J Clin Invest 56:56, 1975.
148. Reichek N, et al.: Noninvasive determination of left ventricular end-systolic stress: validation of the method and initial application. Circulation 65:99, 1982.
149. Quinones MA, et al.: Noninvasive quantification of left ventricular wall stress. Validation of method and application of assessment of chronic pressure overload. Am J Cardiol 45:782, 1980.
150. Kumpuris AG, et al.: Importance of preoperative hypertrophy, wall stress and end-systolic dimension as echocardiographic predictors of normalization of left ventricular dilatation after valve replacement in chronic aortic insufficiency. Am J Cardiol 49:1091, 1982.
151. Mirsky I: Review of various theories for evaluation of left ventricular wall stresses. *In* Mirsky J, Chiston DN, Sander J (eds.): Cardiac Mechanics: Physiological, Chemical and Mathematical Considerations. New York: John Wiley & Sons, 1974.
152. Tomlinson CW: Left ventricular geometry and function in experimental heart failure. Can J Cardiol 3:305, 1987.
153. Janz RF: Estimation of local myocardial stress. Am J Physiol 242:H875, 1982.
154. Segar DS, Moran M, Ryan T: End-systolic regional wall stress-length and stress-shortening relations in an experimental model of normal, ischemic and reperfused myocardium. J Am Coll Cardiol 17:1651, 1991.
155. Downing SE, Sonnenblick EH: Cardiac muscle mechanics and ventricular performance: force and time parameters. Am J Physiol 207:705, 1964.
156. Fifer MA, Braunwald E: End-systolic pressure-volume and stress-length relations in the assessment of ventricular function in man. Adv Cardiol 32: 36, 1985.
157. Weber KT, Janicki JS, Hefner LL: Left ventricular force-length relations of isovolumic and ejecting contractions. Am J Physiol 231:337, 1976.
158. Grossman W, et al.: Contractile state of the left ventricle in man as evaluated from end-systolic pressure-volume relations. Circulation 56:845, 1977.
159. Borow KM, Neumann A, Wynne J: Sensitivity of end-systolic pressure-dimension and pressure-volume relations to the inotropic state in humans. Circulation 65:988, 1982.
160. Colan SD, Borow KM, Gamble WJ, Sanders SP: Effects of enhanced afterload (methoxamine) and contractile state (dobutamine) on the left ventricular late-systolic wall stress-dimension relation. Am J Cardiol 52:1304, 1983.
161. Foult JM, Loiseau A, Nitenberg A: Size dependence of the end-systolic stress/volume ratio in humans: implications for the evaluation of myocardial contractile performance in pressure and volume overload. J Am Coll Cardiol 16:124, 1990.
162. Caidahl K, et al.: Dyspnoea of cardiac origin in 67 year old men: (1). Relation to systolic left ventricular function and wall stress. The study of men born in 1913. Br Heart J 59:319, 1988.
163. Crawford MH, White DH, Amon KW: Echocardiographic evaluation of left ventricular size and performance during handgrip and supine upright bicycle exercise. Circulation 59:1188, 1979.
164. Sugishita Y, Kosekt S: Dynamic exercise echocardiography. Circulation 60:743, 1979.
165. Zwehl W, et al.: Quantitative two dimensional echocardiography during bicycle exercise in normal subjects. Am J Cardiol 47:866, 1981.
166. Ginzton LE, et al.: Noninvasive measurement of the rest and exercise peak systolic pressure/end-systolic volume ratio: a sensitive two-dimensional

echocardiographic indicator of left ventricular function. J Am Coll Cardiol 4:509, 1984.
167. Brion R, et al.: Echocardiographie d'effort et étude du ventricule gauche des sportifs pendant l'effort. Arch Mal Coeur 83:229, 1990.
168. Paulsen WJ, Boughner DR, Friesen A, Persaud JA: Ventricular response to isometric and isotonic exercise. Echocardiographic assessment. Br Heart J 42:521, 1979.
169. Heng MK, Bai JX, Marin J: Changes in left ventricular wall stress during isometric and isotonic exercise in healthy men. Am J Cardiol 62:794, 1988.
170. Perez-Gonzalez JF, Schiller NB, Parmley WW: Direct and noninvasive evaluation of the cardiovascular response to isometric exercise. Circ Res 48:I-138, 1981.
171. Laird WP, Fixler DE, Huffines FD: Cardiovascular response to isometric exercise in normal adolescents. Circulation 59:651, 1979.
172. Erickson HH, Bishop VS, Kardon MB, Horwitz LD: Left ventricular internal diameter and cardiac function during exercise. J Appl Physiol 30:473, 1971.
173. Braunwald E, Goldblatt A, Harrison DC, Mason DT: Studies on cardiac dimensions in intact unanesthetized man. III. Studies of muscular exercise. Circ Res 13:460, 1963.
174. Vatner SF, et al.: Left ventricular response to severe exertion in untethered dogs. J Clin Invest 51:3052, 1972.
175. Rerych SK, et al.: Cardiac function at rest and during exercise in normals and in patients with coronary heart disease: evaluation by radionuclide angiocardiography. Ann Surg 187:449, 1978.
176. Erbel R, et al.: Effects of heart rate changes on left ventricular volume and ejection fraction: a 2-dimensional echocardiographic study. Am J Cardiol 53:591, 1984.
177. Seals DR, et al.: Left ventricular dysfunction after prolonged strenuous exercise in healthy subjects. Am J Cardiol 61:875, 1988.
178. Sullivan J, Hanson P, Rahko PS, Folts JD: Continuous measurement of left ventricular performance during and after maximal isometric deadlift exercise. Circulation 85:1406, 1992.
179. Borow KM, Green LH, Grossman W, Braunwald E: Left ventricular end-systolic stress-shortening and stress-length relations in humans. Normal values and sensitivity to inotropic state. Am J Cardiol 50:1301, 1982.
180. Bonow RO, et al.: The natural history of asymptomatic patients with aortic regurgitation and normal left ventricular function. Circulation 68:509, 1983.
181. St John Sutton M, et al.: Early postoperative changes in left ventricular chamber size, architecture, and function in aortic stenosis and regurgitation and their relation to intraoperative changes in afterload: a prospective two-dimensional echocardiographic study. Circulation 76:77, 1987.
182. St John Sutton MG, Plappert TA, Hirshfeld JW, Reichek N: Assessment of left ventricular mechanics in patients with asymptomatic aortic regurgitation: a two-dimensional echocardiographic study. Circulation 69:259, 1984.
183. Florenzano F, Glantz SA: Left ventricular mechanical adaptation to chronic aortic regurgitation in intact dogs. Am J Physiol 252:H969, 1987.
184. Kawanishi DT, et al.: Cardiovascular response to dynamic exercise in patients with chronic symptomatic mild-to-moderate and severe aortic regurgitation. Circulation 73:62, 1986.
185. Gumbiner CH, Gutgesell HP: Response to isometric exercise in children and young adults with aortic regurgitation. Am Heart J 106:540, 1983.
186. Henry WL, Bonow RO, Rosing DR, Epstein SE: Observations on the optimum time for operative intervention for aortic regurgitation: II. Serial echocardiographic evaluation of asymptomatic patients. Circulation 61:484, 1980.
187. Bonow RO, et al.: Survival and functional results after valve replacement for aortic regurgitation from 1976 to 1983: impact of preoperative left ventricular function. Circulation 72:1244, 1985.
188. Ren JF, et al.: Effect of coronary bypass surgery and valve replacement on left ventricular function: assessment by intraoperative two-dimensional echocardiography. Am Heart J 109:281, 1985.
189. Dubroff JM, et al.: Left ventricular ejection fraction during cardiac surgery: a two-dimensional echocardiographic study. Circulation 68:95, 1983.
190. Gaasch WH, Andrias CW, Levine HJ: Chronic aortic regurgitation: the effect of aortic valve replacement on left ventricular volume, mass and function. Circulation 58:825, 1978.
191. Henry WL, et al.: Observations on the optimum time for operative intervention for aortic regurgitation: I. Evaluation of the results of aortic valve replacement in symptomatic patients. Circulation 61:471, 1980.
192. Bonow RO, et al.: Long-term serial change in left ventricular function and reversal of ventricular dilatation after valve replacement for chronic aortic regurgitation. Circulation 78:1108, 1988.
193. Schuler G, et al.: Serial noninvasive assessment of left ventricular hypertrophy and function after surgical correction of aortic regurgitation. Am J Cardiol 44:585, 1979.
194. Carroll JD, Gaasch WH, Naimi S, Levine HJ: Regression of myocardial hypertrophy: electrocardiographic-echocardiographic correlations after aortic valve replacement in patients with chronic aortic regurgitation. Circulation 65:980, 1982.
195. Schwartz F, et al.: The effect of aortic valve replacement on survival. Circulation 66:1105, 1982.
196. Gaasch WH, Carroll JD, Levine HJ, Criscitiello MG: Chronic aortic regurgitation: prognostic value of left ventricular end-systolic dimension and end-diastolic radius/thickness ratio. J Am Coll Cardiol 1:775, 1983.
197. Bonow RO, et al.: Reversal of left ventricular dysfunction after aortic valve replacement for chronic aortic regurgitation: influence of duration of preoperative left ventricular dysfunction. Circulation 70:570, 1984.
198. Borow KM, Colan SD, Neumann A: Altered left ventricular mechanics in patients with valvular aortic stenosis and coarctation of the aorta: effects on systolic performance and late outcome. Circulation 72:515, 1985.
199. Hess OM, et al.: Asymmetric septal hypertrophy in patients with aortic stenosis: an adaptative mechanism or a coexistence of hypertrophic cardiomyopathy? J Am Coll Cardiol 1:783, 1983.
200. DePace NL, et al.: Correlation of echocardiographic wall stress and left ventricular pressure and function in aortic stenosis. Circulation 67:854, 1983.
201. Horstkotte D, Loogen F: The natural history of aortic valve stenosis. Eur Heart J 9(Suppl E):57, 1988.
202. Zile MR, Gaasch WH, Carroll JD, Levine HJ: Chronic mitral regurgitation: predictive value of preoperative echocardiographic indexes of left ventricular function and wall stress. J Am Coll Cardiol 3:235, 1984.
203. Schuler G, et al.: Temporal response of left ventricular performance to mitral valve surgery. Circulation 59:1218, 1979.
204. Keren G, et al.: Effect of isometric exercise on cardiac performance and mitral regurgitation in patients with severe congestive heart failure. Am Heart J 118:973, 1989.
205. Wong CYH, Spotnitz HM: Systolic and diastolic properties of the human left ventricle during valve replacement for chronic mitral regurgitation. Am J Cardiol 47:40, 1981.
206. Zile MR, Gaasch WH, Levine HJ: Left ventricular stress-dimension-shortening relations before and after correction of chronic aortic and mitral regurgitation. Am J Cardiol 56:99, 1985.
207. Reed D, Abbott RD, Smucker ML, Kaul S: Prediction of outcome after mitral valve replacement in patients with symptomatic chronic mitral regurgitation. The importance of left atrial size. Circulation 84:23, 1991.
208. Shapiro LM, McKenna WJ: Left ventricular hypertrophy. Relation of structure to diastolic function in hypertension. Br Heart J 51:637, 1984.
209. Fouad FM, Slominski JM, Tarazi RC: Left ventricular diastolic function in hypertension: relation to left ventricular mass and systolic function. J Am Coll Cardiol 3:1500, 1984.
210. Papademetriou V, Gottdiener JS, Fletcher RD, Freis ED: Echocardiographic assessment by computer-assisted analysis of diastolic left ventricular function and hypertrophy in borderline or mild systemic hypertension. Am J Cardiol 56:546, 1985.
211. Topol EJ, Traill TA, Fortuin NJ: Hypertensive hypertrophic cardiomyopathy of the elderly. N Engl J Med 312:277, 1985.
212. Moriaka S, Simon G: Echocardiographic evidence for early left ventricular hypertrophy in dogs with renal hypertension. Am J Cardiol 49:1890, 1982.
213. Drayer JIM, Weber MA, DeYoung JL: BP as a determinant of cardiac left ventricular muscle mass. Arch Intern Med 143:90, 1983.
214. Devereux RB, et al.: Left ventricular hypertrophy in patients with hypertension: importance of blood pressure response to regularly occurring stress. Circulation 68:470, 1983.
215. Rowlands DB, et al.: Assessment of left ventricular mass and response to antihypertensive treatment. Lancet 1:467, 1982.
216. Ren J-F, Hakki A-H, Kotler MN, Iskandrian AS: Exercise systolic blood pressure. A powerful determinant of increased left ventricular mass in patients with hypertension. J Am Coll Cardiol 5:1224, 1984.
217. Gosse P, et al.: "White coat" hypertension: no harm for the heart (abstr.). J Am Coll Cardiol 19:85A, 1992.
218. Savage DD, et al.: Echocardiographic comparison of black and white hypertensive subjects. J Nat Med Assoc 71:709, 1979.
219. Dunn FG, et al.: Racial differences in cardiac adaptation to essential hypertension determined by echocardiographic indexes. J Am Coll Cardiol 5:1348, 1983.
220. Hammond IW, et al.: Contrast in cardiac anatomy and function between black and white patients with hypertension. J Nat Med Assoc 76:247, 1984.
221. Logan AG, et al.: Early effects of mild hypertension on the heart. A longitudinal study. Hypertension 3(Suppl 2):187, 1981.
222. Dreslinski GR, et al.: Patterns of left ventricular adaptation in borderline and mild essential hypertension. Echocardiographic findings. Chest 80:592, 1981.
223. Hartford M, et al.: Left ventricular wall stress and systolic function in untreated primary hypertension. Hypertension 7:97, 1985.
224. Guazzi M, et al.: Cardiac load and function in hypertension. Ultrasonic and hemodynamic study. Am J Cardiol 44:1007, 1979.
225. Lutas EM, et al.: Increased cardiac performance in mild essential hypertension. Left ventricular mechanics. Hypertension 7:979, 1985.
226. Karliner JS, et al.: Left ventricular performance in patients with left ventricular hypertrophy caused by systemic arterial hypertension. Br Heart J 39:1239, 1977.
227. Boudoulas H, et al.: Left ventricular mass and systolic performance in chronic systemic hypertension. Am J Cardiol 57:232, 1986.
228. Devereux RB, et al.: Relation of hemodynamic load to left ventricular hypertrophy and performance in hypertension. Am J Cardiol 51:171, 1983.
229. Borer JS, et al.: Left ventricular performance in the hypertensive patient.

Exercise-mediated noninvasive separation of loading influences from intrinsic muscle dysfunction. Chest 83(Suppl.):314, 1983.
230. Aronow WS, Epstein S, Koenigsberg M, Schwartz KS: Usefulness of echocardiographic left ventricular hypertrophy, ventricular tachycardia and complex ventricular arrhythmias in predicting ventricular fibrillation or sudden cardiac death in elderly patients. Am J Cardiol 62:1124, 1988.
231. Cohen A, et al.: Clinical correlates in hypertensive patients with left ventricular hypertrophy diagnosed with echocardiography. Am J Cardiol 47: 335, 1981.
232. Shapiro LM, MacKinnon J, Beevers DG: Echocardiographic features of malignant hypertension. Br Heart J 46:374, 1981.
233. Schlant RC, et al.: Echocardiographic studies of left ventricular anatomy and function in essential hypertension. Cardiovasc Med 2:477, 1977.
234. Liebson PR: Clinical studies of drug reversal of hypertensive left ventricular hypertrophy. Am J Hypertens 3:512, 1990.
235. Fouad FM, et al.: Reversal of left ventricular hypertrophy in hypertensive patients treated with methyldopa. Am J Cardiol 49:795, 1982.
236. Leenen FHH, et al.: Vasodilators and regression of left ventricular hypertrophy. Am J Med 72:969, 1987.
237. Schulman SP, et al.: The effects of antihypertensive therapy on left ventricular mass in elderly patients. N Engl J Med 322:1350, 1990.
238. Sugishita Y, Iida K, Yukisada K, Ito I: Cardiac determinants of regression of left ventricular hypertrophy in essential hypertension with antihypertensive treatment. J Am Coll Cardiol 15:665, 1990.
239. Ferrara LA, et al.: Left ventricular mass reduction during salt depletion in arterial hypertension. Hypertension 6:755, 1984.
240. MacMahon SW, Wilcken DEL, MacDonald GJ: The effect of weight reduction on left ventricular mass. N Engl J Med 314:334, 1986.
241. von Bibra H, Richardson PJ: Left ventricular hypertrophy in patients with moderate essential hypertension: an echocardiographic study. *In* Robertson JIS, Caldwell ADS (eds.): Left Ventricular Hypertrophy in Hypertension. New York, Grune & Stratton, 1979.
242. Liebson PR, Savage DD: Echocardiography in hypertension: a review: I. Left ventricular wall mass, standardization, and ventricular function. Echocardiography 3:181, 1986.
243. Kansal S, Roitman D, Sheffield LT: Interventricular septal thickness and left ventricular hypertrophy. An echocardiographic study. Circulation 60: 1058, 1979.
244. Savage DD, et al.: Disproportionate ventricular septal thickness in hypertensive patients. J Cardiol Ultrasonography 1:79, 1982.
245. Safar ME, et al.: Echocardiographic dimensions in borderline and sustained hypertension. Am J Cardiol 44:930, 1979.
246. Granger CB, et al.: Rapid ventricular filling in left ventricular hypertrophy: I. Physiologic study. J Am Coll Cardiol 5:862, 1985.
247. Douglas PS, OToole ML, Hiller WD, Reichek N: Left ventricular structure and function by echocardiography in ultraendurance athletes. Am J Cardiol 58:805, 1986.
248. Colan SD, Sanders SP, Borow KM: Physiologic hypertrophy: effects on left ventricular systolic mechanics in athletes. J Am Coll Cardiol 9:776, 1987.
249. Fagard R, et al.: Noninvasive assessment of systolic and diastolic left ventricular function in female runners. Eur Heart J 8:1305, 1987.
250. Mickelson JK, et al.: Left ventricular dimensions and mechanics in distance runners. Am Heart J 112:1251, 1986.
251. Ehsani AA, Hagberg JM, Hickson RC: Rapid changes in left ventricular dimensions and mass in response to physical conditioning and deconditioning. Am J Cardiol 42:52, 1978.
252. Martin WH, Coyle EF, Ehsani AA: Effects of physical deconditioning after intense endurance training on left ventricular dimensions and stroke volume. J Am Coll Cardiol 7:982, 1986.

CHAPTER

21

LEFT VENTRICLE II: QUANTIFICATION OF SEGMENTAL DYSFUNCTION

STEFAN MARK NIDORF and ARTHUR E. WEYMAN

Acute coronary occlusion results in almost immediate cessation of myocardial contraction in the region supplied by the obstructed vessel.[1] Once established, the area of abnormal function tends to persist, and repeated injury generally causes progressive deterioration of ventricular function. The characteristic association between loss of regional myocardial blood flow and muscular function permits segmental contraction abnormalities to be used as early and sensitive markers of underlying ischemia and/or infarction.[2] These wall motion abnormalities are particularly significant because they appear within seconds after the onset of ischemia (before any important change in the electrocardiogram or clinical symptoms)[3] and because their extent can be related to overall pump function[4] and, as a result, to subsequent morbidity and mortality.[5]

During the past 15 years, cross-sectional echocardiography has emerged as a potentially ideal noninvasive method to visualize the changes in left ventricular structure and function that occur during myocardial ischemia or following infarction.[6–28] The high spatial resolution and rapid sampling rate of this technique permit these functional changes to be defined at their onset (i.e., immediately following coronary occlusion) and to be followed sequentially over time. Clinical studies using this technique have demonstrated a clear relationship between the location and extent of echocardiographically defined regional dysfunction and electrocardiographic infarct location,[10,14,23,25] pathologic evidence of infarction,[10,15] clinical/hemodynamic patient status,[11,19–21] occurrence of complications,[11,12,19] and survival.[11,12]

In the experimental model, the relationship of segmental wall motion abnormalities to underlying infarct size and perfusion deficit have been even more clearly defined.[9,13,16,17,24,26,27,29] In a variety of studies, an excellent quantitative relationship has been demonstrated between the circumferential extent of abnormal wall motion and histologic infarct size,[9,16] extent of dyssynergy defined by force-gauge mapping,[16] and the area of infarction defined by technetium pyrophosphate scintigraphy.[13] Function along individual radii has further been related to the transmural extent of infarction, with radii intersecting histologically infarcted and normal zones,[17] showing clearly different values for the percentage of wall thickening and the percentage of endocardial excursion.

The available data reinforce the early opinion that this technique would ultimately find its greatest clinical utility in detecting and quantifying the functional sequelae of myocardial ischemia and infarction. All of these relationships, however, depend on some form of measurement of ventricular structure and function. These vary from simple visual assessment and comparison with known patterns of normality to precise quantitative recording of interface position and motion using sophisticated computer algorithms. The purpose of this chapter is to review (1) the characteristics of the ultrasonic imaging technique and display format that effect the spatial and temporal nature of the resulting image and hence the accuracy of measurement of time-related events such as wall motion and thickening and (2) the status and limitations of quantitative methods for defining the extent and degree of regional dysfunction. The next chapter discusses the use of these techniques in assessing the structural and functional sequelae of acute and chronic coronary artery disease.

TECHNIQUE AND IMAGE CHARACTERISTICS

Technique

The techniques for image acquisition and the standard ventricular planes used to assess segmental left ventricular function are the same as those described for routine ventricular imaging in the preceding chapter. However, the need for precision in plane recording and the structural detail required are far greater for the assessment of wall motion than volume or mass because the range of changes being recorded is much smaller. For example, the dimensions used to calculate ventricular volume are generally given in centimeters, whereas the amplitude of contraction is more typically recorded in millimeters. Because the measurements are so small, factors such as fundamental image resolution, ventricular rotation and translation, respiratory changes in position and volume, display of data acquired over a varying period of time in the same image, and observer- and instrument-introduced noise become of critical importance in quantitation.

Imaging Characteristics (Resolution)

Spatial Resolution

As discussed in Chapters 2 and 20, the resolution and display characteristics of individual points along the endocardial and epicardial surface of the ventricle vary depending on the position of the targets relative to the direction of propagation of the ultrasonic beam. Targets that are perpendicular to the beam reflect sound directly back to the transducer and are resolved using the axial resolution of the system, which depends on transducer frequency and pulse duration. Resolution in this dimension is accurate to the millimeter or submillimeter level. Targets that are laterally positioned relative to the scan plane are less highly reflective and depend on the lateral resolution of the system for their definition. Lateral resolution depends on beam width, which in turn varies with position along the beam, degree of focusing, output power, and receiver gain. Because of this characteristic, only points separated laterally by more than the beam width can be resolved as being distinct. Individual targets likewise are laterally broadened to the effective beam width at the target level (point spread function). Figure 21–1 illustrates this phenomenon for a single-point target. The effect of these two characteristics of resolution on the display characteristics of a circular target are illustrated in Figure 20–2.

For parasternal short axis views, targets positioned anteriorly and posteriorly in the ventricle are recorded using the axial resolution of the imaging system, whereas those oriented medially and laterally are imaged using the lateral resolution. For subcostal short axis views, the relationship is shifted by 90°. From the apical window, virtually all endocardial and epicardial targets are imaged with the lateral resolution of the system. Because laterally positioned targets are less clearly recorded, areas of echo dropout frequently occur along the medial and lateral margins of the endocardium and epicardium. In addition, because of the broadening of laterally positioned targets, the black-white (wall-cavity) interface for these targets will always be closer to the center of the chamber than that of anteriorly and posteriorly positioned targets. This will change the denominator in many quantitative methods for determining wall motion and may effect thickening measurements as well, because any increase in the angle of the beam relative to the target also increases the point-spread function. The net effect of these resolution differences is complex. As a rule, however, targets recorded in the apical views, as well as those positioned along the medial and lateral regions of the ventricle in parasternal and subcostal views, are imaged less clearly and appear closer to the center of the ventricle than the same target recorded in parasternal views using the axial resolution of the system.

Temporal Resolution

Because any analysis of wall motion or thickening involves the recording of movement relative to time, it is also important to understand the temporal resolution of an ultrasonic system and its relationship to the temporal-resolving characteristics of the medium on which data are stored. As discussed in Chapters 1 and 2, all two-dimensional images are composed of a series of data lines (B-mode lines), which represent the amplitude-

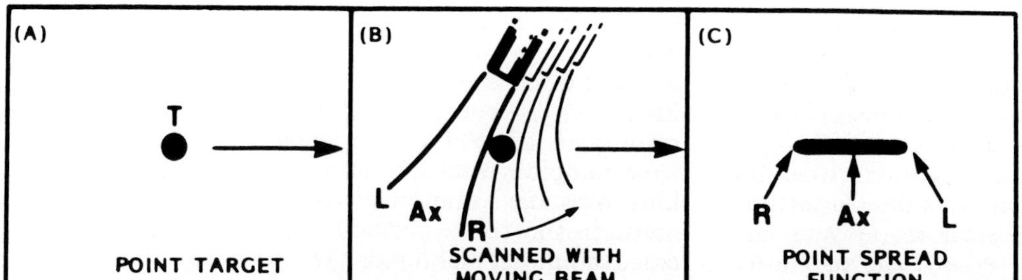

Fig. 21–1. Image produced when a point target **(A)**, is swept by a moving ultrasound beam **(B)**. The target is broadened to the effective beam width, with the result that the circular target is displayed as an ellipse **(C)**. (From Mann DL, Gillam LD, Weyman AE: Cross-sectional echocardiographic assessment of regional left ventricular performance and myocardial perfusion. Prog Cardiovasc Dis 29:1, 1986.)

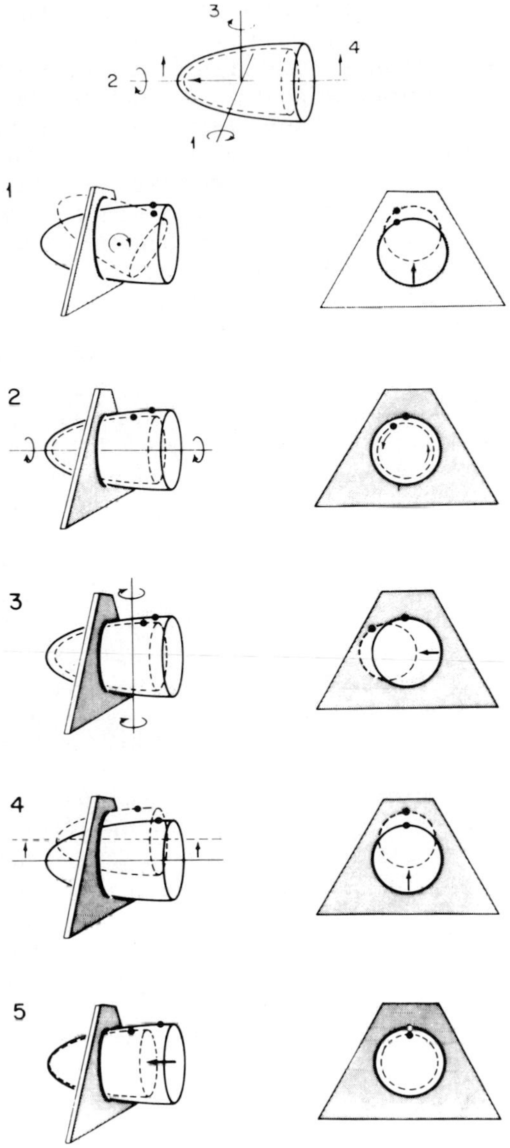

Fig. 21–2. Effects of translation and rotation about each of the three primary axes and base-to-apex shortening on the recording of a short axis image of the ventricle. **1.** Rotation about the horizontal minor axis. **2.** Rotation about the long axis. **3.** Rotation about the ventricular minor axis. **4.** Translation. **5.** Base-to-apex shortening. (From Mann DL, Gillam LD, Weyman AE: Cross-sectional echocardiographic assessment of regional left ventricular performance and myocardial perfusion. Prog Cardiovasc Dis 29: 1, 1986.)

modulated reflections of ultrasonic pulses transmitted as the beam is swept across the precordium. The number of pulses transmitted as the sound beam sweeps through its fixed arc varies depending on the depth of field being examined and the line density within each echo image. In general, the deeper the structures being examined, the longer the transit time for each pulse and thus, for a given line density, the slower the scan rate. If a particular area of the heart is scanned 20 times per second, then the data from the last line will be recorded 50 msec after the data from the first line. These analog data are then converted to a digital format using a digital scan converter (see Chapter 3 for a description of scan converter function). Scan converter speed varies between instruments, as does the pattern in which they update the image. As a rule, only a portion of the image is updated by the scan converter with each output cycle, with the result that the pattern of data in the output image may not be temporally synchronous with the pattern in which it was recorded.

The digitized image is then converted back to an analog format for video display. During conversion to the video format, the image is scanned vertically from top to bottom each $\frac{1}{60}$ of a second to form one video field. Two sequential video fields are then interlaced to form a video frame. Finally, the video data must be replayed for analysis using either a video recorder or video disc. Because individual frames/fields are analyzed, the time interval between frames/fields determines the temporal resolution imposed by the video system. Recorders that advance frame by frame will have a 33-msec interval between individual images. Most recorders that nominally advance in a field-by-field mode actually project one field, skip the interlaced field, and move on to the first field of the next pair. The time interval between displayed fields is, likewise, 33 msec. Disc systems are available, however, that permit interlacing of identical fields and progress without skipping any fields, with the result that the time interval between video data samples is at best 16.5 msec.

In analyzing time-varying wall motion, this heterogeneity in the rate of recording, digitization, and video display may play an important, but not widely appreciated, role in some of the perceived heterogeneity of contraction. It is important to note that even if the scan converter output is synchronous with the recording rate, neither are video synchronous, and hence, in the best case, there may be up to a 33-msec difference in the time at which individual points on the same image were recorded. In most commonly used systems, however, this difference may be 50 msec or more.

The Effects of Rotation and Translation

In addition to the instrumentation-related artifacts described previously, misperception of the true pattern of ventricular contraction can also be introduced by ventricular rotation (motion of the left ventricle about one of its three primary axes) or translation (motion of the entire ventricle in space). The ability to perceive and correct for these movements, which are unrelated to contraction, depends on their orientation relative to the plane being recorded. In addition, ventricular contraction itself may alter the relative position of the imaging plane to the recording myocardium between systole and diastole as a result of base-to-apex shortening. Figure 21–2 illustrates the effects of rotation about the three primary cardiac axes, translation, and base-to-apex shortening on recorded short axis images. Figure 21–3 illustrates the same effects on a representative apical view. In short axis, rotation about the ventricular long axis, the horizontal minor axes, and translation can be directly appreciated. Base-to-apex shortening, however, is less readily detectable. A shift in the point at

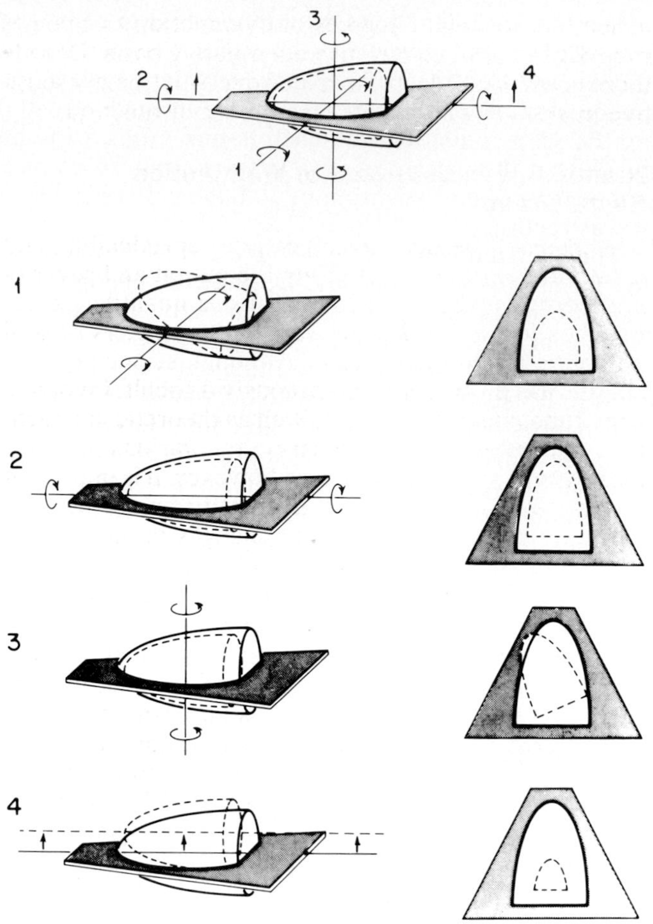

Fig. 21–3. Effects of translation and rotation about the three primary axes on the apical image of the ventricle. **1.** Rotation about the horizontal minor axis. **2.** Rotation about the long axis. **3.** Rotation about the ventricular minor axis. **4.** Translation. In the absence of confounding variables, base-to-apex shortening can be appreciated directly from the image of this projection and, therefore, not illustrated. The pattern would appear similar to that shown in **2.** (From Mann DL, Gillam LD, Weyman AE: Cross-sectional echocardiographic assessment of regional left ventricular performance and myocardial perfusion. Prog Cardiovasc Dis 29:1, 1986.)

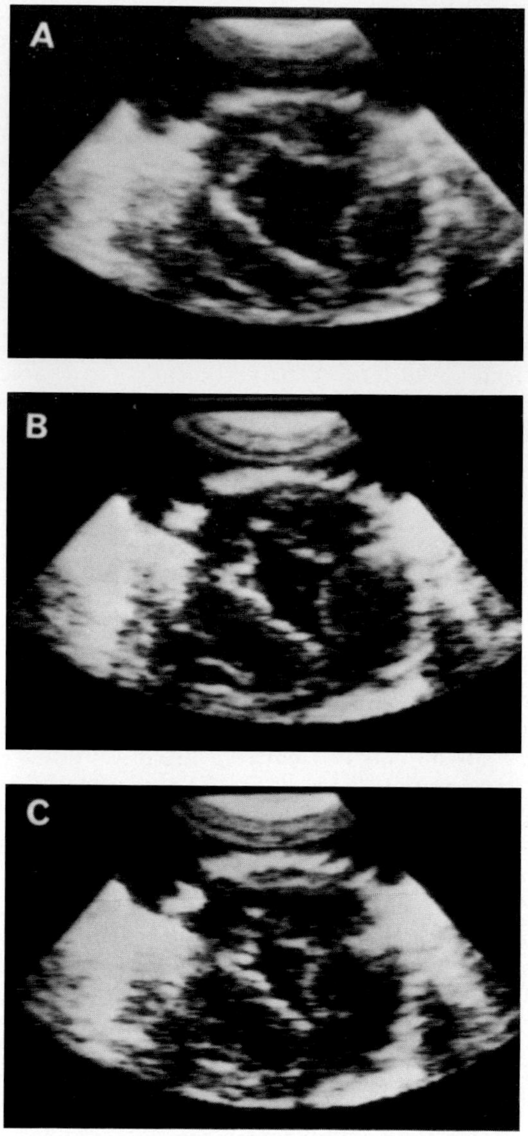

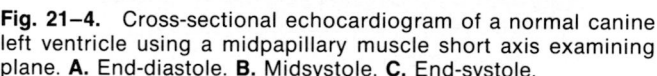

Fig. 21–4. Cross-sectional echocardiogram of a normal canine left ventricle using a midpapillary muscle short axis examining plane. **A.** End-diastole. **B.** Midsystole. **C.** End-systole.

which the plane intersects the ventricle from end-systole to diastole therefore may be misinterpreted as a change in contraction. In the apical views, only rotation about the vertical minor axis and base-to-apex shortening can be appreciated directly from the image. Translation and rotation about the horizontal axis may be perceived as being due to ventricular contraction and, hence, lead to either under- or overestimation of segmental function.

ASSESSMENT OF THE EXTENT AND SEVERITY OF ABNORMAL WALL MOTION WITHIN A SINGLE PLANE: METHODS AND CRITIQUE

All cross-sectional echocardiographic images are by definition planar. Function within individual planes is assessed by the motion of point targets along the endocardium or epicardium between sequentially recorded images or predetermined time points in the cardiac cycle. Figure 21–4 contains a series of short axis recordings that illustrate the appearance and motion of these interfaces during normal systolic contraction in the canine ventricle. As the ventricle contracts, the targets along the endocardial interface move inward toward the center of the ventricle (endocardial excursion). The cavity area decreases (area shrinkage), the cavity perimeter becomes smaller (perimeter shrinkage), and the distance between the endocardial and epicardial interfaces increases (wall thickening). Following coronary occlusion, a local decrease in the amplitude of endocardial excursion and subjacent wall thickening becomes apparent within seconds, in the area supplied by the obstructed vessel.[9] In the previously normal ventricle, these changes are sufficiently distinct that they can be easily visualized in comparison to adjacent normally contracting muscle. Once established, the severity of the contraction abnormality can be defined semiquantitatively—as hypokinetic (normally directed but reduced in magnitude), akinetic (absent motion), or dyskinetic (systolic bulging)—or quantitatively using one of the methods described later. The extent of abnormal wall motion within a single plane can also be determined visually by defining the junctional points between the normally moving myocardium and the abnormal segment or quantitatively by demarcating regions in which some measure of contraction lies outside a previously defined normal range or pattern.

Visual Assessment of Wall Motion (Single Plane)

Visual definition of the extent of abnormal wall motion from a real-time display is clearly the simplest approach. This can be done in one of two ways. First, the plane can be divided into segments based on anatomic references, and function within each segment can be determined semiquantitatively (e.g., normal or hypokinetic).[10,11,14,15,20,25,28,30] Second, the observer can define the margins of the area of dysfunction and express the extent of abnormal function as a fraction of the ventricular perimeter.[9,15,16] Figure 21–5 illustrates visual quantitation of the extent of abnormal wall motion by the latter method. In this example, the diastolic contour of the ventricle is outlined, and the center of this contour is approximated. The hinge points between normal and abnormally moving myocardium are then identified during real-time video playback. The number of degrees separating these hinge points, in this case 90°, is determined and expressed as a percentage of the total 360° ventricular circumference.

Although attractive because of their simplicity, all visual-based approaches depend on the skill and experience of the observer and therefore may lack objectivity. Further, these approaches do not provide truly quantitative data concerning function within abnormal zones and,

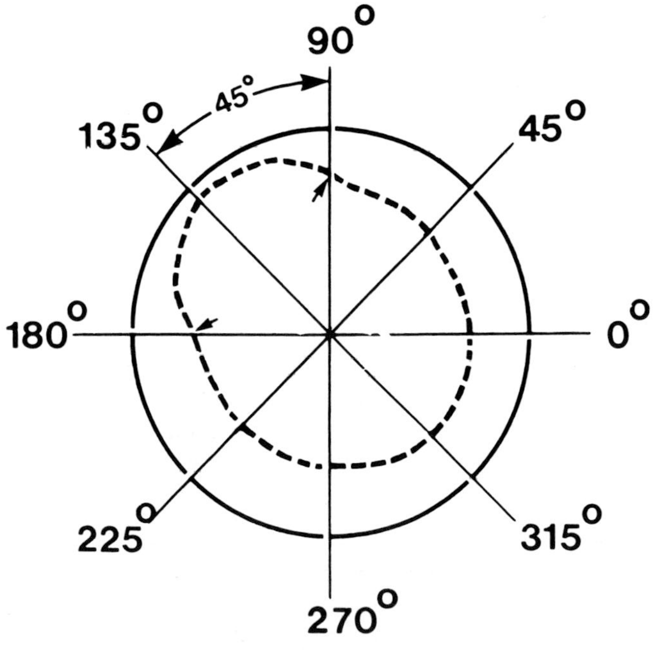

Fig. 21–5. The circumferential extent of an area can be determined visually using a radial coordinate system.

hence, do not relate degrees of dysfunction to changes in perfusion or histology on a quantitative basis. Despite these limitations, the well-trained eye is extremely sensitive in separating abnormal from normal function.

Quantitative Assessment of Wall Motion (Single Plane)

Because of the need for objective, reproducible, and quantitative means of assessing the extent and severity of abnormal regional function, various quantitative approaches for measuring the various parameters of wall motion have been developed. Although seemingly simple, this has proven to be enormously difficult, involving many fundamental choices as well as theoretic and technical problems. Before discussing the various methods for measuring regional function, however, it is important to remember that all of the factors discussed become important because the absolute changes in motion and thickening measured are very small (in the range of 1 to 10 mm). Because function is generally expressed as a percentage of the end-diastolic value for the chosen parameters (normalized), the degree of magnification is determined by the denominator of the fractional expression. Because of these small numbers and the large relative errors they produce, it is important that all the potential sources of error be considered and eliminated for these measurements to be as meaningful as possible.

Definition of Endocardial and Epicardial Interfaces

The first step in any quantitative analysis of wall motion or thickening is to define the endocardial and epicardial interfaces from which all quantitative parameters are derived. These interfaces are not depicted by discrete points but rather by ellipses whose size and eccentricity is determined by the resolving characteristics of the imaging system and whose intensity typically decreases from the center to the edges of the ellipse. It is necessary, therefore, to establish at the outset which portion of the ellipse will be taken to represent the boundary. This is usually defined as the peak of the local intensity gradient or the junction between the peak and one of the descending limbs. Because the peak may be broad and, along the epicardium, may merge with extracardiac reflectors, we prefer to take the junction of the peak and the inner descending limb as the border.

Methods of Tracing Borders

Once the points that comprise the border are established, their position can be recorded by (1) manual tracing directly from the video screen;[9,26,29,31–34] (2) digital tracing using an electronically directed cursor;[35,36–38] (3) positioning points at selected equiangular intervals along the boundary with the interpolation of contours between points;[17,39] or (4) using an automated border-tracking algorithm.[40]

The manual tracing of boundaries directly from the video screen is a relatively crude approach, given the precision in measurement required and the parallax errors inherent in any screen-derived measurement. Trac-

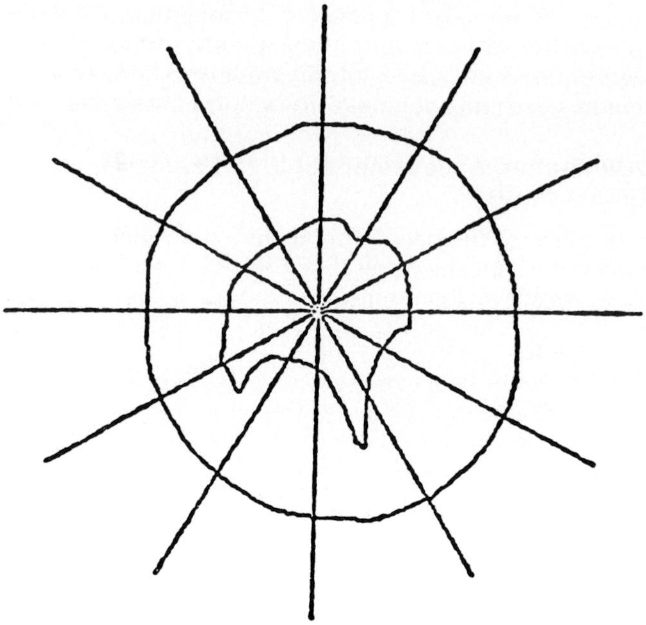

Fig. 21–6. Representative digitized endocardial and epicardial outlines of a single cross-sectional echocardiographic field. The echocardiographic images were recorded in a short axis view at the level of the midpapillary muscles. (From Mann DL, Gillam LD, Weyman AE: Cross-sectional echocardiographic assessment of regional left ventricular performance and myocardial perfusion. Prog Cardiovasc Dis 29:1, 1986.)

ing of boundaries with digital recording of point coordinates is preferred because it removes any parallax error and permits storage of the contours in a form that allows their subsequent reconstruction and manipulation. Because the sampling rate of digitizers is typically constant, while the speed at which the operator can trace the borders varies, the point density of the digitized contours will usually be large and the points unevenly spaced. Points used to define the contour, therefore, are typically filtered and the number of points reduced. This initial reduction has a smoothing effect on the raw data, which will vary with the type of filtering and the degree of point reduction. Figure 21–6 illustrates reconstructed boundaries using one such algorithm. Also displayed are the actual number of stored points used to reconstruct each boundary.

Superimposition of points on the endocardial and epicardial targets at equiangular distances requires the initial approximation of a ventricular contour and calculation of a center of reference from which the equiangular radii can be generated and along which the intersecting points can be identified. The selected points along each interface are then connected using a spline-fitting algorithm or Fourier transform to create a contour.[39] Resulting contours, therefore, are largely composed of nonreal or processed data; however, only the actual target coordinates appear to be used in computations.

While seemingly a trivial point, the difference in these methods (interface tracing and point superimposition) may be of great importance because they define the raw data for all subsequent analyses. Although not critically compared to date, it is likely that these methods differ significantly in terms of ease of identification of individual points along the myocardial border, appropriate or inappropriate observer bias in the selection of point pairs vs. independent digitization of the endocardial and epicardial contours, the effects of the different smoothing algorithms, and the need to define an initial arbitrary center for the point placement approach with the constraints this center places on subsequent point positioning.

Automated methods of border detection are discussed in detail in Chapter 3. While subject to less observer bias,[41] automated methods of boundary detection have not developed to the point where they can be considered sufficiently reliable for routine clinical or experimental use.

Primary Descriptors of Regional Function

Once the endocardial and epicardial interfaces have been stored in a digital format, function can be assessed from their motion and separation. The two primary quantitative descriptors of regional function are wall motion (endocardial excursion) and wall thickening (interface separation). Both of these approaches have major advantages and limitations, which are summarized in Table 21–1. Wall motion relies on a more readily defined interface, the endocardium, and is more easily visualized around the entire circumference or silhouette of the ventricle. Further, it is an easier parameter to compare with other techniques, such as angiography and radionuclide ventriculography, than is wall thickening. Its major

Table 21–1. Advantages and Disadvantages of Methods of Assessing Abnormal Wall Motion[62]

Endocardial Excursion	Wall Thickening
Advantages	
Relies on a more readily defined interface (endocardium)	Independent of a center of reference
More readily measured around the entire circumference of the ventricle	Unaffected by translation or rotation
	Unaffected by shape changes
Disadvantages	
Centroid-dependent	Difficult to measure around the entire circumference of the ventricle due to poor epicardial definition
Affected by translation and rotation	Tends to be an "all-or-none phenomenon"
	Difficult to correlate with results obtained by other imaging modalities (radionuclide or contrast ventriculograms)

(From Mann DL, Gillam LD, Weyman AE: Cross-sectional echocardiographic assessment of regional left ventricular performance and myocardial perfusion. Prog Cardiovasc Dis 29:1, 1986.)

limitations are that endocardial motion must be related to some reference within or surrounding the heart and it is influenced by cardiac translation and rotation, patient and respiratory movement, and ventricular shape changes.

Thickening, in contrast, has the major advantage of being relatively independent of a center of reference and is unaffected by translation, rotation, or changes in ventricular shape. The major limitations of thickening are that it tends to be binary. That is, it is expressed in terms of thickening or thinning, it is difficult to measure around the whole circumference of the ventricle in short axis and apical views as a result of the relatively poor epicardial resolution along the medial and lateral walls; and when quantified, it produces a large percentage of change for very small increments in absolute interface separation.

Methods of Referencing

Having defined the endocardial and epicardial borders of the left ventricle, it is then necessary to select a reference system within which to assess ventricular motion. The two primary choices are the boundaries of the video raster (external) or a reference within the heart (internal).

External Reference-Based Systems. The simplest reference system uses the boundaries of the video raster for the alignment of individual frames. In this format, endocardial and epicardial interface position is compared at end-diastole and end-systole, and the degree of separation is determined around the circumference. Separation is generally expressed in terms of the extent of the circumference over which the contours coincide (akinesis), the diastolic contour extends beyond the systolic one (dyskinesis), or there is an abrupt decrease in the distance between boundaries (hypokinesis). The extent of the region of reduced contour separation can then be measured and expressed in absolute terms or as a percentage of the diastolic ventricular contour.[9,15,16] The amplitude of motion at specific points along the contour can also be measured and compared to reference normal values (see centerline method later).

Superimposition of ventricular contours using the margins on the video raster, however, does not permit correction for translation or rotation, which is a major limitation in any analysis of wall motion. In the absence of rotation, thickening can be measured using this approach; however, measurements of wall thickness should be made perpendicular to the contours, rather than as the difference between radii relative to an arbitrary central point. This is particularly true when assessing wall thickening from apical views or when assessing wall thickening from short axis images in patients with distorted ventricles.

Internal Reference-Based Systems. The second approach is to use a central reference point (centroid) or axis within the ventricle as a reference. The use of an internal reference has the advantage that, if properly selected, it will move with the heart and, hence, offers the potential to correct for cardiac motion unrelated to contraction.[22,23,32,33,37,38,42,43] It also provides a reference around which a contour can be rotated to correct for rotation-induced artifacts and from which radii can be drawn to measure wall thickening or endocardial excursion. Although complex to compute, the internal reference is unquestionably more appropriate for motion analysis than is any external reference system.

Methods for Calculating the Central Reference (Centroid) for an Individual Frame

Unfortunately, there is no true anatomic landmark within the left ventricular cavity that can serve as an internal reference point. Therefore, this point must always be derived. Because all quantitative measurements of endocardial excursion critically depend on the centroid (center of mass) chosen, the identification of a reproducible and reliable centroid becomes extremely important. Two general methods have been suggested.

The first defines the central reference as the bisector of a line running from a fixed point on the ventricular wall (e.g., the posterior junction of the right and left ventricles) to the furthest point on the opposite endocardial surface[22,23] or the bisector of a line running from a fixed external reference (e.g., the midpoint of the interventricular septum) to the opposite free ventricular wall such that it divides the cavity area in half.[26,27,31] The accuracy of these bisecting points as centers of reference for radial measurements of ventricular function has not, to date, truly been tested. Although relatively simple to implement, these approaches appear to have several theoretic limitations. First, the bisecting points have no inherent or consistently demonstrated relationship to the true center of left ventricular tomograms. Second, contraction-induced distortions in ventricular shape will further alter any relationship that might exist between arbitrarily derived points and the actual ventricular centroid; and the effects will vary depending whether the intercepts of the reference line are included in the distortion or not. Further, although any derived centroid by definition will be an approximation, the greater the number of points included in the computation of the reference, the more accurate it should be. Because the volume of data provided by the two-dimensional echocardiogram is now matched by the capacity for computers to handle multiple reference points for each frame, it seems reasonable that theoretically more precise methods of centroid computation are appropriate rather than those employing only two or three arbitrarily selected points.

The second general approach is to compute the center of the left ventricle as the center of the region bounded by one of the margins of the left ventricular tomogram. The tomographic two-dimensional echocardiogram provides several anatomic interfaces or areas from which the central reference can be calculated. Likewise, a variety of mathematical methods can be applied to these anatomic data to derive the central point. Figure 21–7 illustrates the difference in pattern of short axis centroid migration from end-diastole to end-systole produced by using six different methods of centroid calculation. It has been demonstrated[44] that there is significant method-related difference in the reproducibility between

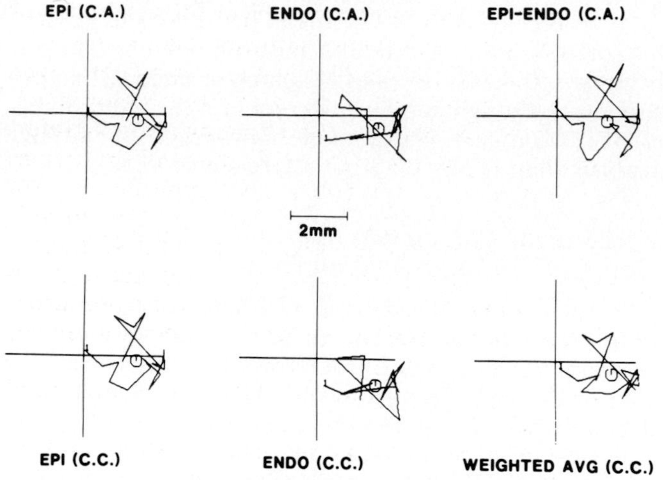

Fig. 21–7. Spatial migration of the centroid for each echocardiographic field from end-diastole to end-systole, plotted using six methods. The spacial average of all points is indicated by the open circle. CA = center of area: CC, center of coordinates. (From Mann DL, Gillam LD, Weyman AE: Cross-sectional echocardiographic assessment of regional left ventricular performance and myocardial perfusion. Prog Cardiovasc Dis 29:1, 1986.)

observers of the calculated centroids, with endocardial-based centers being more reproducible than those that use the epicardium.

Centroids calculated as the center of area appear to be more reproducible than those calculated as the center of coordinates. This difference is to be expected because the center of coordinates is the average of all coordinates on the boundary and therefore is sensitive to differences in single coordinates, each of which contributes equally to the centroid. The center of area, in contrast, is an integral over the entire region bounded by the epicardial or endocardial margin and therefore should be less sensitive to small changes in coordinates on either boundary. Although not specifically tested, the fact that significant differences can be detected between methods, both of which calculate the centroid from large numbers of points, suggests that two-point methods should be even less reproducible.

Centroid for a Contraction Sequence

Once the center for an individual frame is defined, it is next necessary to determine the appropriate center of reference against which to compare motion throughout the contraction sequence. Again, two basic choices are available: (1) the fixed center or fixed axis methods and (2) the floating center or floating axis methods. In a fixed system, all motion throughout the cardiac cycle is referred to the center of a particular frame (end-diastolic or end-systolic) or to the average of the centers of all frames in the contraction sequence (fixed average; see Fig. 21–7). In a floating system, the centers of all frames/fields are calculated independently and superimposed. Fixed internal references are similar in effect to external references; however, they provide an origin for sampling and rotation.

Figure 21–8 illustrates the theoretic considerations involved in this choice. Figure 21–8A diagrammatically depicts normal symmetric short axis contraction of the heart with no translation. Inward motion at all points is similar, and the centers of area of both contours should be identical. Figure 21–8B illustrates the same symmetric pattern of contraction with superimposition of anteriorly directed translation. Because of the translation, the systolic contour is shifted anteriorly and the apparent separation between the anterior portion of the systolic and diastolic contours is reduced, while posteriorly, the separation between the contours is increased. If wall motion is determined from these contours, it will appear to be reduced anteriorly and exaggerated posteriorly. If the center of each contour in Figure 21–8B is calculated and superimposed (floating center of reference), then the end-systolic contour is appropriately repositioned, and calculated motion will again appear symmetric about the circumference. Finally, Figure 21–8C illustrates a combination of translation and dyskinesis. The end-systolic contour, enclosed in the stippled area, is again shifted anteriorly by the translation vector. In this example, however, there is a superimposed dyskinetic segment along the anterior surface. Because of this region of dyskinesis, the calculated end-systolic centroid will shift toward the dyskinetic area, increasing the relative length of end-systolic radii to normal segments and decreasing radial lengths to abnormal regions. If the end-systolic and end-diastolic centroids are superimposed (floating centroid), the resulting fractional excursion in the infarct zone will be spuriously increased while excursion along the opposite wall will be apparently diminished. If a fixed end-diastolic reference is

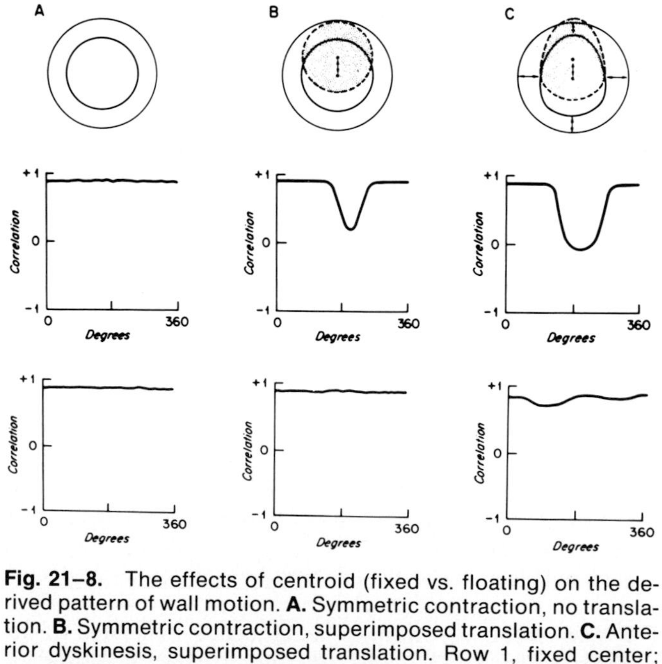

Fig. 21–8. The effects of centroid (fixed vs. floating) on the derived pattern of wall motion. **A.** Symmetric contraction, no translation. **B.** Symmetric contraction, superimposed translation. **C.** Anterior dyskinesis, superimposed translation. Row 1, fixed center; row 2, floating center. (See text for details.) (From Mann DL, Gillam LD, Weyman AE: Cross-sectional echocardiographic assessment of regional left ventricular performance and myocardial perfusion. Prog Cardiovasc Dis 29:1, 1986.)

employed, the abnormal region is appropriately localized but the degree of both normal and abnormal motion is exaggerated by the amount of the translation vector. Thus, in theory, a moving center should appropriately correct for translation in the normal heart while masking the effects and location of dyskinesis in the ischemic ventricle. A fixed center, in contrast, will represent translation as abnormal function in the normal ventricle, will permit correct localization and quantitation of function in the nontranslating ischemic ventricle, and will overestimate both normal and abnormal function in the ischemic translating ventricle.

Once the properties of these different centroids are understood, it is possible to infer the presence or absence of translation and some rotational components from the effects of centroid selection on the calculated pattern of motion. For example, if short axis motion in the normal ventricle is symmetric about both a fixed and floating center, then it can be reasonably assumed that no translation is present. Likewise, if normal contraction is symmetric about only a floating center at all short axis levels, then it can be presumed that translation is present with the magnitude and direction of the translation vector corresponding to that of centroid migration. In contrast, if normal contraction is symmetric about a fixed and floating center at one short axis level but not another—in other words, if the ventricle appears to translate in one tomographic view but not in another—then rotation is implied about a minor axis whose orientation is orthogonal to the apparent "translation" vector in the affected plane (see Figs. 21–3 and 21–4).

The results of most clinical and experimental studies to date have been consistent with this theoretic construct. For example, in patients with established infarction, where dyskinesis should be more prominent than translation, both fixed and floating systems have been shown to detect abnormal segmental function.[23] The floating axis system, however, fails to localize wall motion abnormalities as clearly as the fixed axis system. In contrast, following uncomplicated coronary bypass surgery, where anteromedial translation[32,33] is typical, septal shortening in either the apical four-chamber or parasternal short axis views appears significantly decreased compared to baseline values, and lateral wall motion is exaggerated if a fixed axis system is employed. Correction for translation using a floating center of reference normalizes both septal and lateral wall excursion.

When true dyssynergy complicates translation, as in the patient with postoperative infarction, a fixed axis system tends to be less sensitive in detecting segmental dysfunction because dyssynergy involving the wall opposite the translation vector will tend to be obscured. In this situation, a floating system will detect a greater number of truly abnormal segments and classify a smaller percentage of normal segments as abnormal (Fig. 21–9).

Because the projection of the cardiac translation vector and its effect on wall motion will vary in each view, the most appropriate reference system may also vary with view in the same study.[43] In addition, ventricular rotation around the minor axis may appear as translation at levels above and below the axis of rotation and may require correction that is not necessary at the level of the rotational axis.

In summary, the optimal centroid (fixed vs. floating) for the assessment of wall motion appears to depend on the conditions under which the heart is imaged. While unanimity does not exist[23,42,45,46] with regard to the optimal centroid for determination of wall motion in the clinical setting, experimental data[43] suggest that in the nontranslating model, any "fixed" centroid provides a more accurate assessment of the extent of abnormal wall motion than does a floating centroid. Further, these data would suggest that no one fixed centroid method is better than any other. However, under conditions where excessive translation of the heart occurs, such as might be seen following cardiac surgery,[30,31] a floating axis approach better defines the location of abnormal wall motion. Whether this floating axis approach will also accurately delineate the extent of abnormal wall motion remains to be determined, but it is unlikely that it will ever approach the accuracy of a fixed centroid in a nontranslating model.

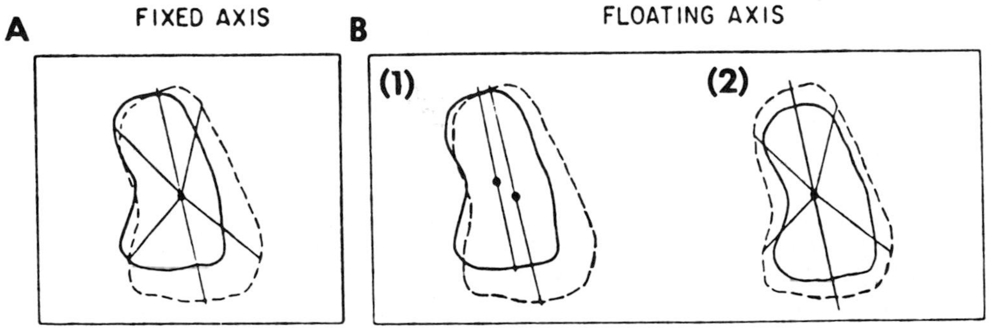

Fig. 21–9. Schematic of fixed **(A)** and floating **(B)** axis systems in the apical four-chamber view. For the fixed system, radii are generated from the midpoint of the end-diastolic centroid (bisector of the end-diastolic long axis). In the floating axis system, the end-diastolic and end-systolic centroids are superimposed to compensate for translation. Thus, the extent of shortening along a given radius is determined by the centroid chosen. (From Force T, et al.: Quantitative two-dimensional echocardiographic analysis of regional wall motion in patients with perioperative myocardial infarction. Circulation 70:233, 1984. Reproduced by permission of the American Heart Association, Inc.)

References used to Define End-Diastole and End-Systole

Once the reference system for individual frames and for the cardiac cycle has been defined, it is necessary to define cardiac motion or separation between fixed reference points in the cardiac cycle. Figure 21–10 illustrates the relationship of such a radial coordinate system to the endocardial intercepts of the left ventricular cavity. In Figure 21–10A, the radii are plotted at 30° intervals for simplicity, and the endocardial intercepts are depicted only at end-diastole and end-systole. Figure 21–10B shows a three-dimensional plot of the change in the distance of the endocardial intercepts for each ray from the ventricular centroid over time for three cardiac cycles. In this idealized example, ventricular contraction and relaxation are assumed to be symmetric, and target motion is represented as a sine wave. At end-diastole, the endocardial intercept along each radius is at its greatest distance from the ventricular centroid, while at end-systole, the endocardial intercept is closest to the centroid and therefore the ray length is shortest. The distance from the peak of each wave to its nadir represents an individual systolic contraction.

In actual practice, however, contraction and relaxation are not truly symmetric, and the radial change along individual rays is not equal. Further, the apparent amplitude of contraction may also vary depending on the references used to define end-diastole and end-systole. Because there is no general agreement concerning the optimal method for defining these references, it is important to understand the variation in the resulting data that individual choices may produce.

The most common method (based on the angiographic precedent) is to assume that the frame with the largest cavity area represents end-diastole, while that with the smallest cavity area represents end-systole.[47–51] The portions of the cardiac cycle that each of these references should include, unfortunately, vary with the model being studied. In the open-chest canine model, the shape of the ventricle tends to become more spherical during isovolumic contraction, while in the closed chest dog, the ventricle shifts toward a more elliptic configuration. These changes in shape are related to ventricular volume, with the ventricle becoming more spherical during isovolumetric systole at lower volumes and more elliptic as ventricular volume increases. Because the open-chest animal is relatively volume-depleted, sphericallization is noted in that preparation. In humans, there appears to be general agreement that the transverse diameter of the endocardial cavity decreases during the pre-ejection phase of systolic contraction,[52–54] while the epicardial transverse diameter increases because of muscular thickening.[55] Thus, the frame with the largest area will differ with the type of image recorded (apical or short axis) and the model (open vs. closed chest) being used.

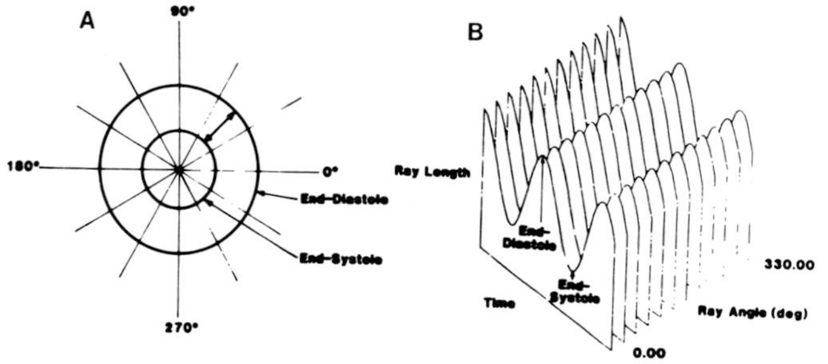

Fig. 21–10. The relationship of the radial coordinate system to the endocardial intercepts of the ventricular cavity. **A.** Radii are plotted at 30° intervals for simplicity, and the endocardial intercepts are depicted only at end-diastole and end-systole. **B.** A three-dimensional plot generated from these data. In this plot, the change in distance of the endocardial intercept of each radius from the ventricular centroid is plotted over time for three cycles. In this idealized example, ventricular contraction and relaxation are assumed to be symmetric and represented as a sine wave. At end-diastole, the endocardial intercept along each ray is at its greatest distance from the ventricular centroid, while at end-systole, the endocardial intercept is closest to the centroid, and therefore the length of the ray is shortest. The distance from the peak of each wave to the nadir represents an individual systolic contraction. (From Mann DL, Gillam LD, Weyman AE: Cross-sectional echocardiographic assessment of regional left ventricular performance and myocardial perfusion. Prog Cardiovasc Dis 29:1, 1986.)

Therefore, in human and closed chest animal studies, defining end-diastole as the frame before the onset of initial inward motion would include isovolumetric systole in the contraction sequence. In the open-chest animal, however, this will likely not be the case because in isovolumetric systole, the ventricle becomes more spheric and increases in cross-sectional area. In apical views, these shape changes can be appreciated, but the relationship of a single-plane area to ventricular volume will still vary.

Other commonly used references for end-diastole include the R wave of the electrocardiogram and the point of mitral valve closure determined from a simultaneous phonocardiogram or M-mode or two-dimensional echocardiographic image. Assuming there is no delay in electromechanical activation, these references should be comparable to the largest cavity area in humans and the closed chest dog. In the open-chest animal, however, these references may result in underestimation of the maximal target distance from the centroid, because the short axis cross-sectional area would be expected to increase during isovolumic contraction in this model.

Selection of the frame with the smallest cavity area to represent end-systole includes the period up to but not including isovolumetric relaxation,[50,56] because a slight but significant increase in ventricular chamber diameter and angiographically measured volume are noted during the isovolumetric phase of ventricular relaxation. The frame with the smallest cavity area should correspond to the time of aortic valve closure, while some increase in cavity area should occur between aortic valve closure and mitral opening, resulting in potential underestimation of excursion if the latter reference is used.

When individual radii or area segments are analyzed, these relationships become more complex because all points around the circumference do not reach their point of maximal excursion simultaneously. As a result, variation in the selection of temporal points for analysis of excursion may produce significant changes in the magnitude of recorded contraction. For example, a difference of two short axis frames at end-systole (66 msec) has been shown capable of causing a greater than 60% difference in the recorded amplitude of contraction for an individual segment.[31] By measuring excursion from the point in the cardiac cycle with the largest segment area of radial length to the smallest, the degree of variability within a given normal subject can be reduced but not eliminated.[31] This also requires digitization of all fields within the systolic contraction sequence as well as those immediately preceding end-diastole and following end-systole. In the apical views, mitral valve motion can be visualized and offers an alternative reference. Again, however, significant variability can be expected around the time of mitral valve opening and closure.

In the ischemic ventricle, visual reference (i.e., the frame with the largest cavity area or frame before the onset of inward motion) is useful only until the dyssynergic portion of the ventricular contour approaches 50%. At that point, all visual ability to discriminate systole from diastole is lost, and some external reference (i.e., valve motion, the electrocardiogram, or phonocardiogram) must be used to define at least one if not both of these points.

Selecting the Parameters to be Measured

Once end-systole and end-diastole have been defined, function can in theory be assessed using any of the excursion-based measurements: (1) the radial change from end-diastole to end-systole; (2) sector area shrinkage from end-diastole to end-systole; (3) perimeter shrinkage between rays; or (4) measurement of wall thickening.

Radial change and sector area shrinkage provide similar information. The major advantage of the area method is its tendency to mean data, making it less subject to local irregularities when large area subdivisions are used. Not surprisingly, the major reported difference in these methods has been in the interobserver variability or accuracy with which these measures can be defined.[22,23,32] For example, it has been reported[22] that the measurement of shortening along a given ray is less sensitive, specific, and accurate than area change methods in detecting the location of abnormal segmental wall motion for divisions up to octants. For smaller divisions, 5 to 45°,[42] on the other hand, no significant difference between area change and radial methods has been noted in the detection of abnormal segmental wall motion. In fact, reported intraobserver variability (day-to-day) has been somewhat less for the radial method (range 7 to 9%) than for the area technique (range 9 to 13%). It appears, therefore, that the resolution required to measure changes in functional infarct size, there should be little difference between methods. It is important to realize that these studies have considered only patients with large infarctions; thus, the actual sensitivity of their methods may be somewhat less than reported, particularly for less extensive myocardial infarctions. Further, the relative accuracy of these methods has been compared only in identifying the location of abnormal wall motion and has not, as yet, been tested in the quantification of (1) the histologic extent of infarction, (2) the degree of abnormal wall motion (i.e., hypokinesis, akinesis, or dyskinesis); or (3) the extent of global left ventricle dysfunction. Thus, the quantitative precision of these methods has not truly been examined.

Although it can be presumed that the length of the perimeter between rays showing normal motion would shrink more than in a region of abnormal contraction, this parameter has not found clinical utility.

Wall thickening can also be measured along radii or can be expressed as a change in the myocardial area within sectors, from diastole to systole. Although both approaches have been used, the latter seems preferable because it would be less sensitive to small irregularities in the digitized contour.

Methods of Measuring the Extent and Severity of Abnormal Wall Motion

Having aligned systolic and diastolic contours using either an internal or external reference system, and decided which parameter of regional function is to be measured, it is necessary to choose a method to quantify the extent and severity of abnormal endocardial motion and/or wall thickening.

Although it is possible to describe the extent of abnormal wall motion by simply measuring the length of the circumference over which the ventricular contours either coincide or overlap,[9,15,16] this method is limited, because it does not allow for accurate quantification of the severity of abnormal wall motion. To quantify regional wall motion, therefore, it is necessary to either construct a series of chords from a reference within the ventricular outline or between contours to consecutive points along the ventricular border. This can be achieved either by (1) constructing radial chords between a centroid and the ventricular contours, (2) constructing perpendicular chords from a reference line drawn within the ventricle to the ventricular contours, (3) constructing both perpendicular and radial chords from a reference line within the ventricle, or (4) constructing perpendicular chords between the ventricular contours.

Construction of Radial Chords Between a Centroid and Ventricular Boundaries. When an internal reference has been defined, it is possible to construct radial chords between the reference point and both systolic and diastolic contours if endocardial excursion is to be measured or between the centroid and endocardial and epicardial boundaries if wall thickening is to be measured (Fig. 21–11A). Although construction of radial chords is simple and ideally suited to the assessment of regional function in short axis views of the ventricle, it is not an ideal method for assessing regional motion from apical views, because it is associated with a wide variation in the range of normal motion, which in turn limits the ability to detect the true extent of regional dysfunction.

Construction of Perpendicular Chords From a Reference Line Drawn Within the Ventricle. Although primarily developed for the assessment of regional wall motion from 30° (RAO) ventriculograms,[47] construction of a series of regularly spaced chords perpendicular to a reference line, drawn between the apex and a point at the

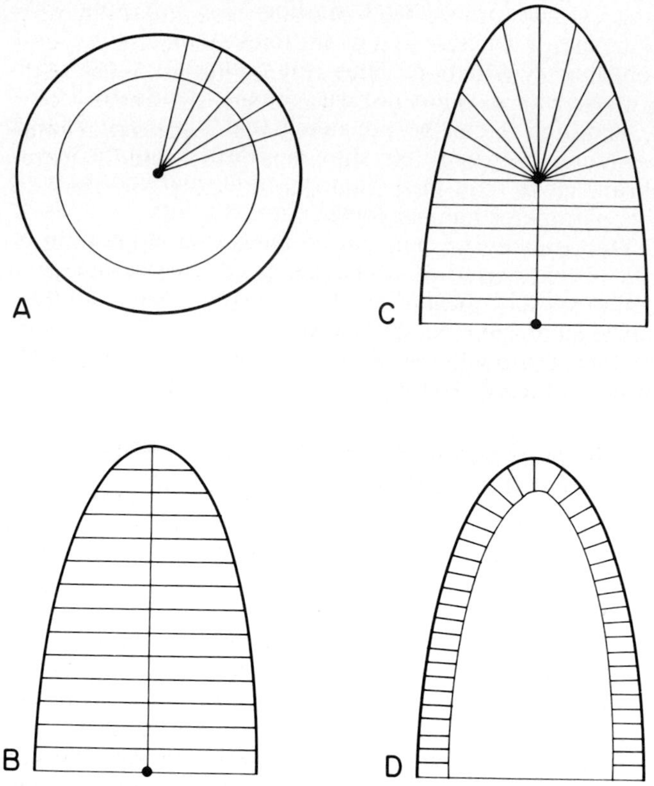

Fig. 21–11. Methods of measuring the extent and severity of abnormal wall motion: **A.** Radial chords, constructed between the centroid and the (inner) end-systolic and (outer) end-diastolic ventricular contours. **B.** A series of parallel, evenly spaced, chords constructed perpendicular to the long axis of the ventricle. **C.** A series of perpendicular chords constructed perpendicular to the long axis of the ventricle, from base to midventricle, and a series of radii constructed from the midpoint of the long axis of the ventricle from the midventricle to apex. **D.** A series of perpendicular chords constructed between the (inner) end-systolic and (outer) end-diastolic ventricular contours.

midbase of the ventricle, has been used to assess regional function from apical two- and four-chamber views (Fig. 21–11B). This method is not suitable for analysis of wall motion from short axis views and tends to result in overestimation of apical wall motion in apical views. The major limitation of this method, therefore, is the high degree of variability in the range of normal apical motion, caused predominantly by the sensitivity of the algorithm to small changes in positioning of the midventricular reference line.

Construction of a Combination of Perpendicular and Radial Chords. In an effort to reduce variability in the range of apical motion as assessed from apical images, an alternate algorithm has been employed in which a combination of perpendicular and radial chords are constructed between a central reference line and the ventricular contours. In this construct, perpendicular chords are used to measure motion at the base of the ventricle, and radial chords are used to measure apical motion (Fig. 21–11C). Although this method reduces the degree of variability in the range of normal motion in the region of the apex and is more sensitive to apical abnormality, it is still limited by the variability encountered when defining the central reference line from which the chords originate and therefore has not been widely used for the echocardiographic assessment of regional function.

Construction of Perpendicular Chords Between Ventricular Boundaries: The Center Line Method. An alternate method of measuring the distance between ventricular boundaries is to construct, and then measure, a series of perpendicular lines between the ventricular contours (Fig. 21–11D). Although this can be achieved manually, chord placement and alignment have been automated using an algorithm that defines a reference line midway between the ventricular contours from which a series of regularly spaced chords are constructed. Although this center line method was developed for quantification of regional wall motion from angiographic images of the left ventricle,[57,58] it has been applied to echocardiographic imaging.

For regional motion to be quantified by the center-line technique, it is necessary to construct a line midway between the end-diastolic and end-systolic endocardial contours. For this "center line" to be derived, the end-diastolic contour is initially smoothed using a sliding point filter. This smoothed contour is then divided into a large number of equidistant points (up to 200). Next, a series of perpendicular lines are constructed to the tangent of an arc passing through each increment of three adjacent points along this smoothed end-diastolic boundary. To avoid chords crossing one another, intercepts along the ventricular contours are sought only from the beginning of the last intercept, over a preset radial arc. If a point on either ventricular contour cannot be found, the intercept is taken to be the same as the previous (adjacent) intercept. Because each perpendicular chord extends through ventricular contours, it is possible to define the length of each chord. The midpoint of each chord is then used to define the initial coordinates of the center line. Once defined, the center line is repeatedly smoothed, and a series of 100 perpendicular chords is then constructed, with the chords drawn at regular intervals along the center line as described previously. The repeated smoothing of the center line is important, because it ensures that each chord is constructed perpendicular to the true end-diastolic and end-systolic contours. Hence, in this way motion at each point along the ventricular contour is defined as the absolute length of each chord constructed along the center line. Because absolute chord length is measured from the end-diastolic contour, inward motion is assigned a positive value, and outward motion (corresponding to areas of dyskinesis) is assigned a negative value (Fig. 21–12).

Use of the center line method to assess wall thickening requires that a center line be constructed between the endocardial and epicardial contours of both the end-diastolic and end-systolic images using the algorithm described previously. The difference in chord length between systole and diastole is taken to represent the degree of regional thickening.

The advantage of the center line technique is that it can be used to measure endocardial excursion or wall thickening with both internal and external reference systems. Further, because assessment of normal motion

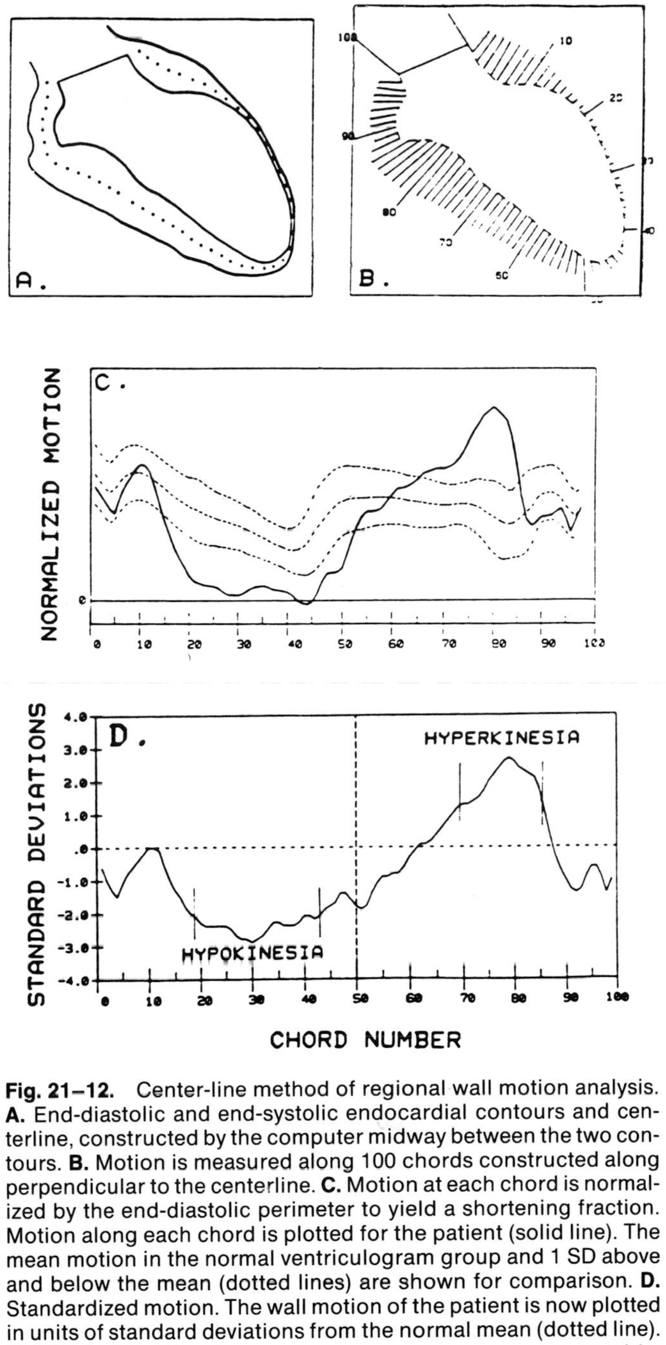

Fig. 21–12. Center-line method of regional wall motion analysis. **A.** End-diastolic and end-systolic endocardial contours and centerline, constructed by the computer midway between the two contours. **B.** Motion is measured along 100 chords constructed along perpendicular to the centerline. **C.** Motion at each chord is normalized by the end-diastolic perimeter to yield a shortening fraction. Motion along each chord is plotted for the patient (solid line). The mean motion in the normal ventriculogram group and 1 SD above and below the mean (dotted lines) are shown for comparison. **D.** Standardized motion. The wall motion of the patient is now plotted in units of standard deviations from the normal mean (dotted line). The normal ventriculogram group mean is now represented by the horizontal zero line. Vertical lines delimit the most hypokinetic and hyperkinetic portions of the anterior and inferior regions of the ventricle. (From Sheehan FH, et al.: Advantages and applications of the centerline method for characterizing regional ventricular function. Circulation 74:293, 1986. Reproduced by permission of the American Heart Association.)

from apical views is associated with less variability than that seen when regional function is assessed using radial chords in these views, this method of measurement may be a more sensitive means of assessing the extent of regional dysfunction. Although the center line approach has been validated for the assessment of wall motion from ventriculographic images, which provide a silhouette of the ventricle, difficulties are encountered when it is used to analyze echocardiographic (tomographic) images, due to the effects of translation and rotation. In an attempt to overcome these problems, some algorithms attempt to correct for noncardiac motion by referencing the end-diastolic and end-systolic images to an arbitrary point, such as the midpoint of the mitral annular plane, or the center of a line constructed between the apex and midbase, and then rotating the contours along these reference lines.

Despite the fact that the center line method is yet to be validated as a means of assessing the true extent of abnormal wall motion, or the extent of infarction, from echocardiographic apical or short axis planes, the algorithm has been incorporated into several commercially available systems used to assess regional function.[59,60]

Defining the Angular Separation Between Radii

There is little agreement or data concerning the degree of angular separation between radii/chords necessary to detect changes in the extent of abnormal wall motion. Although algorithms with the potential to sample up to 200 points have been described, most clinical and experimental studies have used fewer sampling intervals. The computer algorithm used in our laboratory samples target motion at 5° increments around the ventricular circumference and outputs data at 5°- or 10°-intervals. Excluding other potential sources of error or variability, a 10° sampling interval should accurately detect changes involving >5.6% of the ventricular circumference. In contrast, if the ventricle were sampled at 12 points, a change involving 16% of the circumference could, in theory, go undetected. We have assessed changes in functional infarct extent using the correlation methods described later for 6, 24, 48 and 72 hours postinfarction for both individual planes ($n = 50$) and the entire ventricle ($n = 10$) and observed that, after correction for variation in infarct size between animals, a 5.5% global change in the circumferential extent of abnormal wall motion was required to be considered significant.[63] Thus, a sampling interval that will identify changes at this level of spatial resolution appears reasonable; however, this is clearly a question that needs further study.

Criteria for Defining Normal and Abnormal

The goal of all quantitative echocardiographic methods of wall motion analysis is to objectively define the extent and severity of abnormality. A fundamental aspect of the development of quantitative methods, therefore, is the establishment of criteria for normal and abnormal. This can be achieved either (1) by establishing a range of normality and then defining anything that falls outside that range as abnormal[23,24,34,42] or (2) by comparing observed motion to the extent and density of infarction or area of ischemia and then determining the degree of dysfunction that best correlates with the extent of the histologic or flow abnormality.[36]

The establishment of a range of normality is based on the visual perception that normal contraction is characterized by symmetry in amplitude and phase. This being the case, a range of normal function should be definable for the ventricle as a whole or for individual anatomic regions. Unfortunately, both experimental[64] and clinical studies[31,42,34] have demonstrated major regional differences in the normal pattern of contraction recorded by cross-sectional echocardiography with a range of 0 to 100% for fractional area change and 0 to 150% for wall thickening being reported.[31] In addition, virtually all large quantitative studies of normal ventricular contraction have found isolated "normal" segments in which dyskinesis or wall thinning have been recorded. Because these data are derived from preselected normal persons, such segments are usually considered artifacts and discarded from analysis.[31] In a prospective study, however, this would not be possible. In addition, significant intersubject differences have been reported in both mean cavity area change and wall thickening. Further, although reported data are contradictory, variation in the pattern of contraction both around the ventricle and from apex to base has also been reported.[35,36]

Thus, any statistical definition of normality is complicated by the broad range of normal radial contraction and thickening that varies around the perimeter of the ventricle and from apex to base and is influenced by the center of reference selected, the method of measurement (radial vs. perpendicular chords) and changes in loading conditions. In addition, any standard statistical definition of normality (i.e., mean +/− 2 standard deviations [SD]) will result in 5% of normal rays being defined as "abnormal." Given the large number of rays typically sampled in an experimental study, this can lead to an unacceptable number of control rays or segments being classified as abnormal. Increasing the confidence limits to 3 SD, unfortunately, will result in a prohibitive number of abnormal rays being classified as normal. Further studies in our laboratory that defined as abnormal any ray whose end-diastolic-to-end-systolic fractional radial change fell outside 2 SD from the normal mean yielded a very poor correlation between the extent of abnormal motion thus defined and the circumferential extent of histologically defined infarction.[36]

An alternative and more arbitrary approach is to set an absolute threshold below which endocardial excursion will be considered abnormal. This threshold may be optimized by relating the extent of abnormal wall motion thus defined to some independent measure of the extent of left ventricle abnormality (e.g., histochemical or histologic extent of infarction, or circumferential extent of reduced blood flow). In practice, however, this approach has been difficult and the results inconsistent. Although in individual studies it has been possible to define such a threshold, the absolute value has varied from study to study. For example, in one study in the acute experimental model it was found that the best correlation between nitro-blue tetrazolium staining technique (TTC)-defined infarction and the extent of abnormal wall motion at 6 hours postinfarction was obtained using a percentage of radial change of less than 20% to define abnormality.[36] In a second study in a similar model, it was found that a threshold fractional radial change of 10% correlated most closely with the area at risk for infarction defined by myocardial contrast echocardiography at 3 hours postligation.[65] In yet another study, a threshold fractional radial change of 15% yielded the best correlation with histologic infarct span in animals studied at 72 hours.[63] Because contraction depends on heart rate, preload, and afterload, this variability is not surprising. Recognition of the problem, however, makes it no less difficult to deal with, and we currently feel that no absolute threshold between normal and abnormal can be established. Others have suggested that because hypokinesis is undefinable, dyskinesis be used as the threshold for abnormality.[31] Although highly specific for ischemia, this threshold would classify a large number of abnormal rays (i.e., rays intersecting regions of infarct) as normal. Also, when we have quantitatively compared the extent of dyskinesis sampled at 10° intervals to infarct span, we have consistently observed a poor correlation.

As with normal contraction, the definition of abnormal is also complicated by temporal variability of con-

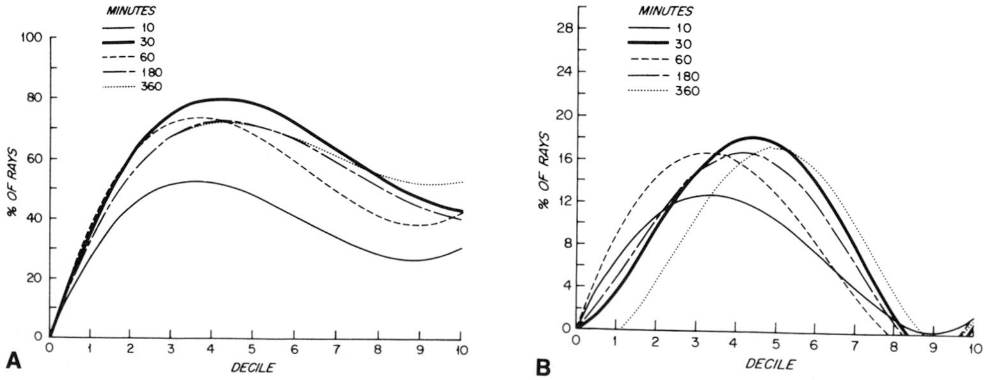

Fig. 21–13. A. The percentage of rays exhibiting dyskinesia per decile following acute coronary occlusion in a canine model. The percentage of rays exhibiting dyskinesia is shown on the y axis, and the time during systole, divided into deciles, is on the x axis. End-diastole is at 0 end-systole is at 10 on the x axis. The fitted polynomial functions for each of the acute study periods are curves 1 to 5. Curve 1 = 10 minutes (solid line); curve 2 = 30 minutes (dark solid line); curve 3 = 60 minutes (dashed line); curve 4 = 180 minutes (dot-dashed line); curve 5 = 360 minutes (dotted line). **B.** Percentage of rays exhibiting maximal amplitude of dyskinesia per decile following acute coronary occlusion. (From Ascah KJ, et al.: Evolution of the temporal contraction sequence after acute experimental myocardial infarction. J Am Coll Cardiol 13:730, 1989. Reprinted with permission from the American College of Cardiology.)

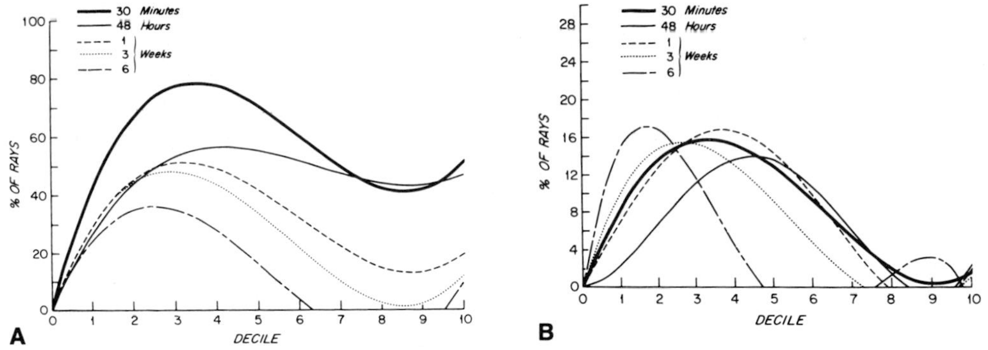

Fig. 21–14. A. The percentage of rays exhibiting dyskinesia per decile in the 6-week period following coronary occlusion in a canine model. The fitted polynomial functions for the chronic study periods are shown in curves 1 to 5. The axes are the same as for the study of acute coronary occlusion (Fig. 21–13). Curve 1 = 30 minutes (dark solid line); curve 2 = 48 hours (single solid line); curve 3 = 1 week (dashed line); curve 4 = 3 weeks (dotted line); curve 5 = 6 weeks (dot-dashed line). The spatial extent of dyskinesia decreased and the temporal pattern of dyskinesia changed progressively from 30 minutes to 48 hours, to 1 week after coronary ligation ($p < .00125$ 30 minutes vs. 48 hours vs. 1 week). **B.** The percentage of rays exhibiting maximal amplitude of dyskinesia per decile in the 6-week period following coronary occlusion. (From Ascah KJ, et al.: Evolution of the temporal contraction sequence after acute experimental myocardial infarction. J Am Coll Cardiol 13:730, 1989. Reprinted with permission from the American College of Cardiology.)

traction within ischemic zones. Early studies revealed that quantitation of endocardial motion from end-diastole to end-systole did not always produce results that corresponded to the visual impression of the degree or extent of abnormality. This observation led to a series of studies to examine the temporal pattern of dyskinetic motion within ischemic zones and its effect on the echocardiographic analysis of abnormal wall motion.[35] As illustrated in Figure 21–13, these studies showed that maximal dyskinesis in animals studied 1 hour after the onset of myocardial infarction occurred most frequently during the fourth decile of the normalized contraction sequence, while at end-systole, only a small percentage of the study rays were at their farthest distance from the center of reference. Figure 21–14 illustrates, how, when studied at multiple points up to 6 weeks, this pattern varies, with both the time and extent of maximal dyskinesis, shifting to an earlier portion of systole as the infarct matures.

Detection of this spatial and temporal variability of contraction in ischemic zones as well as in normal segments requires examination of motion throughout the entire contraction sequence, not just at end-diastole and end-systole. This involves digitization of multiple frames, which when sampled at multiple radial points, yields a large matrix of data such as that illustrated in Figure 21–15. Assuming that 10 fields are digitized from end-diastole to end-systole with target motion sampled at 36 radial points, such a table would contain 360 data points. If thickening is also considered, an additional table with another 360 data points would also be generated. In a natural history study, multiple planes are sampled at multiple periods. which yields an enormous volume of data. One method to define *normal* and *abnormal*

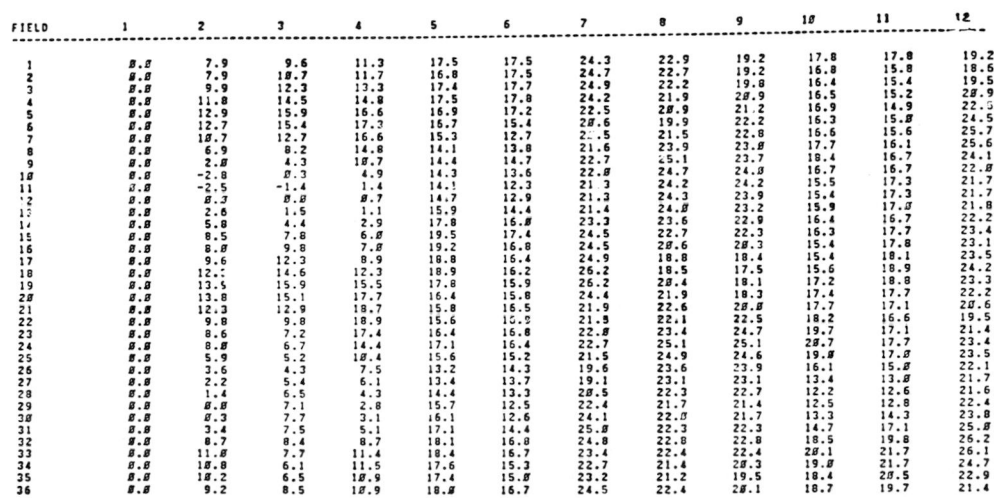

FIELD	1	2	3	4	5	6	7	8	9	10	11	12
1	0.0	7.9	9.6	11.3	17.5	17.5	24.3	22.9	19.2	17.8	17.8	19.2
2	0.0	7.9	10.7	11.7	16.8	17.5	24.7	22.7	19.2	16.8	15.8	18.6
3	0.0	9.9	12.3	13.3	17.4	17.7	24.9	22.2	19.8	16.4	15.4	19.5
4	0.0	11.8	14.5	14.8	17.5	17.8	24.2	21.9	20.9	16.5	15.2	20.9
5	0.0	12.9	15.9	16.6	16.9	17.2	22.5	20.9	21.2	16.9	14.9	22.5
6	0.0	12.7	15.4	17.3	16.7	15.4	20.6	19.9	22.2	16.3	15.0	24.5
7	0.0	10.7	12.7	16.6	15.3	12.7	[illegible]	21.5	22.8	16.6	15.6	25.7
8	0.0	6.9	8.2	14.8	14.1	13.8	21.6	23.9	23.0	17.7	16.1	25.6
9	0.0	2.0	4.3	10.7	14.4	14.7	22.7	25.1	23.7	18.4	16.7	24.1
10	0.0	-2.8	0.3	4.9	14.3	13.6	22.0	24.7	24.0	16.7	16.7	22.0
11	0.0	-2.5	-1.4	1.4	14.1	12.3	21.3	24.2	24.2	15.5	17.3	21.7
12	0.0	0.3	0.0	0.7	14.7	12.9	21.3	24.3	23.9	15.4	17.3	21.7
13	0.0	2.6	1.5	1.1	15.9	14.4	21.4	24.0	23.2	15.9	17.0	21.8
14	0.0	5.8	4.4	2.9	17.8	16.0	23.3	23.6	22.9	16.4	16.7	22.2
15	0.0	8.5	7.8	6.0	19.5	17.4	24.5	22.7	22.3	16.3	17.7	23.4
16	0.0	8.0	9.8	7.0	19.2	16.8	24.5	20.6	20.3	15.4	17.8	23.1
17	0.0	9.6	12.3	8.9	18.8	16.4	24.9	18.8	18.4	15.4	18.1	23.5
18	0.0	12.[illegible]	14.6	12.3	18.9	16.2	26.2	18.5	17.5	15.6	18.9	24.2
19	0.0	13.5	15.9	15.5	17.8	15.9	26.2	20.4	18.1	17.2	18.8	23.3
20	0.0	13.8	15.1	17.7	16.4	15.8	24.4	21.9	18.3	17.4	17.7	22.2
21	0.0	12.3	12.9	18.7	15.8	16.5	21.9	22.6	20.0	17.7	17.1	20.6
22	0.0	9.8	9.8	18.9	15.6	16.9	21.5	22.1	22.5	18.2	16.6	19.5
23	0.0	8.6	7.2	17.4	16.4	16.8	22.0	23.4	24.7	19.7	17.1	21.4
24	0.0	8.0	6.7	14.4	17.1	16.4	22.7	25.1	25.1	20.7	17.7	23.4
25	0.0	5.9	5.2	10.4	15.6	15.2	21.5	24.9	24.6	19.0	17.0	23.5
26	0.0	3.6	4.3	7.5	13.2	14.3	19.6	23.6	23.9	16.1	15.0	22.1
27	0.0	2.2	5.4	6.1	13.4	13.7	19.1	23.1	23.1	13.4	13.0	21.7
28	0.0	1.4	6.5	4.3	14.4	13.3	20.5	22.3	22.7	12.2	12.6	21.6
29	0.0	0.0	7.1	2.8	15.7	12.5	22.4	21.7	21.4	12.5	12.8	22.4
30	0.0	0.3	7.7	3.1	16.1	12.6	24.1	22.0	21.7	13.3	14.3	23.8
31	0.0	3.4	7.5	5.1	17.1	14.4	25.0	22.3	22.3	14.7	17.1	25.0
32	0.0	8.7	8.4	8.7	18.1	16.8	24.8	22.8	22.8	18.5	19.8	26.2
33	0.0	11.0	7.7	11.4	18.4	16.7	23.4	22.4	22.4	20.1	21.7	26.1
34	0.0	10.8	6.1	11.5	17.6	15.3	22.7	21.4	20.3	19.0	21.7	24.7
35	0.0	10.2	6.5	10.9	17.4	15.0	23.2	21.2	19.5	18.4	20.5	22.9
36	0.0	9.2	8.5	10.9	18.0	16.7	24.5	22.4	20.1	18.7	19.7	21.4

Fig. 21–15. Tabular display of fractional radial change recorded for each of the 36 equally spaced endocardial targets during a normal systolic contraction sequence. Target position (from 1 to 36) is listed in the left column. Target 1 corresponds to the midpoint between the papillary muscles. Sampling times (corresponding to echocardiographic field) are represented by successive columns (column 1, end-diastole; column 12, end-systole). In this example, the systolic contraction period consists of 12 echocardiographic fields (=12 × 16.5 msec). (From Mann DL, Gillam LD, Weyman AE: Cross-sectional echocardiographic assessment of regional left ventricular performance and myocardial perfusion. Prog Cardiovasc Dis 29:1, 1986.)

more satisfactorily, to synthesize the resulting data in a usable format, and to output it in a spatially correct graphic display, is the correlation approach described next.[36]

Assessment of Motion for the Entire Contraction Sequence: Correlation Methods for Analyzing Normal and Abnormal Wall Motion (Short Axis Views)

Given that the observed temporal and spatial variability in normal contraction confounds definition of normality when only two frames are sampled, and alternative method of analysis is necessary. One such approach is to assume symmetry of contraction along individual radii or a constant slope of contraction and comparing contraction along an unknown radii to these reference values. This can be achieved by (1) comparing contraction along a given radius (Ro) to the mean of all other radii at comparable time points or (2) by comparing the contractile motion of targets along Ro to established normal data. Comparison of contraction along a radius Ro to the mean contraction of all other radii for the same time interval is valid until roughly 50% of the ventricle becomes abnormal, at which point the mean also becomes abnormal and the observed relationship inverts. For example, if more than 50% of the sampled radii are dyskinetic, then the mean can be dyskinetic or negative, and a positively moving target will be defined as abnormal or oppositely moving relative to the mean. This problem occurs most commonly in short axis planes near the apex, because in these images, it is generally not possible to detect dyskinesia, which is due to the lack of an internal reference to define systole. Definition of the mean contraction slope for pooled radial data from a group of normal subjects and comparison of contraction along radii intersecting regions of "unknown" function to these group data obviates the inversion problem and yields a more stable reference.

This correlation process is described in Figure 21–16. For a given ray, the observed fractional radial change (end-diastole radius minus observed radius divided by end-diastolic radius), measured at sequential times in systole (i.e., every video field, 16.7 msec or frame, 33 msec) is plotted against the pooled normal value at comparable times. By the least squares regression technique, a line is then fitted to the data points, and the correlation coefficient is calculated. In Figure 21–16, three hypothetical situations are considered. For the first, motion along a normal ray at all points throughout systole, the fractional radial change along that radius is similar to that derived from the pooled normal data. Hence, there is a perfect linear fit and the correlation coefficient is 1. The opposite situation, in which there is progressive outward rather than inward motion, is also depicted. Although a straight line can again be fitted to these data points, the correlation coefficient (r) is negative. The real situation in infarcted portions of the ventricle is more accurately represented by the third set of data points. In this case, there is maximal outward motion early in systole with a tendency toward inward motion as systole proceeds. Although a line can be fitted to these points, the fit is poor, and the correlation coefficient is low. In the example illustrated, r = −.4. In general, therefore, the correlation coefficient derived for each ray simply reflects to what extent motion along that ray resembles composite motion along normal rays. An r value of 1 indicates normal motion; a value of 0 implies either random or no motion, and a negative value approaching −1 indicates motion in the opposite direction.

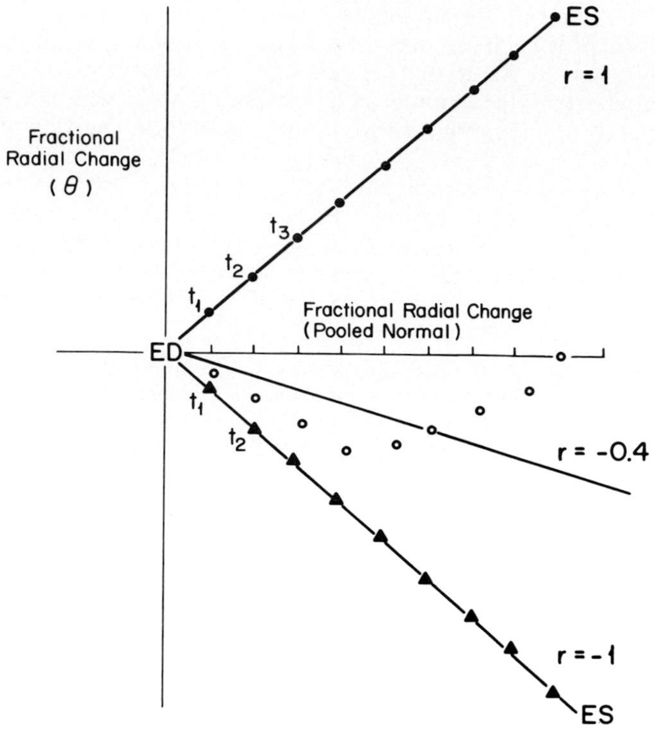

Fig. 21–16. Derivation of the correlation coefficients for individual radii. For each radii, the course of motion of endocardial target along that radius is correlated with the course of normal motion. This is equivalent to selecting a given radius and plotting the fractional radius change at different times during systole vs. pooled data from normal values for comparable points in time. A line is then fitted to these points using standard least squares linear regression techniques, and the associated r^2 statistic is calculated. Three hypothetical situations are depicted. Motion along a normal ray is depicted with closed circles. At all points through systole, the fractional radius change along that radius is the same as that obtained from pooled normal data. Hence, there is a perfect linear fit, and the correlation coefficient is 1.0. In the next situation (depicted by triangles), there is progressive outward rather than inward motion. Although a straight line can again be fitted to these data points, the correlation coefficient is −1.0. The situation in infarcted portions of the ventricle is more accurately represented by the third curve (open circles). In this case, there is maximal outward motion in early systole with a tendency for inward motion during the course of systole. Although a line can be fitted to these data, the fit is poor, and the correlation coefficient is low. In general therefore, the correlation coefficient derived for each ray simply reflects how much the motion along the ray being examined is like composite normal ray motion. A value of 1.0 indicates normal motion; a value of 0 implies either random or no motion, and a negative value implies motion in the opposite direction from normal. (From Mann DL, Gillam LD, Weyman AE: Cross-sectional echocardiographic assessment of regional left ventricular performance and myocardial perfusion. Prog Cardiovasc Dis 29:1, 1986.) ED = end diastole; ES = end systole.

As the next step in this analysis, the correlation coefficients for each ray are plotted against ray location, progressing sequentially around the circumference of the ventricle. This is illustrated in Figure 21–17, where the y axis in each plot represents the correlation coefficient and the x axis represents the ray position from 0 to 360°. Figure 21–17A contains data from the control period in an experimental study: motion around the circumference is uniformly similar to composite normal ray motion, and the correlation coefficients for all rays are near unity (r = .95). Following coronary occlusion, however, plots such as that in Figure 21–17B are obtained. As before, the correlation coefficients for the normal rays (in this example, 0 to 210°) are near unity. When the infarcted portion of the ventricle (210 to 340°) is approached, however, there is an abrupt decrease in the correlation coefficient with values, as in this case, generally becoming negative. To define the circumferential extent of abnormal wall motion by the correlation method, we first defined 95% confidence limits for the correlation coefficient of the baseline normal radii. Radii with correlation coefficients outside these limits were considered abnormal and the circumferential extent of abnormal wall motion thus defined is calculated.

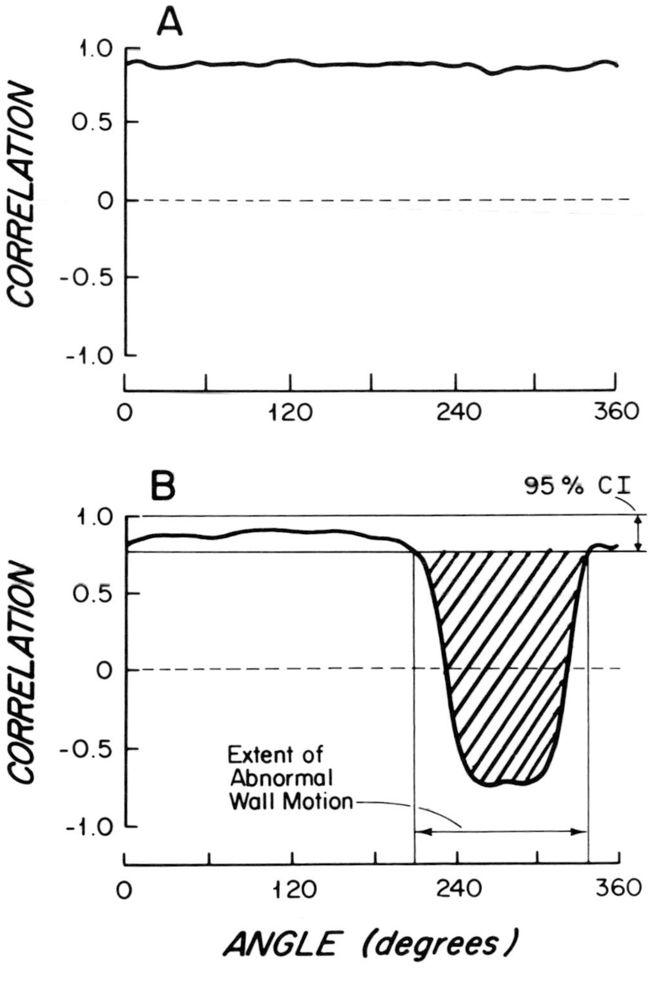

Fig. 21–17. Radially referenced display of the correlation analysis of wall motion in canine ventricles. **A.** Normal. **B.** Infarcted. Correlation coefficients are represented along the y axis, and ray position (degree) along the x axis (0° is a midpoint between papillary muscles). **A.** From a cross-sectional study of a normal animal. Motion around the circumference is uniformly similar to composite normal ray motion, and the correlation coefficients for all rays are near unity—in this example, 0.95. **B.** A representative plot of wall motion following experimental coronary occlusion. As in **A**, the correlation coefficients for the normal rays (in this example, 0° to 210°) are near unity. When one approaches the infarcted portion of the ventricle (210° to 300°), however, there is an abrupt fall in the correlation coefficient with values, as in this case, generally becoming negative. As illustrated, rays whose correlation coefficients fall outside the 95% confidence limits are considered to be abnormal.[62] CI = confidence interval.

Table 21–2. Comparison of Quantitative Methods of Measuring Abnormal Wall Motion/Blood Flow With Histologic Infarction[62]

	Extent of Abnormal Wall Motion/Flow vs. TTC Infarction	
	r	F value
Correlation—95% CL*	0.87	19.21
Correlation—FW†	0.78	10.23
ED-ES < 0.20‡	0.35	1.00
Maximum dyskinesis§	0.37	1.30
NBF < 0.75‖	0.85	17.30

TTC = nitro-blue tetrazolium staining technique.
* Correlation analysis—95% confidence limits.
† Correlation analysis—"full width of half maximum."
‡ End-diastolic to end-systolic excursion <0.20 end-diastolic radius.
§ Extent of dyskinesis at maximal dyskinesis.
‖ Normalized blood flow <0.75 of control.
(From Mann DL, Gillam LD, Weyman AE: Cross-sectional echocardiographic assessment of regional left ventricular performance and myocardial perfusion. Prog Cardiovasc Dis 29:1, 1986.)

Table 21–2 compares the relationship of abnormal wall motion assessed by three different techniques with histologic extent of infarction. The techniques are the correlation method; an end-diastolic to end-systolic excursion absolute threshold method (<20%, percentage radial change being defined as abnormal); and the point in the cardiac cycle at which maximal dyskinesis occurs. As illustrated, the correlation method using the 95% confidence limits for the normal rays as a threshold of normality provided the closest correlation with the extent of histologic infarction.

This method, which requires only that normal motion can be represented by a constant slope, is highly reproducible. The definition of abnormal wall motion it provides has been shown to correlate well with the histochemical and histologic extent of infarction, contrast-defined infarct region, and extent of abnormal blood flow. Although this method is clearly tedious and thus is poorly adapted to clinical implementation, it has yielded important information in the experimental setting. In addition to the correlation coefficient, the analysis also outputs the slope to the correlation. This provides a ray-by-ray comparison of observed with normal function; however, it has proven to be less accurate as a measure of infarct size.

Correction for Cardiac Rotation

Another point that, although seemingly minor, creates difficulties in the quantitative analysis of wall motion is cardiac rotation about the long axis. This rotation creates two problems. First, if the heart rotates 30° as it contracts, then an individual ray will intersect a point at end-systole that is 30° from the point on the perimeter that it intersected at end-diastole. Given the variability in end-diastolic segment lengths, if only end-systole and end-diastole are considered, this shift may make a normal ray appear abnormal or vice versa. Second, rotation can cause significant artifacts in the region of the papillary muscles. If the ventricular contour is not smoothed, rays extending from the centroid to the papillary muscles will have relatively short end-diastolic lengths, while those extending to the ventricular wall at the margins of the papillary muscle will be longer. If rotation causes the papillary muscle to cross one or more rays at end-systole, which were not crossed at end-diastole, then apparently exaggerated contraction of one ray group with apparent dyskinesis of an adjacent group will result. Although these types of artifacts can be recognized and corrected for in the normal ventricle, they frequently obscure the margins of an abnormal zone, and observer interaction in removing these artifacts invariably introduces some bias into the quantitative nature of the analysis. As a result, it is important to identify an internal reference and to rotate the contour of each digitized outline around the computed centroid for that frame until the external references are realigned. Thus, each frame/field is individually corrected for any rotation-induced artifact (Fig. 21–18). The major advantage of rotational correction is in the elimination of spuriously abnormal rays in control and normal studies. It has the further advantage of providing a uniform 0 reference for all the output data. Rotation is of less concern when larger area segments are analyzed and when the ventricular contours are smoothed.

Correction for rotation in apical views can be achieved empirically by rotating contours about a centroid, or by aligning images along an axis. This latter technique usually involves constructing a line between the apex and midbase. Images are then superimposed along this axis. Construction of this line is often a source of variability of measurement, however, especially in situations in which the apex is distorted. Further, error can also occur if the apical image is foreshortened. This variability necessarily widens the range of normal motion for each chord and reduces the ability to detect abnormal wall motion.

Correction for Variation in Heart Size

Because it is difficult to compare absolute numbers across patients of varying size, it is conventional to normalize both wall motion and thickening by dividing the absolute excursion or thickening by the end-diastolic circumference (or end-diastolic length, when apical measurements are made). Although this clearly has the desired effect, it is important when analyzing longitudinal studies to be certain that percentage changes actually reflect a true change in contraction and are not merely an artifact induced either by ventricular dilatation with an increase in the end-diastolic reference or a diminution in ventricular size with a corresponding decrease in this reference.

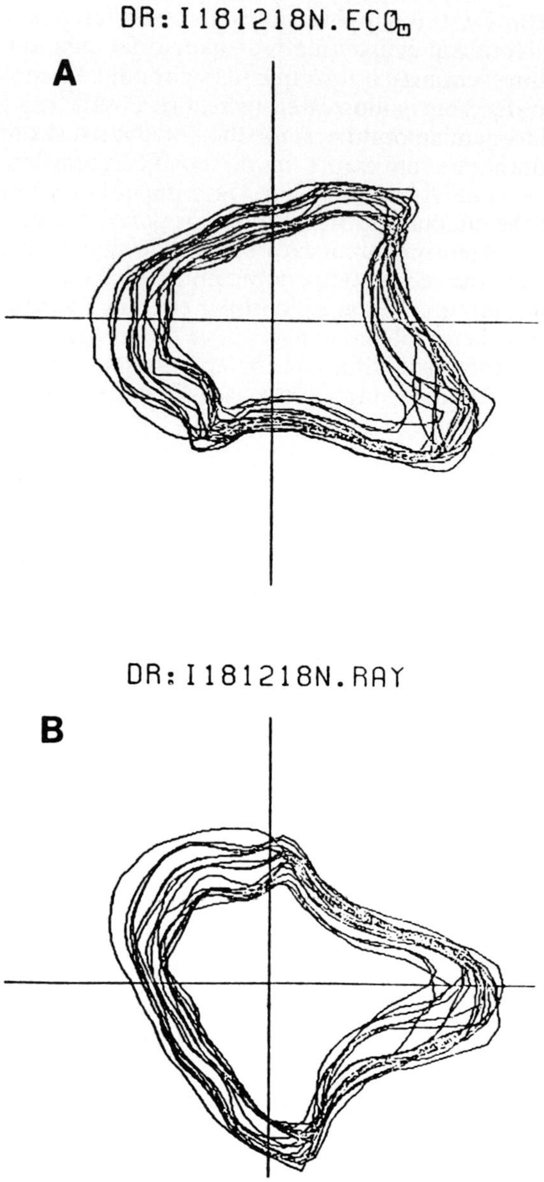

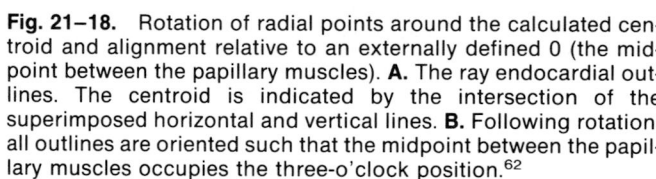

Fig. 21–18. Rotation of radial points around the calculated centroid and alignment relative to an externally defined 0 (the midpoint between the papillary muscles). **A.** The ray endocardial outlines. The centroid is indicated by the intersection of the superimposed horizontal and vertical lines. **B.** Following rotation, all outlines are oriented such that the midpoint between the papillary muscles occupies the three-o'clock position.[62]

Smoothing of Ventricular Contours

As echocardiographic image resolution improves, the irregularities present along the endocardial surface of the ventricle become more prominent. The most obvious of these are the papillary muscles; however, on occasion, large trabecular ridges may also be encountered. The question arises whether these should be included in the digitized endocardial contour or removed using some form of smoothing algorithm. A variety of smoothing approaches have been employed. Some authors have simply manually digitized through the papillary muscles using the endocardial points at their margins to approximate the ventricular curvature.[26,27,66] Using the method of point placement along projected radii, it is possible to approximate the position of the endocardial interface beneath the papillary muscles and then connect points around the circumference using a spline fitting algorithm.[39] Another approach is to use an expanding polynomial or convex-hull algorithm that rejects all points that are not concave toward the center of the left ventricle and therefore cannot contribute to contraction.

All of these methods, however, are heavily weighted by the points at the junction of the bases of the papillary muscles and the endocardium, and when irregularities are removed, the motion of the resulting targets represents highly smoothed or approximate data. Figure 21–19 compares smoothed and unsmoothed contours using the convex-hull algorithm.

For wall thickening, some form of smoothing is essential because irregularities in the endocardial contour will markedly alter the end-diastolic thickness measurement and create large variations in the derived data. For this purpose, some form of sliding filter or spline fitting algorithm would appear essential to maintain appropriate separation of point pairs in the area of the papillary muscles.

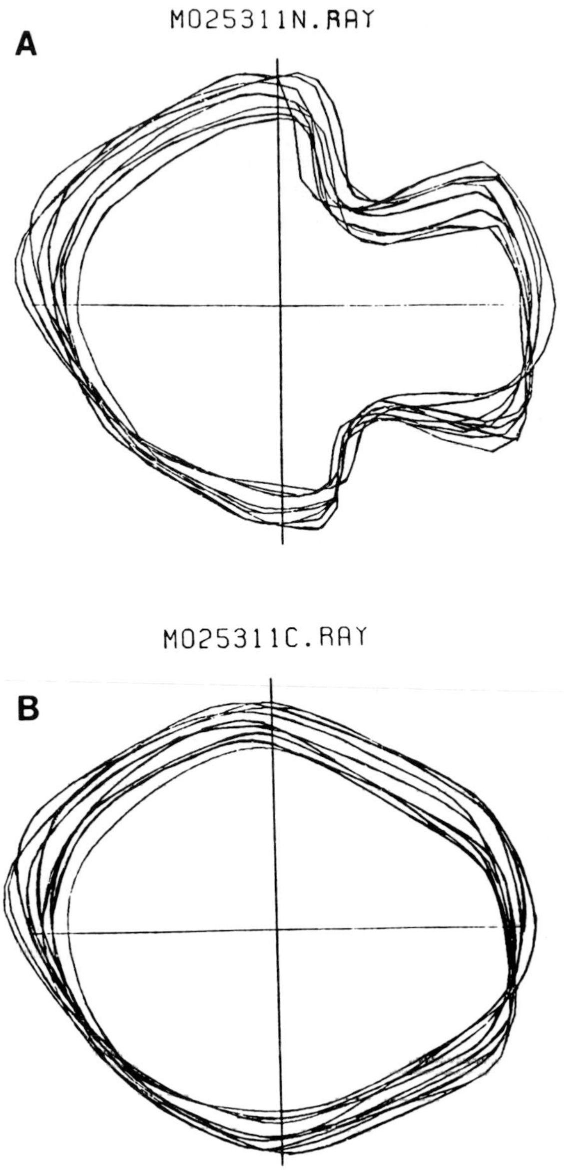

Fig. 21–19. Examples of the convex hull algorithm, which performs a smoothing iteration by removing all points that are not concave toward the center of the ventricle. **A.** The nonsmoothed endocardial outlines. The papillary muscles are easily identified because they project into the left ventricle. **B.** Their smoothed counterparts. The papillary muscles have now been removed.[62]

Summary of Methods

In the preceding section, the visual, quantitative excursion-based, and thickening methods of wall motion analysis were discussed individually. An analysis of the relative merits of these methods is more complex because little comparative data exist. It is further complicated by the fact that the utility of individual approaches varies with the projection to be analyzed, the model being studied, and the specific question posed. For parasternal long and short axis views, data are available using all three methods. For apical views, however, only excursion-based data appear to be reliable, owing to the difficulty in recording complete epicardial and endocardial interfaces around the circumference of the ventricle. Although individual studies have suggested that septal thickening can be measured in the apical four-chamber view, others have opted to record septal thickening in the parasternal projection and assume that this can be applied to the entire septum.

If the investigator seeks to define *normal* in the symmetrically contracting ventricle, visual assessment must be based on the individual's prior experience. Even for the most experienced observer, separation of hypo- or hyperkinesis from normal may be extremely difficult. Both excursion-based and thickening studies show a wide range of normal; however, variability has been consistently lower for the excursion-based parameters than for wall thickening.[31,34] The correlation methods are consistent in their depiction of normal and show little variability but require large amounts of data to be input.[36]

Visual definition of a region of dyssynergy in the ischemic ventricle appears as accurate as most quantitative methods, and at least one quantitative study has relied on visual localization of abnormal motion as the "gold standard" for validating the accuracy of their quantitative algorithm.[42] The eye naturally integrates space and time, and its discriminatory power is difficult to reproduce, much less surpass. As the pattern of ischemic dysfunction becomes more complex, however, visual discrimination becomes more difficult and less accurate. The correlation methods, which also integrate space and time, simulating the visual process, appear to perform better than other excursion-based approaches.

The accuracy of wall thickening in determining the extent of dysfunction has been evaluated only for relatively large sampling intervals (22.5 to 45°).[24,29] At intervals of this magnitude, it is localization rather than quantitation that is being tested, so that the resolution of the method is difficult to define. The accuracy of thickening data appears to be further influenced by the type of analysis performed. Studies based on large area segments, or looking at specific point pairs within the myocardium, have yielded positive results.[17,25] Although it was our initial impression that the independence of thickening from translation would make it an ideal method, we have subsequently found that, when endocardial and epicardial contours are digitized separately and thickening is compared at a larger number of points around the ventricular circumference, there is so much variability in the resulting data that it has proven unreliable for the quantitation of infarct extent. Figure 21–20 compares wall motion defined by the correlation methods, endocardial excursion, and wall thickening to the percentage of transmural infarction for an animal with acute myocardial infarction. The variability in the wall thickening appears to result from difficulties in defining the epicardial interface around the entire circumference of the ventricle and changes in the end-diastolic reference, which when normalized result in large point-to-point changes in thickening.

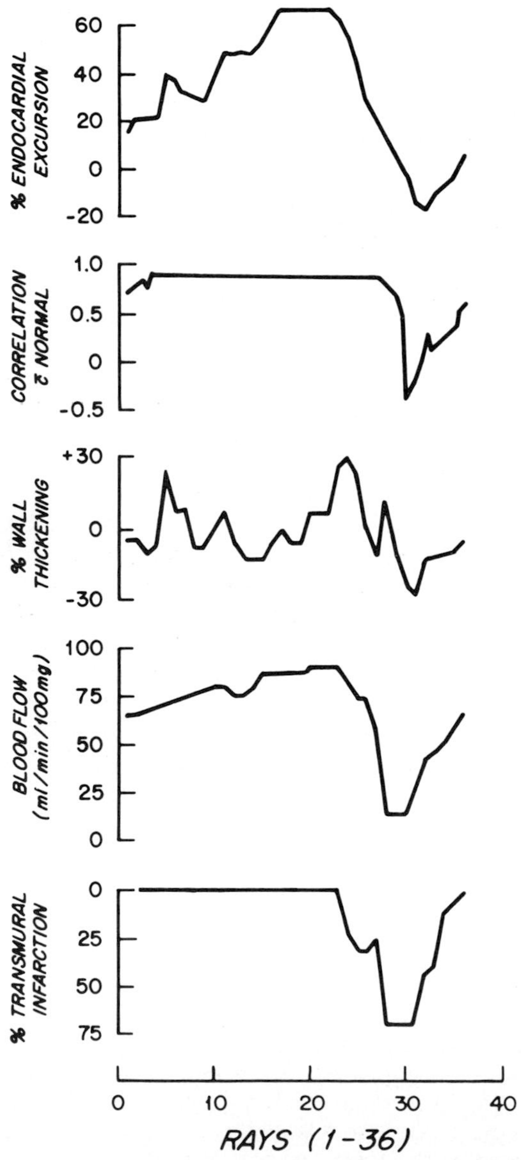

Fig. 21–20. Comparison of the patterns of wall motion assessed by endocardial excursion, correlation with normal and wall thickening, and correlation with transmural extent of infarction for a single low papillary muscle short axis plane, following acute coronary occlusion in a canine model.[62]

Thus, wall thickening, when it can be accurately recorded, has many important advantages, and in experimental studies where resolution is optimal and data are sampled at large intervals or area is integrated, lack of thickening or thinning appears to be an accurate descriptor of ischemia/infarction. When sampled at smaller intervals and in clinical studies where resolution is often suboptimal, it appears less generally useful.

METHODS OF ALIGNING REGIONAL WALL MOTION DATA WITH OTHER FUNCTIONAL AND MORPHOLOGIC PARAMETERS

In all studies that seek to examine the relationship of function to other descriptors of ischemia or infarction, the functional data must be spatially aligned with the gold standard against which they are to be tested. This alignment process is far more complex than it may initially appear. All histologic data are derived from anatomic sections that are fixed and will vary in size depending on the point in the cardiac cycle at which the heart is arrested. Precise alignment of this histologic data with radially oriented functional data requires the establishment of a comparable radial coordinate system and the fixation of a common center of reference. Because the ventricle is no longer distended, the exact relationship between the center of area of the anatomic section and that for the in vivo beating heart cannot truly be defined. However, it is the placement of this point that determines the relationship of the two data sets. This is a particular problem at the margins of an infarct zone where a misalignment of 10 to 20° can markedly affect the resulting assessment of border zone function. In our experience these data sets cannot truly be anatomically registered, despite the preplacement of epicardial markers or the implantation of intramyocardial markers at the time of sacrifice. We have, thus, developed an algorithm for aligning data sets that is based on the presumption that the most severe wall motion abnormalities will be spatially related to the most severe flow and histologic abnormalities. The algorithm shifts corresponding data sets in 5° increments until the optimal correlation between data sets is achieved (Fig. 21–21). This process has resulted in a mean radial shift of roughly 5.7° with a maximal shift of 20°. Although this has little effect on infarct and normal zone data, it appears to be the only reasonable way to analyze function in zones bordering the infarct.

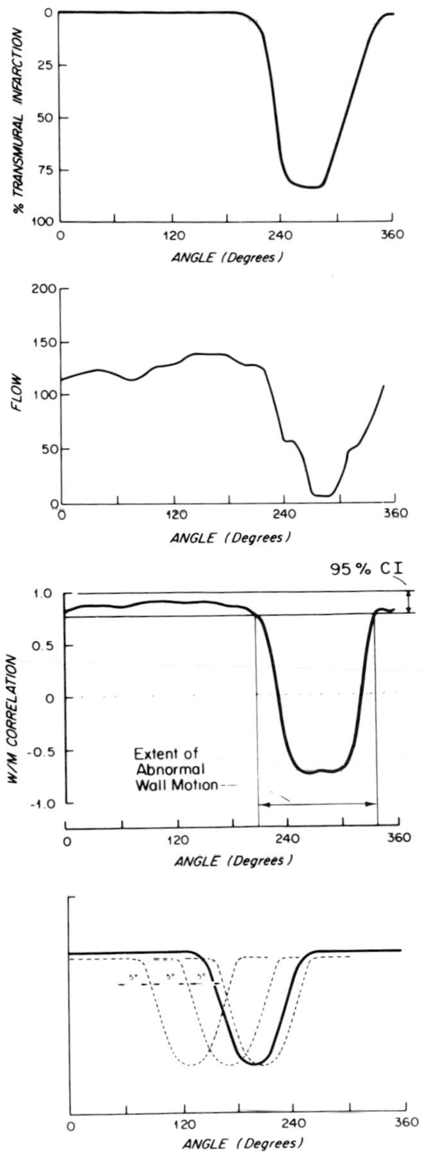

Fig. 21–21. A computer algorithm for shifting data sets until the optimal correlation between curves is achieved. In this format, each curve is shifted in 5° increments until the best fit with the select reference data set, i.e., transmural extent of infarction, is achieved.[62]

METHOD OF ASSESSING VENTRICULAR SIZE AND GEOMETRY IN A SINGLE PLANE

Several early echocardiographic studies examined serial changes in ventricular morphology after myocardial infarction by measuring the length of the anterior and posterior endocardial segments in a single short axis plane at the papillary muscle level[12,21,67,68] (Fig. 21–22). Although this method allows for a simple measure of ventricular size, it has significant limitations that affect its application to the study of the natural history of ventricular remodeling after myocardial infarction. First, because changes in ventricular size are assessed at only one level of the ventricle, the full extent of infarction may be underestimated. Hence, infarct regression or infarct expansion occurring in other regions, such as the apex or base, will not be fully appreciated. Second, it would not be possible to determine whether an increase in size of one segment was due to infarct expansion or infarct extension, because the infarct zone is not measured independently. Third, the use of a "thinning ratio" as an index of infarct expansion is subject to significant error as a result of the variability inherent in accurately measuring the thickness of the posterior free wall and ventricular septum. Finally, and of most importance, interpretation of serial changes in ventricular shape and size are very sensitive to small variations in viewing plane orientation. Standardization of the short axis plane at the papillary level may be impossible when the ventricle becomes deformed as a consequence of infarct expansion. Therefore, although this method has contributed to the understanding of the natural history of ventricular remodeling following myocardial infarction, its potential for error is such that it is unlikely that it will be sensitive or reproducible enough to define less profound changes in ventricular size and shape, which might occur as a consequence of therapy. Hence, alternate, and more sensitive approaches to the assessment of global ventricular size and geometry are required.

ASSESSMENT OF GLOBAL FUNCTION: METHODS AND CRITIQUE

Any assessment of global function must be based on the summation of data from individual echocardiographic planes or portions of planes. This can be achieved using four general approaches: (1) the segmental approach, in which the ventricle is divided into anatomically defined segments and function within each segment is summed to derive an index of global left ventricular performance; (2) the Simpson's rule method, in which data from parallel planes are summed using a Simpson's rule algorithm; (3) the geometric figure approach, in which the endocardial surface of the ventricle is represented as a geometric figure (or combination of figures) and the extent of abnormal wall motion is expressed as a percentage of the total geometric area: and (4) *a mapping algorithm* in which ventricular areas and dimensions are used to construct a planar map of the endocardial surface of the ventricle and the area of dysfunction is superimposed on this planar map to determine a functional infarct size. Each of these approaches has its strengths and weaknesses, and indeed, no one approach is ideal.

Segmental Approach

Using the segmental approach, function within anatomically defined segments of the ventricle is initially determined either semiquantitatively (visually) or quantitatively (see preceding discussion). Function within each segment (e.g., normal, 1; hypokinetic, 2; akinesis, 3; dyskinesis, 4) is then summed, and global function is expressed as the total "score" for all segments or as a wall motion index derived by dividing the sum score by the total number of segments into which the ventricle was initially divided. Segmental systems involving between 5 and 20 segments have been described.[8,10,11,14,

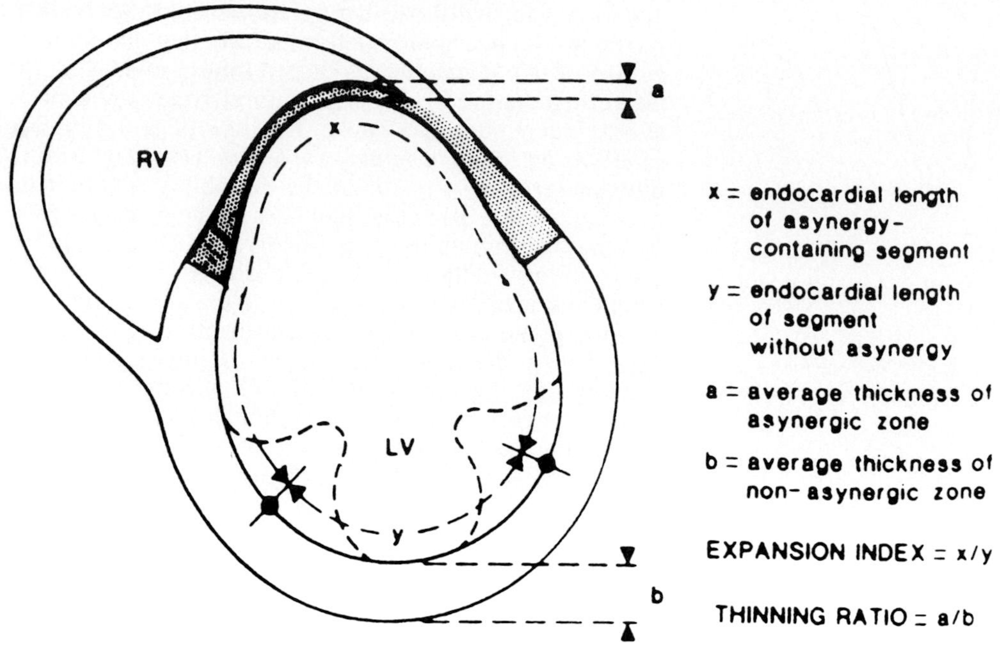

Fig. 21–22. A two-dimensional short axis echocardiogram at midpapillary muscle, indicating the method used to express ventricular enlargement and changes in wall thickness. In this construct, the x/y ratio is used as an index of infarct expansion. See text. RV = right ventricle, LV = left ventricle. (Adapted from Jugdutt BI, Michorowski BL: Role of infarct expansion in rupture of the ventricular septum after acute myocardial infarction. A two-dimensional echocardiographic study. Clin Cardiol 10:641, 1987.)

[20,25,28,44] Figure 21–23 is an example of the segmental system that we use. In this system, the ventricle is divided into three levels (base, midventricle, and apex) along its long axis with the papillary muscles as references. The basal and midventricular levels are then subdivided into eight segments around the short axis circumference, while the apex is divided into four segments. Degrees of dysfunction can then be displayed in their anatomically correct location using a target diagram such as that illustrated in Figure 21–24. This system offers the advantages of relative ease of segmental definition, relatively high global resolution (5%), and ready adaptability to computer systems.

The segmental approach is clearly the easiest of the global methods for defining ventricular performance and is naturally suited to the visual definition of function. Further, it does not require that any plane be completely recorded but only that each segment be visualized in one or more views. This is a major advantage in clinical studies, where recording the entire ventricular silhouette in a given plane may be impossible. Unfortunately, it is also the least precise, its resolution being limited[39] by the number of segments employed. For example, if a ventricle is divided into 10 segments, the maximal spatial resolution of the system would be 10%, and the score assigned to each of the 10 regions must reflect an average function within that large segment. In addition, because all segments receive the same weight, there is no way to correct for their unequal contribution to the ventricular surface. Likewise, if regional dilation occurs following infarction, there is no way to correct for changes in the relative contribution of an individual portion of the ventricle to the segmental construct. For example, if in a segmental system the apex is defined to represent 20% of the left ventricle, then an apical infarct will, by definition, involve 20% of the left ventricle. If the apex were then to expand to represent 40% of the anatomic left

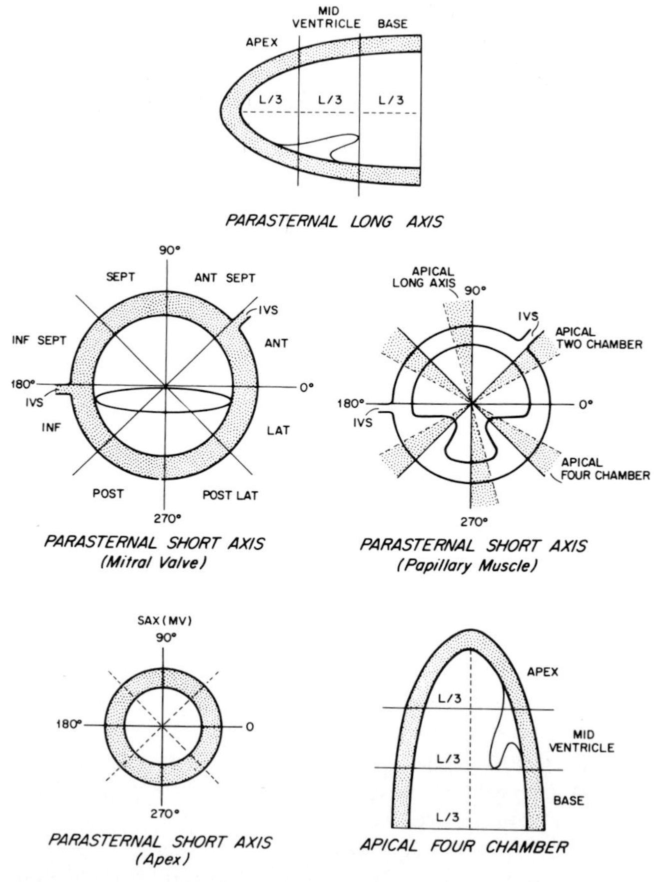

Fig. 21–23. The segmental system used at the Massachusetts General Hospital laboratory. In this construct, there are 20 segments, 8 at the base, 8 at the midventricular level, and four at the apex. (From Mann DL, Gillam LD, Weyman AE: Cross-sectional echocardiographic assessment of regional left ventricular performance and myocardial perfusion. Prog Cardiovasc Dis 29:1, 1986.)

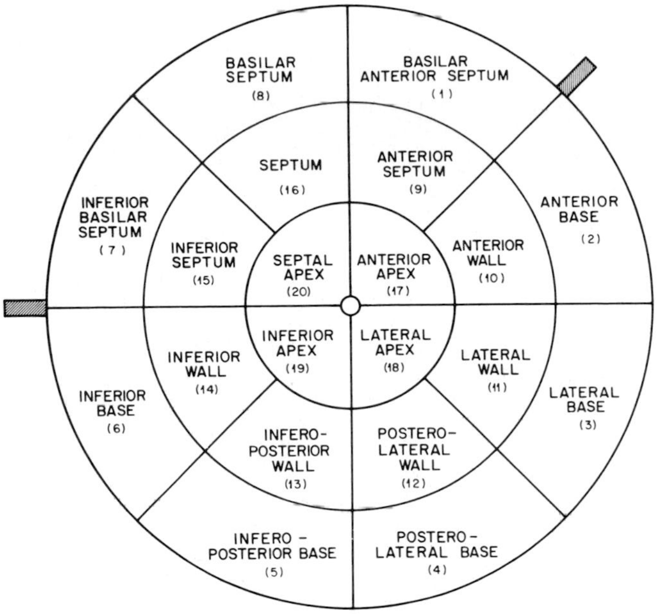

Fig. 21–24. Left ventricular segmental system. Target diagram displaying each of the segments defined in Figure 21–23 in the appropriate spatial positions. The outermost ring contains the basal segments; the middle ring, the midventricular segments; and the center, the apex. This ventricle is thus displayed as if visualized from the apex toward the base.

ventricle, in the segmental construct, it will still account for only 20%. Thus, segmental constructs cannot account for infarct expansion, regression, or ventricular dilation. As a result, any segmental system will necessarily be of limited value in a study designed to examine the natural history of ventricular remodeling after myocardial infarction. Finally, although some authors score motion only in those segments that are well visualized, this is conceptually incorrect, because it may underestimate the extent of regional dysfunction if image acquisition is suboptimal and, at the extreme, could describe ventricular function as the function of a single segment.

Similar Planes: Summation of Data Using Simpson's Rule

A more accurate means of quantifying global left ventricle function is to sum the function from serial short axis planes using a Simpson's rule algorithm. This method is ideally suited for quantitative analysis because it permits the resolution inherent in single-plane short axis analysis to be retained. In addition, it permits the relative contribution of each plane to the endocardial surface to be appropriately calculated and is readily adapted to changes in left ventricle shape.

The requirement that individual short axis planes be recorded at equidistant or known intervals necessitates some mechanical or electronic method for precisely recording plane position (Fig. 21–25). This requires extensive access to the anterior cardiac surface, making the method more suitable for experimental studies where the entire anterior surface of the ventricle can be exposed. Even in the ideal setting, it is not always possible to achieve optimal interface visualization and maintain parallel plane position at the same time. In the normally shaped ventricle, therefore, a compromise is frequently reached in which plane position is defined by anatomic reference and separation estimated based on anatomic precedents. Unfortunately, in the deformed ventricle, there is no alternative to direct measurement of plane position. Another limitation of this method is that it cannot account for the cardiac apex, because the apical cap does not border a cavity that can be appreciated in short axis. Function in the most apical ventricular section must therefore be assumed to reflect the degree of apical

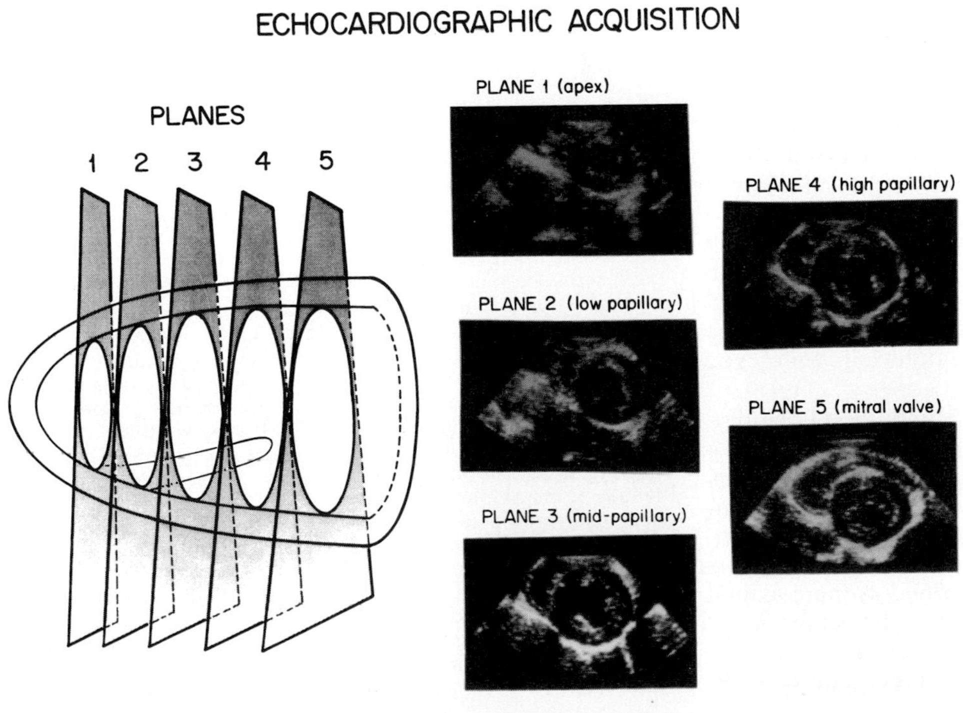

Fig. 21–25. The five parasternal short axis view of the left ventricle most readily identifiable in practice, including the (1) apical level, (2) low papillary muscle, (3) midpapillary, (4) high papillary, and (5) mitral valve.

involvement, or the apex must simply not be considered.[16]

Geometric Figure Approach

In this approach, the ventricle is modeled as a single geometric figure or series of figures, and the endocardial surface area of the ventricle is calculated from the area of the figure(s) employed (Fig. 21–26). Once the surface area of the endocardium is known, the area of dysfunction can be calculated as the area of a subfigure, and the functional infarct size can be derived by determining the percentage of the endocardium that functions abnormally. The geometric figure most frequently employed in calculating the endocardial area of the body of the ventricle has been the truncated cone, while the apex of the ventricle has generally been represented as a truncated ellipse.

The geometric figure approach has been used to define the natural history of acute wall motion abnormalities[13] and to predict survival following acute myocardial infarction.[66] The accuracy of these figures, however, has not yet been truly validated in the experimental setting. Further, the geometric figure method is not easily applied to deformed ventricles.

Endocardial Surface Mapping

Endocardial surface mapping enables one to quantitate and display the area of the endocardium[69] and the extent of abnormal wall[70] motion using standard cross-sectional echocardiographic images.

Geometric Principles

The algorithm used to calculate the ventricular endocardial surface area was developed on three basic assumptions. First, if the endocardial surface of the left ventricle was coated with a thin liner, then the area of this liner would correspond to the endocardial surface area of the ventricle. Second, if the left ventricle was sectioned into four equal quadrants by two perpendicular apex-to-base cuts, then these two cuts would also quadrisect the thin ventricular liner. Third, if the four sections of the ventricular liner were separated from the endocardium and laid flat, they would form a two-dimensional map of the endocardial surface of the left ventricle. In this way, the length of each quadrant of the map would approximate the length of the ventricle, the length of the curved edges would correspond to the sectioned edge of the liner, and the width of each section of the map would correspond to a quarter of the circumference of the ventricle at that level.

Figure 21–27A illustrates how standard echocardiographic imaging planes intersecting a representative ventricle yield dimensions that correspond to those required to describe the area of the ventricular liner. Comparable dimensions of the ventricle are derived from images taken in these planes as follows. The long axis length of the ventricle (LAX) is defined as the maximal distance from the apical epicardium to the center of the mitral annular plane in either the apical two- or four-chamber views. The length of the endocardial base-to-

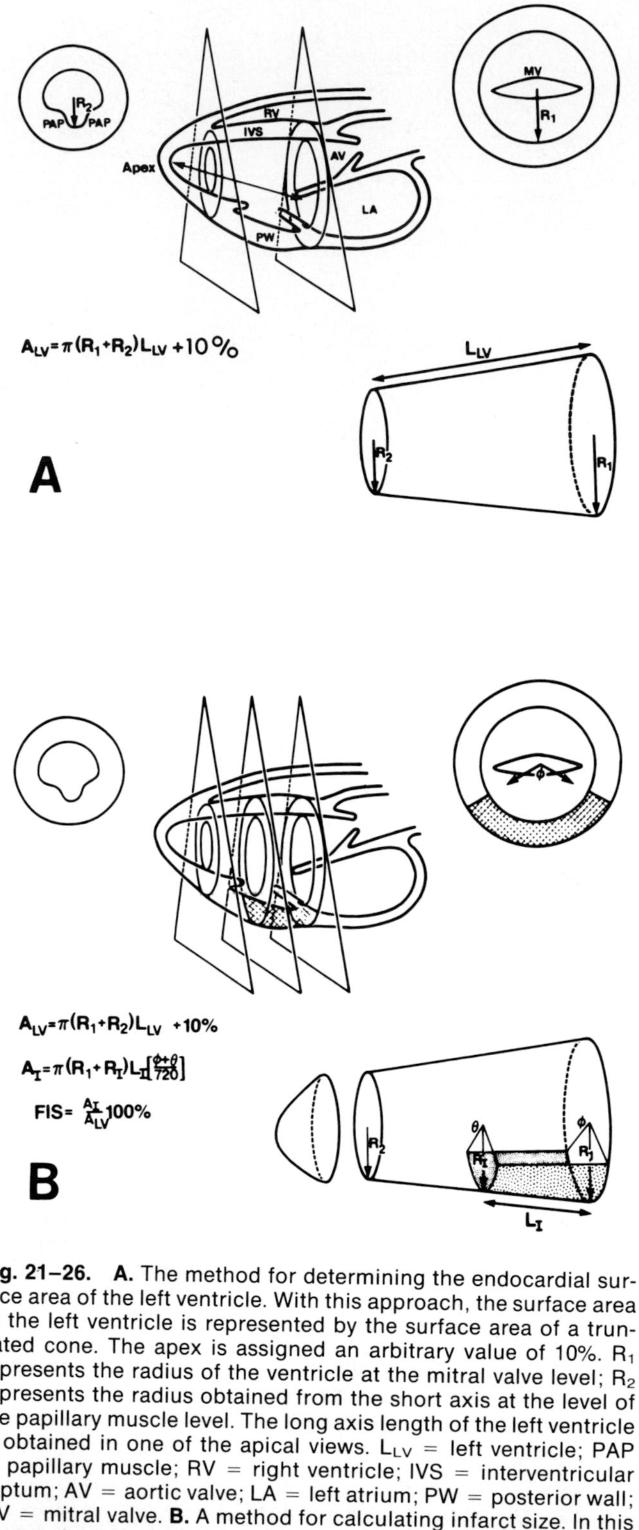

Fig. 21–26. A. The method for determining the endocardial surface area of the left ventricle. With this approach, the surface area of the left ventricle is represented by the surface area of a truncated cone. The apex is assigned an arbitrary value of 10%. R_1 represents the radius of the ventricle at the mitral valve level; R_2 represents the radius obtained from the short axis at the level of the papillary muscle level. The long axis length of the left ventricle is obtained in one of the apical views. L_{LV} = left ventricle; PAP = papillary muscle; RV = right ventricle; IVS = interventricular septum; AV = aortic valve; LA = left atrium; PW = posterior wall; MV = mitral valve. **B.** A method for calculating infarct size. In this format, the endocardial surface area of the left ventricle is initially calculated as in Figure 21–26A. The area of a second figure that encompasses the infarct is then calculated separately. L_I is the length of the asynergic segment; R_1 is the radius of a short axis scan taken at the base of the area of asynergy; R_I is the radius of the scan taken at the apical margin of the asynergic segment. The functionally abnormal area within this subfigure can be calculated from the percentage of the circumference of the short axis scan at the base and apex of the area that demonstrates asynergy. The area of abnormal function can be expressed as a percentage of the total LV endocardial surface area. FIS = functional infarct size.

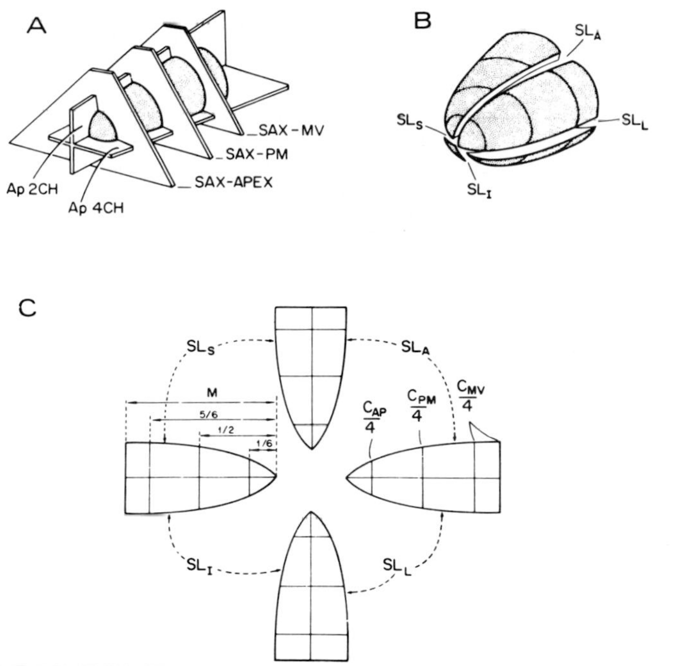

Fig. 21–27. **A.** Relative positions of echocardiographic imaging planes shown as they intersect the left ventricle. Ap 4CH = apical four-chamber plane; Ap 2CH = apical two-chamber plane; SAX-MV = mitral valve short-axis plane; SAX-PM = papillary muscle short axis plane; SAX-APEX = apical short axis plane. **B.** A schematic diagram of the left ventricle that has been quadrisected by two perpendicular apical imaging planes. The transverse lines represent the positions at which short axis planes would intersect the endocardial surface. $SL_{A,I,L,S}$ values represent the endocardial apex to base segment lengths. **C.** A schematic of the planar endocardial surface map obtained of the left ventricle. C_{AP} = circumference at the apex; C_{PM} = circumference at the papillary muscle level; C_{MV} = circumference at the mitral valve level; M = midline dimension of each quadrant. (From Guyer DE, et al.: A new echocardiographic model for quantifying three-dimensional endocardial surface area. J Am Coll Cardiol 8:819, 1986. Reprinted with permission from the American College of Cardiology. Journal of the American College of Cardiology, 1986, 8, 819.)

apex segments of the anterior and inferior portions of the ventricle is determined from the apical two-chamber view, and the length of the lateral and septal portions of the ventricle is determined from the apical four-chamber view. Short axis imaging planes are shown at the mitral valve level (SAX-MV), the midpapillary muscle level (SAX-PM), and at the apical level just below the papillary muscles (SAX-APEX). Short axis circumferences (C) are measured at each of these levels by tracing the endocardial border.

Figure 21–27B and C shows how the idealized left ventricular liner is sectioned into four equal quadrants and shows the corresponding idealized endocardial surface map that can be constructed from these data when the four quadrants are laid flat. Note that the LAX of the ventricle does not appear on this map. This is because the long axis length runs down the center of the ventricle and does not lie along the endocardial surface. Rather, a midline dimension of each quadrant (M), determined by the mapping procedure using a technique of successive approximation, is used as the distance from the apical tip to the basal plane of the map.

The morphologic assumptions that underlie the construction of these points from routine echocardiographic measurements relate to the positions at which each short axis imaging plane intersects the endocardial surface. Specifically, it is assumed that the apical short axis plane intersects the central ventricular axis at one sixth of the apex-to-base length; the midpapillary muscle short axis plane is assumed to intersect the midpoint of the central axis, and the mitral valve plane is assumed to intersect the central axis at five sixths of the apex-to-base length. These positions are all based on the assumption that each of the three short axis planes lies centrally within its respective anatomic third of the left ventricle, as defined by Edwards et al.[71] Finally, it is assumed that the endocardial circumference at the base of the ventricle is substantially the same as the circumference at the mitral valve level.

Quantification and Display of the Endocardial Surface Area

Method. Data for the construction of ventricular maps are obtained as follows. The left ventricular long axis length is taken as the mean of the left ventricular lengths measured in both the apical two- and four-chamber views. Apex-to-base endocardial segment lengths are measured by tracing the endocardial border in these two views. Ventricular circumferences are measured by tracing the endocardial borders at each of the short axis levels. All dimensions are obtained from three separate frames, and the results from each dimension are averaged to obtain a single value.

To construct maps from the echocardiographic data, the quadrant midline (M) is plotted along each of the four major axes of a planar Cartesian coordinate system (+x, −x, +y, −y) using the ventricular long axis as an initial approximation. This length of these axes then forms the spines of the four quadrants, or leaves, of the map. The three short axis circumferences are then divided by four, and the resultant lengths are plotted on each of the long axes at their appropriate location relative to and bisected by the quadrant midline. Next, the apical point is connected to the end of each of the short axis arms using a smoothed (Fig. 21–28) line whose length is equal to the corresponding endocardial segment length.

If the length of the quadrant midline (M) that was initially approximated from the ventricular long axis length falls within predefined tolerance specifications, relative to the midline length determined by the segment lengths, the mapping procedure is complete. Should there be a discrepancy between the estimated vs. measured length of the ventricle, the map is adjusted by altering the quadrant length (M). A flow diagram of the iterative algorithm is shown in Figure 21–29. Using this algorithm, the midline length has been found to converge within three iterations to the same value, irrespective of the initial long axis measurement. Thus, the segment lengths force the map to conform to ventricular geometry irrespective of actual ventricular length. After plotting is complete, the map-derived endocardial surface area is determined by planimetry of the four map quadrants.

Validation of the Endocardial Surfacing Algorithm. The accuracy of the endocardial surface mapping technique was initially tested using computer models that allowed the accuracy of the technique to be examined under conditions in which (1) ventricular shape could be varied by altering the eccentricity of the assumed ellipsoidal surface of the ventricle; (2) the number of transverse circumferences used to plot the endocardial surface maps could be increased or decreased, and (3) the relative apex-to-base positions of each short axis plane within its third of the ventricle could be altered to determine the effect of differences between actual and assumed plane position on the computed endocardial surface area.

The effect of varying eccentricity and number of transverse circumferences on the estimate of true endocardial surface area is summarized in Table 21–3. As seen, the algorithm can accurately quantitate the surface of all hemiellipsoids, with estimates approaching truth, for physiologic shapes (eccentricity = 0.95) when six or more planes are analyzed. Even when the data from only three planes are used, however, the largest error for physiologic shaped hemiellipsoids is less than 2%.

The effect of varying any of the three short axis plane positions within their respective thirds of a hemiellipsoid ventricle on the area ratio (true/estimated) is shown in Figure 21–30. These data were derived from a hemiellipsoid with an eccentricity of 0.95. As expected, moving a short axis plane from the apical to the basal portion of its third of the ventricle increases the area ratio. It should be noted, however, that this effect is likely to be important only if there is marked deviation in the apical or papillary muscle short axis plane position and that inaccuracies in mitral plane position have almost no effect on the estimate of true endocardial surface area.

The accuracy of the endocardial surface mapping technique as a means of measuring the endocardial sur-

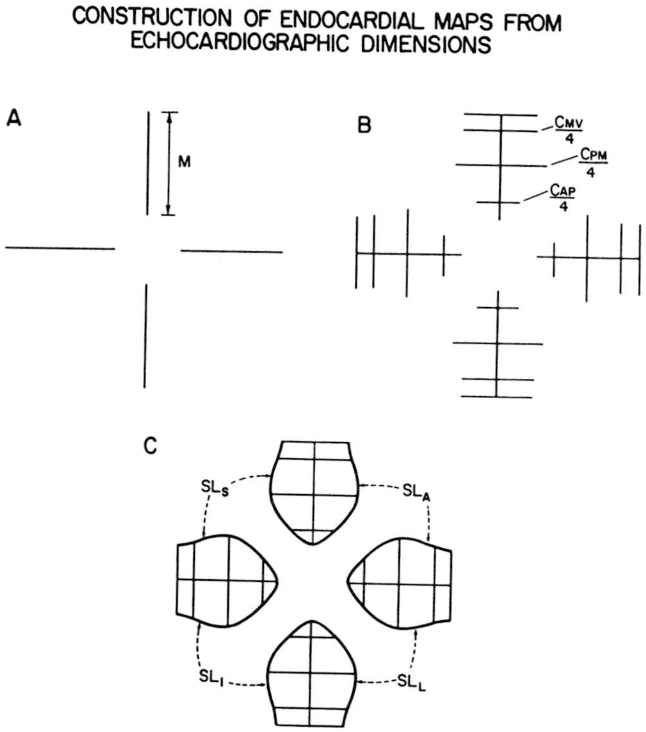

Fig. 21–28. Procedure for plotting an endocardial map from echocardiographic data. **A.** The layout of the quadrant midline dimensions. In the first stage of the plotting sequence, the ventricular long axis dimension is used as the map quadrant midline (M) value. **B.** The short axis data are then plotted at their correct positions along the quadrant midlines. **C.** Smoothed curves are fitted between the ends of the short axis arms and the apex points of each quadrant. CMV/4 = one quarter of the end-diastolic endocardial circumference at the short axis mitral valve level; CPM/4 = one quarter of the end-diastolic endocardial circumference at the short axis papillary muscle level; CAP/4 = one quarter of the end-diastolic endocardial circumference at the short axis apical level. SL = segment length from base to apex; SL_A = anterior; SL_L = lateral; SL_I = inferior; SL_S = septal. (From Guyer DE, et al.: A new echocardiographic model for quantifying three-dimensional endocardial surface area. J Am Coll Cardiol 8:819, 1986. Reprinted with permission from the American College of Cardiology. Journal of the American College of Cardiology, 1986, 8, 819.)

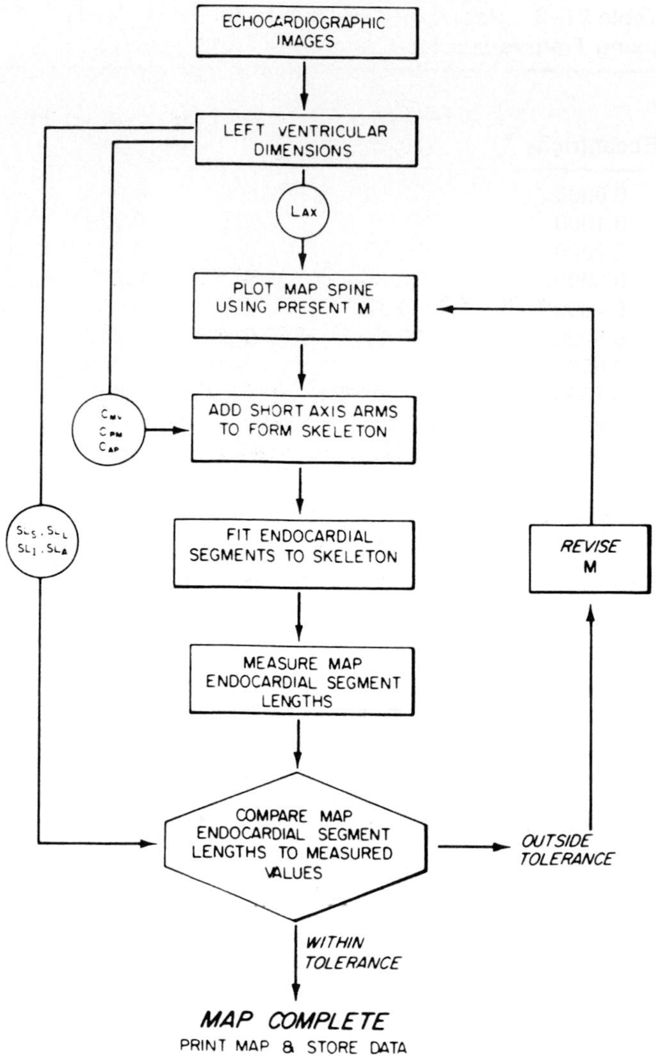

Fig. 21–29. Steps in the iterative mapping procedure for plotting endocardial surface maps. For abbreviations, see Figures 21–26 and 21–27. (From Guyer DE, et al.: A new echocardiographic model for quantifying three-dimensional endocardial surface area. J Am Coll Cardiol 8:819, 1986. Reprinted with permission from the American College of Cardiology.)

Table 21–3. Ratios of Map-Derived to Actual Areas of Ellipsoid Surfaces With Varying Shapes (Eccentricities) and Using Transverse Plane Data From 3 to 10 Levels

Eccentricity	True area (cm^2)	Number of Short-Axis Planes							
		3	4	5	6	7	8	9	10
0.0000	402.12	0.924	0.928	0.930	0.931	0.932	0.932	0.932	0.933
0.1000	399.44	0.925	0.929	0.930	0.932	0.932	0.933	0.933	0.933
0.2000	391.36	0.926	0.930	0.932	0.933	0.934	0.934	0.934	0.935
0.3000	377.77	0.929	0.933	0.935	0.936	0.936	0.937	0.937	0.937
0.4000	358.47	0.933	0.936	0.938	0.940	0.940	0.941	0.941	0.941
0.5000	333.14	0.938	0.942	0.944	0.945	0.945	0.946	0.946	0.946
0.6000	301.19	0.944	0.948	0.950	0.951	0.952	0.952	0.953	0.953
0.7000	261.59	0.942	0.946	0.948	0.950	0.950	0.951	0.951	0.952
0.8000	212.22	0.955	0.960	0.962	0.964	0.964	0.965	0.965	0.966
0.9000	147.24	0.971	0.976	0.979	0.980	0.981	0.982	0.982	0.983
0.9100	139.29	0.973	0.978	0.981	0.982	0.983	0.984	0.984	0.985
0.9200	130.93	0.975	0.980	0.983	0.984	0.985	0.986	0.986	0.987
0.9300	122.08	0.976	0.982	0.984	0.986	0.987	0.988	0.988	0.988
0.9400	112.63	0.978	0.984	0.986	0.988	0.989	0.990	0.990	0.990
0.9500	102.42	0.980	0.985	0.988	0.990	0.991	0.991	0.992	0.992
0.9600	91.24	0.981	0.987	0.990	0.991	0.992	0.993	0.994	0.994
0.9700	78.66	0.983	0.988	0.991	0.993	0.994	0.995	0.995	0.996
0.9800	63.91	0.984	0.990	0.993	0.994	0.996	0.996	0.997	0.997
0.9900	44.95	0.977	0.982	0.985	0.987	0.988	0.989	0.989	0.990
0.9990	14.13	0.984	0.990	0.993	0.995	0.996	0.997	0.997	0.997
0.9999	4.47	0.985	0.991	0.994	0.996	0.997	0.998	0.998	0.998

Each row represents data for one shape or eccentricity that is indicated in column 1. The second column lists the actual or true areas of the hemiellipsoids, and succeeding columns display the area ratios (map area/true area) of the surfaces using transverse or short-axis circumferences from 3 to 10 planes. The actual hemiellipsoid areas are calculated for surfaces with semimajor axis lengths of 8.0 cm.

(From Guyer DE, et al.: A new echocardiographic model for quantifying three dimensional surface area. J Am Coll Cardiol 8:819, 1986. Reprinted with permission from the American College of Cardiology.)

face area of both normal and distorted ventricles has also been examined by comparing the estimated endocardial surface area to the actual endocardial surface area measured directly from latex casts of canine left ventricles[70] (Fig. 21–31) and from human hearts[72] (Fig. 21–32). As seen, there is an excellent correlation between true and estimated endocardial surface area in both canine and human ventricles; however, in both cases the mapping technique tended to overestimate the true surface areas, especially in smaller hearts. This consistent finding is presumably due to shrinkage of the ventricle that occurs during fixation. More recently, the technique has also been demonstrated to compare well with three-dimensional echocardiographic estimates of endocardial surface area.[73]

Intraobserver variability in the measurement of endocardial surface area has been demonstrated to be within 5%. Further, the day-to-day variability in endocardial surface area in normal individuals has also been demonstrated to be within 5%.[74]

Quantification and Display of the Extent of Abnormal Wall Motion

Method. To measure the three-dimensional extent of ventricular dysfunction, one must plot the area of abnormal wall motion on the endocardial surface area map. To achieve this, the extent of dysfunction within each of the standard echocardiographic imaging planes is initially assessed visually. The length of the abnormally moving segments is then defined in each plane, and its location is determined by referencing it to internal landmarks: the distance along the endocardial surface from the mitral valve plane in the apical views and the distance from the medial mitral valve commissure or papillary muscle in the short axis planes. Through this process, the margins of the area of abnormal wall motion are placed at their appropriate location on the endocardial map. These points can then be connected, and the enclosed area can be taken as the region of abnormal wall motion (Fig. 21–33). The percentage of the endocardial surface area that moves abnormally is then calculated as the following ratio:

$$\%AWM = \frac{AWM(cm^2)}{ESA(cm^2)} \times 100$$

where ESA is the endocardial surface area and AWM is the extent of abnormal wall motion.

Validation. The accuracy of the endocardial surface mapping technique in assessing the extent of myocardial

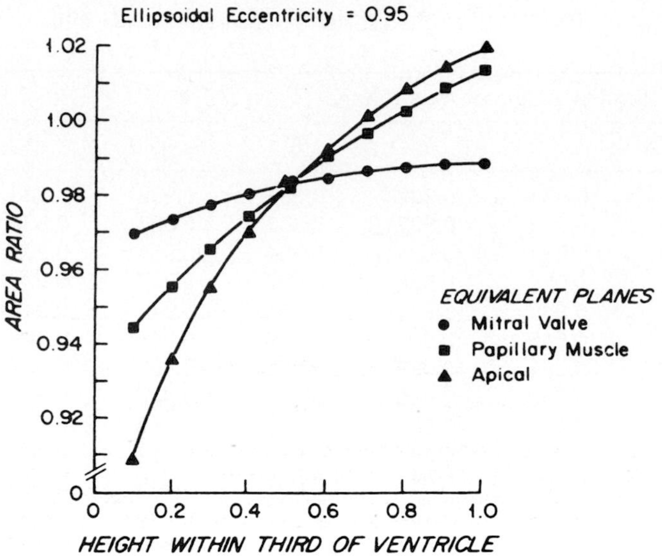

Fig. 21–30. Effect of varying the relative apex-to-base position of each short axis plane on overall accuracy of the map. The x axis represents the height at which the short axis circumference was measured within the appropriate third of the ventricle, with 0.1 being 1/10 of the way from the most apical extreme of the given third to the base. The position of the two short axis planes that are not varied is the correct one: each halfway along its respective third of the central long axis. The relative position of the variable plane within its third of the ventricle is plotted on the y axis. (From Guyer DE, et al.: A new echocardiographic model for quantifying three-dimensional endocardial surface area. J Am Coll Cardiol 8: 819, 1986. Reprinted with permission from the American College of Cardiology.)

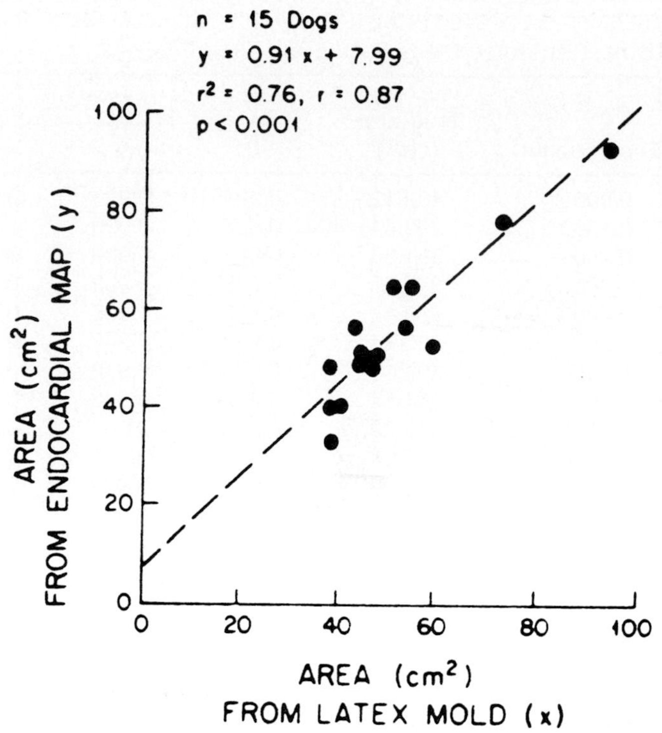

Fig. 21–31. Correlation of endocardial surface area derived from endocardial maps (y axis) with smoothed endocardial surface areas calculated from latex molds (x axis) of 15 excised canine ventricles. (From Guyer DE, et al.: A new echocardiographic model for quantifying three-dimensional endocardial surface area. J Am Coll Cardiol 8:819, 1986. Reprinted with permission from the American College of Cardiology.)

infarction has been evaluated in both canine and human autopsied hearts.[70,72] In both situations, there has been a good correlation between the extent of abnormal wall motion, expressed as a percentage of the total endocardial surface area, and the extent of infarction defined histologically (Figs. 21–34 and 21–35). As with other echocardiographic and angiographic methods, however, the extent of abnormal wall motion tends to result in overestimation of the infarct span and volume determined from histologic sections in acute infarctions. Reasons for this systematic overestimation include the presence of dysfunctional ischemic but noninfarcted myocardium in the region of the infarct, tethering of normal myocardium by adjacent dyskinetic segments, and acute infarct expansion (functional aneurysm formation), which may disappear once intracavity pressure is removed. Despite these differences, it is function, not histology, that determines the effect of infarction on the whole organism and hence is an important parameter in itself. In chronic infarcts, the relationship tends to reverse, and the area of dysfunction underestimates histologic infarct size. This is believed to be due to motion of the margins of the scarred segments in a normal direction as a result of tethering to adjacent normal myocardium.

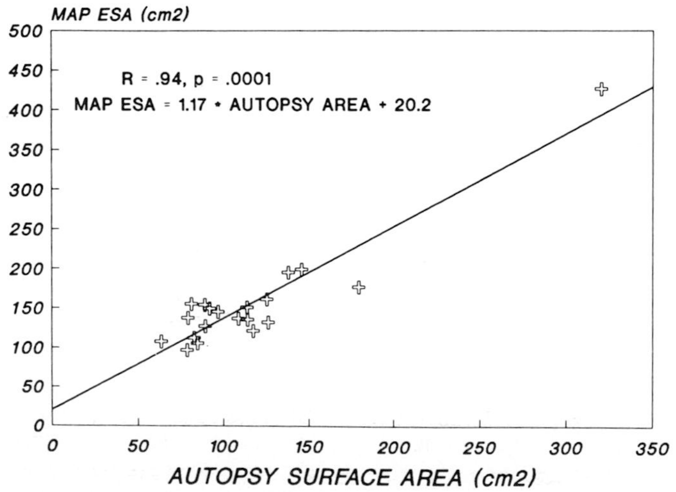

Fig. 21–32. Correlation between the left ventricular endocardial surface area (ESA) in 19 human ventricles measured at autopsy (x axis) and the ESA derived from the echocardiographic map (y axis). (From Wilkins GT, et al.: Correlation between echocardiographic endocardial surface mapping of abnormal wall motion and pathologic infarct size in autopsied hearts. Circulation 77:978, 1988. Reproduced by permission of the American Heart Association, Inc.)

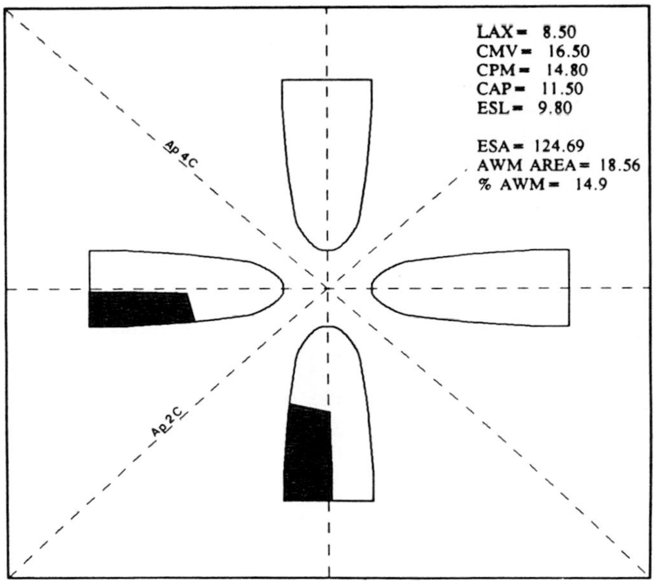

Fig. 21–33. Representative echocardiographic endocardial surface map from a patient with an inferior infarction extending from base to midpapillary muscle (shaded area). The orientation of the septal, anterior, lateral, and inferior apex-to-base axes are displayed. The numeric data in the upper corner include the initial map input dimensions, the calculated map endocardial surface area (ESA, in square centimeters), the map of abnormal wall motion (AWM, in square centimeters), and the percentage of abnormality (%AWM). LAX = long axis length; ESL = endocardial segment length; CMV = circumference at mitral valve level; CPM = circumference at papillary muscle level; CAP = circumference at apex.

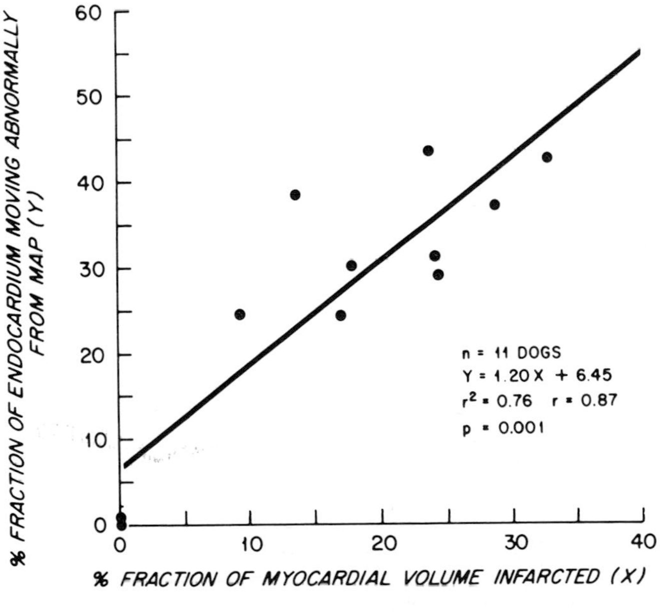

Fig. 21–34. Correlation of the overall extent of abnormal wall motion in canines, determined from endocardial maps (y axis), with the fraction of the endocardial surface overlying histochemical evidence of infarction (x axis). The line of least squares regression is drawn through the data points. (From Guyer DE, et al.: A new echocardiographic model for quantifying three-dimensional endocardial surface area. Reprinted with permission from the American College of Cardiology, J Am Coll Cardicl 8:819, 1986.)

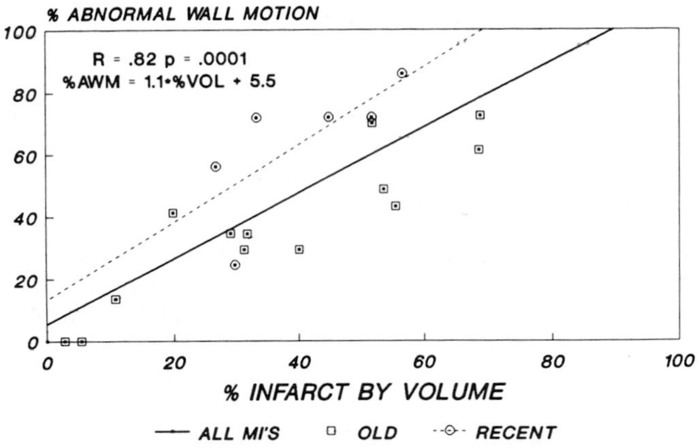

Fig. 21–35. Correlation of the pathologic extent of myocardial infarction (MI) by volume (x axis) with the extent of abnormal wall motion (AWM) derived from the endocardial surface map (y axis). The correlation line (solid line) and regression line for the total group are given. Circles denote those with recent infarcts, and the correlation for this group is shown as a dashed line. Squares denote those with old infarcts. (From Wilkins GT, et al.: Correlation between echocardiographic endocardial surface mapping of abnormal wall motion and pathologic infarct size in autopsied hearts. Circulation 77:978, 1988. Reproduced by permission of the American Heart Association, Inc.)

Advantages and Limitations

The major advantages of the endocardial mapping technique are (1) it is essentially free of geometric assumptions about the shape of the ventricle (except for the relationship of long and short axis planes); (2) it makes use of all available echocardiographic data to provide a quantitative measure of the endocardial surface, the extent of abnormal wall motion, and their relationship; (3) it outputs planar maps of the data, which permit detection of flaws in data entry and facilitate the identification and characterization of serial changes in ventricular and infarct size. This illuminates the processes of ventricular remodeling and helps separate infarct expansion, global dilation, infarct extension, and infarct regression; and (4) it can provide a measure of ventricular volume from the same data set. Further, the accuracy of the technique has been rigorously demonstrated.

Like all quantitative methods currently in use, however, the method requires (1) multiple on-axis images displaying endocardium (2) digitation of multiple frames, and (3) the visual assessment of the extent of abnormal wall motion. In our experience, however, it has been possible to obtain echocardiographic images suitable for quantitative analysis in almost 80% of consecutive patients presenting to the hospital with their first myocardial infarction.

A Simplified Visual Method for Estimating Functional Infarct Size During the Cross-Sectional Examination

Each of the methods described previously in this chapter for infarct quantitation requires detailed analysis of wall motion or extensive calculation. Figure 21–36 illustrates a simplified method by which infarct size can

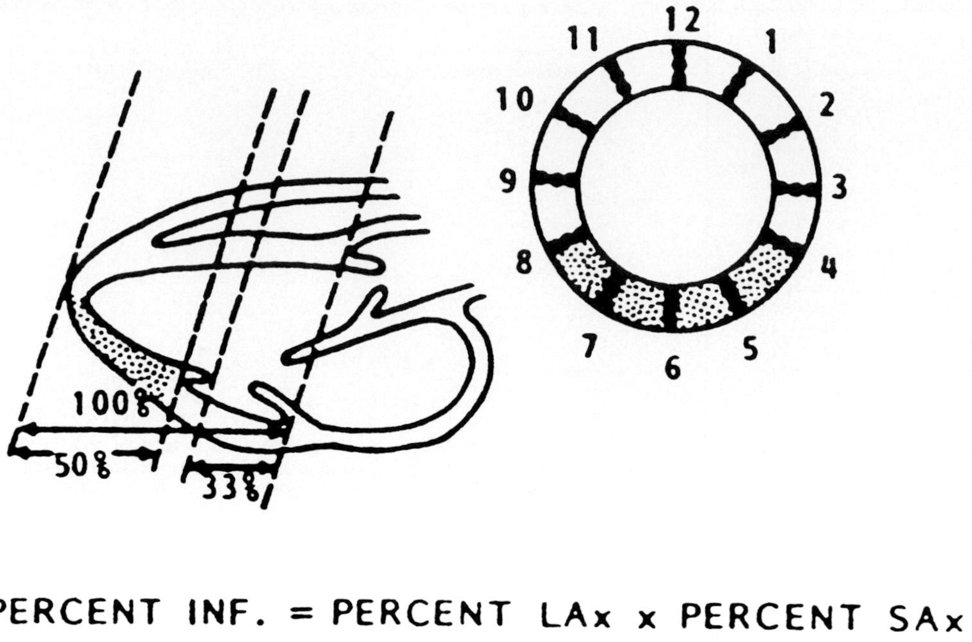

Fig. 21–36. A simplified method for visual calculation of the functional infarct area. In this format, the long axis extent of the asynergic segment is expressed as a percentage of the total long axis (LAx) and is multiplied by the percentage of the circumference in short axis (SAx) that is asynergic, to obtain the overall percentage of the ventricle that shows functional evidence of infarction.

be estimated visually during the course of a cross-sectional examination. With this approach, the maximal long axis extent of the abnormally moving segment is first defined and expressed as a percentage of the total long axis length of the ventricle. In this illustration, for example, the abnormally moving segment, indicated by the stippled region, involves 50% of the posterior wall.

The next step is to determine the maximal short axis extent of the abnormally contracting area. This determination is made by looking at the ventricular short axis as the face of a clock and determining the extent of the infarct area in terms of hours (Fig. 21–36). In Figure 21–36, the abnormally moving segment (stippled area) extends from the four- to the eight-o'clock position, encompassing a 4-hour segment of the 12-hour clock face. Thus, the abnormal segment involves 33% (12 ÷ 4) of the ventricular circumference. The total percentage of infarction is then calculated by multiplying the percentage of long axis involvement (in this example, 50%, or 0.5) by the short axis percentage (33%, or 0.33), to yield the functional infarct size, which in this case is roughly 17% of the ventricle.

This simplified method has been compared with the truncated cone method (Fig. 21–26) for calculating functional infarct size with surprisingly good results. It is particularly useful in the emergency room or coronary care unit, where some numeric estimate of infarct size is frequently helpful and detailed immediate analysis is impractical.

REFERENCES

1. Tennant R, Wiggers CJ: The effect of coronary occlusion on myocardial contraction. Am J Physiol 112:351, 1935.
2. Theroux P, Franklin D, Ross J, Kemper WS: Regional myocardial function during acute coronary artery occlusion and its modification by pharmacologic agents in the dog. Circ Res 35:896, 1974.
3. Pilcher J: Non-invasive assessment of segmental left ventricular wall motion: its clinical relevance in detecting ischemia. Clin Cardiol 1:173, 1978.
4. Herman MV, Heinle RA, Klein MD, Gorlin R: Localized disorders in myocardial contraction. N Engl J Med 277:222, 1967.
5. Burggraf GW, Parker JO: Prognosis in coronary artery disease: angiographic, hemodynamic, and clinical factors. Circulation 51:146, 1975.
6. Teichholz LE, Cohen MV, Sonnenblick BM, Gorlin R: Study of left ventricular geometry and function by B-scan ultrasonography in patients with and without asynergy. N Engl J Med 291:1220, 1964.
7. Weyman AE, et al.: Detection of left ventricular aneurysms by cross-sectional echocardiography. Circulation 54:936, 1976.
8. Kisslo J, et al.: A comparison of real-time, two-dimensional echocardiography and cineangiography in detecting left ventricular asynergy. Circulation 55:134, 1977.
9. Weyman AE, Franklin TD, Egenes KM, Green D: Correlation between extent of abnormal regional wall motion and myocardial infarct size in chronically infarcted dogs. Circulation 56(Suppl. 2):72, 1977.
10. Heger J, et al.: Cross-sectional echocardiography in acute myocardial infarction: detection and localization of regional left ventricular asynergy. Circulation 60:531, 1979.
11. Heger J, et al.: Cross-sectional echocardiographic analysis of the extent of left ventricular asynergy in acute myocardial infarction. Circulation 61:1113, 1980.
12. Eaton L, et al.: Regional cardiac dilatation after acute myocardial infarction. N Engl J Med 300:57, 1979.
13. Meltzer RS, et al.: Two-dimensional echocardiographic quantification of infarct size alteration by pharmacologic agents. Am J Cardiol 44:257, 1979.
14. Nixon JV, Narahara KA, Smitherman TC: Estimation of myocardial involvement in patients with acute myocardial infarction by two-dimensional echocardiography. Circulation 62:1248, 1980.
15. Weiss JL, Bulkley BH, Hutchins GM, Mason SJ: Two-dimensional echocardiographic recognition of myocardial injury in man: comparison with postmortem studies. Circulation 63(2):401, 981.
16. Wyatt HL, et al.: Experimental evaluation of the extent of myocardial dyssynergy and infarct size by two-dimensional echocardiography. Circulation 63:607, 1981.
17. Lieberman AN, et al.: Two-dimensional echocardiography and infarct size: relationship of regional wall motion and thickening to the extent of myocardial infarction in the dog. Circulation 63:739, 1981.
18. Falsetti HL, Marcus ML, Kerber RE, Skorton DJ: Editorial: Quantification of myocardial ischemia and infarction by left ventricular imaging. Circulation 63:747, 1981.
19. Horowitz RS, et al.: Immediate diagnosis of acute myocardial infarction by two-dimensional echocardiography. Circulation 65:323, 1982.
20. Gibson RS, et al.: Value of early two-dimensional echocardiography in patients with acute myocardial infarction. Am J Cardiol 49:1110, 1982.
21. Erlebacher JA, et al.: Late effects of acute infarct dilation on heart size: a two-dimensional echocardiographic study. Am J Cardiol 49:1120, 1982.
22. Moynihan P, Parisi A, Feldman CL: Quantitative detection of regional left ventricular contraction abnormalities by two-dimensional echocardiography: I. Analysis of methods. Circulation 63:752, 1981.
23. Parisi AF, Moynihan P, Folland ED, Feldman CL: Quantitative detection

of regional left ventricular contraction abnormalities by two-dimensional echocardiography: II. Accuracy in coronary artery disease. Circulation 63: 761, 1981.
24. Nieminen M, et al.: Serial evaluation of myocardial thickening and thinning in acute experimental infarction: identification and quantification using two-dimensional echocardiography. Circulation 66:174, 1982.
25. Vizzer CA, et al.: Detection and quantification of acute, isolated myocardial infarction by two-dimensional echocardiography. Am J Cardiol 47:1020, 1981.
26. Pandian NG, Kerber RE: Two-dimensional echocardiography in experimental coronary stenosis: I. Sensitivity and specificity in detecting transient myocardial dyskinesis: comparison with sonomicrometers. Circulation 66: 597, 1982.
27. Pandian NG, Kieso RA, Kerber RE: Two-dimensional echocardiography in experimental coronary stenosis: II. Relationship between systolic wall thinning and regional myocardial perfusion in severe coronary stenosis. Circulation 66:603, 1982.
28. Stamm RB, et al.: Echocardiographic detection of infarct-localized asynergy and remote asynergy during acute myocardial infarction: correlation with the extent of angiographic coronary disease. Circulation 67:233, 1983.
29. Pandian NG, et al.: Serial quantification of myocardial dyskinesis in acute myocardial infarction by two-dimensional echocardiography in dogs. J Am Coll Cardiol 1:619, 1983.
30. Nishimura RA, et al.: Role of two-dimensional echocardiography in the prediction of in hospital complications after acute myocardial infarction. J Am Coll Cardiol 4:1080, 1984.
31. Pandian NG, et al.: Heterogeneity of segmental left ventricular wall thickening and excursion in two-dimensional echocardiograms in normal humans. Am J Cardiol 47:452, 1981.
32. Force T, et al.: Quantitative two-dimensional echocardiographic analysis of motion and thickening of the interventricular septum after cardiac surgery. Circulation 68:1013, 1983.
33. Force T, et al.: Quantitative two-dimensional echocardiographic analysis of regional wall motion in patients with perioperative myocardial infarction. Circulation 70:233, 1984.
34. Haendchen RV, et al.: Quantitation of regional cardiac function by two-dimensional echocardiography. Circulation 67:1234, 1983.
35. Ascah KJ, et al.: Evolution of the temporal contraction sequence after acute experimental myocardial infarction. J Am Coll Cardiol 13:730, 1989.
36. Gillam LD, et al.: A comparison of quantitative echocardiographic methods for delineating infarct-induced abnormal wall motion. Circulation 70:112, 1984.
37. Gillam LD, et al.: Natural history of abnormal wall motion within infarct zones in the acutely infarcted canine ventricle. J Am Coll Cardiol 1:620, 1983.
38. Gibbons EF, et al.: The natural history of regional dysfunction in a canine preparation of chronic infarction. Circulation 61:394, 1985.
39. Garrison JB, et al.: Quantifying regional wall motion and thickening in two-dimensional echocardiography with a computer-aided contouring system. *In* Ostrow H, Ripley K (eds.): Proceedings of Computers in Cardiology, 1977. Long Beach, CA, Institute of Electrical and Electronics Engineers, p. 25, 1977.
40. Geiser EA, et al.: Validation of an algorithm to define 2D echo endocardial borders by comparison to manually defined borders in excellent quality studies: man vs. machine. Clin Res 31:882A, 1983.
41. Oliver L, et al.: Evaluation of an automated border detection algorithm in 2D echo images of varying quality: observer vs. computer variability. J Am Coll Cardiol 3:564, 1984.
42. Schnittger I, et al.: Computerized quantitative analysis of left ventricular wall motion by two-dimensional echocardiography. Circulation 70:242, 1984.
43. Wiske PS, et al.: Echocardiographic definition of the left ventricular centroid: II. Determination of the optimal centroid during systole in the normal and abnormal heart. J Am Coll Cardiol 19:993, 1990.
44. Pearlman JD, et al.: Echocardiographic definition of the left ventricular centroid: I. Analysis of methods for centroid calculation from a single tomogram. J Am Coll Cardiol 16:986, 1990.
45. Sakamaki T, et al.: Comparative validation of two-dimensional echocardiographic segmental wall motion analysis methods. J Am Coll Cardiol 1:581, 1983.
46. Grube E, et al.: Quantitative evaluation of left ventricular wall motion by two-dimensional echocardiography. J Am Coll Cardiol 1:581, 1983.
47. Dodge HT, et al.: The use of biplane and angiocardiography for the measurement of left ventricular volume in man. Am Heart J 60:762, 1960.
48. Hamilton GW, Murray JA, Kennedy JW: Quantitative angiocardiography in ischemic heart disease. The spectrum of abnormal left ventricular function and the role of abnormally contracting segments. Circulation 45:1065, 1972.
49. Hamby RI, et al.: Late systolic bulging of left ventricle in patients with angina pectoris. Chest 65:169, 1974.
50. Ruttley MS, Adams DF, Cohn PF, Abrams HL: Shape and volume changes during "isovolumetric relaxation" in normal and asynergic ventricles. Circulation 50:306, 1974.
51. Clayton PD, et al.: The characteristic sequence for the onset contraction in the normal human left ventricle. Circulation 59:671, 1979.
52. Karliner JS, Bouchard RJ, Gault JH: Dimensional changes of the human heart ventricle prior to aortic valve opening: a cineangiographic study in patients with and without left heart disease. Circulation 44:312, 1971.
53. McDonald IG: The shape and movements of the human left ventricle during systole: a study by cineangiography and by cineradiography of epicardial markers. Am J Cardiol 26:221, 1970.
54. Gibson DG, Brown DJ: Continuous assessment of left ventricular shape in man. Br Heart J 37:904, 1975.
55. Rushmer RF: Physical characteristics of myocardial performance. Am J Cardiol 18:6, 1966.
56. Marier DL, Gibson DG: Limitations of two frame methods for displaying regional left ventricular wall motion in man. Br Heart J 44:555, 1980.
57. Sheehan FH, et al.: Advantages and applications of the centerline method for characterizating regional ventricular function. Circulation 74:293, 1986.
58. Sheehan FH, et al.: Quantitative analysis of regional wall thickening by transesophageal echocardiography. J Thorac Cardioasc Surg 103:347, 1992.
59. Dextra Medical Inc.: System 300 Manual 3-38, 1990.
60. Freeland Medical Division: Cine'View quantifying system. Users guide. 8-8, 1988.
61. Serruys PW, et al.: Preservation of global ventricular and global left ventricular thrombolysis in acute myocardial infarction. J Am Coll Cardiol 7:729, 1986.
62. Mann DL, Gillam LD, Weyman AE: Cross-sectional echocardiographic assessment of regional left ventricular performance and myocardial perfusion. Prog Cardiovasc Dis 29:1, 1986.
63. Mann DL, et al.: Persistence of abnormal wall motion in the canine ventricle after subacute infarction: implications for reperfusion therapy. J Am Coll Cardiol 5:425, 1985.
64. Franklin TD, et al.: Variation in cross-sectional echocardiographic radial target motion relative to a calculated mean centroid of the left ventricle (abstr.) Circulation 62:132, 1985.
65. Kaul S, et al.: Contrast echocardiography in acute myocardial ischemia: III. An in vivo comparison of the extent of abnormal wall motion with the area at risk for necrosis. J Am Coll Cardiol 7:383, 1986.
66. Ormiston JA, Shah PM, Tei C, Wong M: Size and motion of the mitral valve annulus in man: I. A two-dimensional echocardiographic method and findings in normal subjects. Circulation 64:113, 1981.
67. Rogers W, et al.: Predicting survival after myocardial infarction by cross-sectional echo. Circulation 58(Suppl 2):II-233, 1978.
68. Jugdutt BI, Michorowski BL: Role of infarct expansion in rupture of the ventricular septum after acute myocardial infarction; a two-dimensional echocardiographic study. Clin Cardiol 10:641, 1987.
69. Guyer DE, et al.: A new echocardiographic model for quantifying three-dimensional endocardial surface area. J Am Coll Cardiol 8:819, 1986.
70. Guyer DE, et al.: An echocardiographic technique for quantifying and displaying the extent of regional left ventricular dyssynergy. J Am Coll Cardiol 8:830, 1986.
71. Edwards WD, Tajik AJ, Seward JB: Standardized nomenclature and anatomic basis for regional tomographic analysis of the heart. Mayo Clin Proc 56:479, 1981.
72. Wilkins GT, et al.: Correlation between echocardiographic endocardial surface mapping of abnormal wall motion and pathologic infarct size in autopsied hearts. Circulation 77:978, 1988.
73. Picard MH, et al.: Three-dimensional echocardiographic reconstruction and quantitation of the left ventricular endocardial surface area. Circulation (Suppl 2):84:685, 1991.
74. Picard MH, Wilkins GT, Ray PA, Weyman AE: Natural history of left ventricular size and function after acute myocardial infarction: assessment and prediction by echocardiographic endocardial surface mapping. Circulation 82:484, 1990.

CHAPTER

22

LEFT VENTRICLE III: CORONARY ARTERY DISEASE—CLINICAL MANIFESTATIONS AND COMPLICATIONS

SAMUEL C. B. SIU and ARTHUR E. WEYMAN

The assessment of the patient with coronary heart disease is one of the most important clinical applications of echocardiography. The importance of this application lies in the fact that (1) coronary artery disease is the most common form of heart disease and the leading cause of death in the United States and (2) echocardiography plays a diagnostic role at all stages of the disease from the early detection of transient, stress-induced, ischemic dysfunction, through the phase of acute myocardial infarction and its attendant complications, to the development of chronic ischemic heart disease.

As noted in Chapter 21, myocardial ischemia/infarction is manifest echocardiographically as a segmental abnormality in ventricular function. In addition to offering a convenient, noninvasive method for identifying the abnormal wall motion that occurs as a result of ischemia or following acute infarction, echocardiography also permits evaluation of the severity, extent, anatomic location, and natural history of these abnormally contracting segments. It also permits the detection of associated structural changes such as ventricular aneurysms, ventricular septal defect, and mitral regurgitation as well as superimposed complications such as thrombus formation.

Chapter 21 described the various methods by which these contraction abnormalities can be recognized and quantitated. This chapter reviews the sensitivity and specificity of wall motion abnormalities as markers of ischemia/infarction, their relationship to other parameters such as the electrocardiogram (ECG), and their functional significance, natural history, and association with recognized complications. Segmental contraction abnormalities are discussed in the three general settings in which they are encountered: (1) following acute myocardial infarction; (2) in patients with chronic ischemic heart disease, and (3) as a result of transient ischemia induced by exercise or some other form of controlled stress.

ACUTE MYOCARDIAL INFARCTION

Several experimental studies have demonstrated that regional wall motion abnormalities can be visualized echocardiographically within 5 to 10 beats after acute coronary ligation.[1–3] In rigidly controlled experimental studies, functional changes can be observed to precede the development of ECG abnormalities, and in clinical studies of stress-induced ischemia, functional changes precede both the onset of ECG changes and pain. Abnormal wall motion can be observed coincident with the onset of pain in patients with unstable angina; following acute infarction, abnormal wall motion is usually established by the time an examination can be initiated.

These regional contraction abnormalities are characterized by a decreased amplitude and rate of endocardial excursion and an associated decrease in subjacent wall thickening.[1,4–8] When present, they are usually of sufficient magnitude to permit identification by simple visual comparison with adjacent, more normally moving segments.[2,9–13]

Sensitivity and Specificity of Abnormal Wall Motion as an Echocardiographic Marker of Acute Infarction

Available data suggest that some abnormality of left ventric (LV) wall motion can be detected echocardiographically in 89 to 100% of patients with transmural infarction.[9,10,12,14–18] Likewise, in the experimental animal, abnormal wall motion (AWM) can be detected in virtually every case following successful acute coronary ligation.[2] Although, on occasion, individual ventricular segments that do not show evidence of infarction pathologically may move abnormally and areas containing limited or old infarction may appear to move normally,[9,12] no cases of adequately studied, documented transmural infarction have been reported in which no wall motion abnormalities were noted.

When the infarction is nontransmural or subendocardial, AWM is noted less consistently. Although patient groups have been small, the reported occurrence of AWM in nontransmural infarction has ranged from 0 to 100%.[12,14–17,19] If the available data are pooled,[12,14–17,19] 79% (56/71) of nontransmural infarcts demonstrate AWM. In our experience, AWM has been detected in 86% of patients with documented non-Q-wave infarction studied within the first 48 hours of onset of symptoms.[20] The presence or absence of AWM appears to relate to the transmural rather than to the circumferential extent of the subendocardial infarct, with minor degrees of transmural involvement being less likely to produce regional dysfunction.[15] An assessment of wall motion in these patients, therefore, is particularly useful because it distinguishes functionally significant from nonsignificant infarction.

Methods for quantitating the extent of abnormal motion were discussed in Chapter 21, and success rates vary with the requirements of the system of quantitation employed. Recordings that are technically adequate for *segmental* analysis (partial or complete) have been obtained in 73 to 100% of patients examined within 24 hours of symptom onset.[19,21] In earlier clinical studies, complete visualization was felt to be possible in roughly 85% of patients in whom any data could be obtained; however, more recently success rates of 98 and 100% have been reported.[19,22] Quantitation of the extent of infarction within a single plane can be achieved less frequently, and endocardial mapping that requires that the endocardium be recorded around the circumference of the ventricle in multiple orthogonal projections is feasible in ≤80% of patients.[23]

In experimental studies, acoustic access can easily be obtained when appropriate models are used, and in this setting, technical problems relate primarily to acoustic coupling, fine plane positioning, and data registration.

Degree of Abnormal Motion Within Infarcted Segments

Acute transmural infarction generally produces profound changes in regional LV function, with the majority of affected segments (more than 72%) being either akinetic or dyskinetic.[15,24] Hypokinesis, when present, is usually severe, with a mean decrease from normal of 50 to 75% reported Wall motion changes associated with nontransmural infarction are characteristically less severe, with roughly two thirds being hypokinetic and one third dyskinetic. Wall thickening is likewise characteristically decreased in areas of acute ischemia, while frank thinning is not uncommonly noted.[24–28] Direct comparison between wall thickening and transmural extent of pathologic infarct suggests that when the transmural extent of infarction is less than 20%, thickening decreases by roughly 50%, whereas infarction of more than 20% of the thickness of the myocardium is uniformly associated with wall thinning.[24]

The relationship between abnormalities of mechanical function and reduction in coronary blood flow is nonlinear.[29] Therefore, it is difficult to correlate the degree of AWM with the level of decreased coronary blood flow. Wall thinning, however, has been reported only when myocardial blood flow is reduced to greater than 75% of control values.[27] Function, likewise, is not directly related to the degree of coronary stenosis, with normal function being preserved despite the creation of 90% stenosis in the experimental model. When increased afterload or hypotension is superimposed on this degree of stenosis, however, regional dysfunction is produced.[27]

Segmental Dysfunction in Regions Outside the Zone of Ischemia/Infarction

Several studies[9,15,24,30,31] have shown that segments of myocardium adjacent to, but not grossly involved in, the ischemic/infarction process may display major contraction abnormalities. Although the reasons for this "adjacent asynergy" are unknown, they may in part relate to mechanical tethering by adjacent ischemic tissue, adenosine triphosphate (ATP) depletion, or other metabolic abnormalities within the adjacent tissue, or perhaps damage at the ultrastructural level. In addition, remote asynergy from potentially reversible ischemia outside the infarct zone has also been reported.[17,22] Hence, any attempt to quantify the amount of myocardial ischemia/infarction by measuring the extent of AWM is limited to some degree by uncertainty as to the underlying pathologic, physiologic, and metabolic environment that the functional abnormality reflects. It is important to remember that function is an independent marker of the effects of ischemic disease, because it is function rather than histology or local metabolism that determines the effect of ischemia on the organism as a whole.

Recovery of Regional Function Following Reperfusion

The return of myocardial function to normal after the restoration of normal coronary flow is also variable.[32] Regional wall abnormalities may persist for as long as

3 days in dogs subjected to 5 hours of partial coronary occlusion followed by reperfusion. Variable recovery has been reported after 3 hours of total occlusion followed by reperfusion, with loss of the expected correlation between the extent of AWM and infarct span. Shorter occlusion periods of 10 to 15 minutes are associated with recovery times of ½ to 2½ hours. The rate of recovery appears to relate directly to the size of the ischemic zone and the duration of occlusion. In patients who received acute thrombolytic therapy for myocardial infarction, some recovery of wall motion within the infarct zone has been observed from 24 hours to 10 days after treatment.[33–38] Continued recovery, however, can be documented for up to 3 months after myocardial infarction.[39,40]

Other Causes of Segmental Dysfunction

Finally, it is important to remember that myocardial ischemia and infarction are not the only causes of AWM. Abnormal septal motion may be seen in patients with right ventricular volume overload, left bundle branch block, and Wolff-Parkinson-White syndrome, as well as following cardiac surgery. Anterior wall motion may also be abnormal in aortic insufficiency. In the overwhelming majority of these instances, although endocardial excursion is abnormal, wall thickening will be normal, and this distinction permits the identification of these abnormalities as nonischemic. Focal myocarditis is indistinguishable from myocardial ischemia/infarction in that both excursion and myocardial thickening are depressed.[41] Conversely, multiple infarctions resulting in an ischemic cardiomyopathy can be manifested as diffuse left ventricular hypokinesis.[42]

Relationship of the Location and Extent of Dysfunction to Other Parameters for Defining Infarct Location, Patient Status, and Prognosis

Pathologic Infarction

The relationship of AWM to underlying pathologic infarct distribution and transmural extent has been examined both clinically and experimentally for segments, planes, and for the entire LV. In general, there is a good relationship between histologic evidence of infarction and segmental function.[9,15] Segments with morphologic evidence of infarction show abnormal function in greater than 90% of cases and in all cases in which the infarct involves more than 5% of the myocardium.[9,15] In patients dying during the acute phase of their first infarction, histologic evidence of necrosis or scar has been reported in 95% of segments exhibiting AWM.[9] In a mixed population with both acute and chronic infarction, the association was less clear, with roughly 32% of abnormally functioning segments occurring in morphologically normal areas. The majority of these morphologically normal but functionally abnormal segments, however, were adjacent to myocardial scar, and their abnormal motion was presumably due to mechanical traction.[15] The remainder lay in territories supplied by critically narrowed coronary arteries and presumably represent regions that were ischemic during life.

A general relationship has also been noted between the severity of segmental dysfunction and degree of pathologic abnormality. Transmurally infarcted segments most commonly are akinetic or dyskinetic, while hypokinesis is seen more often in nontransmurally infarcted or adjacent normal zones. The presence of normal wall motion, on the other hand, appears to exclude transmural infarction.

Experimentally, the circumferential extent of AWM within individual short-axis sections has been shown to correlate well with both the pathologic infarct area[2] and the linear extent of infarction in comparable anatomic sections.[15] The area of AWM, however, consistently overestimates both the area and the marginal extremes of the underlying infarct.[2,15] Figure 22–1 illustrates the relationship of the extent of AWM, expressed as a percentage of the end-diastolic circumference of the ventricle, to the percentage of the myocardial area that shows evidence of infarction in 47 ventricular sections.

When examined quantitatively, this relationship, however, varies with the level of dysfunction. In our experience, dyskinesis underestimates infarct span, while hypokinesis overestimates the extent of infarction. True akinesis in the intact beating heart virtually never occurs. Studies of global dysfunction reveal similar trends with two-dimensional estimates of dysfunction overestimating histologic extent of infarction, particularly for smaller infarcts.[43]

Loss of wall thickening or wall thinning has also been compared to the extent of underlying infarction, and although the results are less consistent, generally good correlations have been found between the absence of

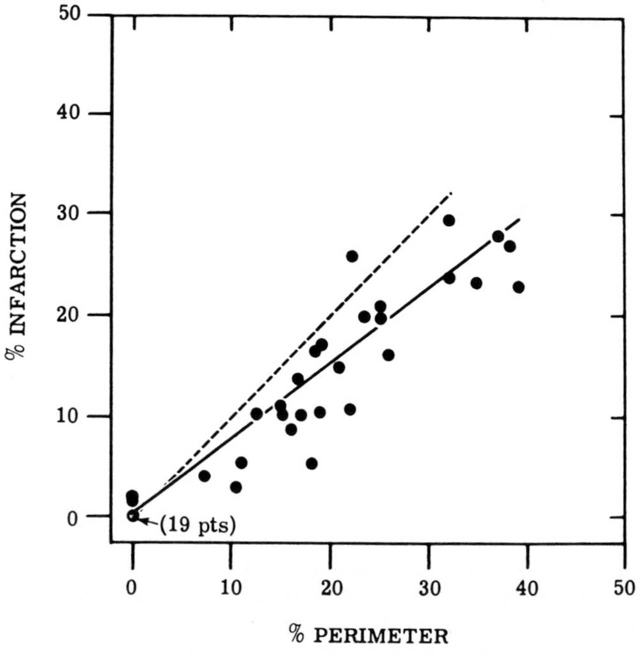

Fig. 22–1. Relationship of the percentage of the ventricle showing asynergy to the percentage of the myocardium in the same section showing evidence of infarction in a series of 47 ventricular sections. The area of abnormal wall motion tends to overestimate consistently the underlying infarct area. Interrupted line = line of unity; solid line = regression line.

wall thickening and infarct size.[25,28] The global infarct size has also been compared to the three-dimensional extent of the region of dysfunction using the echocardiographic mapping technique described in Chapter 21. Figure 22–2 illustrates the results of that comparison.

Relationship of Abnormal Wall Motion to Electrocardiographic Infarct Location

Traditionally, the anatomic site of acute transmural myocardial infarction has been localized clinically by the Q wave distribution on the standard 12-lead ECG. The relationship between infarct location predicted by the ECG and the area of asynergy detected by the echocardiogram has been examined in several studies.[9,14,16,17,19,21,22] Correspondence of the echocardiographic location of dyssynergy with the ECG location of infarction has been found in roughly 95% of reported cases with disagreement generally being caused by the area of dysfunction reported by the echocardiogram extending beyond that predicted by the ECG. These relationships can be described best by using one of the segmental systems. This approach permits direct correlation between events occurring at specific anatomic locations within the ventricle.

Figure 22–3 illustrates a method that has been derived to display these data graphically. This format incorporates the segmental system discussed in Chapter 21 and depicts the heart as a series of three concentric rings.[9] The cardiac apex forms the central ring, and the four segments at the base of the heart form the outer ring. The ventricle is thereby displayed as if viewed from the apex. The interventricular septum is to the viewer's left, the lateral wall is to the right, the anterior wall is positioned superiorly, and the posterior wall is positioned inferiorly.

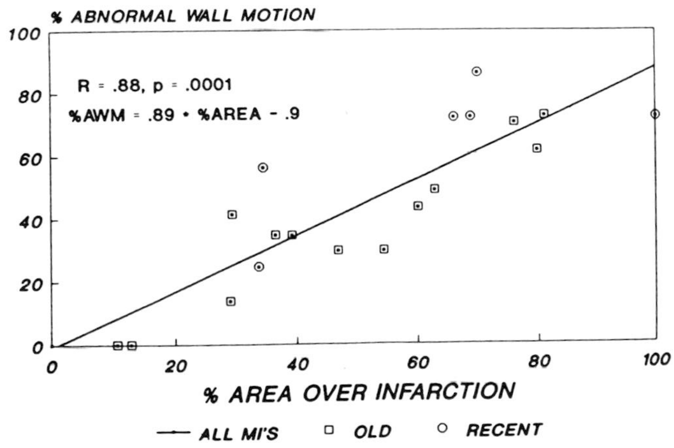

Fig. 22–2. Correlation of the pathologic extent of myocardial infarction by endocardial surface area overlying infarction (% area over infarction) with the extent of abnormal wall motion derived from the echocardiographic endocardial surface map (% AWM). The correlation line (solid line) and regression equation for the total group are given. Circles denote those with recent infarcts and squares denote those with old infarcts. (From Wilkins GT, et al.: Correlation between echocardiographic surface mapping of abnormal wall motion and pathologic infarct size in autopsied hearts. Circulation 77:978, 1988. Reproduced by permission of the American Heart Association, Inc.)

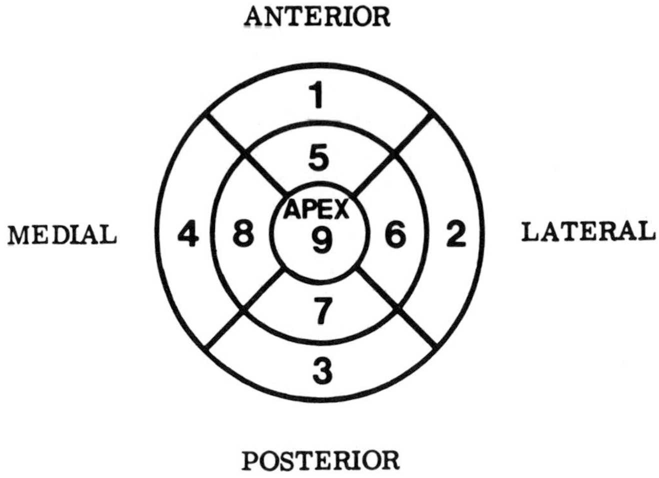

Fig. 22–3. Diagrammatic method for displaying motion within individual segments of the ventricle. The center, or bull's-eye, of the target represents the ventricular apex; the middle concentric ring, the four segments at the midventricular or papillary muscle level; and the outer concentric ring, the four segments at the base of the ventricle. (From Heger J, et al.: Cross-sectional echocardiography in acute myocardial infarction: detection and localization of regional left ventricular asynergy. Circulation 60:531, 1979. Reproduced by permission of the American Heart Association, Inc.)

Inferior Infarction. The patterns of AWM observed in patients with electrocardiographic evidence of isolated inferior, inferoposterior, and inferolateral infarction are illustrated in Figure 22–4. In this series, 95% of patients with electrocardiographic evidence of infarction involving the inferior wall (Q waves and leads 2,3, AVF) had dyssynergy involving at least one of the two posterior segments. When isolated inferior infarction was present electrocardiographically (Fig. 22–4A), asynergy was typically confined to the posterior quadrant and limited to one or, at most, two segments. The specific area of posterior involvement was evenly distributed between the base of the ventricle and the papillary muscle region. When inferior wall infarction was complicated by acute ventricular septal defect (Fig. 22–4B), the region of asynergy uniformly involved the two medial segments, which correspond anatomically to the posterior portion of the interventricular septum. In each instance, septal aneurysm formation was noted.[9] None of these patients had electrocardiographic evidence of septal involvement, and the wall motion abnormality, therefore, was a better predictor of the extent and location of infarction. Patients in the electrocardiographic subgroups of inferoposterior infarction (Fig. 22–4C) had asynergy extending to the lateral segments in addition to their posterior involvement. Those in the electrocardiographic inferolateral group (Fig. 22–4D) had the most extensive involvement, which included the whole posterior quadrant, the lateral wall at the base, and variable involvement of the lateral wall in the midventricle. In this group, AWM was also frequently noted in the cardiac apex, the midanterior wall, and the septum.

Unfortunately, this segmental system is not ideally aligned to depict the anatomic location of inferior infarction. The location of the abnormal inferior wall motion

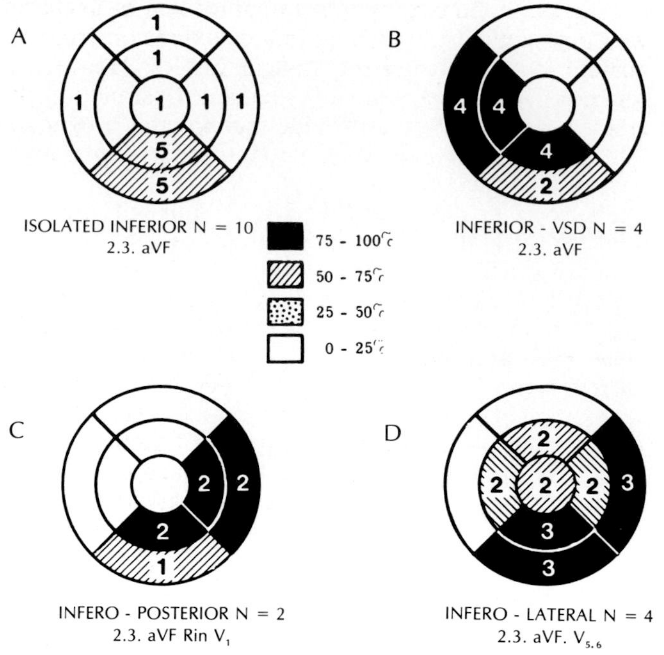

Fig. 22–4. Frequency of segmental asynergy associated with electrocardiogram subgroups of patients with inferior infarction. The shading indicates the percentage of patients within each group who show asynergy in a particular segment. VSD = ventricular septal defect. (From Heger J, et al.: Cross-sectional echocardiography in acute myocardial infarction: detection and localization of regional left ventricular asynergy. Circulation 60:531, 1979. Reproduced by permission of the American Heart Association, Inc.)

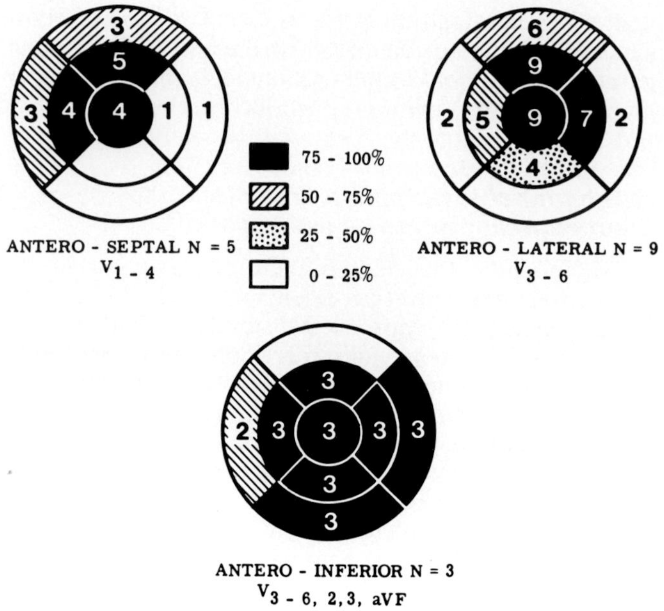

Fig. 22–5. Frequency of segmental asynergy associated with the electrocardiogram subgroups of patients with anterior wall infarction. (From Heger J, et al.: Cross-sectional echocardiography in acute myocardial infarction: detection and localization of regional left ventricular asynergy. Circulation 60:531, 1979. Reproduced by permission of the American Heart Association, Inc.)

in this system is rotated roughly 30° counterclockwise from its true anatomic location, and most inferior infarctions actually involve a portion of the medial and posterior segments.

Anterior Infarction. Figure 22–5 illustrates the patterns of AWM observed in patients in the electrocardiographic subgroups of anterior infarction.[9] In all instances of anterior infarction, one of the anterior segments, either at the base or midventricular level, was abnormal.[9] In patients with anteroseptal infarction, abnormal motion occurred most frequently in the anterior segment at the midventricular level with associated involvement of the cardiac apex and the interventricular septum at the midventricle. The anterobasal and medial-basal segments were also frequently involved but less so than were the more distal portions of the ventricle. Involvement of the base of the ventricle in anteroseptal infarction appears to depend on the level of obstruction to the left anterior descending coronary artery.

When the obstruction occurs proximal to the first septal perforator, the full extent of the anterior wall is abnormal, whereas obstruction below the first septal perforator characteristically spares the basal portions of the anterior wall.[44] In the subgroup of patients with anterolateral infarction, asynergy was observed to involve uniformly the cardiac apex and the anterior segment of the ventricle at the midventricular level. In the majority of these patients, the lateral segment at the midventricular level was also abnormal with an extensive but heterogeneous pattern of involvement of the remainder of the ventricle. Finally, patients with combined anterior and inferior infarction had extensive ventricular motion abnormalities. Only the anterobasal segment was completely spared.

Apical Infarction. The sensitivity and specificity of the 12-lead ECG in localizing left ventricular apical infarction is poorly defined despite numerous electrocardiographic criteria.[45–47] In contrast, the presence and extent of apical dysfunction can be readily visualized and quantitated by two-dimensional echocardiography.[48–50] In a report of 64 patients with apical asynergy from myocardial infarction, it was observed that abnormal Q waves were absent in 37%.[51] In patients with abnormal Q waves and apical asynergy on echocardiography, only 10% had an infarct correctly localized to the apex by recognized electrocardiographic criteria for apical infarction. Although Q-wave distribution was an insensitive predictor of isolated apical dysfunction, the presence of Q waves was associated with a greater extent and degree of apical dysfunction. This association was particularly evident when persistent ST-segment elevation was also present.

These observations are consistent with older pathologic data and suggest that, in general, inferior infarction tends to be oriented more toward the base of the ventricle, whereas anterior infarctions tend to involve the cardiac apex. They also suggest that apical dysfunction is poorly reflected electrocardiographically and that inferior wall infarction may extend into the interventricular septum and may be associated with severe septal damage without electrocardiographic evidence of septal involvement.

In other studies, asynergy in segments remote from

the electrocardiographically predicted site of infarction has been shown to correlate with angiographic evidence of stenosis of the coronary arteries supplying these remote segments.[17,22]

Relationship Between Extent and Site of Abnormal Wall Motion and Electrocardiographic Type of Infarction: Q Versus Non-Q-Wave Infarction

Patients with non-Q-wave infarction generally have a smaller extent of dysfunction than those with Q-wave infarction.[19,20] These findings are consistent with ventriculographic observations that non-Q-wave infarctions are associated with better regional and global left ventricular function than Q-wave infarctions.[52] Thus, the relatively benign in-hospital morbidity and mortality observed in non-Q-wave infarctions may be a result of a more limited functional abnormality.[52–54]

In a study of 115 consecutive patients with documented myocardial infarction, non-Q-wave infarctions more commonly involved the posterolateral region (25%) than Q-wave infarctions (7%).[20] Because coronary angiographic studies fail to note a higher prevalence of right or circumflex arterial involvement in non-Q-wave infarctions,[52,55] this increased prevalence of posterolateral wall motion abnormalities in non-Q-wave infarctions may be a result of (1) inability to detect Q wave in the posterolateral region by 12-lead electrocardiography[56] or (2) protection of the posterolateral wall from transmural injury by collaterals from the distal right and left circumflex coronary arteries.

Relationship of Extent of Dyssynergy to Radionuclide Measures of Infarct Location and Size

Several studies have examined the relationship between echocardiographically defined regional wall motion abnormalities and conventional radionuclide methods for infarct sizing.[14,57,58] A good relationship has been reported between the echocardiographic wall motion scores and thallium-201 and technetium pyrophosphate estimation of infarct size.[14,57,58]

Relationship of Abnormal Wall Motion to Ventricular Performance

The extent and severity of the AWM that is recorded echocardiographically have been compared to both clinical and hemodynamic evidence of ventricular performance in several clinical studies.[10,59,60] In each study, a clear relationship could be established between the degree of AWM, expressed as a wall motion score or score index and patient status. The wall motion score index has been reported to be a better and more stable prognostic indicator for subsequent cardiac events after myocardial infarction than Killip class alone. The wall motion score permitted stratification of patients into those with low or high risk clinical outcomes regardless of electrocardiographic type of infarction (Q vs. non-Q wave) or the timing of the echocardiogram (early vs. predischarge).[19,61–64] In those patients with recurrent chest pain, echocardiographic quantitation of asynergy was better at distinguishing infarct extension from recurrent ischemia than the 12-lead ECG.[65] Hence, the quantitative assessment of regional dysfunction by echocardiography may provide incremental prognostic information to the care of patients after acute myocardial infarction.

Figure 22–6 illustrates the results of one of these studies.[10] In this series, the ventricle was divided into nine segments, as illustrated in Figure 22–3, wall motion within each segment was assigned a numeric value (normal motion = 0, hypokinesis = 1, akinesis = 2, dyskinesis = 3, and hyperkinesis = −1), and the values of each segment were then summed to derive a total score reflecting both the extent and degree of dysfunction. In this format, when all nine segments functioned normally, the total wall motion score equaled 0. When all segments were dyskinetic, the score was 3 (the numeric value for dyskinesis) × 9 (the number of segments), or 27. With this approach, the indices noted in patients with uncomplicated infarctions were significantly lower than those in patients with evidence of pulmonary congestion or peripheral hypoperfusion. Further, in the absence of acute ventricular septal defect or mitral regurgitation, death occurred only in patients with the highest wall motion scores.

When ventricular septal rupture or acute mitral regurgitation complicated infarction, the mean wall motion

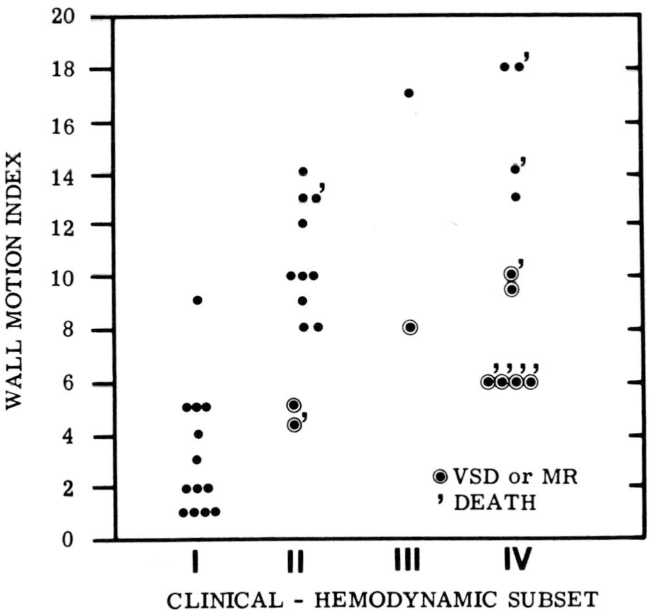

Fig. 22–6. Relationship of extent and severity of abnormal wall motion (expressed as a wall motion index) to the clinical-hemodynamic performance of individual patients. Group I = uncomplicated myocardial infarction; group II = pulmonary congestion without peripheral hypoperfusion; group III = peripheral hypoperfusion without pulmonary congestion; and group IV = cardiogenic shock. (Swan-Forrester classification). VSD = ventricular septal defect; MR = mitral regurgitation. (From Heger J, et al.: Cross-sectional echocardiographic analysis of the extent of left ventricular asynergy in acute myocardial infarction. Circulation 61:1113, 1980. Reproduced by permission of the American Heart Association, Inc.)

score, although still significantly higher than that observed with uncomplicated infarction, was less than expected given the severity of the hemodynamic dysfunction and the high mortality within this group.[10] Apparently, allowance for hyperkinesis in the noninfarcted segments inappropriately weighted the score, and in this setting, areas of apparent compensatory hyperfunction do not favorably affect outcome. As a result of this finding, we no longer weigh hyperkinesis differently from normal.

Others have modified this original system by both increasing the number of segments and dividing the sum score by the total number of segments in the system to derive a wall motion score index.[19,61] Despite variations in approach, however, the overall results have been comparable. Note, however, that the index is only truly valid when the total number of segments in the system is used as the divisor. Division only by the number recorded is incorrect and at the extreme could lead to ventricular function being represented by a single segment.

Relationship of Abnormal Wall Motion to Survival

In addition to providing information about ventricular function in the setting of myocardial ischemic/infarction, several studies suggest that two-dimensional echocardiography can also provide important prognostic information following infarction. To date, such studies have examined the following parameters: functional infarct size,[13] infarct expansion,[66] and the presence of remote asynergy.[17,22] Figure 22–7 illustrates the relationship of survival to functional infarct size derived using the truncated cone formula illustrated in Figure 21–26 and expressed as a percentage of overall left ventricular endocardial surface area. In this group of 32 patients, the mean functional infarct area for survivors was significantly less than the mean for nonsurvivors. Importantly, all patients with functional infarct areas involving 35% or less of the ventricle survived. In the group with infarct areas of greater than 35%, approximately 60% were nonsurvivors. Thus, although patients with large functional infarct sizes (up to 68%) may survive, such patients are at high risk, and survival is associated with major pump dysfunction.[13] Because wall motion becomes abnormal immediately following an acute ischemic event, this method should identify patients at high risk early in their clinical course.

The second parameter that is associated with a significant mortality is infarct expansion.[66] Significant expansion within the infarct area has been reported in 12 to 29% of patients.[23,66] Infarct expansion occurs within minutes after coronary ligation in the experimental animal and has been observed as early as 2 hours after acute infarction in humans.[23,67] The major component of expansion appears to occur acutely and, once initiated, continues at a reduced rate through the first several weeks. Expansion was originally reported to be associated with significant risk of ventricular rupture and death (50%).[66] Subsequent data, however, suggest that these complications occur much less commonly, which is more consistent with our experience.[23,68] In summary,

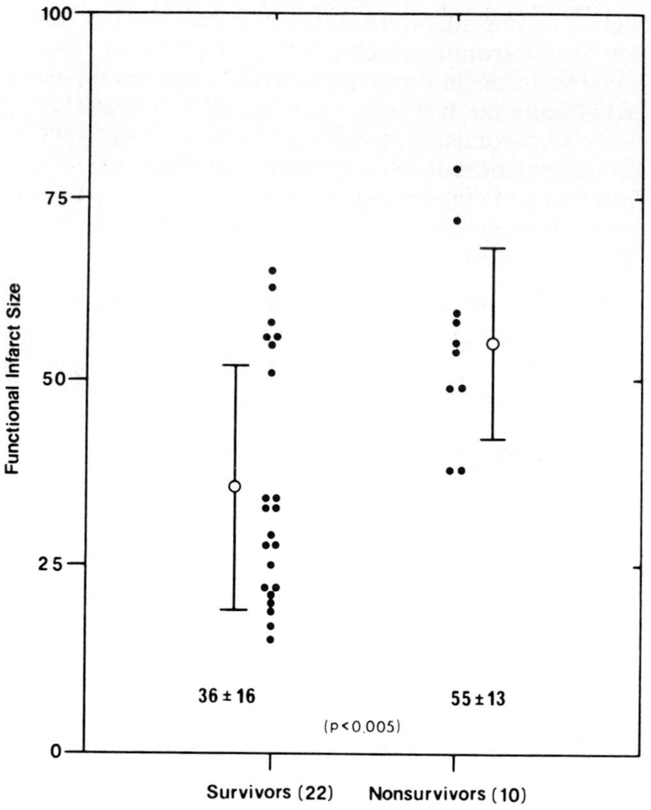

Fig. 22–7. Relationship of functional infarct size, expressed as a percentage of total left ventricular endocardial surface area, to patient survival.

the two-dimensional echocardiographic recognition of infarct expansion in the setting of acute myocardial infarction has been related to a worse short-term patient prognosis and functional classification.

Wall motion abnormalities outside the electrocardiographically predicted infarct zone—remote asynergy—have also been reported to correlate with a greater prevalence of death, cardiogenic shock, progression to a worse Killip class, and reinfarction.[17] This finding has been attributed to the presence of multivessel coronary disease with resulting ischemia or infarction in the vascular territories remote from that of the infarct vessel.[17,22]

Natural History of Abnormal Wall Motion

Despite the clearly defined association between the extent of AWM and the underlying region of ischemia/infarction and the documented importance of these functional changes little data exist about their natural history. This lack of information is predominantly a function of the limitations of the techniques that have been available to study regional function. Angiography, which has been the gold standard for such assessment, is highly invasive and poorly suited to serial studies in the acute infarct patient. Although noninvasive, cumulative radiation dose also limits the frequency with which radionuclide ventriculograms can be obtained. As a result, most clinical studies report only baseline characteristics, which are then related to long-term prognosis.[69–71] However, a clear definition of the natural history of postinfarction ventricular morphology and regional dysfunction remains essential, because it is only on the basis of such knowledge that patients can appropriately be selected for aggressive therapies and the effects of additional interventions to limit infarct size or to modify ventricular remodeling can be assessed.

The introduction of two-dimensional echocardiography appeared to provide an ideal method for defining the natural history of postmyocardial infarction regional dysfunction. Unfortunately, early reports yielded discordant and often misleading results. Studies based on segmental systems, which by their nature cannot describe ventricular expansion or chamber dilation, not surprisingly reported little change in functional infarct sizes over the first days and weeks following the onset of symptoms.[14,19,21,28] At least one study, however, reported a decrease in the extent of segmental dysfunction within the first 48 hours, both adjacent and distant to the site of infarction.[25] In contrast, studies using quantitative segment length measurements derived from midpapillary short axis views suggested that between a quarter and a third of patients develop disproportionate dilation of the endocardial segment length within the infarct zone.[66] This infarct expansion was observed as early as 3 days after infarction, and the segment length continued to expand over a period of days to weeks. On longer follow-up, these patients showed a continued increase in endocardial segment length in both the infarcted and noninfarcted zones.[68] Experimental studies, in which infarct location and size could be better controlled, likewise dlffer in result, with some reporting infarct expansion,[72] while others note a lack of change in the extent of AWM[28] or even regression over the first 48 hours after coronary ligation.[25] This lack of clarity of message appears to relate to (1) the type of measurement system employed; (2) the time points at which the extent of dysfunction was sampled; (3) the nature of the study performed (experimental or clinical); and (4) failure to subdivide populations based on initial entry characteristics (i.e., ventricular size) and infarct subtype (anterior, inferior, apical, or subendocardial).

The more recent development of the endocardial mapping technique (EMT) described in Chapter 21 has permitted ventricular size or endocardial surface area (ESA), the extent of ventricular dysfunction (AWM), and the relationship of the region of dysfunction to the normally functioning zone of myocardium (%AWM) to be assessed over time.[73–75] By simultaneously quantifying the functional infarct size and ventricular size, one can more precisely determine the interaction of ventricular dysfunction and morphology and characterize the subtypes.

Separation of Acute From Chronic Changes

To define the patterns of change in ventricular (ESA) and functional infarct size (AWM), it is necessary to record these parameters at sequential points following the onset of symptoms and then relate changes over time to initial parameters. Acute changes in ventricular morphology and function are generally complete by 3 months. Although in some infarct types, the acute changes may be completed earlier, 3 months appears to be sufficient to allow acute changes to be characterized in all patients. More chronic changes, which are opposite in direction to the acute changes or occur at a different rate, continue for a year or more (Figs. 22–8 and 22–9).

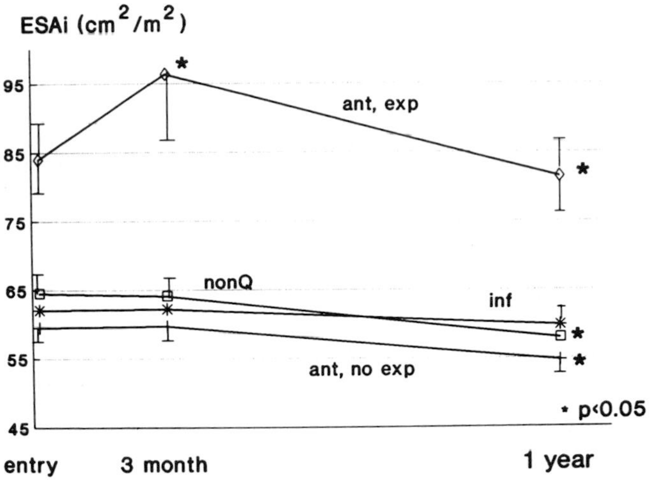

Fig. 22–8. Graph of endocardial surface area index (ESAi) over 1-year observation period for four subgroups. ant, exp = anterior infarction with early infarct expansion; ant, no exp = anterior infarction without early expansion; inf = inferior infarction; nonQ = non Q wave infarction. (From Picard MH, et al.: Progressive changes in ventricular structure and function during the year after acute myocardial infarction. Am Heart J 124:24, 1992.)

Types of Acute Changes Recorded

Serial echocardiographic studies using the EMT reveal five distinct patterns of response to acute infarction

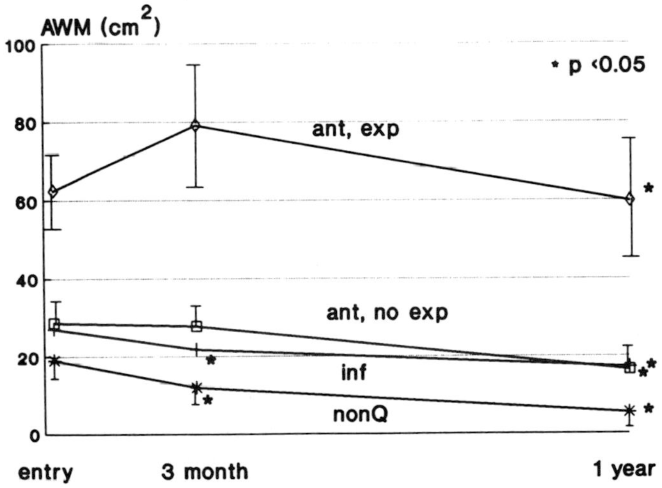

Fig. 22–9. Graph of area of abnormal wall motion (AWM) over 1-year observation period for four subgroups. ant, exp = anterior infarction with early infarct expansion; ant, no exp = anterior infarction without early expansion; inf = inferior infarction; nonQ = non Q wave infarction. (From Picard MH, et al.: Progressive changes in ventricular structure and function during the year after acute myocardial infarction. Am Heart J 124:24, 1992. Reproduced by permission of C.V. Mosby Co.).

(assessed at the 3-month follow-up period).[23] These patterns include the following:

1. *Infarct expansion*—an increase in the infarct area without extension of the infarct or a significant change in the area of normally functioning myocardium (an increase in total ESA of at least 5% accompanied by a greater than 5% increase in the extent, the percentage, of AWM).
2. *Ventricular dilation*—symmetric enlargement of both normal and abnormal endocardial segments (an increase of more than 5% in ESA without a change in the percentage of AWM).
3. *Infarct extension*—an increase in AWM of greater than 5% and extension of the AWM into a previously uninvolved echocardiographic wall segment.
4. *Absence of significant change over time*—variation of less than 5% in the absolute extent of AWM.
5. *Infarct regression*—a 5% decrease in the absolute area of AWM.

Thus, an increase in the region of the left ventricle functioning abnormally can be due to extension of dysfunction to a new territory, expansion or stretching of infarcted myocardium, or an increase in total LV surface area without a change in the percentage of infarct size (Table 22–1). The threshold of 5% is used because this is outside the error of the method. Importantly, because the goal of these studies is to define the natural history of a single infarct, patients with prior infarcts, valvular or primary myocardial disease, mechanical or surgical intervention, or clinical evidence of reinfarction are generally excluded.

Parameters Available at Entry

Three primary parameters can be examined in the initial study and related to natural history: ventricular size (ESA), infarct location, and functional infarct size (AWM).

Natural History Based on Ventricular Size at Entry. Patients presenting with acute infarction can have ventricular surface areas within or above the normal range for body surface area (ESA). The majority of patients with acute infarcts have ESA's slightly below the normal mean; however, none have ventricles below the normal range in the absence of confounding disease. A subgroup of patients have an initial ESA above the normal range, and as discussed later, these patients typically have infarct expansion. Because the total population is composed of a larger group whose ventricles are slightly reduced in size combined with a smaller subgroup whose ventricles have expanded, the mean

Table 22–1. Echocardiographic Characteristics Based on Location of Abnormal Wall Motion

	Anterior (n = 26)	Inferior (n = 43)	Apical (n = 7)
ESA index (cm²/m²)			
Entry	70.5 ± 13.6**	61.4 ± 7.8	59.1 ± 7.9
3 Months	79.6 ± 18.6‡	63.2 ± 8.2	57.7 ± 7.3
%AWM			
Entry	39.6 ± 18.0§‖	23.0 ± 11.5¶	9.9 ± 4.5
3 Months	39.7 ± 20.4	20.9 ± 13.6	6.4 ± 6.0#
Infarct Group			
No change (n)	1	21	1
Regression (n)	3	13	5
Extension (n)	2	6	1
Dilation (n)	11	3	0
Expansion (n)	9	0	0

Seventy-six patients with acute myocardial infarction examined within 48 hours of onset of symptoms (entry) and again at 3 months.

Anterior, inferior, apical = site of abnormal wall motion; ESA index = endocardial surface area index; %AWM = extent of abnormal wall motion expressed as a percentage of the total endocardial surface area; infarct group = pattern of change in ESA index and %AWM between entry and 3 months.

* p < .005 vs. inferior.
† p < .05 vs. apical.
‡ p < .0005 c/w entry.
§ p < .00005 c/w inferior.
‖ p < .00005 vs. apical.
¶ p < .005 vs. apical.
# p < .01 c/w entry.

(From Picard MH, et al.: Echocardiographic assessment of postmyocardial infarction size and function. Heart Failure 7:180, 1991.)

ESA of infarct patients at entry (within hours after the onset of symptoms) does not differ from normal (normal range of ESA, 53 to 78.9 cm^2/m^2).[23]

Patients With an Increase in Ventricular Surface (ESA) at Entry: Infarct Expansion. The subgroup of patients with first infarcts who have normalized ventricular surface areas above the normal range at entry has been demonstrated in both experimental and clinical studies to have infarct expansion.[23,67,76] Infarct expansion is defined as enlargement of the infarct zone without further myocardial necrosis. Members of this subgroup have (1) ESAs that fall outside the normal range at the earliest point of study (2 hours or less), (2) have anterior and apical sites of infarction, and (3) demonstrate continued expansion within the infarct zone for up to 3 months in the absence of intervention (see Figs. 22–8 and 22–9).[23,77]

Infarct expansion is important to identify because it is associated with increased morbidity and mortality and is the substrate for aneurysm formation.[66,68,78–82] The early increase in ESA is due to enlargement of myocardial segments within the infarct zone and occurs primarily at the ventricular apex. The thinning and stretching of the infarct zone observed macroscopically is due to slippage of myocytes and sarcomere stretching.[83,84] In our studies, anteroapical location of myocardial dysfunction, rather than size of infarct alone, was the most important predictor of expansion.[23,67] In reporting an autopsy study, Pirolo et al. stated that infarct expansion may be attenuated by preinfarction ventricular hypertrophy.[85]

The prominence of apical expansion probably relates to the exaggerated changes in wall stress that occur in this region during infarction. Normal apical myocardium is thinner, appropriate to its smaller radius of curvature, than that of other areas of the ventricle.[86,87] The increased myocardial thinning and increase in radius of curvature that occur following ischemia would be expected, by the LaPlace relationship, to lead to a more rapid rise in regional wall stress at the apex compared to other regions of the ventricle and may lead to regional differences in cardiac dilatation.[88] Regional differences in myocardial fiber arrangement, shortening, and the effects of ischemia may also contribute to the increased vulnerability of the cardiac apex to infarct expansion.[89–94]

Establishing the exact timing of the expansion process has implications not only for understanding the mechanism of the initial alterations in ventricular morphology but also in determining whether interventions to prevent or reverse early functional expansion will prevent longstanding infarct expansion. Although clinical studies are limited by the time interval from onset of symptoms to patient presentation, experimental studies suggest that infarct expansion occurs in the first minutes following coronary occlusion, a duration known to cause reversible myocardial cell injury without necrosis.[67,95] In the canine model of ischemia, it has been observed that functional expansion of the endocardial surface is a regional process rather than a diffuse one and is determined primarily by an anterior-apical location of ischemic dysfunction.[67] The size of this anterior region of dysfunction appears to be a secondary factor correlating with the degree of early expansion. In the clinical setting, early infarct expansion manifesting as an increase in endocardial surface area has been detected as early as 2 hours from the onset of the symptoms of myocardial infarction.[23] These observations suggest that immediate reversible morphologic changes in the endocardial surface establish the template for late abnormalities of ventricular shape that becomes fixed as myocytes become necrotic and are later replaced by fibrotic tissue.

During the first week following infarction, further dilation of the endocardial segment in the infarct zone may be observed in patients with anterior infarctions and early infarct expansion.[66] Studies performed at 1 month and 3 months revealed that changes in ventricular size and extent of AWM generally parallel those observed during the first week.[23,68] Thus, patients with acute infarct expansion continue to undergo progressive LV enlargement with an increase in AWM during the first 3 months. Although stretching and elongation of endocardial segments in both infarcted and noninfarcted regions have been reported to be the mechanism of chronic infarct expansion, the relative increases in the two regions are not identical. Patients with early expansion tended to undergo further expansion with a disproportionately greater increase in LV surface area overlying the area of dysfunction.[23] Beyond 3 months, two patterns of evolution have been observed. In our studies, the compensated ventricle generally showed a gradual decrease in ESA and AWM from 3 months to a year.[76] Importantly, both the ESA and the extent of AWM are similar at 1 year to those seen at entry (see Fig. 22–8 and 22–9). This pattern is similar to that seen in experimental models with an extended time course and has been attributed to replacement of the infarct zone by scar tissue and subsequent scar contracture.[72]

Others have reported that ventricular dilation was an ongoing process during the first year following infarction.[96,97] These studies have focused primarily on patients with anterior Q wave infarctions or those with extensive left ventricular dysfunction. Furthermore, left ventricular volume was quantitated without an assessment of the change in the extent of dysfunction relative to the change in ventricular volume. Hence, it is possible that the patients in these studies are experiencing progressive global dilation that is due to a failure of ventricular dilation to restore stroke volume and to normalize wall stress. Indeed, a ventriculographic study reported that patients exhibiting ventricular enlargement within 1 month of myocardial infarction may either undergo progressive ventricular dilation or stabilization of ventricular volume in the following 6 months.[98] In this study, all patients with progressive enlargement had anterior infarction with a greater infarct extent compared to those who had a stabilization of ventricular volume. In another study, these same investigators reported that late patency of the infarct vessel attenuated ventricular dilation following myocardial infarction.[99] Hence, whether acute infarct expansion lead to continual ventricular dilation or stabilization of ventricular size may reflect the balance between scar contraction, patency status, and the status of hemodynamic compensation of the left ventricle. Although the exact time point at which acute expansion in the infarct zone progresses to chronic ventricular dilation is unknown, it is likely that the two processes represent a continuum in the process of ventricular remodeling.

Although the detection of infarct expansion in the first week of hospitalization is associated with a poor prognosis,[23,66] the clinical impact of chronic infarct expansion is not well defined. Studies examining patients with progressive ventricular dilation during the first year have reported a decrease in exercise tolerance and survival compared to those patients with a stable ventricular size.[96,98]

Normal ESA at Entry. When patients with ESAs in the normal range at entry were considered as a whole, there was no mean change in ventricular size over the first 3 months (see Fig. 22–8).[23,77] This lack of change of the mean was due to a balance between those with an interval increase in ESA (35%), those without a significant change (46%), and those whose ESA decreases over time (19%). The group with an increase in ESA is divided relatively equally between patients with anterior and inferior infarcts. The predominant cause of the increase in ventricular size for anterior infarctions presenting with a normal ESA is global ventricular dilation, whereas the major cause for the increase in ESA within the inferior infarct group is infarct extension.

Global Ventricular Dilation. Symmetric dilation of normal and infarcted myocardial segments was observed primarily in large anterior infarcts.[23,77] Although rare with inferior infarctions, when present, global ventricular dilation was observed in patients with extensive inferior wall motion abnormalities extending from the base to the apex of the left ventricle.

The fact that the dilation is not present on the initial examination, occurs independent of location, and develops in patients with large regions of dysfunction supports prior experimental and clinical observations that this is an adaptive process aimed at maintaining adequate stroke volume and reducing wall stress by an increase in ventricular size.[69,98,100–102]

Although patients with anterior or extensive inferoapical infarctions may exhibit significant chronic ventricular dilation with expansion of both the normal and infarcted zones, the degree of expansion of the infarct zone is generally less than that seen in patients with acute infarct expansion.[23]

The complications of ventricular dilation appears to be a function of the progressive nature of increasing LV volume, which adversely affects exercise capacity and subsequent survival.[96,98] Long-term studies reporting the relationship between ventricular volume and prognosis have not distinguished between global dilation and infarct expansion.[69]

Infarct Extension. Clinically, silent infarct extension was noted in approximately 12% of the infarcts studied.[23,77] Infarct extension was most common in inferior infarctions and was associated with a significant increase in ESA. Both the extent of AWM and the ESA in this subgroup at 3 months were similar to values observed in the global dilation group, suggesting that the mechanism responsible for the increase in ventricular size accompanying infarct extension may be similar to that observed with global ventricular dilation. Infarct extension as defined here occurs in the absence of clinical symptoms but is presumably preventable if patients at risk for extension could be identified early. Because there are no obvious distinguishing characteristics at entry, some form of stress testing appears necessary to identify this group.

Absence of Change. The majority of patients with normal-sized ventricles show no significant change in ventricular size over the first 3 months following infarction.[23,77] The majority of these patients had inferior wall infarctions and generally showed some decrease in the extent of AWM during the acute follow-up period. Between 3 months and 1 year, a reduction in both ESA and AWM is observed in patients with a stable ESA during the first 3 months (see Figs. 22–8 and 22–9). This late reduction in both ESA and AWM has been attributed to scar contraction.[76]

Infarct Regression. A significant decrease in the extent of regional dysfunction was observed in 21% of patients with Q-wave infarctions, most of whom had inferior or apical infarcts.[23] Furthermore, patients with non-Q infarctions who did not receive additional interventions generally exhibited infarct regression during the first 3 months.[76] Infarct regression was rarely observed in anterior infarcts. Ventricular size, which was in the normal range at baseline, generally remains unchanged. In some Q-wave infarctions, however, the changes in AWM were accompanied by a decrease in the endocardial surface area of the infarct zone. Although these changes are all statistically significant, they represent variations within the range of normal, and hence their clinical importance is unclear.

The pattern of infarct regression is similar to that observed experimentally with scar contraction or when blood flow is reestablished to ischemic or infarcted territories.[72,103,104] An identical pattern of change has been observed in patients with both anterior and inferior infarctions receiving either successful thrombolytic therapy or coronary angioplasty.[39,40]

In those patients with a stable ESA during the first 3 months, a decrease in both AWM and ESA was observed between 3 months and 1 year.[76] The rate of change of ESA between 3 months to 1 year was not related to infarct site or extent and was also observed in those patients with acute expansion (see Figs. 22–8 and 22–9). The consistency of these late changes suggests a common mechanism such as scar contraction as a major factor in the decrease in ESA and AWM—a process that could be demonstrated by 3 months after the acute event.[105] The late behavior of those patients with a normal ESA at entry who underwent subsequent infarct extension or regression was not clearly defined, because they comprised a relatively small proportion of the study group.

Relationship of Infarct Location to Natural History of Dysfunction. While any of the patterns of response to infarction described previously can be seen with any infarct location, there are characteristic patterns that are more commonly related to specific infarct types (see Figs. 22–8 and 22–9, Table 22–1).

Anterior Wall Infarction. The majority of anterior wall Q-wave infarcts show an increase in ventricular size from onset of 3 months.[23,77] This increase is approximately equally distributed between patients with infarct expansion and those with ventricular dilation, although infarct extension is observed on occasion. These types of changes could be predicted by the entry ESA. An abnormal ESA at entry correctly identified all patients with infarct expansion. Conversely, a normal entry ESA with an infarct size greater than 26% (%AWM) predicted subsequent global dilation.[23] Patients who subsequently showed evidence of infarct extension had normal ESAs at entry and were without other predictive characteristics at rest. Those patients with acute expansion generally have a greater extent of AWM than those with a normal ESA at entry. As discussed previously, these observed trends are in agreement with clinical and postmortem reports that acute infarct expansion predominantly occurs with anterior transmural ischemia or infarction.[66,85] Although some patients with anterior infarctions have a stable ESA and percentage of AWM during the first 3 months following the acute event, infarct regression was seldom observed during this time period.

Regardless of the presence or absence of acute infarct expansion, we have observed a general reduction in AWM and ESA between 3 months and 1 year in those patients with anterior infarctions (Figs. 22–8 and 22–9).[76]

Inferior Wall Infarction. Inferior wall infarcts are at least twice as frequent as anterior wall infarcts.[23,77] The mean ESA for the total patient group with inferior infarcts does not change during the first 3 months after infarction; however, this population is heterogenous (Table 22–1). Although approximately 50% of patients with inferior wall infarctions demonstrate no significant change from entry to 3 months, approximately 30% show infarct regression, 14% infarct extension, and the remainder ventricular dilation.

Infarct patients with a stable ESA generally have areas of dysfunction limited to the base of the LV and show no change over time. This would be expected in infarcts that are small and do not significantly impact on overall LV function. This observation of stable LV size and function in the majority of inferior infarctions is complimentary to those observed using other techniques.[66,98] Infarct regression and extensions are patterns primarily noted with inferior wall infarcts and were discussed previously.

In contrast to patients with anterior infarcts, in patients with inferior infarcts, the major changes in ventricular size and extent of dysfunction occurred early in the acute phase.[76] Although a gradual decrease in AWM continues for up to a year, the absolute long-term changes are generally smaller than those seen acutely (Figs. 22–8 and 22–9).

Apical Infarcts. Infarcts isolated to the true cardiac apex without anterior, inferior, or lateral wall predominance were relatively infrequent.[23,77] Isolated apical infarcts tended to be smaller than those involving the anterior or inferior wall (Table 22–1). ESA in these patients did not generally change with time; however, the majority of patients showed a decrease in the extent of AWM during the first 3 months.

Natural History Based on Infarct Size. Patients with an enlarged ESA at entry and thus defined as having acute expansion have a significantly greater extent of dysfunction (AWM) than those with an initially normal ESA.[23,76,77] All patients with an enlarged ESA at entry subsequently underwent further infarct expansion with a disproportionate increase in their AWM relative to ESA.[23,76] The fact that these patients also had anterior Q-wave myocardial infarction reflects the interaction between infarct size, site, and transmural extent in the pathogenesis of acute infarct expansion.[85] In those patients with an initially normal ESA at entry, global ventricular dilation or further infarct expansion was not observed in those with isolated inferior or apical infarctions. Conversely, extensive inferior infarctions involving the apex exhibited ventricular dilation. Between 3 months and 1 year, the absolute or rate of change in ESA was not significantly influenced by initial infarct size.[76] This apparent contradiction may reflect the relative predominance of two opposing forces. In the first 3 months, structural changes within the infarct zone as well as in the noninfarcted zone favor ventricular enlargement to preserve stroke volume in the setting of extensive myocardial dysfunction. After the first 3 months, scar contraction within the infarct zone leads to a reduction of AWM and ESA regardless of initial infarct site or extent. The influence of an extensive infarction cannot be completely overcome, because patients with acute expansion at entry continue to have an abnormally enlarged ESA at 1 year.

Natural History of Non-Q-Wave Infarcts: Comparison With Q-Wave Infarction. In patients with non-Q-wave infarctions, the initial LV surface area is generally normal and remains stable over the first 3 months, as does the extent of AWM (Figs. 22–8 and 22–9).[76] These patients also have a significantly smaller mean extent of dysfunction at entry than patients with Q-wave infarctions.[20,76] A decrease in the extent of AWM is observed for up to 1 year, although the maximal change is noted during the first 3 months.[76] The stable ESA and infarct regression observed in this patient group may be a result of spontaneous recanalization of the infarct vessel, collateral recruitment, or nontransmural injury.[85,106]

Although the changes between entry and 3 months observed in patients with non-Q-wave infarctions appeared to be more homogeneous than in those with Q-wave infarctions,[23,76,77] late decrease in AWM and ESA from 3 months to 1 year was observed in both patient groups (Figs. 22–8 and 22–9).

When examining the natural history of ventricular structure and function following non-Q-wave infarction, it should be noted that the pattern described previously should not be extrapolated to those patients who experienced recurrent infarction or ischemia following non-Q-wave infarctions. Indeed, the resting echocardiogram may have limited value in predicting subsequent reinfarctions, although one study has suggested that early recovery of function within the infarct zone is associated with a high likelihood of recurrent ischemic events.[107] Furthermore, the natural history of ventricular size and function in these patients with complicated non-Q-wave infarctions remains undefined.

Application of Natural History Data

The proper application of the echocardiographic technique should be the prospective identification on admission to the emergency room of patients with infarct expansion as well as those at risk for other types of abnormal ventricular remodeling. This identification can be based on entry ESA, the location of AWM, and the extent of AWM. The fact that functional expansion can be observed immediately after coronary occlusion during the period when myocardial salvage is possible suggests that at least a portion of the expansion process should be reversible, with restoration of flow in the infarct-related artery. In contrast, patients with smaller infarcts in less critical locations can be managed with the assurance that they will remain hemodynamically stable. Furthermore, patients with equivocal or misleading ECGs can be more appropriately diagnosed and managed. This type of classification seems extremely important in the decision to proceed with aggressive therapy in the presence of relative contraindications or to weight the complications of a particular path of management more heavily when the likelihood of major improvement is small and the mortality, morbidity, and likelihood of adverse functional sequelae low.

Left Ventricular Morphology and Regional Wall Motion Following Interventions

Reperfusion Therapy

Multiple prospective randomized studies have established that the use of acute thrombolytic therapy in the treatment of myocardial infarction reduces mortality and subsequent cardiac complications.[108–111] Some of these clinical benefits of thrombolysis have been attributed to acute myocardial salvage resulting from prompt restoration of antegrade blood flow.[111] In a large echocardiographic study of patients from a randomized trial, treatment with streptokinase was associated with lower left ventricular wall motion index and systolic and diastolic volumes than controls at 2 weeks after myocardial infarction.[112] These differences in volumes and extent of dysfunction associated with thrombolytic therapy are still present 6 months later. Similarly, studies that have stratified outcomes based on the 90-minute coronary angiogram have observed that acute patency of the infarct-related artery is associated with improvement in regional function and decreased likelihood of infarct expansion during initial hospitalization.[33–35] In some studies, this early improvement in ventricular topology and function was also related to the timing of thrombolytic therapy,[33,38,112] a finding that is concordant with observations that the greatest reduction in mortality occurs when thrombolysis is given within the initial hours following the onset of symptoms.[108,109] Despite many reports documenting the benefits of acute thrombolysis on ventricular remodeling during hospitalization, the natural history of ventricular structure and function beyond hospital discharge is less well understood. By examining patients with serial echocardiograms during the year following myocardial infarction, we observed that acute thrombolytic therapy was associated with alterations in the pattern and timing of ventricular remodeling in the year after myocardial infarction.[113] Specifically, thrombolytic therapy was associated with an acceleration in the recovery of regional function independent of location when compared to untreated controls (Fig. 22–10). In anterior infarctions, significant improvement in regional function was observed within 3 months after myocardial infarction, whereas in untreated controls, improvement in regional function was not detected until 1 year. In inferior infarcts, improvement was noted within 1 week after thrombolytic therapy, while a similar change was not evident until 3 months in untreated controls. Furthermore, thrombolytic therapy reversed the process of progressive ventricular dilation in those patients who exhibited early infarct expansion with resulting normalization of left ventricular size by 3 months (Fig. 22–11). In contrast, left ventricular size continued to increase over the first 3 months in those patients with acute infarct expansion who did not receive thrombolytic therapy.

The preceding data suggest that acute thrombolytic therapy benefits ventricular structure and function. However, the effect of late or delayed reperfusion on ventricular remodeling or clinical outcome remains undefined. Experimental evidence indicates that late reperfusion may prevent acute and chronic infarct expansion independent of myocardial salvage.[114,115] It has been hypothesized that infarct expansion is attenuated by the increased tissue turgor resulting from hemor-

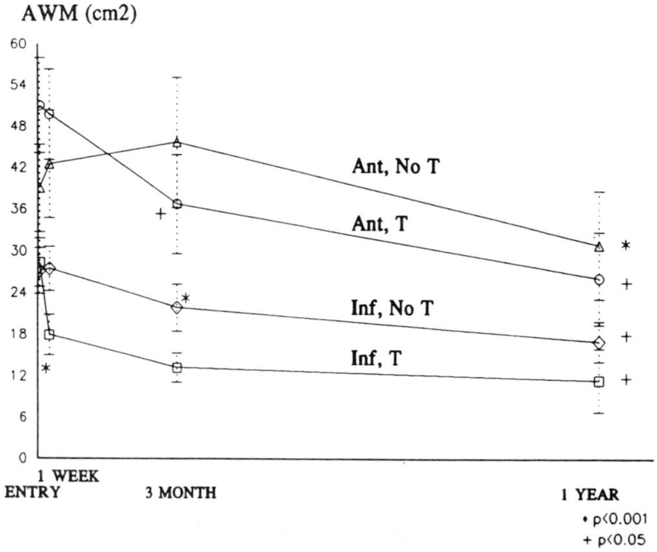

Fig. 22–10. Graph displaying the mean area of abnormal wall motion (AWM) at each time point for the four groups of infarctions: Ant, T = anterior AWM, received thrombolytic therapy; Inf, T = inferior AWM, receiving thrombolytic therapy; Ant, No T = anterior AWM, not receiving thrombolytic therapy; Inf, No T = inferior AWM, not receiving thrombolytic therapy. (From Picard MH, et al.: Left ventricular size and function during the year following acute myocardial infarction. Reprinted with permission from the American College of Cardiology. Journal of the American College of Cardiology, 1991, 17, 2A.)

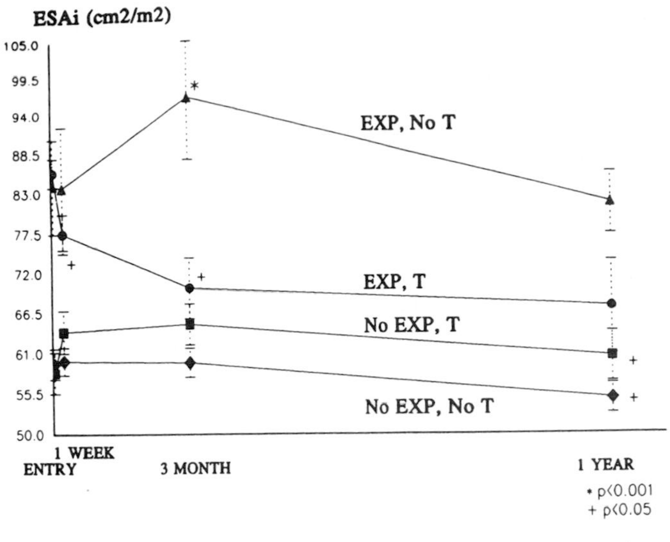

Fig. 22–11. Graph displaying the mean endocardial surface area index (ESAi) at each time point for the four groups of anterior infarctions. EXP T = anterior infarctions with early infarct expansion who received acute thrombolytic therapy; EXP, No T = anterior infarctions with early infarct expansion and not receiving thrombolysis; No EXP, T = anterior infarctions without early infarct expansion who received acute thrombolytic therapy; No EXP, No T = anterior infarctions without early infarct expansion and not receiving thrombolysis. (From Picard MH, et al.: Left ventricular size and function during the year following acute myocardial infarction. Reprinted with permission from the American College of Cardiology. Journal of the American College of Cardiology, 1991, 17, 2A.)

rhage, cellular swelling, and edema associated with reperfusion.[114] Preservation of viable myocardium in the subepicardium and the scaffolding effect of blood-filled vasculature in the infarct zone have also been postulated as mechanisms whereby late reperfusion preserves ventricular morphology.[114,116] In patients with acute myocardial infarction, late patency of the infarct-related coronary artery within days after admission has been associated with improvements in regional function and attenuation of left ventricular dilation in the following months.[39,99] Conversely, in those patients who failed to reperfuse acutely or experienced reocclusions, the ventricular size increased, and regional function did not recover. These echocardiographic observations have been extended to patients with documented spontaneous thrombolysis as well as those who have undergone coronary angioplasty for an occluded infarct-related artery during the days immediately following myocardial infarction.[40] It was observed that patency of the infarct-related artery was associated with stabilization of ventricular size and improvement in regional function between entry and 3 months in both patients who had early (within 6 hours) or late (days) patency of the infarct vessel. Conversely, in those patients who had an occluded infarct vessel, ventricular size increased and regional function failed to improve during the 3-month follow-up period. Restoration of antegrade perfusion to the infarct zone therefore appears to improve regional function, which in turn attenuates LV dilation. Note that these patients were catheterized for ongoing symptoms, and thus the late reperfusion presumably reversed ongoing ischemia. Others have also reported similar findings between admission and 1 year in patients who received either early (<4 hours of onset of symptoms) or late (4 to 8 hours after onset of symptoms) thrombolytic therapy.[117] Despite these encouraging reports of the benefit of late patency on ventricular remodeling, the effects of delayed reperfusion of an occluded infarct-related artery on clinical outcome have yet to be proven.

Pharmacologic Interventions

Intravenous Nitroglycerin. The use of intravenous nitroglycerin during the early hours of myocardial infarction has been associated with limitation of infarct size, reduction of infarct-related complications, and possibly reduction of mortality.[118–121] The proposed mechanisms whereby intravenous nitroglycerin affects myocardial salvage and remodeling include (1) a decrease in myocardial oxygen demand by reduction in preload and afterload, (2) relief of coronary artery spasm, (3) improved collateral flow to the infarct zone, and (4) reduced infarct expansion by decreasing wall stress.[118–122]

In a large study in which patients with acute myocardial infarction were randomized to receive either intravenous nitroglycerin or placebo, it was observed that nitroglycerin administration was associated with a lower echocardiographic extent of LV asynergy, a higher LV ejection fraction, and a lower extent of infarct expansion compared to controls.[121] Intravenous nitroglycerin was also associated with a reduction in the incidence of in-hospital complications such as cardiogenic shock or infarct extensions. At a mean follow-up interval of 43 months, in the subset of patients with anterior infarction, there was a significant lower mortality in the nitroglycerin-treatment group compared with control. Interestingly, it was observed that excessive hypotension (mean arterial pressure <80 mm Hg) attenuated or negated the beneficial effects of intravenous nitroglycerin on ventricular remodeling.

Angiotensin-Converting Enzyme Inhibitor. Studies to date examining the effects of angiotensin-converting enzyme (ACE) inhibition on ventricular remodeling have used captopril or enalapril. By reducing afterload, preload, and systemic vascular resistance, ACE inhibitors maintain cardiac output while attenuating ventricular dilation. In experimental models of infarction and ischemia, treatment with captopril reduces acute functional infarct expansion, improves diastolic relaxation, and is associated with improved long-term survival.[123–125] Several prospective randomized studies have observed a survival benefit with ACE-inhibitor treatment in patients with symptomatic left ventricular systolic dysfunction.[126,127] Other long-term studies (follow-up period, 3 months to 1 year) have observed that captopril treatment in asymptomatic patients with Q-wave myocardial infarctions attenuates LV dilation, preserves ejection fraction, and improves exercise tolerance.[96,97,128]

In summary, compelling experimental and clinical evidence indicates that therapy that reduces ventricular filling pressure while preserving cardiac output may alter the natural history of ventricular size and function following myocardial infarction. Ongoing prospective studies are examining the impact of these therapies on clinical outcome.

The Utility of Two-Dimensional Echocardiography in the Emergency Room Evaluation of Patients with Suspected Myocardial Infarction

Recent studies have reported the utility of two-dimensional echocardiography in the emergency room evaluation of patients with symptoms suggestive of myocardial infarction. At the time of emergency room evaluation, most patients in these studies did not have diagnostic electrocardiographic changes of infarction or ischemia.[16,129–132] The presence of regional asynergy in such patients was of high sensitivity (88 to 93%) but of relatively low specificity (41 to 53%) in the diagnosis of acute myocardial infarction.[130,131] In a prospective study of 180 patients presenting to the emergency room with symptoms of acute myocardial infarction, the echocardiographic assessment of regional wall motion abnormalities was superior to conventional clinical methods in the diagnosis of infarction and in the prediction of its complications.[131] In addition, use of regional dysfunction on echocardiography as a criteria for admission would have reduced the number of unnecessary hospital admissions without discharging additional patients with myocardial infarction. In a parallel study, these investigators reported that in patients presenting with cardiac-related symptoms, the presence of left ventricular systolic dysfunction on echocardiography was predictive of a 27% chance of a major cardiac event in the next 2 years.[132] The evidence to date suggests that echocardiography has a valuable diagnostic and prognostic role in the emergency evaluation of patients who have cardiac-related symptoms but lack definite clinical evidence of myocardial ischemia/infarction.

CHRONIC ISCHEMIC HEART DISEASE

Chronic ischemic changes in the LV that can be appreciated echocardiographically include fixed segmental wall motion abnormalities,[133–137] myocardial scar,[138,139] and ventricular aneurysm.[48,140,141] Regional wall motion abnormalities may be the result of a single small area of infarction or a prior massive event or may be the sum of the multiple small areas of ventricular damage. As such, they vary widely in severity, distribution, and extent. In the past, the left ventricular cineangiogram was the standard clinical method for evaluating regional left ventricular wall motion, and several studies have compared the echocardiographic and angiographic assessment of regional ventricular function. When examining these comparative data, one must first appreciate the relationship of the areas of the ventricle imaged in the more commonly obtained angiographic views to the standard echocardiographic imaging planes.

Figure 22–12 illustrates the path along which the x-ray beam transects the LV in the standard angiographic views and the relationship of the ventricular borders delineated in these angiographic projections to a standard

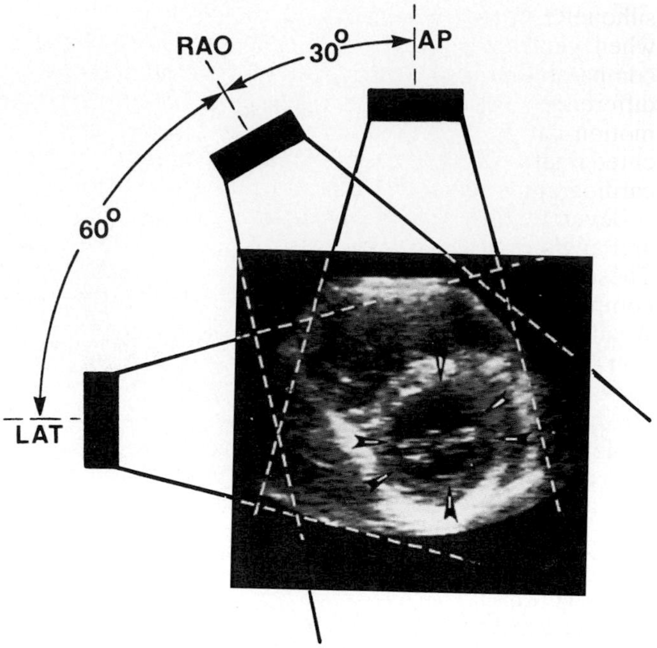

Fig. 22–12. Parasternal short axis recording of the left ventricle indicates the points on the ventricular circumference that are imaged by using the standard cineangiographic anteroposterior (AP), right anterior oblique (RAO), and right lateral projections (LAT). Because the angiogram is a silhouette image, the margins of the ventricle that are projected in each of these standard planes are orthogonal to the direction of the x-ray beam.

echocardiographic short axis cross section. In each of the angiographic projections, the margins of the ventricle that are imaged are orthogonal to the direction of the x-ray beam. The margins of the ventricular wall, which are imaged in the anteroposterior projections, roughly correspond to the 3- and 9-o'clock positions of the short axis plane; the 30° right anterior oblique projection to the 1 and 7-o'clock positions; the 30° left anterior oblique projection to the 11- and 5-o'clock positions; and the left lateral projection to the ventricular borders at 12 and 6 o'clock. Given these relationships, the parasternal long axis view of the LV appears to correspond most closely to the 30° left anterior oblique angiographic projection. The apical four-chamber view images the ventricular walls at a point between the 30 and 60° left anterior oblique projections, and the apical two-chamber view roughly approximates a right anterior oblique (RAO) projection.

When comparing angiographic and echocardiographic data, therefore, one must analyze the views that look at similar areas of the ventricle. In many older studies, comparisons were made between the M-mode assessment of ventricular wall motion and the RAO angiographic projections. These studies, unfortunately, look at different areas of the ventricle. In addition, comparisons between two-dimensional echocardiographic and angiographic analyses of wall motion cannot be made precisely, because different physiologic stresses are imposed by the examinations and because of basic differences in the data obtained. The echocardiographic image is tomographic in nature, whereas the angiogram is a silhouette image, which lies within a single plane only when ventricular geometry is symmetric. Even when comparable areas of the ventricle are examined, some differences in angiographic and echocardiographic wall motion can be expected because the angiogram is oriented relative to the axes of the body, whereas the echocardiogram is aligned relative to the heart.

Several studies have compared echocardiographic and angiographic assessments of regional wall motion. These studies generally employ a segmental system and compare qualitative performance in individual regions. Available data suggest that echocardiographic visualization of at least a portion of the ventricle can be achieved in between 89 and 95% of the patients with chronic ischemic disease.[49,136] Complete visualization of the ventricle can be achieved in from 60 to 88% of patients.[133,136] The percentage of individual segments of the ventricle recorded varies with the segmental system employed; when general areas of interest are considered, 72 to 87% of segments are usually recordable.[133,136] Comparisons of wall motion in areas that are adequately visualized by both techniques have been excellent, and the major sources of discrepancy relate to differences in definition or visual grade.[49,136]

Left Ventricular Scar

Scar formation is common following myocardial infarction. Scar tissue is typically more dense than surrounding muscle, and the ventricular wall in the scarred area is thinner than normal (Fig. 22–13). Echocardiographically, scar is characterized by an increase in echo production from the dense fibrous area and a decrease in diastolic wall thickness (less than 7 mm or 30% less than surrounding normal areas.)[139] Systolic wall motion and thickening are usually decreased in the scarred area. On occasion, however, both motion and thickening may appear normal. Echocardiography appears to be a sensitive and specific method for detecting myocardial scar with surgical or pathologic confirmation being demonstrated in 95% of patients in one series.[139]

Left Ventricular Aneurysms

Left ventricular aneurysms may be acquired or congenital. Acquired aneurysms most commonly develop following acute myocardial infarction, although more rarely they result from trauma or myocardial abscess. Pathologically, left ventricular aneurysms can be divided into true aneurysms; false aneurysms, or pseudoaneurysms; and congenital aneurysms, or diverticula. These types of aneurysms differ in both their clinical significance and their echocardiographic appearance, and therefore, they are discussed separately.

True Aneurysms

By far, the most common type of aneurysm is the true aneurysm. True aneurysms usually develop following acute myocardial infarction and have been noted in as many as 22% of reported cases.[80,142–144] True aneurysms form through gradual expansion and thinning of the myocardium in the infarcted area and characteristically contain all the layers of the ventricular wall.[144] Initially, the wall of the aneurysm is composed predominantly of necrotic muscle and fibrous tissue.[144] With time, fibrosis and, occasionally, calcification increase.[145] Though early rupture of these aneurysms may be noted on rare occasions, late rupture almost never occurs.[138,146] Once formed, ventricular aneurysms may contribute to the development of cardiac decompensation and may underlie such serious secondary complications as refractory congestive heart failure, recurrent ventricular arrhythmias, and systemic emboli.[144] Furthermore, aneurysm formation within the first 5 days of hospitalization has been associated with a high 3-month and 1-year mortality rate.[78,80] Because others have observed that the initial size of the aneurysm may also provide prognostic information on subsequent clinical events,[82] the association between early aneurysm formation and poor long-term survival may be due to the greater extent of regional dysfunction in this patient group.

Echocardiographically, true aneurysms distort the

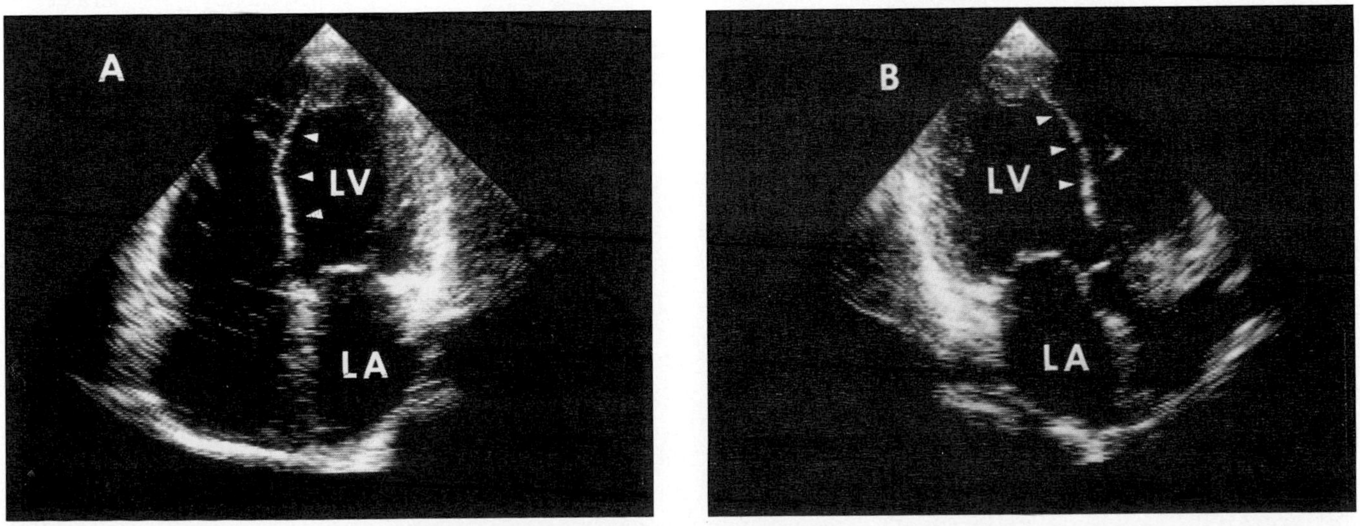

Fig. 22–13. Apical views illustrating an area of anteroseptal scar (arrowheads). **A.** Four chamber. **B.** Long axis. The area of scar is thinner than the normal muscle and in real time was dyskinetic. LV = left ventricle; LA = left atrium.

shape of the LV during both diastole and systole.[48] This definition distinguishes aneurysms from dyskinetic segments (where the distortion in shape is present only during systole). The wall of the aneurysm is typically thin in comparison to the normal myocardium, and motion of the aneurysmal segment is paradoxic. True aneurysms characteristically have a wide neck, and the diameter of the neck is comparable to the maximal diameter of the aneurysm.

The presence of the aneurysm is frequently highlighted by a prominent junction or hinge point between the more normally moving areas of the ventricle and the paradoxic motion of the aneurysmal segment.[48] The sensitivity of the echocardiographic diagnosis of ventricular aneurysms has ranged from 93 to 100%.[48,141] Occasional false-negatives have also been reported.[140,141] These occur most commonly when the aneurysms are small and extend from the tip of the cardiac apex or involve the high anterolateral wall. Between 85 and 95% of true aneurysms involve the cardiac apex, and extension into the anterior wall is common.[48,140,147] Thrombus is frequently present within left ventricular aneurysms and is reported pathologically in 15 to 77% of cases[148,149] and echocardiographically in as many as 34% of patients.[140]

Figure 22–14 is an example of a large anteroapical aneurysm. The aneurysm, indicated by the arrowheads, creates a distortion in the apical segment of the LV. The neck of the aneurysm is wide, and when viewed in real time, the aneurysmal segment moved paradoxically. Figure 22–15 illustrates a second large anteroapical aneurysm. In this example, the aneurysm is larger than the remaining normally functioning ventricle. Despite their predominant apical location, true aneurysms may develop anywhere in the ventricular wall. Figure 22–16, for example, illustrates a large aneurysm arising from the posterolateral surface of the ventricle.

False Aneurysms or Pseudoaneurysms

A rare type of left ventricular aneurysm is the false aneurysm, or pseudoaneurysm.[138,146,150] Pseudoaneurysms result from myocardial rupture, with the extravasated blood being contained by adherent parietal pericardium.[150] The rupture most commonly follows acute myocardial infarction, though it may also result from trauma, laceration, or abscess.[148–150] Pathologically, pseudoaneurysms are characterized by a small, narrow-necked channel that connects the ventricle with a larger aneurysmal sac containing blood and thrombus and lined by fibrous pericardial tissue without any myocardial elements. Pseudoaneurysms may be associated with the same complications noted with true aneurysms but are particularly important because of their greater overall incidence of rupture and because of their tendency for late rupture.[149,150]

Echocardiographically, the pseudoaneurysms appear as large, saccular or globular, echo-free chambers that are external to the left ventricular cavity.[151–154] They are connected to the ventricular cavity by a narrow

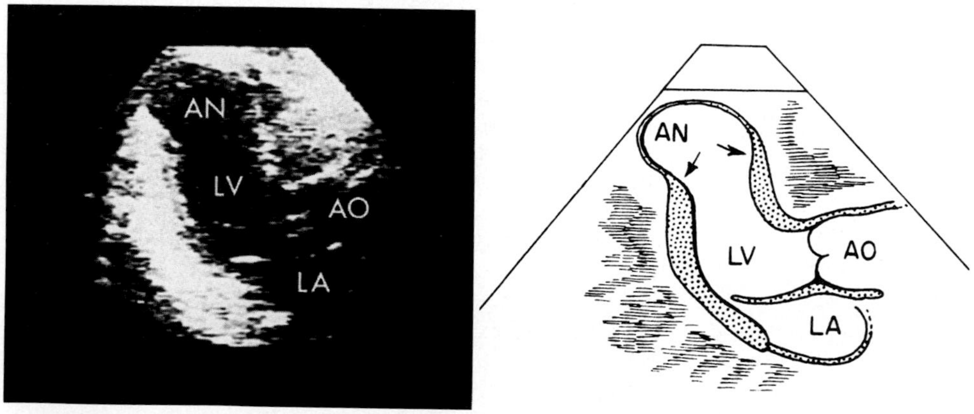

Fig. 22–14. Parasternal long axis recording illustrates a large anteroapical aneurysm (AN). LA = left atrium; LV = left ventricle; AO = aorta.

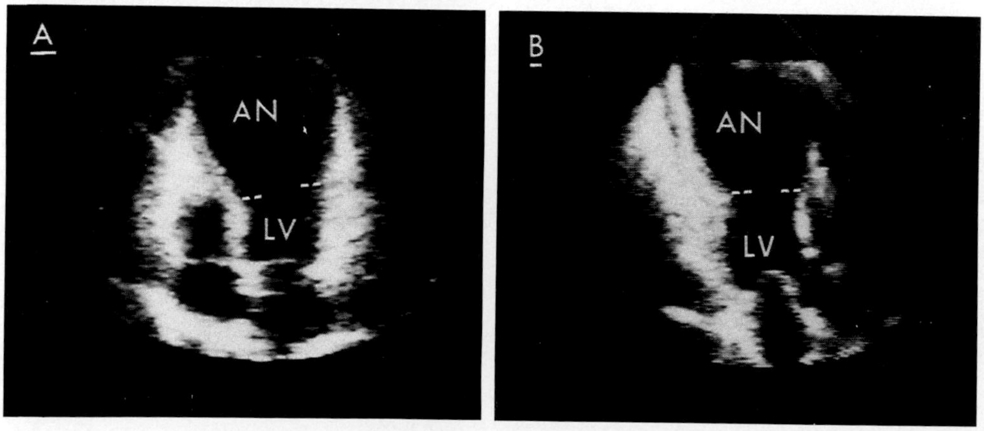

Fig. 22–15. Apical views of the left ventricle (LV) from a patient with a large anteroapical aneurysm (AN). **A.** Four chamber. **B.** Long axis. In this example, the aneurysm is twice the size of the residual left ventricular cavity.

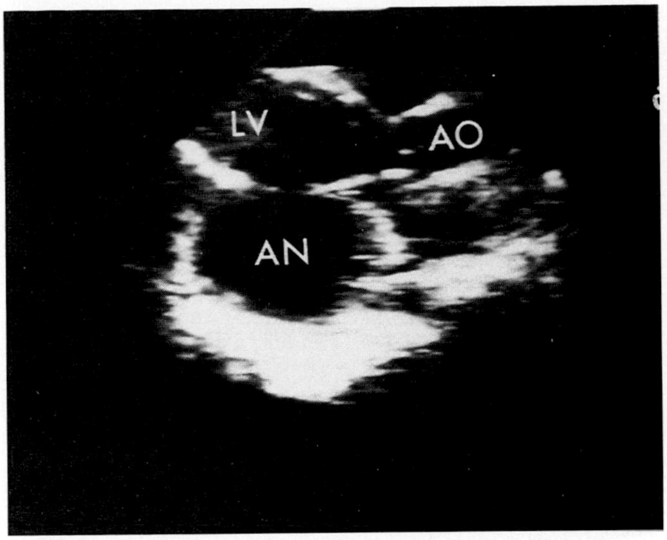

Fig. 22–16. Parasternal long axis recording of a large posterior aneurysm (AN). LV = left ventricle; AO = aorta.

neck, the diameter of which is generally less than 40% of the maximal diameter of the aneurysm.[154] The neck typically produces an abrupt interruption in the ventricular wall in contrast to the gradual tapering of the myocardium into the aneurysm (which is characteristic of a true aneurysm). Although the preceding criteria are generally useful to differentiate true aneurysms from pseudoaneurysms, true aneurysms located in the inferior wall have been falsely diagnosed as being pseudoaneurysm using these echocardiographic criteria.[155] Doppler color flow mapping may provide complementary information by demonstrating the bidirectional blood flow between the pseudoaneurysm and the LV as well as by detecting left-to-right shunting when the pseudoaneurysm communicates with both the right ventricle (RV) and LV.[156–158] Figure 22–17 illustrates a large pseudoaneurysm that appears as an echo-free space external to the lateral wall of the ventricle. This aneurysm was produced by laceration of the ventricle, and the aneurysmal neck is small in comparison to the diameter of the aneurysm.

Left Ventricular Diverticula

Left ventricular diverticula are uncommon but well-recognized congenital cardiac malformations.[159–164] These diverticula are classified as either muscular or fibrous.[161] The muscular type is typically associated with midline thoracoabdominal defects and other cardiac malformations, whereas the fibrous variety usually occurs as isolated ventricular lesions located in the subvalvular or apical regions. Multiple diverticula, familial clustering, and a possible association with hypertrophic cardiomyopathy have also been reported.[165–167] These diverticula, often referred to as *aneurysms*, may be associated with many complications, including mitral incompetence, angina pectoris, cardiac arrhythmias, systemic emboli, and cardiac rupture.[161,163,164] Figure 22–18 illustrates both the angiographic and cross-sectional echocardiographic appearance of a small diverticulum arising from the posterior surface of the LV and communicating with the ventricular cavity. Echocardiographically, the diverticulum appeared as a small, circular, echo-free space behind and apparently communicating with the left ventricular cavity.[168] Figure 22–19 is an example of a large apical diverticulum communicating with the LV via a short neck. Although this was similar in appearance to a false aneurysm, Doppler flow mapping revealed systolic flow from the diverticulum to the LV with a 49-mm Hg systolic pressure gradient (diverticulum > left ventricle) between the two chambers. This pattern of flow is in direct contrast to that seen with a pseudoaneurysm, where systolic flow is from the left ventricle into the pseudoaneurysm.

Ventricular Septal Rupture

Ventricular septal rupture is a rare complication of acute myocardial infarction, occurring in 0.5 to 1.0% of patients.[169] Ventricular septal rupture is associated with a grave prognosis, and death occurs in 54% of the patients within the first week following perforation and in as many as 87% within the first 2 months.[169] Most septal perforations are located in the posteroapical region and are characteristically associated with extensive myocardial infarction. The size of the perforation may vary considerably but is usually less than 4 cm in diameter.[169] Although in the majority of cases, a single perforation is noted, multiple perforations have been reported. Septal perforations can complicate both anterior and inferior infarctions. The interval from the onset of pain to perforation averages 3.5 days; intervals of from several hours to 9 days have been reported.[169,170]

Clinically, septal perforation is heralded by the sud-

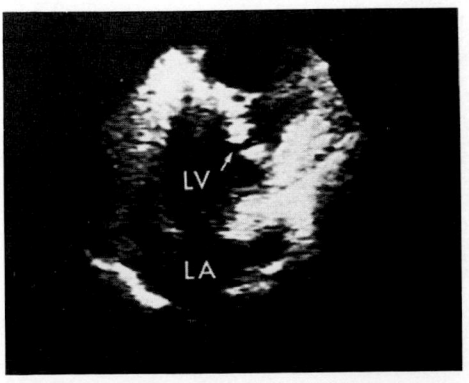

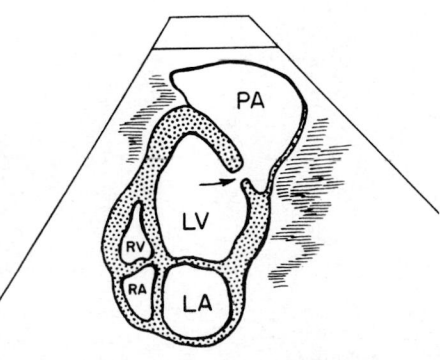

Fig. 22–17. Apical four-chamber recording of a left ventricular pseudoaneurysm (PA). The pseudoaneurysm appears as a large echo-free space anterior and lateral to the apex and lateral wall of the left ventricle (LV). The narrow neck of the aneurysm is indicated by the horizontal arrow. RV = right ventricle, RA = right atrium; LA = left atrium.

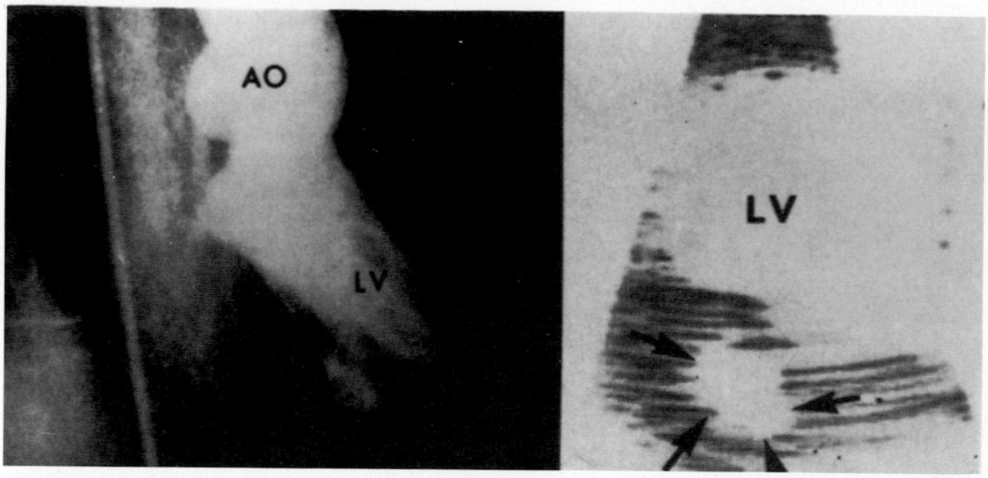

Fig. 22–18. Angiogram and cross-sectional echogram from a patient with a congenital left ventricular diverticulum. The diverticulum echocardiographically appears as a well-circumscribed, echo-free space posterior to the left ventricular cavity, which communicates to the left ventricular chamber through a narrow neck. LV = left ventricle; AO = aorta.

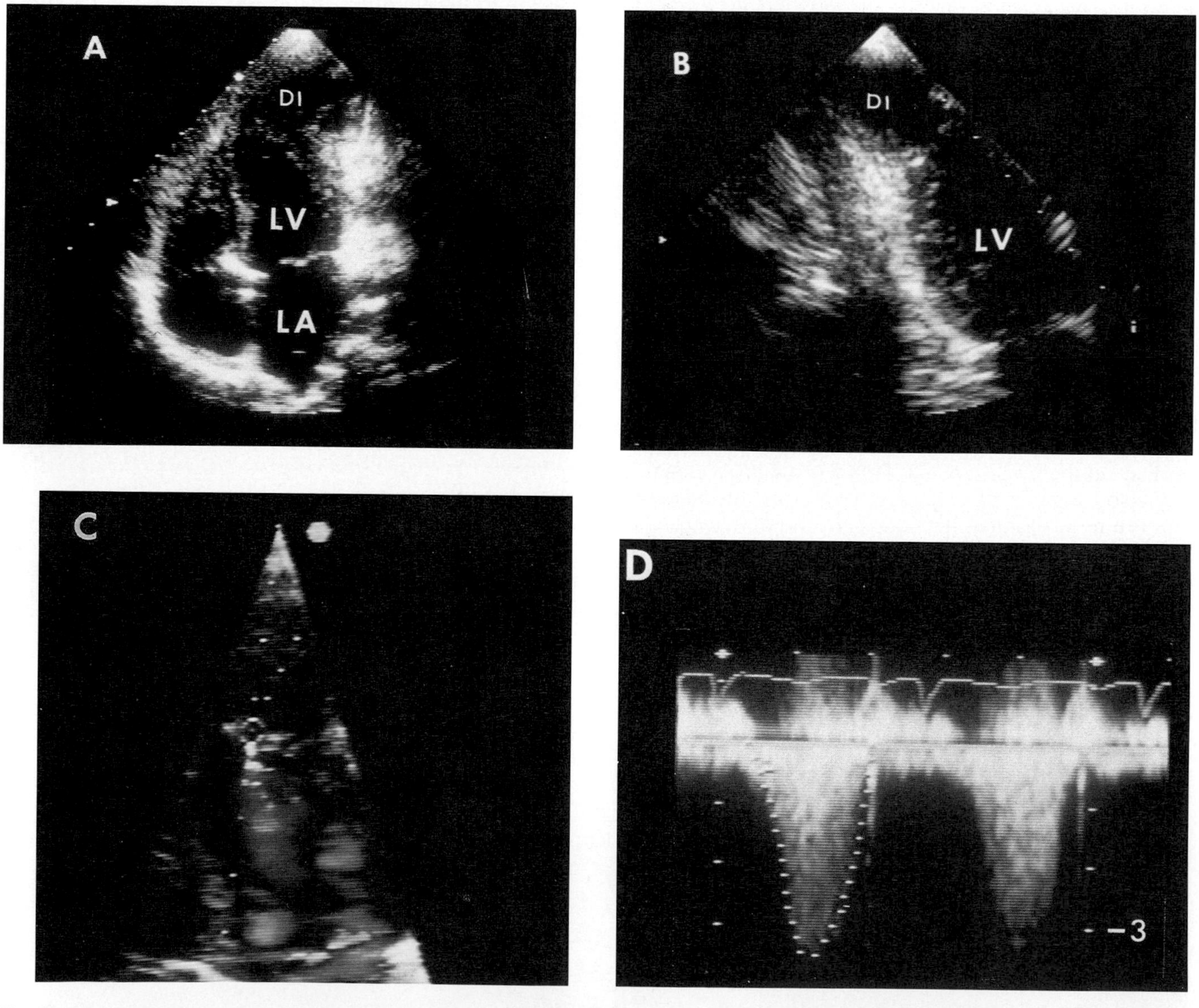

Fig. 22–19. **A** and **B.** Apical four-chamber **(A)** and two-chamber **(B)** views of a left ventricular diverticulum. **C.** During systole, there is flow from the diverticulum into the left ventricular cavity. **D.** Continuous wave Doppler recording showing a peak gradient of 49 mm Hg between the diverticulum and the left ventricle during systole. DI = diverticulum; LV = left ventricle; LA = left atrium.

den appearance of a new systolic murmur and by rapid hemodynamic deterioration. The differential diagnosis in these instances is generally between septal rupture and acute mitral regurgitation that is due to papillary muscle dysfunction or chordal rupture.[169–171]

Echocardiographically, septal perforation is detected primarily through direct visualization of the septal defect.[172–174] These defects appear as abrupt interruptions in the septal musculature and are usually surrounded by an extensive area of asynergy. They are typically located posteriorly in close proximity to the cardiac apex, and associated septal aneurysm formation is common.[174] Their method of formation and echocardiographic appearance are similar to those of a pseudoaneurysm. When septal perforation complicates anterior infarction, anteroapical dyskinesis is characteristically present. When septal rupture complicates inferior infarction, the apex is generally spared, and there is an extensive area of posterior wall dyskinesis.

Variation in the size of the perforation is frequently noted. During systole, the perforation typically expands and may increase by as much as three times its diastolic diameter.[172,174]

Because of the higher left ventricular systolic pressure, shunt flow through these septal perforations is predominantly from left to right.[172] Peripherally injected contrast may be helpful in confirming the diagnosis of ventricular septal perforation. In general, this is based on a negative contrast effect at the right ventricular margin of the defect where the contrast-containing blood in the right ventricular cavity is displaced by the blood flowing from the LV that does not contain contrast.[172]

Pulsed, continuous wave, and color flow Doppler can confirm the left-to-right shunting across the septal perforation.[175–179] The defect size estimated by Doppler color flow imaging has generally correlated closely with the size determined during surgery or at autopsy as well as with the pulmonic-systemic flow ratio measured at cardiac catheterization.[177] Transesophageal imaging may also be useful in cases where the transthoracic images are nondiagnostic.[180]

Additional findings that can be noted with acute ventricular septal rupture are right ventricular dilation, left atrial dilation, and exaggerated contraction of noninfarcted areas of the LV.[170] Paradoxic septal motion, when present, is usually the result of septal dyskinesis. Extensive right ventricular dysfunction has been reported to be a predictor of poor survival.[177,181] In one study, patients with combined right ventricular and septal dysfunction had a 100% mortality rate.[181]

Figure 22–20 is an example of ventricular septal rupture complicating acute myocardial infarction. In this instance, the ventricular septal defect lies at the posterior margin of the interventricular septum, just superior to the posteromedial papillary muscle.

Papillary Muscle Rupture

Papillary muscle rupture is a relatively rare complication of acute myocardial infarction.[182,183] In most cases of papillary muscle rupture, the acute infarction was a first coronary event with a minority of patients having prior infarction or angina pectoris.[183–185] The posteromedial papillary muscle is more frequently involved, presumably because of its more tenuous blood supply. The clinical presentation and natural history of papillary muscle rupture are similar to that of ventricular septal rupture; acute onset of clinical and hemodynamic deterioration with a high likelihood of death in the absence of surgical intervention.[183,186] Typically, only the head of the papillary muscle is ruptured because complete rupture of the trunk is generally considered to be rapidly fatal.[170]

Two-dimensional echocardiography can correctly demonstrate the structural abnormality of the mitral valve (visualizing the flail valve, prolapse, or the ruptured head of the papillary muscle) and also exclude concomitant ventricular septal rupture.[179,187] Pulsed wave and color flow Doppler can permit identification of the presence of mitral regurgitation as well as definition of the specific mitral leaflet abnormality from the direction of the regurgitant jet.[179] Color flow Doppler quantitation of severity of mitral regurgitation generally correlates well with the angiographic grade. Color flow Doppler, however, may underestimate the severity of acute mitral regurgitation in the presence of an eccentric regurgitant jet or a small noncompliant left atrium.[179] As with ventricular septal rupture, transesophageal echocardiography can establish the diagnosis in cases in which the transthoracic images are suboptimal.[180,188]

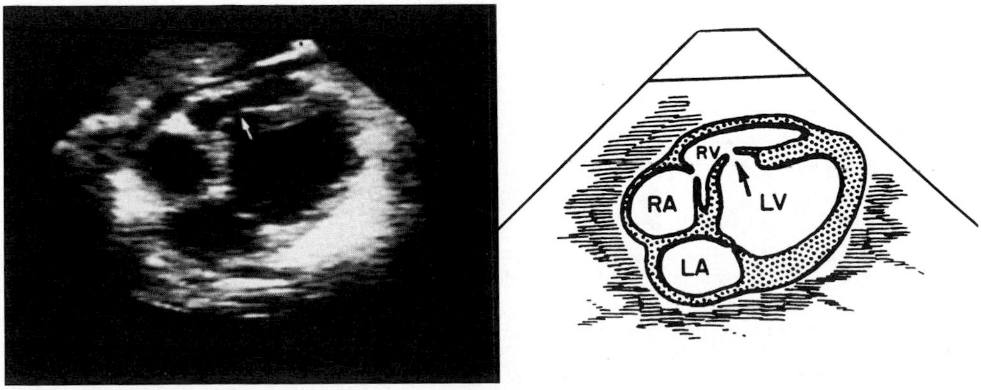

Fig. 22–20. Subcostal long axis recording illustrates ventricular septal rupture complicating acute myocardial infarction. The defect (arrow) is at the tip of a septal aneurysm. RV = right ventricle; RA = right atrium; LV = left atrium; LV = left ventricle.

Left Ventricular Thrombi

Left ventricular mural thrombi are a relatively common complication of acute myocardial infarction, being noted in from 20 to 60% of cases in postmortem series.[143,148,149,189–191] Thrombus formation appears more often with larger infarcts, and the incidence of mural thrombus increases when there is left ventricular aneurysm formation. Detection of these thrombi may be of major clinical importance because they presumably underlie the arterial embolic events noted in as many as 5% of patients following acute infarction.[192–194]

Echocardiographically, mural thrombi appear as focal, echo-producing masses superimposed on and interrupting the normal endocardial contour of the ventricle in regions of akinesis or dyskinesis.[195–203] They may be fixed, pedunculated, and freely mobile or may have a fixed base with mobile filaments extending from the surface. Thrombi characteristically have a speckled appearance and, when organized, may contain areas that are brighter than surrounding myocardium. Thrombi that occur in the presence of aneurysm formation almost invariably involve the cardiac apex. On rare occasions, however, a thrombus may be noted arising from the anterior or anterolateral free wall when no aneurysm is present. Apical thrombi are best visualized in one of the apical views. When thrombus is suspected in an apical view, however, confirmation usually requires its visualization in at least one other projection.

Thrombi generally become visible echocardiographically between the sixth and tenth day following an acute infarction.[201] The natural history of these thrombi is unclear. In small series, however, little change has been noted within the first few months after formation, but regression and ultimate disappearance during long-term observation is possible.[196] Most thrombi have been observed following anterior wall infarction.[202,204–206] This association is not surprising, because anterior infarctions tend to be larger than, and tend to involve the cardiac apex more frequently than, inferior wall infarcts. The critical underlying factors appear to be the size and the severity of the apical wall abnormality (akinesis/dyskinesis).[202,206] Inferior wall infarction with apical dyskinesis is also reported to underlie apical thrombus formation.

The echocardiographic detection of ventricular thrombus within 48 to 72 hours following myocardial infarction has been reported to be associated with a poor prognosis, similar to that of early left ventricular aneurysm formation.[207,208] It is likely that early thrombus formation is an indicator of extensive regional dysfunction. Several prospective studies have reported that patients with ventricular thrombi that are mobile, protrude into the ventricular cavity, or are adjacent to zones of hyperkinetic wall motion are more likely to have an embolic event.[205,206,209]

Figure 22–21A shows a globular thrombus within the cardiac apex of a patient with an established anterior wall myocardial infarction. This thrombus is well defined and has a speckled internal appearance. Figure 22–21B and C provides two examples of laminar thrombus within an apical aneurysm. In Figure 22–21B, the thrombus appears confined to the anterior margin of the aneurysm; however, as the scan is continued inferiorly, a second area of laminar thrombus along the posterior wall of the aneurysm is apparent. The posterior thrombus is more dense and appears better organized than the thrombus that is recorded anteriorly. Figure 22–22 illustrates an anteroapical aneurysm with a large thrombus that protrudes into the left ventricular cavity.

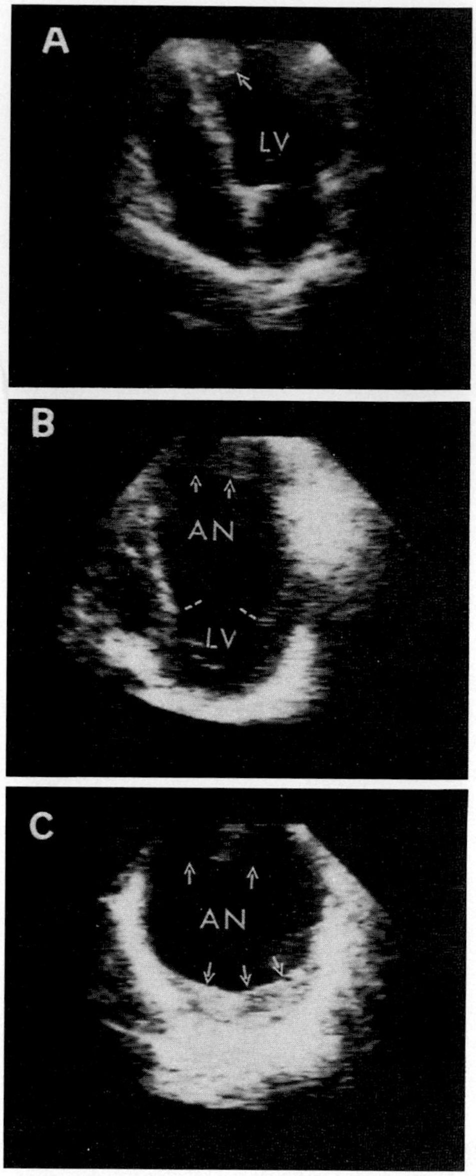

Fig. 22–21. **A.** Apical four-chamber recording illustrates a circumscribed thrombus within the apex of the left ventricle (LV). The thrombus (as indicated by arrows) is clearly demarcated and has a speckled internal pattern. **B.** A recording from a second patient with an anteroapical aneurysm (AN) contains a large laminar thrombus (vertical arrowheads). The origin of the aneurysm from the left ventricle (LV) is indicated by the interrupted lines. **C.** Short axis recording through the aneurysm (AN). Anteriorly, the faint laminar thrombus is apparent, whereas posteriorly, an equally large area of thrombus is more highly reflective, suggesting that it is better organized.

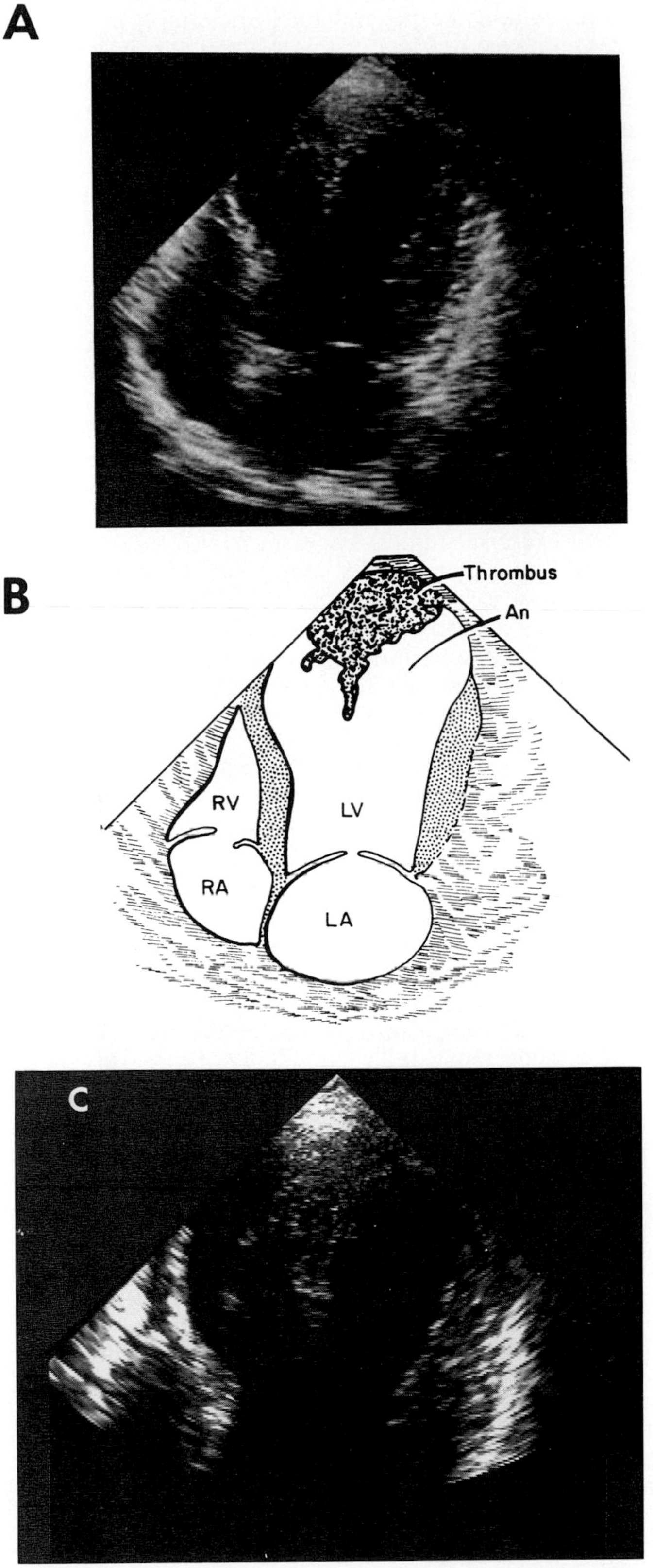

Fig. 22–22. Apical four-chamber view of an anteroapical aneurysm with a large thrombus that protrudes into the left ventricular cavity. An = aneurysm; LV = left ventricle; LA = left atrium; RV = right ventricle; RA = right atrium.

STRESS ECHOCARDIOGRAPHY

Many patients with coronary artery disease and normal left ventricular function develop wall motion abnormalities during exercise in areas that are marginally perfused.[210,211] Echocardiographic studies performed during exercise can identify these transient motion abnormalities. When present, the abnormalities appear to be highly specific for identifying ischemic disease, as evidenced by high-grade coronary obstruction of the vessels supplying the abnormal region and by transient thallium-201 perfusion defects.[210,212] Currently, stress-induced wall motion abnormalities are elicited by either exercise or pharmacologic agents.

Definition of Normal Versus Abnormal Response

A normal response to stress consists of generalized hyperkinesis, an increase in myocardial thickening in all segments, and an increase in ejection fraction.[210,213–215] An abnormal response has been defined as a new AWM or a decrease in ejection fraction during the study. The criteria for diagnosing coronary artery disease have also included a resting AWM that persists or worsens with exercise. Doppler techniques have been used in conjunction with stress to assess changes in global ventricular performance.[216–222] The normal response of the aortic Doppler profile to exercise is an increase in peak acceleration, peak velocity, and the aortic flow velocity integral in proportion to increasing contractility and cardiac output.[220–223] In the presence of significant coronary artery obstruction, a flat or decreasing response is noted in one or more of these Doppler parameters. As with ejection fraction, these abnormal responses are not specific for coronary artery disease and can be seen in cardiomyopathy, valvular heart disease, or in patients receiving cardiac medications in the absence of coronary disease.

Exercise Echocardiography

Most studies of exercise echocardiography have used treadmill[214,215,224–229] or bicycle[210,211,230–237] exercise to induce the stress required to produce ischemia. The choice of treadmill or bicycle exercise is usually determined by laboratory preference. Each form of exercise has advantages and disadvantages when used in conjunction with echocardiographic imaging.

Treadmill Versus Bicycle

When treadmill exercise is used, imaging is performed before and immediately after exercise because it is difficult to image an upright, walking patient. Baseline images are acquired in the supine or left lateral decubitus positions. Most laboratories acquire images in the parasternal short- and long-axis, and apical two- and four-chamber views.[214,215,224–229,234] Patients then perform graded upright treadmill exercise. Immediately after cessation of exercise, patients resume the recumbent position, and imaging is repeated in the same four views described. The use of postexercise imaging is based on observations that exercise-induced regional AWM can persist 1 to 5 minutes after exercise.[210,224] In patients with multivessel coronary artery disease, these abnormalities may last even longer.[225] Nevertheless, image acquisition must be completed within 90 to 120 seconds following exercise termination to ensure optimal diagnostic accuracy.[234] The advantage of treadmill exercise is that it is widely used, is the best standardized, and is most readily accepted by patients.[223] The disadvantage is that information at peak exercise is not available and transient regional wall abnormalities can resolve rapidly following exercise and be missed by postexercise imaging.[234]

Bicycle exercise can be performed either in a supine[210,211,235] or upright[230,232,234,236,237] posture. In addition to the initial four images taken in the parasternal and apical views when the patient is recumbent, images are acquired from the apical two-chamber and four-chamber views when the patient is sitting on the bicycle.[210,211,230,234–237] The exercise protocol is initiated, and apical four- and two-chamber views are acquired and updated before the end of each exercise stage. Some investigators have used subcostal imaging during exercise.[230] Postexercise imaging is performed in the four standard views (four- and two-chamber apical views, parasternal long and short axis views). The potential advantage of continuous imaging during exercise is offset by the more limited imaging windows during exercise and the decreased target resolution of the apical views. Hence, both treadmill and bicycle echocardiographic techniques appear to have equivalent accuracy in the detection of significant coronary obstruction.

Data Analysis: Exercise Echocardiography

Once recorded, there are numerous methods for displaying and interpreting the echocardiographic data. Data analysis can be performed off-line by review of the recorded images from videotape.[210,211,224–226,230,235] This method requires that each view be recorded for a relatively long period and does not allow side-by-side comparison of rest and exercise images. In addition, respiratory artifacts may make interpretation of exercise images difficult. More recent studies of exercise echocardiography have used some form of digital acquisition technique that enables a high quality cardiac cycle from each image plane to be digitized and stored in a continuous loop format.[214,215,227–229,234,236–238] Digitizing of images can be performed either off-line after review of the videotape or on-line during the exercise echocardiographic examination. The digitized images are stored on a floppy disc while the videotape is always available for backup analysis. The digitized recording of the rest and exercise images can then simultaneously be displayed in a "quad screen" format during interpretation of the exercise study.

Although quantitation of indexes of regional and global function have been applied to exercise echocardiography,[226,231,232] most investigators have used qualitative or semiquantitative methods in their analysis of regional wall motion. One approach has been to divide the LV into 12 to 20 segments and to grade the function visually in each segment as normal, hypokinetic, akinetic, or dyskinetic.[210,211,214,215,224,225,227–229,234–237] By relating wall motion abnormalities to ventricular regions that lie within the general territories supplied by the three coronary arteries,[9,22] this segmental approach aids in localizing the "culprit" coronary vessel. Others have combined the individual grades of function from all the segments to generate a wall motion score,[223,226,239] which may be useful in the assessment or comparison of the effect of an intervention on regional ventricular function during exercise.

Diagnosis of Coronary Artery Disease

Early studies of exercise echocardiography reported that in up to 29% of patients the echocardiographic data were inadequate for analysis,[210,211] although the diagnostic accuracy was good in those segments visualized.[210] More recently, with improvements in imaging devices and the availability of digital acquisition capability, over 90% of patients referred for exercise echocardiography had images adequate for analysis.[215,234,237,238] Recent exercise studies report an overall sensitivity of 71 to 97% and specificity of 64 to 100% when significant coronary stenosis was defined as a >50% luminal narrowing on a visually assessed angiogram.[214,227–229,236,238] In these same series, the ability of exercise echocardiography to permit accurate prediction of the presence or absence of coronary artery disease ranged from 81 to 94%. The diagnostic accuracy of exercise echocardiography appeared to be high whether imaging was performed after or during peak exercise. One study that compared imaging at peak with that obtained immediately postexercise reported a lower sensitivity with postexercise imaging, although not all patients underwent coronary angiography.[234]

The excellent sensitivity reported with exercise echocardiography may partially reflect the fact that most patients in these studies are referred for coronary angiography and thus have a high pretest likelihood of disease. Furthermore, most studies included patients with previous myocardial infarctions with resting wall motion abnormalities who were defined as having an abnormal exercise echocardiogram. When patients with prior myocardial infarction or regional wall abnormalities are excluded from analysis, the overall sensitivity of exercise echocardiography varied from 66 to 97%.[215,227–229,238] The sensitivity of exercise echocardiography is lower in patients with single-vessel coronary obstruction (64 to 92%) compared to those with multivessel coronary disease (80 to 100%).[214,226,228,229,236,237] The lower sensitivity in detecting single-vessel coronary obstruction may have resulted from a more transient nature of the wall motion abnormality that resolved rapidly after exercise. False-negative results are also associated with submaximal exercise, moderate (50 to 70% luminal narrowing) stenoses, or collateral supply to the ischemic territory.[229,234,238]

In several studies, investigators reported that exercise echocardiography caused incorrect identification of up to 53% of patients with multivessel coronary obstruction as having single vessel disease.[214,215] In more recent studies, the accuracy of exercise echocardiography in distinguishing single from multivessel coronary disease has varied from 66 to 88%.[228,229] The limited ability to distinguish single-vessel from multivessel disease probably reflects the fact that the onset of ischemia from the most compromised vascular territory is responsible for the termination of exercise protocol. Furthermore, the difference in diagnostic accuracy in determining the extent of coronary disease in the previously mentioned studies may be the result of differences in patient selection, sample size, and proportion of patients with multivessel disease. Several studies have compared the sensitivity and specificity of exercise echocardiography with that of the exercise ECG. Virtually all recent studies comparing the two modalities have reported exercise echocardiography to have greater sensitivity and positive predictive accuracy for coronary disease than exercise electrocardiography.[215,228,229,238] These differences were apparent even when patients with nondiagnostic exercise ECGs were excluded from analysis.[229,238] Indeed, exercise echocardiography may have its greatest incremental diagnostic value in patients with a nondiagnostic exercise ECG or when the false-positive rate with exercise is high.[238] Although the two techniques have a similar specificity, the exercise echocardiogram has a greater negative predictive value than the exercise ECG by virtue of its increased sensitivity.[215,228,229,238]

Isometric handgrip has also been used to elicit AWM.[240–242] In a study of 45 patients, new wall motion abnormalities during handgrip exercise were noted in 65% of patients with coronary artery obstruction.[242] Although the relative insensitivity of the technique may have been a function of the limited imaging planes used in that study,[242] isometric handgrip probably produces a smaller increment in myocardial oxygen demand than treadmill exercise because it has a lesser effect on heart rate.[240]

Assessment of Global Ventricular Function

Several studies have examined changes in indices of global left ventricular function during exercise. Studies examining changes in ejection fraction or aortic Doppler parameters report that patients with coronary artery disease had a blunting or a reversal of the normal response to exercise.[220,221,226] However, an abnormal ejection fraction response was observed in only 70% of patients with coronary artery obstruction.[226] Furthermore, there was a marked heterogeneity in the ejection fraction response to exercise within the patient group with single-vessel coronary disease. Not surprisingly, the patients showing the most marked abnormal response on exercise have extensive multivessel coronary artery disease. Similarly, studies examining aortic Doppler parameters in patients with coronary disease have noted that the most marked abnormal responses to exercise were seen in patients with multivessel disease and/or depressed systolic function at rest.[220,221] Hence, the preceding studies suggest that assessment of regional function may be more useful than global function when applied to patient groups with a diverse spectrum of coronary artery disease.

Prognostic Role of Exercise Echocardiography

Several studies have examined the prognostic value of exercise echocardiography in patients with documented or suspected coronary artery disease. In three studies examining a total of 110 patients with uncomplicated myocardial infarctions, the investigators reported that worsening or new wall motion abnormalities during exercise were present in 63 to 80% of patients who had cardiac events within the next 12 months.[243–245] Conversely, in those patients who had no cardiac events during the follow-up period, 80 to 95% did not have new regional asynergy detected during exercise. These investigators reported that exercise echocardiography provided better stratification of postinfarction patients into low and high risk groups for subsequent cardiac events than the exercise ECG. Although these studies reported that remote asynergy during exercise identified patients with multivessel coronary disease or at risk for subsequent events,[243,244] it is unclear whether worsening of a pre-existing area of dyssynergy during exercise has the same prognostic implication as a new wall motion abnormality.

In a study of 148 patients without a prior myocardial infarction, a normal exercise echocardiogram was associated with a low (4%) rate of nonfatal cardiac complications over the next 28 months.[246] Interestingly, a negative exercise echocardiogram in a patient with good exercise capacity was predictive of an excellent prognosis even if the exercise electrocardiogram was abnormal. Several studies have examined the utility of exercise echocardiography in the functional assessment of coronary artery lesions before angioplasty, in the evaluation of the functional result of a successful angioplasty,[239,247] or in the evaluation of restenosis.[248] Although some have suggested that exercise echocardiography has a greater sensitivity than the exercise ECG in detecting significant stenosis either before or following angioplasty, an independent indicator of myocardial ischemia was not used in these studies.[247,248]

Nonexercise Stress Echocardiography

Other forms of nonexercise stress can also increase myocardial oxygen demand or alter myocardial blood flow. Techniques that increase myocardial oxygen demand involve increasing heart rate and/or blood pressure by infusion of catecholamines or by cardiac pacing.

Techniques That Increase Myocardial Oxygen Demand: Catecholamine Infusion and Cardiac Pacing

Catecholamine Infusion. Catecholamine infusion with isoproterenol or dobutamine has been used to elicit AWM. The diagnostic accuracy of isoproterenol infusion is limited by the fact that increasing heart rate without an increase in blood pressure does not always raise myocardial oxygen demand sufficiently to induce ischemia.[249] More recently, dobutamine has been employed because experimental observations have suggested that it increases myocardial oxygen demand by augmenting heart rate, blood pressure, and contractility.[250–254] Dobutamine is typically administered by infusion pump, beginning with a dose of 2.5 μg/kg/min and then increasing the infusion rate every 3 minutes up to a maximal dose of 30 to 40 μg/kg/min.[252–254] Typically, images are acquired at baseline, low dose infusion (dobutamine 2.5 to 15 μg/kg/min), high dose infusion (20 to 40 μg/kg/min), and 5 minutes after the termination of infusion. End points used by investigators to terminate the dobutamine infusion included (1) administration of a maximal dose of dobutamine, (2) detection of new wall motion abnormality, (3) ischemia detected by electrocardiography, (4) complex ventricular arrhythmia, (5) excessive elevation of systolic or diastolic blood pressure, and (6) intolerable adverse symptoms. Although up to 36% of patients in these studies experienced side effects during dobutamine infusion, almost all patients achieved one of the primary end points and thus had a diagnostic test.[253,254] The two major side effects observed were ischemic chest pain and arrhythmias. Ischemic chest pain usually responded to termination of the infusion or administration of sublingual nitroglycerin, and it occasionally required treatment with a short-acting β-blocker. Transient atrial or ventricular ectopic beats were observed in 15% of patients and usually resolved with termination of dobutamine infusion.

Although the number of studies examining the diagnostic role of dobutamine infusion is limited, the overall sensitivity ranged from 76 to 89%, and specificity ranged from 70 to 95%.[252–255] The use of β-blockers did not affect the diagnostic accuracy of this technique.[253] As was observed with exercise echocardiography, sensitivity was the highest with multivessel or left main coronary disease. The advantage of dobutamine echocardiography is that it simulates the hemodynamic effects of isotonic exercise but does not depend on patient effort. Furthermore, diagnostic images can be obtained in nearly all patients because of absence of patient motion and limited respiratory interference.[253,254]

Cardiac Pacing. Transesophageal pacing is the usual method of cardiac pacing used in conjunction with echocardiographic imaging.[223,256–258] The diagnostic accuracy of this approach is limited by the fact that increasing heart rate alone does not raise myocardial oxygen demand sufficiently to cause myocardial ischemia in many patients with coronary artery obstruction. Furthermore, there is a tendency for Wenckebach heart block to occur at a low heart rate, and some patients have esophageal pain. More recently, the feasibility of simultaneous transesophageal pacing with transesophageal echocardiographic imaging has been described.[259,260] Despite the high sensitivity and specificity initially reported, the clinical utility and incremental benefit of this technique remain to be defined.

Techniques to Alter Coronary Blood Flow: Dipyridamole, Adenosine, Cold Pressor Test

Dipyridamole. Dipyridamole is a potent arterial vasodilator that acts primarily on normal coronary arteries, diverting blood flow away from the vascular territory distal to a coronary obstruction. The resulting flow heterogeneity is the presumed ischemic mechanism responsible for perfusion defects and wall motion abnormalities when dipyridamole is administered in the presence of a coronary artery obstruction.[250,261,262] The resulting systemic vasodilation and the compensatory increase in the heart rate also may lead to a modest increase in myocardial oxygen demand.

Most echocardiographic studies examining this drug have used the intravenous formulation,[263–269] although the use of the oral formulation has been reported.[270] Echocardiographic image acquisition is performed at baseline and during the peak action of the drug (approximately 30 seconds to 4 minutes after the start of intravenous infusion). In early studies 0.56 mg/kg (low dose), of intravenous dipyridamole was administered over 4 minutes.[263,264,267] In more recent studies, 0.84 mg/kg (high dose) intravenous drug was administered over 10 minutes.[265,266,268,269] In these studies, up to 70% of patients reported side effects, although most symptoms were not ischemic (headache, flushing, dyspnea, nausea). Intravenous aminophylline was administered at the termination of the test when the patient experienced chest pain or intolerable side effects or had evidence of myocardial ischemia.

Studies using the low dose (0.56 mg/kg) of dipyridamole reported a sensitivity of 52 to 56% and specificity of 80%.[263,264] These studies reported that the sensitivity of low dose dipyridamole echocardiography was lower than that of the exercise treadmill test performed by the same patients. However, an abnormal response with the low dose of dipyridamole was predictive of a greater reduction of exercise tolerance and severity of underlying coronary disease.[264] Subsequently, investigators have reported that the use of high dose (up to 0.84 mg/kg intravenously) of dipyridamole has increased the sensitivity (74 to 83%) of the test without lowering its specificity.[265,266,269] Unfortunately, the use of this higher dose was associated with a higher incidence of dyspnea in elderly patients.[269] When dipyridamole (high dose) echocardiography and exercise electrocardiography were performed in patients with chest pain, after myocardial infarction, or following coronary angioplasty, the two methods had a similar sensitivity for the detection of the presence of significant coronary disease.[265,266,269,271] However, a higher positive predictive value and specificity were observed with dipyridamole echocardiography. Following myocardial infarction, dipyridamole echocardiography has a higher sensitivity in detecting remote asynergy and multivessel coronary disease than the exercise electrocardiogram.[268] In these studies, dipyridamole echocardiography was not more sensitive at detecting angiographically significant coronary artery disease than the exercise ECG. This finding is concordant with experimental observations that dipyridamole has a greater impact on perfusion than regional function distal to a coronary stenosis.[250]

Little data exist concerning the prognostic role of dipyridamole echocardiography. In a study of 109 patients undergoing peripheral vascular surgery, a new or worsening AWM on a preoperative dipyridamole ECG (high dose) was 88% sensitive and 98% specific for the development of postoperative cardiac complications.[272] In this study, the positive and negative predictive values of dipyridamole echocardiography were 78% and 99%, respectively, suggesting a negative test may be more helpful than a positive result.

Adenosine. Adenosine is a potent vasodilator that alters coronary blood flow through a similar mechanism of action to that of dipyridamole. Because its hemodynamic effects dissipate rapidly, it is administered as a continuous intravenous infusion. Although experience with this agent is limited, in an initial study of 73 patients, investigators reported an overall sensitivity of 85% and a specificity of 93%.[273] Although most patients experienced side effects during the study, the maximal severity of their symptoms occurred predominantly at the maximal infusion dose (140 μg/kg/min) and resolved with the termination of the infusion without the need for intravenous aminophylline.

Cold Pressor Test. Use of the cold pressor response to diagnose ischemic heart disease requires emerging the patient's hand in an ice water bath for 1 to 4 minutes.[274,275] The resultant stimulus produces an α-adrenergic discharge that increases arterial pressure. In normal individuals, the increase in myocardial oxygen demand is met by coronary dilation, whereas in the presence of coronary obstruction, there may be paradoxic vasoconstriction when the adrenergic tone overwhelms the metabolic vasodilation. In a study involving 20 patients, this test demonstrated only modest sensitivity in eliciting regional wall motion abnormalities.[276] Thus, it is of primarily historic interest.

Comparison Between Stress Echocardiographic Techniques

Published studies examining the relative accuracy of various methods in the prediction of angiographically documented coronary disease have involved relatively small numbers of patients. To date, these reports have compared exercise echocardiography (bicycle ergometry) vs. high dose dipyridamole echocardiography,[277] dobutamine vs. high dose dipyridamole echocardiography,[278] or adenosine vs. dipyridamole vs. dobutamine echocardiography.[255] When the diagnostic accuracy of exercise (bicycle) echocardiography was compared to high dose dipyridamole echocardiography, the sensitivity and specificity of the two modalities were similar. Interestingly, only 73% of patients in this study had adequate exercise images for analysis, whereas all patients had adequate images during dipyridamole echocardiography. The lack of difference between the two techniques may be a result of the high proportion of patients with unsuitable exercise images who were excluded from the comparison.

When dipyridamole (high dose) was compared with dobutamine echocardiography, dobutamine echocardiography was more sensitive in detecting single-vessel coronary disease than was dipyridamole echocardiography.[278] Both methods, however, had similar sensitivity in patients with multivessel coronary disease. A lower sensitivity in the detection of single-vessel coronary disease was observed with both modalities. In this study, ventricular arrhythmias were observed in 31% of patients during dobutamine infusion.

A recent study comparing adenosine, dipyridamole, and dobutamine echocardiography observed a higher sensitivity with dobutamine echocardiography than either of the other two techniques.[255] Furthermore, it was reported that more patients required treatment for persistent adverse symptoms following dipyridamole than after dobutamine or adenosine administration.

Comparison of Stress Echocardiography With Radionuclide Techniques

Published studies to date have compared stress echocardiography to either exercise radionuclide ventriculography or myocardial scintigraphy. Two early studies reported that exercise echocardiography was as sensitive[226] or less sensitive[235] than exercise radionuclide ventriculography in the detection of significant coronary disease. A definitive conclusion from these early studies was limited by the fact that in a significant proportion of patients one of the two tests was not feasible or was not performed.

Although no large series have been published that compare stress echocardiography with perfusion imaging, exercise echocardiography has been reported to have roughly the same overall sensitivity and specificity as myocardial scintigraphy.[210,236,237] These studies, however, have also observed that myocardial imaging was more sensitive in detecting single-vessel coronary disease, in localizing the involved vessels, and in distinguishing between single-vessel or multivessel coronary disease.[236,237]

In summary, echocardiography with exercise or pharmacologically induced stress appears to be sensitive and specific for the diagnosis of coronary artery disease and offers prognostic information that is at least as good as or better than that provided by exercise testing alone. Although its role is still being defined, its current main role in diagnosis is in the evaluation of patients with nondiagnostic exercise tests or those who are unable to exercise. Whether pharmacologic stress will become a substitute for exercise testing awaits further experience. Although stress echocardiography is portable and is less expensive than radionuclide techniques, echocardiographic image acquisition is interactive, and there is a significant "learning curve" in interpreting stress echocardiographic studies.[279]

REFERENCES

1. Theroux P, et al.: Regional myocardial function in the conscious dog during acute coronary occlusion and responses to morphine, propranolol, nitroglycerin and lidocaine. Circulation 53:302, 1976.
2. Weyman AE, Franklin TD, Egenes KM, Green D: Correlation between extent of abnormal regional wall motion and myocardial infarct size in chronically infarcted dogs. Circulation (Suppl 2)56:72, 1977.
3. Franklin TD, Jr, et al.: Differentiation of A-mode ultrasound signals from normal and ischemic myocardium by multivariate discriminant analysis of waveform parameters. Am J Cadiol 45:403, 1980.
4. Kerber R, Abboud F: Echocardiographic detection of regional myocardial infarction. Circulation 47:997, 1973.
5. Kerber R, et al.: Effects of acute coronary occlusion on the motion and perfusion of the normal and ischemic interventricular septum. Circulation 54:928, 1976.
6. Corya B, et al.: Echocardiography in acute myocardial infarction. Am J Cardiol 36:1, 1975.

7. Heikkila J, Nieminen M: Echoventriculographic detection, localization, and quantification of left ventricular asynergy in acute myocardial infarction. Br Heart J 37:46, 1975.
8. Heikkila J, Nieminen M: Echoventriculography in acute myocardial infarction. IV. Infarct size and reliability by pathologic anatomic correlations. Clin Cardiol 3:26, 1980.
9. Heger JJ, et al.: Cross-sectional echocardiography in acute myocardial infarction: detection and localization of regional left ventricular asynergy. Circulation 60:531, 1979.
10. Heger J, et al.: Cross-sectional echocardiographic analysis of the extent of left ventricular asynergy in acute myocardial infarction. Circulation 61: 1113, 1980.
11. Visser C, et al.: Quantification and localization of uncomplicated acute myocardial infarction by cross-sectional echocardiography. Circulation 59, 60(Suppl. 2): II–152, 1979.
12. Bloch A, Morard J, Mayor C, Perrenoud J: Cross-sectional echocardiography in acute myocardial infarction. Am J Cardiol 43:387, 1979.
13. Rogers EW, et al.: Predicting survival after myocardial infarction by cross-sectional echo. Circulation 58(Suppl. 2): II–233, 1978.
14. Nixon JV, Narahara KA, Smitherman TC: Estimation of myocardial involvement in patients with acute myocardial infarction by two-dimensional echocardiography. Circulation 62:1248, 1980.
15. Weiss JL, Buckley BH, Hutchins GM, Mason SJ: Two-dimensional echocardiographic recognition of myocardial injury in man: comparison with postmortem studies. Circulation 63:401, 1981.
16. Horowitz RS, et al.: Immediate diagnosis of acute myocardial infarction by two-dimensional echocardiography. Circulation 65:323, 1982.
17. Gibson RS, et al.: Value of early two-dimensional echocardiography in patients with acute myocardial infarction. Am J Cardiol 49:1110, 1982.
18. Drobac M, et al.: Complicated acute myocardial infarction: the importance of two-dimensional echocardiography. Am J Cardiol 43:387, 1979.
19. Nishimura RA, et al.: Role of two-dimensional echocardiography in the prediction of in-hospital complications after acute myocardial infarction. J Am Coll Cardiol 4:1080, 1984.
20. Marshall SA, Picard MH, Ray PA, Weyman AE: Ventricular morphology and function in acute non Q-wave myocardial infarction. Circulation 82(Suppl. 3): III–73, 1990.
21. Visser CA, et al.: Detection and quantification of acute, isolated myocardial infarction by two-dimensional echocardiography. Am J Cardiol 47: 1020, 1981.
22. Stamm RB, et al.: Echocardiographic detection of infarct-localized asynergy and remote asynergy during acute myocardial infarction: correlation with the extent of angiographic coronary disease. Circulation 67:233, 1983.
23. Picard MH, Wilkins GT, Ray PA, Weyman AE: Natural history of left ventricular size and function after acute myocardial infarction: assessment and prediction by echocardiographic endocardial surface mapping. Circulation 82:484, 1990.
24. Lieberman AN, et al.: Two-dimensional echocardiography and infarct size: relationship of regional wall motion and thickening to the extent of myocardial infarction in the dog. Circulation 63:739, 1981.
25. Nieminen M, et al.: Serial evaluation of myocardial thickening and thinning in acute experimental infarction: identification and quantification using two-dimensional echocardiography. Circulation 66:174, 1982.
26. Pandian NG, Kerber RE: Two-dimensional echocardiography in experimental coronary stenosis. I. Sensitivity and specificity in detecting transient myocardial dyskinesis: comparison with sonomicrometers. Circulation 66:597, 1982.
27. Pandian NG, Kieso RA, Kerber RE: Two-dimensional echocardiography in experimental coronary stenosis. II. Relationship between systolic wall thinning and regional myocardial perfusion in severe coronary stenosis. Circulation 66:603, 1982.
28. Pandian NG, et al.: Serial quantification of myocardial dyskinesis in acute myocardial infarction by two-dimensional echocardiography in dogs. J Am Coll Cardiol 1:619, 1983.
29. Vatner SF: Correlation between acute reductions in myocardial blood flow and function in conscious dogs. Circ Res 47:201, 1980.
30. Geltman EM, et al.: The influence of location and extent of myocardial infarction on long-term ventricular dysrhythmia and mortality. Circulation 60:805, 1979.
31. Blumenthal DS, et al.: Impaired function of salvaged myocardium: two-dimensional echocardiographic quantification of regional wall thickening in the open-chest dog. Circulation 67:225, 1983.
32. Matsuzaki M, et al.: Sustained regional dysfunction produced by prolonged coronary stenosis: gradual recovery after reperfusion. Circulation 68:171, 1983.
33. Oh JK, et al.: Effects of acute reperfusion on regional myocardial function: serial two-dimensional echocardiography assessment. Int J Cardiol 22:161, 1989.
34. Widimsky P, et al.: First month course of left ventricular asynergy after intracoronary thrombolysis in acute myocardial infarction. A longitudinal echocardiographic study. Eur Heart J 6:759, 1985.
35. Charuzi Y, et al.: Improvement in regional and global left ventricular function after intracoronary thrombolysis: assessment with two-dimensional echocardiography. Am J Cardiol 53:662, 1984.
36. Bourdillon PDV, et al.: Early recovery of regional left ventricular function after reperfusion in acute myocardial infarction assessed by serial two-dimensional echocardiography. Am J Cardiol 63:641, 1989.
37. Otto CM, et al.: Echocardiographic evaluation of segmental wall motion early and late after thrombolytic therapy in acute myocardial infarction: the western Washington Tissue Plasminogen Activator Emergency Room Trial. Am J Cardiol 65:132, 1990.
38. Touchstone DA, et al.: Effects of successful intravenous reperfusion therapy on regional myocardial function and geometry in humans: a tomographic assessment using two-dimensional echocardiography. J Am Coll Cardiol 13:1506, 1989.
39. Siu SC, et al.: The effect of late patency of the infarct-related coronary artery on left ventricular morphology and regional function following thrombolysis. Am Heart J 124:265, 1993.
40. Nidorf SM, et al.: The benefit of late coronary reperfusion on ventricular morphology and function after myocardial infarction. J Am Coll Cardiol 21:683, 1993.
41. Weyman AE: Cross-Section Echocardiography. Philadelphia, Lea & Febiger, 1982.
42. Medina R, et al.: The value of echocardiographic regional wall motion abnormalities in detecting coronary artery disease in patients with or without a dilated left ventricle. Am Heart J 109:799, 1985.
43. Wyatt HL, et al.: Experimental evaluation of the extent of myocardial dyssynergy and infarct size by two-dimensional echocardiography. Circulation 63:607, 1981.
44. Kan G, Visser CA, Lie KI, Durrer D: Correlation of two-dimensional echocardiography with coronary arteriography and electrocardiogram in anterior wall infarction. Circulation 62(Suppl. 3):III–186, 1980.
45. Sullivan W, et al.: Correlation of electrocardiographic and pathologic findings in healed myocardial infarction. Am J Cardiol 42:724, 1978.
46. Young E, et al.: Vectorcardiographic diagnosis and electrocardiographic correlation in left ventricular asynergy due to coronary artery disease. I. Severe asynergy of the anterior and apical segments. Circulation 51:467, 1975.
47. Bodenheimer MM, et al.: Correlation of pathologic Q waves on the standard electrocardiogram and the epicardial electrogram of the human heart. Circulation 54:213, 1976.
48. Weyman AE, et al.: Detection of left ventricular aneurysms by cross-sectional echocardiography. Circulation 54:936, 1976.
49. Hickman HO, et al.: Cross-sectional echocardiography of the cardiac apex. Circulation 56 (Suppl. 3):589, 1977.
50. Barrett MJ, Charuzi Y, Corday E: Ventricular aneurysms: cross-sectional echocardiographic approach. Am J Cardiol 46:1133, 1980.
51. Errichetti A, Homma S, Guyer DE, Weyman AE: Limitations of the 12-lead electrocardiogram in predicting segmental apical dysfunction: comparison with apical dysfunction by 2-D echocardiography. Circulation 76 (Suppl. 4):IV-226, 1987.
52. Gibson RS: Clinical, functional, and angiographic distinctions between Q wave and non-Q wave myocardial infarction: evidence of spontaneous reperfusion and implications for intervention trials. Circulation 75:V128, 1987.
53. Spokick DH: Q-wave infarction versus S-T infarction. Nonspecificity of electrocardiographic criteria for differentiating transmural and non-transmural lesions. Am J Cardiol 51:913, 1983.
54. Krone RJ, et al.: Long-term prognosis after first Q-wave (transmural) or non-Q-wave (nontransmural) myocardial infarction: analysis of 593 patients. Am J Cardiol 52:234, 1983.
55. Schulze RA, et al.: Coronary angiography and left ventriculography in survivors of transmural and nontransmural myocardial infarction. Am J Med 64:108, 1978.
56. Montague TJ, et al.: Non-Q-wave acute myocardial infarction: body surface potential map and ventriculographic patterns. Am J Cardiol 58:1173, 1986.
57. Feild BJ, et al.: Regional left ventricular performance in the year following myocardial infarction. Circulation 46:679, 1972.
58. Meltzer RS, et al.: Two-dimensional echocardiographic quantification of infarct size alteration by pharmacologic agents. Am J Cardiol 44:257, 1979.
59. Charuzi U, et al.: A quantitative comparison of cross-sectional echocardiography and radionuclide angiography in acute myocardial infarction. Circulation 58 (Suppl. 2):II-52, 1978.
60. Wynne J, Birnholz J, Finberg H, Alpert J: Regional left ventricular wall motion in acute myocardial infarction as assessed by two-dimensional echocardiography. Circulation 55, 56(Suppl. 3):III-152, 1977.
61. Nishimura RA, et al.: Prognostic value of predischarge 2-dimensional echocardiogram after acute myocardial infarction. Am J Cardiol 53:429, 1984.
62. Shina A, et al.: Prognostic significance of regional wall motion abnormality in patients with prior myocardial infarction: a prospective correlative study of two-dimensional echocardiography and angiography. Mayo Clin Proc 61:254, 1986.
63. Kan G, Visser CA, Koolen JJ, Dunning AJ: Short and long term predictive value of admission wall motion score in acute myocardial infarction: a cross sectional echocardiographic study of 345 patients. Br Heart J 56:422, 1986.

64. Berning J, Steensgaard-Hansen F: Early estimation of risk by echocardiographic determination of wall motion index in an unselected population with acute myocardial infarction. Am J Cardiol 65:567, 1990.
65. Isaacsohn JL, Earle MG, Kemper AJ, Parisi AF: Postmyocardial infarction pain and infarct extension in the coronary care unit: role of two-dimensional echocardiography. J Am Coll Cardiol 11:246, 1988.
66. Eaton L, et al.: Regional cardiac dilatation after acute myocardial infarction. N Engl J Med 300:57, 1979.
67. Picard MH, et al.: Immediate regional endocardial surface expansion following coronary occlusion in the canine left ventricle: disproportionate effects of anterior versus inferior ischemia. Am Heart J 121:753, 1991.
68. Erlebacher JA, et al.: Late effects of acute infarct dilation on heart size: a two-dimensional echocardiographic study. Am J Cardiol 49:1120, 1982.
69. White HD, et al.: Left ventricular end-systolic volume as the major determinant of survival after recovery from myocardial infarction. Circulation 76:44, 1987.
70. Nemerovski M, et al.: Radionuclide assessment of sequential changes in left and right ventricular function following acute transmural myocardial infarction. Am Heart J 104:709, 1982.
71. Greenberg H, et al.: Left ventricular dysfunction after acute myocardial infarction: results of a prospective multicenter study. J Am Coll Cardiol 4:867, 1984.
72. Gibbons EF, et al.: The natural history of regional wall motion in the acutely infarcted canine ventricles. Circulation 71:394, 1985.
73. Guyer DE, et al.: A new echocardiographic model for quantifying three-dimensional endocardial surface area. J Am Coll Cardiol 8:819, 1986.
74. Guyer DE, et al.: An echocardiographic technique for quantifying and displaying the extent of regional left ventricular dyssynergy. J Am Coll Cardiol 8:830, 1986.
75. Wilkins GT, et al.: Correlation between echocardiographic endocardial surface mapping of abnormal wall motion and pathologic infarct size in autopsied hearts. Circulation 77:978, 1988.
76. Picard MH, Wilkins GT, Ray PA, Weyman AE: Progressive changes in ventricular structure and function during the year after acute myocardial infarction. Am Heart J 124:24, 1992.
77. Picard MH, Weyman AE: Echocardiographic assessment of post-myocardial infarction left ventricular size and function. Heart Failure 7:180, 1991.
78. Meizlish JL, et al.: Functional left ventricular aneurysm formation after acute anterior transmural myocardial infarction: incidence, natural history, and prognostic complications. N Engl J Med 311:1001, 1984.
79. Schuster EH, Bulkey BH: Expansion of transmural myocardial infarction: a pathophysiologic factor in cardiac rupture. Circulation 60:1532, 1979.
80. Visser CA, et al.: Incidence, timing, and prognostic value of left ventricular aneurysm formation after myocardial infarction: a prospective serial echocardiographic study of 158 patients. Am J Cardiol 57:729, 1986.
81. Hochman JS, Bulkley BH: The pathogenesis of left ventricular aneurysm: an experimental study in the rat model. Am J Cardiol 50:83, 1982.
82. Matsumoto M, et al.: Left ventricular aneurysm and the prediction of left ventricular enlargement studied by two-dimensional echocardiography: quantitative assessment of aneurysm size in relation to clinical course. Circulation 72:280, 1985.
83. Weisman HF, et al.: Cellular mechanisms of myocardial infarct expansion. Circulation 78:186, 1988.
84. Crozatier B, Ashraf M, Franklin D, Ross J: Sarcomere length in experimental myocardial infarction: evidence for sarcomere overstretch in dyskinetic ventricular region. J Mol Cell Cardiol 9:785, 1977.
85. Pirolo JS, Hutchins GM, Moore GW: Infarct expansion: pathologic analysis of 204 patients with a single myocardial infarct. J Am Coll Cardiol 7: 349, 1986.
86. Streeter DD, Hanna WT: Engineering mechanics for successive states in canine left ventricular myocardium: Cavity and wall geometry. Circ Res 33:639, 1973.
87. Streeter DD: Gross morphology and fiber geometry of the heart. *In* Berne RM, Sperelakis N (eds.): Handbook of Physiology, Section 2: The Cardiovascular System. Vol. 1. The Heart. Baltimore: Williams & Wilkins, 1979.
88. Bogen DK, et al.: An analysis of the mechanical disadvantage of myocardial infarction in the canine left ventricle. Circ Res 47:728, 1980.
89. Heyndrickx GR, et al.: Regional myocardial functional and electrophysiological alterations after brief coronary artery occlusion in conscious dogs. J Clin Invest 56:978, 1975.
90. Gallagher KP, et al.: Dissociation between epicardial and transmural function during acute myocardial ischemia. Circulation 71:1279, 1985.
91. Hattori S, et al.: Contrasting ischemic patterns by zone and layer in canine myocardium. Am J Physiol 243:H852, 1982.
92. Greenbaum RA, et al.: Left ventricular fibre architecture in man. Br Heart J 45:248, 1981.
93. LeWinter MM, et al.: Regional differences in myocardial performance in the left ventricle in the dog. Circ Res 37:191, 1975.
94. Rankin JS, et al.: The three-dimensional dynamic geometry of the left ventricle in the conscious dog. Circ Res 39:304, 1976.
95. Erlebacher JA, et al.: Early infarct expansion: structural or functional? J Am Coll Cardiol 6:839, 1985.
96. Pfeffer MA, et al.: Effect of captopril on progressive ventricular dilatation after anterior myocardial infarction. N Engl J Med 319:80, 1988.
97. Sharpe N, Murphy J, Smith H, Hannan S: Treatment of patients with symptomless left ventricular dysfunction after myocardial infarction. Lancet 1:255, 1988.
98. Jeremy RW, Allman KC, Bautovitch G, Harris PJ: Patterns of left ventricular dilation during the six months after myocardial infarction. J Am Coll Cardiol 13:304, 1989.
99. Jeremy RW, et al.: Infarct artery perfusion and changes in left ventricular volume in the month after acute myocardial infarction. J Am Coll Cardiol 9:985, 1987.
100. Kostuk WJ, et al.: Left ventricular size after myocardial infarction: serial changes and their prognostic significance. Circulation 47:1174, 1973.
101. McKay RG, et al.: Left ventricular remodeling after myocardial infarction: a corollary to infarct expansion. Circulation 74:693, 1986.
102. Seals AA, et al.: Relation of left ventricular dilation during acute myocardial infarction to systolic performance, diastolic dysfunction, infarct size, and location. Am J Cardiol 61:224, 1988.
103. Choony CY, et al.: Relationship of functional recovery of scar contraction after myocardial infarction in the canine left ventricle. Am Heart J 117: 819, 1989.
104. Davidoff R, et al.: Ventricular structure and function recovers in a wavefront from base to apex. Circulation 78(Suppl. 2):II-464, 1988.
105. Mallory GK, White PD, Salcedo-Salgar J: The speed of healing of myocardial infarction: A study of the pathologic anatomy in seventy-two cases. Am Heart J 18:647, 1939.
106. Preuss KC, et al.: Spontaneous recovery of left ventricular function following acute anterior myocardial infarction. Clin Cardiol 11:497, 1988.
107. Mahias-Narvarte H, Adams KF, Willis PW: Evolution of regional left ventricular wall motion abnormalities in acute Q and non-Q wave myocardial infarction. Am Heart J 113:1369, 1987.
108. Gruppo Italiano per lo Studio Della Streptochinasi, Nell'Infarto Miocardico (GISSI): Effectiveness of intravenous thrombolytic treatment in acute myocardial infarction. Lancet 1:397, 1986.
109. ISIS-2 (Second International Study of Infarct Survival) Collaborative Study Group: Randomized trial of intravenous streptokinase, oral aspirin, both or neither among 17,187 cases of suspected acute myocardial infarction. Lancet 2:349, 1988.
110. AIMS Trial Study Group: Effect of intravenous APSAC on mortality after acute myocardial infarction: preliminary report of a placebo-controlled clinical trial. Lancet 1:545, 1988.
111. Van de Werf F, Arnold AER, the European Cooperative Study Group for Recombinant Tissue-type Plasminogen Activator (rt-PA): Intravenous rt-PA and size of infarct, left ventricular function and survival in acute myocardial infarction. Br Med J 297:1374, 1988.
112. Marino P, Zanolla L, Zardini P, on behalf of the Gruppo Italiano per Lo Studio Della Streptochinasi Nell'Infarto Miocardico (GISSI): Effect of streptokinase on left ventricular modeling and function after myocardial infarction: The GISSI (Group Italiano perlo Studio della Streptochinase nell'Infarto Miocardico) Trial. J Am Coll Cardiol 14:1149, 1989.
113. Picard MH, Ray P, Weyman AE: Left ventricular size and function during the year following acute myocardial infarction. J Am Coll Cardiol 17:2A, 1991.
114. Hochman JS, Choo H: Limitation of myocardial infarct expansion by reperfusion independent of myocardial salvage. Circulation 75:299, 1987.
115. Force T, Kemper A, Leavitt M, Parisi AF: Acute reduction in functional infarct expansion with late coronary reperfusion: assessment with quantitative two-dimensional echocardiography. J Am Coll Cardiol 11:192, 1988.
116. Braunwald E: Myocardial reperfusion, limitation of infarct size, reduction of left ventricular dysfunction, and improved survival: should the paradigm be expanded? Circulation 79:441, 1989.
117. Bonaduce D, et al.: Effects of late administration of tissue-type plasminogen activator on left ventricular remodeling and function after myocardial infarction. J Am Coll Cardiol 16:1561, 1990.
118. Bussman WD, Passek D, Seidel W, Kaltenbach M: Reduction of CK and CK-MB indexes of infarct size by intravenous nitroglycerin. Circulation 63:615, 1981.
119. Jaffe AS, et al.: Reduction of infarct size in patients with inferior infarction with intravenous glyceryl trinitrate. A randomized study. Br Heart J 49: 452, 1983.
120. Flaherty JT, et al.: A randomized prospective trial of intravenous nitroglycerin in patients with acute myocardial infarction. Circulation 68:576, 1983.
121. Jugdutt BI, Warnica JW: Intravenous nitroglycerin therapy to limit myocardial infarct size, expansion, and complications: effects of timing, dosage, and infarct locations. Circulation 78:906, 1988.
122. Borer JS, et al.: Reduction in myocardial ischemia with nitroglycerin or nitroglycerin plus phenylephyrine administered during acute myocardial infarction. N Engl J Med 293:1008, 1975.
123. Pfeffer JM, Pfeffer MA, Braunwald E: Influence of chronic captopril therapy on the infarcted left ventricle of the rat. Circ Res 57:84, 1985.
124. Pfeffer MA, Pfeffer JM, Steinberg C, Finn P: Survival after an experimental myocardial infarction: beneficial effects of long-term therapy with captopril. Circulation 72:406, 1985.
125. Mehta PM, Alker KJ, Kloner RA: Functional infarct expansion, left ventricular dilation and isovolumic relaxation time after coronary occlusion:

a two-dimensional echocardiographic study. J Am Coll Cardiol 11:630, 1988.
126. The CONSENSUS Trial Study Group: Effects of enalapril on mortality in severe congestive heart failure. N Engl J Med 316:1429, 1987.
127. The SOLVD Investigators: Effect of enalapril on survival in patients with reduced left ventricular ejection fractions and congestive heart failure. N Engl J Med 325:293, 1991.
128. Sharpe N, et al.: Early prevention of left ventricular dysfunction after myocardial infarction with angiotensin-converting-enzyme inhibition. Lancet 337:872, 1991.
129. Oh JK, et al.: Evaluation of acute chest pain syndromes by two-dimensional echocardiography: its potential application in the selection of patients for acute reperfusion therapy. Mayo Clin Proc 62:59, 1987.
130. Peels CH, et al.: Usefulness of two-dimensional echocardiography for immediate detection of myocardial ischemia in the emergency room. Am J Cardiol 65:687, 1990.
131. Sabia P, et al.: Value of regional wall motion abnormality in the emergency room diagnosis of acute myocardial infarction: a prospective study using two-dimensional echocardiography. Circulation 84(Suppl. 1):I-85, 1991.
132. Sabia P, et al.: Importance of two-dimensional echocardiographic assessment of left ventricular systolic function in patients presenting to the emergency room with cardiac-related symptoms. Circulation 84:1615, 1991.
133. Lengyel M, Tajik A, Seward J, Smith H: Correlation of two-dimensional echocardiographic and angiographic segmental wall motion abnormalities in patients with prior transmural myocardial infarction: a prospective double-blind study. Circulation 59, 60(Suppl. 2):153, 1979.
134. Kisslo J: Evaluation of the left ventricle by two-dimensional echocardiography. Acta Med Scand 627(Suppl.):112, 1979.
135. Ross A, Michaelson S: Left ventricular contraction patterns by mechanical, two-dimensional real-time echocardiography. Clin Res 25:250A, 1977.
136. Kisslo J, et al.: A comparison of real-time, two-dimensional echocardiography and cineangiography in detecting left ventricular asynergy. Circulation 55:134, 1977.
137. Jacobs JJ, Feigenbaum H, Corya BC, Phillips JF: Detection of left ventricular asynergy by echocardiography. Circulation 68:263, 1973.
138. VanTassel RA, Edwards JE: Rupture of the heart complicating myocardial infarction: analysis of 40 cases including nine examples of left ventricular false aneurysms. Chest 61:104, 1972.
139. Rasmussen S, Corya B, Feigenbaum H, Knoebel S: Detection of myocardial scar tissue by M-mode echocardiography. Circulation 57:230, 1978.
140. Lengyel M, et al.: Sensitivity and specificity of two-dimensional echocardiography in the detection of left ventricular aneurysms. Am J Cardiol 45: 436, 1980.
141. Rakowski H, et al.: Left ventricular aneurysm: detection and determination of resectability by two-dimensional ultrasound. Circulation 56(Suppl. 3): III-153, 1977.
142. Berman B, McGuire J: Cardiac aneurysms. Am J Med 8:480, 1950.
143. Abrams DL, Edelist A, Luria MH, Miller AJ: Ventricular aneurysm: a reappraisal based on a study of 65 consecutive autopsies cases. Circulation 27:164, 1963.
144. Schiehter J, Hellerstein KH, Katz LN: Aneurysm of the heart: correlative study of 102 proved cases. Medicine 33:43, 1954.
145. Williams TW, Peabody CA, Pruitt RD: Calcified aneurysm of the left ventricular apex associated with intraventricular block of the left bundle branch type. Am Heart J 63:557, 1962.
146. Vlodaver Z, Coe JJ, Edwards JE: True and false aneurysms: propensity for the latter to rupture. Circulation 51:567, 1975.
147. Gorlin R, Klein MD, Sullivan JM: Prospective correlative study of ventricular aneurysms. Am J Med 42:512, 1967.
148. Rao G, et al.: Experience with sixty consecutive ventricular aneurysm resections. Circulation 49, 50(Suppl. 2):149, 1974.
149. Graber JD, et al.: Ventricular aneurysm. An appraisal of diagnosis and surgical therapy. Br Heart J 34:831, 1972.
150. Roberts WC, Morrown AG: Pseudoaneurysm of the left ventricle: an unusual sequel of myocardial infarction and rupture of the heart. Am J Med 43:639, 1967.
151. Katz RJ, et al.: Non-invasive diagnosis of left ventricular pseudoaneurysm: role of two-dimensional echocardiography and radionuclide gated pool imaging. Am J Cardiol 44:372, 1979.
152. Sears TD, Ong YS, Starke H, Forker AD: Left ventricular pseudoaneurysm identified by cross-sectional echocardiography. Ann Int Med 90:935, 1979.
153. Nanda NC, Gatewood RD: Differentiation of left ventricular pseudoaneurysm from true aneurysms by two-dimensional echocardiography. Circulation 60 (Suppl. 2):II-144, 1979.
154. Catherwood E, et al.: Two-dimensional echocardiographic recognition of left ventricular pseudoaneurysm. Circulation 62:294, 1980.
155. Lascault G, Reeves F, Drobinski G: Evidence of the inaccuracy of standard echocardiographic and angiographic criteria used for the recognition of true and "false" left ventricular inferior aneurysm. Br Heart J 60:125, 1988.
156. Olalla JJ, et al.: Color Doppler diagnosis of left ventricular pseudoaneurysm. Chest 94:443, 1988.
157. Roelandt JFTC, Sutherland GR, Yoshida K, Yoshikawa J: Improved diagnosis and characterization of left ventricular pseudoaneurysm by Doppler color flow imaging. J Am Coll Cardiol 12:807, 1988.
158. Chiariello L, et al.: Extracardiac left to right shunt in a patient with biventricular postinfarction rupture and pseudoaneurysm. J Am Coll Cardiol 6: 246, 1985.
159. Skapinker S: Diverticulum of the left ventricle of the heart. Arch Surg 63: 629, 1951.
160. Potts WJ, DeBoer A, Johnson FR: Congenital diverticulum of the left ventricle. Surgery 33:301, 1953.
161. Chesler E, Tucker RBK, Barlow JB: Subvalvular and apical left ventricular aneurysms in the Bantu as a source of systemic emboli. Circulation 35: 1156, 1967.
162. Edgett JW, Jr, et al.: Diverticulum of the heart. Part of the syndrome of congenital cardiac and midline thoracic and abdominal defects. Am J Cardiol 24:580, 1969.
163. Treistman B, Cooley DA, Lufschanowski R, Leachman RD: Diverticulum or aneurysm of left ventricle. Am J Cardiol 32:119, 1973.
164. Kanarek KS, et al.: Clinical aspects of submitral left ventricular aneurysms. S Afr Med J 47:1225, 1973.
165. Tecklenberg PL, Alderman EL, Billingham ME, Shumway NE: Diverticulum of the left ventricle in hypertrophic cardiomyopathy. Am J Med 64: 707, 1978.
166. Shizukuda Y, et al.: Siblings with left ventricular diverticulum and hypertrophic cardiomyopathy. J Cardiol 18:867, 1988.
167. Sanada H, et al.: Two-dimensional echocardiographic and left ventriculographic evaluations of left ventricular diverticula. J Cardiol 19:1107, 1989.
168. Estevez CM, Weyman AE, Feigenbaum H: Detection of left ventricular diverticulum by cross-sectional echocardiography. Chest 69:544, 1976.
169. Sanders RJ, Kern WH, Blount SG: Perforation of the interventricular septum complicating myocardial infarction. Am Heart J 81:736, 1956.
170. Vlodaver Z, Edwards JE: Rupture of ventricular septum or papillary muscle complicating myocardial infarction. Circulation 55:815, 1977.
171. Pagall JC, Pryor R, Blount SG: Systolic murmur following myocardial infarction. Am Heart J 87:577, 1974.
172. Farcot JC, et al.: Two-dimensional echocardiographic visualization of ventricular septal rupture after acute myocardial infarction. Am J Cardiol 45: 370, 1980.
173. Scanlan JG, Seward J, Tajik A: Visualization of ventricular septal rupture utilizing wide-angle two-dimensional echocardiography. Mayo Clin Proc 54:381, 1979.
174. Rogers EW, et al.: Aneurysms of the posterior interventricular septum with post-infarction ventricular septal defect. Echocardiographic identification. Chest 78:741, 1980.
175. Miyatake K, et al.: Doppler echocardiographic features of ventricular septal rupture in myocardial infarction. J Am Coll Cardiol 5:182, 1985.
176. Zachariah ZP, Hsiung MC, Nanda NC, Camarano GP: Diagnosis of rupture of the ventricular septum during acute myocardial infarction by Doppler color flow mapping. Am J Cardiol 59:162, 1987.
177. Helmcke F, et al.: Two-dimensional echocardiography and Doppler color flow mapping in the diagnosis and prognosis of ventricular septal rupture. Circulation 81:1775, 1990.
178. Bansal RC, Eng AK, Shakudo M: Role of two-dimensional echocardiography, pulsed, continuous wave and color flow Doppler techniques in the assessment of ventricular septal rupture after myocardial infarction. Am J Cardiol 65:852, 1990.
179. Smyllie JH, et al.: Doppler color flow mapping in the diagnosis of ventricular septal rupture and acute mitral regurgitation after myocardial infarction. J Am Coll Cardiol 15:1449, 1990.
180. Koenig K, et al.: Transesophageal echocardiography for diagnosis of rupture of the ventricular septum or left ventricular papillary muscle during acute myocardial infarction. Am J Cardiol 59:362, 1987.
181. Moore CA, et al.: Postinfarction ventricular septal rupture: the importance of location of infarction and right ventricular function in determining survival. Circulation 74:45, 1986.
182. Cederqvist L, Soderstrom J: Papillary muscle rupture in myocardial infarction: a study based upon an autopsy material. Acta Med Scand 176:287, 1964.
183. Wei JY, Hutchins GM, Bulkley BJ: Papillary muscle rupture in fatal acute myocardial infarction: a potentially treatable form of cardiogenic shock. Ann Intern Med 90:149, 1979.
184. Nishimura RA, et al.: Papillary muscle rupture complicating acute myocardial infarction: analysis of 17 patients. Am J Cardiol 51:373, 1983.
185. Barbour DJ, Roberts WC: Rupture of left ventricular papillary muscle during acute myocardial infarction: analysis of 22 necropsy patients. J Am Coll Cardiol 8:558, 1986.
186. Sanders RJ, Neubuerger KT, Ravin A: Rupture of papillary muscles: occurrence of rupture of the posterior muscle in posterior myocardial infarction. Dis Chest 31:316, 1957.
187. Eisenberg PR, Barzilai B, Perez JE: Noninvasive detection by Doppler echocardiography of combined ventricular septal rupture and mitral regurgitation in acute myocardial infarction. J Am Coll Cardiol 4:617, 1984.
188. Goldman AP, et al.: Role of echocardiography/Doppler in cardiogenic shock: silent mitral regurgitation. Ann Thorac Surg 52:296, 1991.
189. Yates WM, Welsh PP, Stapleton JF, Clark ML: Comparison of clinical and pathologic aspects of coronary artery disease in men of various age groups: a study of 950 autopsied cases from the Armed Forces Institute of Pathology. Ann Intern Med 34:352, 1951.

190. Jordan RA, Miller RD, Edwards JE, Parker RL: Thrombi embolism in acute and healed myocardial infarction. I. Intracardiac mural thrombus. Circulation 6:1, 1952.
191. Phares WS, Edwards JE, Burchell HB: Cardiac aneurysms: clinicopathologic studies. Mayo Clin Proc 28:264, 1953.
192. Helden T, Iversen K, Rapschou F, Schwartz M: Anticoagulants in acute myocardial infarction. Lancet 2:327, 1961.
193. Report of the Working Party on Anticoagulant Therapy in Coronary Thrombosis to the Medical Research Council: Assessment of short-term anticoagulant administration after cardiac infarction. Br Med J 1:335, 1969.
194. Veterans Administration Hospital Investigators: Anticoagulants in acute myocardial infarction: results of a cooperative clinical trial. JAMA 225: 724, 1973.
195. DeMaria AN, et al.: Left ventricular thrombi identified by cross-sectional echocardiography. Ann Int Med 90:14, 1979.
196. Meltzer RS, et al.: Diagnosis of left ventricular thrombi by two-dimensional echocardiography. Br Heart J 42:261, 1979.
197. Suzuki S, et al.: Cross-sectional echocardiographic findings of left ventricular thrombi in a ten-year old patient with cardiomyopathy. Jpn Heart J 20: 675, 1979.
198. Seward JB, Gura GM, Hagler DJ, Tajik AJ: Evaluation of M-mode echocardiography and wide angle two-dimensional echocardiography in the diagnosis of intracardiac masses. Circulation 57, 58(Suppl. 2):II-234, 1978.
199. Drobac M, et al.: Two-dimensional echocardiographic recognition of mural thrombi: in vivo and in vitro studies. Am J Cardiol 45:435, 1980.
200. Ports FA, Cogan J, Schiller NB, Rapaport E: Echocardiography of left ventricular masses. Circulation 58:528, 1978.
201. Asinger RW, et al.: Serial evaluation for left ventricular thrombus during acute transmural myocardial infarction using two-dimensional echocardiography. Am J Cardiol 45:483, 1980.
202. Asinger RW, Mikell FL, Elsperger J, Hodges M: Incidence of left-ventricular thrombosis after acute transmural myocardial infarction. N Engl J Med 305:297, 1981.
203. Mikell F, et al.: Experimental left ventricular thrombi: early detection by two-dimensional echocardiography. Circulation 62(Suppl. 3):III-330, 1980.
204. Stratton JR, Lighty GW, Jr, Pearlman AS, Ritchie JL: Detection of left ventricular thrombus by two-dimensional echocardiography: sensitivity, specificity, and causes of uncertainty. Circulation 66:156, 1982.
205. Visser CA, et al.: Embolic potential of left ventricular thrombus after myocardial infarction: a two-dimensional echocardiographic study of 119 patients. J Am Coll Cardiol 5:1276, 1985.
206. Keren A, et al.: Natural history of left ventricular thrombi: their appearance and resolution in the posthospitalization period of acute myocardial infarction. J Am Coll Cardiol 15:790, 1990.
207. Spirito P, et al.: Prognostic significance and natural history of left ventricular thrombi in patients with acute anterior myocardial infarction: a two-dimensional echocardiographic study. Circulation 72:774, 1985.
208. Kupper AJF, et al.: Left ventricular thrombus incidence and behavior studied by serial two-dimensional echocardiography in acute anterior myocardial infarction: left ventricular wall motion, systemic embolism, and oral anticoagulation. J Am Coll Cardiol 13:1514, 1989.
209. Jugdutt BI, et al.: Prospective two-dimensional echocardiographic evaluation of left ventricular thrombus and embolism after acute myocardial infarction. J Am Coll Cardiol 13:554, 1989.
210. Wann LS, et al.: Exercise cross-sectional echocardiography in ischemic heart disease. Circulation 60:1300, 1979.
211. Morganroth J, et al: Exercise cross-sectional echocardiographic diagnosis of coronary artery disease. Am J Cardiol 47:20, 1981.
212. DeMaria AN, et al.: Evaluation of left ventricular responses to isometric exertion by two-dimensional echocardiography. Circulation 59, 60(Suppl. 2):II-152, 1979.
213. Feigenbaum H: Exercise echocardiography. J Am Soc Echocardiogr 1: 161, 1988.
214. Armstrong WF, O'Donnell J, Ryan T, Feigenbaum H: Effect of prior myocardial infarction and extent and location of coronary artery disease on accuracy of exercise echocardiography. J Am Coll Cardiol 10:531, 1987.
215. Ryan T, et al.: Exercise echocardiography: detection of coronary artery disease in patients with normal left ventricular function at rest. J Am Coll Cardiol 11:993, 1988.
216. Sabbah HN, et al.: Noninvasive evaluation of left ventricular performance based on peak aortic blood acceleration measured by a continuous-wave Doppler velocity meter. Circulation 74:323, 1986.
217. Wallmeyer K, et al.: The influence of preload and heart rate on Doppler echocardiographic indexes of left ventricular performance. Comparison with invasive indexes in an experimental preparation. Circulation 74:181, 1986.
218. Colocousis JS, Huntsman LL, Curreri PW: Estimation of stroke volume changes by ultrasonic Doppler. Circulation 56:914, 1977.
219. Huntsman LL, et al.: Noninvasive Doppler determination of cardiac output in man. Circulation 67:593, 1983.
220. Bryg RJ, et al.: Effect of coronary artery disease on Doppler-derived parameters of aortic flow during upright exercise. Am J Cardiol 58:14, 1986.
221. Harrison MR, Smith MD, Friedman BJ, DeMaria AN: Uses and limitations of exercise Doppler echocardiography in the diagnosis of ischemic heart disease. J Am Coll Cardiol 10:809, 1987.
222. Daley PJ, et al.: Detection of exercise induced changes in left ventricular performance by Doppler echocardiography. Br Heart J 58:447, 1987.
223. Armstrong WF: Stress echocardiography for detection of coronary artery disease. Circulation 84(Suppl. 1):I-43, 1991.
224. Maurer G, Nanda NC: Two dimensional echocardiographic evaluation of exercise-induced left and right ventricular asynergy: correlation with thallium scanning. Am J Cardiol 48:720, 1981.
225. Robertson WS, et al.: Exercise echocardiography: a clinically practical addition in the evaluation of coronary artery disease. J Am Coll Cardiol 2:1085, 1983.
226. Limacher MC, et al.: Detection of coronary artery disease with exercise two-dimensional echocardiography. Circulation 67:1211, 1983.
227. Armstrong WF, et al.: Complementary value of two-dimensional exercise echocardiography to routine treadmill exercise testing. Ann Intern Med 105:829, 1986.
228. Crouse LJ, et al.: Exercise echocardiography as a screening test for coronary artery disease and correlation with coronary arteriography. Am J Cardiol 67:1213, 1991.
229. Marwick TH, et al.: Accuracy and limitations of exercise echocardiography in a routine clinical setting. J Am Coll Cardiol 19:74, 1992.
230. Ginzton LE, et al.: Exercise subcostal two-dimensional echocardiography: a new method of segmental wall motion analysis. Am J Cardiol 53:805, 1984.
231. Ginzton LE, et al.: Noninvasive measurement of the rest and exercise peak systolic pressure/end-systolic volume ratio: sensitive two-dimensional echocardiographic indicator of left ventricular function. J Am Coll Cardiol 4:509, 1984.
232. Crawford MH, Amon KW, Vance WS: Exercise 2-dimensional echocardiography: quantitation of left ventricular performance in patients with severe angina pectoris. Am J Cardiol 51:1, 1983.
233. Crawford MH, et al.: Comparative value of 2-dimensional echocardiography and radionuclide angiography for quantitating changes in left ventricular performance during exercise limited by angina pectoris. Am J Cardiol 53:42, 1984.
234. Presti CF, Armstrong WF, Feigenbaum H: Comparison of echocardiography at peak exercise and after bicycle exercise in evaluation of patients with known or suspected coronary artery disease. J Am Soc Echocardiogr 1:119, 1988.
235. Visser CA, et al.: Comparison of two-dimensional echocardiography with radionuclide angiography during dynamic exercise for the detection of coronary artery disease. Am Heart J 106:528, 1983.
236. Pozzoli MMA, et al.: Exercise echocardiography and technetium-99m MIBI single-photon emission computed tomography in the detection of coronary artery disease. Am J Cardiol 67:350, 1991.
237. Galanti G, et al.: Diagnostic accuracy of peak exercise echocardiography in coronary artery disease: comparison with thallium-201 myocardial scintigraphy. Am Heart J 122:1609, 1991.
238. Sawada SG, et al.: Exercise echocardiographic detection of coronary artery disease in women. J Am Coll Cardiol 14:1440, 1989.
239. Broderick T, et al.: Improvement in rest and exercise-induced wall motion abnormalities after coronary angioplasty: an exercise echocardiographic study. J Am Coll Cardiol 15:591, 1990.
240. Siegel W, et al.: Use of isometric handgrip for the indirect assessment of left ventricular function in patients with coronary atherosclerotic heart disease. Am J Cardiol 30:48, 1972.
241. Ludbrook P, Karlinger JS, O'Rourke RA: Effects of submaximal isometric handgrip on left ventricular size and wall motion. Am J Cardiol 33:30, 1974.
242. Mitamura H, et al.: Two dimensional echocardiographic analysis of wall motion abnormalities during handgrip exercise in patients with coronary artery disease. Am J Cardiol 48:711, 1981.
243. Jaarsma W, et al.: Usefulness of two-dimensional exercise echocardiography shortly after myocardial infarction. Am J Cardiol 57:86, 1986.
244. Applegate RJ, Dell'Italia LJ, Crawford MH: Usefulness of two-dimensional exercise echocardiography during low-level exercise testing early after uncomplicated acute myocardial infarction. Am J Cardiol 60:10, 1987.
245. Ryan T, Armstrong WF, O'Donnell JA, Feigenbaum H: Risk stratification after acute myocardial infarction by means of exercise two-dimensional echocardiography. Am Heart J 114:1305, 1987.
246. Sawada SG, et al.: Prognostic value of a normal exercise echocardiogram. Am Heart J 120:49, 1990.
247. Labovitz AJ, et al.: The effects of successful PTCA on left ventricular function: assessment by exercise echocardiography. Am Heart J 117:1003, 1989.
248. Aboul-Enein H, et al.: Effect of the degree of effort on exercise echocardiography for the detection of restenosis after coronary artery angioplasty. Am Heart J 122:430, 1991.
249. Mancini GBJ, Friedman HZ, Hramiec JE, Deboe SF: Relation between graded, subcritical impairments of coronary flow reserve and regional myocardial dysfunction induced by isoproterenol infusion in dogs. Am Heart J 113:906, 1987.
250. Fung AY, Gallagher KP, Buda AJ: The physiologic basis of dobutamine as compared with dipyridamole stress interventions in the assessment of critical coronary stenosis. Circulation 76:941, 1987.
251. Mannering D, et al.: The dobutamine stress test as an alternative to exercise testing after acute myocardial infarction. Br Heart J 59:521, 1988.

252. Berthe C, et al.: Predicting the extent and location of coronary artery disease in acute myocardial infarction by echocardiography during dobutamine infusion. Am J Cardiol 58:1167, 1986.
253. Sawada SG, et al.: Echocardiographic detection of coronary artery disease during dobutamine infusion. Circulation 83:1605, 1991.
254. Cohen JL, et al.: Dobutamine digital echocardiography for detecting coronary artery disease. Am J Cardiol 67:1311, 1991.
255. Martin TW, et al.: Comparison of adenosine, dipyridamole, and dobutamine in stress echocardiography. Ann Intern Med 116:190, 1992.
256. Chapman PD, et al.: Stress echocardiography with transesophageal atrial pacing: preliminary report of a new method for detection of ischemic wall motion abnormalities. Circulation 70:445, 1984.
257. Iliceto S, et al.: Detection of coronary artery disease by two-dimensional echocardiography and transesophageal atrial pacing. J Am Coll Cardiol 5: 1187, 1985.
258. Iliceto S, et al.: Comparison of postexercise and transesophageal atrial pacing two-dimensional echocardiography for detection of coronary artery disease. Am J Cardiol 57:547, 1986.
259. Lambertz H, Kreis A, Trumper H, Hanrath P: Simultaneous transesophageal atrial pacing and transesophageal two-dimensional echocardiography: a new method of stress echocardiography. J Am Coll Cardiol 16:1143, 1990.
260. Zabalgoitia M, et al.: Transesophageal stress echocardiography: detection of coronary artery disease in patients with normal resting left ventricular contractility. Am Heart J 122:1456, 1991.
261. Gould KL: Non-invasive assessment of coronary stenoses by myocardial perfusion imaging during pharmacologic coronary vasodilation: I. Physiologic basis and experimental validation. Am J Cardiol 41:268, 1978.
262. Gould KL, Westcott RJ, Albro PC, Hamilton GW: Non-invasive assessment of coronary stenoses by myocardial imaging during pharmacologic coronary vasodilation: II. Clinical methodology and feasibility. Am J Cardiol 41:279, 1978.
263. Picano E, et al.: Dipyridamole-echocardiography test in effort angina pectoris. Am J Cardiol 56:452, 1985.
264. Morgonata A, et al.: Limitations of dipyridamole-echocardiography in effort angina pectoris. Am J Cardiol 59:225, 1987.
265. Picano E, et al.: High dose dipyridamole echocardiography test in effort angina pectoris. J Am Coll Cardiol 8:848, 1986.
266. Masini M, et al.: High-dose dipyridamole-echocardiography test in women: correlation with exercise-electrocardiography test and coronary arteriography. J Am Coll Cardiol 12:682, 1988.
267. Josephson RA, Weiss JL, Becker LC, Shapiro EP: Dipyridamole echocardiography in the detection of vulnerable myocardium in the early postinfarction period. J Am Soc Echocardiogr 2:324, 1989.
268. Bolognese L, et al.: High-dose dipyridamole echocardiography early after uncomplicated acute myocardial infarction: correlation with exercise testing and coronary angiography. J Am Coll Cardiol 14:357, 1989.
269. Ferrara N, et al.: Dipyridamole echocardiography as a useful and safe test in the assessment of coronary artery disease in the elderly. J Am Geriatr Soc 39:993, 1991.
270. Jain A, et al.: Functional significance of myocardial perfusion defects induced by dipyridamole using thallium-201 single-photon emission computed tomography and two-dimensional echocardiography. Am J Cardiol 66:802, 1990.
271. Pirelli S, et al.: Comparison of usefulness of high-dose dipyridamole echocardiography for detection of asymptomatic restenosis after coronary angioplasty. Am J Cardiol 67:1335, 1991.
272. Tischler MD, et al.: Prediction of major cardiac events after peripheral vascular surgery using dipyridamole echocardiography. Am J Cardiol 68: 593, 1991.
273. Zoghbi WA, et al.: Diagnosis of ischemic heart disease with adenosine echocardiography. J Am Coll Cardiol 18:1271, 1991.
274. Hines EA, Brown GE: The cold pressor test for measuring the reactivity of the blood pressure: data concerning 571 normal and hypertensive subjects. Am Heart J 11:1, 1936.
275. Mudge GH, Jr, et al.: Reflex increase in coronary vascular resistance in patients with ischemic heart disease. N Engl J Med 295:1333, 1976.
276. Gondi B, Nanda NC: Cold pressor test during two-dimensional echocardiography: usefulness in detection of patients with coronary disease. Am Heart J 107:278, 1984.
277. Picano E, et al.: Comparison of the high-dose dipyridamole echocardiography test and exercise two-dimensional echocardiography for diagnosis of coronary artery disease. Am J Cardiol 59:539, 1987.
278. Previtali M, et al.: Dobutamine versus dipyridamole echocardiography in coronary artery disease. Circulation 84(Suppl. 3):III-27, 1991.
279. Picano E, et al.: Stress echocardiography and the human factor: the importance of being expert. J Am Coll Cardiol 17:661, 1991.

CHAPTER

23

LEFT VENTRICLE IV: ASSESSMENT OF MYOCARDIAL PERFUSION WITH CONTRAST TWO-DIMENSIONAL ECHOCARDIOGRAPHY

SANJIV KAUL and THOMAS S. FORCE

Contrast echocardiography was first applied to the study of myocardial blood flow in 1980, when it was noted that the injection of CO_2 bubbles into the left main coronary artery of the dog enhanced ultrasonic reflections from the myocardium supplied by that artery.[1] The potential importance of the technique was immediately apparent. For the first time, myocardial perfusion could be assessed in vivo and in real-time with a method that had sufficient resolution to define the perfusion territories of specific vessels and the potential to quantitate regional myocardial blood flow. It could also be used to serially assess changes in perfusion occurring either spontaneously or following specific interventions.

In the years since that initial observation, two major lines of investigation have developed. The first has employed myocardial contrast echocardiography (MCE) to define the perfusion territories of coronary arteries. The major experimental application of such perfusion bed determinations has been to quantify the amount of myocardium that is at risk for necrosis following total occlusion of a coronary artery (risk area). The second and more complex line of investigation has employed MCE to measure regional myocardial blood flow. This chapter provides an in-depth review of these two areas of investigation and examines the current and potential clinical applications of this technique.

PRINCIPLES OF MYOCARDIAL CONTRAST ECHOCARDIOGRAPHY

The application of contrast echocardiography to the examination of intramyocardial blood flow is based on the same physical principles outlined in Chapter 15 for intracavitary contrast echocardiography. The use of ultrasonic contrast (i.e., microbubbles in a carrier solution) to enhance images from the myocardium is based on the increased reflectance of incident sound waves, which occurs when they encounter the multiple gas liquid interfaces presented by microbubbles in the intramyocardial vascular beds.

Following an injection of ultrasonic contrast, the microbubbles travel through the epicardial coronary arteries and eventually reach the myocardial capillary network. If the microbubbles are sufficiently small ($\leq 6\mu m$), they pass through the capillaries unimpeded. Larger microbubbles lodge when they reach a point at which the vessel diameter is less than that of the bubble and then either dissolve and/or break down to smaller microbubbles, which ultimately pass through the capillary bed.

CONTRAST AGENTS

Perfusion Bed Size Determination

To define the perfusion bed of a vessel, a contrast agent should traverse all the major branches of the main artery under study and increase local reflectivity sufficiently to be clearly recorded. Because the perfusion territory of a vessel is generally used to define the area at risk for subsequent infarction, it is important that the agent not cause independent tissue damage or necrosis. In studies relating structure to function, it is also imperative that the contrast agent itself not be a source of permanent functional abnormality.

Contrast agents containing microbubbles of varying size, gaseous content, and dissolved in different carrier solutions have been used experimentally to define the perfusion territories of coronary vessels. Initial experiments used relatively large microbubbles either created by mixing H_2O_2 and blood to produce O_2 bubbles (12 to 100 μm in diameter)[2] or commercially fabricated by gelatin encapsulation of CO_2 to generate microbubbles of a uniform size (76 μm in diameter).[3] These were followed by a series of studies using hand-agitated mixtures of diatrizoate sodium-diatrizoate meglumine (Renografin-76) and saline, which also produced relatively large microbubbles (12 to 15 μm in diameter).[4–6] Although microbubbles produced by hand agitation were shown not to produce any pathologic effects in the myocardium, brain, or kidneys of dogs, they did produce significant, albeit transient, effects on left ventricular and systemic hemodynamics and regional wall thickening.[7] Nevertheless, because the contrast effect of an air-filled microbubble is related to the sixth power of its radius, these relatively large microbubbles produced excellent myocardial opacification.[8] Figure 23–1 illustrates the myocardial opacification produced by intracoronary injection of a hand-agitated mixture of Renografin-76 and 0.9% saline.

In the past 5 years, use of the technique of sonication has resulted in smaller microbubbles (<10 μm in diameter with a mean diameter of 4 to 6 μm).[9] Sonication involves exposing liquid media to high energy sound waves, which transform any air present in the media (or introduced into it) into microbubbles. The size and number of microbubbles are determined by the energy output and the duration of sonication. Using this method, researchers have produced microbubbles in a variety of solutions including Renografin-76 and albumin, the agents used most frequently in experimental and clinical studies. Figure 23–2 is a short axis recording of the left ventricle from a subject with normal coronary arteries following left (Fig. 23–2A) and right (Fig. 23–2B) coronary injections of sonicated Renografin-76.[10] This agent has been shown to be safe in humans, and although it produced minor changes in left ventricular and systemic hemodynamics, these effects could be explained by the hyperosmolarity and calcium chelating properties of Renografin-76.[10,11] Techniques other than sonication have also been used to produce smaller bubbles.[12,13]

Assessing Myocardial Blood Flow

The requirements for contrast agents used to measure myocardial blood flow are more complex than for those used only to define the perfusion territory of a coronary artery. The ideal agent for myocardial perfusion measurements should be able to freely traverse the myocardial capillary network and should remain stable in vivo. It should also be hemodynamically inert, with no independent effects on coronary vascular tone. The most extensively studied agent currently available for the quantification of myocardial blood flow is sonicated al-

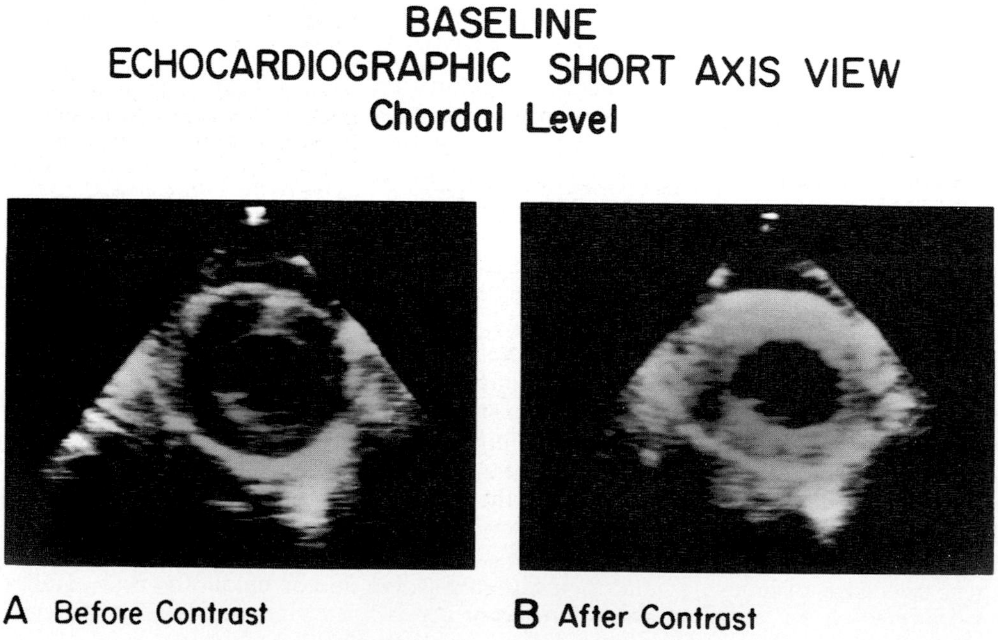

Fig. 23–1. Two-dimensional echocardiographic short axis view of the left ventricle in a dog. **A.** Before intracoronary injection of hand-agitated mixture of Renografin-76 and saline. **B.** After injection. (From Kaul S, et al.: Contrast echocardiography in acute myocardial ischemia: I. In-vivo determination of total left ventricular "area at risk." J Am Coll Cardiol 4:1272, 1984. Reprinted with permission from the American College of Cardiology.)

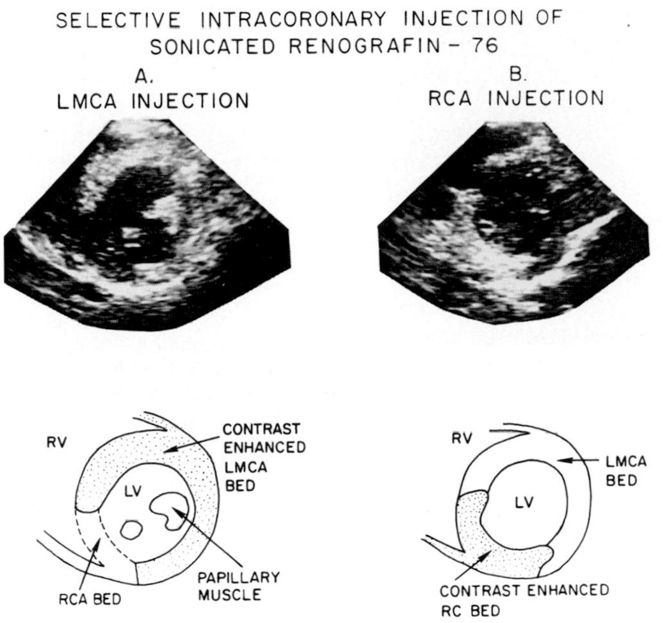

Fig. 23–2. Echocardiograms following intracoronary injection of sonicated Renografin-76 in a human with normal coronary arteries. Note the opacification in the distribution of **(A)** left main coronary artery (LMCA) and **(B)** right coronary artery (RCA). LV = left ventricle; RV = right ventricle. (From Moore CA, Smucker ML, Kaul S: Myocardial contrast echocardiography in humans: I. Safety—a comparison with routine coronary arteriography. J Am Coll Cardiol 8:1066, 1986. Reprinted with permission from the American College of Cardiology.)

bumin. This agent has been demonstrated to be free of any adverse effects on coronary blood flow, systemic hemodynamics, or regional function.[14] Figure 23–3 compares the hemodynamic effects of 5% human albumin, sonicated albumin, and sonicated and hand-agitated Renografin-76 in dogs. Neither 5% human serum albumin, nor the sonicated version affect coronary blood flow, left ventricular end-diastolic pressure, or wall thickening. The effects of sonicated human albumin on left ventricular rate of change in pressure (dP/dt) are minimal.[14] Similar results have been reported in humans.[15] In clinically applicable quantities, sonicated albumin has been shown not to produce any pathologic effects on the heart, brain, or kidneys of rabbits.[14]

The intravascular rheology of albumin microbubbles is very similar to that of red blood cells.[16] Figure 23–4 depicts fluorescein-labeled red blood cells (Fig. 23–4B) and sonicated albumin microbubbles (Fig. 23–4C) during their transit through a branching arteriole of the hamster cheek pouch. The branch point flux, velocity, velocity profile, intravascular distribution, and arteriole-to-venule transit times of red blood cells and sonicated albumin microbubbles were found to be similar.[16] This agent is now being commercially produced and should soon be available for human use. The commercial product has also been found to have no adverse hemodynamic effects when injected into the coronary circulation in amounts adequate for optimal myocardial opacification.[17] Other contrast agents with small microbubbles are also being evaluated.[12,13]

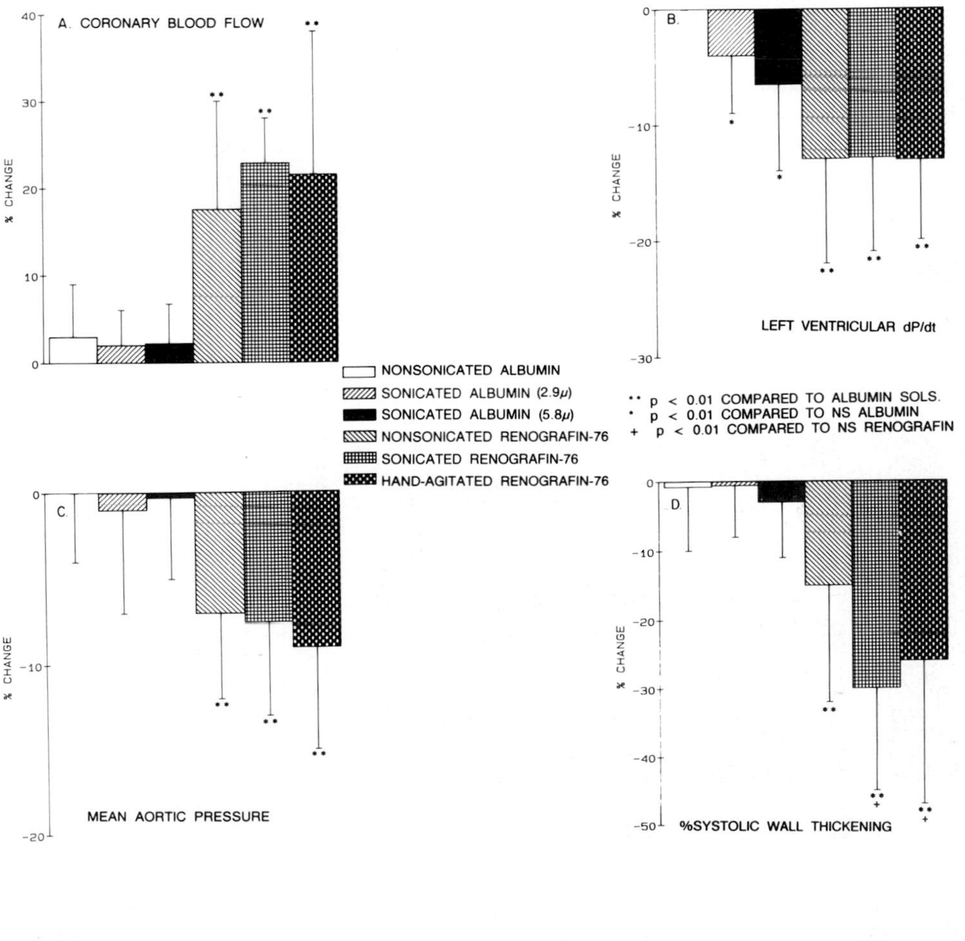

Fig. 23–3. Peak effects in dogs of 5% human albumin, sonicated albumin microbubbles (mean diameter = 2.9 μ), sonicated albumin microbubbles (mean diameter = 5.8 μ), Renografin-76, sonicated Renografin-76, and a hand-agitated mixture of Renografin-76 and 0.9% saline on the following: **A.** Coronary blood flow. **B.** Peak positive left ventricular dp/dt. **C.** Mean arterial pressure. **D.** Regional wall thickening. NS = nonsonicated. (From Kaul S: Assessment of myocardial perfusion with two-dimensional contrast echocardiography. Am J Med Sci 299:113, 1990. With permission of the Southern Society for Clinical Investigation.)

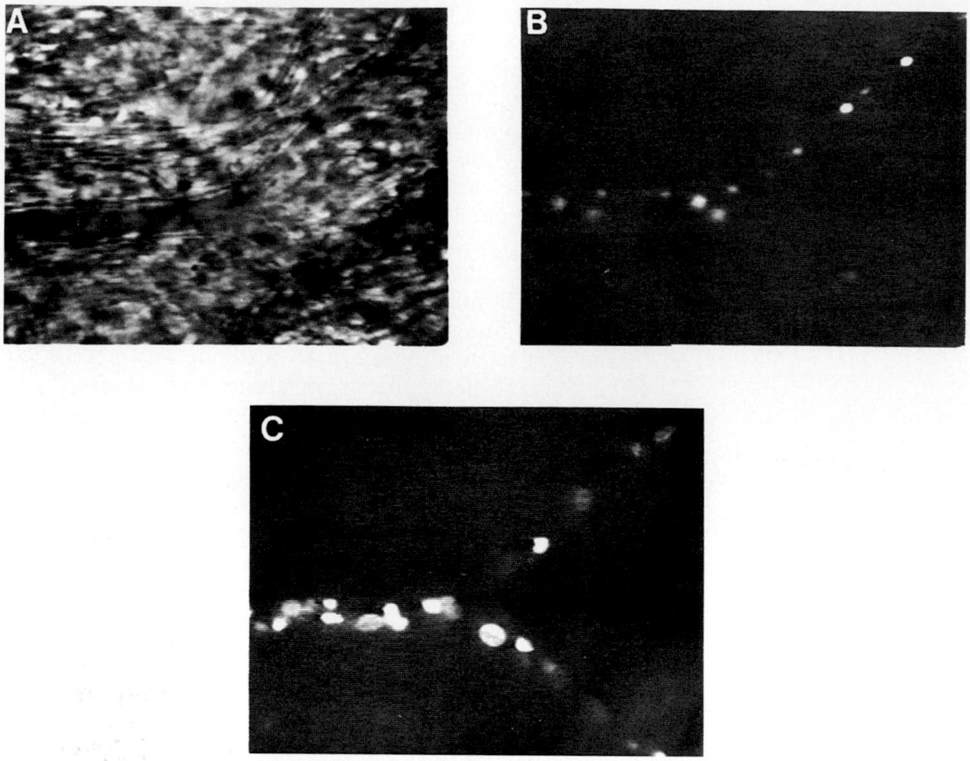

Fig. 23–4. **A.** A branching arteriole in a hamster cheek pouch viewed under transillumination. **B.** The distribution of fluorescein-labeled red blood cells within the same arteriole when viewed during fluorescein microscopy. **C.** The distribution of fluorescein-labeled sonicated albumin microbubbles in the same vessel. (From Keller MW, Segal SS, Kaul S, Duling BR: The behavior of sonicated albumin microbubbles in the microcirculation: a basis for their use during myocardial contrast echocardiography. Circ Res 65: 458, 1989. Reprinted with permission of the American Heart Association.)

ASSESSMENT OF THE PERFUSION TERRITORY OF A CORONARY ARTERY

Perfusion Bed Size (Risk Area) Determination

The initial application of MCE was to define the regions of the myocardium perfused by major coronary arteries and their branches, as well as the size of the hypoperfused region following total coronary occlusion. Determination of the perfusion territory of an occluded vessel was based solely on whether or not the myocardium distal to a coronary ligation demonstrated opacification following injection of contrast. These studies were conducted in the canine model, where total coronary occlusion produces severe transmural ischemia with residual blood flows of $\leq 15\%$ of normal. Because the number of bubbles reaching the myocardium at such low flow rates was insufficient to produce obvious myocardial opacification, myocardial regions beyond a total occlusion were clearly demarcated from areas receiving adequate blood flow.

Risk area determined by MCE has been shown to compare favorably with that measured by both intracoronary injection of colored dyes[2,18] and technetium autoradiography.[5] Figure 23–5 compares the risk areas obtained by MCE and technetium autoradiography at the same short axis level of the left ventricle. The high-resolution MCE images facilitated separation of normal and ischemic zones, permitted the recording of risk area in multiple tomographic planes from which the three-dimensional extent of the perfusion bed could be determined (Fig. 23–6), and allowed risk area to be defined serially in vivo and thus the effects of interventions on the size of the jeopardized perfusion bed to be quantitated.

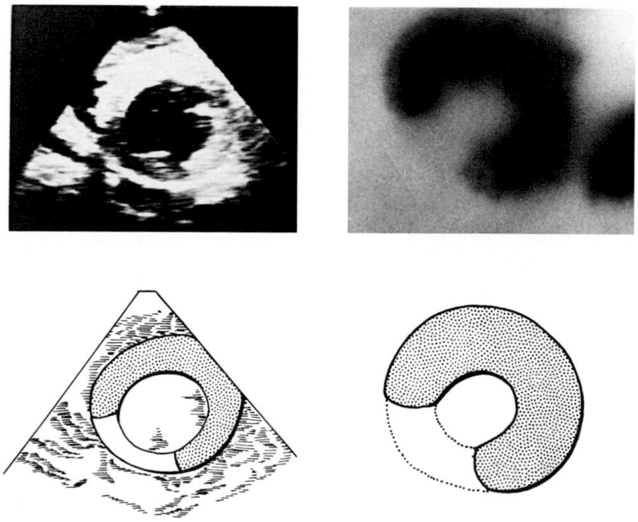

A Contrast Echocardiography **B** Technetium Autoradiography

Fig. 23–5. **A.** Two-dimensional contrast echocardiographic short axis view at the chordal level showing a "risk area" in the posterior left ventricular wall following occlusion of the left circumflex coronary artery. **B.** Technetium autoradiograph showing a "risk area" (cold spot) at the same level as the contrast echo "risk area" illustrated in **A.** (From Kaul S, et al.: Contrast echocardiography in acute myocardial ischemia: I. In vivo determination of total left ventricular "area at risk." J Am Coll Cardiol 4:1272, 1984. Reprinted with permission from the American College of Cardiology.)

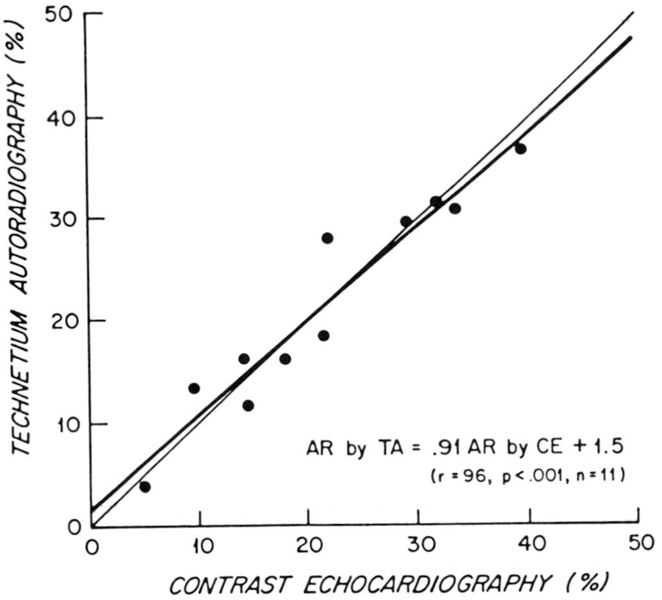

Fig. 23–6. Relationship between total left ventricular "risk area" by contrast echocardiography and technetium autoradiography. The thin line represents the line of identity. AR = area at risk; TA = technetium autoradiography; CE = contrast echocardiography. (From Kaul S, et al.: Contrast echocardiography in acute myocardial ischemia: I. In vivo determination of total left ventricular "area at risk." J Am Coll Cardiol 4:1272, 1984. Reprinted with permission from the American College of Cardiology.)

Many of these features cannot be duplicated by more established postmortem techniques used for the measurement of risk area such as coronary stereoangiography,[19] intracoronary injection of colored dyes,[20] and technetium autoradiography.[21] Both coronary stereoangiography and injection of colored dyes are performed after the heart is excised from the thorax. Even if the injection pressure into the different arteries is controlled, it is often not equal to the antemortem pressure during infarction. Moreover, the risk area can be influenced by the collateral driving pressure[22] and the anterograde flow through the vessels,[23] making it more difficult to reproduce in the postmortem setting. In addition, dyes stain the myocardium beyond the intravascular space, and postmortem shrinkage of tissue introduces additional errors in estimating the size of the risk area. Although the microspheres or albumin macroaggregates used for technetium autoradiography are injected antemortem,[21] this technique, like other postmortem methods, cannot be used serially to assess dynamic changes in the risk area.

"Positive" Versus "Negative" Risk Area

Risk area can be defined using MCE as (1) the area demonstrating contrast enhancement when the contrast agent is injected directly into the coronary artery immediately distal to the site of occlusion ("positive" risk area)[4] or (2) the area failing to show contrast enhancement when contrast is injected proximal to the site of occlusion ("negative" risk area).[2,3] The spatial extent of the risk area measured using these two approaches differs slightly.[6] When other variables such as the perfusion pressure in the nonoccluded bed are within the physiologic range, the "positive" risk area is larger than the "negative" area.[5] In the experimental canine model, the difference between the two areas is predominantly in their epicardial extent, as depicted in Figure 23–7.

The same relationship has been observed using other techniques for the assessment of risk area[24] and has been studied in detail by injecting colored dyes into coronary vessels at and proximal to a site of occlusion.[25,26] The risk area defined by direct injection of dye just distal to the site of occlusion reflects only antegrade perfusion and does not include collateral flow. This risk area has been defined as the *anatomic risk area*,[26] and the *positive risk area* on MCE, therefore, is the in vivo equivalent of the anatomic risk area. When dye is injected proximal to the site of occlusion, the unstained region is the area not supplied by either anterograde flow or collateral flow through adjacent vessels. The risk area defined in this manner has been termed the *functional risk area*.[26] The negative risk area defined by MCE, therefore, is the in vivo equivalent of the functional risk area. Depending on the extent of collateral flow, the functional risk area will invariably be smaller than the anatomic risk area.[26] During MCE, even if there were no collateral blood flow, the point spread function of the echocardiographic instrument will slightly expand the margins of the positive risk area and encroach slightly on the negative risk area, creating a disparity between these two measures.

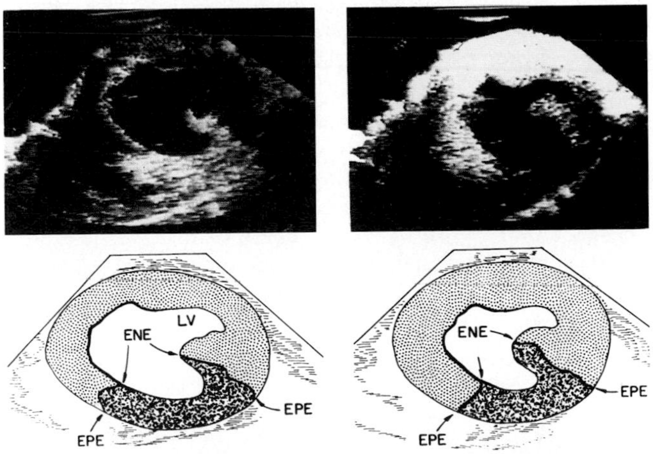

Fig. 23–7. Two-dimensional echocardiographic short axis view at the papillary muscle level of a dog demonstrating risk area after coronary occlusion when contrast is injected locally into the occluded artery showing a "positive" risk area (left), and when it is injected into the nonoccluded artery showing a "negative" risk area (right). The "positive" risk area is larger than the "negative" risk area, especially in its epicardial extent (indicated by arrows). ENE = endocardial extent; EPE = epicardial extent; LV = left ventricle. (See text for details.) (From Kaul S, et al. Contrast echocardiography in acute myocardial ischemia: II. The effect of site of injection of contrast agent on the estimation of "area at risk" for necrosis after coronary occlusion. J Am Coll Cardiol 6:825, 1985. Reprinted with permission from the American College of Cardiology.)

Effects of Anterograde Flow on the Size of the Perfusion Bed

Under stable hemodynamic conditions, the MCE-defined perfusion territory of a coronary artery remains constant following multiple injections and appears to be determined strictly on an anatomic basis. However, selective alteration in antegrade flow changes the size of the risk area, indicating functional as well as anatomic control of the perfusion territory.[23] Figure 23–8 illustrates the left circumflex perfusion bed (positive risk area) defined by MCE at three different anterograde left circumflex artery flow rates in the same animal. In Figure 23–8A, the size of the perfusion bed is 10.1 cm^2, and the anterograde transmural blood flow to it is 1.83 ml/min/g. In Figure 23–8B, the size of the perfusion bed is 8.20 cm^2, and the anterograde transmural blood flow to it is 1.42 ml/min/g. In Figure 23–8C, the size of the perfusion bed is 4.40 cm^2, and the anterograde transmural blood flow to it is 0.12 ml/min/g. The most dramatic change in the size of the perfusion bed occurs at anterograde flows below approximately 30% of baseline, which is probably related to the failure of autoregulation within the vessels supplying the region under study.

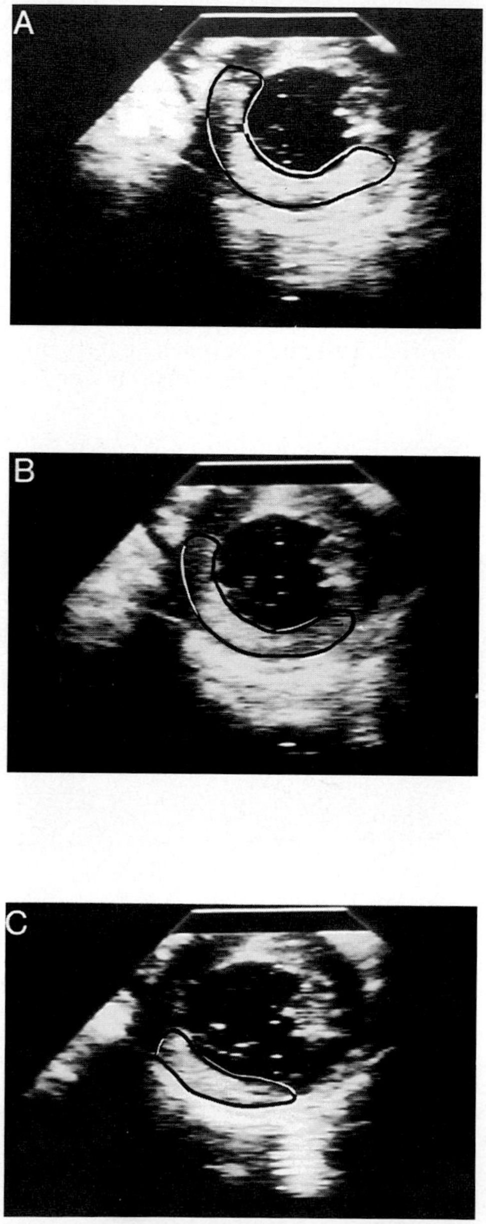

Fig. 23–8. The left circumflex perfusion bed defined by myocardial contrast echocardiography during three different anterograde blood flow rates in a dog. (See text for details.) (From Kaul S, et al.: Submitted, J Am Coll Cardiol 17:1403, 1992. Reprinted with permission from the American College of Cardiology.)

Figure 23–9 illustrates the relationship between the area perfused by the left circumflex artery (expressed as a percentage of the maximum MCE-defined perfusion area in each dog) and anterograde transmural blood flow (normalized to the highest blood flow in each dog). The size of the perfused area is directly related to anterograde blood flow. An approximately 18% decrease in the size of the perfusion bed is noted when anterograde flow is decreased from normal levels (approximately 1 ml/min/g) to 10% of normal. When the flow, however, is reduced from approximately twice normal (mean, 1.9 ml/min/g) to 10% of normal, the decrease in the size of the bed is approximately 40%. Thus, changes in the perfusion territory occur in response to both increasing and decreasing anterograde flow.

These observed changes in the perfusion territory of a coronary vessel in response to changing anterograde flow can be explained by the anatomy of the myocardial vascular bed. It has been demonstrated that capillaries arising from individual vessels form loops at the borders of the vascular beds and do not interconnect with capillaries arising from other vessels (Fig. 23–10).[27] As a result, there is a negligible border zone between infarcted and normal tissue following coronary occlusion in the dog. Although there are no intercapillary connections,

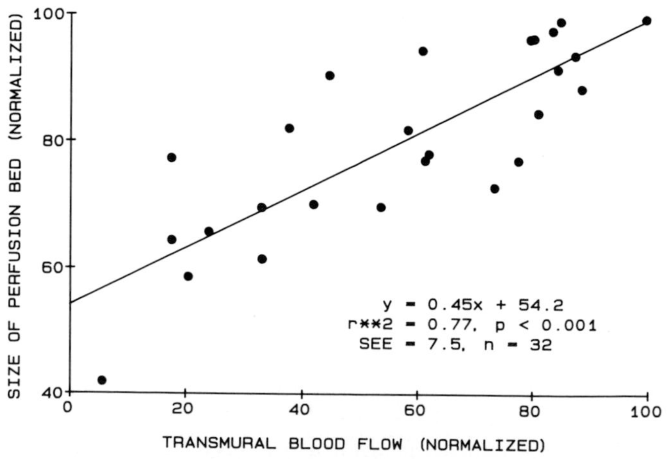

Fig. 23–9. The relationship between transmural blood flow normalized to the highest value in each dog (x axis) and the size of the left circumflex perfusion bed normalized to the largest value in each dog (y axis). The data point on the top right corner represents highest values from all animals superimposed on each other. r**2 = r^2. (See text for details.) SEE = standard error of estimate. (From Kaul S, et al. J Am Coll Cardiol 17:1403, 1992. Reprinted with permission from the American College of Cardiology.)

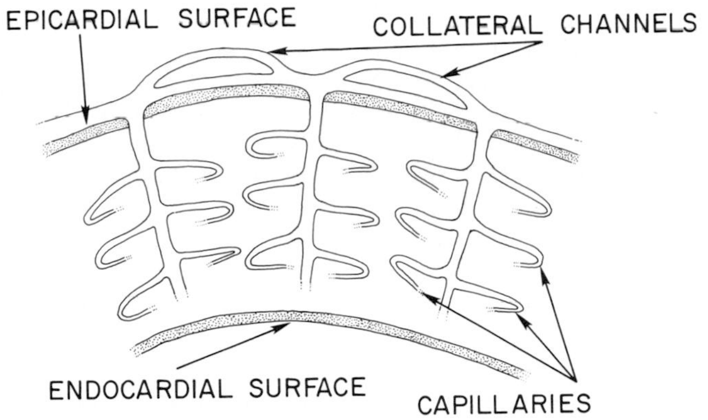

Fig. 23–10. End capillary loops from different arterioles. Although the capillaries arising from different arterioles are not directly interconnected, they are connected to each other via epicardial and endocardial (not shown here) collateral channels. (From Kaul S, et al. J Am Coll Cardiol 17:1403, 1992. Reprinted with permission from the American College of Cardiology.)

depending on the species being studied, there are several connections between vessels in the epicardial and subendocardial regions of the heart (see Fig. 23–10).[28] The relative flow in these connecting vessels at the time of coronary occlusion appears to determine the final line of demarcation between ischemic and healthy tissue. This line can be shifted toward or away from the center of the ischemic bed based on the anterograde flow to this region.

These data also imply that when anterograde flow is reduced, the margins of the region perfused by a coronary vessel become dependent on collateral flow (Fig. 23–11). The degree of collateral dependence should be determined by the systemic pressure, the magnitude of the reduction in anterograde flow, the duration of ischemia, the number and functional state of the collateral vessels, and the collateral driving pressure. In the event that collateral flow is compromised, the marginal zones might not receive enough flow (and may even receive less flow than the central zone supplied by anterograde flow), resulting in ischemia and infarction of the periphery of the ischemic bed. This phenomenon could predispose the patient to infarct extension.[29–31] Not unexpectedly, lower flows and higher mortality have been demonstrated in canine models of coronary artery occlusion where vessels supplying zones remote from the occlusion have severe stenosis.[32]

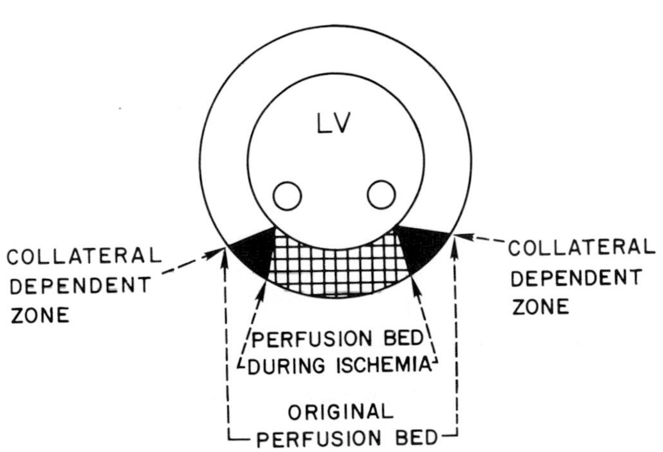

Fig. 23–11. The implications of reduction in the size of the bed perfused by a coronary artery on the peripheral collateral-dependent areas within the bed. LV = left ventricular cavity. (See text for details.) (From Kaul S, et al. J Am Coll Cardiol 17:1403, 1992. Reprinted with permission from the American College of Cardiology.)

Effects of Collateral Flow on Risk Area

Anterograde Flow to Adjacent Arteries

In a canine model of total coronary occlusion where collateral flow to the occluded bed was increased by increasing collateral driving pressure, diminution in the size of the MCE-defined perfusion bed was noted (Fig. 23–12). These results were confirmed by radiolabeled microspheres[22] and are supported by more recent data.[33]

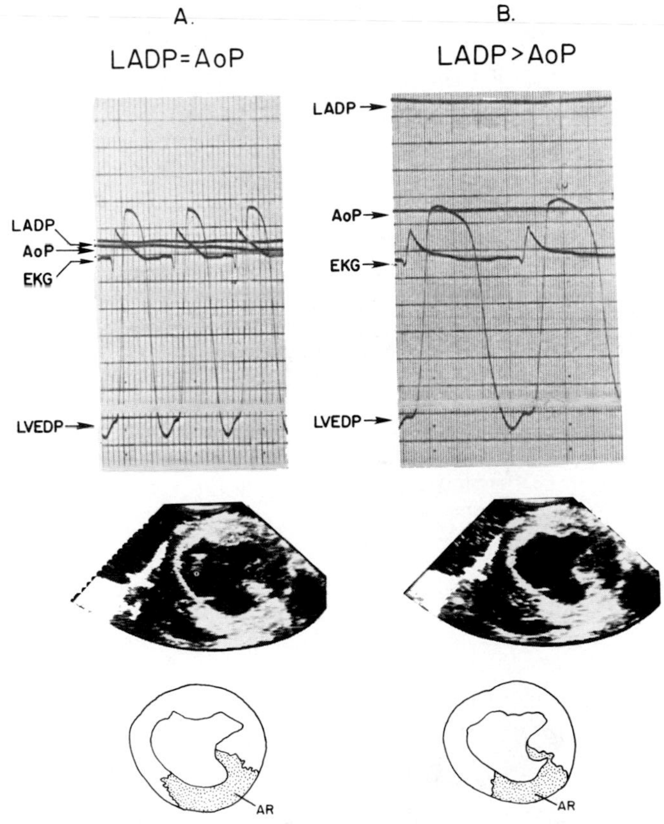

Fig. 23–12. The effect of increasing the pressure in the nonoccluded left anterior descending artery on the size of the occluded left circumflex perfusion bed in the dog (contrast-enhanced area on two-dimensional echocardiography and indicated as "AR" on the accompanying diagram). **A.** Size of the left circumflex arterial bed when left anterior descending arterial pressure (LADP) equals mean aortic pressure (AoP). **B.** Size of the left circumflex arterial bed when LADP. The size of the bed is smaller compared to **A.** EKG = electrocardiogram; LVEDP = left ventricular end-diastolic pressure. (From Kaul S, et al.: The effects of selectively altering the collateral driving pressure on regional perfusion and function in the occluded coronary bed of the dog. Circ Res 61:77, 1987. Reprinted with permission of the American Heart Association.)

Collateral Flow in Chronic Coronary Artery Disease

Normally, collaterals in the dog exceed those found in humans. In patients with chronic coronary artery disease, however, there are abundant collaterals, and these vessels are present in both the epicardium and endocardium.[28] This has not generally been appreciated, because there are no appropriate methods of assessing collateral blood flow in humans. Most collateral vessels are ≤ 100 μm in diameter, and coronary angiography, the most commonly employed clinical technique for assessing the coronary circulation, can only detect vessels ≥ 100 μm in diameter.[28] Because MCE uses microbubbles whose size is similar to that of red blood cells, it should be possible to identify collateral flow in humans that might otherwise be inapparent.[34–37]

Figure 23–13 illustrates an example of a patient with a totally occluded right coronary artery and a recent subendocardial infarction. In Figure 23–13A, sonicated Renografin-76 was injected into the left main coronary artery before angioplasty of the right coronary artery. The entire left ventricular myocardium (including the region normally supplied by the right coronary artery, indicated by an arrow) shows immediate opacification suggesting the presence of abundant collateral flow from the left coronary system. Figure 23–13B shows a left main injection of contrast in the same patient following successful angioplasty of the right coronary artery. Following angioplasty, the right coronary bed (indicated by an arrow) is no longer perfused by the left main coronary artery because there is no longer a gradient between the left and right coronary systems.

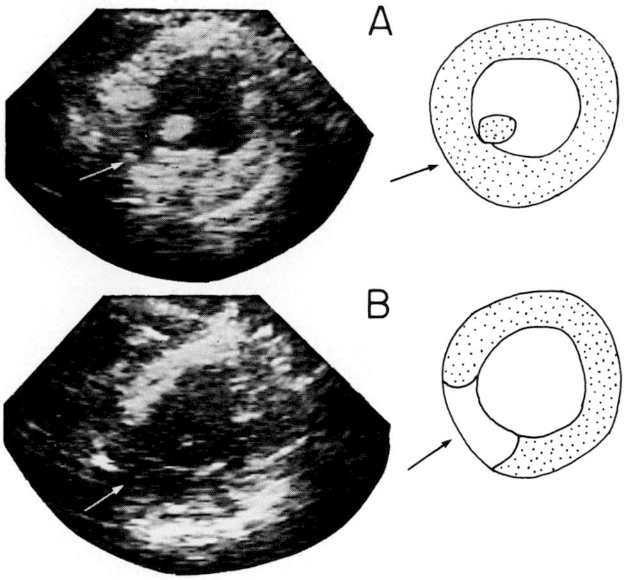

Fig. 23–13. Left main coronary artery injection of a contrast agent in a patient with a recent acute infarction and a totally occluded right coronary artery. **A.** Before angioplasty, the right coronary bed (indicated by arrow) filled at the same time as the left bed indicating abundant collateral flows to the right bed from the left coronary system. **B.** After successful angioplasty of the occluded right coronary artery, left main injection did not opacify the right arterial bed (indicated by arrow), suggesting a gradient no longer existed between the left coronary system and the right arterial bed. (From Sabia PJ, et al.: Functional significance of collateral blood flow in patients with recent myocardial infarction. A study using myocardial contrast echocardiography. Circulation 85:2080, 1992. Reprinted with permission of the American Heart Association.)

Collateral Flow in Acute Myocardial Infarction

The extent of functional recovery after acute infarction is related to the transmural extent of infarction. The transmural extent of infarction, in turn, is related to the duration of coronary occlusion as well as the amount of residual collateral-derived blood flow within the risk area. If there is sufficient residual blood flow to maintain cell viability, the myocardium should remain viable even if the duration of occlusion is prolonged. To test this hypothesis, patients who had suffered a recent (mean = 12 days) acute myocardial infarction with total occlusion of the infarct-related artery were studied by MCE.[38] Contrast was injected into the nonoccluded bed, and the degree of contrast enhancement of the occluded bed (representing collateral flow) was measured. Collateral-derived residual flow was noted in approximately two thirds of patients. Regional function was also assessed within the infarct zone. Coronary angioplasty was then attempted. One month later, regional function was reassessed. Those with collateral flow and successful angioplasty showed improvement in regional function, while those with unsuccessful angioplasty did not show any recovery of function. Importantly, the degree of functional recovery in patients with successful angioplasty was related to the extent of collaterals within the infarct zone.[38]

Figure 23–14 shows the first and seventh end-diastolic frames following left main injection of contrast in a patient with a totally occluded right coronary artery. It can be appreciated that whereas there is very little contrast in the right coronary arterial bed in the first frame (indicated by an arrow), by the seventh frame, the contrast effect in this bed is almost equal to that in the regions supplied by the nondiseased left main artery. These observations indicate that there is significant left-to-right collateral flow in this patient, albeit less than that noted in the patient whose echocardiograms are depicted in Figure 23–13. Both patients showed marked improvement in regional function 1 month after coronary angioplasty. These data suggest that by estimating residual collateral-derived flow within the risk area, MCE enables assessment of myocardial viability.

Interoperative Detection of Collateral Flow

Collateral blood flow can also be detected during intraoperative MCE in humans.[34] For example, opacification of the anterior myocardium (left anterior descending artery territory) has been demonstrated in patients with multivessel disease when contrast was injected into the aorta after right coronary artery bypass but before bypass of the left anterior descending artery. This contrast effect (indicated by an arrowhead in Fig. 23–15) was in addition to the expected opacification noted in the right coronary arterial bed. The contrast seen in the anterior bed frequently far exceeds that anticipated on the basis of preoperative angiographically documented collater-

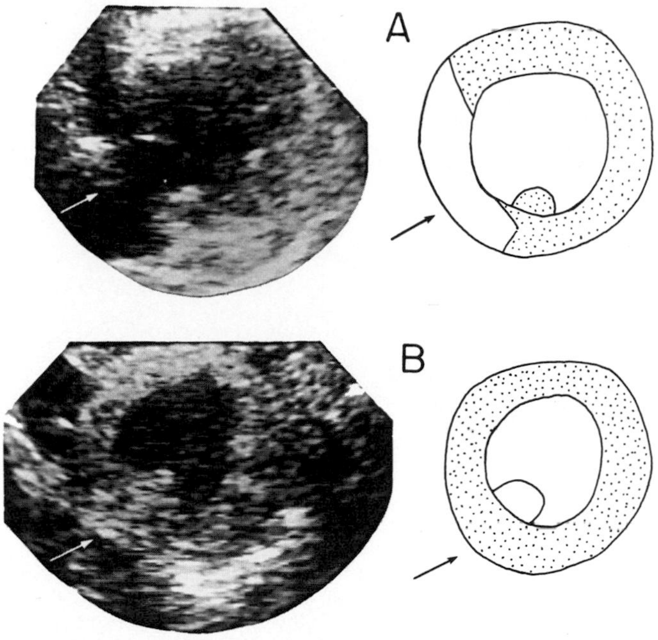

Fig. 23–14. Left main coronary artery injection of a contrast agent in a patient with recent acute infarction and occlusion of the right coronary artery. **A.** First end-diastolic frame after appearance of the contrast agent shows lack of contrast in the right coronary bed (indicated by arrows). **B.** Seven cycles later, contrast effect in the right arterial bed is adequate, indicating significant collateral flow to the right bed, albeit not as abundant as that noted in Figure 23–13. (See text for details.) (From Sabia PJ, et al.: Functional significance of collateral blood flow in patients with recent myocardial infarction. A study using myocardial contrast echocardiography. Circulation 85:2080, 1992. Reprinted with permission of the American Heart Association.)

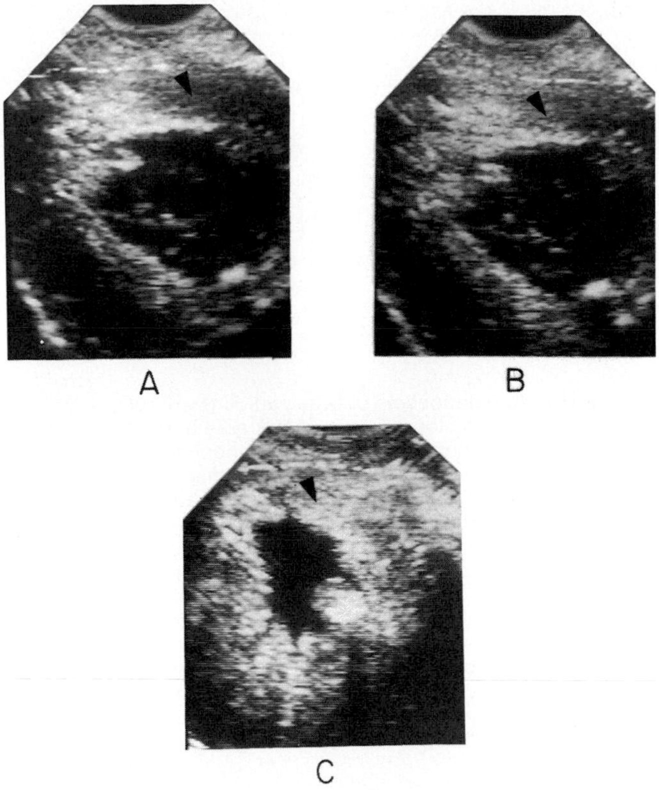

Fig. 23–15. Intraoperative echocardiograms from a patient with severe right coronary and left anterior descending artery disease during cardioplegia delivery. **A.** Before bypass and injection of contrast agent into the aortic root. **B.** After injection. Poor opacification is noted in all myocardial beds. **C.** After bypass to the right coronary artery and no bypass to the left anterior descending artery, opacification is noted not only in the right arterial bed (which would be expected) but also in the left anterior descending arterial bed (indicated by arrow). (See text for details.) (From Spotnitz WD, et al.: Intra-operative demonstration of coronary collateral flow using myocardial contrast echocardiography. Am J Cardiol 65: 1259, 1990. Reprinted with permission.)

als. Several factors may contribute to the improved visualization of collateral flow by intraoperative MCE compared to preoperative angiography. First, as already noted, most collaterals are <100 μm in diameter, whereas angiography can only detect vessels >100 μm in diameter. Second, after right coronary artery bypass, a pressure gradient develops between the right coronary artery and the left anterior descending arterial bed, which could open collapsed collateral vessels. Third, cardioplegia results in vasodilation, which may further enhance collateral blood flow. MCE, therefore, has the potential for assessing the interaction between risk area, collateral flow, and myocardial viability.

Risk Area Versus Infarct Size

Experimental studies have demonstrated that histologic infarct size is consistently smaller than the risk area defined using MCE.[39,40] This occurs because the risk area represents the entire transmural extent of the perfusion territory of the occluded vessel, whereas the area of necrosis typically does not involve the full thickness of the myocardium, which is due to variable sparing of the subepicardial region. Because the transmural extent of infarction increases with the duration of coronary occlusion, the longer the occlusion is maintained, the closer the necrotic area/risk area ratio approaches unity. When the endocardial and epicardial extent of infarction are compared to similar measures of the risk area, the endocardial extent of the risk area corresponds closely with the endocardial extent of the ultimate infarct, while the epicardial extent of the risk area overestimates the epicardial extent of the established infarct. Figure 23–16 compares the size (Fig. 23–16A) and the endocardial extent (Fig. 23–16B) of the risk area immediately after coronary occlusion to the size and the endocardial extent of infarction measured at 6 hours after occlusion. These data confirm that the overestimation of infarct size by risk area is due to differences in transmural rather than subendocardial extent. Figure 23–17 illustrates the spatial difference in risk area determined by MCE and infarct size assessed by 2,3,5-triphenyltetrazolium chloride staining.

The ultimate transmural extent of infarction is highly variable in both animals and humans, being affected by the duration of occlusion and individual differences in collateral-derived blood flow. In general, myocardium within the perfusion bed of an occluded coronary artery that receives collateral flow $\geq 30\%$ of normal can survive for prolonged periods.[40] MCE has been reported to enable detection of collateral-derived blood flow in this

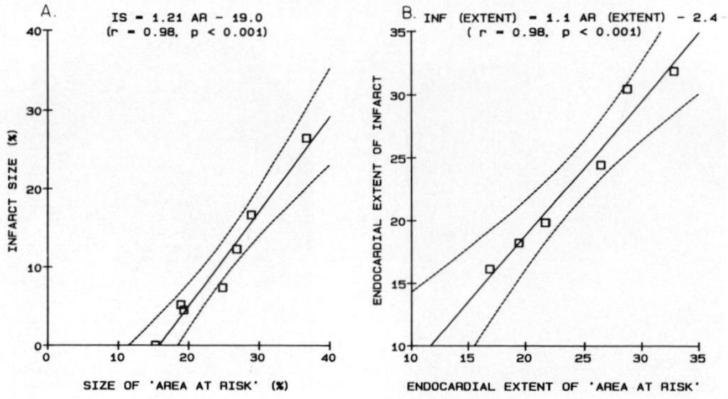

Fig. 23–16. **A.** Relationship between ultimate infarct size 6 hours after coronary occlusion and size of risk area at the time of coronary occlusion. **B.** Relationship between endocardial extent of infarct (percentage of left ventricular endocardial circumference) of infarct 6 hours after occlusion and the endocardial extent of the risk area at the time of coronary occlusion. The size of the risk area at the time of coronary occlusion modestly overestimates the ultimate infarct size, whereas the endocardial extent of the risk area at the time of coronary occlusion more closely predicts the endocardial extent of the ultimate infarct. IS = infarct size; AR = area at risk; INF = infarct. (See text for details.) (From Kaul S, et al.: The importance of defining left ventricular area at risk in vivo during acute myocardial infarction: an experimental evaluation with myocardial contrast two-dimensional echocardiography. Circulation 75:1249, 1987.)

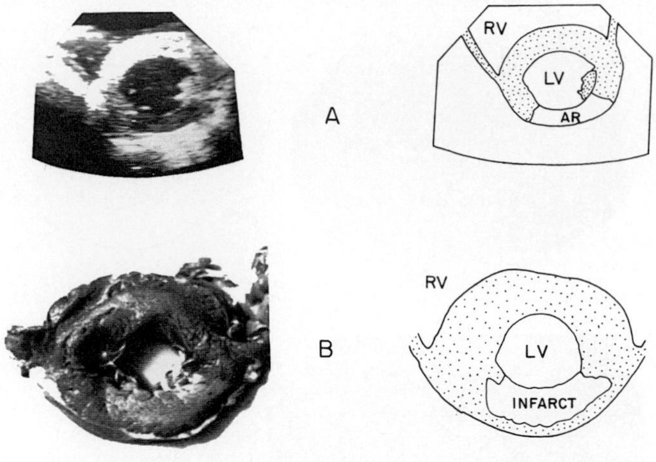

Fig. 23–17. **A.** Short axis view of the left ventricle at the papillary muscle level during myocardial contrast echocardiography showing risk area in the distribution of the left circumflex coronary artery. **B.** Slice of the heart at the same short axis level as in **A**, showing an infarct after staining with 2,3,5-triphenyltetrazolium chloride. AR = area at risk; LV = left ventricle; RV = right ventricle. (From Kaul S, et al.: The importance of defining left ventricular area at risk in vivo during acute myocardial infarction: an experimental evaluation with myocardial contrast two-dimensional echocardiography. Circulation 75:1249, 1987. Reproduced by permission of the American Heart Association, Inc.)

range (based on low levels of opacification a number of cycles after contrast injection) and to differentiate it from lower levels of flow (which fail to produce even delayed opacification) and will not support tissue survival.[40]

Preliminary studies using MCE in patients with recent myocardial infarction also demonstrate a relationship between collateral blood flow and transmural extent of infarction.[37] In patients in whom collaterals extend to the endocardial bed, the infarction is patchy rather than confluent. Figure 23–18 contains two end-diastolic frames from a patient with a recent anterior myocardial infarction and a totally occluded left anterior descending coronary artery. Following right coronary injection (Fig. 23–18A), the contrast effect extends into the anterior interventricular septum (arrows), well beyond the normal perfusion territory of the right coronary. When contrast is injected into the left main artery (Fig. 23–18B), no contrast enhancement is noted in the left anterior descending arterial bed, while the left circumflex bed shows adequate opacification.

After successful angioplasty of the occluded left anterior descending artery (Fig. 23–19), contrast injected into the right coronary artery no longer opacifies the anterior interventricular septum (arrows, Fig. 23–19A), because there is no longer a gradient between the right coronary artery and the left anterior descending arterial bed. When contrast is injected into the left main artery (Fig. 23–19B), perfusion is noted in the portion of the left anterior descending bed, which was supplied by the right coronary artery before angioplasty (Fig. 23–18A). The center of the left anterior descending arterial bed, however, suggests a nontransmural infarction, because perfusion is evident only in a small epicardial rim.

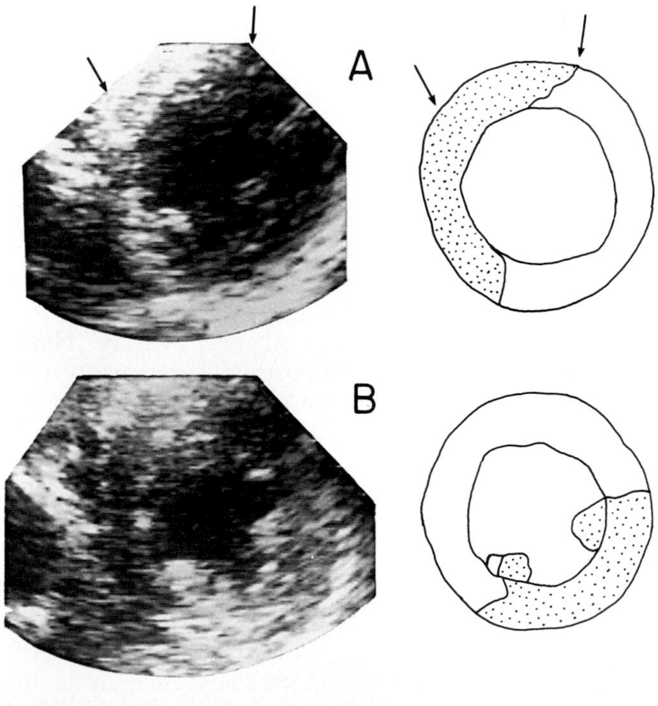

Fig. 23–18. Contrast echocardiograms obtained in a patient with a recent infarction and a totally occluded left anterior descending artery. **A.** An image after right coronary injection. The opacification extends into the anterior interventricular septum as well (indicated by arrows). **B.** An image after left main injection. Contrast is not seen in the left anterior descending arterial bed but is noted in the left circumflex arterial bed. (From Kaul S: Clinical applications of myocardial contrast echocardiography. Am J Cardiol 69: 46H, 1992, reprinted with permission.)

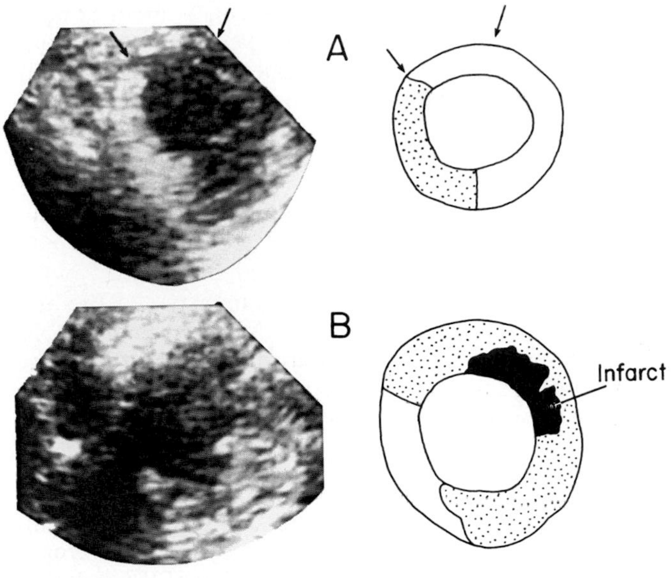

Fig. 23–19. Images from the same patient depicted in Figure 23–18 taken after successful angioplasty of the left anterior descending artery. **A.** Because there is no longer a gradient present between the right and left systems, collateral flow to the anterior interventricular septum (indicated by arrows) is no longer seen after right coronary injection of contrast agent. Instead, contrast effect is limited to the right coronary bed. **B.** After left main injection, contrast is seen in the left anterior descending bed, which was initially supplied from the right collaterals (see Fig. 23–18A). In addition, a subendocardial infarct is noted with no flow within that region. This region is surrounded by an epicardial rim of contrast. (From Kaul S: Clinical applications of myocardial contrast echocardiography. Am J Cardiol 69:46H, 1992, reprinted with permission.)

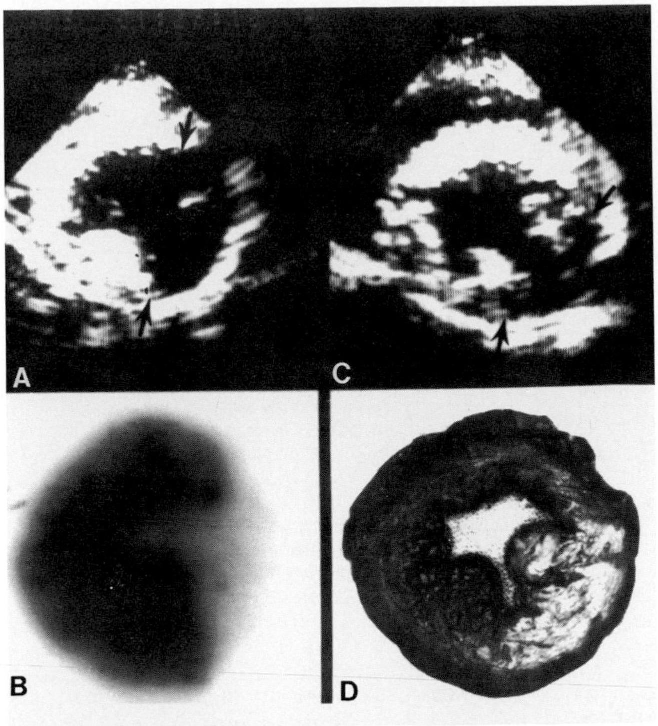

Fig. 23–20. Risk area by contrast echocardiography and technetium autoradiography: **A** and **B**. Two hours after occlusion (left). **C** and **D**. Risk area by contrast echocardiography and infarct after staining with 2,3,5-triphenyltetrazolium chloride following reperfusion. Note that the "risk area" on contrast echocardiography after reperfusion, indicated by arrows in **C**, closely predicts infarct size in **D**. (See text for details.) (From Kemper AJ, et al.: Hydrogen peroxide contrast echocardiography: quantification in vivo of myocardial risk area during coronary occlusion and the necrotic area remaining after myocardial reperfusion. Circulation 70:309, 1984. Reproduced by permission of the American Heart Association, Inc.)

Experimental data also suggest that the pattern of contrast enhancement postreperfusion predicts regions within the ischemic zone that remain viable, based on restoration of normal flow.[41] Thus, areas that failed to opacify during occlusion when the risk area is transmural (indicated by arrows in Fig. 23–20A) but received contrast following reperfusion (indicated by arrows in Fig. 23–20C) are presumably free of necrosis, edema, or hemorrhage; by inference, these areas received adequate collateral flow during the ischemic period to maintain viability. These areas are generally found at both the lateral and epicardial borders of the original risk area. As a result the contrast-free area, postreperfusion, more closely predicts infarct size (Fig. 23–20D) than does the original risk area. The same phenomenon is also noted in the patient whose echocardiograms are illustrated in Figure 23–19, where the size of the infarct was more closely estimated after reperfusion than before.

Risk Area Versus Abnormal Wall Motion

Although the accuracy and reproducibility of MCE in quantifying risk area have been demonstrated repeatedly, there has been controversy regarding the relation of risk area to the extent of abnormal wall motion or thickening. Earlier work suggested a lack of correlation between the extent of the perfusion abnormality and the extent of regional dysfunction.[3] More recent studies, however, have demonstrated a closer relation between these two parameters.[2,4] A detailed study comparing the extent of perfusion abnormality with the extent of abnormal wall motion reported that when the entire systolic contraction sequence is analyzed, the relationship between risk area and extent of abnormal wall motion is closer than when only end-diastolic and end-systolic frames are analyzed (Fig. 23–21).[42] Important regional dysfunction can be missed when only end-diastolic and end-systolic frames are analyzed because dyssynergy may be present at other times during systole.[43]

Assuming that the extent of regional dysfunction correlates with the size of the risk area, one could argue that the region of dysfunction alone could be used to determine the size of the ischemic zone, obviating the need to directly measure the risk area using MCE. There are several reasons for independently determining risk area. First, although the region of dysfunction correlates with infarct size, the precision of separation between ischemic and nonischemic zones does not approach the resolution that can be attained using MCE. Second, although a discrete coronary occlusion can be performed in the canine model, in clinical situations abnormal wall motion can be present in beds other than those supplied by the acutely occluded artery. These beds could represent either old infarction, postischemic ("stunned")

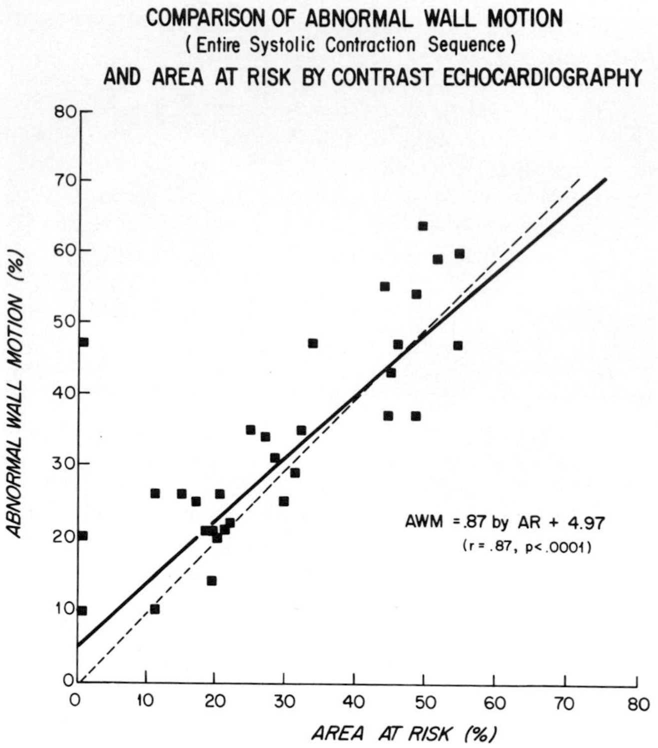

Fig. 23–21. Relationship between abnormal wall motion (assessed using the entire systolic contraction sequence) and size of risk area determined by myocardial contrast echocardiography at the time of coronary occlusion. The dashed line represents the line of identity. AWM = circumferential extent of abnormal wall motion; AR = area at risk. (See text for details.) (From Kaul S, et al.: Contrast echocardiography in acute ischemia: III. An in vivo comparison of the extent of abnormal wall motion with the "area at risk" for necrosis. J Am Coll of Cardiol 7:383, 1986. Reproduced with permission from the American College of Cardiology.)

myocardium, or chronically ischemic ("hibernating") myocardium.[44] Because no established patterns of wall motion can reliably differentiate between these possible causes of abnormal motion, the size of the risk area cannot be definitely established using wall motion analysis alone. Finally, in addition to being influenced by the analytical techniques applied,[45] the relationship between the region of dysfunction and the ischemic/infarcted zone varies with time after occlusion and is independently affected by preload and afterload,[46] while MCE appears to be a more stable measure of the area at risk. Consequently, whereas the assessment of regional and global left ventricular function is very important in the setting of ischemia, an independent estimation of the size of the risk area is also valuable.

Risk Area Versus Hemodynamics

Hemodynamic measurements made during acute myocardial infarction are thought to reflect the status of the left ventricle, and therefore, the size of the ischemic zone/risk area. Based on these assumptions, hemodynamic subsets have been characterized in patients with acute myocardial infarction.[47] However, it has been shown in the canine model, using MCE, that hemodynamic parameters are poor indicators of the size of the ischemic zone (Fig. 23–22).[39] These parameters become abnormal only when the risk area is very large. For example, cardiac output and mean arterial pressure fall significantly only when the risk area is >40% of the entire left ventricle. Similarly, left ventricular end-diastolic pressure becomes abnormal when risk area exceeds 25% of the left ventricle. Mean left atrial pressure shows a trend toward abnormality but does not become significantly abnormal even when risk area exceeds 40% of the

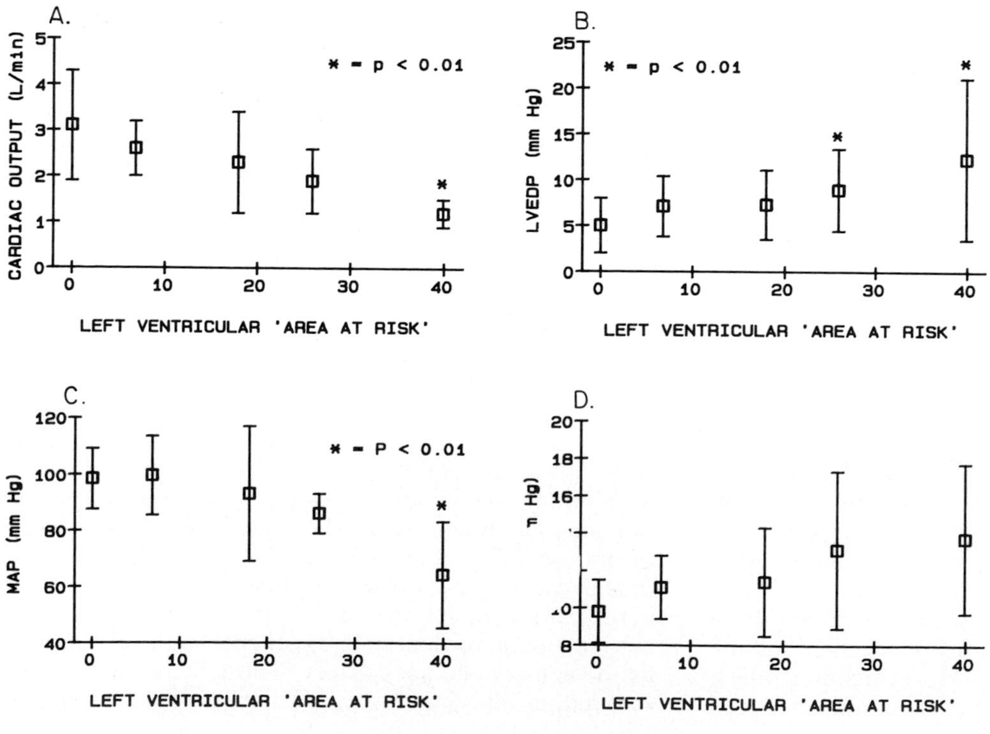

Fig. 23–22. Relationship between hemodynamic parameters and risk area in a canine model of acute coronary occlusion. Hemodynamic parameters: **A.** Cardiac output. **B.** Left ventricular end-diastolic pressure (LVEDP). **C.** Mean arterial pressure (MAP). **D.** Mean left atrial pressure (LAP). (See text for details.) (From Kaul S, et al.: The importance of defining left ventricular areas at risk in vivo during acute myocardial infarction: an experimental evaluation with myocardial contrast two-dimensional echocardiography. Circulation 75:1249, 1987. Reproduced by permission of the American Heart Association, Inc.)

left ventricle. Similar results have been demonstrated in the clinical setting.[48,49]

Risk Area Versus Left Ventricular Systolic Function

Experimental data suggest that when cardiac output and left ventricular ejection fraction are normalized to baseline values, each is inversely and linearly related to risk area (Fig. 23–23).[39] However, without normalization, this relationship is not apparent. Cardiac output and left ventricular ejection fraction cannot, therefore, be used reliably in the clinical setting to determine the size of the risk area during acute myocardial infarction. For example, a left ventricular ejection fraction of 0.50 may represent a drop of 0.15 in a patient with a baseline ejection fraction of 0.65 but may represent a normal left ventricular ejection fraction in another patient. In addition, when risk area is <18% of the left ventricular myocardium, the left ventricular ejection fraction may not change, which is due to compensatory hyperkinesis of other normally perfused regions.[39] In contrast to cardiac output and ejection fraction, mean arterial pressure may even rise above baseline during acute myocardial infarction, which may reflect arterial vasoconstriction that is due to catecholamine response (Fig. 23–23). It is only when risk area is very large (>40% of the left ventricular myocardium) that arterial pressure starts to decline. These observations further underscore the importance of measuring risk area directly using methods such as MCE.

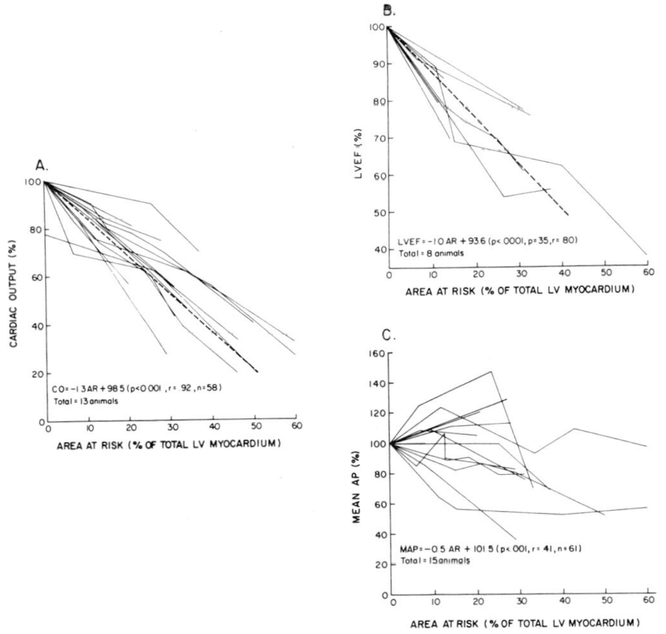

Fig. 23–23. Relationship between risk area and indices of left ventricular systolic function normalized to baseline values in a canine model of acute coronary occlusion. **A.** Cardiac output. **B.** Left ventricular ejection fraction (LVEF). **C.** Mean arterial pressure (AP). LV = left ventricular. (See text for details.) (From Kaul S, et al.: The importance of defining left ventricular area of risk in vivo during acute myocardial infarction: an experimental evaluation with myocardial contrast two-dimensional echocardiography. Circulation 75:1249, 1987. Reproduced by permission of the American Heart Association, Inc.)

Intraoperative Assessment of the Adequacy of Myocardial Perfusion

During coronary artery bypass surgery, flow of cardioplegia solution through the coronary circulation may be impaired by coronary stenosis.[50,51] Insufficient cardioplegia delivery to the regions of the myocardium supplied by stenotic coronary arteries could cause inadequate myocardial protection, resulting in ischemia or infarction. Depending on the sensitivity of the technique used to detect myocardial infarction, perioperative infarction can occur in 4 to 21% of all bypass operations.[52–54] If regions of the myocardium most susceptible to ischemic injury could be identified, the vessels supplying these regions could be bypassed first and cardioplegia delivered earlier; potentially lessening the chance of perioperative infarction.

At present, preoperative coronary angiography provides the cardiac surgeon with a road map to estimate the degree and location of coronary arterial stenosis. The surgeon is thus able to judge where to place bypass grafts to achieve successful revascularization. Coronary angiography, however, frequently does not accurately assess the anatomic[55–57] or the physiologic[58,59] significance of coronary artery stenosis, which has led to the development of other intraoperative techniques for assessing coronary anatomy and blood flow. For example, high resolution intraoperative epicardial echocardiography is capable of imaging coronary arteries and bypass graft anastomosis to evaluate the degree of coronary arterial stenosis and the technical success of a bypass graft.[60] Intraoperative Doppler flow probes can also be used to document and measure bypass graft blood flow to regions of the myocardium.[61] With neither of these techniques, however, is it possible to evaluate multiple perfusion beds simultaneously. Both methods require manipulation of the heart during operations, particularly when trying to interrogate the posterior circumflex coronary arterial bed. Furthermore, they do not provide information regarding either collateral flow or total nutrient flow.

MCE has several potential advantages over these techniques: It allows the physician to measure the size of myocardial perfusion beds; it can be used to determine perfusion to different regions of the myocardium simultaneously; and, it can delineate the degree of collateral flow to underperfused myocardial zones. During coronary artery bypass operations, cardioplegia is delivered to the cross-clamped aortic root through a cannula at controlled flow rates to reduce myocardial temperature and to produce cardiac arrest in order to achieve myocardial preservation. The ideal time to perform MCE is during cardioplegia delivery, because delivery of contrast through the aortic root is possible without interfering with the surgical routine; the aortic root functions as a mixing chamber; and repetition of MCE is possible during each dose of cardioplegia, allowing data acquisition at baseline and after completion of each distal coronary anastomosis.

The capability of MCE to enable confirmation of bypass graft patency has been evaluated in a canine model of left internal mammary artery to left anterior descend-

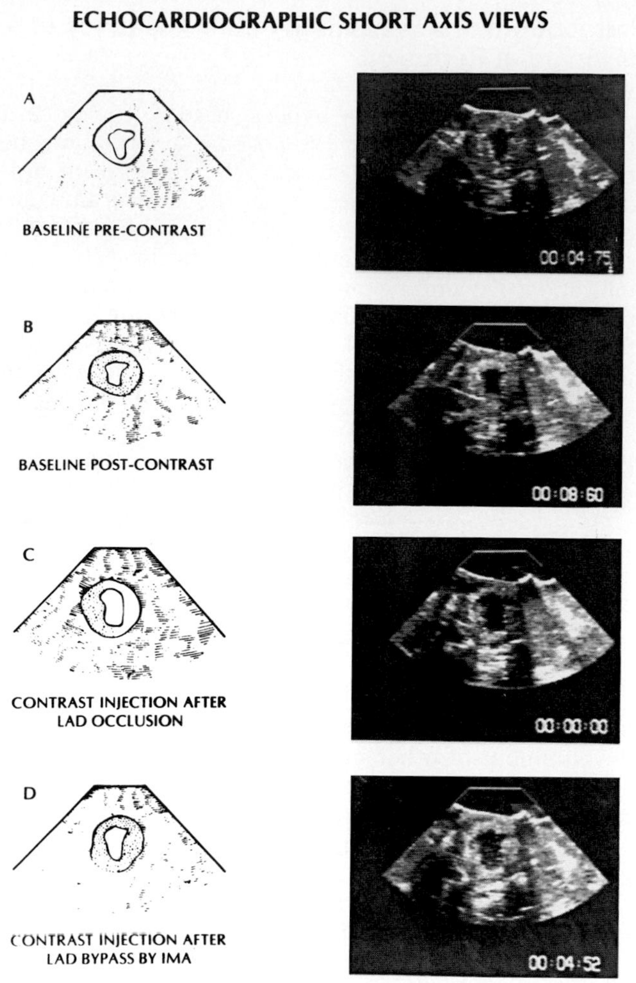

Fig. 23–24. Images from an arrested dog heart receiving cardioplegia solution intraoperatively. **A.** Before contrast injection. **B** to **D.** After contrast injection. **B.** Internal mammary graft (IMA) to the left anterior descending artery (LAD) is occluded, and native left LAD is patent. **C.** Both the LAD and graft are occluded. **D.** The graft is open, but the native LAD is occluded. (See text for details.) (From Spotnitz WD, et al.: Success of internal mammary bypass grafting can be assessed intraoperatively using myocardial contrast two-dimensional echocardiography. J Am Coll Cardiol 12: 196, 1988. Reprinted with permission from the American College of Cardiology.)

ing coronary artery bypass.[62] The aorta was cross-clamped beyond the origin of the internal mammary artery so that cardioplegia entering the cross-clamped aortic root perfused only the coronary arteries and the bypass graft. Figure 23–24 illustrates echocardiograms at the midpapillary muscle short axis level before contrast injection (Fig. 23–24A); after contrast was injected with the left anterior descending artery patent (Fig. 23–24B); lack of anterior wall perfusion with the left anterior descending artery occluded (Fig. 23–24C); and restoration of perfusion with the left anterior descending artery occluded and the bypass graft open (Fig. 23–24D). In 1 of the 11 dogs in this study, no contrast appeared in the anterior wall after the bypass graft was opened. Postmortem inspection revealed that the anastomotic site was narrowed and would not allow passage of a 1.5-mm probe.[62] Thus, MCE documented a technically inadequate bypass that could have been easily revised in the operating room.

The initial use of intraoperative MCE in humans depended on air bubble formation caused by microcavitation during delivery of cardioplegia to the cross-clamped aortic root.[63] Because the bubble size and concentration were not constant, the contrast effect was not easily reproducible. Since then, microbubbles of known sizes have been introduced into the cardioplegia solution and have become the principal means of assessing myocardial perfusion during intraoperative MCE.[64,65]

Retrograde cardioplegia is now used intraoperatively during both bypass and valve surgery. During bypass surgery, it is used to perfuse regions of the myocardium supplied by severely stenosed vessels, which may not receive adequate cardioplegia following aortic root injection. It also provides a clear operative field without having to interrupt the operation repeatedly for cardioplegia delivery. No intraoperative method, however, assesses the intramyocardial distribution of retrogradely delivered cardioplegic solution. This is important because the balloon on the coronary sinus catheter, which is inflated during cardioplegia delivery, has a tendency to obstruct venous tributaries draining into the sinus. A method for assessing the intramyocardial distribution of cardioplegic solution could permit the position of the balloon to be readjusted.

MCE has been used intraoperatively in a canine model to determine the intramyocardial distribution of retrogradely delivered cardioplegia solution.[66,67] Figure 23–25B illustrates a short axis view in which contrast is not present in the interventricular septum (indicated by arrows). Radiolabeled microspheres confirm relative hypoperfusion of this region by cardioplegic solution (also indicated by arrows in Fig. 23–25A). Figure 23–25B also

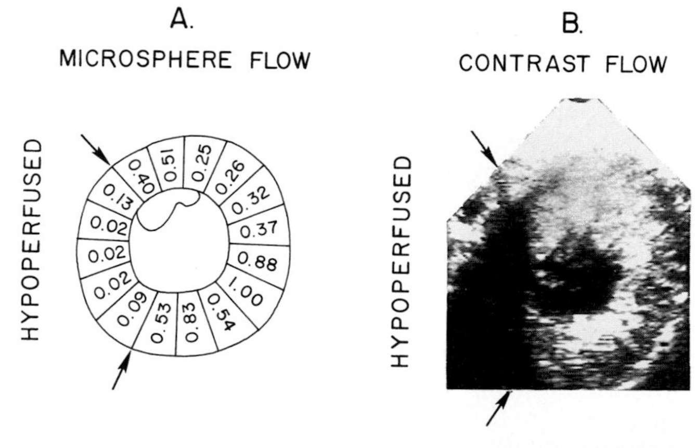

Fig. 23–25. **A.** Radiolabeled microsphere of normalized blood flow data. The arrows depict the regions receiving more than 15% of maximal flow. **B.** Contrast echocardiographic data from a dog in which microspheres and contrast were introduced through the coronary sinus. Echocardiographic data show that absence of contrast is noted in exactly the same regions showing less than 15% of flow. The interventricular septum in the dog is not drained by epicardial coronary veins but, rather, by Thebesian veins. (See text for details.) (From Villanueva FS, et al.: Intraoperative assessment of the distribution of retrograde cardioplegia using myocardial contrast echocardiography. Surg Forum 41:252, 1990. With permission of the American College of Surgeons.)

illustrates the intramyocardial distribution of cardioplegic solution, which appears as spokes of a wheel, consistent with the intramyocardial distribution of veins.[68] Unlike the situation when contrast is injected into the aortic root, contrast is readily noted, even when epicardial coronary arteries are occluded.[67] MCE could, therefore, provide clues to the ideal method of cardioplegia delivery (anterograde vs. retrograde) in patients with severe multivessel disease, in whom intraoperative myocardial preservation may be an issue.

Assessment of Myocardial Perfusion Beds Using Systemic Venous Contrast Injection

For MCE to be used as a routine clinical tool in the outpatient laboratory, it is imperative that myocardial contrast enhancement be achieved following a peripheral venous injection of contrast. Although venous injection of contrast has been demonstrated to cause enhancement of the left ventricular blood pool in humans,[69,70] myocardial opacification has not yet been achieved clinically following venous contrast injection.

Recent data indicate, however, that this may become a reality in the near future. Right atrial injection of sonicated albumin has been demonstrated to reproducibly opacify the left ventricular myocardium in the dog (Fig. 23–26).[71] Figure 23–26A is an end-systolic short axis recording from a canine left ventricle following right atrial contrast injection. The contrast appears as a thin

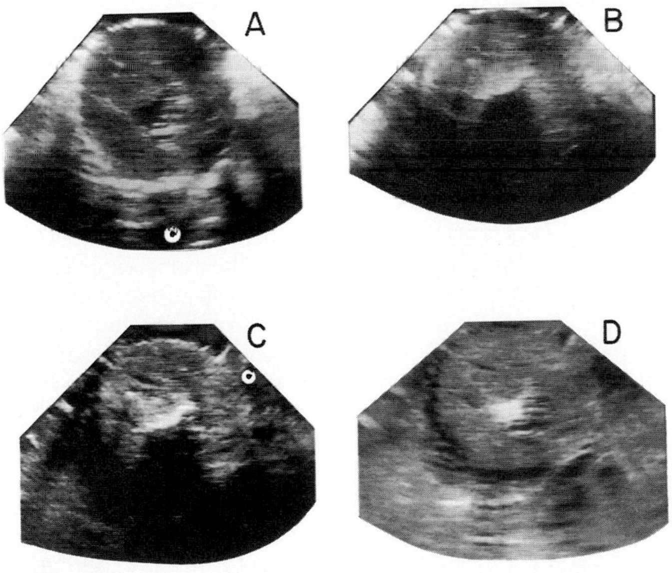

Fig. 23–26. Echocardiograms after right atrial injection of contrast agent in a dog. **A.** Contrast is seen in the right ventricle. **B.** Contrast is seen in the left ventricular cavity and attenuates the posterior myocardium. The myocardium also shows contrast enhancement. **C.** Image obtained after subtracting **A** from **B.** This subtraction image shows clear myocardial opacification that was not as readily noted in the unsubtracted image **(B).** After a few cycles, when contrast in the left ventricular cavity is not enough to attenuate the posterior wall, a subtraction image still shows homogeneous myocardial opacification (panel **D**). (From Villanueva FS: Successful and reproducible myocardial opacification during two-dimensional echocardiography from right heart injection contrast. Circulation 85:1557, 1992, reproduced with permission of the American Heart Association.)

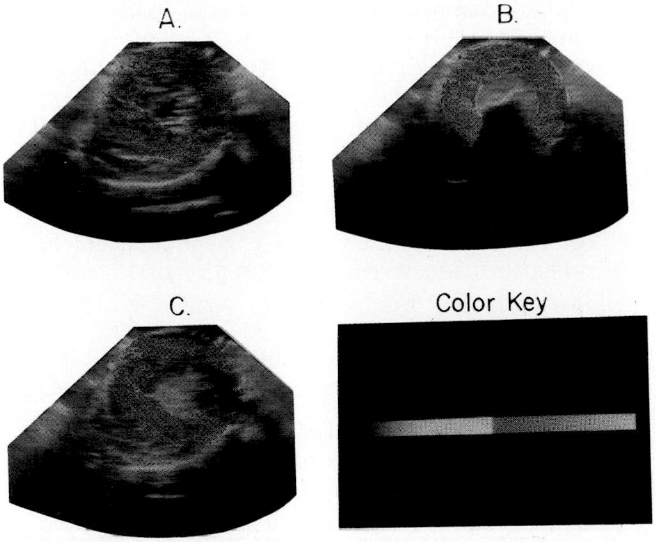

Fig. 23–27. Color coded data from injection sequence similar to that noted in Figure 23–26. All regions except the myocardium have been "masked." The color code is shown in the bar, with red being minimal echo brightness and yellow being more bright. **A.** Image before contrast opacification of the myocardium. The red is homogeneously distributed. This image corresponds to Figure 23–26A. **B.** Image taken during maximal myocardial opacification when the contrast present in the left ventricular cavity is producing posterior wall attenuation. Note the yellow. This image corresponds to Figure 23–26B and C. **C.** Image obtained a few cycles later when posterior wall attenuation is no longer present. Although the myocardial contrast effect is not as great as in **B,** it is still present. This image corresponds to Figure 23–26D. (From Villanueva FS: Successful and reproducible myocardial opacification during two-dimensional echocardiography from right heart injection of contrast. Circulation 85:1557, 1992, reprinted with permission of the American Heart Association.)

sickle-shaped area in the right ventricular cavity. Figure 23–26B, recorded several cycles later, shows opacification of the myocardium of the anterior left ventricular wall. No posterior wall opacification is noted, which is due to attenuation by the contrast in the left ventricle. Figure 23–26C is an image obtained by subtracting Figure 23–26A from 23–26B. The subtraction image defines the myocardial opacification more clearly. Figure 23–26D shows a subtracted image several cycles later, when there was no longer sufficient contrast in the left ventricular cavity to produce posterior wall attenuation. Although the contrast enhancement is less than in Figure 23–26C, it is still clearly present.

It is possible to highlight subtle changes in signal intensity produced by MCE by displaying intensity levels in color rather than black and white because the human eye can appreciate only 16 gray levels but can discriminate several hundred color hues. One such color-coding algorithm is that of a heated object. Consider a piece of iron being heated in a flame. As the iron becomes hotter, it initially turns a faint red hue, which increases in intensity as the temperature continues to rise. Further heating causes the color to change from red to yellow and the brightness to also increase. Figure 23–27 illustrates the effect of color encoding data similar to that in Figure 23–26. All regions except the myocardium have been masked. Figure 23–27A shows a color-coded image before the appearance of contrast in the left ventricular myocardium (equivalent to Fig. 23–26A). Note the hues of red throughout. Figure 23–27B depicts a color-coded image after contrast has appeared in the myocardium, but there is posterior wall attenuation (equivalent to Fig. 23–26B and C). Note the yellow hues in all regions except those from which the signal has been obscured as a result of attenuation. Figure 23–27C illustrates milder hues of yellow when the contrast in the left ventricular cavity is insufficient to cause attenuation of the posterior wall (equivalent to Fig. 23–26D).

Limitations of Myocardial Contrast Echocardiography for the Estimation of Risk Area

Three physical characteristics of ultrasound can potentially limit the accuracy of risk area determinations using MCE: limited lateral resolution, attenuation, and blooming. Because only targets that are separated by more than the width of the ultrasound beam can be seen as distinct, resolution deteriorates as the target is displaced posteriorly and laterally within the scan plane. Deterioration of resolution relative to the center of the sector can potentially expand the area of contrast enhancement in the posterior bed and thus result in underestimation of the size of the area without contrast enhancement.

Attenuation artifacts occur commonly along the lateral walls (see Fig. 23–1) of the ventricle when it is viewed in short axis. These artifacts occur because the echo beam must travel through a longer segment of the myocardium to reach these areas and results in artifactual loss of echoes at the four- and eight-o'clock positions on the short axis images. Although these attenuation artifacts have a very characteristic appearance, they can interfere with risk area determinations, particularly when the margins of the risk area involve either of the lateral walls (see Fig. 23–20). Posterior wall attenuation is noted after right-sided contrast injections as a result of signal loss as the contrast passes through the left ventricular cavity (see Fig. 23–26). This can also become a problem during intraoperative studies when there is regurgitation of contrast through the aortic valve.

Blooming refers to the artifactual increase in gray level immediately adjacent to a region showing contrast enhancement and is most prominent when contrast enhancement is at its peak. It occurs as a result of the increase in electron beam intensity in the region of contrast enhancement, which expands the area of phosphor that is illuminated on the display tube and may result in underestimation of areas without contrast enhancement.

Current and Potential Applications of Risk Area Determination

The current applications of MCE for the determination of risk area have already been discussed. Given the accuracy of MCE for quantifying risk area in experimental animals, it should provide similar information in patients with acute myocardial infarction. Widespread clinical application will, nevertheless, depend on the development of agents capable of transpulmonary passage. Using such agents, it might be possible to immediately diagnose acute myocardial infarction in patients presenting to the emergency room with cardiac-related symptoms. Likewise, absence of perfusion abnormalities can be presumed to exclude infarction. This technique could also improve risk stratification sufficiently in patients with acute infarction to better define those who would benefit most from an intervention and those who could be spared the additional risk.

The ability to detect collateral blood flow into an acutely ischemic region could be of major clinical importance. For instance, patients previously felt not to be candidates for thrombolytic therapy because of prolonged symptoms before presentation might have sufficient collateral flow to delay the onset of irreversible injury. These patients might benefit from treatment. Alternatively, borderline duration of symptoms but total absence of collateral flow might predict a poor result.

QUANTIFICATION OF REGIONAL MYOCARDIAL BLOOD FLOW

Theoretical Considerations

Quantitation of regional myocardial blood flow is far more difficult than simply defining the perfusion territory of a coronary vessel. Several approaches have been employed that are based on the analysis of time-intensity plots obtained from the myocardium following the injection of ultrasonic contrast material. The algorithms for analyzing the time-intensity curves are, in general, adapted from indicator-dilution theory.

To understand the measurement of myocardial blood flow using MCE, one must be conversant with tracer kinetics in different models that resemble actual in vivo situations. These models will be discussed at this point and referred to later when considering actual in vivo situations. First, consider a reservoir filled with 200 ml of water and connected to two pipes (Fig. 23–28A). One pipe delivers water into the reservoir at a rate of 100 ml/min, while the other removes it at the same rate. Let us now inject a tracer (e.g., a dye) into the reservoir as an instantaneous bolus, and let us assume that the tracer is capable of rapidly mixing with the water in the reservoir. Because the water in the reservoir is constantly turning over at a rate of 100 ml/min, the amount of dye in the reservoir will be progressively diluted. There will be 50% of the dye left at the end of the first minute, 25% at the end of the second minute, 12.5% at the end of the third minute, and so on. This logarithmic dilution of the dye can be characterized by fitting a monoexponential function ($e^{-\kappa t}$) to the data where κ is equal to the flow/"tissue" volume and t is time (Fig. 23–28B). As long as the method of injection of dye and the volume of the reservoir remain constant, κ will be directly proportional to flow through the reservoir.

Now let us assume that this reservoir is connected to another reservoir of the same size also filled with water and that the effluent from the first reservoir enters the second reservoir at a known flow rate (Fig. 23–29A). When we inject dye into the first reservoir (reservoir "a"), it will be diluted to a logarithmic manner, as depicted in Figure 23–28B. After a certain interval (which

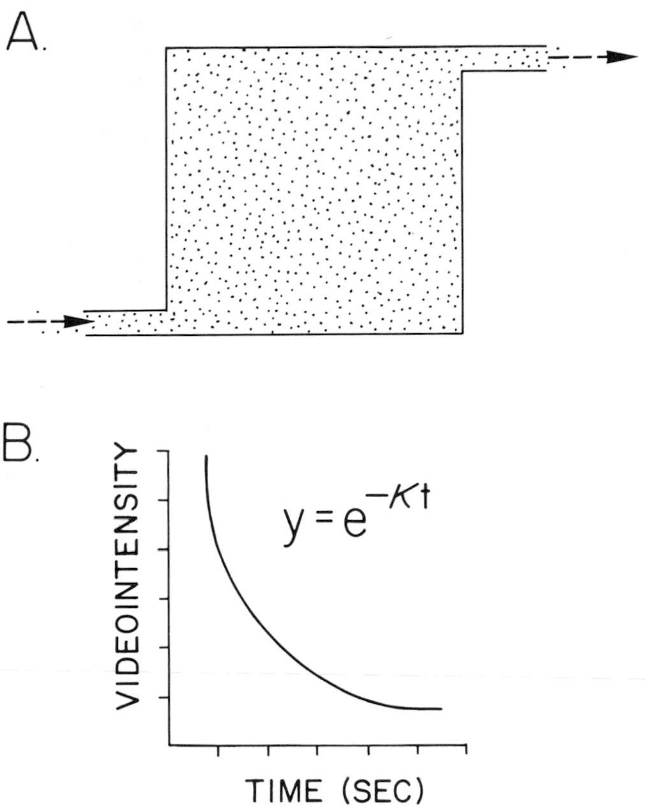

Fig. 23–28. Model to describe dye dilution curve. (See text for details.) (From Kaul S.: Quantitation of myocardial perfusion with contrast echocardiography. Am J Card Imag 5:200, 1991, reproduced with permission.)

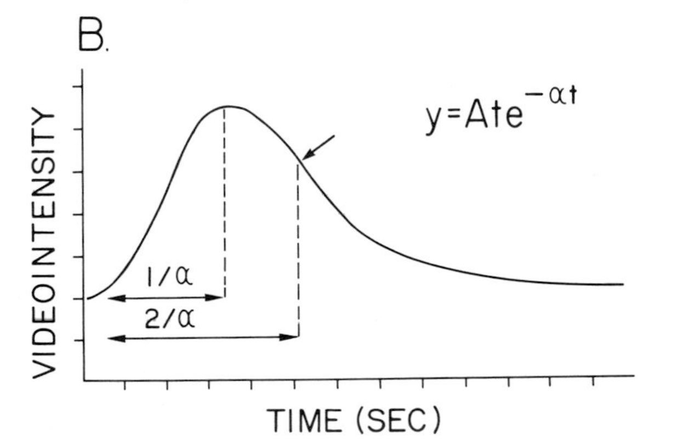

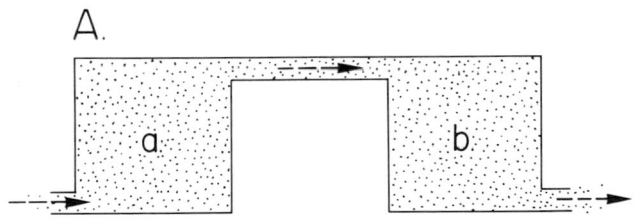

Fig. 23–29. Model to describe the gamma-variate function. (See text for details.) (From Kaul S: Quantitation of myocardial perfusion with contrast echocardiography. Am J Card Imag 5:200, 1991, reproduced with permission.)

depends on the flow as well as the length of the tubing connecting the two reservoirs), the dye will appear in the second reservoir (reservoir "b"), reach a maximal concentration, and then slowly disappear. The concentration of dye over time in reservoir "b" will look like the curve depicted in Figure 23–29B. This curve has a characteristic appearance: There is relatively fast upslope, a peak, and a slower downslope, which is asymptotic. There is also a point on the downslope of this curve (arrow) where the shape of the curve changes from convex to concave. This curve can be mathematically defined by a γ-variate function $y = Ate^{-\alpha t}$, where A is a scaling factor, t is time, and α is flow rate/unit volume; $1/\alpha$ is the time between appearance of dye and the peak intensity of the dye, while $2/\alpha$ is the time between appearance of dye and the point where the downslope of the curve changes its shape from convex to concave (arrow in Fig. 23–29B).[72] The area under the curve represents the amount of dye injected into reservoir "a" and can be derived using the equation A/α^2.

Several factors will influence the appearance of the curve shown in Figure 23–29B. First, the amount of dye injected in reservoir "a" will determine the area under the curve in reservoir "b." If less dye is injected, the area under the curve will be smaller, and vice versa. Second, the shape of the dye dilution curve in reservoir a (input function) will determine the shape of the curve in reservoir "b" (output function). For example, if the same amount of dye is injected over a longer period into reservoir "a," the input function will be more spread out, which will also make the output function (shape of the curve in reservoir "b") more spread out, despite the flow rate remaining constant. Despite this change in shape, if the amount of dye injected into reservoir "a" is constant, the area under the curve obtained from reservoir "b" will be constant.

The manner in which the input function can affect the output function is depicted in Figure 23–30. Figure 23–30A illustrates several reservoirs of the same size connected in series. Water is flowing through them at the same flow rate. If dye is injected as an instantaneous bolus in the first reservoir (reservoir "a"), it will demonstrate a logarithmic decay, as depicted in Figure 23–30B.

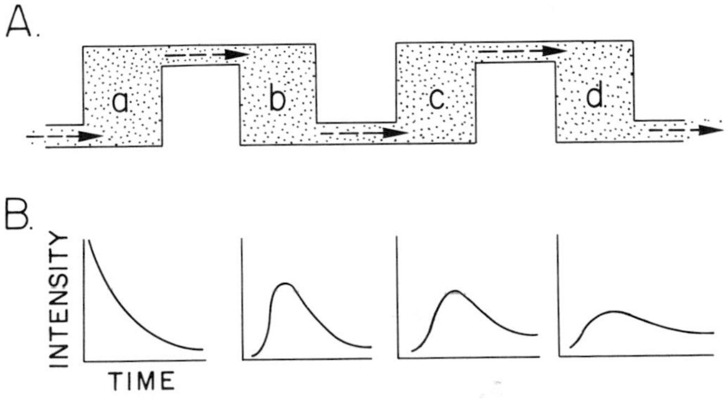

Fig. 23–30. Model to describe the effect of the input function on the output function. (See text for details.) (From Kaul S.: Quantitation of myocardial perfusion with contrast echocardiography. Am J Card Imag 5:200, 1991, reproduced with permission.)

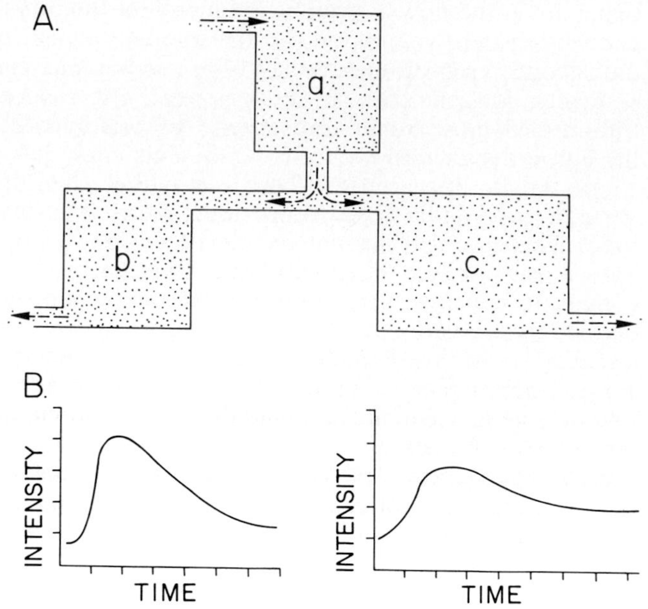

Fig. 23–31. Model to describe the effect of volume on output function. (See text for details.) (From Kaul S: Quantitation of myocardial perfusion with contrast echocardiography. Am J Card Imag 5:200, 1991, reproduced with permission.)

By the time the dye appears in reservoir "b," it will assume a γ-variate form, as illustrated in Figure 23–30B. When the dye enters the third reservoir (reservoir "c"), the form of the curve will be unchanged, but it will be more spread out as shown in Figure 23–30B. The curve spread will be greater in the fourth reservoir (reservoir "d"), as illustrated in Figure 23–30B, and so on. Because the amount of dye entering and leaving each reservoir is the same, the area under each curve will remain the same, but the transit time of the dye will differ for each reservoir despite the flow rate remaining constant. If the input function for each reservoir (which is the output function of the preceding reservoir) were not known, the different shapes of the curves from the different reservoirs could easily be mistaken for different flow rates in those reservoirs, when in fact the different shapes are due to different input functions.

Another factor that can affect the shape of the curve is the volume of the reservoir. Assume that reservoir "a" is connected to two reservoirs "b" and "c," each with a different volume (Fig. 23–31A). Assume also that the flow rates through reservoirs "b" and "c" are identical. For the same input function, the dye dilution curve will be more spread out in the larger reservoir (reservoir "c") than in the smaller reservoir (reservoir "b"), but the areas under the curves will be the same (Fig. 23–31B).

The final factor that affects the shape of the dye dilution curve in reservoir "b" in Figure 23–29 is the flow through the reservoir. For the same input function in reservoir "a" and the same volume in reservoir "b," the width of the dye dilution curve in reservoir "b" will be inversely related to flow through it. The faster the flow, the narrower the curve, and the slower the flow, the wider the curve. In this model, because all dye injected into reservoir "a" has to pass through reservoir "b," the area under the curve will remain the same, irrespective of the flow rate. Because the area under the curve remains the same, and the curve width decreases at higher flows, it follows that the peak intensity will increase at higher flows. Peak intensity can be derived from the γ-variate function using the equation $A/\alpha e$.

Let us now assume that reservoir "b" is connected to various smaller reservoirs of the same size and that the flow rates to these reservoirs differ (Fig. 23–32A). The input function for these reservoirs is the dye dilution curve obtained from reservoir "b" (depicted in Fig. 23–32B). All the smaller reservoirs "see" the same input function. Because all of the dye in reservoir "b"

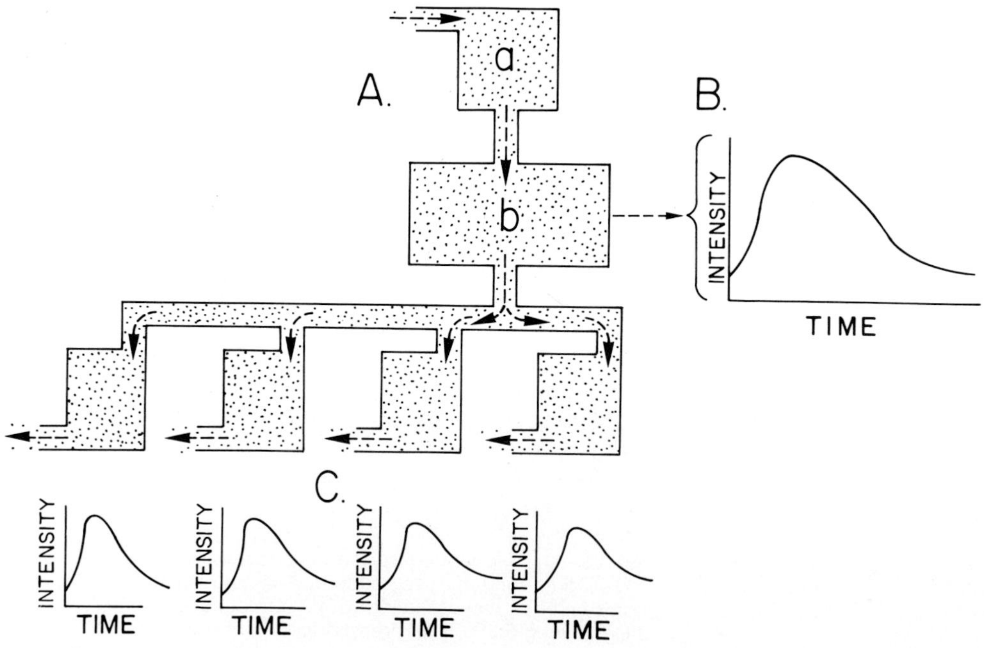

Fig. 23–32. Model to describe the method of quantitating flow when input function is known. (See text for details.) (From Kaul S: Quantitation of myocardial perfusion with contrast echocardiography. Am J Card Imag 5:200, 1991.)

empties into these smaller reservoirs, the sum of the areas under the curves obtained from each of the smaller reservoirs (Fig. 23–32C) should equal the area under the curve in reservoir "b." In this model, if the flow in reservoir "b" is known, and the dye dilution curves from this and the other smaller reservoirs are available, the flow in any of the smaller reservoirs can be calculated. If the dye dilution curve from reservoir "b" is not available, the areas under the curves from the smaller reservoirs can be used to assess relative flow to these smaller reservoirs. Finally, if flow to any of the small reservoirs is known, flow to the other small reservoirs can be calculated.

It is important to appreciate that in these models the γ-variate function describes the entire curve. The upslope and downslope of the curves are obligatorily related, both being defined by the input function, volume, and flow rate. It is thus artificial to analyze the wash-in and wash-out phases of this curve separately. The only situation where the wash-in and wash-out portions of a dye dilution curve should be analyzed separately is when the tracer does not pass freely through the volume of tissue being sampled. This occurs in MCE either when large bubbles are used, which get lodged within the arterioles, or when small bubbles are trapped in tissue for reasons other than their size. In these situations, the time-intensity curve cannot be defined by γ-variate function. The appropriate model will be described later when intraoperative assessment of myocardial flow is discussed.

Once these general principles are understood, the complexities of measuring myocardial blood flow in vivo using MCE (or other techniques using tracers, e.g., digital subtraction angiography or fast Cine-computed tomography) become clearer. Once the in vivo situation is likened to one of the models described in Figures 23–28 to 23–32 (obviously, many more models are possible, but for the sake of clarity, only five have been described), the method of analysis specific to that situation becomes apparent. The situation would have been far more complex if the tracers used for MCE were totally or partially diffusible. Luckily, the microbubbles are true intravascular tracers, which makes the analysis of blood flow using MCE relatively simple. One important issue, as yet not fully resolved, is the stability of the microbubbles during their transit through tissue.[73,74] Obviously, if contrast or bubbles are lost spontaneously during transit, the accuracy of the calculations described previously will be affected.

Data Acquisition, Processing, and Analysis

The steps involved in quantitation of myocardial perfusion during MCE are data acquisition, selection of appropriate frames, alignment of these frames, placement of regions of interest to derive time-intensity plots, applying appropriate curve fits to the data, and derivation of pertinent parameters.[75]

Data Acquisition. A digital echocardiographic system with a broad dynamic range (120 dB) and at least 256 levels of gray would be desirable for data acquisition. Because such a system is not commercially available, analog data from the video output port of the echo system either can be sent directly to a computer for on-line analysis or can be stored on videotape for subsequent off-line analysis. For most current applications, data are analyzed off-line (except for the operating room, which will be discussed later).

Selection of Appropriate Frames. Because coronary blood flow occurs in diastole, and because end-diastolic frames are easy to identify, they have been conventionally used to generate time-intensity plots. There are two approaches to selecting these frames. The first is to employ a gating device (i.e., an R-wave trigger) to select end-diastolic frames on-line and transfer them directly to computer memory. The second is to transfer an entire injection sequence to memory and then select individual end-diastolic frames.

Image Alignment. Translation of the heart between end-diastolic frames often occurs because of respiration. To minimize translation, patients can be asked to hold their breath during an injection. Because the transit of the microbubbles through the myocardium may take as little as 5 to 10 seconds, respiratory gating would not be effective. Despite breath holding, however, some translation can be present, which can be eliminated by computer cross-correlation techniques.

For this purpose, a region of interest is defined in a reference frame that is approximately equal to the area within the epicardial outline (Fig. 23–33). A rectangular area is then defined around the region of interest within which the computer performs a search for the same region of interest in the other frames (Fig. 23–33). The size of this search area is determined by the observer, who examines the degree of translation by viewing the end-diastolic frames in cine-loop format. If the translation is minimal, the search area is smaller.

The cross-correlation is then performed as follows. Let p_i denote the pixel intensity at a particular point i within the region of interest in the reference frame and let q_i denote the pixel intensity at the same location in another frame. If we plot p_i vs. q_i for all the points within the two frames, and the two frames are identical, then the correlation coefficient will be 1 with the use of the following equation:

$$r = \frac{\Sigma p_i q_i}{\sqrt{\Sigma p_i^2 \Sigma q i^2}} \qquad [23.1]$$

If the two frames are not optimally aligned, then the correlation coefficient will be <1. In such a case, the frame to be realigned is translated 1 pixel at a time within the search area, and the correlation coefficient between all the points within the region of interest in both frames is recalculated. The position at which the correlation coefficient is closest to 1 is taken to represent the best alignment.

This method is diagrammatically depicted in Figure 23–34A, illustrating the index image, and 23–34B, illustrating the image to be realigned. A point (i) has a certain location in the index image in terms of the x and y coordinates. The same point is shifted by 10 pixels in both the leftward and downward directions in the image to be

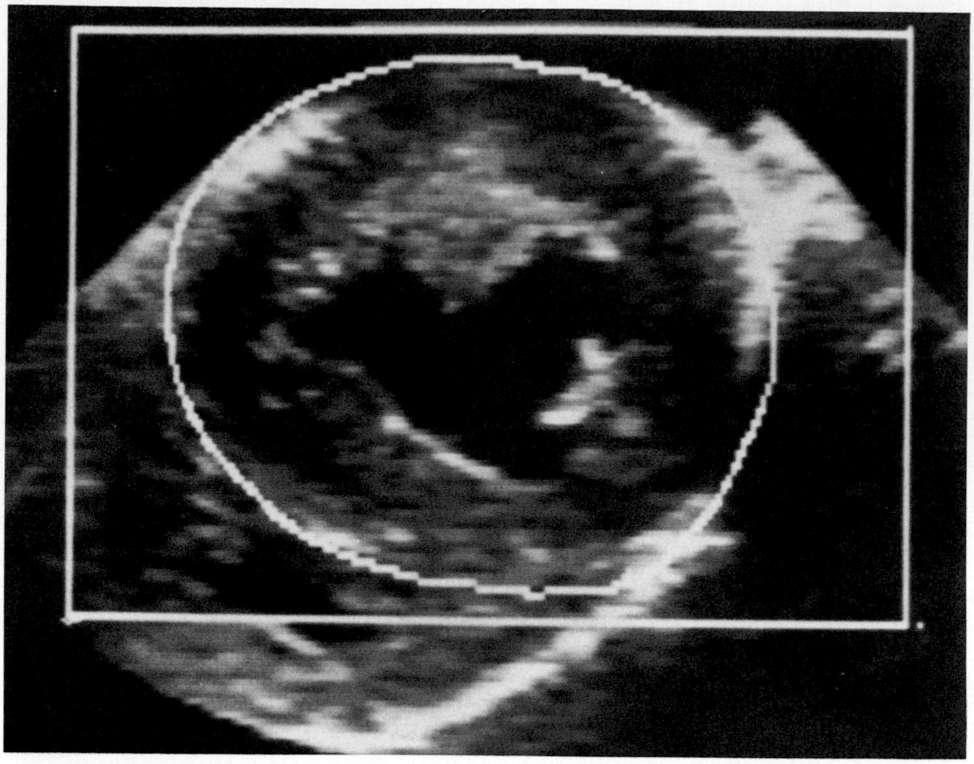

Fig. 23–33. Method of placing region of interest (circular area) and determining the "search area" (rectangular area) for image alignment. (See text for details.) (From Jayaweera AR, et al.: Method for the quantitation of myocardial perfusion during myocardial contrast echocardiography. J Am Soc Echo 3:91, 1990. Reprinted with permission of the American Society of Echocardiography.)

aligned. Additionally, it is also rotated clockwise by 15°. To align these two identical points in the two images, the second image (Fig. 23–34B) must be translated and rotated such that the x and y coordinates as well as the angle are similar to that of the index image. In general, whereas the amount of translation required to align end-diastolic frames varies, the amount of rotation required is usually <2°.

Derivation of Time-Intensity Plots. Once the images are appropriately aligned, regions of interest are selected within the myocardium from which serial changes in intensity produced by contrast injection are measured. Any of the registered images can be used for initial placement of the regions of interest. Care should be taken in this process to ensure that the regions of interest overly only myocardium and do not include the specular reflections from the epicardial and endocardial interfaces. Figure 23–35 illustrates regions of interest placed over the left anterior descending, left circumflex, and right coronary arterial beds. Because the larger the region of interest, the greater the signal/noise ratio, there is an obligate trade-off between the number of regions that can be examined and the quality of the data. Five to six regions in any one view are usually sufficient to differentiate vascular beds without compromising signal quality. The average videointensity within each of these regions is then calculated automatically for every frame starting five to six frames before contrast appearance and continuing until the contrast has completely washed out of the myocardium. The result is a time intensity curve for each region for the duration of contrast passage through the myocardium.

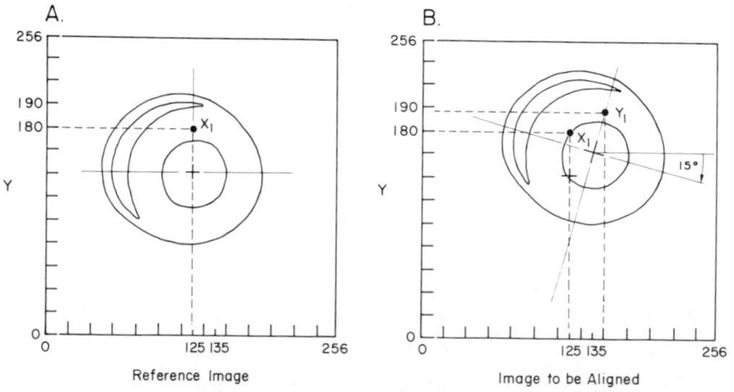

Fig. 23–34. Computer cross-correlation algorithm used for image alignment. (See text for details.) (From Jayaweera AR, et al.: Method for the quantitation of myocardial perfusion during myocardial contrast echocardiography. J Am Soc Echo 3:91, 1990. Reprinted with permission of the American Society of Echocardiography.)

Background Subtraction and Derivation of Parameters. The next step after the generation of the time-intensity plots is background subtraction. Background subtraction is achieved by calculating the average video intensity, for each region of interest, from the five to six frames before contrast appearance and subtracting this value from all subsequent frames.[81] In this manner, videointensity at time 0 (just before contrast appearance in the myocardium), is 0. A least-squares curve (usually γ-variate, except in the operating room, as described later) is then fit to the intensity data and parameters of the curve such as width (or transit time), amplitude, and area under the curve are derived.

Effects of Bubble Size on Myocardial Blood Flow Measurement

Both large and small microbubbles have been shown to have the potential for measuring regional myocardial

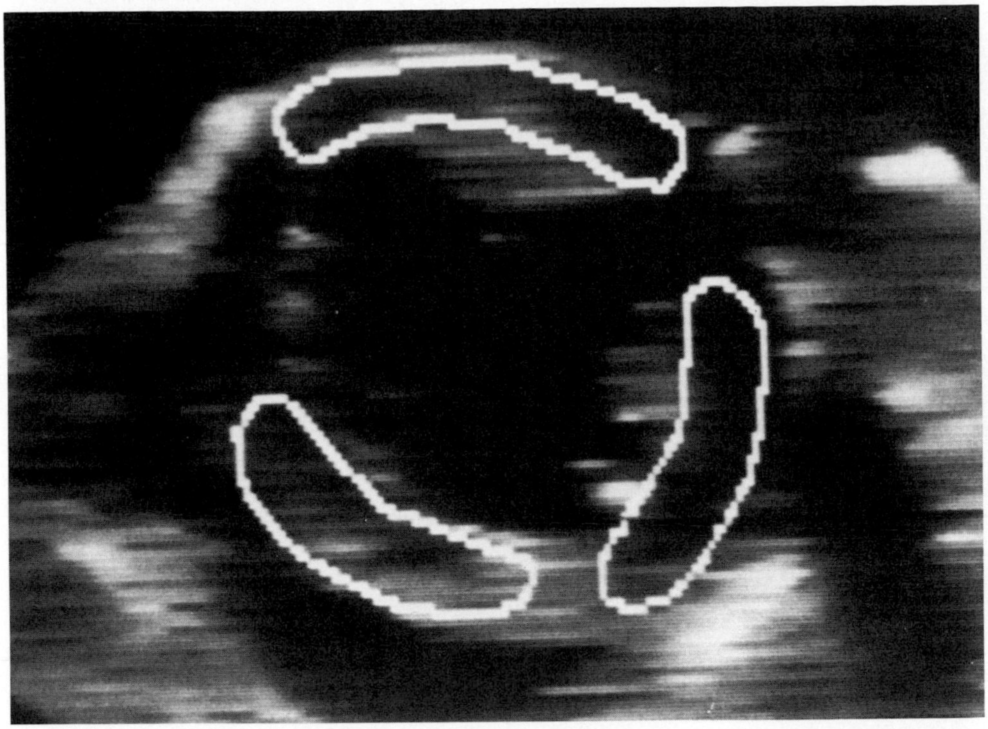

Fig. 23–35. Method of placing regions of interest over vascular territories for generation of time-intensity plots. (See text for details.) (From Jayaweera AR, et al.: Method for the quantitation of myocardial perfusion during myocardial contrast echocardiography. J Am Soc Echo 3:91, 1990. Reprinted with permission of the American Society of Echocardiography.)

blood flow. When large microbubbles are injected into the aortic root (equivalent to the model in Figure 23–32—provided we assume adequate mixing of the bubbles in the aorta before their traveling down the coronaries), they initially lodge in arterioles in a manner similar to radiolabeled microspheres.[76] In theory, therefore, the number of bubbles in any myocardial region should be proportional to the flow to that region; and because more bubbles should lodge in areas with greater flow, they should produce a proportionately greater contrast effect. In experimental studies, the peak contrast intensity produced by large microbubbles has been shown to correlate linearly with actual blood flow measured using radiolabeled microspheres.[77]

Unfortunately, several problems are inherent in the use of large microbubbles. First, they produce independent hemodynamic abnormalities including alterations in coronary blood flow,[7,14] which become more significant in the setting of critical coronary stenosis.[14] Second, because the intensity of the reflected ultrasound is proportional to the sixth power of the bubble radius,[8] large variability in the distribution frequency of bubble sizes can alter the relationship between bubble number and signal amplitude. Thus, a single large bubble entrapped in an arteriole with low flow could result in greater contrast enhancement than many smaller bubbles lodged in an arteriole receiving higher flow. Finally, the relation between video intensity and the amplitude of scattered ultrasound is nonlinear in most ultrasound systems, and the dynamic range is narrow. As a result, even if the amplitude of reflected ultrasound truly represented the number of microbubbles within a region of myocardium, the distortion in the gray scale would produce a nonlinear relation between the number of bubbles and video intensity.

In comparison, because small microbubbles produce no hemodynamic effects[14,15] and behave like red blood cells within the microvasculature,[16] their transit through the myocardium should reflect myocardial blood flow. In experimental studies, the myocardial transit rates of these microbubbles in the beating dog heart have been found to be similar to those of technetium-labeled red blood cells over a wide range of physiologic flows.[78] Because red blood cell transit rate is linearly related to coronary blood flow, these data imply that the myocardial transit rates of small microbubbles should provide information regarding true intravascular myocardial blood flow. This characteristic is important because no other currently used imaging technique can provide similar information.

Intracoronary Injection of Contrast

Data have been generated in vivo by comparing myocardial time-intensity curve parameters to myocardial blood flow measured using radiolabeled microspheres.[79] In one such study, microbubbles and radiolabeled microspheres were injected directly into the left circumflex coronary artery at varying flow rates using a different label for each flow. Figure 23–36 depicts the pattern of opacification during one such injection. In this example, contrast appears in the fourth end-diastolic frame, reaches maximal intensity by the eighth frame, and gradually disappears. This situation is similar to the model depicted in Figure 23–29B, in that the coronary artery acts like reservoir "a" and the myocardium acts like reservoir "b." The only assumption is that the microbubbles mix adequately with blood in the coronary artery.

Figure 23–37A illustrates time-intensity plots ac-

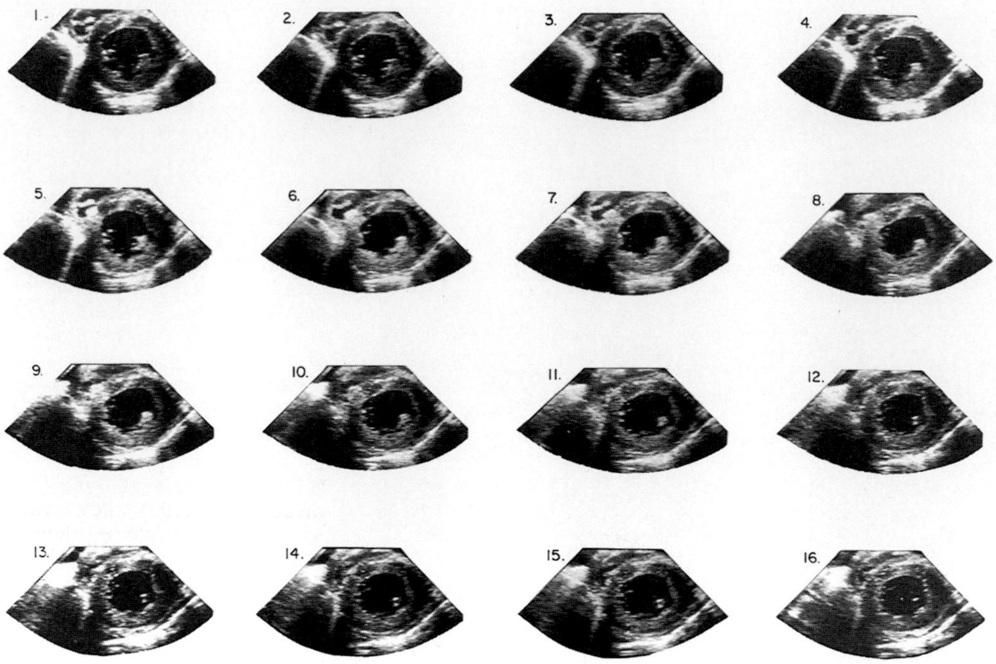

Fig. 23–36. Every other end-diastolic frame at the papillary muscle, short axis level, from the time of injection of contrast agent into a plastic tubing connected to the left circumflex coronary artery until its disappearance from the myocardium. (See text for details.) (From Kaul S, et al.: Assessment of regional myocardial. J Am Coll Cardiol 13:468, 1989. Reprinted with permission from the American College of Cardiology.)

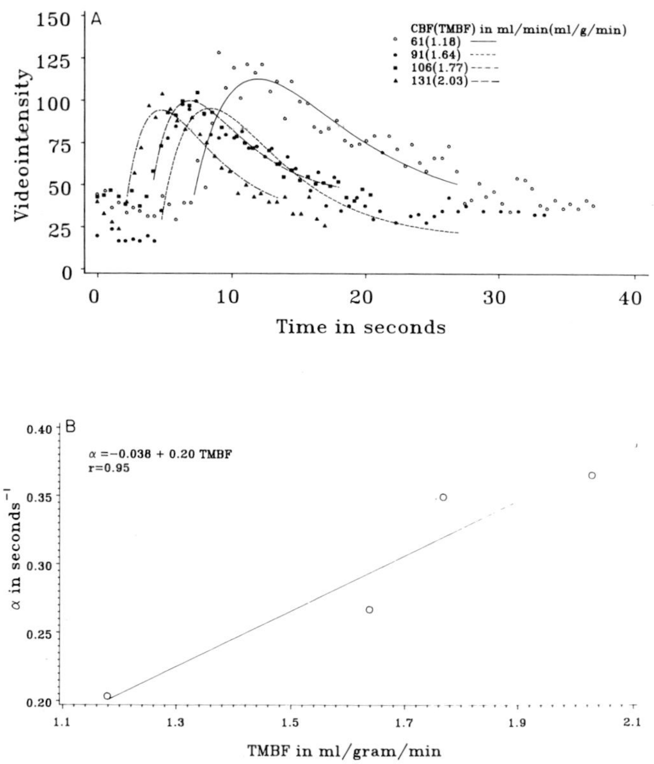

Fig. 23–37. Data from four different stages in the same experiment (different flow rates) when contrast agent is injected subselectively into a coronary artery. **B.** Relation between curve width (reciprocal of α) and transmural blood flow in the four stages shown in **A.** CBF = coronary blood flow; TMBF = transmural blood flow. (See text for details.) (From Kaul S, et al.: Assessment of regional myocardial blood flow with myocardial contrast two-dimensional echocardiography. J Am Coll Cardiol 13:468, 1989. Reprinted with permission from the American College of Cardiology.)

quired from a myocardial region of interest in the perfusion territory of the left circumflex coronary artery at four different flow rates. It can be appreciated that the higher the flow rate, the narrower the curve. Figure 23–37B illustrates the relation between α (reciprocal of curve width) and radiolabeled microsphere determined blood flow at the four different flow rates shown in Figure 23–37A. The relation is linear and close and remains so when the data from eight different experiments are pooled. A linear relation between myocardial blood flow and transit rate of bubbles from different animals suggests that when contrast is injected subselectively into a coronary artery it might be possible to measure actual myocardial blood flow from myocardial time-intensity curves. (Note that in these early studies the number of bubbles injected could not be controlled, so that the area under the curves will not be the same.)

If, instead contrast injected subselectively into the left circumflex artery, it is injected directly into the left main coronary artery, and there is adequate mixing, the number of bubbles going down the left anterior descending artery or circumflex artery would depend on the relative flow to the two arteries. If we assume that the flow to both the left anterior descending and left circumflex arteries is equal at baseline, then the number of microbubbles reaching the left anterior descending coronary artery bed will be half of the total number of microbubbles injected into the left main artery. If the left anterior descending coronary artery flow is reduced by half and the flow in the left main artery is unchanged, the left anterior descending arterial flow will be one third the left circumflex flow. As flow decreases, the number of bubbles reaching the left anterior descending arterial bed should also decrease, and the transit rate of these bubbles should decrease.

Figure 23–38A illustrates the time-intensity curves recorded at five different flow rates through the left ante-

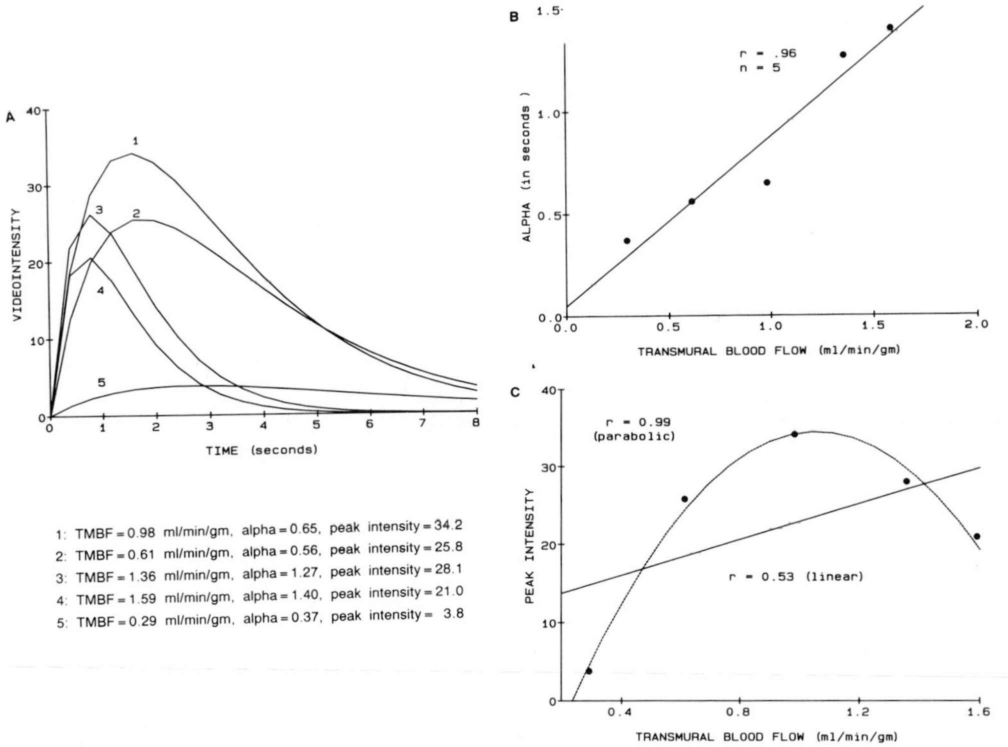

Fig. 23–38. **A.** Time-intensity curves from five different flow rates in the left anterior descending artery with contrast agent being injected into the left main coronary artery. **B.** Relationship between curve width (reciprocal of α) and transmural blood flow for the five stages depicted in **A.** The relationship is linear. **C.** Relationship between peak videointensity and transmural blood flow (TMBF) in the same experiment. The relationship is nonlinear. α = reciprocal of curve width. (See text for details.) (From Kaul S, et al.: Assessment of regional myocardial blood flow with myocardial contrast two-dimensional echocardiography. J Am Coll Cardiol 13:468, 1989. Reprinted with permission from the American College of Cardiology.)

rior descending coronary artery, while Figure 23–38B depicts the relationship between α and myocardial blood flow determined by radiolabeled microspheres. As predicted, the latter relationship is close and linear. In contrast, the relationship between peak video intensity and myocardial blood flow is nonlinear (Fig. 23–38C). At flow rates >1.0 ml/min/g, video intensity decreases as flow increases. This paradoxic decrease in peak intensity at higher flow rates may be due to an increase in destructive interference at higher bubble concentrations.[80]

Although the correlation between α and myocardial blood flow was excellent in individual experiments, when data from all the experiments were pooled, the correlation was no longer observed. This lack of correlation between α and myocardial blood flow when pooled data were examined can be explained on the basis of differences in the input function (Fig. 23–39). When contrast was injected subselectively into the left circumflex artery at each stage (Fig. 23–39A), flow through the myocardium was proportional to flow through the artery, and the width of the bolus in the artery (input function) was always proportional to the width of the time-intensity plot obtained from the myocardium (output function).

In contrast, in the second model (left main coronary artery injection), the relative flow to the myocardium supplied by the left anterior descending coronary artery may have been identical in different experiments (Fig. 23–39B), but flow in the left main artery may have varied widely. Variation in the flow in the left main artery could cause the width of the bolus in the left main artery (input function) to vary. As already discussed, the output function (time-intensity plot derived from the myocardium)

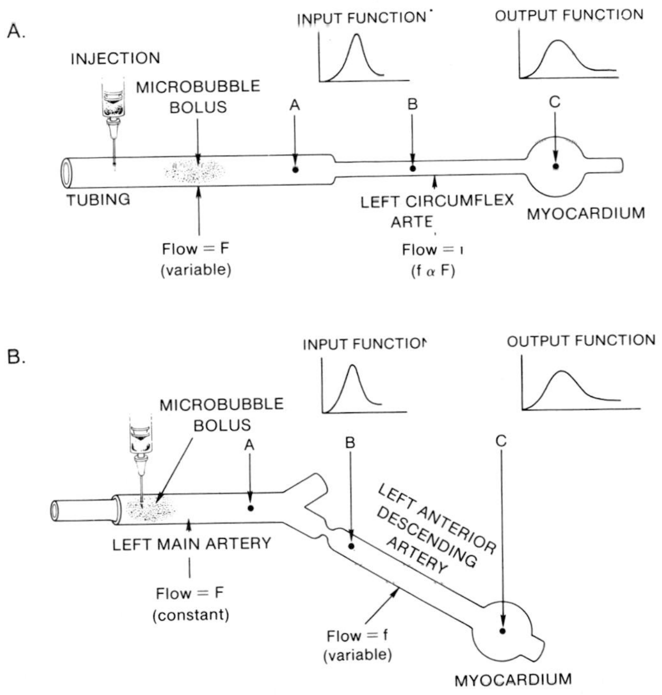

Fig. 23–39. The differences between subselective **(A)** and selective **(B)** coronary injection of contrast agent and its effects on time-intensity curves. (See text for details.) (From Kaul S, et al.: Assessment of regional myocardial blood flow with myocardial contrast two-dimensional echocardiography. J Am Coll Cardiol 13:468, 1989. Reprinted with permission from the American College of Cardiology.)

is influenced both by myocardial blood flow and by the input function (Fig. 23–30); therefore, pooled data (where the input function from different experiments varies) may fail to show a correlation between α and myocardial blood flow. These results suggest that when contrast is injected into the left main coronary artery, it may not be feasible to measure absolute myocardial blood flow, although relative blood flow from different myocardial beds can still be determined.

Assessment of Coronary Blood Flow Reserve

As previously described and illustrated in Figure 23–31, parameters that measure the rate of turnover of an intravascular tracer will accurately represent changes in flow only as long as the vascular volume into which they are injected remains constant. Vasoactive drugs such as papaverine and dipyridamole can significantly alter vascular volume at the same time as they change blood flow. Consequently, when these agents are used, the transit rate of microbubbles through the myocardium may not reflect myocardial blood flow unless correction for changes in vascular volume are also made.

From the model in Figure 23–32, it should be apparent that if the amount of tracer injected into reservoir a remains constant, but the flow through it is increased, flow to all the smaller reservoirs attached to it will also increase. When this occurs, the area under the curves will be the same, but the width of the curves will decrease. Thus, in patients with normal coronary arteries, intracoronary injection of papaverine[81] produced changes in the contrast transit rates in the left anterior descending arterial bed, which correlated linearly with changes in blood flow velocity measured by a Doppler probe in the artery.

The results differ when coronary stenoses are present. Figure 23–40, e.g., illustrates short axis views from a canine left ventricle in a model in which a critical stenosis has been created in the left circumflex coronary artery.[82] Figure 23–40A is a baseline recording before the intracoronary injection of papaverine or contrast. In Figure 23–40B, recorded at the same level after the injection of contrast but not papaverine, there is homogenous opacification of the entire heart, indicating normal blood flow at rest despite a critical stenosis. Figure 23–40C, recorded after injection of both papaverine and contrast, illustrates an obvious decrease in relative opacification of the circumflex territory. This differential opacification permits the areas supplied by the two arteries (indicated by arrows) to be differentiated and quantitated.

Figure 23–41 depicts the contrast time-intensity curves derived from the left anterior descending coronary artery and left circumflex arterial beds before and after the injection of papaverine in the same model of coronary stenosis. The areas under the curves from both perfusion territories are similar before the injection of papaverine. After papaverine injection, however, the area under the curve from the left circumflex bed is significantly smaller than that from the left anterior descending arterial bed. Figure 23–42 illustrates an excellent relationship between the ratio of the areas under the curves from the two beds compared to the ratio of myocardial blood flow in the two beds using radiolabeled microspheres before and after papaverine. This relationship is apparent only when the ratios are compared; when absolute values are compared, the correlation is poor. These data imply that, despite papaverine-induced changes in vascular volume, the ratio of the areas under the time-intensity curves from different perfusion beds corresponds to the relative differences in blood flow, and thus there is no need to correct for vas-

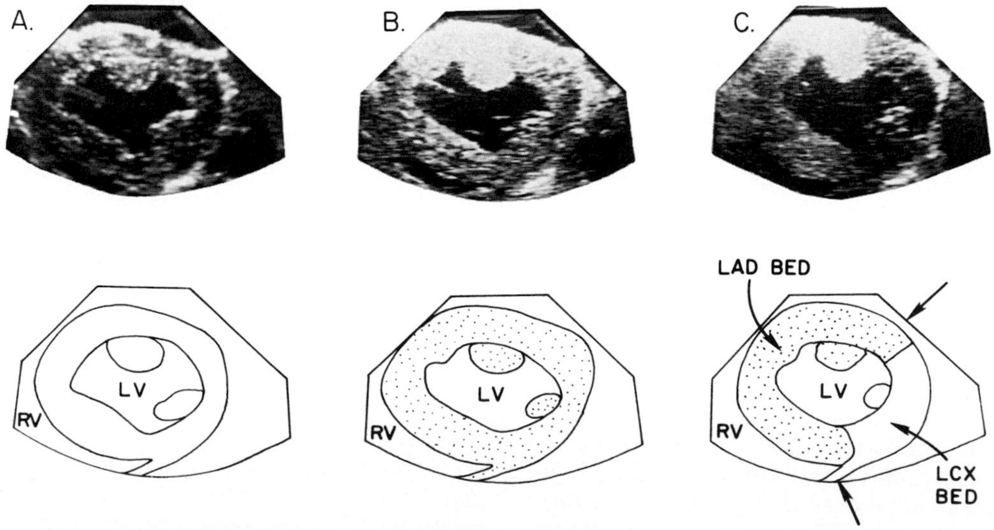

Fig. 23–40. A. Two-dimensional echocardiograms after placement of critical stenosis but before injection of contrast agent. **B.** After injection of contrast alone, showing homogenous opacification of the entire left ventricular myocardium. **C.** After injection of both papaverine and contrast, showing significantly greater opacification in the left anterior descending arterial (LAD) bed. The size of the less opacified left circumflex (LCX) bed (indicated by arrows) can be easily measured. (See text for details.) LV = left ventricle; RV = right ventricle. (From Keller MW, Glasheen W, Gear A, Kaul S: Myocardial contrast echocardiography in humans. II Assessment of coronal blood flow reserve. J Am Coll Cardiol 12:924, 1988. Reprinted with permission from the American College of Cardiology.)

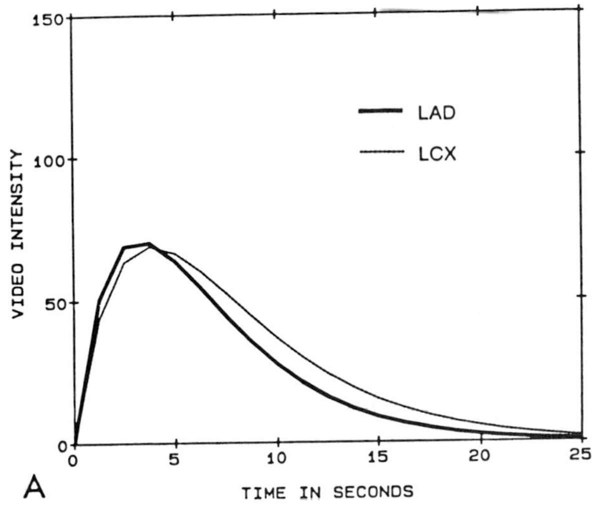

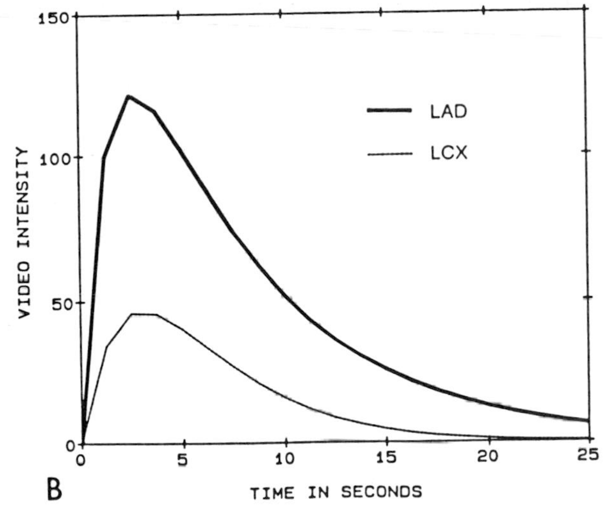

Fig. 23–41. **A.** The time-intensity curves from the left anterior descending (LAD) and left circumflex (LCX) arterial beds before intracoronary injection of papaverine and sonicated renografin. **B.** The same area after injection. (See text for details.) (From Keller MW, Glasheen W, Gear A, Kaul S: Myocardial contrast echocardiography in humans. II-Assessment of coronary blood flow reserve. J Am Coll Cardiol 12:924, 1988. Reprinted with permission of the American College of Cardiology.)

cular volume. It should be remembered, however, that with pharmacologic vasodilators, flow increases only as a result of increase in volume.[83]

These data presented above can be explained as follows: At baseline (with critical stenosis), if flow to the left anterior descending and left circumflex arterial beds is the same, then the number of bubbles traveling down the two arteries will also be the same. Thus, if 100 bubbles are injected into the left main artery, 50 will go down the left circumflex artery, and 50 will travel down the left anterior descending artery. When papaverine is injected, the left anterior descending arterial flow increases by approximately four times, while that in the left circumflex bed does not change. Now, if 100 bubbles

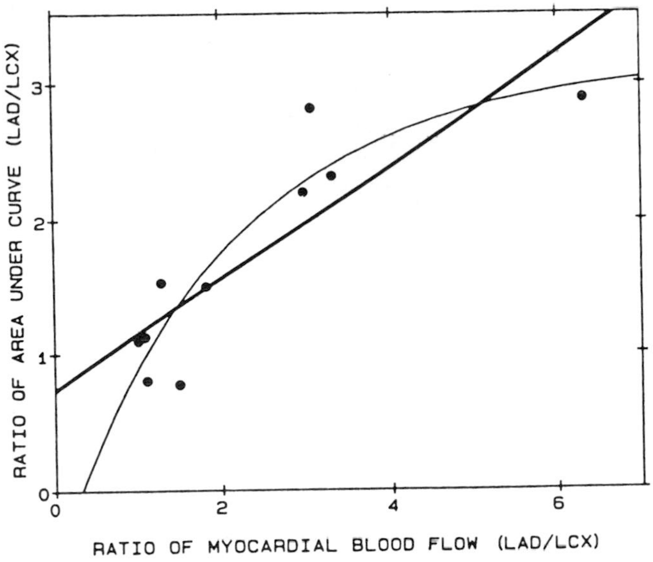

Fig. 23–42. The relationship between the ratio of the areas under the curves derived from the left anterior descending (LAD) and left circumflex (LCX) arterial beds after injection of papaverine, versus the ratio of the blood flow measured in these beds using radiolabeled microspheres. (See text for details.) (From Keller MW, Glasheen W, Gear A, Kaul S: Myocardial contrast echocardiography in humans. II-Assessment of coronary blood flow reserve. J Am Coll Cardiol 12:924, 1988. Reprinted with permission from the American College of Cardiology.)

are injected into the left main artery, 80 will go down the left anterior descending artery, and 20 will go down the left circumflex artery. The ratio of the number of bubbles going down the two arteries, therefore, will be proportional to the ratio of the flow to the two beds. This will occur despite changes in tissue volume induced by paraverine. Because the ratio of the areas under the curves is proportional to the ratio of the total number of bubbles going down both arteries, this ratio is a good indicator of relative blood flow reserve. For absolute changes in blood flow reserve within a single bed, however, MCE cannot be used without correcting for changes in blood volume. (Note: these results are based on knowledge of the absolute number of bubbles injected and differ from those in Fig. 23–37, where the number of bubbles in the injectate was not controlled.)

Coronary blood flow reserve has also been assessed in humans before and following coronary angioplasty.[82,83] Figure 23–43 is an apical short axis recording of the left ventricle from a patient with mid left anterior descending arterial stenosis. Figure 23–43A was recorded at baseline before contrast injection, while Figure 23–43B is a similar recording after contrast injection. Despite a significant left anterior descending arterial stenosis, there is homogeneous opacification of the entire myocardium. After intracoronary injection of papaverine, however, relatively less contrast is apparent in the left anterior descending bed compared to that received by the left circumflex bed (stippled and indicated by arrows in Figure 23–43C). This difference in coronary flow reserve indicates the presence of the critical stenosis in the left anterior descending artery.

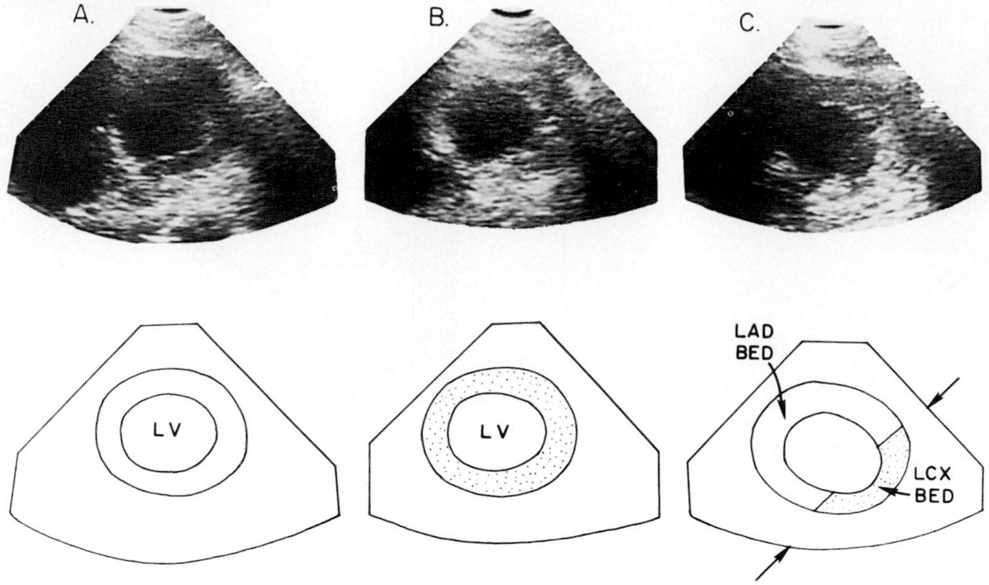

Fig. 23–43. Apical short axis views in a patient with a mid left anterior descending arterial stenosis. **A.** Before injection of contrast agent. **B.** After injection of contrast agent, showing homogeneous opacification of the left ventricular myocardium. **C.** After injection of contrast agent, 45 seconds after intracoronary injection of 9 mg of papaverine hydrochloride showing much greater opacification in the left circumflex (LCX) bed (indicated by arrows and stippling in the accompanying drawing) compared to the left anterior descending arterial (LAD) bed. (See text for details.) LV = left ventricle. (From Keller MW, Glasheen W, Gear A, Kaul S: Myocardial contrast echocardiography in humans. II-Assessment of coronary blood flow reserve. J Am Coll Cardiol 12:924, 1988. Reprinted with permission from the American College of Cardiology.)

Endocardial Versus Epicardial Blood Flow

Although data from several laboratories demonstrate that MCE can reliably assess mean transmural blood flow, there is controversy regarding the ability of this technique to detect differences in the transmural distribution of flow in the ischemic myocardium. A study using hand-agitated Urografin-76 with microbubbles large enough to be trapped in the arterioles[84] showed that during pacing-induced myocardial ischemia, the video intensity in the endocardial bed was less than that noted in the epicardial bed.[85] Unfortunately, this study, performed in humans, provided no independent confirmation of regional myocardial blood flow. Another group has reported that video intensity within the endocardium during MCE decreases after intracoronary injection of papaverine in a canine model of critical coronary artery stenosis in parallel with a decrease in the radiolabeled microsphere-derived endocardial/epicardial ratio.[86] Detailed studies using several models of myocardial ischemia without associated infarction, however, have failed to confirm these observations.[87]

Figure 23–44 illustrates end-diastolic echocardiographic frames from a dog following contrast injection at baseline (Fig. 23–44A) and following creation of a severe left anterior descending artery stenosis (Fig. 23–44B). During the period of severe stenosis, the myocardium supplied by the left anterior descending artery appears thin and the contrast effect appears homogeneously diminished across the bed. Figure 23–44C and D depict time-intensity curves from the endocardium and epicardium during baseline and left anterior descending artery stenosis, respectively. Whereas the peak intensity and the area under the curve are diminished during left anterior descending artery stenosis, the decrease is equal for both the epicardium and endocardium. This lack of differential change in contrast effect occurred despite a 32% decrease in the endocardial/epicardial blood flow ratio measured using radiolabeled microspheres (from 1.1 at baseline to 0.75 during severe left anterior descending artery stenosis).

The earlier observations of differential contrast opacification of the endocardium could, in part, be explained by endocardial attenuation in the left anterior descending arterial bed, which can occur when excessive contrast is injected into the coronary circulation. This is particularly likely when hand agitation is used to prepare bubbles, because the bubble size and number cannot be standardized. Figure 23–45A is an echocardiographic image of the left anterior descending arterial bed at a depth setting of 4 cm before contrast injection. Figure 23–45B shows endocardial attenuation that occurred when a large number of microbubbles were intentionally injected into the left anterior descending artery during entirely normal flow. This effect usually dissipates after a few cardiac cycles (Fig. 23–45C). When a smaller number of bubbles was injected at the same flow rate, endocardial attenuation was not seen (Fig. 23–45D).

Figure 23–46 suggests several additional reasons why MCE, which can accurately assess mean myocardial blood flow, may fail to define the transmural distribution of flow. The first is related to tissue sampling (Fig. 23–46A). Radiolabeled microspheres lodge in precapillary arterioles, while microbubbles traverse the capillaries and venules. The venules in the epicardium also drain endocardial capillaries. Likewise, although not illustrated in this figure, the venules in the endocardium partially drain the epicardial capillaries.[88] Because of this flow pattern, "contamination" of the epicardial and endocardial images can result from microbubbles (unlike

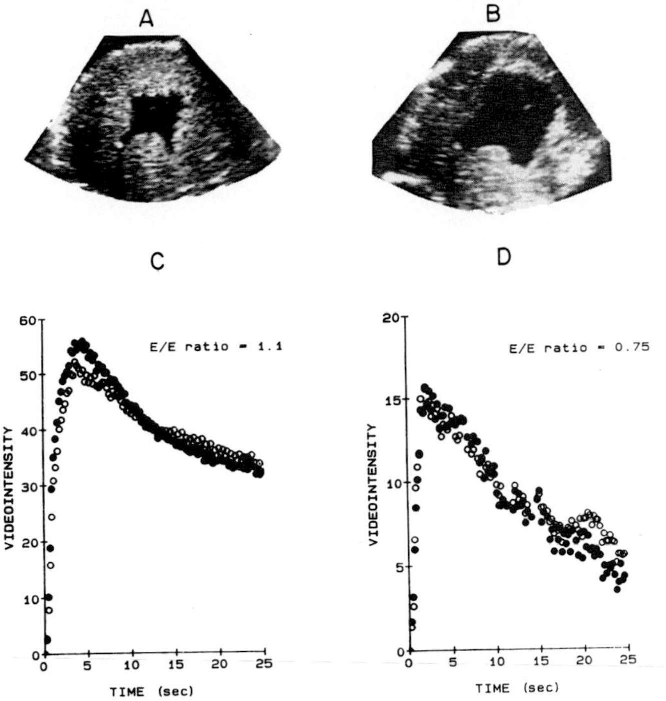

Fig. 23–44. Contrast echocardiographic data from the left anterior descending arterial bed in a dog. **A.** Short axis view of the heart during peak contrast effect following injection of sonicated albumin microbubbles before the creation of a severe left anterior descending artery stenosis. **B.** The same view after creation of stenosis. **C** and **D.** Endocardial and epicardial time-intensity plots obtained at these two stages. **C.** Data correspond to echocardiograms depicted in **A,** where the endocardial to epicardial (E/E) ratio is 1.1. **D.** Data correspond to echocardiograms in **B,** where the ratio is 0.75. (See text for details). The filled circles denote data from the epicardial bed. The open circles denote data from the endocardial bed. See text for details. (From Kaul S, et al.: Myocardial contrast echocardiography and the transmural distribution of flow: A critical appraisal during myocardial ischemia not associated with Infarction. J Am Coll Cardiol 20:1005, 1992. Reprinted with permission of the American College of Cardiology.)

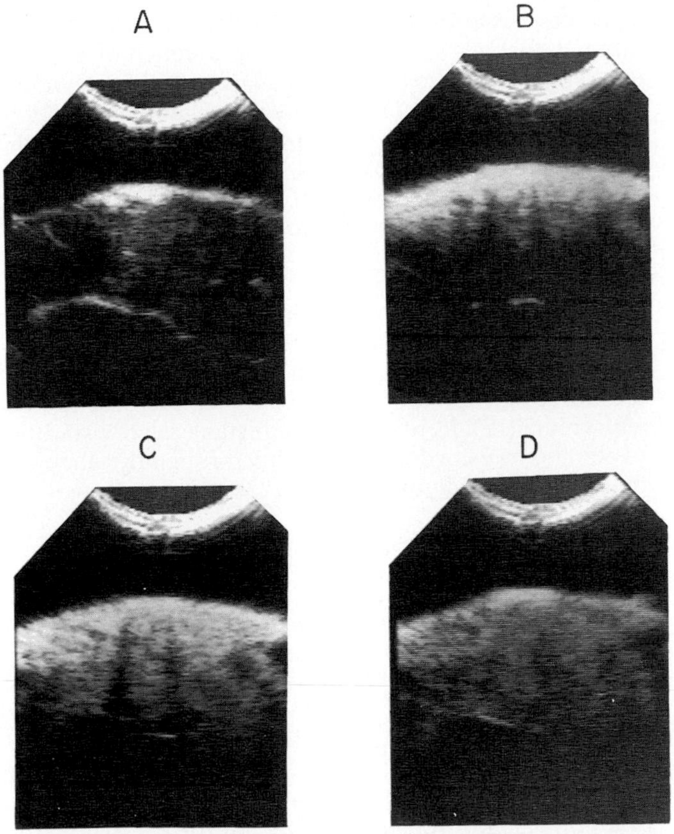

Fig. 23–45. The effect of the amount of contrast agent injected into the coronary circulation during normal blood flow. **A.** The left anterior descending arterial bed imaged at a depth setting of 4 cm before injection of contrast. **B.** An end-diastolic frame immediately after the intentional injection of a large number of microbubbles. Endocardial attenuation is noted. **C.** An end-diastolic frame five cardiac cycles later. The endocardial attenuation has dissipated. **D.** An end-diastolic frame immediately following intracoronary injection of one-third the amount of contrast that was injected in B. (See text for details.) (From Kaul et al.: Myocardial contrast echocardiography and the transmural distribution of flow: A critical appraisal during myocardial ischemia not associated with infarction. J Am Coll Cardiol 20:1005, 1992. Reprinted with permission of the American College of Cardiology.)

the microspheres) traversing regions of the myocardium that they do not initially enter.

The second mechanism deals with bubble "cross-talk." Small microbubbles, unlike large interfaces (represented by the large bubble in Fig. 23–46B), are not reflectors but scatterers of ultrasound.[89] After the injection of microbubbles, thousands of scatterers (depicted as small circles in Fig. 23–46B) are present in the myocardium. Backscatter from one microbubble necessarily interacts with the backscatter from its neighbors, producing fluctuation in the diffraction pattern from otherwise homogeneously perfused region. Of more importance, internal reflections of sound from one bubble to the next can delay the returning signal, producing reverberations that displace signals beyond the depth of origin.

A third mechanism relates to the signal/noise characteristics of the analysis method. As more discrete areas of myocardium are analyzed, the sample size must decrease, and the statistical variability in the data will, of necessity, increase. This makes it much more difficult to define subtle differences such as those between the endocardium and epicardium, than those between perfu-

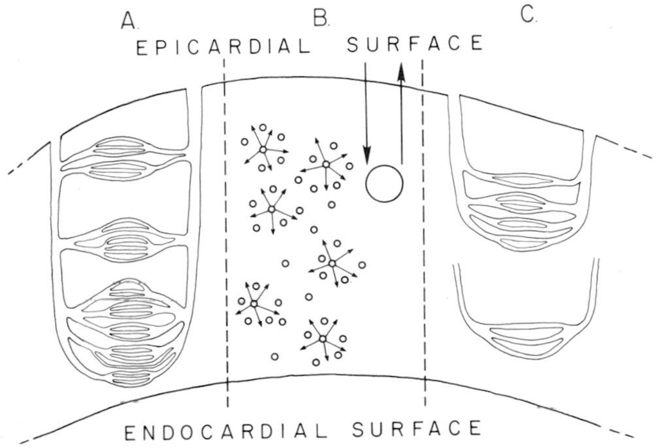

Fig. 23–46. The proposed mechanisms for the inability of myocardial contrast echocardiography to assess the transmural distribution of myocardial blood flow. (See text for details.) (From Kaul et al.: Myocardial contrast echocardiography and the transmural distribution of flow: A critical appraisal during myocardial ischemia not associated with infarction. J Am Coll Cardiol 20:1005, 1992. Reprinted with permission of the American College of Cardiology.)

sion beds. The final mechanism relates to flow-volume interactions. As stated earlier, the kinetics of a tracer are related to both flow and volume. If the volume is constant, the transit of the tracer is related inversely to flow. If the volume changes, transit of the tracer can no longer be related to flow unless an appropriate correction is introduced to account for the volume change. During ischemia, the endocardial flow falls disproportionately relative to the epicardial flow, and it is likely that the endocardial blood volume also decreases because fewer capillaries remain open, which is due to both lower distending pressure and increased myocardial pressure (resulting from increased intracavitary pressure, Fig. 23–46C).[90] This parallel decrease in flow and volume could result in a constant relationship between the transit of microbubbles through the endocardium and epicardium.

Intraoperative Quantification of Myocardial Perfusion

The washout of contrast during cardioplegia is much slower than with blood perfusion. Figure 23–47 illustrates two time-intensity curves at the same myocardial blood flow rate (1.1 ml/min/g). One is from a blood-perfused beating heart, and the other is from a cardioplegia-perfused arrested heart. Although the slower wash-in in the latter situation can be explained by a slower input function, the slower washout of contrast during cardioplegia delivery is related to adherence of the bubbles to the vascular endothelium (mostly the veins), which is not seen during normal blood perfusion[91] and is related to endothelial hypoxia occurring in the absence of blood.

During cardioplegia delivery, therefore, albumin microbubbles do not behave like true intravascular tracers that readily pass through the microcirculation and exhibit a curve of a γ-variate form (curve 1 in Fig. 23–48). They also do not exhibit characteristics of an indicator that is completely entrapped within the microcirculation, as are radiolabeled microspheres. In the latter situation, the time-intensity curve would resemble curve 3 in Figure 23–48, which is proportional to the integral of curve 1. Instead, the time-intensity curves exhibit a mixed behavior akin to curve 2 in Figure 23–48. Despite adherence of bubbles to the endothelium, their influx into the myocardium should be unimpeded. Consequently, parameters that reflect the total flow to the myocardium such as the initial area under the curve and those that reflect the "wash-in" of contrast to the myocardium, such as the initial slope and the slope at 1 second, should show a good correlation with cardioplegia flow. However, because of bubble adherence to the vascular endothelium, the "wash-out" parameters should not correlate with flow.

Therefore, unlike the situation in the beating heart, where the wash-in and wash-out of contrast are obligatorily related, during cardioplegia perfusion, these two aspects of the time-intensity curve are not related to each other in a predictable manner. For this reason, the wash-in and wash-out parameters must be assessed separately. This is best achieved when a general exponential function $f(t) = Ce^{-\alpha t} + De^{-\beta t}$ is applied to the data (Fig. 23–49), where C, D, α, and β are descriptors of the cure, and t is time in seconds.[81] Using these descriptors, the slope of the curve at time t and the initial slope of the curve can be calculated by differentiating f(t) with respect to t: $f't = -\alpha Ce^{-\alpha t} - \beta De^{\beta t}$. Time-to-peak height can be calculated by using the following equation:

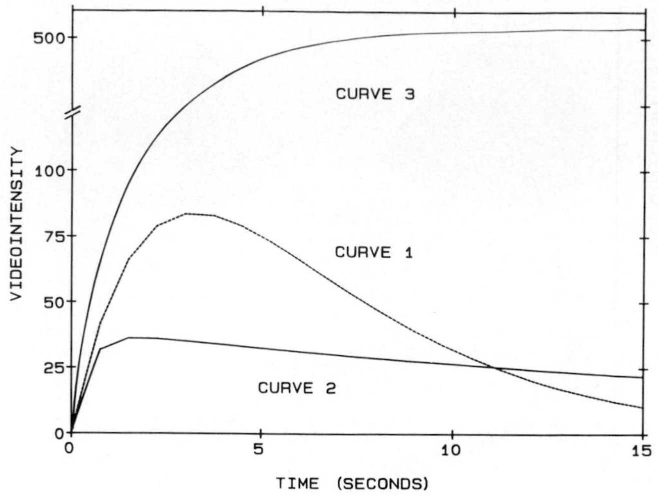

Fig. 23–48. The behavior of microbubbles within the myocardium during cardioplegia delivery (curve 2), compared to an ideal intravascular tracer that travels unimpeded through the myocardium (curve 1) and another tracer that becomes completely entrapped within the myocardium (curve 3). (From Keller MW, et al.: Intraoperative assessment of myocardial perfusion using quantitative myocardial contrast echocardiography: an experimental evaluation. J Am Coll Cardiol 16:1267, 1990. Reprinted with permission from the American College of Cardiology.)

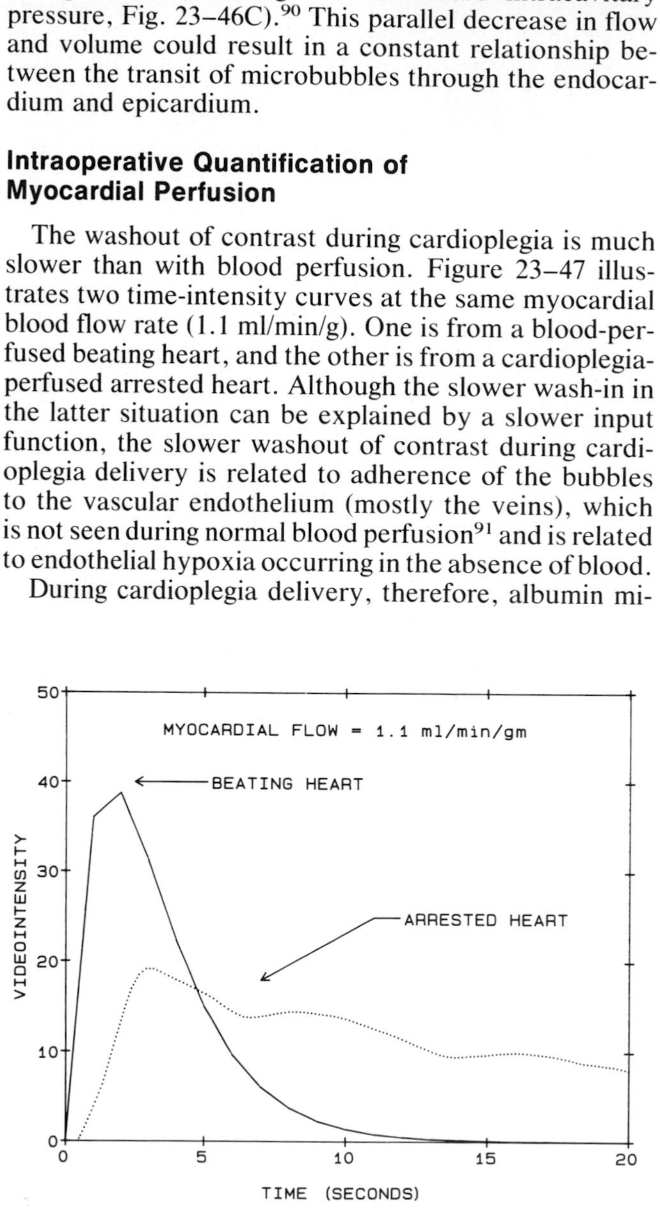

Fig. 23–47. Time-intensity curves from the blood-perfused beating heart and from a cardioplegia-perfused arrested heart at the same flow rate (1.1 ml/min/g). Note the delayed washout of contrast from the cardioplegia-arrested heart compared to the blood perfused beating heart. (See text for details.) (From Keller MW, et al.: Intraoperative assessment of myocardial perfusion using quantitative myocardial contrast echocardiography: an experimental evaluation. J Am Coll Cardiol 16:1267, 1990. Reprinted with permission from the American College of Cardiology.)

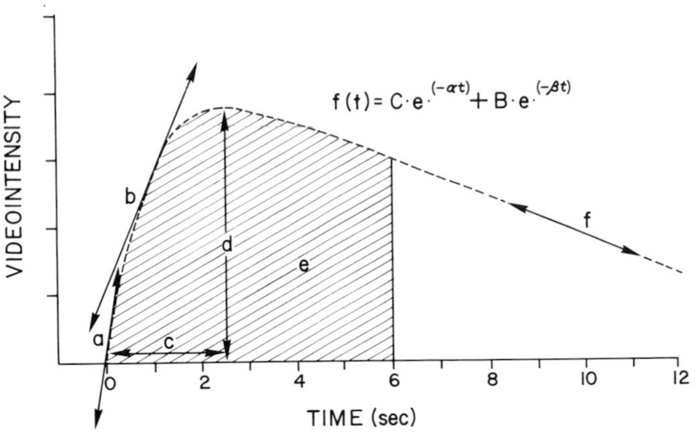

Fig. 23–49. Parameters of the time-intensity curves that are generated after a general exponential fit is applied to echocardiographic data obtained from a cardioplegia-arrested heart. a = initial slope of the curve; b = slope of the curve at 1 second (both denoting appearance of contrast in the myocardium); d = peak contrast effect; e = area under the curve (both denoting total number of bubbles entering the myocardium); f = slope of curve at 10 seconds (denoting washout of contrast from the myocardium). (From Keller MW, et al.: Intraoperative assessment of myocardial perfusion using quantitative myocardial contrast echocardiography: an experimental evaluation. J Am Coll Cardiol 16:1267, 1990. Reprinted with permission from the American College of Cardiology.)

$\mathrm{Ln}(\beta D/\alpha C)/\beta - \alpha$. The peak height of the curve can be calculated by solving f(t) at the time-to-peak height. The area under the curve at time t can be derived from the integral of f(t) with respect to time t using the following equation: $(C/\alpha)(1 - e^{-\alpha t}) + (D/\beta)(1 - e^{-\beta t})$. All these parameters are depicted in Figure 23–49.

In canine experiments performed in a model of graded left anterior descending artery stenosis, cardioplegia was introduced into the aortic root at a constant flow rate. The aorta was cross-clamped at the same site at each stage to provide a constant mixing volume. After 1 minute, when the heart had been arrested, sonicated albumin microbubbles were injected into the aortic root through the cardioplegia line. The degree of contrast opacification seen in the left anterior descending arterial bed varied with the degree of stenosis.[92] Examples of contrast echocardiograms recorded at three different degrees of stenosis are illustrated in Figure 23–50.

Time-intensity curves from one experiment at six different degrees of left anterior descending coronary arterial stenosis are shown in Figure 23–51. It can be appreciated that the higher the flow, the steeper the contrast appearance slopes, the greater the peak of the curve, and the larger the area under the curve. Figure 23–52 illustrates the correlation between myocardial flow and the initial area under the curve for the six time-intensity curves shown in Figure 23–51. Peak curve height demonstrated a good correlation with myocardial flow for individual animals, as did wash-in parameters such as the initial slope and the slope at 1 second. As expected, wash-out parameters such as the slope at 10 seconds did not correlate as well with flow.

Because the time-intensity curves from the myocardium (output function) are influenced not only by myocardial flow but also by the input function, the cardioplegia delivery rate into the aorta and the method of contrast injection are important. Although the cross-clamped aortic volume was constant in each dog, it varied between dogs. The volume of cardioplegia with which the bolus of microbubbles mixed in the aortic root, therefore, was not the same in all dogs. This difference between dogs resulted in varying rates of contrast washout from the aorta and, hence, different input functions. Thus, while there was an excellent correlation between myocardial flow and the parameters of the time-intensity curves in individual experiments (where the aorta was always cross-clamped at the same site and did not alter in size between different stages), pooled data did not yield as good a correlation.[92]

The rate of injection of contrast may have a significant effect on the measurements of regional perfusion, which is important when comparing serial changes in perfusion in a given patient. The method of injection should, therefore, be similar in every patient. Time-intensity curves from the aortic root during cardioplegia delivery by bolus injection using a power injector and by continuous infusion using an infusion pump are shown in Figure 23–53. Although these curves clearly differ, both methods provide good independent correlations between MCE-measured regional perfusion and that estimated using radiolabeled microspheres as long as the method of injection remains consistent.[92]

Intraoperative MCE has been found to be successful

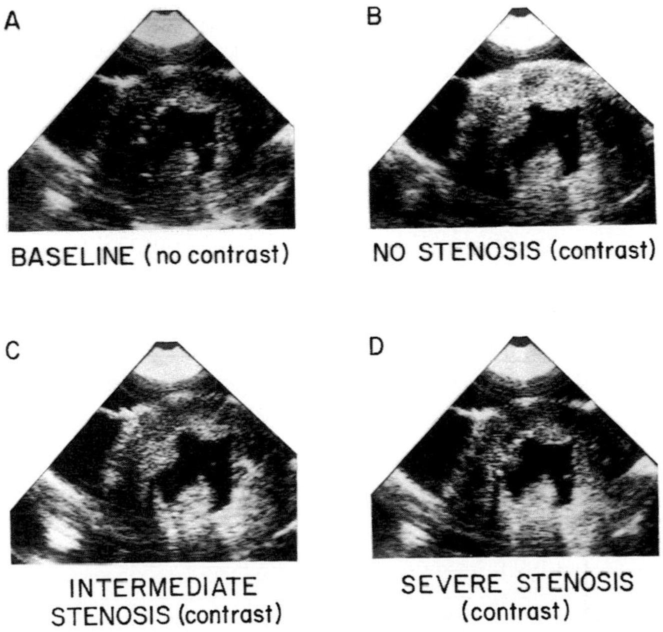

Fig. 23–50. Images obtained intraoperatively during cardioplegia delivery. **A.** At baseline before contrast injection. **B.** At baseline after contrast injection. **C.** After contrast injection in the presence of an intermediate left anterior descending arterial stenosis. **D.** After contrast injection in the presence of a severe left anterior descending artery stenosis. (See text for details.) (From Keller MW, et al.: Intraoperative assessment of myocardial perfusion using quantitative myocardial contrast echocardiography: an experimental evaluation. J Am Coll Cardiol 16:1267, 1990. Reprinted with permission from the American College of Cardiology.)

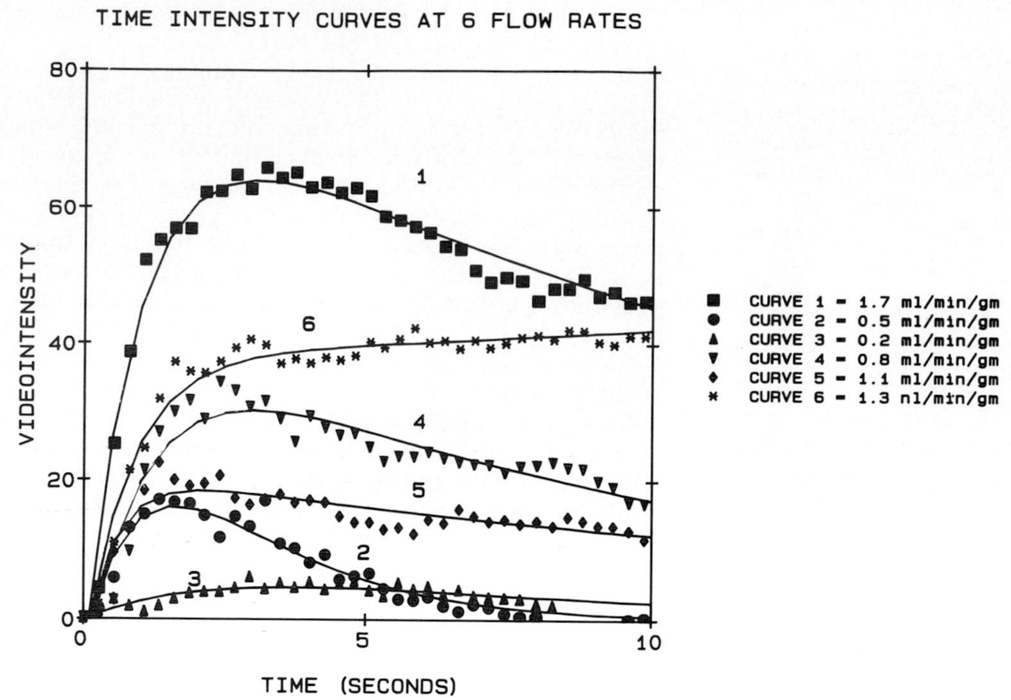

Fig. 23–51. Time-intensity curves generated from the left anterior descending arterial bed at six different flow rates through the left anterior descending coronary artery. Contrast agent was injected at each stage into the cross-clamped aortic root during time of cardioplegia delivery. (See text for details.) (From Keller MW, et al.: Intraoperative assessment of myocardial perfusion using quantitative myocardial contrast echocardiography: An experimental evaluation. J Am Coll Cardiol 16:1267, 1990. Reprinted with permission from the American College of Cardiology.)

for the comparison of myocardial perfusion before and after bypass graft placement.[34,63,65] Although to date, most data have been acquired by intraoperative epicardial recordings, similar information can be obtained using the transesophageal approach.

Measurement of myocardial perfusion can be performed on-line in the operating room using microcomputers.[74,93] Multiple regions of interest can be placed over the myocardium before injection of contrast with the transducer held constant until contrast disappears completely. Because the heart is arrested during cardioplegia delivery, there is no need for image alignment (a computer-intensive technique). A frame grabber is used to capture images from which average video intensity within myocardial regions of interest is calculated. This process is repeated for all images in real-time, and the video intensity data are stored in a file. Background (average video intensity in the regions of interest before the appearance of contrast) is subtracted from each video-in-

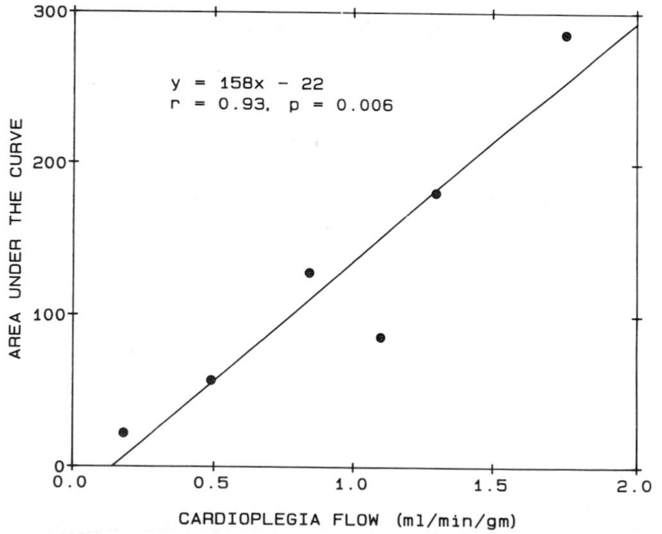

Fig. 23–52. The relationship between the areas under the curves shown in Figure 23–51 and radiolabeled microsphere-measured cardioplegia flow rates through the myocardium during the same stages. (See text for details.) (From Keller MW, et al.: Intraoperative assessment of myocardial perfusion using quantitative myocardial contrast echocardiography: An experimental evaluation. J Am Coll Cardiol 16:1267, 1990. Reprinted with permission from the American College of Cardiology.)

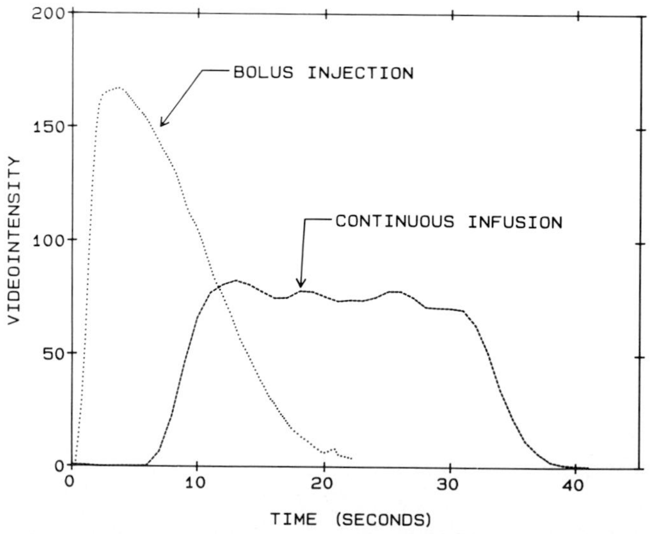

Fig. 23–53. Time-intensity curves obtained from the cross-clamped aortic root during bolus injection and during continuous infusion. The two curves are dissimilar. (See text for details.) (From Keller MW, et al.: Intraoperative assessment of myocardial perfusion using quantitative myocardial contrast echocardiography: An experimental evaluation. J Am Coll Cardiol 16:1267, 1990. Reprinted with permission from the American College of Cardiology.)

tensity value, and background-subtracted time-intensity plots are generated. An exponential function (discussed previously) is applied to the plots, and parameters of the curves are automatically calculated. Prebypass and postbypass curves along with the derived parameters are simultaneously displayed and compared. The entire system is placed on a mobile cart, which can be conveniently located in close proximity to an ultrasound system.

Quantification of Myocardial Blood Flow Using Systemic Venous Contrast Injections

One of the ultimate goals of MCE is to be able to assess region myocardial flow following systemic venous injection. Experience with myocardial opacification following right-sided contrast injections is currently limited to animal studies. Figure 23–54 is an example of a time-intensity curve obtained from the anterior myocardium of a dog in whom contrast was injected into the right atrium.[71] The time-intensity curve is not particularly noisy and has a γ-variate form. Because the contrast is injected into the right heart, the situation can be likened to the model in Figure 23–29 with the injection chamber (reservoir "a") being the right atrium. In this situation, the connection between reservoirs "a" and "b" is long allowing the bolus to spread as it enters the left heart. As a result, the myocardial transit time of the bubbles may be shorter than the bolus length, making it difficult to analyze the transit rate from the myocardium. Furthermore, the width of the curve shown in Figure 23–54 is much smaller than the duration of left ventricular opacification. This occurs because of the limited sensitivity of current echocardiographic instruments, which can detect myocardial activity only when the number of microbubbles within the myocardium exceeds a critical value. Thus, although feasibility has been demonstrated, much work is necessary before this can be translated into a useful clinical tool.

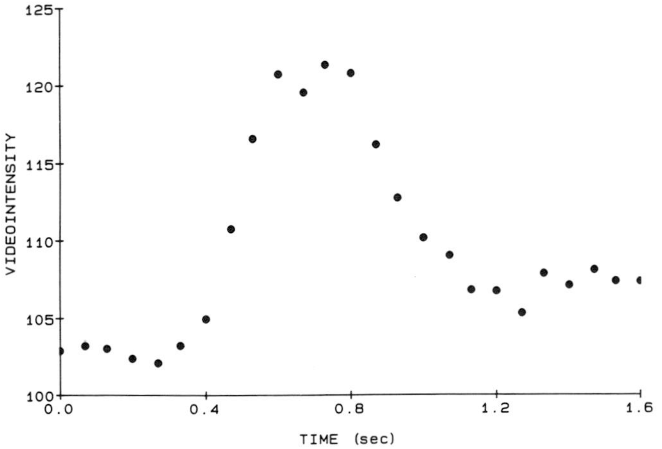

Fig. 23–54. A time-intensity curve obtained from the anterior myocardium after a right atrial injection of contrast agent in a dog. This curve corresponds to data depicted in Figures 23–26 and 23–27. (See text for details.) (Reprinted from Villanueva FS: Successful and reproducible myocardial opacification during two-dimensional echocardiography from right heart injection of contrast. Circulation 85:1557, 1992, with permission of the American Heart Association.)

Limitations of Myocardial Contrast Echocardiography for Quantification of Myocardial Perfusion

Despite the large amount of data acquired and the insights gained from MCE, three factors currently limit the potential of the technique to accurately measure myocardial flow. The limitations are related to the design features of current echocardiographic equipment, the nature of available contrast agents, and the physics of ultrasound.

The analog output of the ultrasound system that forms the basis for generating the time-intensity curve bears little resemblance to the echo amplitudes actually received by the transducer. To produce a visually pleasing image, current systems process the received signal and, in so doing, markedly alter it. Amplitude compression results in a significant loss of dynamic range. Furthermore, translation of this compressed echo signal into video gray levels is nonlinear. To accurately display time-intensity data, these distortions of the echo intensities actually received by the transducer will need to be reduced, and direct digital acquisition will be required. Furthermore, to improve the sensitivity of the system to detect smaller changes in signal (especially following transpulmonary myocardial opacification), a broad dynamic range (theoretically, on the order of 120 dB) will be required. Systems with greater dynamic range are currently in the developmental stages, but it remains to be seen how they will influence the acquisition and processing of echo data. Interest has also been demonstrated in acquiring raw radio frequency data for analysis of time-intensity curves.[94–96] Although theoretically very attractive, because of costs related to redesigning the machines and the need to use powerful computers to reduce the radio frequency data obtained in an entire imaging sequence, this approach is still futuristic.

The time-intensity curves are also affected by the composition of available contrast agents. If the microbubbles are too large to pass readily through the capillaries, the time-intensity plots will not resemble a γ-variate function. If the bubbles disrupt or coalesce during myocardial transit, they will distort the shape of the curves. Additionally, the concentration of the bubbles needs to be constant. During arterial injections, the injected volume should be small enough to limit far-field myocardial attenuation, while during venous injections, it should be large enough to successfully opacify the left ventricular myocardium.

Regional gray level variation, even of an acoustically homogeneous object, is an inherent feature of ultrasound. This is largely due to absorption and scattering of the ultrasound energy as it traverses tissue, resulting in two problems that are particularly troublesome to MCE—lateral dropout and shadowing. The former has already been discussed in the section relating to risk area assessment. *Acoustic shadowing* refers to the loss of gray level of a target located directly behind another highly reflective object. Thus, during standard precordial or anterior epicardial recording, contrast in the anterior wall can diminish the intensity of signals from the posterior wall. Because echo intensity is inherently nonhomogeneous, determining when this variability is due to a physiologic effect and when it is due to physical interactions within the ultrasonic beam or the signal processing characteristics of the instruments is difficult.

Current and Potential Clinical Applications for the Quantitation of Myocardial Flow

Many of the current applications of MCE have already been discussed. These include detecting residual flow in areas of myocardial ischemia/evolving infarction; assessing coronary blood flow reserve during cardiac catheterization before and after coronary angioplasty to predict improvement in regional function following restoration of patency; and intraoperative demonstration of regional perfusion, success of graft placement to hypoperfused regions, and distribution of cardioplegia.

Obviously, the most important potential clinical applications would be the noninvasive detection and quantification of the extent of coronary artery disease. For this application to become a reality, however, myocardial opacification after a peripheral venous injection of contrast would have to be easily and reproducibly achieved in humans. MCE could also have a role in determining the presence of myocardial hypoperfusion in diseases not affecting the epicardial coronary arteries such as aortic stenosis and hypertrophic cardiomyopathy. In this regard, MCE has the potential to compete with, and eventually replace, other myocardial perfusion imaging techniques.

SUMMARY

MCE is a new technique capable of providing information concerning regional myocardial perfusion in vivo and in real-time. Experimental studies have validated the ability of this technique to assess risk area and regional myocardial blood flow. Initial clinical studies from the cardiac catheterization laboratory and the operating room suggest that it can also be used for the assessment of regional myocardial perfusion in humans. The demonstration that myocardial opacification can be achieved following right atrial injection of contrast in experimental animals raises hopes that this technique can be used clinically following peripheral venous injection of contrast. If this proves to be the case, the technique should find increasing use in the noninvasive assessment of regional myocardial perfusion in patients suspected or known to have coronary artery disease. Further technological advances and clinical studies, however, are required before its clinical utility becomes clear.

REFERENCES

1. DeMaria AN, et al.: Echocardiographic visualization of myocardial perfusion by left heart and intracoronary injection of echo contrast agents (abstr.). Circulation 60(Suppl. 3):III–143, 1980.
2. Kemper A, et al.: Hydrogen peroxide contrast-enhanced two-dimensional echocardiography: real-time in-vivo delineation of regional myocardial perfusion. Circulation 68:603, 1983.
3. Armstrong WF, et al.: Assessment of myocardial perfusion abnormalities with contrast enhanced two-dimensional echocardiography. Circulation 66: 166, 1982.
4. Tei C, et al.: Myocardial contrast echocardiography: a reproducible technique of myocardial opacification for identifying regional perfusion defects. Circulation 67:585, 1983.
5. Kaul S, et al.: Contrast echocardiography in acute myocardial ischemia: I. In-vivo determination of total left ventricular "area at risk." J Am Coll Cardiol 4:1272, 1984.
6. Kaul S, Gillam LD, Weyman AE: Contrast echocardiography in acute myocardial ischemia: II. The effect of site of injection of contrast agent on the estimation of "area at risk" for necrosis after coronary occlusion. J Am Coll Cardiol 6:825, 1985.
7. Gillam LD, et al.: Functional and pathologic effects of multiple echocardiographic contrast injections on the myocardium, brain, and kidneys. J Am Coll Cardiol 6:687, 1985.
8. Albers VM: Underwater Acoustic Handbook. State College, The Pennsylvania State University Press, 1960.
9. Feinstein SB, et al.: Two-dimensional contrast echocardiography: I. In vitro development and quantitative analysis of echo contrast agents. J Am Coll Cardiol 3:14, 1984.
10. Moore CA, Smucker ML, Kaul S: Myocardial contrast echocardiography in humans: I. Safety—a comparison with routine coronary arteriography. J Am Coll Cardiol 8:1066, 1986.
11. Lang RM, et al.: Effects of intracoronary injection of sonicated microbubbles on left ventricular contractility. Am J Cardiol 60:166, 1987.
12. Becher H, et al.: Contrast enhanced color Doppler imaging of left heart chambers—first clinical results. Circulation 82(Suppl. 3):III–95, 1990.
13. Shell WE, Dewood M: Echocardiographic contrast enhancement with solid biodegradable microspheres. Circulation 82(Suppl. 3):III–97, 1990.
14. Keller MW, Glasheen W, Gear A, Kaul S: Myocardial contrast echocardiography without significant hemodynamic effects or reactive hyperemia: a major advantage in the imaging of myocardial perfusion. J Am Coll Cardiol 12:1039, 1987.
15. Reisner SA, et al.: Myocardial perfusion imaging by contrast echocardiography with use of intracoronary sonicated albumin in humans. J Am Coll Cardiol 14:660, 1989.
16. Keller MW, Segal SS, Kaul S, Duling BR: The behavior of sonicated albumin microbubbles in the microcirculation: a basis for their use during myocardial contrast echocardiography. Circ Res 65:458, 1989.
17. Keller MW, Glasheen WP, Kaul S: Albunex®: a safe and effective commercially produced agent for myocardial contrast echocardiography. J Am Soc Echocardiogr 2:48, 1989.
18. Sakamaki T, et al.: Verification of myocardial contrast two-dimensional echocardiographic assessment of perfusion defects in ischemic myocardium. J Am Coll Cardiol 3:34, 1984.
19. Schaper W, Frenzel H, Hort W: Experimental coronary artery occlusion: I. Measurement of infarct size. Basic Res Cardiol 74:46, 1979.
20. Factor SM, Okun EM, Kirk ES: The histological lateral border of acute canine myocardial infarction. A function of microcirculation. Circ Res 48: 640, 1981.
21. Kaul S, et al.: Determination of left ventricular "area at risk" with high-resolution single-photon emission computerized tomography in experimental coronary occlusion. Am Heart J 109:1369, 1985.
22. Kaul S, et al.: The effects of selectively altering the collateral driving pressure on regional perfusion and function in the occluded coronary bed in the dog. Circ Res 61:77, 1987.
23. Kaul S, et al.: Relation between anterograde blood flow through a coronary artery and the size of the perfusion bed it supplies: experimental and clinical implications. J Am Coll Cardiol 17:1403, 1992.
24. Marcus ML: Effects of coronary occlusion on myocardial perfusion. *In* The Coronary Circulation in Health and Disease. New York, McGraw-Hill, p. 221, 1983.
25. Lowe JE, Reimer KA, Jennings RB: Experimental infarct size as the function of the myocardium at risk. Am J Pathol 90:363, 1978.
26. Jugdutt BI, Hutchins GM, Bulkley BH, Becker LC: Myocardial infarction in the conscious dog: three dimensional mapping of infarct, collateral flow, and region at risk. Circulation 60:1141, 1979.
27. Okun EM, Factor SM, Kirk ES: End-capillary loops in the heart: an explanation for discrete myocardial infarctions without border zones. Science 206: 565, 1979.
28. Cohen MV: Morphological considerations of the coronary collateral circulation in man. *In* Coronary Collaterals. Clinical and Experimental Observations. New York, Futura Publishing, p. 1, 1985.
29. Buda AJ, et al.: Myocardial infarct extension: prevalence, clinical significance, and problems in diagnosis. Am Heart J 105:744, 1983.
30. Baker JT, et al.: Myocardial infarct extension: incidence and relationship to survival. Circulation 65:918, 1982.
31. Marmour A, Sobel BE, Roberts E: Factors presaging early recurrent myocardial infarction ("extension"). Am J Cardiol 48:603, 1981.

32. Lesnefsky E, et al.: Influence of severity of remote ischemia on mortality during acute left anterior descending occlusion (abstr.). Circulation 70(Suppl. 2):II–86, 1987.
33. Nishioka T, et al.: Assessment of collateral circulation and myocardial salvage during acute coronary occlusion using myocardial contrast echocardiography. Circulation 82(Suppl. 3):III–26, 1990.
34. Spotnitz WD, et al.: Intra-operative demonstration of coronary collateral flow using myocardial contrast echocardiography. Am J Cardiol 65:1259, 1990.
35. Lim Y, et al.: Coronary collaterals assessed with myocardial contrast echocardiography in healed myocardial infarction. Am J Cardiol 66:556, 1990.
36. Grill HP, et al.: Contrast echocardiographic mapping of collateralized myocardium in humans before and after coronary angioplasty. J Am Coll Cardiol 16:1594, 1990.
37. Sabia PJ, et al. Functional significance of collateral blood flow in patients with recent acute myocardial infarction. A study using myocardial contrast echocardiography. Circulation 85:2080, 1992. Circulation 82(Suppl. 3): III–27, 1990.
38. Sabia PJ, et al.: An association between collateral blood flow and myocardial viability in patients with recent myocardial infarction. N Engl J Med 372: 1825, 1992.
39. Kaul S, et al.: The importance of defining left ventricular area at risk in-vivo during acute myocardial infarction: an experimental evaluation with myocardial contrast two-dimensional echocardiography. Circulation 75: 1249, 1987.
40. Kemper AJ, et al.: In-vivo prediction of the transmural extent of experimental acute myocardial infarction using contrast echocardiography. J Am Coll Cardiol 8:143, 1986.
41. Kemper AJ, et al.: Hydrogen peroxide contrast echocardiography: quantification in vivo of myocardial risk area during coronary occlusion and the necrotic area remaining after myocardial reperfusion. Circulation 70:309, 1984.
42. Kaul S, et al.: Contrast echocardiography in acute myocardial ischemia: III. An in-vivo comparison of the extent of abnormal wall motion with the "area at risk" for necrosis. J Am Coll Cardiol 7:383, 1986.
43. Weyman AE, et al.: Importance of temporal heterogeneity in assessing the contraction abnormalities associated with acute myocardial infarction. Circulation 70:102, 1984.
44. Smucker ML, Beller GA, Watson DD, Kaul S: Left ventricular dysfunction in excess of the size of infarction: a possible management strategy. Am Heart J 115:749, 1988.
45. Force T, et al.: Overestimation of infarct size by quantitative two-dimensional echocardiography: the role of tethering and of analytic procedures. Circulation 73:1360, 1986.
46. Wyatt WH, et al.: Contrasting effects of alterations in ventricular preload and afterload upon systemic hemodynamics, function, and metabolism of ischemic myocardium. Circulation 55:318, 1977.
47. Forrester JS, et al.: Medical therapy of acute myocardial infarction by application of hemodynamic subsets. N Engl J Med 295:1356, 1976.
48. Feiring AJ, et al.: The importance of the determination of the myocardial area at risk in the evaluation of the outcome of acute myocardial infarction. Circulation 74:1186, 1987.
49. Touchstone DA, Nygaard TW, Kaul S: Correlation between left ventricular risk area and clinical, electrocardiographic, hemodynamic, and angiographic variables during acute myocardial infarction. J Am Soc Echocardiogr 3:106, 1990.
50. Hilton CJ, et al.: Inadequate cardioplegia protection with obstructed coronary arteries. Ann Thorac Surg 28:323, 1979.
51. Grondin CM, Helias J, Vouhe PR, Robert P: Influence of a critical coronary artery stenosis on myocardial protection through cold potassium cardioplegia. J Thorac Cardiovasc Surg 82:608, 1981.
52. Rose DM, et al.: Analysis of morbidity and mortality in patients 70 years of age and over undergoing isolated coronary artery bypass surgery. Am Heart J 110:341, 1985.
53. Force T, et al.: Quantitative two-dimensional echocardiographic analysis of regional wall motion in patients with perioperative myocardial infarction. Circulation 70:233, 1984.
54. Burns RJ, et al.: Myocardial infarction determined by technetium-99m pyrophosphate single-photon tomography complicating elective coronary artery bypass grafting for angina pectoris. Am J Cardiol 63:1429, 1989.
55. Vlodaver Z, et al.: Correlation of antemortem coronary arteriogram and postmortem specimen. Circulation 47:162, 1973.
56. Schwartz JN, et al.: Comparison of angiocardiographic and postmortem findings in patients with coronary artery disease. Am J Cardiol 36:174, 1975.
57. Arnett EN, et al.: Coronary artery narrowing in coronary heart disease: comparison of cineangiography and necropsy findings. Ann Intern Med 91: 350, 1979.
58. White CW, et al.: Does the visual interpretation of the coronary angiogram predict the physiologic importance of a coronary stenosis? N Engl J Med 310:819, 1984.
59. Khuri SF, et al.: Intraoperative assessment of the physiologic significance of coronary stenosis in humans. J Thorac Cardiovasc Surg 92:71, 1986.
60. Hiratzka LF, et al.: Intraoperative evaluation of coronary artery bypass graft anatamoses with high frequency epicardial echocardiography: experimental evaluation and initial patient studies. Circulation 73:1199, 1986.
61. Greene ER, Reilly PR, Miranda IP: Doppler echocardiographic assessment of left internal mammary grafts in humans (abstr.). Circulation 74(Suppl. 2):II–308, 1986.
62. Spotnitz WD, et al.: Success of internal mammary bypass grafting can be assessed intraoperatively using myocardial contrast two-dimensional echocardiography. J Am Coll Cardiol 12:196, 1988.
63. Goldman ME, Mindich BP: Intraoperative cardioplegic contrast echocardiography for assessing myocardial perfusion during open heart surgery. J Am Coll Cardiol 4:1029, 1984.
64. Kabas JS, et al.: Evaluation of myocardial perfusion during coronary artery bypass grafting using intra-operative contrast echocardiography. Surgical Forum 39:262, 1988.
65. Matthew TL, Keller MW, Kaul S, Spotnitz WD: Assessment of myocardial perfusion during coronary artery bypass graft operations in humans using myocardial contrast echocardiography. Surgical Forum 40:248, 1989.
66. Villanueva FS, et al.: Intraoperative assessment of the distribution of retrograde cardioplegia using myocardial contrast echocardiography. Surg Forum 41:252, 1990.
67. Villanueva FS, et al.: Assessment of intramyocardial distribution of coronary sinus retrograde cardioplegia using myocardial contrast echocardiography. Circulation 82(Suppl. 3):III–26, 1990.
68. Lechleuthner A, v Ludinghausen M: The functional architecture and clinical significance of the cardiac venous system with special reference to venous valves and Thebesian veins. *In* Mohl W, Faxon D, Wolner E (eds.): Progress in Coronary Sinus Interventions. Darmstadt, Streinkopff Verlag, and New York, Springer-Verlag, p. 33, 1986.
69. Berwing K, Schlepper M: Echocardiographic imaging of the left ventricle by peripheral intravenous injection of echo contrast agent. Am Heart J 115: 399, 1988.
70. Feinstein SB, et al.: Safety and efficacy of a new transpulmonary ultrasound contrast agent: initial multicenter clinical results. J Am Coll Cardiol 16:316, 1990.
71. Villanueva FS, et al.: Successful and reproducible myocardial opacification during two-dimensional echocardiography from right heart injection of contrast. Circulation 85:1557, 1992.
72. Thompson MK, Starmer CF, Whorten RE, McIntosh MD: Indicator transit time considered as a gamma variate. Circ Res 14:502, 1964.
73. Mottley J, et al.: Decay of ultrasound integrated backscatter from a saccharide contrast agent is accelerated by increased pressure. Circulation 82 (Suppl. 3):III–28, 1990.
74. Shandas R, et al.: Persistence of Albunex® (ALB) ultrasound contrast agent: in-vitro study of the effects of pressure and acoustic power on particle size, and the duration of contrast and Doppler effect. Circulation 82(Suppl. 3): III–96, 1990 (abstr.).
75. Jayaweera AR, et al.: Method for the quantitation of myocardial perfusion during myocardial contrast echocardiography. J Am Soc Echo 3:91, 1990.
76. Heyman MA, Payne BD, Hoffman JI, Rudolf AM: Blood flow measurements with radionuclide-labeled particles. Prog Cardiovas Dis 20:55, 1977.
77. Kemper AJ, et al.: Contrast echocardiographic estimation of regional myocardial blood flow after acute coronary occlusion. Circulation 72:1115, 1985.
78. Edwards N, et al.: Myocardial contrast two-dimensional echocardiography can be used to measure myocardial red cell transit time in-vivo. Circulation 82(Suppl. 3):III–96, 1990 (abstr.).
79. Kaul S, et al.: Assessment of regional myocardial blood flow with myocardial contrast two-dimensional echocardiography. J Am Coll Cardiol 13:468, 1989.
80. Powsner SM, Keller MW, Saniie J, Feinstein SB: Quantitation of echo contrast effects. Am J Physiol Imag 1:124, 1986.
81. Porter TR, et al.: Myocardial contrast echocardiography for the assessment of coronary blood flow reserve. Validation in humans. J Am Coll Cardiol 21:349, 1993.
82. Keller MW, et al.: Myocardial contrast echocardiography in humans: II. Assessment of coronary blood flow reserve. J Am Coll Cardiol 12:925, 1988.
83. Kaul S, Jayaweera AR: Myocardial contrast echocardiography has the potential for the assessment of coronary microvascular reserve. J Am Coll Cardiol 21:356, 1993.
84. Cheirif J, et al.: Assessment of myocardial perfusion in humans by myocardial contrast echocardiography: I. Evaluation of regional coronary reserve by peak contrast intensity. J Am Coll Cardiol 11:735, 1988.
85. Lim YJ, et al.: Visualization of subendocardial myocardial ischemia with myocardial contrast echocardiography in humans. Circulation 79:233, 1989.
86. Cheirif J, et al.: Assessment of regional myocardial perfusion by contrast echocardiography: II. Detection of changes in transmural and sub-endocardial perfusion during dipyridamole-induced hyperemia in a model of critical coronary stenosis. J Am Coll Cardiol 14:1555, 1989.
87. Kaul S, et al.: Myocardial contrast echocardiography and the transmural distribution of flow: A critical appraisal during myocardial ischemia not associated with infarction. J Am Coll Cardiol 200:1005, 1992.
88. Tschabitscher M: Anatomy of coronary veins. *In* Mohl W, Wolner E, Glogar D (eds.): The Coronary Sinus. Darmstadt, Steinkopff Verlag, p. 8, 1984.

89. Reisner SA, Shapiro JR, Amico AF, Meltzer RS: Contrast agents for myocardial perfusion studies. Mechanisms, state of the art, and future prospects. *In* Meerbaum S, Meltzer R (eds.): Myocardial contrast two-dimensional echocardiography. Dordrecht, Kluwer Academic Publishers, p. 45, 1989.
90. Wusten B: Biophysics of myocardial perfusion. *In* Schaper W (ed.): The Pathophysiology of Myocardial Perfusion. Amsterdam, Elsevier/North Holland Biomedical Press, p. 199.
91. Keller MW, et al.: Manifestations of reperfusion injury in the microcirculation following perfusion with hyperkalemic, hypothermic, cardioplegic solutions and blood perfusion: Effects of adenosine. Circulation 84:2485, 1991.
92. Keller MW, et al.: Intraoperative assessment of myocardial perfusion using quantitative myocardial contrast echocardiography: an experimental evaluation. J Am Coll Cardiol 16:1267, 1990.
93. Villanueva FS, et al.: On-line intraoperative quantitation of regional myocardial perfusion during coronary artery bypass graft operations with myocardial contrast two-dimensional echocardiography. J Thorac Cardiovasc Surg 104:1524, 1992.
94. Monaghan MJ, et al.: Digital subtraction contrast echocardiography: a new method for the evaluation of regional myocardial perfusion. Br Heart J 59: 12, 1988.
95. de Jong N, Mittertreiner WH, Ligtvoet KM, Ten Cate FJ: A computerized system that uses high-frequency data for analysis of myocardial contrast echocardiograms. J Am Soc Echocardiogr 3:99, 1990.
96. Lombardi M, et al.: Flow quantitation by contrast echocardiography: radiofrequency or videodensitometric analysis? Circulation 82(Suppl. 3):III–96, 1990.

CHAPTER

24

LEFT VENTRICLE V: DIASTOLIC FUNCTION—ITS PRINCIPLES AND EVALUATION

CHRISTOPHER Y. CHOONG

The clinical importance of the diastolic function of the heart is unquestioned. It is increasingly recognized that impairment of left ventricular diastolic function produces significant hemodynamic abnormalities, which may be fully responsible for or contribute substantially to the pathophysiology of many cardiac diseases.[1-3] In conditions such as pressure-load left ventricular hypertrophy and hypertrophic or restrictive cardiomyopathy, diastolic dysfunction may lead to frank cardiac failure even when systolic function is normal. During acute myocardial ischemia, diastolic dysfunction occurs before systolic dysfunction, electrocardiographic changes of ischemia and angina and may contribute significantly to the development of cardiac failure.

Questions concerning the precise meaning of diastolic function and its evaluation are complex. Unlike systolic function, which represents the properties and effects of myocardial contraction alone, diastolic function encompasses several distinct hemodynamic phases which are fundamentally different in their properties. A large number of parameters have been used to measure many aspects of diastolic function, and this diversity itself reflects the absence of a single index that is ideal or universally applicable. These parameters of diastolic function often differ markedly from one another, and their relationships to each other remain poorly understood.

Research into diastolic function has often been conducted within relatively confined areas of interest, such as the evaluation of ventricular passive stiffness, active relaxation, pressure-volume relations, or filling patterns. As a result of these focused approaches, the presentation of a unified view of diastolic function is uncommon. Considering the complex nature of this topic, all those engaged in the noninvasive evaluation of diastolic function must familiarize themselves not only with the measurement techniques in their field but also with the fundamental concepts that lie outside their chosen disciplines. This broader approach is essential for a balanced perspective of the many indices of diastolic function that exist and for a careful understanding of their implications and limitations.

Accordingly, the basic physiologic principles of diastole and commonly employed invasive measurements of diastolic function are summarized in the first part of this chapter. This is followed by a more detailed description of noninvasive measurements of diastolic function related to echocardiography. Special attention is paid to the evaluation of ventricular filling by the Doppler technique, which has attracted considerable attention in recent years. For more thorough accounts of the general principles of diastolic function and its invasive evaluation, the reader is referred to comprehensive reviews of the subject.[4-8]

DEFINITION OF DIASTOLE

Diastole, from the Greek word διαστολη meaning "a drawing asunder or expansion," was defined by Wiggers in physiologic terms as a process extending from the opening of the mitral valve, i.e., the onset of ventricular filling, to the onset of contraction (Fig. 24–1). Later, this definition was modified for clinical application so that diastole commenced at the onset of the second heart sound, indicating closure of the aortic valve, and ended with the first heart sound, indicating closure of the mitral valve. More recently, another definition of diastole was proposed in which the heart was viewed functionally as an integrated pump instead of just a contracting organ. In this approach, which offers advantages in the understanding of muscle mechanics, contraction and relaxation were grouped together under the definition of systole. This was based on the notion that active myocardial tension is present (either increasing or dissipating) during that period.[5] By this definition, diastole was confined to only the duration of the cardiac cycle when the myocardium was fully relaxed (Fig. 24–1). In this chapter, the more conventional definition of diastole is used, so that relaxation is still considered as a diastolic event.

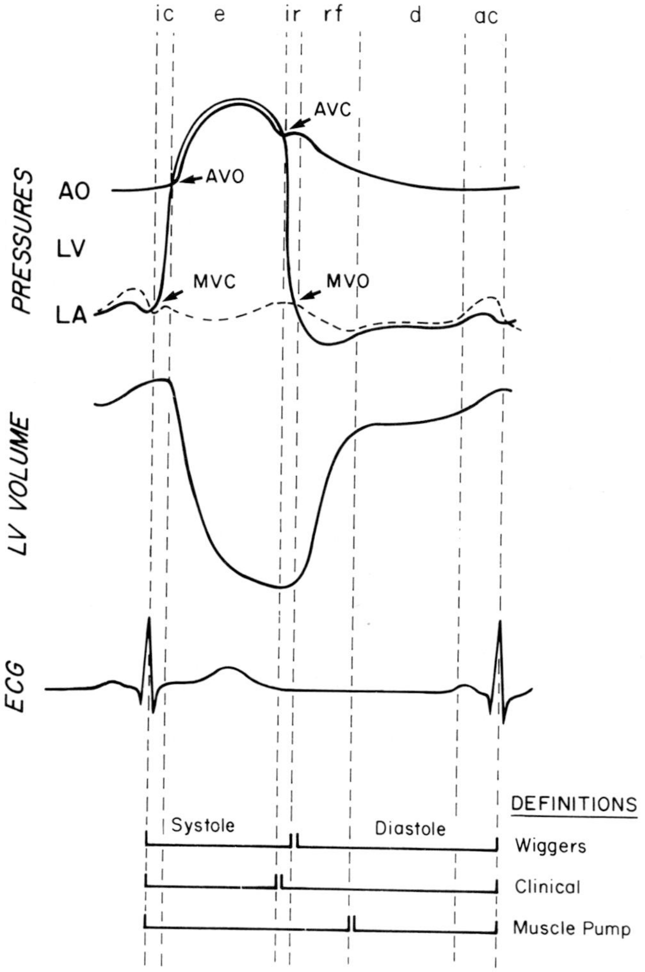

Fig. 24–1. The changes in left ventricular, left atrial and aortic pressures, left ventricular volume, and the electrocardiogram during one cardiac cycle. The timing of aortic and mitral valve opening and closure is indicated by arrows. The various definitions of diastole according to Wiggers, clinical criteria, and the more recent muscle pump concept are shown at the bottom of the figure (see text). ac = atrial contraction; AO = aortic; AVC = aortic valve closure; AVO = aortic valve opening; d = diastasis; e = ejection period; ic = isovolumic contraction; ir = isovolumic relaxation; LA = left atrial; LV = left ventricular; MVC = mitral valve closure; MVO = mitral valve opening; rf = rapid filling period.

HEMODYNAMIC PHASES DURING DIASTOLE

Isovolumic Relaxation

The initiation of the process of relaxation occurs around the time of peak left ventricular systolic pressure.[5] This process is manifested physiologically as a decline in left ventricular pressure from its peak value generated during systole by myocardial contraction. When left ventricular pressure falls below aortic pressure, the ejection of blood from the ventricle into the aorta ceases, and the aortic valve closes. At this stage, the mitral valve is still closed as left ventricular pressure exceeds left atrial pressure. Thus, left ventricular volume remains constant as left ventricular pressure continues to fall with further myocardial relaxation, hence the term *isovolumic relaxation* (Fig. 24–1). Changes in ventricular shape may occur even though absolute volume remains constant. The isovolumic phase ends when left ventricular pressure falls below left atrial pressure, and the mitral valve opens, initiating ventricular filling.

Rapid Filling Phase

During the early or rapid filling phase of the ventricle, blood leaves the left atrium and enters the ventricle passively down a pressure gradient generated by continued ventricular relaxation. This phase is therefore commonly termed the *passive filling phase* of the ventricle, even though relaxation is an active, i.e., an energy-requiring process. It has been suggested that the ventricle actually exerts a sucking effect through the generation of negative pressures during relaxation.[6] Left atrial pressure decreases as the atrial chamber empties but at a slower rate than the active decline in left ventricular pressure. The atrioventricular pressure gradient reaches a maximal level, at which time (or more accurately, shortly after which, because of the influence of inertial forces) the peak rate of ventricular filling occurs. Under normal conditions, the left ventricle fills most rapidly at this time, which explains the widespread use of the term *rapid filling phase*.

As the ventricle fills and ventricular volume increases, ventricular pressure also tends to increase, purely as a result of the physicomechanical properties of the chamber. This effect on pressure opposes the tendency for the pressure to fall as a result of continuing relaxation. Because the rate of relaxation decreases with time, its effect on lowering ventricular pressure decreases correspondingly. Also, as the left atrium empties, its volume decreases, and left atrial pressure progressively declines. This is reflected in the y descent of the left atrial pressure trace. As a result of these three processes—namely, ventricular relaxation, ventricular filling, and atrial emptying—the atrioventricular pressure gradient decreases until a point is reached when the pressures in both chambers equilibrate, and ventricular filling stops.

Diastasis

The term *diastasis* is applied to the phase in diastole when left atrial and left ventricular pressures are essentially in equilibrium following the rapid filling phase, and little or no filling occurs. Flow from the pulmonary veins may continue to contribute slightly to ventricular filling, with the left atrium acting as a passive conduit. The duration of this period depends importantly on the heart rate, and its presence is abolished at heart rates of more than 100 to 110 beats per minute.

Late Filling Phase

In the presence of sinus rhythm, synchronous electrical activation of the left atrium is followed by atrial contraction and the ejection of a further amount of blood into the left ventricle. Naturally, this phase of left ventricular filling is absent in atrial fibrillation. Normally, very little retrograde flow of blood into the pulmonary veins occurs, and practically all of the blood ejected by the atrium enters the ventricle. In health, left atrial contraction contributes from around 10 to 30% or more to the total filling volume of the ventricle.[9] This wide physiologic variation depends largely on age, and this proportion is increased in a variety of pathologic conditions described later in this chapter.

PROPERTIES OF THE LEFT VENTRICLE DURING DIASTOLE

The functional properties of the ventricle during diastole have mostly been described in terms of either the rate at which it relaxes in early diastole or its stiffness when it is fully relaxed in the latter part of diastole. By definition, these two properties are manifested at times that are mutually exclusive of one another. The relationship of one property to the other remains poorly defined.

Relaxation

Relaxation may be defined broadly as the process by which muscle returns from its contracted state to that which existed before the initiation of contraction. Abnormalities of relaxation may occur with myocardial ischemia or hypoxia, myocardial hypertrophy, hypothyroidism, hypothermia, aging, and a variety of other conditions discussed later. Our understanding of the control of relaxation has been greatly aided by detailed studies of isolated muscle twitch preparations. Three main controlling mechanisms have been identified. These are inactivation, load, and in the case of the intact ventricle, heterogeneity of inactivation of the ventricular chamber.[5]

Inactivation

Inactivation refers to the disengagement of actin-myosin cross bridges within the myocardial cell, the prior formation of which is the subcellular mechanism responsible for myocardial contraction. At a molecular level, this process commences with the cessation of the slow inward calcium current across the sarcolemma that is responsible for the plateau phase of membrane depolarization and with the initiation of active, energy (adenosine triphosphate [ATP])-dependent uptake of calcium ions from the cytosol into the sarcoplasmic reticulum.[10] As a result of these two processes, the concentration of calcium ions in the cytosol decreases from around 10^{-5} to 10^{-7} M, and calcium detaches from its binding site on the troponin-actin-myosin complex on the myocardial filaments. This separation of calcium from troponin-C initiates the disengagement of cross bridges between actin and myosin filaments, resulting in myocardial relaxation. The inactivation process is influenced by many factors, which include the concentration of intracellular calcium, sympathomimetic stimulation and blockade, and the availability of ATP.

Load

Independent of the process of inactivation, many loading conditions that are imposed on isolated muscle as well as the intact ventricle exert important effects on relaxation. The various loading conditions that have been demonstrated or postulated to occur are listed in Table 24–1. Relaxation loads are those loads that are present during the period of relaxation. Of these, internal restoring forces refer to the intrinsic forces created by deformation of myocardial geometry resulting from contraction. These forces are relatively unimportant at the level of individual muscle cells because these cells seldom contract to less than their slack lengths. In the intact ventricle, however, internal restoring forces may

Table 24–1. Determinants of Left Ventricular Relaxation Rate in the Intact Heart

A. Loading
   1. Internal restoring forces (cardiac fiber)
   2. External restoring forces (intact heart)
      - Configurational loading: end ejection pressure-volume relation
   3. Hemodynamic loading (cardio-circulatory system)
      - Arterial impedance
      - Transmission of pressure wave in coronary circulation
      - Laplace relationship during rapid filling phase
      - Pericardial, right ventricular hemodynamics

B. Inactivation
   1. Modulators
      - Metabolic control: coronary circulation
      - Neurohumoral control: catecholamines

C. Nonuniformity
   1. Spatial and temporal distribution of force and loading inactivation

(From Brutsaert DL, et al.: Analysis of relaxation in the evaluation of ventricular function of the heart. Prog Cardiovasc Dis 28:143, 1985.)

play a more important role, particularly when end-systolic volume is small.

The term *external restoring forces*, as the name implies, refers to those forces acting on the myocardium from outside the myocardium itself. Muscle twitch experiments have demonstrated that an abrupt increase in load in late systole causes contraction to be abbreviated and relaxation to occur sooner, whereas an abrupt increase in load during relaxation causes relaxation to proceed at a faster rate.[5] In the intact ventricle, three main factors contribute to the external restoring forces. They are (1) the aortic pressure waveform, which changes with alteration in aortic impedance produced by disease or pharmacologic intervention; (2) coronary turgor or coronary erectile effect, produced by the distending pressure within the coronary vasculature, giving rise to a stiffening effect on the ventricle; and (3) the increase in ventricular wall stress that accompanies ventricular filling, in accordance with Laplace's law.

When changes in load are imposed in early-systole, the effects of these changes on relaxation are directly opposite to those produced by loads imposed during late-systole or relaxation. For example, an increase in load in early-systole causes a prolongation of relaxation (delayed relaxation) as well as a reduced rate of relaxation. In the intact heart, this is seen as a reduction in the rate of relaxation when aortic systolic pressure is increased. This influence has been termed *contraction load* in contradistinction to *relaxation load* described previously.

Heterogeneity of Relaxation

When different segments of the ventricle relax asynchronously, some segments may commence relaxation when others are almost fully relaxed. The resulting effect is a reduction in chamber or global relaxation rate. The magnitude of this effect depends on the extent of the inhomogeneity of regional relaxation. Such heterogeneity of regional relaxation may occur because of regional ischemia or infarction in coronary artery disease or as a result of an abnormal sequence of electrical depolarization and repolarization seen with ventricular pacing or intraventricular conduction defects.

Indices of Relaxation

Relaxation is expressed hemodynamically as the decline in left ventricular chamber pressure from its peak level generated by myocardial contraction. The measurement of left ventricular pressure has been possible for many years and can be made relatively easily and accurately. It is not surprising, therefore, that descriptions of the left ventricular pressure waveform have been used traditionally and continue to be used most commonly to describe the relaxation process. Several indices have been employed for this purpose.

Isovolumic Relaxation Period. The isovolumic relaxation period is the time from aortic valve closure to mitral valve opening, when left ventricular volume is constant (Fig. 24–1). The timing of these two events may be determined directly from phonocardiography (for the aortic valve closure sounds) and M-mode echocardiography (for mitral valve opening), or from Doppler echocardiography (by timing the cessation of transaortic blood flow and commencement of transmitral blood flow). The use of two-dimensional echocardiography for this purpose is limited by the relatively slow frame rate of the technique. The isovolumic relaxation period is prolonged in many conditions in which the rate of relaxation is reduced.[11] As may be seen in Fig. 24–1, however, the rate of decline of the left ventricular pressure is only one of several factors that determine this period. The aortic diastolic and left atrial pressures determine the timing of aortic valve closure and mitral valve opening, respectively, and must also influence the isovolumic relaxation period. A lower aortic diastolic pressure or higher left atrial pressure will shorten this period independently of the relaxation rate. Therefore, although this parameter has the advantage of being relatively easy to measure, its interpretation must be made cautiously. For obvious reasons, the presence of mitral or aortic regurgitation negates the occurrence of a true isovolumic relaxation period.

Peak Negative dP/dt. The peak negative rate of change of pressure (dP/dt) is the maximal rate of decline of left ventricular pressure during relaxation and is usually taken as the lowest value of the first derivative of this pressure (Fig. 24–2). For the accurate measurement of this parameter, left ventricular pressure must be measured using a transducer system with a high frequency response, such as provided by micromanometer-tipped catheters.

The peak negative dP/dt occurs at or around the time of aortic valve closure. It is decreased (less negative) in conditions associated with impaired relaxation, such as myocardial ischemia, and increased with enhanced relaxation, for example, during sympathomimetic stimulation. It must be remembered, however, that the peak negative dP/dt occurs at just one point in time and cannot

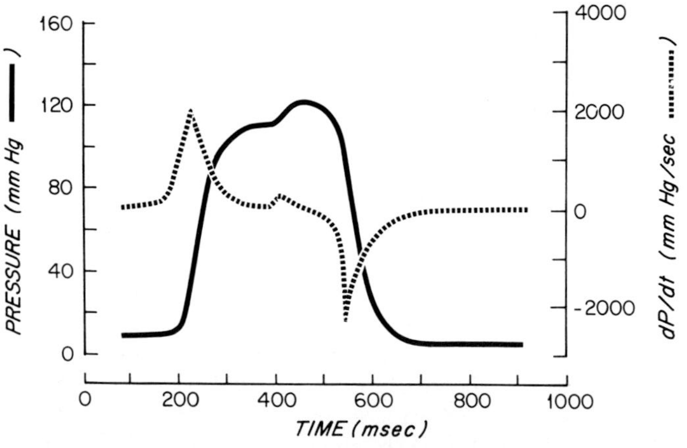

Fig. 24–2. Schema of a left ventricular pressure trace and the first derivative of this trace, dP/dt. The peak negative dP/dt has been used to measure relaxation rate but is limited by two main disadvantages. It describes just one instant in the relaxation phase of the ventricle and is highly sensitive to left ventricular systolic pressure. The peak negative dP/dt occurs close to the time of the aortic valve closure and conveniently has been used to indicate the start of isovolumic relaxation when analyzing left ventricular pressure traces.

fully represent all events occurring during relaxation. It also depends highly on left ventricular or aortic systolic pressure, which is a major disadvantage of this measurement.[12] An increase in left ventricular systolic pressure increases peak negative dP/dt independently of the influence of relaxation. As a result of this load dependence, peak negative dP/dt may change in a direction opposite to that of other measures of relaxation, such as the time constant of relaxation (T).

Time Constant of Relaxation. The decline in left ventricular pressure during the isovolumic relaxation period approximates an exponential decay curve, and therefore, its slope may be expressed by a time constant called tau, or T. This measurement is usually derived from that portion of the left ventricular pressure waveform that starts at the time of peak negative dP/dt (used to represent the time of aortic valve closure) and ends at an arbitrary point on the downslope of the pressure trace, which is 5 mm Hg higher than the left ventricular end-diastolic pressure (chosen to precede the time of mitral valve closure). As in the case of the peak negative dP/dt, high fidelity transducer systems must be used for these measurements.

Two basic methods are used to calculate the time constant of relaxation. In the method first described by Weiss et al. in 1976,[13] left ventricular pressure is assumed to decline exponentially to zero in the absence of ventricular filling. Isovolumic pressure is thus fitted to the simple exponential equation $P = P_0 * e^{At}$, where P is left ventricular pressure at time t, P_0 is left ventricular pressure at time 0, i.e., at peak negative dP/dt, t is time after peak negative dP/dt, and A is a constant.

The application of natural logarithm to both sides of the equation yields $\text{Log } P = At + \text{Log } P_0$, which is a linear equation. In practice, therefore, the natural logarithm of isovolumic left ventricular pressure is plotted against time, and a straight line is fitted to the data points. In general, these points closely approximate a straight line, with some minor downward deviation at the lower end of the line.[14] The slope of the line, A, has a negative value. The negative reciprocal of the slope, $-1/A$, is the exponential decay time constant of isovolumic relaxation, T_L (Fig. 24–3). This parameter remains today a widely accepted, although imperfect, measurement of the rate of relaxation.

The time constant may be considered as the time it takes for isovolumic left ventricular pressure to decline by 1/e of any initial value, and it is usually expressed in units of milliseconds. By definition, therefore, it takes 3.5 T_L msec for the left ventricular pressure to decline to 3% of its initial value, by which time relaxation may be considered to be practically complete. Given that the normal value of T_L is around 25 to 40 msec, relaxation is practically complete by approximately 140 msec after the start of isovolumic relaxation. In most instances, this occurs well before the end of diastole. However, in some situations, such as when T_L is large or when heart rate is fast and the diastolic period therefore is short, relaxation may still be incomplete at the end of diastole.[15]

A modification of the method of Weiss et al.[13] was subsequently introduced, in which left ventricular pressure is not assumed to decline to an asymptote of zero pressure but is allowed to decline exponentially to a variable asymptote determined by extrapolation of the data points recorded during the isovolumic period.[14] The equation may be written thus: $P = (P_0 * e^{At}) + P_B$, where P is left ventricular pressure at time t, P_0 is initial left ventricular pressure at time zero, P_B is asymptotic pressure to which P declines, and A is a constant (see Fig. 24–3). This equation is similar to that for the derivation of T_L and differs only with the addition of P_B. Applying the first derivative to both sides of the equation yields the equation $dP/dt = A * (P_0 * e^{At})$. As $(P_0 * e^{At})$ is equal to $(P - P_B)$ from the first equation, substitution into the second equation yields $dP/dt = A * (P - P_B)$. Thus, a plot of dP/dt against P mathematically yields a straight line with a slope of A, which always has a negative value (see Fig. 24–3). As in the derivation of T_L, the time constant of relaxation, T_D (D is derivative), is the negative reciprocal of the slope of the line, i.e., $-1/A$.

The pressure asymptote, P_B, is obtained from the x-axis intercept of the fitted straight line, i.e., when dP/dt is zero. It often possesses a negative value and has been claimed to represent residual tone in the ventricle

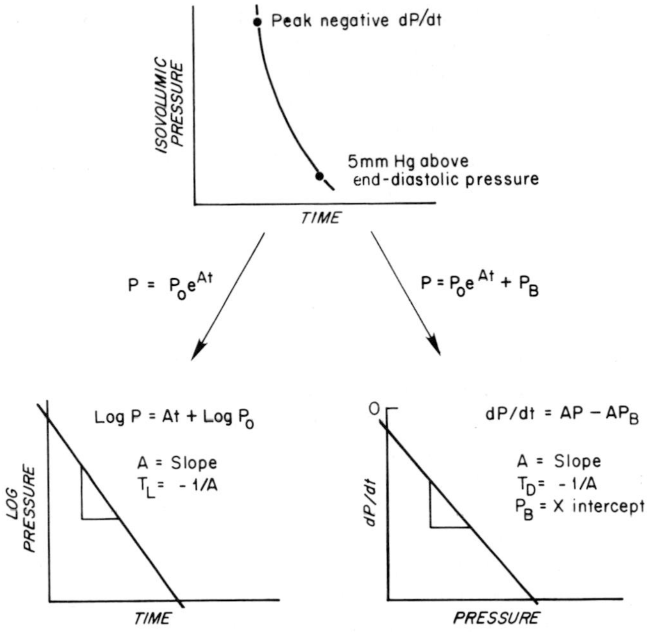

Fig. 24–3. The two usual methods for calculating the time constant of relaxation, T (tau). Top. The portion of the left ventricular pressure trace corresponding to isovolumic relaxation. By convention, the initial point is the time when the peak negative dP/dt occurs, approximating aortic valve closure. The lower point is taken at 5 mm Hg above the end-diastolic pressure, approximating mitral valve opening. Bottom left. The logarithmic method of Weiss et al.,[13] which assumes that left ventricular isovolumic pressure decays exponentially to zero. The corresponding time constant is called T_L. It is the negative reciprocal of the slope of the line relating the natural logarithm of ventricular pressure to time. Bottom right. The "derivative method," which allows the isovolumic left ventricular pressure to decline to a variable asymptote, P_B. The corresponding time constant is called T_D. It is the negative reciprocal of the slope of the line relating dP/dt to ventricular pressure. P_B is the value on the x axis when the y axis value (dP/dt) is zero. See text for a more detailed explanation.

after relaxation is complete. Figure 24–4 illustrates how changes in T_D and P_B affect the slopes and positions of the left ventricular pressure trace. P_B has been shown to increase (become less negative) during myocardial ischemia and is attributed to incomplete relaxation that is due to the persistence of cross-bridge linkages between actin and myosin filaments.[16] Although the use of T_D instead of T_L imposes less assumptions on the behavior of the left ventricular pressure trace, and may therefore be seen as advantageous in this regard, the physiologic significance of P_B remains uncertain.

Both T_L and T_D may be calculated more directly by fitting the unmodified digitized left ventricular pressure trace to the appropriate exponential functions. Using this method, any deviation of data points from an exponential function at the lower end of the left ventricular pressure curve is not amplified, unlike the case when a straight line is fitted to a logarithmically transformed pressure curve. Some workers have found a closer fit of the raw pressure data to a sixth-order polynomial function than to the conventional exponential functions and have chosen to derive T in this way.[17]

The time constant of relaxation is relatively independent of preload but is altered by afterload.[14,18–20] The extent of the latter effect in vivo is unclear but is less than the effect of afterload on the peak negative dP/dt. A limitation of the use of the isovolumic time constant of relaxation is that isovolumic left ventricular pressure decay is not always a perfectly simple exponential decay function.[14] Actual ventricular pressure often tends to fall faster during the latter part of isovolumic relaxation than predicted from a purely monoexponential decay function. It must be remembered also that the ventricular relaxation rate measured in this way is derived solely from the observed behavior of the isovolumic ventricle, but it is not uncommon for extrapolations to be made from these measurements to describe ventricular behavior during the subsequent filling phase. It has recently been shown that relaxation during the rapid filling phase of the ventricle may proceed at a different rate from that measured during the isovolumic relaxation phase, presumably because of alterations in loading conditions during ventricular filling.[21] Despite these limitations, however, the time constant of isovolumic relaxation remains the most widely accepted and used index of ventricular relaxation at the present time.

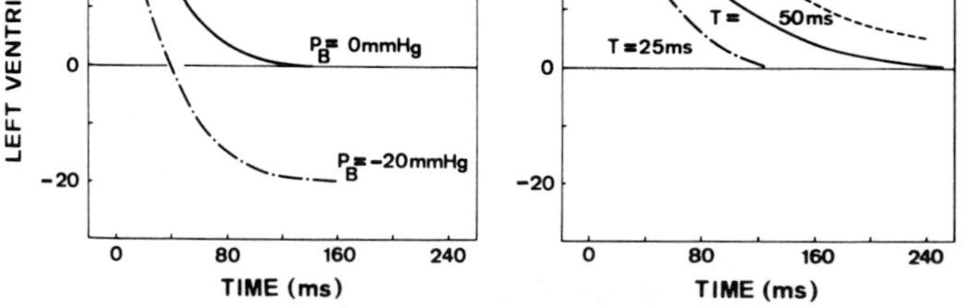

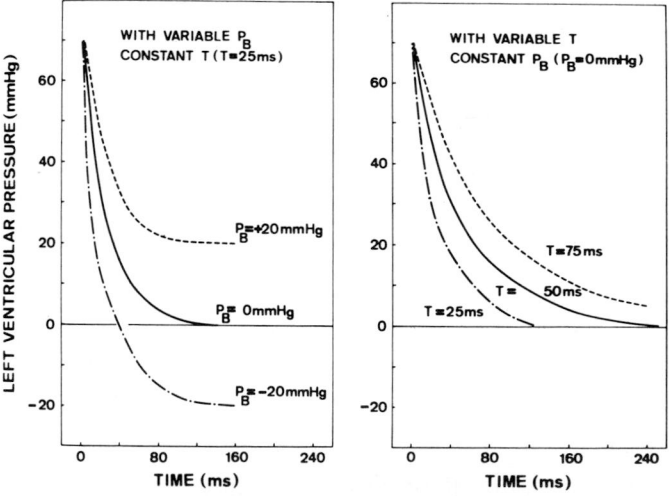

Fig. 24–4. Left. The independent effect of the left ventricular asymptotic pressure, P_B, on the slope and position of the left ventricular pressure trace with a fixed time constant of isovolumic relaxation, T_D. Right. The independent effect of the time constant of isovolumic relaxation, T_D, on ventricular pressure decay with a fixed asymptotic pressure, P_B.[16] (From Carroll JD, Hess OM, Hirzel HO, Krayenbuehl HP: Exercise induced ischemia: the influence of altered relaxation on early diastolic pressures. Circulation 67:521, 1983. Reproduced by permission of the American Heart Association, Inc.)

Passive Diastolic Properties of the Left Ventricle

The passive properties of the left ventricle describe its stiffness or elasticity when the myocardium is fully relaxed. The passive properties of myocardium should be distinguished from those of the ventricular chamber itself.

Passive Properties of Myocardium

The passive properties of myocardium are best described by its stress-strain relationships. Much information in this area has been obtained from detailed studies of isolated muscle strips. Several terms need to be defined. *Stress* is force applied per unit cross-sectional area, and its units are usually expressed as grams or dynes per square centimeter. *Strain* is the change in dimension produced by the application of stress and is usually expressed as a proportional change from the unstressed dimension. Two definitions of strain are often employed. *Lagrangian strain* refers to the proportional change in dimension relative to the dimension at zero stress, i.e., $(l - l_0)/l_0$, where l is length at a particular stress and l_0 is length at zero stress. Because zero stress and strain are technically difficult to measure, l_0 is often incorrectly substituted by the end-diastolic length. *Natural strain,* on the other hand, is the natural logarithm of the ratio of the length at a particular stress to the length at zero stress, i.e., $\text{Log}_e(l/l_0)$. Use of natural strain is more appropriate for biologic material and has the advantage that the dimension at zero stress is not strictly required.

Any material that exhibits a linear relation between the application of stress and the resultant strain obeys Hooke's law, and is described as being Hookian. Most biologic tissue, however, exhibits a curvilinear relation between stress and strain that is nearly exponential.[6] The slope of the curve relating stress to strain, i.e., the slope of the tangent at any point on the curve, describes the rate at which one parameter changes with the other and is termed the *myocardial elastic stiffness* (Fig. 24–5). As can be seen in Figure 24–5, an increase in stress or strain is accompanied by an increase in the slope of the curve, so that the stiffness of the same myocardium varies with the amount of stress applied. By virtue of the exponential relationship between stress and strain, the relationship between elastic stiffness and stress is necessarily linear, and the slope of this line is therefore constant and is termed the *myocardial stiffness constant,* or k_m. Use of the myocardial stiffness

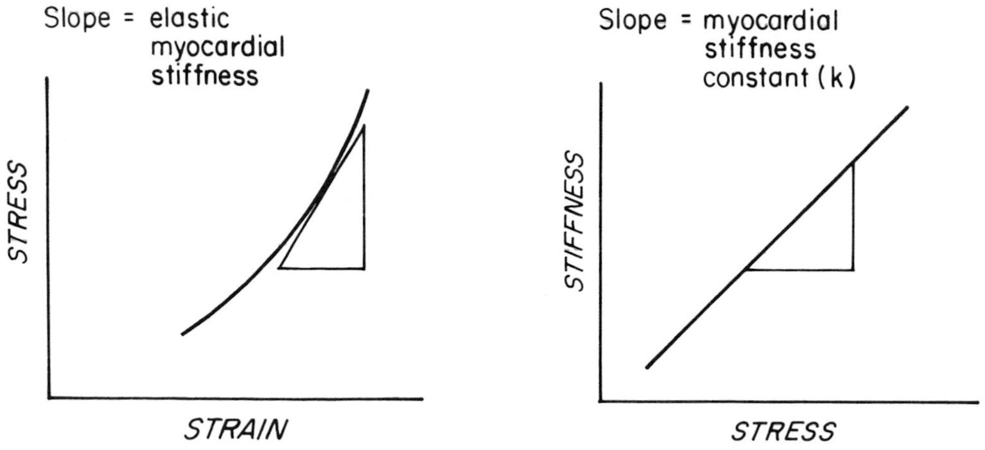

Fig. 24–5. The exponential relationship between myocardial stress and strain. Left. The slope of this curvilinear plot is the elastic myocardial stiffness. Right. By its exponential nature, a plot of elastic myocardial stiffness against stress yields a straight line whose slope is the modulus of elasticity or myocardial stiffness constant, k. Unlike the slope of the stress-strain relationship, which changes with changes in stress, the slope of the stiffness-stress relationship is constant with changes in stress.

constant to compare the stiffness of different myocardial samples avoids the problems presented by the dependence of elastic stiffness on different levels of stress and strain. Figure 24–6 demonstrates the relationship between elastic stiffness and stress for two quite different curves. On the left, stress is plotted against strain for curves 1 and 2. The stiffness or slope of curve 1 measured at point C is identical to that of curve 2 measured at point B, despite the curves being obviously different. The stiffness or slope of curve 2 at point A, which has the same stress as at point C, is appropriately lower. On the right, the two straight lines represent plots of stiffness vs. stress for curves 1 and 2. The slopes of the two lines represent the myocardial stiffness constants and clearly differ from each other, with the steeper line representing stiffer myocardium.

With elastic material, the relation between stress and strain may be altered by the rapid application of stress. The term *stress relaxation* describes the gradual decline in stress at constant length after an elastic material has been stretched rapidly. The term *creep* refers to the gradual increase in length at constant stress after the

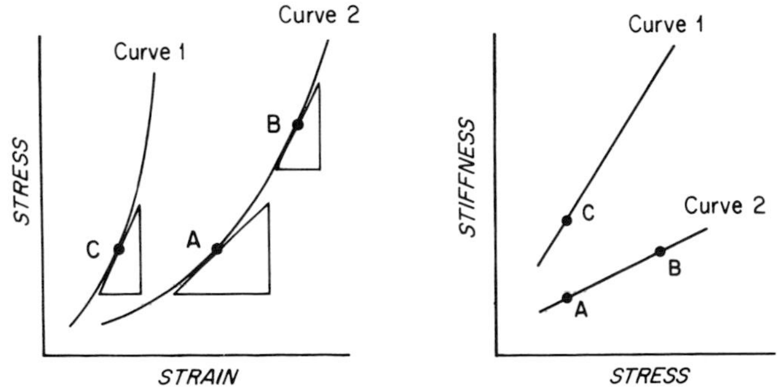

Fig. 24–6. The importance of stress on measurements of the elastic myocardial stiffness. Left. Two quite different curves, 1 and 2, are shown. The slopes of the curves, i.e., myocardial stiffness, at points C and B are equal but occur at different stresses. When the slopes are measured at the same stress, namely points C and A, respectively, myocardial stiffness is clearly lower in curve 2. Right. Plots of myocardial stiffness against stress are shown for the two curves. The slopes of the two curves, i.e., the myocardial stiffness constants, are now quite different irrespective of the level of stress.

rapid application of stress. Both phenomena have been described in canine heart preparations under nonphysiologic conditions and do not appear to play any important part in normal cardiac mechanics. Viscous elements in the myocardium produce the property of *viscoelasticity*. This property of myocardium causes the amount of stress in the myocardium to be greater during rapid lengthening than predicted from static stress-strain relationships (Fig. 24–7). The effects of viscoelasticity have been described during rapid ventricular filling that is due to atrial contraction and may also occur during passive rapid ventricular filling. However, the practical importance of these effects remains controversial.[6]

Passive Properties of the Ventricular Chamber

The passive properties of the ventricular chamber are described by its end-diastolic pressure to end-diastolic volume relationship, which, like the stress-strain relationship, is curvilinear and approximates an exponential function.[6] *Chamber stiffness* is the slope (the change of pressure per unit change in volume [dP/dV]) of this relationship and varies with volume and pressure for a given chamber (Fig. 24–8). The term *compliance* is the rate of change in volume per rate of change in pressure and is the reciprocal of chamber stiffness, i.e., dV/dP. As the relationship of pressure to volume is exponential or near-exponential, the relationship between its slope (chamber stiffness) and pressure is linear. The slope of this straight line is the *modulus of chamber stiffness*, k_v (Fig. 24–8).

In ventricles with high end-diastolic pressure, particularly in chronically dilated hearts, the relationship between pressure and volume may lose its monoexponential nature. Thus, the description of the passive properties of a ventricle by its chamber stiffness or modulus of chamber stiffness should always be qualified by the pressure at which the measurements are made.

Clearly, a change in chamber stiffness may result from a change in volume along the same pressure-volume relationship (Fig. 24–8). Alternatively, it may result from a shift to a different pressure-volume relationship. Therefore, comparisons of chamber stiffness between different ventricles, especially those with very different volumes, should be made using normalized values (VdP/

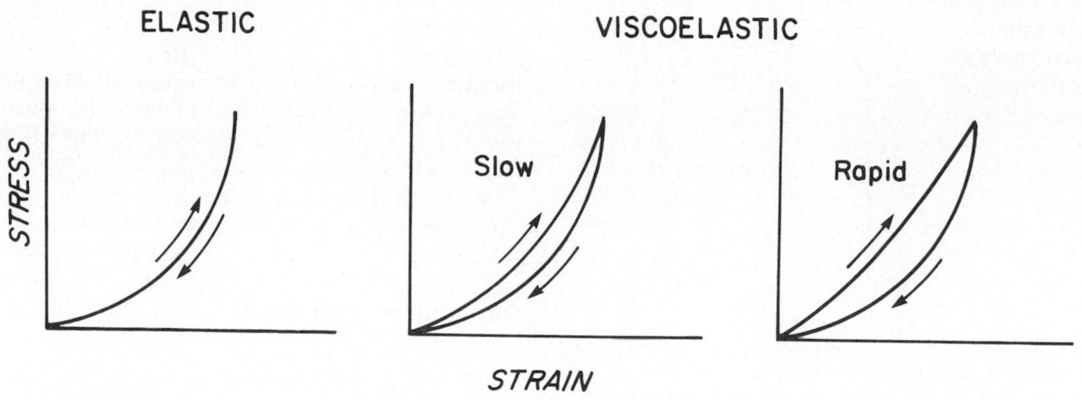

Fig. 24–7. The properties of viscoelasticity. Left. The stress-strain relation for a simple elastic material. The relation is not altered by the speed at which stress and strain are altered. Middle and right. The stress-strain relation for a viscoelastic material, which is altered by the speed at which stress and strain are altered. A slow increase in stress (middle) produces less effect on the stress-strain relation than a rapid change (right).

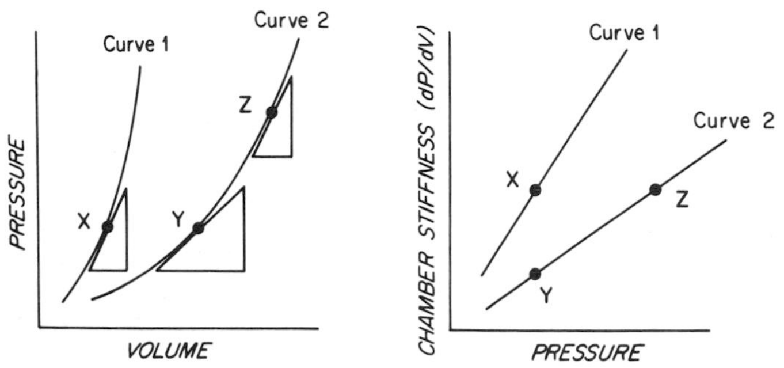

Fig. 24–8. Left. The exponential relation between ventricular end-diastolic pressure and end-diastolic volume. The chamber stiffness is defined as the rate of change in pressure per unit change in volume (dP/dV) and is derived from the instantaneous slope of the exponential curve. It is obvious that for a given chamber, chamber stiffness increases as pressure or volume increase. An increase in chamber stiffness may result from a rightward shift along the same pressure-volume relation (a preload-dependent change) represented by points Y and Z, or by a change to a different pressure volume relation, represented by points Y and X. Right. The relation between chamber stiffness and pressure is linear, and the slope of this line is the modulus of chamber stiffness, k_v, which is independent of pressure and volume.

dV), also called the *volume elasticity*. The reciprocal of this term, dV/dP, is called the *specific compliance*. One should be aware that the effects of acute changes in ventricular loading on the pressure-volume relationship may differ from the effects of more chronic changes. With acute changes in ventricular volume, the curve of the pressure-volume relationship tends to remain relatively constant, whereas with chronic changes, such as sustained volume loading in aortic regurgitation or the creation of an arteriovenous shunt, the pressure-volume curve may shift rightward.[22] As a result of this rightward shift, a progressive increase in end-diastolic volume is not accompanied by a corresponding increase in end-diastolic pressure beyond that caused by the initial acute volume load.

While ventricular pressure-volume relationships for the assessment of passive stiffness should strictly be obtained from serial measurements of end-diastolic pressure at several end-diastolic volumes, some workers have attempted to evaluate pressure-volume relationships from measurements made during the diastolic phase of one cardiac cycle. This approach should be treated with caution, because the left ventricle may not be fully relaxed for a considerable portion of that curve and viscoelastic effects may operate during atrial contraction and possibly also during the rapid filling phase.

Relationship Between Left Ventricular Chamber Stiffness and Myocardial Stiffness

Characteristics of myocardial stiffness may be calculated from myocardial stress-strain relationships derived from measurements made in the intact ventricle. As described previously, wall stress, usually designated by σ, is the force measured in dynes acting on a unit of cross-sectional area of myocardium measured in square centimeters. Stress acting on the ventricular wall may be measured in three orthogonal planes, namely, radial, circumferential, and meridional. Because myocardial fibers at the midventricular level are organized in a circumferential pattern, the stress on individual muscle fibers is often calculated as the circumferential midwall stress. Radial and meridional stress act perpendicular to the longitudinal direction of the myocardial fibers at this level. Circumferential wall stress is also the strongest force acting at the equator of the ventricle. From measurements of the inner radius of the ventricular chamber, wall thickness, and intraventricular pressure, midwall circumferential stress may be calculated using a simple application of Laplace's law, as follows:

$$\text{Stress } (\sigma) = (P * a)/(2 * h) \text{ for a spherical ventricle, or}$$
$$= (P * b/h) * (1 - b^2)/2 * c^2 \text{ for an ellipsoid ventricle}$$

where a is the inner radius at the endocardium; b and c are semiminor and semimajor axes, respectively, at the endocardium; h is wall thickness; and P is intraventricular pressure. More complex formulas for calculating wall stress have been suggested.[23]

The relationship of chamber stiffness to chamber volume, myocardial mass, and myocardial elastic stiffness may be described mathematically.[24] Chamber stiffness is directly proportional to $E/V(1 + V/M)$, where E is myocardial elastic stiffness, V is ventricular volume, and M is myocardial mass. Because myocardial elastic stiffness is equal to the product of the myocardial stiffness constant (k_m) and wall stress (σ), chamber stiffness is directly proportional to $k_m * \sigma/V(1 + V/M)$. Thus, VdP/dV (normalized chamber stiffness or volume elasticity) is directly proportional to $k_m * \sigma/(1 + V/M)$ or $E/(1 + V/M)$.

In other words, for any given myocardial stiffness, normalized chamber stiffness is increased by a reduction in the chamber volume/mass ratio. A ventricle with thick walls, a large mass, and a normal volume (a low volume/mass ratio) will have increased normalized chamber stiffness despite having normal myocardial stiffness. Thus, the volume/mass ratio may be a useful index for assessing the contribution of chamber geometry to chamber stiffness.

External Factors That Modify Chamber Stiffness

Besides ventricular volume and myocardial mass and stiffness, other factors external to the ventricle act to modulate chamber stiffness. Right ventricular pressure, pericardial pressure, pleural pressure, and coronary turgor have all been shown to play roles in altering net chamber stiffness. In the absence of a pericardium, for example, volume infusion or reduction slides the pressure-length relationship along the same pressure-length curve, and the chamber stiffness constant, k_v, is unaltered.[25] With the pericardium intact, however, volume infusion shifts the pressure-length relation up to a different curve, while volume unloading shifts the pressure-length relation down to a different curve. The chamber stiffness constant is altered little, but chamber pressure for any given volume is increased or decreased, as the case may be. Because the right and left ventricles share the same septum, it is not surprising that right ventricular diastolic pressures may affect the stiffness of the left ventricle. This ventricular interaction appears more prominent in the presence of an intact pericardium. An increase in the volume of the coronary vasculature, whether by an increase in coronary perfusion pressure or by vasodilation, also increases left ventricular wall thickness and stiffness. This effect appears to be greater when the ventricle is adequately loaded, i.e., on the steep portion of the pressure-volume curve, and is enhanced by the presence of an intact pericardium. The actual importance of this phenomenon remains controversial.

Measurement of Regional Wall Stress

Recent attempts have been made to characterize regional diastolic function by measuring regional wall stress. In one such technique, left ventricular pressure decay is derived from an exponential fit of pressure during isovolumic relaxation, extrapolated, and subtracted from measured and uncorrected left ventricular pressure to yield "residual pressure." Because measured left ventricular pressure is equal to but negative in sign to radial stress at the endocardium, "residual pressure," which is independent of relaxation, may be considered to represent residual radial stress. By plotting residual pressure against the logarithm of wall thickness, radial stiffness modulus is obtained from the slope of the plot.[26] Using this technique, radial stiffness modulus was found to increase in the posterior left ventricular wall during pacing induced ischemia, contributing to the upward shift in left ventricular pressure-wall thickness and pressure-volume relationships in this condition.

Functional Performance of the Left Ventricle During Diastole

Studies of myocardial relaxation and the passive characteristics of the ventricle provide valuable information about the two important functional properties of the ventricle in diastole. This information, however, does not describe the performance of the ventricle in a way that can be easily translated into a practical or clinical context. For example, there is no a priori reason why a ventricle that relaxes slowly should necessarily be undesirable to the patient, and it is not possible at the present time to predict the impact of a particular relaxation rate or a change in this rate on a patient's clinical status. Similarly, it is difficult to interpret quantitatively or even semiquantitatively what a particular measurement of ventricular stiffness means in terms of functional impairment to the patient.

In functional terms, therefore, it is more useful to consider simply the ventricular diastolic pressure that occurs in a patient at a particular ventricular diastolic volume or preload. This parameter is the one that is the most directly relevant to the patient in terms of the tendency for cardiac failure to develop. In keeping with well-established observations, an increase in ventricular preload is favorable for ventricular systolic function because of the augmentation of stroke volume through the Frank Starling mechanism. This benefit to systolic function carries an undesirable cost in diastole, because there is an obligatory increase in diastolic pressure and hence in pulmonary venous pressure. The extent of this trade-off between the potential for preload reserve to improve systolic function and the cost in the tendency to develop backward cardiac failure depends on the diastolic performance of the ventricle and epitomizes the important role of diastolic function in disease.

The functional performance of the ventricle in diastole may best be described by the position of its pressure-volume relation during diastole over one or more cardiac cycles. This curve should not be confused with the end-diastolic pressure-volume relationship, which describes measurements taken only at end-diastole under varying loading conditions. If an intervention or disease slides the new pressure-volume curve along the control curve, the ventricle is considered not to have changed its distensibility but merely to have undergone a preload-dependent change in the pressure-volume relationship.[27] On the other hand, when a pressure-volume curve is shifted upward or downward from its control position, the ventricle is considered to have become less or more "distensible," respectively (Fig. 24–9). Some workers have applied the terms *compliance* and *stiffness* to describe such shifts in the pressure-volume relationship. This practice should be discouraged to avoid confusion with the conventional and strict definitions of these terms discussed earlier.

An upward shift in the pressure-volume relation has been observed in conditions such as acute myocardial ischemia, hypertrophic cardiomyopathy, pericardial tamponade, pericardial constriction, and right ventricular dilation. A downward shift has been described with nitroglycerin infusion and during nitroprusside infusion in patients with cardiac failure. The mechanisms of the shifts in the positions and slopes of the pressure-volume curves remain incompletely understood. The parallel downward shift in the pressure-volume curve seen with nitroglycerin infusion has been attributed to a reduction in right ventricular pressure acting on the left ventricle through ventricular interaction.[28] The parallel upward shift seen following the induction of cardiac tamponade in dogs provides another example of an extrinsic factor producing a parallel shift in the pressure-volume relationship. Other situations are less easily explained. For example, a downward shift in the pressure-volume curve (i.e., improved distensibility) is seen during nitroprusside infusion in patients with cardiac failure, but this is accompanied paradoxically by an increase in the slope of the curve, suggesting increased chamber stiffness.[27]

A variety of factors both intrinsic and extrinsic to the left ventricle have been implicated in the determination of left ventricular chamber distensibility.[27] These factors generally resemble those described earlier in the modulation of chamber stiffness. Many other factors besides those that govern chamber stiffness, however, determine the exact position of the pressure-volume relationship of a ventricle in diastole. These factors include, among others, the end-systolic volume, end-systolic pressure, and relaxation rate, so that passive chamber stiffness is only one of the determinants.[29] At the present time, our understanding of how active relaxation and the passive stiffness of the ventricular chamber interact to influence the position and shape of the pressure-volume curve is still inadequate and remains a potentially fruitful area of research.

THE NONINVASIVE EVALUATION OF DIASTOLIC FUNCTION

Noninvasive techniques have the obvious advantage over invasive ones in being safer. They are therefore eminently suited for the investigation of large numbers of patients, especially those in whom the risks of invasive procedures cannot be justified. Serial studies also can be performed more easily by noninvasive means. It follows that a number of noninvasive modalities have been evaluated for their ability to measure the diastolic function of the left ventricle. These include radionuclide ventriculography, M-mode echocardiography with or without phonocardiography, two-dimensional echocardiography, and more recently, Doppler echocardiography. In one way or another, these various techniques measure the timing of diastolic events or the pattern of

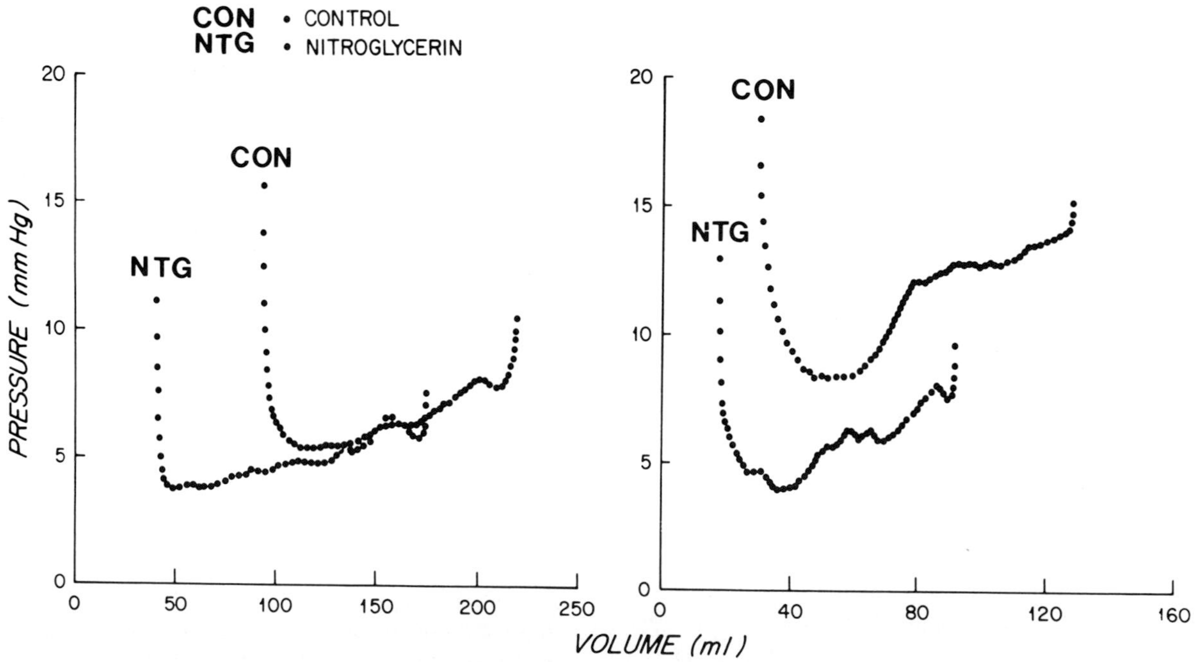

Fig. 24–9. Instantaneous diastolic pressure-volume relations measured during single cardiac cycles of two different ventricles (left and right) before and after the administration of nitroglycerin. The positions of the ventricular pressure-volume relations displayed in this way provide clinically meaningful information about ventricular diastolic performance. Left. Nitroglycerin has produced a leftward and downward slide along the same pressure-volume curve without a change in ventricular distensibility. This change has been called a *preload-dependent change.* Right. Nitroglycerin has shifted the pressure-volume relation downward, indicating an increase in ventricular distensibility and an improvement in diastolic function. The ventricle can now operate at the same volume or preload but at a lower diastolic pressure. An upward shift in the pressure-volume relation would have indicated a decrease in ventricular distensibility.

dimensional changes or filling of the left ventricle. From changes in the diastolic time intervals or the pattern of ventricular filling, inferences are made about ventricular diastolic function.

It should be remembered, however, that diastolic filling and diastolic function are not synonymous, and these terms should not be used loosely or interchangeably. Although a variety of patterns of ventricular filling have been described in normal hearts and in many different diseases, the precise relationships between parameters of diastolic filling and the diastolic properties of the ventricle remain incompletely understood.

Determinants of the Filling Pattern of the Left Ventricle: Theoretical Considerations

It is important for those who measure the pattern of left ventricular filling in research or for clinical purposes to understand first what these measurements mean in relation to other standard parameters of diastolic function described earlier in this chapter. The filling pattern of the ventricle depends on a complex and continuous interaction of multiple factors, of which only some relate directly to the diastolic properties of the ventricle itself. Other factors relate purely to hemodynamic conditions imposed on the ventricle.

From fundamental hydrodynamic principles, the pressure gradient (or loss in pressure energy) across an orifice (the mitral orifice in this case) produces work in three essential ways. These are convective acceleration, flow acceleration, and viscous losses. The first two terms represent an increase in kinetic energy, while the third represents the generation of heat that is due to friction between adjacent fluid layers. *Convective acceleration* refers to the increase in velocity of fluid particles (kinetic energy) when they traverse a region of reduced cross-sectional area while maintaining a constant volumetric flow rate. *Flow acceleration* refers to the increase in velocity of fluid particles that results from an increase in the volumetric flow rate itself. From the Law of Conservation of Energy, total hydraulic energies on both sides of the equation are balanced:

$$P1 - P2 = 1/2 * \rho(V_2^2 - V_1^2) + m * \int d\vec{V}/dt * d\vec{s}) + R * \vec{V}$$

In the specific case of left ventricular filling; P1 is left atrial pressure; P2 is left ventricular pressure; ρ is mass density of blood; V1 is velocity of blood in the left atrium; V2 is velocity of blood in the left ventricle; $d\vec{v}/dt$ is flow acceleration; s is distance in the ventricle along which change in kinetic energy that is due to flow acceleration is measured; and R is resistance of the mitral valve from viscous effects. This equation has been called the Bernoulli equation,[30] and is discussed in greater detail in Chapter 9.

The Rapid Filling Phase

By analyzing the determinants of left atrial and left ventricular pressures separately, the factors that govern the atrioventricular pressure gradient, and hence the velocity of blood flow across the mitral annulus (i.e., the filling of the ventricle), may be derived from first principles. The three phases of diastole have been outlined previously in this chapter.

During left ventricular relaxation, a point is reached at which left ventricular pressure descends below left atrial pressure, and the mitral valve opens and ventricular filling begins. The left atrial-left ventricular pressure gradient starts at zero and then rapidly increases as left ventricular pressure decreases faster than left atrial pressure. This rapid increase in the pressure gradient results in the acceleration of the early filling or E wave, according to the Bernoulli equation. In addition to the *convective forces* represented by the simplified Bernoulli equation, *inertial forces* play a part when blood is accelerated or decelerated. Energy loss that is due to friction (*viscous losses*) also occurs but is negligible in this situation.

The peak atrioventricular pressure gradient usually occurs just before minimum left ventricular pressure.[31] With filling proceeding after attainment of minimum left ventricular pressure, ventricular pressure rises as its volume increases while atrial pressure continues to fall as it empties, so that the atrioventricular pressure gradient decreases. Because of the brief persistence of a positive atrioventricular pressure gradient after the peak pressure gradient is reached and as a result of the inertia of blood, the peak flow velocity occurs after the onset of the peak pressure gradient. In one study, the peak flow velocity coincided with the first crossover pressure point between the rising left ventricular pressure and falling left atrial pressure[31] (Fig. 24–10). Following this first cross-over pressure point, left ventricular pressure transiently exceeds atrial pressure and hastens the deceleration of the early filling phase. Thus, flow may actually take place against a pressure gradient because of the inertia of blood. Several subsequent crossover points may occur between left atrial and left ventricular pressures as the two pressures oscillate about one another until full equilibrium is reached (see later). An important point to remember when making such fine temporal discriminations is that an obligatory time delay occurs in the derivation of Doppler velocity signals (approximately 10 msec or less, depending on the ultrasound scanner). This technical limitation must be borne constantly in mind when comparing the timing of pressure and velocity events.

To aid our understanding of the behavior of the atrioventricular pressure gradient, the determinants of instantaneous left atrial and left ventricular pressures may be considered separately. As the left atrial chamber empties into the ventricle, its volume decreases by an amount equal to that which has left the chamber minus the relatively smaller amount that has entered simultaneously from the pulmonary veins. At this time, the left atrium is fully relaxed and behaves as a passive chamber. Its pressure therefore declines with its volume according to the pressure-volume relationship, in a manner analogous but directionally opposite to the filling of a fully relaxed ventricle. The configuration of the left atrial pressure-volume relationship has not been fully studied but has been described alternatively as curvilin-

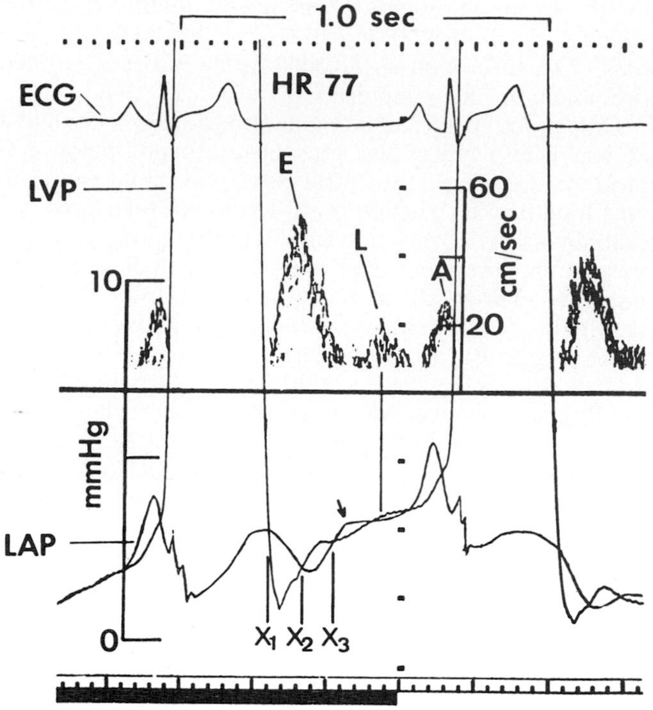

Fig. 24–10. High fidelity left ventricular (LVP) and left atrial pressures (LAP) and simultaneous Doppler transmitral flow velocities measured in a closed chest canine preparation, demonstrating the timing of flow velocities in relation to hemodynamic events. Mitral valve opening and initiation of transmitral flow occurs at the first LAP-LVP crossover point (X_1). The peak flow velocity of the early filling (E) wave occurs at or close to the second pressure crossover point (X_2). The duration of the Doppler flow velocity E wave is similar to the period from X_1 to the third pressure crossover point (X_3). In animals with heart rates between 49 and 90 beats per minute, a mid-diastolic left atrial-left ventricular positive pressure gradient follows the third pressure crossover point (X_3) and is associated with an L wave on the Doppler flow velocity profile. In late diastole, atrial contraction follows the electrocardiographic P wave and produces a left atrial-left ventricular positive pressure gradient corresponding to the Doppler flow velocity A wave.[31] ECG = electrocardiogram; HR = heart rate. (From Courtois M, Kovacs SJ, Jr, Ludbrook PA: Transmitral pressure-flow velocity relation: importance of regional pressure gradients in the left ventricle during diastole. Circulation 1988:78, 661. Reproduced by permission of the American Heart Association, Inc.)

ear by some[32] and linear by others.[33] Whichever the case, left atrial compliance is an important determinant of the atrioventricular pressure gradient because it influences the amount of change in atrial pressure for any given decrease in volume.[34]

The *initial left atrial pressure* when the mitral valve opens is also an important factor governing the subsequent behavior of the atrioventricular pressure gradient. This pressure has been called the *crossover pressure* because it occurs when the left ventricular pressure trace crosses the left atrial trace. Following the crossover point, left atrial pressure always declines more slowly than ventricular pressure, and a higher crossover point allows a larger peak atrioventricular pressure gradient to develop. This major determinant of transmitral flow velocities is discussed in more detail later in the chapter.

During isovolumic relaxation, left ventricular pressure declines in an exponential or near exponential manner according to its rate of relaxation. After the commencement of filling, ventricular pressure declines further but now comes under the influence of two opposing processes, as previously discussed. If we are to imagine that the mitral valve does not open and no filling occurs, left ventricular pressure would continue to decline at a progressively slower rate, as a result of the dissipation of relaxation until an asymptotic pressure is reached. With the occurrence of left ventricular filling, however, the increase in ventricular volume tends to increase intracavitary pressure. The magnitude of this tendency to raise pressure depends on the increase in ventricular volume and the slope of the pressure-volume relationship of the ventricle at that instant.

To develop the idea of an instantaneous pressure-volume relationship further, consider the left ventricular chamber from a theoretical standpoint as having a unique pressure-volume relationship at any moment during contraction and relaxation, not just when fully relaxed. Relaxation is represented by a descent of the pressure-volume relation over time, and the rate at which the pressure-volume curves descend during relaxation is determined by the relaxation rate (Fig. 24–11). From basic principles, left ventricular pressure, at any time during rapid filling, is a function of the pressure-volume relationship at that particular instant (not to be confused with the passive pressure-volume relationship) as well as the ventricular volume. The instantaneous pressure-volume relationship in turn depends on the relaxation rate and the pressure-volume relationship of the ventricle at the onset of relaxation, i.e., the starting point of the relaxation process.

As discussed earlier in the chapter, not only does chamber pressure depend on volume but so does chamber stiffness. The instantaneous ventricular volume during filling is the sum of the initial volume at the time of mitral valve opening (end-systolic volume) and the increase in volume arising from ventricular filling. The stiffness of the ventricle at the initiation of filling depends on the end-systolic volume as well as on the pressure-volume relation at the time. The end-systolic volume is therefore a determinant of the operating stiffness of the ventricle during diastole and hence of the pattern of ventricular filling. Because left ventricular contractility is a major determinant of the end-systolic volume, it is potentially an important determinant of the pattern of left ventricular filling. This mechanism of action, which exerts its effects through the operating chamber stiffness, is independent of the other mechanism linking contractility to diastolic filling, namely, the influence of internal restoring forces on relaxation rate through its load dependence (described earlier in discussion of relaxation).

The mitral orifice area should not be forgotten as a theoretically important determinant of the transmitral flow pattern because it governs the relation between flow velocities generated by the pressure gradients and volumetric flow rates. The latter then directly determine changes in the volumes of the atrial and ventricular chamber. Changes in mitral orifice area theoretically

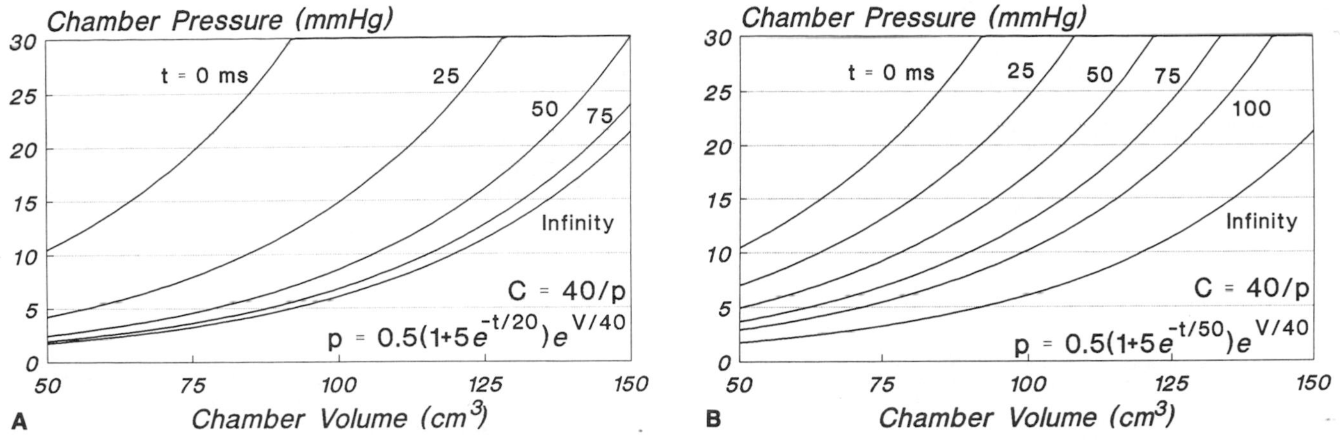

Fig. 24–11. Conceptual representation of instantaneous left ventricular pressure-volume relations during ventricular relaxation. This theoretical approach allows the effects of ventricular relaxation rate, chamber stiffness, and the effect of chamber filling on ventricular pressure to be represented simultaneously. The pressure-volume plots have been generated by a computer model and indicate sequential exponential pressure-volume relations at 25-msec intervals for a ventricle with rapid relaxation (T = 20 msec, **A**) and one with slow relaxation (T = 50 msec, **B**). Other variables have been held constant. The progressive flattening of the pressure-volume curves from t = 0 msec to t = infinity (fully relaxed ventricle) represents the progressive lowering of the stiffness constants of the ventricular chambers that is due to relaxation. The difference between the rates at which these curves change is obvious. Initially, when relaxation proceeds in an isovolumic manner before mitral valve opening (not shown), ventricular pressure declines vertically in the graph but exponentially over time, with the pressure point advancing to successively flatter curves. With the onset of ventricular filling, the ventricular pressure point moves rightward and upward along each instantaneous pressure-volume curve while continuing to migrate to successive pressure-volume curves as a result of progressive relaxation. (Courtesy of Dr. James D. Thomas.)

may also affect viscous flow resistance, but this should be unimportant in normal valves.

The situation in vivo is clearly more complicated than that described here. The effects of viscous resistance in the ventricular wall and the inertia of blood in motion, for example, may need to be considered. Also, regional pressure gradients occur between the apex and base of the left ventricle during ventricular filling, which must modulate the pattern of blood flow within the chamber.[31] The fact that the ventricle draws in or sucks blood from the atrium during the early filling phase while the atrium pushes out blood into the ventricle during the late filling phase may explain the subtle differences in patterns of intraventricular pressure gradients that occur during these periods.

Diastasis

As described earlier, left ventricular pressure increases from its nadir to equilibrate with left atrial pressure during the early filling phase. Often, it exceeds left atrial pressure as flow continues momentarily across the mitral valve against a pressure gradient. In other words, because of the inertial effects of blood, flow has to decelerate to zero even when the pressure gradient has reversed. The pressure gradient may reverse itself a few more times during diastasis, which is due to repetitions of the preceding hemodynamic events. This produces fine oscillations in left atrial and ventricular pressures until true equilibrium is reached.[31]

During diastasis, the left atrium acts mainly as a passive conduit, transferring pulmonary venous flow into the left ventricle. Very little left ventricular filling occurs during this period because left atrial and left ventricular pressures are essentially in equilibrium. Under certain conditions, however, a small and brief transmitral flow wave may be detected at this point. This wave, the L wave, is thought to follow from the diastolic or K wave of pulmonary venous inflow (see following discussion). As the K wave fills the left atrium in early diastole, it re-establishes a positive pressure gradient between the left atrium and ventricle after the occurrence of a reversed pressure gradient during the later part of the early filling phase.[35,36] This new positive pressure gradient results in the L wave.

The L wave produces an equivalent deflection in the anterior mitral leaflet on the M-mode echocardiogram, and its occurrence is predicted by computer modeling of transmitral flow. It may be seen in normal subjects and is expected to be more prominent when flow deceleration of the early filling phase is rapid, such as when ventricular stiffness is increased or ventricular relaxation is rapid.[36] Figure 24–12 shows an example of prominent L waves in the Doppler transmitral flow velocity profile.

Pulmonary Venous Flow

The pattern of pulmonary venous flow has recently been described by pulsed Doppler echocardiography and has attracted much attention. Early studies have generally employed the transthoracic approach using the apical window.[35–37] Here, the pulmonary veins are in the far field of the ultrasound beam, and optimal Doppler signals are not infrequently difficult to obtain in adults. From the apex, blood flow from the right inferior pulmonary vein is directed closest in line with the Doppler ultrasound beam and generally offers the most optimal signals for analysis. The advent of transesophageal echocardiography brings the entrance of the pulmonary

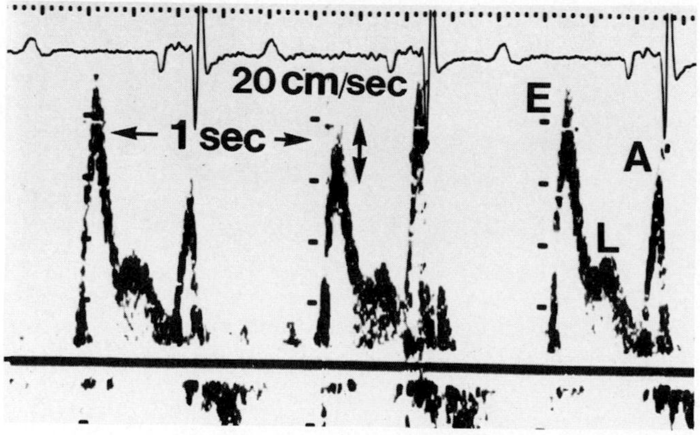

Fig. 24–12. A Doppler transmitral flow velocity profile with a prominent L wave (L). The patient is a middle-aged woman with hypertension, coronary artery disease, moderate concentric left ventricular hypertrophy, and normal left ventricular systolic function. The genesis of the L wave is discussed in the text. Early filling (E) and atrial contraction (A) waves are labeled.

veins much closer to the transducer and has provided excellent opportunities for more detailed studies of pulmonary venous flow.

Although the right ventricle generates the pressure (i.e., potential energy) for pulmonary venous flow, the actual pattern of pulmonary venous flow is determined largely by hemodynamic events in the left atrium, more so than by events in the pulmonary artery or right ventricle. The pulsatility of blood flow in the pulmonary artery does not affect the pattern of pulmonary venous flow, as demonstrated in patients who have had Fontan surgical procedures (right atrial to pulmonary artery anastomoses) performed or Glen shunts (superior vena cava to pulmonary artery communications) inserted.

There are essentially two major forward flow waves, one systolic and the other diastolic, termed by some workers the J and K waves.[35–37] This nomenclature has not been standardized or universally accepted. The systolic wave occurs with atrial relaxation immediately following atrial contraction and also accompanies ventricular systole. It often consists of two discrete flow waves, giving rise in total to a triphasic pulmonary venous forward flow pattern.[38] The first component of the systolic wave is considered to result directly from atrial relaxation. The notch between the first and second components may be the Doppler correlate of the C wave of the left atrial pressure trace. The second component, or late systolic wave, which occurs with ventricular contraction, has been suggested by some to result from or be aided by the descent of the mitral annulus toward the ventricular apex during contraction, producing a suction effect. The exact importance of this suggested mechanism of atrial filling is unclear. In an early report, the entire systolic wave was observed to be absent in three patients with atrial fibrillation but reappeared after cardioversion to sinus rhythm, suggesting that ventricular contraction was not the only factor involved in its generation.[39] Similarly, in the same study, two patients with atrioventricular sequential pacemakers did not demonstrate systolic waves during ventricular pacing (VVI mode). These waves were restored with resumption of sequential atrioventricular (DDD) pacing. More recent studies have helped the understanding of these changes, and these are discussed later in this section.

The diastolic wave occurs in early diastole and accompanies the rapid filling phase of the ventricle. It is produced by the creation of a positive pressure gradient between the pulmonary veins and the left atrium as atrial pressure decreases with early ventricular filling. With short R-R intervals, the systolic and diastolic wave may fuse to produce a monophasic pattern.[38] A very small amount of reversed flow in the pulmonary veins is seen during atrial contraction in the majority of normal patients. This reversed flow is accentuated when there is resistance to left ventricular filling, such as occurs in mitral stenosis, left ventricular hypertrophy, or pericardial constriction. Recently, a late flow reversal wave has been described in patients with atrial fibrillation and without mitral regurgitation, which occurs slightly later than that seen in patients in sinus rhythm.[40] This later wave may be due to the movement of a minimal volume of blood into the left atrium that is trapped by the mitral leaflets during ventricular contraction.

Thus, pulmonary venous flow may be considered to have four distinct flow waves, three forward and one reverse. Figure 24–13 shows a typical pulmonary venous flow profile containing these four waves recorded from the transesophageal approach. Several recent studies exploiting the advantages of transesophageal echocardiography in obtaining high quality flow signals in the near field (2 to 4 cm) have contributed importantly to our understanding of pulmonary venous flow in health and disease and deserve further elaboration here. Signals from the transesophageal approach are far superior to those from the transthoracic approach but also differ qualitatively. In one study, flow reversal during atrial contraction could be observed in only 37% of normal subjects compared to 100% of subjects from the transesophageal approach.[38] Biphasic systolic forward flow

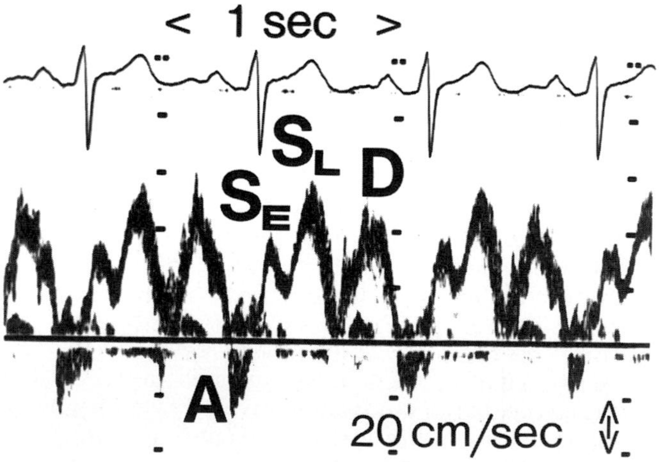

Fig. 24–13. Typical example of a pulmonary venous flow velocity profile containing four waves, three forward, and one reverse. The recording was taken from the left superior pulmonary vein using the transesophageal approach. S_E = early systolic wave; S_L = late systolic wave; D = diastolic wave; A = atrial flow reversal wave.

was not observed in any subject from the transthoracic approach compared to 73% of subjects from the transesophageal approach. In another study, a biphasic systolic forward flow pattern was seen in only 30% of normal subjects with the transthoracic approach.[41]

Quantitatively similar pulmonary venous flow velocities are recorded from the right pulmonary vein by both transthoracic and transesophageal tracings.[38] Systolic flow velocities may be higher in the right upper pulmonary vein (transthoracic or transesophageal) than left upper pulmonary vein (transesophageal), but diastolic flow velocities are similar.[38] The standardization of sampling depth is important. As the sample volume is moved distally into the pulmonary vein, signal quality worsens, and spectral broadening increases markedly when the sample volume is positioned 1 cm or more into the vein. The biphasic nature of systolic flow may be lost, and while systolic flow velocities are not altered significantly, diastolic flow velocities tend to decrease.[38] For research and clinical recordings, a depth of 0.5 to 1 cm is recommended.

In a recent study, the manipulation of loading conditions produced changes in the peak velocities and deceleration time of the pulmonary venous diastolic flow wave that correlated directly with changes in the transmitral early (E) filling wave, suggesting that diastolic flow velocity in the pulmonary vein was determined by the same factors that determined early left ventricular filling.[42] The systolic pulmonary venous flow velocity changed in direct proportion to cardiac output. In this study, pulmonary venous flow reversal at atrial contraction correlated best with the pulmonary capillary wedge pressure.

Others investigating the usefulness of the pulmonary venous flow pattern for estimating left atrial pressure have found that the systolic fraction (i.e., the systolic velocity-time integral expressed as a fraction of the sum of systolic and early-diastolic velocity-time integral) correlated most strongly (but negatively) with mean left atrial pressure ($r = -0.88$). This was due to both a reduction in systolic flow velocity and an increase in diastolic flow velocity as left atrial pressure increased.[43] Mitral flow variables correlated less well with left atrial pressure than pulmonary venous flow variables. Similarly, changes in the systolic fraction produced by interventions correlated best with changes in the mean left atrial pressure.[44] In normal subjects, the systolic forward flow is dominant (systolic fraction 68 ± 6% standard deviation [SD]), but in patients without mitral regurgitation who have pulmonary capillary wedge pressures ≥15 mm Hg, diastolic flow is dominant (systolic fraction 42 ± 15%). Neither left atrial expansion nor descent of the mitral annulus seemed to influence the relationship between pulmonary venous flow and pulmonary capillary wedge pressure, but left ventricular fractional shortening confounded this relationship.

Results from a more recent study in dogs caution against the indiscriminate use of pulmonary venous flow pattern to assess left atrial pressure.[45] An increase in left atrial pressure with volume loading was associated with an increase rather than decrease in the pulmonary venous systolic velocity/diastolic velocity ratio and the systolic velocity time integral/diastolic velocity from integral ratio. This was due to an increase in systolic velocities and a decrease in diastolic velocities. By contrast, when left atrial pressure was increased by impairing left ventricular contractility, there was no such correlation. The systolic and diastolic velocities both fell, and there was a nonsignificant tendency for the systolic velocity time integral to fall. Independent correlates of the pattern of pulmonary venous flow were found to be atrial systolic shortening, aortic systolic pressure, heart rate, and left ventricular end-systolic dimension. Apart from these matters concerning load, the confounding effect of age must also be borne in mind. In normal subjects, increasing age produces an increase in systolic flow velocity and ratio of systolic to diastolic flow velocity, a decrease in diastolic flow velocity, and an increase in flow reversal during atrial contraction, at least partly reflecting altered left ventricular diastolic function and filling.[41]

Another important recent application of the pulmonary venous flow profile has been in the estimation of mitral regurgitation severity. In one study, patients with no significant mitral regurgitation had a higher peak systolic velocity (55 ± 16 cm/sec) and lower peak diastolic velocity (43 ± 13 cm/sec) than those with significant mitral regurgitation (−4 ± 16 cm/sec, $p < .0001$; 59 ± 17 cm/sec, $p < .01$).[46] Thus, the peak systolic/diastolic velocity ratio was higher in those without than with significant regurgitation (1.4 ± 0.5 vs. 0.4 ± 1.3, $p < .0001$). The same trend was found for systolic and diastolic velocity integrals. The peak systolic velocity and velocity-time integral decreased, and peak diastolic velocity and velocity-time integral increased as mitral regurgitation increased. In patients with severe (4+) mitral regurgitation, systolic flow reversal occurred with a sensitivity of 90%, specificity of 100%, and positive predictive value of 98% for severe regurgitation. Others have found similarly a high sensitivity of 93% and specificity of 100% when using transesophageal color flow mapping as a gold standard for severe mitral regurgitation, but they have found a sensitivity of 86% and specificity of 81% when using nonsimultaneous cardiac catheterization.[47] Discordant flows were observed between the left superior and right superior pulmonary veins in 24% of patients, with the left vein usually showing blunted systolic flow (ratio of peak systolic to diastolic flow velocities between 0 and 1) and the right showing reversed systolic flow. The reason for this discordance remains speculative but is likely to be due to differences in regurgitant jet direction. Although the systolic flow velocity and peak systolic/diastolic velocity ratio decreased and diastolic flow velocity increased as mitral regurgitation severity worsened, the presence of blunted systolic flow itself did not allow reliable discrimination between the various grades of severity. To date, few patients have been evaluated, and larger studies are awaited.

Left Atrial Contraction Phase

Left atrial function has not been studied as well as has left ventricular function. It is clinically less important than left ventricular function and is less easily measured but is by no means unimportant. The left atrium contracts in a manner similar to the Frank Starling mechanism described for the left ventricle.[48] Thus, a higher left atrial volume just before atrial contraction is expected to generate a higher left atrial stroke volume and peak pressure. In ways similar to the left ventricle, left atrial systolic function also depends on the contractility of the atrial myocardium as well as the resistance to atrial emptying offered by the left ventricle.[48,49] This resistance depends on the pressure of the ventricle and on the stiffness characteristics of the ventricle, because a stiffer ventricle is expected to exhibit a higher pressure at any particular volume and, furthermore, to raise its pressure more for any given amount of filling during atrial contraction.

The heart rate and the atrioventricular (or electrocardiographic PR) time interval determine the period available for diastolic flow and the temporal relation between the early filling and atrial contraction flow waves. They are therefore expected to strongly influence the transmitral flow velocity profile.

A summary of the various primary factors involved in the determination of the transmitral flow velocity profile is given in Figure 24–14. Experimental studies of these factors are discussed in further detail in the section of Doppler echocardiography in this chapter. The whole situation in vivo can be considerably more complex and may involve various secondary factors that modify the interactions between the primary factors described here. For example, right-to-left ventricular interactions and pericardial influences may alter atrial or ventricular loading and pressure-volume relationships. In valvular disease, mitral regurgitation, among other effects, increases left atrial and therefore crossover pressure; aortic regurgitation, by increasing left ventricular volume and pressure, decreases the atrioventricular pressure gradient independently of flow across the mitral orifice; mitral stenosis not only increases the crossover pressure but alters the normal relation between transmitral flow velocity and flow volume.

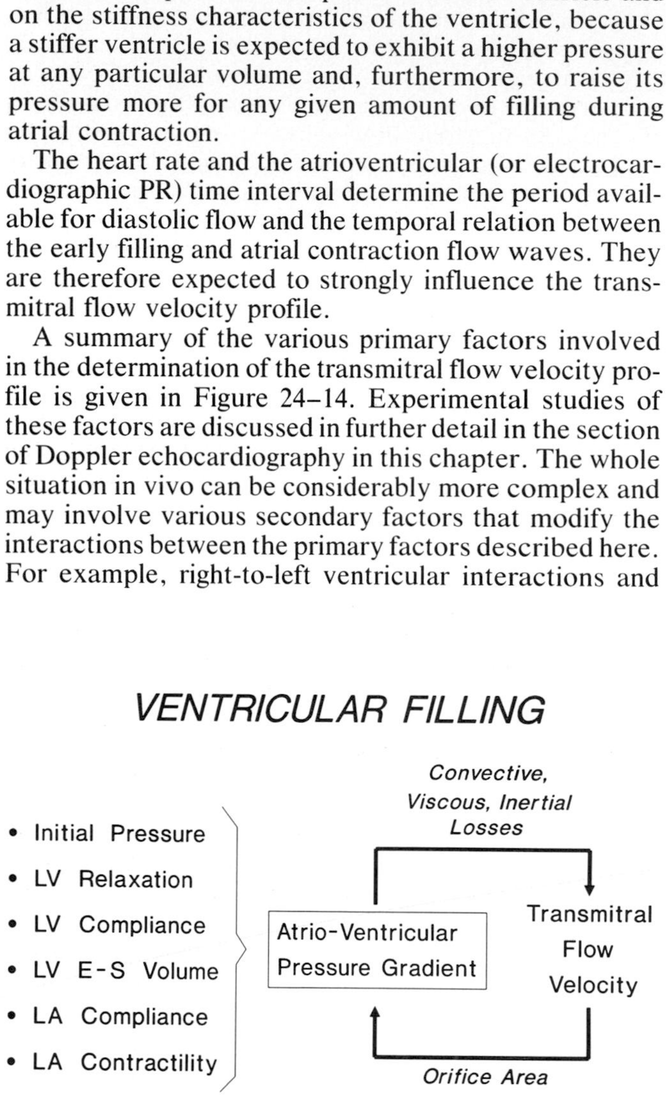

Fig. 24–14. Summary of the multiple determinants of the transmitral flow velocity profile. A complex and continuous interaction occurs among all the factors. Interactions among the factors listed in the left column primarily determine the left atrial to left ventricular pressure gradient. This gradient represents the potential hydraulic energy available to generate the transmitral flow velocity. Energy losses from convective, inertial, and viscous resistance modulate this relationship. The flow orifice area determines volumetric flow rate for any given transmitral flow velocity, and in turn influences the rate of change of the atrial and ventricular volumes. In this simplified model, phasic pulmonary venous flow into the left atrium during diastole is ignored. Heart rate is not listed and may be considered a secondary factor. It affects the flow velocity profile by determining the timing of atrial contraction, modifying loading conditions and possibly by altering contractility (see text). E-S = end-systolic; LA = left atrial; LV = left ventricular.

ECHOCARDIOGRAPHIC MEASUREMENTS OF THE FILLING CHARACTERISTICS OF THE LEFT VENTRICLE

M-Mode Echocardiography

M-mode echocardiography has been employed extensively to evaluate the diastolic properties of the left ventricle. Two types of measurements are made: static measurements, which describe dimensions taken at one point only in the cardiac cycle, usually end-diastole, and dynamic measurements, which describe the pattern of motion of the ventricle in diastole.

Static Measurements

The thickness of the myocardium in diastole, reflecting the degree of ventricular hypertrophy, is a useful guide to its diastolic function, although this parameter in itself is not strictly a measure of function. As discussed previously in this chapter, a nondilated ventricle with thick walls may be expected to have increased chamber stiffness even if the stiffness of individual myocardial elements is normal. M-mode echocardiography is ideally suited for the measurement of wall thickness because endocardial and epicardial borders can often be clearly demarcated. By convention, septal and posterior wall thickness are measured at a level in the ventricle just beyond the tips of the mitral leaflets in the parasternal long axis view, as described elsewhere in this book. Measurements of diastolic wall thickness antemortem have been found to correlate poorly with autopsy measurements, largely because the hearts at autopsy are usually in a state of contracture.[50] Diastolic measurements of wall thickness by M-mode echocardiography correlate better with measurements at surgery, while systolic measurements by M-mode echocardiography correlate better with autopsy measurements.[51]

If the internal diameter of the ventricle is also measured and geometric assumptions are made about the shape of the ventricle, the volume of myocardium can be calculated. From this volume and with knowledge of the density of myocardium, myocardial mass can also be calculated. Myocardial mass is a more direct measure of myocardial hypertrophy than wall thickness alone. Various methods for measuring myocardial mass by M-mode echocardiography have been proposed. These differ from one another in the positions where measurements are taken for the septal and ventricular borders and whether corrections are made for alterations in ventricular shape with increases in ventricular size. Satisfactory validation against autopsy data has been obtained.[52] Details of these methods are described in Chapter 14 on M-mode echocardiography.

As discussed previously, the evaluation of wall stress provides useful information about the load placed on individual myocardial elements. The measurement of wall stress requires intraventricular radius, wall thickness, and intraventricular pressure to be known. Because circumferential wall stress is approximated by the product of pressure and radius, divided by twice the wall thickness (Laplace's law), an increase in wall thickness is seen as a compensatory mechanism whereby the ventricle can restore wall stress, i.e., the load imposed on individual myocardial elements, to normal levels in the face of elevated systolic pressures.[53] The ratio of wall thickness to radius has been used to determine whether a degree of hypertrophy is appropriate for a given increase in pressure.

A great deal of valuable clinical information has been derived from studies using M-mode measurements of ventricular hypertrophy. Such measurements are more sensitive than and at least as specific as if not more specific than the standard criteria used in electrocardiography.[50,54] A large body of information has been accumulated on the development, progression, and regression of wall thickness and myocardial mass in a variety of pressure overload, volume overload, and primary forms of hypertrophy.[55] The deleterious effects of hypertrophy on the development of myocardial ischemia, arrhythmias, and diastolic dysfunction are well recognized. With the introduction of a host of medications capable of causing regression of pressure load hypertrophy, greater reliance than ever before has been placed on the ability of echocardiographic techniques to quantitate ventricular hypertrophy accurately. In the calculation of wall mass, caution must be exercised when the ventricle is not symmetric or is particularly large, because geometric assumptions may be highly inaccurate in these situations. Two-dimensional echocardiography has been used and has the advantage of allowing a much larger portion of the ventricle to be viewed but is limited by poorer temporal resolution. Calculations of mass with this technique still must rely on assumptions about ventricular geometry that may or may not be valid.

Dynamic Parameters

Time-varying events during diastole may be characterized in detail using M-mode echocardiography. The high axial (<1 mm) and temporal (pulse repetition frequency 1000 Hz) resolutions of the technique and the display of time on the x axis are major advantages in making these measurements. Such measurements may be divided into those that measure time periods, often termed *diastolic time intervals*, and those that measure rates of change of various dimensions.

Among the more commonly used parameters are the isovolumic relaxation period, the peak rate of increase in left ventricular dimension, the peak rate of ventricular wall thinning, and the atrial filling fraction (the proportion of total dimensional increase accounted for by atrial contraction), all of which have been used to reflect the diastolic function of the ventricle. Many other measurements have been reported and are listed later at the end of this section.

The isovolumic relaxation period is measured from aortic valve closure to mitral valve opening. Because aortic and mitral valve traces are not recorded from the same cardiac cycle on an M-mode echocardiogram (unless two transducers or dual M-line systems are used), the point of aortic valve closure is usually taken from the onset of the aortic valve closure sound recorded simultaneously by phonocardiography. Measurement of the isovolumic relaxation period is facilitated by superimposing the phono signal on the M-mode echocardiographic trace showing mitral leaflet motion.

Alternatively, the isovolumic relaxation period may be approximated by measuring the duration from minimal left ventricular dimension at the end of systole to mitral valve opening, obviating the need for phonocardiography. This measurement, the relaxation time index, is usually shorter than measurements derived from the aortic valve closure, because aortic valve closure precedes the time of minimal left ventricular dimension.[56] Although a relatively good correlation exists between the isovolumic relaxation period and the relaxation time index, caution should be exercised with the use of the relaxation time index because the two indices are not interchangeable. For example, in some instances, mitral valve opening may start before minimal left ventricular dimension occurs.[57] Normal values for the relaxation time index have been reported to be 13 ± 15 msec (range -29 to $+35$ msec)[57] and even as low at 1 ± 6 msec,[56] values that are substantially lower than those for the true isovolumic relaxation period (62 ± 10 msec).[58] The relatively late and variable occurrence of the minimal left ventricular dimension in these M-mode measurements may be related to the placement of the M-mode beam closer to the base of the ventricle than is the standard practice when measuring ventricular dimensions. This shift in the M-line position is made to obtain clearer records of mitral leaflet opening. The ultrasound beam in this situation may therefore transect the membranous interventricular septum and the posterolateral wall at the base, probably one of the last regions of the ventricle to be excited.

Apart from the echocardiographic parameters mentioned previously, many other descriptive measurements of diastolic events have been derived from M-mode echocardiographic tracings. These include the peak rate of posterior wall motion in diastole (which is very susceptible to distortion by cardiac translation),[59] the duration of the rapid filling phase (represented arbitrarily by the time from minimum left ventricular dimension to the moment when the rate of increase in dimension has decreased to 20% or 50% of its maximum value),[57,60] and the time to peak filling rate (represented by the time from minimum left ventricular dimension to the moment of peak rate of increase in dimension).[59] The time from the Q wave on the electrocardiogram to the point at which the rate of wall thinning is maximal, the time from the Q wave to the end of the period of diastolic thinning during the rapid filling phase, and the total filling period have also been used.[61] Abnormalities in these measurements have been found in a wide range of cardiac diseases (see later), but their relative usefulness for evaluating diastolic function remains undetermined.

Methodologic Considerations

Ideally, the diastolic time intervals and rates of increase in left ventricular dimension and wall thinning are measured from M-mode traces with the M-line positioned across the left ventricle just at the level of the tips of the mitral leaflets. Data should be recorded at relatively high paper speeds, at least 50 mm/sec, or preferably 100 mm/sec. It is important that the M-line be positioned perpendicular to the endocardium of the interventricular septum and posterior wall. If this is not done, distances recorded along the M-line and measured on the tracing will exceed the true dimensions.[62]

Analysis of such data is greatly facilitated by tracing the right and left sides of the interventricular septum and the endocardium and epicardium of the posterior left ventricular wall using a digitizing system interfaced to a computer. Hand tracing the raw information with a pencil first before digitization with a cursor is recommended to reduce noise that is due to hesitation and tremor. Several consecutive beats (at least three in sinus rhythm) should be traced and the results averaged. In most systems that have been used, the absolute values of ventricular diameter (D) and wall thickness (T) and their rates of change (obtained from the first derivatives, dD/dt and dT/dt, respectively) are automatically computed and displayed as a function of time[63] (Fig. 24–15). The peak rates of increase in ventricular dimension and of wall thinning are obtained from the peak values of dD/dt and dT/dt, respectively.[64]

Uncertainties in the measurement of time intervals and dimensions may be calculated from the formulae

$$\Delta T = \Delta M \times \sqrt{(2/P)} \quad \text{and} \quad \Delta D = \Delta M \times \sqrt{(2/S)}$$

where ΔT is the uncertainty in time, ΔD is the uncertainty in distance, ΔM is digitizer resolution, P is paper speed, and S is depth scale (millimeters per centimeter of tissue). Thus, the error in the calculation of the rate of change in dimension depends on the paper speed, the depth scale, the digitizer resolution, and the sampling rate of the digitizing system for dimension and resampling rate for change in dimension.[61] Unprocessed traces showing ventricular dimension and wall thickness are usually smoothed first using various techniques, such as a sixth-order polynomial fit,[65,66] a five-point smoothing filter,[61] or a three-point triangular fit.[60]

Echocardiographic measurements of dD/dt have been validated against measurements obtained from contrast[60,67] and radionuclide angiography.[68] Various methods have been proposed for normalizing these echocardiographic measurements. The peak rate of increase in dimension has been normalized to the end-diastolic dimension,[69] the instantaneous diastolic dimension,[60] and the total change in dimension from systole to diastole.[65] If normalization is considered necessary, there are persuasive theoretical grounds for using the third method.[65] Unlike the first and second methods, normalization to

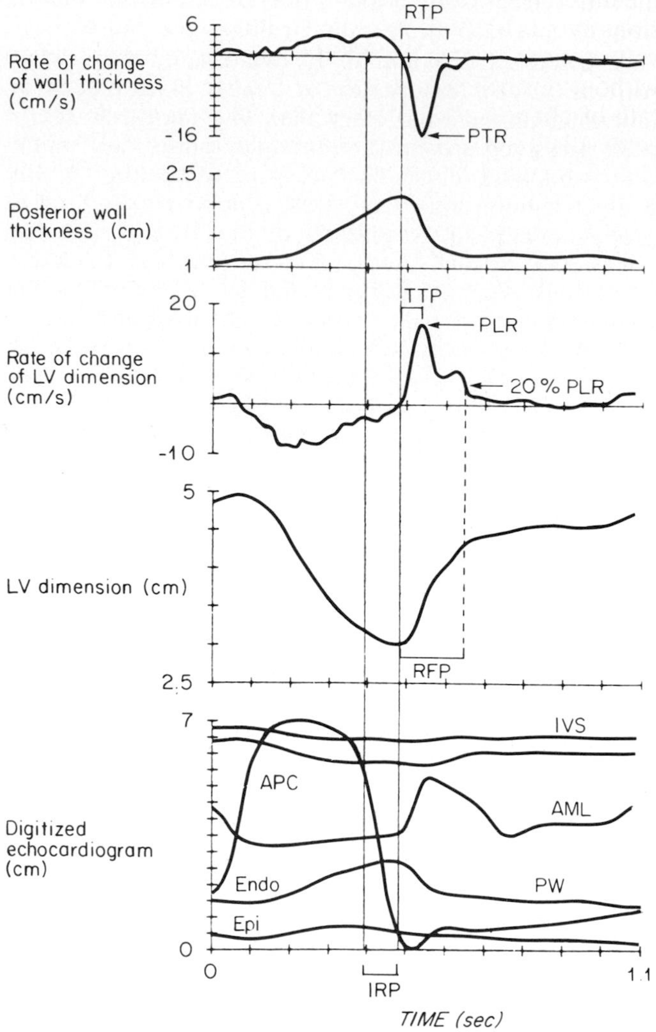

Fig. 24–15. An example of computer-generated M-mode echocardiographic indices of left ventricular diastolic function recorded in a normal subject. Bottom. Digitized traces of the endocardial (Endo) and epicardial (Epi) surfaces of the posterior wall (PW) of the left ventricle and both endocardial surfaces of the interventricular septum (IVS) are obtained from M-mode echocardiographic recordings. Instantaneous parameters are calculated automatically and plotted with the raw data. The figure shows, from top to bottom, the rate of change in PW thickness, PW thickness, rate of change in left ventricular (LV) internal dimension, LV internal dimension, and the traced endocardial borders of the IVS, endocardial and epicardial borders of the posterior ventricular wall, the anterior mitral leaflet (AML), and an apexicardiogram (APC). The vertical lines on the left demonstrate the time of aortic valve closure derived from the aortic second sound (phonocardiogram not shown) and on the right demonstrate the onset of mitral valve opening derived from the M-mode echocardiograph. In this subject, minimal LV dimension and mitral valve opening occurred together, but this is often not the case in others. Commonly measured indices of diastolic function are indicated. IRP = isovolumic relaxation period; PLR = peak lengthening rate, i.e., peak rate of increase in left ventricular internal dimension; PTR = peak thinning rate; RFP = rapid filling period, taken as the time from minimal left ventricular dimension to the point at which the lengthening rate has decreased to 20% of its peak value; RTP = rapid thinning period; TTP = period from minimal left ventricular dimension to the time of peak lengthening rate.[63] (From Trail TA, Gibson DG, Brown DJ: Study of left ventricular wall thickness and dimension changes using echocardiography. Br Heart J 40:162, 1978.)

the difference between the systolic and diastolic dimensions avoids the automatic generation of low normalized values when ventricles are dilated. Furthermore, even without normalization, a given change in dimension or rate of change in dimension in a large ventricle represents a larger volumetric change than in a small ventricle. Normalization of dimensional change using division by the absolute dimension therefore underestimates volumetric changes even more.

The approach using systolic-to-diastolic differences for normalization is further supported by the finding that the maximal lengthening velocity of isolated canine papillary muscle (dL/dt_{max}) is linearly related to the extent of muscle shortening.[70] The maximal lengthening velocity normalized in this way appears to be independent of preload, afterload, contractile state, and contraction frequency. Also, the maximal lengthening rate of rat papillary muscle is directly related to its extent of shortening, regardless of whether it has been obtained from normal or chronic pressure- or volume-loaded ventricles.[71] Finally, in normal humans, filling rate measured from contrast angiography correlates directly with stroke volume.[72]

Echocardiographic measurements of the rate of ventricular wall thinning have also been normalized to various parameters. Some workers have chosen to normalize these measurements to maximal wall thickness,[61] while others have chosen to use instantaneous thickness[56] or the total change in thickness from systole to diastole.[65] There is no consensus on which method is most correct.

Several important geometric considerations should be recognized when M-mode echocardiographic measurements are used to describe the filling characteristics of the left ventricle, simply because linear dimensions rather than volumes are measured. As mentioned earlier, the rate of change in ventricular volume for a given rate of change in dimension depends on the actual dimension of the ventricle itself as well as the geometry of the ventricular chamber. Thus, the rate of change in volume is higher in a larger chamber and lower in a smaller one for a given rate of change in dimension.[73] On the other hand, in a ventricle that is dilated, the chamber assumes a more spheroidal shape and at the same time changes less in shape as it contracts. This is due to relatively less shortening of the longitudinal dimension produced by apical contraction. As a result, for any given decrease in the anteroposterior dimension that occurs during contraction, ventricular volume decreases less without a change in shape than with a normal change in shape.[73]

With these considerations in mind, it is important to realize that changes in echocardiographic measurements of chamber dimensions or wall thickness do not equate directly with ventricular filling, although there clearly must be a relationship between them. Further evidence supporting this point comes from observations that changes in ventricular dimensions and wall thickness may occur during the isovolumic relaxation period when ventricular volume is strictly constant. These changes presumably are due to alterations in ventricular shape. Although such changes are very small in normal subjects, they may be grossly exaggerated in patients with ischemic heart disease or ventricular hypertrophy.[57,74]

Simultaneous measurements of ventricular dimension and volume derived from contrast cineangiography indicate that peak rates of increase in dimension occur at least 40 to 60 msec before peak rates of increase in volume. This discrepancy probably results from the ventricle assuming a more spherical shape during rapid filling.[75] The duration of the rapid filling phase, however, is usually similar when measured by the two techniques. It should be noted that in normal subjects, the contribution of atrial contraction to left ventricular filling measured as a dimensional change of the ventricle is smaller than that derived from measurements of volume change (5 vs. 20%).[73]

Normal Values

Published normal values for the M-mode echocardiographic measurements of diastolic events have generally been based on small numbers of subjects. Earlier reports gave mean values for subjects over a wide range of ages, but it has more recently been appreciated that age exerts significant influences on these measurements.[65,76] In one study, peak filling rate (normalized to total change in dimension) and peak thinning rate (normalized to the total change in thinning) correlated negatively with age, peak left ventricular systolic pressure, and wall thickness. Peak left ventricular systolic pressure and end-diastolic wall thickness correlated positively with age, and it has been suggested, therefore, that the effects of age on diastolic function are mediated at least in part by age-related increases in systolic pressure and wall thickness.[65] These observations are supported by another study that involved 165 normal subjects aged from 6 to 62 years. The author found an increase in left ventricular wall thickness and mass, a prolongation of the left ventricular isovolumic relaxation period, and a decrease in the peak rates of increase in left ventricular dimension and wall thinning with increasing age of the subjects. These age-related changes were associated with a delay in the occurrence of the physiologic third heart sound as well as a diminishing amplitude and, eventually, a complete disappearance of the sound.[76]

Changes in heart rate may also alter diastolic time intervals but have not been shown to significantly affect measurements of peak rates of increase in ventricular dimension or of wall thinning.[65,77] Spontaneous variations in normal left ventricular systolic function, as represented by the shortening fraction, are also associated with the rate of increase in ventricular dimension.[77] Inotropic stimulation with dobutamine in normal subjects raises the peak rates of increase in left ventricular dimension and of wall thinning and causes them to occur earlier.[78] From a mechanistic viewpoint, it is important to understand that these diastolic changes may occur not only through alterations in contractility per se (an increase in contractility decreases the left ventricular end-systolic volume and hence the ventricular volume and chamber stiffness at the initiation of filling—see previous discussion in this chapter) but also as a result of a concurrent increase in relaxation rate produced by the sympathomimetic stimulation. The effects of loading conditions have recently been described.[77,78] Increased preload produces higher peak rates of increase in left ventricular dimension and of wall thinning without any apparent change in their times of occurrence. Increased afterload delays the occurrence of both these events and in this study did not significantly alter their peak rates of change.[78]

Some published normal values of M-mode echocardiographic diastolic measurements that take into consideration age differences are given in Tables 24–2 and 24–3. The numbers of subjects studied in each age group were relatively small, and these values should serve only as general guidelines.

Clinical Observations From Diastolic M-Mode Measurements

From the measurements described previously, a variety of abnormal patterns of left ventricular filling have been described in many cardiac diseases. A brief summary only is provided here.

Coronary Artery Disease. Compared to normal control subjects of similar age, patients with coronary artery disease have been reported to show a reduced peak rate of early increase in left ventricular dimension, a reduced proportion of total left ventricular filling resulting from the rapid filling phase, an unaltered peak rate of increase in left ventricular dimension resulting from atrial contraction, and an increased proportion of total left ventricular filling resulting from atrial contraction. In many patients, these findings are present even in regions where systolic function remains normal.[79]

Mitral and Aortic Valve Disease. Patients with mitral stenosis have a reduced peak rate of increase in left ventricular dimension, which persists throughout diastole. The duration of the early filling period is correspondingly prolonged. In patients with mixed mitral disease, the duration of filling is also prolonged, but peak rates of increase in dimension may be normal because of coexisting mitral regurgitation.[60] Patients with aortic regurgitation have been reported to show a reduced peak rate of increase in left ventricular dimension, increased time from minimum left ventricular dimension to peak filling rate, and increased duration of rapid filling (time from minimum left ventricular dimension to 20% of peak filling rate).

Hypertrophic Cardiomyopathy. Patients with hypertrophic cardiomyopathy show a heterogeneous filling pattern on M-mode echocardiography and can be divided into three main groups on this basis. Such patients may have either increased, normal, or reduced peak filling rates, which are related essentially to the rate of posterior wall thinning.[56] The presence of mitral regurgitation may be an important confounding factor because this may increase the peak rate of ventricular filling. Variations in the severity of mitral regurgitation alone, however, do not appear to be the entire explanation for the differences in filling rates. A reduction in peak filling rate has been associated with progressive asynchrony of septal and posterior wall contraction and an increased incidence of atrial fibrillation and perhaps also of angina.[56] A markedly prolonged relaxation time index

Table 24–2. Normal Values of M-Mode Echocardiography Measurements During Diastole Separated by Age Groups

	Age (Years)	HR (bpm)	IVRP (msec)	Dd (mm)	Ds (mm)	STd (mm)	PWd (mm)	LV Mass (gm)	max dD/dt/D (sec^{-1})	max dPW/dt/PW (sec^{-1})	FS%
Group I (n = 20)	6.1 ± 0.8	89.6 ± 12.9	53.8 ± 5.1	37.7 ± 2.8	25.1 ± 2.3	6.0 ± 0.7	5.3 ± 0.7	54.6 ± 9.0	6.5 ± 1.3	20.5 ± 6.3	33.5 ± 3.2
Group II (n = 18)	12.1 ± 0	77.0 ± 12.2	56.4 ± 5.0	43.3 ± 3.6	28.5 ± 2.7	7.2 ± 0.8	7.0 ± 0.7	83.0 ± 11.8	6.5 ± 1.0	18.5 ± 4.7	34.2 ± 3.4
Group III (n = 21)	19.2 ± 0.8	73.5 ± 13.4	57.8 ± 6.4	48.4 ± 3.8	31.9 ± 2.7	8.3 ± 0.9	8.2 ± 1.1	110.5 ± 17.0	5.5 ± 1.1	13.3 ± 3.2	34.1 ± 2.6
Group IV (n = 19)	24.1 ± 0.7	68.7 ± 13.7	62.7 ± 5.9	50.3 ± 2.9	34.1 ± 3.4	7.6 ± 1.0	7.7 ± 1.2	105.7 ± 17.3	5.2 ± 0.7	14.1 ± 2.7	32.3 ± 4.1
Group V (n = 21)	29.2 ± 0.9	66.9 ± 9.1	73.0 ± 7.9	49.8 ± 2.9	32.4 ± 2.3	8.3 ± 1.4	8.1 ± 1.1	113.6 ± 19.2	5.1 ± 1.0	12.3 ± 3.9	34.9 ± 4.2
Group VI (n = 22)	35.6 ± 1.0	67.0 ± 7.9	78.3 ± 8.1	51.6 ± 4.5	33.4 ± 3.2	8.1 ± 0.9	7.8 ± 1.1	114.7 ± 22.7	5.2 ± 1.2	12.1 ± 4.2	35.4 ± 2.6
Group VII (n = 44)	47.7 ± 6.0	66.4 ± 8.9	82.1 ± 11.1	49.2 ± 4.5	30.6 ± 3.6	9.3 ± 1.5	8.9 ± 1.3	127.1 ± 25.9	5.2 ± 1.2	10.5 ± 2.5	37.9 ± 4.3
F		12.91^B	52.51^B	34.8^B	21.4^B	23.0^B	27.3^B	36.0^B	6.6^B	20.5^B	7.3^b
r		-0.48^B	0.75^B	0.54^B	0.30^B	0.66^B	0.66^B	0.71^B	-0.33^B	-0.60^B	0.41^B
F′		0.3 (NS)	21.2^B	1.8 (NS)	6.6^B	9.6^B	6.7^B	4.6^A	0.1 (NS)	6.0^B	9.7^B
r′		−0.11 (NS)	0.48^B	−0.10 (NS)	-0.36^B	0.52^B	0.49^B	0.43^B	0.05 (NS)	-0.38^B	0.47^B

HR = heart rate; IVRP = isovolumic relaxation period; Dd and Ds = left ventricular internal diameter at end-diastole and end-systole, respectively; STd = left ventricular septal thickness at end-diastole; PWd = left ventricular posterior wall thickness at end-diastole; LV = left ventricular; max dD/dt/D = peak increase of dimension in early diastole normalized to instantaneous dimension; max dPW/dt/PW = peak thinning rate of the posterior wall in early diastole normalized to instantaneous thickness; FS = fractional shortening; r, r′ = linear correlation coefficients with age for all groups and for groups IV to VII, respectively; F, F′ = F ratio for all groups and for groups IV to VII, respectively.

[A] $p < .01$.

[B] $p < .001$.

(From Van der Werf F, et al.: The mechanism of disappearance of the physiologic third heart sound with age. Circulation 73:877, 1986. Reproduced by permission of the American Heart Association, Inc.)

Table 24–3. Normal Values of M-Mode Echocardiographic Measurements During Diastole in Two Groups of Different Ages

	Group 1 (n = 19)	Group 2 (n = 19)
Age (yr)	15 ± 7	54 ± 10*
HR (beats/min)	77 ± 18	74 ± 11
LVPSP (mm Hg)	111 ± 9	127 ± 15*
h_{ed} (mm)	7.7 ± 1.5	9.3 ± 1.5
D_{ed} (mm)	42 ± 7	44 ± 4
% delta D	35 ± 3	37 ± 4
dD/dt (mm/sec)	168 ± 38	143 ± 46
dD/dt/delta D (sec^{-1})	11.5 ± 3.0	8.7 ± 2.7*
dPW/dt (mm/sec)	129 ± 32	100 ± 38*
dPW/dt/delta PW (sec^{-1})	22.5 ± 4.6	14.7 ± 4.2*

* $p < 0.0125$ vs. group 1.

Subjects in Group 1 were 26 years old or less, and those in Group 2 were 40 years or older.

HR = heart rate; LVPSP = left ventricular peak systolic pressure; h_{ed} = end-diastolic posterior wall thickness; D_{ed} = end-diastolic dimensions; % delta D = percent fractional shortening; dD/dt = peak rate of early diastolic increase in left ventricular dimension; dD/dt/delta D = peak rate of early diastolic increase in left ventricular dimension normalized to change in dimension between systole and diastole; dPW/dt = peak early diastolic posterior wall thinning rate; dPW/dt/delta PW = peak early diastolic posterior wall thinning rate normalized to change in wall thickness between systole and diastole.

(From Fifer MA, Borow KM, Colan SD, Lorell BH: Early diastolic left ventricular function in children and adults with aortic stenosis. J Am Coll Cardiol 5:1147, 1985. Reprinted with permission from the American College of Cardiology.

(minimum left ventricular dimension to mitral valve opening), shortened rapid filling phase, and smaller increase in ventricular dimension during the rapid filling phase have all been found in patients with hypertrophic cardiomyopathy and those with chronic pressure overload hypertrophy.[57] In one study, patients with chronic pressure overload hypertrophy had a greater augmentation of left ventricular dimension during atrial contraction, whereas those with hypertrophic cardiomyopathy did not demonstrate this finding.[60] In another study, the severity of the abnormalities in diastolic wall motion appeared to be related to the magnitude of the ventricular hypertrophy. Diastolic wall motion abnormalities, however, were also found in patients with only mild hypertrophy involving just one segment of the ventricle and could be detected in segments that were not hypertrophied.[59]

Pressure Load Left Ventricular Hypertrophy. As mentioned earlier, patients with chronic left ventricular pressure overload from hypertension or aortic stenosis have a prolonged left ventricular relaxation time index (minimal left ventricular dimension to mitral valve opening) and a marked increase in left ventricular dimension during this period, which probably is due to an abnormal change in ventricular shape during isovolumic relaxation.[57] The increase in left ventricular dimension during the rapid filling phase is reduced compared to that in normal control subjects. This is compensated for by a greater increase in left ventricular dimension during atrial contraction. Others have found a reduced atrial emptying index (decrease in left atrial diameter during the first third of diastole as a percentage of total decrease during diastole), reflecting a reduction in the early filling phase of the left ventricle. These changes may occur even when left ventricular wall thickness and the radius/thickness ratio are normal. Left atrial size and left ventricular mass were larger than values in normal controls but were still within usual normal ranges.[80] Children and adults with aortic stenosis have a reduced peak rate of increase in left ventricular dimension and of posterior wall thinning compared to normal subjects.[65] Peak filling rate (normalized to the total change in dimension) and peak thinning rate (normalized to the total change in thinning) were found to correlate negatively with age, peak left ventricular systolic pressure, and wall thickness, similar to findings in normal subjects.

Restrictive Cardiomyopathy. Patients with restrictive cardiomyopathy from amyloid heart disease characteristically have, among other echocardiographic abnormalities, small or normal-sized left ventricular chambers, increased wall thicknesses, prolonged isovolumic relaxation periods, decreased peak rates of increase in left ventricular dimension, and decreased peak rates of septal and posterior wall thinning (normalized to instantaneous thickness). In addition to abnormalities of diastolic filling, systolic function measured from fractional shortening, peak velocity of circumferential shortening, and peak rate of systolic wall thickening may be impaired. When compared to patients with aortic stenosis who have similar left ventricular sizes and wall thicknesses, patients with amyloidosis appear to have more impaired systolic and diastolic function, suggesting that factors other than left ventricular geometry alone are responsible for the abnormal systolic and diastolic function seen in patients with cardiac amyloidosis.[56] In a study of five children with restrictive cardiomyopathy, the isovolumic relaxation period was normal, the change of left ventricular dimension during the rapid filling period was reduced, and the time between the maximal anterior movement of the posterolateral wall and the minimum of its first derivative was shortened.[81] There was no difference in the maximum velocity of circumferential fiber lengthening (VCF_{min}) and normalized rate of posterior wall thinning between these patients and those with primary and secondary left ventricular hypertrophy.

Pericardial Constriction. The diagnosis of pericardial constriction is often difficult to distinguish from myocardial restriction clinically or even by hemodynamic assessment in the catheterization laboratory. Not uncommonly, there exists simultaneously a combination of the two processes. Most studies of diastolic abnormalities in these two diseases have involved very small numbers of patients. In one such study, which compared four patients with pericardial constriction with three patients with restrictive myocardial disease, the total duration of filling was reduced in constrictive and increased in restrictive disease. The time from the minimum left ventricular dimension to the peak rate of increase in dimension was shorter in constrictive disease, and the peak rate of posterior wall thinning in constrictive disease was more than double that in restrictive disease.[61] A review of data pooled from several studies found relatively poor sensitivity and specificity for all echocardiographic features of pericardial constriction.[82]

Other Approaches Using Measurements From M-Mode Echocardiography

More recently, some studies have focused not just on rates of increase in left ventricular dimension and volume, as has traditionally been the case, but also on the lengthening properties of the myocardial unit represented at the midwall circumference. It has been suggested that because the inner (subendocardial) half of the ventricular wall contributes more to thickening and thinning than the outer (subepicardial) half, a modified approach to the measurement of standard midwall circumference should be adopted that does not assume that a theoretical midwall fiber remains at the midwall throughout the cardiac cycle.[83] The peak rate of increase in ventricular dimension and midwall fiber length were decreased in patients with hypertrophy compared to normal controls. Conventional methods used to measure peak fiber velocity overestimated "true" velocity, both in patients with hypertrophy and in normal subjects, but overestimated it more in the patients with hypertrophy.

M-mode echocardiographic measurements of left ventricular dimension and wall thickness may be combined with simultaneous pressure measurements to calculate wall stress, as described earlier. Angiographic and M-mode echocardiographic measurements of wall stress correlate well with those derived from contrast angiography,[84–87] and left ventricular stress-strain curves may be derived by combined invasive and noninvasive techniques. Echocardiographic-pressure data may also be presented as pressure-dimension loops, which are similar to those studied in animals using epicardial strain gauges and sonomicrometers.[73]

Two-Dimensional Echocardiography

The application of two-dimensional echocardiography to the measurement of diastolic function has theoretical advantages over M-mode echocardiography in providing global views of the ventricle from multiple windows. Intraventricular end-diastolic areas and lengths can be measured in various planes, and by adopting reasonable geometric assumptions, ventricular volumes can be calculated from one of the several formulas available. Simultaneous pressure data may be plotted against end-diastolic volume and area measurements to yield end-diastolic pressure-volume and pressure-area curves. These measurements should reflect the global characteristics of the ventricle more faithfully than equivalent M-mode measurements, particularly in asymmetric ventricles.

The calculation of left ventricular wall mass using two-dimensional echocardiography has been reported by several workers, and the technique has been well validated in animal experiments and human autopsy studies.[88–91] Mathematical models for calculating wall mass that incorporate directly measured left ventricular longitudinal lengths are felt to be more accurate than those models that assume a certain ventricular length, such as the cube formula used in M-mode echocardiography.[89] Also, mass models that incorporate directly measured left ventricular cross-sectional areas are thought to be more accurate than those that employ linear dimensions, such as those found in M-mode echocardiography. In a study of ill patients just before death, many of whom had distorted left ventricles, ventricular mass measured by two-dimensional echocardiography was found to be more accurate than those derived from M-mode echocardiography.[91] A more detailed discussion of left ventricular volume and wall mass measurements by two-dimensional echocardiography is offered in Chapter 20.

The calculation of the rate of change of left ventricular volume using two-dimensional images obtained in multiple planes is theoretically possible and should yield more accurate data in asymmetric ventricles compared to M-mode echocardiography. An important disadvantage of two-dimensional echocardiography, however, is that spatial and temporal resolution are both reduced compared to the M-mode technique. As a result, the delineation of endocardial borders is less precise. Because the frame rate in two-dimensional echocardiography is relatively slow (30 frames per second compared to a pulse repetition frequency of 1000/sec in M-mode echocardiography), rates of change in dimension or areas cannot be followed with high fidelity. Furthermore, incongruities in temporal relationships are introduced during the conversion of digital information to analog video data by the digital scan converter. This phenomenon leads to a mismatching of events on the screen, which may produce misleading video images with regard to the timing of events.

The absence of an automatic display of data with time on the x axis necessitates the manual digitization of endocardial borders frame by frame or field by field, which is exceedingly laborious. Furthermore, the generation of random noise from the manual tracing of individual video frames results in highly erratic rates of change in the derived parameters. Preliminary experience using this technique to measure regional filling rates in the left ventricle of dogs has found significant heterogeneity in the measured pattern of filling between the short axis slices through the base, midventricular level and apex, as well as between eight segments within each slice.[92] The application of smoothing techniques, such as spatial and temporal smoothing by two-dimensional Fourier analysis[93] may yield more optimal data by eliminating the high frequency components in the signal that are due to noise. However, care must be taken not to eliminate the physiologic high frequency signals representing peak rates of change of the various parameters. The reliability of measurements of rates of change during diastole from two-dimensional data remains unestablished. With all these difficulties, use of two-dimensional echocardiography for this purpose has not been commonly accepted.

Doppler Echocardiography

Principles of the Measurement

The principles of pulsed and continuous wave Doppler echocardiography are described in earlier chapters. Unlike other measurements of the left ventricular filling pattern based on M-mode and two-dimensional echocardiography, Doppler measurements provide unique information about the velocity of blood flow across the mitral valve into the ventricle. As discussed earlier, this velocity is a complex function of the pressure gradient across the mitral valve, described in the Law of Conservation of Energy equation. Therefore, flow velocity represents the intermediate link between hemodynamic conditions indicated by instantaneous left atrial and left ventricular pressures and the volumetric filling characteristics of the ventricle. The latter parameter is obtained by multiplying the instantaneous flow velocity across the mitral valve by the orifice area through which the blood is traveling at that particular instant (Fig. 24–16). Measurements are simplified because blood flow here is laminar and has reasonable spatial uniformity (plug flow).[94–96]

Details of volumetric flow assessments are provided elsewhere in this book (Chapter 30), but a few principles may be noted here. Individual differences in mitral orifice area may be significant. For example, when peak volumetric filling rates derived from the Doppler technique and contrast ventriculography were compared, correlation was improved with the measurement of individual orifice areas compared to the use of a common area.[97] A circular shape for the mitral orifice is usually assumed, although some have chosen an ellipse.[98–100] The mitral annulus area increases by approximately 15% from early to late diastole and then decreases substantially with atrial contraction.[101] For simplicity, a single measurement of the annulus is made at the time of maximal leaflet opening in early diastole. Other workers have measured mitral orifice area at the leaflet tips using M-mode measurements.[102] Good correlations with roller pump blood flow measurements were obtained in dogs,[102] but subsequent studies have suggested poorer results in humans.[103]

Figure 24–17 illustrates how volumetric flow-time curves may be generated simply by multiplying the instantaneous flow velocity by the mitral annulus area. Integration of the volumetric curve yields a cumulative

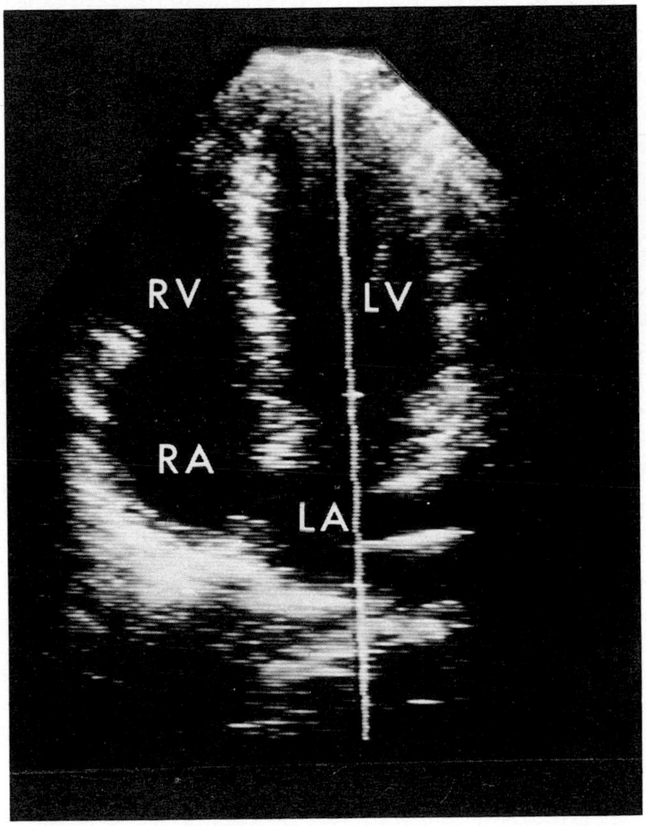

Fig. 24–16. Apical four-chamber view of the left ventricle, which is used most commonly to measure the transmitral flow velocity profile with the pulsed Doppler technique. The two-dimensional image is first adjusted to yield the widest mediolateral dimension of the mitral annulus. The Doppler ultrasound beam is directed to lie perpendicular to the mitral annular plane and bissect it. The Doppler sample volume, denoted here by the short cross bar on the Doppler beam, is positioned to sit just within the left ventricle to early diastole. Fine adjustments are then made to the transducer angulation to obtain the highest transmitral flow velocities. It should be noted that some workers position the same volume at the level of the mitral leaflet tips. Flow velocities at this level are higher than those at the mitral annular plane. The relative advantages and disadvantages of each method are discussed in the text. LA = left atrium; LV = left ventricle; RA = right atrium; RV = right ventricle.[121] (From Choong CY, Herrmann HC, Weyman AE, Fifer MA: Preload dependence of Doppler-derived indexes of left ventricular diastolic function in humans. J Am Coll Cardiol 10:800, 1987. Reprinted with permission from the American College of Cardiology.)

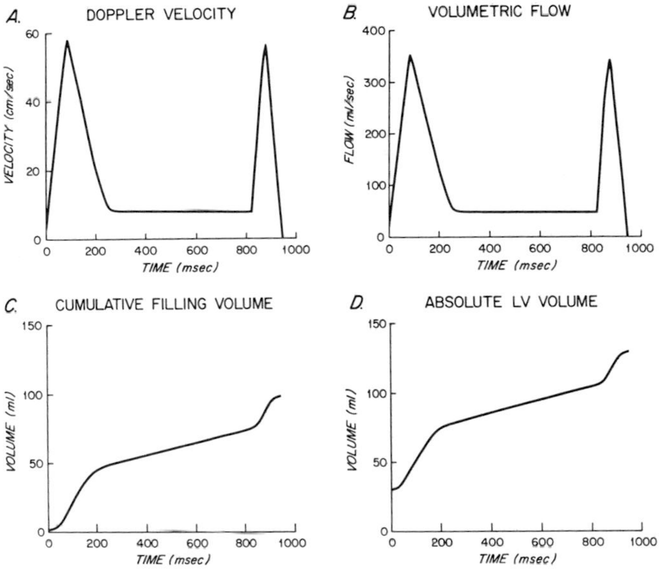

Fig. 24–17. How left ventricular volume-time curves may be derived from a combination of the transmitral flow velocity profile and two-dimensional echocardiographic measurement of mitral annular size. **A.** A typical transmitral flow velocity profile, which has been digitized. **B.** The velocity is integrated over time. **C.** The mitral annular area derived from two-dimensional echocardiographic measurements is multiplied to the value obtained in **B** to yield a cumulative volume-time curve of ventricular filling. **D.** To generate a ventricular volume-time curve, the end-diastolic volume is measured by two-dimensional echocardiography, and the entire filling volume-time curve is offset so that the largest volume now equals the measured end-diastolic volume. LV = left ventricular.

volume-time curve of ventricular filling. If the end-diastolic volume is known, e.g., from two-dimensional echocardiographic measurements, then the entire curve may be offset to the appropriate end-diastolic volume to produce a ventricular volume-time curve in diastole. Volume-time curves generated in this manner closely resemble those derived from contrast ventriculography and are potentially useful for monitoring the effects of intervention. If pressure-time measurements are also available, accurate pressure-volume curves can be generated relatively easily by combining the volume-time and pressure-time curves (Fig. 24–18).[104]

At the present time, the comparative importance of using volumetric flow rates or flow velocities to represent ventricular diastolic function remains unresolved. There is general acceptance that for the purpose of evaluating the diastolic characteristics of the ventricle, transmitral flow velocities alone are adequate markers, and there is no need to further derive volumetric flow rates.

Measurements of the transmitral flow velocity profile are best made in the apical four-chamber, two-chamber, or long axis views of the ventricle. Most workers use the four-chamber view alone. With the pulsed Doppler technique, some workers place the sample volume just within the ventricle next to the plane of the mitral annulus. Because the mitral annulus moves toward the apex during ventricular systole and back toward the base during diastole, an arbitrary time during diastole, usually early diastole when the mitral leaflets open maximally, has to be chosen to represent the position of the mitral annulus plane (Fig. 24–16). The Doppler ultrasound beam is directed to bisect the annulus plane and is aligned as close to perpendicular to the plane as possible. Once the sample volume is in the correct anatomic position, minor adjustments are made to the transducer angulation regardless of the two-dimensional image to obtain the highest peak velocity of the early or E wave.

Some workers have chosen to position the Doppler sample volume at the level of the leaflet tips rather than close to the mitral annulus. Velocities recorded at this level often differ significantly from those taken at the annulus, and the numeric details of these differences are discussed later in this chapter. The choice of each level has its own advantages and limitations, and it is important to consider the purpose for which the measurements are made.

When the description of the pattern or temporal distribution of transmitral flow is of greater interest than the description of the actual maximal flow velocities, the use of the annulus level is advantageous, owing to the greater stability of the mitral orifice area at the annulus compared to the leaflet tips. A potential advantage of recording flow velocities at the leaflet tips is that it yields higher velocities than at the annulus. Knowledge of the highest flow velocities that are present in the ventricular chamber provides unique information about the maximal performance of the "hydraulic system" in terms of its ability to generate pressure gradient and flow velocities. Whether this knowledge offers additional useful information about diastolic ventricular function beyond that obtained from the annulus plane, however, remains unestablished. It should be noted that maximal velocities of the early (E) and late (A) flow waves do not necessarily occur exactly at the leaflet tips nor at the same sample volume position, and this may vary between individuals. If indeed detecting maximal velocities is the main objective, the continuous wave Doppler technique may be the most appropriate one to use here. With this technique, however, contributions to the peak velocity signals may arise from different depths along the ultrasound beam during the course of diastole, and so may not truly reflect the ventricular filling pattern.

In practice, for describing diastolic processes, it is probably more important that a standard convention for making these measurements be widely adopted than

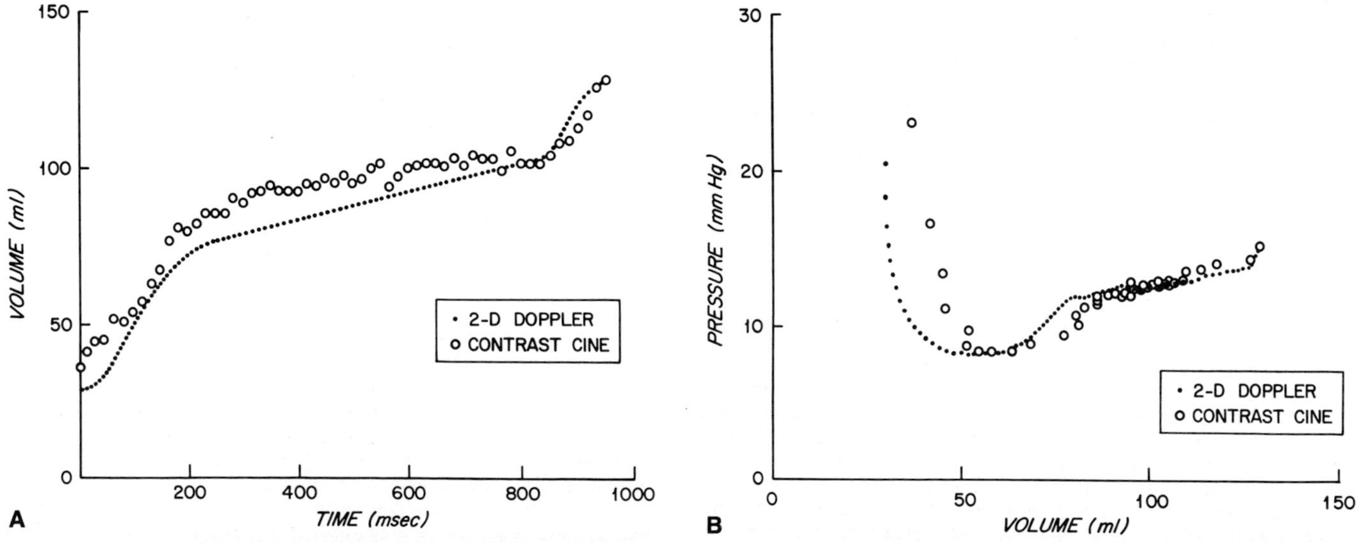

Fig. 24–18. Examples of left ventricular volume-time curves **(A)** and pressure-volume curves **(B)** derived from combined two-dimensional and Doppler echocardiographic measurements compared to the same parameters derived from contrast cineangiography. Details of the echocardiographic method are described in the text and illustrated in Figure 24–17. The close resemblance between measurements by the two techniques is evident.

which particular method is chosen. Considering the advantages and limitations of the different methods, one may argue that the pulsed Doppler technique be used with the sample volume placed in the ventricular chamber, where the peak E wave velocity is highest, regardless of the exact relation to the mitral annulus or leaflet tips. In most instances, the sample volume will be found closer to the leaflet tips than the annulus. Guidance from the color flow map is often helpful.

THE DOPPLER TRANSMITRAL FLOW VELOCITY PROFILE

Two distinct phases in the transmitral flow velocity profile can be easily identified, namely, the E wave and the A wave (Fig. 24–19). These phases represent the flow velocities of the early filling phase and the atrial contraction phase, respectively, and generally appear as well-defined triangles. The slopes of the sides of each triangle define the acceleration (upslope) and deceleration (downslope) of the wave, and the height of the triangle represents the peak velocity. At relatively slower heart rates, diastasis separates the E and A waves, and generally appears as a flat, low velocity signal, which is often obscured in part or in whole by the low velocity ("wall") filter. Under certain situations, a brief wave of slightly higher velocity may be seen at the beginning of diastasis, the L wave, which, as stated earlier, is felt to represent a wave of pulmonary venous flow passing directly through the left atrium into the left ventricle.[36] At higher heart rates, diastole is shortened, and diastasis is abolished. The A wave commences at the foot of the descending limb of the E wave, and with progressively increasing heart rates, climbs further up the descending limb of the E wave, until the peaks of both waves coincide.

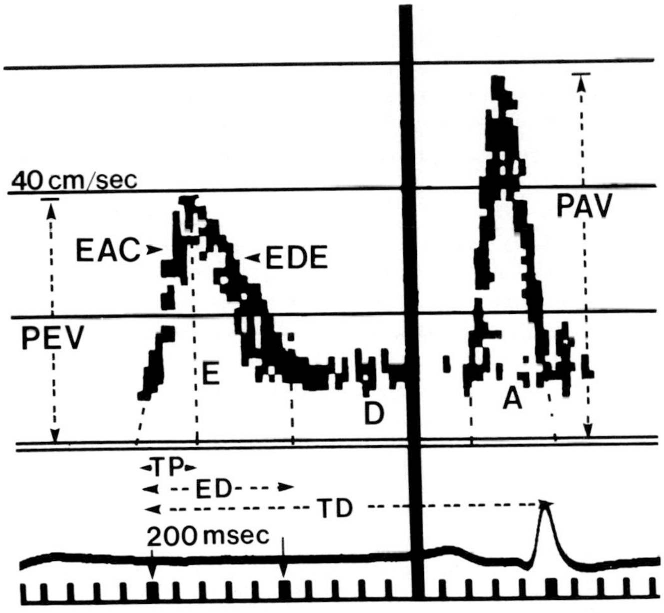

Fig. 24–19. A normal spectral Doppler transmitral flow velocity profile. The profile is generally divided into three phases, namely, the early filling or E wave, diastasis, and the atrial contraction or A wave. With faster heart rates, diastasis shortens and may be eliminated completely. The flow velocity pattern may be characterized in several ways, as indicated by the abbreviations in the figure. A = A wave resulting from atrial contraction; D = diastasis; E = E wave representing the early filling phase; EAC = E wave acceleration rate; ED = E wave duration; EDE = E wave deceleration rate; PAV = peak A wave velocity; PEV = peak E wave velocity; TD = total filling duration; TP = time from onset of transmitral flow to the peak E wave velocity. Other characteristics used include the ratios of the peak velocities and velocity-time integrals of the E and A waves, the proportion of the total velocity-time integral supplied by the A wave, and the proportion of the total velocity-time integral occurring in the first one third of diastole.[121] (From Choong CY, Herrmann HC, Weyman AE, Fifer MA: Preload dependence of Doppler-derived indexes of left ventricular diastolic function in humans. J Am Coll Cardiol 10:800, 1987. Reprinted with permission from the American College of Cardiology.)

Characterization of the Transmitral Flow Velocity Profile

For descriptive purposes, the Doppler flow velocity profile may be characterized by the use of a variety of parameters, including the peak velocities, acceleration and deceleration rates, and areas (velocity-time integrals) of the E and A waves, as well as the ratios of the peak velocities and velocity-time integrals of these two waves. The velocity-time integrals of each wave may also be expressed as percentages of the total velocity-time integral, which when given a relatively constant mitral annular area throughout diastole, reflect the relative contribution of the early filling phase (for the E wave) and atrial contraction (for the A wave) to the total filling volume. The first third and first half filling fractions, i.e., the proportion of the total velocity-time integral occurring during the first third and first half of the diastolic filling period, have also been examined. Various time intervals have been measured, including the time from cessation of transaortic flow or aortic valve closure to the onset of mitral flow (the isovolumic relaxation time); the time from the onset of filling to the peak velocity of the E wave (or acceleration time); the time from the peak velocity of the E wave to the cessation of the E wave (or deceleration time); and the duration of the E and A waves (Fig. 24–19).

Normal values of some commonly used Doppler indices of diastolic function have been extracted from multiple sources and are summarized in Table 24–4. Many physiologic and methodologic factors influence these values, and some of the more important ones are specified in the table where available. These factors are discussed in greater detail later in the chapter and should always be kept in mind when comparing measurements taken from different sources. A large study of normal Doppler values is presently not available. Most of the quoted reports involve relatively few subjects used in control groups in specific research projects. Unfortunately, most of the measurements have not been stratified according to such potentially important physiologic variables as age and heart rate.

Demarcation of the Various Phases of the Transmitral Flow Velocity Profile

Several methods have been used to divide the transmitral flow velocity profile into its various phases, and

Table 24–4. Normal Values for Characteristics of the Pulsed Doppler Transmitral Flow Velocity Profile (Mean ± SD)

Study Source	N	Sex (Years)	Age (Years)	SV Pos	Loc	HRate (bts/min)	PEV (cm/sec)	E Decel (cm/sec^2)	E VTI (cm)	PAV (cm/sec)	A VTI (cm)	E/A Vel	A/E Vel	E/A VTI	0.33/T VTI	A/Total VTI	A2-D (msec)	D-F (msec)
1a.	35	48 M, 38 F for three groups	22 ± 3 (≤29)	Highest	Modal	m58 for three groups	69 ± 12	550 ± 12		27 ± 7	—	2.7 ± 0.7	—	—	—	—	72 ± 12	218 ± 30
1b.	33		40 ± 5 (30–49)	Velocity	Modal		62 ± 14	470 ± 110		33 ± 7	—	2.0 ± 0.6	—	—	—	—	80 ± 12	220 ± 27
1c.	18		57 ± 6 (≥50)	Present	Modal		59 ± 14	420 ± 120		46 ± 13	—	1.2 ± 0.4	—	—	—	—	84 ± 12	221 ± 33
2a.	8	6 M, 2 F	(21–30)	Tips	Modal	n.a.		—		41 ± 7	—	—	0.6 ± 0.1	—	—	—	—	—
2b.	18	4 M, 14 F	(61–70)	Tips	Modal	n.a.	66 ± 11	—		55 ± 11	—	—	1.2 ± 0.3	—	—	—	—	—
							45 ± 10											
3.	47	26 M, 21 F	13 ± .9 (12–14)	Tips	Modal	74 ± 12	73 ± 12	730 ± 160	6.5 ± 1.4	39 ± 7	2.2 ± 0.5	—	0.73 ± 0.16	—	—	—	—	—
4.	16	6 M, 10 F	m38 (19–60)	Tips	Modal	66 ± 9	60 ± 9	399 ± 110		38 ± 8	—	—	0.66 ± 0.19	—	—	—	—	—
5a.	52	24 M, 28 F	m49 (21–78)	An-Tip*	Modal	67 (50–88)	54 ± 12	—		47 ± 11	—	—	0.94 ± 0.4	—	—	—	—	—
5b.	40	(n.a.; subgroup of 5a)		LA × ×	Modal	n.a.	43 ± 12	—		36 ± 7	—	—	0.91 ± 0.3	—	—	—	—	—
6a.	10	18 M, 14 F for three groups	m26 (20–29)	Annulus	Modal	—	108 ± 10	—		58 ± 15	—	1.98 ± 0.53	—	—	—	—	—	—
6b.	12		m36 (30–49)	Annulus	Modal	— —	103 ± 16	—		71 ± 17	—	1.52 ± 0.36	—	—	—	—	—	—
6c.	10		m57 (50–68)	Annulus	Modal		91 ± 16	—		80 ± 15	—	1.07 ± 0.41	—	—	—	—	—	—
7.	17	10 M, 7 F	m39 (29–60)	Annulus		—	62 ± 9	482 ± 99		40 ± 8	—	1.61 ± 0.39	—	—	—	—	—	—
									59 ± 14									
8.	24	10 M, 14 F	m51 (42–76)	Annulus	Highest	n.a.	68 ± 12	—	8.6 ± 1.8	48 ± 11	3.6 ± 1.0	1.5 ± 0.32	—	2.5 ± 0.69	0.53 ± 0.06	0.26 ± 0.07	—	—

Significant variations in imaging and measurement techniques exist. The references have been listed according to sample volume position and the presence of age stratification. For reasons that are not readily apparent, the measurements from Bryg et al.[149] are higher compared to other studies.

0.33/T VTI = velocity-time integral during first third of diastole/total velocity-time integral; A2-D = isovolumic relaxation period; Accel = acceleration; Decel = deceleration; D-F = duration of E wave; HRate = heart rate; Loc = location for identifying peak velocities (modal velocity vs. highest velocities seen); m = mean; PAV = peak A-wave velocity; PEV = peak E-wave velocity; SV Pos = sample volume position; n.a. = not available; Vel = velocity; VTI = velocity-time integral.

* Between annulus and leaflet tips.

† In left atrium 1 cm from annulus.

References: 1. Ref. 177; 2. ref. 150; 3. ref. 164; 4. ref. 175; 5. ref. 107; 6. ref. 149; 7. ref. 166; 8. ref. 187.

no consensus exists on which is most correct (Fig. 24–20). The wall filter often obscures the initial point of upslope of the E wave on the time axis. This initial point may be identified either by extrapolating the relatively straight upslope of the E wave down to the baseline, or by dropping a vertical line from the origin of the velocity signal at the top of the wall filter. The former method has advantages, because it is independent of the wall filter setting and appears more representative of actual flow events. The point of mitral valve opening may occasionally be indicated by a vertical valve signal, which may be used to identify the time of onset of transmitral flow.

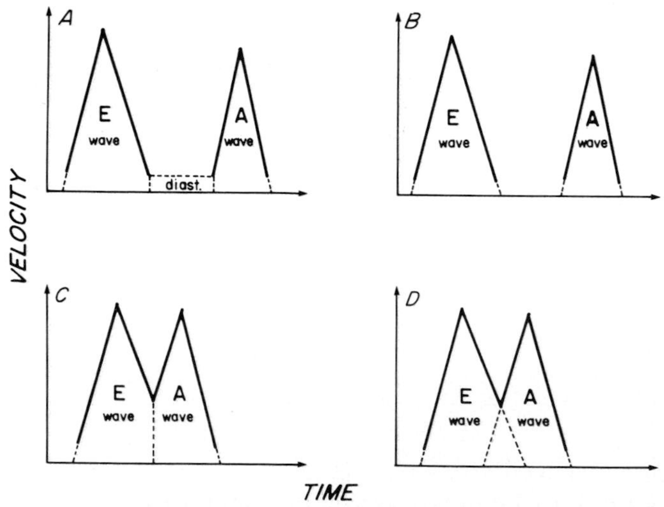

Fig. 24–20. Some of the various ways that may be used to demarcate the transmitral flow velocity profile into its different phases. A discussion of the relative advantages and disadvantages of each method is given in the text.

Similar considerations apply to timing the cessation of the A wave. Extrapolation of the descending limb of the A wave to the baseline is preferred to dropping a vertical line at the top of the wall filter. Guidance may be obtained, where available, from a vertical mitral valve closure signal.

The methods used to separate the E and A waves have been similarly variable. In the absence of a diastasis period, the A wave arises at the foot of the E wave or on its descending limb, depending on the heart rate. The demarcation of the two waves in the former situation is clear, because they naturally separate themselves. In the latter situation, the end of the E wave may be considered as the point at which the two waves meet, and a vertical line dropped from that point to the baseline separates the two waves adequately. Others have considered that the A wave artificially truncates the E wave in this situation and have extrapolated the descending limb of the E wave down to the baseline to describe it, ignoring the A wave entirely. The A wave may then be considered as that portion of the velocity spectrum that remains, or it may be demarcated similarly by extrapolating its ascending limb to the baseline and ignoring the E wave entirely.

These various methods clearly give very different results for measurements of velocity-time integrals and time intervals, although peak velocities and acceleration and deceleration rates are the same with all methods. The validity of each method depends mainly on the purpose of the analysis. If one is interested only in describing actual events in diastole, the method that employs a vertical line is more appropriate, because regardless of the modification of one wave by the other, this method describes directly the events that have occurred. If one is interested in understanding the physiologic mechanisms underlying the actual events, however, then extrapolation of the slopes of each wave to the baseline without regard to the other wave may provide useful additional information.

Whichever method is used, the interpretation of measurements made when E and A waves merge is unclear and should be made very cautiously. It cannot be simply assumed that characteristics of the E or A wave can be measured meaningfully by extrapolating the inner side of the wave as though the other wave did not exist, because the two waves do not behave independently of one another. This interdependence of the E and A waves can be understood when considering the physiologic mechanisms that generate each wave, discussed later in this chapter. It should be realized also that this interdependence is not related to heart rate alone. In patients with dual-chamber pacemakers, alteration of the timing of the A wave by changing the A-V interval significantly modifies the characteristics of the E wave even though heart rate is constant.[105]

The situations described previously dealt with conditions in which heart rates were sufficiently fast so that diastasis did not occur. In the presence of a diastasis period, several methods also have been used to demarcate diastasis from the two waves. Very little left ventricular filling, if any, occurs during diastasis, because pressures in the two chambers are at or close to equilibrium. Velocity signals are either very low or nonexistent. Depending on the setting of the wall filter, either no velocity signal is recorded above the wall filter, or occasionally, a very low velocity signal may be seen just above the wall filter, especially in the earlier part of diastasis. Complete elimination of the wall filter is usually not helpful because low velocity noise is shown, which cannot be easily differentiated from true velocity signals.

Some workers have extrapolated the descending limb of the E wave and the ascending limb of the A wave across the wall filter onto the baseline and have arbitrarily assigned the velocity during diastasis to zero. A major advantage of this method is its simplicity, but a disadvantage is that extrapolation is made to points that do not exist in reality, because low velocity signals are not uncommonly detected early in diastasis. Others, including ourselves, have dropped vertical lines at the intersection of the descending limb of the E wave with the highest velocity signals occurring during early diastasis or with the top of the wall filter. The same technique is applied to the ascending limb of the A wave. The rationale for this method is that in the presence of detectable flow velocities in early diastasis, this point in fact represents the time when the E wave actually ends and diastasis begins. In this situation, the selection of the velocity during diastasis is often arbitrary. The presence of clear velocity signals is helpful, but in the absence of such data, the velocity during diastasis may be assumed to be zero or the maximal velocity of the wall filter, or indeed, any intermediate velocity between the two. This is a major problem with the method, but fortunately, any flow velocities occurring during diastasis tend to be very low and diastasis is usually brief, so that any error incurred tends to be minimal. There is no accepted convention, and one approach has been to use the top of a standardized wall filter setting. It is also simplest to assume that this nominated velocity is uniform throughout diastasis, even though it may not be so in practice. Other approaches have been used to divide up the velocity profile. These include demarcation of the A wave by horizontal extrapolation of the maximal diastasis velocity so as to exclude the base of the A wave. This has been one of the methods used to calculate atrial contribution to ventricular filling.[106]

The continued existence of multiple methods to demarcate the transmitral velocity profile reflects the absence of one which is both obviously correct and widely accepted. This lack of convention leads to difficulties when comparing results between studies that employ different methods. Caution must be exercised when heart rates are slow and diastasis prolonged, because an overestimation of flow velocity during diastasis may produce a substantial exaggeration of its true velocity-time integral and therefore of the total velocity-time integral. By the same token, when examining the effects of interventions that alter heart rate or when comparing groups with different heart rates, the assumption of an arbitrary velocity during diastasis creates the possibility of falsely creating or exaggerating differences in total velocity-time integrals that are due purely to differences in the length of diastasis.

A lack of standardization also exists for locating the peak velocities of the E and A waves on the velocity spectrum. Some workers have used the highest velocity seen on the spectral profile. This method has the disadvantage that the highest velocity signals sometimes appear smeared and poorly represented and are susceptible to alterations in gain settings. Others have chosen instead to use the highest velocity represented by the darkest portion of the velocity spectrum, often termed the *modal velocity*.[107] This point is less susceptible to alterations in gain settings, and although this is strictly not the true peak velocity found, it nevertheless represents the peak velocity of most of the blood within the sample volume. On balance, therefore, the second method seems preferred. Differences in measurements by the two methods are usually relatively small, but care should still be taken to standardize the method within studies.

Finally, in tracing the velocity profile for measuring the slopes and calculating the velocity-time integrals of the E and A waves, some workers have approximated the slopes of the two waves to straight lines, while others have traced accurately along the recorded velocities. In most instances, the actual slopes themselves are fairly straight so that little discrepancy occurs between the two methods. When the slopes are curved, especially seen on the downslope of the E wave, significant differences may be obtained. Where facilities for digitizing exist, tracing along the true slope is preferred because this describes the events that actually occurred.

Measurements of Left Ventricular Filling by Doppler Echocardiography Compared to Other Techniques

The measurement of left ventricular filling by Doppler echocardiography has several important advantages over other methods. Unlike radionuclide and contrast ventriculography, the Doppler method does not cause exposure to radioactivity, and being safer, measurements may be made repeatedly. Unlike contrast ventriculography, no geometric assumptions are required if only flow velocities are analyzed. Also, unlike contrast ventriculography, the technique does not produce hemodynamic changes, which can alter measurements when these are repeated at close intervals.

Pulsed Doppler echocardiography has a temporal resolution of approximately 10 msec or less, depending on the ultrasound scanner used, and the more modern machines have much higher resolution. This relatively high temporal resolution is important for faithfully recording the rapid changes in flow velocities that occur in normal and pathologic states. It is superior to that found in radionuclide methods, where a relatively slow frame rate is a major disadvantage. Doppler echocardiography also allows the measurement of beat-by-beat changes, unlike gated radionuclide techniques, which need to sum multiple cardiac cycles over several minutes to accumulate sufficient radioactive counts for analysis.

Another major advantage of Doppler echocardiography is the relative ease with which reliable measurements can be made. Compared to radionuclide and contrast cineangiographic measurements, which are laborious and usually require considerable processing of the raw data, Doppler information is acquired immediately. This easy access has been crucial in encouraging its exploitation for research and clinical application.

Disadvantages of the Doppler technique must also be clearly recognized. In some patients, ultrasound signals of adequate quality cannot be obtained. The technique depends highly on the competence of the operator, and the transmitral flow velocity profile depends highly on changes in the position of the sample volume, which therefore, must be carefully standardized.

There are fundamental differences between the nature of Doppler measurements and those made by the other techniques. For example, the Doppler technique yields flow velocities whereas radionuclide ventriculography yields radioactive counts normalized to end-diastolic counts, and contrast ventriculography yields blood volume derived from the planimetry of the ventricular silhouette. Not surprisingly, the comparison between techniques of measurements that refer to precisely the same parameters have yielded close correlations, whereas the comparison of measurements of nonidentical parameters have often yielded weaker results, as illustrated later.

In a comparison of Doppler echocardiographic with radionuclide angiographic measurements, fractional filling in early diastole ($r = .84$) and during atrial contraction ($r = .83$), diastolic filling period ($r = .94$), and duration from end-diastole to the peak velocity of the E wave or peak filling rate ($r = .88$) correlated well. The peak filling rate normalized to end-diastolic volume did not correlate well ($r = .46$, $p < .05$) between the two techniques, probably because of inaccuracies introduced by the measurement of mitral annular area and end-diastolic volume using echocardiography and inaccuracies inherent in the radionuclide measurements.[108]

The normalization of peak filling rate to stroke volume is equivalent in Doppler echocardiography to dividing the peak velocity by the velocity-time integral. This approach obviates the need to calculate mitral annular area and end-diastolic volume from two-dimensional echocardiography and is free from geometric assumptions except for one, that the mitral annular area does not change significantly during diastole. In one study, measurements of the peak E wave velocity normalized to the velocity-time integral correlated well with measurements of peak filling rate normalized to stroke volume measured by radionuclide angiography ($r = .85$, standard error of estimate [SEE] $= 1.2$, $y = 0.95x + 0.52$).[109]

In another study, there was a good correlation between the time from aortic valve closure (S2) to the end of the Doppler E wave and the time from end-systole to the end of rapid filling measured by radionuclide angiography.[110] The deceleration rate of the E wave correlated with the radionuclide peak filling rate (normalized to end-diastolic volume) ($r = .79$). The ratio of peak E-wave velocity to peak A-wave velocity correlated well with the ratio of fractional filling during rapid filling to fractional filling during atrial contraction by radionuclide ventriculography ($r = .76$). The two techniques were in agreement in diagnosing normal and abnormal filling patterns in 21 (84%) of 25 patients with cardiac disease.

A significant correlation has also been reported between Doppler two-dimensional echocardiographic and contrast angiographic peak filling rate ($r = .87$, SEE $= 91.5$ ml/sec) and between Doppler two-dimensional echocardiographic and angiographic peak filling rate normalized to end-diastolic volume ($r = .83$, SEE $= .52\ sec^{-1}$). As discussed earlier in the chapter, the peak E wave velocity correlated less well with angiographic peak filling rate ($r = .64$), which is probably due to a significant variation in mitral annular sizes between patients.[105] The peak E-wave velocity to peak A-wave velocity ratio and the half-filling fraction by Doppler echocardiography correlated relatively well with angiographic parameters of filling (peak filling rate, peak filling rate normalized to end-diastolic volume, first half-filling fraction), but only when the diastolic filling periods were similar during both measurements.

The relationship between M-mode and Doppler echocardiographic measurements of ventricular filling has not been fully examined. In one study, children with mild systemic hypertension who had no left ventricular hypertrophy had abnormal filling patterns by Doppler echocardiography but normal parameters of filling (dL/dt, dL/dt/L) by M-mode echocardiography.[111] In another study, the ratio of the peak to mean E-wave velocity, the ratio of the peak E-wave velocity to peak A-wave velocity, the ratio of the E-wave velocity-time integral to the A-wave velocity-time integral, and the Doppler-derived peak filling rate were all lower, and the peak A-wave filling rate was higher in patients with left ventricular hypertrophy compared to normal control subjects.[112] The peak rate of increase in ventricular dimension by M-mode echocardiography and the measurement normalized to the instantaneous dimension remained normal in these patients. These studies suggest that Doppler echocardiographic measurements may be more sensitive than M-mode echocardiographic measurements for detecting abnormalities of diastolic function, at least in patients with hypertension with or without left ventricular hypertrophy. In the latter study, there was no correlation between the peak rate of increase in left ventricular dimension by M-mode echocardiography and the peak filling rate by Doppler and two-dimensional echocardiography. This lack of correlation emphasizes the fact that these two measurements are not strictly equivalent, the first being one-dimensional and the second being volumetric or three-dimensional. The conversion of rate of change in one dimension to rate of change in volume requires knowledge of the absolute dimension, a value that may vary substantially between patients. Thus, for a particular rate of change in one dimension, the rate of change in volume is greater in a bigger ventricle and less in a smaller one. When these measurements were normalized to instantaneous dimension (for M-mode measurements) and end-diastolic volume (for Doppler and two-dimensional measurements), respectively, they correlated more strongly but still only modestly ($r = .56$, $p < .001$).

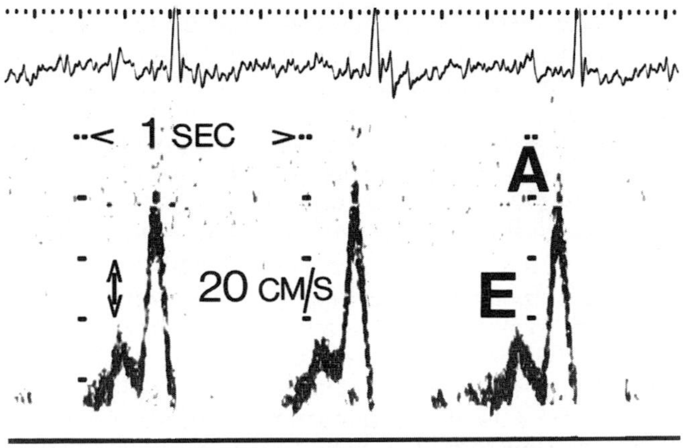

Fig. 24–21. Transmitral flow velocity profile taken from a 57-year-old man with moderately severe aortic stenosis, single-vessel coronary artery disease, moderate concentric left ventricular hypertrophy, and normal left ventricular systolic function. The peak velocity of the E wave is reduced, with a relative increase in the peak velocity of the A wave so that the ratio of the peak velocities of the E and A waves is reduced. The proportion of the total velocity-time integral occupied by the A wave is increased, indicating increased contribution of atrial contraction to ventricular filling.

Characteristics of the Transmitral Flow Velocity Profile Found to Reflect Abnormal Left Ventricular Diastolic Function

Alterations in a large number of characteristics of the Doppler transmitral flow velocity profile have been described in many conditions associated with left ventricular diastolic dysfunction. These alterations in the velocity profile are not specific for any particular disease but are seen in diseased states that share the same abnormal diastolic properties, such as reduced relaxation rate, increased passive chamber stiffness, or more usually, both together. Common examples of such conditions are left ventricular hypertrophy, chronic coronary artery disease, acute myocardial ischemia, and dilated cardiomyopathy. Typical alterations in the velocity profile include a reduction in the peak velocity of the E wave, an increase in the peak A-wave velocity, a decrease in the ratio of the peak velocities of the E and A waves, and an increase in the relative contribution of the A wave to total diastolic filling (Fig. 24–21). Such abnormal patterns may be very striking on occasions. Figure 24–22 shows a grossly abnormal velocity profile in which the E wave is miniscule, and the A wave is highly dominant, contributing almost totally to ventricular filling.

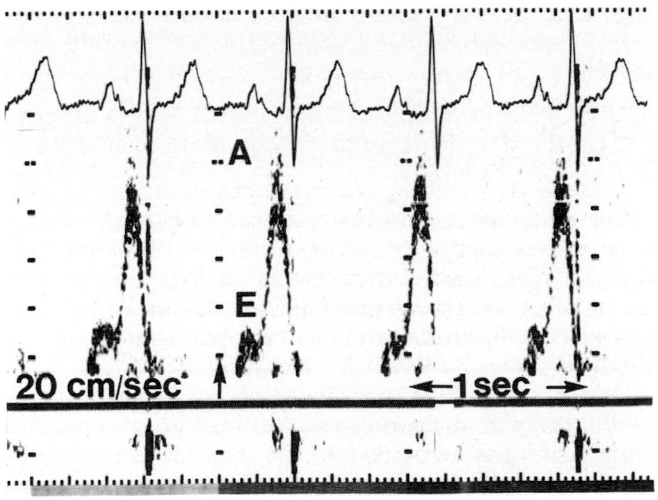

Fig. 24–22. Striking example of a markedly abnormal transmitral flow velocity profile taken from an 82-year-old woman with severe aortic stenosis, moderate concentric left ventricular hypertrophy, and normal left ventricular systolic function. The E wave is miniscule, and the A wave is large, contributing almost totally to left ventricular filling.

Other alterations in the velocity profile that have been described include decreases in the acceleration and deceleration rates of the E wave, an increase in the acceleration time of the E wave (time from onset of transmitral flow to the peak E-wave velocity) and decreases in the first third and first half-filling fractions, which refer to the proportions of total velocity-time integral occurring in the first one-third and the first half, respectively, of the diastolic filling period. In all these parameters, a relatively wide scatter of Doppler measurements is found in both normal and diseased states, and there is usually a broad overlap of individual data points between the two groups, even though group means may differ statistically. This calls into question the practicality of applying simple and inflexible criteria for diagnosing and quantifying abnormality in the individual patient. Which of these Doppler characteristics alone or in combination are the most discriminating for detecting abnormal diastolic function remains unresolved.

It is important to realize that diastolic dysfunction does not result from one universal diastolic functional abnormality, and there is no single abnormal transmitral flow velocity pattern that typifies all conditions with diastolic dysfunction. Differences in velocity patterns are expected to occur between different functional states.

For example, a reduced deceleration rate of the E wave has been found to reflect impaired ventricular relaxation, whereas an enhanced deceleration rate is seen with myocardial restriction.[113] In a recent study, impaired ventricular relaxation and increased chamber stiffness constant were found to produce directionally opposite changes in the transmitral flow velocity profile.[114] Differences in left atrial pressure, however, may have accounted for some of these results. In patients with dilated cardiomyopathy compared with those with pressure load hypertrophy, differences in atrial systolic function (impaired in dilated cardiomyopathy) may produce differences in the A-wave velocity.[115] Characteristic respiratory variations in transmitral flow velocities occur in certain conditions such as pericardial constriction and tamponade and may be used to support their diagnoses.

In summary, present evidence indicates that the transmitral flow velocity profile relates more to ventricular diastolic function and hemodynamic conditions than to particular diseases. Thus, it is possible for a single pathologic entity to produce different types of flow velocity patterns and for several types of diseases to manifest identical flow patterns. A more detailed description of the typical transmitral flow velocity profiles seen in different pathologic conditions is given later in this chapter.

In Vivo Relationships of Transmitral Flow Velocity Characteristics to Hemodynamic Measurements of Diastolic Function

The potential factors that may be expected to determine the velocity and pattern of transmitral blood flow have been outlined earlier in this chapter. In this and the next section, investigations into the nature and importance of these factors will be examined in greater detail.

Sparse information is available on the correlation between Doppler measurements of ventricular diastolic filling and invasive hemodynamic measurements representing diastolic function. A preliminary study in 20 patients found fairly good correlations between the ratio of the peak E-wave velocity to peak A-wave velocity and dV/VdP (r = .60), the ratio of the E-wave velocity-time integral to A-wave velocity-time integral and dV/VdP (r = .68), and the time to the peak E-wave velocity and peak negative dP/dt (r = .81).[116] Subsequent studies by the same and other workers, however, have not substantiated these early and encouraging results.

In one study, no correlation was found in 52 patients between the modulus of chamber stiffness, k_v, and the peak E-wave velocity to peak A-wave velocity ratio and the E-wave velocity-time integral to A-wave velocity-time integral ratio.[117] A peak E-wave velocity/peak A-wave velocity ratio of less than 1 was sensitive (83%) but not specific (30%) for detecting abnormal left ventricular compliance defined by the modulus of chamber stiffness. On the other hand, an abnormal E-wave velocity-time integral/A-wave velocity-time integral of less than 1 was insensitive (33%) but specific (73%) for detecting abnormal compliance. Accuracy was not improved by using both Doppler criteria together. Although a mild abnormality of left ventricular compliance was associated with increased peak A-wave velocities, a severe reduction in compliance was associated paradoxically with decreased A-wave velocities. The presumed explanation was that a marked decrease in ventricular compliance produced a very high left ventricular end-diastolic pressure, which increased resistance to left ventricular filling from atrial contraction.

In a study of 15 patients with coronary artery disease, many Doppler parameters (acceleration half-time, deceleration half-time, deceleration rate, and peak velocity of the E wave, peak velocity of the A wave, and ratio of the peak velocities of the E wave and A wave) were compared with catheterization measurements considered to reflect diastolic function (left ventricular end-diastolic pressure, peak negative dP/dt, time constant of relaxation).[118] Measurements of many of these Doppler parameters differed from those found in 14 normal subjects (the peak velocity, acceleration half-time, deceleration half-time, and deceleration rate of the E wave and peak E-wave velocity/peak A-wave velocity ratio). However, the only significant correlations demonstrated between Doppler and catheterization parameters in the patients were modest ones between the deceleration rate of the E wave and the peak negative dP/dt (r = .53) and between the peak velocity of the A wave and the peak negative dP/dt (r = .65). In this small study, the deceleration rate was found to be the most sensitive Doppler predictor of abnormal relaxation represented either by the time constant (sensitivity 60%) or peak negative dP/dt (sensitivity 62%). Their specificities were 100% and 60%, respectively.

Other studies have similarly demonstrated disappointing correlations in vivo between changes in Doppler indices of diastolic function and hemodynamic parameters of diastolic function.[119] A recent report throws light on this complex matter. Eleven normal controls demonstrated significant correlations between the left ventricular chamber stiffness constant (derived from M-mode and pressure measurements) and several Doppler parameters, including the peak E-wave velocity (r = .73), peak E-wave/A-wave velocity ratio (r = .82), E-wave/A-wave velocity-time integral ratio (r = .70), A-wave velocity-time integral (r = −.73) and the percentage of atrial contribution to total filling (r = −.64).[114] In 10 patients with coronary artery disease and "complete" ventricular relaxation (defined as the elapse of three or more time constants of relaxation by the time minimal ventricular pressure occurred), chamber stiffness constant also correlated positively with the peak E-wave velocity (r = .68), E-wave velocity-time integral (r = .65), and E-wave/A-wave velocity-time integral ratio (r = .74). In these normal subjects and patients, significant correlations were not found between the time constant of relaxation and Doppler parameters. In 14 patients with coronary artery disease and "incomplete" relaxation (defined as the elapse of less than three time constants by the time minimal ventricular pressure occurred), however, the chamber stiffness constant did not correlate with Doppler parameters, but the time constant of relaxation correlated negatively with the peak E-wave velocity (r = −.71) and the acceleration rate of the E wave (r = −.79) and correlated positively with the percentage of atrial contribution to total filling (r = .56).[114] These observations suggest that in a relatively uncontrolled setting in vivo, increased chamber stiffness constant and depressed relaxation rate—diastolic abnormalities that often occur together in cardiac disease—may exert directionally opposite effects on the pattern of left ventricular filling. The resultant flow profile therefore depends on the relative dominance of one abnormality over the other. It should be noted that theoretical predictions (see following section on computer modeling) indicate that reduced relaxation rate and increased chamber stiffness should produce directionally similar changes in the peak E-wave velocity, and many of the differences observed in vivo may have been due to secondary changes in left atrial pressure.

The findings of another recent study serve to illustrate further the complexity of Doppler hemodynamic correlations found in vivo.[120] In patients with normal left ventricular ejection fraction, the deceleration half-time of the E wave correlated with the time constant of relaxation. In patients with depressed ejection fraction, however, peak A-wave velocity and peak A-wave/peak E-wave velocity ratio correlated with chamber stiffness, but deceleration half-time no longer correlated with relaxation, reflecting the confounding influence of additional factors. For similar reasons, in patients with normal ejection fraction and impaired relaxation, the deceleration time of the E wave was longer compared to normal controls, but in patients with depressed ejection fraction and similarly impaired relaxation, it was shorter than in normal controls.

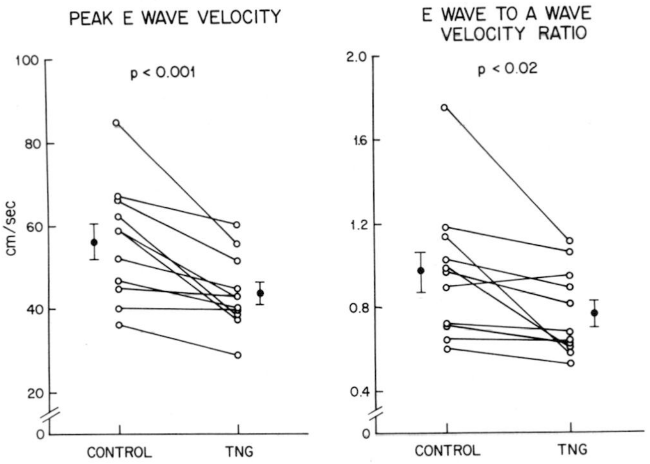

Fig. 24–23. Individual measurements of characteristics of the transmitral flow velocity profile commonly used as indices of diastolic function. Changes in these parameters have been produced by a reduction in left atrial pressure following nitroglycerin infusion (TNG). The Doppler changes mimicked an impairment of diastolic function that in fact did not occur.[121] (From Choong CY, Herrmann HC, Weyman AE, Fifer MA: Preload dependence of Doppler-derived indexes of left ventricular diastolic function in humans. J Am Coll Cardiol 10:800, 1987. Reprinted with permission from the American College of Cardiology.)

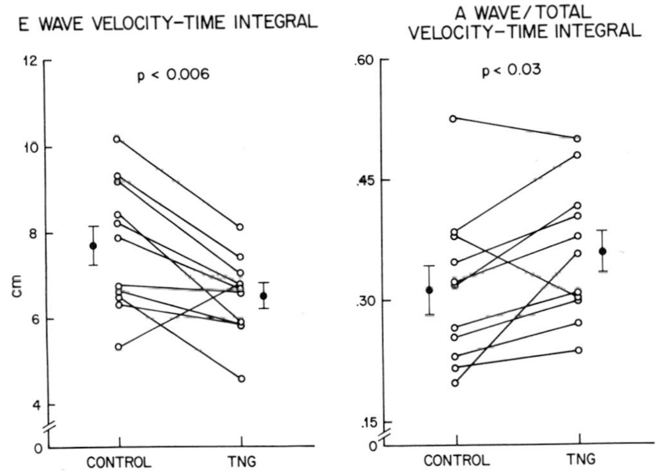

Fig. 24–24. Individual measurements of characteristics of the transmitral flow velocity profile commonly used as indices of diastolic function. Changes in these parameters have been produced by a reduction in left atrial pressure following nitroglycerin infusion (TNG). The Doppler changes mimicked an impairment of diastolic function, which in fact did not occur.[121] (From Choong CY, Herrmann HC, Weyman AE, Fifer MA: Preload dependence of Doppler-derived indexes of left ventricular diastolic function in humans. J Am Coll Cardiol 10:800, 1987. Reprinted with permission from the American College of Cardiology.)

In Vivo Interventional Studies of Factors That Determine the Transmitral Flow Velocity Profile

The generally poor correlation between single-Doppler and hemodynamic indices of diastolic function results from the complex relationship between the pattern of blood flow across the mitral annulus and the many determinants of this process. The failure to consider simultaneous variations in other important factors unrelated to diastolic function may lead to the misleading interpretation of changes in the transmitral flow velocity profile. The correct use of Doppler measurements to represent diastolic function depends first on the clear identification of the many factors that determine the transmitral flow velocity profile as well as the relative importance of their effects in vivo.

We have demonstrated in patients that a reduction in left atrial (i.e., ventricular filling) pressure by intravenous nitroglycerin reduces the peak velocity, acceleration rate, deceleration rate, and velocity-time integral of the E wave, without affecting the A wave significantly.[121] There is a resultant reduction in the peak E-wave/peak A-wave velocity ratio and an increase in the A-wave velocity-time integral/total velocity-time integral ratio (relative contribution of atrial contraction to left ventricular filling) (Figs. 24–23 and 24–24). These Doppler changes mimic an impairment of diastolic function (Fig. 24–25), when in fact, there is no hemodynamic evidence for such a deterioration. Examination of the pressure traces demonstrates that as the left atrial pressure at mitral valve opening is lowered by nitroglycerin, the nadir of the left ventricular pressure trace is also lowered but by a lesser extent than the left atrial pressure. The peak left atrial to left ventricular pressure gradient is therefore reduced. A schematic representation of the effect of increasing left atrial pressure on the subsequent time courses of the left atrial and left ventricular

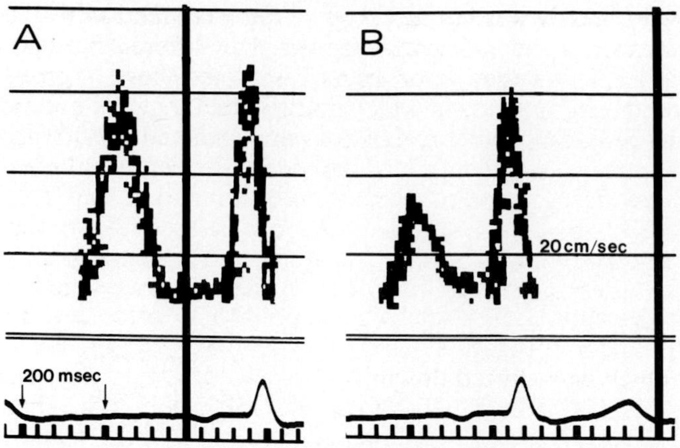

Fig. 24–25. Transmitral flow velocity profiles taken from a patient before **(A)** and after **(B)** the administration of nitroglycerin given to reduce left atrial pressure. Changes in the flow velocity profile produced by a reduction in ventricular filling pressure resemble those produced by a worsening of diastolic function, as illustrated in Figure 24–21.[121] (From Choong CY, Herrmann HC, Weyman AE, Fifer MA: Preload dependence of Doppler-derived indexes of left ventricular diastolic function in humans. J Am Coll Cardiol 10:800, 1987. Reprinted with permission from the American College of Cardiology.)

pressures and thus the transmitral pressure gradient is depicted in Figure 24–26.

Other workers have shown that an acute reduction in left ventricular filling pressure in humans by alternative means—such as vertical tilt, inflation of a balloon catheter in the inferior vena cava, and lower body negative pressure—similarly alter the flow velocities of the E wave without much change to the A wave.[122,123] These results corroborate and expand on the earlier demonstration in dogs that the peak filling rate of the left ventricle measured by electromagnetic flow probes depends on left atrial pressure.[34]

We and others have observed similar effects on the Doppler E-wave velocity profile in dogs with a reduction

INCREASE IN LEFT ATRIAL PRESSURE

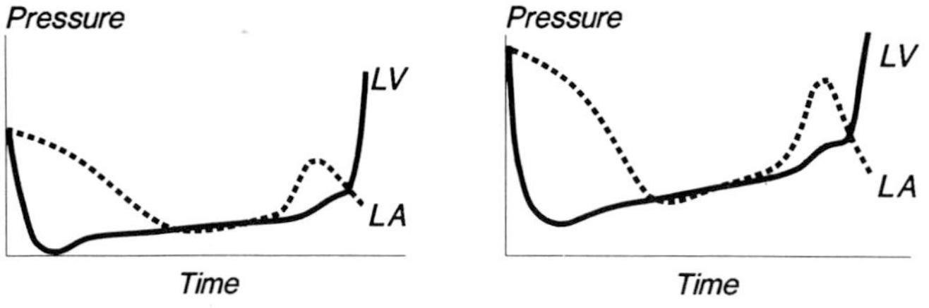

Fig. 24–26. The effect of an increase in left atrial (LA) pressure on the subsequent time courses of the LA and left ventricular (LV) pressures during diastole. The Left. The control state. Right. The pressure at which the mitral valve opens, or "crossover" pressure, increases. The nadir of the LV pressure, i.e., the minimal pressure, also increases but by a smaller amount than the elevation in LA pressure. The peak LA-to-LV pressure gradient therefore increases and results in a higher peak E-wave velocity. If the increase in LA pressure and volume (preload) before atrial contraction is sufficiently large, an increase in the peak atrioventricular pressure gradient in late diastole may occur and result in a higher peak A-wave velocity.

in left ventricular filling pressure, either by reducing roller pump flow in a right heart bypass model[124] or by transient occlusion of the inferior vena cava.[125] In both these studies, however, the peak velocity of the A wave also fell with a reduction in filling pressure. If left atrial preload is reduced sufficiently just before atrial contraction, a reduction in the peak A-wave velocity may be expected to occur. This discrepancy between the human and animal studies may have occurred for various reasons, including differences in experimental design (anesthetized dogs vs. conscious humans), a greater reduction in filling pressure, and stricter control of heart rate in the animal experiments.

As discussed earlier, a close relationship between Doppler parameters and hemodynamic measurements of diastolic function such as relaxation rate and chamber compliance has been difficult to demonstrate in vivo. Ventricular relaxation rate is expected to play an important role in modifying the E wave, because the ventricle is still relaxing during the rapid filling phase. The ventricular chamber may be seen to have a compliance characteristic (i.e., a relation between pressure and volume) during this relaxation phase, which continually changes, becoming less stiff as the ventricle relaxes. This dynamic or active compliance must not be confused with the passive compliance of the ventricle, which is manifested only after the ventricle has fully relaxed. Strictly, passive compliance is not manifested hemodynamically during the early filling phase but during the atrial contraction phase in late diastole. Thus, the passive compliance of the ventricle is expected to exert important effects on the A wave. It probably has an effect on the early filling phase also because of an indirect influence on the active pressure volume relation during relaxation. Put simply, it may be argued that, given the same relaxation rate, a ventricle with a lower passive compliance (a stiffer ventricle) should also have a lower active compliance during the latter part of relaxation (when early filling occurs). The relative importance of passive compliance vs. relaxation rate in the determination of the E wave in vivo, however, remains poorly described.

Difficulties with the strict control of multiple hemodynamic conditions in humans require studies that critically examine relationships between Doppler and hemodynamic parameters to be conducted in animal models. In our laboratory, we employed an open-chest right-heart bypass canine model, in which we could alter left atrial pressure by adjusting the rate of blood flow into the pulmonary artery, and simultaneously and independently alter aortic and left ventricular systolic pressure (representing afterload) by pumping blood into or out of the femoral artery through a second roller pump.[124] Heart rate was kept constant by crushing and pacing the sinus node. In individual dogs, the peak velocity of the E wave increased linearly with left atrial pressure at constant left ventricular pressure and heart rate (Fig. 24–27). The correlation was high, and the effect of atrial pressure was relatively great. At constant left atrial pressure and heart rate, there was a significant but weaker negative correlation between the peak velocity of the E wave and left ventricular systolic pressure (Fig. 24–28). Because left ventricular systolic pressure is a self-evi-

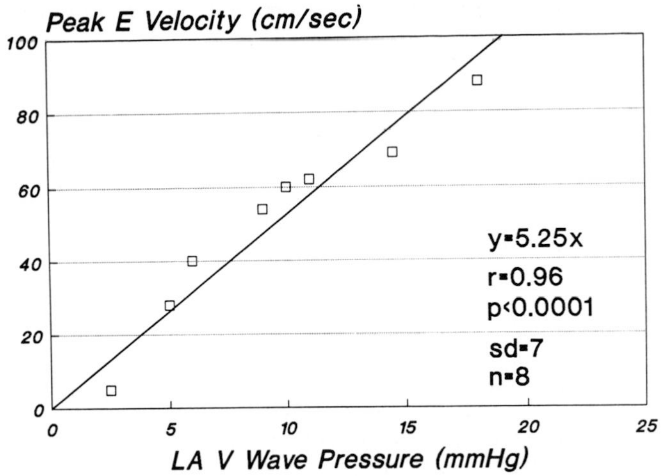

Fig. 24–27. Relation between the peak velocity of the E wave and left atrial (LA) V-wave pressure measured at constant heart rate and left ventricular systolic pressure in an individual dog. A right heart bypass experimental preparation was used, which allowed independent control of heart rate, left atrial pressure, and left ventricular systolic pressure. A positive linear correlation is clearly seen.[124] (From Choong CY, et al.: Combined influence of ventricular loading and relaxation on the transmitral flow velocity profile in dogs measured by Doppler echocardiography. Circulation 78: 672, 1988. Reproduced by permission of the American Heart Association, Inc.)

dent systolic event, this relationship must be mediated through secondary mechanisms, which may include changes in relaxation rate (which is afterload dependent) and changes in left ventricular end-systolic volume (also afterload dependent).

When data were pooled from all dogs, the relationships between Doppler and hemodynamic parameters were much weaker, a result of the introduction of unmeasured but influential factors that differed between dogs. This situation probably resembled those in group studies of humans in which multiple factors were uncontrolled and poor correlations were obtained. Multivariate analysis of the pooled data identified left atrial pressure first, followed next by relaxation rate and then weakly by left ventricular systolic pressure as significant hemodynamic determinants of the peak E-wave velocity. Compliance characteristics were not measured in this study. There was a positive linear relationship between the peak E-wave velocity and left atrial pressure, which was shifted downward by an increase in the time constant of relaxation (reduced relaxation rate) (Fig. 24–29 and 24–30). In essence, a decrease in the relaxation rate was accompanied by a higher nadir of the left ventricular pressure (minimal pressure) in early diastole, and given other factors being equal, this change reduced the pressure gradient between the left atrium and left ventricle and hence the magnitude of the transmitral flow velocities. As a corollary, there was a negative relationship between the peak E-wave velocity and the time constant of relaxation, which was shifted upward by an increase in left atrial pressure (Fig. 24–31). Generally, various parameters of the E wave, such as the velocity-time integral and deceleration rate, behaved similarly to the peak velocity of the E wave. A schematic representation of the effects of a reduction in ventricular relaxation rate on the time courses of the left atrial and left ventricular pressures and the resultant transmitral pressure gradient is shown in Figure 24–32. Proportional changes in peak filling rate measured by electromagnetic flow probes have been shown to correlate negatively to

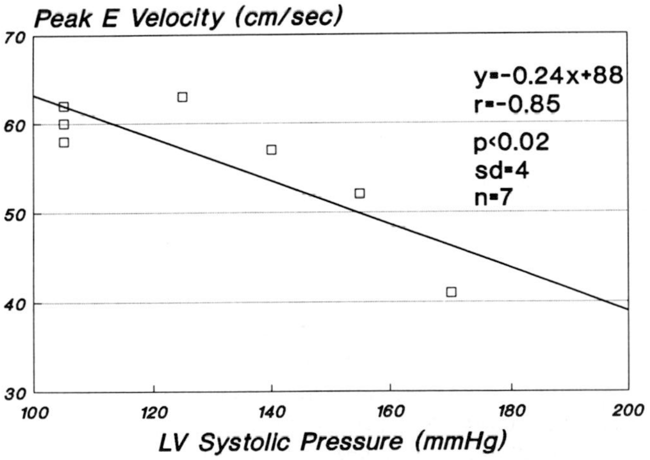

Fig. 24–28. Relation between the peak velocity of the E wave and left ventricular (LV) systolic pressure at constant heart rate and left atrial V-wave pressure in an individual dog. A right heart bypass experimental preparation was used, which allowed independent control of heart rate, left atrial pressure, and LV systolic pressure. A negative correlation is seen. The influence of LV systolic pressure is relatively smaller than that of left atrial pressure seen in Fig. 24–27.[124] (From Choong CY, et al.: Combined influence of ventricular loading and relaxation on the transmitral flow velocity profile in dogs measured by Doppler echocardiography. Circulation 78:672, 1988. Reproduced by permission of the American Heart Association, Inc.)

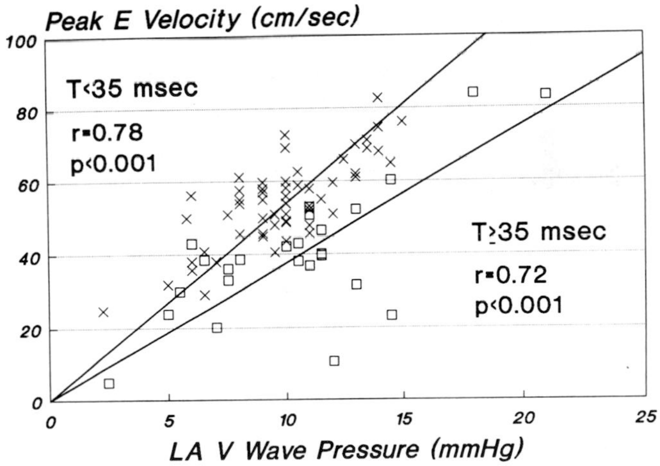

Fig. 24–29. Relation between the peak velocity of the E wave and left atrial (LA) V-wave pressure for all experimental stages in all dogs studied. Data points have been stratified according to whether the time constant of relaxation (T_L) is <35 msec (crosses) or ≥35 msec (squares). Regression lines are fitted through the origin. The slope of the relation between peak E-wave velocity and LA V-wave pressure is shifted downward by higher values of T_L. For T_L less than 35 msec, $y = 5.39x$. For T_L equal to or more than 35 msec, $y = 3.76x$.[124] (From Choong CY, et al.: Combined influence of ventricular loading and relaxation on the transmitral flow velocity profile in dogs measured by Doppler echocardiography. Circulation 78:672, 1988. Reproduced by permission of the American Heart Association, Inc.)

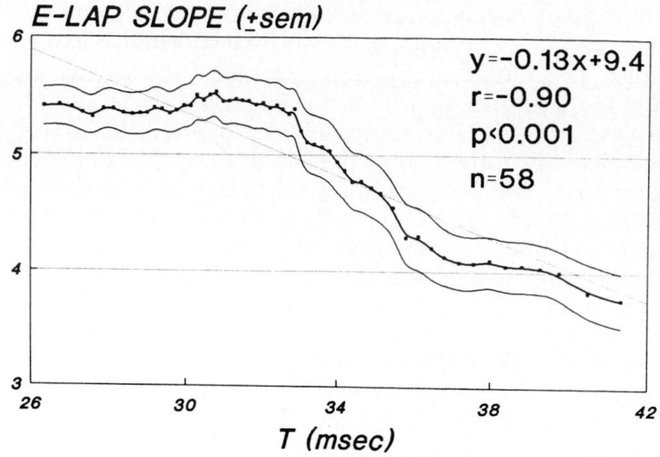

Fig. 24–30. Plot of the slope of the relation between peak E-wave velocity and left atrial V-wave pressure (y axis) against increasing values of the time constant of relaxation (T_L) (x axis). Calculations have been derived from the same data set as in Figure 24–29. The fine lines on either side of the data points represent ±1 SEM. The slope of the relation between peak E-wave velocity and left atrial pressure (LAP) decreases with an increase in T_L over a fairly wide range of T_L.[124] (From Choong CY, et al.: Combined influence of ventricular loading and relaxation on the transmitral flow velocity profile in dogs measured by Doppler echocardiography. Circulation 1988:78, 672. Reproduced by permission of the American Heart Association, Inc.)

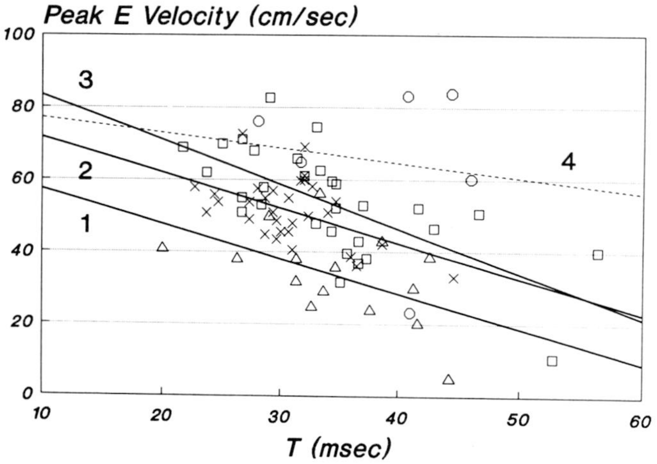

Fig. 24–31. Relation between the peak velocity of the E wave and the time constant of relaxation (T_L) taken from the same data set shown in Figure 24–29. There is a negative correlation between the peak E-wave velocity and T_L, which is shifted upward by an increase in left atrial V-wave pressure. Triangles and regression line 1 represent left atrial V-wave pressures ≤ to 7 mm Hg; crosses and regression line 2 represent left atrial V wave pressures >7 mm Hg and ≤10 mm Hg; squares and regression line 3 represent left atrial pressures >10 mm Hg and ≤14 mm Hg; circles and regression line 4 represent left atrial pressures >14 mm Hg. Correlations for lines 1, 2, and 3 were statistically significant. Line 1: $y = -0.95x + 67$, $p < .05$, $r = .51$, SD = 11 cm/sec, n = 15; Line 2: $y = -0.98x + 81$, $p < .004$, $r = .50$, SD = 8 cm/sec, n = 31; Line 3: $y = -1.23x + 96$, $p < .001$, $r = .67$, SD = 11 cm/sec, n = 30; Line 4: $y = -0.42x + 81$, p = NS, $r = .14$, SD = 25 cm/sec, n = 6.[124] (From Choong CY, et al.: Combined influence of ventricular loading and relaxation on the transmitral flow velocity profile in dogs measured by Doppler echocardiography. Circulation 78:672, 1988. Reproduced by permission of the American Heart Association, Inc.)

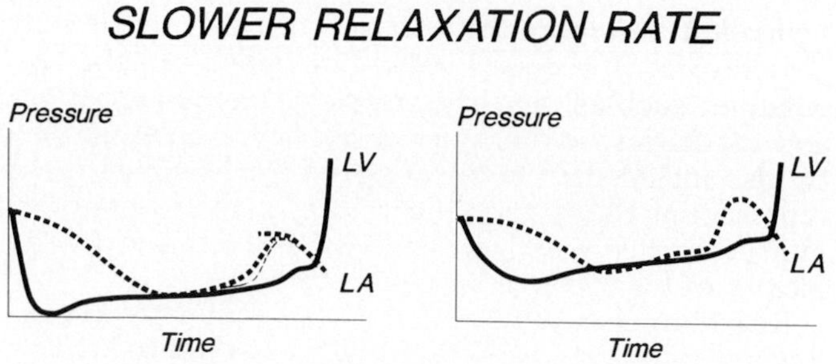

Fig. 24–32. The effect of a reduction in left ventricular (LV) relaxation rate on the time courses of the left atrial (LA) and LV pressures. Left. The control state. Right. At the same crossover pressure when the mitral valve opens, the LV pressure descends more slowly and reaches a nadir that is higher than in the control state. Left atrial pressure also descends more slowly as the rate of atrial emptying is reduced. The peak atrioventricular pressure gradient is reduced and, accordingly, the peak E-wave velocity is lowered. If LA pressure and volume (preload) remain higher before atrial contraction, the peak atrioventricular pressure gradient in late diastole may increase, resulting in a higher peak A-wave velocity.

proportional changes in the time constant of relaxation in conscious dogs,[34] suggesting that these Doppler observations extend to the conscious closed chest situation.

A detailed Doppler and hemodynamic study in dogs has demonstrated a significant relation between the peak velocity of the E wave and the left ventricular end-systolic volume ($r = -.63$, $p < .009$).[126] This important in vivo observation corroborates the theoretical prediction of a link between systolic function and diastolic function because the end-systolic volume dimension is determined primarily by left ventricular contractility and afterload. The manner by which end-systolic volume alters transmitral flow has already been discussed in this chapter. This link between systolic function and the transmitral peak E-wave velocity was recently demonstrated in humans with an examination of the effects of the postextrasystolic potentiation of left ventricular systolic function on transmitral flow.[127]

Very few detailed combined Doppler echocardiographic and hemodynamic studies have been performed. Much more work is needed in animals and humans before we will be able to understand fully the relative importance of the many determinants of the transmitral flow velocity profile and discover which Doppler parameters, if any, are more representative of diastolic properties and less dependent on loading conditions.

Computer Studies of Factors That Determine the Transmitral Flow Velocity Profile

Our current understanding of the complex and continuous interactions of these multiple hemodynamic factors has been greatly aided by the use of computer models to describe the processes during the early and late filling phases. Most workers have employed lumped parameter models, which contain hydraulic elements such as compliance, inertance, and resistance represented by mathematical descriptors. Depending on the complexity of the model that is required, representation of the pulmonary veins, left atrium, mitral valve, and left ventricle may be sufficient. If required, other components of the vasculature, such as the right ventricle, pulmonary artery and capillaries, aorta, and peripheral vasculature may be also included. Additional terms, for example, those representing the viscoelastic properties of the ventricle, may be applied with increasing sophistication and complexity of the model.

Relaxation has been modeled by some workers by allowing systolic (active) elastance, a linear pressure-volume function, to decay at an exponential rate to zero on a background of a constant passive elastance.[128] When active elastance reaches zero, the operative elastance becomes the passive elastance (stiffness) of the ventricle. Alternatively, relaxation has been modeled by generating exponential pressure-volume curves during relaxation, which continually decrease in their stiffness constants at an exponential rate until relaxation ceases, when the pressure-volume curve then becomes the passive pressure-volume relation of the ventricle (previously illustrated in Fig. 24–11).[129] Changes in relaxation rate (T) may thus be represented by altering the rate of decline of active elastance or stiffness constant, respectively. The continuous interaction of all these processes is described by the simultaneous solving of several linear and nonlinear differential equations in the model. An example of a relatively simple but useful model has been devised in our laboratory that solves three coupled first-order differential equations simultaneously:

$$dQ/dt = P_a(t) - P_v(t) - R_v * Q(t) - R_c * Q^2(t)/M \quad [24.1]$$

$$dP_a/dt = -Q(t)/C_a(P_a) \quad [24.2]$$

$$dP_v/dt = Q(t)/C_v(P_v,t) \quad [24.3]$$

where C_a is left atrial plus pulmonary venous bed compliance, C_v is left ventricular compliance, M is inertance of blood column, P_a is left atrial pressure, P_v is left ventricular pressure, Q is transmitral volumetric blood flow, R_c is convective resistance, R_v is viscous resistance, and t is time.

Equation 24.1 is analogous to the Bernoulli equation,[30] as described previously and in other chapters and differs only in the expression of blood flow in terms of volumetric flow rate rather than velocity. Equations 24.2 and 24.3 are based essentially on the definitions of combined left atrial-pulmonary venous bed and left ventricular compliances, respectively. Equation 24.2 describes the rate of change in left atrial pressure as a function of blood flow leaving the left atrium and the instantaneous compliance of the combined left atrial-pulmonary venous bed (itself a function of left atrial pressure). Equation 24.3 describes the rate of change in left ventricular pressure as a function of blood flow entering the left ventricle from the left atrium and the instantaneous compliance of the left ventricle (itself a function of left ventricular pressure as well as time, to represent active relaxation) (Fig. 24–33).

To execute the model, values for some specific parameters, such as left atrial compliance or mitral orifice resistance and inertance, must be taken from in vivo experiments. Instantaneous time-varying pressure and transmitral flow curves generated from these models have been shown to closely resemble actual pressures and flows measured in vitro and in vivo (Fig. 24–34). The computer models are used to predict the effects of alterations in individual parameters, such as relaxation rate, atrial compliance, left atrial pressure, and others on various characteristics of transmitral flow. Examples of how alterations in left atrial pressure, left ventricular relaxation rate, ventricular chamber compliance, and end-systolic volume are predicted to influence instantaneous left atrial and left ventricular pressures and early transmitral flow velocities are shown in Figure 24–35. The results of these individual changes on the left ventricular pressure-volume relationship are plotted in Figure 24–36.

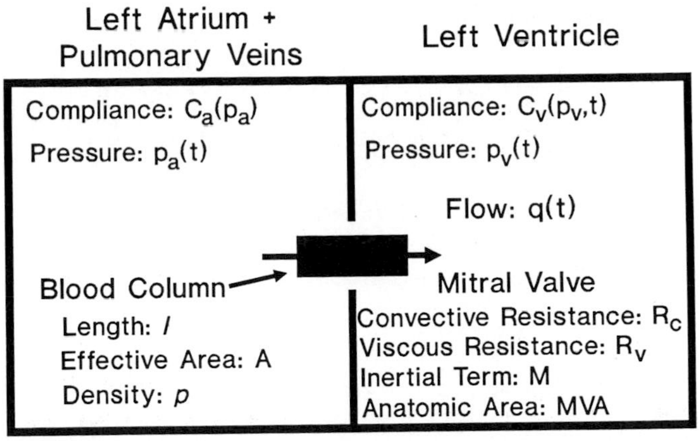

Fig. 24–33. Computer model of left ventricular filling that essentially incorporates two chambers, a combined left atrial-pulmonary venous bed chamber, and a left ventricle, connected by a mitral orifice. The chambers are described by compliance properties that are constant for the left atrial-pulmonary venous bed chamber and are time-varying (to represent relaxation) for the ventricle. The mitral orifice is described by resistive and convective components. An inertance term is included to account for volumetric flow acceleration and deceleration of the blood column. See text for details. (Courtesy of Dr. James D. Thomas.)

The effects of simultaneous alterations in left atrial pressure and the time constant of relaxation on various flow characteristics of the early filling phase are shown in Figure 24–37. The peak velocity of transmitral flow decreases with increasing time constant of relaxation (decreasing relaxation rate) and increases with increasing left atrial pressure. In agreement with the open-chest dog experiment described earlier,[124] the positive relationship between peak flow velocity and left atrial pressure is shifted up by an increase in relaxation rate.[130–132] Of interest and underscoring how complex these interactions can be, the influence of relaxation rate is greater at higher left atrial pressure, and the influence of left atrial pressure is greater at faster relaxation rates.

Figure 24–38 illustrates the effects of simultaneous changes in left atrial pressure and the left ventricular chamber volume constant (the reciprocal to the modulus of stiffness) on the same flow characteristics as described for Figure 24–37. A decrease in volume constant (equivalent to increased stiffness) produces a marked

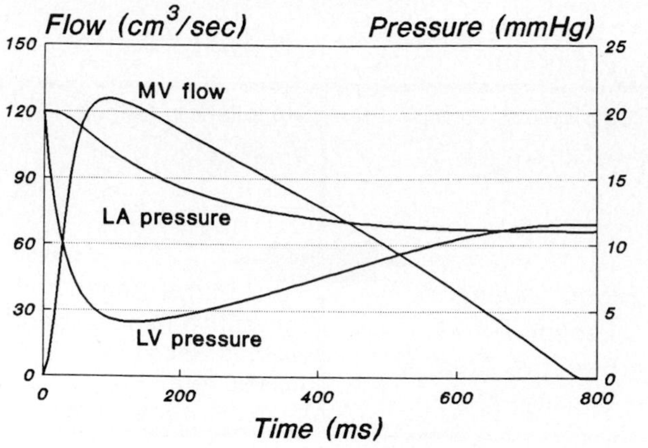

Computer Simulation

Input values

$p_a(0)$: 20 mmHg
$p_v(0)$: 20 mmHg
MV area: 0.7 cm^2
Inertial mass: 3

Pressure-volume curves

LA: $p = 3e^{V/60}$
LV: $p = 2(1+5e^{-t/30})e^{V/60}$

Output values

Stroke volume: 55 cm^3
Peak flow: 126 cm^3/sec
Peak velocity: 180 cm/sec
Acceleration time: 94 ms
Pressure half-time: 242 ms
Peak gradient: 13 mmHg
Minimum LV pressure: 4.1 mmHg
Zero gradient: 664 ms
Zero flow: 774 ms

Fig. 24–34. Computer-generated predictions of instantaneous left atrial (LA) and left ventricular (LV) pressures and the resultant transmitral flow velocities occurring during the early filling phase of diastole. The model and equations used to derive these predictions are described in the text and illustrated in Figure 24–33. (MV = mitral valve; $p_a(0)$ = atrial pressure; $p_v(0)$ = ventricular pressure. (Courtesy of Dr. James D. Thomas.)

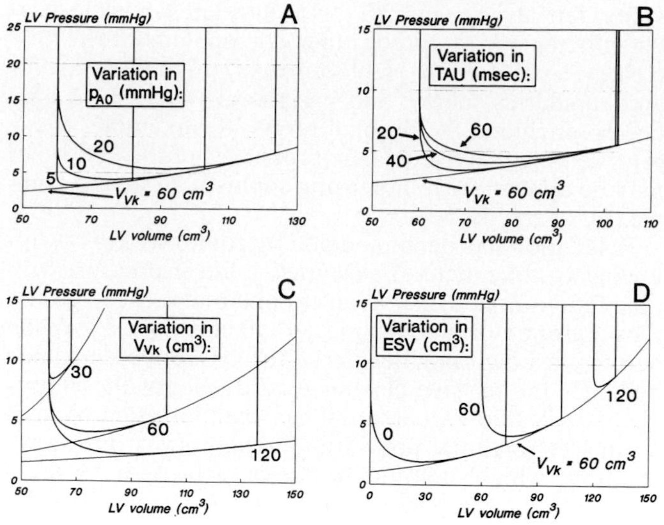

Fig. 24–36. Computer-generated left ventricular (LV) diastolic pressure-volume curves corresponding to the conditions shown in Figure 24–35. **A** to **D.** The effects of variations in initial left atrial pressure, relaxation rate, ventricular volume constant (reciprocal to the modulus of stiffness), and ventricular end-systolic volume (ESV), respectively. The middle curves represent identical conditions, the same as those found in Figure 24–35E. The other two curves show the effects of changes in the respective parameters and correspond to each pair of diametrically opposite panels shown in Figure 24–35. The exponential pressure-volume curves of the fully relaxed ventricles are also shown. Note that the x and y axes are not identical in the four panels. P_{AO} = initial left atrial pressure; TAU = time constant of isovolumic relaxation; V_{Vk} = ventricular chamber volume constant. (Courtesy of Dr. James D. Thomas.)

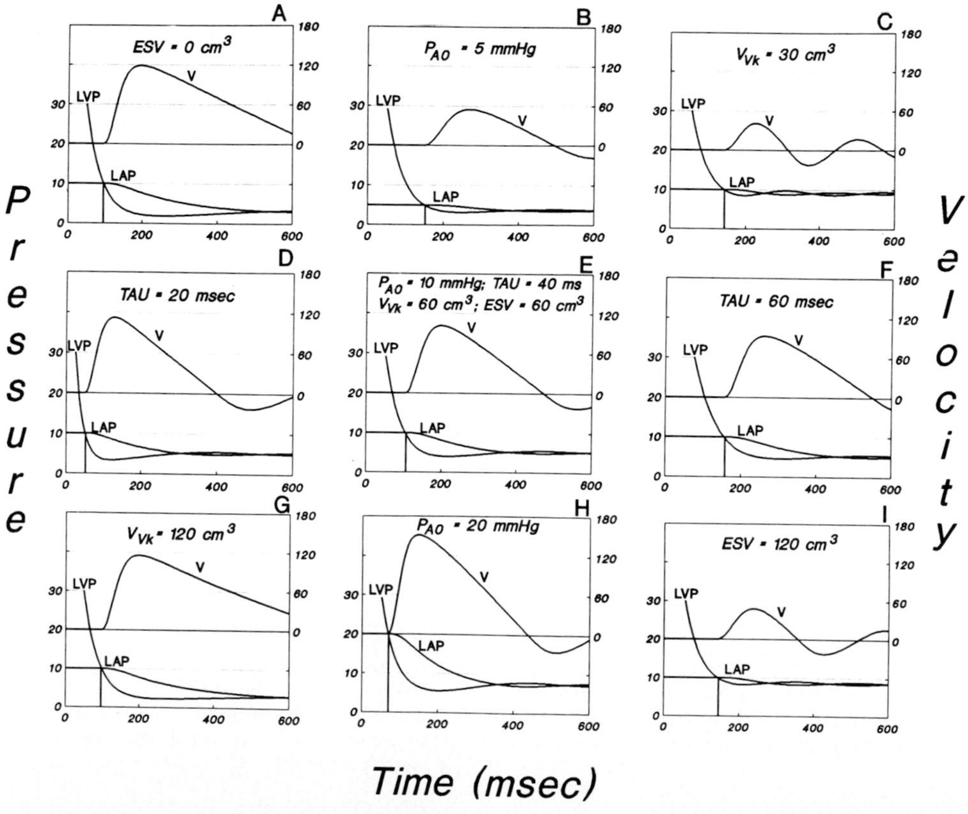

Fig. 24–35. Computer-generated predictions of left atrial and left ventricular pressures and transmitral flow velocities plotted as functions of time for changes in the left ventricular end-systolic volume **(A, E, and I),** initial left atrial pressure **(B, E, and H),** ventricular

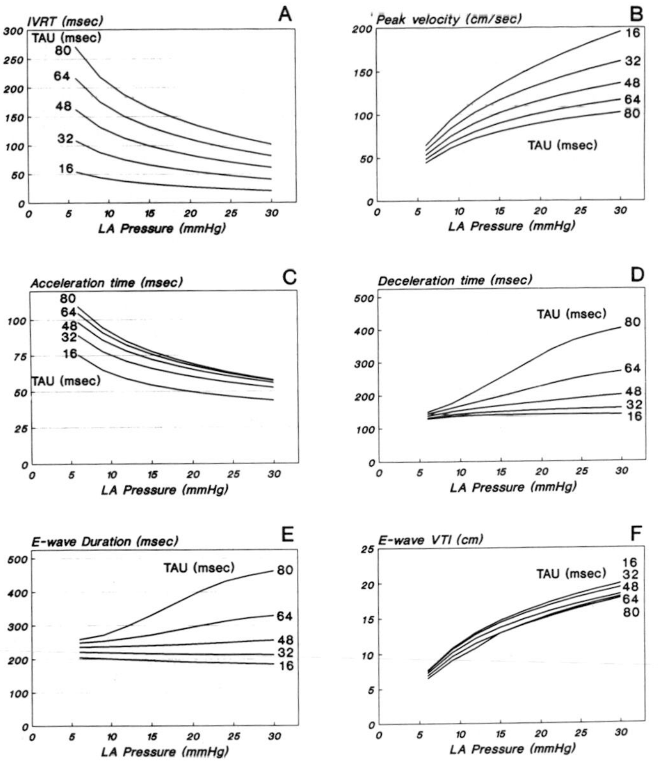

Fig. 24–37. Computer-generated predictions of the effects of simultaneous changes in the time constant of isovolumic relaxation (TAU) and initial left atrial (LA) pressure (at mitral valve opening) on commonly measured transmitral flow velocity parameters. **A.** Isovolumic relaxation time (IVRT). **B.** Peak E-wave velocity. **C.** E-wave acceleration time. **D.** E-wave deceleration time. **E.** E-wave duration. **F.** E-wave velocity-time integral (VTI). For this and Figures 24–38 to 24–40, the input variables are held constant unless specified along the x axis or are stratifying variables: A = 4 cm^2; M = 2 g/cm^2; P_{AO} = 20 mm Hg; TAU = 40 msec; V_{Ak} = 60 cm^3; and ESV = 60 cm^3. **B.** The positive relation between the peak E-wave velocity and left atrial pressure is shifted upward by decreasing TAU, i.e., faster relaxation. The curves diverge upward indicating that the influence of relaxation is small when left atrial pressure is low and larger when the latter is higher. **D.** A slower rate of relaxation (higher TAU) increases the deceleration time, but this effect is more pronounced at higher than at lower left atrial pressures. Also, the effect of relaxation rate is nonlinear so that the difference in deceleration time between TAU of 64 and 80 msec is greater than that between TAU of 16 and 32 msec. Abbreviations same as in Figure 24–35. (Courtesy of Dr. James D. Thomas.)

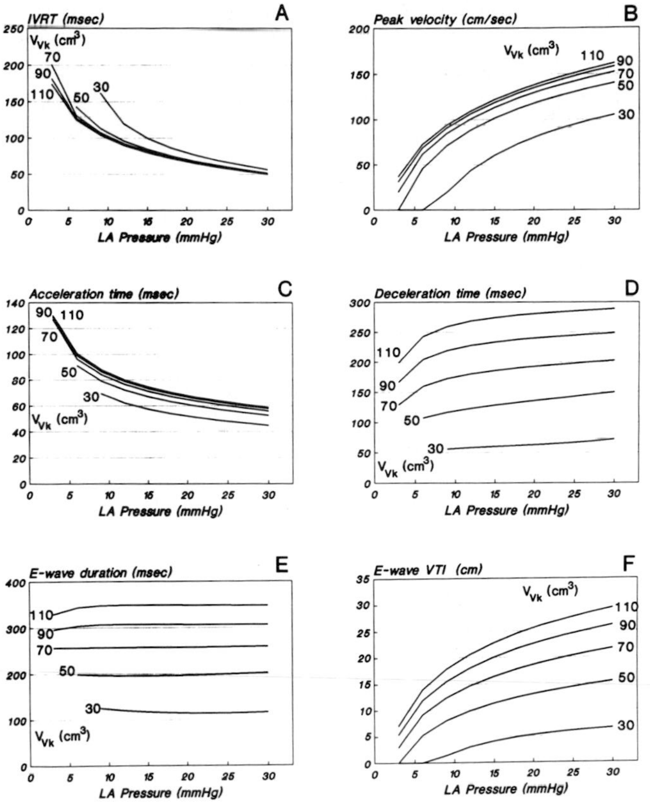

Fig. 24–38. Computer-generated predictions of the effects of simultaneous changes in the left ventricular chamber volume constant (V_{Vk}, the reciprocal to the modulus of stiffness) and initial left atrial (LA) pressure on the same flow characteristics shown in Figure 24–37. Values for other input variables are listed in the legend to Figure 24–37. A decrease in the chamber volume constant (equivalent to a stiffer ventricle) produces a marked decrease in the E-wave deceleration time, in keeping with in vivo observations in patients with restrictive cardiomyopathy and marked ventricular hypertrophy (see text). A decrease in the chamber volume constant also reduces the peak E-wave velocity, opposite to the effects suggested by some workers to occur in vivo. Simultaneous changes in other variables in vivo may explain this apparent discrepancy (see text). IVRT = isovolumic relaxation time; VTI = velocity-time integral. (Courtesy of Dr. James D. Thomas.)

volume constant **(C, E,** and **G),** and ventricular relaxation rate **(D, E,** and **F). E.** Contains the baseline parameters (additionally, A = 2 cm^2, M = 2 g/cm^2, and V_{Ak} = 60 cm^3). All other panels change only the parameter indicated. The vertical lines represent the isovolumic relaxation time, with aortic valve closing pressure assigned to be 100 mm Hg in all instances. A = effective mitral valve area; ESV = left ventricular end-systolic volume; LAP = left atrial pressure; LVP = left ventricular pressure; M = inertial mass accelerated within mitral apparatus normalized to effective orifice area; P_{AO} = initial left atrial pressure, i.e., at mitral valve opening; TAU = time constant of isovolumic relaxation; V_{Ak} = atrial chamber volume constant; V_{Vk} = ventricular chamber volume constant. The chamber volume constant describes the compliance property of the chamber from the exponential equation $p = p_k e^{V/V_k}$, where p = chamber pressure, V = chamber volume, and p_k = pressure when volume is 0. It is the reciprocal to the modulus of stiffness of the chamber. By definition, if V_k cm^3 of blood is added to the chamber, its pressure increases by a factor of e (2.71828). Thus, a lower V_k indicates a stiffer ventricle. (Courtesy of Dr. James D. Thomas.)

decrease in the deceleration time, consistent with observations in patients with restrictive cardiomyopathy and marked chamber hypertrophy (see later discussion). Given unaltered relaxation rate and left atrial pressure, note that, as chamber volume constant decreases, the peak flow velocity decreases, a change directionally opposite to that observed in vivo.[114] This discrepancy may be a result of concomitant changes in loading or other conditions in vivo, notably a compensatory increase in left atrial pressure with increasing ventricular stiffness.

Figure 24–39 shows the effects of simultaneous changes in left atrial pressure and left ventricular end-systolic volume. The model predicts a substantial influence of the end-systolic volume, in turn a function of ventricular contractility and afterload, on many early filling parameters, including peak velocity, deceleration time, velocity-time integral and duration. This potential influence of ventricular contractility and afterload on ventricular filling has only recently been recognized.

The last figure in this series shows the effects of simultaneous alterations in left atrial and left ventricular chamber volume constants on the flow characteristics (Fig. 24–40). A decrease in left atrial volume constant (increased stiffness constant) shifts the peak flow velocity vs. ventricular volume constant relation downward, producing a lower peak flow velocity for a given ventricular volume constant. As in many of the relationships predicted earlier, this effect is nonlinear, so that the difference in peak velocity seen between atrial volume constants of 30 and 50 cm^2 is greater than that between 50 and 70 cm^2.

Abnormalities in diastolic function are usually accompanied by secondary elevations in left atrial pressure. These increases in pressure modify the transmitral flow profile and may mask abnormal flow patterns that might otherwise occur. This phenomenon of pseudonormalization can be demonstrated with computer modeling. Figure 24–41 shows how the early transmitral flow profile changes in the presence of diastolic functional impairment when left atrial pressure is allowed to rise to keep stroke volume constant.[131]

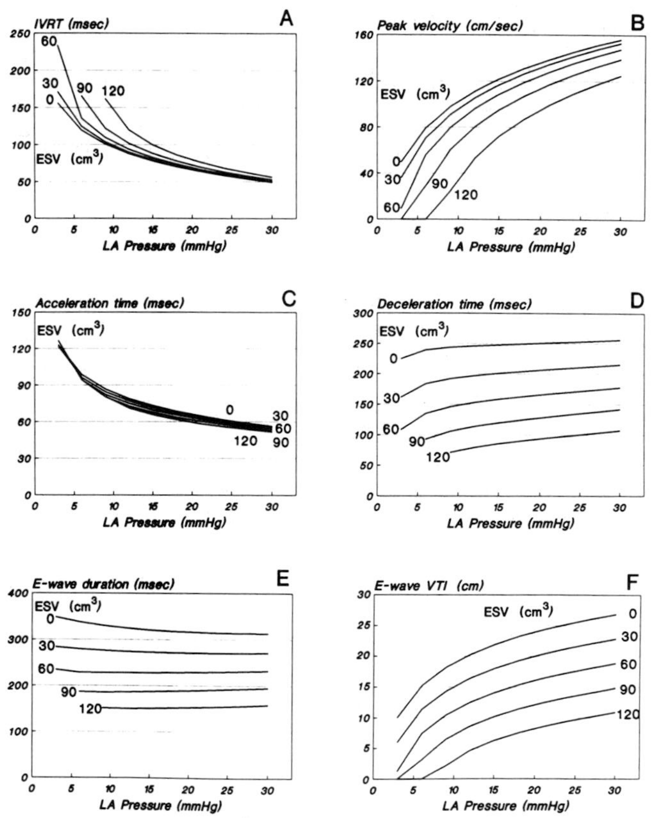

Fig. 24–39. Computer-generated predictions of the effects of simultaneous changes in the left ventricular end-systolic volume (ESV) and initial left atrial pressure (LA) on the same flow characteristics shown in Figure 24–37. Values for other input variables are listed in the legend to Figure 24–37. Note that the ESV has substantial influence on the peak velocity, deceleration time, duration, and velocity-time integral of the E wave, effects not previously well recognized. Because the ESV is determined largely by the contractility and afterload of the ventricle, these latter factors may be important determinants of the pattern of ventricular filling in vivo, independent of their known relationships to relaxation rate. IRVT = isovolumic relaxation time; VTI = velocity-time integral. (Courtesy of Dr. James D. Thomas.)

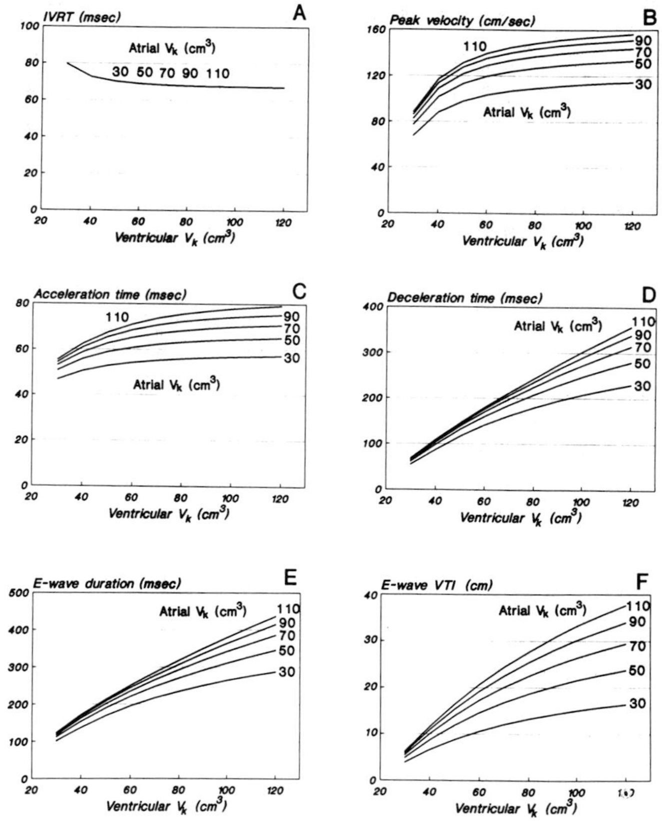

Fig. 24–40. Computer-generated predictions of the effects of simultaneous changes in the left atrial chamber volume constant (atrial V_K, the reciprocal to the modulus of stiffness) and left ventricular chamber volume constant (ventricular V_K) on the same flow characteristics shown in Figure 24–37. Values for other input variables are listed in the legend to Figure 24–37. The effects of the ventricular chamber volume constant have been demonstrated previously, in Figure 24–38. Note that a decrease in the atrial chamber volume constant shifts the positive relationship between peak E-wave velocity and the ventricular chamber volume constant downward. In other words, as the atrial chamber becomes stiffer, with all other factors held constant, the peak E-wave velocity falls. Similar findings apply to the E-wave deceleration time, duration, and velocity-time integral (VTI). IVRT = isovolumic relaxation time. (Courtesy of Dr. James D. Thomas.)

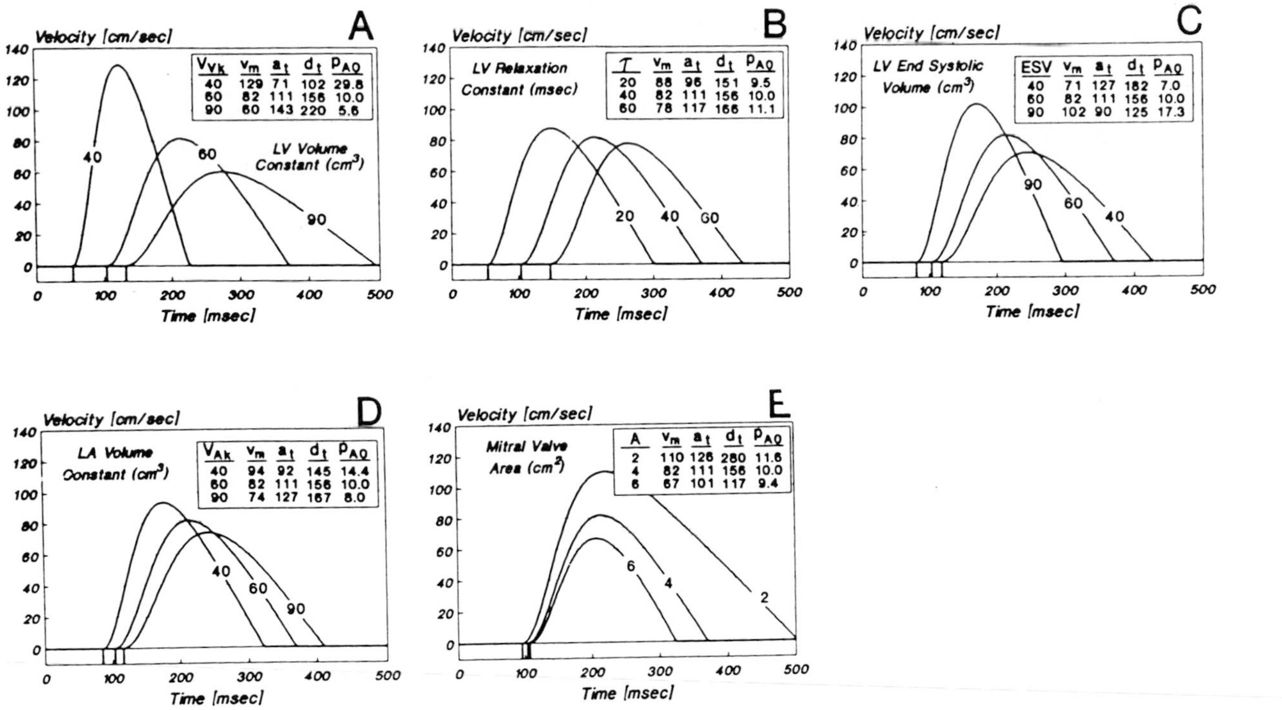

Fig. 24–41. Computer-generated predictions of changes in the early transmitral flow profile with variation in the following parameters: **A.** Left ventricular (LV) volume constant. **B.** Left ventricular relaxation constant. **C.** Left ventricular end-systolic volume. **D.** Left atrial (LA) volume constant. **E.** Mitral valve area. In each case, LA pressure has been allowed to vary simultaneously to keep stroke volume constant. A pseudonormalization effect may be seen as left atrial pressure increases. a_t = acceleration time; d_t = deceleration time; ESV = left ventricular end-systolic volume; P_{AO} = left atrial pressure at mitral valve opening; T = isovolumic relaxation time constant; V_{Ak} = left atrial volume constant; V_m = peak velocity; V_{Vk} = left ventricular volume constant.[131] (From Thomas J, Choong C, Flachskampf F, Weyman A: Analysis of the early transmitral Doppler velocity curve: effect of primary physiologic changes and compensatory preload adjustment. J Am Coll Cardiol 16:644, 1990. Reprinted with permission from the American College of Cardiology. Journal of the American College of Cardiology.)

This area of study is clearly complicated, and the following statements summarize the more important predictions of the computer model.[131,132] Transmitral flow velocity is affected fundamentally by two principal physical determinants, the transmitral pressure gradient and the net atrioventricular compliance (i.e., the instantaneous difference between atrial and ventricular compliance). Mitral valve impedance exerts an influence to a lesser extent. The peak E velocity is most strongly related to the initial left atrial pressure and is lowered by prolonged relaxation, low atrial and ventricular compliance, and systolic dysfunction. The peak acceleration rate correlates directly with atrial pressure and inversely with the time constant of relaxation, with little influence from compliance. The deceleration rate may be described by the mitral valve area divided by the instantaneous atrioventricular compliance at the end of the E wave. If relaxation is incomplete at this time, a longer time constant of relaxation also slows the deceleration rate. A recent in vitro study has shown encouragingly that net atrioventricular compliance may be calculated noninvasively and quantitatively from mitral valve area and the deceleration slope of the E wave.[133]

As vividly demonstrated previously, dynamic interactions among the mechanisms of transmitral blood flow are enormously complex. The computer predictions are a clear endorsement of how computer modeling can provide extremely valuable insights into intricate physiologic processes and greatly enhance our understanding of these matters. It should not be forgotten, of course, that computer models employ many inherent assumptions, and modeling does not dictate but only serves as a guide to the actual processes that take place. Ultimately, these predictions must be verified by in vivo observations. For a more detailed discussion of the computer modeling of transmitral flow and theoretical considerations of its determinants, the following references are recommended.[131,132,134]

The Influence of Methodologic Technique and Physiologic Conditions on the Transmitral Flow Velocity Profile

Effects of Sample Volume Position

The transmitral flow velocity profile is highly dependent on the site of sampling within the ventricle or atrium. In 52 normal subjects, with the Doppler sample volume placed in the left atrium 1 cm from the mitral annulus, peak E-wave and A-wave velocities were, respectively, around 25 and 22% lower compared to velocities recorded with the sample volume placed in the left ventricle between the mitral annulus and the tips of the mitral leaflets. The peak E-wave velocity/peak A-wave velocity ratio was not significantly different between the two positions.[107]

In a study that comprised 16 normal subjects and 46

Table 24–5. Influence of Pulsed Doppler Sample Volume Position on the Transmitral Flow Velocity Profile

	Position			
	LA 0.5 cm[a]	Annulus[b]	LV 0.5 cm[c]	LV 1.0 cm[d]
Total VTI (cm)	10.5 ± 3.7	12.0 ± 3.8*	13.4 ± 4.1†	14.6 ± 4.8‡
Peak E Vel (cm/sec)	44 ± 15	53 ± 18*	61 ± 22†	64 ± 24‡
Peak A Vel (cm/sec)	45 ± 13	52 ± 16*	58 ± 20*	58 ± 22†
Peak E/A Vel Ratio	1.02 ± 0.41	1.12 ± 0.55	1.20 ± 0.64*	1.28 ± 0.71†
E/A VTI Ratio	2.04 ± 1.02	2.02 ± 0.90	2.16 ± 0.95	2.32 ± 1.07†

[a] Sample volume in left atrium 0.5 cm from mitral annulus.
[b] Sample volume at mitral annulus.
[c] Sample volume in left ventricle 0.5 cm from mitral annulus.
[d] Sample volume in left ventricle 1.0 cm from mitral annulus, close to leaflet tips.
* $p < .05$ vs. a.
† $p < .05$ vs. a and b.
‡ $p < .05$ vs. a, b, and c.
Vel = velocity; VTI = velocity-time integral.

The study population consisted of 29 subjects (14 M, 15 F) with a mean age of 50 years (range 22 to 80). Fourteen were normal, 13 had mitral regurgitation of varying degrees and causes, and 2 had wall motion abnormalities without mitral regurgitation.

(From Pearson AC, et al.: Effect of sampling volume location on pulsed Doppler-echocardiographic evaluation of left ventricular filling. Am J Cardiac Imag 2:40, 1988.)

patients with cardiac disease, the peak velocities of the E and A waves were both higher (33 and 13%, respectively) at the level of the leaflet tips than at the annulus, but as the peak E-wave velocity was proportionately higher, the peak E-wave velocity/peak A-wave velocity ratio was correspondingly higher.[135] In another study of a mixed population of normal subjects and cardiac patients, peak E-wave and peak A-wave velocities, peak E-wave/peak A-wave velocity ratio, total velocity-time integrals and the ratio of the E-wave to A-wave velocity-time integrals increased as the Doppler sample volume was moved from the left atrium (0.5 cm from the mitral annulus) to the annulus plane and then to two levels in the left ventricle (0.5 cm and 1.0 cm from the annulus).[136] In some of these Doppler parameters, small shifts in sample volume positions of just 0.5 cm resulted in statistically significant changes in the measurements (Table 24–5). The presence or absence of mitral regurgitation did not appear to affect these positional changes. Figure 24–42 illustrates typical examples of changes in the Doppler flow velocity profiles when recorded at different sample volume locations.

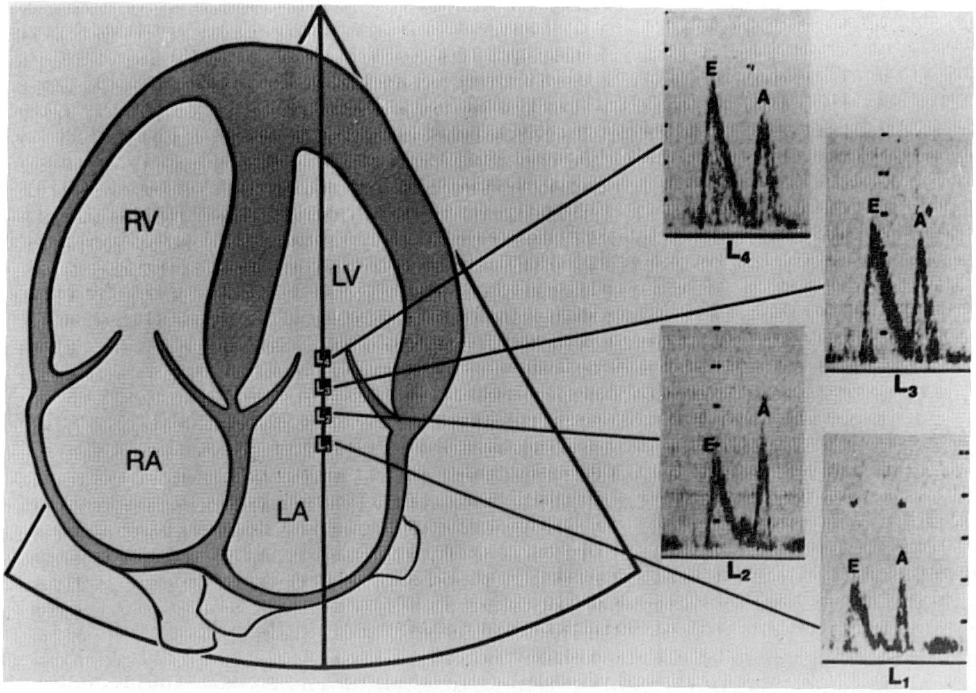

Fig. 24–42. Doppler transmitral flow velocity profiles recorded at various levels in the same patient. The figure demonstrates typical changes in absolute flow velocities and the distribution of flow velocities between early and late diastole seen at these various levels (see text and Table 24–5).[136] LA = left atrium; LV = left ventricle; RA = right atrium; RVG = right ventricle. (From Pearson AC, et al.: Effect of sample volume location on pulsed Doppler-echocardiographic evaluation of left ventricular filling. Am J Cardiac Imag 1988:2, 40.

As a result of the relatively large changes in the transmitral flow velocity profile at different sample volume locations, the position of the sample volume must be standardized within studies, and comparisons of results between studies should always consider this as a potential confounding factor. Furthermore, in any study where an intervention alters left ventricular size, the depth setting of the sample volume must be altered appropriately to maintain the same relation of the sample volume to the mitral annulus plane or leaflet tip, whichever is the chosen reference point.

Pulsed Wave Versus Continuous Wave Doppler Measurements

As pointed out earlier, transmitral flow velocity profiles recorded by the continuous wave Doppler technique represent the highest velocities occurring anywhere along the Doppler ultrasound beam. As such, they do not reflect the filling pattern of the ventricle as accurately as those obtained by the pulsed Doppler technique, which records the flow velocities at one specific level. Any comparison of measurements of transmitral flow velocity profiles between studies must take into consideration this important difference between the pulsed and continuous wave Doppler techniques.

Peak E-wave and peak A-wave velocities measured by the continuous wave Doppler technique are higher than those measured by the pulsed wave Doppler technique whether recorded at the level of the mitral annulus or at the leaflet tips.[135] However, the peak E-wave velocity/peak A-wave velocity ratio measured by the continuous wave Doppler technique appears similar to that measured by the pulsed Doppler technique at the leaflet tips.[135] Correspondingly, the velocity-time integrals of the E wave and A wave when measured by the continuous wave Doppler technique are larger than those measured by the pulsed wave Doppler technique at either the mitral annulus or leaflet tip levels. The ratio of the E-wave/A-wave velocity-time integrals by continuous wave Doppler examination is similar to that measured by the pulsed wave technique at the leaflet tips.

Effects of Imaging View of the Left Ventricle

When using the transthoracic approach, the apical window is required for the accurate recording of transmitral flow velocities as the direction of the inflow jet generally points toward the apex. Little information is available on the differences in transmitral flow velocities obtained from different apical views of the left ventricle. Any difference is expected to be minimal, because deviation of the Doppler ultrasound beam from the true direction of blood flow in any one view is likely to be small. As discussed in Chapter 7, angle correction of Doppler flow velocities is performed by dividing the recorded velocities by the cosine of the angle between the Doppler ultrasound beam and the actual direction of blood flow. The cosine of an angle of 0° is 1, and this value decreases in a curvilinear function to 0 as the angle increases to 90°. The cosine remains relatively large for small angles so that angle-correction may usually be ignored until the angle exceeds 20°. At this angle, the cosine is 0.94, and angle correction therefore produces a 6.4% increase in flow velocities. In one study, peak E-wave and peak A-wave velocities tended to be slightly higher (by approximately 4%) when recorded in the apical four-chamber view compared to the apical two-chamber view, but differences of this magnitude are unlikely to be of clinical significance.[107]

Effects of Respiration

During inspiration, the peak velocity and duration of the E wave decrease compared to expiration. The peak velocity of the E wave has been reported to decrease by 4% and as much as 10%, and the E-wave velocity-time integral may decrease by as much as 20%. There is no change in the peak velocity or duration of the A wave.[137,138] Ratios of the E-wave to A-wave peak velocities and velocity-time integrals may decrease by around 12 and 14%, respectively.[138] Other workers have not found any effect of respiration on the transmitral peak E/peak A velocity ratio.[139] These Doppler respiratory variations agree with the well-established observation that systolic blood pressure and stroke volume normally decrease slightly with inspiration and suggest that these changes are brought about at least partly by an inspiratory reduction in ventricular preload. The effects of respiration on flow velocities across the tricuspid valve are very different from those across the mitral valve. Inspiration produces substantial increases in the peak velocities of both E and A waves, reflecting enhanced venous return.[138] As a result, the ratio of these velocities is not altered.

Because of the variation in transvalvular flow velocities with respiration, the respiratory phase during Doppler recordings should be standardized. Patients should be asked to breathe quietly, and analyses should be made of beats taken during unforced end-expiration. An advantage of using the end-expiratory phase is that variability in transmitral flow velocities due to variations in inspiratory effort are avoided. Furthermore, in apical views, higher quality two-dimensional images and Doppler signals are usually obtained during expiration rather than inspiration.

Recent work has suggested that characteristics of the respiratory variation in mitral and tricuspid flow velocity may aid the diagnosis of certain pathologic states, such as pericardial constriction and tamponade. These changes are discussed in the following appropriate sections.

Effects of Heart Rate

Heart rate plays an important role in the pattern of transmitral blood flow. It must be appreciated that artificial changes to heart rate in a resting patient do not represent the same hemodynamic situation as when heart rate changes "naturally," such as during exercise. Hemodynamic studies of atrial pacing indicate that as heart rate is artificially increased in patients at rest, cardiac output generally stays unchanged, stroke volume falls, and ventricular volume often decreases. During exercise, the increase in heart rate is accompanied by an increase in cardiac output and stroke volume, and peak flow velocities are correspondingly higher. It must also be appreciated that changes in heart rate at constant stroke volume represent a different hemodynamic situation from changes in heart rate with atrial pacing. The former allows a purer study of the effects of heart rate alone but is much more difficult to produce experimentally, especially in humans, and its effects have not been well described.

The mechanisms by which changes in heart rate alter transmitral flow velocities involve not only the timing of the A wave in relation to the preceding E wave (by definition) but also other factors, most notably loading conditions such as left atrial pressure. A sudden increase in heart rate may also increase myocardial contractility through the Bowditch staircase phenomenon or Treppe effect. The importance of this effect here is unknown.

In a preliminary study, an increase in heart rate from 60 to 90 beats per minute by atrial pacing progressively decreased the velocity-time integral of the E wave and increased the peak velocity and velocity-time integral of the A wave. The peak velocity of the E wave and the ratio of the peak E-wave velocity to peak A-wave velocity decreased slightly but not statistically significantly. These changes occurred even though the E and A waves did not merge. At heart rates of 100 beats per minute and higher, the E and A waves fused.[140] In another preliminary study involving patients with DDD (atrioventricular) pacemakers, peak E-wave velocity and velocity-time integral, peak E-wave/peak A-wave velocity ratio, and E-wave/A-wave velocity-time integral ratio decreased progressively, and the peak A velocity and velocity-time integral increased progressively as heart rate was increased from 60 to 100 beats per minute at 5 beats per minute stages with a constant atrioventricular delay.[141] Similar results with dual-chamber pacing have been reported by others.[142]

In a more recent study using transesophageal atrial pacing to increase heart rate in normal volunteers, the peak velocity and velocity time integral of the E wave did not change with an increase in heart rate in contrast to earlier studies, but the peak velocity and velocity-time integral of the A wave increased. For each increase in heart rate by 10 beats per minute, peak A velocity increased by 8 cm/sec.[143] A more detailed study in dogs yielded similar results and provided insightful hemodynamic correlates of the observed Doppler changes.[144] Regardless of whether heart rate was increased by right atrial pacing, atropine, or isoproterenol, qualitatively similar changes in mitral flow velocity and transmitral pressure gradient occurred as heart rate increased. At any particular heart rate, however, mitral flow velocity parameters and late diastolic pressure gradients often differed markedly between interventions, and this was due largely to their different effects on the PR interval and, to a lesser extent, on relaxation rate.

In summary, the effects of heart rate must be carefully considered when assessing any transmitral flow velocity profile, when examining the results of interventions that also alter heart rate (such as β-adrenergic blockade) or when studying conditions characterized by altered heart rates (such as heart failure, which is often associated with tachycardia). Figure 24–43 shows an example of changes in the transmitral flow velocity profile produced by progressive increases in heart rate in a patient with a dual-chamber pacemaker.

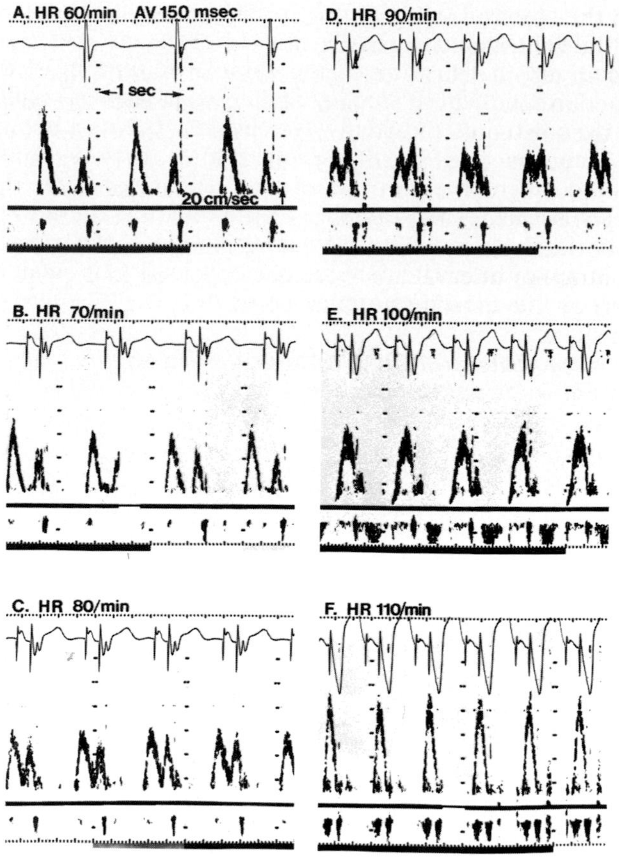

Fig. 24–43. Effects of alterations in heart rate (HR) at rest on the transmitral flow velocity profile. The patient is a 35-year-old woman with idiopathic degeneration of the conduction system. Left and right ventricular systolic function are normal, and there is no valvular disease. She has a dual-chamber AV sequential pacemaker (DDD), which was repeatedly reprogrammed to pace AV synchronously at increasing heart rates. **A.** The transmitral flow velocity profile at her ambient heart rate of 60 beats per minute with sinus rhythm. The right atrium is sensed, and the right ventricle is paced after a preset AV interval of 150 msec. **B** to **F.** The flow velocity profiles with the right atrium paced at increasing rates of 70, 80, 90, 100, and 110 beats per minute. The right ventricle is paced after a fixed AV interval of 150 msec. With increasing heart rates, there is a progressive merging of the E and A waves as the diastasis period shortens and then is obliterated. Initially, the peak velocity of the E wave decreases slightly as heart rate increases. The peak velocity of the A wave does not change much initially until it merges with the end of E wave at a rate of 80 beats per minute, when it starts to rise. With further increases in the heart rate, the two waves fuse and the velocity peaks converge, producing increasing peak velocities and decreasing total flow duration. Note that if the AV interval had been allowed to shorten with increasing heart rates, the E wave would have occurred progressively earlier relative to the following A wave, and fusion of the two waves would have been delayed. Some workers have reported no change or only a minimal decrease in the peak E-wave velocity with an increase in heart rate (see text).

Effects of Atrioventricular Interval

Even when the heart rate is constant, changes in the duration of the atrioventricular interval (the PR interval on the electrocardiogram) may affect the filling pattern of the ventricle. An increase in the atrioventricular interval in effect delays the occurrence of ventricular contraction following atrial contraction and hence the onset of the subsequent E wave. At a constant heart rate, i.e., a constant electrocardiographic P wave/P wave or Doppler A-wave/A-wave interval, an increase in the atrioventricular interval takes the E wave closer to the following A wave. The effects of changes to the atrioventricular interval are therefore expected to depend in part on the existing heart rate and thus the duration of diastasis.

In patients with dual chamber pacemakers, an increase in the atrioventricular interval from 74 to 150 msec and then 250 msec at constant heart rate produced progressive decreases in the diastolic filling period and the peak E-wave velocity and a progressive increase in the atrial contribution to ventricular filling without any change in the stroke volume.[105] These findings are supported by previous observations in calves where electromagnetic flow probes sewn onto the mitral annulus indicated progressively lowered flow rates during early ventricular filling with increases in the atrioventricular interval.[145] In a more detailed report of patients with dual-chamber pacemakers and normal ventricular function, however, changes to the electrocardiographic PQ interval ranging from 75 to 175 msec at a constant rate of 80 beats per minute did not alter peak E- or A-wave velocities. At a PQ interval of 250 msec, the E and A waves merged with summation of their velocities.[146] Reasons for the different findings between these two studies are unclear.

Figure 24–44 shows the transmitral flow velocity profiles of the same patient with a dual-chamber pacemaker as in Figure 24–43. At an atrial pacing rate of 70 beats per minute, there was no significant change in the flow velocity profile when the atrioventricular interval was increased from 100 to 175 msec. At higher preset atrioventricular intervals in this patient, atrioventricular node conduction supervened with a bundle branch block pattern. There was no accompanying change in the flow velocity profile.

Figure 24–45 shows transmitral flow velocity profiles taken from a middle-aged man in sinus rhythm with first-degree atrioventricular block and an electrocardiographic PR interval of 300 msec. In sinus rhythm, only one flow wave is seen, and it is unclear how much of this wave represents the E or A waves. The situation is clarified with the occurrence of blocked and also conducted atrial premature beats, which produce separation of the subsequent E and A waves. An interesting variety of flow profiles is seen, which may be explained by carefully examining the timing of the P waves and the durations of the PR intervals.

Effects of Age

Age is an important determinant of the transmitral flow velocity profile in the normal population and may be a major confounding factor when comparing patient groups that are uncontrolled for age. An early study of 69 healthy subjects aged from 22 to 69 years indicated that the peak velocity of the E wave tended to decrease and that the peak velocity of the A wave tended to increase with increasing age. Consequently, the ratio of the peak velocity of the E wave to the peak velocity of the A wave decreased significantly with increasing age.[147] Figure 24–46 illustrates examples of the striking changes in the transmitral flow velocity profile that can occur with normal aging.

The influence of age on six Doppler diastolic parameters were studied in 86 normal subjects aged 20 to 74

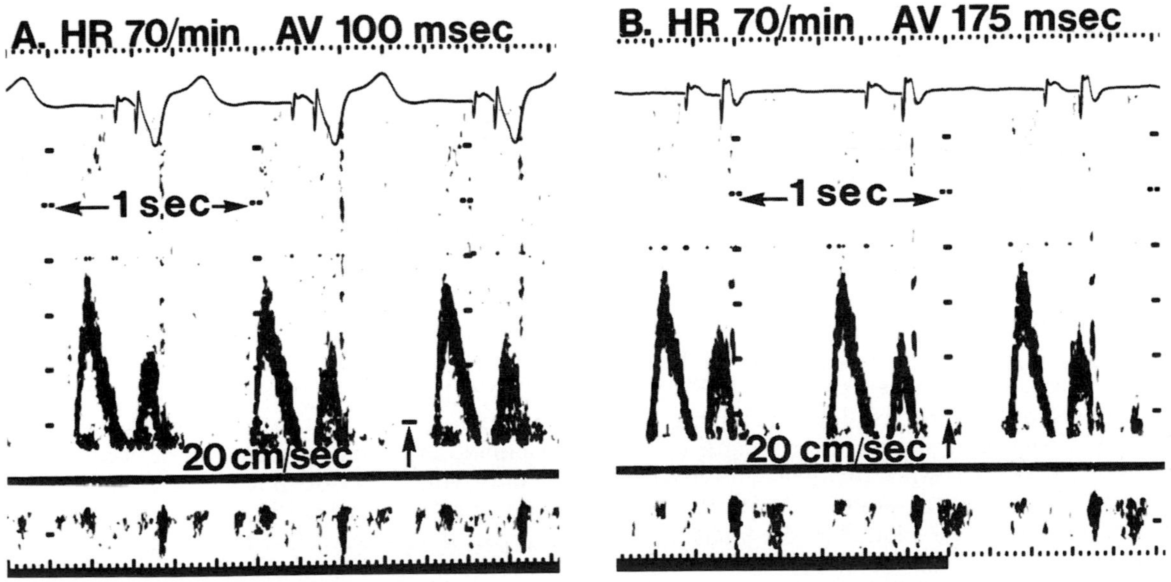

Fig. 24–44. Transmitral flow velocity profiles of the same patient with a dual-chamber pacemaker as in Figure 24–43. The atrial pacing rate is kept constant at 70 beats per minute, and the atrioventricular (AV) interval is increased from 100 msec **(A)** to 175 msec **(B)**. In this patient, there is no significant change in the flow velocity profile within this range of AV intervals. At an AV interval of 200 msec (not shown), the patient's natural atrioventricular node conduction supervenes with a bundle branch block pattern on the electrocardiogram. There is also no significant change in the flow velocity profile in this setting. See text for further discussion.

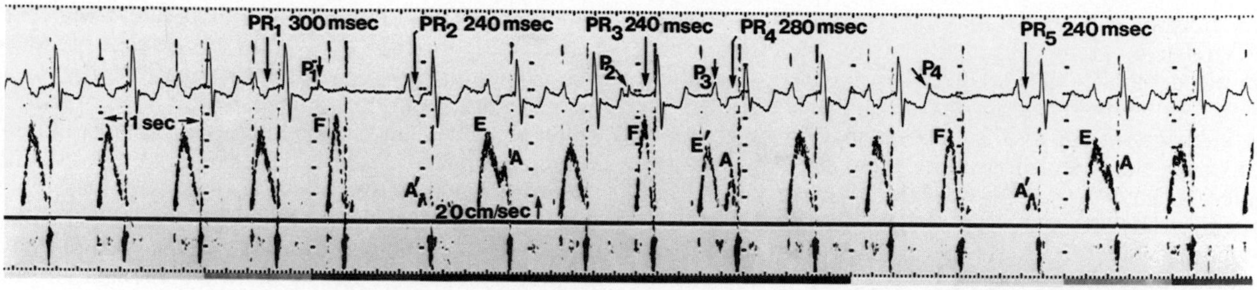

Fig. 24–45. Transmitral flow velocity profiles taken from a 68-year-old man with hypertension, concentric left ventricular hypertrophy, and normal left ventricular systolic function. The patient is in sinus rhythm with a rate of 84 beats per minute and has first-degree atrioventricular block with a PR interval of 300 msec (PR_1). The first few cycles from the left show single transmitral flow waves. From these cycles alone, the respective contributions of the E and A waves to the single flow wave cannot be determined. The situation is clarified following the occurrence of atrial premature beats. A variety of patterns of transmitral flow are seen, which may be explained by carefully considering the timing of the different P waves and the durations of the PR intervals. The first atrial premature beat (P_1) is not conducted by the atrioventricular node. The following transmitral flow wave (F) is narrower and taller because of a closer superimposition of the premature A wave on the preceding E wave. The following flow wave is a miniscule A wave (A′), which results from the atrium's contracting into a ventricle that has a higher volume and pressure than usual, not having had the chance to eject after the preceding E and A waves. The PR interval (PR_2) immediately following this premature P wave is shorter (240 msec) than usual, which causes the subsequent E wave to occur earlier. The result is a clear separation of the peaks of the following E and A waves. The next premature atrial beat (P_2) is conducted to the ventricle. A closely fused E- and A-flow wave (F) is seen for the same reasons described earlier. The associated PR interval (PR_3) is shortened (240 msec). The following E wave (E′) is premature, because it originates from a premature atrial beat and also follows a shortened PR interval. The following P wave (P_3) and corresponding A wave are slightly delayed when timed from the preceding ectopic P wave (P_2). The combination of these factors results in the clear separation of the corresponding E and A waves. The PR interval of the next cycle (PR_4) increases to 280 msec, and the following flow wave becomes single again. These Doppler sequences are reproducible with subsequent premature beats (P_4) indicating that they are not from artifacts in the Doppler recording.

years.[148] The peak E-wave velocity, the deceleration rate of the E-wave velocity and the ratio of the peak E-wave to peak A-wave velocity all correlated negatively with age (respectively, $r = -.40$, $r = -.42$, $r = -.66$, $p < .001$), while the isovolumic relaxation period, the duration of the E wave and the peak A-wave velocity correlated directly with age (respectively, $r = .40$, $r = .32$, $r = .63$, $p < .001$). With subdivision of the patients into three age groups (20 to 29, 30 to 49, 50 to 74 years), the isovolumic relaxation period was longer, deceleration rate of the E wave was slower, and ratio of the peak E-wave to peak A-wave velocities was lower in the older compared to the younger subjects. Similar results involving these and other Doppler filling parameters, such as reduced ratio of the E-wave to A-wave velocity-time integrals and increased atrial contribution to total ventricular filling with age have been reported by others.[149,150] Correlations of Doppler-derived peak volumetric filling rate and of the E-wave/A-wave velocity-time integral ratio with age were lost in the presence of left ventricular hypertrophy, presumably because ventricular hypertrophy itself acted as an independent modifier of the transmitral flow velocities.[112]

Several reasons may be proposed for the alteration in left ventricular filling pattern with increasing age. It is known that left ventricular wall thickness and mass increase with age in the normal population.[151–153] These morphologic changes are a plausible explanation because of increased ventricular stiffness. In one study, although the peak E-wave velocity, the ratio of the peak E-wave to peak A-wave velocity and the atrial filling fraction correlated well with age in normal subjects ($r = .91$, $r = .82$ and $r = .81$, respectively),[151] these age-related "physiologic" changes in flow velocity profile did not correlate with the radius/thickness ratio of the left ventricle. This finding prompted the authors to suggest that alterations in intrinsic myocardial fiber stiffness, perhaps from an increase in fibrous content, rather than or in addition to ventricular geometry, were responsible for the altered filling patterns. The effect of aging on ventricular relaxation in the normal heart has not been closely examined. As mentioned earlier, the isovolumic relaxation period is known to lengthen with age, and any reduction in relaxation rate with aging may reduce the peak velocity of the early filling phase even in the absence of changes in ventricular geometry or myocardial passive stiffness. Blood pressure tends to increase with age, even in the normotensive population. The contribution of increased diastolic and systolic blood pressure to this phenomenon also remains poorly understood. There are theoretical grounds for implicating at least a contributory role. For example, higher diastolic pressure may increase coronary turgor; higher systolic pressure, representing ventricular afterload, may slow relaxation rate and increase ventricular end-systolic volume.

Recently, a group of workers were unable to detect any differences in left ventricular mass, heart rate, contractility, and loading conditions between young and old healthy volunteers despite marked differences in their transmitral flow velocity profiles. Relaxation rate and myocardial stiffness, however, were not measured.[154]

A recent interesting report indicated that "abnormalities" in the transmitral flow velocity profile in normal elderly subjects are improved by calcium channel blockade with diltiazem.[155] Clinical correlates of this improvement in left ventricular filling pattern are as yet unknown.

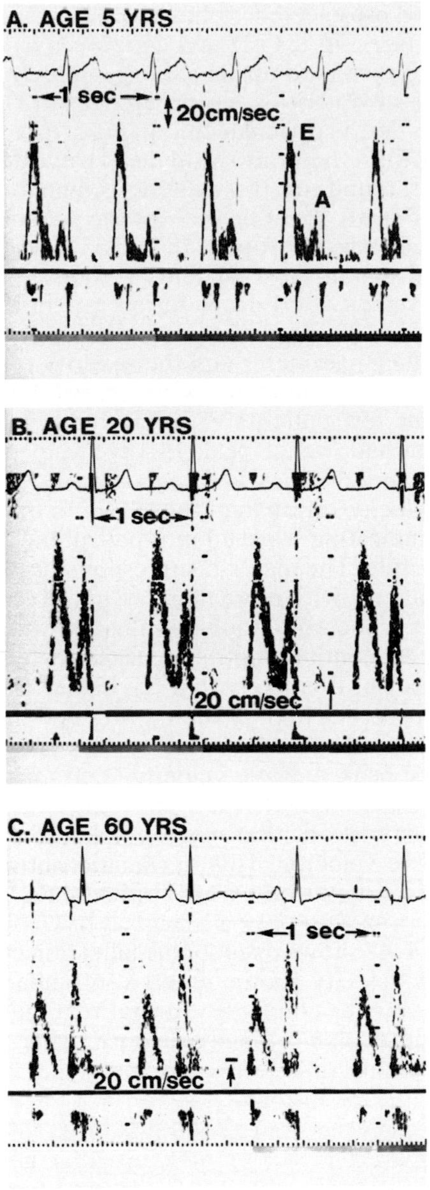

Fig. 24–46. Transmitral flow velocity profiles in normal subjects of different ages showing the dramatic effects of normal aging on these profiles. **A.** Age 5 years. **B.** Age 20 years. **C.** Age 60 years. Characteristically, as age increases, the peak velocity of the E wave decreases, the peak velocity of the A wave increases, the ratio of the peak E-wave to peak A-wave velocities decreases, and atrial contribution to total ventricular filling (A wave velocity-time integral/total velocity-time integral ratio) increases. Note that a wide scatter of normal values occurs in each of various age ranges, so that the patterns shown here are meant to illustrate the classic changes and not to represent strictly normal shapes for the different age groups. The y axes of the panels are not identical.

Studies in Fetuses and Neonates

The examination of fetal intracardiac blood flow is in its infancy and is an area with great potential for research and clinical applications. Recent studies have indicated that in the fetus, the peak velocity of the A wave is consistently higher than that of the E wave,[156] a finding that has been attributed to decreased left ventricular compliance.[157] As gestation proceeds, the peak E-wave velocity does not change, while the peak A-wave velocity decreases, so that the ratio of the peak E-wave to peak A-wave velocities increases significantly although the A wave remains dominant.[158]

The peak E-wave/peak A-wave velocity ratio increases from the in utero to the neonatal period because of proportionately greater increases in the peak E-wave velocity than the peak A-wave velocity.[159] These changes have been attributed to a postnatal increase in left atrial pressure that is due to an increase in pulmonary venous flow, with or without an accompanying increase in left ventricular compliance. These changes in the transmitral flow velocity profile after birth contrast with the absence of significant changes in the transtricuspid flow velocity profile. Neonates have reduced peak E-wave/peak A-wave velocity ratios for transtricuspid flow, which may reflect reduced right ventricular compliance as a result of intrauterine dominance.[160] No significant difference was found in transmitral flow velocities between preterm and full-term neonates, but transtricuspid velocities were slightly lower in the preterm neonates.[161]

Other Physiologic Parameters

No effect of body surface area (range, 1.40 to 2.14 m^2) or gender was found on Doppler transmitral flow velocity measurements in 66 normal subjects (28 men, 38 women, ages from 21 to 78 years).[107] A thorough study in which potentially confounding physiologic factors have been well controlled has not been reported.

MEASUREMENTS OF LEFT VENTRICULAR FILLING IN PATHOLOGIC STATES BY DOPPLER ECHOCARDIOGRAPHY

Abnormalities in the Doppler transmitral flow velocity profile have been described in many cardiac diseases. These abnormalities are generally interpreted as representing abnormalities in diastolic function, and in the majority of situations, this is probably correct when the conclusions are applied to the patient group as a whole. Left atrial pressure is increased in most cardiac diseases, and except in a few instances, cannot be held responsible for the abnormal filling patterns observed. In fact, the elevated left atrial pressures may mask or cause an underestimation of underlying diastolic abnormalities.

In individual patients, variations in left atrial pressure and other factors such as left atrial compliance modulate the transmitral flow velocity and distort the relation between the degree of Doppler abnormality and the severity of diastolic functional abnormality. The "physiologic" influences of age and heart rate are important and must be considered carefully. Systolic blood pressure may also play a role. Patients are often studied on cardiovascular medications, which may alter the Doppler velocity profile independently of alterations in diastolic function. Most studies demonstrate considerable scatter of individual Doppler echocardiographic data in normal controls as well as study patients, with substantial overlap between the two groups. This scatter and overlap reflect random variation in the many factors involved in determining the transmitral flow profile and not just variation in the severity of the underlying diastolic abnormality. Minor discrepancies in results are not uncommon among studies and often reflect differences in methodology, severity of the disease, and sometimes the small numbers of patients studied. These points should be borne in mind when considering the many abnormalities of transmitral flow described in diseased states, summarized in the following pages.

Pressure Load Left Ventricular Hypertrophy

Children with mild systemic hypertension may have an abnormal pattern of left ventricular filling by Doppler echocardiography even in the absence of ventricular hypertrophy or abnormal peak rates of increase in ventricular dimension by M-mode echocardiography.[162] Increased peak velocity and velocity time integral of the A wave and proportion of the total velocity-time integral occupied by the A wave in these patients reflect a shift of ventricular filling to the atrial contraction phase. The proportion of velocity-time integral occurring during the first third of diastole is correspondingly reduced. However, there was no statistical change in the peak velocity or velocity-time integral of the E wave or in the peak E-wave/peak A-wave velocity ratio. Another study has found abnormal left ventricular filling in 22% of subjects with untreated early essential hypertension, which predated the development of detectable left ventricular hypertrophy. These abnormal filling changes could be related to supine systolic blood pressure and age.[163]

In a study of healthy normotensive adolescents, diastolic blood pressure correlated negatively with the peak velocity, velocity-time integral, and deceleration rate of the E wave and the ratio of the peak E-wave to the peak A-wave velocities.[164] Diastolic blood pressure did not correlate with echocardiographic left ventricular mass, while systolic blood pressure correlated with left ventricular mass but not with any of the Doppler parameters. The explanation for these results remains unclear. Although the authors postulated a possible prehypertensive state in the children with higher diastolic blood pressures, physiologic variations in loading conditions may have been responsible for the observed Doppler correlations. The same authors have also found, in young normotensive men with a family history of hypertension, a shift in the transmitral flow pattern toward that found in hypertensive patients.[165]

In adults with hypertension, the peak E-wave velocity is reduced, and this is accompanied by reduced mitral leaflet excursion in early diastole on M-mode echocardiography.[166] The peak A-wave velocity is increased and the ratio of peak E-wave/peak A-wave velocities is reduced. Others have also found a reduced ratio of the peak E-wave velocity to the peak A-wave velocity in patients with mild-to-moderate hypertension but no statistical difference in the peak velocity, deceleration rate, and time to peak velocity of the E wave or peak velocity of the A wave.[167] An increased atrial filling fraction has been described.[106]

More obvious Doppler abnormalities are found when patients are preselected to have actual ventricular hypertrophy (see Fig. 24–21 and 24–22). In a study of 49 patients with isolated aortic stenosis distributed over a wide range of severities, no differences in Doppler parameters of left ventricular filling (peak E-wave and A-wave velocities, their ratios and the E-wave deceleration rate) were found in the patients compared to age-matched controls.[168] In the 67% of the patients who had left ventricular hypertrophy, the peak A-wave velocity was higher than in those patients without hypertrophy. The peak velocity and deceleration rate of the E wave did not differ. There was no correlation between any Doppler filling parameter and the severity of aortic stenosis assessed by valve area or pressure gradient. Interestingly, the few patients with left ventricular systolic dysfunction had higher peak E-wave velocities, lower peak A-wave velocities and higher peak E-wave/peak A-wave velocity ratios than those with normal systolic function, indicating a pseudonormalization of the flow velocity profile. The mechanism responsible was not examined. Patients with more than 1+ mitral regurgitation by Doppler echocardiographic evaluation were not studied so that concomitant mitral regurgitation was unlikely to be the cause. It is likely that the higher end-diastolic pressures observed in the patients with systolic dysfunction increased resistance to left atrial contraction and reduced the peak A-wave velocity. Left atrial pressure was not measured, but if it were higher in those with systolic dysfunction, that would explain the increased peak E-wave velocity. This explanation of pseudonormalization is supported by experimental findings in animals.[169]

Figure 24–47 shows pseudonormalization of the transmitral flow velocity profile in left ventricular hypertrophy that is due to concurrent mitral regurgitation. The flow velocity profile is taken from an 82-year-old patient with severe concentric left ventricular hypertrophy, nor-

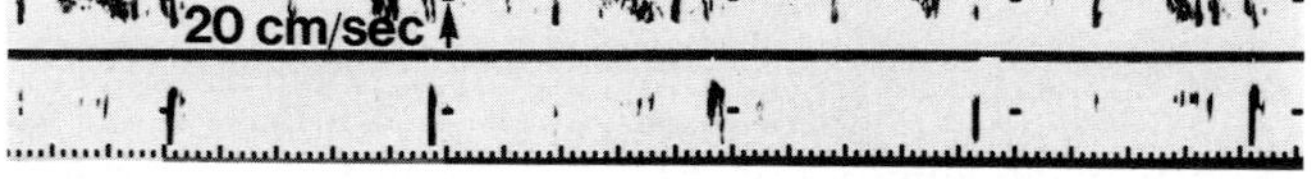

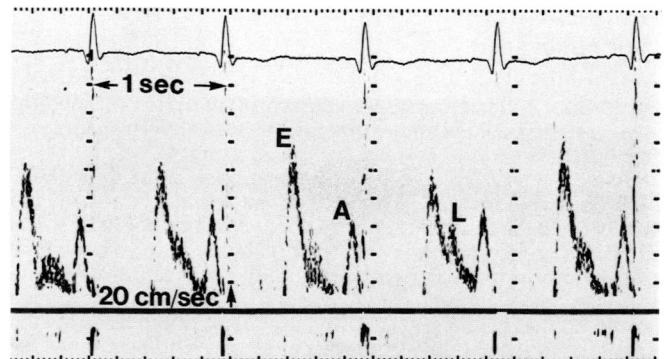

Fig. 24–47. Transmitral flow velocity profiles taken from an 82-year-old patient with severe concentric left ventricular hypertrophy, normal systolic function, and mitral regurgitation of moderate severity. Despite advanced age and marked ventricular hypertrophy, the peak E-wave (E) velocity is relatively high, and the peak E-wave velocity/peak A-wave (A) velocity ratio is substantially above 1. In this patient, the mechanism for this apparent discrepancy or pseudonormalization is, at least partly, an elevation of the left atrial V-wave pressure caused by mitral regurgitation. The effects of this pressure change on the flow velocity profile have been discussed previously. Note that a diastolic L wave (L) is also seen, which may be related to increased ventricular chamber stiffness (see the section on diastasis in the text).

mal left ventricular systolic function, and mitral regurgitation of moderate severity. Despite advanced age and severe ventricular hypertrophy, the peak E-wave velocity is relatively high, and the E-wave/A-wave peak velocity ratio is substantially above 1. In this patient, the likely explanation is an elevation of the left atrial V wave pressure by mitral regurgitation, which raises the atrial pressure at mitral valve opening. The effects of such a change in filling pressure have been discussed previously.

In 24 patients with left ventricular hypertrophy, including 6 with hypertrophic cardiomyopathy, the peak volumetric filling rate derived from Doppler echocardiographic measurements was lower than in normal subjects. This difference in the peak flow rate was detectable even when M-mode echocardiographic measurements of the peak rate of increase in ventricular dimension (with or without normalization to instantaneous dimension) did not differ.[112] The rapid filling index (ratio of the peak E-wave velocity to the mean velocity), the ratio of the peak E-wave velocity to peak A-wave velocity, the ratio of the E-wave velocity-time integral to the A-wave velocity-time integral were all significantly lower, and the peak A-wave filling rate was higher in the hypertrophy group compared to the control group. There was no demonstrable relationship between left ventricular mass and any of the Doppler parameters. There was also no correlation between the peak rate of increase in left ventricular dimension by M-mode echocardiography and the peak filling rate, probably for the reasons discussed previously in the M-mode echocardiography section of this chapter. Normalized measurements (to instantaneous dimension and end-diastolic volume, respectively), however, correlated poorly but significantly ($r = .56$, $p < .001$).

Elderly patients with isolated systolic hypertension have a higher prevalence of left ventricular hypertrophy and abnormal left ventricular filling pattern (higher peak A velocity and lower peak E-wave to A-wave velocity ratio) than age-matched controls.[170] There are some elderly patients, predominantly female and black, who have marked concentric left ventricular hypertrophy grossly out of proportion to any degree of hypertension present. This condition has been termed *hypertensive hypertrophic cardiomyopathy of the elderly* and has a pathophysiology similar to that found in hypertrophic cardiomyopathy. Patients with this condition have been reported to have a significantly higher peak A-wave velocity and lower peak E-wave/peak A-wave velocity ratio compared to normal age-matched controls.[171] The peak E-wave velocity was not different despite the presence of marked ventricular hypertrophy. Some of the patients also had elevated left ventricular outflow tract flow velocities indicating elevated intraventricular pressure gradients. Obesity, even when unassociated with hypertension, may produce eccentric left ventricular hypertrophy and exhibit an abnormal left ventricular filling pattern similar to that seen in pressure load concentric hypertrophy.[172,173]

The Doppler abnormalities seen in patients with hypertrophy have been related to indices of ventricular chamber architecture. In a heterogenous group of patients with left ventricular hypertrophy or dilated cardiomyopathy, the peak E-wave velocity, the ratio of the peak E-wave velocity to A-wave velocity and the atrial filling fraction correlated moderately with the radius/wall thickness ratio of the ventricle ($r = .63$, $r = .75$, and $r = .63$), but not with age.[151] This contrasted with the findings in the normal controls, where the same Doppler parameters correlated highly with age ($r = -.91$, $r = .82$, and $r = .81$) but not with the radius/wall thickness ratio. In a small study of patients with left ventricular hypertrophy that was due to aortic stenosis or dilated cardiomyopathy, the peak E-wave velocity was similar in both groups and in normal controls, but the peak A-wave velocity was much higher in the aortic stenosis group than in the dilated cardiomyopathy and normal groups.[56] The peak A velocity in the patients and normal subjects correlated well with left ventricular architecture represented by the ventricular mass/volume ratio but not with left ventricular mass or volume.

Changes in transmitral blood flow after balloon valvuloplasty for aortic stenosis have been reported. Immediately after the procedure, diastolic filling dynamics are unchanged, but at 24 hours, there is an increase in the peak E velocity and peak E-wave/A-wave velocity ratio with further increases at 3 to 6 months. These increases were not seen in patients who also had mitral regurgitation, presumably because a decrease in mitral regurgitation secondary to left ventricular afterload reduction may have masked the changes that were due directly to afterload reduction and regression of ventricular hypertrophy.[174]

The relative contribution of various factors involved in producing the abnormal Doppler flow velocity pattern in left ventricular hypertrophy—namely, increased ventricular chamber stiffness, decreased relaxation rate, and increased afterload—is largely unexplored and remains an interesting area for research.

Hypertrophic Cardiomyopathy

Patients with hypertrophic cardiomyopathy have a varied range of transmitral flow velocity profiles. In one study, patients with systolic anterior motion of the mitral valve had flow velocity profiles similar to those in normal subjects. However, patients without systolic anterior motion tended to have lower peak E-wave velocities, higher peak A-wave velocities, lower peak E-wave/A-wave velocity ratios and lower E-wave deceleration rates, reflecting impaired diastolic function.[175] A plausible explanation is that in patients with systolic anterior motion of the mitral valve, mitral regurgitation and elevated left atrial pressure—with which this echocardiographic abnormality is associated—mask any abnormal filling pattern. Other workers have also found no abnormality in the ratio of the peak E-wave/peak A-wave velocities in those patients with hypertrophic cardiomyopathy who have systolic anterior motion of the mitral valve. However, when only the patients without mitral regurgitation were examined, the peak E-wave/peak A-wave velocity ratio was significantly reduced (0.99 ± 0.52 vs. 1.47 ± 0.40, $p < .01$).[176]

In a large study of 111 patients with hypertrophic cardiomyopathy, the time from aortic closure to onset of transmitral flow (isovolumic relaxation period) and the time from onset of transmitral flow to the peak E-wave velocity were longer, the peak E-wave velocity and the ratio of peak E-wave/peak A-wave velocity were lower, and the peak A-wave velocity was higher compared to 86 normal controls.[177] The great majority of the patients (82%) had at least one abnormal Doppler parameter of diastolic function listed previously, with normal ranges defined by the 95% confidence limits of normal controls of similar age. Abnormal diastolic parameters occurred with similar frequency in those patients with or without left ventricular outflow tract obstruction (defined by catheterization or by M-mode echocardiographic evidence of systolic anterior motion of the mitral leaflets) and also in those with or without symptoms. Patients without obstruction, however, had more marked changes in Doppler parameters than those with obstruction, supporting the results of the other studies. Others have also found no relationship between Doppler indices of left ventricular filling and symptoms.[178]

As discussed earlier in this chapter, the transmitral flow velocity profile is determined in a complex manner by multiple factors, so that the characteristics of the profile do not necessarily reflect only the diastolic properties of the ventricle. Figure 24–48 shows an intriguing example of a boy with severe familial hypertrophic cardiomyopathy. Despite the presence of marked asymmetric left ventricular hypertrophy and the absence of mitral regurgitation, the transmitral flow velocity profile remains normal. Considering the markedly abnormal morphologic appearance of the left ventricle, it is very likely that gross abnormalities of diastolic function are present. The reason for the discrepancy between the Doppler and two-dimensional echocardiographic findings is unclear. It is probably related to the presence of a very high left ventricular end-diastolic pressure coupled with a high filling pressure, producing a pseudonormalization pattern. This example highlights the great caution one must adopt when using Doppler indices of diastolic function to predict diastolic function in individual patients.

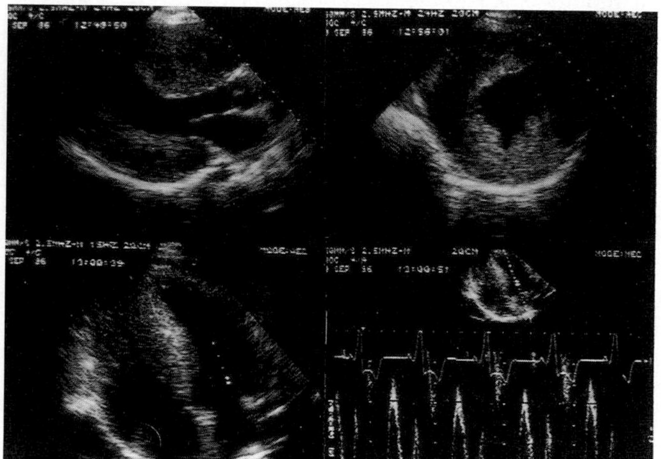

Fig. 24–48. A transmitral flow velocity profile of a boy with severe familial hypertrophic cardiomyopathy. Despite the presence of marked asymmetric left ventricular hypertrophy and the absence of mitral regurgitation, the velocity profile intriguingly remains normal. It is highly likely that significant abnormalities of diastolic function are present, judging from the gross morphologic abnormalities seen in the left ventricle. The explanation of this apparent discrepancy in the Doppler echocardiographic findings is speculative. Probably, a very high left ventricular end-diastolic pressure (increased resistance to atrial contraction) has suppressed the peak A-wave velocity, and a high left atrial pressure has increased the peak E-wave velocity, resembling the situation reported in some cases of restrictive physiology. This example highlights the great caution one must adopt when using Doppler indices of diastolic function to predict actual diastolic function in an individual patient.

Physiologic Hypertrophy

The concept of *physiologic hypertrophy* has been proposed to represent the ventricular hypertrophy that occurs in athletes. Physiologic hypertrophy allegedly does not produce the same pathophysiologic consequences as pathologic hypertrophy. In a study of normal subjects and cyclists with left ventricular hypertrophy, there was no difference in the peak E-wave and peak A-wave velocities or ratio of peak E-wave to peak A-wave velocities between normal controls and cyclists. The peak E-wave/A-wave velocity ratio was not related to left ventricular internal dimension, wall thickness, or mass, but by multiple regression analysis, it was significantly and independently related to age, systolic blood pressure, and heart rate. The multiple r value of .82 implied that 68% of the variance in the velocity ratio could be attributed to a combination of the three factors.[179]

Twenty-six intensively trained triathletes were found to have similar left ventricular systolic and diastolic dimensions compared to normal sedentary subjects, but they had increased left ventricular wall thickness, thickness/chamber radius ratio and myocardial mass.[180] Of interest, left ventricular mass correlated well with mean exercise blood pressure during an 8-hour exercise test performed by 14 of the athletes. Digitized M-mode echocardiographic measurements showed no differences between athletes and controls in the peak rates of cavity enlargement and wall thinning, while Doppler echocardiographic measurements demonstrated no difference in the peak E-wave velocity and a slightly higher peak E-wave/peak A-wave velocity ratio in the athletes.

A study of competitive weight lifters revealed significantly higher end-diastolic left ventricular volumes, dimensions, and posterior wall thicknesses compared to normal control subjects. These differences were eliminated after correction for body surface area.[181] The weight lifters, however, had higher left ventricular mass and mass index. There was no difference between the weight lifters and controls in Doppler measurements of peak volumetric filling rate, peak volumetric filling rate normalized to end-diastolic volume, the peak E-wave/peak A-wave velocity ratio, the E-wave/A-wave velocity-time integral ratio, or the rapid filling index (ratio of peak velocity to mean velocity). The peak atrial rate, however, was slightly but significantly higher in the weight lifters. None of the Doppler parameters correlated with left ventricular mass index.

It has been suggested that the absence of marked changes in the transmitral flow velocity profile of athletes with ventricular hypertrophy implies a physiologic form of hypertrophy. The validity of this concept remains incompletely established. Of interest, the results of a small study suggested that athletes who took anabolic steroids had more abnormalities in the transmitral flow velocity profile than those who did not.[181] However, a subsequent larger study of 23 weight lifters (of whom 12 were using anabolic steroids) found no difference in left ventricular hypertrophy, transmitral flow velocities, and fractional shortening between those who did and did not use steroids.[182]

Coronary Artery Disease

Experimental Coronary Occlusion

Many studies have demonstrated changes in the transmitral flow velocity profile after experimental coronary occlusion. These findings most likely reflect changes in the diastolic properties of the ventricle. The underlying mechanisms are complex and probably relate to alterations in relaxation rate that are due to myocardial ischemia and asynchronous relaxation, as well as alterations in chamber stiffness characteristics resulting from myocardial ischemia, changes in ventricular volume, and alterations in coronary turgor.

In an early report, the peak E-wave velocity, ratio of the peak E-wave to peak A-wave velocity, E-wave velocity-time integral, and E-wave deceleration rate decreased while the peak velocity and velocity-time integral of the A wave and the time to peak E-wave velocity increased after experimental coronary occlusion in dogs. These Doppler changes paralleled the worsening of diastolic function represented by the peak negative dP/dt, left ventricular end-diastolic pressure, and the time constant of isovolumic relaxation, T, but did not correlate well with them. The Doppler changes returned to baseline after the restoration of coronary flow.[183,184] The changes may occur early. For example, the peak E-wave/peak A-wave velocity ratio decreased within 5 minutes of left anterior descending artery occlusion in one study. The magnitude of the decrease, however, did not correlate well with the extent of infarction of the ventricle.[185] In dogs with infarcts involving more than 28% of the left ventricle, however, the E wave was totally abolished, and left ventricular filling occurred only with atrial contraction.

Studies of the effects of experimental coronary reperfusion are few. In a study that examined the early and late effects of a 2-hour period of coronary occlusion of the mid-left anterior descending artery in dogs followed by reperfusion, the peak E-wave/peak A-wave velocity ratio decreased, and the atrial filling fraction (ratio of A-wave velocity-time integral to total velocity-time integral) increased at 1 hour after coronary occlusion, remained abnormal 2 hours following reperfusion, and returned only partially to baseline values at 1 week after reperfusion.[186]

Chronic Coronary Artery Disease and Myocardial Infarction in Humans

In 34 patients with a history of typical angina that was due to obstructive coronary artery disease (documented as at least 70% diameter narrowing of at least one major coronary artery or a large branch) and normal global left ventricular function (left ventricular ejection fraction >50%), the peak E-wave velocity, ratio of peak E-wave/peak A-wave velocity, ratio of E-wave velocity-time integral to A-wave velocity-time integral, 0.33 velocity-time integral/total velocity-time integral and E velocity-time integral/total velocity-time integral were all lower than in age-matched control subjects.[187] Patients with and without segmental wall motion abnormalities did not differ in Doppler velocities and velocity-time integrals. Likewise, all Doppler measurements in those with single-vessel disease did not differ from those with multiple-vessel disease.

In another study, patients with anterior, inferior, and lateral myocardial infarction showed abnormal filling patterns of the left ventricle, with prolongation of the acceleration half-time and deceleration half-time of the E wave and with reduction in the ratio of the peak E-wave velocity/peak A-wave velocity.[188] Similar abnormalities in right ventricular filling were seen in those with myocardial infarction who had obstructive lesions in the right coronary artery. Patients with anterior infarction who had obstruction of the proximal left anterior descending artery involving the first septal perforator but patent right coronary artery also had a similar abnormal right ventricular filling pattern. Possibly, infarction of the interventricular septum altered right ventricular relaxation and compliance.

Patients with inferior infarction have been reported to have lower peak E-wave/peak A-wave velocity ratios of the transtricuspid flow velocity profile than patients with anterior infarcts, patients with angina but no left ventricular dyssynergy, and normal subjects.[189] The tricuspid E-wave deceleration time, normalized to the square root of the R-R interval, is also longer in the patients with inferior infarction. Further, the patients with inferior infarction who have right ventricular end-diastolic pressures of more than 8 mm Hg have peak E-wave/peak A-wave velocity ratios, which are lower than those with end-diastolic pressures of less than 8 mm Hg. This ratio is also lower in those with proximal right coronary artery occlusion than those with distal occlusion.

The clinical application of Doppler information in myocardial infarction remains uncertain. A preliminary report of 60 patients undergoing first myocardial infarction found a significant trend toward a higher Killip class with decreasing peak E-wave/peak A-wave velocity ratios.[190] Also, the patients with cardiogenic shock tended to have the lowest peak E-wave/peak A-wave velocity ratios. A more recent study, however, found a direct correlation between larger myocardial infarction size and higher peak E-wave velocity, lower peak A-wave velocity, and higher peak E-wave/A-wave velocity ratio, which is possibly due to elevated left ventricular end-diastolic pressure and left atrial pressure in those with large infarcts.[191] Much more information therefore is required before the Doppler transmitral flow velocity profile can be used as a reliable prognostic index in myocardial infarction.

Acute Myocardial Ischemia

In patients with coronary artery disease, myocardial ischemia produced by increasing myocardial oxygen demand, such as during exercise or atrial pacing, may theoretically produce different effects on diastolic function compared to ischemia produced by reducing myocardial oxygen supply, such as during acute coronary occlusion. The effects of exercise-induced ischemia are difficult to study with Doppler echocardiography because tachycardia produces a fusion of the E and A waves. Relatively little information is available on this topic, and a brief discussion is given later in this chapter in a section on exercise. Myocardial ischemia produced by atrial pacing in patients with coronary artery disease results in a reduction in the peak E-wave velocity and ratio of the peak E-wave/peak A-wave velocities immediately after cessation of pacing.[192] There is an increase in the relative contribution of atrial contraction to ventricular filling so that cardiac output may remain unchanged. The Doppler changes gradually return to baseline values, and recovery is complete 1 minute after the cessation of pacing.

The effects of coronary angioplasty-induced transient myocardial ischemia on the transmitral flow velocity profile in humans have been well described. One study included 17 angioplasties of the left anterior descending artery, 13 of the right coronary artery and 2 of the circumflex artery. The ratio of the peak E-wave velocity to peak A-wave velocity, the ratio of the peak E-wave velocity to the mean velocity, the ratio of the E-wave velocity-time integral to A-wave velocity-time integral and the first third filling fraction decreased within 15 seconds of coronary occlusion and preceded two-dimensional echocardiographic evidence of new systolic dysfunction, electrocardiographic changes, and chest pain. Diastolic and systolic abnormalities returned to baseline within 15 seconds of balloon deflation.[193]

Others workers similarly reported a reduction in the peak rapid filling rate and the ratio of the peak early to late filling rate 15 to 20 seconds after balloon inflation in the left anterior descending artery, which returned to baseline values 15 to 20 seconds after balloon deflation.[194] Unlike the previous study, however, these Doppler changes were not seen during angioplasty of the right coronary or left circumflex arteries. A reduction in the peak E-wave/A-wave velocity ratio has been reported as early as 8 seconds after balloon occlusion of the left anterior descending artery.[195] Other Doppler abnormalities that have been described during angioplasty include an increase in the proportion of ventricular filling that is due to atrial contraction and a prolongation of the time to the peak E-wave velocity normalized to the diastolic filling period.[196]

Improvement in the pattern of ventricular filling has been seen as early as 2 days after angioplasty for unstable angina and postinfarction ischemia.[197] The longer-term effects of coronary angioplasty have also been studied. No improvement in the transmitral flow velocity profile was detected 24 hours after successful coronary angioplasty compared to the measurements before angioplasty.[198] However, increases in the peak E-wave velocity and the ratio of the peak E-wave velocity to the peak A-wave velocity were found 2 days after successful coronary angioplasty compared to measurements before angioplasty, with further increases noted 9 days after angioplasty.[199] These changes in the transmitral flow velocity profile were greater in patients with more severe coronary stenoses before angioplasty and may reflect improvement in diastolic function in myocardial segments that were previously chronically ischemic.

Right Ventricular Pressure and Volume Overload

Patients with primary pulmonary hypertension have reduced ratios of peak E-wave to peak A-wave velocities compared to normal control subjects and have a markedly reduced percentage of the velocity-time integral occurring in the first half of diastole.[200] These changes are associated with prolongation of the left ventricular isovolumic relaxation time and abnormal flattening of the interventricular septum toward the left ventricle at end-systole, which persists during early diastolic filling and ends before end-diastole. The lower peak E-wave velocity in the patients and the abnormal redistribution of filling to late diastole may be due in part to low filling (left atrial) pressures as well as altered relaxation and increased stiffness of the left ventricular chamber brought about by the elevated right ventricular pressures and septal distortion. In right ventricular volume overload that is due to severe tricuspid regurgitation, maximal leftward ventricular septal shift occurs at end-diastole, and there is a reduction in atrial systolic contribution to ventricular filling but no influence on the left ventricular isovolumic relaxation time. Approximately 78% of left ventricular filling occurs in early diastole compared with 52% in patients with right ventricular pressure overload ($p < .001$).[201]

Dilated Cardiomyopathy

Patients with dilated cardiomyopathy have abnormal transmitral flow velocity profiles, which, however, may be masked by the presence of mitral regurgitation. In a study comparing 21 patients with dilated cardiomyopathy and mitral regurgitation against 12 patients with dilated cardiomyopathy without mitral regurgitation and 19 normal subjects, the peak E-wave velocity, peak A-wave velocity, and ratio of peak E-wave to peak A-wave velocities did not differ in the patients with mitral regurgitation compared to the normal subjects. The deceleration half-time of the E wave, however, was shorter in these patients. In contrast, the peak velocity of the E wave and the ratio of the peak E-wave velocity to peak A-wave velocity were lower in the patients without mitral regurgitation compared to normal subjects and to the patients with mitral regurgitation. The peak velocity of the A wave and E-wave deceleration half-time in the patients without mitral regurgitation did not differ from normal.[202] Other workers have found a reduced peak E-wave velocity and an unaltered peak A-wave velocity in patients with dilated cardiomyopathy. The peak E-wave/peak A-wave velocity ratio was slightly but not significantly reduced.[203]

It is not surprising that the transmitral flow velocity profile in this condition is very heterogeneous. In the individual patient, the flow velocity profile theoretically will depend on the degree of impairment of ventricular relaxation and chamber stiffness, on left atrial pressure (which varies with many factors including the severity of left ventricular impairment, blood volume, therapy, and the severity of mitral regurgitation); on the degree of atrial involvement in the disease process; on the left ventricular end-systolic volume; and on the left ventricular end-diastolic pressure (which acts as an impediment to atrial contraction). A recent study has found that, in practice, the pattern of left ventricular filling in patients with dilated cardiomyopathy is determined largely by left atrial pressure and by the severity of mitral regurgitation. Filling indices correlated better with functional class than did indices of left ventricular systolic function.[204] In patients with dilated cardiomyopathy who had similarly elevated left ventricular volumes and impaired systolic fractional shortening, those with an increase in left ventricular filling pressure had higher peak E-wave velocity and higher ratio of E-wave to total velocity-time integrals than patients with normal filling pressures and normal subjects. The presence of mitral regurgitation in each patient group increased peak E-wave velocity further without significantly altering the distribution of the flow velocity-time integral during diastole.[205] Figure 24–49 shows a striking example of an abnormal transmitral flow velocity profile of a patient with dilated cardiomyopathy. The mitral leaflet opening artifact can be seen to occur relatively late, just before the onset of the P wave, so that the E wave is practically nonexistent. The A wave is large and contributes almost totally to ventricular filling.

Insulin-dependent diabetics with no clinical evidence of heart disease may have abnormal Doppler transmitral flow patterns compared to age- and sex-matched controls.[206,207] In one study, the peak E-wave velocity and ratio of the peak E-wave to peak A-wave velocities were decreased, and the peak A-wave velocity and atrial contribution to total ventricular filling were increased in diabetic patients.[206] These filling abnormalities did not correlate with the duration of diabetes or presence of retinopathy, nephropathy, and peripheral neuropathy. Using the 95% confidence limits of the distribution of normal control values as normal limits, 6 of the 21 patients (29%) had at least two abnormal Doppler parameters.

A recent report suggests that Doppler measurements of transmitral flow velocities may aid in the diagnosis of acute cardiac rejection after cardiac transplantation.[208] In a group of 25 patients with rejection based on histopathologic evidence, the left ventricular isovolumic relaxation time and pressure half-time of the transmitral E wave decreased during rejection compared to before rejection. The peak velocity of the E wave and two-dimensional echocardiographic measurements of left ventricular systolic function did not change. These abnormalities returned to baseline values after immunosuppressive therapy. A group of 30 transplant patients without histologic evidence of rejection did not demonstrate these abnormalities. With a 20% decrease in the half-time of the E wave used as the diagnostic criterion for rejection, the sensitivity, specificity, and predictive value in this early series were 88%, 87%, and 85%, respectively.

Other workers have found reductions in the isovolumic relaxation period and pressure half-times of the mitral and tricuspid E waves in transplant patients who had hemodynamic evidence of restriction-constriction.[209] These patients also had significantly higher peak E-wave velocities of the mitral and tricuspid valves and lower mean aortic flow velocities and acceleration rates. These findings were associated with a higher incidence of graft rejection. The abrupt increases in early ventricular diastolic pressures seen with restrictive-constrictive physiology may have been responsible for the shortened Doppler pressure half-times, and increased atrial pressures may have shortened the isovolumic relaxation period and increased the peak E-wave velocities.

Pericardial Tamponade

The two-dimensional echocardiographic features of pericardial tamponade are described elsewhere in this book (Chapter 35). Doppler features of tamponade may

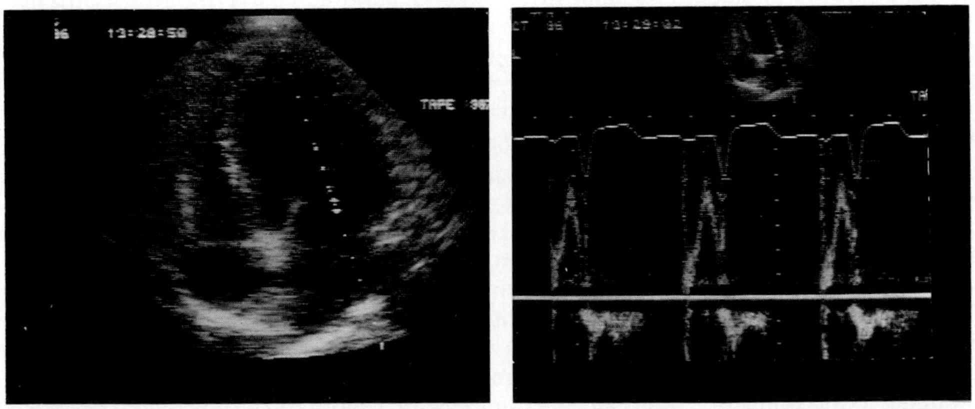

Fig. 24–49. A striking example of a grossly abnormal transmitral flow velocity profile of a patient with dilated cardiomyopathy. The vertical line representing the mitral leaflet opening artifact may be seen. This event occurs very late in diastole and just precedes the P wave on the electrocardiogram. The E wave is practically nonexistent while the A wave is large and contributes almost entirely to ventricular filling. A variety of transmitral flow profiles may be seen in dilated cardiomyopathy (see text).

help provide useful complementary information for the diagnosis of this condition. It is important to remember that the process of tamponade should be considered as a continuum and not an all-or-none phenomenon.

In experimental pericardial tamponade produced in closed chest spontaneously breathing dogs, markedly exaggerated increases in transtricuspid flow velocity and decreases in transmitral flow velocity are seen during inspiration, compared to the much smaller changes seen in pericardial effusion without tamponade and in normal control subjects.[210] The same preliminary report included three patients with tamponade, in whom transtricuspid flow velocity increased by 100%, and transmitral flow velocity decreased by 42% during inspiration. These flow abnormalities disappeared after pericardiocentesis.

In a larger study involving 11 patients with pericardial tamponade, exaggerated changes were found in the flow velocity-time integrals across all four valves during inspiration.[211] The tricuspid and pulmonary velocity-time integrals increased by 80 and 96%, respectively, during inspiration compared to expiration, and the mitral and aortic velocity-time integrals decreased by 35 and 33%, respectively. In normal controls, on the other hand, directionally similar changes were found, but their magnitudes were much smaller (+5%, +9%, −8%, −3%, respectively). The abnormal respiratory changes in the flow velocity-time integrals were markedly reduced after pericardiocentesis.

Similar results have been reported by others. In seven patients with severe pericardial tamponade requiring emergency pericardiocentesis, respiratory variations in transvalvular flow velocities, left ventricular ejection times, and isovolumic relaxation time were markedly increased compared to measurements made after pericardiocentesis and in normal subjects.[212] During inspiration, the left ventricular isovolumic relaxation time increased by 85%, the transmitral peak E-wave velocity decreased by 43%, and the transmitral peak A-wave velocity decreased by 25% compared with values at expiration. The corresponding respiratory variations after pericardiocentesis and in normal subjects were less than 10%. Also, during inspiration in the tamponade group, the transtricuspid peak E-wave velocity increased by 85%, and the transtricuspid peak A velocity increased by 58%, compared to corresponding changes of less than 25% after pericardiocentesis and in normal subjects. Changes in velocity-time integrals generally paralleled those in peak velocity. Other Doppler abnormalities in the tamponade group included exaggerated inspiratory decreases in left ventricular ejection time and peak transaortic flow velocity and an exaggerated increase in the peak transpulmonary flow velocity.[212] In 14 patients with pericardial effusion without marked hemodynamic compromise, seven had respiratory variations in Doppler measurements that were generally intermediate between the tamponade group and normal subjects, while the remaining seven had results similar to those in the normal subjects. These Doppler observations provide useful insights into the mechanisms of pulsus paradoxus seen in this condition.

Abnormal flow patterns were also seen in the superior vena cava and hepatic veins of patients with pericardial tamponade.[212] In normal subjects, on the one hand, venous flow was biphasic, with flow velocities in systole higher than in diastole during all phases of respiration. A small reversal of flow was usually seen during atrial contraction. On inspiration, systolic and diastolic flow velocities increased in most normal subjects, and at the onset of expiration, diastolic flow velocity did not decrease compared with apnea. In patients with tamponade, on the other hand, there was a marked predominance of systolic flow during apnea. With the first beat of inspiration, only minimal increases in systolic and diastolic flow velocities were seen that were less than the inspiratory increases found in normal subjects. On the first beat after the onset of expiration, all tamponade patients had a decrease or reversal of diastolic flow velocities and occasionally of systolic flow velocities compared to measurements during apnea, unlike the normal subjects. After pericardiocentesis, all patients showed increased forward flow velocities in the superior vena cava during apnea, and abnormal flow patterns with respiration generally improved or reverted to normal.

Studies of hemodynamic and Doppler correlations in tamponade have been reported using animal experiments and confirm that abnormal filling dynamics in tamponade result from altered relations between intracardiac and intrathoracic pressures during respiration.[213] More specifically, with an acute increase in pericardial pressure, left ventricular diastolic pressure changes less than left atrial pressure during respiration, and this leads to a transmitral pressure gradient that is smaller on inspiration and larger on expiration. Corresponding variations in transmitral flow velocity ensue. In a model of acute pericardial effusion, abnormal transmitral flow (increased respiratory variation of the peak E-wave velocity and of left ventricular isovolumic relaxation time) occurred as soon as pericardial pressure increased and persisted throughout all stages of increasing pericardial effusion.[213] The abnormal respiratory variation occurred before equalization of intracardiac pressures and before the onset of unequivocal right heart collapse. Importantly, the magnitude of the respiratory change did not predict pericardial pressure or the severity of hemodynamic compromise, raising potential limitations to its clinical applications. In another animal study, a quantitative relationship was found between increases in respiratory variations in peak aortic and pulmonary flow velocities and increases in intrapericardial pressure.[214]

Pericardial Constriction and Myocardial Restriction

The M-mode and two-dimensional echocardiographic features of pericardial constriction and myocardial restriction are relatively insensitive and nonspecific. A difficulty often encountered with studies in this area is the inexact distinction between patients with constrictive and those with restrictive physiology; not uncommonly, a combination of both conditions exist. There has been great interest in examining whether Doppler parameters of ventricular filling are able to aid in making these diagnoses. Very important preliminary work has been performed, but only relatively small numbers of patients have been studied. These early results must be confirmed by larger prospective studies before the Doppler technique can be used confidently to predict or exclude constrictive and restrictive physiology in individual patients.

In a study of 14 patients with "restrictive" physiology (7 of whom also had pericardial thickening on echocardiography), transmitral and transtricuspid flow velocity patterns were found to differ from those in normal control subjects.[215] The deceleration times of the E waves across the mitral and tricuspid valves were shortened, reflecting abrupt cessation of filling of both ventricles. These Doppler abnormalities corresponded to the diastolic dip and plateau contour of the ventricular pressure tracings. Abnormal reversals of flow in the hepatic vein and superior vena cava during inspiration and diastolic mitral and tricuspid regurgitation were also observed.

The differentiation between the Doppler features of pericardial constriction and myocardial restriction remains under investigation. An important study has found that differences in the response of the mitral and tricuspid flow velocity profiles to respiration may be helpful in separating these two conditions. In a report of 7 patients with pericardial constriction, 12 with myocardial restriction, and 20 normal control subjects, the isovolumic relaxation time, and the peak E-wave and A-wave velocities across the mitral and tricuspid valves in the patients with constriction did not differ from controls during apnea.[216] The mitral and tricuspid E-wave deceleration times tended to be lower, but the differences were not statistically significant. In the patients with restriction, the mitral and tricuspid peak A-wave velocities were lower, and the E-wave deceleration times were markedly shorter during apnea than in the normal controls. However, no parameter differed significantly between patients with restriction and constriction.

An observation of potential practical importance was that in the patients with restrictive cardiomyopathy and the normal controls, changes in the isovolumic relaxation time and the peak E-wave velocity with respiration were very small (mean changes less than 5%), while in the patients with constrictive physiology, marked changes with respiration were found. In those patients, the isovolumic relaxation time increased by 50%, and the mitral peak E-wave velocity decreased by 33% from expiration to inspiration. The peak E- and A-wave velocities across the tricuspid valve increased from expiration to inspiration in all three patient groups, but the increase was much larger in those with constriction. This increase occurred because of a marked decrease in flow velocities during expiration in the patients with constriction. In these patients, the largest changes in E- and A-wave peak velocities occurred on the first beat after the onset of expiration or inspiration, and the changes were directionally opposite in the mitral and tricuspid valves. These abnormal respiratory variations in flow velocities were abolished after pericardiectomy.

Another preliminary report by the same authors suggested that in patients with restriction, diastolic forward flow in the superior vena cava and hepatic vein during apnea was greater than systolic forward flow. On the other hand, in patients with constriction, diastolic forward flow during apnea was either equal to or less than systolic forward flow.[217] Patients with restriction had an abnormal decrease in systolic forward flow with or without increased flow reversal on the first or second inspiratory beat, while patients with constriction had a normal increase in systolic and diastolic forward flow and a decrease in flow reversal on the first inspiratory beat. The second inspiratory beat, however, was abnormal in the patients with constriction, with a decrease in systolic or diastolic flow, or with increased flow reversal. During expiration, patients with restriction had flow velocity patterns similar to those during apnea, while patients with constriction had a marked decrease in diastolic forward flow compared to apnea. These very interesting and complex Doppler observations reflect the intricate interplay between extrathoracic, intrathoracic, intrapericardial, and intracardiac pressures seen during different phases of respiration in patients with pericardial constriction and myocardial restriction. Classic patterns have been described; their reliability and clinical applicability depend on the documentation of sensitivity and specificity information from larger studies.

A further level of complexity may arise from the nature of the disease process itself. Patients with primary systemic amyloidosis have recently been shown to have a spectrum of abnormal left ventricular filling patterns, which could be related to the degree of left ventricular hypertrophy and hence the extent of cardiac involvement by the disease process.[218] In the patients with mild-to-moderate hypertrophy (left ventricular wall thickness >12 mm but <15 mm) representing early involvement, the isovolumic relaxation time was prolonged, the peak E-wave velocity was decreased, the peak A velocity was increased, and the peak E-wave to peak A-wave velocity ratio was decreased compared to data in normal control subjects, findings similar to those seen in patients with secondary left ventricular hypertrophy or hypertrophic cardiomyopathy. The E-wave deceleration time was unaltered. The patients with wall thicknesses of ≤12 mm had similar abnormal findings. Such Doppler changes have also been reported in patients with familial amyloid polyneuropathy and either mild or no left ventricular hypertrophy.[219] A key observation in the former study[218] was that the group of patients with left ventricular wall thicknesses of >15 mm representing advanced involvement had markedly shortened E-wave deceleration times and slightly but not significantly higher peak E-wave velocities compared to the normal controls, changes that the authors attributed to restrictive pathophysiology. The isovolumic relaxation time, peak A-wave velocity, and peak E-wave to peak A-wave velocity ratio did not differ from control measurements. Measurements of pulmonary venous flow demonstrated markedly decreased peak systolic and increased peak diastolic venous flow velocities in the patients with advanced disease. This "restrictive" pattern was shown later to confer poor prognosis, with a 1-year survival of 49% in those with a restrictive pattern (E-wave deceleration time ≤150 msec) compared to 92% in those without.[220]

Evaluation of Pacemaker Hemodynamics

Although not strictly concerned with evaluating diastolic function, the Doppler echocardiographic examination of left ventricular filling in patients with pacemakers has a potentially valuable role in assessing hemodynamic status. Differences in forward stroke volume between ventricular (VVI) pacing and atrioventricular sequential (DDD) pacing modes may be measured relatively easily and may be used to identify those patients who benefit more from dual-chamber pacing.[221–223] This technique may also be used to optimize pacemaker settings such as the atrioventricular interval, particularly in those individuals who depend most on this adjustment.[222,223]

Evaluation of the Transmitral Flow Velocity Profile During Exercise

Although exercise has been studied extensively for its ability to test the systolic functional reserve of the heart, its potential for evaluating diastolic functional reserve has not been fully explored. As with systolic dysfunction, symptoms that are due to diastolic dysfunction may occur during exercise before they become clearly expressed at rest. It is possible, therefore, that hemodynamic manifestations of diastolic dysfunction that are absent at rest may become revealed during exercise. Physiologic principles support this idea. Dynamic exercise, particularly when conducted in the upright rather than supine position, employs an increase in left ventricular end-diastolic volume as an important means to increase stroke volume via the Frank-Starling mechanism. This increase in diastolic volume raises diastolic pressure along the passive pressure-volume curve of the ventricular chamber. A less compliant ventricle has a steeper pressure-volume relation and so generates a greater rise in ventricular pressure for any given usage of preload reserve.

Unfortunately, an important limitation of the evaluation of the transmitral flow velocity profile during exercise is the fusion of the E and A waves when the heart rate exceeds 90 to 110 beats per minute. This phenomenon limits our ability to analyze transmitral flow velocity profiles reliably with present criteria.

An early study of 10 normal subjects demonstrated that the increase in stroke volume during bicycle exercise was produced by increases in the mean transmitral flow velocity and mitral annular area.[224] These changes occurred despite a reduction in the diastolic flow time/cycle length and a decrease in the transmitral velocity-time integral. The increase in transmitral flow velocities during exercise must be mediated by an increase in the left atrial-to-left ventricular pressure gradient. During normal supine bicycle exercise, this increase in the gradient has been shown to occur because of a decrease in the left ventricular minimal pressure, or nadir. This, in turn, is produced by an increase in ventricular relaxation rate and consequently a more complete state of relaxation when the minimal pressure occurs.[225] In this study, left atrial pressure did not increase significantly to contribute to the augmented pressure gradient. Other studies, however, have reported substantial increases in left ventricular filling pressures during normal supine and sitting exercise,[226] so that this may be additionally an important adaptive mechanism of ventricular filling to exercise.

In a study of 18 patients with coronary artery disease and normal resting left ventricular function, the peak E-wave/peak A-wave velocity-time integral ratio decreased by 34% during exercise compared to resting values. In 8 normal control subjects, by contrast, there was no change in this parameter.[227] This difference between study groups appeared to result mainly from a difference in the response to exercise of the duration of the A wave, which decreased in the normal group but did not change in the patients. The peak E-wave and peak A-wave velocities increased during exercise in both groups, and the increases did not differ between the two groups. In another study, patients with coronary artery disease and exercise-induced ischemia were compared to those with coronary artery disease without ischemia using Doppler measurements made at rest and immediately after exercise.[228] Peak E-wave and A-wave velocities increased from rest to postexercise in both the ischemic and nonischemic groups, but the ischemic groups demonstrated a greater increase in peak E velocity. The peak E-wave to peak A-wave velocity ratio increased slightly from rest to postexercise in the ischemic group but fell slightly in the nonischemic group. The authors suggested that an increase in left atrial pressure by ischemia resulted in pseudonormalization of the flow profile. This theory is supported by a separate study of patients with coronary artery disease before and immediately after bicycle exercise. Any increase in peak E-wave/peak A-wave velocity ratio immediately after exercise was associated with a marked increase in pulmonary artery wedge pressure at peak exercise. In those whose peak E-wave/peak A-wave velocity ratio fell, the pulmonary artery wedge pressure increased only very slightly.[229]

Some workers have used isometric (handgrip) exercise to study patients with previous myocardial infarction.[230] In normal control subjects during handgrip exercise, peak E-wave velocity did not change significantly, peak A velocity increased, and peak E-wave/peak A-wave velocity ratio decreased. In postinfarct patients with normal left ventricular end-diastolic pressures at rest, the end-diastolic pressure increased by 2 mm Hg from 11 to 13 mm Hg, the peak E-wave velocity fell, the peak A-wave velocity increased, and the peak E-wave/A-wave velocity ratio decreased. In postinfarct patients with elevated end-diastolic pressures at rest, by contrast, end-diastolic pressures increased more (by 7 mm Hg from 23 to 30 mm Hg), and peak E-wave velocity increased and peak A-wave fell, so that the peak E-wave/peak A-wave velocity ratio actually increased. This is another example of how changes in hemodynamic conditions may produce a pseudonormalization pattern unrelated to any change in diastolic function. Age may also exert a significant influence on the response of transmitral flow to isometric exercise in normal subjects.[231]

In one of the few reports available on the effects of exercise and drug therapy on the transmitral flow velocity profile, patients with hypertrophic cardiomyopathy and normal subjects were compared before and immediately after bicycle exercise.[232] The cardiomyopathy patients were restudied after 1 or 2 weeks' therapy with diltiazem. Heart rate in the patients and subjects were similar, and diltiazem did not affect heart rate at rest or after exercise. In the normal subjects, peak E-wave and peak A-wave velocities after exercise were substantially higher, and peak E-wave/peak A-wave velocity ratio and the E-wave pressure half-time were slightly lower compared to before exercise. At rest, the hypertrophic patients had lower peak E-wave velocity and peak E-wave/peak A-wave velocity ratio and higher E-wave pressure half-time than the normal subjects. After exercise, Doppler parameters in the patients changed in the same direction as in the normal subjects except for the E-wave pressure half-time, which did not change in the postexercise period. Diltiazem shifted these Doppler parameters toward normal values both at rest and during the post-exercise period. The authors discounted any increase in left atrial pressure by diltiazem as the explanation for the Doppler changes because this agent had been shown by others to reduce exercise-induced elevations in pulmonary artery pressure.[233] They therefore implicated an improvement in ventricular diastolic function.

SUMMARY

The study of left ventricular filling by Doppler echocardiography in health and disease remains an exciting area that continues to develop. Diastolic function is a multifaceted phenomenon that is complex and still poorly understood but nevertheless clinically important. Doppler echocardiography has a potentially valuable role in its evaluation and, arguably, is the best technique currently available for measuring the pattern of ventricular filling in humans.

It is important to remember that *diastolic filling* and *diastolic function* are not synonymous. Theoretical considerations and empirical observations dictate that the pattern of the transmitral flow velocity profile does indeed reflect the diastolic properties of the left ventricle. The simultaneous influence of loading conditions, however, is also well established, and these effects must be considered carefully in any interpretation of flow velocity profiles in diseased states or after interventions.

Many difficult problems must be resolved. The phenomenon of pseudonormalization of the velocity profile—whether occurring through an elevation of left atrial pressure (that is due to or independent of mitral regurgitation) or an elevation of left ventricular end-diastolic pressure, or both—is a critically important one that must be overcome. This problem is not related to the Doppler technique itself but to all measurements of ventricular filling in general. The reliability of any technique is seriously jeopardized when markedly abnormal pathophysiology can yield normal results. It is hoped that in the future, the simultaneous evaluation of pulmonary venous flow patterns may help to identify patients with this phenomenon.

Another difficult area is the lack of standardization of methodology for acquiring and analyzing the transmitral flow velocity profile. Its implementation would greatly aid the comparison of results between studies and would reduce confusion in this area. Comprehensive normal ranges derived from large numbers of subjects and stratified according to important physiologic and technical variables are surprisingly lacking. Whether specific Doppler parameters or combinations of parameters can be identified that are more sensitive or specific for diagnosing particular diastolic hemodynamic abnormalities remains to be determined. Success here would markedly improve the application of the technique as a diagnostic tool. The quantification of diastolic dysfunction rather than just its diagnosis is clearly preferable but remains elusive. Left ventricular filling patterns in atrial fibrillation and flutter remain largely unstudied, even though these arrhythmias are found in many patients with diastolic dysfunction. Characteristics of early left ventricular filling found in patients with sinus rhythm cannot be applied to those with atrial fibrillation or flutter, as demonstrated clearly in Figure 24–50. The difference

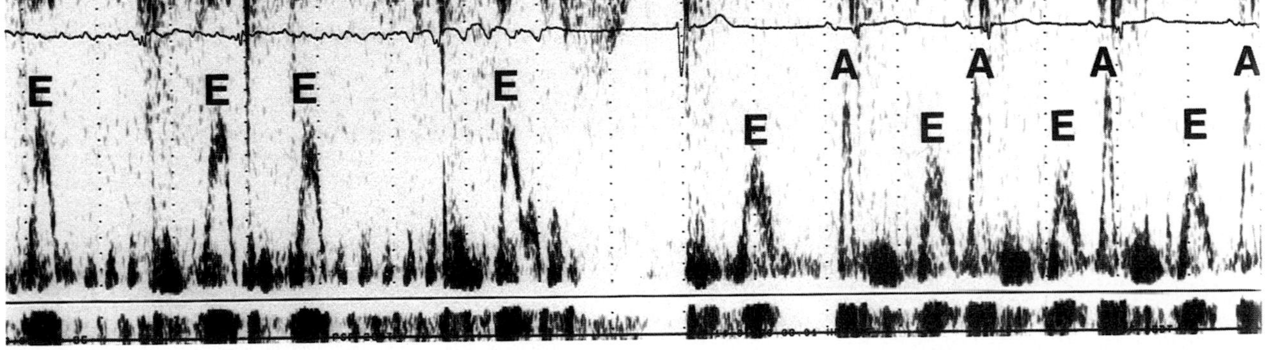

Fig. 24–50. Transmitral flow velocity profile of a patient with atrial flutter with spontaneous reversion to sinus rhythm. Note the change in the E wave although no change in left ventricular diastolic function has occurred. The most likely explanation is a reduction in left atrial pressure with the change in rhythm. A = A wave; E = E wave.

between the flow profiles is not simply the absence of the A wave in atrial fibrillation, because E wave changes also occur. The evaluation of filling patterns in these situations awaits further study.

By now, the enormous value of Doppler echocardiography as a research tool for measuring transmitral flow velocities has been clearly demonstrated. Through the application of this technique, our understanding of the complexities of left ventricular filling has advanced greatly from the simplistic notions of earlier years. Nevertheless, it is still appropriate now to caution against the natural tendency to oversimplify for clinical application what is essentially a very complex area. Differences in mean Doppler values between study groups have provided valuable information about differences in diastolic function between the groups and have offered new insights into the pathophysiologic mechanisms of many diseases. At the present time, however, the clinical role of Doppler echocardiography for evaluating diastolic function in *individuals* remains unestablished. The influence of factors unrelated to diastolic function cannot be weighed easily in any one person. Descriptions of "classic" transmitral flow profiles in specific pathophysiologic conditions do not justify their widespread and uncritical adoption for clinical diagnosis unless satisfactory data on sensitivity, specificity, and predictive accuracy are available.

Until more information is obtained, our present knowledge allows us to make these basic statements. In clinical practice, markedly abnormal transmitral flow profiles associated with reduced E-wave velocities and deceleration rates (with or without raised A-wave velocities) usually signify abnormal diastolic function *if* filling pressures are not low and systolic function is normal. Conversely, abnormally high E-wave velocities usually reflect abnormal elevations in left atrial pressure, while associated reductions in A-wave velocities usually indicate concomitant elevations in left ventricular end-diastolic pressure (regardless of whether the cause is systolic or diastolic dysfunction). Importantly, normal transmitral flow profiles can never be used to exclude diastolic dysfunction because of the potential for pseudonormalization to occur. At a clinical level, this limitation, more than any other, has hindered the widespread adoption of Doppler echocardiography for the routine evaluation of diastolic function. The discovery of a practical and reliable application of transmitral flow measurements for this purpose remains a major challenge in echocardiography.

REFERENCES

1. Dougherty AH, et al.: Congestive heart failure with normal systolic function. Am J Cardiol 54:778, 1984.
2. Topol EJ, Traill TA, Fortuin NJ: Hypertensive hypertrophic cardiomyopathy of the elderly. N Engl J Med 312:277, 1985.
3. Soufer R, et al.: Intact systolic left ventricular function in clinical congestive heart failure. Am J Cardiol 55:1032, 1985.
4. Mirsky I: Assessment of passive elastic stiffness of cardiac muscle: mathematical concepts, physiologic and clinical considerations, directions of future research. Prog Cardiovasc Dis 18:277, 1976.
5. Brutsaert DL, et al.: Analysis of relaxation in the evaluation of ventricular function of the heart. Prog Cardiovasc Dis 28:143, 1985.
6. Gaasch WH, Apstein CS, Levine HJ: Diastolic properties of the left ventricle. *In* Levine HJ, Gaasch WH (eds.): The Ventricle: Basic and Clinical Aspects. Boston, Martinus Nijhoff Publishing, p. 143, 1985.
7. Grossman W, Lorell BH (eds.): Diastolic Relaxation of the Heart. Boston, Martinus Nijhoff Publishing, 1988.
8. Gilbert JC, Glantz SA: Determinants of left ventricular filling and the diastolic pressure-volume relation. Circ Res 64:827, 1989.
9. Arora RR, et al.: Atrial kinetics and left ventricular diastolic filling in the healthy elderly. J Am Coll Cardiol 9:1255, 1987.
10. Braunwald E, Sonnenblick EH, Ross J Jr.: Mechanisms of cardiac contraction and relaxation. *In* Braunwald E (ed.): Heart Disease. Philadelphia, WB Saunders, p. 383, 1988.
11. Gamble WH, et al.: A critical appraisal of diastolic time intervals as a measure of relaxation in left ventricular hypertrophy. Circulation 68:76, 1983.
12. Weisfeldt ML, et al.: Hemodynamic determinants of maximum negative dP/dt and periods of diastole. Am J Physiol 227:613, 1974.
13. Weiss JL, Frederiksen JW, Weisfeldt ML: Hemodynamic determinants of the time-course of fall in canine left ventricular pressure. J Clin Invest 58: 751, 1976.
14. Raff GL, Glantz SA: Volume loading slows left ventricular isovolumic relaxation rate. Circ Res 48:813, 1981.
15. Weisfeldt ML, Frederiksen JW, Yin FCP, Weiss JL: Evidence of incomplete left ventricular relaxation in the dog. J Clin Invest 62:1296, 1978.
16. Carroll JD, Hess OM, Hirzel HO, Krayenbuehl HP: Exercise induced ischemia: the influence of altered relaxation on early diastolic pressures. Circulation 67:521, 1983.
17. Lorell BH, et al.: Modification of abnormal diastolic properties by nifedipine in patients with hypertrophic cardiomyopathy. Circulation 65:499, 1982.
18. Gaasch WH, et al.: Myocardial relaxation: II. Hemodynamic determinants of rate of left ventricular isovolumic pressure decline. Am J Physiol 239(Heart Circ Physiol 8):H1, 1980.
19. Starling MR, Montgomery DG, Mancini GBJ, Walsh RA: Load independence of the rate of isovolumic relaxation in man. Circulation 76:1274, 1987.
20. Brutsaert DL, et al.: Ventricular relaxation. *In* The Ventricle: Basic and Clinical Aspects. Boston, Martinus Nijhoff Publishing, p. 123, 1985.
21. Nikolic S, et al.: Passive properties of canine left ventricle: diastolic stiffness and restoring forces. Circ Res 62:1210, 1988.
22. McCullagh WH, Covell JW, Ross J Jr.: Left ventricular dilatation and diastolic compliance changes during chronic volume overloading. Circulation 45:943, 1972.
23. Mirsky I: Elastic properties of the myocardium: a quantitative approach with physiological and clinical applications. *In* Berne RH (ed.): Handbook of Physiology, Section 2, The Cardiovascular System, Volume 1, The Heart. Bethesda, Md, American Physiological Society, p. 497, 1979.
24. Mirsky I: Assessment of diastolic function: suggested methods and future considerations. Circulation 69:836, 1984.
25. Ross J Jr.: Acute displacement of the diastolic pressure-volume curve of the left ventricle: role of the pericardium and the right ventricle. Circulation 59:32, 1979.
26. Bourdillon PD, et al.: Increased regional myocardial stiffness of the left ventricle during pacing induced angina in man. Circulation 67:317, 1983.
27. Grossman W: Evaluation of systolic and diastolic function of the myocardium. *In* Grossman W (ed.): Cardiac Catheterization and Angiography. Philadelphia, Lea & Febiger, p. 301, 1986.
28. Ludbrook PA, Byrne JD, McKnight RC: Influence of right ventricular hemodynamics on left ventricular diastolic pressure-volume relations in man. Circulation 59:21, 1979.
29. Thomas J, Newell J, Choong C, Weyman A: Physical and physiological determinants of transmitral velocity: numerical analysis. Am J Physiol 260(Heart Circ Physiol 29):H1718, 1991.
30. Hatle L, Angelsen B: Doppler Ultrasound in Cardiology. Philadelphia, Lea & Febiger, p. 24, 1985.
31. Courtois M, Kovacs SJ Jr., Ludbrook PA: Transmitral pressure-flow velocity relation: importance of regional pressure gradients in the left ventricle during diastole. Circulation 78:661, 1988.
32. Matsuda Y, et al.: Importance of left atrial function in patients with myocardial infarction. Circulation 67:566, 1983.
33. Meisner JS, Pajaro OE, Yellin EL: Investigation of left ventricular filling dynamics: development of a model. Einstein Q J Biol Med 4:47, 1986.
34. Ishida Y, et al.: Left ventricular filling dynamics: influence of left ventricular relaxation and left atrial pressure. Circulation 74:187, 1986.
35. Keren G, et al.: Pulmonary venous flow pattern—its relation to cardiac dynamics. Circulation 71:1105, 1985.
36. Keren G, et al.: Interrelationship of mid-diastolic mitral valve motion, pulmonary venous flow, and transmitral flow. Circulation 74:36, 1986.
37. Smallhorn JF, Freedom RM, Olley PM: Pulsed Doppler echocardiographic assessment of extraparenchymal pulmonary vein flow. J Am Coll Cardiol 9:573, 1987.
38. Castello R, Pearson A, Lenzen P, Labovitz A: Evaluation of pulmonary venous flow by transoesophageal echocardiography in subjects with a normal heart: comparison with transthoracic echocardiography. J Am Cardiol 18:65, 1991.

39. Keren G, et al.: Atrial contraction is an important determinant of pulmonary venous flow. J Am Coll Cardiol 7:693, 1986.
40. Pasierski T, Alton M, Pearson A: Transoesophageal echocardiographic characterization of pulmonary vein flow not due to atrial contraction or mitral regurgitation. Am J Cardiol 68:415, 1991.
41. Masuyama T, et al.: Pulmonary venous flow velocity pattern as assessed with transthoracic pulsed Doppler echocardiography in subjects without cardiac disease. Am J Cardiol 67:1396, 1991.
42. Nishimura R, Abel M, Hatle L, Tajik A: Relation of pulmonary vein to mitral flow velocities by transoesophageal Doppler echocardiography. Effect of different loading conditions. Circulation 81:1488, 1990.
43. Kuecherer H, et al.: Estimation of mean left atrial pressure from transoesophageal pulsed Doppler echocardiography of pulmonary venous flow. Circulation 82:1127, 1990.
44. Kuecherer H, et al.: Am Heart J 122:1683, 1991.
45. Hoit B, Shao Y, Gabel M, Walsh R: Influence of loading conditions and contractile state on pulmonary venous flow. Validation of Doppler velocimetry. Circulation 86:651, 1992.
46. Castello R, Pearson AC, Lenzen P, Laboritz A: Effect of mitral regurgitation on pulmonary venous velocities derived from transoesophageal echocardiography color-guided pulsed Doppler imaging. J Am Coll Cardiol 17: 1499, 1991.
47. Klein A, et al.: Transoesophageal Doppler echocardiography of pulmonary venous flow: a new marker of mitral regurgitation severity. J Am Coll Cardiol 18:518, 1991.
48. Williams JF, Sonnenblick EH, Braunwald E: Determinants of atrial contractile force in the intact heart. Am J Physiol 209:1061, 1965.
49. Greenberg B, et al.: The influence of left ventricular filling phase on atrial contribution to cardiac output. Am Heart J 98:742, 1979.
50. Maron BJ, Henry WL, Roberts WC, Epstein SE: Comparison of echocardiographic and necropsy measurements of left ventricular wall thickness in patients with and without disproportionate septal thickening. Circulation 55:341, 1977.
51. Larkin H, et al.: Anatomical accuracy of echocardiographically assessed left ventricular wall thickness. Clin Sci 57:55S, 1979.
52. Liebson PR, Savage DD: Echocardiography in hypertension: a review. I. Left ventricular wall mass, standardization, and ventricular function. Echocardiography 3:181, 1986.
53. Grossman W, Jones D, McLaurin LP: Wall stress and patterns of hypertrophy in the human left ventricle. J Clin Invest 56:56, 1975.
54. Woythaler JN, et al.: Accuracy of echocardiography versus electrocardiography in detecting left ventricular hypertrophy: comparison with postmortem mass measurements. J Am Coll Cardiol 2:305, 1983.
55. Belkin RN, Kisslo J: Clinical applications of echocardiography in myocardial and ventricular heart disease. Prog Cardiovasc Dis 29:81, 1986.
56. St. John Sutton MG, et al.: Echocardiographic assessment of left ventricular filling and septal and posterior wall dynamics in idiopathic hypertrophic subaortic stenosis. Circulation 57:512, 1978.
57. Hanrath P, Mathey DG, Siegert R, Bleifeld W: Left ventricular relaxation and filling pattern in different forms of left ventricular hypertrophy: an echocardiographic study. Am J Cardiol 45:15, 1980.
58. Rahko PS, Shaver JA, Salerni R, Uretsky BF: Noninvasive evaluation of systolic and diastolic function in severe congestive heart failure secondary to coronary artery disease or dilated idiopathic cardiomyopathy. Am J Cardiol 57:1315, 1986.
59. Spirito P, et al.: Diastolic abnormalities in patients with hypertrophic cardiomyopathy: relation to magnitude of left ventricular hypertrophy. Circulation 72:310, 1985.
60. Gibson DG, Brown DJ: Measurement of instantaneous left ventricular dimension and filling rate in man using echocardiography. Br Heart J 35: 1141, 1973.
61. Janos GG, et al.: Differentiation of constrictive pericarditis and restrictive cardiomyopathy using digitized echocardiography. J Am Coll Cardiol 1: 541, 1983.
62. Pollick C, Fitzgerald P, Popp RL: Variability of digitized echocardiography: size, source and means of reduction. Am J Cardiol 51:576, 1983.
63. Trail TA, Gibson DG, Brown DJ: Study of left ventricular wall thickness and dimension changes using echocardiography. Br Heart J 40:162, 1978.
64. St. John Sutton MG, Reichek N, Kastor JA, Giuliani ER: Computerized M-mode echocardiographic analysis of left ventricular dysfunction in cardiac amyloid. Circulation 66:790, 1982.
65. Fifer MA, Borow KM, Colan SD, Lorell BH: Early diastolic left ventricular function in children and adults with aortic stenosis. J Am Coll Cardiol 5: 1147, 1985.
66. Lorell BH, et al.: Modification of abnormal left ventricular diastolic properties by nifedipine in patients with hypertrophic cardiomyopathy. Circulation 65:499, 1982.
67. Gibson DG, Brown DJ: Measurement of peak rates of ventricular wall motion in man. Comparison of echocardiography with contrast angiography. Br Heart J 37:677, 1975.
68. Bryhn M: Abnormal left ventricular filling in patients with sustained myocardial relaxation: assessment of diastolic parameters using radionuclide angiography and echocardiography. Clin Cardiol 7:639, 1984.
69. Parameswaran R, Kotler MN, Parry W, Goldman AP: Echocardiographic analysis of left ventricular filling in isolated pure chronic aortic regurgitation. Am J Cardiol 58:794, 1986.
70. Tamiya K, Sugawara M, Akurai Y: Maximum lengthening velocity during isotonic relaxation at preload in canine papillary muscle. Am J Physiol 237: H83, 1979.
71. Le Carpentier Y, Martin JL, Gastineau P, Hatt PY: Load dependence of mammalian heart relaxation during cardiac hypertrophy and heart failure. Am J Physiol 242:H855, 1982.
72. Hammermeister KE, Warbasse JR: The rate of change of left ventricular volume in man. II. Diastolic events in health and disease. Circulation 49: 739, 1974.
73. Upton MT, Gibson DG: The study of left ventricular function from digitized echocardiograms. Prog Cardiovasc Dis 20:359, 1978.
74. Gibson DG, Traill TA, Brown DJ: Changes in left ventricular free wall thickness in patients with ischemic heart disease. Br Heart J 39:1312, 1977.
75. Gibson DG, Brown DJ: Continuous assessment of left ventricular shape in man. Br Heart J 37:904, 1975.
76. Van der Werf F, et al.: The mechanism of disappearance of the physiologic third heart sound with age. Circulation 73:877, 1986.
77. Bahler RC, Vrobel TR, Martin P: The relation of heart rate and shortening fraction to echocardiographic indexes of left ventricular relaxation in normal subjects. J Am Coll Cardiol 2:926, 1983.
78. Colan SD, Borow KM, Neumann A: Effects of loading conditions and contractile state (methoxamine and dobutamine) on left ventricular early diastolic function in normal subjects. Am J Cardiol 55:790, 1985.
79. Lawson WE, et al.: A new use for M-mode echocardiography in detecting left ventricular diastolic dysfunction in coronary artery disease. Am J Cardiol 58:210, 1986.
80. Dreslinski G, et al.: Echocardiographic diastolic ventricular abnormality in hypertensive heart disease: atrial emptying index. Am J Cardiol 47:1087, 1981.
81. Hausdorf G, Gravinghoff I, Sieg K, Keck EW: Echocardiographic characteristics of diastolic function dysfunction in restrictive cardiomyopathy in childhood (abstr.). J Am Coll Cardiol 5:528A, 1985.
82. Engel PJ, et al.: M-mode echocardiography in constrictive pericarditis. J Am Coll Cardiol 6:471, 1985.
83. Shimizu G, Zile MR, Blaustein AS, Gaasch WH: Left ventricular chamber filling and midwall lengthening in patients with left ventricular hypertrophy: overestimation of fiber velocities by conventional midwall measurements. Circulation 71:266, 1985.
84. Brodie BR, McLaurin LP, Grossman W: Combined hemodynamic-ultrasonic method for studying left ventricular wall stress: comparison with angiography. Am J Cardiol 37:864, 1976.
85. Ratshin RA, Rackley CE, Rusell RO Jr.: Determination of left ventricular preload and afterload by quantitative echocardiography in man. Circ Res 34:711, 1974.
86. Spotnitz HM, et al.: Effects of open heart surgery on pressure-diameter relative of the human left ventricle. Circulation 59:662, 1979.
87. Hess OM, Grimm J, Krayenbuehl HP: Diastolic single elastic and viselastic properties of the left ventricle in man. Circulation 59:1178, 1979.
88. Schiller NB, et al.: Canine left ventricular mass estimation by two-dimensional echocardiography. Circulation 68:210, 1983.
89. Wyatt HL, et al.: Cross-sectional echocardiography: I. Analysis of mathematical models for quantifying mass of the left ventricle in dogs. Circulation 60:1104, 1979.
90. Helak JW, Reichek N: Quantitation of human left ventricular mass and volume by two-dimensional echocardiography: in vitro anatomic validation. Circulation 63:1398, 1981.
91. Reichek N, et al.: Anatomic validation of left ventricular mass estimates from clinical two-dimensional echocardiography: initial results. Circulation 67:348, 1983.
92. Funai JT, Pandian NG, Salem DN, Levine HJ: Heterogeneity of regional diastolic filling dynamics in normal left ventricle. Experimental two-dimensional echocardiographic studies (abstr.). J Am Coll Cardiol 5:426A, 1985.
93. Thomas JD, et al.: Improved accuracy of echocardiographic endocardial borders by spatio temporal filtered Faurier reconstruction: description of the method and optimization of filter cutoffs. Circulation 77:415, 1988.
94. Taylor DEM, Whamond JS: Velocity profile and impedance of the healthy mitral valve. In Kalmanson D (ed.): The Mitral Valve, A Pluridisciplinary Approach. Acton, MA: Publishing Scientific Group, p. 127, 1976.
95. Samstad S, et al.: Cross-sectional early mitral flow velocity profiles from color Doppler. Br Heart J 62:177, 1989.
96. Samstad S, et al.: Cross-sectional early mitral flow-velocity profiles from color Doppler in patients with mitral valve disease. Circulation 86:748, 1992.
97. Rokey R, et al.: Determination of parameters of left ventricular diastolic filling with pulsed Doppler echocardiography: comparison with cineangiography. Circulation 71:543, 1985.
98. Goldberg S, Dickinson DF, Wilson N: Evaluation of an elliptical area technique for calculating mitral blood flow by Doppler echocardiography. Br Heart J 54:68, 1985.
99. Lewis JF, et al.: Pulsed Doppler echocardiographic determination of stroke volume and cardiac output: clinical validation of two new methods using the apical window. Circulation 70:425, 1984.

100. Gillam CD, et al.: Which cardiac valve provides the best Doppler estimate of cardiac output in man? (abstr.) Circulation 72(Suppl. 3):III-99), 1985.
101. Ormiston JA, Shah PM, Tei C, Wong M: Size and motion of the mitral valve annulus in man. 1. A two-dimensional echocardiographic method and findings in normal subjects. Circulation 64:113, 1981.
102. Fisher DC, et al.: The mitral valve orifice method for noninvasive two-dimensional echo Doppler determination of cardiac output. Circulation 67: 872, 1983.
103. Loeber CP, Goldberg SJ, Allen HD: Doppler echocardiographic comparison of flows distal to the four cardiac valves. J Am Coll Cardiol 4:268, 1984.
104. Choong CY, Herrmann HC, Weyman AE, Fifer MA: Left ventricular diastolic pressure-volume relation in man derived from Doppler and two-dimensional echocardiography (abstr.). Circulation 74(Suppl. 2):II-46, 1986.
105. Rokey R, et al.: Influence of atrial emptying on early left ventricular filling dynamics (abstr.). J Am Coll Cardiol 5:510A, 1985.
106. Kuo LC, et al.: Quantification of atrial contribution to left ventricular filling by pulsed Doppler echocardiography and the effect of age in normal and diseased hearts. Am J Cardiol 59:1174, 1987.
107. Gardin JM, et al.: Effect of imaging view and sample volume location on evaluation of mitral flow velocity pulsed by Doppler echocardiography. Am J Cardiol 57:1335, 1986.
108. Freidman BJ, et al.: Assessment of left ventricular diastolic function: comparison of Doppler echocardiography and gated blood pool scintigraphy. J Am Coll Cardiol 8:1348, 1986.
109. Bowman LK, et al.: Validation of Doppler echocardiographically derived peak filling normalized to stroke volume: a comparison with radionuclide angiographic techniques (abstr.). J Am Coll Cardiol 9:16A, 1987.
110. Spirito P, Maron BJ, Bonow RO: Noninvasive assessment of left ventricular diastolic function: comparative analysis of Doppler echocardiographic and radionuclide angiographic techniques. J Am Coll Cardiol 7:518, 1986.
111. Snider AR, et al.: Doppler evaluation of left ventricular diastolic filling in children with systemic hypertension. Am J Cardiol 56:921, 1985.
112. Pearson AC, et al.: Assessment of diastolic function in normal and hypertrophied hearts: comparison of Doppler echocardiography and M-mode echocardiography. Am Heart J 113:1417, 1987.
113. Appleton CP, Hatle LK, Popp RL: Relation of transmitral flow velocity patterns to left ventricular diastolic function: new insights from a combined hemodynamic and Doppler echocardiographic study. J Am Coll Cardiol 12:426, 1988.
114. Stoddard MF, et al.: Left ventricular diastolic function: comparison of pulsed Doppler echocardiographic and hemodynamic indexes in subjects with and without coronary artery disease. J Am Coll Cardiol 13:327, 1989.
115. St. John Sutton M, Plappert T: Relation between instantaneous Doppler velocity across the mitral valve and changes in left ventricular volume in normal, dilated and hypertrophied hearts (abstr.). J Am Coll Cardiol 7: 227A, 1986.
116. Drinkovic N, et al.: Assessment of diastolic left ventricular function by Doppler: comparison with catheterization measurements (abstr.). J Am Coll Cardiol 7:227A, 1986.
117. Drinkovic N, et al.: Sensitivity and specificity of transmitral flow velocity measurements in detecting impaired left ventricular compliance (abstr.). Circulation 74(Suppl. 2):II-46, 1986.
118. Lin S, et al.: Comparison of Doppler echocardiographic and hemodynamic indexes of left ventricular diastolic properties in coronary artery disease. Am J Cardiol 62:882, 1988.
119. David D, et al.: Reliability of Doppler derived indices of left ventricular diastolic function in patients with dilated cardiomyopathy: comparison with simultaneously obtained left atrial and ventricular micromanometer pressures (abstr.). J Am Coll Cardiol 11:119A, 1988.
120. Himura Y, et al.: The assessment of left ventricular diastolic function with Doppler transmitral flow velocity recording. J Am Coll Cardiol 18:753, 1991.
121. Choong CY, Herrmann HC, Weyman AE, Fifer MA: Preload dependence of Doppler-derived indexes of left ventricular diastolic function in humans. J Am Coll Cardiol 10:800, 1987.
122. Takahashi T, et al.: Left ventricular early filling flow is sensitive to changes in left atrial pressure: a study of lower body negative and positive pressure (abstr.). Circulation 74(Suppl 2):II-477, 1986.
123. Leeman DE, et al.: Effects of decreases in preload on pulsed Doppler indices of left ventricular filling (abstr.). Circulation (Suppl 2):II-46, 1986.
124. Choong CY, et al.: Combined influence of ventricular loading and relaxation on the transmitral flow velocity profile in dogs measured by Doppler echocardiography. Circulation 78:672, 1988.
125. Courtois M, et al.: The transmitral pressure-flow velocity relation. Effect of abrupt preload reduction. Circulation 78:1459, 1988.
126. Courtois M, Mechem C, Barzilai B, Ludbrook P: Factors related to end-systolic volume are important determinants of peak entry diastolic transmitral flow velocity. Circulation 85:1132, 1992.
127. Miki S, et al.: Dependence of Doppler echocardiographic transmitral early peak velocity in left ventricular systolic function in coronary artery disease. Am J Cardiol 67:475, 1991.
128. Meisner JS, Pajaro OE, Yellin EL: Investigation of left ventricular filling dynamics: development of a model. Einstein Q J Biol Med 4:47, 1986.
129. Thomas JD, Weyman AE: Fluid dynamics model of mitral flow: description with in vitro validation. J Am Coll Cardiol 13:221, 1989.
130. Thomas JD, et al.: A quantitative model for transmitral blood flow: description with in vitro verification (abstr.). J Am Coll Cardiol 9:(Suppl. A):212A, 1987.
131. Thomas J, Choong C, Flachskampf F, Weyman A: Analysis of the early transmitral Doppler velocity curve: effect of primary physiologic changes and compensatory preload adjustment. J Am Coll Cardiol 16:644, 1990.
132. Thomas J, Newell J, Choong C, Weyman A: Physical and physiological determinants of transmitral velocity: numerical analysis. Am J Physiol 260(Heart Circ Physiol 29)H1718, 1991.
133. Flachskampf F, Weyman A, Guerrero J, Thomas J: Calculation of atrioventricular compliance from the mitral flow profile: analytic and in vitro study. J Am Coll Cardiol 19:998, 1992.
134. Thomas J, Weyman A: Echocardiographic Doppler evaluation of left ventricular diastolic function. Physics and physiology. Circulation 84:977, 1991.
135. Drinkovic N, et al.: Influence of sampling site upon the ratio of atrial to early diastolic transmitral flow velocities by Doppler (abstr.). J Am Coll Cardiol 9:16A, 1987.
136. Pearson AC, et al.: Effect of sample volume location on pulsed Doppler-echocardiographic evaluation of left ventricular filling. Am J Cardiac Imag 2:40, 1988.
137. Dabestani A, et al.: Effects of spontaneous respiration on left ventricular filling assessed by pulsed Doppler echocardiography. Am J Cardiol 61: 1356, 1988.
138. Riggs TW, Snider AR: Respiratory influence on right and left ventricular diastolic function in normal children. Am J Cardiol 63:858, 1989.
139. Uiterwal C, et al.: The effect of respiration on diastolic blood flow velocities in the human heart. Eur Heart J 10:108, 1989.
140. Herzog CA, et al.: Effect of atrial pacing on left ventricular diastolic filling measured by pulsed Doppler echocardiography. J Am Coll Cardiol 9(Suppl. A):197A, 1987.
141. Gillam LD, et al.: The influence of heart rate on Doppler mitral inflow patterns (abstr.). Circulation 76(Suppl. 4):IV-123, 1987.
142. Crouse LJ, Parsonnet V, Lighty GW Jr.: Doppler evaluation of the effect of heart rate on transmitral blood flow in patients with dual-chambered pacemakers (abstr.). Circulation 70(Suppl 2):II-408, 1984.
143. Harrison M, Clifton G, Pennell A, DeMaria A: Effect of heart rate on left ventricular diastolic transmitral flow velocity patterns assessed by Doppler echocardiography in normal subjects. Am J Cardiol 67:622, 1991.
144. Appleton C, Carucci M, Henry C, Olajos M: Influence of incremental changes in heart rate on mitral flow velocity: assessment of lightly sedated, conscious dogs. J Am Coll Cardiol 17:227, 1991.
145. Nolan SP, Dixon SH, Fisher RD, Morrow AG: The influence of atrial contraction and mitral valve mechanics on ventricular filling. Am Heart J 77:784, 1969.
146. Freedman RA, Yock PG, Echt DS, Popp RL: Effect of variation in PQ interval on patterns of atrioventricular valve motion and flow in patients with normal ventricular function. J Am Coll Cardiol 7:595, 1986.
147. Miyatake K, et al.: Augmentation of atrial contribution to left ventricular inflow with aging as assessed by intracardiac Doppler flowmetry. Am J Cardiol 53:586, 1984.
148. Spirito P, Maron BJ: Influence of aging on left ventricular diastolic function as assessed by Doppler echocardiography (abstr.). J Am Coll Cardiol 9: 16A, 1987.
149. Bryg RJ, Williams GA, Labovitz AJ: Effect of aging on left ventricular diastolic filling in normal subjects. Am J Cardiol 59:971, 1987.
150. Gardin JM, et al.: Doppler transmitral flow velocity parameters: relationship between age, body surface area, blood pressure and gender in normal subjects. Am J Noninvas Cardiol 1:3, 1987.
151. Sartori MP, Quinones MA, Kuo LC: Relation of Doppler-derived left ventricular filling parameters to age and radius/thickness ratio in normal and pathologic states. Am J Cardiol 59:1179, 1987.
152. Van de Werf F, et al.: The mechanism of disappearance of the physiologic third heart sound with age. Circulation 73:877, 1986.
153. Matsumoto M, Sekimoto H: Geriatric echocardiography: I. Review of stueies of the normal aging heart. Echocardiography 5:87, 1988.
154. Kitzman D, et al.: Age related alterations of Doppler left ventricular filling in normal subjects are independent of left ventricular mass, heart rate, contractility and loading conditions. J Am Coll Cardiol 18:1243, 1991.
155. Manning W, et al.: Reversal of changes in left ventricular diastolic filling associated with normal aging using diltiazem. Am J Cardiol 67:894, 1991.
156. Reed K, et al.: Cardiac Doppler flow velocities in human fetuses. Circulation 73:41, 1986.
157. Romero T, Covell J, Friedman WF: A comparison of pressure-volume relations of the fetal, newborn and adult heart. Am J Physiol 222:1285, 1972.
158. Reed K, et al.: Doppler echocardiographic studies of diastolic function in the human fetal heart: changes during gestation. J Am Coll Cardiol 8:391, 1986.
159. Wilson N, et al.: Doppler echocardiographic observations of pulmonary and transvalvular changes after birth and during the early neonatal period. Am Heart J 113:750, 1987.

160. Riggs T, et al.: Doppler echocardiographic evaluation of right and left ventricular diastolic function in normal neonates. J Am Coll Cardiol 13:700, 1989.
161. Johnson G, Moffett C, Noonan J: Doppler echocardiography studies of diastolic filling patterns in premature infants. Am Heart J 116:1568, 1988.
162. Snider AR, et al.: Doppler evaluation of left ventricular diastolic filling in children with systemic hypertension. Am J Cardiol 56:921, 1985.
163. Phillips R, et al.: Determinants of abnormal left ventricular filling in early hypertension. Am J Cardiol 14:979, 1989.
164. Graettinger WF, Weber MA, Gardin JM, Knoll ML: Diastolic blood pressure as a determinant of Doppler left ventricular filling indexes in normal adolescents. J Am Coll Cardiol 10:1280, 1987.
165. Graettinger W, Neutel J, Smith D, Weber M: Left ventricular diastolic filling alterations in normotensive young adults with a family history of systemic hypertension. Am J Cardiol 68:51, 1991.
166. Douglas PS, Berko BA, Iolo A, Reichek N: Variable responses of mitral valve motion and flow in systemic hypertension and in idiopathic dilated cardiomyopathy. Am J Cardiol 60:363, 1987.
167. Belkin RN, et al.: Doppler derived indices of diastolic filling in mild to moderate hypertension (abstr.). Circulation 74(Suppl. 2):II-47, 1986.
168. Otto CM, Pearlman AS, Amsler LC: Doppler echocardiographic evaluation of left ventricular diastolic filling in isolated valvular aortic stenosis. Am J Cardiol 63:313, 1989.
169. Myreng Y, Smiseth O, Risoe C: Left ventricular filling at elevated diastolic pressures: relationship between transmitral Doppler flow velocities and atrial contribution. Am Heart J 119:620, 1990.
170. Pearson A, et al.: Echocardiographic evaluation of cardiac structure and function in elderly subjects with isolated systolic hypertension. J Am Coll Cardiol 17:422, 1991.
171. Pearson AC, Gudipati CV, Labovitz AJ: Systolic and diastolic flow abnormalities in elderly patients with hypertensive hypertrophic cardiomyopathy. J Am Coll Cardiol 12:989, 1988.
172. Chakko S, et al.: Abnormal left ventricular diastolic filling in eccentric left ventricular hypertrophy of obesity. Am J Cardiol 68:95, 1991.
173. Grossman F, Oren S, Messerli F: Left ventricular filling in the systemic hypertension of obesity. Am J Cardiol 68:57, 1991.
174. Stoddard M, et al.: Valvuloplasty on left ventricular diastolic function and filling in humans. J Am Cardiol 14:1218, 1989.
175. Takenaka K, et al.: Left ventricular filling in hypertrophic cardiomyopathy: a pulsed Doppler echocardiographic study. J Am Coll Cardiol 7:1263, 1986.
176. Bryg RJ, Pearson AC, Williams GA, Labovitz AJ: Left ventricular systolic and diastolic flow abnormalities determined by Doppler echocardiography in obstructive hypertrophic cardiomyopathy. Am J Cardiol 59:925, 1987.
177. Maron BJ, et al.: Noninvasive assessment of left ventricular diastolic function by pulsed Doppler echocardiography in patients with hypertrophic cardiomyopathy. J Am Coll Cardiol 10:733, 1987.
178. Nihoyannopoulos P, et al.: Diastolic function in hypertrophic cardiomyopathy: relation to exercise capacity. J Am Coll Cardiol 19:536, 1992.
179. Fagard R, et al.: Assessment of stiffness of the hypertrophied left ventricle of bicyclists using left ventricular inflow Doppler velocimetry. J Am Coll Cardiol 9:1250, 1987.
180. Douglas PS, O'Toole ML, Hiller DB, Reichek N: Left ventricular structure and function by echocardiography in ultraendurance athletes. Am J Cardiol 58:805, 1986.
181. Pearson AC, et al.: Left ventricular diastolic function in weight lifters. Am J Cardiol 58:1254, 1986.
182. Thompson P, et al.: Left ventricular function is not impaired in weight-lifters who use anabolic steroids. J Am Coll Cardiol 19:278, 1992.
183. Armstrong WF, Ryan T, Feiganbaum H: Doppler evaluation of left ventricular inflow during transient myocardial ischaemia (abstr.). J Am Coll Cardiol 9:213A, 1987.
184. Fisher DC, Voyles WF, Sikes W, Greene ER: Left ventricular filling patterns during ischaemia: an echo/Doppler study in open chest dogs (abstr.). J Am Coll Cardiol 5:426A, 1986.
185. Rosoff M, Funai J, Wang SS, Pandian N: Left ventricular diastolic filling dynamics in acute myocardial infarction: immediate effects of ischemia time course in first six hours and relation to infarct size (abstr.). J Am Coll Cardiol 7:227A, 1986.
186. Ridner ML, et al.: Alterations in Doppler indexes of diastolic function following coronary artery reperfusion (abstr.). Circulation 74(Suppl. 2):II-47, 1986.
187. Wind BE, et al.: Pulsed Doppler assessment of left ventricular diastolic filling in coronary artery disease before and immediately after coronary angioplasty. Am J Cardiol 59:1041, 1987.
188. Fujii J, et al.: Noninvasive assessment of left and right ventricular filling in myocardial infarction with a two-dimensional Doppler echocardiographic method. J Am Coll Cardiol 5:1155, 1985.
189. Isobe M, et al.: Right ventricular filling detected by pulsed Doppler echocardiography during the convalescent stage of interior wall acute myocardial infarction. Am J Cardiol 59:1245, 1987.
190. Visser CA, et al.: Pulsed Doppler-derived mitral inflow velocity in acute myocardial infarction: an early prognostic indicator (abstr.). J Am Coll Cardiol 7:136A, 1986.
191. Johannessen K, Cerqueria M, Stratton J: Influence of myocardial infarction size on radionuclide and Doppler echocardiographic measurements of diastolic function. Am J Cardiol 65:692, 1990.
192. Iliceto S, et al.: Doppler echocardiographic evaluation of the effect of atrial pacing-induced ischemia on left ventricular filling in patients with coronary artery disease. J Am Coll Cardiol 11:953, 1988.
193. Labovitz AJ, et al.: Evaluation of left ventricular systolic and diastolic dysfunction during transient myocardial ischaemia produced by angioplasty. J Am Coll Cardiol 10:748, 1987.
194. Bowman LK, et al.: Evaluation of left ventricular diastolic filling during coronary angioplasty during Doppler echocardiography (abstr.). J Am Coll Cardiol 9:213A, 1987.
195. Raisarro A, et al.: Doppler evaluation of left ventricular diastolic filling function during angioplasty (abstr.). J Am Coll Cardiol 9:213A, 1987.
196. Klodnicki W, et al.: Doppler evaluation of left ventricular filling dynamics during coronary angioplasty (abstr.). J Am Coll Cardiol 9:213A, 1987.
197. Snow F, et al.: Doppler echocardiographic evaluation of left ventricular diastolic function after percutaneous transmitral coronary angioplasty for unstable angia pectoris or acute myocardial inspiration. Am J Cardiol 65: 840, 1990.
198. Wind BE, et al.: Pulsed Doppler assessment of left ventricular diastolic filling in coronary artery disease before and immediately after coronary angioplasty. Am J Cardiol 59:1041, 1987.
199. Masuyama T, et al.: Effects of changes in coronary stenosis on left ventricular diastolic filling assessed with pulsed Doppler echocardiography. J Am Coll Cardiol 11:744, 1988.
200. Louie EK, Rich S, Brundage BH: Doppler echocardiographic assessment of impaired left ventricular filling in patients with right ventricular pressure overload due to primary pulmonary hypertension. J Am Coll Cardiol 8: 1298, 1986.
201. Louie F, Rich S, Levitsky S, Brundage B: Doppler echocardiographic demonstration of the differential effects of right ventricular pressure and volume overload on left ventricular geometry and filling. J Am Coll Cardiol 19:84, 1992.
202. Takenaka K, et al.: Pulsed Doppler echocardiographic study of left ventricular filling in dilated cardiomyopathy. Am J Cardiol 58:143, 1986.
203. Douglas PS, Berko BA, Iola A, Reichek N: Variable responses of mitral valve motion and flow in systemic hypertension and in idopathic cardiomyopathy. Am J Cardiol 50:363, 1987.
204. Vanoverschelde J, Raphael D, Robert A, Cosyns J: Left ventricular filling in dilated cardiomyopathy: relation to functional class and hemodynamics. J Am Coll Cardiol 15:1288, 1990.
205. Lavine S, Arends D: Importance of the left ventricular filling pressure on diastolic filling in idiopathic dilated cardiomyopathy. Am J Cardiol 64:61, 1989.
206. Zarich SW, et al.: Diastolic abnormalities in young asymptomatic diabetic patients assessed by pulsed Doppler echocardiography. J Am Coll Cardiol 12:114, 1988.
207. Riggs T, Transue D: Doppler echocardiographic evaluation of left ventricular diastolic function in adolescents with diabetes mellitus. Am J Cardiol 65:899, 1990.
208. Desruennes M, et al.: Doppler echocardiography for the diagnosis of acute cardiac allograft rejection. J Am Coll Cardiol 12:63, 1988.
209. Valantine HA, et al.: A hemodynamic and Doppler echocardiographic study of ventricular function in long-term cardiac allograft recipients. Circulation 79:66, 1989.
210. Pandian NG, et al.: Doppler echocardiography in cardiac tamponade. Abnormalities in tricuspid and mitral flow response to respiration in experimental and clinical tamponade (abstr.). J Am Coll Cardiol 5:485A, 1985.
211. Leeman DE, Riley MF, Carl LV, Come PC: Doppler echocardiography in cardiac tamponade. Exaggerated respiratory variation in transvalvular blood flow velocity integrals (abstr.). J Am Coll Cardiol 9:17A, 1987.
212. Appleton CP, Hatle LK, Popp RL: Cardiac tamponade and pericardial effusion: respiratory variation in transvalvular flow velocities studied by Doppler echocardiography. J Am Coll Cardiol 11:1020, 1988.
213. Gonzalez M, et al.: Experimental pericardial effusion: relation of abnormal respiratory variation in mitral flow velocity to hemodynamics and diastolic right heart collapse. J Am Coll Cardiol 17:239, 1991.
214. Picard M, et al.: Quantitative relation between increased intrapericardial pressure and Doppler flow velocities during experimental cardiac tamponade. J Am Coll Cardiol 18:234, 1991.
215. Appleton C, Hatle L, Popp R: Demonstration of restrictive ventricular physiology by Doppler echocardiography. J Am Cardiol 11:757, 1987.
216. Hatle LK, Appleton CP, Popp RL: Differentiation of constrictive pericarditis and restrictive cardiomyopathy by Doppler echocardiography. Circulation 79:357, 1989.
217. Appleton CP, Hatle LK, Popp RL: Central venous flow velocity in patterns can differentiate constrictive pericarditis from restrictive cardiomyopathy (abstr.). J Am Coll Cardiol 9:119A, 1987.
218. Klein AL, et al.: Doppler characterization of left ventricular diastolic function in cardiac amyloidosis. J Am Coll Cardiol 13:1017, 1989.
219. Kinoshita O, et al.: Impaired left ventricular diastolic filling in patients with familial amyloid polyneuropathy: a pulsed Doppler echocardiographic study. Br Heart J 69:198, 1989.

220. Klein A, et al.: Prognostic significance of Doppler measures of diastolic function in cardiac amyloidosis. Circulation 83:808, 1991.
221. Stewart WJ, et al.: Doppler ultrasound measurement of cardiac output in patients with physiologic pacemakers. Am J Cardiol 54:308, 1984.
222. Iwase M, et al.: Evaluation by pulsed Doppler echocardiography of the atrial contribution to left ventricular filling in patients with DDD pacemakers. Am J Cardiol 58:104, 1986.
223. Pearson AC, et al.: Prediction of hemodynamic of physiologic pacing from baseline Doppler-echocardiographic parameters. PACE 10:438A, 1987.
224. Rassi A Jr., Richards KL, Miller JF, Crawford MH: Echo/Doppler assessment of mitral blood flow during exercise (abstr.). Circulation 74(Suppl. 2):II-47, 1987.
225. Nonogi H, Hess OM, Ritter M, Krayenbuehl HP: Diastolic properties of the normal left ventricle during supine exercise. Br Heart J 60:30, 1988.
226. Thadani U, Parker JO: Haemodynamics at rest and during supine and sitting exercise in normal subjects. Am J Cardiol 41:52, 1978.
227. Kuecherer HF, Ruffmann K, Schaefer E, Kuebler W: Doppler echocardiographic assessment of left ventricular filling dynamics in patients with coronary heart disease and normal systolic function. Euro Heart J 9:649, 1988.
228. Presti C, et al.: Influence of exercise induced myocardial ischemia on the pattern of left ventricular diastolic filling: a Doppler echocardiographic study. J Am Coll Cardiol 18:75, 1991.
229. Iwase M, et al.: Non-invasive detection of exercise induced markedly elevated left ventricular filling measure by pulsed Doppler echocardiography in patients with coronary artery disease. Am Heart J 118:947, 1989.
230. Hayashi K, et al.: Evaluation of preload reserve during isometric exercise testing in patients with old myocardial infarction: Doppler echocardiographic study. J Am Coll Cardiol 17:106, 1991.
231. Swinne C, Shapiro E, Lima S, Fleg S: Age associated changes in left ventricular diastolic performance during isometric exercise in normal subjects. Am J Cardiol 69:823, 1992.
232. Iwase M, et al.: Effects of diltiazem on left ventricular diastolic behaviour in patients with hypertrophic cardiomyopathy: evaluation with exercise pulsed Doppler echocardiography. J Am Coll Cardiol 9:1099, 1987.
233. Nagao M, et al.: Diltiazem-induced decrease of elevated pulmonary arterial diastolic pressure in hypertrophic cardiomyopathy patients. Am Heart J 102:789, 1981.

CHAPTER

25

ECHOCARDIOGRAPHIC ASSESSMENT OF THE CARDIOMYOPATHIES

ROBERT A. LEVINE

Cardiomyopathy is most simply defined as disease of the heart muscle.[1] The most widely accepted use of this term in practice refers to diseases that are intrinsic to the heart muscle or are systemic, as opposed to those that can be attributed to abnormalities of other components of the cardiovascular system, in particular, coronary artery disease, valvular disease, congenital anomalies, and systemic or pulmonary hypertension.[1–8] There are three generally recognized forms of cardiomyopathy distinguished by their functional and morphologic features: hypertrophic, congestive or dilated, and restrictive or infiltrative.

HYPERTROPHIC CARDIOMYOPATHY

Definition

Hypertrophic cardiomyopathy (HCM) is defined as unexplained hypertrophy of a nondilated left ventricle.[9,10] In its classic description, this disorder is familial, transmitted in an autosomal dominant fashion,[11,12] and characterized by focal or asymmetric myocardial hypertrophy that preferentially involves the interventricular septum.[10,13–19] Histologically, the area of hypertrophy is generally composed of large numbers of bizarrely shaped, disorganized cardiac muscle cells.[1,19–23] The hypertrophied segment typically encroaches on the left ventricular cavity and, when the septum is involved, on the left ventricular outflow tract.[24] Obstruction, when present, is in most cases associated with systolic anterior motion of the mitral valve into the narrow outflow space[25–31] and is the most widely studied example of functional (as opposed to fixed) subvalvular aortic stenosis. Patients with obstruction can be classified as having *hypertrophic obstructive cardiomyopathy (HOCM),* also referred to as *idiopathic hypertrophic subaortic stenosis (IHSS).*[13,32–37]

Prevalence

Because hypertrophic cardiomyopathy is often asymptomatic, its prevalence in the general population is difficult to determine, with estimates ranging from 0.2% by electrocardiographic screening[38] to at least 1.6% and possibly as high as 4.9% with echocardiographic screening.[39] Our experience favors the intermediate number.

Echocardiographic Features

Echocardiography has emerged as the procedure of choice for establishing this diagnosis because of its ability to measure wall thickness, to display its regional variations, to describe the dynamic relations of the mitral valve to surrounding structures, and to measure intracardiac pressure gradients noninvasively.

The two primary echocardiographic features of hypertrophic cardiomyopathy, asymmetric hypertrophy of the interventricular septum (ASH)[16,40,41] and systolic anterior motion (SAM) of the mitral valve, are illustrated in Figures 25–1 to 25–4. In addition, various other abnormalities, mainly nonspecific, are frequently noted in hypertrophic cardiomyopathy, including anterior displacement of the mitral valve apparatus within the left ventricle,[24] a decrease in left ventricular cavity size,[24] an unusual reflective pattern from the area of hypertro-

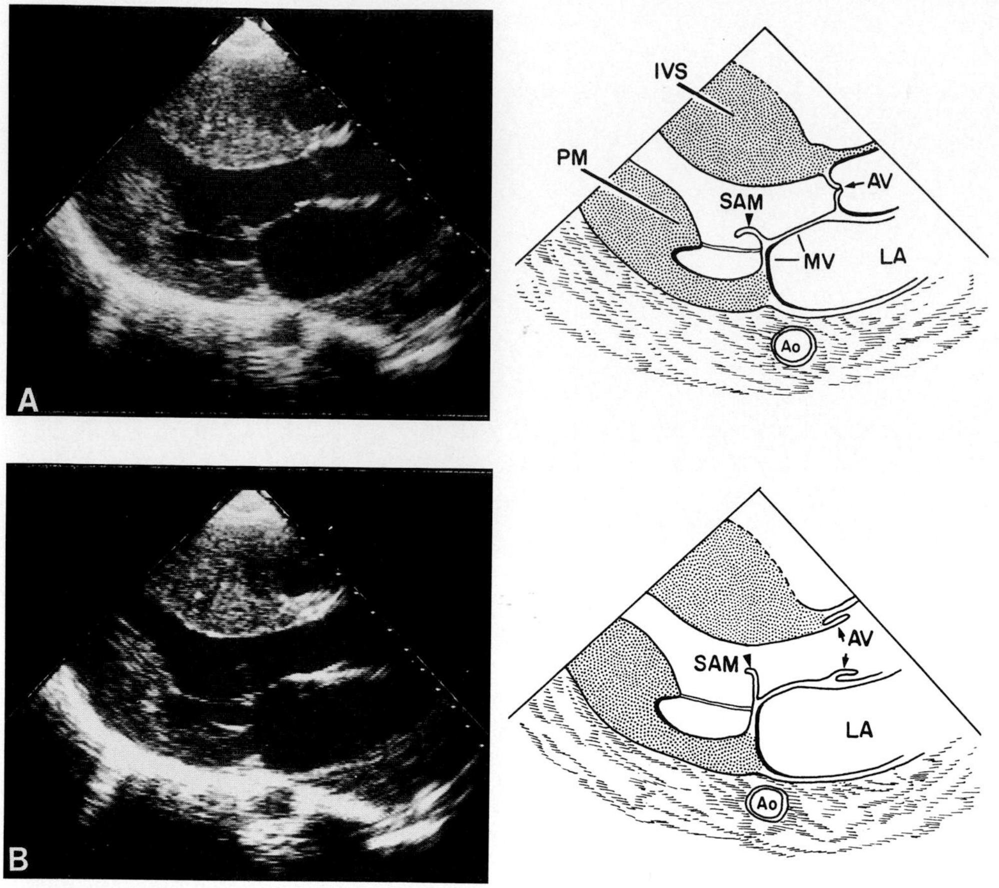

Fig. 25–1. Asymmetric hypertrophy of the interventricular septum (IVS) and systolic anterior motion (SAM) of the mitral valve (MV) in parasternal long axis views of a patient with hypertrophic cardiomyopathy. **A.** The onset of SAM early in systole, before aortic valve (AV) opening, and representing the first video frame after the peak of the ECG QRS complex. **B.** Progressive anterior motion with aortic valve opening. Ao = aorta; LA = left atrium; PM = papillary muscle. (From Jiang L, Levine RA, King ME, Weyman AE: An integrated mechanism to explain the systolic anterior motion of the mitral valve in hypertrophic cardiomyopathy based on echocardiographic observations. Am Heart J 113:633, 1987.)

phied myocardium,[41] left atrial enlargement, abnormal systolic motion of the aortic valve,[29,42] and pericardial effusions that do not appear to have functional significance.

Evaluation of Hypertrophy

Asymmetric Septal Hypertrophy: Definition and Specificity. ASH, defined as thickening of the interventricular septum that produces a septal/free-wall thickness ratio of 1.3 : 1 or greater, was initially felt to be so characteristic of hypertrophic cardiomyopathy that it could be used to identify not only affected patients but also asymptomatic carriers.[11,16,43] Subsequently, it has been shown that concentric left ventricular hypertrophy with symmetric thickening of the septum and left ventricular free wall may, on occasion, be seen in patients with hypertrophic cardiomyopathy whereas asymmetric or disproportionate septal hypertrophy may be found in a variety of congenital and acquired lesions in the absence

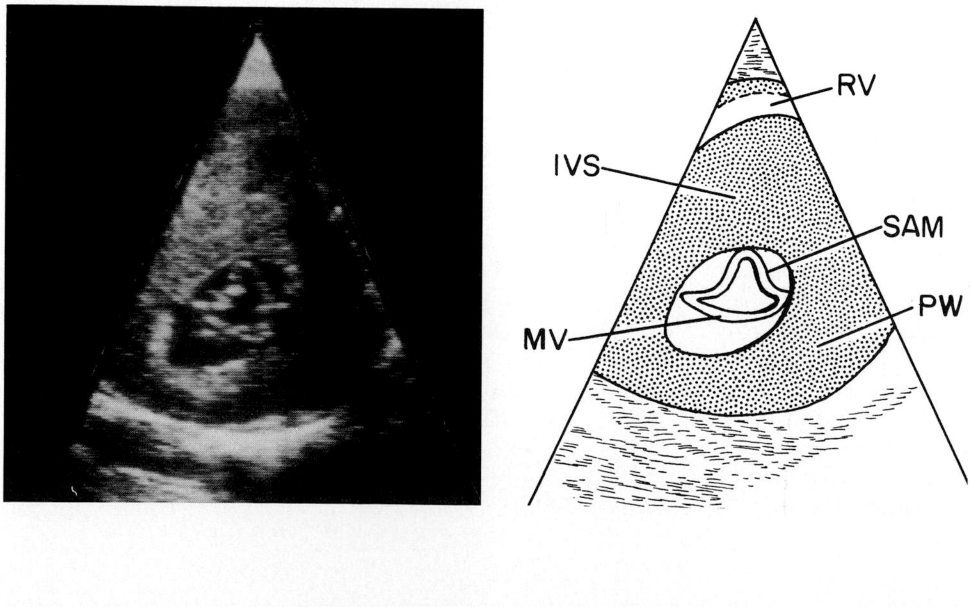

Fig. 25–2. Systolic anterior motion (SAM) of the mitral valve (MV) in a short axis view of the left ventricle in a patient with hypertrophy of the interventricular septum (IVS) extending into the anterolateral walls. Leaflet-septal contact occurs at the center of the valve, while the lateral leaflet portions remain relatively posterior. PW = posterior wall; RV = right ventricle. (From Jiang L, Levine RA, King ME, Weyman AE: An integrated mechanism to explain the systolic anterior motion of the mitral valve in hypertrophic cardiomyopathy based on echocardiographic observations. Am Heart J 113:633, 1987.)

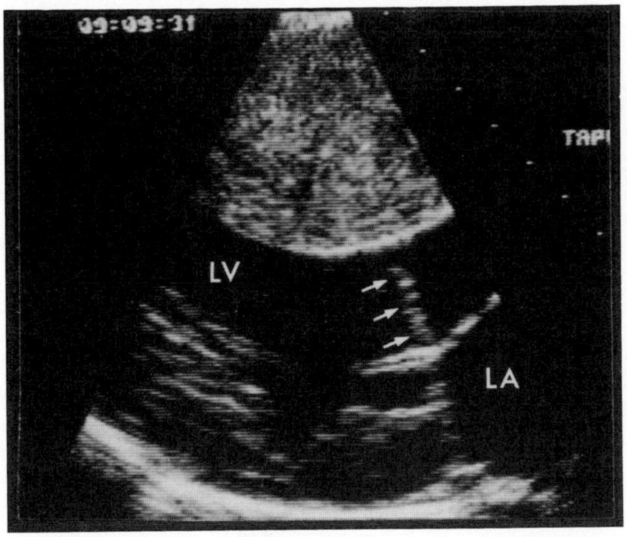

Fig. 25–3. Close-up view of systolic anterior motion of the mitral valve (arrowheads) approaching the interventricular septum in a parasternal long axis view. The highly reflective acoustic texture of the septum can be appreciated. LV = left ventricle; LA = left atrium.

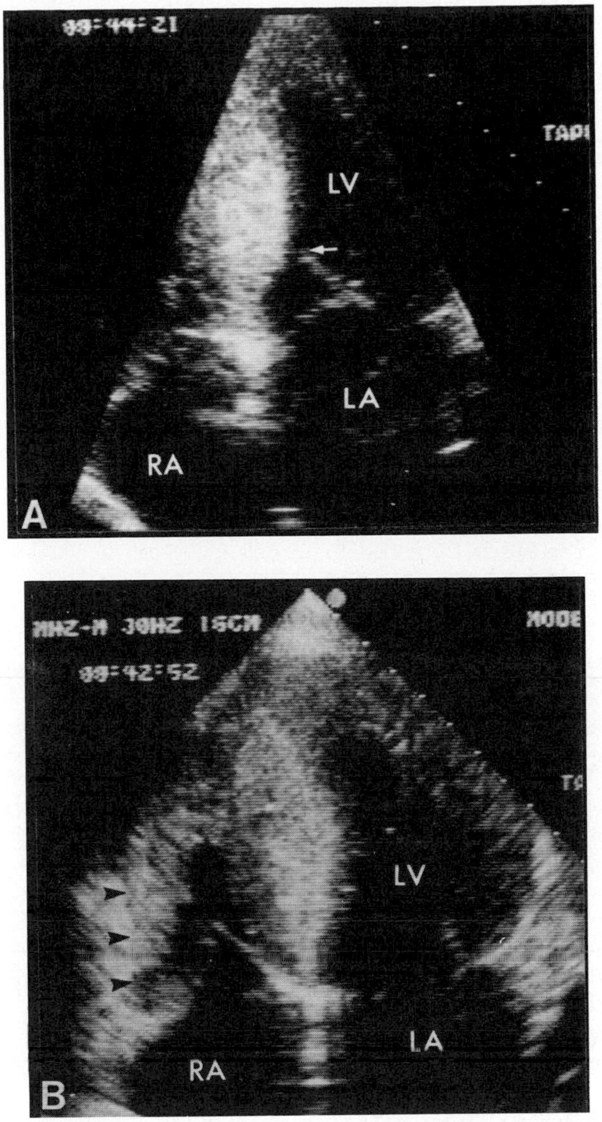

Fig. 25–4. A. Systolic anterior motion (arrow) in an apical four-chamber view, moving to contact the subaortic interventricular septum. **B.** Right ventricular as well as left ventricular hypertrophy demonstrated in this view. LA = left atrium; LV = left ventricle; RA = right atrium; RV = right ventricle.

of hypertrophic cardiomyopathy.[9,10,19,44–46] Disproportionate septal hypertrophy appears to be a normal finding in the fetus and disappears by the age of 1 to 2 years.[47] Although hypertrophic cardiomyopathy occurs in infants,[48] it must be distinguished from a transient condition in infants born to insulin-dependent diabetic mothers, which is characterized by ASH, functional subaortic obstruction, and heart failure.[49,50] In the older child and adult, disproportionate septal hypertrophy may be seen with lesions producing long-standing right ventricular hypertension, such as valvular pulmonary stenosis and primary pulmonary hypertension, as well as in D-transposition of the great arteries.[51–53] It may also be seen, albeit less frequently, in patients with aortic stenosis, systemic hypertension, Eisenmenger's syndrome, and a variety of other conditions, including septal sarcomas, amyloidosis, glycogen and mucopolysaccharide storage diseases, Freidreich's ataxia, and myxedema (in which reversible changes have been described).[44,46,51–61] Coexisting concentric hypertrophy and free wall infarction can also produce the appearance of ASH without prominent septal hypertrophy or obstructive physiology. Thus, although the reported specificity of ASH as an echocardiographic marker of hypertrophic cardiomyopathy remains high (90%, e.g., in a large series[46]), in individual cases one may not be able to distinguish reliably between secondary disproportionate septal thickening and a primary hypertrophic cardiomyopathy on the basis of the simple echocardiographic measurement alone.[46] The distribution and extent of hypertrophy, however, may provide additional diagnostic information. Localized areas of marked hypertrophy or right ventricular free wall involvement (Fig. 25–4) are clearly more specific for a hypertrophic myopathy than is generalized septal thickening.[17,62] Practically—because asymmetric hypertrophy is generally primary in nature[18,46]—in the absence of other obvious causes (particularly congenital), it can be described as consistent with hypertrophic cardiomyopathy. If hypertrophy is truly concentric in two-dimensional views,[18] hypertrophic cardiomyopathy can be listed in the differential diagnosis, particularly if the hypertrophy is prominent; evidence favoring that diagnosis, such as systolic anterior motion of the mitral valve and right ventricular hypertrophy, should be noted.[46,62]

Distribution of Hypertrophy. Hypertrophic cardiomyopathy is characterized by its pleomorphism. Hypertrophy most commonly involves the interventricular septum and anterolateral wall, although in substantial numbers of patients, only the septum or its anterior segments are involved.[10,17,19] (Figs. 25–5 and 25–6). Hypertrophy is noted most frequently in the upper and middle

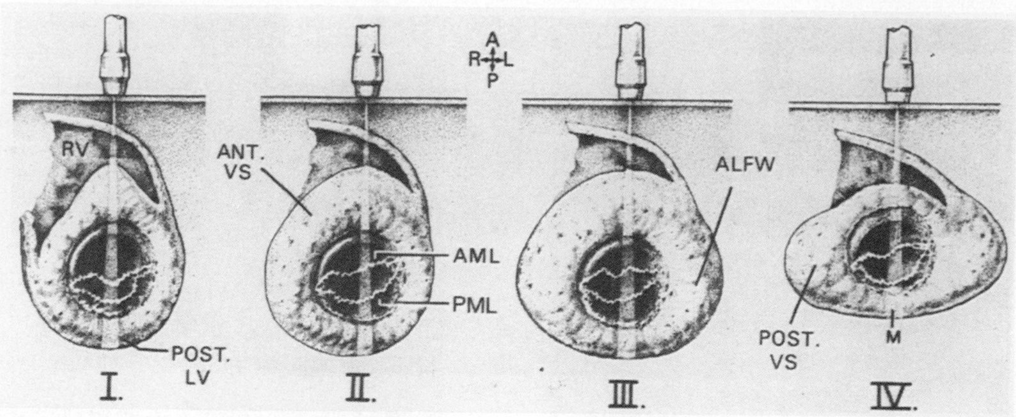

Fig. 25–5. Four major patterns of asymmetric hypertrophy seen in patients with hypertrophic cardiomyopathy, including anteroseptal (I) and panseptal (II) hypertrophy, more extensive involvement sparing the posterior wall (III), and a relatively rare medial and lateral form (IV). Note that the M-mode beam (M) does not portray the full distribution of hypertrophy seen in these cross-sectional views at the mitral valve level. ALFW = anterolateral free wall; AML = anterior mitral leaflet; ANT VS = anterior ventricular septum; PML = posterior mitral leaflet; POST LV = posterior left ventricular wall; RV = right ventricle. (From Maron BJ: Asymmetry in hypertrophic cardiomyopathy: the septal to free wall ratio revisited. Am J Cardiol 55:835, 1985. With permission of the author and Cahners Publishing Co.)

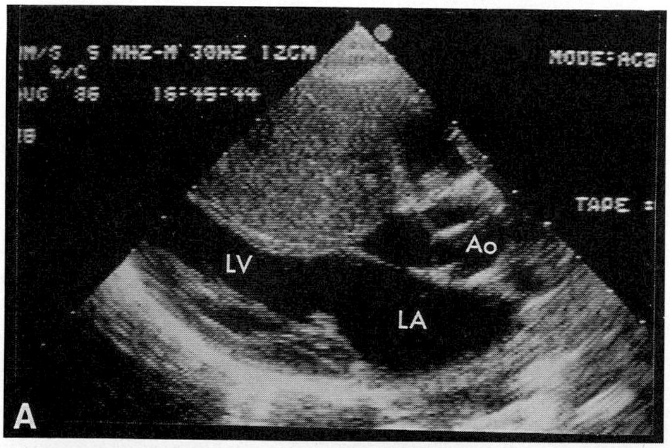

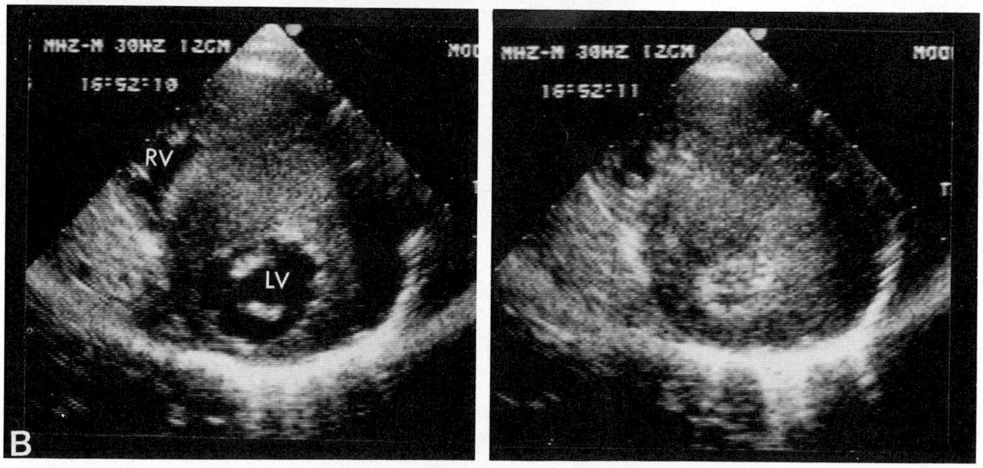

Fig. 25–6. **A.** Severe hypertrophy of the entire ventricular septum with sparing of the left ventricular (LV) free wall as seen in a long axis view. **B.** Corresponding diastolic (left) and systolic (right) short axis views at the mitral valve level illustrating the marked asymmetry of hypertrophy and systolic cavity obliteration. Ao = aorta; LA = left atrium; RV = right ventricle.

portions of the septum; hypertrophy of the lower third of the septum is less common.[17,19,41] Involvement of the entire septum, creating a crescentic residual left ventricular cavity, has been described, particularly in younger patients with severe hypertrophy often involving the right ventricle.[63] Few patients have predominant hypertrophy of the inferior and lateral segments or the posterobasal free wall[17,64,65] (Figs. 25–7 and 25–8). Apical hypertrophy, originally described in Japan but subsequently found in non-Japanese patients as well,[66–69] produces a characteristic spade-like appearance of the left ventricle that is due to systolic obliteration of the apical

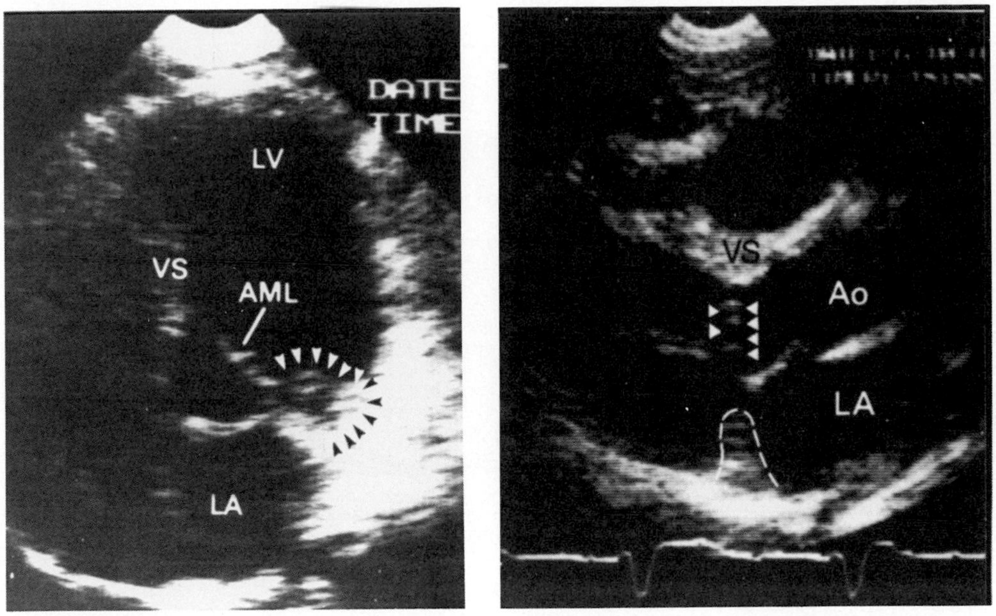

Fig. 25–7. Localized posterobasal hypertrophy seen in the apical four-chamber view (left; arrowheads) and parasternal long axis view (right; dotted line) in systole. Despite normal thickness of the ventricular septum (VS), there is prominent systolic anterior motion of the anterior mitral leaflet (AML; arrows, right). Ao = aorta; LA = left atrium; LV = left ventricle. (From Maron BJ, Spirito P, Chiarella F, Vecchio C: Unusual distribution of left ventricular hypertrophy in obstructive hypertrophic cardiomyopathy: localized posterobasal free wall thickening in two patients. J Am Coll Cardiol 5:1474, 1985. Reprinted with permission from the American College of Cardiology. Journal of the American College of Cardiology. 1985, 5, 1474.)

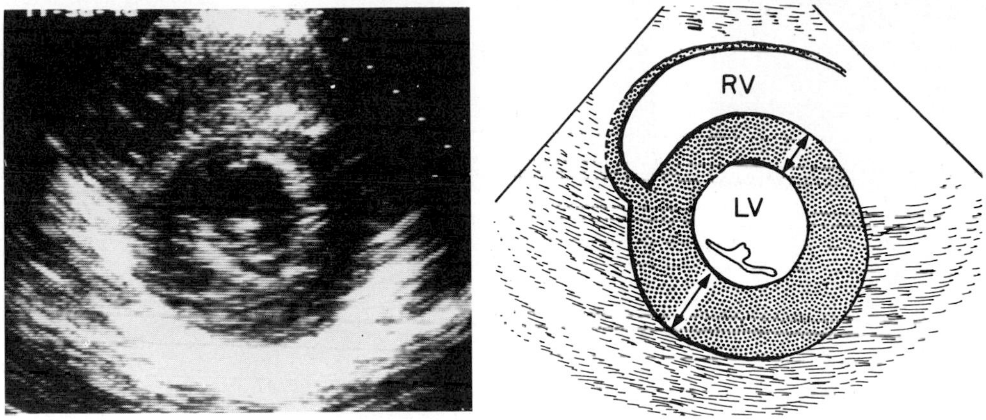

Fig. 25–8. Parasternal short axis view showing greater hypertrophy of the inferoposterior wall (lower arrow) than the anterior wall (upper arrow), an unusual finding. LV = left ventricle; RV = right ventricle.

cavity; as a rule, it is unassociated with outflow obstruction unless the hypertrophy also extends toward the outflow tract (Fig. 25–9). Atypical patterns may also be noted, such as midventricular constricting rings and medial-lateral dumbbell-like areas of hypertrophy producing systolic midcavity obstruction[70–72a] (Fig. 25–10). Apical infarction with localized aneurysm formation (Fig. 25–11) has been described in association with such midventricular hypertrophy[72] and has been ascribed to increased wall stress in the obstructed apical segment, possibly combined with underlying small vessel coronary disease.[73] Truly concentric hypertrophy in hypertrophic cardiomyopathy (Fig. 25–12) is now felt to be less common than previously thought, given the improved ability of two-dimensional echocardiography to display segmental asymmetries not previously apparent by M-mode studies[10,17–19] (Fig. 25–13).

Extent of Hypertrophy and Its Significance. In general, the more extensive the involvement, the more severe the functional impact and the outflow obstruc-

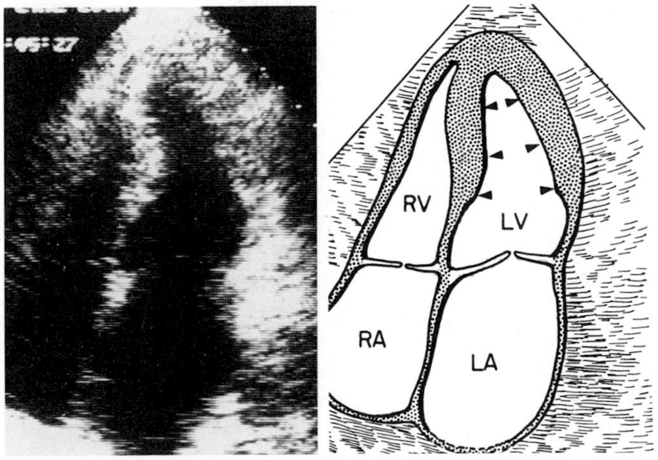

Fig. 25–9. Apical predominance of hypertrophy as seen in an apical four-chamber view, with normal thickness of the basal myocardium. LA = left atrium; LV = left ventricle; RA = right atrium; RV = right ventricle.

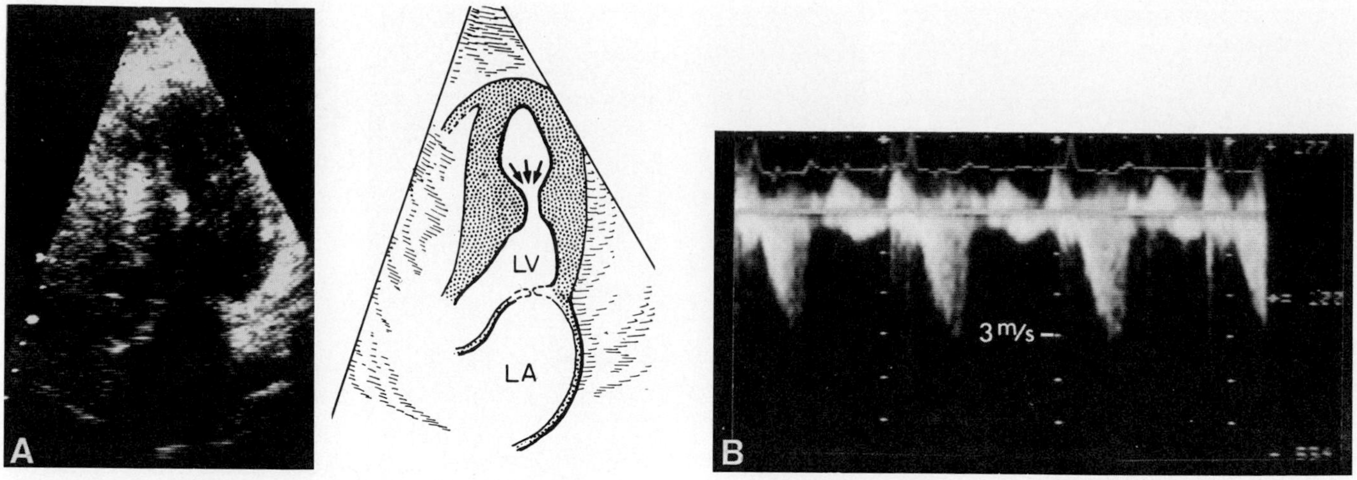

Fig. 25–10. **A.** Apical view showing a midventricular constricting ring, with flow exiting from the apex indicated by arrows in the line drawing. **B.** Late-peaking systolic velocities created by this dynamic stenosis, which progressively narrows the area available for flow. LA = left atrium; LV = left ventricle.

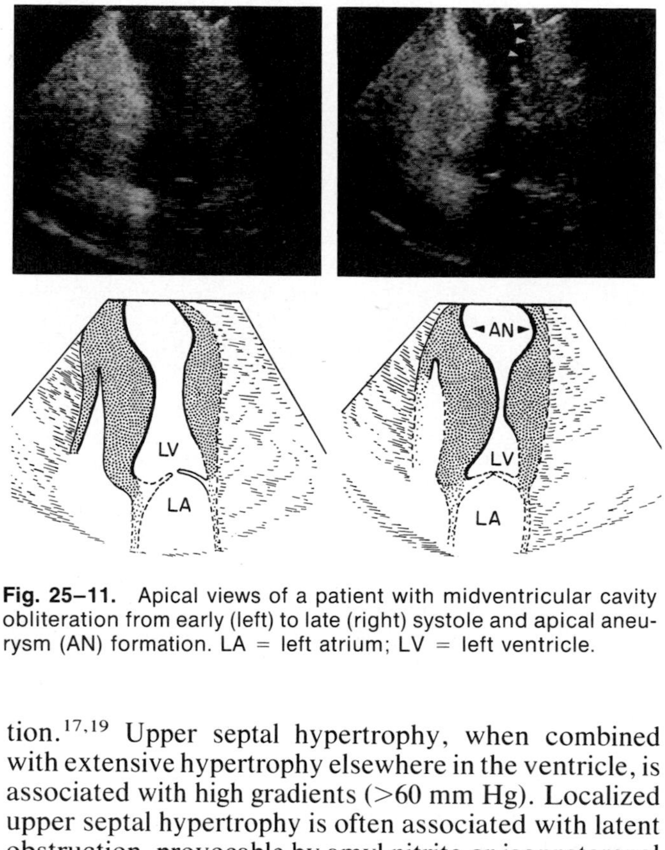

Fig. 25–11. Apical views of a patient with midventricular cavity obliteration from early (left) to late (right) systole and apical aneurysm (AN) formation. LA = left atrium; LV = left ventricle.

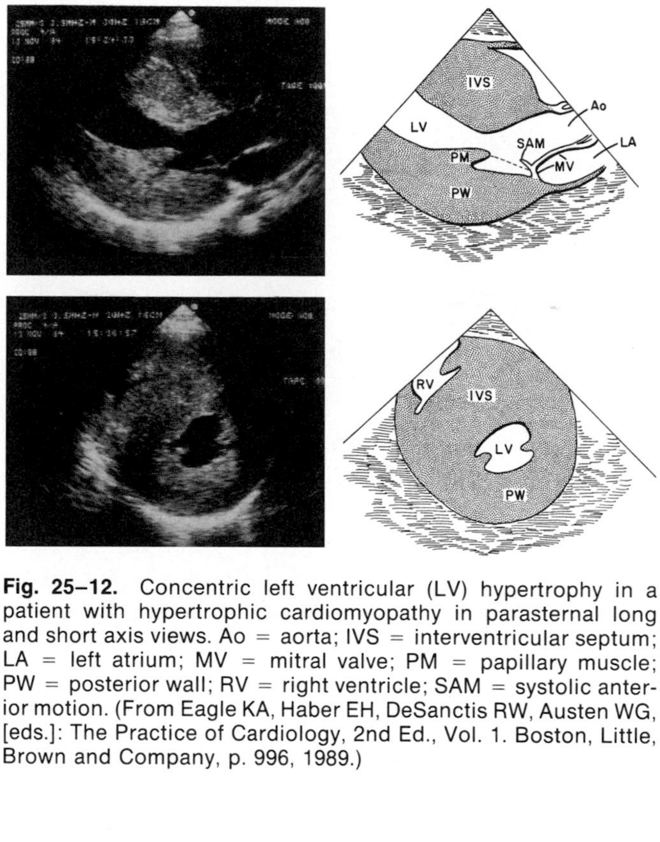

Fig. 25–12. Concentric left ventricular (LV) hypertrophy in a patient with hypertrophic cardiomyopathy in parasternal long and short axis views. Ao = aorta; IVS = interventricular septum; LA = left atrium; MV = mitral valve; PM = papillary muscle; PW = posterior wall; RV = right ventricle; SAM = systolic anterior motion. (From Eagle KA, Haber EH, DeSanctis RW, Austen WG, [eds.]: The Practice of Cardiology, 2nd Ed., Vol. 1. Boston, Little, Brown and Company, p. 996, 1989.)

tion.[17,19] Upper septal hypertrophy, when combined with extensive hypertrophy elsewhere in the ventricle, is associated with high gradients (>60 mm Hg). Localized upper septal hypertrophy is often associated with latent obstruction, provocable by amyl nitrite or isoproterenol infusion.[19] In asymptomatic or mildly symptomatic adult patients, sudden death appears to bear a relationship to the extent of hypertrophy and is uncommon in those with mild hypertrophy.[74] Changes in the pattern of diastolic mitral inflow, on the other hand, could not be related to the degree of hypertrophy in a recent study[75]; the determinants of these patterns, however, are complex (see following discussion).

Technical Factors in the Diagnosis of ASH. M-mode scanning can produce a spurious appearance of ASH if the beam passes obliquely through the septum but remains perpendicular to the posterior left ventricular wall.[76–78] This artifact is particularly common with the transducer located in a lower intercostal space.[76,79] The two-dimensional study is not immune from such artifacts in parasternal short axis views; asymmetry should therefore be confirmed in long axis views. Precise demarcation of the septal borders and correct recognition of left parasternal bands (Fig. 25–14) and right-sided papillary muscles as discrete from the septum are best accomplished with cross-sectional scanning:[80] such longitudinal structures, which could be interpreted as ASH in

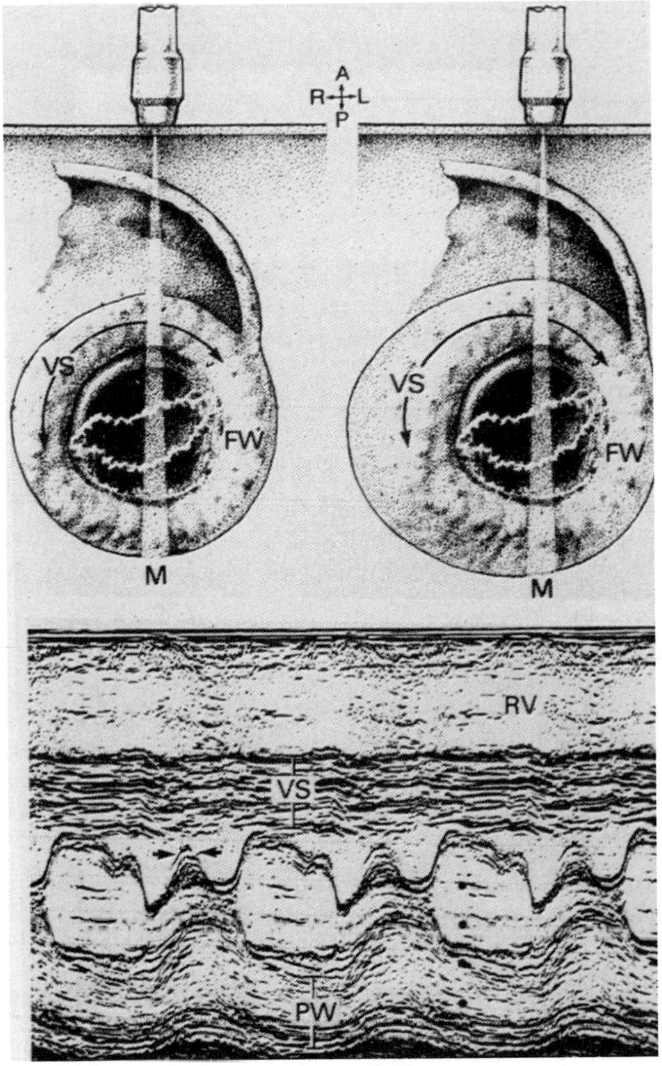

Fig. 25–13. Appreciation of ventricular hypertrophy. The M-mode technique (M) portrays both patients in the upper panel as having equal thickness of the ventricular septum (VS) and free wall (FW); only the two-dimensional scan can display the asymmetry on the right. The improved temporal resolution of the M-mode, on the other hand, allows the duration of mitral approach to the septum to be measured (arrows, below). A = anterior; P = posterior; PW = posterior wall; RV = right ventricle. (From Maron BJ: Asymmetry in hypertrophic cardiomyopathy: the septal to free wall ratio revisited. Am J Cardiol 55:835, 1985. With permission of the author and Cahners Publishing Co.)

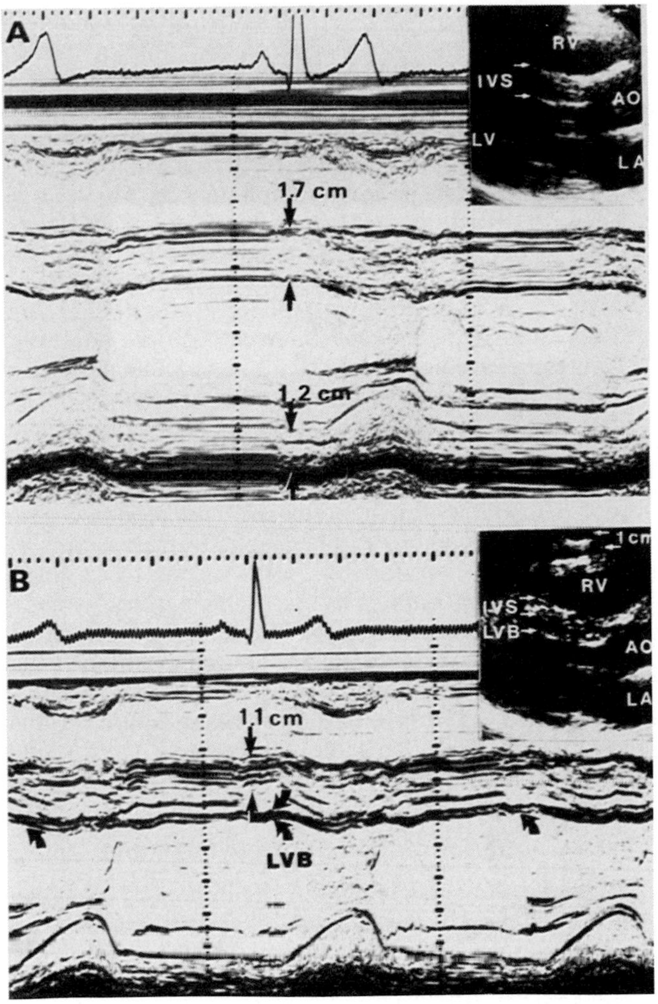

Fig. 25–14. In making the diagnosis of asymmetric septal hypertrophy, one must exclude paraseptal bands. In this patient, asymmetric hypertrophy was suggested by the initial M-mode and two-dimensional study **(A),** but on closer scrutiny **(B)** could be resolved as a septum (IVS) of *normal* thickness with a distinct left ventricular band (LVB) posterior to it. RV = right ventricle; Ao = aorta; LA = left atrium. (From Keren A, Billingham ME, Popp RL: Echocardiographic recognition of paraseptal structures. J Am Coll Cardiol 6:913, 1985. Reprinted with permission from the American College of Cardiology.)

long axis views, will have only a limited circumferential extent on short axis views.

Acoustic Texture of the Septum. The area of focal hypertrophy frequently has a speckled acoustic texture resembling ground glass, which has been noted as an adjunct feature in the diagnosis of hypertrophic cardiomyopathy[41] (Fig. 25–3). A similar but more diffuse pattern is also encountered in infiltrative disorders, such as cardiac amyloidosis.[59] (See later discussion of tissue characterization.) This unusual reflection pattern may represent an echocardiographic expression of the abnormal myocardial architecture. Recent studies, however, have shown that the presence of a finely granular texture in the septum and its absence in the posterior wall in parasternal long axis views do not necessarily imply that architectural changes are *limited* to the septum.[81,82] This discrepancy has, in fact, been reproduced with phantoms, which display a granular texture in the near field but not in the far field of the transducer, where the granular reflections are broadened into arcs by the point-spread function of the beam at the increased depth.

Epidemiologic Considerations in the Evaluation of Hypertrophy. The discussion to this point has dealt largely with the classic forms of the disease, characterized by prominent left ventricular hypertrophy. It is important to keep in mind, however, that most of our knowledge of this disease has been derived from studying patients sufficiently affected to present to medical attention and to be referred to several large specialized centers. The extent of hypertrophy is, in fact, often milder in screened relatives of such patients,[83–85] and the disease has a more benign prognosis in patients identified by routine screening of students and workers.[86]

Genetics of Hypertrophy. The echocardiographer is often asked to screen families for hypertrophic cardiomyopathy after one or more of their members have come to medical attention. It is important to be aware, therefore, that the inheritance patterns of this condition appear to be as variable as its morphologic manifestations. While initial echocardiographic referral studies suggested familial occurrence in over 90% of patients,[11] more recent studies have shown a familial pattern in only 56% of patients, with sporadic occurrence in the remainder.[84,85] The majority of familial patterns are consistent with autosomal dominance, but other patterns are evident, with incomplete penetrance. Markedly different distributions of hypertrophy can be noted even within families demonstrating genetic transmission.[83–85] This variability is consistent with recent DNA probe studies that show familial hypertrophic cardiomyopathy to be a genetically heterogeneous disease.[87] Both genetic studies and counseling are limited by the fact that the disease may not become apparent until adolescence or afterward, even in kindreds showing familial transmission.[49,88] After the adolescent growth spurt, however, progression of hypertrophy is rare.[89]

Systolic Anterior Motion of the Mitral Valve

Dynamic Subaortic Stenosis: Evolution of the Concept. Beginning in the late 1950s, several groups were surprised to find patients with pressure gradients across the left ventricular outflow tract but no identifiable fixed anatomic cause of obstruction. These included patients who had undergone surgery for fixed valvular aortic stenosis and had persistent pressure gradients postoperatively and patients with concentric and asymmetric left ventricular hypertrophy.[13,33,34,90–92] In some of these patients, the "functional aortic stenosis"[92] was relieved by removing small amounts of myocardium from the upper interventricular septum.[93] The initial concept, therefore, evolved that systolic contraction of the hypertrophied muscle itself caused obstruction, explaining the patency of the outflow tract to probing in vivo[92] and the absence of an identifiable fixed obstruction. Subsequently, however, the focus shifted to the mitral valve when angiographic studies in patients with functional outflow obstruction demonstrated left ventricular filling defects, which were tentatively identified as portions of the mitral leaflets moving anteriorly in systole to contact the interventricular septum and obstruct outflow.[35,94–99] The precise nature and timing of this motion was clarified by echocardiography beginning in the late 1960s, with identification of the moving element as the distal mitral valve.[24–27,41,100,101]

Anterior Mitral Valve Motion. The actual functional outflow obstruction in hypertrophic cardiomyopathy is produced by independent anterior displacement of the mitral valve (with attached chordae tendinea) into the left ventricular outflow tract during systole. This anterior motion involves the distal mitral valve from the coaptation point to the tip,[101] with the coapted body of the leaflet held in position by the pressure difference between the left atrium and left ventricle. Systolic anterior motion may involve either or both leaflets,[102,103]

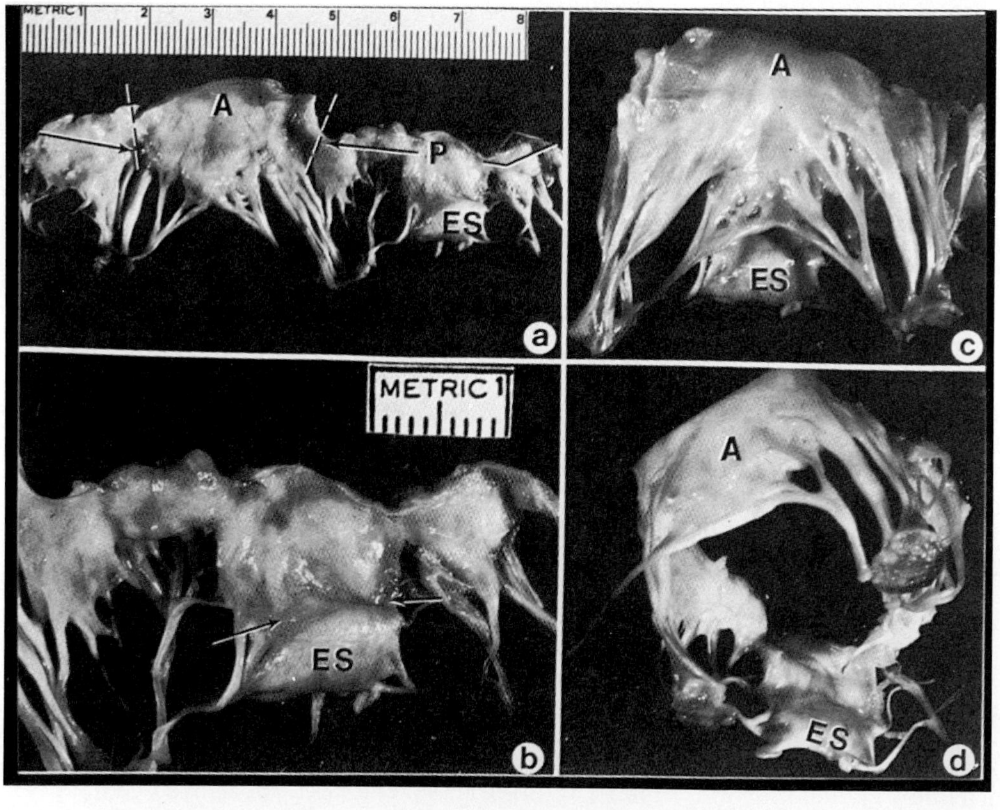

Fig. 25–15. Mitral valve removed at operation from a patient with hypertrophic cardiomyopathy and systolic anterior motion of the posterior mitral leaflet (P), which has an elongated central scallop (ES) that is relatively free to move anteriorly in the V-shaped space between the normal chordal insertions to the anterior mitral leaflet (A), as suggested by Figure **C. B.** The groove is felt to indicate the line of leaflet coaptation. (From Maron BJ, et al.: Systolic anterior motion of the posterior mitral leaflet: a previously unrecognized cause of dynamic subaortic obstruction in patients with hypertrophic cardiomyopathy. Circulation 68:282, 1983. Reproduced by permission of the American Heart Association, Inc.)

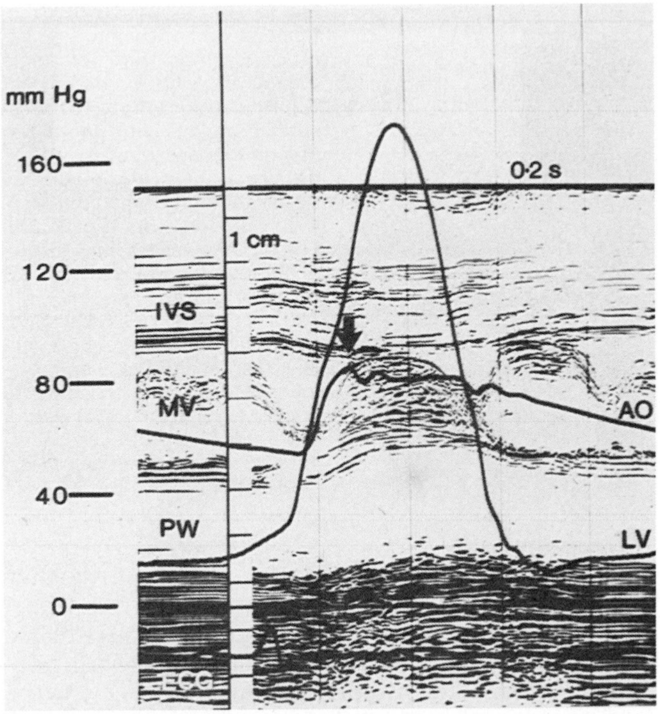

Fig. 25–16. Simultaneous recordings of left ventricular pressure (LV), central aortic pressure (AO), and mitral valve (MV) motion showing a marked increase in outflow tract gradient with mitral-septal contact (arrow). IVS = interventricular septum; PW = posterior wall. (From Pollick C, et al.: Muscular subaortic stenosis: the temporal relationship between systolic anterior motion of the anterior mitral leaflet and the pressure gradient. Circulation 66: 1087, 1982. Reproduced by permission of the American Heart Association, Inc.)

with posterior leaflet SAM appearing to involve an elongated central scallop of the posterior leaflet that moves anteriorly in a gap between the chordal connections to the anterior leaflet[102] (Fig. 25–15). Figures 25–1 to 25–4, and 25–13 show examples of this abnormal systolic motion.

Systolic Anterior Motion as Evidence of Obstruction. Close approach or contact of the mitral valve with the septum is temporally correlated with both significant gradient development and abrupt deceleration of flow in the aortic root (Figs. 25–16 and 25–17).[30,31,104,105] The severity of obstruction has been related to both the absolute reduction in outflow tract size and the degree and duration of SAM of the mitral valve. An outflow tract diameter of less than 20 mm has been reported in as many as 66% of patients with obstruction but was not observed in normal persons and occurred rarely in patients with nonobstructive hypertrophic cardiomyopathy.[24] The magnitude and duration of the SAM has been demonstrated to correlate with the severity of the intraventricular gradient, both under basal conditions and with provocative maneuvers (Fig. 25–18) and to vary in parallel from beat to beat in atrial fibrillation.[28–31,106,107] In general, obstruction occurs if the mitral valve contacts the septum for 30% or more of systole.[28–31] Maneuvers that decrease ventricular volume or increase contractility can prolong the duration of mitral-septal contact in the same patient, with an associated increase in gradient.[31]

Technical Factors in the Evaluation of Systolic Anterior Motion. In any consideration of the systolic motion of the mitral valve, one must remember that the coapted mitral leaflets are fixed at the papillary muscle level and

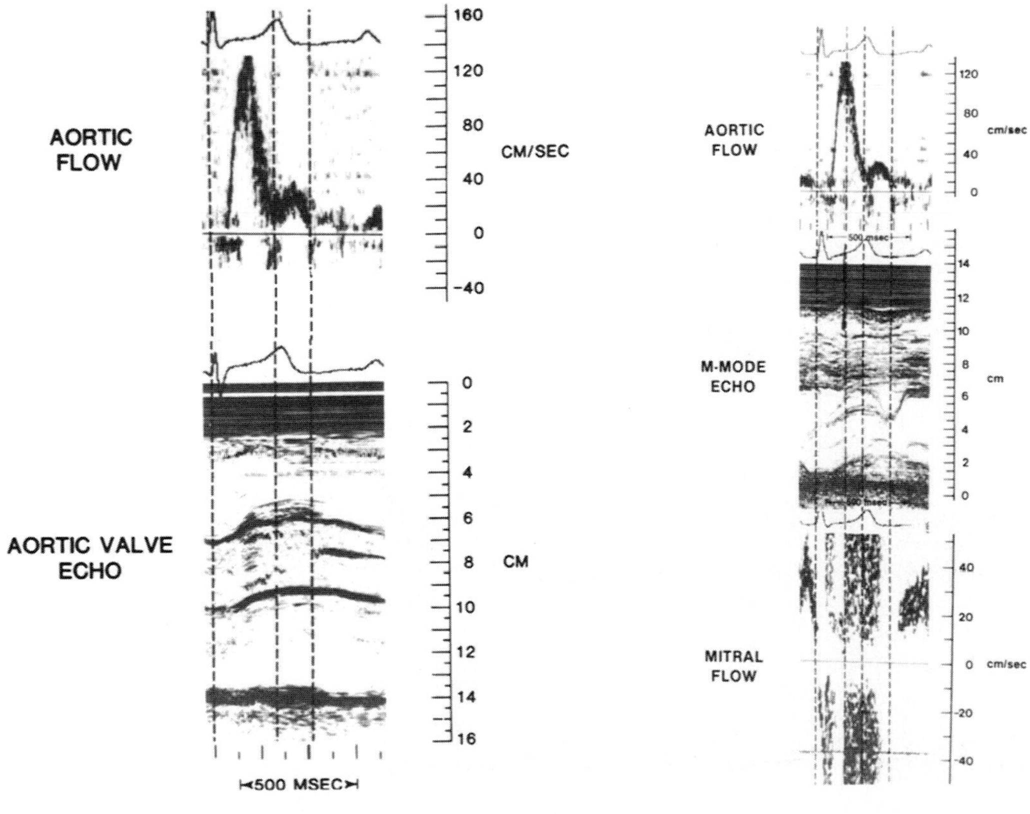

Fig. 25–17. Correspondence between deceleration of forward flow in the aorta, midsystolic partial aortic valve closure (left), and mitral-septal contact (right). (The lower right panel shows turbulent flow in the left atrium indicating mitral regurgitation.) (From Gardin JM, et al.: Echocardiographic and Doppler flow observations in obstructed and non-obstructed hypertrophic cardiomyopathy. Am J Cardiol 56:614, 1985. With permission of the authors and Cahners Publishing Co.)

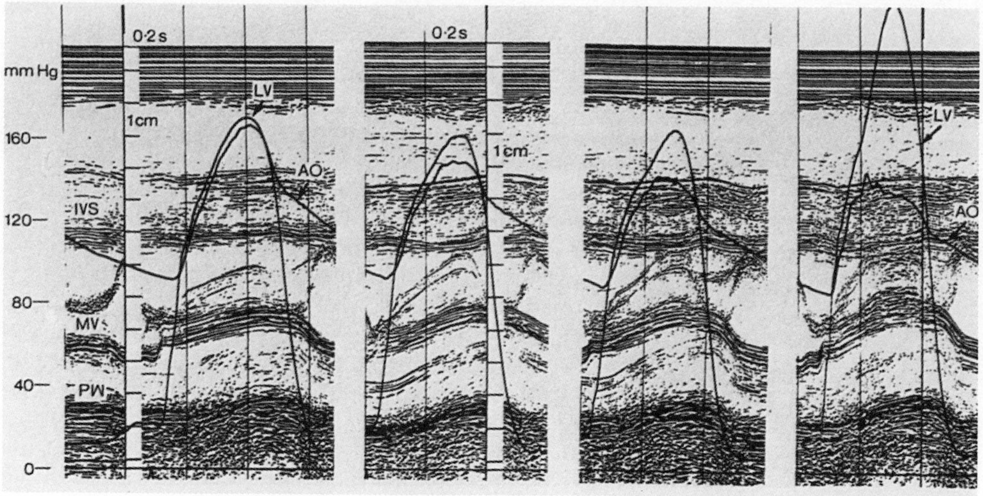

Fig. 25–18. Four sets of simultaneous hemodynamic and M-mode tracings from the same patient showing increasing left ventricular-aortic (LV-AO) pressure gradient with increased magnitude and duration of mitral-septal contact created by pharmacologic manipulation. IVS = interventricular septum; MV = mitral valve; PW = posterior wall; LV = left ventricle; AO = aorta. (From Pollick C, Rakowski H, Wigle ED: Muscular subaortic stenosis: the quantitative relationship between systolic anterior motion and the pressure gradient. Circulation 69:43, 1984. Reproduced by permission of the American Heart Association, Inc.)

at the mitral valve ring. During systole, therefore, the mitral apparatus normally moves anteriorly in unison with the anterior motion of the posterior left ventricular wall, annulus, and papillary muscles. Any phenomenon that exaggerates the normal systolic anterior motion of these points of mitral valve attachment will, of necessity, increase the anterior motion of the coapted leaflets. It is not surprising, therefore, that increased systolic motion of the mitral apparatus has been described in conditions associated with exaggerated left ventricular posterior wall motion, such as left ventricular aneurysm, anterior wall myocardial infarction, and left ventricular volume overload.[46,108] This mitral valve motion is not, by itself, abnormal, but merely represents the obligatory anterior motion of the mitral apparatus in unison with the exaggerated movement of its points of attachment.

The most common form of SAM seen on routine studies involves only chordal structures,[109] reflecting a normal degree of chordal laxity, which presumably allows the valve to adapt to changing ventricular volume. Practically, chordal SAM involves structures that appear thinner than the leaflet bodies on the echocardiogram and that can most clearly be differentiated from leaflet SAM in the short axis view, where one or more isolated chordae, as opposed to a continuous leaflet structure, can be seen moving into the outflow tract (Fig. 25–19). Two-dimensional echocardiography can also differentiate anterior motion of linear leaflet structures from that of more rounded or irregular masses or vegetations attached to the mitral leaflets; such masses can move anteriorly during systole if not sufficiently restrained.[19]

In assessing the duration of mitral-septal contact by the M-mode technique, it must be remembered that the proximity of the two structures involved will be underestimated if the beam does not pass through the point of maximal anterior leaflet motion at the distal leaflet tip. Also, the degree of contact varies across the mediolateral width of the leaflet (Fig. 25–2).[110] Because the degree of obstruction is determined by the cross-sectional area between the mitral valve and the septum,[111] a single M-mode tracing can overestimate the degree of obstruction if there is uneven mitral-septal contact, such as may

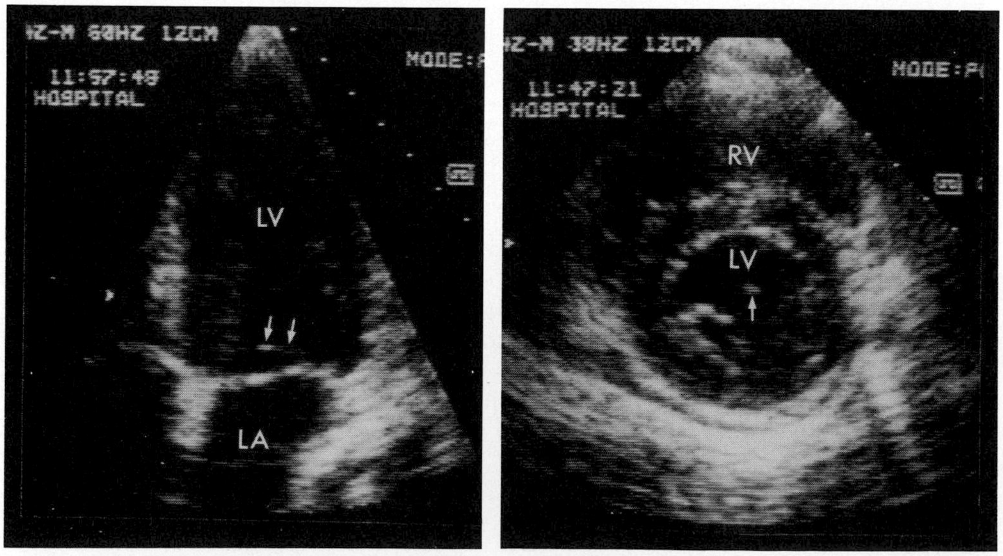

Fig. 25–19. Left. Chordal systolic anterior motion (arrows) in an apical four-chamber systolic image. Right. In the parasternal short axis view, the anterior motion can be seen to involve only an isolated chord (arrow), as opposed to a continuous leaflet surface. LV = left ventricle; LA = left atrium; RV = right ventricle.

occur in milder degrees of SAM involving only the center of the leaflet, or with persistent systolic anterior motion following myomectomy.[112]

Aortic Valve Motion

Partial midsystolic closure of the aortic valve is another, currently subsidiary, form of evidence for subaortic obstruction[29,42] and appears to reflect the abrupt decrease in aortic blood flow that occurs halfway to three-quarters of the way through the systolic ejection period.[104,105] Only one or two cusps exhibit this partial closure, which may be explained by an asymmetric post-stenotic outflow tract jet that maintains the opening of the cusps against which it is directed and fails to support the others. The unsupported cusps may also be drawn centrally by the Venturi effect created by this high velocity jet. This finding, however, is not pathognomonic for obstruction and can be noted when the upper septum inserts into the aortic root below and posterior to the right coronary cusp of the aortic valve (Fig. 25–20). The septal protuberance deflects flow into the posterior aortic lumen, and the right coronary cusp is unsupported by flow and returns to a more posterior position after its initial opening (determined by a small early-systolic pressure difference between the left ventricle and aorta). Milder degrees of this motion have also been described with mitral regurgitation, mitral prosthesis, ventricular septal defect, and aortic root dilation, reflecting altered flow patterns in the outflow tract or aortic sinuses.[42,113,114] Aortic valve closure in discrete subaortic stenosis occurs earlier in systole and tends to be more complete.

Functional Characteristics of the Hypertrophied Muscle

The percentage of systolic septal thickening in hypertrophic cardiomyopathy has been reported to be decreased,[115,116] although this may reflect the prominent diastolic thickness (large denominator). It has recently been suggested that the percentage of thickening is normal if measured at a consistent location within the septum on the two-dimensional study and that previous underestimates were caused by the M-mode tracings' traversing different portions of the contracting septum at different points within the cardiac cycle.[117]

Although ventricular function has often been described as hyperdynamic in hypertrophic cardiomyopathy, this may relate, at least in part, to the small end-diastolic cavity size, which will produce a higher ejection fraction for a given stroke volume. It has also been shown that the normal relationship between wall stress and ejection fraction prevails in patients with hypertrophic cardiomyopathy: Wall stress is decreased by the hypertrophy, and the ejection fraction is commensurately higher.[118] Progression of hypertrophic cardiomyopathy to a dilated hypokinetic state is rare.[119–124]

Doppler Evaluation of Hypertrophic Cardiomyopathy

Outflow Tract Obstruction

Outflow Velocities and Pressure Gradient. Currently, Doppler ultrasound provides the most reliable assessment of left ventricular outflow obstruction, overcoming the previously noted limitations of the M-mode evaluation of mitral-septal contact and aortic valve closure. The modified Bernoulli equation (pressure gradient = 4 × velocity^2), which assumes negligible viscous losses, can successfully predict the pressure gradient across the outflow tract both at rest and following maneuvers such as verapamil administration.[125–129] In practice, the left ventricular outflow tract is scanned from an apical window by moving a sample volume from the midventricular cavity to the region where the mitral valve approaches the septum to detect the rise in velocity at that site, indicating stenosis.[130] A continuous-wave Doppler beam is then directed into the outflow tract to detect the high velocity jet, which accelerates in mid- to late-systole and parallels the development and progression of mitral-septal contact (Fig. 25–21).[127,128,130,131] Color Doppler flow mapping can facilitate and guide this examination by visually demonstrating flow acceleration proximal to the region of mitral-septal contact and the

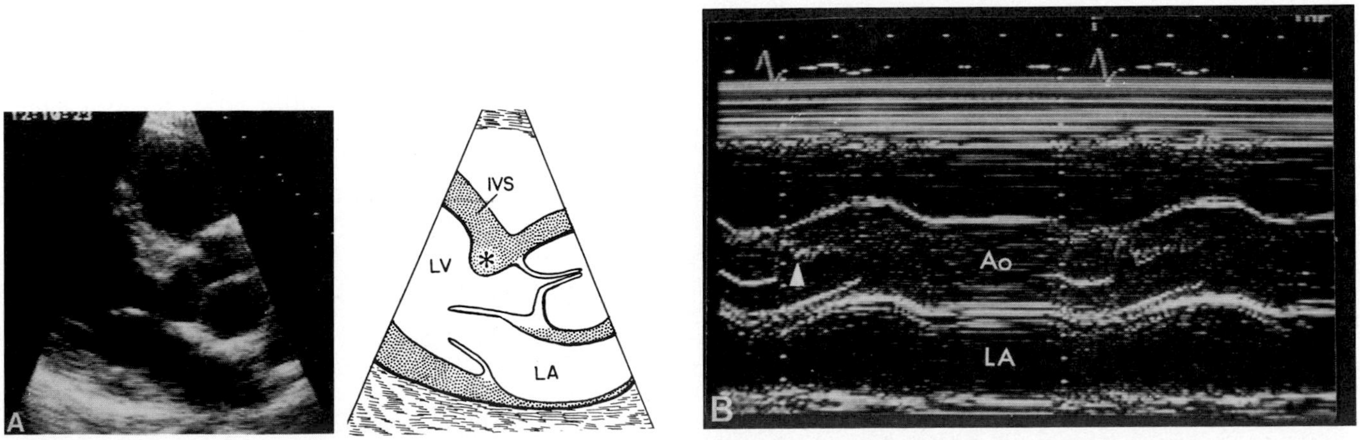

Fig. 25–20. Midsystolic partial closure of the right coronary cusp of the aortic valve (**B,** arrow) in a patient with insertion of the upper septum below and posterior to that cusp (**A,** asterisk) but no Doppler evidence of outflow tract obstruction. Ao = aorta; IVS = interventricular septum; LA = left atrium; LV = left ventricle.

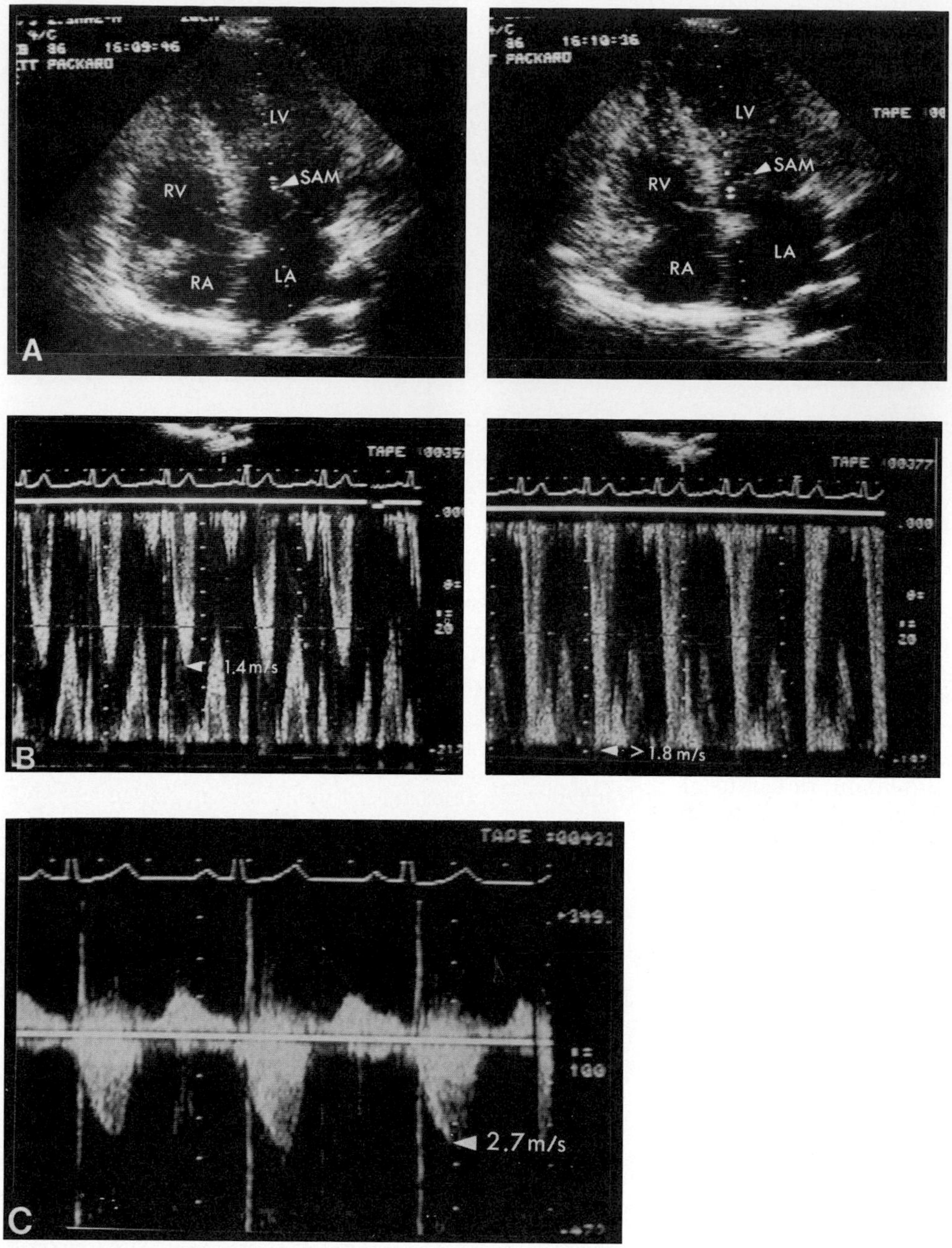

Fig. 25–21. Doppler evaluation of left ventricular outflow tract obstruction. Velocities are scanned from an apical window by pulsed Doppler. With the sample volume just at or proximal to the region of systolic anterior motion (SAM)- septal contact (**A,** left), a velocity of 1.4 m/sec can be resolved by pulsed Doppler (**B,** left). When the sample volume is moved superiorly (**A,** right), aliasing occurs (**B,** right). **C.** Continuous wave Doppler shows a late-peaking pattern going up to 2.7 m/sec. LV = left ventricle; LA = left atrium; RA = right atrium; RV = right ventricle.

turbulent post-stenotic jet, which may be eccentrically and posteriorly directed within the outflow tract (Fig. 25–22).[132,133]

Technical Considerations. Maximum velocities are, in general, obtained from the apical window. It is important to scan medially and laterally to distinguish the contiguous high velocity jets of left ventricular outflow and mitral regurgitation that commonly occur together[97–99,131,134–136] (Figs. 25–22 and 25–23). Mitral regurgitation can be distinguished by its earlier onset during isovolumic systole and earlier attainment of high velocities, as opposed to the late-peaking outflow tract velocities[127,128,130,131] (Fig. 25–24). It is also useful to note that, in general, the velocity of the outflow tract jet will be lower than that of the regurgitant jet because the driving pressure for the outflow tract jet (ventricular minus aortic pressure) is smaller than that of the regurgitant jet (ventricular minus left atrial pressure). As with aortic stenosis, only the same measure of gradient, such as instantaneous peak or mean, can be compared in the Doppler and catheterization studies. Doppler may underestimate the catheter-derived gradient if the beam is not optimally aligned with the outflow tract jet, or if the late-systolic high-velocity signals are weak because relatively few reflectors (red blood cells) are moving at that time.

Physical Factors: Pressure Recovery. Despite the technical reasons that may cause Doppler to underestimate invasively derived gradients, Doppler more commonly provides slightly higher values.[127,128] In one study, for

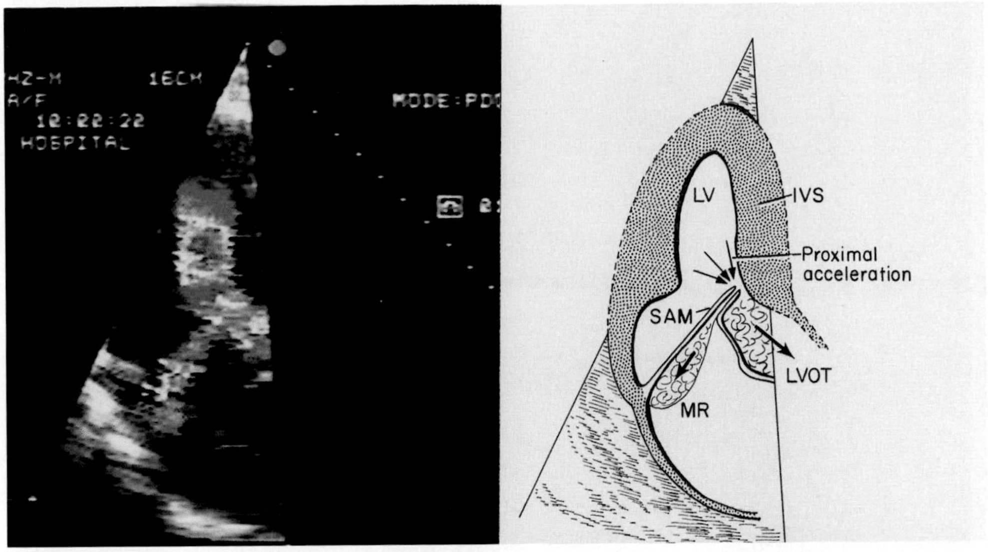

Fig. 25–22. Apical long axis view with color flow map showing acceleration of flow proximal to the site of mitral-septal contact (blue going to yellow coded velocities) and admixture of colors consistent with turbulent jets in the left ventricular outflow tract (LVOT) and left atrium (mitral regurgitation, MR). IVS = interventricular septum; SAM = systolic anterior motion.

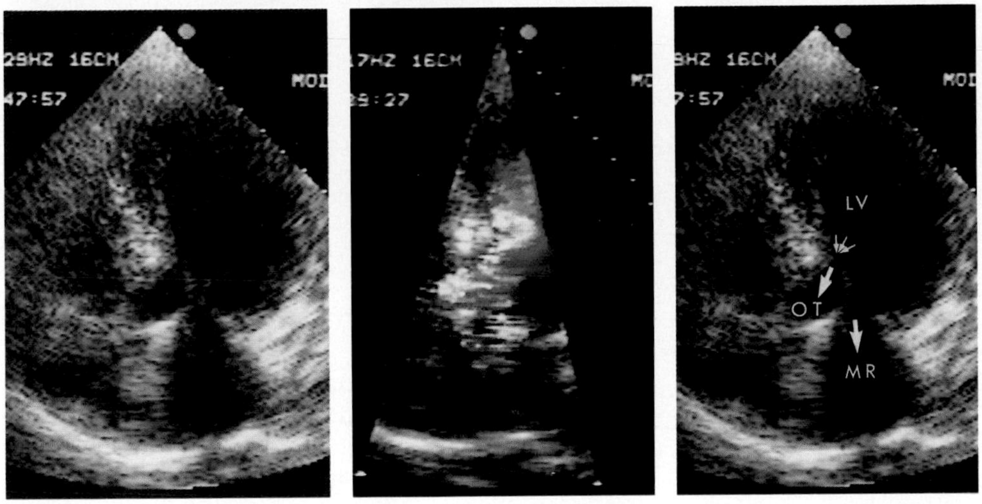

Fig. 25–23. Apical views of a patient with outflow tract obstruction and mitral regurgitation (MR) showing contiguous outflow tract (OT) and regurgitant jets distal to the region of mitral-septal contact, with proximal acceleration (small arrows). The continuous wave Doppler beam must be scanned in different directions to record the velocity of each jet. LV = left ventricle.

example, Doppler gradients measured at the time of operation exceeded those measured simultaneously between needle taps in the left ventricle and ascending aorta in 79% of patients studied (27 out of 34), often by 15 to 25 mm Hg.[127] These observations can potentially be explained by the phenomenon of pressure recovery distal to stenosis[126,137,138] (Fig. 25–25). Doppler detects the highest velocity of red cells passing through the orifice and the region where the streamlines of flow are most narrowly constricted (the vena contracta), and it therefore measures the maximal gradient, which best reflects the anatomic stenosis. The catheter or needle tap, on the other hand, measures pressures in the aorta, several centimeters downstream from the vena contracta. In the intervening distance, the post-stenotic jet has had an opportunity to re-expand, with a corresponding decrease in velocity. By conservation of energy, as the velocity and, therefore, the kinetic energy of the blood decrease, its potential energy, reflected in lateral pressure, must increase, so that the total energy of the blood remains constant; in other words, pressure is recovered downstream. The pressure in the aorta will therefore be higher than at the limiting orifice, and the catheter-derived gradient will be lower than the maximal gradient at the vena contracta, as determined by Doppler.[126,137] Pressure recovery is frequently limited by turbulent interactions of the jet with surrounding stagnant fluid, which cause energy to be lost. However, the geometry of obstruction in hypertrophic cardiomyopathy may increase the amount of pressure recovery, particularly if there is a relatively long region of mitral-septal contact that gradually tapers outward into the subaortic outflow tract (Fig. 25–26). Such tapering, unlike the abrupt exit from a discrete stenotic orifice, may allow flow to re-expand, at first, in a streamlined fashion, relatively protected from turbulent interaction with stagnant fluid and may therefore favor pressure recovery (Fig. 25–27).[126]

Spectrum of Dynamic Outflow Abnormalities. Not all increases in velocity along the pathway of left ventricular outflow result from mitral-septal contact. In some patients, upper septal hypertrophy can cause localized

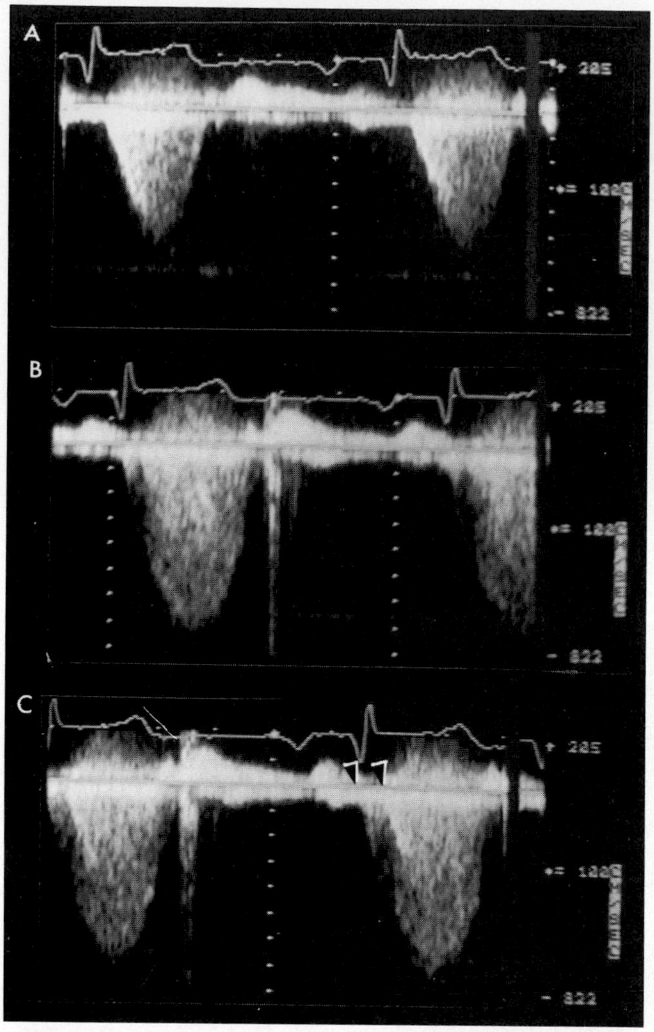

Fig. 25–24. **A.** Continuous wave Doppler recording of late-peaking outflow tract jet in a patient with hypertrophic obstructive cardiomyopathy. **B.** Higher-velocity, earlier-peaking mitral regurgitant jet. **C.** Intermediate beam location encompassing portions of both jets. The onset of the regurgitant jet occurs before the rise in outflow tract velocities (arrowheads).

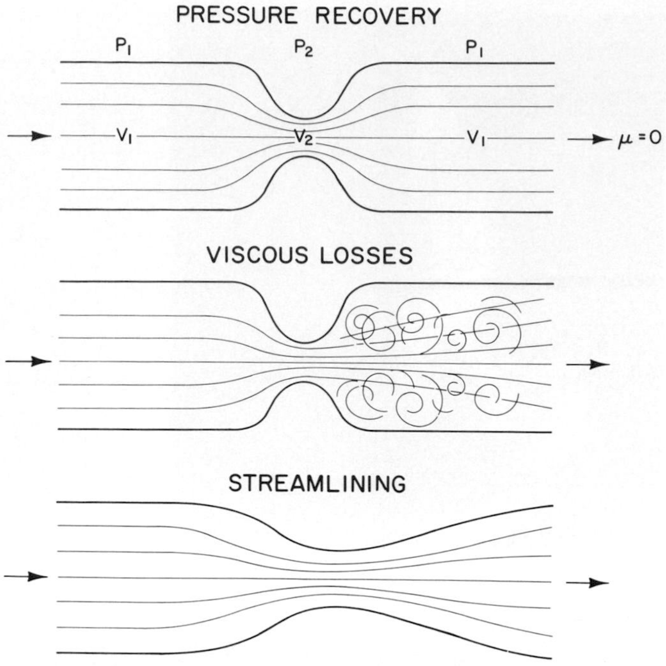

Fig. 25–25. Pressure recovery. Top. Complete recovery of pressure (P) for inviscid flow (mu = 0), where velocity (v) increases and then decreases to its prestenotic value. In reality, pressure recovery is limited by turbulence distal to the stenosis (middle), which can be minimized by streamlining the stenosis (bottom) to minimize separation of flow from adjacent walls. (From Levine RA, et al.: Pressure recovery distal to stenosis: potential cause of gradient "overestimation" by Doppler. J Am Coll Cardiol 13:706, 1989. Reprinted with permission from the American College of Cardiology.)

but generally mild increases in outflow tract velocity (Fig. 25–28). (Such patients may have a variant of hypertrophic cardiomyopathy or an unrelated finding that may be seen in the elderly.[139]) Although there will be a localized drop in pressure at the site of flow acceleration, as predicted by Bernoulli's equation, the absence of a turbulent post-stenotic jet and the relatively smooth, streamlined nature of the stenosis make pressure recovery likely to occur.[126] No important gradient, therefore, is likely to be measured by catheters within the left ventricle and aorta, distal to the site of hypertrophy, implying that little additional work is required to achieve flow across the outflow tract despite the localized acceleration.[140] These patients also do not develop SAM of the mitral valve, despite the elevated outflow tract velocities, because their mitral valves are normally restrained by the papillary muscles.

Midcavity muscular obstruction[70–72a] will elevate velocities at a more apical level at a time, when the myocardial walls have had an opportunity to approach one another and narrow the cavity. Although this typically produces steep late-systolic increases in velocity (Fig. 25–29), velocity will rise earlier when muscular rings narrow the cavity at the onset of systole.[70–72a] (Fig. 25–29). A late-systolic pattern may also be recorded throughout most of the ventricular cavity in patients with diffuse hypertrophy, small cavity size, and hyperdynamic contraction causing late-systolic cavity obliteration. In such patients, the color Doppler flow map in an apical view may show a thin line of aliased flow extending from the apex toward the base in late systole, reflecting the diffuse acceleration of blood out of the remaining cavity (Fig. 25–30). The simplified Bernoulli equation no longer adequately describes the relationship between velocity and pressure gradient in this situation, because it describes gradients caused by an increase in velocity along a streamline of flow (convective acceleration). In the case of cavity obliteration, a column of blood is being accelerated out of the ventricle all along its length by the inward contraction of the myocardial walls. Pressure differences will therefore relate more to the local (temporal) acceleration term in the complete Bernoulli equation (dv/dt; see Chapter 9) and to frictional losses at the borders of the long, narrowed lumen.[137]

The Physiologic Significance of Obstruction. Doppler and imaging echocardiography have helped resolve the

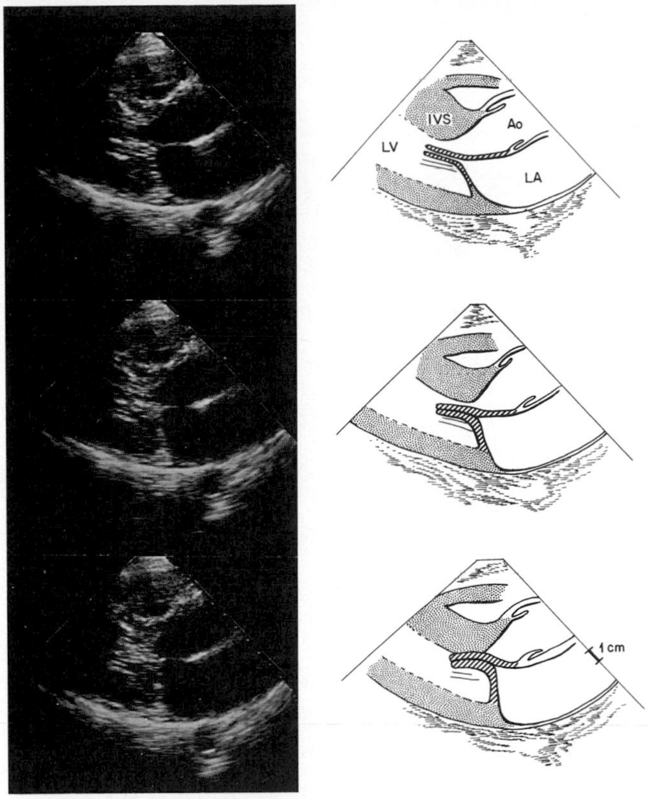

Fig. 25–26. Longitudinally prolonged region of mitral-septal contact in three successive systolic long-axis views in a patient with hypertrophic obstructive cardiomyopathy. Ao = aorta; LA = left atrium; LV = left ventricle; IVS = interventricular septum. (From Levine RA, et al.: Pressure recovery distal to stenosis: potential cause of gradient "overestimation" by Doppler. J Am Coll Cardiol 13:706, 1989. Reprinted with permission from the American College of Cardiology.)

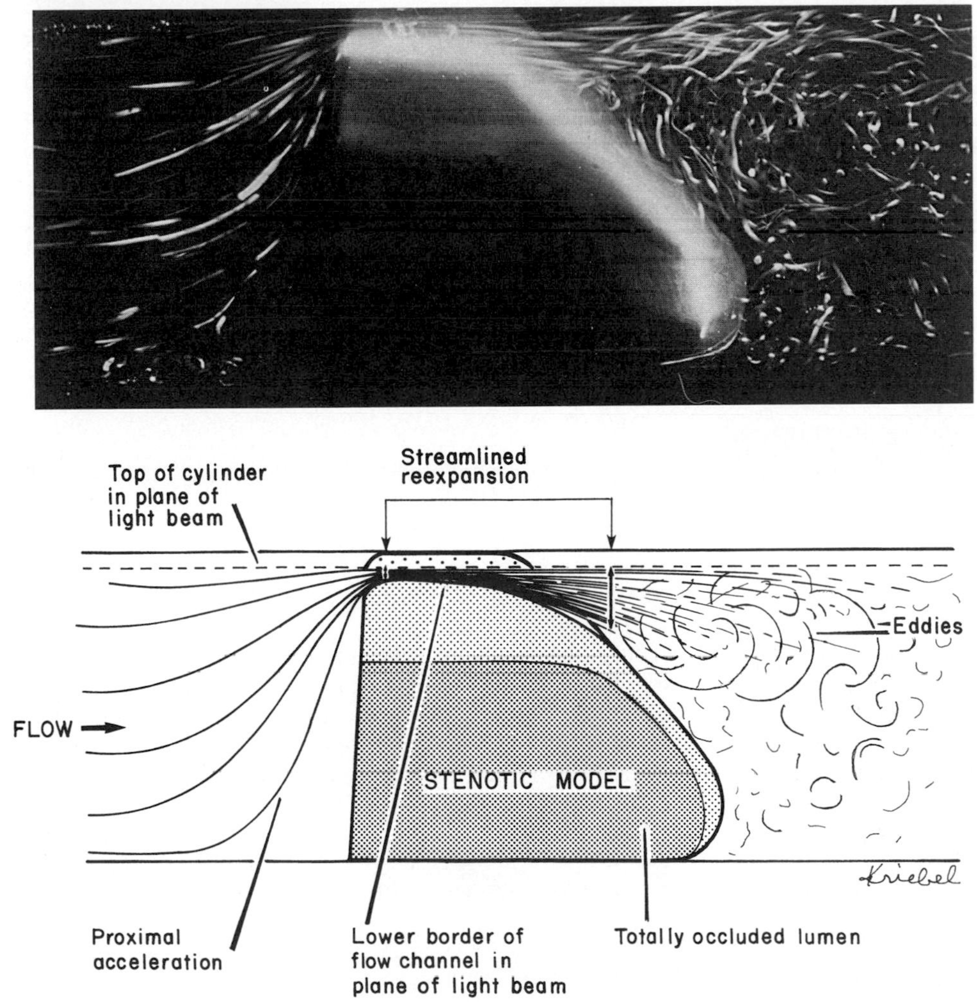

Fig. 25–27. Flow visualization of stenotic model with longitudinal prolongation creating a tunnel-like component that gradually tapers outward. Flow accelerates proximal to the stenosis and can expand considerably. Bottom. Turbulent eddies invade the jet (streamlined effort). Therefore, at a flow rate of 3.5 L/min, marked pressure recovery (68 mm Hg, or 60% of the maximal gradient) was observed. (From Levine RA, et al.: Pressure recovery distal to stenosis: potential cause of gradient "overestimation" by Doppler. J Am Coll Cardiol 13: 706, 1989. Reprinted with permission from the American College of Cardiology.)

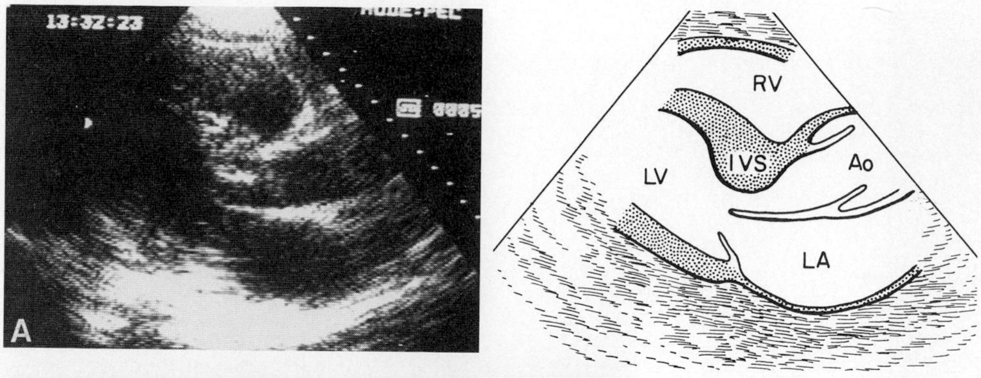

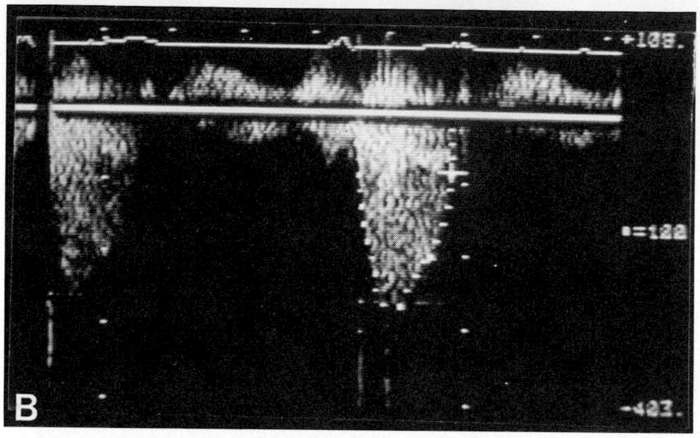

Fig. 25–28. **A.** Localized upper septal hypertrophy in a parasternal long axis view. **B.** Continuous wave Doppler tracing showing an elevated outflow velocity (2.7 m/sec). Despite this, no systolic anterior motion was observed in the presence of a normal papillary-mitral apparatus. RV = right ventricle; Ao = aorta; LA = left atrium; LV = left ventricle; IVS = interventricular septum.

long-standing historical debate concerning the significance of outflow tract gradients in hypertrophic cardiomyopathy, thereby providing a rationale for continuing to measure such gradients in routine practice. In the debate concerning obstruction, one school maintained that a physiologically significant impediment to ejection was present,[35,141,142] while another claimed that the gradient simply reflected obliteration of a virtually empty chamber after the bulk of ejection had been completed because of hyperdynamic contraction in early systole.[143–146] Echocardiography has provided the following insights into this issue:

1. Because Doppler ultrasound can measure both volumetric flow (from velocities at the aortic root level) and pressure gradient (from subaortic jet velocities), it has been able to provide a simple criterion for physiologic subaortic obstruction, namely, the existence of a pressure gradient that is present during the period of systolic ejection and therefore increases the work load on the left ventricle. The magnitude of obstruction can be as-

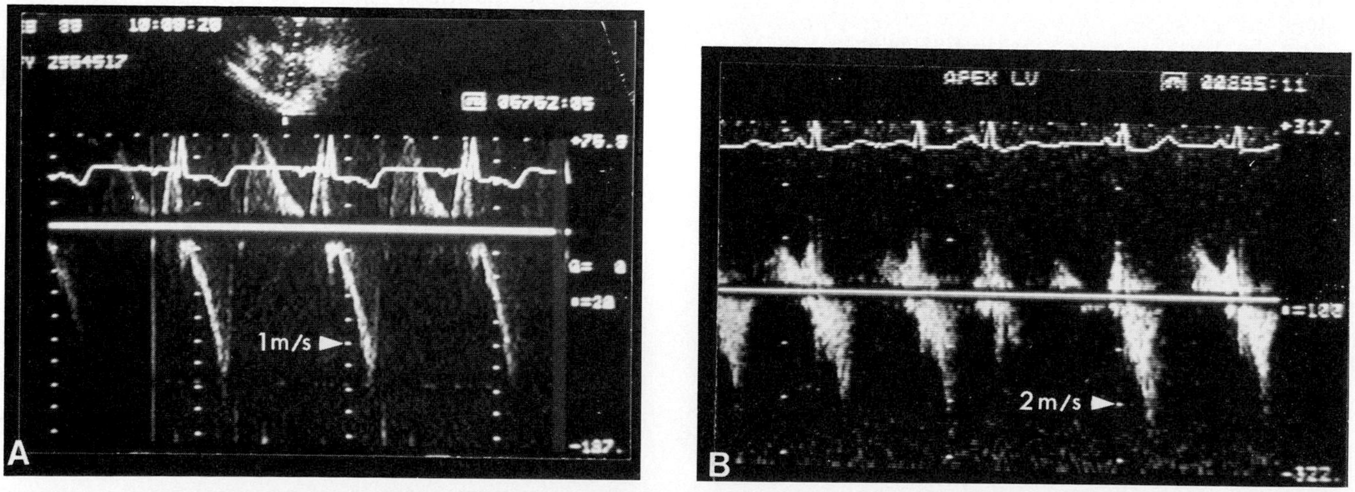

Fig. 25–29. Late-peaking systolic velocities in patients with midcavity obliteration, reflecting progressive decrease in area available for flow during systole. **A.** Pulsed Doppler tracing of the midventricular level, where flow velocities are normally well below 1 m/sec. **B.** Continuous wave Doppler tracing in another patient.

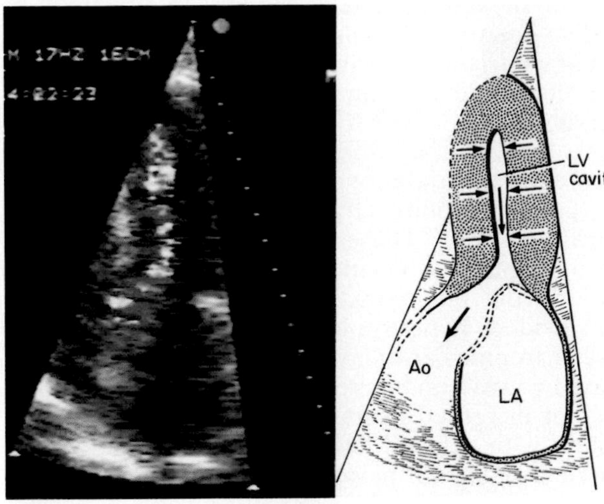

Fig. 25–30. Apical view of a patient with diffuse left ventricular (LV) hypertrophy showing near-cavity obliteration and flow acceleration (aliasing from blue to yellow) spanning the length of the ventricle. Ao = aorta; LA = left atrium.

sessed in terms of the fraction of forward flow ejected in the presence of a subaortic gradient.[104,147] Simultaneous catheterization-Doppler and echo-Doppler studies have, in fact, shown that an average of 58% of forward aortic flow is ejected while a gradient or mitral-septal contact (predicting a gradient) is present.[104] Further, the left ventricle visibly continues to shorten and empty well after the onset of a gradient.[104] Similar findings have been described by other groups using echo-Doppler,[105] catheterization,[19] and radionuclide angiography with simultaneous pressure measurements.[148]

2. Left ventricular ejection time is prolonged in patients with hypertrophic cardiomyopathy and subaortic pressure gradients,[104,133,149–151] consistent with the presence of physiologic obstruction.

3. The high velocities detected in the outflow tract during mid- to late-systole are consistent with continued ejection through a stenosis[131] and are inversely proportional to the anatomic orifice area between the mitral valve and the septum, which can be visualized by two-dimensional echocardiography.[111] In addition to these echocardiographic insights, studies that show symptomatic improvement and resolution of pacing-induced lactate production with relief of obstruction add further support to the concept that subaortic obstruction constitutes a physiologically significant load on the left ventricle and therefore merits evaluation by echocardiography.[19,49,152–161]

Mitral Regurgitation

Mitral regurgitation[35,97–99] virtually always accompanies obstruction created by SAM.[134–136] For example, in one study of 100 consecutive patients with hypertrophic cardiomyopathy and a resting pressure gradient, mitral regurgitation was uniformly present.[134,162,163] In that study, increasing the outflow tract gradient with isoproterenol or amyl nitrite consistently increased the degree of regurgitation in the individual patient.[134] Abolishing the gradient with angiotensin greatly reduced or abolished the regurgitation in 80% of the patients to whom it was administered; in those patients, myomectomy, when successful, eliminated both the gradient and the regurgitation.[162,163] In 20% of the patients, however, mitral regurgitation persisted with gradient abolition both by angiotensin and by surgery,[162,163] suggesting a more fixed leaflet deformity. Reversible regurgitation has also been demonstrated by other groups[164] as well as in animal models of reversible SAM.[165–167] In patients without obstructive SAM, on the other hand, regurgitation is variable and, as a rule, mild.[134–136]

The occurrence of regurgitation is not surprising, because SAM demonstrates the disruption of the normal coaptational geometry of the mitral leaflets, which are then exposed to the increased pressures created by obstruction. Although regurgitation, like SAM, begins early in systole,[29,131,136] its magnitude is greatest in mid- to late-systole, when the driving pressures are greatest, as demonstrated by the outflow tract velocity profile.[132,168]

Left Ventricular Diastolic Filling

Heart failure in hypertrophic cardiomyopathy can in part be attributed to elevated filling pressures caused by delayed relaxation of the myopathic ventricle and increased chamber stiffness (potentially reflecting both increased *myocardial* stiffness and an elevated mass/volume ratio, which increases *chamber* stiffness). Digitized M-mode echocardiography has provided one means of demonstrating decreased rates of left ventricular filling and myocardial thinning, reflecting delayed myocardial relaxation[169–173] (Chapter 24, Fig. 24–14). The Doppler pattern of mitral inflow velocities, which reflects the pattern of volumetric left ventricular filling,[174,175] might also be expected to yield valuable information regarding altered relaxation and stiffness. Based on patients with mitral inflow patterns clearly different from normal, the initial concept evolved that hypertrophic cardiomyopathy is accompanied by a low velocity of early mitral inflow (E wave), reflecting delayed ventricular relaxation and increased chamber stiffness, which elevate left ventricular diastolic pressures and thereby diminish the pressure gradient between the atrium and ventricle (the prime determinant of the E-wave velocity) (Fig. 25–31). Delayed relaxation also prolongs the isovolumic relaxation time between aortic valve closure and mitral valve opening and may account for a delayed deceleration of the E-wave velocity by prolonging the duration of the atrioventricular pressure gradient (Chapter 24, Fig. 24–32). The velocity of late-diastolic filling following atrial contraction (the A wave) tends to be higher, possibly because the atrium, having failed to empty fully in early diastole, is at a higher point in its Starling curve. The net result is a decrease in the ratio of peak E-wave to peak A-wave velocities (the E/A ratio).[75,175,176]

This pattern has been reproduced experimentally in a model of hypertensive hypertrophy.[177] Nevertheless, this pattern does not uniformly occur in patients with

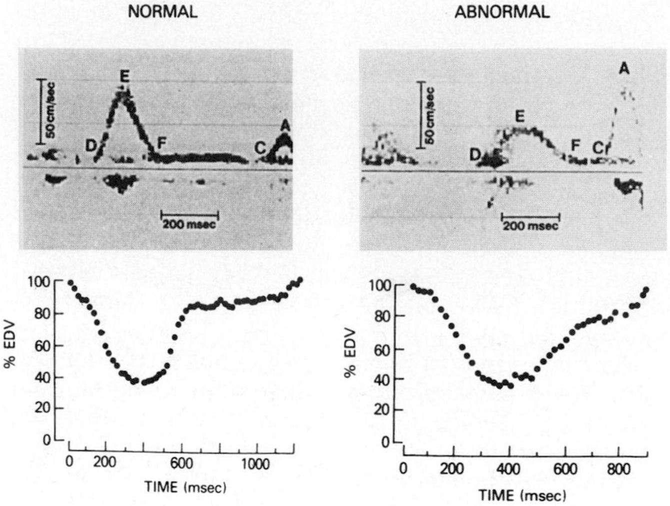

Fig. 25–31. Classic illustration of altered left ventricular filling pattern caused by delayed relaxation. In contrast to the normal subject, the patient with delayed relaxation has an E wave (early inflow velocity) lower than the A wave in late diastole, with prolonged E-wave deceleration. The Doppler patterns (top) parallel to radionuclide angiographic time-activity curves (bottom). (From Spirito P, Maron BJ, Bonow RO: Noninvasive assessment of left ventricular diastolic function: comparative analysis of Doppler echocardiographic and radionuclide angiographic techniques. J Am Coll Cardiol 7:518, 1986. Reprinted with permission from the American College of Cardiology.)

hypertrophic cardiomyopathy, nor is it specific for that condition. In one study, for example, the classic pattern occurred primarily in patients *without* subaortic obstruction, but a relatively normal pattern occurred in patients *with* obstruction.[178] This can potentially be understood on the basis of the mitral regurgitation associated with subaortic obstruction, which can raise left atrial pressure and, therefore, early inflow velocities[178] (see also Chapter 24, Fig. 24–47). Similar findings or trends have been noted by other groups.[176,179] Even in studies demonstrating significant differences in peak mitral inflow velocities between patients with hypertrophic cardiomyopathy and normal persons, overlap is considerable.[176,180] For example, in one study of 111 patients with hypertrophic cardiomyopathy and 86 control subjects, peak E velocity was $.5 \pm .2$ m/sec in hypertrophic cardiomyopathy vs. $.6 \pm .1$ in normals, with a peak A velocity of $.4 \pm .3$ m/sec vs. $.3 \pm .1$ (both significant at $p<.001$ because of the large numbers studied). There was, however, a better separation of E/A-wave ratios ($1.4 \pm .8$ vs. $2.1 \pm .9$).[176] On the other hand, the classic pattern of low E-wave and E/A-wave ratio can be mimicked in patients *without* hypertrophic cardiomyopathy by nitroglycerin infusion, which lowers the filling pressure and therefore the gradient which drives the E-wave[181] (Chapter 24, Fig. 24–25). Similar changes can also be produced by increasing the heart rate or simply by varying the position of the Doppler sample volume in the vicinity of the mitral annulus[182–185] (Chapter 24, Figs. 24–42 and 24–43). Finally, a subset of patients with hypertrophic cardiomyopathy appear to have a restrictive-type inflow pattern, with rapid early diastolic inflow and decreased filling during atrial systole.[19,186] This pattern can be thought of as representing the effects of increased myocardial stiffness, causing more rapid equilibration of ventricular and atrial pressures (rapid E-wave deceleration), and causing compensatory increases in left atrial pressure, which increase peak E-wave velocity.

The observed variability of inflow patterns is not surprising, given the complexity of factors determining ventricular filling.[187–189] These factors must be understood before attempting to diagnose diastolic abnormalities, particularly out of context—for example, in patients without evident hypertrophy. Practically, in a patient with hypertrophic cardiomyopathy, a classic pattern of decreased E-wave and increased E/A-wave ratio, in the absence of increased heart rate, can be interpreted as consistent with delayed left ventricular relaxation and increased chamber stiffness. This assumes that left atrial pressure is not reduced. On the other hand, a normal filling pattern in a patient with hypertrophic cardiomyopathy cannot necessarily be taken to imply the absence of intrinsic left ventricular diastolic abnormalities (Chapter 24, Fig. 24–48).

Finally, the clinical significance of the Doppler findings in asymptomatic patient groups is unknown. Inflow velocity changes have been described in 84% of patients with asymptomatic hypertrophic cardiomyopathy in a referral population[176] as well as in asymptomatic individuals with hypertrophic cardiomyopathy identified by routine health screening.[86] In this context it is important to remember that the diastolic mitral inflow velocities also do not provide the absolute pressures in the atrium and ventricle; they provide only the differences between them, so that a decreased E/A-wave ratio, e.g., does not necessarily imply that left-sided filling pressures are elevated or that diastolic dysfunction is present, with resultant heart failure.

Functional Subvalvular Aortic Stenosis and the Mechanism of Systolic Anterior Motion

Functional Subvalvular Aortic Stenosis

Outflow tract obstruction in hypertrophic cardiomyopathy is only one form of a broader pathophysiologic abnormality, *functional subvalvular aortic stenosis*. This term encompasses a heterogeneous group of disorders with common features, including (1) anatomic narrowing of the left ventricular outflow tract in the region between the interventricular septum and the anterior mitral leaflet and (2) variable anterior systolic displacement of the mitral valve into this narrowed outflow space, producing obstruction. The functional component of this type of obstruction, SAM of the mitral valve, has been reported to have a 97% specificity for hypertrophic cardiomyopathy in one referral population[46,190] but has been described in a variety of other conditions as well. Situations in which SAM occurs can be classified under three major headings: (1) Narrowing of the outflow tract by asymmetric or disproportionate septal hypertrophy, as in hypertrophic cardiomyopathy, D-transposition of the great arteries,[52,53,191–193] or subaortic stenosis of the fibromuscular type;[194] (2) hypercontractile states such as hypovolemia and anemia;[195–201] and (3) congenital or acquired abnormalities of the mitral valve and papillary muscles,[202–205] e.g., following mitral valve repair and insertion of a Carpentier ring for mitral valve prolapse with regurgitation.[206–211] The variety of conditions in which SAM occurs raises the question of whether a unified mechanism can explain the occurrence of SAM in such diverse situations.

The Mechanism of Systolic Anterior Motion

Initial Proposals. Two mechanisms initially proposed to explain SAM have been excluded by echocardiographic studies. The first was based on the angiographic impression that the papillary muscles actively pulled the mitral valve anteriorly.[97,212,213] Two-dimensional echocardiography showed that SAM occurs at a right angle to a line drawn from the free edges of the mitral leaflets to the tips of the papillary muscles and cannot therefore be caused directly by the force of papillary muscle contraction.[41] The second mechanism proposed that hyperdynamic contraction of the basal posterior wall of the left ventricle pushed the leaflets anteriorly.[214] Echocardiographic studies showed that SAM followed an independent and more rapid time course than posterior wall motion, which could therefore not be the primary cause of SAM.[24,30]

The Venturi Mechanism. This mechanism states that outflow tract narrowing, possibly combined with hyperdynamic left ventricular ejection, increases flow velocity above the mitral valve. By Bernoulli's equation, as the velocity and kinetic energy of the blood increase, its potential energy, or pressure, must decrease because energy is conserved, so that the pressure above the mitral valve must fall below that on its posterior surface. The valve consequently moves anteriorly in the same way that an airplane rises when it achieves sufficient lift.[162] This mechanism is supported by the correlation between outflow tract size (or upper septal thickness) and the presence and extent of SAM[24,28,106,215,216] and by the reduced severity of obstruction produced by surgical widening of the outflow tract[106,155–160,217] and negative inotropic agents.[218,219] This mechanism, however, cannot explain the observed occurrence of SAM at or near the onset of systole,[28,105,110] when outflow tract velocities are relatively low[220,221] (Fig. 25–1); and it cannot explain how the mitral leaflet can be drawn into the left ventricular cavity, because normally, both the force of ventricular pressure and the restraint of the papillary muscles hold the leaflets in a posterior and closed position. SAM, in fact, fails to occur in patients with localized upper septal hypertrophy and elevated outflow tract velocities but normally restrained mitral valves (see Fig. 25–28). Experimentally, graded septal thickening produced by saline infusion into an implanted balloon failed to produce obstructive SAM of a normal mitral valve despite outflow tract velocities of up to 2.3 m/sec.[166] Only at extremes of septal thickening with isoproterenol infusion producing virtual cavity obliteration could obstructive SAM be induced, suggesting that other causative or contributory factors must be considered to explain obstruction in patients who, in general, do not have such infusions or such extreme hypertrophy.

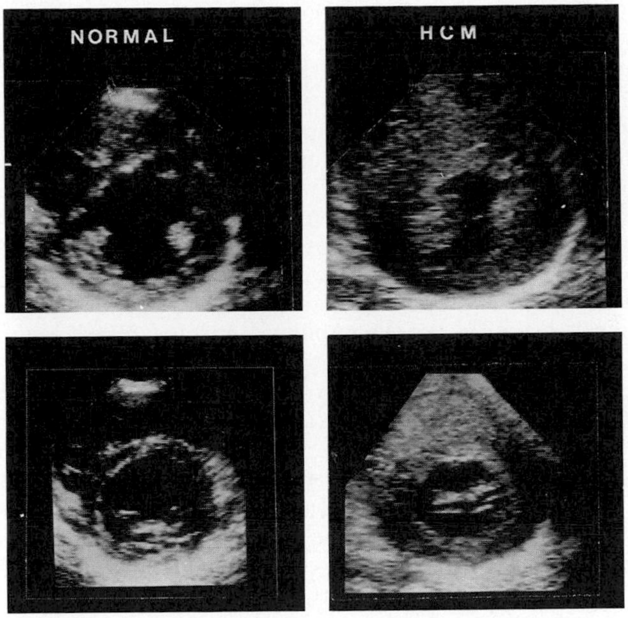

Fig. 25–32. Anterior and inward (central) displacement of the papillary muscles (top) in hypertrophic cardiomyopathy (HCM) compared to normal, with anterior shift of the coapted mitral leaflets (bottom), which normally lie above the posterior left ventricular wall.

An Integrated Mechanism Based on Mitral Valve Mechanics. Echocardiographic observations of patients with subaortic obstruction provide insight into how SAM might occur based on considerations of the effects of papillary muscle position and chordal tension on mitral leaflet closure[110,201] (see Chapter 17, discussion of papillary muscle dysfunction). Specifically, in patients with hypertrophic obstructive cardiomyopathy, the hypertrophied papillary muscles are displaced anteriorly and toward the center of the ventricular cavity (Figs. 25–32 and 25–33).[24,98,99,102,110,212–213,222–225] The mitral valve apparatus is likewise in a relatively anterior position

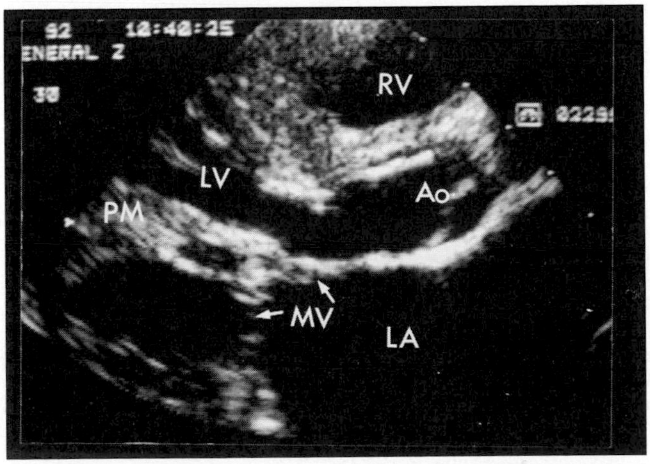

Fig. 25–33. Parasternal long axis view showing anterior malposition of the papillary muscle (PM), with a parallel anterior shift of mitral valve (MV) coaptation in hypertrophic cardiomyopathy. RV = right ventricle; Ao = aorta; LV = left ventricle.

within the ventricle at the onset of systole, and the degree of anterior displacement has been related to the severity of obstruction.[24,41,101,102,110,223] In addition, the mitral leaflets in such patients are typically elongated, measuring up to 1.7 cm longer than normal,[110,225a] consistent with pathologic observations.[95,226,227]

Anterior displacement of the papillary muscles should decrease the relative tension on the chordae to the body of the anterior mitral leaflet (Figs. 25–34 and 25–35B, top).[201] (This situation is the converse of that in ischemic disease of the papillary muscle regions, in which posterior displacement of the papillary muscles increases tension in this area.) This decrease in tension should be even more prominent when the distance from the papillary muscle tips to the leaflet is decreased by a combination of myocardial hypertrophy at the base of the papillary muscles, reduced cavity size, and increased leaflet length. Anterior displacement may interpose the leaflets into the streamlines of flow, causing them to be pushed anteriorly and superiorly by the stream of blood rushing through the outflow tract (Fig. 25–34).[24,110,201] The valve, in this sense, resembles an unfurling sail, filling out with left ventricular ejection, which generates drag forces parallel to flow.[228,229] Anterior displacement of the papillary muscles may also pull the posterior leaflet anteriorly so that it meets the anterior leaflet closer to the annulus and creates a long, overlapping residual leaflet, which has been described as a prerequisite for SAM (unlike the leaflet body, it is unrestrained by the pressure difference between the left atrium and ventricle) (Fig. 25–34).[101,110]

Displacement of the papillary muscles toward the center of the left ventricular cavity should also increase tension at the margins of the leaflets compared with that exerted at their midportion (Fig. 25–35B, bottom).[201] (This situation, again, is the exact opposite of that in papillary muscle dysfunction.) This combination of forces should produce redundancy or relative slack of the midportion of the affected leaflets, thereby predisposing them to be drawn anteriorly by Venturi forces or pushed anteriorly by drag forces.[110,230] The altered distribution of tension could also cause anterior buckling of the central leaflet portions even during isovolumic systole, as soon as the papillary muscles generate force, causing SAM to occur near the onset of systole, as noted.

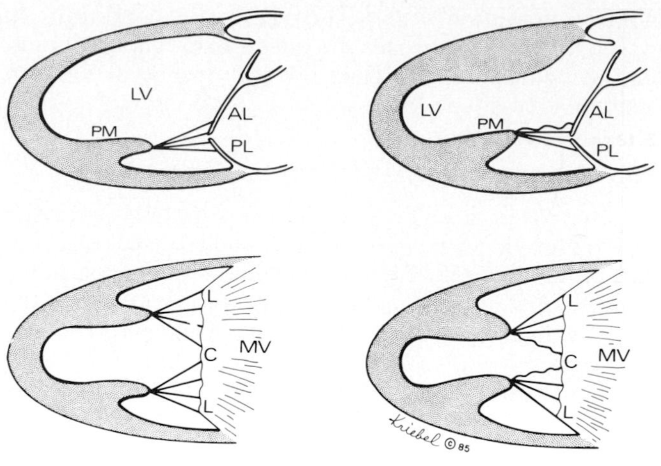

Fig. 25–35. Diagrams of chordal geometry illustrating effects of papillary muscle malposition on distribution of tension to the mitral leaflets (**A** to **B**). The mitral apparatus is viewed from the side in the upper diagrams and from above in the lower. In hypertrophic cardiomyopathy (HCM) with systolic anterior motion, the papillary muscle (PM) tips are displaced anteriorly and toward one another. This geometry can be predicted to produce relative chordal slack in the central and anterior leaflet portions. This is indicated by the relatively lax chordae (wavy lines) that are longer than the distance between their papillary and mitral insertions. MV = mitral valve; L = lateral edge; C = central portion; AL = anterior leaflet; PL = posterior leaflet; LV = left ventricle. (From Jiang L, Levine RA, King ME, Weyman AE: An integrated mechanism to explain the systolic anterior motion of the mitral valve in hypertrophic cardiomyopathy based on echocardiographic observations. Am Heart J 113:633, 1987.)

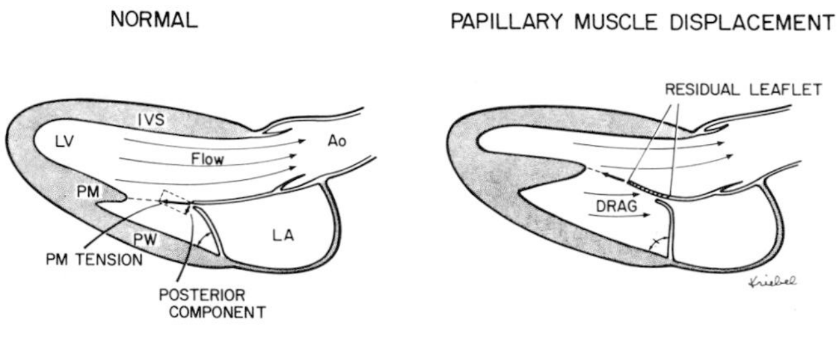

Fig. 25–34. Possible mechanisms for systolic anterior motion with anterior displacement of the papillary muscles (PM): (1) the normal posterior component of PM tension (its component along the short axis ventricular diameter at that level) is reduced or eliminated by anterior displacement of the muscle tips; (2) interposing the mitral leaflets into the streamlines of flow causes drag forces with an anterior component; and (3) pulling up the posterior leaflet so that it meets the anterior leaflet closer to its base creates a long, overlapping *residual leaflet,* as seen clinically. This leaflet portion is relatively free to move anteriorly, unlike the coapted leaflet bodies that are restrained by the balance of ventricular and atrial pressures acting across them. Ao = aorta; IVS = interventricular septum; LA = left atrium; LV = left ventricle; PW = posterior wall.

This mechanism integrates mitral valve mechanics with flow-related forces. It allows for the possible contribution of lift or Venturi forces, particularly once SAM has begun and the outflow tract is acutely narrowed. However, it emphasizes the role of papillary-mitral geometry in permitting the initiation of SAM in early systole, when outflow velocities are low.

This integrated mitral valve mechanism can be illustrated by a simple flow model in which a flexible membrane moves anteriorly with release of chordal tension to its midportion and assumes a configuration similar to that observed clinically (Figs. 25–36 and 25–37).[229] Anterior displacement of the chordal attachments potentiates this effect by permitting anterior motion at lesser degrees of chordal laxity. Flow visualization studies demonstrate the importance of drag forces caused by particles hitting the undersurface of the membrane in causing anterior motion (Fig. 25–38). Similar results have been demonstrated in vitro using an excised mitral valve in a ventricular chamber: When normally tethered, no anterior motion occurred despite velocities up to 3.5

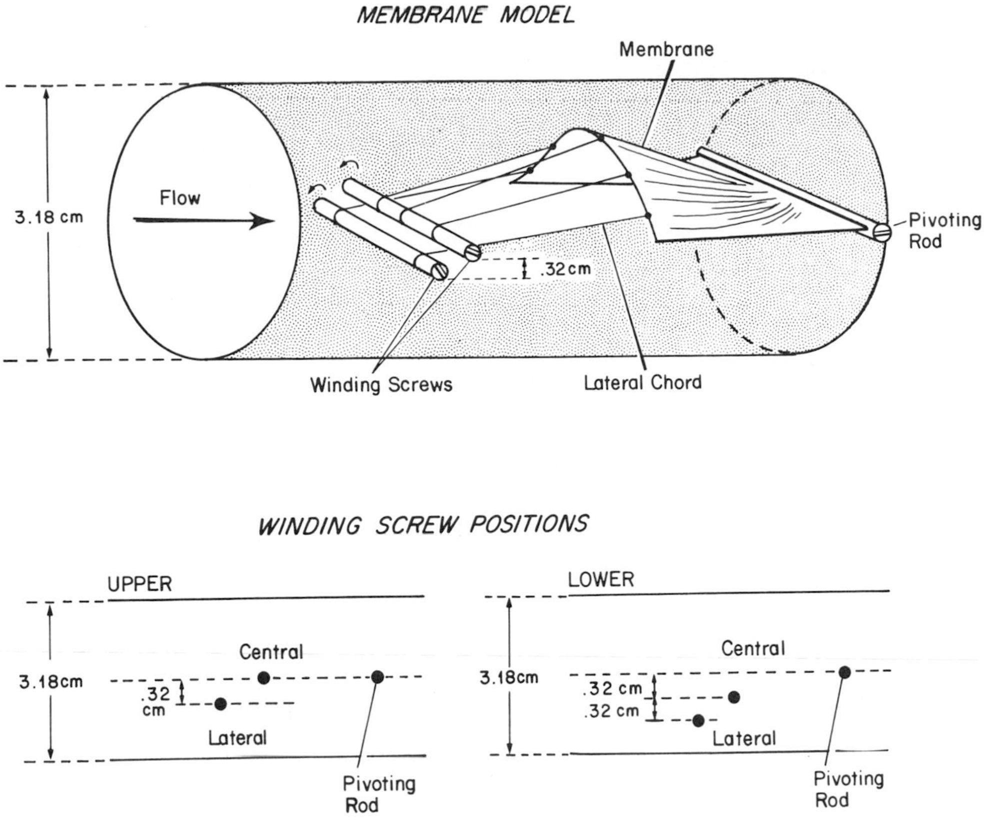

Fig. 25–36. Flow model with a flexible membrane (reflecting the mitral leaflet) and tethering chords which allow the tension on the leaflet center and its edges to be varied independently. Slack of the central or lateral leaflet portions is created by unwinding the chords using the winding screws. The bottom diagrams show how the anteroposterior position of these screws could be varied. (From Cape EG, et al.: Chordal geometry determines the shape and extent of systolic anterior mitral motion: *in vitro* studies. J Am Coll Cardiol 13:1438, 1989. Reprinted with permission from the American College of Cardiology.)

m/sec above the valve, whereas anterior and central papillary muscle displacement combined with chordal slack produced progressive anterior motion.[231–234] Obstructive SAM has also been created in a canine model of anterior papillary muscle displacement by attached sutures.[167,235]

Clinical Implications of This Mechanism. The previously described mechanism explains several unusual clinical features of SAM:

1. The observed geometry of anterior motion, which is greatest at the center of the valve (Fig. 25–2):[110,230] Based on the Venturi mechanism, SAM should be great-

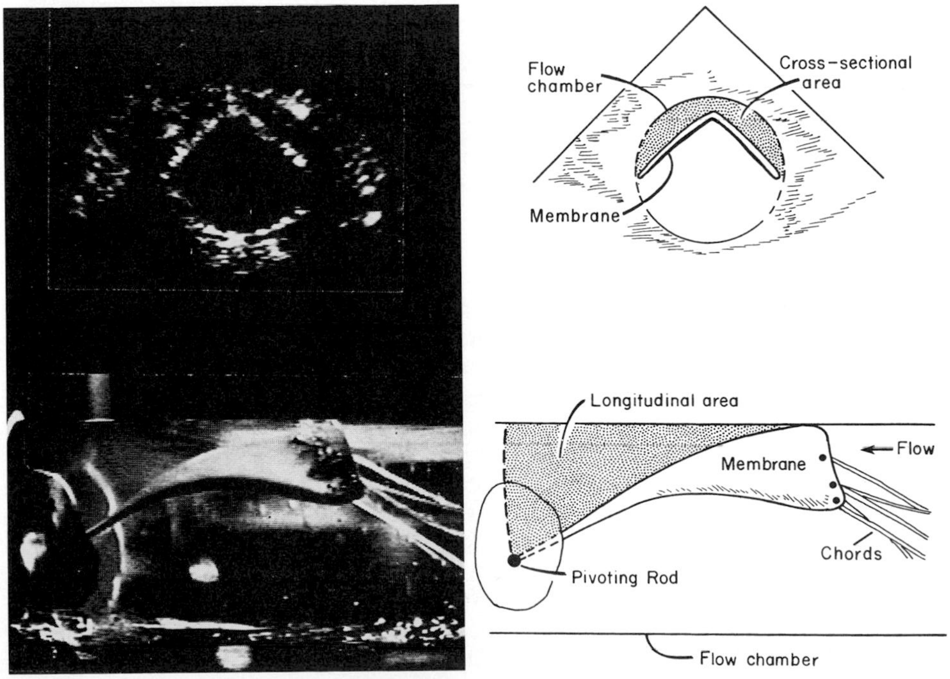

Fig. 25–37. Releasing the tension on the central membrane portion allows it to move anteriorly in the flow field, creating a cross-sectional echo image similar to that shown in the upper figures and an upward curving membrane resembling systolic anterior motion (SAM) in a videotaped longitudinal view (lower figures). (From Cape EG, et al.: Chordal geometry determines the shape and extent of systolic anterior mitral motion: *in vitro* studies. J Am Coll Cardiol 13:1438, 1989. Reprinted with permission from the American College of Cardiology.) Compare this with Figure 25–35B, in which an imbalance of tension across the leaflet is proposed as a mechanism for SAM.

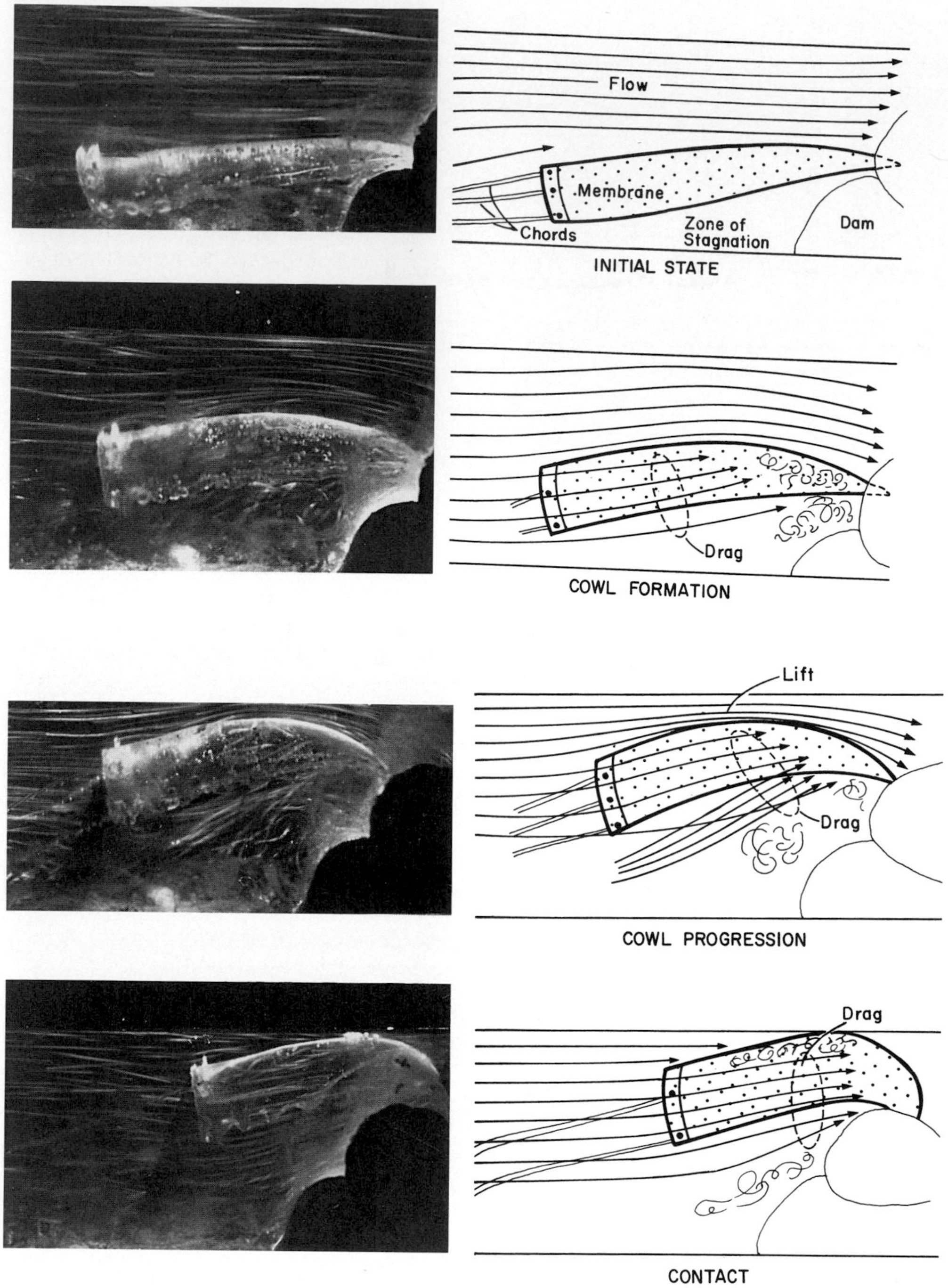

Fig. 25–38. Flow visualization studies using laser-illuminated particles in the membrane model, showing how anterior motion of the membrane is promoted by drag forces from flow hitting the leaflet undersurface, even before there is important lift from flow acceleration above the valve. (From Cape EG, et al.: Chordal geometry determines the shape and extent of systolic anterior mitral motion: *in vitro* studies. J Am Coll Cardiol 13: 1438, 1989. Reprinted with permission from the American College of Cardiology.)

est at the leaflet margins, where the outflow tract is narrowest.

2. The early systolic onset of anterior motion,[110,220,221] which may result from an imbalance of chordal tension during isovolumic contraction: Late-diastolic prepositioning of the leaflets into the outflow tract[221] by pre-ejection flow (mitral inflow turning around the apex[236,237]) may relate to anterior malposition of the leaflets combined with their diastolic slackness.[238]

3. The importance of relatively free leaflet portions and papillary-mitral anomalies in causing SAM: The distal residual leaflet, for example, which is relatively free to move anteriorly, has been described as a geometric prerequisite for SAM.[101] Subaortic obstruction has been observed in association with relatively free or anteriorly malpositioned mitral structures[202–205,239] and, in a previously normal heart, following tumor infiltration of the posterior wall, causing anterior displacement of the papillary muscles.[205,240] The integrated mitral valve mechanism can also explain the development of SAM in patients with anterior displacement of the mitral apparatus caused by dense annular calcification,[241–244] localized posterobasal hypertrophy,[65] and anteriorly positioned papillary muscles in the absence of important septal hypertrophy.[245]

4. The relationship between mitral valve prolapse and

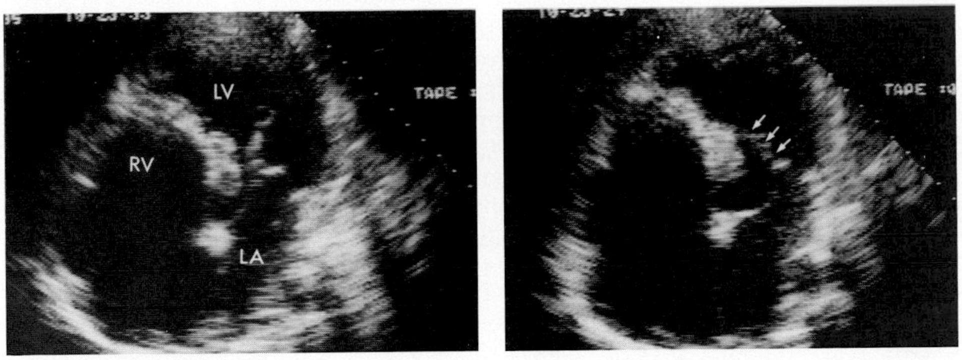

Fig. 25–39. Contribution of leaflet redundancy to systolic anterior motion (SAM). These apical four-chamber views correspond to initial mitral valve closure and early SAM (arrows) in a patient with Ebstein's anomaly, with compression of the septum toward the posterior wall. Although septal geometry may alter the flow field so as to promote anterior leaflet motion, the marked leaflet elongation allows the valve to respond to those forces. LV = left ventricle; LA = left atrium; RV = right ventricle.

SAM: Leaflet slack or redundancy, created by papillary muscle displacement and mitral leaflet elongation, plays a key role in the development of SAM by allowing the leaflets to move in response to flow-related forces (Fig. 25–39). In that sense, SAM resembles primary mitral valve prolapse, in which leaflet slack or redundancy also increases leaflet excursion. In prolapse, the leaflets move superiorly into the left atrium but retain their posterior position. In SAM, anterior malposition of the papillary muscles and mitral valve directs the superior motion anteriorly into the left ventricular outflow tract. This relationship may explain the frequently noted association between SAM and mitral valve prolapse in patients.[246,247] It can also explain the occasional transformation of prolapse into SAM following mitral valve repair and insertion of a Carpentier ring: residual leaflet redundancy and anterior malposition created by ring geometry may combine to cause SAM of the mitral valve. Figure 25–40 shows a patient who at times manifests SAM, at others mitral valve prolapse, illustrating the close relation between the two. Finally, in occasional patients with prosthetic mitral valve replacement, retention of the anterior mitral leaflet in the outflow tract renders it entirely redundant to coaptation and allows it to move anteriorly and obstruct outflow.[248]

Other Forms of Functional Outflow Obstruction

Mitral leaflet motion must reflect a balance between flow-related forces and papillary muscle restraint (Fig. 25–41). It might therefore be anticipated that for any given ejection velocity, functional subvalvular obstruction would occur any time the distance between the interventricular septum and the anterior mitral leaflet reached a critical point, assuming that there is sufficient flexibility of the mitral valve apparatus to permit anterior leaflet motion. Given these relationships, any factor that increases ejection velocity, decreases the space between the anterior mitral leaflet and septum, or increases leaflet redundancy should increase the tendency for obstruction.[201]

Three clinical settings in which functional subvalvular obstruction often develops illustrate this physiology. The first is the elderly patient, usually a woman with long-standing hypertension, who is admitted to the hospital with hypovolemia resulting from gastrointestinal bleeding or excessive diuresis. A harsh systolic murmur prompts an echocardiographic examination that typically reveals concentric left ventricular hypertrophy, a small left ventricular cavity, and SAM, which resolves with volume replacement or correction of the anemia.[199,201] The combination of anemia and hypovolemia in such patients presumably increases ejection velocity and decreases the outflow space, thereby producing obstruction. In general, an association between hypertensive hypertrophy in the elderly and functional subaortic obstruction has been noted.[90,91,201,249–254] Whether such hypertrophy represents a primary myopathy or an exuberant response to the increased afterload,[253,255–257] its practical significance is that treatment with afterload-reducing agents, thus further narrowing the outflow tract, often causes marked hypotension; negative inotro-

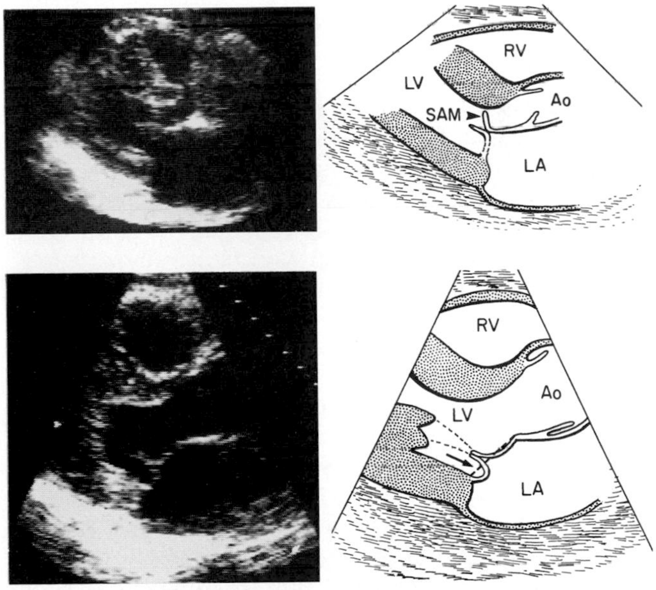

Fig. 25–40. Two parasternal long axis views of the same patient separated by 2 years, illustrating a dynamic change from systolic anterior motion (SAM) (top) to prolapse of the posterior mitral leaflet (bottom). In both cases, leaflet motion is excessive, but its anteroposterior component varies depending on the relationship between the leaflets and the flow field. RV = right ventricle; Ao = aorta; LA = left atrium; LV = left ventricle.

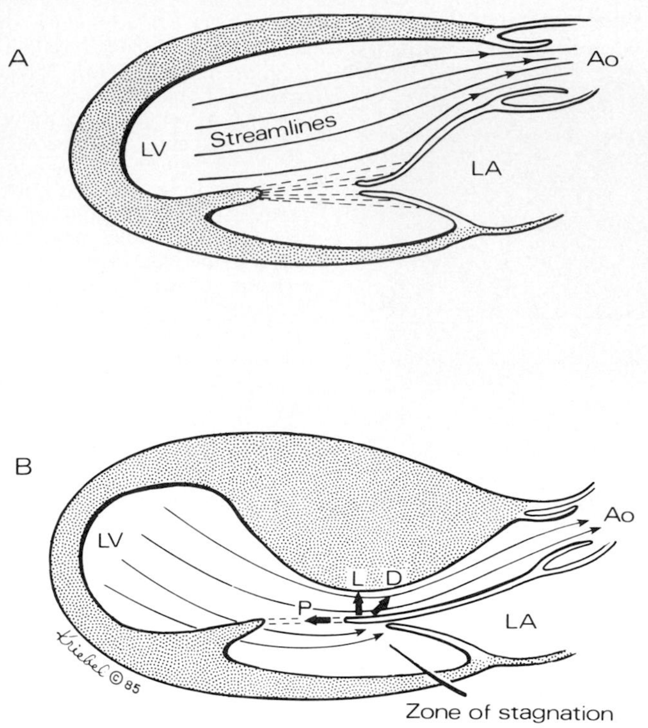

Fig. 25–41. Schematic parasternal long axis views of left ventricle (LV) in normal individual **(A)** and in a patient with hypertrophic cardiomyopathy **(B),** demonstrating forces acting on the distal leaflet. Increased velocity in the narrowed outflow tract causes a lift force (L) capable of producing anterior mitral motion. Diversion of flow around the septum interposes the distal leaflet in the path of flow, generating drag forces (D), which act anteriorly. Ao = aorta; P = papillary muscle tension; LA = left atrium; LV = left ventricle. (From Jiang L, Levine RA, King ME, Weyman AE: An integrated mechanism to explain the systolic anterior motion of the mitral valve in hypertrophic cardiomyopathy based on echocardiographic observations. Am Heart J 113:633, 1987.)

pic agents such as β-blockers are therefore the treatment of choice for the hypertension.[253]

The second setting in which functional subvalvular obstruction occurs involves patients with fixed outflow obstruction at the subvalvular, valvular, or supravalvular level with secondary left ventricular hypertrophy. Following surgical relief of the outflow obstruction, these patients develop functional obstruction at the ventricular level, which is commonly transient.[90,92,258] Relief of the fixed obstruction may allow ejection velocity to increase, and given the narrowed outflow space, functional subvalvular obstruction may result.

The third setting involves patients with D-transposition of the great arteries.[51–53,192,193] SAM in such patients may relate to curvature of the prominent septum, which indents the left ventricular outflow tract, causing blood to curve beneath the mitral leaflets to exit and thereby creating drag forces that cause SAM.

Functional subvalvular aortic stenosis, therefore, appears to develop in response to a series of geometric and hemodynamic alterations within the left ventricle and, as such, seems to be a functional derangement with multiple causes.

Summary

Imaging and Doppler echocardiography are therefore powerful noninvasive techniques for assessing the anatomy and physiology of hypertrophic cardiomyopathy and related conditions. They have provided important insights into the mechanism and physiologic significance of obstruction in this condition and in functional subvalvular obstruction in general. Ultimately, they should provide a means of validating hypotheses relating to responsible genetic defects and to the progression of morphologic and functional changes in models based on such new knowledge.

DILATED OR CONGESTIVE CARDIOMYOPATHIES

Definition and Cause

The congestive or dilated cardiomyopathies are fundamentally defined by a generalized disease in systolic pump function.[3,4,259,260] The term *dilated cardiomyopathy* is used by some to emphasize the earlier and predominant feature of dilation as opposed to the generally later clinical manifestation of heart failure (congestive cardiomyopathy).[261] Depending on the population studied, frequent causative associations include excessive alcohol consumption and antecedent influenza-like illnesses.[261] Some patients have had rheumatic fever several years earlier without apparent involvement of the cardiac valves.[261] Less commonly, dilated cardiomyopathy occurs on a familial or postpartum basis; as part of the spectrum of hemochromatosis and transfusional iron overload[262–264]; as a dose-related adverse effect of adriamycin therapy; or as a result of deficiencies of essential metabolites or nutrients, such as carnitine or selenium.[265]

Salient Echocardiographic Features

The reduction in contractile function as evaluated echocardiographically is typically symmetric,[266] involving both ventricles, and is associated with an increase in both systolic and diastolic chamber volumes (Fig. 25–42). Wall thickness is usually normal but may be increased or decreased; when increases in wall thickness do occur, they are not proportionate to the increase in chamber volume.[267] Overall cardiac mass, on the other hand, is almost invariably increased.[1,2] Diastolic mitral valve excursion is reduced (Fig. 25–42A) and the E-point septal separation is usually increased, reflecting the low output.[268,269] Left and right atrial dilation are common. The echocardiographic features of these myopathies, however, provide little insight into the underlying cause, and the congestive pattern represents a final common pathway for a variety of disorders.

Differential Diagnosis

Congestive changes are generally not subtle, at least in the referral population, and care must be taken not to diagnose this condition solely because the left ventricular internal dimension exceeds the 95% confidence limits of normal. This may be the case, e.g., in patients

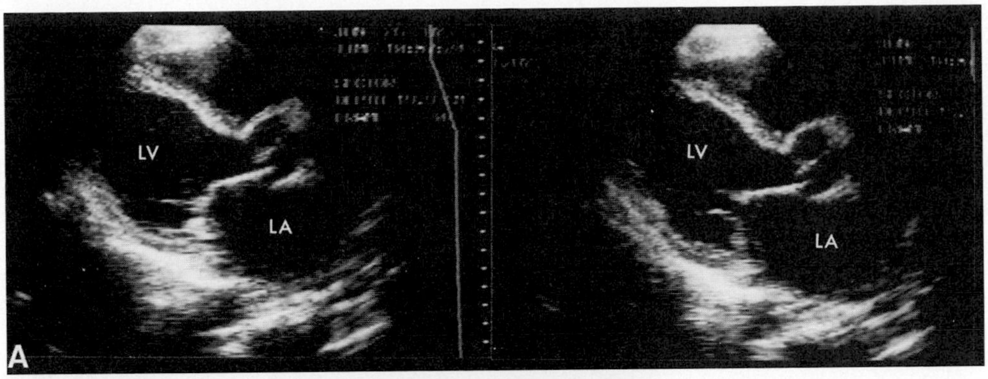

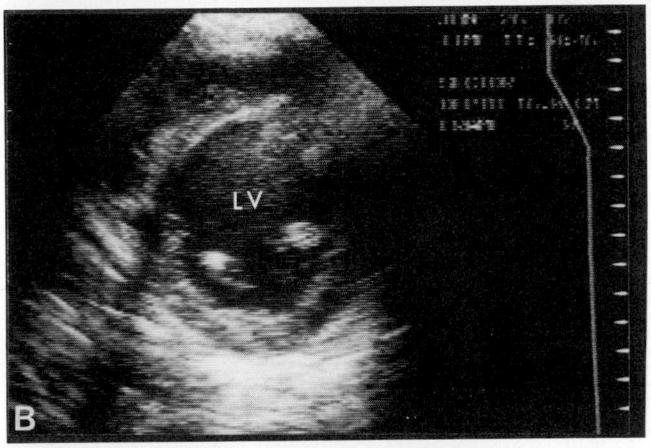

Fig. 25–42. Diffuse dilation of the left ventricle (LV) as well as left atrium (LA) in a patient with dilated cardiomyopathy. **A.** Parasternal long axis view: left, systole, showing large end-systolic volume; right, diastole, showing limited mitral valve excursion reflecting decreased cardiac output. **B.** Parasternal short axis view. **C.** Apical four-chamber view, showing tenting of the mitral valve (MV) toward the dilated left ventricular apex, away from the dashed line connecting the annular hinge points. RA = right atrium; RV = right ventricle.

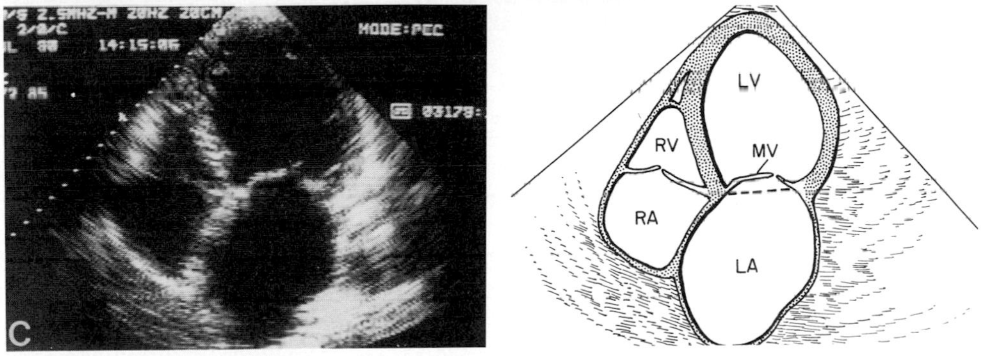

with large body surface areas or in aerobically trained athletes, who may have mildly dilated ventricles and diminished fractional shortening of the left ventricular internal diameter.[6] Major elements in the differential include the following:

1. *Ischemic heart disease*. As a rule, wall motion is symmetrically reduced in the cardiomyopathy, whereas wall motion abnormalities are typically segmental in ischemic heart disease.[266] Diffuse hypokinesis involving the right ventricle as well is also a differential point in favor of cardiomyopathy. Exceptions occur, however. For example, segmental wall motion abnormality has been described in dilated cardiomyopathy without angiographic coronary lesions,[270,271] such as that which may occur following transient myocarditis.[272] Segmental abnormalities, in particular apical aneurysms, are, in fact, the classic presentation of chronic Chagas' disease (Trypanosoma cruzi infestation).[273] On the other hand, ischemic heart disease may manifest as diffuse wall motion abnormality,[271,274] reflecting the widespread nature of the vascular lesions, although segmental variability in function often persists. The increased afterload created by dilation of infarcted segments (Laplace's law: increased radius producing increased wall stress) could also potentially create more diffuse hypokinesis by decreasing the fractional shortening of noninfarcted segments to which the vascular supply is compromised.

2. *Volume overload lesions*. Diffuse left ventricular dysfunction can occur secondary to chronic volume overload, which can be recognized on the Doppler study as prominent aortic or mitral insufficiency, for example, or rarely, as an uncorrected ductal or ventricular shunt without right-sided outflow or vascular obstruction. Dilated cardiomyopathy, however, may itself cause vary-

ing degrees of mitral regurgitation;[275] therefore, when chronic, severe mitral regurgitation and ventricular dysfunction coexist, it may not be obvious which is primary, although therapeutic options may be limited in either event. Valvular morphology can, of course, be helpful, with apical tethering of the mitral valve (the incomplete closure pattern; see following discussion) occurring in dilated cardiomyopathy and intrinsic abnormalities occurring in primary valvular disease.

3. In the *pediatric* range, concomitant dilation and hypertrophy can suggest carnitine deficiency,[265] while anomalous origin of the left coronary from the pulmonary artery is suggested by a characteristic distribution of wall motion abnormality and visualization of the coronary anomaly (see Chapter 34).

Variants

The term *mildly dilated cardiomyopathy* has been used to describe a generally familial condition manifesting severe left ventricular dysfunction, often leading to transplantation, but with left ventricular internal diameters $<$ 10 to 15% above the normal range.[276] Histologically, such patients have little or no myofibrillar loss, possibly explaining their failure to dilate, in contrast to patients with the more typical dilated myopathy, in whom myofibrillar loss is prominent.[276,277] Failure without fiber loss may relate to defects of energy generation (at the mitochondrial or adenosine triphosphatase level) or of activation (at the sarcolemmal level).

Right Ventricular Involvement

Right ventricular involvement generally parallels global cardiac dilation; occasional patients, however, have predominant or exclusive right ventricular dilation (e.g., after some instances of Coxsackie B virus infection).[278,279] Such patients retain normal right ventricular wall thickness, unlike those with Uhl's anomaly (Osler's "parchment heart"), in whom replacement of myocardium with adipose and fibrous tissue creates the echocardiographic appearance of regional wall thinning with wall motion abnormality.[279]

Evaluation of Ventricular Function

Systolic Function

Fundamental to the diagnosis of congestive cardiomyopathy is the ability to measure left ventricular pump function and establish that it lies below the range of normal. Because of the typically symmetric reduction in wall motion, this can generally be accomplished from end-systolic and end-diastolic measurements of the left ventricular internal dimension below the tips of the mitral leaflets from the M-mode or two-dimensional recording, with calculation of the percentage of fractional shortening or a derived ejection fraction (see Chapter 20). Doppler echocardiography also permits direct calculation of cardiac output, e.g., by integrating pulsed Doppler aortic outflow velocities and multiplying by cross-sectional area at the same level, subject to measurement limitations[280] (see Chapter 30). Several studies have attempted to simplify this procedure by using peak aortic flow velocity only. Initial results were promising using pulsed Doppler scans from the suprasternal window, with good separation between normal subjects (72 to 120 cm/sec) and patients with dilated cardiomyopathy (35 to 62 cm/sec, $p < .001$).[281] Subsequent studies, however, have shown a good correlation only between changes in peak velocity and changes in stroke volume with afterload manipulation, while absolute velocities correlated poorly with stroke volume in both patients and experimental animals,[282,283] perhaps because of variability in outflow tract area and in the time course of left ventricular ejection, which also affect these velocities. More recently, it has been recognized that peak aortic flow velocity is not only a function of intrinsic left ventricular contractile function but depends on loading conditions and heart rate as well.[284]

Such limitations have motivated attempts to develop other measures of left ventricular contractility. In patients with mitral regurgitation, left ventricular dP/dt (the first derivative of chamber pressure) can be calculated from the continuous-wave Doppler tracing of the regurgitant jet because of the relationship between pressure gradient and the square of the velocity (the simplified Bernoulli equation)[285,286] (see Chapter 9). Both the percentage of fractional shortening of the left ventricular internal dimension and the velocity of fractional shortening (V_{cf}) derived from digitized M-mode tracings vary inversely and linearly with left ventricular end-systolic circumferential or meridional wall stress, which reflects afterload.[287] Therefore, one might suppose that a myopathic decrease in contractility could be demonstrated by a decreased fractional shortening for any given end-systolic wall stress, compared with normal ventricles. For the same end-systolic wall stress, however, fractional shortening also increases with increasing preload (initial fiber stretch; Starling's Law), and therefore this measure cannot be used alone to assess contractility. In contrast, the line relating the velocity of fractional shortening (corrected for heart rate) to end-systolic wall stress is preload independent and shifts upward with increasing inotropic state. The location of this line relative to normal can therefore be considered an index of contractility.[287] Both V_{cf} and end-systolic wall stress can be estimated noninvasively from an M-mode echocardiogram and a carotid pulse tracing calibrated from brachial cuff pressures.[287] Although not in routine clinical use, this index has recently been used in young diabetics with a decrease in exercise ejection fraction to demonstrate the absence of a myopathic decrease in inotropic state. Their V_{cf}/end-systolic wall stress relation fell within normal limits and responded appropriately to dobutamine administration.[288]

Diastolic Function

As discussed previously, the Doppler pattern of diastolic mitral inflow directly reflects left ventricular filling but is influenced by a complex combination of loading conditions, heart rate and atrial characteristics in addition to intrinsic left ventricular diastolic properties. It is not surprising, therefore, that a spectrum of inflow patterns has been described in dilated cardiomyopathy depending on hemodynamic presentation. The first pattern has a decreased velocity of early diastolic inflow (E wave) and a relatively increased velocity of inflow following atrial contraction (A wave).[289,290] This pattern is characteristic of delayed ventricular relaxation, which has been demonstrated by other methods in this condition.[291] Delayed relaxation delays and diminishes the development of the early diastolic atrioventricular pressure gradient, which drives inflow and therefore prolongs the isovolumic relaxation time (IVRT) and decreases the peak E-wave velocity, with a presumably compensatory increase in atrial contribution (Chapter 24, Figs. 24–32 and 24–49). This pattern has been described in patients with clinically milder disease (New York Heart Association classes I and II) and those without mitral regurgitation.[289,290] It is potentially important in assessing the importance of the atrial contribution to ventricular filling, e.g., in deciding whether to institute dual-chamber pacing. On the other hand, patients with mitral regurgitation and those with a more severe clinical presentation (NYHA class III–IV) have shown a normalization of the peak E velocity and a relatively smaller A-wave.[289,290] Potential factors causing normalization of the inflow pattern include (1) increased left atrial pressure caused by mitral regurgitation or as a compensatory response to raise cardiac output by increasing filling pressure.[189] This will cause left ventricular pressure to fall below left atrial pressure sooner after aortic valve closure, decreasing the IVRT, and it will raise the early diastolic atrioventricular pressure gradient and, therefore, the corresponding inflow velocity (Chapter 24, Fig. 24–26). In a recent study, in fact, peak E-wave velocity varied directly with the pulmonary capillary wedge pressure in patients with dilated cardiomyopathy, and IVRT varied inversely with wedge pressure.[290] (2) Another potential factor is increased left ventricular stiffness (slope of the pressure-volume curve) that is due to fibrosis (causing an increase in the exponential stiffness constant describing that curve)[292] and ventricular dilation (shifting the ventricle to steeper portions of the curve). This will cause left ventricular diastolic pressure to rise more rapidly and the atrioventricular pressure gradient to fall more rapidly, as diastole progresses, causing a more rapid E-wave deceleration, as described in such patients with more severe heart failure.[290] Peak A-wave velocities are also decreased because of increased atrial afterload (higher ventricular end-diastolic pressures). The development of this pattern therefore suggests increased filling pressures that are due to mitral regurgitation or progressive ventricular dysfunction. Although practical clinical applications of these findings have yet to be described, such as restrictive-type pattern might suggest limitation to ventricular filling that could be alleviated by agents that decrease left ventricular size.[282,293]

Complications and Prognosis: Ultrasound Evaluation

Mortality

Imaging and Doppler echocardiography can evaluate the basic predictors of mortality in dilated cardiomyopathy, such as increased heart size, decreased cardiac index[261] and decreased ejection fraction[260] (see Chapters 20 and 30). These measures can also be monitored during therapy[262,293] or prophylactically during adriamycin administration.[265] The ratio of left ventricular wall thickness to cavity size has also been proposed as a prognostic index, reflecting the adequacy of hypertrophy in response to increased wall stress in the dilated ventricle[267]; the prognostic value of this ratio has been confirmed in a recent multicenter Veterans' Administration study of 390 patients.[260] (While a smaller study of 36 patients found this ratio did not distinguish survivors from nonsurvivors, both groups in the latter study had ratios at the lower end of the overall range seen in the Veterans' Administration trial.[294])

Mitral Regurgitation. Myopathic ventricular dilatation may produce the incomplete mitral valve closure pattern,[295,296] in which apical displacement of the papillary muscles puts increased tension on the leaflets and, in turn, displaces their coaptation apically (Figures 25–42c and 25–43).[297,298] A similar pattern is observed in ischemic heart disease with dilatation of myocardial segments lying below the papillary muscles.[295] This apical tenting impairs the ability of the mitral valve to achieve a competent closure (Fig. 25–44) by causing the leaflets to coapt at or near their tips rather than by apposition of their rough zones. When right ventricular dilation is marked, similar changes in the tricuspid valve may also be noted.[299] The role of mitral annular dilation in this process has been debated. Pathology of the fixed heart suggests that the mitral, unlike the tricuspid annulus, remains normal in these myopathies.[1,300] One echocardiographic study, while showing an increase in annu-

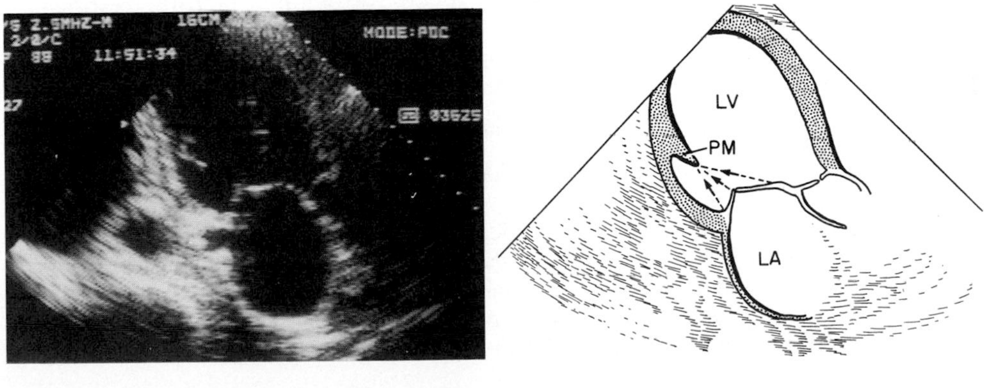

Fig. 25–43. The incomplete mitral valve closure pattern in an apical long-axis view. Tethering of the mitral leaflets by the apically and posteriorly displaced papillary muscles (PMs) tents them as shown, creating a characteristic angulation in the anterior leaflet contour. LV = left ventricle; LA = left atrium.

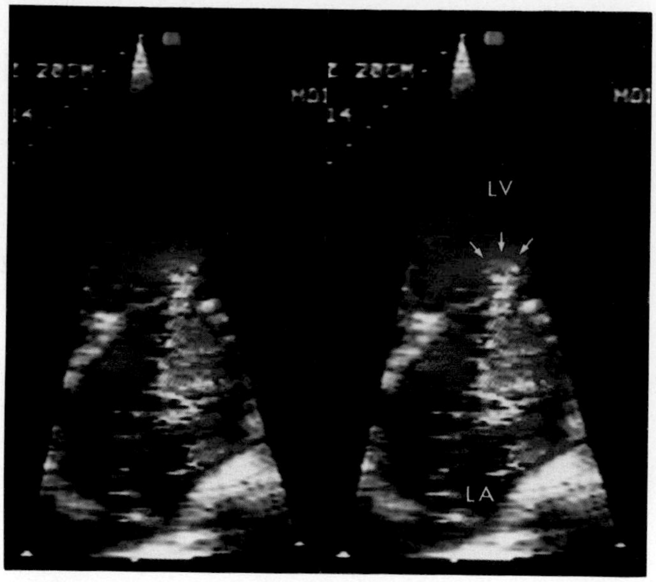

Fig. 25–44. Mitral regurgitation in a patient with dilated cardiomyopathy and incomplete mitral valve closure, with proximal acceleration (arrows) on the ventricular (LV) side of the leaflets and a turbulent jet within the left atrium (LA).

lar diameter in dilated cardiomyopathy, did not find it predictive of angiographic regurgitation;[301] in contrast, another showed that annular area was greater in patients with dilated cardiomyopathy and a murmur of mitral regurgitation than in those without such a murmur, paralleling left atrial dilation in the patients with a murmur.[302] Whether the annular dilation, in fact, caused regurgitation or resulted from it could not be resolved by such studies. A potential role for dilation of the dynamic annulus, however, is not inconsistent with the unified mechanism of incomplete mitral valve closure proposed in Chapter 17, in that (1) both apical papillary muscle displacement and annular dilation geometrically act on opposite ends of the leaflets to create the tented incomplete closure configuration; and (2) annular dilation increases the area that must be occluded by the leaflets, thereby increasing the likelihood of incomplete coaptation.[302]

Thromboembolic Complications

Thrombi commonly form within the dilated chambers, most often in the left ventricle and least often in the left atrium.[1] Two-dimensional echocardiography can detect left ventricular thrombi with reasonable sensitivity and specificity (>80 to 90% each), although false-positives may relate to near-field reverberatory artifacts (which have less distinct ventricular interfaces) and false tendons (which are linear and surrounded by fluid)[259,303,304] (see Chapter 36). Swirling patterns of echogenic blood corresponding to regional stasis (''smoke'') can also be demonstrated and are felt to imply the potential for thrombosis.[305,306] Unfortunately, however, the ability to predict either thrombus formation or embolization in the individual patient has not been achieved to date. A proposed method for predicting thrombus formation based on low apical velocities by pulsed Doppler[307] requires prospective testing in larger populations, in whom anticoagulant therapy may represent a confounding variable. Two critical points must be emphasized, however, in practical considerations: (1) the incidence of embolization in one large clinical review of dilated cardiomyopathy was 18% in patients without anticoagulation vs. 0% in anticoagulated patients;[261] (2) in another study, of 96 patients with dilated cardiomyopathy, the incidence of presumed systemic embolization was the same in patients with and without left ventricular thrombi by two-dimensional echocardiography and was comparable for mobile, pedunculated, and flat thrombi,[308] despite a report to the contrary.[309] Such data have led some to recommend prophylaxis unless contraindicated,[261] at least until risk can be more clearly determined.

In summary, echocardiography can directly identify the dilated myopathic state and evaluate its severity and effect on ventricular size, output, and filling. It can demonstrate complications such as regurgitation and thrombus formation and can evaluate the results of therapy.

RESTRICTIVE AND INFILTRATIVE CARDIOMYOPATHIES

Definitions and Salient Features

Restrictive cardiomyopathies are characterized by a myopathic process that restricts ventricular filling, resulting in elevated ventricular filling pressures with typically normal or only mildly reduced systolic function.[2–4,310–312] Ventricular chamber size is normal or slightly reduced, and biatrial dilation is common. This hemodynamic classification overlaps to a large extent with the pathologic classification of *infiltrative cardiomyopathies,* in which abnormal interpolation of material between myocytes or metabolite storage within them creates the restrictive constellation, with prominently thickened myocardial walls that often have a highly abnormal acoustic texture.[313–323] Restriction, however, is not an invariable consequence of infiltration. The degree to which infiltration produces the clinical and hemodynamic picture of restriction depends on the nature and extent of the infiltrative process,[316,324,325] while some infiltrative processes can produce a dilated picture in certain patients (iron deposition) or regional wall motion abnormality in others (sarcoidosis).[313] The term *obliterative cardiomyopathy* has also been used to describe conditions in which endomyocardial disease processes and deposits produce a restrictive picture.[8]

In contrast to the dilated cardiomyopathies, with their common final pathway, the unique features of individual restrictive and infiltrative conditions require separate consideration.

Infiltrative Cardiomyopathies

Amyloidosis

Amyloidosis is a disease characterized by the deposition of an abnormal eosinophilic fibrous protein in various tissues and organs of the body.[326] Cardiac involvement is common, and amyloidosis is reported to account for between 5 and 10% of noncoronary cardiomyopathies.[327] In patients with amyloidosis, heart failure is the most common cause of death and is noted in as many as 20% of patients.[328,329]

Pathology. In amyloidosis, the abnormal protein is deposited between the myocardial fibers, which it may surround, compress, and finally replace.[1,327,330,331] It may also be found in the papillary muscles, conduction system, pericardium, and coronary artery walls. Amyloid deposition in the left atrium and particularly the atrial septum has been reported, and atrial involvement may be useful echocardiographically in differentiating amyloidosis from other infiltrative myopathies.[313,320] Endocardial involvement of both the atrium and ventricles is not uncommon and may be associated with overlying thrombus. Amyloidosis also frequently causes focal or diffuse thickening of the cardiac valves, but valvular dysfunction is not a predominant characteristic. There are four principal forms of amyloidosis:

1. Primary amyloidosis, which occurs independent of other systemic diseases and in which the tissue involvement is localized primarily to the heart, tongue, skin, gastrointestinal tract, and carpal ligaments:[328] The amyloid protein in this form is identical to the immunoglobulin light chain (AL type),[329,332] which can also produce amyloid deposits in patients with multiple myeloma.[313]
2. Secondary amyloidosis, which usually occurs in association with chronic disorders, such as rheumatoid arthritis or tuberculosis, and in which tissue involvement is primarily localized to the spleen, kidney, liver, and adrenals: The amyloid protein in this form is protein AA,[333] and cardiac involvement, although reported, is rare.[334]
3. Familial amyloidosis, of which multiple varieties have been described that differ in either clinical presentation or primary organ involvement:[335] Primary involvement of the heart has been felt to be rare in familial amyloidosis[335,336] but may be more common than previously suspected. It is reportedly common, on the other hand, in familial amyloidosis with polyneuropathy.[319]
4. Senile amyloidosis, which appears to be a clinically distinct form of primary amyloidosis and is characterized by the advanced age of the affected person and the almost entirely cardiac location of the amyloid deposits, which consist of prealbumin-related protein:[330,337–339] Available data suggest that senile amyloidosis may be the most common form of amyloid, and its incidence can be expected to increase as the average age of the population increases. Senile amyloidosis has been reported at autopsy in 2 to 15% of the population over the age of 80, and its incidence is three to four times greater in patients dying of heart failure than in those without overt cardiac disease.[330,337]

Echocardiographic Features. The classic echocardiographic picture of amyloidosis is a constellation of increased right and left ventricular wall thickness, typically symmetric with a speckled or granular sparkling appearance, and normal or small ventricular cavity size[313–324,340–341] (Figs. 25–45 to 25–47). Left ventricular systolic function may be normal or reduced, and biatrial enlargement is common, reflecting the elevated filling pressures.[313–316,318] Other distinctive features include diffuse valvular thickening and evidence of atrial infiltration by the amyloid deposits[316,320,341] (Figs. 25–48 and 25–49). Valvular regurgitation, typically mild, is present in the majority of patients, more commonly across the mitral and tricuspid valves than the aortic and pulmonary valves.[313,318] Small-to-moderate pericardial effusions are common.[313,314,316,318]

Spectrum of Findings and Clinical Correlations. Although the preceding features were frequently found in the initial echocardiographic studies of patients who mainly presented with advanced disease,[314–316] more recent studies of a broader range of patients have revealed a wide spectrum of wall thickness and systolic function.[318,324] Echocardiography, e.g., can demonstrate abnormalities (primarily increased wall thickness) in patients with systemic amyloidosis even before there is clinical evidence of cardiac involvement. The spectrum of echocardiographic wall thickness also has its clinical and functional correlates.[318] In particular, a study of 132

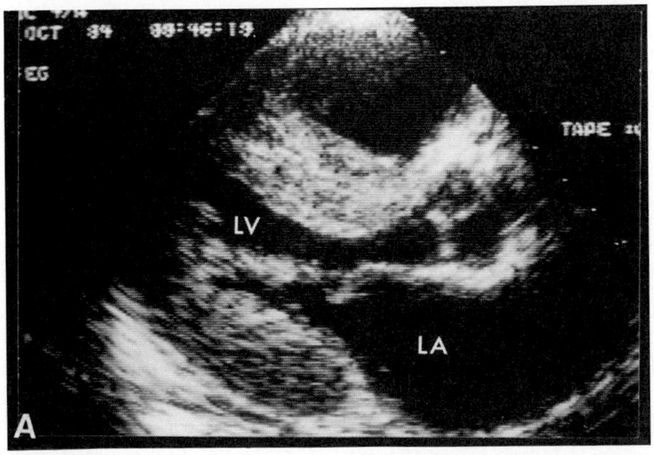

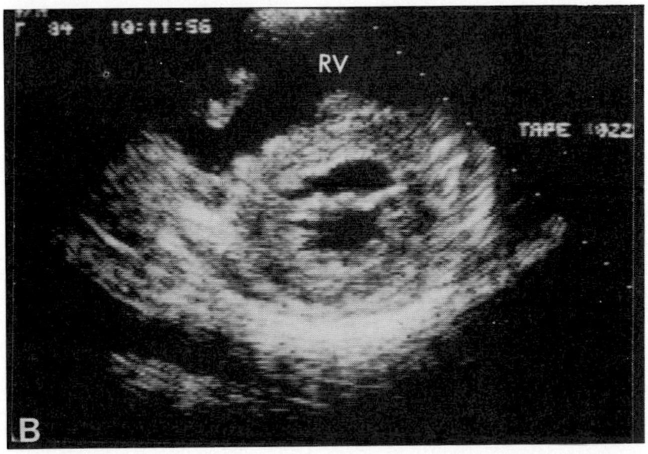

Fig. 25–45. Parasternal long axis and short axis views of a patient with cardiac amyloidosis, showing concentric left ventricular hypertrophy and mild, diffuse thickening of the aortic and mitral valves. LV = left ventricle; LA = left atrium; RV = right ventricle.

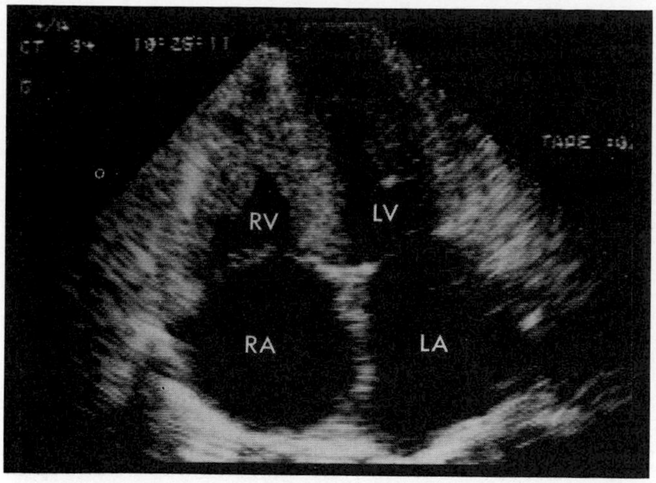

Fig. 25–46. Biventricular hypertrophy in amyloidosis. RV = right ventricle; LV = left ventricle; LA = left atrium; RA = right atrium.

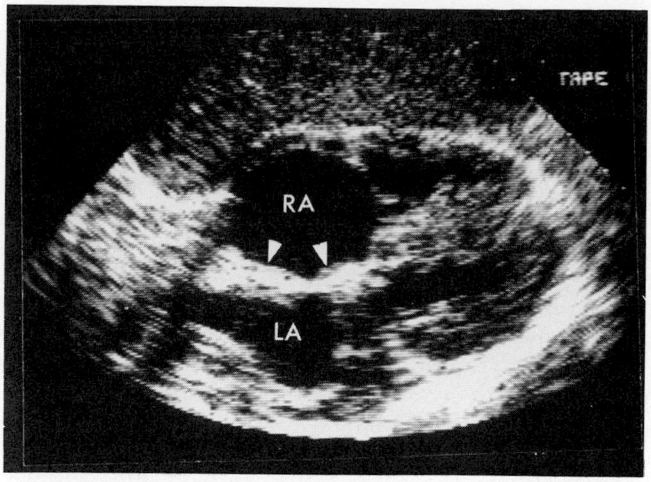

Fig. 25–49. Bilobed thickening of the atrial septum (subcostal view) in a patient with cardiac amyloidosis. RA = right atrium; LA = left atrium.

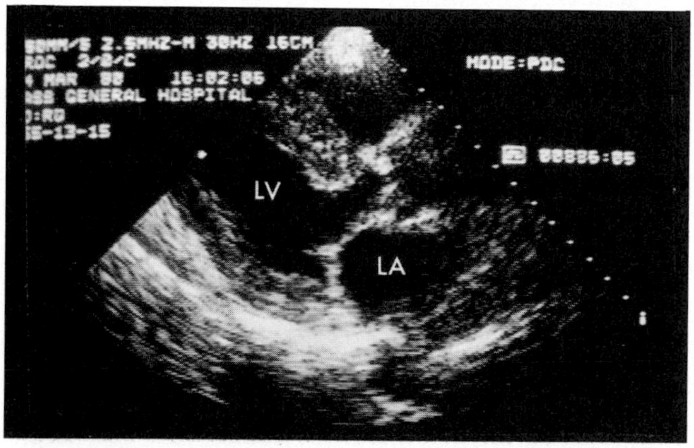

Fig. 25–47. Sparkling granular myocardial texture in amyloidosis. LV = left ventricle; LA = left atrium.

patients with biopsy-proved systemic amyloidosis showed that median survival was longest (2.4 years) in patients with mean wall thickness (average of septal and posterior wall thickness) $\leq$ 12 mm; none of these patients had decreased systolic function (defined as fractional shortening of the left ventricular internal diameter $<$ 30%)[318] (Table 25–1). Median survival was shorter (1.3 years) in patients with mean wall thickness between 12 and 15 mm, 35% of whom had systolic dysfunction, and decreased to 0.4 years in those with mean wall thickness $\geq$ 15 mm, 71% of whom had systolic dysfunction as well. A corresponding graded increase was seen in the frequency of granular sparkling myocardial texture, left atrial enlargement, and clinical congestive heart failure (Table 25–1). In patients who had serial echocardiographic examinations, clinical deterioration corresponded to progressive increases in left and right ventricular wall thickness. Both increased wall thickness and decreased systolic function made independent

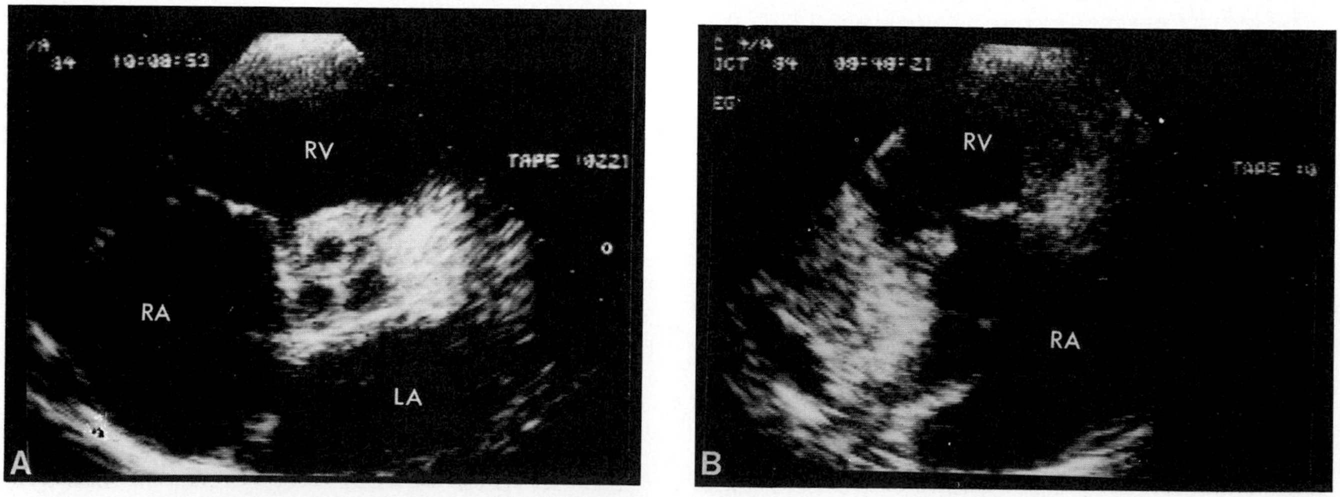

Fig. 25–48. Diffuse thickening of the aortic **(A)** and tricuspid **(B)** valves in cardiac amyloidosis. RV = right ventricle; LA = left atrium; RA = right atrium.

Table 25–1. Primary Systemic Amyloidosis: Echocardiographic and Clinical Variables

	MWT ≤ 12	12 < MWT < 15	MWT ≥ 15	Atypical	Total
Number	34	23	68	7	132
CHF	24%	52%	80%	43%	58%
Systolic dysfunction (FS < 30%)	0%	35%	71%	100%	48%
LV dilation (LVID > 55 mm)	0%	0%	0%	71%	4%
Granular sparkling	0%	48%	72%	29%	47%
Dilated left atrium	21%	41%	83%	67%	61%
Normal echocardiogram	74%	0%	0%	0%	19%
Median actuarial survival (years)	2.4	1.3	0.4	0.5	1.1

CHF = congestive heart failure; FS = fractional shortening; LVID = left ventricular internal dimension; MWT = mean left ventricular wall thickness (in mm).

Adapted from Cueto-Garcia L, et al.: Serial echocardiographic observation in patients with primary systemic amyloidosis: an introduction to the concept of early (asymptomatic) amyloid infiltration of the heart. Mayo Clin Proc 59:589, 1984.

and additive contributions to the adverse prognosis. Despite the frequency of systolic dysfunction, however, only 5% (7) of the patients studied had left ventricular dilation (internal diameter ≥ 55m) or segmental wall motion abnormalities; at autopsy, 3 of these atypical patients had amyloid involvement confined to the coronary arteries, suggesting a potential vascular cause for their left ventricular dysfunction.[318] There is therefore a broad correspondence between the spectrum of echocardiographic, clinical, and prognostic features of cardiac amyloidosis, and echocardiography has become the procedure of choice for its noninvasive diagnosis and assessment.

Differential Diagnosis. Several features can be helpful in differentiating amyloidosis from other conditions causing increased ventricular wall thickness, most notably hypertrophic cardiomyopathy: (1) The increased wall thickness in amyloidosis is typically symmetric, as opposed to the classic asymmetry of hypertrophic cardiomyopathy. Although occasional instances of asymmetric septal hypertrophy with SAM of the mitral valve have been reported with pathologically confirmed cardiac amyloidosis,[59,342–344] the amyloid infiltration could also make it difficult to diagnose a coexisting hypertrophic cardiomyopathy pathologically by demonstrating myocardial fiber disarray. (2) The speckled or granular sparkling appearance of the myocardium in amyloidosis is a potentially useful differential point. Acoustic speckling, which results from the constructive and destructive interference of ultrasound reflected from small structures,[322] has been attributed to acoustic mismatch between amyloid material and adjacent myocytes,[316] although such a difference in acoustic impedance has yet to be demonstrated. In the series shown in Table 25–1, which includes a broad spectrum of cardiac amyloidosis, speckling occurred in approximately half of patients, with a higher frequency in those with more severe involvement.[318] In a review of 2000 consecutive echocardiograms from patients not initially known to have amyloidosis, 11 of 15 (73%) patients with speckling subsequently had positive gingival biopsies for amyloid, although 15 other patients refused biopsy.[317] While abnormal texture clearly occurs in amyloidosis, the specificity of this finding remains uncertain, given similar observations in patients with hypertrophic cardiomyopathy, chronic renal failure, and less common storage conditions such as Pompe's disease,[41,321,322] but not in hypertensive hypertrophy. Some have felt that textural changes are less diffuse in hypertrophic cardiomyopathy, being localized primarily to the interventricular septum;[316] others have claimed its virtual absence in that condition.[319] A recent tissue characterization study, which did not routinely note abnormal texture visually in any of eight patients with hypertrophic cardiomyopathy, did note quantitative abnormalities in backscatter and run-length statistics derived from the returning acoustic signal.[323] Nevertheless, abnormal texture has been reported in hypertrophic cardiomyopathy,[41] consistent with our routine clinical experience. Practically, although speckling is currently a subjective assessment with incomplete specificity, *abnormal texture of a symmetrically hypertrophied myocardium is useful in suggesting the diagnosis of amyloidosis as opposed to hypertensive hypertrophy.*[320] (3) Diffuse valvular thickening and (4) atrial involvement are characteristic of amyloidosis,[316,320,341] although bilobed thickening of the atrial septum (sparing the foramen ovale) is also seen in lipomatous hypertrophy (a common finding, particularly in the older population). (5) Systolic dysfunction without ventricular dilation is characteristic of progessive amyloid infiltration,[314,316,318] which may replace large areas of myocardium;[1] in contrast, systolic function in hypertrophic cardiomyopathy is typically normal or hyperdynamic, whereas the unusual patients who develop dysfunction generally dilate as well. (6) Increased right ventricular free wall thickness, although occurring in hypertrophic cardiomyopathy, is more commonly associated with amyloidosis.[316,324,340] (7) Echocardiographic information has also been combined with electrocardiographic voltage, based on the observation that voltage is diminished by the infiltrative condition;[319] in one study, a value < 1.5 for the ratio of the S-wave in V_1 + R-wave in V_5 or V_6/myocardial cross-sectional area at the base was over 80% sensitive and specific for amyloidosis as opposed to hypertrophic cardiomyopathy and hypertensive hypertrophy.[320]

In summary, therefore, several echocardiographic features strongly suggest the diagnosis of amyloidosis and help differentiate it from other conditions in which myocardial thickness is increased. Only biopsy (initially gingival), however, can provide a definitive diagnosis, particularly in the early stages of the disease when wall thickness is only mildly increased and textural changes are generally absent.[318]

Hemochromatosis

Hemochromatosis is a systemic disorder characterized by increased deposition of iron in tissue, causing heart failure, hepatic cirrhosis, diabetes mellitus, and involvement of other organs, such as the pituitary, gonads, and skin.[262,313,345] Hemochromatosis may be primary (idiopathic or hereditary) or secondary to chronic anemia (with or without transfusional iron overload), to congenital or acquired defects of erythrocytes or their production, or to excess oral iron intake.[345] Cardiac iron deposition is common in hemochromatosis but is virtually never seen without iron accumulation in other tissues.[1,345] Unlike amyloid deposits, which infiltrate between myocytes, iron deposits are stored within the muscle cells, typically around the nuclei but also extending to occupy much of the fiber.[345] They are most common in the working tissues of the heart, particularly the left ventricular myocardium; and are greatest in the subepicardial region, intermediate in the subendocardium, and papillary muscles; and are least prominent in the middle myocardial wall. Atrial involvement occurs later and is less marked, and in contrast to amyloid, there are no valvular deposits.[1] The myocardial iron deposits appear to cause fiber degeneration, and fibrosis can result in congestive heart failure. Both phenomena appear related to the severity of the iron deposition.[1,346]

A spectrum of echocardiographic findings has been described in this condition. In primary hemochromatosis, cardiac involvement, which is the leading cause of death, typically takes the form of left ventricular dilation, with moderate-to-severe global systolic dysfunction and biatrial enlargement.[347–349] Such findings were seen in 37% of a series of 24 patients with primary hemochromatosis and no other valvular, ischemic, or hypertensive heart disease.[347] Neither these patients nor those in other in vivo and autopsy series showed increased wall thickness, regional wall motion abnormalities, or primary valvular changes.[347–350] A restrictive physiology has rarely been reported.[351] Dilated cardiomyopathy has also been described in patients with secondary hemochromatosis,[262,264,346] although at least some M-mode reports have observed increased wall thickness as the major abnormality, possibly at an early stage of the disease.[264,315,352] Regional wall motion abnormalities have been described in patients with β-thalassemia,[353,354] although these abnormalities may relate to microcirculatory effects as opposed to iron deposition. In addition to identifying myocardial involvement, echocardiography has been useful in evaluating the beneficial effects of chelation therapy on systolic function.[262,263,348,349] Abnormal mitral inflow patterns have been described in limited studies of patients with cardiac involvement, but as in amyloidosis (see following discussion), no consistent or unique pattern has been noted,[313] reflecting the variable spectrum of disease and loading conditions.

Sarcoidosis

Sarcoidosis is a disease characterized by noncaseating granulomas involving the lungs, skin, eyes, heart, and other organs.[1] Autopsy studies have demonstrated cardiac infiltration in 20 to 25% of patients with sarcoidosis, most frequently in the left ventricular free wall, the upper interventricular septum (with associated conduction abnormalities), and the papillary muscles (with associated mitral regurgitation).[1,355,356] Sarcoidosis with clinically apparent cardiac involvement also involves other organs;[1] nevertheless, the earliest cardiac manifestation of this process may be sudden death.[355,356]

The most common echocardiographic abnormality in patients with myocardial involvement is left ventricular dilation with segmental or diffuse wall motion abnormalities.[313,357,358] (Coronary artery disease, however, has also been found in several patients with sarcoidosis and segmental defects.[357]) The interventricular septum may be increased or decreased in thickness,[357] and left ventricular aneurysms have occasionally been reported following corticosteroid therapy,[359] although their occurrence does not appear to be the rule.[357] Cor pulmonale caused by pulmonary sarcoidosis may increase the free wall thickness of the right ventricle and decrease its systolic function because of increased afterload.[360] Pericardial effusions have also been reported as well as left ventricular thrombi (as in other patients with dilated cardiomyopathy).[355,358] A restrictive pattern caused by extensive myocardial infiltration has also been described but is rare.[361]

Glycogen, Lipid, and Mucopolysaccharide Storage Diseases

Abnormal metabolites may accumulate within the cardiac myocytes in several storage diseases created by inborn errors of metabolism, which are generally autosomal recessive. Echocardiographic studies of these conditions have been limited by their infrequent occurrence and by chest wall deformities occurring in the mucopolysaccharidoses.[58]

In Pompe's disease (type II glycogen storage disease), cardiac hypertrophy involving both ventricles is typically seen; similar findings occur less commonly in type III (Cori's) disease[265,362–364] (Fig. 25–50). Occasionally, prominent and asymmetric septal hypertrophy is seen in Pompe's disease, along with obstructive SAM of the mitral valve.[55,56,365]

Asymmetric hypertrophy has also been reported in Fabry's disease (angiokeratoma corporis diffusum universale), a rare sex-linked disorder of lipid metabolism in which ceramide trihexoside accumulates in many tissues, producing, e.g., characteristic angiokeratomas on the lower trunk.[57] The cardiac picture in Fabry's disease is similar to that in cardiac amyloidosis, including promi-

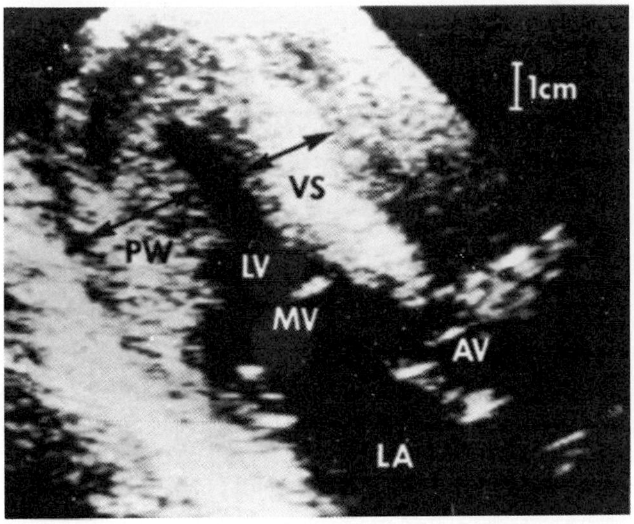

Fig. 25–50. Diffuse left ventricular (LV) hypertrophy of the ventricular septum (VS) and posterior wall (PW) in a patient with type III glycogen storage disease (apical long axis view). MV = mitral valve; AV = aortic valve; LA = left atrium. (From Olson LJ, et al.: Cardiac involvement in glycogen storage disease III: morphologic and biochemical characterization with endomyocardial biopsy. Am J Cardiol 53:900, 1984.)

nent biventricular hypertrophy, a granular sparkling texture, normal ventricular size with reduced systolic function, and pericardial effusion.[366,367] Occasional patients with upper septal thickening have also been described in the mucopolysaccharide storage diseases (Hurler-Scheie, Sanfilippo, and Morquio); mitral leaflet thickening, however, appears to be the most common lesion in such conditions and may be associated with mitral regurgitation.[58]

Endomyocardial Disease

Endocardial Fibroelastosis

Endocardial fibroelastosis is a disorder of infants and young children characterized by diffuse hyperplasia of the endocardium caused by proliferation of collagenous and elastic tissue.[368,369] This disorder may be primary or secondary. The primary form is unassociated with other congenital cardiac defects and involves the left ventricle almost exclusively.[370–373] The endocardium is thicker, and the area of involvement is greater than in the secondary variety. Primary endocardial fibroelastosis can be subdivided on the basis of left ventricular size into the dilated and contracted forms.[368,369] The dilated form, in which the ventricular chamber is enlarged and the walls hypertrophied, is the more common. Fibrosis and thickening of the aortic and mitral leaflets with chordal shortening and fibrosis are also common and may lead to mitral regurgitation.[369]

Secondary endocardial fibroelastosis is pathologically indistinguishable from the primary form. In general, however, the secondary variety is more focal in nature, and the endocardial proliferation is less marked. Mural thrombi commonly complicate both varieties.[374] The secondary form is most commonly associated with obstruction to left ventricular outflow, particularly aortic stenosis[375] and coarctation of the aorta[376] but may be observed in a variety of other conditions, including anomalous origin of the left coronary artery from the pulmonary artery and hypoplastic left heart syndrome. Echocardiographically, subendocardial fibroelastosis appears as a focal or diffuse area of increased echo production arising from the endocardial interface. This dense band of echoes is usually homogeneous and may be several millimeters thick.[377] It stands out in sharp contrast to the normal epicardial echoes. Figure 25–51 is a parasternal long axis recording from a patient with subendocardial fibroelastosis and illustrates the endocardial predominance.

Löffler's Endocarditis and Endomyocardial Fibrosis

Löffler's endocarditis (eosinophilic endomyocardial disease) is a rare form of endocardial fibrosis that is characteristically associated with a chronic persistent elevation in circulating eosinophils.[378–382] At greatest risk are patients with the idiopathic hypereosinophilic syndrome,[383,384] in whom this cardiac manifestation occurs predominantly in males over the age of 15.[382,385] Similar pathologic findings occur less commonly in patients with secondary hypereosinophilia related to parasitic disease, hypersensitivity, and tumors,[383,384] although patients with such secondary hypereosinophilias do not generally manifest cardiac disease by two-dimensional echocardiography, even when the hypereosinophilia is prolonged.[386,387] A similar process was originally described by Davies as endomyocardial fibrosis,[388] occurring primarily in tropical countries with only variable hypereosinophilia, often indistinguishable from that

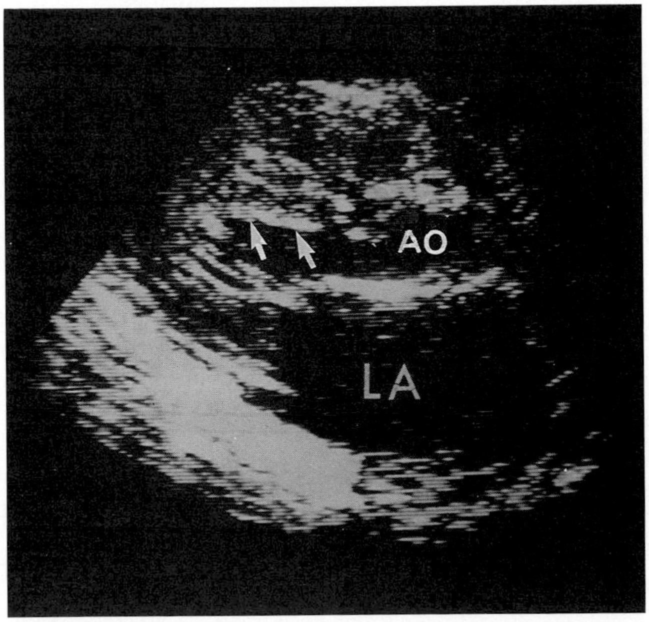

Fig. 25–51. Parasternal long axis view of a patient with subendocardial fibroelastosis illustrating the highly reflective layer, particularly evident along the left septal surface (arrows). AO = aorta; LA = left atrium.

in the surrounding unaffected population.[384,386] Subsequent analysis has shown that the tropical and nontropical processes are pathologically identical,[389,390] leading to the concept that they represent a single disease entity,[387–392] with the absence of hypereosinophilia in tropical patients reflecting clinical presentation at a late fibrotic stage following an initial necrotic stage with acute eosinophilic myocarditis.[387]

In these conditions, the endocardial fibrosis usually involves the mitral and tricuspid subvalvular areas and cardiac apex and, when pronounced, may cause valvular insufficiency that is due to thickening of the chordae tendineae and interference with their normal function.[378–382,389,393–395] Mitral and tricuspid stenosis may also occur and appear to result from entrapment of the subvalvular apparatus in the fibrous material.[396–398] Superimposed thrombus formation occurs frequently.[378,382,393] Pathologically, the endocardium is thickened with hyaline fibrosis. Inflammatory cells and dilated blood vessels lie between the endocardium and underlying myocardium. Degranulated eosinophils in the peripheral blood smear are a clue to this process,[384,386] and the contents of these granules have been demonstrated to have cardiac toxicity in experimental studies.[386]

Two-dimensional echocardiography is the most useful technique for evaluating this condition.[384,386,387,398–402] The endocardial deposits cause an increase in wall thickness with layering of the endocardial echoes[398,399] (Figs. 25–52 and 25–53). This is most evident at the apex of one or both ventricles, which are obliterated by the deposits, and in the region of the papillary muscles and

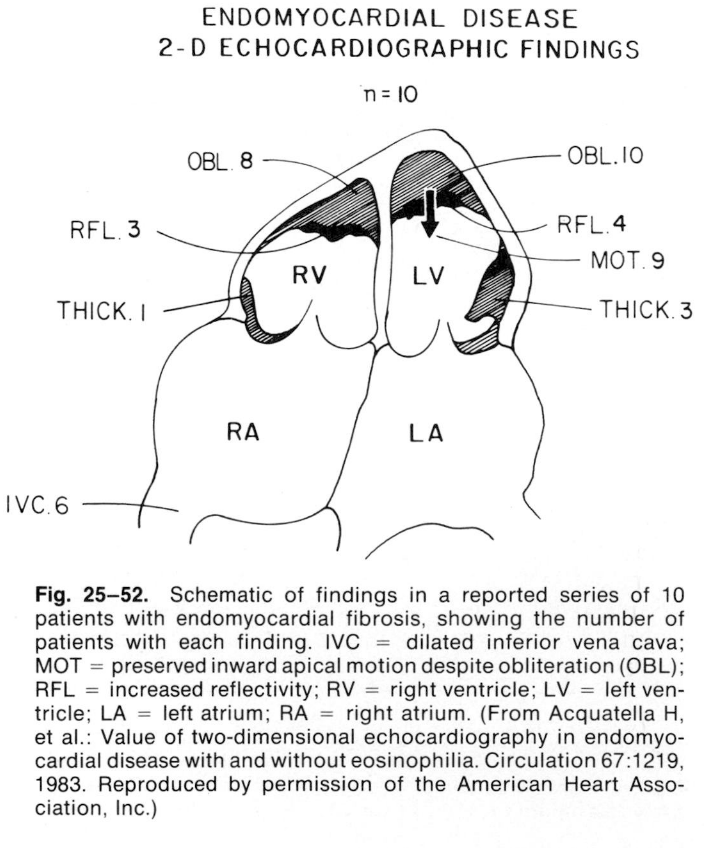

Fig. 25–52. Schematic of findings in a reported series of 10 patients with endomyocardial fibrosis, showing the number of patients with each finding. IVC = dilated inferior vena cava; MOT = preserved inward apical motion despite obliteration (OBL); RFL = increased reflectivity; RV = right ventricle; LV = left ventricle; LA = left atrium; RA = right atrium. (From Acquatella H, et al.: Value of two-dimensional echocardiography in endomyocardial disease with and without eosinophilia. Circulation 67:1219, 1983. Reproduced by permission of the American Heart Association, Inc.)

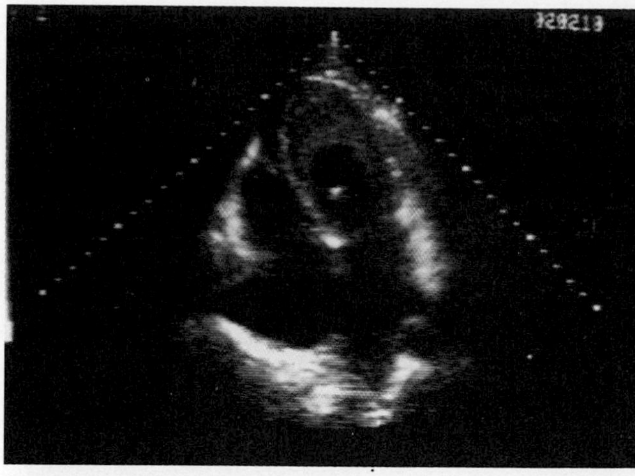

Fig. 25–53. Reported North American patient with echogenic deposits obliterating the left ventricular apex. The patient presented with biventricular failure and eosinophilia. (From Acquatella H, Schiller NB: Echocardiographic recognition of Chagas' disease and endomyocardial fibrosis. J Am Soc Echocardiogr 1:60, 1988.)

the posterior mitral and anterior tricuspid valve leaflets, causing regurgitation of those valves, which can be severe.[386,398] The endocardial border of the deposits may appear bright and specular, suggesting calcification, as seen radiographically in the chronic phase. The ventricular chambers are generally normal or small with dilated atria, although ventricular dilation occasionally occurs as a result of an eosinophilic myocarditis.[386] An important differential point is that ventricular function is, as a rule, preserved, with inward systolic motion of the obliterated left ventricular apex, as opposed to the dyskinesis seen in ischemia and Chagas' disease.[386,387] Pericardial effusions have also been reported.[386,399] Figure 26–14 is an example of Löffler's endocarditis that presented as mitral and tricuspid stenosis. In this example, there is focal accumulation of echogenic material along the endocardial surface of the right ventricular free wall and reduced tricuspid valve opening.

Diastolic Filling Patterns in Restrictive Disease

The classic description of a restrictive cardiomyopathy is one in which ventricular filling pressures are elevated with normal or nearly normal systolic function.[310] Ventricular pressure in such conditions declines prominently at the onset of diastole and then rises abruptly because of decreased chamber compliance, producing a dip and plateau or "square-root sign" in the ventricular pressure tracing.[310] One would expect that such a distinctive pattern of ventricular filling would find its counterpart in the Doppler patterns of mitral and tricuspid inflow velocities. In fact, patients with restrictive cardiomyopathy *selected* to have the dip and plateau pattern hemodynamically had a corresponding mitral inflow pattern characterized by rapid deceleration of the early filling (E) wave and a diminished velocity of late-diastolic filling following atrial contraction (A-wave)[403] (Fig. 25–54). The rapid E-wave deceleration corresponded to a rapidly rising ventricular pressure early in diastole,

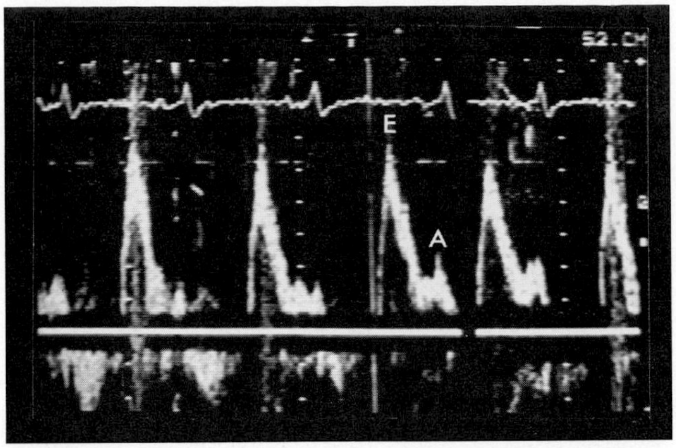

Fig. 25–54. Classic restrictive-type mitral inflow pattern in a patient with cardiac amyloidosis (also shown in Figs. 25–45 and 25–46). There is a tall E wave that rapidly decelerates and a relatively small A wave.

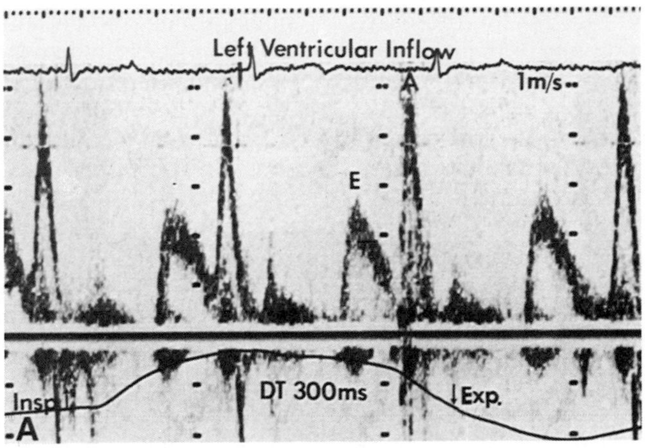

Fig. 25–55. Decreased E/A wave ratio (0.5) and prolonged deceleration time (DT) of 300 msec in a patient with early cardiac amyloidosis, suggesting delayed relaxation. (From Klein AL, et al.: Doppler characterization of left ventricular diastolic function in cardiac amyloidosis. J Am Coll Cardiol 13:1017, 1989. Reprinted with permission from the American College of Cardiology.)

which rapidly decreased the atrioventricular pressure difference driving transmitral flow. The small A wave can be thought of as reflecting increased ventricular late-diastolic pressure, which opposes atrial contraction. Note, however, that only 7 of the 14 patients in the study referred to had an echocardiographic pattern consistent with pericardial thickening, raising the possibility of superimposed constriction.

A far more variable picture emerges from studies of diastolic filling in amyloidosis, which is the most common infiltrative cardiomyopathy examined.[325] Hemodynamically, the classic restrictive dip and plateau may be absent;[404–406] instead, there may be evidence of the "stiff heart syndrome," characterized by elevations in both early and late ventricular diastolic pressures because of delayed relaxation and reduced chamber compliance.[404] Ventricular filling patterns may also depart from the classic restrictive pattern of increased peak filling rate and decreased time from the onset of diastole to peak filling rate. Both decreased peak filling rate and increased time to peak filling rate have, in fact, been demonstrated in patients with amyloidosis by digitized left ventriculography,[407] radionuclide ventriculography,[408,409] and digitized M-mode echocardiography, looking at the peak rate of ventricular wall thinning and internal diameter increase.[410,411] Further, a wide variety of mitral and tricuspid inflow velocity patterns have been described in patients with echocardiographically evident amyloid involvement of the heart, ranging from the normal contour to the classic restrictive pattern described previously (rapid E-wave deceleration, small A wave) as well as the converse pattern seen with delayed relaxation (relatively small E-wave with prolonged deceleration)[324,412,413] (Fig. 25–55).

A convenient basis for beginning to understand this variability is provided by classifying patients into subgroups on the basis of mean ventricular wall thickness, which serves as an index of the degree of myocardial involvement and corresponds to other echocardiographic and clinical expressions of the disease (see Table 25–1).[318] In a study of 53 patients with primary systemic amyloidosis, patients with milder involvement (mean wall thickness between 12 and 15 mm) had mitral inflow patterns most consistent with delayed relaxation: a decreased peak E-wave velocity and increased peak A-wave velocity compared to normal control subjects (E/A-wave ratio of 1.2 ± .6 vs. 1.6 ± .5 in normal control subjects), with a prolonged isovolumic relaxation time (IVRT) (87 ± 15 vs. 73 ± 13 ms). In patients with more severe involvement (mean wall thickness ≥ 15 mm), a more typically restrictive pattern was seen, with an increased E/A wave ratio (2.0 ± 1.2), a rapid E-wave deceleration (deceleration time of 148 ± 50 vs. 199 ± 32 ms), and no prolongation of the IVRT. Similar differences in tricuspid inflow velocity patterns have also been demonstrated in a similar population divided on the basis of right ventricular free wall thickness < 7 mm or ≥ 7 mm.[324]

These patterns can be understood in terms of the determinants of ventricular filling described in Chapter 24. In patients with milder involvement, the predominant abnormality affecting ventricular filling appears to be delayed relaxation, which can prolong IVRT and decrease peak E-wave velocity (delayed relaxation increases the time it takes for ventricular pressure to fall below atrial pressure and decreases the early diastolic atrioventricular pressure gradient) (Chapter 24, Fig. 24–32). There is a corresponding and possibly compensatory increase in the peak A-wave velocity. With more severe involvement, initial atrial pressure may rise for several reasons: to compensate for decreased filling; because of atrial involvement and decreased atrial compliance;[325] and as a result of superimposed mitral or tricuspid regurgitation. This will decrease the time it takes for ventricular pressures to fall below atrial pressure at the onset of diastole (shorter IVRT) and will increase the early diastolic transvalvular pressure gradient, causing an increase in E wave relative to the A wave (Chapter 24, Fig. 24–26). Increased chamber stiffness (potentially reflecting both increased myocardial stiffness and an increased mass/volume ratio as a determinant of chamber stiffness) will also cause the E wave to decelerate more rapidly, reflecting the early filling of a less compliant ventricle. The increased ventricular end-diastolic pressure, transmitted back to the atrium, may also diminish the gradient, driving venous return into the atrium during the subsequent systole, consistent with the decreased systolic pulmonary vein and superior vena cava flow seen in patients with more severe involvement.[324,412] Based on this reasoning, it is not surprising that transitions from normal or delayed relaxation-type mitral inflow patterns to the restrictive pattern can be observed over time in patients with amyloidosis and often correspond to the development of clinical symptoms.[414]

Although this reasoning is of value in understanding the variety of Doppler inflow patterns seen in patients with amyloidosis, it must be emphasized that, in reality, the interplay of factors may be more complex. Although statistically significant differences in velocity patterns can be identified between different patient subgroups, there is great overlap between velocities and other Doppler measurements in individual patients. Individual variability may result from the particular amyloid protein involved,[325] the degree of atrial involvement, the presence and severity of superimposed valvular regurgitation, and the effects of heart rate, medical therapy, and sample volume location on the observed Doppler inflow velocities. It should be evident that some combination of decreased relaxation rate, increased chamber stiffness, and counterbalancing increased atrial pressure can result in an apparently normal filling pattern despite abnormalities of intrinsic ventricular properties. Similarly, the nonuniqueness of the Doppler mitral inflow pattern is highlighted by the occurrence of a similar "restrictive" pattern in patients with acute severe aortic regurgitation, in whom increased left atrial pressures and rapidly rising left ventricular diastolic pressures generate a tall E-wave that decelerates rapidly.[189,415]

Practically, therefore, care must be exercised to avoid unwarranted interpretation of normal or abnormal inflow patterns. Nevertheless, there appears to be an emerging consensus that informed interpretation of these patterns guided by the results of computational models and in vitro simulations can allow us to extract meaningful pathophysiologic insights from them.[189,324,325,412,413] In particular, in a patient with prominent, symmetrically thickened ventricular walls and a texture suggestive of amyloidosis, the presence of a tall mitral E wave, an increased E/A-wave ratio and a rapid E-wave deceleration can allow us to infer the presence of increased left atrial pressure at the onset of diastole, reflecting restrictive physiology with or without superimposed mitral regurgitation. In contrast, if the E/A-wave ratio is prominently decreased (without an increased heart rate that could otherwise decrease it), with a delayed E-wave deceleration, one can suggest the presence of either (1) a milder stage of the disease with predominant evidence of delayed relaxation or (2) the absence of an initially high transmitral gradient because of medical therapy (lower left atrial pressure) or because of markedly elevated early diastolic ventricular pressure[404] without a compensatory rise in atrial pressure.

Restrictive Versus Constrictive Physiology

The ability of echocardiography to display correlates of restrictive physiology has led to the question of whether this technique can be useful in distinguishing restrictive from constrictive physiology. This differentiation is difficult even with invasive hemodynamic measurements;[416] it is further complicated by the potential coexistence of both restrictive and constrictive abnormalities[409] and by the absence of an echocardiographic pattern completely diagnostic of pericardial thickening.[417] Two potential echocardiographic approaches have been advocated with promising, albeit preliminary, results.

The first approach presumes that limitation of diastolic ventricular filling occurs earlier in constriction than restriction because of the fixed volume within the constricting pericardium. On the other hand, in restriction, unlike constriction, myocardial relaxation is prolonged by the underlying muscle disease. Data consistent with this postulate have been obtained in limited numbers of patients with constrictive pericarditis and a variety of restrictive disorders studied by digitized left ventriculography, radionuclide angiography, and digitized M-mode echocardiography.[407,409–411] In the M-mode studies, the major left ventricular filling period (from minimum to maximum internal dimension) was abnormally prolonged in restriction, and the rate of posterior wall thinning was diminished. In constriction, on the other hand, the major filling period was shorter than normal, with no significant change in posterior wall thinning rate.[411] It should be noted, however, that these studies presuppose a uniformly decreased rate of early diastolic filling in restrictive cardiomyopathy, which is not invariably present, as shown by the Doppler studies discussed previously. Elevated atrial pressures and advanced disease can increase the rate of early diastolic filling, with rapid deceleration and early cessation of such filling;[324,403,412,418] these changes should be reflected in the M-mode tracing of left ventricular diameter. Therefore, the digitized M-mode can be useful in identifying restrictive cardiomyopathy if peak filling rate is, in fact, decreased, but is unlikely to be specific otherwise.

The second approach proposed to differentiate constriction and restriction relates to the fixed value of total intrapericardial volume in constriction, so that any change in right ventricular filling, as with respiration, must be accompanied by a comparable and opposite change in left ventricular filling. Pure restriction, in contrast, imposes no such limitation. Thus, in one recent study, inspiration raised right ventricular systolic pressure and decreased left ventricular systolic pressure in patients with classic constriction, whereas both pressures fell on inspiration in patients with restriction.[419] In addition, the gradient between pulmonary capillary wedge pressure and left ventricular pressure (i.e., the gradient driving left ventricular diastolic filling) varied with respiration only in constriction. These hemodynamic findings had Doppler correlates: (1) In constriction, there was marked respiratory variation of left ventricular (IVRT) and peak E-wave velocity. The inspiratory and expiratory values of these measures differed by 25% or more in all patients, with a mean of >30%. The greatest changes in these values occurred in the first beat following inspiration or expiration. In restriction, respiratory changes in these variables averaged <5%, and were <15% in any given patient, comparable to the variations seen in controls. Further, the constrictive changes resolved following pericardiectomy. (2) In constriction, there were also reciprocal respiratory changes in mitral and tricuspid inflow velocities. Peak tricuspid inflow velocity decreased prominently during expiration, producing a 44 ± 22% variation from inspiration to expiration in constriction, as opposed to 17 ± 16% in restriction ($p < .05$).[419] The diagnostic value of these findings must ultimately be tested in further prospective studies and clinical practice including patients with varying depths of respiration.

In summary, therefore, echocardiography provides a detailed representation of the effects of cardiomyopathy on cardiac structure and function. Although microscopic disease may be inapparent, echocardiography can often detect morphologic alterations before they are clinically apparent. Although biopsy remains the ultimate method for biochemical and histologic diagnosis, individual diseases have distinctive and suggestive ultrasound appearances. Doppler inflow patterns are not unique to any condition but provide insight into the complex interaction between intrinsic myocardial properties and loading conditions and their effect on the time course and extent of left ventricular filling.

REFERENCES

1. Waller BF: Pathology of the cardiomyopathies. J Am Soc Echocardiogr 1:4, 1988.
2. Report of the WHO/ISFC task force on the definition and classification of cardiomyopathies. Br Heart J 44:672, 1980.
3. Goodwin JF: Congestive and hypertrophic cardiomyopathies: a decade of study. Lancet 1:73, 1970.
4. Goodwin JF, Oakley CM: The cardiomyopathies. Br Heart J 34:545, 1972.
5. Goodwin JF: Clarification of the cardiomyopathies. Mod Concept Cardiovasc Dis 41:41, 1972.
6. Leitl GP, McDonald: The echocardiographic assessment of cardiomyopathy: diagnosis, classification and problems. Aust NZ J Med 11:394, 1981.
7. Wynne J, Braunwald E: The cardiomyopathies and myocarditides. *In* Braunwald E, (ed.): Heart Disease. Philadelphia, WB Saunders, p. 1412, 1984.
8. Abelmann WH: Classification and natural history of primary myocardial disease. Prog Cardiovasc Dis 27:73, 1984.
9. Maron BJ, Epstein SE: Hypertrophic cardiomyopathy: a discussion of nomenclature. Am J Cardiol 43:1242, 1979.
10. Shapiro LM, McKenna WJ: Distribution of the left ventricular hypertrophy in hypertrophic cardiomyopathy: a two-dimensional echocardiographic study. J Am Coll Cardiol 2:437, 1983.
11. Clark CE, Henry WL, Epstein SE: Familial prevalence and genetic transmission of idiopathic hypertrophic subaortic stenosis. N Engl J Med 289: 709, 1973.
12. Jarcho JA, et al.: Mapping a gene for familial hypertrophic cardiomyopathy to chromosome 14q1. N Engl J Med 321:1372, 1989.
13. Teare D: Asymmetrical hypertrophy of the heart in young adults. Br Heart J 20:1, 1958.
14. Menges H Jr, Brandenburg RO, Brown AL JR: The clinical, hemodynamic and pathological diagnosis of muscular subvalvular aortic stenosis. Circulation 24:1126, 1961.
15. Roberts WC: Valvular, subvalvular and supravalvular aortic stenosis: morphological features. Cardiovasc Clin 5:97, 1973.
16. Henry WL, Clark CE, Epstein SE: Asymmetric septal hypertrophy: echocardiographic identification of the pathognomonic anatomic abnormality of IHSS. Circulation 47:225, 1973.
17. Maron BJ, Gottdiener JS, Epstein SE: Patterns and significance of distribution of left ventricular hypertrophy in hypertrophic cardiomyopathy: a wide angle, two dimensional echocardiographic study of 125 patients. Am J Cardiol 48:418, 1981.
18. Maron BJ: Asymmetry in hypertrophic cardiomyopathy: the septal to free wall ratio revisited. Am J Cardiol 55:835, 1985.
19. Wigle ED, et al.: Hypertrophic cardiomyopathy: the importance of the site and the extent of hypertrophy: a review. Prog Cardiovasc Dis 28:1, 1985.
20. Van Noorden S, Olsen EGJ, Pearse AGE: Hypertrophic obstructive cardiomyopathy, a histological, histochemical, and ultrastructural study of biopsy material. Cardiovasc Res 5:118, 1971.
21. Ferrans VJ, Morrow AG, Roberts WC: Myocardial ultrastructure in idiopathic hypertrophic subaortic stenosis: a study of operatively excised left ventricular outflow tract muscle in 14 patients. Circulation 45:769, 1972.
22. Maron BJ, Roberts WC: Quantitative analysis of cardiac muscle cell disorganization in the ventricular septum of patients with hypertrophic cardiomyopathy. Circulation 59:689, 1979.
23. Bulkley BH, Weisfeldt ML, Hutchins GM: Isometric cardiac contraction: a possible cause of the disorganized myocardial pattern of idiopathic hypertrophic subaortic stenosis. N Engl J Med 296:135, 1977.
24. Henry WL, Clark CE, Griffith JM, Epstein SE: Mechanism of left ventricular outflow obstruction in patients with obstructive asymmetric septal hypertrophy (idiopathic hypertrophic subaortic stenosis). Am J Cardiol 35: 337, 1975.
25. Shah PM, Gramiak R, Kramer DH: Ultrasound location of left ventricular outflow obstruction in hypertrophic obstructive cardiomyopathy. Circulation 40:3, 1969.
26. Popp RL, Harrison DC: Ultrasound in the diagnosis and evaulation of therapy of idiopathic hypertrophic subaortic stenosis. Circulation 40:905, 1969.
27. Shah P, Gramiak R, Adelman AG, Wigle ED: Role of echocardiography in diagnostic and emodynamic assessment of hypertrophic subaortic stenosis. Circulation 44:891, 1971.
28. Henry WL, Clark CE, Glancy DL, Epstein SE: Echocardiographic measurement of the left ventricular outflow gradient in idiopathic hypertrophic subaortic stenosis. N Engl J Med 288:898, 1973.
29. Gilbert BW, Pollick C, Adelman AG, Wigle ED: Hypertrophic cardiomyopathy: subclassification by M mode echocardiography. Am J Cardiol 45: 861, 1980.
30. Pollick C, et al.: Muscular subaortic stenosis: the temporal relationship between systolic anterior motion of the anterior mitral leaflet and the pressure gradient. Circulation 66:1087, 1982.
31. Pollick C, Rakowski H, Wigle ED: Muscular subaortic steonsis: the quantitative relationship between systolic anterior motion and the pressure gradient. Circulation 69:43, 1984.
32. Braunwald E, et al.: Idiopathic hypertrophic subaortic stenosis: clinical, hemodynamic and angiographic manifestations. Am J Med 29:924, 1960.
33. Goodwin JF, Hollman A, Cleland WP, Teare D: Obstructive cardiomyopathy simulating aortic stenosis. Br Heart J 22:403, 1960.
34. Braunwald E, et al.: Idiopathic hypertrophic subaortic stenosis: I. A description of the disease based upon an analysis of 64 patients. Circulation 30(Suppl. 4):IV–3, 1964.
35. Ross J Jr, et al.: The mechanism of the intraventricular pressure gradient in idiopathic hypertrophic subaortic stenosis. Circulation 34:558, 1966.
36. Braunwald E, Brockenbrough EC, Morrow AG: Hypertrophic subaortic stenosis—a broadened concept. Circulation 26:161, 1962.
37. Cohen J, et al.: Hypertrophic obstructive cardiomyopathy. Br Heart J 26: 16, 1964.
38. Jada Y, et al.: Prevalence of hypertrophic cardiomyopathy in a population of adult Japanese workers as detected by electrocardiographic screening. Am J Cardiol 59:183, 1987.
39. Agnarsson U, Hardaron T, Sigfusson N: Hypertrophic cardiomyopathy identified by echo-screening: prevalence and clinical significance (abstr.). Circulation 78(Suppl. 2):II–584, 1988.
40. Abbasi AS, MacAlpin RN, Eber LM, Pearce ML: Echocardiographic diagnosis of idiopathic hypertrophic cardiomyopathy without outflow obstruction. Circulation 46:897, 1972.
41. Martin RP, Rakowski H, French J, Popp RL: Idiopathic hypertrophic subaortic stenosis viewed by wide-angle, phased-array echocardiography. Circulation 59:12, 1979.
42. Krajcer Z, et al.: Early systolic closure of the aortic valve in patients with hypertrophic subaortic stenosis and discrete subaortic stenosis. Am J Cardiol 41:823, 1978.
43. Epstein SE, et al.: Asymmetric septal hypertrophy. Ann Intern Med 81: 650, 1974.
44. Maron BJ, et al.: Prevalence and characteristics of disproportionate ventricular septal thickening in patients with acquired or congenital heart disease: echocardiographic and morphologic findings. Circulation 55:489, 1977.
45. Maron BJ, et al.: Left ventricular outflow tract obstruction due to systolic anterior motion of the anterior mitral leaflet in patients with concentric left ventricular hypertrophy. Circulation 57:527, 1978.

46. Maron BJ, Epstein SE: Hypertrophic cardiomyopathy: recent observations regarding the specificity of three hallmarks of the disease: asymmetric septal hypertrophy, septal disorganization and systolic anterior motion of the anterior mitral leaflet. Am J Cardiol 45:141, 1980.
47. Maron B, Verter J, Kapur S: Disproportionate ventricular septal thickening in the developing normal human heart. Circulation 57:520, 1978.
48. Maron BJ, et al.: Hypertrophic cardiomyopathy in infants: clinical features and natural history. Circulation 65:7, 1982.
49. Maron BJ, Cannon RO III, Leon MB, Epstein SE: Hypertrophic cardiomyopathy: interrelations of clinical manifestations, pathophysiology, and therapy. N Engl J Med 16:780, 1987.
50. Gutgesell HP, Speer ME, Rosenberg HS: Characterization of the cardiomyopathy in infants of diabetic mothers. Circulation 61:441, 1980.
51. Somerville J, Becu L: Congenital heart disease associated with hypertrophic cardiomyopathy. Br Heart J 40:1034, 1978.
52. Robinson PJ, Wyse RKH, Macartney FJ: Left ventricular outflow tract obstruction in complete transposition of the great arteries with intact ventricular septum: a cross sectional echocardiography study. Br Heart J 54: 201, 1985.
53. Riggs T, Hirschfeld S, Rajai H: The pediatric spectrum of dynamic left ventricular obstruction. Am Heart J 99:301, 1980.
54. Ackroyd RS, Finnegan JA, Green SH: Friedreich's ataxia. Arch Dis Child 59:217, 1984.
55. Bulkley BH, Hutchins GM: Pompe's disease presenting as hypertrophic cardiomyopathy with Wolff-Parkinson-White syndrome. Am Heart J 96: 246, 1977.
56. Shapir Y, Roguin N: Echocardiographic findings in Pompe's disease with left ventricular obstruction. Clin Cardiol 8:181, 1985.
57. Tanaka H, et al.: Four cases of Fabry's disease mimicking hypertrophic cardiomyopathy. J Cardiol 18:705, 1988.
58. Gross DM, et al.: Echocardiographic abnormalities in the mucopolysaccharide storage diseases. Am J Cardiol 61:170, 1988.
59. Sedlis SP, Saffitz JE, Schwab VS, Jaffe AS: Cardiac amyloidosis simulating hypertrophic cardiomyopathy. Am J Cardiol 53:969, 1984.
60. Santos AD, et al.: Echocardiographic characterization of the reversible cardiomyopathy of hypothyroidism. Am J Med 68:675, 1980.
61. Shenoy MM, Goldman JM: Hypothyroid cardiomyopathy: echocardiographic documentation of reversibility. Am J Med Sci 294:1, 1987.
62. McKenna WJ, Kleinebenne A, Nihoyannopoulos P, Foale R: Echocardiographic measurement of right ventricular wall thickness in hypertrophic cardiomyopathy: relation to clinical and prognostic features. J Am Coll Cardiol 11:351, 1988.
63. Lever HM, Karam RF, Currie PJ, Healy BP: Hypertrophic cardiomyopathy in the elderly: Distinctions from the young based on cardiac shape. Circulation 79:580, 1989.
64. Maron BJ, Gottdiener JS, Bonow RO, Epstein SE: Hypertrophic cardiomyopathy with unusual location of left ventricular hypertrophy undetectable by M-mode echocardiography: identification by wide-angle two-dimensional echocardiography. Circulation 67:1227, 1983.
65. Maron BJ, Spirito P, Chiarella F, Vecchio C: Unusual distribution of left ventricular hypertrophy in obstructive hypertrophic cardiomyopathy: localized posterobasal free wall thickening in two patients. J Am Coll Cardiol 5:1474, 1985.
66. Sakamoto T, et al.: Giant T wave inversion as a manifestation of asymmetrical apical hypertrophy (AAH) of the left ventricle echocardiographic and ultrasono-cardiotomographic study. Jpn Heart J 17:611, 1976.
67. Yamaguchi H, et al.: Hypertrophic nonobstructive cardiomyopathy with giant negative T waves (apical hypertrophy): ventriculographic and echocardiographic features in 30 patients. Am J Cardiol 44:401, 1979.
68. Louie EK, Maron BJ: Apical hypertrophic cardiomyopathy: clinical and two-dimensional echocardiographic assessment. Ann Intern Med 106:663, 1987.
69. Webb JG, et al.: Apical hypertrophic cardiomyopathy: clinical follow-up and diagnostic correlates. J Am Coll Cardiol 15:83, 1990.
70. Falicov RE, Resnekov L, Bharati S, Lev M: Midventricular obstruction: a variant of obstructive cardiomyopathy. Am J Cardiol 37:432, 1976.
71. Sheikhzadeh A, et al.: Midventricular obstruction—a form of hypertrophic obstructive cardiomyopathy—and systolic anterior motion of the mitral valve. Clin Cardiol 9:607, 1986.
72. Gordon EP, Henderson MA, Rakowski H, Wigle ED: Midventricular obstruction with apical infarction and aneurysm formation (abstr.). Circulation 70:145, 1984.
72a. Schwammenthal E, et al: Prediction of the site and severity of obstruction in hypertrophic cardiomyopathic by color flow mapping and continuous wave Doppler echocardiography. J Am Coll Cardiol 20:964, 1992.
73. Maron BJ, Wolfson JK, Epstein SE, Roberts WC: Intramural ("small vessel") coronary artery disease in hypertrophic cardiomyopathy. J Am Coll Cardiol 8:545, 1986.
74. Spirito P, Maron BJ: Relation between extent of left ventricular hypertrophy and occurrence of sudden cardiac death in hypertrophic cardiomyopathy. J Am Coll Cardiol 15:1521, 1990.
75. Spirito P, Maron BJ: Relation between extent of left ventricular hypertrophy and diastolic filling abnormalities in hypertrophic cardiomyopathy. J Am Coll Cardiol 15:808, 1990.
76. Fowles RE, Martin RP, Popp RL: Apparent asymmetric septal hypertrophy due to angled interventricular septum. Am J Cardiol 46:386, 1980.
77. Allen JW, Kim SJ, Edmiston WA, Venkatarman K: Problems in ultrasonic estimates of septal thickness. Am J Cardiol 42:89, 1978.
78. Popp RL, Filly K, Brown GR, Harrison DC: Effect of transducer placement on echocardiographic measurement of left ventricular dimensions. Am J Cardiol 35:537, 1975.
79. Keren A, Billingham ME, Popp RL: Echocardiographic recognition of paraseptal structures. J Am Coll Cardiol 6:913, 1985.
80. Bernstein RF, Tei C, Child JS, Shah PM: Angled interventricular septum on echocardiography: anatomic anomaly or technical artifact? J Am Coll Cardiol 2:297, 1983.
81. Skorton DJ, et al.: Range- and azimuth-dependent variability of image texture in two-dimensional echocardiograms. Circulation 68:834, 1983.
82. Kawamura K, et al.: Analysis of myocardial texture in two-dimensional echocardiographic images. J Cardiol 18:619, 1988.
83. Ciro E, Nichols PF III, Maron BJ: Heterogeneous morphologic expression of genetically transmitted hypertrophic cardiomyopathy: two-dimensional echocardiographic analysis. Circulation 67:409, 1983.
84. Maron BJ, et al.: Patterns of inheritance in hypertrophic cardiomyopathy: assessment by M-mode and two-dimensional echocardiography. Am J Cardiol 53:1087, 1984.
85. Maron BJ, Mulvihill JJ: The genetics of hypertrophic cardiomyopathy. Ann Intern Med 106:610, 1986.
86. Spirito P, et al.: Clinical course and prognosis of hypertrophic cardiomyopathy in an outpatient population. N Engl J Med 320:749, 1989.
87. Solomon SD, et al.: Familial hypertrophic cardiomyopathy is a genetically heterogeneous disease. J Clin Invest 86:993, 1990.
88. Maron BJ, Spirito P, Wesley Y, Arce J: Development and progression of left ventricular hypertrophy in children with hypertrophic cardiomyopathy. N Engl J Med 315:610, 1986.
89. Spirito P, Maron BJ: Absence of progression of left ventricular hypertrophy in adult patients with hypertrophic cardiomyopathy. J Am Coll Cardiol 9:1013, 1987.
90. Brock R: Functional obstruction of the left ventricle (acquired aortic subvalvular stenosis). Guy's Hosp Rep 106:221, 1957.
91. Bercu BA, et al.: Pseudoaortic stenosis produced by ventricular hypertrophy. Am J Med 25:814, 1958.
92. Morrow AG, Braunwald E: Functional aortic stenosis: a malformation characterized by resistance to left ventricular outflow without anatomic obstruction. Circulation 20:181, 1959.
93. Cleland WP: The surgical management of obstructive cardiomyopathy. J Cardiovasc Surg 4:489, 1963.
94. Nordenstrom B, Ovenfors CO: Low subvalvular aortic and pulmonic stenosis with hypertrophy and abnormal arrangement of the muscle bundles of the myocardium. Acta Radiol 57:321, 1962.
95. Fix P, Moberg A, Soderberg H, Karnell J: Muscular subvalvular aortic stenosis: abnormal anterior mitral leaflet possibly primary factor. Acta Radiol 2:177, 1964.
96. Wigle ED, Heimbecker RO, Gunton RW: Idiopathic ventricular septal hypertrophy causing muscular subaortic stenosis. Circulation 26:325, 1962.
97. Dinsmore RE, Sanders CA, Harthorne JW: Mitral regurgitation in idiopathic hypertrophic subaortic stenosis. N Engl J Med 275:1225, 1966.
98. Simon AL, Ross J, Gault JH: Angiographic anatomy of the left ventricle and mitral valve in idiopathic hypertrophic subaortic stenosis. Circulation 36:857, 1967.
99. Adelman AG, et al.: Left ventricular cineangiographic observations in muscular subaortic stenosis. Am J Cardiol 24:689, 1969.
100. Shah PM, Gramiak R, Adelman AG, Wigle ED: Echocardiographic assessment of the effects of surgery and propranolol on the dynamics of outflow obstruction in hypertrophic subaortic stenosis. Circulation 45:516, 1972.
101. Shah P, Taylor RD, Wong M: Abnormal mitral valve coaptation in hypertrophic obstructive cardiomyopathy: proposed role in systolic anterior motion of mitral valve. Am J Cardiol 48:258, 1981.
102. Maron BJ, et al.: Systolic anterior motion of the posterior mitral leaflet: a previously unrecognized cause of dynamic subaortic obstruction in patients with hypertrophic cardiomyopathy. Circulation 68:282, 1983.
103. Spirito P, Maron BJ: Patterns of systolic anterior motion of the mitral valve in hypertrophic cardiomyopathy: assessment by two-dimensional echocardiography. Am J Cardiol 54:1039, 1984.
104. Maron BJ, et al.: Dynamic subaortic obstruction in hypertrophic cardiomyopathy: analysis by pulsed Doppler echocardiography. J Am Coll Cardiol 6:1, 1985.
105. Gardin JM, et al.: Echocardiographic and Doppler flow observations in obstructed and non-obstructed hypertrophic cardiomyopathy. Am J Cardiol 56:614, 1985.
106. Spirito P, Maron BJ, Rosing DR: Morphologic determinants of hemodynamic state after ventricular septal myotomy-myectomy in patients with obstructive hypertrophic cardiomyopathy: M-mode and two-dimensional echocardiographic assessment. Circulation 70:984, 1984.
107. Come PC, Riley MF, Miklozek CL: Echocardiographic evidence of increased obstruction following long cycle lengths in atrial fibrillation in patients with hypertrophic cardiomyopathy. J Clin Ultrasound 13:241, 1984.
108. Greenwald J, Yap JF, Franklin M, Lichtman AM: Echocardiographic mi-

tral systolic anterior motion in left ventricular aneurysm. Br Heart J 37: 684, 1975.
109. Gardin JM, et al.: Systolic anterior motion in the absence of asymmetric septal hypertrophy: a buckling phenomenon of the chordae tendineae. Circulation 63:181, 1981.
110. Jiang L, Levine RA, King ME, Weyman AE: An integrated mechanism to explain the systolic anterior motion of the mitral valve in hypertrophic cardiomyopathy based on echocardiographic observations. Am Heart J 113:633, 1987.
111. Levine RA, Laznicka H: Further evidence for physiologic significance of systolic anterior motion in hypertrophic cardiomyopathy: inverse relationship between outflow velocity and orifice area (abstr.). Circulation 76(Suppl. 4):IV–316, 1987.
112. King JF, et al.: Markedly abnormal mitral valve motion without simultaneous intraventricular pressure gradient due to uneven mitral-septal contact in idiopathic hypertrophic subaortic stenosis. Am J Cardiol 34:360, 1974.
113. Eldar M, et al.: Systolic closure of aortic valve in patients with prosthetic mitral valves. Br Heart J 48:48, 1982.
114. Gardin J, Tommaso CL, Talano JV: Echocardiographic early systolic partial closure (notching) of the aortic valve in congestive cardiomyopathy. Am Heart J 107:135, 1984.
115. Ciro E, Maione S, Giunta A, Maron BJ: Echocardiographic analysis of ventricular septal dynamics in hypertrophic cardiomyopathy and other diseases. Am J Cardiol 53:187, 1984.
116. Rossen RM, Goodman DJ, Ingham RE, Popp RL: Ventricular systolic septal thickening and excursion in idiopathic hypertrophic subaortic stenosis. N Engl J Med 291:1317, 1974.
117. Kaul S, Tei C, Shah PM: Interventricular septal and free wall dynamics in hypertrophic cardiomyopathy. J Am Coll Cardiol 1:1024, 1983.
118. Pouleur H, et al.: Force-velocity-length relations in hypertrophic cardiomyopathy: evidence of normal or depressed myocardial contractility. Am J Cardiol 52:813, 1983.
119. Ciro E, et al.: Relation between marked changes in left ventricular outflow tract gradient and disease progression in hypertrophic cardiomyopathy. Am J Cardiol 53:1103, 1984.
120. Spirito P, Maron BJ, Bonow RO, Epstein SE: Occurrence and significance of progressive left ventricular wall thinning and relative cavity dilatation in hypertrophic cardiomyopathy. Am J Cardiol 59:123, 1987.
121. Fighali S, Krajcer Z, Edelman S, Leachman RD: Progression of hypertrophic cardiomyopathy into a hypokinetic left ventricle: higher incidence in patients with midventricular obstruction. J Am Coll Cardiol 9:288, 1987.
122. Ten Cate FJ, Roelandt J: Progression to left ventricular dilatation in patients with hypertrophic obstructive cardiomyopathy. Am Heart J 97:762, 1979.
123. Ando H, et al.: Apical segmental dysfunction in hypertrophic cardiomyopathy: subgroup with unique clinical features. J Am Coll Cardiol 16:1579, 1990.
124. Iwami G, et al.: Hypertrophic cardiomyopathy with left ventricular dilatation. J Cardiol 18:319, 1988.
125. Levine RA, et al.: The simplified Bernoulli equation correctly predicts outflow tract pressure gradients in hypertrophic cardiomyopathy: an *in vitro* study (abstr.).J Am Coll Cardiol 9:237, 1987.
126. Levine RA, et al.: Pressure recovery distal to stenosis: potential cause of gradient "overestimation" by Doppler. J Am Coll Cardiol 13:706, 1989.
127. Stewart WJ, et al.: Intraoperative Doppler echocardiography in hypertrophic cardiomyopathy: correlations with the obstructive gradient. J Am Coll Cardiol 10:327, 1987.
128. Sasson Z, et al.: Doppler echocardiographic determination of the pressure gradient in hypertrophic cardiomyopathy. J Am Coll Cardiol 11:752, 1988.
129. Cooper M, Shaddy R, Silverman N, Enderlein M: Usefulness of Doppler echocardiography for determining hemodynamic improvement with intravenous verapamil in hypertrophic cardiomyopathy. Am J Cardiol 56:201, 1985.
130. Hatle L, Angelsen B: Doppler Ultrasound in Cardiology. 2nd Ed. Philadelphia, Lea & Febiger, p. 205, 1985.
131. Yock PG, Hatle L, Popp RL: Patterns and timing of Doppler-detected intracavitary and aortic flow in hypertrophic cardiomyopathy. J Am Coll Cardiol 8:1047, 1986.
132. Nishimura RA, Tajik AJ, Reeder GS, Seward JB: Evaluation of hypertrophic cardiomyopathy by Doppler color flow imaging: initial observations. Mayo Clin Proc 61:631, 1986.
133. Hoit BD, Penonen E, Dalton N, Sahn DJ: Doppler color flow mapping studies of jet formation and spatial orientation in obstructive hypertrophic cardiomyopathy. Am Heart J 117:1119, 1989.
134. Wigle ED, Adelman AG, Auger P, Marquis Y: Mitral regurgitation in muscular subaortic stenosis. Am J Cardiol 24:698, 1969.
135. Kinoshita N, et al.: Mitral regurgitation in hypertrophic cardiomyopathy; noninvasive study by two-dimensional Doppler echocardiography. Br Heart J 49:574, 1983.
136. Jiang L, et al.: Systolic anterior motion as a predictor of mitral regurgitation in IHSS (abstr.). Circulation 70(Suppl. 2):II–71, 1984.
137. Pasipoularides A: Clinical assessment of ventricular ejection dynamics with and without outflow obstruction. J Am Coll Cardiol 15:859, 1990.
138. Baumgartner H, et al.: Discrepancies between Doppler and catheter gradients in aortic prosthetic valves in vitro: a manifestation of localized gradient and pressure recovery. Circulation 82:1467, 1990.
139. Shapiro LM, Howat AP, Crean PA, Westgate CJ: An echocardiographic study of localized subaortic hypertrophy. Eur Heart J 7:127, 1986.
140. Sugawara M, Kajiya F, Kitabatake A, Matsuo H (eds.): Blood Flow in the Heart and Large Vessels. Tokyo, Springer-Verlag, p. 97, 1989.
141. Wigle ED, Marquis Y, Auger P: Muscular subaortic stenosis: initial left ventricular inflow tract pressure in the assessment of intraventricular pressure differences in man. Circulation 35:1100, 1967.
142. Pierce GE, Morrow AG, Braunwald E: Idiopathic hypertrophic subaortic stenosis: III. Intraoperative studies of the mechanism of obstruction and its hemodynamic consequences. Circulation 30(Suppl. 4):IV–152, 1964.
143. Hernandez RR, Greenfield JC Jr, McCall BW: Pressure-flow studies in hypertrophic subaortic stenosis. J Clin Invest 43:401, 1964.
144. Criley JM, Lewis KB, White RJ, Ross RS: Pressure gradients without obstruction: a new concept of "hypertrophic subaortic stenosis." Circulation 32:881, 1965.
145. Murgo JP, et al.: Dynamics of left ventricular ejection in obstructive and nonobstructive hypertrophic cardiomyopathy. J Clin Invest 66:1369, 1980.
146. Criley JM, Siegel RJ: Has "obstruction" hindered our understanding of hypertrophic subaortic cardiomyopathy? Circulation 72:1148, 1985.
147. Levine RA, Weyman AE: Dynamic subaortic obstruction in hypertrophic cardiomyopathy: criteria and controversy. J Am Coll Cardiol 6:16, 1985.
148. Bonow RO, et al.: Left ventricular ejection dynamics in hypertrophic cardiomyopathy: comparison with valvular aortic stenosis (abstr.). J Am Coll Cardiol 5:394, 1985.
149. Jenni R, et al.: Dynamics of aortic flow in hypertrophic cardiomyopathy. Eur Heart J 6:391, 1985.
150. Sasson Z, et al.: Causal relation between the pressure gradient and left ventricular ejection time in hypertrophic cardiomyopathy. J Am Coll Cardiol 13:1275, 1989.
151. Bonow RO: Left ventricular ejection dynamics and outflow obstruction in hypertrophic cardiomyopathy. J Am Coll Cardiol 13:1280, 1989.
152. Cannon RO, et al.: Differences in coronary flow and myocardial metabolism at rest and during pacing between patients with obstructive and patients with nonobstructive hypertrophic cardiomyopathy. J Am Coll Cardiol 10:53, 1987.
153. Cannon RO, et al.: Effect of surgical reduction of left ventricular outflow obstruction on hemodynamics, coronary flow, and myocardial metabolism in hypertrophic cardiomyopathy. Circulation 79:766, 1989.
154. Adelman AG, et al.: The clinical course in musuclar subaortic stenosis—a retrospective and prospective study of 60 hemodynamically proved cases. Ann Intern Med 77:515, 1972.
155. Morrow AG, et al.: Operative treatment in hypertrophic subaortic stenosis: techniques and the results of pre- and postoperative assessments in 83 patients. Circulation 52:88, 1975.
156. Schapira JN, et al.: Single and two-dimensional echocardiographic visualization of the effects of septal myectomy in idiopathic hypertrophic subaortic stenosis. Circulation 58:860, 1978.
157. Maron BJ, Epstein SE, Morrow AG: Symptomatic status and prognosis of patients after operation for hypertrophic obstructive cardiomyopathy: efficacy of ventricular septal myotomy and myectomy. Eur Heart J 4(Suppl. F):175, 1983.
158. Beahrs MM, et al.: Hypertrophic obstructive cardiomyopathy: ten- to 21-year follow-up after partial septal myectomy. Am J Cardiol 51:1160, 1983.
159. Fighali S, Krajcer Z, Leachman RD: Septal myomectomy and mitral valve replacement for idiopathic hypertrophic subaortic stenosis: Short- and long-term follow-up. J Am Coll Cardiol 3:1127, 1984.
160. Krajcer Z, et al.: Mitral valve replacement and septal myomectomy in hypertrophic cardiomyopathy: ten-year follow-up in 80 patients. Circulation 78(Suppl. 1):I–35, 1988.
161. Wigle ED: Hypertrophic cardiomyopathy: a 1987 viewpoint. Circulation 75:311, 1987.
162. Wigle ED, Adelman AG, Silver MD: Pathophysiological considerations in muscular subaortic stenosis. *In* Wolstenholme GEW, O'Connor M (eds.): Hypertrophic Obstructive Cardiomyopathy. CIBA Foundation Study Group No. 37. London: J&A Churchill, p. 63, 1971.
163. Wigle ED, Adelman AG, Felderhof CH: Medical and surgical treatment of cardiomyopathy. Circ Res 35(Suppl. 2):II–196, 1974.
164. Whalen RE, Cohen AI, Sumner RG, McIntosh HD: Demonstration of the dynamic nature of idiopathic hypertrophic subaortic stenosis. Am J Cardiol 11:8, 1963.
165. Hasegawa I, et al.: Correlation of left ventricular outflow obstruction with mitral regurgitation. J Cardiol 18:339, 1988.
166. Levine RA, et al.: An experimental model for studying systolic anterior motion of the mitral valve in idiopathic hypertrophic subaortic stenosis (abstr.). J Am Coll Cardiol 5:424, 1985.
167. Levine RA, Vlahakes G, Weyman AE: Anterior papillary muscle displacement causes systolic anterior motion of the mitral valve in the absence of septal hypertrophy (abstr.). J Am Coll Cardiol 11:74A, 1988.
168. Hasegawa I, et al.: Relationship between mitral regurgitation and left ventricular outflow obstruction in hypertrophic cardiomyopathy. J Am Soc Echocardiogr 2:177, 1989.
169. St. John Sutton MG, et al.: Echocardiographic assessment of left ventricu-

lar filling and septal and posterior wall dynamics in idiopathic hypertrophic subaortic stenosis. Circulation 57:512, 1978.
170. Hanrath P, Mathey DG, Siegert R, Bleifeld W: Left ventricular relaxation and filling pattern in different forms of left ventricular hypertrophy: an echocardiographic study. Am J Cardiol 45:15, 1980.
171. Suwa M, Hirota Y, Kawamura K: Improvement in left ventricular diastolic function during intravenous and oral diltiazem therapy in patients with hypertrophic cardiomyopathy. Am J Cardiol 54:802, 1984.
172. Bryhn M: Echocardiographic assessment of left ventricular diastolic function in a normal population and a group of patients with myocardial hypertrophy. Clin Cardiol 7:335, 1984.
173. Spirito P, et al.: Noninvasive assessment of left ventricular diastolic function: comparative analysis of pulsed Doppler ultrasound and digitized M-mode echocardiography. Am J Cardiol 58:837, 1986.
174. Rokey R, et al.: Determination of parameters of left ventricular diastolic filling with pulsed Doppler echocardiography: comparison with cineangiography. Circulation 71:543, 1985.
175. Spirito P, Maron BJ, Bonow RO: Noninvasive assessment of left ventricular diastolic function: comparative analysis of Doppler echocardiographic and radionuclide angiographic techniques. J Am Coll Cardiol 7:518, 1986.
176. Maron BJ, et al.: Noninvasive assessment of left ventricular diastolic function by pulsed Doppler echocardiography in patients with hypertrophic cardiomyopathy. J Am Coll Cardiol 10:733, 1987.
177. Douglas PS, Berko B, Lesh M, Reichek N: Alterations in diastolic function in response to progressive left ventricular hypertrophy. J Am Coll Cardiol 13:461, 1989.
178. Takenaka K, et al.: Left ventricular filling in hypertrophic cardiomyopathy: a pulsed Doppler echocardiographic study. J Am Coll Cardiol 7:1263, 1986.
179. Bryg RJ, Pearson AC, Williams GA, Labovitz AJ: Left ventricular systolic and diastolic flow abnormalities determined by Doppler echocardiography in obstructive hypertrophic cardiomyopathy. Am J Cardiol 59:925, 1987.
180. Gidding SS, et al.: Left ventricular diastolic filling in children with hypertrophic cardiomyopathy: assessment with pulsed Doppler echocardiography. J Am Coll Cardiol 8:310, 1986.
181. Choong CY, Hermann HC, Weyman AE, Fifer MA: Preload dependence of Doppler-derived indexes of left ventricular diastolic function in humans. J Am Coll Cardiol 10:800, 1987.
182. Gardin JM, et al.: Effect of imaging view and sample volume location on evaluation of mitral flow velocity by pulsed Doppler echocardiography. Am J Cardiol 57:1335, 1986.
183. Drinkovic N, et al.: Influence of sampling site upon the ratio of atrial to early diastolic transmitral flow velocities by Doppler (abstr.). J Am Coll Cardiol 9:16A, 1987.
184. Appleton CP, with the technical assistance of Carucci MJ, Henry CP, Olajos M: Influence of incremental change in heart rate on mitral flow velocity: assessment in lightly sedated, conscious dogs. J Am Coll Cardiol 17:227, 1991.
185. Harrison MR, Clifton GD, Pennell AT, DeMaria AN: Effect of heart rate on left ventricular diastolic transmitral flow velocity patterns assessed by Doppler echocardiography in normal subjects. Am J Cardiol 67:622, 1991.
186. Felderhof CH, et al.: Left ventricular function in cardiomyopathy. Can Med Assoc J 107:42, 1972.
187. Grossman W, McLaurin LP: Diastolic properties of the left ventricle. Ann Intern Med 84:316, 1976.
188. Ishida Y, et al.: Left ventricular filling dynamics: influence of left ventricular relaxation and left atrial pressure. Circulation 74:187, 1986.
189. Levine RA, Thomas JD: Insights into the physiologic significance of the mitral inflow velocity pattern. J Am Coll Cardiol 14:1718, 1989.
190. Maron BJ, Gottdeiner JS, Perry LW: Specificity of systolic anterior motion of anterior mitral leaflet for hypertrophic cardiomyopathy. Br Heart J 45: 206, 1981.
191. Aziz K, et al.: Clinical manifestations of dynamic left ventricular outflow tract stenosis in infants with d-transposition of the great arteries with intact ventricular septum. Am J Cardiol 44:290, 1979.
192. Vitarelli A, D'Addio AP, Gentile R, Burattini M: Echocardiographic evaluation of left ventricular outflow tract obstruction in complete transposition of the great arteries. Am Heart J 108:531, 1984.
193. Moro E, et al.: Doppler and two-dimensional echocardiographic observations of systolic anterior motion of the mitral valve in d-transposition of the great arteries: an explanation of the left ventricular outflow tract gradient. J Am Coll Cardiol 7:889, 1986.
194. Khan MM, Varma MPS, Cleland J: Discrete subaortic stenosis. Br Heart J 46:421, 1974.
195. Boughner DR, Rakowski HE, Wigle D: Mitral valve systolic anterior motion in the absence of hypertrophic cardiomyopathy (abstr.). Circulation 58(Suppl. 2):II–235, 1978.
196. Bulkley BH, Fortuin NJ: Systolic anterior motion of the mitral valve without asymmetric septal hypertrophy. Chest 69:694, 1976.
197. Wei JY, Weiss JL, Bulkley BH: The heterogeneity of hypertrophic cardiomyopathy: an autopsy and one-dimensional echocardiographic study. Am J Cardiol 45:24, 1980.
198. Come PC, et al.: Hypercontractile cardiac states simulating hypertrophic cardiomyopathy. Circulation 55:901, 1977.
199. Levisman JA: Systolic anterior motion of the mitral valve due to hypovolemia and anemia. Chest 70:687, 1976.
200. Mintz GS, Kotler MN, Segal BL, Parry WR: Systolic anterior motion of the mitral valve in the absence of asymmetric septal hypertrophy. Circulation 57:256, 1978.
201. Weyman AE: Cross-Sectional Echocardiography. Philadelphia, Lea & Febiger, p. 256, 1982.
202. Bjork VO, Hultquist G, Lodin H: Subaortic stenosis produced by an abnormally placed anterior mitral leaflet. J Thorac Cardiovasc Surg 41:659, 1961.
203. Gomes AS, et al.: Accessory flaplike tissue causing ventricular outflow obstruction. J Thorac Cardiovasc Surg 80:211, 1980.
204. Alboliras ET, et al.: Cases from the Mayo Clinic: accessory mitral valve tissue in association with discrete subaortic stenosis: a two-dimensional echocardiographic diagnosis. Echocardiography 2:191, 1985.
205. O'Shea JP, Danchin N, Weyman AE, Levine RA: Pathogenesis of systolic anterior motion of the mitral valve—can the papillary-mitral apparatus play a primary role clinically? (abstr.) J Am Coll Cardiol 13:88, 1989.
206. Gallerstein PE, et al.: Systolic anterior motion of the mitral valve and outflow obstruction after mitral valve reconstruction. Chest 83:819, 1983.
207. Kronzon I, Cohen L, Winer HE, Colvin SB: Left ventricular outflow obstruction: a complication of mitral valvuloplasty. J Am Coll Cardiol 4:825, 1984.
208. Kreindel MS, Schiavone WA, Lever HM, Cosgrove D: Systolic anterior motion of the mitral valve after Carpentier ring valvuloplasty for mitral valve prolapse. Am J Cardiol 57:408, 1986.
209. Galler M, et al.: Long-term follow-up after mitral valve reconstruction: incidence of postoperative left ventricular outflow obstruction. Circulation 74(Suppl. 1):I–99, 1986.
210. Schiavone WA, et al.: Long-term follow-up of patients with left ventricular outflow tract obstruction after Carpentier ring mitral valvuloplasty. Circulation 78(Suppl. 1):I–60, 1988.
211. Mihaileanu S, et al.: Left ventricular outflow obstruction after mitral valve repair (Carpentier's technique): proposed mechanisms of disease. Circulation 78(Suppl. 1):I–78, 1988.
212. Reis RL, et al.: Anterior superior displacement of papillary muscles producing obstruction and mitral regurgitation in idiopathic hypertrophic subaortic stenosis. Operative relief by posterior-superior realignment of papillary muscles following ventricular septal myectomy. Circulation 49, 50 (Suppl. 2):II–101, 1973.
213. Rodger JC: Motion of mitral apparatus in hypertrophic cardiomyopathy with obstruction. Br Heart J 38:732, 1976.
214. Udoshi M, Shah A, Fisher VJ, Dolgin M: Systolic anterior motion of the mitral valve with and without asymmetric septal hypertrophy. Cardiology 66:147, 1980.
215. Henry WL, Clark CE, Roberts WC, Epstein SE: Differences in distribution of myocardial abnormalities in patients with obstructive and nonobstructive asymmetric septal hypertrophy (ASH): echocardiographic and gross anatomic changes. Circulation 50:447, 1974.
216. Spirito P, Maron BJ: Significance of left ventricular outflow tract cross-sectional area in hypertrophic cardiomyopathy: a two-dimensional echocardiographic assessment. Circulation 67:1100, 1983.
217. Pollick C, Williams WG, Rakowski H, Wigle ED: Post ventriculomyectomy eccentric SAM: further evidence for the Venturi mechanism (abstr.). J Am Coll Cardiol 3:492, 1984.
218. Pollick C: Muscular subaortic stenosis. Hemodynamic and clinical improvement after disopyramide. N Engl J Med 307:997, 1982.
219. Sherrid M, Delia E, Dwyer E: Oral disopyramide therapy for obstructive hypertrophic cardiomyopathy. Am J Cardiol 62:1085, 1988.
220. Levine RA, et al.: Systolic anterior motion of the mitral valve in hypertrophic cardiomyopathy can begin with low outflow tract velocities (abstr.). Circulation 78(Suppl. 2):II–28, 1988.
221. O'Shea JP, Castellani S, Harrigan P, Levine RA: Anterior motion of the mitral valve—onset before systolic ejection: a Doppler-echocardiographic study (abstr.). Circulation 78(Suppl. 2):II–548, 1988.
222. King JF, et al.: Echocardiographic assessment of idiopathic hypertrophic subaortic stenosis. Chest 64:723, 1973.
223. Cohen MV, Teichholz LE, Gorlin R: B-scan ultrasonography in idiopathic hypertrophic obstructive cardiomyopathy: proposed role in systolic anterior motion of mitral valve. Am J Cardiol 48:258, 1981.
224. DeMaria A, Bommer W, Lee G, Mason DT: Value and limitations of two dimensional echocardiography in assessment of cardiomyopathy. Am J Cardiol 46:1224, 1980.
225. Nagata S, et al.: Mechanism of systolic anterior motion of mitral valve and site of intraventricular pressure gradient in hypertrophic obstructive cardiomyopathy. Br Heart J 49:234, 1983.
225a. Grigg LE, et al.: Transesophageal Doppler echocardiography in obstructive hypertrophic cardiomyopathy: clarification of pathophysiology and importance in intraoperative decision making. J Am Coll Cardiol 20;42, 1992.
226. Corday SR, Virmani R, Waller B, Shah PM: Necropsy evaluation of anterior mitral leaflet elongation in cardiomyopathies: possible role in hypertrophic cardiomyopathy (abstr.). Circulation 60(Suppl. 2):II–243, 1979.
227. Klues HG, Dollar AL, Roberts WC, Maron BJ: Diversity of structural mitral valve alterations in hypertrophic cardiomyopathy. Circulation 85: 1651, 1992.
228. Fox RW, McDonald AT: Introduction to Fluid Mechanics. 2nd Ed. New York, John Wiley, p. 424, 1970.

229. Cape EG, et al.: Chordal geometry determines the shape and extent of systolic anterior mitral motion: *in vitro* studies. J Am Coll Cardiol 13:1438, 1989.
230. Hasegawa I, et al.: Mechanism of systolic anterior motion and left ventricular outflow obstruction in hypertrophic cardiomyopathy. J Cardiogr 15: 655, 1985.
231. Levine RA, et al.: New insights into the mechanism of obstruction in hypertrophic cardiomyopathy: experimental models (abstr.). Circulation 80(Suppl 2):II–662, 1989.
232. Levine RA, et al.: Increased outflow tract velocity fails to produce SAM of a normally restrained mitral valve *in vitro* (abstr.). Circulation (Suppl. 2):II–662, 1989.
233. Lefebvre X, et al.: Reproduction of systolic anterior motion of the mitral valve in a pulsatile flow model (abstr.). Circulation 82(Suppl. 3):III–396, 1990.
234. Lefebvre XP, Yoganathan AP, Levine RA. Insights from in vitro flow visualization into the mechanism of systolic anterior motion of the mitral valve in hypertrophic cardiomyopathy under steady flow conditions. J Biomech Eng 114:406, 1992.
235. O'Shea JP, et al.: Mechanism of obstruction in hypertrophic cardiomyopathy: increasing septal thickness potentiates the effect of SAM in an experimental echocardiographic model (abstr.). Circulation 80(Suppl. 2):II–269, 1989.
236. Mizushige K, et al.: Pre-ejection flow in the left ventricular outflow tract elucidated by pulsed Doppler technique. J Cardiogr 14:507, 1984.
237. Panayiotou H, Byrd BF III: Origin and significance of diastolic Doppler flow signals in the left ventricular outflow tract. J Am Coll Cardiol 16: 1625, 1990.
238. Salisbury PF, Cross CE, Rieben PA: Chorda tendinea tension. Am J Physiol 205:385, 1963.
239. Morais P, Westaby S, Hallidie-Smith KA: Left ventricular outflow tract obstruction due to anomalous mitral valve: successful mitral valve replacement in a four month old infant. Br Heart J 56:385, 1986.
240. Danchin N, et al.: Two-dimensional echocardiographic recognition of extra-cardiac masses and cardiac metastases. (Submitted for publication.)
241. Lewis JF, Maron BJ: Elderly patients with hypetrophic cardiomyopathy: a subset with distinctive left ventricular morphology and progressive clinical course late in life. J Am Coll Cardiol 13:36, 1989.
242. Krasnow N: An acquired disease component in hypertrophic cardiomyopathy: new clinical clarifications. J Am Coll Cardiol 13:46, 1989.
243. Wanderman K, Margulis G: Coexistence of hypertrophic obstructive cardiomyopathy and mitral annular calcification: proposed etiologic relationship. Isr J Med Sci 15:422, 1979.
244. Lindvall K, Herrlin B: Mitral annulus calcification, systolic anterior motion of the anterior mitral leaflet and outflow obstruction in two patients without hypertrophic cardiomyopathy. Acta Med Scand 209:513, 1981.
245. Maron BJ, et al.: Obstructive hypertrophic cardiomyopathy associated with minimal left ventricular hypertrophy. Am J Cardiol 53:377, 1984.
246. Rubenstein S, et al.: Coexisting hypertrophic heart disease and mitral valve prolapse: a continuum of hereditary cardiac disease. Chest 78:51, 1980.
247. Panza JA, Maron BJ: Simultaneous occurrence of mitral valve prolapse and systolic anterior motion in hypertrophic cardiomyopathy. Am J Cardiol 67:404, 1991.
248. Come PC, et al.: Dynamic left ventricular outflow tract obstruction when the anterior leaflet is retained at prosthetic mitral valve replacement. Ann Thorac Surg 43:561, 1987.
249. Pomerance A, Davies MJ: Pathological features of hypertrophic obstructive cardiomyopathy (HOCM) in the elderly. Br Heart J 37:305, 1975.
250. Kransow N, Stein RA: Hypertrophic cardiomyopathy in the aged. Am Heart J 96:326, 1979.
251. Berger M, Rethy C, Goldberg E: Unsuspected hypertrophic subaortic stenosis in the elderly diagnosed by echocardiography. J Am Geriatr Soc 27: 178, 1979.
252. Petrin TJ, Tavel ME: Idiopathic hypertrophic subaortic stenosis as observed in the large community hospital: relation to age and history of hypertension. J Am Geriatr Soc 27:43, 1979.
253. Topol EJ, Traill TA, Fortuin NJ: Hypertensive hypertrophic cardiomyopathy of the elderly. N Engl J Med 312:277, 1985.
254. Pearson AC, Gudipati CV, Labovitz AJ: Systolic and diastolic flow abnormalities in elderly patients with hypertensive hypertrophic cardiomyopathy. J Am Coll Cardiol 12:989, 1988.
255. Wicker P, et al.: Prevalence and significance of asymmetric septal hypertrophy in hypertension: an echocardiographic and clinical study. Eur Heart J 4(Suppl. G):1, 1983.
256. Karam R, Lever HM, Healy BP: Hypertensive hypertrophic cardiomyopathy or hypertrophic cardiomyopathy with hypertension?: A study of 78 patients. J Am Coll Cardiol 13:580, 1989.
257. Lewis JF, Maron BJ: Diversity of patterns of hypertrophy in patients with systemic hypertension and marked left ventricular wall thickening. Am J Cardiol 65:874, 1990.
258. Schwinger ME, O'Brien F, Freedberg RS, Kronzon I: Dynamic left ventricular outflow obstruction after aortic valve replacement: a Doppler echocardiographic study. J Am Soc Echocardiogr 3:205, 1990.
259. Louie EK: Congestive cardiomyopathy: Doppler echocardiographic assessment of structure and function. Echocardiography 4:119, 1987.
260. Shah PM: Echocardiography in congestive or dilated cardiomyopathy. J Am Soc Echocardiogr 1:20, 1988.
261. Fuster V, et al.: The natural history of idiopathic dilated cardiomyopathy. Am J Cardiol 47:525, 1981.
262. Rahko PS, Salerni R, Uretsky BF: Successful reversal by chelation therapy of congestive cardiomyopathy due to iron overload. J Am Coll Cardiol 8: 436, 1986.
263. Easley RM, Schreiner BJ, Yu PN: Reversible cardiomyopathy associated with hemochromatosis. N Engl J Med 287:866, 1972.
264. Henry WL, et al.: Echocardiographic abnormalities in patients with transfusion-dependent anemia and secondary myocardial iron deposition. Am J Med 64:547, 1978.
265. Meyer RA: Cardiomyopathy in the young. J Am Soc Echocardiogr 1:88, 1988.
266. Corya BC, Feigenbaum H, Rasmussen S, Black MJ: Echocardiographic features of congestive cardiomyopathy compared with normal subjects and patients with coronary artery disease. Circulation 49:1153, 1974.
267. Benjamin IJ, Schuster EH, Bulkley BH: Cardiac hypertrophy in idiopathic dilated congestive cardiomyopathy: a clinicopathologic study. Circulation 64:442, 1981.
268. Massie BM, Schiller NB, Ratshin RA, Parmley WW: Mitral-septal separation: new echocardiographic index of left ventricular function. Am J Cardiol 39:1008, 1977.
269. Child JS, Krovokapich J, Perloff JK: Effect of left ventricular size on mitral E-point to ventricular septal separation in assessment of cardiac performance. Am Heart J 101:797, 1981.
270. Wallis DE, O'Connell JB, Henkin RE, Costanzo-Nordin MR, Scanlon PJ: Segmental wall motion abnormalities in dilated cardiomyopathies: a common finding and good prognostic sign. J Am Coll Cardiol 4:674, 1984.
271. Medina R, et al.: The value of echocardiographic regional wall motion abnormalities in detecting coronary artery disease in patients with or without a dilated left ventricle. Am Heart J 109:799, 1985.
272. Pasquini JA, Gottdiener JS, Cutler DJ, Fletcher RD: Myocarditis with transient left ventricular apical dyskinesis. Am Heart J 109:371, 1985.
273. Acquatella H, et al.: M-mode and two-dimensional echocardiography in chronic Chagas' heart disease: a clinical and pathologic study. Circulation 62:787, 1980.
274. Fujiwara T, Tarumoto T, Kudo K: Echocardiography of ischemic heart disease simulating dilated cardiomyopathy, with special reference to abnormal wall movement on the short axis. J Cardiogr 13:89, 1983.
275. McDonald IG: Echocardiographic assessment of left ventricular function in mitral valve disease. Circulation 53:865, 1976.
276. Keren A, Billingham ME, Popp RI: Features of mildly dilated congestive cardiomyopathy and typical dilated cardiomyopathy. J Am Soc Echocardiogr 1:78, 1988.
277. Keren A, et al.: Mildly dilated congestive cardiomyopathy: use of prospective diagnostic criteria and description of the clinical course withiout heart transplantation. Circulation 81:506, 1990.
278. Fitchett DH, Sugrue DD, MacArthur CG, Oakley CM: Right ventricular dilated cardiomyopathy. Br Heart J 51:25, 1984.
279. Ribeiro PA, et al.: Echocardiographic features of right ventricular dilated cardiomyopathy and Uhl's anomaly. Eur Heart J 8:65, 1987.
280. Ascah KJ, Stewart WJ, Levine RA, Weyman AE: Doppler-echocardiographic assessment of cardiac output. Radiol Clin North Am 23:659, 1985.
281. Gardin JM, et al.: Evaluation of dilated cardiomyopathy by pulsed Doppler echocardiography. Am Heart J 106:1057, 1983.
282. Elkayam U, et al.: The use of Doppler flow velocity measurement to assess the hemodynamic response to vasodilators in patients with heart failure. Circulation 67:377, 1983.
283. Wallmeyer K, et al.: The influence of preload and heart rate on Doppler echocardiographic indexes of left ventricular performance: comparison with invasive indexes in an experimental preparation. Circulation 74:181, 1986.
284. Gardin JM: Doppler measurements of aortic blood flow velocity and acceleration: load-independent indexes of left ventricular performance? Am J Cardiol 15:935, 1989.
285. Bargiggia GS, et al.: A new method for estimating left ventricular dP/dt by continuous wave Doppler-echocardiography: validation studies at cardiac catheterization. 80:1287, 1989.
286. Chen C, et al.: Noninvasive estimation of the instantaneous first derivative of left ventricular pressure using continuous-wave Doppler echocardiography. Circulation 83:2101, 1991.
287. Colan SD, Borow KM, Neumann A: Left ventricular end-systolic wall stress-velocity of fiber shortening relation: a load-independent index of myocardial contractility. J Am Coll Cardiol 4:715, 1984.
288. Borow KM, et al.: Myocardial mechanics in young adult patients with diabetes mellitus: effects of altered load, inotropic state and dynamic exercise. J Am Coll Cardiol 15:1508, 1990.
289. Takenaka K, et al.: Pulsed Doppler echocardiographic study of left ventricular filling in dilated cardiomyopathy. Am J Cardiol 58:143, 1986.
290. Vanoverschelde J-LJ, Raphael DA, Robert AR, Cosyns JR: Left ventricular filling in dilated cardiomyopathy: relation to functional class and hemodynamics. J Am Coll Cardiol 15:1288, 1990.
291. Grossman W, McLaurin LP, Rolett EL: Alterations in left ventricular re-

laxation and diastolic compliance in congestive cardiomyopathy. Cardiovasc Res 13:514, 1979.
292. Bortone AS, et al.: Functional and structural abnormalities in patients with dilated cardiomyopathy. J Am Coll Cardiol 14:613, 1989.
293. Waagstein F, et al.: Long-term beta-blockade in dilated cardiomyopathy: effects of short- and long-term metroprolol treatment followed by withdrawal and readministration of metroprolol. Circulation 80:551, 1989.
294. Douglas PS, Morrow R, Ioli A, Reichek N: Left ventricular shape, afterload and survival in idiopathic dilated cardiomyopathy. J Am Coll Cardiol 13:311, 1989.
295. Godley RW, et al.: Incomplete mitral leaflet closure in patients with papillary muscle dysfunction. Circulation 63:565, 1981.
296. Godley RW, et al.: Relation of incomplete mitral leaflet closure to the site of dyssynergy in patients with papillary muscle dysfunction. Circulation 60(Suppl. 2):204, 1979.
297. Levy MJ, Edwards JE: Anatomy of mitral insufficiency. Prog Cardiovasc Dis 5:119, 1962.
298. Burch GE, DePasquale NP, Phillips JH: The syndrome of papillary muscle dysfunction. Am Heart J 75:399, 1968.
299. Gibson TC, Foale RA, Guyer DE, Weyman AE: Clinical significance of incomplete tricuspid valve closure seen on two-dimensional echocardiography. J Am Coll Cardiol 4:1052, 1984.
300. Waller BF: Rheumatic and nonrheumatic conditions causing valvular heart disease. *In* Frankl WS, Brest AN (eds.): Valvular Heart Disease. Philadelphia, FA Davis, p. 3, 1985.
301. Ballester M, et al.: The mechanism of mitral regurgitation in dilated left ventricle. Clin Cardiol 6:333, 1983.
302. Boltwood CM, Tei C, Wong M, Shah PM: Quantitative echocardiography of the mitral complex in dilated cardiomyopathy; the mechanism of functional mitral regurgitation. Circulation 68:498, 1983.
303. Takamoto T, et al.: Comparative recognition of left ventricular thrombi by echocardiography and cineangiography. Br Heart J 53:36, 1985.
304. Stratton JR, Lighty GW, Pearlman AS, Ritchie JL: Detection of left ventricular thrombus by two-dimensional echocardiography: sensitivity, specitivity, and causes of uncertainty. Circulation 66:156, 1982.
305. Mikell FL, et al.: Regional stasis of blood in the dysfunctional left ventricle: echocardiographic detection and differentiation from early thrombosis. Circulation 66:755, 1982.
306. Beppu S, et al.: Abnormal blood pathways in left ventricular cavity in acute myocardial infarction: experimental observations with special reference to regional wall motion abnormality and hemostasis. Circulation 78:157, 1988.
307. Maze SS, Kotler MN, Parry WR: Flow characteristics in the dilated left ventricle with thrombus: qualitative and quantitative Doppler analysis. J Am Coll Cardiol 13:873, 1989.
308. Gottdiener JS, et al.: Frequency and embolic potential of left ventricular thrombus in dilated cardiomyopathy: assessment by 2-dimensional echocardiography. Am J Cardiol 52:1281, 1983.
309. Kinney EL: The significance of left ventricular thrombi in patients with coronary heart disease: a retrospective analysis of pooled data. Am Heart J 109:191, 1985.
310. Benotti JR, Grossman W, Cohn PF: Clinical proflie of restrictive cardiomyopathy. Circulation 61:1206, 1980.
311. Meaney E, et al.: Cardiac amyloidosis, constrictive pericarditis and restrictive cardiomyopathy. Am J Cardiol 38:547, 1976.
312. Gaasch WH, Zile MR: Evaluation of myocardial function in cardiomyopathic states. Prog Cardiovasc Dis 27:115, 1984.
313. Klein AL, et al.: Two-dimensional and Doppler echocardiographic assessment of infiltrative cardiomyopathy. J Am Soc Echocardiogr 1:48, 1988.
314. Child JS, Levisman JA, Abbasi AS, MacAlpin RN: Echocardiographic manifestations of infiltrative cardiomyopathy. A report of seven cases due to amyloid. Chest 70:726, 1976.
315. Borer JS, Henry WL, Epstein SE: Echocardiographic observation in patients with systemic infiltrative disease involving the heart. Am J Cardiol 39:184, 1977.
316. Siqueira-Filho AG, et al.: M-mode and two-dimensional echocardiographic features in cardiac amyloidosis. Circulation 63:188, 1981.
317. Nicolosi GL, et al.: Prospective identification of patients with amyloid heart disease by two-dimensional echocardiography. Circulation 70:432, 1984.
318. Cueto-Garcia L, et al.: Serial echocardiographic observation in patients with primary systemic amyloidosis: an introduction to the concept of early (asymptomatic) amyloid infiltration of the heart. Mayo Clin Proc 59:589, 1984.
319. Eriksson P, et al.: Differentiation of cardiac amyloidosis and hypertrophic cardiomyopathy. Acta Med Scand 221:39, 1987.
320. Falk R, et al.: Sensitivity and specificity of the echocardiographic features of cardiac amyloidosis. Am J Cardiol 59:418, 1987.
321. Bhandari AK, Nanda NC: Myocardial texture characterization by two-dimensional echocardiography. Am J Cardiol 50:817, 1983.
322. Skorton DJ, Collins SM: Clinical potential of ultrasound tissue characterization in cardiomyopathies. J Am Soc Echocardiogr 1:69, 1988.
323. Chandrasekaran K, et al.: Feasibility of identifying amyloid and hypertrophic cardiomyopathy with the use of computerized quantitative texture analysis of clinical echocardiographic data. J Am Coll Cardiol 13:832, 1989.
324. Klein AL, et al.: Comprehensive Doppler assessment of right ventricular diastolic function in cardiac amyloidosis. J Am Coll Cardiol 15:99, 1990.
325. Plehn JF, Friedman BJ: Diastolic dysfunction in amyloid heart disease: restrictive cardiomyopathy or not? J Am Coll Cardiol 13:54, 1989.
326. Briggs GW: Amyloidosis. Ann Intern Med 55:943, 1961.
327. Buja LM, Khol NB, Roberts WC: Clinically significant cardiac amyloidosis: clinicopathologic findings in 15 patients. Am J Cardiol 26:394, 1975.
328. Kyle RA, Baynd ED: Amyloidosis; review of 236 cases. Medicine 54:271, 1975.
329. Kyle RA, Greipp PR: Amyloidosis (AL): clinical and laboratory features in 229 cases. Mayo Clin Proc 58:665, 1983.
330. Pomerance A: Senile cardiac amyloidosis. Br Heart J 27:711, 1965.
331. Roberts WC, Waller BF: Cardiac amyloidosis causing cardiac dysfunction: analysis of 54 necropsy patients. Am J Cardiol 52:137, 1983.
332. Smith TJ, Kyle RA, Lie JT: Clinical significance of histopathologic pattern of cardiac amyloidosis. Mayo Clin Proc 59:547, 1984.
333. Wright JR, Calkins E, Humphrey RL: Potassium permanganate reaction in amyloidosis. A histologic method to assist in differentiating forms of this disease. Lab Invest 36:274, 1977.
334. Simons M, et al.: Noninvasive evaluation of cardiac amyloidosis. Echocardiography 2:401, 1985.
335. Mahloudji M, et al.: The genetic amyloidoses. Medicine 48:1, 1969.
336. Frederiksen T, et al.: Familial primary amyloidosis with severe amyloid heart disease. Am J Med 33:328, 1962.
337. Pomerance A: Pathology of the heart with and without cardiac failure in the aged. Br Heart J 27:697, 1965.
338. Pomerance A: The pathology of senile cardiac amyloidosis. J Pathol Bacteriol 91:357, 1966.
339. Cornwell GG III, et al.: Frequency and distribution of senile cardiovascular amyloidosis. Am J Med 75:618, 1983.
340. Child JS, Krivokapich AJ, Abbasi AS: Increased right ventricular wall thickness on echocardiography in amyloid infiltrative cardiomyopathy. Am J Cardiol 44:1391, 1979.
341. Cunha CLP, et al.: Characteristic two-dimensional echocardiographic appearance of amyloid heart disease (abstr.). Circulation (Suppl. 2):II–18, 1979.
342. Griffiths BE, Hughes P, Dowdle R, Stephens MR: Cardiac amyloidosis with asymmetrical septal hypertrophy and deterioration after nifedipine. Thorax 37:711, 1982.
343. Weston LT, et al.: Primary amyloid heart disease presenting as hypertrophic obstructive cardiomyopathy. Cathet Cardiovasc Diagn 12:176, 1986.
344. Oh JK, et al.: Dynamic left ventricular outflow tract obstruction in cardiac amyloidosis detected by continuous-wave Doppler echocardiography. Am J Cardiol 59:1008, 1987.
345. Buja LM, Roberts WC: Iron in the heart, etiology and clinical significance. Am J Med 51:209, 1971.
346. Olson LJ, et al.: Endomyocardial biopsy in hemochromatosis: clinicopathologic correlates in six cases. J Am Coll Cardiol 13:116, 1989.
347. Olson LJ, Baldus WP, Tajik AJ: Echocardiographic features of idiopathic hemochromatosis. Am J Cardiol 60:885, 1987.
348. Candell-Riera J, et al.: Cardiac hemochromatosis: beneficial effects of iron removal therapy. An echocardiographic study. Am J Cardiol 52:824, 1983.
349. Dabestani A, et al.: Primary hemochromatosis: anatomic and physiologic characteristics of the cardiac ventricles and their response to phlebotomy. Am J Cardiol 54:153, 1984.
350. Olson LJ, et al.: Cardiac iron deposition in idiopathic hemochromatosis: histologic and analytic assessment of 14 hearts from autopsy. J Am Coll Cardiol 10:1239, 1987.
351. Cutler DJ, et al.: Hemochromatosis heart disease: an unemphasized cause of potentially reversible restrictive cardiomyopathy. Am J Med 69:923, 1980.
352. Arnet EN, et al.: Massive myocardial hemosiderosis: a structure function conference at the National Heart and Lung Institute. Am Heart J 90:777, 1975.
353. Leon MB, et al.: Detection of early cardiac dysfunction in patients with severe beta-thalassemia and chronic iron overload. N Engl J Med 301: 1143, 1979.
354. Valdes-Cruz LM, et al.: Preclinical abnormal segmental cardiac manifestations of thalassemia major in children in transfusion-chelation therapy; echocardiographic alterations of left ventricular posterior wall contraction and relaxation patterns. Am Heart J 103:505, 1982.
355. Roberts WC, McAllister HA Jr, Ferrans BJ: Sarcoidosis of the heart. A clinicopathologic study of 35 necropsy patients (group I) and review of 78 previously described necropsy patients (group II). Am J Med 63:86, 1977.
356. Silverman KJ, Hutchins GM, Bulkley BH: Cardiac sarcoid. A clinicopathologic study of 84 unselected patients with systemic sarcoidosis. Circulation 58:1204, 1978.
357. Lewin RF, et al.: Echocardiographic evaluation of patients with systemic sarcoidosis. Am Heart J 110:116, 1985.
358. Fry ETA, Barzilai B, Waggoner AD: Echo assessment of dilated cardiomyopathy due to sarcoidosis. Cardio August:99, 1990.
359. Lull RJ, et al.: Ventricular aneurysm due to cardiac sarcoidosis with surgical cure of refractory ventricular tachycardia. Am J Cardiol 30:282, 1972.

360. Rizzato G, et al.: Right heart impairment in sarcoidosis: hemodynamic and echocardiographic study. Eur J Respir Dis 64:121, 1983.
361. Wenger NK, Goodwin JF, Roberts WC: Cardiomyopathy and myocardial involvement in systemic disease. *In* Hurst JW (ed.): The Heart. New York, McGraw-Hill, p. 1218, 1985.
362. Hwang B, Meng CCL, Lin CY, Hsu HC: Clinical analysis of five infants with glycogen storage disease of the heart: Pompe's disease. Jpn Heart J 27:25, 1986.
363. Olson LJ, et al.: Cardiac involvement in glycogen storage disease: III. Morphologic and biochemical characterization with endomyocardial biopsy. Am J Cardiol 53:900, 1984.
364. Gussenhoven WJ, Busch HFM, Kleijer WJ, De Villeneuve VH: Echocardiographic features in the cardiac type of glycogen storage disease II. Eur Heart J 4:41, 1983.
365. Rees A, Elbl F, Minhas K, Solinger R: Echocardiographic evidence of outflow tract obstruction in Pompe's disease (glycogen storage disease of the heart). Am J Cardiol 37:1103, 1976.
366. Cohen IS, Fluri-Lundeen J, Wharton TP: Two-dimensional echocardiographic similarity of Fabry's disease to cardiac amyloidosis: a function of ultrastructural analogy? JCU 11:437, 1983.
367. Bass J, et al.: The M-mode echocardiogram in Fabry's disease. Am Heart J 100:807, 1980.
368. Edwards JE, Carey LS, Neufeld HN, Lester RG: Congenital Heart Disease. Philadelphia, WB Saunders, 1965.
369. Moller JH, et al.: Endocardial fibroelastosis. Circulation 30:759, 1964.
370. Fisher JH: Primary endocardial fibroelastosis: a review of 15 cases. Can Med Assoc J 87:105, 1962.
371. Kelly J, Andersen DH: Congenital endocardial fibroelastosis: clinical and pathologic investigation of those cases without associated cardiac malformations including report of 2 familial instances. Pediatrics 18:539, 1956.
372. Manning JA, Keith JD: Fibroelastosis in children. Prog Cardiovasc Dis 7: 172, 1964.
373. Still WJS: Endocardial fibroelastosis. Am Heart J 61:579, 1961.
374. Branch CL, Castle RF: Thromboembolic complications in primary endocardial fibroelastosis. J Pediatr 69:250, 1966.
375. DuShane JW, Edwards JE: Congenital aortic stenosis in association with endocardial sclerosis of the left ventricle. Mayo Clin Proc 29:102, 1954.
376. Hallidie-Smith KA, Olsen EGJ: Endocardial fibroelastosis, mitral incompetence, and coarctation of the abdominal aorta. Br Heart J 30:850, 1968.
377. Yoshida Y, et al.: Ultrasonic studies on endocardial fibroelastosis. Tohoku J Exp Med 123:329, 1977.
378. Loeffler W: Endocarditis parietalis fibroplastica mit Bluteosinophilie. Ein eigenartiges Krankheitsbild. Schweiz Med Wochenschr 66:817, 1936.
379. Benvenisti DS, Ultmann JE: Eosinophilic leukemia. Report of five cases and review of literature. Ann Intern Med 71:731, 1969.
380. Odenberg B: Eosinophilic leukemia and disseminated eosinophilic collagen disease—a disease entity. Acta Med Scand 177:129, 1965.
381. Hardy WR, Anderson RE: The hypereosinophilic syndromes. Ann Intern Med 68:1220, 1968.
382. Chusid MJ, Dale DG, West BC, Wolff SM: The hypereosinophilic syndrome: analysis of fourteen cases with review of the literature. Medicine 54:1, 1975.
383. Olsen EGJ, Spry CJF: The pathogenesis of Loffler's endomyocardial disease, and its relationship to endomyocardial fibrosis. *In* Yu PN, Goodwin JF (eds.): Progress in Cardiology. Vol. 8. Philadelphia, Lea & Febiger, p. 281, 1979.
384. Olsen EGJ, Spry CJF: Relation between eosinophilia and endomyocardial disease. Prog Cardiovasc Dis 27:241, 1985.
385. Davies J, et al.: Cardiovascular features of eleven patients with eosinophilic endomyocardial disease. Q J Med 52:23, 1983.
386. Acquatella H, et al.: Value of two-dimensional echocardiography in endomyocardial disease with and without eosinophilia. Circulation 67:1219, 1983.
387. Acquatella H, Schiller NB: Echocardiographic recognition of Chagas' disease and endomyocardial fibrosis. J Am Soc Echocardiogr 1:60, 1988.
388. Davies J: Endocardial fibrosis in Africans. East Afr Med J 25:10, 1948.
389. Brockington IF, Olsen EGJ: Loffler's endocarditis and Davies' endomyocardial fibrosis. Am Heart J 85:308, 1973.
390. Roberts WC, Ferrans VJ: Pathologic anatomy of the cardiomyopathies. Idiopathic dilated and hypertrophic types, infiltrating types and endomyocardial disease with and without eosinophilia. Hum Pathol 6:287, 1975.
391. Davies J, Spry CJF, Vijayaraghavan G, DeSouza JA: A comparison of the clinical and cardiological features of endomyocardial disease in temperate and tropical regions. Postgrad Med J 59:179, 1983.
392. Roberts WC, Buja LM, Ferrans VJ: Loffler's fibroplastic parietal endocarditis, eosinophilic leukemia and Davies' endomyocardial fibrosis. The same disease at different stages? Pathol Microbiol 35:90, 1970.
393. Blair HT, Breaux P: Unusual hemodynamics in Loffler's endomyocarditis. Am J Cardiol 34:606, 1974.
394. Roberts WC, Liegler DG, Carbone PP: Endomyocardial disease and eosinophilia. A clinical and pathologic spectrum. Am J Med 46:28, 1969.
395. Bell JA, Jenkins BS, Webb-Peploe MM: Clinical, hemodynamic and angiographic findings in Loffler's eosinophilic endocarditis. Br Heart J 38:541, 1976.
396. Mumme C: Zur Klinik und Pathologie der Endokarditis und Aortitis fibroplastica sowie Thromboendarteriitis obliterans mit hochgradiger Eosinophilie im Blut, Knochenmark and in den Organen. Z Klin Med 138:22, 1940.
397. Hoffman FG, Rosenbaum D, Genovese PD: Fibroplastic endocarditis with eosinophilia (Loffler's endocarditis parietalis fibroplastica): case report and review of literature. Ann Intern Med 42:668, 1955.
398. Weyman AE, Rankin R, King H: Loffler's endocarditis presenting as mitral and tricuspid stenosis. Am J Cardiol 40:438, 1977.
399. Parrillo JE, et al.: The cardiovascular manifestations of the hypereosinophilic syndrome: prospective study of 26 patients, with review of the literature. Am J Med 67:572, 1979.
400. Davies J, et al.: Echocardiographic features of eosinophilic endomyocardial disease. Br Heart J 48:434, 1982.
401. Vijayaraghavan G, et al.: Echocardiographic features of tropical endomyocardial disease in South India. Br Heart J 50:450, 1983.
402. Gottdiener JS, et al.: Two-dimensional echocardiographic assessment of the idiopathic hypereosinophilic syndrome. Anatomic basis of mitral regurgitation and peripheral embolization. Circulation 67:572, 1983.
403. Appleton CP, Hatle LK, Popp RL: Demonstration of restrictive ventricular physiology by Doppler echocardiography. J Am Coll Cardiol 11:757, 1988.
404. Chew C, Ziady GM, Raphael MJ, Oakley CM: The functional defect in amyloid heart disease. The "stiff heart" syndrome. Am J Cardiol 36:438, 1975.
405. Meaney E, et al.: Cardiac amyloidosis, constrictive pericarditis and restrictive cardiomyopathy. Am J Cardiol 38:547, 1976.
406. Swanton RH, et al.: Systolic and diastolic ventricular function in cardiac amyloidosis: studies in six cases diagnosed with endomyocardial biopsy. Am J Cardiol 39:658, 1977.
407. Tyberg TI, et al.: Left ventricular filling in differentiating restrictive amyloid cardiomyopathy and constrictive pericarditis. Am J Cardiol 47:791, 1981.
408. Hongo M, Fujii T, Hirayama J, Kinoshita O, Tanaka M, Okubo S: Radionuclide angiographic assessment of left ventricular diastolic filling in amyloid heart disease: a study of patients with familial amyloid polyneuropathy. J Am Coll Cardiol 13:48, 1989.
409. Aroney CN, et al.: Differentiation of restrictive cardiomyopathy from pericardial constriction: assessment of diastolic function by radionuclide angiography. J Am Coll Cardiol 13:1007, 1989.
410. St. John-Sutton MJ, Reichek N, Kastor JA, Giuliani ER: Computerized M-mode and echocardiographic analysis of left ventricular dysfunction in cardiac amyloid. Circulation 66:790, 1982.
411. Janos GG, et al.: Differentiation of constrictive pericarditis and restrictive cardiomyopathy using digitized echocardiography. J Am Coll Cardiol 1: 541, 1983.
412. Klein AL, et al.: Doppler characterization of left ventricular diastolic function in cardiac amyloidosis. J Am Coll Cardiol 13:1017, 1989.
413. Kinoshita O, et al.: Impaired left ventricular diastolic filling in patients with familial amyloid polyneuropathy: a pulsed Doppler echocardiographic study. Br Heart J 69:198, 1989.
414. Klein AL, et al.: Serial Doppler echocardiographic follow-up of left ventricular diastolic function in cardiac amyloidosis. J Am Coll Cardiol 16:1135, 1990.
415. Oh JE, et al.: Characteristic Doppler echocardiographic pattern of mitral inflow velocity in severe aortic regurgitation. J Am Coll Cardiol 14:1712, 1989.
416. Schoenfeld MH, et al.: Restrictive cardiomyopathy versus constrictive pericarditis: role of endomyocardial biopsy in avoiding unnecessary thoracotomy. Circulation 75:1012, 1987.
417. Schnittger I, Bowden RE, Abrams J, Popp RL: Echocardiography: pericardial thickening and constrictive pericarditis. Am J Cardiol 42:388, 1978.
418. Appleton CP, Hatle LK, Popp RL: The relationship of transmitral flow velocity patterns to left ventricular diastolic function: new insights from a combined hemodynamic and Doppler echocardiographic study. J Am Coll Cardiol 12:426, 1988.
419. Hatle LK, Appleton CP, Popp RL: Differentiation of constrictive pericarditis and restrictive cardiomyopathy by Doppler echocardiography. Circulation 79:357, 1989.

CHAPTER

26

RIGHT VENTRICULAR INFLOW TRACT

The right ventricular inflow tract includes (1) the tricuspid valve and supporting apparatus, (2) the right atrium, and (3) the great systemic veins (the inferior and superior vena cava). This region of the heart collects the returning venous blood from the systemic capillary beds and transports it to the right ventricle for subsequent ejection into the pulmonary vessels. The tricuspid valve, in addition to permitting unimpeded flow from the right atrium to the right ventricle during diastole, prevents systolic regurgitation and helps to direct ejected blood toward the right ventricular outflow tract. The coronary sinus, which is also a tributary of the right atrium, might functionally be considered a part of the right ventricular inflow tract. Because the coronary sinus is anatomically incorporated into the posterior wall of the left atrium and is uniformly recorded with this structure, it is included in the discussion of the left, rather than the right, ventricular inflow tract.

THE TRICUSPID VALVE

Historically, the tricuspid valve was one of the most difficult structures to record using the M-mode echocardiographic technique.[1] This difficulty occurred because of its location immediately beneath the sternum and its plane of motion relative to the anterior chest wall. The improved visualization of the right side of the heart provided by the cross-sectional method, however, has facilitated tricuspid valve recording, and an evaluation of this structure along with the other areas of the right ventricular inflow tract should now be a routine part of the echocardiographic examination.[2–4] Doppler recording of tricuspid flow should also be routine and is not only of diagnostic value in assessing the integrity of the valve but also depicts the hydrodynamic changes that characterize several other disorders that effect right ventricular filling.[5–9]

Anatomy

The tricuspid valve is a complex anatomic structure composed of leaflet tissue, chordae tendineae, papillary muscles, and the supporting annular ring and right ventricular myocardium.[10,11] The tricuspid valve is larger and structurally more complicated than the mitral valve. The orifice it must occlude is likewise larger and more irregular than the mitral orifice.[11] The tricuspid leaflets are actually a continuous veil of thin fibrous tissue with a basal portion that is attached around the entire circumference of the tricuspid annulus. This fibrous tissue veil can be separated into three distinct leaflets by indentations along its free edge; however, these areas of separation are less distinct than those that characterize the mitral valve.[11] The three major tricuspid leaflets—the anterior, septal, and posterior—are of unequal size. The anterior leaflet is the largest and stretches from the infundibular region anteriorly to the inferolateral wall posteriorly. The septal leaflet stretched posteriorly along the interventricular septum from the infundibulum to the posterior ventricular border, attaching to both the membranous and muscular portions of the septum. The insertion of the septal leaflet of the tricuspid valve is characteristically inferior or apical relative to the septal insertion of the anterior mitral leaflet. The posterior leaflet attaches along the posterior margin of the annulus from the septum to the inferolateral wall. These relationships can be visualized in both the parasternal and subcostal short axis views.

Three papillary muscles or muscle groups typically support the tricuspid leaflets and lie beneath each of the three commissures.[10,11] The anterior papillary muscle is the largest and lies beneath the commissure between the anterior and posterior leaflets. It arises from both the moderator band and the free anterolateral wall of the right ventricle. The posterior papillary muscle lies inferior to the junction of the posterior and septal leaflets, whereas a small, septal papillary muscle, originating from the septal border of the infundibulum, tethers the anterior and septal leaflets high against the infundibular wall. At times, this papillary muscle may be virtually absent, and the chordae tendineae then arise from small tendinous connections to the infundibulum.[11] The chordae arising from each of these papillary muscles attach to the free edges and the proximal ventricular surfaces of both of the leaflets supported by the papillary muscle.

The tricuspid valve has several unique morphologic features that distinguish it from the mitral valve and frequently aid in identifying the anatomic right ventricle with which it is uniformly associated. These features include (1) the trileaflet configuration; (2) the presence of three separate papillary muscles; (3) the partial origin of the anterior papillary muscle from the moderator band; and (4) the inferior or apical insertion point of the septal leaflet of the tricuspid valve relative to the anterior leaflet of the mitral valve. These points of distinction are particularly valuable when ventricular situs is in question and are discussed further in Chapter 31.

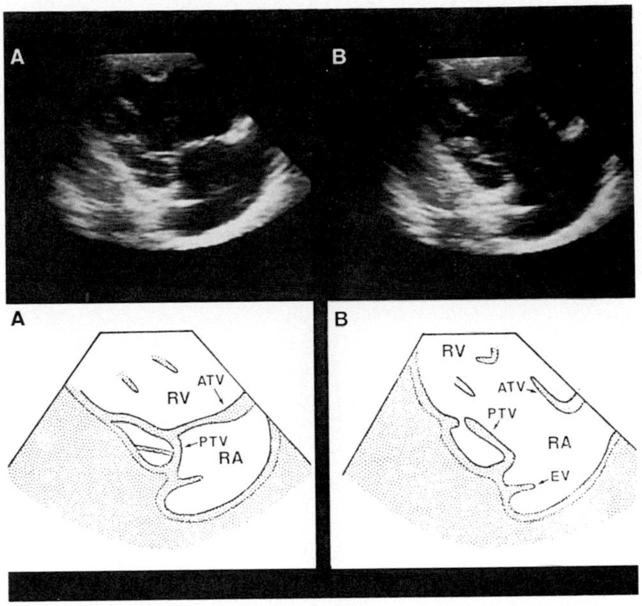

Fig. 26–1. Parasternal long axis recording of a normal tricuspid valve during systole **(A)** and diastole **(B).** The right ventricular apex is displayed anteriorly and to the left, and the right atrium appears to the right and posteriorly. The tricuspid leaflets separate these two cavities. RV = right ventricle; RA = right atrium; ATV = anterior leaflet of tricuspid valve; PTV = posterior leaflet of tricuspid valve; EV = Eustachian valve. Fragments of the anterior and posterior right ventricular papillary muscles are also evident in the apical segment of the right ventricular cavity.

Methods of Cross-Sectional Examination

The tricuspid valve is examined using three primary cross-sectional imaging planes. These include (1) the parasternal long axis of the right ventricular inflow tract,[2] (2) the parasternal short axis of the right ventricular inflow tract at the tricuspid valve level, and (3) the apical four-chamber view.[3] The tricuspid valve can also be recorded in both the subcostal long axis view of the right ventricle and the subcostal long axis of the right ventricular outflow tract.[4] In addition, multiple short axis views of the tricuspid valve can be independently obtained from the subcostal transducer location. The subcostal views, however, place the valve in the far field of the scan plane and, except in infants, do not provide the image quality available from the parasternal or apical transducer locations.

The parasternal long axis view of the right ventricular inflow tract transects the anterior and posterior tricuspid leaflets from their points of annular insertion to their free edges. It also includes the proximal chordal attachments to these leaflets and the anterior and posterior extremes of the tricuspid annulus (Fig. 26–1). Although the right ventricular papillary muscles normally are not visualized, one or more of the papillary muscles may be visible when the ventricle is hypertrophic or dilated. This imaging plane records the motion of the anterior and posterior tricuspid leaflets; their systolic and diastolic positions and spatial configurations; the anteroposterior tricuspid annular diameter; the motion pattern of the tricuspid annulus in both a superior-inferior and anteroposterior direction; and the temporal and spatial positions of the tricuspid leaflets in relation to the right ventricular cavity, annulus, and atrium. It is also one of the principle views for Doppler recording of tricuspid regurgitation. This view is difficult to standardize because there are not enough reference points to fix precisely the examining plane in space. As a rule, no left-sided structure should be recorded, and the tricuspid annulus should be visualized in a plane that passes through its maximal diameter. The maximal separation of the tricuspid leaflets at their free edges should likewise be recorded (see Chapter 5).

The parasternal short axis of the right ventricle at the tricuspid level is recorded by angling the imaging plane rightward from the parasternal short axis of the left ventricle at the mitral valve level. Because the tricuspid annulus lies at a more acute angle to the anterior chest wall than does the mitral annulus, the imaging plane must generally be tilted toward the cardiac apex, and on occasion, the transducer must be moved superiorly one interspace. Figure 26–2 illustrates the configuration of the tricuspid valve in the parasternal short axis view. In normal persons, this type of image is difficult to obtain. Fortuitously, most diseases affecting the right side of the heart cause the right ventricle to dilate and/or to change shape, thereby making short axis tricuspid recording easier. This view is particularly useful because it permits direct visualization of the tricuspid orifice. It likewise permits the extent of circumferential involvement in focal disorders to be defined.

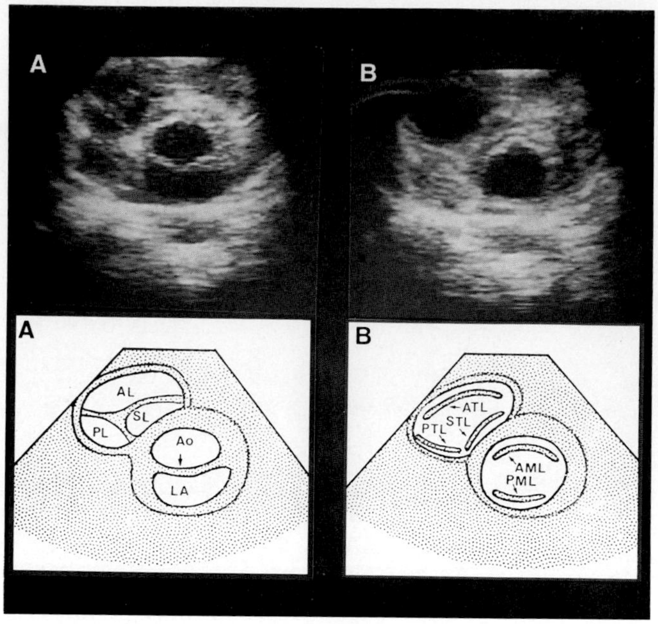

Fig. 26–2. Parasternal short axis recording of a normal tricuspid valve during systole **(A)** and diastole **(B)**. **A.** The commissures separating the three leaflets are recorded, and their relationships can be appreciated. AL = anterior tricuspid leaflet; SL = septal tricuspid leaflet; PL = posterior tricuspid leaflet; Ao = aortic inlet; LA = left atrium. The vertical arrow in the accompanying diagram indicates the echo from the anterior mitral leaflet, which is transected just below the aortic valve. **B.** The three tricuspid leaflets are recorded adjacent to the endocardial margins of the right ventricular cavity. The open mitral valve leaflets can also be visualized within the left ventricular cavity. AML = anterior mitral leaflet; PML = posterior mitral leaflet; ATL = anterior tricuspid leaflet; STL = septal tricuspid leaflet; PTL = posterior tricuspid leaflet.

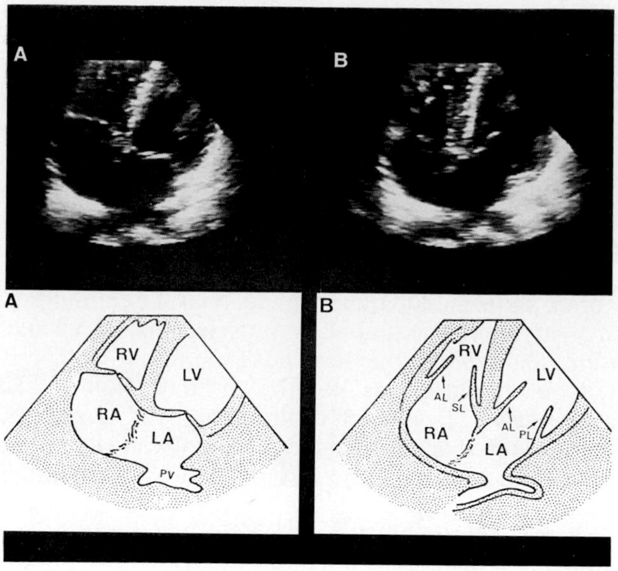

Fig. 26–3. Apical four-chamber view of a normal tricuspid valve during systole **(A)** and diastole **(B)**. **A.** The slightly apical insertion of the septal tricuspid leaflet relative to the insertion of the anterior mitral leaflet is evident. In addition, the relationship of the coapted tricuspid leaflets to the tricuspid annulus can be appreciated. **B.** The leaflets are fully open and lie in close proximity to the endocardial surface of the right ventricle. AL = anterior leaflet of both the tricuspid and mitral valves; SL = septal leaflet of the tricuspid valve; PL = posterior leaflet of the mitral valve; RV = right ventricle; LV = left ventricle; RA = right atrium; LA = left atrium; PV = pulmonary veins.

The apical four-chamber view passes through the tricuspid orifice along a line extending from roughly the 10-o'clock to the 4-o'clock positions relative to the corresponding short axis plane transecting the anterior and septal tricuspid leaflets. The anterior leaflet is displayed laterally, and the septal leaflet is displayed medially (Fig. 26–3). This plane is ideal for determining the position of the right-sided atrioventricular ring and for defining the plane of leaflet closure relative to this anatomic landmark. It is also useful for defining the level at which the septal tricuspid leaflet inserts into the interventricular septum and for comparing this insertion point to that of the corresponding anterior mitral leaflet. The apical four-chamber view is also the primary view for Doppler recording of tricuspid inflow and for assessing the size and distribution of regurgitant jets.

Normal Tricuspid Leaflet Motion

Long Axis

The normal tricuspid leaflets are thin, pliable structures that move passively in response to the forces acting on their surfaces. During diastole, overall leaflet movement represents the combination of the independent leaflet motion in response to phasic flow into the right ventricle and the motion of the tricuspid annulus to which the leaflets are attached. During systole, no independent leaflet motion occurs, and the observed movement of the leaflets represents the motion of the tricuspid annulus and papillary muscles to which these leaflets are attached. Figure 26–4 depicts the normal patterns of tricuspid leaflet motion observed in the long axis view.

Short Axis

The motion of the tricuspid leaflets in short axis is illustrated in Figure 26–5. In this example, the imaging plane passes through the right ventricle just beneath the tricuspid annulus and the left ventricle at the mitral valve level. Because the plane is optimized to record the right-sided structures, it is oblique to the left ventricle and mitral valve, and they appear distorted.

Apical Four-Chamber View

The normal motion of the tricuspid valve in the apical four-chamber view is depicted in Figure 26–6. In addition to demonstrating the pattern of tricuspid leaflet motion, this view allows comparison of the timing of tricuspid leaflet movement with mitral leaflet movement because both valves are recorded in the same imaging plane. Tricuspid closure normally lags behind mitral closure, and as illustrated in Figure 26–6F, the tricuspid leaflets may fail to close completely until the mitral valve has been closed for one or more frames.

The diastolic motion of the tricuspid leaflets is more

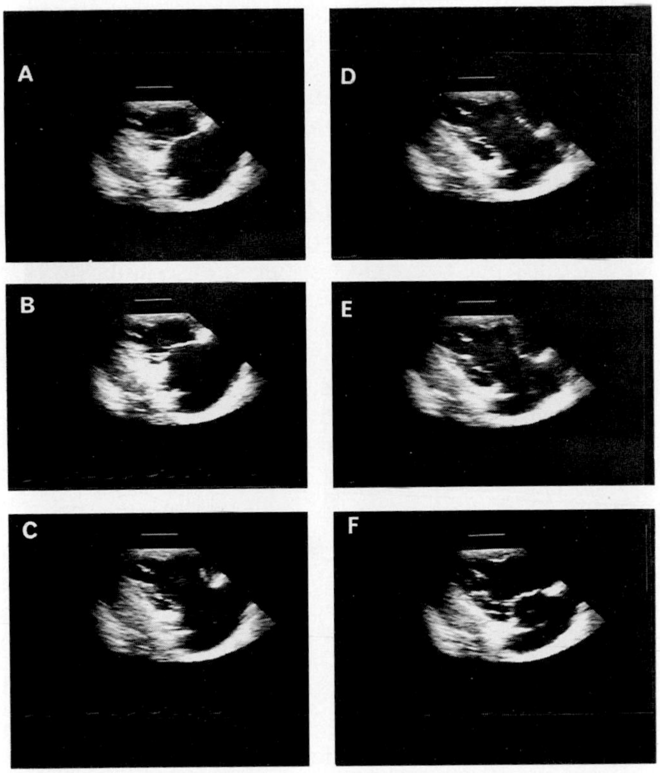

Fig. 26–4. Normal pattern of tricuspid leaflet motion in the parasternal long axis view. **A.** Recorded at end-systole just before tricuspid leaflet opening. The right ventricular cavity is small, and the right atrium is maximally dilated. **B.** The initial downward motion of the tricuspid leaflets into the right ventricular cavity during isovolumic relaxation. **C.** The leaflets fly widely apart during rapid right ventricular filling, and at their maximal point of separation, the distance between the leaflet tips exceeds the diameter of the tricuspid annulus. **D.** The position of the valve during the slow-phase right ventricular filling. The leaflets lie parallel to one another and at right angles to the margins of the tricuspid annulus. **E.** Following atrial systole, the leaflet tips further separate. **F.** Atrial relaxation initiates leaflet closure, which is then completed by ventricular contraction. In the absence of an appropriately timed ventricular systole, however, leaflet closure is normally completed by atrial relaxation. Throughout the diastolic filling period, the tricuspid annulus moves posteriorly and superiorly and, at the onset of ventricular systole, is in its most posterior and superior position.

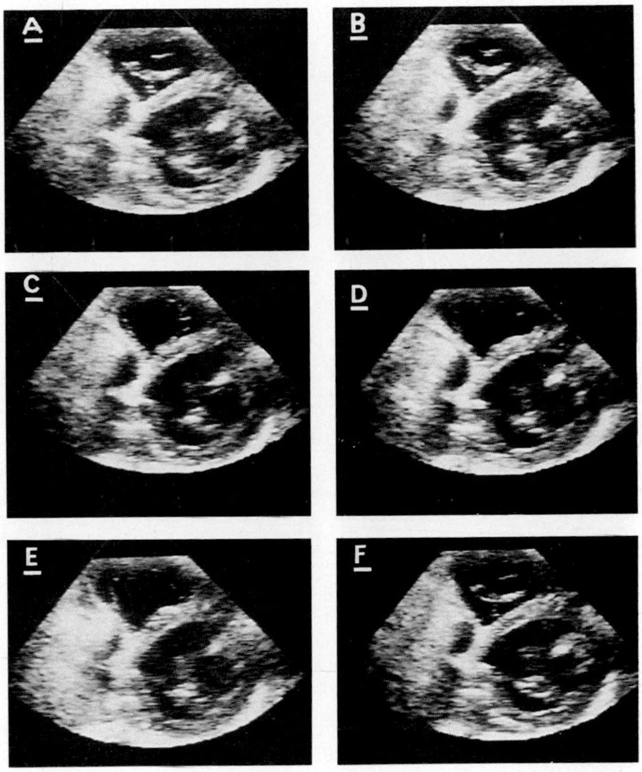

Fig. 26–5. Normal tricuspid leaflet motion in the parasternal short axis view. **A.** The three commissures of the tricuspid valve within the right ventricular cavity recorded during systole. The anterior tricuspid leaflet is positioned anteriorly, the posterior leaflet is positioned to the left and posteriorly, and the septal leaflet is positioned to the right posteriorly. **B.** Recorded at the end of the ventricular systole. Right ventricular size decreases with continued appearance of the three leaflet commissures. **C.** At the onset of diastole, the leaflets separate widely and lie against the triangular margins of the right ventricular cavity. **D.** Recorded slightly later in diastole, this figure illustrates the leaflets against the margins of the right ventricle. **E.** Recorded at end-diastole just before the tricuspid leaflet closure. The apparent decrease in right ventricular cavity size reflects the motion of the right ventricular cavity superiorly through the imaging plane and the relatively lower level of the right ventricle recorded at this point in the cardiac cycle. **F.** Recorded following initial systolic closure of the valve. This panel is similar in configuration to **A,** although recorded slightly earlier in the cardiac cycle.

difficult to analyze in the apical four-chamber view than in either the long or short axis projections. This difficulty occurs because the leaflets are oriented parallel to the path of the ultrasonic beam during diastole and, hence, are poorly visualized. During systole, however, the leaflets lie perpendicular to the path of the beam and are well recorded. In addition, the plane of the tricuspid annulus is visualized more readily in this view than in any other imaging plane, and hence, this particular projection is optimal for recording systolic leaflet position relative to the plane of the annulus.

Factors Affecting the Timing, Amplitude, and Rate of Tricuspid Leaflet Motion

The factors that govern the timing, amplitude, and rate of tricuspid leaflet motion have been less well studied than those that determine the corresponding movement of the mitral valve. Because these parameters and their effects are presumably similar, however, the discussion in Chapter 17 of the relationship of pressure and flow to mitral leaflet motion should also apply to the tricuspid valve.

Several differences in the timing of tricuspid and mitral motion, however, should be noted. First, tricuspid opening normally precedes mitral opening.[12] This earlier opening of the tricuspid valve occurs because the peak systolic pressure in the right ventricle is normally below that in the left ventricle, and the time required for right ventricular pressure to fall to the level of right atrial pressure, therefore, is much less than the corresponding time period on the left side of the heart. This leads to a shorter right ventricular isovolumic relaxation and an earlier tricuspid opening. Second, tricuspid closure oc-

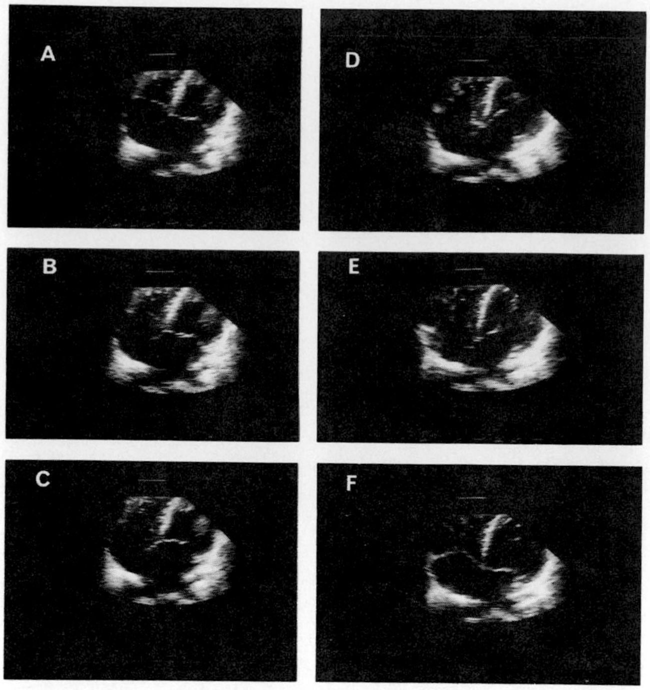

Fig. 26–6. Normal pattern of tricuspid leaflet motion in the apical four-chamber view. **A.** The position of the closed tricuspid leaflets at end of ventricular systole. **B.** Recorded during isovolumic relaxation, this panel demonstrates the initial downward displacement of the tricuspid valve leaflets into the right ventricle just before rapid leaflet opening. **C.** Recorded at the point of peak leaflet excursion. As demonstrated here, tricuspid leaflet opening precedes mitral leaflet opening, and the tricuspid leaflets are in a fully opened position before the onset of mitral leaflet motion. **D.** Recorded during the diastasis phase. Both the mitral and tricuspid leaflets can be visualized in a neutral or resting position within the respective ventricular cavities. **E.** Recorded following atrial systole; the reopening of the tricuspid leaflets in response to atrial contraction. **F.** The position of the tricuspid leaflets following atrial relaxation just before ventricular systole. At this point, the tricuspid leaflets have not reached their fully closed position, whereas the mitral valve is already closed. This view is particularly well suited for making comparisons between events on the right and left sides of the heart.

curs after mitral closure because electrical activation of the left ventricle precedes that of the right ventricle. This earlier contraction of the left ventricle results in earlier initial systolic pressure generation on the left side and, thus, earlier mitral valve closure. Finally, right atrial contraction and relaxation precede corresponding left atrial contraction and relaxation. The tricuspid valve A wave, therefore, should precede the mitral valve A wave, and because the tricuspid valve closes after the mitral valve, the AC interval (duration from peak of the A wave (A) to the point of leaflet closure (C) on the right side should normally be longer than the corresponding interval on the left side.

Tricuspid Valve flow

The flow field leading to and exiting from the tricuspid valve is highly complex, with the instantaneous velocities in the right atrium and ventricle varying both spatially and temporally in response to locally changing pressure gradients. To simplify analysis, flow through the tricuspid valve is generally represented by the mean spatial velocity at the vena contracta recorded at sequential time points during diastolic filling. These mean velocities are usually recorded by pulsed Doppler with the transducer located at the cardiac apex and the sample volume positioned to record the peak inflow velocities, which generally occur near the tips of the tricuspid leaflets.[13] Tricuspid inflow occurs during right ventricular diastole. The tricuspid flow profile is similar to that of the mitral valve (Fig. 26–7); however, tricuspid flow, like leaflet movement, begins slightly before and ends slightly after mitral inflow. Tricuspid flow can also be recorded from the parasternal and subcostal windows, but the angle between the flow vector and the ultrasonic beam is usually greater than that from the apex.

Normal Flow

The impetus for blood to move from the right atrium to the right ventricle through the tricuspid valve is the development of the diastolic atrioventricular pressure gradient, and the velocity of flow generally follows this gradient. Immediately after tricuspid valve opening, blood accelerates in response to the rapidly increasing gradient (RA > RV); reaches a peak (E point) following the peak gradient and then decelerates toward the baseline. Following atrial contraction, a positive gradient RA > RV is reestablished, and the forward flow velocity again accelerates (A wave) to a peak and then deceler-

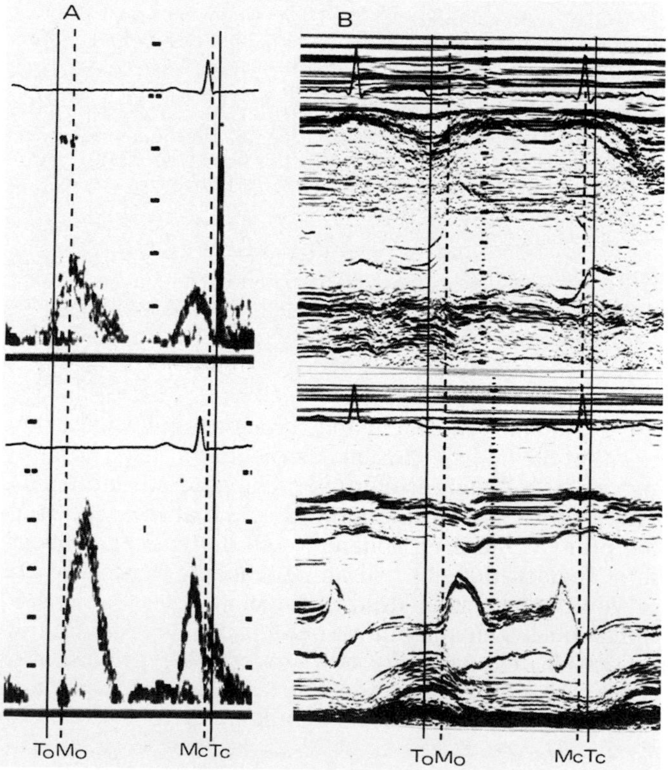

Fig. 26–7. Comparison of normal mitral and tricuspid Doppler transvalvular flow and M-mode leaflet motion. T_o = tricuspid opening; M_o = mitral opening; M_c = mitral closure; T_c = tricuspid closure.

ates as the atrium relaxes. At normal PR intervals, flow terminates with ventricular contraction; however, in patients with varying degrees of heart block, a reversal of the gradient (RV > RA) can occur at end-diastole in association with diastolic tricuspid regurgitation (see following discussion). Some forward motion can occasionally be recorded by continuous wave Doppler during systole, but this represents apical displacement of the valve and surrounding blood pool as the ventricle contracts and not actual flow through the valve.

Factors Affecting the Development of the Transvalvular Gradient and Tricuspid Valve Flow Profile

The determinants of the various components of the early diastolic tricuspid velocity profile have not been studied as extensively as those that determine mitral valve flow, but the same physical principles should apply.[14,15] Thus, flow acceleration during initial diastole should be determined primarily by the rate at which the atrioventricular pressure gradient increases following tricuspid valve opening. This in turn should be governed by the initial right atrial pressure, the rate of right ventricular relaxation, and the resistance to flow offered by the tricuspid valve apparatus. Increasing right atrial pressure augments the atrioventricular pressure gradient for any ventricular relaxation rate and increases both flow acceleration and peak velocity. An increase in ventricular relaxation rate shortens the time to peak gradient and likewise increases flow acceleration, while decreasing ventricular relaxation rate has the opposite effect. Opposing acceleration is the mass of blood that must be set in motion. This has been shown experimentally to be the equivalent of a column whose length is equal to roughly twice the orifice diameter.[16] Thus, as the orifice area decreases (i.e., in tricuspid stenosis), acceleration increases. The rate of deceleration of tricuspid valve flow should be determined by the rate at which the atrial and ventricular pressures approach each other following the peak atrioventricular pressure gradient. This in turn is governed by the net stiffnesses or compliances of the two chambers and the resistance of the tricuspid valve (see Chapters 17 and 24). Stiffness and compliance are altered by factors that either change the basic pressure-volume relationship of the chamber or alter the location of the pressure-volume curve at which the chamber is operating. Changes in the intrinsic properties of the atrium or ventricle that increase stiffness (or decrease compliance) will increase the rate of flow deceleration, as will an increase in atrial pressure or ventricular end-systolic volume.

The peak tricuspid inflow velocity likewise should be increase by factors that increase acceleration and should be decreased by factors that increase deceleration. Peak velocity should be most directly affected by initial right atrial pressure. It should be lowered somewhat by prolonged relaxation, low atrial pressure, and systolic dysfunction.

The atrial filling wave should be determined by (1) the right atrial volume at the time of contraction (Starling's law of the atrium); (2) the contractility of the atrium; (3) the compliance of the ventricle (the less compliant the ventricle, the more blood will be ejected retrograde into the systemic veins; and (4) the systolic function of the ventricle, which determines the point on the pressure volume curve at which the ventricle is operating when it begins to fill.

Differences Between the Tricuspid and Mitral Flow Profiles

Normally, tricuspid flow acceleration during early-diastole, the peak E-wave velocity, and E-wave deceleration are all lower than comparable mitral valve measurements. Acceleration is slower because right atrial pressure is normally lower than left atrial pressure, and the inertia offered by the column of blood that must be accelerated is greater because the tricuspid orifice is larger than the mitral. Tricuspid E-wave deceleration is likewise prolonged because of the greater compliance of the right ventricle vs. the left. The peak tricuspid E-wave velocity is decreased primarily because of the relatively lower right atrial pressure. Despite the general reduction in tricuspid velocities, constant tricuspid and mitral flow is maintained because of the larger tricuspid valve orifice.

Effects of Respiration on Normal Tricuspid Valve Flow

Respiration also has a greater effect on normal tricuspid flow than on mitral flow. During inspiration, all components of the tricuspid inflow profile increase proportionally, and flow is often evident throughout diastole. In normal children, the tricuspid E-wave velocity increases by a mean of 26% from expiration to inspiration, and the mean A-wave velocity increases by 18%. The E/A-wave ratio, however, remains the same.[17] In adults, the peak E-wave velocity increases by a mean of 14%, and the peak A-wave velocity increases by a mean of 13% from expiration to inspiration. The E/A-wave ratio is again unchanged.[18]

Changes in Tricuspid Flow Patterns as the Heart Develops

Although the tricuspid E-wave velocity is greater than the A-wave velocity in normal children and adults, this relationship is reversed in the normal fetus and during the early postnatal period.[19] The diminished peak E-wave velocity and reversed E/A ratio in the fetus and newborn presumably relate to delayed right ventricular relaxation that is due to right ventricular hypertrophy, because atrial pressure must be slightly higher on the right side than the left. The ratio of peak E/A wave velocity increases with gestational age, with mean values of 0.52 and 0.84 being reported in one study at 20 weeks and 40 weeks, respectively (see also Chapter 33).[19]

THE ABNORMAL TRICUSPID VALVE ECHOGRAM

Normal function of the tricuspid valve permits unimpeded flow of blood from the right atrium into the right ventricle during diastole and prevents regurgitation into the right atrium during systole. On the basis of these functional requirements, tricuspid valve lesions can be divided into (1) those that restrict diastolic inflow into the right ventricle and are characterized echocardiographically by decreased diastolic leaflet excursion, (2) those that primarily affect the systolic competence of the valve and are associated with abnormalities of leaflet closure on either a functional or a structural basis, and (3) miscellaneous disorders of the tricuspid valve not primarily associated with either stenosis or regurgitation.

Right Ventricular Inflow Obstruction

Obstruction to right ventricular inflow may result from an acquired or congenital deformity of the tricuspid valve or may develop as a functional disorder associated with tumors, vegetations, or thrombi that partially occlude the tricuspid orifice.[20] Acquired tricuspid stenosis is seen most commonly in patients with rheumatic heart disease but may also develop in association with a malignant carcinoid, endocardial fibroelastosis,[21] and endomyocardial fibrosis. Stenosis can also be caused by loculated pericardial effusion and focal constriction.[22] Congenital tricuspid stenosis associated with a normal right ventricle is rare and is characterized by leaflets that are fused at their commissures but are otherwise relatively normal.[23,24] A profound reduction in tricuspid valve size—tricuspid atresia—is commonly associated with hypoplasia of the right ventricle and pulmonary atresia.[12] This combination of disorders is discussed in Chapter 32. Tumors and thrombi that produce functional right ventricular inflow obstruction usually arise within the right atrium; however, metastatic tumors from the great veins[25] and tumors of leaflet origin may on occasion be obstructive.

Rheumatic Tricuspid Stenosis

Rheumatic fever is, by far, the most common cause of acquired valvular tricuspid stenosis. Rheumatic inflammation of the tricuspid valve produces scarring and fibrosis of the valve leaflets, fusion of the commissures, and associated fibrosis and thickening of the chordae tendineae.[26,27] These abnormalities combine to limit tricuspid leaflet mobility and to reduce the size of the tricuspid orifice, thereby obstructing right ventricular filling. Rheumatic tricuspid stenosis occurs less frequently than, but is almost invariably associated with, mitral stenosis and is reported in 2 to 22% of patients with rheumatic mitral involvement.[28–34] In a study of 147 patients with rheumatic heart disease examined in our laboratory, tricuspid stenosis was present in 9.5%.[35] When mitral stenosis is accompanied by tricuspid stenosis, the mitral lesion is typically more severe and predominates clinically.[32,33,36] Detection of concomitant tricuspid stenosis is important, however, because the tricuspid lesion may lead to chronic elevation of right atrial pressure and low cardiac output despite successful surgical relief of the left-sided valvular disease.[32,37]

Imaging. Tricuspid stenosis is characterized echocardiographically by (1) an increase in echo production from the thickened deformed tricuspid leaflets, (2) abnormal diastolic leaflet motion, and (3) a reduction in the tricuspid valve orifice size.[35,38]

The increase in echo production from the deformed tricuspid leaflets is due to leaflet thickening and fibrosis and occurs most commonly along their free edges. It is typically less pronounced than that seen with mitral stenosis, and the chordae, likewise, are less severely involved. Calcification is rarely noted.

The abnormal diastolic leaflet motion and reduced opening excursion result both from fibrosis and commissural fusion, which prevent normal leaflet tip separation in a manner similar to that observed with mitral stenosis. The bodies of the leaflets, in contrast, are more freely mobile and separate widely. This dissociation of movement between the leaflet tips and bodies results in a prominent doming of the valve toward the right ventricle. Doming of the anterior leaflets is most prominent, while the septal and posterior leaflets generally show restricted motion with or without doming.

In normal persons, reclosure of the leaflets begins immediately on reaching their point of maximal excursion. When tricuspid stenosis is present, the gradient across the valve holds the leaflets in a fully open or domed position, and the normal initial diastolic closing movement (E-F slope) is either diminished or absent. As diastole progresses and the right ventricle fills, the tricuspid annulus moves superiorly and posteriorly. This annular movement draws the leaflets in a similar direction, thereby producing movement relative to the anterior chest wall. Independent leaflet motion, however, does not occur until the distending pressure dissipates and the leaflets are allowed to fall backward toward a closed position.

Figure 26–8 is a parasternal long axis recording illustrating the systolic and diastolic appearance of rheumatic tricuspid stenosis. During systole, the coapted leaflets are normally positioned and show only a slight increase in reflectivity, suggesting leaflet thickening. In diastole, there is no movement of the posterior tricuspid leaflet, which is thickened and deformed, as are its chordal attachment. The body of the anterior leaflet moves more freely. Motion of both leaflet tips, however, is obviously reduced, producing prominent diastolic doming of the anterior leaflet. Figure 26–9 is an example of a patient with both tricuspid stenosis and insufficiency. In diastole, there is valve doming and restriction of leaflet motion. In systole, the leaflets appear contracted and fail to coapt. The massive right atrial dilation is consistent with a mixed valvular lesion. The characteristic tricuspid leaflet diastolic doming and inflow obstruction can also be seen in both the apical four-chamber (Fig. 26–10) and subcostal four-chamber views (Fig. 26–11). In each of these examples, the leaflets appear slightly thickened. The most prominent and consistent features, however, are the lack of complete leaflet opening and the diastolic leaflet doming that results in narrowing of the tricuspid orifice.[35]

Tricuspid valve recording is usually easier in patients with rheumatic heart disease than in normal persons, because the right heart tends to dilate as a result of associated tricuspid regurgitation, pulmonary hypertension, and/or pulmonary regurgitation. Successful leaflet visu-

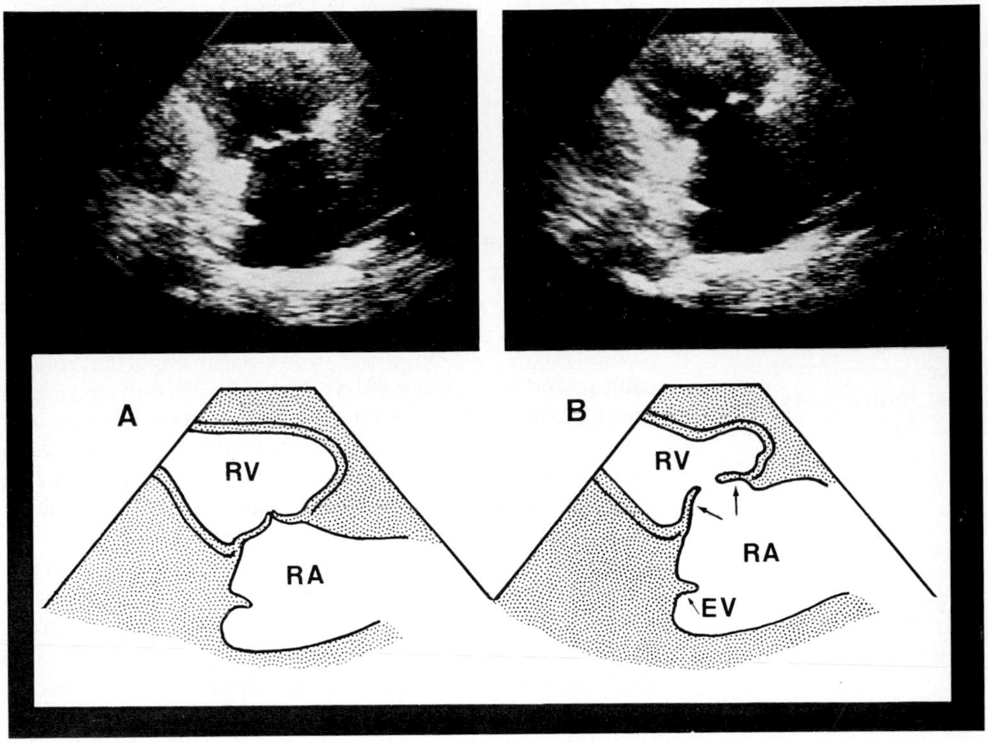

Fig. 26–8. Parasternal long axis recording of a stenotic tricuspid valve. **A.** During ventricular systole, leaflet reflectivity is slightly increased; however, the leaflets otherwise appear normal. Right atrial dilation is obvious. **B.** During diastole, both the anterior and posterior tricuspid leaflets arc or dome downward into the right ventricular cavity. The tricuspid orifice diameter is reduced, and reflectivity from the free edges of the stenotic leaflets is increased. The chordae extending from the ventricular surface of the posterior leaflet to the posterior papillary muscle are prominent. RV = right ventricle; RA = right atrium; EV = Eustachian valve.

alization is most common in the apical four-chamber view (95%), followed by the parasternal long axis (68%) and the subcostal long axis views (39%). Successful leaflet visualization can almost always be obtained in at least one view and in two orthogonal views in 78% of patients.[35] The combination of imaging planes permits each of the three tricuspid leaflets to be independently recorded in at least two projections and thus allows their configuration and motion pattern to be studied in detail.[35]

Several studies have reported virtually uniform agreement between the echocardiographic and hemodynamic

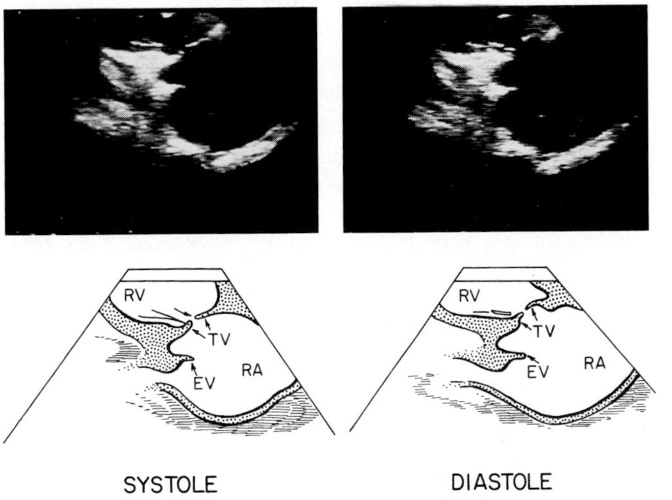

Fig. 26–9. Parasternal right ventricular inflow view from a patient with severe, mixed tricuspid valve disease. The right atrium (RA) is markedly enlarged. In systole, the tricuspid valve (TV) leaflet tips do not meet, and severe tricuspid regurgitation was present. In diastole, the posterior leaflet is immobile and the anterior cusp moves only slightly, while the body of the leaflet domes. EV = Eustachian valve; RV = right ventricle. (From Guyer DE, et al.: Comparison of the echocardiographic and hemodynamic diagnosis of rheumatic tricuspid stenosis. J Am Coll Cardiol 3:1135, 1984. Reprinted with permission from the American College of Cardiology.)

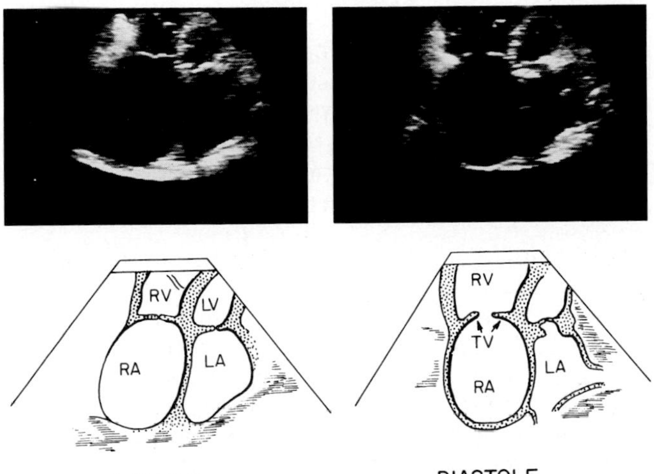

Fig. 26–10. Apical four-chamber recording of tricuspid stenosis. The tricuspid valve (TV) leaflets are brightly echo-reflecting. They separate only slightly in diastole, and the bodies of the leaflets dome. There is marked right atrial (RA) enlargement. LA = left atrium; LV = left ventricle; RV = right ventricle. (From Guyer DE, et al.: Comparison of the echocardiographic and hemodynamic diagnosis of rheumatic tricuspid stenosis. J Am Coll Cardiol 3: 1135, 1984. Reprinted with permission from the American College of Cardiology.)

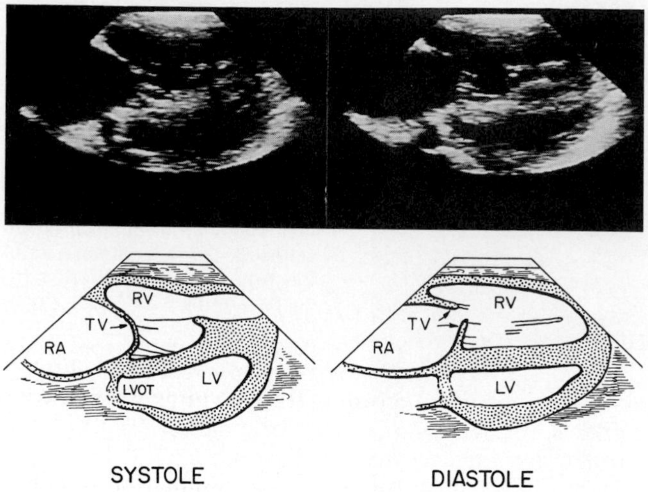

Fig. 26–11. Subcostal four-chamber view of tricuspid stenosis. The tricuspid valve (TV) leaflets are thickened. These leaflets do not open fully in diastole, and they obstruct the right ventricular inflow tract. The right atrium (RA) is enlarged. LVOT = left ventricular outflow tract; RV = right ventricle; LV = left ventricle. (From Guyer DE, et al.: Comparison of the echocardiographic and hemodynamic diagnosis of rheumatic tricuspid stenosis. J Am Coll Cardiol 3:1135, 1984. Reprinted with permission from the American College of Cardiology.)

diagnosis of tricuspid stenosis when right atrial and ventricular pressure are measured simultaneously.[35,38] In another report, however, the two-dimensional criteria for stenosis were found to have a low predictive value.[39] These differences probably reflect minor differences in both the echocardiographic and hemodynamic criteria for diagnosis. As a rule, doming of the anterior leaflet must be present for hemodynamic evidence of tricuspid stenosis to be evident. Thickening and restricted motion of the posterior leaflet alone can occur in the absence of hemodynamic evidence of stenosis. This pattern is generally seen with rheumatic tricuspid regurgitation and appears analogous to that seen in patients with isolated mitral regurgitation. Patients can also be seen with isolated doming of the septal leaflet or both the septal and posterior leaflet with normal motion of the anterior leaflet and no evidence of a gradient. Thus, only patients with doming of the anterior leaflet, which invariably occurs in association with doming of the other two leaflets, and a reduction in tricuspid orifice diameter can be expected to have a hemodynamically detectable gradient.[35]

Doppler. Although the diagnosis of tricuspid stenosis generally can be made by imaging alone, Doppler studies are occasionally necessary for confirmation and are always required to determine the transvalvular gradient and the valve area. The Doppler diagnosis of tricuspid stenosis rests on the characteristic changes the stenosis produces on the magnitude and pattern of the inflow velocities.[13] Because velocity must increase to maintain flow constant across the stenosis, the peak velocity will generally be greater than normal and will increase in proportion to the degree of stenosis. The decrease in valve area will likewise increase the acceleration rate of tricuspid inflow and will decrease flow deceleration by prolonging the duration of the positive RA > RV pressure gradient. Figure 26–12 is a continuous wave Doppler recording from a patient with tricuspid stenosis illustrating the characteristic increase in peak velocity, prolongation of the deceleration slope, and increase in acceleration. Color flow mapping can also aid in diagnosis by demonstrating the narrowing of the flow stream as it passes through the restrictive orifice and the turbulent free jet distal to the stenotic orifice (Fig. 26–13).

Assessment of Severity

Transvalvular Gradient. The transvalvular gradient can be calculated from the instantaneous velocity of flow through the valve at any point in diastole using the simplified Bernoulli equation ($\Delta P = 4V^2$). Commonly reported gradients are the peak, mean, and end-diastolic gradient. Mean gradients have been shown to correlate closely with those reported at catheterization in both native and stenotic prosthetic tricuspid valves when both data sets are recorded simultaneously.[40,41] Doppler recording during exercise can also be useful to assess the lability of the gradient and to relate these changes to symptoms.

Valve Area. Direct short axis recording of the stenotic tricuspid valve orifice has proven more difficult than short axis recording of the mitral valve orifice. This diffi-

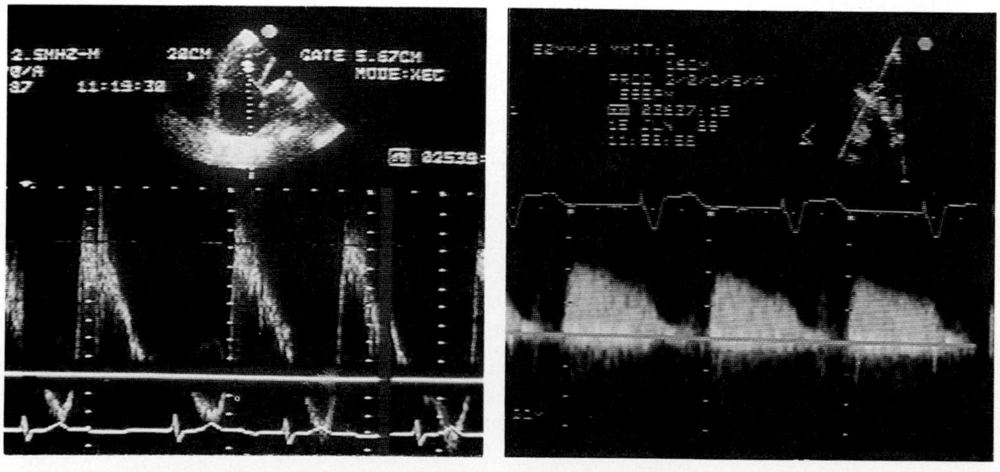

Fig. 26–12. Left. Pulsed Doppler recording of tricuspid valve inflow from a patient with mild tricuspid stenosis. The peak velocity is roughly 1.7 m/sec and rapidly falls to 0 m/sec by end-diastole. Right. Continuous wave Doppler recording from a second patient with more severe tricuspid stenosis. Note the increase in the rate of flow acceleration, increased peak velocity (2 m/sec) and slow rate of flow deceleration.

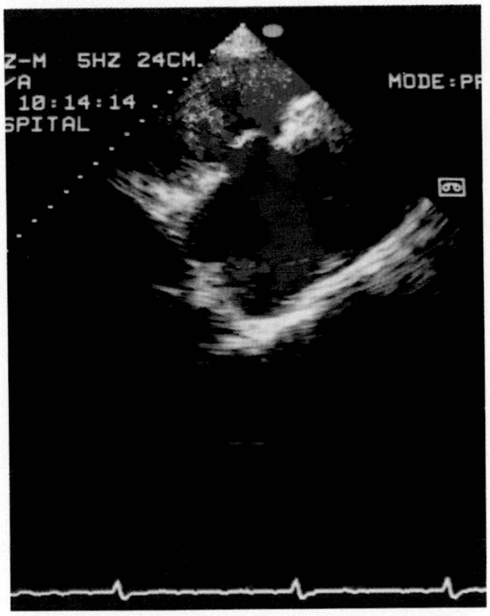

Fig. 26–13. Parasternal long axis, color Doppler recording of the turbulent flow stream (red-blue mosaic) in the right ventricle distal to a stenotic tricuspid valve. The solid red flow in the right atrium represents inflow from the inferior vena cava. (Courtesy of Dr. Leng Jiang.)

culty occurs because of the position of the tricuspid valve orifice beneath the sternum and its orientation relative to the anterior chest wall. These factors combine to prevent positioning of the imaging plane across the valve orifice in most cases. To date, although the tricuspid valve orifice has been recorded in individual patients with tricuspid stenosis, there are insufficient data to correlate the echocardiographic orifice areas with either hemodynamic, surgical, or pathologic measurements of tricuspid valve area. Thus, although the accuracy of this approach can be inferred from the experience gained with mitral valve orifice measurements in mitral stenosis, it has not been confirmed.

Tricuspid valve area is also difficult to calculate by Doppler, although several approaches are possible. In the rare patient without tricuspid regurgitation, the continuity equation should be valid, with reference flow taken as flow across any other competent valve; valve area may be calculated as

$$A_E = \text{Stroke volume } (A_1 \times V_1)/\text{TVI}$$

Where A_E is the effective valve area in square centimeters, stroke volume is in milliliters, and the tricuspid velocity integral is in centimeters.[42] Another approach might be to determine the dimensions of flow stream passing through the orifice (Fig. 26–13) from color flow recordings in two orthogonal planes and to calculate the orifice area using the formula for the area of an ellipse, as has been described for the mitral valve.[43,44] Use of the half-time method is problematic, because the appropriate constant for the tricuspid valve has not been determined, and simple extrapolation of the constant used for the mitral valve is not theoretically sound. In one study, the constant 190 was used, and a good correlation (r = .81) was reported with catheterization data;[45] however, results have varied.[42]

Tricuspid Stenosis in Endomyocardial Fibrosis (Löffler's Endocarditis)

A group of acquired disorders—endomyocardial fibrosis, endocardial fibroelastosis, and malignant carcinoid—is characterized by deposition of fibrinous or fibroelastic material on the endocardial and valvular surfaces of the right ventricular inflow tract. This deposition of fibrinous material may lead to restriction of tricuspid leaflet motion and tricuspid stenosis. Figure 26–14 is a long axis recording from a young woman with Löffler's endocarditis. The tricuspid leaflets and chordae are thickened, and diastolic leaflet doming is obvious. In addition, there is an accumulation of echogenic material along the anterior endocardial surface of the right ventricle beneath the anterior tricuspid leaflet. Although differences in the appearance of the stenotic valve in this example and of the rheumatic valve in Figure 26–8 are obvious, these lesions are uncommon, and hence, sufficient experience is not available to permit differentiation on an echocardiographic basis alone. The clinical setting in which these lesions arise, however, should suggest their cause.

Tricuspid Regurgitation

Normal closure of the tricuspid valve depends on the integrated function of the tricuspid leaflets, chordae tendineae, papillary muscles, and subjacent area of right ventricular myocardium. Improper function of any of these components can cause the tricuspid leaflets to close improperly and can lead to valvular insufficiency. Tricuspid insufficiency is most commonly functional and occurs in the setting of right ventricular dilation with an associated increase in tricuspid annular size, decrease in the normal systolic diminution in annular area, and inappropriate contraction of the papillary muscles.[20] Organic causes of tricuspid regurgitation include rheumatic heart disease,[26] tricuspid prolapse,[46] bacterial endocarditis,[47–49] carcinoid syndrome,[50] trauma,[20] and more rarely, congenital disorders.[51] The congenital disorders include incomplete cusp differentiation and chordal development, which prevent normal closure,[51] and Ebstein's anomaly.[52–54]

Diagnosis

Tricuspid regurgitation is characterized by the presence of retrograde flow from the right atrium to the right ventricle. The retrograde flow generally originates from a small defect at the junction of the three leaflets or along one of the tricuspid commissures and takes the form of a free turbulent jet in the right atrium. Tricuspid regurgitation is most commonly systolic, although diastolic regurgitation can occur in patients with arrhythmias. Tricuspid regurgitation can be readily detected by any of the Doppler techniques, and these form the primary method for both diagnosis and assessment of severity.

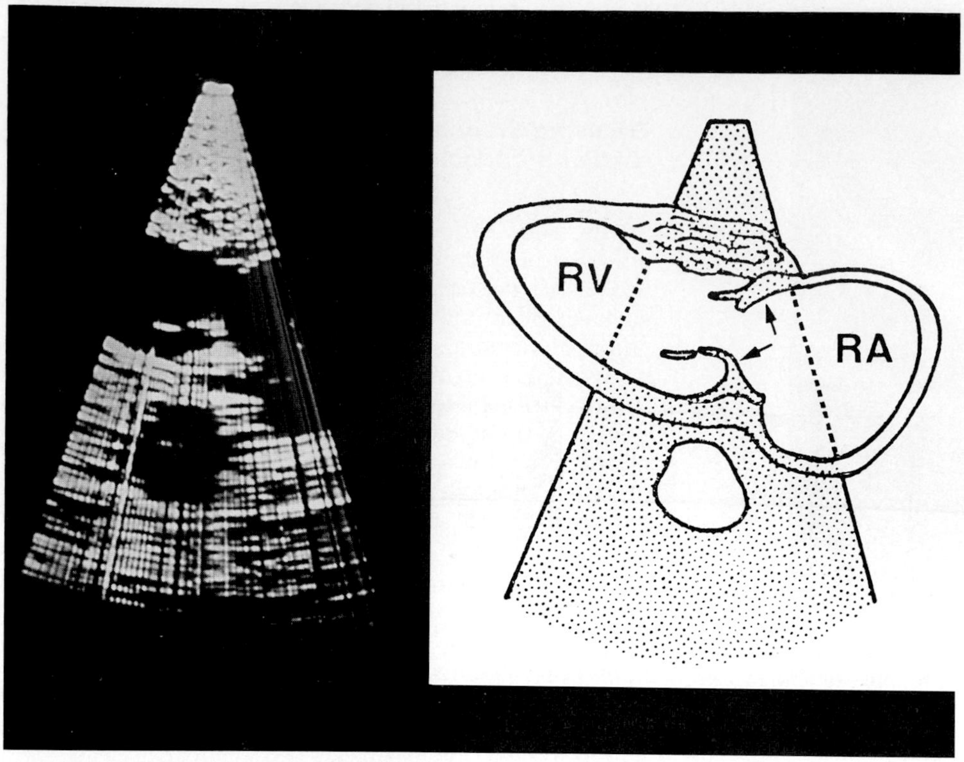

Fig. 26–14. Parasternal long axis recording of the tricuspid valve from a patient with Löffler's endocarditis (eosinophilic endomyocardial disease) and valvular tricuspid stenosis. This frame, recorded during diastole, illustrates prominent doming of both the anterior and posterior tricuspid leaflets into the right ventricular cavity. This configuration is associated with a decrease in tricuspid orifice diameter and restriction to right ventricular inflow. A prominent accumulation of echogenic material appears along the anterior right ventricular wall just above the anterior tricuspid leaflet. The chordae tendineae from both the anterior and posterior leaflets extend toward the respective papillary muscles. The arrowheads in the accompanying diagram point to the stenotic tricuspid leaflets. The echo-free space beneath the right ventricle (RV) probably represents the descending aorta coursing behind the right heart. RA = right atrium.

Doppler. The Doppler diagnosis of tricuspid regurgitation is based on the presence of an abnormal, wide-bandwidth, systolic flow disturbance in the right atrium behind the tricuspid valve. Tricuspid regurgitant flow is best recorded from the apex or a low parasternal window. The velocity of the regurgitant jet reflects the pressure difference between the right ventricle and atrium and hence may vary from 2 to 2.6 m/sec in normal persons (corresponding to pressure differences of 16 to 27 mm Hg) to >5 m/sec in patients with right ventricular pressures at systemic levels.[55] Figure 26–15A is a color Doppler recording from a patient with tricuspid regurgitation and elevated right ventricular systolic pressures. The regurgitant jet is relatively narrow but extends from the valve to the superior wall of the atrium. Figure 26–15B is a continuous wave Doppler recording from the same patient illustrating high velocity, holosystolic flow with a peak right ventricle-right atrium gradient of 117 mm Hg and a mean gradient of 68.4 mm Hg (see following discussion). The rate of rise of the regurgitant jet velocity reflects the rate of increase in right ventricular systolic pressure. Thus, in patients with right ventricular failure, the regurgitant velocities rise more slowly than in those with normal systolic function.[55]

Although tricuspid regurgitant jets usually have a symmetric teardrop shape on color flow images, the complex flow patterns in the right atrium can often distort their appearance. Figure 26–16A, for example, illustrates a jet that remains narrowly collimated as it courses through the atrium and then splays out against the superior atrial wall. Figure 26–16B illustrates another jet, which divides shortly after exiting from the regurgitant orifice and spreads out in two different directions in the atrium.

Contrast. Tricuspid regurgitation can also be diagnosed from M-mode recordings of the direction and timing of contrast movement in the right atrium and inferior vena cava following peripheral injection in the supine, quietly breathing patient. Regurgitation is considered to be present if contrast is observed to stream posteriorly in the right atrium or to reflux into the inferior vena cava during systole[56–60] (Chapter 15). However, because of the greater sensitivity and ease of grading provided by the Doppler method,[61] use of peripheral contrast has largely been abandoned for this purpose. In patients with indwelling right ventricular catheters, however, detection of contrast in the right atrium following right ventricular injection is a sensitive sign of tricuspid regurgitation.

Sensitivity and Specificity. Doppler techniques have been reported to have a sensitivity of between 74 and 100% and a specificity of between 85 and 100% for the diagnosis of tricuspid regurgitation. True sensitivity and specificity are difficult to assess because the gold standards used in these studies all have major limitations. General experience, however, suggests that the Doppler method is exquisitely sensitive for detecting tricuspid regurgitation and is likewise highly specific. Greater difficulty occurs in determining when regurgitation is clinically important than in determining its presence.

Assessment of Severity

Qualitative Methods

Jet Size. The general approaches to the assessment of the severity of tricuspid and mitral regurgitation are similar. However, much less information is available concerning their accuracy when applied to the right-

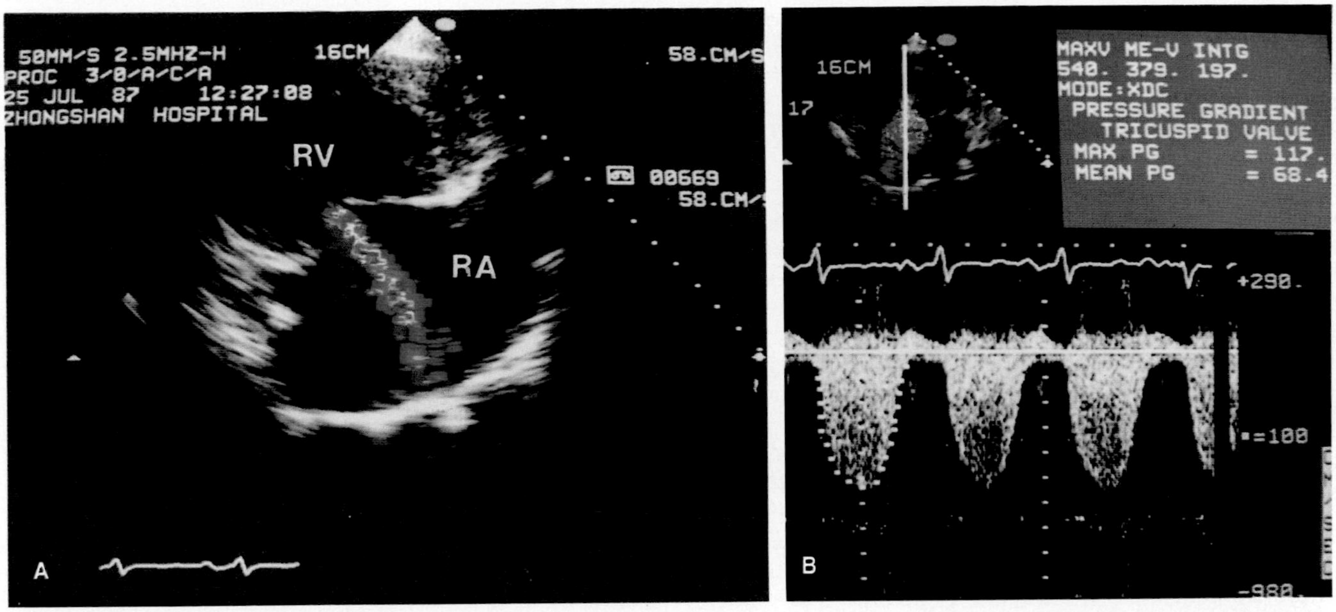

Fig. 26–15. **A.** Parasternal long axis color Doppler recording illustrating a free turbulent tricuspid regurgitant jet (blue-red mosaic) extending from the center of the coaptation line to the superior wall of the right atrium. **B.** Continuous wave Doppler recording of the peak flow velocities contained in this jet. In this example the velocities exceed 5 m/sec, and the calculated peak gradient is 117 mm Hg. RV = right ventricle; RA = right atrium. (Courtesy of Dr. Leng Jiang.)

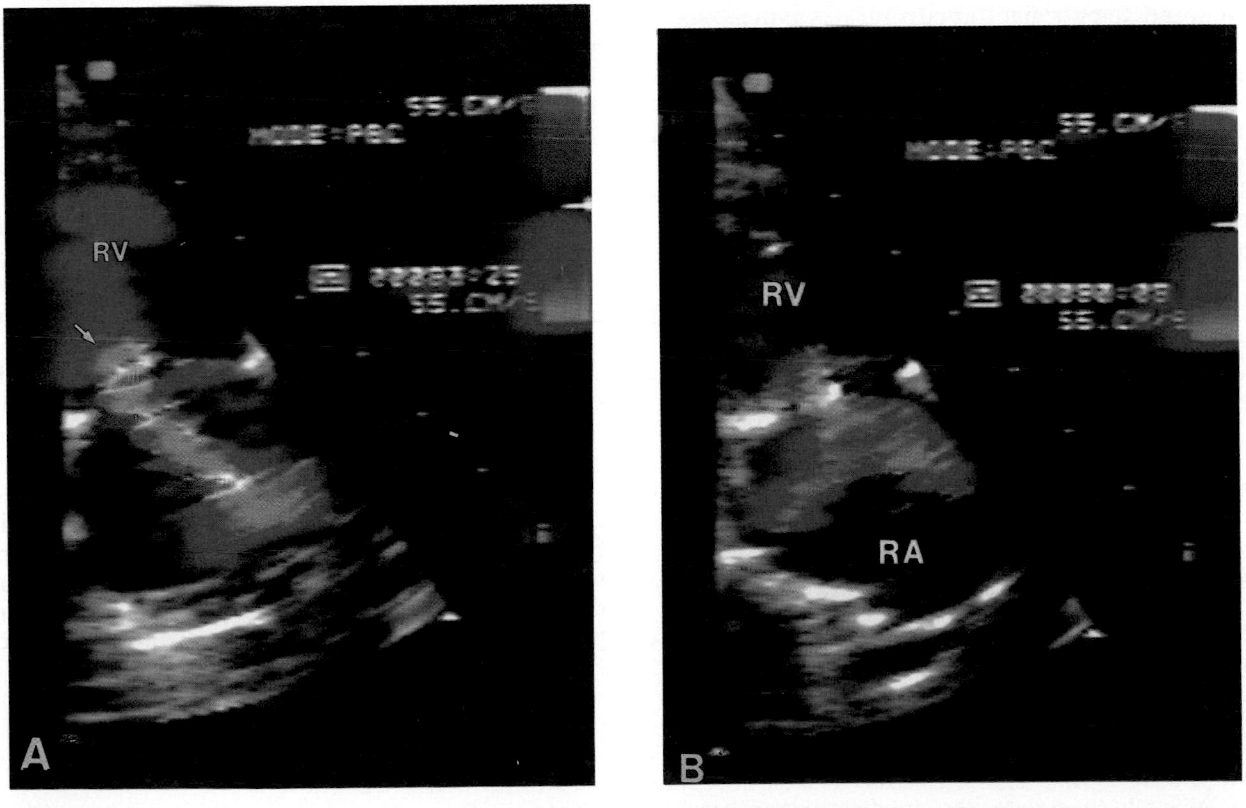

Fig. 26–16. Parasternal long axis right ventricular inflow recordings illustrating different tricuspid regurgitant jet configurations. **A.** A long narrow jet, which strikes and splays out along the superior wall of the right atrium. A proximal acceleration zone is also evident in the right ventricle (RV) leading into the regurgitant valve orifice. **B.** A jet that expands almost immediately after leaving the regurgitant orifice and then splits into two branches, which course independently within the right atrium (RA).

sided lesion because of the lack of an accurate, readily available gold standard. Absolute jet length and area have been shown to correlate reasonably well with angiographic grade, r = .75 and r = .74, respectively[62] (Fig. 26–17). As discussed in detail in Chapter 13, however, jet area and length are not simply related to regurgitant volume but rather to momentum, which is the product of flow and velocity. This is important because right ventricular pressure is typically less than left ventricular pressure with the result that a tricuspid regurgitant jet generally will represent a greater regurgitant volume than will a mitral regurgitant jet of the same absolute area. As a result, one cannot simply extrapolate criteria used to quantitate mitral jets size to the tricuspid valve.

Hepatic Vein and Caval Flow Profiles. Another qualitative approach for assessing severity is based on the pattern of flow in the vena cavae and hepatic veins. This can be most easily assessed by recording proximal hepatic vein flow (which is similar to inferior vena caval flow) from the subcostal transducer position. Normally, the hepatic vein drains into the inferior vena cava and right atrium during systole in response to the fall in right atrial pressure that is due to atrial relaxation and inferior motion of the tricuspid annulus. In patients with severe tricuspid regurgitation, right ventricular ejection causes sustained retrograde flow through the right atrium and back up into the inferior vena caval system, with the result that systolic flow reversal is recorded in the hepatic vein (see later discussion). In patients with moderate regurgitation, frank reversal of flow may not be recorded, but the normal forward flow is typically absent or diminished.

Quantitative Methods for Measuring Regurgitant Volume. The quantitative methods for measuring regurgitant volume, the difference in flow volumes, proximal acceleration, and conservation of momentum all appear applicable to the tricuspid valve. Use of the difference between tricuspid flow and that across a reference nonregurgitant valve as a measure of regurgitant volume

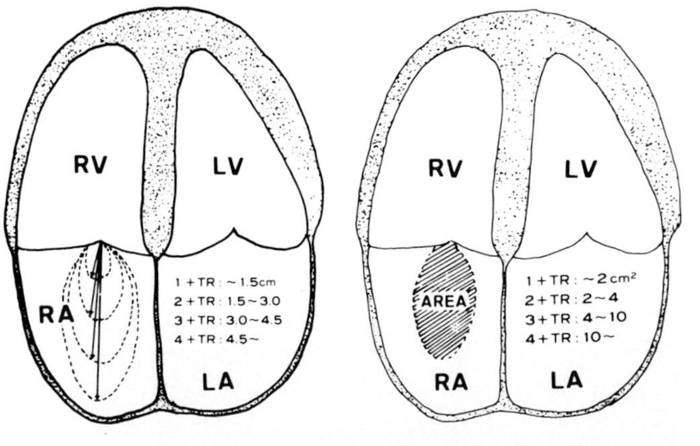

Fig. 26–17. Method for quantitating tricuspid regurgitant (TR) jet area and volume. LV = left ventricle; LA = left atrium; RV = right ventricle; RA = right atrium. (From Miyatake K, et al.: Evaluation of tricuspid regurgitation by pulsed Doppler and two-dimensional echocardiography. Circulation 66:777, 1982. Reproduced by permission of the American Heart Association, Inc.)

is complicated by the fact that the significant tricuspid regurgitation so frequently occurs in the setting of polyvalvular disease or intracardiac shunt. Further, in less severe cases, the error in the combined calculations is often greater than the regurgitant volume. Despite these limitations, when the flows can be appropriately calculated, the measurements should be valid.[63] Proximal acceleration and conservation of momentum are both reasonable approaches for quantitating regurgitation (see Chapters 13 and 17), and the measurement of momentum flux should be facilitated by the lack of aliasing in low velocity tricuspid jets. Further work, however, is necessary to validate these approaches.

Tricuspid Regurgitation in Otherwise Normal Patients

Minor degrees of tricuspid regurgitation are commonly observed in patients with structurally normal hearts with a reported prevalence of between 17 and 95%.[64–68] The prevalence of "normal" regurgitation appears to increase with age.[67,69] In one study, tricuspid regurgitation was found in only 8% of subjects with otherwise normal hearts under the age of 20, increasing to 30% in subjects over the age of 60 years.[67] It is also associated with physical conditioning, being found in 93% of highly trained atheletes and in only 24% of sedentary control subjects. The size of these jets is usually small. Using the pulsed wave technique, "normal" regurgitant jets do not typically extend more than 1 cm into the atrium. Somewhat higher values have been found using color flow mapping (up to 2.5 cm); however, the jet area/right atrial area ratio was consistently less than 18%.[70]

Secondary Abnormalities Commonly Associated With Tricuspid Regurgitation. Tricuspid regurgitation increases the volume of blood that must be borne by all the chambers of the right side of the heart. This increased volume causes dilation of the right ventricle, the right atrium, and the venous tributaries that drain into the right atrium. The right atrium appears to dilate early in the course of tricuspid regurgitation, as does the inferior vena cava.[20] In addition to dilation, there may be abnormal systolic expansion of the inferior vena cava resulting from the combined forward and regurgitant systolic flow into the vessel.

The increased volume load on the right ventricle, in addition to enlarging this chamber, also alters its shape by shifting the diastolic position of the interventricular septum toward the left ventricle.[71] This alteration causes the right ventricle to become more circular and the septum to move paradoxially during systole.[71,72]

The right ventricular volume overload pattern is nonspecific (see Chapters 28 and 29) and can be seen with other lesions that impose a volume load of the right heart such as atrial septal defect, anomalous pulmonary venous return, and ventricular septal defect with left ventricular-to-right atrial shunting. Pulmonary insufficiency rarely causes marked right atrial or vena caval dilation in the absence of tricuspid regurgitation or right-heart failure.

Acquired Lesions Associated With Tricuspid Regurgitation

Functional Tricuspid Regurgitation. *Functional tricuspid regurgitation* is a term used to describe valvular incompetence that is due to dilation of the right ventricle in the absence of any primary structural abnormality of the tricuspid valve. Functional tricuspid regurgitation is seen most commonly with left-sided valvular lesions leading to pulmonary hypertension or with primary pulmonary hypertensive disease. It can also occur in patients with right ventricular dilation that is due to myocardial or ischemic dysfunction.

The primary echocardiographic abnormality is right ventricular dilation. This is associated with tricuspid annular dilation and both apical and lateral displacement of the papillary muscles. The annular dilation decreases the degree of leaflet overlap at the tips. Apical displacement of the leaflets as a result of the malposition of the papillary muscles further decreases the leaflet area available for coaptation.[73] As the process progresses, a point is reached at which the leaflets fail to seal the orifice at some point along the closure line—usually, in the center of the orifice. Once the valve becomes incompetent, tricuspid regurgitation develops, which further augments the right ventricular volume overload, and a vicious cycle can be established. Not surprisingly, the severity of tricuspid regurgitation has been shown to relate to (1) the degree of tricuspid annular dilation; (2) the degree of apical leaflet displacement; (3) malcoaptation of the tricuspid leaflets (one tricuspid leaflet tip deviated anteriorly relative to the other in the apical four-chamber view); and (4) loss of coaptation (separation between the tips of the leaflets).[74,75]

Annuloplasty is the primary surgical treatment for functional tricuspid regurgitation. Several retrospective studies have suggested that the size of the tricuspid regurgitant jet and valve annulus are significantly larger in patients felt on clinical grounds to require tricuspid annuloplasty. Comparison of maximal color Doppler regurgitant jet area in the apical four-chamber view, normalized for right atrial area, showed a ratio of ≥34% in 96% of patients requiring annuloplasty and <34% in 95% of those not clinically felt to require annuloplasty.[76]

Tricuspid Valve Prolapse. *Tricuspid valve prolapse* can be defined as the anatomic displacement of one or more of the tricuspid leaflets into the right atrium during right ventricular systole. The echocardiographic diagnosis of tricuspid prolapse reflects this definition and is based on the demonstration of abnormal superior movement or arcing of one or more of the tricuspid leaflets above the plane of the tricuspid annulus at peak systolic excursion. Both tricuspid leaflet motion and the plane of the tricuspid leaflet annulus can be well defined in both the parasternal long axis view of the right ventricular inflow tract[2] and in the apical four-chamber view.[3] In the parasternal view, the anterior and posterior leaflets are visualized, whereas in the apical four-chamber view, the anterior and septal leaflets are recorded. Figure 26–18 illustrates prolapse of the tricuspid valve in the parasternal long axis view. In this example, the anterior tricuspid leaflet arcs above the plane of the tricuspid annulus at the point of peak systolic excursion.

Isolated tricuspid prolapse occurs rarely.[77] The reported incidence of tricuspid prolapse in patients with mitral valve prolapse has varied from greater than 50%[78] to less than 6%.[77] In our experience, tricuspid valve prolapse is found in 23% of patients with classic mitral valve prolapse.[79] It is also a common finding in patients with Marfan's syndrome. Tricuspid prolapse appears to involve the septal and anterior leaflets primarily[78] and has not been noted to occur in patients with right ventricular volume overload.[77] The latter finding is in contrast to the increased incidence of mitral valve prolapse noted in the presence of right ventricular volume overload.[56,80–83] This finding is not unexpected, however, because right ventricular dilation should increase the ventricle/valve size ratio on the right and thus retard tricuspid leaflet closure. In contrast, the altered geometry and relative decrease in size of the left ventricle should decrease this ratio on the left side, resulting in mitral valve prolapse.

Tricuspid Vegetations. Endocarditis involving the tricuspid valve is relatively infrequent and has a mean inci-

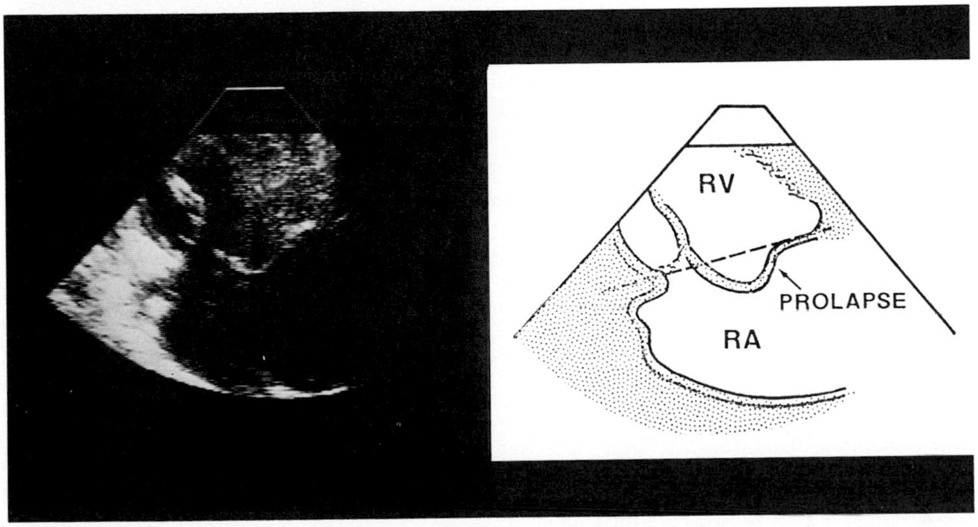

Fig. 26–18. Parasternal long axis recording of the tricuspid valve illustrates anterior tricuspid leaflet prolapse. In this recording, taken at the point of peak systolic superior displacement of the tricuspid valve, the anterior leaflet arcs superiorly into the right atrium (RA) beyond the plane of the tricuspid annulus. The RA is dilated. Clinical and hemodynamic evidence of tricuspid regurgitation was present. RV = right ventricle.

dence of only 2% in reported series.[47] Tricuspid endocarditis is typically an acute rather than subacute process.[47] Staphylococcus aureus is the most common infecting organism.[47,48,84] Predisposing factors include intravenous drug abuse, alcohol abuse, virulent skin infections, and infected venous catheters.

The clinical diagnosis of tricuspid endocarditis is suggested by the triad of fever, narcotic addition, and multiple lung lesions.[85] A pathologic murmur, which generally alerts the clinician to the possibility of endocarditis in lesions involving the left side of the heart, is frequently absent with isolated tricuspid valve involvement. In one series, a murmur was absent in 65% of patients with isolated right-sided endocarditis,[47] whereas in another series, the murmur of tricuspid insufficiency went undetected in 16 of 42 patients with proven tricuspid involvement.[84] Although significant tricuspid leaflet destruction and ruptured chordae are fairly common, the low pressure gradient between the right ventricle and right atrium may be responsible for the absence of a murmur.[48] This frequent lack of clinical signs directing attention to the tricuspid valve makes the routine echocardiographic examination of this valve imperative in instances of suspected endocarditis.

The cross-sectional echocardiographic diagnosis of tricuspid endocarditis is based on visualization of the bacterial vegetations that are characteristic of this disorder. Tricuspid vegetations generally appear as fairly large, echo-producing masses that disrupt the normally smooth, thin contour of the tricuspid leaflets (Fig. 26–19).[86,87] The echoes from these vegetations have been described as thick and "shaggy," and when leaflet destruction is present, may be associated with high-frequency oscillatory motion of part of the disrupted leaflet or of the vegetations themselves.[86] Tricuspid vegetations are usually larger than corresponding left-sided lesions and tend to involve the atrial surface of the involved leaflets. Abrupt disappearance of a vegetation is generally associated with pulmonary embolism and infarction.[86]

Figure 26–20 is an example of a large tricuspid vegetation attached to the atrial surface of the anterior tricuspid leaflet. There has been extensive destruction of the anterior leaflet, and the remaining leaflet tissue has been incorporated into the mass. Consequently, visualization of discrete leaflet tissue is no longer possible. Figure 26–21 is an angiogram from the same patient and illustrates extensive contrast displacement by the large vegetative mass. Figure 26–22 is a pathologic specimen showing the vegetation depicted in Figures 26–20 and 26–21 occluding the pulmonary artery following spontaneous embolization. Large tricuspid vegetations may be difficult to differentiate from atrial tumors. Their uniform association with the affected leaflet and their movement in unison with leaflet motion, however, aid in their identification.[86] When vegetations arise on a stalk, their motion may be more erratic. In these situations, their point of origin should aid in their recognition.

When vegetations cause extensive destruction of leaflet tissue, a portion of the leaflet may become flail and

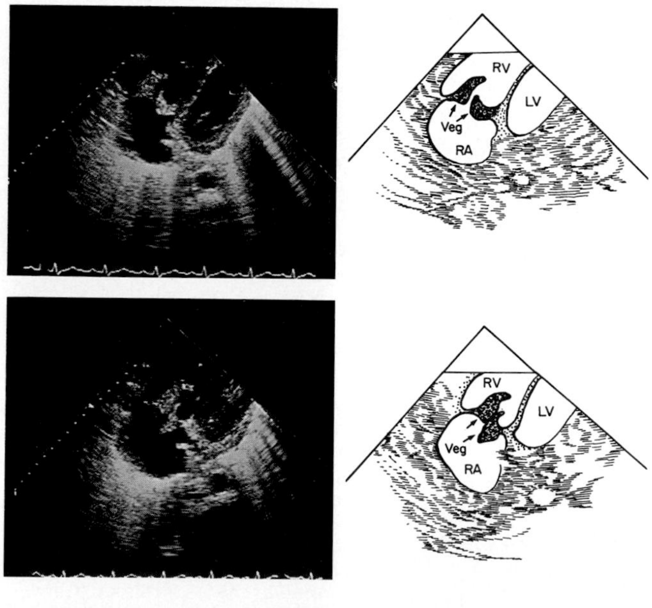

Fig. 26–19. Apical four-chamber recordings during diastole (top) and systole (bottom) in a patient with staphylococcal endocarditis and vegetations involving all of the tricuspid leaflets. During diastole, the large vegetations partially fill the tricuspid orifice, while during systole, a portion of the vegetation attached to the septal leaflet prolapses in the right atrium (RA). RV = right ventricle; LV = left ventricle.

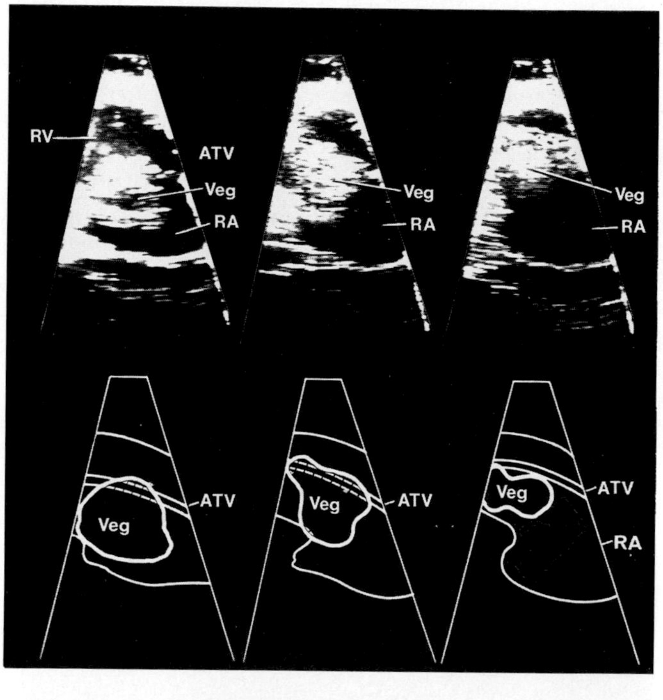

Fig. 26–20. Parasternal long axis recording of a large tricuspid valve vegetation. The vegetation (Veg) appears as a large echo-producing mass that is attached to the atrial surface of the anterior tricuspid leaflet and moves in unison with this leaflet. Left. Recorded during ventricular systole, the vegetative mass lies within the right atrial cavity, and the tricuspid valve is closed. In the center panel, recorded at the onset of valve opening, the vegetation shifts down into the tricuspid orifice as the leaflet opens. Right. Recorded during mid-diastole, the vegetation is displaced into the right ventricle (RV) and almost completely fills the tricuspid valve orifice. ATV = anterior leaflet of tricuspid valve; RA = right atrium.

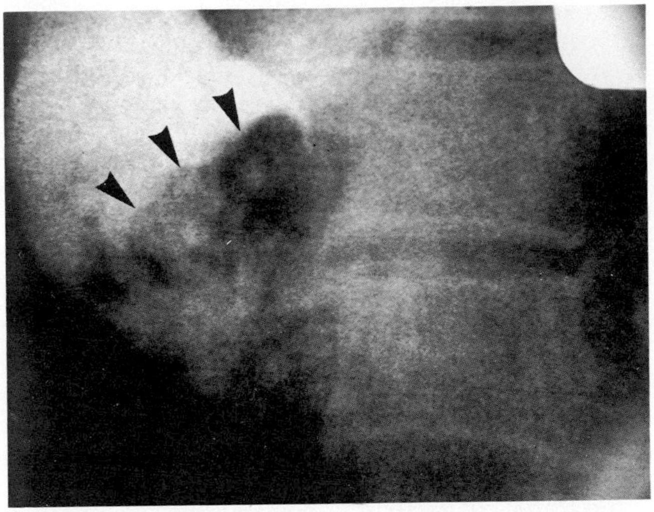

Fig. 26–21. Right atrial and ventricular angiogram from the patient discussed in Figure 26–20. The tricuspid vegetation produces a large area of contrast displacement indicated by the arrowheads in the region of the tricuspid annulus.

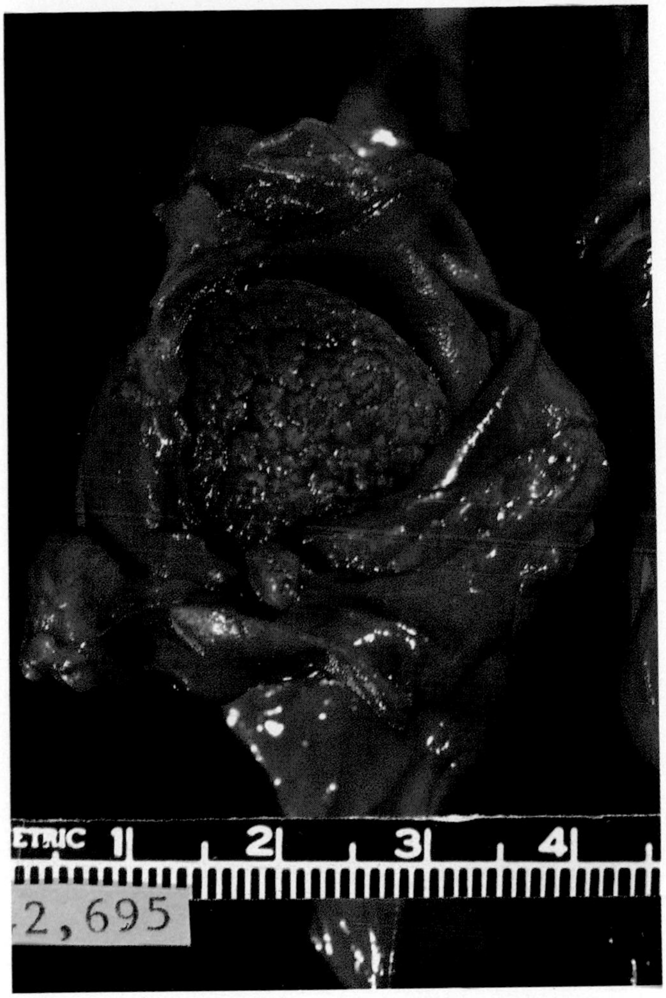

Fig. 26–22. Pathologic specimen illustrating the large vegetation demonstrated in Figures 26–20 and 26–21 following spontaneous embolization with total occlusion of the pulmonary artery.

evert into the right atrium during systole.[87] Marked valvular incompetence is usually associated with a right ventricular volume overload pattern.[87]

Carcinoid Heart Disease. Malignant carcinoid tumors with hepatic metastases frequently present with a clinical syndrome characterized by episodic flushing, diarrhea, and bronchospasm.[50] In addition, more than half of these patients develop extensive fibrous deposits on the endocardial surfaces of the right side of the heart. These deposits interfere with normal myocardial and valvular function; as a result, heart failure is the leading cause of death. This fibrous tissue deposition appears to result from endocardial damage produced by a hormonal substance(s) secreted by the tumor. This substance apparently circulates through the right side of the heart and is inactivated in the lungs, because in the absence of right-to-left shunting, left-sided lesions are uncommon. Both serotonin and kinin peptides have been implicated as the injury-inducing agent.

The reported echocardiographic features of carcinoid heart disease include thickening and shortening of the tricuspid valve leaflets with variable degrees of diastolic leaflet immobility; failure of complete systolic leaflet coaptation; and on occasion, total fixation of the leaflets in a partially open position.[88,89] Thickening of the right atrial wall, particularly the endothelial layer, has also been reported.[90] Figure 26–23 illustrates a thickened immobile tricuspid valve in a patient with carcinoid syndrome.

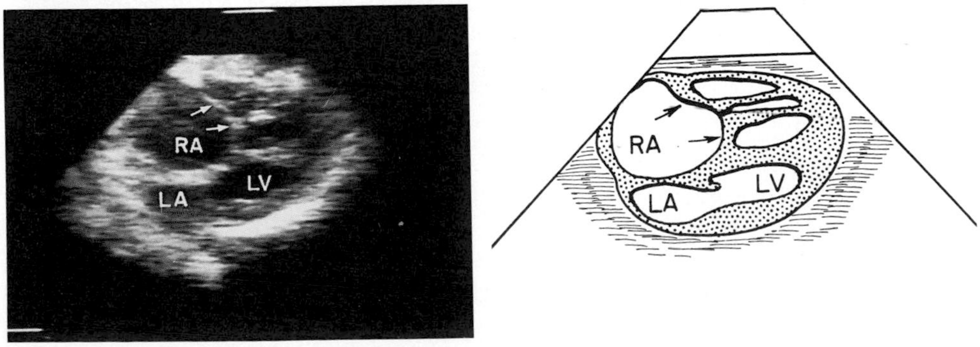

Fig. 26–23. Subcostal long axis recording of the tricuspid valve in carcinoid syndrome. The valve leaflets (horizontal arrows) and chordae are thickened, and in this diastolic frame, there is no evidence of valve opening. In real time, the valve appeared completely fixed and stenotic with no observable motion from diastole to systole. The right atrium (RA) is dilated. LV = left ventricle; LA = left atrium.

Congenital Anomalies Associated With Tricuspid Regurgitation

Tricuspid Valve Dysplasia. Tricuspid valve dysplasia is due to the incomplete development of either chordal or leaflet tissue and is usually manifest by significant valvular regurgitation in a young patient without other evidence of cardiac disease. On occasion, leaflet thickening, chordal or leaflet shortening, or focal leaflet malposition can be appreciated during careful scanning of the valve in multiple views. More often, however, this is a diagnosis of exclusion based on the presence of moderate or severe tricuspid regurgitation in a young person with no other obvious cause.

Ebstein's Anomaly. Ebstein's anomaly is a congenital deformity characterized by downward displacement of part or all of a malformed tricuspid valve into the right ventricular cavity with associated alteration of the architecture of the chamber.[91,92] Anatomic variability in the degree of displacement and the presence of associated anomalies results in a broad spectrum of clinical presentation ranging from asymptomatic to lethal.

The tricuspid leaflets typically attach in part to the tricuspid annulus and in part to the right ventricular endocardium, either directly or by multiple thick chordae. The portion of the ventricle above the displaced tricuspid valve is thin walled and functions as a reservoir rather than contributing to the pumping ability of the right ventricle. Although an intracavitary right ventricular electrogram is recorded in this chamber, the intracavitary pressure is similar to that of the right atrium, and hence, it is referred to as *atrialized*.[93–95]

The septal and posterior leaflets are characteristically deformed in Ebstein's anomaly, and either or both may be rudimentary or absent. The anterior tricuspid leaflet is the largest and the least affected.[91,96,97] The right atrium is almost always dilated, and an associated atrial septal defect is common. The degree of right ventricular dysfunction relates to (1) the degree of deformity of the tricuspid leaflets and the presence or absence of tricuspid regurgitation; (2) the size of the atrialized portion of the right ventricle that not only fails to contribute to right ventricular contraction but may expand in an aneurysmal fashion during atrial systole, further impairing right ventricular filling; and (3) the absolute decrease in right ventricle chamber size and resulting decrease in right ventricle output.

The characteristic feature of Ebstein's anomaly (downward displacement of the malformed tricuspid valve) can be best visualized in the apical four-chamber view.[98] Apical displacement of the septal leaflet in this view has been shown to be the single most diagnostic feature of the anomaly.[96,99–103] Normally, in the apical four-chamber view, the septal leaflet of the tricuspid valve inserts into the interventricular septum slightly (<1 cm) apical to the septal insertion of the anterior mitral leaflet. In Ebstein's anomaly, this separation increases. In one large series, apical displacement of the septal leaflet in Ebstein's anomaly ranged from 7 to 50 mm; whereas in patients with a normal tricuspid valve, secundum atrial defect, and severe tricuspid regurgitation, displacement ranged from 0 to 10 mm, 2 to 14 mm and 2 to 15 mm, respectively. When these values were indexed for body surface area (Fig. 26–24), however, a displacement index of ≥8 mm/m² appeared to more clearly separate patients with Ebstein's anomaly from normal subjects and patients with other forms of right ventricular volume overload.[103] The ratio of the mitral valve-left ventricular apex distance to the corresponding tricuspid valve-right ventricular apex distance has also been used to identify patients with Ebstein's anomaly. In normal persons and in patients with right ventricular volume overload, this ratio is reported to range from 1:1.2:1 (mean, 1.09:1) vs. 1.8:3.2:1 in a group of patients with documented Ebstein's anomaly.[96]

The morphology of septal leaflet displacement is also variable. The septal leaflet has been reported to be absent in 12% of patients; to originate near its annulus but

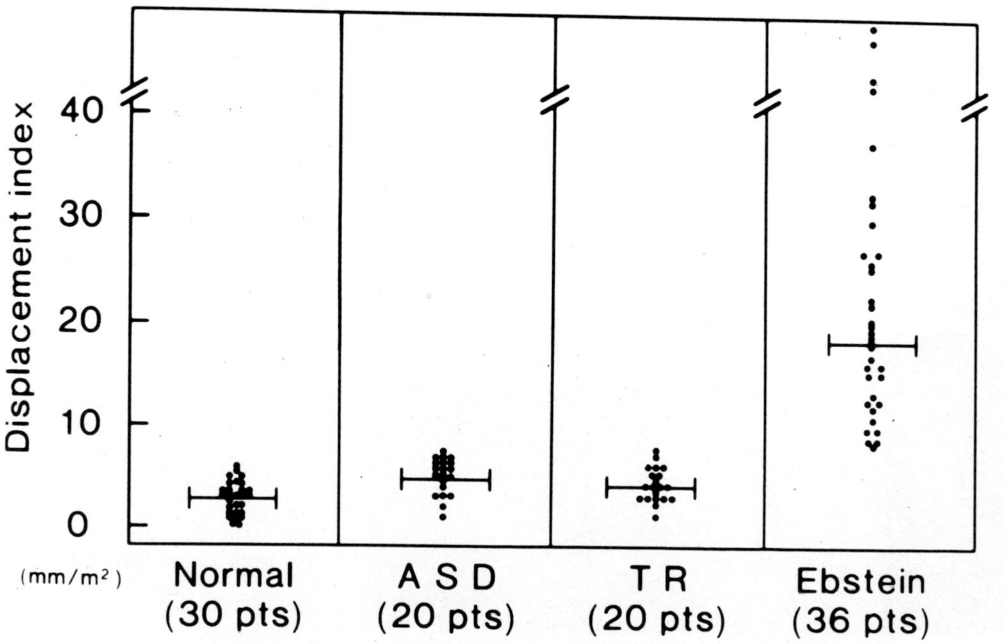

Fig. 26–24. Septal tricuspid valve displacement index for normal subjects and patients with atrial septal defect (ASD), tricuspid regurgitation (TR) and Ebstein's anomaly. (From Shiina A, et al.: Two-dimensional echocardiographic spectrum of Ebstein's anomaly: detailed anatomic assessment. J Am Coll Cardiol 3:356, 1984. Reprinted with permission from the American College of Cardiology.)

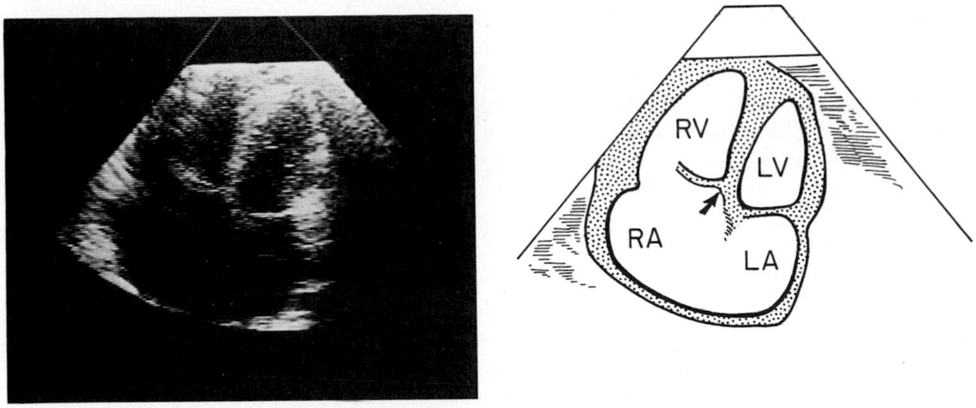

Fig. 26–25. Apical four-chamber recording illustrates minimal apical displacement of the septal tricuspid leaflet in a patient with a mild form of Ebstein's anomaly and tricuspid regurgitation. The increased separation between the anterior mitral and septal tricuspid leaflets is indicated by the arrowhead. The right atrium (RA) and right ventricle (RV) are dilated. LA = left atrium; LV = left ventricle.

to be tethered to the septum with its free edge apically displaced in 22%; and to be intimately adherent to the ventricular septum and originate from an apically displace position in the remaining 66%.[103] Dysplasia of the septal leaflet was noted in roughly 60% of patients.[103]

Displacement of the anterior leaflet is less common, occurring in roughly 13% of patients in the apical four-chamber view; however, some degree of tethering of this leaflet is present in roughly 85% of patients. Elongation and whiplike motion of the anterior leaflet is also noted in roughly 85% of patients but is a nonspecific finding.[103,104] Eccentric leaflet coaptation occurs in roughly 73% of patients with Ebstein's anomaly and is most pronounced in patients with a dysplastic septal leaflet.[103] Fenestrations and clefts in the anterior mitral leaflet are poorly appreciated on two-dimensional echocardiography.

Figures 26–25 to 26–27 illustrate various degrees of tricuspid displacement in Ebstein's anomaly. In Figure 26–25, the septal tricuspid leaflet in a patient with hemo-

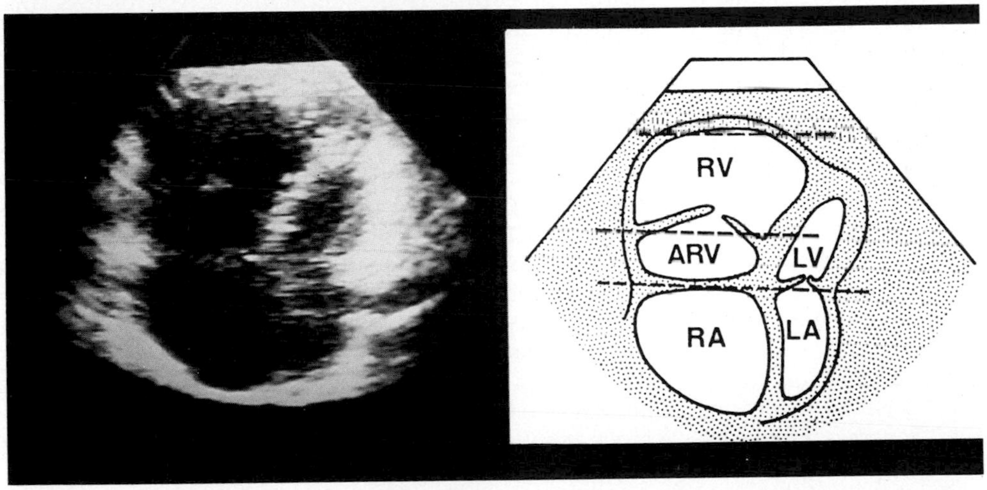

Fig. 26–26. Apical four-chamber recording illustrates a moderately severe degree of tricuspid displacement in another patient with Ebstein's anomaly. Both the displaced tricuspid leaflets and the tricuspid annulus are visible. The diagram to the right illustrates the relative sizes of the residual right ventricle (RV), extending from the right ventricular apex to the plane of insertion of the displaced tricuspid leaflets, and the atrialized right ventricle (ARV), which includes the area from the plane of insertion of the displaced tricuspid valve to the tricuspid annulus. RA = right atrium; LV = left ventricle; LA = left atrium.

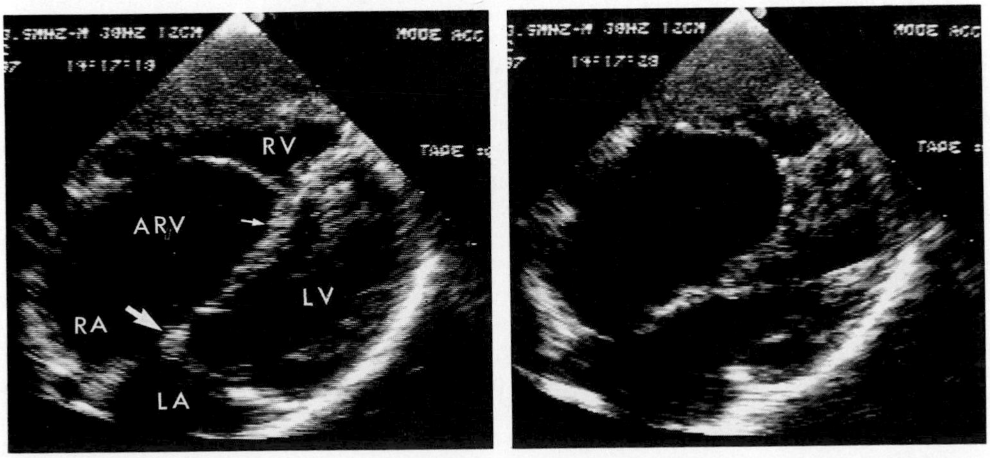

Fig. 26–27. Subcostal four-chamber recording illustrates an example of Ebstein's anomaly with marked apical displacement (small arrow) of the septal leaflet of the tricuspid valve (large arrow indicates the normal insertion point of the leaflet). Left. Systole. Right. Diastole. In this person, the atrialized portion of the right ventricle is much larger than the residual right ventricular cavity. ARV = atrialized right ventricle; RV = right ventricle; LV = left ventricle; LA = left atrium; RA = right atrium.

dynamically confirmed Ebstein's anomaly and tricuspid regurgitation inserts farther below the anterior mitral leaflet than is normal. In Figure 26–26, the tricuspid valve is further displaced toward the apex and separates the right ventricular cavity into an atrialized chamber and a true muscular right ventricle. Figure 26–27 is a still more severe example in which the tricuspid valve is displaced well into the apical segment of the right ventricle and the atrialized portion of the ventricular chamber is much larger than the residual ventricle.

Quantitation of Severity. The anatomic and functional severity of Ebstein's anomaly can be assessed by determining the absolute and relative sizes of the functional right ventricle and atrialized portion of the right ventricular cavity (Fig. 26–26). The size of the functional right ventricle should most appropriately be defined by the volume encompassed by the closed tricuspid leaflets and the apical right ventricular myocardium, whereas the atrialized portion of the ventricle is the volume from the anatomic valve annulus to the valve leaflets. Because such volume measurements have not generally been available, chamber lengths have conventionally been used to measure relative size. The overall right ventricular length is taken as the distance from the anatomic annular plane to the ventricular apex. The extent of the atrialized portion of the ventricle has then been defined as the distance from the anatomic annulus to either the plane of coaptation of the dysplastic valve or the coapted valve leaflets at the center of the closure line. The functional right ventricle is then described by the difference between these two values (right ventricle length minus the atrialized right ventricle length). Although there is no consensus, it seems reasonable, because normal left and right ventricular volumes are measured at end-diastole, that these dimensions likewise be measured as close to end-diastole as possible (i.e., in the first frame following valve closure). The anatomic tricuspid annulus is readily defined because it maintains its normal position and can be identified as a band of linear echoes that divides the right side of the heart at a level that approximates the plane of the mitral annulus and corresponds roughly to the point of mitral leaflet insertion. The right atrium extends from the tricuspid annulus to the superior wall of the right atrial cavity. Studies comparing the length of the atrialized right ventricle measured echocardiographically with that quantitated angiographically have shown a good correlation and confirm the ability of the cross-sectional echogram to define this relationship.[94] Likewise, correlations between two-dimensional echocardiographic descriptions of valve and chamber morphology and size have been highly correlated with those observed at surgery or autopsy.[103]

Although the apical four-chamber view is the primary echocardiographic view for assessing Ebstein's anomaly, changes in tricuspid leaflet structure and right atrial and ventricular size can also be visualized in the parasternal long axis and short axis views. The long axis view is most useful for assessing posterior leaflet involvement because this leaflet is not recorded in the apical four-chamber view. The parasternal short axis view is ideal for assessing right ventricular outflow tract size with a right ventricular outflow tract/aortic root diameter ratio of ≥2:1 being considered diagnostic of aneurysmal dilation of the outflow tract. When right ventricular volume overload is present, paradoxic motion of the interventricular septum may be noted.

Morphologic characteristics associated with lower functional classification include (1) a small functional right ventricle (atrialized/functional right ventricle ratio of >0.5); (2) extreme septal leaflet displacement; (3) absent septal leaflet; (4) displaced anterior tricuspid leaflet; (5) tethering of the anterior leaflet; and (6) aneurysmal dilation of the right ventricular outflow tract. Moderate or severe tricuspid regurgitation is also associated with a lower function classification.

Clinical status is the primary determinant of the need for surgery in patients with Ebstein's anomaly. However, two-dimensional echocardiography may be useful in separating patients in whom valve repair is feasible from those who will require valve excision.[105] In general, valve excision is required in patients in whom there is extensive tethering of the free edges of the tricuspid valve leaflets to the underlying myocardium, resulting in severe restriction of motion. Particularly important is the anterior leaflet because its immobilization reduces the likelihood that the surgeon will be able to construct a competent unicuspid valve by plastic repair.[105] Patients with a small functional right ventricular cavity (ratio of functional to total right ventricular cavity of less then 35%) are also more likely to require valve replacement.[105] The technique is also of value in assessing postoperative repair and in evaluating the efficacy of various procedures.[106]

Ebstein's anomaly has also been diagnosed by M-mode echocardiography based on an increased amplitude of motion of the anterior tricuspid leaflet, an increase in right ventricular cavity dimension, paradoxic septal motion, and delayed closure of the tricuspid valve in relation to the mitral valve (Fig. 26–28). Although delayed closure of the tricuspid valve relative to the mitral (>65 msec) has generally been considered the most reliable sign of Ebstein's anomaly, none of these criteria have proven to be specific.[101,107,108] As a result, the M-mode method is no longer used to assess this anomaly.[96,103]

Diastolic Tricuspid Regurgitation

Diastolic tricuspid regurgitation is recorded in any condition in which there is a reversal (RV > RA) of the normal atrioventricular pressure gradient during diastole. Diastolic regurgitation occurs most commonly in patients with heart block when atrial contraction is not followed by a normally timed ventricular systole.[109] In this situation, atrial contraction raises diastolic right ventricular pressure (A wave), and this pressure remains high as the atrium relaxes. The elevated ventricular pressure in the face of a relaxing atrium reverses the normal pressure gradient, and if an appropriately timed ventricular systole does not cause complete valve closure, it will produce diastolic regurgitation. The delay from the onset of the P wave to the onset of diastolic regurgitation ranges from .25 to .30 seconds. A similar

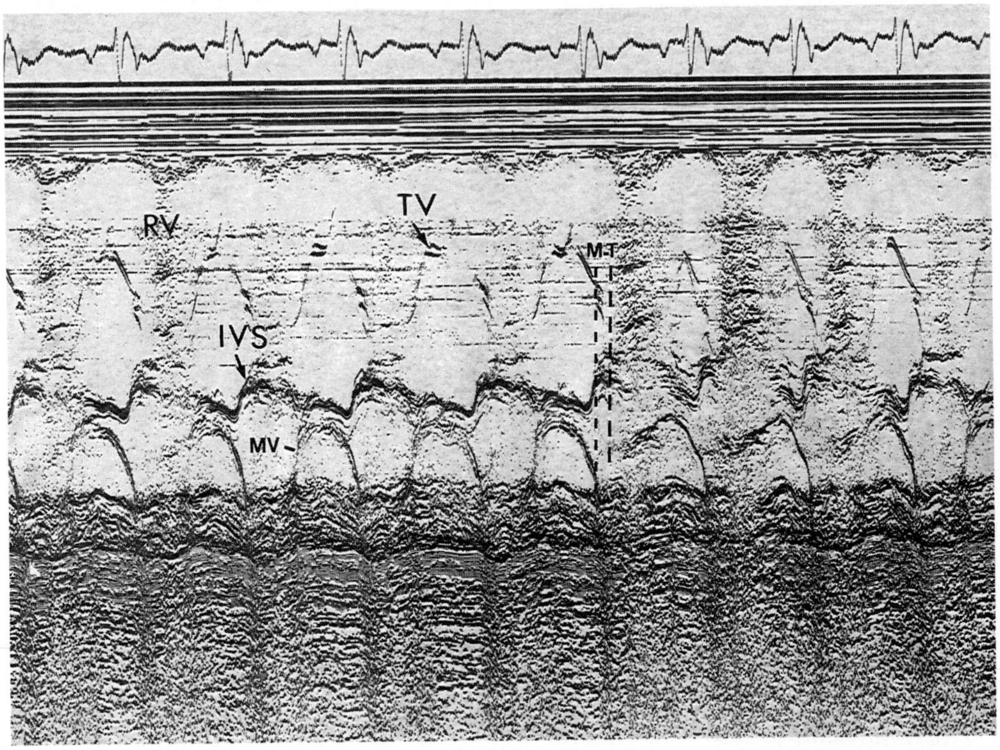

Fig. 26–28. M-mode recording from a patient with Ebstein's anomaly. Note dilated right ventricle (RV), the broad excursion of the anterior tricuspid leaflet (TV); paradoxic motion of the interventricular septum (IVS); and the delayed closure of the tricuspid valve relative to that of the mitral valve (M-T). MV = mitral valve.

reversal of the pressure gradient (RV > RA)[109] can also occur in patients with mechanically effective atrial fibrillation, atrial flutter, severe pulmonic regurgitation, and restrictive cardiomyopathy. Systolic tricuspid regurgitation is also recorded in the majority of patients with diastolic regurgitation but is not necessary for diastolic regurgitation to occur (see also Chapters 17 and 40).

Estimation of Right Ventricular Systolic Pressure From the Tricuspid Regurgitant Jet Velocity

In patients with tricuspid regurgitation, the pressure gradient between the right ventricle and right atrium during systole can be estimated from the peak velocities in the regurgitant jet using the simplified Bernoulli equation ($\Delta P = 4V^2$).[55,110–112] To estimate absolute right ventricular systolic pressure, some estimate of right atrial pressure is necessary, because the absolute pressure is the sum of the gradient and the simultaneous right atrial systolic pressure. In the absence of a significant gradient across the pulmonary valve or right ventricular outflow tract, the right ventricular systolic pressure is equivalent to the pulmonary artery systolic pressure.

Percentage of Patients With Tricuspid Regurgitation. Although tricuspid regurgitation can be recorded in normal subjects and is frequently observed in patients with valvular heart disease, it is not invariably present. Fortunately, the prevalence of tricuspid regurgitation increases as right ventricular systolic and pulmonary artery pressures increase (Fig. 26–29), and hence, the measurement is most frequently available in patients in whom the data are of greatest importance. In one series, tricuspid regurgitation was observed in 80% of patients with right ventricular systolic pressures >35 mm Hg and in roughly 96% of patients with systolic right ventricular pressures >50 mm Hg.[111] In studies of patients with clinically suspected right ventricular systolic hypertension, between 84 and 90% have had tricuspid regurgitation by Doppler.[110,112]

Method of Measurement. Unfortunately, not all patients with detectable tricuspid regurgitation will have

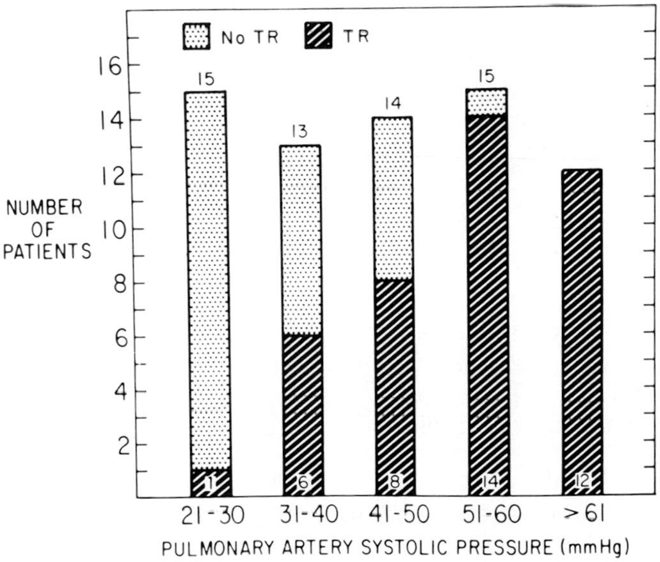

Fig. 26–29. The relationship between pulmonary artery systolic pressure and the presence of tricuspid regurgitation (TR). (From Berger M, et al.: Quantitative assessment of pulmonary hypertension in patients with tricuspid regurgitation using continuous-wave Doppler ultrasound. J Am Coll Cardiol 6:359, 1985. Reprinted with permission from the American College of Cardiology.)

regurgitant velocity profiles suitable for measurement. The reported percentage of patients with tricuspid regurgitation with measurable peak velocities has ranged from 75,[112] to 96%.[110] The maximum velocity of regurgitant flow is taken as the average of the peak velocities derived from beats that produce the most complete envelopes and have the greatest representation of high velocity flows in the spectral envelope. In patients with weak signals, the peripheral injection of small amounts of contrast can significantly improve the signal/noise ratio.[113–115] Because right-sided velocities vary with respiration and cycle length (Fig. 26–30), we generally average at least 5 beats in patients in sinus rhythm and 10 beats in patients in atrial fibrillation.

Correlation of Doppler and Catheter Measurement of Gradient. Correlations between Doppler- and catheter-derived gradients have been excellent, with reported correlation coefficients of $r = .95$ and $r = 0.96$ (Fig. 26–31). In patients in whom gradients were measured simultaneously and then repeated several days later, the correlation for the nonsimultaneous gradients was lower ($r = .87$, standard error of estimation [SEE] = 12) than for the simultaneously recorded gradients ($r = .97$, SEE = 6 mm Hg).

Doppler-derived gradients have also been compared to directly measured pulmonary artery pressures, and an excellent correlation has been reported ($r = .97$) (Fig. 26–32). In these patients there was a proportional underestimation of the pulmonary artery pressure by the gradient ($y = 1.23 \times -0.09$). This suggests the right atrial pressure increases in proportion to the pulmonary artery pressure, so that a constant relationship between the gradient and pulmonary artery pressure is maintained.

Errors in the Doppler-derived peak velocity of the tricuspid regurgitant jet are similar to those that affect all Doppler velocity measurements and include (1) a non-

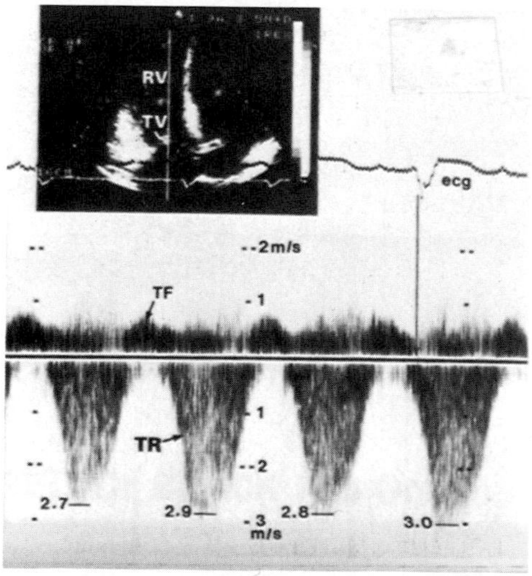

Fig. 26–30. Continuous wave Doppler recording illustrating the cycle-to-cycle variation in tricuspid regurgitant (TR) velocity. TF = tricuspid inflow. (From Yock PG, Popp RL; Noninvasive estimation of right ventricular systolic pressure by Doppler ultrasound in patients with tricuspid regurgitation. Circulation 70:657, 1984. Reproduced by permission of the American Heart Association, Inc.)

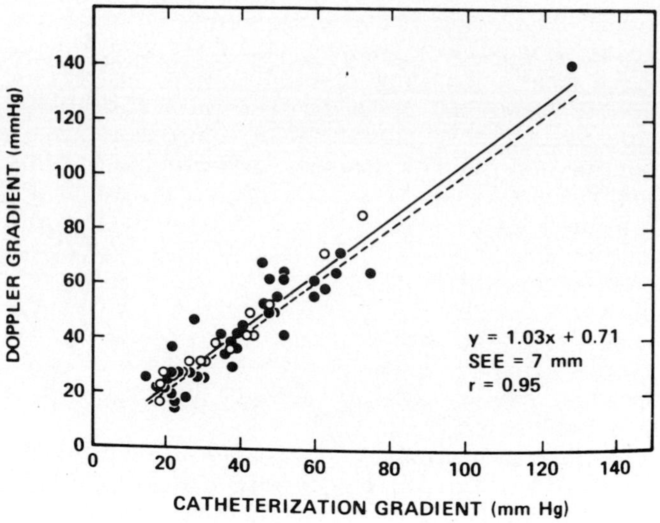

Fig. 26–31. The correlation between the peak catheterization and Doppler-derived gradients across the tricuspid valve. SEE = standard error of estimate. (From Yock PG, Popp RL: Noninvasive estimation of right ventricular systolic pressure by Doppler ultrasound in patients with tricuspid regurgitation. Circulation 70:657, 1984. Reproduced by permission of the American Heart Association, Inc.)

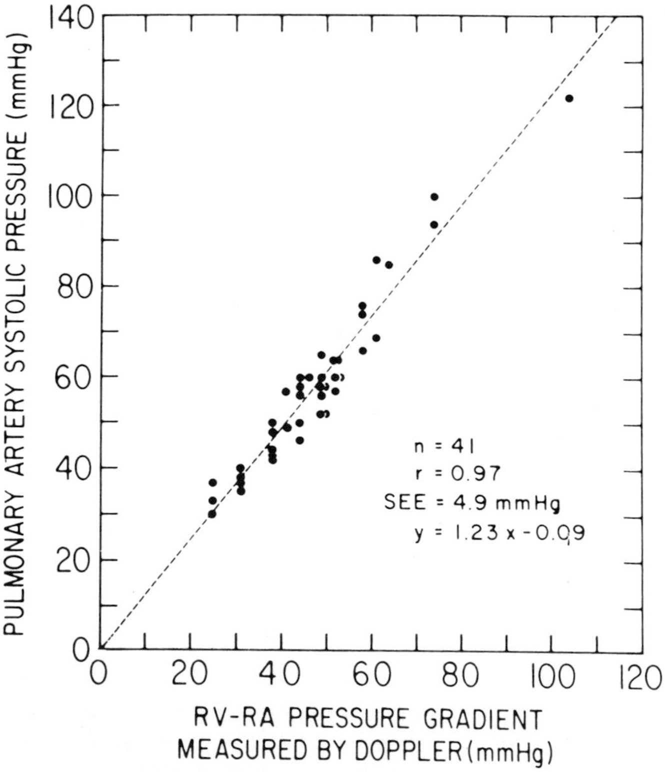

Fig. 26–32. The correlation between the right ventricle-right atrium pressure gradient measured by Doppler and the pulmonary artery systolic pressure. SEE = standard error of estimate. (From Berger M, et al.: Quantitative assessment of pulmonary hypertension in patients with tricuspid regurgitation using continuous-wave Doppler ultrasound. J Am Coll Cardiol 6:359, 1985. Reprinted with permission from the American College of Cardiology.

parallel relationship between the ultrasonic beam and the direction of the regurgitant jet and (2) inaccurate or biased measurement that is due to a poor signal/noise ratio. Changes in signal/noise ratio on a beat-to-beat basis are caused by patient and/or transducer motion, differing cardiac cycle lengths, and respiratory variation. The possibility of systematic error in the estimation of mean gradient occurs in the latter two categories if good quality signals are recorded only during certain cycle lengths (e.g., with longer R-R intervals) or at certain phases of the respiratory cycle (e.g., only during inspiration).[110] Despite these and other potential sources of error, accurate gradients can generally be obtained through careful attention to the general principles of Doppler flow recording.

Intra- and Interobserver Variability. Interobserver variability for peak jet velocity measurements has been low. The mean interobserver difference in calculated gradients has been reported to be 1.8 mm Hg (standard deviation, [SD] 4.9 mm Hg). Intraobserver variation is even lower, with a mean difference of 0.2 mm Hg (SD, 3.4 mm Hg). In another study, the average coefficient of variation was 2.8% for velocity and 5.4% for the gradient.

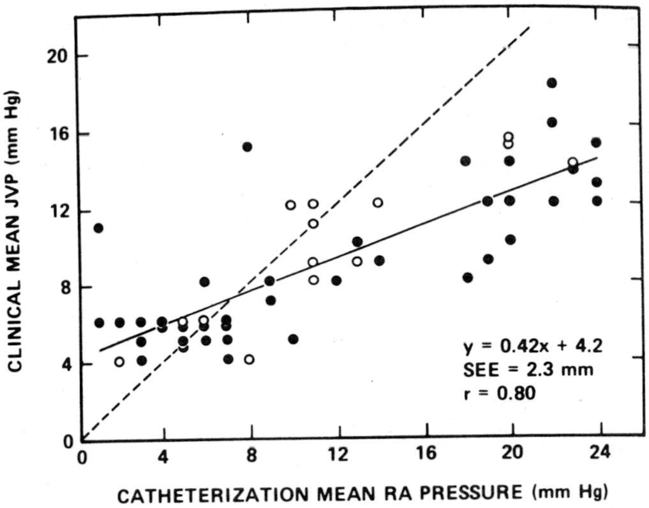

Fig. 26–33. The relatively poor correlation between the mean right atrial (RA) pressure estimated clinically from the jugular venous pressure (JVP) and that determined by catheterization. SEE = standard error of estimate. (From Yock PG, Popp RL: Noninvasive estimation of right ventricular systolic pressure by Doppler ultrasound in patients with tricuspid regurgitation. Circulation 70: 657, 1984. Reproduced by permission of the American Heart Association, Inc.)

Estimation of Right Atrial Pressure

Because right ventricular systolic pressure is equal to the transvalvular gradient plus the right atrial pressure, it is necessary to estimate right atrial pressure to determine systolic right ventricular or pulmonary artery pressure. Four general approaches have been explored: (1) clinical estimation of right atrial pressure from the mean jugular venous pressure; (2) use of a linear regression equation to convert the transvalvular gradient to the absolute pressure; (3) estimation of right atrial pressure from inferior vena caval diameter and diameter change with respiration and (4) use of an assumed right atrial pressure (e.g., 10 mm Hg), irrespective of right ventricular pressure. The clinical estimation of right atrial pressure from the jugular venous pulse is not available in all patients, particularly small children and the obese. Even when the right atrial pressure can be measured from the jugular venous pressure, the correlation with actual catheter measurement is poor (Fig. 26–33).[110,112] Reasonable correlation has been reported between the inspiratory pressure required to decrease the inferior vena caval diameter to ≥85% of the difference between its maximal and minimal values and mean right atrial pressure (r = .87). Unfortunately, this approach requires specialized equipment and is sufficiently time-consuming that it is unlikely to prove generally useful.

Application of regression data to correct for the difference between transvalvular gradients and right ventricular or pulmonary artery pressure is reasonable, but several different equations have been reported. At least one approach requires a different equation for high and low atrial pressures, which must still be separated clinically. The use of an absolute value for right atrial pressure is simple and does not require that a physician be present during the Doppler examination to determine the mean jugular venous pressure. In addition, because the right atrial pressure is small relative to the transvalvular gradient, small differences between the actual and estimated right atrial pressure will have a limited impact on the ventricular pressure estimate.

Figure 26–34 compares the difference in correlation

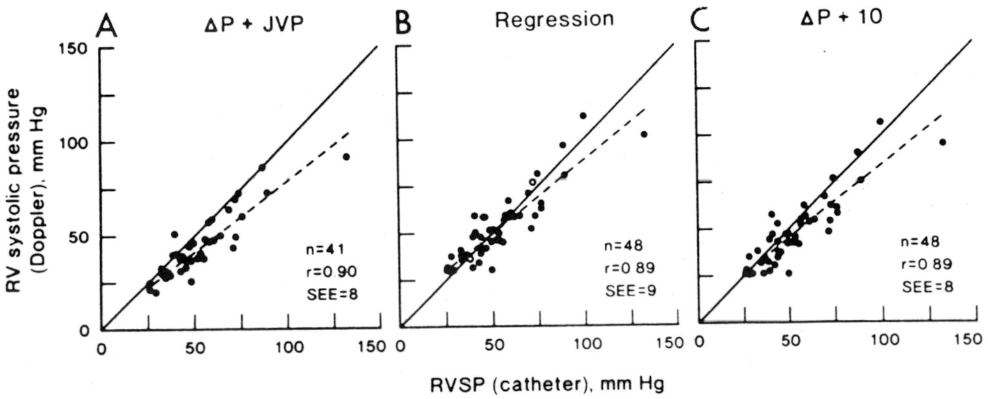

Fig. 26–34. Comparison of right ventricular systolic pressure (RVSP) determined using three methods for estimating the right atrial pressure. JVP = jugular venous pressure; SEE = standard error of estimate. (From Currie PJ, et al.: Continuous-wave Doppler determination of right ventricular pressure: a simultaneous Doppler-catheterization study in 127 patients. J Am Coll Cardiol 6:750, 1985. Reprinted with permission from the American College of Cardiology.)

between right ventricular systolic pressure measured using the pressure gradient and right atrial pressure estimated from the jugular venous pressure (Fig. 26–34A); the right ventricular systolic pressure derived from the gradient using a regression equation (Fig. 26–34B); and the correlation derived by adding a constant value of 10 mm Hg to the pressure gradient (Fig. 26–34C). Note that all of the correlation coefficients are similar. Although the regression equation method was slightly more accurate in this group, it adds complexity to the calculation, and as a result, we prefer to simply estimate the right atrial pressure at 10 mm Hg.

Miscellaneous Disorders of the Tricuspid Valve

Tricuspid Annular Calcification

Although mitral annular calcification is commonly observed in the elderly, tricuspid annular calcification is a relatively rare finding.[116–118] Few echocardiographic data are available describing the prevalence of tricuspid annular calcification; however, in one study it was observed in 1 of 80 patients with mitral annular calcification.[119] The echocardiographic features of tricuspid annular calcification are similar to those of mitral annular calcification, and both lesions are characterized by an intense echo-producing mass in the myocardium at the base of the valve leaflets visible in multiple views and associated with acoustic shadowing.[119,120] Anterior tricuspid annular calcification must be distinguished from right coronary and aortic root calcification.[119] Tricuspid annular calcification is usually found in patients with long-standing right ventricular pressure or with volume overload secondary to pulmonic stenosis,[117] atrial septal defect, or cor pulmonale; however, its clinical significance is unclear.

Tricuspid Leaflet Tumors

Tricuspid leaflet tumors are rare and may arise from any of the cellular elements normally present in the leaflets or chordae. Myxomas (see Chapter 36) and fibroelastomas are the most frequent. Papillary fibroelastomas are small (<1 cm) and benign masses. They are most commonly found on the tricuspid valve in children and are rarely if ever associated with symptoms. In adults, they are more commonly found on the left side of the heart, but tricuspid valve involvement is reported. Figure 36–19 (Chapter 36) illustrates a small papillary fibroelastoma of the tricuspid valve in an adult.

Tricuspid Valve Fluttering

High-frequency fluttering of the tricuspid valve can be detected by M-mode recording during both systole and diastole. Systolic fluttering can be seen with leaflet disruption and regurgitation that is due to bacterial endocarditis or penetrating trauma;[121,122] high membranous ventricular septal defects[123] with the jet directed against the septal leaflet; ventricular septal defect with a membranous aneurysm;[124] or left ventricular-to-right atrial shunts passing through the septal tricuspid leaflet.[125] Diastolic fluttering can be seen with severe pulmonary regurgitation, atrial septal defect, coronary arteriovenous fistula[126] and as a result of turbulent flow through a fenestrated Chiari network.[127]

THE RIGHT ATRIUM

Anatomy

The right atrium is a thin-walled (slightly thinner than the left), irregularly shaped chamber that occupies the majority of the right superior quadrant of the heart. The posterior and superior borders of the right atrium lie at the same level as, and are continuous with, those of the left atrium. The interatrial septum, which separates these two chambers, forms its left margin, while inferiorly it is bounded by the tricuspid annulus. The anterior wall, which is covered by the right atrial appendage, lies directly beneath the anterior chest wall. The free right border, which typically parallels the right side of the sternum, forms the majority of the right margin of the heart. There are four principal openings in the right atrial walls. These include (1) the orifice of the inferior vena cava, which is found along the right posterior margin of the inferior wall; (2) the insertion of the superior vena cava, which interrupts the right anterior portion of the superior wall; (3) the tricuspid orifice, which angles from anterior to posterior and superior to inferior along the inferior atrial border; and (4) the ostium of the coronary sinus, which is found posteriorly beneath the lower border of the interatrial septum and just superior to the posterior margin of the tricuspid annulus.[11,12]

Functionally, the right atrium serves as a reservoir for systemic venous blood returning to the heart during ventricular systole, as a conduit during the majority of diastolic filling, and as a contractile chamber to augment right ventricular filling just before tricuspid valve closure. Its volume increases throughout the systolic reservoir phase and is greatest at end-systole just before tricuspid valve opening.[12]

The right atrium has no natural long or short axes, and as a result, these axes, like those of the left atrium, are defined relative to the axes of surrounding structures, particularly, the right ventricle. The long axis of the right atrium, therefore, is considered to lie in the same plane as that of the right ventricle and, thus, to extend from the tricuspid annulus to the superior atrial border. The short axis lies within a plane perpendicular to the long axis and runs from the interatrial septum to the free right atrial wall. Both of these axes should roughly bisect the corresponding geometric areas of the atrium.

Examining Planes and Linear Dimensions

The right atrium can be recorded in several of the standard imaging planes or modifications thereof, including (1) the apical four-chamber view, (2) the subxiphoid long axis, (3) the parasternal long axis of the right ventricular inflow tract, and (4) a parasternal short axis at the aortic valve level, which is angled rightward to record the right atrial chamber. The primary view for recording atrial dimensions and estimating volume changes has been the apical four-chamber view (Fig. 26–35). In this image orientation, the scan plane transects

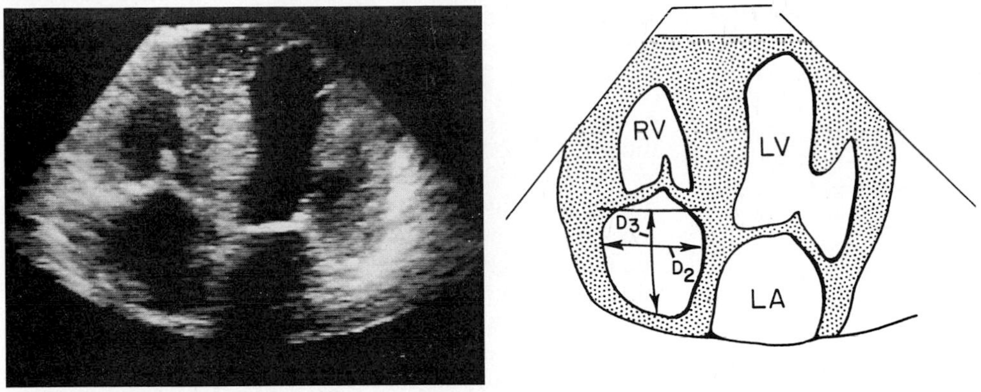

Fig. 26–35. Apical four-chamber view illustrates a method for obtaining right atrial linear dimensions. The inferior-superior dimension (D_3) is taken from the tricuspid annulus to the superior wall of the atrium. The medial-lateral dimension (D_2) is taken as the length of the line that extends from the interatrial septum to the free lateral atrial wall. This dimension roughly bisects D_3. RV = right ventricle; LV = left ventricle; LA = left atrium.

the atrium from the tricuspid annulus to the superior atrial wall, with the X-axis parallel to a line running from the interatrial septum medially to the free right atrial wall laterally. Two axes or dimensions of the right atrium can be defined in the apical four-chamber view. These axes are illustrated in Figure 26–35 and include an inferior-superior dimension or long axis (D_3)*, which extends from the midpoint of the tricuspid annulus to the superior border of the right atrium and should roughly bisect the geometric area of this chamber. The second dimension (D_2) is taken from the medial to lateral aspects of the atrium in a plane that is perpendicular to the long axis. Because the atrium is relatively circular in this view, the minor dimension (D_2) should roughly bisect both the long axis and the geometric area of the atrium and represents the longest medial-lateral dimension that can be obtained in this plane. Other methods for obtaining the right atrial long axis have been suggested and include a maximal superior-inferior dimension[98] and a dimension from the medial insertion of the tricuspid valve drawn along the right margin of the interatrial septum to the posterior atrial wall.[104] I prefer to relate these linear dimensions to the axes of the ventricle and, hence, to draw them such that they roughly bisect the atrium. This method is also consistent with the method for obtaining left atrial dimensions.

Linear dimensions used to estimate atrial size are, by convention, taken at the point of maximal atrial volume or at end-ventricular systole. In normal persons, the reported mean superior-inferior dimension of the right atrium at end-systole is 4.2 ± 0.4 cm.[128] The end-systolic right atrial medial-to-lateral dimension (short axis) appears slightly smaller, averaging 3.7 ± 0.4 cm.[128] The normal area of the right atrium has been reported to average 13.5 ± 2 cm^2.[128] The change in right atrial size that occurs during systolic atrial filling is primarily due to apical displacement of the tricuspid annulus. The long axis or superior-inferior dimension, therefore, increases throughout systole, whereas the medial-lateral dimension remains fairly constant.

The right atrium has been reported to dilate in both right ventricular volume and pressure overload states.[98] This dilation is characteristically symmetric, with an increase in both the inferior-superior and medial-lateral dimensions.[104] Figure 26–36 compares the right atrial long and short axis dimensions in a group of normal patients with patients with right ventricular volume overload that is due to both tricuspid regurgitation and atrial septal defect.

A comparable orthogonal image of the right atrium can also be recorded in the subcostal long axis view.[4] In this orientation, the imaging plane transects the atrium from the free right atrial wall to the interatrial septum. The x axis of the imaging plane is oriented parallel to a line running from the tricuspid annulus to the superior atrial border. The linear dimensions recorded in this plane are the same as those observed in the apical four-chamber view. In children, the right atrium may be more easily visualized in the subcostal orientation, and hence, this view offers a preferred alternative to the four-chamber view. In adults, however, the image quality is rarely as good from the subcostal transducer location, and although comparable dimensions can be obtained, the four-chamber view is clearly preferred.

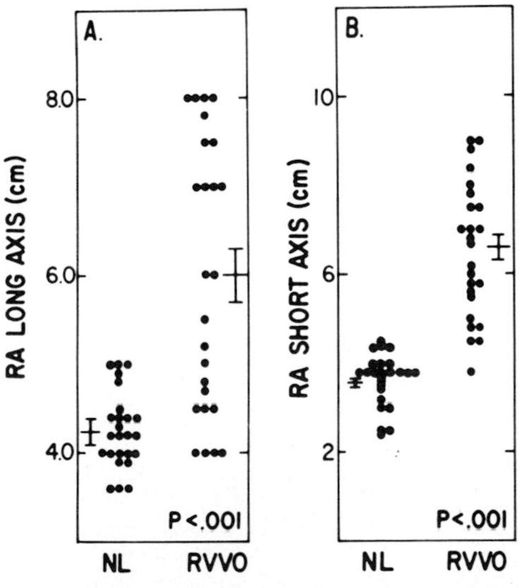

Fig. 26–36. Comparisons of the means and ranges of right atrial (RA) dimensions in normal persons (NL) and patients with right ventricular volume overload (RVVO). (From Bommer W, et al.: Determination of right atrial and right ventricular size by two-dimensional echocardiography. Circulation 60:91, 1979. Reproduced with permission of the American Heart Association, Inc.)

* The designation of these dimensions is intended to correspond to the method used to denote the corresponding left atrial dimensions. A standardized method for recording a right atrial anteroposterior dimension (D_1) has not yet been defined.

The right atrium can also be recorded in a parasternal long axis view of the right ventricular inflow tract (Fig. 26–37). In this view, the imaging plane passes obliquely through the atrium from the left anterior to the right posterior borders. Both oblique anteroposterior and superior-inferior dimensions of the atrium can be obtained in this projection; however, their relationship to right atrial size and their reproducibility have not been evaluated. The oblique orientation of this plane relative to the right atrium suggests that the four-chamber or subcostal views are preferred.

The parasternal short axis view of the right atrium is even less valuable because the free right border of the atrium can rarely be recorded from this transducer location. The primary role of this view is in defining the anteroposterior orientation of the interatrial septum. The aorta and anterior insertion of the interatrial septum may become displaced to the left in patients with right atrial dilation, thereby shifting the orientation of the interatrial septum toward the left shoulder. This change in position of the aorta and interatrial septum can be seen only in the short axis view (see Chapter 29).

Right Atrial Volume

Little information is available concerning the calculation of right atrial volume. This is due to the lack of a readily available, accurate gold standard and a theoretically sound echocardiographic approach to volume calculation. Right atrial volume can be calculated from the apical four-chamber view using a length-diameter ellipsoid formula assuming that the two minor axes are approximately equal. It could also be approximated by taking the measured length and diameter from the apical four-chamber view and measuring or calculating an orthogonal minor axis from the parasternal long axis view of the atrium. Unfortunately, all of these methods require some fundamental assumption, and as a result, none can be recommended without reservation. Clearly, the most accurate method in the future will be by three-dimensional reconstruction of the atrium. Figure 26–38 illustrates a three-dimensional reconstruction of the canine right atrium with the rest of the heart outlined. Once the boundaries of the chamber are outlined, volume can be calculated automatically using several surfacing algorithms.

Anomalies Resulting From Lack of Normal Regression of the Embryonic Right or Inferior Valve of the Sinus Venosus

During early cardiac development, the right horn of the sinus venosus is guarded by two valves, the right and left venous valves. The right valve normally regresses between the ninth and fifteenth week of gestation, with the superior portion forming the crista terminalis and the inferior portion developing into the eustachian valve of the inferior vena cava and the thebesian valve of the coronary sinus. The inferior or right sinus valve is responsible for directing blood toward the atrial septum and accounts for the fact that a significant portion of the inferior vena caval return crosses the atrial septum to the left atrium. Lack of normal regression of the right valve of the sinus venosus can result in abnormalities ranging from partial septation of the right atrium by a prominent eustachian valve to complete division of the right atrium (cor triatriatum dexter). Alternatively, the right valve of the sinus venosus may form a pendulous wind-sock-like structure. Depending on the length of the stalk and where it is carried by blood flow, the wind sock may obstruct the tricuspid orifice, right ventricular outflow tract, inferior vena cava, or atrial septal defect. Extensive fenestration of the right venous valve can result in a weblike Chiari network.

The Eustachian Valve

The eustachian valve, or the valve of the inferior vena cava, is frequently visualized within the right atrium. This valve is formed by a fold of endocardium that arises from the lower end of the crista terminalis and stretches across the posterior margin of the inferior vena cava to become continuous with the border of the fossa ovalis.[11] The eustachian valve is most obvious in the parasternal long axis view of the right ventricular inflow tract,[129] in which it appears as a horizontal linear echo arising along the inferior border of the atrium just below the lower margin of the tricuspid annulus. The eustachian valve is evident in Figures 26–1, 26–8, and 26–9. When large, the eustachian valve may show considerable (2 cm) rapid movement within the right atrial cavity[129] and has been confused on M-mode studies with right atrial catheters, vegetations, and tumors. This structure can be

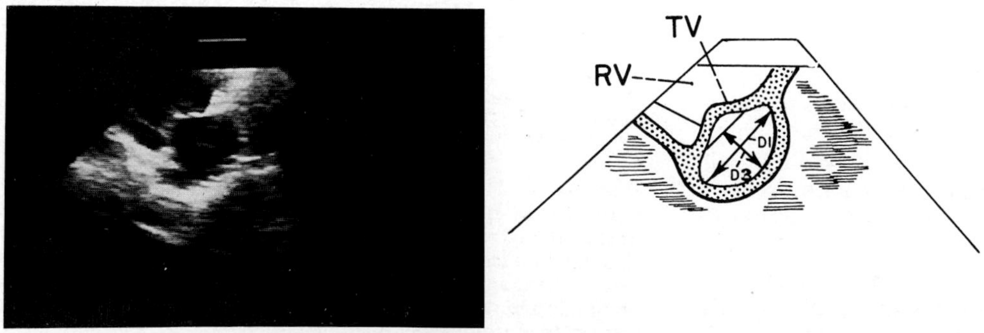

Fig. 26–37. Parasternal long axis recording of a normal right atrium. As indicated in the accompanying diagram, both an anteroposterior dimension (D_1) and a superior-inferior dimension (D_3) can be obtained from this view. Because the plane obliquely transects the atrium, the significance of dimensions obtained in this projection remains to be established. TV = tricuspid valve; RV = right ventricle.

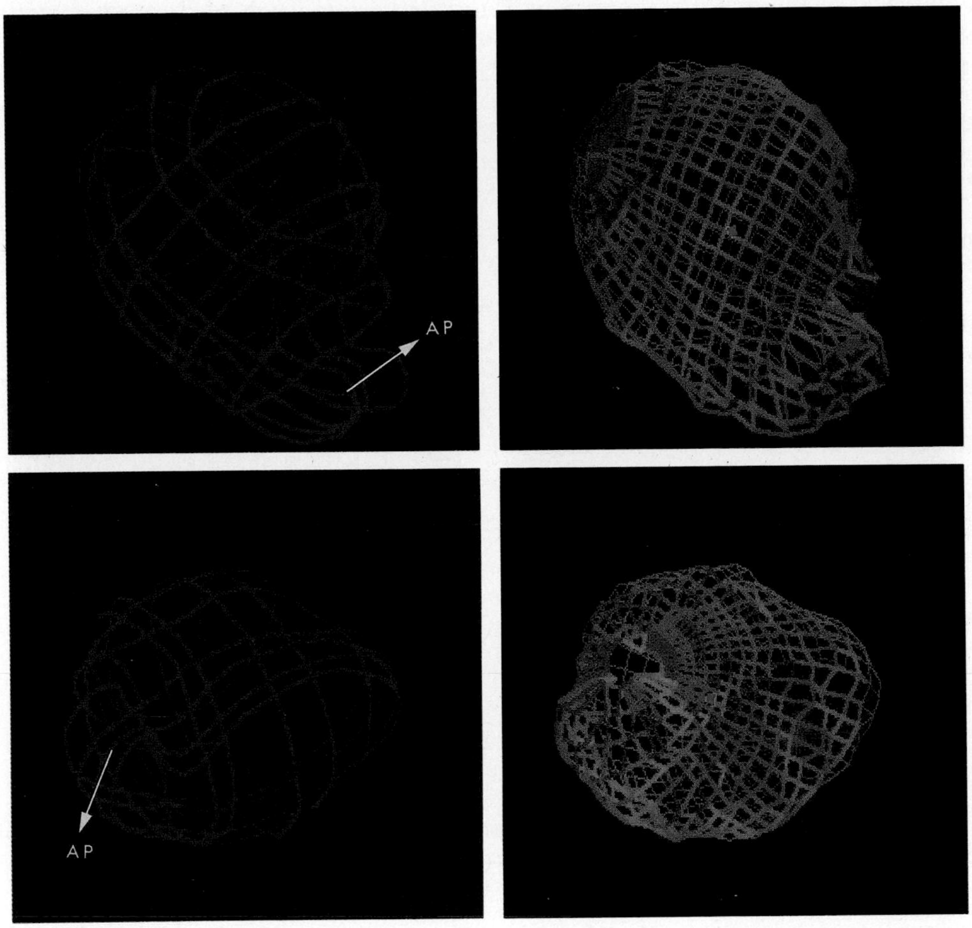

Fig. 26–38. Three-dimensional reconstruction of the canine right atrium recorded in two different projections. Left. Digitized tracings form a wire frame. AP = appendage. Right. Computer surfacing.

readily identified on cross-sectional examination, however, by its origin from the margin of the inferior vena cava and its characteristic orientation within the atrium.[129]

Chiari Network

A Chiari network is a membranous structure that is similar to but generally more extensive than a eustachian valve. The membranous Chiari network is usually fenestrated and like the eustachian valve is associated with the orifice of the inferior vena cava.[130] There is, however, variability in the primary origin of the network with attachment to the right atrial wall, coronary sinus, and interatrial septum being observed pathologically.[131] Figure 26–39 illustrates a Chiari network excised at surgery. This honeycombed membrane was attached near the orifice of the inferior vena cava.

Echocardiographically, a Chiari network appears similar to but is more extensively attached than a Eustachian valve. It presents as one or more highly mobile curvilinear echoes in the right atrium that can move toward but generally not through the tricuspid valve during diastole. The largest excursion toward the tricuspid orifice occurs with atrial contraction, followed by a rapid posterior motion toward the posterior right atrial wall at the onset of systole.[127] The Chiari network can be visualized in any of the standard views of the right atrium and is commonly recorded in multiple planes.[127,132]

This congenital remnant is seldom of clinical importance but has been reported to be a site of thrombus formation as well as a site of entrapment for right-heart catheters.[133]

Cor Triatriatum Dexter

Cor triatriatum dexter is a rare cardiac malformation that results from persistence of the embryonic right

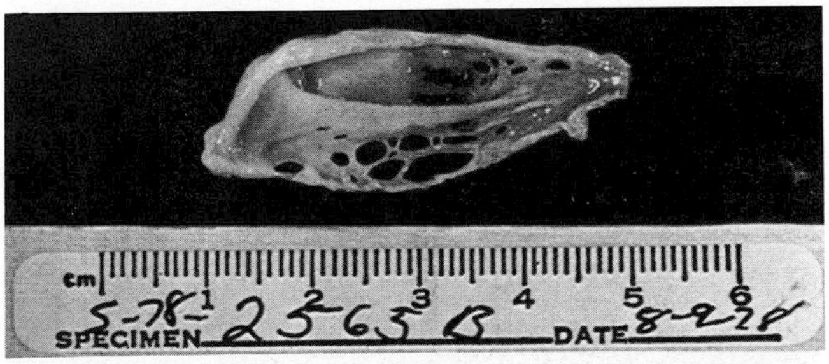

Fig. 26–39. Pathologic specimen excised at surgery from the right atrium, attached near the orifice of the inferior vena cava. Note the honeycombed or "network-like" appearance of this structure. (From Werner JA, et al.: Echocardiographic appearance of the Chiari network: differentiation from right-heart pathology. Circulation 63:1104, 1981. Reproduced by permission of the American Heart Association, Inc.)

valve of the sinus venosus and its division of the right atrium into two separate chambers. The upstream chamber receives superior and inferior vena caval flow, while the downstream chamber incorporates the right atrial appendage. In this situation, venous flow is directed to the upstream chamber and subsequently across an atrial septal defect to the left atrium, resulting in a right-to-left shunt. As the membrane is usually perforated, there is also some flow across the membrane into the downstream chamber and through the tricuspid orifice into the right ventricle.

Echocardiographically, the anomalous membrane is best imaged in the subcostal views, although apical imaging should provide similar information. The membrane is generally seen running from the inferior vena cava to the superior vena cava, separating the right atrial appendage and tricuspid valve from the great veins. The coronary sinus usually empties into the upstream chamber, but exceptions do occur. Right-to-left shunting through the atrial septal defect can be demonstrated by contrast or pulsed or color flow Doppler. In addition, flow can be recorded transversing the membrane and entering the lower chamber and passing through the tricuspid valve. A normal tricuspid orifice and right ventricle are typically present, which serves to distinguish this lesion from tricuspid atresia. Normal motion of the tricuspid valve also should distinguish this entity from tricuspid stenosis.

Large eustachian valves and the valve of cor triatriatum dexter have been reported to increase right-to-left shunting in patients with atrial septal defect by directing inferior vena caval flow through the defect into the left atrium. This finding is important because it can produce cyanosis in the absence of an elevated right atrial pressure.[134–136]

Right Atrial Tumors

A variety of tumors, either primarily or secondarily, involve the right atrium (see also Chapter 36). These tumors may be intracavitary, mural, or extramural. The most common primary intracavitary tumors are right atrial myxomas and sarcomas (particularly angiosarcomas). Secondary extension into the right atrium may be seen with hypernephroma, hepatoma, sarcomas of the testes, and other less common lesions, such as the leiomyosarcoma of the inferior vena cava.

The right atrium is the site of origin of approximately 15% of cardiac myxomas. Right atrial myxomas typically arise from the right side of the interatrial septum in the region of the fossa ovalis. They may occur alone or may be associated with left atrial myxomas. Right atrial myxomas may be solitary or multiple, stationary or mobile. They may be small or may grow to almost completely fill the atrial cavity.

The echocardiographic appearance of right atrial myxomas is similar to the appearance of those arising in the left atrium. They are typically spherical or globular with well-defined borders and multiple internal reflective interfaces that give a speckled appearance to the tumor mass.[86] Right atrial myxomata are usually mobile, moving toward or into the tricuspid orifice during diastole, and being thrust back into the right atrial cavity at the onset of ventricular systole. When large, they may obstruct the tricuspid orifice, thereby producing functional tricuspid stenosis (Figs. 36–11 to 36–13 illustrate the M-mode and two-dimensional echo appearance of right atrial myxomas). The tumor appears as a ball-like mass of echoes lying within the right atrial cavity during systole and prolapsing downward into the tricuspid orifice during diastole.

A variety of tumors secondarily involve the right atrium by extension from the inferior vena cava. Figure 26–40 illustrates a large, echo-producing mass growing out of the inferior vena cava into the right atrium, which subsequently proved to be a hepatoma. The intra-atrial portion of the mass was mobile, and during diastole, the leading edge extended through the tricuspid orifice.

Mural right atrial tumors may arise primarily from the atrial wall or may result from secondary invasion. Figure 26–41 is an example of a metastatic tumor that has invaded the atrial and proximal ventricular walls in the region of the tricuspid annulus. In this example, the tumor is characterized by a focal increase in echo production and regional thickening of the atrial wall. Both mural and intracavitary metastatic tumors may also produce an irregular distortion in the normally smooth margins of the atrium, thereby highlighting their presence and facilitating their detection (see also Chapter 36). Compression of the right atrium can also be observed as a result of loculated postoperative hematoma (see Chapter 35).[137,138] Rupture of the right atrium with blood flow into the pericardial space and loculated hematoma

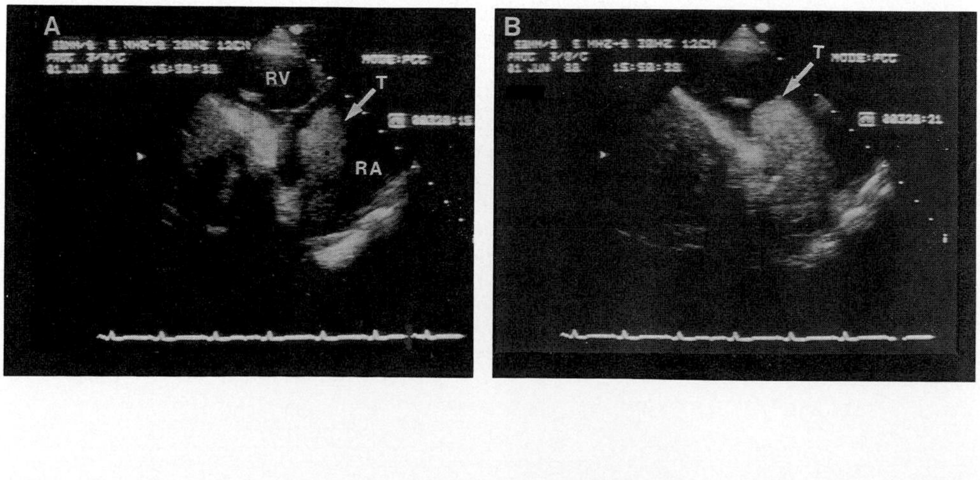

Fig. 26–40. Systolic **(A)** and diastolic **(B)** parasternal long axis inflow views illustrating a large tumor (T) extending from the inferior vena cava into the right atrium (RA). During diastole the tumor extends into the tricuspid valve orifice partially obstructing inflow. (RV = right ventricle.)

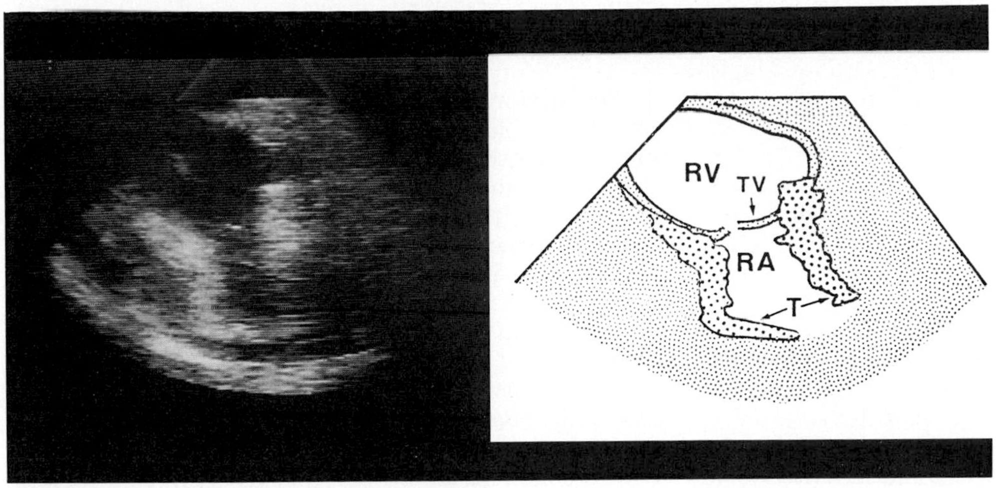

Fig. 26–41. Parasternal long axis recording of the right ventricular inflow region from a patient with metastatic adenocarcinoma. An increase in echo density from the walls of the right atrium (RA) and tricuspid annulus is consistent with tumor infiltration (T). The area of increased echo production is indicated by the stippled area in the accompanying diagram. A pericardial effusion is also present. RV = right ventricle; TV = tricuspid valve.

has also been reported in a patient with a right atrial angiosarcoma.[139]

Right Atrial Thrombi

Both fixed and freely mobile thrombi can be recorded in the right atrium.[140,141] Fixed thrombi usually originate in the right atrium, have a broad-based attachment to the atrial wall, and show little movement.[142] Fixed thrombi are usually found in patients with low cardiac output, dilated right atrium, and relative stasis of blood. They may also arise from the presence of foreign bodies or following endocardial trauma (e.g., catheter-induced abrasion).[143] Peripherally arising thromboemboli, in contrast, are usually freely mobile, show no obvious attachment to the right atrial wall, and may remain within the atrial cavity or move back and forth across the tricuspid valve. Thromboemboli tend to have a rotational pattern of motion in the right atrium. On occasion, right-sided intracavitary thromboemboli can become wedged in or pass through a patent foramen ovale. They can also become trapped within the tricuspid valve apparatus.[141] Freely mobile thromboemboli may on occasion be evident in the right atrium for several days[141,144] and are commonly associated with pulmonary emboli.[145] Thromboemboli can also be detected extending from the inferior vena cava into the right atrium. This topic is discussed and illustrated in more detail in Chapter 36.

Venous Catheters

A variety of venous catheters can be visualized within the right ventricular inflow tract. The most common of these are transvenous pacing catheter and Swan-Ganz catheters. These catheters typically appear as elongated, thin, linear echoes that course through the inflow tract and may be detected in the right ventricle, right atrium, or right ventricular outflow tract. Their movement is comparable in timing and direction to that of the anterior tricuspid leaflet; however, it is typically damped when compared with leaflet motion. The catheter echoes may be single or associated with multiple linear reverberations that can be visualized posterior to the catheter. When the catheter is visualized, the source of these reverberations is readily apparent. On occasion, reverberations from a catheter may be detected within the left side of the heart, even though the right-heart catheter is not recorded. Recognition of the source of these abnormal echoes requires that the examiner be familiar with this potential artifact as well as with the clinical setting in which the study was recorded. Figure 26–42 is an example of a pacing catheter coursing through the right atrium. This catheter appears as a thin, strand-like echo arcing gradually through the posterior portion of the right atrium toward the tricuspid orifice.

Cross-sectional echocardiography may be helpful in demonstrating the position of right ventricular pacing catheters[146] and biopsy forceps. Coronary sinus cathe-

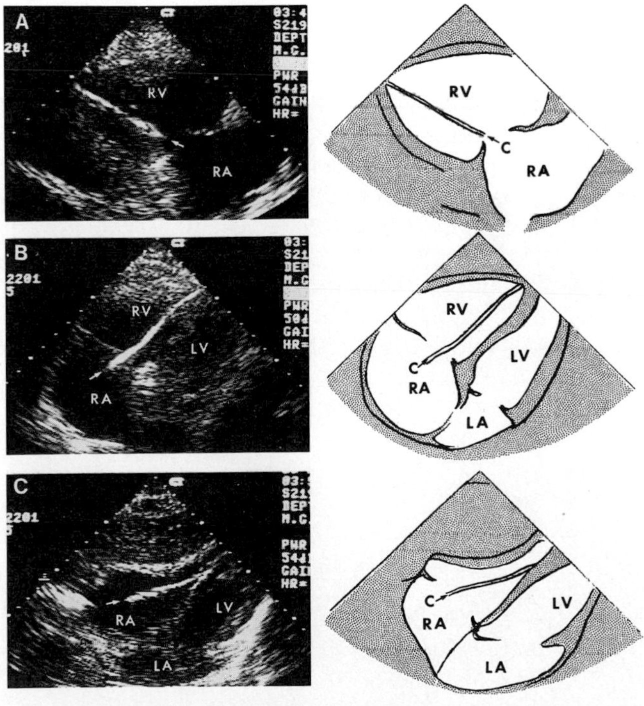

Fig. 26–42. Parasternal long axis **(A)**, modified apical four-chamber view **(B)**, and subcostal four-chamber views **(C)** illustrating a bright, thin linear echo arising from a transvenous pacing catheter (C) coursing through the right atrial and ventricular cavities to the right ventricular apex. RA = right atrium; RV = right ventricle; LA = left atrium; LV = left ventricle.

ters can also be demonstrated near the base of the atrial septum and within the sinus.[146]

Right Atrial Flow

Flow in the right atrium is complex because it originates from the inferior vena cava, the superior vena cava, and the coronary sinus. Near the orifices of each of these sources of inflow, the velocity patterns are similar to those in the vessel from which it originates and are determined by the pressure gradient between the right atrium and the venous reservoir. Between the orifice and the tricuspid valve, these flow streams must combine to form the flow pattern across the valve. Figure 26–43 is a color flow recording that illustrates the flow streams arising from the inferior and superior venae cavae joining during diastole and the combined flow volume crossing the tricuspid valve. An atrial septal defect adds an additional source of flow to the right atrium, whose pattern varies with the pressure gradient between the left and right atria. Although color Doppler can often identify the source of flow entering the right atrium, the timing of the flow velocities by pulsed Doppler is occasionally necessary for accurate separation. This is particularly true in the infant and small child with an atrial septal defect where the superior vena caval and left-to-right shunt are close together and can be difficult to separate. Figure 26–44 summarizes the various flow patterns that can be seen entering the right atrium. Each of these patterns is discussed in detail in the appropriate section.

THE VENAE CAVAE

The Inferior Vena Cava

The inferior vena cava arises from the confluence of the common iliac veins anterior to the fifth lumbar vertebra and courses superiorly to penetrate the diaphragm and insert into the inferior border of the right atrium.[11] In the adult, this vessel extends roughly 8 inches and receives numerous tributaries, the most important of which (from an echocardiographic standpoint) are the hepatic veins. The hepatic veins insert into the anterior border of the inferior vena cava just proximal to the diaphragm.

The inferior vena cava is oriented parallel to the long axis of the body. It normally lies to the right of the midline and is anterior to the abdominal aorta, from which it must be differentiated. Echocardiographic differentiation of the inferior vena cava from the aorta is achieved by noting the absence of typical arterial pulsations, by observing the insertions of the hepatic veins into its anterior border, by following its course into the right atrium, and by Doppler recording of the characteristic biphasic venous profile directed toward the heart.

The inferior vena cava is typically recorded in both long and short axis projections with the transducer placed over the anterior abdominal wall or in the subcostal region. Because the vessel runs parallel to the long axis of the body, the imaging plane orientations roughly parallel the corresponding anatomic planes. Because only soft tissue is interposed between the vena cava and abdominal walls, this vessel is easily recorded and should be available for examination in almost every pa-

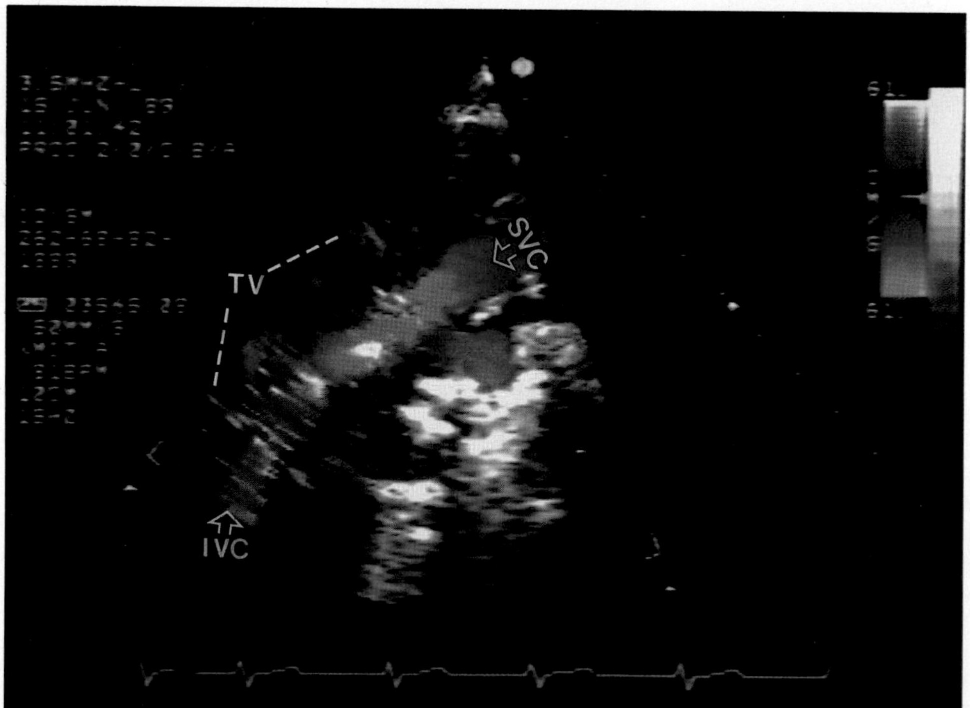

Fig. 26–43. Right parasternal long axis recording illustrating the confluence of superior vena caval flow (blue) and inferior vena caval flow (red) in the right atrium. The flow streams join in the posterior portion of the atrium, and in this systolic frame, there is recirculation (darker red) in the anterior portion of the chamber. The tricuspid valve (TV) plane is indicated by the interrupted lines. SVC = superior vena cava; IVC = inferior vena cava.

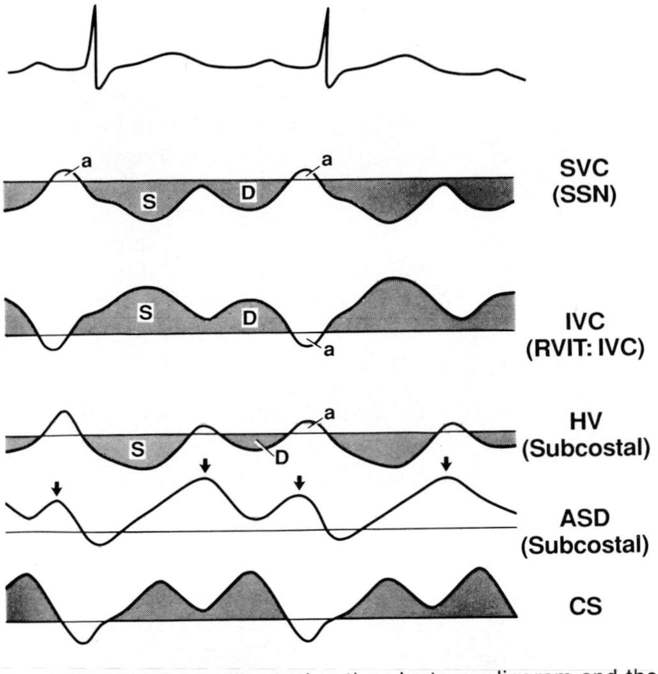

Fig. 26–44. Diagram illustrating the electrocardiogram and the normal pulsed wave Doppler spectral waveforms for right atrial venous inflow as well as the spectral waveform for an uncomplicated atrial septal defect (ASD). Note the similarities in the timing of the peak flow velocities for the superior vena cava (SVC), inferior vena cava (IVC), and hepatic vein (HV), which occur in midsystole and early diastole (shaded areas of SVC, IVC, and HV). To differentiate normal venous and right atrial inflow from uncomplicated ASD, it is important to note that the peak flow velocity in an ASD occurs during late systole and with atrial contraction (arrows). The nadir of ASD flow occurs in early ventricular systole, whereas venous inflow begins to peak. Also, remember that in response to inspiration, flow will decrease across an ASD whereas venous flow will increase (not illustrated). SSN = suprasternal notch; RVIT = right ventricular inflow tract; CS = coronary sinus; S = systolic flow; D = diastolic flow. (From Reynolds T, Appleton CP: Doppler flow velocity patterns of the superior vena cava, inferior vena cava, hepatic vein, coronary sinus, and atrial septal defect: A guide for the echocardiographer. J Am Soc Echocardiogr 4:503, 1991.)

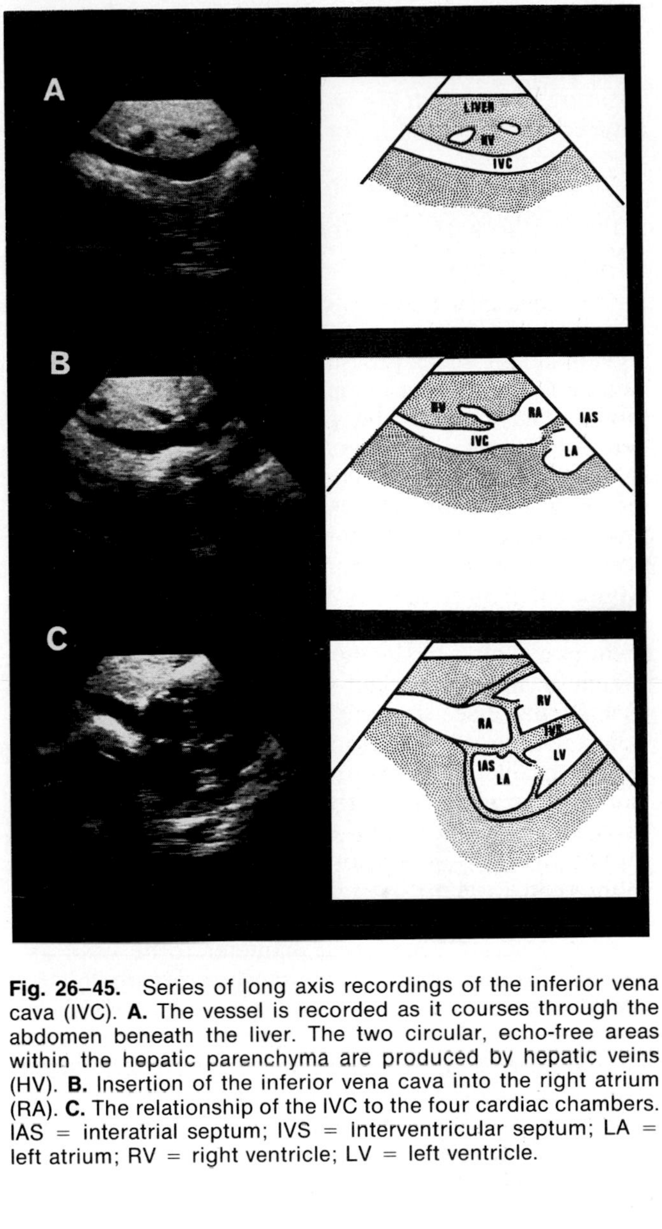

Fig. 26–45. Series of long axis recordings of the inferior vena cava (IVC). **A.** The vessel is recorded as it courses through the abdomen beneath the liver. The two circular, echo-free areas within the hepatic parenchyma are produced by hepatic veins (HV). **B.** Insertion of the inferior vena cava into the right atrium (RA). **C.** The relationship of the IVC to the four cardiac chambers. IAS = interatrial septum; IVS = interventricular septum; LA = left atrium; RV = right ventricle; LV = left ventricle.

tient. Long axis views are conventionally displayed with the superior margin of the vessel to the right of the display, whereas short axis views are displayed as if viewed from below with the left margin of the vena cava positioned to the right of the display. Figure 26–45 illustrates the long axis appearance of the inferior vena cava in the abdominal cavity beneath the liver (Fig. 26–45A), as it courses through the diaphragm and inserts into the right atrial cavity (Fig. 26–45B), and as it relates to the other cardiac chambers (Fig. 26–45C).

In the long axis projection, the vessel appears as a broad, linear, nonpulsatile, echo-free space with parallel margins and smooth borders. The hepatic veins join the vena cava from above, inserting at approximately a 30° angle. They are smaller in diameter and can be seen arising from within the parenchyma of the liver. In short axis, the inferior vena cava appears circular. The insertion points of multiple hepatic veins can frequently be recorded if the short axis plane is positioned at the appropriate level.

Inferior Vena Caval Physiology

The proximal inferior vena cava is a thin-walled, highly compliant vessel that changes its diameter and cross-sectional area in parallel with changes in the blood volume and central venous pressure. Respiration and changes in intra-abdominal pressure have also been observed to rapidly influence the volume of the inferior vena cava. Because the inferior vena cava acts as a reservoir, increased return of blood to the right side of the heart during inspiration is accompanied by caval emptying and a decrease in both diameter and area.[147] The degree of emptying is determined by both the inferior vena cava-right atrium pressure gradient, which in turn varies with the mean right atrial pressure and the chamber/vessel compliance. It has been reported that an inspiratory decrease in inferior venal caval diameter of <50% has a predictive value 87% for a right atrial mean pressure of ≥10 mm Hg, while an index of ≥50% has a predictive value of 82% for a right atrial mean pressure of ≤10 mm Hg.

Abnormalities of the Inferior Vena Cava and Hepatic Veins

Abnormalities of the inferior vena cava and hepatic vein include (1) nonspecific dilation in patients with an elevated right atrial pressure; (2) loss of normal vena caval collapse during inspiration (3) inferior vena cava dilation that is due to abnormal venous inflow in infants with total anomalous pulmonary venous connection to the inferior vena cava or one of its tributaries;[148] (4) interrupted inferior vena cava (see Chapter 31); and (5) primary or secondary tumors and thrombi of the inferior vena cava with or without extension into the right atrium.

The inferior vena caval diameter increases in patients with an elevated mean right atrial pressure that is due to right heart failure, right ventricular hypertension, tricuspid valve disease, pericardial tamponade, or pericardial constriction.[149] Often, inferior vena caval and hepatic vein dilation provide one of the earliest anatomic marks of an increase in right atrial pressure. A rough correlation between vena caval diameter measured by M-mode and two-dimensional echocardiography and absolute right atrial pressure has been observed.[147,150] Unfortunately, this relationship has not been strong enough to allow inferior vena caval diameter to be used as a predictor of mean right atrial pressure. Figure 26–46 illustrates the long and short axis appearance of the inferior vena cava in a patient with cardiomyopathy and combined right and left ventricular failure. Dilation of both the vena cava and hepatic veins is prominent, and the points of insertion of the distended hepatic veins into the vena cava are clearly evident.

Relationship of Cyclic and Respiratory Changes in Inferior Vena Caval Size to Specific Disease States. Abnormal changes in the diameter of the inferior vena cava during the cardiac and respiratory cycle can be observed in specific disease states. For example, in patients with severe tricuspid regurgitation, not only dilation but also systolic expansion of the vessel may be evident.[150,151] Loss of the normal inspiratory decrease in inferior vena cava size can be observed in both tamponade and constrictive pericarditis. A change in diameter of <50% has been reported to be a sensitive but nonspecific marker of tamponade in patients with moderate or large pericardial effusion.[151]

Tumors and Thrombi of the Inferior Vena Cava. A variety of tumors can extend into the inferior vena cava from the organs it drains, causing partial or total obstruction. The most common are the hypernephroma, hepatoma, Wilm's tumor, lymphosarcoma, and leiomyosarcoma. Extramural tumors within the abdomen can also compress the vessel. Intraluminal tumors often extend into the right atrium and can cause tricuspid inflow obstruction (Fig. 26–40). Thrombi can also develop within the vena cava, particularly when there is stenosis from some other cause. Peripheral thromboemboli pass through the vena cava but are most often visualized when they pause or become entrapped in the right atrium.

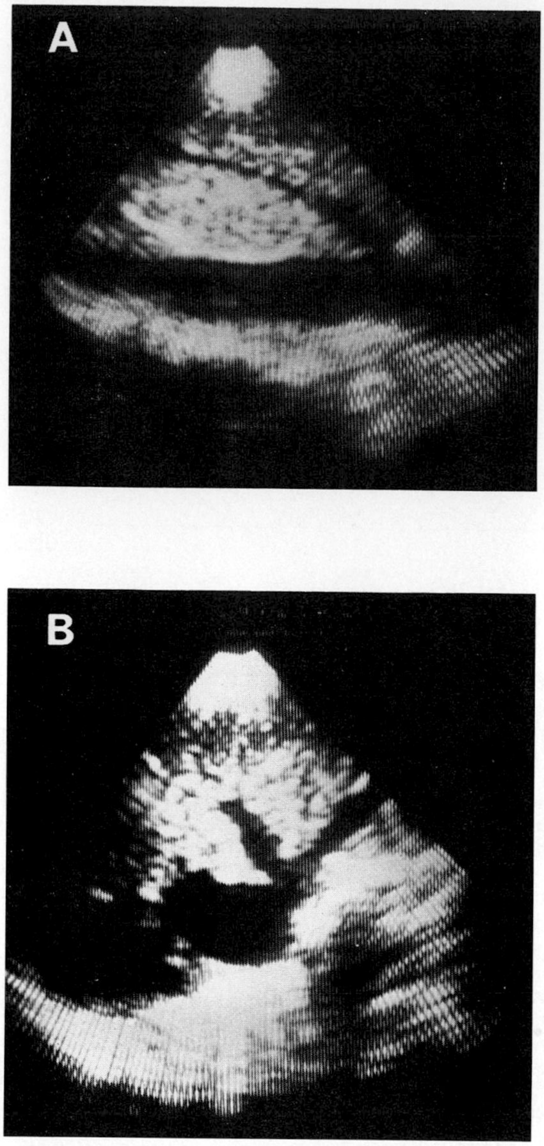

Fig. 26–46. Long and short axis recordings of a dilated inferior vena cava. **A.** In the long axis, the dilated vessel is recorded as it passes beneath the liver to its penetration through the diaphragm at the right margin of the scan. A single hepatic vein inserts into the anterior margin of the vessel just proximal to the level of the diaphragm. **B.** In short axis, the dilated circular vessel, with two hepatic veins entering its anterior margin, can be seen.

Inferior Vena Caval and Hepatic Vein Flow

The patterns of flow in the inferior vena cava and hepatic veins are similar and are best recorded from a subcostal transducer location. Because the ultrasonic beam is easily aligned parallel to hepatic vein flow from this transducer location but intersects the inferior vena cava at a more acute angle, Doppler sampling of hepatic flow velocities near the junction of the two vessels is usually used to represent flow in both vessels. Figure 26–47A illustrates normal flow recorded by pulsed Doppler in the hepatic vein. There is flow toward the right atrium (away from the transducer) during both systole and diastole. A small retrograde flow wave is typically recorded following atrial systole and at end ventricular systole. The forward flow during systole is in response to the fall in atrial pressure that accompanies atrial relaxation and the downward displacement of the tricuspid annulus as the right ventricle contracts. Forward diastolic flow is due to the fall in atrial pressure that accompanies ventricular filling.

Major respiratory changes can be seen in the right-sided venous flow patterns in normal subjects and in patients with various disease entities.[152] During inspiration, forward flow velocity is increased and reversal is

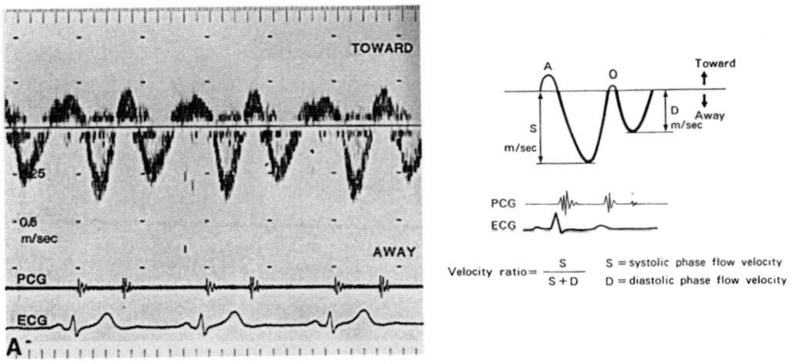

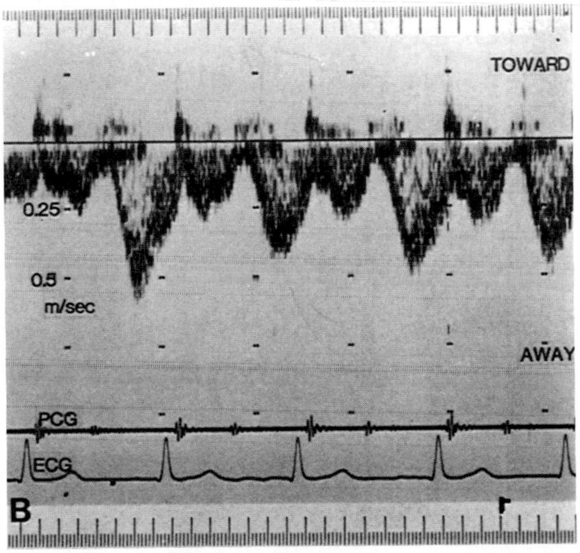

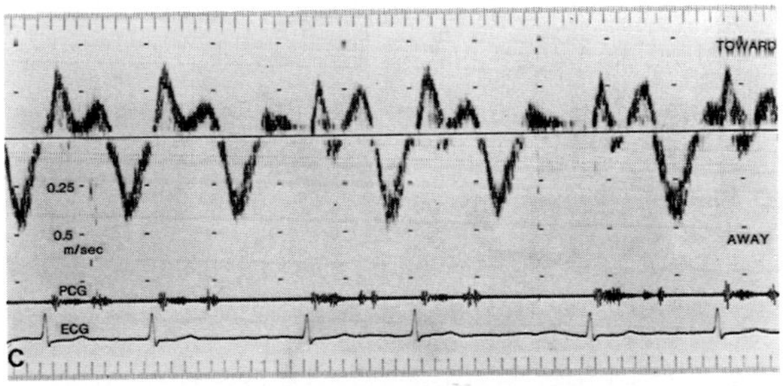

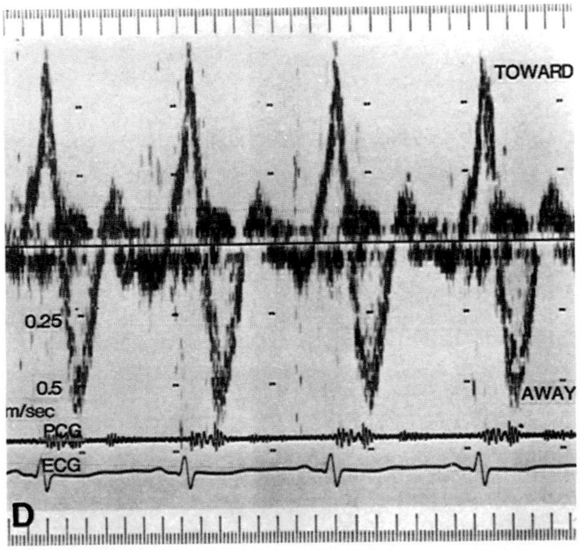

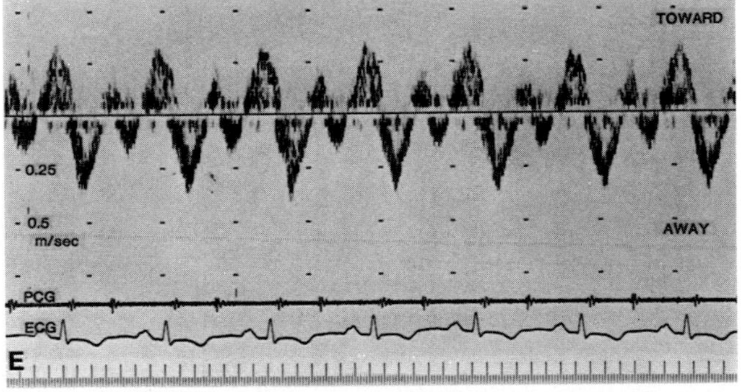

Fig. 26–47. Hepatic vein flow in patients with a variety of abnormalities. **A.** Normal. There is minimal reversed flow during atrial systole (A wave) and forward flows during ventricular systole (S wave) and diastole (D wave). The relationship between systolic flow velocity (S) and diastolic flow velocity (D) is expressed as the velocity ratio [S/(S + D)]. **B.** Atrial fibrillation. The systolic flow velocity is less than the diastolic flow velocity. **C.** Severe tricuspid regurgitation. Reversed flow is present during ventricular systole. **D.** Pulmonary hypertension. Reversed flow during atrial systole is prominent. **E.** Constrictive pericarditis. Prominent reversed flow during atrial systole. ECG = electrocardiogram; PCG = phonocardiogram. (From Sakoda S, Mitsunami K, Kinoshita M: Evaluation of hepatic venous flow patterns using a pulsed Doppler technique. J Cardiol 20:193, 1990.)

diminished. With the onset of expiration, increased reversal can be observed, and forward velocity is slightly less than during apnea.[152] Abnormalities of venous flow are seen in patients with atrial fibrillation, tricuspid regurgitation, abnormalities of right ventricular relaxation, and decreased compliance.

In patients with atrial fibrillation, the normal flow reversal seen during atrial relaxation is absent (Fig. 26–47B). Systolic forward flow velocity is also diminished, because it is partially due to atrial relaxation. Severe tricuspid regurgitation causes a large retrograde systolic flow volume from the right ventricle into the right atrium and vena cava, reversing the normal antegrade direction of systolic flow (Fig. 26–47C). Because all forward flow occurs during diastole, antegrade diastolic velocities are typically increased. Patients with lesser degrees of tricuspid regurgitation may have only a reduction in or cessation of the systolic forward flow velocity.[152] Note that the pattern of hepatic vein and vena caval flow depends not only on the degree of tricuspid regurgitation but also on atrial size and compliance as well as atrial and ventricular function. When tricuspid regurgitation occurs in conjunction with atrial fibrillation, the degree of flow reversal will be greater than when tricuspid regurgitation occurs alone.

Abnormal right ventricular relaxation decreases the forward flow velocity during diastole (Fig. 26–47D). When relaxation abnormalities are severe, diastolic forward flow may be absent completely. When there is a decrease in compliance such as that seen with restrictive myopathy, the first finding is an increase in retrograde velocity during atrial contraction (Fig. 26–47E). With further progression of disease, systolic filling can be completely lost, and all forward flow may occur during diastole. In the later stages, rapid cessation of diastolic filling is noted, and reversed flow can occur before the onset of atrial contraction.[152] The point at which diastolic filling comes to predominate over systolic filling is determined by atrial contractility, right ventricular diastolic pressure, right ventricular systolic function, and coexistent tricuspid regurgitation. Respiratory changes are also noted in patients with restrictive cardiomyopathy. Typically, there is an increase in forward velocity during inspiration. In contrast to normal subjects, however, there is a greater degree of reversal during atrial contraction and ventricular systole. Holosystolic flow reversal can be seen, which is due to blending of these two retrograde components.[152]

The Superior Vena Cava

The superior vena cava is formed by the confluence of the right and left innominate veins beneath the first intercostal space and descends vertically to join the superior border of the right atrium at the level of the third right costal cartilage.[11] The superior vena cava can be recorded from the suprasternal notch or from the subcostal, transesophageal (Fig. 26–48), or parasternal win-

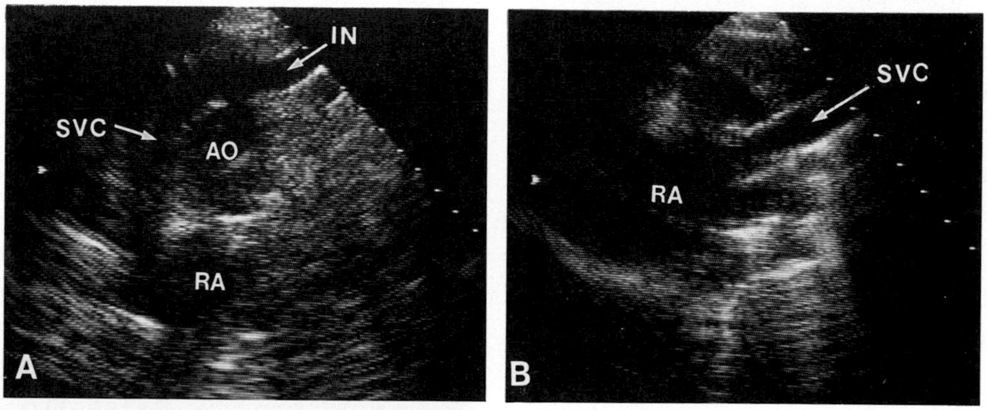

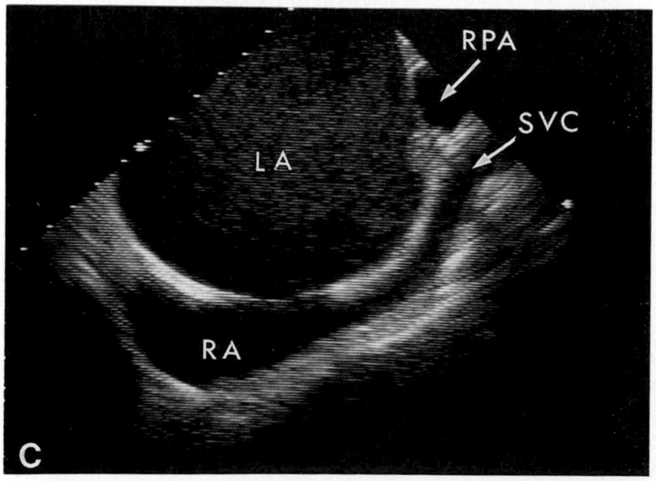

Fig. 26–48. **A.** Suprasternal notch recording of the superior vena cava (SVC) from its junction with the innominate vein (IN) to its insertion into the right atrium (RA). **B.** Superior vena cava and its insertion into the right atrium from the subcostal long axis view. **C.** Transesophageal long axis recording of the inferior vena cava and superior left atrium. AO = aorta; LA = left atrium; RPA = right pulmonary artery.

dows. The most direct approach is from the suprasternal notch with the transducer initially positioned to record a short axis view of the aortic arch. From this position, slight clockwise rotation and rightward angulation will bring the superior vena cava into view (Fig. 26–48A). Alternatively, the transducer can be positioned in the right supraclavicular window and directed inferiorly. Starting with the transducer parallel to the sagittal plane of the body, slight rotation of the transducer should permit the superior vena cava to be recorded. This plane orientation is also ideal for Doppler recording of superior venal caval flow.

The superior vena cava can also be recorded using a subcostal long axis view, which will display the vessel entering the superior margin of the right atrium and usually permits the great vein to be recorded for varying distances upstream (Fig. 26–48B).[4] In this plane orientation, the superior vena cava lies parallel and slightly anterior to the path of the ascending aorta. Transesophageal long axis recordings of the superior vena cava provide excellent resolution and structure definition of both the superior vena cava and right atrium (Fig. 26–48C).

Figure 26–49 illustrates the configuration of the superior vena cava in the parasternal long axis view of the right ventricular inflow tract. In this orientation, the vena cava courses from right to left, entering the anterosuperior margin of the right atrial cavity. If the scan plane is angled farther to the right in the parasternal long axis view, the anterior and posterior borders of the inferior and superior vena cava appear to join, forming two parallel arcuate echoes. The more anterior of these echoes is formed by the right margin of the tricuspid annulus, whereas the posterior echo appears to arise from a ridge, the crista terminalis, joining the posterior borders of the two great veins (Fig. 26–50). The right atrium lies beneath the posterior margin of this ridge. The superior vena cava can also be recorded from the esophagus.

Abnormalities of the Superior Vena Cava

Abnormalities of the superior vena cava that have been described to date includes (1) dilation, (2) anomalous superior vena caval drainage, (3) tumors, (4) thrombi and vegetations, and (5) persistence of the left superior vena cava.

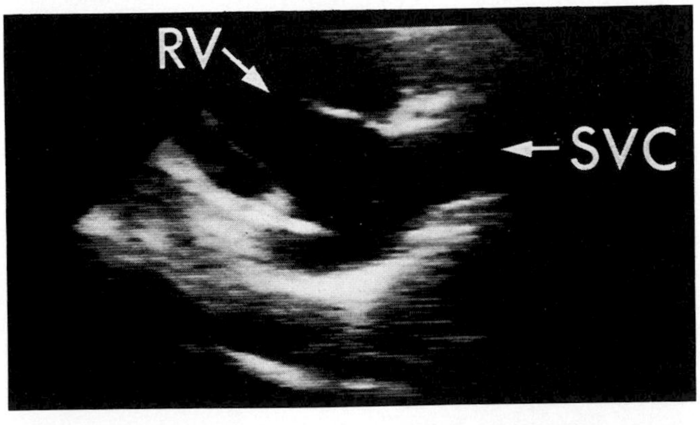

Fig. 26–49. Parasternal long axis recording of the right ventricular inflow tract illustrates the insertion of the superior vena cava into the superior right atrial wall. SVC = superior vena cava; RV = right ventricle.

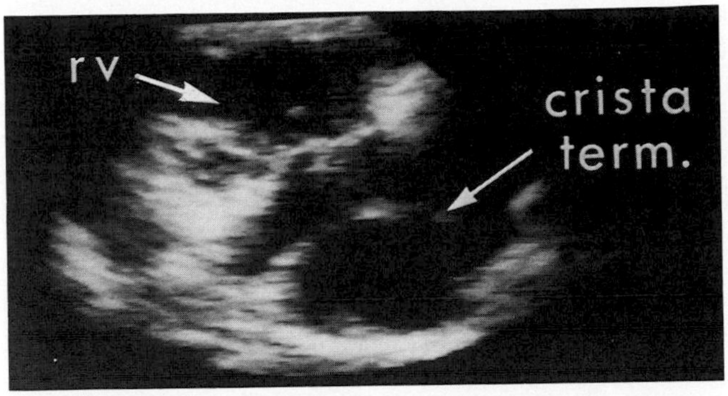

Fig. 26–50. Parasternal long axis scan of the right ventricular inflow tract. The scan plane is angled to the right toward the lateral wall of the right atrium. In this scan position, an arcuate groove is often recorded along the lateral wall of the right atrium between the tricuspid annulus and the crista terminalis. The lateral recess of the right atrium is also evident beneath the crista terminalis. RV = right ventricle.

Dilation. Abnormal dilation occurs in patients with elevated right atrial pressure resulting from tricuspid valve disease, right-heart failure, pericardial restriction, constriction, or tamponade. In addition, superior vena caval dilation is seen in infants with total anomalous pulmonary venous connection draining into the right atrium via the superior vena cava.[148]

Anomalous Superior Vena Caval Drainage. There have been several reports of isolated superior vena caval connection to the left atrium presenting in children as arterial desaturation in the absence of other cardiac findings.[153–155] This anomaly must be differentiated from pulmonary arteriovenous fistula, pulmonary artery connection to the left atrium, and persistent left superior vena caval connection to the left atrium. This differentiation can be made using contrast echocardiography and is discussed and illustrated in Chapter 15.

Tumors Involving the Superior Vena Cava. Tumors of the lungs, breast, and mediastinum can either compress the superior vena cava or extend into the heart via this venous tributary. Figure 26–51 is an example of a thymoma involving the superior vena cava, which extends into the right atrium. Tumors that partially or completely obstruct the superior vena cava alter the path of blood return to the heart and can lead to the development of the superior vena caval syndrome. Abnormal venous return from the upper extremities can be detected by contrast echocardiography (see Chapter 15).

Superior Vena Caval Thrombus and Vegetations. Thrombosis of the superior vena cava can occur spontaneously or result from trauma. Spontaneous thrombosis usually occurs in the setting of right ventricular infarction, congestive heart failure, malignancies, or polycythemia vera.[156] Traumatic thrombosis is usually caused by intimal irritation and abrasion caused by indwelling catheters. Increasing use of intravascular devices such as transvenous pacemakers, hyperalimentation catheters, central venous lines, and Swan-Ganz

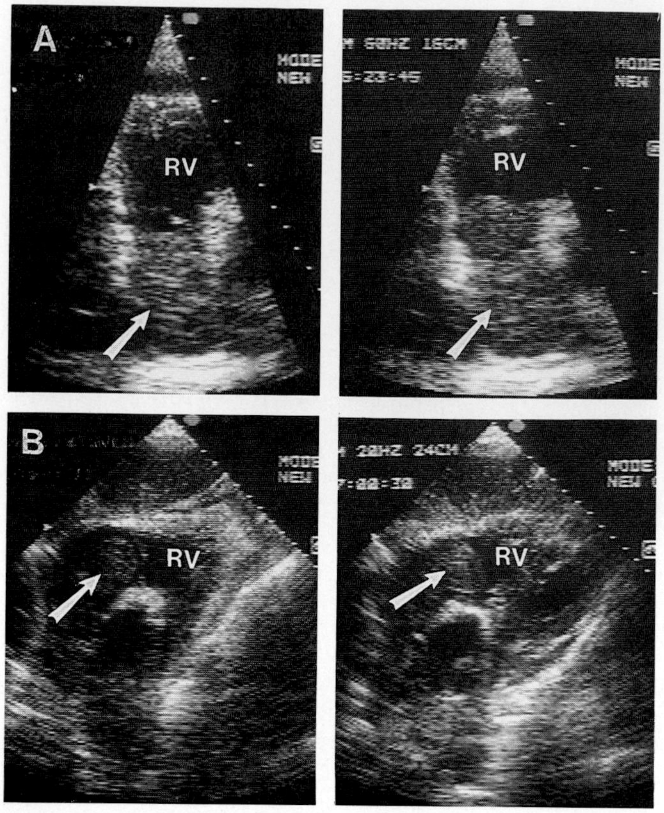

Fig. 26–51. A malignant thymoma (arrows) extending into the right atrium. **A** and **B.** Left. Systolic recordings illustrating the tumor extending into the right atrium from the superior vena cava. Right. The tumor extends through the tricuspid orifice during diastole. Upper recordings were made from a precordial transducer location; lower recordings, from a subcostal window. All views are nonstandard. RV = right ventricle.

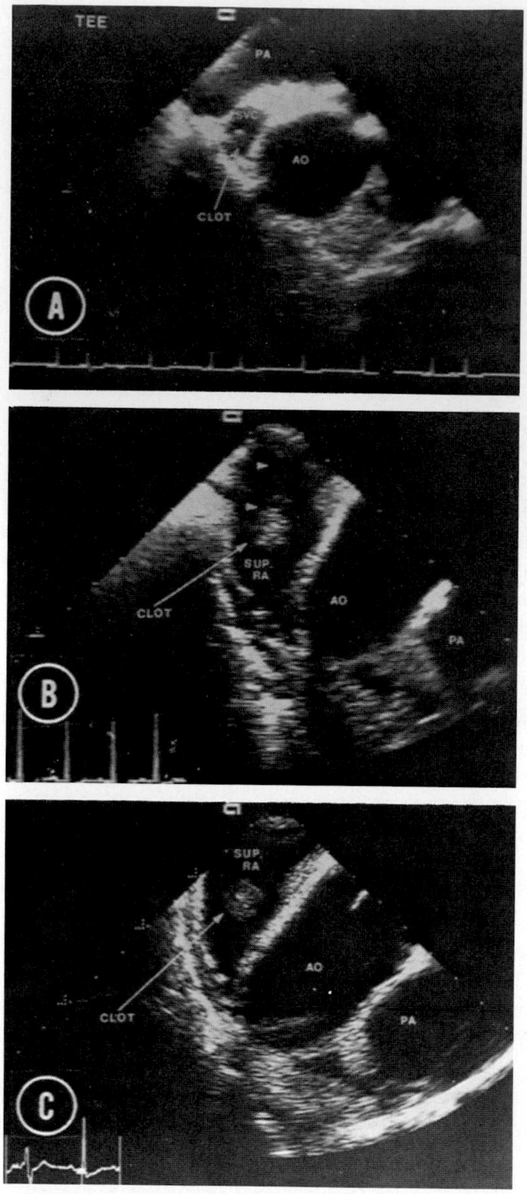

Fig. 26–52. Transesophageal short axis recording of the pulmonary artery (PA), aorta (AO); and superior vena cava (SVC) from a patient with a permanent atrioventricular sequential pacemaker. **A.** An infected thrombus (CLOT) is recorded in the superior vena cava. The mass can be visualized extending into the superior portion **(B)** and body of the right atrium (RA) **(C).** (From Podolsky LA, et al.: Superior vena caval thrombosis detected by transesophageal echocardiography. J Am Soc Echocardiogr 4:189, 1991.)

catheters has led to an increasing incidence of superior vena cava thrombus and vegetation with partial or complete obstruction of the larger thoracic veins. Many superior vena caval thrombi occur just above its entrance into the right atrium. This may be due to the fact that catheters curve as they leave the superior vena cava and enter the right atrium. This curve may press against the vessel wall and with continual cardiac motion may lead to endothelial irritation and thrombosis, which if infected develops superimposed vegetation.

Masses in this location can often be best visualized by transesophageal echocardiography (Fig. 26–52), which provides enhanced resolution and permits a more extensive area of the superior vena cava to be visualized.

Persistence of the Left Superior Vena Cava. When there is persistence of the left superior vena cava, this anomalous vessel commonly drains into the right atrium by way of the coronary sinus. This drainage causes coronary sinus dilation and can be detected by contrast injection into the left arm. (This anomaly is discussed further in Chapter 18.)

Superior Vena Caval Flow

Normal superior vena caval flow is similar to that of the inferior vena cava and hepatic veins because it is governed by the same forces. Superior vena caval flow consists of three primary phases: (1) ventricular systolic forward flow that is due to the fall in atrial pressure caused by atrial relaxation and inferior displacement of the tricuspid annulus during systolic contraction. (2) Diastolic forward flow during rapid ventricular filling, and (3) retrograde flow during atrial contraction (Fig. 26–53). The atrial wave is small in normal individuals and may be absent on occasion. Inspiration normally increases the magnitude of the systolic and diastolic forward flow and decreases the flow reversal during atrial

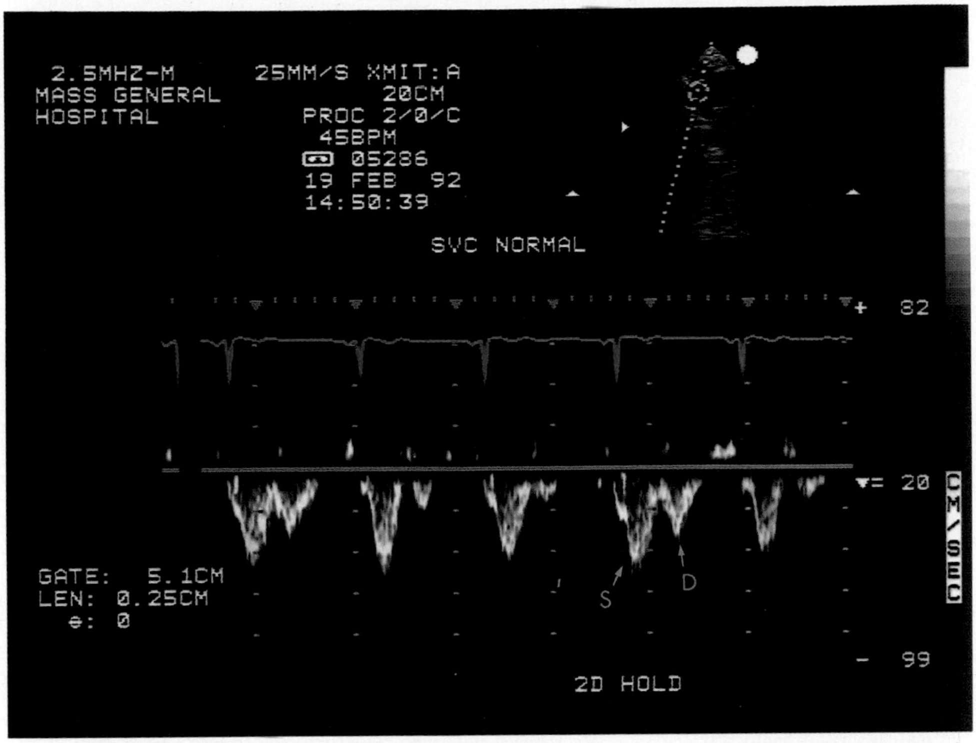

Fig. 26–53. Pulsed Doppler recording of normal superior vena caval (SVC) flow. Flow is similar to that seen in the hepatic vein with forward flow during systole (S) and diastole (D). Retrograde flow can often be seen following atrial contraction but is less apparent than that seen in the hepatic vein.

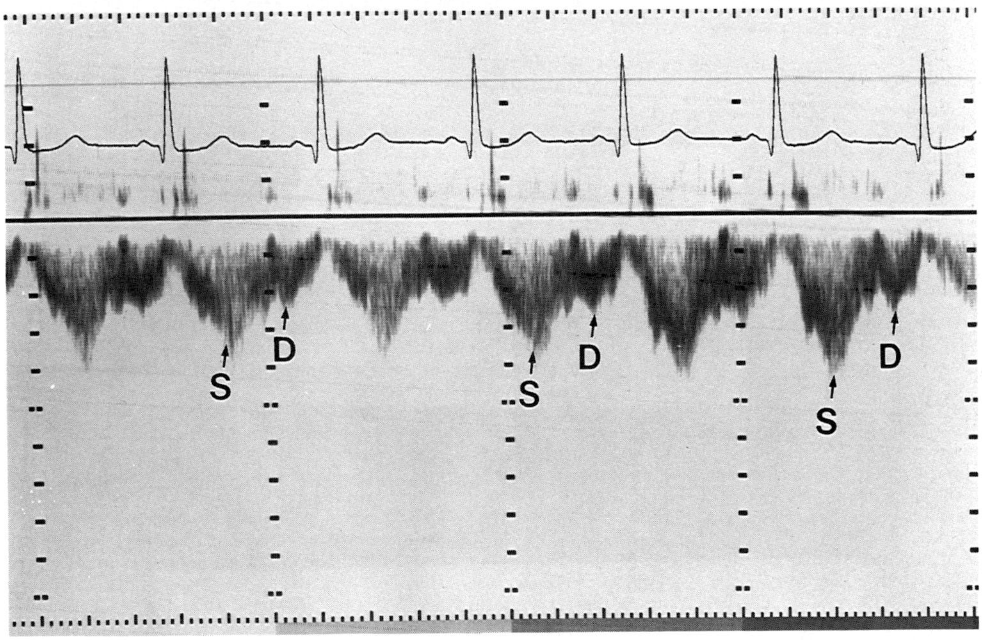

Fig. 26–54. Pulsed Doppler recording of flow in a persistent left superior vena cava connected to the coronary sinus. Flow in this anomalous vessel is similar to that in the right-sided superior vena cava. S = systolic flow toward the right atrium; D = diastolic flow toward the right atrium.

systole. However, because inspiration also increases the size of the superior vena cava, flow velocity may stay the same or even decrease, despite the fact that absolute flow is increasing.

The systolic flow wave is normally greater than the diastolic flow wave. Like hepatic vein and inferior vena caval flow, the systolic forward flow wave decreases with atrial fibrillation, tricuspid regurgitation, right ventricular failure, pericardial tamponade, and restrictive myopathy, and after pericardiectomy. Flow in a persistent left superior vena cava connected to the right atrium via the coronary sinus is similar to that in the right superior vena cava (Fig. 26–54).

REFERENCES

1. Feigenbaum H: Echocardiography. Philadelphia, Lea & Febiger, 1976.
2. Tajik AJ, et al.: Two-dimensional real-time ultrasonic imaging of the heart and great vessels. Mayo Clin Proc 53:271, 1978.

3. Silverman NH, Schiller NB: Apex echocardiography. A two-dimensional technique for evaluating congenital heart disease. Circulation 57:503, 1978.
4. Lange LW, Sahn DJ, Allen HD, Goldberg SJ: Subxiphoid cross-sectional echocardiography in infants and children with congenital heart disease. Circulation 59:513, 1979.
5. Hoit B, Sahn DJ, Shabetai R. Doppler-detected paradoxus of mitral and tricuspid valve flows in chronic lung disease. J Am Coll Cardiol 8:706, 1986.
6. Leeman DE, Levine MJ, Come PC: Doppler echocardiography in cardiac tamponade: Exaggerated respiratory variation in transvalvular blood flow velocity integrals. J Am Coll Cardiol 11:572, 1988.
7. Appleton CP, Hatle LK, Popp RL: Cardiac tamponade and pericardial effusion: respiratory variation in transvalvular flow velocities studied by Doppler echocardiography. J Am Coll Cardiol 11:1020, 1988.
8. Appleton CP, Hatle LK, Popp RL. Demonstration of restrictive ventricular physiology by Doppler echocardiography. J Am Coll Cardiol 11:757, 1988.
9. Nishimura RA, Hatle LK, Tajik AJ: Assessment of diastolic function of the heart: background and current applications of Doppler echocardiography. Part II. Clinical studies. Mayo Clin Proc 64:181, 1989.
10. Gray H: Gray's Anatomy. CM Goss (ed.). Philadelphia, Lea & Febiger, p. 589, 1974.
11. Grant JCB, Basmajian JV: Grant's Method of Anatomy. Baltimore, Williams & Wilkins, 1965.
12. Hurst JW: The Heart. New York, McGraw-Hill, 1974.
13. Hatle L, Angelsen B: Doppler Ultrasound in Cardiology: Physical Principles and Clinical Applications. 2nd Ed. Philadelphia, Lea & Febiger, 1985.
14. Thomas JD, Newell JB, Choong CYP, Weyman AE: Physical and physiological determinants of transmitral velocity: numerical analysis. Am J Physiol 260(Heart Circ Physiol 29):H1718, 1991.
15. Thomas JD: Flow in the descending aorta. A turn of the screw or a sideways glance? Circulation 82:2263, 1990.
16. Flachskampf RA, Rodriguez L, Chen C, Thomas JD: Calculation of mitral inertial mass: a factor critical to extracting relaxation from Doppler filling properties; an *in vitro* study. Circulation 80:II-567, 1989.
17. Riggs TW, Snider AR: Respiratory influence on right and left ventricular diastolic filling in normal children. J Am Coll Cardiol 13:205, 1989.
18. Hatle LK, Appleton CP, Popp RL: Differentiation of constrictive pericarditis and restrictive cardiomyopathy by Doppler echocardiography. Circulation 79:357, 1989.
19. Kenny JF, et al.: Changes in intracardiac blood flow velocities and right and left ventricular stroke volumes with gestational age in the normal human fetus: a prospective Doppler echocardiographic study. Circulation 74:1208, 1986.
20. Friedberg CW: Diseases of the Heart. Philadelphia, WB Saunders, 1966.
21. Dennis JL, Hansen AE, Corpening TN: Endocardial fibroelastosis. Pediatrics 12:130, 1953.
22. Baruchin MA, Hecht SR, Berger M: Reversible tricuspid stenosis. Demonstration with two-dimensional echocardiography and continuous wave Doppler. Chest 100:852, 1991.
23. Sapirstein W, Baker CB: Isolated tricuspid stenosis. Report of a surgically treated case. N Engl J Med 269:236, 1963.
24. Gibson RV, Wood P: The diagnosis of tricuspid stenosis. Br Heart J 17: 552, 1955.
25. Sethi KK, Nair M, Khanna SK: Primary fibrosarcoma of the heart presenting as obstruction of the tricuspid valve: diagnosis by cross-sectional echocardiography. Int J Cardiol 24:228, 1989.
26. Hollman A: The anatomic appearance of tricuspid valve disease. Br Heart J 19:211, 1957.
27. Wood P: Chronic rheumatic heart disease. *In* Diseases of the Heart and Circulation. 3rd Ed. Philadelphia: JB Lippincott, 1968.
28. Austen WG, DeSanctis RW, Sanders CA, Scannell JG: Surgical treatment of acquired trivalvular disease. J Thorac Cardiovasc Surg 49:640, 1965.
29. Cooke WT, White PD: Tricuspid stenosis: with particular reference to diagnosis and prognosis. Br Heart J 3:147, 1941.
30. Smith JA, Levine SA: The clinical features of tricuspid stenosis. Am Heart J 23:739, 1942.
31. Aceves S, Carral R: The diagnosis of tricuspid valve disease. Am Heart J 34:114, 1947.
32. Gibson R, Wood P: The diagnosis of tricuspid stenosis. Br Heart J 17:552, 1955.
33. Goodwin JF, Rab SM, Sinha AK, Zoob M: Rheumatic tricuspid stenosis. Br Med J 2:1383, 1957.
34. Kitchin A, Turner R: Diagnosis and treatment of tricuspid stenosis. Br Heart J 26:354, 1964.
35. Guyer DE, et al.: Comparison of the echocardiographic and hemodynamic diagnosis of rheumatic tricuspid stenosis. J Am Coll Cardiol 3:1135, 1984.
36. Perloff JK, Harvey WP: Clinical recognition of tricuspid stenosis. Circulation 22:346, 1960.
37. Yu PN, et al.: Clinical and hemodynamic studies of tricuspid stenosis. Circulation 13:680, 1956.
38. Nanna M, et al.: Value of two-dimensional echocardiography in detecting tricuspid stenosis. Circulation 67:221, 1983.
39. Daniels SJ, Mintz GS, Kotler MN: Rheumatic tricuspid valve disease: two dimensional echocardiographic, hemodynamic and angiographic correlations. Am J Cardiol 51:493, 1983.
40. Perez JE, Ludbrook PA, Ahumada GG: Usefulness of Doppler echocardiography in detecting tricuspid valve stenosis. Am J Cardiol 55:601, 1985.
41. Wilkins GT, et al.: Validation of continuous-wave Doppler echocardiographic measurements of mitral and tricuspid prosthetic valve gradients: simultaneous Doppler-catheter study. Circulation 74:786, 1986.
42. Karp K, Teien D, Eriksson P: Doppler echocardiographic assessment of the valve area in patients with atrioventricular valve stenosis by application of the continuity equation. J Intern Med 225:261, 1989.
43. Kawahara T, et al.: Application of Doppler color flow imaging to determine valve area in mitral stenosis. J Am Coll Cardiol 18:85, 1991.
44. Monterroso VH, et al.: Estimation of mitral valve area by color Doppler flow mapping. Circulation 80(Suppl. 2):II-167, 1989.
45. Fawzy ME, et al.: Doppler echocardiography in the evaluation of tricuspid stenosis. Eur Heart J 10:985, 1989.
46. Osborn JR, Jones RC, Jahnke EJ: Traumatic tricuspid insufficiency: hemodynamic data and surgical treatment. Circulation 30:217, 1964.
47. Bain TC, Edwards JE, Scheifley CH, Geraci JE: Right-sided bacterial endocarditis and endarteritis. Am J Med 24:98, 1958.
48. Roberts WC, Buchbinder NE: Right-sided valvular infective endocarditis. Am J Med 53:7, 1972.
49. Banks T, Fletcher R, Ali N: Infective endocarditis in heroin addicts. Am J Med 55:444, 1973.
50. Roberts WC, Sjoerdsma A: The cardiac disease associated with the carcinoid syndrome. Am J Med 36:5, 1964.
51. Reisman M, Hipona FA, Bloor CM, Talner NS: Congenital tricuspid insufficiency: a cause of massive cardiomyopathy and heart failure in the neonate. J Pediatr 66:869, 1965.
52. Kumar A, Fyler D, Miettinen O, Nadas A: Ebstein's anomaly: clinical profile and natural history. Am J Cardiol 28:84, 1971.
53. Bialostozky D, Horwitz S, Espino-Vela J: Ebstein's malformation of the tricuspid valve. A review of 65 cases. Am J Cardiol 29:826, 1972.
54. Watson H: Natural history of Ebstein's anomaly of tricuspid valve in childhood and adolescence. Br Heart J 36:417, 1972.
55. Skjaerpe T, Hatle L: Diagnosis and assessment of tricuspid regurgitation with Doppler ultrasound. *In* Risterborgh H (ed.): Echocardiology. The Hague, The Netherlands, Martinus Nijoff, p. 299, 1981.
56. Lieppe W, Behar VS, Scallon R, Kisslo JA: Detection of tricuspid regurgitation with two-dimensional echocardiography and peripheral vein injections. Circulation 57:128, 1979.
57. Meltzer RS, et al.: Diagnosis of tricuspid regurgitation by contrast echocardiography. Circulation 63:1093, 1981.
58. Meltzer RS, et al.: Diagnosing tricuspid regurgitation by direct imaging of the regurgitant flow in the right atrium using contrast echocardiography. Am J Cardiol 52:1050, 1983.
59. Wise NK, et al.: Contrast M-mode ultrasonography of the inferior vena cave. Circulation 63:1100, 1981.
60. Tei C, Shah PM, Ormiston JA: Assessment of tricuspid regurgitation by directional analysis of right atrial linear reflux echoes with contrast M-mode echocardiography. Am Heart J 103:1025, 1982.
61. Curtius JM, Thyssen M, Breuer HM, Loogen F: Doppler versus contrast echocardiography for diagnosis of tricuspid regurgitation. Am J Cardiol 56:333, 1985.
62. Miyatake K, et al.: Evaluation of tricuspid regurgitation by pulsed Doppler and two-dimensional echocardiography. Circulation 66:777, 1982.
63. Meijboom EJ, et al.: A Doppler echocardiographic method for calculation volume flow across the tricuspid valve: correlative laboratory and clinical studies. Circulation 71:551, 1985.
64. Kostucke W, Vandenbossche JL, Friart A, Englert M: Pulsed Doppler regurgitant flow patterns of normal valves. Am J Cardiol 58:309, 1986.
65. Pollak SJ, et al.: Cardiac evaluation of women distance runners by echocardiographic color Doppler flow mapping. J Am Coll Cardiol 11:89, 1988.
66. Yock PG, Naasz C, Schnittger I, Popp RL: Doppler tricuspid and pulmonic regurgitation in normals: is it real? Circulation 70(Suppl. 2):II-40, 1984.
67. Choong CY, et al.: Prevalence of valvular regurgitation by Doppler echocardiography in patients with structurally normal hearts by two-dimensional echocardiography. Am Heart J 117:636, 1989.
68. Berger M, Hecht SR, Van-Tosh A, Lingam U. Pulsed and continuous wave Doppler echocardiographic assessment of valvular regurgitation in normal subjects. J Am Coll Cardiol 13:1540, 1989.
69. Akasaka T, et al.: Age-related valvular regurgitation: a study by pulsed Doppler echocardiography. Circulation 76:262, 1987.
70. Kral J, Hradec J, Petrasek J: Valvular regurgitations in healthy young people. Cor-Vasa 31:485, 1989.
71. Weyman AE, et al.: Mechanism of abnormal septal motion in patients with RV volume overload. Circulation 54:169, 1976.
72. Louie EK, Bieniarz T, Moore AM, Levitsky S: Reduced atrial contribution to left ventricular filling in patients with severe tricuspid regurgitation after tricuspid valvectomy: a Doppler echocardiographic study. J Am Coll Cardiol 16:1617, 1990.
73. Gibson TC, Foale RA, Guyer DE, Weyman AE: Clinical significance of incomplete tricuspid valve closure seen on two-dimensional echocardiography. J Am Coll Cardiol 4:1052, 1984.
74. Garcia-Dorado D, et al.: Diagnosis of functional tricuspid insufficiency by pulsed-wave Doppler ultrasound. Circulation 66:1315, 1982.
75. Mikami T, et al.: Mechanisms for development of functional tricuspid re-

gurgitation determined by pulsed Doppler and two-dimensional echocardiography. Am J Cardiol 53:160, 1984.
76. Chopra HK, et al.: Can two-dimensional echocardiography and Doppler color flow mapping identify the need for tricuspid valve repair. J Am Coll Cardiol 14:1266, 1989.
77. DeMaria AN, et al.: Evaluation of tricuspid valve prolapse by two-dimensional echocardiography (abstr.). Am J Cardiol 43:385, 1979.
78. Mardelli TJ, Morganroth J, Meixell LL, Vergel J: Enhanced diagnosis of tricuspid valve prolapse by cross-sectional echocardiography (abstr.). Am J Cardiol 43:385, 1979.
79. Marks AR, et al.: Identification of high-risk subgroups of patients with mitral-valve prolapse. N Engl J Med 320:1031, 1989.
80. Pocock WA, Barlow JB: An association between the billowing posterior mitral leaflet syndrome and congenital heart disease, particularly atrial septal defect. Am Heart J 81:720, 1971.
81. Betriu A, Wigle D, Felderhof LH, McLoughlin MJ: Prolapse of the posterior leaflet of the mitral valve associated with secundum atrial septal defect. Am J Cardiol 35:363, 1975.
82. Victorica BE, Elliott LP, Gessner IH: Ostium secundum atrial septal defect associated with balloon mitral valve in children. Am J Cardiol 33:668, 1974.
83. Leachman RD, Cokkinos DV, Cooley DA: Association of ostium secundum atrial septal defects with mitral valve prolapse. Am J Cardiol 38:167, 1976.
84. Banks T, Fletcher R, Ali N: Infective endocarditis in heroin addicts. Am J Med 55:444, 1973.
85. Wright JS, Glennie JS: Excision of tricuspid valve with later replacement in endocarditis of drug addiction. Thorax 33:518, 1978.
86. Come PC, Kuurland GS, Vine HS: Two-dimensional echocardiography in differentiating right atrial and tricuspid valve mass lesions. Am J Cardiol 44:1207, 1979.
87. Kisslo J, Von Ramm OT: Echocardiographic evaluation of tricuspid valve endocarditis: an M-mode and two-dimensional study. Am J Cardiol 38:502, 1976.
88. Rakowski H, et al.: Cardiac carcinosis: a new method of diagnosis. Circulation 58(Suppl. 2):II-237, 1978.
89. Himelman RB, Schiller NB: Clinical and echocardiographic comparison of patients with the carcinoid syndrome with and without carcinoid heart disease. Am J Cardiol 63:347, 1989.
90. Lundin L, Landelius J, Andren B, Oberg K: Transesophageal echocardiography improves the diagnostic value of cardiac ultrasound in patients with carcinoid heart disease. Br Heart J 64:190, 1990.
91. Edwards JE, et al.: Congenital Heart Disease. Philadelphia, WB Saunders, 1965.
92. Vacca JB, Bussmann DW, Mudd JG: Ebstein's anomaly. Complete review of 108 cases. Am J Cardiol 2:210, 1958.
93. Brown JW, Heath D, Whitaker W: Ebstein's disease. Am J Med 20:322, 1956.
94. Ellis K, et al.: Ebstein's anomaly of the tricuspid valve. Angiocardiographic considerations. Am J Roentgenol 92:1338, 1964.
95. Kezdi R, Wennemark J: Ebstein's malformation: clinical findings and hemodynamic alterations. Am J Cardiol 2:200, 1958.
96. Ports TA, Silverman NH, Schiller NB: Two-dimensional echocardiographic assessment of Ebstein's anomaly. circulation 58:336, 1978.
97. Sahn DJ, et al.: The comparative utilities of real-time cross-sectional echocardiographic imaging systems for the diagnosis of complex congenital heart disease. Am J Med 63:50, 1977.
98. Kushner FG, Lam W, Morganroth J: Apex sector echocardiography in evaluation of the right atrium in patients with mitral stenosis and atrial septal defect. Am J Cardiol 42:733, 1978.
99. Matsumoto M, et al.: Visualization of Ebstein's anomaly of the tricuspid valve by two-dimensional echocardiography and standard echocardiography. Circulation 53:69, 1976.
100. Hirschklau MJ, et al.: Cross-sectional echocardiographic features of Ebstein's anomaly of the tricuspid valve. Am J Cardiol 40:400, 1977.
101. Gussenhoven WJ, Spitaels SEC, Bom N, Becker AE: Echocardiographic criteria for Ebstein's anomaly of tricuspid valve. Br Heart J 43:31, 1980.
102. Kambe T, et al.: Apex and subxiphoid approaches to Ebstein's anomaly using cross-sectional echocardiography. Am Heart J 100:53, 1980.
103. Shiina A, et al.: Two-dimensional echocardiographic spectrum of Ebstein's anomaly: detailed anatomic assessment. J Am Coll Cardiol 3:356, 1984.
104. Bommer W, et al.: Determination of right atrial and right ventricular size by two-dimensional echocardiography. Circulation 60:91, 1979.
105. Shiina A, et al.: Two-dimensional echocardiographic-surgical correlation in Ebstein's anomaly: preoperative determination of patients requiring tricuspid valve plication vs replacement. Circulation 68:34, 1983.
106. Marino JP, et al.: Echocardiography and color-flow mapping evaluation of a new reconstructive surgical technique for Ebstein's anomaly. Circulation 80:1197, 1989.
107. Daniel W, et al.: Value of M-mode echocardiography for non-invasive diagnosis of Ebstein's anomaly. Br Heart J 43:38, 1980.
108. Farooki ZQ, Henry JG, Green EW: Echocardiographic spectrum of Ebstein's anomaly of the tricuspid valve. Circulation 53:63, 1976.
109. Schnittger I, Appleton CP, Hatle LK, Popp RL: Diastolic mitral and tricuspid regurgitation by Doppler echocardiography in patients with atrioventricular block: new insight into the mechanism of atrioventricular valve closure. J Am Coll Cardiol 11:83, 1988.
110. Yock PG, Popp RL: Noninvasive estimation of right ventricular systolic pressure by Doppler ultrasound in patients with tricuspid regurgitation. Circulation 70:657, 1984.
111. Berger M, et al.: Quantitative assessment of pulmonary hypertension in patients with tricuspid regurgitation using continuous wave Doppler ultrasound. J Am Coll Cardiol 6:359, 1985.
112. Currie PJ, et al.: Continuous wave Doppler determination of right ventricular pressure: a simultaneous Doppler-catheterization study in 127 patients. J Am Coll Cardiol 6:750, 1985.
113. Goldberg SJ, et al.: Range gated ultrasound detection of contrast echographic microbubbles for cardiac and great vessel blood flow patterns. Am Heart J 101:302, 1983.
114. Waggoner AD, Barzilai B, Perez JE: Saline contrast enhancement of tricuspid regurgitant jets detected by Doppler color flow mapping. Am J Cardiol 65:1368, 1990.
115. Beppu S, et al.: Contrast enhancement of Doppler signals by sonicated albumin for estimating right ventricular pressure. Am J Cardiol 67:1148, 1991.
116. Rogers JV Jr, Chandler NW, Franch RH. Calcification of the tricuspid annulus. Am J Radiol 106:550, 1969.
117. Arnold JR, Grahramani AR, Hernandez FA, Sommer LS: Calcification of annulus of tricuspid valve: observation in two patients with congenital pulmonary stenosis. Chest 60:229, 1971.
118. Malkawki K, Bouchard F, Maurice P: Calcification of the tricuspid annulus. Arch Mal Coeur 4:487, 1981.
119. Mattleman S, et al.: Calcification of the tricuspid annulus diagnosed by two-dimensional echocardiography. Am Heart J 107:986, 1984.
120. Zema MJ, Caccavano M: Calcification of the tricuspid annulus: diagnosis by two-dimensional echocardiography. J Cardiovasc Ultrasonogr 2:19, 1983.
121. Watanabe T, et al.: Ruptured chordae tendineae of the tricuspid valve due to nonpenetrating trauma. Echocardiographic findings. Chest 80:751, 1981.
122. Kawaratani H, Narita M, Kurihara T, Usami Y: A case of traumatic tricuspid insufficiency. J Cardiogr 7:393, 1977.
123. Alam M, Folger GM, Golstein S: Tricuspid valve fluttering: echocardiographic features of ventricular septal defect. Chest 77:517, 1980.
124. Snider AR, Silverman NH, Schiller NB, Parts TA. Echocardiographic evaluation of ventricular septal aneurysms. Circulation 59:920, 1979.
125. Nanda NC, Gramiak R, Manning JA: Echocardiography of the tricuspid valve in congenital left ventricular-right atrial communication. Circulation 51:268, 1975.
126. Nair T, Joy MV, Subramanyan R, Venkitachalam CG: Two-dimensional and Doppler echocardiographic study of coronary arteriovenous fistulas. Indian Heart J 42:149, 1990.
127. Werner JA, et al.: Echocardiographic appearance of the Chiari network: differentiation from right-heart pathology. Circulation 63:1104, 1981.
128. Triulzi MO, et al.: Normal adult cross-sectional echocardiographic values: linear dimensions and chamber areas. Echocardiography 1:403, 1984.
129. Bommer WJ, Kwan OL, Mason DT, DeMaria AN: Identification of prominent eustachian valves by M-mode nd two-dimensional echocardiography: differentiation from right atrial masses. Am J Cardiol 45:402, 1980.
130. Chiari H: Ueber Netzbildungen im rechten Vorhofe des Herzens. Beitr Pathol Anat 22:1, 1897.
131. Edwards JE: Congenital malformations of the heart and great vessels. Malformations of the atrial septal complex. *In* Gould SE (ed.): Pathology of the Heart and Blood Vessels. Springfield, IL, Charles C Thomas, p. 60, 1968.
132. Cloez JL, et al.: Echocardiographic rediscovery of an anatomical structure: the Chiari Network. Apropos of 16 cases. Arch Mal Coeur 76:1284, 1983.
133. Goldschlager A, Goldschlager N, Brewster H, Kaplan J: Catheter entrapment in a Chiari network involving an atrial septal defect. Chest 62:345, 1972.
134. Doucette J, Knoblich R: Persistent right valve of the sinus venosus. Arch Pathol 75:117, 1963.
135. Jones RN, Niles NR: Spinnaker formation of sinus venosus valve: case report of a fatal anomaly in a ten-year-old boy. Circulation 38:468, 1968.
136. Thomas JD, Tabakin BS, Ittleman FP: Atrial septal defect with right to left shunt despite normal pulmonary artery pressure. J Am Coll Cardiol 9: 221, 1987.
137. Simpson IA, Munsch C, Smith EE, Parker DJ: Pericardial haemorrhage causing right atrial compression after cardiac surgery: role of transoesophageal echocardiography. Br Heart J 65:355, 1991.
138. Kochar GS, Jacobs LE, Kotler MN: Right atrial compression in postoperative cardiac patients: detection by transesophageal echocardiography. J Am Coll Cardiol 16:511, 1990.
139. Satou Y, et al.: Cardiac angiosarcoma with ruptured right atrium diagnosed by echocardiography. Chest 100:274, 1991.
140. Rosenzweig MS, Nanda NC: Two-dimensional echocardiographic detection of circulating right atrial thrombi. Am Heart J 103:435, 1981.
141. Starkey IR, DeBono DP: Echocardiographic identification of right-sided cardiac intracavitary thromboembolus in massive pulmonary embolism. Circulation 66:1322, 1982.

142. Lim SP, Hakim SZ, Van der Bel-Kahn: Two-dimensional echocardiography for detection of primary right atrial thrombus and pulmonary embolism. Am Heart J 106:1547, 1984.
143. Manno BV, et al.: Two-dimensional echocardiographic detection of right atrial thrombi. Am J Cardiol 51:615, 1983.
144. Mallory PC, et al. Transient right atrial thrombus resulting in pulmonary embolism detected by two-dimensional echocardiography. Am Heart J 106: 1047, 1984.
145. Goldberg SM, Pizzarello RA, Goldman MA, Padmanabhan VT: Echocardiographic diagnosis of right atrial thromboembolism resulting in massive pulmonary embolization. Am Heart J 108:1371, 1984.
146. Reeves WC, Nanda NC, Barold SS: Echocardiographic evaluation of intracardiac pacing catheters: M-mode and two-dimensional studies. Circulation 58:1049, 1978.
147. Simonson JS, Schiller NB: Sonospirometry: a new method for noninvasive estimation of mean right atrial pressure based on two-dimensional echographic measurements of the inferior vena cava during measured inspiration. J Am Coll Cardiol 11:557, 1988.
148. Bierman FZ, Williams RG: Subxiphoid two-dimensional echocardiographic diagnosis of total anomalous pulmonary venous return in infants. Am J Cardiol 43:401, 1979.
149. Ettinger E, Steinberg I: Angiographic measurement of the cardiac segment of the inferior vena cava in health and in cardiovascular disease. Circulation 26:508, 1962.
150. Mintz GS, et al.: Real-time inferior vena caval ultrasonography: normal and abnormal findings and its use in assessing right-heart function. Circulation 64:1018, 1981.
151. Himelman RB, Kircher B, Rockey DC, Schiller NB: Inferior vena cava plethora with blunted respiratory response: a sensitive echocardiographic sign of cardiac tamponade. J Am Coll Cardiol 12:1470, 1988.
152. Nishimura R, Abel M, Hatle L, Tajik AJ: Assessment of diastolic function of the heart: background and current applications of Doppler echocardiography: II. Clinical studies. Mayo Clin Proc 64:195, 1989.
153. King RE, Plotnick GD: Isolated right superior vena cava into the left atrium detected by contrast echocardiography. Am Heart J 122:583, 1991.
154. Schick EC, Lekakis J, Rothendler JA, Ryan TJ: Persistent left superior vena cava and right superior vena cava drainage into the left atrium without arterial hypoxemia. J Am Coll Cardiol 5:374, 1985.
155. Truman AT, Rao PS, Kulangara RJ: Use of contrast echocardiography in diagnosis of anomalous connection of right superior vena cava to left atrium. Br Heart J 44:718, 1980.
156. Podolsky LA, et al.: Superior vena caval thrombosis detected by transesophageal echocardiography. J Am Soc Echocardiogr 4:189, 1991.

CHAPTER

27

RIGHT VENTRICULAR OUTFLOW TRACT

The right ventricular outflow tract extends from the crista supraventricularis to the bifurcation of the main pulmonary artery. It arises from the anterosuperior margin of the right ventricle and courses superiorly and leftward above the anterior border of the aorta. After crossing the aorta, it continues in a posterior arc along the left aortic border, bifurcating into the right and left pulmonary arteries at the level of the posterior aortic wall just above the superior margin of the left atrium. The right ventricular outflow tract has three major structural components: (1) the pulmonary valve; (2) the subvalvular conus arteriosus or infundibulum; and (3) the main pulmonary artery.

The specific methods for examining the individual segments of the right ventricular outflow tract are discussed in the appropriate section. In general, the right ventricular outflow tract, like all tubular structures, is optimally recorded with the imaging plane oriented parallel to its long axis. This orientation can be achieved from either the parasternal or subcostal transducer locations.[1,2] The parasternal location is preferred, in most adults, because it places the areas of primary interest (the distal portion of the infundibulum, the pulmonary valve, and the main pulmonary artery) in close proximity to the transducer and within the focal zone of the scan plane. In infants and small children, subcostal imaging is often superior.[3–5]

Figure 27–1 is a parasternal long axis recording of the right ventricular outflow tract and illustrates its three major components. The subvalvular, or infundibular, region lies anterior to the aortic root and extends from the tricuspid annulus to the pulmonary valve. The coapted pulmonary leaflets are recorded within the outflow tract anteriorly and to the right at approximately the 1:30 (clock) position relative to the circular aorta. The pulmonary artery courses vertically along the left margin of the aorta to its point of bifurcation. The long axis of the right ventricular outflow tract is optimally recorded when the dimensions of this tubular structure are maximal throughout the region of interest. Image orientation is achieved with reference to the pulmonary valve, the proximal inflow region, and the pulmonary artery bifurcation (see Chapter 4).

A limited segment of the subvalvular portion of the right ventricular outflow tract can also be viewed in short axis from the parasternal transducer location with the imaging plane aligned parallel to the long axis of the aorta (Fig. 27–2A). This view, however, is difficult to standardize and has proved to be of little clinical value to date. If this plane is angled leftward, however, an orthogonal long axis view of the pulmonary artery and valve can be obtained, and the crossing pattern of the aorta and descending pulmonary artery can be better appreciated (Fig. 27–2B).

From the subcostal transducer location, it is possible to align the scan plane parallel to the long axis of the entire outflow tract from the infundibulum to the main pulmonary artery branches in children and some adults (Fig. 27–3). Unfortunately, in many adults, the pulmonary valve is in the far field of a subcostally positioned transducer and hence is difficult to record. In subcostal recordings, the walls of the outflow tract are imaged using the lateral resolution of the transducer, which can significantly affect the accuracy of measurements of vessel size. This is especially important in infants and children where small absolute errors in outflow tract dimensions can result in large percentage errors.

Doppler recording of flow velocity in the different sec-

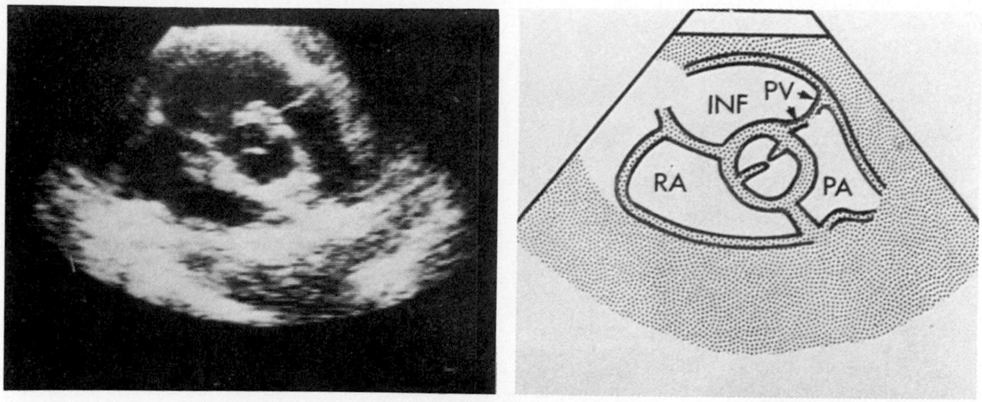

Fig. 27–1. Parasternal long axis recording of the right ventricular outflow tract. The outflow tract extends from the crista supraventricularis, at the left margin of the scan, to the bifurcation of the pulmonary artery (PA), to the right and posteriorly. It includes the pulmonary infundibulum, the pulmonic valve, and the main PA. INF = infundibulum; PV = pulmonary valve; RA = right atrium.

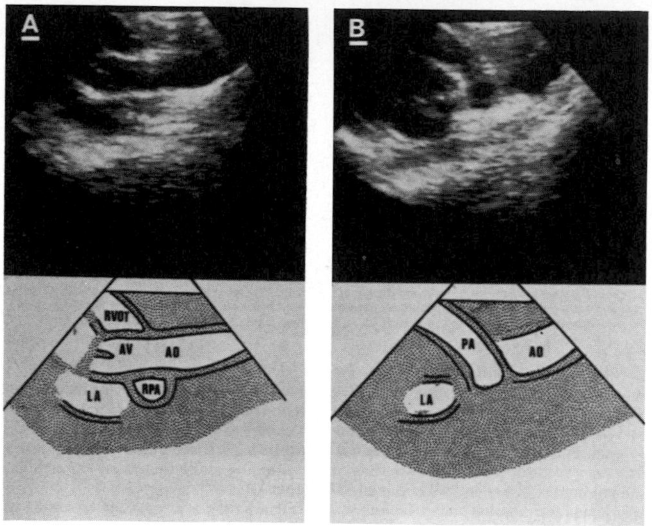

Fig. 27–2. A. Parasternal long axis recording of the ascending aorta, which transects the right ventricular outflow tract (RVOT) in a plane roughly parallel to its short axis as it courses above the aortic root. The right pulmonary artery (RPA) can also be visualized beneath the aorta (AO) as it swings underneath this vessel. **B.** The plane has been angled slightly to the left to record the descending sweep of the pulmonary artery (PA). By combining these figures, the course of the pulmonary artery (across the top of the proximal aorta and down its left margin to the point of bifurcation) and the return of the right pulmonary artery (beneath the AO posteriorly at the level of the superior margin of the left atrium [LA]), can be appreciated. AV = aortic valve.

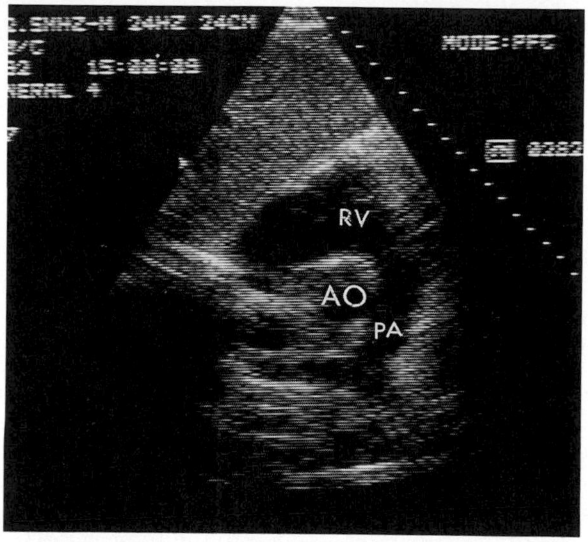

Fig. 27–3. Subcostal recording of right ventricular outflow tract. RV = right ventricle; AO = aorta; PA = pulmonary artery.

tions of the right ventricular outflow tract is more complex because the outflow tract curves more than 90° from the crista supraventricularis to the bifurcation of the pulmonary artery and more than 180° if the right pulmonary artery is included. Flow in the distal infundibulum, across the pulmonary valve, and in the main and proxi-

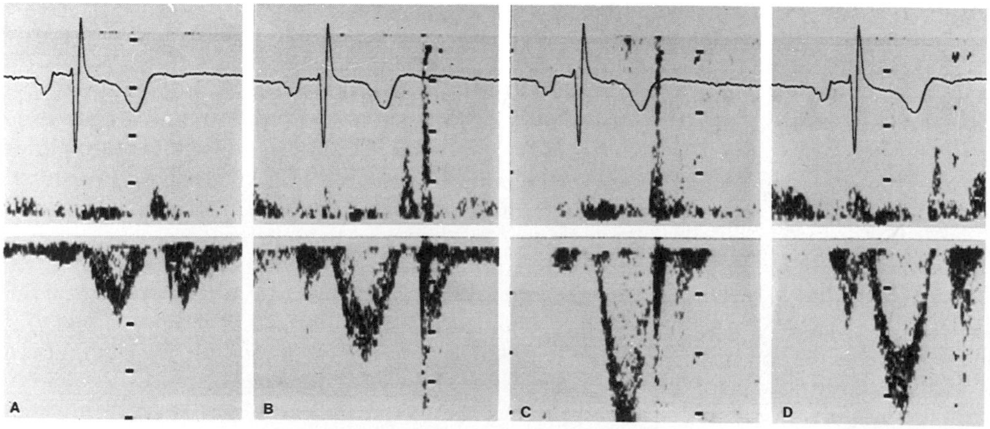

Fig. 27–4. Flow velocity changes from the crista supraventricularis to the pulmonary artery bifurcation. **A.** The right ventricle, proximal to the crista supraventricularis. **B.** Right ventricular outflow tract, proximal to the pulmonic valve. **C.** At the pulmonic valve. **D.** In the pulmonary artery, proximal to its bifurcation. (Velocities are not angle corrected.)

mal branch pulmonary arteries is generally recorded from the precordium because the ultrasonic beam is relatively parallel to the flow vector from this location and signal sensitivity is excellent. In contrast, flow in the proximal and midinfundibulum and in the right pulmonary artery is better recorded from the subcostal window, from which the ultrasonic beam can be more closely aligned parallel to the direction of flow through these regions. Figure 27–4 contains Doppler recordings of outflow tract velocities from the crista supraventricularis to the pulmonary artery bifurcation.

THE PULMONARY VALVE

Normal Orientation and Motion

The pulmonary valve lies anterior, superior, and to the left of the aortic valve and, thus, is the most anteriorly positioned of the principal cardiac structures. Anatomically, the pulmonary valve has three semilunar cusps (the anterior, right posterior, and left posterior), which face leftward superiorly and slightly posteriorly.

Imaging

The pulmonary valve is best recorded from the parasternal transducer location with the imaging plane aligned parallel to the long axis of the right ventricular outflow tract and the central ray angled slightly leftward toward the left shoulder. Figure 27–5 illustrates the relationship of a 30° scan to the pulmonary artery and pulmonary valve. Although this type of transducer angulation might appear unnecessary with instruments that provide larger scan areas, detection of the subtle changes noted in disorders such as pulmonary stenosis as a rule require fairly precise plane angulation and positioning of the central ray through the valve.

Figure 27–6 is a long axis recording of a normal pulmonary valve. During diastole, the coapted pulmonary leaf-

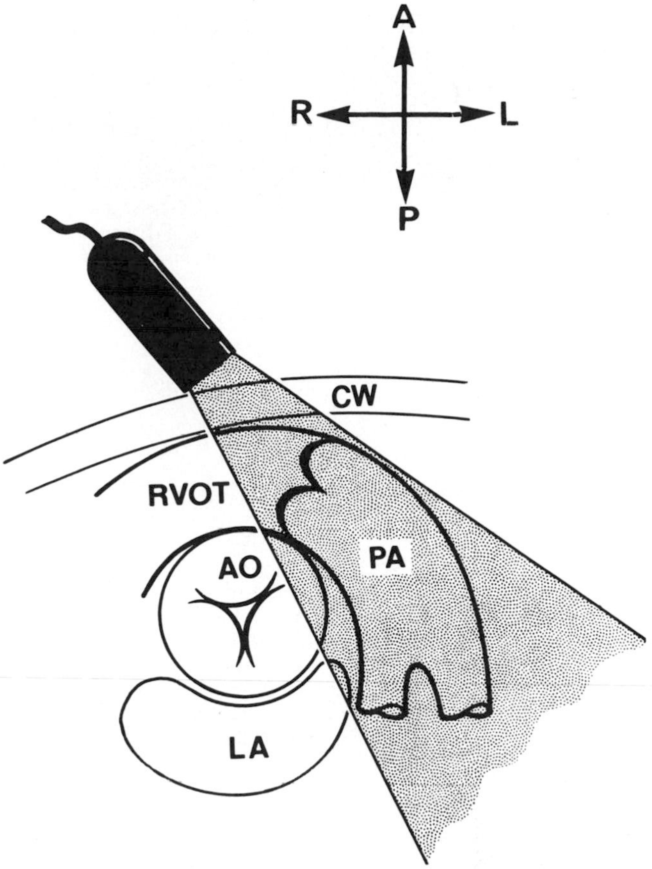

Fig. 27–5. The transducer orientation used to record the pulmonary valve. CW = chest wall; RVOT = right ventricular outflow tract; PA = pulmonary artery; AO = aorta; LA = left atrium. (From Weyman AE, et al.: Cross-sectional echocardiographic visualization of the stenotic pulmonary valve. Circulation 56:769, 1977. Reproduced by permission of the American Heart Association, Inc.)

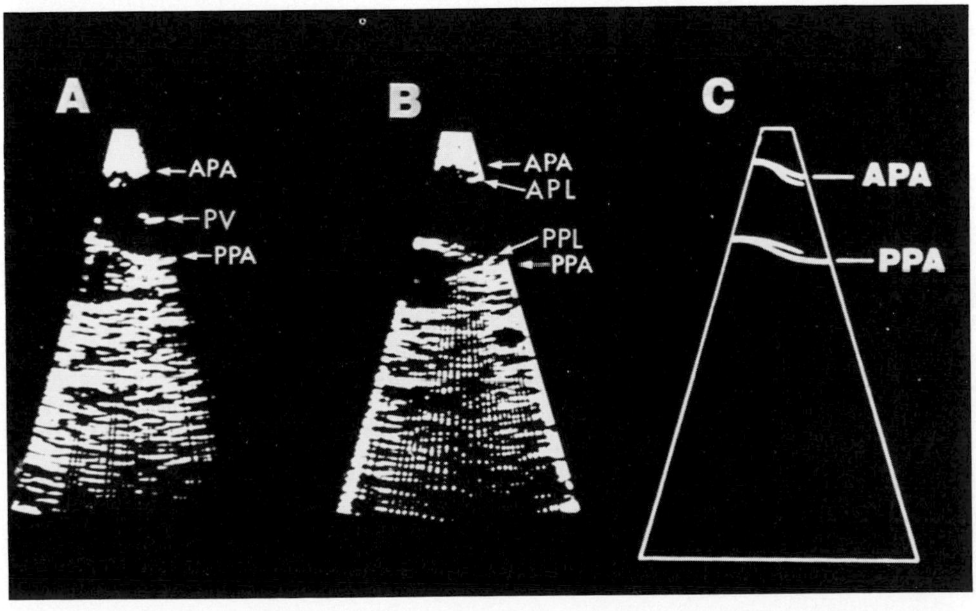

Fig. 27–6. Parasternal long axis recording of a normal pulmonary valve. **A.** The coapted pulmonary leaflets appear as a linear echo midway between the anterior and posterior margins of the pulmonary artery. **B.** Recorded during systole, the full open pulmonary leaflets lie parallel and close to the anterior and posterior margins of the pulmonary artery. **C.** The position of the fully open pulmonary leaflets. APA = anterior margin of the pulmonary artery; PPA = posterior pulmonary artery; PV = coapted pulmonary leaflets during diastole; APL = anterior pulmonary leaflet; PPL = posterior pulmonary leaflet. (From Weyman AE, et al.: Cross-sectional echocardiographic visualization of the stenotic pulmonary valve. Circulation 56:769, 1977. Reproduced by permission of the American Heart Association, Inc.)

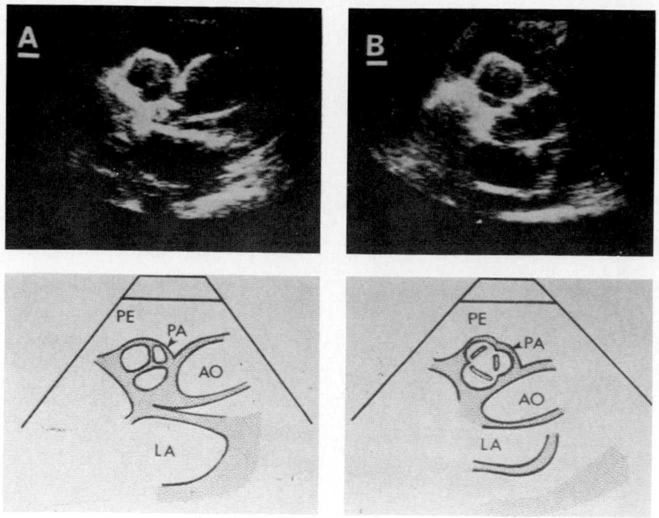

Fig. 27–7. Parasternal short axis recording of a normal pulmonary valve during diastole **(A)** and systole **(B).** In the diastolic frame, the three commissures of the coapted semilunar pulmonary leaflets can be visualized. During systole, the leaflets separate widely, and the anterior leaflets and one posterior leaflet can be seen lying against the margins of the pulmonary arterial wall. The large echo-free area anterior to the pulmonary artery represents a large pericardial effusion. PE = pericardial effusion; PA = pulmonary artery; AO = aorta; LA = left atrium.

lets appear as a thin, linear echo lying within the pulmonary artery midway between the anterior and posterior margins of the vessel. This echo represents the line of coaptation between the anterior and one of the posterior leaflets. The cusps themselves are oriented parallel to the path of the scan plane and, thus, are rarely visualized. At the onset of systole, this single linear echo separates into two discrete linear echoes, which move rapidly away from each other toward the margins of the pulmonary artery. The echo from the posterior leaflet can usually be recorded lying parallel and in close apposition to the posterior wall of the pulmonary artery. The echo from the anterior leaflet, however, is generally lost within the dense mass of echoes originating from the anterior chest wall.[6]

The pulmonary valve is far more difficult to record in short axis from the parasternal transducer location. This difficulty occurs because the pulmonary annulus in its normal orientation lies at an approximate 60° angle to the path of the imaging plane. Short-axis recordings of the pulmonary valve are possible in several situations, however. The most common of these occurs with large pericardial effusion and counterclockwise rotation of the base of the heart. Other conditions that shift the heart rightward can also displace the pulmonary valve beneath the parasternal window, thereby permitting short axis recording. Figure 27–7 is a short axis view of a normal pulmonary valve. The valve orifice in this example is oriented as if viewed from the left shoulder with the ascending aorta recorded beneath the pulmonary artery coursing to the viewer's right. Unfortunately, this type of image can be obtained so infrequently that it has more curiosity value than clinical utility.

The pulmonary valve can also be recorded in the subcostal outflow tract view (Fig. 27–3) and from the cardiac apex by elevating the scan plane until the central ray passes through the pulmonary valve and then rotating the transducer until the plane transects the long axis of the pulmonary artery (Fig. 27–8).

M-mode studies permit more detailed analysis of pulmonary valve motion. Figure 27–9 illustrates the characteristic motion of the posterior leaflet of the normal pulmonary valve recorded throughout several cardiac cycles. In the first complex surrounded by the box, the systolic and diastolic movements are lettered to denote specific components of valve motion. The lettering system is similar to that used to describe mitral and tricuspid valve motion. The "a" wave, which begins at the end of the P wave of the electrocardiogram, reflects the effect of atrial contraction on the pulmonary valve. That this deflection is due to atrial contraction is confirmed by its temporal relation to the P wave of the electrocardiogram, its disappearance during atrial fibrillation, and the constant relation to the P wave throughout diastole during complete heart block (Fig. 27–10). After atrial contraction, the leaflet usually returns to the base line before ventricular systole.

Point b represents the position of the valve at the onset of ventricular systole. In the normal subject, a definite inspiratory increase in the depth of the "a" wave can usually be demonstrated. In some normal subjects, particularly when the "a" wave is deep or the P-R interval

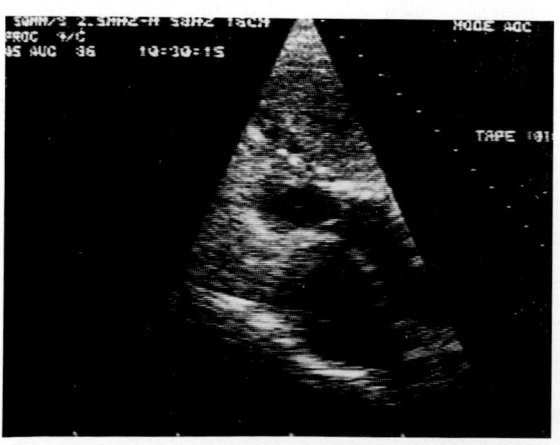

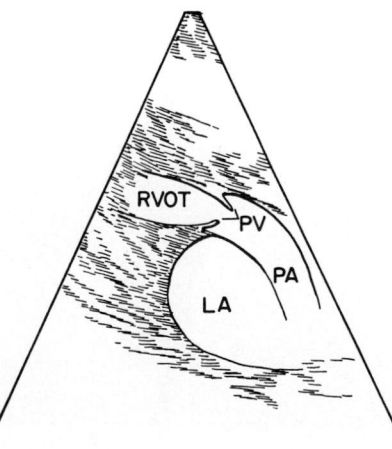

Fig. 27–8. Pulmonary valve recording from the cardiac apex/low parasternal window. The partially opened leaflets lie along the beam axis and are clearly recorded in this view. RVOT = right ventricular outflow tract; PV = pulmonary valve; PA = pulmonary artery; LA = left atrium.

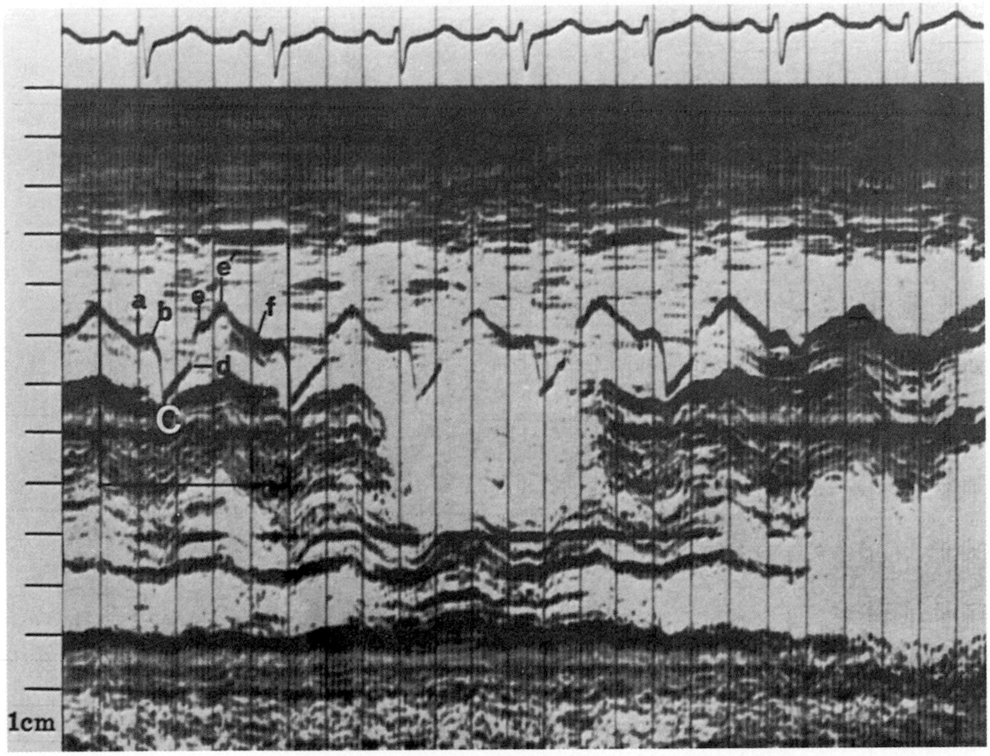

Fig. 27–9. A normal pulmonary valve recorded during several cardiac cycles. On the left, the valve is seen within the echo-free pulmonary artery moving between 5 and 7 cm beneath the chest wall. The dense mass of echoes reflected from the chest wall can be seen above the valve. Immediately beneath the valve, another dense mass of echoes is recorded from the potential space between the pulmonary artery and left atrium. As the scan is followed to the right, the aorta appears with the left atrium behind it. In the first complex on the left (surrounded by the box), the various components of leaflet motion are lettered to facilitate discussion. The a wave beginning at the end of the P wave of the electrocardiogram represents leaflet motion in response to atrial systole. Point b indicates the position of the valve at the onset of ventricular systole; the b-c segment represents rapid systolic opening of the valve; the c-d segment represents the leaflet in the open position during systole; d-e indicates rapid diastolic closure; e-f represents the leaflets in the closed position during diastole; e-e′ is a variable finding and probably represents transmitted aortic pulsations. (From Weyman AE, Dillon JC, Feigenbaum H, Chang S: Echocardiographic patterns of pulmonary valve motion in valvular pulmonary stenosis. Am J Cardiol 34:644, 1974. Reproduced with permission of Cahners Publishing Co.)

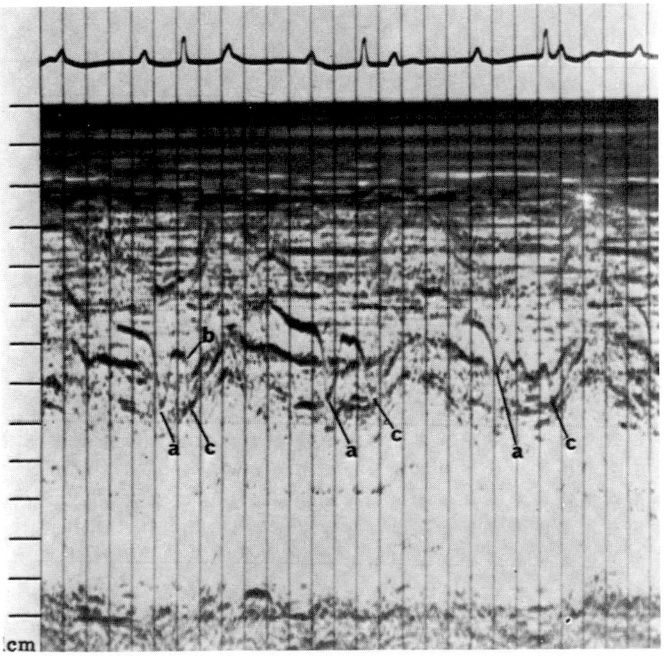

Fig. 27–10. Pulmonary echogram from a patient with a complex congenital lesion, including an atrial septal defect, pulmonary stenosis, pulmonary hypertension, and complete heart block. This figure illustrates the constant relation of the pulmonary valvular "a" wave to the P wave of the electrocardiogram and confirms the fact that the "a" wave is caused by atrial contraction. a = valve opening caused by atrial systole; b = position of the valve at the onset of ventricular systole; c = valve in the fully open position following ventricular systole. In the first two complexes on the left, it can be seen that atrial systole causes as great a degree of valvular motion as ventricular systole, suggesting complete valvular opening or doming in response to atrial systole. (From Weyman AE, Dillon JC, Feigenbaum H, Chang S: Echocardiographic patterns of pulmonary valve motion in valvular pulmonary stenosis. Am J Cardiol 34:644, 1974. Reproduced with permission of Cahners Publishing Co.)

short, the leaflet will not have time to return to the base line during inspiration, and ventricular systole will occur while it is still in a posterior or in some cases partially open position. Figure 27–11 illustrates the variation in the position of the valve at the onset of ventricular systole (point b) in a normal patient with a short P-R interval. After the onset of ventricular systole (point B), which occurs at or slightly after (0.04 seconds) the peak of the R wave of the electrocardiogram, the leaflet moves rapidly posteriorly and reaches a fully open position at point c (see Fig. 27–9). During systole, there is a gradual anterior movement of the leaflet, c–d, followed by rapid diastolic closure of the valve, d–e. During diastole, the leaflet moves gradually posteriorly to a point f, which precedes the onset of atrial systole. The anterior systolic c–d and posterior diastolic e–f slopes of the leaflet probably represent pulsatile movement of the pulmonary artery and valvular apparatus. In Figure 27–9, there is further anterior motion from point e to e′. This is a variable finding and appears to represent transmitted pulsations from the aorta. Figure 27–9 illustrates the movements of the posterior leaflet throughout the cardiac cycle. In many normal tracings, the leaflet echo is lost during systole (c–d) and rapid diastolic closure (d–e). Figure 27–12 illustrates both the anterior and posterior pulmonic leaflets. When the anterior leaflet is recorded, it moves in a direction opposite to that of the posterior leaflet during ventricular systole, producing a box-like pattern similar to the systolic configuration of the aortic valve.

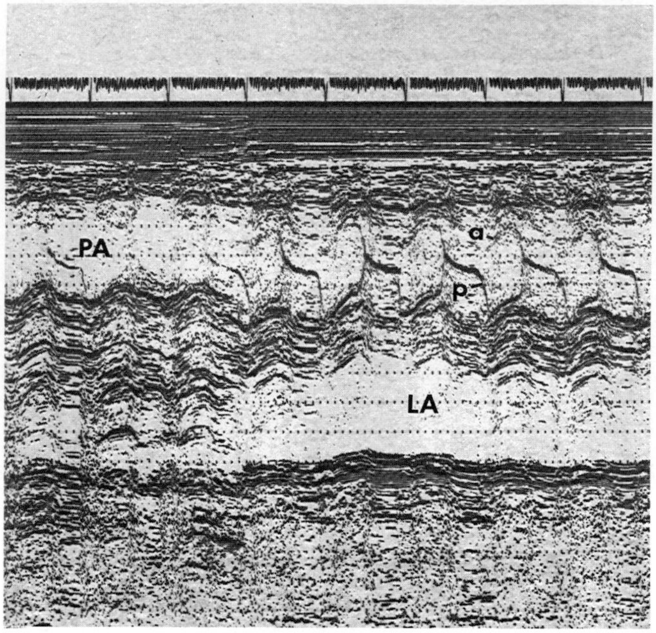

Fig. 27–12. M-mode scan illustrating normal motion of both the anterior and posterior pulmonary leaflets. The left portion of the scan illustrates the posterior pulmonary leaflet and pulmonary artery. Moving to the right, the transducer is scanned slightly inferiorly, and the anterior leaflet becomes apparent with the left atrium (LA) recorded beneath the atriopulmonic sulcus. PA = pulmonary artery; a = anterior pulmonary leaflet; p = posterior pulmonary leaflet.

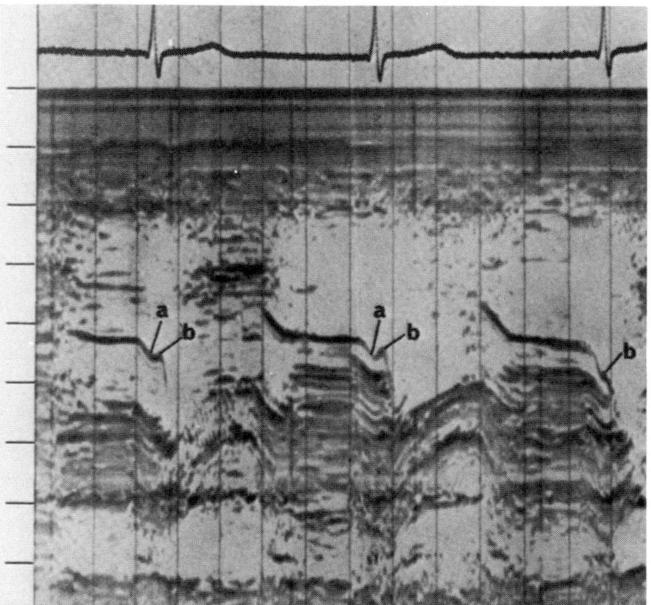

Fig. 27–11. Normal respiratory variation in the position of the leaflet at the onset of ventricular systole (point b). In the middle complex recorded during expiration, the leaflet returns almost to the base line before ventricular systole. In the complex on the right, recorded in early inspiration, the leaflet is in a posterior or partially open position at the onset of ventricular systole. The complex on the left, recorded at the end of the previous inspiration, is an intermediate complex. (From Weyman AE, Dillon JC, Feigenbaum H, Chang S: Echocardiographic patterns of pulmonary valve motion in valvular pulmonary stenosis. Am J Cardiol 34:644, 1974. Reproduced with permission of Cahners Publishing Co.)

Doppler

Flow across the pulmonary valve is normally laminar (see following discussion) with a velocity profile that peaks in midsystole. The velocity of flow is less than that across the aortic valve because the valve area is slightly larger. Normal velocities for adults range from 0.6 to 0.9 m/sec (mean 0.75) and for children from 0.7 to 1.1 m/sec (mean 0.9). Age-related changes occur during growth and development, with peak velocities in newborns being significantly lower (0.68 ± 0.09) than those recorded in older children (0.80 ± 0.12 m/sec).[7] Diastolic forward flow across the valve following atrial contraction can be recorded during inspiration in children and young adults, particularly when the heart rate is slow.[8]

Abnormalities of the Pulmonary Valve

Abnormalities of the pulmonary valve can be categorized as (1) congenital anomalies of leaflet number; (2) those associated with valvular pulmonic stenosis; (3) those that produce valvular insufficiency; and (4) lesions associated with premature opening of the pulmonic valve. Obstructive lesions involving the right ventricular outflow tract and pulmonary tree occur in 25% to 30% of all patients with congenital heart disease. Regurgitation is even more common, being seen with both normal and diseased valve but is rarely of functional significance.

Abnormalities of Leaflet Number

Pulmonary, like aortic valves, are normally tricuspid; however, bicuspid, unicuspid (acommissural and unicommissural), and quadricuspid valves also occur. The most common congenital anomaly of the pulmonary valve is the quadricuspid valve. However, the reported frequency of appreciable dysfunction of quadricuspid valve is low, ranging between 4%[9] and 6%.[10] Unicuspid valves, although less common, are generally associated with valvular stenosis and/or insufficiency.

Valvular Pulmonary Stenosis

Valvular pulmonary stenosis is almost invariably congenital, although acquired stenosis is occasionally encountered. Congenitally stenotic valves may be bicuspid, tricuspid, unicuspid (acommissural or unicommissural), or atretic. The most common type associated with isolated congenital pulmonary stenosis is the acommissural unicuspid valve,[11] although malformed tricuspid valves were noted more frequently in one surgical series. Stenotic valves are characterized by conical or dome-like fusion of the valve cusps with a central perforation at the apex.[12] All congenital forms have some degree of cusp thickening; however, the leaflets generally remain thin and pliable and can move easily toward either the right ventricle or the pulmonary artery in responses to small differences in the pressures acting on their surfaces.[13] Calcification is generally not a feature of valvular pulmonary stenosis.

Acquired valvular pulmonary stenosis is most commonly due to carcinoid disease, followed by rheumatic heart disease and active infective endocarditis.[14] Although microscopic inflammation of the pulmonary valve is common in patients with rheumatic heart disease, stenosis is rare. Both intramural and extramural tumors obstructing left ventricular outflow at the pulmonary valve level have also been reported.[15]

Valvular pulmonary stenosis also occurs in association with more complex anomalies of the right heart such as tetralogy of Fallot, double-outlet right ventricle, univentricular heart, and complete atrioventricular canal. Pulmonary stenosis associated with complex congenital lesions is discussed in Chapter 32.

Diagnosis.

Imaging. Echocardiographically, pulmonary stenosis is characterized by (1) systolic doming of the stenotic leaflets into the pulmonary artery,[6] (2) abnormal initial systolic leaflet motion,[6] and (3) opening or doming following atrial systole but before ventricular systole in more severe cases.[6,16]

Figure 27–13 illustrates the cross-sectional appearance of valvular pulmonary stenosis. During diastole, the coapted leaflets appear as a single linear echo within the pulmonary artery that is indistinguishable from that seen with a normal valve. During systole, however, the leaflets arc into the lumen of the vessel and do not lie flat against the walls of the pulmonary artery. Consequently, a domed configuration is produced, and the pulmonary valve orifice is effectively narrowed.[6]

Figure 27–14 is a recording from a second patient with valvular pulmonary stenosis and again demonstrates the characteristic systolic doming of the pulmonary leaflets. In the majority of cases (64%), careful inspection of the valve permits demonstration of doming of both the anterior and posterior leaflets.[6] Only the posterior leaflet, however, must be recorded to establish the diagnosis of pulmonary stenosis. Figure 27–15 illustrates such an example. The posterior leaflet arcs into the pulmonary

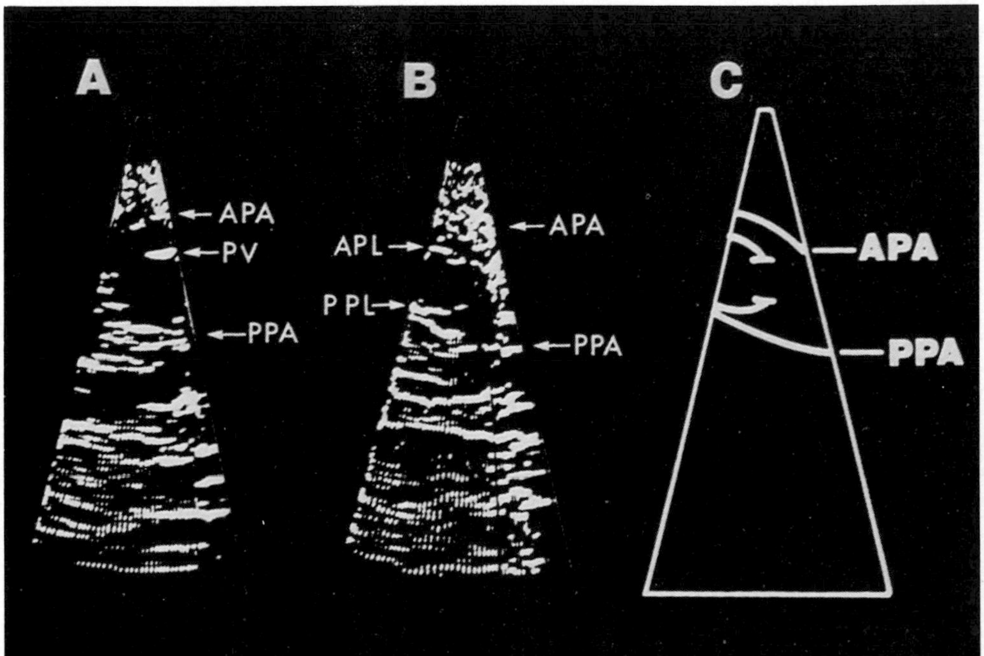

Fig. 27–13. Parasternal long axis recording of the pulmonary artery and pulmonic valve illustrates valvular pulmonary stenosis. **A.** Recorded during diastole, the single linear echo arising from the coapted pulmonary leaflets is evident in the midportion of the artery. **B.** The domed systolic configuration of the stenotic pulmonary leaflets. **C.** The domed systolic appearance of the leaflets in **B.** APA = anterior margin of the pulmonary artery; PV = pulmonary valve; PPA = posterior pulmonary artery; APL = anterior pulmonary leaflet; PPL = posterior pulmonary leaflet. (From Weyman AE, et al.: Cross-sectional echocardiographic visualization of the stenotic pulmonary valve. Circulation 56:769, 1977. Reproduced by permission of the American Heart Association, Inc.)

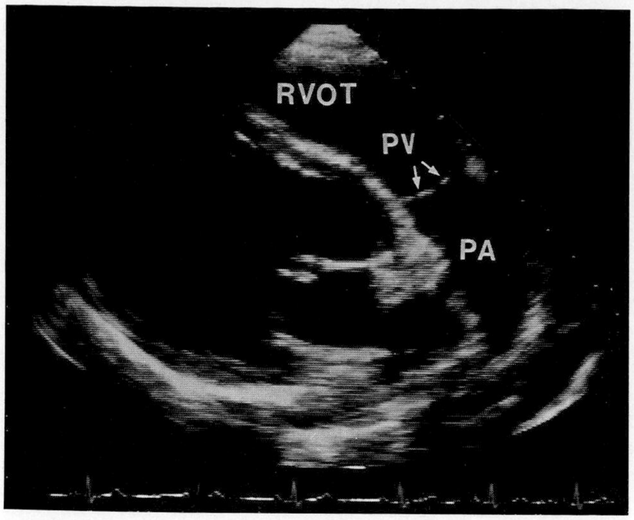

Fig. 27–14. Parasternal long axis recording from a patient with valvular pulmonary stenosis. Again, the pulmonary leaflet echoes (PV) arc inward toward the center of the pulmonary artery, thereby producing a significant narrowing of the vascular lumen. The posterior pulmonary leaflets are evident. RVOT = right ventricular outflow tract; PA = pulmonary artery.

artery during systole, and the hook-like configuration of this leaflet alone suffices to establish the presence of leaflet doming and, hence, the appropriate diagnosis.

The systolic opening motion of the stenotic pulmonary valve also differs from normal. In normal persons, the leaflet echoes remain parallel to each other and to the walls of the pulmonary artery as they separate.[6] In patients with valvular pulmonary stenosis, the proximal portion of the leaflet echoes separates and swings through a wide arc, whereas the distal tips of the leaflets remain relatively close. This motion causes the angle between the leaflet echoes and the margins of the pulmonary artery to become increasingly obtuse, finally terminating in full leaflet doming. When viewed in real time, this abrupt tipping of the leaflet echoes as they begin to open alerts the examiner to the possible presence of pulmonary stenosis. More detailed frame-by-frame analysis is generally necessary to demonstrate the domed systolic configuration. Figure 27–16 illustrates the difference between the opening sequence of the normal and stenotic pulmonary valve.

Two-dimensional imaging has a reported specificity of 97% for pulmonic stenosis but only a 77% sensitivity

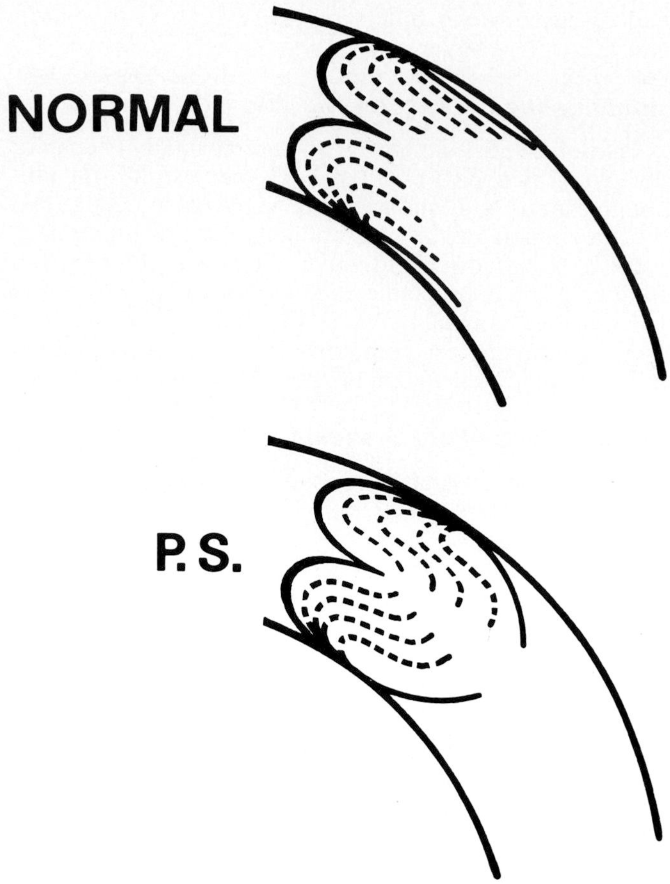

Fig. 27–16. Diagram comparing the opening patterns of a normal and a stenotic pulmonary valve. In the normal valve, the leaflets move away from each other while maintaining their relative parallel orientation. In the stenotic valve, the free edges of the pulmonary leaflets angle abruptly away from each other. This motion pattern creates an increasingly more obtuse angle between the leaflet echoes as they open and highlights the presence of valvular stenosis when viewed in real time. (From Weyman AE, et al.: Cross-sectional echocardiographic visualization of the stenotic pulmonary valve. Circulation 56:769, 1977. Reproduced by permission of the American Heart Association, Inc.)

in patients with all types of congenital heart lesions.[17] In our experience the sensitivity is much higher in patients with isolated pulmonary stenosis while the specificity remains excellent.

Doppler. Although valvular pulmonary stenosis is usually diagnosed by two-dimensional imaging, Doppler

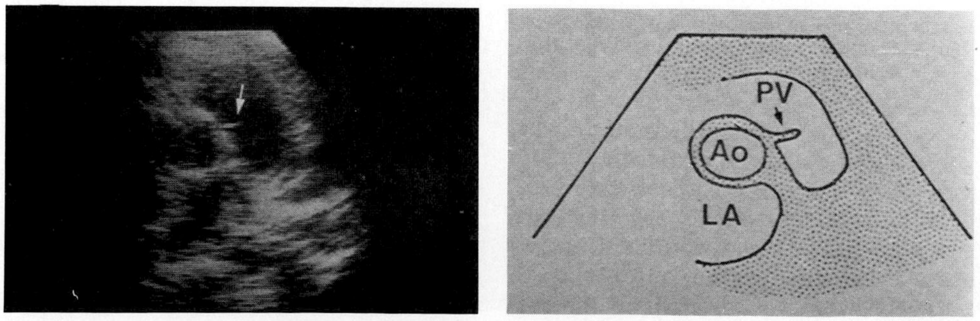

Fig. 27–15. Parasternal long axis recording of the pulmonary artery and valve (PV) illustrates the characteristic appearance of valvular pulmonary stenosis when only one leaflet can be recorded. Although the entire valve is not visible, a diagnosis can be established based on the hook-like systolic configuration of the single leaflet. AO = aorta; LA = left atrium.

methods may be of value when the diagnosis is unclear and are always necessary to determine severity. The Doppler diagnosis of pulmonic stenosis, like that of stenotic lesions elsewhere in the cardiovascular system, is based on (1) demonstration of an increase in flow velocity through the stenotic valve, (2) a decrease in the flow area at the valve level, and (3) an area of turbulence distal to the flow-restricting orifice (Fig. 27–17).

The local increase in flow velocity at the stenosis can be demonstrated either by pulsed or color flow Doppler. Generally, flow proximal to the valve is laminar and its velocity is normal. Within a centimeter of the valve orifice, convective acceleration begins and flow velocity increases, reaching its maximum just distal to the orifice at the vena contracta. Narrowing of the flow stream at the orifice can be visualized by color Doppler (Fig. 27–17), and a close relationship was observed in one patient between jet diameter by multigate Doppler and valve orifice diameter measured at surgery.[18]

Demonstration of the local increase in velocity at the valve level is important for several reasons. First, as the pulmonary artery curves around the aorta, the beam becomes increasingly more parallel to the flow vector. Therefore, using pulsed Doppler, without precise angle correction, the recorded velocity will increase gradually without any actual change in the rate of flow. Second, in infants, the velocity in the left pulmonary artery can be greater than that in that across the valve, and blind continuous wave recording can suggest a gradient when there is no abnormality.

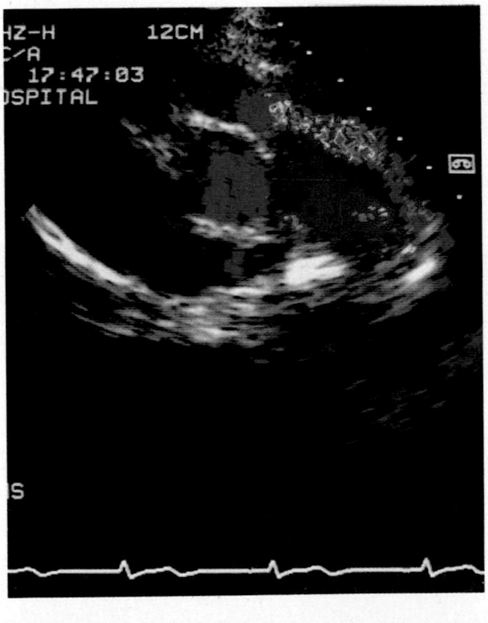

Fig. 27–17. Parasternal color Doppler recording of the pulmonary valve and pulmonary artery in long axis from a patient with severe valvular pulmonary stenosis. Just proximal to the valve, flow accelerates (blue to red) and becomes turbulent (blue red mosaic) as it passes through the stenotic orifice. Just distal to the orifice, the flow stream reaches its narrowest diameter and then re-expands slightly in the pulmonary artery. The free jet extends into the left pulmonary artery. The main pulmonary artery is dilated, and there is an extensive area of recirculation (red) along the medial wall of the vessel. (Courtesy of Dr. Leng Jiang.)

Distal to the valve, a free turbulent jet develops (Fig. 27–17), whose size, shape, depth, and direction of penetration are determined by the severity of stenosis and the unique geometry of the pulmonary artery.[19] As the severity of stenosis increases, the diameter of the jet decreases, its velocity and turbulent intensity increase, it is directed more toward the left pulmonary artery, and its point of impact extends further down the left pulmonary artery. The decrease in jet diameter causes a corresponding increase in the size of the adjacent region of low axial flow between the jet and the pulmonary arterial wall (see Fig. 27–17). Increased flow directed toward the left pulmonary artery can alter the relative volume of flow in left and right branches. Normally, flow is divided evenly between the right and left pulmonary arteries; however, this ratio may increase to 70:30 (left/right) in patients with severely stenotic valves.[20]

Turbulence alone is not diagnostic of valvular pulmonary stenosis, because turbulence in the region of the valve can also be seen with infundibular stenosis, supracristal ventricular septal defect, and sinus of Valsalva aneurysm rupture into the right ventricular outflow tract.

Atriogenic Opening of the Pulmonary Valve. In many patients with pulmonic stenosis, the pulmonary leaflets shift to an open or domed position at end-diastole following atrial contraction but before ventricular systole (Fig. 27–18). This presystolic opening movement results from the abnormal end-diastolic pressure relationships that frequently occur in valvular pulmonary stenosis.[13,21] Specifically, the decreased compliance of the right ventricle and resulting increased force of right atrial contraction may increase peak right ventricular end-diastolic pressure to a level that exceeds simultaneous pulmonary artery pressure. This produces a positive gradient across the valve and results in both presystolic valve opening or doming and presystolic flow (Fig. 27–19). The presystolic doming motion is responsible for the enlarged A waves seen on the M-mode echocardiogram in many patients with moderate or severe pulmonary stenosis as well as the characteristic inspiratory decrease in the systolic ejection click of pulmonary valve stenosis (Fig. 27–20).[16]

Quantitation of Severity.

Transvalvular Gradient. The pressure gradient across a stenotic pulmonary valve can be determined from the maximal flow velocity at the vena contract using the modified Bernoulli equation where $\Delta P = 4\,v^2$. Because the pulmonic valve is relatively close to the anterior chest wall, the Doppler sensitivity is excellent and the beam can be aligned parallel to the flow vector without great difficulty. In children, jet velocities can also be recorded from the subcostal window. Even in adults where sensitivity is limited the highest velocities will occasionally be recorded form this window. Correlations between Doppler and catheterization values for transpulmonary gradients have been excellent, with correlation coefficients ranging from .95 to .98 and standard errors between 6.5 and 8 mm Hg.[22–25] In patients in whom the jet is more difficult to record, proper alignment can be facilitated by color flow mapping. In some cases, gradient measurement is simplified because the

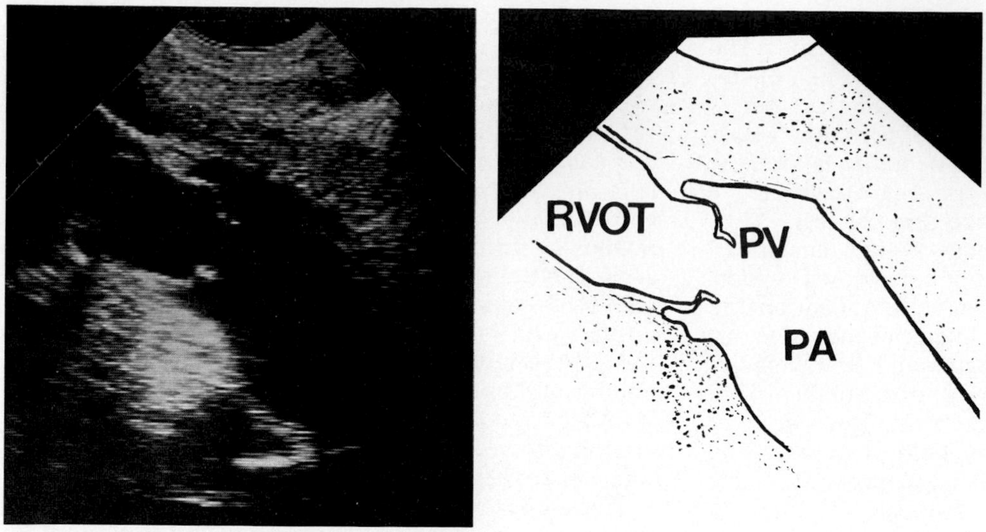

Fig. 27–18. Parasternal long axis recording of the pulmonary artery and pulmonary valve. The recording was obtained following atrial but before ventricular systole. Opening or doming of the pulmonary leaflets in response to atrial contraction is evident. This presystolic opening or doming of the valve corresponds to the enlarged A waves noted in earlier M-mode studies and suggests deranged hemodynamics reflective of a more severe valvular lesion. RVOT = right ventricular outflow tract; PV = pulmonary valve; PA = pulmonary artery.

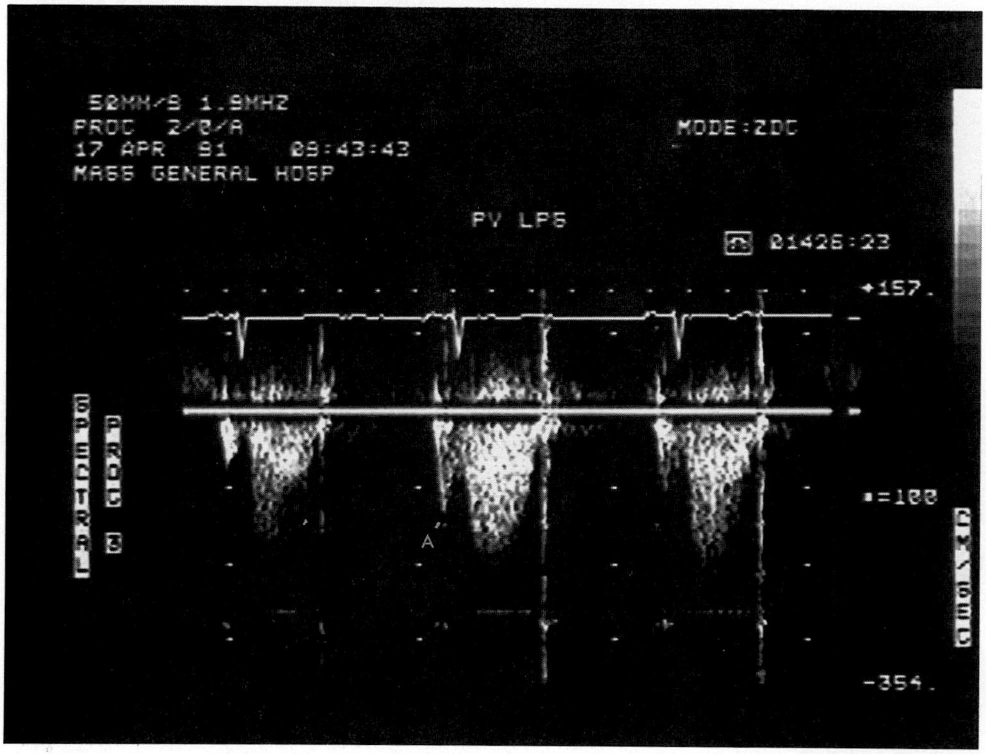

Fig. 27–19. Doppler recording of presystolic flow across the pulmonary valve in valvular pulmonary stenosis. In this example, the velocity of the presystolic flow is almost equal to the maximal velocity recorded during systole.

catheter instantaneous and peak-to-peak pressure gradients are often similar; however, the Doppler peak gradient will still overestimate the peak-to-peak gradient in many cases.[25] In calculating the Doppler gradient, it is rarely necessary to consider the proximal velocity because most lesions that increase volume flow also cause the outflow tract to dilate. The presence of a subvalvular ventricular septal defect, however, may increase the proximal velocity, and this must be considered in gradient calculation. Sedation can alter gradients in children, with the result that precatheterization gradients may be significantly higher than measurements recorded at catheterization. Doppler-derived gradients are frequently used to assess the efficacy of percutaneous balloon valvuloplasty for pulmonary stenosis. Immediately postvalvuloplasty, the gradient may be significantly higher than that recorded several days later as a result of associated infundibular stenosis.[26] In some cases, the velocity waveform will show a fixed and superimposed higher velocity dynamic component immediately after the procedure. In this situation, the fixed component is the better estimate of long-term results.[26] Because of this early fluctuation in gradient, the results of balloon valvuloplasty are best assessed at least a day after the procedure.

Valve Area. Although the pulmonary artery gradient is usually an accurate measure of pulmonary stenosis, this may not be the case in patients with severe right

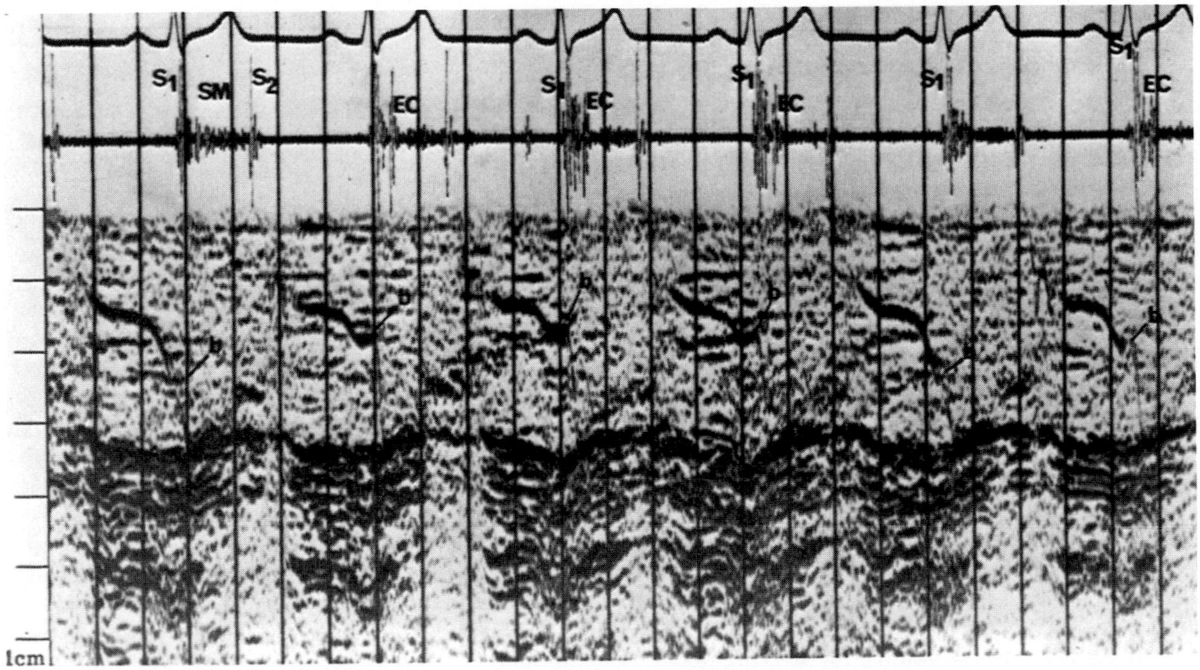

Fig. 27–20. Echocardiogram and phonocardiogram illustrating the relation of the position of the pulmonary valve at the onset of ventricular systole (point b) to the intensity of the pulmonary ejection click (EC). In the first complex from the left, recorded during inspiration, the valve is in a partially open position at the onset of ventricular systole (point b), and the ejection click is barely recordable. In the next three complexes, during expiration, the valve is in a baseline or closed position at the onset of systole, and a prominent ejection click is recorded. In the fifth complex, during inspiration, the valve is again in a partially open position at the onset of systole, and the ejection click is markedly diminished. (From Weyman AE, Dillon JC, Feigenbaum H, Chang S: Echocardiographic patterns of pulmonary valve motion in valvular pulmonary stenosis. Am J Cardiol 34:644, 1974. Reproduced with permission of Cahners Publishing Co.)

heart failure. In such cases, calculation of valve area using the continuity equation may provide a better estimate of severity. Kosturakis and co-workers[27] used Doppler-derived flow and velocity measurements to calculate stenotic valve area in 11 children with pulmonary stenosis.

Pulmonary Atresia. Pulmonary atresia is generally characterized by a dense band of echoes stretching across the pulmonary artery at the level of the pulmonary valve annulus. The annulus may be either normal or hypoplastic. On occasion, an atretic pulmonic valve may show some motion that can be misinterpreted as indicating a perforate valve. Absence of antegrade or retrograde flow across the valve by Doppler should indicate the appropriate diagnosis.

Functional Pulmonary Atresia. Functional pulmonary atresia is the absence of systolic valve opening and forward flow from the right ventricle into the pulmonary artery despite a functional pulmonary valve. Functional atresia occurs in neonates with severe tricuspid regurgitation and grossly impaired right ventricular function (e.g., severe Ebstein's anomaly, Uhl's anomaly, or right ventricular ischemia). The pulmonary valve generally fails to open in these cases because ductal flow into the constricted pulmonary circulation elevates pulmonary artery pressure above the maximal pressure that the abnormal right ventricle can generate. Functional atresia can be differentiated from anatomic atresia by the echocontrast or Doppler demonstration of retrograde flow passing through the pulmonary valve. This regurgitation occurs primarily during mid- to late-systole with lesser amounts of diastolic regurgitation noted.[28]

Pulmonary Regurgitation

Pulmonary regurgitation is characterized by the retrograde flow of blood from the pulmonary artery, through the closed pulmonary valve, and into the right ventricular outflow tract. Pulmonary regurgitation is almost invariably diastolic; however, in unusual disorders (i.e., functional pulmonary atresia), it may also occur during systole. Pulmonary regurgitation can be either congenital or acquired. Congenital regurgitation may be due to anomalies of cusp number (quadricuspid, or bicuspid valves) or development (hypoplasia, dysplasia, or absence of the pulmonary valve). Acquired pulmonary regurgitation is most often seen in patients with pulmonary hypertension, which may be primary or secondary to vascular changes that are due to mitral stenosis, ventricular septal defect, atrial septal defect, or other congenital defects. It also occurs in association with infective endocarditis, trauma, carcinoid, tertiary syphilis, after pulmonary valvotomy, following pulmonary valve prolapse through a ventricular septal defect, and in patients with idiopathic dilation of the pulmonary artery. Trivial pulmonary regurgitation is also noted frequently in patients with presumably normal pulmonary valves (see later discussion). Pulmonary regurgitation alone generally has a benign course, with the natural history determined by that of associated lesions.[29] Severe pulmonary regurgitation, however, is often associated with an increase in right ventricular size, paradoxic septal motion, and occasionally, fluttering of the tricuspid valve. On rare occasions, severe isolated pulmonary regurgitation may lead to congestive heart failure and even death in the neonate.

Diagnosis. Pulmonary regurgitation is detected primarily by Doppler echocardiography,[8,30–33] although contrast techniques have also been described.[34,35] The Doppler diagnosis is based on the demonstration of regurgitant flow in the pulmonary artery and right ventricular outflow tract by pulsed Doppler or by the color Doppler demonstration of a free turbulent jet in the right ventricular outflow tract beginning at the line of leaflet coaptation and extending backward toward the right ventricle.[36] Color Doppler is optimally suited to assess jet size and spatial orientation; pulsed Doppler, to determine jet temporal characteristics; and continuous wave Doppler, to determine maximal jet velocity in patients with pulmonary hypertension. The size, extent, and duration of the jet are determined by the driving pressure (gradient between the pulmonary artery and the right ventricle) and the regurgitant volume (i.e., the jet momentum). In patients with normal pulmonary artery pressures and small regurgitant orifices, the regurgitant jets are usually small, have their highest velocity immediately after pulmonary valve closure when the pulmonary artery to right ventricular gradient (PA > RV) is at its peak, and then decrease in velocity and size as diastole progresses and the gradient decreases. A posterior deflection in the regurgitant velocity profile (decreased jet velocity) is often recorded following atrial contraction because the associated increase in right ventricular pressure decreases the right ventricle/pulmonary artery pressure gradient. In patients with normal pulmonary artery pressures, peak regurgitant jet velocity ranges from 1.2 to 1.9 m/sec.[37] Figure 27–21 illustrates the spatial distribution of a small low velocity jet. In patients with small, narrow jets, pulsed Doppler may demonstrate only regurgitant flow during the period of diastole when the moving jet (the jet moves superiorly with the pulmonary artery and valve as the ventricle fills) falls within the fixed sample volume. This phenomenon can often creates the incorrect appearance of pulmonary regurgitation being present only during the later portion of diastole.

In patients with elevated pulmonary artery pressures, jet velocities tend to remain high throughout diastole and spatial distribution increases even though the regurgitant orifice remains small. Figure 27–22 illustrates the spatial distribution of the regurgitant jet and the peak jet velocities in a patient with pulmonary hypertension. The instantaneous pulmonary artery-to-right ventricular diastolic pressure gradient can be calculated from the velocity of regurgitant flow using the modified Bernoulli equation ($\Delta P = 4V^2$). Adding clinically assessed or estimated right atrial pressure yields an estimate of pulmonary artery diastolic pressure. Pulmonary artery diastolic pressures estimated by Doppler-echocardiography have been found to correlate closely with those recorded at catheterization (r = .94 mean absolute difference 3.3 mm Hg). The noninvasive estimate of pulmonary artery diastolic pressure also correlates closely with the wedge pressure (r = .87, mean absolute difference 3.8 mm Hg).[38] Doppler-derived end-diastolic pressure gradients have also been observed to correlate closely with catheterization measurements before and after vasodilator therapy.[39]

When the regurgitant volume is large, regurgitant flow can be recorded by color Doppler extending from the valve, through the outflow tract, and into the right ventricle. In these cases, subcostal recordings may be re-

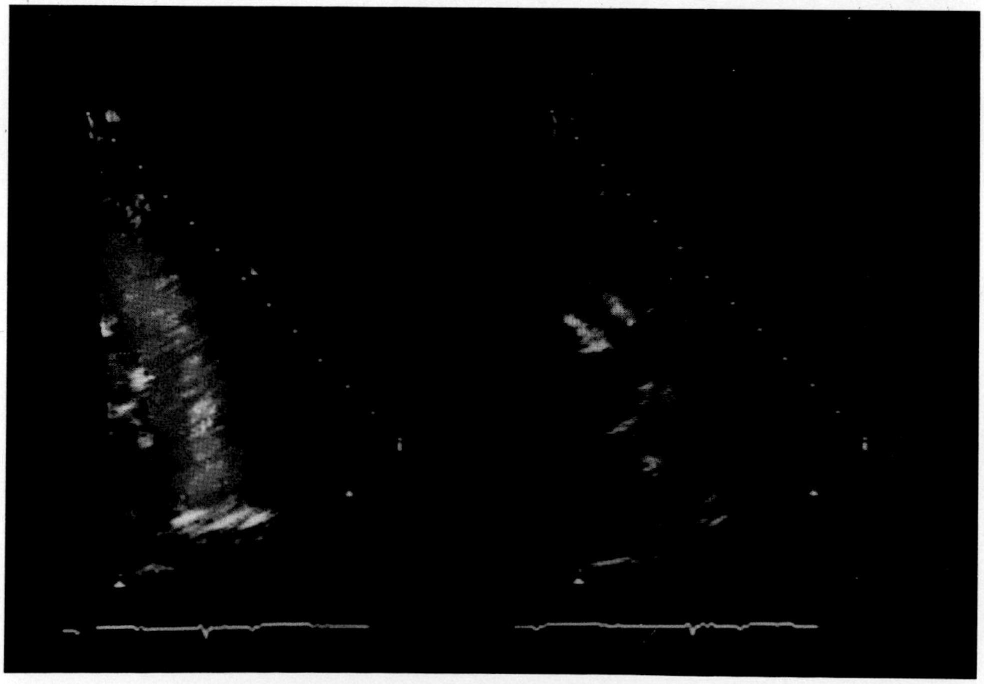

Fig. 27–21. Color Doppler recording of the distal right ventricular outflow tract, pulmonic valve, and pulmonary artery during systole (left) and diastole (right). During systole, normal flow away from the transducer (blue) is recorded. During diastole, a small spindle-shaped area of regurgitant flow (red) is recorded arising at the plane of leaflet closure and extending roughly 1.5 cm into the outflow tract.

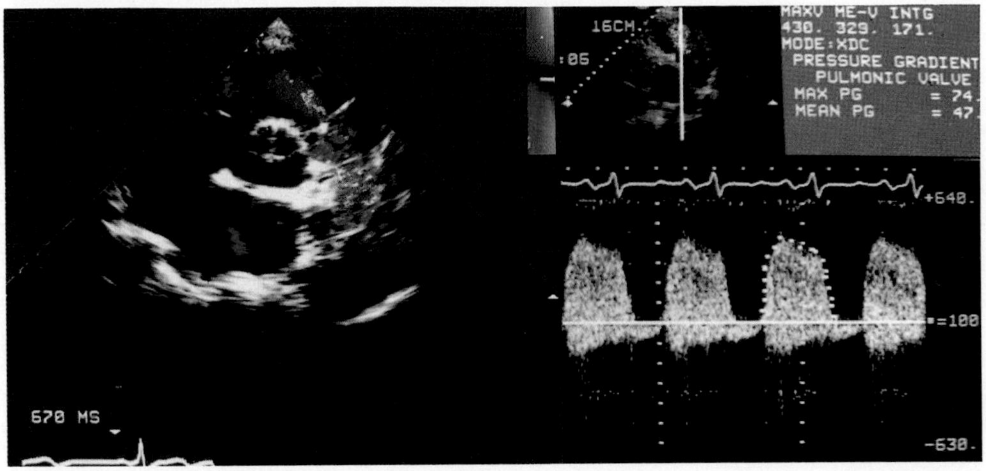

Fig. 27–22. Left. Color Doppler recording from a patient with pulmonary hypertension and pulmonary regurgitation. The regurgitant jet (red) arises from the center of the valve leaflets and extends into the right ventricular outflow tract. Right. Continuous wave Doppler recording of peak jet velocities. In this example, the peak gradient from the pulmonary artery to the right ventricle was 74 mm Hg, while the mean gradient was 47.7 mm Hg. (Courtesy of Dr. Leng Jiang.)

quired to visualize the full extent of the jet (Fig. 27–23). Significant regurgitation also causes an increase in the forward flow velocity during systole and a rapid fall in diastolic regurgitant velocities with regurgitation ending before end-diastole (Fig. 27–24). This pattern indicates equilibration of right ventricular and pulmonary artery pressures before end-diastole, and in these cases forward flow can be observed following atrial contraction.[8] The largest regurgitant jets occur when the regurgitant orifice is larger and the pulmonary artery pressure is elevated.

Retrograde or disturbed flow in the outflow tract can also be caused by tricuspid inflow, which can create a circular flow pattern with blood directed toward the pulmonic valve in the anterior and central parts of the outflow tract and away from the valve along its septal margin.[36] Although this retrograde flow has caused confusion on pulsed Doppler recordings, color Doppler can easily distinguish this normal circular flow pattern from true regurgitation.

Estimation of Severity. The severity of pulmonary regurgitation, like that of other valves, can be determined both semiqualitatively and quantitatively. Early studies suggested that a regurgitant jet length of 10 mm or less was indicative of trivial regurgitation. Jets of >10 mm were seen in patients with heart disease; however, only those with jets of ≥20 mm had an audible murmur.[36]

The planimetered jet area indexed for body surface area has also been used as a measure of severity. When compared to angiographic grade, a pulmonary regurgitant area index (cm^2/m^2) of 0.64 ± 0.60 was seen with mild, 1.07 ± 0.63 with moderate, and 2.2 ± 1.67 with

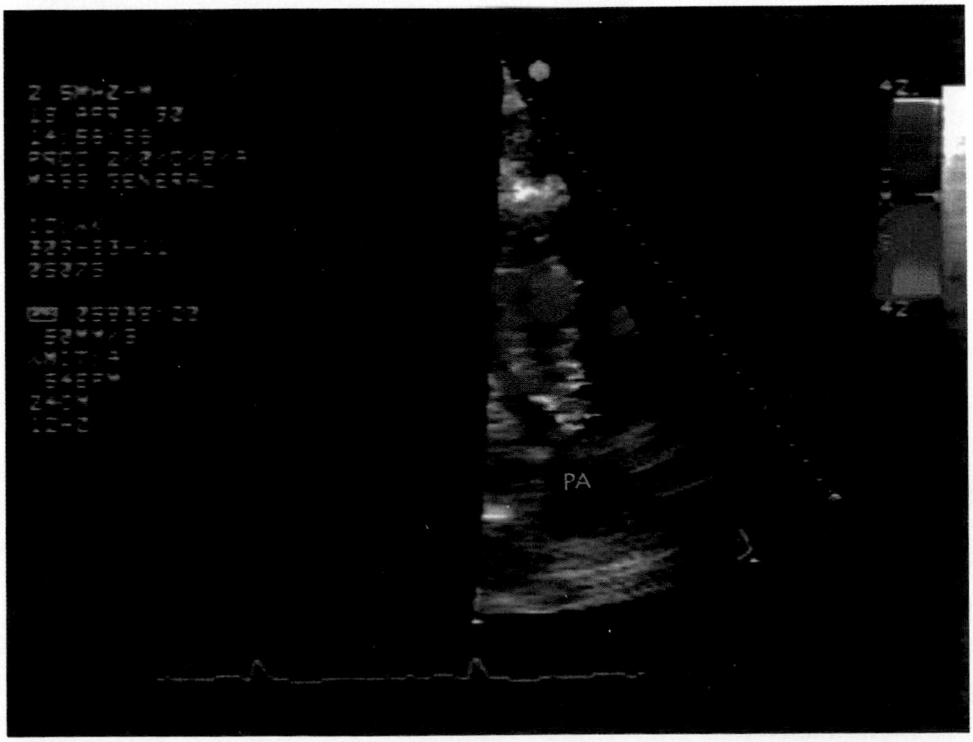

Fig. 27–23. Elevated subcostal long axis color Doppler recording of the pulmonary artery (PA) illustrating free pulmonary regurgitation extending from the valve leaflets to the free wall of the right ventricle.

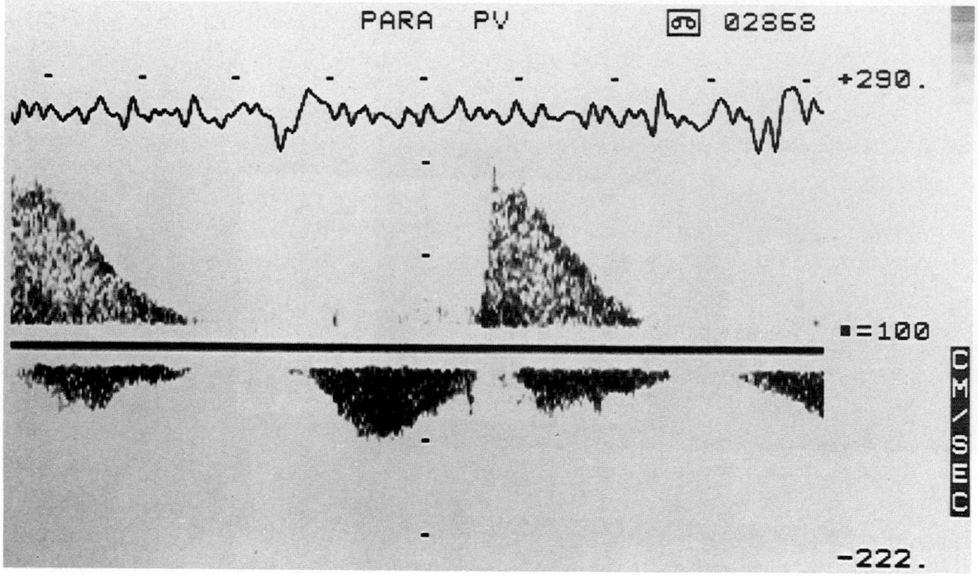

Fig. 27–24. Pulsed Doppler recording of the velocity profile of a low pressure, high volume pulmonary regurgitant jet. Immediately after pulmonary valve (PV) closure, regurgitant flow begins to accelerate, reaches a peak velocity of roughly 1.8 m/sec, and then rapidly decelerates until flow ceases roughly 240 msec before the next systole. This rapid equilibration of pressures is seen both in patients with significant regurgitation, which produces a rapid rise in right ventricular pressure and fall in pulmonary artery pressure, and in normal persons with a low pulmonary artery end-diastolic pressure. PARA = parasternal.

severe regurgitation. The regurgitant index also showed a strong correlation with pulmonary regurgitant fraction by videodensitometric techniques (r = .84).

Finally, regurgitant volume and fraction have been calculated as the difference between forward and reverse flow in the pulmonary artery[40,41] (Fig. 27–25). Using this approach, forward (total) flow is calculated as the product of the stroke velocity integral recorded at the midpulmonary artery level and the arterial diameter measured at the level of the sample volume. Regurgitant flow is similarly calculated from the regurgitant velocity integral and vessel diameter. Subtracting regurgitant flow from total forward flow yields the net forward flow. The net forward flow should equal the aortic flow in the absence of aortic regurgitation, and comparison of these values is a useful cross check of measurement accuracy.[40] Using this method, a relationship has been observed between regurgitant fraction and clinical severity of disease.[40] Although imperfectly validated, a regurgitant fraction of <40% has been associated with mild, 40 to 60% with moderate, and >60% with severe clinically estimated regurgitation.[41] Even in preliminary studies, however, overlap between groups was apparent.[40]

The method is not valid in patients with pulmonary stenosis because mean systolic velocities cannot be obtained from the turbulent post-stenotic jet. However, diastolic regurgitant velocities should be accurate. Accuracy requires the following: velocities must be sampled in the main pulmonary artery (distal to the region of flow acceleration toward the regurgitant orifice); sample volume position must be altered to optimally record forward and regurgitant flow; mean velocity must be computed from a number of cardiac cycles, diameters must be measured at the sample volume site, and net flow must be computed and compared with flow in a normal portion of the heart. The method may not be applicable in patients with multiple lesions in whom there is no

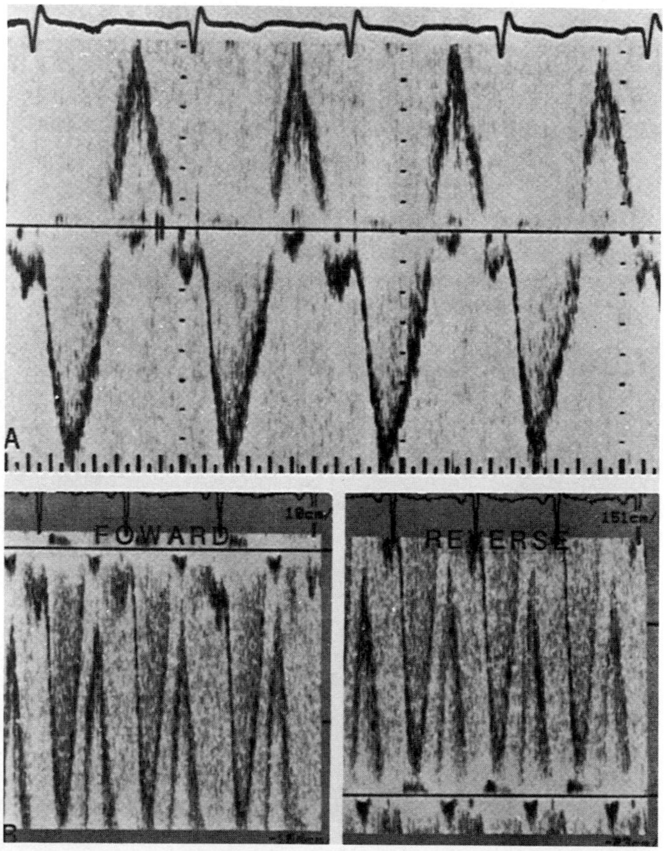

Fig. 27–25. Pulsed Doppler recording of flow in the main pulmonary artery from a patient with pulmonary regurgitation. Anterograde flow is away from the transducer and thus displayed below the baseline, while retrograde flow is displayed above the baseline. (From Marx GR, Hicks RW, Allen HD, Goldberg SJ: Noninvasive assessment of hemodynamic responses to exercise in pulmonary regurgitation after operations to correct pulmonary outflow obstruction. Am J Cardiol 61:595, 1988. Reproduced with permission of Cahners Publishing Co.)

reference for true output, and as described, it assumes that the pulmonary artery diameter is constant in diastole and systole.[40] If the diameter is assumed to be constant, then the ratio of the forward and reverse integrals can be used by themselves. Although the ratio can be computed without the diameter, the internal accuracy check is no longer available.[40]

Lesions Commonly Associated With Pulmonary Regurgitation.

Congenital Absence of the Pulmonary Valve. Congenital absence of the pulmonary valve is a rare cardiac malformation usually associated with tetralogy of Fallot; however, isolated absence of the valve can also be observed. Two-dimensional imaging generally reveals a markedly dilated pulmonary artery and local ridges or masses of tissue at the level of the annulus that extend several millimeters into the lumen. However, there is no evidence of obvious leaflet structure or motion.[42,43] The right ventricle is dilated, and there is generally paradoxic septal motion. Isolated absence of the pulmonary valve is associated with free pulmonary regurgitation and massive dilation of the pulmonary artery and right ventricle. Figure 27–26 is an M-mode sweep from the right ventricle through the infundibulum into the pulmonary artery from a patient with isolated congenital absence of the pulmonary valve.[44]

Pulmonary Valve Endocarditis. Infective endocarditis involving the pulmonary valve is relatively rare,[45,46] although echocardiographic visualization of pulmonary valve vegetations has been reported in growing number of cases.[47–50] Pulmonary valve vegetations have a similar appearance to vegetations involving the other cardiac valves and are described as globular or shaggy, mobile masses of echoes that adhere to the valve leaflets (Fig. 27–27). Pulmonary vegetations may be single or multiple. When there is disruption of the valve, the area of involvement may appear more irregular and may be associated with rapid oscillatory movement of the free edges of the damaged tissue[47] (Fig. 27–27A). Figure 27–27B is a parasternal long axis recording of a pulmonary valve from one such case. In this example, small globular masses of echoes were attached to the posterior pulmonary leaflet, which were noted to move in unison with the leaflet during opening and closure. Following

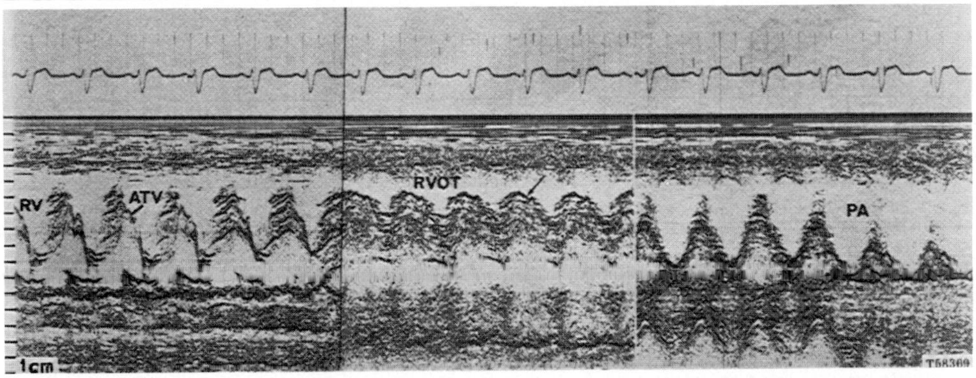

Fig. 27–26. Composite scan from right ventricle (RV) through right ventricular outflow tract (RVOT) into pulmonary artery (PA) in a patient with congenital absence of the pulmonary valve. Distinct dilation of right ventricle (8 cm) is observed along with fluttering of anterior leaflet of the tricuspid valve (ATV), suggesting pulmonary regurgitation. The RVOT appears to be of normal size. There is massive dilation of the PA with pronounced systolic expansion consistent with severe pulmonary regurgitation. A structure in the RVOT at the level of the normal pulmonary valve (arrow, center) with a pattern of motion somewhat similar to the pulmonary valve suggests the possibility of a rudimentary valve structure. (From Weyman AE, Dillon JC, Feigenbaum H, Chang S: Pulmonary valve echo motion in pulmonary regurgitation. Br Heart J 37:1184, 1975. Reproduced with permission of the British Medical Association.)

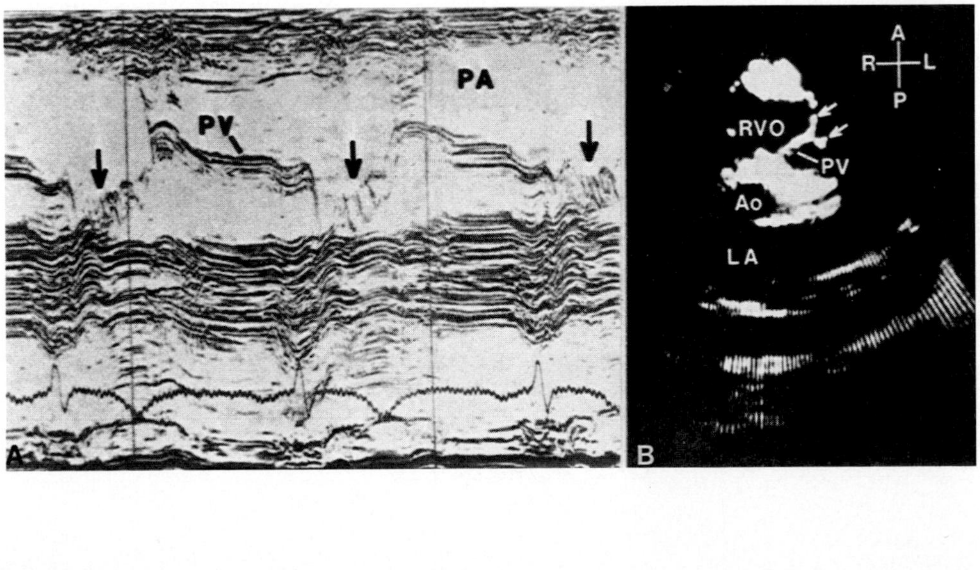

Fig. 27–27. A. M-mode recording showing coarse systolic fluttering (arrows) of the pulmonary valve (PV) in a patient with PV vegetations. **B.** Two-dimensional echogram demonstrating two small vegetations of the posterior leaflet of the PV. PA = pulmonary artery. (From Berger M, et al.: M-mode and two-dimensional echocardiographic findings in pulmonic valve regurgitation. Am Heart J 107:391, 1984.)

treatment, pulmonary vegetation size may remain constant, decrease, or disappear completely.[47,51] Rapid disappearance of a vegetation has been associated with pulmonary embolism;[50] however, emboli can also occur without change in vegetation size.

Bacterial endocarditis can cause rupture of a pulmonary leaflet with loss of basal support. In these cases, the flail leaflet typically prolapses into the right ventricular outflow tract during diastole and is thrust into the pulmonary artery during systole (Fig. 27–28).[48,50,52–54] Patients with pulmonary valve vegetations generally have pulmonary regurgitation detectable by Doppler techniques.[50,51] Premature opening of the pulmonic valve can also be noted.[48,51]

In addition to valvular involvement, endocarditis can be seen in the right ventricular outflow tract at the outlet of a high membranous or bulbar ventricular septal defect or arising from the opposite wall at the site of a jet lesion.[55]

Pulmonary Regurgitation in Patients with Presumably Normal Valves. Pulmonary regurgitation has been reported in between 40% and 78% of patients with morphologically normal pulmonic valves and no other evidence of structural heart disease.[56] Normal regurgitant jets are usually small and spindle shaped and originate from the central coaptation point of the pulmonary leaflets and extend less than a centimeter into the outflow tract.[36] The maximal velocity of regurgitant jets in healthy subjects ranges from 1.2 to 1.9 m/sec,[37] which by the modified Bernoulli equation corresponds to pressure difference of between 6 to 14 mm Hg.

Several mechanisms have been suggested to explain the common occurrence of regurgitation across normal pulmonary valves when leakage of the morphologically similar aortic valve is rare in the absence of disease. First, although the tricuspid configuration of the pulmonary valve is ideally suited to occlude a round orifice, the pulmonary artery is often not perfectly circular as it drapes across the top of the aorta. Second, the pressure in the pulmonary artery is low relative to that in the aorta and hence does not force the leaflets together creating a tight seal. These two factors appear to result in incomplete coaptation at the leaflets at their tips, which permits a small degree of leakage of the right-sided semilunar valve. The fact that the noncircular shape of the pulmonary artery is not a function of age, the pulmonary artery pressure remains low, and the valve is not subject to the same wear and tear as other cardiac valves may explain why the prevalence of "normal" pulmonary regurgitation appears to be independent of age.

Pulmonary Hypertension

Several approaches have been suggested for the noninvasive estimation of pulmonary artery pressure including (1) Doppler-derived gradients, (2) changes in pulmonic valve motion and pulmonary artery flow profiles, and (3) measurement of the right ventricular isovolumic relaxation time. While the data required for all of these measurements are not available in every patient, at least one measure of pulmonary artery pressure can be obtained in up to 98% of patients with a broad range of disease states.[57]

Doppler-Derived Pressure Gradients. Pulmonary artery pressure can be estimated from (1) the right ventricular-right atrial pressure gradient in patients with tricuspid regurgitation, (2) the left ventricular-right ventricular pressure gradient in patients with ventricular septal defect, (3) the aorta-pulmonary artery gradient in patients with aortopulmonary connections, and (4) from the pulmonary artery-right ventricular gradient in patients with

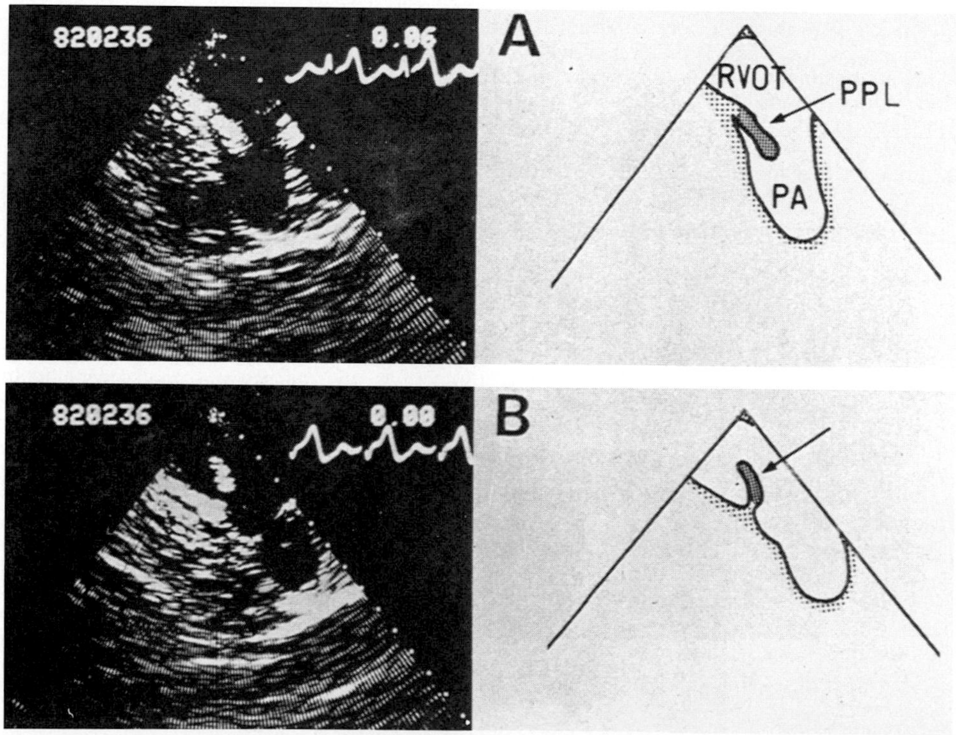

Fig. 27–28. Two-dimensional echocardiographic recordings of the pulmonic valve during diastole and systole. **A.** In the systolic frame, there is marked thickening of the posterior leaflet. **B.** During diastole, the flail posterior leaflet prolapses backward into the outflow tract. RVOT = right ventricular outflow tract; PPL = posterior pulmonary leaflet; PA = pulmonary artery. (From Harasawa Y, et al.: Two-dimensional echocardiographic demonstration of flail pulmonic valve due to infective endocarditis. Am Heart J 108: 1552, 1984.)

pulmonary regurgitation. The most common approach is to estimate pulmonary artery systolic pressure from right ventricular pressure (assuming no pulmonic stenosis) determined as the sum of the right ventricular-right atrial pressure gradient and either an assumed or clinically determined right atrial pressure.[58,59] It has also been demonstrated that pulmonary artery pressure bears a direct relationship to the tricuspid valve gradient (r = .99, standard error of estimation [SEE] = 4.9 mm Hg) and thus can be derived from the pressure gradient alone using the regression equation [pulmonary artery systolic pressure (PASP) = 1.23 * gradient − 0.09]. In patients with pulmonic stenosis, the pulmonary artery pressure is equal to the right ventricular systolic pressure less the transpulmonic gradient. Although this approach requires the presence of tricuspid regurgitation, measurable regurgitant velocities are present in roughly 72%[60] of adult cardiac patients with pulmonary hypertension and in virtually all patients (96%) in whom the pulmonary artery systolic pressure exceeds 50 mm Hg. Tricuspid regurgitation is also present in roughly 25% of normal and in 50% of preterm infants, permitting early changes in pulmonary artery pressure to be monitored.[61]

In patients with ventricular septal defects, right ventricular pressure can be determined as the peak aortic pressure (measured by sphygmomanometer), which is equal to the left ventricular systolic pressure minus the gradient across the defect. With associated pulmonary stenosis, the pulmonary artery pressure will equal the right ventricular pressure minus the transpulmonary gradient. When a ventricular septal defect and pulmonary stenosis coexist, the combined calculated pressure differences may exceed the true gradient between the left ventricle and the pulmonary artery by 10 to 15 mm Hg, because the velocity peaks can occur at different points in systole.[8]

When there is a direct systemic to pulmonary artery connection (i.e., a patent ductus arteriosus, Waterston shunt, Blalock-Taussig shunt, left pulmonary artery-aorta anastomosis or an aortopulmonary window), the pulmonary pressure will equal the systemic cuff pressure minus the gradient. The pressure difference across these shunts when related to blood pressure gives information about both systolic and diastolic pressures in the pulmonary artery. Echo or color flow mapping is necessary to characterize the type and location of the shunt, with continuous wave Doppler usually being required to measure peak velocity. Although alignment of the Doppler beam parallel with flow through these diverse shunts can be difficult, a success rate of 95% has been reported for accurate flow velocity measurement.[62] Inability to record the peak velocity across the shunts leads to overestimation of the pulmonary artery pressure. Underestimation can occur when the cuff pressure is less than that directly measured in the aorta. Despite these potential problems, an excellent correlation (r = .92, SEE = .08) between Doppler and catheter gradients has been reported.[62] Finally, in patients with pulmonary regurgitation, the maximal velocity in the regurgitant jet approximates the diastolic pressure in the pulmonary artery except when the right ventricular diastolic pressure is elevated.[8]

Changes in Pulmonary Valve Motion and Transpulmonary Flow Profiles. Pulmonary hypertension alters the timing of pulmonic valve opening and closure, the pattern of pulmonary valve motion, and the shape of the pulmonary flow velocity profile. As illustrated in Figure 27–29, when pulmonary hypertension is present, pulmonary artery end-diastolic pressure exceeds right ventricular pressure, reducing or eliminating any effect of atrial contraction on pulmonary valve motion. As pulmonary artery pressure increases, the time required for the right ventricular pressure to rise to the level of end-diastolic pulmonary pressure will increase and the valve will open later than normal. The rate of rise of right ventricular pressure dP/dT at the time of valve opening is generally greater than normal, with the result that valve opening and flow acceleration are more rapid. Pulmonary valve closure occurs slightly earlier than normal, and the time for right ventricular pressure to fall to the level of right atrial pressure increases.

Figure 27–30 illustrates the classic M-mode pattern of pulmonic valve motion observed in patients with pulmonary hypertension. The characteristic features include diminution or complete absence of the "a" wave; prolongation of the time from the onset of the Q wave of the electrocardiogram to the valve opening (the right ventricular pre-ejection period, RPEP); an increase in the rate of pulmonary valve opening (b–c slope); a de-

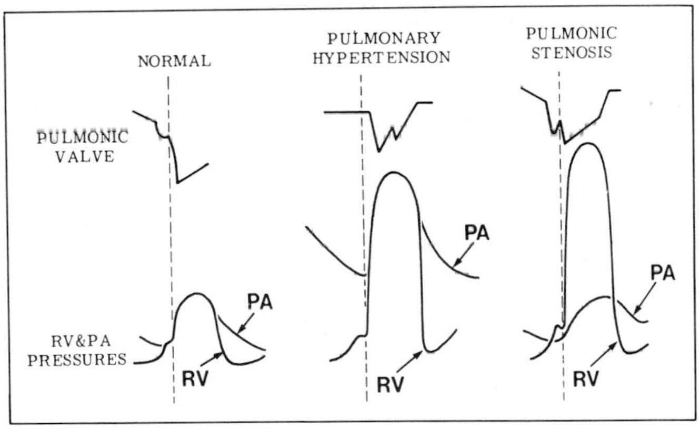

Fig. 27–29. The relationship of the pattern of pulmonary valve echo motion to simultaneous right ventricular and pulmonary artery (PA) diastolic pressures. Normally, there is a very small difference between simultaneous right ventricular and pulmonary artery end-diastolic pressure. In this situation the small increase in right ventricular end-diastolic pressure produced by atrial contraction may produce a slight posterior deflection or opening movement of the pulmonary valve. In patients with pulmonary hypertension (center), there is usually a significant difference between pulmonary artery and right ventricular end-diastolic pressures. In this situation, the slight increase in right ventricular end-diastolic pressure produced by atrial contraction is not sufficient to elevate the right ventricular pressure to a level approaching simultaneous pulmonary artery pressure; hence, no motion of the pulmonary valve is produced. Conversely, in patients with valvular pulmonary stenosis, the decrease in right ventricular compliance and increased force of right atrial contraction together with a normal or low pulmonary artery pressure frequently results in a positive gradient across the valve at end-diastole. This pressure gradient across the valve may produce presystolic opening of the valve following atrial contraction, which is reflected by a marked increase in the depth of the A wave. RV = right ventricle. (From Feigenbaum H: Echocardiography. 2nd Ed. Philadelphia, Lea & Febiger, 1976.)

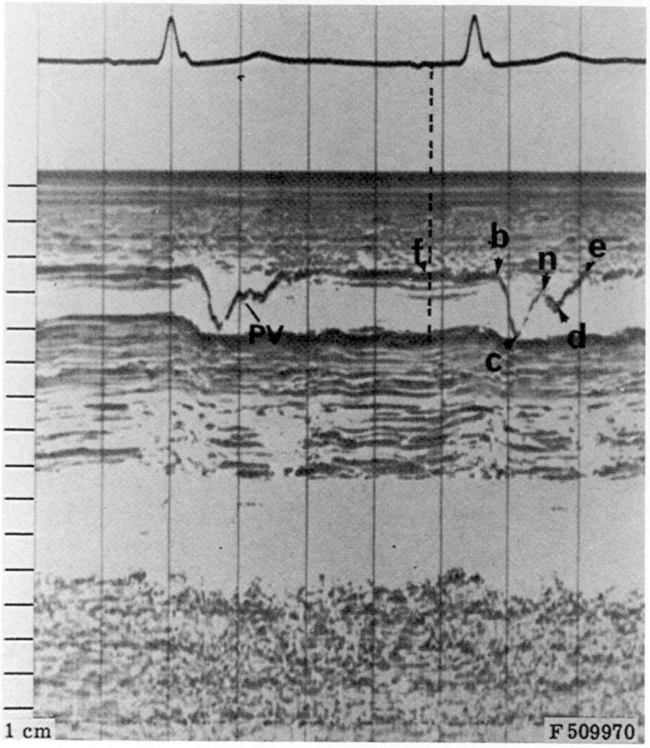

Fig. 27–30. Pulmonary valve echogram demonstrating the characteristic features seen with pulmonary hypertension. Following the P wave of the electrocardiogram (interrupted vertical line) (point f), there is no posterior deflection of the leaflet echo (A wave) in response to atrial contraction. Systolic opening of the pulmonary valve (PV) is delayed, resulting in prolongation of the Q to B interval (pre-ejection period). The diastolic or e to f slope is markedly flattened. In addition, there is a very prominent midsystolic notch (n). f = position of the leaflet at the onset of atrial systole; b = the position of the leaflet at the onset of ventricular systole; c = full opening of the valve following ventricular systole; n = midsystolic closure of the valve; d = the position of the valve at the onset of diastolic closure; e = the expected position of the coapted leaflet with diastolic closure of the valve. (From Weyman AE: Pulmonary valve echo motion in clinical practice. Am J Med 62:843, 1977. Reproduced with permission of Cahners Publishing Co.)

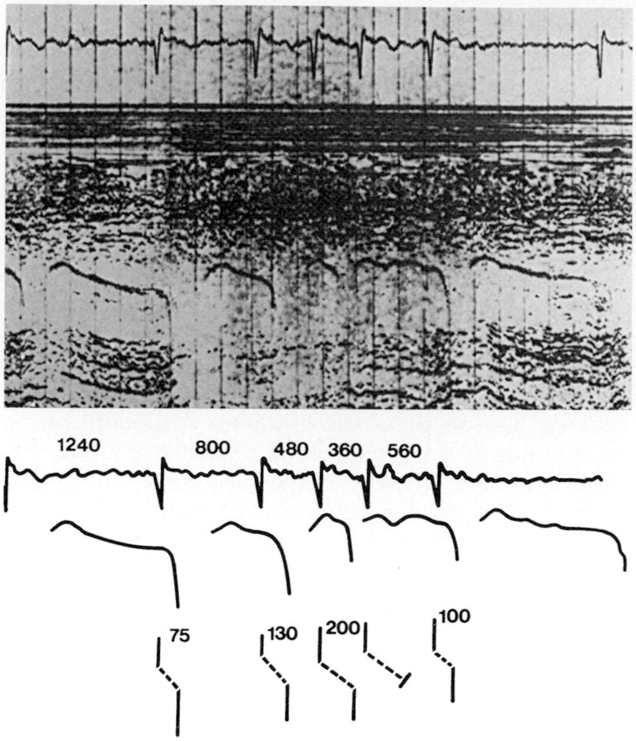

Fig. 27–31. **A** and **B.** Pulmonary valve echogram from a patient with pulmonary hypertension and atrial fibrillation. This recording demonstrates a gradual lengthening of the right ventricular pre-ejection period (Q to B interval), with decreasing cycle lengths. Following the fifth QRS complex in the series, the pulmonary valve fails to open entirely. This creates a relatively long diastolic pause, which is followed by shortening of the RVPEP in the subsequent complex. The upper line shows the approximate cycle lengths in milliseconds superimposed above the electrocardiogram, a corresponding diagram of the pulmonary valve echo (middle line drawing), and finally, a ladder diagram (bottom) indicating the approximate duration of the pre-ejection period in milliseconds. The upper solid vertical line in the ladder diagram corresponds to the Q wave of the electrocardiogram, the lower solid vertical line to the B point, and the oblique interrupted line connecting these two to the Q-B interval or RVPEP. There is gradual lengthening of the pre-ejection period with decreasing cycle lengths until complete failure of the valve opening occurs. This Wenckebach-type periodicity of the pulmonic valve is an unusual finding, which to date has been seen only with pulmonary hypertension. (From Weyman AE: Pulmonary valve echo motion in clinical practice. Am J Med 62:843, 1977. Reproduced with permission of Cahners Publishing Co.)

crease in the diastolic or e–f slope; and a midsystolic interruption or notch in the normally linear systolic echo. The notch is generally followed by late-systolic reopening of the leaflet with final closure at the onset of diastole. Unfortunately, none of these features is sufficiently sensitive or specific to be considered diagnostic. A waves are typically absent in patients with atrial fibrillation; both clinical and animal studies have shown a variable relation between the opening rate (b–c slope) and pulmonary artery pressure; and the e–f slope is affected by heart rate and flow across the valve in addition to pulmonary artery pressure. Even the midsystolic notch, which is the most specific feature, is insensitive, occurring in roughly 40% of patients with pulmonary hypertension, and has been reported in patients with idiopathic dilation of the pulmonary artery with normal pressures.[63] Other more subtle signs have been described in pulmonary hypertension such as a paradoxic increase in the RPEP with decreasing cycle length (Fig. 27–31) and reappearance of the "a" wave following prolonged diastolic filling periods (Fig. 27–32). Findings of this type unfortunately are rare.

Figure 27–33 compares the normal Doppler flow pattern in the pulmonary artery with that seen in patients with pulmonary hypertension. In normal persons, (Fig. 27–33A) flow accelerates gradually, peaks in midsystole, and then decelerates smoothly, terminating just before pulmonary valve closure. Flow into the pulmonary artery following atrial systole ("a" wave) is infrequently recorded, but when present, indicates a normal pulmonary artery pressure.[60] In pulmonary hypertension (Fig. 27–33B), there is a more rapid increase in velocity following valve opening, an earlier peak velocity, an earlier decrease in velocity, and less flow or even flow reversal

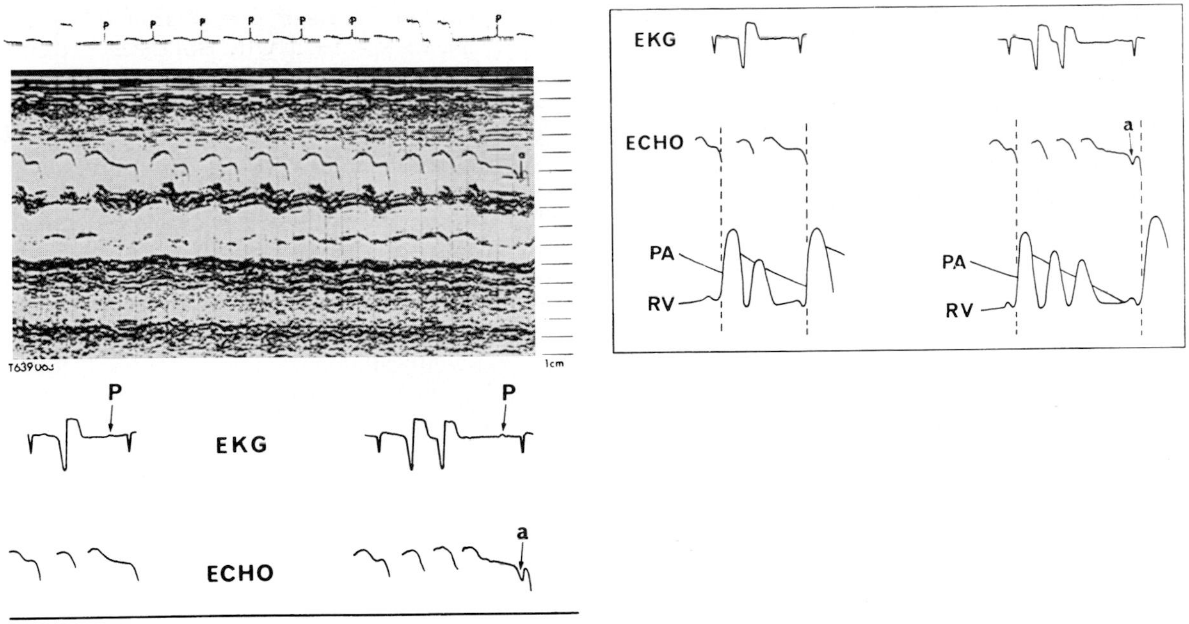

Fig. 27–32. Pulmonary valve echogram from a patient with pulmonary hypertension and multiple premature ventricular beats. Left. The echocardiographic and phonocardiographic recordings. Beneath the graphic records are line drawings of the pertinent segments. In the left side of the recording, there is a premature ventricular contraction followed by a relatively long diastolic pause. Following the long diastolic pause, the P wave or atrial contraction of the subsequent complex fails to produce any opening motion of the pulmonary valve or A wave. Right. Two premature ventricular contractions with a more prolonged diastolic pause. Following this increase in diastolic duration, the subsequent P wave or atrial contraction produces a prominent A wave on the pulmonary valve echogram. This recording demonstrates that a very prolonged diastolic period was required for pulmonary artery end-diastolic pressure to fall to a level approaching right ventricular end-diastolic pressure, permitting the valve motion in response to atrial contraction. Bottom. The relationship of the simultaneous pulmonary artery and right ventricular diastolic pressure (indicated diagrammatically) to the pulmonary valve echogram (ECHO) and simultaneous electrocardiogram (EKG). PA = pulmonary artery; RV = right ventricle. (From Weyman AE: Pulmonary valve echo motion in clinical practice. Am J Med 62:843, 1977. Reproduced with permission of Cahners Publishing Co.)

in late systole. Despite changes in the pattern of flow, the peak velocity does not usually differ from normal.

An abrupt midsystolic decrease in velocity, coincident in timing to the midsystolic notch of the posterior pulmonary leaflet noted on M-mode recordings, can also be observed (Fig. 27–33C). This notch is present in roughly 40 to 50% of patients with pulmonary hypertension and is usually associated with more severe disease. The notch appears to be related to a transient reversal of the right ventricular-pulmonary artery pressure gradient (PA > RV). This reversed gradient appears to results from a decrease in pulmonary artery compliance and an increase in main pulmonary artery size, impedance, and the transmission time of the velocity wave, which com-

DOPPLER PULMONARY ARTERIAL VELOCITY PROFILES

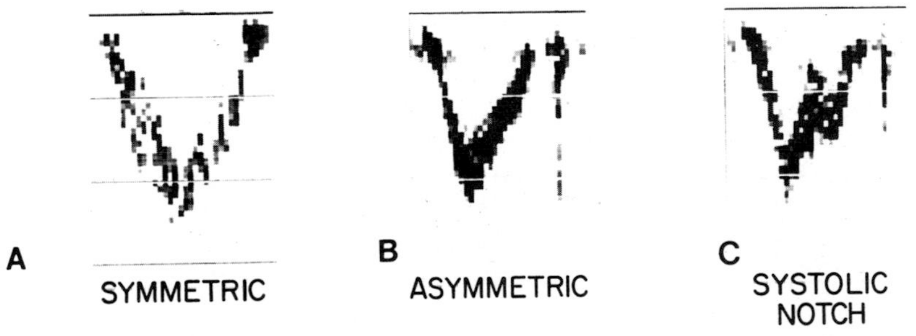

	SYMMETRIC	ASYMMETRIC	SYSTOLIC NOTCH
NORMAL (18)	16	2	0
PULMONARY HYPERTENSION (16)	0	16	8

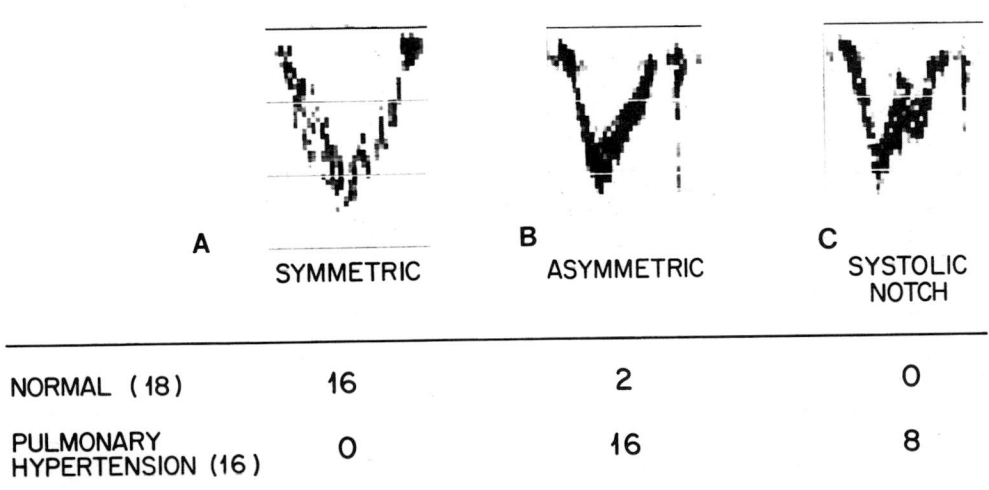

Fig. 27–33. Comparison of pulmonary flow patterns in a group of 18 normal pulmonary artery pressures and in 16 patients with documented pulmonary hypertension. A symmetric flow pattern is generally seen only in patients with normal pulmonary artery pressures. An asymmetric pattern predominates in patients with pulmonary hypertension. A midsystolic notch is highly specific for pulmonary hypertension.

bine to produce vortex formation along the medial wall with retrograde flow and an increase in pressure beneath the posterior leaflet during midsystole.

As described in Chapter 13, the normal pattern of pulmonary flow varies with sample volume location, with the result that many of the features of pulmonary hypertension can be reproduced in normal persons by sampling along the medial border of the pulmonary artery. Although this problem can be avoided by careful positioning of the sample volume in the center of the pulmonary artery, some authors have recommended sampling in the right ventricular outflow tract, where the velocity profile is more consistent.

Severe tricuspid regurgitation and idiopathic dilation of the pulmonary artery can produce a pulmonary artery flow pattern similar to that seen in pulmonary hypertension. In contrast, the flow pattern is often normal in patients with large left-to-right shunts, which increase pressure without increasing vascular resistance.[8] In patients with pulmonary regurgitation and pulmonary hypertension, the early peak velocity may be pronounced, but the calculated resistance may be lower than predicted because of the decrease in pulmonary artery diastolic pressure.[8]

Right Ventricular Systolic Time Intervals

To quantitate the time-related changes in valve motion and flow, specific portions of the M-mode recording or pulmonary artery flow profile have been measured and related to pulmonary artery pressure. The intervals usually measured include the RPEP, the acceleration time (AcT), and the right ventricular ejection time (RVET) (Fig. 27–34). The RPEP is measured from the onset of the Q wave of the electrocardiogram to pulmonary valve opening on the M-mode recording or the beginning of the pulmonary artery Doppler systolic flow signal. The right ventricular AcT, by M-mode recording is the time from the onset of valve opening to the point of peak leaflet displacement, and by Doppler it is the time from the onset of flow to peak velocity. Finally, the ejection

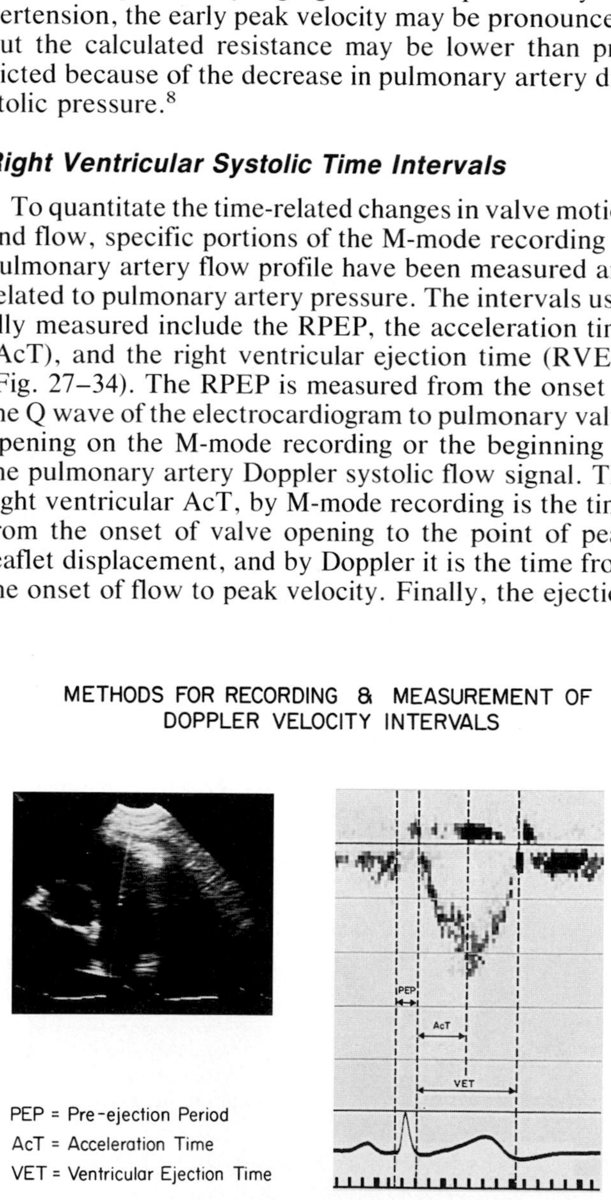

Fig. 27–34. Doppler-derived systolic time intervals.

time by M-mode recording is the time from valve opening to valve closure, while by Doppler it is the time from the onset to the termination of flow. Note that the RPEP and RVET should be approximately the same by M-mode and Doppler recordings, provided that the onset and termination of flow can be accurately measured by both techniques. The acceleration times, however, may differ because the point of peak valve opening and peak flow velocity are not specifically related. It was recognized in the late 1970s that Doppler measurement of the onset and termination of pulmonary artery flow provided an easier and more consistent method for estimating right ventricular systolic time intervals than M-mode recordings of valve motion.[64] As a result, the M-mode approach has been largely abandoned. M-mode recordings, however, can still be useful to confirm the time of valve opening and closure when the onset or termination of flow is unclear. A clearly defined pulmonary artery flow velocity profile can be recorded in 85 to 90% of patients.[60,65]

The interval that correlates most closely with pulmonary artery pressure is the AcT.[65–72] The AcT decreases as pulmonary pressure increases. In normal persons, the reported AcT has varied from 130 ± 15 msec[72] to 137 ± 24,[65] decreasing to 97 ± 20 in patients with mean pulmonary artery pressures between 20 and 39 mm Hg and to 65 ± 14 in patients with mean pulmonary artery pressures ≥40 mm Hg.[65] In one study, an AcT of <100 msec was reported to have a predictive value of 97% for pulmonary hypertension,[73] while in another, an AcT of ≤106 msec had a sensitivity of 79% and a specificity of 100% for an abnormal pulmonary artery systolic pressure.[74] Others, however, have found adequate predictive accuracy only when the AcT was <80 msec.[70] Correlations between AcT and pulmonary artery pressure have ranged from −0.87 to −0.65. Although it has been suggested that the correlation improves slightly when AcT is compared to Log_{10} mean pulmonary artery pressure, this has not been confirmed.[60,68] Figure 27–35A illustrates the correlation between AcT and mean pulmonary artery pressure in a group of 34 patients studied at the time of catheterization.[75] It has been suggested that the AcT should be measured from right ventricular outflow velocities because pulmonary artery waveforms vary with sample volume location. Correction of AcT for heart rate $[(AcT/\sqrt{R{-}R})]$ appears necessary only at rates in excess of 120 beats per minute (bpm). Several regression equations have been used to relate AcT to mean pulmonary artery pressure (MPAP = 78 − 0.52 (AcT)[72] and MPAP = 79 − 0.45 AcT) with variable results. Inter- and intraobserver variabilities have been moderately good (r = .86, SEE = 8.1). Although AcT correlates with pulmonary artery pressure at rest, changes in AcT did not correlate with changes in pulmonary vascular resistance or pulmonary artery systolic pressure during 10 minutes of oxygen breathing.[76]

Although AcT clearly correlates with pulmonary artery pressure, the absolute changes are small; the interval varies with heart rate (the precise heart rate at which correction becomes necessary is unclear); and the reported standard errors are not insignificant. As a result, several ratios have been developed to improve correla-

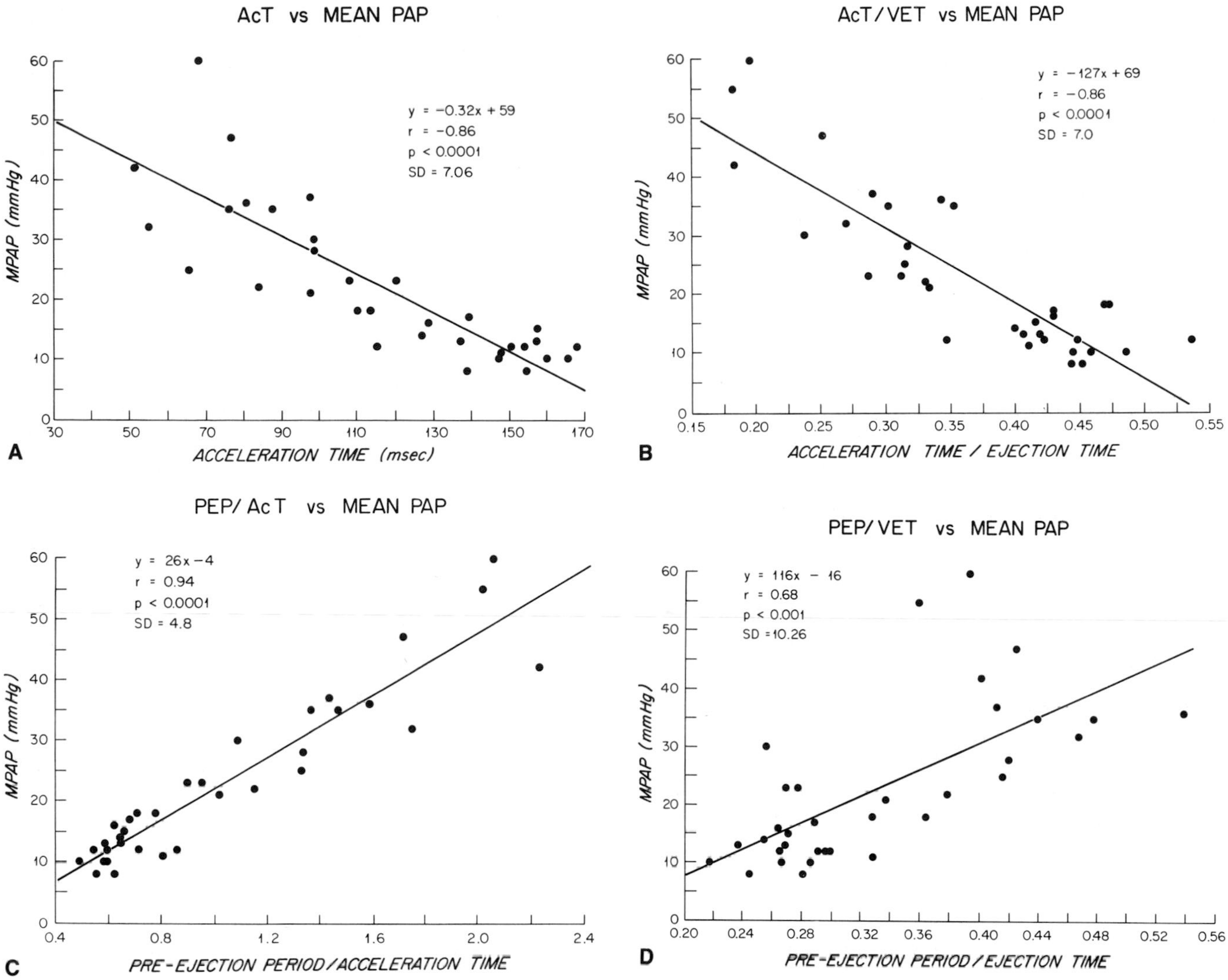

Fig. 27–35. Scatter plots comparing the following parameters to mean pulmonary artery pressure (MPAP) in a group of 34 patients studied at the time of catheterization: **A.** Acceleration time (AcT). **B.** The ratio of acceleration time to ejection time (AcT/VET). **C.** The ratio of pre-ejection time to acceleration time (PEP/AcT). **D.** The ratio of the pre-ejection period to the ejection time (PEP/VET). (Data from Jiang L, Stewart WJ, King ME, Weyman AE: An improved method for estimation of pulmonary artery pressure using Doppler velocity time intervals. J Am Coll Cardiol 3:613, 1984.)

tion and reduce variation. The most commonly employed ratios are the AcT/RVET and the RPEP/AcT. The AcT/RVET, or acceleration time index, varies inversely with pulmonary artery pressure, with reported normal values of 46% ± 3.1% and 45% ± 5% decreasing to 34% ± 5% for mean pulmonary artery pressures between 20 and 39 mm Hg and to 26% ± 2% in patients with pulmonary artery pressures ≥40 mm Hg. Correlations between AcT/RVET and mean pulmonary artery pressure have been similar to those reported for AcT alone, although in several studies the ratio performed less well, which was due to difficulties in measuring the termination of systolic flow.[60,72,74] In addition, at very high pulmonary artery pressures, flow may terminate early, inappropriately shifting the ratio toward normal.[8] Figure 27–35B compares the AcT/VET ratio to mean pulmonary artery pressure. Note that the correlation and standard deviation of the regression are almost identical to those for the AcT alone.[75] The AcT/RVET has also correlated well with beat-to-beat variation in pulmonary artery systolic pressure and with changes in mean pulmonary artery pressure caused by hypoxic breathing.

An alternative to the AcT/RVET is the ratio of the pre-ejection period to the AcT. This ratio appears preferable because the PEP and AcT vary in opposite directions as pulmonary artery pressure increases and hence cannot cancel at high pulmonary artery pressures. Figure 27–35C compares the PEP/AcT ratio to mean pulmonary artery pressure. Note that correlation is higher and the standard deviation less than that for the AcT alone or the AcT/VET ratio in the same patient group. Others have found a similar relationship[66,77] although experience has varied.[72]

The PEP and RVET have also been tested as markers of pulmonary artery pressure. Although the pre-ejection period increases and the ejection time shortens[78] as pulmonary artery pressure increases,[65] neither of these intervals alone has proven useful in predicting pulmonary artery pressure.[70,71,74] The limited correlation of these intervals with pulmonary artery pressure undoubtedly relates to the fact that the PEP is also effected by heart rate and conduction disturbances while the RVET is independently altered by heart rate and flow.

Although the PEP and RVET alone are not reliable determinants of pulmonary pressure, their ratio (PEP/VET) performs slightly better. Figure 27–35D compares the ratio of PEP/VET to mean pulmonary artery pressure. In this population, the correlation (r = .68) was less good than for the AcT, AcT/VET, or PEP/AcT, and the standard deviation was larger. This Doppler correlation, however, was similar to the values found in the original M-mode studies (.69 to .72).[79,80] Over the narrow range of pulmonary artery pressures found in normal subjects at rest, none of the Doppler indices correlates significantly with mean pulmonary artery pressure or pulmonary vascular resistance.

Combinations of Ratios. Because the components of each of these ratios are influenced by factors other than pulmonary artery pressure, it has been suggested that several ratios be considered in combination.[8] For example, in one study, no patient had pulmonary hypertension if both the RPEP/RVET and ACT/RVET ratios were normal, whereas when both were abnormal, pulmonary hypertension was invariably present.

Right Ventricular Isovolumic Relaxation Time. The right ventricular isovolumic relaxation time (RV-IVRT) has also been reported to be an accurate measure of pulmonary artery pressure. The IVRT, or the time from pulmonary valve closure to tricuspid valve opening ($P_c - T_o$),[81] varies directly with pulmonary artery pressure, because (for a constant relaxation rate) an increase in pulmonary artery pressure will increase the time required for the right ventricular pressure at pulmonary valve closure to fall to the level of right atrial pressure. Because this interval is also inversely related to heart rate, a nomogram has been developed that relates both heart rate and the RV-IVRT to systolic pulmonary artery pressure (Fig. 27–36). Pulmonary artery pressures estimated from this nomogram have correlated well with those obtained at cardiac catheterization in patients with pulmonary hypertension of varying causes.[81,82] The relationship has been consistent in noninvasive studies in which pulmonary closure and tricuspid valve opening have been measured by phonocardiography and noninvasive pulse tracings, from M-mode echocardiographic measures of pulmonary closure and tricuspid opening,[83] or by Doppler recordings of the interval from the termination of pulmonary outflow to the onset of tricuspid inflow. The Doppler method appears the least cumbersome and most accurate of these approaches. Success rates have ranged from 21% to >95% of patients.[60,70,82] Because the method is complex, success undoubtedly relates to the diligence with which it is pursued. In Doppler studies, it is essential to record valve movement together with the flow velocity curve because in patients with pulmonary hypertension and early cessation or reversal of flow, the velocity profile alone may be misleading. Because the interval varies slightly with respiration,

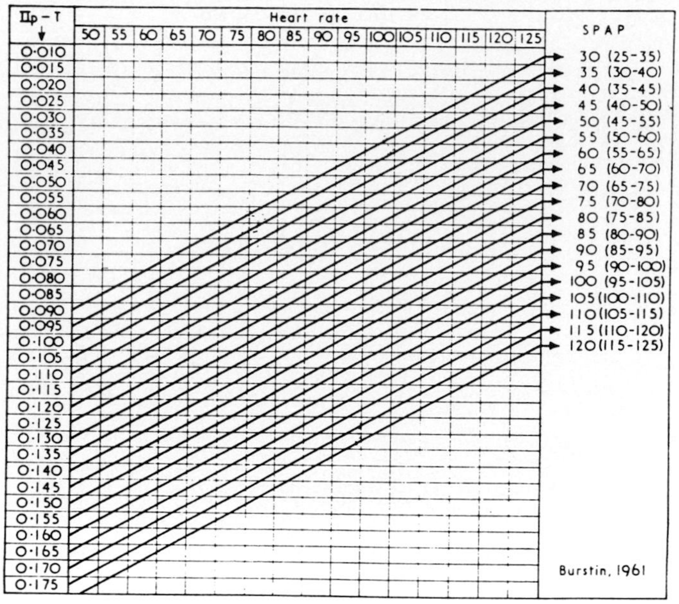

Fig. 27–36. This nomogram illustrates how systolic pulmonary arterial pressure (SPAP) can be calculated from the IIp-T interval heart rate. (From Burstin L: Determination of pressure in the pulmonary artery by external graphic recordings. Br Heart J 29:396, 1967. Originally published in Proceedings of 4th World Congress of Cardiology, 1962. Reproduced with permission of the British Medical Association.)

10 beats are generally averaged in normal sinus rhythm and 20 in patients in atrial fibrillation. Because pulmonary closure and tricuspid opening are not usually measured simultaneously, some common reference (phonocardiogram or electrocardiogram) is necessary to relate these two points, particularly in patients with atrial fibrillation. Although the published nomogram extends only to heart rates of 125 bpm, extrapolation above this limit appears reliable.[82]

Although the method rests on the assumptions that the right atrial pressure is constant or can be ignored and that the RV-IVRT is constant at varying pulmonary artery pressures, neither are uniformly correct. An increase in right atrial pressure will shorten the RV-IVRT because the tricuspid valve will open earlier and pulmonary artery pressure will be underestimated. This occurs most commonly with severe tricuspid regurgitation but can also be seen in patients with right ventricular failure and pericardial constriction. Although assumed to be constant, right ventricular pressure has been shown to fall more rapidly in patients with pulmonary artery hypertension than in normal subjects. These results would invalidate the method; however, the increased rate of pressure decline appears to be offset by earlier cessation of flow and closure of the pulmonary valve.[82] Two other sources of potential error are the presence of pulmonary regurgitation—which causes flow toward the transducer and on blind recordings may be incorrectly interpreted as tricuspid inflow—and severe cardiac failure where tricuspid valve opening may be apparent only following atrial contraction.

In summary, pulmonary artery pressure can be estimated in most patients (>95%) using one of the methods described previously. Measurement of tricuspid regurgitant jet velocities appears preferable because it provides a direct, ordered estimate of pressure. In patients with congenital heart disease, several shunts are often present, allowing multiple values to be obtained and validated. In patients without tricuspid regurgitation or intracardiac shunting, pulmonary systolic time intervals such as the PEP/AcT, AcT, or AcT/RVET are useful. Because of their relatively large standard errors, however, measurements of these intervals cannot be considered more than an estimation. The RV-IVRT is a complex measurement, but when appropriately recorded, it appears more accurate than any of the right ventricular systolic time intervals.

Premature Pulmonary Valve Opening

Pulmonary valve opening occurs when right ventricular pressure exceeds pulmonary artery pressure. Normal pulmonary valve opening occurs with the onset of ventricular systole, although valve opening can also be seen following atrial contraction in patients with valvular pulmonic stenosis and in normal subjects at slow heart rates, particularly during inspiration. Premature opening of the pulmonary valve is defined as an opening movement that occurs before ventricular or atrial systole and implies that right ventricular diastolic pressure exceeds simultaneous pulmonary artery pressure before atrial contraction. Premature opening may be present throughout the respiratory cycle or only during inspiration. This phenomenon is generally associated with conditions that either (1) restrict right ventricular filling, causing a rapid rise in early diastolic pressure (e.g., constrictive pericarditis, restrictive myopathy, Löffler's endocarditis, or right ventricular infarction) or that impose an extreme volume load on the right ventricle (e.g., sinus of Valsalva aneurysm rupture into the right atrium, absence of the tricuspid valve, severe tricuspid insufficiency, combined atrial septal defect and pulmonary insufficiency, and Ebstein's anomaly).[84–88] Figure 27–37 is a pulmonic valve echogram from a patient with rupture of an aneurysm of the sinus of Valsalva into the right atrium. Figure 27–37A illustrates opening of the pulmonic valve well before atrial contraction. Figure 27–37B is a postoperative study following repair of the aneurysm and demonstrates normal opening of the pulmonary valve following ventricular systole. In this case, the large flow volume entering the right heart during diastole produced an early increase in diastolic right ventricular pressure, which exceeded pulmonary artery pressure and produced valve opening. This phenomenon, therefore, is not specific for any disease entity but rather reflects the pressure relationship across the pulmonary valve in early diastole.

THE SUBVALVULAR RIGHT VENTRICULAR OUTFLOW TRACT: THE CONUS ARTERIOSUS OR INFUNDIBULUM

The pulmonary infundibulum extends from the crista supraventricularis to the pulmonary valve. The crista supraventricularis is a thick, rounded, muscular ridge that lies in the angle between the body of the right ventricle and the infundibulum, separating the tricuspid and pulmonary valve orifices. The infundibulum is a muscular conduit composed of two primary muscle layers. The superficial layer, which is the more complex, has a superior-inferior orientation and mechanically appears to shorten the proximal outflow tract. The deeper layer is simpler, horizontally oriented, and on constriction, appears to narrow the outflow tract.[89]

Failure of one or more muscle groups in the infundibular region to develop results in a defect in the interventricular septum in the region separating the right and left ventricular outflow tracts, whereas hypertrophy of these muscles may result in subvalvular obstruction.[12] Infundibular hypertrophy has been attributed either to an overgrowth of muscular tissue resulting from injury to the predifferentiated bulbar primordia or to a secondary adaptation to hemodynamic stress. The muscular hypertrophy, when present, may be confined to the area immediately beneath the valve,[90] may be located in the outflow tract farther below the valve and associated with a small subvalvular chamber,[13] or may arise in the right ventricle dividing this cavity into two chambers.[91,92]

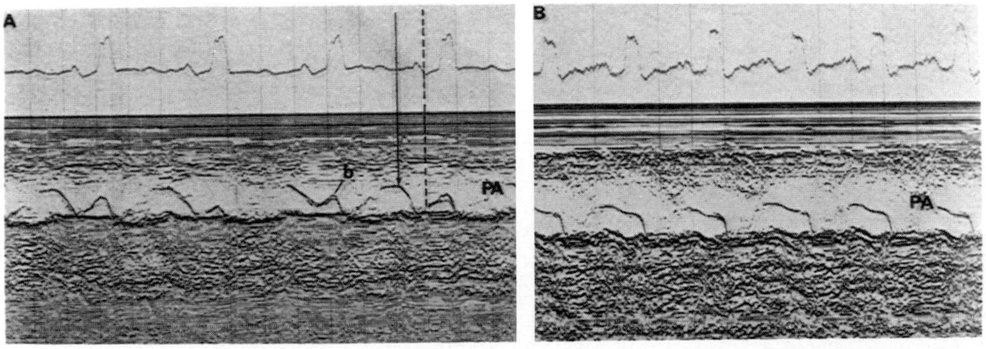

Fig. 27–37. A pre- and postoperative recording from a patient with an aneurysm of the sinus of Valsalva that ruptured into the right atrium. **A.** Premature opening of the pulmonary valve (i.e., opening before either atrial or ventricular systole) in response to the rapid initial increase in diastolic pressure in the right ventricle produced by the aorta to right atrial fistula. **B.** A postoperative recording demonstrating the return to relatively normal pulmonary valve motion. In this case, there is a minimal opening motion or A wave of the pulmonary valve following atrial contractions suggesting postoperative pulmonary hypertension. PA = pulmonary artery. (From Weyman AE, et al.: Premature pulmonic valve opening following sinus of Valsalva aneurysm rupture into the right atrium. Circulation 51:556, 1975. Reproduced with permission of the American Heart Association, Inc.)

Normal flow in the infundibulum is primarily systolic with a slight increase in velocity recorded from the inlet to the pulmonary artery and with inspiration. Proximal to the pulmonary valve, forward flow can usually be recorded following atrial contraction, and in small children and young adults, the rapid filling wave can also be detected.

Infundibular Pulmonary Stenosis

Infundibular pulmonary stenosis can be congenital or acquired. Congenital infundibular stenosis can occur as an isolated lesion or more commonly in association with other anomalies, particularly ventricular septal defect. Acquired infundibular obstruction can be seen in patients with idiopathic hypertrophic subaortic stenosis (IHSS), infiltrative disorders such as Pompe's disease, or outflow tract tumor. Acute acquired obstruction can occur following pulmonary valvuloplasty or surgical valvotomy.[93] Infundibular stenosis can be visualized in the parasternal long axis view of the pulmonary outflow tract or in subcostal views oriented to display the outflow tract[4] and the inlet septum.[94] Isolated congenital infundibular stenosis can be diffuse or local or can present as a discrete membrane located immediately beneath the valve, a more extensive area of fibromuscular hyperplasia, or malposition and hypertrophy of the inlet septum. Figure 27–38 illustrates a discrete membrane located immediately beneath the pulmonary valve. The membrane presents as thick linear echoes arising from the anterior and posterior margins of the outflow tract narrowing the vascular lumen. Figure 27–39 shows a more diffuse area of isolated fibromuscular hyperplasia characterized by hypertrophy and increased echo production from the anterior and posterior margins of the outflow tract with inward bending of the echoes from the vascular walls and narrowing of the lumen. Distal to the area of obstruction, the outflow tract returns to a more normal diameter, resulting in an hourglass-type deformity. Similar changes in outflow tract diameter have been noted in patients with tetralogy of Fallot; however, in this setting, the outflow tract deformity is frequently more extensive, and the inlet septum generally is involved (see Chapter 32).[95] In studies performed before and after repair, an excellent correlation has been demonstrated (r = .93) between the cross-sectional echocardiographic and angiographic assessment of infundibular size during both diastole and systole (Fig. 27–40).[96]

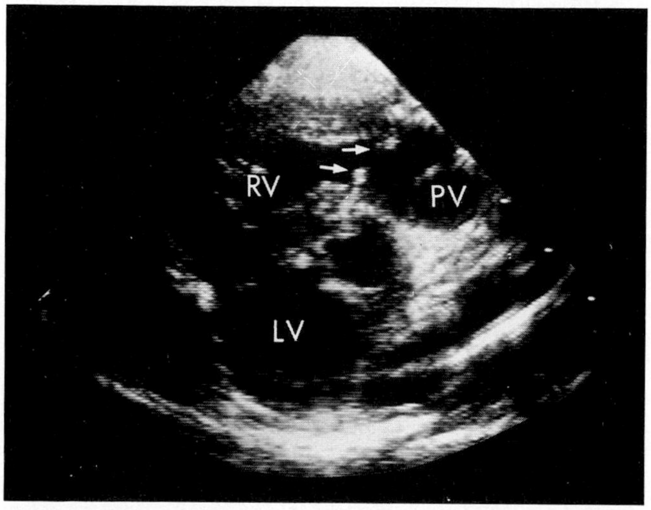

Fig. 27–38. Parasternal view of the left ventricle (LV) and right ventricle (RV) optimized to demonstrate the long axis of the right ventricular outflow tract. The patient is a 2-year-old child with a muscular ventricular septal defect and right ventricular outflow obstruction who demonstrated a discrete ridge of tissue (arrows) in the infundibulum beneath the pulmonary valve (PV). RV = right ventricle. (From Liberthson RR, King ME, O'Rourke RA: Congenital heart disease. *In* Pohost GM, O'Rourke RA (eds.): Principles and Practice of Cardiovascular Imaging. Boston, Little, Brown and Company, 1991.)

Infundibular stenosis produces a high velocity turbulent jet, which strikes the pulmonary valve leaflets, causing high frequency systolic fluttering and early closure of the valve leaflets with the fluttering often extending into diastole. This pattern is similar to that of aortic leaflet motion in patients with subvalvular aortic stenosis, although fluttering of the left-sided leaflets is never present in diastole.[97,98] Figure 27–41 is an M-mode recording from a patient with infundibular stenosis illustrating the characteristic early closure and high frequency fluttering of the valve. In contrast to left-sided lesions, where the pattern of early leaflet closure and fluttering differ with the depth and nature of the obstruction, the pulmonary valve pattern appears similar irrespective of the cause or location of the obstruction. Fluttering may be absent

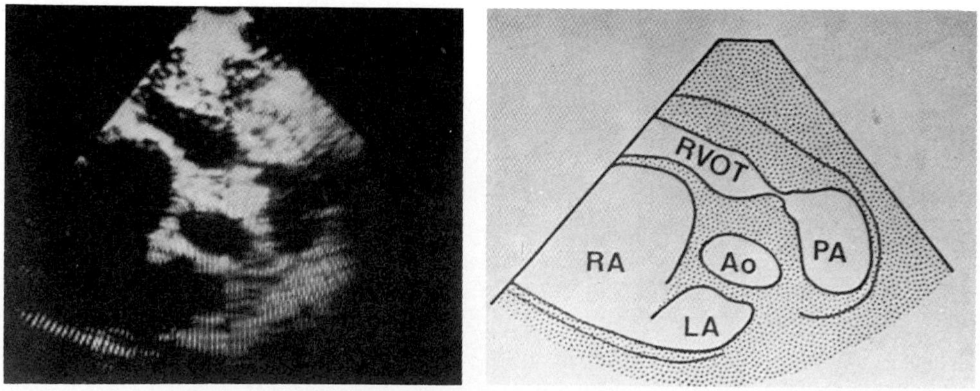

Fig. 27–39. Parasternal long axis recording of the right ventricular outflow tract (RVOT) illustrates isolated infundibular pulmonary stenosis. Echo production from the anterior and posterior walls of the outflow tract in the infundibular region is increased, and the vascular lumen is narrowed. Distal to this hourglass-shaped area of obstruction, the vessel returns to a normal diameter. Right atrial dilation is also evident. PA = pulmonary artery; Ao = aorta; RA = right atrium; LA = left atrium.

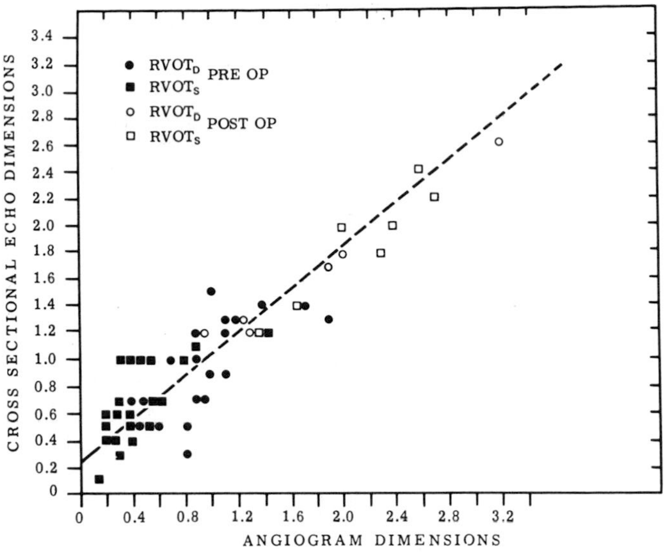

Fig. 27–40. Correlation between the cross-sectional echocardiographic and angiographic measurements of right ventricular outflow tract diameter at end-systole ($RVOT_S$) and end-diastole ($RVOT_D$) recorded before and after operative correction in patients with tetralogy of Fallot. (From Caldwell RL, et al.: Right ventricular outflow tract assessment by cross-sectional echocardiography in tetralogy of Fallot. Circulation 59:395, 1979. Reproduced by permission of the American Heart Association, Inc.)

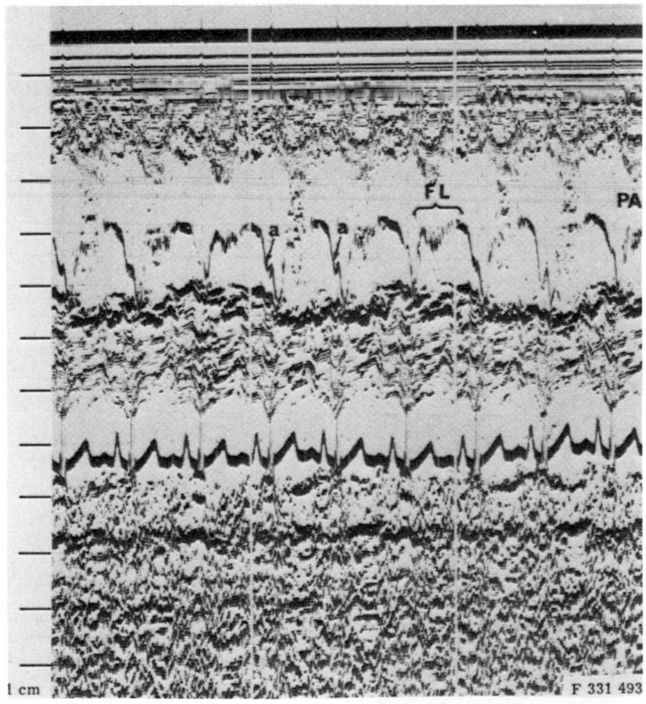

Fig. 27–41. Recording from a patient with infundibular pulmonary stenosis demonstrating prominent A waves as well as marked prolonged diastolic fluttering of the pulmonary leaflets, suggesting turbulent flow crossing the leaflet during systole. The duration of this fluttering extends beyond the T wave of the electrocardiogram, suggesting continuation of leaflet vibration into the diastolic period. PA = pulmonary artery; FL = flutter. (From Weyman AE: Pulmonary valve echo motion in clinical practice. Am J Med 62:843, 1977. Reproduced with permission of Cahners Publishing Co.)

when valvular and infundibular stenosis coexist or when valve motion is restricted by tumor.[98]

The gradient across the region of infundibular obstruction can be determined from the peak flow velocities recorded by continuous wave Doppler using the modified Bernoulli equation ($\Delta P = 4V^2$). Flow in the infundibulum is generally perpendicular to an ultrasonic beam originating from the parasternal window. Therefore, to record outflow velocities accurately, it is often necessary to roll the patient into an extreme left lateral position or alternatively to record flow from the subcostal transducer location. The subcostal window is preferred in children and may also yield the highest velocities in adults. Although some authors have reported excellent correlation between hemodynamic and Doppler-derived gradients when all right-sided obstructions are grouped together, others have observed either greater scatter in the data than seen with valvular stenosis or frank Doppler overestimation resulting from downstream pressure recovery.[99,100] These inconsistencies presumably relate to the wide variation in the morphology of individual subvalvular lesions.

THE PULMONARY ARTERY

The main pulmonary artery extends only a short distance from its origin at the pulmonary valve to its bifurcation into the left and right pulmonary arteries. After bifurcation, the left pulmonary artery courses posterior and leftward for several centimeters before entering the hilum of the left lung. The right pulmonary artery bends more sharply to the right and passes beneath the aorta adjacent to the superior margin of the left atrium. After passing beneath the aorta, it generally gives off a superior branch before disappearing into the hilum of the right lung.

Imaging

The main pulmonary artery is most consistently imaged from the parasternal window in adults and from either the parasternal or subcostal window in children. The right and left branches are most easily recorded from the suprasternal or supraclavicular window. The diameter of the main pulmonary artery is larger than that of the aorta but is often difficult to measure precisely because the arterial walls are parallel to the direction of the scan plane in most image orientations. Pulmonary size increases during systole. Quantitative studies have focused on the right pulmonary artery because it is most easily measured from two-dimensional images and its size is critical for surgical planning in many patients with complex congenital heart disease (i.e., pulmonary atresia-ventricular septal defect). Echocardiographic measurements of right pulmonary artery diameter have correlated closely with those measured by angiography or at surgery in normal persons, in patients with increased volume flow into the pulmonary artery, and in those with tetralogy of Fallot.[101] Correlations have been equally good for systolic and diastolic measurements.

Flow

Flow in the pulmonary artery normally begins at pulmonary valve opening, accelerates to a gradual peak, and then decelerates slowly to terminate at pulmonary valve closure (see Fig. 27–33). The systolic flow profile is normally laminar with a relatively flat spatial velocity distribution (Fig. 27–42). As discussed earlier, the profile is altered by pulmonic stenosis, and pulmonary hypertension and some regional variation in the temporal flow velocity pattern is normally noted when the sample volume is moved from the lateral to the medial wall of the artery. Normal flow velocity in the pulmonary artery in adults ranges from 0.6 to 0.9 m/sec and in children from 0.7 to 1.1 m/sec.[8] Reported velocities during the first 3 days of life are slightly lower: day 1, 71.8 ± 11.4; day 2, 72.6 ± 7.1; day 3, 67.8 ± 9.2 cm/sec.

Pulmonary artery flow normally increases during inspiration. In normal subjects, flow increases by roughly 15%, while in pericardial tamponade, the flow velocity can increase by 50% or more. An exaggerated increase in inspiratory flow velocity (mean 35%) is also noted following the Fontan procedure.

Abnormalities of the Pulmonary Artery

Many disorders of the pulmonary artery and its proximal branches have been detected by echocardiography, including (1) anomalies of pulmonary artery origin; (2) pulmonary artery stenosis (supravalvar and branch); (3) pulmonary artery hypoplasia in patients with tetralogy of Fallot; (4) pulmonary artery bands; (5) pulmonary artery dilation); (6) coronary artery A–V fistula connecting to the pulmonary artery; and (7) tumors of the pulmonary trunk.

Abnormal Origin of the Left and Right Pulmonary Arteries

Three primary anomalies of pulmonary artery origin have been described: (1) origin of the left pulmonary artery from the right pulmonary artery—the pulmonary artery sling, (2) origin of the right pulmonary artery from the ascending aorta,[102,103] and (3) complete absence of the right pulmonary artery.

Pulmonary artery sling is an unusual anomaly in which the left pulmonary artery arises from the right pulmonary artery and passes posteriorly and then leftward between the trachea and esophagus to reach the hilum of the left lung. This places the trachea within a vascular ring with the main pulmonary artery anterior, the left pulmonary artery to the right and posterior, and the ductus arteriosus or ductal ligament on the left. The anomaly usually presents as respiratory distress during infancy, although adults with minimal or no symptoms have been reported.

Approximately half of all infants with pulmonary artery sling have associated anomalies, particularly complete cartilaginous rings and associated hypoplasia of the distal trachea and bronchi. Associated cardiovascular anomalies include patent ductus arteriosus, atrial septal defect, persistent left superior vena cava, and ventricular septal defect. Conotruncal abnormalities are rare. Mortality remains high despite current surgical techniques.[104]

The anomalous origin and course of the left pulmonary artery can be observed in subcostal long axis, short axis, and parasternal short axis views. Figure 27–43 is a parasternal short axis recording illustrating the main and right pulmonary arteries in their normal positions.

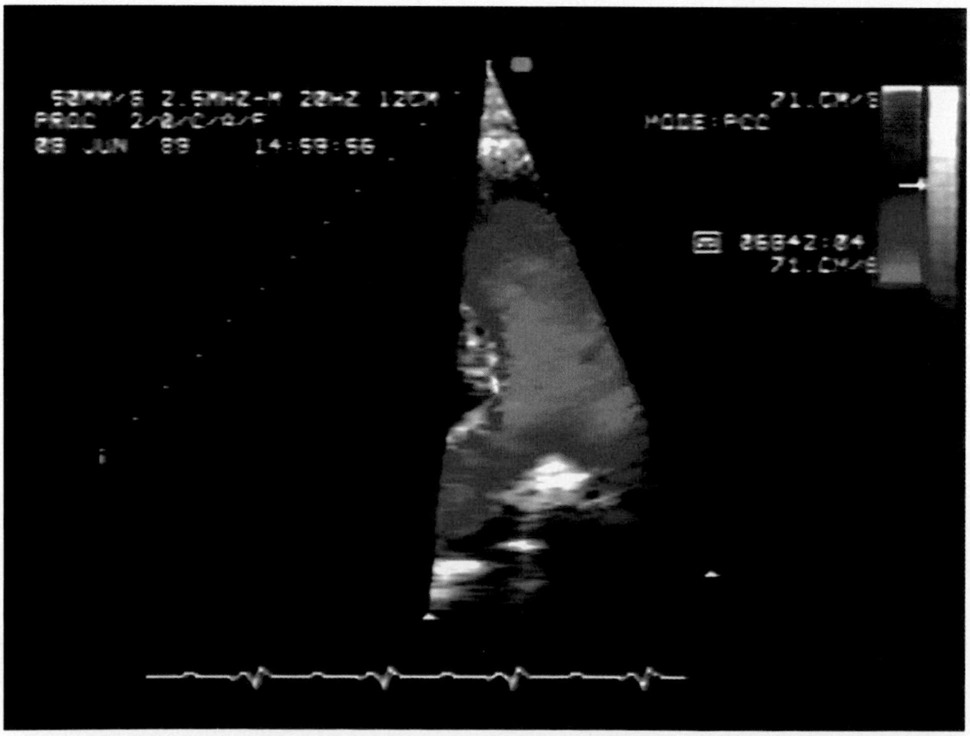

Fig. 27–42. Long axis, color Doppler of normal pulmonary artery systolic flow. Flow in this view is away from the transducer. The flow profile is generally flat with a slight increase in velocity (lighter blue) along the medial wall.

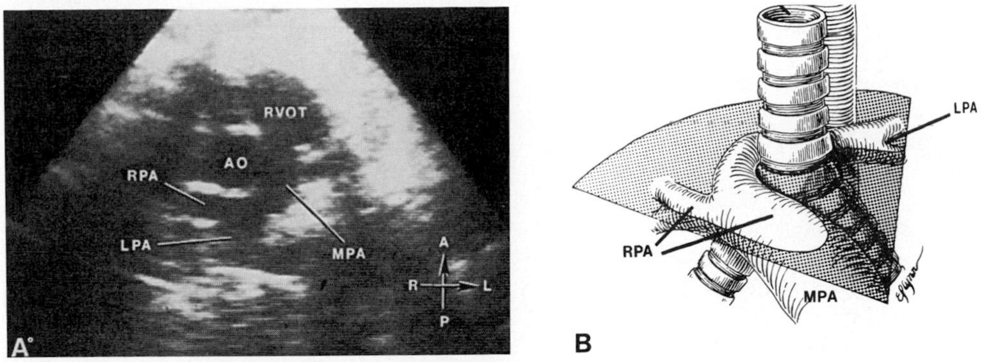

Fig. 27–43. Echocardiographic image **(A)** and graphic representation **(B)** of a pulmonary artery sling. The left pulmonary artery (LPA) is seen arising from the right pulmonary artery (RPA) and coursing posteriorly (P) and leftward (L). The main pulmonary artery does not bifurcate in the usual fashion, and the left pulmonary artery is absent from its usual location. AO = aorta; RVOT = right ventricular outflow tract; MPA = main pulmonary artery; A = anterior; T = trachea; E = esophagus. (From Yeager SB, Chin AJ, Sanders SP: Two-dimensional echocardiographic diagnosis of pulmonary artery sling in infancy. J Am Coll Cardiol 7:625, 1986. Reprinted with permission from the American College of Cardiology.)

The left pulmonary artery can be visualized originating from the right pulmonary artery and sweeping posteriorly and leftward. The retrotracheal portion of the left pulmonary artery generally cannot be visualized in any view, being obscured by the intervening air column.[104] Suprasternal and particularly transesophageal imaging should also be of value in diagnosing the anomaly. Color Doppler flow imaging also helps delineate the anomalous course of the vessel.[105] Pulmonary artery sling must be distinguished from delayed origin of the left pulmonary artery that is due to clockwise rotation of the heart. If the left pulmonary artery can be followed from its origin to the hilum of the left lung (i.e., it does not pass behind the trachea), a sling is not present.[106]

The right pulmonary artery may arise anomalously from the aorta or may be absent completely. Anomalous origin of the right pulmonary artery from the aorta hemodynamically mimics truncus arteriosus; however, the great vessels and semilunar valves are typically normal. Echocardiographically, the main pulmonary artery is normal and continues into a normal left pulmonary artery. The distal right pulmonary artery can be recorded superior to the left atrium, but rather than continuing to join the main pulmonary artery, it courses slightly anterior to attach to the posterolateral wall of the aorta.[102,103,107] In the suprasternal long axis view, the right pulmonary artery is not present beneath the aorta. Doppler recordings reveal continuous flow in the right pulmonary artery with retrograde diastolic flow in the aorta. Elevated arterial pressures in the left lung are common.[106]

In patients with complete absence of the right pulmonary artery, the right lung is supplied by bronchial collateral vessels. Echocardiographically, there is no evidence of a right pulmonary artery beneath the aorta in the suprasternal long axis view. The lesion is differentiated from anomalous origin of the right pulmonary artery by the absence of a vessel to the right of the aorta superior to the left atrium.

Congenital unilateral absence of the left pulmonary artery has also been reported.[108] This lesion is typically associated with hypoplasia of the left lung, a shift of the heart to the left side of the chest, and posterior cardiac displacement.[109] Because of the unusual cardiac position, echocardiographic recordings were obtainable only from the back.[108] Specific features of the lesion, however, were not described.

Supravalvular Pulmonary Arterial Stenosis

Supravalvular pulmonary artery stenosis may involve the main pulmonary trunk, its right or left branches, or smaller segmental arteries. Multiple areas of stenosis are commonly present. The stenosis may present as a discrete membrane or more extensive tubular hypoplasia. Pulmonary arterial stenosis may be sporadic, familial, or may occur in patients with rubella syndrome or supravalvular aortic stenosis with or without Williams syndrome.[110] It may occur alone or in combination with other cardiac anomalies, most commonly, pulmonic valve stenosis, atrial and ventricular septal defect, patent ductus arteriosus, or tetralogy of Fallot. The natural history of isolated pulmonary artery stenosis is benign, and the gradient usually decreases with time.[111] Complications can occur, however, including pulmonary hypertension, right ventricular failure, pulmonary artery thrombosis, and post-stenotic aneurysmal dilation with rupture and hemoptysis.[112–114]

Main Pulmonary Artery Stenosis. Stenosis of the main pulmonary artery may present as a discrete thick, fibrous ring or diaphragm located just beyond the pulmonary sinuses or as elongated tubular hypoplasia of the main pulmonary segment. Discrete supravalvular stenosis is not typically associated with stenoses in the pulmonary artery branches. Pulmonary valve stenosis, however, is frequently present.

Supravalvular stenosis can be recorded in either a parasternal or subcostal long axis view of the pulmonary artery. The discrete membranous type presents as a thick band of echoes arising from the medial and lateral walls of the vessel, which partially occlude the vessel lumen (Fig. 27–44).[115] Tubular hypoplasia of the main pulmonary artery is characterized by an extensive region of vessel narrowing (Fig. 27–45). The severity of

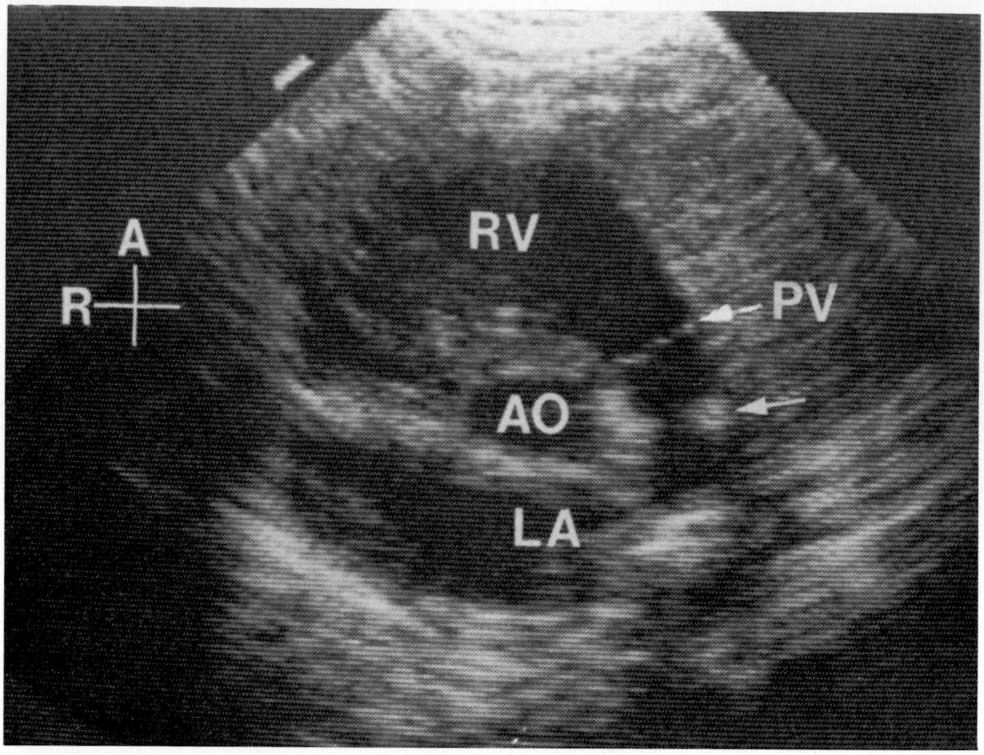

Fig. 27–44. Long axis recording of the pulmonary artery from a child with supravalvular pulmonary stenosis caused by a discrete diaphragm (arrow) in the main pulmonary artery. A = anterior; AO = aorta; LA = left atrium; PV = pulmonary valve; R = right; RV = right ventricle. (From Snider AR, Serwer GA: Echocardiography in Pediatric Heart Disease. Chicago, Year Book Medical Publishers, 1990. Reproduced with permission.)

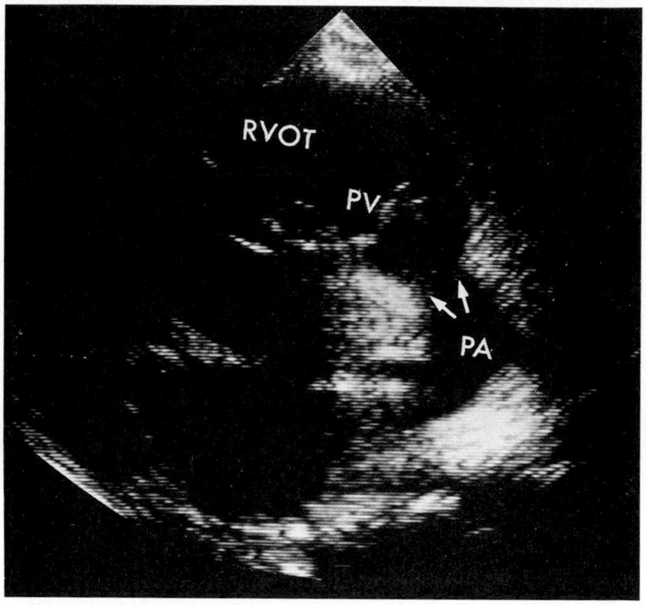

Fig. 27–45. Long axis recording of the right ventricular outflow tract (RVOT); pulmonary valve (PV); and the pulmonary artery (PA) illustrating a diffuse hourglass-type narrowing of the mid- and main pulmonary artery (arrows).

stenosis can be assessed from the peak velocity of flow across the stenosis using the modified Bernoulli equation ($\Delta P = 4V^2$). In patients with tubular stenosis, Doppler-derived gradients may underestimate measure gradients, presumably as a result of the viscous losses encountered as blood flows through the long region of narrowing.[106]

Branch Pulmonary Artery Stenosis. Branch pulmonary stenosis may also present as a discrete membrane, an area of tubular hypoplasia, or focal stricture. Localized branch stenoses are easily recognized by two-dimensional echocardiography because they appear as discrete areas of narrowing with post-stenotic dilation (Fig. 27–46). Diffuse bilateral hypoplasia is more difficult to diagnose. This is a particular problem in the neonate, where the right and left branches are normally con-

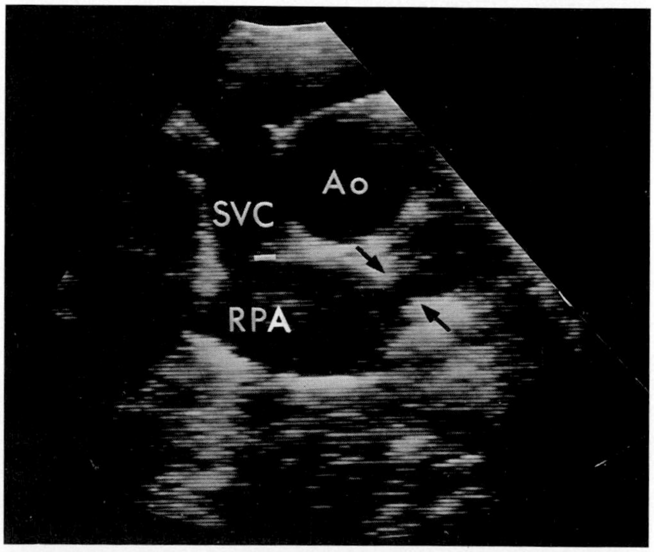

Fig. 27–46. Long axis recording of the right pulmonary artery (RPA) illustrating a discrete area of stenosis (arrows) just distal to the origin of the vessel with post-stenotic dilation beyond to the obstruction. SVC = superior vena cava; Ao = aorta.

siderably smaller than the main pulmonary artery because of the diversion of blood away from the lungs in the fetus. When there is uniform hypoplasia of both pulmonary artery branches, the diagnosis depends on accurate echocardiographic measurement of the branch pulmonary artery diameter and on comparison of this measurement with normal values (Fig. 27–47).

The entire length of the right pulmonary artery (from its origin from the main pulmonary artery to its entry into the hilum of the right lung) can usually be imaged using a combination of parasternal, subcostal, and suprasternal views of the long axis of the vessel. The left pulmonary artery, in contrast, can be seen for only a short distance before it reaches the hilum of the left lung.[116] In infants, long segments of both pulmonary artery branches can be visualized for a high left parasternal position.

In most cases, echocardiographic findings correlate well with those seen at angiography when the lesions are proximal. Stenosis of secondary branches are difficult to identify, while tertiary branches are generally obscured by lung parenchyma.[116]

Additional features that suggest branch pulmonary artery stenosis even when the lesion(s) cannot be directly identified include unexplained severe right ventricular hypertrophy and marked pulsation of the proximal pulmonary artery branches. Exaggerated pulsations of the proximal pulmonary arteries are caused by the continued runoff of blood into the peripheral pulmonary circulation during diastole, which in turn causes a low pulmonary artery diastolic pressure, wide pulse pressure, and bounding pulmonary artery pulsations.

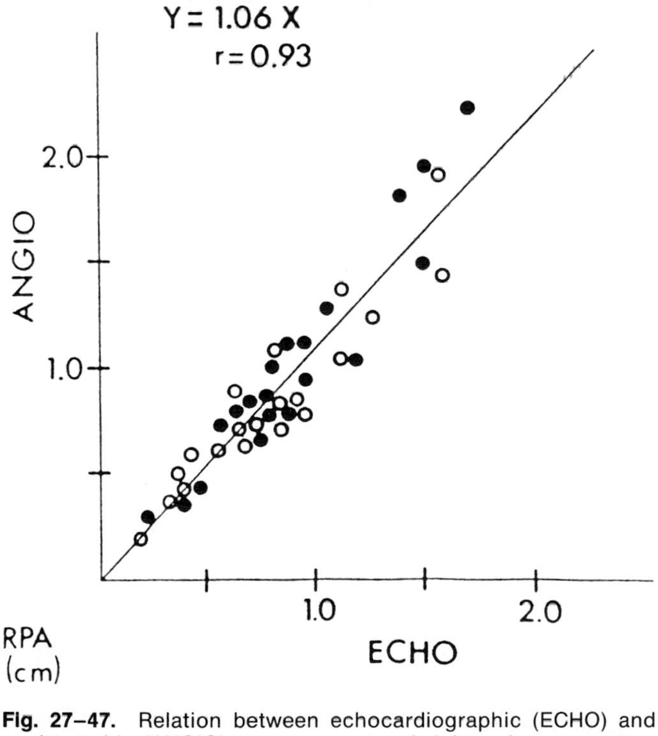

Fig. 27–47. Relation between echocardiographic (ECHO) and angiographic (ANGIO) measurements of right pulmonary artery (RPA) diameter obtained from 20 patients. The open circles represent diastole, and the closed circles represent systole. The data from systole and diastole were pooled because their individual regression formulas were not significantly different. (From Lappen RS, et al.: Two-dimensional echocardiographic measurement of right pulmonary artery diameter in infants and children. J Am Coll Cardiol 2:121, 1986. Reprinted with permission from the American College of Cardiology.)

Doppler echocardiography can be useful for both diagnosing and estimating the severity of supravalvular pulmonary stenosis. Color flow mapping is particularly helpful in diagnosis because local acceleration in flow and turbulence at the site of the stenosis draws attention to the lesion and helps confirm the imaging impression. This is particularly valuable in detecting mild degrees of stenosis that cannot be clearly visualized by two-dimensional echocardiography. Normal color Doppler flow in regions of spurious luminal narrowing that are due to vessel tortuosity can also help eliminate false-positives.

Doppler echocardiography can also help in assessing the severity of the lesion based on the peak velocities in the stenotic jet. Alignment of the Doppler beam parallel to flow in the right pulmonary is difficult from any echocardiographic window, although left pulmonary artery stenosis is more easily recorded. Color Doppler flow mapping may be helpful in obtaining the best alignment for continuous wave recording of jet flow; however, angle correction may still be necessary. In newborns, it is common to record a slight increase in velocity as the sample volume is moved from the main pulmonary artery into the right or left branch. This is probably because of the discrepancy in size between the main pulmonary artery and the pulmonary artery branches that normally exists at birth (physiologic peripheral pulmonary stenosis). With severe obstruction in a peripheral artery, the jet velocity typically peaks in systole, but high velocity flow extends into diastole because of persistence of the pressure gradient.[106]

Pulmonary Arterial Identification and Sizing in Children With Pulmonary Atresia and Ventricular Septal Defect

Patients with pulmonary atresia and ventricular septal defect (tetralogy of Fallot) can have hypoplastic confluent pulmonary arteries, hypoplastic nonconfluent arteries, or less commonly, absence of true pulmonary arteries. The presence and size of the pulmonary arteries are of particular importance in children with pulmonary atresia and ventricular septal defect because these factors determine whether surgery is feasible and, if so, whether a palliative procedure should be performed to promote pulmonary blood flow, and it is hoped, to stimulate pulmonary arterial growth, or for complete intracardiac repair. Although angiography is the primary tool for assessing pulmonary artery size, echocardiography can be very useful in preliminary diagnosis and in following pulmonary artery growth following a first-stage repair. The right pulmonary artery has been successfully imaged by two-dimensional echocardiography in 85% of patients with this complex, and the left pulmonary artery, in 25%.[117] Detection is possible in the vast majority of patients with confluent pulmonary arteries, and the presence of a proximal right pulmonary artery appears to be a reliable marker of confluence.[117] Echocardiographic measurement of the right pulmonary artery yielded values that were slightly smaller than those reported by angiography; however, the correlation coefficient was r = .95 with a standard error of 1.3 mm. Failure to record the pulmonary arteries can be due to severe scoliosis, other chest wall deformity, or prior thoracic surgery, which distorts cardiac anatomy. False-positives can occur if large systemic-to-pulmonary collaterals are misinterpreted as pulmonary arteries.[117]

Pulmonary Artery Bands

Ventricular septal defects with large left-to-right shunts may lead to severe pulmonary hypertension and to its associated morbidity and mortality. Experiments of nature, such as tetralogy of Fallot, have demonstrated that narrowing of the pulmonary outflow tract may control the degree of shunting through a ventricular septal defect and may exert a protective effect on the pulmonary vasculature. This principle has been used surgically by placing a constricting band around the pulmonary artery in patients with large ventricular septal defects in an attempt to decrease shunting and to protect the pulmonary vascular bed.[5,118] Although the use of pulmonary artery banding has decreased in favor of complete repair at an early age, many of these bands are still in place and may be evident during the course of a cross-sectional study.

Echocardiographically, pulmonary artery bands appear as a focal narrowing in the proximal pulmonary artery just beyond the pulmonary valve. There may be a fairly extensive area of surrounding scar tissue, which varies the extent of the arterial narrowing produced by the band. Figure 27–48 is a recording of the right ventricular outflow tract and pulmonary artery from a child with a banded pulmonary artery. The band produces a fairly large, hourglass-type narrowing just distal to the level of the pulmonary valve. Distal to the band, the vessel returns to a more normal size.

Knowledge of the pressure gradient across a pulmonary artery band is crucial for the clinician in assessing its efficacy. The pressure gradient across the band-induced stenosis can be calculated from the peak flow velocities recorded by Doppler using the modified Bernoulli equation. The accuracy of this approach has been validated in animal models and human studies.[119–121]

Pulmonary Artery Dilation

Dilation of the pulmonary artery may be observed in disorders that increase flow into the pulmonary vascular bed[122] or produce pulmonary hypertension.[123] In addition, pulmonary artery dilation may occur as an idiopathic lesion[124–127] that is due to a developmental defect in pulmonary arterial elastic tissue or as a part of the complex of vascular abnormalities seen in Marfan's syndrome.[128] Post-stenotic dilation of the pulmonary artery may also be noted in valvular pulmonary stenosis.[18]

Figure 27–49 is an example of a massively dilated vessel in a patient with idiopathic dilation of the pulmonary artery. The increase in size of the pulmonary artery can usually be appreciated by simple comparison to the aorta.

Coronary Artery Fistula to the Pulmonary Artery

Coronary A-V fistulas arising from a small left anterior descending or circumflex branch can occasionally be visualized emptying into the pulmonary artery.[129] Figure 27–50 is a color Doppler recording illustrating a small diastolic jet from an A-V fistula arising from the lateral wall of the main pulmonary artery midway between the pulmonary valve and the bifurcation. This jet was obvious during diastole but was obscured by pulmonary outflow during systole. The retrograde direction of the jet toward the pulmonic valve is similar to that seen with a patent ductus arteriosus, but the timing, velocity, and character of flow serve to differentiate the two lesions.

Tumors of the Pulmonary Artery

Primary tumors of the pulmonary trunk are rare, with myomas and sarcomas being reported most commonly.

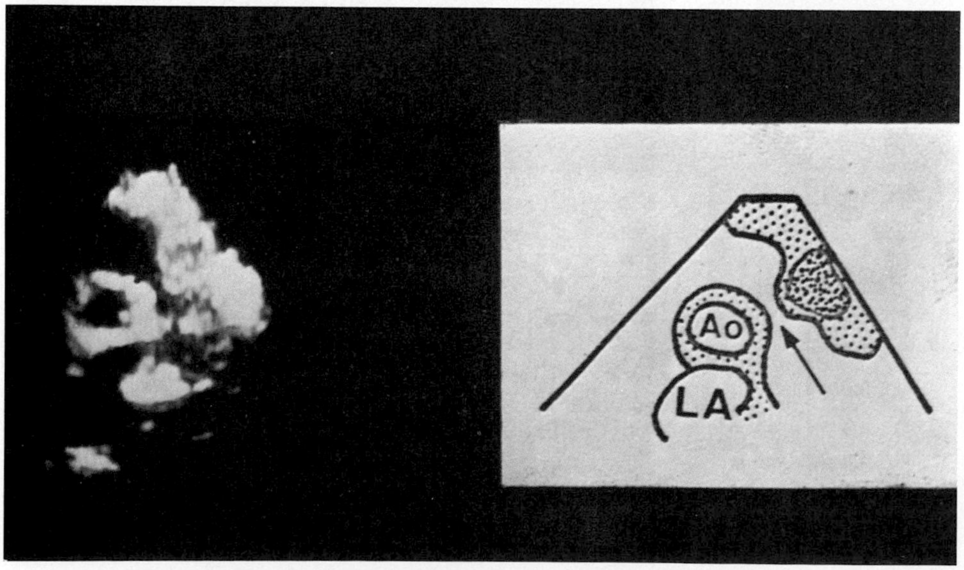

Fig. 27–48. Parasternal long axis recording of the pulmonary artery illustrates a pulmonary artery band. The band produces an area of arterial narrowing just distal to the pulmonary valve (approximately the 2:30 position relative to the circular aorta [Ao]). There is an increase in echo production from the arterial wall in the region of the band. This increase probably reflects local scarring caused by the band. Beyond the banded area, the arterial lumen returns to a more normal diameter. LA = left atrium.

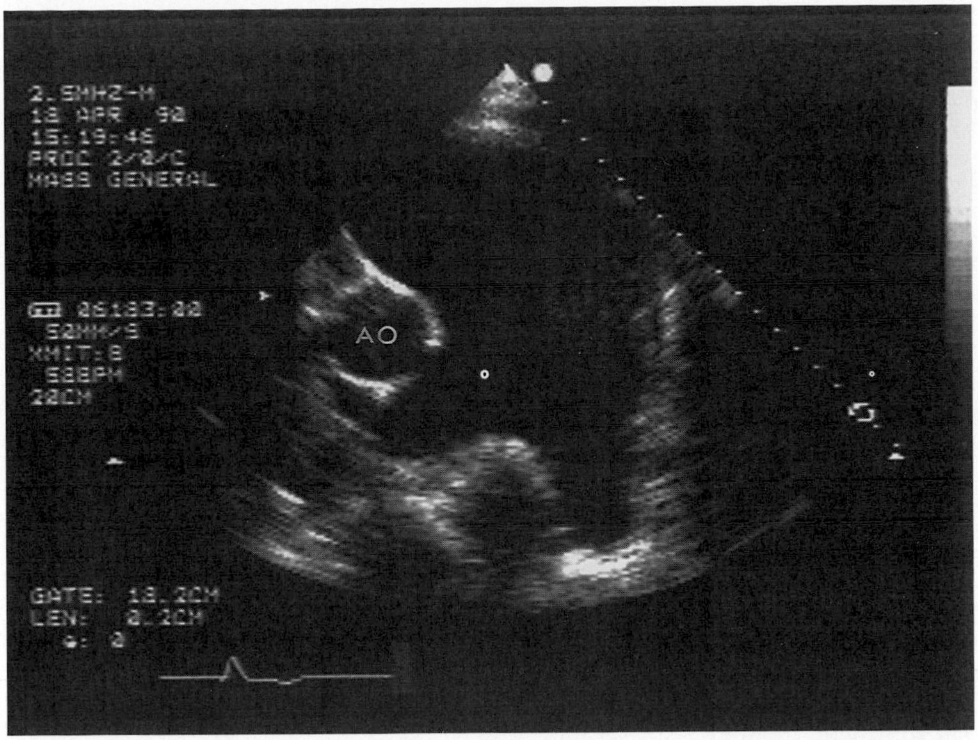

Fig. 27–49. Long axis recording of the pulmonary artery from a patient with idiopathic dilation of the vessel. AO = aorta.

Figure 27–51 is an example of a large myxoma arising from the medial wall of the pulmonary artery just beneath the pulmonary valve. Primary sarcomas are generally multinodular tumors, fixed at the level of the pulmonary valve or base of the pulmonary trunk. The tumor may fill the vessel and often extends to and beyond the bifurcation of the main pulmonary artery.[130] Multiple microscopic patterns have been described including

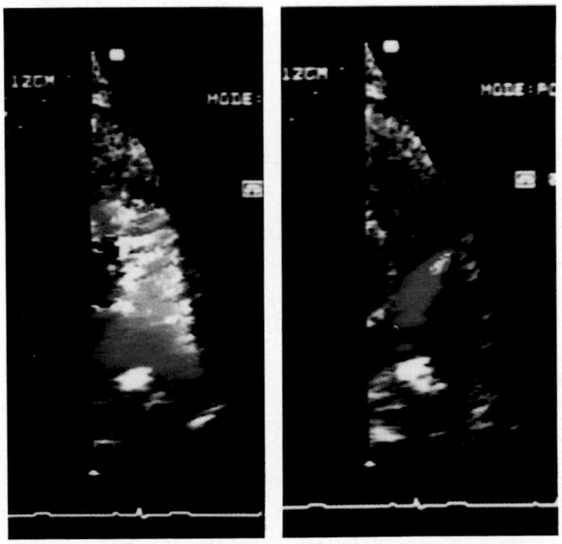

Fig. 27–50. Long axis, color Doppler recordings of the pulmonary artery during systole (left) and diastole (right). During systole, the pulmonary artery flow profile appears normal. During diastole, there is a small low velocity jet, which originates from the lateral wall of the main pulmonary artery. This jet arises from a small coronary arteriovenous fistula, which drains into the pulmonary artery.

undifferentiated pleomorphic sarcoma, leiomyosarcoma, rhabdomyosarcoma, fibrosarcoma, and myxosarcoma.[131–134]

Pulmonary A-V Fistula

See Chapter 15.

Generalized Abnormalities of the Right Ventricular Outflow Tract

In addition to abnormalities involving specific areas of the right ventricular outflow tract, the entire outflow

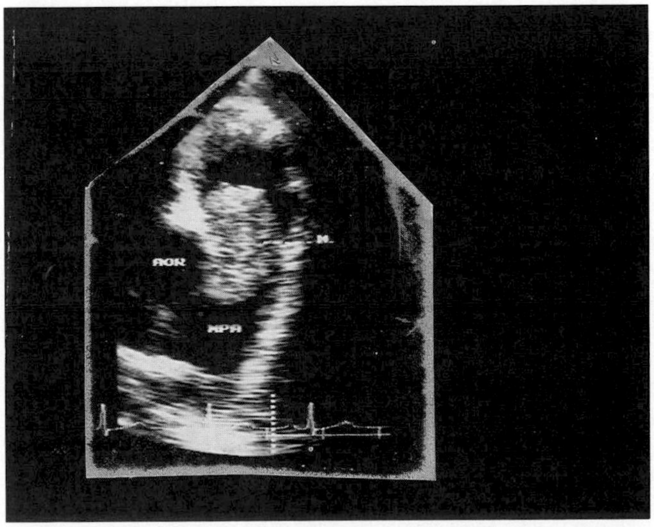

Fig. 27–51. Long axis recording of the pulmonary artery illustrating a large myxoma partially obstructing the pulmonary artery. AOR = aorta; MPA = main pulmonary artery. (Courtesy of Dr. George Xie.)

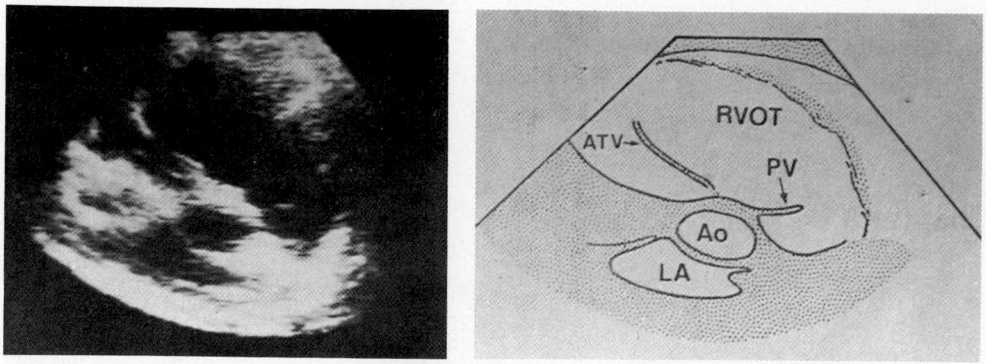

Fig. 27–52. Parasternal long axis recording of the right ventricular outflow tract (RVOT) illustrates diffuse outflow tract dilation. This nonspecific pattern may be seen in patients with large left-to-right shunts or with other lesions associated with the right ventricular volume overload pattern. ATV = anterior tricuspid valve leaflet; PV = pulmonary valve; Ao = aorta; LA = left atrium.

region may be hypoplastic or atretic in lesions, such as pulmonary atresia and pseudo-truncus arteriosus (see Chapter 32), or it may dilate nonspecifically because of increased flow into the pulmonary artery, such as occurs with atrial septal defect and anomalous pulmonary venous connection or with disorders that increase right ventricular volume. Figure 27–52 is an example of a dilated right ventricular outflow tract from a patient with Ebstein's anomaly and right ventricular volume overload. The aortic root in this example is displaced posteriorly and appears small in comparison to the dilated right ventricular outflow tract.

PATENT DUCTUS ARTERIOSUS

In the fetus, the ductus arteriosus provides a normal connection from the pulmonary artery to the descending aorta, diverting flow from the developing pulmonary vascular bed. At birth, the lungs expand, pulmonary flow increases, pulmonary artery pressure falls, and the ductus begins to constrict spontaneously. In normal newborns, the ductus typically closes by the third day of life, with ductal flow being reported in 91% of newborns on the first postnatal day and 18% on the second day of life. The significance of a patent ductus arteriosus therefore varies with the clinical setting. In premature infants, patency of the ductus is normal, and closure is maturation dependent. The clinical and therapeutic importance of the ductus in this group is determined by shunt size and its effect on cardiac performance. In older patients, the presence of an uncomplicated ductus is usually an indication for surgical intervention.[135]

Persistent patency of the ductus arteriosus is a common cardiac anomaly that can occur as an isolated lesion or in association with other congenital cardiac defects. A patent ductus arteriosus is found in roughly 10% of all children with congenital cardiovascular disease and in 0.3 to 0.7% of all live births. The medical and surgical management of patent ductus arteriosus requires knowledge of the magnitude and direction of the ductal shunt and the pulmonary artery pressure. In many instances, the duct can be directly recorded by two-dimensional imaging with Doppler techniques confirming the diagnosis. Doppler techniques also provide a method for diagnosing shunts that are too small to be imaged; for determining the direction, timing, and magnitude of shunt flow; and for estimating pulmonary artery pressure.

Imaging

Patent ductus arteriosus is usually imaged from a high left parasternal or suprasternal window with the scan plane aligned to record the long axis of the pulmonary artery. From the parasternal window, the ductus is usually seen arising from the main pulmonary artery between the right and left pulmonary branches and connecting to the descending thoracic aorta. With slight rotation of the transducer toward the long axis of the aorta, a greater extent of the descending thoracic aorta and the entire length of the patent ductus arteriosus can usually be visualized. Small ducts may be inapparent in this view because the vessel is positioned vertically within the scan plane and hence is imaged with the lateral resolution of the system. Doppler recording of the associated shunt flow should confirm the presence of the patent ductus (Fig. 27–53).

In the suprasternal long axis view, the ductus can be seen connecting the descending aorta (just beyond the left subclavian artery) and the main pulmonary artery.[136,137] In many cases, it is necessary to tilt the scan plane anteriorly toward the left pulmonary artery to image the duct. In this imaging plane, the ductus is seen between the origin of the left pulmonary artery and the descending aorta. Ductal length has been reported to vary from 5.5 mm to 13 mm (mean, 8 mm), and the aortic orifice size may range from 1.5 to 13 mm (mean, 7.5 mm).[138] Confusion can arise if the left pulmonary artery is misinterpreted as the ductus when it crosses in front of the aorta. The ductus is also difficult to record in a single plane when it is long and tortuous. In infants, aneurysms of the ductus arteriosus can be observed that can rupture spontaneously or regress over time.[139]

Flow

Doppler techniques are useful for detecting small ducts that are not visualized during routine two-dimensional imaging; for assessing the location, direction, and quality of shunt flow; for measuring the pressure gradient from the aorta to the pulmonary artery; and for quantitating the volume of the shunt flow. Because pressure in the aorta is normally higher than that in the pulmonary artery, flow through the ductus is usually from left to right (aorta to pulmonary artery). Figure 27–53 (right) is a color flow recording from a patient with a small ductus arteriosus illustrating the characteristic

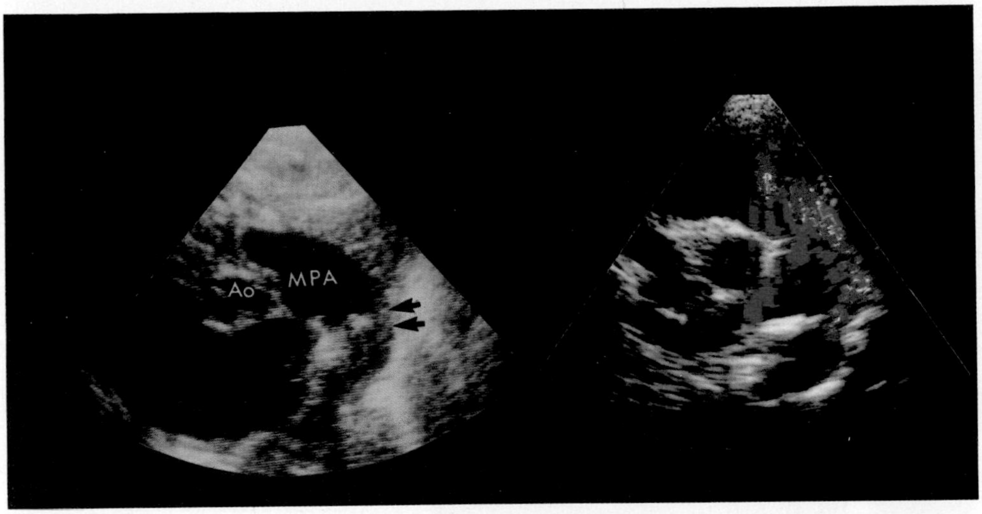

Fig. 27–53. Left. Suprasternal long axis recording of a ductal connection (arrows) between the main pulmonary artery (MPA) and the descending aorta (PAo). Right. Color flow recording of flow through the ductus from the descending aorta to the pulmonary artery. The small flow area in the right ventricular outflow tract distal to the valve represents pulmonary regurgitation.

high velocity, turbulent jet arising from the ductus during diastole and extending along the lateral wall of the pulmonary artery. As the jet approaches the pulmonary valve, flow is deflected back along the medial wall of the artery, producing an antegrade diastolic flow pattern in this region.[140] During systole, the normal antegrade flow stream in the pulmonary artery deflects the jet downward toward the right pulmonary artery, and retrograde flow in the pulmonary artery is no longer apparent. Figure 27–54 is a color flow recording from a patient with a larger ductus arteriosus. In this example, ductal flow fills the central portion of the pulmonary artery with only a small area of counter flow apparent along the medial wall. When the ductus is very large (Fig. 27–55), shunt flow may completely fill the pulmonary artery with resultant loss of any obvious secondary flow patterns in the pulmonary artery.

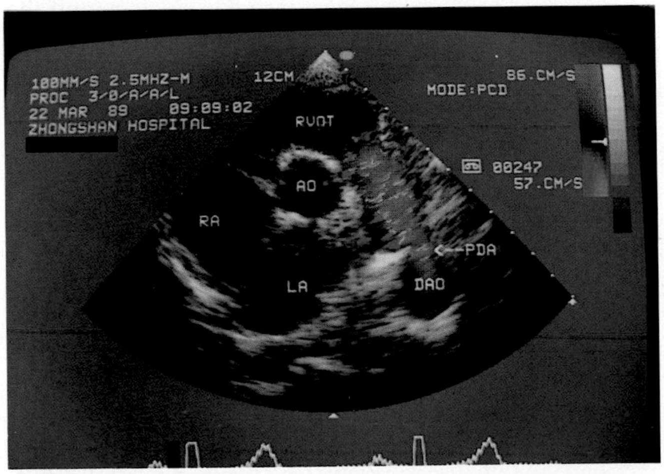

Fig. 27–54. Color flow recording from a patient with a moderately large patent ductus arteriosus (PDA) illustrating a large centrally directed flow stream, which fills most of the pulmonary artery with only a small area of counter flow along the medial wall of the vessel. Proximal acceleration of flow into the ductus is evident in the descending thoracic aorta. RVOT = right ventricular outflow tract; DAO = descending thoracic aorta; AO = aorta; RA = right atrium; LA = left atrium. (Courtesy of Dr. Leng Jiang.)

Positioning a pulsed Doppler sample volume at the mouth of the ductus reveals disturbed flow during both diastole and systole. If the pulmonary artery pressure is low, the pressure gradient between the aorta and pulmonary artery will be large and the flow velocity will be high. If the sample volume is positioned closer to the pulmonary valve, the systolic component of flow will be normal and only the diastolic retrograde component of ductal flow will be apparent. If the sample volume is placed in the midportion of the pulmonary artery close to the medial wall, antegrade flow may be apparent during both diastole and systole. In some patients with small or restrictive ducts, flow may be directed along the medial wall of the pulmonary artery, creating a clockwise flow pattern.[141,142] Because the ductal shunt is distal the pulmonary valve, flow in the right ventricular outflow tract proximal to the valve should be normal.

Doppler sampling within the duct permits ductal flow to be independently assessed and helps to differentiate this lesion from other anomalies associated with abnormal pulmonary artery diastolic flow. It further permits identification of right-to-left shunting that is inapparent in the pulmonary artery. In subjects with an isolated left-to-right shunt, flow through the duct is continuous, is directed toward a transducer in a parasternal location, and has a peak velocity in late systole (Fig. 27–56). Patients with isolated right-to-left ductal shunting (as can occur in infants with aortic arch interruption or severe pulmonary hypertension) show continuous flow from the pulmonary artery to the aorta (away from a parasternally located transducer), which peaks in early systole. Bidirectional ductal shunting is detectable in infants with a patent ductus arteriosus and severe pulmonary arterial hypertension. The right-to-left shunt causes retrograde (PA to AO) flow beginning in late systole and extending into late diastole. As shunt size increases, peak shunt flow generally occurs later in the cardiac cycle. In patients with bidirectional shunts and pulmonary pressures at or below systemic levels, right-to-left shunting has been reported to occupy $<60\%$ of systole, whereas in patients with suprasystemic pulmonary artery pressure, right-to-left shunting continued for $\geq 60\%$ of systole. As

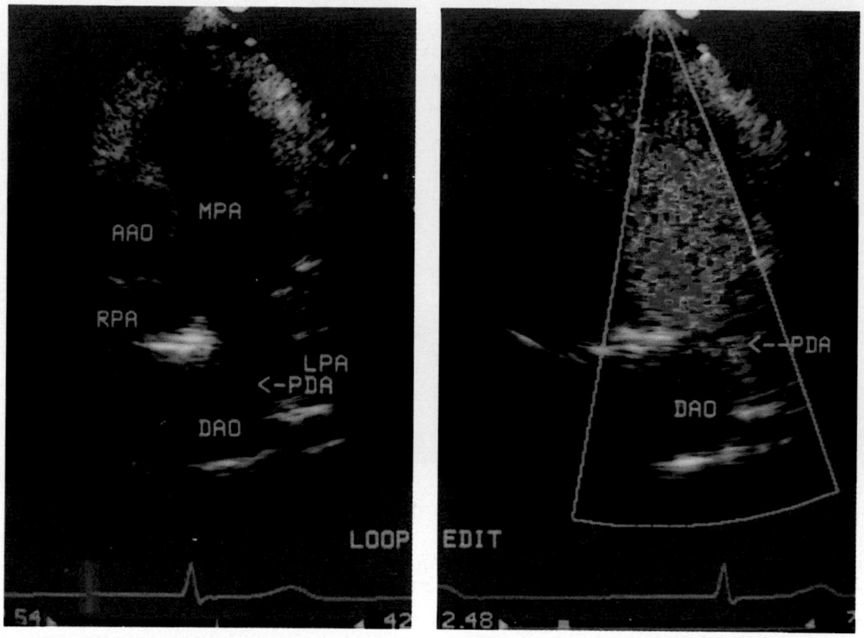

Fig. 27–55. Two-dimensional image of a large patent ductus arteriosus (PDA) (left) and color Doppler recording of ductal shunt flow (right). In this example, the ductus is large, and the shunt flow fills the pulmonary artery from the ductal orifice to the pulmonary valve. Proximal acceleration of flow into the ductus is also evident in the descending thoracic aorta (DAO). MPA = main pulmonary artery; AAO = ascending aorta; RPA = right pulmonary artery; LPA = left pulmonary artery. (Courtesy of Dr. Leng Jiang.)

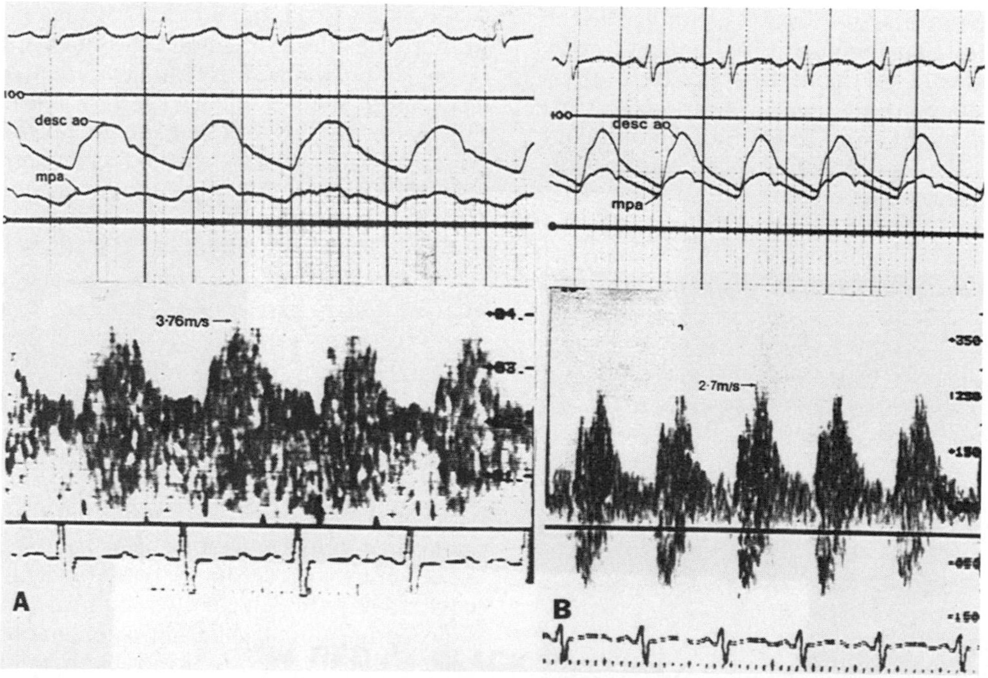

Fig. 27–56. Characteristic Doppler velocity profiles of patent ductus arteriosus (PDA) flow in a patient with isolated left-to-right shunting. **A.** Restrictive PDA with high pressure gradients. The superimposed simultaneous pressure tracing (top) shows a continuous gradient from aorta to main pulmonary artery (mpa). Peak Doppler velocity of 3.76 m/sec corresponded to a peak instantaneous pressure gradient of 53 mm Hg. Minimum Doppler velocity (2.3 m/sec) occurred at end-diastole and corresponded to a minimum pressure gradient of 26 mm Hg. The mean Doppler-derived gradient (41 mm Hg) corresponded to a mean catheter-derived gradient of 40 mm Hg. **B.** Hypertensive PDA with low pressure gradients. Peak instantaneous systolic pressure gradient was 30 mm Hg, corresponding to a maximum Doppler velocity of 2.7 m/sec. Mean gradient was 14 mm Hg from pressure bearings and 12 mm Hg from Doppler velocity. Flow below the 0 line was simultaneously recorded from the descending aorta by the continuous wave Doppler transducer. ao = aorta. (From Musewe NN, et al.: Validation of Doppler-derived pulmonary arterial pressure in patients with ductus arteriosus under different hemodynamic states. Circulation 76:1081, 1987. Reproduced with permission of the American Heart Association, Inc.)

the pulmonary artery pressure increases, the jet arising from the ductus is far less extensive and is often localized to the ductus and the immediately adjacent region of the main pulmonary artery. As a result, the region of ductal insertion must be carefully sampled to detect ductal flow. In normal infants, ductal flow is usually bidirectional during the first hours of life, rapidly changing to continuous left-to-right flow before complete closure.[143] Shunt velocity also increases before ductal closure. Figure 27–57 illustrates the changes in the pattern of flow across the duct in an infant with pulmonary hypertension during maneuvers designed to vary relative pulmonary artery and aortic pressures.

Peak systolic gradients can be calculated from the peak velocity of shunt flow using the simplified Bernoulli equation. Doppler gradients have correlated closely with catheterization measurements of the peak instantaneous systolic gradient.[138] If blood pressure is measured at the time of the Doppler examination, the pulmonary artery systolic pressure can be calculated as the systolic cuff pressure minus the Doppler peak gradient (see preceding discussion). Color flow mapping can be particularly useful in aligning the ultrasonic beam parallel to the direction of flow for accurate Doppler velocity recording.

In assessing peak velocities of a patent ductus arteriosus using pulsed Doppler, it is important to remember that the maximal velocities of left-to-right shunts are recorded with the sample volume at the pulmonary end of the ductus while the maximal velocities of right-to-left shunts are detected at the aortic outlet.

Doppler examination of the descending thoracic aorta can often demonstrate retrograde flow in the region around the entrance into the duct during diastole. This retrograde flow is best detected by pulsed Doppler with the sample volume positioned just distal to the duct or by the demonstration of a local area of convergent flow toward the entrance into the duct during diastole by color flow mapping (Figs. 27–53 to 27–55). When shunt flow is large, reverse diastolic flow can also be recorded on Doppler tracings from the brachial, femoral, subclavian, carotid, and cerebral arteries.[144–147]

The finding of retrograde flow in the descending aorta is not specific for a patent ductus arteriosus and can be seen in any condition in which diastolic run-off of blood from the aorta occurs (i.e., aortic insufficiency).

The magnitude of the ductal shunt can be calculated as the difference between the pulmonary and systemic blood flow. Because the shunt occurs beyond the pulmonary valve, calculation of flow volume across the pulmonary valve provides a measure of systemic flow (not pulmonary flow, which is the sum of systemic and shunt flow), whereas measurement of flow volume across the aortic valve is equal to pulmonary flow. Close correlations have been found between the Doppler and catheterization estimates of pulmonary/systemic flow ratio in infants with a patent ductus arteriosus.[148]

In newborns and premature infants, the Doppler method may be less reliable because of the errors inherent in measuring the diameter of small vessels. In these cases, other secondary findings may be more helpful in identifying infants with significant shunts.

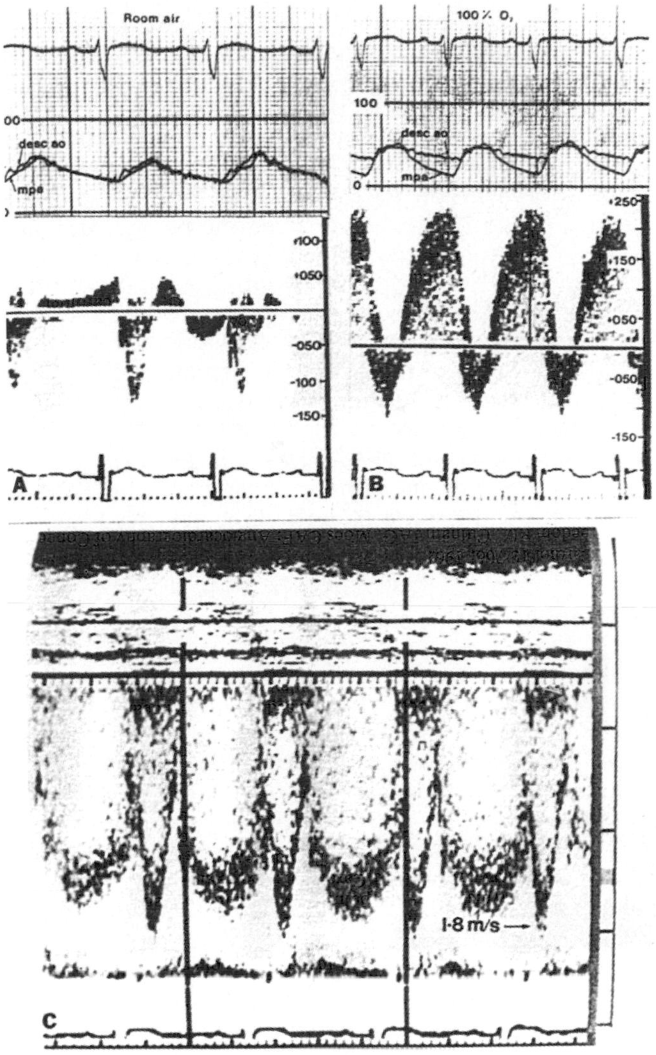

Fig. 27–57. Bidirectional flow across the patent ductus arteriosus (PDA) in a patient with bidirectional shunting. Simultaneous pressure measurements (top) and Doppler velocity spectral displays are shown. Flow toward the transducer (aorta to main pulmonary artery [MPA]) is above the 0 line. **A.** Pressure and Doppler measurements obtained in room air. There was no mean pressure gradient between the aorta and MPA either in systole or diastole. Pulsed Doppler recordings show systolic right-to-left flow and very low velocity variable left-to-right flow in diastole. **B.** In 100% oxygen, the MPA diastolic and mean pressures have decreased, and the Doppler velocity in diastole has correspondingly increased to reflect the higher pressure gradient between the aorta and MPA. Arrows indicate peak instantaneous pressure gradient between the aorta and the MPA (20 mm Hg), and maximum Doppler velocity, both in diastole (2.5 m/sec, equivalent to 25 mm Hg). The Doppler velocity of the right-to-left flow (1 m/sec, equivalent to 4 mm Hg) does not change between the two states. **C.** Doppler recording from the same patient obtained the day before cardiac catheterization. All shunting was right to left. The patient was moderately heavily sedated and became mildly cyanotic. (From Musewe NN, et al.: Validation of Doppler-derived pulmonary arterial pressure in patients with ductus arteriosus under different hemodynamic states. Circulation 76:1081, 1987. Reproduced with permission of the American Heart Association, Inc.)

Associated Findings

Left-to-right shunt flow through the ductus arteriosus leads to increased pulmonary blood flow, increased pulmonary venous return, and consequently, left atrial and left ventricular volume overload. In premature infants with compliant left atria, the left atrial/aortic root measured from the M-mode echocardiogram has been suggested as an indirect assessment of the size of the ductal shunt[149–151] with an LA/AO ratio of >1.3 indicating a significant shunt. However, given the recognized variability of M-mode measurement in distorted hearts, confirmation of atrial dilation by two-dimensional recording is important. The left ventricle is also enlarged and hypercontractile because of the increased preload. The end-systolic volume is usually normal. Because of the large run-off of blood in diastole from the descending aorta to the main pulmonary artery through the patent ductus arteriosus, the aortic pulse pressure is widened, and the descending aortic pulsation in the subcostal views are increased. An increase in aortic flow velocity is generally present in patients with a significant shunt.

Differential Diagnosis

Although the diagnosis of patent ductus arteriosus is generally straightforward, a variety of other conditions can produce abnormal diastolic flow in the pulmonary artery and have been confused with ductal flow. These include aortopulmonary window, anomalous origin of a coronary artery,[152–154] pulmonary regurgitation, coronary A-V fistula (see preceding discussion), coronary blood flow, and surgically created shunts.[61] In the aortopulmonary window, the connection between the aorta and the pulmonary artery is usually located along the medial pulmonary arterial wall. The jet usually enters the pulmonary artery perpendicular to its long axis and expands rapidly. Retrograde pulmonary flow is uncommon, and there is typically a flow disturbance in the aorta at the site of the fenestration. In patients with anomalous origin of a coronary artery (usually the left) from the pulmonary artery, the anomalous vessel generally arises from one of the sinuses of the pulmonary valve. If a left-to-right shunt develops from the normal right coronary artery through anastomotic connections, a flow disturbance may be detectable at the orifice of the left coronary artery.[152,154] These flow disturbances are usually localized to the valve sinuses and do not extend into the main pulmonary artery.[153] Pulmonary regurgitation can cause confusion on pulsed Doppler recordings if the sample volume shifts above the valve; however, this can be eliminated by care in recording. Occasionally, normal left coronary arterial flow can be misinterpreted as ductal flow because of a beam width artifact. Color flow mapping should eliminate this confusion because coronary flow is not found deep within the pulmonary artery, is nonturbulent, and is directed away from the aorta. Finally, surgically created shunts tend to have flow patterns similar to those of a patent ductus, but the abnormal flow is localized to the site of the shunt, which is usually remote from the origin of the ductus arteriosus.[135]

REFERENCES

1. Tajik AJ, et al.: Two-dimensional real-time ultrasonic imaging of the heart and great vessels. Mayo Clin Proc 53:271, 1978.
2. Lange LW, Sahn DJ, Allen HD, Goldberg SJ: Subxiphoid cross-sectional echocardiography in infants and children with congenital heart disease. Circulation 59:513, 1979.
3. Bierman FZ, Williams RG: Prospective diagnosis of transposition of the great arteries in neonates by subxiphoid two-dimensional echocardiography. Circulation 60:1496, 1979.
4. Silove ED, de Giovanni JV, Shiu MF, Yi MM: Diagnosis of right ventricular outflow obstruction in infants by cross sectional echocardiography. Br Heart J 50:416, 1983.
5. Lange LW, Sahn DJ, Allen HD, Goldberg SJ: Subxiphoid cross-sectional echocardiography in infants and children with congenital heart disease. Circulation 59:513, 1979.
6. Weyman AE, et al.: Cross-sectional echocardiographic visualization of the stenotic pulmonary valve. Circulation 56:769, 1977.
7. Grenadier E, et al.: Normal intracardiac and great vessel Doppler flow velocities in infants and children. J Am Coll Cardiol 4:343, 1984.
8. Hatle L, Angelson B: Doppler Ultrasound in Cardiology: Physical Principles and Clinical Applications. Philadelphia, Lea & Febiger, 1985.
9. Hurwitz LE, Roberts WC: Quadricuspid semilunar valves. Am J Cardiol 31:623, 1973.
10. Cavia JE, DeCastro CM, McAllister HA, Jr: Quadricuspid semilunar valves. Chest 72:186, 1977.
11. Gikonyo BM, Lucas RV, Edwards JE: Anatomic features of congenital pulmonary valvar stenosis. Pediatr Cardiol 8:109, 1987.
12. Friedberg C: Diseases of the Heart. Philadelphia, WB Saunders, 1966.
13. Hultgren HN, Reeve R, Cohn K, McLeod R: The ejection click of valvular pulmonic stenosis. Circulation 40:631, 1969.
14. Waller BF: The operatively excised pulmonary valve—a forgotten entity (editorial). Mayo Clin Proc 64:1452, 1989.
15. Fox R, et al.: Detection by Doppler echocardiography of acquired pulmonic stenosis due to extrinsic tumor compression. Am J Cardiol 53:1475, 1984.
16. Weyman AE, Dillon JC, Feigenbaum H, Chang S: Echocardiographic patterns of pulmonary valve motion in valvular pulmonary stenosis. Am J Cardiol 34:644, 1974.
17. Gutgesell HP, et al.: Accuracy of two-dimensional echocardiography in the diagnosis of congenital heart disease. Am J Cardiol 55:514, 1985.
18. De Knecht S, Daniels O, Reneman RS: Non-invasive assessment of pulmonary valve stenosis with a multigate pulsed Doppler system. Br Heart J 50:592, 1983.
19. Philpot E, et al.: In-vitro pulsatile flow visualization studies in a pulmonary artery model. J Biomed Eng 107:368, 1985.
20. Chen JTT, Robinson AE, Goodrich JK, Lester RG: Uneven distribution of pulmonary blood flow between the left and right lungs in isolated valvular pulmonary stenosis. Am J Roentgenol 107:343, 1969.
21. Reeve R: Variations of the ejection click in valvular pulmonic stenosis. Clin Res 14:129, 1966.
22. Lima CO, et al.: Noninvasive prediction of transvalvular pressure gradient in patients with pulmonary stenosis by quantitative two-dimensional echocardiographic Doppler studies. Circulation 67:866, 1983.
23. Johnson GL, et al.: Accuracy of combined two-dimensional echocardiography and continuous wave Doppler recordings in the estimation of pressure gradient in right ventricular outlet obstruction. J Am Coll Cardiol 3:1013, 1984.
24. Murphy DJ, Ludomirsky A, Danford DA, Huhta JC: Doppler echocardiography in pulmonary stenosis. Echocardiography 4:187, 1987.
25. Aldousany AW, et al.: Doppler estimation of pressure gradient in pulmonary stenosis: maximal instantaneous vs peak-to-peak, catheter gradient. Pediatr Cardiol 10:145, 1989.
26. Lim MK, et al.: Variability of the Doppler gradient in pulmonary valve stenosis before and after balloon dilatation. Br Heart J 62:212, 1989.
27. Kosturakis D, et al.: Noninvasive quantification of stenotic semilunar valve areas by Doppler echocardiography. J Am Coll Cardiol 3:1256, 1984.
28. Smallhorn JF, Izukawa T, Benson L, Freedom RM: Noninvasive recognition of functional pulmonary atresia by echocardiography. Am J Cardiol 54:925, 1984.
29. Hamby RI, Gulotta SJ: Pulmonic valvular insufficiency: etiology, recognition, and management. Am Heart J 74:110, 1967.
30. Chandraratna PA, et al.: Invasive and noninvasive assessment of pulmonic regurgitation: clinical, angiographic, phonocardiographic, echocardiographic, and Doppler ultrasound correlations. Clin Cardiol 5:360, 1982.
31. Waggoner AD, et al.: Pulsed Doppler echocardiographic detection of right-side valve regurgitation. Am J Cardiol 47:279, 1981.
32. Miyatake K, et al.: Pulmonary regurgitation studied with the ultrasonic pulsed Doppler technique. Circulation 65:969, 1982.
33. Patel AK, et al.: Pulsed Doppler echocardiography in diagnosis of pulmonary regurgitation: its value and limitations. Am J Cardiol 49:1801, 1982.
34. Gullace G, et al.: Contrast echocardiographic features of pulmonary hypertension and regurgitation. Br Heart J 46:369, 1981.

CHAPTER

28

RIGHT VENTRICLE

LENG JIANG, SUSAN E. WIEGERS, and ARTHUR E. WEYMAN

The right ventricle is a structurally complex chamber that forms the majority of the anterior surface of the heart and overlies the anteromedial border of the left ventricle. When viewed from the side, the right ventricle appears triangular, whereas in cross section, it is normally crescent shaped. Its medial wall is formed by the thick, convex, interventricular septum, whereas laterally, it is bordered by the thinner, concave, free right ventricular wall. In addition to the main right ventricular chamber, the infundibular portion of the right ventricular outflow tract is considered both structurally and functionally as a part of the right ventricle, further complicating its anatomic description.

The inner walls of the right ventricle are irregular, being lined by numerous small muscle bundles, the trabeculae carneae. In addition to forming multiple ridges along the inner surfaces of the chamber, the trabeculae occasionally cross from one wall to another. A large muscle bundle, the moderator band, is noted in approximately 60% of persons and stretches from the lower interventricular septum to the anterior right ventricular wall, where it joins the anterior papillary muscle.

Functionally, the right ventricle provides the energy to propel the systemic venous blood returning from the right atrium through the pulmonary vascular bed. Because the resistance in the pulmonary circuit is normally low, the right ventricle is not required to generate high intracavitary pressures. The shape of the right ventricle, with a large surface area relative to the intracavitary volume, is therefore ideally suited to eject large volumes of blood with minimal amounts of myocardial shortening.

The right ventricle has been likened to a fireplace bellows in which the sides are large in comparison to the space between them. A slight movement of the sides toward each other causes displacement of a large volume from within.

The right ventricle normally contracts by three separate mechanisms: (1) contraction of the spiral muscles, which shortens the long axis and draws the tricuspid annulus toward the apex; (2) inward movement of the right ventricular free wall, which produces the bellows effect; and (3) traction on the margins of the free right ventricular wall at their points of attachment to the left ventricle resulting from left ventricular contraction. The inward movement of the right ventricular free wall is the primary mechanism by which blood is ejected. The amplitude of this motion is not great; however, because of the shape of the right ventricle, this motion is sufficient to eject a relatively large volume.

Although the shape of the right ventricle is well suited to eject a large volume of blood with little muscular contraction, it is poorly suited to contract against high pressure. If the normal right ventricle were suddenly required to provide the intraventricular pressure developed by the left ventricle, the right ventricular myocardium would have to develop tension many times as great as that in the left ventricle. As will be demonstrated later, the right ventricle frequently adapts to an acquired pressure load by altering its shape to a more efficient configuration.

The pattern of right ventricular ejection also differs from that of the left ventricle. The velocity of right ventricular ejection increases more gradually, peaks later, and decreases more slowly than that noted on the left side. Ejection also persists longer in the right ventricle.

Some of this delay can be attributed to the relatively late contraction of the infundibulum, which prolongs the ejection phase of the right ventricle.

RIGHT VENTRICULAR EXAMINING PLANES AND LINEAR DIMENSIONS

The right ventricle can be recorded in (1) a parasternal long axis view of the right ventricular inflow tract; (2) a parasternal short axis view of the right ventricle at the tricuspid valve level; (3) the apical four-chamber view; and (4) the subcostal long axis view of the right ventricle. In addition, portions of the right ventricle can be visualized in the subcostal long axis of the right ventricular outflow tract, and multiple short axis cuts of the right ventricle can be obtained from the subcostal location if necessary.

The apical four-chamber view of the right ventricle has been the most extensively studied and appears to provide the most useful information. In this orientation, the imaging plane transects the right ventricle from the apex to the base and with its x axis oriented obliquely across the chamber from the free right ventricular wall laterally to the interventricular septum medially. This plane includes a long axis of the right ventricle from the ventricular apex to the tricuspid annulus and passes through a ventricular short axis. It also permits an area measurement, which is comparable to, but clearly not the same as, an angiographic left anterior oblique (LAO) view.

It has been suggested, based on comparative measurements of right ventricular casts, that the right ventricular long axis in the four-chamber view should be drawn from the apical tip to the medial insertion of the tricuspid leaflet. Figure 28–1 compares the shape of the normal right ventricle to that seen with right ventricular volume overload and marked right ventricular hypertrophy. In normal persons, the right ventricular long axis can be appropriately drawn along the right-hand margin of the interventricular septum; however, in the latter two instances, this measurement is better taken from the tip of the apex to the plane of the tricuspid annulus through the ventricular cavity. The long axis, therefore, may be best defined as the maximal distance between parallel lines passing through the tricuspid annulus and the right ventricular apex rather than drawn along the margin of the interventricular septum.

Two dimensions have also been defined that are parallel to the short axis plane of the right ventricle. These dimensions include a mid- and maximal right ventricular minor dimension (short axis). The mid-right ventricular dimensions is measured from the right septal to the free wall endocardial intercepts of a line drawn perpendicular to and bisecting the right ventricular long axis. The maximal dimension (short axis) is defined as the longest distance that can be measured in the four-chamber view between the septal and free wall endocardium in a plane perpendicular to the long axis. Right ventricular linear measurements can be taken at any point in the cardiac cycle. When a single measurement is used to express right ventricular size, however, it is conventionally taken at end-diastole when the ventricle is largest. These dimensions are illustrated in Figure 28–1. Each of these linear dimensions and the planimetered right ventricular area have been shown to relate directly to right ventricular cast volumes. The best correlations, however, have been obtained using the maximal short axis dimension and the planimetered area.

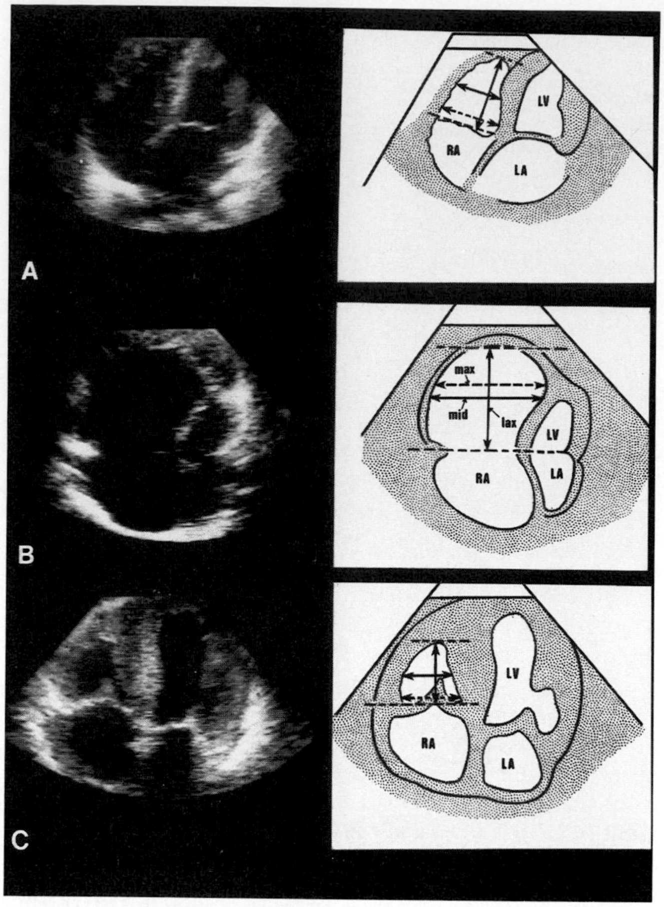

Fig. 28–1. Series of apical four-chamber recordings comparing the size and shape of the right ventricle. **A.** Normal right ventricle. **B.** The volume-overloaded right ventricle. **C.** The hypertrophied right ventricle. The variation in linear dimensions in each of these settings is indicated in the accompanying diagrams. The right ventricular long axis (lax), taken as the distance between parallel lines intersecting the right ventricular apex and tricuspid annulus, increases slightly in right ventricular volume overload **(B)** and may be reduced in cases of marked right ventricular hypertrophy **(C)**. The two minor dimensions that can be obtained in this view are also indicated in the diagrams. These dimensions include a midventricular short axis (mid), which is perpendicular to and bisects the long axis (solid line), and a maximal short axis (max), which is the longest dimension that can be obtained in a plane that is perpendicular to the long axis (interrupted line). In both the normal and hypertrophied ventricle, the maximal dimension is recorded close to the tricuspid annulus. In contrast, the maximal dimension in the patient with right ventricular volume overload is positioned apical to the midventricular dimension. LV = left ventricle; RA = right atrium; LA = left atrium.

The other standard views of the right ventricle have, to this point, proved less useful. The parasternal long axis of the right ventricular inflow tract, which is of primary value for recording the tricuspid valve, provides less information about the right ventricle. This plane transects the ventricle obliquely from its anterior to its posterolateral surfaces and, as such, is difficult to standardize. Although theoretically orthogonal to the apical four-chamber view, the apex of the ventricle is rarely recorded in this imaging plane, and hence, a ventricular area and/or reproducible dimensions are not available.

Figure 28–2 is a parasternal long axis of the right ventricle recorded at end-diastole just as the tricuspid leaflets coapt. Although the tricuspid valve is well visualized, the ventricular border is poorly recorded. The apex is not clearly visualized, and the anterior wall is interrupted by the origin of the right ventricular outflow tract. The only landmark available to standardize this view is the tricuspid valve, which is insufficient to fix the plane in space.

The parasternal short axis view at the base is likewise limited in its ability to encompass the entire ventricle (Fig. 28–3). This limitation occurs because the free wall of the right ventricle at this level lies beneath the sternum and is difficult to record consistently. When the entire ventricle is visualized, however, the parasternal short axis provides a ventricular area at the base and should permit recording of a more accurate maximal right ventricular short axis dimension than can the apical four-chamber view. This occurs because of the crescent shape of the right ventricle and because the four-chamber plane may not truly pass through the maximal thickness of the crescent. The short axis view, however, should allow this point to be defined and the measurement to be determined more appropriately. Figure 28–3 illustrates comparable parasternal short axis recordings in a normal person and in a patient with right ventricular volume overload. In the latter example, the right ventricle is dilated and has rotated above the left ventricle such that the maximal dimension lies in a roughly anteroposterior plane. This difference in orientation can be appreciated only in the short axis view.

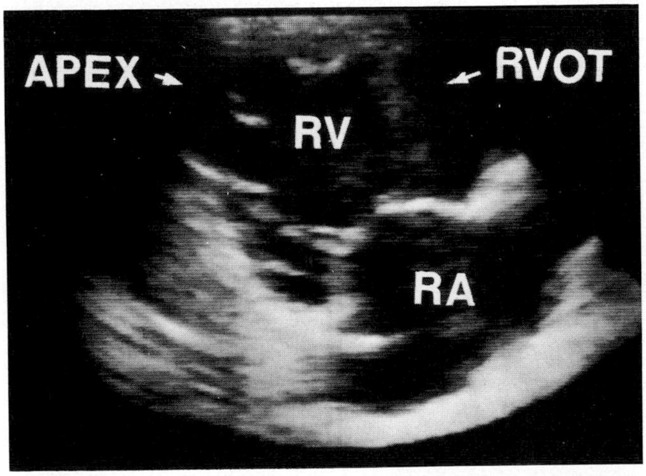

Fig. 28–2. Parasternal long axis diastolic recording of the right ventricle (RV) and tricuspid valve. Although of primary importance in evaluating tricuspid valve motion and structure, this plane transects the right ventricular cavity obliquely; consequently, any measured right ventricular dimensions are difficult to standardize. In addition, the complete apex is rarely recorded, the anterior wall is poorly visualized, and the continuity of the anterior wall is interrupted by the origin of the right ventricular outflow tract (RVOT). This view, therefore, contains little quantitative information concerning right ventricular size or configuration. The motion of the anterior right ventricular wall and right ventricular apex, however, can be assessed, and gross changes in right ventricular contraction can be appreciated. RA = right atrium.

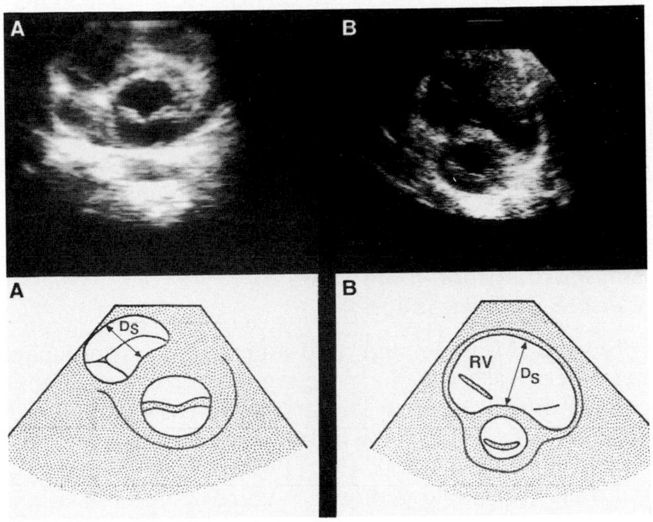

Fig. 28–3. Parasternal short axis recording of the right ventricle. **A.** Normal right ventricle. **B.** Volume-overloaded right ventricle. The volume-overloaded ventricle (RV) is dilated and rotated clockwise relative to the normal right ventricle. The minor axis (D_S) shifts in the same direction, and its true position within the ventricle can be appreciated only in this short axis view.

The subcostal four-chamber view of the right ventricle is often equated with, but is actually slightly oblique to, the apical four-chamber view. This plane can be compared to the parasternal long axis of the left ventricle in that it passes through one of the lateral horns of the crescent rather than through its true center. This plane can be useful in defining right ventricular chamber size in infants but, to date, has played only a minor role in examining adults. Measurements of the right ventricle derived from this plane vary greatly with plane elevation and are difficult to standardize, except with reference to the tricuspid valve.

Finally, the subcostal long axis of the right ventricular outflow tract should be mentioned. This plane transects the right ventricle from the free lateral wall to the pulmonary valve, passing through the center of the infundibular region. This plane provides a long axis right ventricular dimension, which bisects the infundibulum and extends from the pulmonary valve to the free right ventricular lateral wall. This dimension is readily available in this view and, although orthogonal, is similar to the long axis dimension measured in the apical four-chamber view. A comparable dimension taken from the right anterior oblique (RAO) angiographic projection has been used in angiographic right ventricular volume calculations. In addition, this plane includes a right ventricular area at the base of the ventricle, which has proven useful in area-length geometric volume models.

RIGHT VENTRICULAR VOLUME MEASUREMENTS

The right ventricle is both technically and conceptually more difficult to study in a quantitative manner than the left ventricle. The right ventricle is crescent shaped in cross section, asymmetric, and heavily trabeculated. These characteristics defy description in terms of a simple geometric model. In addition, any such model would have to allow for the changes in right ventricular shape that occur with volume and pressure loads and for the contribution of the infundibular portion of the ventricle to overall chamber volume.

Echocardiographic Methods of Volume Determination

Several M-mode and two-dimensional approaches have been taken to measure right ventricular volume echocardiographically. These include (1) estimation of volume from single-plane dimensions and areas; (2) the Simpson's rule method; (3) representation of the right ventricle by simple geometric figures or combinations of figures, the so-called area-length method; (4) determination of volume as the difference between the crescentic shells formed by the septum and free wall; and (5) three-dimensional reconstruction.

Single Plane Measurements

The simplest, and most routinely used, echocardiographic method for assessing right ventricular size relies on dimensions and areas obtained for single tomographic planes transecting the chamber. These parameters yield an index that may correlate with but cannot be used to determine right ventricular volume.

Estimation of Right Ventricular Size From the Parasternal Long and Short Axis Views of the Left Ventricle

Parasternal Long Axis View. Historically, the first echocardiographic measurement of right ventricular size was derived from the standard M-mode recording of the left ventricle (see Chapter 14). Although these recordings were by definition positioned with reference to left ventricular structures and geometry, a rough correlation was observed between a dimension taken from the intersection of the M-mode beam with the endocardium of the right ventricular free wall to its intersection with the right side of the interventricular septum and right ventricular size (Fig. 28–4). Because the path of the beam in the standard M-mode recording of the left ventricle corresponds to the orientation of the central ray of the scan plane in the parasternal long axis view of the left ventricle, a similar dimension can be derived from the two-dimensional image. Unfortunately, the parasternal long axis view of the left ventricle transects the lateral horn of the crescentic right ventricle, and thus the recorded right ventricular diameter will be affected by right ventricular shape (i.e., whether the crescent is flat and wide or thick and narrow), by the degree of right ventricular rotation in the chest, and by patient position. For example, rolling the patient from the supine into the left lateral decubitus position may increase the right ventricular dimension by up to 40%.[4] Further, because this right ventricular dimension is not and cannot be fixed relative to any structure in the right ventricle and bears no consistent relationship to right ventricular geometry, it cannot be considered standard.

As a result, evaluation of the size of the right ventricle in the parasternal long axis view of the left ventricle is useful only to alert the examiner to the possibility of right ventricular dilation or hypoplasia and hence that the right ventricle needs to be examined more closely in other views.

Despite all of these limitations, this view provides the first impression of the right ventricle, and the dimension derived from it is the only measure of right ventricular size reported by many, if not most, laboratories.

Parasternal Short Axis View. Although still imperfect, the parasternal short axis view of the right ventricle at the base provides a more consistent dimension than the long axis view. Based on normative data generated in our laboratory (Appendix A), the end-diastolic dimen-

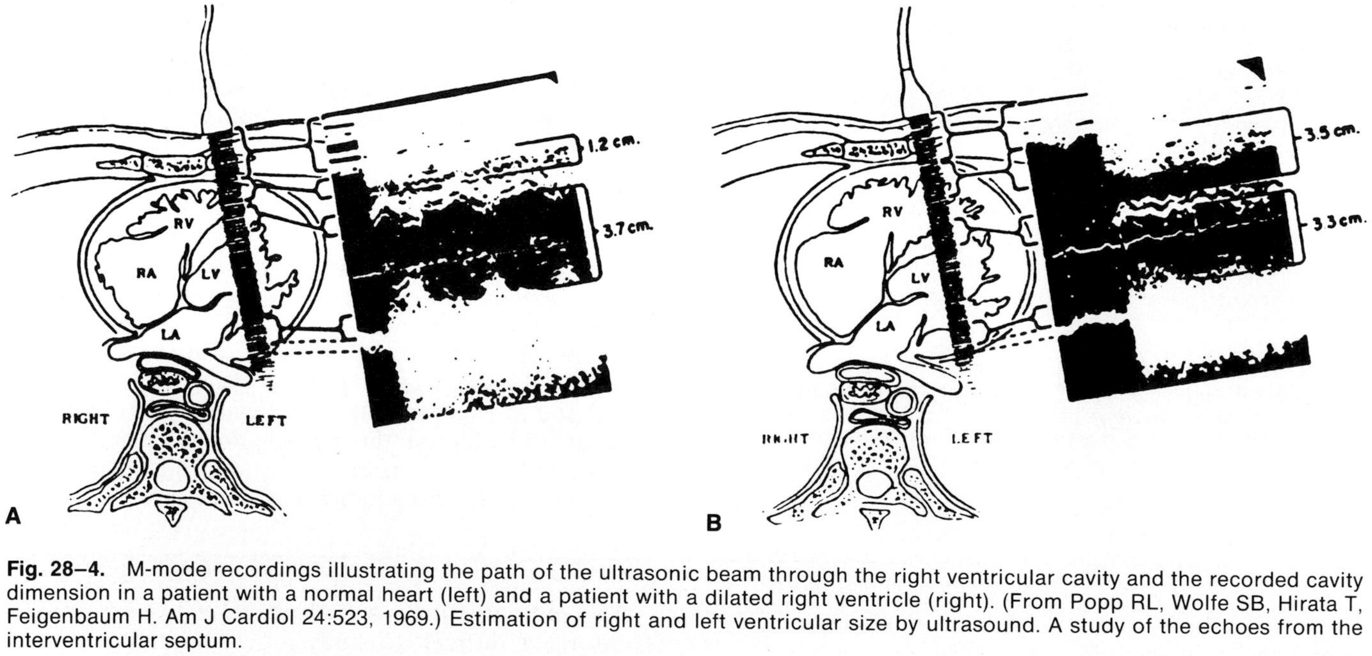

Fig. 28–4. M-mode recordings illustrating the path of the ultrasonic beam through the right ventricular cavity and the recorded cavity dimension in a patient with a normal heart (left) and a patient with a dilated right ventricle (right). (From Popp RL, Wolfe SB, Hirata T, Feigenbaum H. Am J Cardiol 24:523, 1969.) Estimation of right and left ventricular size by ultrasound. A study of the echoes from the interventricular septum.

sion of the right ventricle measured in the parasternal short axis view should be approximately 60% of the equivalent left ventricular dimension.

Dimensions and Areas Derived From the Apical Four-Chamber View. In patients with right ventricular volume overload, the area of the right ventricle in the apical four-chamber view as well as the midventricular and maximal short axis dimensions are larger than those in normal subjects. However, there is a significant overlap between the two groups[1] (Fig. 28–5), and neither of these measurements reliably identifies enlarged right ventricles. Similarly, correlation between the long axis of the right ventricle in the apical four-chamber view and angiographically measured volume is poor (r = .25). The correlation between the short axis in this view and angiography is better (r = .6) but still not clinically useful.[2] Correlations between chamber areas and angiographic end-diastolic and end-systolic volumes and the percentage of volume change (ejection fraction) have been better than for simple dimensions (Table 28–1).[3,4] Results have been less good (r = .44) when echocardiographic area change is compared to radionuclide ventriculograms; however, the reference standard is also less accurate.[5] Comparison of relative right and left ventricular size may also be useful: We have found that in the apical four-chamber view, the normal end-diastolic right ventricular chamber area should be ≤⅔ that of the left ventricle.

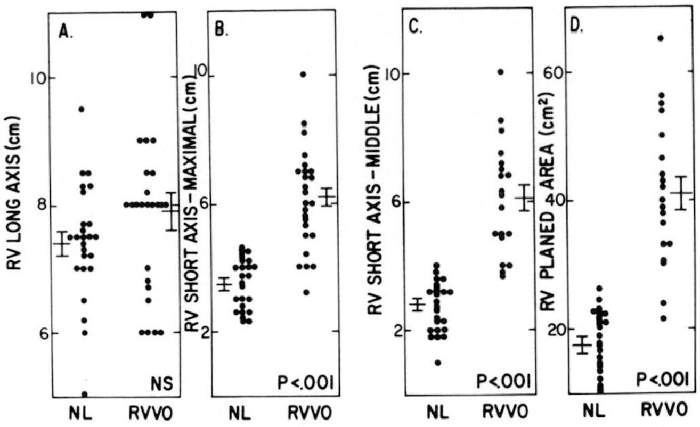

Fig. 28–5. Comparison of the means and averages for right ventricular (RV) long axis, maximal short axis, midventricular minor dimension, and planimetered right ventricular area in normal persons (NL) with patients with right ventricular volume overload (RVVO). (From Bommer W, et al.: Determination of right atrial and ventricular size by two-dimensional echocardiography. Circulation 60:91, 1979. Reproduced by permission of the American Heart Association, Inc.)

It has also been reported that tricuspid annular excursion in the apical four-chamber view (measured from the tip of the scan plane to the tricuspid free wall margin of the tricuspid annulus) correlates well with right ventricular ejection fraction (r = .92). This method, while intui-

Table 28–1. Single Plane: Area and Length Method

Authors	Study Population	Echo Views	Formula	Reference		Results
Hiraishi[3]	22 children (CHD)	A4C	$V = (1.061 * CA_{ap} * CA_{lat})/CL_{ap}$	Angiogram	EDV	r = .92 y = .96x − 1.14
					ESV	r = .84 y = 0.94x − 0.27
					EF	r = .78 y = 1.03x − 0.01
			$V = (0.849 * CA_{ap} * CA_{lat})/CL_{lat}$		EDV	r = .91 y = 0.97x − 0.32
					ESV	r = .83 y = 1.02x − 0.74
					EF	r = .74 y = 0.90 + 0.07
			$V = (1.316 * CA_{lat}^2)/CL_{lat}$		EDV	r = .93 y = 0.93x + 1.46
					ESV	r = .88 y = 0.94x + 0.33
					EF	r = .77 y = 0.87x + 0.33
Silverman[4]	20 children (CHD)	A4C	V = 0.849 A/L	Angiogram	EDV	r = .81 y = 0.62x + 7.0
					ESV	r = .85 y = 0.82x + 1.4
					EF	r = .82 y = 0.66x + 17.8

A = area; CHD = congenital heart disease; A4C = apical four-chamber view; CA = corrected echo area; CL = corrected echo long axis length; ap = anteroposterior plane of angiogram; lat = lateral plane of angiogram; EDV = end-diastolic volume; ESV = end-systolic volume; EF = ejection fraction; L = length.

tively attractive, is based on an external reference system, fails to account for any base-to-apex motion of the entire heart as it contracts, and will yield differing results in proportion to the angle between the transducer and the annular point of motion.

Limitations are also found in the accuracy of dimensions measured in the apical four-chamber view. The right ventricle may be foreshortened by transducer position despite apparently correct positioning of the transducer in relation to the left ventricle. In addition, methods that compare the right ventricle to the left may mask enlargement of the former if left ventricular enlargement is also present. Because of the obvious limitations encountered when trying to estimate right ventricular volume from single plane areas and dimensions, approaches have been sought to measure the volume of the right ventricle more directly.

Use of Simpson's Rule to Determine Right Ventricular Volume

Using the Simpson's rule approach, the right ventricular chamber is divided into a series of slices of equal thickness. This volume of each slice is calculated using the general formula:

$$\text{volume} = \text{area} \times \text{length (height)} \qquad [28.1]$$

and the volume of the entire chamber is obtained by summing the volumes of the individual slices. Alternatively, each slice can be represented by a simple geometric figure, and the volumetric formula for that figure is used to calculate slice volume. Figure 28–6[6] illustrates how the volume of a large figure can be derived from the sum of the volumes of its components. To obtain these slices of the right ventricle, the chamber must first be imaged in two orthogonal projections/sections. Conventionally, the slices are then made perpendicular to a long axis that is common to both projections/sections. In its original application, this technique was applied to frontal and lateral or RAO and LAO projections of right ventriculograms and the slices considered to be elliptic cylinders (see Fig. 28–7). The volume of this figure is given by the following formula:

$$V = \pi \left(\frac{D_1}{2}\right)\left(\frac{D_2}{2}\right) H \qquad [28.2]$$

The height of each elliptic cylinder, H, can be determined by dividing the measured long axis into a number of segments of even length or by arbitrarily defining the figure such that each segment has a predetermined length and the number of segments depends on the length of the long axis. The borders of the cylinder are defined by the projections of the right ventricle in orthogonal planes or the chamber margins in tomographic sections. D_1 and D_2 are then the distances between the contralateral borders of the image along lines drawn perpendicularly to the long axis in each of the orthogonal imaging planes at the specified segment length H. When using the ellipsoid-cylinder formula, the volume of the right ventricle would be

$$V = \frac{\pi}{4} H \sum_{0}^{n} D_1 D_2 \qquad [28.3]$$

Others have shown that triangular, rectangular, or elliptic volume elements give similar results.[7–10] In vivo, right ventricular volume obtained in this manner correlates with stroke volume measured with a flowmeter in dogs; it also correlates with right ventricular stroke volume obtained by measuring left ventricular stroke volume angiographically and assuming equality in the steady state.[9–12] In general, however, these calculations overestimate right ventricular volume by as much as 40%.[12] The overestimation has been related to the failure of the method to allow for the volume displaced by the trabeculae, papillary muscles, and the convex interventricular septum. The error, however, appears to be consistent, and with appropriate correction using derived regression equations, the correlation between angiographically estimated and measured volumes has been good.

While yielding useful angiographic volume data, application of Simpson's rule is cumbersome, requiring some form of correction to convert measured to true volumes as well as a computer for calculation.

Application of Simpson's rule to echocardiographic images is further complicated by the need to identify two appropriate orthogonal views of the right ventricle with a common long axis. The right ventricular long axis can be readily defined from the apical four-chamber view; however, a second orthogonal plane with a common long axis is difficult to record. The parasternal long axis view would be a potential orthogonal imaging plane,

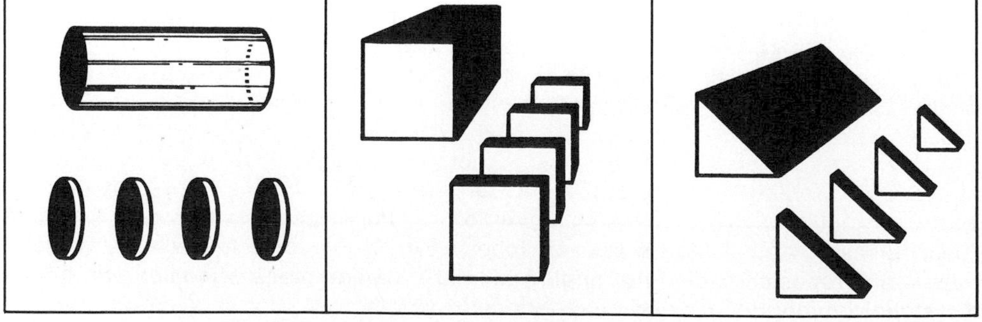

Fig. 28–6. Simpson's rule method of volume calculation, in which the volume of a larger figure is determined from the sum of the volumes of a series of comparable smaller figures. (From Rogers EW, Feigenbaum H, Weyman AE: Echocardiography for quantitation of cardiac chambers. *In* Yu PN, Goodwin JF (eds.): Progress in Cardiology. Philadelphia, Lea & Febiger, 1979.)

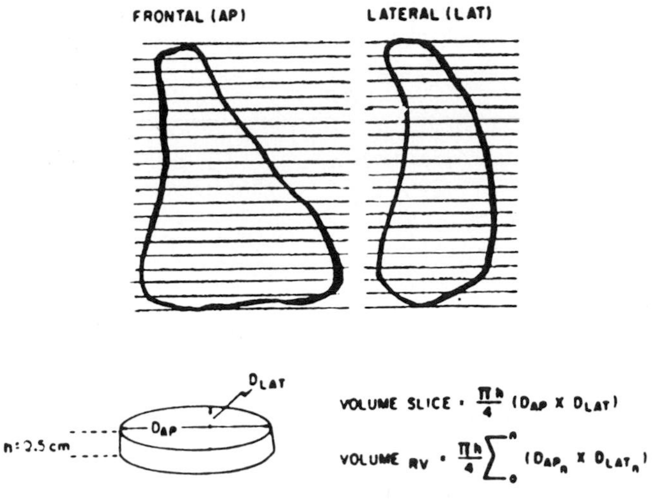

Fig. 28–7. Simpson's rule reconstruction of the right ventricular volume from the frontal (AP) and lateral (LAT) angiographic projections. (From Gentzler RD, Briselli MF, Gault JH: Angiographic estimation of right ventricular volume in man. Circulation 50:324, 1974. Reproduced by permission of the American Heart Association, Inc.)

however, visualization of the apex is rarely possible from this view. The subcostal four-chamber view is almost parallel rather than perpendicular. The parasternal short axis view is orthogonal, but the common axis with the apical-four chamber view is a short axis. One novel approach has been to record an apical long axis view of the right ventricle, (the right ventricular apical two-chamber view), which although difficult to obtain and standardize, does contain diameters that are orthogonal about the right ventricular long axis. Unfortunately, any volumes calculated from an apical four-chamber and right ventricular apical two-chamber view will fail to include the infundibulum. Theoretically, the combinations of apical four-chamber long axis dimensions and multiple parasternal short axis areas could be used to calculate right ventricular volume, as is done for the left ventricle. However, the asymmetry and lack of appropriate internal landmarks make it a practical impossibility to obtain multiple short axis slices of the right ventricle at known separations.

Nevertheless, Simpson's rule has been used widely in echocardiographic studies to determine right ventricular volume. Orthogonal views used have included the subcostal four-chamber and the subcostal outflow in a pediatric population;[13] the apical four-chamber and multiple parasternal short axis views;[14] the apical four-chamber and subcostal four-chamber;[15] and the apical four-chamber and a nonstandard two-chamber right ventricular view.[2] Table 28–2 summarizes the results of the echocardiographic studies of right ventricular volumes calculated using the Simpson's rule approach.[13–17] In all of these studies, the echocardiographic analysis underestimated or correlated poorly with right ventricular volume as measured by angiography[2,13,14] or nuclear angiography.[15] This is most likely because of difficulty identifying the true long axis of the right ventricle in two echo views as well as poor endocardial definition and failure to include the infundibulum. Clearly, however, the gold standards are imperfect. Correlation with right ventricular ejection fraction was much better in these studies, as might be expected, because any error in the volume measurements would presumably be systematic (i.e., present in both the diastolic and systolic volumes).

Determination of Right Ventricular Volume Based on Simple Geometric Figures

The complexity and limitations of the Simpson's rule method have led to the evaluation of a series of simpler geometric figures as possible models from which right ventricular volumes could be calculated. Again, this approach is based on angiographic methods that have used the prolate ellipse,[9,18] and the parallelepiped,[18] the prism,[10] and the pyramid with a triangular base,[19] as well as combinations of figures as models from which to calculate right ventricular volume. The volumes of these figures are all given in the form

$$\text{volume} = c \times \text{area}_1 \times \text{length}_2 \qquad [28.4]$$

where c is the appropriate constant, area_1 is the area of any face, and the length_2 is the long axis dimension taken in a plane perpendicular to the area. Applying the area-length method to estimate right ventricular volumes again requires two orthogonal views with a common long axis, whether these are obtained echocardiographically (Table 28–3)[13,15,17,20,22] or angiographically.

Approximation of the Right Ventricle as an Ellipsoid. The ellipsoid figure has been examined as a basis for right ventricular volume calculations in several angiographic studies.[9,18] Volumes are calculated using the

Table 28–2. Biplane: Simpson's Rule

Authors	Study Population	Echo View	Formula	Reference		Results
Saito[8]	31 children (CHD)	SCF/SCL	$V = \frac{\pi h}{3}\left(\sum^{odd} A_iB_i + \sum^{even} \frac{1}{2} A_j B_j\right)$	Angiogram	EDV	r = .85 y = 0.91x + 7.35
Ninomiya[9]	24 children (CHD)	PSA/A4C	" "	Angiogram	EF	r = .98 y = 0.97x + 0.02
Panidis[10]	39 patients (CHD)	A4C/A2C	" "	Radionuclide	EF	r = .78 y = 0.78x + 4.1
		A4C/SC4C	" "		EF	r = .74 y = 0.66x + 6.2
Trowitzseh[11]	19 patients (CHD)	SCLA/SCSA	$V = \frac{L}{20} * \frac{\pi}{4} * \sum_{i=1}^{20} a_i b_i$	Angiogram	EDV ESV EF	r = .65 r = .56 r = .83 y = 0.94x + 4.43

CHD = congenital heart disease; SCF = subcostal frontal view; SCL = subcostal lateral view; PSA = parasternal short axis; A4C = apical four-chamber view; A2C = RV apical two-chamber view; SC4C = subcostal four-chamber view; SCLA = subcostal long axis; SCSA = subcostal short axis; EDV = end-diastolic volume; ESV = end-systolic volume; EF = ejection fraction.

*This modified Simpson's formula approximates the sum of the segmental volumes ($V = \pi(D_1/2)*(D_2/2)*H$). Further modifications of Simpson's rule for the calculation of segmental volume have also been reported but have not been included because their derivation and validation are poorly documented.

Table 28–3. Biplane: Area and Length Method

Authors	Study Population	Echo Views	Geometric Formula	Reference		Results
Saito[13]	31 children (CHD)	SCF/SCL	Ellipsoid $V = \frac{8A_1A_2}{3\pi L}$	Angiogram	EDV	r = .86 y = 1.32x − 7.39
Panidis[15]	39 patients (CHD)	A4C/A2C	Ellipsoid $V = \frac{8A_1A_2}{3\pi L}$	Radionuclide	EF	r = .76 y = 0.71x + 8.2
		A4C/SC4C			EF	r = .76 y = 0.69x + 11.4
Wann[12]	13 patients (CAD, COPD, or CMP)	A4C/PSA	Ellipsoid $V = \frac{4}{3\pi} a \times b \times c$	Radionuclide	EF	r = .84 y = 0.82x + 6.4
Levine[20]	12 human casts	A4C/SCOT	$V = \frac{2}{3} \times A_{(A4C)} \times L_{(SCOT)}$	Cast volume	Volume	r = .95 y = 1.1x − 3.9
			$V = \frac{2}{3} \times A_{(SCOT)} \times L_{(A4C)}$		Volume	r = .95 y = 1.02x − 2.1
Starling[22]	19 patients (COPD)	SC inflow/ SC outflow	Pyramid $V = A\frac{H}{3}$	Radionuclide	EDV	r = .76 y = 1.54x + 21
					ESV	r = .82 y = 1.71x + 10
					EF	r = .83 y = 0.74x + 12
Wann[17]	13 patients (CAD, COPD, or CMP)	A4C/PSA	Pyramid $V = A\frac{H}{3}$	Radionuclide	EF	r = .79 y = 0.69x + 11
			Prism* $V = \frac{h}{2}(AA \times BB)$		EF	r = .62 y = 0.72x + 10

* Although originally described and subsequently referred to as an example of Simpson's rule, the stated formula actually calculates the volume of a prism with a triangular base.

AA = area of the base; BB = height of the base; h = height from the apical 4-chamber view; CHD = congenital heart disease; COPD = chronic obstructive pulmonary disease; CAD = coronary artery disease; CMP = cardiomyopathy; SCF = subcostal frontal view; SCL = subcostal lateral view; SCOT = subcostal right ventricle outflow view; A4C = apical four-chamber view; A2C = right ventricle apical two-chamber view; SC4C = subcostal four-chamber view; PSA = parasternal short axis; EDV = end-diastolic volume; ESV = end-systolic volume; EF = ejection fraction.

formula

$$V = \frac{4}{3}\pi\left(\frac{D_1}{2}\right) \times \left(\frac{D_2}{2}\right) \times \left(\frac{L}{2}\right) \qquad [28.5]$$

where D is

$$\frac{4A}{\pi L_{max}}$$

and where L_{max} equals the longer of the of the two major axes, and where the areas A_1 and A_2 in these studies were derived from the frontal and lateral radiographic projections of right ventricular casts. This approach overestimated measured right ventricular volume; however, in each instance, an excellent correlation with true volumes was obtained, and reasonably accurate estimates of calculated volume were possible after appropriate correction.

To allow for the two-chamber configuration of the right ventricle, a modification of this method has also been examined in which the right ventricular inflow chamber is expressed as an ellipse and the outflow chamber is considered separately as a cylinder.[9] The total right ventricular volume then is the sum of the volume of the outflow chamber (V_o) and the inflow chamber (V_i), where

$$V_o = \pi r_o^2 L \qquad [28.6]$$

and

$$V_i = \frac{4}{3}\pi r_i^2 \frac{LL}{2} \qquad [28.7]$$

This method uses only the lateral angiogram and divides the right ventricle at the level of the superior aspect of the tricuspid valve into inflow and outflow segments. This approach again yielded a good correlation with measured volumes; however, it was associated with a greater percentage error than was the simple area-length method.[9] The additional calculations, therefore, did not appear warranted.

Echocardiographic studies designed to define the optimal relationship between right ventricular area, length, and volume have also revealed that the constant ⅔ provides the optimal correlation with known volume.[20,21] This constant is the same as that for the area-length ellipsoid volume of the left ventricle and supports the concept of modeling the right ventricle as an ellipsoid of revolution. The two orthogonal views used in these validation studies were the apical four-chamber and the intersecting subcostal view of the right ventricular outflow tract (Fig. 28–8). Using the planimetered area from either of these views and the maximal length from the other (Fig. 28–9), volume was calculated using the formula

$$\text{volume} = 2/3 \text{ area} \times \text{length} \qquad [28.8]$$

This simple product of a cross-sectional area and an in-

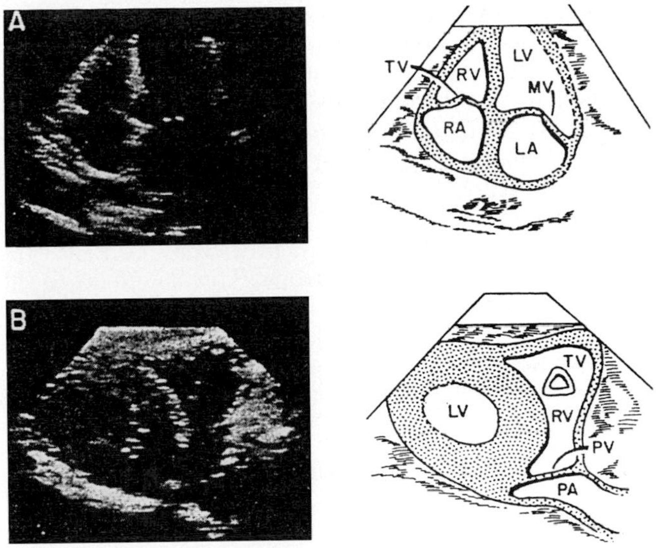

Fig. 28–8. Echocardiographic views comparable to the planes used in vitro in this study. **A.** Apical four-chamber view. **B.** Right ventricular outflow tract. LA = left atrium; LV = left ventricle; MV = mitral valve; PA = pulmonary artery; RA = right atrium; RV = right ventricle; TV = tricuspid valve. (From Levine RA, et al.: Echocardiographic measurement of right ventricular volume. Circulation 69:497, 1984. Reproduced by permission of the American Heart Association, Inc.)

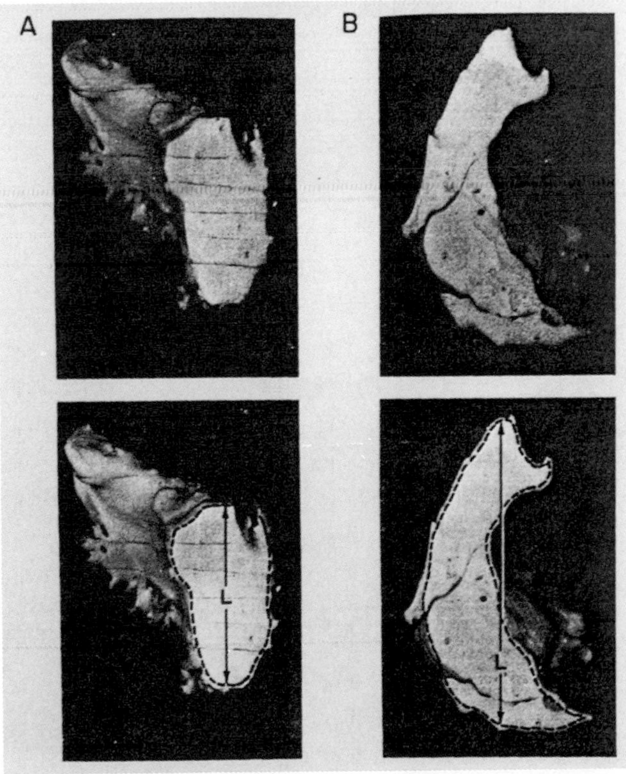

Fig. 28–9. Cut surfaces of the casts illustrating the measurements made in the apical four-chamber **(A)** and right ventricular outflow tract **(B)** views. L = long axis length. (From Levine RA, et al.: Echocardiographic measurement of right ventricular volume. Circulation 69:497, 1984. Reproduced by permission of the American Heart Association, Inc.)

tersecting length yielded a correlation of r = .95 when compared to human right ventricular cast measurements (Fig. 28–10). Besides its simplicity, one of the major advantages of this technique is that it evaluates the infundibular contribution to volume.

Thus, whereas the shape of the right ventricle is clearly not ellipsoid, the ellipsoid formula shifts the outflow tract area/diameter to the middle of the apex to base long axis or vice versa and thereby converts the chamber to a more elliptic shape. This is similar to the manner in which the area-length ellipsoid formula performs in the "worst case" left ventricle (see Fig. 20–22), in which the shape of the chamber is altered by the ellipsoid formula but the relationship of calculated to true

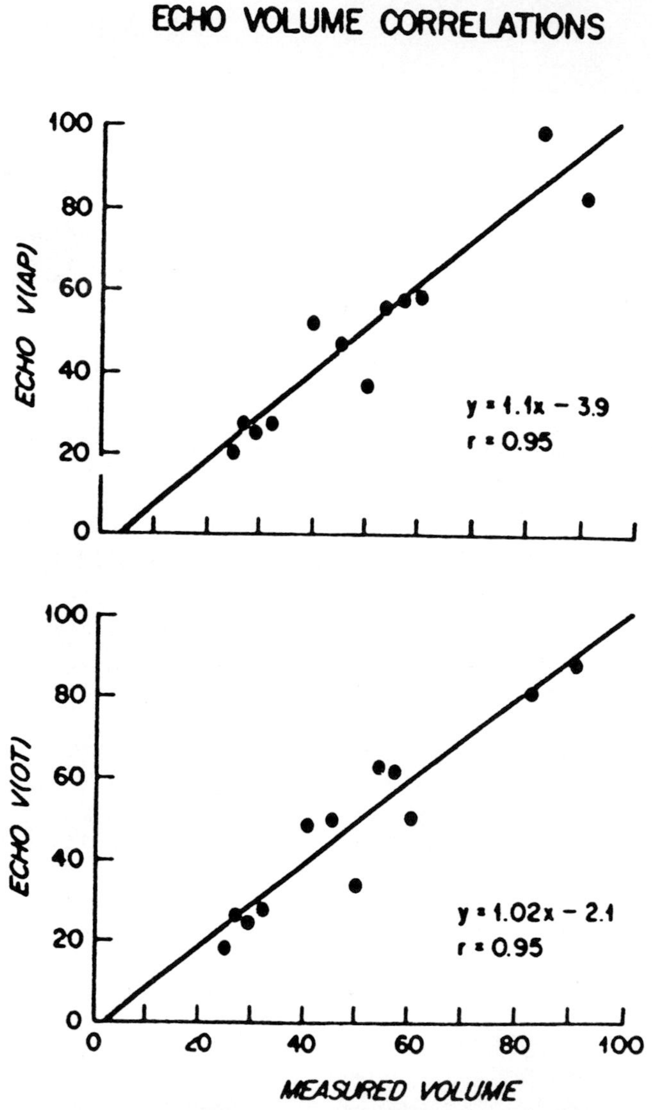

Fig. 28–10. Comparison of volumes calculated from echocardiographic views of latex molds with actual cast volumes, together with the line of regression. The standard error of estimate is 5.2 ml for the overall repeated-measures analysis. V(AP) = the volume calculated from the area in the apical four-chamber view and the length in the outflow tract view; V(OT) = the volume calculated from the area in the outflow tract view and the length in the apical view. (From Levine RA, et al.: Echocardiographic measurement of right ventricular volume. Circulation 69:497, 1984. Reproduced by permission of the American Heart Association, Inc.)

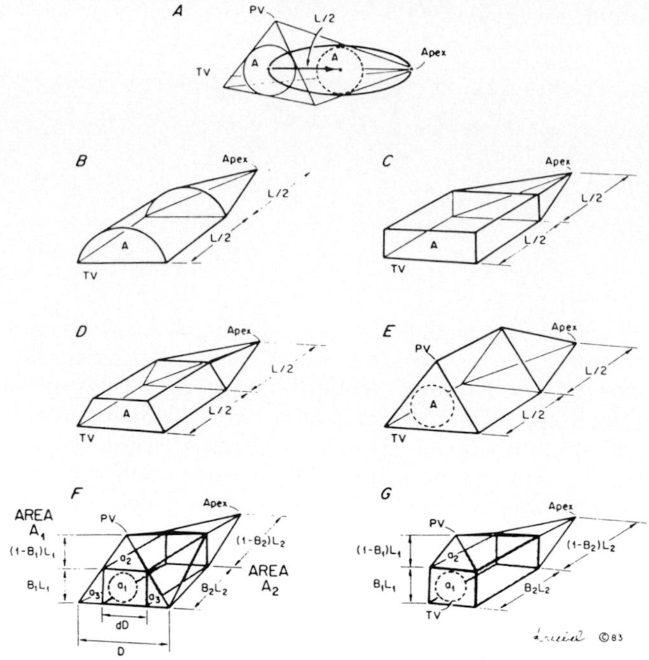

Fig. 28–11. Geometric models with volumes of 2 A L/3. **A.** Prolate ellipsoid constructed by moving the area of the outflow tract back to the center of the right ventricular long axis. **B.** Half-cylindric, half-conical structure. **C** through **E**. Tapering structures with rectangular **(C)**, trapezoidal **(D)**, and triangular **(E)** bases. **F.** Flexible right ventricular model. **G.** Similar model without flanking structures that taper. A = area; a_{1-3} = fractions of area A_1 contributed by different portions of the model; $b_{1,2}$ = fractions of lengths $L_{1,2}$ contributed by the rectangular portion of the model; d = the fraction of width D contributed by the rectangular portion; PV = pulmonic valve; TV = tricuspid valve. (From Levine RA, et al.: Echocardiographic measurement of right ventricular volume. Circulation 69:497, 1984. Reproduced by permission of the American Heart Association, Inc.)

volume appears to remain relatively constant. Figure 28–11 illustrates the various figures that can be constructed using the constant ⅔ and the generic area-length formula.

In a study comparing the echocardiographic area-length (derived from the apical four-chamber and "orthogonal" subcostal views) and Simpson's rule methods of determining ejection fraction to nuclear angiography, both echocardiographic methods had a similar correlation to the first-pass radionuclide ventriculogram. The similarity of these methods was also demonstrated using the apical four-chamber and the nonstandard apical two-chamber view.[15]

Because the right ventricle is obviously not a true ellipse, three other figures have been examined as possible geometric models in angiographic studies because they appeared to correspond more closely to the actual shape of the right ventricle. These figures are illustrated in Figure 28–12.

The Parallelepiped. The first of these figures is the parallelepiped or three-dimensional parallelogram. The volume of this figure is simply expressed by

$$V = \text{length} \times \text{width} \times \text{height} \qquad [28.9]$$

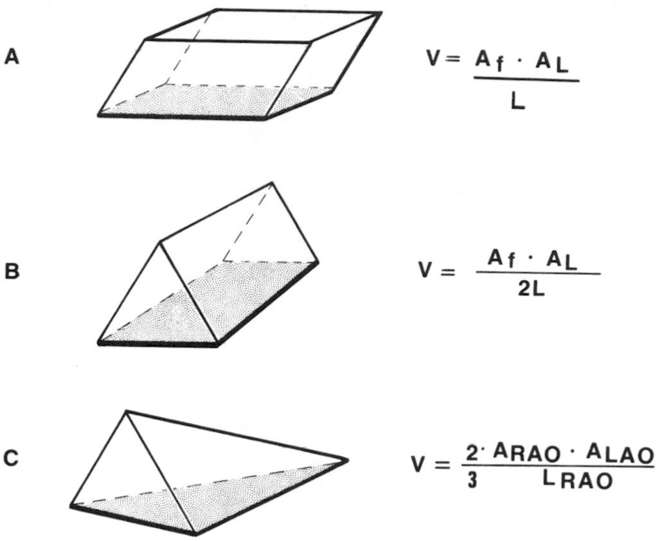

Fig. 28–12. The simple geometric figures that have been used to represent the right ventricle and the formulas for their volumes. **A.** The three-dimensional parallelogram, or the parallelepiped. **B.** The prism. **C.** The pyramid with the triangular base. V = volume; A_f = angiographic area in the frontal projection; A_L = angiographic area in the lateral projection; A_{RAO} = angiographic area in the right anterior oblique projection; A_{LAO} = angiographic area in the left anterior oblique projection. (From Rogers EW, Feigenbaum H, Weyman AE: Echocardiography for quantitation of cardiac chambers. *In* Yu PN, Goodwin JF (eds.): Progress in Cardiology. Philadelphia, Lea & Febiger, 1979.)

When derived from angiographic images, imaginary rectangles are constructed with surface areas identical to those of the ventricular images recorded in the frontal and lateral planes and with lengths equal to a superior-inferior dimension in the lateral plane. The area of the right ventricle can then be equated with length times width in the frontal plane, whereas the height can be determined by dividing the area in the lateral projection by the maximal length. The angiographic volume, therefore, is expressed by

$$V = \frac{\text{area}_{\text{frontal}} \times \text{area}_{\text{lateral}}}{\text{LL}} \qquad [28.10]$$

This method has been used in both in vitro comparisons between right ventricular casts and cast angiograms[18] and in pediatric studies, with good correlations consistently observed.[20] Note that the general form of this figure is similar to all others with the constant in this case being 1. However, in in vitro echocardiographic studies, this constant resulted in values that consistently overestimated measured cast volumes.

The Prism With a Triangular Base. The next figure whose shape has been compared with that of the right ventricle is the prism with a triangular base. The volume of such a prism is expressed as follows:

$$V = \text{area}_{\text{triangle}} \times \text{height}$$

$$V = \frac{\text{L(base)} \times \text{W(base)}}{2} \times \text{H} \qquad [28.11]$$

By assuming that the frontal and lateral angiographic projections form the sides of the triangular prism, the volume can then be calculated from

$$V = \frac{\text{area}_{\text{frontal}} \times \text{area}_{\text{lateral}}}{2\text{L}} \qquad [28.12]$$

This angiographic method, as with the previous figures, correlates well with cast-determined volumes, but this model slightly underestimated the actual measured volume.[14] Using this figure, the constant in the area-length equation would be ½, which in echocardiographic validation studies has likewise been shown to yield volumes consistently below those of cast volumes. In the one echocardiographic study that used this formula, volume was likewise underestimated.[17]

The Pyramid With a Triangular Base. The final figure is the pyramid with the triangular base. In this model, the triangular base is assumed to be formed by the base of the right ventricle (including the right ventricular outflow tract), whereas the long axis or height of the pyramid is the long axis of the right ventricle from the base to the apex. The volume of such a figure is expressed by

$$V = \text{area}_{\text{base}} \times \frac{\text{H}}{3} \qquad [28.13]$$

The base of the pyramid cannot be directly visualized angiographically; however, this value can be calculated from the RAO and LAO projections of the right ventricle and ventricular volume, calculated as

$$V = \frac{2}{3} \times \frac{\text{area}_{\text{RAO}} \times \text{area}_{\text{LAO}}}{\text{L}_{\text{RAO}}} \qquad [28.14]$$

Thus, although the angiographic formula was motivated by the theoretical model of a pyramid of volume ($\frac{1}{3}$ A_1L_2), the actual formula used to fit the data was $V = \frac{2}{3} \times A_1 \times A_2/L$, similar to the constant ⅔ found in echocardiographic studies.

The validity of this angiographic method has also been confirmed in vitro and applied to patients with coronary artery disease. This method has also been adapted to single-plane ventriculograms and, therefore, represents the first method for right ventricular volume calculations that does not require biplane images.[21] By assuming that the area of the LAO projection approximates two thirds of the area in the RAO projection, the formula can be simplified to

$$V = 0.4\,\frac{(\text{area}_{\text{RAO}})^2}{\text{L}_{\text{RAO}}} + 3.9 \qquad [28.15]$$

These single-plane volumes have been shown to correlate well with biplane volumes.

This theoretic formula ($V = \frac{1}{3}\ A_1/L_2$) has been applied in studies comparing echocardiographic volumes (calculated as the product of right ventricular area in the subcostal four-chamber view and the length in the subcostal outflow tract view[5]) to end-diastolic and end-systolic counts and ejection fraction measured from a right ventricular nuclear angiogram in a small group of selected patients with chronic obstructive pulmonary disease. Although reasonable correlations between counts and volume were observed at end-diastole (r = .76) and end-systole (r = .82) as well as for ejection fraction (r = .83), the validity of the constant could not be tested, because actual volumes were not compared.[22]

Determination of Volume as the Difference Between Crescentic Shells Formed by the Septum and Right Ventricular Free Wall

A recent crescentic method modeled the cross-sectional area of the right ventricle using the arcs of two intersecting circles, defined by the right ventricular free wall and the interventricular septum. The width of the crescentic area is defined as the distance between two parallel tangents to these areas. The right ventricular body may then be divided into two parts: the basal portion of length (L_1), where the width of the crescentic area is constant, and the apical portion of length (L_2), where the width decreases progressively toward the apex. The basal volume is obtained by multiplying the crescentic area by the length (L_1). If the ventricular width begins to decrease from the tricuspid annulus, L_1 is taken as zero. The apical volume is obtained by integration of the crescentic area, with the width decreasing progressively along a parabolic line toward the apex (Fig. 28–13). The sum of these two volumes provides the right ventricular body volume. A good correlation has been demonstrated between this method and the measured volumes of casts of canine hearts; however, the method ignored the infundibulum, and as a result underestimated the measured volume by 25%. In addition, as should be apparent from Figure 28–1, separation of the tapering from the nontapering portion of the right ventricle is not always trivial; the crescent model has not been validated in the volume- or pressure-loaded chamber where the septum may be deviated to the left; the short axis plane, which is the basis of the model, is standardized with reference to the left and not the right ventricle; the calculations are complex; and the results suggest little improvement over the methods previously described.[23]

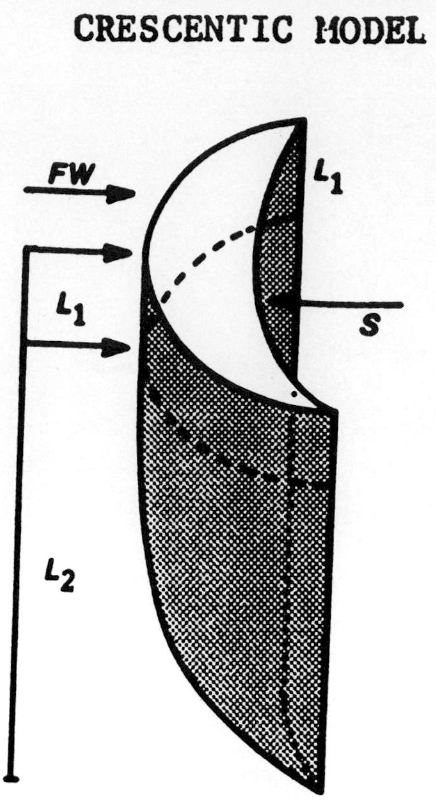

Fig. 28–13. The method for calculating the volume of the right ventricle from the crescent-shaped figure where the base is assumed to have a constant shape and the apical segment to taper in a parabolic fashion. L_1 = length from base to onset of tapering portion; L_2 = length from the onset of the tapering portion of the ventricle to the apex; S = septum; FW = free wall. (From Aebischer NM, Czegledy F: Determination of right ventricular volume by two-dimensional echocardiography with a crescentic model. J Am Soc Echocardiogr 2:110, 1989.)

To date, none of the echocardiographic methods described here have undergone extensive clinical validation. The multiplicity of methods reflects the fact that none is perfect and that all are cumbersome and subject to significant operator error because of the difficulty in obtaining appropriate views and in tracing the endocardium. Injection of agitated saline has been used to improve endocardial definition and may also be helpful in the measurement of right ventricular areas by digital subtraction.[17,24]

Three-Dimensional Reconstruction of Right Ventricular Volumes

Three-dimensional reconstruction, by providing the correct spatial relationship of individual two-dimensional images from different tomographic views, can eliminate the need for geometric assumptions and can provide more reliable volume measures. The precise spatial location of imaging planes can be determined by spark gap, electromagnetic, or mechanical positioning devices. Using a specially designed transducer-locating system and multiple, nonparallel two-dimensional echocardiographic images, three-dimensional reconstructions of the right ventricle were successfully generated in an in vitro study.[25] Right ventricular volume calculation was performed by remapping traced endocardial contours into a set of border points on a series of equally spaced parallel planes and by integrating all the area estimations. The correlation with reference volumes was excellent both for animal ventricles, with volumes ranging from 30 to 166 ml ($r = .98$), $y = 1.35\times - 20$, standard error of estimation [SEE] = 8.7) and for human ventricles, with volumes ranging from 5 to 166 ml ($r = .97$, $y = 0.88\times + 0.42$, SEE = 1.2).

We have recently developed a fully integrated system for three-dimensional reconstruction, which automatically integrates images and positional data in real time. Volume is automatically calculated from traced endocardial contours using an expanding spheroid to define the ventricular surface; the total volume is equal to the sum of the volume of trapezoid segments defined by

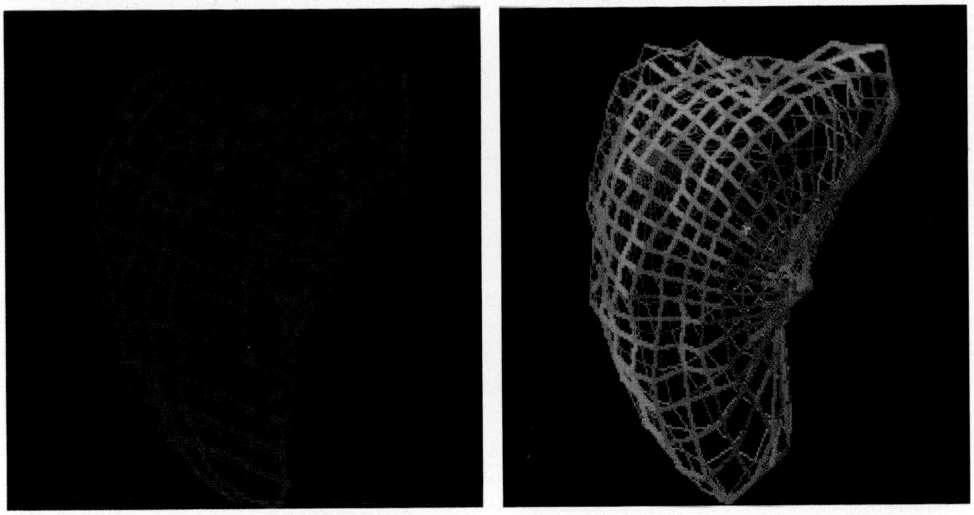

Fig. 28–14. Left. Wire-frame diagram of the right ventricle assembled from random spatially oriented images of a human right ventricular cast in short and long axis. Right. Expanding spheroid model has been fitted to the raw data and volume calculated automatically.

equally spaced radii emanating from the center of the sphere. A preliminary in vitro study demonstrated that this algorithm can successfully describe the shape of the right ventricle (Fig. 28–14). In these studies, a strong linear correlation was demonstrated ($r = .99$, $y = 1.05\times - 1.9$, SEE = 3.0) between volumes calculated using the three-dimensional echocardiographic technique and the volume measured by water displacement of human right ventricular agarose casts, with volumes ranging from 18 to 74 ml (Fig. 28–15). Subsequent in vivo studies have demonstrated similar accuracy for end-diastolic, end-systolic, and stroke volumes in the canine model. Further improvements in equipment, processing, and design should permit accurate noninvasive three-dimensional reconstruction of right ventricular volume in the clinical setting.

To summarize the approach to assessing the size of the right ventricle, in the average study, visual inspection or measurement of single plane indices should suffice. However, the major goal is to develop a reproducible area or dimension that will allow for inter- or intracase comparison. To measure the volume or ejection fraction, an area-length method or Simpson's rule approach is needed. Simpson's rule assumes an elliptic symmetry present in the left ventricle but not in the right ventricle. Application of the area-length method to the subcostal outflow tract and apical four-chamber views is by far the most practical approach. Three-dimensional imaging promises to be the most accurate method for volume calculation and in the future should be the standard for research and many clinical applications.

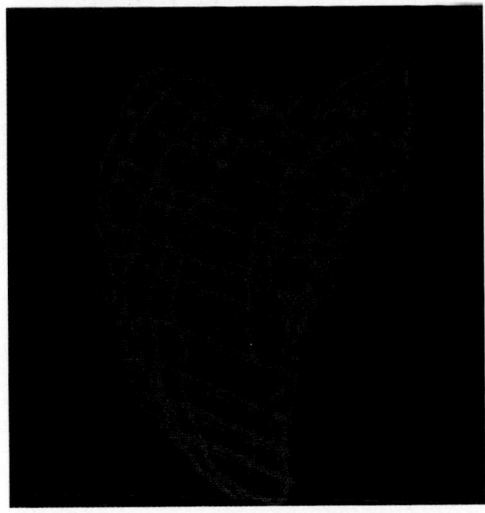

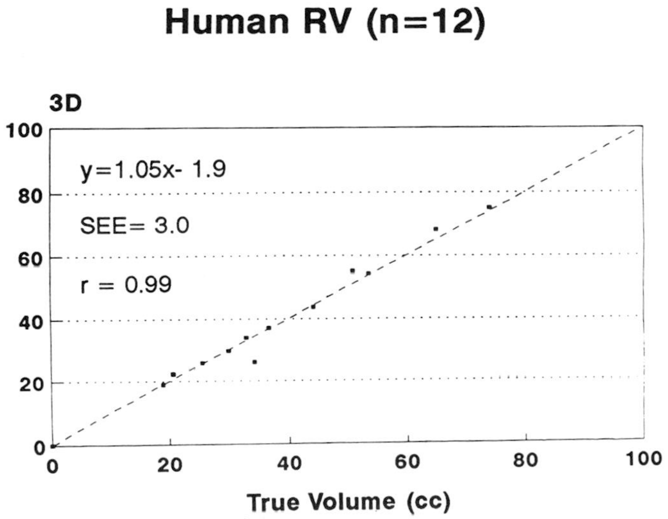

Fig. 28–15. The correlation between measured and three-dimensionally reconstructed volumes of a human right ventricular cast (RV). SEE = standard error of estimate.

RIGHT VENTRICULAR VOLUME OVERLOAD

The lesions associated with right ventricular volume overload include the regurgitant lesions of tricuspid and pulmonary insufficiency as well as shunt lesions including atrial septal defect (ASD), partial or total anomalous pulmonary venous connection, the far less common ventricular septal defect with left ventricular-to-right atrial shunting, and sinus of Valsalva rupture or coronary artery fistula communication with the right atrium or ventricle. Ventricular septal defect without ventriculoatrial communication is not typically a cause of right ventricular volume overload.[10]

Right ventricular volume overload can alter both the size and the shape of the right ventricle. Figure 28–16 is an example of a massively dilated right ventricle recorded in both parasternal long and short axis projections during diastole and systole. In the long axis, the dilated ventricle expands in both an anteroposterior and superior-inferior direction. The right ventricular apex is distal to the left ventricular apex, and the right ventricular cavity is much larger than the left. In short axis, the right ventricle is no longer crescent shaped but appears more oval. During diastole, the interventricular septum is displaced toward the left ventricular cavity, further smoothing the posterior surface of the ventricle. With systolic contraction, however, the increase in left ventricular systolic pressure pushes the septum in toward the right ventricle and makes the left ventricle more circular.[26] While the primary sign of right ventricular vol-

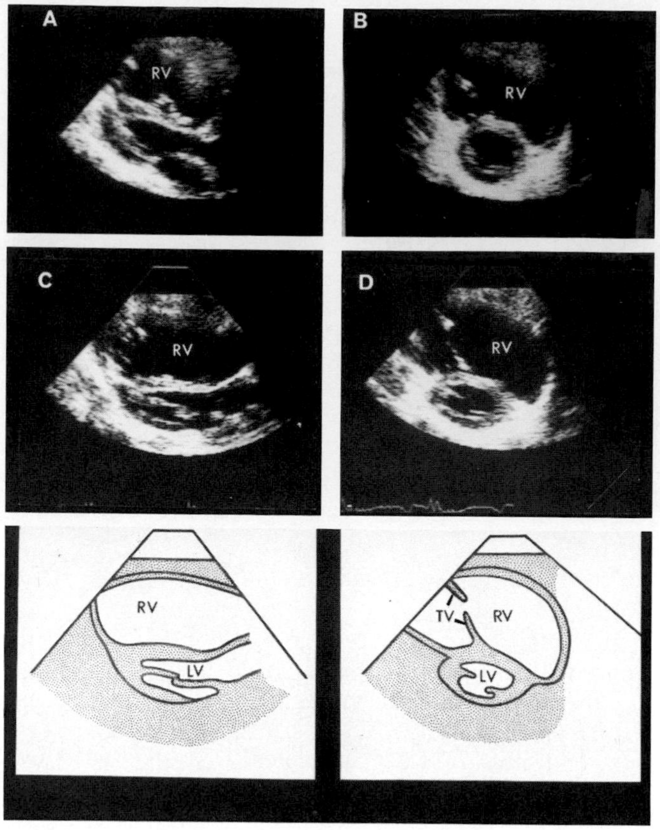

Fig. 28–16. Parasternal long and short axis recordings of the right ventricle (RV) illustrate right ventricular volume overload. In the long axis projection, the ventricle is expanded in both the anteroposterior and the apex-to-base dimensions. The right ventricle occupies the cardiac apex, and the left ventricle (LV) and the interventricular septum are displaced posteriorly. In the short axis view, the right ventricle is enlarged and rotated in a clockwise direction above the left ventricle. During diastole (**C** and **D**), the interventricular septum is displaced posteriorly, and the left ventricle is flattened in its short axis configuration. During systole (**A** and **B**), the septum shifts anteriorly or paradoxically, and the ventricle becomes more circular. The diagrams at the bottom of the figure correspond to the diastolic frames, **C** and **D**.

ume overload is obviously an enlarged right ventricle, diastolic septal flattening is also an important echocardiographic feature.[27–29] This sign has also been shown to occur in normal subjects during the Mueller maneuver, which causes a transient increase in right ventricular volume.[30]

RIGHT VENTRICULAR HYPERTROPHY

The right ventricle may hypertrophy in a variety of conditions that increase the chamber's afterload. Such conditions include valvular, infundibular, and supravalvular pulmonary stenosis; tetralogy of Fallot and longstanding pulmonary hypertension, which may be primary or secondary to left ventricular dysfunction; mitral stenosis; veno-occlusive disease; chronic pulmonary emboli; or Eisenmenger's physiology. Right ventricular hypertrophy is generally assessed by measuring the thickness of the free wall. Although the interventricular septum may also hypertrophy with right ventricular pressure overload, the septum is primarily a functional component of the left ventricle. Septal hypertrophy is more commonly associated with disorders of the left ventricle or may exhibit independent hypertrophy, such as in idiopathic hypertrophic subaortic stenosis. This makes it of minimal value as a predictor of right ventricular wall thickness.

Although the right ventricular free wall may be viewed in many projections, it probably is best recorded from the parasternal long axis position. This orientation places the endocardial and epicardial surfaces in the near field, perpendicular to the beam axis, and should provide the best resolution. Because the right ventricle lies immediately beneath the anterior chest wall, precise near-gain adjustment is necessary to separate this structure from the highly reflective chest wall. An alternative view is the subcostal long axis, in which a wide extent of the diaphragmatic right ventricular wall is available for examination. This view may be particularly useful in infants and children with congenital heart disease because this region of the heart is more accessible.

Normal right ventricular wall thickness has been shown to be 2.4 ± 0.5 mm in a group of 25 normal subjects.[31] Because of the vagaries of this measurement, an end-diastolic wall thickness of less than 5 mm is considered to be normal. Good correlation exists between measurement of right ventricular wall thickness by echo and postmortem study.[32] M-mode measurements have a sensitivity of 93% and a specificity of 95% for detecting right ventricular hypertrophy when compared to autopsy data.[32] Echocardiographic measurements of right ventricular free wall thickness have been shown to be superior to electrocardiographic diagnosis of right ventricular hypertrophy in several studies.[32,33] However, the correlation between right ventricular free wall thickness and right ventricular mass is only moderate in postmortem studies.[34] Some have suggested that this is because the right ventricle increases its mass by dilating rather than by developing an increased thickness of the wall.[34,35] Others have suggested that the unavoidable inclusion of epicardial fat in the weight makes the mass measurement less accurate.[36] It should be noted that right ventricular hypertension that is present at birth results in right ventricular hypertrophy without significant right ventricular enlargement. On the other hand, right ventricular hypertension acquired after the involution of the right ventricle results in a chamber enlargement as well as hypertrophy of the walls.

The degree of right ventricular hypertrophy correlated to the pulmonary artery pressure (r = .75) in one study. This improved slightly by correcting the wall thickness measurement for body surface area (r = .85).[31] In another study of patients with chronic lung disease, the correlation was poorer, but adequate echoes were not obtained for all patients.[37]

It should be kept in mind that not all increases in right ventricular wall thickness are the response to an increased pressure load. Infiltrative diseases such as amyloid and hypertrophic cardiomyopathy involving the

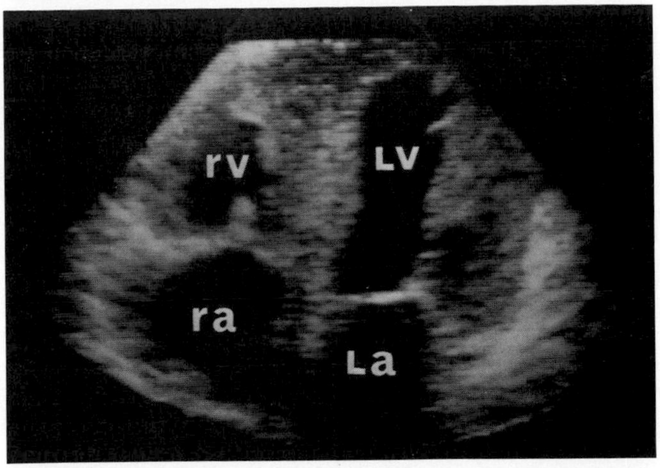

Fig. 28–17. Apical four-chamber recording illustrates diffuse cardiac infiltration and right ventricular hypertrophy in a patient with hereditary amyloidosis. rv = right ventricle; ra = right atrium; Lv = left ventricle; La= left atrium.

right ventricle may result in marked increases in free wall thickness.[38,39] Figure 28–17 is a recording from a patient with hereditary amyloidosis and diffuse infiltration of the myocardium and the cardiac valvular tissue. There is an increase in both right and left ventricular wall thickness as well as thickening of the atrial walls and interatrial septum. Endocardial fibroelastosis of the right ventricle simulating right ventricular hypertrophy has also been described.[40]

CHRONIC RIGHT VENTRICULAR PRESSURE OVERLOAD

Right ventricular hypertrophy is not the only echocardiographic sign of right ventricular pressure overload. Dilation of the right ventricle occurs primarily in acquired pressure overload. As tricuspid regurgitation ensues, the added volume overload may cause marked right ventricular enlargement. Even in the absence of tricuspid or pulmonic regurgitation, however, the right ventricular volume may increase. As the right ventricular pressure overload takes its toll on the chamber, right ventricular failure ensues. In this case, hypokinesis of the free wall will be a sign of severe pressure overload.[41]

Interventricular Septal Motion

Abnormal interventricular septal motion can be used to distinguish right ventricular volume overload from pressure overload. Although the interventricular septum is thought of primarily as a functional component of the left ventricle, the motion of the septum is influenced by several factors. The state of the musculature contraction is a primary determinant. Contraction of the septum between its fixed insertion points tends to straighten the septum in systole. The opposing factor, the pressure gradient between the ventricles, normally tends to push the septum rightward and reverse the tendency toward flattening. In the normal heart where the systolic pressure gradient strongly favors the left ventricle, the left ventricle is a nearly perfect circle.[27] During diastole, there is also a normal positive gradient from the left to right ventricle, maintaining an approximately circular shape of the left ventricle. A decrease or reversal of either of these gradients, however, will alter the position of the septum and the shape of the two chambers during the period when the gradient change is present. Thus an increase in right ventricular diastolic pressure (RV > LV) will shift the septum to the left and cause the right ventricle to become more circular. A decrease or reversal of the systolic gradient will have the same effect during this period of the cardiac cycle. A combination of a right ventricular pressure and volume overload will result in an abnormal septal position during both diastole and systole, with instantaneous changes in position reflecting simultaneous fluctuations in the gradient (see Chapter 29 for additional discussion).[42,43]

ACUTE RIGHT VENTRICULAR PRESSURE OVERLOAD

Pulmonary embolism is, by far, the most common cause of acute right ventricular pressure overload. An embolus obstructing 25% of the pulmonary vasculature causes elevated pressures. However, any acute pulmonary process with hypoxia may cause a rise in pulmonary artery pressures. This can occasionally lead to overt right heart failure, usually in the setting of chronic right ventricular pressure overload. A previously normal right ventricle can only generate peak systolic pressures of roughly 40 mm Hg before it begins to fail.[44] The physiologic responses to increased pulmonary pressures are easily detected by echocardiography. The signs include right ventricular dilation and subsequent development of tricuspid regurgitation. Hypokinesis develops as right ventricular failure ensues. The right atrium, inferior vena cava, and pulmonary artery may also dilate. Thrombus or filling defects in the main pulmonary artery or its branches by contrast echocardiography have been reported.[45] Marked systolic and diastolic flattening of the interventricular septum will be evident.[46] A decrease in left ventricular size may also occur, resulting in an increased right ventricle/left ventricle ratio. All of these findings have been reported to be reversed after successful thrombolysis[41] or in follow-up after recovery from the acute event.[46] Decreased pulmonary artery pressures may be documented by a decrease in the tricuspid regurgitation jet velocity, if it is indeed still present after recovery.[41,46]

RIGHT VENTRICULAR INFARCTION

Right ventricular infarction has now been recognized as a distinct clinical entity, although in the past, controversy existed regarding the right ventricle's contribution to overall cardiac function.[47] Right ventricular infarction presents with systemic hypotension, which may progress to cardiogenic shock, elevated jugular venous pressure, and clear lung fields. It occurs almost exclusively in the setting of inferior myocardial infarction. Hemodynamic criteria required for the diagnosis include a mean right atrial pressure >10 mm Hg. A ratio of mean right atrial pressure to pulmonary capillary wedge pressure of >0.8 is also diagnostic, as long as the pulmonary capillary wedge pressure is >15 mm Hg.[47]

Estimates of the incidence of right ventricular involvement in an inferior infarction vary depending on the criteria used to establish the diagnosis. The classic clinical presentation represents an extreme in the spectrum from subtle right ventricular involvement without significant hemodynamic alteration to severe dysfunction. Autopsy series have demonstrated pathologic evidence of right ventricular involvement 24%[48] to 90%[49] of inferior left ventricular infarctions. Clinical recognition of the syndrome of right ventricular infarction occurs far less frequently, being reported in as few as 3% of acute inferior infarctions.[50] Echocardiographic recognition of right ventricular infarction occurs with an intermediate frequency that ranges in different studies from 20%[51] to 50%.[52]

Unlike the left ventricle, however, where the walls contract symmetrically toward the center of mass, the irregularity and asymmetry of right ventricular geometry together with the reduced amplitude of normal contraction (relative to the left ventricle) make the determination of minor changes in local contraction (hypokinesis) more difficult. Therefore, many studies require definite akinesis or dyskinesis to make the diagnosis of right ventricular infarction.[52–54] Once identified, the region and extent of dysfunction must be expressed in some formal construct. Figure 28–18 illustrate one such system.

Right ventricular akinesis is an extremely sensitive indicator of right ventricular infarction, and wall motion abnormalities have been demonstrated in practically all

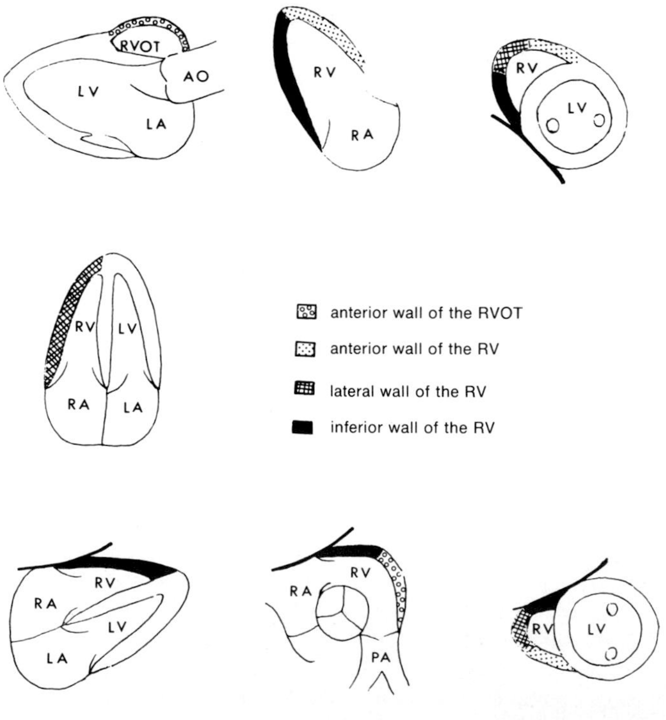

Fig. 28–18. Segmental system for localizing and quantitating regional right ventricular asynergy. RV = right ventricle; RVOT = right ventricular outflow tract; AO = aorta; LA = left atrium; LV = left ventricle; PA = pulmonary artery.

patients with clinical[53,54] or hemodynamic[55] evidence of right ventricular infarction. In the only study comparing hemodynamic criteria and echocardiography for the diagnosis of right ventricular infarction, the sensitivity and specificity of echocardiography was found to be 82% and 62%, respectively. The same study found the sensitivity of nuclear ventriculography to be 92% and the specificity 82%, compared to hemodynamic measurements.[52] Hemodynamic criteria also identified many patients as abnormal without the clinically recognizable syndrome of right ventricular infarction. It has been shown that there is a correlation between the degree of echocardiographic right ventricular involvement (as measured by the number of involved segments) and the presence of hemodynamic abnormalities.[54] When compared to nuclear ventriculography, the sensitivity-specificity of echocardiography has been found to be 82% and 93%[56] in one study and 92% and 79% in another.[57] The specificity is less than the sensitivity because wall motion abnormalities are frequently identified in patients with acute inferior infarction without other evidence of right ventricular involvement.[52,55] These abnormalities, however, are uncommon in patients with anterior infarctions or in normal control subjects.[58]

The demonstration of free wall asynergy in patients without hemodynamic criteria of right ventricular infarction represents a degree of right ventricular involvement that is not extensive enough to produce functional alteration. The extent of involvement necessary to produce clinically significant dysfunction has not been established. Some cases of right ventricular asynergy may represent myocardial stunning rather than completed infarction, although this is controversial.

The right coronary artery is the primary coronary supply to the right ventricle. The left anterior descending the conus branch may supply a small portion of the right anterior free wall.[47] Small segmental wall motion abnormalities of the anterior right ventricular wall or distal right ventricular apex have been described in anterior left ventricular infarctions.[49,54] However, the right ventricular diaphragmatic wall is the most commonly involved[48,53,59] and is associated with infarction of the inferior septum in most cases.[44] Involvement may extend to the lateral and anterior free walls of the right ventricle. Figure 28–19 is an apical four-chamber recording of both the right and left ventricular apices in a patient with a large anterior wall infarction.

Right ventricular hypertrophy may predispose patients to infarction in the setting of decreased perfusion. An association between right ventricular hypertrophy and infarction has been demonstrated,[60,61] although this has been disputed.[48] Chronic obstructive pulmonary disease has been shown to be more common in patients who develop right ventricular involvement with inferior infarcts.[36] Presumably, this is on the basis of the associated right ventricular hypertrophy.

Beside abnormal wall motion, other echocardiographic signs associated with right ventricular infarction are less specific because they occur in many other disease states. Right ventricular dilation is a common finding in most[53,55,59] but not all studies.[57] Dilation of the chamber and papillary muscle dysfunction lead to tricus-

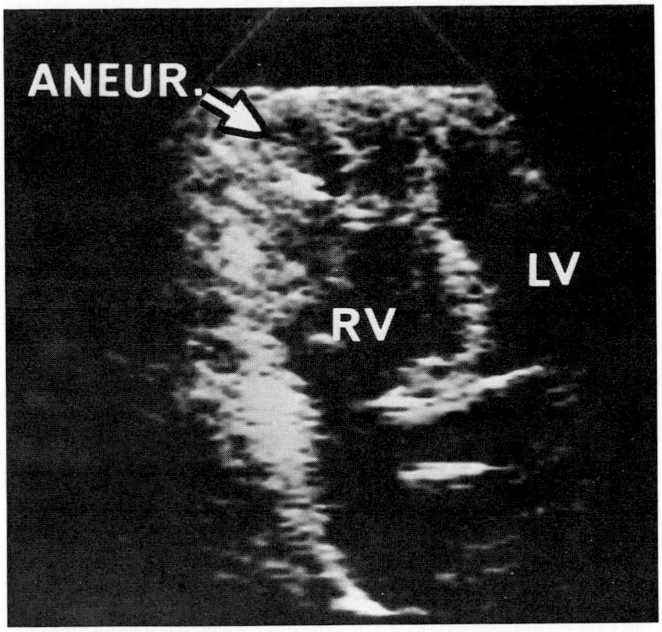

Fig. 28–19. Apical four-chamber recording illustrates aneurysmal dilation of the right ventricular apex in a patient with a large anteroapical left ventricular myocardial infarct and clinical evidence of associated right ventricular infarction. During the real time study, the right ventricular apex and anterior wall were dyskinetic. ANEUR. = aneurysm; RV = right ventricle; LV = left ventricle.

pid regurgitation, which frequently accompanies right ventricular infarction.[53,59] This may in turn lead to paradoxic septal motion, another common finding.[54,62] In an animal model that produced right ventricular free wall infarction in closed chest dogs, paradoxic septal motion was shown to occur in the absence of tricuspid insufficiency.[63] Although the right ventricular end-diastolic pressure changed only slightly, the gradient between the left and right ventricles at end-diastole shifted from a slightly positive to a slightly negative value. These investigators postulate that the systolic motion of the septum toward the dyskinetic free wall "provided mechanical assistance" to right ventricular ejection.[63] Septal infarction and the associated dyskinesis may also contribute to the appearance of paradoxic septal motion in some patients.[62]

Echocardiography plays an important role in the diagnosis of the complications of acute infarctions that involve the right ventricle. Ventricular septal rupture after inferior myocardial infarction has a higher mortality if extensive right ventricular involvement is identified echocardiographically at the onset of rupture (Fig. 28–20).[64] Complete heart block is more likely to complicate inferior infarcts involving the right ventricle.[47] Placement of a temporary pacemaker at the right ventricular apex may be problematic when this area is infarcted. Puncture of the right ventricle by the pacing wire and resultant tamponade have been easily diagnosed by echocardiography[65,66] (see Fig. 36–75). Right ventricular thrombi have been demonstrated in some patients with infarction.[48] These thrombi may calcify and appear as highly reflective echo-dense masses at the right ventricular apex.[67] The true incidence of right-sided thrombi is unknown. One echocardiographic study showed a remarkable 41% incidence of right ventricular thrombi in right-sided infarction. Sixty percent of these patients had evidence of pulmonary embolus.[59] The finding of left ventricular thrombus in 35% of these patients with inferior infarctions is much higher than in other studies.[68] Remember, however, that unless the right ventricle is completely visualized from several planes, apical thrombus will be missed. Doppler studies have replaced contrast in identifying tricuspid regurgitation after right ventricular infarction. By transesophageal echocardiography, right-to-left shunting through a patent foramen ovale, the result of an elevated end-diastolic pressure secondary to right ventricular dysfunction, may also be demonstrated, and occlusion by a balloon catheter may be confirmed.[69]

Chronic Ischemia

Substantial recovery of right ventricular wall motion abnormalities has been shown in some[56] but not all[59] studies of survivors of right ventricular infarction. Similarly, right ventricular asynergy, dilation, and decreased ejection fraction are more common in survivors of inferior compared to anterior infarctions.[51,58] As expected, right ventricular function at rest is normal in patients

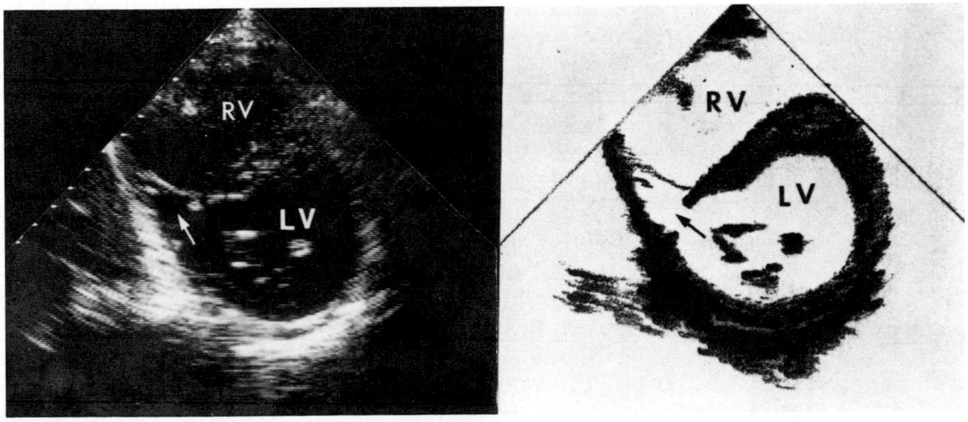

Fig. 28–20. Parasternal short axis recording of the right and left ventricles illustrating a ventricular septal defect in a patient with inferoposterior left ventricular myocardial infarction and associated right ventricular infarction. RV = right ventricle; LV = left ventricle.

without previous infarction who have significant right coronary artery obstructions.[51]

Given the circulatory supply to the right ventricle, isolated ischemia of the right ventricle is rare. However, spasm of the right coronary artery involving right ventricular branches has been shown to occur.[70] In occasional patients, thallium exercise testing may miss isolated right ventricular ischemia that can be documented by exercise echocardiographic testing.[70,71] It has been suggested that evaluation for right ventricular ischemia be undertaken in patients with a typical exertional or Prinzemetal's anginal syndrome if initial evaluation of the left ventricle is normal. It has also been shown that thrombolysis may, on occasion, dramatically improve right ventricular function without a change in left ventricular performance.[72]

RIGHT VENTRICULAR DYSPLASIA

Arrhythmogenic right ventricular dysplasia is a relatively rare cardiac disorder that can have a variety of clinical and pathologic presentations. The primary pathophysiologic process involves the replacement of the right ventricular myocardium by adipose or collagenous tissue.[73,74] The myocardium may be affected focally or diffusely throughout the right ventricular free wall. The wall may be of normal thickness if adipose deposition predominates, or it may be markedly thinned. The affected patients present with recurrent ventricular tachycardia. The cause is unknown. Familial occurrences of the disease have been reported,[75–77] but it is frequently sporadic. Uhl's anomaly, or parchment right ventricle, has been considered to be the extreme manifestation of this entity. Recent observations suggest that the myocardial atrophy may not be due to abnormal embryogenesis, and the term right ventricular cardiomyopathy has been suggested. Its association with sudden death in young people is well recognized. The clinical diagnosis of this disorder is usually based on the documentation of recurrent right ventricular tachycardia in association with verification of right ventricular morphologic changes.

In infancy, the condition presents with severe right-sided heart failure. This presentation is less common in adults but can occur.[78] Recurrent ventricular tachycardia, usually with a left bundle branch block pattern, most often brings the adolescent or adult patients to medical attention. Less frequently, an asymptomatic increase in the cardiac silhouette may be noted on chest radiograph.[78,79] The association between sudden death in young people and dilated right ventricular cardiomyopathy has recently been recognized.[80]

Echocardiography plays an important role in the diagnosis both by demonstrating the features of arrhythmogenic right ventricular dysplasia and by eliminating other causes of right ventricular enlargement. Echocardiographic criteria for the diagnosis include right ventricular enlargement and either diffuse or focal asynergy of the ventricular free wall. As previously noted, the free wall may be normal or thinned. Localized outpouchings or aneurysms have been considered to be a hallmark of the disease (Fig. 28–21) but are not present in every

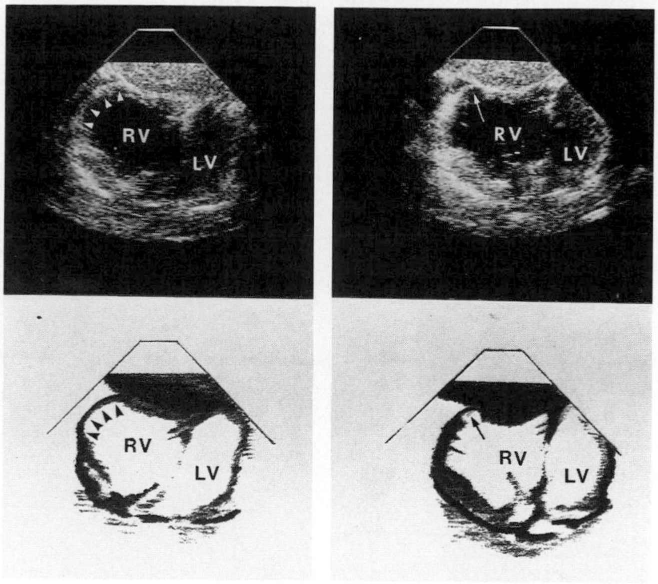

Fig. 28–21. Subcostal four-chamber recording. Left. An area of focal aneurysm dilation and akinesis of the right ventricular free wall (arrowheads) characteristic of right ventricular dysplasia. Right. Arrow indicates a small secondary aneurysm superimposed on the larger region of dysfunction. RV = right ventricle; LV = left ventricle.

patient.[81] They occur most commonly in the anterior infundibular and basal inferior walls and the apex.[78] Structural changes of the moderator band and trabecular disarrangement are also noted.[82,83] The echocardiogram has been demonstrated to be completely normal in some patients who subsequently develop the disease.[84] In addition, right ventricular abnormalities may progress over time.[85]

Until recently, angiography has been the mainstay of diagnosis, but it is often not definitive. Deep fissuring of the free wall and slow dye evaluation from the right ventricle are neither sensitive nor specific.[86] All of the angiographic findings have been demonstrated in normal patients.[87] Considerable subjectivity has been noted in the visual assessment of right ventricular changes by angiography,[87] making comparison of sensitivity and specificity with echocardiography difficult in this rare disease. Several studies have demonstrated agreement between echocardiography and angiography in detecting the presence of ventricular enlargement, localized involvement, and hypokinesis. However, there was a lack of uniform concordance in the location of the lesions.[81] In one small study in which right ventricular dysplasia was diagnosed by angiography, echocardiography failed to show diffuse or segmental abnormalities in all patients. The sensitivity of the echocardiogram was 80%, but the specificity was 100%.[79]

In the absence of clearly defined right ventricular structural and functional abnormalities, arrhythmogenic right ventricular dysplasia is primarily a diagnosis of exclusion. Biopsy can be extremely dangerous because of the thinned and abnormal wall. Echocardiography is used to distinguish this disease from the other causes of right ventricular enlargement. These include Ebstein's anomaly, atrial septal defect, partial anomalous venous return and right-sided valvular lesions. Congenital partial absence of the left pericardium may cause apparent right ventricular enlargement,[88] and the rarer absence of the right pericardium may simulate right ventricular outpouchings.[89] This is a difficult lesion to exclude using any technique. Right ventricular infarction is a potentially confounding diagnosis. In arrhythmogenic right ventricular dysplasia, however, the left ventricle has been found to be normal by most[90] but not all[91] groups, while segmental left ventricular asynergy will almost always be present in the setting of right ventricular infarction.

RIGHT VENTRICULAR MASSES

Differential diagnosis of masses involving the right ventricle includes primary and metastatic tumors, thrombi, vegetations, and artifacts. Routine exams must be specifically directed to include optimal views of the entire right ventricle, or important lesions may be missed. Heavy trabeculations, the moderator band, and prominent muscle bundles or redundant papillary muscles may also be confused for pathologic lesions.

Right ventricular tumors are uncommon, and echocardiographic experience is, therefore, limited. The most commonly observed right ventricular tumor appears to be the myxoma.[92,93] Rhabdomyoma involves the right ventricle more frequently than the left and is usually associated with tuberous sclerosis.[94,95] Metastatic tumors, particularly melanoma, have been reported.[92,96] Tumors may cause right ventricular failure as a result of cavity obliteration,[92,97] may involve the tricuspid valve to restrict its motion,[92] or may prolapse into the right ventricular outflow tract, causing outflow obstruction.[98,99] The right ventricle may be enlarged with paradoxic septal motion. Echocardiography is superior to angiography in defining the points of attachment of the tumor and its intramyocardial extent,[92,100] often rendering angiography unnecessary before surgery.[93,101]

Thrombi involving the right ventricular cavity may be present in congestive cardiomyopathy, Löffler's endocarditis, and right ventricular infarction. In addition, emboli originating in the systemic venous system may become trapped in the right heart. Right atrial thrombi that prolapse into the right ventricle and right ventricular thrombi detected in cases of recurrent pulmonary embolism have been reported.[67,102,103]

Right ventricular vegetations are extremely rare but have been reported in association with tricuspid valve endocarditis, infected pacemakers, or catheters and ventricular septal defects.[104]

RIGHT VENTRICULAR BIOPSY

Percutaneous biopsy of the right ventricle has proven useful in several conditions and has become particularly important in the management of cardiac transplantation.[105] Echocardiography has been used to direct the bioptome forceps and to minimize complications.[106] Visualization of the forceps can be accomplished in most patients from the apical four-chamber view. The subcostal view may also be useful. The bioptome forceps can be seen crossing the tricuspid valve and directed to minimize trauma to the valvular apparatus. In addition, the forceps can be directed to different portions of the right ventricle and can allow for the sampling of many more sites than is possible with fluoroscopy. Multiple samples are extremely important in the diagnosis of rejection post-transplantation.[105] In some centers, biopsies are performed with echocardiographic guidance alone. In the largest published series of 910 biopsies done in 58 cardiac transplant patients, there was a total complication rate of 0.2% with a mean of 5 to 6 samples removed at each biopsy.[107] Sampling of the free wall was routinely accomplished without perforation of the right ventricle. In addition, echocardiography allows avoidance of inadvertent biopsy of the moderator band, which may decrease the incidence of arrhythmias.[107]

REFERENCES

1. Bommer W, et al.: Determination of right atrial and right ventricular size by two-dimensional echocardiography. Circulation 60:91, 1979.
2. Watanabe T, et al.: Estimation of right ventricular volume with two-dimensional echocardiography. Am J Cardiol 49:1946, 1982.
3. Hiraishi S, et al.: Two-dimensional echocardiographic assessment of right ventricular volume in children with congenital heart disease. Am J Cardiol 50:1368, 1982.
4. Silverman NH, et al.: Determination of left ventricular volume in children: echocardiographic and angiographic comparisons. Circulation 62:548, 1980.
5. Kaul S, Tei C, Hopkins JM, Shah PM: Assessment of right ventricular function using two-dimensional echocardiography. Am Heart J 107:526, 1984.
6. Feigenbaum H: Echocardiography. 4th Ed. Philadelphia, Lea & Febiger, p. 158, 1986.
7. Goerke RJ, Carlsson E: Calculation of right and left ventricular volumes; method using standard computer equipment and biplane angiograms. Invest Radiol 2:360, 1967.
8. Mullins CB, Jones DC, Freeborn WA: Comparison of models for measurement of right ventricular volume (abstr.). Clin Res 18:321, 1970.
9. Graham TP, Jarmakani JW, Atwood GF, Canent RV: Right ventricular volume determinations in children. Circulation 47:144, 1973.
10. Fisher EA, DuBrow IW, Hastreiter AR: Right ventricular volume in congenital heart disease. Am J Cardiol 36:67, 1975.
11. Mullins CB, Knapp RS: Three cineangiographic models for measurement of right ventricular stroke volume (abstr.). Clin Res 19:330, 1971.
12. Gentzler ED, Briselli MF, Gault JH: Angiographic estimation of right ventricular volume in man. Circulation 50:324, 1974.
13. Saito A, Ueda K, Nakano H: Right ventricular volume determinations by two-dimensional echocardiography. J Cardiogr 11:1159, 1981.
14. Ninomiya K, et al.: Right ventricular ejection fraction and volumes after Mustart repair: correlation of two-dimensional echocardiograms and cineangiograms. Am J Cardiol 48:317, 1981.
15. Panidis IP, et al.: Two dimensional echocardiographic estimation of right ventricular ejection fraction in patients with coronary artery disease. J Am Coll Cardiol 2:911, 1983.
16. Trowitzsch E, Colan SD, Sanders SP: Two-dimensional echocardiographic estimation of right ventricular area change and ejection fraction in infants with systemic right ventricle (transposition of the great arteries or hypoplastic left heart syndrome). Am J Cardiol 55:1153, 1985.
17. Wann LS, Stickels KR, Bamrah VS, Gross CM: Distal processing of contrast echocardiograms: a new technique for measuring right ventricular ejection fraction. Am J Cardiol 53:1164, 1984.
18. Arcilla RA, Tsai P, Thilenius OG, Ranniger K: Angiographic method for volume estimation of right and left ventricles. Chest 60:446, 1971.
19. Ferlinz J, Gorlin R, Cohn PF, Herman MV: Right ventricular performance in patients with coronary artery disease. Circulation 52:608, 1975.
20. Levine RA, et al.: Echocardiographic measurement of right ventricular volume. Circulation 69:497, 1984.
21. Gibson TC, et al.: Methods for estimating right ventricular volume by planes applicable to cross-sectional echocardiography: correlation with angiographic formulas. Am J Cardiol 55:1584, 1985.
22. Starling MR, Crawford MH, Sorensen SG, O'Rourke RA: A new two-dimensional echocardiographic technique for evaluating right ventricular size and performance in patients with obstructive lung disease. Circulation 66:612, 1982.
23. Aebischer NM, Czegledy F: Determination of right ventricular volume

by two-dimensional echocardiography with a crescentic model. J Am Soc Echocardiogr 2:110, 1989.

24. Lange PE, et al.: Value of image enhancement—injection of contrast medium for right ventricular volume determination by two-dimensional echocardiography in congenital heart disease. Am J Cardiol 55:152, 1985.
25. Linker DT, Moritz WE, Pearlman AS: A new three-dimensional echocardiographic method of right ventricular volume measurement. In vitro validation. J Am Coll Cardiol 8:101, 1986.
26. Weyman AE, Wann LS, Feigenbaum H, Dillon JC: Mechanism of abnormal septal motion in patients with right ventricular volume overload. Circulation 54:179, 1976.
27. Ryan T, et al.: An echocardiographic index for separation of right ventricular volume and pressure overload. J Am Coll Cardiol 5:918, 1985.
28. King ME, et al.: Interventricular septal configuration as a predictor of right ventricular systolic hypertension in children: a cross-sectional echocardiographic study. Circulation 68:68, 1983.
29. Feneley M, Garagham T: Paradoxical and pseudoparadoxical interventricular septal motion in patients with right ventricular volume overload. Circulation 74:230, 1986.
30. Brinker JA, et al.: Leftward septal displacement during right ventricular loading in man. Circulation 61:626, 1980.
31. Tsuda T, et al.: Echocardiographic measurement of right ventricular wall thickness in adults by anterior approach. Br Heart J 44:55, 1980.
32. Prakash R: Determination of right ventricular wall thickness in systole and diastole. Br Heart J 40:1257, 1978.
33. Cacho A, Prakash R, Sarma R, Kaushik VS: Usefulness of two-dimensional echocardiography in diagnosing right ventricular hypertrophy. Chest 84:154, 1983.
34. Baker BJ, Scovil JA, Kane JJ, Murphy MG: Echocardiographic detection of right ventricular hypertrophy. Am Heart J 105:611, 1983.
35. Devereux RB, Gottlieb GJ, Alonso DR: Echocardiographic detection of right ventricular hypertrophy (abstr.). Circulation 62 (Suppl. 3):33, 1980.
36. Kopelman HA, et al.: Right ventricular myocardial infarction in patients with chronic lung disease: possible role of right ventricular hypertrophy. J Am Coll Cardiol 5:1302, 1985.
37. Weitzenblum E, Moyses B, Dickele M, Methlin G: Detection of right ventricular pressure overloading by thallium-201 myocardial scintigraphy. Chest 85:164, 1984.
38. Child JS, Krivokapich J, Abbasi AS: Increased right ventricular wall thickness on echocardiography in amyloid infiltrative cardiomyopathy. Am J Cardiol 44:1391, 1979.
39. Falk RH, et al.: Sensitivity and specificity of the echocardiographic features of cardiac amyloidosis. Am J Cardiol 59:418, 1987.
40. Larson JE, et al.: Isolated endocardial fibroelastosis of the right ventricle associated with pulmonary hypertension. Am Heart J 107:1286, 1984.
41. Come PC, et al.: Early reversal of right ventricular dysfunction in patients with acute pulmonary embolism after treatment with intravenous tissue plasminogen activator. J Am Coll Cardiol 10:971, 1987.
42. Krayenbuehl HP, Turina J, Hess O: Left ventricular function in chronic pulmonary hypertension. Am J Cardiol 41:1150, 1978.
43. Stool EW, Mullins CB, Leshin SJ, Mitchell JH: Dimensional changes of the left ventricle during acute pulmonary arterial hypertension in dogs. Am J Cardiol 33:868, 1974.
44. Braunwald E: Heart Disease. 3rd Ed. Philadelphia, WB Saunders, p. 1579, 1988.
45. Kasper W, et al.: Echocardiographic findings in patients with proved pulmonary embolism. Am Heart J 112:1284, 1986.
46. Jardin F, et al.: Quantitative two-dimensional echocardiography in massive pulmonary embolism: emphasis on ventricular interdependence and leftward septal displacement. J Am Coll Cardiol 10:1201, 1987.
47. Wilson BC, Cohn JN: Right ventricular infarction: clinical and pathophysiologic considerations. Adv Intern Med 33:295, 1988.
48. Isner JM, Roberts WC: Right ventricular infarction complicating left ventricular infarction secondary to coronary heart disease. Am J Cardiol 42: 885, 1978.
49. Anderson HR, Falk E, Nielsen D: Right ventricular infarction: frequency, size and topography in coronary heart disease. J Am Coll Cardiol 10:1223, 1987.
50. Lorell B, et al.: Right ventricular infarction. Am J Cardiol 43:465, 1979.
51. Panidis IP, et al.: Right ventricular function in coronary artery disease as assessed by two-dimensional echocardiography. Am Heart J 107:1187, 1984.
52. Dell-Italia LJ, et al.: Right ventricular infarction: identification by hemodynamic measurements before and after volume loading and correlation with noninvasive techniques. J Am Coll Cardiol 4:931, 1984.
53. D'Arcy B, Nanda NC: Two-dimensional echocardiographic features of right ventricular infarction. Circulation 65:167, 1982.
54. Lopez-Sendon J, et al.: Segmental right ventricular function after acute myocardial infarction: two-dimensional echocardiographic study in 63 patients. Am J Cardiol 51:390, 1983.
55. Baigrie RS, et al.: The spectrum of right ventricular involvement in inferior wall myocardial infarction: a clinical, hemodynamic and noninvasive study. J Am Coll Cardiol 1:1396, 1983.
56. Bellamy GR, et al.: Value of two-dimensional echocardiography, electrocardiography and clinical signs in detecting right ventricular infarction. Am Heart J 112:304, 1986.
57. Arditti A, et al.: Right ventricular dysfunction in acute inferoposterior myocardial infarction. Chest 87:307, 1985.
58. Kaul S, Hopkins JM, Shah PM: Chronic effects of myocardial infarction on right ventricular function: a noninvasive assessment. J Am Coll Cardiol 2:607, 1983.
59. Jugdutt BI, Sussex BA, Sivaram CA, Rossall RE: Right ventricular infarction: two-dimensional echocardiographic evaluation. Am Heart J 107:505, 1984.
60. Forman MB, et al.: Right ventricular hypertrophy is an important determinant of right ventricular infarction complicating acute inferior left ventricular infarction. J Am Coll Cardiol 10:1180, 1987.
61. Horan LG, Flowers NC, Havelda CJ: Relation between right ventricular mass and cavity size: an analysis of 1500 human hearts. Circulation 64: 135, 1981.
62. Mikell FL, Asinger RW, Hodges M: Functional consequences of interventricular septal involvement in right ventricular infarction: echocardiographic, clinical and hemodynamic observations. Am Heart J 105:393, 1983.
63. Sharkey SW, et al.: M-mode and two-dimensional echocardiographic analysis of the septum in experimental right ventricular infarction: correlation with hemodynamic alterations. Am Heart J 110:1210, 1985.
64. Moore CA, et al.: Postinfarction ventricular septal rupture: the importance of location of infarction and right ventricular function in determining survival. Circulation 74:45, 1986.
65. Owensby DA: Corticosteroid therapy and late right ventricular rupture after temporary pacing. Am J Cardiol 58:558, 1986.
66. Gondi B, Nanda N: Real-time, two-dimensional echocardiographic features of pacemaker perforation. Circulation 64:97, 1981.
67. Patel AK, et al.: Multiple calcified thrombi (Rocks) in the right ventricle. J Am Coll Cardiol 2:1224, 1983.
68. Asinger RW, Mikell FL, Elsperger J, Hodges M: Incidence of left ventricular thrombis after acute transmural myocardial infarction. N Engl J Med 305:297, 1981.
69. Gudipati CV, et al.: Transesophageal echocardiographic guidance for balloon catheter occlusion of patent foramen ovale complication right ventricular infarction. Am Heart J 121:919, 1991.
70. Parodi O, et al.: Transient right ventricular ischemia caused by coronary vasospasm. Circulation 70:170, 1984.
71. Maurer G, Nanda NC: Two-dimensional echocardiographic evaluation of exercise induced left and right ventricular asynergy: correlation with thallium scanning. Am J Cardiol 48:720, 1981.
72. Schuler G, et al.: Effect of successful thrombolytic therapy on right ventricular function in acute inferior wall myocardial infarction. Am J Cardiol 54: 951, 1984.
73. Maron BJ: Right ventricular cardiomyopathy: another cause of sudden death in the young. N Engl J Med 318:178, 1988.
74. Fitchett D, Sugrue DD, MacArthur CG, Oakley CM: Right ventricular dilated cardiomyopathy. Br Heart J 51:25, 1984.
75. Hoback J, et al.: A report of Uhl's disease in identical adult twins. Chest 79:306, 1981.
76. Diggelmann U, Baur HR: Familial Uhl's anomaly in the adult. Am J Cardiol 53:1402, 1984.
77. Nava A, et al.: A polymorphic form of familial arrhythmogenic right ventricular dysplasia. Am J Cardiol 59:1405, 1987.
78. Marcus FI, et al.: Right ventricular dysplasia: a report of 24 adult cases. Circulation 65:384, 1982.
79. Manyari DE, et al.: Usefulness of noninvasive studies for diagnosis of right ventricular dysplasia. Am J Cardiol 57:1147, 1986.
80. Theine G, et al.: Right ventricular cardiomyopathy and sudden death in young people. N Engl J Med 318:129, 1988.
81. Robertson JH, et al.: Comparison of two-dimensional echocardiographic and angiographic findings in arrhythmogenic right ventricular dysplasia. Am J Cardiol 55:1506, 1985.
82. Jiang L, Zhu HJ, Shi YF. The morphological features of arrhythmogenic right ventricular dysplasia in echocardiograms. Chinese Circulation 6:191, 1991.
83. Kisslo J: Two-dimensional echocardiography in arrhythmogenic right ventricular dysplasia. Eur Heart J 10(Suppl. D):22, 1989.
84. Bewick DJ, Chandler BM, Montague TJ: Dilated right ventricular cardiomyopathy: Uhl's disease. Chest 90:300, 1986.
85. Higuchi S, et al.: Sixteen-year follow-up of arrhythmogenic right ventricular dysplasia. Am Heart J 108:1363, 1984.
86. Daubert C, et al.: Critical analysis of cineangiographic criteria for diagnosis of arrhythmogenic right ventricular dysplasia. Am Heart J 115:448, 1988.
87. Blomstrom-Undqvist C, et al.: Cardioangiographic findings in patients with arrhythmogenic right ventricular dysplasia. Br Heart J 59:556, 1988.
88. Nicolosi GL, et al.: M-mode and two-dimensional echocardiography in congenital absence of the pericardium. Chest 81:610, 1982.
89. Minocha G, Falicov RE, Nijensohn E: Partial right-sided congenital pericardial defect with herniation of right atrium and right ventricle. Chest 76: 484, 1979.

90. Rossi P, Massumi A, Gillette P, Hall RJ: Arrhythmogenic right ventricular dysplasia: clinical features, diagnostic techniques and current management. Am Heart J 103:415, 1982.
91. Manyari DE, et al.: Arrhythmogenic right ventricular dysplasia: a generalized cardiomyopathy? Circulation 68:251, 1983.
92. Ports TA, Schiller NB, Strunk BL: Echocardiography of right ventricular tumors. Circulation 56:439, 1977.
93. Viswanathan B, Luber JM, Bell-Thomson J: Right ventricular myxoma. Ann Thorac Surg 39:280, 1985.
94. Farooki ZQ, Henry JG, Arciniegas E, Green E: Ultrasonic pattern of ventricular rhabdomyoma in two infarcts. Am J Cardiol 34:842, 1974.
95. Gutierrez deLoma J, et al.: Rhabdomyoma of the heart. J Cardiovasc Surg 23:149, 1982.
96. Kutalek SP, et al.: Metastatic tumors of the heart detected by two-dimensional echocardiography. Am Heart J 109:343, 1985.
97. Allen HD, et al.: Echocardiographic demonstration of a right ventricular tumor in a neonate. J Pediatr 84:854, 1974.
98. Roelandt J, et al.: Ultrasonic demonstration of right ventricular myxoma. J Clin Ultrasound 5:191, 1977.
99. Nanda NC, et al.: Echocardiographic features of right ventricular outflow tumor prolapsing into the pulmonary artery. Am J Cardiol 40:272, 1977.
100. Stern MJ, Cohen MV, Fish B, Rosenthal R: Clinical presentation and noninvasive diagnosis of right heart masses. Br Heart J 46:552, 1981.
101. Chia BL, Lim CH, Sheaves JH, Choo MH: Echocardiographic findings in right ventricular myxoma. Am J Cardiol 58:663, 1986.
102. Ouyang P, et al.: Intracavitary thrombi in the right heart associated with multiple pulmonary emboli. Chest 84:296, 1983.
103. Cameron J, et al.: Right heart thrombus: recognition, diagnosis and management. J Am Coll Cardiol 5:1239, 1985.
104. Agathangelon NE, DosSantos LA, Lewis BS: Real-time two-dimensional echocardiographic imaging of right-sided cardiac vegetations in ventricular septal defect. Am J Cardiol 52:420, 1983.
105. Fowles RE, Mason JW: Role of cardiac biopsy in the diagnosis and management of cardiac disease. Prog Cardiol Dis 27:153, 1984.
106. Williams GA, et al.: Clinical experience with two-dimensional echocardiography to guide endomyocardial biopsy. Clin Cardiol 8:137, 1985.
107. Miller LW, et al.: Echocardiography-guided endomyocardial biopsy. Circulation 78(Suppl. 3)III-99, 1988.

CHAPTER

29

INTERATRIAL AND INTERVENTRICULAR SEPTA

PIETER M. K. VANDERVOORT and ARTHUR E. WEYMAN

The interatrial and ventricular septa partition the fetal atrioventricular canal and thereby provide the framework for the separation of the pulmonary and systemic circulations in the fully developed heart.[1,2] In addition, these membranes form a significant portion of the muscular walls of the atria and ventricles and contribute to their contractile function. Normally, the septa appear to favor, both geometrically and functionally, the left-sided cardiac chambers, which bear the major workload of the heart. A variety of disorders, however, alter the configuration, motion, and structural integrity of the septa. These abnormalities form the basis of this chapter.

Before discussing the septa individually, it is important to note that each of these membranes is situated between dynamic chambers in which intracavitary pressures and volumes are continuously changing.[3] The observed shape and movement of the respective septa, therefore, depend on the relative magnitude and timing of events acting on their opposite surfaces.[4,5] In addition, loss of structural integrity of a part of one septum may affect the shape and movement of the other,[6] whereas more complex lesions may involve both.[7] Therefore, although the shape, motion, and integrity of both the interatrial and interventricular septa are considered separately, all of these factors are of necessity interrelated.

THE INTERATRIAL SEPTUM

Anatomy

Anatomically, the interatrial septum is a thin muscular membrane that separates the right and left atrial chambers.[1,2] It stretches from the posteromedial margin of the aortic root posteriorly and slightly rightward to the common posterior atrial wall and from the midportion of the superior atrial border to its junction with the upper margin of the interventricular septum. An oval depression in the midportion of the septum, the fossa ovalis, corresponds to the position of the foramen ovale in the fetal heart.[1,2]

Development

Embryologically, the interatrial septum develops in several stages (Fig. 29–1). Initially, an anteroposterior partition, the septum primum, grows downward from the superior border of the primitive common atrial chamber and divides the chamber into right and left halves (Fig. 29–1A).[1] Before its lower end reaches the anterior and posterior endocardial cushions, which have already fused and divide the common primitive atrioventricular canal into the mitral and tricuspid orifices, its connection with the superior margin of the atrium is severed (Fig. 29–1B). Consequently, the superior border of the septum primum is free. A second partition, the septum secundum, then grows downward from the atrial roof to the right of the septum primum until their edges overlap.[1,2] These overlapping membranes form a flap valve between the two atria (Fig. 29–1C). Before birth, right atrial pressure exceeds left atrial pressure, thereby holding this valve open and permitting blood flow from right to left. After birth, with the establishment of the normal pulmonary circulation, the pressure gradient between the right and left atria is reversed, closing the flap valve. When closed, the free edge of the septum

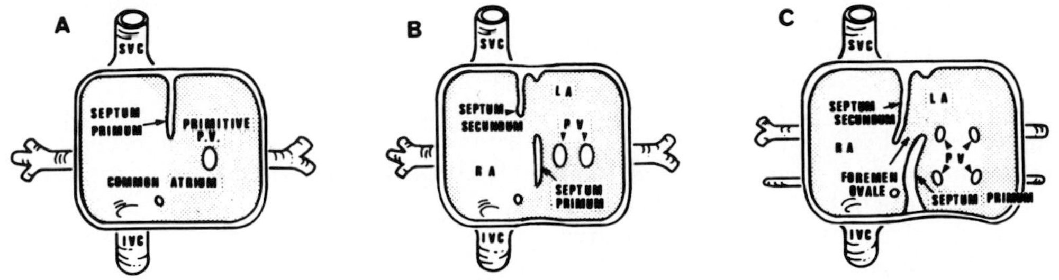

Fig. 29–1. The development of the interatrial septum. **A.** The primitive septum primum initially grows downward from the superior border of the common atrium. **B.** Before reaching the floor of the atrium, the septum primum separates from its original point of attachment to the atrial roof. A second membrane, the septum secundum, then grows downward from the superior border of the atrium to the right of the septum primum. **C.** In the fetal heart, the free edge of the septum secundum overlaps the superior border of the septum primum, thereby forming a flap valve, the foramen ovale, which permits blood flow from the right to the left atrium. SVC = superior vena cava; IVC = inferior vena cava; LA = left atrium; PV = pulmonary vein.

secundum becomes the crescentic upper margin of the foramen ovale. In about 75% of individuals, the opposed surfaces of the two septa fuse.[1] In the remaining 25%, the opposed surfaces fail to fuse; as a result, the foramen is patent anatomically but closed physiologically. In these situations, should right atrial hypertension develop, the flap valve will reopen and physiologic right-to-left shunting will occur.

Examining Planes

Transthoracic Echocardiography

Using standard transthoracic echocardiography, the interatrial septum can be visualized using four principal views. These views include (1) a parasternal short axis view at the aortic level (Fig. 29–2A);[8,9] (2) the apical four-chamber view (Fig. 29–2B);[10,11] (3) a subcostal long axis view optimized to the interatrial septum (Fig. 29–2C);[12,13] and (4) a right parasternal long axis view of the interatrial septum (Fig. 29–2D).[4,5]

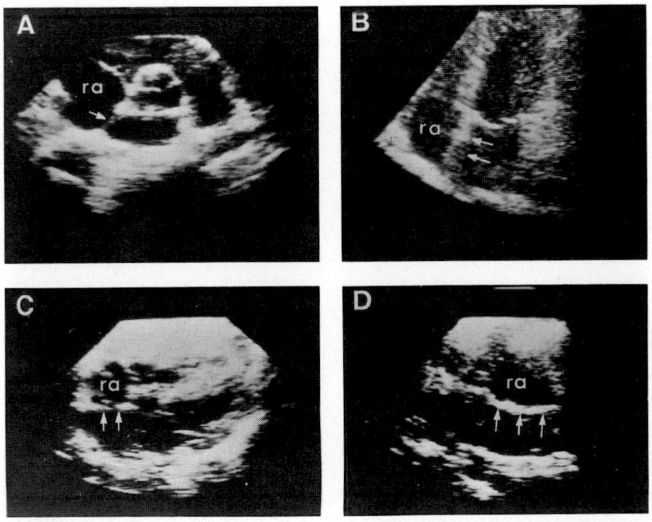

Fig. 29–2. Primary examining planes used in recording the interatrial septum. In each case, the position of the interatrial septum is indicated by the arrows. **A.** The parasternal short axis view at the aortic valve level. **B.** The apical four-chamber view. **C.** The subcostal long axis view optimized to the interatrial septum. **D.** The right parasternal long axis of the interatrial septum. ra = right atrium.

In the parasternal short axis view, the imaging plane transects the interatrial septum from its anterior insertion into the aortic root to its posterior junction with the common atrial wall. The y axis of the imaging plane is perpendicular to the superior-inferior or long axis of the septum. Figure 29–2A illustrates the appearance of the interatrial septum in this orientation. The septum normally arises from the posterior aortic wall at approximately the 7-o'clock position. It then courses vertically (posteriorly) and slightly rightward through a gradual arc curving away from the left atrium. It usually joins the posterior atrial wall at a point almost directly beneath the medial margin of the aorta. Success in recording the atrial septum in this plane has varied from 83[8] to 90%.[9] Because the path of the ultrasonic beam is normally parallel to the plane of the septum, echo "dropout" in the midportion of the septum occurs frequently and was noted in 50% of normal patients in one study.[9]

This problem can be partially alleviated by shifting the transducer leftward on the chest and angling the imaging plane back toward the septum. This change in transducer position frequently shifts the orientation of the scan plane sufficiently to permit complete septal recording. This view is primarily important for recording the relative anteroposterior and medial-lateral orientation of the septum and for defining the changes in septal orientation that occur in the presence of right and left atrial volume overloads. Septal defects can also be recorded; however, the high incidence of false-positives makes other views preferable for that purpose.

The apical four-chamber view is probably the most useful plane for imaging the interatrial septum in the adult. In this orientation, the imaging plane transects the septum from its inferior junction with the interventricular septum to its superior border. Figure 29–2B illustrates the configuration of the septum in this view. Normally, the atrial septum is not a straight-line extension of the interventricular septum but is displaced slightly toward the left atrium.[11] This view is ideal for determining the relative sizes of the atria and also for permitting visualization of septal defects.[10,11,14] Unfortunately, the path of the imaging plane in the four-chamber view is also parallel to the interatrial septum and makes complete recording difficult.[11,12] In addition, when this plane is angled posteriorly, echo dropout is commonly noted in the region of the fossa ovalis.[11] Anterior plane angulation more frequently results in complete septal visualization without thinning or dropout; however, this plane orientation bypasses the location of the typical ostium secundum defect. Thus, both false-positive and false-negative atrial septal defects can be produced using this view, and septal echo dropout as an isolated finding must be interpreted with caution.

The subcostal long axis is theoretically the ideal view for recording the interatrial septum.[12,13,15] In this orientation, the septum is perpendicular to the path of the scan plane and can be visualized throughout its superior-inferior extent (see Fig. 29–2C). Using this view, the interatrial septum was adequately displayed in one study in 87 of 88 infants with a variety of congenital disorders,[13] whereas in a second study, satisfactory imaging was obtained in each of 118 consecutive infants and children.[12] In adults, the subcostal long axis view is more difficult to obtain because of the distance of the interatrial septum from the transducer face. In a large group consisting predominantly of adults with a mean age of 31 years (ranging from 2 months to 74 years), satisfactory images of the interatrial septum could be obtained in 154 of 163 patients studied.[15] When the septum can be recorded from this transducer location, it should be considered the optimal plane for evaluating its structural integrity.

An additional plane has been described and has proved useful for evaluating interatrial septal motion.[4,5] This plane, which is termed here the right parasternal long axis of the interatrial septum (see Fig. 29–2D), is recorded with the transducer located to the right of the sternum in the third, fourth, or fifth intercostal spaces. The x axis of the imaging plane then appears to be aligned parallel to the superior-inferior axis of the interatrial septum, and the plane is then angled sharply to the left until it passes through the septum from right to left atria. This orientation should result in the imaging plane transecting the anterior third of the septum along a line running from the interventricular septum to the superior atrial border.

Transesophageal Echocardiography

With the introduction of transesophageal echocardiography, a new window for imaging the interatrial septum became available[16,17] (Fig. 29–3). The close proximity of the esophagus to the left and right atria allows superior quality images of the interatrial septum to be obtained. Both the limbus and the thin membrane of the fossa ovalis can be evaluated (Fig. 29–3A). In one study, the interatrial septum could be imaged by the transesophageal approach in each of 138 consecutive patients.[17] With the more recent biplane transesophageal technique, an additional longitudinal, or "vertical," cross section of the atrial septum can be obtained[18] (Fig. 29–3B). In this scanning plane, the interatrial septum can be visualized from its superior border near the entry of the superior vena cava to its inferior border near the entry of the inferior vena cava. Incremental rotation of the endoscope from this position provides sequential vertical cross-sectional images of the atrial septum, the foramen ovale, and the limbus. Transesophageal echocardiography is discussed in more detail in Chapter 16.

Spatial Orientation of the Interatrial Septum

The normal spatial orientation and shape of the interatrial septum can be altered by changes in the relative volumes and pressures within the right and left atria. Changes in both septal orientation and shape can be appreciated and have been described in each of the standard septal imaging planes.[4,5,8,13] Figure 29–4 compares the normal short axis configuration of the interatrial septum with that seen in left and right atrial volume overloads and right atrial hypertension. Normally, the septum bows slightly toward the right atrium (Fig. 29–4A). As the left atrial volume increases, the anteroposterior length of the septum also increases, and it bows more prominently toward the right atrium (Fig. 29–4B).

As a rule, when the left atrial dilation is chronic (i.e., in mitral stenosis), the percentage of change in atrial volume from diastole to systole is small, and there is prominent septal bowing toward the right atrium during both diastole and systole. When the left atrial volume overload is acute (i.e., with chordal rupture), the cyclic change in left atrial volume may be great, with the septum bowing toward the right atrium at end-systole but returning to a more normal, flat, or even slightly convex orientation relative to the left atrium at end-diastole.[5]

When there is a right atrial volume overload, the structures at the base of the heart often rotate in a clockwise direction and the interatrial septum becomes more horizontally positioned and tends to bow inward toward the left atrium (Fig. 29–4C). This convexity is present at end-diastole and increases during systolic right atrial filling, thereby resulting in paradoxic motion of the interatrial septum. Right atrial hypertension reverses the normal curvature of the septum, displacing it toward the left atrium without significantly increasing its length (Fig. 29–4D).

Interatrial Septal Motion

The interatrial septum is a relatively thin membrane that separates two dynamic chambers. Motion of the septum, therefore, would be expected to reflect the relative pressures to which it is exposed during various phases of the cardiac cycle.[3,5] When viewed in short axis, the normal curvature of the septum causes the structure to appear confluent with the other borders of the left atrium and, hence, to form a part of this chamber. This septal orientation may reflect the fact that left atrial pressure normally exceeds that in the right atrium and, therefore, represents the major influence on septal configuration.[3] Detailed studies of atrial septal movement, however, suggest a more complex relationship. These studies have been conducted primarily from the right parasternal transducer location. As a result, the imaging plane transects the septum at approximately the 10:30-o'clock position relative to the short axis of the left atrium.[4,5] The motion recorded in this view, therefore, is comparable to that along a vector oriented roughly

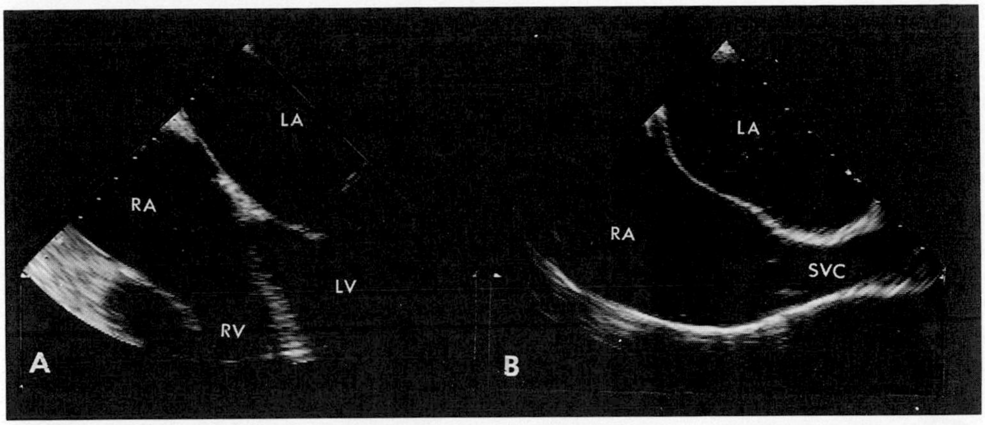

Fig. 29–3. Biplane transesophageal imaging views. **A.** A transverse, or horizontal, cross-section of the interatrial septum illustrating the limbus and the thin membrane of the fossa ovalis. **B.** A longitudinal, or vertical, scanning view shows the interatrial septum from its superior border near the entry of the superior vena cava (SVC) to its inferior border. LA = left atrium; RA = right atrium; LV = left ventricle; RV = right ventricle.

midway between the anteroposterior (D_1) and medial-lateral (D_3) axes of the left atrium. Because the largest component of motion in this plane normally is due to the anteroposterior expansion of the atrium, this component should predominate.

Figure 29–5 illustrates the imaging plane orientation used to record septal motion in the right parasternal view as well as the normal septal motion pattern. These M-mode recordings are taken from the midpoint of the septum, where maximal movement has been observed. Septal events are identified at eight points labeled "a" through "h." These points can be related to specific points in the cardiac cycle. The initial downward movement toward the left atrium ("a") has been attributed to right atrial contraction, which normally precedes left atrial contraction and thus may reverse or decrease the left-to-right pressure gradient.[5] This downward movement is followed by a series of small movements ("b,c,d") that have been related to the pressure fluctuations that result from the dissociation between left and right atrial and ventricular contraction and ejection.[5] The septum then moves anteriorly toward the right atrium as the left atrium fills ("d,e"). At the end of atrial filling, rightward movement increases slightly ("e,f"). The increase has been explained by the fact that the tricuspid valve opens before the mitral valve, thus increasing the left-to-right gradient and shifting the septum further toward the right atrium.[5] During rapid left ventricular filling, the septum moves inward toward the left atrium ("f,g"), and little movement occurs during mid-diastole. These characteristic movements are diminished with chronic left atrial volume overload (mitral stenosis); exaggerated with acute left atrial volume overload (acute mitral regurgitation); and may show a reversal in direction with right atrial volume overload (tricuspid insufficiency). These patterns are summarized in Figure 29–5. Because the left atrium is less compliant and has a smaller venous capacity than the right atrium, an equal change in volume in the two atria will result in a more marked change in pressure in the left atrium than in the right atrium. So it has been postulated that the interatrial septal motion predominantly reflects changes in the left atrial volume.[19] Although there appears to be a great deal of information in the analysis of septal motion, the role of this type of measurement in the clinical setting remains to be defined.

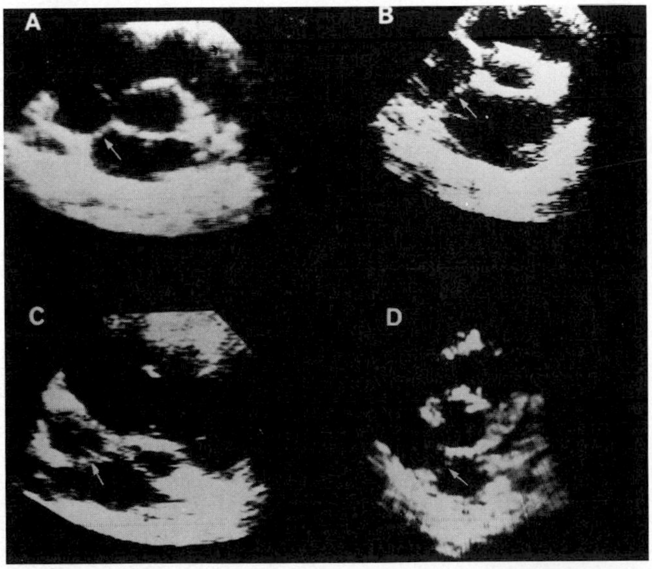

Fig. 29–4. Parasternal short axis recordings. **A.** The normal configuration of the interatrial septum. **B.** The interatrial septum in left atrial volume overload states. **C.** The interatrial septum in right ventricular volume overload. **D.** The interatrial septum in right atrial hypertension. The interatrial septum in each instance is indicated by the arrow.

Atrial Septal Defects

Anatomy

Uncomplicated atrial septal defect is one of the more common forms of congenital heart disease, representing from 7 to 15% of all cases in children. It is the most common congenital lesion (excluding the bicuspid aortic valve) encountered after the age of 20.[20]

Atrial septal defects are classified on the basis of their position in the septum and their embryologic origin into four different types: ostium primum, ostium secundum, sinus venosus, and coronary sinus[20–23] (Fig. 29–6).

The most common is the ostium secundum type, which represents roughly 70% of all defects in the atrial septum.[21] Ostium secundum defects are located in the region of the fossa ovalis and result from incomplete development of the septum secundum.

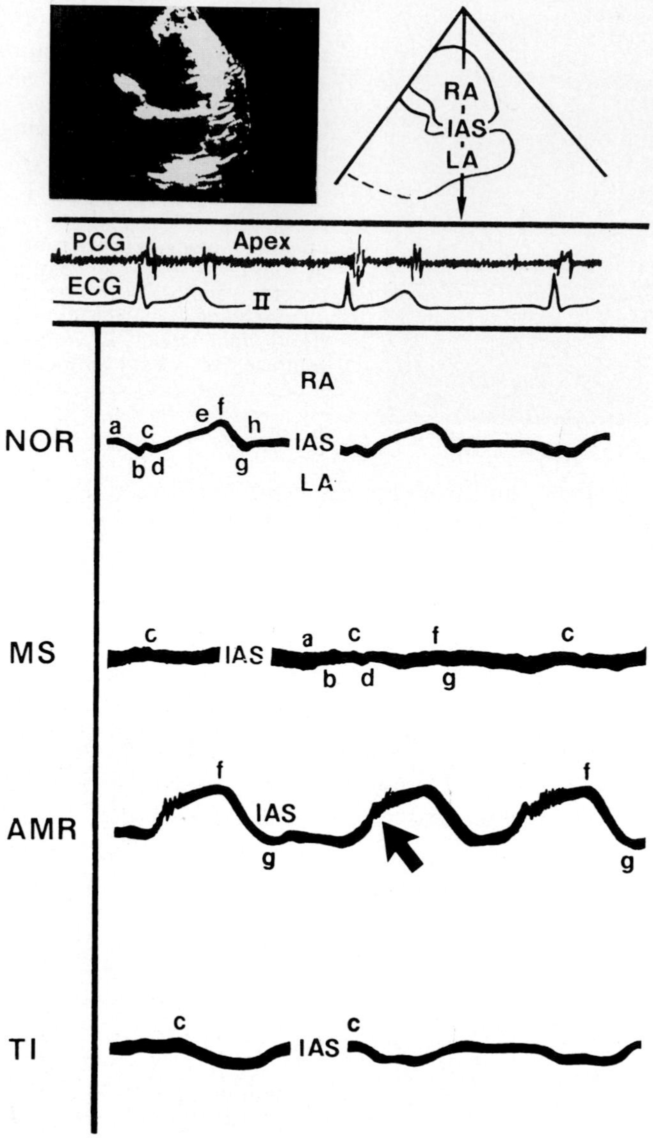

Fig. 29–5. Top. Cross-sectional scan of the interatrial septum (IAS) recorded from the right parasternal transducer location. As indicated in the accompanying diagram, the imaging plane transects the septum from the right atrium (RA) to the left atrium (LA). The y axis is aligned parallel to the long axis of the septum. Bottom. Serial redrawn M-mode recordings depict the "M-mode" pattern of the septal motion sampled from the midseptum (area indicated by the vertical arrow in the top, right diagram). The arrowhead in the example of acute mitral regurgitation points to an area of early, systolic, high-frequency, septal fluttering produced by the turbulent jet of blood (from the regurgitant lesion) that strikes the septum. NOR = normal; MS = mitral stenosis; AMR = acute mitral regurgitation; TI = tricuspid insufficiency. (Redrawn from Tei C: Echocardiographic analysis of interatrial septal motion. Am J Cardiol 44:472, 1979.)

Ostium primum defects are less common (approximately 20%) and are positioned in the lower portion of the septum in continuity with the atrioventricular valves. Ostium primum defects result from incomplete fusion of the septum primum with the endocardial cushions and are considered a partial form of the common atrioventricular canal. This type of atrial septal defect is discussed in more detail in Chapter 32.

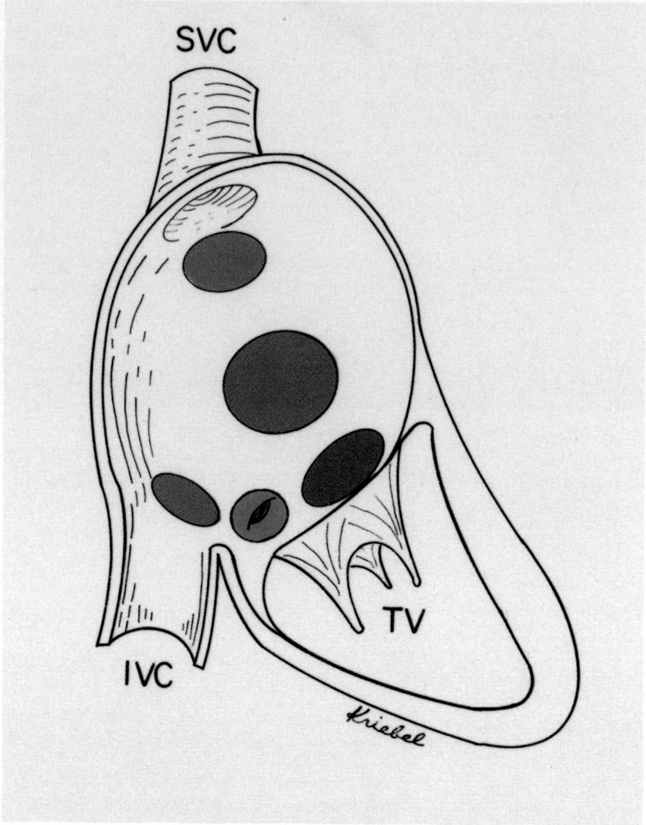

Fig. 29–6. Diagram of the interatrial septum, viewed from the right atrial side, illustrating the location of a "primum" atrial septal defect (red); a "secundum" atrial septal defect (green); superior and inferior sinus venosus defects (orange); and a coronary sinus defect (blue). TV = tricuspid valve; IVC = inferior vena cava. (Modified from Higgins CB, Silverman NH, Kersting-Sommerhoff BA, Schmidt K: Congenital Heart Disease: Echocardiography and Magnetic Resonance Imaging. New York, Raven Press, 1990.)

Sinus venosus defects constitute 6 to 8% of all defects in the interatrial septum and can be subdivided in superior and inferior sinus venosus defects depending on location. The majority of sinus venous defects are superior sinus venosus defects. They are positioned high in the interatrial septum in close proximity to the entrance of the superior vena cava and are frequently associated with anomalous drainage of the right upper pulmonary vein.[21] Inferior sinus venosus defects are more rare and have been described in the mouth of the inferior vena cava, often in association with anomalous attachment of the right lower pulmonary vein.[24]

Coronary sinus defects are even less common and are seen in association with an unroofed coronary sinus. Coronary sinus defects are located at the site of origin of the coronary sinus and are usually associated with a persistent left superior vena cava that connects to the left atrium.[15]

Echocardiographic and Doppler Evaluation

Echocardiographically, atrial septal defects are usually suspected on the basis of the nonspecific changes they produce in right ventricular and right atrial size and in interventricular septal motion (the right ventricular volume overload pattern).[25–28] Their presence can then be confirmed either by direct echocardiographic visualization of the defect,[7–9,12,13,29,30] by the detection of abnormal turbulent flow across the atrial septum by pulsed Doppler or color flow Doppler,[31–35] or by abnormalities in the pattern of echocardiographic contrast flow through the atria that result from the defect.[36–38] Using Doppler and two-dimensional echocardiography, systemic (Q_s) and pulmonary blood flow (Q_p) can be measured to calculate Q_p/Q_s and to estimate shunt flow ($Q_p - Q_s$) across the atrial septal defect.[39–41]

The right ventricular volume overload pattern occurs in atrial septal defect because of the characteristic tendency for shunt flow to occur from left to right.[42–46] In uncomplicated atrial septal defects, left-to-right shunting predominates because the major determinants of the degree and direction of shunting are (1) the size of the defect and (2) the instantaneous pressure difference between the two atria. The determinants of the interatrial pressure difference are the relative compliances of the atria and their associated venous reservoirs, the effective atrioventricular orifice area, and the relative compliance of the ventricles.[47] Because the thin-walled right ventricle is normally more compliant than the thicker left ventricle, predominant shunting is toward the right and imposes an increased volume load on the right atrium and ventricle. Increased right ventricular diastolic volume also displaces the interventricular septum posteriorly toward the left ventricle. During systole, the increased left ventricular pressure shifts the interventricular septum anteriorly or paradoxically as a result of the reestablishment of a more normal ventricular shape[6] and/or the anterior displacement of the centroid of the left ventricle.[48]

Right ventricular dilation is almost invariably noted in patients with an uncomplicated atrial septal defect.[25–28] It also has been noted to develop experimentally with shunts measuring as small as 500 ml/min and to resolve following cessation of the abnormal flow pattern.[49] In cross-sectional studies, the reported incidence of abnormal septal motion has varied from 38[50] to 100%.[6,51] The relatively low incidence reported in the former study may be due to the fact that septal movement was examined at the papillary muscle level (where this abnormality is less evident). The right ventricular volume overload pattern is illustrated in Chapter 28, Figure 28–16; paradoxic interventricular septal motion is illustrated and discussed later in this chapter.

Qualitative Assessment of Atrial Septal Defects

Two-Dimensional Echocardiographic Imaging. Direct visualization of atrial septal defects can be achieved in each standard view of the interatrial septum. Defects appear as discontinuities or areas of focal dropout in the normal linear band of echoes arising from the interatrial septum.[8–15] In ostium secundum defects, this area of dropout is located in the midportion of the septum (Fig. 29–7A), whereas with ostium primum defects, the dropout is located in the lower atrial septum just superior to the crest of the interventricular septum and insertions of the atrioventricular valves (Fig. 29–7B). In sinus venosus defects, the area of dropout is located at the entry of the superior vena cava (Fig. 29–7C) or, less commonly, near the mouth of the inferior vena cava. Two-dimensional echocardiographic studies suggest that areas of focal echo dropout can be observed almost uniformly in patients with atrial septal defect, providing that the septum itself is recorded.[8,9,11–13,15] False-negatives theoretically can occur when the cross-sectional plane transects the interatrial septum at a level above or below the defect. In one study, a defect was not visualized (false-negative response) in 12 (11%) of 105 patients with a secundum ostium defect and in 9 (56%) of 16 patients with a sinus venosus defect using the subcostal imaging window.[15] False-positives that are due to the presence of an artifactual echo dropout in the region of the interatrial septum may represent a problem in the short axis and apical views in which the scan plane is oriented parallel to the path of the septum. Earlier studies have reported an incidence of false-positives ranging from 27% for the apical view to 50% for the short axis

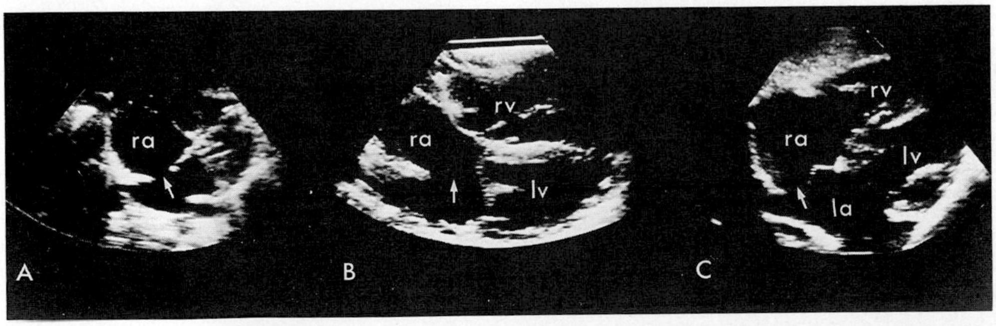

Fig. 29–7. Subcostal views demonstrating atrial septal defects. **A.** An ostium secundum atrial septal defect is noted with echo dropout in the midportion of the interatrial septum (arrow). **B.** A large ostium primum septal defect, which encompasses the inferior portion of the interatrial septum adjacent to the atrioventricular valves (arrow). **C.** A sinus venosus atrial septal defect is demonstrated with absence of the interatrial septal reflections along the superior rim of the septum (arrow). Note the entry of the right superior pulmonary vein adjacent to the defect. rv = right ventricle; ra = right atrium; la = left atrium; lv = left ventricle. (From Levine RA, et al.: Echocardiography: principles and clinical applications. *In* Eagle KA, Halser E, DeSanctis RW, Austen WG (eds.): The Practice of Cardiology. Boston, Little, Brown and Company, 1989.)

view.[9] However, as image quality has improved, the incidence of this artifactual echo dropout has decreased significantly.

One sign that helps to differentiate true defects from false-positives is the characteristic echo broadening that is frequently noted at the margins of a true defect. Echo broadening is caused by the more highly reflective blood-tissue interface at the defect margin. Because of the high incidence of false-positive defects noted in the apical and short axis views, the subcostal imaging plane, which places the interatrial septum perpendicular to the path of the scan plane, has been stressed as the view of choice for recording the interatrial septum. Using this transducer location, the sensitivity and specificity of the technique have improved markedly,[12,13,15] and in infants, differentiation of patent foramen ovale from true ostium secundum atrial septal defect has also been possible in the majority of cases.[13] From this subcostal approach, 93 (89%) of 105 ostium secundum atrial septal defects, all 32 (100%) ostium primum defects, and 7 (44%) of the 16 sinus venosus defects could be successfully visualized in a group of patients with ages ranging from 2 months to 74 years (mean, 31 years).[15]

Transesophageal echocardiography is particularly advantageous for assessing atrial septal defects because the ultrasound transducer is located very close to the atrial septum and the scan plane is oriented nearly perpendicular to the septum.[17,52] This approach provides detailed anatomic information on the atrial septum and has proven to be a very sensitive technique to detect atrial septal defects.[16]

Doppler Examination. Doppler echocardiography is a very sensitive technique for detecting flow across an atrial septal defect.[32,53] The Doppler examination is especially useful to confirm the presence of shunt flow when the atrial septal defect cannot be imaged by two-dimensional echocardiography and is also extremely helpful in differentiating artifactual echo dropout from a true atrial septal defect. The pulsed Doppler examination provides additional information on the direction of shunt flow, instantaneous flow velocity, and changes in velocity throughout the cardiac cycle.[31] A Doppler examination can be performed from each of the previously described imaging windows; however, the subcostal and right parasternal positions provide the best approach for alignment of the Doppler interrogation beam parallel with the shunt flow.[32] The currently available echocardiographs combine two-dimensional imaging and Doppler capabilities permitting accurate positioning of the pulsed Doppler sample volume at the level of the defect. Optimal flow velocity recordings are obtained with the sample volume positioned immediately distal to the defect in the direction of the expected shunt flow (this is near the surface of the interatrial septum in the right atrium when predominantly left-to-right shunt flow is present).[32]

With the introduction of two-dimensional color flow mapping, direct visualization of disturbed flow velocities in the cardiac chambers has become possible. Color Doppler flow mapping has been shown to be a very sensitive technique to detect shunt flow across an atrial septal defect.[33] Figure 29–8 illustrates the color Doppler display of left-to-right shunt flow in a patient with a secundum atrial septal defect, obtained from a parasternal (Fig. 29–8A), apical (Fig. 29–8B), and subcostal (Fig. 29–8C) transducer position. Color flow Doppler is particularly useful to distinguish between a true defect and artifactual echo dropout or to detect the presence of multiple fenestrations in the fossa ovalis membrane (Fig. 29–9). From a subcostal imaging window, left-to-right flow across the atrial septum is displayed as an area of low velocity turbulent flow originating at the right atrial side of the defect. Color Doppler flow mapping has been reported to have a higher sensitivity than contrast echo-

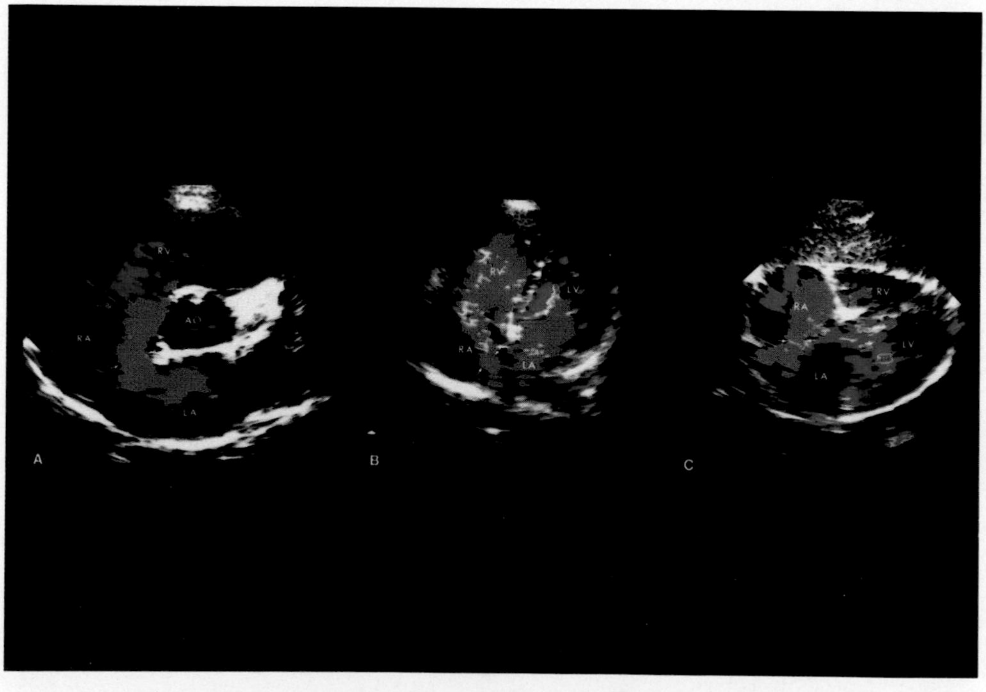

Fig. 29–8. Color Doppler flow images illustrating left-to-right shunt flow, represented as a red color, through a secundum atrial septal defect (white arrows). **A.** Parasternal short axis view. **B.** Apical four-chamber view. **C.** Subcostal four-chamber view. RV = right ventricle; LV = left ventricle; RA = right atrium; LA = left atrium; AO = aorta.

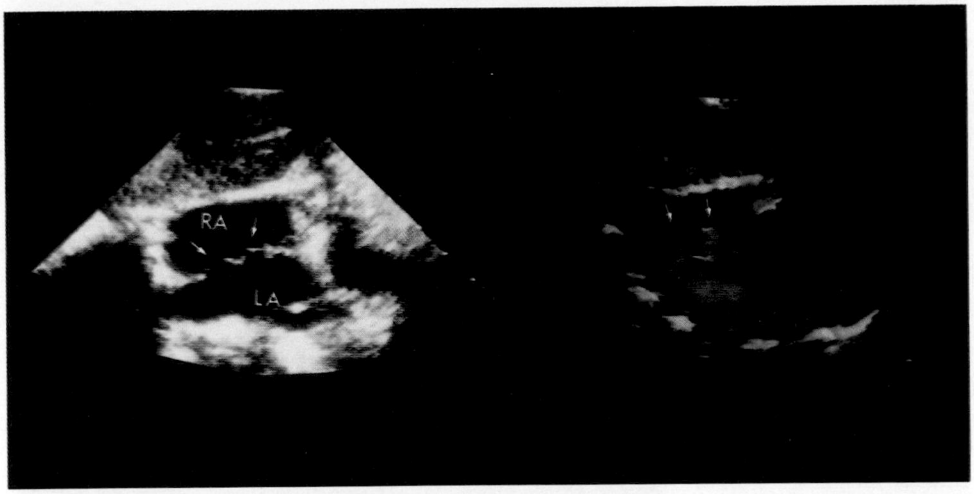

Fig. 29–9. Color flow mapping permits one to discriminate separate flow streams, as illustrated in this example from an infant with two discrete fenestrations in the interatrial septum. Left. This example suggests two small defects in the septum. Right. The color flow map confirms these defects with two orange jets passing through these apparent defects. LA = left atrium; RA = right atrium. (From Levine RA, et al.: Echocardiography. Principles and clinical applications. *In* Eagle KA, Haber E, DeSanctis RW, Austen WG (eds.): The Practice of Cardiology. Boston, Little, Brown and Company, 1989.)

cardiography in demonstrating left-to-right shunt flow through an atrial septal defect.[33] In addition, color Doppler flow imaging provides real-time information on the location and the direction of the disturbed velocities in the right atrium. Pulsed Doppler and color Doppler flow imaging obtained by the transesophageal approach further increase the diagnostic information.[54]

Normal Atrial Septal Defect Flow Velocity Pattern. The characteristic flow velocity pattern through an uncomplicated atrial septal defect shows predominantly left-to-right shunt flow, and the Doppler spectrum has a typical biphasic pattern, as is shown in Figure 29–10. The Doppler examination shows disturbed flow toward the transducer (from a right parasternal or subcostal position) starting at early-to-midventricular systole, peaking in late-systole, and extending into early-diastole. A second period of left-to-right shunting occurs at the time of atrial contraction.[31,32,34] In addition, a short period of right-to-left flow can usually be recorded at the beginning of systole.[31,34] This flow velocity pattern is consistent with the instantaneous cyclic pressure differences between the left and the right atrium.[47,55] Simultaneous pressure measurements have shown that the greatest difference in left and right atrial pressures and the largest shunt flow occurs in late systole at the peak of the left atrial V wave.[55] This pressure gradient (LA > RA) decreases with opening of the atrioventricular valves and increases again with atrial systole. The maximum velocity usually recorded across an atrial septal defect is 1 to 1.3 m/sec, indicating a peak pressure difference of 5 mm Hg. A short reversal of the pressure difference and a minimal right-to-left shunt occurs at the onset of systole, which is due to a more prominent fall in left atrial pressure.[34,55] A small amount of right-to-left shunt flow in uncomplicated septal defects is regularly seen with contrast echocardiography in which a few contrast bubbles generally appear in the left cavities. Two-dimensional color Doppler flow mapping, however, may not demonstrate this transient right-to-left shunting at the onset of systole.[33,34] The flow velocity patterns of atrial shunting were detected using pulsed Doppler in 30 of 31 patients in one study[32] and in all of 15 patients with an uncomplicated secundum atrial septal defect in another study.[34] Doppler patterns suggesting an atrial left-to-right flow were not found in 15 normal patients.[32] The presence of positive left-sided contrast demonstrating right-to-left shunt flow has been reported in 50[34] to 96%[32] of patients with an uncomplicated secundum atrial septal defect with predominant left-to-right shunting.

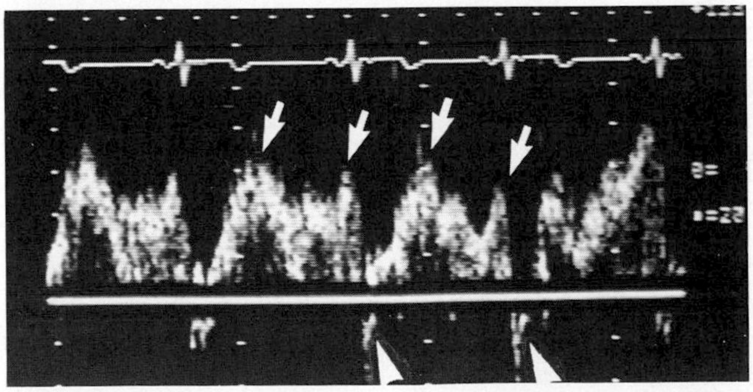

Fig. 29–10. Pulsed wave Doppler tracing of shunt flow through an uncomplicated atrial septal defect obtained from a subcostal scanning position. This velocity tracing illustrates the biphasic pattern of left-to-right shunt flow (toward the transducer) with a first period of shunt flow, peaking at late systole, extending into diastole, and a second period of left-to-right shunting at the time of atrial contraction (white arrows). There is a short period of shunt flow reversal with right-to-left shunting (away from the transducer) at the onset of systole (white arrowheads).

Conditions Affecting Normal Atrial Septal Defect Flow Velocity Patterns

Respiratory Variation. The normal flow velocity pattern across an atrial septal defect will vary with respiration. During inspiration, a decrease in the pressure difference between the two atria at end-systole has been shown to result in decreased left-to-right shunting. Likewise, the reversal of shunt flow at the onset of systole is accentuated during inspiration. Right-to-left atrial shunt flow often must be distinguished from superior vena cava inflow, which may have a similar direction and flow velocity pattern. Caval inflow, however, has a different location and shows an increase in flow velocities during inspiration.

Associated Lesions. The typical flow velocity pattern across an uncomplicated atrial septal defect will also be affected by the presence of concomitant cardiac lesions that alter the normal phasic variation in instantaneous pressure differences between the atria (e.g. atrial fibrillation, mitral or tricuspid stenosis, the presence of significant mitral or tricuspid regurgitation). With the development of pulmonary hypertension, pressures on the right side increase and left-to-right shunt flow decreases. In patients with Eisenmenger's syndrome and severe pulmonary hypertension, no shunt flow or predominantly right-to-left shunting across the atrial septal defect may be recorded.[32]

Intra-atrial Structures. Extremely rarely, intra-atrial structures can deviate caval inflow, and right-to-left shunt flow may be present despite normal pulmonary artery pressures. This has been reported in a patient with an atrial septal defect in which a prominent eustachian valve and a redundant flap of the septum secundum acted like a spinnaker and preferentially shunted blood from the inferior vena cava into the left atrium.[56]

Echocardiographic Contrast. When direct anatomic visualization of a defect cannot be achieved or when the question of a false-positive remains, echocardiographic contrast can be used to confirm the diagnosis.[36–38] The contrast technique involves the injection of such substances as saline or indocyanine green (Cardio-Green) dye, which contain multiple microbubbles, into a peripheral arm vein and following the path of contrast flow through the right side of the heart. Normally, contrast passes through the right atrium into the right ventricle and then out into the pulmonary arterial system. The microbubbles are totally filtered out at the pulmonary capillary level, and no contrast should flow into the left side of the heart. In normal persons, the contrast completely fills the right atrium and outlines the borders of the interatrial septum. This sharply defined contrast margin can also be used to confirm the presence of the dividing membrane and to rule out a false-positive defect even when the interatrial septum itself is not visualized. When an atrial septal defect is present with right-to-left shunting, contrast can be seen immediately flowing into the left atrium, thereby confirming the presence and location of the defect and the direction of the shunt.[36–38] Even in patients with predominant left-to-right shunts, mixing at the atrial level frequently results in the recording of microbubbles in the left atrium, thus providing defect confirmation (Fig. 29–11). When right-to-left shunting is not present, however, observation of the displacement of the contrast-containing blood from the right atrial side of the septal defect by non-contrast-containing blood flowing through the defect from left to right (the negative contrast effect) can be used to confirm the presence of the defect (Fig. 29–11).[37] One must be cautious however, because a negative contrast effect can also originate from inferior vena cava inflow or prominent coronary sinus flow. The use of echocardiographic contrast is discussed in detail in Chapter 15.

Semiquantitative Assessment of Atrial Septal Defects

Atrial septal defects with left-to-right shunting will increase tricuspid and pulmonary flow velocities, especially when compared with flow velocities across the mitral and aortic valves. The ratio between velocities in the right and the left heart could be used to provide some estimate of the shunt flow.[31] In the absence of any shunt flow, the ratio between right- and left-sided velocities is usually 0.6 for both the atrioventricular valves and the great arteries. In the presence of an atrial septal defect, tricuspid flow velocities become as high or even higher than mitral flow velocity and pulmonary flow velocity may be 2 times as high as that in the aorta.[31]

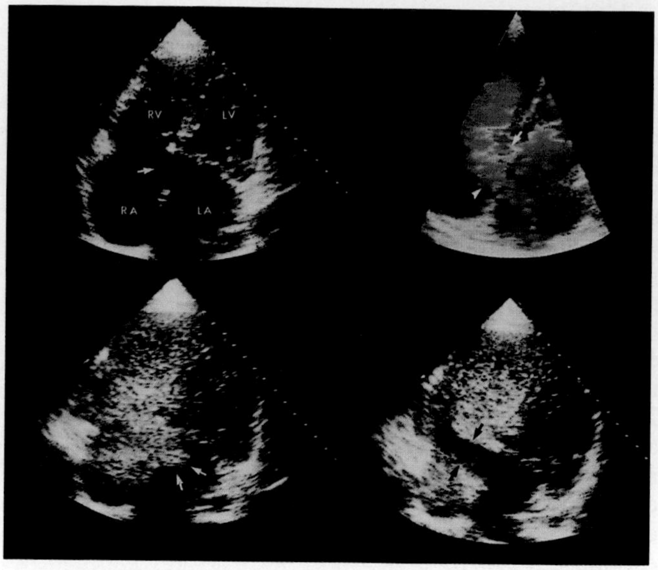

Fig. 29–11. A series of apical four-chamber images from a 16-year-old with a large ostium primum atrial septal defect. The images depict a large area of echo dropout in the atrial septum (arrow, top, left) and left-to-right shunt-flow streaming through the defect on the color flow mapping (arrows, top, right). Saline contrast images show positive contrast appearing in the left atrium (arrows, bottom, left) and negative contrast created by unopacified blood streaming left-to-right across the septal defect (arrows, bottom, right). LA = left atrium; RA = right atrium; LV = left ventricle; RV = right ventricle. (From Levine RA, et al.: Echocardiography. Principles and clinical applications. *In* Eagle KH, Haber E, DeSanctis RW, Austen WG (eds.): The Practice of Cardiology. Boston, Little, Brown and Company, 1989.)

Quantitative Assessment of Atrial Septal Defects

Quantitative echo-Doppler measures of transvalvular flow provides a more accurate assessment of shunt flow, calculated as the difference between right- and left-sided volume flow rates. The ratio of pulmonary to systemic flow rate (Q_p/Q_s) calculated by echo-Doppler methods has been validated in experimental studies[57,58] and has been shown to correlate closely with the ratio of pulmonary to systemic flow measured at cardiac catheterization.[40,41] The use of echo-Doppler in volume flow measurements is discussed in more detail in Chapter 30.

Color Doppler flow imaging of the atrial septal defect jet has also been used to assess directly the shunt size in atrial septal defects. In one study, a reasonable correlation was reported between measurements of maximum jet width and maximum jet area in the right atrium and Q_p/Q_s and shunt flow (Q_p-Q_s).[59] However, the spatial and temporal resolution of two-dimensional color Doppler flow mapping are limited, and thus its ability to detect relatively small and rapid changes in atrial shunt flow is limited. In addition, a major difficulty in quantifying shunt flow by simple jet parameters is that the appearance of a turbulent jet in the color flow image is affected by several physical and instrument factors other than flow rate itself. This limitation is discussed in more detail in Chapter 12.

Although it is the amount of shunt flow and not the physical size of the defect that is of importance in the hemodynamic assessment of an atrial septal defect,[60] exact sizing of the defect may become very important in the decision to use transcatheter closure techniques. The assessment of defect size by the transesophageal approach has been shown to be more accurate than the measurements obtained by conventional transthoracic echocardiography. Both direct measurement of the largest diameter of the defect by two-dimensional transesophageal echocardiography and measurements of the width of the shunt flow by color flow Doppler at the level of the defect have shown good correlations with surgical measurements of the major axis.[35,54]

A preliminary report[60a] has suggested the ability to image and accurately size atrial septal defects by a catheter-based intracardiac ultrasound system in an experimental setup. However, further validation of this new technique in vivo is necessary, and the incremental value of this approach remains to be proven.

Patent Foramen Ovale

The foramen ovale is an opening in the midportion of the fetal atrial septum at the junction of the septum primum and septum secundum. This foramen is normally covered by a thin flap of septum primum. Before birth, it is kept open by flow from the right to left atrium. After birth, the establishment of the normal pulmonary circulation increases the left atrial pressure and presses the flap of septum primum against the foramen ovale, closing the opening. This flap may then fuse with the septum secundum to close the orifice permanently or may remain separate such that the orifice can reopen if the left-to-right pressure gradient should reverse.

Several studies in infants have demonstrated that the foramen ovale and covering flap of septum primum can be visualized from a subcostal transducer location.[12,13] Movement of this flap has also been observed in response to cyclic cardiac and respiratory motion.[12,13] In the majority of infants with right-sided volume overload, the septal flap has been observed to bulge into the left atrium, while the remainder of the atrial septum remains flat.[13] This configuration is usually associated with a right-to-left shunt. A small associated defect may be seen at the superior aspect of the foramen ovale and has been attributed to separation of the superior rim of the septum primum from the septum secundum.[13]

A similar small defect associated with incompetence of the flap is noted in infants with left ventricular volume and pressure overloads where the entire atrial septum and the thinner, septum primum-covered foramen ovale bow into the right atrium.[13]

Effects of Balloon Atrial Septostomy and Surgical Septectomy on the Interatrial Septum

Enlargement of the foramen ovale is frequently necessary in infants with transposition of the great vessels to permit increased mixing of blood at the atrial level. This enlargement is usually achieved by balloon atrial septostomy (tearing a larger hole in the septum by pulling an inflated balloon through the foramen ovale) or, when this is unsuccessful, by surgical septectomy. The septostomy defect is located in the midportion of the septum, and the rhythmic movement of blood through the defect can be observed to impart corresponding motion to the torn margins of the septum primum.[13] Successful septostomies have been reported to produce defects that occupy more than 30% of the total septal length, whereas smaller defects (less than 30%) are frequently associated with persistent desaturation and require early surgical intervention.[61] The surgical septectomy defect is larger and includes both the original defect and the surgically created defect in the posterior septum. Figure 29–12 summarizes the principal atrial septal defect locations and associated patterns of septum primum movement relative to the foramen ovale in each of these disorders.

Atrial Septal Aneurysms

An atrial septal aneurysm was first reported at autopsy in 1934.[62] Although the first in vivo diagnosis was made by angiography,[63] it was not until the development of two-dimensional echocardiography that the presence of an atrial septal aneurysm could be diagnosed routinely in patients.[64–67] Recently, interest in atrial septal aneurysms has increased because they have been identified as potential cardiac sources of cerebrovascular and peripheral embolic events.[66–69] Atrial septal aneurysms have also been reported to be associated with pulmonary emboli,[63] atrial tachyarrhythmias,[70] atrial septal defects,[71] and prolapse of the atrioventricular valves.[72]

In a series of 1578 consecutive autopsy studies, 16 patients (1%) were identified with the pathologic findings of a fossa ovalis aneurysm.[73] None of these aneurysms had been diagnosed during life, and all were clinically asymptomatic. The reported prevalence of atrial septal aneurysms by conventional two-dimensional echocardiography has varied from 0.12%[74] to 0.52%.[69] Aneurysms of the interatrial septum are more commonly identified by transesophageal echocardiography and were observed in 3%[67] to 8%[75] of patients undergoing transesophageal echocardiography for a variety of reasons. In 20 patients (15%) of 133 patients with stroke, an interatrial septal aneurysm was detected by transesophageal echocardiography.[75] Interatrial septal aneurysms occur more often as an isolated abnormality than in association with other cardiac malformations.

The criteria of an atrial septal aneurysm diagnosed by two-dimensional echocardiography include a diameter at the base of the aneurysm of 15 mm and an excursion of 11 mm into either atrial chamber from the plane of the atrial septum, obtained from a parasternal, apical, subcostal, or transesophageal transducer position.[75] Other authors require that the aneurysms protrude at least 15 mm beyond the plane of the atrial septum or

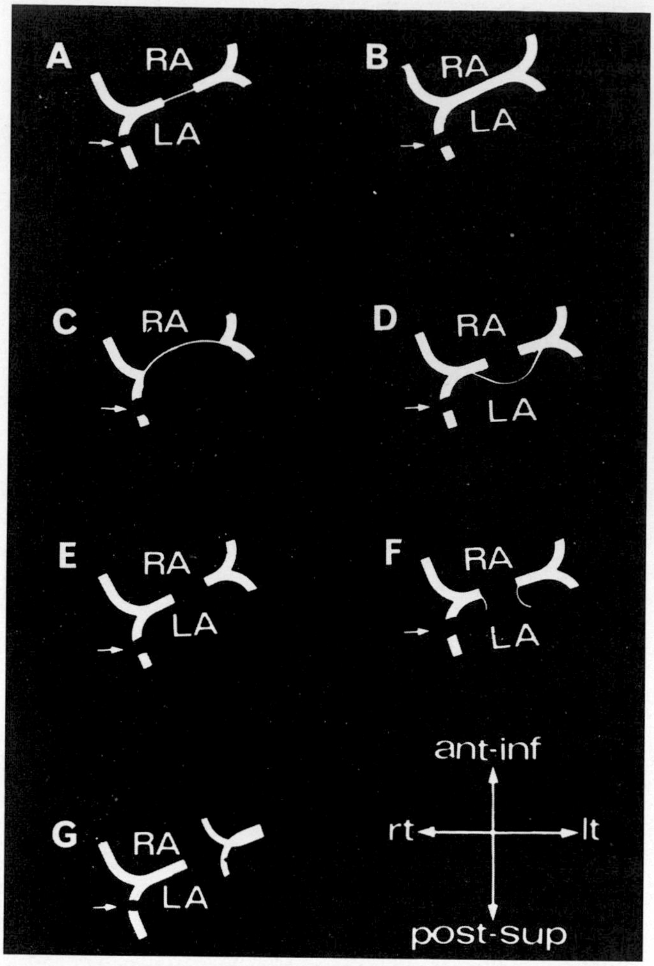

Fig. 29–12. The position and appearance of the atrial septum, recorded from the subcostal transducer location, in a variety of common disorders. **A.** Normal, undeviated interatrial septum shows thinning in the region of the foramen ovale. The horizontal arrow indicates the position of insertion of the right pulmonary vein. **B.** Normal septal position with septal thickening in the region of the septum primum. **C.** Deviation of the interatrial septum toward the right atrium (RA) with left atrial volume overload. **D.** Right ventricular volume overload with opening of the flap valve of septum primum covering the foramen ovale. **E.** Ostium secundum atrial septal defect illustrates the absence of septal echoes in the region of the foramen ovale. **F.** Flail remnants of septum primum at the margins of an atrial septal defect created by balloon atrial septostomy. **G.** Ostium primum atrial septal defect located in the inferior portion of the septum and bounded inferiorly by the atrioventricular valves. LA = left atrium. (From Bierman FZ, Williams RG: Subxiphoid two-dimensional imaging of the interatrial septum in infants and neonates with congenital heart disease. Circulation 60:80, 1979. Reproduced by permission of the American Heart Association, Inc.)

show phasic excursion during the cardiorespiratory cycle exceeding 15 mm.[66] Of interest, however, is that these commonly used criteria are based on an autopsy series of asymptomatic patients[73] and that none of these criteria have been independently validated.

On the basis of their appearance, atrial septal aneurysms can be divided into two distinct groups where (1) the aneurysm involves only the region of the fossa ovalis (fossa ovalis aneurysm), (2) the aneurysm involves the entire interatrial septum.

Fossa Ovalis Atrial Septal Aneurysm

Fossa ovalis aneurysms are usually an isolated abnormality in patients without complex congenital heart disease and accounted in one study for 84% of all cases of atrial septal aneurysms.[66] Figure 29–13 illustrates a patient with a small mobile aneurysm involving the region of the fossa ovalis. Some authors have subclassified fossa ovalis aneurysms according to the direction of the maximal protrusion and the mobility of the aneurysmal membrane during the cardiorespiratory cycle. This two-dimensional echocardiographic classification may have clinical implications because it reflects the transatrial septal pressure gradient and its variation with the cardiorespiratory cycle. A mobile aneurysmal membrane is frequently associated with an atrial septal defect and the presence of atrial shunt flow (Fig. 29–13C). The motion of the interatrial septal has been discussed in more detail earlier in this chapter. Figure 29–14 is an example of a larger atrial septal aneurysm that partially fills the right atrium. In this example, contrast has been injected into the opposite atrial chamber to highlight the presence of the lesion.

Transesophageal echocardiography is superior to transthoracic echocardiography in evaluating the interatrial septum, especially in patients with poor conventional imaging windows. In one study,[67] the presence of multiple fenestrations in the aneurysmal membrane in four patients and the presence of thrombotic material within an atrial septal aneurysm in two patients was diagnosed only by transesophageal echocardiography.

Aneurysm of the Entire Atrial Septum

Aneurysm of the entire atrial septum appears to be an anatomically distinct group of atrial septal aneurysms and is typically seen in patients with associated congenital malformations. Infants with either right ventricular inflow or outflow obstruction often require patency of the interatrial septum, either in the form of an atrial septal defect or a patent foramen ovale, to survive. When there is restricted right-to-left shunting, aneurysmal dilation of the interatrial septum may develop, and the thinned septum may bulge prominently into the left atrium.[76,77] These septal aneurysms may grow to a point where they partially obstruct the mitral orifice.

Atrial Septal Thickness

In adults, an abnormally thick septum may be seen in amyloidosis, mural atrial thrombus, infiltrating benign and malignant tumors, or lipomatous hypertrophy. Lipomatous hypertrophy is the most common cause of abnormal atrial septal thickness in the elderly and has been associated with supraventricular arrhythmias.[78] The following echocardiographic criteria for diagnosis of lipomatous hypertrophy have been proposed: (1) a bilobed or dumbbell-shaped appearance of the interatrial septum because the globular thickening of the limbus spares the

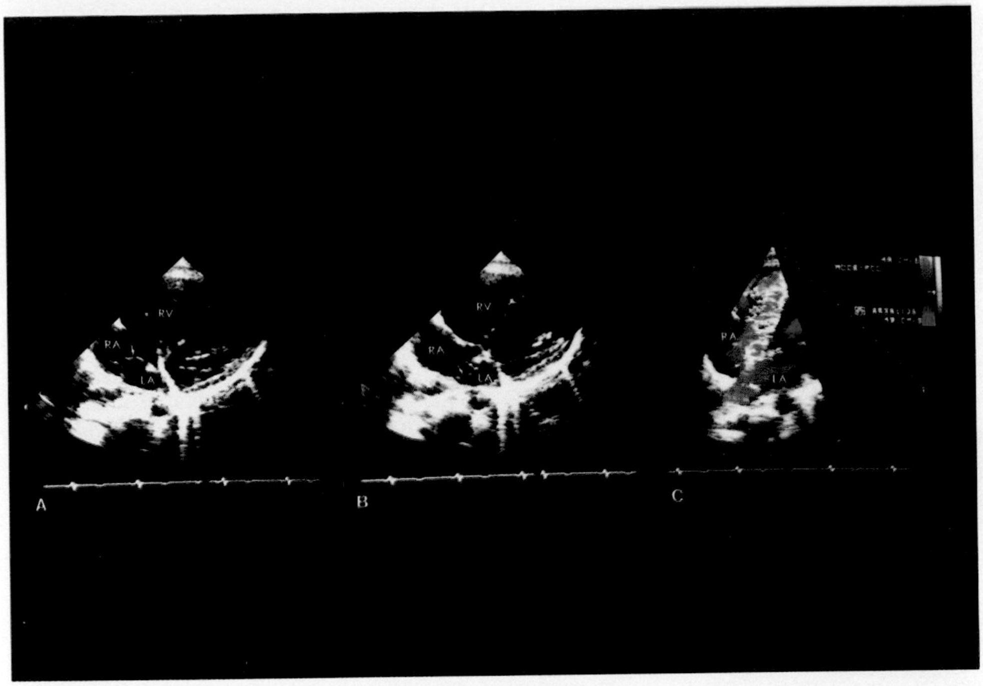

Fig. 29–13. Off-axis four-chamber view illustrating a small mobile fossa ovalis atrial septal aneurysm. **A.** The aneurysm (white arrows) protrudes throughout most of the cardiac cycle into the right atrium (RA). **B.** There is a very short reversal of the curvature of the aneurysm with protrusion into the left atrium (LA) (white arrows) at early systole. **C.** Color Doppler flow image illustrating the associated left-to-right shunt flow (white arrows). The limited temporal resolution of two-dimensional color Doppler flow mapping did not allow identification of the presence of very short reversal of shunt flow. RV = right ventricle.

membrane of the fossa ovalis, (2) an absolute atrial septal thickness of 15 mm* or more, excluding the valve of the fossa ovalis;[79,80] and (3) the absence of any other explanation for the abnormal septal thickness[81] (Fig. 29–15).

An abnormally thick atrial septum may also be seen in amyloidosis. This is usually a late finding, occurring in association with increased thickening of the other walls of the heart and cardiac valves. Figure 29–16 is a subcostal long axis view of the interatrial septum from a patient with hereditary amyloidosis and demonstrates the generalized increase in cardiac and interatrial septal thickness.

In infants, apparent thickening of the interatrial septum that is due to loss of the normal central thinning characteristic of the foramen ovale has been reported in two cases and, in both, was associated with torrential pulmonary blood flow and left ventricular volume overload.[13]

The most common cause of an apparently thickened atrial septum in infants, however, is a surgical patch covering a repaired atrial septal defect. These patches appear thicker and more highly reflective than the normal septum and do not show the same elastic motion that is characteristic of the normal septum. Figure 29–17 illustrates the increase in reflectivity and width of a surgical patch covering a defect in the atrial septum. Rarely, increased atrial septal thickness may be due to the presence of an atrial septal defect closure device. Figure 29–18 shows a patient with a secundum atrial septal defect before (Fig. 29–18A) and after (Fig. 29–18B) percutaneous closure of the defect with a clamshell device. The struts can be clearly seen on both sides of the septum.

Echocardiographic Guidance During Transeptal Interventions

During transeptal cardiac catheterization or balloon mitral valvuloplasty, transthoracic[82] and transesophageal[83] imaging are useful to visualize the transeptal

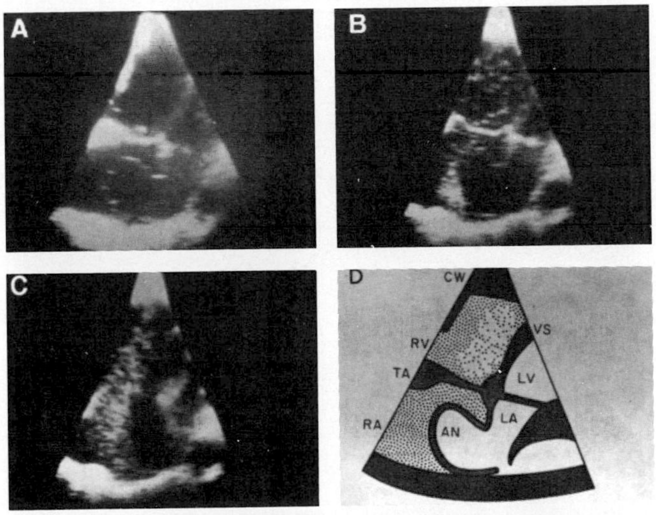

Fig. 29–14. Apical four-chamber recording of an atrial septal aneurysm (AN). **A.** In this example, the aneurysm bulges into the right atrium (RA). **B** and **C.** Contrast has been injected peripherally and fills the RA, outlining the AN. **D.** The relationship of the AN to surrounding structures. CW = chest wall; VS = ventricular septum; RV = right ventricle; LV = left ventricle; TA = tricuspid annulus; LA = left atrium. (From Nanda NC: Contrast echocardiography. *In* Yu PN, Goodwin JF (eds.): Progress in Cardiology. Philadelphia, Lea & Febiger, 1979.)

* In a series of 54 normal hearts in older children and adults, it was observed that the maximal septal thickness was 3.4 mm (range, 1.5 to 6.0 mm).[79] In a series of unselected hearts from elderly patients (age ranging from 61 to 90 years) the average maximal septal thickness was 12.5 mm (range, 2 to 25 mm).[80]

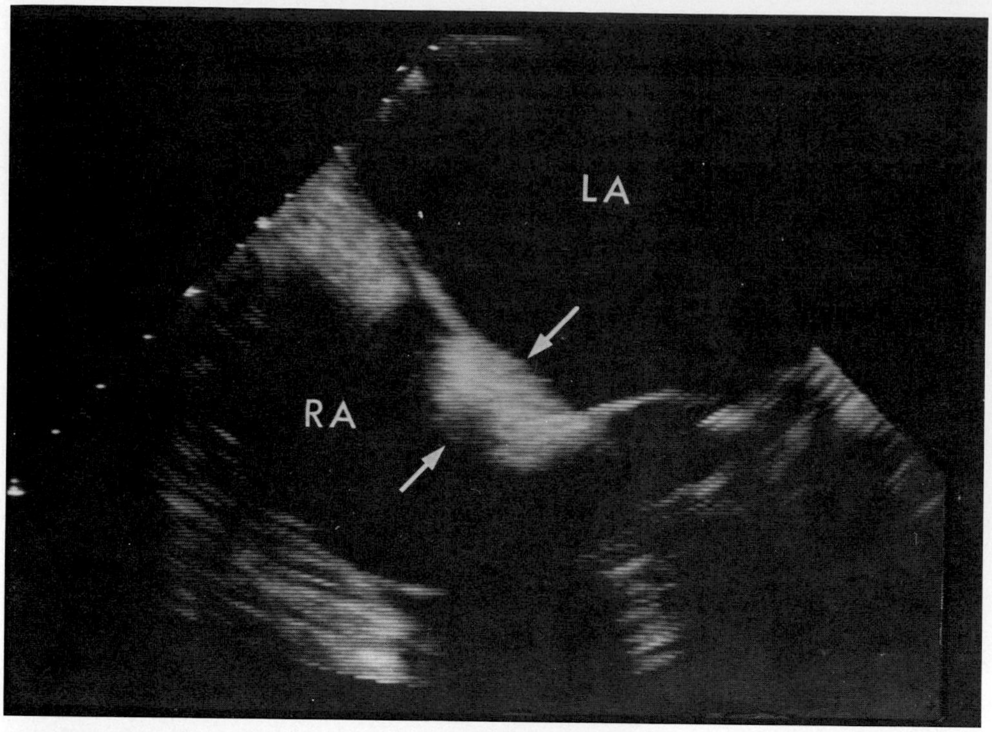

Fig. 29–15. Transverse transesophageal view of lipomatous hypertrophy of the interatrial septum in an elderly patient, showing the increased thickness of the limbus (arrows) and sparing of the membrane of the fossa ovalis. LA = left atrium; RA = right atrium.

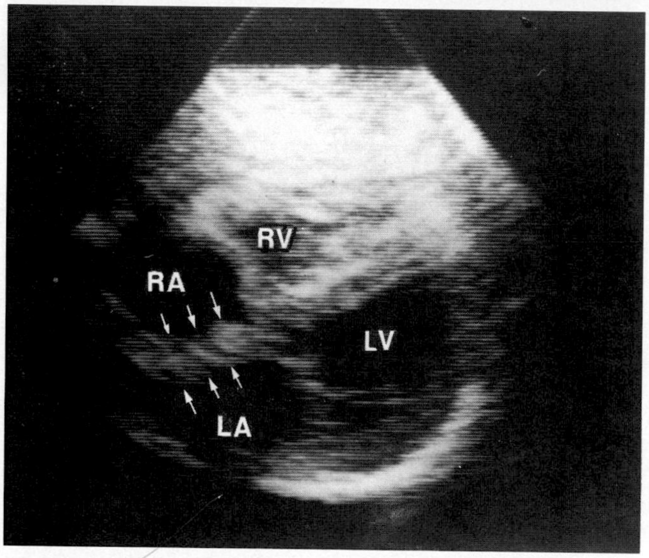

Fig. 29–16. Subcostal long axis recording of the interatrial septum in hereditary amyloidosis. An increase in atrial septal thickness is associated with generalized hypertrophy of the cardiac valves and the ventricular myocardium. The thickened interatrial septum is indicated by the arrowheads. RA = right atrium; RV = right ventricle; LV = left ventricle; LA = left atrium.

needle and catheter and to assess their position relative to other cardiac structures, in particular, the aortic root.

THE INTERVENTRICULAR SEPTUM

Anatomy

The interventricular septum is a thick, triangular, muscular wall that separates the left and right ventricles.[1] Normally, this septum is both an anatomic and a functional component of the left ventricle and accounts for roughly one-third of the muscle mass of that chamber.[1] Its radius of curvature is similar to that of the free wall of the left ventricle; consequently, it is concave toward the left ventricle and convex toward the right. The majority of the septum is muscular, with the exception of a small membranous segment located at its superior border just beneath the right and noncoronary cusps of the aortic valve.

Development

Embryologically, the interventricular septum develops from three different sources.[84] The major component, the muscular septum, originates as a median partition along the floor of the common ventricle. This partition grows superiorly as the ventricles enlarge. It has the form of a crescentic plate with two horns that join the respective dorsal and ventral endocardial cushions. For a short time, the primitive interventricular septum is an incomplete partition that only partially divides the common ventricle. The remaining communication between the ventricles, situated above the superior margin of the muscular septum is called the *interventricular foramen*. This foramen is bounded (1) inferiorly by the interventricular septum; (2) anteriosuperiorly by the proximal bulbar septum, which continues downward from the longitudinally dividing bulbus; and (3) posteriosuperiorly by the fused middle portion of the endocardial cushions. Final closure of the interventricular foramen is the result of tissue proliferation from each of these sources but especially from the endocardial cushions. The resulting thin membrane that completes this partition is the membranous septum.[84]

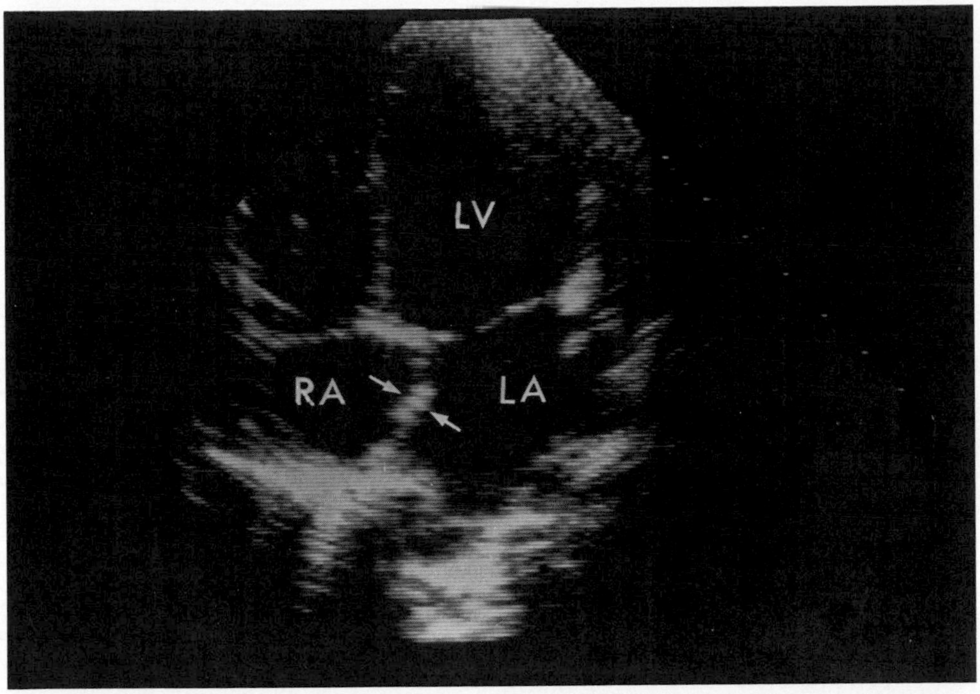

Fig. 29–17. Apical four-chamber recording of the interatrial septum illustrates the presence of a septal patch. The patch (arrows) is thicker and more highly reflective than the normal septum. The movement of the patch is restricted, and the normal diastolic decrease in anteroposterior septal length is diminished. LV = left ventricle; LA = left atrium; RA = right atrium.

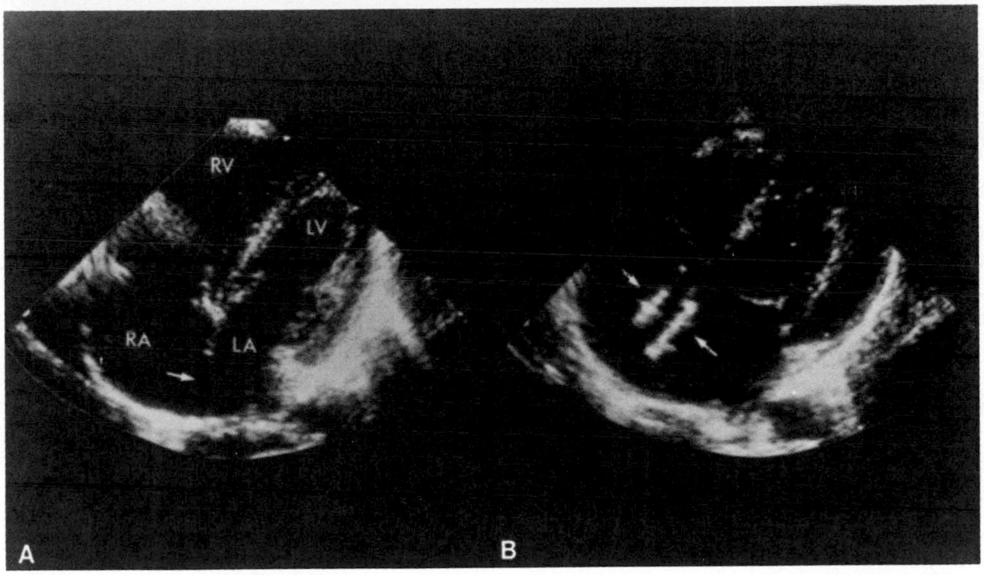

Fig. 29–18. Off-axis apical four-chamber views. **A.** A patient with a secundum atrial septal defect (arrow) before it has been closed using a clamshell device. **B.** The same patient after closure (arrows). LA = left atrium; RA = right atrium; LV = left ventricle; RV = right ventricle.

Examining Planes

The interventricular septum is primarily recorded in (1) the parasternal long axis view of the left ventricle (Fig. 29–19A); (2) a parasternal short axis, which can be swept from the cardiac apex to the basal insertion of the septum into the atrioventricular groove (Fig. 29–19B); (3) the apical four-chamber view (Fig. 29–19C); and (4) the subcostal long-axis views (Fig. 29–19D). Portions of the septum can also be recorded in the apical long axis view, and serial short axis scans can be obtained from the subcostal transducer location. The long and short axes of both interventricular and interatrial septa are defined relative to those of the surrounding chambers.

The parasternal long axis view transects the interventricular septum between the 11- and 12-o'clock positions (relative to the left ventricular short axis) along a line from its junction with the anterior aortic root to a point just proximal to its apical termination. This plane is ideally suited for (1) evaluating septal motion in an anteroposterior direction; (2) relating septal motion to aortic root motion, which is normally in the opposite direction; and (3) defining the hinge point at which these oppositely directed movements intersect.[85] This plane also permits the junction of the interventricular septum and anterior

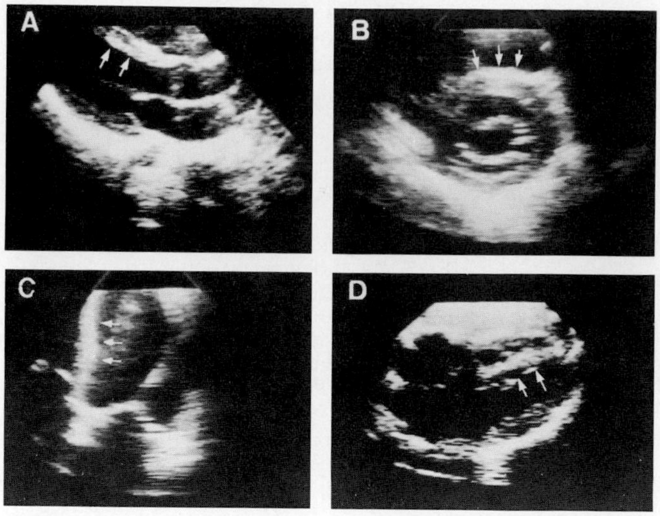

Fig. 29–19. Primary cross-sectional views used to record the interventricular septum. A. Parasternal long axis view. B. Parasternal short axis view. C. Apical four-chamber view. D. Subcostal long axis view. The position of the interventricular septum in each frame is indicated by the arrowheads.

aortic root to be recorded and larger defects in the membranous or bulbar septum to be visualized (particularly those associated with aortic overriding). Finally, this view is useful for defining diffuse and/or focal abnormalities of interventricular septal thickness.

The parasternal short axis view displays the anteroposterior arc of the septum and, as such, is the primary plane for recording changes in septal position and configuration as well as for detecting relative changes in left and right ventricular shape. Parasternal short axis recordings can be taken at any level from the base of the left ventricle to the apical extreme of the septum; however, changes in ventricular shape are most obvious at the base. This view is useful for visualizing the apically positioned interventricular septal aneurysms and septal defects associated with acute myocardial infarction and for recording the membranous aneurysms associated with congenital defect closure. The circumferential extent of septal involvement in ischemic heart disease is also best defined using this plane.

In the four-chamber view, the interventricular septum is visualized from the cardiac apex to its insertion into the interatrial septum at the base of the right and left ventricles. This plane is ideal for recording septal defects in the region of the atrioventricular canal as well as for recording the larger defects in the muscular septum. Muscular defects that are located toward the apex of the ventricle and are associated with acute myocardial infarction can, on occasion, also be recorded in this plane. The four-chamber view is also useful for defining the superior-inferior extent of dyssynergy in the midseptal plane.

The subcostal long-axis view of the interventricular septum is ideal for visualizing defects in the muscular portion of this membrane. In this view, the imaging plane is perpendicular to the path of the interventricular septum, and hence, defects should be clearly visualized. Because of the difficulty in locating small defects in the muscular septum, rotating the plane 90° and sweeping the interventricular septum from apex to base may be necessary. This combination of subcostal planes should provide the most detailed evaluation of the interventricular septum and should offer the greatest sensitivity for detection of muscular defects.

Interventricular Septal Thickness, Thickening, and Scar

The normal thickness of the interventricular septum (mean, 9 mm; range, 7 to 12 mm) is approximately the same as that of the left ventricular free wall[86] (mean, 10 mm; range, 7 to 12 mm) and is roughly three times that of the right ventricle.[1] The thickness of the septum is conventionally measured during mid-diastole between the rapid phase of diastolic relaxation and atrial contraction.[86] During systolic contraction, septal thickness normally increases. The peak systolic thickness of the septum can be compared to the diastolic measurement, and a percentage of thickening or thinning can be determined. The thickening characteristics of the septum can then be related to local myocardial performance.[86–88]

The diastolic thickness of the septum may increase with the rest of the left ventricle in response to chronic pressure loads, such as systolic hypertension or left ventricular outflow obstruction. Septal thickness may also increase in some of the infiltrative myopathies, including amyloidosis and hemochromatosis.

An increase in septal thickness disproportionate to that of the remainder of the left ventricle may also be noted. This increase is most frequently described in patients with idiopathic hypertrophic subaortic stenosis and has been considered the anatomic basis for that disorder.[89–91] The septum may also hypertrophy disproportionately to the left ventricular free wall in association with right ventricular hypertrophy.[91] Septal hypertrophy has also been reported occasionally in association with several other uncommon disorders including the glycogen storage disease Kearns-Sayre syndrome,[92] hypereosinophilic syndrome,[93] and acromegaly.[94] Abnormally thickened septum has been seen to result from the presence of a septal hematoma, localized abscess, echinococcus cyst, and septal fibroma. As a result, its diagnostic value as an isolated finding is limited.[91] Most of the specific causes of septal hypertrophy are discussed in detail elsewhere (see Chapter 25) and, therefore, are only mentioned in this section.

An abnormally thin septum is less common and, when noted, suggests septal scar formation following myocardial infarction.[95] The criteria for septal scar include (1) a mid-diastolic septal thickness of less than 7 mm; (2) an increase in echo production from the thinned septal area in comparison either to surrounding, more normal areas of septum or to the opposite ventricular wall; and (3) myocardium in the scarred area that is 30% thinner than adjacent areas. Using these criteria, scar was detected by echocardiography in 52 of 182 patients with coronary artery disease and was confirmed either pathologically or surgically in 95% of patients.[95] Surprisingly, in the absence of frank scar formation, the diastolic thickness of the septum remains within the normal range in most patients with both acute and chronic coronary artery disease and in congestive cardiomyopathy.[86,95]

In addition to baseline measurements of septal thickness, the thickening characteristics of the septum may provide useful information concerning regional left ventricular function. Left ventricular thickening may be determined at specific points along the ventricular wall or along serial radii drawn around the ventricular circumference.[96] Thickening measurements are particularly useful because they are generally independent of motion and are less critically dependent on the centroid placement in radial systems.

M-mode studies have shown that normal septal thickening averages 36% (range, 15 to 57%). Septal thickening has been reported to increase slightly in some patients with atrial septal defect[86] and was likewise noted to increase in 20% of patients with inferior wall infarcts.[86]

Septal thinning apparently occurs only with acute ischemia and has been reported in 30% of patients with acute infarcts.[86] Experimentally, systolic thinning is noted more frequently. In one study, systolic thinning was observed in 30 of 37 animals following acute coronary occlusion; reduced thickening was present in the remaining 7 animals.[87] This difference in clinical and experimental data probably represents the more precise sampling from the center of the ischemic region that can be achieved in the experimental setting. Figure 29–20 compares the normal pattern of septal motion and thickening to the decreased thickness and thickening seen in acute ischemic disease.

Decreased systolic thickening without actual thinning is frequently noted in patients with coronary artery disease and a history of prior myocardial infarction. It is also seen in patients with congestive cardiomyopathy. Abnormal thickening, however, is less common in patients *without* prior infarct histories, despite the angiographic presence of coronary artery disease.[86]

A decrease in the percentage of septal thickening has also been reported in idiopathic hypertrophic subaortic stenosis.[97,98] In view of the marked increase in baseline septal thickness, however, these abnormal changes may be less reflective of septal function.

Interventricular Septal Motion

The unique position of the interventricular septum between the right and left ventricles causes both septal orientation and movement to depend on the relative forces acting on its opposite surfaces. Normally, the interventricular septum is oriented and contracts such that it forms an integral part of the left ventricle, and its function in this context is discussed in Chapters 20 to 22. On occasion, however, the relative dynamics of the right and left ventricles may alter the movement and/or configuration of the septum such that it functions either partly or totally independent of the left ventricle or, at the extreme, as part of the right ventricle. Any analysis of septal movement may be further complicated by the fact that the septum may be primarily influenced by one chamber or set of forces during one portion of the cardiac cycle and by a completely different dynamic milieu at another. It is not surprising, therefore, that many different patterns of abnormal septal motion have been observed and that many clinical settings have been noted in which abnormal motion can occur.[99]

To recognize and understand the factors that underlie the various abnormal patterns of septal motion, one must first become familiar with the general mechanisms by which septal movement occurs. The septum can move (1) in response to the contraction and relaxation of the septal musculature; (2) as a result of motion of the left ventricle in space; and (3) in response to factors that change the position of the septum relative to the two ventricles and, therefore, change the shape of the ventricles themselves.

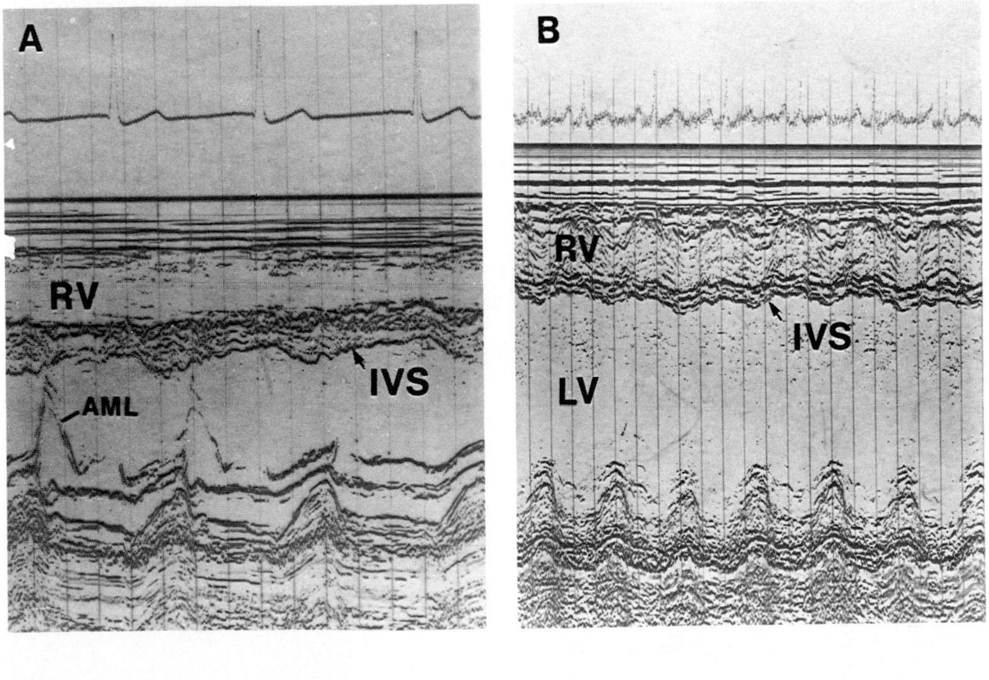

Fig. 29–20. M-mode recordings. **A.** The normal pattern of interventricular septal motion, thickness, and thickening. **B.** The decreased thickness, thickening, and excursion noted in a patient with acute anterior wall infarction. IVS = interventricular septum; RV = right ventricle; LV = left ventricle; AML = anterior mitral leaflet.

Before considering septal motion further, two additional points must be noted. First, this motion is considered relative to a fixed external reference (i.e., the anterior chest wall or transducer face). As discussed in Chapter 21, analysis of endocardial motion relative to the centroid of the left ventricle is preferred; however, this type of motion analysis is not currently practical in most laboratories, and the principles discussed in this section should apply irrespective of the reference used.

Second, motion does not always imply function. Thus, infarcted or scarred muscles may be pulled in a normal direction by surrounding normally contracting areas,[95] whereas normally contracting muscle may appear to move abnormally through one of the mechanisms discussed later.[6,100] As described in the preceding section, however, normal muscle thickens when it contracts, and its function can be inferred from its thickening characteristics. Once its functional status is determined, the reasons for a particular pattern of movement can then usually be elucidated.

Normal Septal Motion

Normal motion of the interventricular septum can best be appreciated in the short axis view of the left ventricle at the mitral valve level. In this view, the left ventricle appears circular, and the septum forms an arc representing approximately two-fifths of its circumference. Normal systolic contraction of the septal musculature displaces this arc inward toward its center of curvature, thereby contributing to the overall decrease in left ventricular circumference and cavity area. This direction of contraction is mandated by the concave orientation of the septum relative to the ventricular cavity because, if any muscle or series of muscles is fixed at both ends and positioned in an arc, muscular contraction must, by geometric necessity, displace the arc toward its center of curvature.

Figure 29–21B illustrates diagrammatically the normal short axis contraction sequence of the left ventricular endocardium from end-diastole to end-systole. Figure 29–21A is a comparable M-mode recording from contralateral points on the septum and posterior wall. In each of these figures, it is evident that the systolic excursion of the septum and that of the posterior wall are not equal. The difference in excursion is attributable to the second factor determining net septal motion (i.e., the spatial displacement of the left ventricle). Figure 29–22A illustrates the relative effects of myocardial contraction and the spatial motion of the heart on the recorded excursion of individual points on the anterior (septal) and posterior endocardial surfaces of the left ventricle. Because both of these components of motion have amplitude and direction, they can be represented as vectors. Thus, in this figure, a contraction vector (C) represents the amplitude and direction of endocardial motion resulting from active muscular contraction. Because both the anterior and posterior walls move inward toward the center of curvature of the ventricle, the contraction vectors of each wall are equal in amplitude but opposite in direction.

Also, a spatial vector (s) represents the overall motion of the left ventricle in space and has the same amplitude and direction relative to both the anterior and posterior walls. The net vector (N) represents the sum of the spatial and contraction vectors and, thus, the actual motion perceived from the anterior chest wall.

Normally, both the anterior and posterior walls contract equally (Fig. 29–22A); however, because the ventricle as a whole moves anteriorly in space, the spatial vector is added to the posterior wall contraction vector and is subtracted from the septal contraction vector. The net septal motion, therefore, is less than the corresponding posterior wall motion.

During diastole, this sequence is reversed; the septum moves anteriorly or away from the center of the left

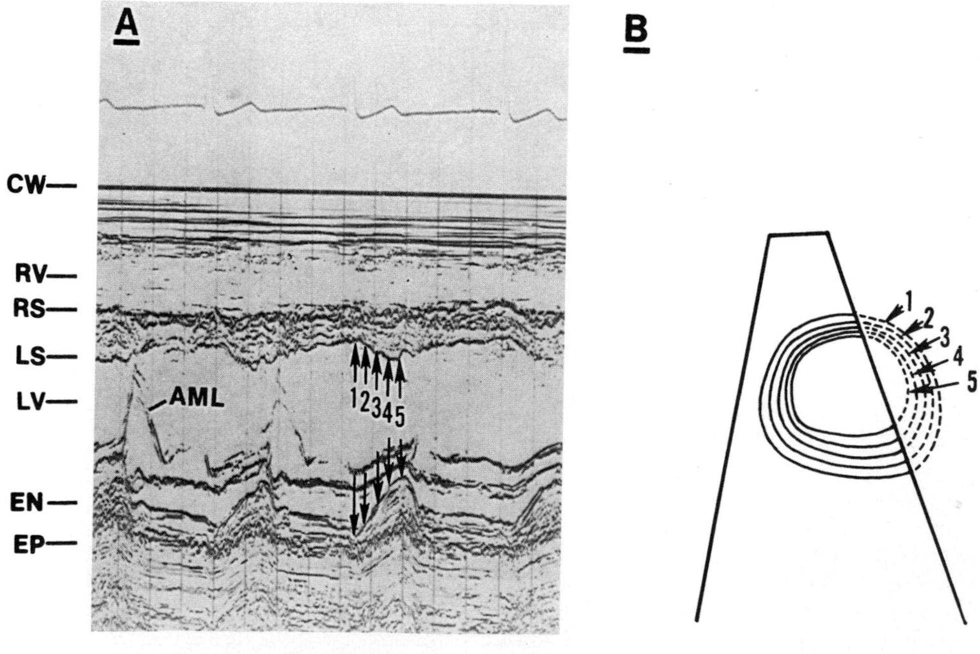

Fig. 29–21. **A.** M-mode recording of a normal left ventricle (LV) illustrates the patterns and the relative amplitudes of motion of the septum and posterior wall during normal ventricular contraction and relaxation. The vertical arrows indicate five selected points during the contraction sequence from end-diastole (1) to end-systole (5). **B.** A corresponding diagram illustrates the position of the left ventricular endocardium, viewed in short axis, at corresponding points in the contraction sequence. CW = chest wall; RV = right ventricle; RS = right septal interface; LS = left septal interface; EN = endocardium; EP = epicardium; AML = anterior mitral leaflet.

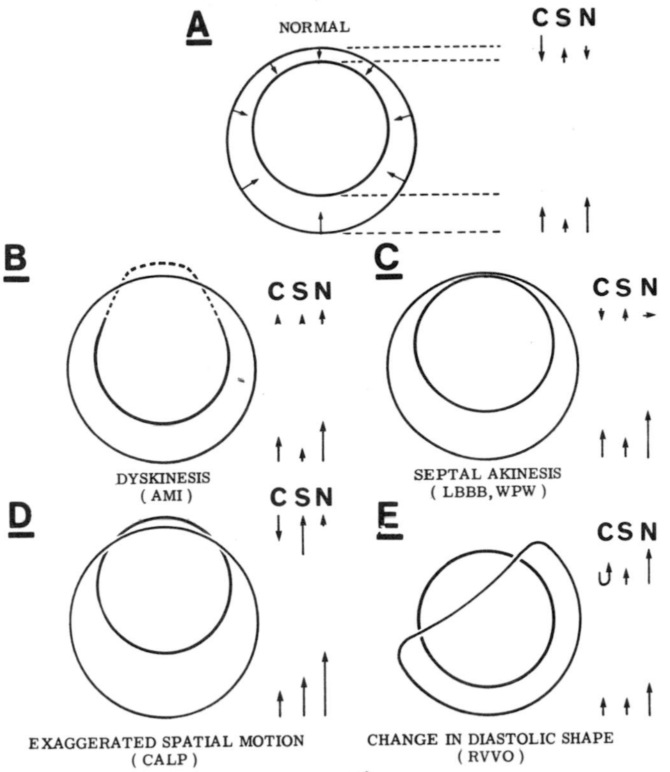

Fig. 29–22. Series of diagrams depicts the factors (expressed as vectors) that determine recorded interventricular septal motion. **A.** Normal contraction. **B.** Septal dyskinesis, as in anterior wall myocardial infarction (AMI). **C.** Septal akinesis, as in a left bundle branch block (LBBB) or Wolff-Parkinson-White (WPW) syndrome. **D.** Abnormal septal motion that is due to exaggerated anterior displacement of the left ventricle in space, as in congenital absence of the left pericardium (CALP) or large pericardial effusion. **E.** Abnormal septal motion that is due to a change in ventricular shape and septal position, as occurs in right ventricular volume overload (RVVO). C = contraction vector; S = spatial vector, which corresponds to the overall spatial movement of the heart; N = the net vector or sum of the spatial and contraction vectors.

ventricle, and its radius of curvature increases. Spatial movement of the left ventricle is posterior and, therefore, is again subtracted from the absolute septal displacement, thereby decreasing apparent or recorded septal motion.

Throughout the normal contraction and relaxation sequences, the ventricle retains its circular configuration, and the radius of curvature of the septum corresponds to that of the free wall. Changes of ventricular shape or septal position, therefore, do not affect normal contraction.

Abnormal Septal Motion

Abnormal septal motion may fall into one of three categories: (1) exaggerated or abnormally increased septal motion (septal hyperkinesis); (2) diminished or absent septal motion (hypokinesis or akinesis); or (3) paradoxic septal motion. Paradoxic septal motion is defined as motion that is opposite to the normally expected direction of septal movement. Thus, paradoxic systolic motion is anterior rather than posterior, whereas paradoxic diastolic motion is posterior rather than anterior. Dyskinetic motion may be classified as paradoxic, but the converse is not always true, because *dyskinesis* implies an abnormality of muscular function that is not inherent in the concept of paradoxic motion.

Exaggerated Septal Motion

Exaggerated septal motion occurs in two primary settings: (1) left ventricular volume overload and (2) compensatory hypercontraction in response to reduced function elsewhere in the ventricle. In left ventricular volume overload states, the primary increase in septal motion is due to an increase in muscular contraction. Note, however, that the amplitude of septal excursion frequently exceeds the corresponding motion of the posterior wall. This is the reverse of the normal relationship and suggests that the spatial vector has shifted and that systolic motion of the centroid of the left ventricle is now posterior. Consequently, the spatial vector is added to the septal contraction vector.

Exaggerated septal motion occurring as a compensation for reduced motion elsewhere is most frequently seen in ischemic heart disease and has been noted in as many as 65% of patients with acute inferior wall infarction.[86] Exaggerated septal motion also commonly occurs in children with anomalous origin of the left coronary artery and produces a characteristic left ventricular contraction pattern. This pattern includes hyperkinesis of the basal septum in association with extensive anterolateral hypokinesis. This prominent dissociation in regional motion draws attention to the underlying abnormality and is the primary echocardiographic sign suggestive of anomalous coronary artery (see Chapter 34). Likewise, in adults with diffuse ischemic disease and severe left ventricular dysfunction, a small area of the basal septum is frequently hyperdynamic. This small area of preserved function permits the segmental or ischemic cause of the dysfunction to be defined and a generalized cardiomyopathy to be excluded.

Diminished Septal Motion

Decreased septal excursion can be observed in a variety of disorders, including ischemic heart disease, various forms of cardiomyopathy, and infiltrative disease of the septum, and as a result of delayed or asynchronous septal contraction caused by abnormal electrical activation. In each of these disorders, the decrease in septal movement represents a decrease in the contraction vector (Fig. 29–22C). The spatial motion of the ventricle is rarely abnormal, and the position or shape of the interventricular septum is not markedly distorted. In the majority of these cases, there is corresponding hypofunction of other areas of the ventricle. In some patients, however, diminished septal motion may represent one end of a spectrum in which severe expression is characterized by paradoxic septal motion. The operative factors in this situation are discussed in the next section.

Paradoxic Septal Motion

If contraction of the normal concave interventricular septum must be inward toward the diastolic center of septal curvature (or posteriorly relative to the anterior chest wall), paradoxic motion must be passive and can theoretically occur in only one of three ways: (1) as a result of septal dyskinesis; (2) as a result of exaggerated motion of the entire left ventricle in space; or (3) as a result of change in septal shape or configuration from diastole to systole.

Both mechanisms (1) and (3) may be associated with a change in ventricular shape. In the former, however, the affected muscle does not function normally, whereas in the latter, a normally functioning septum is compelled to move in an abnormal direction by a shift in its spatial configuration.

Paradoxic movement of the septum is generally viewed as a systolic phenomenon because the functional activity of the septum occurs during systole. There is generally also a diastolic component, which, in the instances of dyskinesis and exaggerated motion of the ventricle in space, merely reflects return of the septum to the normal basal position. When septal and ventricular shape change, however, the diastolic abnormality may be predominant, and the paradoxic systolic movement is then merely a secondary response. *As a general rule, any movement of the septum that is more rapid than the peak velocity of normal systolic muscular contraction is passive and is associated with some change in septal position and, hence, ventricular shape.*

In several situations, paradoxic septal motion may be confined to a specific portion of the cardiac cycle (usually diastole) and may not be associated with any alteration in systolic motion or function.

Septal Dyskinesis (Systole). Septal dyskinesis resulting from myocardial ischemia is the simplest situation and is illustrated in Figure 29–22B. In this setting, the septum fails to contract actively and is pushed outward by the developing left ventricular intracavitary pressure. The "contraction vector," therefore, is anterior or paradoxic. The ischemic muscle is stretched, and the wall either fails to thicken normally or thins slightly, indicating that the muscle is functioning abnormally. The left ventricle moves anteriorly in space, and the spatial vector is anteriorly directed and normal in amplitude. The spatial vector, therefore, is added to the anterior or paradoxic movement of the ischemic region and to the normal anteriorly directed contraction vector of the posterior wall, thereby increasing the apparent movement of both regions.

A similar, though less dramatic example, occurs with septal akinesis or hypokinesis (Fig. 29–22C). In this setting, septal contraction is diminished or absent, and the contraction vector is also absent or decreased. The anterior motion of the left ventricle in space, however, persists. When the anterior spatial motion equals the diminished septal contraction, no motion is perceived relative to the anterior chest wall. When the contraction vector exceeds the spatial vector, slight or hypokinetic movement may be noted, whereas spatial motion in excess of septal contraction results in paradoxic septal motion relative to the external reference point.

Paradoxic Septal Motion as a Result of Exaggerated Motion of the Left Ventricle in Space. Exaggerated motion of the left ventricle in space is apparent in such conditions as moderate or large pericardial effusion and congenital absence of the left pericardium in which the normal pericardial restraint on the heart is lost. In these disorders, although contraction of both the anterior and posterior walls is normal, the increase in spatial cardiac movement is so marked that the spatial vector greatly exceeds contraction, and net septal motion is, therefore, anterior or paradoxic (Fig. 29–22D). The fact that the septal musculature is contracting normally despite its abnormal movement in space can be determined by the normal pattern of systolic muscular thickening.

Increased spatial cardiac movement has also been postulated to at least partially underlie the paradoxic septal motion noted following open-heart surgery.[101] Studies of the overall excursion of the posterior wall epicardium suggest exaggerated anterior motion of the entire heart in space with resulting paradoxic septal motion. This has been related to sternal adhesions, which fix the anterior right ventricular wall and cause the heart to assume a "teardrop" shape during diastole and an exaggerated anterior motion during systole as it returns to a more normal configuration. This hypothesis, however, does not explain the more recent observation of paradoxic septal motion occurring within 15 minutes to hours after surgery[102,103] or the tendency toward resolution with time.[104,105] Alternatively, the disruption of the structures in the anterior mediastinum following median sternotomy has been postulated to allow the entire heart to shift anteriorly during systole.[106] The development of postoperative adhesions could gradually replace the loss of extracardiac restraint and account for the resolution of the abnormal septal motion with time. In a 1990 study, interventricular septal motion was monitored by using continuous transesophageal echocardiographic imaging during cardiac surgery.[103] This study showed that median sternotomy, sternal retraction, or pericardiotomy did not induce altered septal motion. However, after discontinuation of cardiopulmonary bypass and before chest closure, markedly decreased or paradoxic septal motion and hyperkinesis of the posterolateral segments were noted, consistent with anterior translation of the heart. This suggests that abnormal postoperative interventricular septal motion may be related to events occurring during cardiopulmonary bypass rather than resulting from removal of restraining forces of the pericardium or anterior mediastinum. The role of localized septal ischemia in the pathogenesis of this phenomenon is unclear; however, most studies do not report electrocardiographic changes or increased myocardial enzyme release in the vast majority of the patients studied.[103,107] Thus, postoperative septal motion is a complex and multifactorial problem that remains poorly understood.

Paradoxic Septal Motion Due to Changes in Left Ventricular Shape. Paradoxic motion of the interventricular septum resulting from a change in the left ventricular shape may affect both the systolic and diastolic phases of the cardiac cycle or be confined to diastole alone. Functionally, isolated paradoxic diastolic septal motion (and by interference and abnormal shape change) should affect only ventricular compliance, whereas paradoxic systolic and diastolic motion may affect both compliance and systolic function.

Paradoxic Systolic and Diastolic Motion. The final method by which the interventricular septum can move paradoxically during systole is through the rearrangement of a shape abnormality that originated during the diastolic filling phase.[6,108–110] During diastole, when the ventricle is fully relaxed, the interventricular septum essentially behaves as a passive membrane between two fluid-filled chambers. Normally, left ventricular diastolic pressure exceeds right ventricular diastolic pressure (LVP > RVP), and the interventricular septum is convex toward the right ventricle. However, when the diastolic interventricular pressure gradient decreases or reverses (RVP > LVP), diastolic bulging of the upper portion of the interventricular septum toward the left ventricle occurs.[108] The degree of end-diastolic displacement of the interventricular septum has been demonstrated to correlate closely with the end-diastolic transeptal gradient.[109] This phenomenon occurs most frequently in right ventricular volume overload and is diagrammed in Figure 29–22E and illustrated in Figure 29–23. This example shows marked right ventricular volume overload that is due to pulmonary insufficiency. During diastole, the increased right ventricular volume displaces the interventricular septum away from the right ventricle and causes it to bow inward toward the left ventricle (Fig. 29–23A and B). This leftward shift of the interventricular septum at end-diastole is determined by the decrease or reversal of the normal transeptal pressure gradient. At the onset of systole, the left ventricular intracavitary pressure rises rapidly and exceeds simultaneous right ventricular intracavitary pressure. This positive left-to-right pressure gradient shifts the septum toward a more normal orientation, which is concave toward the left ventricle, and causes the left ventricle to return to a more circular configuration (in the absence of right ventricular systolic hypertension) (Fig. 29–23C). This rearrangement of ventricular shape has the effect of thrusting the septum into the right ventricular cavity (paradoxically) and might theoretically contribute to right ventricular ejection.

Figure 29–24A is an M-mode recording that demonstrates this type of paradoxic septal motion. Figure 29–24B illustrates the left ventricular endocardial contraction sequence underlying this motion. These companion figures suggest that the primary rearrangement in shape occurs early in systole during isovolumic abrupt upward movement of the interventricular septum. During the later phases of systole, anterior movement of the ventricle continues as a result of an exaggeration of the spatial vector. The fact that the septal myocardium functions normally can again be ascertained by observing the preserved pattern of septal thickening.

Several points should be emphasized about this type of systolic change in ventricular shape. First, as previously mentioned, the primary abnormality is diastolic not systolic. The apparent abnormal systolic motion merely represents a rearrangement or normalization of left ventricular shape. This rearrangement corrects a distortion that occurred during diastole because of the unequal filling of the two ventricles, resulting in a decrease or reversal of the normal diastolic transeptal gradient. Second, the degree of distortion appears to have some

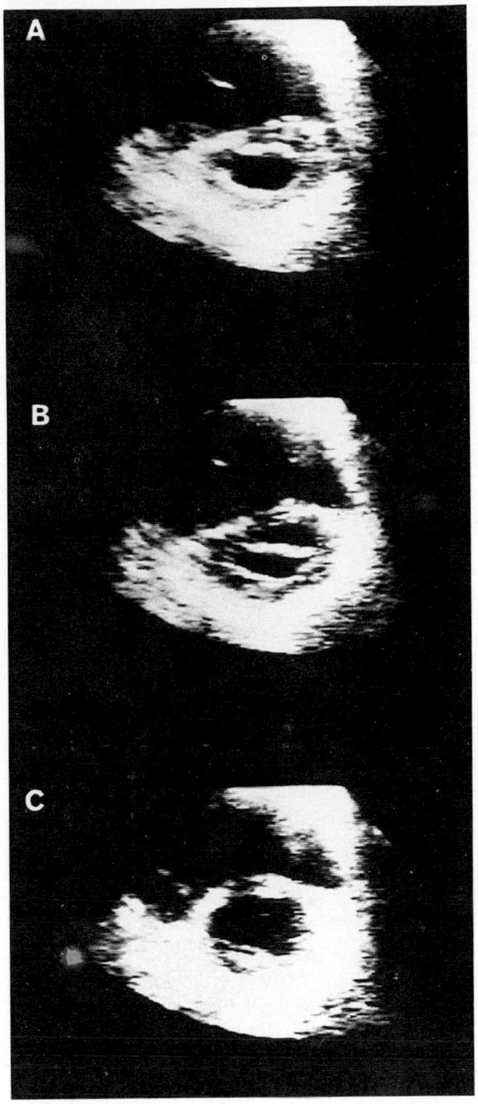

Fig. 29–23. Short axis, cross-sectional recording of the left ventricle at the mitral valve level illustrates the variation in ventricular shape and septal position from diastole to systole. Such variation is characteristic of a right ventricular volume overload. **A.** Recorded during initial diastole. The right ventricle is dilated, and the septum is displaced to the left and flattened. The mitral valve is fully open. **B.** Recorded later in diastole. The left ventricular cavity area is slightly larger. The mitral valve is in a resting position, and the septum remains flattened and displaced to the left. **C.** Recorded during ventricular systole. The left ventricle is more circular, the mitral valve is closed, and the septum has shifted to the right (paradoxically) and is now more convex toward the right ventricle.

relationship to both the degree and the type of right ventricular volume overload. In patients with isolated right ventricular volume overloads, such as tricuspid insufficiency and pulmonary insufficiency, the septum appears to be more markedly displaced, and the left ventricle appears more distorted. The septal distortion may not be as great in the right ventricular volume overload associated with atrial septal defect. It has been suggested that the atrial septal defect itself may play a protective role, because as the right ventricle becomes deformed, right ventricular compliance decreases. As a result,

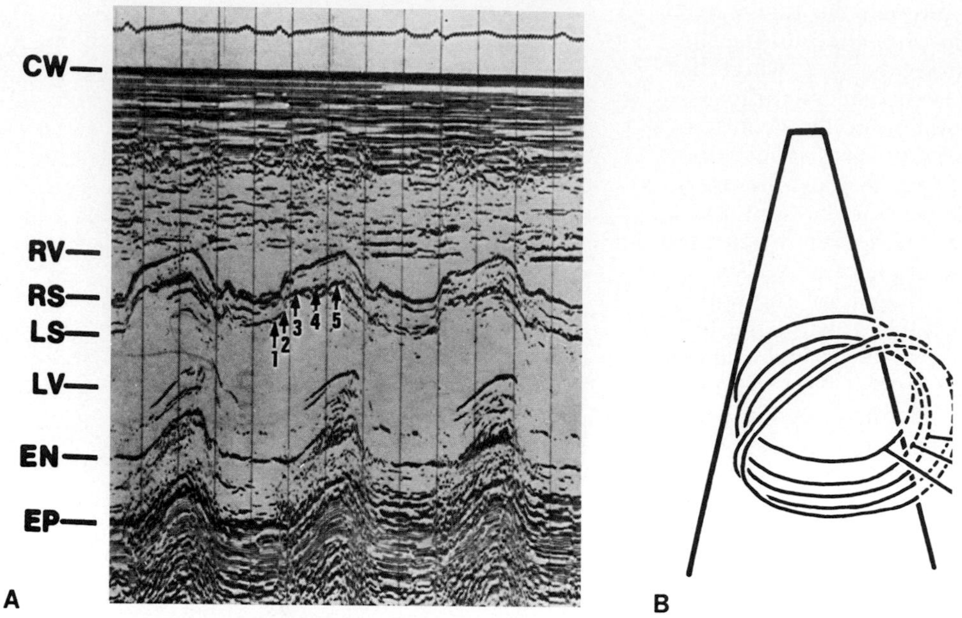

Fig. 29–24. **A.** M-mode recording illustrates paradoxic septal motion in a patient with right ventricular volume overload. An abrupt, initial, anterior (paradoxic) motion of the septum corresponds to the change in ventricular shape that occurs in early systole. This initial rapid movement is followed by a more gradual continued anterior or paradoxic septal motion. The septal muscle thickness normally, indicating preservation of myocardial function. **B.** Diagram illustrates the corresponding short axis motion from end-diastole (1) to end-systole (5). CW = chest wall; RV = right ventricle; RS = right septal interface; LS = left septal interface; LV = left ventricle; EN = endocardium; EP = epicardium. (From Weyman AE, et al.: Mechanism of abnormal septal motion in patients with right ventricular volume overload. Circulation 54:9, 1976. Reproduced by permission of the American Heart Association, Inc.)

more blood is preferentially shunted into the left ventricle, and further septal deformity is retarded. Third, the position and shape of the interventricular septum at end-diastole are determined by the transeptal pressure gradient. A decrease in, or reversal of this gradient causes a leftward shift of the interventricular septum at end-diastole and results in paradoxic septal motion as it returns to its normal configuration during systole.[108,109]

In systole, however, the degree to which the septum returns to normal relates roughly to the relative pressures in the two ventricles. Thus, with right-sided systolic hypertension, the septum appears to retain much of its abnormal diastolic configuration and to remain flattened during systole (Fig. 29–25).[111] A quantitative relationship has been demonstrated between the alteration in septal configuration, expressed as a normalized septal

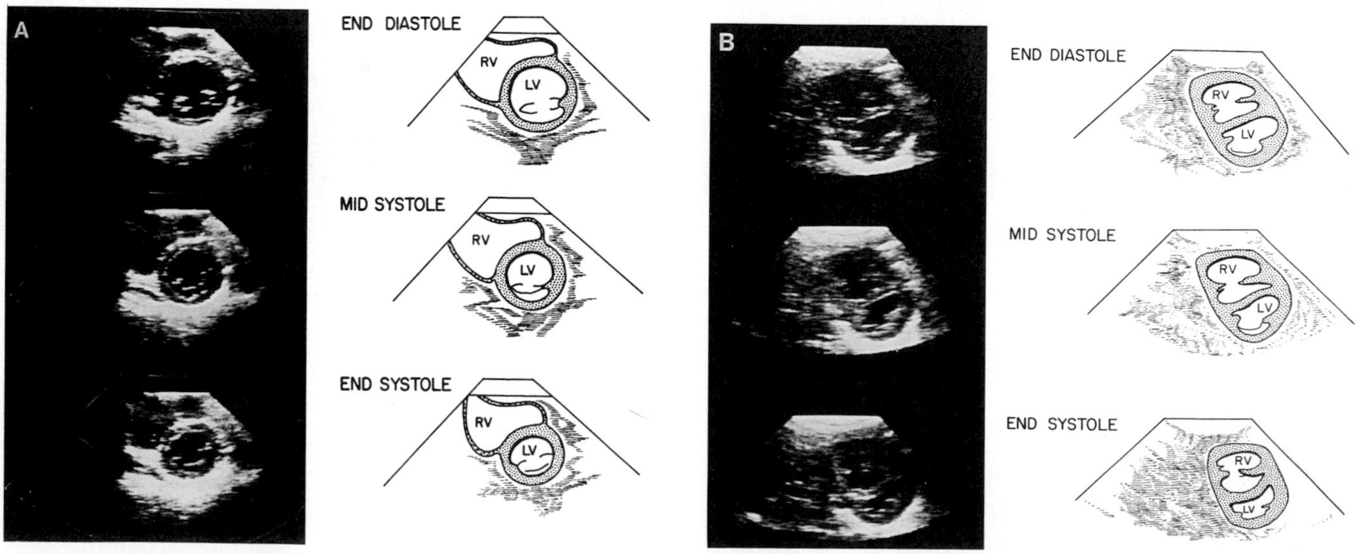

Fig. 29–25. **A.** Parasternal short axis stop-frame images of the left ventricle in a normal person at end-diastole, midsystole, and end-systole. The typical rounded configuration of the interventricular septum is demonstrated throughout the cardiac cycle. **B.** Parasternal short axis images of the left ventricle in a patient with suprasystemic right ventricular pressures. The interventricular septum is flattened at end-diastole, and at end-systole it reverses its curvature to become convex toward the left ventricle. LV = left ventricle; RV = right ventricle. (From King ME, et al.: Interventricular septal configuration as a predictor of right ventricular systolic hypertension in children: a cross-sectional echocardiographic study. Circulation 68:68, 1983. Reproduced by permission of the American Heart Association, Inc.)

curvature, $1/(r/r_i)$, and the severity of right ventricular systolic hypertension.[112] A slight leftward shift and flattening of the interventricular septum occurs in the course of normal contraction (Fig. 29–25A). However, marked exaggeration of this configurational change occurs in patients with right ventricular systolic hypertension, with progressive loss of septal curvature from end-diastole to end-systole (Fig. 29–25B). The normalized septal curvature at end-systole showed a good correlation (r = .86) with the relative right ventricular systolic pressure.

A shift in septal position has also been noted during Müller's maneuver (forced inspiration against a closed airway).[113,114] This maneuver causes a transient increase in right ventricular loading and a decrease in left-to-right ventricular transeptal gradient throughout diastole. This decreased diastolic transeptal gradient is associated with a leftward shift in interventricular septal position. In this setting, the septum also transiently fails to return to a normal systolic configuration despite a large left-to-right ventricular systolic pressure gradient, thereby implying an altered systolic relationship between the two chambers.[113,114] Finally, the degree of deformity is greatest at the base of the heart and decreases toward the apex. This predominant basal deformity is illustrated in Figure 29–26 and can be explained by the simple relationship: force = pressure × area. Because the area at the base is greatest, it has the greatest force acting on it and should, therefore, show the greatest degree of deformity.

Paradoxic Diastolic Septal Motion. Isolated paradoxic diastolic septal motion is seen in several conditions, the most common of which are mitral stenosis and aortic insufficiency.

Mitral Stenosis. Isolated paradoxic diastolic septal motion occurs most prominently in patients with mitral stenosis.[115,116] Figure 29–27 is an M-mode recording from a patient with mitral stenosis. In this example, the septum moves abruptly, paradoxically or posteriorly, at the onset of diastole. This motion is more rapid than the peak rate of normal septal contraction and, thus, according to the concepts discussed previously, should be passive. Such movement also results in a decrease in the transverse diameter of the left ventricle when the ventricle should be actively filling. This disparity suggests that the geometric shape of the ventricle must be changing for one of the minor ventricular axes to decrease while ventricular volume is increasing.

Figure 29–28 contains a series of short axis cross-sectional scans of the left ventricle from initial diastole to end-diastole from a patient with mitral stenosis. This figure illustrates this predicted change in shape. At end-

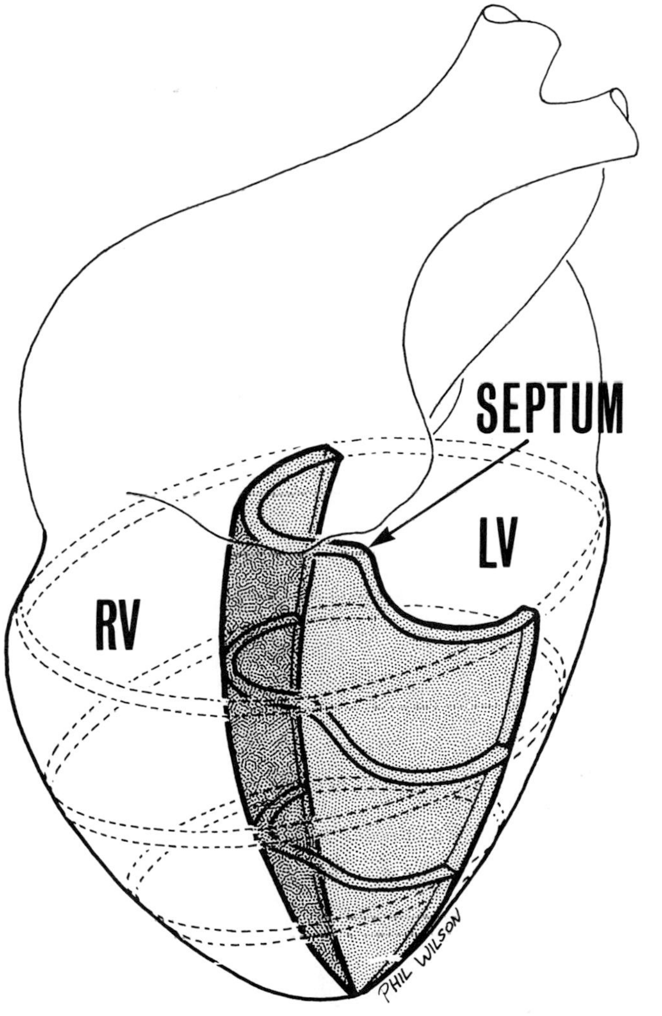

Fig. 29–26. Comparison of the relative degree of septal displacement at the base and apex of the heart in right ventricular volume overload states. The degree of septal displacement and corresponding change in left ventricular shape is relatively greater at the base and gradually decreases toward the apex. RV = right ventricle; LV = left ventricle. (From Weyman AE, et al.: Mechanism of abnormal septal motion in patients with right ventricular volume overload. Circulation 54:9, 1976. Reproduced by permission of the American Heart Association, Inc.)

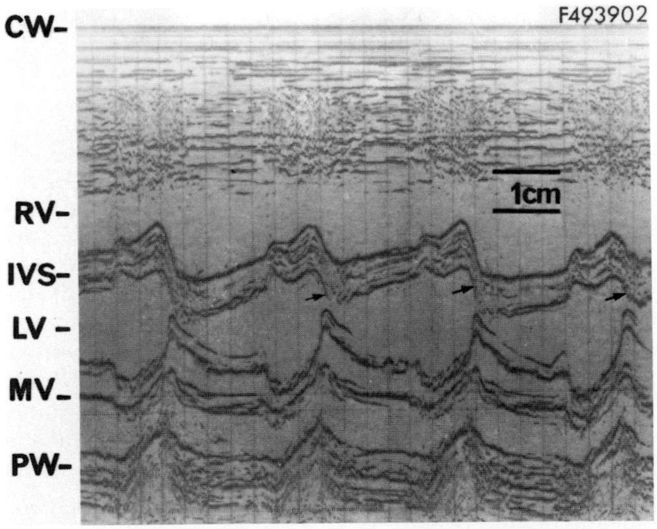

Fig. 29–27. M-mode recording of the left ventricle (LV) and the interventricular septum (IVS) from a patient with mitral stenosis illustrates prominent initial paradoxic diastolic septal motion (arrows). This motion corresponds to mitral valve (MV) opening and exceeds the peak posterior excursion of the septum during systolic contraction. CW = chest wall; RV = right ventricle; PW = posterior wall.

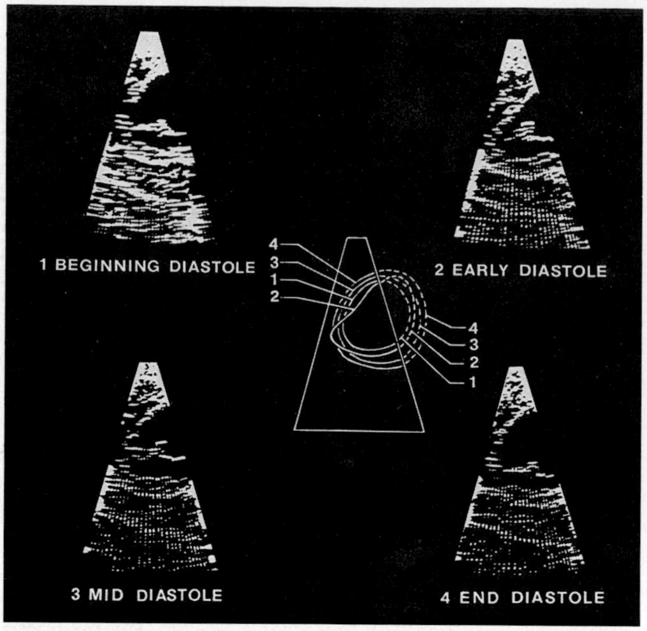

Fig. 29–28. Serial, diastolic, short axis, cross-sectional recordings of the left ventricle from a patient with mitral stenosis and prominent septal motion abnormality. **1.** At end-systolic or beginning-diastole, the left ventricle has a relatively circular configuration. **2.** In the initial portion of diastole, immediately after opening of the mitral valve, the position of the interventricular septum shifts away from the right ventricle and toward the left ventricle. This movement alters the shape of the left ventricle during initial diastole. **3** and **4.** Throughout the remainder of diastole, the left ventricle gradually fills, and septal position shifts back toward the right ventricle and away from the left ventricle. At end-diastole, the ventricle has returned to its normal circular configuration. Systolic contraction then proceeds in a normal fashion. Center. The relative positions of the endocardial surface of the left ventricle are outlined from end-systole to end-diastole. Between positions 1 and 2, left ventricular diastolic shape changes abruptly. In positions 3 and 4, the ventricle gradually returns toward its normal circular configuration. (From Weyman AE, et al.: Mechanism of paradoxical early diastolic septal motion in patients with mitral stenosis: a cross-sectional endocardiographic study. Am J Cardiol 40:691, 1977.)

systole, the ventricle is circular. At the onset of diastole, however, the septum abruptly shifts inward toward the center of the left ventricular cavity and returns toward a more normal position. By end-diastole, the ventricular shape is circular, and systolic contraction proceeds in a normal sequence and direction.

The position of the septum throughout diastole in patients with mitral stenosis is highly correlated with the instantaneous transeptal pressure gradient.[116] The initial diastolic shift in the position of the septum in mitral stenosis has been demonstrated to result from an inequality in filling of the two ventricles during early diastole.[115] This inequality occurs because the stenotic mitral valve delays left ventricular filling, whereas the right ventricle fills at a normal rate. This produces a relative right ventricular volume overload with a relative increase in right ventricular pressure and shifts the septum to the left. Because the volume that can be accepted by one ventricle at any given filling pressure has been shown to be related directly to the degree of filling of the other, the initial diastolic compliance of the right ventricle may increase because of the partially empty left ventricle.[117] This may create not only a relative but also an absolute right ventricular volume overload. As the left ventricle slowly fills, the normal transeptal gradient is reestablished, and the septum returns toward a more normal position.[116] Left ventricular filling, however, occurs when the right ventricle is already fully distended. Left ventricular compliance, therefore, may be relatively decreased, and a greater filling pressure may be required to introduce a normal diastolic volume.

The degree of initial diastolic septal displacement in mitral stenosis has been shown to relate to the severity of the stenotic lesion and to be absent with tricuspid stenosis.[115] Figure 29–29 shows the relationship between varying rates of the left ventricular filling and the severity of this paradoxic septal movement. Figure

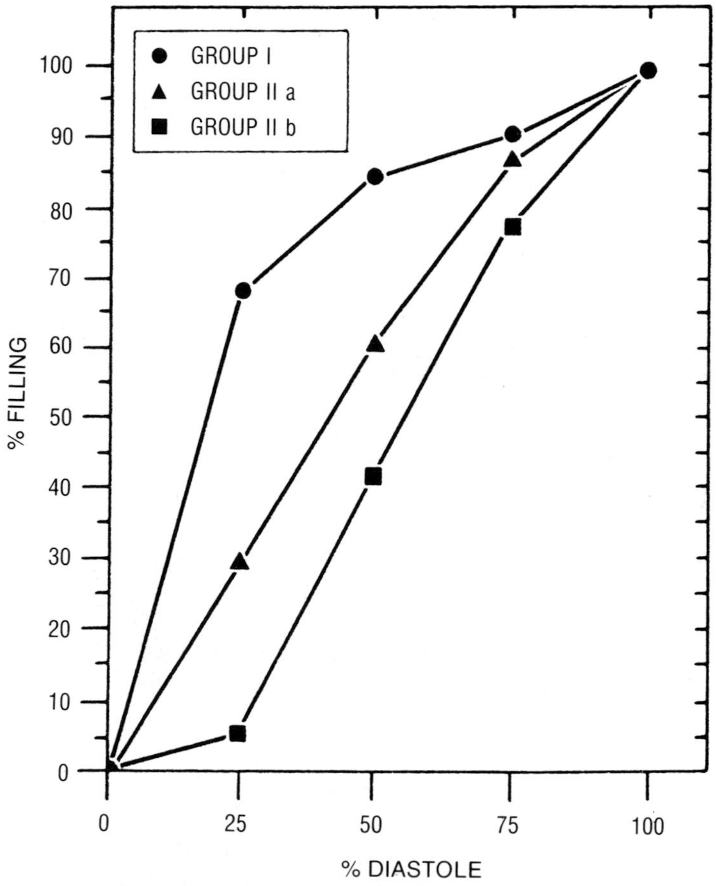

Fig. 29–29. Relative rates of left ventricular filling in normal patients (group I), patients with mitral stenosis with minimal septal motion abnormality (group IIa), and patients with mitral stenosis with more severe septal motion abnormality (group IIb). The rate of diastolic filling of the left ventricle is significantly different between group I and groups IIa and IIb at each of the first three quarters of diastole. In addition, the difference between groups IIa and IIb is significant in the first quarter of diastole. (From Weyman AE, et al.: Mechanism of paradoxical early diastolic septal motion in patients with mitral stenosis: a cross-sectional endocardiographic study. Am J Cardiol 40:691, 1977.)

29–30 compares the right and left ventricular angiographic filling rates for each quarter of diastole (normalized to 100%) to septal motion in a patient with both mitral stenosis and a right ventricular volume overload. In each example the interdependence of septal motion on right and left ventricular filling patterns is evident.

Aortic Insufficiency. Another disorder associated with a unique pattern of paradoxic diastolic septal motion is aortic insufficiency. In aortic insufficiency, there is frequently an abrupt anterior movement of the septum at end-systole followed by a second downward or paradoxic displacement at the onset of ventricular diastole (Fig. 29–31). Both of these movements are more rapid than can be accounted for by active contraction and, therefore, should be passive. It has been suggested that the initial upward movement is due to the regurgitant flow through the aortic valve, which begins immediately following aortic valve closure. This flow causes the left ventricular cavity to expand during left-sided isovolumic relaxation before tricuspid valve opening. Once the tricuspid valve opens and right ventricular filling begins, the septum is then displaced toward the left ventricle. This paradoxic septal displacement may appear unusual in the setting of a left ventricular volume overload; however, one must remember that the total left ventricular volume in aortic insufficiency accumulates throughout diastole. Initial diastolic inflow, therefore, may represent a relatively smaller than normal percentage of end-diastolic ventricular volume. Thus, there may be a comparative right ventricular volume overload in initial diastole because the initial right ventricular inflow represents a greater percentage of end-diastole right ventricular volume than does the comparable initial left ventricular inflow.

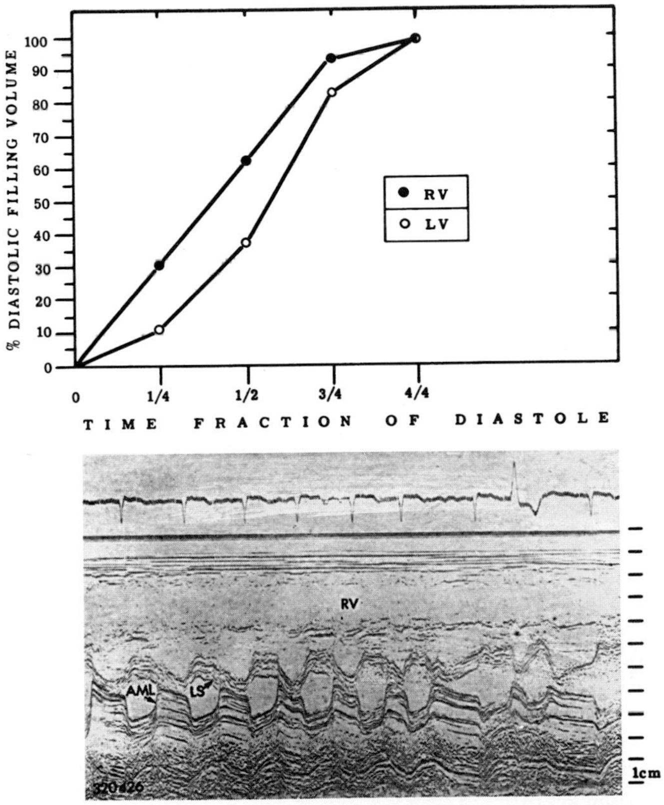

Fig. 29–30. Top. Comparative right and left ventricular filling rates (at each quarter of diastole) normalized to 100% filling in a patient with combined mitral stenosis and right ventricular overload. Bottom. An M-mode echocardiographic recording from the same patient illustrates the abnormal septal motion that occurs as a result of this discrepancy in relative ventricular filling. AML = anterior mitral leaflet; LS = left septal interface; RV = right ventricle; LV = left ventricle.

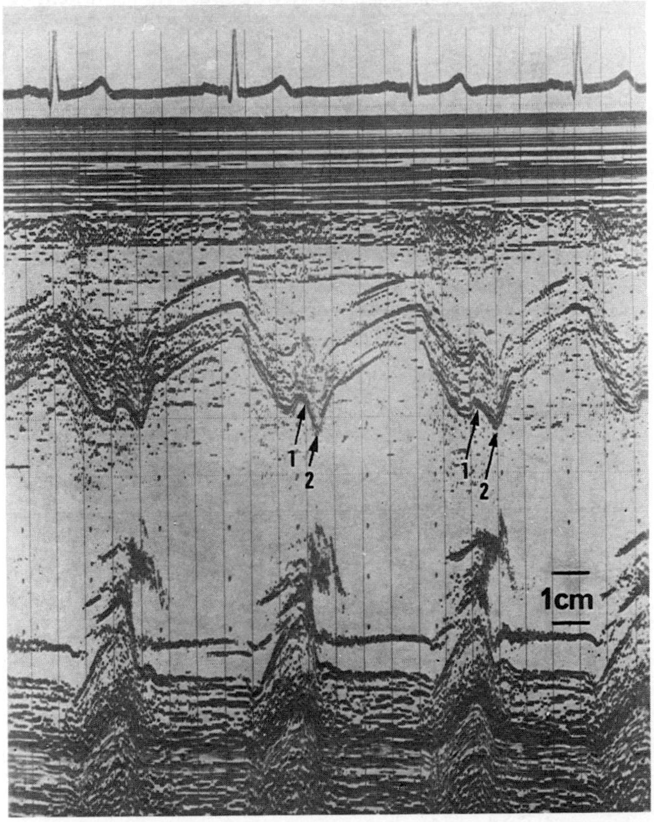

Fig. 29–31. M-mode recording of the interventricular septum and aortic insufficiency. The characteristic pattern in these cases is an abrupt anterior motion of the septum at end-ventricular systole (arrow 1) followed by a rapid downward or paradoxic motion of the septum at the onset of ventricular diastole (vertical arrow 2).

Left Bundle Branch Block

These principles can be used to approach other abnormalities of septal motion. In left bundle branch block, for example, a characteristic feature is an abrupt downward or posterior movement of the interventricular septum almost coincident with the onset of the QRS complex (the so-called septal beak).[118,119] This movement is usually small and occurs at a rate beyond that associated with active contraction. If one assumes that, because of the conduction delay, isovolumic contraction in the right ventricle precedes isovolumic contraction in the left ventricle, this motion may represent passive movement of the septum in response to the unopposed initial increase in right ventricular pressure. Once the left ventricle contracts, this minimal derangement of shape is rapidly corrected, and septal motion then depends on the relative magnitudes of the contraction and spatial vectors.

Discussion of all the possible ways in which the septum can move paradoxically or abnormally is clearly beyond the scope of this text. It is hoped, however, that these simple principles will aid the reader in analyzing the various components of abnormal septal motion when it is encountered. Although most of these phenomena have been described and are best depicted using the M-mode format, they can be seen interrupting the normally symmetric contraction and relaxation sequence of the left ventricle during cross-sectional studies. An understanding of the mechanisms underlying these abnormal movements therefore appears warranted.

Ventricular Septal Defects

Ventricular septal defect is the most common congenital malformation of the heart, occurring in between 1.3 and 2.4% of live births.[120] These defects may occur as isolated lesions; may form an integral part of a more complex anomaly, such as tetralogy of Fallot or truncus arteriosus; or may be associated with, but not anatomically related to, other cardiac anomalies.[121] Isolated ventricular septal defects represent approximately 23% of all instances of congenital heart disease, but ventricular septal defects are present in approximately 50% of all congenital anomalies of the heart.[120]

Anatomy

Anatomically, ventricular septal defects are conventionally divided at the level of the crista supraventricularis into supracristal and infracristal defects. The supracristal defects (also called infundibular defects), lie immediately below the pulmonary valve, and the valve typically forms the superior margin of the defect (Fig. 29–32). They appear in an area of the interventricular septum that is normally closed by downward growth of the bulbar septum and represent incomplete development of this membrane. Viewed from the left side of the heart, they are positioned immediately inferior to the commissure between the left and right aortic cusps.[120] Infracristal defects, as a group, are found inferior and posterior to the crista and can be subdivided into those that encompass or are contiguous with the membranous septum (the membranous septal defects), those within the muscular septum that are completely surrounded by muscular tissue (muscular septal defects), and those that arise in the site that the defect would occupy if it were part of an endocardial cushion malformation (inlet septal defects) (Fig. 29–32).

The most common of these defects is the membranous defect. Although referred to as *membranous* because of their anatomic association with the membranous septum, these defects generally include a portion of the muscular septum. This loss of muscular tissue may constitute the major portion of the lesion.[121] When viewed from the left side of the heart, membranous defects lie beneath the commissure between the right and noncoronary aortic cusps. Muscular defects may arise anywhere in the muscular septum. They may be small or large, single or multiple. On occasion, the septum may be thin and may contain multiple sieve-like fenestrations. In other instances, small sinoidal passages may be threaded among the septal trabeculae. From a functional standpoint, multiple small defects appear to have the same significance as do single large defects.[122,123]

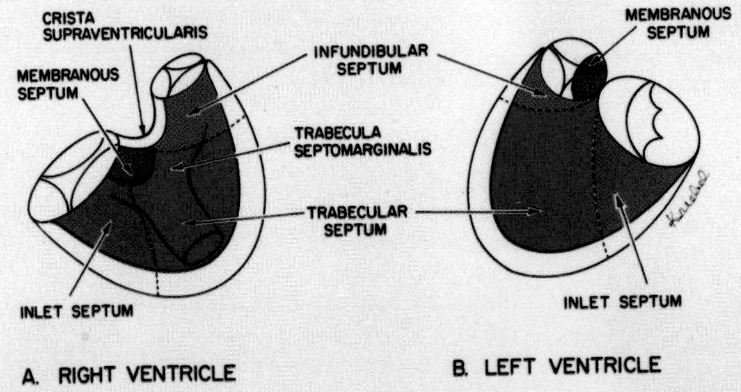

Fig. 29–32. The interventricular septum. **A.** Viewed from the right ventricular side. **B.** The left ventricular side. The muscular septum colored in blue, the atrioventricular inlet septum in green, the membranous septum in red, and the infundibular or supracristal septum in orange.

An uncommon form of ventricular septal defect (the Gerbode defect) is characterized by an abnormal communication between the left ventricle and the right atrium with left ventricular-to-right atrial shunt flow. This rare septal defect can occur as a result of the more apical location of the tricuspid annulus versus the annulus of the mitral valve and is sometimes seen as a complication after mitral or tricuspid valve surgery. It is also unique among ventricular septal defects in that it produces an obligatory right ventricular volume overload because the entire shunt volume is returned to the right ventricle during diastole.

Although the majority of ventricular septal defects are congenital, acquired ventricular communications can occur as a complication following myocardial infarction.[124] These defects are almost always located in the muscular septum, and differentiation from mitral regurgitation due to papillary muscle dysfunction in acute myocardial infarction is essential. Acquired ventricular septal defects have also been seen after penetrating chest trauma and have been reported to be due to septal perforation with a pacing wire.

Echocardiographic and Doppler Evaluation

Ventricular septal defects are often clinically apparent, and the echocardiographic examination, therefore, is directed toward defining their location, size, and association with other lesions. Nonspecific assessment of the presence of the defect based on the sequelae of the left-to-right shunt (the left ventricular volume overload pattern), therefore, is of secondary diagnostic importance. In contrast, the atrial septal defect is itself clinically silent, and its presence must be initially inferred from the effects of the lesion on the right ventricle and atrium (the right ventricular volume overload pattern).[6,25–27] Once recorded, however, the echocardiographic appearance of defects in both the atrial and ventricular septa are similar and are characterized by a focal discontinuity or area of "dropout" in the normally continuous linear band of echoes arising from the intact septum.

Qualitative Assessment of Ventricular Septal Defects

Two-Dimensional Echocardiographic Imaging. Echocardiographic ventricular septal defect recording can be achieved in a variety of imaging planes; however, the parasternal long axis, the apical four-chamber, and the subcostal long axis views are the most commonly used for this purpose (Fig. 29–33). Supracristal defects are probably best visualized in a parasternal short axis view because of their atypical leftward position.

Success rates for visualization of isolated ventricular septal defects by two-dimensional echocardiography have ranged from 74[125] to 88%[126] in prospective studies and from 88[127] to 100%[128] in patients with known ventricular septal defect. False-negatives have been noted primarily in patients with small defects[125–127] and/or as a result of failure to visualize a second lesion in a patient with multiple defects.

The relative value of individual views in recording de-

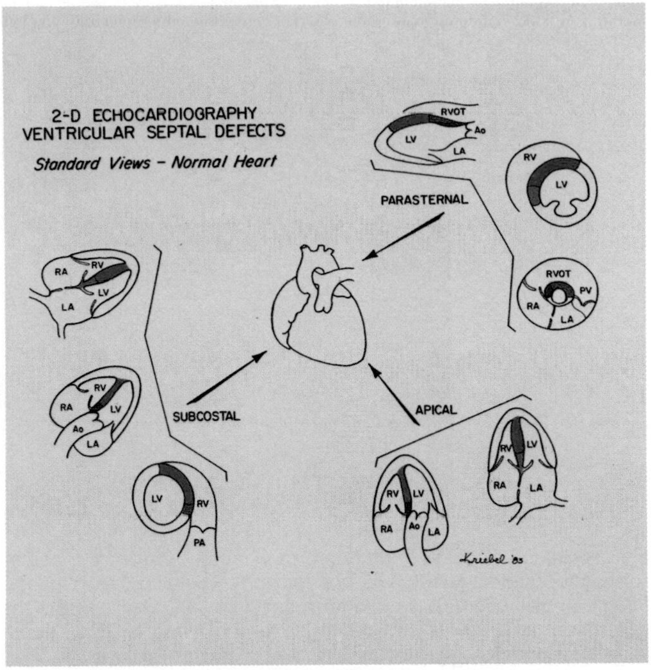

Fig. 29–33. This diagrammatic representation of the multiple echocardiographic views of the interventricular septum marks the subdivisions of the septum in color. Blue denotes the muscular septum; green, the atrioventricular inlet septum; red, the perimembranous septum; and orange, the infundibular or supracristal portion of the ventricular septum. Thus, the appropriate echocardiographic views to diagnose the various types of septal defects can be determined. LA = left atrium; LV = left ventricle; RA = right atrium; RV = right ventricle; Ao = Aorta; RVOT = right ventricular outflow tract; PA = pulmonary artery; PV = pulmonary valve. (From Levine RA, et al.: Echocardiography: Principles and Clinical Applications. *In* Eagle KA, Haber E, DeSanctis RW, Austen WG (eds.): The Practice of Cardiology. Boston, Little, Brown and Company, 1989.)

fects has varied in reported series. In one study, for example, 91% of recorded defects were visualized in the parasternal long axis view,[127] whereas in another, only 46% were apparent in this view.[128] Similarly, from the subcostal location, reported success rates have varied from 42[128] to 88%.[126] This wide variability undoubtedly reflects the large anatomic variation in defect size and location. In general, however, the subcostal views are more successful in infants and children, whereas the parasternal and apical views are more useful in adults with complicated lesions.

False-positives have also been noted with imaging alone, in as many as 12% of normal persons.[125,128] False-positives are encountered more frequently in the apical four-chamber view; 70% of false-positives occur in this one plane.[128] The highest specificity has been noted in the subcostal view (92% in one series and 100% in another). Importantly, when the long axis, apical four-chamber, and subcostal views were all recorded, no false-positives were consistently imaged in all views.[128]

Figure 29–34 illustrates direct visualization of different types of ventricular communications by two-dimensional echocardiographic imaging. Figure 29–34A is an example of an apical four-chamber view illustrating a complete atrioventricular canal-type ventricular septal

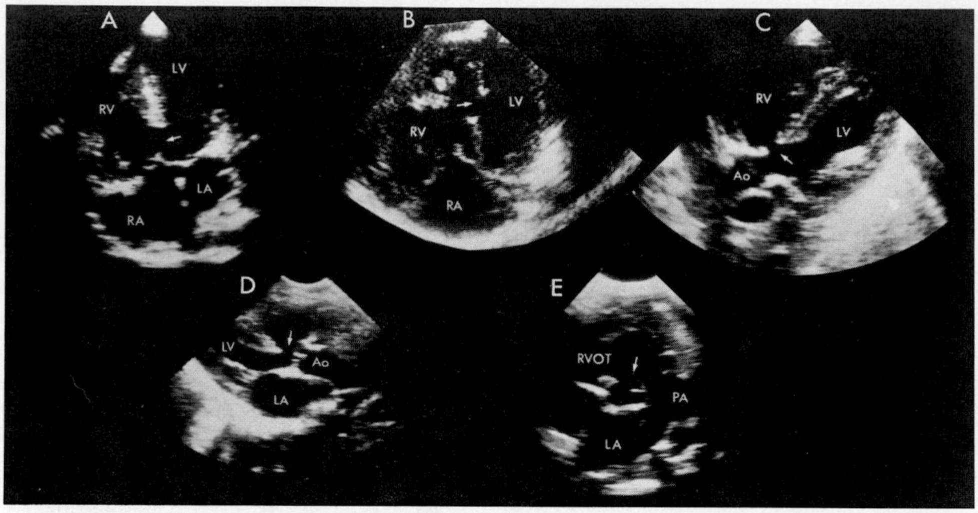

Fig. 29–34. Typical two-dimensional echocardiograms in patients with the following defects: **A.** A complete atrioventricular canal-type ventral septal defect (VSD) (apical four-chamber view). **B.** A muscular VSD (apical four-chamber view). **C.** A membranous defect (subcostal five-chamber view). **D.** A malalignment-type VSD viewed from the parasternal long axis position. **E.** A supracristal VSD viewed from the short axis parasternal view of the aorta (arrows). RVOT = right ventricular outflow tract; LV = left ventricle; RV = right ventricle; LA = left atrium; RA = right atrium; Ao = aorta; PA = pulmonary artery. (From Liberthson RR: Congenital heart disease in the child, adolescent, and adult. *In* (ed.): The Practice of Cardiology. Boston, Little, Brown and Company, 1989.)

defect with a ventricular communication in the inlet septum. Endocardial cushion defects are discussed in more detail in Chapter 32. A muscular ventricular septal defect is shown in Figure 29–34B. In this figure, a prominent area of discontinuity in the trabecular interventricular septum is evident. Figure 29–34C illustrates a membranous ventricular septal defect recorded in a subcostal five-chamber view. This defect is positioned at the superior margin of the muscular septum. Figure 29–34D shows a parasternal long axis view of a malalignment-type ventricular septal defect in a patient with tetralogy of Fallot. The defect separates the septum from its normal point of junction with the anterior aortic root. Ventricular septal defects associated with complex congenital heart disease are discussed in Chapter 32. An example of a supracristal or infundibular ventricular septal defect imaged in a parasternal short axis view is shown in Figure 29–34E.

Doppler Examination. In ventricular septal defects with left-to-right shunting (LVP > RVP), an abnormal flow signal in the right ventricle can virtually always be recorded using Doppler echocardiography.[31] Doppler is of particular importance when the defect is too small to be seen by two-dimensional echocardiography but can also help eliminate false-positives. In combination with imaging, pulsed Doppler sampling can help to localize and often visualize small ventricular septal defects. The sensitivity and specificity of combined imaging and pulsed Doppler to diagnose ventricular septal defects are 96 and 99%, respectively.[53]

With the introduction of two-dimensional color Doppler flow mapping, disturbed shunt-flow velocities in the ventricular cavities can easily be highlighted as an abnormal mosaic color display, superimposed on a two-dimensional image.[129] Figure 29–35 illustrates the two-dimensional color Doppler display of left-to-right shunt flow in a patient with a perimembranous ventricular septal defect imaged from a parasternal long axis view (Fig. 29–35A) and a parasternal short axis view (Fig. 29–35B); with a muscular ventricular septal defect (low parasternal long axis view) (Fig. 29–35C); and with a supracristal ventricular septal defect (parasternal short axis view) (Fig. 29–35D). Whereas combined two-dimensional and Doppler echocardiography have a high sensitivity and specificity for the detection of isolated perimembranous ventricular septal defects, color Doppler flow mapping has been shown to significantly increase sensitivity for detection of multiple ventricular septal defects or small muscular defects. In one study, the sensitivity of detecting multiple ventricular septal defects increased from 38% by combined imaging and pulsed Doppler echocardiography to 72% using color Doppler flow mapping.[130] Color Doppler flow mapping has also been shown to be highly sensitive (100%) and specific (100%) for differentiation between ventricular septal rupture and acute mitral regurgitation after myocardial infarction.[131] However, in the presence of a large defect with equalization of right and left ventricular pressures, there may be virtually no shunt flow, and no flow velocities will be recorded by Doppler. These large defects, however, are easily identified by two-dimensional echocardiography.

In general, the pressure difference between the left and right ventricles is large, and continuous wave Doppler is often necessary to determine the peak velocity of the shunt flow. Color Doppler is valuable in displaying the direction of the jet passing through a ventricular septal defect and allows for aligning the continuous wave Doppler interrogation beam with the direction of the flow. Shunt flow through a perimembranous septal defect can be interrogated from a parasternal transducer position. Sampling from this position, left-to-right shunt flow is directed toward the transducer, and several beam

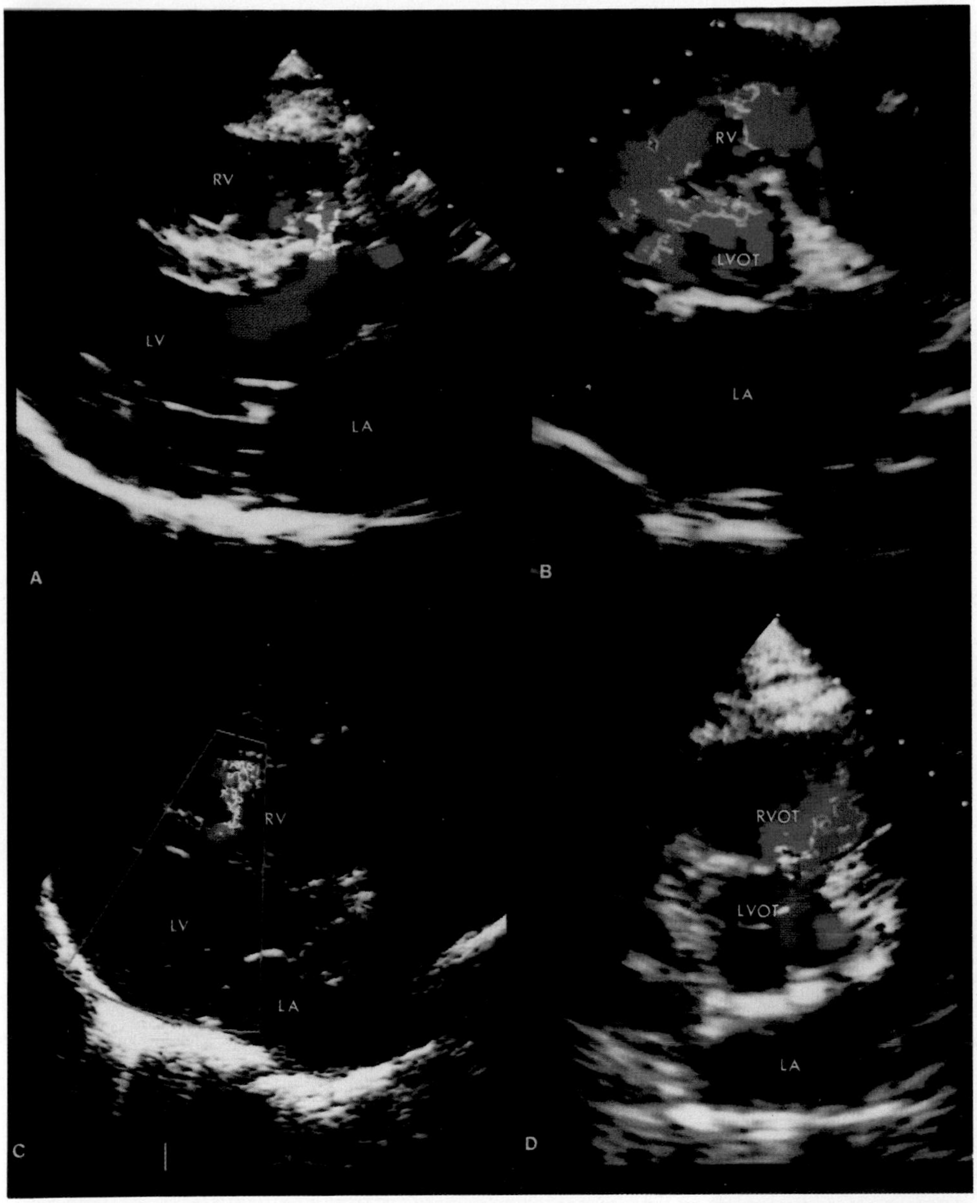

Fig. 29–35. Color Doppler flow images illustrate left-to-right shunt flow (white arrows) in a patient with a perimembranous ventricular septal defect. **A.** Parasternal long axis view. **B.** Parasternal short axis view. **C.** Muscular ventricular septal defect located at midseptal level (low parasternal long axis view). **D.** Infundibular or supracristal ventricular septal defect (parasternal short axis view). LV = left ventricle; RV = right ventricle; LVOT = left ventricular outflow tract; RVOT = right ventricular outflow tract; LA = left atrium.

directions should be attempted to find the signal with highest velocities. Apical septal defects should be interrogated from a low parasternal or subcostal position.

Applying the simplified Bernoulli equation ($\Delta P = 4v^2$), the systolic pressure difference between the right and left ventricles can be calculated from the maximal jet velocity.[132] Subtracting the gradient from a peripheral blood pressure measurement (in the absence of left ventricular outflow obstruction) gives an accurate assessment of the absolute right ventricular systolic pressures.

The typical velocity spectrum of a ventricular septal defect with left-to-right shunt flow starts very early in systole and may continue past the closure of the semilunar valves because pressure in the left ventricle is still higher than in the right (Fig. 29–36). Diastolic left-to-right shunt flow through a ventricular septal defect can frequently be recorded, especially when diastolic left ventricular pressures are elevated, as seen in patients with ventricular septal rupture complicating acute myocardial infarction.[133] Diastolic shunt flow often shows a biphasic pattern, with one peak in early diastole and a second peak in late diastole following atrial contraction (Fig. 29–36). Sometimes, shunt flow through a ventricular septal defect is only recorded in early systole. This type of velocity spectrum almost only occurs in small muscular ventricular septal defects, which presumably close during the later portion of systole.

Semiquantitative Assessment of Ventricular Septal Defect

The apparent size of the defect may vary in different views. This variance has been attributed to the asymmetric anatomic shape of many defects and to the resulting variations in the defect diameter presented to a particular imaging plane. Because of the wide variability in patient size, the absolute dimensions of a ventricular septal defect have little meaning. Therefore, defect size

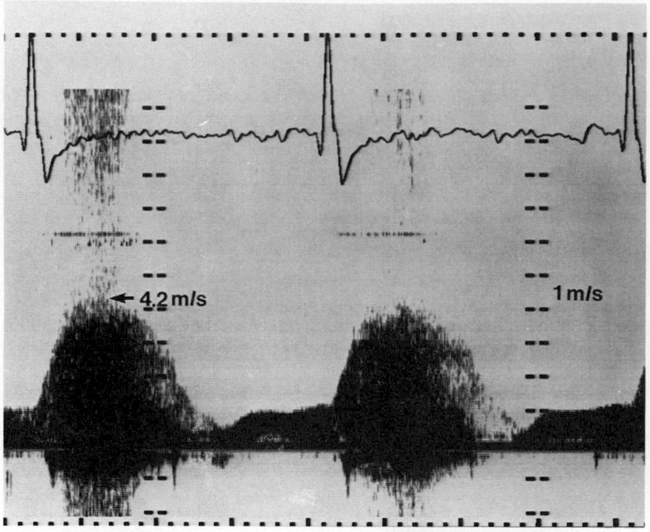

Fig. 29–36. Continuous wave Doppler velocity spectrum obtained from a parasternal transducer position in a patient with a perimembranous ventricular septal defect and left-to-right shunt flow (toward the transducer). This Doppler velocity tracing shows the increase in velocities starting very early in systole and continuing past the closure of the semilunar valves. Also shown is the biphasic low velocity left-to-right shunt flow present during diastole. The peak systolic shunt flow velocity is 4.2 m/sec. Using the simplified Bernoulli equation, the peak systolic pressure difference between the two ventricles can be calculated as $4v^2 = 4(4.2)^2 = 71$ mm Hg.

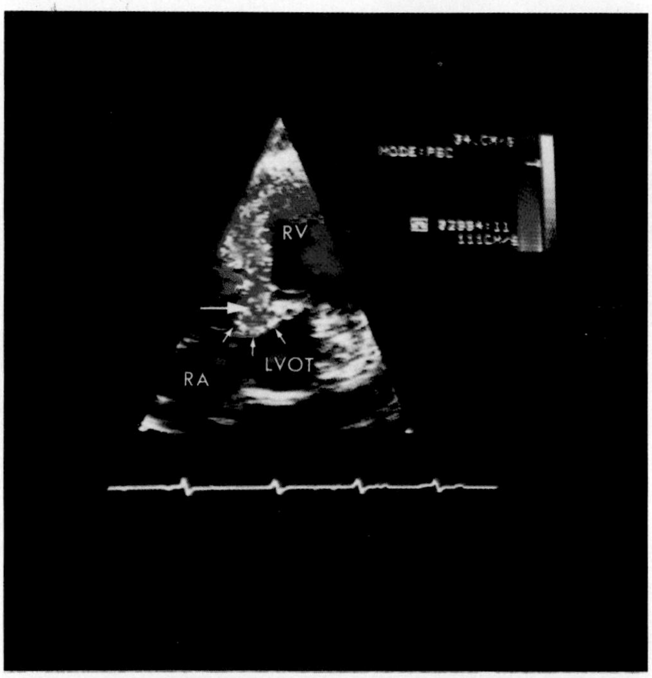

Fig. 29–37. Parasternal short axis color Doppler flow image of a perimembranous ventricular septal defect illustrating the converging flow field (small white arrows) in the left ventricular outflow tract proximal to the defect (large white arrow) and the turbulent jet directed into the right ventricle. To highlight the proximal flow convergence zone, the aliasing velocity has been lowered by shifting the color baseline upward (in the direction of the flow). The red-to-blue aliasing contour corresponds to a velocity of 34 cm/sec. LVOT = left ventricular outflow tract; RA = right atrium; RV = right ventricle.

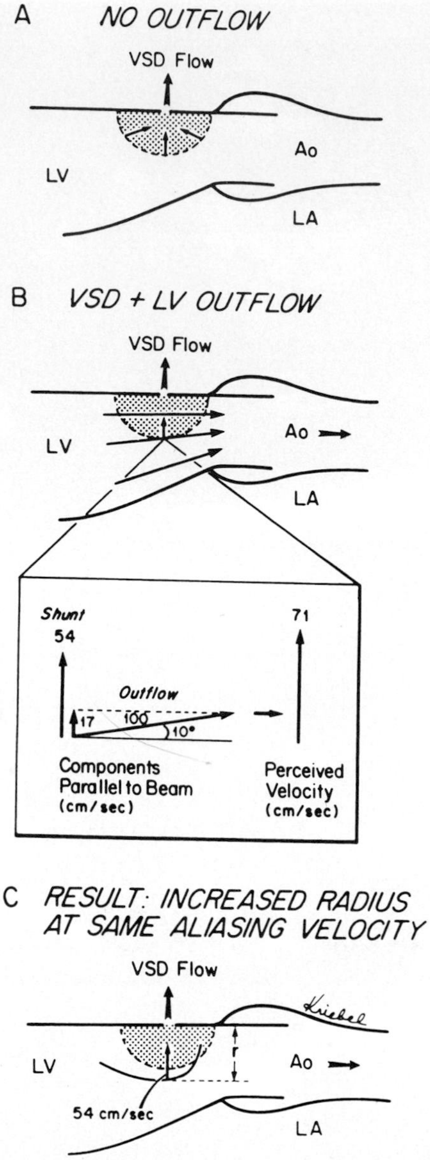

Fig. 29–38. **A.** Schematic of shunt flow through a membranous ventricular septal defect (VSD) in the idealized case of no left ventricular (LV) outflow. A particular isovelocity shell defined by an aliasing velocity of 54 cm/sec is indicated. All flow entering the shell passes through the defect. **B.** Superimposed LV outflow can pass through the aliasing boundary without entering the defect. The component of outflow velocity parallel to the Doppler beam (inset) will increase the apparent velocity of flow toward the defect at the point where the radius of the flow convergence region is measured (along the central axis of the flow). For example, an outflow velocity of 100 cm/sec that makes an angle of 10° toward the beam will augment the recorded flow by (100 cm/sec) (sin 10°) = 17 cm/sec so that the velocity at the surface defined in **A** is increased from 54 to 71 cm/sec at the point shown. **C.** Therefore, the aliasing border (velocity = 54 cm/sec) is displaced farther from the defect as shown (solid curve), and r, the axial distance from the defect to the aliasing boundary, is increased. In that case, the shunt flow rate, calculated as $2\pi r2 \times 54$ cm/sec will overestimate the actual flow rate by a factor of $54/(54-17) = 1.46$. Ao = aorta; LA = left atrium. (From Levine RA: Doppler color mapping of the proximal flow convergence region: a new quantitative physiologic tool. J Am Coll Cardiol 18:833, 1991. Reprinted with permission from the American College of Cardiology. Journal of the American College of Cardiology, 1991, 18, 833.)

is customarily normalized by relating it to the aortic root diameter (VSD/AO).[121,134] Using this ratio, a weak but consistent relationship between echocardiographic defect size and Q_p/Q_s, has been observed.[128] Defect size also decreases from diastole to systole. A mean decrease of almost 50% has been reported.[128] In individual patients, a decrease in defect size of as much as 90% has been noted.[128]

Quantitative Assessment of Ventricular Septal Defect

To evaluate the hemodynamic significance of shunt flow across the ventricular septal defect, the ratio of pulmonic versus systemic blood flow (Q_p/Q_s) and shunt flow (Q_p-Q_s) can be calculated using the combined Doppler/two-dimensional echocardiographic method. This method is discussed in more detail in Chapter 30. Recently, the analysis of the proximal converging flow field on the left ventricular side of the septal defect using color Doppler flow mapping has been described as a promising approach to estimate the defect shunt flow[135] (Fig. 29–37). A good correlation was found between instantaneous flow rate calculated by color Doppler and invasive measurements of Q_p/Q_s and shunt flow (Q_p-Q_s). Although the proximal flow convergence method is potentially capable of providing direct measures of shunt flow, flow calculations by this method may be significantly affected by concomitant outflow present in the left ventricular outflow tract during systole, by effects of orifice size, by surrounding geometry, and by instrument settings[136,137] (Fig. 29–38).

Ventricular Septal Defects Forming an Integral Part of More Complex Congenital Anomalies

Ventricular septal defects may form an integral part of a variety of complex congenital anomalies of the heart, including tetralogy of Fallot, truncus arteriosus, double outlet right ventricle, D- and L-transposition, and endocardial cushion defects.[120,121] These defects can be generally subdivided into those that are associated with aortic overriding or malposition (Fig. 29–34D) and those that arise in the region of the closing endocardial cushions (Fig. 29–34A). These defects are considered in more detail in Chapter 32 and, therefore, are only briefly discussed here.

Defects associated with aortic overriding occur in either the bulbar of the membranous septa. When the lesion involves primarily the bulbar septum, as in truncus arteriosus, it is typically high, anterior, and limited by the semilunar valves of the truncus superiorly and the crest of the ventricular septum posteriorly. When it involves the membranous septum, the bulbar septum extending below the semilunar valve is present and limits the defect superiorly. These defects are usually large, easily recognized, and are best recorded in the parasternal long axis view of the left ventricle.

Figure 29–39 is an example of a large ventricular septal defect associated with truncus arteriosus. In this example, the large separation between the superior margin of the interventricular septum and the anteriorly positioned anterior border of the aortic root is clearly evident. The presence of these defects is highlighted by the associated aortic overriding. Success rates for defect recording are better for this group (93 to 95%)[128,138] than those reported for isolated defects. With the combined use of two-dimensional imaging and pulsed Doppler or color Doppler flow mapping, the success rate is even better.

Ventricular Septal Aneurysms

Two primary types of aneurysms involve the ventricular septum: the discrete membranous ventricular septal

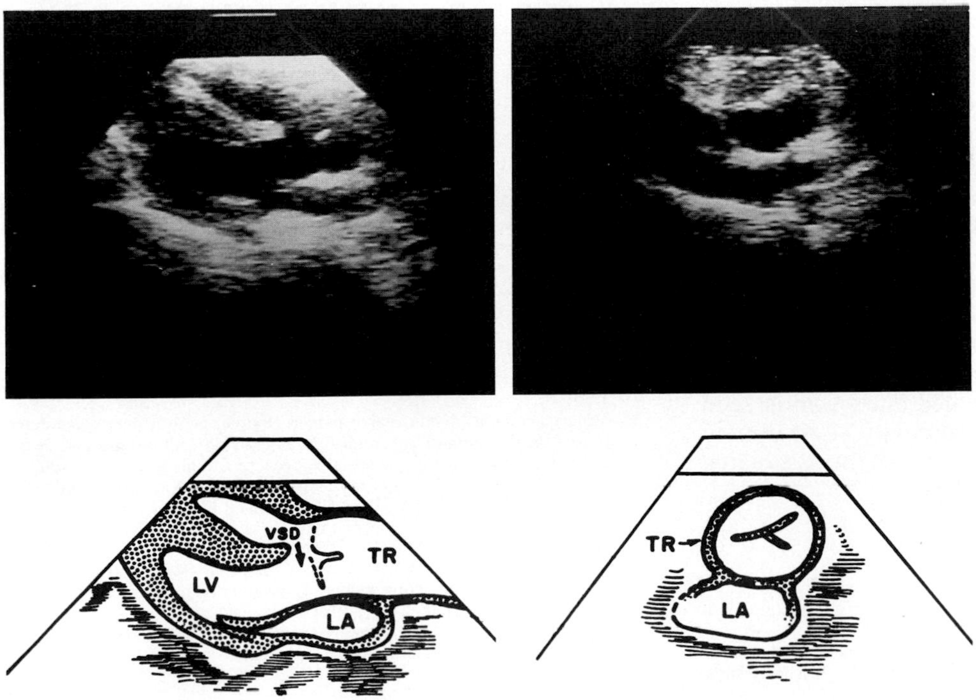

Fig. 29–39. Parasternal long axis recording of a large ventricular septal defect (VSD) associated with aortic overriding in a patient with truncus arteriosus. The defect is indicated by the vertical arrow. LV = left ventricle; LA = left atrium; TR = truncus arteriosus.

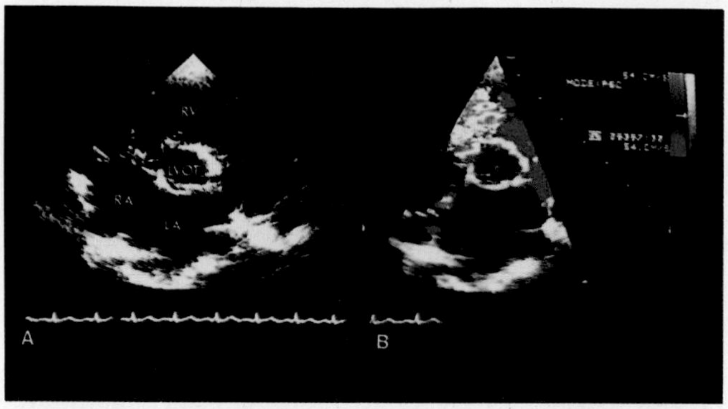

Fig. 29–40. **A.** Parasternal short axis recording illustrates a small membranous ventricular septal aneurysm (white arrows). The aneurysm is thin walled and protrudes into the right ventricular cavity just proximal to the junction of the membranous septum and anterior aortic root. **B.** Color Doppler flow image shows the presence of left-to-right shunt flow through the associated ventricular septal defect (white arrows). RV = right ventricle; LVOT = left ventricular outflow tract; LA = left atrium; RA = right atrium.

aneurysms, which develop as part of the natural process of closure of congenital ventricular septal defects, and the large septal aneurysms, which complicate acute myocardial infarction and underlie ventricular septal perforation. This section deals with the small, congenital, ventricular septal aneurysm. The infarct-associated aneurysms are discussed under complications of acute myocardial infarction in Chapter 22.

Studies of the natural history of ventricular septal defects suggest a continuing rate of spontaneous closure throughout childhood.[139–141] Aneurysm formation has been well documented as one mechanism by which this defect closure occurs.[142–144] The initial formation of a ventricular septal aneurysm is frequently associated with partial defect closure and decrease in the size of the left-to-right shunt. After complete closure, the aneurysm may remain as the only evidence of a prior defect. In addition to suggesting the presence of an earlier defect, the aneurysm may also offer a possible nidus for infection in bacterial endocarditis. Membranous ventricular aneurysms are generally visualized in the right ventricular outflow tract, anterior to the junction of the anterior aortic root and muscular septum. They are typically small and thin-walled and show little mobility. They can usually be recorded in either a parasternal long axis view of the left side of the heart or a short axis view of the left ventricular outflow tract recorded below the level of the aortic valve. Figure 29–40A illustrates a membranous ventricular septal aneurysm recorded in a parasternal short axis view. The thin-walled aneurysm is seen protruding into the right ventricular cavity. Two-dimensional color Doppler flow mapping shows the associated left-to-right shunt flow (Fig. 29–40B).

REFERENCES

1. Grant JCB, Basmajian JV: Grant's Method of Anatomy. Baltimore, Williams & Wilkins, 1965.
2. Bloor CM: Cardiac Pathology. Philadelphia, JB Lippincott, 1978.
3. Braunwald TE, Fishman AP, Cournand A: Time relationship of dynamic events in the cardiac chambers, pulmonary artery and aorta in man. Circ Res 4:100, 1956.
4. Tei C, et al.: Real-time cross-sectional echocardiographic evaluation of the interatrial septum by right atrium-interatrial septum-left atrium direction of ultrasonic beam. Circulation 60:539, 1979.
5. Tei C, et al.: Echocardiographic analysis of interatrial septal motion. Am J Cardiol 44:472, 1979.
6. Weyman AE, Wann LS, Feigenbaum H, Dillon JC: Mechanism of abnormal septal motion in patients with right ventricular volume overload. Circulation 54:179, 1976.
7. Hagler DJ, et al.: Real-time wide angle sector echocardiography: atrioventricular canal defects. Circulation 59:140, 1979.
8. Dillon JC, et al.: Cross-sectional echocardiographic examination of the interatrial septum. Circulation 55:1, 1977.
9. Schapira JN, Martin RP, Fowles RE, Popp RL: Single and two-dimensional echocardiographic features of the interatrial septum in normal subjects and patients with an atrial septal defect. Am J Cardiol 43:816, 1979.
10. Silverman NH, Schiller NB: Apex echocardiography. A two-dimensional technique for evaluating congenital heart disease. Circulation 57:503, 1978.
11. Tajik AJ, et al.: Two-dimensional real-time ultrasonic imaging of the heart and great vessels. Mayo Clin Proc 53:271, 1980.
12. Lange LW, Sahn DJ, Allen HD, Goldberg SJ: Subxiphoid cross-sectional echocardiography in infants and children with congenital heart disease. Circulation 59:513, 1979.
13. Bierman FZ, Williams RG: Subxiphoid two-dimensional imaging of the interatrial septum in infants and neonates with congenital heart disease. Circulation 60:80, 1979.
14. Kushner FG, Lam W, Morganroth J: Apex sector echocardiography in evaluation of the right atrium in patients with mitral stenosis and atrial septal defect. Am J Cardiol 42:733, 1978.
15. Shub C, et al.: Sensitivity of two-dimensional echocardiography in the direct visualization of atrial septal defect utilizing the subcostal approach: experience with 154 patients. J Am Coll Cardiol 2:127, 1983.
16. Hanrath P, et al.: Detection of ostium secundum atrial septal defects by transesophageal cross-sectional echocardiography. Br Heart J 49:350, 1983.
17. Schwinger ME, Gindea AJ, Freedberg RS, Kronzon I: The anatomy of the interatrial septum: a transesophageal echocardiographic study. Am Heart J 119:1401, 1990.
18. Nanda NC, Pinheiro L, Sanyal RS, Storey O: Transesophageal biplane echocardiographic imaging: technique, planes and clinical usefulness. Echocardiography 7:771, 1990.
19. Lin CS, Chen HY, Jan YI: The interatrial septal echocardiogram: relationship to left atrial volume change in the normal and diseased heart. Am Heart J 107:519, 1984.
20. Friedberg CK: Diseases of the Heart. Philadelphia, WB Saunders, 1966.
21. Hurst JW: The Heart. New York, McGraw-Hill, 1978.
22. Perloff JK: The Clinical Recognition of Congenital Heart Disease. Philadelphia, WB Saunders, 1978.
23. Higgins CB, Silverman NH, Kersting-Sommerhoff B, Schmidt KG (eds.): Congenital Heart Disease: Echocardiography and Magnetic Resonance Imaging. New York: Raven Press, p. 99, 1990.
24. Becker AE, Anderson RH (eds.): Cardiac Pathology: An Integrated Text and Colour Atlas. New York: Raven Press, 1983.
25. Diamond MA, et al.: Echocardiographic features of atrial septal defect. Circulation 43:129, 1971.
26. McCann WD, Harbold NB, Giuliani BR: The echocardiogram in right ventricular overload. JAMA 221:1243, 1972.
27. Tajik AJ, Gau GT, Ritter D, Schattenberg TT: Echocardiographic pattern of right ventricular diastolic volume overload in children. Circulation 46: 36, 1972.
28. Pernod J, Terdjman M, Kermarec J, Haguenauer G: Myocardial contraction. Study by ultrasonic echocardiography (results in 200 normal patients). Nouv Presse Med 2:2393, 1973.
29. Matsumoto M: Ultrasonic features of interatrial septum: its motion analysis and detection of its defect. Jpn Circ J 37:1383, 1973.
30. Nimura Y, et al.: Interatrial septum in ultrasonocardiotomogram and ultrasoundcardiogram. Med Ultrasonics 9:58, 1971.
31. Hatle L, Angelson B (eds.): Doppler Ultrasound in Cardiology: Physical Principles and Clinical Applications. Philadelphia, Lea & Febiger, p. 228, 1985.
32. Minagoe S, et al.: Noninvasive pulsed Doppler echocardiographic detection of the direction of the shunt flow in patients with atrial septal defect: usefulness of the right parasternal approach. Circulation 71:745, 1985.
33. Suzuki Y, et al.: Detection of intracardiac shunt flow in atrial septal defect using a real-time two-dimensional color-coded Doppler flow imaging system and comparison with contrast two-dimensional imaging. Am J Cardiol 56:347, 1985.
34. Lin FC, Fu M, Yeh SJ, Wu D: Doppler atrial shunt flow patterns in patients with secundum atrial septal defect: determinants, limitations and pitfalls. J Am Soc Echocardiogr 1:141, 1988.
35. Faletra F, et al.: Color Doppler echocardiographic assessment of atrial septal defect size: correlation with surgical measurements. J Am Soc Echocardiogr 4:429, 1991.

36. Seward JB, Tajik AJ, Spangler JG, Ritter DG: Echocardiographic contrast studies: initial experience. Mayo Clin Proc 50:3, 1975.
37. Weyman AE, et al.: Negative contrast echocardiography: a new method for detecting left-to-right shunts. Circulation 59:498, 1979.
38. Valdes-Cruz LM, Pieroni DR, Roland JM, Varghese PJ: Echocardiographic detection of right-to-left shunts following peripheral vein injections. Circulation 54:558, 1976.
39. Valdez-Cruz LM, et al.: A pulsed Doppler echocardiographic method for calculating pulmonary and systemic blood flow in atrial level shunts: validation studies in animals and initial human experience. Circulation 69:80, 1984.
40. Kitabatake A, et al.: Noninvasive evaluation of the ratio of pulmonary to systemic flow in atrial septal defect by duplex Doppler echocardiography. Circulation 69:73, 1984.
41. Dittmann H, et al.: Accuracy of Doppler echocardiography in quantification of left to right shunts in adult patients with atrial septal defect. J Am Coll Cardiol 11:338, 1988.
42. Dow JW, Dexter L: Circulatory dynamics in atrial septal defect. J Clin Invest 29:809, 1950.
43. Dexter L: Atrial septal defect. Br Heart J 18:209, 1956.
44. Hull E: Cause and effects of flow through defects of atrial septum. Am Heart J 38:350, 1949.
45. Mathew R, Thilenius OG, Arcilla RA: Comparative responses of right and left ventricles to volume overload. Am J Cardiol 38:209, 1974.
46. Rowe GG, et al.: Atrial septal defect and the mechanism of shunt. Am Heart J 61:369, 1961.
47. Alexander AJ, Rembert JC, Sealy WC, Greenfield JC, Jr: Shunt dynamics in experimental atrial septal defects. J Appl Physiol 39:281, 1975.
48. Pearlman AJ, et al.: Determinants of ventricular septal motion. Circulation 54:84, 1976.
49. Kerber RE, Dippel WF, Abbound FM: Abnormal motion of the interventricular septum in right ventricular volume overload. Experimental and clinical echocardiographic studies. Circulation 48:86, 1973.
50. Lieppe W, Scallion R, Behar VS, Kisslo JA: Two-dimensional echocardiographic findings in atrial septal defect. Circulation 56:447, 1977.
51. Schreiber TL, Weyman AE, Feigenbaum H, Stewart J: Effects of atrial septal defect repair on left ventricular geometry and degree of mitral valve prolapse. Circulation 61:888, 1980.
52. Seward JB, et al.: Transesophageal echocardiography: technique, anatomic correlations, implementation and clinical applications. Mayo Clin Proc 63:649, 1988.
53. Nanda NC (ed.): Doppler echocardiography. Tokyo, Igaku-Shoin, p. 408, 1985.
54. Morimoto K, et al.: Diagnosis and quantitative evaluation of secundum-type atrial septal defect by transesophageal Doppler echocardiography. Am J Cardiol 66:85, 1990.
55. Levin AR, et al.: Atrial pressure-flow dynamics in atrial septal defects (secundum type). Circulation 37:476, 1968.
56. Thomas JD, Tabakin BS, Ittleman FP: Atrial septal defect with right to left shunt despite normal pulmonary artery pressure. J Am Coll Cardiol 9: 221, 1987.
57. Valdez-Cruz LM, et al.: A pulsed Doppler echocardiographic method for calculation of pulmonary and systemic flow: accuracy in a canine model with ventricular septal defect. Circulation 68:597, 1983.
58. Meijboom EJ, et al.: A two-dimensional Doppler echocardiographic method for calculation of pulmonary and systemic blood flow in a canine model with a variable-sized left-to-right extra cardiac shunt. Circulation 68:437, 1983.
59. Pollick C, Sullivan H, Cujec B, Wilansky S: Doppler color-flow imaging assessment of shunt size in atrial septal defect. Circulation 78:522, 1988.
60. Forfar JC, Godman MJ: Functional and anatomical correlates in atrial septal defect. An echocardiographic analysis. Br Heart J 54:193, 1985.
60a. Sanzobrino BW, et al.: Intracardiac two-dimensional ultrasonic assessment of atrial septal defects: human studies. Circulation 82(suppl):III–31, 1990.
61. Williams RG, Bierman FZ: Evaluation of balloon atrial septostomy by subxiphoid two-dimensional echocardiography. Am J Cardiol 43:401, 1979.
62. Lang FJ, Posselt A: Aneurysmatische Vorwolbung der Fossa ovalis in den linken Vorhof. Wien Med Wochenschr 84:392, 1934.
63. Thompson JI, Phillips LA, Melmon KL: Pseudotumor of the right atrium: report of a case and review of its etiology. Ann Intern Med 64:665, 1966.
64. Sahn DJ, Allen HD, Anderson R, Goldberg SJ: Echocardiographic diagnosis of atrial septal aneurysm in an infant with hypoplastic right heart syndrome. Chest 73:227, 1978.
65. Gondi B, Nanda NC: Two-dimensional echocardiographic features of atrial septal aneurysm. Circulation 63:452, 1981.
66. Hanley PC, et al.: Diagnosis and classification of echocardiography: report of 80 consecutive cases. J Am Coll Cardiol 6:1370, 1985.
67. Schneider B, Hanrath P, Vogel P, Meinertz T: Improved morphologic characterization of atrial septal aneurysm by transesophageal echocardiography: relation to cerebrovascular events. J Am Coll Cardiol 16:1000, 1990.
68. Grosgogeat Y, et al.: Aneurysme de la cloison interauriculaire revele par une embolie cerebrale. Arch Mal Coeur 66:169, 1973.
69. Belkin RN, Hurwitz BJ, Kisslo J: Atrial septal aneurysm: association with cerebrovascular and peripheral embolic events. Stroke 18:856, 1987.
70. Ong LS, Nanda NC, Falkoff MD, Barold SS: Interatrial septal aneurysm, systolic click and atrial tachyarrhythmia—a new syndrome? Ultrasound Med Biol 8:691, 1982.
71. Belkin BN, Waugh RA, Kisslo J: Interatrial shunting in atrial septal aneurysm. Am J Cardiol 57:310, 1986.
72. Abinader EG, et al.: Prevalence of atrial septal aneurysm in patients with mitral valve prolapse. Am J Cardiol 62:1139, 1988.
73. Silver MD, Dorsey JS: Aneurysms of the septum primum in adults. Arch Pathol Lab Med 102:62, 1978.
74. Longhini C, et al.: Atrial septal aneurysm: echopolycardiographic study. Am J Cardiol 56:653, 1985.
75. Pearson AC, et al.: Atrial septal aneurysm and stroke: a transesophageal echocardiographic study. J Am Coll Cardiol 18:1223, 1991.
76. Freedom R, Rowe R: Aneurysm of the atrial septum in tricuspid atresia: diagnosis during life. Am J Cardiol 38:265, 1976.
77. Sahn DJ, Allen HD, Anderson R, Goldberg SJ: Echocardiographic diagnosis of atrial septal aneurysm in an infant with hypoplastic right heart syndrome. Chest 73:227, 1978.
78. Hutter AM, Jr, Page DL: Atrial arrhythmias and lipomatous hypertrophy of the cardiac interatrial septum. Am Heart J 82:16, 1971.
79. Rosenquist GC, Sweeney LJ, Ruckman RN, McAllister HA: Atrial septal thickness and area in normal heart specimens and in those with ostium secundum atrial septal defects. J Clin Ultrasound 7:345, 1979.
80. Page DL: Lipomatous hypertrophy of the cardiac interatrial septum: its development and probable clinical significance. Hum Pathol 1:151, 1970.
81. Fyke FE, Tajik AJ, Edwards WD, Seward JB: Diagnosis of lipomatous hypertrophy of the atrial septum by two-dimensional echocardiography. J Am Coll Cardiol 1:1352, 1983.
82. Kronzon I, Glassman E, Cohen M, Winer H: Use of two-dimensional echocardiography during transseptal cardiac catheterization. J Am Coll Cardiol 4:425, 1984.
83. Ballal RS, Mahan EF, Nanda NC, Dean LS: Utility of transesophageal echocardiography in interatrial septal puncture during percutaneous mitral balloon commissurotomy. Am J Cardiol 66:230, 1990.
84. Goor OA, Edwards JW, Lillehei CW: The development of the interventricular septum of the human heart: correlative morphogenetic study. Chest 58:453, 1970.
85. Hagan AD, et al.: Ultrasound evaluation of systolic anterior septal motion in patients with and without right ventricular volume overload. Circulation 50:248, 1974.
86. Corya BC, et al.: Systolic thickening and thinning of the septum and posterior wall in patients with coronary artery disease, congestive cardiomyopathy, and atrial septal defect. Circulation 55:109, 1977.
87. Kerber RE, Marcus ML, Ehrhardt J, Abbound FM: Effect of increases in afterload on the systolic thickening of acutely ischemic myocardium: an experimental echocardiographic study. Acta Med Scand 205(627):142, 1978.
88. Kerber RE, Martins JB, Marcus ML: Effect of acute ischemia, nitroglycerin and nitroprusside on regional myocardial thickening, stress, and perfusion. Circulation 60:121, 1979.
89. Henry WL, Clark CE, Epstein SE: Asymmetric septal hypertrophy: the unifying link in the IHSS disease spectrum: observations regarding its pathogenesis, pathophysiology and course. Circulation 47:827, 1973.
90. Henry WL, Clark CE, Epstein SE: Asymmetric septal hypertrophy: echocardiographic identification of the pathognomonic anatomic abnormality of IHSS. Circulation, 47:225, 1973.
91. Maron BJ, Epstein SE: Hypertrophic cardiomyopathy: recent observations regarding the specificity of three hallmarks of the disease: asymmetric septal hypertrophy, septal disorganization and systolic anterior motion of the anterior mitral leaflet. Am J Cardiol 45:141, 1980.
92. Kupari M: Assymmetric septal hypertrophy in Kearns-Sayre syndrome. Clin Cardiol 7:603, 1984.
93. Nunoda S, Genda A: A case of hypereosinophilic syndrome with asymmetric septal hypertrophy. Heart Vessels 6:116, 1991.
94. Csanady M, Haspar L, Hogye M, Gruber N: The heart in acromegaly: an echocardiographic study. Int J Cardiol 2:349, 1983.
95. Rasmussen S, Corya BC, Feigenbaum H, Knoebel SB: Detection of myocardial scar tissue by M-mode echocardiography. Circulation 57:230, 1978.
96. Garrison JB, et al.: Quantifying regional wall motion and thickening in two-dimensional echocardiography with a computer. Aided contouring system. *In* Ostrow H, Ripley K (eds.): Proccedings of Computers in Cardiology. Long Beach, CA, IEEE, 1977.
97. Rossen RM, Goodman DJ, Ingham RE, Popp RL: Ventricular septal thickening and excursion in idiopathic hypertrophic subaortic stenosis. Circulation, 50:29, 1974.
98. Smith ER, Flemington CS: Systolic muscle thickening and excursion in patients with asymmetric septal hypertrophy. Circulation 52:141, 1975.
99. Feigenbaum H: Echocardiography. Philadelphia, Lea & Febiger, 1976.
100. Kerber RE, et al.: Correlation between echocardiographically demonstrated segmental dyskinesis and regional myocardial perfusion. Circulation 52:1097, 1975.
101. Kerber RE, Duty D: Abnormalities of interventricular septal motion following cardiac surgery. Cross-sectional echocardiographic studies. Am J Cardiol 41:372, 1978.

102. Feneley M, et al.: Mechanisms of the development and resolution of paradoxical interventricular septal motion after uncomplicated cardiac surgery. Am Heart J 114:106, 1987.
103. Lehmann KG, et al.: Onset of altered interventricular septal motion during cardiac surgery. Assessment by continuous intraoperative transesophageal echocardiography. Circulation 82:1325, 1990.
104. Kerber RE, Litchfield R: Postoperative abnormalities of interventricular septal motion: two-dimensional and M-mode echocardiographic correlations. Am Heart J 104:263, 1982.
105. Schroeder E, Marchandise B, Schoevaerdts JC, Kremer R: Paradoxical ventricular septal motion after cardiac surgery. Analysis of M-mode echocardiograms and follow-up in 324 patients. Acta Cardiol 40:315, 1985.
106. Force T, et al.: Quantitative two-dimensional echocardiographic analysis of motion and thickening of the interventricular septum after cardiac surgery. Circulation 5:1013, 1983.
107. Ribeiro P, et al.: Role of transient ischaemia and perioperative myocardial infarction in the genesis of new septal wall motion abnormalities after coronary bypass surgery. Br Heart J 54:140, 1985.
108. Tanaka H, et al.: Diastolic bulging of the interventricular septum toward the left ventricle. Circulation 62:558, 1980.
109. Kingma I, Tyberg JV, Smith ER: Effects of diastolic transseptal pressure gradient on ventricular septal position and motion. Circulation 68:1304, 1983.
110. Fenely M, Gavaghan T: Paradoxical and pseudoparadoxical interventricular septal motion in patients with ventricular volume overload. Circulation 74:230, 1986.
111. Lieppe W, Scallion R, Behar VS, Kisslo JA: Two-dimensional echocardiographic findings in atrial septal defect. Circulation 56:447, 1977.
112. King ME, et al.: Interventricular septal configuration as a predictor of right ventricular systolic hypertension in children: a cross-sectional echocardiographic study. Circulation 68:68, 1983.
113. Brinker JA, et al.: Leftward septal displacement during right ventricular loading in man. Circulation 61:626, 1980.
114. Guzman PA, et al.: Transseptal pressure gradient with leftward septal displacement during the Muller's manoeuvre in man. Br Heart J 46:657, 1981.
115. Weyman AE, et al.: Mechanism of paradoxical early diastolic septal motion in patients with mitral stenosis: a cross-sectional echocardiographic study. Am J Cardiol 40:691, 1977.
116. Thompson CR, et al.: Transseptal pressure gradient and diastolic ventricular septal motion in patients with mitral stenosis. Circulation 76:974, 1987.
117. Taylor RR, Covell JW, Sonnenblick EH, Ross J: Dependence of ventricular distensibility on filling of the opposite ventricle. Am J Physiol 213:711, 1967.
118. McDonald IG: Echocardiographic demonstration of abnormal motion of the interventricular septum in left bundle branch block. Circulation 48:272, 1973.
119. Dillon JC, Chang S, Feigenbaum H: Echocardiographic manifestations of left bundle branch block. Circulation 49:876, 1974.
120. Keith JD, Rowe RD, Vlad P: Heart Disease in Infancy and Childhood. New York, Macmillan, 1978.
121. Beca LM, et al.: Anatomic and pathologic studies in ventricular septal defect. Circulation 14:349, 1956.
122. Saab NG, Burchell HB, DuShane JW, Titus JL: Muscular ventricular septal defects. Am J Cardiol 18:713, 1966.
123. Perloff JH: The Clinical Recognition of Congenital Heart Disease. Philadelphia, WB Saunders, 1970.
124. Campion BC, et al.: Ventricular septal defect after myocardial infarction. Ann Intern Med 1969;70:251–255.
125. Cheatham JP, Latson LA, Gutgesell HP: Ventricular septal defect in infancy: detection by two-dimensional echocardiography. Circulation 60(2): 112, 1979.
126. Bierman FZ, Williams RG: Prospective diagnosis of ventricular septal defects in infants by subxyphoid two-dimensional echocardiography. Circulation 60(2):112, 1979.
127. Seward JB, Tajik AJ, Hagler DJ, Mair DD: Visualization of isolated ventricular septal defect by wide-angle two-dimensional sector echocardiography. Circulation 58(2):202, 1978.
128. Canale JM, et al.: Factors affecting real-time cross-sectional echocardiographic imaging of perimembranous ventricular septal defects. Circulation 63:689, 1981.
129. Ortiz E, et al.: Localization of ventricular septal defects by simultaneous display of superimposed color Doppler and cross-sectional echocardiographic images. Br Heart J 54:53, 1985.
130. Ludomirsky A, et al.: Color Doppler detection of multiple ventricular septal defects. Circulation 74:1317, 1986.
131. Smyllie JH, et al.: Doppler color flow mapping in the diagnosis of ventricular septal rupture and actue mitral regurgitation after myocardial infarction. J Am Coll Cardiol 15:1449, 1990.
132. Murphy DJ Jr, Ludomirsky A, Huhta JC: Continuous wave Doppler in children with ventricular septal defect: noninvasive estimation of interventricular pressure gradient. Am J Cardiol 57:428, 1985.
133. Miyatake K, et al.: Doppler echocardiographic features of ventricular septal rupture in myocardial infarction. J Am Coll Cardiol 5:182, 1985.
134. Selzer A: Defect of the ventricular septum: summary of twelve cases and review of the literature. Arch Intern Med 84:798, 1949.
135. Moises VA, et al.: A new method for noninvasive estimation of ventricular septal defect shunt flow by color Doppler flow mapping: imaging of the laminar flow convergence region on the left septal surface. J Am Coll Cardiol 18:824, 1991.
136. Levine RA: Doppler color mapping of the proximal flow convergence region: a new quantitative physiologic tool. J Am Coll Cardiol 18:833, 1991.
137. Vandervoort PM, Thoreau DH, Weyman AE, Thomas JD: Wall filtering significantly increases Doppler velocities in proximal flow convergence (abstr.). Circulation 84(Suppl. 2):II–104, 1991.
138. Caldwell RL, et al.: Right ventricular outflow tract assessment by cross-sectional echocardiography in tetralogy of Fallot. Circulation 59:395, 1979.
139. Freedom RM, et al.: The natural history of the so-called aneurysm of the membranous ventricular septum in childhood. Circulation 49:375, 1974.
140. Hoffman JEI, Rudolph AM: The natural history of ventricular septal defects in infancy. Am J Cardiol 634, 1965.
141. Bloomfield K: The natural history of ventricular septal defects in patients surviving infancy. Circulation 29:914, 1964.
142. Lambert ME, et al.: Natural history of ventricular septal defects associated with ventricular septal aneurysms. Am Heart J 88:566, 1974.
143. Varghese PJ, Rowe RD: Spontaneous closure of ventricular septal defects by aneurysmal formation of the membranous septum. J Pediatr 75:700, 1969.
144. Miora KP, et al.: Aneurysm of the membranous ventricular septum: a mechanism for spontaneous closure of ventricular septal defect. N Engl J Med 283:58, 1970.

CHAPTER

30

DOPPLER ESTIMATION OF VOLUMETRIC FLOW

SHANE A. MARSHALL and ARTHUR E. WEYMAN

For centuries physicians have been searching for practical and reliable methods for quantifying blood flow within the heart and great vessels. The most important and extensively studied measure of blood flow is the cardiac output, which is the primary indicator of the effectiveness of the heart as a pump. Additional knowledge of the blood volumes moving through individual cardiac chambers, if available, could be used to quantify regurgitant and shunt flows and to assess differential hemodynamic responses to therapeutic interventions.

The first steps toward estimating blood flow were made by William Harvey (1578 to 1657), who calculated the "cardiac output" by measuring the volume of blood in the heart (an observation from cadavers) and multiplying it by a representative heart rate. He supported these speculations by measuring the blood expelled in unit time from the severed main artery of sheep.[1] Over time, the techniques available for quantifying blood flow have increased in both number and sophistication. At present the most common clinical approaches to measuring cardiac output include the Fick, indicator dilution, and angiographic methods. All of these approaches require the insertion of catheters into the central circulation, which limits the frequency with which these measurements can be made, out of respect for patient comfort and safety. Furthermore, each of these invasive techniques operates on many theoretical assumptions and have practical constraints,[2] which limit their value as "gold standards" of volumetric flow.

In 1972, the first clinical estimates of blood flow by Doppler echocardiography were made.[3] In these studies, blood velocity in the aortic arch was determined by continuous wave Doppler and was shown to vary appropriately in response to maneuvers known to alter cardiac output. Subsequently, it has been shown that Doppler flow velocity measurements combined with echocardiographic imaging can be reliably used to measure volumetric flow at specific locations within the heart and great vessels.

The advantages of such a technique for quantifying blood flow are considerable. Because patients are examined at rest and unsedated, Doppler studies provide information about basal hemodynamics, which invasive measurements of blood flow may not accurately reflect as a result of the attendant patient anxiety and discomfort. In addition, because Doppler studies are noninvasive and nontoxic, they may be repeated as often as necessary and can provide information concerning hemodynamic status and response to interventions on a beat-to-beat basis. Finally, the ability of the Doppler method to noninvasively measure flow through the mitral, aortic, pulmonic, and tricuspid valves offers the potential not only to determine the cardiac output but also to quantify shunt flow and regurgitant volumes based on comparisons of flow through individual valves.

As with any quantitative measurement, reliability of results is operator dependent. Measurements of volumetric flow rely on a combination of imaging and flow data, each of which have inherent sources of error. Use of flows through different valves as interchangeable measures of cardiac output or as references from which to calculate flow differences between vascular beds or cardiac chambers also requires that the relative accuracy and sources of error for measurement at each valve be understood.

This chapter summarizes the theory and practical methods for calculating cardiac flows by Doppler-echocardiography, examines the accuracy and potential sources of error of the technique, and describes its current and potential applications.

THEORETIC CONSIDERATIONS

In its simplest form, blood flow through the cardiovascular system can be likened to the flow of fluid through a tube of constant diameter. Flow (Q) is defined as volume per unit time. As illustrated in Figure 30–1, flow is equal to the product of the cross-sectional area of the tube and the mean velocity of the fluid moving through the tube. In this example, if the fluid column moves forward 5 cm during a 1-second period, the velocity equals 5 cm/sec. If the cross-sectional area of the tube is 10 cm^2, the flow would be equal to 50 cm^3/sec. In the case of cardiovascular flow measurements, the "fluid" is blood, and the "tube" is the vessel or valve through which flow is occurring.

Of course, in the beating heart, the velocity of blood changes with each systole and diastole. Figure 30–2 illustrates this more complex situation in which velocity is changing. In this case, the "instantaneous" velocity can be measured for time t_1 and multiplied by the "instantaneous" cross-sectional area to calculate forward flow during the interval t_1, where t is sufficiently small that the velocity is effectively constant during it. Similarly, instantaneous velocity and derived flow can be calculated at times t_2, t_3, and so on. For a pulsatile system such as the heart, if the flows for each time period are added or, for continuous sampling, integrated as t approaches zero, the volume per pulse can be calculated. In a conduit whose cross-sectional area does not change significantly during the period of forward flow, total blood flow (stroke volume) can be calculated as the integral over time of the instantaneous velocities multiplied by the mean cross-sectional area.

$$SV = CSA \times TVI \qquad [30.1]$$

where SV is stroke volume, CSA is cross-sectional area, and TVI is time-velocity integral.

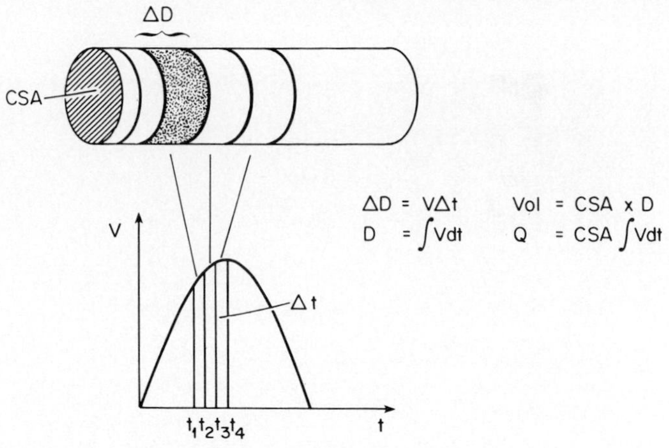

Fig. 30–2. Calculation of volumetric flow with changing velocity. This illustration shows the more complex situation in which velocity is changing. Distance traveled (D) is the product of velocity and time. The distance traveled over a time period (Δt) equals the product of Δt and the mean velocity, which is assumed constant over this small time interval. The volume of flow during this period is the product of the cross-sectional area (CSA) and the distance traveled: CSA × D. The cumulative distance is therefore the integral of the instantaneous velocity over the time period during which flow occurs: D × ∫V dt. Volumetric flow (Q) is then the product of the velocity integral and the CSA: Q = CSA × ∫V dt. (From Ascah KJ, et al.: Doppler echocardiographic assessment of cardiac output. Radiol Clin North Am 23:661, 1985.)

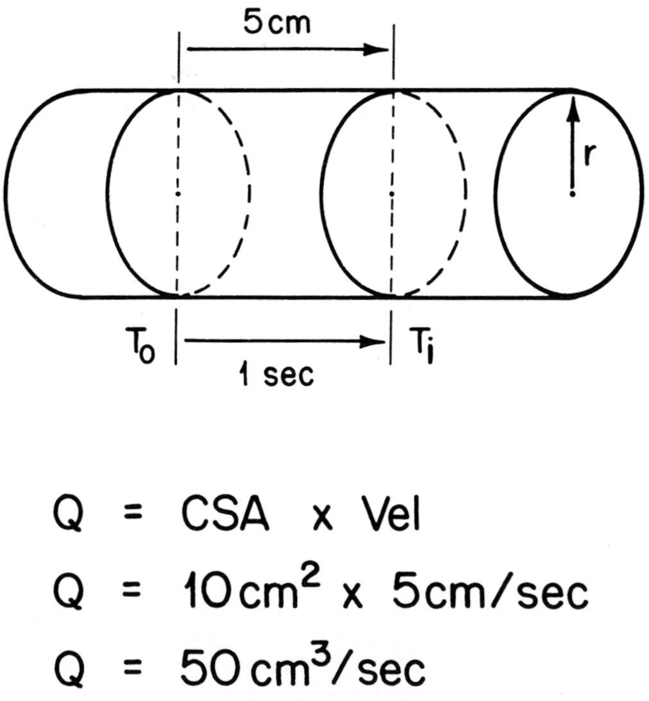

Fig. 30–1. Calculation of volumetric flow. Volumetric blood flow (Q) is the product of cross-sectional area (CSA) and the linear flow velocity (Vel) when the CSA is fixed and Vel is constant. In this example, Q = 10 cm^2 × 5 cm/sec, or 50 cm^3/sec. (From Ascah KJ, et al.: Doppler echocardiographic assessment of cardiac output. Radiol Clin North Am 23:660, 1985.)

DOPPLER-ECHOCARDIOGRAPHIC CALCULATION OF VOLUMETRIC FLOW

Figure 30–3 illustrates how the Doppler-echocardiographic method provides the data necessary to calculate volumetric flow. Figure 30–3 contains a cross-sectional echocardiographic recording of the distal right ventricular outflow tract, pulmonary valve, and main pulmonary artery. This recording is obtained with the scan plane aligned parallel to the long axis of the pulmonary artery. In this view the vessel diameter can be measured at the pulmonary annulus, and the vessel area can be calculated from the diameter as

$$\text{Area} = \pi(D/2)^2 \qquad [30.2]$$

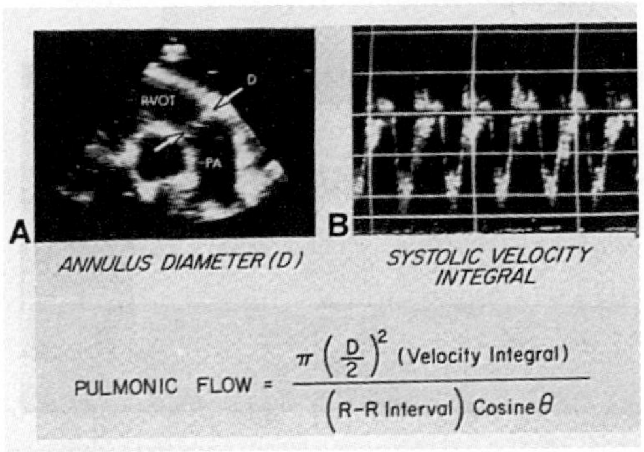

Fig. 30–3. Echocardiographic Doppler-derived date for the measurement of pulmonary valve flow. **A.** A long axis recording of the pulmonary artery (PA) extending from the right ventricular outflow tract (RVOT) to the bifurcation of the pulmonary artery. The point of measurement of the vessel diameter (D) is indicated by the oblique arrows. **B.** A series of representative pulmonary artery flow velocity profiles. The equation used to calculate pulmonary flow is included below the illustration. (From Stewart WJ, et al.: Variable effects of changes in flow rate through the aortic, pulmonary, and mitral valves on valve area and flow velocity: impact on quantitative Doppler flow calculations. J Am Coll Cardiol 6:655, 1985. Reprinted with permission from the American College of Cardiology. Journal of the American College of Cardiology, 1985, 6, 655.)

Figure 30–3, right, contains a representative Doppler recording of blood flow velocity in the pulmonary artery. The Doppler data report velocity per unit time, conventionally in centimeters per second. When integrated over the time interval during which flow occurs (i.e., cm/sec × seconds), the result is the distance traveled by the blood column (in centimeters) during each systole. If this systolic velocity integral or stroke distance is multiplied by the cross-sectional area of the vessel, the result is the stroke volume (milliliters per beat). The stroke volume (SV) may then be multiplied by heart rate (HR) to determine pulmonary artery flow which, in the absence of pulmonary regurgitation or intracardiac shunts, will equal the cardiac output (CO).

$$CO = SV \times HR \qquad [30.3]$$

Alternatively, the mean linear flow velocity (centimeters per second) can be calculated by dividing the velocity integral by the R-R interval. The cardiac output (in liters per minute) is then the product of the mean velocity (in centimeters per second) × 60 (seconds per minute) times the cross-sectional area of the vessel. When the heart rate is variable, as in the presence of frequent atrial or ventricular premature beats or atrial fibrillation, the stroke volume and mean linear velocities change on a beat-to-beat basis. In these instances, velocity measurements must be averaged over a number of beats to obtain an appropriate estimate of cardiac output.

Although, conceptually, the Doppler-echocardiographic calculation of volumetric flow is relatively straightforward, in practice, several potential sources of error exist in the measurement of both the area and velocity that must be recognized and understood.

Assumptions and Potential Sources of Error in the Determination of Cross-Sectional Area

The cross-sectional area of a vessel (or valve) through which blood is flowing can be calculated either from the vessel diameter, as illustrated in Figure 30–3, or from the short axis area of the vessel. Both approaches have advantages and limitations.

Calculation of Area From Vessel/Orifice Diameter(s)

Assumption of Geometric Shape. Calculation of vessel or orifice areas from their diameter(s) assumes these human cardiac structures can be represented as conduits with geometrically "perfect" shapes in cross-section, e.g., a perfect circle or perfect ellipse.

In the case of the aorta, the assumption of a circular geometry seems appropriate, and a diameter taken from a plane that includes the long axis of the vessel should normally permit accurate calculation of vessel area at that level. The pulmonary artery deviates slightly from circularity as it courses above the aorta, but the assumption that the vessel is circular still yields reasonably accurate estimates of area. For the mitral valve, on the other hand, the situation is more complex because a flow area can be measured at either the leaflet tips (the valve orifice) or the valve annulus. The valve orifice changes in both area and shape throughout the diastolic filling period, and the assumption of circular annular geometry, although applied widely and validated clinically,[4] does not appear to be anatomically correct. The shape of the tricuspid valve and its influence on the calculation of flow have been even less well studied.[5]

Compounding of Error That Is Due to Diameter Measurements. When using a diameter to derive the area of a circular vessel or orifice, the percentage of error in the diameter measurement is roughly doubled in the process of area calculation. For instance, a measurement error of 2 mm, when applied to a vessel whose true diameter is 20 mm, will result in an over- or underestimation of the true cross-sectional area of roughly 20%.* A measurement error as small as 1 mm in the same vessel will result in an over- or underestimation of the area by roughly 10% percent. The percentage of error can be expressed by the equation

$$\frac{\Delta A}{A} = \frac{2\Delta d}{d} + \left(\frac{\Delta d}{d}\right)^2 \qquad [30.4]$$

where d is the measured diameter, Δd is the error in diameter measurement, A is the cross-sectional area of vessel or orifice, and ΔA is the error in area measurement.

The error in calculated volume flow is also given by this equation and is shown plotted as a function of $\Delta d/d$ in Figure 30.4. Color flow mapping has been used to outline the flow area within the two-dimensional image

* Based on Equation 30.4, a ±2-mm error in the measurement of the diameter of a 20-mm vessel will yield a 21% error (2 × .10 or .20 or 20% + $(.10)^2$ or .01 or 1% = 21%). For simplicity, in this discussion we ignore the higher order term because its contribution to the overall error is relatively small.

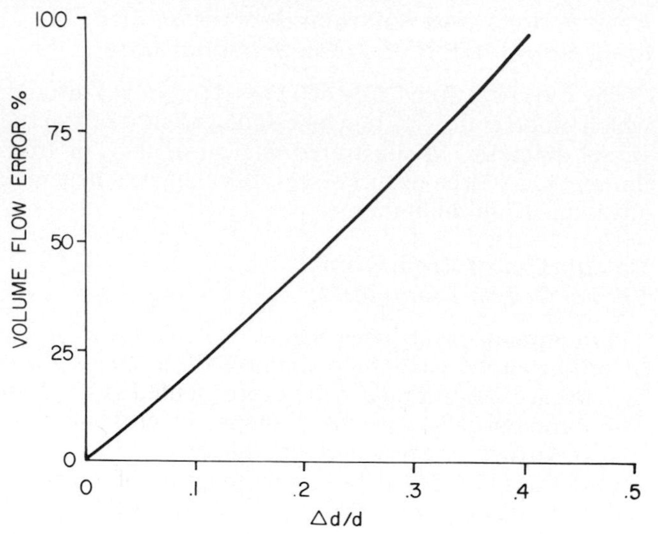

Fig. 30–4. The percentage of error in volume flow caused by error in diameter measurement. (From Baker DW, Forster FK, Daigle RE: Doppler principles and techniques. *In* Fry FJ (ed.): Ultrasound: Its Application in Medicine and Biology. New York, Elsevier Scientific Publishing, 241, 1978.)

in an attempt to better assess effective vessel diameter, but this approach has not improved the measurement of vessel area.[6]

As indicated in Equation 30.4, the percentage of error in calculating flow from the diameter of a circular vessel is inversely related to the size of the vessel. Because the accuracy with which linear dimensions can be measured from echocardiographic images is relatively constant, the percentage of error will increase as the vessel size decreases. For example, in the adult with a 2-cm aorta, a ±1-mm accuracy in the measurement of the vessel diameter would result in a potential error in the area and volume calculation of roughly 10%; for a child with a 10-mm aorta, the error would increase to roughly 20%, while for a neonate or fetus with a 5-mm aorta, the error would exceed 40%. In the adult, diameter measurements can be made with sufficient accuracy to generate a reasonable cross-sectional area. In the very small child, however, the percentage of measurement error may be so large as to limit the validity of the method.

Dynamic Geometry of Cardiac Structures

Effects of Phasic Flow on Instantaneous Vessel Area. Blood does not flow through tubes of fixed diameter but rather through elastic vessels that change in shape and area during the flow period and whose size is itself a function of flow volume. For instance, it is known that aortic area depends on intra-aortic pressure and may increase by as much as 11% during systole.[7–9] The systolic variation in pulmonary artery cross-sectional area is even greater (up to 18%). Thus, even if the area of the vessel/valve can be accurately represented by a simple geometric shape and measured using basic geometric assumptions, the result would represent only the area at the point of temporal sampling. It is necessary, therefore, either to measure the area at each point in time when flow occurs or to identify a "mean" value that represents the vessel area throughout the flow period.

An attempt has been made to account for aortic distention during systole by planimetering the M-mode echocardiogram of the aortic root to obtain the average of the time-integrated systolic diameters;[10] this average systolic diameter is then used to calculate the aortic cross-sectional area. Although of theoretical merit, this effort has proven too time-consuming and impractical for routine use.

Fortunately, the major increase in aortic area occurs at the onset of systole, while most left ventricular outflow occurs later when the vessel is maximally distended and the aortic valve fully open. Because variation in aortic cross-sectional area during the ejection period is relatively small, it can be neglected without importantly altering the calculation of aortic blood flow.

The same approach is typically applied to the pulmonary artery. The greater area change, however, combined with the recognized difficulty in defining the lateral margin of the vessel may account for poorer correlations with invasively determined flows when this vessel is used as the site of measurement.[11–13]

The flow-related fluctuations in the diastolic area of the atrioventricular valves are much greater than for the great vessels and approaches to correcting for these changes are more complex (see following discussion).

Effects of Changes in Absolute Flow on Mean Vessel Area. In addition to the instantaneous changes in vessel area that occur in response to phasic changes in blood flow, mean vessel/orifice size may also vary in response to acute changes in total flow. Figure 30–5, for example,

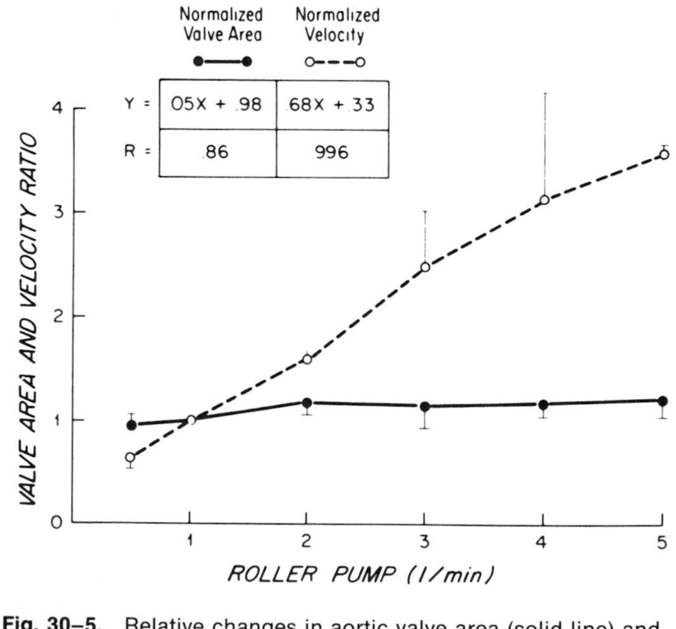

Fig. 30–5. Relative changes in aortic valve area (solid line) and velocity ratio (interrupted line) for a series of experimental studies. Each measurement is normalized to the value at 1 liter/min and presented as the mean percentage of increase or decrease relative to the 1 liter/min value in all animals. (Error bars represent 1 standard deviation from the mean). (From Stewart, WJ, et al.: Variable effects of changes in flow rate through the aortic, pulmonary, and mitral valves on valve area and flow velocity: impact of quantitative Doppler flow calculations. J Am Coll Cardiol 6:658, 1985. Reprinted with permission from the American College of Cardiology. Journal of the American College of Cardiology, 1985, 6, 658.)

illustrates the relative changes in aortic area and velocity integral observed to occur as output was increased from 0.5 to 5 liters/min in our experimental model. Vessel area increases as absolute flow is increased from 0.5 to 2 liters/min, but little further change occurs over the range from 2 to 5 liters/min. For the mitral valve, the changes in valve area are more striking (Fig. 30–6), being proportionally equal to those observed in the velocity integral over the entire range of outputs studied. The effects of increased flow on pulmonary artery cross-sectional area and systolic mean velocity are illustrated in Figure 30–7. For the pulmonary artery, there was a consistent increase in pulmonary annulus diameter with increasing flow throughout the entire range of cardiac outputs. Flow velocity also increased, but the percentage of increase was slightly less than for either the mitral or aortic valve. These observations are important for serial studies in the same patient, because they indicate that the area cannot be routinely measured once and assumed to remain constant as flow is varied; in many cases, the area must be measured separately at each flow level.

Selection of Appropriate Site for Cross-Sectional Area Determination. Because volumetric flow can theoretically be measured at any point along a vessel at which both area and velocity can be recorded, it is important to define the optimal location at which to calculate cross-sectional area. For instance, the "aortic cross-sectional area" can be calculated from a diameter taken within the left ventricular outflow tract, at the orifice valve annulus, the aortic leaflet tips, the sinotubular junction, or the proximal ascending aorta. Several studies have looked specifically at this problem and have arrived at conflicting conclusions.[7,13–15] Our experimental data indicate that diameter measurements taken at the aortic annulus correlate best (r = .97) with roller pump deter-

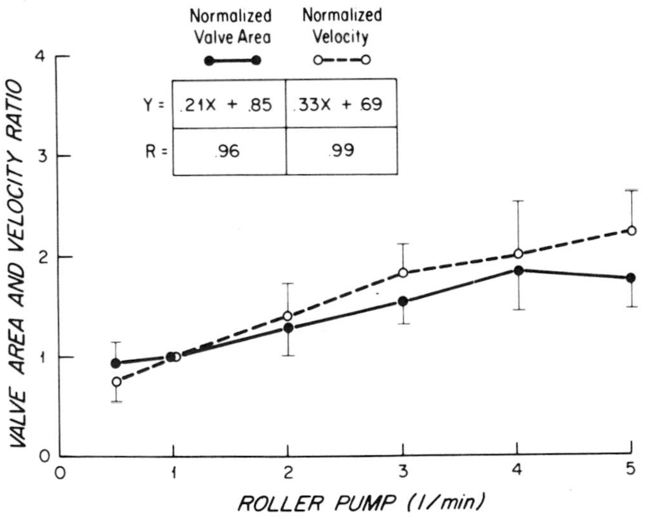

Fig. 30–6. Relative effects of increasing roller pump output on mitral valve area (solid line) and transmitral flow velocity (interrupted line). (From Stewart WJ, et al.: Variable effects of changes in flow rate through the aortic, pulmonary, and mitral valves on valve area and flow velocity: impact on quantitative Doppler flow calculations. J Am Coll Cardiol 6:658, 1985. Reprinted with permission from the American College of Cardiology. Journal of the American College of Cardiology, 1985, 6, 658.)

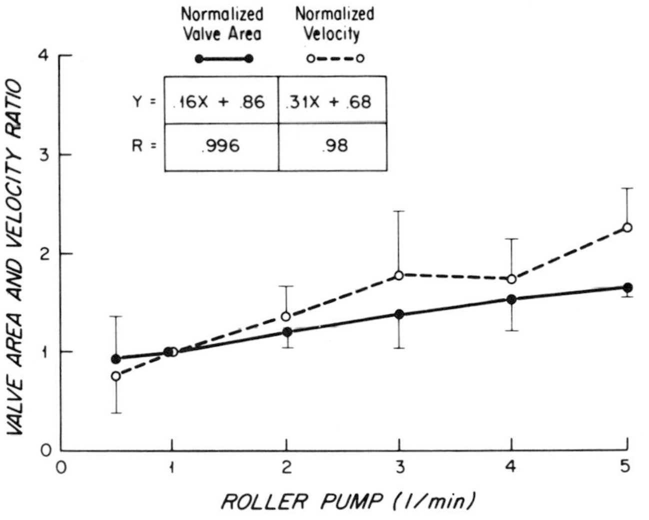

Fig. 30–7. Relative effects of increasing roller pump output on pulmonary valve area (solid line) and transmitral flow velocity (interrupted line). (From Stewart WJ, et al.: Variable effects of changes in flow rate through the aortic, pulmonary, and mitral valves on valve area and flow velocity: impact on quantitative Doppler flow calculations. J Am Coll Cardiol 6:659, 1985. Reprinted with permission from the American College of Cardiology. Journal of the American College of Cardiology, 1985, 6, 659.)

minations of flow.[16] Other theoretical and practical advantages of using this site are (1) the fibrous nature of the annulus, which likely minimizes potential errors as a result of changing orifice area during the cardiac cycle; (2) the easy recognition of the aortic annulus on two-dimensional images, which allows for reproducible diameter measurements with minimal inter- and intraobserver variability; and (3) the fact that the annulus normally represents the narrowest point along the outflow tract and thus is the level at which the peak velocity should occur. This facilitates integration of nonsimultaneously acquired flow and area data. (The appropriate locations to measure the areas of other vessels/valves are discussed later.)

Direct Measurement of Valve or Vessel Area

To avoid the problems encountered in determining the area of a vessel from its diameter, it might seem more accurate to planimeter area directly from short axis views of the structure of interest. In practice, however, the accuracy of this method has been limited by rotational errors in plane alignment, imprecision in plane positioning relative to the limiting orifice, the potential for the heart to shift relative to the short axis plane of view in the period during which flow occurs, and the inaccuracy of planimetry relative to simple diameter measurement.[16] Further, in many instances short axis areas simply cannot be recorded. For example, no view includes a short axis area of the main pulmonary artery or permits reproducible short axis recording of the tricuspid valve area.

These limitations in direct measurement of cross-sectional area have led most investigators to calculate area using a vessel or valve orifice diameter or diameters.

An exception is the measurement of mitral valve area using the orifice method, which is discussed later.

Assumptions and Potential Sources of Error in the Measurement of Velocity

All Doppler calculations of blood flow are based on the measurement of velocity within the region encompassed by the ultrasonic beam. For continuous wave systems, flow is sampled along the entire length of the beam; it is therefore necessary to assume that the maximum velocity recorded corresponds to the velocity at the level where the cross-sectional area has been measured. For pulsed systems, flow is sampled at a predetermined depth selected by the time or range gate. The actual spatial volume sampled by a pulsed system is equal in axial dimension to the length of the time gate, and in lateral dimension, to the width of the beam at the selected sampling level.* Because the depth of flow is known using pulsed Doppler, velocity can be recorded at the same level at which cross-sectional area is measured.[16–18]

Assumption of a Uniform Spatial Velocity

To determine the mean spatial velocity, the velocities recorded within the sample volume must be assumed to represent the velocity distribution across the entire cross-sectional area of the vessel. This is most easily achieved in areas in which the velocity profile is flat. If the velocity profile varies across the width of a vessel (i.e., is parabolic or skewed), then a centrally positioned sample volume may not accurately reflect the mean velocity.

The spatial velocity profile depends on flow acceleration, viscous forces, and geometric factors.[19] Acceleration and convergence of flow, in particular, result in a relatively flat profile, so that flow in the ventricular outflow tracts and in immediate proximity to the semilunar valves has a relatively uniform spatial flow profile in both animals[20,21] and humans.[22] On the other hand, divergence of the flow stream, which occurs within a ventricular chamber or in a dilated aortic root, results in a more parabolic flow profile. Alterations in vessel geometry, such as curvature of the aorta and asymmetry of the outflow tract, may cause the location of peak flow velocities to shift from the center of the flow stream to one side or the other of center (see Chapter 9, Figs. 9–7 and 9–8). This causes the flow field to deviate toward a more parabolic shape and the peak to diverge further from the mean.

Thus, in normal subjects, if flow is measured at a vessel inlet or valve orifice, the velocity profile can be assumed to be flat, and a local sample will be representative of the mean.[23] Likewise, in the absence of turbulence, the mean and the peak velocities will give similar measures of flow.

* Although sample volumes are commonly quoted as being 2 to 4 mm in length, this is the minimal value obtainable at the half-power level at the focal zone of the beam. In clinical studies, the actual sample volume size may be much larger. For example, at a frequency of 3 MHz and a burst duration of 12 cycles, the sample volume will be 6 mm in axial length. Likewise, when sampling the aorta from the apex, the beam will be well beyond the focal zone, and although effective beam width will vary with gain, the beam may easily exceed a centimeter in diameter. Although this results in a loss of spatial resolution, it allows for a more representative acquisition of velocity profiles across the orifice.

Selection of the Appropriate Component of the Spectral Profile to Represent Velocity

Even in areas where the flow profile is relatively flat, there will still be some heterogeneity in the velocities output by the spectrum analyzer. Ideally, the mean flow velocity should be used to calculate flow volume. In practice, however, this value is highly unstable (see Chapter 10) because it is influenced by both system noise and signal sensitivity. The modal velocity (i.e., the velocity that is recorded most frequently) yields a close correlation with independent measures of volumetric flow and is theoretically more stable than the mean. This measure of flow is also the most easily identified because it is represented by the darkest portion of the spectral output. As a result, the modal velocity is most often used in cardiac output determinations.

Determination of Three-Dimensional Spatial Velocity Vector

The basic Doppler equation requires either that the interrogating ultrasound beam be aligned parallel to the direction of blood flow or that the spatial angle between the flow vector and the sound beam (angle Θ) be determined to correct for the difference between the recorded and true velocity. Visual steering of the ultrasound beam permits its alignment parallel to the expected direction of blood flow within the plane of the image. The addition of color Doppler recording of the direction of flow may improve on this visual estimate in cases where the flow stream deviates markedly from its expected path, but this situation is unusual. However, because two-dimensional guidance does not report the relationship between the flow vector and the ultrasonic beam in the orthogonal (elevational) plane, slight adjustments in transducer angulation or in the sample volume axial location or both may be required to obtain the best spectral display. Fortunately, as long as the angle between the ultrasound beam and the spatial vector of blood flow is less than 20°, the error introduced into the Doppler measurement of peak flow velocity is less than 6%[24] (see Fig. 7–21). Thus, although of theoretic concern, this potential error has not proven to be of clinical significance when the beam is initially aligned parallel to the center of the visually defined flow stream and then repositioned to record the highest local velocity with the narrowest spectral bandwidth.

Signal Strength

A final source of error is failure to record the entire Doppler velocity profile as a result of lack of signal strength (low signal/noise ratio). This potential source of error exists in any quantitative Doppler measurement and can be avoided by measuring only spectra in which a clearly defined laminar flow profile is present.

Potential Error Introduced by Combining Nonsimultaneously Recorded Flow and Area Data

In most cases, area and flow measurements are not recorded simultaneously and often are not even acquired in the same plane. For example, the aortic annular diameter is typically determined from a parasternal long axis view, which images the vessel using the axial resolution of the system, while aortic flow velocity is recorded from the cardiac apex, which places the beam parallel to the flow vector. Thus, the two data sets cannot be acquired simultaneously, and it must be assumed that the vessel area has not changed during the interval necessary to acquire the velocity data or vice versa. As a rule, this interval is too short for major hemodynamic changes to occur. In patients with arrythmias, however, it is necessary to acquire the data during similar cycle lengths or to mean both the area and the velocity values for several cycles (particularly, when flow across the A-V valves is being measured in patients with atrial fibrillation).

Assumption of Continuity of Flow

To use volumetric flow measurements to represent the total cardiac output, measurements of blood flow must be taken at sites across which the total stroke volume passes. For example, Doppler estimates of stroke volume taken in the ascending aorta (at or above the sinotubular junction) do not take into account coronary blood flow, which originates proximal to the level of measurement of aortic cross-sectional area and also proximal to the level of measurement of aortic Doppler flow velocity. A more obvious example would be estimating stroke volume from area and velocity measurements taken in the descending aorta, which does not account for the proportion of cardiac output delivered to the arch vessels.

This potential limitation, however, can be used to one's advantage when estimating left-to-right shunt flows. Although flow across the aortic valve cannot be assumed to represent total left ventricular stroke volume in the presence of a ventricular septal defect, it does represent systemic blood flow in this condition and hence can be compared to flow across the pulmonic or mitral valve to estimate shunt ratio.

CLINICAL AND EXPERIMENTAL VALIDATION

Experimental Studies

Because of the many theoretic limitations in the Doppler-echocardiographic measurements of volumetric flow described in the preceding section, early studies were designed to validate the feasibility and accuracy of the method. Although the first of these validation studies were clinical, the variability of clinical measures of flow and output is such that the ultimate accuracy of the method could only be determined from experimental models in which flow could be precisely controlled and measured. The majority of these experimental studies compared volumetric flow determined by the echo-Doppler method with the output of roller pumps in right heart bypass or more complex models (Fig. 30–8), which permitted precise control of flow at specific locations or through the entire heart. The roller pump model was used because it represents the currently accepted gold standard for measurement of volumetric flow in the experimental setting.

Figure 30–9 compares the results of Doppler flow through the aortic, mitral, and pulmonic valves with roller pump cardiac output from a series of seven experiments. For the aortic valve, there is an excellent correlation (r = .98) between the Doppler-echocardiographic measurement and roller pump output, with a slope close to unity (1.06) and a standard deviation of 0.3 liter/min.[16] The correlation between Doppler-echocardiographic mitral valve flow, using the orifice method (see following discussion)[25] and roller pump output was equally good (r = .97) with a slope approximating unity (.98) and a standard deviation of 0.3 liter/min. Correlation between calculated pulmonary valve flow and roller pump output, although still good (r = .93), was not as high as those for the aortic and mitral valves. Likewise, the slope of the regression was less than unity, and the standard deviation (0.5 liter/min) was greater than that noted for either of the previous Doppler-echocardiographic measurements.

In a similar study, flow was recorded with the Doppler technique at several sites in the aortic arch, resulting in correlation coefficients of 0.98 to 0.99 with roller pump outputs and a mean standard error of 0.23 liter/min.[17] The same group found an excellent correlation (r = .97) between Doppler-derived mitral flow and roller pump

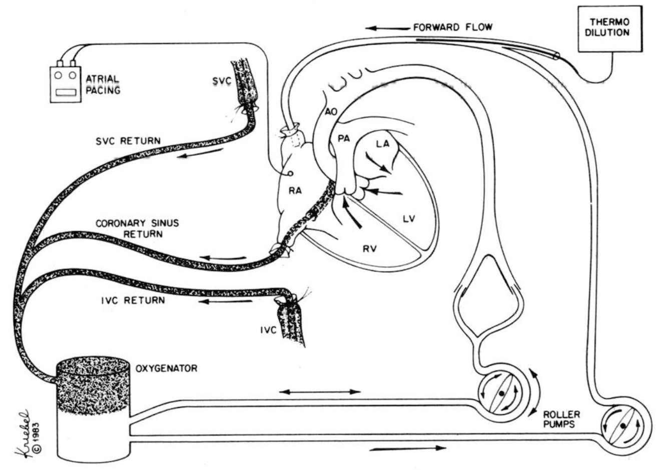

Fig. 30–8. The roller pump model used in volumetric flow studies. Systemic venous return (dark stippled areas) is collected from the superior vena cava (SVC), inferior vena cava (IVC), and the coronary sinus and returned to a membrane oxygenator. Oxygenated blood is reinfused into the right atrium (RA) at a controlled rate using a roller pump. Arterial pressure is controlled by infusion or withdrawal of blood from the femoral arteries using a second roller pump. Heart rate can be controlled by atrial pacing. AO = aorta; LA = left atrium; LV = left ventricle; PA = pulmonary artery; RV = right ventricle. (From Stewart WJ, et al.: Variable effects of changes in flow rate through the aortic, pulmonary, and mitral valves on valve area and flow velocity: impact on quantitative Doppler flow calculations. J Am Coll Cardiol 6:654, 1985. Reprinted with permission from the American College of Cardiology. Journal of the American College of Cardiology, 1985, 6, 654.)

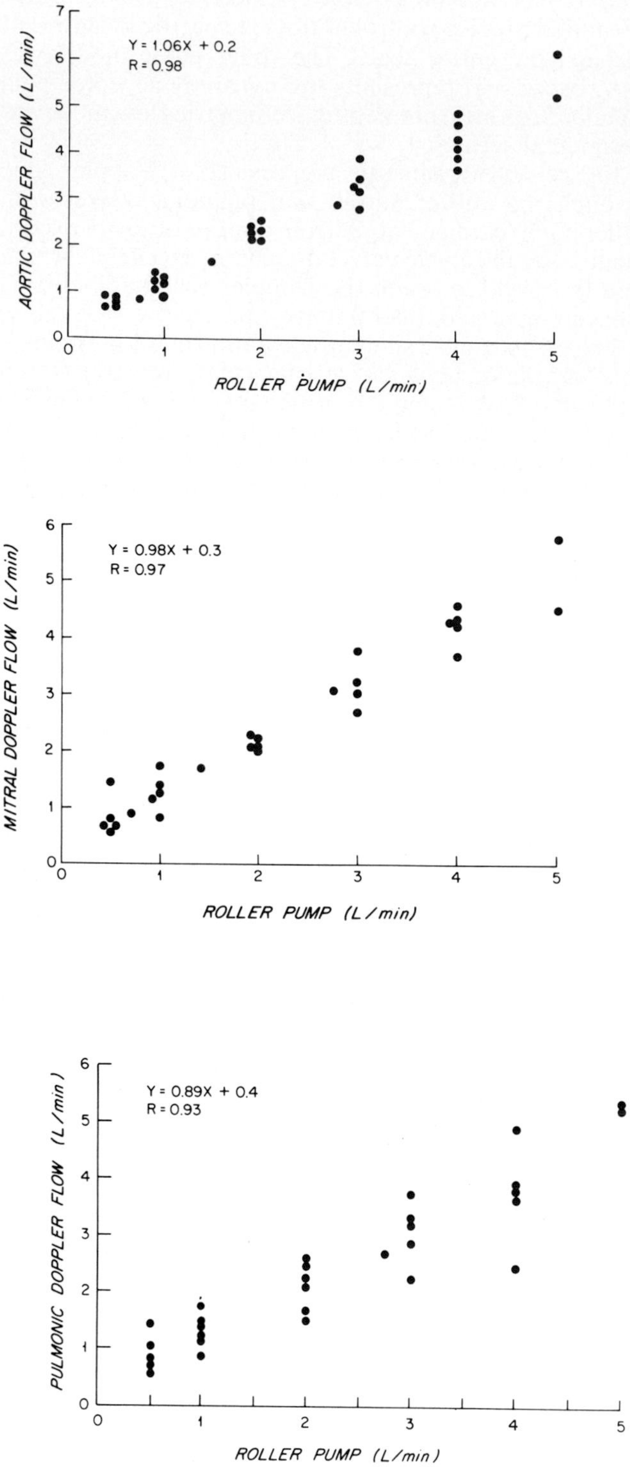

Fig. 30–9. Comparison of the results of Doppler flow through the aortic, mitral, and pulmonic valves with roller pump output. Top. Doppler cardiac output through the aortic valve demonstrates an excellent correlation with roller pump flow (r = 0.98). Middle. Doppler mitral valve flow also correlates well with roller pump flow (r = 0.97). Bottom. Pulmonic flow, however, showed a lesser degree of correlation with roller pump output. (From Stewart WJ, et al.: Variable effects of changes in flow rate through the aortic, pulmonic, and mitral valves on valve area and flow velocity: impact on quantitative Doppler flow calculation. J Am Coll Cardiol 6:653, 1985. Reprinted with permission from the American College of Cardiology.

output over a range of cardiac outputs from 1.0 to 5 liters/min.[17] Likewise, in a more complex experimental model of ventricular septal defect, an excellent correlation was found between Doppler-derived mitral valve flow and pulmonary artery flow measured by an electromagnetic flow probe.[26] These data validated the accuracy of the echo-Doppler method in the ideal experimental setting and provided valuable insight into the optimal methods and locations of measurement.

Clinical Studies

The development of instruments that combine Doppler velocity recording with echocardiographic measurement of vessel area using both the M-mode and two-dimensional techniques also led to a host of clinical studies to test the accuracy of the Doppler method of volumetric flow determination. Clinical validation of the Doppler method has necessarily relied on comparisons with invasive standards of flow measurement, which are each imperfect approximations of a gold standard for volumetric flow. Nonetheless, Doppler estimates of volumetric flow seem to compare as favorably with the traditional invasive methods of assessing cardiac output as these methods compare among themselves.

APPROACHES TO MEASURING VOLUMETRIC FLOW AT INDIVIDUAL INTRACARDIAC SITES

Aortic Valve and Aortic Arch Flow

Early studies demonstrate that aortic flow velocity could be recorded in human subjects by the continuous wave Doppler method, and this approach was termed "aortovelography."[27] These flow velocity recordings were subsequently demonstrated to be proportional to cardiac output in both clinical and experimental studies and to vary appropriately in response to stimuli designed to increase or decrease stroke volume.[18–30] When tested on a beat-to-beat basis in the experimental model (Fig. 30–10), the Doppler velocity integral showed a strong correlation with flows recorded by an electromagnetic flow probe.[24]

These early observations were followed by numerous studies testing the accuracy of the Doppler method of measuring flow across the aortic valve. Minor variations in individual studies arise from the use of continuous wave vs. pulsed Doppler and, more importantly, from the selection of different sites from which to measure aortic diameter for use in area calculation. Good correlations (r = .75 to .98) seem to be achieved regardless of the site chosen for aortic diameter measurement when compared with Fick[7,31–33] or thermodilution[5,7,10,13,15,34–43] methods of measuring cardiac output. These determinations can be accomplished with less than 5% interobserver variability.[44] Clinical correlations that appear better than those that can be achieved in the ideal experimental setting are likely fortuitous, and in general, one might expect clinical results to approach but not exceed those that can be obtained with the transducer directly on the heart.

Figure 30–11 contains early data comparing echo-

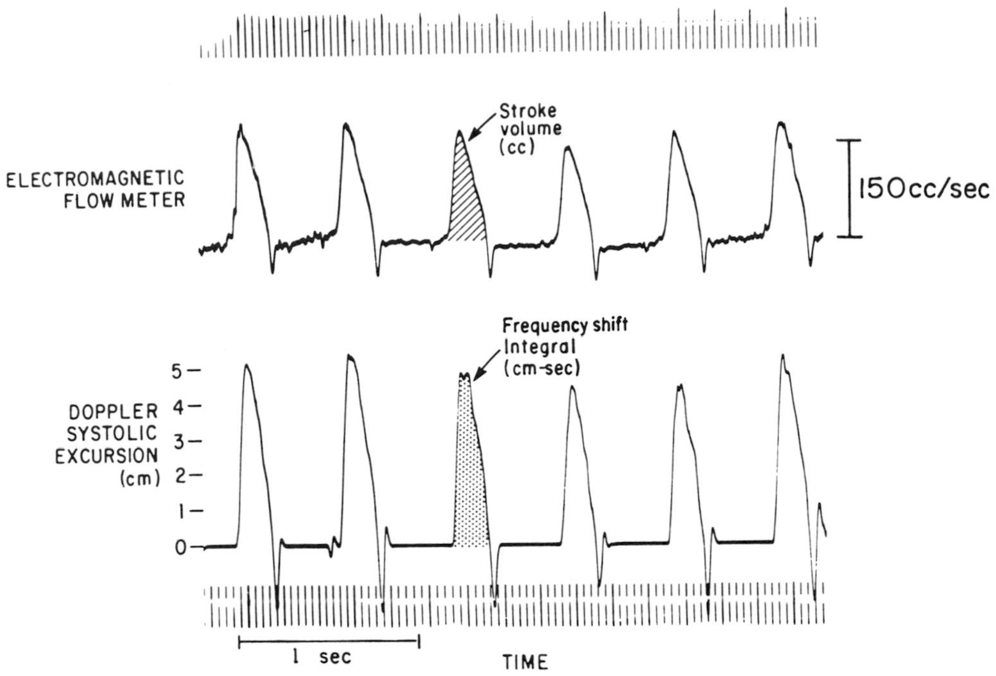

Fig. 30–10. Simultaneous electromagnetic flowmeter and pulsed Doppler recordings from the ascending aorta of a dog illustrate the similarity of these two measures of velocity. The Doppler output is expressed as stroke distance (i.e., centimeters per beat). (From Steingart R, et al.: Pulsed Doppler echocardiographic measurement of beat-to-beat changes in stroke volume in dogs. Circulation 62: 544, 1980. Reproduced by permission of the American Heart Association, Inc.)

Doppler measurements of cardiac output with those obtained by thermodilution. Although methods have been refined and equipment improved significantly since this study, the results appear representative of what the experienced operator can expect to obtain in routine clinical studies. Correlations may be somewhat better in carefully controlled research studies (Fig. 30–12A) performed under ideal conditions and can be expected to be less good in the intensive care setting where patient access and cooperation are necessarily limited. In any case, the operator must be able to recognize the quality of the recorded data and hence the expected accuracy of the result.

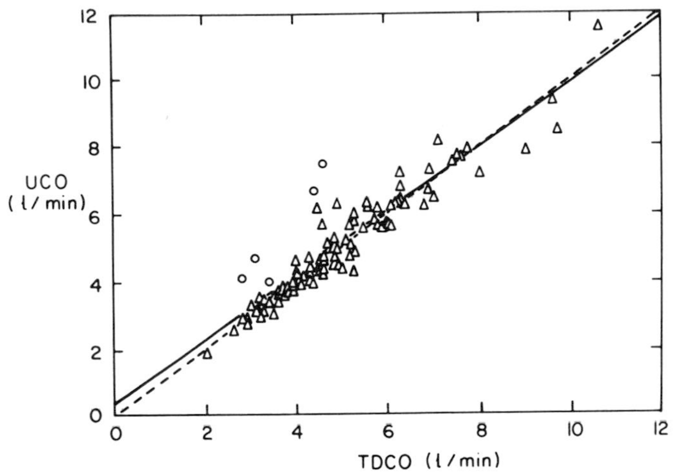

Fig. 30–11. Correlation of ultrasonic and thermodilution cardiac output (UCO and TDCO) measurements. The line of identity (dashed) and the least-squares regression line (solid) are shown. The regression line is described by: UCO = 0.98 TDCO + 0.17 (r = 0.96, SEE = 0.44, n = 105). Triangles = data points. (Modified from Huntsman LL, et al.: Noninvasive Doppler determination of cardiac output in man: clinical validation. Circulation 67:599, 1983. Reproduced by permission of the American Heart Association, Inc.) UCO = ultrasound cardiac output; TDCO = thermodilution cardiac output.

Doppler estimates of cardiac output have also been validated in children, with reported correlation coefficients of 0.94 to 0.98[45,46] when compared to invasive measures of cardiac output. As in adults, the best correlations are obtained when the area measurement at the aortic annulus is used in calculating Doppler cardiac outputs.[47,48] Volumetric determinations in children are aided somewhat in that two-dimensional images are often of higher quality than those obtained in many adults. All diameter measurements, however, are more critical in small infants and children because the error of measurement introduces an increasingly greater percentage of error in cardiac output with decreasing vessel diameter.

Based on available data, we measure the aortic diameter at the level of the aortic valve annulus, which is easily recognized in parasternal images and whose size does not change significantly during the cardiac cycle. Ascending aortic velocity waveforms are best recorded by pulsed Doppler with the sample volume placed just beyond the valve annulus in the proximal ascending aorta using the apical five-chamber or apical long axis view (Fig. 30–13). Although other echocardiographic windows may be used, the recommended views usually allow acquisition of aortic flow velocity recordings with an angle Θ of less than 20°. The velocity waveforms should be traced through the modal velocity, which represents the velocity most frequently found in the sampling site, and is manifested as the darkest output in the spectral display. In tracing the velocity waveform, the components after systole should be ignored, because they result primarily from wall reflections and elastic recoil. If the beginning and end of systole cannot be clearly recorded, it is acceptable practice to extrapolate

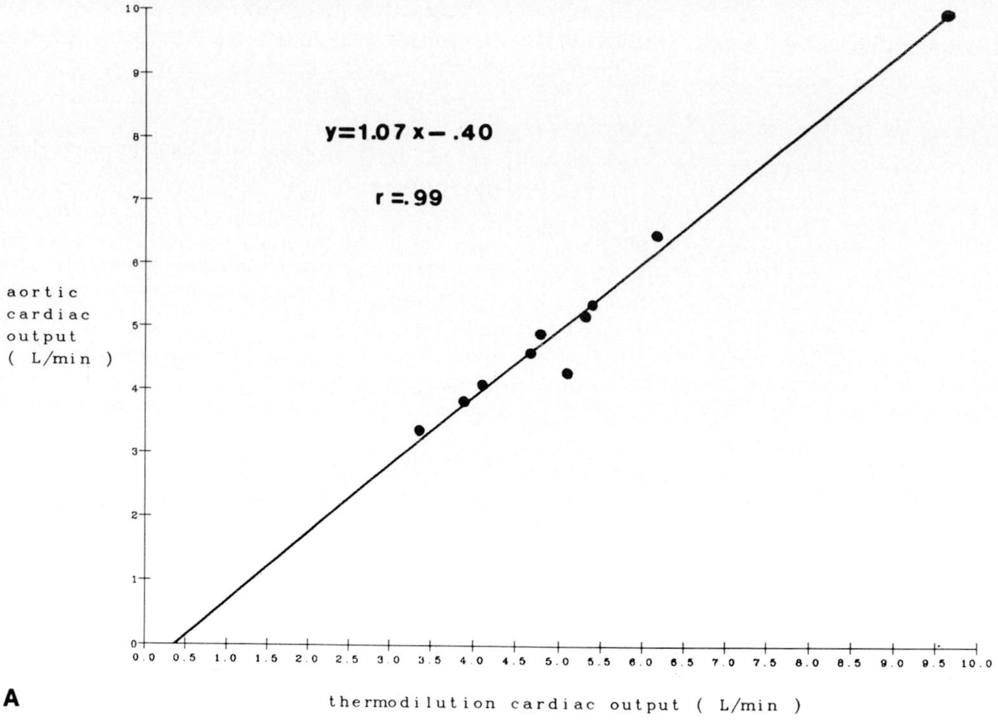

A

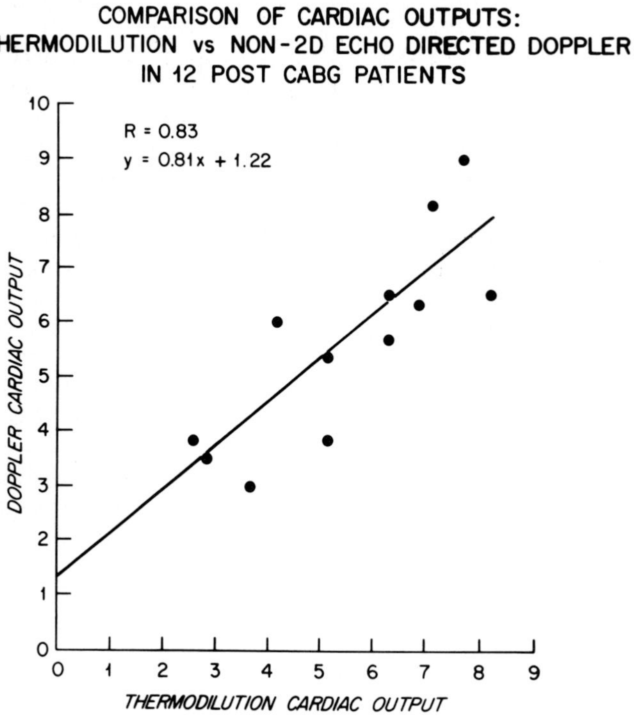

B

Fig. 30–12. A. Comparison of Doppler cardiac output with thermodilution cardiac output in the controlled research environment. Doppler cardiac outputs calculated using the aortic valve (y axis) compare well with thermodilution cardiac outputs (x axis) in the group of patients studied (r = .99). **B.** Comparison of Doppler cardiac output with thermodilution cardiac output in the intensive care unit. Doppler cardiac outputs (aortic valve) on the y axis compare less well with thermodilution cardiac outputs (x axis) in the intensive care unit setting (r = 0.83), where patient access and cooperation are limited. CABG = coronary artery bypass graft. (From Ascah KJ, et al.: Doppler echocardiographic assessment of cardiac output. Radiol Clin North Am 23:664, 1985.)

the acceleration and deceleration phases of the systolic velocity to zero flow.

Mitral Valve Flow

Clinical assessment of mitral flow[4,25,49] has proven more difficult than that of the aortic valve, and the results are more variable. Difficulties relate to the phasic pattern of diastolic filling and the associated variation in effective flow area. Measurement of the velocity integral is appropriately made at the point at which the peak E- and A-wave velocities are recorded. This generally occurs between the annulus and the leaflet tips, and the precise location can be identified by incrementally moving the sample volume between these two reference points and radially scanning outward from the center of the orifice at each sample volume location. Experimental evidence indicates that the velocity profile across the mitral valve is flat except for a zone of high shear at the margin of the anterior leaflet in mid- and end-diastole.[50]

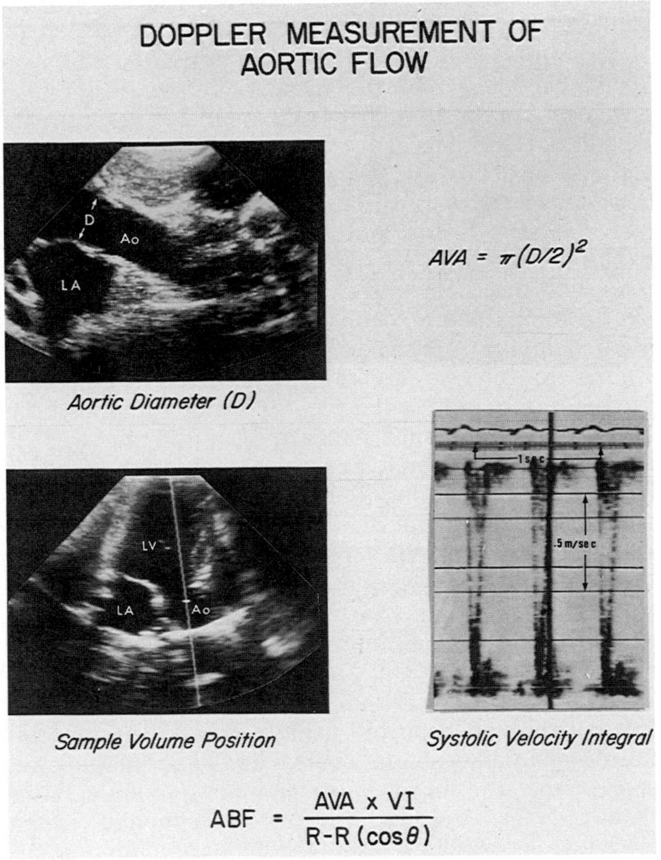

Fig. 30–13. Doppler measurement of aortic flow. D = left ventricular outflow track diameter; R = R wave of the EKG; AO = aorta; LA = left atrium; AVA = Aortic Valve Area; LV = left ventricle; ABF = aortic blood flow; VI = velocity interval. (See text for details.)

Although flow accelerates from the atrium to the valve and decelerates within the ventricle, the spatial extent of the peak velocity at the time of the E wave is relatively long, so that a representative velocity is not difficult to acquire (Fig. 30–14).

As in the case of the aortic valve, controversy exists concerning the optimal method for determining the cross-sectional area of the mitral valve. Two principal alternatives have been suggested: (1) measurement of the valve area at the leaflet tips (orifice method), with correction by the mean-to-maximum leaflet separation to derive a mean flow area, and (2) measurement of annular diameter(s) with area calculated assuming either a circular or elliptic annular shape.

Mitral Orifice Method

Doppler quantification of left ventricular inflow was first obtained by measuring the mean orifice area at the mitral leaflet tips. The mean area was determined by planimetry of the largest mitral valve orifice recorded using parasternal short axis views in open-chest dogs.[25] To convert this maximal valve area to a mean flow area, the ratio of the mean-to-maximal leaflet separation (Fig. 30–15) was derived from an M-mode recording through the leaflet tips. When the maximal two-dimensional planimetered area was multiplied by this ratio, it yielded a mean mitral valve area for diastole. The product of this mean area and the mitral diastolic velocity integral then yielded the transmitral flow. Using this method, which inherently assumed an elliptic mitral orifice, excellent correlation (r = .97) was found between Doppler measurements and roller pump flows over cardiac outputs from 1 to 5 liters/min. We have subsequently verified these findings in the experimental animal model.[16]

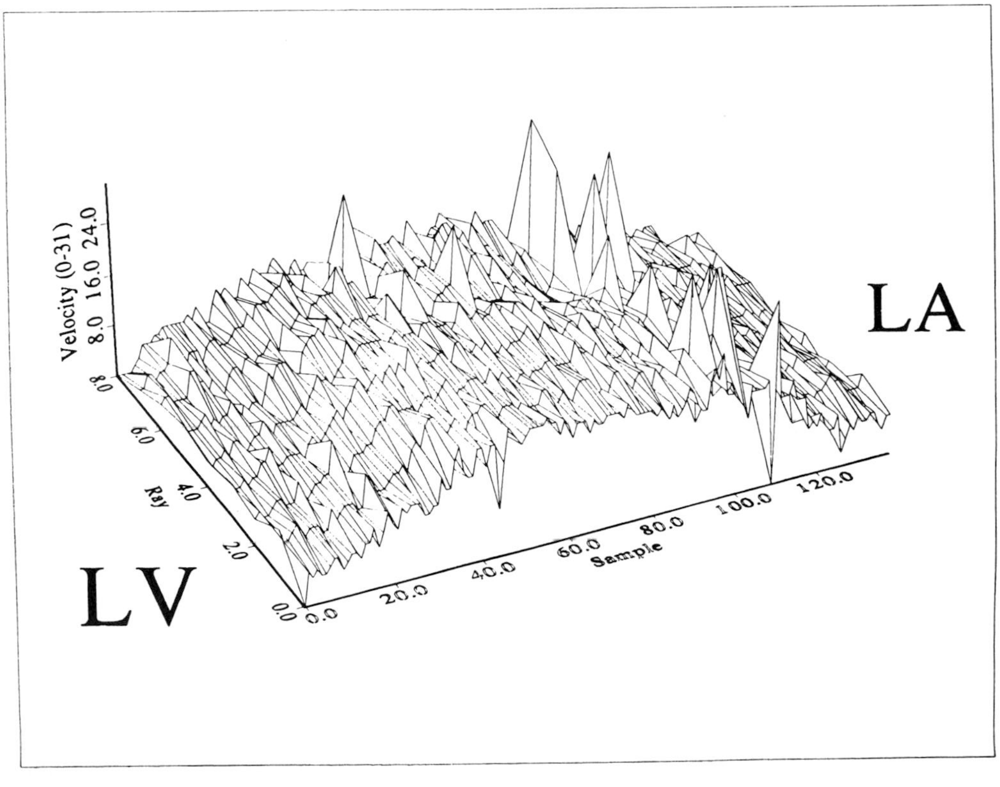

Fig. 30–14. Digitized velocity field across the mitral valve at the peak of the E wave. Sample length extends from the middle of the left ventricle (LV) (0.0) to the middle of the left atrium (LA) (right margin). Digitized flow field extends from the posterior (Ray 0) to anterior mitral leaflet (Ray 8.0). Note the relatively flat velocity profile over an extensive area between the mitral leaflets.

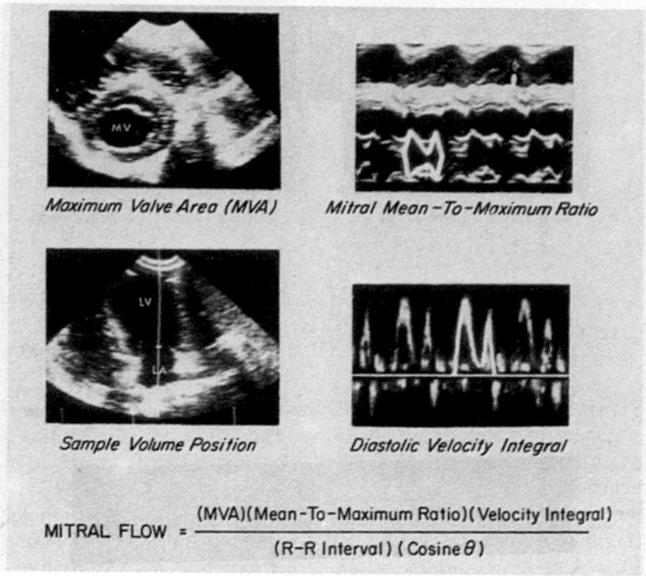

Fig. 30.15. Echocardiographic Doppler-derived data used to measure mitral valve flow. Top, left. A short axis cross-sectional scan through the mitral valve leaflets at the point of maximal leaflet opening. Top, right. An M-mode recording taken through the valve leaflets at the point of maximal excursion. Superimposed on the second M-mode complex is the area encompassed by the mitral valve echogram as outlined by the video digitizer. Bottom, left. The relation of the Doppler cursor to the mitral inlet with the transducer positioned at the cardiac apex and the sample volume just proximal to the mitral valve annulus. Bottom, right. Diastolic flow through the mitral valve with the modal components outlined by the video digitizer in the central complex. Below the illustrations is the formula used in calculating mitral valve flow. LA = left atrium; LV = left ventricle; MV = mitral valve. (From Stewart WJ, et al.: Variable effects of changes in flow rate through the aortic, pulmonary, and mitral valves on valve area and flow velocity: impact on quantitative Doppler flow calculations. J Am Coll Cardiol 6:655, 1985. Reprinted with permission from the American College of Cardiology.

Since these initial animal experiments, conflicting data have appeared regarding the feasibility and reliability of this method in human adults.[42,49,51] Several investigators have modified this approach by using only M-mode diameter measurements[52] or by employing both instantaneous flow and instantaneous orifice measurements[53] in attempts to simplify measurements or improve correlation with invasive determinations of cardiac output. These variations of the original method enjoy similar high correlations with thermodilution cardiac outputs (r = .93 to .94).

Mitral Annulus Method

An alternative to the measurement of the mitral valve orifice is to measure area at the mitral annulus. The area at the annulus can be determined from a single diameter assuming a circular configuration or from two orthogonal diameters with area calculated as the area of an ellipse. Regardless of the method used, it is necessary to correct for the change in annular size that occurs during diastole. This is achieved by measuring the annular diameter(s) several frames (typically two) after valve opening, which is assumed to provide a mean diastolic value.

Assumption of a Circular Orifice. Experimental studies[54] have determined the mitral valve annulus area by measuring the maximal diastolic diameter between the medial and lateral insertions of the anterior and posterior leaflets, respectively, in the apical four-chamber view. Assuming a circular orifice, mitral valve area was calculated as $\pi(D/2)^2$. This method has been validated in the experimental model by comparison to roller pump outputs with excellent correlations reported (r = .99).[25] When compared to results obtained using the orifice method in the same model, overall correlations with control flow measurements by both methods of area approximation were similar.[25] The orifice method, however, showed a smaller standard error and thus was felt to be more reproducible and more accurate than the annular method assuming a circular orifice. Flow calculated using the annular diameter with a circular approximation also correlated surprisingly well (r = .98) with thermodilution cardiac outputs in children.[54] Other clinical studies assuming a circular mitral orifice have also demonstrated excellent correlations with thermodilution measurements.[5]

Assumption of an Elliptic Orifice. Despite the excellent correlations reported using a circular assumption for mitral annulus shape, clinical and experimental data suggest that the mitral valve annulus is elliptic rather than circular. Further, in the experimental canine model, areas calculated from the major and minor annular diameters using an elliptic assumption (area = $\pi \times d_1/2 \times d_2/2$) resulted in a more accurate measurement of transmitral flow than did those calculated using a circular assumption.[55] Clinical studies assuming an elliptic orifice[3] have also resulted in good correlation with both Doppler aortic flows and Fick methods of measuring cardiac output.

Thus, despite numerous studies seeking to validate mitral valve flow measurements, questions remain concerning the best method for determining the orifice area. The mitral orifice method, although theoretically attractive and highly accurate in the experimental model, has proven difficult for many to apply clinically. These difficulties, which appear to relate to the accuracy with which the short axis area of the valve can be measured from clinical recordings, have limited widespread use. Although the annular diameter is clearly easier to measure than the orifice area, the appropriate formula to use in the annular area calculation remains unclear. Assumption of an elliptic orifice seems to provide the best correlations with roller pump determinations of cardiac output in the experimental preparation, while methods assuming a circular orifice, although anatomically inaccurate, have repeatedly achieved high correlations with invasive measures of cardiac output in the clinical setting. The potential inaccuracies introduced by using the circular approximation to calculate the area of an ellipse are illustrated in Figure 30–16. This apparent paradox of good results being achieved by an apparently inappropriate model can be explained by two factors. First, the diameter measured in the apical four-chamber view is not the maximal diameter of the annulus, and therefore,

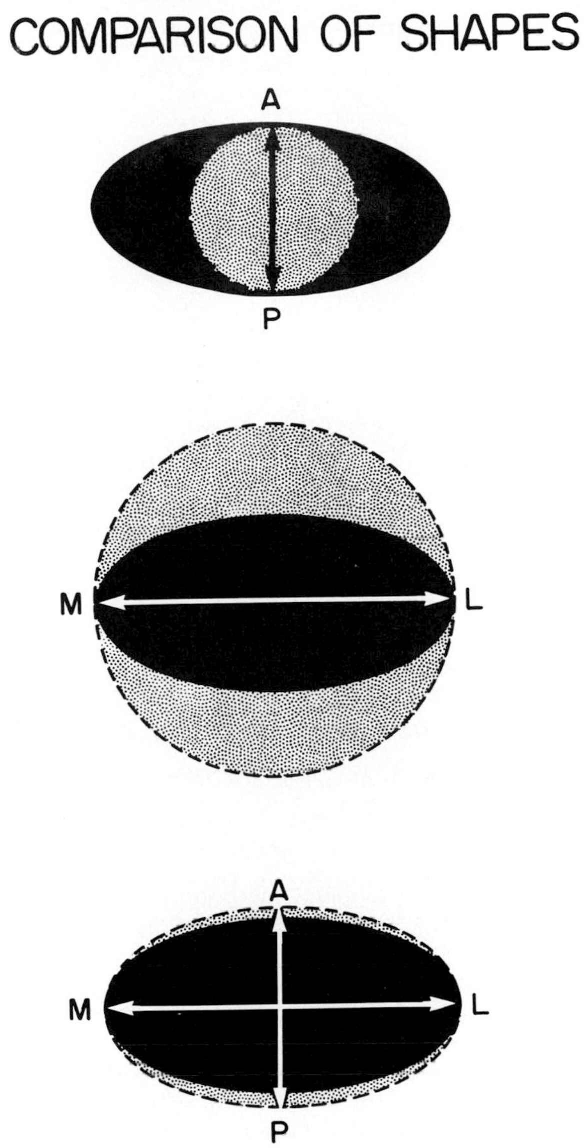

Fig. 30–16. Comparison of models for calculating effective mitral valve orifice. Top. When the mitral annulus was assumed to be circular, effective valve area was underestimated when the anteroposterior dimension was used. Middle. Valve area was overestimated when the mediolateral dimension was used. Bottom. When the annulus was modeled as an ellipse, close approximation of initial annular area was obtained. (From Ascah KJ, et al.: Calculation of transmitral flow by Doppler echocardiography: a comparison of methods in a canine model. Am Heart J 117:408, 1989.)

a circle calculated from this diameter will fall between that which would be calculated using the major or minor dimensions alone. Second, the annular images recorded from the apex will be narrowed, which is due to the point-spread function encountered in the far field of the image. These factors probably combine to produce a diameter that falls between the major and minor diameters of the annulus and from which a circular area will result that approximates the true area of the annulus.

Because reliance on errors' canceling is dangerous in individual cases, we prefer to use the mitral orifice method in patients in whom image quality allows accurate measurements. Area calculations from the annulus diameter assuming a circular shape can be used in patients with suboptimal short axis images as long as the potential limitations are recognized.

Pulmonic Valve Flow

Pulmonic valve flow has been less well studied clinically, and results have been variable, with correlation coefficients ranging from 0.72 to >0.9 when compared to independent measures of flow.[11,13,16,56,57] The major source of this variability in echo-Doppler calculations of pulmonary flow, as with aortic flow determination, appears to be in the measurement of pulmonary artery diameter. The pulmonary artery diameter is often difficult to measure accurately, which is due to poor visualization of the lateral wall of the main pulmonary artery. The importance of this source of error is supported by the observation that correlation of Doppler flows with clinical measures of cardiac output improves significantly when the angiographic diameter of the pulmonary artery is used to calculate the cross-sectional area of the vessel instead of using the echocardiographic diameter.[11] These data also confirm the general observation that the major source of error in flow measurements is the area determination as opposed to the velocity measurement.

We measure the systolic diameter of the main pulmonary artery from the parasternal window at the level of the valve annulus from inner edge to inner edge, in the frame following maximal systolic leaflet separation. Pulmonary blood flow velocity should be measured in the main pulmonary artery at the pulmonary leaflet tips. Averaging several beats is especially important when determining cardiac outputs at the pulmonic valve because respiratory variation may be substantial.

Tricuspid Valve Flow

Quantitation of tricuspid valve flows has been less well studied; most investigators have assumed a circular orifice and a constant diameter throughout diastole for the tricuspid valve. Excellent correlations ($r = .93$ to $.98$) have been reported between tricuspid valve flow and thermodilution cardiac output in clinical studies with the assumption of a circular orifice.[5,57]

Despite these encouraging results, one must remain skeptical when correlations in the clinical situation exceed values obtained for the same valve orifice under carefully controlled experimental conditions. As a result, the routine clinical use of tricuspid flow measurements cannot be recommended at this time. As more is learned, and less is assumed, about the geometry and function of the tricuspid valve, it is likely that reliable and reproducible methods of determining cardiac output across this valve will follow.

VALIDATION DURING HEMODYNAMIC INTERVENTIONS

Although absolute flow determined by the Doppler-echocardiographic method has been shown to correlate with measured flow in both experimental and clinical studies over a wide range of cardiac outputs, there is clearly variability in the Doppler measurements. This measurement error might be sufficient to preclude detection of small but real changes that are due to physiologic or therapeutic interventions. Therefore, several investigators have sought to extend validation to measurements made during clinical interventions that change cardiac output. Most of these studies have involved cardiac output measured in the ascending aorta and have reported the relationship between change in output measured by Doppler to that obtained using an independent standard. These types of studies are important because they suggest that the errors in absolute Doppler measurements are consistent and hence permit relatively small serial changes to be observed and that useful data concerning serial changes in flow may be obtained even in settings where absolute values may differ. They also suggest that serial measurement of the aortic flow velocity integral may be used to determine the percentage of change in aortic flow (because aortic area is less influenced by flow over the physiologic range than that of other valves), thereby avoiding the area measurement that contains the greatest source of error in the Doppler flow calculation.

In a study designed to measure the effects of vasodilator therapy in patients with congestive heart failure,[35] a close correlation between the percentage changes in systolic velocity integral and stroke volume by thermodilution was found (r = .88).

Subsequent comparisons between Doppler measurements of aortic flow and thermodilution outputs in patients with coronary artery disease before, during, and after dobutamine infusion achieved good correlation (r = .92), suggesting that Doppler-echo could reliably follow *changes* in stroke volume.[58]

A significant correlation between cardiac output measurements by pulsed Doppler and thermodilution (r = .88) has also been demonstrated during incremental pacing, inotropic stimulation, and systemic vasodilation.[40] Although paired values for cardiac output by the two techniques differed by up to 0.9 liter/min in individual patients, the *changes* in output in response to hemodynamic interventions were directionally similar in the two techniques.

In 1987, comparisons of Doppler outputs with the CO_2 rebreathing method and the dye dilution method of cardiac output determination were made in a small group of normal subjects at rest and after a variety of interventions designed to alter the cardiac output or heart rate either together or separately.[59] Excellent correlation (r = .99) was found when mean cardiac output values of the group for each intervention were compared.

Other studies have yielded poorer correlations with invasive methods of cardiac output determination. For example, Doppler-echocardiography has been compared with Fick cardiac outputs in assessing the hemodynamic response to felodipine and metoprolol in hypertensive patients.[60] Although there was poor agreement between the two methods, both determinations of cardiac output rose significantly with felodipine and reached their highest values after 30 minutes.

Thus, good correlation has generally been demon-

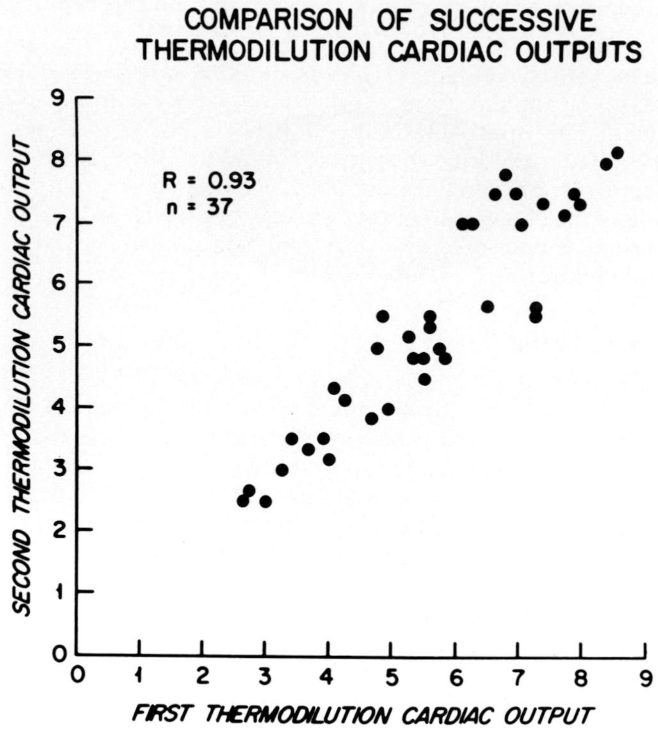

Fig. 30–17. Correlation of consecutive thermodilution cardiac outputs. (See text for details.)

strated between the Doppler method of cardiac output determination and traditional invasive measures, both at rest and during interventions designed to alter cardiac output. Although both Doppler and invasive methods will yield similar results, their correlations with each other must be viewed in the context of the recognized errors in the measured components of each method. Figure 30–17 illustrates the correlation of paired consecutive thermodilution cardiac output measurements over a range extending from 2.5 to 9 liters/min. Despite careful repeated measurements, the best correlation we could achieve for one thermodilution cardiac output compared to a second thermodilution measurement was r = .93. It would appear unlikely that any invasive measure of cardiac output would show a better correlation with an independent measure of output than it does with itself.

CLINICAL APPLICATIONS

The Doppler technique for measuring blood flow has a variety of potential clinical applications including the baseline and serial assessment of cardiac output, calculation of the magnitude of intra- and extra-cardiac shunts, quantifying valvular regurgitation, and calculating the orifice area of stenotic valves.

Baseline and Serial Assessment of Cardiac Output

Doppler-echocardiography is particularly well suited to the serial evaluation of cardiac function and the assessment of interventions because it is noninvasive and provides information on a beat-to-beat basis. Changes in stroke volume and cardiac output are expected to be determined more accurately than are absolute flows, because any systematic error such as that introduced by vessel or annular diameter measurements would be negated. This approach has been used clinically to assess the effects of drug therapy, to evaluate the hemodynamic response to different types of pacemakers, to document the changes in output during pregnancy and in the peripartum period, and to determine outputs in neonates and children.

Drug Therapy

Doppler-echocardiography has been used to study the effects of vasodilator therapy in patients with congestive heart failure.[35] The peak systolic flow velocity showed a strong inverse correlation (r = .89) with systemic vascular resistance, and it was concluded that these measurements could be helpful in the evaluation and management of subjects with heart failure in whom afterload reduction is being considered.

Doppler-echocardiography has also been used to determine noninvasively the serial hemodynamic effects (cardiac output and systemic vascular resistance) of a new antihypertensive, rilmenidine.[61]

Pacemakers

The hemodynamic response to various pacing modes is an important consideration in the selection and programming of implantable pacemakers. We[62] and others[63,64] have demonstrated a significant increase in cardiac output, determined by Doppler-echocardiography, in response to atrioventricular (DDD) versus ventricular (VVI) pacing in groups of patients with a variety of cardiac disorders (Fig. 30–18). Doppler-derived estimates of cardiac output have also been used to determine optimal atrioventricular delays in patients with programmable dual-chamber pacemakers.[63,65] These studies suggest that quantitative Doppler-echocardiography may be useful in the selection of patients likely to benefit from DDD pacing and for the optimization of pacemaker settings.

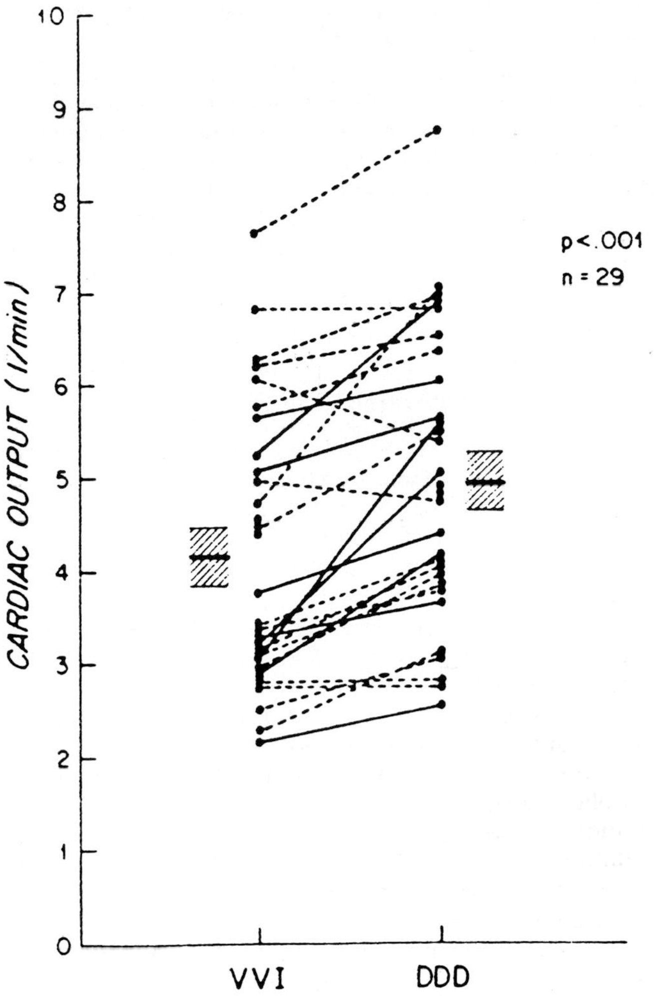

Fig. 30–18. Comparison of cardiac output in VVI and DDD pacing modes. In patients with either ventriculoatrial conduction or the pacemaker syndrome, the data points are connected by a solid line. Data points from patients with neither ventriculoatrial conduction nor the pacemaker syndrome are connected with dashed lines. Hash-marked areas denote the group mean ± standard error of the mean. (From Stewart WJ, et al.: Doppler ultrasound measurement of cardiac output in patients with physiologic pacemakers. Am J Cardiol 54:309, 1984.)

Pregnancy

Two thirds of maternal deaths from heart disease occur during or shortly after labor,[66] but the changes in cardiac output during these times were not well studied until the late 1980s. The echo-Doppler method of calculating cardiac output in the ascending aorta has been validated in pregnant patients with pulmonary artery catheters in place.[67,68] Excellent correlations (r = .91 to .94) were achieved when compared to thermodilution cardiac outputs.

Doppler-derived estimates of flow across the pulmonary valve have also been used to evaluate hemodynamic changes in the pregnant patient during labor and the early puerperium.[69] Pulmonary artery diameter was measured during systole at the level of the pulmonary annulus, and it was assumed that pulmonary artery cross-sectional area did not change appreciably during labor. It was demonstrated that basal cardiac output increased from prelabor values to time of cervical dilation of >8 cm as a result of an increase in stroke volume and increased further during uterine contractions as a result of increases in both stroke volume and heart rate. One hour after delivery, heart rate and cardiac output had returned to normal. This same group has extended these hemodynamic observations to demonstrate that cardiac output continued to fall postpartum by 27 to 29% by 2 weeks after delivery.[70] Of interest, they also noted that aortic, pulmonary artery, and mitral valve areas all declined throughout the postnatal period by 8%, 11%, and 12%, respectively.

Premature Infants, Neonates, and Children

Although not compared with invasive methods, Doppler-derived cardiac output measurements have been used to define normal standards in newborns and older children.[71–76] These methods have also been used to follow cardiac outputs in children before and after medical or surgical closure of patent ductus arteriosus, to evaluate the effects of dopamine administration on cardiac output in newborns with myocardial dysfunction,[77] to correlate cardiac output with septal thickness in infants of diabetic mothers,[78] to assess the effects of theophylline administration on cardiac output in preterm infants,[79] to assess the effects of phototherapy for hyperbilirubinemia on cardiac output,[80] and to evaluate the effects of positive end-expiratory pressure on systemic and pulmonary blood flows in premature infants with the respiratory distress syndrome.[81]

Assessment of Cardiac Shunts

The magnitude of systemic-to-pulmonary shunts can be quantitated by determining the ratio of pulmonary to systemic blood flow. This information can be obtained by Doppler-echocardiography, with the sites used to measure individual flows varying according to the level of the shunt.

The validity of this approach has been evaluated in canine models of ventricular septal defect. It has been demonstrated that Doppler-echocardiographic estimates the pulmonary to systolic flow ratio of (Q_P/Q_S) correlate well with those determined by flow meter (r = .91 to .96), with slopes of regression approaching unity.[26,82]

Good correlation of Q_P/Q_S ratios obtained by Doppler-echocardiography with those measured invasively has been achieved in groups containing both adult and pediatric patients with atrial (r = .92)[83] and ventricular (r = .97)[84] septal defects. A lesser degree of correlation has been reported in pediatric patients alone with a variety of cardiac lesions (r = .85) and in children with atrial septal defects (r = .82) (Fig. 30–19) and ventricular septal defects (r = .79).[85] Differences in the degree of correlation between studies may reflect the use of different sites for measuring flow, with mitral orifice methods being potentially less accurate than those involving the great vessels. Other potential sources of error include underestimation of cardiac output during high flow states, which is due to exaggerated changes in vessel area,[86] aliasing in the proximal pulmonary artery that is due to high velocity ventricular septal defect flow, and a greater percentage of inaccuracies in vessel diameter determinations in children. It has recently been shown that peak aortic and pulmonary flow velocity signals could be substituted for the respective systolic flow velocity integrals in the calculation of the Q_p/Q_s ratio, while still preserving the excellent correlation of these measurements with thermodilution outputs (r = .93).[87]

Attempts have also been made to quantify left-to-right shunts in atrial septal defects using systolic time intervals derived from pulsed Doppler.[88] Pre-ejection period and ejection times were measured in the pulmonary artery and ascending aorta. "Hemodynamic ratios" (pre-ejection period/ejection time) were calculated for each ventricle. The ratio of left hemodynamic ratio/right hemodynamic ratio correlated well (r = .80) when compared to Q_p/Q_s determined by the Fick oxygen method. Although the right hemodynamic ratio decreased with large shunts, the presence of pulmonary hypertension is known to reverse this change, limiting the application of this method in a population of patients predisposed to the development of pulmonary vascular changes.

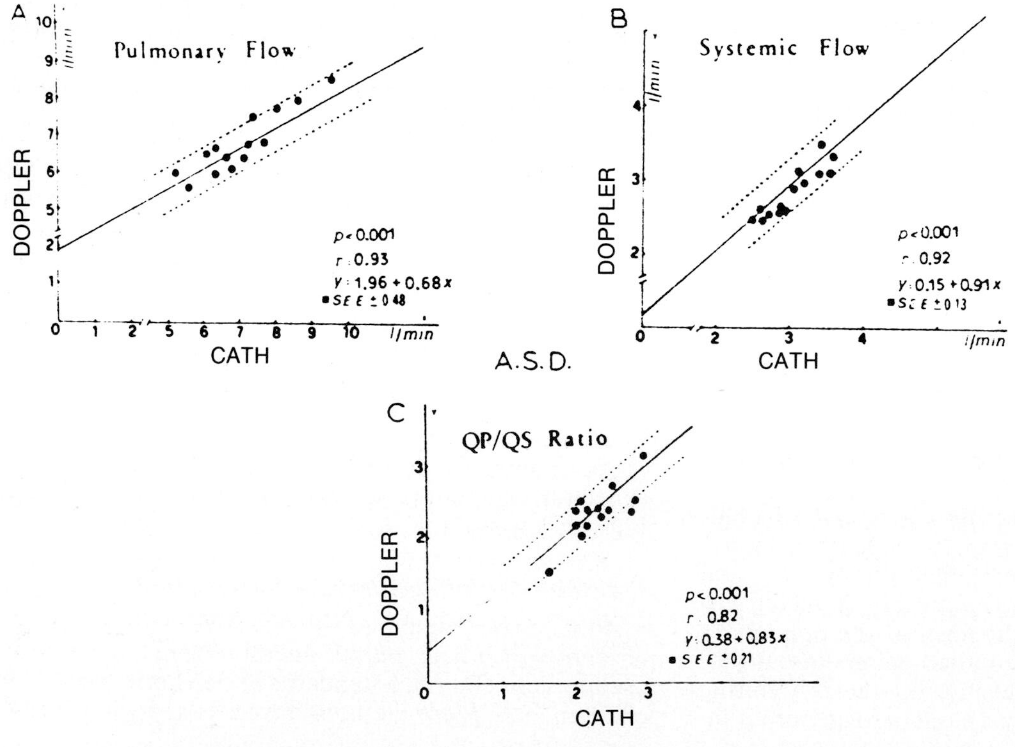

Fig. 30–19. Regression analysis correlating pulmonary **(A)** and systemic **(B)** Doppler flows to the flows obtained by cardiac catheterization in patients with atrial septal defect, along with the derived pulmonary to systemic flow ratio **(C)**. The 5% and 95% confidence limits for the data points are shown as dotted lines. (From Cacciapuoti F, et al.: Noninvasive evaluation of the left-to-right shunts by pulsed Doppler echocardiography. Int J Cardiol 13:64, 1986.)

Quantitation of Regurgitant Flow

The ability to quantify flow across individual cardiac valves and great vessels provides echo-Doppler with the unique opportunity to calculate not only shunt flows but also regurgitant volumes.

Mitral Regurgitation

Early attempts to assess the severity of mitral regurgitation involved determining the ratio of the area under the first half of the aortic flow curve to the total area under that curve (the systolic velocity integral).[89] This measurement was based on the observation that with increasingly severe mitral regurgitation, the aortic blood velocity became skewed leftward with a proportionately greater flow occurring in early systole than normal. The reported correlation coefficient between this Doppler-derived index and an angiographic estimate of severity of mitral regurgitation was .84. Although of interest, this approach has found limited clinical applicability.

A more direct approach is to calculate mitral regurgitation as the difference between mitral inflow, which includes both forward and regurgitant flow, and aortic outflow, which represents only forward flow (Fig. 30–20). This approach has been validated in the experimental canine model by comparison with electromagnetic flowmeter measures of regurgitant volume. Despite the narrow range of regurgitant volumes obtainable in this model, a good correlation between Doppler estimates of regurgitant volume and flowmeter measurements was obtained with standard errors similar to those observed for forward flow alone. ($r = .84$; $y = .97 \times + .05$; standard deviation [SD] = .36) (Fig. 30–21).

This approach has also been applied in humans for the quantitation of mitral regurgitation.[90] Doppler stroke volume was calculated across the aortic valve and across the mitral valve. Aortic blood velocity was measured from the suprasternal position, and aortic diameter was measured at the level of attachment of the aortic cusps by leading edge methodology. The maximal mitral orifice area in diastole was obtained from the two-dimensional parasternal short axis view and multiplied by the mitral orifice opening ratio obtained from the mitral M-mode. Regurgitant fraction correlated well ($r = .82$) with the semi-quantitative standard grading system (grades I to IV) for mitral regurgitation used at cardiac catheterization. The major limitation of this method is that it can be used only in cases of pure mitral regurgitation.

Two-dimensional echo estimates of ventricular volume can also be combined with Doppler-echocardiographic determinations of aortic flow to calculate regurgitant fraction in patients with mitral regurgitation.[91] Left ventricular (total) stroke volume (LVSV) can be calculated by measuring systolic and diastolic volumes using two-dimensional echo. The forward stroke volume (FSV) can be obtained from the product of aortic valve area and ascending aortic flow velocity integral assessed by Doppler. Regurgitant fraction is then calculated as LVSV − FSV/LVSV. This method has been compared to regurgitant fraction measured by cardiac catheterization ($r = .82$) and by scintigraphy ($r = .89$).[91]

This method has been used to determine the effects of intravenous nitroglycerin on forward flow and regurgitant fraction in patients with functional mitral regurgitation that is due to dilated cardiomyopathy.[92] Intravenous nitroglycerin administration resulted in improved forward flow, manifested by increased forward stroke

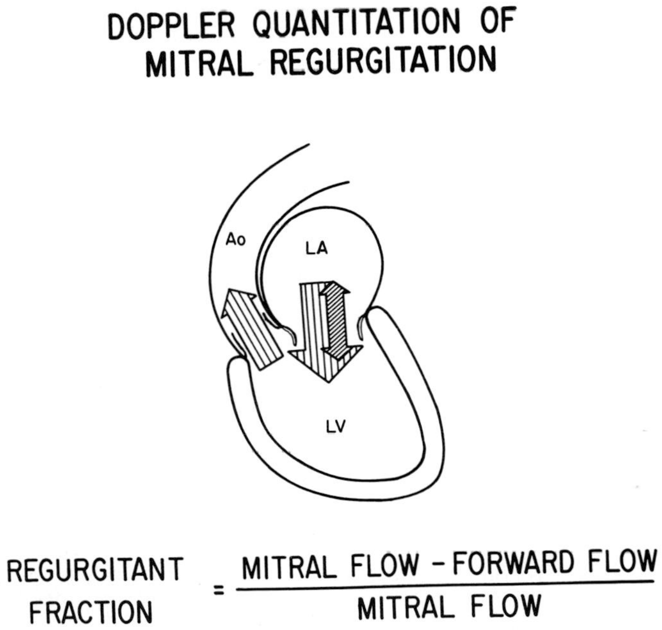

Fig. 30–20. The calculation of regurgitant volume. Total mitral inflow equals the forward flow through the aorta plus the mitral regurgitant flow. Mitral regurgitant flow is therefore the mitral inflow minus aortic outflow. AO = aorta; LA = left atrium; LV = left ventricle.

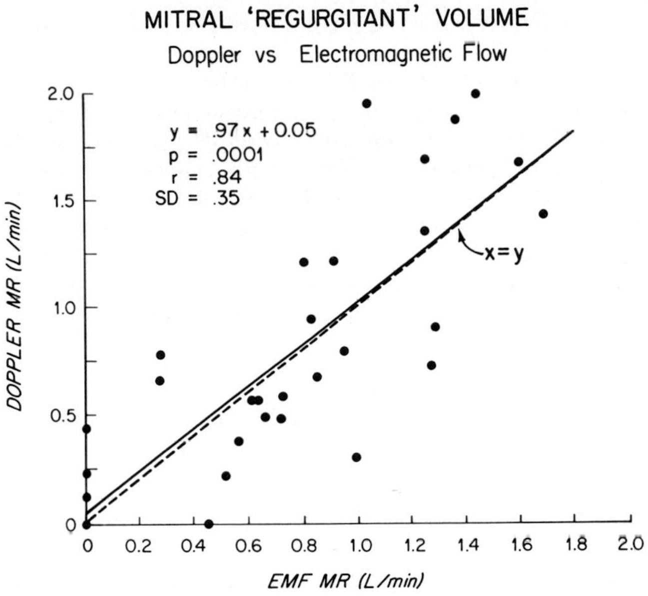

Fig. 30–21. Comparison of mitral regurgitant (MR) volume by the Doppler method vs. electromagnetic flowmeter (EMF) measurements. (See text for details.) (From Ascah KG, et al.: A Doppler two-dimensional echocardiographic method for quantitation of mitral regurgitation. Circulation 72:381, 1985. Reproduced by permission of the American Heart Association, Inc.)

volume and decreased regurgitant volume, without a change in total LVSV.

Different echo-Doppler methods of calculating mitral regurgitant fraction seem to correlate well with each other in patients with dilated cardiomyopathy.[93] Mitral regurgitant volume calculated as the difference between two-dimensional total stroke volume (measured from the apical four-chamber view using Simpson's rule) and forward aortic volume obtained by Doppler correlated well ($r = .90$) with regurgitant volume calculated as the difference between mitral valve inflow (assuming a circular geometry) and forward aortic flow, both determined by Doppler-echocardiography. Assumption of a circular geometry for the mitral orifice was felt to be valid in patients with dilated cardiomyopathy in whom the mitral annulus is dilated, more circular, and less dynamic.[94]

Aortic Regurgitation

The first attempts to quantify aortic regurgitant volumes using Doppler ultrasound took advantage of reverse flow signals in the descending aorta seen in patients with clinically or echocardiographically detectable aortic insufficiency (Fig. 30–22). Excellent correlation ($r = .91$) between the ratio of the diastolic to the systolic flow velocity integrals (DVI/SVI), measured in the descending aorta, and the angiographic regurgitant fraction has been reported in patients with various degrees of aortic insufficiency.[95] A modification of this approach has been used to measure regurgitant volume through the semilunar valves as the product of the reverse flow integral in the great artery, distal to the valve, multiplied by the cross-sectional area of that vessel.[18] Although a good correlation was reported with angiographic and clinical assessments of severity, these determinations do not take into account coronary diastolic flow, changes in aortic diameter that are due to elastic recoil of the aorta, and the possibility that reverse aortic diastolic flow does not have the same flat velocity profile seen with forward aortic flow. Hence, this method cannot be considered to accurately reflect aortic regurgitant volume.

A method for the volumetric determination of aortic regurgitation using both Doppler-derived and two-dimensional volume measurements has also been described.[96] The transmitral volumetric flow was obtained by multiplying the corrected mitral orifice area by the diastolic velocity integral, and the total LVSV was derived by subtracting the left ventricular end-systolic volume from the end-diastolic volume with volume calculated using the single-plane ellipsoid formula (see Chapter 20). This calculation was based on the premise that in aortic regurgitation left ventricular diastolic inflow comes from both the aortic and mitral valves, and hence left ventricular stroke volume will be greater than mitral diastolic inflow by a volume equal to the aortic regurgitant volume. The aortic regurgitant fraction (RF) is thus calculated as $RF = 1 - MF/SV$. Transmitral volumetric flow (MF) measured in patients without aortic valve disease were compared to those in patients with aortic regurgitation. There was good agreement between the regurgitant fractions determined by Doppler-echocardiography and radionuclide ventriculography.

The major advantage of this method of calculating regurgitant fraction is that the volume measurement by two-dimensional echo of the left ventricle is not affected by concomitant aortic stenosis or by mitral regurgitation. Thus, the difference between LVSV and the transmitral volumetric flow will equal the aortic regurgitant volume, whether the aortic insufficiency is isolated or associated with other valvular regurgitations. Note that all of these complex measurements contain independent sources of error and that, although correlations over wide ranges will generally be good, in individual cases, absolute values should be interpreted cautiously.

Pulmonary Regurgitation

Quantitation of pulmonary regurgitation has not generated as much interest as left-sided regurgitant lesions. One proposed method of determining pulmonary regurgitant fraction involves multiplying the reverse flow integral in the pulmonary artery by the cross-sectional area of the pulmonary artery.[18] This method has been used

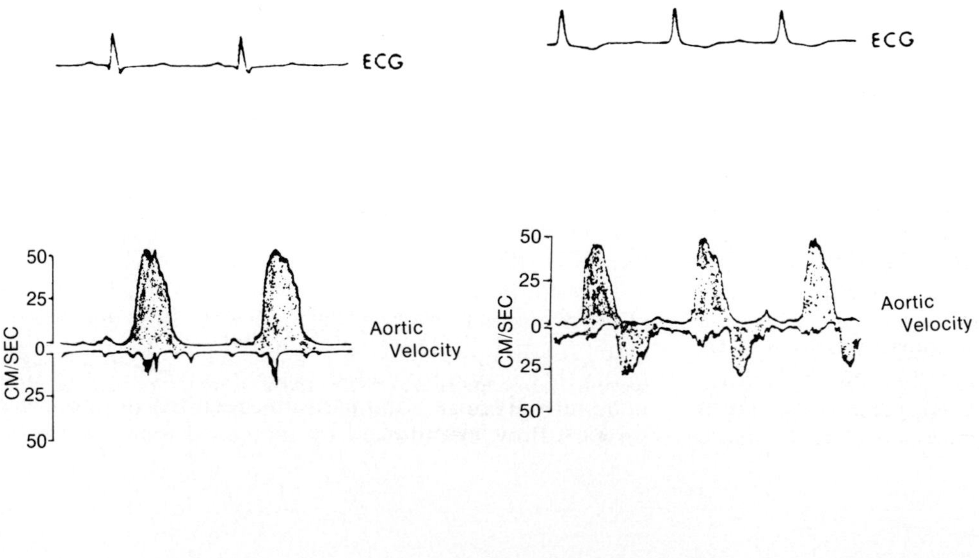

Fig. 30–22. Left. Descending aortic velocity profiles from a normal individual. Blood velocity away from the transducer is plotted upright, and flow toward the transducer is inverted. Forward aortic velocity is the shaded area. Right. Taken from a patient with moderately severe aortic insufficiency, regurgitant fraction is 54%. The shaded areas represent aortic arch velocity in systole and diastole. Planimetry of forward and reverse flow areas provided an estimate of regurgitation. (Modified from Boughner D: Assessment of aortic insufficiency by transcutaneous Doppler ultrasound. Circulation 52:875, 1975. Reproduced by permission of the American Heart Association, Inc.)

to estimate pulmonary regurgitant fraction following corrective surgery for pulmonary outflow obstruction.[97] Pulsed Doppler was used to obtain pulmonary forward and regurgitant velocities by placing the sample volume in the midpulmonary artery, right ventricular outflow tract patch, or conduit. A computer program determined the positive and negative mean velocity by dividing the area under the time velocity curve by distance along the time axis. The percentage of pulmonary regurgitation was derived as regurgitant mean velocity/forward mean velocity × 100. By using Doppler-derived estimates of cardiac output in the ascending aorta during exercise, it was possible to demonstrate that patients with severe pulmonary regurgitation had markedly low cardiac output responses during submaximal exercise testing compared to patients with lesser degrees of pulmonary regurgitation.

Calculation of Valve Area

Calculation of aortic valve area represents the single most widely used clinical application of volumetric flow analysis. Although Doppler-echocardiography can estimate pressure gradients across stenotic valves with excellent correlation[98–102] with catheterization data, it is also desirable to determine valve area, because the gradient depends strongly on cardiac output and will be low when the cardiac output is depressed.

Initial efforts to determine aortic valve area employed a combination of data from both Doppler recordings and thermodilution cardiac outputs.[103,104] It is now possible, however, for Doppler-echocardiography to provide a completely noninvasive determination of valvular cross-sectional area. This has represented a significant advance in following patients with aortic stenosis because cardiac catheterization has a small but definite risk, particularly if a transseptal approach to the left ventricle becomes necessary to measure aortic valve area.

Using Doppler-echocardiography, one can determine the area of a stenotic valve by employing the *continuity equation* (Fig. 30–23). This equation is simply an extension of the law of conservation of mass and states that because flow is continuous, flow across the left ventricular outflow tract will be identical to flow across the aortic valve (unless there is a high ventricular septal defect) and can be expressed mathematically by the equation

$$A_1 v_1 = A_2 v_2$$

or rearranged to calculate aortic valve area (A_2) as

$$A_2 = A_1 v_1 / v_2$$

where A_1 = the area of the left ventricular outflow tract measured 0.5 to 1.0 cm below the aortic valve in midsystole, i.e., just proximal to the site of prestenotic flow acceleration. The left ventricular outflow tract diameter is measured in the parasternal long axis view, and the left ventricular outflow tract diameter is assumed to be circular so that $A_1 = \pi(D/2)^2$); v_1 is the left ventricular outflow tract velocity measured using pulsed wave from the apical view. One must be careful not to measure subvalvular velocities from within the zone of proximal acceleration, which is usually located 0.5 to 1.5 cm proximal to the stenotic valve. v_2 is the highest aortic stenotic jet velocity measured by continuous wave Doppler from the apical, right parasternal, or suprasternal windows.

An advantage of the continuity equation is that it can calculate aortic valve areas accurately, regardless of whether the cardiac output is abnormally low, as with concomitant left ventricular dysfunction, or abnormally high, as with coexisting aortic insufficiency.

Several investigators[99,105–108] have validated this completely noninvasive approach to measuring aortic valve area by comparing results obtained using this method to those reported by the standard Gorlin formula employed at cardiac catheterization and have achieved

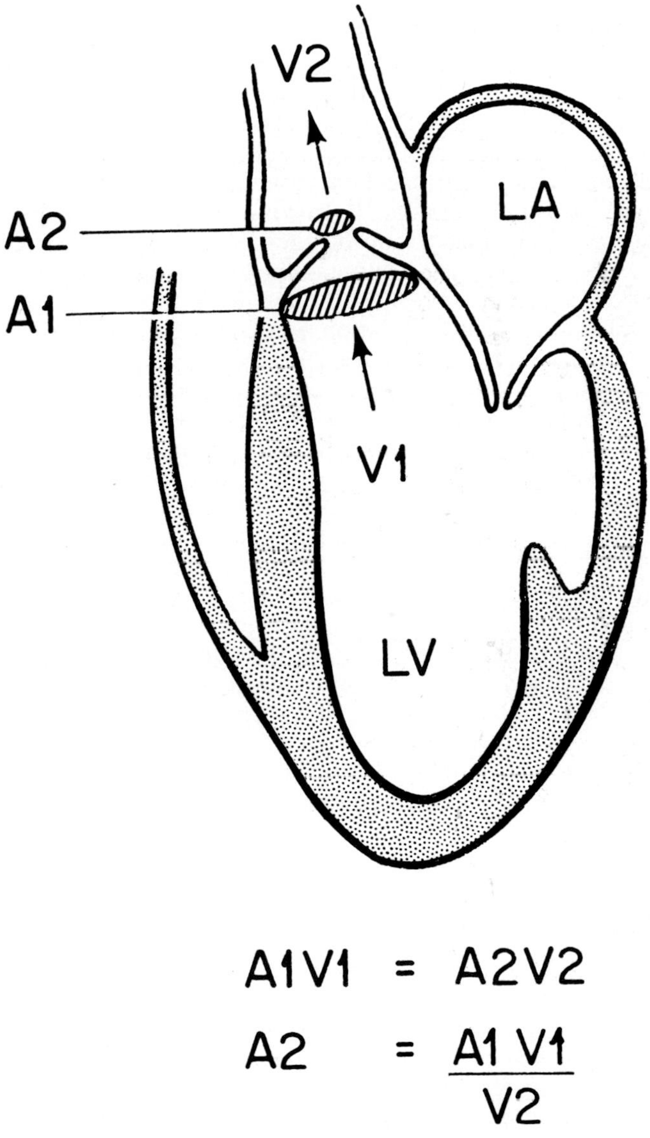

Fig. 30–23. The continuity equation for estimation of aortic valve area. A1 = the area of the LVOT measured 0.5 to 1.0 cm below the aortic valve; V1 = mean LVOT velocity measured using pulsed wave from the apical view; A2 = aortic valve area (unknown); V2 = aortic stenosis jet measured by continuous wave; LA = left atrium; LV = left ventricle.

correlation coefficients of 0.83 to 0.89 over a very narrow range of values. Because the continuity equation is instantaneously applicable, using peak flow velocities instead of the time-velocity integrals will not significantly affect the good correlations achieved with invasive data.[99,106,109]

Several investigators have employed variations of the continuity equation and the Gorlin formula[101,107] or combined data from Doppler measurements and carbon dioxide rebreathing[110] or electrical bioimpedance[98] estimates of flow to improve correlation with invasive data. Although reported correlation coefficients tend to be somewhat higher with these alternate methods (r = .87 to .94), they require additional equipment, expertise, and operating time to obtain measurements.

Special Applications

Transesophageal Doppler Echocardiography

Several recent attempts have been made to measure descending aortic blood flow with specially designed intraesophageal echo-Doppler probes.[31,111] The intraesophageal method has been validated in an in vitro roller pump model with excellent correlations between true and measured outputs.[111] In vivo validation was performed in a small group of unconscious ventilated patients, by comparing intraesophageal measurements of cardiac output with those obtained by thermodilution, and an excellent correlation was obtained (r = .98)

Despite these encouraging preliminary results, transesophageal determinations of cardiac output from the descending aorta suffer from major theoretical and practical limitations, including inability to align the Doppler ultrasound beam parallel to descending aortic flow, and the fact that descending aortic flow measurements do not account for the percentage of stroke volume "lost" to the arch vessels. Attempts have been made to correct for the difference between cardiac output measured in the proximal aorta and descending aortic flow by establishing a baseline ratio between the two, which is used to convert flows measured in the descending aorta during interventions to absolute flow. This unfortunately assumes that the relationship of resistance and flow above and below the site of measurement remains constant in settings in which changes in these parameters are likely.

Fetal Doppler Echocardiography

In the fetus, the right and left circulations work in parallel, and right-to-left shunting occurs at the atrial level (through the foramen ovale) and at the ductal level. Doppler characterization of fetal blood flow patterns is of potential benefit in our understanding of fetal circulatory physiology and in assessing abnormalities of fetal hemodynamics. Such studies may lead to potential clinical applications such as the selection of optimal therapy for the treatment of heart failure and of arrhythmias in utero.

Fetal intracardiac Doppler flow patterns were first studied in 1984.[112] Pulsed Doppler studies of the fetus were performed during the third trimester of pregnancy (28 to 36 weeks). Right ventricular stroke volume could be calculated in 6 of 15 fetuses in whom the inner pulmonary artery width could be measured. Greater Doppler frequency shifts were noted in the right atrium than in the left atrium, in keeping with known fetal physiology.

More recent studies have used Doppler-echocardiography to quantify and compare RVSV and LVSV in normal human fetuses.[113,114] These studies have demonstrated that RVSV consistently exceeds LVSV, reflecting right ventricular dominance in utero. These and other[115,116] normative fetal data may be helpful in interpreting results from fetuses with structural heart disease or cardiac arrhythmias.

The fact that attempts to measure stroke volume by the Doppler technique have now been extended to include the fetus is encouraging. Unfortunately, in this population, the accuracy of output determinations is left open to considerable question. Fetal position often restricts the operator's ability to align the ultrasound beam parallel to flow. Of equal or greater concern is the inability to accurately measure very small vessel and valvular diameters, given the resolution of currently available commercial equipment. Considerable work must be done in this area before quantitative flow measurements can be applied with confidence in prenatal care.

Exercise Doppler Echocardiography

Doppler echocardiography, being noninvasive, has facilitated the evaluation of normal physiologic responses to exercise that previously could be ascertained only by invasive study. Most of these studies examine exercise-related changes in stroke volume or cardiac output based on aortic flow measurements. Typically, the aortic diameter is measured at rest and assumed not to change significantly during exercise.[117] Measuring the aortic diameter at the level of the aortic orifice (part of the fibrous skeleton of the heart) probably minimizes changes in aortic diameter that are due to intraluminal aortic pressure elevation during exercise. Aortic blood flow velocities are obtained by pulsed or continuous wave Doppler recordings from the suprasternal notch, because this window fixes the transducer and allows Doppler recordings, which are relatively free of motion artifacts and respiratory interference during exercise.

Doppler estimates of cardiac output at rest and during exercise have been validated in clinical studies of normal subjects in comparison with a variety of standards including the N_2O rebreathing method,[10] the indirect[118] and direct[117] Fick method, and thermodilution[36] with good correlations (r = .78 to .98). Doppler-derived outputs have allowed several important hemodynamic observations to be made in normal subjects during exercise. For instance, it has been demonstrated that the increase in stroke volume during exercise occurs earlier in the upright position than in the supine position[119] and that although stroke volume is lower at rest in the upright position than in the supine position, they equalize at peak exercise.[120]

Doppler-echocardiography has also been used to determine the mechanisms by which flow is increased in the ascending aorta and across the mitral valve orifice during isotonic exercise.[121] Aortic blood velocity was determined by continuous wave from the suprasternal notch during steady state at each stage of exercise, and changes in aortic cross-sectional area were measured just distal to the valve leaflets during exercise from the parasternal window. Mitral inflow velocities were recorded from the apical four-chamber view during steady state at each stage of exercise, and the corrected mitral valve orifice[25] was measured at rest and during exercise. The increase in stroke volume with exercise measured at the aortic level was accomplished by an increase in the time-velocity integral, with little change in the aortic cross-sectional area (5% supine and 0% upright, p = NS). The increase in stroke volume with exercise at the mitral valve was mainly due to an increase in mean diastolic mitral orifice area (29% supine and 34% upright, $p < .05$); the time-velocity integral did not increase significantly (−10% supine and 4% upright, p = NS). We have previously shown a similar relationship for aortic valve area in the experimental model. In the experimental setting, however, heart rate was controlled, and the mitral velocity integral also increased in parallel with the area change (see Fig. 30–5).[4] In the exercising patient, the increase in heart rate and decrease in diastolic filling period appear to hold the mitral velocity integral constant despite an increase in total flow. These observations support the use of changes in time-velocity integral as an indicator of stroke volume at the aortic valve level but also stress the importance of serial area measurements at the mitral orifice level in assessing changes in stroke volume with exercise or other maneuvers that alter cardiac output or heart rate.

Validation of the exercise-Doppler method in patients with coronary artery disease has been performed by comparing Doppler-derived stroke volume at rest and during supine and sitting exercise with thermodilution cardiac outputs.[122,123] As with validations of the Doppler-echo method at rest, considerable variation between absolute results obtained by Doppler and those obtained by thermodilution may be seen, but systematic differences are not usually found.

Several studies have suggested that exercise cardiac output responses might be used to diagnose the presence of coronary artery disease. It has been observed that the mean increase in stroke index and cardiac index during exercise is significantly smaller in patients with coronary artery disease than in normal subjects.[124] This observation has been confirmed by comparing two-dimensional measurements of ejection fraction, visualization of wall motion abnormalities, and Doppler-derived measurements of cardiac output in normals and in patients with coronary artery disease.[125] Although ejection fraction increased significantly in normal subjects from resting to peak exercise, the response was blunted in patients with coronary artery disease. Likewise, stroke index and cardiac index, although similar in both groups at rest, was significantly higher in normals at peak exercise than in patients with coronary artery disease.

The hypothesis that Doppler measurement of ascending aortic blood flow could detect exercise-induced changes in left ventricular performance during exercise in patients suspected of having coronary artery disease has recently been tested prospectively.[126] Pulsed and continuous wave recordings were made from the sternal notch as patients underwent simultaneous exercise radionuclide ventriculography. The diameter of the aortic annulus was measured using leading edge methodology at the onset of the QRS and the peak of the T wave and averaged to calculate the cross-sectional area. Doppler-derived stroke volume increased in patients with normal radionuclide ejection fractions whose ejection fraction rose by >5% with exercise. Stroke volume was seen not to rise in groups of patients in whom the radionuclide ejection fraction was abnormal at rest or did not increase by ≥5% with exercise.

Doppler determinations of cardiac output have also been used to evaluate the hemodynamic effects of orally administered propranolol and verapamil during exercise[127] and to determine the effect of left ventricular function on the exercise hemodynamics of demand (VVI) vs. variable rate (VVIR) pacemakers.[128]

Exercise Doppler echocardiography represents a potentially useful adjunct to routine exercise testing in selected patients. Given its noninvasive nature and good correlation with invasive standards, it should be of value in both the research and clinical settings. However, the technique requires a great deal of expertise; machines designed to yield automated output measures when used by inexperienced personnel have yielded predictably poor results, ultimately delaying progress in this area.

CONCLUSIONS

Both clinical and experimental data suggest that the Doppler-echocardiographic approach can generate accurate measures of volumetric flow at specific locations within the heart and great vessels. Doppler-echocardiography, like all other methods for measuring volumetric flow, has many theoretic limitations and potential sources of error. Once these are understood, however, reliable data can be obtained by the experienced observer.

The technique has great potential value because it is noninvasive, provides beat-to-beat information, and permits measurement of both absolute and relative flows. To be of quantitative value, however, the component measurements must be made with great care and accuracy, and considerable experience is necessary before meaningful data can be derived.

As greater experience leads to greater acceptance, it seems likely that Doppler-echocardiography will replace the invasive hemodynamic methods for assessing flow in many patients with valvular disease and selected forms of congenital heart disease. Measurement of flows proximal to, and velocity at, sites of stenosis now allows the determination of the area of stenotic valves without the aid of cardiac catheterization. Furthermore, the ability of Doppler-echocardiography to measure flow at multiple sites within the heart makes the calculation of intracardiac shunt flow ratios and regurgitant flow volumes possible. These applications define Doppler-echocardiography as a powerful quantitative tool that greatly enhances the strength of noninvasive evaluation in cardiac diagnosis and management.

REFERENCES

1. Harvey W: Exercitatio de Motu Cordis et Sanguinis in Animalibus. Frankfurt, W. Fitzer, 1628. *In* Willis R (trans.): The Works of William Harvey, M.D. London, Sydenham Society, 1847.
2. Schuster AH, Nanda NC: Doppler echocardiography. Part I: Doppler cardiac output measurements: perspective and comparison with other methods of cardiac output determination. Echocardiography 1:45, 1984.
3. Light LH, Cross G: Cardiovascular data by transcutaneous aortovelography. *In* Roberts C (ed): Blood Flow Measurement. London, Sector Publishing, p. 60, 1972.
4. Lewis JF, et al.: Pulsed Doppler echocardiographic determination of stroke volume and cardiac output: clinical validation of two new methods using the apical window. Circulation 70:425, 1984.
5. Meijboom EJ, et al.: A Doppler echocardiographic method for calculating volume flow across the tricuspid valve: correlative laboratory and clinical studies. Circulation 71:551, 1985.
6. Valdes-Cruz LM, et al.: Comparison of cardiac flows calculated with color coded Doppler flow mapping and conventional Doppler techniques: validation studies in an open chest animal model. J Am Coll Cardiol 5:452, 1985.
7. Ihlen H, et al.: Determination of cardiac output by echocardiography. Br Heart J 51:54, 1984.
8. Merillon J, et al.: Evaluation of the elasticity and characteristic impedance of the ascending aorta in man. Cardiovasc Res 12:401, 1978.
9. Greenfield J, Patel D: Relation between pressure and diameter in the ascending aorta of man. Circ Res 10:778, 1962.
10. Mehta, N, et al.: Validation of a Doppler technique for beat-to-beat measurement of cardiac output. Clinical Science 69:377, 1985.
11. Goldberg SJ, et al.: Evaluation of pulmonary and systemic flow by 2-dimensional Doppler echocardiography using fast Fourier transform spectral analysis. Am J Cardiol 50:1394, 1982.
12. Greenfield JC, Griggs DM: Relation between pressure and diameter in the main pulmonary artery of man. Circ Res 10:557, 1962.
13. Labovitz AJ, et al.: The effects of sampling site on the two-dimensional echo-Doppler determination of cardiac output. Am Heart J 109:327, 1985.
14. Bouchard A, et al.: Measurement of left ventricular stroke volume using continuous wave Doppler echocardiography of the ascending aorta and M-mode echocardiography of the aortic valve. J Am Coll Cardiol 9:75, 1987.
15. Gardin J, et al.: Superiority of two-dimensional measurement of aortic vessel diameter in Doppler echocardiographic estimates of left ventricular stroke volume. J Am Coll Cardiol 6:66, 1985.
16. Stewart WJ, et al.: Variable effects of changes in flow rate through the aortic, pulmonary and mitral valves on valve area and flow velocity: impact on quantitative Doppler flow calculations. J Am Coll Cardiol 6:653, 1985.
17. Fisher DC, et al.: The effect of variations on pulsed Doppler sampling site on calculations of cardiac output: an experimental study in open-chest dogs. Circulation 67:370, 1983.
18. Goldberg SJ, et al.: Quantitative assessment by Doppler echocardiography of pulmonic or aortic regurgitation. Am J Cardiol 56:131, 1985.
19. Skjaerpe RM, Hegrenaes L, Ihlen H: Cardiac output. *In* Hatle L, Angelsen B (eds.): Doppler Ultrasound in Cardiology. Philadelphia, Lea & Febiger, p. 306, 1985.
20. Newhouse VL, Bendick PJ: Analysis of random signal blood flow measurement. *In* de Klerk J (ed.): Proceedings: IEEE Ultrasonics Symposium. New York, IEEE, p. 94, 1979.
21. Ling SC, et al.: Application of heated-film velocity and shear probes to hemodynamic studies. Circ Res 23:789, 1968.
22. Schultz DL, et al.: Velocity distribution and transition in the arterial system. *In* Wolstenholme GEW, Knight J (eds.): Circulatory and Respiratory Mass Transport. London, J & A Churchill, p. 172, 1969.
23. Lucas CL, et al.: The velocity profile in the canine ascending aorta and its effects on the accuracy of pulsed Doppler determinations of mean blood flow velocity. Cardiovasc Res 18:282, 1984.
24. Steingart R, et al.: Pulsed Doppler echocardiographic measurement of beat to beat changes of stroke volume in dogs. Circulation 62:542, 1980.
25. Fisher DC, et al.: The mitral valve orifice method for non-invasive two-dimensional echo Doppler determinations of cardiac output. Circulation 67:872, 1983.
26. Valdes-Cruz LM, et al.: A pulsed Doppler method for calculation of pulmonary and systemic flow: accuracy in a canine model with ventricular septal defect. Circulation 68:597, 1983.
27. Sequeira RF, et al.: Transcutaneous aortovelography: a quantitative evaluation. Br Heart J 38:443, 1976.
28. Angelsen BAJ, Brubakk AO: Transcutaneous measurement of blood flow velocity in the human aorta. Cardiovasc Res 10:368, 1976.
29. Colocousis JS, Huntsman LL, Curreri PW: Estimation of stroke volume changes by ultrasonic Doppler. Circulation 56:914, 1977.
30. Huntsman LL, et al.: Transcutaneous determination of aortic blood flow velocities in man. Am Heart J 89:605, 1975.
31. Mark JB, et al.: Continuous noninvasive monitoring of cardiac output with esophageal Doppler ultrasound during cardiac surgery. Anesth Analg 65: 1013, 1986.
32. Loeppky JA, Hoekenga DE, Greene ER, Luft UC: Comparison of noninvasive pulsed Doppler and Fick measurements of stroke volume in cardiac patients. Am Heart J 107:339, 1984.
33. Magnin PA, et al.: Combined Doppler and phased-array echocardiographic estimation of cardiac output. Circulation 63:388, 1981.
34. Chandraratna PAN, et al.: Determination of cardiac output by transcutaneous continuous-wave ultrasonic Doppler computer. Am J Cardiol 53:234, 1984.
35. Elkayam U, et al.: The use of Doppler flow velocity measurement to assess the hemodynamic response to vasodilators in patients with heart failure. Circulation 67:377, 1983.
36. Huntsman LL, et al.: Non-invasive Doppler determination of cardiac output in man: clinical validation. Circulation 67:593, 1983.
37. Rose JS, et al.: Accuracy of determination of changes in cardiac output by transcutaneous continuous-wave Doppler computer. Am J Cardiol 54: 1099, 1984.
38. Vandenbogaerde J, et al.: Comparison between ultrasonic and thermodilution cardiac output measurements in intensive care patients. Crit Care Med 14:294, 1986.
39. Nishimura R, et al.: Noninvasive measurement of cardiac output by continuous wave Doppler echocardiography: initial experience and review of the literature. Mayo Clin Proc 59:484, 1984.
40. Bojanowski L, Timmis A, Najm Y, Gosling R: Pulsed Doppler ultrasound compared with thermodilution for monitoring cardiac output responses to changing left ventricular function. Cardiovasc Res 21:260, 1987.
41. Lang-Jensen T, Berning J, Jacobsen E: Stroke volume measured by pulsed ultrasound Doppler and M-mode echocardiography. Acta Anaesthesiol Scand 27:464, 1983.
42. Dittman H, Voelker W, Karsch KR, Seipel L: Influence of sampling site and flow area on cardiac output measurements by Doppler echocardiography. J Am Coll Cardiol 10:818, 1987.
43. Levy BI, et al.: Noninvasive ultrasonic cardiac output measurement in intensive care unit. Ultrasound in Med Biol 11:841, 1985.
44. Gardin JM, et al.: Are Doppler aortic blood flow velocity measurements reproducible? Studies on day-to-day and interobserver variability in normal subjects. J Am Coll Cardiol 1:657, 1983.
45. Alverson DC, et al.: Noninvasive pulsed Doppler determinants of cardiac output in neonates and children. J Pediatr 101:46, 1982.
46. Goldberg SJ, et al.: Evaluation of pulmonary and systemic blood flow by 2-dimensional Doppler echocardiography using fast Fourier transform spectral analysis. Am J Cardiol 50:1394, 1982.
47. Rein MJ, et al.: Cardiac output estimates in the pediatric intensive care unit using a continuous-wave Doppler computer: validation and limitations of the technique. Am Heart J 112:97 1986.
48. Mellander M, et al.: Doppler determination of cardiac output in infants and children: comparison with simultaneous thermodilution. Pediatr Cardiol 8: 241, 1987.
49. Loeber CP, Goldberg SJ, Allen HD: Doppler echocardiographic comparison of flows distal to the four cardiac valves. J Am Coll Cardiol 4:268, 1984.
50. Taylor DEM, Whamond JS: Velocity profile and impedance of the healthy mitral valve. *In* Kalmanson D (ed.): The Mitral Valve. A Pluridisciplinary Approach. London, Edward Arnold, p. 127, 1976.
51. Zhang Y, Nitter-Hauge S, Ihlen H, Myhre E: Doppler echocardiographic measurement of cardiac output using the mitral orifice method. Br Heart J 53:130, 1985.
52. Hoit BD, et al.: Calculating cardiac output from transmitral volume flow using Doppler and M-mode echocardiography. Am J Cardiol 62:131, 1988.
53. Zuttere D, et al.: Doppler echocardiographic measurement of mitral flow volume: validation of a new method in adult patients. J Am Coll Cardiol 11:343, 1988.
54. Meijboom E, et al.: A simplified mitral valve method for two-dimensional echo Doppler blood flow calculation: validation in an open-chest canine model and initial clinical studies. Am Heart J 113:335, 1987.
55. Ascah KJ, et al.: Calculation of transmitral flow by Doppler echocardiography: a comparison of methods in a canine model. Am Heart J 117:402, 1989.
56. Sanders SP, et al.: Measurement of systemic and pulmonary blood flow and Qp/Qs ratio using Doppler and two-dimensional echocardiography. Am J Cardiol 51:952, 1983.
57. Kolev N, Lazarova M, Lengyel M: Doppler two-dimensional echocardiographic determinations of right ventricular output and diastolic filling. J Cardiography 16:659, 1986.
58. Ihlen H, et al.: Changes in left ventricular stroke volume measured by Doppler echocardiography. Br Heart J 54:378, 1985.
59. Hinderliter A, Fitzpatrick A, Schork N, Julius S: Research utility of noninvasive methods for measurement of cardiac output. Clin Pharmacol Ther 41:419, 1987.
60. Fagard R, Staessen J, Amery A: The use of Doppler echocardiography to assess the acute hemodynamic response to felodipine and metoprolol in hypertensive patients. J Hypertension 5:143, 1987.
61. N'Guyen Van Cao A, Levy B, Slama R: Noninvasive study of cardiac structure and function after rilmenidine for essential hypertension. Am J Cardiol 61:72D, 1988.

62. Stewart W, et al.: Doppler ultrasound measurement of cardiac output in patients with physiologic pacemakers. Am J Cardiol 54:308, 1984.
63. Faerestrand S, Ohm O: A time-related study of the hemodynamic benefit of atrioventricular synchronous pacing evaluated by Doppler echocardiography. PACE 8:838, 1985.
64. Masuyama T, et al.: Beneficial effects of atrioventricular sequential pacing on cardiac output and left ventricular filling assessed with pulsed Doppler echocardiography. Jpn Circ J 50:799, 1986.
65. Forfang K, Otterstad JE, Ihlen H: Optimal atrioventricular delay in physiological pacing determined by Doppler echocardiography. PACE 9:17, 1986.
66. Conradsson TB, Werko L: Management of heart disease in pregnancy. Prog Cardiovasc Dis 16:407, 1974.
67. Lee W, Rokey R, Cotton DB: Noninvasive maternal stroke volume and cardiac output determinations by pulsed Doppler echocardiography. Am J Obstet Gynecol 158:505, 1988.
68. Easterling TR, Watts DH, Schmucker BC, Benedetti TJ: Measurement of cardiac output during pregnancy: validation of Doppler technique and clinical observations in preeclampsia. Obstet Gynecol 69:845, 1987.
69. Robson SC, Dunlop W, Boys RJ, Hunter S: Cardiac output during labor. Br Med J 295:1169, 1987.
70. Robson SC, Hunter S, Moore M, Dunlop W: Hemodynamic changes during the puerperium: a Doppler and M-mode echocardiographic study. Br J Obstet Gynecol 94:1028, 1987.
71. Walther FJ, et al.: Pulsed Doppler determinations of cardiac output in neonates: normal standards for clinical use. Pediatrics 76:829, 1985.
72. Walther FJ, Siassi B, King J, Wu P: Blood flow in the ascending and descending aorta in term newborn infants. Early Hum Dev 13:21, 1986.
73. Walther FJ, Siassi B, Wu PY: Echocardiographic measurement of left ventricular stroke volume in newborn infants: a correlative study with pulsed Doppler and M-mode echocardiography. J Clin Ultrasound 14:37, 1986.
74. Sholler GF, Celermajer JM, Whight CM, Bauman AE: Echo Doppler assessment of cardiac output and its relation to growth in normal infants. Am J Cardiol 60:1112, 1987.
75. Sholler GF, Celermajer JM, Whight CM: Doppler echocardiographic assessment of cardiac output in normal children with and without innocent precordial murmurs. Am J Cardiol 59:487, 1987.
76. Hirsimaki H, et al.: Doppler-derived cardiac output in healthy newborn infants in relation to physiological patency of the ductus arteriosus. Pediatr Cardiol 9:79, 1988.
77. Walther FJ, Siassi B, Ramadan NA, Wu PY: Cardiac output in newborn infants with transient myocardial dysfunction. J Pediatr 107:781, 1985.
78. Walther FJ, Siassi B, King J, Wu PY: Cardiac output in infants of insulin-dependent diabetic mothers. J Pediatr 107:109, 1985.
79. Walther FJ, Sims ME, Siassi B, Wu PY: Cardiac output changes secondary to theophylline therapy in preterm infants. J Pediatr 109:874, 1986.
80. Walther FJ, Wu PY, Siassi B: Cardiac output changes in newborns with hyperbilirubinemia treated with phototherapy. Pediatrics 76:918, 1985.
81. Hausdorf G, Hellwege H: Influence of positive end-expiratory pressure on cardiac performance in premature infants: Doppler-echocardiography study. Crit Care Med 15:661, 1987.
82. Meijboom EJ, et al.: A two-dimensional Doppler echocardiographic method for calculation of pulmonary and systemic blood flow in a canine model with variable-sized left-to-right extracardiac shunt. Circulation 68: 437, 1983.
83. Kitabatake A, et al.: Noninvasive evaluation of the ratio of pulmonic to systemic flow in atrial septal defect by duplex Doppler echocardiography. Circulation 69:73, 1984.
84. Kurokawa S, et al.: Noninvasive evaluation of the ratio of pulmonary to systemic flow in ventricular septal defect by means of Doppler two-dimensional echocardiography. Am Heart J 116:1033, 1988.
85. Cacciapuoti F, et al.: Noninvasive evaluation of left-to-right shunts by pulsed Doppler echocardiography. Int J Cardiol 13:57, 1986.
86. Barron JV, et al.: Clinical utility of two-dimensional Doppler echocardiographic techniques for estimating pulmonary to systemic flow ratios in children with left to right shunting, atrial septal defect, ventricular septal defect, and patent ductus arteriosus. J Am Coll Cardiol 3:169, 1984.
87. Cloez JL, Schmidt KG, Birk E, Silverman NH: Determination of pulmonary to systemic blood flow ratio in children by a simplified Doppler echocardiographic method. J Am Coll Cardiol 11:825, 1988.
88. Veyrat C, et al.: Quantification of left to right shunt in atrial septal defect using systolic time intervals derived from pulsed Doppler velocimetry. Br Heart J 52:633, 1984.
89. Nichol PM, Boughner DR, Persaud J: Noninvasive assessment of mitral insufficiency by Doppler ultrasound. Circulation 54:656, 1976.
90. Zhang Y, et al.: Quantification of mitral regurgitation by Doppler echocardiography. Eur Heart J 8:59, 1987.
91. Blumlein S, et al.: Quantitation of mitral regurgitation by Doppler echocardiography. Circulation 74:306, 1986.
92. Keren G, Bier A, LeJemtel T: Improvement in forward cardiac output without a change in ejection fraction during nitroglycerin therapy in patients with functional mitral regurgitation. Can J Cardiol 2:206, 1986.
93. Keren G, et al.: Noninvasive quantification of mitral regurgitation in dilated cardiomyopathy: correlation of two Doppler echocardiographic methods. Am Heart J 116:758, 1988.
94. Boltwood CM, Chuwa T, Wong M, Shah PM: Quantitative echocardiography in the mitral complex in dilated cardiomyopathy. The mechanism of functional mitral regurgitation. Circulation 68:498, 1983.
95. Boughner DR: Assessment of aortic insufficiency by transcutaneous Doppler ultrasound. Circulation 52:874, 1975.
96. Zhang Y, et al.: Measurement of aortic regurgitation by Doppler echocardiography. Br Heart J 55:32, 1986.
97. Marx GR, Hicks RW, Allen HD, Goldberg SJ: Noninvasive assessment of hemodynamic responses to exercise in pulmonary regurgitation after operations to correct pulmonary outflow obstruction. Am J Cardiol 61:595, 1988.
98. Goli VD, et al.: Noninvasive evaluation of aortic stenosis severity utilizing Doppler ultrasound and electrical bioimpedance. J Am Coll Cardiol 11:66, 1988.
99. Oh JE, et al.: Prediction of the severity of aortic stenosis by Doppler aortic valve area determination: prospective Doppler-catheterization correlation in 100 patients. J Am Coll Cardiol 11:1227, 1988.
100. Currie PJ, et al.: Continous-wave Doppler echocardiographic assessment of severity of calcific aortic stenosis: a simultaneous Doppler-catheter correlative study in 100 adult patients. Circulation 71:1162, 1985.
101. Holmvang G, McConville B, Tomlinson CW: Noninvasive determination of valve area in adults with aortic stenosis using Doppler echocardiography. Cathet Cardiovasc Diagn 12:9, 1986.
102. Nitta M, Takamoto T, Taniguchi K, Hultgren HN: Diagnostic accuracy of continuous wave Doppler echocardiography in severe aortic stenosis in the elderly. Jpn Heart J 29:169, 1988.
103. Kosturakis D, et al.: Noninvasive quantification of stenotic semilunar valve areas by Doppler echocardiography. J Am Coll Cardiol 3:1256, 1984.
104. Warth DC, et al.: A new method to calculate aortic valve area without left heart catheterization. Circulation 70:978, 1984.
105. Otto CM, et al.: Determination of the stenotic aortic valve area in adults using Doppler echocardiography. J Am Coll Cardiol 7:509, 1986.
106. Skjaerpe T, Hegrenaes L, Hatle L: Noninvasive estimation of valve area in patients with aortic stenosis by Doppler ultrasound and two-dimensional echocardiography. Circulation 72:810, 1985.
107. Teirstein P, et al.: Doppler echocardiographic measurement of aortic valve area in aortic stenosis: a noninvasive application of the Gorlin formula. J Am Coll Cardiol 8:1059, 1986.
108. Come PC, et al.: Prediction of severity of aortic stenosis: accuracy of multiple noninvasive parameters. Am J Med 85:29, 1988.
109. Come PC, Riley MF, McKay RG, Safian R: Echocardiographic assessment of aortic valve area in elderly patients with aortic stenosis and of changes in valve area after percutaneous balloon valvuloplasty. J Am Coll Cardiol 10:115, 1987.
110. Ohlsson J, Wranne B: Noninvasive assessment of valve area in patients with aortic stenosis. J Am Coll Cardiol 7:501, 1986.
111. Lavandier B, et al.: Noninvasive aortic blood flow measurement using an intraesophageal probe. Ultrasound Med Biol 11:451, 1985.
112. Maulik D, Nanda NC, Saini VD: Fetal Doppler echocardiography: methods and characterization of normal and abnormal hemodynamics. Am J Cardiol 53:572, 1984.
113. Kenny JF, et al.: Changes in intracardiac blood flow velocities and right and left ventricular stroke volumes with gestational age in the normal human fetus: a prospective Doppler echocardiography study. Circulation 74:1208, 1986.
114. De Smedt M, Visser G, Meijboom EJ: Fetal cardiac output estimated by Doppler echocardiography during mid- and late gestation. Am J Cardiol 60:338, 1987.
115. Allan LD, et al.: Doppler echocardiographic evaluation of the normal human fetal heart. Br Heart J 57:528, 1987.
116. Kenny J, et al.: Effects of heart rate on ventricular size, stroke volume, and output in the normal human fetus: a prospective Doppler echocardiographic study. Circulation 76:52, 1987.
117. Christie J, et al.: Determination of stroke volume and cardiac output during exercise: comparison of two-dimensional and Doppler echocardiography, Fick oximetry, and thermodilution. Circulation 76:539, 1987.
118. Marx GR, Hicks RW, Allen HD, Kinzer SM: Measurement of cardiac output and exercise factor by pulsed Doppler echocardiography during supine bicycle ergometry in normal young adolescent boys. J Am Coll Cardiol 10:430, 1987.
119. Loeppky JA, et al.: Beat-by-beat stroke volume assessment by pulsed Doppler in upright and supine exercise. J Appl Physiol 50:1173, 1981.
120. Daley PJ, Sagar KB, Wann LS: Doppler echocardiographic measurement of flow velocity in the ascending aorta during supine and upright exercise. Br Heart J 54:562, 1985.
121. Rassi A, Crawford MH, Richards KL, Miller JF: Differing mechanisms of exercise flow augmentation at the mitral and aortic valves. Circulation 77: 543, 1988.
122. Ihlen H, Endresen K, Golf S, Nitter-Hauge S: Cardiac stroke volume during exercise measured by Doppler echocardiography; comparison with the thermodilution technique and evaluation of reproducibility. Br Heart J 58: 455, 1987.

123. Nanna M, et al.: Noninvasive cardiac output monitoring during exercise stress test. Can J Cardiol 4:165, 1988.
124. Bryg JB, et al.: Effect of coronary artery disease on Doppler-derived parameters of aortic flow during upright exercise. Am J Cardiol 58:14, 1986.
125. Mehdirad AA, et al.: Evaluation of left ventricular function during upright exercise: correlation of exercise Doppler with postexercise two-dimensional echocardiographic results. Circulation 75:413, 1987.
126. Daley PJ, et al.: Detection of exercise induced changes in left ventricular performance by Doppler echocardiography. Br Heart J 58:447, 1987.
127. Harrison MR, et al.: Use of exercise Doppler echocardiography to evaluate cardiac drugs: effects of propranolol and verapamil on aortic blood flow velocity and acceleration. J Am Coll Cardiol 11:1002, 1988.
128. Buckingham TA, et al.: Effect of ventricular function on the exercise hemodynamics of variable rate pacing. J Am Coll Cardiol 11:1269, 1988.

CHAPTER

31

COMPLEX CONGENITAL HEART DISEASE I: A DIAGNOSTIC APPROACH

The evaluation of the patient with complex congenital heart disease is one of the most challenging and rewarding areas in echocardiography. The echocardiographer's approach to these patients should be like the clinician's approach to the physical examination in that the echocardiographic examination must be conducted in an organized and orderly fashion. The precise sequence in which the examination is conducted is not as important as the presence of order and the compilation of data sufficient to answer all relevant diagnostic questions. Without such an organized approach, even the most experienced observer frequently becomes fascinated by one or two striking abnormalities and fails to record all the information necessary to describe the anatomic and functional characteristics of a particular lesion completely.

This chapter describes an approach that I have found helpful in examining these patients. With this method, the examination is conducted to answer a series of questions. These questions are directed toward determining (1) atrial location or *situs*; (2) ventricular number, size, orientation, and identity; (3) atrioventricular (AV) connection; (4) great vessel orientation and identity; (5) the pattern by which the great vessels are connected to the ventricular chambers; (6) the presence and direction of intracardiac shunts; and (7) the presence, location, and severity of outflow obstruction. These echocardiographic data can then be combined to describe the pathophysiology of a complex lesion using any of the standard segmental systems.[1-4]

The information necessary to answer these questions is contained in views comparable to the standard imaging planes. In the patient with complex congenital heart disease, however, the primary cardiac structures used to align these planes may be far removed from their normal position or relationships, and the appearance and identity of structures within these views may be greatly dissimilar to those normally encountered. Therefore, here more than in any other circumstance, these planes must be aligned relative to specific intracardiac structures rather than to groups of structures or external references.

The relative importance of individual examining planes is also significantly different from their importance in the routine examination and differs still further depending on whether an adult or a child is studied. In the routine examination, for example, the majority of information is obtained from the parasternal long axis view. In the patient with complex congenital heart disease, in contrast, the parasternal short axis, apical four-chamber, and subcostal views provide more information. In the adult, the parasternal short axis and apical four-chamber views, which define the orientation of the interventricular septum, AV valve structure, and great vessel orientation, are of primary importance, whereas in the child, almost the entire examination can usually be recorded from the subcostal transducer location. Despite these generalities, standard views are usually less meaningful when one is examining the malformed, malpositioned heart, and for this reason, the examination is directed toward answering specific questions rather than toward obtaining a series of routine views.

VARIATIONS IN CARDIAC POSITION AND SITUS

Cardiac Position and Situs

Before discussing the echocardiographic examination in patients with congenital heart disease, one must be familiar with (1) the potential locations of the heart in the chest (cardiac position), (2) the various relationships of the heart with the other unpaired organs of the body (situs), and (3) anomalies associated with specific disorders of cardiac position and situs. Although the segmental approach to the diagnosis of congenital heart disease is independent of cardiac position, determining position is important, to relate echocardiographic data to data obtained from other techniques and to benefit from predictions concerning pathophysiology that can be made from the position of the heart.

Cardiac position is defined relative to the midline of the thorax, with the result that the heart can lie in the right chest (dextrocardia), the left chest (levocardia), or in the midline (mesocardia). Situs, in contrast, refers to the right-left position of the unpaired organs of the body (i.e., the heart, lungs, liver, spleen, and intestines). When these organs are in their normal positions, the morphologic right lung and liver are to the right, and the morphologic left lung, heart, spleen, and stomach are to the left. This relationship is termed *situs* (position or location) *solitus* (usual or accustomed). In 1 in 5000 to 1 in 10,000 individuals, the right-left orientation of the unpaired viscera including the heart is inverted, a condition known as *situs inversus*.[5] In situs inversus the heart, stomach, spleen, and morphologic left lung lie to the right, and the morphologic right lung and liver are to the left. Cardiac situs is determined by the position of the atria because they bear the most consistent relation to the situs of the viscera.

The heart normally lies predominantly in the left chest (levocardia), with the morphologic right atrium and ventricle to the right and the morphologic left atrium and ventricle to the left ((situs solitus) (Fig. 31–1). In some cases, however, the heart may be found in the right chest, and definition of the cause of this dextrocardia may be the referring echocardiographic question. Dextrocardia has three primary causes. The first is mechanical, owing to a general shift in mediastinal structures caused by either a space-occupying lesion in the left chest or a lack of normal lung volume in the right chest. This form of dextrocardia is usually termed *dextroposition*. The second cause is situs inversus. The term "mirror-image dextrocardia" has also been applied to this condition because the cardiac chambers are a mirror image of their normal location (Fig. 31–1). The final form of dextrocardia is known as *dextroversion*. In the early fetus the position of the cardiac apex is opposite to that of later fetal and adult life. In normal hearts (situs solitus), the apex rotates from right to left to reach its ultimate left-sided position. Dextroversion occurs because the apex fails to rotate normally during fetal development and so remains in the right chest. The position of the cardiac chambers in the dextroverted heart can be better appreciated if one imagines grasping the normal heart by the apex and rotating it to the right around its valvular pedicle until the apex passes the midline. At this point, the right atrium and ventricle will still be to the right and the left ventricle and atrium to the left. Depending on the degree of rotation, however, the left ventricle may be slightly anterior to the right ventricle, the interventricular septum vertical relative to the anterior chest wall and the pulmonic valve displaced to the right and posteriorly as it is rotated around the aorta. In dextroversion of the heart, the right ventricle occupies the cardiac apex. Because dextroversion represents isolated failure of apical rotation, the heart remains in situs solitus (Fig. 31–1). The same failure of apical rotation can occur in patients with situs inversus, resulting in levoversion[6] (Fig. 31–1). Mesocardia is simply the midline arrest of normal cardiac rotation in situs solitus or situs inversus. Failure to complete normal apical rotation is particularly common with discordant AV relationships, as in physiologically corrected transposition.[4,5]

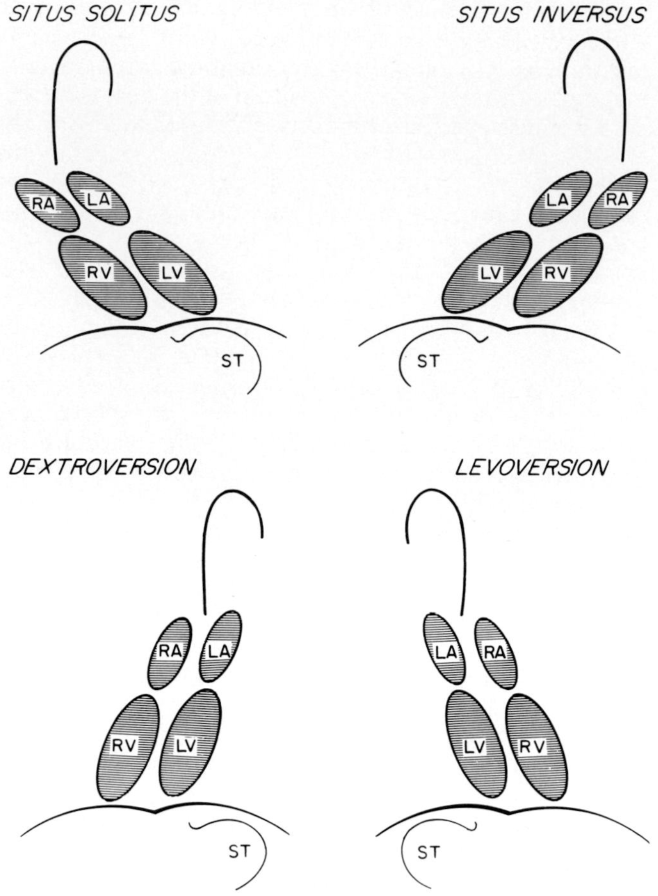

Fig. 31–1. The position of the atria and ventricles in situs solitus, situs inversus, dextroversion, and levoversion. Visceral situs is indicated by the location of the stomach (ST), the normal side of the aortic arch. LA = left atrium; RA = right atrium; LV = right ventricle; RV = right ventricle.

Situs Ambiguus, Asplenia, and Polysplenia

In addition to the orderly arrangement of organs seen in patients with situs solitus and situs inversus, one may see varying degrees of visceral disorder (heterotaxia) ranging from situs solitus with isolated malrotation of the bowel, through isolated cardiac malposition relative to situs (dextroversion and levoversion), to reduplication of the organs of one side of the body with associated suppression of those with opposite-sidedness. These more symmetric body configurations in which lateralization is incomplete and situs is no longer clearly defined are collectively termed *situs ambiguus*. Patients with situs ambiguus are classified based on the presence and location of the spleen. Splenic abnormalities are intimately associated with malposition of the heart and viscera because splenic primordia differentiate during the early weeks of fetal life at approximately the same time as the truncal and conal regions of the heart and at the same time that body situs is determined.[7] Two symmetric body configurations have been associated with splenic abnormalities.[4] The first is the *asplenia* syndrome, which, in addition to absence of the spleen, is characterized by bilateral right-sidedness or duplication of right-sided structures including bilateral morphologic right lungs, bilateral morphologic right atria (right atrial insomerism), a liver that is symmetric and horizontal, and a stomach near the midline.[4,8,9] In this syndrome, no left-sided structures are present and hence the spleen, morphologic left atrium, and lung are absent. The second is the *polysplenia syndrome*, which is characterized by a tendency toward bilateral left-sidedness and typically includes multiple spleens on both sides of the abdomen, bilateral morphologic left atria*, and bilateral morphologic left lungs.[4,10,11] The abdominal organs tend less toward symmetry than in asplenia. Although the liver may have two roughly equal halves, the major portion often lies to one side of the abdomen. Similarly, the stomach is seldom midline, and considerable abdominal heterotaxia is often present. Although rarely seen beyond infancy because of the high early mortality (79 to 94% by 1 year for asplenia[11,12]), patients with these abnormalities have been reported to represent as many as 10% of admissions to pediatric cardiac units. In general, the more severely disordered the visceroatrial relationships, the greater the tendency for associated congenital heart disease. Asplenia is always associated with a complex cardiac malformation; polysplenia shows a more variable pattern with an occasional normal heart at one end of the spectrum and severe cardiac malformation at the other.[7,13–15]

Recognized Associations Between Disorders of Cardiac Position and Cardiac Abnormalities

In the majority of patients with congenital heart disease, cardiac position and situs are normal. Although malpositions are uncommon, their importance lies in their frequent association with congenital heart disease. Dextrocardia occurs in roughly 1.6% of patients with congenital heart disease.[16] In situs inversus with mirror-image dextrocardia, about 90 to 95% of patients have otherwise normal hearts; however, in large groups of patients with known congenital heart disease, the incidence of situs inversus is about 0.8%, a frequency much higher than in the general population. If a congenital defect does exist, it is most likely to be corrected transposition.[17] Other defects may also coexist, but with no prevailing pattern. Patients with dextroversion almost invariably have additional congenital malformations. The commonest associated abnormalities include corrected transposition, pulmonic stenosis, hypoplasia and atresia of the pulmonary artery, tricuspid valve abnormalities, and ventricular or atrial septal defect. Visceral heterotaxia with asplenia or polysplenia is also seen. Levoversion with an otherwise normal heart is virtually nonexistent; the associated abnormalities are similar to those seen with dextroversion.

Patients with asplenia syndrome may have a normally positioned heart, but mesocardia and dextrocardia are more common. Associated cardiac anomalies include (1) anomalous systemic venous return; (2) large atrial septal defects resulting from absence of the septum primum or endocardial cushions (both left-sided structures); (3) AV canal; (4) common ventricle or a large ventricular septal defect as part of the AV canal; (5) ventricular inversion; (6) transposition of the great vessels; (7) severe pulmonic stenosis or atresia; and (8) anomalous pulmonary venous connection. In patients with polysplenia syndrome, the heart may be right- or left-sided, but mesocardia is rare.[4] Common cardiac malformations include (1) anomalous systemic venous connection; (2) anomalous pulmonary venous connection; (3) atrial septal defects; (4) ventricular septal defects; (5) double outlet right ventricle; and (6) left-sided obstructive lesions. In contrast to asplenia, transposition of the great vessels and pulmonic stenosis are unusual.[4] Interruption of the inferior vena cava with azygos continuation to the superior vena cava is highly suggestive of polysplenia.[4]

INITIAL APPROACH TO THE HEART

The initial approach to the heart differs with the population studied and the available historical data. Because the heart is normally positioned (levocardia in situs solitus) in such a overwhelming preponderance of routine studies (including patients with congenital heart disease), it is common practice in most laboratories to assume that cardiac position and situs are normal (i.e., the heart is in the left chest and the atrium that connects to the left-sided ventricle is the left atrium) and to begin all examinations by attempting to record the routine parasternal long and short axis views. Once the presence of complex congenital heart disease is apparent, these views are then modified and the examination conducted to answer specific questions as indicated later (beginning with the determination of ventricular morphology). If the heart cannot be located in the left chest, dextrocardia either from dextroposition or from situs inversus should be suspected and the transducer moved to the right chest in an attempt to record valvular motion. If cardiac location, orientation, or situs remains unclear after this initial precordial screening, it is necessary to shift the transducer to the subcostal position to locate the heart, determine its major axis, and identify atrial situs before proceeding. Once the heart is located, the examination again proceeds as outlined later (beginning with the identification of the atria).

In laboratories that deal with large numbers of pa-

* The association of bilateral "right-sidedness" with asplenia and "bilateral left-sidedness" with polysplenia are useful conceptually but imprecise anatomically. There is some cross-over between syndromes, and although both atria in polysplenia typically have morphologic features of left atria, a heart with truly bilateral left atria with four pulmonary veins entering each side and two septa prima forming the septal surface on each side has not been described.

tients with complex congenital heart disease in whom anomalies of cardiac position or situs are frequent, it is common practice to begin the examination in the subcostal window and determine cardiac position and atrial situs before proceeding to the examination of the ventricles.

Cardiac position can be defined relative to the midline of the body by placing the transducer immediately beneath the xyphoid process and aligning the central ray parallel to the midsagittal plane of the body. As a general rule, patients with situs solitus have a central cardiac axis directed between 30 and 45° to the left of this plane, whereas those with levoversion have a central axis that lies between 0 and 30° to the left of the midline. In patients with dextrocardia from dextroposition, the central cardiac axis remains normal (i.e., leftward relative to the midline) despite the abnormal position. Dextrocardia resulting from situs inversus results in a central cardiac axis that is the opposite of normal (i.e., 30 to 45° to the right of the central sagittal plane), whereas in those with dextroversion the central axis lies between 0 and 30° rightward. Patients with mesocardia by definition have a central cardiac axis roughly parallel to that of the body.

ATRIAL SITUS AND VISCEROATRIAL RELATIONS

Atrial Identity and Location (Where Are the Atria and Which Is Which?)

Two direct approaches have been suggested to determine atrial identity and thus atrial situs. The first is based on the insertion of the inferior vena cava (IVC). and the second on atrial morphology. When present, the IVC almost always returns to the morphologic right atrium,[18,19] and in both situs solitus and situs inversus, the IVC lies on the side of the spine opposite the abdominal aorta (Fig. 31–2). In cases in which visceral situs and atrial situs are discordant, the IVC typically switches sides at the liver to enter the morphologic right atrium.[18] In the asplenia syndrome, both the IVC and abdominal aorta characteristically lie on the same side of the spine (right or left) (Fig. 31–3 top), but the IVC remains a reliable indicator of the basic type of visceroatrial situs. In patients with the polysplenia syndrome with bilateral morphologic left atria, the portion of the chamber that receives the IVC can be considered the systemic venous atrium.[18] When the suprarenal-to-subhepatic segment of the IVC is absent, the IVC usually connects to the superior vena cava (SVC) through an azygos extension.[20] In such cases, the side of the azygos

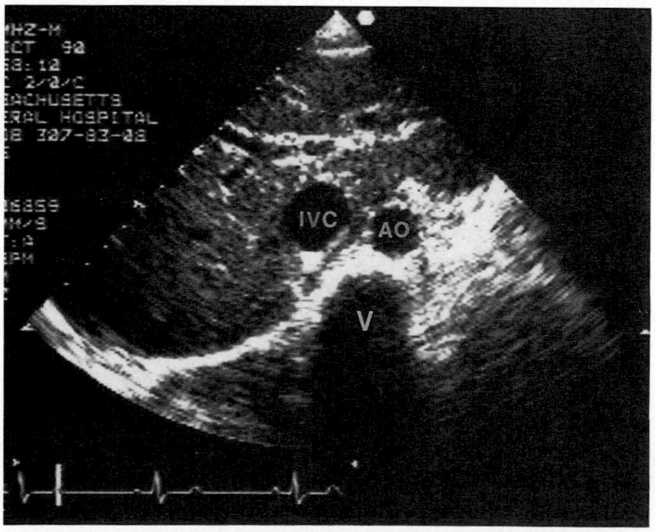

Fig. 31–2. Subcostal short axis view illustrating the normal relationship of the inferior vena cava (IVC) and abdominal aorta (AO). In this example, the inferior vena cava lies to the right of the midline defined by the vertebral body (V) and the abdominal aorta lies to the left.

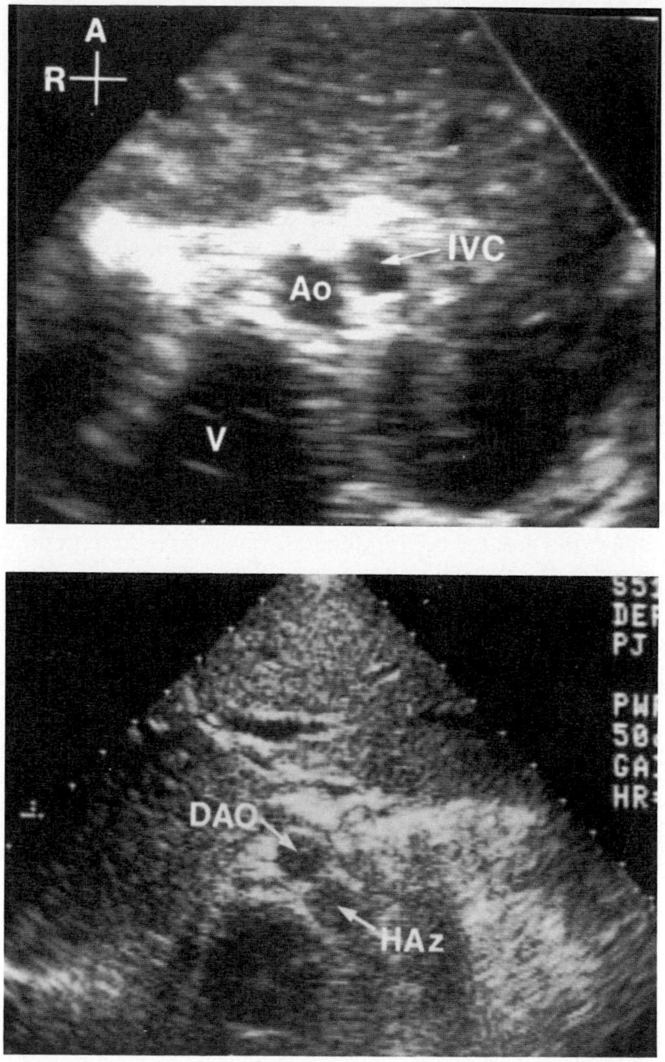

Fig. 31–3. Top. Subcostal short-axis recording of the inferior vena cava (IVC) and abdominal aorta (AO) in a patient with asplenia. The aorta and IVC both lie to the left of the midline, and the IVC is anterior and lateral to the aorta. Bottom. Same recording in a patient with polysplenia. In this condition, there is frequently subhepatic interruption of the inferior vena cava, which continues via a hemiazygos connection to the superior vena cava. In this case the hemiazygos vein (HAz) and aorta (DAO) again lie on the same side of the spine, but the hemiazygos vein is posterior and lateral to the aorta. V = vertebral body. (From Snider AR, Serwer GA: Echocardiography in Pediatric Heart Disease. Chicago, Year Book Medical Publishers, 1990.)

extension appears to correspond to that of the IVC, thereby indicating atrial situs (Fig. 31–3 bottom). In cases of so-called absence of the IVC, the hepatic segment of the IVC is not absent and the hepatic vein(s) can be visualized entering the atrium. Use of the hepatic segment of the IVC as a marker of atrial situs appears controversial. The SVC is of little help in atrial localization because it may open into either atrium or it may be duplicated.[18]

The assessment of atrial situs from chamber morphology is based on pathologic and surgical precedent but has proved far less reliable in echocardiographic studies.[21] The morphologic right atrium has a septal surface that receives the tendinous insertion of the eustachian valve and contains the limbus of the fossa ovalis. The eustachian valve crosses the floor of the right atrium from the orifice of the inferior vena and inserts into the septum primum. In real time, the eustachian valve moves rapidly back and forth in the right atrium and can be visualized in virtually all infants and in many older children and adults.[22] The left atrial septal surface has the flap valve of the fossa ovalis. This is the septum primum tissue that covers the foramen ovale and seals it closed after birth. On the two-dimensional echocardiogram, the flap valve can be seen protruding into the left atrium in the fetus when the foramen ovale is open. This sign is not foolproof, however, because high left atrial pressure can cause the septum primum to herniate into the right atrium.[23] Atrial appendage morphology also differs; the right atrium has a short, broad, pyramidal appendage, whereas the left atrial appendage is long and fingerlike. Unfortunately, the morphology of the atrial appendages has been of marginal value in identifying the atria by echocardiography.[24]

Atrial Isomerism

When atrial isomerism is present, the IVC defines the systemic venous atrium, but the basic identity of the isomeric atria must be determined by morphology or by associated lesions. In right and left atrial isomerism, the vena cava and abdominal aorta both lie on the same side of the spine (Fig. 31–3), In right atrial isomerism, the inferior vena cava is positioned anteriorly, whereas in left atrial isomerism, the major vein is often posterior to the aorta (i.e., the azygos connection of the IVC) (see Fig. 31–3). In the asplenia syndrome, the isomeric right atria have typical pyramidal appendages. Two types of atrial septal defect also commonly coexist. The first is an atrial septal defect of the foramen ovale type. The fossa ovalis a right-sided structure is usually present, but the valve of the foramen ovale (a left-sided structure) is absent. The second typical defect is the atrial portion of a complete AV canal. Both defects are usually large and are separated by only a strand of septal tissue. In left atrial isomerism, both atria have windsocklike appendages. The septum primum is usually present, and the right-sided foramen ovale is absent.

Abdominal Situs—Visceroatrial Discordance

Although visceroatrial concordance is the rule, visceroatrial discordance occurs on rare occasions and is associated with a high incidence of severe complex congenital heart disease. In most cases of visceroatrial discordance, the subhepatic IVC defines abdominal situs lying to the right in abdominal situs solitus and to the left in situs inversus of the viscera. To enter the right atrium in these cases, the IVC changes sides at the level of the liver.[18] An exception is the syndrome of isolated atrial inversion in which both the IVC and aorta are left-sided and the viscera are in their normal situs solitus position. Location of the stomach bubble and position of the liver may aid in determining abdominal situs in these cases.

Note that when the IVC is used to determine cardiac situs, only two types are possible, situs solitus and situs inversus. Functionally, this simplified categorization is appropriate because it achieves the goal of defining the systemic venous atrium. Definition of abdominal situs is important in predicting associated abnormalities, but it does not independently relate to cardiac function or surgical repair.

VENTRICULAR NUMBER, SIZE, ORIENTATION, AND IDENTITY

The second step in the evaluation of the patient with complex congenital heart disease is to determine ventricular number, size, orientation, and identity.

What Is a Ventricle?

Before describing how ventricles are numbered and identified, it is important to define what constitutes a ventricle. A chamber is generally considered a ventricle if it receives more than 50% of the ventricular inlet or fibrous ring of an AV valve.[25] The valve itself need not be patent for the chamber to be considered a ventricle (e.g., mitral or tricuspid atresia). A chamber need not be connected to an outlet (great vessel) to be considered a ventricle. Chambers that do not receive 50% of an inlet are termed rudimentary chambers. The two types of rudimentary chambers are outlet chambers and trabecular pouches. Outlet chambers receive less than 50% of an inlet but underlie more than 50% of a outlet (i.e., the aorta or pulmonary artery). A trabecular pouch is a rudimentary chamber that receives less than 50% of an inlet and underlies less than 50% of an outlet.

How Many Ventricles Are Present?

Ventricular number, that is, whether one or two separate ventricular chambers exist, is determined by the presence or absence of an interventricular septum. The normal interventricular septum is best visualized in the parasternal short axis, apical four-chamber, and subcostal long and short axis views (see Chapter 29). The same views are used in the patient with complex congenital disease to confirm or exclude the presence of a septum.

Figure 31–4 compares the appearance and orientation of the interventricular septum in the normal biventricular heart to the single large chamber and the complete absence of septum, which characterize the single ventricle. In both the apical four-chamber and subcostal long axis views, the interatrial septum helps to define the

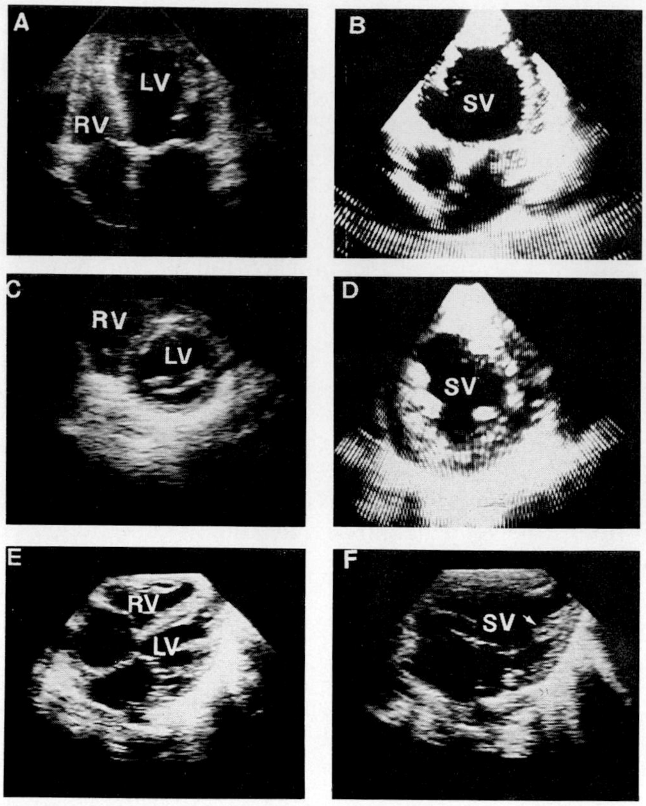

Fig. 31–4. This series of recordings compares the appearance and orientation of the interventricular septum of the normal biventricular heart with the single ventricular heart, which is characterized by a large chamber and complete absence of the septum. **A.** Apical four-chamber recording illustrating the division of the normal heart into two separate ventricles by the interventricular septum. **B.** Apical four-chamber view of a single ventricle. There is no septum and only one large chamber. **C.** Normal appearance of the two ventricles and interventricular septum in the parasternal short axis view. **D.** Large, circular, single ventricle in short axis view. **E.** Subcostal long axis (four-chamber) views of a normal heart. **F.** Subcostal long axis recording of a single ventricle in which a large papillary muscle arises from the posterolateral ventricular wall (oblique arrow). LV = left ventricle; RV = right ventricle.

expected point of insertion and orientation of the interventricular septum and further highlights the absence of this structure. On occasion, as illustrated in Figure 31–4F, single or multiple large papillary muscles may give the appearance of a rudimentary septum, particularly in the subcostal long axis view. These papillary muscles can be distinguished from a rudimentary septum in short axis by the demonstration of ventricular cavity surrounding the papillary muscle head. It might also be expected that chordal origin could be used to differentiate a papillary muscle from septum. This differential point may be misleading, however, because in certain disorders, such as AV canal defect, chordae tendineae may arise directly from the interventricular septum.

In some patients, a rudimentary muscular shelf can be observed extending outward from the ventricular wall in a position that, if further extended, would roughly bisect the large ventricular chamber. Figure 31–5 illustrates the short axis appearance of such a muscular shelf. These rudimentary septa are important anatomically because they differentiate the biventricular heart with a large ventricular septal defect from a single ventricle. From a functional standpoint, however, these rudimentary septa appear to have little significance.[6,25]

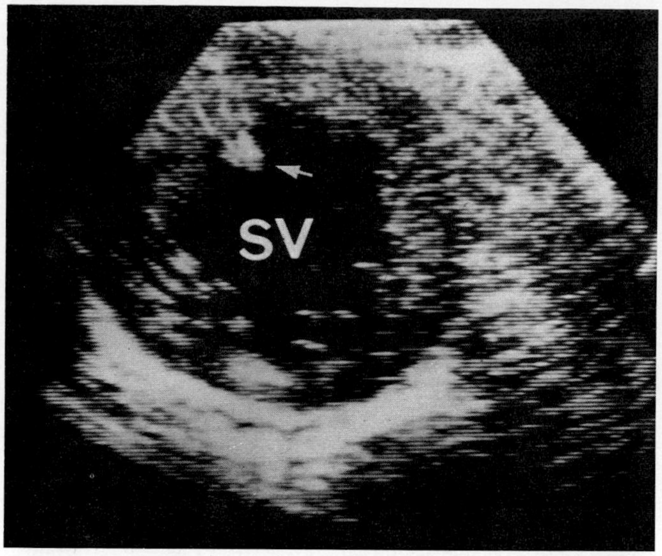

Fig. 31–5. Parasternal short axis view records a single large ventricular chamber (SV) with a rudimentary interventricular septum arising from the ventricular wall at roughly 11 o'clock (horizontal arrow).

Finally, when confronted with a single ventricle, one must determine whether an outflow chamber is present.[1,26] These outflow chambers represent the infundibular portion of the right ventricle and, when the great vessels are transposed, are always found at the base of the anteriorly positioned aorta. In the uncommon situation in which the great vessels are normally oriented, the outflow chamber is associated with the anterior pulmonary artery.[1]

Figure 31–6 illustrates the appearance of an outflow chamber at the base of the anteriorly positioned aorta in a patient with a single ventricle and D-transposition of the great vessels. (The pathophysiology of single ventricle is discussed in detail in the next chapter).

What Is the Relative Size of the Two Ventricles, and Are They Both Morphologically Intact?

Once the presence of two ventricular chambers has been established, the next step is to determine their relative size and structural integrity. Normally, the two ventricles are approximately equal in size. Marked disproportion in ventricular size may occur because the larger ventricle is subject to an abnormal volume load, because flow into the smaller ventricle is obstructed, or because the smaller ventricle is hypoplastic.

Figure 31–7 compares the appearance of the left and right ventricles of three infants younger than 2 months of age. Figure 31–7A is recorded from a normal infant and illustrates the appropriate size and configuration of the left and right ventricles. In Figure 31–7B, the left ventricle is much smaller than the right, and the inter-

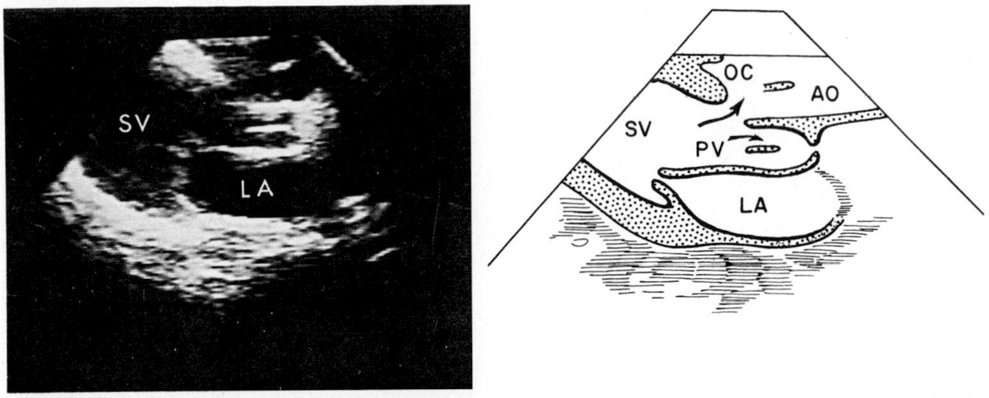

Fig. 31–6. Parasternal long axis recording from a patient with a single ventricle and D-transposition of the great vessels illustrates the appearance of a subaortic outflow chamber. The longer curved arrow illustrates the path of blood flow from the single ventricle (SV) into the anteriorly positioned aorta (AO). The apparent abrupt termination of the posteriorly positioned pulmonary artery is caused by a pulmonary artery band positioned just above the pulmonary valve (PV). OC = outflow chamber, LA = left atrium.

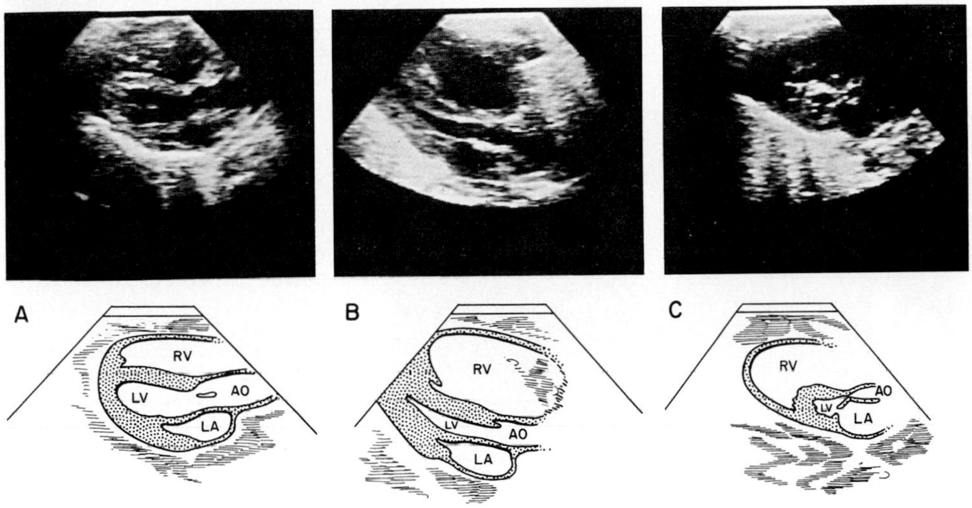

Fig. 31–7. Parasternal long axis recordings of the left (LV) and right (RV) ventricles. **A.** A normal infant. **B.** An infant with a severe reduction in left ventricular size caused by right ventricular volume overload and obstructed left ventricular inflow. **C.** An infant with a hypoplastic left ventricle. AO = aorta; LA = left atrium.

ventricular septum is displaced posteriorly. The aortic root is also considerably smaller than normal. In this example, the decrease in left ventricular size was the result of reduced left ventricular inflow because of a left atrial membrane or cor triatriatum. Figure 31–7C is a recording from a patient with a hypoplastic left ventricle with associated mitral and aortic hypoplasia. The size of the left ventricle in Figures 31–7 B and C is below the lower limit of normal for a patient of such age, and because the obstructing membrane in the patient with cor triatriatum cannot be appreciated in this view, it was initially questioned whether this might not also be an example of a hypoplastic left heart. A truly hypoplastic left ventricle, however, can usually be differentiated from a ventricle that is abnormally small because of reduced inflow or compression by a dilated right ventricle by examining AV valve structure. In the hypoplastic ventricle, the associated AV valve is characteristically smaller, structurally deformed, and moves poorly, if at all. In the morphologically normal ventricle, the AV valve is normally formed and typically moves freely despite the reduced ventricular size or limited inflow from the left atrium. Figure 31–8 is a comparable example of the hypoplastic right ventricle and fixed immobile tricuspid valve of tricuspid atresia. In this example, the interatrial septum is absent, and hence, there is a common atrium.

Which Is the Morphologic Right and Which Is the Morphologic Left Ventricle?

In many instances in which the ventricles are malpositioned or ventricular inversion is suspected, one must determine which is the morphologic right ventricle and which is the morphologic left ventricle. Normally, the ventricles are differentiated by their position, their shape, and the thickness of their muscular walls. In complex congenital heart disease, however, all these features may be misleading. In Figure 31–9A, for example, one sees a large, circular, anterior ventricle and a smaller, flat, posterior ventricle. The walls of both ventricles are thick, and the septum, in real time, appeared to contract with the anterior ventricle. The identity of these ventricles can be established by determining which ventricle contains the mitral valve and which contains the tricuspid valve because the mitral valve is always associated with the anatomic left ventricle and the tricuspid valve with the anatomic right ventricle.

Five features help to distinguish the tricuspid valve and anatomic right ventricle from the mitral valve and

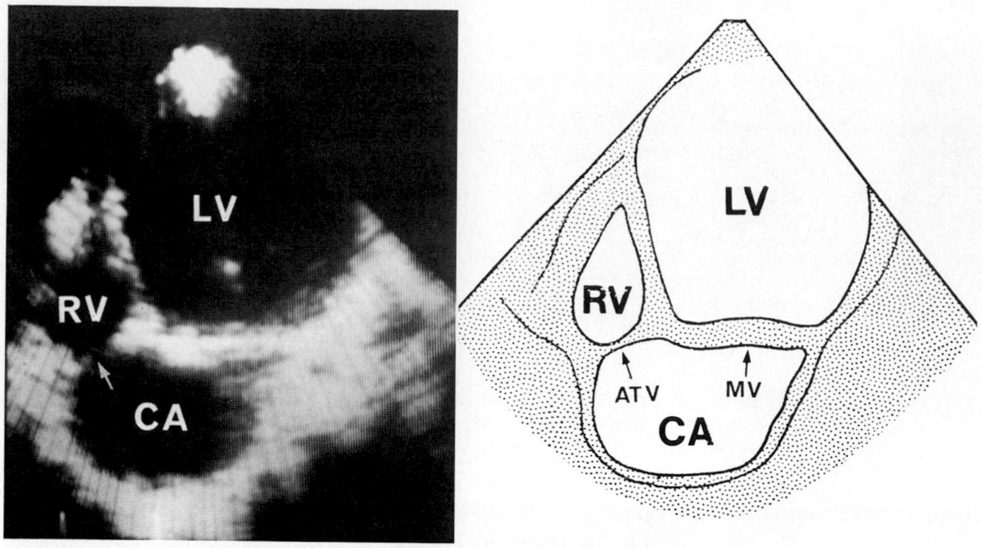

Fig. 31–8. Apical four-chamber view illustrates tricuspid atresia. The left ventricle (LV) is dilated, and the right ventricle (RV) is small. During diastole, tricuspid valve movement was not apparent, whereas the mitral valve orifice (MV) was large. Interatrial septum was not present. ATV = atretic tricuspid valve; CA = common atrium. The vertical white arrow points to the tricuspid valve.

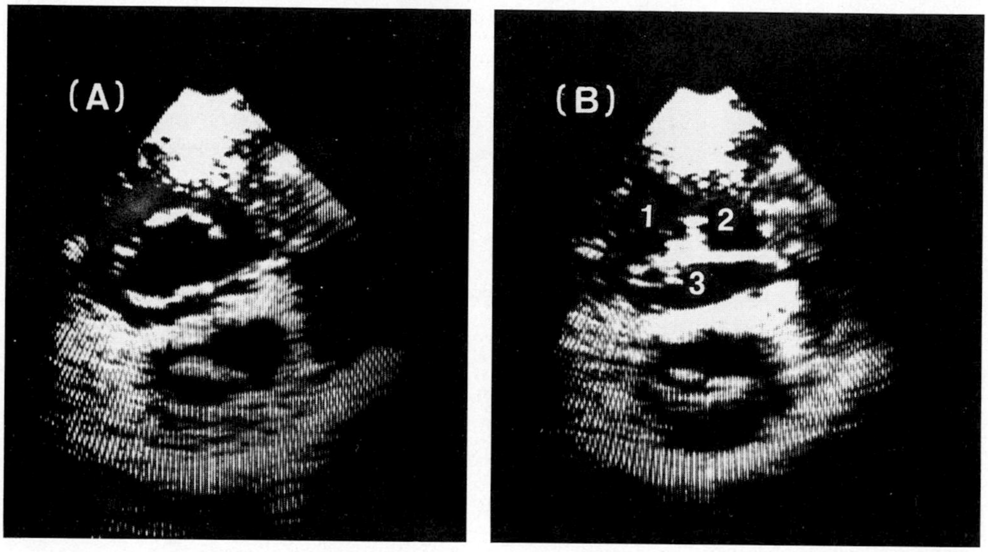

Fig. 31–9. Parasternal short axis scans of a biventricular heart. **A.** A large, circular, anterior ventricle and a smaller, flattened, posterior ventricle. The walls of both ventricles are thick, and in this diastolic frame, both atrioventricular valves are open. **B.** During systole, the trileaflet tricuspid valve can be observed within the anterior ventricle (1, 2, 3). It can thereby be confirmed that the anterior ventricle is the morphologic right ventricle, and the posterior ventricle must be the anatomic left ventricle.

associated left ventricle. The simplest method for distinguishing the mitral valve from the tricuspid valve is to determine the number of leaflets the valve contains. (The tricuspid valve normally has three leaflets, whereas the normal mitral valve has only two.[27,28] Figure 31–9B illustrates this leaflet structure. In this example, the AV valve associated with the anterior ventricle has three distinct leaflets and therefore must be an anatomic tricuspid valve. The posterior valve is not as well visualized, but by exclusion, can be assumed to be the mitral valve. By this simple method, the anterior ventricle can be determined to be the anatomic right ventricle, whereas the posterior ventricle then becomes the anatomic left ventricle.

Figure 31–10 is a second example in which the two AV valves are side by side and no interventricular septum is recorded. In this example, the left-sided AV valve has three clearly defined commissures and therefore is the anatomic tricuspid valve, whereas the right-sided valve has only two commissures and therefore is the mitral valve. (In this example, right and left are used to refer to the patient's rather than the viewer's right and left.) By identifying AV valve structure, the ventricles in this example can be determined to be inverted. Confusion occasionally arises when the patient has a cleft mitral valve; however, in these instances, there are still only two commissures and the systolic configuration is that of an anatomic mitral valve. Greater difficulty occurs in those cases with ventricular inversion in which the inlet valve of the morphologic right ventricle has only two leaflets,[29] and in such cases other criteria must be used.

The second method for identifying the AV valves is through their relative level of insertion into the interventricular septum. The septal leaflet of the tricuspid valve normally inserts slightly inferior (apical) (5 to 10 mm) to the insertion of the anterior mitral leaflet.[30] This occurs because the mitral AV groove is normally slightly superior to the tricuspid groove. The anterior leaflet of the mitral valve therefore inserts into the left AV sulcus near the superior end of the membranous septum, whereas the septal leaflet of the tricuspid valve inserts near the mid portion of the membranous septum.[30]

Figure 31–11 illustrates the relative points of septal insertion of the mitral and tricuspid valves in the normal

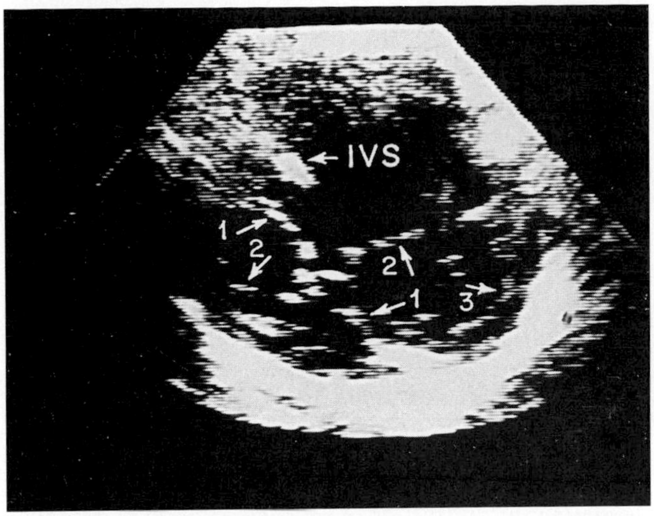

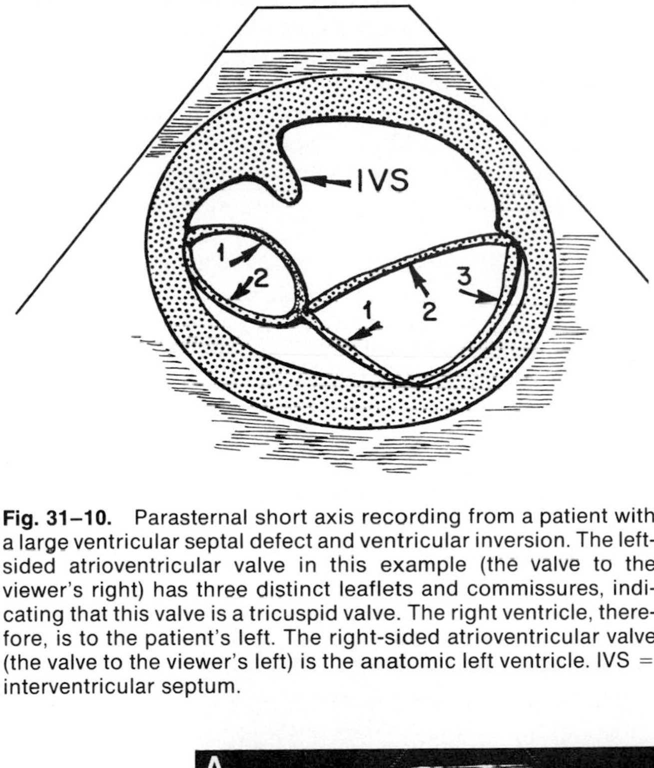

Fig. 31–10. Parasternal short axis recording from a patient with a large ventricular septal defect and ventricular inversion. The left-sided atrioventricular valve in this example (the valve to the viewer's right) has three distinct leaflets and commissures, indicating that this valve is a tricuspid valve. The right ventricle, therefore, is to the patient's left. The right-sided atrioventricular valve (the valve to the viewer's left) is the anatomic left ventricle. IVS = interventricular septum.

patient (Fig. 31–11A) and in a patient with ventricular inversion (Fig. 31–11B). The relative position of leaflet insertion is frequently easier to define than the number of valve leaflets and is not affected by a cleft mitral valve or alterations in expected leaflet number.[31] This highly specific sign is the most frequently used marker of ventricular morphology. The one situation in which the level of septal leaflet insertion cannot be used to define ventricular morphology is in patients with large perimembranous ventricular septal defects with absence of an extensive portion of the inlet septum. In these patients, both AV valve septal leaflets insert into the central fibrous body and thus lie at the same level. When the tricuspid valve inserts more than 10 mm inferior to the mitral valve, Ebstein's anomaly should be considered.

The third feature that allows one to differentiate between the morphologic right and left ventricles is the number and orientation of the papillary muscles associated with each chamber. The anatomic left ventricle usually has two papillary muscles of relatively equal size that arise from the medial and lateral free walls of the ventricle at the junction of the apical and middle thirds of the chamber. These muscles lie parallel to, and slightly below, the line of mitral leaflet coaptation. The right ventricle, in contrast, normally contains three papillary muscles that vary in size and site of origin. Figure 31–12 compares the two-papillary-muscle configuration of the anatomic left ventricle with the three papillary muscles that typify the anatomic right ventricle.

The fourth feature that distinguishes the anatomic right ventricle is the large muscular moderator band.[31] The moderator band is found only in the right ventricle, where it stretches from the lower interventricular septum to the anterior right ventricular wall, at which point it joins the base of the anterior papillary muscle. The moderator band, within an inverted right ventricle, can be appreciated in Figure 31–11B.

The final feature that characterizes the right ventricle is the pattern of chordal insertion. In patients with two discrete AV valves, the morphologic right ventricle has an inlet valve that has at least one chordal insertion to the interventricular septum, whereas the morphologic

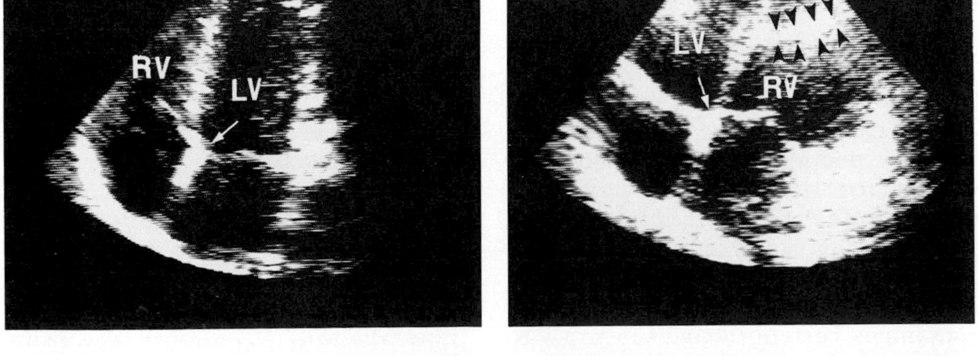

Fig. 31–11. **A.** Apical four-chamber view illustrates normal ventricular orientation. **B.** Ventricular inversion. Differentiation of the right (RV) and left ventricles (LV) can be achieved by determining the identity of the tricuspid and mitral valves. The septal leaflet of the tricuspid valve has an apical or inferior point of insertion into the ventricular septum, relative to the insertion point of the mitral valve. The superior insertion point of the mitral valve is indicated by the oblique arrow in **A.** When the ventricles are inverted, as in **B,** the mitral valve and anatomic left ventricle reverse their position, and the right-sided atrioventricular valve then has a relatively superior point of insertion into the interventricular septum, as indicated by the oblique arrow.

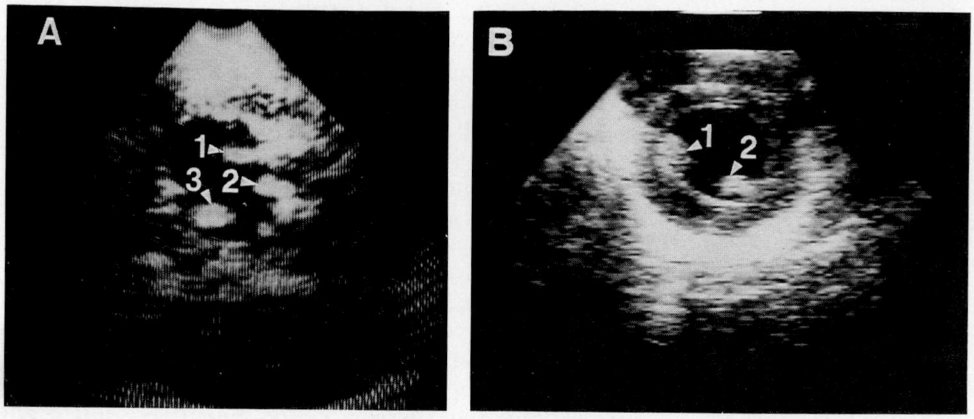

Fig. 31–12. **A.** Short axis scans illustrating the characteristic three-papillary-muscle configuration of the right ventricle. **B.** The same scan shows the two papillary muscles that typify the left ventricle.

left ventricle normally has chordae tendineae that insert into papillary muscles arising from the free wall.[29]

Although in individual cases one or more of these features may be absent, when considered together, they usually make it possible to define the morphologic ventricles confidently.

ATRIOVENTRICULAR CONNECTIONS

The third step in this sequential analysis is to determine the pattern of AV connection. AV connections are considered concordant when the morphologic right atrium connects to the morphologic right ventricle and the morphologic left atrium connects to the morphologic left ventricle. When the converse is true and the morphologic right atrium connects to the morphologic left ventricle while the morphologic left atrium connects to the morphologic right ventricle, AV discordance is present. When situs ambiguus is present, one AV relationship must be discordant.

AV discordance is seen most commonly in patients with physiologically corrected transposition. Other rare disorders characterized by AV discordance, include isolated atrial inversion, isolated ventricular inversion, and corrected malposition, all discussed later in this chapter.

GREAT VESSEL ORIENTATION AND IDENTITY

Are the Great Vessels Normally Related or Transposed?

The fourth step in evaluating a patient with complex congenital heart disease is to determine the orientation and identity of the great vessels. Customarily, great vessel orientation is defined first because, if the vessels are normally oriented, their identity can be presumed. Normally oriented vessels cross obliquely as they exit from the right and left ventricles. The right ventricular outflow tract lies anterior to the aorta and intersects it as approximately a 45° angle. After crossing the aorta, the outflow tract then curves posteriorly as the main pulmonary artery and continues posteriorly and superiorly to its point of bifurcation into the right and left pulmonary arteries. These normal relationships are best illustrated in the subcostal long axis view of the right ventricular outflow tract (Fig. 31–13). Because the great vessels normally cross at their origin, an imaging plane aligned parallel to the short axis of one great vessel is, of necessity, oblique to the short axis or more closely parallel to the long axis or the other crossing vessel.[32] The vessel that the imaging plane transects parallel to its short axis appears circular by definition, whereas the vessel that is transected obliquely appears as an elongated oval or has a more ''sausagelike'' shape.[32] Similarly, if the plane is oriented parallel to the long axis of one vessel, it must be oblique to the short axis of the other. Thus, as illustrated in Figure 31–13, a plane passing through the long axis of the right ventricular outflow tract and pulmonary artery is slightly oblique to the short axis of the aorta when these vessels cross normally.

When the great vessels are transposed, they maintain a parallel orientation as they leave the heart. When vessels are parallel, any plane oriented such that it passes through the short axis of one vessel must, of necessity, be parallel to the short axis of the second.[32] Both the aorta and pulmonary artery therefore appear circular in short axis when the vessels exit from the heart in parallel fashion.[32–35] Figure 31–14 illustrates this double-circle appearance of the transposed vessels in patients with D-transposition (Fig. 31–14A), L-transposition (Fig. 31–14B), and double-outlet right ventricle (Fig. 31–14C). Although the double circle configuration can be uniformly demonstrated in patients with transposi-

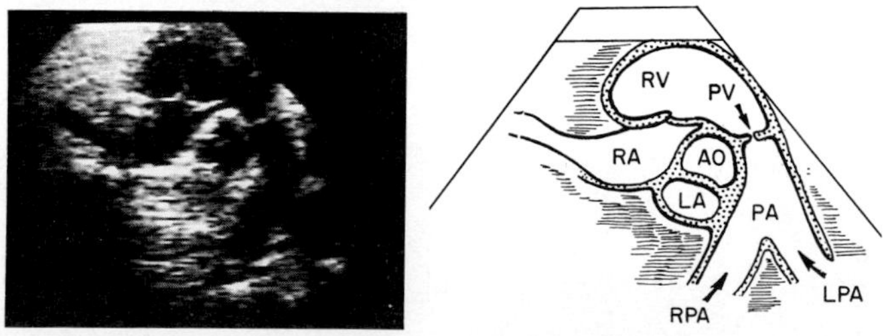

Fig. 31–13. Subcostal long axis recording of the right ventricular outflow tract illustrates the normal crossing pattern of the great vessels. The pulmonary artery (PA), viewed in the long axis, crosses the aorta (AO) and then sweeps posteriorly to its bifurcation into the left (LPA) and right pulmonary arteries (RPA). Because the vessels cross at their origin, the same plane transects the aorta oblique to its short axis, and this vessel appears roughly circular. RV = right ventricle; PV = pulmonary valve; RA = right atrium; LA = left atrium.

tion of the great vessels, a similar configuration can, on occasion, be produced in patients with normally crossing great vessels. Figure 31–15 illustrates two examples in which normally crossing great vessels are recorded such that they both appear circular. Figure 31–15A is a recording from a patient with primary pulmonary hypertension in whom the pulmonary artery is dilated and is significantly larger than the aorta. When the imaging plane was aligned parallel to the short axis of the pulmonary artery, a configuration looking much like D-transposition of the great vessels was produced. Figure 31–15B is a second example in which the short axis great vessel appearance is similar to that of L-transposition. In this example, the origin of the great vessels was also normal, and the vessel anterior and to the left is the pulmonary artery. When the examination is easily performed and the pulmonary artery and aorta are readily identified, these patterns cause little confusion. In limited examinations, however, they may lead to incorrect diagnoses. In such situations, the observation that the anterior vessel is the pulmonary artery makes the presence of one of the transposition complexes unlikely. When the great vessels have a directly anteroposterior relationship, the term A-transposition has been used.

The final great vessel pattern is produced by the truncus arteriosus. When a truncus is present, orientation of the short axis imaging plane through the base of the ventricle results in the display of a single, large, circular vessel. Figure 31–16 illustrates the appearance of the truncus arteriosus in both the long axis and parasternal short axis views.

Figure 31–17 summarizes the different short axis configurations of the great vessels. In the left-hand panel,

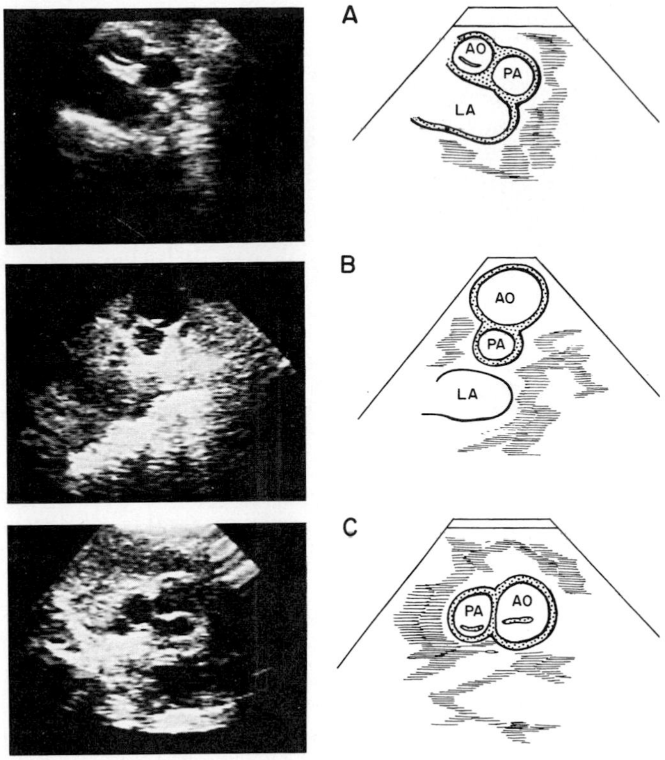

Fig. 31–14. These parasternal short axis recordings illustrate the typical double circle appearance of the great vessels when they leave the heart parallel to one another. **A.** A recording from a patient with D-transposition of the great vessels in which the anterior aorta is positioned to the patient's right. **B.** An L-transposition in which the anterior aorta is to the patient's left. **C.** A double-outlet right ventricle in which the two great vessels lie side by side. AO = aorta; PA = pulmonary artery; LA = left atrium.

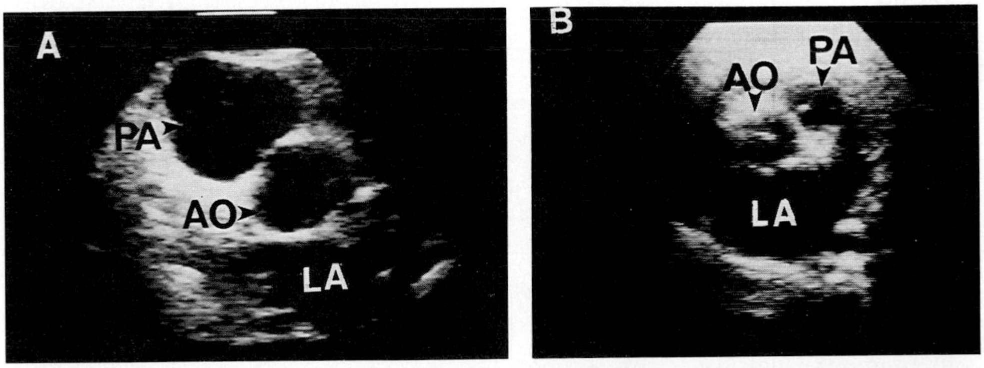

Fig. 31–15. Two cases in which normal-crossing great vessels show a double circle configuration that might be confused for transposition. **A.** The anterior vessel is positioned to the patient's right and simulates D-transposition. **B.** The anterior vessel is to the left, simulating an L-transposition. In each case, however, the anterior vessel is the pulmonary artery (PA), which makes the diagnosis of transposition highly unlikely. AO = aorta; LA = left atrium.

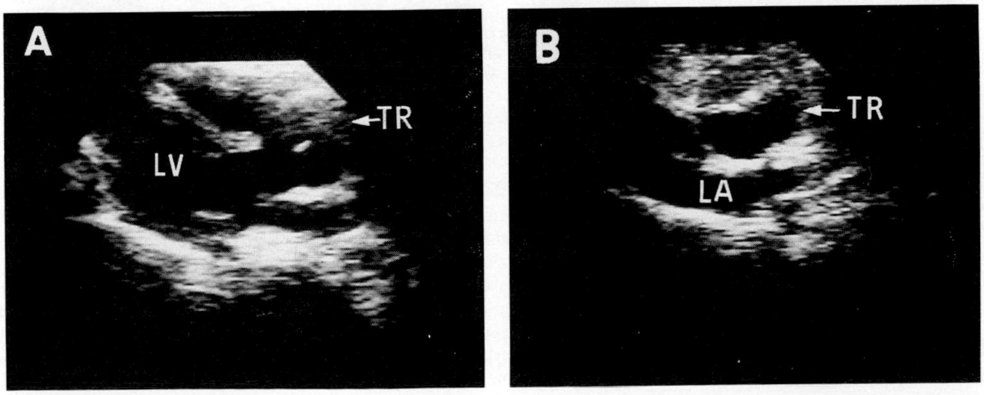

Fig. 31–16. A. Parasternal long axis view of a patient with truncus arteriosus (TR). A single, large vessel overrides a large ventricular septal defect. **B.** Parasternal short axis view of the same patient. The vessel appears as a single large circle without evidence of either a second parallel vessel or an anterior crossing vessel. LA = left atrium; LV = left ventricle.

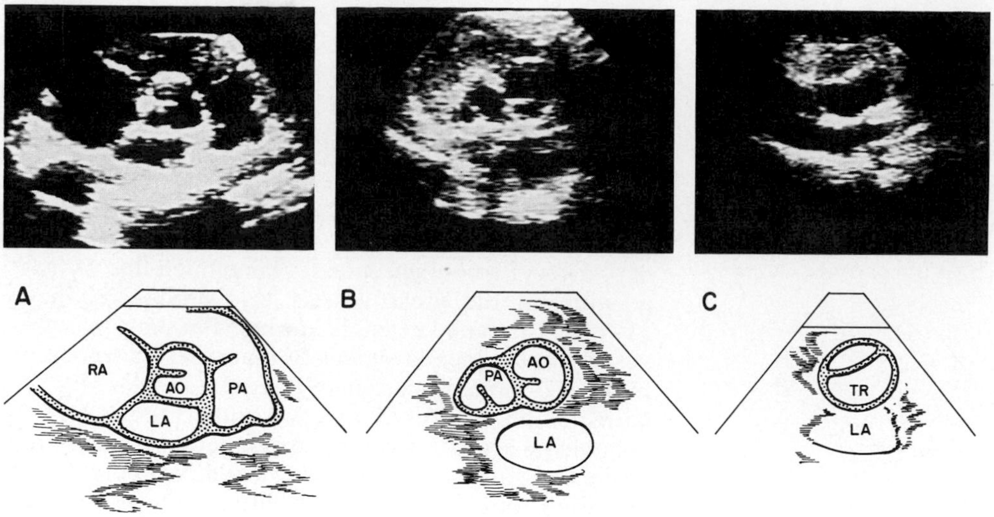

Fig. 31–17. Parasternal short axis recordings summarize the primary great vessel orientation. **A.** Normal crossing pattern. The aorta (AO) appears as a single circle, and the cylindric pulmonary artery (PA) courses above and to the right of the aortic root. **B.** Transposed great vessels in which both the AO and the PA are transected parallel to their short axes and, therefore, appear circular. **C.** The single large circle that characterizes the truncus arteriosus (TR). LA = left atrium; RA = right atrium.

the normally crossing vessels are oriented such that when the imaging plane is aligned parallel to the short axis of the aorta, it must be oblique to the short axis of the pulmonary artery or must more closely approximate its long axis. The aorta therefore appears circular, whereas the pulmonary artery looks like an oval or curved cylinder crossing anteriorly above the aorta. The center panel depicts the configuration observed when the great vessels exit the heart in a parallel or transposed orientation. Here, the imaging plane is parallel to the short axis of both the aorta and the pulmonary artery, and thus, they both appear circular. Finally, the right-hand panel illustrates the single large circular vessel characteristic of the truncus arteriosus.[32]

When the examining plane can be passed directly through the long axes of both great vessels, their parallel orientation can be directly defined. Figure 31–18 illustrates this parallel orientation in both the parasternal long axis (Fig. 31–18A) and subcostal long axis (Fig. 31–18B) views. In Figure 31–18A, one sees a large anterior aorta and a slightly smaller posterior pulmonary artery. The aorta originates from the anterior ventricular chamber and the pulmonary artery from the posterior chamber. The larger aorta courses more superiorly into the neck and, by varying the imaging plane, can be observed to give rise to the neck vessels. The smaller posterior vessel appears to terminate more quickly and, by following its branching pattern in short axis, could be identified as the pulmonary artery. Figure 31–18B is an example of a double-outlet right ventricle with an L-loop in which both great vessels exit from the left-sided ventricle, which is the anatomic right ventricle. Here, again, the parallel orientation of the great vessels (with the two semilunar valves positioned at an identical level) confirms that the great vessels are transposed.

If Two Great Vessels Are Visible, Which Is the Aorta and Which Is the Pulmonary Artery?

Once the relationship of the great vessels has been defined, the examiner must then determine which is the aorta and which is the pulmonary artery. When the great vessels cross at their origin, the anterior vessel is always the pulmonary artery and the posterior vessel is always the aorta. When the great vessels are transposed and one vessel is anterior to the other, the anterior vessel is almost invariably the aorta, and the posterior vessel, the pulmonary artery. When the great vessels lie beside one another, as illustrated in Figure 31–19A, identification of the aorta and pulmonary artery may be more difficult. When there is a question, the great vessels can be identified by following their course superiorly and observing their branching patterns and distribution.[36] The vessel that courses posteriorly into the thorax and bifurcates is always the pulmonary artery, whereas the vessel that courses into the neck and gives off multiple branches to the upper extremities is always the aorta.[36]

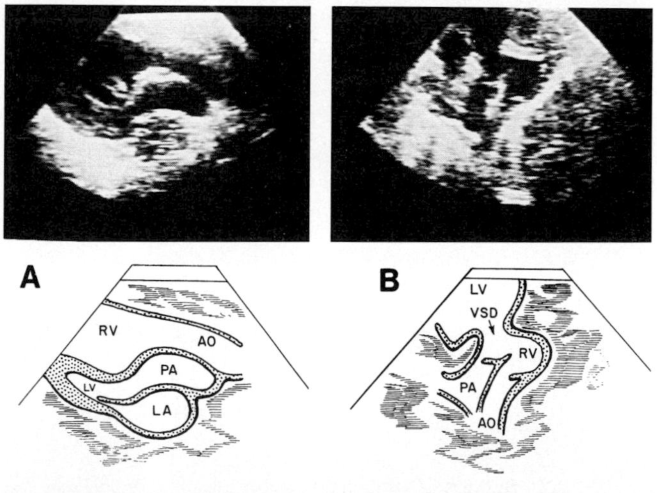

Fig. 31–18. Parasternal **(A)** and subcostal long axis **(B)** views of parallel transposed great vessels recorded with the scan plane simultaneously directed through the long axis of both vessels. **A.** D-transposition with an anterior aorta (AO) and posterior parallel pulmonary artery (PA). **B.** Double outlet right ventricle (RV) and ventricular inversion again illustrate the parallel orientation of the two great vessels as they exit from the left-sided cardiac chamber. LV = left ventricle; LA = left atrium; VSD - ventricular septal defect.

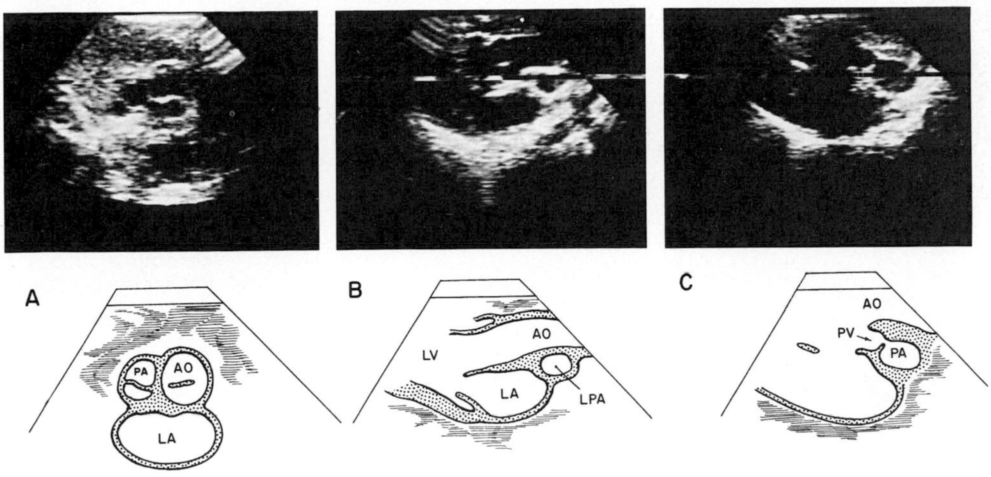

Fig. 31–19. **A.** Short axis recording of transposed, side-by-side vessels. **B.** Long axis recording demonstrates that the larger vessel courses anteriorly and superiorly toward the neck and, therefore, is the aorta (AO). This conclusion can further be confirmed by the presence of the left pulmonary artery (LPA) sweeping beneath this anterior vessel. **C.** Long axis scan of the smaller vessel, which angles posteriorly and bifurcates, thereby indicating that it is the pulmonary artery (PA). Systolic doming of the pulmonary valve (PV) and associated supravalvular narrowing are apparent. LV = left ventricle; LA = left atrium.

Figure 31–19B and C illustrates the characteristic features of the aorta and pulmonary artery in the parasternal long axis view. In Figure 31–19B, the larger of the two transposed vessels can be observed to curve anteriorly and to continue toward the neck. If the scan is continued superiorly, branches to the upper extremities can be identified. The anterior path and superior extension of this vessel suggest that it is the aorta. In addition, the left pulmonary artery can be visualized just superior to the left atrium, crossing beneath the larger aorta. In Figure 31–19C, the scan plane has been aligned parallel to the long axis of the smaller vessel. At its origin, there is stenosis of the semilunar valve and an additional area of supravalvular narrowing. Distal to the area of stenosis, the vessel dilates transiently and then appears to end abruptly. This apparent point of vessel termination actually represents the bifurcation of a pulmonary artery and illustrates a second general rule: when the scan plane is aligned such that it follows the long axis of transposed great vessels superiorly, the vessel that appears to end first is the pulmonary artery.

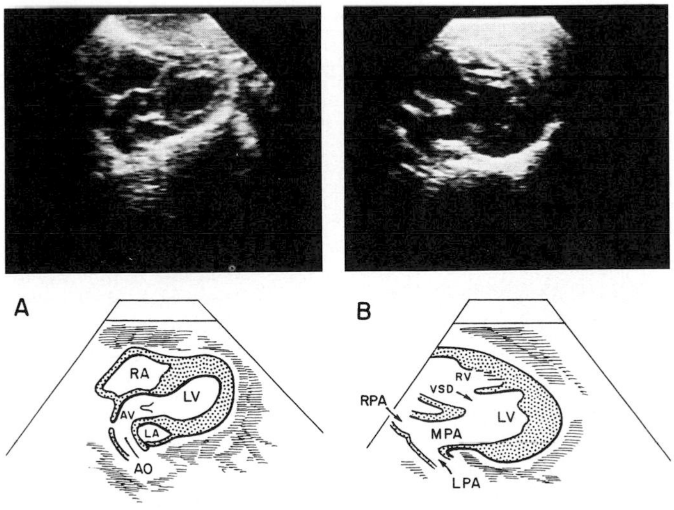

Fig. 31–20. Subcostal long axis recordings illustrate how the course and branching patterns of the aorta and pulmonary artery can be used to identify these vessels. **A.** The aorta (AO) arises normally from the left ventricle (LV) and then sweeps to the left, giving off smaller branches to the neck. **B.** Unlike the aorta, a transposed pulmonary artery courses directly superiorly and bifurcates into two branches of equal size. RPA = right pulmonary artery; LPA = left pulmonary artery; AV = aortic valve; LA = left atrium; RA = right atrium; MPA = main pulmonary artery; VSD = ventricular septal defect; RV = right ventricle.

The course and branching pattern of the great vessels can frequently be better visualized from the subcostal transducer location than from the anterior chest wall. Figure 31–20 contrasts the appearance of a normal aortic arch arising from the left-sided ventricle (Fig. 31–20A) with that of a left-sided or transposed pulmonary artery in a patient with D-transposition of the great vessels (Fig. 31–20B). The normal aorta courses leftward in a gradual arc after leaving the left-sided ventricle and gives off several small branches to the upper extremities. The pulmonary artery (Fig. 31–20B), in contrast, follows a straighter path and bifurcates after several centimeters into two large vessels of approximately equal size.

VENTRICULAR-GREAT VESSEL RELATIONSHIPS—HOW ARE THE GREAT VESSELS AND VENTRICLES CONNECTED?

The fifth step in approaching the patient with complex congenital heart disease is to define the interrelationship of the ventricles and the great vessels. The relationship of the great vessels with the ventricular chambers is defined relative to the plane of the interventricular septum. The two general methods for determining the relationship of the great vessels with the septal plane are: the short axis approach, in which the short axis orientation of the septum and great vessels relative to the transducer are compared;[37] and the long axis method, in which the scan plane is simultaneously directed through the long axes of both great vessels and the septum. In the short axis approach, the short axis plane of the interventricular septum is first defined. Without changing the orientation of the scan plane, the transducer is then angled superiorly to determine the spatial orientation of the great vessels. The relationship of the great vessels with the septal plane can then be determined by marking the plane of the septum on the video screen,[37] superimposing photographic outlines of the septum and great vessels, or simply scanning rapidly back and forth from one area to the other to visually establish their relative positions.

Figure 31–21 compares the most common septal-great vessel relationships. Figure 31–21A depicts the normal pattern in which the great vessels cross at their origin, and the plane of the septum. In Figure 31–21B (tetralogy of Fallot), the great vessels cross normally at their origin, and the pulmonary artery is above the aorta. Because of aortic overriding, the septal plane lies well below the anterior margin of the aorta. Figure 31–21C, the double-outlet right ventricle, the great vessels are

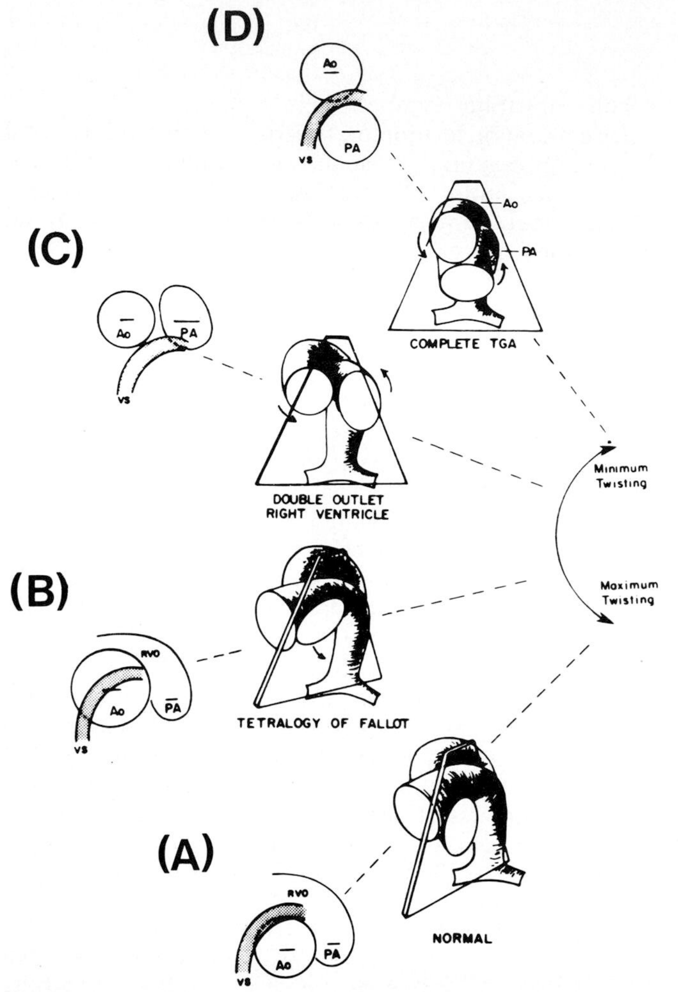

Fig. 31–21. The relationship of the great vessels to the short axis plane of the interventricular septum in the more common complex congenital anomalies. **A.** The normal pattern. The great vessels cross at their origin, and the septal plane is at roughly the same level as the anterior margin of the aorta. **B.** In tetralogy of Fallot, aortic overriding occurs, and the anterior margin of the aortic root is displaced above the plane of the septum. **C.** The double-outlet right ventricle in which the aorta and pulmonary artery are parallel and rise above the septal plane. **D.** In D-transposition of the great vessels, both vessels appear circular because they leave the heart parallel to one another. The septal plane is below the anterior aorta and above the posterior pulmonary artery. Ao = aorta; PA = pulmonary artery; TGA = transposition of the great arteries; RVO = right ventricular outflow tract. (From Henry WL, et al.: Cross-sectional echocardiography in the diagnosis of congenital heart disease. Circulation 56:267, 1977. Reproduced with permission of the American Heart Association, Inc.)

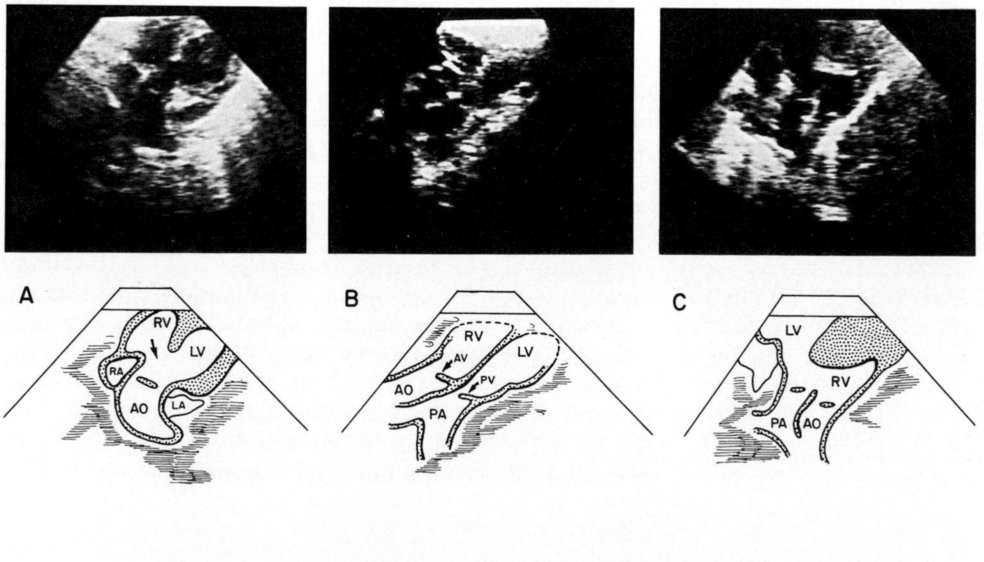

Fig. 31–22. The relationship of the great vessels to the interventricular septum can be directly visualized in long axis. **A.** A recording from a patient with pulmonary atresia where the large aorta (AO) overrides the plane of the interventricular septum. **B.** D-transposition in which the great vessels are parallel as they leave the right (RV) and left (LV) ventricles and originate from opposite sides of the interventricular septum. **C.** A recording from a patient with double-outlet right ventricle and ventricular inversion where both great vessels arise from the left-sided chamber or from the left of the septal plane. RA = right atrium; LA = left atrium; AV = aortic valve; PV = pulmonary valve.

transposed; consequently, both appear circular in short axis and both originate from the right ventricle, anterior and to the right of the plane of the interventricular septum. The final example (Fig. 31–21D) illustrates the relationship of the great arteries with the septum in D-transposition. Here, again, the great vessels appear circular in short axis because they are transposed. The aorta in D-transposition is anterior to the plane of the interventricular septum, and the pulmonary artery is posterior to the septal plane.

In the long axis method, the scan plane is oriented such that it passes through the long axis of the great vessels and interventricular septum simultaneously and thereby permits direct visualization of their relationship. Figure 31–22 illustrates three examples, recorded in the subcostal long axis view, in which the relation of the great vessels to the interventricular septum can be directly appreciated. In Figure 31–22A, a single, large vessel straddles the plane of the septum at its origin and curves superiorly and leftward into the neck, thereby indicating that this vessel is the aorta. No pulmonary artery is evident. This example, which illustrates aortic overriding, was obtained from a patient with pulmonary atresia. In Figure 31–22B, both great vessels are parallel as they leave the ventricles and therefore are transposed. The left-sided great vessel, which bifurcates in this example, is the pulmonary artery and arises totally to the left of the interventricular septum. The right-sided aorta, in contrast, originates from the right-sided ventricle. The septum is intact, and because the aorta is to the patient's right and the vessels are transposed, this pattern must represent D-transposition. In the final example (Figure 31–22C), both great vessels again are parallel or transposed and both arise from the left-sided ventricular chamber. A defect in the interventricular septum is present, but both vessels are clearly positioned to the left of the septal plane. In this example, the ventricles are also inverted and therefore represent an example of a double-outlet right ventricle with an L-loop. Simultaneous visualization of the great vessels and of the septum obviously is the preferred method for determining the pattern by which they are connected. When a vessel overrides the plane of the interventricular septum, the rule of 50% again applies, and if more than 50% of the area of the vessel lies above the ventricle, it is considered to arise from that ventricle.

PRESENCE AND LOCATION OF INTRACARDIAC SHUNTS—ARE ANY INTRACARDIAC SHUNTS PRESENT, AND WHAT IS THE DIRECTION OF SHUNT FLOW?

The sixth step in the evaluation of the patient with complex congenital heart disease is to determine whether any intracardiac shunts are present, and if so, to determine their location and the direction of the shunt flow. Intracardiac shunts occur when a defect is present in one of the walls of the heart or great vessels that separate the left and right sides of the circulation or when an arteriovenous communication bypasses the pulmonary or myocardial capillary beds. The most common and best-studied intracardiac shunts are those associated with defects in the atrial or ventricular septa (see Chapter 29) and persistence of the ductus arteriosus (see Chapter 27). The presence of an intracardiac shunt is initially suggested during the imaging examination by enlargement of the chambers receiving the increased, shunt-related flow. In patients with an atrial septal defect, the right atrium, right ventricle, and pulmonary artery are typically dilated, whereas in patients with a ventricular septal defect or patent ductus arteriosus, the left atrium, left ventricle, and pulmonary artery receive the increased volume. Note that uncomplicated ventricular septal defect is not associated with right ventricular volume overload because there is no increase in right ventricular diastolic volume.

Direct demonstration of an atrial or ventricular septal defect is based on the visualization of an interruption in the normal continuous septal barrier. When the margins of the defect are perpendicular to the path of the sound beam, they are often highlighted because of the point spread function of the imaging system. The ductal communication between the pulmonary artery and the aorta can also be recorded in some patients (predominantly in infants), but this finding is inconsistent. Large defects and those associated with major structural distortion or with malalignment are easily diagnosed from the image alone. Because the diagnosis of smaller defects depends on the absence of echoes arising from a particular region of the heart, false-positive results are frequent. In these cases, confirmation of the presence of a defect requires the demonstration of abnormal shunt flow through the area of echo-dropout. Similarly, exclusion of a false-positive result may require that septal integrity be confirmed by an independent method. Furthermore, when a defect is recorded, it is usually not possible to determine the direction or volume of shunt flow from the image alone. This section therefore is concerned with the documentation of the presence and direction of abnormal blood flow through these apparent defects.

The presence and direction of abnormal blood flow through a defect in the interatrial or interventricular septum or persistence of the ductus arteriosus can usually be demonstrated by the use of color flow mapping techniques, conventional pulsed and continuous wave Doppler, and echocardiographic contrast. Color flow mapping permits direct visualization of abnormal shunt flow crossing a suspected defect and in many cases can call attention to a small defect that may have been initially inapparent on a routine imaging study. In patients with atrial septal defect, the area of the color flow jet has been reported to have a rough correlation with shunt flow, and the diameter of the jet as it traverses the defect has been shown to correlate closely with the diameter of the defect measured at surgery.

Pulsed Doppler recordings may be useful in timing the shunt-related flow and in separating shunt flow from complex normal flow streams in chambers such as the right atrium. In low velocity shunts (i.e., those whose velocity does not exceed the Nyquist limit), pulsed Doppler can also be used to determine the gradient across the defect (using the modified Bernoulli equation: $\Delta P = 4v^2$) and hence the pressure difference between the chambers feeding and receiving the shunt. When the shunt velocity is high, as in a ventricular septal defect with normal right-sided pressures or across a patent ductus arteriosus, continuous wave Doppler recordings are required to resolve flow velocities accurately.

Despite the variety of Doppler techniques available to record shunt flow, echo-contrast remains a valuable tool in shunt detection. Echo-contrast is particularly useful when Doppler sensitivity is poor, shunt velocity is low and difficult to record, or shunt flow is small and cannot be distinguished from surrounding flow streams. In patients with an atrial septal defect, contrast has been reported to be more sensitive than color Doppler, particularly in patients with small shunts and those with a patent foramen ovale. The echocardiographic contrast effect is the result of multiple intense reflections arising from microbubbles that are included with or develop during the injection of a variety of media into the vascular stream (see Chapter 15). The gaseous material within these microbubbles is a strong, omnidirectional, ultrasonic reflector, and the reflections arising from these microbubbles can be used to follow their path and, by inference, to follow the path of the blood with which the bubbles mix as it passes through the heart.[38–41] Contrast-producing agents can be injected into a peripheral vein or directly into the heart through a catheter. When the contrast material is injected peripherally, the microbubbles normally follow the path of blood flow into the right atrium and then continue through the tricuspid valve into the right ventricle and then into the pulmonary artery.

Figure 31–23 is a short axis scan at the aortic root level that illustrates the normal pattern of contrast flow through the right side of the heart. Figure 31–23A is recorded before peripheral vein contrast injection and illustrates the normal, relatively echo-free appearance of the blood pool within each cardiac chamber. After the injection of indocyanine green (Cardio-Green) dye (Figure 31–23B), multiple bright echoes fill the right atrium and right ventricular outflow tract. These echoes are recorded as the contrast medium flows through the right side of the circulation. The aorta and left atrium, in this example, are echo free because the microbubbles producing the contrast effect are too large to pass through the pulmonary capillary bed and consequently are trapped at this level.

The pattern of contrast flow in patients with intracardiac shunts varies depending on the location and the direction of the shunt. When the patient has a right-to-left shunt at either the atrial or the ventricular level, a portion of the peripherally injected contrast medium travels with the shunted blood and appears on the left side of the heart in the chamber into which the shunt empties.[40–42] When the right-to-left shunt is at the atrial level, contrast is initially visualized in the left atrium and then flows through the mitral valve into the left ventricle. When the right-to-left shunt is at the ventricular level, contrast initially appears in the left ventricle, and no contrast is evident in either the left atrium or the mitral valve orifice (see also Chapter 15).

Figure 31–24 illustrates the patterns of contrast flow through a defect in the interatrial septum. Figure 31–24A illustrates the preinjection appearance of the right and left atria and the atrial septal defect (vertical arrow). In Figure 31–24B, recorded immediately following contrast injection, one sees opacification of both the right and left atria because of contrast flow through the defect. In this example, contrast medium was injected into the left atrium, and flow was from left to right. A similar pattern would have been observed if a right-to-left shunt had been present and contrast medium had been injected into the right side of the circulation. Detection of contrast on the left side of the heart after right-sided injection is highly specific for a right-to-left shunt, and when this pattern of contrast flow is evident, no further study is necessary to confirm the presence of the shunt.[41–45]

Detecting a predominant left-to-right shunt using the echocardiographic contrast method may prove more difficult. Left-to-right shunts may be detected in two ways. In patients with a predominant left-to-right shunt with a small right-to-left component, some passage of contrast across the plane of the atrial or ventricular septum may be observed during the period of right-to-left

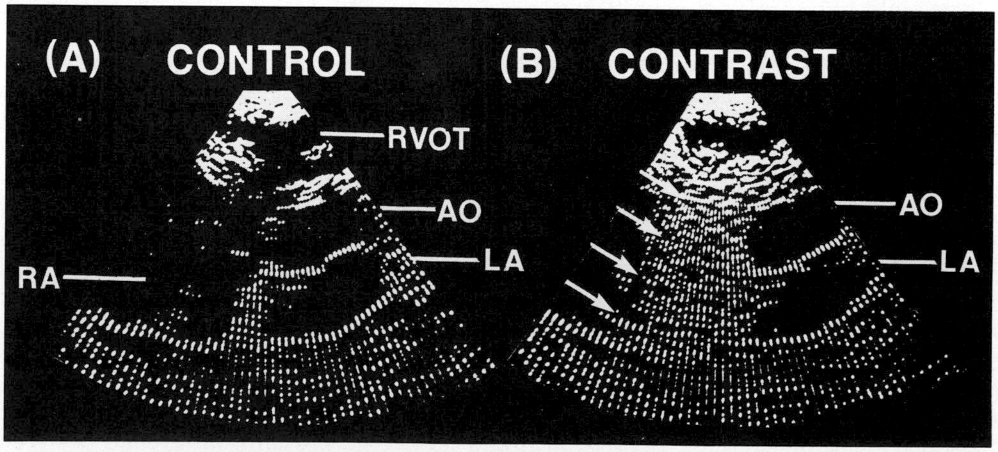

Fig. 31–23. Parasternal short axis recordings of the left (LA) and right atria (RA). **A.** Before peripheral contrast injection. **B.** After injection. The contrast (horizontal arrows in **B**) creates a dense cloud of echoes that completely opacifies the RA and right ventricular outflow tract (RVOT) as they pass through the right heart. The aorta (AO) and LA remain echo-free because the microbubbles are filtered out in the pulmonary capillary bed and do not cross to the left side of the heart. (From Weyman AE, et al.: Negative contrast echocardiography: a new method for detecting left-to-right shunts. Circulation 59: 498, 1979. Reproduced by permission of the American Heart Association, Inc.)

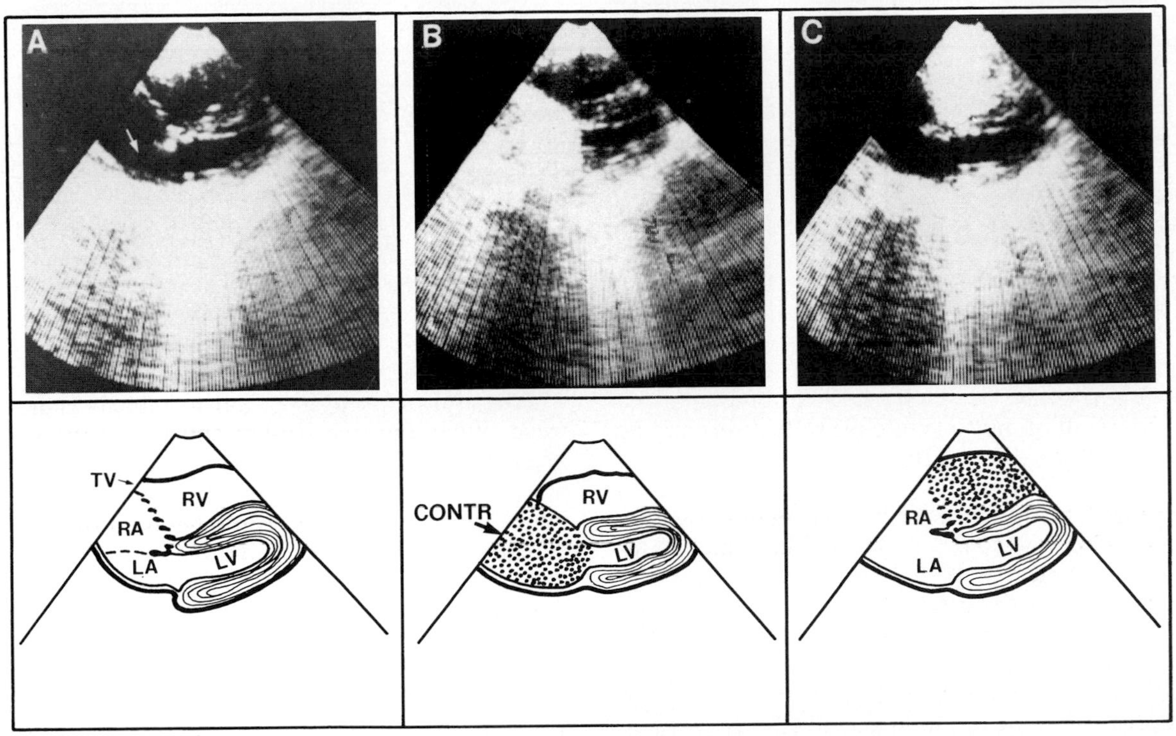

Fig. 31–24. Subcostal long axis recordings illustrate the patterns of contrast flow through the left and right atria in a patient with an atrial septal defect and predominant left-to-right shunting. **A.** The defect is indicated by the vertical arrow. **B.** Contrast medium has been injected into the left atrium and flows from left to right through the defect, indicating the presence of a left-to-right shunt. Contrast flow in the opposite direction is observed when contrast is injected into the right atrium and the patient has a right-to-left shunt. **C.** Contrast medium has been injected peripherally, and a cloud of bubbles can be seen in the right ventricle but not in the right atrium. The contrast is displaced from the right atrial side of the interatrial septum by non-contrast-containing blood that flows from left to right through the defect, thereby producing an area of negative contrast. TV = tricuspid valve; RV = right ventricle; RA = right atrium; LA = left atrium; LV = left ventricle. (From Weyman AE, et al.: Negative contrast echocardiography: a new method for detecting left-to-right shunts. Circulation, 59:498, 1979. Reproduced by permission of the American Heart Association, Inc.)

shunting.[44,45] Alternatively, when no right-to-left shunting is apparent, a left-to-right shunt can still be inferred from the area of "negative contrast," which occurs when non-contrast-containing blood passing from left to right through the septal defect displaces the contrast-containing blood from the right side of the lesion.[46,47]

Figure 31–24C is an example of this negative contrast phenomenon. This recording was obtained following peripheral injection of contrast material and demonstrates a large accumulation of contrast within the right ventricular cavity. One sees no contrast, however, within the right atrium to the right of the atrial septal defect. This occurs because the contrast-containing blood entering the atrium from the SVC is displaced above and below the level of the atrial septal defect. The atrium to the immediate right of the defect therefore appears free of contrast because flow into this area is predominantly composed of non-contrast-containing blood entering the right atrium through the atrial septal defect.

When a catheter is already present in the peripheral venous system or within the heart, use of contrast is further facilitated. On occasion, a catheter is placed fortuitously such that a shunt can be detected directly. Figure 31–25A is a recording from a young infant with an atrial septal defect who has left-to-right shunting at the atrial level. In this example, an umbilical vein catheter has inadvertently been passed through the right atrium and the atrial septal defect and lies along the superior border of the left atrium. In Figure 31–25B, recorded while the catheter was being flushed, a stream of bubbles flows from the tip of the catheter through the atrial septal defect into the right atrium. This pattern of contrast flow confirms the presence of the atrial septal defect and indicates that predominant shunting is from left to right. Combining both direct visualization of defects in the interatrial and interventricular septum and an assessment of the pattern, location, and direction of shunt flow, as evidenced by the pattern of Doppler or contrast flow through and around these lesions, should represent an accurate and minimally invasive method for determining the direction, location, and volume of intracardiac shunting in patients with complex congenital disease.

Contrast can also be used more simply to confirm or to exclude a defect in patients with "echo-dropout" in the interatrial or interventricular septum. Figure 31–26A illustrates an example in which echoes could not be recorded from a portion of the interatrial septum, thereby simulating an atrial septal defect. Following peripheral contrast injection (Fig. 31–26B), the right atrium is completely opacified, and the separation between right and left atria is clearly demonstrated. The separation of the contrast within the right atrium and the echo-free blood of the left atrium confirms the integ-

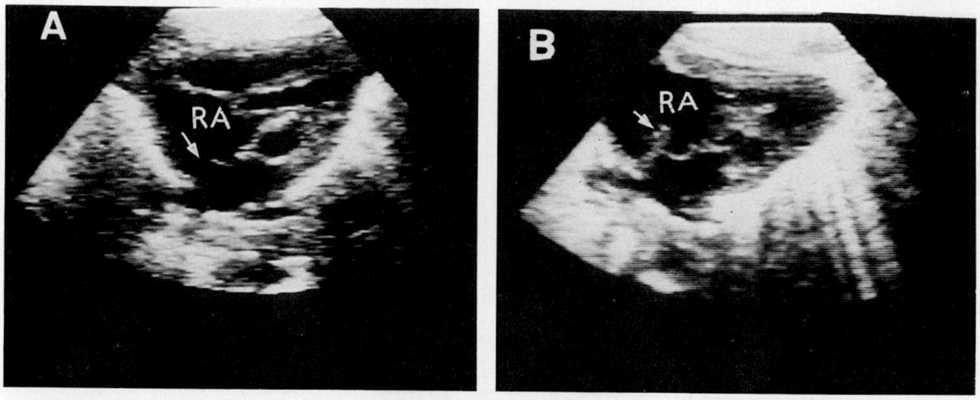

Fig. 31–25. Subcostal long axis recording obtained from a patient with a hypoplastic left ventricle and an atrial septal defect (vertical arrow). **A.** An umbilical vein catheter has been passed through the defect and lies along the superior wall of the left atrium. **B.** As the catheter is flushed, a stream of bubbles flows from the tip of the catheter back through the defect from the left atrium to the right (RA). This pattern of contrast flow serves to confirm the presence of the defect and indicates that the direction of the shunt is from left to right.

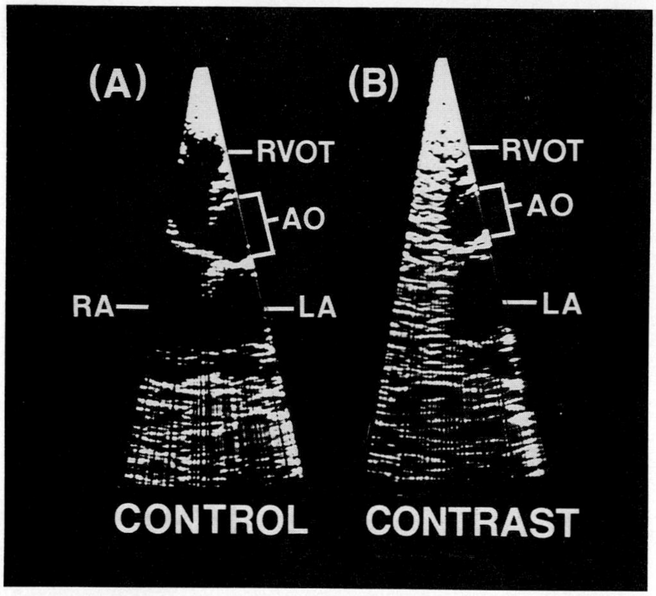

Fig. 31–26. Parasternal short axis recordings of the right (RA) and left atria (LA) obtained before and after peripheral contrast injection. **A.** Recorded before contrast injection, an apparent defect in the interatrial septum is noted. **B.** Following contrast injection, the atrium is homogeneously opacified, and the contrast pool outlines the position of the interatrial septum even though the septum itself cannot be visualized. No contrast flows from right to left, and displacement of contrast from the right side of the apparent defect does not occur. Contrast, therefore, can be used to confirm the integrity of the septum, even when the membrane itself cannot be visualized. AO = aorta; RVOT = right ventricular outflow tract. (From Weyman AE, et al.: Negative contrast echocardiography: a new method for detecting left-to-right shunts. Circulation 59:498, 1979. Reproduced by permission of the American Heart Association, Inc.)

rity of the septum even though the membrane itself cannot be visualized.

Figure 31–27 contains a series of apical four-chamber recordings that summarize the primary methods used for shunt detection in patients with complex congenital heart disease. In Figure 31–27A, one notes a defect in the atrial septum that is suggestive of an ostium primum atrial septal defect. Figure 31–27B is a color flow recording illustrating a large left-to-right shunt crossing the area of echo-dropout and confirming the presence and size of the defect and the predominant direction of shunt flow. Figure 31–27C is a peripheral contrast injection. In this frame, a small portion of the contrast bolus can be observed crossing the defect from right to left. Figure 31–27D illustrates the negative contrast effect produced by the large left-to-right shunt that corresponds both in size and location to the color jet recorded in Figure 31–27B.

LOCATION AND PRESENCE OF OUTFLOW OBSTRUCTION

The final step in evaluation of the patient with complex congenital heart disease is to determine the presence and location of left or right ventricular outflow obstruction. The general appearance of individual obstructive lesions in patients with complex congenital disease is similar to that observed in patients with isolated lesions. In patients with complex disease, however, the degree of outflow tract deformity tends to be more marked, and obstruction at multiple levels is common. Further, when the great vessels are transposed or malpositioned, the location of obstructing lesions may be far removed from that which might be expected if the great vessels were normally oriented. Figure 31–28, for example, illustrates a complex type of left ventricular outflow obstruction in which one sees an elongated area of subvalvular narrowing consistent with a subvalvular tunnel and an extensive area of aortic annular hypoplasia. Distal to this prolonged area of obstruction, the aorta begins to dilate to a more normal diameter. Marked left ventricular hypertrophy is also present, and the left atrium is dilated. Figure 31–29A to F, compares the normal parasternal long axis appearance of the left ventricular outflow tract with the severely deformed hypoplastic outflow tract of a patient with normally oriented great vessels and aortic hypoplasia. In the hypoplastic aorta, diffuse outflow tract narrowing begins in the subvalvular region and continues superiorly into the aortic arch. The aortic valve is deformed, and a valvular motion is restricted. Figure 31–29D and E compare the appearance of the normal aortic arch with this hypoplastic aortic arch in the subcostal long axis view. Again, obstruction involving the entire sweep of the vessels can be appreciated. When the great vessels are transposed, similar pat-

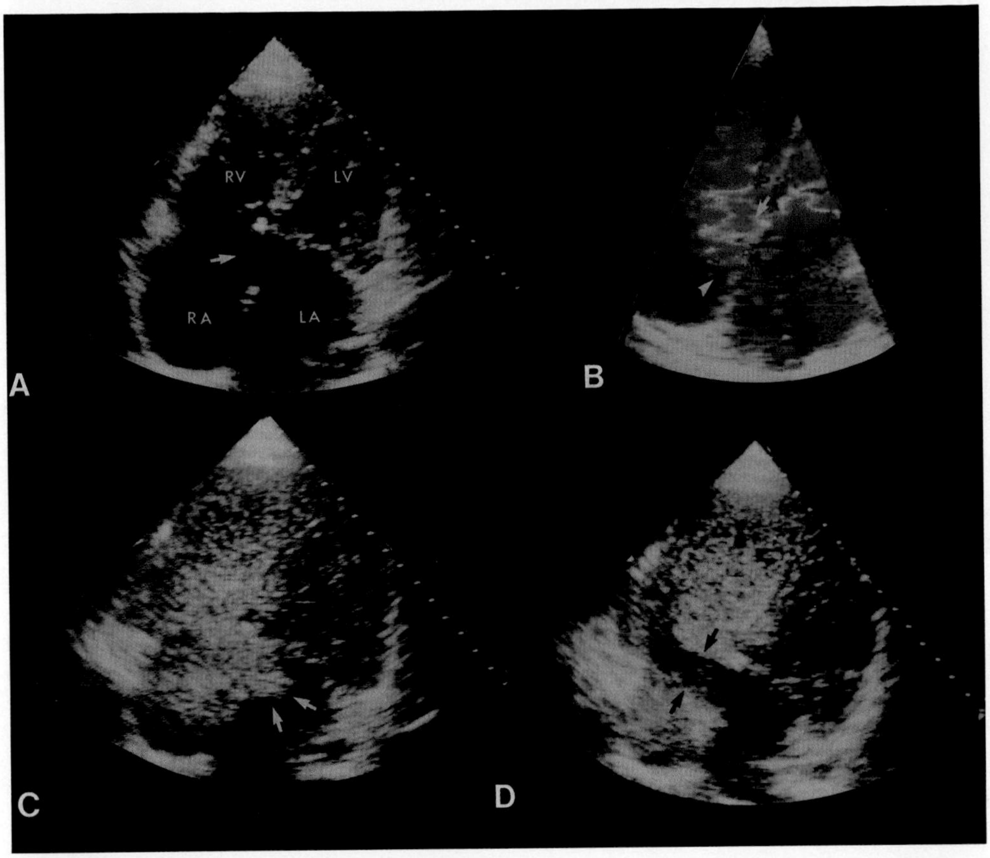

Fig. 31–27. Series of apical four-chamber views illustrating the methods of shunt detection in a patient with an ostium primum atrial septal defect. **A.** The defect (arrow) is directly visualized. **B.** Color Doppler recording demonstrating the left-to-right shunt flow (red) traversing the defect (arrows) and entering the right atrium and ventricle. **C** and **D.** Recorded after peripheral injection of a bolus of echocontrast. **C.** A portion of the contrast bolus passes from right to left in the left atrium (arrows) and ventricle, indicating a right-to-left component to the shunt. **D.** During peak left-to-right shunt flow, a bolus of non-contrast-containing blood passes through the defect from left to right, creating an area of negative contrast, which corresponds to the area of shunt flow indicated in the color flow Doppler recording. (From Levine RA, et al.: Echocardiography: principles and clinical applications. In Eagle KA, Haber E, DeSanctis RW, Austen GA (eds.): The Practice of Cardiology. Boston, Little, Brown and Company, 1989.)

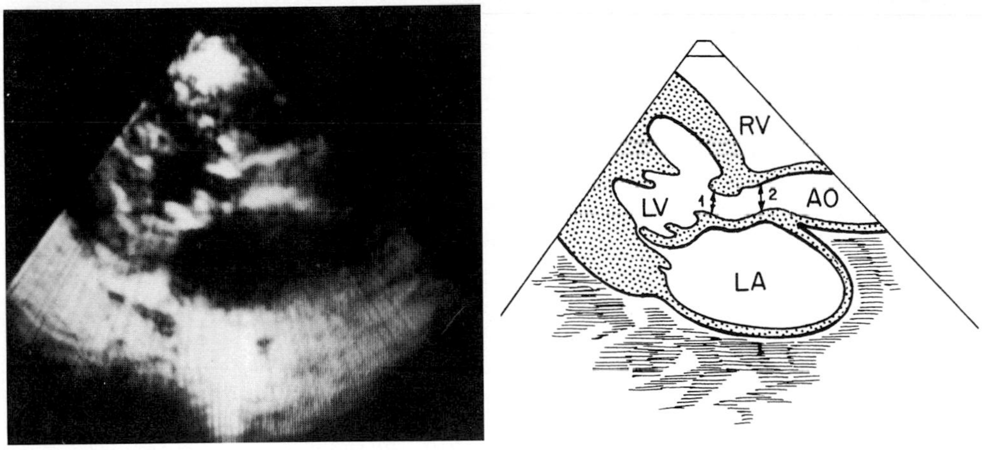

Fig. 31–28. Parasternal long axis recording of the left ventricular outflow tract illustrates subvalvular aortic stenosis and aortic root hypoplasia. The two areas of maximal narrowing are indicated by the vertical arrows in the accompanying diagram. RV = right ventricle; LV = left ventricle; AO = aorta; LA = left atrium.

terns of outflow obstruction can be appreciated. Figure 31–30, for example, illustrates a small pulmonary artery with narrowing at the annulus, doming of the pulmonary valve indicating stenosis at the valvular level, and a decrease in vascular size distal to the area of valvular stenosis in a patient with D-transposition of the great vessels. The individual components of these complicated outflow lesions are not greatly dissimilar to those of isolated obstruction at each level; however, their appearance in groups or in series is more characteristic of the complicated malformation.

Gradients across localized areas of obstruction can, in general, be determined by continuous wave Doppler using the same principles that apply to isolated valvular stenoses (i.e., the modified Bernoulli equation where $\Delta P = 4v^2$). When multiple stenoses occur in series, the total pressure loss is equal to the sum of the pressure loss encountered at each site of stenosis. Two points must be remembered when multiple stenoses occur in series. First, continuous wave Doppler will only record the highest velocity present and not the sum of the gradients. Thus, each gradient must be evaluated separately as the difference between the proximal and distal velocity using pulsed Doppler techniques. In cases where the velocities exceed the Nyquist limit of the pulsed Doppler system, it may be necessary to use high pulse repetition

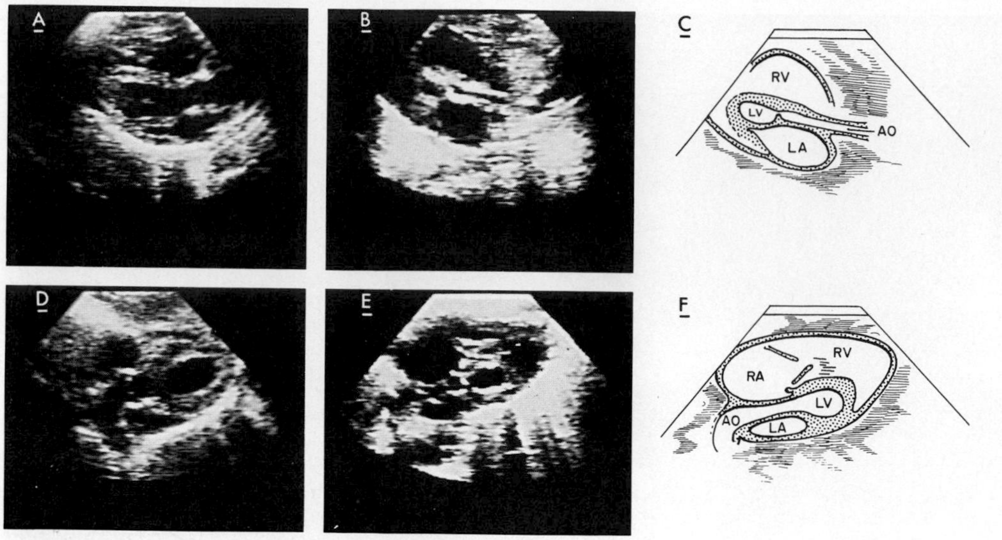

Fig. 31–29. Series of illustrations compares the normal configuration of the aortic root in the parasternal long axis **(A)** and subcostal long axis **(D)** views with that of a hypoplastic aorta **(B** and **E).** These recordings were obtained from children of comparable size. The accompanying diagrams **(C** and **F)** correspond to the parasternal long axis **(B)** and the subcostal long axis **(E)** recordings of the hypoplastic vessel. RV = right ventricle; LV = left ventricle; LA = left atrium; AO = aorta; RA = right atrium.

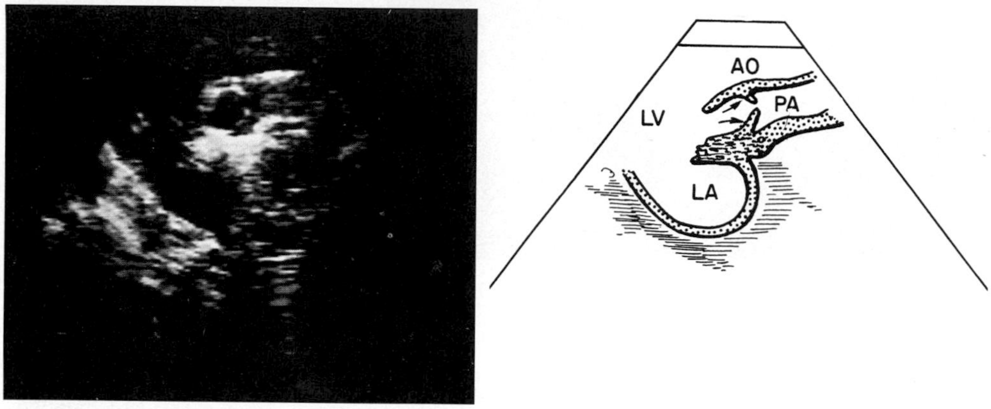

Fig. 31–30. Parasternal long axis recording from a patient with D-transposition illustrates combined annular, valvular, and supravalvular narrowing of the posterior pulmonary artery (PA). The pulmonary valve is domed and obviously stenotic. The overall size of the vessels is reduced, and there is further narrowing at the annulus and in the supravalvular area. AO = aorta; LV = left ventricle; LA = left atrium.

frequency (HiPRF) Doppler (see Chap. 8), and the analysis of stenoses in series represents one of the only applications in which the HiPRF approach is uniquely necessary. Second, to resolve the stenotic jets as separate, the Doppler sample volume length must be shorter than the distance between the two lesions. If this is not the case, the two intense, high velocity signals produced at the discrete sites of stenosis may become mixed in the Doppler sample volume, and any intervening fall in velocity indicating a pressure drop and energy loss at the proximal lesion will be obscured. This can lead to overestimation of the gradient if the peak velocity is presumed to correspond to the degree of obstruction at both levels or underestimation if only a single increase in velocity is reported. Finally, gradients are instantaneously additive. For example, if both fixed valvular and functional subvalvular obstruction are present, the gradient across the fixed obstruction may reach its peak in midsystole, whereas the gradient across the functional obstruction may reach its peak at end-systole. In this case the true peak gradient is not the sum of the two peaks, but rather the peak instantaneous sum. Thus, if the peak transvalvular gradient is 80 mm Hg at a time when the subvalvular gradient is only 10 mm Hg, then the instantaneous peak is 90 mm Hg. If the subvalvular gradient later rises to 65 mm Hg while at the same time the valvular component falls to 12 mm Hg, the instantaneous peak at that point will be 77 mm Hg. The absolute peak is the highest instantaneous gradient, not the sum of the two peaks, that is, 90 mm Hg and not 155 mm Hg.

ESTIMATION OF ABSOLUTE INTRACARDIAC PRESSURES

In some cases, one may need to determine or at least approximate absolute intracardiac pressures. This can be particularly important in patients with suspected pulmonary hypertension where the level of pulmonary pressure may determine the suitability for surgery. As a rule, if the pressure in any chamber or vessel can be measured or estimated, then the pressures in all chambers in direct communication should also be calculable. For example, if the aortic systolic pressure is measured by sphygmomanometer, this measurement should approximate the left ventricular systolic pressure in the absence of aortic stenosis. If aortic stenosis is present, then the left ventricular systolic pressure should equal the aortic pressure plus the Doppler-derived transvalvular gradient. If the patient also has a ventricular septal defect, then the right ventricular systolic pressure will equal the left ventricular pressure minus the gradient across the defect.

Once right ventricular pressure is known, the pulmonary artery systolic pressure should equal right ventricular systolic pressure in the absence of pulmonic stenosis. If pulmonic stenosis is present, then the pulmonic systolic pressure will equal the right ventricular pressure minus the transpulmonic gradient. It is often possible to validate pressures using other references. For example, in the case described previously, if tricuspid regurgitation is also present, then the right ventricular pressure can be measured from the transtricuspid gradient by assuming a right atrial pressure (usually 10 mm Hg) and compared to that backcalculated from the aortic pressure. Once one begins filling in known and calculable pressures, it is often surprising how consistent the prediction of chamber pressures becomes and how often one can validate a confusing or complex gradient.

UNUSUAL ATRIOVENTRICULAR AND VENTRICULOARTERIAL RELATIONSHIPS

Criss-Cross Hearts

The term *criss-cross heart* is used to describe a rare abnormality in which the right-sided atrium connects to the left-sided ventricle and the left-sided atrium connects to the right-sided ventricle.[48] Because of this pattern of connection, the systemic and pulmonary venous streams cross at the AV level without mixing. The ventricles are usually positioned in an anteroposterior manner, and the defect can be found with concordant (morphologic right atrium to morphologic right ventricle) or discordant (morphologic right atrium to morphologic left ventricle) AV relationships. A ventricular septal defect is invariably present, and discordant ventriculoarterial connections are common, as are associated atrial septal defects.[49]

The cross-sectional echocardiographic features of criss-cross hearts have been described in detail.[50–52] When recorded in standard parasternal views, the AV valves have an anteroposterior relationship, and thus the tricuspid valve is recorded in front of, rather than to the right of, the mitral valve. Because of their crossing relationship, a plane intersecting one valve parallel to its long axis passes through the short axis of the other. Normal apical or subcostal four-chamber views may reveal only one AV valve, and from these windows the plane must be swept in an anteroposterior arc to reveal the true nature of the lesion. The diagnosis of criss-cross heart should be suspected when the normal parallel arrangement of the AV valves and ventricular inflow regions cannot be found in the standard subcostal and apical four-chamber views.

The subcostal views in general are best for imaging the connections and spatial relationships of the cardiac chambers and great arteries.[49,50] Using a posteriorly displaced subcostal long axis view, one can see the left-sided atrium communicating by way of an AV valve to the right-sided ventricle (Fig. 31–31). In the usual situation, the left-sided atrium is a morphologic left atrium connected to a right-sided morphologic left ventricle. However the morphologic left ventricle is posterior, inferior, and rightward. Hence, flow through the posterior

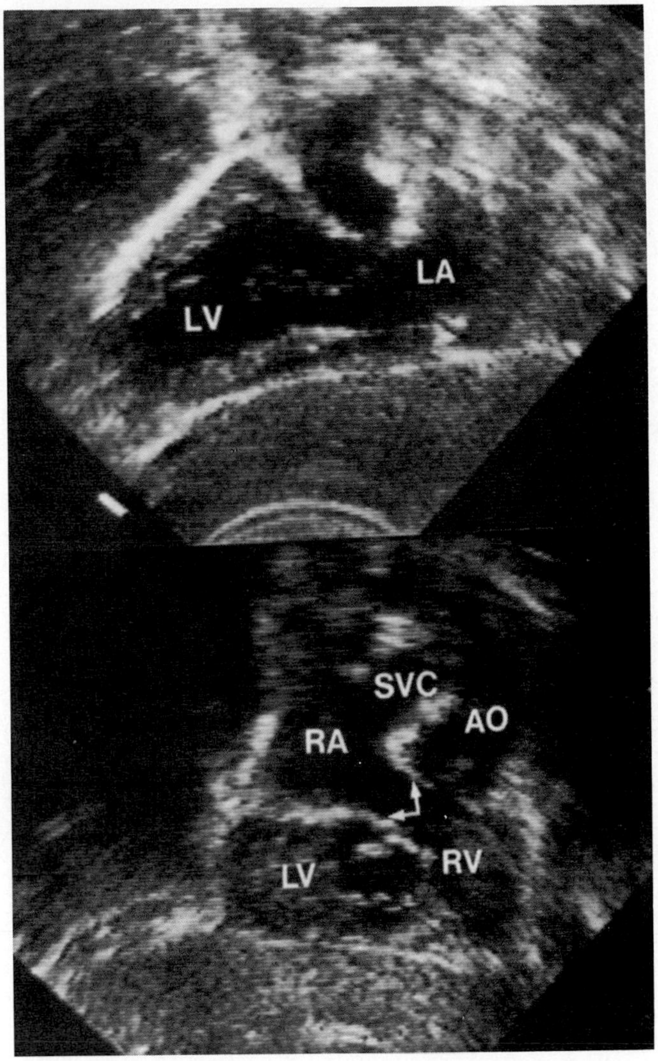

Fig. 31–31. Subcostal long axis recordings from a patient with criss-cross heart. Top. The connection of the left-sided morphologic left atrium (LA) to the right-sided morphologic left ventricle (LV). Bottom. The scan plane has been tilted anteriorly to illustrate the connections from the right-sided atrium (RA) to the left-sided morphologic right ventricle (RV). The right-sided morphologic RA receives the drainage from the superior vena cava (SVC); the morphologic RV gives rise to a leftward and anteriorly positioned aorta (AO). (From Snider AR, Serwer GA: Echocardiography in Pediatric Heart Disease. Chicago, Year Book Medical Publishers, 1990.)

mitral valve is directed rightward inferiorly and anteriorly. As the subcostal long axis plane is tilted farther anteriorly, the connection from the right-sided atrium to the left-sided ventricle can be visualized. In the usual situation, the right-sided morphologic right atrium is connected to a morphologic right ventricle that is anterior, superior, and leftward. Flow through the tricuspid valve is directed from right to left and from posterior to anterior. Tilting the scan plane further anteriorly permits the entire anterior ventricle and its outflow portion to be visualized. In the example illustrated in Figure 31–31, the anterior superior ventricle is the morphologic right ventricle that gives rise to a transposed aorta.

Associated defects are common in criss-cross hearts.

Ventricular septal defects are invariably present and usually involve the inlet septum. When the ventriculoarterial connections are discordant and the pulmonary valve is posterior, subvalvular stenosis and valvular pulmonary stenosis commonly occur. Straddling AV valves are also frequently encountered.[22]

Isolated Ventricular Inversion

Isolated ventricular inversion is a rare congenital malformation in which ventricular inversion occurs without transposition (i.e., AV discordance and ventriculoarterial concordance).[53] Because isolated ventricular inversion causes a physiologic state identical to that of complete transposition of the great arteries, most patients with this defect are symptomatic in infancy with cyanosis and congestive heart failure.

On the two-dimensional echocardiogram, patients with isolated ventricular inversion have AV discordance. In the typical case, one sees atrial situs solitus with inversion of the ventricles such that the morphologic left ventricle is to the right and the morphologic right ventricle is to the left (Fig. 31–32). The ventriculoarterial connections are normal. Thus, a posterior aorta usually arises from a right-sided morphologic left ventricle and is in fibrous continuity with a right-sided mitral valve. An anterior pulmonary artery arises from the left-sided morphologic right ventricle and is separated from the left AV valve by a persistent subpulmonary conus. The great arteries maintain a relatively normal relationship with each other, with the aortic valve rightward, posterior, and inferior to the pulmonary valve and the great arteries coiled about one another at their origin.[54]

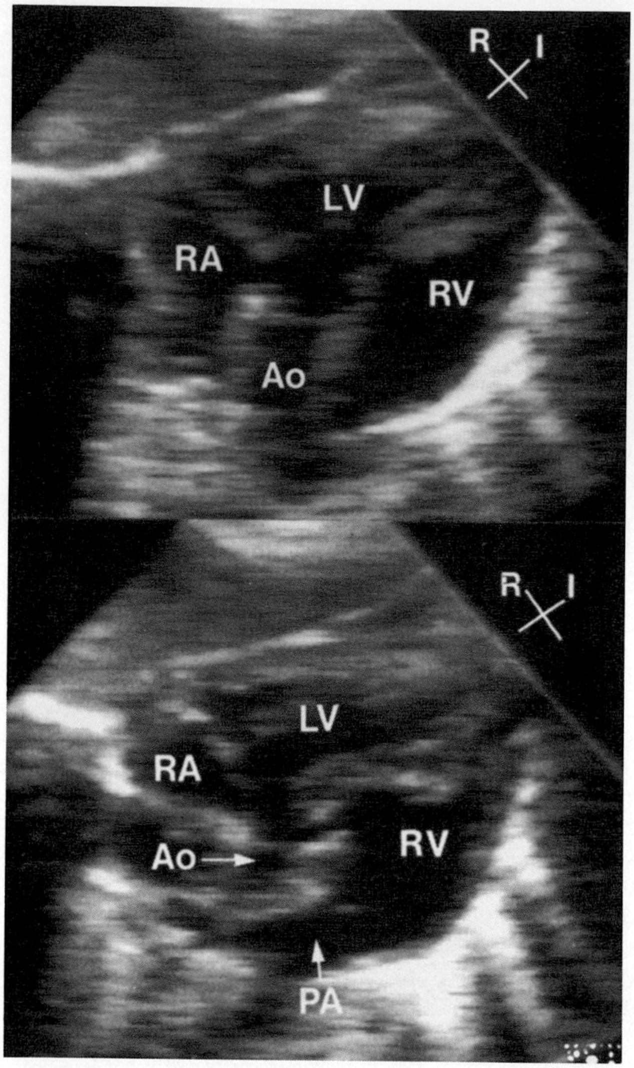

Fig. 31–32. Subcostal long axis views illustrating discordant atrioventricular connections and ventriculoarterial concordance in a patient with isolated ventricular inversion. Bottom. With slightly more elevation of the scan plane, the anteriorly positioned pulmonary artery (PA) can be seen arising from the left-sided morphologic right ventricle (RV). The great vessels are normally related. LV = morphologic left ventricle; Ao = aorta; RA = morphologic right atrium. (From Snider AR, et al.: Isolated ventricular inversion: Two-dimensional echocardiographic findings and a review of the literature. Pediatr Cardiol 5:27, 1984.)

Anatomically Corrected Malposition

Another rare defect is anatomically corrected malposition. This disorder is also characterized by AV discordance and ventriculoarterial concordance. The echocardiographic diagnosis of the AV and ventriculoarterial relationships is similar to that of the conditions previously described. The unique aspect of anatomically corrected malposition is an abnormal relationship between the aorta and the AV canal such that mitral-aortic continuity does not occur (i.e., bilateral conus). In addition, although the great vessels arise above the correct chamber, the aortic valve is anterior to the pulmonary valve and the great vessels exit the heart in a parallel fashion (i.e., in a pattern similar to that seen with corrected transposition[55]).

Isolated Atrial Inversion

Isolated atrial inversion is an example of visceroatrial discordance in which the viscera are in situs solitus, the atria are in situs inversus, the ventricles are in situs solitus, and the great arteries are normally interrelated.[56] Because the venae cavae and aorta both are left-sided, whereas the pulmonary veins and artery both are right-sided, the systemic and pulmonary circulations are parallel, as in transposition of the great arteries.

In summary, if a patient with complex congenital disease is approached in the fashion described in this chapter, even the inexperienced examiner should be able to piece together all the components of the lesion. Once the various elements of a particular disorder are recorded, it is relatively simple to determine the pathologic entity with which one is dealing. Other functional disorders such as valvular regurgitation and ventricular dysfunction can then be included to complete the diagnostic description.

REFERENCES

1. Van Praagh R: The segmental approach to diagnosis in congenital heart disease. *In* Bergsma D (ed.): Birth Defects: Original Article Series. Baltimore, Williams & Wilkins, p. 4, 1972.
2. Shinebourne EA, Macartney FJ, Anderson RH: Sequential chamber locali-

zation: logical approach to diagnosis in congenital heart disease. Br Heart J 38:327, 1976.
3. Van Praagh R: Terminology of congenital heart disease: glossary and commentary. Circulation 56:139, 1977.
4. Stanger P, Rudolph AM, Edwards JE: Cardiac malpositions: an overview based on study of sixty-five necropsy specimens. Circulation 56:159, 1977.
5. Moller TH, Neal WA: Heart Disease in Infancy. New York, Appleton-Century-Crofts, 1978.
6. Perloff JK: The Clinical Recognition of Congenital Heart Disease. Philadelphia, W.B. Saunders, 1980.
7. Ivemark B: Implications of agenesis of the spleen on the pathogenesis of conotruncus anomalies in childhood. Acta Paediatr Scand 44:590 and Suppl. 104, 1955.
8. Van Mierop LHS, Patterson PR, Reynolds RW: Two cases of congenital asplenia with isomerism of the cardiac atria and the sinoatrial nodes. Am J Cardiol 13:407, 1964.
9. Ruttenberg HD, et al. Syndrome of congenital cardiac disease with asplenia: distinction from other forms of congenital cyanotic cardiac disease. Am J Cardiol 13:387, 1964.
10. Moller JH, Nakib A, Anderson RC, Edwards JE: Congenital cardiac disease associated with polysplenia. Circulation 36:789, 1967.
11. Van Mierop LHS, Gessner IH, Schiebler GL: Asplenia and polysplenia syndromes. Birth Defects. VIII:36, 1972.
12. Rose V, Izukawa T, Moes CAF: Syndromes of asplenia and polyspenia: a review of cardiac and non-cardiac malformations in 60 cases with special reference to diagnosis and prognosis. Br Heart J 37:840, 1975.
13. Putschar WG, Manion WC: Congenital absence of the spleen and associated anomalies. Am J Clin Pathol 26:429, 1956.
14. Polhemus DW, Schafer WB: Congenital absence of the spleen: syndrome with atrioventricularis and situs inversus. Pediatrics 9:696, 1952.
15. Polhemus DW, Schafer WB: Congenital absence of the spleen. Pediatrics 16:495, 1955.
16. Arey JB: Cardiovascular Pathology in Infants and Children. Philadelphia, W.B. Saunders, 1984.
17. Campbell M, Deuchar DC: Dextrocardia and isolated levocardia. II. Situs inversus and isolated dextrocardia. Br Heart J 28:472, 1966.
18. Keith A: The Hunterian lectures on malformations of the heart. Lecture II. Lancet 2:433, 1909.
19. de la Cruz MV, Polansky BJ, Navarro-Lopez F: The diagnosis of corrected transposition of the great vessels. Br Heart J 24:483, 1962.
20. Leachman RD, Cokkinos DV, Zamalloa O: Discordance of the suprahepatic inferior vena cava and right atrium from liver situs: report of 2 cases with dextrocardia and clinical implications. Chest 63:926, 1973.
21. Sanders SP: Echocardiography and related techniques in the diagnosis of congenital heart defects. I. Veins, atria and interatrial septum. Echocardiography 1:185, 1984.
22. Snider AR, Serwer GA: Echocardiography in Pediatric Heart Disease. Chicago, Year Book, 1990.
23. Bierman FZ, Williams RG: Subxiphoid two-dimensional imaging of the interatrial septum in infants and neonates with congenital heart disease. Circulation 60:80, 1979.
24. Huhta JC, Smallhorn JF, Macartney FJ: Two-dimensional echocardiographic diagnosis of situs. Br Heart J 48:97, 1982.
25. Anderson RH, et al.: Definition of cardiac chambers. *In* Anderson RH, Shinebourne EA (eds.): Paediatric Cardiology 1977. Edinburgh, Churchill Livingstone, p. 5, 1978.
26. Seward JB, Tajik AJ, Hagler DJ, and Mair DD: Cross-sectional echocardiography in common ventricle utilizing 80° phased array sector scanning. Circulation 55–56:III–41, 1977.
27. Sahn DJ, et al.: The comparative utilities of real-time cross-sectional echocardiographic imaging systems for the diagnosis of complex congenital heart disease. Am J Med 63:50, 1977.
28. Henry WL, et al.: Evaluation of A-V valve morphology in congenital heart disease by real-time cross-sectional echocardiography. Circulation 52:120, 1975.
29. Sutherland GR, et al.: Atrioventricular discordance: cross-sectional echocardiographic-morphologic correlative study. Br Heart J 50:8, 1983.
30. Tajik AJ, et al.: Two-dimensional real-time ultrasonic imaging of the heart and great vessels: technique, image orientation, structure identification and validation. Mayo Clin Proc 53:271, 1978.
31. Hagler DJ, et al.: Wide angle two-dimensional echocardiographic criteria for ventricular morphology (abstr.) Am J Cardiol 45:466, 1980.
32. Henry WL, et al.: Differential diagnosis of anomalies of the great arteries by cardiac ultrasonography. Radiology 107:181, 1973.
33. King DL, Steeg CN, and Ellis K: Demonstration of transposition of the great arteries by cardiac ultrasonography. Radiology 107:181, 1973.
34. Sahn DJ, Terry R, O'Rourke R, and Friedman WF: Multiple crystal cross-sectional echocardiography in the diagnosis of cyanotic congenital heart disease. Circulation 50:230, 1974.
35. Foale RA, Stefanine L, Richards AF, and Somerville J: Two-dimensional echocardiographic features of corrected transposition. Am J Cardiol 45:466, 1980.
36. Bierman FZ, and Williams RG: Prospective diagnosis of D-transposition of the great arteries in neonates by subxyphoid, two-dimensional echocardiography. Circulation 60:1496, 1979.
37. Henry WL, Maron BJ, and Griffith JM: Cross-sectional echocardiography in the diagnosis of congenital heart disease: identification of the relations of the ventricles and great arteries. Circulation 56:267, 1977.
38. Gramiak R, Shah DM, and Kramer DH: Ultrasound cardiography: contrast studies in anatomy and function. Radiology 92:939, 1969.
39. Feigenbaum H, et al.: Identification of ultrasound echoes from the left ventricle using intracardiac injections of indocyanine green. Circulation 41:615, 1970.
40. Seward JB, Tajik AJ, Spangler JG, and Ritter PG: Echocardiographic contrast studies: initial experience. Mayo Clin Proc 50:163, 1975.
41. Seward JB, Tajik AJ, Hagler DJ, and Ritter DG: Peripheral venous contrast echocardiography. Am J Cardiol 39:202, 1977.
42. Valdes-Cruz LM, Pieroni DR, Roland JMA, and Varghese DJ: Echocardiographic detection of intracardiac right-to-left shunts following peripheral vein injection. Circulation 54:558, 1976.
43. Serreuys PW, VanDenBrand M, Hugenholtz PD, and Roelandt J: Intracardiac right-to-left shunts demonstrated by two-dimensional echocardiography after peripheral vein injection. Br Heart J 42:429, 1979.
44. Fraker TD, Harris PJ, Behar VS, and Kisslo JA: Detection and exclusion of interatrial shunts by two-dimensional echocardiography and peripheral venous injection. Circulation 59:379, 1979.
45. Gilbert BW, Drobac M, and Rakowski H: Contrast two-dimensional echocardiography and peripheral venous injection (abstr.) Am J Cardiol 45:402, 1980.
46. Weyman AE, et al.: Negative contrast echocardiography: a new method for detecting left-to-right shunts. Circulation 59:498, 1979.
47. Kronik G, Hutterer B, Mosslacher H: Diagnosis of atrial left-to-right shunts by cross-sectional contrast echocardiography. Z Kardiol 70:138, 1981.
48. Anderson RH, Shinebourne EA, Gerlis LM: Criss-cross atrioventricular relationships producing paradoxical atrioventricular concordance or discordance: their significance to nomenclature of congenital heart disease. Circulation 50:176, 1974.
49. Robinson PJ, Kumpeng V, Macartney FJ: Cross-sectional echocardiographic and angiographic correlation in criss cross hearts. Br Heart J 54: 61, 1985.
50. van Mill G, et al.: Subcostal two-dimensional echocardiographic recognition of a criss-cross heart with discordant ventriculoarterial connections. Pediatr Cardiol 3:319, 1982.
51. Marino B, et al.: Two-dimensional echocardiographic anatomy in criss cross heart. Am J Cardiol 58:325, 1986.
52. Carminati M, et al.: Cross sectional echocardiographic study of criss-cross hearts and superoinferior ventricles. Am J Cardiol 59:114, 1987.
53. Van Praagh R, Van Praagh S: Isolated ventricular inversion: a consideration of the morphogenesis, definition and diagnosis of nontransposed and transposed great arteries. Am J Cardiol 17:395, 1985.
54. Snider AR, et al.: Isolated ventricular inversion: two-dimensional echocardiographic findings and a review of the literature. Pediatr Cardiol 5:27, 1984.
55. Pasquini L, et al.: Echocardiographic and anatomic findings in atrioventricular discordance with ventriculoarterial concordance. Am J Cardiol 62:1256, 1988.
56. Clarkson PM, Brandt PWT, Barratt-Boyes BG, Neutze JM: "Isolated atrial inversion." Visceral situs solitus, visceroatrial discordance, discordant ventricular d-loop without transposition, dextrocardia: diagnosis and surgical correction. Am J Cardiol 29:877, 1972.

CHAPTER

32

COMPLEX CONGENITAL HEART DISEASE II: A PATHOLOGIC APPROACH

MARY ETTA E. KING

The majority of congenital heart defects occur as isolated abnormalities and have been described elsewhere in this text under the specifically affected cardiac system. Some occur as regularly associated groups of lesions, discussed here under the heading of complex congenital heart disease.

VENTRICULAR ABNORMALITIES

Univentricular Heart

The presence of a single ventricle represents 1 to 1.5% of all congenital heart defects and occurs in approximately 4% of neonates with congenital heart disease.[1,2] Debate continues on the proper terminology for this group of cardiac malformations in which both atria connect with one ventricular chamber.[3] The term *single ventricle* expresses simply the functional state, not necessarily the anatomic reality. The majority of these patients do in fact have another ventricular mass, albeit hypoplastic. *Univentricular atrioventricular connection* has emerged as the most precise classification,[4] although it is a cumbersome term. For ease of usage in this chapter I therefore choose the simpler term *univentricular heart*. The classic entities of hypoplastic left heart syndrome and tricuspid atresia, which may have only one functional ventricle, are excluded from this classification and are considered separately.

The basic element of the univentricular heart is communication of both atria or a common atrium with a single main ventricular chamber. The important aspects to ascertain echocardiographically in patients with this anomaly are: (1) the presence and location of an accessory chamber; (2) the number and functional status of the atrioventricular (AV) valves; (3) the number and orientation of the great vessels and their relation to the main or accessory chamber; (4) the presence and severity of outflow obstruction, most often obstruction to pulmonary blood flow; (5) the functional performance of the systemic ventricle; and (6) the nature and adequacy of venous return in the case of atresia of one of the atrioventricular valves.

Accessory Chambers

The accessory chamber represents the abortive second ventricle in patients with univentricular heart. These chambers are generally small and do not receive atrioventricular valve inflow. An anteriorly positioned accessory chamber, termed an *outflow chamber* because it gives rise to one or more great vessels, represents the infundibulum of the rudimentary right ventricle. The main chamber, then, is of left ventricular morphology. This group of univentricular hearts of left ventricular type is the most common form, comprising 65 to 78% of those documented in several large published series.[5–9] The main chamber communicates with the outlet chamber through the outlet (or bulboventricular) foramen (Fig. 32–1 and 32–2). When an accessory chamber is located posteriorly, it is referred to as a *blind*

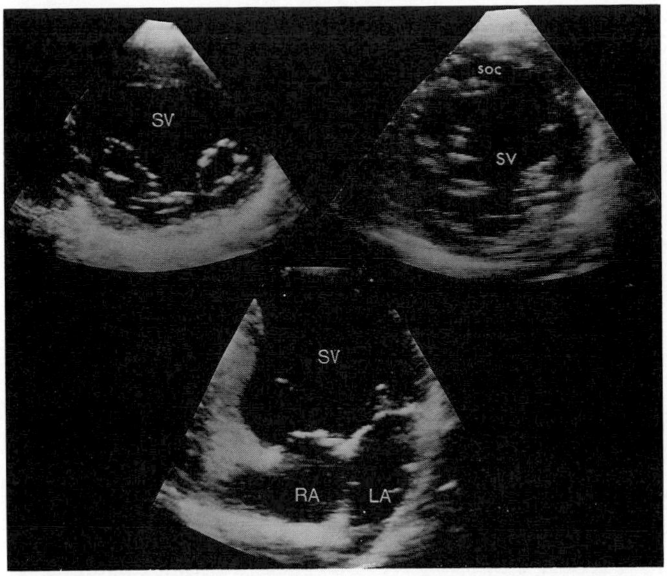

Fig. 32–1. Echocardiographic views of a univentricular heart of left ventricular type with two atrioventricular valves. Top. The cross-sectional view at the ventricular level shows two atrioventricular orifices of equal size within the single ventricular chamber. Scanning toward the base of the heart, the bulboventricular foramen is noted anteriorly and to the left, leading into an anterior small outlet chamber (top, right). Bottom. From the apex, both atria communicate with the single ventricular chamber with no evidence of an interventricular septum. LA = left atrium; RA = right atrium; soc = small outlet chamber; SV = single ventricle. (From Liberthson RR: Congenital heart disease in the child, adolescent, and adult. *In:* The Practice of Cardiology. Boston, Little Brown and Company, 1989.)

trabecular pouch and denotes the remnant left ventricle. The main chamber in this instance is of right ventricular morphology. This subgroup makes up about 10 to 15% of all patients with univentricular heart. An additional 10 to 20% of patients have no definable accessory chamber, thereby acquiring the classification of "indeterminate type" of univentricular heart (Fig. 32–3).

Echocardiographic assessment of these morphologic subgroups is most reliably made by identifying and locating the position of the accessory chamber. The secondary supporting features of ventricular morphology—trabeculation, moderator band, number of papillary muscles—are helpful when present, but they may prove to be too variable for accurate prediction of ventricular subgrouping.[7,8,10] When surgical management was aimed at palliative procedures alone, the importance of ventricular morphology was primarily academic. As more aggressive management is contemplated, knowledge of the main chamber morphology may be more clinically relevant. Some authors have intimated that the morphology of the main chamber is a useful predictor of immediate postoperative and long-term ventricular function. For example, inadequate hypertrophic response of an anatomic right ventricle has been suggested as an explanation for the less satisfactory operative results in the subgroup of patients with univentricular hearts with a main chamber of right ventricular origin.[11,12]

Atrioventricular (AV) Valves

Atrioventricular inflow may occur through two valves, a common AV orifice, or a single valve with absence of the second connection (Fig. 32–4). *Double-inlet* anatomy occurs most frequently (55 to 70%). Although it may be possible in some instances to distin-

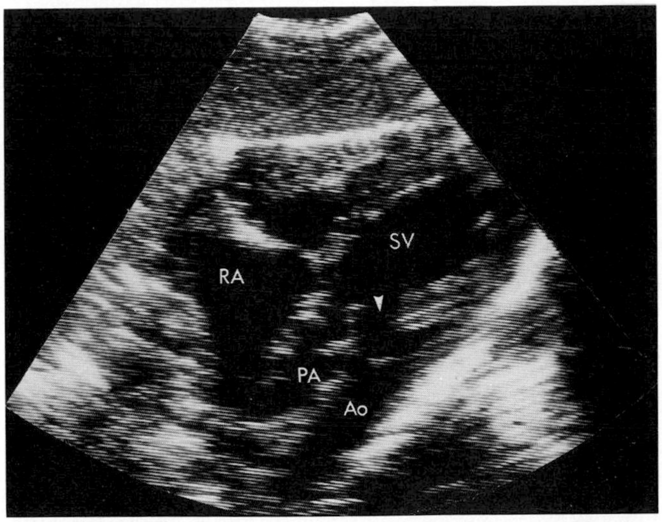

Fig. 32–2. Subcostal echocardiographic view of a univentricular heart in which the aorta arises from the small outlet chamber on the left anterior surface of the heart. The bulboventricular foramen is marked with a single arrowhead. The pulmonary artery (PA) originates from the main ventricular chamber and demonstrates subpulmonary obstruction. The muscular ridge within the ventricle is a large papillary muscle and should not be mistaken for an interventricular septum. Ao = aorta; RA = right atrium; SV = single ventricular chamber.

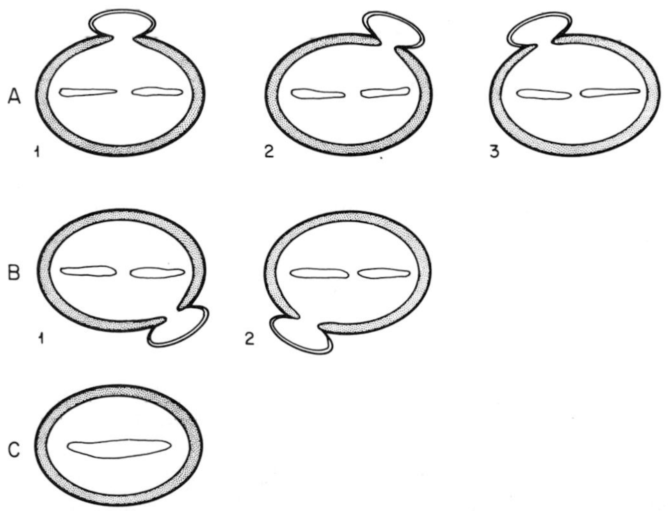

Fig. 32–3. Morphologic subgroups of univentricular heart. **A.** The univentricular heart of left ventricular type, with an anterior outflow chamber, which may be directly anterior (1), to the left (2), or to the right (3). **B.** The univentricular heart of right ventricular type with a blind posterior pouch, which lies to the left (1) or to the right (2). **C.** The univentricular heart of indeterminate morphology with neither an outflow chamber nor a blind pouch. This form often has a single atrioventricular valve.

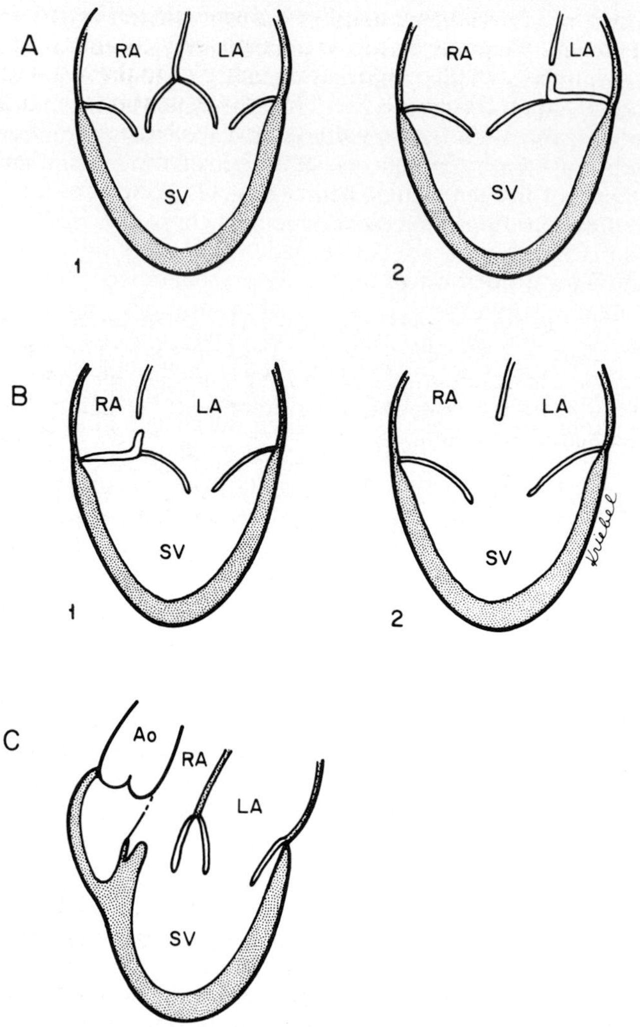

Fig. 32–4. Atrioventricular valves in the univentricular heart. **A.** Inflow occurs across two equally developed atrioventricular valves (1), or across a large right-sided atrioventricular valve with atresia of the left-sided valve (2). **B**(2). Alternatively, the right-sided atrioventricular valve may be atretic with a large left-sided valve. In single inlet with atresia of the right- or left-sided valve, note that venous return from the side of the atretic orifice must pass through the atrial septum to return to the circulation. **B**(2). The form of univentricular heart with a common atrioventricular orifice. A large atrial septal defect or common atrium is present to allow both atrial chambers to communicate with the single ventricular chamber. **C.** One of the atrioventricular valves straddles into the outlet chamber. Ao = aorta; RA = right atrium; LA = left atrium; SV = single ventricular chamber.

guish between the anatomic characteristics of mitral valves and those of tricuspid valves, the two AV valves often have a variable number of leaflets and papillary muscles and thus are referred to as "right" or "left" rather than mitral or tricuspid. Usually, the right AV valve lies in a slightly anterior plane to the left AV valve, and both AV valves are of equivalent size,[13] in the same plane, with diastolic apposition of the medial cusps of each valve. In some cases, however, the valves may vary in size and lie in different anteroposterior or superoinferior planes. A cursory echocardiographic examination might result in a diagnosis of single-inlet anatomy, but apical and subcostal views will clarify the correct number and orientation of both AV orifices.

The AV valve structure should be carefully evaluated echocardiographically for the presence of straddling of chordal structures into the small outflow chamber or for the interdigitating of chordae tendineae to contralateral papillary muscles within the main ventricular chamber (Fig. 32–4C). Because the double-inlet type of univentricular heart lends itself to possible subdivision into two ventricular chambers, the presence of chordal straddling would have obvious surgical implications. Significant AV valve incompetence is of concern as a potential contraindication to definitive repair by the Fontan procedure,[14] and it should be carefully assessed by pulsed Doppler and/or color flow mapping.

The *single-inlet* univentricular heart generally has one normal AV valve and one that is atretic. The right or left atrium thus terminates blindly in a fibrous or membranous ridge, with the interatrial septal communication as the only egress for venous return to that atrium (Fig. 32–4B). This phenomenon is best appreciated from apical or subcostal echocardiographic views. In some cases, the nonfunctioning AV valve may be imperforate, rather than completely atretic, with rudimentary tensor apparatus on the ventricular aspect of the valve tissue. This type of AV valve anatomy may be difficult to appreciate angiographically, and the blind atrial chamber may be difficult to define during cardiac catheterization. Echocardiography thus contributes substantially to accurate anatomic diagnosis and surgical planning.

The third mode of AV connection in univentricular hearts is through a *common AV* valve. This occurs less often than either double- or single-inlet anatomy (5 to 15%) and is always associated with a primum atrial septal defect (ASD) or common atrium, in order for both atria to connect by a common valve to the main ventricular chamber. Atrial isomerism, situs ambiguus, and anomalies of systemic and pulmonary venous return are also commonly associated with univentricular hearts of this type.[15] The common valve generally has one large central leaflet flanked by two smaller lateral leaflets. Chordal connections again are variable, with straddling into the outlet chamber or attachment to the outlet septal crest. This is less problematic, however, than with double-inlet ventricles because surgical management would not be directed toward creating two ventricular chambers. The competency of the common AV valve must be assessed by pulsed Doppler or color flow mapping if a Fontan repair is contemplated.

Great Vessels

Great vessel orientation and relationships are another important feature of the univentricular heart that one can reliably diagnose echocardiographically.[10] The possibilities are myriad, but can be condensed to the following: (1) normal ventriculoarterial connection, in which the pulmonary artery arises from the small outlet chamber and the aorta arises from the main ventricular chamber; (2) transposed great arteries, in which the aorta arises from the small outlet chamber and the pulmonary artery arises from the main chamber; the outlet chamber may be either to the right (D-loop) or to the left (L-loop); (3) double-outlet anatomy, in which both great vessels originate from either the main chamber or the outlet chamber; and (4) single-outlet anatomy, in which one great vessel arises from either the outlet chamber or the main chamber, and the other is atretic (Fig. 32–5).

As in other forms of complex congenital heart disease, the echocardiographic identification of the great vessels is made from long and short axis planes and relies on recognition of the characteristic branching pattern of each vessel—the simple bifurcation of the pulmonary artery into right and left branches, or the arch configuration of the aorta with its brachiocephalic vessels (see Chapter 31). In the majority of patients with univentricular heart, the great vessels are transposed; the anteriorly positioned aorta lies either to the right or to the left with nearly equal frequency.[6,8,10] The infrequent occurrence of univentricular heart with normally related great vessels (with the pulmonary artery arising from the outflow chamber and the aorta from the main chamber) has been termed the *Holmes heart*.[16]

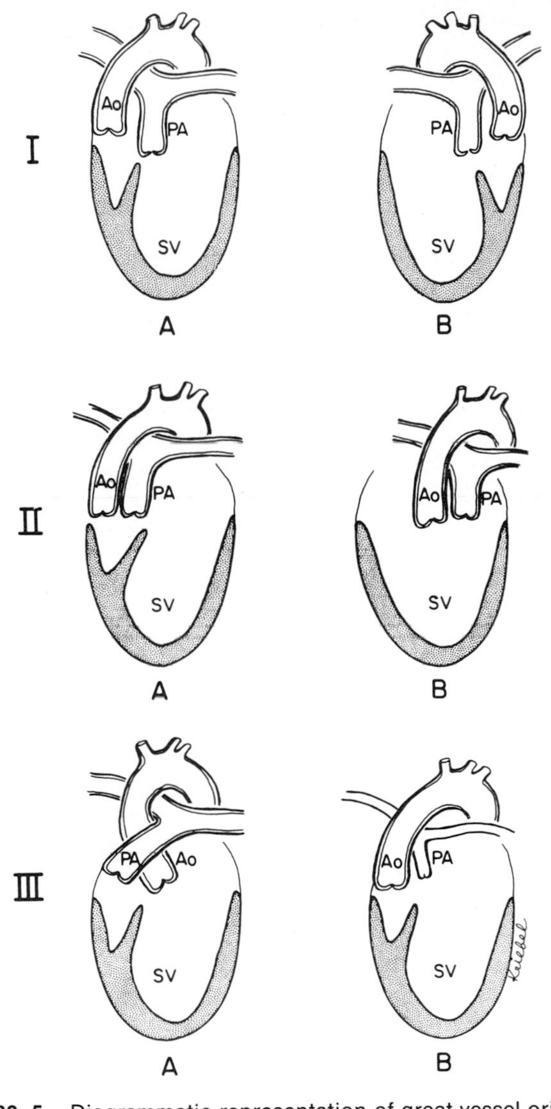

Fig. 32–5. Diagrammatic representation of great vessel orientation in the univentricular heart. **I.** Origin of the aorta from the small outlet chamber and the pulmonary artery from the main ventricular chamber. This may occur with the outlet chamber and aorta to the right **(A)** or to the left **(B)**. **II.** The great vessels may both arise from the small outlet chamber **(A)** or from the main ventricular chamber **(B)**. **III(A).** The so-called "Holmes heart," with normally oriented great vessels, the pulmonary artery originating from the small outlet chamber and the aorta from the main ventricular chamber. **III(B).** Occasionally, the pulmonary artery is hypoplastic or atretic. Ao = aorta; PA = pulmonary artery; SV = single ventricle.

Outflow Obstruction

The clinical presentation and long-term outcome of the patient with univentricular heart depend on the presence or absence of obstruction to pulmonary blood flow. This frequent concomitant finding can be accurately evaluated with echocardiographic imaging and Doppler study to localize the type and level of obstruction, whether subvalvular or valvular, stenotic, or atretic. In cases where both valvular and subvalvular obstruction are present, it is usually not possible to quantitate accurately the severity of each obstruction individually because of its proximity to the other. With continuous wave Doppler, however, the gradient across the entire outflow tract can be estimated.

Outflow obstruction may also occur in univentricular hearts at the level of the bulboventricular foramen. Because the aorta usually arises from the outlet chamber, systemic flow thus depends on an adequate communication between the main chamber and the outflow chamber. Obstruction at this level may be present from the start or it may develop subsequent to muscular hypertrophy of the main ventricular chamber in response to pulmonary stenosis or pulmonary artery banding (Fig. 32–6). Echocardiographic assessment of the univentricular heart should always enable one to establish that the outlet foramen is greater than half the aortic root diameter and that no significant gradient exists between the main chamber and the outlet chamber by Doppler examination.[17] Some investigators have advocated an isoproterenol challenge in the cardiac catheterization or echocardiography laboratory at the time of initial evaluation, to uncover potential cases of subaortic obstruction.[18]

Ventricular Function

The main ventricular chamber in univentricular heart must perform systolic work for both pulmonary and systemic circulations. This is usually accomplished successfully in the early years of life, but with advancing age or with associated lesions that contribute to the volume or pressure overload, ventricular failure supervenes. A noninvasive estimate of ventricular function is important both preoperatively and after palliative or corrective surgery. The geometry of the main ventricular chamber does not fit the usual elliptic models from which formulas for left ventricular volumes have been derived. A Simpson's rule technique from an apical or subcostal projection thus may be the most accurate means of quantifying ventricular ejection fraction echocardiographically. Most studies of ventricular function in univentricular hearts have used angiographic or radionuclide methods for calculating ejection fraction, and

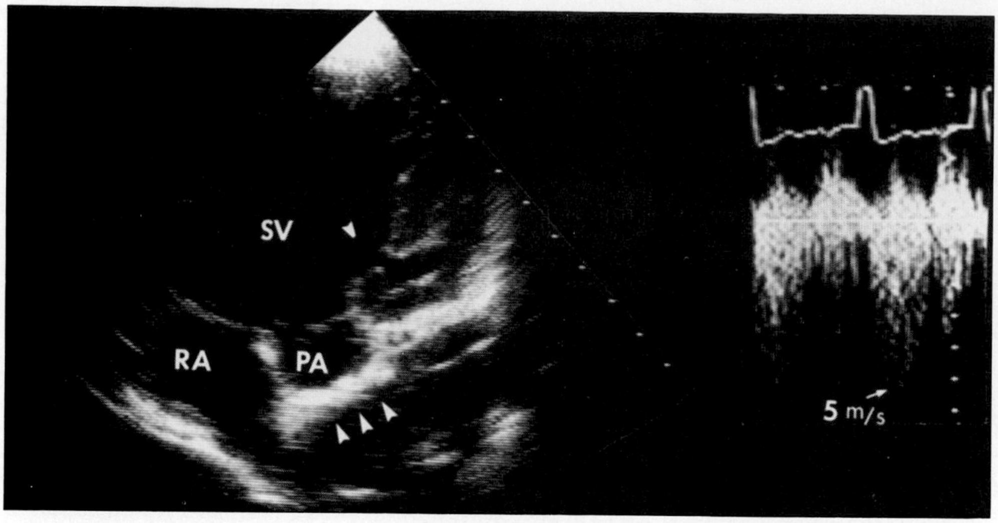

Fig. 32–6. Echocardiographic view from the apex in a child with univentricular heart following pulmonary artery banding (triple arrowheads). The small outlet chamber can be seen as a muscular chamber high on the left lateral wall. The outlet foramen from the main ventricular chamber (single arrowhead) has become restricted as a result of progressive hypertrophy after band placement. The continuous wave Doppler tracing on the right demonstrates a peak velocity of 5 m/sec across this restriction, indicating an outflow gradient of 100 mm Hg. PA = pulmonary artery; RA = right atrium; SV = single ventricular chamber.

few data are available on which echocardiographic methods are best for quantifying ventricular function or on "normal" values for echocardiographic ejection fraction in this group of patients. Significant depression of ventricular function is a contraindication for the Fontan repair because elevated filling pressures inhibit passive forward flow from the right atrium through the lungs. In late follow-up studies after Fontan repair, outcome was adversely affected by preoperative ventricular dysfunction.[19,20]

Abnormalities of Venous Return

Abnormalities of systemic and pulmonary venous return are also of concern in the patient with univentricular heart. The subgroups of indeterminate ventricles or right ventricular main chamber morphology with a common AV valve more frequently have abnormalities of atrial situs and anomalies of systemic and pulmonary venous drainage, including total anomalous pulmonary venous connection. These anomalies may add to the difficulty of separating the pulmonary and systemic venous returns at the time of definitive repair and thus should be assessed as carefully as possible echocardiographically and angiographically. (See Chapters 15, 18, and 26 for discussions of pulmonary and systemic venous abnormalities.)

In patients with absence or atresia of one of the AV valves, it is critical that the venous return to the associated atrium have an adequate outlet through an atrial septal defect or a widely patent foramen ovale. In the case of a restrictive atrial septal communication, flow velocities across the defect detected by pulsed Doppler are abnormal in peak velocity and flow pattern.[21] A peak velocity of 1.5 to 2 m/sec or greater with continuous nonphasic flow is indicative of a restrictive interatrial defect requiring an emergency balloon septostomy or surgical septectomy (Fig. 32–7).

Surgical Management

Aortopulmonary Shunt. Although a few patients with univentricular heart have a fortunate balance of intracardiac streaming and pulmonic stenosis that allows them to survive well into adult years with minimal symptoms, the long-term prognosis of patients with unoperated univentricular hearts is grim. In one of the largest series of such patients (n = 83),[22] a 50% mortality was reported within 15 years of diagnosis for the subgroup with an outflow chamber and a 50% mortality within 4 years of diagnosis for the subgroup with no outflow chamber. This series did not include infants diagnosed in the newborn period and hence portrays more optimistic figures than otherwise expected because of prior natural selection.

Until recent years, the surgical management of univentricular heart was limited to palliative measures. In patients whose pathophysiologic features are primarily those of inadequate pulmonary blood flow, a systemic-to-pulmonary artery shunt is performed to relieve severe cyanosis. The most common anastomosis has been the Blalock-Taussig shunt, a subclavian-to-pulmonary artery connection, or a central prosthetic interposition shunt to control shunt size and to ensure patency.[23] The hospital mortality for this procedure is quite low (2%), and Taussig's original series showed a 10-year survival of 72%; 50% of these patients were alive at 20-year follow-up.[24] More recent figures show that 85% survive 10 years after a simple shunt procedure, with some patients requiring additional shunting procedures.[25] The advantages of low operative risk and reasonable long-term survival must be weighed against the chronic volume overload imposed on the ventricle that predisposes it to early ventricular failure and the potential development of pulmonary vascular obstructive disease from long-term shunt flow at high pressure. In addition, the patient who requires an early shunt procedure will likely need additional shunt flow with growth during later childhood and in early adulthood. Distortion of the pulmonary artery at the shunt site often creates peripheral pulmonary stenosis, which must be surgically corrected with angioplasty before complete repair is possible.

Echocardiographic assessment of the patient with a systemic-to-pulmonary shunt relies on detection of turbulent shunt flow at the site of the shunt or in the receiv-

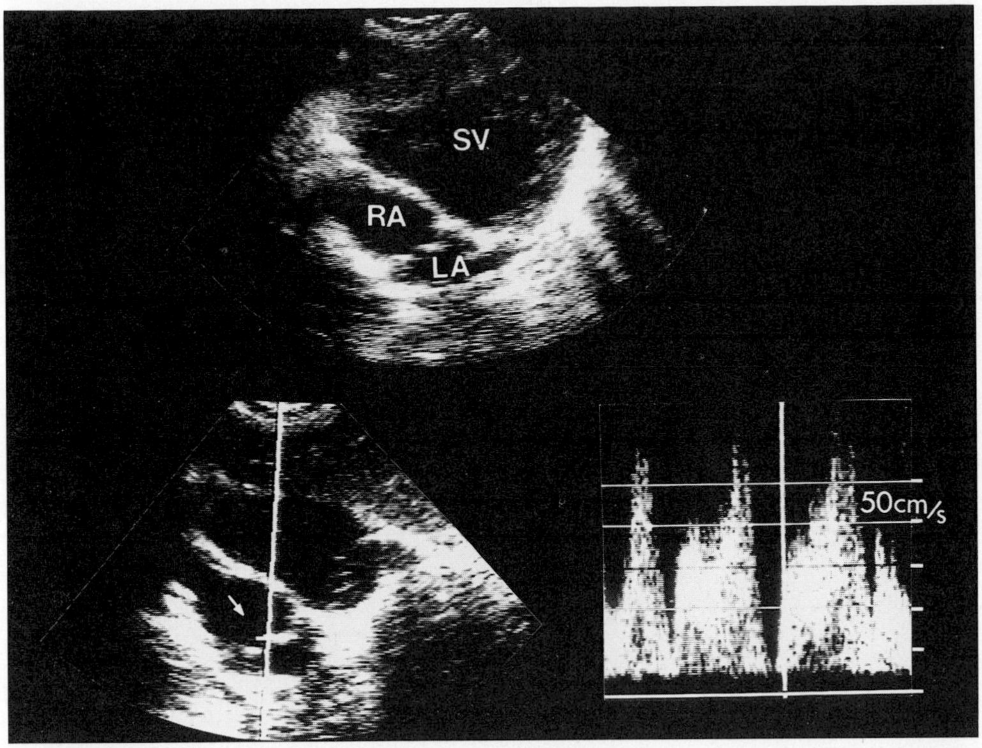

Fig. 32–7. Echocardiographic subcostal view in an infant with a univentricular heart and atresia of the left atrioventricular valve. Top. The left atrium is small, and a minute defect in the interatrial septum can be seen. Bottom, left. Placement of the Doppler sample volume along the right side of the atrial defect is seen. Bottom, right. This spectral tracing indicates a peak velocity in excess of 2.5 m/sec. (The calibrations are shown in 50-cm/sec increments.) LA = left atrium; RA = right atrium; SV = single ventricular chamber.

ing pulmonary vessel. Color flow mapping clearly portrays the presence and location of this shunt flow. Retrograde runoff flow from the aorta at or near the site of the shunt is also supportive evidence of shunt patency. Figure 32–8 illustrates the most frequent sites for aortopulmonary anastomoses. Often, a right Blalock-Taussig shunt can be imaged from a suprasternal notch or right parasternal approach focusing on the distal right pulmonary artery just lateral to the superior vena cava. A prominent right subclavian artery can be appreciated when one follows the innominate artery from the aorta, often with turbulent flow on color flow mapping (Fig. 32–9). Detecting the presence of pulmonary vascular obstructive disease secondary to exces-

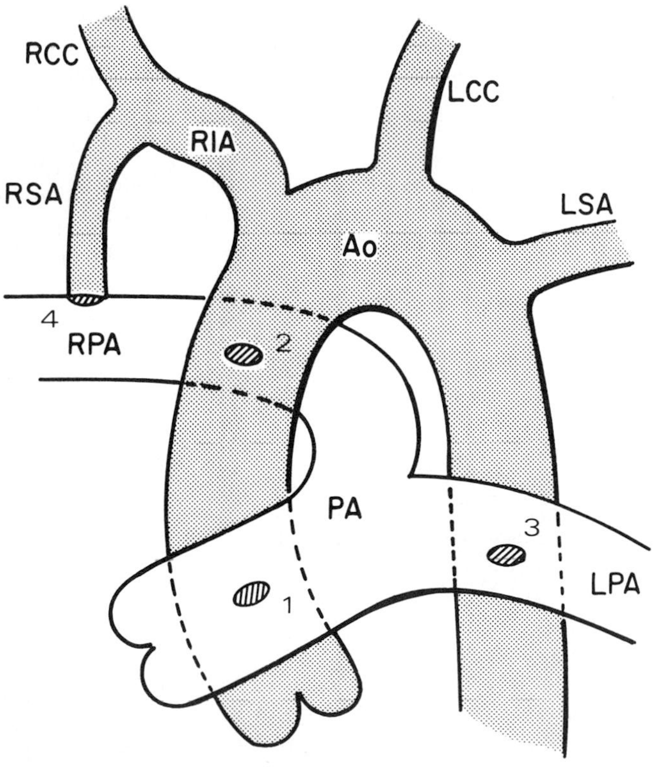

Fig. 32–8. The major sites of aortopulmonary anastomoses. The aorta and pulmonary artery are shown as they intertwine, with possible shunt sites indicated with small cross-hatched circles. The most proximal connection (1) is the central Waterston shunt between main pulmonary artery and ascending aorta. A right Waterston shunt (2) can be created between aorta and right pulmonary artery where the latter passes under the ascending aortic root. The Potts shunt is made between descending aorta and left pulmonary artery (3). A Blalock-Taussig shunt is created by anastomosing either right or left subclavian artery to its ipsilateral pulmonary artery (4). Ao = aorta; LCC = left common carotid artery; LPA = left pulmonary artery; LSA = left subclavian artery; PA = pulmonary artery; RCC = right common carotid artery; RIA = innominate artery; RSA = right subclavian artery.

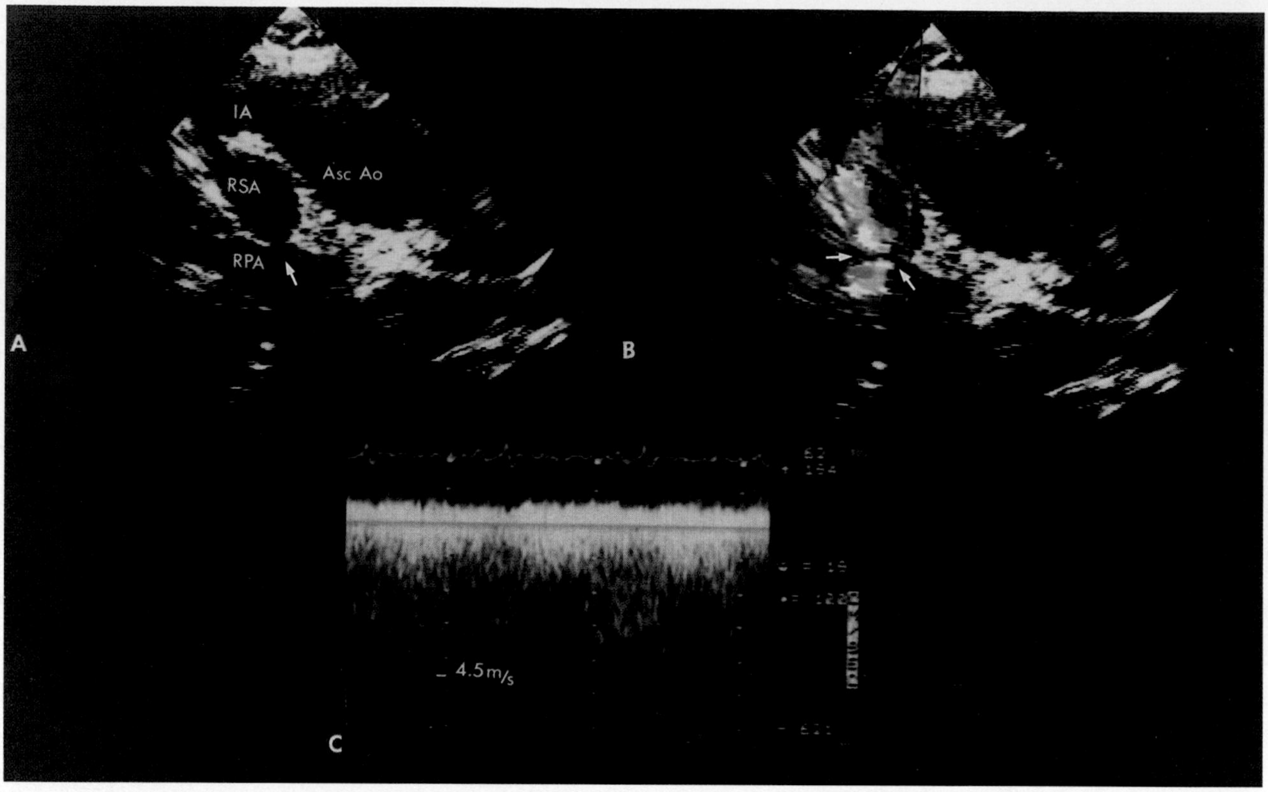

Fig. 32–9. Echocardiographic views of a right Blalock Taussig shunt. **A.** A suprasternal notch echocardiographic view of the ascending aorta demonstrates the origin of the innominate artery and the point where the right subclavian artery has been turned down and anastomosed to the right pulmonary artery. The anastomotic site is restrictive (small arrow). **B.** Color flow Doppler is superimposed on the two-dimensional image. The flow stream narrows at the restricted anastomosis (double arrow). **C.** A continuous wave Doppler spectral profile of the shunt flow, with peak velocities of 4.5 m/sec, indicating a gradient of 80 mm Hg between aorta and right pulmonary artery. Asc Ao = ascending aorta; IA = innominate artery; RSA = right subclavian artery; RPA = right pulmonary artery.

sive shunt flow is an important part of the evaluation of univentricular heart, both as a guide to clinical management and as a determinant of future surgical options. Because the pulmonary arteries may be difficult to enter through the Blalock shunt during catheterization, a noninvasive method for assessing pulmonary artery pressures would be desirable. Continuous wave Doppler has been reported to be helpful in allowing one to predict the gradient between the systemic and pulmonary circuits.[26] The continuous wave probe is positioned over the right subclavicular area and is angled toward the right pulmonary artery as one searches for the highest velocity of continuous shunt flow (Fig. 32–9B). The same procedure can be applied over the left chest in the case of a left Blalock shunt and can be more centrally positioned for central shunts. With current instrumentation, an image-directed steerable continuous wave Doppler cursor helps with optimal alignment of the interrogating Doppler beam with the direction of the color flow jet through the shunt. The peak velocity obtained can then be used in the modified Bernoulli equation to estimate the pressure gradient between aortic and pulmonary circuits. It is obviously critical to ascertain the highest velocity present in the shunt flow because an underestimation in the peak velocity causes one to estimate a falsely high pulmonary artery pressure that might exclude a patient from further surgical consideration.

Pulmonary Artery Banding. Banding of the pulmonary artery has been the palliative procedure for patients with univentricular heart whose pathophysiologic feature is that of a large central mixing lesion with no restriction to pulmonary blood flow. The operative mortality is negligible and a 10-year survival of 74% has been reported with this procedure alone.[25] As results of newer operative procedures improve, the use of pulmonary artery banding for prolonged palliation in univentricular heart is coming under closer scrutiny.[18] At issue is the degree of hypertrophy that occurs in response to banding. Increasing hypertrophy of the main ventricular chamber leads to a stiffer, less compliant chamber with impaired diastolic function. This in turn creates a higher risk of a poor result if a subsequent Fontan procedure is contemplated[27,28] (see the discussion later in this chapter). In addition, muscular hypertrophy surrounding the outlet foramen can lead to progressive obstruction to outflow from the main ventricle to the great vessel that arises from the outlet chamber, most often the aorta. This complication is difficult to remedy primarily at the time of surgery and often requires a two-stage procedure to enlarge the ventricular septal defect (VSD) or a complex procedure anastomosing the proximal pulmonary artery to the ascending aorta to provide a vessel of adequate size for systemic outflow.[17]

Two-dimensional and Doppler echocardiography can

enable one to assess the band position and to determine the adequacy of restriction by estimating the peak gradient. Complications of banding such as pseudoaneurysm formation or branch pulmonary artery obstruction can also be detected echocardiographically.[29,30]

Septation. In attempting more corrective than palliative surgical approaches, some centers have used ventricular septation for the treatment of certain subgroups of univentricular heart. This procedure, in which an artificial septum is supplied to subdivide the single chamber into two separately functioning ventricles, requires that the patient have two AV valves or a common valve that can be subdivided. The initial in-hospital mortality has been high (36 to 45%),[25,31] and most patients require a permanent pacemaker for surgically induced complete heart block. The in-hospital mortality falls to more acceptable levels (6%)[6] if only ideal candidates are selected: those with a single left ventricle of moderate size with two competent AV valves, a left-sided aorta, and not enough pulmonary stenosis to require a conduit.

Fontan Procedure. In 1971, Fontan and Baudet first reported a procedure for right ventricular exclusion with direct connection of systemic venous return to the pulmonary artery for correction of tricuspid atresia.[32] Modifications of this approach are advocated as the most physiologically desirable long-term means of correction for univentricular hearts. As currently performed, the modified Fontan procedure diverts right atrial venous return through a direct anastomosis or a nonvalved conduit to the pulmonary artery, with the exact mode of connection dictated by the individual patient's anatomy (Fig. 32–10). When two AV valves are present, the right AV valve may be oversewn or patch occluded, allowing the blind right atrium to serve as a reservoir for systemic venous return. The proximal pulmonary artery is oversewn, and the distal pulmonary circuit is connected with the right atrium. The systemic and pulmonary circuits are thereby completely separated, removing the adverse effects of arterial desaturation and ventricular volume overload. In this configuration, pulmonary blood flow must perforce occur without a ventricular pump and must rely on right atrial pressure, with or without atrial contraction, changes in intrathoracic pressure during respiration, and a low pulmonary vascular resistance to achieve forward flow.

More recent modifications of Fontan's procedure have been made and are referred to as a bicaval pulmonary anastomosis or total cavopulmonary connection. This modification can be made in two steps, to exclude the right ventricle in stages, or in one step with a fenestrated atrial channel to allow decompression of the systemic venous pathway.[33] In this surgical approach, the main pulmonary artery is transected, and the superior vena cava is anastomosed to the right pulmonary artery to create a bidirectional Glenn shunt. This allows venous return from the head and upper extremities to flow directly into the pulmonary artery, thereby relieving a portion of the volume load on the ventricle. The junction of the superior vena cava and the right atrium is temporarily occluded with a patch. Inferior caval return still

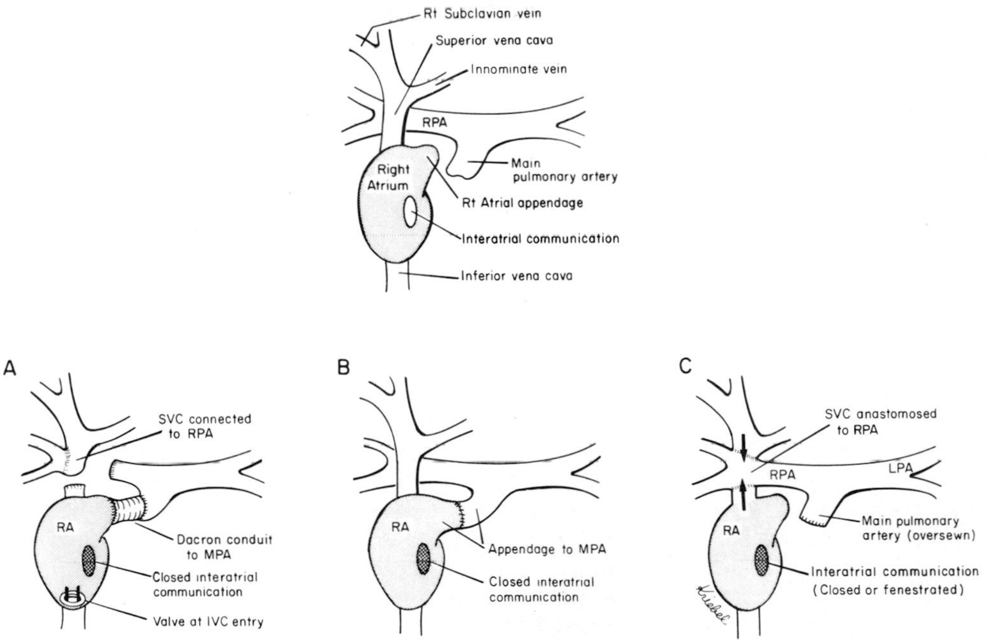

Fig. 32–10. Methods for right ventricular exclusion used in the Fontan procedure. Top. The normal relationships of right atrium (RA), venae cavae, and pulmonary artery. **A.** The original Fontan procedure is depicted employing a Glenn shunt, a valve at the inferior vena caval (IVC) entry to the RA and a prosthetic conduit to connect the RA to the pulmonary artery. This technique was modified to that shown in **B,** requiring no prosthetic materials but utilizing the right atrial appendage to create a passage for flow from RA to the pulmonary circuit. **C.** A more recent modification that may be performed in stages, referred to as a *bicaval-pulmonary artery anastomosis.* The superior vena cava (SVC) is first connected to the right pulmonary artery (RPA) similar to a bidirectional Glenn shunt. In the second stage, the inferior caval flow is then directed through the RA, into the SVC, and thence into the RPA. IVC = inferior vena cava; MPA = main pulmonary artery; LPA = left pulmonary artery. (Modified from Sapire DW: Understanding and Diagnosing Pediatric Heart Disease. Norwalk, CT, Appleton & Lange, 1991.

enters the right atrium and the single ventricle at this stage. The second stage then consists of creating a channel within the right atrium to direct inferior vena caval flow to the pulmonary artery through the junction of the superior vena cava and the right atrium once the temporary patch is removed. When two AV valves are present, the interatrial septum is widely resected so pulmonary venous flow can pass unobstructed through either AV valve (Fig. 32–11A).

Evaluation of the patient with univentricular heart thus must address the potential for a successful Fontan palliation: adequate pulmonary artery size and confluence, low pulmonary artery pressures, competent systemic AV valves, good ventricular function with low ventricular end-diastolic pressure, and no obstruction to ventricular outflow at the outlet foramen.[14]

Echocardiographic and Doppler evaluation of postoperative anatomy and physiology is also important after a Fontan procedure. Persistent pericardial and pleural effusions are common in the early postoperative period because filling pressures must be kept high in the right atrium to facilitate forward pulmonary blood flow. The blind right atrium is frequently dilated, with deviation of the interatrial septum into the left atrium. The oversewn or patch-closed tricuspid orifice should be inspected for persistent communication or patch dehiscence because this would be a source of systemic desaturation. In the case of an intra-atrial channel, one can also detect residual shunts by color flow Doppler by carefully searching the interface between systemic and pulmonary venous circuits. The communication between right atrium and pulmonary artery may be visualized echocardiographically in modified parasternal, right parasternal, and suprasternal views; one seeks the plane in which the right atrial appendage or anterior right atrial surface interfaces with the main pulmonary artery or its bifurcation (Fig. 32–11B). Subcostal windows visualizing the right atrium and distal pulmonary artery are also

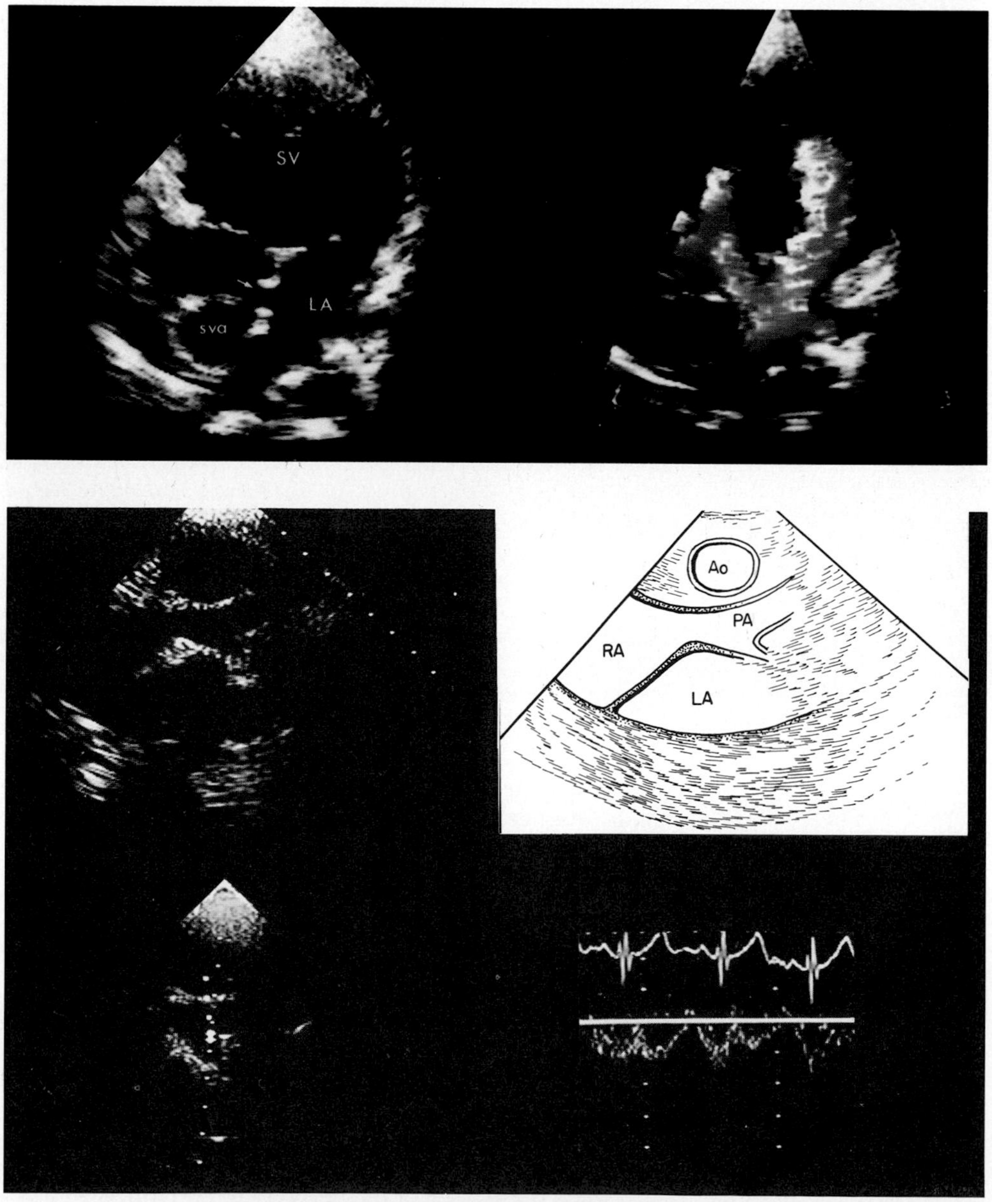

Fig. 32–11. A. Apical echocardiographic view of a child with univentricular heart following a modified Fontan repair. Left. A tunnel within the right atrium (sva) directs the systemic venous return from the inferior vena cava through the right atrium toward the superior vena cava. An atrial septal defect (arrow) was created to allow pulmonary venous flow to pass unimpeded through either right or left atrioventricular valve, as shown in color on the right. SV = single ventricular chamber, LA = left atrium; sva = systemic venous atrium. **B.** Parasternal echocardiographic view of a patient with univentricular heart following the Fontan procedure. Beneath the ascending aorta, the connection between right atrial appendage and pulmonary artery can be seen (top, left). Bottom, left. The pulsed Doppler sample volume is placed in the left pulmonary artery and detects the low velocity forward flow. The biphasic pattern includes forward flow with atrial contraction, a return to baseline, and then a smaller additional forward flow component with ventricular systole. Ao = aorta; LA = left atrium; RA = right atrium; PA = pulmonary artery.

useful in smaller children. Right parasternal views of the superior vena cava and right pulmonary artery are needed to assess the staged Fontan procedure.

Because of the many possible individual anatomic variations, it is critical to know the specific details of each surgical repair to successfully evaluate the patient postoperatively. Pulsed Doppler flow profiles in the pulmonary artery with a normally functioning Fontan repair show a biphasic forward flow pattern in the pulmonary artery beginning in early ventricular diastole (end of T wave) and peaking during atrial systole (end of P wave), with a second peak during ventricular systole[34,35] (Fig. 32–11B). Thus, pulmonary flow occurs because of active atrial contraction in atrial systole and passive flow during atrial diastole, the latter perhaps assisted by mechanical movement of the underlying ventricle. Considering the absence of a valve to prevent reverse flow, surprisingly little pulmonary regurgitation is seen. Some degree of pulmonary regurgitant flow has been detected using intracardiac velocity probes following the R wave on the ECG, but the flow is low in velocity and may be missed with pulsed Doppler sampling.[34]

Hypoplastic Right Heart Complex

Hypoplasia of the right heart encompasses a spectrum of abnormal right ventricular development that may affect any of the three segments of the right heart: (1) the tricuspid valve and inlet portion of the ventricle; (2) the trabecular or muscular apical segment of the ventricle; and (3) the outlet or infundibular portion and pulmonary valve. In its mildest expression, one sees generalized hypoplasia of the right ventricle with a small tricuspid annulus and relatively normal infundibulum and pulmonary valve.[36,37] The most extreme form of this complex includes the well-known entities of pulmonary atresia with intact ventricular septum and tricuspid atresia (Fig. 32–12). (Tricuspid atresia is discussed as a separate entity under AV valve abnormalities later in this chapter.)

The hemodynamic and clinical findings in this complex vary with the size of the right ventricle and the relative degree of obstruction to inflow and outflow. Nearly all patients have a restriction to right ventricular filling from a small tricuspid annulus, from tricuspid stenosis, or from a hypertrophied noncompliant ventricle. In addition, an interatrial communication is almost invariably present, allowing right-to-left shunt and resultant cyanosis.

Echocardiographic evaluation requires careful assessment of the presence and size of the three components of the right ventricle, the adequacy of the interatrial communication, the exact nature of the pulmonary valve obstruction, the size and confluence of the distal pulmonary arteries, and the patency of the ductus arteriosus or other aortopulmonary collaterals supplying flow to the pulmonary bed (Fig. 32–13).

Right Ventricle

The size of the right ventricle and the presence or absence of each of the three components of that chamber are important to assess echocardiographically because they affect the type of surgical procedure that is possible

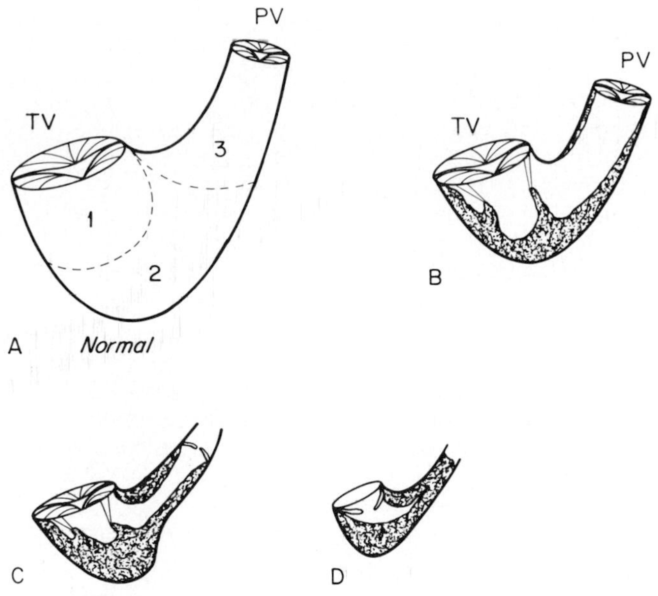

Fig. 32–12. Degrees of hypoplasia of the right ventricle. **A.** The three segments of the normal right ventricle are demonstrated: (1) the inlet portion, (2) the trabecular segment, and (3) the infundibular portion. **B.** Hypoplasia of the trabecular segment with a relatively normal inlet and outlet segment. **C.** The trabecular and infundibular segments are hypoplastic with valvular pulmonic stenosis. **D.** The most severe form with pulmonic valvular and infundibular atresia and a hypoplastic tricuspid valve. PV = pulmonic valve; TV = tricuspid valve.

and the potential for postoperative growth of the right ventricle. The right ventricular sinus is a relatively smooth-walled portion of the chamber that incorporates the tricuspid valve apparatus and whose size correlates closely with tricuspid annular size. The trabecular portion of the ventricle contains the papillary muscles and the apical musculature. This portion is often deficient by virtue of muscular hypertrophy that effectively obliterates the apical section.[38] The infundibulum or outlet portion of the right ventricle constitutes that segment between the crista supraventricularis and the pulmonary valve. The extent to which this portion is functionally patent is a crucial determinant of the ability to achieve forward flow through the right heart surgically.

Quantifying the degree of hypoplasia of the right ventricle has been attempted in several ways. One method has used the Simpson's rule formulation to right ventricular angiograms in patients with pulmonary atresia/intact ventricular septum for determination of right ventricular volumes and has compared their results to predicted norms.[39,40] Other investigators have made the observation that tricuspid annular size correlates well with right ventricular size and have made angiographic[38] or echocardiographic[41] measurements of tricuspid annular dimensions as an indication of deviation from expected normal. Despite the availability of quantitative methods to assess the degree of hypoplasia, no accepted minimal ventricular volume ensures the ability of the right ventricle to handle the entire cardiac output successfully. The functional status of the tricuspid valve and the compliance of the severely hypertrophied cham-

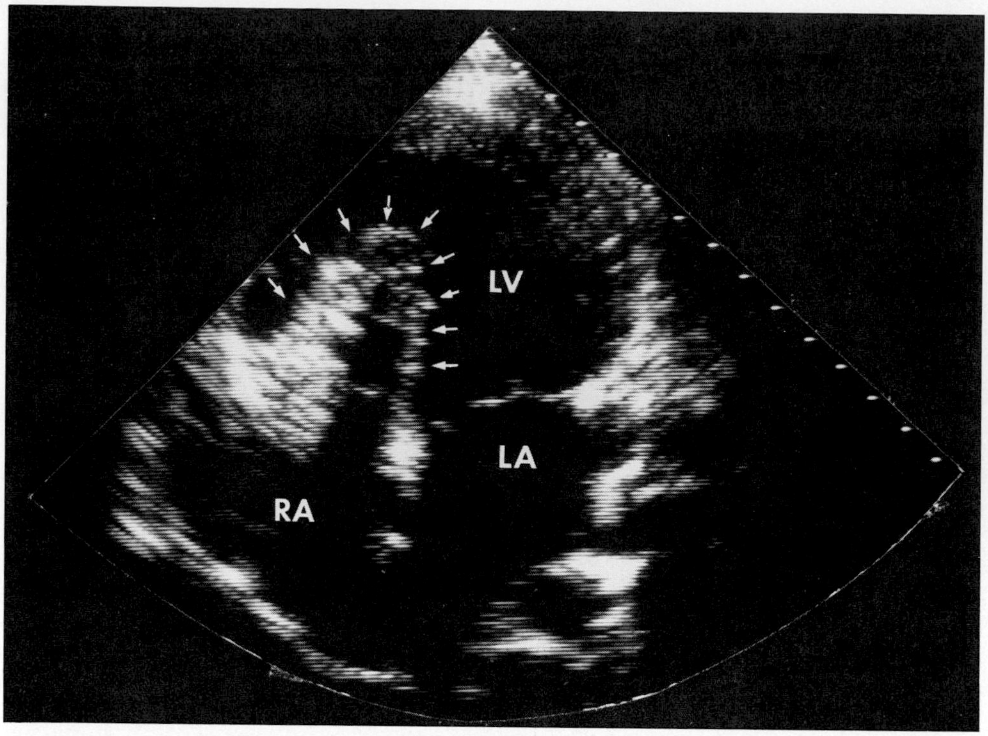

Fig. 32–13. Apical echocardiographic view in a patient with hypoplastic right ventricle. The tricuspid valve is minute with a tiny inlet portion of the right ventricle present. The trabecular portion is hypertrophied. The left ventricle has become distorted in shape and forms a diverticulum around the nubbin of a right ventricular chamber (arrows). LA = left atrium; LV = left ventricle; RA = right atrium.

ber may contribute as significantly to the adequacy of right ventricular function as the absolute volume. Adding to the hypertrophic component of compliance is the frequent finding of endocardial fibroelastosis and sclerosis. Early surgical relief of pulmonary atresia and decompression of the hypertensive ventricle may help to minimize the degree of endocardial fibrosis.[42]

Myocardial Sinusoids

About 35% of patients with hypoplastic right heart have prominent sinusoidal channels that may end blindly within the myocardium but also may connect the right ventricular chamber and the coronary arterial circulation.[43–45] Those hearts with an atretic or severely stenotic pulmonary valve and a competent tricuspid valve are most likely to have sinusoid formation because of the striking hypertension in the obstructed right ventricle. When ventriculocoronary communication is present, it is often to the more distal ramifications of the left anterior descending coronary artery. Physiologically, this situation results in retrograde flow of systemic venous blood from the right ventricle through the sinusoids and into the left coronary system during systole. Areas of coronary stenosis and dysplasia also contribute to the high incidence of ischemia and infarction in this group of patients.[43] One case report has described an infant with extensive ventriculocoronary connections who developed right ventricular necrosis and cardiac rupture.[46] Several cases have been described in which the proximal coronary arterial system was absent, and all coronary perfusion derived from ventriculocoronary sinusoidal channels.[43,47,48] There are as yet no echocardiographic reports of visualization of sinusoids, ventriculocoronary connections, or absent proximal coronary arteries. With the increasing sophistication of this technique, however, especially color flow Doppler, it should be possible to detect such abnormal channels and to note anomalies of the proximal coronary vessels. In fact, diagnosis of ventriculocoronary communication might be made by injecting intravenous agitated saline and then echocardiographically monitoring the patient for myocardial contrast in the affected regions.

Tricuspid Valve

The tricuspid valve in hypoplastic right heart complex is often small but has the usual leaflet and chordal architecture and frequently is competent.[49] Although the structure may appear normal, the diminutive annulus, shortened chordae tendineae, and hypoplastic papillary muscles can present a major impediment to right ventricular filling, and sometimes constitute the limiting lesion despite surgical relief of outflow obstruction at the pulmonic valve level.[42] In some instances, the leaflet margins are thickened and rolled with shortened or fused chordae, resulting in moderate or severe tricuspid regurgitation. The presence of tricuspid insufficiency causes right ventricular volume loading and consequently a larger ventricular size than in hearts with a competent valve. A few patients may have an Ebsteinlike malformation with a variable degree of apical displacement of leaflet attachment and adherence of leaflets to the myocardium[50] (Fig. 32–14). Two-dimensional echocardiography allows one clearly to define the anatomic details of the tricuspid apparatus,[41] and pulsed and color flow Doppler techniques demonstrate valve patency and the presence of regurgitation.

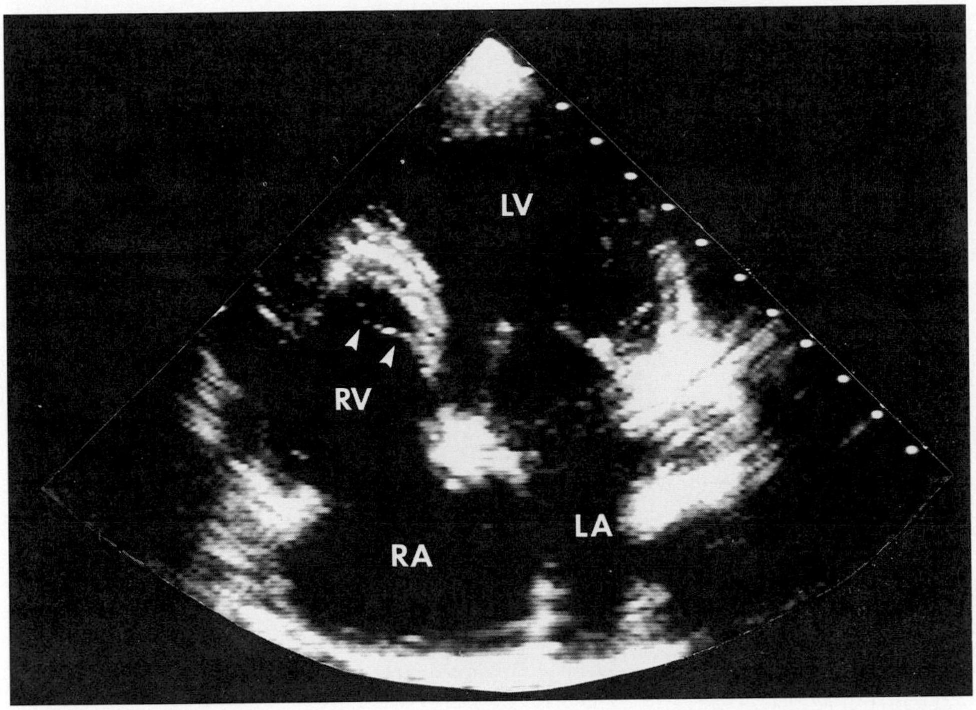

Fig. 32–14. Apical echocardiographic view in a patient with hypoplastic right ventricle and Ebstein's malformation of the tricuspid valve. The tricuspid leaflets are markedly displaced into the right ventricle and bound to the septum and lateral wall (double arrowheads). LA = left atrium; LV = left ventricle; RA = right atrium; RV = right ventricle.

Pulmonary Artery and Valve

The pulmonary valve varies from normal to completely atretic. In about one third of patients with pulmonary atresia, pulmonary valve leaflets are identifiable but not patent. In the remainder, a solid fibrous ridge or a thick fibromuscular segment forms the terminus of the right ventricular infundibulum[51] (Fig. 32–12). Two-dimensional imaging and Doppler flow assessment of the patency of the right ventricular outflow tract and pulmonic valve provide valuable information for surgical planning. The main pulmonary artery segment and branches are generally present and confluent, although diminutive. Their size is often larger than in severe tetralogy of Fallot with pulmonary atresia. The main pulmonary artery and branches can be accurately measured from two-dimensional images obtained in parasternal and suprasternal notch views.[52,53] In the normal term neonate, the main pulmonary artery is usually 6 to 12 mm, and the right and left branches are 4 to 8 mm in diameter.[52]

Pulmonary artery size and, of course, neonatal survival are determined by the presence of a patent ductus arteriosus, which provides the entire pulmonary blood supply. Ductal flow is readily assessed by color flow mapping from parasternal, suprasternal, or subcostal views in which the pulmonary arteries and aortic arch are imaged. The ductus is often a long, tortuous channel that may be difficult to visualize in its entirety in a single plane.

Atrial Septum

Right-to-left shunting at the atrial level is necessary for survival in patients with hypoplastic right ventricle and severe or complete obstruction to pulmonary blood flow. The interatrial shunt occurs through a stretched patent foramen ovale or secundum ASD in the majority of cases. In some instances, the atrial communication may be too small and may thereby restrict flow.[36] The resultant aneurysmal deviation or herniation of the foramen flap can be clearly imaged echocardiographically and may result in increased flow velocities by pulsed Doppler[21] (Fig. 32–15). Rarely, the atrial septum is intact, in which case a fenestration between coronary sinus and left atrium allows right-to-left shunting.[36] Another frequently associated feature is a prominent eustachian valve within the enlarged hypertrophied right atrium. This feature has led several investigators to postulate that excessive diversion of caval blood across the foramen ovale by this eustachian valve in early fetal life may be responsible for resultant hypoplasia of the right heart.[54,55]

Surgical Management

The initial surgical approach to patients with hypoplastic right ventricle is directed at increasing pulmonary blood flow, preferably by creating continuity from right ventricle to pulmonary artery. This approach provides the best opportunity for subsequent right ventricular and pulmonary artery growth. In recent years, the use of prostaglandins to maintain ductal patency has contributed significantly to the improvement in early surgical mortality.[56] Prostaglandins stabilize the infant's condition before surgery and, in the perioperative period, can continue to provide a temporary supplemental source of pulmonary flow through the ductus.

When all three portions of the ventricle are present, and when the tricuspid annulus is of adequate size to transport total systemic venous return, a complete re-

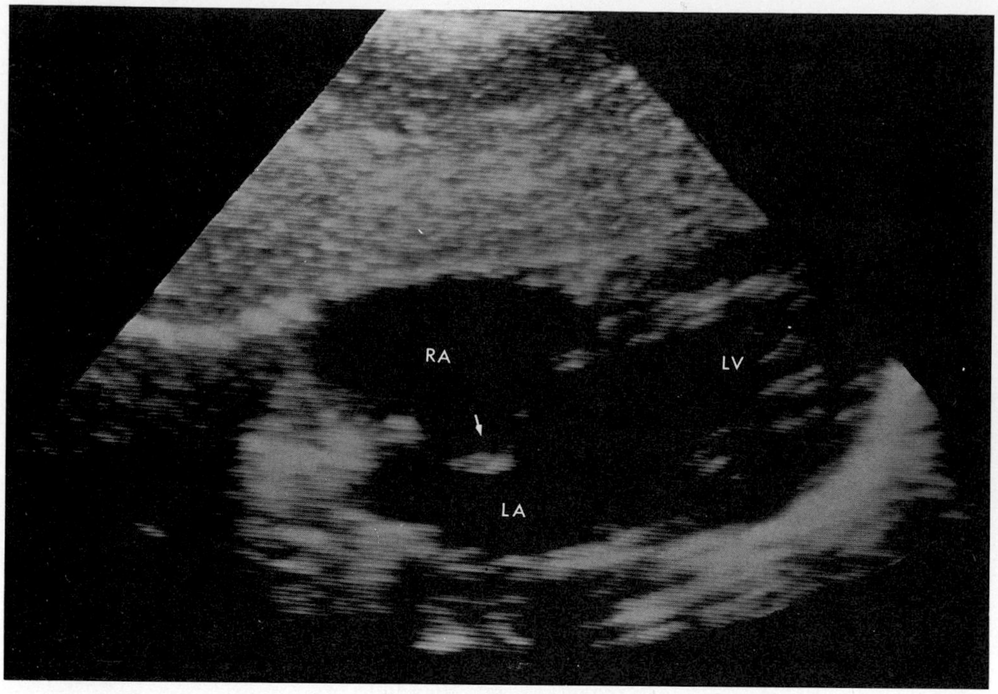

Fig. 32–15. Subcostal view of the interatrial septum in a patient with hypoplasia of the right ventricle. The flap of the foramen ovale bows markedly into the left atrium (LA) (arrow), reflecting right atrial hypertension and right-to-left shunt. LV = left ventricle; RA = right atrium.

pair can be performed in infancy, consisting of pulmonary valvotomy, patch enlargement of the right ventricular infundibulum, ASD closure, and ductal ligation.

If the right ventricle is tripartite but of insufficient size to support pulmonary blood flow independently, a pulmonary valvotomy along with a systemic-to-pulmonary shunt (Blalock-Taussig or central shunt) will provide increased pulmonary blood flow through the shunt while also promoting forward flow through the right heart. If the right ventricle grows, definitive repair can be attempted later.

The usual surgical method of valvotomy for the atretic or severely stenotic pulmonary valve has been a closed transventricular approach or a transpulmonary approach under direct vision. The development of balloon valvuloplasty techniques has promoted recent interest in balloon dilatation of the pulmonary valve in patients with a relatively discrete, membranous form of atresia or severe pulmonic stenosis. Intraoperative balloon dilatation to establish continuity from right ventricle to pulmonary artery has been successfully reported as an initial procedure in neonates.[57]

In infants in whom right heart hypoplasia is severe and the infundibulum is absent, systemic-to-pulmonary shunting alone is the only surgical alternative. If subsequent pulmonary flow is adequate without being excessive, the child may then be considered for a Fontan procedure at a later date.

Two-dimensional and Doppler echocardiography in the perioperative and postoperative period should address the status of blood flow through the small right ventricle and across the surgically widened outflow tract. Pulsed and color flow Doppler can also assist in verifying the patency of aortopulmonary shunts and in detecting tricuspid regurgitation. When the foramen ovale has been left open as a potential relief for postoperative right heart failure, Doppler assessment of shunting and saline contrast study to document right-to-left shunt contribute to an understanding of the complex hemodynamics immediately after surgery.

Serial volumetric assessments of the right ventricle and tricuspid valve annular dimensions by two-dimensional echocardiography are important in the long-term follow-up of survivors of initial palliative procedures. If right heart growth occurs and right ventricular volumes and tricuspid annular size approach 50% of normal, complete repair of the palliated state will be indicated. Patients whose ventricles fail to grow after palliation would then be potential candidates for a surgical treatment that excludes the right ventricle, such as the Fontan procedure.[39,56] Echocardiographic assessment of the Fontan procedure was discussed previously in this chapter.

Hypoplastic Left Heart

Hypoplastic left heart syndrome is a spectrum of disorders associated with underdevelopment of the inflow and outflow portions of the left heart. Its expression varies in severity from aortic and mitral atresia with only a slitlike left ventricular chamber to milder degrees of mitral and aortic stenosis and aortic coarctation. Investigators have speculated that premature closure or inhibited flow across the foramen ovale in fetal life might be responsible for such hypoplasia of the left heart,[58] although preliminary echo-Doppler observations of fetuses with hypoplastic left heart have not consistently shown premature closure of the foramen.[59]

The classic constellation of features in hypoplastic left heart syndrome includes aortic atresia, mitral atresia or hypoplasia, a diminutive left ventricle, and severe hypoplasia of the ascending aorta. The infant usually is seen within the first 24 to 36 hours of life with tachypnea, tachycardia, cardiomegaly, and progressive cardiogenic shock. The work of the entire circulation is performed by the right ventricle; perfusion to the head and coronary arteries is retrograde to the ascending aorta through the ductus arteriosus, and perfusion to the lower body is anterograde through the ductus to the descending aorta. Physiologic closure of the ductus leads to rapid deterioration. The prognosis is uniformly fatal within hours to days, but longer periods of survival are possible with lesser degrees of hypoplasia or continued ductal patency. Until recent years, little could be done for such infants other than supportive care. Because limited success has now been reported with palliative surgery, however, several centers are actively including these patients as surgical candidates.[60–64] In addition, because of the progress made in cardiac transplantation in children, hypoplastic left heart syndrome is now an indication for receipt of a donor organ.[65]

Left Ventricle

The accurate identification of all the component anomalies in this complex becomes more critical because of the surgical options available. In the earliest period of noninvasive diagnosis, M-mode echocardiography allowed detection of the small left ventricular cavity, diminutive aortic root, and presence or absence of aortic and mitral valve leaflet motion.[66,67] Criteria for hypoplasia were an internal dimension smaller than 9 mm for the left ventricle and smaller than 6 mm for the aorta. The M-mode echocardiogram thus allowed one to differentiate rapidly between the neonate in congestive heart failure or shock due to hypoplastic left heart syndrome from the neonate whose condition had other causes such as severe coarctation, critical aortic stenosis, sepsis, or cardiomyopathy, because the latter group of disorders is characterized by normal to large left ventricles when assessed by M-mode measurement.

Two-dimensional echocardiography and Doppler can now provide additional precision in diagnosing hypoplastic left heart syndrome. The left ventricle may be slitlike and difficult to locate on standard parasternal long axis views because of the dominant right ventricle. Care must be taken to avoid mistaking large hypertrophied right ventricular muscle bundles for the interventricular septum (Fig. 32–16). A parasternal cross section at the ventricular level often demonstrates more clearly a thick-walled walnut-sized cavity appended to the posterolateral aspect of the markedly dilated right ventricle (Fig. 32–17A). On occasion, the absolute internal dimension of the left ventricle, as measured in the standard parasternal long axis view, falls in the range of normal. This finding causes some consternation in deciding whether such an infant belongs in the hypoplastic left heart category, particularly when the patient has a patent aortic valve and only mild hypoplasia of the aortic root. Two-dimensional imaging often demonstrates a foreshortening of the left ventricular cavity from apex to base, thickened myocardium with reduced contractility, and echogenic endocardium suggestive of endocardial fibroelastosis, however (Fig. 32–17B). This finding has led to the recommendation to use left ventricular cavity area as the criterion for determining hypoplasia;[68] ventricles measuring less than 1.6 cm^2 in parasternal long axis area are of insufficient size for long-term survival, and those measuring 1.6 to 1.8 cm^2 are marginally capable of sustaining a systemic workload.

Mitral Valve

Mitral valve morphology in this syndrome varies from mitral atresia to congenital mitral stenosis to a diminu-

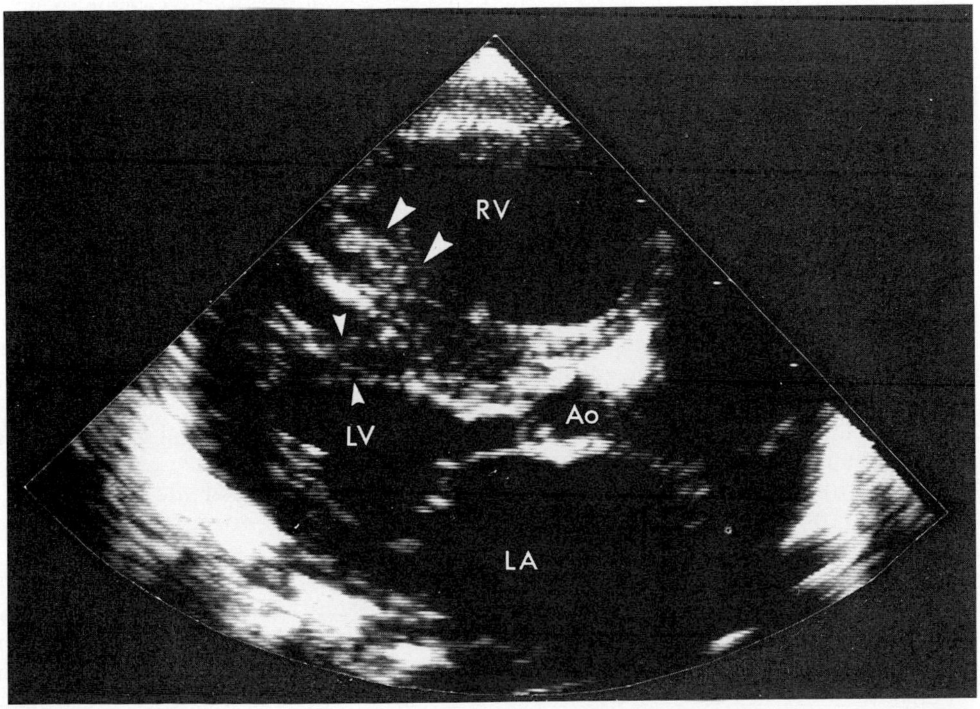

Fig. 32–16. Echocardiographic illustration of hypoplastic left ventricle. In this parasternal long axis projection, the left ventricle, left ventricular outflow tract, aortic annulus, and ascending aorta are all hypoplastic. The right ventricle is enlarged with a prominent muscle band (large double arrowheads), which might be mistaken for the interventricular septum (small double arrowheads). Ao = aorta; LA = left atrium; LV = left ventricle; RV = right ventricle.

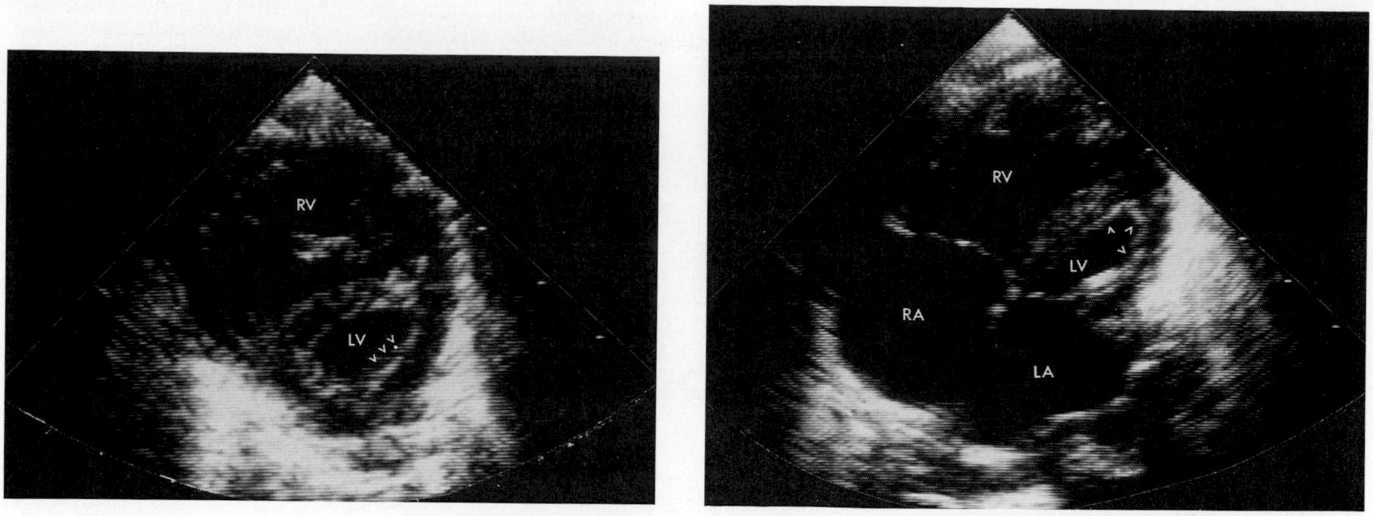

A B

Fig. 32–17. Echocardiographic images in a patient with a hypoplastic left ventricle. **A.** A cross-sectional view at the ventricular level showing marked discrepancy between right and left ventricular sizes. The endocardium of the left ventricle is echo dense, consistent with endocardial fibroelastosis (small arrowheads). **B.** An apical view demonstrating the foreshortening of the left ventricular cavity and, again, endocardial thickening (arrowheads). LA = left atrium; LV = left ventricle; RA = right atrium; RV = right ventricle.

tive but normal valve apparatus. Two-dimensional imaging accurately depicts valve motion and chordal and papillary muscle configuration.[69] Pulsed Doppler and color flow mapping can allow one to detect forward flow across a patent mitral valve and regurgitant flow, which often occurs when the patient has aortic atresia with no egress for blood from the hypoplastic ventricle. In milder forms of left ventricular hypoplasia, the detection of hemodynamic manifestations of mitral stenosis on initial echocardiographic evaluation may be problematic. Thickened valve leaflets, shortened chordae, and close apposition of leaflets to the papillary muscles are the morphologic basis for congenital mitral stenosis and are present at the outset. Classic pulsed Doppler patterns of increased peak and mean velocities and prolonged velocity half-time may not be present in the neonate, however. Severe outflow obstruction and small left ventricular stroke volumes may delay the appearance of these typical features of mitral stenosis until aortic stenosis or coarctation has been relieved.

Aortic Valve

The aortic valve in the majority of instances is atretic,[70] with a membranous covering across a small aortic annulus or miniature valve cusps that are fused. The valve can be mobile in response to underlying cardiac events, yet not be patent. Pulsed Doppler techniques allow one to detect the presence of and direction of flow in the ascending aorta. In patients with a markedly hypoplastic aorta, sampling within the root is difficult, and forward flow from the adjacent large pulmonary artery can be mistakenly perceived as aortic flow. Color flow mapping often clarifies the ambiguity by displaying a turbulent jet if forward aortic flow is present, by showing low velocity retrograde flow from the ductus in the case of aortic atresia, and also be clearly defining the pulmonary artery flow stream. Additional caution is advised to avoid mistaking a large innominate vein and superior vena cava for the ascending aorta and transverse arch (Fig. 32–18).

When the aortic valve is not atretic, it may be bicuspid (45%), tricuspid (30%), or unicuspid (25%), with varying degrees of stenosis. Severe stenosis with hypoplastic annulus and ascending aorta does not lend itself to any specific therapy directed to the aortic valve. In patients with less severe hypoplasia, balloon valvuloplasty has been used either to improve clinical status preoperatively or as a primary therapeutic procedure. Despite a higher risk in these critically ill neonates, a recent series reports more than half the newborns with congenital aortic stenosis achieved a greater than 50% reduction in gradient with only a modest increase in aortic regurgitation.[71]

Aortic Arch

The ascending aorta exhibits tubular hypoplasia and appears stringlike (Fig. 32–19). At the level of the transverse arch, the aorta widens as it receives retrograde flow from the ductus destined for the brachiocephalic vessels. The prevalence of true coarctation in hypoplastic left heart syndrome varies with the criteria applied for diagnosing coarctation. Nearly all patients have isthmic narrowing at the site of ductal entry that may become hemodynamically significant after ductal closure. The presence of a posterior ledge extending across the aortic lumen is less frequent. Regardless of the type of constriction, it is usually necessary to enlarge the aortic isthmus as part of surgical palliation.[72,73]

In echocardiographic evaluation, attention should also be directed to the right ventricle and pulmonary arteries. Dysfunction of the right ventricle or tricuspid and pulmonary valves significantly impairs the chances for success of a surgical procedure in which the right ventricle assumes systemic work.

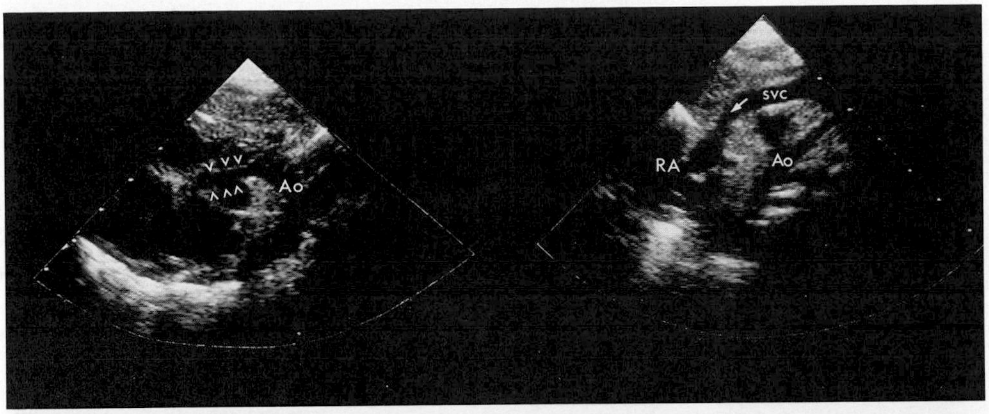

Fig. 32–18. Echocardiographic views of the aorta from the suprasternal window. Left. The hypoplastic ascending aorta is demarcated by arrowheads. The caliber of the arch increases at the brachiocephalic vessels and descending aorta as a result of retrograde flow provided by the ductus. Right. The large innominate vein and superior vena cava (arrow) can be misinterpreted as an ascending aorta. The transverse and descending aorta can be seen in a more posterior plane. Ao = aorta; RA = right atrium; SVC = superior vena cava.

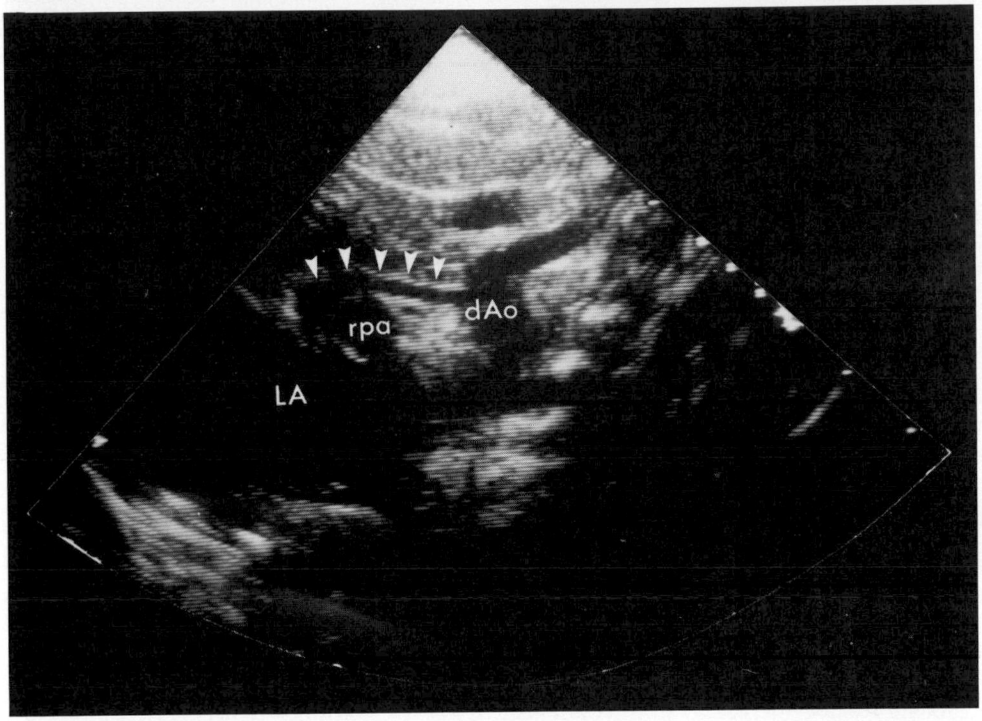

Fig. 32–19. Suprasternal echocardiographic view of the aorta in hypoplastic left heart syndrome. The ascending aorta is stringlike (arrowheads) but expands in its transverse and descending portions. dAo = descending aorta; LA = left atrium; rpa = right pulmonary artery.

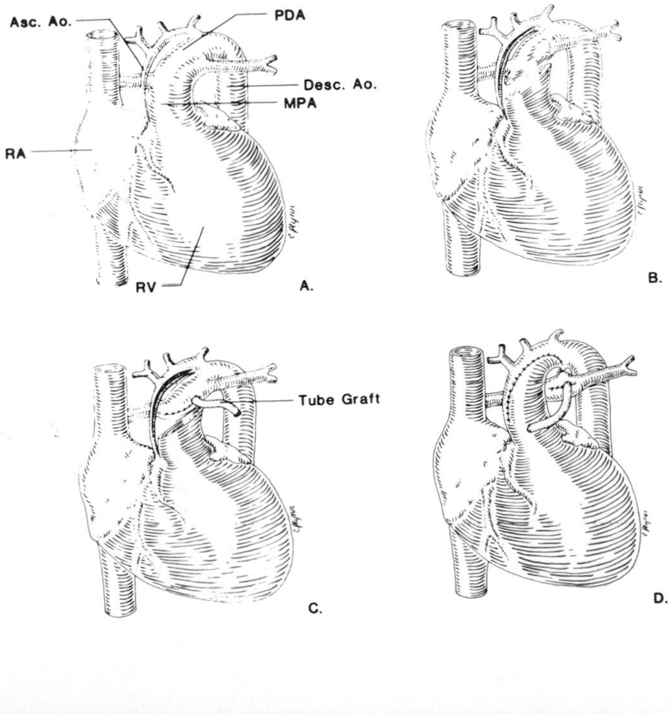

Fig. 32–20. The first stage of surgical repair of hypoplastic left heart syndrome. **A.** The hypoplastic ascending aorta is shown adjacent to the dilated main pulmonary artery. The large ductus arteriosus forms a continuum directly from pulmonary trunk to descending aorta. **B.** A longitudinal incision is made in the ascending aorta, and the main pulmonary artery is transsected. **C.** The branch pulmonary arteries are segregated from the main pulmonary artery, and a central tube graft is sewn into their confluence. **D.** The proximal main pulmonary artery is sutured to the filleted ascending aorta, and the remaining end of the tube graft is attached to the new ascending aorta. Asc Ao = ascending aorta; Desc Ao = descending aorta; MPA = main pulmonary aorta; PDA = patent ductus arteriosus; RA = right atrium; RV = right ventricle. (From Lang P, Norwood WI: Hemodynamic assessment after palliative surgery for hypoplastic left heart syndrome. Circulation 68:104, 1983. Reproduced by permission of the American Heart Association, Inc.)

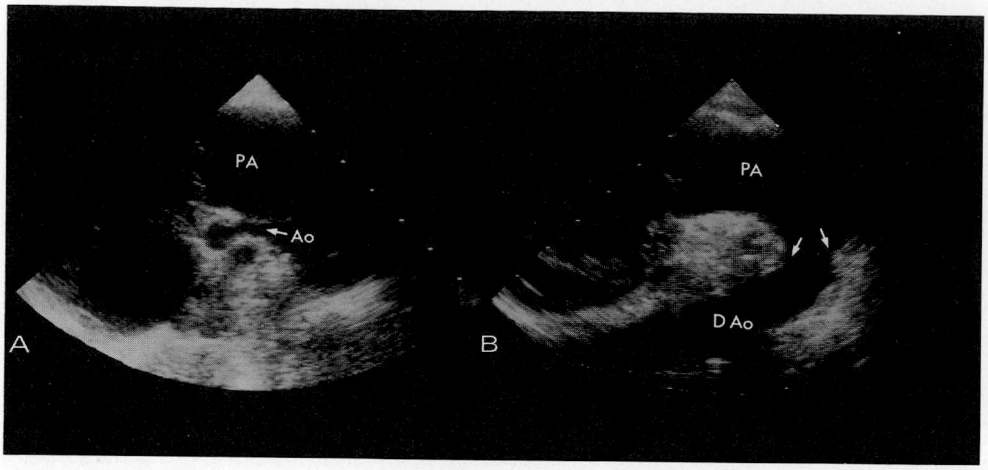

Fig. 32–21. Parasternal echocardiographic views of the neoaorta following the Norwood procedure for repair of hypoplastic left heart syndrome. **A.** The pulmonary artery and pulmonic valve now serve as the systemic semilunar valve and root. The hypoplastic proximal aorta can be seen posteriorly as it merges with the posterior border of the pulmonary artery. **B.** The anastomosis between proximal pulmonary artery (augmented with supplemental patch material) and descending aorta is shown (arrows). There is no obstruction at this point, and the "aortic arch" has a remarkably normal appearance. Ao = aorta; DAo = descending aorta; PA = pulmonary artery.

Surgical Management

Efforts to provide surgical relief of hypoplastic left heart syndrome are directed toward using the right ventricle as the systemic pump, appropriating the main pulmonary artery as a replacement for the hypoplastic aorta, and providing for pulmonary blood flow passively from the right atrium directly to the branch pulmonary arteries in a Fontan-type procedure. The ability to perfuse the pulmonary circuit in this way, however, requires a low pulmonary vascular resistance, which is not present until later in infancy. Thus, the surgical approach is a two-stage procedure. In the first stage, the atrial septal communication is enlarged, allowing complete mixing of venous return. The main pulmonary artery is transected and the proximal portion anastomosed to the hypoplastic ascending aorta. The ductus arteriosus is closed, and a controlled central aortopulmonary shunt to the isolated branch pulmonary arteries is performed, to provide pulmonary blood flow (Figs. 32–20 and 32–21). The second stage, performed when the patient is about 12 to 24 months old, consists of removing the aortopulmonary shunt, ensuring unobstructed left atrial return to the tricuspid valve, and anastomosing the systemic venous return to the pulmonary arteries.[74] Because mortality for both stages of this procedure remains high (approximately 52% 1-year mortality for the first stage, 35% for the second[61,75]), surgical techniques for this lesion continue to evolve.

ABNORMALITIES OF ATRIOVENTRICULAR VALVES

Atrioventricular Septal Defects

AV septal defects, also known as AV canal or endocardial cushion defects, comprise a group of abnormalities characterized by a deficiency in the AV septum and aberrant formation of the AV valves. During embryologic development, the common AV canal of the primitive heart divides into separate left and right orifices by fusion of the superior and inferior endocardial cushions, which then join the developing atrial and ventricular septa to complete the division of the heart into its four distinct chambers. The mitral and tricuspid valve leaflets are then formed by contributions from the superior and inferior cushions, along with left and right lateral cushion components.[76] Failure of these events to follow their expected course results in anomalies that can be grouped into three categories: (1) complete AV canal defects, comprising about 20% of the total group; (2) partial AV canal defects, representing the majority of cases within this spectrum; and (3) transitional AV defects.

Complete Atrioventricular Canal

In the complete form of this malformation, the patient usually has a large ostium primum atrial septal defect. The remainder of the atrial septum is frequently normal, but ostium secundum defects and patency of the foramen ovale may occur. Common atrium is described in approximately 10% of patients with AV septal defects,[77,78] usually in association with the more complex forms of AV canal defects seen in asplenia or polysplenia syndromes.[79]

The inlet ventricular septum is deficient, with a "scooped out" appearance creating a large discrepancy between the lengths of the inlet and outlet septa. The VSD is large in the complete form of AV canal and may extend anteriorly to variable degrees into the membranous septum. Associated muscular VSD occur in 2 to 15% of cases and should be carefully searched for by echo-Doppler examination and/or angiography.[80]

The common AV orifice between atria and ventricles is oriented in a more directly anteroposterior and equiplanar fashion than are the mitral and tricuspid annuli in the normal heart. A five-leaflet valve surrounds the common orifice, consisting of a posterior bridging leaflet, a right lateral leaflet, left lateral leaflet, and two anterior leaflet components (Fig. 32–22). The posterior leaflet is common to both ventricles and has chordal attachments to the posteromedial papillary muscle on the left and the posterior papillary muscle on the right.

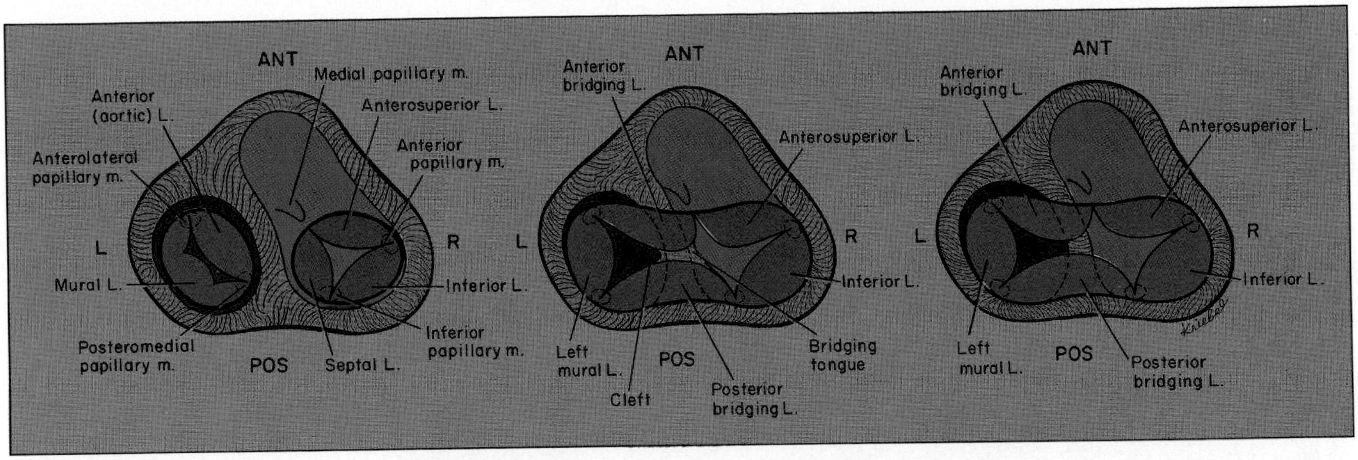

Fig. 32–22. The atrioventricular valve anatomy in the normal heart (left), the partial atrioventricular canal defect (middle), and the complete atrioventricular canal defect (right). The valves are presented as though viewed from the atria, looking into the ventricles. (The left ventricle is depicted in red, the right ventricle in purple, the interventricular septum and myocardium in brown). Left. Note the completed development of two separate atrioventricular valves. The mitral and tricuspid annuli are oriented at an angle to one another, and the anterior mitral leaflet has no association with the interventricular septum. Right. A complete atrioventricular canal defect, with both an anterior and posterior bridging leaflet which are shared between the two ventricles. The anterior leaflet has two components, the anterior and anterosuperior leaflets. There is a lateral portion of the common atrioventricular valve contributed from each ventricle—the left lateral and right lateral leaflets. Note that the plane of the atrioventricular orifice is horizontal, with equiplanar mitral and tricuspid annuli. Middle. A partial atrioventricular canal in which a tongue of tissue has connected the anterior and posterior bridging leaflets (shown in white), thereby creating two distinct atrioventricular orifices but without complete fusion of the anterior and posterior components of the mitral valve and without separation of the anterior leaflet from its attachment to the underlying interventricular septum. (Modified from Hurst JW, Anderson RH, Becker AE, Wilcox BR: Atlas of the Heart. New York, McGraw-Hill, 1988.)

It frequently has chordal attachments along the crest of the inlet septum.[81] This leaflet may be rudimentary, with thickened or curled edges, and thus may be responsible for severe AV valve regurgitation and problematic for the surgeon attempting to fashion a competent mitral valve. The left and right lateral leaflets are generally well developed and attach to the anterior and posterior papillary muscles in the appropriate ventricles in a normal manner. The left lateral leaflet corresponds to the posterior mitral leaflet of a normal valve, and the right lateral leaflet corresponds to the posterior tricuspid leaflet.[82]

The configuration of the two anterior leaflets has been used to classify complete AV canal into subgroups, the Rastelli types A, B, and C[83] (Fig. 32–23). In the type A pattern, the right and left anterior leaflets are equivalent

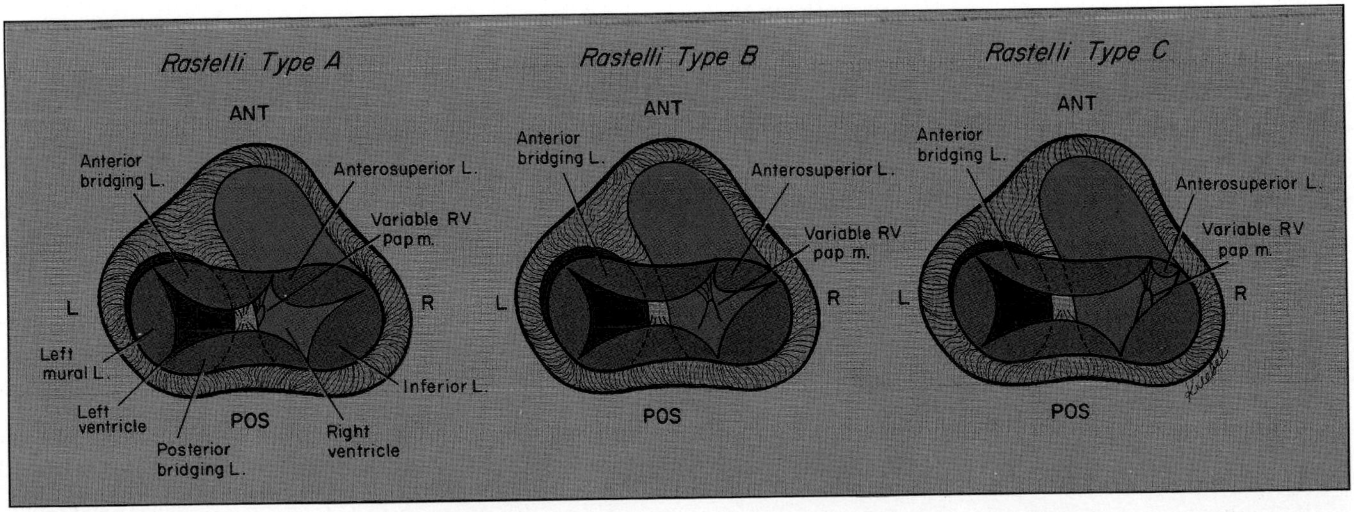

Fig. 32–23. Diagrammatic representation of the subclassification of complete atrioventricular canal defect based on the morphologic variations of the anterior bridging leaflet, the Rastelli typing. Left. The type A arrangement, with the two components of the anterior leaflet being of relatively equal size. Chordal attachments from each component insert onto the crest of the underlying interventricular septum. Middle. The type B atrioventricular canal shows a discrepancy in size of the two anterior leaflet portions, with the anterosuperior leaflet being underdeveloped. The larger portion is now attached by chordae to a papillary muscle within the body of the right ventricle. Right. The anterosuperior leaflet is vestigial, leaving the anterior leaflet as a large bridging leaflet with no chordal attachments to the septum but inserting onto an anterolateral papillary muscle in each ventricle, the type C form of atrioventricular canal. (Modified from Hurst JW, Anderson RH, Becker AE, Wilcox BR: Atlas of the Heart, New York, McGraw-Hill, 1988.)

in size, each committed to its respective ventricle, and their medial contiguous aspects have chordal attachments to the underlying septal crest. This pattern is the most common leaflet arrangement, seen in about two thirds of complete AV septal defects. The type B pattern is uncommon and results from a larger left anterior leaflet bridging the ventricular septum and inserting into a papillary muscle within the right ventricle. In Rastelli type C, the left anterior leaflet is the predominant component of the two anterior leaflets, with the right anterior component vestigial or absent. The type C leaflet configuration is recognized by its free floating motion with no chordal attachments to the septum, but only to the anterior papillary muscles in each ventricle.

Partial Atrioventricular Canal

The term partial AV canal has generally included those hearts with only an atrial defect and cleft mitral valve. The partial form is the result of partial fusion of the anterior and posterior common leaflets such that distinct right and left AV orifices are created (Fig. 32–22). The AV septal defect is anatomically identical to that of the complete AV canal; however, the fused leaflets often attach directly or with dense chordal structures to the crest of the interventricular septum and effectively obliterate the interventricular communication. Thus, the partial AV canal consists of an ostium primum ASD and cleft mitral valve.

Transitional Atrioventricular Canal

The term transitional AV canal has been applied to an intermediate form in which separate mitral and tricuspid orifices have been created by fusion of the anterior and posterior cushion components, but the AV valve leaflets have not fused with the septal crest, leaving both the ASD and VSD.[84] This and other variants, such as VSD with cleft mitral valve, or isolated cleft mitral valve, are examples of the broad spectrum of misadventure in these malformations.

Echocardiographic Assessment

The anatomic features of the AV valves in AV septal defects can be accurately discerned by careful echocardiographic evaluation.[78,85,86] Details of leaflet number, papillary muscle size and position, and chordal insertions can be better determined by ultrasound than by angiography.

In standard parasternal long axis views, the atypical nature of the anterior mitral leaflet is readily apparent. The left anterior leaflet demonstrates mitral-aortic continuity, but with medial angulation, the appearance of the left posterior leaflet tissue within the outflow tract and attached to the rim of the ventricular septum can be appreciated. Parasternal short axis views clearly show the ostium primum (ASD) beneath the aorta, and at the ventricular level, the defect of the inlet septum with the common AV valve leaflets spanning the defect. In partial AV canal malformations, the ventricular septum appears intact in this view, but the mitral cleft and chordal attachments to the ventricular septum can be appreciated (Fig. 32–24). Particular attention should be paid in the short axis views to the number, position, and size of the papillary muscles, to exclude a parachute mitral valve or a double-orifice mitral valve. Color flow Doppler in the short axis sweep from base to apex confirms the presence of the inlet ventricular defect when present and also assists in detecting small, muscular VSDs.

The apical and subcostal views have classically afforded the clearest view of AV valvular anatomy[78,86,87] (Fig. 32–25A). Atrial and ventricular defects can be well defined from this vantage point, and the exact nature of the common or divided AV apparatus can be elucidated. It is critical to sweep the scanning plane anteriorly and posteriorly through the AV valve leaflets to distinguish the anterior from the posterior common leaflet, because their position relative to the septum and the lateral leaflets is the same from the apical window. The posterior leaflet nearly always has septal chordal attachments, so one must be certain that the anterior leaflet is scanned before commenting on its type of chordal insertions.

Pulsed and color flow Doppler echocardiography from the apical or subcostal window allows one to detect the presence and severity of AV valve incompetence, as well as the direction of the regurgitant jet. Valvular insufficiency often occurs at several points through the common valve leaflets; left ventricle to left atrial, right ventricle to right atrial, left ventricle to right atrial and right ventricle to left atrial jets are possible.

The presence and direction of shunt flow across the atrial and ventricular septum by pulsed or color flow Doppler can be confirmed from the apical and subcostal positions. In differentiating between partial and transi-

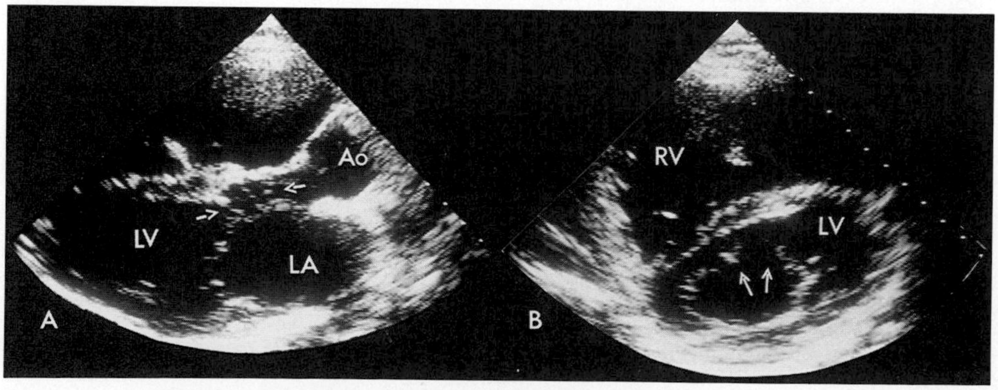

Fig. 32–24. Parasternal echocardiographic views of the mitral valve in a patient with a partial atrioventricular canal. **A.** The chordal attachments of the mitral leaflet to the septum can be seen crossing the left ventricular outflow tract (arrows). **B.** The short axis view of the left ventricle at the mitral valve level clearly shows the bifid appearance of the cleft anterior leaflet (arrows). Ao = aorta; LA = left atrium; LV = left ventricle; RV = right ventricle.

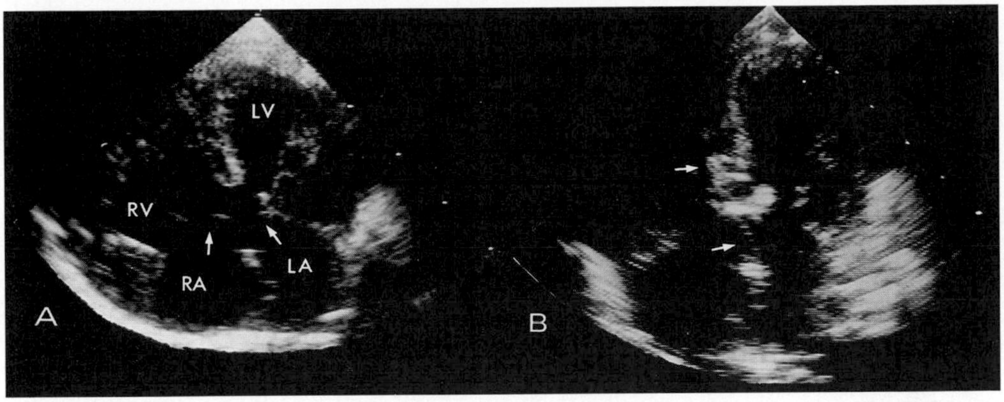

Fig. 32–25. Apical echocardiographic views of a type C atrioventricular canal. **A.** The anterior central bridging leaflet of the common atrioventricular valve is seen (arrows) spanning the large defect in the atrioventricular septum. This leaflet has no chordal attachments to the crest of the interventricular septum but inserts onto papillary muscles within the left and right ventricles. **B.** The large patch (arrows) that has been placed surgically to close the atrial and ventricular defects is visible. The central bridging leaflet has been subdivided and reattached to the patch. Note the increased thickness of the mitral aspect of the reattached leaflet, which represents postoperative change but makes associated endocarditis difficult to detect. LA = left atrium; LV = left ventricle; RA = right atrium; RV = right ventricle.

tional defects, color flow Doppler is particularly sensitive to shunts through small defects that may appear by imaging to be closed by chordal or fibrous tissue. Shunts across the large inlet ventricular defect in a complete canal are often low in velocity and bidirectional because of associated pulmonary hypertension.

Pulsed Doppler sampling in the left ventricular outflow tract and aorta assists one in detecting outflow tract obstruction created by discrete subaortic stenosis or coarctation.

Associated Abnormalities

Mitral Valve Anomalies. About 10% of patients with AV septal defect have additional anomalies of the left AV valve that increase the difficulty of surgical repair and consequently increase surgical mortality.[77,80] Double-orifice mitral valve occurs in approximately 5% of patients with AV septal defects and is more often present in the partial or transitional forms, but has been documented in complete AV canal defects as well.[88,89] This unusual malformation results from a bridge of tissue connecting the left lateral leaflet with either the left anterior leaflet or the posterior common leaflet. Typically, one orifice has its own chordae that connect to one papillary muscle, whereas the chordae of the second orifice attach to the other papillary muscle. The secondary orifice may function normally, but it also may be stenotic or regurgitant (see Chapter 17).

A single left ventricular papillary muscle creates the opportunity for a parachute mitral valve after surgical repair of the septal defects and suture of the mitral cleft. In 8 to 10% of AV septal defects, the posteromedial papillary muscle is severely hypoplastic or absent, leaving all the chordal apparatus assigned to a solitary, large anterolateral muscle.[90] As long as the cleft in the anterior leaflet is present, the mitral orifice is unrestricted, but should the potential parachute anatomy be unsuspected, the closure of the cleft at surgery will create significant mitral stenosis. Some cases of this type have been described with both papillary muscles present, but with all the chordal insertions directed to the anterolateral muscle.[91] Hence one must establish echocardiographically not only the number of papillary muscles, but also the chordal attachments to both muscles.

Left Ventricular Outflow Obstruction. As a part of the developmental abnormality of AV canal defects, the aortic annulus does not get tucked between the mitral and tricuspid annuli, but is displaced anteriorly. The left ventricular outflow tract (LVOT) is elongated and narrowed, giving the familiar "gooseneck" deformity described angiographically and echocardiographically.[92] Left ventricular outflow is further compromised by the medial mitral leaflet attachment to the ventricular septal crest. These features alone are usually not sufficient to create a significant hemodynamic obstruction, but 4 to 7% of patients have either discrete subaortic stenosis or coarctation of the aorta.[93,94] Discrete subaortic obstruction has been described preoperatively by echocardiography and angiography,[95–97] yet in some cases it seems to develop postoperatively in patients who had no evidence of stenosis before repair.[93,98] Coarctation occurs with and without subaortic stenosis and is usually preductal.[93]

Ventricular Dominance. Most AV septal defects are of the balanced type with the common orifice equally committed to each ventricle. Usually, one sees a normal-to-enlarged left ventricle and an enlarged right ventricle.[99,100] In some instances, however, the AV orifice is primarily oriented over one ventricle with resulting hypoplasia of the other ventricle.[79] Surgical mortality is exceedingly high during attempts to repair either right dominant or left dominant ventricles, so preoperative assessment of ventricular size is critically important.[77,100,101] This can be achieved by calculation of angiographic volumes or of two-dimensional echocardiographic volume estimates and comparison with predicted normal values.[99] Although clear minimal limits have not been established, a left ventricular volume of less than 20 ml/m^2 or an RV/LV ratio of 1.5 to 2:1 is indicative of inadequate left ventricular development.[77,80,100]

Other Associated Defects. The majority of complete AV septal defects occur as isolated defects without associated major cardiac malformations. Patent ductus arteriosus (10%) and tetralogy of Fallot (6.5%) are among the most common associated malformations[77] Down's syndrome is a well recognized association, occurring in 50 to 60% of series with complete AV canal.[77,79]

Surgical Management

Surgical attention is devoted to closing the ASD and VSD, fashioning two distinct competent AV valves, and avoiding the AV node. Hospital mortality figures with current surgical techniques indicate a minimal surgical risk for uncomplicated partial AV canal defects (<1%). With complete AV canal defects, which usually require repair at a younger age, hospital mortality for patients with mild AV valve incompetence is 5 to 6%, increasing to 13% when complicated by significant left AV valve insufficiency.[77,80,102]

Septal defect closure can be performed using a one- or two-patch technique. The left anterior and posterior leaflets are sandwiched between the two patches or are divided and stitched to the single patch. If the left anterior leaflet bridges the septum and inserts onto a papillary muscle along the right septal surface, the ventricular patch may sometimes be attached further down along the right septal surface, thus leaving the bridging leaflet and its chordae unaltered,[102] provided this maneuver does not unduly narrow the right ventricular inflow tract. Another approach divides the left anterior and posterior bridging leaflets at the level of the septum by incising the leaflets from their free edge to the annulus and then reattaches them to the AV septal defect patch.[80] Further manipulation of the mitral and tricuspid orifices is individualized to each patient, with partial closure of the cleft or annuloplasty performed if needed to ensure AV valve competence.

Echocardiographic assessment postoperatively should address: (1) AV valve competence or stenosis; (2) residual septal defects; and (3) left ventricular outflow obstruction. From apical and subcostal views, the dense septal patch material is readily apparent, with the tricuspid and mitral leaflets attached midway. These structures often create a dense crosslike structure at the crux of the heart (Fig. 32–25B). Color flow mapping or pulsed Doppler imaging displays residual atrial or ventricular defects and residual AV valve regurgitation (Fig. 32–26). In short axis parasternal views, the anterior leaflet may still appear cleft and will continue to show evidence of its medial chordal attachments to the ventricular septum. Careful imaging and pulsed Doppler sampling should be performed to detect subaortic obstruction.

Tricuspid Atresia

Tricuspid atresia is a malformation, comprising 1 to 3% of congenital heart defects,[1,103] in which the AV valve of the morphologic right ventricle is absent or imperforate. The majority of patients have normal atrial and ventricular situs. Invariably, an atrial septal communication is present, and the right ventricle is underdeveloped. The left heart is compensatorily enlarged. Although the obligatory right-to-left shunt at the atrial level causes arterial desaturation, the degree of clinical cyanosis is determined by the presence or absence of pulmonary outflow obstruction. A VSD is also a standard feature of this complex if those patients with tricuspid atresia with intact septum are relegated to the hypoplastic right heart syndrome, as discussed earlier in this chapter under hypoplastic right heart complex. The

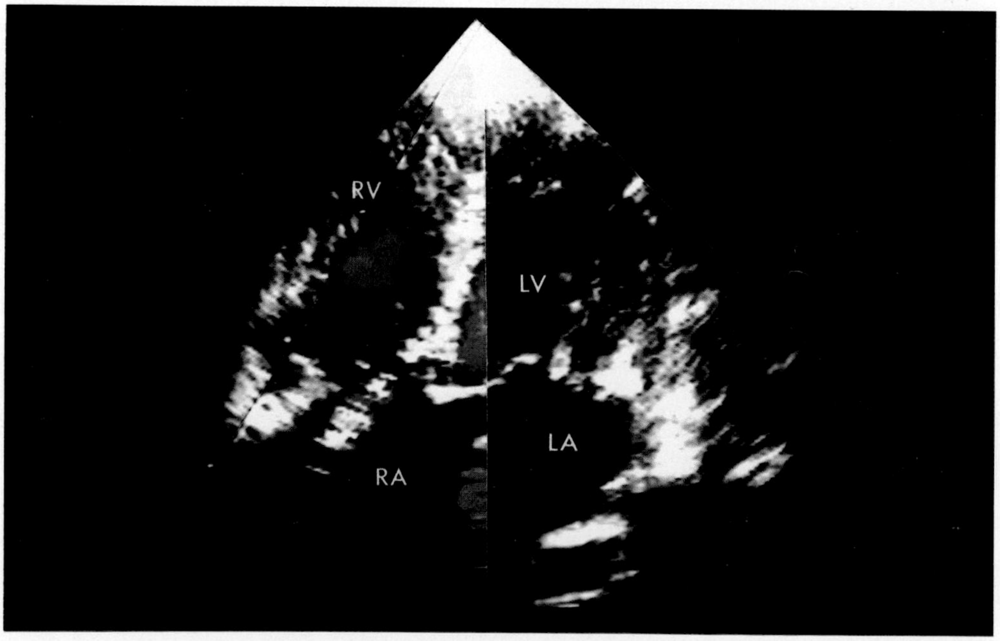

Fig. 32–26. Apical echocardiographic view of complete atrioventricular canal defect following repair. Color flow mapping detects a stream of regurgitant flow passing from left ventricle to right atrium. LA = left atrium; LV = left ventricle; RA = right atrium; RV = right ventricle.

great vessels may be normally related or transposed, with or without obstruction to pulmonary blood flow. This variety of combinations makes for considerable complexity in this entity and thus requires careful echocardiographic analysis of the component parts.

Tricuspid Valve

In place of the tricuspid valve is a thick band of fibromuscular tissue, sometimes with a central dimple marking the intended tricuspid orifice. In some cases, one sees a thinner membranous band or, rarely, formed leaflets that are imperforate. Ebstein's anomaly with an imperforate valve orifice is occasionally seen.[104] Echocardiographically, the atretic valve is a thick, echo-dense band at the level of the tricuspid annulus (Fig. 32–27). A thinner membrane or formed leaflets and chordal structures can be accurately distinguished from the fibromuscular form of atresia by two-dimensional imaging,[105] and absence of flow across the valve can be confirmed with pulsed and color flow Doppler.

Atrial Septum

The right atrium is enlarged and thick-walled, with a prominent eustachian valve. An interatrial communication is virtually always present, either as a widely patent foramen ovale (66%) or a secundum ASD (33%).[103] Occasionally, the atrial septum is absent. Rarely, the only interatrial communication is through an unroofed coronary sinus. Because the entire cardiac output must pass through the atrial defect, any degree of restriction has adverse clinical effects. Evidence of distention of the interatrial septum to the left by two-dimensional imaging is suggestive of a pressure gradient between the atria. Pulsed Doppler sampling of peak velocity of flow across the septum from any view that is optimally aligned with the direction of shunt flow allows estimation of the pressure gradient between right and left atrium. Although it is unusual to find a restrictive ASD in tricuspid atresia with normally oriented great vessels, it is common in the forms with transposed great arteries (50% or more).[104] Any restriction to flow at the atrial level requires a balloon septostomy as part of the initial management of this lesion.

Right Ventricle

Varying degrees of hypoplasia of the right ventricle exist, depending on the location and size of the VSD. In patients with an intact septum or insignificant VSD, the ventricle may be slitlike. When the VSD is small or lies in the outlet septum, there is little or no right ventricular sinus or trabecular portion, but a well-developed infundibular chamber. In patients with a larger septal defect, the right ventricle may develop to more nearly normal size.

Echocardiographic assessment of the size of the right ventricle contributes to surgical decision making, because patients with an adequate right ventricular infundibulum may be considered for right atrial to right ventricular anastomosis (provided no pulmonary stenosis is present), rather than right atrial to pulmonary artery anastomosis. Postoperative functional results appear to be better when a portion of the right ventricle is included in the repair,[106,107] although some groups have shown no hemodynamic advantage to the incorporation of the right ventricle after a Fontan procedure.[108,109]

Ventricular Septal Defect

The interventricular septal defect may lie in the perimembranous region or the muscular septum. The size of the VSD is related not only to the development of the right ventricle, as previously mentioned, but also to the size of the great vessel arising from the right ventricle.

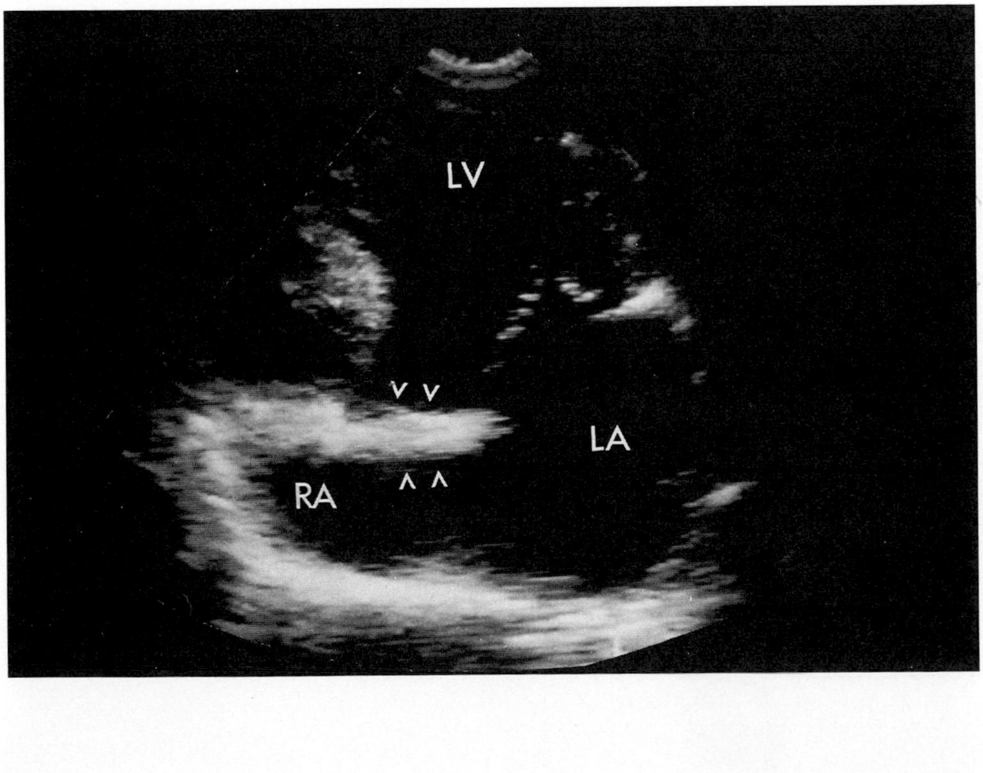

Fig. 32–27. Echocardiographic image from the apical window in a patient with tricuspid atresia showing a thick band of fibrous tissue at the tricuspid annulus (arrowheads). The left ventricle is dilated, and the mitral valve is elongated and redundant. LA = left atrium; LV = left ventricle; RA = right atrium.

When the VSD is small, the artery that receives its flow through the VSD may be underdeveloped.

In nearly half these patients, the VSD is restrictive at the outset or becomes restrictive over time, by progressive hypertrophy of surrounding musculature, membranous septal aneurysm formation, or adhesion of mitral valve apparatus to the defect.[110] Restriction is usually expressed as a VSD diameter smaller than the diameter of the outlet vessel arising from the right ventricle.[104] Two-dimensional imaging can provide one with comparative diameters to indicate the potentially restrictive ventricular defect. Pulsed Doppler flow velocities greater than 1.5 to 2 m/sec indicate a restriction to flow. When the great vessels are normally oriented, the VSD size is less critical in the long term because surgical treatment routes the systemic venous circuit from right atrium to right ventricular outflow tract or pulmonary artery, closing or ignoring the VSD. When the great vessels are transposed, however, the aorta arises from the right ventricle, and systemic output depends on flow through the VSD from the left ventricle.

Progressive spontaneous closure of the interventricular septal defect has been well documented, with catastrophic outcome if the patient is not carefully monitored.[110] Noninvasive ultrasound evaluation can provide serial data on defect size and peak flow velocity, thus allowing prediction of impending closure.

Great Vessels

The origin and relationship of the great vessels in tricuspid atresia runs the gamut of possibilities and forms the basis for the classification system for this lesion. In 60 to 70% of cases, the arteries are normally related (type I), with the pulmonary artery arising from the small right ventricle and the aorta from the larger left ventricle. Transposition of the great arteries (TGA) occurs in 30 to 40%, with D-transposition (type II) representing the large majority and L-transposition (type III) the minority.[103,111] Isolated cases of double-outlet left or right ventricle or truncus arteriosus have also been reported.[103,112,113]

Obstruction to pulmonary blood flow is common (75%) in type I tricuspid atresia (normally related great arteries). This occurs at the VSD, the infundibulum, the pulmonary valve, or a combination of all three. Pulmonary atresia is present in a few cases. Patients with transposed great vessels (types II and III) are less likely to have obstruction to the pulmonary artery (which arises from the large left ventricular chamber) and thus usually have normal or excessive pulmonary blood flow. About one third of this subgroup does have subpulmonary stenosis or pulmonary atresia, however.

A more frequent association in tricuspid atresia with transposed vessels is obstruction to systemic outflow, in the form of subaortic or valvular aortic stenosis, aortic hypoplasia, coarctation, or arch interruption.[103,112] Left juxtaposition of the atrial appendages occurs in about 10% of patients with tricuspid atresia with transposition[114] (see Chapter 18).

Echocardiographic study in the patient with tricuspid atresia must focus on the presence, size, and origin of the aorta and pulmonary artery. Further investigation by imaging and Doppler should then establish whether obstruction to pulmonary outflow is present at any level and, in those with transposition, whether there is systemic outflow obstruction at any level. A high degree of suspicion for coarctation and/or arch interruption is needed in this second group, sometimes implied by a small proximal aorta. A sizable patent ductus is a necessary concomitant.

Surgical Management

The clinical presentation and surgical management of tricuspid atresia are dictated by the two major physiologic subsets: obstructed versus unobstructed pulmonary blood flow.

In the group with normal or excessive pulmonary blood flow, congestive heart failure ensues when neonatal pulmonary resistance falls. Placement of a pulmonary artery band is required in the first 6 months of life to relieve congestive heart failure and to protect the pulmonary vascular bed. Band placement should avoid distortion and deformity of the distal main and branch pulmonary arteries, to preserve these arteries for a subsequent Fontan procedure at 2 to 5 years of age. Echo-Doppler assessment of these patients after pulmonary artery banding should address: (1) band position on the pulmonary artery; (2) band gradient; (3) serial VSD size and transdefect gradient; (4) atrial defect size and transatrial gradient; and (5) left ventricular function and mitral valve competency. Evidence of progressive closure of the VSD may require additional surgical procedures to enlarge the VSD or more complex surgery (Damus-Kaye-Stancil procedure) to bypass the defect.

Severe cyanosis is the hallmark of the infant with tricuspid atresia and significant obstruction to pulmonary blood flow. A systemic-to-pulmonary shunt is required in early infancy, using either a controlled central aortopulmonary shunt or a Blalock-Taussig shunt (see the discussion earlier in this chapter on aortopulmonary shunts). Long-term survival after shunting alone is good,[115,116] but additional shunts are needed as the patient grows, and by the second decade of life, the chronic volume overload leads to progressive left ventricular failure.[113]

In the past, the Glenn procedure was used to provide pulmonary blood flow and ostensibly to relieve a portion of the left ventricular volume load. This shunt requires transection of the superior vena cava near its junction with the right atrium and transection of the distal right pulmonary artery with subsequent end-to-end anastomosis of these two vessels (Fig. 32–10A). In this way, the systemic venous return from the upper body is diverted directly to the right lung. Although many centers still use this procedure for tricuspid atresia, surgical preference seems to be moving toward the Fontan procedure at age 2 to 3 years after an initial systemic-to-pulmonary shunt.[116,117]

Diversion of right atrial blood to the right ventricular outflow tract (RVOT) or to the main pulmonary artery (Fontan procedure) is considered the definitive procedure for physiologic correction of tricuspid atresia.

When the right ventricle, pulmonary valve, and pulmonary arteries are well developed, this procedure can be accomplished by placement of a nonvalved or valved homograft conduit between right atrium and RVOT. Right ventricular contraction thus provides some benefit to pulmonary flow. In patients with obstructed pulmonary outflow, a direct anastomosis is made to the pulmonary artery using the right atrial appendage or graft material, or the newer bicaval-pulmonary anastomoses (see the discussion earlier in this chapter on univentricular heart).

Echocardiographic assessment of the patient who has undergone the modified Fontan procedure is discussed in the section of this chapter on univentricular heart. In patients with a right atrial to right ventricular conduit, surveillance for conduit degeneration and obstruction is necessary (see the next section of this chapter).

ABNORMALITIES OF THE GREAT VESSELS

Tetralogy of Fallot

Although tetralogy of Fallot has long been considered a tetrad of anomalies—VSD, infundibular pulmonary stenosis, overriding aorta, and right ventricular hypertrophy—it might more appropriately be considered a "monology" with sequelae.[118] The basic abnormality in this entity is underdevelopment of the subpulmonary infundibulum. Malalignment and deviation of the parietal band result in obstruction to pulmonary outflow and a large subaortic VSD. Valvular pulmonic stenosis or atresia and hypoplastic pulmonary arteries are the natural consequences of the impeded transpulmonary flow in utero. The aorta is enlarged reciprocally, in part because of increased flow through the VSD. Right ventricular hypertrophy follows predictably from significant obstruction to pulmonary outflow.

Ventricular Septal Defect

The deviation of the right ventricular parietal band is a hallmark feature that distinguishes tetralogy of Fallot from other forms of VSD and pulmonic stenosis, and one that is clearly demonstrable echocardiographically (Fig. 32–28). The resulting VSD is large and subaortic but generally not due to a deficiency of the membranous septum, thus most appropriately termed a malalignment VSD. The septal defect is usually well appreciated in parasternal long axis views; the aortic root straddles the ventricular septum and receives flow from both ventricles (Fig. 32–29). Apical and subxyphoid long axis and five-chamber views also depict the relationship of aorta to ventricular chambers and the VSD size and position. Color flow mapping demonstrates the flow streams exiting through the aorta from both high pressure ventricles. When right ventricular outflow obstruction is minimal, shunting occurs from left to right across the VSD.

In 3 to 15% of patients, additional muscular VSDs are present,[119] and rarely an inlet or canal-type VSD. These defects should be excluded by careful screening with pulsed or color flow Doppler. In a much smaller number of cases, the VSD in tetralogy of Fallot is restrictive, with suprasystemic right ventricular pressures. The septal defect in these cases becomes obstructed either by marked septal hypertrophy surrounding the defect or by redundant accessory tricuspid valve tissue.[120–122] Parasternal long and short axis imaging enables one to detect mobile tissue along the right septal surface that obstructs the VSD in systole and may prolapse into the LVOT. Pulsed or color flow Doppler demonstrates a right-to-left shunt in systole. This variant of tetralogy carries a high operative mortality and is not always clearly defined by angiography, so echocardiographic diagnosis is particularly important.[120]

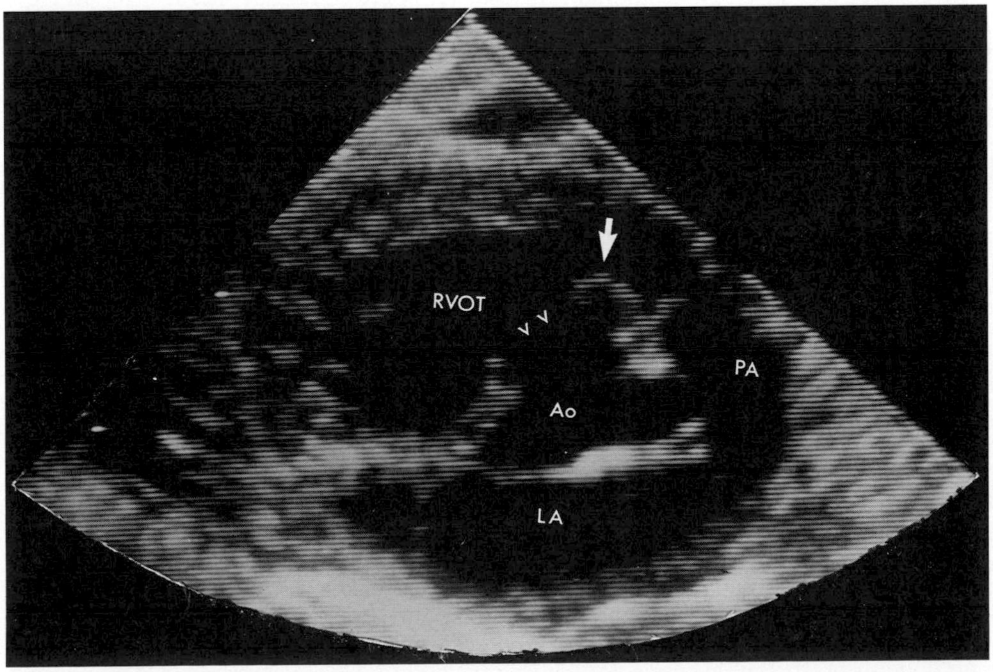

Fig. 32–28. Parasternal short axis echocardiographic image at the base of the heart, demonstrating the anterior deviation of the parietal band (large arrow) into the right ventricular outflow tract, which narrows the subpulmonary infundibulum and leaves a large malalignment ventricular septal defect (small arrowheads). Ao = left ventricular tract just below the aorta; LA = left atrium; PA = pulmonary artery; RVOT = right ventricular outflow tract.

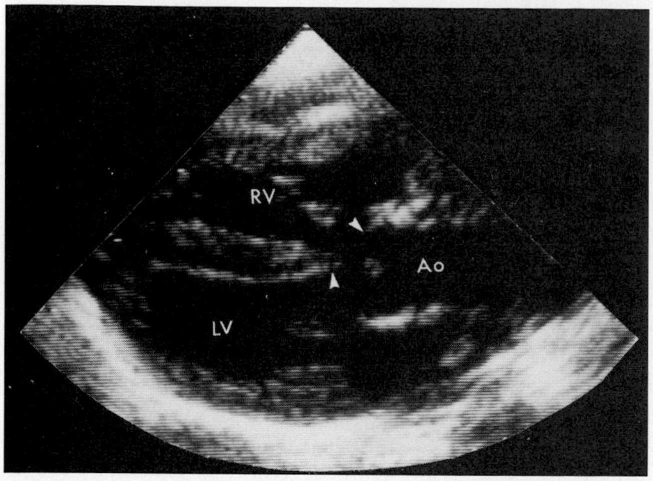

Fig. 32–29. Parasternal long axis view of the left ventricle (LV) in a patient with tetralogy of Fallot, demonstrating a malalignment ventricular septal defect and overriding of the septum by the large aorta. The anterior border of the aortic root is displaced toward the right, with the tip of the interventricular septum oriented toward the coaptation point of the aortic leaflets (arrows). Ao = aorta; RV = right ventricle.

Right Ventricular Outflow Tract

The degree and location of right ventricular outflow obstruction in tetralogy of Fallot are variable. In all instances, the superior, anterior, and leftward positioning of the parietal band produces some element of infundibular stenosis. Infants with so-called "pink" tetralogy have mild obstruction with well-developed pulmonary annulus, valve, main and branch pulmonary vessels. Shunt flow is from left to right, and the transpulmonary gradient is low. In time, however, right ventricular hypertrophy progresses, causing more severe infundibular narrowing and reversal of shunt flow with increasing cyanosis.

Most commonly, infundibular stenosis is significant, with associated valvular pulmonic stenosis and hypoplastic pulmonary arteries. Two-dimensional imaging in the parasternal long and short axis planes details the specific features of the RVOT. Hypertrophied right ventricular infundibular muscle and thickened domed pulmonic leaflets are apparent. Color flow mapping demonstrates acceleration of flow velocities with aliasing that begins at the subvalvular level. Pulsed Doppler sampling may allow distinction of the gradients at the infundibular and valvular levels, but often velocities are too high for resolution by the pulsed technique and require continuous wave Doppler assessment of peak velocity across the entire pulmonary outflow tract. Comparison of continuous wave Doppler-derived gradients with catheter-determined gradients has been favorable in this group of patients with mixed subvalvular and valvular obstruction.[123] When the RVOT and main pulmonary artery are diminutive, they may be difficult to detect in standard parasternal views. Suprasternal imaging frequently demonstrates tiny pulmonary vessels beneath the large ascending aorta, with a "mustache" appearance of the small confluent vessels. Subxyphoid views of the RVOT in infants and children are additionally helpful, to resolve the anatomic details of the hypoplastic infundibulum and pulmonary artery.

An additional level of RVOT obstruction may exist in the form of a low-lying hypertrophied muscle bundle at the junction between the right ventricular sinus and the infundibulum, creating a "double-chambered right ventricle." Subcostal views of the RVOT are particularly helpful in detecting this phenomenon because the standard parasternal long axis views of the RVOT may not extend far enough down toward the sinus to detect this muscular ridge. Pulsed Doppler sampling assists in determining whether hemodynamic obstruction exists at this point.[124]

At the extreme end of the spectrum of RVOT obstruction in tetralogy of Fallot are infants with infundibular or valvar pulmonic atresia. Acquired pulmonary atresia is also seen in older patients who have undergone palliative shunt procedures and whose infundibular stenosis has progressed over time to complete atresia. In either the congenital or acquired type, the RVOT is completely obstructed by hypertrophied muscle. In the congenital forms, the pulmonary valve may also be imperforate. Pulmonary blood supply depends on ductal shunt flow or large aortopulmonary collaterals. As previously discussed, echocardiographic evaluation is directed toward establishing the length and nature of infundibular obstruction, the presence and size of a main pulmonary vessel, and continuity of right and left pulmonary branches.[125] Pulsed Doppler and color flow mapping provide confirmation that no forward flow is occurring across the infundibulum and allow one to detect the presence of continuous shunt flow in the distal pulmonary vessels from the ductus or collaterals. This subgroup of tetralogy of Fallot has been referred to as "pseudotruncus," but it can be distinguished from persistent truncus arteriosus by the presence of an RVOT that ends blindly and by the lack of direct origin of pulmonary arteries from the proximal aorta.[126,127] Because palliative aortopulmonary shunting is performed in some centers without cardiac catheterization, it is crucial that echocardiographic study provide accurate detail of branch pulmonary artery size, confluence of right and left branches, and the position of the aortic arch[53,128] (see later).

The syndrome of absent pulmonary valve occurs in about 10% of cases of tetralogy of Fallot.[129] The pulmonary valve consists of nubbins of vestigial valve tissue, which are freely regurgitant. The pulmonary annulus, however, is hypoplastic and therefore still restricts forward flow. The stenotic flow jet and the wide open regurgitation result in marked pulmonary artery dilatation, the latter often constituting the major source of clinical disability because of compression of surrounding pulmonary airways.[130]

Echocardiographic imaging in this syndrome is remarkable for the typical features of tetralogy of Fallot but incongruously large pulmonary arteries (Fig. 32–30). The term *absent pulmonary valve* is a misnomer in that valvular tissue is often apparent echocardiographically; however, the presence of significant pulmonary regurgitation shown by pulsed Doppler or color flow mapping

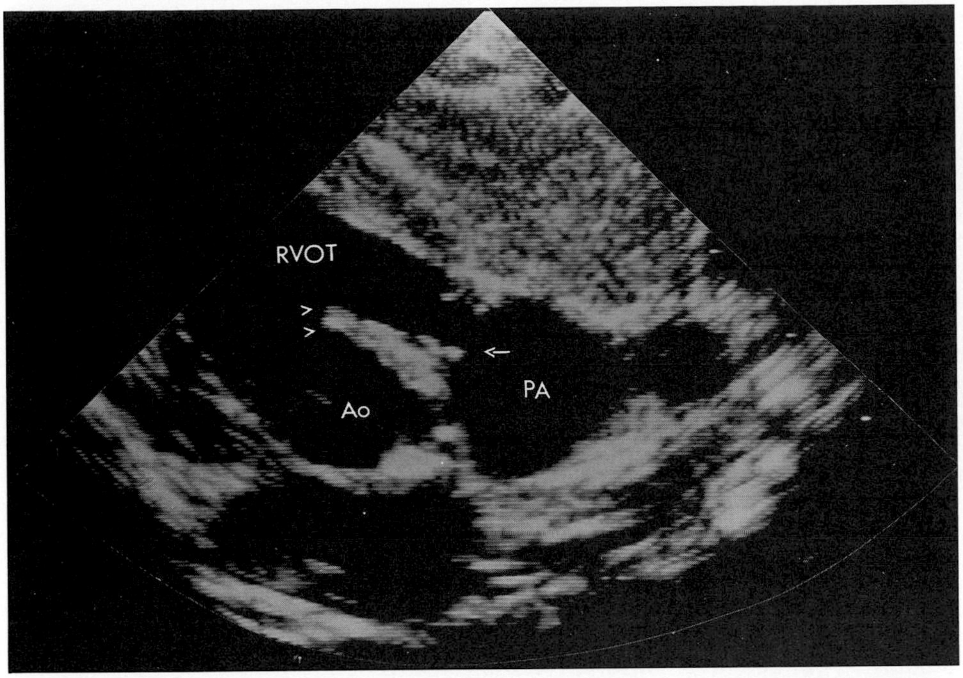

Fig. 32–30. Parasternal long axis view of the right ventricular outflow tract (RVOT) in a patient with absent pulmonary valve syndrome. The parietal band is deviated into the right ventricular outflow tract (double arrowheads), and the pulmonary annulus is hypoplastic. There are vestigial nubbins of pulmonary valve tissue (arrow) and marked dilation of the main pulmonary artery and branches. Ao = aorta; PA = pulmonary artery; RVOT = right ventricular outflow tract.

and of dilated pulmonary branches should identify the appropriate pathophysiologic entity.

Pulmonary Arteries

Diffuse hypoplasia of the main pulmonary artery and its branches is the rule in tetralogy of Fallot. Several additional abnormalities of the pulmonary arterial tree are possible, however, particularly in the subgroup of patients with pulmonary atresia. Focal stenoses of the main pulmonary artery and of the branch vessels at their origin may occur. Long-segment atresia of either branch pulmonary artery or absence of the left pulmonary artery also complicates tetralogy of Fallot and contributes to increased surgical mortality.[131] These abnormalities should be considered in echocardiographic study and are best demonstrated from parasternal and suprasternal views or subcostally in younger infants.

Coronary Artery Anomalies

An abnormal origin or course of a coronary artery with passage of a major branch anteriorly across the RVOT can interfere with ventriculotomy and transannular patching in patients with tetralogy of Fallot. This may occur when the origin of the left anterior descending branch is the right coronary artery or with bilateral anterior descending branches, one of which arises from the right coronary and courses anteriorly. Such anomalies occur in 5 to 9% of cases, and generally root aortography or selective coronary arteriography has been required to screen patients preoperatively. With increasing experience in imaging coronary vessels with two-dimensional echocardiography, it is possible to diagnose these coronary anomalies noninvasively, at least in younger patients.[132] Careful attention should be paid to cross-sectional lumina seen anterior to the RVOT in high parasternal views and anteriorly coursing vessels arising from the proximal right coronary artery. Coronary fistulas are occasionally noted in patients with tetralogy of Fallot and may be suspected when one sees a dilated fistulous channel and continuous fistulous flow on pulsed Doppler or color flow mapping[132,133] (see Chapter 34).

Associated Lesions

About 25% of patients with tetralogy of Fallot have a right aortic arch. This is often evident from plain chest films, but it should be assessed routinely by two-dimensional echocardiography in all patients with this diagnosis. The arch situs can be inferred by the presence or absence of the descending aorta behind the left atrium in parasternal long or short axis views of the left heart.[134,135] Difficulty in obtaining a complete long axis image of the aortic arch and descending aorta from the usual suprasternal window also suggests a nonstandard arch position. If one pays careful attention to the degree of rotation of the transducer in this window, the right aortic arch will be better visualized with counterclockwise rotation and angulation toward the right. More specific localization is possible from the suprasternal notch views, visualizing the ascending aorta in cross section and noting the presence of the descending aorta to the right or left in cross section behind the left atrium (Fig. 32–31). Tracking the branching pattern of the brachiocephalic vessels is also useful in diagnosing a right aortic arch, assuming the patient has no anomalies of the origins of brachiocephalic vessels. The first vessel arising from a right aortic arch is a left innominate artery, which can be traced into the left neck. The second branch is the right carotid artery, and the third arch vessel is the right subclavian artery.

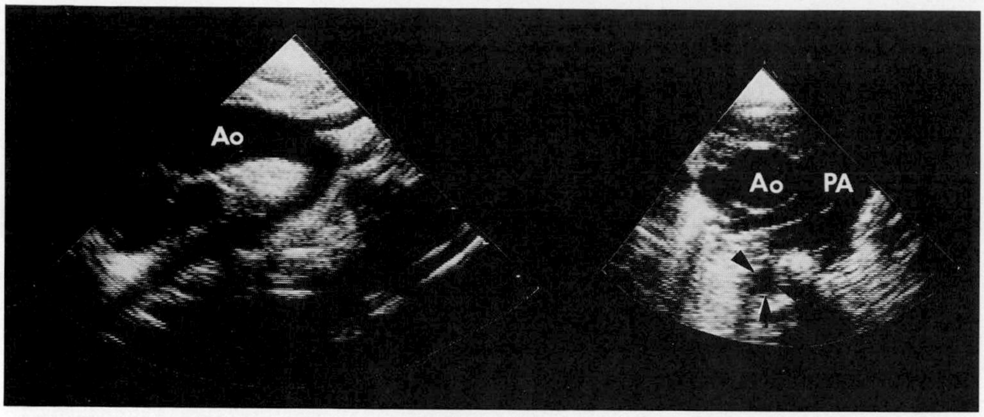

Fig. 32–31. Echocardiographic views of a right aortic arch in a patient with tetralogy of Fallot. Left. An enlarged ascending aorta that arches and begins to descend out of the plane of the usual leftward angulation for this scan. Only with angulation and rotation toward the right is the descending aorta clearly seen. Right. The large ascending aorta is shown in cross section from a suprasternal view with a small right pulmonary artery passing beneath it. The superior vena cava can be seen in cross section lying immediately to the right of the aorta. In the far field of this image, the descending aorta is shown in cross section lying well to the right of its usual location (black arrows). Ao = aorta; PA = pulmonary artery.

A secundum ASD creates a "pentalogy of Fallot" in about 25% of patients and is readily diagnosed on standard two-dimensional imaging. Patent ductus arteriosus is present in infancy, most often in the subgroup of patients with pulmonary atresia. Discrete left-sided obstructive lesions are infrequent concomitant findings, either as discrete subaortic stenosis or as supramitral ring (Fig. 32–32). Complete AV canal defect, which occurs in about 1.5% of patients with tetralogy of Fallot,[136] is an important associated defect to diagnose echocardiographically because catheterization may fail to permit detection of the canal abnormality unless left ventricular angiography is routinely performed. Mortality rates with this combination of lesions are significantly higher than with either lesion alone (17 to 29%).[136,137]

Surgical Management

The basic operative intent in tetralogy of Fallot is to establish an unobstructed RVOT in continuity with the pulmonary artery and to close the interventricular septal communication. When the outflow obstruction is solely infundibular, repair can be accomplished by a right ventriculotomy with excision of muscular bundles and placement of an outflow patch to relieve obstruction. Associated valvular pulmonic stenosis is addressed with pulmonary valvotomy. In patients with more diffuse hypoplasia of the infundibulum and pulmonary artery, an outflow tract patch extending across the pulmonary annulus is required. This is generally constructed from Dacron or pericardium. A transannular patch renders the

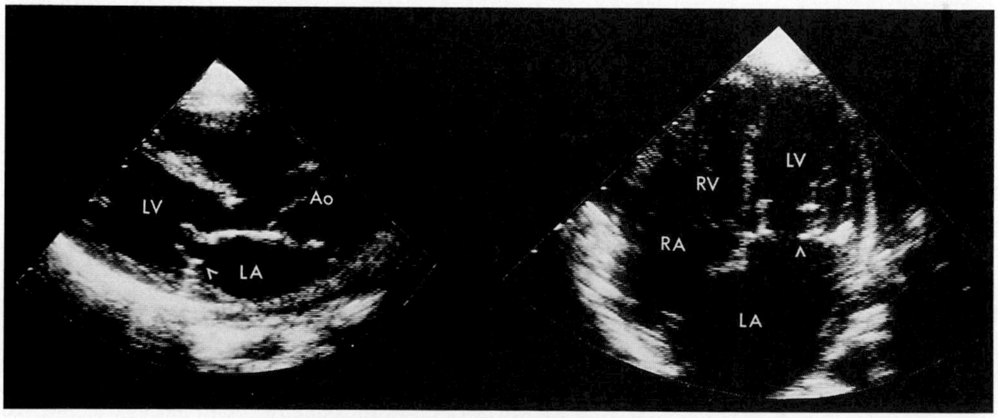

Fig. 32–32. Echocardiographic views of a child with tetralogy of Fallot and supramitral ring. Left. The large malalignment ventricular septal defect and overriding aorta are characteristic of tetralogy of Fallot. The mitral leaflets open without doming at the valve tips, but leaflet excursion is limited by a circumferential ring, which projects as a discrete density along the midportion of the anterior and posterior leaflets (arrowhead). Right. From an apical projection, the left atrium is disproportionately enlarged for an uncomplicated tetralogy of Fallot, and in diastole, the supramitral ring is apparent, projecting from the base of the mitral leaflets into the left ventricular inflow tract (arrowhead). Ao = aorta; LA = left atrium; LV = left ventricle; RA = right atrium; RV = right ventricle.

pulmonic valve incompetent, but mild degrees of pulmonary insufficiency are well tolerated for many years.[138,139] In a few patients with residual outflow obstruction, peripheral pulmonary stenoses, or pulmonary hypertension, significant pulmonary regurgitation causing unremitting right heart failure may require pulmonary valve replacement.[140]

Surgical management of tetralogy of Fallot with pulmonary atresia has traditionally been a two-stage procedure. An initial aortopulmonary shunt is placed in infancy to relieve cyanosis and to promote growth of the small pulmonary arterial tree. The second stage may be delayed until the patient is 3 to 5 years old, when placement of a valved conduit from right ventricle to main pulmonary artery is performed (Rastelli procedure). The higher mortality in this group of patients and the problems related to shunt-created stenoses and conduit degeneration have led to alternate approaches. One such alternative involves a first-stage reconstruction of the RVOT using extensive outflow patch or conduit, leaving the ventricular septal defect open. With subsequent growth of the pulmonary arteries, a complete repair can be attempted at the second stage.[141,142]

One of the most important factors in choosing a surgical approach is the size and confluence of the main pulmonary artery and its branches. Several methods have been suggested by which to derive a quantitative index predictive of adequate pulmonary artery capacity for accepting total forward pulmonary blood flow.[141,143,144] Although these indices have been determined from angiographic measurements, they can also be derived noninvasively from two-dimensional echocardiography and thus can be followed serially to assess growth in the pulmonary vessels after first-stage palliation.[53] One such index (the McGoon ratio) uses the sum of the diameters of right and left pulmonary arteries normalized by the diameter of the descending thoracic aorta at the diaphragm: (D rpa + D lpa)/D Ao. A normal ratio falls between 1.5 and 2.5, whereas a ratio of 0.5 or less suggests pulmonary arteries that are too small to accept complete repair.[144] An alternative method (the Nakata index) normalizes for body surface area rather than aortic diameter and sums the cross-sectional area of the right and left pulmonary arteries: RPA area (mm^2) + LPA area (mm^2)/BSA (m^2). The normal range for this method is 300 to 400 mm^2/m^2. The minimal index for successful total correction of tetralogy of Fallot is suggested to be 100 mm^2/m^2.[145]

Currently, the majority of patients with tetralogy of Fallot undergo complete repair of their cardiac defects in early childhood. There are still patients, however, who have survived into early adult years with either untreated or palliated tetralogy of Fallot. These patients are potentially candidates for complete repair, provided their systemic-to-pulmonary anastomoses have not created irreversible pulmonary vascular obstructive disease or severe focal pulmonary artery stenosis. Several clinical series have documented acceptable mortality figures for complete repair of tetralogy of Fallot in the adult with no increase in surgical risk from prior aortopulmonary shunt.[146–149] All groups report an improvement in functional class, with resolution of cyanosis and polycythemia.

Echocardiographic study in the older patient with tetralogy of Fallot adds considerable anatomic and functional data to the preoperative considerations. Technically, these patients are a challenge because longstanding cardiac disease often creates chest wall deformities that make transthoracic access more difficult. By combining multiple views, and with the addition of transesophageal study, the most information can be derived. The VSD size and location and the direction of shunt flow are assessed as previously discussed. The RVOT should be evaluated for level of obstruction and for patency because acquired infundibular atresia is frequent in older patients with tetralogy of Fallot. Size and confluence of pulmonary arteries are again important features to determine echocardiographically. Color flow mapping is helpful in enabling one to detect aortopulmonary shunt flow either from surgical shunts or from larger central collaterals. Right and left ventricular function may be depressed by longstanding pressure overload on the right heart and longstanding volume overload on the left heart after shunt palliation. Acquired aortic valve disease is another issue of concern in the adult with tetralogy of Fallot, and one that two-dimensional and Doppler echocardiography are ideally suited to evaluate.

After total correction of tetralogy of Fallot, possible residual defects can be followed and quantified by echo-Doppler study. Residual VSD have been reported in 10 to 25% of patients in postoperative follow-up, only a small percentage of whom require reoperation for defect closure.[139,150] Pulsed and color flow Doppler interrogation of the patch margins generally permits detection of even the smallest residual shunt (Fig. 32–33). The examiner need be aware, however, that systolic turbulence in the RVOT may be caused by residual outflow obstruction and not from shunt flow across the VSD. Doppler flow velocities with residual VSD should be relatively high (in accordance with the expected interventricular pressure gradient), and color flow mapping should demonstrate crossing of shunt flow from left to right through the septum to avoid misdiagnosing residual shunts. Occasionally, the ventricular septal patch becomes detached along a large margin and is visible echocardiographically as it moves in and out of the LVOT. The prosthetic patch material is normally more echodense than the native myocardium. Because of this density, the diagnosis of associated endocarditis may be difficult to exclude unless mobile vegetative masses are present or unless a previous study is available for comparison.

Mild right ventricular outflow obstruction is common after surgical repair; 70 to 80% of patients have residual gradients of 25 to 40 mm Hg.[150] Pulmonary regurgitation is also present in the majority of patients who have required valvotomy and transannular patching. These sequelae are readily detected during standard echo-Doppler study. If significant residual obstruction to right ventricular outflow exists, the likelihood of aneurysmal bulging of the outflow patch is high. This complication

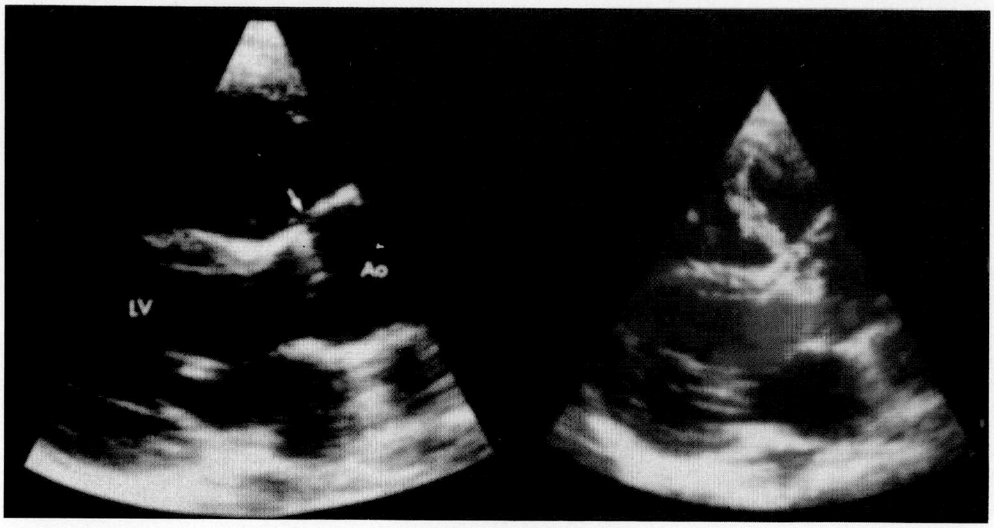

Fig. 32–33. Parasternal long axis echocardiographic view of the left ventricle in a patient following repair of tetralogy of Fallot. The ventricular septal defect patch is an echo-dense structure between the interventricular septum and anterior aortic root. Color flow mapping demonstrates a red jet of left-to-right shunt flow across a residual interventricular communication. LV = left ventricle; Ao = aorta.

can be easily demonstrated echocardiographically in parasternal and subcostal views of the RVOT (Fig. 32–34).

Patients requiring an RVOT conduit must be serially followed for the development of obstruction or degeneration.[151,152] In the early days of conduit placement, the Dacron tube with a porcine heterograft valve was preferred; however, porcine valve leaflets frequently calcify or degenerate. Conduit obstruction may occur at any of four levels: (1) the anastomotic origin of the conduit from the anterior right ventricular wall; (2) the prosthetic valve; (3) the tubular conduit, which may form a pseudointimal "peel;" and (4) the distal attachment of conduit to pulmonary artery.[153,154]

Imaging of outflow tract conduits has generally been difficult because of their substernal position. The proximal anastomosis with the right ventricular anterior wall can usually be visualized from the parasternal views of the right ventricular inflow tract, as one carefully scans the high anterior free wall. Obstruction to flow at this point can be appreciated during pulsed and color flow Doppler imaging. Superficial angulation from the parasternal long axis view of the RVOT may demonstrate the highly reflective "corrugated" appearance of the woven Dacron tube (Fig. 32–35). An intimal peel appears as irregular echodensities narrowing the lumen of the conduit. The mobile prosthetic leaflets may be visible, but pulsed and color flow Doppler are essential in assisting one to diagnose prosthetic stenosis or regurgitation. The conduit course from this view is usually horizontal, placing it perpendicular to ultrasound sampling. This course facilitates imaging, but complicates attempts to sample Doppler flow velocities. Once the conduit has been localized, however, minor shifts in imaging angle from the high right or left parasternal windows project the outflow tract into a position where pulsed or continuous wave Doppler sampling can be performed accurately.

Subcostal long axis views of the RVOT may allow imaging and Doppler access to the conduit if the plane can be angled superficially enough. This window often allows more parallel access to proximal flow in the conduit. A peak outflow gradient of up to 20 mm Hg has been considered normal for conduits; gradients above 40 mm Hg are usually seen when significant conduit stenosis exists.[151,154] The distal insertion of the conduit into the pulmonary artery is difficult to image. Suprasternal views of the pulmonary branches and bifurcation provide the closest access to flow from the distal conduit,

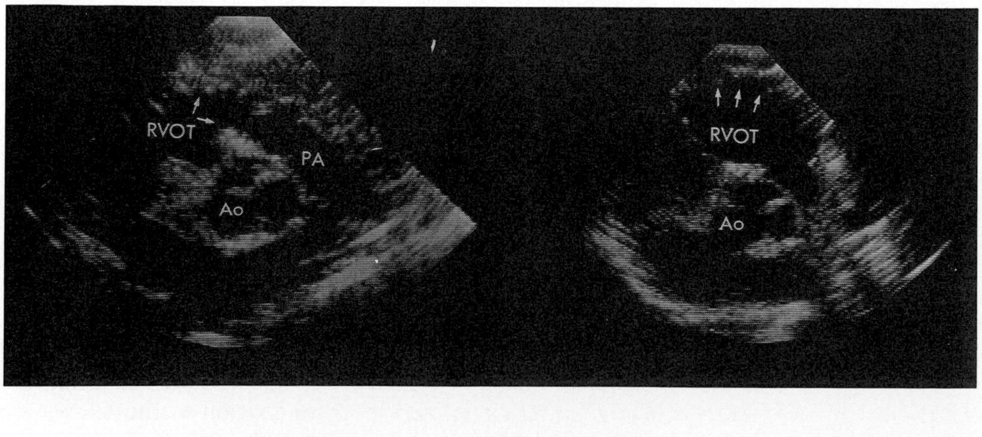

Fig. 32–34. Parasternal echocardiographic views of the right ventricular outflow tract in a child with tetralogy of Fallot. Left. The infundibulum is narrowed (arrows), and the main pulmonary artery is small. Right. Demonstrates the marked widening of the right ventricular outflow tract (RVOT) following placement of an anterior outflow tract patch (triple arrows). Ao = aorta; PA = pulmonary artery. (From Liberthson RR: Congenital heart disease in the child, adolescent, and adult. *In:* The Practice of Cardiology. Boston, Little, Brown and Company, 1989.)

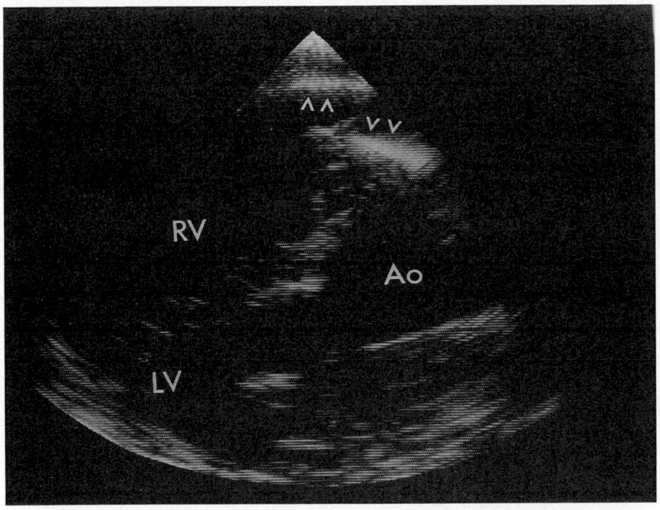

Fig. 32–35. Long axis echocardiographic view of the right ventricular outflow tract in a child with a Dacron conduit. Note the ridged appearance of the woven Dacron tube (arrowheads). The porcine heterograft leaflets are faintly seen (between the arrowheads).

and in some patients, subcostal images may permit interrogation of the distal conduit at the pulmonary bifurcation. Pulsed or color flow Doppler studies may show high velocity turbulent flow in the right or left pulmonary artery to indicate stenosis proximal to the branches.

Transesophageal study provides an excellent view of the base of the heart and therefore increases the likelihood of imaging the conduit insertion into the distal main pulmonary artery or the confluence of branch pulmonary arteries. When imaging of the conduit is not possible, the diagnosis of obstruction may have to rely on indirect signs such as right ventricular and right atrial enlargement and systolic flattening of the interventricular septum. If tricuspid regurgitation is present, estimation of elevation of right ventricular systolic pressure from the peak tricuspid regurgitant jet velocity allows prediction of the degree of outflow obstruction.

In recent years, a preference has developed for cryopreserved aortic or pulmonary homografts over the Dacron conduit. The use of autologous tissue seems to stimulate less intimal peel and thus less degeneration and obstruction than the prosthetic material.[155,156] When an aortic homograft is used, the anterior mitral valve leaflet may be used to augment the entrance into the conduit from the right ventricular free wall. Thus, the echocardiographic appearance of this type of RVOT reconstruction may include a prominent subvalvular chamber. Doppler examination of these conduits frequently shows mild valvular regurgitation and may demonstrate obstruction more commonly at the ends of the homograft than at the valve level.[157]

Complete Transposition of the Great Arteries

The literal translation of the term *transposition* is "to place across," meaning that the aorta and pulmonary artery are displaced across the ventricular septum from their normal positions such that the aorta arises from the right ventricle and the pulmonary artery originates from the left ventricle. The term *complete transposition* has classically been used to distinguish this cardiac anomaly from other abnormalities of conotruncal development, such as double-outlet right ventricle, which have been labeled incomplete or partial transpositions, or more appropriately, *malpositions* of the great arteries.

In complete TGA, atrioventricular concordance and ventriculoarterial discordance occur; that is, the right atrium connects to the right ventricle but then gives rise to the aorta, whereas the left atrium empties into the left ventricle but directs its output into the pulmonary artery. In the majority of instances, the atria and ventricles are normally positioned (situs solitus). The arrangement of intracardiac blood flow in this entity creates two circuits in parallel, with no means for oxygenation of systemic blood supply unless an opportunity for mixing occurs at the atrial, ventricular, or ductal level. Such infants are severely cyanotic at birth. Complete TGA occurs with a frequency of about 1 in 4000 live births and constitutes 10% of all serious heart disease in infants in the first year of life.[158,159]

Evaluation of a patient with suspected transposition requires attention to the following features critical to this lesion: (1) great vessel orientation and ventricular relationship; (2) status of the interatrial septal communication; (3) location and size of VSD; (4) ductal patency; (5) subaortic or subpulmonic outflow obstruction; (6) coronary anatomy; and (7) anomalies of the tricuspid and mitral valves.

Great Vessels

The great arteries in transposition arise in parallel at the base of the heart, instead of the usual wrapping of the pulmonary artery around the aorta. This results in the typical echocardiographic appearance of parallel vessels in the long axis views of the great arteries and in the "owl's-eye" pattern in short axis views, where both semilunar valves are seen in cross section in the same plane[160] (Fig. 32–36). Generally, the aortic valve is anterior, to the right, and slightly superior to the pulmonary valve (D-TGA, or dextrotransposition). The aorta arises from the right ventricular infundibulum. The pulmonary artery originates directly above the LVOT, with fibrous continuity between the mitral and pulmonic valves. Variant forms of complete transposition are occasionally seen, however, where the aorta is directly anterior, leftward, or even posterior to the pulmonary artery.[161,162] Echocardiographic evaluation of infants with TGA should clearly determine the relative position of the great arteries with respect to each other because this bears significantly on the choice of surgical procedure. Variants with direct side-by-side positioning or with the aorta in a posterior position present more anatomic difficulties for the arterial switch or Jatene procedure. Regarding the diagnosis of TGA based on the short axis appearance of these arteries, one caveat should be mentioned: When the pulmonary artery is enlarged, it is possible to obtain a view in which both semilunar valves are visualized in cross section at the same time

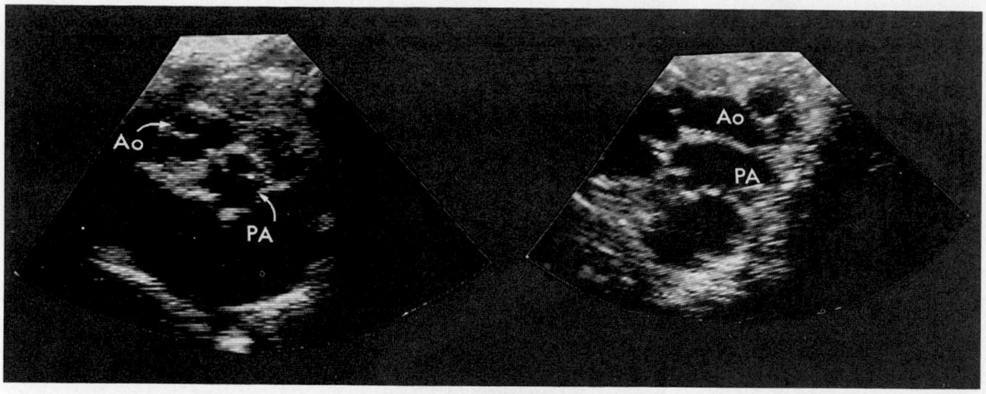

Fig. 32–36. Echocardiographic views at the base of the heart in an infant with complete transposition of the great vessels. Left. The typical appearance of both semilunar valves seen in cross section in the same plane. The aorta is anterior and to the right (D-transposed) of the pulmonary artery. Right. The parallel course of both great vessels in the parasternal long axis view. Ao = aorta; PA = pulmonary artery. (From Levine RA et al: Echocardiography. Principles of clinical applications. *In:* The Practice of Cardiology. Boston, Little, Brown and Company, 1989.)

even with normally oriented great vessels. Hence this criteria should not be used in isolation for making an echocardiographic diagnosis of transposition.

Establishing the relationship of the great arteries with the ventricles by echocardiography is easily done with low parasternal long axis or apical and subcostal long axis views.[163,164] The vessel arising from the right ventricle courses anteriorly and gives rise to the brachiocephalic vessels, whereas the posterior course and early bifurcation of the artery arising from the left ventricle identifies this as a pulmonary artery.

Ventricular Septal Defect

Whereas most patients with TGA have an intact interventricular septum, 30 to 40% have defects in the ventricular septum.[158,165] One third of these are perimembranous defects. An occasional patient has an extension of this perimembranous defect posteriorly into the inlet septum, resulting in a defect of the AV canal type.[166] The percentage of septal defects in the muscular septum is smaller, and they may be single or multiple. Another important type of VSD seen in TGA is a malalignment VSD, where the conal septum fails to close the outlet portion of the interventricular septum properly because of deviation either toward the RVOT or the LVOT. When the deviation is toward the left, muscular subpulmonic obstruction results (see the next section of this chapter). If displacement occurs to the right, the subaortic area may be compromised.

Careful two-dimensional imaging of all aspects of the interventricular septum is essential in enabling one to detect defects, and color flow mapping is immensely beneficial to assist one in quickly detecting shunt flow. In the first few hours of life, flow across VSD in transposition may be from the left ventricle to the right ventricle, or it may be bidirectional. As pulmonary resistance drops, left ventricular pressures fall, and the right ventricle retains systemic pressure, thus reversing shunt direction from right ventricle to left ventricle.

Interatrial Septal Communication

The interatrial septum allows mixing between the pulmonary and systemic circuits through the foramen ovale, with a true secundum ASD of any size present only rarely. Shunt flow in TGA with an intact interventricular septum occurs from left atrium to right atrium during ventricular systole and from right atrium to left atrium during ventricular diastole. If an associated VSD or patent ductus arteriosus is present, increased pulmonary blood flow will lead to higher left atrial pressure and consequently to left-to-right shunt flow during a longer portion of the cardiac cycle.[167]

Enlarging the interatrial septal communication has been standard procedure as the initial management of infants with TGA to ensure maximal mixing at the atrial level. This practice has changed with the movement toward earlier surgical repair, particularly if the arterial switch procedure is chosen. When arterial P_{O_2} and pH are acceptable ($P_{O2} > 25$, pH > 7.30) and neonatal repair is planned, atrial septostomy may not be necessary.[168] If surgical management calls for repair later in infancy, then balloon atrial septostomy is performed after echocardiographic diagnosis.

Balloon septostomy is often accomplished under echocardiographic guidance, either in the cardiac catheterization laboratory or in the neonatal intensive care unit.[169–171] Subcostal imaging of the right and left atria and of the interatrial septum permits visualization of the balloon catheter as it is passed through the atrial defect. If the catheter should terminate in the atrial appendage, in the pulmonary vein, or across the mitral valve, that fact can be readily established and the catheter can be withdrawn before balloon inflation. The adequacy of the balloon septostomy is initially assessed by an increase in oxygen saturation and a decrease in pressure gradient between the atria at catheterization. If balloon septostomy merely stretches the foramen ovale, however, the interatrial communication may return to its initial restrictive size soon after the procedure, with a fall in arterial oxygen saturations. Echocardiographic evaluation can assist in determining the success of balloon septostomy in several ways, by demonstrating: (1) the defect size; (2) the presence of a mobile tag of septal tissue that flails from side to side; (3) the neutral position of the interatrial septum between the two atrial chambers; and (4) Doppler evidence of bidirectional flow of low velocity indicating lack of a pressure difference across the atrial septum (Fig. 32–37). The size of the newly created ASD alone does not always ensure adequate atrial mixing, because atrial mixing is strongly influenced by relative right and left ventricular compliance, volume status, and pulmonary artery pressure and resistance. When echocardiography is used at the time of balloon septostomy, if a septal tear is not apparent, an additional attempt can be made during the same procedure and thus avoid a repeat study or the need to proceed to surgical septectomy.

Left Ventricular Outflow Obstruction

Obstruction to left ventricular emptying is seen in 20 to 30% of patients with TGA and can be fixed or dynamic. Dynamic LVOT obstruction, one of the most common forms of outflow obstruction, occurs most often in the presence of an intact ventricular septum. As the left ventricular pressures fall after birth, the right ventricle retains systemic pressure and the interventricular septum shifts toward the left, becoming concave toward the right ventricle (Fig. 32–38). The encroachment of the septum on the left ventricle pancakes the LVOT and may result in mitral chordal or leaflet apposition to the septum in systole similar to that seen in idiopathic hypertrophic subaortic stenosis.

Echocardiographic detection of dynamic outflow obstruction can be made using parasternal, apical, and subcostal long axis views.[172] Frame by frame video playback is of great help in infants, whose rapid heart rates and compressed left heart chambers make the distinction between fixed and dynamic obstruction difficult. When one samples flow velocities in the LVOT, the typical late peaking acceleration of flow velocities by pulsed Doppler resembles that in idiopathic hypertrophic sub-

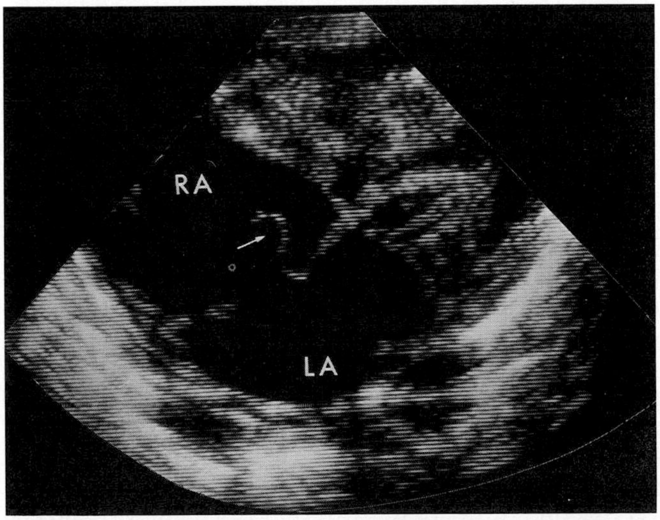

Fig. 32–37. Subxyphoid echocardiographic view of the interatrial septum in a patient with complete transposition following balloon septostomy. The arrow demonstrates the flail portion of atrial septum, which in real time will be seen moving freely into left or right atria. LA = left atrium; RA = right atrium. (From Liberthson RR: Congenital heart disease in the child, adolescent and adult. *In:* The Practice of Cardiology. Boston, Little, Brown & Company, 1989.)

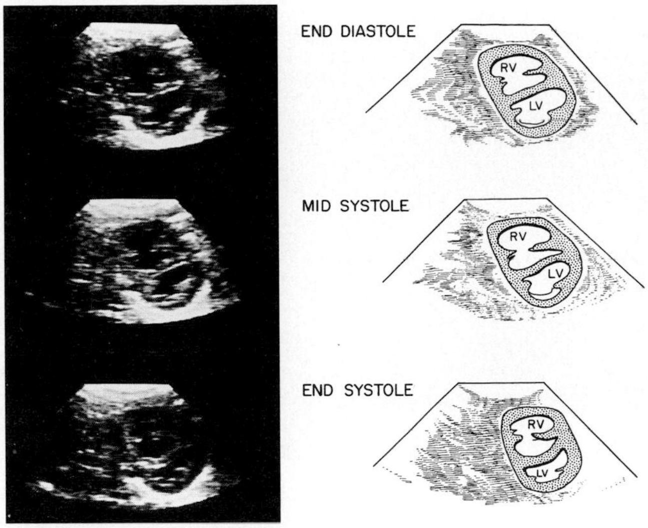

Fig. 32–38. Parasternal short axis echocardiographic views of the right and left ventricle in a patient with complete transposition of the great arteries during three phases of the cardiac cycle. The right ventricle is enlarged with a rounded configuration, and the interventricular septal curvature is reversed from its normal concave orientation toward the left ventricle. In diastole, the interventricular septum is in a neutral position between the ventricles. During systole, it bows toward the lower pressure chamber. LV = left ventricle; RV = right ventricle. (From King ME, et al.: Interventricular septal configuration as a predictor of right ventricular systolic hypertension in children: a cross-sectional echocardiographic study. Circulation 68:68, 1983. Reproduced by permission of the American Heart Association, Inc.)

aortic stenosis. Dynamic obstruction develops during the first week after birth but usually moderates or disappears after intra-atrial repair, when flow ratios across the systemic and pulmonary circuits are equalized. It is, of course, neutralized after arterial switch because the left ventricle assumes systemic work and septal curvature reverts to normal.

Fixed LVOT obstruction can occur at several levels, either singly or in combination[173,174] (Fig. 32–39). Most patients with fixed subpulmonic obstruction have an associated VSD. Valvar pulmonic stenosis is the least prevalent form, comprising only 11% of cases with pulmonary outflow obstruction in one large angiographic series.[174] A hypoplastic pulmonary annulus may accompany valvar stenosis. Two-dimensional imaging clearly portrays leaflet doming in systole in the posterior semilunar root and defines the number of cusps and the degree of commissural separation in the cross-sectional plane. Pulsed and continuous wave Doppler imaging techniques add the hemodynamic data for estimating the severity of obstruction. Awareness of functional abnormality of the pulmonary valve is critical for surgical decision making, because the pulmonary valve becomes the systemic semilunar valve after an arterial switch operation.

A discrete membranous diaphragm in the LVOT also constitutes a form of outflow obstruction in TGA. Similar to discrete subaortic membranes, the thin fibrous ridge also attaches to the base of the anterior mitral leaflet. Echocardiographically, this structure appears as a

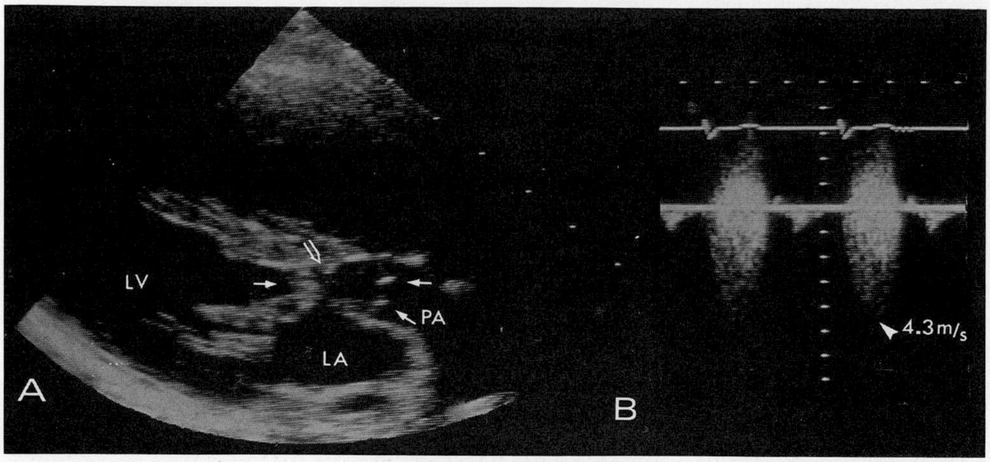

Fig. 32–39. Parasternal long axis echocardiographic view of the left ventricle (LV) and left ventricular outflow tract in a child with complete transposition of the great arteries. The interventricular septum bows posteriorly toward the left ventricle. Multiple levels of obstruction are present in the outflow tract—valvar (double arrows), fixed fibrous (open arrow), and dynamic chordal motion (single arrow). **B.** The spectral continuous wave Doppler tracing with a peak systolic velocity of 4.3 m/sec predicting a peak gradient across the entire outflow tract of 74 mm Hg. LA = left atrium; PA = pulmonary artery.

bright, linear echo immediately beneath the pulmonary leaflets in parasternal, apical, or subxyphoid views. Pulsed Doppler sampling in the LVOT reflects a velocity step up in the outflow tract proximal to the pulmonary valve. During color flow mapping, aliasing occurs within the outflow tract because of acceleration of flow across the stenosis proximal to the valve leaflets.

The most common type of fixed LVOT obstruction is the subpulmonary fibromuscular tunnel. This subgroup represented about 40% of all TGA with LVOT obstruction in the previously mentioned angiographic series. Muscular tissue beneath the pulmonary valve results from either posterior displacement of the infundibular septum or from residual conal tissue beneath the pulmonary artery, in which case there is muscle around the entire circumference of the LVOT and lack of mitral and pulmonic fibrous continuity. Echocardiographically, the LVOT is elongated, with fibromuscular and muscular elements contributing to the obstruction.

An unusual form of left ventricular outflow obstruction in TGA is herniation of a septal aneurysm through a membranous VSD, protruding into the subpulmonary region. Echocardiographically, this appears as a windsock of fibrous tissue and tricuspid valve apparatus that expands into the LVOT in systole.[175] Finally, accessory mitral leaflet tissue and/or septal attachments of a cleft anterior mitral leaflet may impede pulmonary flow within the outflow tract. These septal attachments are rarely an independent cause of severe obstruction.

Right Ventricular Outflow Obstruction

Deviation of the infundibular septum toward the right occurs rarely in TGA. The result, however, is muscular subaortic stenosis and often more distal outflow obstruction as well, in the form of aortic hypoplasia, coarctation, or arch interruption. This type of RVOT obstruction is nearly always associated with a VSD as a result of the displacement of the infundibular septum. When the interventricular septum is intact, RVOT obstruction may still occur because of hypertrophied or aberrant muscle bundles at the entrance to the RVOT.[176,177] Subaortic obstruction may be difficult to detect echocardiographically in the parasternal views because of the extreme anterior substernal placement of the aorta and the RVOT. Apical and subcostal long axis projections place the RVOT in a more favorable position to note subaortic muscular tunnels or obstructive muscle bundles.[172] Doppler sampling enables one to confirm increased flow velocities across the outflow tract. The distal aorta should be carefully searched for associated coarctation or arch interruption.

Patent Ductus Arteriosus

Nearly half of all infants with TGA have a patent ductus arteriosus on presentation to the physician, although only 10 to 15% of these defects persist beyond the first month of life. A large ductal shunt complicates medical management of these infants by increasing pulmonary resistance, thus discouraging mixing at the atrial level, and by contributing to earlier development of fixed pulmonary vascular obstructive disease.[178,179] Two-dimensional imaging of the ductus and color flow mapping or pulsed Doppler confirmation of shunt flow are readily performed in the same fashion as in patients with normally related great vessels (see Chapter 27).

Coronary Artery Anatomy

As more centers choose anatomic correction of TGA by surgically repositioning the great vessels and reimplanting the coronary arteries, the exact origin and course of the coronary arteries become vital preoperative information. The presence of a single right coronary artery or an inverted pattern increases the operative risk.[180] Accurate echocardiographic visualization of the coronary anatomy, possible in a high percentage of infants,[181] is aided by knowledge of the variations expected (Fig. 32–40). Although the anatomic features are variable, a few common patterns are easily recognized. The expected coronary anatomy in TGA has the origin of a coronary artery from each of the two posterior aortic sinuses. In this instance, two coronary ostia should be visible in the short axis parasternal images: the left main exiting from the left posterior sinus, the right coronary from the right posterior sinus. When some or all of the left coronary system arises from the right coronary ar-

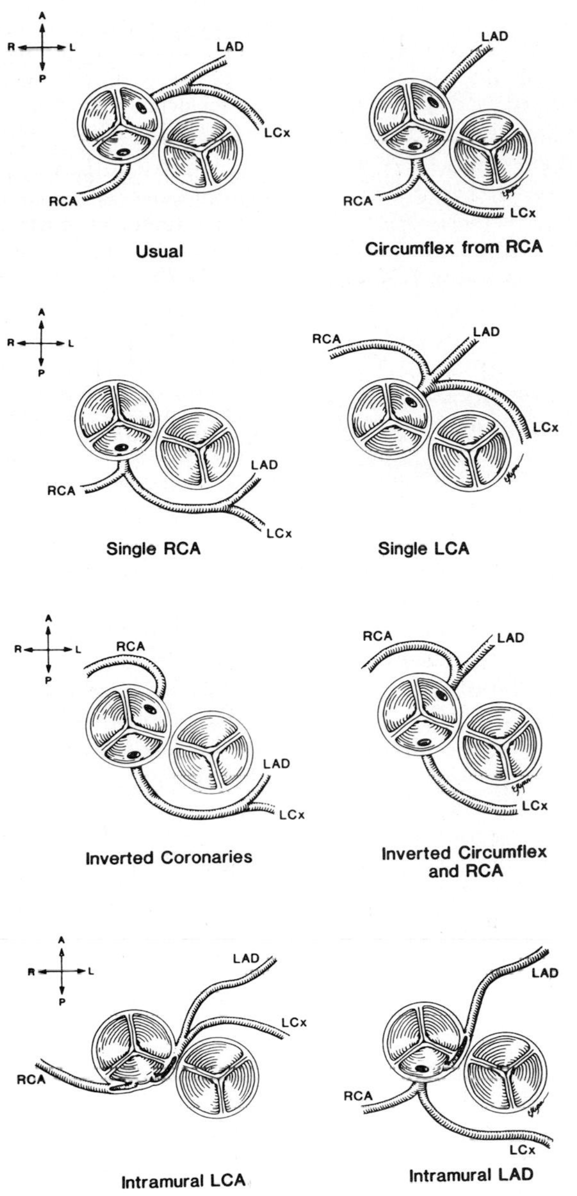

Fig. 32–40. Diagrammatic depiction of the variety of coronary arterial patterns in complete transposition of the great arteries. The semilunar valves are shown when viewed from below, as with a typical short axis echocardiographic scan. LAD = left anterior descending; LCx = left circumflex; RCA = right coronary artery. (From Mayer JE, et al.: Coronary artery pattern and outcome of arterial switch operation for transposition of the great arteries. Circulation 82(Suppl 4):IV-139, 1990. Reproduced by permission of the American Heart Association, Inc.)

tery, a vessel can be seen coursing beneath the pulmonary artery in the cross-sectional plane. In the remaining variant, a single coronary artery arises from the left posterior aortic sinus, in which case the absence of a right coronary ostium is noted echocardiographically.

Additional Associated Abnormalities

A variety of abnormalities of the tricuspid valve described in TGA have particular significance if the tricuspid valve will be the systemic AV valve after a Mustard or Senning atrial switch operation.[182] As the right ventricle assumes systemic work, the tricuspid annulus may become dilated and the tricuspid valve regurgitant. Severe tricuspid incompetence may occur if the tricuspid leaflets are dysplastic. Chordal insertions from the tricuspid apparatus to the margins of a perimembranous or malalignment VSD may complicate surgical closure of the ventricular defect. A few patients with TGA also have mitral valve anomalies, including cleft anterior leaflets, parachute mitral valves, and redundant valve apparatus. Careful two-dimensional imaging and pulsed or color flow Doppler examination should permit one to assess the presence of significant mitral or tricuspid valve disease. Juxtaposition of the atrial appendages is a rare congenital anomaly that occurs in association with complex forms of TGA. Left juxtaposition of the right atrial appendage is seen most commonly.[183,184] The displacement of the right atrial appendage results in a loss of effective area of the right atrial wall that complicates surgical attempts to rechannel venous return by either the Mustard or Senning procedure. Echocardiographic delineation of this malformation is discussed in Chapter 18.

Surgical Management

The present surgical management of complete TGA is in evolution. Until recently, the standard approach to the infant with TGA was balloon atrial septostomy at the time of diagnosis, with elective surgical repair to redirect venous return at the atrial level (Mustard or Senning procedure) at about 1 year of age. The initial surgical mortality with this approach is low;[185–187] however, long-term follow-up of patients after atrial repair has shown considerable morbidity and mortality from pulmonary and systemic venous obstruction, atrial arrhythmias, and late right ventricular (systemic) dysfunction.[188] These results have led to a resurgence of interest in the arterial switch procedure, which had been attempted in the earliest surgical efforts to repair TGA but was abandoned because of excessive mortality.[189] In this so-called anatomic repair, the aorta and pulmonary artery are transected above the semilunar valves. The coronary arteries are excised from the original aorta with a button of aortic root tissue and repositioned above the neoaortic valve (previously the pulmonic valve). The distal aorta is then reattached above the newly implanted coronary ostia. The main pulmonary artery is flipped anteriorly and is anastomosed to the former aortic stump.

Many centers are now electively performing the arterial switch procedure within the first few weeks of life,[190,191] and some prefer to do this "anatomic correction" as a two-stage procedure, even in older infants.[192] When the arterial switch is performed in the first week of life before pulmonary vascular resistance falls, the left ventricle has not yet become a "pulmonary ventricle" and so is able to assume its job as the systemic pump postoperatively. In the older infant, it is necessary to prepare the left ventricle before surgery by first-stage placement of a pulmonary artery band, which is then removed at the second-stage definitive repair, after sufficient time has elapsed for left ventricular pressure loading. Although initial learning curve mortality with the arterial switch has been high, modifications of surgical technique and more appropriate selection of patients have made the anatomic correction a more desirable alternative to atrial repair. Short and midterm follow-up after one-stage arterial switch in infancy has shown normal left ventricular mechanics, no significant arrhythmias, and no resting coronary insufficiency despite angiographic evidence of silent coronary occlusions in some patients.[180,193,194] Short-term problems have included supravalvular pulmonic stenosis at the anastomotic site requiring reoperation.[194,195] Longer-term studies will be needed to assess later complications from coronary reimplantation.[196]

Intra-atrial Repair. After intra-atrial repair, the anatomy of the great vessels remains unchanged. In short axis views at the ventricular level, the right ventricle is enlarged and globular in configuration, whereas the left ventricle assumes the crescent shape of the low pressure pump. Interventricular septal curvature is reversed with its convexity toward the left (see Fig. 32–38). Older patients may manifest depressed right ventricular function.[197] Systemic venous return and pulmonary venous return are redirected within the atrium. The Mustard procedure does this by removal of much of the interatrial septum and placement of a complex Dacron or pericardial baffle. The Senning procedure uses more native atrial tissue in constructing the interatrial pathway, and as such is believed to provide greater opportunity for normal growth, less damage to conduction pathways, and fewer complications from baffle obstruction to venous return.[185]

The venous pathways created by either type of atrial baffle are most readily appreciated from modified apical and subcostal echocardiographic views. Inferior and superior caval flows are directed by the baffle through the midatrium toward the mitral valve. This pathway has an hourglass shape, broadest at the caval entry and at the mitral valve, with a narrow midsection. Pulmonary venous return is channeled across the roof of the atria toward the tricuspid valve, wrapping in horseshoe fashion around the midatrial systemic venous channel.[198] Doppler flow patterns through both venous pathways displays some turbulence or nonlaminarity, because the baffle channels are inherently obstructive to some degree. Flow should remain phasic, however, mirroring the atrial pressure trace, and low in velocity if no significant baffle obstruction exists.[199,200]

Caval obstruction (>5 mm Hg mean pressure gradient) has been reported in as many as 37% of patients from a composite of various surgical series,[188] only a small percentage of whom were symptomatic and required surgical revision. This complication was noted more often when Dacron material was used for the baffle and occurred more frequently with the Mustard than with the Senning technique. The most common site of obstruction was the junction of the superior vena cava with the right atrium near the excision of the superior rim of the interatrial septum. Although two-dimensional imaging of this region is possible suprasternally or subcostally,[198] it may be difficult to establish clearly the degree of narrowing by imaging alone. Loss of phasic flow and increased flow velocity within the midbaffle channel are useful diagnostic features. Peripheral venous saline contrast has also been used successfully to demonstrate lack of contrast in the systemic venous pathway from the superior vena cava with late appearance of contrast through the inferior vena cava from collateral pathways.[201] Pulmonary venous obstruction occurs either at the midbaffle region or as an isolated pulmonary vein stenosis. The midatrial channel appears restrictive, and Doppler flow demonstrates loss of phasic flow in the pulmonary veins and a turbulent high velocity flow across the stenotic site (Fig. 32–41). Peak flow velocity of >2 m/sec is indicative of significant obstruction, but flow velocities >1.5 m/sec should also be suspect.[21,200] A point of caution, however, is the increase in flow velocity created by increased pulmonary blood flow from a residual left-to-right shunt that might be mistaken for obstructed baffle flow.

Residual atrial shunts are noted commonly around the superior limb of the baffle during routine postoperative cardiac catheterization.[188] These are rarely of clinical significance; however, they may be detected as bidirectional or pulmonary venous-to-systemic venous atrial shunts by color flow mapping. Saline contrast echocardiography or contrast from intravenous lines may demonstrate residual shunting in the postoperative period.

Arterial Switch. True to its name, the "anatomic repair" results in a heart that appears echocardiographically normal. Abnormal echocardiographic findings noted after the arterial switch procedure are generally confined to the anastomotic sites on the great vessels and mild degrees of semilunar valve regurgitation.[202] The initial courses of the ascending aorta and the proximal pulmonary artery are slightly distorted. Suture lines are appreciated in the supra-aortic region, but significant supravalvular aortic stenosis is unusual. The suprapulmonary region, however, is more likely to demonstrate significant supravalvar stenosis because of substantial loss of the root tissue when the coronary arteries are removed for reimplantation.[194] Marked differences in size of the great vessels also create difficulty in fashioning the new aortic and pulmonary roots to a uniform caliber. Pulsed and continuous wave Doppler are important adjuvants for diagnosing and quantifying supravalvar stenosis (Fig. 32–42).

Congenitally Corrected Transposition

The term congenitally corrected transposition refers to a specific congenital complex in which the great vessels are transposed—arising from the opposite ventricle—but the circulation is physiologically corrected because the ventricles are inverted and discordant relative to the atria. Hence atrioventricular discordance and ventriculoarterial discordance occur. This double switch results in normal physiologic flow from left atrium through right ventricle to aorta and from right atrium through left ventricle to pulmonary artery (Fig. 32–43). Whereas the majority of patients have situs solitus of the viscera and atria, it is possible to have corrected transposition with situs inversus, in which case the path of blood flow

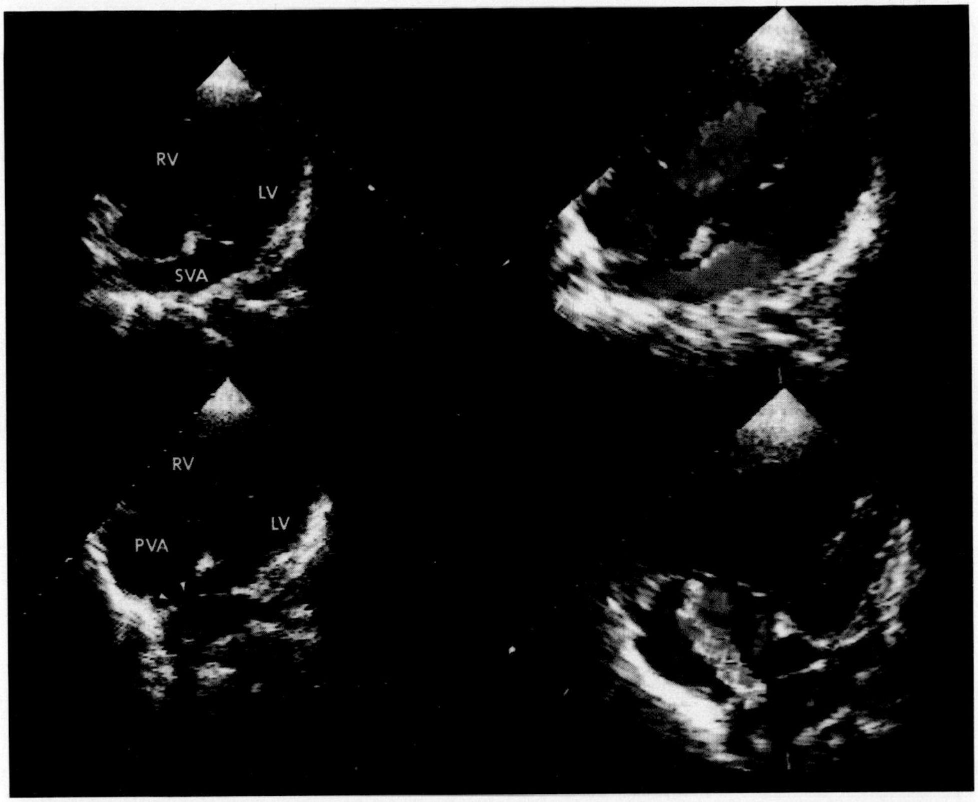

Fig. 32–41. Modified apical echocardiographic views of a patient with complete transposition of the great arteries following the Mustard procedure. Top, left. The systemic venous pathway directing flow from the inferior vena cava across to the mitral valve and into the left ventricle (LV). Top, right. The color flow image shows low velocity flow without significant narrowing of the flow stream at the midbaffle region. Bottom, left. Delineates the pulmonary venous atrium directing flow from the pulmonary veins across to the tricuspid valve and right ventricle. The small arrowheads point to a narrow neck in the midbaffle portion. Bottom, right. The color flow map shows a narrow, turbulent stream of flow across this small orifice. Peak Doppler flow velocity across this obstruction was 1.8 m/sec at rest, and the patient was asymptomatic. LV = left ventricle; PVA = pulmonary venous atrium; RV = right ventricle; SVA = systemic venous atrium.

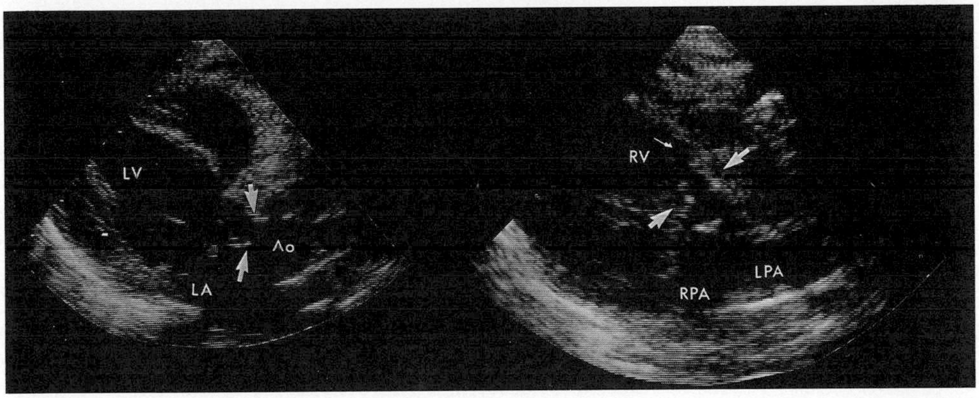

Fig. 32–42. Parasternal echocardiographic views of the long axis of the left and right ventricular outflow tracts following the arterial switch procedure for complete transposition of the great vessels. Left. A discrete narrowing of the ascending aorta is noted at the site of surgical anastomosis (double arrows). A more severe degree of luminal restriction is apparent on the right (double arrows) above the pulmonary valve (single arrow). Ao = aorta; LA = left atrium; LPA = left pulmonary artery; LV = left ventricle; RPA = right pulmonary artery; RV = right ventricle.

is the same, but the right-left orientation of each chamber is reversed.[203] In the absence of associated lesions, corrected transposition may go clinically unnoticed and is entirely compatible with a normal life span.[204] This situation is uncommon, however, because most patients with this anomaly come to a physician's attention because of: (1) ventricular septal defect; (2) pulmonary stenosis; (3) systemic AV valve dysfunction; and/or (4) conduction disturbances.

Ventricular Chambers

Because of abnormal looping of the primitive cardiac tubes, the anatomic right ventricle assumes a left-sided position with the anatomic left ventricle lying on the right side of the heart. The ventricular chambers lie in a side-by-side configuration or with the anatomic right ventricle slightly anterior to the left ventricle. This places the interventricular septum in an anteroposterior plane directly beneath the sternum. The typical course of a parasternal ultrasound beam therefore runs parallel to the septum rather than perpendicular to it, and this configuration explains the difficulty of optimally imaging the interventricular septum in parasternal views of this anomaly.

Echocardiographic establishment of ventricular identity allows accurate prospective diagnosis of ventricular inversion (see Chapter 31). The presence of a moderator band, trileaflet AV valve, and papillary muscle or other large trabeculations on the surface of the interventricu-

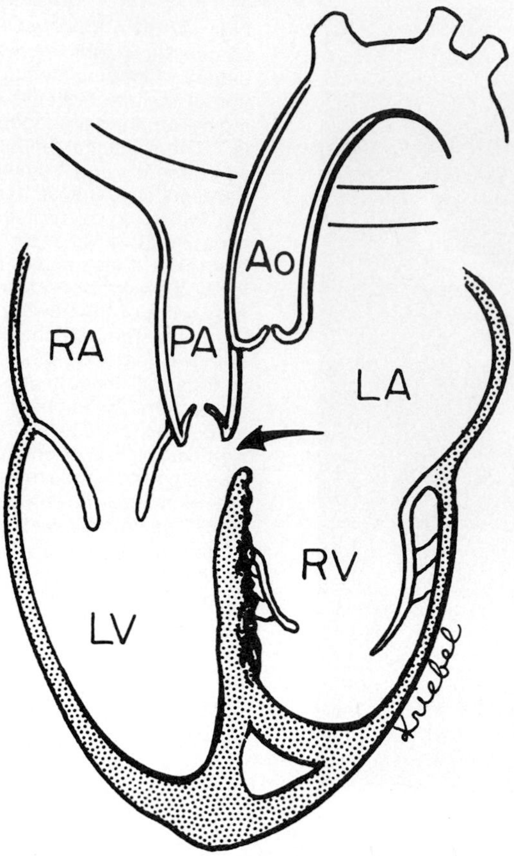

Fig. 32–43. Congenitally corrected transposition. The atrial situs is normal, but the ventricular orientation is inverted, with the anatomic right ventricle lying to the left and receiving flow from the left atrium. The anatomic left ventricle is right-sided and receives flow from the right atrium. The great arteries are transposed and arise in parallel from the base of the heart: the aorta lying to the left and arising from the anatomic right ventricle, the pulmonary artery lying to the right and arising from the anatomic left ventricle. Note the moderator band in the right ventricular apex, the trabeculations and septal leaflet insertion on the right ventricular septal surface, and the smooth left ventricular septal surface, all of which assist in assigning anatomic chamber identity. As is often the case, there is a subpulmonic ventricular septal defect (arrow) and valvular pulmonic stenosis. Ao = aorta; LA = left atrium; LV = left ventricle; PA = pulmonary artery; RA = right atrium; RV = right ventricle.

lar septum will indicate the anatomic right ventricle. The anatomic left ventricle is designated by a bileaflet AV valve, two distinct papillary muscles, and a smooth interventricular septal surface. One key distinguishing feature of the right ventricle is the apical displacement of the septal tricuspid leaflet relative to the mitral anterior leaflet.[205] This is best visualized echocardiographically from the apical four-chamber view (Fig. 32–44). In the presence of a VSD involving the inlet septum, however, both mitral and tricuspid valves attach at the same point, and other features must be used to determine ventricular morphology.[206]

Great Artery Position

Classically corrected transposition usually has L-transposed great arteries; that is, the vessels arise in parallel from the base of the heart, with the aorta anterior and to the left of the pulmonary artery (Fig. 32–45). (The extreme anterior and leftward position of the aorta creates the typical x-ray appearance of a straight upper left heart border and the accentuated aortic component of the second heart sound on auscultation in corrected transposition.) Depending on the exact degree of rotational abnormality in ventricular looping, however, the great vessels may lie in a more side-by-side relationship, directly anteroposterior, or even with the aorta to the right of the pulmonary artery.[207] Parasternal short axis views of the great vessels are most helpful in establishing right-left and anteroposterior relationships. Long axis views are needed from parasternal, apical, or subcostal projections to relate the great vessels appropriately to their respective ventricles. Because of the extreme leftward origin of the aorta in classically corrected transposition, the parasternal long axis view that best demonstrates systemic ventricular inflow and outflow must be obtained by placing the transducer further to the left and orienting the sector more vertically in a plane perpendicular to the left clavicle.

Ventricular Septal Defect

Nearly 80% of patients with corrected transposition have a VSD.[207,208] These defects are usually perimembranous, with variable degrees of extension into the inlet and outlet septum. Two-dimensional imaging readily permits one to detect the ventricular defects from nearly all vantage points. Color flow mapping quickly enables one to detect flow from the systemic (anatomic right ventricle) to pulmonary (anatomic left ventricle) circuits. Additional muscular defects are also easily located with color flow imaging.

Pulmonary Outflow Obstruction

In the abnormal development of the heart that occurs in corrected TGA, the interventricular septum is malaligned with the interatrial septum and the conal septum. As a result, the pulmonary valve is wedged between the mitral and tricuspid annuli, and the pulmonary outflow tract lies in an oblique or transverse plane, particularly susceptible to obstruction. In some cases, obstruction is caused by valvar pulmonic stenosis. More often, as VanPraagh has poetically stated, "all the woe lies below."[209] Subpulmonary obstruction may take the form of a discrete membrane, muscular collar, fibrous tag from the mitral apparatus, or herniated sacs of tricuspid tissue (Fig. 32–46). Pulmonary atresia also occurs occasionally.[208,210]

Echocardiographic evaluation of the pulmonary outflow tract is of critical importance because the nature and extent of outflow obstruction has considerable surgical relevance. Discrete membranes, isolated valvular stenosis, and tissue tags lend themselves to surgical removal, whereas more extensive or complex forms of obstruction require a conduit from the anatomic left ventricle to the distal pulmonary artery. In most instances, apical and subcostal windows permit clear visualization of the anatomic LVOT, and pulsed or continuous wave Doppler allows estimation of overall outflow gradients.

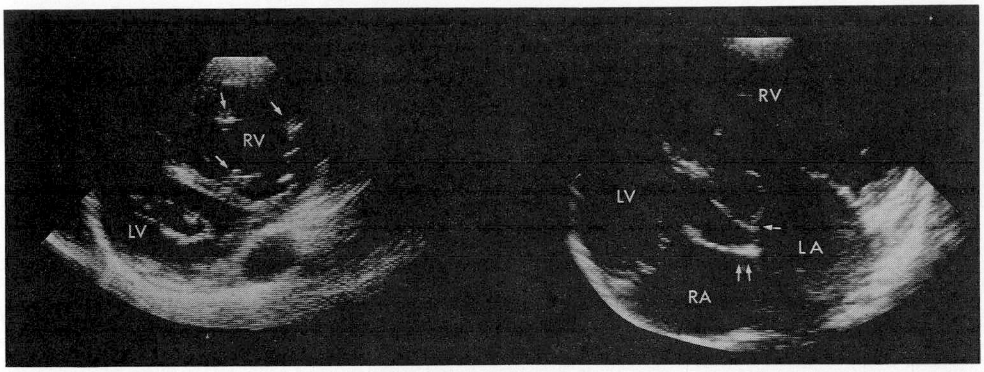

Fig. 32–44. Echocardiographic views of a patient with corrected transposition of the great arteries. Left. A parasternal short axis view of the ventricles depicting the larger systemic right ventricle (RV) anteriorly and to the left of the anatomic left ventricle (LV). The right-sided ventricle has a bileaved atrioventricular valve and a smooth septal surface indicating an anatomic LV. The three papillary muscles of the left-sided anatomic RV are noted by arrows. Right. An apical projection shows the relative insertion points of the atrioventricular valves along the interventricular septum. The mitral leaflet (double arrows) arises closer to the base of the heart, while the septal leaflet of the tricuspid valve inserts more apically (single arrow). LA = left atrium; RA = right atrium.

Ebstein's Malformation

Anatomic malformation of the left-sided tricuspid valve is another common abnormality in corrected transposition. The most common form is an Ebsteinlike anomaly with apical displacement and tethering of the tricuspid leaflets. The posterior and septal leaflets are similar to their right-sided Ebsteinoid counterparts; however, there are several differences from the Ebstein's anomaly that affect the right-sided tricuspid valve. First, the anterior leaflet is small rather than large and sail-like. It may also be cleft. With its origin along the anterior tricuspid valve annulus, when apically displaced, it is obstructive to flow streaming from the inlet to outlet portions of the systemic ventricle. The tricuspid annulus in left-sided Ebstein's anomaly is not dilated, and the systemic ventricle may be hypoplastic.[211,212] Functionally, about one third of left-sided tricuspid valves in corrected transposition are regurgitant.[207] Occasionally, this insufficiency of the systemic AV valve is severe enough to require surgical intervention (Fig. 32–47). Because annular dilatation is not a

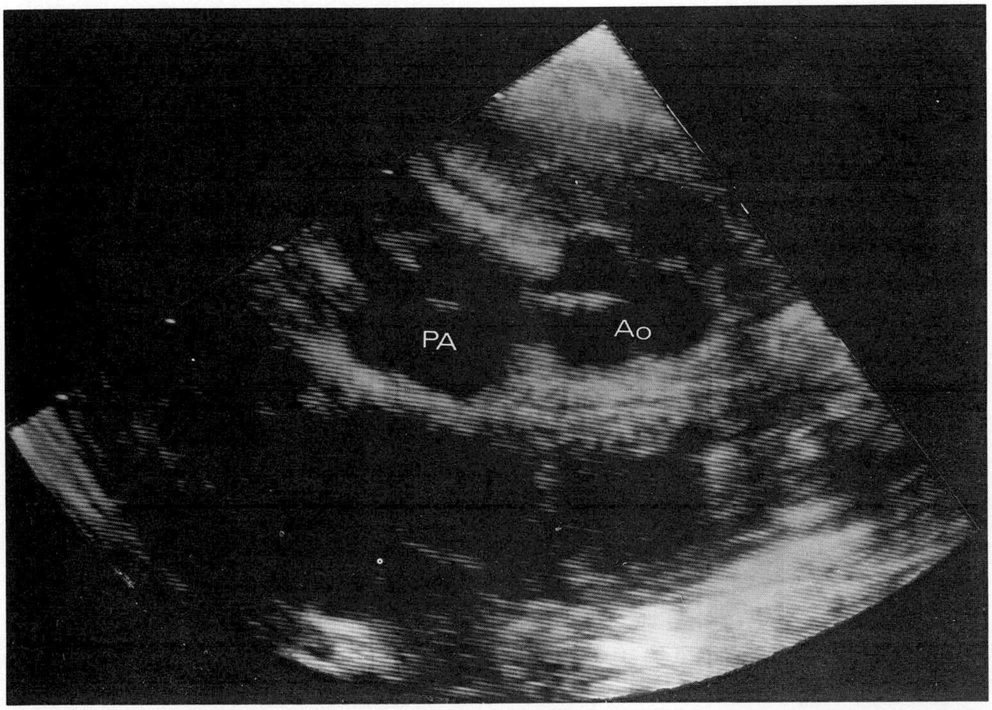

Fig. 32–45. Parasternal short axis echocardiographic view of the great vessels in congenitally corrected transposition of the great vessels. Both semilunar valves are imaged in cross section in the same plane. The aorta lies slightly anterior and to the left of the pulmonary artery. Ao = aorta; PA = pulmonary artery.

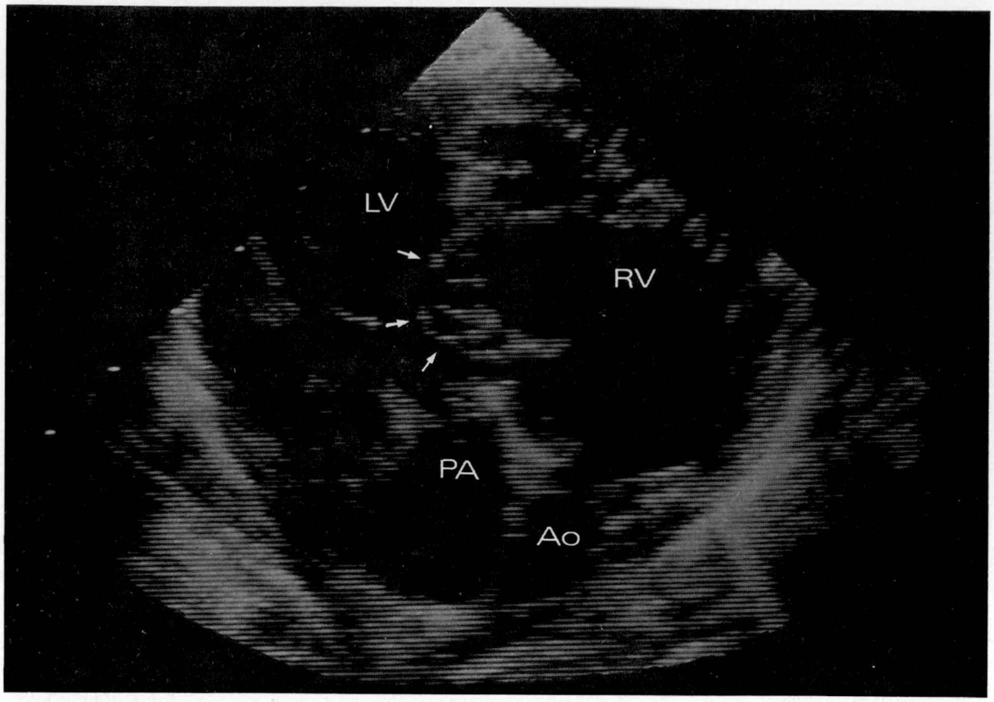

Fig. 32–46. Apical echocardiographic view from a patient with congenitally corrected transposition. A large ventricular septal defect permits herniation of tricuspid valve tissue into the left ventricular outflow tract (arrows), causing dynamic subpulmonary obstruction (and in addition, severe tricuspid insufficiency). Ao = aorta; LV = left ventricle; PA = pulmonary artery; RV = right ventricle.

contributing feature in the pathophysiology of this disorder, annuloplasty and valve repair are rarely successful and valve replacement is necessary.[213,214]

The echocardiographic delineation of the tricuspid valve in corrected transposition should establish the attachment of the valve leaflets, whether normal or apically displaced, and any restriction of leaflet excursion caused by chordal thethering. Pulsed and color flow Doppler permit one to detect the presence and severity of tricuspid (systemic AV valve) regurgitation. Herniation of septal tricuspid tissue through the VSD should be sought, and chordal attachment to the rim of the VSD or straddling of the leaflet into the opposite ventricle noted.

Hypoplasia of the systemic right ventricle may accompany Ebstein's malformation. Requiring the small right ventricle to support the systemic circulation independently by closure of a large VSD has disastrous results. Thus, noninvasive determination of a hypoplastic right ventricle dictates palliative rather than corrective surgery. Noninvasive quantitation of right ventricular volume and function can be performed in the same manner as for the systemic right ventricle in complete TGA.[39,215,216] A right ventricular volume less than 60%

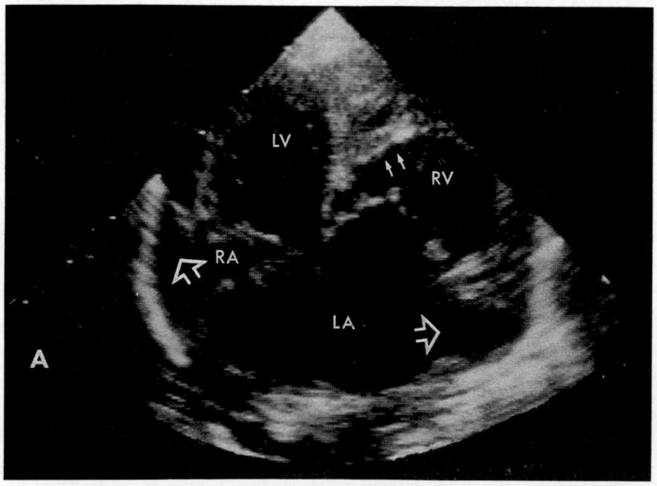

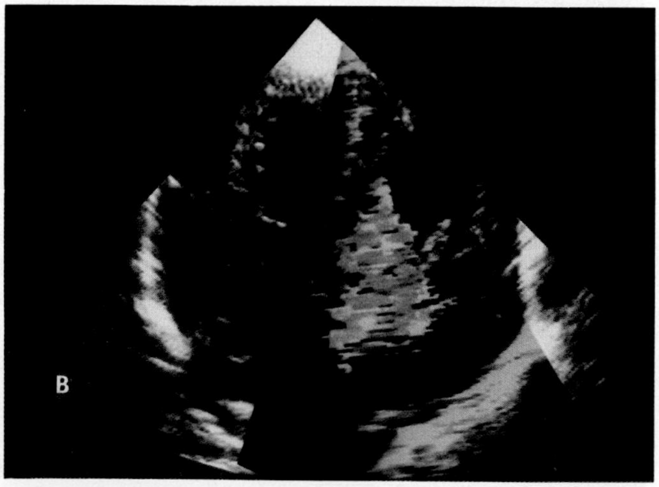

Fig. 32–47. Apical echocardiographic view of a child with corrected transposition with severe tricuspid (systemic atrioventricular valve) insufficiency. **A.** Note the markedly enlarged left atrium (LA) with deviation of the interatrial septum into the right atrium (RA). Double arrows mark the moderator band in the anatomic right ventricle (RV). The open arrows denote the atrial appendages; the left atrial appendage has a more narrow neck and is more tubular in shape than the broader right atrial appendage. **B.** The broad jet of tricuspid regurgitation by color flow Doppler. LV = left ventricle.

of normal will likely be unable to function as the systemic pump.[212]

Conduction Abnormalities

The normal course of conduction is disturbed in corrected TGA because of the malalignment of interatrial, interventricular, and conal septa and because of the inverted ventricular chamber orientation. Complete heart block is a frequent concomitant finding, either present from birth (5 to 10% of cases) or developing over time spontaneously or after invasive diagnostic or therapeutic procedures (up to 30% of cases).[217] Wolff-Parkinson-White syndrome coexists frequently in this group of patients.[218] Physicians who refer children with complete heart block, or Wolff-Parkinson-White syndrome for echocardiographic study to exclude structural heart disease often are seeking this known association with corrected transposition. The intimate relationship between the AV penetrating bundle with the pulmonary annulus and VSD has made heart block a common postsurgical complication.

Coronary Arteries

Just as the ventricular masses are inverted in this lesion, so too the coronary arterial supply is the inverse of the normal coronary pattern. This situation requires that the left main coronary artery arise from the right posterior aortic sinus, and the right coronary arterial supply arise from the left posterior sinus. The most anterior aortic sinus then is the noncoronary sinus. Of the variant patterns, the most common pattern in corrected transposition is a single coronary artery from the right sinus, which then divides into right and left branches.[219]

Surgical Management and Post-operative Assessment

Surgical intervention in corrected transposition is primarily focused on closure of significant interventricular septal communication, relief of significant pulmonary outflow obstruction, and repair or replacement of a malfunctioning systemic AV valve. During patch repair of a VSD, one must avoid stitch placement into the conduction system, which leads to postoperative heart block. Straddling chordal or leaflet tissue complicates VSD repair as well.

Primary relief of pulmonary outflow obstruction is performed when possible, including pulmonary valvotomy, subpulmonary membrane resection, or removal of obstructing fibrous tags. Frequently, the outflow obstruction is complex, and the diffusely narrowed oblique outflow tract makes direct repair difficult, especially with the additional risk of surgical trauma to the conduction tissue. In this instance, the main pulmonary artery is oversewn, and an extracardiac conduit, preferably a homograft, is placed between the right-sided anatomic left ventricle and the distal pulmonary artery.

The systemic AV valve may be repaired primarily or replaced if tricuspid regurgitation is clinically significant. Some patients who do not require tricuspid valve replacement during their initial procedure develop hemodynamically important valvular insufficiency secondary to leaflet alteration by the VSD patch or secondary to late right ventricular failure.[213] Postoperative echocardiographic evaluation should address residual ventricular shunting, residual pulmonary outflow obstruction, tricuspid (systemic AV valve) function whether native or prosthetic, conduit obstruction, and right ventricular (systemic ventricular) function. When an extracardiac conduit has been implanted and the main pulmonary artery oversewn, the native pulmonary valve continues to be visualized echocardiographically, with forward and reverse flow shown by pulsed or color flow Doppler across the valve.

Double-Outlet Right Ventricle

As its name implies, double-outlet right ventricle is an anomaly in which both great arteries arise either entirely or mostly from the right ventricle. The left ventricle must eject blood through a VSD to the right-sided aorta and pulmonary artery. This congenital complex is uncommon and has a variable expression both anatomically and physiologically, depending on the placement of the VSD in relation to the great arteries and depending on the presence or absence of obstruction to pulmonary blood flow[220] (Fig. 32–48). The clinical presentation may be simply that of a large VSD, or it may be similar to complete transposition with VSD. When pulmonary stenosis is present, the clinical picture is indistinguishable from that of tetralogy of Fallot. About one third of patients with double-outlet right ventricle have no additional major cardiac malformations; however, this disorder is frequently part of other complex malformations such as univentricular heart, heterotaxy syndromes with indeterminate situs, and complete AV canal defects.[221] This discussion focuses primarily on evaluation of the patient with double-outlet right ventricle as the primary abnormality.

Echocardiographic diagnosis requires determination of: (1) great vessel origin and relative position; (2) ventricular septal defect size and commitment; (3) obstruction to pulmonary blood flow; (4) coarctation of the aorta; and (5) associated AV valve anomalies.

Great Vessels

The aorta and pulmonary artery arise in parallel from the right ventricle, as seen in other transposition complexes. The aorta frequently lies to the right in a side-by-side relationship with the pulmonary artery, but it may also be posterior and rightward (normal semilunar valve relationship), anterior and to the right (D-transposed), directly anterior, or anterior and to the left (L-transposed).[222] Parasternal short axis echocardiographic views delineate the relative position and size of the great vessels accurately[223] (Fig. 32–49). Because in most types of double-outlet right ventricle the aorta is to the right, the leftward vessel in the short axis views is most often the pulmonary artery. This places the pulmonary valve in closest proximity to the mitral valve. The identity of the great arteries can be confirmed by determining which vessel bifurcates and which ascends to the arch.

The other characteristic feature of double-outlet right

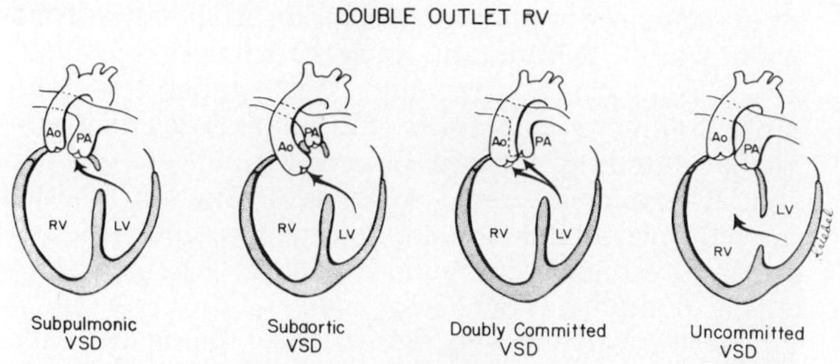

Fig. 32–48. The subtypes of double-outlet right ventricle (RV). The arrows demonstrate the direction of flow through the ventricular septal defect (VSD) in its different locations. With a subpulmonic VSD, left ventricular flow passes primarily into the pulmonary artery (PA), giving a physiology more akin to complete transposition. With a subaortic VSD, flow is directed into the aorta, and if pulmonary stenosis is associated, the physiology resembles tetralogy of Fallot. With a doubly committed defect, flow will stream preferentially to the lower resistance circuit, resulting in pulmonary congestion and systemic desaturation. Flow across the uncommitted defect will again seek the path of least resistance with varying degrees of pulmonary overcirculation and systemic desaturation. Ao = aorta; LV = left ventricle.

ventricle is the lack of fibrous continuity between the mitral valve and its nearest semilunar valve (usually pulmonic). Subarterial conus (or infundibulum) is frequently present beneath both vessels, thus separating both semilunar valves from the AV valves. In the parasternal long axis plane, this feature is apparent as a muscular separation between the base of the mitral leaflet and whichever semilunar valve is more posterior and leftward[222,223] (Fig. 32–49). The amount of conal tissue is variable, however, and may even be absent beneath one or both great arteries. In these instances, conal tissue cannot be appreciated echocardiographically, so double-outlet right ventricle is difficult to distinguish from tetralogy of Fallot with extreme aortic overriding or from complete transposition with VSD and pulmonary overriding.[126,127]

Ventricular Septal Defect

Although there are a few reported cases of double-outlet right ventricle with intact ventricular septum,[224,225] nearly all patients with this disorder have a VSD that allows for egress of blood from the left ventricle. The size and particularly the location of the defect with respect to the great vessels determine the clinical presentation and the type of surgical repair. Four general types of VSD are recognized: (1) subaortic (68%); (2) subpulmonic (22%) (the Taussig-Bing heart); (3) doubly-committed (3%); and (4) uncommitted or remote (7%).[226] The subaortic and subpulmonic defects commit the major flow from the left ventricle to the aorta or pulmonary artery, respectively, and that vessel usually overrides the ventricular septum (see Fig. 32–48). A doubly committed defect lies immediately beneath both great vessels, with no conal septal tissue. Remote or uncommitted defects may be large, muscular VSD or posterior inlet defects, including AV canal defects.

Detecting the VSD and its shunt flow is simple with good diagnostic two-dimensional imaging and Doppler techniques. Evaluating the commitment of the VSD to the great arteries can be more difficult because of the complex three-dimensional relationship of the ventricular septum and great arteries. Using a combination of parasternal or subcostal short axis sweeps from ventri-

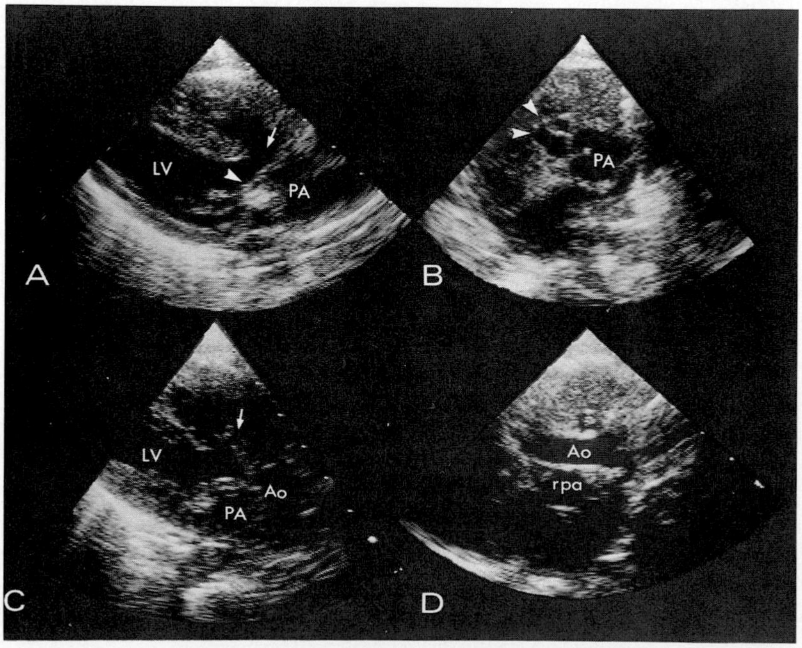

Fig. 32–49. Echocardiographic views from a patient with double-outlet right ventricle with anterior deviation of conal septum resulting in subaortic obstruction and subsequent hypoplasia and coarctation of the aorta. **A.** A parasternal long axis view outlines the subpulmonary ventricular septal defect (small arrow) and the subpulmonary conus (large arrow), which separates the pulmonary valve from the mitral valve. **B.** The parasternal short axis view at the base is shown, with a parallel and relatively side-by-side relationship of aorta (arrows) and pulmonary artery (PA). The aorta is hypoplastic. **C.** A parasternal long axis projection in which the conal septum (arrow) is noted deviating anteriorly impinging on the aortic outflow tract. **D.** The result of the proximal limitation of flow is noted. A coarctation of the aorta (Ao) is present. LV = left ventricle; rpa = right pulmonary artery.

cles to great vessels, one can infer the location of the septal defect with respect to the semilunar valves.[160] The defect is considered committed to the great vessel that is most readily imaged in the same or immediately adjacent short axis plane.[227] Parasternal or subcostal long axis views with medial-lateral angulation also help one to define the position of the interventricular septum, septal defect, and semilunar valves.

The VSD in double-outlet right ventricle is usually generous in size and provides little restriction to outflow from the left ventricle. In rare instances, the defect may be restrictive primarily or may become secondarily compromised by muscular hypertrophy or obstructing AV valve apparatus.[228,229] Serial echocardiographic and Doppler study should facilitate the diagnosis of restrictive VSD by noting changes in the defect's size and increases in Doppler flow velocities. Provided ventricular function is normal, the peak flow velocity across the VSD is predictive of the pressure drop from left ventricle to right ventricle and can therefore be used to determine the degree of VSD restriction. Peak velocities higher than 2 to 2.5 m/sec should be suspect.

Pulmonary Outflow Obstruction

Pulmonary outflow obstruction is a common feature of double-outlet right ventricle that occurs in approximately 60% of cases.[222,223,230] Pulmonary stenosis occurs most often in those hearts with a subaortic VSD, so this morphologic subgroup is both anatomically and physiologically similar to tetralogy of Fallot. Patients with a doubly committed VSD also commonly have pulmonic stenosis, whereas those with a subpulmonic or remote VSD generally do not. Infundibular stenosis results from conal septal impingement on the outflow tract. Valvular stenosis, annular narrowing, and peripheral stenosis all contribute to complex forms of pulmonary outflow obstruction (Fig. 32–50). When subvalvular or valvular atresia occurs, it is sometimes impossible to assign a chamber of origin to the pulmonary artery.

As with other transposition complexes, the pulmonary valve is easily imaged echocardiographically in both long axis and cross section and is readily accessible to sampling by pulsed and continuous wave Doppler. In patients with complex stenoses, the long axis parasternal or subcostal views provide the most complete view of each level of obstruction. Echocardiographic description of the presence and type of outflow obstruction is critical in determining whether simple primary repair is possible or more complex surgery is indicated requiring insertion of an RVOT conduit or right ventricular exclusion with a Fontan procedure.[231]

Coarctation of the Aorta

In double-outlet right ventricle with subpulmonary VSD (the Taussig-Bing malformation), the pulmonary artery is large and overrides the interventricular septum. When the aorta lies in a side-by-side relationship, the conal musculature is well developed beneath both great arteries and may cause subaortic obstruction with hypoplasia of the ascending aorta and distal coarctation or arch interruption.[232] This situation occurs in as many as one third of patients with Taussig-Bing anatomy and contributes to the higher mortality noted in this subgroup of patients.[220] Echocardiographically, particular attention should be focused on the aortic arch when subaortic conus is present and the proximal aorta appears smaller than the main pulmonary artery (see Fig. 32–49). Subaortic stenosis may progress over time, with further hypertrophy of conal tissue and right ventricular muscle bundles. This change should be sought by Doppler sampling of the subaortic region.

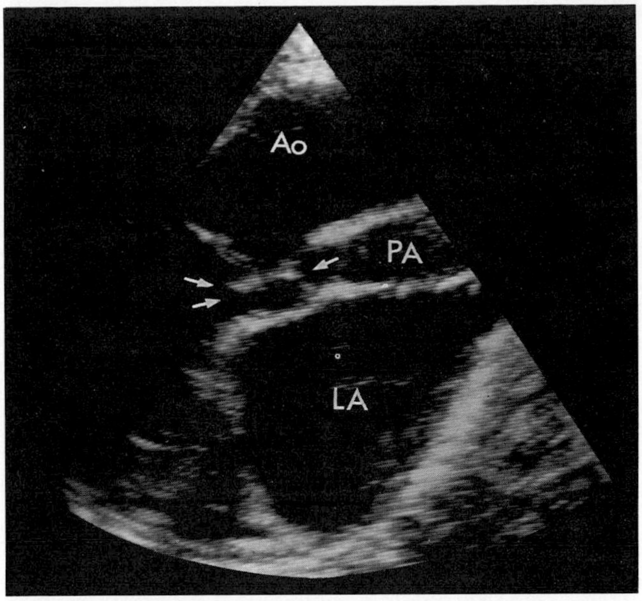

Fig. 32–50. Parasternal long axis echocardiographic view of the great vessels in double-outlet right ventricle. The aorta (Ao) is enlarged and anterior. The pulmonary artery (PA) lies beneath the aorta and demonstrates infundibular stenosis (double arrows), a small pulmonary annulus, and valvular pulmonary stenosis (single arrow). LA = left atrium.

Atrioventricular Valve Abnormalities

Many anomalies of the AV valves have been reported in double-outlet right ventricle, most commonly in the subgroups without pulmonary stenosis.[220,222,223] These include: (1) chordal attachment from either valve to the rim of the VSD or to the conal septum; (2) overriding or straddling of the mitral or tricuspid valve;[233] (3) mitral atresia; and (4) cleft mitral valve or complete AV canal. Echocardiography is uniquely suited to the diagnosis of these abnormalities, and their detection will influence both the type of surgical procedure and operative risk. For example, simple closure of the VSD may not be feasible if a major degree of AV valve straddling is present, thus committing the patient to a palliative procedure, a valve replacement, or a Fontan repair.[233] During echocardiographic study, parasternal short axis views demonstrate a cleft in the mitral leaflet, and apical and subcostal views provide the best perspective of the AV valves and intracardiac septa to detect straddling or overriding.

Surgical Management

The goal of surgical treatment is relief of pulmonary stenosis when present and closure of the VSD to connect the left ventricle to the aorta and to leave the left ventricle as the systemic pump whenever possible. These goals are obviously achieved in different ways, depending on the type of double-outlet right ventricle.[231]

Subaortic VSD and Doubly Committed VSD without Pulmonic Stenosis. These patients have the physiologic features of a large, unrestricted VSD. Surgical results in this group are generally excellent. VSD repair is recommended within the first 6 months of life and is accomplished by a VSD patch angled across to the anterior rightward aorta, creating an intraventricular tunnel. If the VSD is large and the aortopulmonary relationship is optimal, then the left ventricular outflow tunnel can be created without obstructing flow passing around the tunnel from the right ventricle into the pulmonary artery. If the VSD is small, the defect can be surgically enlarged, but the intraventricular tunnel will likely compromise the RVOT, necessitating an RVOT patch or conduit.

Subaortic VSD with Pulmonary Stenosis. These patients are physiologically similar to those with tetralogy of Fallot and are managed according to the same timetable. The VSD is closed and right ventricular outflow obstruction is relieved by valvotomy, a transannular outflow tract patch, or an extracardiac homograft conduit.

Subpulmonic VSD. Surgical repair of the Taussig-Bing malformation is more problematic than that of the other subgroups and carries a higher risk. Earlier approaches to this malformation involved VSD closure, leaving the pulmonary artery originating from the left ventricle. This procedure converted the patient from double-outlet right ventricle to complete transposition, thus necessitating an intra-atrial Mustard or Senning procedure to normalize the circulation. High mortality rates have discouraged routine use of this repair.[231] Two major approaches have emerged for this entity: (1) VSD closure followed by an arterial switch;[232,234] and (2) intraventricular tunnel closure of the VSD connecting the left ventricle to the aorta with an extracardiac conduit from the right ventricle to the pulmonary artery if needed.

Remote or Uncommitted VSD. Because the anatomic features of this group are variable, the surgical management must be individualized and often is complex. If the VSD can be closed by a tunneled patch connecting the left ventricle to the aorta, this is preferred. VSD closure and arterial switch may be used if an intraventricular tunnel is not feasible and if pulmonary outflow obstruction is absent. In patients with remote VSD and pulmonic stenosis, a Fontan procedure may be the best alternative.

Postoperative Echocardiographic Assessment

As with most congenital heart lesions, knowledge of the exact method of surgical repair greatly enhances the ability of the echocardiographer to evaluate the postoperative patient fully. This is especially true in double-outlet right ventricle, where the range of pathologic features is so wide.

Because of the complexity of patch placement, residual VSD is not uncommon and has prompted re-operation in up to 20% of patients for significant degrees of shunting.[230,235,236] Patch dehiscense has also been reported.[231,237] Two-dimensional imaging depicts the echo-dense VSD patch, which should firmly adhere to its points of attachment. In apical and subcostal views, the patch can be seen angled obliquely from the septal crest to the right and anteriorly (Fig. 32–51). Color flow mapping and pulsed Doppler imaging assists one in detecting residual shunt flow.

Pulmonary stenosis, either residual or acquired after creation of the intraventricular tunnel, should be assessed by pulsed and continuous wave Doppler. Postoperative echocardiographic assessment of extracardiac conduits is discussed in the section of this chapter on tetralogy of Fallot.

Another potential problem area is the tunneled outflow tract from the left ventricle to the aorta. Subaortic obstruction can be created by the elongated intraventricular channel that has been surgically fashioned, especially if the VSD size and location with respect to the aorta are suboptimal. The restrictive site is most often at the original VSD in the most proximal portion of the tunnel. Even when the VSD has been generously widened, the placement of the patch material and subsequent proliferation of fibrous tissue at the anastomosis

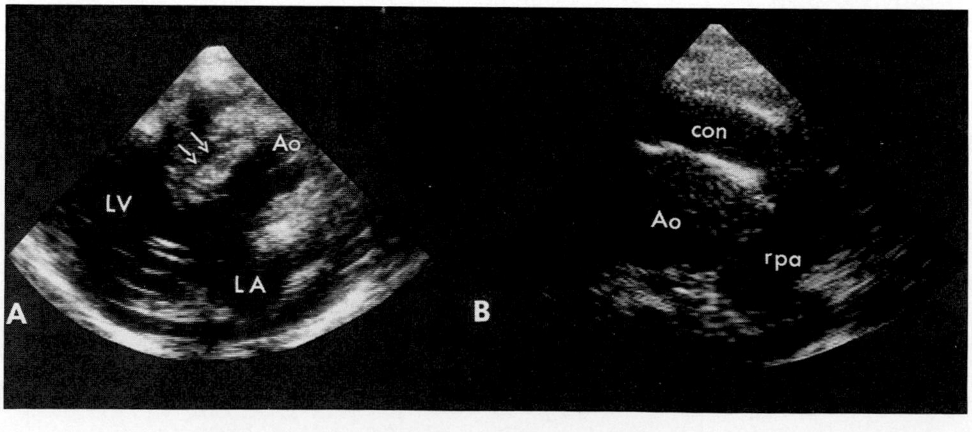

Fig. 32–51. Parasternal long axis echocardiographic view of the left ventricle following repair of double-outlet right ventricle. **A.** The angled ventricular septal defect patch (arrows) connects the left ventricle (LV) to the anteriorly positioned aorta (Ao). **B.** A Dacron conduit (con) was placed between the right ventricle and distal pulmonary artery. Ao = aorta; con = conduit; rpa = right pulmonary artery; LA = left atrium.

can lead to progressive narrowing of the left ventricular outlet.[238]

AV valve regurgitation occasionally becomes clinically significant postoperatively. This may be from preexisting valvular malformations, such as cleft mitral valve, or from distortion or disruption of valve function secondary to VSD patching. Pulsed Doppler and color flow mapping can assist in detecting and roughly quantifying the degree of regurgitation.

In patients who undergo the arterial switch procedure, postoperative evaluation should be directed to the vessel anastomoses and ventricular function, as discussed in the section of this chapter on TGA.

Truncus Arteriosus

Persistent truncus arteriosus is a rare malformation (2% of patients with congenital cardiac anomalies[239]) in which a single arterial trunk arising from the heart supplies the coronary, pulmonary, and systemic circulations. A large VSD is invariably present. Embryologically, this malformation has been attributed to improper septation of the primitive arterial trunk, although another hypothesis attributes the anomaly to infundibular and pulmonary atresia with subsequent failure of truncal septation, making persistent truncus arteriosus a close relative of tetralogy of Fallot.[240]

Several commonly recognized patterns of truncus arteriosus are seen, and these are currently classified as diagrammed in Figure 32–52.[240] This classification supersedes the older and perhaps more familiar classification of Collett and Edwards from 1949.[241] Classification depends upon where the pulmonary arteries arise from the truncus and whether the arch is interrupted. Nearly 50% of cases are represented by type I, in which a short segment of main pulmonary artery arises from the posterolateral wall of the truncus before branching into right and left pulmonary arteries. In the next most common type (type II, approximately 20%), the right and left pulmonary arteries originate independently from the trunk either adjacent to each other posteriorly or from their respective lateral aspects of the common root. In a small percentage of cases (type IV, 12%), the aortic component of the truncus is underdeveloped, with coarctation or arch interruption. In this type, once the pulmonary arteries branch from the common trunk, a large ductus continues on to the descending aorta. The least common pattern is that in which one of the pulmonary arteries is absent (type III, 8%), most often the left pulmonary artery. The ipsilateral lung is supplied by collateral vessels or by a persistent ductus.[242]

Echocardiographic identification relies on demonstration of the typical findings of truncus arteriosus: (1) a large, single great vessel that overrides an outlet VSD; (2) absence of a RVOT and pulmonary valve; and (3) branching of the main pulmonary artery or its independent branches from the large common arterial trunk. These features can be reliably determined on parasternal long and short axis views, with superior angulation of these planes. Suprasternal views may help to demonstrate pulmonary artery origin and course. Subcostal or apical long and short axis views also demonstrate the classic features of truncus arteriosus (Fig. 32–53).[243–245] Tetralogy of Fallot with pulmonary atresia may appear anatomically similar to truncus arteriosus. Clear demonstration of the origin of the pulmonary arteries directly from the main arterial trunk as well as the large, frequently abnormal truncal valve assist one in differentiating these two entities.

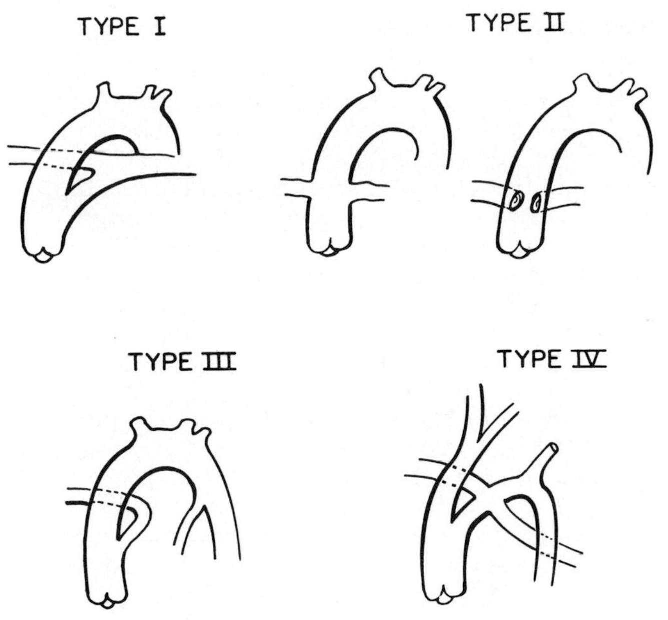

Fig. 32–52. The subtypes of truncus arteriosus. The most common form is type I, in which a short segment of main pulmonary artery is present, arising from the posterolateral wall of the truncus. Type II has no main pulmonary artery but direct and separate origin of the branch pulmonary arteries from the lateral or posterior wall of the truncus. Type III occurs infrequently and consists of the absence of one branch pulmonary artery (often the left) with circulation to the affected lung by aortopulmonary collateral vessels or a persistent ductus. Type IV is also uncommon, with underdevelopment of the aortic component of the truncus and coarctation or arch interruption. The pulmonary arteries arise from the proximal truncal root, and a large ductus arteriosus continues on to supply the descending thoracic aorta.

Truncal Valve

The semilunar valve of the common arterial trunk is frequently abnormal.[246] The valve leaflets are thickened, nodular, and myxomatous. The valve may have two (8%), three (61%), four (31%) or more cusps (0 to 2%).[242,246] About 20% of patients have truncal regurgitation, which adds further hemodynamic burden to the volume-loaded left ventricle. Both absolute and relative valvar stenoses have been described in more than one third of patients, although gradients are usually low. Significant dysfunction is more common with bicuspid or quadricuspid valves.

Because the truncal valve becomes the systemic semilunar valve after surgical repair, it is important to establish its functional status as part of the preoperative noninvasive assessment. Two-dimensional imaging can permit one to determine the number of valve leaflets, valvular doming or prolapse, and significant leaflet thickening. Pulsed and color flow Doppler examination

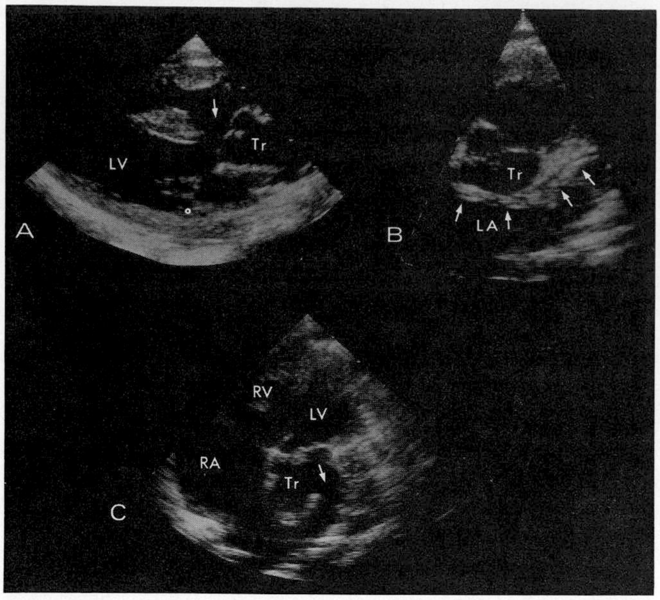

Fig. 32–53. Echocardiographic views of truncus arteriosus (Tr) type I. **A.** The parasternal long axis view of the left ventricle (LV) and overriding truncal root. The large subarterial ventricular septal defect is noted by an arrow. **B.** A parasternal short axis view of the truncal valve with abnormal origin of the left coronary artery from the noncoronary sinus (arrows). **C.** An apical five-chamber view of the heart, demonstrating the large truncal root in the center, with the main pulmonary artery arising from the lateral border of the root (arrow). LA = left atrium; RA = right atrium; RV = right ventricle.

will enable one to detect truncal regurgitation and to estimate the degree of truncal stenosis (Fig. 32–54). Obviously, the need for valve replacement influences the timing, type, and overall risk of surgical repair.[247]

Ventricular Septal Defect

The VSD in truncus arteriosus results from absence or underdevelopment of the conal or infundibular septum, similar to that in tetralogy of Fallot. The defect lies immediately below the truncal valve and is usually large. The truncal root commonly straddles the interventricular septum and gives it a biventricular origin. In 40% of patients, however, the truncus may arise predominantly from the left ventricle and in 15 to 25% predominantly from the right ventricle.[248] The VSD is readily imaged echocardiographically in long and short axis views directly beneath the truncal valve. Pulsed Doppler and color flow mapping demonstrate low velocity bidirectional flow across the defect, with systolic streams from both ventricles exiting through the truncal valve. In rare instances, the VSD is small and restrictive.[249]

Pulmonary Arteries

The pulmonary arteries are well developed and originate from the main arterial vessel just distal to the semilunar valve, either from a short main pulmonary stump (type I) or independently (type II). When the main pulmonary artery is short, it may be impossible to differentiate types I and II either echocardiographically or angiographically. The high left parasternal and suprasternal imaging planes have been of most value in visualizing the anatomy of the pulmonary artery origins and course.

In most cases, pulmonary blood flow is unrestricted and exposes the lungs to high volume flow under systemic pressures. This situation leads initially to severe

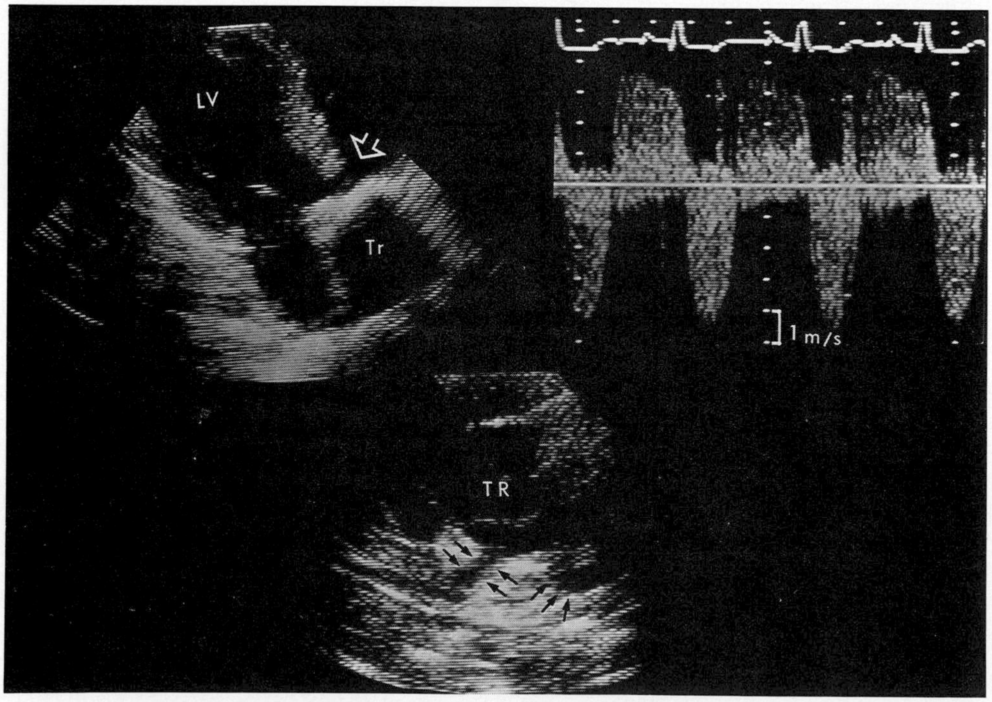

Fig. 32–54. Echocardiographic and Doppler tracings from a patient with truncus arteriosus (Tr) and severe truncal valve stenosis. Top, left. An apical long axis view of the left ventricle (LV) demonstrating the subarterial ventricular septal defect (open arrow) and, just above this, the markedly thickened and calcified truncal valve. Top, right. A continuous wave Doppler spectral trace indicating a peak outflow gradient of about 80 mm Hg. Truncal regurgitation is shown as the diastolic flow above the baseline. Bottom. A short axis view of the truncal root above the level of the truncal valve. Branch pulmonary arteries could be seen emerging from the posterior wall of the root (black arrows). m/s = meters per second. (From Liberthson RR: Congenital heart disease in the child, adolescent and adult. *In:* The Practice of Cardiology. Boston, Little, Brown & Company, 1989.)

congestive heart failure and soon thereafter to pulmonary vascular obstructive disease. Occasionally, branch pulmonary stenosis creates some degree of natural protection to the pulmonary bed. These infants have less severe heart failure and more severe cyanosis than patients with unrestricted pulmonary blood flow. Ostial narrowing may be apparent by two-dimensional imaging of the branch pulmonary vessels, and color flow mapping and pulsed Doppler demonstrate turbulent, high velocity flow. Exact quantitation of gradient is occasionally difficult because of the inability to align the Doppler beam parallel to the flow stream.

One other unusual mode of pulmonary stenosis has been described in truncus arteriosus. An elongated leaflet of the truncal valve adjacent to the pulmonary artery ostium may occlude the vessel orifice in systole.[242]

Unilateral complete absence of a pulmonary artery is seen in a small number of patients (type III) (see Fig. 32–52). The absent pulmonary artery is usually from the same side as the aortic arch; that is, with a left aortic arch, the left pulmonary artery is absent; with a right arch, the right pulmonary artery is missing.[250] A patent ductus or bronchial collateral vasculature supplies flow to the affected lung.

Coronary Arteries

The coronary arteries have an abnormal origin in about a third of patients with truncus arteriosus.[251] Either the right or left coronary may originate from the noncoronary sinus, or there may be a single coronary ostium. Of more physiologic concern is the abnormal positioning of the coronary ostia at or slightly above a valve commissure with a slitlike orifice that is functionally stenotic (see Fig. 32–53). This may lead to ischemia or infarction of the left ventricle, which is already compromised by the large pulmonary shunt, decreased oxygen saturation, and truncal valve regurgitation.

Aortic Arch

A right aortic arch occurs more commonly in patients with truncus arteriosus than in those with other congenital cardiac lesions. This is another similarity that this disorder shares with tetralogy of Fallot. Hypoplasia and coarctation or interruption of the aortic arch are present in 12 to 19% of cases (type IV). A reciprocal relationship appears to exist between the development of the ascending aorta and transverse arch (derived from the embryonic fourth arch) and the ductus arteriosus (derived from the embryonic sixth arch).[240] When the ascending aorta and arch are well developed, the patient usually has no persistent ductus arteriosus. When the ascending aorta is hypoplastic and severe coarctation or interruption occurs, the ductus is large and connects the proximal truncus to the descending aorta. Echocardiographically, this type of truncus arteriosus may be difficult to diagnose if the hypoplastic ascending segment is overlooked and the brachiocephalic vessels are not carefully examined. The large ductal continuation creates the appearance of a continuous aortic arch.

Associated Defects

A secundum ASD has been noted in 10% of cases, and a variety of mitral valve abnormalities have been reported in about 10%, including mitral stenosis, mitral atresia, and double-orifice mitral valve.[252] Another common association with truncus arteriosus is DiGeorge syndrome[253] or thymic aplasia; hence any infant in whom truncus arteriosus is diagnosed should be further evaluated for thymic dysfunction.

Surgical Management

The natural history of this lesion is an abbreviated one, with mean age of death at 5 weeks and a 70 to 85% mortality by 1 year of age. A few patients manage to survive into older childhood or adulthood with irreversible pulmonary hypertension. Obvious preference exists, therefore, for surgical approaches to management. Once medical decongestive measures have been taken, one needs to restrict excessive pulmonary blood flow. Earlier practice recommended initial palliative pulmonary artery banding in infancy—of the main pulmonary artery segment in type I or the individual branches in type II—followed by complete surgical correction at several years of age. Problems with insufficient banding, occlusion or distortion of proximal branch pulmonary arteries, worsening truncal valve regurgitation, and mortality in the range of 30 to 50%, however, led to the recommendation for complete repair of the defect in infancy.[254]

Corrective repair entails patch closure of the VSD, removal of the portion of the common truncus where the main or branch pulmonary ostia originates, and oversewing or patching the defect so created in the truncal root wall. If the truncal valve is significantly dysfunctional, a prosthetic aortic valve or homograft valve is placed at the base of the truncal root. A conduit is then inserted between the right ventricle and the pulmonary artery. Performing such a repair in the infant necessitates reoperation at least once during childhood for conduit replacement. One hopes that using valved homograft conduits will extend the reoperation-free interval, but growth alone will eventually mandate reoperation. Mortality for primary repair of this defect in the first year of life remains high, but in some centers it is as low as 16%.

Postoperative Evaluation

Noninvasive investigation after corrective surgery for truncus arteriosus includes attention to: (1) residual VSD; (2) progressive truncal valve stenosis or regurgitation or prosthetic aortic valve dysfunction; and (3) RVOT conduit deterioration. Because most conduits have a 4- to 5-year life span, the development of increasing evidence of right ventricular pressure overload (right ventricular enlargement and systolic interventricular septal flattening) can be noted on two-dimensional imaging, and increasing gradients during pulsed or continuous wave Doppler can be detected across the conduit (see the section of this chapter on tetralogy of Fallot).

ABNORMALITIES OF VENOUS RETURN: TOTAL ANOMALOUS PULMONARY VENOUS DRAINAGE

Failure of the pulmonary veins to communicate directly with the left atrium results in the congenital complex known as total anomalous pulmonary venous return (TAPVR) or total anomalous pulmonary venous drainage (TAPVD). The pulmonary veins connect instead with one of the systemic venous tributaries (superior and inferior vena cava, azygous vein, or coronary sinus) or directly with the right atrium. A significant right ventricular volume overload results from return of all the pulmonary venous inflow to the right heart. An interatrial septal communication permits the left heart to receive venous return. Although it does occur in association with complex congenital cardiac anomalies (particularly those with atrial situs ambiguus), TAPVR is most commonly seen as an isolated aberration. This malformation represents only 1 to 2% of congenital heart defects in large autopsy series.[255,256]

In its clinical presentation, TAPVR mimics many other diseases of the newborn. It may be difficult to diagnose unless it is consciously sought, and without proper diagnosis and management it is generally lethal.

Because many forms of TAPVR cause obstruction to the pulmonary venous pathway,[257] the clinical presentation is usually that of pulmonary venous hypertension in the first few weeks of life, with marked tachypnea, a small heart, and no significant murmurs. Neonatal pneumonia, transient tachypnea of the newborn, myocarditis, and persistent fetal circulation all have similar clinical features and muddy the clinical waters when one attempts to diagnose the critically ill neonate. In this context, the echocardiographer is frequently summoned to exclude a diagnosis of structural heart disease. In those forms of TAPVR without obstruction to venous return, the clinical presentation occurs later in infancy or even later in childhood, with a predominant right ventricular volume overload pattern similar to that seen in a large ASD. The degree of systemic oxygen desaturation depends on the type and size of the atrial communication and on the pulmonary vascular resistance.

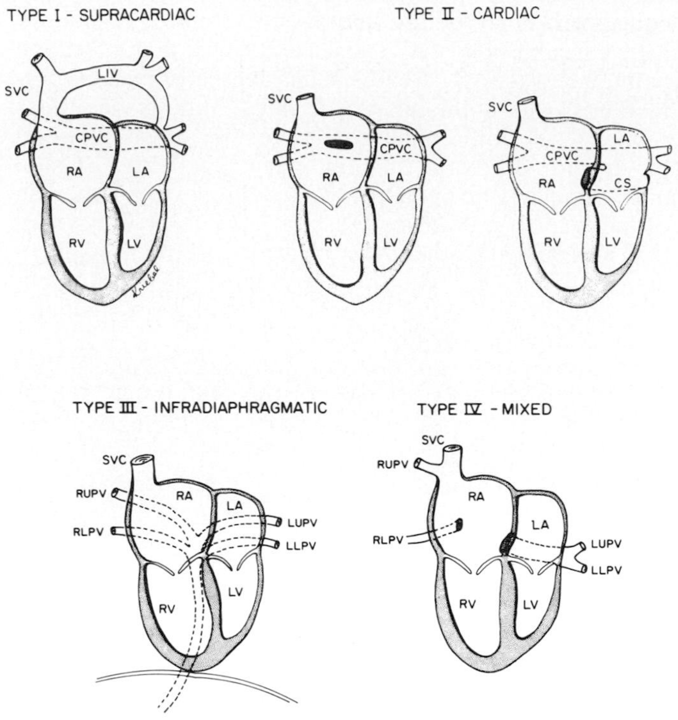

Fig. 32–55. The subtypes of total anomalous pulmonary venous return (TAPVR). In type I, the pulmonary veins return to a common pulmonary venous channel behind the left atrium (LA) and then drain via an ascending vertical vein into the left innominate vein (LIV) and hence into the superior vena cava (SVC). The enlargement of this venous pathway creates a circular shadow on the chest radiograph at the base of the heart, which is responsible for the "snowman" configuration of this type of TAPVR. In type II, return is directly to the right heart, either by an ostium in the common pulmonary venous chamber into the right atrium (RA) or by communication of the common chamber with the coronary sinus (CS). Type III return is below the diaphragm, usually with a "reverse Christmas tree" appearance of the pulmonary veins as they join into a descending vertical vein passing through the diaphragm. Type IV is mixed drainage and is here illustrated with the right upper vein entering the SVC, the left veins draining into the CS, and the right lower vein entering the RA directly. CPVC = common pulmonary venous chamber; LLPV = left lower pulmonary vein; LV = left ventricle; LUPV = left upper pulmonary vein; RLPV = right lower pulmonary vein; RV = right ventricle; RUPV = right upper pulmonary vein.

Venous Return

TAPVR has been classified according to the site of drainage of the pulmonary veins: type I, supracardiac; type II, cardiac; type III, infracardiac; and type IV, mixed.

Supracardiac drainage is most common, comprising 40 to 50% of cases (Fig. 32–55).[256–259] In this form, the right and left pulmonary veins enter a common pulmonary venous chamber that lies along the posterior and superior aspect of the true left atrium. A single venous channel, the ascending vertical vein, then ascends to join the innominate vein, the superior vena cava, or the azygos vein.

The next most frequent site of venous return is the coronary sinus or the right atrium (type II) (Fig. 32–55). Pulmonary venous return in this group of patients is usually to a common venous chamber, which then communicates directly with either the right atrium or the coronary sinus. Infradiaphragmatic drainage is less common, but it occurs in the majority of critically ill neonates with this defect because of the nearly universal presence of venous obstruction in this anatomic subset.[260] In this group, the right and left pulmonary veins drain in a "reverse Christmas tree" fashion into a small inferior venous chamber that continues through the diaphragm as the descending vertical vein to join the inferior vena cava, the portal venous system or the ductus venosus. The rarest form of TAPVR is the mixed type (type IV), in which the pulmonary veins individually return to different sites. The possible combinations and permutations are many; for example, the left veins may join and drain to the coronary sinus or the left vertical vein, whereas the right veins drain to the superior vena cava or directly to the right atrium.

Pulmonary Venous Obstruction

Virtually all infants with infradiaphragmatic TAPVD and about 50% of those with supradiaphragmatic types of the disorder have pulmonary venous obstruction.[257] These obstructions may take several forms: (1) stenosis of the pulmonary veins at the entry to the venous chamber; (2) single or multiple discrete stenoses of the ascending or descending vertical vein; or (3) obstruction at the entry of the vertical vein or common chamber with the receiving systemic vein. Two other forms of obstruction to venous return are found in TAPVR, which drains below the diaphragm. Specific to the infradiaphragmatic type that returns to the portal circuit is a diffuse obstruction presented by the hepatic microcirculation. If the descending vertical vein enters the ductus venosus, the infant will be at risk of complete pulmonary venous obstruction when normal postnatal closure of the ductus venosus occurs. An unusual form of supracardiac stenosis is the "hemodynamic vice,"[261] wherein the ascending vertical vein becomes squeezed between the pulmonary artery and the mainstem bronchus on either the left or the right side.

In all these forms of venous obstruction, echocardiographic and angiographic studies often demonstrate localized constrictions and pinpoint sites of stenosis. Pulsed and color flow Doppler imaging may permit one to detect turbulent, continuous flow of higher velocity than that proximal to the obstruction.[262,263] Attempts have been made to use balloon dilation angioplasty on those vessels accessible by catheter.[257,264] With early definitive surgical management, however, the nature and location of these stenoses are less critical. Patients in whom a simple repair cannot be performed, whose stenoses are at the individual pulmonary vein ostium, or in whom surgical repair must be delayed, still provide a challenge to the interventional cardiologist.

Interatrial Septum

The passage of pulmonary venous flow to the left heart must occur through the interatrial septum. A patent foramen ovale performs this function in the majority of cases, whereas a secundum atrial septal defect is present in the remaining 25%.[256] Restriction to flow across the atrial defect may occur de novo or may develop as the infant grows and the foramen ovale becomes insufficient to accommodate systemic blood flow. This, then, presents another site for physiologic pulmonary venous obstruction. Balloon or blade septostomy is occasionally performed to stabilize a critically ill infant's condition before surgical repair is undertaken, or is used as a temporizing measure in a patient for whom definitive repair must be delayed.[265]

Left Atrium and Ventricle

The left atrium in hearts with TAPVR is small secondary to the absence of the pulmonary venous component. This relative hypoplasia has been implicated in adverse outcomes after surgery.[266] Postoperatively, however, left atrial volumes return to normal and appear to grow appropriately along with the patient.[267,268] The left ventricle is also of small relative volume and occasionally is frankly hypoplastic,[268,269] but it generally assumes normal volume and ejection fraction after surgical correction.[267]

Associated Lesions

Most patients with TAPVR have no associated cardiac defects other than a patent ductus arteriosus. In about one third of patients, however, major congenital cardiac lesions are seen in conjunction with anomalous venous drainage. Complex anomalies with atrial situs ambiguus frequently have anomalous pulmonary and systemic venous drainage. Occasionally, tetralogy of Fallot, double-outlet right ventricle, and interrupted aortic arch may keep company with anomalous pulmonary venous drainage.[259]

Echocardiographic Evaluation

Echocardiographic assessment of the patient with suspected total anomalous pulmonary venous connection should be focused on the following: (1) establishing the absence of pulmonary venous return to the left atrium; (2) detecting right ventricular volume and/or pressure overload; (3) determining the site into which the common pulmonary vein enters; (4) assessing the nature of the interatrial communication; (5) searching the anomalous pathway for sites of obstruction; and (6) noting associated defects.

The most obvious finding on initial inspection of the patient with TAPVR is enlargement of the right atrium and ventricle. In patients with obstructed pulmonary venous return, pulmonary hypertension develops with enlargement of the pulmonary artery, marked leftward shift of the interventricular septum, and small, underfilled left atrial and left ventricular chambers. The foramen ovale or ASD shunts right to left on pulsed or color flow Doppler sampling.

Careful examination of the posterolateral wall of the left atrium in the parasternal long axis, apical, and subcostal four-chamber views usually reveals a small chamber that does not communicate with the true left atrium, but lies directly adjacent to it (Fig. 32–56). Sufficient depth of field should be used to distinguish this chamber from the descending thoracic aorta. Although the normal descending thoracic aorta also appears as a vascular channel adjacent to the left atrium, it should lie in close proximity to the thoracic vertebrae and should have systolic pulsatile flow visible during pulsed Doppler or color flow mapping. In contrast, the common pulmonary venous channel has a low velocity venous flow pattern on Doppler interrogation and lies more anteriorly in the chest than the descending aorta. Suprasternal notch views also help to demonstrate the common pulmonary venous channel running in parallel and posterior to the right pulmonary artery (Fig. 32–57).

Identification of the site of drainage requires considerable effort on the part of the echocardiographer, aided by foreknowledge of the likely pathways. One helpful clue is provided by the receiving systemic vein, which is often dilated from the additional pulmonary venous

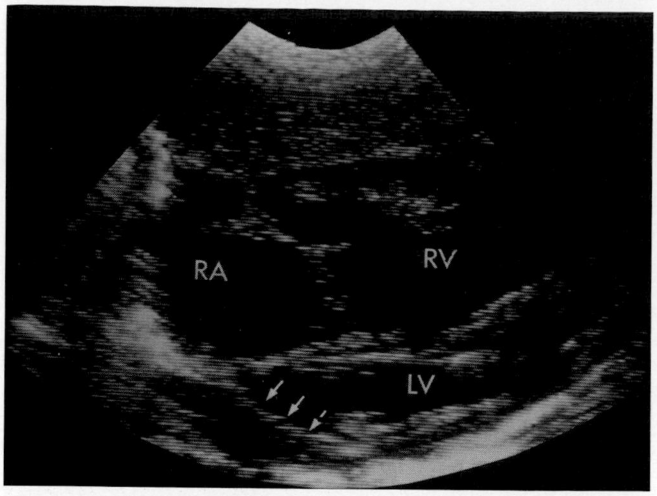

Fig. 32–56. Subxyphoid echocardiographic view of the heart in a patient with total anomalous pulmonary venous return. The right atrium (RA) and right ventricle (RV) are markedly enlarged, and the left atrium and left ventricle (LV) are small. Along the superior aspect of the left atrium is the common pulmonary venous chamber, which is separated from the true left atrium by an imperforate wall (arrows). (From Liberthson RR: Congenital heart disease in the child, adolescent and adult. *In:* The Practice of Cardiology. Boston, Little, Brown & Company, 1989.)

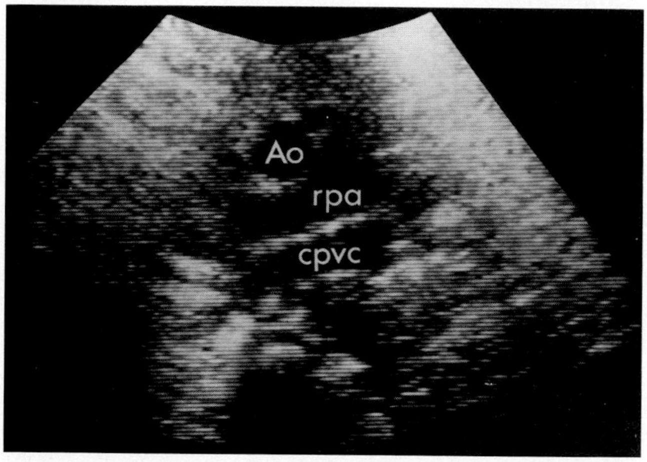

Fig. 32–57. Suprasternal echocardiographic view of the ascending aorta (Ao) and right pulmonary artery (rpa). The common pulmonary venous channel (CPVC) runs parallel to the rpa, carrying the right pulmonary venous flow to join the left pulmonary veins and ascend toward the innominate vein. (From Liberthson RR: Congenital heart disease in the child, adolescent and adult. *In:* The Practice of Cardiology. Boston, Little, Brown & Company, 1989.)

inflow. Thus, supracardiac drainage enlarges the innominate vein or the superior vena cava, and anomalous return to the coronary sinus causes that structure to become markedly dilated. In patients with infradiaphragmatic drainage, the inferior vena cava may not be significantly enlarged because of obstruction within the common descending vein before its junction with the inferior cava. Direct return to the right atrium can be suspected when the common pulmonary venous chamber lies more superiorly and rightward.[270]

When a common pulmonary venous chamber has been identified, the course of the common pulmonary vein should be sought. Color flow mapping is helpful in this process;[271] one traces the venous flow pattern either superiorly or inferiorly. In patients with supracardiac drainage, the common vein may be followed as it ascends along the left heart border to join the innominate vein. In some cases, the ascending vein may cross obliquely and enter the superior vena cava or azygos vein. In either instance, Doppler flow in the unobstructed vertical vein should be phasic and low in velocity, directed toward the transducer from the suprasternal or high parasternal vantage point.[272,273]

In infradiaphragmatic pulmonary venous return, the smaller and slightly more inferior venous chamber can be followed echocardiographically as it descends behind the left heart, through the diaphragm to its connection with hepatic vein or the inferior vena cava. Imaging the short axis of the inferior vena cava and the abdominal aorta at the level of the diaphragm may demonstrate the cross section of an additional vessel anterior to the aorta and leftward of the inferior vena cava. In its long axis, this vessel runs roughly parallel to the abdominal aorta as it connects the common pulmonary venous channel to the inferior vena cava or hepatic circuit. Before the widespread availability of Doppler technology, saline contrast injection in a lower extremity was used to define the inferior vena cava and the descending aorta, because both these structures opacified with contrast medium, whereas the descending pulmonary venous channel remained unopacified.[274] Pulsed Doppler or color flow mapping now allows one to distinguish pulsatile aortic flow from the venous flow in the anomalous venous channel. The latter is nonphasic continuous flow, which is affected by the respiratory cycle.[275] At the site of an obstruction, the venous flow becomes turbulent and higher in velocity.[272] Echo-Doppler delineation of drainage to the coronary sinus relies on dilation of the coronary sinus and turbulence of flow entering it.

Direct visualization of the interatrial septal defect should determine whether a patent foramen ovale or a secundum ASD is present and the approximate size of the defect. Color flow and pulsed Doppler sampling of the right-to-left shunting will permit one to detect high velocity turbulent continuous flow in the presence of a restrictive ASD.

Several studies have recorded excellent sensitivity (97 to 100%) and specificity (99 to 100%) in the diagnosis of total anomalous pulmonary venous return with two-dimensional echocardiography.[276–278] In skilled hands, the ability to pinpoint the exact site of drainage accurately is also good.[276,277] Most difficult are patients with mixed drainage and atrial isomerism.

Surgical Management

Surgical restoration of pulmonary venous flow to the left atrium should provide an excellent long-term outlook in patients with TAPVR because the remaining cardiac anatomy is usually normal. Current operative mortality rates are estimated at 9 to 13%,[268,279,280] with higher risk figures for acutely ill infants with subdiaphragmatic and mixed-type drainage. Surgery is recommended at the time of diagnosis for infants with evidence of obstructed pulmonary venous return, and it is planned electively for those with unobstructed pulmonary venous drainage.[268]

The usual operative approach is through a left thoracotomy, in which the heart is lifted to expose the posterior common venous channel and the true left atrial wall. These two structures are joined to one another with as wide an anastomosis as possible (Fig. 32–58), and the ascending or descending vertical vein is ligated. Repair of TAPVR with drainage to the coronary sinus or right atrium usually requires an intra-atrial approach with baffling to direct the pulmonary venous flow to the left of the atrial septum. The interatrial septal defect is usually closed, but occasionally it is left open as a means of decompression in the perioperative period for patients with severe preoperative pulmonary hypertension.[280] Discussion of the operative management of patients with mixed TAPVR or associated complex lesions is beyond the scope of this text.

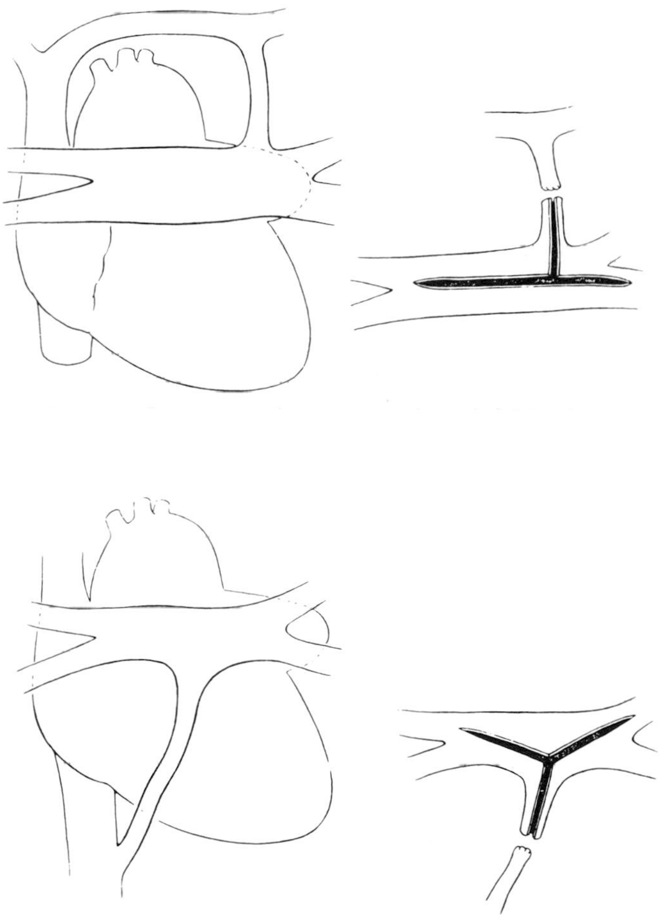

Fig. 32–58. The posterior aspect of the heart in total anomalous pulmonary venous return. Top. Supracardiac drainage from the common pulmonary venous chamber. Top, right. The venous chamber is surgically incised with a "T"-shaped incision, which can then be widely opened and anastomosed to the adjacent left atrial wall. The ascending vertical vein is ligated. Bottom, left. A patient with infradiaphragmatic return. In this Instance, the surgical repair uses a "Y"-shaped incision to achieve the widest possible anastomosis with the left atrium. The descending vertical vein is ligated near its origin from the common pulmonary venous chamber. (From Yee ES, Turley K, Hsieh WR, Ebert PA: Infant total anomalous pulmonary venous connection: factors influencing timing of presentation and operative outcome. Circulation 76(Suppl 3):III-83, 1987. Reproduced by permission of the American Heart Association, Inc.)

Postoperative Evaluation

Recurrent or residual obstruction to pulmonary venous return is the most common problem following repair of TAPVR. This obstruction may occur at the site of anastomosis of the common pulmonary venous chamber with the left atrium or at individual pulmonary vein ostia. Echo-Doppler study enables one to detect turbulent high velocity flow at the site of obstruction easily.[21,281,282] Peak velocity across the restricted area higher than 2 m/sec is indicative of severe inflow obstruction. Lower velocities may also indicate significant obstruction, but the flow pattern is continuous or nonphasic.[21]

Additional postoperative problems include residual atrial septal shunt flow and residual anomalous venous return in cases where mixed drainage was unsuspected preoperatively or was unable to be surgically repaired. Residual right ventricular volume overload and atrial shunting should be detectable by two-dimensional imaging and pulsed and color flow Doppler.

REFERENCES

1. Nadas AS, Fyler DC: Pediatric Cardiology. Philadelphia, W.B. Saunders, 1972.
2. Kidd BSD: Single ventricle. *In* Keith JD, Rowe RD, Vlad P (eds.): Heart Disease in Infancy and Childhood. 3rd Ed. New York, Macmillan, 1978.
3. Anderson RH, et al.: The univentricular atrioventricular connection: getting to the root of a thorny problem. Am J Cardiol 54:822, 1984.
4. Anderson RH, et al.: Univentricular atrioventricular connection: single ventricle trap unsprung. Pediatr Cardiol 4:273, 1983.
5. VanPraagh R, Ongley PA, Swan HJC: Anatomic types of single or common ventricle in man: morphologic and geometric aspects of 60 necropsied cases. Am J Cardiol 13:367, 1964.
6. Kirklin JW, Barrett-Boyes BG: Univentricular atrioventricular connection (single ventricle). *In* Kirklin JW, Barrett-Boyes BG (eds.): Cardiac Surgery. New York, John Wiley and Sons, p. 1301, 1986.
7. Rigby ML, et al.: Two dimensional echocardiographic categorisation of the univentricular heart: ventricular morphology, type, and mode of atrioventricular connection. Br Heart J 46:603, 1981.
8. Sahn DJ, et al.: Cross-sectional echocardiographic diagnosis and subclassification of univentricular hearts: imaging studies of atrioventricular valves, septal structures, and rudimentary outflow chambers. Circulation 66:1070, 1982.
9. Girod DA, et al.: Double-inlet ventricle: morphologic analysis and surgical implications in 32 cases. J Thorac Cardiovasc Surg 88:590, 1984.
10. Huhta JC, et al.: Two-dimensional echocardiographic spectrum of univentricular atrioventricular connection. J Am Coll Cardiol 5:149, 1985.
11. Kuroda O, et al.: Analysis of the effects of the Blalock-Taussig shunt on ventricular function and the prognosis in patients with single ventricle. Circulation 76(Suppl. III):III-24, 1987.
12. Matsuda H, et al.: Problems in the modified Fontan operation for univentricular heart of the right ventricular type. Circulation 76(Suppl. III):III-45, 1987.
13. Bevilaqua M, et al.: Double-inlet single left ventricle: echocardiographic anatomy with emphasis on the morphology of the atrioventricular valves and ventricular septal defect. J Am Coll Cardiol 18:559, 1991.
14. Choussat A, et al.: Selection criteria for Fontan's procedure. *In* Anderson RH, Shinebourne EA (eds.): Pediatric Cardiology, Edinburgh, Churchill Livingstone, p. 559, 1978.
15. Smallhorn JF, Tommasini G, Macartney FJ: Two-dimensional echocardiographic assessment of common atrioventricular valves in univentricular hearts. Br Heart J 46:30, 1981.
16. Holmes AF: Case of malformation of the heart. Trans Med Chir Soc Edinburgh 1:252, 1824.
17. Rothman A, et al.: Surgical management of subaortic obstruction in single left ventricle and tricuspid atresia. J Am Coll Cardiol 10:421, 1987.

18. Freedom RM: The dinosaur and banding of the main pulmonary trunk in the heart with functionally one ventricle and transposition of the great arteries: a saga of evolution and caution. J Am Coll Cardiol 10:421, 1987.
19. Laks H, et al.: Experience with the Fontan procedure. J Thorac Cardiovasc Surg 88:939, 1984.
20. Driscoll DJ, et al.: Five- to fifteen-year follow-up after Fontan operation. Circulation 85:469, 1992.
21. Vick GW, et al.: Pulmonary venous and systemic ventricular inflow obstruction in patients with congenital heart disease: detection by combined two-dimensional and Doppler echocardiography. J Am Coll Cardiol 9:580, 1987.
22. Moodie DS, Ritter DG, Tajik AJ, O'Fallon WM: Long-term follow-up in the unoperated univentricular heart. Am J Cardiol 53:1124, 1984.
23. McKay R, et al.: Postoperative angiographic assessment of modified Blalock-Taussig shunt using expanded polytetrafluoroethylene (Gore-Tex). Ann Thorac Surg 30:137, 1980.
24. Taussig HB: Long-time observations on the Blalock-Taussig operation. IX. Single ventricle (with apex to the left). Johns Hopkins Med J 139:69, 1976.
25. Stefanelli G, et al.: Early and intermediate-term (10 year) results of surgery for univentricular atrioventricular connection ("single ventricle"). Am J Cardiol 54:811, 1984.
26. Marx GR, Allen HD, Goldberg SJ: Doppler echocardiographic estimation of systolic pulmonary artery pressure in patients with aortic-pulmonary shunts. J Am Coll Cardiol 7:880, 1986.
27. Kirklin JK, et al.: The Fontan operation: ventricular hypertrophy, age, and date of operation as risk factors. J Thorac Cardiovasc Surg 92:1049, 1986.
28. Freedom RM, et al.: Subaortic stenosis, the univentricular heart and banding of the pulmonary artery: an analysis of the course of 43 patients with univentricular heart palliated by pulmonary artery banding. Circulation 73: 758, 1986.
29. Foale RA, et al.: Pseudoaneurysm of the pulmonary artery following the banding procedure: cross-sectional echocardiographic description. J Am Coll Cardiol 3:371, 1984.
30. Verel D, Taylor DG, Emery JL: Failure of pulmonary artery banding due to migration of the band. Thorax 25:126, 1970.
31. Feldt RH, et al.: Current status of the septation procedure for univentricular heart. J Thorac Cardiovasc Surg 82:93, 1981.
32. Fontan F, Baudet E: Surgical repair of tricuspid atresia. Thorax 26:240, 1971.
33. DeLeval MR, et al.: Total cavopulmonary connection: a logical alternative to atriopulmonary connection for complex Fontan operations. J Thorac Cardiovasc Surg 96:682, 1988.
34. Nakazawa M, et al.: Dynamics of right heart flow in patients after Fontan procedure. Circulation 69:307, 1984.
35. DiSessa TG, et al.: Systemic venous and pulmonary arterial flow patterns after Fontan's procedure for tricuspid atresia or single ventricle. Circulation 70:898, 1984.
36. Freedom RM, Moes CAF: The hypoplastic right heart complex. Semin Roentgenol 20:169, 1985.
37. Okin JT, et al.: Isolated right ventricular hypoplasia. Am J Cardiol 24:135, 1969.
38. Bull C, et al.: Pulmonary atresia and intact ventricular septum: a revised classification. Circulation 66:266, 1982.
39. Graham TP, Jarmakani JM, Atwood GF, Canent RV: Right ventricular volume determinations in children. Circulation 47:144, 1973.
40. Graham TP, et al.: Increase in right ventricular volume following valvotomy for pulmonary atresia or stenosis with intact ventricular septum. Circulation 50 (Suppl. II):II-69, 1974.
41. Gutgesell HP, et al.: Atrioventricular valve abnormalities in infancy: two-dimensional and angiocardiographic comparison. J Am Coll Cardiol 2:531, 1983.
42. Patel RG, et al.: Right ventricular volume determinations in 18 patients with pulmonary atresia and intact ventricular septum. Circulation 61:428, 1980.
43. Fyfe DA, Edwards WD, Driscoll DJ: Myocardial ischemia in patients with pulmonary atresia and intact ventricular septum. J Am Coll Cardiol 8:402, 1986.
44. O'Connor WN, et al.: Ventriculocoronary connections in hypoplastic right heart syndrome: autopsy serial section study of six cases. J Am Coll Cardiol 11:1061, 1988.
45. Lauer RM, et al.: Angiographic demonstration of intramyocardial sinusoids in pulmonary valve atresia with intact ventricular septum and hypoplastic right ventricle. N Engl J Med 271:68, 1964.
46. Hubbard JF, et al.: Right ventricular infarction with cardiac rupture in an infant with pulmonary valve atresia with intact ventricular septum. J Am Coll Cardiol 2:363, 1983.
47. Lenox CC, Briner J: Absent proximal coronary arteries associated with pulmonic atresia. Am J Cardiol 30:66, 1972.
48. Ueda K, Saito A, Nakano H, Hamazaki Y: Absence of proximal coronary arteries associated with pulmonary atresia. Am Heart J 106:596, 1983.
49. Davignon AL, Grenwold WE, DuShane JW, Edwards JE: Congenital pulmonary atresia with intact ventricular septum: clinicopathologic correlation of two anatomic types. Am Heart J 62:591, 1969.
50. Freedom RM, Dioche MR, Rowe RD: The tricuspid valve in pulmonary atresia and intact ventricular septum. Arch Pathol Lab Med 102:28, 1978.
51. Bharati S, et al.: Anatomic variations in underdeveloped right ventricle related to tricuspid atresia and stenosis. J Thorac Cardiovasc Surg 72:383, 1976.
52. Snider AR, Enderlein MA, Teitel DF, Juster RP: Two-dimensional echocardiographic determination of aortic and pulmonary artery sizes from infancy to adulthood in normal subjects. Am J Cardiol 53:218, 1984.
53. Huhta JC, et al.: Two-dimensional echocardiographic detection and measurement of the right pulmonary artery in pulmonary atresia-ventricular septal defect: angiographic and surgical correlation. Am J Cardiol 49:1235, 1982.
54. Doucette J, Knoblich R: Persistent right valve of the sinus venosus. Arch Pathol 75:105, 1963.
55. Kauffman SL, Andersen DH: Persistent venous valves, maldevelopment of the right heart, and coronary artery-ventricular communications. Am Heart J 66:664, 1963.
56. Weldon CS, Hartmann AF, McKnight RC: Surgical management of hypoplastic right ventricle with pulmonary atresia or critical pulmonary stenosis and intact ventricular septum. Ann Thorac Surg 37:12, 1984.
57. Hamilton JRL, et al.: Operative balloon dilatation for pulmonary atresia with intact ventricular septum. Br Heart J 58:374, 1987.
58. Lev M, et al.: Premature narrowing or closure of the foramen ovale. Am Heart J 65:638, 1963.
59. Sharland GK, et al.: Left ventricular dysfunction in the fetus: relationship to aortic valve anomalies and endocardial fibroelastosis. Br. Heart J. 66: 419, 1991.
60. Norwood WI, Kirklin JK, Sanders SP: Hypoplastic left heart syndrome: experience with palliative surgery. Am J Cardiol 45:87, 1980.
61. Murdison KA, et al.: Hypoplastic left heart syndrome: outcome after initial reconstruction and before modified Fontan procedure. Circulation 82(Suppl. IV):IV-199, 1990.
62. Doty DB, Knott HW: Hypoplastic left heart syndrome: experience with operation to establish functionally normal circulation. J Thorac Cardiovasc Surg 74:624, 1977.
63. Doty DB, Marvin WJ, Shieken RM, Lauer RM: Hypoplastic left heart syndrome. J Thorac Cardiovasc Surg 80:148, 1980.
64. Levitsky S, et al.: Surgical palliation in aortic atresia. J Thorac Cardiovasc Surg 79:456, 1980.
65. Allen HD: Is cardiac transplantation in children an experimental procedure? Am J Dis Child 140:1105, 1986.
66. Meyer RA, Kaplan S: Echocardiography in the diagnosis of hypoplasia of the left or right ventricles in the neonate. Circulation 46:55, 1972.
67. Farooki ZQ, Henry JG, Green EW: Echocardiographic spectrum of the hypoplastic left heart syndrome. Am J Cardiol 38:337, 1976.
68. Latson LA, Cheatham JP, Gutgesell HP: Relation of the echocardiographic estimate of left ventricular size to mortality in infants with severe left ventricular outflow obstruction. Am J Cardiol 48:887, 1981.
69. Lange LW, et al.: Cross sectional echocardiography in hypoplastic left ventricle: echocardiographic and angiographic anatomic correlations. Pediatr Cardiol 1:287, 1980.
70. Bharati S, Lev M: The surgical anatomy of hypoplasia of aortic tract complex. J Thorac Cardiovasc Surg 88:97, 1984.
71. Sholler GF, et al.: Balloon dilation of congenital aortic valve stenosis. Circulation 78:351, 1988.
72. Bash SE, et al.: Hypoplastic left heart syndrome: is echocardiography accurate enough to guide surgical palliation? J Am Coll Cardiol 7:610, 1986.
73. Hawkins JA, Doty DB: Aortic atresia: morphologic characteristics affecting survival and operative palliation. J Thorac Cardiovasc Surg 88:620, 1984.
74. Lang P, Norwood WI: Hemodynamic assessment after palliative surgery for hypoplastic left heart syndrome. Circulation 68:104, 1983.
75. Norwood WI, Pigott JD, Murphy JD, Raphaely RC: Modified Fontan reconstructive surgery for hypoplastic left heart syndrome. Circulation (Suppl. IV):IV-73, 1987.
76. Van Mierop LHS: Embryology of the atrioventricular canal region and pathogenesis of endocardial cushion defects. *In* Feldt RH (ed.): Atrioventricular Canal Defects. Philadelphia, W.B. Saunders, p. 1, 1976.
77. Studer M, et al.: Determinants of early and late results of repair of atrioventricular septal (canal) defects. J Thorac Cardiovasc Surg 84:523, 1982.
78. Hagler DJ, et al.: Real-time wide-angle sector echocardiography: atrioventricular canal defects. Circulation 59:140, 1979.
79. Bharati S, Lev M: The spectrum of common atrioventricular orifice (canal). Am Heart J 86:553, 1973.
80. Castaneda AR, Mayer JE, Jonas RA: Repair of complete atrioventricular canal in infancy. World J Surg 9:590, 1985.
81. Piccoli GP, et al.: Morphology and classification of complete atrioventricular defects. Br Heart J 42:633, 1979.
82. Titus JL, Rastelli GC: Anatomic features of persistent common atrioventricular canal. *In* Feldt RH (ed.): Atrioventricular Canal Defects. Philadelphia, W.B. Saunders, p. 13, 1976.
83. Rastelli GCC, Kirklin JW, Titus JL: Anatomic observations on complete form of persistent common atrioventricular canal with special reference to atrioventricular valves. Mayo Clin Proc 41:296, 1966.

84. Wakai CS, Edwards JE: Pathologic study of persistent common atrioventricular canal. Am Heart J 56:779, 1958.
85. Minich LL, Snider AR, Vermilion RP, Bove EL: Echocardiographic evaluation of atrioventricular valve orifice anatomy in children with atrioventricular septal defects. J Am Coll Cardiol 17(Suppl. A):48A, 1991.
86. Smallhorn JF, et al.: Assessment of atrioventricular septal defects by two dimensional echocardiography. Br Heart J 47:109, 1982.
87. Silverman NH, Schiller NB: Apex echocardiography: a two-dimensional technique for evaluating congenital heart disease. Circulation 57:503, 1978.
88. Warnes C, Somerville J: Double mitral valve orifice in atrioventricular defects. Br Heart J 49:59, 1983.
89. Ilbawi MN, et al.: Unusual mitral valve abnormalities complicating surgical repair of endocardial cushion defects. J Thorac Cardiovasc Surg 85:697, 1983.
90. Chin AJ, et al.: Sybxyphoid 2-dimensional echocardiographic identification of left ventricular papillary muscle anomalies in complete common atrioventricular canal. Am J Cardiol 51:1695, 1983.
91. David I, Castaneda AR, VanPraagh R: Potentially parachute mitral valve in common atrioventricular canal. J Thorac Cardiovasc Surg 84:178, 1982.
92. Yoshidda H, et al.: Subxiphoid cross-sectional echocardiographic imaging of the "goose-neck" deformity in endocardial cushion defect. Circulation 62:1319, 1980.
93. Gow RM, et al.: Coarctation of the aorta or subaortic stenosis with atrioventricular septal defect. Am J Cardiol 53:1421, 1984.
94. Piccoli GP, et al.: Left-sided obstructive lesions in atrioventricular defects. J Thorac Cardiovasc Surg 83:453, 1982.
95. Spanos PK, Fiddler GI, Mair DD, McGoon DC: Repair of atrioventricular canal associated with membranous subaortic stenosis. Mayo Clin Proc 52: 121, 1977.
96. Braunwald NS, Morrow AG: Incomplete persistent atrioventricular canal. J Thorac Cardiovasc Surg 51:71, 1966.
97. Heydarian M, Griffith BBP, Zuberbuhler JR: Partial atrioventricular canal associated with discrete subaortic stenosis. Am Heart J 109:915, 1985.
98. Taylor NC, Somerville J: Fixed subaortic stenosis after repair of ostium primum defects. Br Heart J 45:689, 1981.
99. Thanopoulos BD, Fisher EA, DuBrow IW, Hastreiter AR: Right and left ventricular volume characteristics in common atrioventricular canal. Circulation 57:991, 1978.
100. Mehta S, Hirshfeld S, Riggs T, Liebman J: Echocardiographic estimation of ventricular hypoplasia in complete atrioventricular canal. Circulation 59:888, 1979.
101. Clapp SK, et al.: Surgical and medical results of complete atrioventricular canal: a ten year review. Am J Cardiol 59:454, 1987.
102. Kirklin JW, Barrett-Boyes BG: Atrioventricular canal defects. *In* Kirklin JW, Barrett-Boyes BG (eds.): Cardiac Surgery. New York, John Wiley and Sons, p. 541, 1986.
103. Vlad P: Tricuspid atresia. *In* Keith JD, Rowe RD, Vlad P (eds.): Heart Disease in Infancy and Childhood. 3rd Ed. New York, Macmillan, 1978.
104. Weinberg PM: Anatomy of tricuspid atresia and its relevance to current forms of surgical therapy. Ann Thorac Surg 192:382, 1980.
105. Rigby ML, et al.: Recognition of imperforate atrioventricular valves by two-dimensional echocardiography. Br Heart J 47:329, 1982.
106. Laks H, et al.: Results of right atrial to right ventricular and right atrial to pulmonary artery conduits for complex congenital heart disease. Ann Surg 192:382, 1980.
107. Coles JG, et al.: Repair of tricuspid atresia: utility of right ventricular incorporation. Ann Thorac Surg 45:384, 1988.
108. Nakazawa M, et al.: A quantitative analysis of hemodynamic effects of the right ventricle included in the circulation of the Fontan procedure. Circulation 83:822, 1991.
109. Lee C-N, et al.: Comparison of atriopulmonary versus atrioventricular connections for modified Fontan/Kreutzer repair of tricuspid valve atresia. J Thorac Cardiovasc Surg 92:1038, 1986.
110. Rao PS: Further observations on the spontaneous closure of physiologically advantageous ventricular septal defects in tricuspid atresia: surgical implications. Ann Thorac Surg 35:121, 1983.
111. Tandon R, Marin-Garcia J, Moller JH, Edwards JE: Tricuspid atresia with L-transposition. Am Heart J 88:417, 1974.
112. Tandon R, Edwards JE: Tricuspid atresia: a re-evaluation and classification. J Thorac Cardiovasc Surg 67:530, 1974.
113. Dick M, Fyler DC, Nadas AS: Tricuspid atresia: clinical course in 101 patients. Am J Cardiol 36:327, 1975.
114. Bharati S, et al.: Anatomic variations in underdeveloped right ventricle related to tricuspid atresia and stenosis. J Thorac Cardiovasc Surg 72:383, 1976.
115. Burx J, et al.: Tricuspid atresia: results of treatment in 115 children. J Thorac Cardiovasc Surg 85:440, 1983.
116. Cleveland DC, et al.: Surgical treatment of tricuspid atresia. Ann Thorac Surg 38:447, 1984.
117. Kirklin J, Barrett-Boyes B: Tricuspid atresia. *In* Kirklin JW, Barrett-Boyes BG (eds.): Cardiac Surgery. New York, John Wiley and Sons, p. 857, 1986.
118. Van Praagh R, et al.: Tetralogy of Fallot: underdevelopment of the pulmonary infundibulum and its sequellae. Am J Cardiol 26:25, 1970.
119. Fellows KE, Smith J, Keane JF: Preoperative angiocardiography in infants with tetrad of Fallot: review of 36 cases. Am J Cardiol 47:1279, 1981.
120. Flanagan MF, et al.: Tetralogy of Fallot with obstruction of the ventricular septal defect: spectrum of echocardiographic findings. J Am Coll Cardiol 11:386, 1988.
121. Musewe NN, et al.: Echocardiographic evaluation of obstructive mechanism of Tetralogy of Fallot with restrictive ventricular septal defect. Am J Cardiol 61:664, 1988.
122. Neufeld HN, McGoon DC, DuShane JW, Edwards JE: Tetralogy of Fallot with anomalous tricuspid valve simulating pulmonary stenosis with intact septum. Circulation 22:1083, 1960.
123. Houston AB, et al.: Doppler ultrasound in the estimation of the severity of pulmonary infundibular stenosis in infants and children. Br Heart J 55:381, 1986.
124. Matina D, et al.: Subxyphoid two-dimensional echocardiographic diagnosis of double-chambered right ventricle. Circulation 67:885, 1983.
125. Smyllie JH, Sutherland GR, Keeton BR: The value of Doppler color flow mapping in determining pulmonary blood supply in infants with pulmonary atresia with ventricular septal defect. J Am Coll Cardiol 14:1759, 1989.
126. Hagler DJ, et al.: Wide angle two-dimensional echocardiographic profiles of conotruncal abnormalities. Mayo Clin Proc 55:73, 1980.
127. Sanders SP, Bierman FZ, Williams RG: Conotruncal malformations: diagnosis in infancy using subxiphoid 2-dimensional echocardiography. Am J Cardiol 50:416, 1982.
128. Ueda K, et al.: Modified Blalock-Taussig shunt operation without cardiac catheterization: two-dimensional echocardiographic preoperative assessment in cyanotic infants. Am J Cardiol 54:1296, 1984.
129. Kirklin JW, Barrett-Boyes B: Ventricular septal defect and pulmonary stenosis or atresia. *In* Kirklin JW, Barrett-Boyes B (eds.): Cardiac Surgery. New York, John Wiley and Sons, p. 701, 1986.
130. Miller RA, Lev M, Paul MH: Congenital absence of the pulmonary valve: the clinical syndrome of tetralogy of Fallot with pulmonary regurgitation. Circulation 26:293, 1962.
131. Kirklin JW, et al.: Surgical results and protocols in the spectrum of tetralogy of Fallot. Ann Surg 198:251, 1981.
132. Berry JM, Einzig S, Krabill K, Bass JL: Evaluation of coronary artery anatomy in patients with tetralogy of Fallot by two-dimensional echocardiography. Circulation 78:149, 1988.
133. Chen CC, et al.: Recognition of coronary artery fistula by Doppler 2-dimensional echocardiography. Am J Cardiol 53:392, 1984.
134. Huhta JC, Gutgesell HP, Latson LA, Huffines FD: Two-dimensional echocardiographic assessment of the aorta in infants and children with congenital heart disease. Circulation 70:417, 1984.
135. Celano V, Pieroni DR, Gingell RL, Roland JA: Two-dimensional echocardiographic recognition of the right aortic arch. Am J Cardiol 51:1507, 1983.
136. Uretzky G, et al.: Complete atrioventricular canal associated with tetralogy of Fallot: morphologic and surgical considerations. J Thorac Cardiovasc Surg 87:756, 1984.
137. Nath PH, et al.: Tetralogy of Fallot with atrioventricular canal: an angiographic study. J Thorac Cardiovasc Surg 87:421, 1984.
138. Bender HW, et al.: Experimental pulmonic regurgitation. J Thorac Cardiovasc Surg 45:451, 1963.
139. Katz NM, et al.: Late survival and symptoms after repair of Tetralogy of Fallot. Circulation 65:403, 1982.
140. Misbach GA, Turley K, Ebert PA: Pulmonary valve replacement for regurgitation after repair of tetralogy of Fallot. Ann Thorac Surg 36:684, 1983.
141. Millikan JS, et al.: Staged surgical repair of pulmonary atresia, ventricular septal defect, and hypoplastic, confluent pulmonary arteries. J Thorac Cardiovasc Surg 91:818, 1986.
142. Freedom RM, et al.: Palliative right ventricular outflow tract construction for patients with pulmonary atresia, ventricular septal defect, and hypoplastic pulmonary arteries. J Thorac Cardiovasc Surg 86:24, 1983.
143. Blackstone EH, et al.: Preoperative prediction from cineangiograms of post repair right ventricular pressure in tetralogy of Fallot. J Thorac Cardiovasc Surg 78:542, 1979.
144. Piehler JM, et al.: Management of pulmonary atresia with ventricular septal defect and hypoplastic pulmonary arteries by right ventricular outflow construction. J Thorac Cardiovasc Surg 80:552, 1980.
145. Nakata S, et al.: A new method for the quantitative standardization of cross sectional areas of the pulmonary arteries in congenital heart diseases with decreased pulmonary blood flow. J Thorac Cardiovasc Surg 88:610, 1984.
146. Mattila S, et al.: Total correction of tetralogy of Fallot in adults. Scand J Thorac Cardiovasc Surg 18:23, 1984.
147. Kreindel MS, Moodie DS, Sterba R, Gill CC: Total repair of tetralogy of Fallot in the adult. Cleve Clin Q 52:375, 1985.
148. Hughes CF, et al.: Total intracardiac repair of tetralogy of Fallot in adults. Ann Thorac Surg 43:634, 1987.
149. Hu DCK, et al.: Total correction of tetralogy of Fallot at age 40 years and older: long-term follow-up. J Am Coll Cardiol 5:40, 1985.
150. Oku H, Shirotani H, Sunakawa A, Yodoyama T: Postoperative long-term results in total correction of tetralogy of Fallot: hemodynamics and cardiac function. Ann Thorac Surg 41:41, 413, 1986.
151. Ciaravella JM, et al.: Experience with the extracardiac conduit. J Thorac Cardiovasc Surg 78:920, 1979.
152. Agarwal KC, et al.: Clinicopathological correlates of obstructed right-sided

porcine-valved extracardiac conduits. J Thorac Cardiovasc Surg 81:591, 1981.
153. Miller DC, et al.: The durability of porcine xenograft valves and conduits in children. Circulation 66(Suppl. I):I-172, 1982.
154. Reeder GS, et al.: Extracardiac conduit obstruction: initial experience in the use of Doppler echocardiography for noninvasive estimation of pressure gradient. J Am Coll Cardiol 4:1006, 1984.
155. Radley-Smith R, Yacoub M: Late results of homograft reconstruction of right ventricular outflow tract in infants and children. Br Heart J 37:554, 1975.
156. Moodie DS, et al.: Aortic homograft obstruction. J Thorac Cardiovasc Surg 72:553, 1976.
157. Meliones JN, et al.: Doppler evaluation of homograft valved conduits in children. Am J Cardiol 64:354, 1989.
158. Fyler DC: Report of the New England Regional Infant Cardiac Program. Pediatrics 65:375, 1980.
159. Liebman J, Cullum L, Belloc NB: Natural history of transposition of the great arteries. Circulation 40:237, 1969.
160. Henry WL, Maron BJ, Griffith JM: Cross-sectional echocardiography in the diagnosis of congenital heart disease: identification of the relation of the ventricles and great arteries. Circulation 56:267, 1977.
161. VanPraagh R, et al.: Transposition of the great arteries with posterior aorta, anterior pulmonary artery, subpulmonary conus and fibrous continuity between aortic and atrioventricular valves. Am J Cardiol 28:621, 1971.
162. Beland MJ, Paquet M: Two-dimensional echocardiographic features of complete transposition of the great arteries with posterior aorta. J Am Soc Echocardiogr 1:463, 1988.
163. Sanders SP, Bierman FZ, Williams RG: Conotruncal malformations: diagnosis in infancy using subxiphoid two-dimensional echocardiography. Am J Cardiol 50:1361, 1982.
164. Hagler DJ, et al.: Wide-angle two-dimensional echocardiographic profiles of conotruncal abnormalities. Mayo Clin Proc 55:73, 1980.
165. Kidd BSL, Tyrell MJ, Pickering D: Transposition 1969. *In* Kidd BSL, Keith JD (eds.): The Natural History and Progress in Treatment of Congenital Heart Defects. Springfield, IL, Charles C Thomas, 1971.
166. Kirklin JW, Barrett-Boyes BG: Transposition of the great arteries. *In* Kirklin JW, Barrett-Boyes BG (eds.): Cardiac Surgery. New York, John Wiley and Sons, p. 1129, 1986.
167. Satomi G, et al.: Blood flow pattern of the interatrial communication in patients with complete TGA: a pulsed Doppler echocardiographic study. Circulation 73:95, 1986.
168. Castaneda AR, et al.: Primary anatomic repair of transposition of the great arteries with intact interventricular septum in the neonate. *In* Doyle EF, et al. (eds.): Pediatric Cardiology: Proceedings of the Second World Congress. New York, Springer-Verlag, 1986.
169. Lin AE, DiSessa TG, Williams RG: Balloon and blade atrial septostomy facilitated by two-dimensional echocardiography. Am J Cardiol 57:273, 1986.
170. Allan LD, et al.: Balloon septostomy under two-dimensional echocardiographic control. Br Heart J 47:41, 1982.
171. Perry LW, et al.: Echocardiographically assisted balloon atrial septostomy. Pediatrics 70:403, 1982.
172. Marino B, et al.: Complete transposition of the great arteries: visualization of left and right ventricular outflow tract obstruction by oblique subcostal two-dimensional echocardiography. Am J Cardiol 55:1140, 1985.
173. Shrivastava S, Tadavarthy SM, Fukuda T, Edwards JE: Anatomic causes of pulmonic stenosis in complete transposition of the great arteries. Circulation 54:154, 1976.
174. Sansa M, Tonkin IL, Bargeron LM, Elliott LP: Left ventricular outflow tract obstruction in transposition of the great arteries: an angiographic study of 74 cases. Am J Cardiol 44:88, 1979.
175. Riggs TW, et al.: Two-dimensional echocardiographic and angiocardiographic diagnosis of subpulmonary stenosis due to tricuspid valve pouch in complete transposition of the great arteries. J Am Coll Cardiol 1:481, 1983.
176. Moene RJ, Oppenheiner-Dekker A, Bartelings MM: Anatomic obstruction of the right ventricular outflow tract in transposition of the great arteries. Am J Cardiol 51:1701, 1983.
177. Schneeweiss A, Motro M, Shem-Tov A, Neufeld HN: Subaortic stenosis: an unrecognized problem in transposition of the great arteries. Am J Cardiol 48:336, 1981.
178. Newfeld EA, Paul MH, Muster AJ, Edriss FS: Pulmonary vascular disease in complete transposition of the great arteries: a study of 200 patients. Am J Cardiol 34:75, 1974.
179. Waldman JD, et al.: Transposition of the great arteries with intact ventricular septum and patent ductus arteriosus. Am J Cardiol 39:232, 1977.
180. Mayer JE, et al.: Coronary artery pattern and outcome of arterial switch operation for transposition of the great arteries. Circulation 82(Suppl. IV): IV-139, 1990.
181. Pasquini L, Sanders SP, Parness IA, Colan SD: Diagnosis of coronary artery anatomy by two-dimensional echocardiography in patients with transposition of the great arteries. Circulation 75:557, 1987.
182. Huhta JC, Edwards WD, Danielson GK, Feldt RH: Abnormalities of the tricuspid valve in complete transposition of the great arteries with ventricular septal defect. J Thorac Cardiovasc Surg 83:569, 1982.
183. Wood AE, Freedom RM, Williams WG, Trusler GA: The Mustard procedure in transposition of the great arteries associated with juxtaposition of the atrial appendages with and without dextrocardia. J Thorac Cardiovasc Surg 85:451, 1983.
184. Melhuish BPP, VanPraagh R: Juxtaposition of the atrial appendages: a sign of severe cyanotic congenital heart disease. Br Heart J 30:269, 1968.
185. Bender HW, et al.: Comparative operative results of the Senning and Mustard procedures for transposition of the great arteries. Circulation 62(Suppl. I):I-197, 1980.
186. Mahoney L, Turley K, Ebert P, Heymann MA: Long-term results after atrial repair of transposition of the great arteries in early infancy. Circulation 66:253, 1982.
187. DeLeon VH, et al.: Results of the Senning operation for transposition with intact ventricular septum in neonates. Circulation 70(Suppl. I):I-21, 1984.
188. Graham TP: Hemodynamic residual and sequelae following intra-atrial repair of transposition of the great arteries: a review. Pediatr Cardiol 2:203, 1982.
189. Mustard WT, et al.: A surgical approach to transposition of the great arteries with extracorporeal circuit. Surgery 36:39, 1954.
190. Castaneda AR, et al.: Transposition of the great arteries and intact ventricular septum: anatomical repair in the neonate. Ann Thorac Surg 38:438, 1984.
191. Radley-Smith R, Yacoub MH: One stage anatomic correction of simple transposition of the great arteries in neonates. Circulation 70(Suppl. II): II-26, 1984.
192. Yacoub MH, Radley-Smith R, Maclaurin R: Two-stage operation for anatomical correction of transposition of the great arteries with intact ventricular septum. Lancet 1:1275, 1977.
193. Colan SD, et al.: Myocardial performance after arterial switch operation for transposition of the great arteries with intact ventricular septum. Circulation 78:132, 1988.
194. Wernovsky G, et al.: Midterm results after the arterial switch operation for transposition of the great arteries with intact ventricular septum: clinical, hemodynamic, echocardiographic, and electrophysiologic data. Circulation 77:1333, 1988.
195. Lange PE, et al.: Up to 7 years of follow-up after two-stage anatomic correction of simple transposition of the great arteries. Circulation 74(Suppl. I):I-47, 1986.
196. Goor DA, ShemTov A, Neufeld MN: Impeded coronary flow in anatomic correction of transposition of the great arteries: prevention, detection, and management. J Thorac Cardiovasc Surg 83:747, 1982.
197. Borow KM, Keane JF, Castaneda AR, Freed MD: Systemic ventricular function in patients with tetralogy of Fallot, ventricular septal defect and transposition of the great arteries repaired during infancy. Circulation 64: 878, 1981.
198. Chin AJ, et al.: Two-dimensional echocardiographic assessment of caval and pulmonary venous pathways after the Senning operation. Am J Cardiol 52:118, 1983.
199. Stevenson JG, et al.: Pulsed Doppler echocardiographic detection of obstruction of systemic venous return after repair of transposition of the great arteries. Circulation 60:1091, 1979.
200. Smallhorn JF, et al.: Pulsed Doppler echocardiographic assessment of the pulmonary venous pathway after the Mustard or Senning procedure for transposition of the great arteries. Circulation 73:765, 1986.
201. Silverman NH, et al.: Superior vena caval obstruction after Mustard's operation: detection by two-dimensional contrast echocardiography. Circulation 64:392, 1981.
202. Quinones JA, et al.: Two-dimensional and Doppler echocardiographic assessment of anatomic correction for D-transposition of the great arteries. *In* Doyle EF, et al. (eds.): Pediatric Cardiology: Proceedings of the Second World Congress. New York, Springer-Verlag, 1986.
203. De Albuquerque AT, et al.: The spectrum of atrioventricular discordance: a clinical study. Br Heart J 51:498, 1984.
204. Lieberson AD, Schumacher RR, Childress RH, Genovese PD: Corrected transposition of the great vessels in a 73-year-old man. Circulation 39:96, 1969.
205. Hagler DJ, et al.: Atrioventricular and ventriculoarterial discordance (corrected TGA): wide-angle two-dimensional echocardiographic assessment of ventricular morphology. Mayo Clin Proc 56:591, 1981.
206. Smallhorn JF, Sutherland GR, Anderson RH, Macartney FJ: Cross-sectional echocardiographic assessment of conditions with atrioventricular valve leaflets attached to the atrial septum at the same level. Br Heart J 48:331, 1982.
207. Allwork SP, et al.: Congenitally corrected transposition of the great arteries: morphologic study of 32 cases. Am J Cardiol 38:910, 1976.
208. Sutherland GR, et al.: Atrioventricular discordance: cross-sectional echocardiographic-morphological correlative study. Br Heart J 50:8, 1983.
209. Van Praagh R: What is congenitally corrected transposition? N Engl J Med 282:1097, 1970.
210. Anderson RH, Becker AE, Gerlis LM: The pulmonary outflow tract in classically corrected transposition. J Thorac Cardiovasc Surg 69:747, 1975.
211. Anderson KR, Danielson GK, McGoon DC, Lie JT: Ebstein's anomaly of the left-sided tricuspid valve. Circulation 58(Suppl. I):I-87, 1978.
212. Erath HG, Graham TP, Hammon JW, Smith CW: Hypoplasia of the sys-

temic ventricle in discordant atrioventricular connection. J Thorac Cardiovasc Surg 79:770, 1980.
213. McGrath LB, et al.: Death and other events after cardiac repair in discordant atrioventricular connection. J Thorac Cardiovasc Surg 90:711, 1985.
214. Williams WG, et al.: Repair or major intracardiac anomalies associated with atrioventricular discordance. Ann Thorac Surg 31:527, 1981.
215. Trowitzsch E, Colan SD, Sanders SP: Global and regional RV function in normal infants and infants with transposition of the great arteries after Senning operation. Circulation 72:1008, 1985.
216. Hagler DJ, et al.: Right and left ventricular function after the Mustard procedure in transposition of the great arteries. Am J Cardiol 44:276, 1979.
217. Huhta JC, et al.: Complete AV block in patients with atrioventricular discordance. Circulation 67:1374, 1983.
218. Swiderski J, Lees MH, Nadas AS: The Wolff-Parkinson-White syndrome in infancy and childhood. Br Heart J 24:561, 1962.
219. Kirklin JW, Barrett-Boyes BG: Congenitally corrected transposition of the great arteries. *In* Kirklin JW, Barrett-Boyes BG (eds.): Cardiac Surgery. New York, John Wiley and Sons, p. 1263, 1986.
220. Sondheimer HM, Freedom RM, Olley PM: Double outlet right ventricle: clinical spectrum and prognosis. Am J Cardiol 39:709, 1977.
221. VanPraagh S, et al.: Double outlet right ventricle: anatomic types and developmental implications based on a study of 101 autopsied cases. Coeur 13:389, 1982.
222. Macartney FJ, et al.: Double outlet right ventricle: cross-sectional echocardiographic findings, their anatomical explanation, and surgical relevance. Br Heart J 52:164, 1984.
223. Hagler DJ, et al.: Double-outlet right ventricle: wide-angle two-dimensional echocardiographic observations. Circulation 63:419, 1981.
224. MacMahon HE, Lipa M: Double-outlet right ventricle with intact interventricular septum. Circulation 30:745, 1964.
225. Edwards JE, Janes JW, DuShane JW: Congenital malformation of the heart: origin of transposed great vessels from right ventricle associated with atresia of the left ventricular outlet, double orifice of the mitral valve and single coronary artery. Lab Invest 1:197, 1952.
226. Sridaromont S, et al.: Double-outlet right ventricle anatomic and angiocardiographic correlations. Mayo Clin Proc 53:555, 1978.
227. Sanders SP: Echocardiography and related techniques in the diagnosis of congenital heart defects. Part III. Conotruncus and great arteries. Echocardiography 1:443, 1984.
228. Marin-Garcia J, et al.: Double-outlet right ventricle with restrictive ventricular septal defect. J Thorac Cardiovasc Surg 76:853, 1978.
229. Lavoie R, et al.: Double outlet right ventricle with left ventricular outflow tract obstruction due to small ventricular septal defect. Am Heart J 82: 290, 1971.
230. Luber JM, Castaneda AR, Lang P, Norwood WI: Repair of double outlet right ventricle: early and late results. Circulation 68(Suppl. II):II-144, 1983.
231. Kirklin JW, et al.: Current risks and protocols for operations for double-outlet right ventricle. J Thorac Cardiovasc Surg 92:913, 1986.
232. Yacoub MH, Radley-Smith R: Anatomic correction of the Taussig-Bing anomaly. J Thorac Cardiovasc Surg 88:380, 1984.
233. Rice MJ, et al.: Straddling atrioventricular valve: two-dimensional echocardiographic diagnosis, classification, and surgical implications. Am J Cardiol 55:505, 1985.
234. Kanter KR, et al.: Anatomic correction for complete transposition and double-outlet right ventricle. J Thorac Cardiovasc Surg 90:690, 1985.
235. Judson JP, et al.: Double-outlet right ventricle. J Thorac Cardiovasc Surg 85:32, 1983.
236. Pacifico AD, Kirklin JK, Colvin EV, Bargeron LM: Intraventricular tunnel repair for Taussig-Bing heart and related cardiac anomalies. Circulation 74(Suppl. I):I-53, 1986.
237. Mazzucco A, et al.: Surgical management of double-outlet right ventricle. J Thorac Cardiovasc Surg 90:29, 1985.
238. Rocchini AP, et al.: Subaortic obstruction after the use of an intracardiac baffle to tunnel the left ventricle to the aorta. Circulation 54:957, 1976.
239. Langford Kidd BS: Persistent Truncus Arteriosus. *In* Keith JD, Rowe RD, and Vlad P (eds.): Heart Disease in Infancy and Childhood. 3rd Ed. New York, Macmillan, 1978.
240. VanPraagh R, VanPraagh S: The anatomy of common aorticopulmonary trunk (truncus arteriosus communis) and its embryologic implications. Am J Cardiol 166:406, 1965.
241. Collett RW, Edwards JE: Persistent truncus arteriosus: a classification according to anatomic types. Surg Clin North Am 29:1245, 1949.
242. Calder L, et al.: Truncus arteriosus communis: clinical, angiocardiographic and pathologic findings in 100 patients. Am Heart J 92:23, 1976.
243. Houston AB, Gregory NL, Murtagh E, Coleman EN: Two-dimensional echocardiography in infants with persistent truncus arteriosus. Br Heart J 46:492, 1981.
244. Rice JM, et al.: Definitive diagnosis of truncus arteriosus by two-dimensional echocardiography. Mayo Clin Proc 57:476, 1982.
245. Riggs TW, Paul MH: Two-dimensional echocardiographic prospective diagnosis of common truncus arteriosus in infants. Am J Cardiol 50:1380, 1982.
246. Crupi G, Macartney FJ, Anderson RH: Persistent truncus arteriosus: a study of 66 autopsy cases with special reference to definition and morphogenesis. Am J Cardiol 40:569, 1977.
247. Ebert PA, et al.: Surgical treatment of truncus arteriosus in the first six months of life. Ann Surg 200:451, 1984.
248. Bharati S, et al.: The surgical anatomy of truncus arteriosus communis. J Thorac Cardiovasc Surg 67:501, 1974.
249. Rosenquist GC, Bharati S, McAllister HA, Lev M: Truncus arteriosus communis truncal valve anomalies associated with small conal or truncal septal defects. Am J Cardiol 37:410, 1976.
250. Mair DD, et al.: Selection of patients with truncus arteriosus for surgical correction: anatomic and hemodynamic considerations. Circulation 49:144, 1974.
251. Shrivasta S, Edwards JE: Coronary arterial origin in persistent truncus arteriosus. Circulation 55:551, 1977.
252. Kirklin JW, Barrett-Boyes BG: Truncus arteriosus. *In* Kirklin JW, Barrett-Boyes BG (eds.): Cardiac Surgery. New York, John Wiley and Sons, p. 911, 1986.
253. Raatikka M, et al.: Familial third and fourth pharyngeal pouch syndrome with truncus arteriosus. Pediatrics 67:173, 1981.
254. Singh AL, deLeval MR, Pincott JR, Stark J: Pulmonary artery banding for truncus arteriosus in the first year of life. Circulation 53-54(Suppl. III): III-17, 1976.
255. Darling RC, Rothney WB, Craig JM: Total pulmonary venous drainage into the right side of the heart: report of 17 autopsied cases not associated with other major cardiovascular anomalies. Lab Invest 6:44, 1957.
256. Rowe RD: Anomalies of venous return. *In* Keith JD, Rowe RD, Vlad P (eds.): Heart Disease in Infancy and Childhood. 3rd Ed. New York, Macmillan, 1978.
257. Lucas RV, Lock JE, Tandon R, Edwards JE: Gross and histologic anatomy of total anomalous pulmonary venous connections. Am J Cardiol 62:292, 1988.
258. Burroughs JT, Edwards JE: Total anomalous pulmonary venous connection. Am Heart J 59:913, 1960.
259. Delisle G, et al.: Total anomalous pulmonary venous connection: report of 93 autopsied cases with emphasis on diagnostic and surgical considerations. Am Heart J 91:99, 1976.
260. Gathman GE, Nadas AS: Total anomalous pulmonary venous connection: clinical and physiologic observations of 75 pediatric patients. Circulation 42:143, 1970.
261. Elliott LP, Edwards JE: The problem of pulmonary venous obstruction in total anomalous pulmonary venous connection to the left innominate vein (editorial). Circulation 25:913, 1962.
262. Smallhorn JF, Freedom RM: Pulsed Doppler echocardiography in the preoperative evaluation of total anomalous pulmonary venous connection. J Am Coll Cardiol 8:1413, 1986.
263. Casta A, Wolf WJ: Echo Doppler detection of external compression of the vertical vein causing obstruction in total anomalous pulmonary venous connection. Am Heart J 116:1045, 1988.
264. Rey C, Marache P, Francart C, Dupuis C: Percutaneous balloon angioplasty in an infant with obstructed total anomalous pulmonary venous return. J Am Coll Cardiol 6:894, 1985.
265. Ward KE, et al.: Restrictive interatrial communication in total anomalous pulmonary venous connection. Am J Cardiol 57:1131, 1986.
266. Parr GVS, et al.: Cardiac performance in infants after repair of total anomalous pulmonary venous connection. Ann Thorac Surg 17:561, 1974.
267. Hammon JW, et al.: Total anomalous pulmonary venous connection in infancy. J Thorac Cardiovasc Surg 80:544, 1980.
268. Whight CM, et al.: Total anomalous pulmonary venous connection: long-term results following repair in infancy. J Thorac Cardiovasc Surg 75:52, 1978.
269. Bharati S, Lev M: Congenital anomalies of the pulmonary veins. Cardiovasc Clin 5:23, 1973.
270. Sahn DJ, Allen HD, Lange LW, Goldberg SJ: Cross-sectional echocardiographic diagnosis of the sites of total anomalous pulmonary venous drainage. Circulation 60:1317, 1979.
271. Satomi G, et al.: Detection of the draining site in total anomalous pulmonary venous connection by two-dimensional color Doppler echocardiography. *In* Doyle EF, et al. (eds.): Pediatric Cardiology: Proceedings of the Second World Congress. New York, Springer-Verlag, 1986.
272. Smallhorn JF, Freedom RM: Pulsed Doppler echocardiography in the preoperative evaluation of total anomalous pulmonary venous connection. J Am Coll Cardiol 8:1413, 1986.
273. Skovranek J, Tuma S, Urbancova D, Samanek M: Range-gated pulsed Doppler echocardiographic diagnosis of supracardiac total anomalous pulmonary venous drainage. Circulation 61:841, 1980.
274. Snider AR, Silverman NH, Turley K, Ebert PA: Evaluation of infradiaphragmatic total anomalous pulmonary venous connection with two-dimensional echocardiography. Circulation 66:1129, 1982.
275. Cooper MJ, Teitel DF, Silverman NH, Enderlein MA: Study of the infradiaphragmatic total anomalous pulmonary venous connection with cross-sectional and pulsed Doppler echocardiography. Circulation 70:412, 1984.
276. Huhta JC, Gutgesell HP, Nihill MR: Cross sectional echocardiographic diagnosis of total anomalous pulmonary venous connection. Br Heart J 53: 525, 1985.
277. Chin AJ, Sanders SP, Sherman F, et al.: Accuracy of subcostal two-dimen-

sional echocardiography in prospective diagnosis of total anomalous pulmonary venous connection. Am Heart J 113:1153, 1987.
278. Smallhorn JF, Sutherland DR, Tommasini G, et al.: Assessment of total anomalous pulmonary venous connection by two-dimensional echocardiography. Br Heart J 46:613, 1981.
279. Oelert H, Schafers H-J, Stegmann T, et al.: Complete correction of total anomalous pulmonary venous drainage: experience with 53 patients. Ann Thorac Surg 41:392, 1986.
280. Yee ES, Turley K, Hsieh WR, Ebert PA: Infant total anomalous pulmonary venous connection: factors influencing timing of presentation and operative outcome. Circulation 76(Suppl 3):III-83, 1987.
281. Leung MP, Mok CK, Cheung DLC, Lau KC: Echocardiographic diagnosis of anastomotic stricture following surgical correction of supracardiac total anomalous pulmonary venous connection. Am Heart J 1145:1518, 1987.
282. Smallhorn JF, Burrows P, Wilson G, et al. Two-dimensional and pulsed Doppler echocardiography in the postoperative evaluation of total anomalous pulmonary venous connection. Circulation 76:298, 1987.

CHAPTER

33

FETAL ECHOCARDIOGRAPHY

One of the newer and more exciting applications of echocardiography is the study of the fetal heart in utero. Although the recording of placental blood flow was one of the earliest applications of Doppler ultrasound, and M-mode studies of the fetus have been feasible for many years, not until the development of combined two-dimensional imaging and Doppler systems did a sufficiently large body of knowledge become available for this area of study to warrant separate consideration. This is now clearly appropriate because these combined technologies have made possible detailed noninvasive examination of human fetal cardiac anatomy and blood flow. Using these techniques, it is possible to identify and study fetal cardiac structure and function from the sixteenth week of gestation to delivery and to detect virtually every form of cardiac disorder in utero.[1–7]

Because it enables one to define both normal and abnormal cardiac morphology and function, fetal echocardiography has several important applications. First, it permits screening of high risk pregnancies in the previable period (18 to 22 weeks) for the presence of congenital cardiac defects in the fetus. Detection of serious anomalies in utero permits delivery to be planned at an institution where appropriate treatment is readily available. Second, in patients considered to be at high risk, demonstration of normal cardiac morphology and function can reassure the parents and can thereby ease the burden of pregnancy enormously. Third, in the fetus with an arrhythmia, an accurate diagnosis can be made in almost every case. Such diagnosis is important because in utero medical therapy is available for treatment of these arrhythmias. Finally, fetal echocardiography provides scientific information about the growth patterns of the normal fetus and the developmental dynamics of cardiac defects. Although insufficient data exist to determine the role of this information in treating serious anomalies, these data are clearly a necessary foundation for such treatment.[8,9]

BACKGROUND

Fetal Anatomy

To place fetal imaging and Doppler data in proper perspective, it is necessary to appreciate: (1) the pattern and timing of development of the fetal cardiovascular system; (2) the unique characteristics of the fetal circulation that persist throughout gestation; and (3) the changes in the circulation in the immediate postnatal period. Current knowledge of fetal growth and development is derived from many sources, including postmortem studies of human fetuses, studies of fetal animals (most commonly the fetal sheep), and more recently, studies of the human fetus in utero. These data are limited by methods of study, availability of subjects, and species differences, but they nonetheless form a useful foundation for understanding the structure and function of the fetal cardiovascular system.

The cardiovascular system is not the first organ system to make its appearance in the embryo, but it reaches a functional state long before any of the others. The first appearance of the circulatory system, as scattered masses of angiogenic cells, generally occurs in the presomite embryo at about 20 days' gestation. Within roughly 3 days from this first appearance of vasculogenesis, the endocardial tube has formed and the heart begins to beat. The endocardial tube then undergoes rotation and differential development, and by roughly the twenty-seventh day of gestation is ready for septation to begin. This process lasts approximately 10 days, so the intrauterine structural development of the heart is essentially completed by about 6 weeks. The size of the embryo at this stage, however, is only about 20 mm, and hence cardiac visualization with current echocardiographic techniques is impractical.

By the sixteenth week of gestation, however, when the fetus has grown sufficiently to permit reliable recording, the ventricles and atria are fully formed, the atrioventricular (AV) and semilunar valves are functional and competent, and the basic connections between the ventricles and great vessels are completed. Although differences exist between fetal cardiac anatomy and that of the neonate and adult (i.e., the foramen ovale and ductus arteriosus are normally patent, the right ventricle is slightly larger than the left, and right and left ventricular wall thicknesses are roughly equal), the heart is sufficiently well formed by the time it can be visualized echocardiographically to allow the diagnostic criteria used in the neonate to be applied to the fetus.[10,11] Similarly, because the normal growth of the fetal cardiac chambers and great vessels has been shown to correlate with increasing fetal weight, abnormalities in the development of individual cardiac structures can be recognized.

Fetal Circulation

Although the structure of the heart in the fetus is similar to that of the neonate, the pattern of the circulation differs considerably. As illustrated anatomically in Figure 33–1 and diagrammatically in Figure 33–2, blood is oxygenated in the placenta and returns to the fetus through the umbilical vein, which enters through the umbilicus and joins the portal vein to form the portal venous sinus. A variable proportion of the blood from the portal venous sinus traverses the ductus venosus to enter the inferior vena cava directly, whereas the remainder passes through the liver before rejoining the inferior vena cava through the hepatic vein. Inferior vena caval blood flow, which derives from the lower fetal body, the umbilical veins, and the portal vein, represents about 65 to 70% of the total venous return to the heart. In the right atrium, the crista dividens, the crescentic lower rim of the septum secundum, projects over the upper margin of the inferior vena cava and directs roughly 25% of the inferior vena caval return through the foramen ovale into the left atrium. Here it is joined by the pulmonary venous blood, which contributes about 8% of total venous return to the heart. Left atrial blood then passes into the left ventricle, from which it is distributed to the coronary circulation, the forelimbs, and the head.

Blood returning from the superior vena cava contributes about 22 to 25% of the total venous return to the heart. In the normal fetus, only minute portions of the superior vena caval blood cross the foramen ovale to the left atrium; most passes through the tricuspid valve into the right ventricle in conjunction with the streams from the inferior vena cava and coronary sinus. The majority of the right ventricular blood, which is ejected into the pulmonary trunk, traverses the ductus arteriosus to join

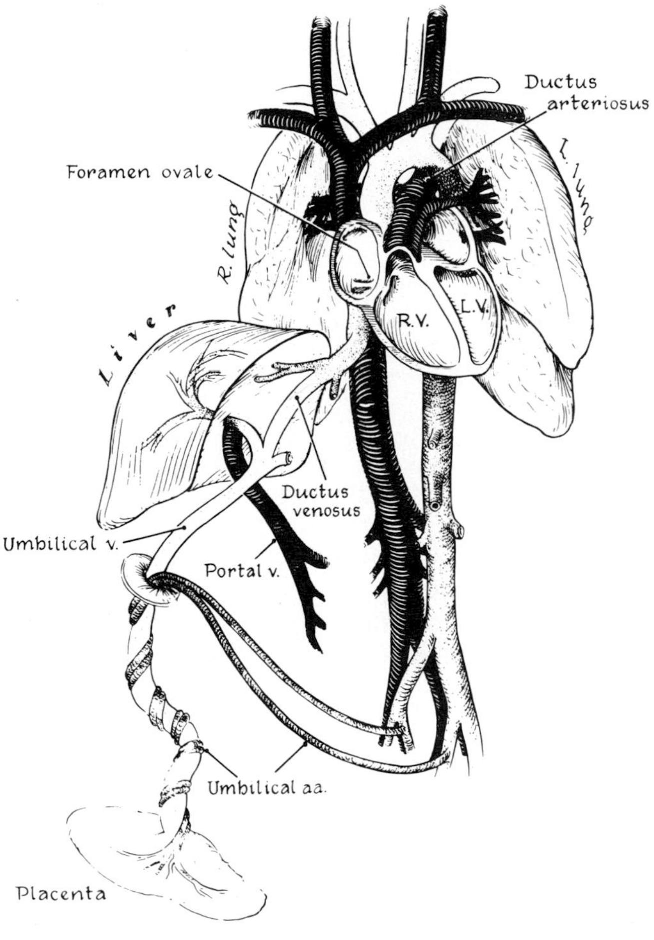

Fig. 33–1. Anatomy of the fetal circulation. Intensity of dots within vessels indicates degree of oxygen desaturation of hemoglobin. Note possible course of blood from the placenta through the liver or through the ductus venosus to the inferior vena cava and then to the heart. Note major sites of mixing of blood streams of varying oxygen content: portal vein, hepatic vein, inferior vena cava, foramen ovale, and ductus arteriosus. RV = right ventricle; LV = left ventricle. (From Adams FH, Emmanouilides GC (eds.): Moss' Heart Disease in Infants, Children, and Adolescents. 3rd Ed. Baltimore, Williams & Wilkins, p. 12, 1983.)

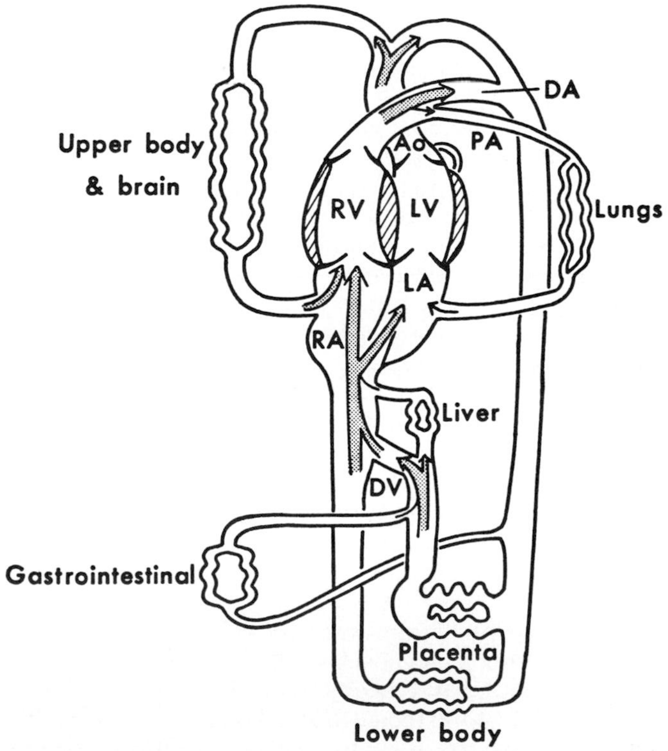

Fig. 33–2. The general course of the mammalian fetal circulation. DA = ductus arteriosus; Ao = aorta; PA = pulmonary artery; RV right ventricle; LV = left ventricle; RA = right atrium; LV = left atrium; DV = ductus venosus. (From Rudolph AM: Congenital Diseases of the Heart. Chicago, Year Book Medical Publishers, 1974.)

the stream of blood that crosses the isthmus of the aorta from the arch. This supplies the abdominal organs, the lower body, and the placenta. The remainder of the blood ejected by the right ventricle (roughly 5 to 10%) enters the pulmonary circulation, returning to the left atrium. Mean pressures in the aorta and pulmonary trunk are almost identical throughout fetal life, and blood flow to various organs is determined by local changes in the vascular resistance.[12]

In the adult, blood passes in series through the right atrium, right ventricle, and pulmonary artery; it returns to the left heart and is ejected into the aorta and peripheral circulation. The cardiac output therefore is expressed as the volume of blood flowing through the heart per unit time, and it represents the volume of blood ejected by each ventricle. In the fetus, blood distributed to the various parts of the body and to the placenta is derived from the systemic venous return as well as the umbilical venous return, and the ventricles effectively act in parallel. As a result, blood flow to many organs is derived from both ventricles, and the cardiac output in the fetus is typically expressed as the combined ventricular output, which represents the total volume of blood ejected by the left and right ventricles and includes pulmonary and coronary flows. It is important therefore, to remember that if comparisons of cardiac output in the fetal and postnatal animal or infant are made, the cardiac output in the fetus customarily is expressed as combined ventricular output, whereas cardiac output after birth represents the output of one ventricle. In the fetus, it is convenient to consider the flows through the cardiac chambers and great vessels in terms of the proportions of combined ventricular output, and these are illustrated graphically for the fetal lamb in Figure 33–3. As depicted in Figure 33–3, the right ventricle receives and ejects roughly 66% of the combined ventricular output, whereas the left ventricle ejects only about 34%. The disparity between right and left ventricular outputs is less marked in the human fetus, in which the brain receives a considerably higher percentage (15 to 20%) of the combined ventricular output than the approximately 3% it receives in the fetal lamb.[13]

The proportions of combined ventricular output traversing the major arteries is reflected in the relative diameters of these vessels. As a result, the pulmonary trunk is extremely large and the ascending aorta much narrower. The descending aorta is also wide, whereas the isthmus of the aorta is much narrower than the ascending or descending aorta or the ductus arteriosus.

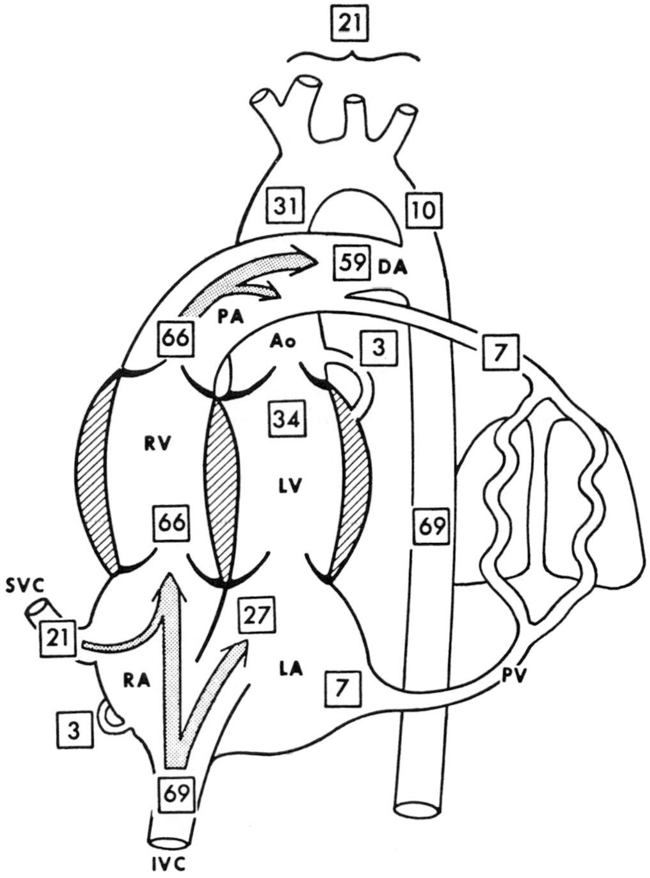

Fig. 33–3. Percentages of the combined ventricular output that return to the fetal heart, which are ejected by each ventricle and that flow through the main vascular channels. Figures are those obtained from late gestation lambs. DA = ductus arteriosus; PA = pulmonary artery; Ao = aorta; RV = right ventricle; LV = left ventricle; SVC = superior vena cava; RA = right atrium; LA = left atrium; IVC = inferior vena cava. (From Rudolph AM: Congenital Diseases of the Heart. Chicago, Year Book Medical Publishers, 1974.)

Myocardial Development and Function

Histologic studies of myocardium from fetal, neonatal, and adult hearts have shown a striking difference in the amount of contractile tissue. In the adult myocardium, the muscle cells are arranged in a well-organized parallel order, and little intercellular connective tissue is present. There is relatively little nuclear substance, and the nuclei are small and pyknotic. In the fetal heart, in contrast, considerable loose areolar tissue is present between muscle cells, and the cells are less well organized; the nuclei are large, and many cells are multinucleated. The result of these differences is that the total number of sarcomeres per unit mass of fetal myocardium is considerably smaller than in the adult. The functional effect of these structural differences is that the fetal myocardium develops considerably greater tension at rest when stretched than does adult myocardium (decreased compliance), and when stimulated, it develops less tension at any resting length. The fetal ventricle therefore has a limited capacity to increase stroke volume or to maintain stroke volume in the face of increased afterload. As a result, the fetus can increase cardiac output to only a limited degree, and mainly by increasing rate, as compared to the adult heart's ability to increase both rate and stroke volume. Because of this obligatory relationship between cardiac output and heart rate, fetal cardiac output is sensitive to decreases in heart rate.[14]

Changes in the Circulation After Birth

Sudden and dramatic changes in the circulation occur within the first few minutes after birth as the function of

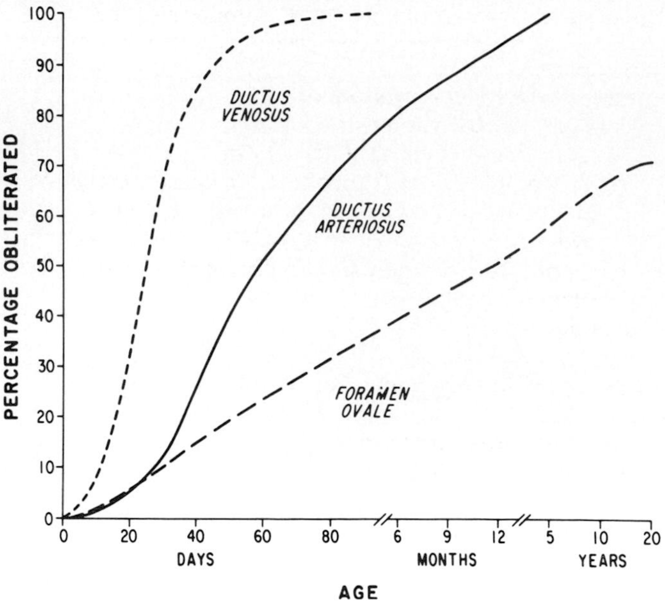

Fig. 33–4. Average percentages of obliterated fetal blood passages according to age. (From Adams FH: Closure of the ductus arteriosus and foramen ovale. *In* Cassels DE (ed.): Heart and Circulation in the Newborn and Infants. New York, Grune & Stratton, 1966.)

gas exchange is transferred from the placenta to the lungs. Clamping the umbilical cord removes the very low-resistance placental vascular bed, which in the fetus had received 40% of the combined ventricular output. This change causes a large increase in vascular resistance on the systemic side of the circulation and results in a marked reduction in inferior vena caval return to the heart. Concurrent with the cessation of umbilical placental flow is a rapid reduction in pulmonary vascular resistance and a marked increase in pulmonary blood flow associated with the onset of respiration and expansion of the lungs with air.

The increase in pulmonary flow increases venous return to the left atrium and raises left atrial pressure slightly while inferior vena caval flow and pressure are decreasing. The simultaneous increase in left atrial pressure and the reduction in vena caval pressure results in apposition of the valve of the foramen ovale against the edge of the crista dividens; resulting in functional closure of the foramen ovale. Initially, any disturbance that results in a higher pressure in the right atrium than the left allows the foramen to reopen and permits venous blood to flow from the right to the left atrium. Over the course of several months, the valve becomes adherent to the margins of the atrial septum, and permanent closure results. As illustrated in Figure 33–4, the foramen re-

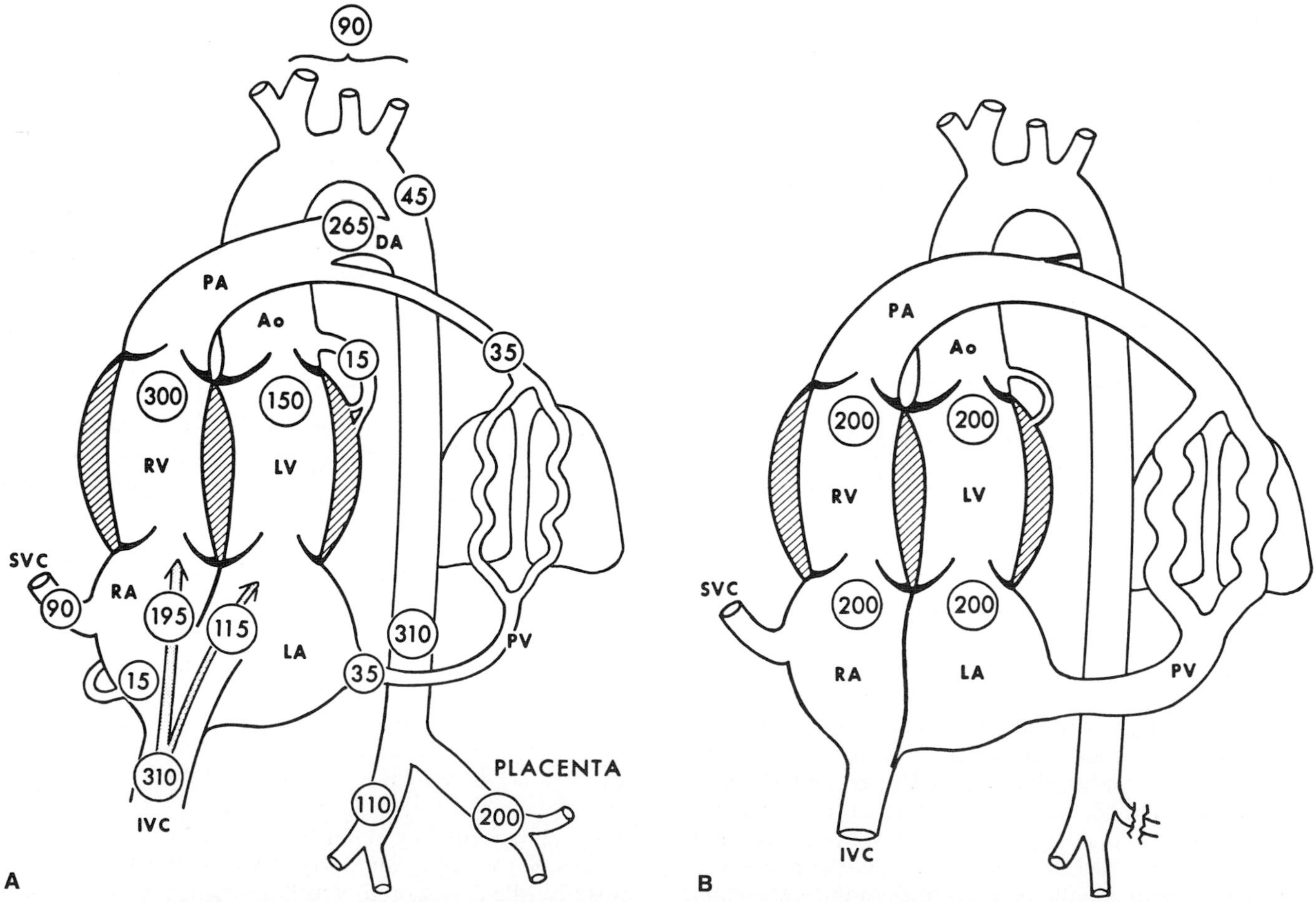

Fig. 33–5. **A.** Volumes of blood in ml/min/kg body weight (figures in circles) that flow through various chambers and vessels in the late gestation fetal heart. **B.** Volumes of blood ejected by each ventricle and returning to each atrium postnatally. DA = ductus arteriosus; PA = pulmonary artery; Ao = aorta; RV = right ventricle; LV = left ventricle; SVC = superior vena cava; RA = right atrium; LA = left atrium; PV = pulmonary vein; IVC = inferior vena cava. (From Rudolph AM: Congenital Diseases of the Heart. Chicago, Year Book Medical Publishers, 1974.)

mains nonadherent and capable of opening into adult life in roughly 20% of normal subjects.

In the fetus, the ductus arteriosus is a large channel with a thick medial muscular coat that is capable of contraction, to close the lumen completely. The ductus is constricted by an increase in P_{O_2} in the environment, and the rise in systemic arterial P_{O_2} that occurs after birth probably is the main factor responsible for ductal closure. If the arterial P_{O_2} does not rise normally after birth because of either inadequate lung expansion or a low oxygen fraction in the inspired air, the ductus arteriosus may remain open for a long period. In the normal mature infant, however, the ductus is functionally closed within 10 to 15 hours after birth. Because the ductus is initially closed by muscular constriction, it can be reopened if systemic arterial P_{O_2} falls, but there appears to be a progressive decrease in responsiveness after birth. Within a few days, small intimal hemorrhages are noted, and thrombosis and fibrosis of the intima and also the media occur, resulting in permanent closure. In full-term infants, complete closure occurs within 10 to 21 days. Premature infants frequently have persistent patency of the ductus arteriosus because the constrictor response is not developmentally mature.

When the infant is separated from the umbilical-placental circulation, the blood flow from the portal veins through the liver is reduced as the contribution from the umbilical veins to the hepatic circulation is removed. The flow through the ductus venosus also falls instantaneously, and this channel, like the foramen ovale and the ductus arteriosus, also closes soon after birth (3 to 7 days) (Fig. 33–4).

Figure 33–5A and B compares the absolute volumes of blood flowing through the through the heart and great vessels in the immediate preterm fetus (Fig. 33–5A) with those observed in the neonate with an established adult circulatory pattern (Fig. 33–5B). Note that with the elimination of placental flow and closure of the foramen ovale and ductus arteriosus, the circulatory pattern shifts from one in which the ventricles work in parallel to one in which they pump in series and the output of each chamber is equal.

ECHOCARDIOGRAPHIC EXAMINATION OF THE HUMAN FETUS

Indications for Fetal Echocardiography

Congenital heart disease is relatively rare, occurring in roughly 8 of 1000 live births, in only 25% of which is it both serious and likely to be diagnosed in utero. Selection of fetuses for echocardiographic study therefore should be based on specific risk factors because the yield would otherwise be prohibitively small. These risk factors are generally considered to fall into three categories (Table 33–1): (1) those related to the fetus; (2) factors related to the mother; and (3) factors involving the family. Fetal risk factors include growth retardation, fetal cardiac arrhythmia, hydrops (right ventricular dilatation, skin edema, abdominal ascites, and when severe, pleural and pericardial fluid), other developmental defects known to be associated with cardiac disorders, and decreased fetal movement. Maternal risk factors include maternal congenital heart disease, polyhydramnios, Rh sensitization, presence of diabetes mellitus, known connective tissue disorders, pre-eclampsia, and a history of exposure in early pregnancy to known cardiac teratogens such as lithium, steroids, phenytoin, or rubella virus. Familial risk factors include a history of congenital heart disease or a genetic syndrome known to be associated with congenital heart disease. A prior pregnancy with a cardiac defect increases the risk to the fetus to 1 in 50, and a defect in a parent may increase the risk to as high as 1 in 10.[15–17]

Table 33–1. Indications for Fetal Echocardiography

Fetal factors
Intrauterine growth retardation
Fetal cardiac arrhythmia
Fetal somatic anomalies (ultrasound)
hydrocephalus, microcephaly, holoprosencephaly, agenesis of the corpus callosum, Meckel-Gruber syndrome, esophageal atresia, duodenal atresia, diaphragmatic hernia, omphalocele, renal dysplasia[17]
Hydrops fetalis
Abnormal genetic screen
Decreased fetal movement
Maternal factors
Congenital heart disease
Polyhydramnios
Rh sensitization
Diabetes mellitus
Collagen vascular disease
Drug exposure (alcohol, anticonvulsants, lithium, etc.)
Pre-eclampsia
Familial factors
Congenital heart disease
Genetic syndromes

Locating the Fetal Heart

During the examination of the fetal heart, the mother is placed in a comfortable supine position. The transducer is applied directly to the anterior abdominal wall, and the uterus is initially scanned in two-dimensional mode to determine fetal location, number, and lie. The abdominal circumference and cranial biparietal dimensions are initially recorded to establish fetal age. Once fetal position is known, the spatial orientation of the thorax and the position of the fetal heart can then be determined.

To record the fetal heart, the echo beam must pass through the abdominal wall of the mother, the uterine wall and cavity contents, and the fetal thorax. The soft tissues of the maternal abdominal wall and uterus attenuate sound minimally and hence provide an ideal acoustic window to the fetus. Similarly, because the lungs of the fetus are filled with fluid, nearly unlimited access to the fetal heart and major vessels can be anticipated from the time the heart first becomes visible (about 16 weeks) until the spine and ribs begin to calcify.

Despite this relatively unimpeded access, the fetal heart is still much smaller than that of the infant and requires high resolution imaging to be clearly recorded. In addition, it does not lie directly beneath the transducer, but is separated by a large standoff (i.e., the mother's abdominal wall, placental structures, and uterine contents). Thus, fetal imaging requires high resolution at depths that often limit the quality of the available images.

Timing of Examination

The optimum time for fetal imaging is between 23 and 26 weeks' gestation. During this period, the fetal heart is large enough to be studied in detail, and fetal movement may facilitate the examination by offering a variety of positions in which the heart can be studied. Imaging closer to term can be hampered by both increased density of the ribs and the higher prevalence of occiput anterior position.[18] Earlier imaging (20 to 22 weeks) is favored by some authors, to facilitate genetic counseling.[19]

General Examination Technique

Once the heart is located and its orientation determined, it can then be studied using any or all of the major echocardiographic techniques: two-dimensional imaging, Doppler, and/or M-mode. Occasionally, fetal lie is unsatisfactory (spine upwards), and the heart cannot be clearly visualized. In these cases, it may be necessary to rotate the mother onto one side or the other or to elevate her head or feet to image the fetus in a slightly different position. If these maneuvers fail, having the mother walk around for a few minutes often results in a change in fetal position. In most cases (90 to 95%), a successful examination can be anticipated on the first attempt. If the first examination is unsatisfactory, normal fetal repositioning within the uterus over a period of days generally shifts the heart to a new location and permits a successful repeat study. Other limiting factors include maternal obesity and hydrops with polyhydramnios, both of which increase the distance from the anterior abdominal wall to the heart and decrease image quality.

Two-Dimensional Examination

Virtually all fetal cardiac examinations begin with a two-dimensional imaging study to assess the structural integrity of the heart. In studying the fetus, the same principles of two-dimensional imaging described in Chapter 4 apply. In fetal studies, these principles are particularly important, however, because one has no external references to help orient the scan plane, and all plane positions must be defined relative to cardiac structures.

Five standard planes are typically recorded in the fetal two-dimensional examination. These include a four-chamber view, a short axis view through the base of the heart including the origins of the great vessels, a short axis view through the base of the ventricles, a long axis view of the left ventricle and aorta, and an arch view. The four-chamber and short axis great vessel views are the most important for fetal cardiac evaluation because they permit cardiac chamber and valve structures as well as the two great arteries to be viewed in detail. Because of limited access and because the fetus may turn during examination, individual views should be recorded as they are identified, rather than obtained in a set sequence similar to the conventional method used after birth.[19]

The four-chamber view (Fig. 33–6) permits visualization of (1) left and right ventricular size, function, and wall thickness; (2) atrial size; (3) the junction of the interatrial and interventricular septa at the crux of the heart; (4) the normal offset of the septal insertion of the two AV valves (ventricular identification) and their motion patterns; and (5) the defect in the atrial septum caused by the open foramen ovale. The eustachian valve, which is prominent in the fetus, can often be identified within the right atrium, where it may function to direct highly saturated blood toward the left atrium and the upper body. In addition, the primum component of the atrial septum can be identified in the left atrium. The phasic motion of the primum component of the septum demonstrates the interatrial dynamics in utero.[20]

The short axis great vessel view (Fig. 33–7A) defines the initial course of the great vessels and their pattern of insertion into the ventricles. The bifurcation of the pulmonary artery can be identified, although in the fetus

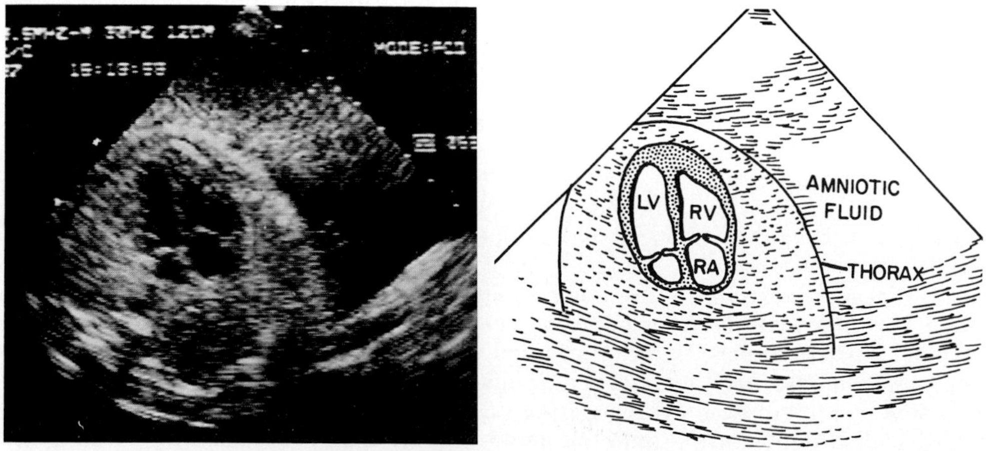

Fig. 33–6. Inverted apical four-chamber view of the fetal heart. Note the distal end of the septum secundum projecting into the right atrium and patent foramen ovale. LV = left ventricle; RV = right ventricle; RA = right atrium.

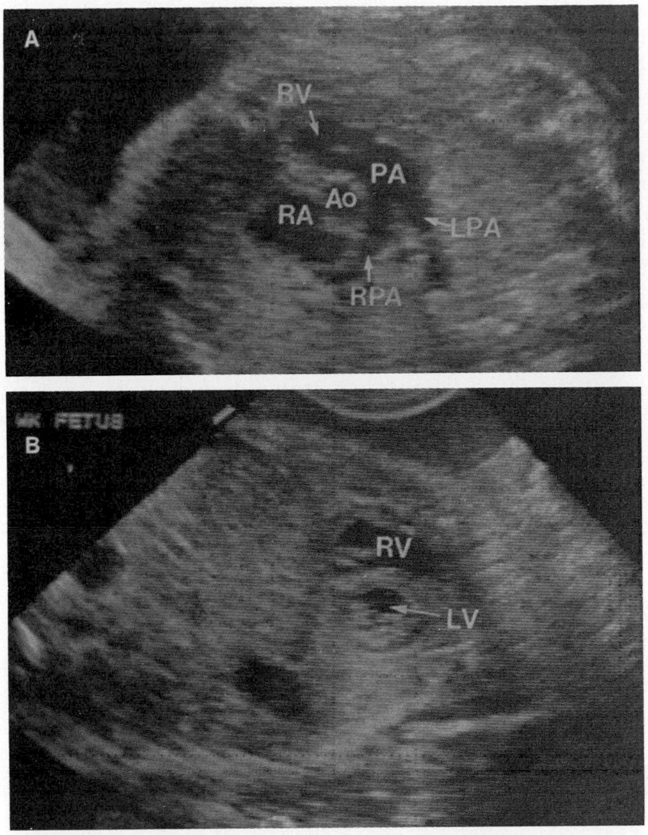

Fig. 33–7. **A.** Parasternal short axis view through the origins of the great vessels. **B.** Parasternal short axis view through the base of the heart. RV = right ventricle; PA = pulmonary artery; Ao = aorta; RA = right atrium; RPA = right pulmonary artery; LPA = left pulmonary artery; RV = right ventricle; LV = left ventricle. (From Snider AR, Serwer GA: Echocardiography in Pediatric Heart Disease. Chicago, Year Book Medical Publishers, p. 68, 1990.)

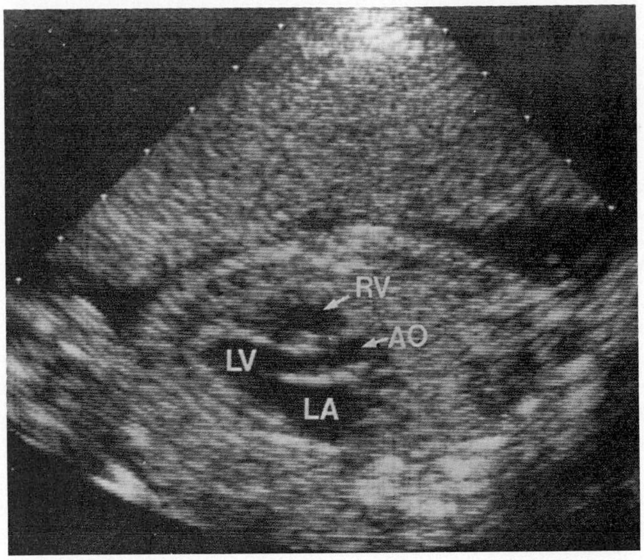

Fig. 33–8. Parasternal equivalent long axis view of the left ventricle (LV), left atrium (LA), and aorta (AO) of the fetus. RV = right ventricle. (From Snider AR, Serwer GA: Echocardiography in Pediatric Heart Disease. Chicago, Year Book Medical Publishers, p. 67, 1990).

the pulmonary branches are small. The ductus arteriosus can also be identified and traced into the descending aorta. Both the aortic and pulmonary valves can be identified from this plane. With slight caudal angulation, a short axis view through the base of the ventricles (Fig. 33–7B) can also be obtained. The short axis view at the base of the ventricles is typically used for measuring chamber diameters and wall thicknesses and to position the M-mode cursor through the center of the ventricular chambers. The short axis and four-chamber views can both be obtained in 95 to 100% of studies.[21]

The long axis view of the left heart (Fig. 33–8) aids in determining the relationship of the interventricular septum with the great vessels, whereas the arch view (Fig. 33–9) is important in identifying the head and neck vessels, to distinguish the arch from the ductal connection to the descending aorta when great vessel identity is in question. This distinction is based on the recognition that the head and neck vessels always arise from the aorta and the ductal connection takes a wider curve and lies below the arch in a different plane of section. These views may not all be attainable with the fetus in one position, and it is occasionally necessary to turn the mother to either side to influence fetal lie.

The fetal examination is obviously more limited in

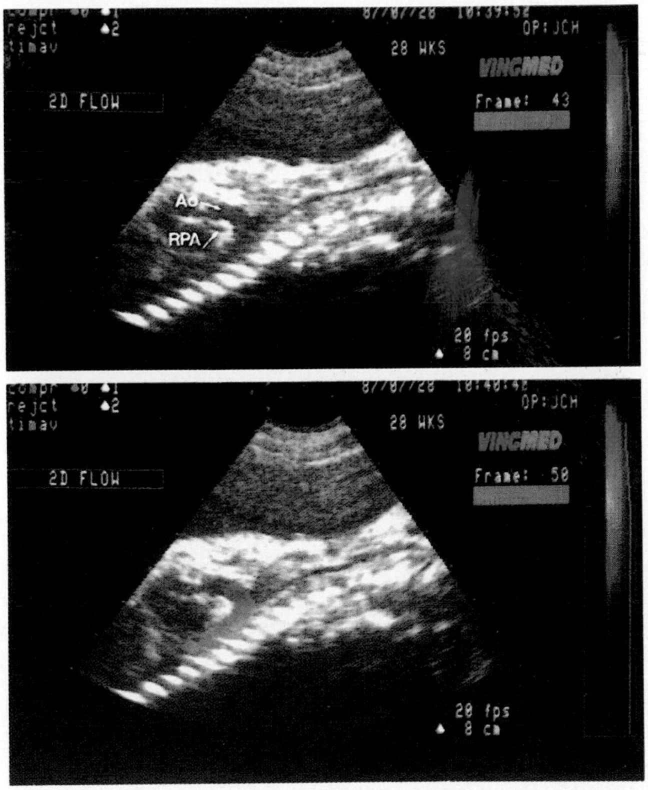

Fig. 33–9. Long axis recording of the ascending aorta, aortic arch with the origins of the head and neck vessels and descending thoracic aorta. Ao = aorta; RPA = right pulmonary artery. (From Huhta JC, Helton JG, Wood DC: Color Doppler in the fetal examination. Echocardiography 6:393, 1989.)

terms of the number of images recorded than that typically performed in the adult or child. Less detailed imaging is necessary for several reasons: (1) The diagnostic questions in the fetus are generally more limited (i.e., determining atrial situs, AV connections, and ventriculoarterial connection), and abnormalities of interest are usually associated with more profound changes in cardiac morphology than in the adult; (2) the fetal heart is much smaller than that of the adult, and it is generally possible to obtain far more information in a single view (i.e., the full sweep of the aorta can generally be recorded in a single view in the fetus, whereas in the adult several images are required to record the same information); and (3) although there is no evidence that ultrasound is toxic to the fetus, it is prudent to limit exposure to the minimum necessary to record the desired data.

M-Mode Examination

M-mode echocardiographic recordings from the fetus were first demonstrated in 1972.[22] In the absence of spatial orientation, however, the variable and constantly changing position of the fetus in the uterus made such "stand-alone" M-mode studies difficult to record and interpret and limited their general utility. The subsequent availability of two-dimensionally derived M-mode recording methods, however, has made it possible to record reproducible M-mode studies from specific locations within the fetal heart and has made the technique of particular value in several diagnostic areas. These include the recording of time-related changes in ventricular function and the sequence of contraction of the ventricles and atria in patients with arrhythmias. Two-dimensionally derived M-mode studies are also often used for measurements of fetal cardiac chamber size because of the simplicity with which these measurements can be made.

Derived M-mode studies of the left ventricle are best obtained from a parasternal equivalent short axis view of the ventricular chamber. The aortic root and left atrium are similarly best recorded in a short axis projection of the aortic root.

Doppler Examination

Doppler echocardiographic studies can also be successfully conducted in the human fetus, thus offering the potential for assessing intracardiac hemodynamics and cardiac output in utero.[5,6,19,23–25] Fetal Doppler studies, like fetal M-mode studies, are generally two-dimensionally directed because the relatively small size of the fetal heart and great vessels makes it almost impossible to obtain reproducible studies in the absence of imaging guidance. The Doppler frequencies used typically vary from 3.5 to 5 MHz, with lower frequencies occasionally required because of the distance of the fetal heart from the maternal abdominal wall.

The technical considerations for fetal Doppler studies are similar to those for any Doppler examination. The small size of the fetal great vessels, however, may make diameter and area measurements relatively less accurate than in the child or adult and hence may limit the role of quantitation. Similarly, the position of the fetus may make it impossible to align the ultrasonic beam parallel to the flow vector and may introduce the need for angle correction.

At present, Doppler flow sampling is primarily used to detect AV valve regurgitation; however, all Doppler parameters are potentially available, including aortic and pulmonary flow velocities, mitral and tricuspid inflow patterns, umbilical arterial and venous flow, and flow across the foramen ovale (Fig. 33–10). Some investigators have also tried to measure cardiac output from pulmonary artery and aortic diameters and systolic velocity integrals; however, given the small vessel diameters of the fetus, such measurements should be viewed with caution (see Chapter 30). Changes in systolic velocity integrals have also been used to assess changes in ventricular performance. Because such measurements are independent of vessel area, they are probably more reliable measures of response to specific interventions.

Systolic aortic Doppler velocity profiles in the fetus appear similar to those in the neonate and adult. Although one would anticipate that the pulmonary artery systolic velocity integral would differ in shape because of the higher pulmonary artery pressure in the fetus, this has not been specifically studied.

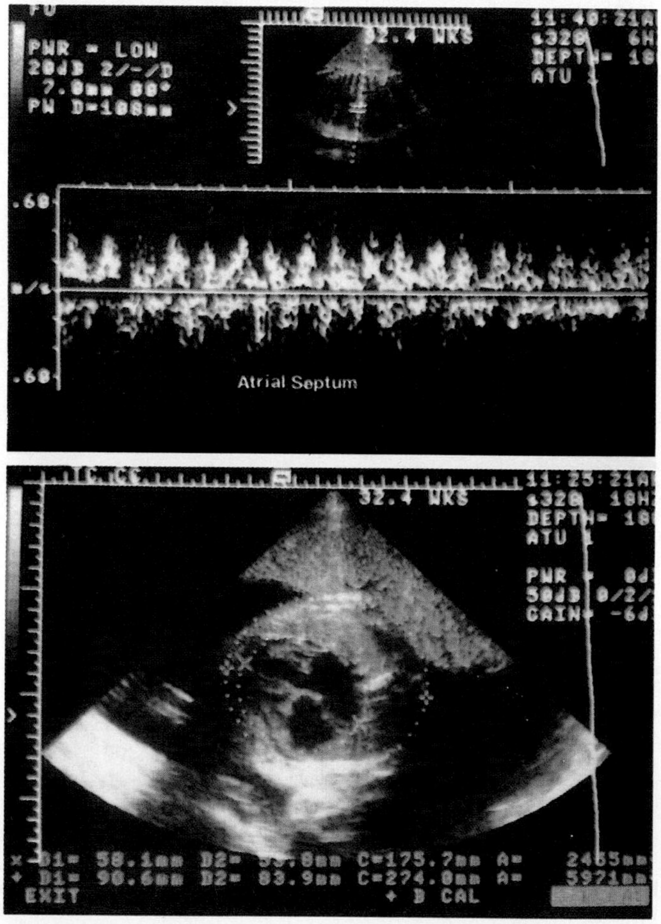

Fig. 33–10. Doppler recording of flow at the atrial septum (fossa ovalis) from a fetus with a supraventricular tachycardia. (From Huhta JC, Helton JG, Wood DC: Color Doppler in the fetal examination. Echocardiography 6:393, 1989.)

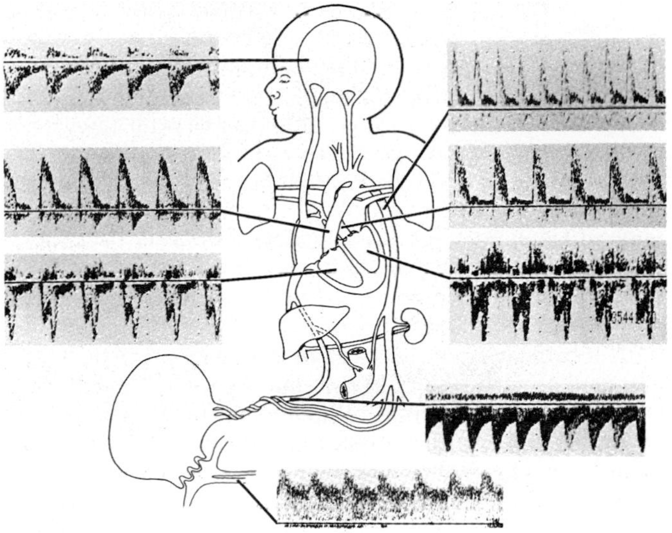

Fig. 33–11. Summary of Doppler recordings, clockwise from bottom left: tricuspid valve, pulmonary valve, intracerebral arteries, descending aorta, aortic valve, mitral valve, umbilical artery and vein, and maternal vessels. (From Reed KL, Anderson CF, Shanker L: Fetal Echocardiography: An Atlas. New York, Alan R. Liss, p. 110, 1988.)

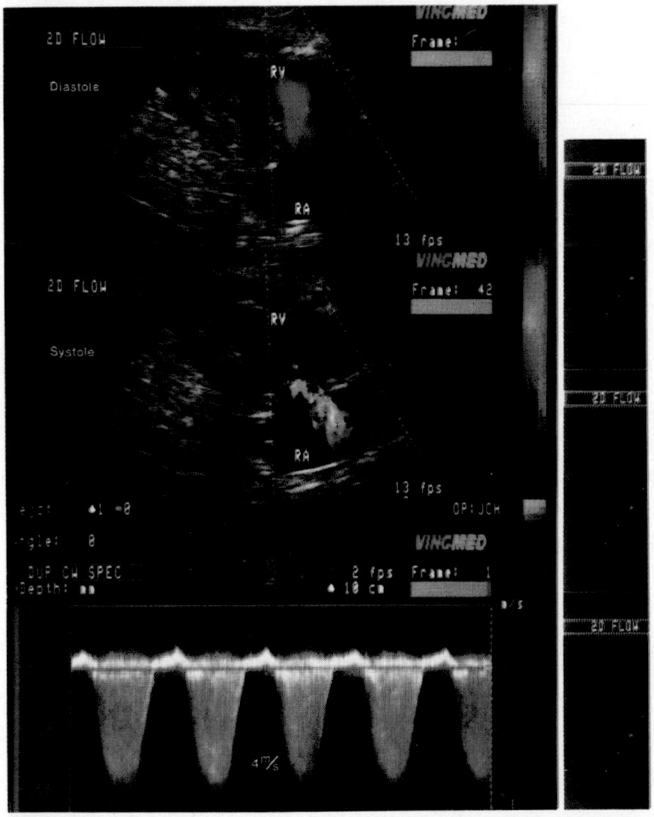

Fig. 33–12. Color and continuous wave Doppler of a fetus with tricuspid valve regurgitation late in gestation. Top. The diastolic frame shows forward flow (red) from the right atrium (RA) to the right ventricle (RV). Middle. Systolic regurgitant flow from the RV to the RA. Bottom. Continuous wave Doppler shows a peak velocity of 4 m/sec. (From Huhta JC, Helton JG, Wood DC: Color Doppler in the fetal examination. Echocardiography 6:393, 1989.)

Diastolic flow patterns through the AV valves vary with valve studied and gestational age. Tricuspid valve flow in general is greater than mitral flow, and this is reflected in a larger tricuspid velocity integral. In contrast, peak flow velocity across the mitral valve in early diastole is greater than that across the tricuspid valve. A/E ratios across both valves are constantly above unity,[6] but decrease from 17 to 42 weeks. This pattern appears to be related to the decreased ventricular compliance during gestation, compared to that after birth, but it may also reflect a lower initial diastolic pressure.[6] Figure 33–11 summarizes many of the typical Doppler flow patterns recorded in the normal fetus.

The primary abnormality uniquely detected by Doppler in the fetus is AV valve insufficiency. AV valvular regurgitation (Fig. 33–12) is associated with a poor prognosis (see later) and is almost uniformly associated with fetal hydrops. Therefore, all infants with hydrops should be examined for AV valve insufficiency.

ECHOCARDIOGRAPHIC MEASUREMENT OF CHAMBER SIZE IN THE NORMAL DEVELOPING FETUS

Before the advent of echocardiography, most of our knowledge of fetal growth and development came from animal studies, with limited additional data obtained from human abortuses. Although they offer important insights into fetal physiology, these studies do not provide the normative values necessary to recognize abnormalities in the pattern of growth of the fetal cardiac chambers and great vessels in vivo, which are the basis for diagnosing many important congenital disorders. Such data, of necessity, must be derived from echocardiographic studies themselves. Unfortunately, few studies have been directed toward quantitative assessment of cardiac chamber size,[1,2,7] and these appear to present conflicting results with regard to the relative sizes of the right and left ventricles and growth patterns of the cardiac chambers.[1,2] Despite the apparent conflicts in these data, the actual numeric differences are small (i.e., in the millimeter range) and hence the absolute data are useful as a point of reference. The reported differences undoubtedly reflect that (1) echocardiographic measurements are affected by factors other than simple biologic variability; (2) a slight difference in data distribution can result in changes in the optimal approach to statistical modeling; and (3) similar dimensions recorded in different views may suggest different results when the absolute numbers are small.

Longitudinal studies of fetal growth and development from 20 weeks' gestation to term show the left and right ventricles to be roughly equal in size (Table 33–2), with a linear growth pattern in both chambers.[7,26] Figure 33–13 illustrates the patterns of normal growth of the right and left ventricles, aorta, and left atrium from 20 weeks' gestation to birth. Right and left ventricular diameters more than double in size during this period, and a clear linear relationship exists, with a good correlation between gestational age and chamber size. Figure 33–14 illustrates the ratio of right ventricular to left ventricular diameter, relative wall thickness (wall thickness/chamber radius),

Table 33–2. Changes in Fetal Chamber Sizes and Ventricular Function from 20 to 40 Weeks' Gestation

Dimension (in cm.)	Gestational Age	
	20 weeks (cm)	40 weeks (cm)
RVd	0.70 ± 0.10	1.40 ± 0.20
RVs	0.45 ± 0.10	1.00 ± 0.20
LVd	0.70 ± 0.10	1.55 ± 0.25
LVs	0.50 ± 0.10	1.05 ± 0.10
RVwth-d	0.20 ± 0.05	0.30 ± 0.05
RVwth-s	0.30 ± 0.05	0.45 ± 0.05
IVSth-d	0.20 ± 0.05	0.35 ± 0.05
IVSth-s	0.25 ± 0.05	0.45 ± 0.05
LVwth-d	0.20 ± 0.05	0.35 ± 0.05
LVwth-s	0.30 ± 0.05	0.45 ± 0.05
RV% ∧ Δ	36% ± 8%	35% ± 4%
LV% ∧ Δ	36% ± 6%	32% ± 5%
Aod	0.50 ± 0.05	0.90 ± 0.10
LAd	0.65 ± 0.10	1.00 ± 0.10
LA/Ao	~1.2 ± 1.0	
LV-MASS (g)	0.86 ± 0.09	7.47 ± 2.43

RVd = right ventricular diameter (diastole); RVs = right ventricular (systole); LVd = left ventricular diameter diastole; LVs = left ventricular (systole); RVwth-d = right ventricular wall thickness diastole; RVwth-s = right ventricular wall thickness systole; IVSth-d = interventricular septum thickness diameter; IVSth-s = interventricular septum thickness (systole); LVwth-d = left ventricular wall thickness diastole; LVwth-s = left ventricular wall thickness systole; RV% ∧ Δ = right ventricular percent change in diameter from diastole to systole; LV% ∧ Δ = left ventricular percent change in diameter from diastole to systole; Aod = aortic diameter; LAd = left atrial diameter; LA/Ao = left atrial/aortic ratio; LVmass = left ventricular mass.

(Data from St. John Sutton MG, et al.: Quantitative assessment of growth and function of the cardiac chambers in the normal fetus: a prospective longitudinal study. Circulation 69:645, 1984.)

and the left atrial/aortic ratio for the same period. Right and left ventricular diameters are similar and increase in parallel, so the ratio of maximum right ventricular to left ventricular diameter is close to unity.[27] Left atrial and aortic diameters also increase linearly,[28,29] so the left atrial/aortic ratio, which is often used as a postnatal indicator of ductal shunting, varies between 1.35 and 1.15 throughout gestation. Figure 33–15 illustrates the increase in left ventricular mass from 20 to 40 weeks' gestation. The echocardiographic left ventricular mass increased by almost 10-fold over this period, which is similar to that expected in total body weight[30] and corresponding closely to postmortem weights recorded over the same period.

The patterns of intrauterine growth of the septum and right and left ventricular wall thicknesses, echocardiographic left ventricular mass, and postmortem left ventricular weight were linear over the period of gestation studied and were similar to those of ventricular chamber diameters. Regardless of the increasing left ventricular chamber size and muscle mass, however, the relationship between cavity radius and relative wall thickness did not change with age and varied over the range observed in adults and children. Left and right ventricular function as manifested by fractional shortening remained constant for both ventricles.

Thus, in the fetus, chamber dimensions, wall thicknesses, and ventricular muscle mass increase linearly with gestational age. The ratios of right ventricular to left ventricular diameters and of left atrial to aortic diameters, relative wall thickness, and left ventricular fractional shortening remain relatively constant throughout gestation. Echocardiographic measures of left ventricular mass in the fetus correspond closely with postmortem anatomic weights.

METHODS OF ASSESSING FETAL CARDIAC PERFORMANCE

The assessment of fetal ventricular performance is complicated by the small size of fetal cardiac structures and the differences in fetal ventricular shape in comparison to the newborn or adult. The small chamber size has the effect of greatly magnifying any measurement errors. For example, if the end-systolic dimension of the left ventricle of the 20-week fetus is 5 mm, then a 1-mm error in measurement will result in roughly a 100% difference in the volume calculated using the D^3 formula (see Chapter 20).

The shape of the fetal right and left ventricles differs from that in the newborn and adult because the loading conditions on the two ventricles in utero are similar and the septum therefore assumes a neutral or midline position rather than being concave toward the left ventricle, as occurs after birth.[31,32] This shift in septal position causes the left ventricle to be relatively flattened, whereas the right ventricle has the shape of a cone bisected from apex to base. These considerations are important because they can make echocardiographic assessment of left ventricular contractility and volume based on standard geometric models unreliable. Thus, although M-mode echocardiographic linear dimensions have been converted to ejection fraction, stroke volume, and cardiac output using standard ellipsoid models, such applications in the fetus are theoretically flawed.

Shortening Fraction

The shortening fraction, which simply measures the percentage of change in left and right ventricular minor dimensions from diastole to systole, is without any true geometric assumptions and hence should be a valid measure of ventricular contraction (assuming that the geometry of the two fetal ventricles remains constant throughout gestation). Because of the differences in ventricular shape, however, the absolute numbers do not have the same meaning in the fetus as in the neonate or adult. Because the small absolute numbers in these calculations also introduce the potential for significant

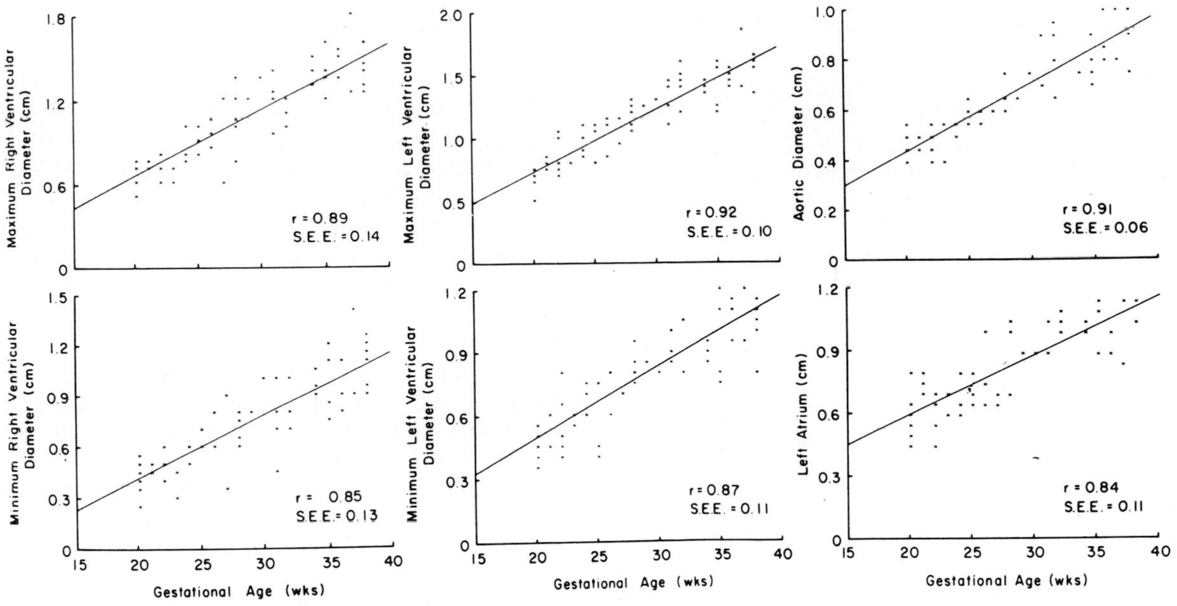

Fig. 33–13. Pattern of normal growth of the right and left ventricles, aorta, and left atrium from 20 weeks of gestation to birth. (From St. John Sutton MG, et al.: Quantitative assessment of growth and function of the cardiac chambers in the normal fetus: a prospective longitudinal study. Circulation 69:645, 1984. Reproduced by permission of the American Heart Association, Inc.)

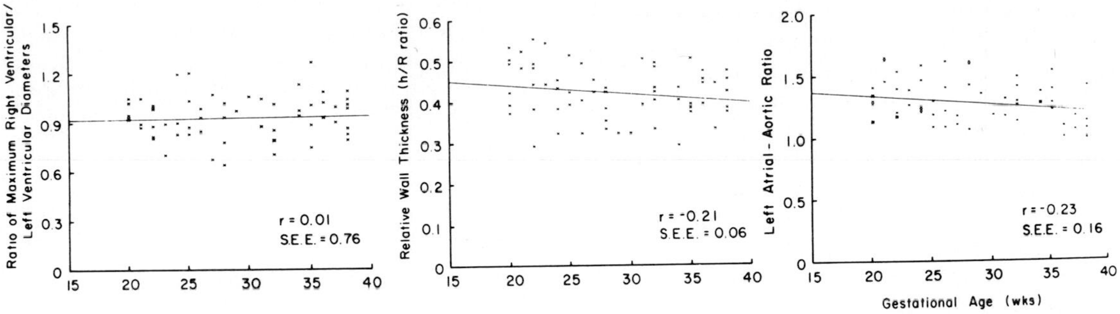

Fig. 33–14. Ratio of right ventricular to left ventricular diameter, relative wall thickness (wall thickness/chamber radius), and the left atrial/aortic ratio from 20 weeks of gestation to birth. (From St. John Sutton MG, et al.: Quantitative assessment of growth and function of the cardiac chambers in the normal fetus: a prospective longitudinal study. Circulation 69:645, 1984. Reproduced by permission of the American Heart Association, Inc.)

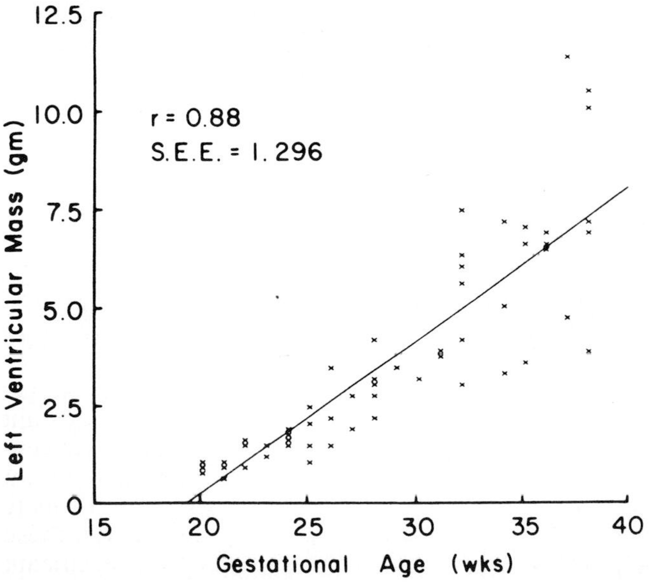

Fig. 33–15. Increase in left ventricle mass from 20 to 40 weeks of gestation. (From St. John Sutton MG, et al.: Quantitative assessment of growth and function of the cardlac chambers in the normal fetus: a prospective longitudinal study. Circulation 69:645, 1984. Reproduced by permission of the American Heart Association Inc.)

error, it is likely that such measurements have their greatest value in assessing longitudinal changes in function in response to some intervention, as opposed to comparisons between individuals. Time-related indices such as peak systolic wall velocity, which are also free of geometric assumptions, may also prove to have value.

Systolic Time Intervals

Systolic time intervals have been used in the infant and adult as a noninvasive technique for the evaluation of systolic ventricular performance and vascular impedance. The most commonly used systolic time intervals are the pre-ejection period (PEP), which extends from the beginning of the QRS complex of the electrocardiogram to the onset of ventricular ejection (consisting of electromechanical activation and isovolumic contraction), the ventricular ejection time (ET), which is the period between semilunar valve opening and closure, and the PEP/ET ratio. The duration of these intervals depends on five factors: (1) preload; (2) afterload; (3) contractility; (4) heart rate; and (5) the sequence of ventricular activation. Systolic time interval can be obtained in the fetus using M-mode echocardiographic recordings of the fetal semilunar valves and simultaneously inscribed fetal electrocardiographic signals obtained using electrodes placed on the maternal abdominal wall.[33] In the fetus, the PEP/ET ratio is independent of heart rate, but is positively correlated with gestational age.[34] These age-related changes are due to variation of the PEP with little change in the ET. The ejection times of the two ventricles have also been observed to differ slightly; however, the reported direction of the differences has been inconsistent. Practical applications of fetal systolic time intervals to date have been limited. Although further study is clearly warranted, limitations of these indices are recognized in postnatal life, and there is no reason to think that these should be any different in the fetus.[33] Moreover, fetal systolic time intervals are more difficult to obtain, largely because of the low success rate in recording adequate transabdominal fetal electrocardiograms against the background interference from the maternal heart.

Doppler Cardiac Output

Doppler echocardiography may prove to be the most reliable method for assessing fetal blood flow. Initial experience with these techniques is encouraging,[19,24,25,35] because flow estimates have been reproducible and quantitatively similar to flows reported using other measurement techniques.[24] Doppler permits an estimate of stroke volume, cardiac output (ventricular output), and stroke distance. Studies of normal fetuses from 19 to 40 weeks suggest a positive relationship between stroke volume and gestational age. Right ventricular stroke volume increased exponentially from a mean of 0.7 ml at 20 weeks to a mean of 7.6 ml at 40 weeks, whereas during the same period, left ventricular stroke volume increased from a mean of 0.7 ml to a mean of 5.2 ml. In 44% of fetuses, it was possible to quantitate both right and left ventricular stroke volume, and in these cases there was a close correlation between the volumes ejected by the two chambers ($r = 0.96$), with right ventricular stroke volume exceeding left ventricular stroke volume by 28%.[36] Similarly, a directionally appropriate decrease in the velocity integral has been noted with premature beats.

The measurement of flow by Doppler, however, requires clear visualization of the vessel walls, and potential errors in Doppler flow measurements are substantial. The first source of error relates to the apparent decrease in flow velocity that occurs as the angle between the sound beam and the flow vector increases. In the child and adult, one can generally keep this angle small and hence avoid the need for angle correction. In the fetus, the relation of the sound beam to the flow vector often cannot be controlled, and angle correction is frequently necessary. In the small vessels examined, the actual direction of flow at the point of sampling may be difficult to determine accurately, and correction therefore is likely to be imprecise. Similarly, in the active fetus, it may not be possible to ensure a constant angle of intersection. In addition, because the vessel diameters are so small, any error in measurement of the vessel lumen causes substantial error in the flow calculation. These concepts are discussed in greater detail in Chapter 30, but it is conceptually unlikely that flow measurements in the fetus can attain the degree of accuracy possible in the newborn or infant. A further problem is that, although values for stroke volume and other parameters have been recorded and published, at present no way exists to confirm their accuracy.

CARDIAC MORPHOLOGIC AND FUNCTIONAL ABNORMALITIES DETECTABLE IN THE FETUS

Morphologic Abnormalities

Nearly every possible example of congenital heart disease has been recognized in prenatal life, with the exception of abnormalities of pulmonary venous drainage. These include ventricular septal defect (Fig. 33–16),[19,37] atrial septal defect,[28] AV canal (Fig. 33–17),[37–39] single ventricle, Ebstein's anomaly (Fig. 33–18),[40] tetralogy of Fallot, double-outlet right ventricle,[39] transposition of the great arteries[40] (Fig. 33–19), corrected transposition, hypoplastic left heart syndrome,[28,41] coarctation of the aorta,[39,42] critical aortic stenosis associated with endocardial fibroelastosis[39,43] (Fig. 33–20), pulmonary atresia and right ventricular hypoplasia (Fig. 33–21),[31,40] tricuspid atresia, pulmonary artery aneurysm,[25] rhabdomyoma (Figs. 33–22 and 33–23), ectopia cordis, myocardial infarction,[2,37] hypertrophic cardiomyopathy, and dilated cardiomyopathy.[1,28,37] Reported sensitivities approach 90%, with false-negative diagnoses occurring in patients with small ventricular septal defects and coarctation of the aorta.

The diagnosis of isolated ventricular septal defect is difficult in the fetus because of the relatively small size of these defects compared to the lateral resolution of the imaging system. For example, between 24 and 26 weeks' gestation, the aortic root is generally between 0.5 and 0.7 cm in diameter, and although a defect greater than half the size of the aortic root and therefore of potential

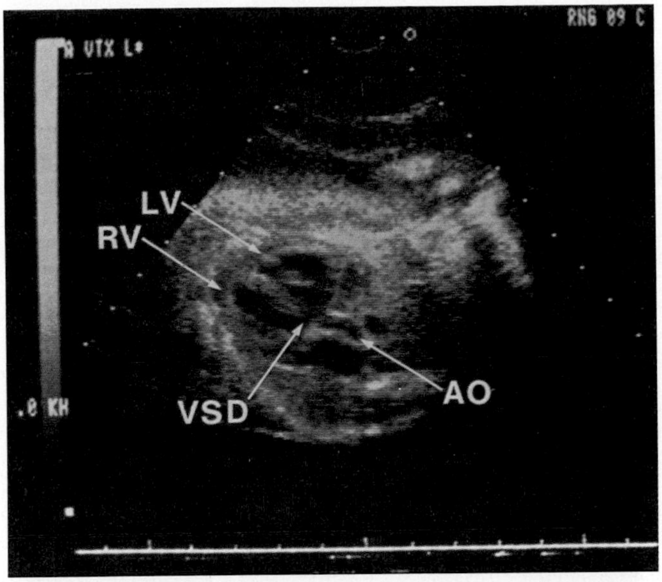

Fig. 33–16. Four-chamber view of a fetus with an interrupted aortic arch. There is slight disproportion between the two ventricles, a ventricular septal defect (VSD) with slight overriding of a small aorta (AO), and subaortic stenosis. RV = right ventricle; LV = left ventricle. (From Reed KL, Anderson CF, Shanker L: Fetal Echocardiography: An Atlas. New York, Alan R. Liss, p. 79, 1988.)

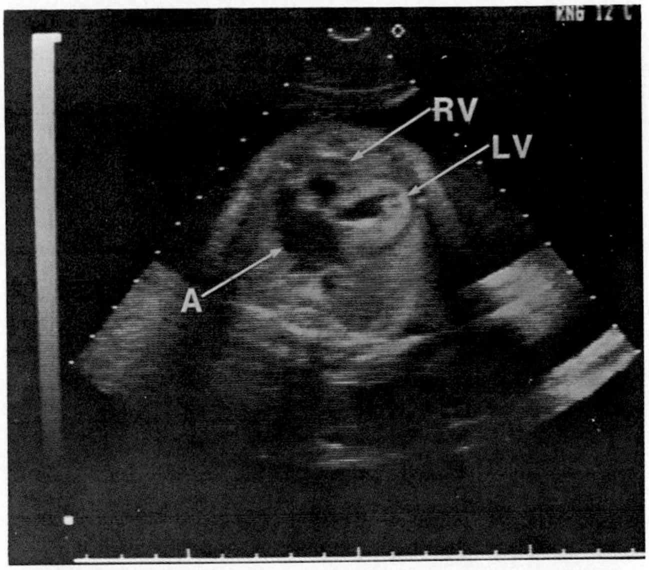

Fig. 33–17. Atrioventricular canal defect in utero. There is a single atrium (A) and a canal-type ventricular septal defect. RV = right ventricle; LV = left ventricle. (From Reed KL, Anderson CF, Shanker L: Fetal Echocardiography: An Atlas. New York, Alan R. Liss, p. 69, 1988.)

functional significance should be visible, precise plane positioning would be required. In the smaller fetal heart, defects of half the aortic diameter may be easily overlooked.[40] Doppler unfortunately is of no help in the diagnosis of ventricular septal defect because the pressures in the two ventricles are similar, and any blood that does cross the defect is unlikely to create enough of a flow disturbance to be detected. False-positive diagnoses of this defect may also occur because of echo dropout in one view. Thus, as in the postnatal examination, all apparent defects must be confirmed in a second view. When ventricular septal defects occur in combination with other anomalies, particularly when malalignment exists between the septum and the aorta (see Fig. 33–16), their detection becomes much easier.

Direct examination of the aortic arch often cannot exclude coarctation. When the diagnosis of coarctation of the aorta has been made in intrauterine life, the clues

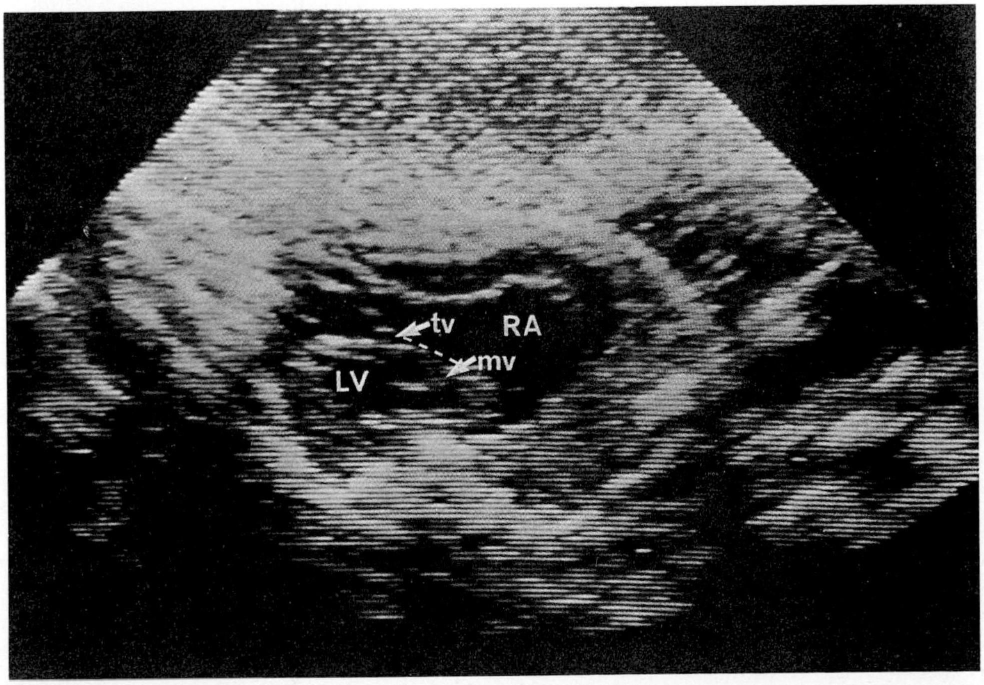

Fig. 33–18. Oblique four-chamber view (apex to left) illustrating Ebstein's anomaly in the fetus. RA = right atrium; tv = tricuspid valve; LV = left ventricle; mv = mitral valve. (From Allan LD, A review of fetal echocardiography. Echocardiography 2: 351, 1985.)

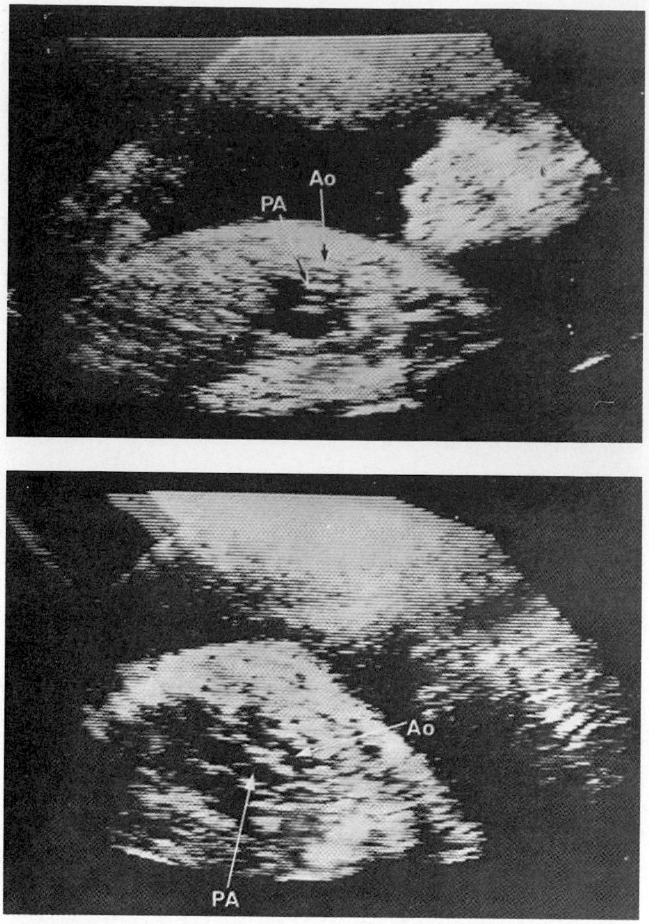

Fig. 33–19. Top. Short axis recording of transposed great vessels in the fetus. The aorta (Ao) is anterior to the pulmonary artery (PA), and both great vessels appear circular in this tomographic slice. Bottom. Long axis recording of the parallel great vessels. The upper vessel in this plane is again the Ao, and the lower vessel is the PA. (From Allan LD: A review of fetal echocardiography. Echocardiography 2:351, 1985.)

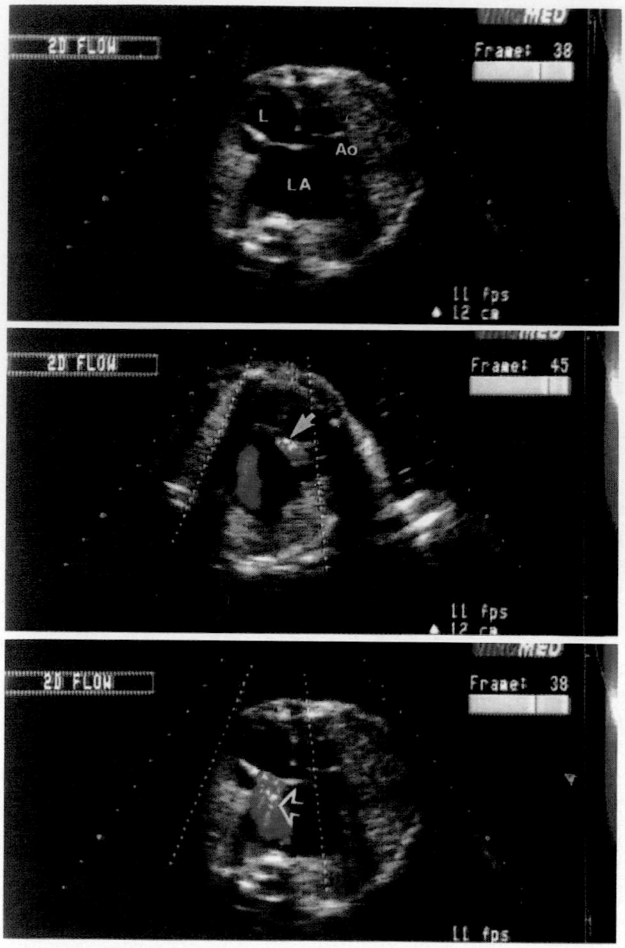

Fig. 33–20. Top. Parasternal equivalent long axis recording of the left heart. Middle. The critical aortic stenosis (arrow). Bottom. Mitral regurgitation (arrow). L = left ventricle; LA = left atrium; Ao = aorta. (From Huhta JC, Helton JG, Wood DC: Color Doppler in the fetal examination. Echocardiography 6:393, 1989.)

have been from cardiac findings, namely, right ventricular and pulmonary artery dilation. The reasons for these findings are unclear, but they probably represent altered hemodynamics resulting in increased right ventricular output.[8] Decreased flow in the aorta is frequently recorded by spectral Doppler imaging, but this is also nonspecific. Relative underdevelopment of the left heart may also be seen with diaphragmatic hernia, and this condition should be excluded before coarctation is inferred.

To date, although available data are limited, the greater problem of false-positive diagnoses has not been encountered for most major structural defects.

Fetal echocardiography can also be used to detect pericardial effusion in utero (Fig. 33–24).[28] Because of its limited potential space, the pericardial sac appears to become distended with fluid before ascites, pleural effusions, or soft tissue edema is detectable on ultrasound. Thus, pericardial effusion appears to be an early sign of hydrops.[44] Pericardial effusion can be observed in association with complete heart block at roughly 20 to 24 weeks' gestation. These effusions tend to resolve spontaneously when there is no associated structural heart defect.[45]

Premature Closure of the Ductus Arteriosus and Foramen Ovale

Premature closure of the ductus arteriosus in the fetus has been related to the treatment of the mother for premature labor using prostaglandin synthetase inhibitors, most notably indomethacin. Premature ductal closure is thought to increase pulmonary arterial pressure and flow,[47–48] which in turn lead to right ventricular dysfunction and tricuspid regurgitation. Increasingly severe constriction of the fetal lamb ductus arteriosus has been shown to result in increasing diastolic pulmonary to aortic pressure gradients, and as a result, the severity of obstruction can be related to the elevation in diastolic transductal velocity.[48] Doppler recorded velocities in the normal ductus arteriosus increase with gestational age, and the maximal systolic and diastolic velocities are 140 and 35 cm/sec, respectively.[49] Figure 33–25 shows continuous wave Doppler tracings from a fetus with

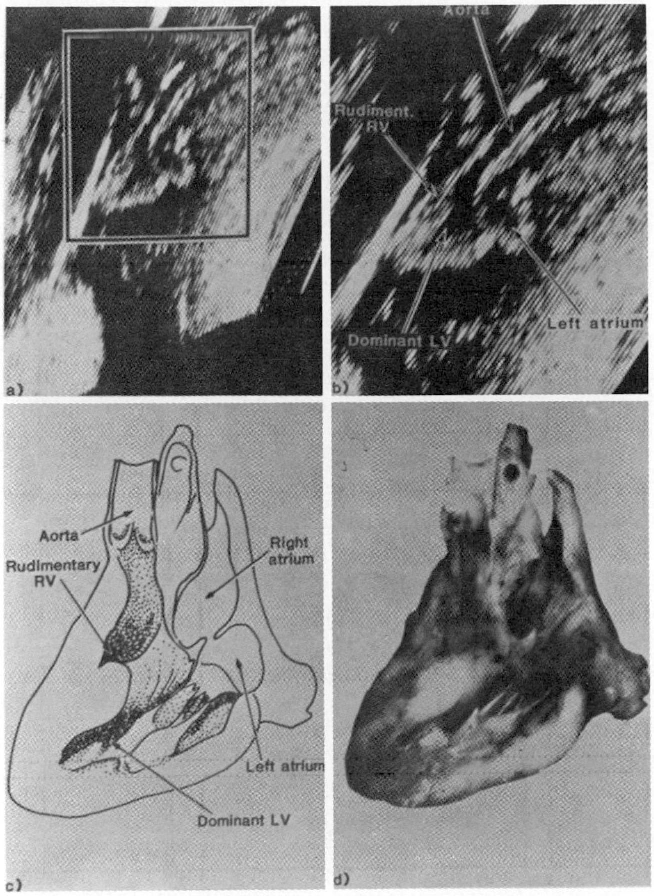

Fig. 33–21. Aorta overriding a rudimentary right ventricle (RV) in this example of absent right atrioventricular connection. LV = left ventricle. (From Allan LD, Crawford DC, Anderson RH, Tynan MJ: Echocardiographic and anatomical correlations in fetal congenital heart disease. Br. Heart J 52:542, 1984.)

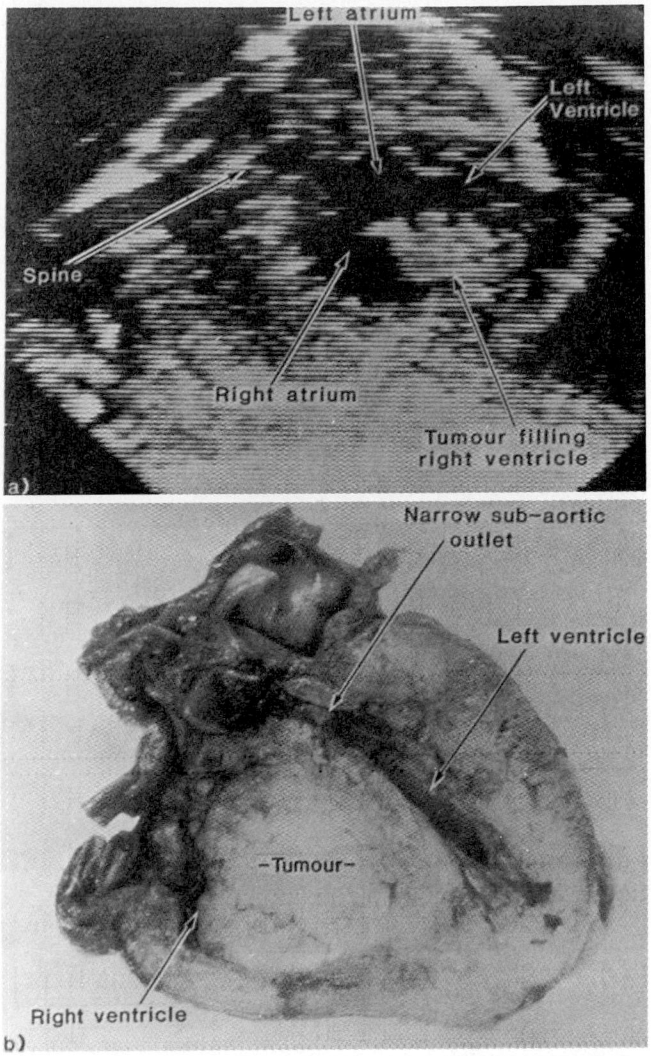

Fig. 33–22. Rhabdomyoma filling the right ventricular cavity. (From Allan LD, Crawford DC, Anderson RH, Tynan MJ: Echocardiographic and anatomical correlations in fetal congenital heart disease. Br. Heart J 52:542, 1984.)

marked elevation in both systolic and diastolic ductal velocities during indomethacin administration to the mother. Tricuspid regurgitation also developed de novo in association with the ductal constriction. When administration of the drug was discontinued, ductal velocities returned to normal, and the tricuspid regurgitation disappeared. As a rule, indomethacin-induced constriction of the ductus is reversible on withdrawal of the drug.

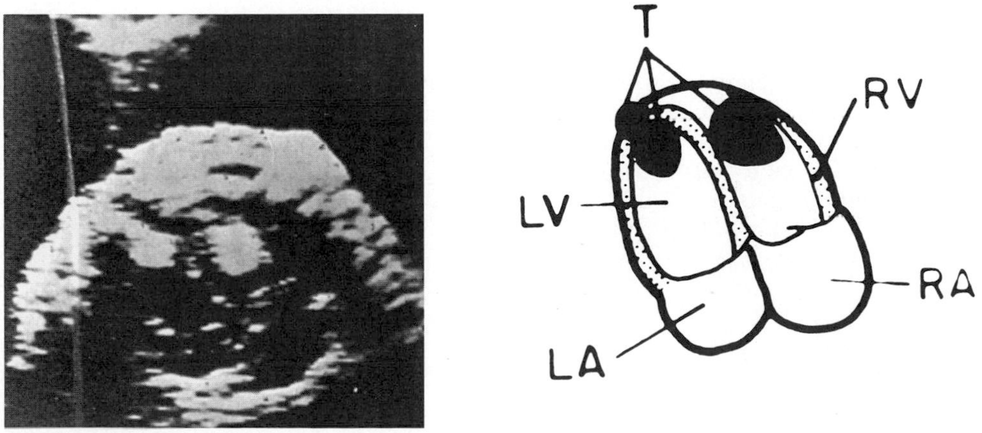

Fig. 33–23. Rhabdomyoma. T = tumor; RV = right ventricle; RA = right atrium; LA = left atrium; LV = left ventricle. (From Birnbaum S, McGahan JP, Janos GG, Meyers M: Fetal tachycardia and intramyocardial tumors. J Am Coll Cardiol 6: 1358, 1985.)

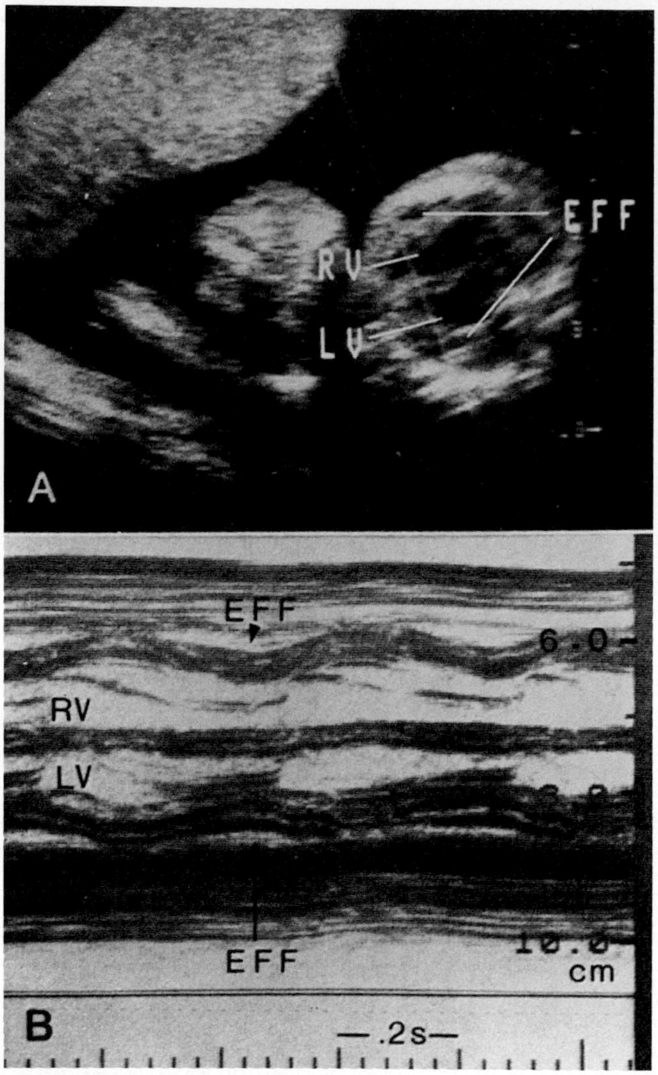

Fig. 33–24. **A.** M-mode cursor line placed through the ventricles demonstrating that the cardiomegaly is almost equal to the entire thoracic diameter. **B.** Resultant M-mode demonstrates the dimensions of the ventricles and the presence of a pericardial effusion (EFF). RV = right ventricle; LV = left ventricle. (From Silverman NH, Schmidt KG: Ventricular volume overload in the human fetus: observations from fetal echocardiography. J Am Soc Echocardiogr 3:20, 1990.)

Premature restriction of the foramen ovale is an unusual cardiac abnormality with potentially serious consequences for the developing fetus. In restrictive foramen ovale, the normal biphasic movement of the septum primum is reduced or absent on M-mode study.[50,51] In some cases, there is an aneurysm of the fossa ovalis with a partially or completely obstructed foramen. In isolated restrictive foramen ovale, this aneurysm consistently bulges into the left atrium.[51,52] When left atrial pressure is elevated as in mitral inflow obstruction, however, the aneurysm may bulge toward the right atrium.[53] Doppler studies in premature restriction are limited, but suggest an increase in flow velocity in fetuses with partial restriction and absent flow when restriction is complete.[52] More clearly established is the use of normal Doppler velocities and color flow recordings without aliasing or variance to exclude restriction even when an atrial septal aneurysm is present.[51]

Various associated abnormalities have been described in the fetus with premature restriction of the foramen. These abnormalities include right atrial enlargement, right ventricular dilation and hypertrophy, dilation of the tricuspid valve annulus, and an enlarged pulmonary artery and ductus arteriosus. Abnormalities of the left heart have also been reported, ranging from moderate reduction in left heart chamber size to hypoplastic left heart syndrome with mitral and aortic atresia. Other frequently encountered abnormalities include nonimmune hydrops fetalis and supraventricular tachycardia.[41,50,52,54]

Cardiac Abnormalities in the Nonimmune Hydropic Fetus

Nonimmune hydrops fetalis is presumably caused by the combination of systemic venous hypertension and the low colloid osmotic pressure typical of the fetus. Echocardiographic studies to date suggest that a cardiac cause can be identified in roughly 40% of these cases.[55] Structural heart disease is the cause in roughly two thirds of cases, and tachyarrhythmia is the cause in the remaining third.

The combination of fetal hydrops, AV valve regurgitation, and a structural cardiac defect (see Figs. 33–12 and 33–20) is a particularly ominous finding, with a reported fetal mortality higher than 90%.[56] Although the mortality of nonimmune hydrops fetalis alone was known to be high before the availability of Doppler studies, its association with AV valvular insufficiency was not recognized. AV valvular regurgitation is an important complication of structural heart disease because the fetal heart has only a limited ability to increase its output in response to an increase in ventricular filling pressure. In addition, the foramen ovale provides a large communication at the atrial level, and volume loading from the regurgitation causes or increases systemic venous hypertension regardless of whether it is mitral, tricuspid, or due to a common AV valve. The systemic venous hypertension and the low colloid osmotic pressure during fetal life lead to edema and hydrops. AV valve insufficiency thus may distinguish the hydropic fetus from the nonhydropic fetus with the same primary cardiac lesion.

Although hydrops and AV regurgitation are most often due to ventricular failure, a relatively small subgroup of patients develop hydrops fetalis primarily from AV valve insufficiency, rather than from systolic pump failure (i.e., absent pulmonary valve syndrome, Ebstein's anomaly, and atrial isomerism with AV canal defects). When hydrops occurs in these cases, transplacental therapeutic intervention or early delivery may be considered.

In contrast, the response of the fetal circulation to obstructive lesions such as hypoplastic left heart syndrome with aortic atresia or pulmonary atresia is to redistribute flow, thereby bypassing the obstruction.

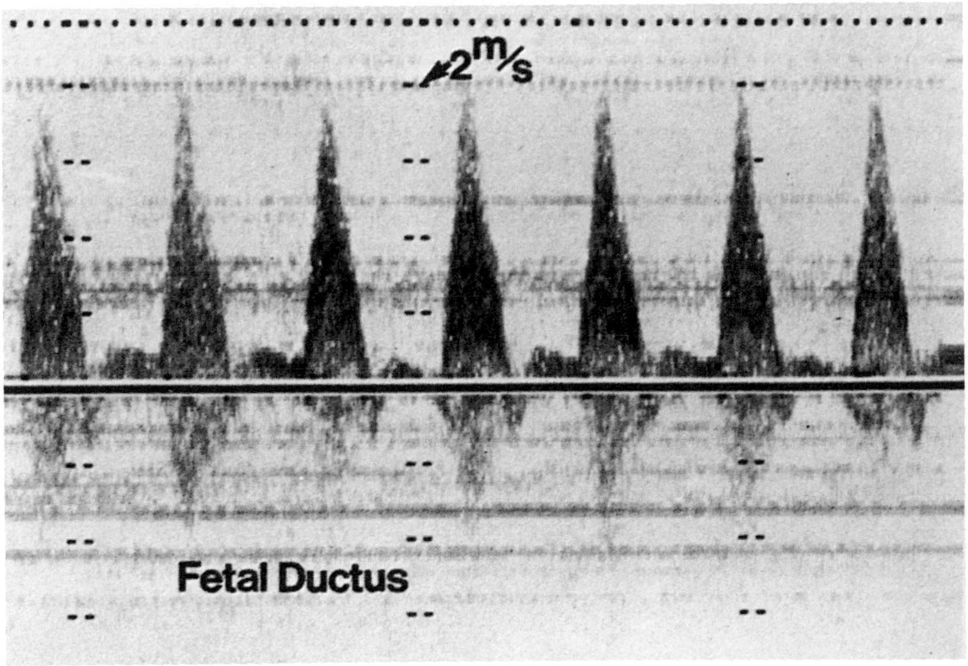

Fig. 33–25. Echocardiographic imaging-directed continuous wave Doppler showing the increased systolic velocities consistent with increased flow in the ductus and not typical of constriction of the ductus. *m/s.*, Meters per second. (From Huhta JC, Cohen AW, Wood DC: Premature constriction of the ductus arteriosus. J Am Soc Echocardiogr 3:31, 1990.)

Thus, cardiac failure and hydrops in this group are uncommon findings at birth.

FETAL ARRHYTHMIAS

Detection of fetal arrhythmias by electrocardiogram is difficult because of the interference of the maternal electrical field. Although the fetal QRS complex can often be recorded, fetal P waves are virtually impossible to detect. Several studies have suggested that M-mode echocardiographic recording of atrial and ventricular contraction can be used to diagnose and monitor fetal arrhythmias.[57–61] This end is most readily achieved by positioning the M-mode cursor through the aortic root in short axis with the left atrium behind. The relationship between atrial contraction from atrial wall motion and ventricular contraction, as inferred from the aortic valve opening, can then be observed. If atrial contraction is difficult to record directly, it can often be determined from the timing of the A wave of the AV valves. In the normal heart, atrial contraction precedes ventricular contraction by a fixed time interval of less than 80 msec, and changes in the temporal relationship and sequence of contraction can be used to diagnose arrhythmias.

Fetal arrhythmias fall into three groups: (1) irregular rhythms; (2) bradycardias; and (3) tachycardias. Irregular rhythms are most often caused by premature atrial or ventricular contractions. When associated with a structurally normal heart, such ectopic beats usually have no significance and disappear near term. Short episodes of sinus bradycardia are also common, particularly in early pregnancy; however, a sustained rhythm of less than 100 beats per minute merits specialized investigation because this is often associated with partial or complete heart block (Fig. 33–26). In a study of 13 patients referred for evaluation of bradycardia, all had complete heart block, which was isolated in 7 and associated with structural heart disease in 6. In the patients with isolated complete heart block, all mothers had serologic evidence of connective tissue disease, a known association.[57,62,63] Each of the 6 patients with structural heart disease had complete AV septal defects and left atrial isomerism. Two had additional anomalies of the

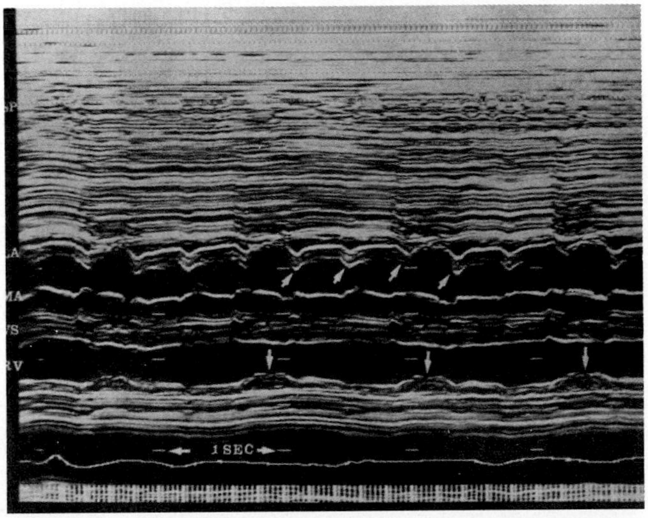

Fig. 33–26. M-mode echocardiogram recorded with the beam directed through the left atrium (LA), mitral annulus (MA), ventricular septum (VS), and right ventricle (RV) in a fetus with heart block with an atrial rate of 120 beats per minute and a ventricular rate of 50/min. The oblique arrows show the contractions of the atrial wall, and the vertical arrows denote systolic inward motion of the right ventricular wall. (From Maulik D, et al.: Application of Doppler echocardiography in the assessment of fetal cardiac disease. Am J Obstet Gynecol 151:951, 1985.)

great arteries. The combination of heart block with the congenital cardiac defect has been recognized as lethal, particularly with AV canal.[8]

Tachyarrhythmia in the fetus is defined as a heart rate above 200 beats per minute. Atrial fibrillation, atrial flutter (Fig. 33–27), supraventricular tachycardia (Fig. 33–28), and ventricular tachycardia have all been described in utero.[64,65]

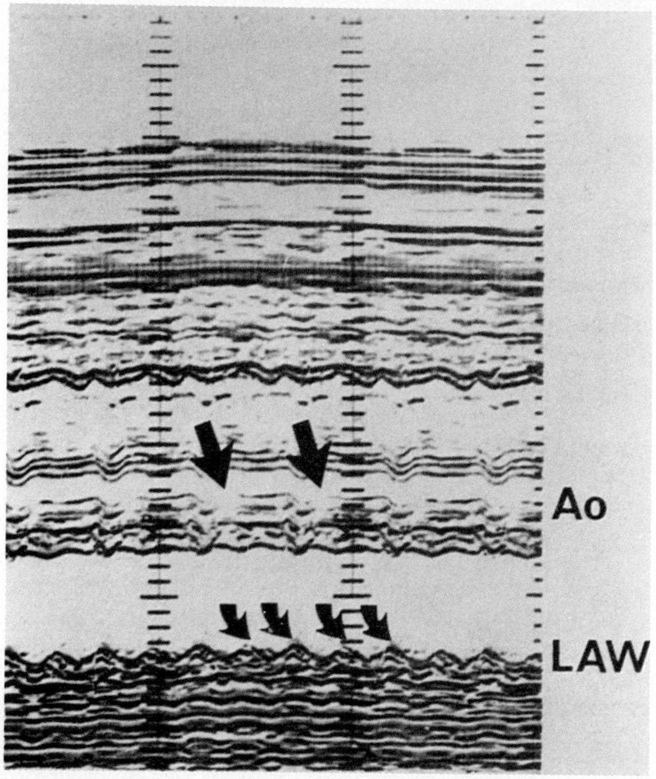

Fig. 33–27. A fetus with atrial flutter with 2:1 block. In this case, the atrial rate is excessive, but ventricular contraction is within normal limits. Ao = aorta, LAW = left atrial wall. (From Allan LD: A review of echocardiography. Echocardiography 2:351, 1985.)

RISKS ASSOCIATED WITH FETAL ECHOCARDIOGRAPHY

The most obvious concern in the use of prenatal echocardiography is that some untoward biologic effect of ultrasound will harm the developing fetus. Despite extensive use of ultrasound in obstetrics, no harmful effects in humans have been confirmed to date. Although a few investigators have reported harmful biologic effects in animal studies, the use of ultrasound in those studies has little or no resemblance to clinical practice. A single report claimed that in vitro exposure of human leukocytes to ultrasound, at power levels used clinically, resulted in an increased rate of chromosome breakage and sister chromatid exchange. This probably resulted from a peculiarity of the experimental setup that significantly magnified the power density of the ultrasound beam. Several other groups have been unable to duplicate these results. Thus, available data suggest that ultrasound in the currently used power range is without harmful biologic effects to the fetus.[9]

In addition to physical effects there are clear psychologic effects on the mother caused by the prenatal diagnosis of severe congenital heart disease, particularly when this becomes apparent at a point where it is no longer possible to terminate the pregnancy. This problem should be more than counterbalanced, however, by the far more frequent definition of normality in patients at risk and the possibility of medical and other planning for the delivery and care of the infant with known disease.

RELATIONSHIP BETWEEN IN UTERO DETECTION OF CARDIAC DEFECTS AND PROGNOSIS

The prognosis for long-term survival for patients with serious cardiac defects detected in utero is poor. In pregnancies that progress to term, studies to date suggest an intrauterine or neonatal death rate exceeding 85%.[8,40] Extracardiac anomalies and intrauterine heart failure are especially poor prognostic signs.

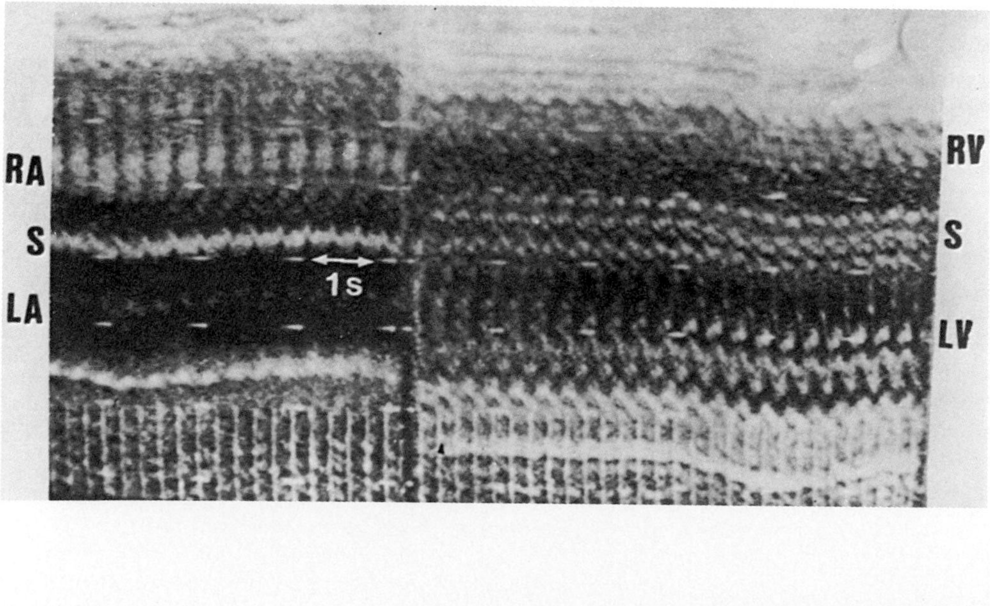

Fig. 33–28. A fetus with paroxysmal and supraventricular tachycardia with 1:1 conduction. In this case both atrial and ventricular rates are excessive. RA = right atrium; S = septum; LA = left atrium; RV = right ventricle; LV = left ventricle. (From Buis-Liem TN, Ottenkamp J, Meerman RH, Verwey R: The concurrence of fetal supraventricular tachycardia and obstruction of the foramen ovale. Prenat Diagn 7:425, 1987. Copyright © 1987 by John Wiley & Sons, Ltd. Reprinted by permission of John Wiley & Sons, Ltd.)

REFERENCES

1. Sahn DJ, et al.: Quantitative real-time cross-sectional echocardiography in the developing normal human fetus and newborn. Circulation 62:588, 1980.
2. Allan LD, et al.: Echocardiographic and anatomical correlates in the fetus and newborn. Br Heart J 44:444, 1980.
3. Wladimiroff JW, McGhie J: Ultrasonic assessment of cardiovascular geometry and function in the human fetus. Br J Obstet Gynaecol 88:870, 1981.
4. De Vore GR, et al.: Fetal echocardiography. I. Normal anatomy as determined by real time directed M-mode ultrasound. Am J Obstet Gynecol 144: 249, 1982.
5. Reed KL, et al.: Cardiac Doppler flow studies in human fetuses. Circulation 73:41, 1986.
6. Reed KL, et al.: Doppler Echocardiographic studies of diastolic function in the human fetal heart: changes during gestation. J Am Coll Cardiol 8:391, 1986.
7. St. John Sutton MG, et al.: Quantitative assessment of growth and function of the cardiac chambers in the normal fetus: a prospective longitudinal study. Circulation 69:645, 1984.
8. Huhta JC: Fetal echocardiography: fulfilling the potential. Echocardiography 2:341, 1985.
9. Sanders S: Fetal echocardiography. Echocardiography 2:343, 1985.
10. Azancot A, et al.: Analysis of ventricular shape by echocardiography in normal fetuses, newborns and infants. Circulation 68:1201, 1983.
11. Versprille A, et al.: Functional interaction of both ventricles at birth and the changes during the neonatal period in relation to the changes in geometry. *In* Longo LD, Reneau DD (eds.): Fetal and Newborn Cardiovascular Physiology. Vol 1. New York, Garland STPM Press, p. 399, 1978.
12. Rudolph AM, Heymann MA: Fetal and neonatal circulation and respiration. Annu Rev Physiol 38:187, 1974.
13. Rudolph AM, et al.: Studies on the circulation of the previable human fetus. Pediatr Res 5:452, 1971.
14. Rudolph AM: Congenital Diseases of the Heart. Chicago, Year Book Medical Publishers, 1983.
15. Emmanuel R, et al.: Evidence of congenital heart disease in the offspring of parents with atrioventricular defects. Br Heart J 49:144, 1983.
16. Whittemore R, Hobbins JC, Engle MA: Pregnancy and its outcome in women with and without surgical treatment of congenital heart disease. Am J Cardiol 50:641, 1982.
17. Copel JA, Pilu G, Kleinman CS: Congenital heart disease and extracardiac anomalies: associations and indications for fetal echocardiography. Am J Obstet Gynecol 154:1121, 1986.
18. Friedewald V: Fetal echocardiography: an interview with James C. Huhta, M.D. Echocardiography 2:347, 1985.
19. Silverman NH, Golbus MS: Echocardiographic techniques for assessing normal and abnormal fetal cardiac anatomy. J Am Coll Cardiol 5:20s, 1985.
20. Copel JA, et al.: Fetal echocardiographic screening for congenital heart disease: the importance of the four-chamber view. Am J Obstet Gynecol 157:648, 1987.
21. Lange LW, et al.: Qualitative real-time cross-sectional echocardiographic imaging of the human fetus during the second half of pregnancy. Circulation 62:799, 1980.
22. Winsberg F: Echocardiography of the fetal and newborn heart. Invest Radiol 7:152, 1972.
23. Allan LD, et al.: Doppler echocardiographic evaluation of the normal human fetal heart. Br Heart J 57:528, 1987.
24. Maulik D, Nanda NC, Saini VD: Fetal Doppler echocardiography: methods and characterization of normal and abnormal hemodynamics. Am J Cardiol 53:572, 1984.
25. Maulik D, et al.: Application of Doppler echocardiography in the assessment of fetal cardiac disease. Am J Obstet Gynecol 151:951, 1985.
26. Shine J, Gresser CD, Rakowski H: Quantitative two-dimensional echocardiographic assessment of fetal cardiac growth. Am J Obstet Gynecol 154: 294, 1986.
27. DeVore GR, Siassi B, Platt LD: Fetal echocardiography. IV. M-mode assessment of ventricular size and contractility during the second and third trimesters of pregnancy in the normal fetus. Am J Obstet Gynecol 150:981, 1984.
28. Shine J, Bertrand M, Hagen-Ansert S, Rakowski H: Two-dimensional and M-mode echocardiography in the human fetus. Am J Obstet Gynecol 148: 679, 1984.
29. DeVore GR, Siassi B, Platt LD: Fetal echocardiography. V. M-mode measurements of the aortic root and aortic valve in second and third trimester normal human fetuses. Am J Obstet Gynecol 152:543, 1985.
30. Langman J: Medical Embryology. 3rd Ed. Baltimore, Williams & Wilkins, p. 82, 1975.
31. Kleinman CS, et al.: Echocardiographic studies of the human fetus: prenatal diagnosis of congenital heart disease and cardiac dysrhythmias. Pediatrics 65:1059, 1980.
32. Azancot A, et al.: Analysis of ventricular shape by echocardiography in normal fetuses, newborns, and infants. Circulation 68:1201, 1983.
33. DeVore GR, Donnerstein RL, Kleinman CS, Hobbins JC: Real time directed M-mode echocardiography: a new technique for accurate and rapid quantitation of the fetal pre-ejection period and ventricular ejection time of the right and left ventricles. Am J Obstet Gynecol 141:470, 1981.
34. Kleinman CS, Donnerstein RL: Ultrasonic assessment of cardiac function in the intact human fetus. J Am Coll Cardiol 5:84s, 1985.
35. Eik-Nes SH, Brubakk AO, Ulstein MK: Measurement of human fetal blood flow. Br Med J 280:283, 1980.
36. Kenny JF, et al.: Changes in intracardiac blood flow velocities and right and left ventricular stroke volumes with gestational age in the normal human fetus: a prospective Doppler echocardiographic study. Circulation 74:1208, 1986.
37. Kleinman CS, et al.: Fetal echocardiography for evaluation of in utero congestive heart failure. N Engl J Med 306:568, 1982.
38. Reed KL, Anderson CF, Shenker L: Fetal Echocardiography: An Atlas. New York, Alan R. Liss, 1988.
39. Allan LD, Tynan M, Campbell S, Anderson RH: Identification of congenital cardiac malformations by echocardiography in midtrimester fetus. Br Heart J 46:358, 1981.
40. Allan LD: A review of fetal echocardiography. Echocardiography 2:351, 1985.
41. Sahn DJ, et al.: Prenatal ultrasound diagnosis of hypoplastic left heart syndrome in utero associated with fetal hydrops. Am Heart J 104:1368, 1982.
42. Allan LD, et al.: Coarctation of the aorta in prenatal life: an echocardiographic, anatomical, and functional study. Br Heart J 59:356, 1988.
43. Huhta JC, Helton JG, Wood DC: Color Doppler in the fetal examination. Echocardiography 6:393, 1989.
44. DeVore GR, et al.: Fetal echocardiography II. The diagnosis and significance of a pericardial effusion in the fetus using real-time-directed M-mode ultrasound. Am J Obstet Gynecol 144:693, 1982.
45. Martin GR, Ruckman RN: Fetal echocardiography: a large clinical experience and follow-up. J Am Soc Echocardiogr 3:4, 1990.
46. Levin DL, et al.: Constriction of the fetal ductus arteriosus after administration of indomethacin to the pregnant ewe. J Pediatr 94:647, 1979.
47. Friedman WR, Printz MP, Kirkpatrick SE, Hoskins EJ: The vasoactivity of the fetal lamb ductus arteriosus studied in utero. Pediatr Res 17:332, 1983.
48. Huhta JC, Cohen AW, Wood DC: Premature constriction of the ductus arteriosus. J Am Soc Echocardiogr 3:30, 1990.
49. Huhta JC, et al.: Detection and quantitation of constriction of the fetal ductus arteriosus by Doppler echocardiography. Circulation 75:406, 1987.
50. Redel DA, Hansmann M: Fetal obstruction of the foramen ovale detected by two-dimensional Doppler echocardiography. *In* Rijsterborgh H (ed.): Echocardiography. The Hague, Martinus Nijhoff, p. 425, 1981.
51. Stewart PA, Wladimiroff JW: Fetal atrial arrhythmias associated with redundancy/aneurysm of the foramen ovale. J Clin Ultrasound 16:643, 1988.
52. Chobot V, Hornberger LK, Hagen-Ansert S, Sahn DJ: Prenatal detection of restrictive foramen ovale. J Am Soc Echocardiogr 3:15, 1990.
53. Personen E, Haavisto H, Ammala P, Teramo K: Intrauterine hydrops caused by premature closure of the foramen ovale. Arch Dis Child 58:1015, 1983.
54. Stewart PA, Tonge HM, Wladimiroff JW: Arrhythmias and structural abnormalities of the fetal heart. Br Heart J 50:550, 1983.
55. Allan LD, Crawford DC, Sheridan R, Chapman MG: Aetiology of non-immune hydrops: the value of echocardiography. Br J Obstet Gynaecol 88: 223, 1986.
56. Silverman NH, et al.: Fetal atrioventricular valve insufficiency associated with non-immune hydrops: a two-dimensional echocardiographic and pulsed Doppler ultrasound study. Circulation 72:825, 1985.
57. Madison JP, Sukhum P, Williamson DP, Campion BC: Echocardiography and fetal heart sounds in the diagnosis of fetal heart block. Am Heart J 98: 505, 1979.
58. Kleinman CS, et al.: Fetal echocardiography. A tool for evaluation of in utero cardiac arrhythmias and monitoring of in utero therapy: analysis of 71 patients. Am J Cardiol 51:237, 1983.
59. Allan LD, et al.: Evaluation of fetal arrhythmias by echocardiography. Br Heart J 50:240, 1983.
60. Silverman NH, et al.: Recognition of fetal arrhythmias by echocardiography. J Clin Ultrasound 13:255, 1985.
61. Kleinman CS, et al.: In utero diagnosis and treatment of fetal supraventricular tachycardia. Semin Perinatol 9:113, 1985.
62. McCue CM, et al.: Congenital heart block in newborns of mothers with connective tissue disease. Circulation 56:82, 1977.
63. Scott JS, et al.: Connective tissue disease, antibodies to ribonucleoprotein and congenital heart block. N Engl J Med 309:209, 1983.
64. Belhassen B, et al.: Intrauterine and postnatal atrial fibrillation in the Wolf-Parkinson-White syndrome. Circulation 66:1124, 1982.
65. Shenker L: Fetal cardiac arrhythmias. Obstet Gynecol Surv 34:561, 1979.

CHAPTER

34

CORONARY ARTERIES

VIVIAN M. ABASCAL, JANE E. MARSHALL, and ARTHUR E. WEYMAN

Cross-sectional echocardiographic visualization of the left main coronary artery was first described in 1976.[1] The same report also noted that areas of left main coronary narrowing and aneurysmal dilation similar to those seen at angiography could be recorded in selected patients. Because atherosclerotic coronary artery disease is the leading cause of death in the Western world, and lesions affecting the proximal coronary arteries have the greatest pathologic importance, this observation raised hopes that echocardiography might permit noninvasive diagnosis or at least exclusion of proximal coronary stenoses. As a result, major early effort was directed toward developing improved methods of transthoracic coronary imaging and diagnosis in the hope of providing a noninvasive alternative to angiography.[2–14] Unfortunately, the small size and technical difficulties encountered in imaging the coronary arteries transthoracically have made this an elusive goal, although the diagnosis of other abnormalities such as coronary aneurysms, arteriovenous fistulas, and anomalous coronary origins have evolved as important clinical applications of the technique. In addition, the development of high frequency epicardial imaging transducers has permitted detailed description of coronary anatomy experimentally and during surgery, whereas intravascular imaging catheters offer the potential for direct visualization of native coronary lesions and of the morphologic effect of various forms of ablative therapy. Various methods for recording coronary flow velocity have also been developed. Epicardial and intravascular Doppler studies have provided significant insights into the physiology of the coronary circulation, have helped to define the functional significance of coronary stenoses, and have provided a unique tool for monitoring responses to therapeutic interventions. Thus, although the initial goal of generalizable transthoracic diagnosis of coronary stenoses has not, as yet, been achieved, other techniques and application have made ultrasonic coronary diagnosis an exciting area in terms of both clinical application and research potential.

CORONARY ANATOMY

Anatomically, the left and right coronary arteries arise from their corresponding sinuses of Valsalva just superior to the insertions of the aortic leaflets. Figure 34–1 diagrammatically illustrates the relationship of these arteries with the aortic root and surrounding structures. This diagram corresponds to an imaging plane passing through the aortic root roughly parallel to its short axis just above the aortic annulus. In this projection, the left coronary artery originates from the posterolateral wall of the aorta near the base of the left coronary cusp of the aortic valve. The left main segment of the left coronary artery is a relatively short vessel that extends leftward from the ostium approximately 1 cm before dividing. Angiographically, the length of the left main segment has been reported to range from 4 to 15 mm (mean of 10.5 mm),[15] whereas pathologically, the length of the left main coronary artery segment has varied from 0 to 40 mm (mean of 9.5 mm).[15,16] Significantly, from the standpoint of echocardiographic visualization, the left main coronary artery segment is less than 2 cm long in more than 95% of patients. The diameter of the left main segment ranges from 3 to 10 mm.[17,18] In most cases (66%), the left main coronary artery segment bifurcates into a left anterior descending branch, which courses leftward and anteriorly, and a left circumflex branch, which runs posteriorly following the path of the mitral annulus (Fig. 34–1). Frequently (31%), a third vessel,

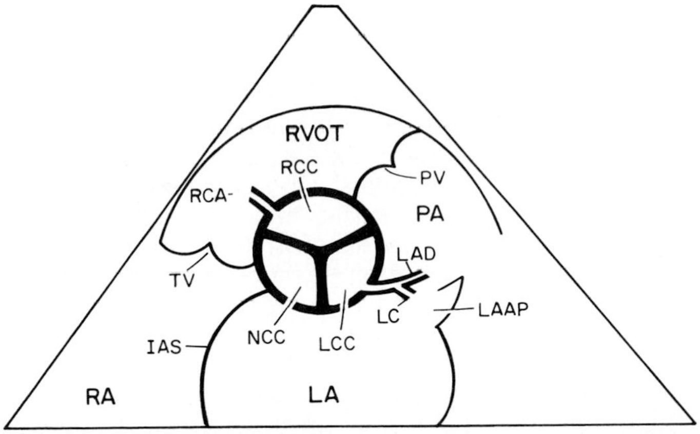

Fig. 34–1. Short axis view of the aortic root illustrates the relative positions of origin of the left and right coronary arteries. The left main coronary artery (LCC) arises from the aortic root at approximately the 4-o'clock position and courses laterally and slightly anteriorly. After traveling approximately 1 cm, it bifurcates into a left anterior descending (LAD) and a left circumflex (LC) branch. The right coronary artery (RCA) arises from approximately the 11-o'clock position and courses to the right and anteriorly. The three aortic cusps, the right coronary (RCC), the left coronary (LCC), and the noncoronary (NCC), insert slightly inferior to the origins of the coronary arteries; however, they are included for orientation. Likewise, the pulmonary valve (PV) is directly superior to the origin of the coronaries and is included to indicate its relative position. RA = right atrium; LA = left atrium; LAAP = left atrial appendage; IAS = interatrial septum; RVOT = right ventricular outflow tract; PA = pulmonary artery; TV = tricuspid valve.

the intermediate branch, also arises at this dividing point, and on occasion (2.4%), a fourth branch is present.[19]

The left main coronary artery normally lies in a relatively fixed anatomic position in relation to the left ventricle and great vessels. It is bordered anteriorly by the right ventricular outflow tract as it crosses the root of the aorta, superiorly by the pulmonary artery (the pulmonic valve lies anterior, superior, and to the left of the left main coronary artery), inferiorly by the superior margin of the left ventricle, and posteriorly by a portion of the left atrium. The left main coronary artery immediately abuts the posterior wall of the pulmonary artery, and hence anomalous insertion of this vessel into the pulmonary artery involves a shift in its ostial position of only a few millimeters.

The right coronary artery originates from the anteromedial border of the aortic root at a level parallel to or slightly superior to the origin of the left coronary artery (Fig. 34–1). It initially courses slightly anteriorly and rightward along the superior margin of the right ventricular outflow tract and then almost directly rightward parallel to the anterior chest wall until it disappears into the atrioventricular groove beneath the right atrial appendage. No anatomic landmarks in the right coronary system compare to the bifurcation of the left main coronary artery. It is therefore more difficult to define the precise position of abnormalities in the right coronary system, except with reference to the ostium. Similarly, fewer external anatomic references are available to help to locate the origin of the right coronary artery or to determine its path. The right ventricular outflow tract defines its inferior boundary; however, no structures either anterior or superior to the vessel are useful in further defining its position in space. The right coronary ostium normally ranges from 2 to 3 mm in diameter at pathologic study.[18]

EXAMINING PLANES

The coronary arterial tree is a complex three-dimensional structure, and a variety of echocardiographic imaging planes are needed to record the different portions of the coronary arteries. These planes are conveniently divided into those used to record the ostia and proximal coronary arteries and those used to image the more distal coronary vessels.

Coronary Ostia and Proximal Coronary Arteries

The echocardiographic examining planes commonly used for imaging the ostia and proximal coronary arteries are as follows: (1) a parasternal long axis plane of the left and right coronary arteries (this plane is comparable to a parasternal short axis of the aortic valve but is rotated to be specifically aligned parallel to the long axis of the vessel to be examined); (2) an apical long axis plane of the left main, proximal right, and circumflex coronary arteries (this plane is a modification of the apical five-chamber view but is specifically aligned to record the coronary arteries); and (3) a long axis plane of the proximal right and left main coronary arteries from the subcostal window. Additional views to image the peripheral coronary arteries are used when abnormal coronary anatomy is suspected such as coronary aneurysms, coronary arteriovenous fistulas, or dilated coronary branches (e.g., arteries feeding tumors, arteriovenous malformations, or other lesions requiring increased local blood flow). These imaging planes are discussed in the following section.

To record the left main coronary artery from the parasternal transducer location, the imaging plane is initially aligned parallel to the short axis of the aorta at the aortic valve level. The artery is then located by angling the imaging plane in a superior-inferior arc to define the superior margin of the left ventricle and the descending portion of the pulmonary artery. These reference points represent the upper and lower limits of the area in which the left main coronary artery should lie.[1] During the course of the sweep, a relatively dense mass of echoes originating along the left, inferior border of the aorta and extending leftward beneath the right ventricular outflow tract can be visualized. This mass of echoes corresponds to the dense echoes normally seen behind the pulmonary artery during routine examination of the pulmonary artery and valve and has been termed the atriopulmonic sulcus.[20] The left main coronary artery lies within this mass of echoes. When one has located the area in which the left main coronary artery lies, one rotates the transducer clockwise approximately 30° in an attempt to align it parallel to the long axis of the left main coronary segment. The probe is then swept back and forth within the previously described boundaries. The aorta is maintained in the left-hand margin of the scan until the coronary ostium or left main coronary artery itself is located. Fine changes in the rotation of the transducer are required to align the scan plane parallel to the long axis of the vessel. Although this process is difficult to describe, the area of the left main coronary artery is relatively easy to locate, and with experience, the entire process can be accomplished in minutes. If the left main coronary artery can be clearly recorded, fine changes in plane position will often reveal its bifurcation along with the proximal left anterior descending and proximal circumflex coronary branches.

The left main coronary artery also can be recorded from the cardiac apex.[3,4] When one records the vessel from the cardiac apex, one locates the transducer over the apical impulse, and the central ray of the beam is angled superiorly and anteriorly to record the aortic root. The plane is initially aligned in a five-chamber view of the heart and is then rotated "clockwise" until the coronary ostium and left main coronary artery are visualized. This imaging plane views the left coronary artery in an orthogonal orientation to the short axis scan and hence may permit better detection of lesions that are poorly visualized from the anterior chest wall. This plan has the theoretic disadvantages of placing the structures to be examined in the far field of the scan plane, where lateral resolution is poorer and penetration of the sound beam is diminished. In addition, the anatomic landmarks used from the cardiac apex are less well defined than those available from the left sternal border. Nevertheless, several authors have reported more frequent visualization of the left main coronary artery from the apex when compared to the short axis view.[3,4]

Certain technical considerations must be kept in mind when attempting to record the left main coronary artery or other segments of the coronary tree. First, several structures in the area of the left coronary artery produce horizontal linear echoes. To be sure one is visualizing the left coronary artery, one must record its origin from the aorta and the continuity between the lumina of the two vessels. Second, because the artery does not remain in the field of vision throughout the cardiac cycle but rather moves in and out of the plane of the cross-sectional scan, frame by frame analysis of several frames may be required to locate the few frames that clearly depict the main coronary structures. Thus, high quality still frames are necessary.

The left main coronary artery, although relatively short, may curve such that it cannot be recorded entirely in one examining plane. Slight changes in transducer angulation and modification of the standard views may therefore be required to record the coronary ostium, the body of the left main coronary artery, and the bifurcation. Thus, individual areas of the vessel may need to be evaluated separately.

The origin of the right coronary artery is recorded from the left parasternal location using the same basic imaging plane used to record the left coronary artery. Location of the right coronary artery is more difficult in adults because of the lack of well-defined anatomic landmarks bracketing the vessel. In children, however, the vessel is relatively prominent and is easier to record.[21]

The right coronary artery lies slightly superior to the plane of the left main coronary artery and requires superior angulation of the imaging plane to be visualized. This requires angulation of the imaging plane in a superior-inferior arc from the aortic valve upward to the superior portion of the right coronary sinus of Valsalva; while one focuses on the right superior margin of the aortic root until an interruption in the aortic wall at the base of the right coronary cusp is visualized. This corresponds to the level at which the anterior tricuspid leaflet merges with the tricuspid valve ring.[21] This interruption usually appears between the ten- and eleven-o'clock positions relative to the short axis of the aorta. Fine positioning of the plane parallel to the long axis of the right coronary can then be achieved by alternately rotating the plane in a clockwise-counterclockwise pattern until the parallel linear echoes from the walls of the artery are optimally recorded. Occasionally, the origin of the right coronary artery from the aortic root and its proximal segment can also be imaged in the apical five chamber view.

Subcostal imaging has also been found useful in the evaluation of the proximal coronary arteries. From the subcostal transducer location, the four-chamber view is first recorded and the transducer is then tilted anteriorly until the aortic root is imaged. From this position, the transducer is angled through a narrow anteroposterior arc until the proximal left and right coronary arteries are visualized as they arise from the aorta.

The parasternal examining planes appear optimal for recording both the left and right coronary arteries because they place these vessels perpendicular to the path of the scan plane and in the near field of the transducer; however, longer segments of the proximal vessels are typically recorded in the apical and subcostal views.

Distal Coronary Arteries

To study the distal coronary arteries in detail, multiple variations on standard views are required (Table 34–1). Conceptually, during such an examination the coronary tree must be divided into segments and each segment examined separately by sweeping the scan plane through the area of interest using a single or multiple standard plane(s) as reference. Figure 34–2 diagrammatically depicts the major coronary arteries along with their location in selected standard planes. In this illustration the peripheral vessels are arbitrarily divided into proximal, middle, and distal thirds to better describe the different imaging planes used to examine specific portions of the arteries.

Left Anterior Descending Coronary Artery

The proximal third of the left anterior descending coronary artery can often be selectively imaged using a modified parasternal long axis view in which the transducer is placed in the third or fourth intercostal space, angled 10 to 30° superiorly and laterally toward the pulmonary artery, and then rotated approximately 10°

Table 34–1. Echocardiographic Examination of the Coronary Arteries

	Proximal Third (view)	Middle Third (view)	Distal Third (view)
Left anterior descending	Parasternal long axis	Elevated subcostal four-chamber	Elevated subcostal four-chamber
Left circumflex	Apical five-chamber	Parasternal short axis	Depressed apical four-chamber
	Parasternal short axis	Subcostal short axis	Parasternal short axis
	Subcostal short axis	Apical four-chamber	Depressed subcostal four-chamber
Right	Parasternal short axis	Subcostal short axis	Depressed apical four-chamber
	Subcostal short axis	Apical four-chamber	Subcostal short axis
	Elevated apical four-chamber		Parasternal right ventricular inflow

clockwise until the parallel linear echoes representing the left anterior descending coronary artery are recorded.[11] It is also possible to record the proximal, middle, and distal thirds of the left anterior descending coronary artery from the subcostal position by elevating the transducer from the subcostal four-chamber view until the scan plane transects the anterior interventricular groove, which contains the anterior descending artery. Although the normal vessel is difficult to visualize because of its small diameter and motion with the heart, dilated or aneurysmal portions of the left anterior descending coronary artery should be apparent. The left anterior descending artery is also present in all parasternal short axis views of the left ventricle at the epicardial junction of the left and right ventricles (Fig. 34–2D).

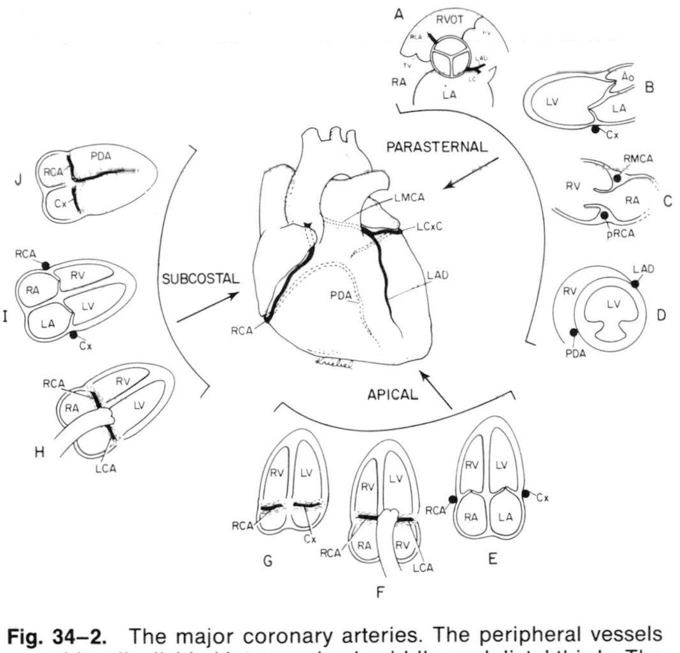

Fig. 34–2. The major coronary arteries. The peripheral vessels are arbitrarily divided into proximal, middle, and distal thirds. The appropriate echocardiographic views to image the different segments of the coronary arteries are shown. RVOT = right ventricular outflow tract; PV = pulmonary valve; LAD = left anterior descending artery; LC = left circumflex artery; LA = left atrium; RA = right atrium; TV = tricuspid valve; RCA = right coronary artery; Ao = aorta; LA = left atrium; LV = left ventricle; RMCA = right main coronary artery; pRCA = posterior right coronary artery; RV = right ventricle. PDA = posterior descending coronary artery; Cx = circumflex coronary artery; LCA = left coronary artery. (See text for details.)

Left Circumflex Coronary Artery

After it originates from the left main coronary artery, the circumflex coronary artery lies in the left atrioventricular groove, and this landmark defines the region of search. The proximal third of the circumflex artery is best approached from the apical five-chamber view by rotating the transducer slightly clockwise to direct the imaging plane posteriorly and inferiorly until the parallel linear echoes from the walls of the vessel appear (Fig. 34–2F).[11] To locate the proximal third of the circumflex coronary artery from the parasternal approach, a short axis view at the level of the aorta is obtained, and the transducer is then rotated approximately 10° clockwise and is angled slightly superiorly (Fig. 34–2A). When diffusely dilated, the artery can be followed distally from the bifurcation; however, when one is seeking focal aneurysms, the area of search must be defined by the atrioventricular groove. The middle third of the circumflex artery can also be imaged from the four-chamber view by sweeping the transducer in an anteroposterior arc while focusing on the lateral atrioventricular groove (Fig. 34–2E), and the distal third can be seen with a depressed apical four-chamber (Fig. 34–2G), subcostal four-chamber (Fig. 34–2J), or parasternal short axis view of the posterior atrioventricular groove. The distal portion of the vessel also is present in short axis in the routine parasternal long axis view of the left ventricle (Fig. 34–2B) and can be scanned by sweeping the transducer from the left to the right margin of the left ventricle.

Right Coronary Artery

The proximal third of the right coronary artery can be imaged in long axis from the parasternal short axis view at the level of the aorta (Fig. 34–2A), or from an elevated apical (Fig. 34–2F) or subcostal four-chamber view (Fig. 34–2H). The proximal portion of the right coronary artery can also be imaged on occasion using a subcostal short axis view. The middle portion of the right coronary artery can be recorded by sweeping an apical (Fig. 34–2E) or subcostal four-chamber view (Fig. 34–2J) along the right lateral atrioventricular groove, or on occasion from a subcostal short axis view parallel to the atrioventricular groove. The distal segment of the right coronary artery can be recorded in long axis from a depressed apical (Fig. 34–2G) or subcostal four-cham-

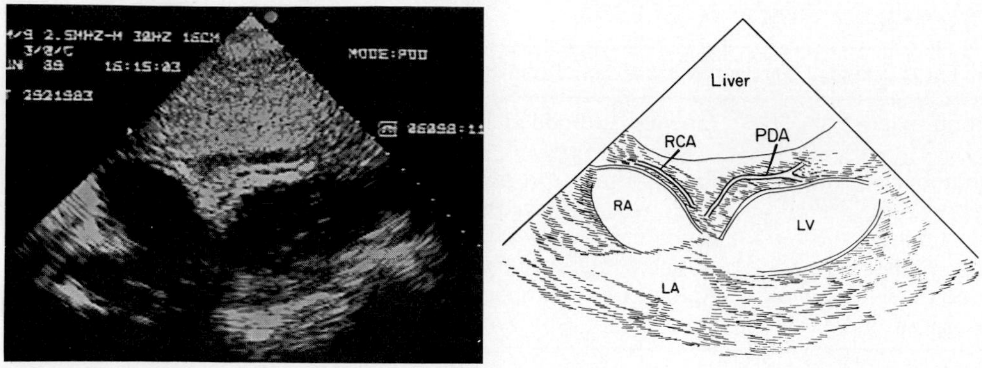

Fig. 34–3. Recording of the posterior descending coronary artery (PDA) from a depressed subcostal four-chamber view. The distal portion of the right coronary artery (RCA) is also visualized. RA = right atrium; LA = left atrium; LV = left ventricle.

ber view (Fig. 34–2J) and in short axis by sweeping the parasternal right ventricular inflow view from the medial to the lateral wall of the right ventricle (Fig. 34–2C). Figure 34–3 shows the posterior descending coronary artery from a depressed subcostal four-chamber view. In the same image, the distal portion of the right coronary artery is also recorded.

NORMAL ECHOCARDIOGRAPHIC ANATOMY

Figures 34–4 and 34–5 illustrate the normal echocardiographic appearance of the left and right coronary arteries. The left coronary ostium normally appears as a funnel-shaped structure that originates from the posterolateral wall of the aorta between the four- and five-o'clock positions.[1] The vessel then continues laterally as two parallel linear echoes separated by a distance of several millimeters. After coursing laterally beneath the posterior wall of the pulmonary artery for approximately 1 cm, the parallel linear echoes arising from the left main coronary segment bifurcate into two pairs of parallel echoes, one of which continues laterally and anteriorly while the other courses more posteriorly (Fig. 34–4). In vitro studies have confirmed that the anteriorly coursing pair of linear echoes originates from the left anterior descending branch of the left coronary artery, whereas the posterior pair arises from the left circumflex branch.[2]

Throughout the cardiac cycle, there is both anteroposterior and superior-inferior motion of the aortic root. Because the left main coronary segment is attached to the aorta, it follows this motion. At end-diastole, the aorta is in its most posterior position. At this point, the left main coronary artery generally follows a lateral and slightly anterior course after leaving the aorta. During systole, the aorta moves anteriorly and reaches its most anterior position at approximately end-systole. From this aortic position, the left main coronary segment generally pursues a directly lateral course. The superior-inferior motion of the vessel follows the motion of the base of the heart. During systolic contraction, the base of the heart moves inferiorly, whereas during diastole, it moves superiorly. The left coronary artery therefore is in its most anterior and inferior position at end-systole and in its most posterior and superior position at end-diastole.

The normal appearance of the proximal right coronary artery is illustrated in Figure 34–5. The ostium of the proximal right coronary lies at approximately the eleven-o'clock position relative to the short axis of the aorta. The right coronary ostium, in general, is less well defined and not as funnel shaped as the left coronary artery. The right coronary artery appears as two parallel linear echoes that leave the aortic root and course rightward and slightly anteriorly. The spatial motion of the right coronary artery follows that of the aortic root and is similar in timing and direction to that of the left coronary artery.

That these parallel linear echoes represent the coronary vessels has been confirmed in several ways. The first method was by direct injection of contrast medium into the vessels during cardiac catheterization.[1] Figure 34–6 is an example of such a study. Figure 34–6A, the

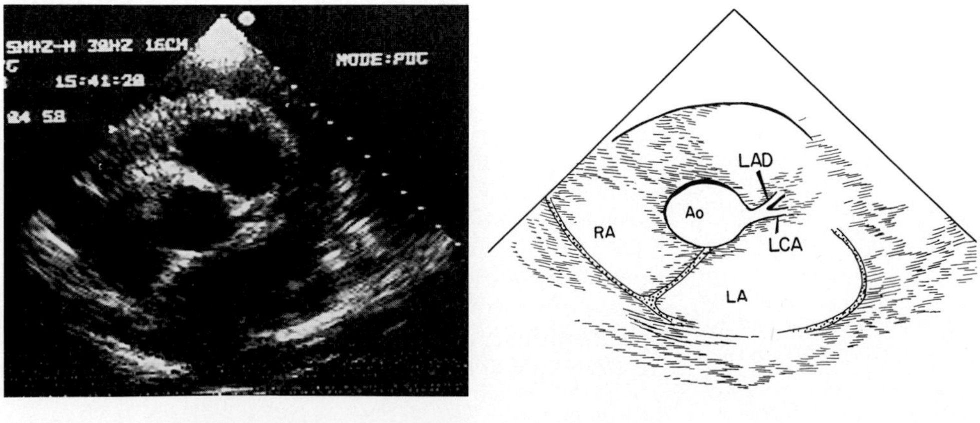

Fig. 34–4. The proximal left coronary artery in long axis. The left main coronary artery can be seen originating from a posterolateral wall of the aorta at approximately the 4-o'clock position. It then courses laterally roughly 1 cm and bifurcates into left anterior descending and left circumflex branches. Ao = aorta; LA = left atrium; LAD = left anterior descending coronary artery; LCA = left circumflex coronary artery.

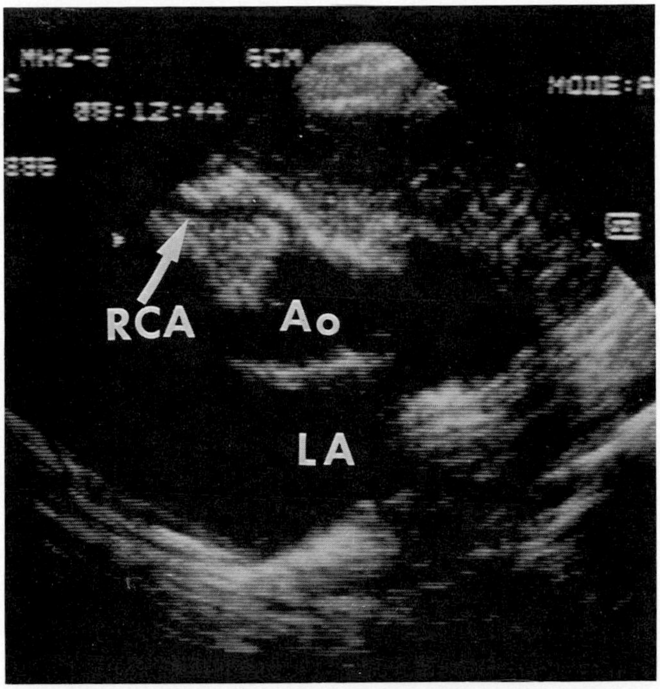

Fig. 34–5. The proximal right coronary artery (RCA) in long axis. This scan plane is aligned roughly parallel to a short axis of the aorta. It is then repositioned to record the long axis of the RCA arising from the aorta at approximately the 11-o'clock position and coursing anteriorly and to the right. The vessel appears as two parallel linear echoes with an echo-free space interposed. Ao = aorta; LA = left atrium.

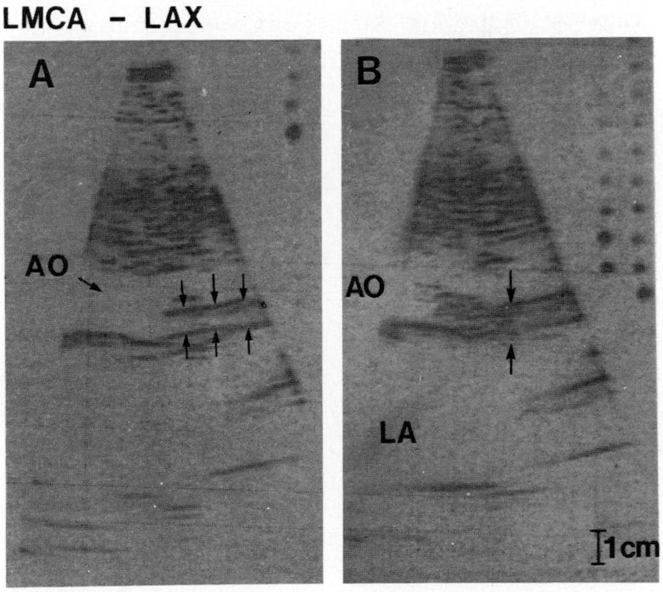

Fig. 34–6. **A.** Cross-sectional recording of a normal left main coronary artery (LMCA). The artery, which appears as two parallel linear echoes (indicated at the tips of the vertical arrows), arises from the inferolateral border of the aorta (AO) and extends slightly anteriorly and to the left. The relatively echo-free space between these linear echoes represents the lumen of the vessel. **B.** Recording from the same patient during injection of indocyanine green dye (Cardio-Green) directly into the left main coronary artery. The dye produces a cloud of echoes that completely fills the space between the original parallel linear echoes, confirming that this is the arterial lumen. AO = aorta; LA = left atrium; LAX = long axis. (From Weyman AE, et al.: Noninvasive visualization of the left main coronary artery by cross sectional echocardiography. Circulation 54:169, 1976. Reproduced by permission of the American Heart Association, Inc.)

left main coronary artery is visualized prior to contrast injection. In Figure 34–6B, indocyanine green (Cardio-Green) dye is injected directly into the left main coronary artery and opacifies the area between the two parallel linear echoes, thereby confirming their identity as a coronary vessel. In addition, the coronary arteries have been visualized during extensive studies of excised hearts, and their ostia have been recorded during serial catheter insertions and multiple contrast injections.[2] Finally, lesions such as coronary aneurysms have been detected within the coronary arteries, and their presence has been used to confirm that the structures from which they originate are the coronary vessels.[1,7,8]

Recording Frequency for Coronary Vessels

The reported frequency with which various segments of the coronary arteries have been visualized echocardiographically is summarized in Table 34–2. The ostium of the left coronary has been recorded in 90 to 99% of adult patients with coronary artery disease,[5,22] as well as in nearly all pediatric patients.[9,23] The left main coronary segment has been slightly more difficult to visualize, and success rates have varied from 58 to 99% in adult patients (mean 78%).[10–12,24] Success in imaging the bifurcation has also varied, being reported in 57 to 75% of cases.[11] In general, success rates for visualizing the proximal left coronary decrease as one moves distally.

The proximal right coronary artery has generally been more difficult to visualize than the left. In adults, success rates of 46 and 48% have been reported. In children, however, the right coronary artery should be recorded in virtually all cases.

Few data are available on the frequency with which the more distal coronary vessels can be imaged. In the one available report, a study of 35 patients, the left anterior descending coronary artery was recorded in 30 (mean length 3.9 ± 2.3 cm, maximal length 7.5 cm), the left circumflex artery in 11 (mean length 1.1 ± 1.0 cm, maximal length 3.0 cm), and the right coronary artery in 32 (mean length 5.6 ± 2.6 cm, maximal length 12 cm).

Unfortunately, data on the frequency with which the distal coronary arteries can be recorded are less meaningful because they relate to the visualization of subsegments of relatively long vessels, and the ability to record a specific region of a nondilated vessel in any given case is unpredictable.

Echocardiographic Vessel Size

The normal echocardiographic luminal diameters of the proximal left and right coronary arteries have been reported in children.[25] These diameters showed little variation in the first centimeter from the ostium and ranged from 2 mm in infants to 5 mm in older children and adolescents. Normal measurements in adults are less well defined. In a heterogeneous group of 35 adults,

Table 34–2. Reported Success Rate for Echocardiographic Visualization of Coronary Arteries

Author	Year	Number	Ostium of Left Coronary Artery	Left Main coronary Segment	Bifurcation/ Left Anterior Descending Artery	Circumflex Artery	Proximal Right Cornary Artery
Ogawa et al.[3]	1980	65	—	55(85%)	26(40%)	—	—
Chen et al.[4]	1979	73	—	52(71%)	—	—	—
Rogers et al.[5]	1980	100	90(90%)	—	—	—	—
Friedman et al.[6]	1982	37	—	30(81%)	—	—	—
Yoshikawa et al.[7]	1979	37	37(100%)	29(78%)	—	—	17(46%)
Malergue et al.[34]	1983	41	—	40(98%)	18(44%)	—	—
Aronow et al.[10]	1979	93	—	54(58%)	—	—	—
Rink et al.[12]	1980	72	71(99%)	71(99%)	—	—	—
Presti et al.[36]	1987	128	—	—	/90(70%)	—	—
Vered et al.[33]	1986	100	—	92(92%)	—	—	—
Ryan et al.[13]	1986	119	—	100(84%)	—	—	—
Douglas et al.[11]	1988	35	—	30(86%)	15(43%)/30(86%)	11(31%)	17(49%)

mean diameters for the left anterior descending coronary artery were 4.7 mm (proximal) and 4.6 mm (distal); for the left circumflex artery they were 2.8 mm, and for the right coronary they were 3.1 mm (proximal), 3.1 mm (middle), and 2.7 mm (distal).[11]

BLOOD FLOW MEASUREMENT BY PULSED DOPPLER ECHOCARDIOGRAPHY

Doppler measurements of coronary artery blood flow velocity and flow reserve capacity have enhanced our understanding of the coronary circulation, have helped to define the physiologic significance of coronary stenoses, and have permitted monitoring of the functional response to therapeutic interventions. The Doppler approach is particularly useful because it permits changes in blood flow velocity to be determined instantly and provides on-line recording and display of the flow data. In addition, miniaturization of the flow sensing apparatus has permitted precise intravascular and epicardial blood flow velocity recording in both experimental and clinical settings (Fig. 34–7). Intravascular and epicardial pulsed Doppler and laser Doppler techniques have been used extensively to assess coronary artery blood flow under normal and altered hemodynamic conditions.[26] The pattern of flow in the coronary arteries differs from that in other parts of the body because the relatively high pressure exerted by myocardial contraction on the intramyocardial vessels, arrests forward systolic flow and displaces the majority of coronary filling to diastole. As a result, normal blood flow velocity in the epicardial coronary arteries is observed to peak in early diastole and then to decrease gradually as aortic diastolic pressure drops until the onset of systole, when it falls abruptly. During systole, the flow profile in the epicardial vessels is parabolic, peaking in midsystole at roughly half the peak diastolic velocity. In the intramyocardial vessels, systolic flow is retrograde, so the positive systolic flow in the epicardial arteries reflects the capacitance of these vessels. As might be expected, the ratio of systolic to diastolic coronary blood flow velocity for the right coronary artery is significantly higher than that for the left (0.67 vs. 0.17).[27]

More recently, the transthoracic measurement of coronary artery blood flow using two-dimensional and pulsed Doppler echocardiography has been described.[28,29] In one report,[28] blood flow through the left

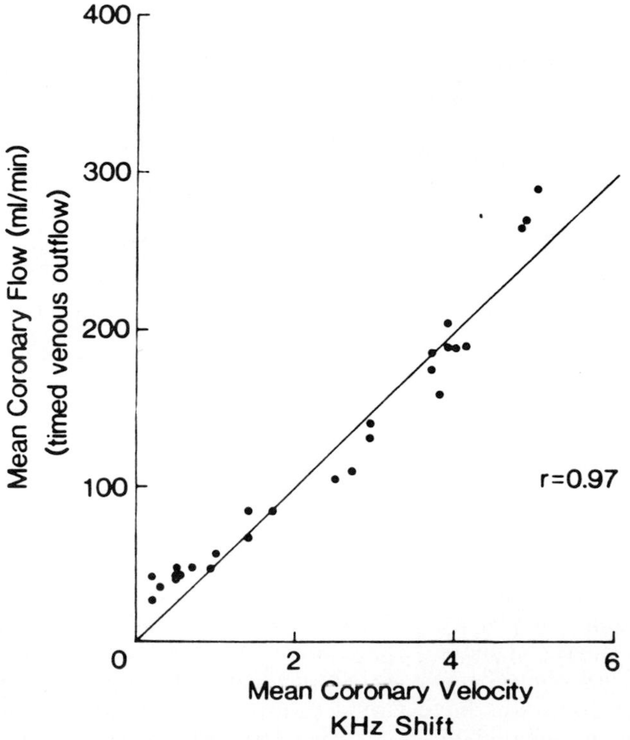

Fig. 34–7. Relationship between changes in mean coronary flow measured by timed coronary sinus venous collection and mean flow velocity measured with an epicardial Doppler probe. (From Marcus ML, et al.: Measurements of coronary velocity and reactive hyperemia in the coronary circulation of humans. Circ Res 49:877, 1981.)

anterior descending coronary artery was detected in 7 of 20 normal subjects (35%) and in 40 of 80 patients (50%) with different cardiovascular diseases. The blood flow pattern recorded transthoracically was biphasic, similar to that reported using other techniques.[29] The average recorded peak diastolic velocity in the left anterior descending coronary artery was 33.5 ± 5.1 cm/sec for the normal subjects and 56 ± 26.8 cm/sec for the group with heart disease. In patients with coronary artery disease without critical stenoses, blood flow patterns in the left anterior descending coronary artery remained biphasic, but with higher diastolic velocities. In patients with severe left anterior descending coronary artery stenoses (presumably flow limiting), however, flow velocity measured distal to the stenosis was low and sustained throughout the cardiac cycle with an early systolic peak.[29] An increase in velocity was consistently noted after coronary angioplasty. Velocities in patients with bypass grafts depended on the site of sampling (native vessel or graft) and the degree of stenosis of the native vessel.[28] Flow velocities in internal mammary bypass grafts were similar in profile but much higher in velocity than those in saphenous vein grafts.[29]

Despite these encouraging observations concerning flow velocity, in the left anterior descending artery, major limitations to the transthoracic measurement of coronary flow remain. First, blood flow can be recorded in only limited portions of the coronary arteries because of their small size and the difficulties in imaging the more distal segments of the arteries. Second, the recorded velocity of flow is influenced by the angle between the Doppler beam and the long axis of the coronary artery imaged by two-dimensional echocardiography, and optimal orientation of the artery for Doppler interrogation is not always possible. Third, the movement of the coronary arteries with the heart frequently shifts the area of interest in and out of the stationary sample volume or imaging plane and causes cyclic interruptions in the recorded signal. Finally, the precise measurement of luminal diameter in these small vessels is extremely difficult, and hence only flow velocity can be practically recorded, and this parameter is of limited value as an isolated measurement. Thus, although preliminary clinical data are interesting, the ultimate diagnostic role of transthoracic or esophageal coronary flow recording based on the pulsed Doppler method remains to be defined.

CORONARY ARTERY STENOSIS

Artherosclerosis is, by far, the most common cause of coronary artery stenosis. Atherosclerotic coronary lesions are characterized by a focal accumulation of lipids, fibrous tissue, and frequently, calcium deposits, which both deform the arterial wall and narrow the vascular lumen.[30]

Two characteristic echocardiographic abnormalities noted in patients with atherosclerotic coronary artery disease correspond to the pathologic nature of the process. These abnormalities are (1) a focal decrease in the size of the arterial lumen and (2) an increase in the local reflectivity of the vascular walls. The luminal narrowing is typified by an increase in the echoes from either the anterior or the posterior margin of the vessel, with loss of their normal parallel orientation and a decrease in or total disruption of the continuous echo-free space characteristic of the vascular lumen. Figure 34–8, an echocardiogram from a patient with a lesion of the left main coronary artery, illustrates this type of abnormality. Figure 34–9 is the corresponding angiogram demonstrating the relationship in both configuration and location with the angiographic obstruction.

The abnormal increase in echo intensity occurs at specific points along the vessel, presumably because of the histologic composition of the atherosclerotic lesions. Importantly, this increased reflectance may occur with or without associated vascular narrowing. Figure 34–10 is an echocardiogram of a patient with left main coronary artery disease. In Figure 34–10B, increased reflectivity and luminal narrowing are seen at the level of the left coronary artery. Figure 34–10C illustrates how the increased echo density can be made more obvious by lowering the system gain. A similar effect can be achieved by other modes of signal processing that amplify high intensity echoes and suppress lower amplitude signals.

The true sensitivity and specificity of these criteria for detecting coronary lesions are difficult to assess. Although some studies have addressed these questions, they have often used different types of instrumentation, examining techniques, criteria for diagnosing coronary

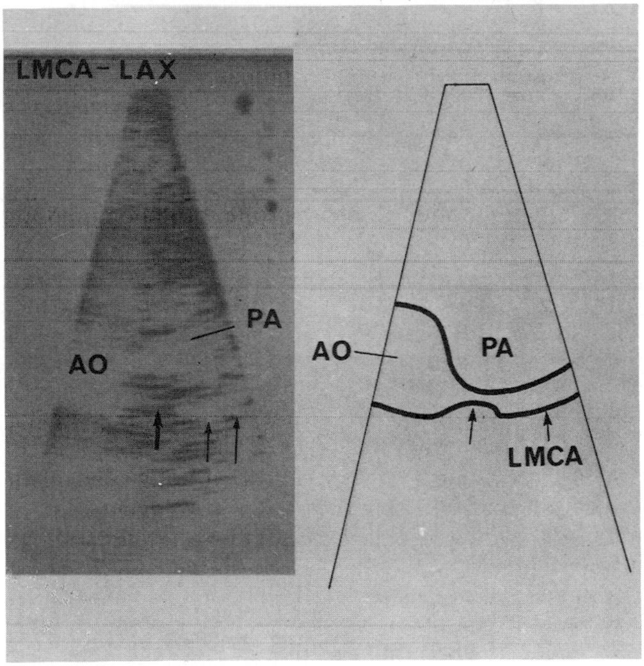

Fig. 34–8. Cross-sectional echogram from a patient with obstruction of the proximal left main coronary artery (LMCA). A fairly extensive area of luminal narrowing begins just distal to the coronary ostium and produces almost complete obliteration of the artery (large vertical arrow). A relatively normal arterial lumen is recorded distal to the area of obstruction (small vertical arrows). PA = pulmonary artery; AO = aorta; LAX = long axis. (From Weyman AE, et al.: Noninvasive visualization of the left main coronary artery by cross-sectional echocardiography. Circulation 54: 169, 1976. Reproduced by permission of the American Heart Association, Inc.)

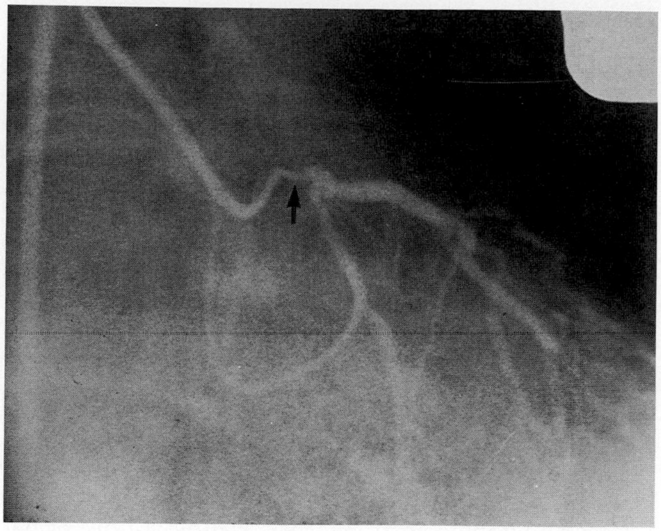

Fig. 34–9. Coronary cineangiogram corresponding to the cross-sectional study illustrated in Figure 34–8. Narrowing of the left main coronary segment (arrow) is significant, extending from the catheter tip to the bifurcation of the left main coronary artery. (From Weyman AE, et al.: Noninvasive visualization of the left main coronary artery by cross-sectional echocardiography. Circulation 54:169, 1976. Reproduced by permission of the American Heart Association, Inc.)

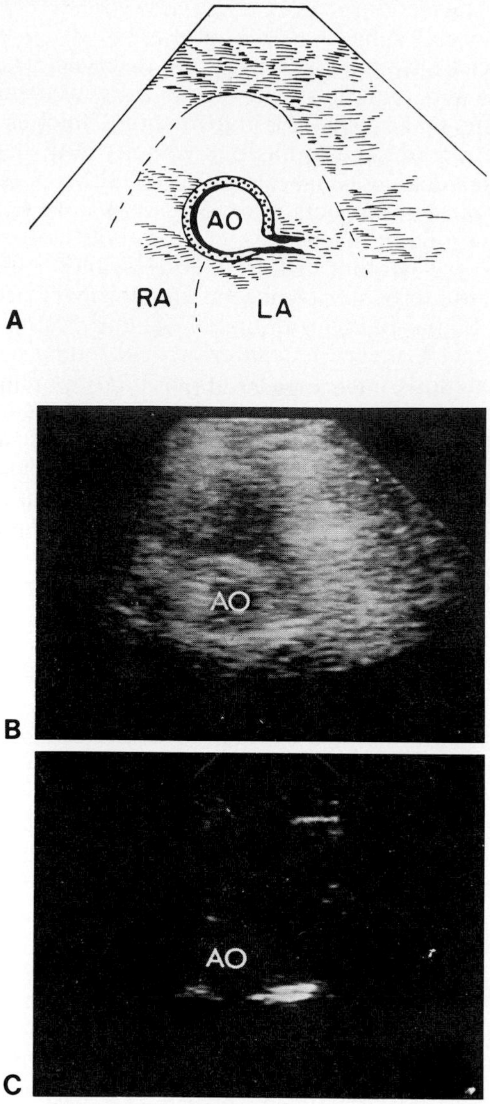

Fig. 34–10. **A.** Diagram illustrating origin of left main coronary artery from the aorta. **B.** Cross-sectional echocardiogram of a patient with left main coronary artery disease. Increased reflectivity and luminal narrowing are seen at the level of the left coronary artery. **C.** The increased echo density is more obvious when the gain setting is lowered. AO = aorta; LA = left atrium; RA = right atrium.

lesions, and methods of image processing. Despite these limitations, there is enough consistency in the results to suggest some general patterns.

Lesions in the left main coronary artery are the easiest to record and have been the most extensively studied. The sensitivity of two-dimensional echocardiography in the detection of left main coronary artery disease has varied from 67 to 100%,[4–6,31,32] whereas the specificity has ranged from 65 to 97%.[4,5,24,33,34] Table 34–3 summarizes the available data on visualization of left main coronary artery lesions using the criteria of luminal narrowing and increased regional reflectivity with standard echocardiographic signal processing.[1,3,4,6,10,12] These studies suggest that lesions of the left main coronary artery can be detected in the majority of patients. Few false-negative results have been reported,[6] whereas false-positive results occur frequently. The highest sensitivity appears to be achieved by using both criteria together. When luminal narrowing was used alone in one study, only four of eight left main coronary lesions were detected, whereas when the combination of luminal narrowing and increased echo intensity was used, all eight lesions were correctly identified.[4] Unfortunately, using echo intensity alone increases the number of false-positive results.

Several prospective studies have examined the relationship of high intensity paracoronary echoes with atherosclerotic disease.[5,6] In 144 patients, of whom 27 had left main coronary artery disease detectable by angiographic study, the sensitivity for detecting stenotic le-

Table 34–3. Comparison of Echocardiographic and Angiographic Detection of Left Main Coronary Stenosis Using Standard Echocardiographic Signal Processing

		ECHO		
		+	–	Total
ANGIO	+	49	13	62
	–	31	294	325
	Total	80	307	

Sensitivity = 49/62(79%); specificity = 294/325(90%); PV+ = 49/80(61%).

sions of the left main artery by echocardiographic examination was 100%, but the specificity was only 54%, yielding a low predictive value (33%). These results suggest that high intensity echoes are highly sensitive indicators of lesions of the left main coronary artery. False-positive results may be due to the presence of atherosclerotic lesions elsewhere in the proximal left coronary system or to lesions that do not produce stenosis and therefore cannot be detected angiographically.[12] They may also indicate other abnormalities that increase local reflectivity, such as valvular or annular calcification or increased epicardial fat overlying the left coronary artery.[2]

Investigators have suggested that these high intensity echoes might be related to the presence of calcification in the atherosclerotic lesions. Although high intensity echoes are almost invariably noted in patients with fluoroscopic evidence of calcified coronary arteries, many patients with high intensity echoes and angiographic evidence of stenosis do not appear to have calcified coronary arteries. In the group of 53 patients with stenotic lesions of the proximal left coronary system, only 30 had fluoroscopic evidence of coronary calcification, whereas 50 had high intensity echoes. Thus, high intensity echoes appear to be far more sensitive detectors of coronary artery disease than coronary calcifications. When fluoroscopic calcification and high intensity echoes were observed together (N = 28), significant coronary stenoses were invariably present.

The effects of calcific valvular heart disease and valve prostheses on the genesis of high intensity echoes have been less well studied. In a group of eight patients with calcific valvular disease (seven aortic and one mitral), high intensity echoes were noted in six. Three of these patients had angiographically evident coronary artery stenoses, and the rest had normal coronary arteries. In the two other patients in whom high intensity echoes were not recorded, angiographic studies were normal. Thus, of the six patients without coronary artery disease, high intensity echoes were detected in three. Although the number of patients studied was small, the results suggest that the specificity of two-dimensional echocardiography for coronary artery disease is reduced in the presence of calcific valvular disease or valve prosthesis.[5]

Other areas of the proximal coronary arteries are more difficult to record and have been less extensively studied. In one report, the left anterior descending branch of the left coronary artery was visualized in 27 of 35 patients. In 20 normal patients, there was no interruption of the vascular lumen, whereas in 7 patients with echocardiographic luminal interruptions, 5 patients had proximal left anterior descending disease and 2 had insignificant lesions of that artery in corresponding areas.[3]

To determine with confidence that an area of luminal narrowing represents a stenotic lesion, one must visualize the lumen of the vessel both proximal and distal to the narrowed area. If the lumen is not visible distal to the area of apparent stenosis, the vessel may merely have curved out of the scan plan so the plane crosses the vascular wall, and thus, the lumen would no longer be recorded. When lesions occur near the bifurcation, viewing the distal vessel may be more difficult, and a higher incidence of false-positive results must be expected.[24]

In addition, no blood-containing structure is ever completely echo free. Fine transient echoes are frequently seen in the left ventricle, the left atrium, and the aorta. Transient echoes that appear to fill the arterial lumen may also be seen in the proximal coronary arteries. Intra-arterial echoes must be fixed in position, consistent from cycle to cycle, and of greater intensity than surrounding structures to be considered indicative of a lesion.

The detection of changes in luminal diameter and the variation in intensity of the echoes from the arterial wall obviously require clear visualization of the vessels. Direct visualization of the coronary arteries is difficult for several reasons. First, the coronary vessels are near the limits of resolution of currently available cross-sectional echocardiographic equipment when they are of normal size. When the lumen becomes further narrowed by atherosclerotic changes, a clear definition of the change in caliber may be difficult to appreciate. Second, variations in normal coronary anatomy are well recognized and may simulate obstructive lesions. Third, the vessels move throughout the cardiac and respiratory cycles and hence may only pass through the plane of the ultrasonic beam transiently, thereby making their identification and visualization even more difficult.

Recent improvements in image resolution and advances in image processing have been reported to improve coronary visualization. The use of annular phased-array transducer technology,[35] more sophisticated computer-based digital processing, and cine loop recall are some of the technologic advances that have facilitated the study of coronary artery disease by echocardiography. In a study of 100 patients, an off-line real-time digital processing technique allowed postprocessing of the images to enhance high intensity echoes.[13] By this method, 15 of 16 patients with left main coronary artery obstruction were correctly identified, resulting in a sensitivity of 94%. Digital echocardiography enabled investigators to identify correctly 78 of 84 patients without significant left main coronary artery obstruction, yielding a specificity of 93%.

Digital two-dimensional echocardiography has also been used to detect coronary artery lesions other than left main coronary artery disease. In another study of 95 patients, digital two-dimensional echocardiography enabled investigators to identify correctly 44 of 45 patients with proximal left anterior descending coronary artery disease, yielding a sensitivity of 98%. Specificity was lower, however, only 67%.[36]

Despite all these data, to date, echocardiographic coronary imaging for the assessment of atherosclerotic disease has generated little widespread enthusiasm. This relates to the high incidence of false-positive results, the failure to quantitate the severity of lesions, and the inability to consistently visualize the entire coronary tree. Although important information about coronary anatomy can be obtained using the epicardial and intravascular approaches (see later), major advances in instrumentation will be necessary before reliable transthoracic evaluation of coronary stenoses becomes a clinical reality.

CORONARY ARTERY ANEURYSMS

Aneurysms of the coronary arteries may be single, multiple, fusiform, or saccular.[37] They involve predominantly the left coronary artery, but may be found anywhere in the coronary tree. Generally, coronary aneurysms are asymptomatic and thus are unsuspected unless complicated by thrombosis, rupture, or embolism from the aneurysm itself.[38] The majority of coronary artery aneurysms are associated with atherosclerotic disease; however, they may also occur in patients with the mucocutaneous lymph node syndrome, polyarteritis, syphilis, infection, rheumatic disease or after trauma.

Cross-sectional echocardiographic recording of aneurysms located within the proximal coronary systems has been extensively described.[1,7,8] These aneurysms appear echocardiographically either as an abrupt focal separation in the echoes from the anterior and posterior walls of the coronary artery or as a diffuse increase in the diameter of the vessel, producing a large echo-free space between the arterial margins. Figure 34–11 illustrates the angiographic appearance of a single saccular aneurysm recorded in a patient with atherosclerotic coronary artery disease. The aneurysm lies at the distal end of the left main coronary artery and involves the origins of the left anterior descending and left circumflex branches. Figure 34–12, a cross-sectional recording of the same patient, illustrates the large, well-circumscribed, echo-free space characteristic of the saccular arterial aneurysm. In addition, the left main coronary segment, with its origin from the aortic root and entrance into the proximal margin of the aneurysm, can be appreciated.

LMCA – LAX

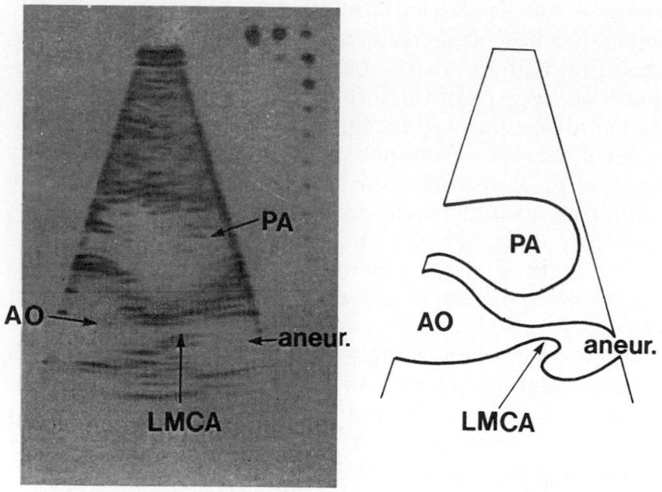

Fig. 34–12. Cross-sectional echocardiogram corresponds to the cineangiogram illustrated in Figure 34–11. The left main coronary artery (LMCA) appears to arise from the inferolateral margin of the aorta (AO) and to extend laterally to communicate with a large, circular, echo-free space representing the aneurysm. PA = pulmonary artery. LAX = long axis; PA = pulmonary artery. (From Weyman AE, et al.: Noninvasive visualization of the left main coronary artery by cross-sectional echocardiography. Circulation 54:169, 1976. Reproduced by permission of the American Heart Association, Inc.)

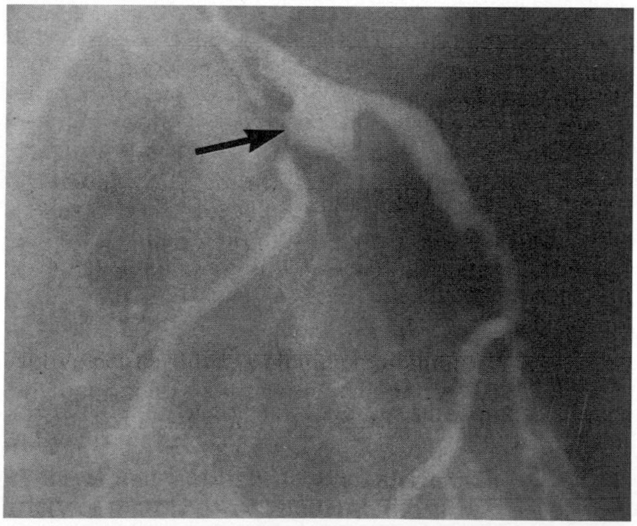

Fig. 34–11. Coronary cineangiogram demonstrates a large aneurysm involving the distal portion of the left main coronary segment (arrow). Both the anterior descending and the circumflex coronary arteries arise from the aneurysm. (From Weyman AE, et al.: Noninvasive visualization of the left main coronary artery by cross-sectional echocardiography. Circulation 54:169, 1976. Reproduced by permission of the American Heart Association, Inc.)

Although initially described for atherosclerotic disease, recent reports suggest a high incidence of coronary aneurysms in children with the mucocutaneous lymph node syndrome.[7,8,39–47] This syndrome, first described by Kawasaki in 1967,[42] and generally referred to as Kawasaki's disease, is an acute inflammatory vasculitis of unknown origin that affects skin, mucous membranes, and multiple other body systems. Patients have fever, rash, and oral and ocular mucosal manifestations. The disease is rarely seen after the age of 10 years and occurs most commonly in children under 2 years of age. Although first described in Japan, the disease has been reported to occur in infants and children of various races in North America, Europe, and Asia.[43–47]

Of the various complications, coronary aneurysm or ectasia is the most important, occurring in 10 to 20% of patients.[48] These aneurysms are most frequently located in the proximal left and right coronary arteries. Thrombosis of the aneurysm and coronary artery stenosis may occur and may cause myocardial infarction, sudden death, or chronic coronary artery insufficiency. Rupture of the aneurysm has also been reported.[47]

Coronary aneurysms usually develop during the second week of the illness, attain maximal size at 3 to 8 weeks, and regress slowly after that. Small aneurysms tend to resolve completely within several months, whereas those of intermediate size may regress in 1 to 2 years. Large aneurysms may remain for many years and are prone to thrombosis with subsequent myocardial ischemia.[52–54] The ability to record these aneurysms appears better in children younger than 1 year of age at the onset of the illness than in those who are older, and it is superior in girls compared to boys. Aneurysms are also more likely to resolve if they are fusiform rather than saccular, and those located distally appear to regress more rapidly than those located proximally.[55]

Cross-sectional echocardiography has been used successfully for the noninvasive evaluation of the coronary arteries in patients with the mucocutaneous lymph node syndrome.[7,8,23,25,49–52] Proximal aneurysms of the coronary arteries are commonly visualized from the parasternal short axis view of the aortic root at the level of the coronary arteries. Figure 34–13A and B demonstrates aneurysms involving the proximal portions of both the right and left coronary arteries in a patient with the mucocutaneous lymph node syndrome. In these examples, one sees extensive areas of luminal dilation just distal to the ostia of both coronary vessels. The communication of both vessels with the aneurysms and the aortic root is detectable. Figure 34–13C shows the proximal aneurysms of the right and the left coronary arteries imaged from the apex. Although these aneurysms most commonly occur in the proximal coronary arteries, any segment of the coronary tree may be involved. Thus, a complete examination requires imaging of all the major coronary branches using the planes described earlier and illustrated in Figure 34–2.[49–51]

Figure 34–14 demonstrates the coronary arteriogram and cross-sectional echocardiogram of a patient with Kawasaki's disease and aneurysmal dilation of the left

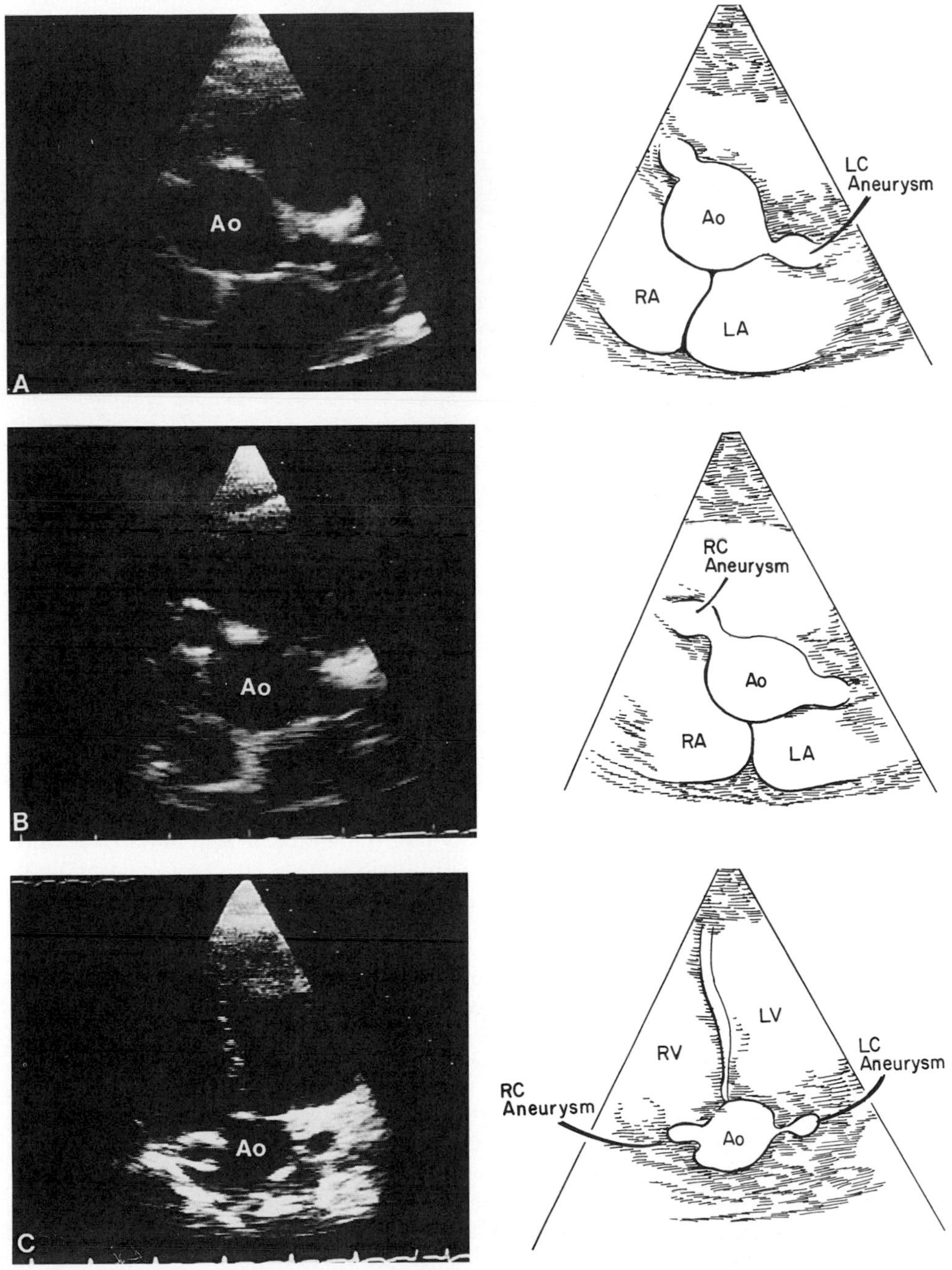

Fig. 34–13. **A.** Cross-sectional echograms from a patient with the mucocutaneous lymph node syndrome demonstrate large aneurysms of the proximal left coronary artery. **B.** The same patient's proximal right coronary artery. **C.** Apical five-chamber view illustrating the proximal aneurysms of both right and left coronary arteries. Ao = aorta; LA = left atrium; RA = right atrium; LV = left ventricle; RV = right ventricle; LC = left coronary; RC = right coronary.

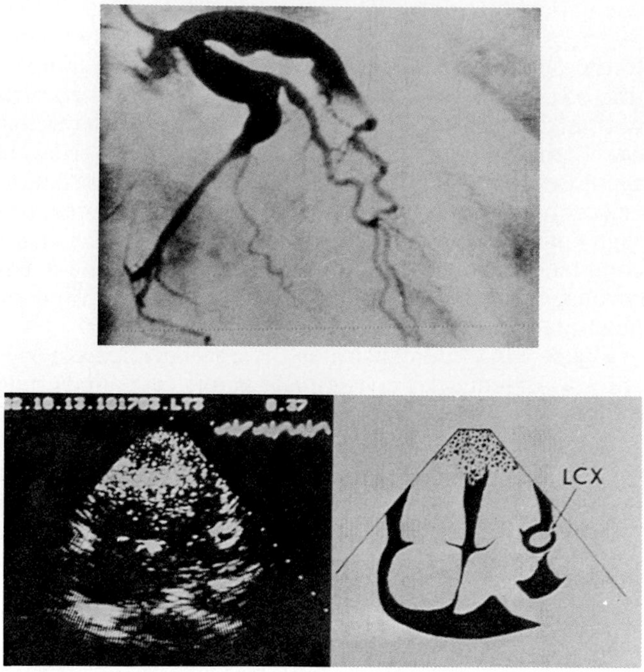

Fig. 34–14. Coronary arteriogram and cross-sectional echocardiogram of a patient with Kawasaki's disease and aneurysmal dilation of the left circumflex coronary artery (LCX). The aneurysm is seen in the apical four-chamber view along the lateral atrioventricular groove between the left ventricle and left atrium. (From Satomi G, et al.: Visualization of coronary arteries by two-dimensional echocardiography in children and infants: evaluation in Kawasaki's disease and coronary arteriovenous fistulas. Am Heart J 107:497, 1984.)

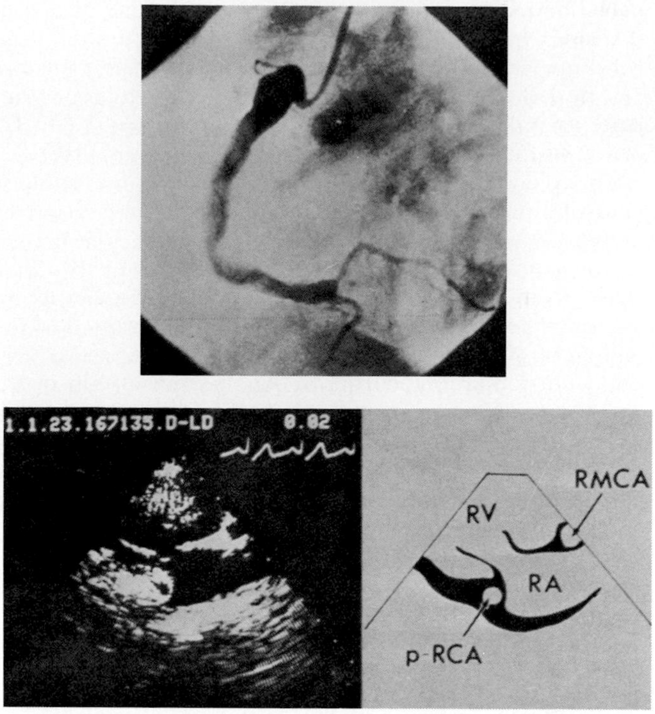

Fig. 34–15. Coronary angiogram **(A)** and cross-sectional echocardiogram **(B)** of a patient with diffuse dilation of the right coronary artery. **B.** The parasternal inflow view of the right ventricle (RV). In this view, the main portion of the right coronary artery just distal to its origin and the more peripheral segment in the posterior atrioventricular groove are imaged in short axis. RMCA = right main coronary artery; p-RCA = peripheral right coronary artery; RA = right coronary artery. (From Satomi G, et al.: Visualization of coronary arteries by two-dimensional echocardiography in children and infants: evaluation in Kawasaki's disease and coronary arteriovenous fistulas. Am Heart J 107:497, 1984.)

circumflex coronary artery. The aneurysm is seen in the apical four-chamber view along the lateral atrioventricular groove between the left ventricle and the left atrium.[49] Figure 34–15 shows the coronary angiogram and cross-sectional echocardiogram of a patient with diffuse dilation of the right coronary artery. Figure 34–15B shows the parasternal inflow view of the right ventricle. In this view, the proximal segment of the dilated right coronary artery just distal to its origin and the distal segment within the posterior atrioventricular groove are imaged in short axis.

The sensitivity of cross-sectional echocardiography in detecting aneurysms in the proximal left and right coronary arteries has been reported to be high (up to 100%).[23] The reported sensitivity for distal portions of the coronary system is lower, varying from 83% for the left anterior descending coronary artery to lower values for the distal right coronary artery. Despite the lower sensitivity for detecting aneurysms in the distal parts of the coronary arterial tree, the overall sensitivity of two-dimensional echocardiography in the identification of coronary artery aneurysms in Kawasaki's disease remains high because distal aneurysms tend to occur in association with proximal lesions.[23]

The specificity of cross-sectional echocardiography in the diagnosis of coronary artery aneurysms varies from 96 to 100%.[8,23,53] False-positive results tend to occur in the proximal segments of the coronary arteries and may result from difficulties in distinguishing between normal arteries whose dimensions are near the upper limits of normal and those that contain a small fusiform aneurysm.[25] It is therefore important to relate the size of the aneurysm to the adjacent coronary artery diameter, because normal arteries maintain a uniform caliber throughout their extent.

Cross-sectional echocardiography may also be useful in the follow-up of patients with Kawasaki's disease. In approximately half the children who initially develop abnormalities of the coronary arteries, angiographic study 1 or 2 years later reveals persistent aneurysms with or without stenosis or tortuosity. The vessels appear normal in the remainder of patients.[52,54,55] Angiography cannot be repeated frequently, however, and the noninvasive examination of the coronary aneurysms by two-dimensional echocardiography is ideal for defining the morphologic changes in these lesions over time.

Aneurysms of the proximal coronary arteries diagnosed during two-dimensional echocardiography and subsequently confirmed by angiography have been recently reported in adults. Some investigators have suggested that the aneurysms might be sequelae of unrecognized Kawasaki's disease that had occurred in childhood.[57,58]

ANOMALOUS ORIGIN FROM THE PULMONARY ARTERY

The left or right coronary arteries or both may originate anomalously from the pulmonary trunk.[37] As indicated in Figure 34–1, the pulmonary trunk lies immediately adjacent to the proximal segments of both the left and right coronary systems, so anomalous insertion of either vessel involves displacement of the coronary ostia by only a few millimeters. When both coronary arteries arise from the pulmonary trunk, survival beyond the neonatal period is generally not possible because normal pulmonary artery pressure is inadequate to perfuse the left ventricular myocardium. Anomalous origin of the left coronary artery from the pulmonary trunk is roughly 10 times as frequent as pulmonary origin of the right coronary artery.[62] Even rarer are isolated origin of the left anterior descending and circumflex arteries from the pulmonary artery. When the left coronary artery arises from the pulmonary trunk, the pressure in the left coronary system is much lower than that in the right, which maintains its normal continuity with the aorta and hence is perfused at systemic pressures. This pressure gradient between the pulmonary and systemic circulations typically leads to reversal of flow in the left coronary system, producing, in effect, an arteriovenous fistula. Once retrograde flow is established in the left coronary artery, intracoronary anastomoses effectively bypass the capillary bed, resulting in myocardial ischemia in the area of ventricle supplied by the anomalously inserted artery.

The manifest clinical disorder in anomalous left coronary artery therefore is left ventricular failure secondary to extensive myocardial ischemia. As a result, children with anomalous left coronary arteries are generally referred to the echocardiographic laboratory to define the cause of their left ventricular dysfunction. The differential diagnosis includes congestive cardiomyopathy, myocarditis, or an anomalous coronary artery. An anomalous coronary artery is suspected when an ischemic pattern of left ventricular contraction is observed. This ischemic pattern is usually characterized by an extensive area of anterolateral hypokinesis or akinesis, myocardial thinning, and decreased systolic muscular thickening. The area of hypofunction may be made more obvious by compensatory hyperfunction, often observed at the base of the septum in a region supplied by the normal coronary artery.[9] Although not uniformly present, the area of relative hyperfunction is of diagnostic aid when apparent.

Children with congestive cardiomyopathy typically have uniform dilation of the left and right ventricles with diffuse hypokinesis. Myocarditis may produce either diffuse or focal left ventricular dysfunction. When a specific area of the left ventricle is involved, however, it is rarely isolated to the anterolateral wall and is rarely associated with hyperfunction of the remainder of the ventricle.

The observation of severe left ventricular dysfunction, particularly a pattern consistent with left ventricular ischemia, in an infant or small child therefore should alert the examiner to the possibility of the presence of an anomalously arising coronary artery. This diagnosis may be confirmed by directly examining the coronary arteries. An anomalous origin of a coronary vessel is characterized by the following: (1) failure to demonstrate a connection between the abnormally arising vessel and the aortic lumen; (2) dilation of the opposite normally inserting vessel; and (3) retrograde flow from the anomalously arising vessel within the pulmonary artery. In some situations, the insertion of the anomalous coronary artery into the pulmonary trunk may be seen; however, this feature of the disorder is more difficult to demonstrate and its presence is not required to confirm the diagnosis.

Figure 34–16 is a cross-sectional echocardiogram from a patient with an anomalous left coronary artery arising from the pulmonary artery. Figure 34–17 illustrates a dilated right coronary artery, characteristic of the syndrome. Figure 34–18 demonstrates serial cross-sectional recordings of the area of expected origin of the left coronary artery in a third patient with an anomalously arising vessel. Figure 34–18B shows an apparent connection of the left coronary artery with the aortic

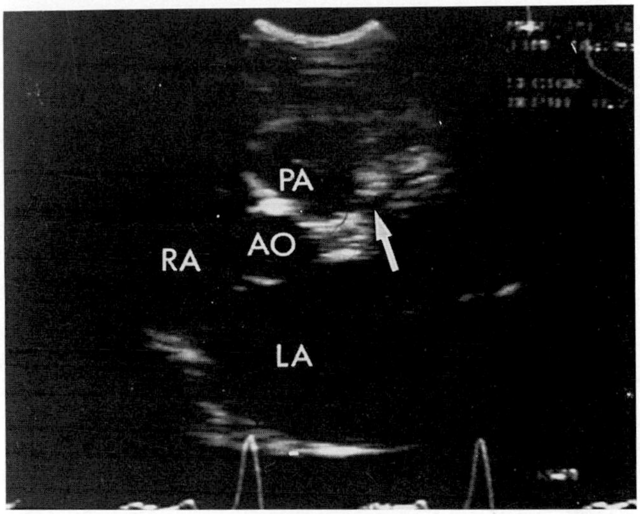

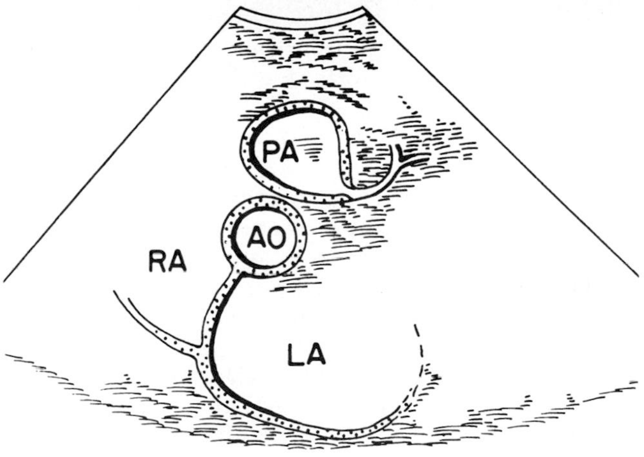

Fig. 34–16. Cross-sectional recording from a patient with anomalous left coronary artery. The anomalous left coronary artery is imaged as it arises from the pulmonary artery in the parasternal short axis view. PA = pulmonary artery; AO = aorta; RA = right atrium; LA = left atrium.

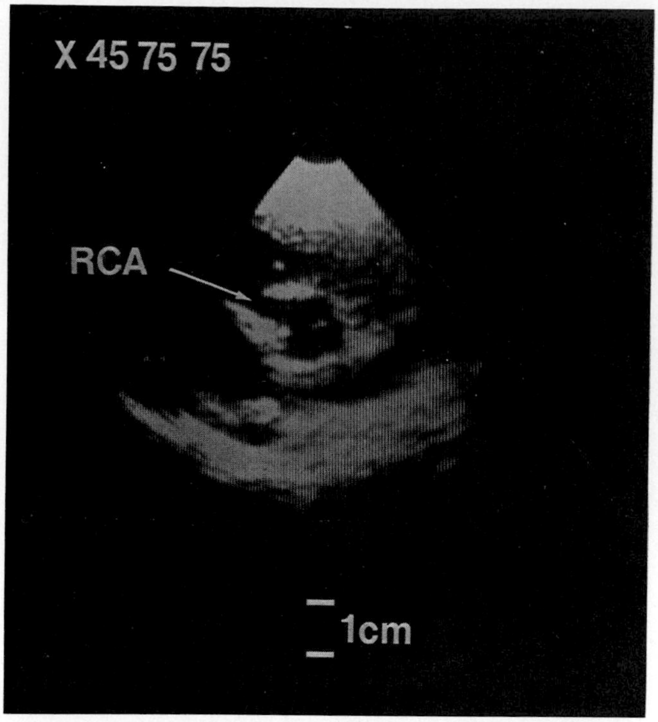

Fig. 34–17. Cross-sectional recording of the right coronary artery (RCA) in a patient with an anomalous left coronary artery arising from the pulmonary artery. There is significant dilation of the RCA which must now bear the entire circulation of the heart. The left coronary artery is not visualized in this plane.

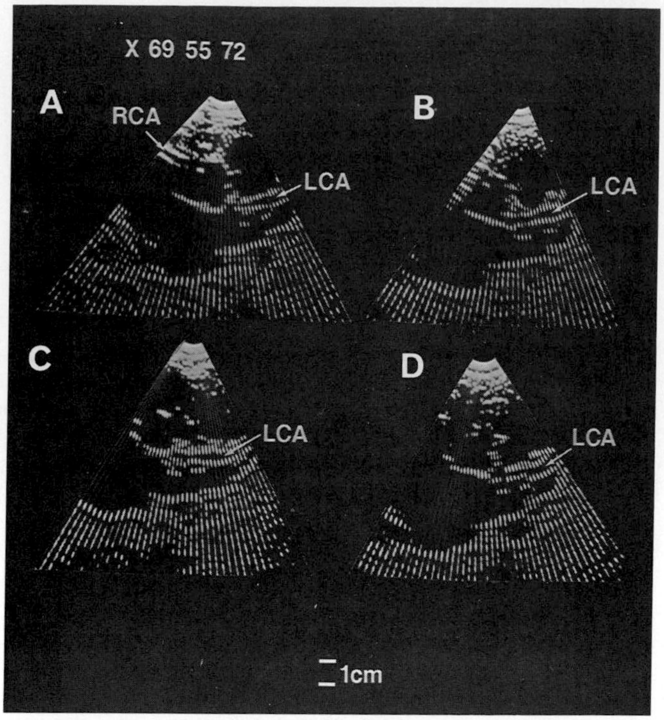

Fig. 34–18. Serial cross-sectional recordings of the area of expected origin of the left main coronary artery (LCA) in a third patient with an anomalously arising left coronary artery. This figure clearly illustrates the close proximity of the left main coronary system to the pulmonary artery. **A.** No continuity between the left coronary artery (LCA) and aorta is evident. **B.** The LCA appears to connect directly to the aortic root. **C.** and **D.** This continuity is no longer apparent. It has been stated that a vessel can be considered to arise normally from the aorta only when it is demonstrated to be continuous with the aortic lumen on three consecutive frames. The difficulties inherent in this type of assessment, however, should be obvious, making the need for abnormal left ventricular function and a dilated right coronary artery (RCA) even more valuable as integral components of this total disease complex.

lumen. This apparent connection is evident in only this one frame, however, not in the preceding (Fig. 34–18A) or in subsequent (Fig. 34–18C and D) frames. It appears that for a vessel to be considered to arise normally from the aorta, it must be demonstrated to be continuous with the aortic lumen on multiple consecutive frames.[9,59]

Figure 34–19A and B shows pre- and postoperative recordings, respectively, from another child with an anomalous left coronary artery. In the preoperative study, the left coronary artery can be visualized arising from the inferior border of the pulmonary artery. In the postoperative study, the reinserted left coronary artery is continuous with the aorta, but it arises at a level anterior to its normal position.

Pulsed Doppler and, more recently, color flow mapping have been useful in the detection of the left-to-right shunt in the pulmonary artery that occurs as a consequence of the anomalous coronary artery.[60,61] Figure 34–20 shows an example of an anomalous left coronary artery arising from the pulmonary artery. In this case, retrograde blood flow entering the pulmonary artery from the anomalous left coronary artery was detected with pulsed Doppler. Figure 34–21 illustrates the same phenomenon using color flow mapping. In this example, retrograde flow from the left coronary artery is shown in yellow as it enters the pulmonary artery. Antegrade flow, shown in blue, indicates forward systolic flow in the pulmonary artery. Color flow mapping has also been helpful in intraoperative and follow-up assessment of these patients.[61]

Anomalous origin of the right coronary artery from the pulmonary artery is a less common condition. Although these patients are generally asymptomatic and the lesion is frequently undetected until later in life, this anomaly may cause cardiac arrest and sudden death. Therefore, surgical intervention is recommended.[62] Early diagnosis is desirable and may be made by demonstrating the anomalous origin of the right coronary artery from the pulmonary artery using cross-sectional echocardiography.[63] Figure 34–22 contains a series of cross-sectional scans from a patient with anomalous origin of the right coronary artery that was recorded while the transducer was swept from the superior margin of the right coronary artery sinus to the aortic annulus. In these sequential frames, the right coronary artery artery initially appears along the right anterior margin of the aorta, coursing leftward and posteriorly toward the aorta (Fig. 34–22A). It then curves anteriorly around the anterior margin of the aortic root, where its lumen appears to be continuous with that of the pulmonary artery (Fig. 34–22B). Normal connection of the right coronary artery with the aorta is not visualized (Fig. 34–22C and D).

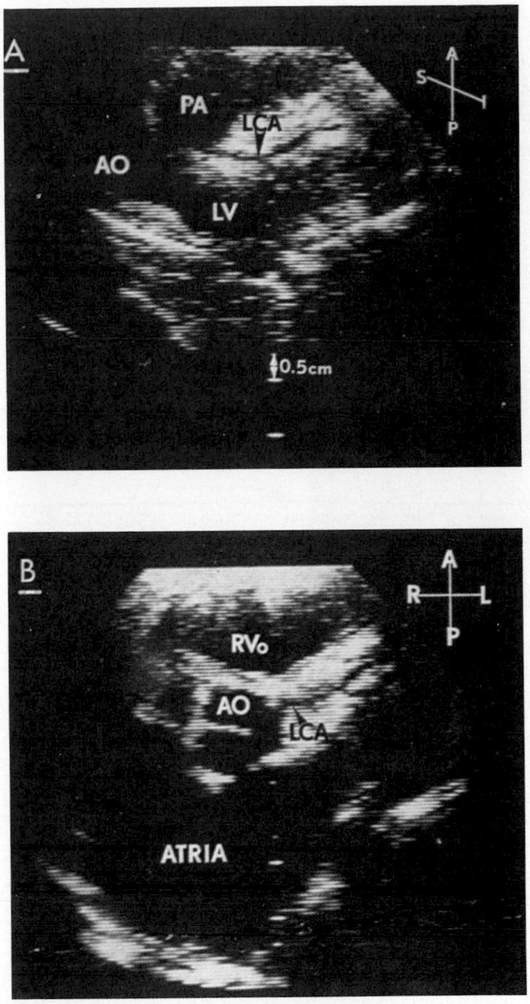

Fig. 34–19. Pre- and postoperative recordings of an anomalous left coronary artery (LCA) **A.** The anomalous vessel before the operation originates from the inferior border of the pulmonary artery (PA). **B.** After the surgical procedure, the anomalous LCA has been reinserted into the aortic root. However, the point of origin is abnormally high, and the vessel courses to the left at an angle more anterior than usual. AO = aorta; LV = left ventricle; RVo = right ventricular outflow tract. (From Fisher EA, et al.: Two-dimensional echocardiographic visualization of the left coronary artery in anomalous origin of the left coronary artery from the pulmonary artery: pre and postoperative studies. Circulation 63:698, 1981. Reproduced by permission of the American Heart Association, Inc.)

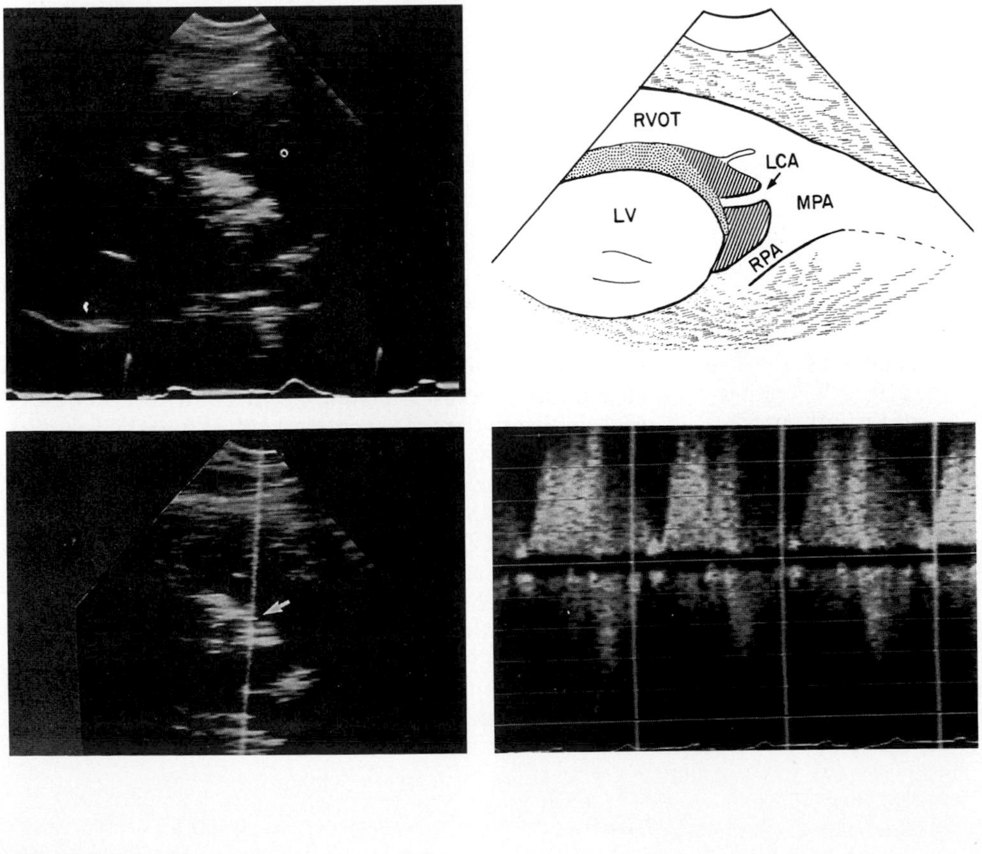

Fig. 34–20. Cross-sectional echocardiogram of a patient with an anomalous coronary artery arising from the pulmonary artery. In this case, the Doppler sample volume was placed at the origin of the anomalous left coronary artery (LCA), and retrograde blood flow entering the pulmonary artery from the anomalous artery is recorded by pulsed Doppler. RVOT = right ventricular outflow tract; MPA = main pulmonary artery; RPA = right pulmonary artery; LV = left ventricle.

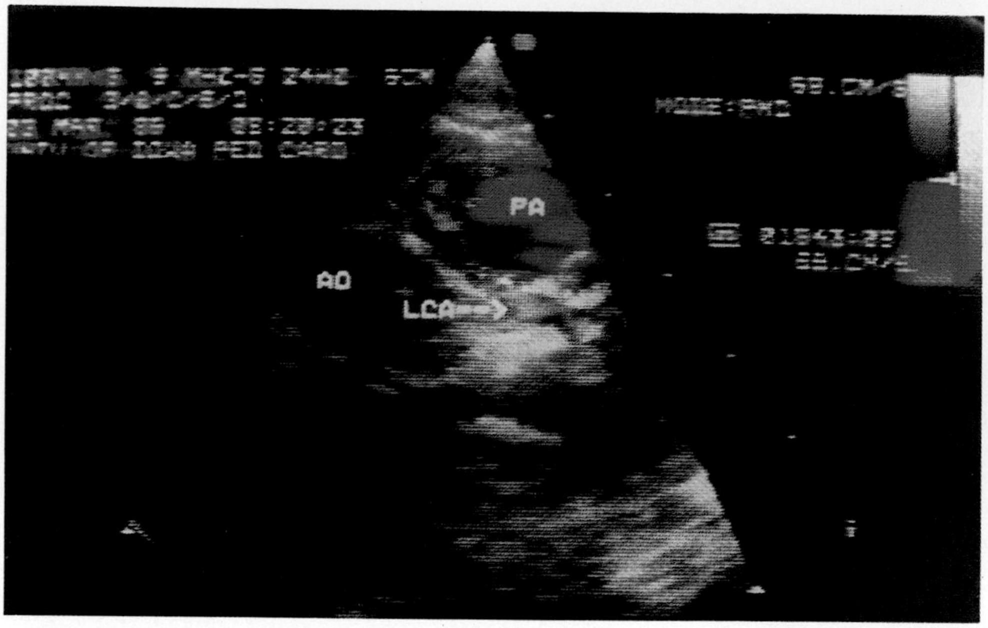

Fig. 34–21. Retrograde flow from the left coronary artery in yellow as it enters the pulmonary artery. Antegrade flow, shown in blue, indicates forward systolic flow in the pulmonary artery. PA = pulmonary artery; LCA = left coronary artery; AO = aorta. (From Baldwin HS, et al.: Color flow mapping of anomalous origin of the left coronary artery from the pulmonary artery. Echocardiography 5:179, 1988.)

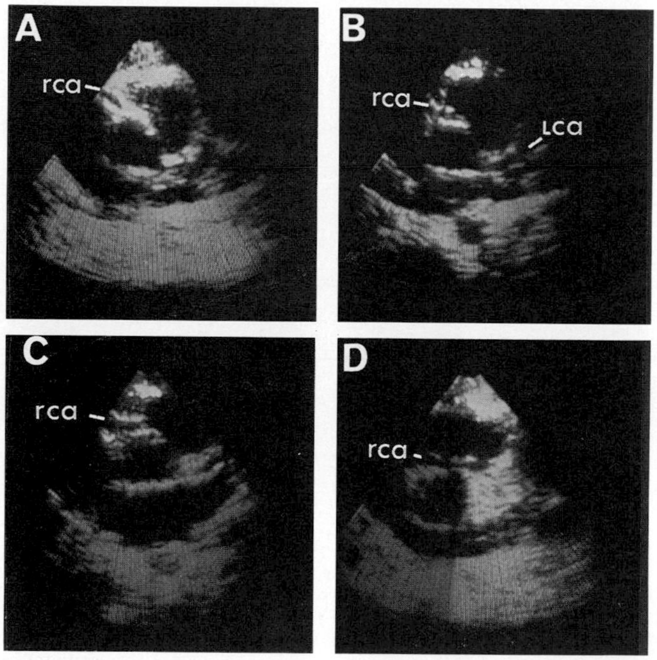

Fig. 34–22. Serial cross-sectional scans from the superior margin of the right coronary sinus of Valsalva to the aortic annulus in a patient with an anomalously arising right coronary artery (rca). **A.** The rca can be visualized in the upper left margin of the scan (horizontal arrow) coursing to the left and posteriorly. **B.** The rca bends slightly to the left. **C.** The rca crosses the top of the aortic root. **D.** The rca continues over the top of the aortic root. In both **C** and **D,** the rca appears to be continuous with the lumen of the pulmonary artery. At no point is it observed to connect with the aortic root. lca = left coronary artery. (Courtesy of Dr. RL Caldwell.)

Left-to-right shunt flow into the pulmonary artery can be variable in size and may be demonstrated by Doppler color flow mapping at the site where the jet enters the pulmonary artery trunk.[64] Dilation of the opposite coronary artery also occurs in anomalous right coronary insertion.

ANOMALOUS ORIGIN FROM THE AORTA

Anomalous sites of origin of either the right or left coronary artery from the aorta are reported in roughly 0.5% of patients undergoing coronary cineangiography. Clinically, anomalous origin of the left main coronary artery from the right coronary sinus or right coronary artery is the most important of these anomalies because it is frequently associated with ischemia, arrhythmias, and sudden death. Anomalous origin of the left circumflex coronary artery from the right sinus of Valsalva or the right coronary artery is noted most commonly (0.3%), but it is usually benign. Anomalous origin of the right coronary artery occurs less frequently.[65] Aberrantly arising left main coronary arteries can be subdivided into those in which the abnormally arising vessel passes (1) above both the aorta and right ventricular outflow tract, (2) beneath the aorta, (3) within the ventricular septum beneath the right ventricular infundibulum, or (4) between the two great vessels. When the left main coronary artery passes anterior to the pulmonary trunk, symptoms of myocardial ischemia do not occur unless significant atherosclerosis is present. The same, with rare exceptions, can be said for vessels that course beneath the aorta. When the anomalous arterial branch connecting the left circumflex and left anterior descending systems with the aorta courses between the infundibulum and the anterior aortic wall, a significant incidence of sudden death has been reported.[65] Sudden death occurs most commonly in young males, predominantly after vigorous physical exertion. The precise mechanism by which anomalously arising left coronary arteries that pass between the aorta and pulmonary trunk cause myocardial ischemia is unclear; however, three mechanisms have been proposed. The first relates to the path of the vessel at its origin. Normal coronary arteries course directly away from the center of the aorta at their origin, whereas these anomalous vessels turn abruptly to follow the wall of the aorta toward the left, thus creating a right-angle bend at the origin of the vessel. This may predispose the vessel to kinking as the aorta and pulmonary artery expand to accommodate increased flow during exercise. Second, the ostium of the anomalous vessels is often slitlike, in contrast to the normal coronary orifice, which is round. This feature may reduce the ability of the artery to increase flow in response to exercise. Finally, the firmly anchored root of the pulmonary trunk together with the expanding aorta may compress the anomalous vessel in a "hemodynamic vise" during vigorous exercise. Because the left main coronary artery is the equivalent of two arteries (the left anterior descending and the circumflex), any narrowing of the vessel is particularly perilous, and any potential compromise of this vessel would be exacerbated by physical exertion.[62]

The ability to detect this condition by means of two-dimensional echocardiography has been described.[66] This is of particular importance because this technique allows the noninvasive screening of young patients having exertional chest pain, syncope, or ventricular tachycardia. In this situation, the diagnosis of anomalous origin of the left coronary artery can be established if the abnormally arising vessel is visualized or ruled out if a normal origin of the artery is found. If the condition is recognized or suspected, selective contrast cineangiography is indicated. Figure 34–23 is an example of an anomalous left coronary system arising from the right coronary artery just distal to the coronary ostium. The anomalous left coronary artery then courses rightward and slightly posteriorly between the pulmonary infundibulum and aorta. After passing beyond the lateral margin of the aorta, it bifurcates into the left anterior descending and left circumflex branches.

Anomalous origin of the circumflex artery from the right coronary sinus of Valsalva or the right coronary artery is generally without clinical significance. The anomalous artery typically passes beneath the aorta, and ischemia is unusual in the absence of associated atherosclerotic disease. Detection of this anomaly is important when surgery is planned, however, because failure to recognize the second ostium arising from the right coronary sinus or placement of the perfusion cannula in the right coronary artery beyond the take-off of the left circumflex artery can result in ischemia of the myocardium perfused by the vessel. Figure 34–24 illustrates the origin and course of an anomalous circumflex coronary artery arising from the right coronary sinus of Valsalva.

Anomalous origin of the right coronary artery from the left sinus of Valsalva is an uncommon abnormality. Usually, the anomalous coronary artery arises anterior to the left main coronary artery and passes between the aorta and the pulmonary artery to reach the right atrioventricular groove. Although this abnormality was previously considered benign, it has recently been associated with cardiac dysfunction including myocardial infarction and sudden death.[67] The mechanism of myocardial ischemia appears to be the same as in those patients in whom the left coronary artery arises from the right sinus of Valsalva and courses between the aorta and pulmonary artery. Myocardial infarction in the absence of atherosclerosis has also been described in patients with anomalous origin of the right coronary artery from the left sinus of Valsalva, even when the aberrant coronary artery courses posterior to the aorta or anterior to the pulmonary artery.[68] Figure 34–25 shows an example of a right coronary artery originating from the aorta, slightly anterior to the normal site of origin of the left main coronary artery. The aberrant artery courses superiorly and toward the right, passing between the aorta and the right ventricular outflow tract.

The left anterior descending and the left circumflex coronary arteries may originate from two separate ostia in the left sinus of Valsalva. In this case, the origin of the right coronary artery should be imaged at its normal site in the right sinus of Valsalva. This anomaly is common and has been reported in approximately 1% of cases

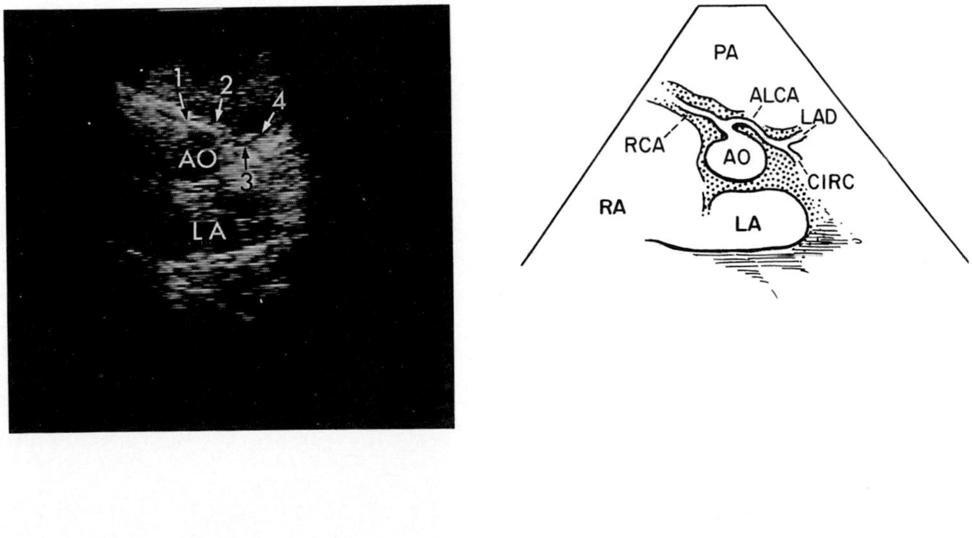

Fig. 34–23. Parasternal recording with the scan plane aligned oblique to the short axis of the aorta (AO) and left atrium (LA) illustrates an anomalous left coronary artery (ALCA) arising from the right coronary artery (RCA). Arrow 1 points to the origin of the ALCA from the proximal RCA. The left coronary artery then courses between the aorta and right ventricular infundibulum (arrow 2). After crossing beneath the pulmonary artery (PA), it then bifurcates (arrow 3) into the left anterior descending (LAD) (4) and circumflex (CIRC) branches. RA = right atrium.

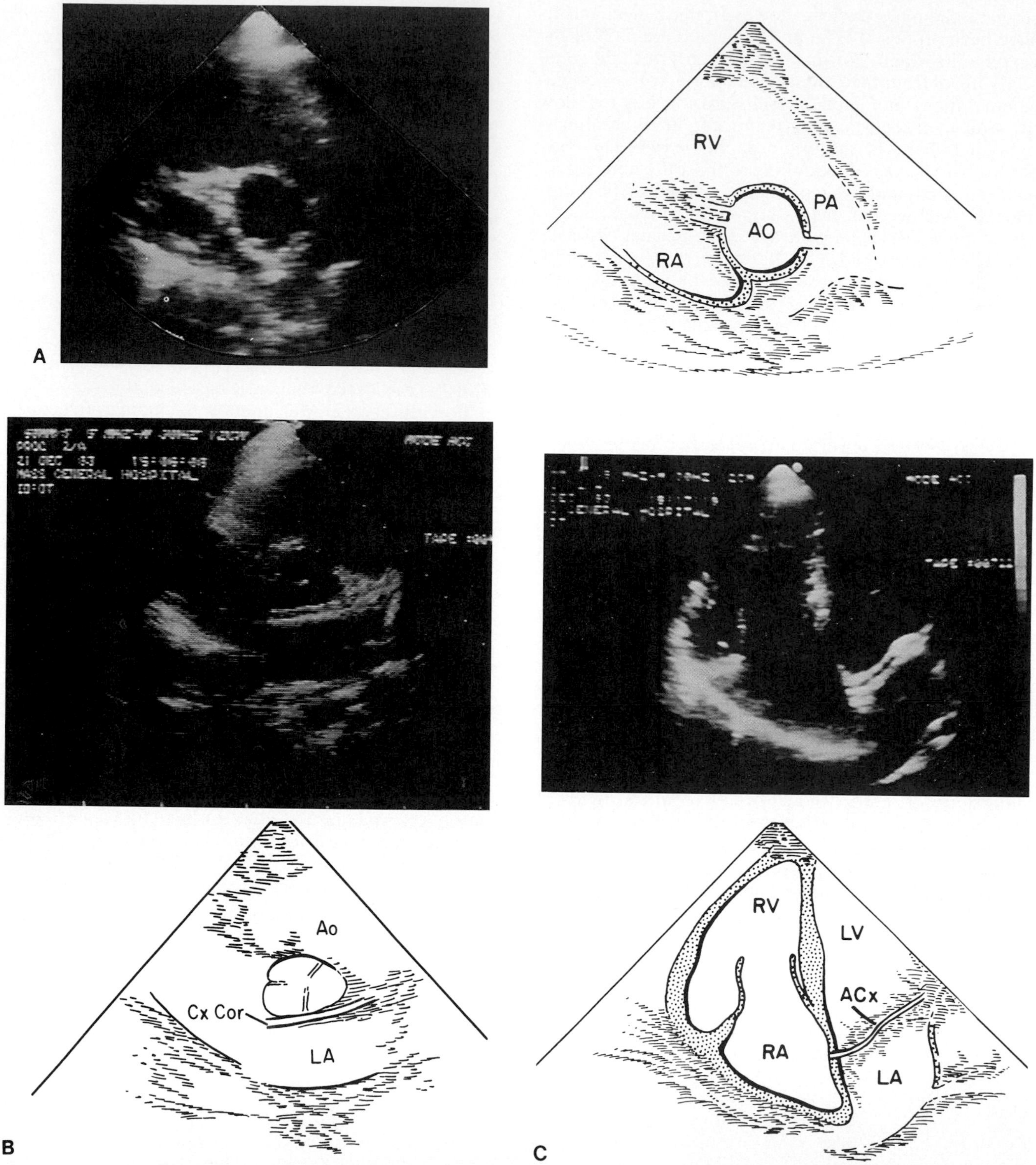

Fig. 34–24. Cross-sectional echocardiograms of a patient with an anomalous circumflex coronary artery arising from the right coronary sinus. **A.** Origin of the right coronary artery (superior) and circumflex from the right coronary sinus of Valsalva. **B.** The anomalous circumflex coronary artery (Cx Cor) coursing beneath the aorta. **C.** The anomalous circumflex coronary artery (ACx) from the apical four-chamber view as it passes beneath the aorta to enter the left atrioventricular groove. PA = pulmonary artery; RV = right ventricle; RA = right atrium; AO = aorta; LA = left atrium; LV = left ventricle; LA = left atrium.

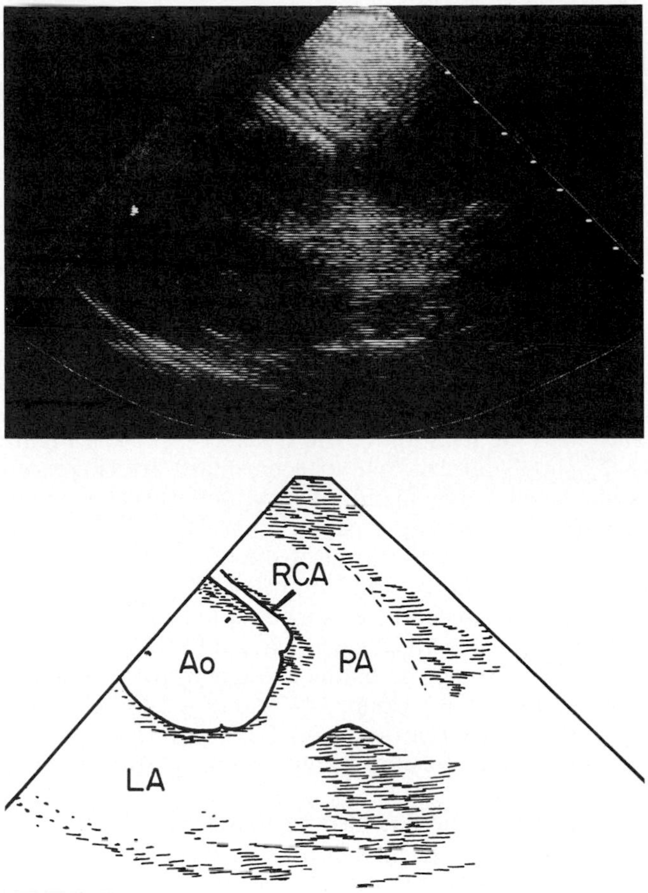

Fig. 34–25. Long axis recording of a right coronary artery artery (RCA) originating from the left coronary sinus of Valsalva, slightly anterior to the normal site of origin of the left main coronary artery. The aberrant artery courses superiorly and toward the right, passing between the aorta (Ao) and the right ventricular outflow tract. PA = pulmonary artery; LA = left atrium.

at necropsy. It does not appear to have any clinical significance.[62] Figure 34–26 shows the left anterior descending and the left circumflex coronary arteries originating from two separate orifices at the left sinus of Valsalva.

CORONARY ARTERY FISTULAS

Coronary artery fistula is a rare anomaly in which a direct precapillary communication exists between a coronary artery and a cardiac chamber, the pulmonary artery, the coronary sinus, or the superior vena cava. Congenital coronary fistulas result from the persistence of embryonic intertrabecular spaces or sinusoids or, in the case of the pulmonary artery, from connections through small accessory conal arteries between the proximal left or right coronary arteries and the main pulmonary artery. Although most coronary artery fistulas are congenital, they may occur after penetrating or nonpenetrating (blunt) chest trauma or as a result of repeat endomyocardial biopsies in recipients of orthotopic heart transplant.[69,70,70a,b]

Coronary artery fistulas are reported in 0.2% of angiograms and become apparent clinically in 0.07% of patients with congenital heart disease.[71,71a] They form the most common group of hemodynamically significant congenital coronary artery anomalies.[72] These lesions are usually isolated, but in approximately 3% of cases, the contralateral coronary artery may be absent.[73] Of 363 cases reviewed, 50% arose from the right coronary artery or its branch, 42% from the left anterior descending or circumflex arteries or their branches, and 5% from multiple vessels.[72] Most commonly, fistulas drain into the right ventricle (41%), followed by the right atrium (26%), pulmonary artery (17%), coronary sinus (7%), left atrium (5%), left ventricle (3%), and superior vena cava (1%). Thus, left-to-right shunt flow occurs in more than 90% of these lesions.

In most cases, the shunt size is small and myocardial blood flow is not compromised.[74] The majority of patients are asymptomatic and are seen because of a murmur detected incidentally, which is often loud, continuous, and superficial. The murmur is loudest at the distal drainage site of the fistula. In one series, half the patients developed symptoms of ventricular dysfunction or angina with increasing age,[74] although these complications have not been as common in the experience of other investigators.[67] Complications of coronary artery fistulas include large left-to-right shunt flow producing pulmonary hypertension and congestive heart failure, thrombosis, infective endocarditis, rupture of the fistula

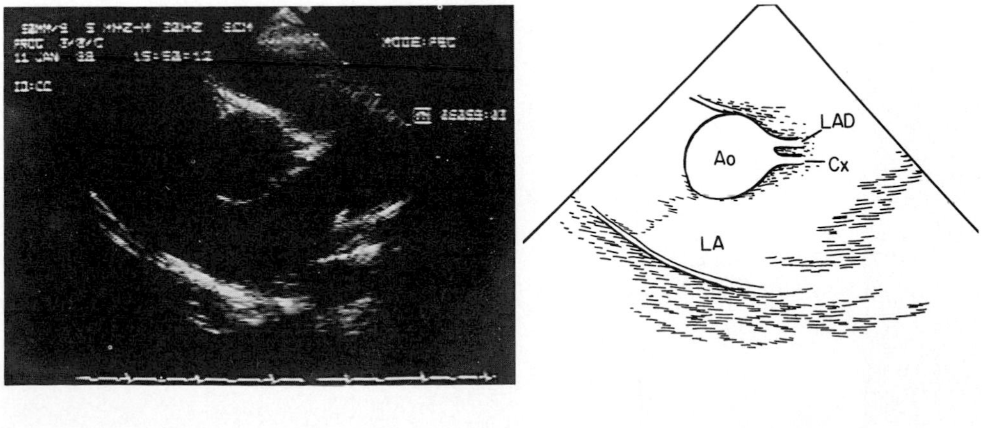

Fig. 34–26. Separate origin of left anterior descending (LAD) and the left circumflex coronary (Cx) arteries from the left sinus of Valsalva. Ao = aorta; LA = left atrium.

or an associated aneurysm, myocardial ischemia, and less commonly, myocardial infarction.[74–76]

Coronary arteriography has been used for the definitive diagnosis of this condition because it allows the precise delineation of the entire extent of the fistula, including its proximal and distal drainage sites. The proximal portion of the coronary artery up to the fistula is usually dilated because of increased blood flow from shunting. The size of the artery generally is related to the size of the shunt. Distal to the origin of the fistula, the size of the coronary artery is usually normal.

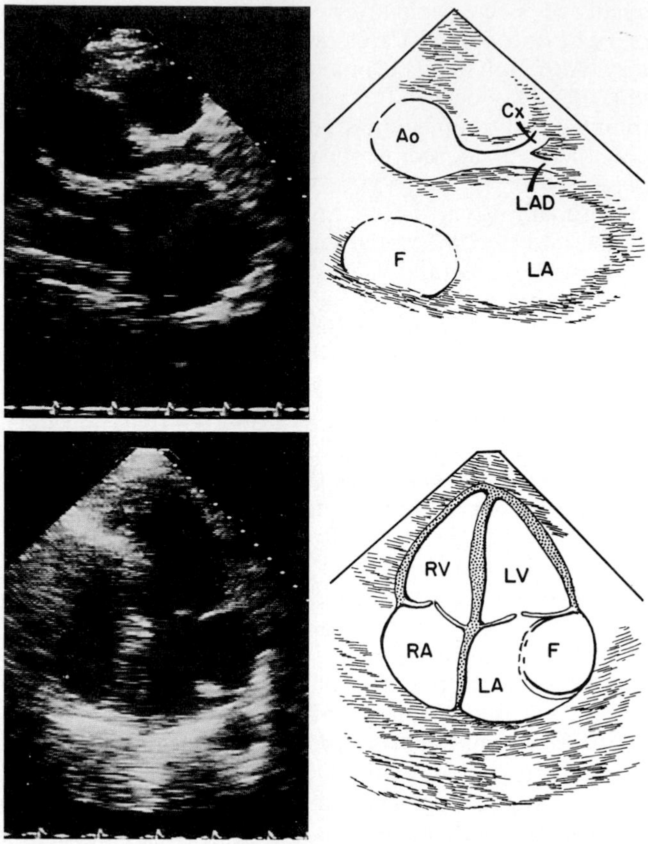

Fig. 34–27. Parasternal and apical recordings of a coronary arteriovenous fistula. Top. Dilated left main circumflex (Cx) and left anterior descending (LAD) coronary arteries. In addition, an echo-free space representing the large coronary fistula is recorded protruding into the left atrium (LA). Bottom. The fistula is imaged from the apical four-chamber view encroaching on the LA. Ao = aorta; F = coronary arteriovenous fistula; RV = right ventricle; RA = right atrium; LV = left ventricle.

More recently, two-dimensional echocardiography has been used to evaluate patients with coronary artery fistulas.[77–81] The usual findings are significant dilation of the coronary artery supplying the fistula and a normal contralateral artery. As a rule, these changes are best visualized at the origins of the arteries from the aorta using a parasternal view.[77–79,82,83] Distal portions of the dilated coronary artery may also be visualized in most cases. The appropriate views depend on the coronary artery and the location of the fistula.[69,78,81,82,84] Figure 34–27 shows an example of a coronary arteriovenous fistula diagnosed by means of two-dimensional echocardiography. In the upper panel, a parasternal short axis echocardiogram at the level of the aorta shows dilated left main, circumflex, and left anterior descending coronary arteries. An echo-free space representing the coronary fistula is also visualized adjacent to the left atrium. In the lower panel, the fistula is imaged from the apical four-chamber view. Figure 34–28 shows another example of a coronary arteriovenous fistula. In this case, the fistula originates from the right coronary artery, which is also dilated.

In some cases, it may also be possible to visualize the distal portion of the fistula and its drainage site. The appropriate echocardiographic views obviously depend on the structure into which drainage occurs. If the left-to-right shunt is sufficiently large, the chambers and vessels receiving the increased flow will also be dilated (Fig. 34–29A and B).

Pulsed Doppler echocardiography enables one to see abnormal blood flow velocity patterns associated with many coronary artery fistulas.[85–87] Sampling in the proximal dilated portion of the fistula may demonstrate continuous unidirectional blood flow with accentuation during diastole.[85] In some cases, abnormal turbulent flow is present as during systole.[86]

If a coronary artery fistula is suspected, Doppler examination of potential receiving chambers or vessels (i.e., right ventricle, right atrium, pulmonary artery, and superior vena cava) should be performed meticulously.

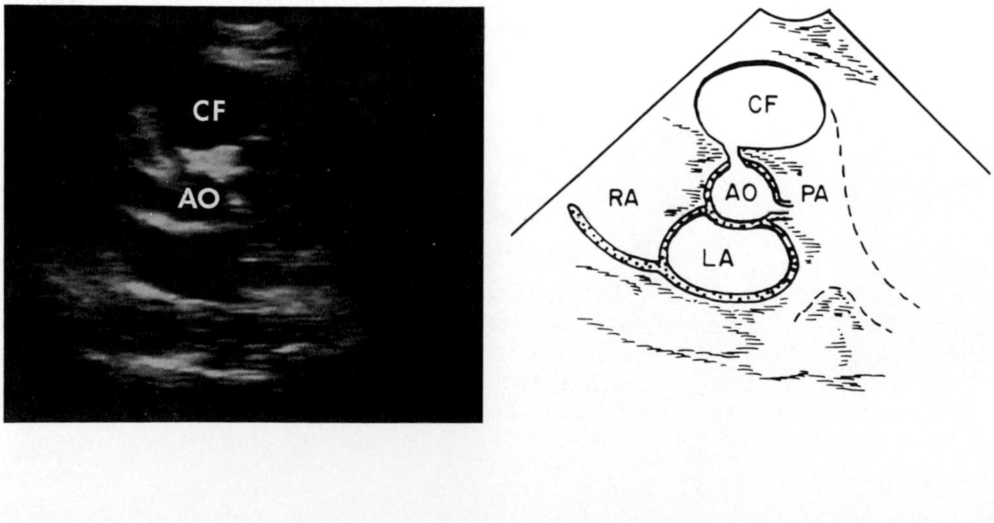

Fig. 34–28. Coronary arteriovenous fistula originating from the right coronary artery. CF = coronary fistula; AO = aorta; PA = pulmonary artery; RA = right atrium; LA = left atrium.

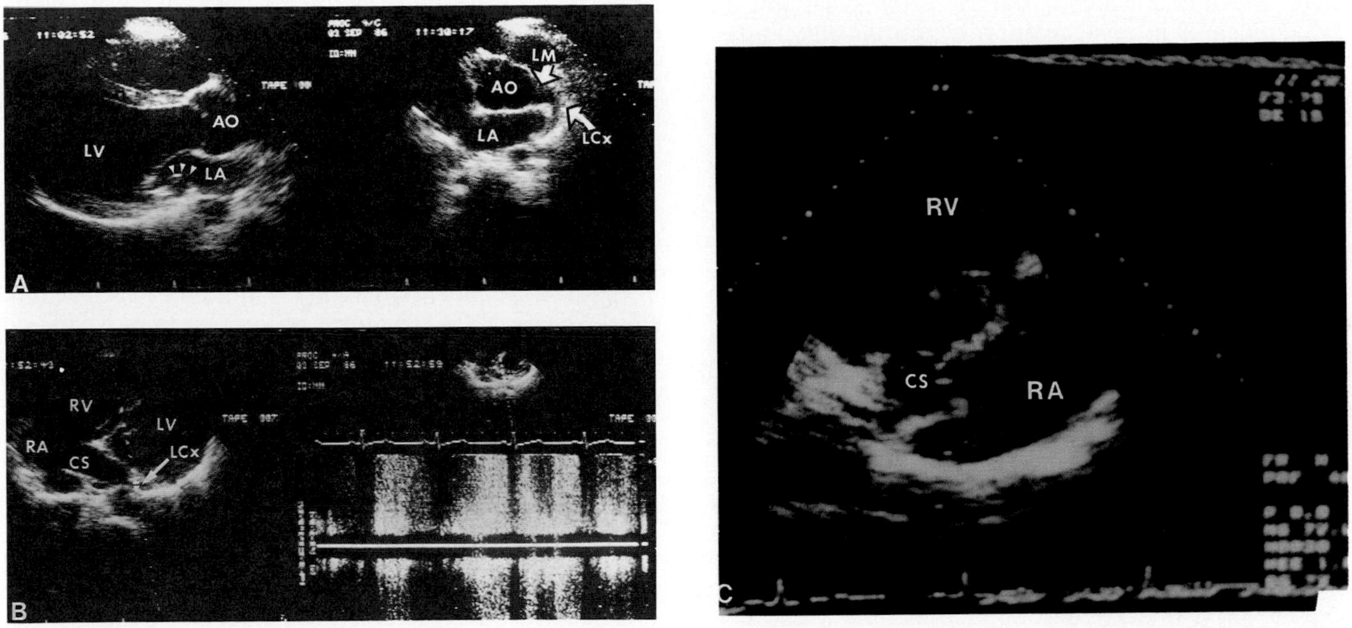

Fig. 34–29. Coronary arteriovenous fistula draining into the coronary sinus. **A.** Left. Arrowheads indicate a dilated coronary sinus imaged in the parasternal long axis view. Right. Short axis view at the level of the aorta (AO) shows dilated left main (LM) and circumflex (LCx) coronary arteries that feed the fistula. LV = left ventricle; LA = left atrium. **B.** Left. Modified apical four-chamber view shows the distal portion of the fistula as it drains into the coronary sinus (CS). A continuous flow velocity signal originating from the fistula was obtained at the site of drainage. RV = right ventricle; RA = right atrium. **C.** Color flow recording of high velocity blood flow from the partially obstructive CS into the RA.

Turbulent flow is usually found at the site of opening of the fistula.[81,85,87] Color flow mapping greatly facilitates this process. Figure 34–29C is an example of high velocity blood flow from the coronary sinus through a relatively restrictive orifice into the right atrium. Figure 27–50 illustrates drainage of a small arteriovenous fistula into the pulmonary artery.

Surgical closure of a coronary artery fistula is indicated when the shunt flow exceeds 1.5:1 or when the patient has symptoms of heart failure.[48] The prognosis after surgery is excellent, but the coronary artery may remain dilated for many years thereafter. Spontaneous closure of a fistula has been reported in young patients. In the adult, this may occur as a result of atherosclerosis.[67]

DIFFERENTIAL DIAGNOSIS OF DILATED CORONARY ARTERIES

The previous sections of this chapter describe several causes of coronary artery dilation. These include coronary artery aneurysms, dilation of the contralateral vessel in patients with anomalous origin of a coronary artery from the pulmonary trunk, and coronary arteriovenous fistula. The coronary arteries may also be dilated in patients with increased left ventricular mass, particularly in association with left ventricular dilation such as occurs in volume overload. The differentiation of these conditions is simple. Aneurysms are generally focal, may be multiple, involve the proximal vessels preferentially, and are not typically associated with increased flow, abnormal drainage, or abnormal left ventricular function. In anomalous origin of a coronary artery, the left ventricle is dilated and function is severely impaired. The anomalous vessel can often be visualized arising from the pulmonary artery, and retrograde flow from the anomalous vessel can be recorded in the pulmonary artery. Coronary arteriovenous fistulas produce the most striking coronary dilation, generally affect only one vessel (i.e., the left or right coronary artery), are associated with increased flow, and may cause dilation of the receiving chambers. Left ventricular function is usually normal. Coronary dilation from increased left ventricular mass and excessive contractile demand is symmetric and involves both proximal and distal vessels. Although the coronary dilation may be striking, the ventricular abnormality typically predominates.

Recent Developments in the Assessment of Coronary Arteries and Flow

Several recent developments have significantly extended the role of echocardiography in assessing the coronary arteries. They include the use of high frequency epicardial echocardiography to image the coronary arterial wall and lumen intraoperatively, visualization of coronary anatomy and flow from the esophagus, and the development of intravascular probes for the direct imaging of the coronary arteries from within the vascular lumen.[88,89] These techniques are discussed in detail in Chapter 16, and hence only the potential clinical applications are reviewed in this section.

HIGH FREQUENCY EPICARDIAL ECHOCARDIOGRAPHY (HFEE)

Epicardial coronary imaging is generally performed in the operating room by the surgeon. To image the coronary arteries, a sterilized, high frequency (12- to 20-MHz) two-dimensional echocardiographic transducer is placed directly against the epicardial surface of the heart in a region overlying the artery of interest. Two-dimensional imaging and pulsed and color flow Doppler recordings can all be obtained. Excellent agreement has been found between coronary arterial luminal diameter and wall thickness measured by this technique when compared with histologic specimens and in vivo data obtained with implanted sonomicrometers.[90] The percentage of reduction in luminal diameter from coronary stenoses measured by this technique also correlates well with that obtained by coronary angiography.[90] Because this technique allows the direct quantification of the extent of coronary atherosclerosis in patients undergoing coronary artery bypass surgery, the nature and precise location of atherosclerotic plaques may be readily determined by the surgeon at the time of operation. The identification of arterial segments free of disease may also help to improve the selection of anastomotic sites for the insertion of bypass grafts. High frequency epicardial echocardiography may also be used to image and identify coronary arteries when a major portion of the artery is embedded in fat or obscured by myocardial bridging or epicardial scarring, thus avoiding time-consuming exploration at the time of surgery.

In addition to the foregoing applications, this technique permits the immediate assessment of coronary bypass anastomoses intraoperatively. Long and short axis images of graft anastomoses permit the measurement of the maximal luminal diameter at the anastomotic site. It is thus possible immediately after the attachment of a coronary bypass graft to detect technical errors that may not be recognized by external inspection alone.[89] This detection allows immediate correction of any mechanical problems and avoids potential complications in the early postoperative period.

Epicardial echocardiography is limited by cardiac motion, which causes structures of interest to move in and out of the imaging plane. Stop-frame analysis may therefore be necessary. This problem may also be overcome by imaging the arteries while the heart is fibrillating and the patient is supported by cardiopulmonary bypass. The coronary arteries are partially collapsed during bypass, however, and this situation prevents reliable measurement of the degree of stenosis due to atherosclerotic lesions. Another limitation of the technique is that the probe, by virtue of its size, does not permit imaging of the right coronary artery, the posterior portion of left circumflex artery, or grafts to those vessel segments without retraction of the heart.

The use of pulsed Doppler echocardiography in conjunction with epicardial two-dimensional echocardiography has been described experimentally and intra-operatively in assessing blood flow velocities in coronary arteries and bypass grafts. This information complements that obtained from two-dimensional imaging alone and permits the monitoring of steady-state flow as well as changes in blood flow in response to interventions. More recently, epicardial color flow mapping has emerged as a tool for evaluating the pattern and physiologic responses of flow in normal and stenotic coronary arteries (Fig. 34–30). The role of high frequency epicardial echocardiography for intraoperative assessment of coronary anatomy and blood flow continues to be of major interest for future investigation.

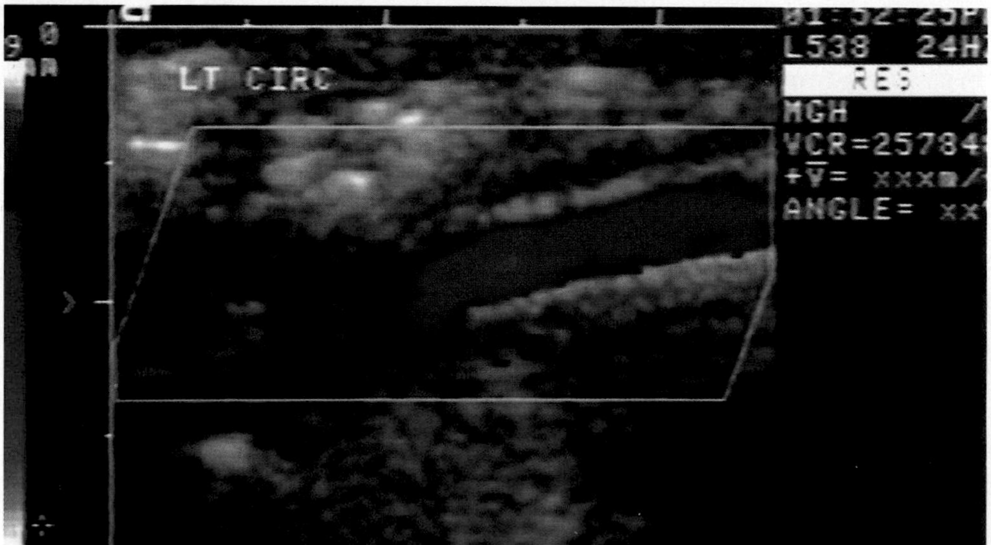

Fig. 34–30. High frequency epicardial color flow image of a normal left circumflex coronary artery in long axis.

TRANSESOPHAGEAL IMAGING

Transesophageal two-dimensional and Doppler echocardiography permit study of the heart and great vessels in great detail because of the proximity of these structures to the esophagus. From this approach, it is possible to image the proximal portions of the coronary arteries as they originate from the aortic root. The technical aspects and examination technique of transesophageal echocardiography are described in detail in Chapter 16.

Visualization of the proximal coronary arteries is possible using the esophageal short axis view of the aortic valve. To image the left coronary artery, the transducer is positioned superior to the aortic valve cusps and is rotated slightly to the left and is angulated anteriorly until the left main coronary artery becomes apparent. With slight rotation and withdrawal of the transducer upward in the esophagus, the left main coronary artery can be followed distally and its bifurcation into the left anterior descending and circumflex arteries imaged. The circumflex and left anterior descending coronary arteries can then be followed for several centimeters beyond the bifurcation.

In an early study of 39 patients in a hospital intensive care unit, the left main and left anterior descending coronary arteries could be imaged from the esophagus in 30 patients (77%) and the circumflex artery in 21 (54%).[91] In another report, the proximal left coronary artery was visualized in all 50 patients studied prospectively,[92] whereas in another study that included patients with normal coronary anatomy and patients with coronary stenoses and previous aortocoronary bypass surgery, the proximal left coronary artery was visualized in 96% of 46 patients.[93]

In a group of 18 prospectively studied patients with angiographically defined proximal coronary artery disease, the left main and circumflex coronary arteries were visualized in all 18, but the left anterior descending coronary artery was seen in only 3. Echocardiographic visualization of left main and circumflex coronary artery disease was excellent; however, the echocardiogram caused an overestimation of the degree of stenosis in 5 of 13 patients.[94]

To record the right coronary artery, the endoscope is withdrawn 1 or 2 cm and is tilted anteriorly until the scan plane transects the artery. The origin of the right coronary artery was imaged in only 10 of 39 (25%) patients in one retrospective study,[91] but in all 50 patients in another prospective study.[92] This finding suggests that, when a deliberate search is made, the proximal right coronary artery can usually be readily imaged.

Recently, pulsed and color Doppler capabilities have been added to transesophageal systems and allow the detection of coronary blood flow velocity. Color flow mapping of coronary blood flow may aid in the identification of the proximal and more distal segments of the coronary arteries and in the placement of the pulsed Doppler sample volume for quantitating flow velocities. Figure 34–31 is a transesophageal color flow recording at the aortic valve level illustrating flow in the left main coronary artery. Figure 34–32 is a color flow recording of the left coronary bifurcation and the left anterior descending coronary artery running anteriorly along the interventricular septum.

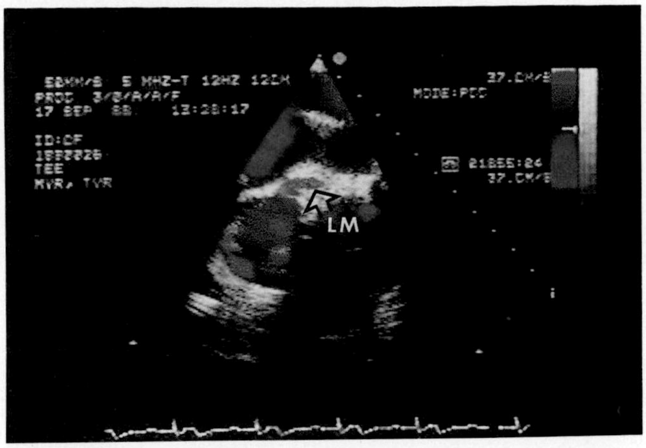

Fig. 34–31. Transesophageal color flow recording of flow within the left main coronary artery (LM) (arrow). Color in the artery is blue, indicating aliased flow.

In preliminary reports, coronary blood flow in the left anterior descending coronary artery was recorded from the esophagus by means of the pulsed Doppler technique in 75 to 90% of patients,[91] with the peak diastolic flow velocities ranging from 40 ± 14 cm/sec to 68 ± 33 cm/sec.[93] In contrast, quantitative right coronary artery flow was obtained in only 26% of patients in whom the right coronary artery was imaged.

Although the noninvasive evaluation of coronary blood flow by the transesophageal pulsed Doppler technique is promising, methodologic problems remain to be solved. The movement of the heart prevents the stable positioning of the sample volume, and the angle of the ultrasound beam with respect to the direction of blood flow is often large. Difficulties in obtaining adequate im-

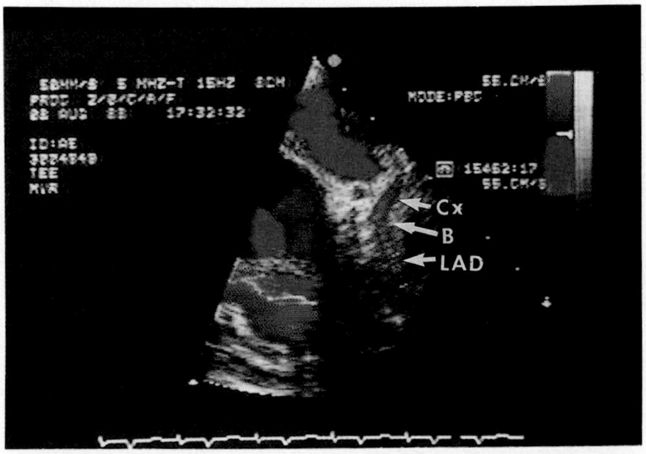

Fig. 34–32. Color flow recording of the bifurcation (B) of the left coronary artery with the left anterior descending (LAD) traveling posterior in the scan planes (away from the transducer in the esophagus) and the circumflex (Cx) anteriorly (toward the transducer).

ages and flow signals from the right coronary artery are common.

INTRA-ARTERIAL ECHOCARDIOGRAPHIC ASSESSMENT OF CORONARY ARTERY LUMEN

Currently, the standard assessment of coronary artery anatomy and the quantification of the severity of coronary stenoses are based on coronary angiography. The limitations of this technique as a "gold standard" for assessing the severity of coronary stenoses are increasingly apparent. These include the large interobserver variability in grading the severity of stenosis, the fact that angiography provides only silhouette images of the coronary arteries in long axis, with the result that eccentric atherosclerotic plaques may cause significant over- or underestimation of stenosis, and the lack of correlation between angiographic assessment of severity and physiologic measures of the significance of obstruction, such as depression of the hyperemic response to transient occlusion.[95–97] Coronary wall thickness, luminal area, and the extent of atherosclerosis would be better assessed if the artery were imaged in its cross section. Intra-arterial imaging of the arteries in cross section has been reported using high frequency transducers (20–30MHz) located at the tips of catheters. Several prototype devices for direct cross-sectional intravascular imaging have been described (see Chapter 16).[98–100] In preliminary studies of normal and pathologic specimens, correlations have been excellent between in vitro and histologic measurements of wall thickness, luminal diameter, and area.[100–102] These images should be of practical utility in guiding techniques such as balloon, laser, and thermal angioplasty of the coronary arteries. The measurements may also be of help in cardiac surgery because if the anatomy of the vessels is precisely defined before the procedure, the morphology and location of the established lesions can easily be reproduced in the operating room, using either epicardial or intravascular imaging. Further technologic improvements such as three-dimensional reconstruction of the tomographic images should aid in the diagnosis and evaluation of coronary artery disease in isolation or in association with therapeutic interventions using catheter-based devices.

In summary, transthoracic coronary imaging is a technically demanding, but fascinating and clinically valuable, technique. To date, the major clinical applications have been in children and adults with congenital anomalies of the coronary arteries or with diseases associated with coronary dilation, rather than in the more prevalent stenotic lesions. The development of new and varied ultrasonic approaches to coronary imaging and flow measurement, however, suggest that echocardiography will play an increasingly important role in the assessment of coronary structure and function.

REFERENCES

1. Weyman AE, et al.: Noninvasive visualization of the left main coronary artery by cross-sectional echocardiography. Circulation 54:169, 1976.
2. Rogers EW, et al.: Evaluation of coronary artery anatomy in vitro by cross-sectional echocardiography. Circulation 62:782, 1980.
3. Ogawa S, et al.: A new approach to visualize the left main coronary artery using apical cross-sectional echocardiography. Am J Cardiol 45:301, 1980.
4. Chen CC, et al.: Differential density and luminal irregularities as criteria to detect disease in the left main coronary artery by apex phased array cross-sectional echocardiography. Am J Cardiol 43:386, 1979.
5. Rogers EW, et al.: Possible detection of atherosclerotic coronary calcification by two-dimensional echocardiography. Circulation 62:1046, 1980.
6. Friedman MJ, et al.: High predictive accuracy for detection of left main coronary artery disease by antilog signal processing of two-dimensional images. Am Heart J 103:194, 1982.
7. Yoshikawa J, et al.: Cross-sectional echocardiographic diagnosis of coronary artery aneurysms in patients with the mucocutaneous lymph node syndrome. Circulation 59:133, 1979.
8. Hiriashi S, Yashiro K, Kusano S: Noninvasive visualization of coronary arterial aneurysm in infants and young children with mucocutaneous lymph node syndrome with two-dimensional echocardiography. Am J Cardiol 43: 1225, 1979.
9. Caldwell RL, et al.: Two-dimensional echocardiographic differentiation of anomalous left coronary artery from congestive cardiomyocardiopathy. Am Heart J 106:710, 1983.
10. Aronow WS, et al.: Left main coronary artery patency assessed by cross-sectional echocardiography and coronary arteriography. Circulation 60(Suppl. II): II-145, 1979.
11. Douglas PS, et al.: Echocardiographic visualization of coronary artery anatomy in the adult. J Am Coll Cardiol 11:565, 1988.
12. Rink LD, et al.: Improved echocardiographic technique for examining the left main coronary artery (abstr.). Am J Cardiol 45:435, 1980.
13. Ryan T, Armstrong WF, Feigenbaum H: Prospective evaluation of the left main coronary artery using digital two-dimensional echocardiography. J Am Coll Cardiol 7:807, 1986.
14. Yoshikawa J, et al.: Ultrasonic features of anomalous origin of the left coronary artery from the pulmonary artery. Jpn Heart J 19:46, 1978.
15. Penther PH, et al.: The length of the left main coronary artery: pathologic features. Am Heart J. 94:705, 1977.
16. Fox C, Davies MJ, Webb-Peploe MM: Length of left main coronary artery. Br Heart J 35:795, 1973.
17. James TM: Anatomy of the Coronary Arteries. Hagerstown, MD, Harper & Row, 1961.
18. James TN: Anatomy of the coronary arteries in health and disease. Circulation 32:1020, 1965.
19. Baraldi G, Scamaggoni G: Coronary Circulation in the Normal and the Pathologic Heart. Washington, DC, U.S. Government Printing Office, 1967.
20. Gramiak R, Nanda NC, Shah PM: Echocardiographic detection of pulmonary valve. Radiology 102:153, 1972.
21. Meyer RA: Echocardiography in assessing cardiac anatomy. J Am Coll Cardiol 5:44S, 1985.
22. Yoshikawa J, et al.: Cross-sectional echocardiographic diagnosis of coronary aneurysms in patients with the mucocutaneous lymph node syndrome. Circulation 59:133, 1979.
23. Capannari TE, et al.: Sensitivity, specificity and predictive value of two-dimensional echocardiography in detecting coronary artery aneurysm in patients with Kawasaki disease. J Am Coll Cardiol. 7:355, 1986.
24. Rink LD, et al.: Echocardiographic detection of left main coronary artery obstruction. Circulation 65:719, 1982.
25. Arjunan K, et al.: Coronary artery caliber in normal children and patients with Kawasaki disease but without aneurysms: an echocardiographic and angiographic study. J Am Coll Cardiol 8:1119, 1986.
26. Marcus ML: The Coronary Circulation in Health and Disease. New York, McGraw-Hill, 1983.
27. Marcus ML, et al.: Measurements of coronary velocity and reactive hyperemia in the coronary circulation of humans. Circ Res 49:877, 1981.
28. Fusejima K: Noninvasive measurement of coronary artery flow using combined two-dimensional and Doppler echocardiography. J Am Coll Cardiol 10:1024, 1987.
29. Fusejima K: Non-invasive analysis of coronary stenotic flow using two dimensional Doppler echocardiography (abstr.). Circulation 78(Suppl. II): 419, 1988.
30. Roberts W: Coronary heart disease: a review of abnormalities observed in the coronary arteries. Cardiovasc Med 2:29, 1977.
31. Chandraratna PAN, Aronow WS: Left main coronary arterial patency assessed with cross-sectional echocardiography. Am J Cardiol 46:91, 1980.
32. Ronderos R, et al.: Value and limitations of two dimensional echocardiography for the detection of left main coronary artery disease. Cleve Clin Q 51:7, 1984.
33. Vered Z, et al.: Two dimensional echocardiographic analysis of proximal left main coronary artery in humans. Am Heart J 112:972, 1986.
34. Malergue MC, et al.: Visualisation par échocardiographie bidimensionnelle du tronc de la coronaire gauche. Arch Mal Coeur Vaiss 76:753, 1983.
35. Ryan T, et al.: Annular array technology: application to cardiac imaging. Echocardiography 4:203, 1987.
36. Presti CF, et al.: Digital two dimensional echocardiographic imaging of the proximal left anterior descending coronary artery. Am J Cardiol 60:1254, 1987.
37. Hurst JW: The Heart. 3rd Ed. New York, McGraw-Hill, 1974.
38. Perloff JK: The Clinical Recognition of Congenital Heart Disease. Philadelphia, W.B. Saunders, 1970.
39. Fujiwara H, Hamashimi Y: Pathology of the heart in Kawasaki disease. Pediatrics 61:100, 1978.

40. Asai T, et al.: Cardiac lesions in Kawasaki's disease: indications for coronary angiography. Jpn J Pediatr 29:1086, 1976.
41. Haba S, et al.: The relationships of coronary artery aneurysm to clinical symptoms and therapy in patients with mucocutaneous lymph node syndrome. Report presented to the Japanese Pediatric Society, Tokyo, 1978.
42. Kawasaki T: Acute febrile mucocutaneous syndrome with lyphoid involvement with specific dequamation of the fingers and toes: clinical description of 50 cases. Jpn J Allergy 16:178, 1967.
43. Stephenson SR: Kawasaki disease in Europe. Lancet 1:373, 1977.
44. Turner-Gomes S, et al.: High persistence rate of established coronary artery lesions secondary to Kawasaki disease among a panethnic Canadian population. J Pediatr 108:928, 1986.
45. Kawasaki T, et al.: A new infantile acute febrile mucocutaneous lymph node syndrome (MLNS) prevailing in Japan. Pediatrics 54:271, 1974.
46. Melish ME, Hicks RM, Larson EJ: Mucocutaneous lymph node syndrome in the United States. Am J Dis Child 130:599, 1976.
47. Chung KJ, et al.: Cardiac and coronary arterial involvement in infants and children from New England with mucocutaneous lymph node syndrome (Kawasaki disease). Am J Cardiol 50:136, 1982.
48. Braunwald E: Heart Disease: A Textbook of Cardiovascular Medicine. 2nd Ed. Philadelphia, W.B. Saunders, 1984.
49. Satomi G, et al.: Systematic visualization of coronary arteries by two-dimensional echocardiography in children and infants: evaluation in Kawasaki's disease and coronary arteriovenous fistulas. Am Heart J 107:497, 1984.
50. Maeda T, et al.: Subcostal 2-dimensional echocardiographic imaging of peripheral left coronary artery aneurysms in Kawasaki disease. Am J Cardiol 52:48, 1983.
51. Yoshida H, et al.: Subcostal two dimensional echocardiographic imaging of periferal right coronary artery in Kawasaki disease. Circulation 65:956, 1982.
52. Yanagisawa M, et al.: Coronary aneurysms in Kawasaki disease: follow-up observation by two-dimensional echocardiography. Pediatr Cardiol 6: 11, 1985.
53. Shimazu S, et al.: Two-dimensional echocardiography of coronary arterial lesions with MCLS in special reference to the comparison with coronary angiography. Acta Paediatr Jpn 83:1632, 1979.
54. Kato H, et al.: Fate of coronary aneurysm in Kawasaki disease: serial coronary angiographic and long-term follow-up study. Am J Cardiol 48: 1758, 1982.
55. Takahashi M, Mason W, Lewis AB: Regression of coronary aneurysms in patients with Kawasaki syndrome. Circulation 75:387, 1987.
56. Nakano H, et al.: Repeated quantitative angiograms in coronary arterial aneurysm in Kawasaki disease. Am J Cardiol 56:846, 1985.
57. Brecker SJD, Gray HH, Oldershaw PJ: Coronary artery aneurysms and myocardial infarction: adult disease or Kawasaki disease? Br Heart J 59: 509, 1988.
58. Oliveira DBG, Foale RA, Bensaid J: Coronary artery aneurysms and Kawasaki disease in an adult. Br Heart J 51:91, 1984.
59. Robinson PJ, et al.: Anomalous origin of the left coronary artery from the pulmonary trunk: potential for false negative diagnosis with cross-sectional echocardiography. Br Heart J 52:272, 1984.
60. Baldwin HS, et al.: Color flow mapping of anomalous origin of the left coronary artery from the pulmonary artery. Echocardiography 5:179, 1988.
61. Swensson RE, et al.: Non invasive Doppler color flow mapping for detection of anomalous origin of the left coronary artery from the pulmonary artery and for evaluation of surgical repair. J Am Coll Cardiol 11:659, 1988.
62. Roberts WC: Major anomalies of coronary arterial origin seen in adulthood. Am Heart J 111:941, 1986.
63. Worsham C, Sanders SP, Bulger BM: Origin of the right coronary artery from the pulmonary trunk: diagnosis by two-dimensional echocardiography. Am J Cardiol 55:232, 1985.
64. Shah RM, et al.: Identification of anomalous origin of the right coronary artery from pulmonary trunk by Doppler color flow mapping. Am J Cardiol 57:366, 1986.
65. Liberthson RR, et al.: Aberrant coronary artery origin from the aorta: diagnosis and clinical significance. Circulation 50:774, 1974.
66. Liberthson RR, et al.: Aberrant origin of the left coronary artery from the proximal right coronary artery: diagnostic features and pre- and postoperative course. Clin Cardiol 5:377, 1982.
67. Douglas JS, Franch RH, King SB: Coronary artery anomalies. *In* King SB, Douglas JS (eds): Coronary Arteriography and Angioplasty. New York, McGraw-Hill, 1985.
68. Chaitman BR, et al.: Clinical and angiographic hemodynamic findings in patients with anomalous origin of the coronary artery. Circulation. 53:122, 1976.
69. Kronzon I, Winer HE, Cohen M: Non-invasive diagnosis of left coronary arteriovenous fistula communicating with the right ventricle. Am J Cardiol 49:1811, 1982.
70. Bravo AJ, et al.: Traumatic coronary arteriovenous fistula: a 20 year follow-up with serial hemodynamic and angiographic studies. Am J Cardiol 27:673, 1971.
70a. Sandler JS, et al.: Coronary artery fistula in the heart transplant patient: a potential complication of endomyocardial biopsy. Circulation 79:350, 1989.
70b. Locke TJ, Furniss SS, McGregor CGA: Coronary artery-right ventricular fistula after endomyocardial biopsy. Br Heart J 60:81, 1988.
71. Keith JD, Rowe RD, Vlad P: Heart Disease in Infancy and Childhood. 3rd Ed. New York, Macmillan, p. 1014, 1978.
71a. Hobbs RE, et al.: Coronary artery fistulae: a 10-year review. Cleve Clin Q 49:191, 1982.
72. Levin DC, Fellows KE, Abrams HL: Hemodynamically significant primary anomalies of the coronary arteries: angiographic aspects. Circulation 58:25, 1978.
73. Oldham HN Jr, et al.: Surgical management of congenital coronary artery fistula. Ann Thorac Surg 12:503, 1971.
74. Liberthson RR, et al.: Congenital coronary arteriovenous fistula. Circulation 59:849, 1979.
75. Trejo JFG, et al.: Fistula arteriovanosa coronaria: estudio de 14 casos. Arch Inst Cardiol Mex 55:153, 1985.
76. Bishop JO, Mathur VS, Gwinn GA: Congenital coronary artery fistula and myocardial infarction. Chest 65:233, 1974.
77. Yoshikawa J, et al.: Noninvasive visualization of the dilated main coronary arteries in coronary artery fistulas by cross-sectional echocardiography. Circulation 65:600, 1982.
78. Chen CC, et al.: Recognition of coronary arterial fistula by Doppler 2-dimensional echocardiography. Am J Cardiol 53:392, 1984.
79. Piot JD, et al.: Echocardiographie bidimensionelle des fistules coronaro-cavitaires. Arch Mal Coeur 78:248, 1985.
80. Agatson AS, et al.: Diagnosis of a right coronary artery-right arterial fistula using two-dimensional and Doppler echocardiography. Am J Cardiol 54: 238, 1984.
81. Sahasakul Y, Chaithiraphan S, Sriyoschati S: Diagnosis of a right coronary artery-left ventricular fistula by cross sectional and Doppler echocardiography. Br Heart J 59:593, 1988.
82. Rodgers DM, et al.: Two-dimensional echocardiographic features of coronary arteriovenous fistula. Am Heart J 104:872, 1982.
83. Slater J, et al.: Doppler echocardiography and computed tomography in diagnosis of coronary arteriovenaous fistula. J Am Coll Cardiol 6:1290, 1985.
84. Reeder GS, et al.: Visualization of coronary artery fistula by two-dimensional echocardiography. Mayo Clin Proc 55:185, 1980.
85. Mitayake K, et al.: Doppler echocardiographic features of coronary arteriovenous fistula. Br Heart J 51:508, 1984.
86. Chin BL, et al.: Two dimensional and pulsed Doppler echocardiographic abnormalities in coronary artery-pulmonary artery fistula. Chest 86:901, 1984.
87. Rein AJJT, Yatsiv I, Simcha A: An unusual presentation or right coronary artery fistula. Br Heart J 59:598, 1988.
88. McPherson DD, et al.: HFE for CA evaluation: in vivo and in vitro validation of arterial lumen and wall thickness measurements. J Am Coll Cardiol 8:600, 1986.
89. Hiratza LF, et al.: The role of intraoperative high-frequency epicardial echocardiography during coronary artery revascularization. Circulation 76(Suppl. V):V–33, 1987.
90. McPherson DD, et al.: Deliniation of the extent of coronary atherosclerosis by high frequency epicardial echocardiography. N Engl J Med 316:304, 1987.
91. Yamagishi M, et al.: Assessment of coronary blood flow by transesophageal two-dimensional pulsed Doppler echocardiography. Am J Cardiol 62: 641, 1988.
92. Zwicky P, et al.: Imaging of coronary arteries by color coded transesophageal Doppler echocardiography. Am J Cardiol 62:639, 1988.
93. Kyo S, et al.: Transesophageal 2-dimensional echo-Doppler visualization of left main coronary arterial anatomy and flow (abstr.). J Am Coll Cardiol 9(Suppl.):179A, 1987.
94. Taams MA, et al.: Detection of proximal left coronary artery stenoses by transesophageal echocardiography (abstr.). Circulation 78(Suppl. II): II-419, 1988.
95. Fisher LD, et al.: Reproducibility of coronary arteriographic reading in the coronary artery surgery study (CASS). Cathet Cardiovasc Diagn 8:565, 1982.
96. White CW, et al.: Does visual interpretation of the coronary arteriogram predict the physiologic importance of coronary stenosis? N Engl J Med 310:819, 1984.
97. Harrison DG, et al.: The value of lesion cross-sectional area determined by quantitative coronary angiography in assessing the physiologic significance of proximal left anterior descending coronary arterial stenosis. Circulation 69:1111, 1984.
98. Bom N, et al.: Ein Weg zur intraluminaren Echoarteriographie. Ultraschall Med 8:233, 1987.
99. Tobis JM, et al.: Intravascular ultrasound visualization before and after balloon angioplasty. Circulation 78(Suppl. II):II-84, 1988.
100. Yock PG, et al.: Real-time, two dimensional catheter ultrasound: a new technique for high-resolution intravascular imaging (abstr.). J Am Coll Cardiol 11:130A, 1988.
101. Pandian NG, et al.: Ultrasound angioscopy: real time, two-dimensional, intraluminal ultrasound imaging of blood vessels. Am J Cardiol 62:493, 1988.
102. Mallery JA, et al.: Intravascular ultrasound imaging catheter assessment of normal and atherosclerotic arterial wall thickness (abstr.). J Am Coll Cardiol 11:22A, 1988.

CHAPTER

35

PERICARDIAL DISEASE

ANTHONY J. SANFILIPPO and ARTHUR E. WEYMAN

The bedside evaluation of pericardial disease remains, as it was in the nineteenth century, one of the most demanding challenges to the clinical cardiologist.[1] As a result, major roles have evolved for two-dimensional and Doppler echocardiography in the timely and accurate diagnosis of these often life-threatening conditions.

In this chapter, a discussion of relevant anatomic considerations is followed by a review of the recommended approach to the echocardiographic examination. The evaluation of pericardial disease is then described in several parts. First, the morphologic features of disease states are presented; this largely involves two-dimensional imaging. This section is followed by discussions of the assessment of elevated intrapericardial pressure and pericardial constriction; these involve integration of all echocardiographic techniques. The chapter concludes with descriptions of several uncommon disorders of the pericardium and of the role of echocardiography in guiding pericardiocentesis.

ANATOMIC CONSIDERATIONS

The pericardium is a thick, fibrous membrane that covers the external surface of the heart and separates it from other intrathoracic structures.[2,3] A pair of serous membranes, the visceral and parietal pericardia, is interposed between this outer fibrous covering and the external border of the heart. The parietal pericardium lines the outer fibrous capsule, whereas the inner, visceral pericardium or epicardium directly overlies the external surface of the heart. Between the two serous membranes is the pericardial cavity. This cavity is normally a potential space and contains only enough fluid to allow the serous membranes to slide smoothly over one another and thus to permit free motion of the heart within the pericardial sac.[2,3]

The pericardial space is limited superiorly by sleevelike attachments of the pericardium to the great arteries just distal to their origins. Posteriorly, the pericardial space is also fixed at the insertions of the pulmonary veins and venae cavae. This posterior series of venous attachments forms a U-shaped arc that is concave inferiorly and creates a blind cul-de-sac behind the left atrium (the oblique pericardial sinus). Between the superior margin of this venous arc and the arterial attachments is a pericardium-lined passage, the transverse sinus (Fig. 35–1). In a variety of disease states, fluid may exude into the pericardium, thereby enlarging the pericardial cavity. The pericardial cavity can expand medially, laterally, and apically; however, it is restrained posteriorly at the atrial level by the venous pericardial attachments and superiorly by the arterial attachments that limit fluid accumulation in these areas.

NORMAL PERICARDIAL PHYSIOLOGY

Because surgical resection and congenital absence of the pericardium are not known to result in any functional impairment, the purpose of this structure has been the topic of considerable debate and conjecture. Both mechanical and membranous functions have been described.[4,5] Mechanically, the pericardium probably limits ventricular filling and therefore affects chamber compliance. The right ventricle has been shown to be influenced by these pericardial restraining forces to a greater degree than the left.[6] This mechanical constraint

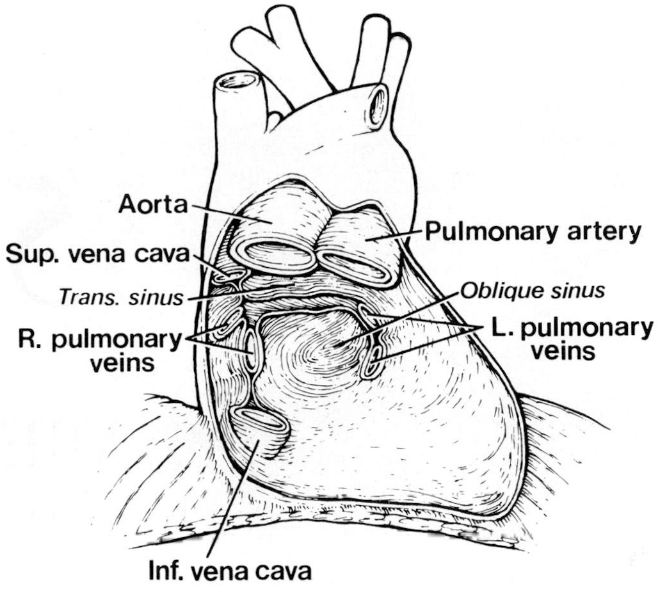

Fig. 35–1. The arterial and venous pericardial attachments.

also limits the extent to which the cardiac chambers are capable of dilating acutely and has been postulated to protect against excessive ventriculoatrial regurgitation. Further, the pericardium may act to distribute pressure evenly over both ventricles, thus tending to balance left and right heart output.[7,8] Maintenance of the thin fluid layer between the parietal and visceral pericardia reduces friction caused by cardiac movement. The pericardium may also be an important barrier to infection, both directly and by containing active immunologic agents.

Normal pericardial pressure is generally subatmospheric throughout the cardiac cycle, when measured by fluid-filled monitoring lines. Cycle-related fluctuations in intrapericardial pressure are closely related to the pressures in adjacent chambers, and the concepts of *transmural and transpericardial pressure* or *pressure gradient* are useful in considering these relationships. The pressure gradient across the free wall of any cardiac chamber (the transmural gradient) is actually the distending pressure on that wall and can be calculated as the difference between intracavitary pressure and intrapericardial pressure. The normal subatmospheric (i.e., negative) intrapericardial pressure results in a *positive transmural gradient* that tends to maintain the chamber open (i.e., the wall directed outward). In certain disease states, pericardial fluid volume and intrapericardial pressure increase. As a result, the absolute transmural gradient, or distending pressure, decreases, and ultimately intrapericardial pressure exceeds the nadir of intracavitary pressure. At this point, the local gradient becomes negative and the wall of the cavity moves inward. Such pressure-related changes in the position of the cardiac walls reflect, and can be used to diagnose, the abnormal intrapericardial pressures discussed in the section of this chapter on cardiac tamponade.

ECHOCARDIOGRAPHIC EXAMINATION OF THE PERICARDIUM

Because the pericardium covers the entire external surface of the heart, portions of these membranes are recorded in all the standard cross-sectional cardiac imaging planes. Similarly, a thorough evaluation of the pericardium involves a detailed study that uses multiple views from different vantage points. Fortunately, most disorders of the pericardium are associated with pericardial effusion or involve the pericardium diffusely. Increased pericardial fluid tends to collect initially behind the posterior wall of the left ventricle just distal to the atrioventricular groove. In this location, the fluid is easily recorded in the parasternal long axis view of the left ventricle. This view is therefore the primary imaging plane used to evaluate the pericardium. Generalized pericardial thickening or fibrosis can also typically be appreciated in the long axis view, and even such characteristically focal disorders as neoplastic invasion of the pericardium appear to have a predilection for this region. As a result, when the pericardium appears normal in the parasternal long axis and routine short axis views of the left ventricle, a high index of suspicion is necessary to pursue the examination of the pericardium further.[9]

When fluid is present behind the left ventricle or when a localized disorder is suspected, a more extensive examination is necessary to determine the location and extent of these abnormalities.[10] This examination includes the following:

1. The parasternal long axis view.
2. Serial short axis scans from the base of the heart to the apex. These scans permit the medial and lateral aspects of the left ventricle to be examined and the extent of fluid accumulation in these areas to be defined.
3. An apical study in the four-chamber orientation and, from this transducer position, a sweep of the scan plane downward toward the patient's left hip until the apical portion of the pericardial space is imaged. This sequence allows the magnitude of apical fluid accumulation to be determined and any intrapericardial abnormality in the apical region to be recorded.
4. With the transducer at the apex and the x axis of the imaging plane in an anteroposterior orientation, angulation of the scan plane medially to visualize the posteromedial and anterolateral recesses of the pericardial space.
5. Placement of the transducer in the subcostal position to evaluate the pericardium surrounding the right ventricular and atrial free walls.[10]

This detailed examining sequence is difficult both to describe and to perform; however, it may be necessary to record localized intrapericardial fibrous bands, thrombi, focal tumor implants, or areas of loculated effusion.[10] As discussed in the section on congenital heart disease (Chapter 31), when the examination is complex, it must be performed in a routine standardized fashion, so atypically positioned or unusual abnormalities are not overlooked.

Visualization of the right ventricular and right atrial free walls is of great importance in the evaluation of pericardial tamponade (see later) and particular care should be devoted to recording the right-sided chambers when cardiac tamponade is suspected.

The importance of respiratory variation in transvalvular flow velocities as a sign of pericardial tamponade and constriction is recognized. Careful recording of maximal Doppler flow at the annular level of at least one right-sided and one left-sided valve may be extremely useful in confirming the presence of elevated intrapericardial pressure. These analyses must be made from spectral Doppler recordings obtained at a rapid paper speed and require simultaneous recording of respiration to be of greatest value.

MORPHOLOGIC FEATURES OF PERICARDIAL DISEASE

Normal Pericardium

The normal epicardium and pericardium are in almost direct contact, with only a thin fluid layer separating their opposing surfaces. Echocardiographically, these contiguous layers appear as a single, highly reflective, linear band of echoes that completely surrounds the external surface of the heart. This single echo layer is generally referred to as the epicardium, although it originates from the combined epicardial and pericardial interfaces.[11] Figure 35–2A is a long axis recording of a normal left ventricle illustrating the bright, single, linear epicardial echo covering the external surface of the posterior ventricular wall. The epicardial echo also extends over the external surface of the left atrium; however, the atrial walls are usually so thin that appreciation of this layer as separate is difficult.

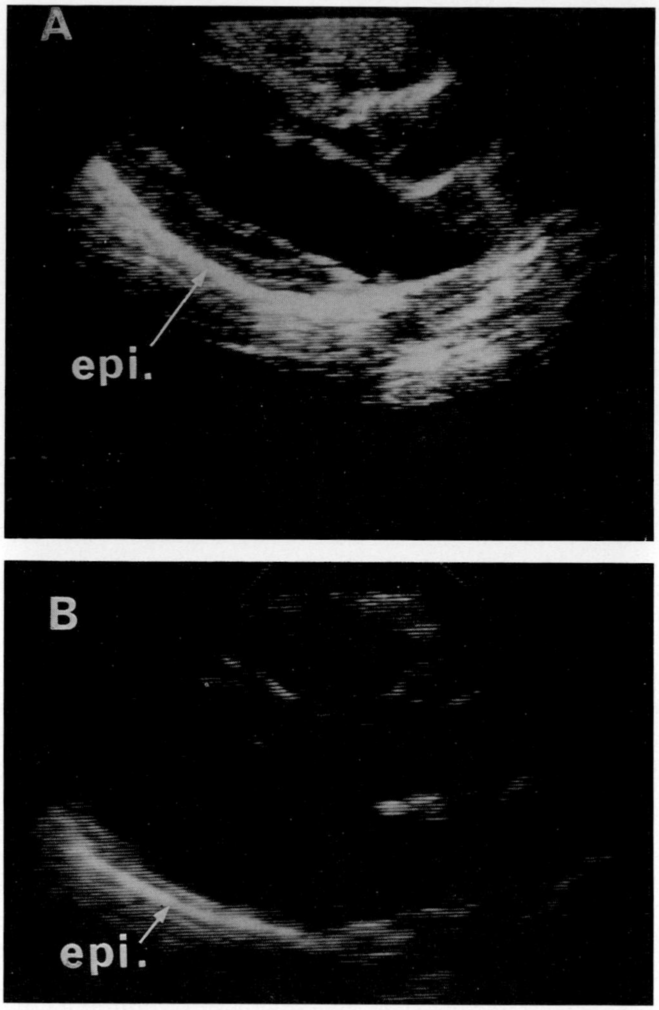

Fig. 35–2. A. Long axis recording of a normal left ventricle illustrates the single dominant linear epicardial echo, which normally covers the external surface of the posterior left ventricular wall. epi = epicardium. **B.** A similar long axis recording from the same patient with increased damping of the output signal. In this example, the surrounding, less intense echoes are significantly reduced, and the stronger pericardial-epicardial interface stands out in greater contrast.

The reflections from the epicardial interface are normally so dominant that they can be separated from other, less-intense echoes in the same area by either decreasing the strength of the transmitted pulse (damping) or decreasing the receiver gain.[11] Each of these maneuvers decreases the amplitude of the surrounding less-intense endocardial and myocardial echoes while still permitting visualization of the stronger epicardial-pericardial reflection. Figure 35–2B is a second long axis recording with an input signal that is more heavily damped. In this figure, the epicardial echo is still well visualized but now stands out in even greater contrast to the surrounding less-visible echoes.

Pericardial Effusion

The pericardial cavity normally contains approximately 20 to 30 ml of fluid that is similar in composition to lymph and originates from the subepicardial lymphatics.[4] These lymphatics normally drain the myocardium and ultimately transport myocardial lymph to the mediastinum and right heart cavities. The amount of pericardial fluid may increase in a variety of disorders, including pericardial inflammation, neoplastic invasion of the pericardium, hypothyroidism, mediastinal irradiation, and trauma[12] (Table 35–1). In addition, conditions that increase cardiac work without directly involving the pericardium may also increase pericardial fluid.[11] The increase in fluid in these diverse disorders results either from interference with myocardial venous and lymphatic drainage because of elevated central venous pressure or from inflammation extending from the visceral pericardium, which interferes with subepicardial drainage and causes loss of interstitial fluid to the pericardium.[4]

Pericardial effusion is detected on the cross-sectional echogram by the following: (1) separation of the visceral and parietal pericardial surfaces (epicardium and pericardium) with an "echo-free" space interposed between these two reflective interfaces; (2) decrease in the motion of the parietal pericardium; and (3) swinging of the entire heart within the pericardial sac when the effusion is large.

Table 35–1. Conditions Associated with Pericardial Effusion

Acute idiopathic or nonspecific (F)
Congestive heart failure
Hypoalbuminemia
Acute myocardial infarction (F)
Postmyocardial infarction syndrome (F)
Trauma, penetrating or nonpenetrating (F)
Cardiac surgery (F)
Connective tissue disease (F)
Rheumatoid arthritis
Rheumatic fever
Systemic lupus erythematosus
Scleroderma
Infectious disease (F)
Bacterial infection
Tuberculosis
Fungal infection; histoplasmosis, actinomycosis, nocardiosis
Viral (Coxsackie B, influenza, ECHO)
Amebiasis
Toxoplasmosis
Neoplasms (primary and metastatic) (F)
Leukemia and lymphoma
Radiation (F)
Uremia (F)
Aortic aneurysm (rupture or leakage of dissecting or nondissecting aneurysm into the pericardial sac)
Drugs
Hydralazine
Procainamide (F)
Chylopericardium
Neoplastic lymph obstruction
Myxedema

(F) = may be associated with serofibrinous pericarditis.

Separation of the epicardium and pericardium occurs because the increase in pericardial fluid enlarges the pericardial space, thereby changing it from a potential space to a fluid-filled cavity. The single linear echo from the normally contiguous pericardial membranes consequently divides into two discrete linear echoes. Each echo arises from one of the now separate borders of the fluid-filled pericardial space. The degree of separation of these echoes, as expected, is related to the amount of fluid accumulated. The fluid itself is relatively echo free and appears as a clear space between the epicardial and pericardial echoes.[9–11]

The location and distribution of fluid vary with the size of the effusion. Figure 35–3 shows long axis recordings from three patients with different sizes of effusions. With small effusions (less than 100 ml),[9,11,13] the fluid tends to be localized behind the posterior left ventricular wall just distal to the atrioventricular ring. As a rule, no fluid is detectable anteriorly, laterally, or apically. On occasion, an anterior, echo-free space is noted in patients with a small posterior effusion; however, this echo-free space is not typically caused by pericardial fluid and is not continuous with the pericardial space. Its exact cause is unclear; however, epicardial fat or accumulated connective tissue appears most likely.[9]

At normal gain settings, small effusions may be obscured by the multiple, low intensity reflections frequently recorded from the region posterior to the left ventricle or by echoes arising from the pericardial fluid itself. Decreasing the receiver gain or damping the output signal usually reduces these extraneous echoes to a point where the stronger epicardial and pericardial reflections become clearly visible. Figure 35–3A is a recording from a patient with a small pericardial effusion illustrating the typical echo-free space behind the left ventricular posterior wall.

With moderate effusions (100 to 500 ml), more fluid accumulates posteriorly; however, in these instances, fluid is also found laterally, apically, and anteriorly and thus is more evenly distributed around the heart.[9] Figure 35–3B is a recording from a patient with a moderate pericardial effusion. In this example, the damping has

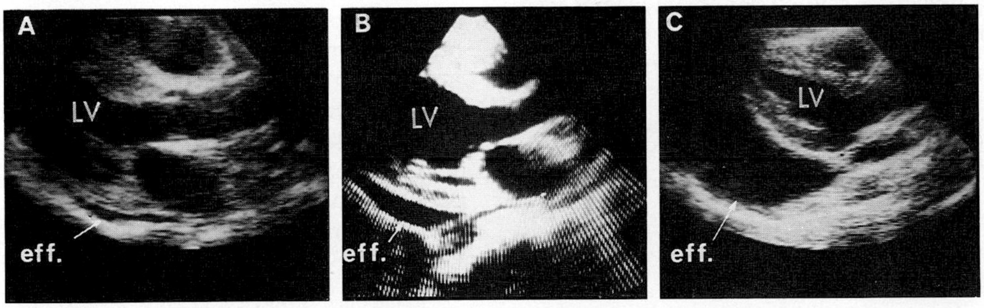

Fig. 35–3. Long axis, cross-sectional recordings from three patients with pericardial effusions of varying size and distribution. **A.** A small pericardial effusion (eff), which is characterized by a discrete echo-free space behind the posterior wall of the left ventricle (LV) separating the epicardium and pericardium. This echo-free space is narrow and extends only from the atrioventricular ring to the midposterior ventricular wall. **B.** A larger pericardial effusion in which the characteristic echo-free space between the posterior left ventricular wall and pericardial interface is wider, and the fluid extends farther toward the cardiac apex. **C.** A large pericardial effusion with an extensive accumulation of fluid posteriorly and apically. The fluid is limited at the atrioventricular ring and fails to extend behind the left atrium because of the venous attachments of the pericardium in this region.

been increased to highlight the pericardial and epicardial echoes. A more extensive clear space is noted behind the left ventricle with greater apical extension. This fluid is limited superiorly by the venous pericardial attachments behind the left atrium and hence does not spread in a superior direction. Figure 35–4A and B are short axis and subcostal long axis recordings from a second patient with a moderately large effusion and illustrate the pattern of fluid spread medially and rightward around the free wall of the right ventricle.

With large effusions (greater than 500 ml), fluid continues to accumulate posteriorly (see Fig. 35–3C); however, in these instances, there is relatively greater expansion of the pericardial space laterally, apically, and anteriorly.[9] Figures 35–5A and B are long and short axis recordings, respectively, from a patient with a large effusion illustrating the typical anterior, lateral, and apical accumulations of this excess fluid.

When the pericardium and epicardium are in their normal, closely apposed position, they characteristically move in unison and follow the movement of the external surface of the heart. During systole, this motion is inward (toward the center of the heart), whereas during diastole, motion is outward (away from the center of the heart) (Fig. 35–6A). In some normal patients, slight systolic separation of the visceral and parietal layers may be recorded by M-mode (Fig. 35–6B). Persistence of this separation beyond the rapid filling phase of the left ventricle is taken to indicate an abnormal increase in fluid, however. As fluid continues to increase in the pericardial space and the membranes separate, the motion of the pericardial layer gradually decreases as an increasingly greater area of contact with the epicardium is lost (Fig. 35–6C). In contrast, the epicardium, which remains attached to the external surface of the heart, continues to move in unison with the cardiac border. This dissociation between the movements of the pericardium and those of the epicardium helps to draw attention to the presence of pericardial effusion.[11]

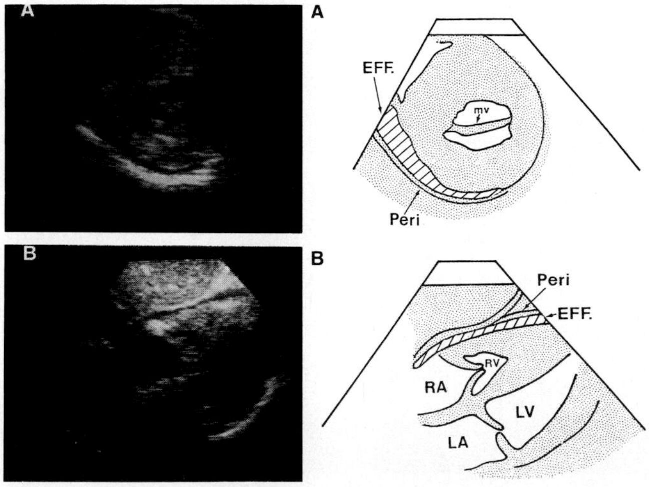

Fig. 35–4. A. Short axis recording from a patient with a moderate size pericardial effusion (EFF), which depicts the posterior and rightward extension of the fluid. **B.** Subcostal recording from the same patient illustrates the pattern of fluid spread medially and to the right around the free wall of the right ventricle (RV). LA = left atrium; LV = left ventricle; MV = mitral valve; Peri = pericardium; RA = right atrium.

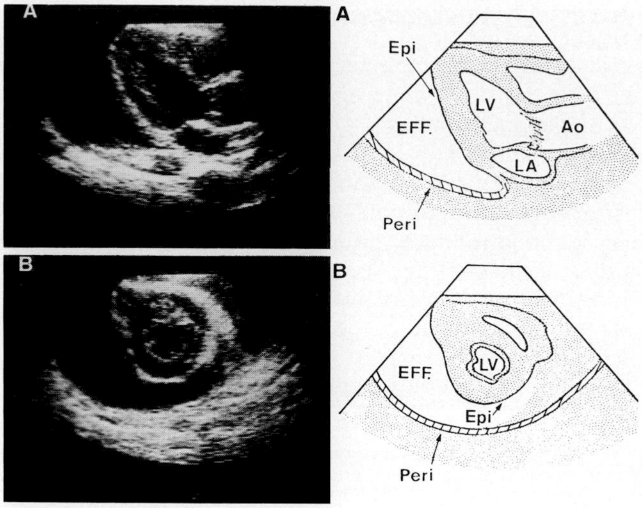

Fig. 35–5. A. Long axis recording from a patient with a large pericardial effusion (EFF) illustrates the apical and posterior fluid spread. **B.** Short axis recording from the same patient illustrates the extensive anterior, medial and lateral fluid accumulation. Epi = epicardium; Peri = pericardium; LV = left ventricle; AO = aorta; LA = left atrium.

In patients with large fluid accumulations, the entire heart may swing dramatically within the pericardial space. This movement occurs in both anteroposterior and mediolateral directions and may include an exaggerated twisting of the heart around its long axis (Fig. 35–7).[14] These abnormal swings may be confined to a single cardiac cycle or may spread over two or more cycles.* This swinging motion has been related to the electrocardiographic phenomenon of electrical alternans, and a clear association can be demonstrated between the position of the heart within the pericardial sac at the onset of electrical systole and the amplitude of the externally recorded QRS deflection.[15–17]

Pericardial effusion may be serous, serosanguineous, serofibrinous, hemorrhagic, chylous, cholesterol-laden, or purulent. Although an increase in the reflectivity of the pericardial fluid might be expected as the protein, fat, and/or cellular content increases,[18] separation of effusion type based on echocardiographic appearance is generally not possible, and specific fluid characteristics can only be inferred from historical or clinical data. Fibrin deposited on the epicardial surface of the heart or collecting to form intrapericardial bands or adhesions tends to have a characteristic appearance, as do intrapericardial thrombi (see later). Even in these cases, however, mixed disease processes may be present.

* In the older M-mode literature, a variety of "pseudo" abnormalities were described (i.e., pseudoprolapse, pseudo-SAM, etc.) that reflected motion of cardiac structures relative to the fixed M-mode transducer parallel to the abnormal motion of the heart as a whole. With the advent of two-dimensional imaging, which permits the relative spatial relationships of cardiac structure to be defined, correct diagnosis of abnormalities such as prolapse can be made despite the abnormal motion of the heart, and thus, these older "pseudo" designations should be abandoned.

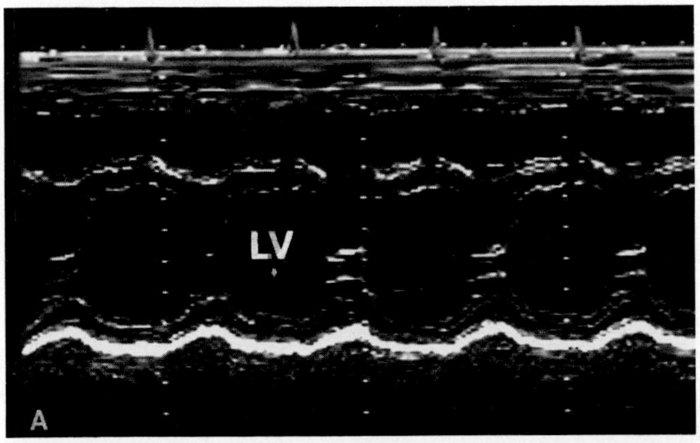

Fig. 35–6. **A.** M-mode recording from a patient with no evidence of pericardial effusion. The echoes from both the epicardium and pericardium are contiguous and do not separate during diastole or systole. **B.** M-mode recording from another patient with no evidence of significant pericardial fluid accumulation. In this example, there is slight separation of the epicardium and pericardium during peak systolic contraction, which is not present during diastole. Such a finding is generally not considered to represent an abnormal accumulation of pericardial fluid and thus can be considered a normal variant. **C.** M-mode recording from a patient with frank pericardial effusion (EFF). In this example, there is clear separation between the epicardial and pericardial layers, with loss of motion of the pericardium. LV = left ventricle; LA = left atrium.

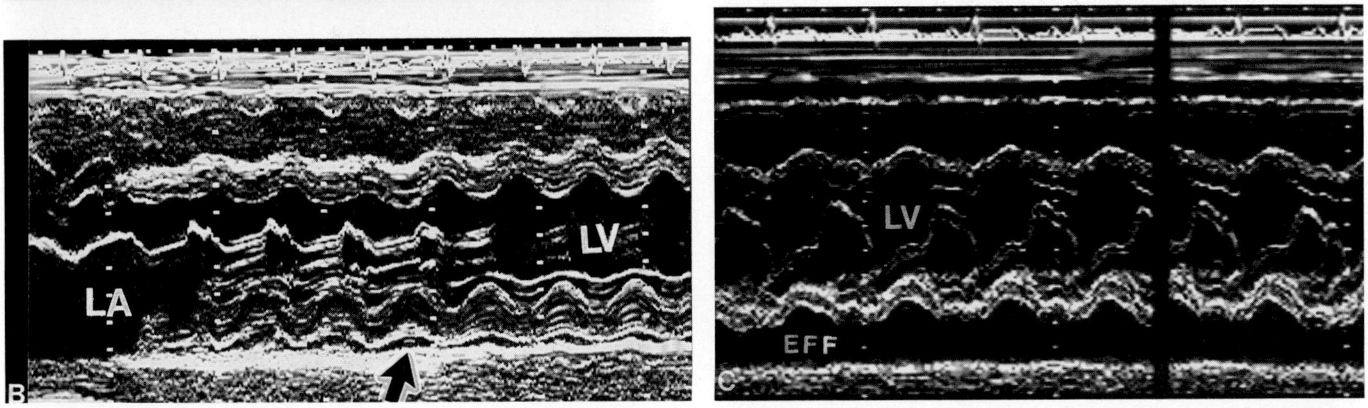

Investigators have suggested that the amount of pericardial fluid can be calculated as the difference between the cubed diameters of the pericardium and epicardium recorded along an anteroposterior line through the center of the heart at end-diastole.[13] This measurement assumes that the pericardial fluid is uniformly distributed around the heart; unfortunately, such is not always the case. The greatest variation appears to occur in patients with small and large effusions, whereas relative symmetry is noted in those with moderate-sized fluid collections.[9] Although such measures should be considered estimates of fluid volume, they may prove valuable in serial comparisons of effusion size and in assessments of the adequacy of pericardiocentesis.[19,20]

Pericardial effusion is common after cardiac surgery, occurring in roughly 85% of postoperative patients. The size of the postoperative effusion varies with time, but in 93% of cases it has peaked by the tenth postoperative

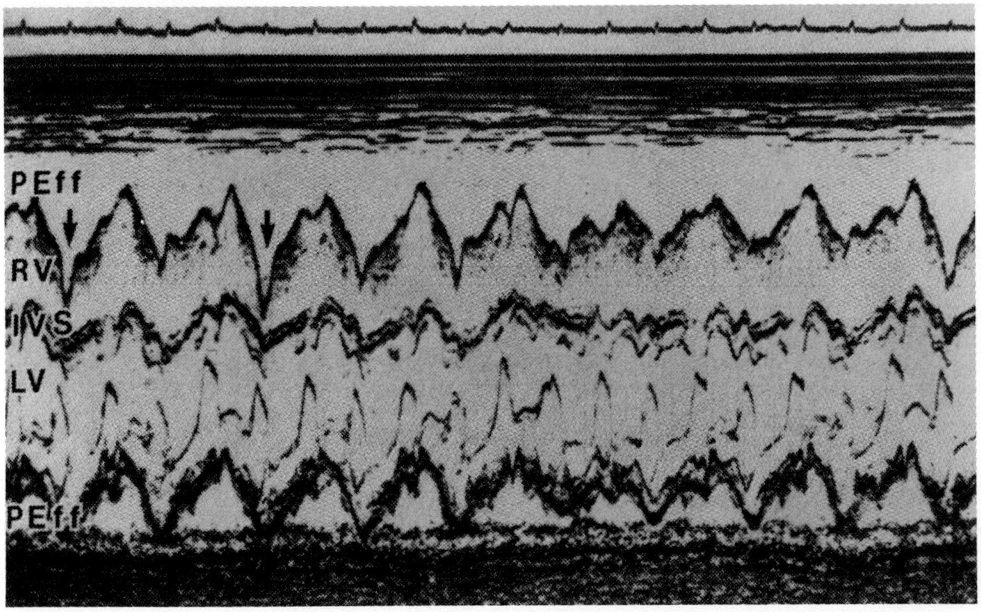

Fig. 35–7. Swinging heart associated with a large pericardial effusion (PEff). The electrocardiogram shows evidence of electrical alternans with the peak QRS voltage occurring when the heart is immediately beneath the anterior chest wall and a decrease in voltage as the heart swings more posteriorly. (↓) RV = right ventricle; IVS = interventricular septum; LV = left ventricle. (From Gaffney FA, et al.: Pathophysiologic mechanism of cardiac tamponade and pulsus alternans. Am J Cardiol 53:1662, 1984.)

day.[21] Pericardial effusion may also be seen in the late stages of pregnancy, particularly in women with increased fluid retention. These effusions typically resolve spontaneously post partum.[22]

Effects of Positional Change on Pericardial Fluid Distribution

The effects of positional change on the distribution of fluid in the pericardial space have also been examined.[9] In patients with moderate and large effusions, fluid is redistributed toward the cardiac apex after 2 minutes in the sitting position.[9] This redistribution does not occur in patients with small effusions, and the absence of this characteristic fluid shift has been observed in patients with compartmentalization of the pericardium by fibrous adhesions between the pericardial layers and in those with loculated pericardial effusions.[10] Demonstration of an apical shift in pericardial fluid may therefore be useful before pericardiocentesis is performed, to exclude a diagnosis of entrapment or loculation of fluid.

Fibrinous Pericarditis

Patients with chronic pericardial inflammation and effusion frequently develop a fibrinous exudate on the pericardial surface. This fibrinous or serofibrinous pericarditis may occur in a variety of cardiac disorders including acute myocardial infarction, as well as in trauma, infection, neoplasm, systemic disease, or without obvious cause (see Table 35–1). Histologically, organization results in the deposition of delicate, threadlike fibrin strands on the surface of the heart. Echocardiographically, the delicate fibrin layer has the appearance of "soap suds" covering the visceral pericardium Figure 35–8. The fibrinous exudate is most often noted along the anterior cardiac surface but may extend to involve the pericardium diffusely.

This form of fibrinous exudate is common in many types of pericardial inflammation, and it should not be confused with metastatic involvement of the pericardium, although the two conditions may occur together. Fibrinous pericarditis may also accompany pericardial infection. Figure 35–9, for example, contains two apical recordings from a child with purulent pericarditis due to Haemophilus influenzae. The large, intrapericardial, tissuelike structure proved to be a fibropurulent epicardial peel. Although the clinical setting in this case suggested the appropriate diagnosis, similar echocardiographic findings can be seen with organizing fibrin or thrombus.[23]

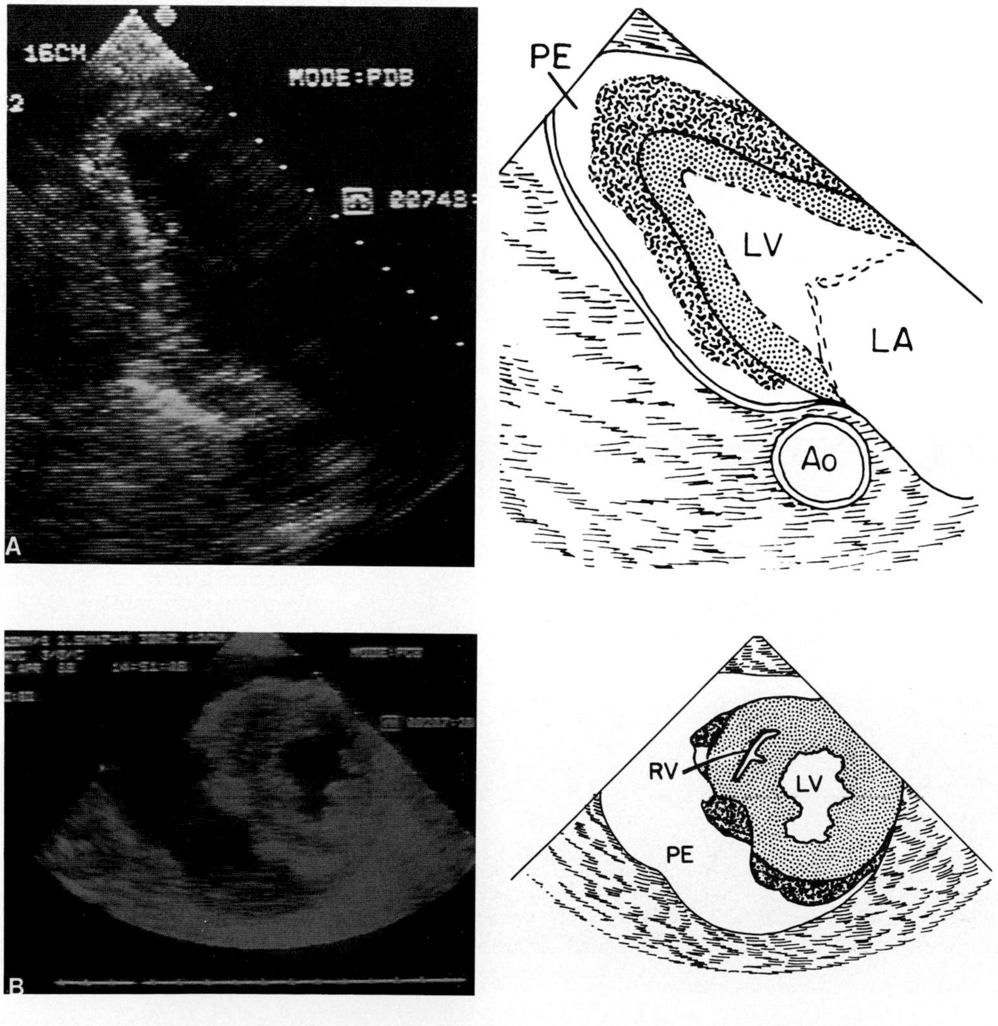

Fig. 35–8. **A.** Apical long axis recording illustrating a dense accumulation of fibrin surrounding the left ventricular apex. The fibrin layer is roughly 1 cm thick and extends from the atrioventricular groove posteriorly around the apex to the full visualized extent of the anterior wall. **B.** Parasternal short axis recording from a second patient with significant accumulation of fibrin at multiple locations on the epicardial surface. The fibrin appears as an increased accumulation of echo-reflective material and is most predominant along the anterior wall and in the posterior interventricular groove and along the posterior surface of the left ventricle (LV). The heart is adherent to the pericardium along its lateral border. LA = left atrium; AO = aorta; PE = pericardial effusion; RV = right ventricle.

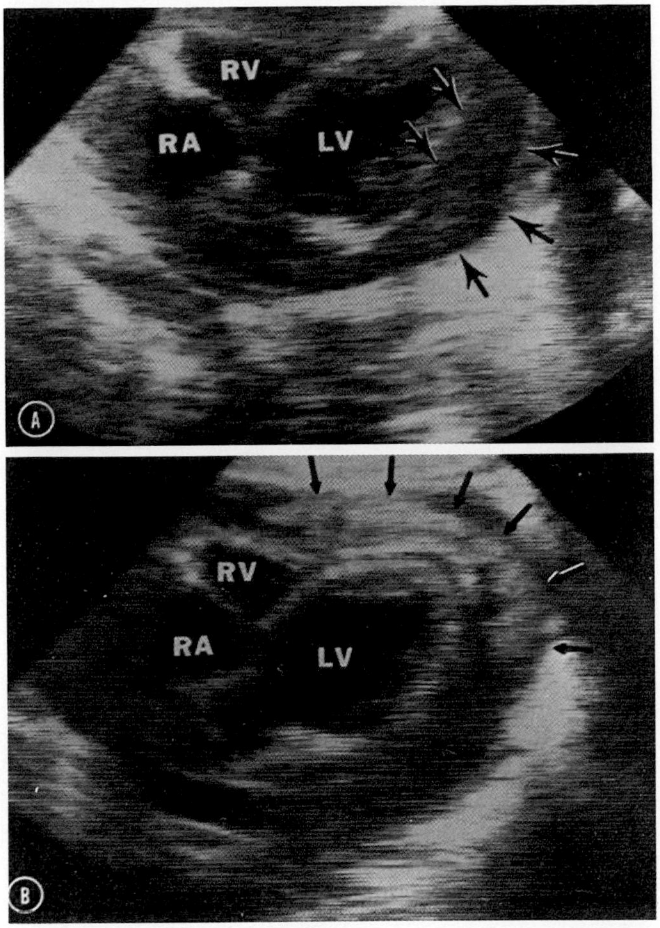

Fig. 35–9. Subcostal long axis recording from a child with purulent pericarditis. **A.** The fibropurulent peel is imaged behind the left ventricle (LV). **B.** With anterior angulation, the peel is shown to extend around the cardiac apex and to abut the right ventricle (RV). (From Wolf WJ: Echocardiographic features of a purulent pericardial peel. Am Heart J 111:990, 1986.) RA = right atrium.

Intrapericardial Fibrous Bands

Fibrinous pericarditis may progress to the formation of intrapericardial fibrous bands (see later) extending from the visceral to the parietal pericardial layer.[10] The characteristics of intrapericardial fibrous bands are illustrated in Figure 35–10. They typically appear as a series of linear, strandlike echoes of varying thickness that frequently bridge the parietal and visceral pericardial surfaces and appear to divide the pericardial space into a series of compartments. On occasion, individual bands do not stretch completely across the pericardial space, and their free ends demonstrate an undulant motion synchronous with the movement of the heart.

When these bands are present, fluid shifts in response to changes in position are typically absent. This finding may imply that the bands are associated with loculation of the pericardial fluid, or alternatively, that they simply retard fluid movement by preventing further local separation of the pericardial membranes without causing actual loculation.

Echo-producing fibrinous bands similar to those described in the pericardium may also be seen in patients with long-term extrapericardial fluid collection. Figure 35–11 is a recording from a patient with a large extrapericardial inflammatory pulmonary cyst located immediately adjacent to the left pericardial border. This cyst contained several filamentous bands that projected into the cavity of the cyst and demonstrated an undulating motion apparently in response to the motion of the heart (Fig. 35–12).

Pericardial Thickening and Adhesions

Chronic pericardial inflammation and effusion may evolve to pericardial fibrosis and longstanding thickening with adhesion between the visceral and parietal pericardial layers.[24] Echocardiographically, pericardial fibrosis (i.e., replacement of the pericardial space by fibrous tissue) is characterized by the following: (1) sep-

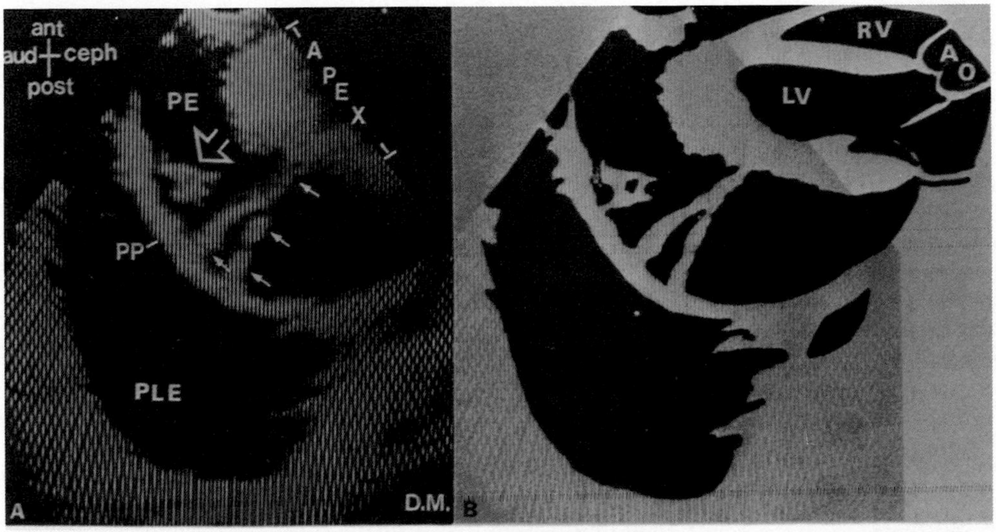

Fig. 35–10. **A.** Long axis cross-sectional scan taken in the region of the cardiac apex illustrates both pericardial and pleural effusion. A series of intrapericardial fibrinous bands (horizontal arrows) extends from the visceral pericardium to the parietal pericardium. **B.** Diagram relating the position of the fibrinous bands to the left ventricular long axis. PE = pericardial effusion; PLE = pleural effusion; PP = parietal pericardium; LV = left ventricle; RV = right ventricle; AO = aorta. (From Martin RP, Bowden R, Filly K, Popp RL: Intrapericardial abnormalities in patients with pericardial effusion: findings by two-dimensional echocardiography. Circulation 61:568, 1980. Reproduced by permission of the American Heart Association, Inc.)

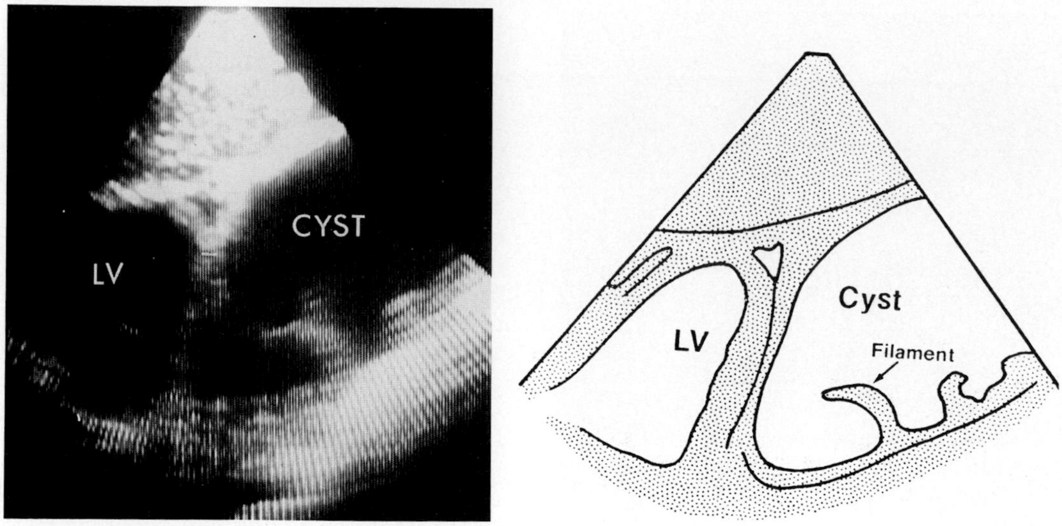

Fig. 35–11. Apical recording from a patient with a large extrapericardial inflammatory cyst. A small portion of the left ventricular apex (LV) is evident in the left portion of the figure. The large, fluid-filled cyst with mobile fibrous filaments is recorded to the right of the scan.

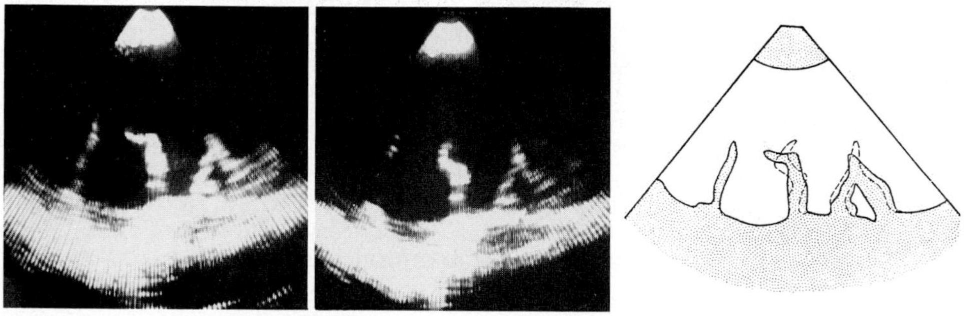

Fig. 35–12. Direct recording of the inflammatory cyst shown in Figure 35–11 shows the mobility of these filaments. The diagram to the right indicates the position and undulant motion of the filaments during different points in the cardiac cycle.

aration between the pericardial and epicardial layers, which is fairly constant around the entire external surface of the heart; (2) an increase in echo production from the fibrous tissue between these two membranes; and most important, (3) parallel motion of the visceral and parietal layers, which implies that they are adherent.[11]

Figure 35–13 is from a patient with a thickened, adherent pericardium. Figure 35–13A is a short axis recording that demonstrates the even separation between the pericardial and epicardial layers around the anterior, lateral, and posterior extremes of the cardiac border. Figure 35–13B and C are diastolic and systolic frames recorded in the apical four-chamber view. These images demonstrate failure of the separation between the membranes to increase during systole, thus suggesting that they are adherent.

Loculated Pericardial Effusion

When excess pericardial fluid is localized to a specific area of the heart, it may be more difficult to detect. Nevertheless, several reports have described the appearance and distribution of isolated anterior effusion, as well as a posterolateral effusion.[25,26]

Identification of loculated effusions is important in view of the recent experimental demonstration that isolated compression of any of the four heart chambers can result in hemodynamic compromise.[27]

Pericardial Calcification

Pericardial calcification may develop as a further degenerative change complicating chronic pericardial inflammation.[24] Pericardial calcification is nonspecific and may be observed in patients with bacterial, tuberculous, or traumatic pericarditis and on occasion may occur without demonstrable cause.[24] The calcium may form discontinuous plates or may completely surround the heart. It tends to involve both parietal and visceral layers of the pericardium and is generally associated with pericardial adhesions and partial or complete obliteration of the pericardial space. Pericardial calcification appears echocardiographically as an increase in reflectivity of the pericardial membranes. This increase in reflectivity may be focal or generalized and is not typically associated with free fluid in the pericardium.

Figure 35–14 is a recording from a patient with extensive pericardial calcification. In this example, one sees an increase in the intensity and width of the pericardial echo in all the standard views. Unfortunately, this increase in reflectivity cannot be differentiated from dense

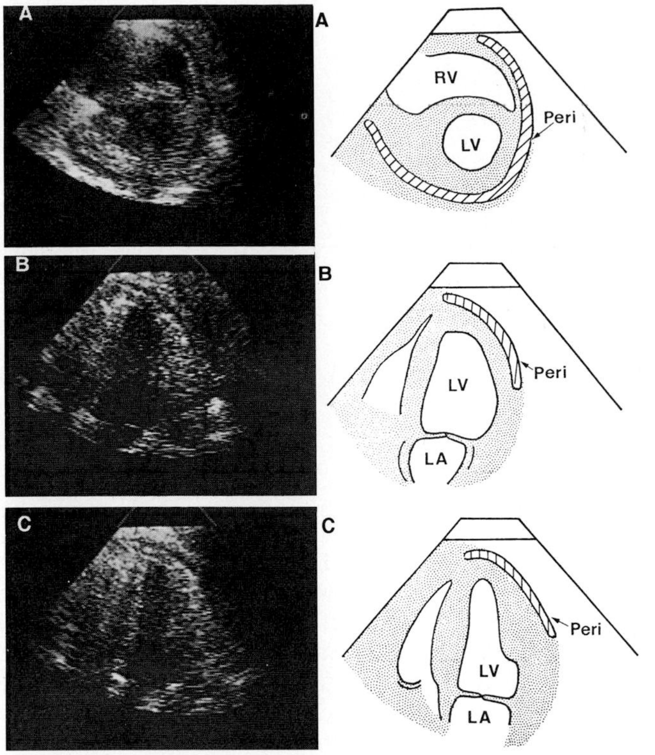

Fig. 35–13. **A.** Short axis recording from a patient with a thickened, adherent pericardium (Peri). Relatively symmetric separation of the visceral and parietal pericardia is apparent around the entire external margin of the left (LV) and right ventricles (RV). **B** and **C.** Diastolic and systolic frames illustrate the lack of systolic separation between the parietal and visceral pericardia, suggesting that these layers are adherent. LA = left atrium.

fibrosis, and when this differentiation is considered essential, a roentgenographic examination is probably preferable. When calcium is noted on a roentgenogram of the chest, however, the spatial resolution of the echogram may aid in defining its location.

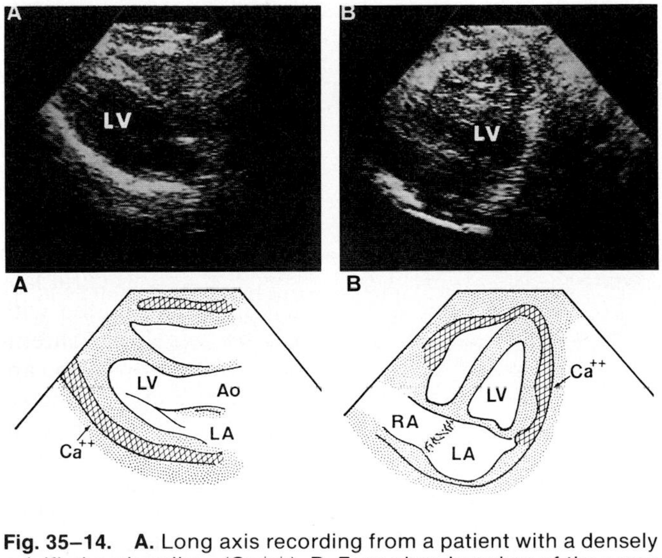

Fig. 35–14. **A.** Long axis recording from a patient with a densely calcified pericardium (Ca^{++}). **B.** Four-chamber view of the same heart. In this example, a significant increase in reflectivity from the calcified pericardium is apparent in both projections. LV = left ventricle; LA = left atrium; Ao = aorta; RA = right atrium.

Pericardial Hematoma

Localization pericardial hematoma may occur early or late after open heart surgery or after cardiac laceration or rupture. Postoperatively, collection of blood is commonly localized anterior and lateral to the right atrial free wall, but it may be found anywhere around the heart. The appearance of the hematoma depends on the extent of thrombus formation and may vary from an entirely echo-free intrapericardial fluid collection to a highly reflective intrapericardial mass. Hematomas typically impinge on adjacent cardiac structures and produce varying degrees of deformity ranging from local concavity to almost complete chamber obliteration. Chamber compression is particularly common when hematomas abut the atria.[28]

Differentiation of an intrapericardial hematoma that compresses the atrium from an intra-atrial thrombus may be difficult. The characteristic location of hematomas along the superolateral wall of the right atrium, encapsulation of the hematoma by the smooth atrial wall, and the occasional echo-free center of the hematoma may be helpful. Figure 35–15 illustrates a hematoma within the pericardial space lateral to the right atrial wall. The hematoma causes inversion of the right atrial free wall and produces a pattern virtually identical to that seen in patients with pericardial tamponade. In this case however, the wall is fixed rather than mobile, as is the case with free fluid, and the hematoma has a granular appearance suggesting organized thrombus. Hematomas adjacent to the left ventricle may cause cavity deformity during diastole that reverts to normal during systole, as the intracavitary pressure rises. When the hematoma is adjacent to lower pressure chambers, the deformity generally persists throughout the cardiac cycle.

Relationship of Pericardial Effusion with Pericarditis

Many patients with chest pain or other features of pericarditis are referred for echocardiographic study in the hope that pericardial effusion or thickening will be detectable. The association between effusion and pericarditis, however, is imprecise. In a large population of uremic patients, 27% of patients without a clinical evidence of pericarditis had a pericardial effusion visible echocardiographically.[29] More important, 33% of patients with clinical evidence of pericarditis and a pericardial friction rub on auscultation did not have a demonstrable pericardial effusion.[29] The size of the effusion, however, did appear to have some prognostic significance because surgical intervention was necessary only in patients with moderate or large effusions.[29]

Differentiation of Pleural and Pericardial Effusion

Large posterior fluid collections may represent either pericardial or pleural effusions or a combination of both. The position of the descending thoracic aorta in the parasternal long axis view is particularly useful in differentiating these conditions. Normally, in this view, the descending aorta is imaged in short axis immediately behind the left atrium just superior to the atrioventricu-

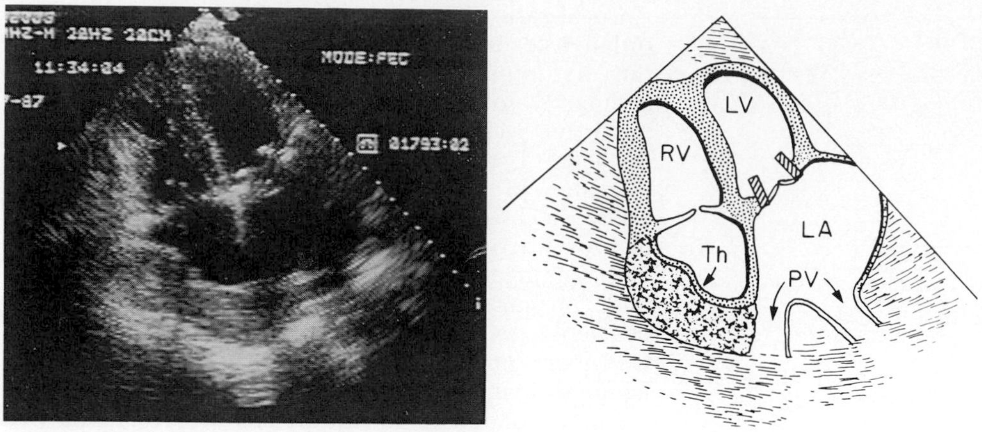

Fig. 35–15. Apical four-chamber view recorded following cardiac surgery and mitral valve replacement. There is a dense collection of echoes superior and lateral to the right atrial free wall, which fills the pericardial space and causes chamber compression. This pattern is typical of a pericardial hematoma. Postoperative thrombus most commonly accumulates outside the right atrium, although it can be seen anywhere along the external surface of the heart or it can surround the heart diffusely. RV = right ventricle; LV = left ventricle; LA = left atrium; Th = pericardial thrombus or hematoma; PV = pulmonary veins.

lar groove. Large pericardial effusions typically expand behind the left atrium, displacing the extrapericardial aorta posteriorly and creating an echo-free space between the left atrial wall and the artery (Fig. 35–16A). In contrast, when a pleural effusion is present, the aorta retains its position immediately beneath the atrium, and the fluid is predominantly posterior and inferior to the vessel (Fig. 35–16B).

Often, pleural effusions lateral to the left ventricle, particularly those containing collapsed lung tissue, are confused with pericardial effusions with intrapericardial tumor (Fig. 35–17). The appropriate diagnosis can be made by the typical triangular appearance of the lung tissue and its location adjacent to the lateral left ventricular wall, and one can demonstrate in multiple views that the fluid is pleural.

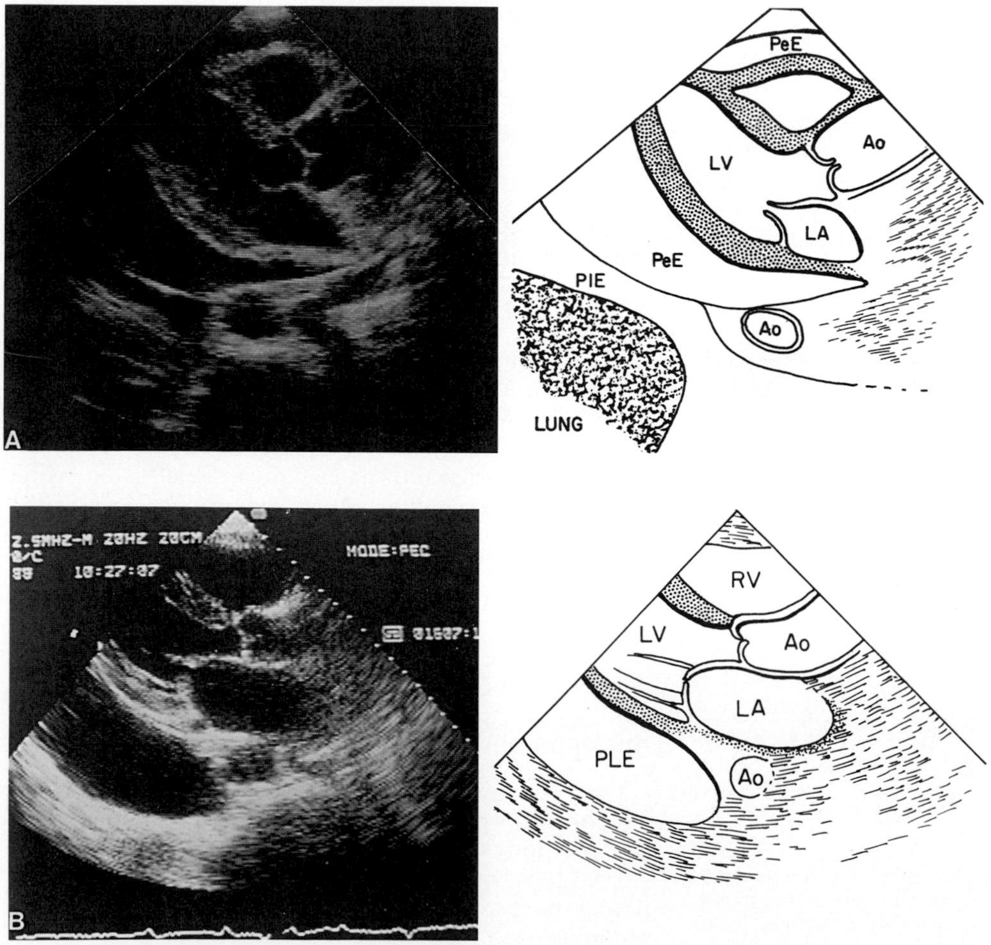

Fig. 35–16. The role of the descending thoracic aorta in differentiating pericardial and pleural effusion. **A.** Large anterior and posterior pericardial effusion (PeE) that extends behind the left atrium (LA) and displaces the descending thoracic aorta (Ao) posteriorly. The posterior pericardium extends from the pericardial reflection at the insertion of the pulmonary veins, courses anterior to the circular Ao (viewed in short axis), and continues toward the left margin of the scan plane. Fluid anterior to the descending Ao, therefore, is pericardial in origin. A pleural effusion (PLE) also occurs posterior to the pericardial effusion. LV = left ventricle. **B.** A large posterior echo space that is predominantly caused by pleural effusion. In this case, the anterior margin of the space begins at the inferior margin of the descending thoracic Ao and extends posteriorly. There is no separation of the Ao from the posterior wall, which serves to differentiate the pleural from the pericardial fluid in **A.** PLE = pleural effusion.

Other Disorders Simulating Pericardial Effusion

A variety of other conditions have been reported to simulate pericardial effusion including pericardial fat, anterior mediastinal tumors, ascites, and giant left atrium with extension beneath the left ventricular posterior wall.

Epicardial Fat

Excess subepicardial fat deposition is one of the most common conditions mimicking pericardial effusion. The amount of subepicardial fat normally increases with age and is characteristically most extensive over the anterior portion of the heart.[30] Excessive fat accumulation is most common in older, obese, diabetic patients, usually women. It may also be seen in patients with exogenous or endogenous steroid excess.[31]

Because of its characteristic distribution, excess subepicardial fat most commonly appears as an anterior echo-free space in the absence of a posterior echo-free space. Fat may accumulate anywhere around the epicardial surface of the heart, however, and may present more diagnostic difficulty when it is recorded posteriorly. In one large study, posterior echo-free spaces simulating pericardial effusion were noted in 370 of 5652 (6.5%) subjects. The prevalence ranged from <1% in subjects 20 to 30 years of age to more than 15% for those in their eighties. These posterior echo-free spaces tended to be more common in older, obese women with high blood sugar levels and hypertension. The spaces tended to be small, with only 18 (0.3%) subjects having moderate-sized echo-free spaces. Patients with small echo-free spaces had no overt evidence of heart disease.[30] In comparative studies in which unexplained echo-free spaces have been examined by computed tomographic (CT) scanning, fat has virtually always been the cause.[32–34] Thus, the possibility that a small or moderate-sized echo-free space at the myocardial-pericardial interface represents fat rather than fluid should always be considered.

Echocardiographic differentiation of fat from fluid is subtle and is usually based on location—anterior rather than posterior (except as noted previously); mobility—fat is slightly less mobile than fluid and the surrounding epicardial and pericardial layers move less freely; and texture—fat is usually slightly more echogenic or granular than fluid. If necessary, differentiation of fat from fluid can be made definitively with a limited CT scan of the chest.[35]

Anterior Mediastinal Tumor

Anterior mediastinal tumors may also suggest loculated pericardial effusion, particularly tumors of hematogenous origin. Fortunately, most such tumors are more echo dense than free fluid or fat; they are not usually associated with posterior effusion despite a large size, and they displace the heart posteriorly, aiding in their identification. Two-dimensional imaging helps one to distinguish tumors outside the pericardium with associated effusion from intrapericardial tumors with effusion.[36–38]

Peritoneal Fluid (Ascites)

Subcostal echocardiography in patients with ascites often reveals an echo-free space anterior to the heart that may be mistaken for a loculated anterior pericardial effusion or pericardial cyst. Ascites can be recognized as the cause of the space by its contour, by its relation to the liver, and by the distinctive midline appearance of the falciform ligament of the peritoneum bisecting the echo-free space. Less frequently, ascitic fluid inferior to the left ventricle and superior to the spleen can mimic a posterior pericardial or pleural effusion on M-mode and even long axis two-dimensional echocardiography, but the definition of the space as ascites is evident on other two-dimensional views.[39,40]

In stand-alone M-mode studies, giant left atria, which dissect beneath the left ventricular posterior wall, often created a posterior echo-free space reported as a cause of false-positive effusion.[41] With the advent of two-dimensional imaging, conditions such as giant atrium should no longer cause diagnostic confusion.

Pericardial Tumors and Masses

Metastatic Tumors

The pericardium is a frequent site of tumor spread in a variety of neoplastic disorders. Pericardial infiltration is most commonly seen in carcinoma of the lung and breast; however, it may also occur in malignant melanoma, lymphoma, and leukemia.[24] With the exception of renal failure, by far the most common cause of an unsuspected moderate or large pericardial effusion is malignant disease. In many instances, this association

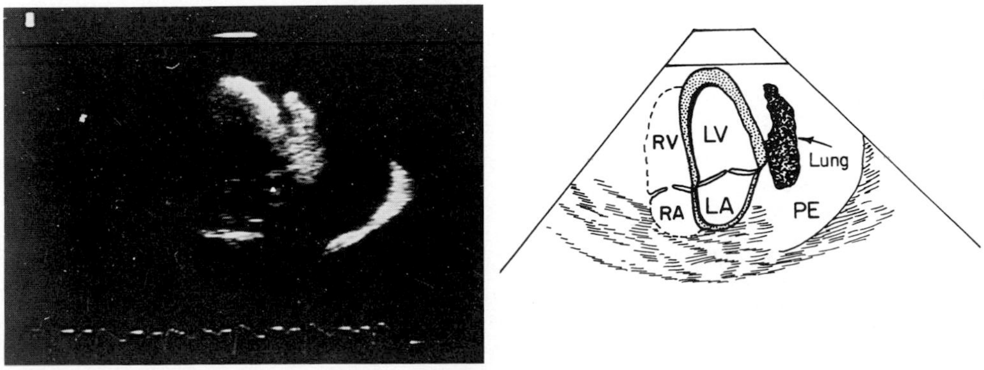

Fig. 35–17. Apical four-chamber recording illustrating a large left pleural effusion that contains a portion of collapsed left lung. Recognition of this pattern is important because it is often confused for a large pericardial effusion with intrapericardial tumor. PE = pleural effusion; LV = left ventricle; LA = left atrium; RV = right ventricle; RA = right atrium.

remains only statistical until the primary tumor site is defined, the pericardial fluid is directly analyzed, or the pericardium itself is examined by biopsy. In other instances, however, tumor implants can be directly visualized on the parietal or visceral pericardial surfaces. When present, the area of neoplastic infiltration is typically more highly reflective than surrounding regions, and it disrupts the normally smooth borders of the pericardium.

Figure 35–18 represents images from a patient with a metastatic adenocarcinoma with extensive tumor invasion of the epicardium. Figure 35–18A is a long axis image that demonstrates tumor within the pericardial space beneath the posterior wall of the left ventricle just distal to the atrioventricular ring. In addition to the encroachment on the pericardial space, tumor can also be seen invading the left ventricular myocardium. Figure 35–18B is a short axis image that illustrates the multiple bright echoes produced by these malignant implants anterolaterally in the region of the anterior interventricular groove, posteriorly beneath the cavity of the left ventricle, and medially beneath the tricuspid ring. In each view, the tumor is easily visualized because of the associated presence of pericardial effusion. In the areas where the tumor directly invades the left ventricular wall, the normal linear epicardial echoes are no longer evident and are replaced by the less well-defined masses of tumor echoes. In contrast to the focal involvement illustrated in Figure 35–18, other metastatic tumors, particular end-stage solid tumors, lymphomas, and leukemia, may infiltrate the pericardial space diffusely (Fig. 35–19).

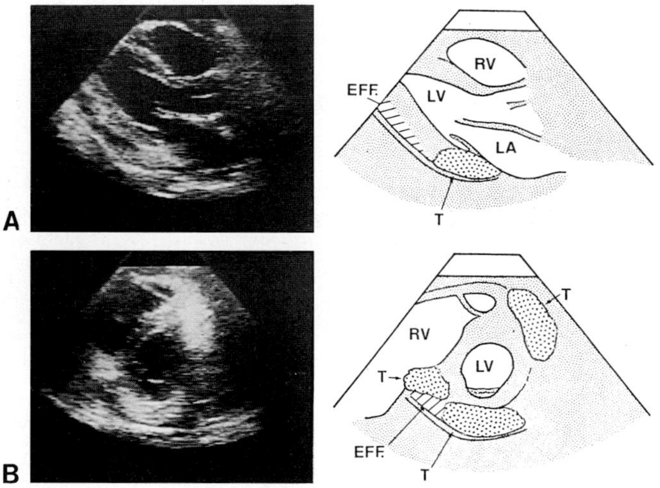

Fig. 35–18. **A.** A long axis image from a patient with metastatic adenocarcinoma with extensive tumor invasion (T) of the myocardium and pericardium. In this view, tumor invasion is evident at the base of the posterior wall in the region of the atrioventricular ring with extension into the pericardial space. The stipple in the accompanying diagram indicates the area of tumor involvement. **B.** A short axis image from the same patient illustrates extensive areas of tumor involvement (T) of the anterior left (LV) and right (RV) ventricular free walls and the interventricular septum. There is also involvement of the posterior left and right ventricular walls adjacent to the interventricular groove. The areas of tumor involvement are indicated by the stippled areas in the diagram to the right. Accompanying pericardial effusion is evident in both images. LA = left atrium; EFF = effusion.

Primary Pericardial Tumors

Although less common, primary pericardial neoplasms may also occur and typically appear as a solid, solitary tumor mass,[42] an angiomatous plexus on the surface of the pericardium, or a cystic structure that is usually of little functional consequence but may be associated with obstruction of intrapericardial vessels.[43,44] The most common primary tumors are mesothelioma, sarcoma, teratoma, fibroma, lipoma, and angioma (Table 35–2).[45]

Pericardial mesothelioma may first appear as pericarditis with fever and chest pain, as constrictive pericarditis, or as cardiac tamponade. The tumor may involve any portion of the pericardium and may infiltrate the myocardium (Fig. 35–20).[46]

Intrapericardial Hematic Cysts

During embryonic development, the left superior vena cava may fail to be completely obliterated and may give rise to an intrapericardial cystic mass. This venous rem-

Table 35–2. Classification of Primary Pericardial Tumors

- Stromal
  - Fibroma
  - Fibrosarcoma
  - Mesothelioma
    - Benign
      - Solitary
      - Diffuse
    - Malignant
      - Solitary
      - Diffuse
- Vascular
  - Lymphangioma
  - Lymphangioepithelioma
  - Hemangioma
  - Malignant hemangioepithelioma
  - Hamartoma
- Developmental rest
  - Intrapericardial bronchogenic cyst
  - Teratoma
    - Benign
    - Malignant
  - Dermoid cyst
  - Thymoma
  - Accessory thyroid
  - Pericardial cyst
- Miscellaneous
  - Leiomyoma
  - Lipoma
  - Neuroma
  - Neurofibroma
  - Rhabdomyosarcoma
  - Granular cell myoblastoma

(From Cohen JJ: Neoplastic pericarditis. *In* Spodick DH (ed.): Pericardial Disease. Philadelphia, F.A. Davis, 1976.)

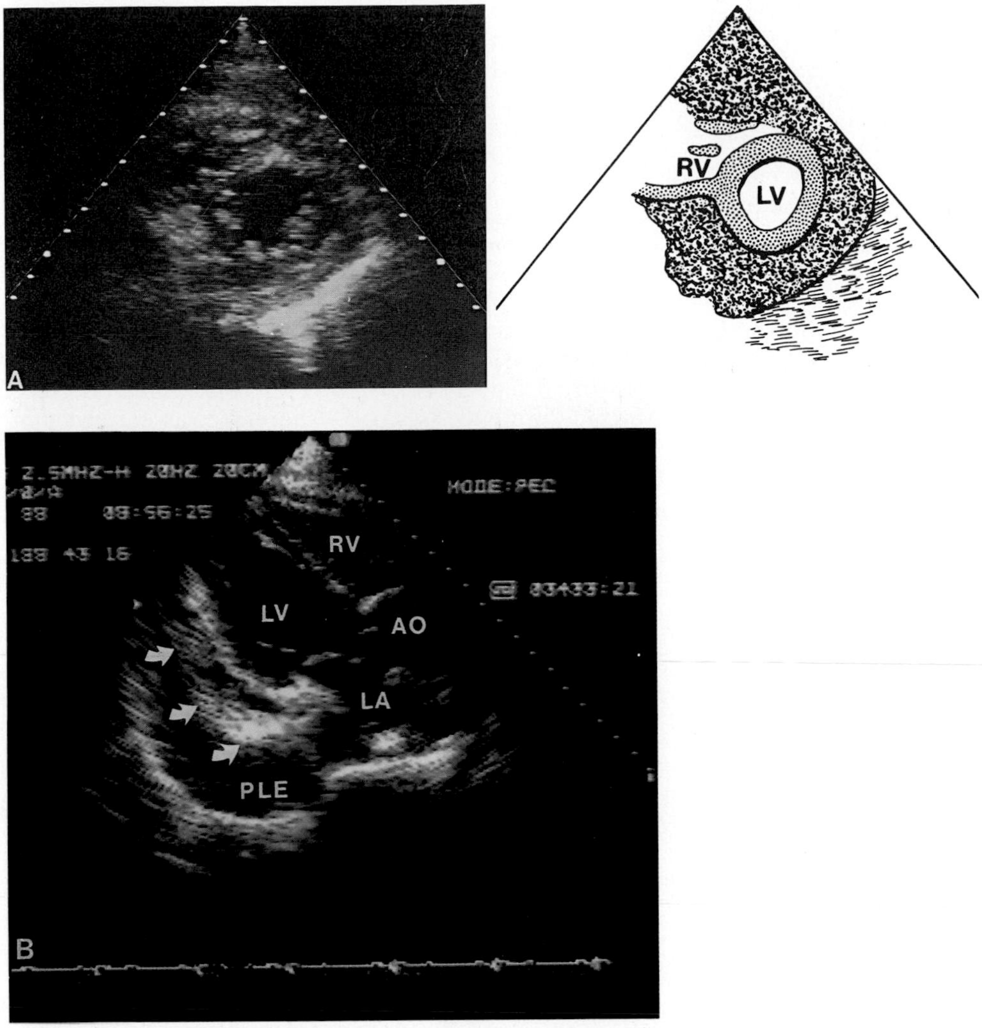

Fig. 35–19. A. Parasternal short axis recording from a second patient with metastatic adenocarcinoma of the breast. In this case, the tumor fills the pericardial space, rigidly encasing the heart. This pattern was associated with end-stage disease and resulted in restriction in ventricular filling. RV = right ventricle; LV = left ventricle. **B.** Parasternal long axis recording from a patient with diffuse involvement of the pericardial space secondary to a malignant lymphoma. The tumor surrounds the heart diffusely but contains numerous echo-free spaces, giving a "moth-eaten" appearance to the mass. There is also a large left pleural effusion (PLE). LA = left atrium; AO = aorta. Curved arrows indicate the lymphoma within the pericardial space.

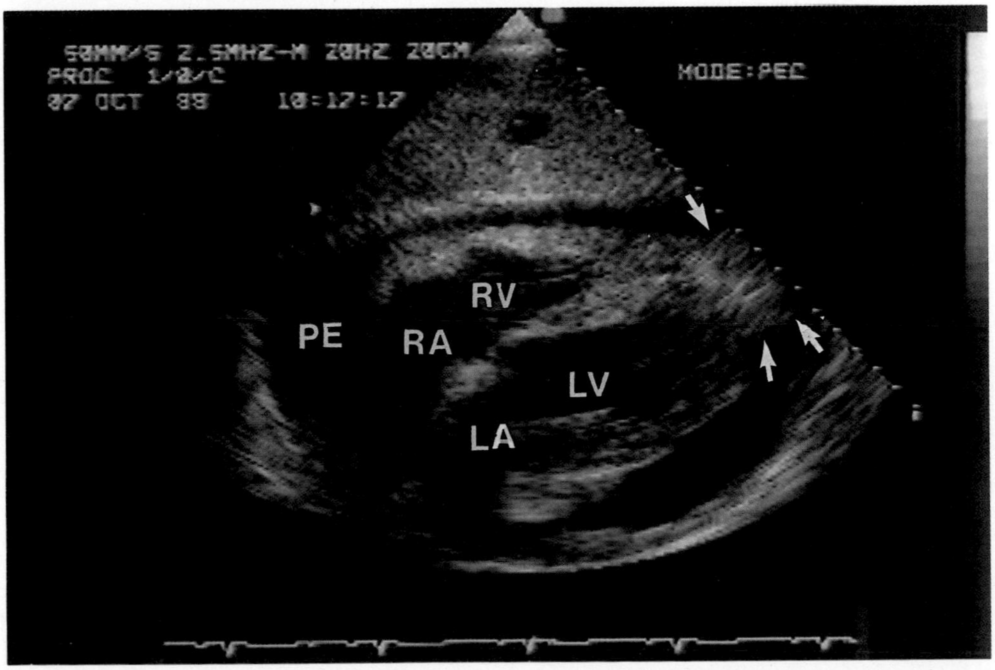

Fig. 35–20. Subcostal long axis recording from a patient with a large pericardial effusion and primary pericardial mesothelioma located at the cardiac apex (arrows). LV = left ventricle; LA = left atrium; RV = right ventricle; RA = left atrium; PE = pericardial effusion.

nant may retain a connection to the left innominate vein and may appear as a cyst within a large pericardial effusion during infancy. Figure 35–21 is an example of a hematic cyst with a large pericardial effusion.[47]

CARDIAC TAMPONADE

Cardiac tamponade is an impairment of diastolic filling caused by an abnormal rise in intrapericardial pressure. This rise in the pericardial pressure may occur as a result of the rapid accumulation of a small amount of intrapericardial fluid, such as occurs in the catheterization laboratory after laceration of the heart, or it may develop more slowly from the gradual accumulation of large amounts of fluid, as in chronic uremic pericarditis. Regardless of cause, cardiac tamponade should be thought of as a continuum ranging from pericardial effusion with minimal hemodynamic involvement that may be asymptomatic to effusion with severe cardiac compression and circulatory collapse. For the purpose of this chapter, the term *tamponade* is used to describe the full range of abnormally elevated intrapericardial pressures, extending from the level just sufficient to cause a compensatory increase in venous pressure to the extreme elevations associated with circulatory collapse. The term *clinical tamponade,* in contrast, refers to the classic changes in heart rate and systemic arterial pressure (i.e., an exaggerated inspiratory fall in arterial pressure >10mm Hg, [the paradoxic pulse] and a fall in mean arterial pressure) that occur at the extreme end of the pericardial pressure volume curve.

Relationship of Intrapericardial Fluid Volume and Pressure

Pericardial pressure is determined by the compliance characteristics of the pericardium and the total intrapericardial volume.[48] The total intrapericardial volume consists of the pericardial fluid and heart volumes. When there is an abnormal accumulation of pericardial fluid, the total pericardial volume increases while cardiac volume remains constant or decreases slightly until the rising pericardial pressure becomes equal to the venous pressure.[48] Beyond this point, the pressure volume curve of the pericardium is equal to or steeper than that of the ventricles, and cardiac filling shifts from the ventricular to the pericardial compliance curve. In short-term experimental studies, intrapericardial pressure does not begin to increase until one has infused 60 to 80 ml of fluid into the pericardial space.[49,50] Beyond this point, however, further injection of fluid causes the slope of the pressure curve to increase rapidly (Fig. 35–22).[50] Cardiac volume can only be maintained if the necessary filling pressure required by the tense pericardium is generated by the venous bed. If the compensatory rise in venous pressure is insufficient to maintain cardiac volume, then the stroke volume will decrease in spite of the rise in venous pressure. Thus, in cardiac tamponade, the absolute pericardial pressure is passively determined by venous pressure, and the two mean pressures are identical. Ordinarily, left ventricular filling pressure is higher than right ventricular filling pressure, but the difference is small. Therefore, as cardiac tamponade progresses, rising pericardial and right ventricular diastolic pressures quickly equilibrate with left ventricular filling pressure.[48]

Because both ventricles must fill against the same pericardial stiffness, the relative filling of these chambers is determined by their respective filling pressures. When left ventricular pressure is markedly elevated before cardiac tamponade, the compensatory rise in systemic venous pressure during tamponade may fail to maintain cardiac output before right ventricular end-diastolic pressure (RVEDP) rises to the level of left ventricular end-diastolic pressure (LVEDP). In this situation, cardiac compression is largely restricted to the right side of the heart.[48]

When pericardial pressure is reduced as a result of pericardiocentesis, the opposite sequence of events is observed. As illustrated in Figure 35–23, when pericardial fluid is removed in 50-ml aliquots, right atrial end diastolic pressures, RVEDP, and LVEDP fall in parallel, and stroke volume and systolic arterial pressure increase.[48] Once pericardial pressure falls below right atrial pressure or RVEDP, however, changes in stroke volume and systolic arterial pressure are no longer significant.[48] Although pericardial pressure continues to decline after this separation occurs, right atrial pressure shows essentially no further change.[48]

Effects of Respiration and Cardiac Contraction on Intrapericardial, Intracavitary, and Transmural Pressures

During normal inspiration, the chest cavity expands, as does the adherent pleura, causing intrapleural pres-

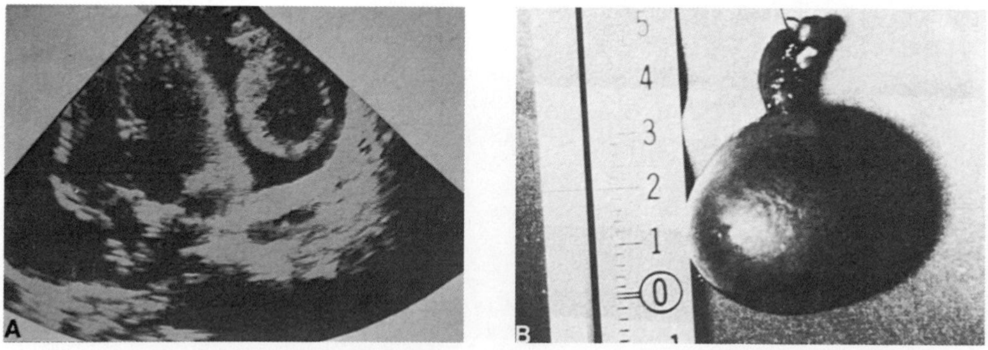

Fig. 35–21. A. Apical four-chamber recording illustrating a large circular cystic mass within the left pericardial space produced by a hematic cyst or venous ectasia. **B.** The morphologic appearance of the cyst following resection. (From Martinez D, et al.: Differential diagnosis of intrapericardial mass identified as venous ectasia. Texas Heart Inst J 13:209, 1986.)

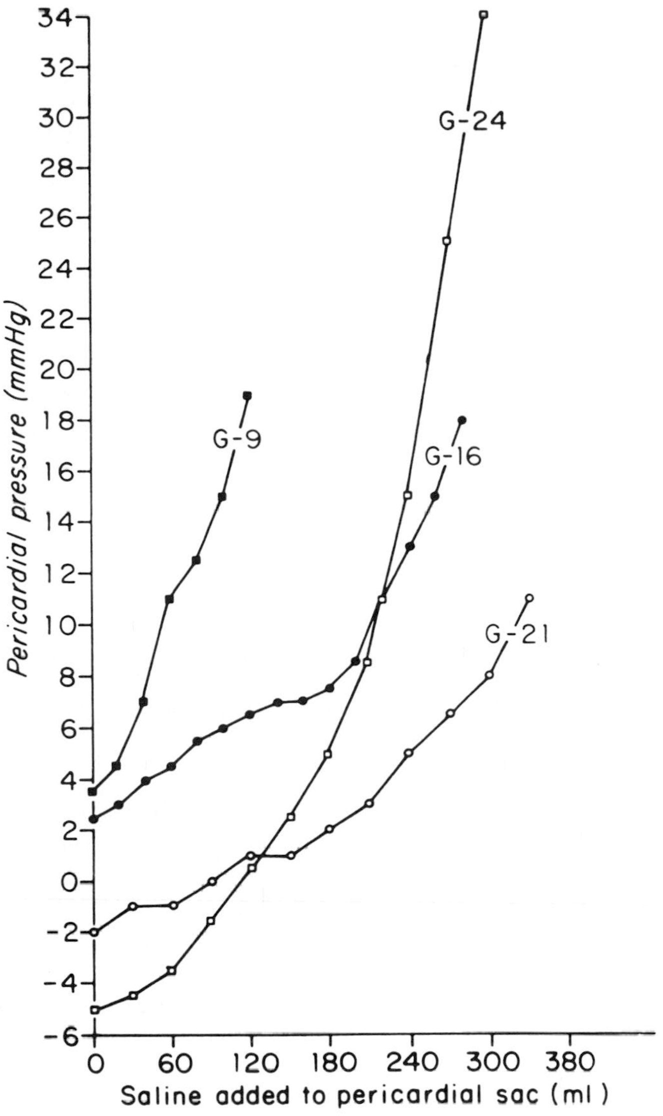

Fig. 35–22. Relationship of pericardial fluid volume to intrapericardial pressure during instillation of saline in 30-ml increments into the pericardial space. At small intrapericardial volumes, there is little change in intrapericardial pressure; however, as volume increases, the pressure rises exponentially, resulting in a large increase in pressure for a small increase in volume. Each curve depicts the pressure volume relationship observed in one experimental animal. (From Morgan BC, Guntheroth WG, Dillard DH: Relationship of pericardial to pleural pressure during quiet respiration and cardiac tamponade. Circ Res 16:493, 1965. Reproduced by permission of the American Heart Association, Inc.)

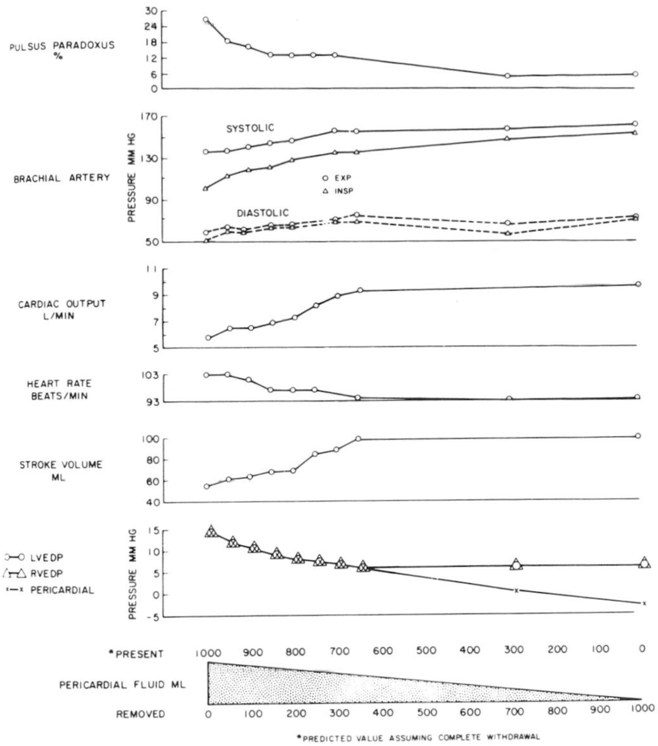

Fig. 35–23. Relation of intrapericardial pressure, right ventricular end-diastolic pressure (RVEDP) and left ventricular end-diastolic pressure (LVEDP) to stroke volume, heart rate, cardiac output, brachial artery pressure, and the percentage of pulsus paradoxicus during incremental removal of fluid by pericardiocentesis. Note that as fluid is withdrawn, intrapericardial pressure drops and hemodynamic parameters improve in parallel until pericardial pressure falls below the left and right ventricular end-diastolic pressures. At this point, the heart shifts from the pericardial pressure volume curve to the ventricular pressure volume curve, and there is little further influence of pericardial pressure or fluid volume on cardiac performance. (From Reddy P, et al.: Cardiac tamponade: hemodynamic observations in man. Circulation 58: 265, 1978. Reproduced by permission of the American Heart Association, Inc.)

sure to become more negative. This change, transmitted to the pericardium, results in a slight inspiratory reduction (roughly 7 mm Hg) in intrapericardial pressure.[49] This, in turn, augments the positive transmural gradient, which favors expansion of the right atrium and right ventricle.

Most studies comparing directly measured intrapericardial and intrapleural pressures have shown little difference in the respiratory fluctuations of these pressures in cardiac tamponade when compared to normal.[50,51] In severe tamponade, however, intrapericardial pressure may follow intrathoracic pressure less faithfully than in mild tamponade. As a result of the inspiratory decrease in pericardial pressure, right atrial and ventricular filling pressures fall and venous return increases. During expiration, the opposite changes occur; intrapericardial pressure rises, as do right atrial and ventricular filling pressures and venous return falls (Fig. 35–24). Because the fluctuations in pericardial pressure are determined by respiration and venous pressure passively follows pericardial pressure, slight phase delays may occur that accentuate any negative transmural pressure gradients that may be present (see later).

Cardiac cycle-related changes in intracardiac pressure and flow also produce transient fluctuations in the transmural pressure gradient (Fig. 35–25). During acute cardiac tamponade, caval flow is reduced and systemic venous pressure is increased. One sees a prominent fall in vena caval and right atrial pressure at the onset of ventricular systole (x descent) and a corresponding peak of flow in the superior and inferior vena cava. The normal rapid drop in pressure at the onset of diastole (y descent) is usually absent, and right heart filling be-

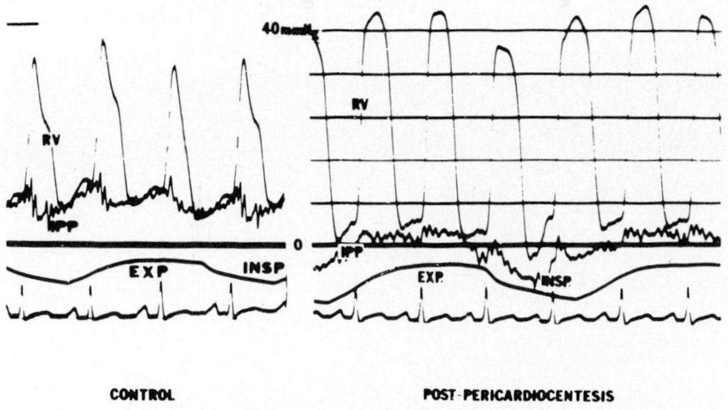

Fig. 35–24. Right ventricular (RV) and intrapericardial pressures (IPP) during cardiac tamponade and following pericardiocentesis. Before pericardiocentesis, the right ventricle (RV) and pericardial pressures are essentially equal during ventricular diastole. Following fluid aspiration, both diastolic pressures fall significantly and are no longer equilibrated. (From Reddy P, et al.: Cardiac tamponade: hemodynamic observations in man. Circulation 58:265, 1978. Reproduced by permission of the American Heart Association, Inc.)

comes monophasic with forward flow confined to ventricular systole. Although mean right atrial pressure does not appear to fall below intrapericardial pressure, transient reversal of the right atrial-pericardial and right ventricular-pericardial pressure gradients do occur.[52] As will be discussed later in this chapter, these transient reversals in transmural pressure gradient appear to cause, and their presence is confirmed by, transient passive compression-inversion of the atrial and ventricular walls, particularly those of the right-sided chambers. The magnitude of these negative gradients varies; the cardiac and respiratory cycles are most prominent at the nadir of the right atrial and ventricular pressure curves (i.e., at the onset of ventricular systole and diastole, respectively) at the point in the respiratory cycle when intrapericardial pressure is highest (i.e., at end-expiratory apnea).[48] Because the atria and right ventricle are more compliant than the left ventricle, they show the most obvious effects of these small, transient, negative pressure gradients.

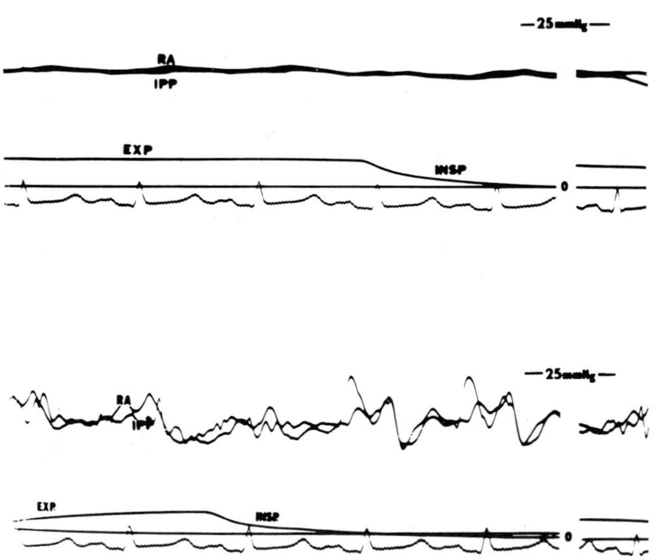

Fig. 35–25. Relationship between intrapericardial pressure (IPP) and right atrial pressure (RA) in a patient with tamponade and pulsus paradoxicus. Mean and phasic pressures are shown in the upper and lower panels, respectively. During both inspiration and expiration, mean RA and IPP pressures are essentially equal; however, there is marked phasic variation in both RA and IPP following atrial contraction, which is modified by respiration-induced changes in intrapleural pressure. (From Reddy P, et al.: Cardiac tamponade: hemodynamic observations in man. Circulation 58: 265, 1978. Reproduced by permission of the American Heart Association, Inc.)

Effects on Arterial Pressure

Cardiac tamponade also causes an increase in the normal inspiratory fall in arterial pressure, the so-called pulsus paradoxus, originally described by Kussmaul.[53] The mechanism of pulsus paradoxus has been investigated by several groups,[54–57] and it provides information of relevance to the echo-Doppler assessment of cardiac tamponade. Experiments using a canine model of cardiac tamponade have shown that the inspiratory increase in systemic venous return in normal subjects is maintained in cardiac tamponade.[51] Further, pulsus paradoxus can be abolished when venous return is kept constant or when the right heart is bypassed. Finally, aortic pressure can be shown to decrease transiently (that is, simulate pulsus paradoxus) when systemic venous return is augmented with a bolus of fluid, even during apnea. Observations such as these have led to the conclusion that the inspiratory augmentation of venous return is critical to the development of pulsus paradoxus. In cardiac tamponade, expansion of the cardiac chambers is limited by the elevated pericardial pressure. During inspiration, enhanced venous return leads to an increase in right ventricular volume that necessarily compromises the left ventricle. This ''competition'' between the ventricles caused by the pericardial constraint leads to a decrease in left ventricular output during inspiration. This effect is probably augmented by the normal increase in left heart flow that occurs four to five cardiac cycles after inspiration as a result of the arrival of this augmented venous return to the left heart after transit through the pulmonary circuit.

Echocardiographic Diagnosis

The changes in transmural pressure and intracardiac flow in cardiac tamponade are reflected in several useful and easily detectable echocardiographic signs that have been described in this disorder. These signs include inversion of the right atrial and ventricular free walls resulting from reversal of the transmural pressure gradient, exaggerated respiratory variation in blood flow through the right and left heart, and generalized compression of the right heart at extremely high intrapericardial pressures.

Diastolic Inversion of the Right Ventricular Free Wall

Probably the most useful echocardiographic sign of cardiac tamponade is right ventricular diastolic inversion or collapse (RVDC). This phenomenon is characterized by a persistent posterior or inward motion of the right ventricular free wall after mitral valve opening (i.e., during diastole). This inward movement produces a localized concavity of the right ventricular free wall, which is present in orthogonal two-dimensional views (Fig. 35–26). Because indentation of a muscular wall cannot be produced by active muscular contraction, diastolic inversion must be passive and reflect a local negative transmural pressure gradient (i.e., pericardial pressure higher than intracavitary). In the supine patient, RVDC most commonly involves the anterior right ventricular free wall and proximal infundibulum, although in upright experimental animals, collapse has been noted in other areas of the ventricle.[58] This difference presumably reflects changes in gravitational pressure as a result of changes in position. Because of its characteristic location in the supine patient, RVDC is best visualized clinically in the standard parasternal long or short axis view of the left ventricle at the base of the heart, and its duration can be appreciated on a routine M-mode recording of the left ventricle. RVDC may be transient or may persist throughout diastole, but it is usually terminated by atrial systole. Figure 35–27 is an M-mode recording illustrating the timing of RVDC. An imprecise relation-

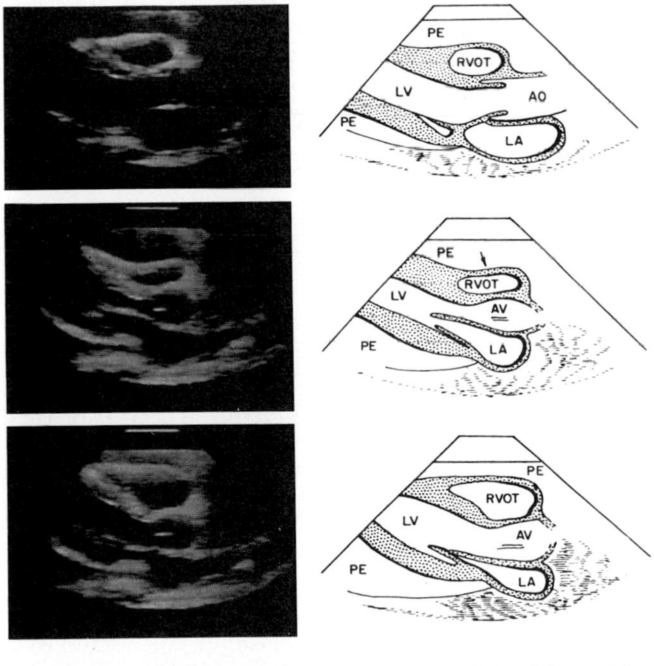

Fig. 35–26. Parasternal long axis recording of the right ventricular outflow tract (RVOT) during systole (top), early diastole (middle), and late diastole (bottom) from a patient with a large pericardial effusion and cardiac tamponade. During systole, the anterior border of the RVOT is curved slightly anteriorly; however, at the onset of diastole, the outflow tract is compressed from without, causing it to become concave anteriorly (downward pointing arrow—middle diagram). As diastole progresses, the outflow tract curvature gradually reverses so that by end-diastole (bottom) the configuration of the outflow tract is again normal. This pattern of diastolic inversion of the RVOT is characteristic of tamponade and is caused by passive local compression of the heart, secondary to transient reversal of the local transmural pressure gradient. PE = pericardial effusion; Ao = aorta; AV = aortic valve; LV = left ventricle; LA = left atrium.

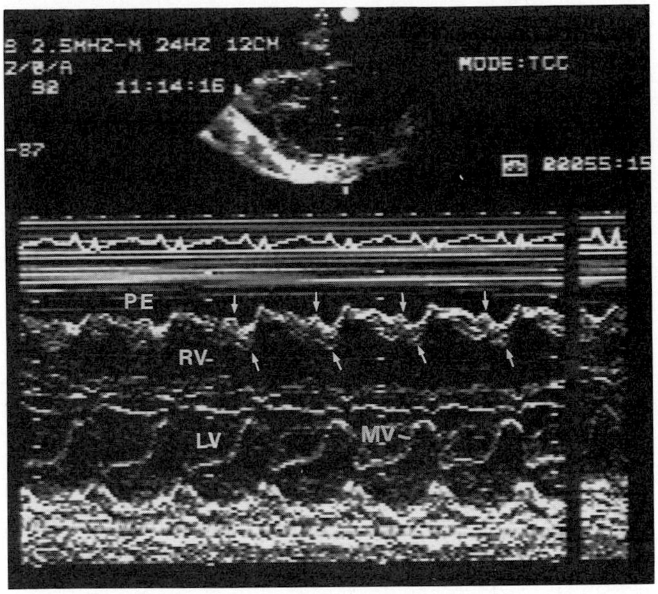

Fig. 35–27. M-mode recording illustrating right ventricular diastolic collapse. In this illustration, there is a large anterior pericardial effusion (PE) with a smaller posterior component. The right ventricular wall moves posteriorly and thickens normally during right ventricular systole; however, immediately following mitral valve opening (diastole), the right ventricular free wall moves abruptly posteriorly (downward pointing arrows), consistent with right ventricular diastolic collapse, and then gradually returns toward a normal diastolic position following atrial contraction (upward pointing arrows). RV = right ventricle; MV = mitral valve; LV = left ventricle.

ship appears to exist between the degree and duration of inversion and the severity of tamponade (i.e., the degree of elevation of intrapericardial pressure).[59]

RVDC appears to occur at a critical level of intrapericardial pressure because, in experimental studies, researchers have noted that "the appearance of RVDC was so striking and its onset frequently so abrupt that the volume of pericardial fluid causing it to occur could often be determined within 5 ml."[58] At the first appearance of RVDC, right ventricular and intrapericardial pressures are equalized.

The relationship of RVDC with intrapericardial pressure, heart rate, mean arterial pressure, cardiac output, and stroke volume has been studied in detail in the experimental animal. Figure 35–28 illustrates the results from one such experiment. Note that in this short-term experiment, RVDC occurs after instillation of 100 ml of fluid into the pericardium and persists during continued fluid injection to the point of circulatory collapse.[58] Figure 35–29 summarizes data from a series of experiments. Note that RVDC first occurs at a mean intrapericardial pressure of 10 ± 4 mm Hg. By the time RVDC is first observed, the cardiac output has already decreased by a mean of 21% and stroke volume has fallen significantly, but mean arterial pressure is essentially unchanged. Thus, RVDC occurs after the onset of cardiac tamponade, as defined by a rise in intrapericardial and venous pressure, but before the onset of clinical tamponade, as defined by a fall in mean arterial pressure and the development of pulsus paradoxus. Once established,

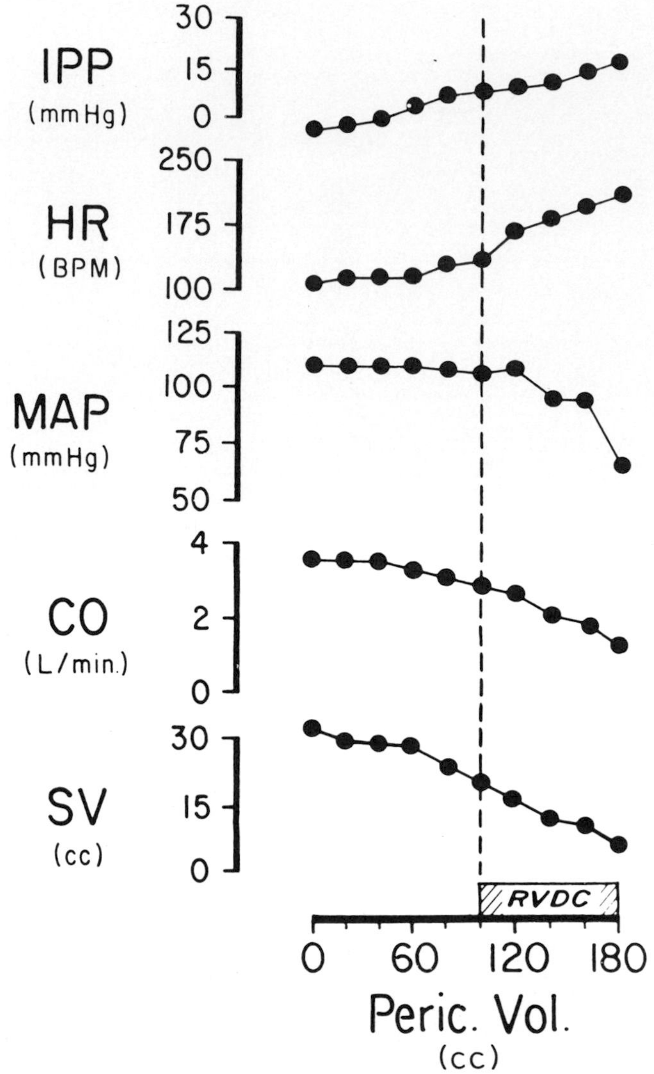

Fig. 35–28. Hemodynamic changes recorded during experimental cardiac tamponade from a representative experimental study. Pericardial volume (peric. vol) was continuously increased at a rate of 10 ml/min. Mean intrapericardial pressure (IPP), heart rate (HR), mean aortic pressure (MAP), cardiac output (CO), and two-dimensional echocardiograms were recorded at 2-minute intervals. Right ventricular diastolic collapse (RVDC) was first observed at a pericardial volume of 100 ml and persisted to the end of the experiment (MAP less than 70% of control). Cardiac output and stroke volume declined consistently as tamponade progressed. Mean aortic pressure, however, was well maintained at the time RVDC was first observed and fell rapidly during the course of tamponade. SV = stroke volume. (From Leimgruber PP, et al.: The hemodynamic derangement associated with right ventricular diastolic collapse in cardiac tamponade: an experimental echocardiographic study. Circulation 68:612, 1983. Reproduced by permission of the American Heart Association, Inc.)

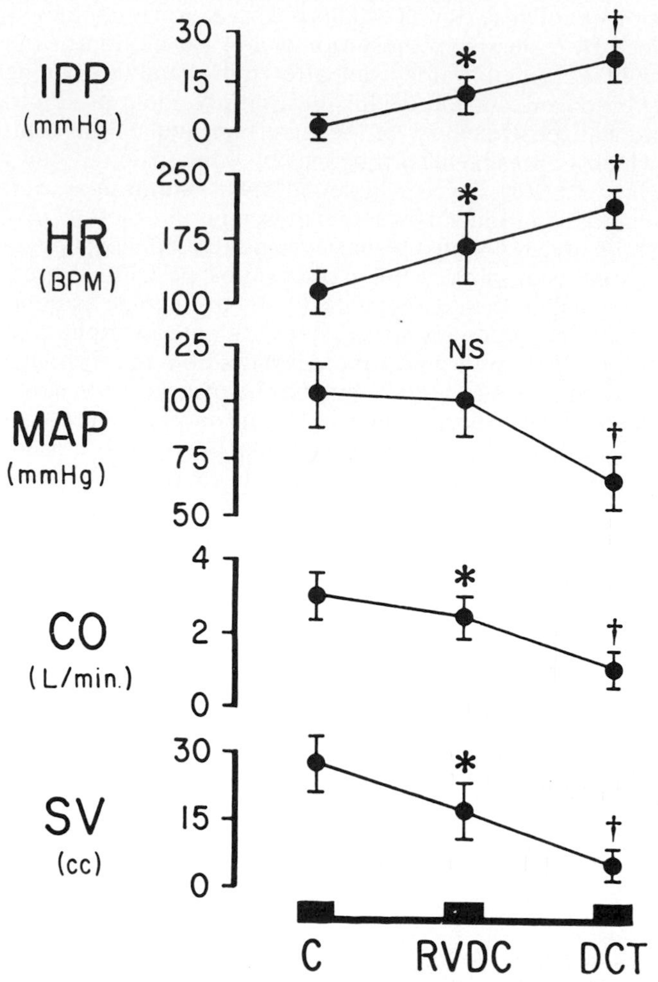

Fig. 35–29. Mean intrapericardial pressure (IPP), heart rate (HR), aortic pressure (MAP), cardiac output (CO), and stroke volume (SV) with empty pericardial space (C) at the first occurrence of right ventricular diastolic collapse (RVDC) and in decompensated cardiac tamponade (DCT) during the induction of experimental tamponade in a group of animals. When RVDC is first seen, CO and SV are substantially reduced, but there is no significant change in MAP. Data are expressed as mean ± SD. NS = no significant change vs. C. *P= < .01 vs. C. +P= < .01 vs. C and/or RVDC. (From Leimgruber P, et al.: The hemodynamic derangement associated with right ventricular diastolic collapse in cardiac tamponade: an experimental echocardiographic study. Circulation 68: 612, 1983. Reproduced by permission of the American Heart Association, Inc.)

RVDC persists and becomes more prominent as the intrapericardial pressure continues to rise, and it remains present to the point of circulatory collapse. In severe cardiac tamponade, the right ventricular cavity is almost completely obliterated, and RVDC persists throughout diastole.[58]

Effects of Intravascular Volume, Right Ventricular Pressure, and Chamber Compliance on Right Ventricular Diastolic Collapse. The level of intrapericardial pressure required to cause RVDC and the hemodynamic status of the patient when it occurs are directly related to intravascular volume, right ventricular pressure, and chamber compliance.

Intracavitary Volume. Conditions that affect the right ventricular filling pressure have been shown to influence the progression of cardiac tamponade and the onset of RVDC. In canine models of acute cardiac tamponade, volume loading has been associated with improved cardiac output, increased arterial blood pressure, and in some instances improved perfusion of major organs. Similarly, studies of the effects of intravascular volume on the onset of RVDC have shown that volume status has a significant influence on the intrapericardial pressure, mean aortic pressure (Fig. 35–30A), and cardiac output (Fig. 35–30B) at which this phenomenon occurs.[60,61]

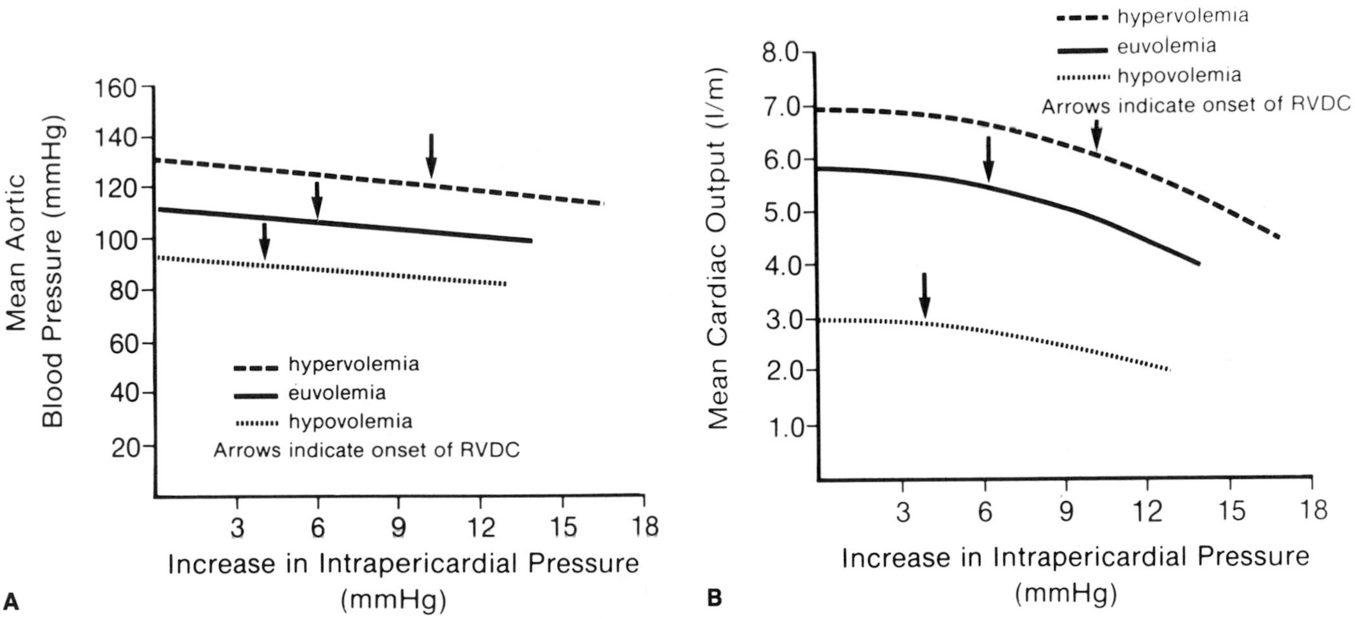

Fig. 35–30. **A.** Relationship of mean aortic blood pressure and intrapericardial pressure (observed intrapericardial pressure minus initial intrapericardial pressure) during cardiac tamponade for a variety of intraventricular volume states. The curves are significantly different from each other ($p < .001$) for any comparison, and the point of onset (arrow) of right ventricular diastolic collapse (RVDC) is different for each volume state ($p < .001$ for any comparison). **B.** Relationship of mean cardiac output and intrapericardial pressure for each intravascular state. The curves all differ significantly from each other ($p < .05$ for any comparison). The cardiac output at the onset (arrows) of right ventricular diastolic collapse (RVDC) during euvolemia differs from that during hypovolemia ($p < .001$) and hypervolemia ($p < .05$). (From Klopfenstein HS, et al.: Alterations in intravascular volume affect the relation between right ventricular diastolic collapse and the hemodynamic severity of cardiac tamponade. Reprinted with permission from the American College of Cardiology. Journal of the American College of Cardiology 1986, 6, 1057.)

Right Ventricular Pressure. Sudden elevation of pulmonary artery pressure with a hydraulic occluder results in a corresponding rise in right ventricular diastolic pressure and elimination of or marked reduction in RVDC.[58] Thus, patients with right ventricular hypertrophy or pulmonary hypertension from any cause would be expected to manifest RVDC relatively later in the disease process or at high intrapericardial pressures. Similarly, in the presence of acute left ventricular pressure overload, right ventricular filling pressures and intrapericardial pressure rise, and RVDC occurs at higher intrapericardial pressure and smaller intrapericardial volumes.[62]

Chamber Compliance. The effects of the transmural gradient on chamber shape is also modulated by chamber stiffness. Thus, despite equal intrapericardial pressures, alterations in left ventricular shape are minimal compared to those seen in the atria or right ventricle, and these differences can be attributed to different chamber stiffnesses.

Sensitivity and Specificity of Right Ventricular Diastolic Collapse as a Sign of Cardiac Tamponade. The sensitivity of RVDC as a sign of cardiac tamponade varies with the population studied. In medical patients, RVDC has generally been a reliable sign of cardiac tamponade.[63–67] Importantly, RVDC occurs when the intrapericardial and right ventricular pressures are equilibrated and hence may herald clinical decompensation.[64,68] In patients studied after cardiac surgery, trauma, or laceration, sensitivity has been poorer, ranging from 48 to 77%.[69,70] RVDC may be absent in these patients because of adhesion of the right ventricular free wall to the parietal pericardium (Fig. 35–31),[69] fluid loculation, or small intrapericardial volumes that do not permit the fluid shifts necessary to produce localized phasic collapse.

Specificity is more difficult to determine because it largely depends on the definition of cardiac tamponade. If tamponade is diagnosed as a fall in systemic arterial pressure and a pulsus parodoxus, then RVDC occurring before a drop in arterial pressure may appear nonspe-

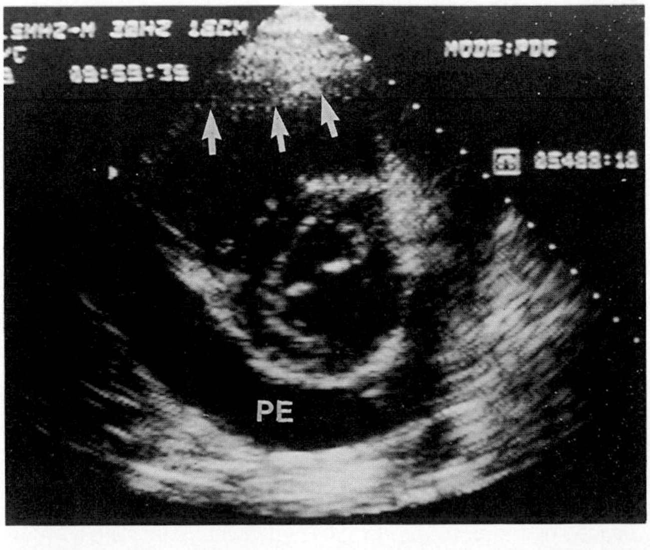

Fig. 35–31. Parasternal short axis recording from a patient with a large pericardial effusion and cardial tamponade. In this example, the anterior right pericardial wall is adherent to the pericardium (arrows), preventing ventricular diastolic collapse from developing. PE = pericardial effusion.

cific because reversal of local transmural pressure gradients occurs before the fall in arterial pressure. If RVDC is used as a marker of an elevated intrapericardial pressure, however, then it becomes highly specific. Thus, as with many Doppler findings described later in this chapter, RVDC reflects local pressure changes rather than specific pathologic processes; and hence, its presence or absence must be interpreted in its specific clinical context.

Right Atrial Compression

The right atrial free wall is normally rounded throughout the cardiac cycle, reflecting the normal positive right atrial to intrapericardial pressure gradient (Fig. 35–32). Any invagination of the right atrial free wall is therefore indirect evidence of elevated intrapericardial pressure and a transient reversal of the normal gradient. Right atrial inversion has been reported by several investigators in patients with pericardial effusion and tamponade,[69,71,72] and it is illustrated in Figures 35–33 and 35–34. The right atrial inversion that occurs in cardiac tamponade typically begins in late diastole and continues into ventricular systole for a variable period before normalizing. When present, this abnormality can be recorded in any view in which the right atrial wall is well visualized (i.e., the subcostal long axis, apical four-chamber, or parasternal short axis view). Right atrial inversion by itself is an extremely sensitive sign of cardiac tamponade; however, its specificity is only 82% and its predictive value is roughly 50%.[69,71] Assessment of the degree of inversion fails to separate patients further; however, when the duration of inversion (the right atrial inversion time index [RAITI] = total number of frames showing inversion/the total number of frames in the cycle) is calculated, groups of patients are more clearly

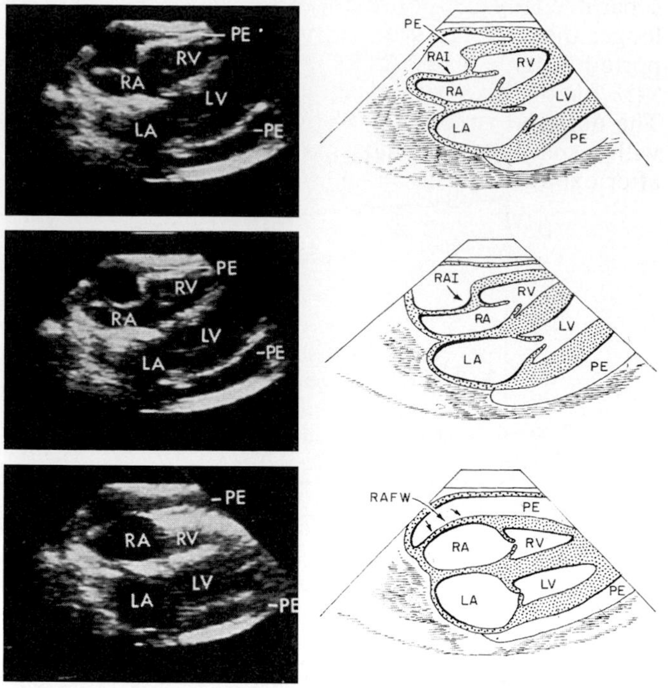

Fig. 35–33. Subcostal long axis cross-sectional echocardiogram from a patient with right atrial inversion (RAI). Inversion is initiated at end-diastole (top) and continues through early systole (middle). By end-systole (bottom), the configuration of the right atrial free wall (RAFW) has normalized. RA = right atrium; RV = right ventricle; LA = left atrium; LV = left ventricle; PE = pericardial effusion. (From Gillam LD: Hemodynamic compression of the right atrium: a new echocardiographic sign of cardiac tamponade. Circulation 68:294, 1983. Reproduced by permission of the American Heart Association, Inc.)

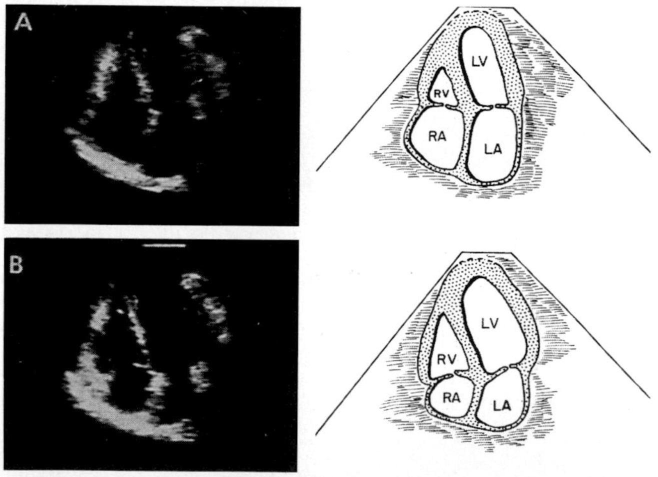

Fig. 35–32. Normal apical four-chamber, cross-sectional echocardiogram. **A.** At end-systole, the right atrium (RA) is maximally filled, and its free wall has a rounded configuration. **B.** At end-diastole, although the RA is relatively empty, the free wall remains rounded. RV = right ventricle; LV = left ventricle; LA left atrium. (From Gillam LD: Hemodynamic compression of the right atrium: a new echocardiographic sign of cardiac tamponade. Circulation 68:294, 1983. Reproduced by permission of the American Heart Association, Inc.)

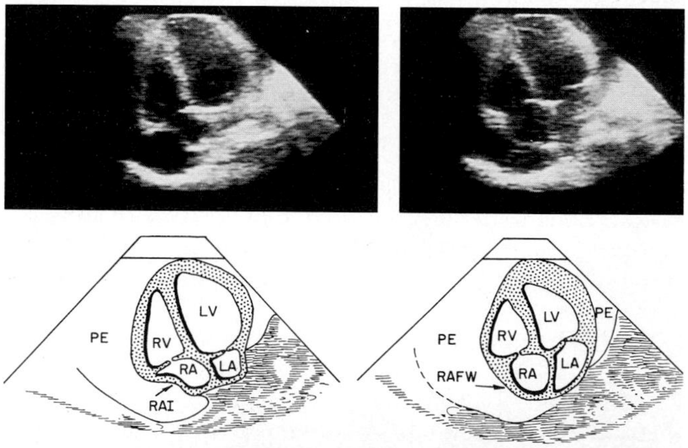

Fig. 35–34. Apical four-chamber cross-sectional echocardiogram demonstrates right atrial inversion (RAI). Left. In early systole, the right atrial free wall (RAFW) is strikingly inverted. Right. By end-systole, the right atrium (RA) has filled and the RAFW contour is normally rounded. RV = right ventricle; LA = left atrium; LV = left ventricle; PE = pericardial effusion. (From Gillam LD: Hemodynamic compression of the right atrium: a new echocardiographic sign of cardiac tamponade. Circulation 68:294, 1983. Reproduced by permission of the American Heart Association, Inc.)

separated (Fig. 35–35). Right atrial inversion lasting for longer than one-third of the cardiac cycle has been reported to have a specificity of 100% and sensitivity of 94% for the presence of clinical cardiac tamponade.[71] The duration and degree of right atrial inversion vary, with respiration being most marked during the first beats after expiration (Fig. 35–36).

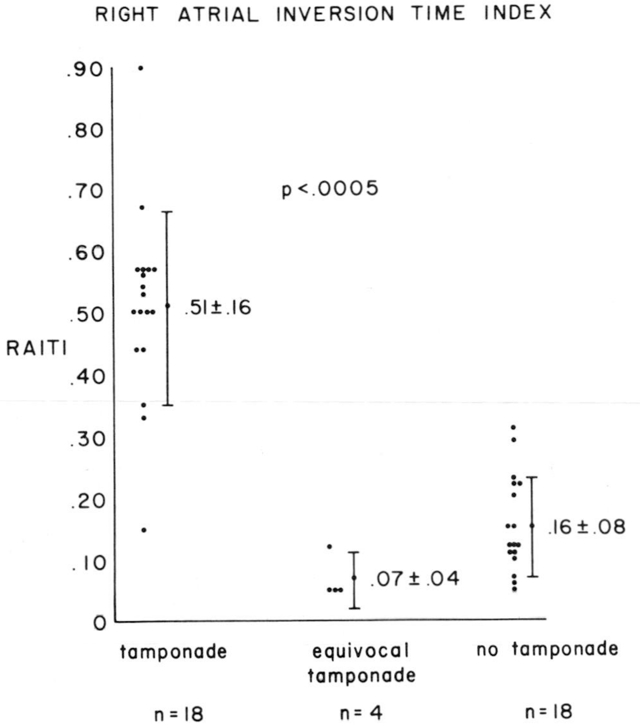

Fig. 35–35. Right atrial inversion time index (RAITI) calculated from patients with right atrial inversion and definite, equivocal, or no tamponade. The difference of means between patients with definite and no cardiac tamponade is highly significant ($p < .0005$), and if a cut off of 0.34 is used, there is little overlap between patient groups. (From Gillam LD: Hemodynamic compression of the right atrium: a new echocardiographic sign of cardiac tamponade. Circulation 68:294, 1983. Reproduced by permission of the American Heart Association, Inc.)

The presence of sinus rhythm is not required for prolonged atrial inversion. Ventricular pacing, however, may affect the accuracy of this sign because the only false-negative result occurred in a patient with a paced rhythm. Although less extensively studied, the same factors that interfere with RVDC should also prevent or diminish atrial collapse (i.e., adhesions involving the right atrial wall, loculated effusion, increased atrial stiffness, and small volume-high pressure tamponade after laceration or trauma).

Comparative Value of Right Atrial and Ventricular Inversion

The value of right atrial and right ventricular collapse has been compared in a group of patients with hemodynamic evidence of cardiac tamponade by performing continuous two-dimensional echocardiography as pericardiocentesis was done.[72] Right atrial inversion occurred earlier in the progression of hemodynamic compromise than right ventricular diastolic inversion, likely because the nadir of the right ventricular pressure curve tends to be higher than the nadir of the right atrial curve. Despite this finding, right ventricular inversion still occurred before systemic blood pressure had decreased.

At extreme levels of intrapericardial pressure, marked diastolic compression of both right-sided chambers may occur, severely limiting both diastolic filling and systolic emptying (Fig. 35–37).[58] This degree of compression is usually associated with arterial hypotension and can be appreciated during both two-dimensional and M-mode recordings.[73]

In most cases, effusions do not extend behind the left atrium because of the tethering effect of the pulmonary veins. In a subset of patients, however, the pericardial reflection may extend sufficiently superiorly to allow part of the left atrial wall to fall under the influence of pericardial pressure. In the setting of cardiac tamponade, invagination of this portion of the left atrial wall can occur,[69] as illustrated in Figure 35–38.[69,74] If present, this finding should correlate well with clinical cardiac tamponade, but it is clearly less sensitive than previously described signs.

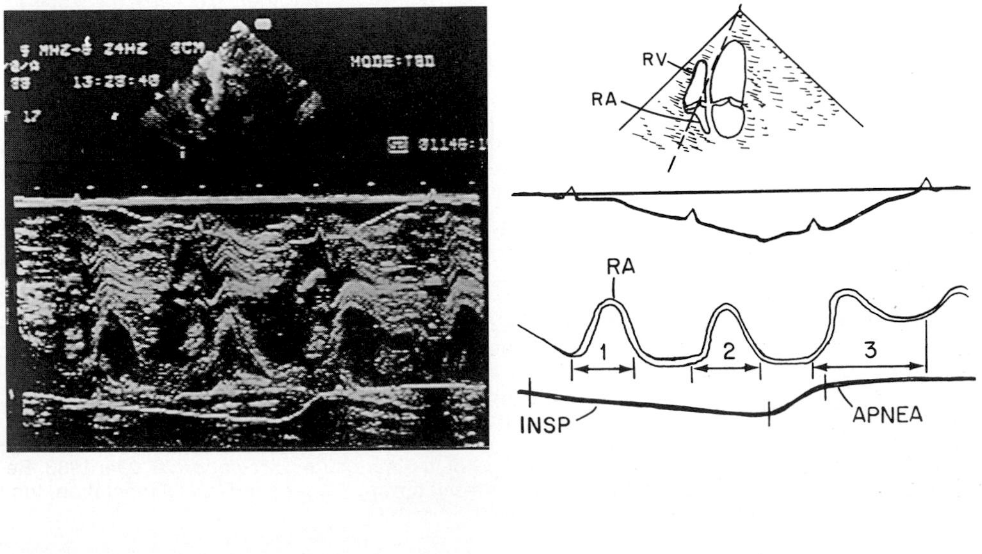

Fig. 35–36. M-mode recording of the right atrial free wall (RA), illustrating both the timing and duration of right atrial inversion. Right atrial inversion begins at the onset of the horizontal arrows in the accompanying diagram (end-diastole immediately following atrial systole) and persists throughout ventricular systole (end of horizontal arrows). The degree and duration of right atrial inversion is most significant in the first beats after the onset of apnea (complex 3). Recordings are obtained from a closed chest, spontaneously breathing experimental model of the cardiac tamponade, and respiration is measured as change in intrapleural pressure. RV = right ventricle.

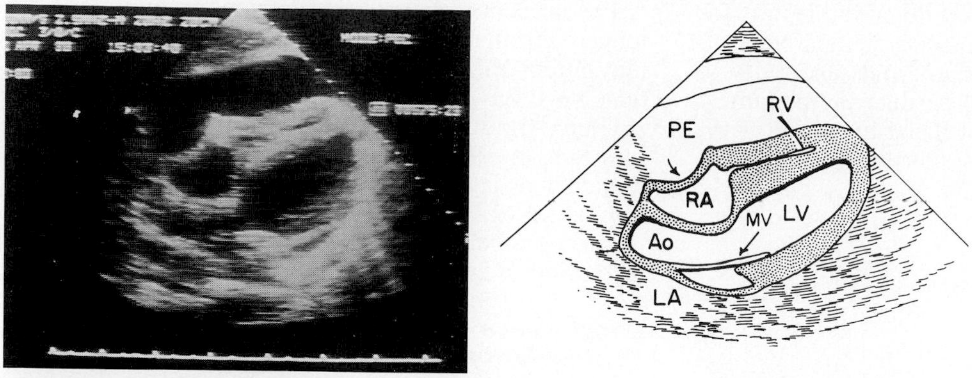

Fig. 35–37. Subcostal long axis recording illustrating compression of both the right ventricle (RV) and right atrium (RA) caused by severe cardiac tamponade. This degree of right-sided compression is usually associated with marked depression in cardiac output and circulatory collapse. Curved arrow in accompanying diagram indicates point of right atrial free wall inversion. PE = pericardial effusion; AO = aorta; MV = mitral valve; LV = left ventricle; LA = left atrium.

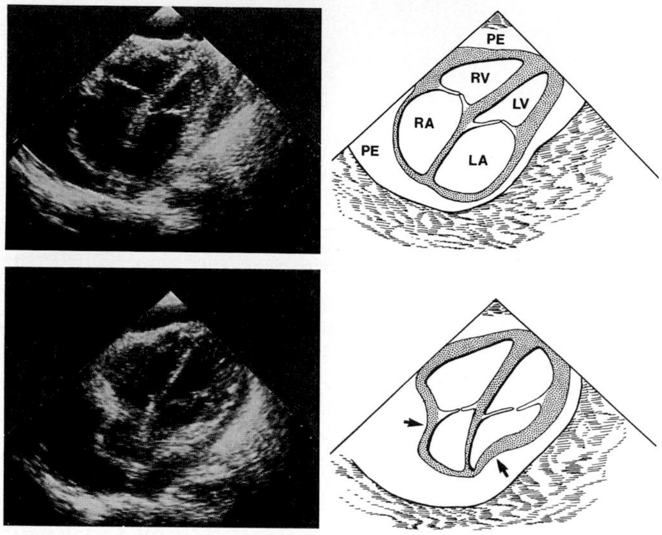

Fig. 35–38. Subcostal four-chamber recordings from a patient with a large pericardial effusion and cardiac tamponade. Top. Recorded at end-ventricular systole, the right and left atria are filled, and the walls of both chambers curve symmetrically outward. Bottom. Recorded during early systole, there are both right and left atrial collapse (arrows), characteristic of cardiac tamponade. RA = right atrium; RV = right ventricle; LA = left atrium; LV = left ventricle; PE = pericardial effusion.

Additional M-Mode and Two-Dimensional Echocardiographic Signs

Additional findings have been reported in cardiac tamponade that are, in general, manifestations of the exaggerated respiratory variations in intracardiac flow known to occur in this condition,[49] and they are most easily identified on M-mode recordings.[75–80] For example, mitral valve opening has been shown to decrease with inspiration, resulting in decreased excursion of the anterior leaflet and a diminished E-F slope.[78–80] Moreover, right and left ventricular diameters vary in a reciprocal fashion during respiration[73,78,80] (Fig. 35–39), and they reflect increased right heart filling during inspiration with secondary compromise of left heart flow, as discussed previously. Decreased phasic changes in the diameter of the inferior vena cava have been described in patients with hemodynamically confirmed pericardial tamponade.[70] A maximum-to-minimum diameter ratio of $<50\%$ (''plethora'') was found to predict the presence of tamponade with 97% sensitivity, but only 40% specificity.

Doppler Findings

More recently, the development of Doppler echocardiography has made quantitation of left- and right-sided

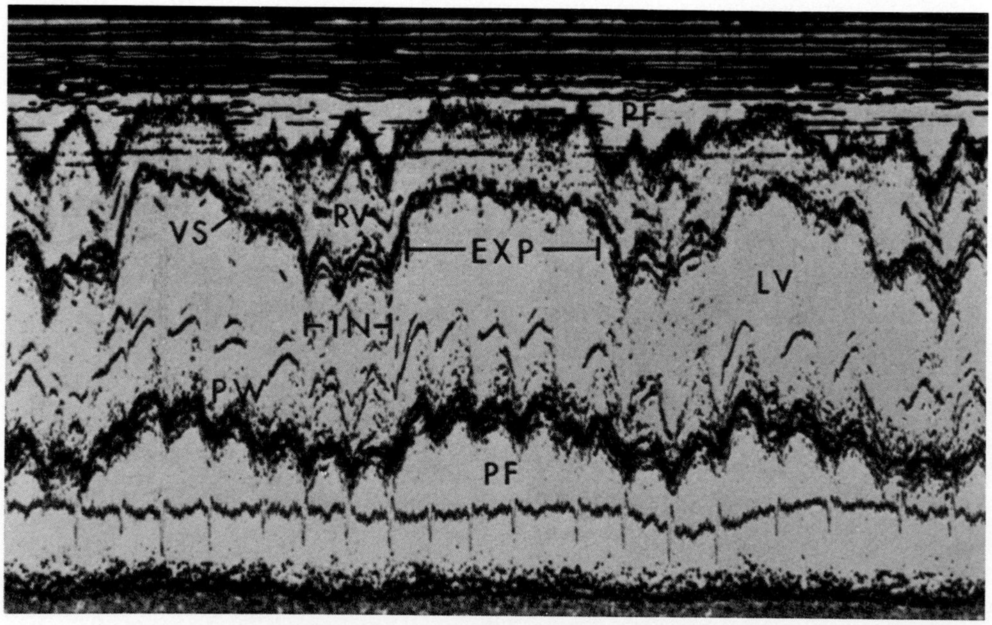

Fig. 35–39. M-mode echocardiogram from a patient with a large pericardial effusion, demonstrating pronounced variation in cardiac dimensions with respiration. During inspiration (IN), the dimension of the right ventricle (RV) appears to increase, whereas that of the left ventricle decreases. The opposite change occurs during expression (EXP). A large posterior and a moderate anterior pericardial effusion are present. PF = pericardial fluid; VS = ventricular septum; LV = left ventricle. (From Tajik AJ: Echocardiography and pericardial effusion. Am J Med 63:29, 1977.)

transvalvular flow velocities possible. In normal patients or during baseline recordings in experimental models, mitral flow velocity decreases by up to 10% during inspiration, and tricuspid flow increases by up to 17%. The changes in aortic and pulmonic flow are smaller, but aortic flow consistently decreases slightly during inspiration (Fig. 35–40A), and pulmonic flow increases (Fig. 35–41A). In the presence of pericardial effusion, these changes in flow velocity remain qualitatively the same but increase in magnitude, even in the absence of hemodynamic markers of cardiac tamponade (Figs. 35–40B and 35–41B). When hemodynamic tamponade occurs, these respiratory variations become much more marked. Inspiratory decreases in mitral and aortic flow in the range of 40% have been consistently recorded (Fig. 35–40C). Right-sided flows vary more dramatically, and inspiratory increases in flow velocities of over 80% from expiratory values have been consistently observed (Fig. 35–41C).[81–84] The results of these studies are summarized in Table 35–3.

When the degree of respiratory variation was assessed at known increments in pericardial pressure, a clear relationship between the percentage of inspiratory change in aortic and pulmonic flow velocity and pericardial pressure, cardiac output, aortic pressure, and pulsus paradoxus was observed (Fig. 35–42). Although a roughly linear relationship existed between intrapericardial pressure and the percentage of change in both aortic and pulmonic flow velocity, the effect on right-sided flow velocities was more than twice that seen on the left (Fig. 35–43). When respiratory effort was considered, the absolute decrease in intrapleural pressure paralleled

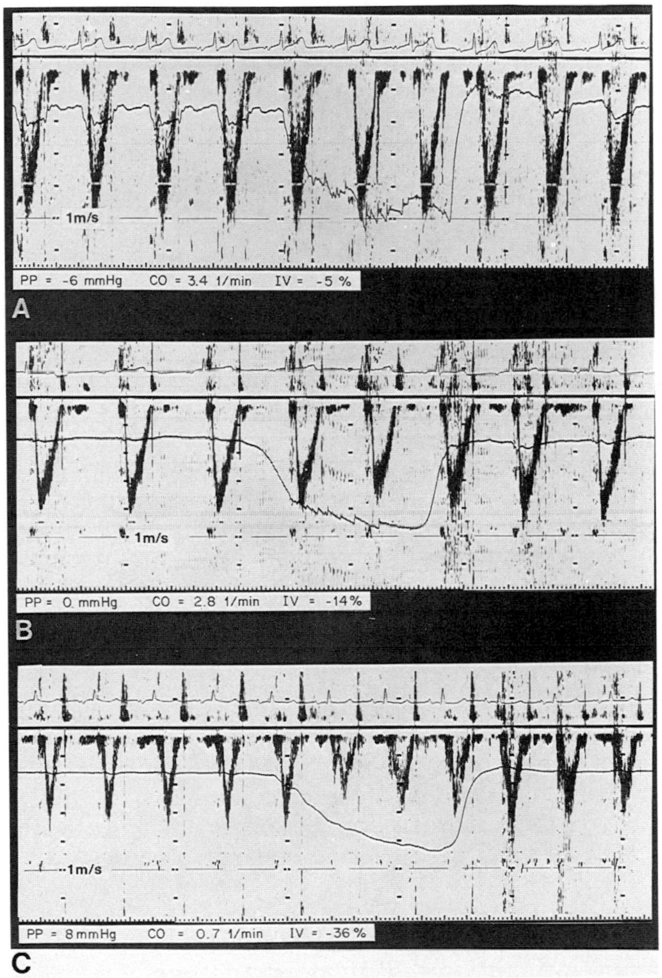

Fig. 35–40. Doppler recordings illustrating the changes in aortic flow velocity: **A.** Changes during inspiration at baseline with normal pericardial pressure and no pericardial effusion. **B.** and **C.** Changes with increasing intrapericardial pressure (PP) produced by instillation of fluid into the pericardial space. During inspiration, indicated by a downward deflection of the respiratory tracing, there is a slight decrease in aortic flow velocity at baseline, which increases in both magnitude and duration as PP is increased. CO = cardiac output; IV = inspiratory variation. From Picard, MH, et al., Quantitative Relation between increased intrapericardial pressure and Doppler flow velocities during experimental cardiac tamponade. J Am Coll Cardiol; 18:234, 1991. Reprinted with permission of the American College of Cardiology.

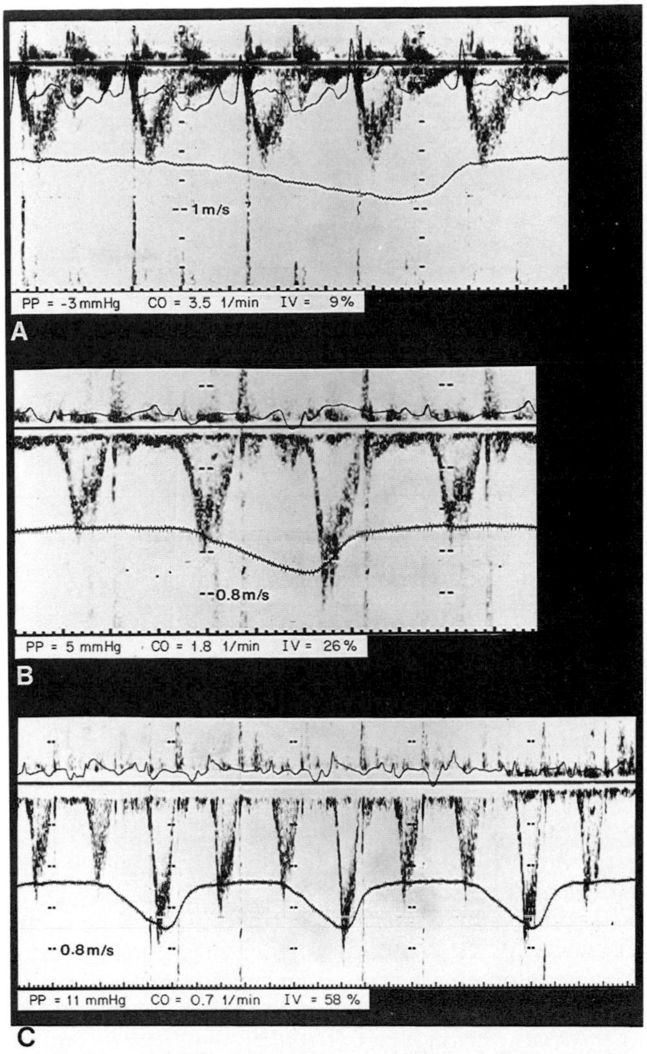

Fig. 35–41. Spectral Doppler recordings of pulmonary flow from a spontaneously breathing experimental model of pericardial tamponade. **A.** At baseline, there is little change in pulmonary flow velocity during inspiration. **B** and **C.** As intrapericardial (PP) pressure is increased to 5 mm Hg **(B)** and 11 mm of Hg **(C)**, cardiac output falls from 3.5 L/min, respectively, and inspiratory variation (IV) in flow velocity increases from 9 to 26 and 58%. From Picard, MH, et al., Quantitative Relation between increased intrapericardial pressure and Doppler flow velocities during experimental cardiac tamponade. J Am Coll Cardiol; 18:234, 1991. Reprinted with permission of the American College of Cardiology.

Table 35–3. Respiratory Variations in Doppler Flow Velocity (all values given are % change with inspiration)

	Pandian[81]	Leeman[83]	Appleton[84]
Control			
Mitral	−10	−8	−4
Tricuspid	17	5	14
Aortic	—	−3	−4
Pulmonic	—	9	5
Effusion			
Mitral	−12	−3	−5*, −31†
Tricuspid	17	21	32*, 74†
Aortic	—	−7	−17
Pulmonic	—	11	49
Tamponade			
Mitral	−42	−35	E −43 ± 9%; A −28 ± 12%
Tricuspid	117	80	E 85 ± 53%; A 58 ± 25%
Aortic	—	−33	−26
Pulmonic	—	86	40 ± 25%
Left ventricular isovolumic relaxation time	—	—	85 ± 14%
Left ventricular ejection time	—	—	−21 ± 3%

* Subgroup with pericardial effusion but no tamponade and no respiratory variation in flow.
† Subgroup with pericardial effusion and no tamponade but respiratory variation in flow.
E = peak E-wave velocity; A = peak A-wave velocity.

the right-sided changes (Fig. 35–44), suggesting that intrapleural pressure was more directly transmitted to the right heart chambers.

In studies of patients with cardiac tamponade requiring emergency pericardiocentesis, variations in certain other parameters of ventricular ejection and relaxation in addition to transvalvular velocities were reported.[84] Respiratory variation in left ventricular ejection and isovolumic relaxation times were markedly increased compared to measurements made after pericardiocentesis and in normal subjects. During inspiration, the left ventricular isovolumic relaxation time increased by 85%, the transmitral peak E-wave velocity decreased by 43%, and the transmitral peak A-wave velocity decreased by 25% compared with values during expiration. After pericardiocentesis, these values fell to normal (i.e., <10%). Also during inspiration in the group with cardiac tamponade, the transtricuspid peak E-wave velocity increased by 85% and the transtricuspid peak A-wave velocity increased by 58%, compared to corresponding changes of less than 25% after pericardiocentesis and in normal subjects. Changes in velocity-time integrals generally paralleled those in peak velocity, with the largest respiratory variation occurring in the patients with cardiac tamponade. As well as serving as markers of clinical cardiac tamponade, these Doppler observations provide useful insights into the mechanisms underlying the pulsus paradoxus seen in this condition.

Abnormal flow patterns were also seen in the superior vena cava and hepatic veins in patients with pericardial tamponade.[76] In normal subjects, venous flow was biphasic, with flow velocities in systole higher than in diastole during all phases of respiration (Fig. 35–45). A small reversal of flow was usually seen during atrial contraction. On inspiration, there was an increase in systolic and diastolic flow velocities in most normal subjects, and at the onset of expiration, there was no decrease in diastolic flow velocity compared with apnea. Patients with cardiac tamponade, on the other hand, had a marked predominance of systolic flow during apnea. During the first beat of inspiration, only minimal increases in systolic and diastolic flow velocities were seen that were less than the inspiratory increases found in most normal subjects. On the first beat after the onset of expiration, all patients with cardiac tamponade had a decrease or reversal of diastolic flow velocities and occasionally systolic flow velocities compared to measurements during apnea, unlike in normal subjects. After pericardiocentesis, all patients showed increased forward flow velocities in the superior vena cava during apnea, and abnormal flow patterns during respiration generally improved or reverted to normal. The clinical utility of these intricate Doppler observations in the diagnosis of cardiac tamponade remains to be proved.

Cardiac Tamponade Associated with Acute Intrapericardial Hemorrhage and Loculated Effusion

When cardiac tamponade results from cardiac laceration, trauma, or intrapericardial hemorrhage after surgery or aortic dissection, the pericardial pressure may rise abruptly despite only a small increase in intrapericardial volume. In such cases, many of the classic signs of tamponade described previously (i.e., right atrial and ventricular inversion, septal motion abnormalities, etc.) are typically absent, and the only diagnostic feature is

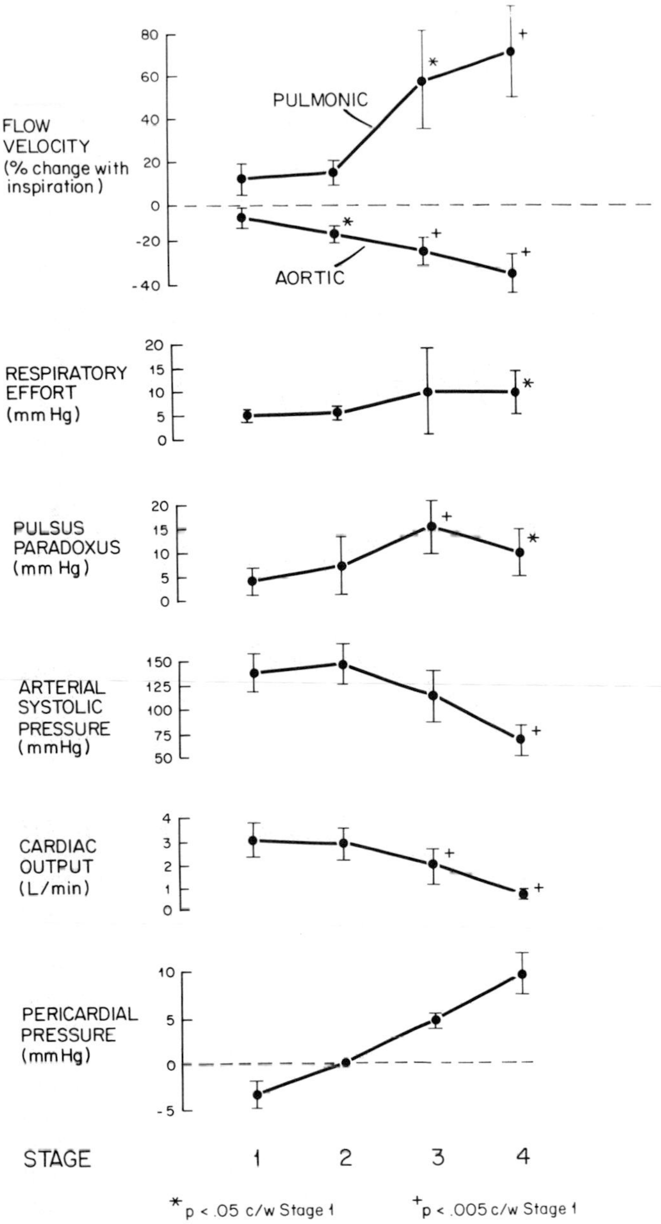

Fig. 35–42. Effects of increasing pericardial pressure on pulmonary and aortic flow velocity, degree of pulsus paradoxus, arterial systolic pressure, and cardiac output. As pericardial pressure increases, the percentage of change in pulmonic flow velocity increases while the percentage of change in aortic pressure falls in a roughly linear fashion. The percentage of decrease in arterial blood pressure or pulsus paradoxus gradually increases to stage 3 and then drops as systemic arterial pressure falls. Arterial pressure and cardiac output both decrease as intrapericardial pressure increases, with the drop in both parameters becoming significant at the point of fully developed tamponade. From Picard, MH, et al., Quantitative relation between increased intrapericardial pressure and Doppler flow velocities during experimental cardiac tamponade. J Am Coll Cardiol; 18:234, 1991. Reprinted with permission of the American College of Cardiology.

the new accumulation of fluid. As a result, the diagnosis of cardiac tamponade can only be presumed, and it is necessary that a control study be available to confirm that the fluid accumulation is actually new.

In patients with loculated effusion, physiologic features of cardiac tamponade may also be present without many of the classic imaging signs previously described. This situation usually occurs postoperatively or after cardiac trauma and is frequently associated with some indentation of the heart caused by the fluid, which is under pressure. When the loculated fluid is adjacent to the left ventricle, the pericardial space may appear to decrease in size during systole when chamber pressure

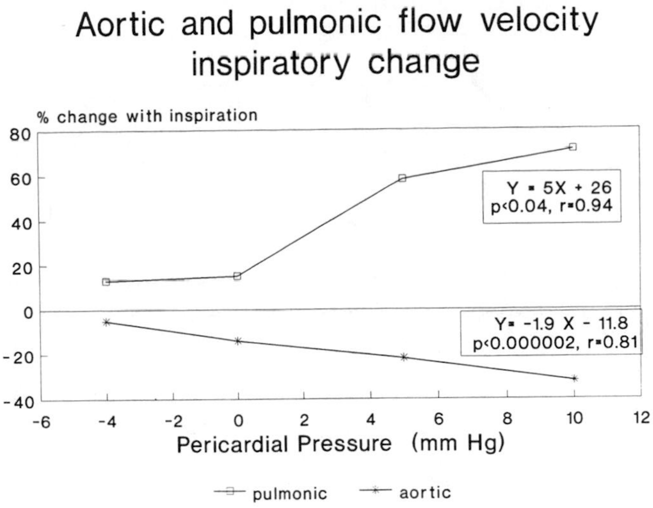

Fig. 35–43. The percentage of change in aortic and pulmonic flow velocity vs. increase in pericardial pressure. Note that the effects of intrapericardial pressure on pulmonic flow are roughly double those recorded for aortic flow.

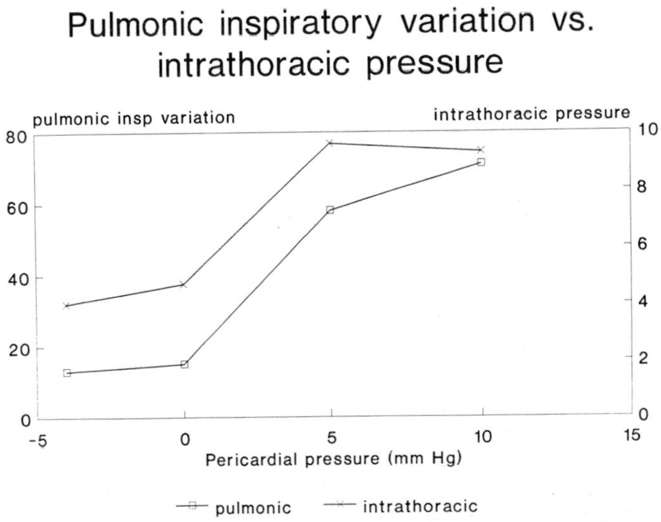

Fig. 35–44. Demonstration of parallel changes in pulmonic flow velocity variation and the absolute change in intrathoracic pressure at varying pericardial pressure. Respiratory effort, as measured by changes in intrathoracic pressure, has a significant effect on pulmonary flow velocity and is the primary determinant of the percentage change in pulmonary flow velocity. Respiratory effort, however, has little effect on aortic flow velocity, suggesting that change in aortic flow velocity may be a more predictable measure of changes in the pericardial pressure.

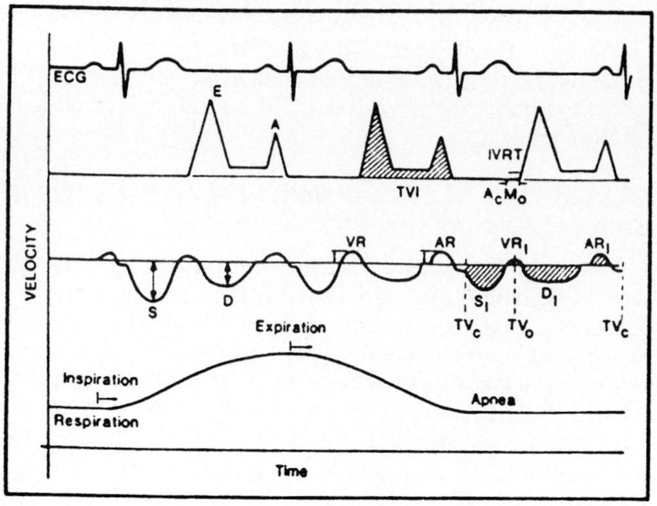

Fig. 35–45. The methods of analysis of mitral and tricuspid flow velocities (top) and hepatic venous flow velocities (bottom). Diagrammatic Doppler profiles are similar to those that would be recorded from the cardiac apex, and their timing can be related both to an electrocadiogram (ECG) and a respiratory tracing. For hepatic vein flow, displacement of the flow profile below the baseline represents flow toward the heart. A = peak atrial filling velocity; A_C = aortic closure; AR = reverse flow during atrial systole (atrial "a" wave); AR_1 = the integral of AR; D = diastolic forward flow velocity; E = peak early mitral or tricuspid filling velocity; IVRT = isovolumic relaxation time; M_o = mitral opening; S = systolic forward flow velocity; S_i = the integral of S; TV_c = tricuspid valve closure; TVI = time velocity integral; TV_o = tricuspid valve opening; VR = reverse flow and end-systole (atrial "v" wave); VR_i = interval of VR. (From Burstow DJ, et al.: Cardiac tamponade: Characteristic Doppler observations. Mayo Clin Proc 64:312, 1989.)

is high and increase during diastole when intracavitary pressure falls below local intrapericardial pressure.[85]

Localized effusion adjacent to the right atrium or ventricle may lead to partial or subtotal cavity obliteration, whereas fluid accumulation above the right ventricle outflow tract may cause outflow obstruction.[86]

CONSTRICTIVE PERICARDITIS

Pathophysiology

Pericardial constriction occurs when the pericardium becomes rigid because of inflammation, fibrosis, calcification, or neoplasm and impedes diastolic filling. Most cases of pericardial constriction probably begin as pericardial inflammation with exudation of fluid into the pericardial sac. This is resorbed, and the visceral and parietal pericardial layers then fuse. A variety of disorders may cause the initial inflammation (Table 35–4), but in most cases no underlying cause is evident clinically or histologically.[87] Constrictive pericarditis occurs in roughly 0.2% of patients after cardiac surgery even though the pericardium is left open.[88]

The typical hemodynamic picture consists of markedly elevated ventricular diastolic pressures with a characteristic pattern of rapid early diastolic ventricular filling that stops abruptly as the limit of ventricular expansion is achieved. This situation results in an early dip in the right ventricular pressure tracing, followed quickly by an equally rapid pressure rise and subsequent plateau as the limitation of filling is reached. This pattern of rapid descent, rise, and plateau of ventricular pressure has the form of the mathematic square root sign and has generally been referred to as such.

Because of the dense pericardial encasement, respiratory fluctuations in pleural pressure are not transmitted to the heart. As a result, inspiration does not enhance right heart inflow, and systemic blood pressure may not vary significantly. Inspiration, however, does decrease pulmonary wedge pressure and, by inference, pulmonary venous pressure. This decreases the left atrial pressure at mitral valve opening and therefore increases left ventricular isovolumic relaxation time and decreases peak mitral inflow velocity.

Because constrictive pericarditis limits cardiac filling to a relatively fixed diastolic volume, events in one ventricle are closely coupled to those in the contralateral chamber. Thus, the respiratory decrease in left ventricular filling is associated with a corresponding increase in right ventricular filling. This ventricular coupling is also reflected by reciprocal respiratory fluctuation in ventricular dimensions, peak systolic pressures, ejection times, and aortic and pulmonary flow velocities. As discussed later in this chapter, these specific pressure and flow patterns can be used to advantage in the echo-Doppler characterization of constrictive pericarditis.

The process causing constriction usually affects the pericardium diffusely and equally. Occasionally, however, one may see a localized area of constriction, most often in patients with previous inadequate pericardiectomies, but rarely without a history of heart surgery. The clinical presentation in cases of focal constriction is typically one of inflow or outflow obstruction of the right or left heart in association with clinical features of typical pericardial constriction.

Table 35–4. Causes of Constrictive Pericarditis

Hereditary disorder
Mulibrey nanism
Infectious diseases
Bacterial
Fungal
Viral
Parasitic
Connective tissue disorders
Rheumatoid arthritis
Systemic lupus erythematosus
Polyarteritis nodosa
Metabolic disorder
Uremia
Trauma
Blunt or penetrating thoracic trauma
Surgery
Radiation therapy
Neoplastic disease
Benign or malignant pericardial tumors
Metastatic malignant disease

Echocardiographic Diagnosis

The echocardiographic signs of pericardial constriction are generally indirect and have proved less sensitive and specific than those previously described for cardiac tamponade. As a rule, cardiac and ventricular size are normal and diastolic function is normal or slightly reduced. The atria may be normal in size or slightly enlarged. The inferior vena cava and hepatic veins are generally prominently dilated. Both morphologic abnormalities (such as pericardial thickening) and signs of altered diastolic filling (such as altered ventricular wall motion and diastolic regurgitation) have been described, but no consistent diagnostic picture has emerged.

Pericardial Thickening

Although pericardial constriction and thickening would appear to be uniformly associated surgically and pathologically, the use of echocardiography to detect and quantitate pericardial thickening has not been completely defined. Investigators who conducted M-mode studies report pericardial thickening in 53%[89] to 100%[90] of patients with documented pericardial constriction. In two-dimensional imaging studies, the association has been more consistent, but the number of patients studied has been small. The relationship of apparent pericardial thickness determined by echocardiography with pathologic measures of pericardial thickness has also been inconsistent. In a retrospective M-mode study of patients with pericardial thickening who subsequently underwent surgery or autopsy, only 76% had pericardial thickening confirmed by direct observation.[92] In an experimental model where constrictive pericarditis was induced in dogs by instillation of a pericardial irritant mixture, the two-dimensional echocardiographic measurement of pericardial thickness was found to correlate only modestly ($r = 0.58$) with measurement at autopsy.[91]

Even when clearly present, pericardial thickening and constriction are not uniformly associated.[90,92] Thus, in a study of patients with pericardial thickening who subsequently underwent cardiac catheterization, only 38% had hemodynamic findings of pericardial constriction.[90] No consistent pattern of pericardial thickening has emerged as diagnostic for pericardial constriction.

The lack of reliability of pericardial thickening as a marker of pericardial constriction may relate to the primary disease process or to technical difficulties in studying these patients. Anatomically, pericardial fibrosis tends to obscure the well-defined anatomic borders of the heart and may involve myocardium and surrounding structures. In addition, the thickness of the pericardium may vary widely at different points around the heart or may involve isolated areas, complicating qualitative or quantitative description. Technically, pericardial constriction is frequently difficult to image, and extremely high gain settings are required to record intracardiac structures. Use of high instrument gain may obscure the fine detail often necessary to characterize the pericardium or to produce the appearance of pericardial thickening when none is present. Thus, an adequate examination generally requires some suspicion of pericardial disease, as well as extreme care in image optimization and gain setting. Transesophageal imaging may permit more precise measurement of pericardial thickness (Fig. 35–46); however, sensitivity and specificity remain to be determined.

M-Mode and Two-Dimensional Echocardiographic Signs of Abnormal Ventricular Filling

Probably more helpful in the assessment of constrictive pericarditis are signs attributable to the abnormal pattern of diastolic ventricular filling that occurs in this condition (see also Chapter 24). Abnormal filling is manifested by a pattern of abrupt early diastolic ventricular expansion, followed by abrupt cessation of further outward motion of the wall with little further expansion for the remainder of diastole. This pattern is often referred to as left ventricular posterior wall "flattening,"[93,94] and it has been reported in 85% of patients with pericardial constriction, but unfortunately it is also seen in 18% of normal subjects.

Abnormalities in both position and motion of the interventricular and interatrial septum have also been described.[95–97] Septal position varies with respiration, and during inspiration, both the interatrial and interventricular septa deviate to the left.[94] Septal motion abnormalities range from an early diastolic "bounce" involving a brisk rightward displacement of the basal septum to frank paradoxic motion. An "atrial systolic notch," consisting of abrupt motion of the septum toward the left ventricle after electrocardiographic evidence of atrial activation, has also been described,[98] as well as an "early diastolic notch."[99] These abnormalities of motion must be caused by transient reversals in the transseptal pressure gradient that become magnified by

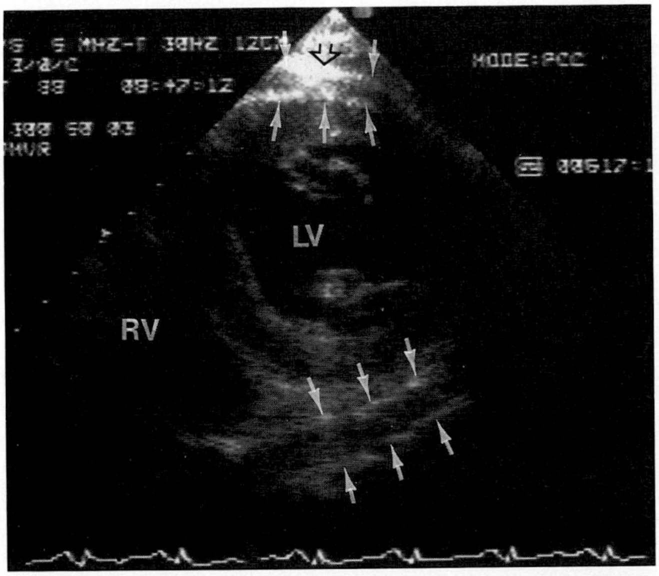

Fig. 35–46. Transesophageal echocardiographic recording of patient with constrictive pericarditis. In this short axis image of the left ventricle, the thickened pericardium can be clearly appreciated both anterior and posterior to the heart and the thickness of the pericardium measured (arrows). The physiologic correlate of this anatomic abnormality, however, must be determined using other approaches. RV = right ventricle; LV = left ventricle.

the relative redundancy of the septum as it seeks to relax within the rigid pericardial shell. Unfortunately, these findings are present in fewer than 50% of patients with pericardial constriction and may be seen in both normal subjects and patients with other cardiac disorders.

Premature diastolic opening of the pulmonic valve has also been observed in patients with pericardial constriction,[100] and it is more prominent during inspiration.[101] Premature pulmonic valve opening reflects the early rapid rise in right ventricular diastolic pressure to a level exceeding pulmonary artery pressure. This sign is nonspecific, however, reported in a variety of other disorders including right ventricular infarction,[75] restrictive myopathy, rupture of a sinus of Valsalva aneurysm into the right atrium,[102] and other conditions that cause abnormally elevated right ventricular mid-diastolic pressure.

Finally, blunting of the normal respiratory variation in the diameter of the inferior vena cava has been observed in pericardial constriction,[103,104] and sensitivity of 79% and specificity of 80% have been reported.[103]

Despite these numerous reports and the variety of signs described, no single two-dimensional or M-mode finding or combination of findings has been proved to be completely reliable in clinical diagnosis.

Doppler Findings

Doppler studies of patients with pericardial constriction report a variety of alterations in intracardiac flow velocity. Early reports noted an increase in early diastolic filling velocities (E wave), followed by a rapid deceleration and a shortened filling period.[105,106] These findings, however, would be expected with any cause of diastolic dysfunction with a compensatory increase in left atrial pressure and are therefore not specific for constrictive pericarditis. More recently, detailed analysis of Doppler flow patterns reported striking respiratory changes in intracardiac flow patterns that reflect the abnormal pressure relationships and increased ventricular interdependence that result from the constrictive process.[76] These include the following: (1) marked respiratory variation in the left ventricular isovolumic relaxation time (i.e., a roughly 50% increase from expiration to inspiration) and a marked inspiratory fall in peak mitral E-wave velocity (mean >30% from expiration) (Fig. 35–47); the largest decrease in mitral valve E-wave velocity and largest increase in left ventricular isovolumic relaxation time are reported to occur in the first beat after the onset of inspiration, compared with the apnea value; these changes reflect the exaggerated respiratory variation in left atrial pressure seen in pericardial constriction; (2) a reciprocal change in tricuspid flow velocity, with the largest increase in velocity occurring in the first beat of inspiration and the largest decrease in velocity in the first beat after the onset of expiration (Fig. 35–47); (3) shortening of the mitral and tricuspid deceleration time with no further decrease during inspiration; (4) a greater mean inspiratory decrease in aortic flow velocity and a left ventricular ejection time longer than typically occurs in normal subjects is seen in the beats immediately after those in which changes in mitral and tricuspid flow velocity were observed; and (5) blood flow from the right ventricle into the pulmonary artery during diastole in roughly 60% of patients.

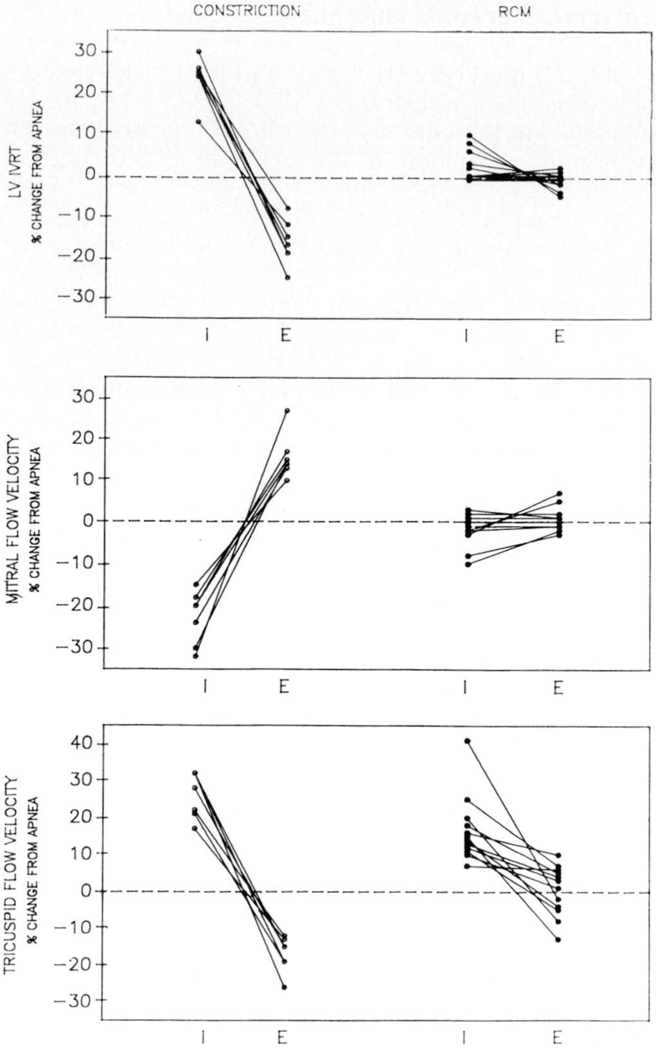

Fig. 35–47. Plots of individual values for respiratory variation (expressed as a percentage of change from apnea) of left ventricular isovolumic relaxation time (LV IVRT), peak early mitral flow velocity, and peak early tricuspid flow velocity in patients with constrictive pericarditis (n = 7) and restrictive cardiomyopathy (RCM) (n = 12). I = inspiration; E = expiration. (From Hatle LK, et al.: Differentiation of restrictive pericarditis and restrictive cardiomyopathy by Doppler echocardiography. Circulation 79:357, 1989. Reproduced by permission of the American Heart Association, Inc.)

Differentiation of Constriction from Restriction

Restrictive cardiomyopathy, irrespective of origin, is characterized by a reduction in myocardial compliance, resulting in an abnormally large increase in early diastolic ventricular pressures for small increments in volume, a pattern similar to that seen in pericardial constriction. Doppler flow patterns have also been reported to be helpful in differentiating patients with pericardial constriction from those with restrictive cardiac physiologic features. Specific differential points include the following: (1) lack of the marked respiratory variation in left ventricular isovolumic relaxation time and mitral E-wave velocity seen in constrictive pericarditis (Fig. 35–47); (2) markedly shortened mitral and tricuspid deceleration times in restriction when compared to normal subjects and patients with pericardial constriction; (3) inspiratory shortening of the tricuspid and sometimes the mitral deceleration time; (4) diastolic mitral and tricuspid regurgitation;[107] and (5) reduced mitral and tricuspid A waves during apnea when compared to normal subjects.

Blood flow from the right ventricle to the pulmonary artery during diastole is seen in roughly 50% of patients with restriction; it is usually associated with inspiration and seen before as well as after atrial contraction. Thus, premature pulmonic valve opening and diastolic flow reflect hemodynamic relationships rather than any specific disease state.

EFFUSIVE-CONSTRICTIVE PERICARDITIS

Although pericardial disease that results in compression of the heart is usually classified as either pericardial constriction or cardiac tamponade, a mixed "effusive-constrictive" form may also occur.[108,109] These patients have constriction of the heart by the visceral pericardium in association with tense effusion in a free pericardial space. The degree of thickening of the visceral pericardium and the extent of its adherence to the underlying myocardium vary from patient to patient, and these disorders occur in different areas of the heart.[110] The visceral constriction is often more severe over the right side of the heart than elsewhere and usually extends to involve the venae cavae.[110] The effusive and constrictive components combine to raise right atrial pressure to a higher level than that found in isolated constriction. The most common causes of effusive-constrictive disease are idiopathic pericarditis, radiation, neoplastic involvement of the pericardium, and tuberculosis.

The diagnosis is established by persistent evidence of pericardial compression after removal of pericardial effusion. Although intrapericardial pressure returns to normal after successful pericardiocentesis, right atrial pressure remains elevated, and its pattern changes from one with a dominant x descent to one with a predominant y descent (Fig. 35–48). Similarly, before pericardiocentesis, the right ventricular pressure curve shows a blunted early diastolic or y descent, whereas after fluid removal the early diastolic pressure dip returns and the right ventricular pressure curve assumes the classic "square root" pattern of constrictive pericarditis. It is therefore necessary to keep a high index of suspicion for constrictive changes in any hemodynamically compromised patient with pericardial disease.

Moreover, patients may convert from a pattern of effusive constrictive pericarditis to a pattern of classic constriction without associated effusion and may do so within several months.[110] This conversion entails resorption of pericardial fluid in association with continued formation of pericardial fibrous tissue.

Echocardiographic features in effusive-constrictive disease are poorly defined, but thickening of the visceral pericardium and frequently associated pericardial effusion are most frequent.[92] Moreover, when constriction and tamponade coexist, RVDC may not be present because the decreased compliance caused by the constriction may elevate right ventricular diastolic pressure above intrapericardial pressure.[63]

MISCELLANEOUS DISORDERS OF THE PERICARDIUM

Congenital Absence of the Pericardium

Total congenital absence of the pericardium is a rare disorder that is usually asymptomatic. Patients are referred for echocardiographic examination because of a

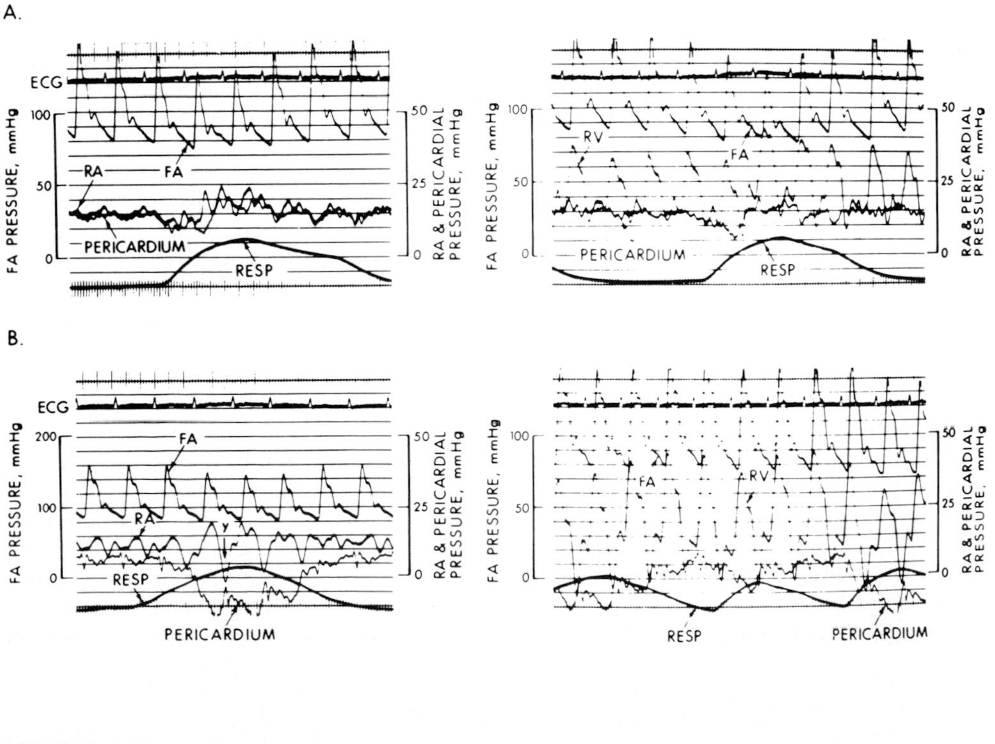

Fig. 35–48. Femoral arterial (FA), right atrial (RA), right ventricular (RV), and pericardial pressure tracings before **(A)** and after **(B)** pericardiocentesis. Left. After pericardiocentesis, the right atrial pressure remains elevated and develops a prominent y descent that is accentuated by inspiration. The late inspiratory rise (Kussmaul's sign) persists after pericardiocentesis. Right. A prominent right ventricular early diastolic pressure dip with a persistently elevated end-diastolic pressure develops after pericardiocentesis. (From Mann, DL, et al.: Effusive-constrictive hemodynamic pattern due to neoplastic involvement of the pericardium. Am J Cardiol 41:781, 1978.

heart murmur, an abnormal electrocardiogram, or marked leftward displacement of the cardiac silhouette and pulmonary artery on a chest roentgenogram. Two-dimensional echocardiography may show apparent right ventricular dilation in the parasternal long axis views, and a derived M-mode study will also show an increase in right ventricular internal dimension. This apparent chamber enlargement is generally not real, however, but reflects leftward malposition of the right ventricle that causes the scan plane to transect a larger portion of the crescent-shaped right ventricle than is normally the case. The interventricular septum may also appear to move paradoxically (i.e., arteriorly during systole); however, septal thickening is normal in the absence of associated disease, and the anterior systolic motion reflects cardiac translation rather than primary septal abnormality.[111]

Partial congenital absence of the pericardium also occurs, and in these patients the left atrial appendage can herniate through the pericardial defect. Marked enlargement of the left atrial appendage is noted in both the parasternal long axis and apical four-chamber views, and the condition may be difficult to differentiate from congenital aneurysm of the atrial appendage.[112]

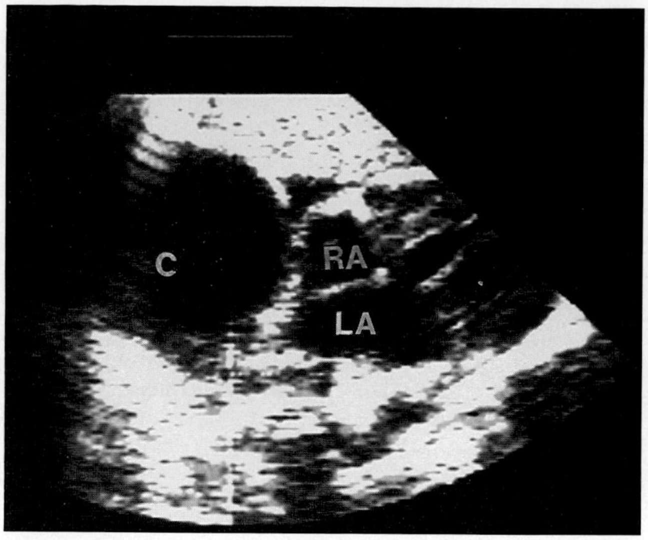

Fig. 35–49. A large cystic structure lateral to the right atrium (RA) within the right chest typical of that usually seen with pericardial cysts. In this case, however, the cyst was caused by a pancreatic pseudocyst that had penetrated the diaphragm and appeared lateral to the right heart. This example emphasizes the importance of considering the full differential diagnosis even when the echocardiographic findings appear classic. RA = right atrium; LA = left atrium; pancreatic pseudocyst simulating a pericardial cyst.

Pericardial Cysts

Pericardial cysts are benign intrathoracic lesions that occur in roughly 1 per 100,000 persons, but they represent approximately 7% of all mediastinal tumors. The diagnosis is usually suggested by the roentgenographic appearance of a round, sharply demarcated mass along the right cardiac silhouette in an asymptomatic patient. Pericardial cysts are typically located at the right costophrenic angle (70%) or the left costophrenic angle (10 to 40%), but they are occasionally seen along the upper mediastinum, hila, or left cardiac border. In one patient whose cyst was visualized by two-dimensional echocardiography, the cyst appeared as an ovoid echo-free space, slightly larger than the right heart, lying superolateral to the right atrial wall in the apical four-chamber view[113] (Fig. 35–49).

ECHOCARDIOGRAPHIC GUIDANCE OF PERICARDIOCENTESIS

Two-dimensional echocardiography may be of particular value in guiding pericardiocentesis because it can be used anywhere in the hospital and provides a unique and potentially simultaneous view of the heart, surrounding fluid, and the exploring needle. It can also be used to monitor catheter position during prolonged drainage and to separate free from loculated fluid by contrast injection.

When performing a pericardiocentesis under echocardiographic guidance, one usually places the patient in a supine or left lateral position. If the patient cannot lie flat because of dyspnea, both the echocardiographic study and pericardiocentesis can be performed with the patient seated. The optimal site for needle insertion—determined by two-dimensional echocardiographic examination—is the point at which the pericardial fluid is closest to the transducer and from which the needle track will avoid the heart and any underlying vital structures. Although the subcostal location is most commonly used for needle insertion in blind pericardiocentesis, in one series of 132 echocardiographically guided procedures, the subcostal location proved optimal in only 25%, whereas the chest wall was the preferable site of entry in 64%.[26] Although a variety of entry sites on the chest wall were used, including left and right parasternal, midclavicular line, and posterior chest, the apex (fifth to sixth intercostal space at the anterior axillary line) was most often the site of choice.

In patients with loculated effusion, multiple entry sites are often necessary. Once the optimal site of needle insertion is defined, the procedure can be performed either under direct echo guidance or by marking the desired point of insertion and defining the appropriate orientation for the needle track. The second procedure is simpler and is successful, with minor complications (right ventricular puncture and pneumopericardium) reported in only 2% of cases.[26]

Once the location and direction of needle insertion are determined, pericardiocentesis is usually performed using a short (2- to 4-cm) 16- to 18-gauge, Teflon-sheathed Intracath needle. When the pericardium is entered and fluid can be withdrawn, the Teflon sheath is advanced and the needle is withdrawn. The removal of fluid can be monitored from a remote transducer location (Fig. 35–50). When any question arises about needle position, echo-contrast can be injected to differentiate an intracavitary from an intrapericardial or intramural location of the needle tip.[114]

For prolonged drainage, a pigtail catheter can be

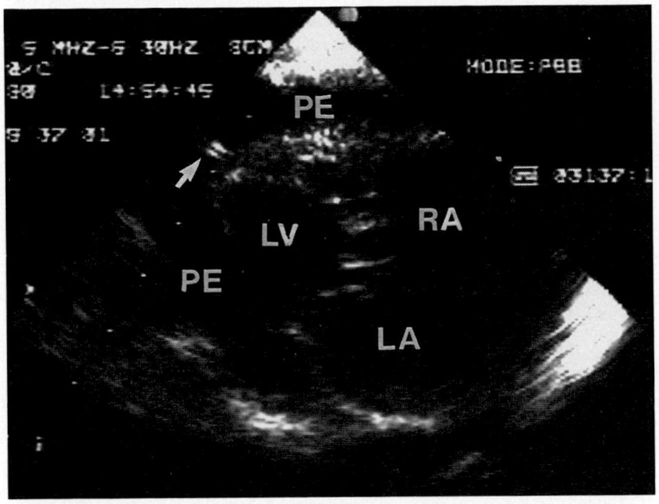

Fig. 35–50. Recording of an intrapericardial catheter (arrow) before pericardiocentesis. LV = left ventricle; LA = left atrium; RA = right atrium, PE = pericardial effusion.

placed in the pericardial space by inserting a guide wire through the Teflon sheath and removing the sheath and needle. A dilator and introducer sheath are then advanced over the guide wire into the pericardial space. The pigtail catheter is then introduced through the sheath and is attached to a closed system for continuous drainage.

After pericardiocentesis, two-dimensional imaging may also be useful for monitoring fluid resorption or reaccumulation, for detecting thrombus occurring de novo, and for observing the development of pericardial fibrosis.[115]

REFERENCES

1. Spodick DH: Medical history of the pericardium: the hairy hearts of hoary heroes. Am J Cardiol 26:447, 1970.
2. Goss CM (ed.): Gary's Anatomy of the Human Body. 29th Ed. Philadelphia, Lea & Febiger, 1973.
3. Gardner E, Gray DJ, O'Rahilly R: Anatomy: A Regional Study of Human Structure. 4th Ed. Philadelphia, W.B. Saunders, 1975.
4. Spodick DH: The normal and diseased pericardium: current concepts of pericardial physiology, diagnosis and treatment. J Am Coll Cardiol 1:240, 1983.
5. Shabetai R: The pericardium: an essay on some recent developments. Am J Cardiol 42:1036, 1978.
6. Tyson GS, et al.: Pericardial influences on ventricular filling in the conscious dog: an analysis based on pericardial pressure. Circ Res 54:173, 1984.
7. Glantz SA, et al.: The pericardium substantially affects the left ventricular diastolic pressure-volume relationship in the dog. Circ Res 42:433, 1978.
8. Janicki JS, Weber KT: Functional significance of the pericardium (abstr.). Circulation 55,56(Suppl. III): III-52, 1977.
9. Martin RP, Rakowski H, French JW, Popp RL: Localization of pericardial effusion with wide-angle phased array echocardiography. Am J Cardiol 42: 904, 1978.
10. Martin RP, Bowden R, Filly K, Popp RL: Intrapericardial abnormalities in patients with pericardial effusion: findings by two-dimensional echocardiography. Circulation 61:568, 1980.
11. Feigenbaum H: Echocardiography. 2nd Ed. Philadelphia, Lea & Febiger, 1976.
12. Hurst JW: The Heart. 3rd Ed. New York, McGraw-Hill, 1974.
13. Horowitz MS, et al.: Sensitivity and specificity of echocardiographic diagnosis of pericardial effusion. Circulation 50:239, 1974.
14. Matsuo H, et al.: Rotational excursion of the heart in massive pericardial effusion studied by phased-array echocardiography. Br Heart J 41:513, 1979.
15. Feigenbaum H, Zaky A, Grabhorn L: Cardiac motion in patients with pericardial effusion: a study using ultrasound cardiography. Circulation 34: 611, 1966.
16. Gabor GE, Winsberg F, Bloom HS: Electrical and mechanical alternation in pericardial effusion. Chest 59:341, 1971.
17. Yuste P, Torres-Carballada MA, Miguel-Alonso JL: Mechanism of electric alternans in pericardial effusion: study with ultrasonics. Arch Inst Cardiol Mex 45:197, 1975.
18. Lopez-Sendon J, et al.: Identification of blood in the pericardial cavity in dogs by two-dimensional echocardiography. Am J Cardiol 53:1194, 1984.
19. Parameswaram R, Goldberg H: Echocardiographic quantitation of pericardial effusion. Chest 83:767, 1983.
20. Prakash R, Moorthy K, Del Vicario L, Aronow WS: Reliability of echocardiography in quantitating pericardial effusion: a prospective study. J Clin Ultrasound 5:398, 1977.
21. Weitzman LB, et al. The incidence and natural history of pericardial effusion after cardiac surgery: an echocardiographic study. Circulation 69:506, 1984.
22. Haiat R, Helphen C: Silent pericardial effusion in late pregnancy: a new entity. Cardiovasc Intervent Radiol 7:267, 1981.
23. Wolf WJ: Echocardiographic features of a purulent pericardial peel. Am Heart J 111:990, 1986.
24. Friedberg CK: Diseases of the Heart. Philadelphia, W.B. Saunders, 1966.
25. Friedman MJ, Sahn DJ, Haber K: Two-dimensional echocardiography and B-mode ultrasonography for the diagnosis of loculated pericardial effusion. Circulation 60:1644, 1979.
26. Callahan JA, et al.: Two-dimensional echocardiographically guided pericardiocentesis: experience in 117 consecutive patients. Am J Cardiol 55: 476, 1985.
27. Fowler NO, Gabel M, Buncher CR: Cardiac tamponade: a comparison of right versus left heart compression. J Am Coll Cardiol 12:187, 1988.
28. Fyke FE III, et al.: Detection of intrapericardial hematoma after open heart surgery: the role of echocardiography and computer tomography. J Am Coll Cardiol 5:1496, 1985.
29. Luft FC, Gilman JK, Weyman AE: Pericarditis in the patient with uremia: clinical and echocardiographic evaluation. Nephron 25:160, 1980.
30. Savage DJ, et al: Prevalence and correlates of posterior extra echocardiographic spaces in a free-living population-based sample (the Framingham Study). Am J Cardiol 51:1207, 1983.
31. Spodick DH: Pericardial Disease. Philadelphia, F.A. Davis, p. 814, 1976.
32. Wada T, Honda M, Matsuyama S: Extra echo spaces: ultrasonography and computerised tomography correlations. Br Heart J 47:430, 1982.
33. Rifkin RD, Isner JM, Carter BL, Bankoff MS: Combined posteroanterior subepicardial fat simulating the echocardiographic diagnosis of pericardial effusion. J Am Coll Cardiol 3:1333, 1984.
34. Isner JM, Carter BL, Roberts WC, Bankoff MS: Subepicardial adipose tissue producing echocardiographic appearance of pericardial effusion. Am J Cardiol 51:565, 1983.
35. Ansari A, Rholl AO: Pseudopericardial effusion: echocardiographic and computerized tomographic correlations. Clin Cardiol 9:551, 1986.
36. Millman A, et al.: Pericardiol tumor and fibrosis mimicking pericardial effusion by echocardiography. Ann Intern Med 86:434, 1977.
37. Candeo MI, Otken L, Stefadouros MA: Echocardiographic features of cardiac compression by a thymoma simulating tamponade and obstruction of the superior vena cava. Br Heart J 39:1038, 1977.
38. Gottdiener JS, Maron BJ: Posterior cardiac displacement by anterior mediastinal tumor. Chest 77:784, 1980.
39. Bream R, et al. Subdiaphragmatic fluid mimicking loculated pericardial effusion on echocardiography. Am J Cardiol 54:1388, 1984.
40. D'Cruz IA: Echocardiographic simulation of pericardial effusion by ascites. Chest 85:93, 1984.
41. Chen CC, et al.: Pseudoposterior pericardial effusion due to enlarged left atrium. Am Heart J 108:1044, 1984.
42. Poole-Wilson PS, Farnsworth A, Brainbridge MU, Pambakian H: Angiosarcoma of pericardium: problems in diagnosis and management. Br Heart J 38:240, 1976.
43. Gomes MN, Hufnagel CA: Intrapericardial bronchogenic cysts. Am J Cardiol 36:817, 1975.
44. Gibson JY: A large intrapericardial cyst presenting as a cardiac abnormality. Radiology 119:219, 1976.
45. Cohen JJ: Neoplastic pericarditis. *In* Spodick DH (ed.): Pericardial Disease. Philadelphia, F.A. Davis, p. 257, 1976.
46. Agatston AS, et al.: Echocardiographic findings in primary pericardial mesothelioma. Am Heart J 111:986, 1986.
47. Martinez D, Del Capo A, Chariza M, Agosti J: Differential diagnosis of intrapericardial mass identified as venous ectasia. Tex Heart Inst J 13:209, 1986.
48. Reddy PS, Curtis EI, O'Toole JD, Shaver JA: Cardiac tamponade: hemodynamic observations in man. Circulation 58:265, 1978.
49. Kerner HM, Wood EH: Intrapericardial, intrapleural, and intracavitary pressures during acute heart failure in dog studies without thoracotomy. Circ Res 19:1071, 1966.
50. Morgan BC, Guntheroth WG, Dillard DH: Relationship of pericardial to pleural pressure during quiet respiration and cardiac tamponade. Circ Res 16:493, 1965.

51. Shabetai R, Fowler NO, Fenton JC, Masangkay M: Pulsus paradoxus. J Clin Invest 44:1882, 1965.
52. Fowler ND, Shabetai R, Braunstein JR: Transmural ventricular pressures in experimental cardiac tamponade. Circ Res 7:773, 1959.
53. Kussmaul A: Uber schwielige Mediastino-perikarditis und den paradoxen Puls. Berlin Klin Wochenschr 10:433, 1873.
54. Dornhorst A, Howard P, Leathart GC: Pulsus paradoxus. Lancet 1:746, 1952.
55. Sharp JT, et al.: Hemodynamics during induced cardiac tamponade in man. Am J Med 29:640, 1960.
56. Golinko RJ, Kaplan N, Rudolph AM: The mechanism of pulsus paradoxus during acute pericardial tamponade. J Clin Invest 42:249, 1963.
57. Guntheroth WG, Morgan BC, Mullins GL: Effect of respiration on venous return and stroke volume in cardiac tamponade: mechanism of pulsus paradoxus. Circ Res 20:381, 1967.
58. Leimgruber PP, Klopfenstein S, Wann SL, Brooks HL: The hemodynamic derangement associated with right ventricular diastolic collapse in cardiac tamponade: an experimental echocardiographic study. Circulation 68:612, 1983.
59. Gaffney FA, et al.: Pathophysiologic mechanism of cardiac tamponade and pulses shown by echocardiography. Am J Cardiol 53:1662, 1984.
60. Cogswell TL, et al. Effects of intravascular volume state on the value of pulsus paradoxus and right ventricular diastolic collapse in predicting cardiac tamponade. Circulation 72:1076, 1985.
61. Klopfenstein HS, et al.: Alterations in intravascular volume affect the relation between right ventricular volume affect the relation between right ventricular diastolic collapse and the hemodynamic severity of cardiac tamponade. J Am Coll Cardiol 6:1057, 1985.
62. Cogswell TL, et al.: The shift in the relationship between intrapericardial fluid pressure and volume induced by acute left ventricular pressure overload during cardiac tamponade. Circulation 74:173, 1986.
63. Armstrong WF, et al.: Diastolic collapse of the right ventricle with cardiac tamponade: an echocardiographic study. Circulation 65:1491, 1982.
64. Shiina A, Yagianuma T, Kondo K: Echocardiographic evaluation of impending tamponade. J Cardiogr 9:555, 1979.
65. Ditchey R, et al: The role of the right heart in acute cardiac tamponade in dogs. Circ Res 48:701, 1981.
66. Singh S, et al.: Usefulness of right ventricular diastolic collapse in diagnosing cardiac tamponade and comparison to pulsus paradoxus. Am J Cardiol 57:652, 1986.
67. Engel PJ, Hon H, Fowler NO, Plummer S: Echocardiographic study of right ventricular wall motion in cardiac tamponade. Am J Cardiol 50:1018, 1982.
68. Naggar CZ, Dillon WD, Butterly JR, Malacoff RF: Echocardiographic manifestations of tense pericardial effusion. J Am Coll Cardiol 6:467, 1985.
69. Kronzon I, Cohen ML, Winer HE: Diastolic atrial compression: a sensitive echocardiographic sign of cardiac tamponade. J Am Coll Cardiol 4:770, 1983.
70. Himelman RB, Kircher B, Rockey DC, Schiller NB: Inferior vena cava plethora with blunted respiratory response: a sensitive echocardiographic sign of cardiac tamponade. J Am Coll Cardiol 12:1420, 1988.
71. Gillam LD, et al.: Hydrodynamic compression of the right atrium: a new echocardiographic sign of cardiac tamponade. Circulation 68:294, 1983.
72. Singh S, et al.: Right ventricular and right atrial collapse in patients with cardiac tamponade: a combined echocardiographic and hemodynamic study. Circulation 6:966, 1984.
73. Schiller NB, Botvinick EH: Right ventricular compression as a sign of cardiac tamponade: an analysis of echocardiographic ventricular dimensions and their clinical implications. Circulation 56:774, 1977.
74. Kidner PH, Kakkar VV, Callum PA, Armstrong P: Left atrial tamponade: report of a case after right heart catheterization. Br Heart J 35:464, 1973.
75. Doyle T, Troup PJ, Wann LS: Mid-diastolic opening of the pulmonary valve after right ventricular infarction. J Am Coll Cardiol 5:366, 1985.
76. Nishimura RA, Able MD, Hatle LK, Tajik AT: Assessment of diastolic function of the heart: background and current applications for Doppler echocardiography. Part II. Clinical studies. Mayo Clin Proc 64:181, 1989.
77. Roberts WC, Spray TL: Pericardial heart disease. Curr Probl Cardiol 2: 17, 1977.
78. D'Cruz IA, Cohen HC, Prabhu R, Glick G: Diagnosis of cardiac tamponade by echocardiography: changes in mitral valve motion and ventricular dimensions, with special reference to paradoxical pulse. Circulation 52:460, 1975.
79. Vignola PA, Pohost GM, Curfman GD, Myers GS: Correlation of echocardiographic and clinical findings in patients with pericardial effusion. Am J Cardiol 37:701, 1976.
80. Settle HP, et al.: Echocardiographic study of cardiac tamponade. Circulation 56:951, 1977.
81. Pandian NG, et al.: Doppler echocardiography in cardiac tamponade: abnormalities in tricuspid and mitral flow response to respiration in experimental and clinical tamponade (abstr.). J Am Coll Cardiol 5:485, 1985.
82. Bommer WJ, et al.: Is Doppler echocardiography better than 2D echo in the detection of cardiac tamponade (abstr.) Clin Res 35:101A, 1987.
83. Leeman DE, Riley MF, Carl LV, Come PC: Doppler echocardiography in cardiac tamponade: exaggerated respiratory variation in transvalvular blood flow velocity integrals (abstr.) J Am Coll Cardiol 9:17A, 1987.
84. Appleton CP, Hatle LK, Popp RL: Cardiac tamponade and pericardial effusion: respiratory variation in transvalvular flow velocities studied by Doppler echocardiography. J Am Coll Cardiol 11:1020, 1988.
85. D'Cruz IA, et al.: Two-dimensional echocardiography in cardiac tamponade occurring after cardiac surgery. J Am Coll Cardiol 5:1250, 1985.
86. Phillips TF, Rodriguez A, Cowley RA: Right ventricular outflow obstruction secondary to right-sided tamponade following myocardial trauma. Ann Thorac Surg 36:353, 1983.
87. Hirschmann, JV: Fundamentals of clinical cardiology. Am Heart J 96:110, 1978.
88. Kutcher MA, et al.: Constrictive pericarditis as a complication of cardiac surgery: recognition of an entity. Am J Cardiol 50:742, 1982.
89. Engel PJ, et al.: M-mode echocardiography in constrictive pericarditis. J Am Coll Cardiol 6:471, 1985.
90. Chandraratna PAN, Aronow WS, Imaizumi T: Role of echocardiography in detecting the anatomic and physiologic abnormalities of constrictive pericarditis. Am J Med Sci 283:141, 1982.
91. Pandian NG, Skorton DJ, Kieso RA, Kerber RE: Diagnosis of constrictive pericarditis by two-dimensional echocardiography: studies in a new experimental model and in patients. J Am Coll Cardiol 4:1164, 1984.
92. Schnittger I, Bowden RE, Abrams J, Popp RL: Echocardiography: pericardial thickening and constrictive pericarditis. Am J Cardiol 42:388, 1978.
93. Voelkel AG, et al.: Echocardiographic features of constrictive pericarditis. Circulation 58:871, 1978.
94. Lewis BS: Real time two dimensional echocardiography in constrictive pericarditis. Am J Cardiol 49:1789, 1982.
95. Pool PE, et al.: Echocardiographic manifestations of constrictive pericarditis. Chest 68:684, 1975.
96. Sutton FJ, Whitley NO, Applefeld MM: The role of echocardiography and computed tomography in the evaluation of constrictive pericarditis. Am Heart J 109:350, 1985.
97. Gibson TC, et al.: An echocardiographic study of the interventricular septum in constrictive pericarditis. Br Heart J 38:738, 1976.
98. Tei C, Child JS, Tanake H, Shah PM: Atrial systolic notch on the interventricular septal echogram: an echocardiographic sign of constrictive pericarditis. J Am Coll Cardiol 1:907, 1983.
99. Candell-Riera J, Garcia-del Castillo H, Permanyer-Miralda G, Soler-Soler J: Echocardiographic features of the interventricular septum in chronic constrictive pericarditis. Circulation 57:1154, 1978.
100. Wann LS, Weyman AE, Dillon JC: Premature pulmonary valve opening. Circulation 55:128, 1977.
101. Vandenbossche JL, et al.: Significance of inspiratory premature opening of pulmonic valve in constrictive pericarditis. Am Heart J 110:896, 1985.
102. Weyman AE, Dillon JL, Feigenbaum H, Chang S: Premature pulmonic valve opening following series of valsalva aneurysm rupture into the right atrium. Circulation 51:586, 1975.
103. Himelman RB, Lee E, Schiller NB: Septal bounce, vena cava plethora and pericardial adhesion: informative two-dimensional echocardiographic signs in the diagnosis of pericardial constriction. J Am Soc Echocardiogr 1:333, 1988.
104. Mintz GS, et al.: Real time inferior vena caval ultrasonography: normal and abnormal findings and its use in assessing right heart function. Circulation 64:1018, 1981.
105. Agatston AS, Rao A, Price RJ, Kinney EL: Diagnosis of constrictive pericarditis by pulsed Doppler echocardiography. Am J Cardiol 54:929, 1984.
106. Tyberg TI, et al.: Left ventricular filling in differentiating restrictive amyloid cardiomyopathy and constrictive pericarditis. Am J Cardiol 47:791, 1981.
107. Isobe M, et al.: Transmitral reversed blood flow during mid- and end diastole in constrictive pericarditis. Am Heart J 112:855, 1986.
108. Spodick DH: Chronic and Constrictive Pericarditis. New York, Grune and Stratton, p. 174, 1964.
109. Spodick DH, Kumar S: Subacute constrictive pericarditis. Dis Chest 54: 62, 1968.
110. Hancock EW: Subacute effusive-constrictive pericarditis. Circulation 43: 183, 1971.
111. Kansal S, et al.: Two-dimensional echocardiography of congenital absence of pericardium. Am Heart J 109:912, 1985.
112. Ruys F, et al.: Expansion of left atrial appendage is a distinctive echocardiographic feature of congenital defect of the pericardium. Eur Heart J 4: 738, 1983.
113. Hynes JK, et al.: Two-dimensional echocardiographic diagnosis of pericardial cyst. Mayo Clin Proc 58:60, 1983.
114. Chandraratna PA, et al.: Application of 2-dimensional contrast studies during pericardiocentesis. Am J Cardiol 52:1120, 1983.
115. Schuster AH, Nanda NC: Pericardiocentesis-induced intrapericardial thrombus: detection by two-dimensional echocardiography. Am Heart J 104:308, 1982.

CHAPTER

36

CARDIAC TUMORS AND MASSES

ANNMARIE ERRICHETTI and ARTHUR E. WEYMAN

Before the advent of echocardiography, the detection of cardiac masses was limited to angiography or to direct inspection at surgery or necropsy. Early M-mode studies established the ability of echocardiographic imaging to show intracardiac tumors and masses as small as 1 to 2 mm and in many cases to give one insight into associated complications. Two-dimensional echocardiography has made it possible to define the spatial extent, structural relationships, and mobility of both intracardiac and extracardiac masses, and this technique has become the method of choice for evaluating patients with primary or secondary tumors of the heart.[1–5] The addition of Doppler techniques to the echocardiographic examination has refined diagnosis and has permitted quantitation of tumor-related stenosis and regurgitation.[1–5] Importantly, echocardiography not only permits early diagnosis but also offers an ideal means of defining the natural history of cardiac masses, of identifying potential complications, and of assessing the response to therapy.

Despite the wide-ranging diagnostic capabilities of echocardiography, one must remember that, although the technique can enable one to detect the presence of cardiac masses, it cannot define their histologic composition. By providing information about the size and shape of a mass, its location, consistency, mobility, and associated heart disease, however, echocardiography can be used to formulate a differential diagnosis and often to suggest the most likely diagnosis.

In this chapter we discuss the echocardiographic features of intra- and extracardiac masses, including primary and metastatic cardiac tumors, pericardial tumors and cysts, mediastinal tumors and cysts, intracardiac thrombi, and miscellaneous findings that may mimic intracardiac masses.

PRIMARY CARDIAC TUMORS

Primary cardiac tumors are rare, with an autopsy incidence between 0.001 and 0.33%.[6] Approximately 25% of all primary cardiac tumors and cysts are malignant (Table 36–1). Malignant tumors are much less common in children and account for fewer than 10% of all tumors and cysts of the heart and pericardium in pediatric patients.[6,7] Cardiac tumors produce few characteristic signs or symptoms unless they interfere with cardiac function. Only 5 to 10% of all cardiac neoplasms are diagnosed on clinical grounds.[6,8,9]

Tumors involving the heart may be intracavitary, intramural, or extracardiac. Most atrial tumors are intracavitary, whereas ventricular tumors are more commonly intramural.[6,8,10] Intracavitary tumors are recognized echocardiographically as clusters of echoes partially filling one or more cardiac chambers, whereas intramural tumors most commonly cause localized thickening or nodularity of one or more heart walls.

Benign Primary Tumors

Myxomas

General Characteristics. In adults, the most common intracardiac tumor is the myxoma, which accounts for 30 to 50% of all benign cardiac tumors and roughly 25% of all primary tumors and cysts of the heart and pericardium.[6,10–12] Myxomas can occur at any age, but are more common between 30 and 60 years.[6,8,10,13,14] A nearly equal sex distribution has been reported in most published series; however, in individual studies, a female predominance of up to threefold has been

Table 36–1. Relative Incidence of Primary Tumors of the Heart

Type	Number	Percentage (%)
Benign		
Myxoma	130	30.6
Lipoma	45	10.6
Papillary fibroelastoma	42	9.9
Rhabdomyoma	36	8.5
Fibroma	17	4.0
Hemangioma	15	3.5
Teratoma	14	3.3
Mesothelioma of the atrioventricular node	12	2.8
Granular cell tumor	3	0.7
Neurofibroma	3	0.7
Lymphangioma	2	0.5
Subtotal	319	75.1
Malignant		
Angiosarcoma	39	9.2
Rhabdomyosarcoma	26	6.1
Fibrosarcoma	14	3.3
Malignant lymphoma	7	1.6
Extraskeletal osteosarcoma	5	1.2
Neurogenic sarcoma	4	0.9
Malignant teratoma	4	0.9
Thymoma	4	0.9
Leiomyosarcoma	1	0.24
Liposarcoma	1	0.24
Synovial Sarcoma	1	0.24
Subtotal	106	24.9
TOTAL	425	100.00

(Modified from McAllister HA, Fenoglio JJ: Tumors of the cardiovascular system. *In* Atlas of Tumor Pathology. Washington, D.C., Armed Forces Institute of Pathology, Fascicle 15, Series 2, p. 1, 1978.)

noted.[3,6,8,15] Myxomas are rare in children.[3,7] Although uncommon, familial occurrence has been reported.[16–18]

Myxomas can occur on the endocardial surface of all cardiac chambers and rarely the heart valves.[6] Approximately 75% of myxomas occur in the left atrium, and most of the remainder originate in the right atrium.[6,10] These tumors involve the right or left ventricle in about 5% of cases.[6,10] Myxomas arising from the mitral valve have been reported.[19–22] Myxomas have also been reported to arise from the inferior vena cava.[23]

Atrial myxomas typically originate from the interatrial septum in the region of the fossa ovalis. As they grow, they characteristically expand into the atrial cavity, but they remain attached to the septum by a stalk. The pedicle may be short, allowing little motion, or it may be long, enabling the tumor to move back and forth from atrium to ventricle during the cardiac cycle. About 10% of atrial myxomas arise from other sites in the atria including, in descending order of frequency, the posterior and anterior walls and the atrial appendage.[2,6,10,14] Right atrial myxomas tend to be broader based than left-sided tumors and involve a larger area of the atrial wall or septum.[3,6,10] Ventricular myxomas may originate on the ventricular free wall or interventricular septum and may be sessile or pedunculated.[24–26]

Multiple myxomas have been reported in approximately 5% of patients.[3,6,10,27] These multiple tumors may be found in the same chamber or in different chambers. The most common pattern is biatrial, representing growth in both directions from a single focus in the interatrial septum.[27–29] Complete examination of all four chambers is therefore warranted in each patient.

Recurrent myxomas have been reported in 5 to 14% of patients after resection of the initial tumor.[30,31] Recurrence can occur at the site of the original tumor,[32,33] at multiple intracardiac sites,[34] or at sites outside the heart. Serial echocardiographic studies provide the best means of screening for tumor recurrence.[3,35]

Morphology. On gross examination, myxomas have a soft, mucoid, gelatinous appearance with some lobulation.[6,10,36] The tumors are generally 5 to 6 cm in diameter, with a range of 1 to 15 cm. They may contain areas of hemorrhage and calcification.[6,10,36] Microscopically, myxomas consist of a myxoid matrix composed of acid mucopolysaccharide and scattered polygonal cells. Ultrastructurally, the tumor cells resemble multipotential mesenchymal cells.[10,36]

Regardless of location, myxomas are similar in gross and microscopic appearance. Most tumors are pedunculated, with a short, broad-based stalk, although they may occasionally be sessile.[6,10] Pedunculated tumors tend to be soft, friable, and papillary, whereas sessile myxomas tend to be firm and round or polypoid.[6,10] Atrial myxomas may become secondarily infected.[31,37,38]

Clinical Signs and Symptoms. The clinical presentation of a cardiac myxoma depends on the cardiac chamber involved by the tumor.[6,10,39] A classic triad of symptoms relates to the obstructive, embolic, and constitutional effects of the tumor.[3,8,39,40] Combinations of two or more of this triad are more likely to suggest the diagnosis of myxoma. Symptoms, murmurs, and arterial blood pressure often vary with positional changes. In approximately 90% of patients, cardiac myxomas mimic a systemic illness consisting of fever, weight loss, joint pain, an elevated erythrocyte sedimentation rate, and raised levels of serum immunoglobulins.[3,8,39,40]

At first, the patient with left atrial myxoma is often presumed to have mitral valve disease (either stenosis or regurgitation).[3,15,39,41] The most common presenting symptoms are related to obstruction of the mitral valve and include dyspnea, fatigue, and weakness, although disruption of the valve apparatus by continual pounding of the tumor may result in mitral regurgitation. Clinical features that suggest a left atrial myxoma include rapid progression of signs and symptoms of heart failure out of proportion to the evidence of mitral valve disease, syncope, intermittent fever, positional variation in symptoms and cardiac murmurs, and unexplained systemic emboli, particularly in a young patient.[3,8,39,40] Larger tumor size, as determined echocardiographically, has been correlated with the clinical presentation.[5] In particular, the risk of embolization appears to be inversely related to tumor size but directly related to tumor consistency, with the highest incidence in highly deformable, mobile tumors.[5]

Right atrial myxomas most commonly obstruct the tricuspid valve, causing signs and symptoms of right heart failure.[3,8,13,39] Right atrial tumors may clinically mimic constrictive pericarditis, tricuspid stenosis, rheumatic tricuspid regurgitation, Ebstein's malformation, pulmonary thromboembolic disease, and superior vena cava obstruction.[3,8,13,14,39]

Because ventricular myxomas are more often sessile, they are less likely to cause obstructive symptoms unless the tumors are located in the ventricular outflow tract, simulating pulmonic[42,43] or aortic stenosis.[26,44] Narrowing of the left ventricular outflow tract by tumor may mimic hypertrophic cardiomyopathy.[9] The rate of embolization from left-sided tumors may be as high as 64%.[24] Emboli from right-sided tumors occur in only 10% of cases but may be a cause of recurrent pulmonary emboli and pulmonary hypertension.[45,46]

Echocardiographic Features. Effert and Domanig first described the M-mode echocardiographic features of a left atrial myxoma in 1959.[47] Although the first actual recording of an atrial myxoma was by Edler and Hertz in 1956 (Fig. 36–1), a report of this case was not published until 1962. Since these early reports, numerous descriptions of cardiac myxomas of varying size, location, and morphology have appeared. Despite individual variability, myxomas typically appear as homogenous masses of echoes arising within a cardiac chamber or from the leaflet tissue or supporting apparatus of a heart valve. The tumors generally have a jellylike, globular appearance. Echo-free spaces may be present within the mass that correspond to areas of hemorrhage or necrosis. Areas of calcification may also appear within the tumor mass. Although all the original echocardiographic descriptions of myxomas were based on M-mode recordings, two-dimensional imaging more accurately defines tumor size, motion pattern, attachments, and relationship with surrounding structures. Two-dimensional imaging is of particular value in the detection of right-sided myxomas or sessile tumors.[1,2] M-mode recordings remain useful for relating the movement of the tumor to that of surrounding structures. False-positive and false-negative studies have been reported, although more commonly with M-mode echocardiography.[2,48–51] Even large mobile tumors may be inapparent in one standard two-dimensional view or from one echocardiographic window, however, and a complete examination as described in Chapter 5 is essential to fully describe or completely exclude an intracardiac myxoma.

Because of the superiority of two-dimensional echocardiography to angiography in the diagnosis of myxoma, surgery can often be performed without preoperative catheterization, particularly in younger patients in whom the presence of coronary artery disease is unlikely.[1–3,52]

Left Atrial Myxomas. M-mode echocardiography was the primary noninvasive technique for the diagnosis of left atrial myxoma for nearly two decades, and there have been numerous descriptions of the M-mode findings in patients with these tumors.[53–55] Figure 36–2 illustrates the typical M-mode features of a left atrial myxoma. The tumor appears as a mass of echoes that completely fills the left atrium in systole. During diastole, the tumor prolapses into the mitral valve orifice, and the mass of echoes appears behind the anterior mitral leaflet. Motion of the tumor generally lags behind that of the mitral valve, so the valve usually opens fully before the tumor swings into the valve orifice. This slight time lag between the motion of the valve and that of the tumor creates an echo-free space behind the anterior mitral leaflet at the onset of diastole (Fig. 36–3). Because the tumor partially obstructs the mitral valve orifice, the mitral E-F slope is decreased, suggesting a persistent gradient across the valve and impaired left ventricular filling. This pattern may mimic the M-mode pattern of mitral stenosis, except the valve leaflets are not thickened and posterior leaflet motion is normal. All other echocardiographically derived measurements, including left atrial size, are usually within normal limits.[52] In patients with nonprolapsing tumors, the E-F slope is normal.[52] M-mode echocardiography is less sensitive in the detection of myxomas when the tumor mass is sessile or restricted in motion.[49–52]

Two-dimensional echocardiography, with its expanded field of vision and spatial orientation, has improved the sensitivity and specificity of echocardiography in the diagnosis of myxomas. Echocardiographic

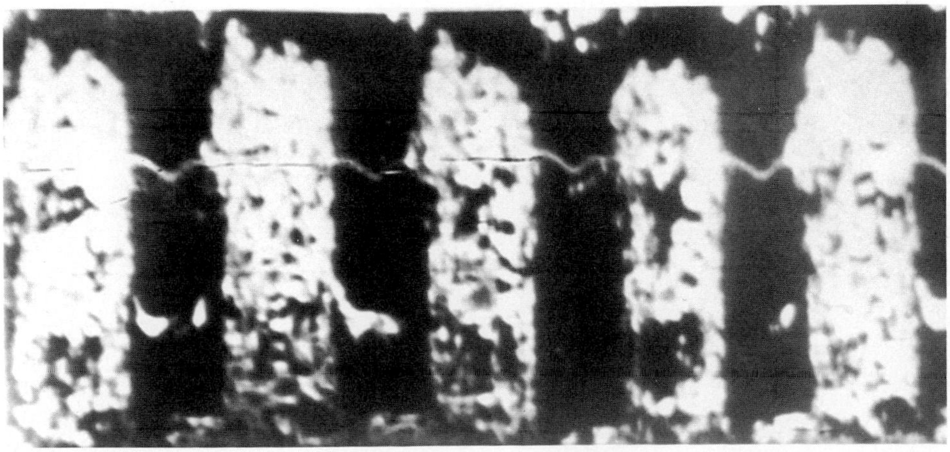

Fig. 36–1. Original M-mode recording of a left atrial myxoma. (Courtesy of Dr. Inge Edler.)

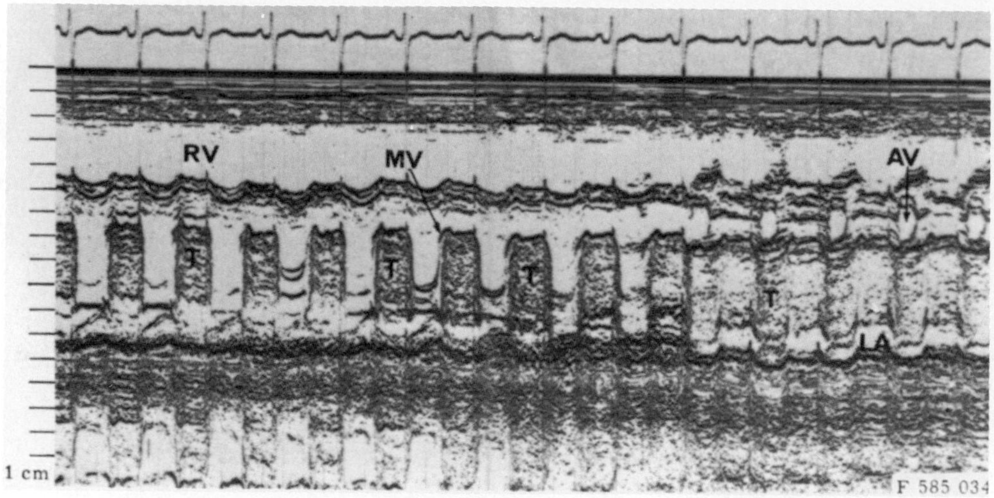

Fig. 36–2. M-mode scan from the left ventricle (left) to left atrium (LA) and aorta (right) from a patient with a left atrial myxoma. The tumor echoes can be seen behind the mitral valve during diastole and almost fill the LA during systole. RV = right ventricle; MV = mitral valve; AV = aortic valve; T = tumor. (From Chang S: M-Mode Echocardiographic Techniques and Pattern Recognition. Philadelphia, Lea & Febiger, p. 34, 1976.)

features are determined by tumor size, pattern of reflectivity, and site of origin. Left atrial myxomas characteristically appear echocardiographically as mobile, rounded, or ovoid echogenic masses that lie completely within the atrial cavity during systole and prolapse into or through the mitral valve during diastole (Figs. 36–4 to 36–6). The tumors most commonly arise from the interatrial septum, and their point of attachment is best demonstrated in an apical, subcostal, or transesophageal four-chamber view (Fig. 36–6). Large prolapsing myxomas generally interfere with left ventricular inflow and mitral valve diastolic motion, whereas small myxomas can cross the mitral valve without obstructing inflow or altering valve motion.[56] Even though myxomas in the atrium often appear larger than the mitral annulus, they readily change shape as they enter the valve. Rarely, a large myxoma cannot enter the mitral orifice because of its size and appears echocardiographically as a nonprolapsing mass of echoes filling the left atrium. Even large, nonprolapsing myxomas usually shift position slightly from systole to diastole, however, and this shift facilitates their recognition. If the myxoma is sessile, the appearance of a cluster of echoes attached to the interatrial septum may be the only clue to the presence of the tumor (Fig. 36–7).

Although most myxomas arise from the interatrial septum, these tumors may originate from any location in the atrium. Figure 36–8, for example, illustrates a myxoma arising from the lateral wall in the region of the atrial appendage. In addition to the unusual location of this tumor, its windsock-like shape contrasts sharply with the typical ovoid myxoma.

Because of their histologic composition, myxomas typically have multiple internal reflective interfaces that give the tumor a finely speckled appearance and make the body of the tumor as reflective as its margins.[57,58]

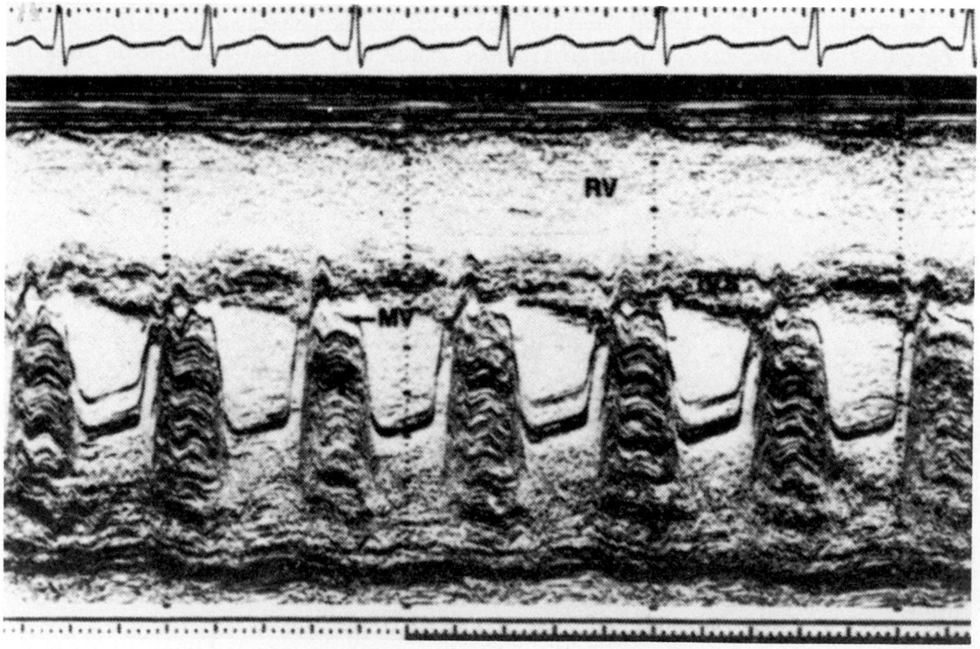

Fig. 36–3. M-mode recording of the left ventricle and mitral valve from a patient with a prolapsing left atrial myxoma. The tumor echoes appear in the mitral valve orifice roughly 40 msec after valve opening and fill the region behind the valve for the remainder of diastole. RV = right ventricle; MV = anterior mitral leaflet. (From Nomeir A, et al.: Intracardiac myxomas: twenty-year echocardiographic experience with review of the literature. J Am Soc Echocardiol 2:139, 1989.)

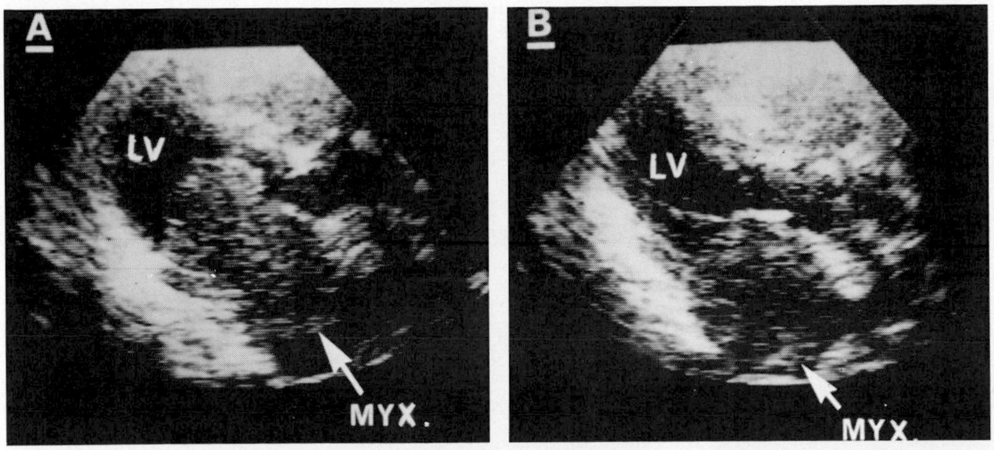

Fig. 36–4. Parasternal long axis recording from a patient with a left atrial myxoma (MYX). The tumor appears as a circular mass of echoes with the confines of the left atrial cavity during systole **(B).** During diastole **(A),** the tumor prolapses through the mitral orifice in the left ventricular cavity, completely filling the valve orifice. LV = left ventricle.

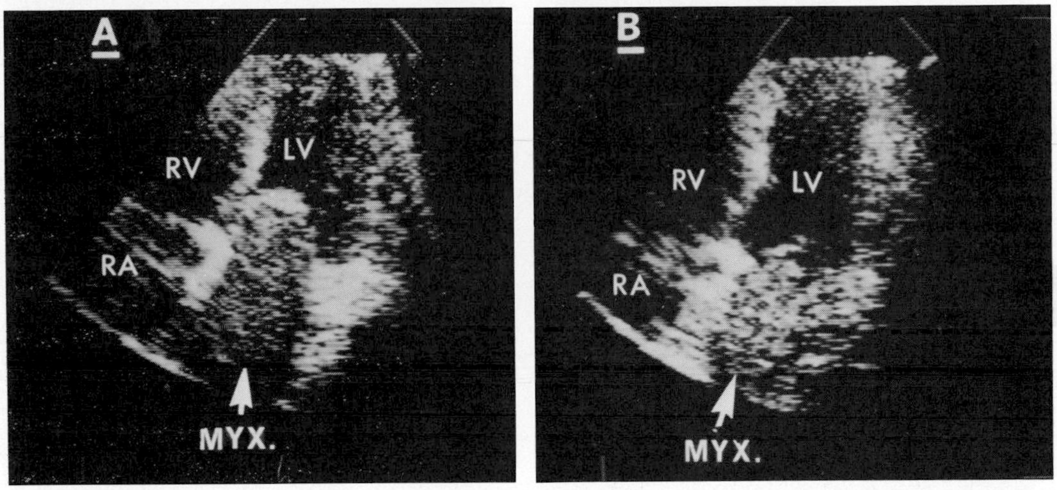

Fig. 36–5. Apical four-chamber view of the tumor demonstrated in Figure 36–4. **Left.** Diastolic frame with the tumor in the mitral valve orifice. **Right.** Recorded just after the onset of ventricular systole showing the anterior mitral leaflet closing behind the tumor as it shifts back into the left atrium. RV = right ventricle; LV = left ventricle; RA = right atrium; MYX = myxoma.

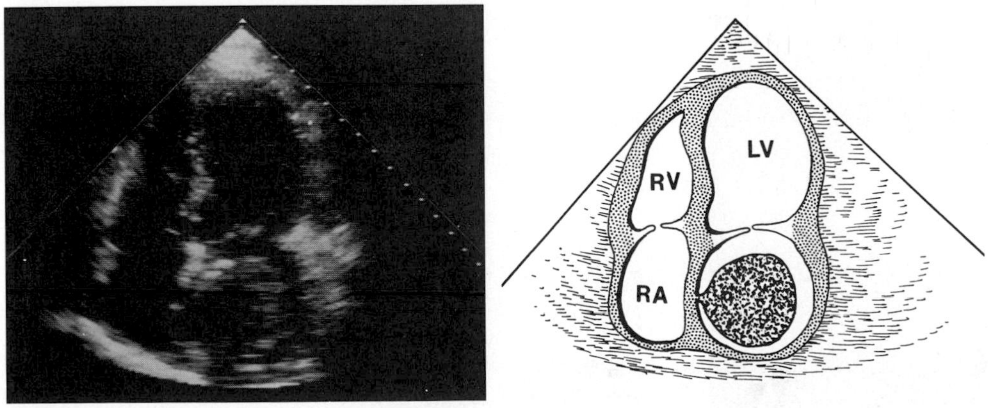

Fig. 36–6. Apical four-chamber recording of a left atrial myxoma illustrating the characteristic origin of the tumor from the interatrial septum in the region of the fossa ovalis. LV = left ventricle RV = right ventricle; RA = right atrium.

Localized calcifications may produce bright echoes, and hemorrhages may produce echo-free zones (Fig. 36–9). Visualization of an echo-free region in a left atrial mass may be a useful feature in differentiating myxoma from thrombus or vegetation.[57] The appearance of echo-free areas may vary with transducer position because hemorrhages and calcifications are not symmetrically located.[48,57] Although one should be able to diagnose virtually all left atrial myxomas by echocardiography, recognition of some tumors may depend on transducer position and angulation. In addition, if a tumor is extremely vascular, it may be less reflective, because its

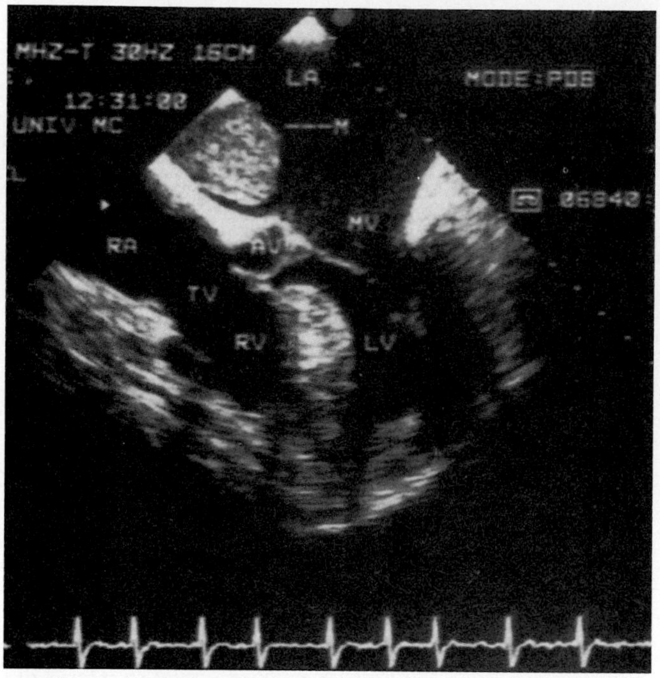

Fig. 36–7. Transesophageal four-chamber view showing a nonprolapsing myxoma. LA = left atrium; LV = left ventricle; M = myxoma; MV = mitral valve; RV = right ventricle; TV = tricuspid valve; RA = right atrium; AV = aortic valve. (From Chandrasekaran K, et al.: Impact of transesophageal color flow Doppler in current practice. Echocardiography 7:136, 1990.)

acoustic properties will be similar to those of blood in the atrial cavity.[48]

Doppler echocardiography can provide useful additional information regarding the hemodynamic consequences of left atrial myxomas by demonstrating the transvalvular gradient produced by mitral orifice obstruction and the degree of regurgitation caused by tumors that interfere with normal valve closure (Fig. 36–10).[59–62]

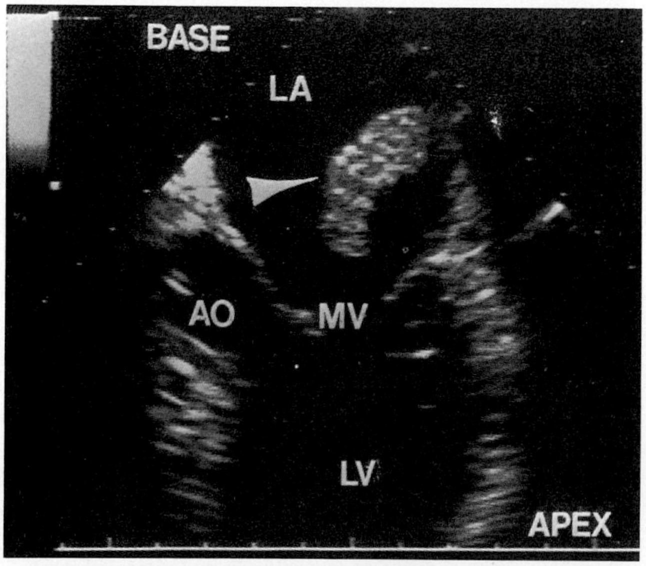

Fig. 36–8. Myxoma arising from the lateral wall of the left atrium (LA). The tumor has a narrow base and a long windsock-like appearance. MV = mitral valve; LV = left ventricle; AO = aorta. (From Chandrasekaran K, et al.: Impact of transesophageal color flow Doppler in current practice. Echocardiography 7:137, 1990.)

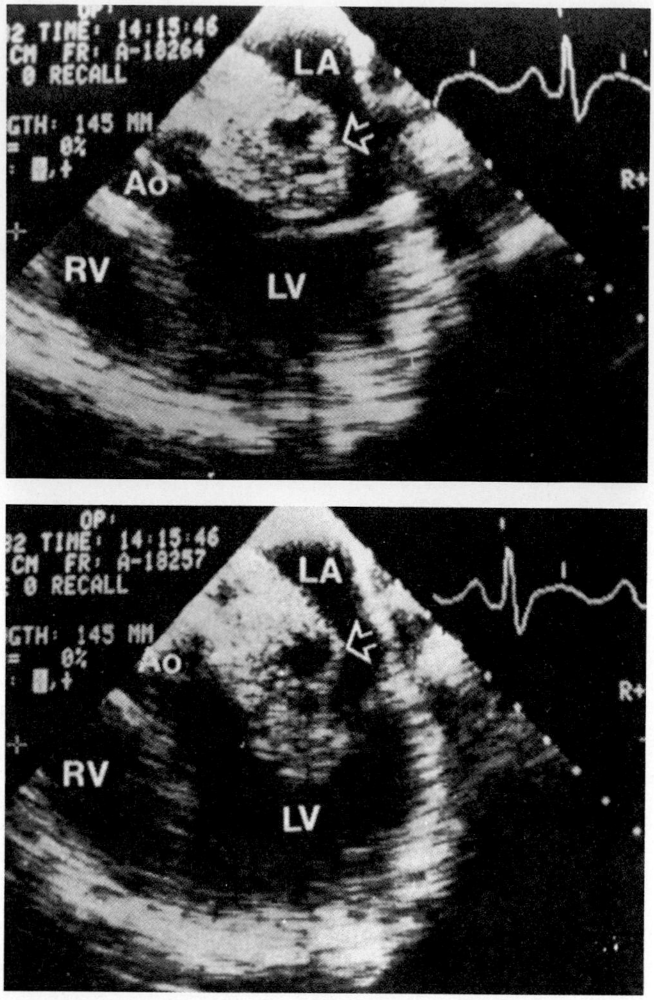

Fig. 36–9. Transesophageal echocardiographic recordings of a left atrial myxoma during systole (top) and diastole (bottom). Two echo-free areas are noted within the tumor (arrows), which proved to be cysts filled with clear serous fluid. LA = left atrium; LV = left ventricle; Ao = aorta; RV = right ventricle. (From Thier [Aschenberg] W, et al.: Cysts in left atrial myxomas identified by transesophageal cross-sectional echocardiography. Am J Cardiol 51:1793, 1983.)

Left atrial myxomas must be differentiated from vegetations, atrial thrombi, malignant tumors, and less commonly, mural tumors.[2,48] The characteristic appearance, motion, and site of origin of most myxomas distinguish them from the majority of atrial and valvular masses. Myxomas that arise from other locations in the atrium, have an unusual shape, and are nonprolapsing may be more difficult to identify correctly, however, and the diagnosis in these cases is often one of exclusion. Valvular vegetations are distinguished echocardiographically by their attachment to the valve leaflets, by the associated valvular disruption, and by the clinical setting. Differentiation of left atrial myxomas from mural thrombi may be more difficult. Often, the clinical setting aids in the distinction because atrial thrombi tend to occur in

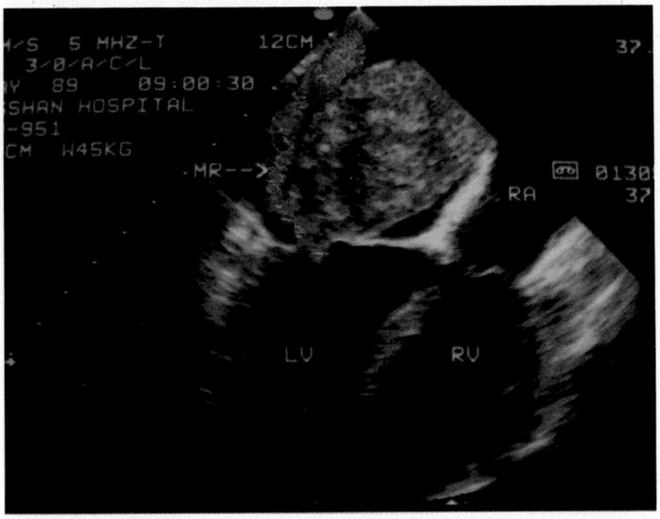

Fig. 36–10. Reversed transesophageal four-chamber color flow recording of left atrial myxoma with associated mitral regurgitation (MR). RA = right atrium; RV = right ventricle; LV = left ventricle. (Courtesy of Dr. Leng Jiang.)

the setting of mitral valve disease or dilated cardiomyopathy and are frequently localized to the atrial appendage. Most intracavitary left atrial thrombi are laminated and immobile, with a broad base of attachment usually to the posterior wall of the left atrium. Atrial thrombi may be pedunculated and mobile, however, and they can arise from the interatrial septum, a situation that makes differentiation difficult and in some cases impossible.

Metastatic tumors may extend into the left atrium from the lungs and can simulate a myxoma, although they can usually be distinguished by their extension into the pulmonary veins, as discussed later in this chapter. Mural tumors are uncommon but are usually smooth, symmetric, immobile masses that protrude from the atrial wall into the body of the chamber. They are frequently calcified, as illustrated in Figure 18–18, which shows calcified left ventricular fibroma that expanded into the cavity of the left atrium above the mitral annulus.

Right Atrial Myxomas. The M-mode echocardiographic appearance of right atrial myxomas (Fig. 36–11) is similar to that of myxomas arising in the left atrium.[63] The M-mode echocardiogram gives one the greatest likelihood of detecting a right atrial mass if the tumor protrudes through the tricuspid valve into the right ventricle, but the M-mode technique is less sensitive to small or nonprolapsing masses.[63,64] Two-dimensional echocardiography, on the other hand, enables one to visualize masses easily within the right atrium in locations other than behind the tricuspid valve.[63,64] The subcostal, apical four-chamber, and long axis views of the right heart are most useful in detecting a right atrial mass, including its site of attachment.

Like left atrial tumors, right atrial myxomas are typically spherical or globular with well-defined borders and multiple internal reflective interfaces that give a speckled appearance to the tumor mass. The tumors are usually mobile, moving toward or into the tricuspid orifice during diastole and back into the right atrial cavity at the onset of ventricular systole (Fig. 36–12). When obstructive, the tumors may interfere with flow through the tricuspid valve and may alter the motion of the tricuspid leaflets. When right atrial myxomas cause tricuspid stenosis or regurgitation, they may be associated with right atrial and ventricular dilation (Fig. 36–13) and paradoxic motion of the interventricular septum, although these features are variably present.[65]

A variety of cardiac structures, masses, and foreign bodies may be confused with right atrial myxomas.[66] Cardiac structures that may be confused with myxomas include congenital variants, such as a Chiari network or persistent eustachian valve, that appear as linear serpiginous echoes in the right atrium but lack the globular shape and bulk typical of a myxoma.[2,67,68] Atrial septal aneurysms may appear as a prominent membranous linear bulge arising from the interatrial septum in the region

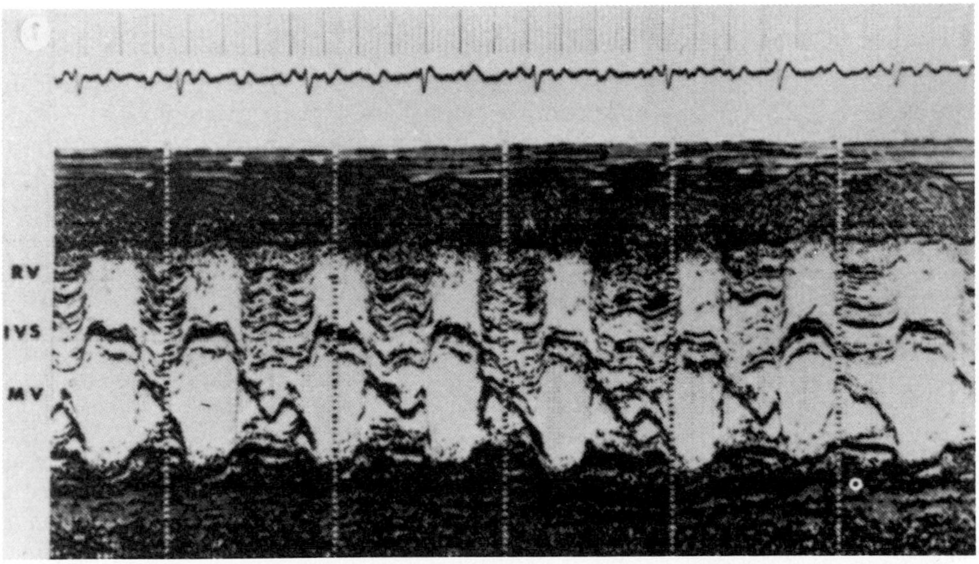

Fig. 36–11. M-mode echocardiographic recording of the right ventricle from a patient with a right atrial myxoma showing a dense mass of echoes in the right ventricle during diastole arising from the prolapsing tumor and paradoxic septal motion. RV = right ventricle; IVS = interventricular septum; MV = mitral valve. (From Nomeir A, et al.: Intracardiac myxomas: twenty-year echocardiographic experience with review of the literature. J Am Soc Echocardiol 2:139, 1989.)

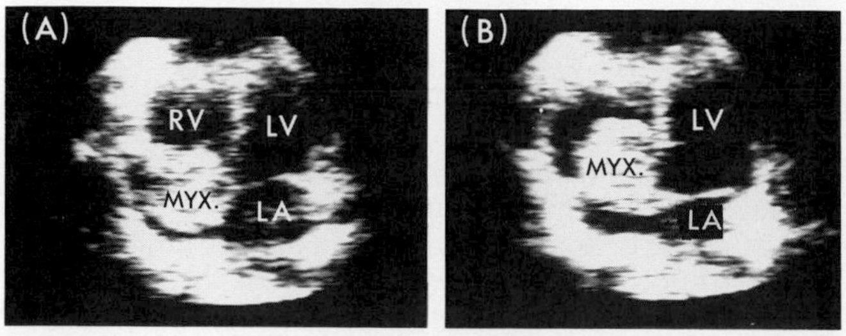

Fig. 36–12. Apical four-chamber recording of a right atrial myxoma (MYX). The tumor appears as a circular echo-producing mass with multiple internal reflections. **A.** During systole, the large tumor mass almost completely fills the right atrium. **B.** In diastole, the tumor prolapses through the tricuspid orifice into the right ventricle (RV). LV = left ventricle; LA = left atrium.

of the foramen ovale and oscillating into the right atrium in diastole (see Chapter 29).[69] These aneurysms frequently create confusion when viewed in only long axis planes (see later), but their appropriate diagnosis generally becomes apparent when they are imaged in orthogonal short axis and apical views.

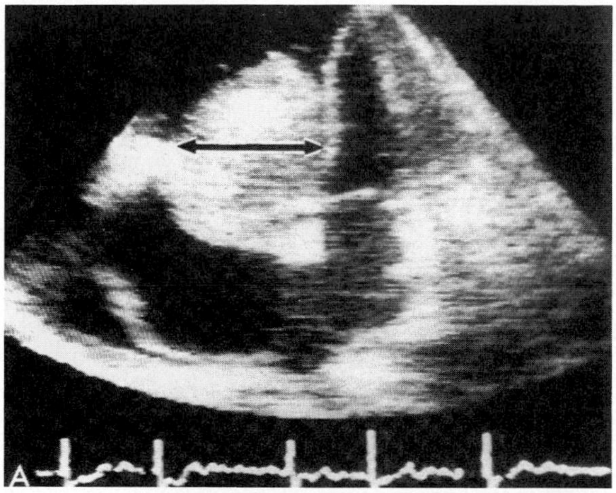

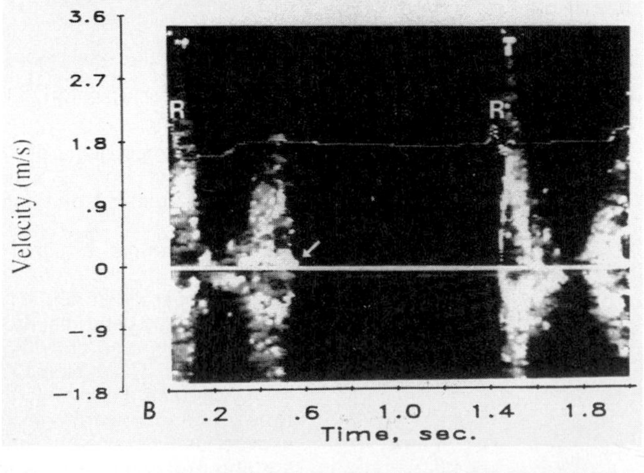

Fig. 36–13. Apical four-chamber recording of a large right atrial myxoma with significant right ventricular and atrial dilation. (From Goli VD, et al.: Doppler echocardiographic profiles of obstructive right and left atrial myxomas. J Am Coll Cardiol 9:701, 1987. Reprinted with permission from the American College of Cardiology.)

Cardiac masses that may resemble myxomas include right atrial thrombi, malignant tumors extending into the right atrium from the inferior vena cava, and vegetations.[63–65] Mural right atrial tumors arise primarily from the posterior atrial wall or may result from secondary invasion from the inferior vena cava. These masses can usually be differentiated from myxomas by their site of origin and their appearance.[64] In addition, foreign bodies including right heart catheters and pacemaker wires may mimic a right-sided mass, particularly when they develop superimposed thrombus. In these cases, recognition of the foreign body is the key to appropriate diagnosis.[66]

Ventricular Myxomas. Most right ventricular myxomas originate in the free wall or in the interventricular septum or, less commonly, on the pulmonic valve, pulmonary ring, or tricuspid valve.[70,71] Mobile right ventricular myxomas typically appear as masses of echoes that lie within the body of the right ventricle during diastole and extend toward the right ventricular outflow tract or even prolapsing through the pulmonic valve during systole.[25,70,72,73] Exaggerated paradoxic septal motion is often noted because of right ventricular distension by the tumor.[72] Differential diagnosis of masses within the right ventricular cavity includes thrombi, tumors of other origin, vegetations, prominent moderator band, and foreign bodies including Swan-Ganz catheters and transvenous pacemakers.[66,74,75] An intracardiac goiter resulting from ectopic thyroid tissue has also been reported to mimic a tumor obstructing the right ventricular outflow tract.[76]

Myxomas of the left ventricle are extremely rare.[25,26,77] Figure 36–14 demonstrates a left ventricular myxoma arising from the left ventricular posterior wall, extending into the body of the left ventricle and outflow tract during diastole, and prolapsing through the aortic valve in systole. Left ventricular myxomas must be differentiated from other left ventricular tumors, thrombi (which are usually apical and associated with akinesis or dyskinesis), false tendons, and prominent or calcified papillary muscles.

Valvular Myxomas. Although rare, myxomas may also arise from cardiac valves. The presentation of valvular myxomas varies, depending on their size and location. Figure 36–15 illustrates a myxoma arising from the ventricular surface of the anterior mitral valve leaflet and chordae tendineae that prolapsed into the left ventricular outflow tract during systole. The clinical presentation in this case was similar to that of idiopathic hypertrophic subaortic stenosis with a systolic ejection murmur and variable outflow tract gradient.

Lipomas

Cardiac lipomas occur throughout the heart including the pericardium, although they are located most frequently in the left ventricle or right atrium.[6,10] These benign tumors occur at all ages and with equal frequency in both sexes.[6] Most tumors are sessile or polypoid and vary in size from 1 to 15 cm, although some have been reported to weigh more than 2 kg.[6,10] Cardiac lipomas may be subepicardial or subendocardial. Subepicardial

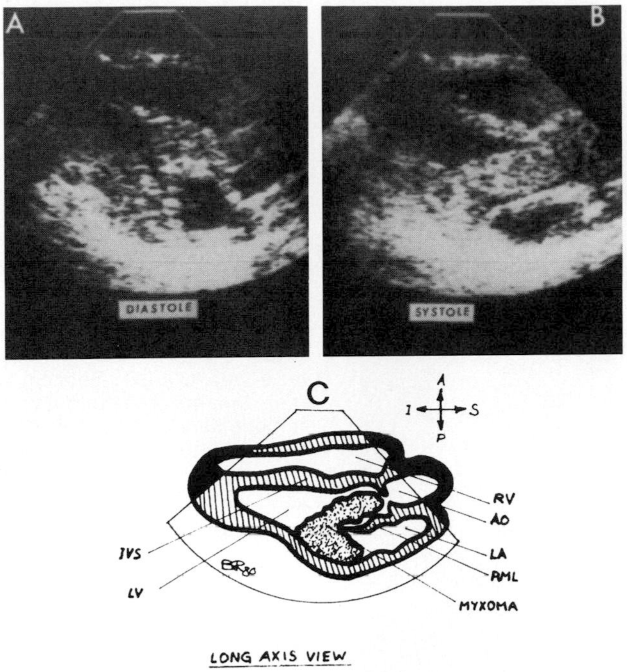

Fig. 36–14. Parasternal long axis recordings of a left ventricular myxoma during diastole **(A)** and systole **(B).** The tumor arises from the left ventricular posterior wall, filling the base of the ventricular chamber during diastole and prolapsing into the left ventricular outflow tract during systole. RV = right ventricle; Ao = aorta; LA = left atrium; AML = anterior mitral leaflet; LV = left ventricle; IVS = interventricular septum. (From Mazer M, Harrigan P: Left ventricular myxoma: M-mode and two-dimensional echocardiographic features. Am Heart J 104:875, 1982.)

tumors are large, smooth, and often pedunculated, whereas subendocardial lipomas are typically sessile.[6] About 25% of lipomas are completely intramyocardial.[6,10] Microscopically, lipomas are well encapsulated and consist of mature fat cells, often with fibrous (fibrolipoma) or muscle (myolipoma) components.[10]

Most lipomas are clinically silent, although arrhythmias, conduction disturbances, and symptoms from mechanical interference have been reported.[78,79] Figure 36–16 depicts a large left ventricular mass in a 57-year-old man with presyncope. A left ventricular lipoma was confirmed by biopsy. Lipomas differ from left ventricular myxomas in that lipomas are less mobile and generally more echo dense.

Valvular lipomas are rare but have been described on the mitral and tricuspid valves.[80–82] Figure 36–17 is an unusual case of multiple mitral valve lipomas, appearing as a dense mass of echoes arising from the posterior mitral leaflet and a second discrete tumor mass in the posterior papillary muscle. A valvular lipoma is not easily differentiated from other valvular tumors such as myxomas, papillary fibroelastomas, or fibromas, or from valvular vegetations. Magnetic resonance imaging may aid in confirming the fatty nature of the tumor.

Cardiac lipomas must be distinguished from lipomatous hypertrophy of the interatrial septum (interatrial lipoma), which is characterized by accumulation of excessive adipose tissue in the atrial septum.[83] Examination from the subcostal transducer position demonstrates globular thickening of the interatrial septum with central sparing that gives the atrial septum a bilobed or

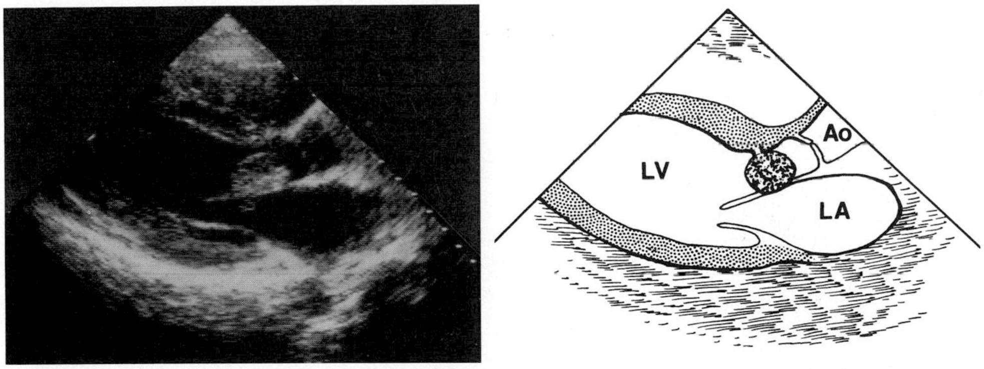

Fig. 36–15. Parasternal long axis recording of a mitral valve myxoma. Ao = aorta; LA = left atrium; LV = left ventricle.

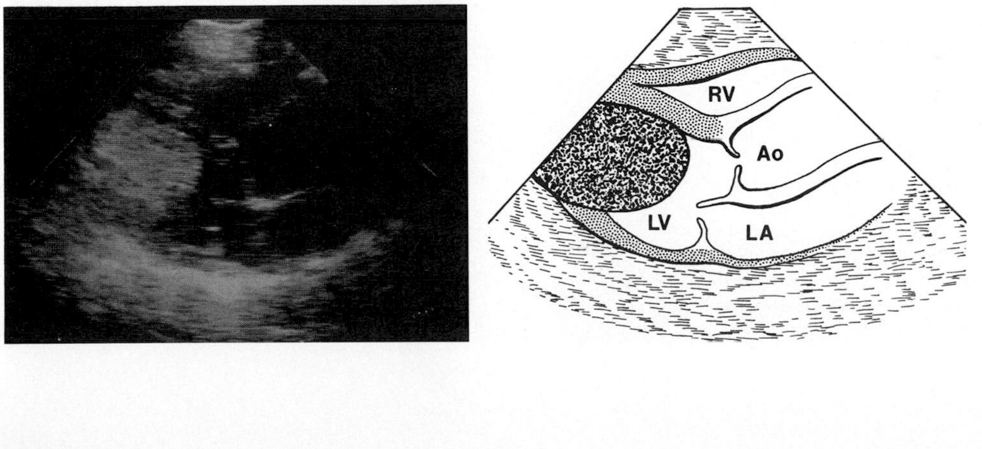

Fig. 36–16. Parasternal long axis recording of a large left ventricular apical lipoma. LV = left ventricle; RV = right ventricle; Ao = aorta; LA = left atrium.

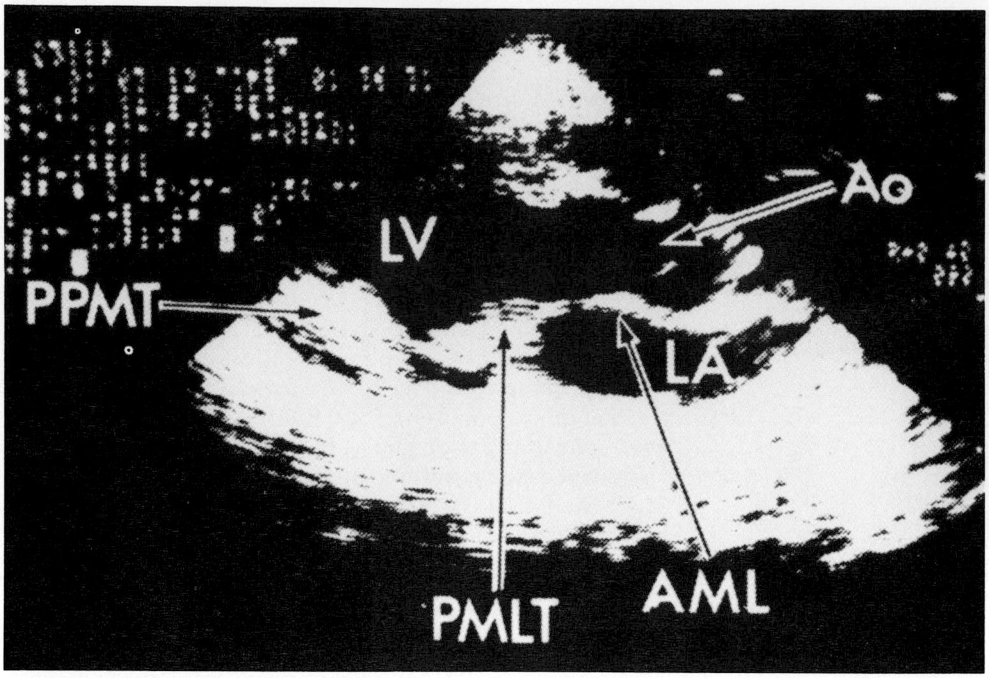

Fig. 36–17. Parasternal long axis recording illustrating lipomas arising separately in the posterior papillary muscle (PPMT) and posterior mitral valve leaflet (PMLT). LV = left ventricle; Ao = aorta; LA = left atrium; AML = anterior mitral valve leaflet. (From Behnam R, et al.: Lipoma of the mitral valve and papillary muscle. Am J Cardiol 51:1459, 1983.)

dumbbell shape (Fig. 36–18). This mass of adipose tissue may bulge from beneath the atrial septal endocardium into the right atrial cavity and may thereby simulate a right atrial tumor.

Papillary Fibroelastomas

Papillary fibroelastomas or papillomas are benign tumors that may be found anywhere in the heart but most frequently arise from valvular endocardium.[6,84] Although these tumors occur in all age groups, they are most commonly seen in patients over 60 years of age.[6]

On gross inspection, papillary fibroelastomas are usually small (1 cm or less), have a characteristic gelatinous appearance, and consist of multiple papillary fronds attached to the endocardium by a short stalk.[6,85] Histologically, these tumors have a central core of dense connective tissue surrounded by an acid mucopolysaccharide matrix, smooth muscle cells, collagen, and elastic fibers and are covered by endothelium.[6] Whether papillomas

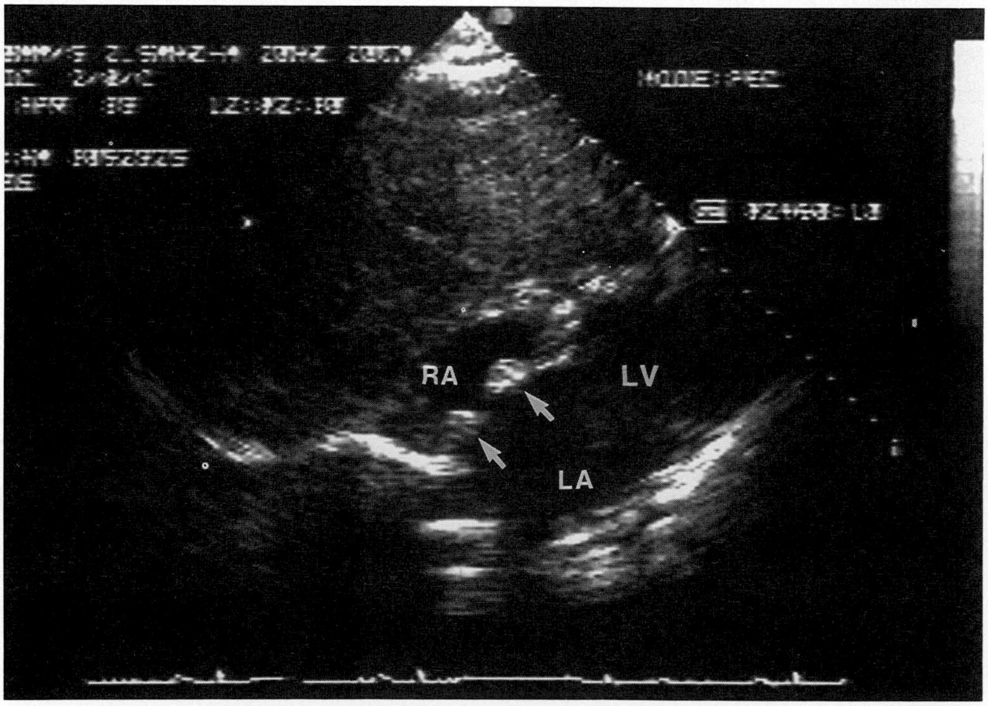

Fig. 36–18. Modified subcostal four-chamber view of the interatrial septum showing the dumbbell-shaped masses in the interatrial septum (arrows) characteristic of lipomatous hypertrophy of the septum. RA = right atrium; LA = left atrium; LV = left ventricle.

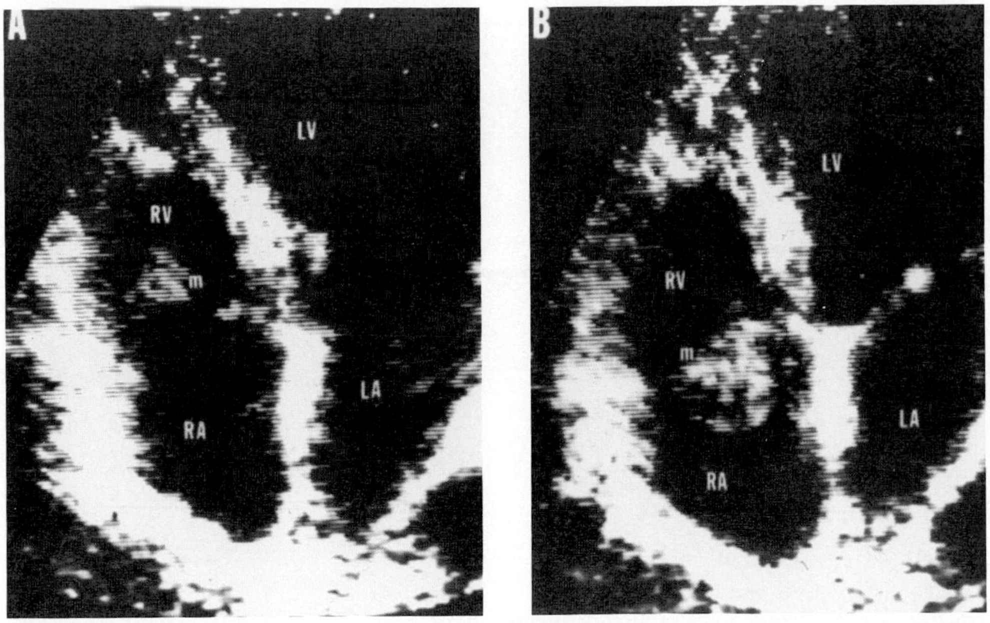

Fig. 36–19. Apical four-chamber recording from a patient with a papillary fibroelastoma of the tricuspid valve. **A.** Diastole. **B.** Systole. LV = left ventricle; LA = left atrium; RA = right atrium; MV = mitral valve; TV = tricuspid valve; RV = right ventricle. (From Frumin H, et al.: Two-dimensional echocardiographic detection and diagnostic features of tricuspid papillary fibroelastoma. J Am Coll Cardiol 2:1016, 1983. Reprinted with permission of the American College of Cardiology.)

are true neoplasms or hamartomas* has been debated.[6] These tumors may represent a degenerative wear-and-tear process, particularly because the fronds resemble chordae tendineae histologically.[6]

Left- and right-sided tumors occur with nearly equal frequency.[6] The ventricular surface of the semilunar valves and the atrial surface of the atrioventricular valves are most commonly affected.[10] The aortic valve is most frequently involved in adults, and the tricuspid valve in children.[6,84,86,87] These tumors may be present less commonly on papillary muscles, chordae tendineae, and atrial or ventricular endocardium.[85,86,88] Occasionally, papillary fibroelastomas are multiple.[6]

Before the introduction of two-dimensional echocardiography, papillary fibroelastomas, which are rarely associated with cardiac dysfunction, were incidental findings at autopsy or at cardiac surgery.[84] Symptoms, which have occurred almost exclusively in patients with aortic valve tumors, result occasionally in clinically significant valvular dysfunction or rarely in angina or sudden cardiac death from coronary ostial occlusion by tumor fronds.[6,84]

On two-dimensional echocardiographic examination, papillary fibroelastomas are homogeneous, rounded, well-demarcated masses attached to the cardiac valves. Figure 36–19 is an example of a papillary fibroelastoma arising from the tricuspid valve. During diastole, the tumor prolapses into the ventricular cavity, whereas in systole, it is located at the point of coaptation of the valve leaflets. The point of attachment to the valve leaflets helps to distinguish papillary fibroelastomas from intracavitary tumors such as myxomas, but differentiation from other valvular tumors and even valvular vegetations may be difficult.

Figure 36–20 is an example of an unusual left ventricular papillary fibroelastoma detected by an examination using two-dimensional echocardiography. In this case, the mobile tumor was attached by a short stalk to the posterior wall of the ventricle just inferior to the papillary muscle. Prominent fluttering of the tumor surface in real time was due to the undulation of the gelatinous mass in the ventricular outflow tract. The appearance of the tumor is similar to that of a left ventricular myxoma.

Rhabdomyomas

Rhabdomyomas are the most common primary cardiac tumor in the pediatric age group.[6,7] In the series compiled by the Armed Forces Institute of Pathology, 78% of rhabdomyomas occurred in children under 1 year of age, and only one patient was more than 15 years of age at diagnosis.[89] Tuberous sclerosis is the most frequently associated lesion, occurring in 30 to 50% of reported cases.[89,90]

Rhabdomyomas are derived from cardiac muscle cells and resemble hamartomas rather than true neoplasms.[89] Histologically, these tumors are characterized by so-called spider cells, which consist of a central nucleus surrounded by fine fibrillar processes radiating to the periphery.[89]

Ninety percent of rhabdomyomas are multiple.[6] They are primarily ventricular tumors with nearly equal frequency in the right and left ventricles. These tumors infrequently involve the atria.[89] In 50% of patients, at least one of the ventricular tumors is intracavitary, resulting in obstruction of ventricular filling or outflow.[6] Rhabdomyomas are associated with a high mortality rate in infants and children, most often because of mechanical outflow obstruction or sudden cardiac death from arrhythmias.[7,89,91–93] Older children and adolescents with tuberous sclerosis more frequently have intramural tumors without overt cardiac symptoms.[90]

Although the diagnosis of rhabdomyoma may often be

* Hamartoma: a localized abnormality comprising an abnormal mixture of fibrous and elastic tissue, fat, and blood vessels that differs from a neoplasm in that it grows at a normal rate and is thus unlikely to compress adjacent normal tissue.

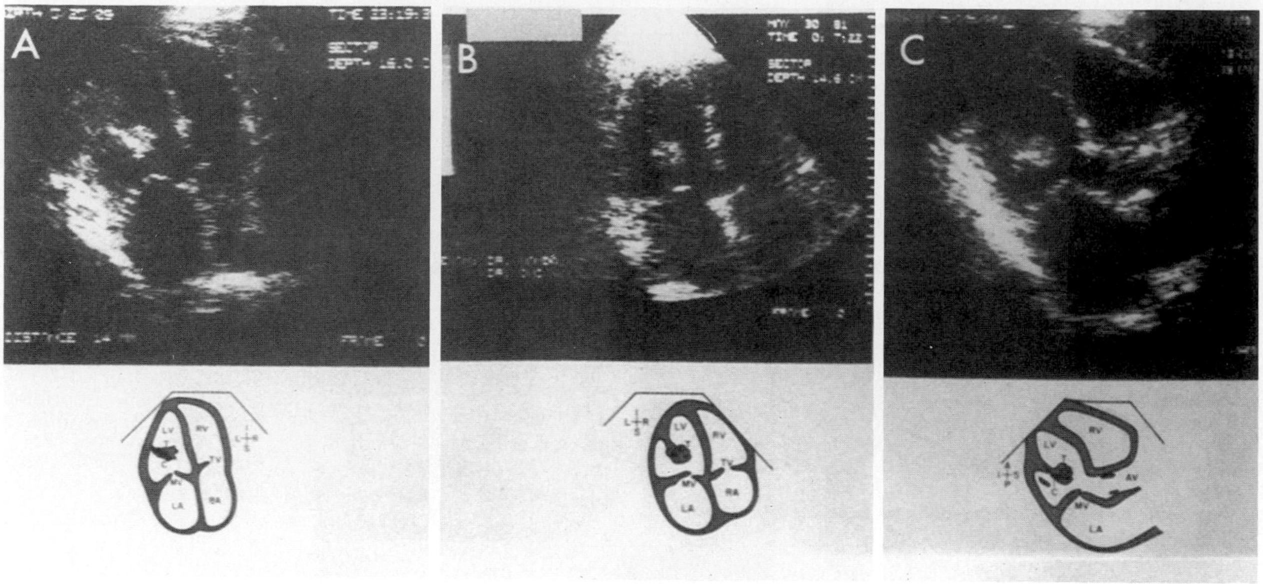

Fig. 36–20. Series of apical recordings from a patient with a left ventricular papillary fibroelastoma attached by a short stalk to the posterior wall just inferior to the papillary muscle. Multiple projections are seen on the tumor (T) surface. The dense white band running through the tumor represents the collagen core (C), which is a typical histologic finding in fibroelastoma. RV = right ventricle; RA = right atrium; LA = left atrium; MV = mitral valve; LV = left ventricle. (From Ong LS, et al.: Two-dimensional echocardiographic detection and diagnostic features of left ventricular papillary fibroelastoma. Am Heart J 103:917, 1982.)

suspected clinically, two-dimensional echocardiography is diagnostic. The presence of multiple nodular masses in several chambers of the heart suggests rhabdomyoma rather than myxoma, fibroma, or other benign tumors. A rhabdomyoma may also appear echocardiographically as a single intramural echo-dense mass in the interventricular septum or ventricular free wall.[90,94] Figure 36–21 shows multiple rhabdomyomas involving the interventricular septum, apex, and left ventricular outflow tract. Tumors may also protrude into one or more of the cardiac chambers or may appear as an intracavitary pedunculated mass, as illustrated in Figure 36–22.

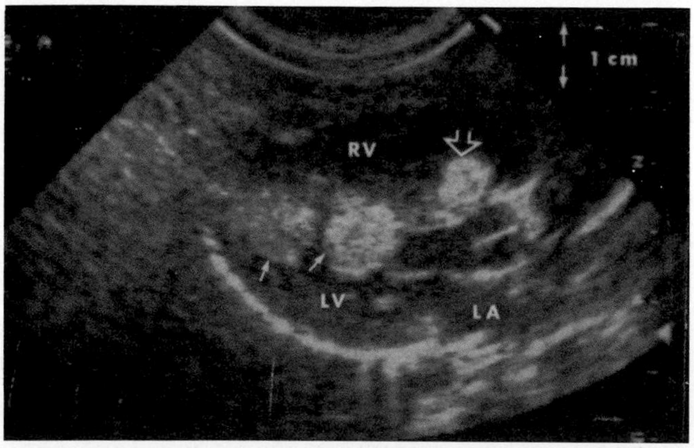

Fig. 36–21. Parasternal long axis view from a patient with multiple rhabdomyomas. Two tumors (closed arrows) are visible in the left ventricle (LV): one at the apex and another in the outflow tract. Both tumors measured approximately 1.5 cm in diameter. A third tumor (open arrow) is present in the outflow tract of the right ventricle (RV). LA = left atrium. (From Murphy DJ, et al.: Multiple cardiac tumors in an infant. Echocardiography 5:253, 1988.)

Two-dimensional echocardiography not only provides the diagnosis, but also is useful in guiding the management of patients with rhabdomyomas and often obviates the need for invasive studies or surgery in infants and children with multiple tumors.[67,94,95] When outflow obstruction is present or suspected, pulsed and continuous wave Doppler can determine the presence of outflow gradients (Fig. 36–23). In critically ill infants requiring urgent surgical intervention, surgical removal of echocardiographically defined tumors has been performed without prior cardiac catheterization.[67] Serial studies may be used to detect changes in size or location of masses and can be used postoperatively to document tumor resolution.[4,94] Spontaneous regression of rhabdomyomas has been documented by echocardiography.[67,94] Two-dimensional echocardiography is also a useful noninvasive method of screening asymptomatic infants and children with tuberous sclerosis for the presence of cardiac tumors.[90] Multiple cardiac rhabdomyomas have been diagnosed in utero by two-dimensional echocardiography during evaluation of a fetus with tachycardia, thereby directing prenatal management and postnatal care (see Chapter 33).[96]

Fibromas

Cardiac fibromas are benign tumors that occur predominantly in infants and children, although they may be found in any age group.[6] They represent the second most common primary ventricular neoplasm, after rhabdomyomas. These tumors are firm and nonencapsulated, ranging in size from 3 cm to more than 10 cm in diameter.[10] Central calcification is frequent.[97]

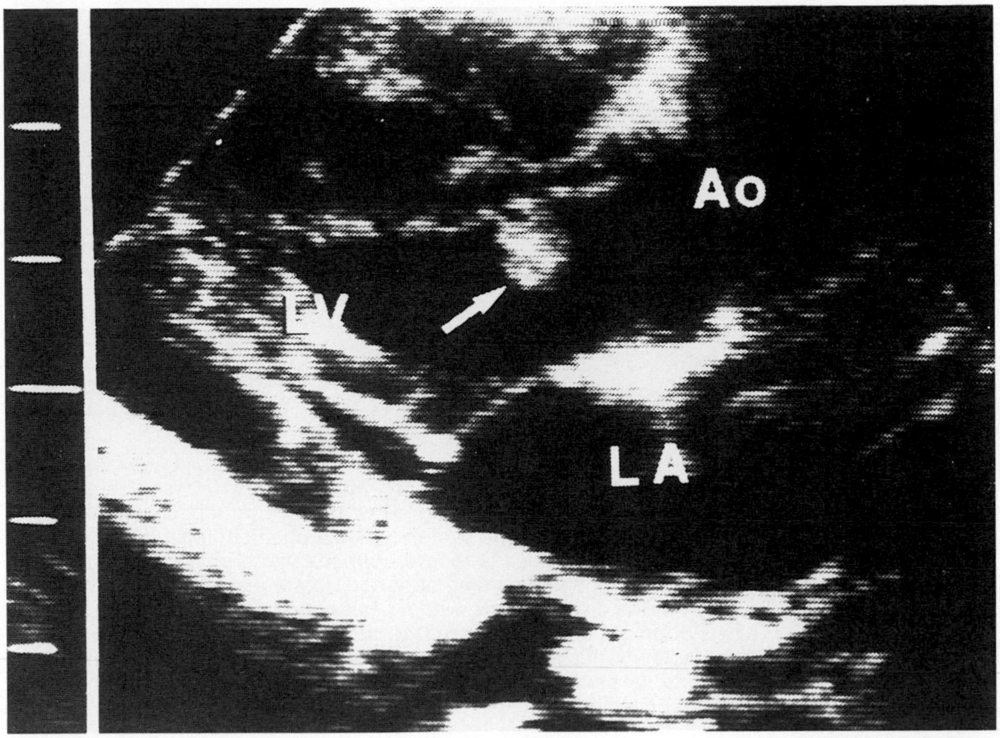

Fig. 36–22. Parasternal long axis recording illustrating a small mobile rhabdomyoma extending from the interventricular septum into the left ventricular outflow tract. LA = left atrium; LV = left ventricle; Ao = aorta. (From Bass JL, et al.: Echocardiographic incidence of cardiac rhabdomyoma in tuberous sclerosis. Am J Cardiol 55: 1379, 1985.)

Cardiac fibromas are found primarily in ventricular myocardium, most frequently within the interventricular septum or anterior free wall of the left ventricle.[10,97] An unusual right atrial fibroma arising from the interatrial septum has been reported in a neonate, associated with pericardial effusion.[98] Figure 36–24 is an example of a calcified left ventricular fibroma at the base of the atrioventricular ring that expanded superiorly into the left atrial cavity. The tumor partially obstructed the mitral valve orifice and produced significant obstruction to inflow.

Clinical manifestations are protean and are determined by the size of the tumor and its location. Approximately 70% of patients at some time demonstrate signs or symptoms of mechanical outflow tract obstruction,[99,100] congestive heart failure, or arrhythmias.[97,101] Sudden cardiac death has also been reported.[97,101]

Right ventricular fibromas may simulate cyanotic congenital heart disease, as in the case of a neonate who was found, during two-dimensional echocardiographic study, to have a massive tumor causing right ventricular outflow obstruction (Fig. 36–25).[102] The apical four-chamber view demonstrated a huge mass of echoes nearly filling the entire right ventricular cavity, displacing the septum against the free wall of the left ventricle and shifting the tricuspid valve backward toward the right atrium.

Because fibromas are solitary and large, they may simulate a rhabdomyoma, particularly if intracavitary; however, their characteristic location within the interventricular septum (Fig. 36–26),[103] or within the ventricular free wall (Fig. 36–27),[104] often aids in the appropriate diagnosis. Two-dimensional echocardiography may be useful in planning surgical therapy.[4,103]

Hemangiomas

Benign vascular tumors of the heart include hemangiomas, lymphangiomas, hemangioendotheliomas, and angioreticuloma, with hemangioma the most common.[6] Anatomically, hemangiomas may occur at any site in the heart including the epicardium, often in association with a pericardial effusion.[6,105] These tumors are usually solitary but may be multiple.[6,105] They may be either intracavitary or intramural. Intramural tumors occur most commonly on the right side of the heart, particularly in the interventricular septum.[6,105] Atrial hemangiomas have been reported, but they are rare.[6,64,105]

Grossly, hemangiomas are small, subendocardial, bluish nodules ranging in size from 2 mm to 3.5 cm in diameter.[6] They are sessile or polypoid. Microscopically, they are vascular tumors composed of endothelium-lined spaces forming channels of blood, lymph, or occasionally thrombi.[6] They are classified according to the predominant type of vascular channel.

In more than 50% of patients, hemangiomas are incidental findings at the time of surgery or autopsy.[6] Clinical signs and symptoms, when they occur, depend on the location of the tumor. The presenting feature of large intracavitary tumors may be congestive heart failure, usually on the right side because of restricted filling of right heart chambers.[64,105] The tumors may simulate infundibular pulmonic stenosis when they involve the upper portion of the interventricular septum.[106] Recurrent pericardial effusion is a frequent presentation.[105,107,108]

Figure 36–28 is a recording from a 15-year-old girl referred for echocardiographic examination for suspected infundibular pulmonic stenosis. The patient was

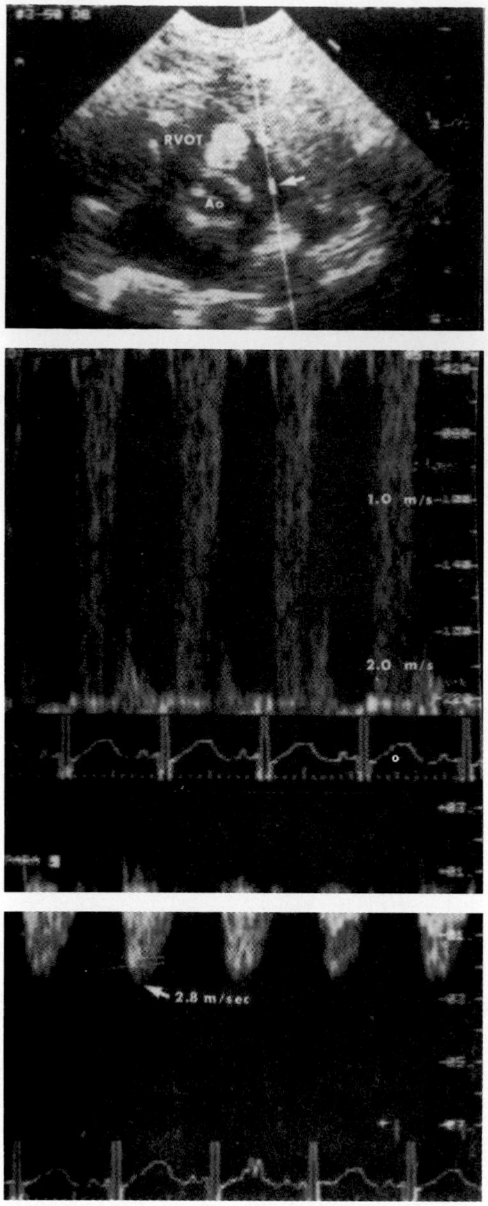

Fig. 36–23. Top. Parasternal long axis recording of the right ventricular outflow tract (RVOT) and pulmonary artery from a patient with partial obstruction of the outflow tract by a rhabdomyoma. A Doppler cursor with the sample volume position illustrated by the arrows is positioned to record pulmonary artery flow. Middle. The pulsed Doppler recording obtained from the main pulmonary artery shows disturbed flow with a peak velocity exceeding 2.2 m/sec. Bottom. Continuous wave Doppler through the main pulmonary artery yields a peak instantaneous velocity of 2.8 m/sec. Ao = aorta. (From Murphy DJ, et al.: Multiple cardiac tumors in an infant. Echocardiography 5:253, 1988.)

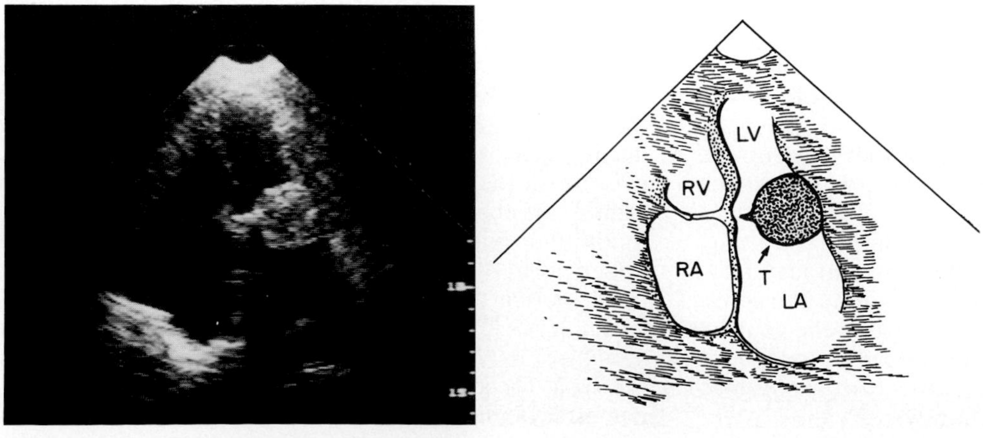

Fig. 36–24. Apical four-chamber recording of a large fibroma (T) arising from the left ventricular myocardium in the region of the posterolateral atrioventricular groove. LA = left atrium; LV = left ventricle; RA = right atrium; RV = right ventricle.

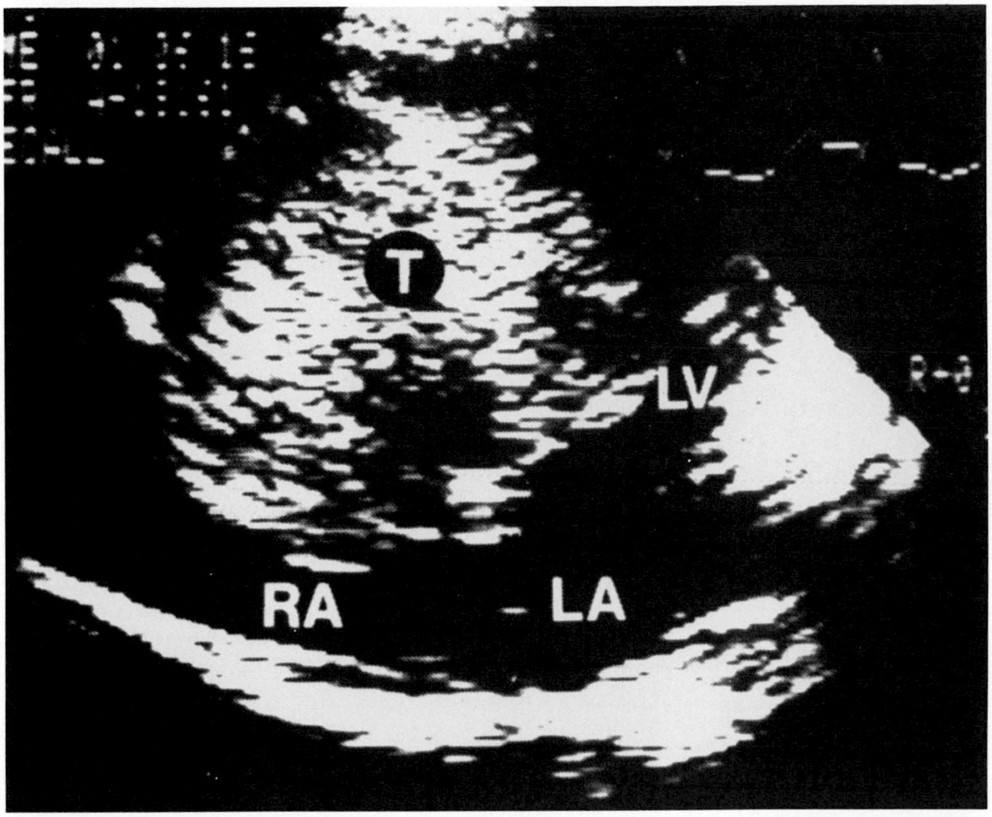

Fig. 36–25. Apical four-chamber view from a newborn with extensive invasion of the right ventricular free wall and septum and obliteration of the right ventricular cavity by a right ventricular fibroma. The tumor (T) displaces the ventricular septum against the free wall of the left ventricle (LV). LA = left atrium; RA = right atrium. (From Marin-Garcia J, et al.: Primary right ventricular tumor (fibroma) simulating cyanotic heart disease in a newborn. Journal of the American College of Cardiology, 3: 868, 1984. Reprinted with permission from the American College of Cardiology.)

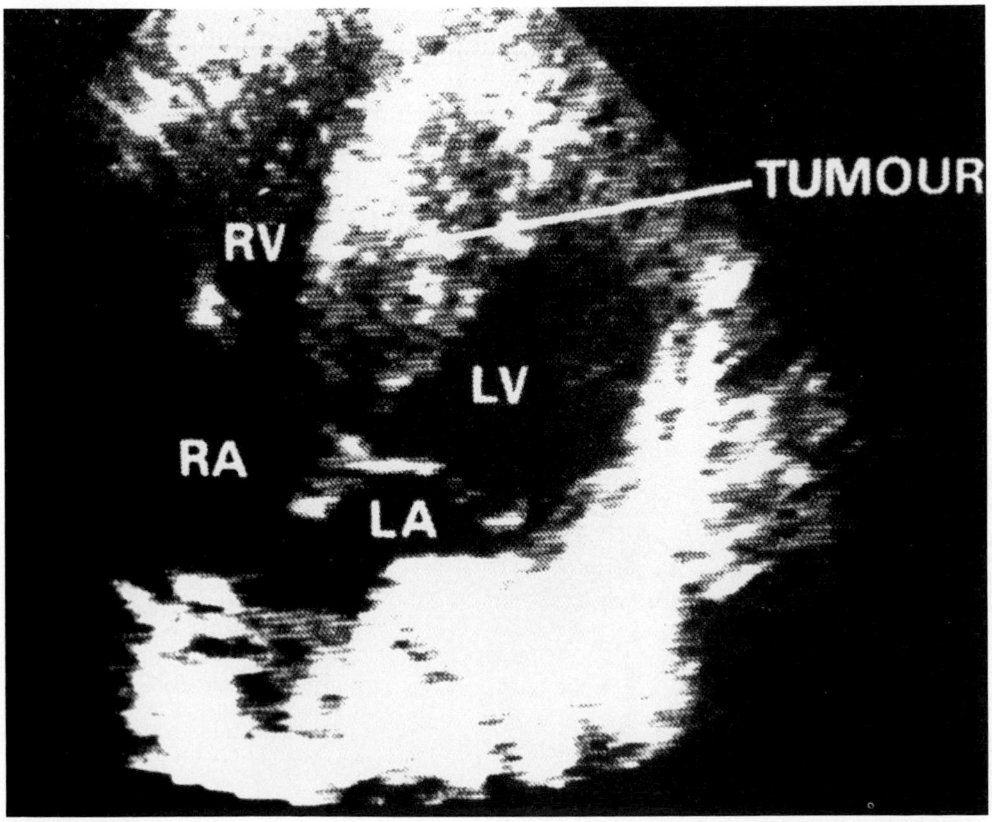

Fig. 36–26. Apical four-chamber recording from an infant with a huge interventricular septal fibroma. RV = right ventricle; LV = left ventricle; LA = left atrium; RA = right atrium. (From Reece IJ, et al.: Interventricular fibroma: echocardiographic diagnosis and successful surgical removal in infancy. Br Heart J 50:590, 1983.)

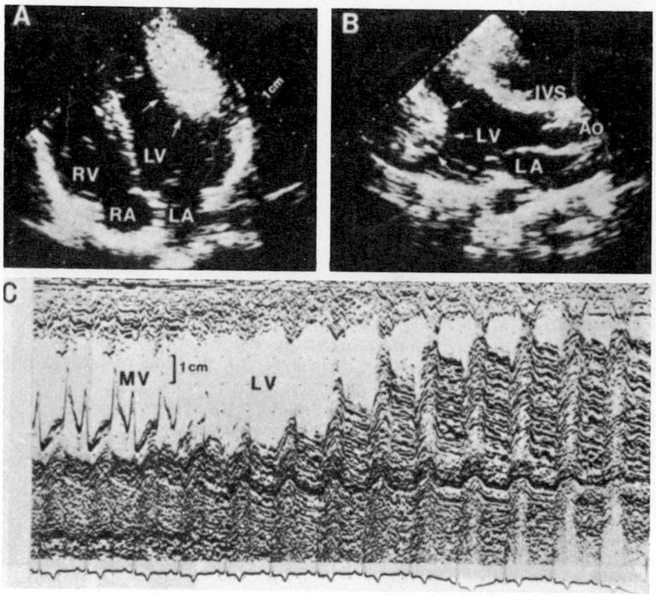

Fig. 36–27. **A.** Apical four-chamber view showing a large fibroma (arrows) in the posterolateral aspect of the left ventricle. **B.** Parasternal long axis view of the same ventricle. **C.** M-mode scan from mitral valve to the apex showing thickened left ventricular posterior wall. Ao = aorta; IVS = interventricular septum; LA = left atrium; MV = mitral valve; RA = right atrium; RV = right ventricle. (From Takahashi K, et al.: Echocardiographic demonstration of an asymptomatic patient with left ventricular fibroma. Am J Cardiol 53:981, 1984.)

found to have an echogenic mass along the right side of the interventricular septum involving the upper portion of the septum and extending into the right ventricular outflow tract. The tumor mass contained echo-free areas representing vascular channels or cavernous lakes. The tumor was sessile and nonencapsulated, and it resulted in intracavitary obstruction. The finding of such a solitary, nonpedunculated, nonhomogeneous right-sided mass, particularly when associated with a pericardial effusion, is more suggestive of hemangioma than myxoma, rhabdomyoma, or any other primary intracardiac tumor.

Figure 36–29 illustrates a large, nonhomogeneous tumor within the right atrium in an infant with a hemangioendothelioma. The tumor was unusual in that it was adherent to the interatrial septum and filled most of the right atrial cavity; it produced signs and symptoms of right-sided heart failure.

Spontaneous regression of a large cavernous hemangioma over a 2-year period has been documented by serial echocardiographic studies.[109]

Cystic Masses

Cystic masses of the heart are rare. They include epithelium-lined cystic tumors, intracardiac teratomas, blood cysts, and echinococcal cysts.

Benign epithelium-lined cystic tumors include mesotheliomas and bronchogenic cysts. Mesotheliomas are small cystic lesions occurring most commonly in the region of the atrioventricular node and often producing atrioventricular block.[6,110,111] Bronchogenic cysts most likely represent embryonic remnants of the respiratory tract and are rarely of clinical significance.[6] Neither of these entities has been described echocardiographically.

By definition, a teratoma contains all three germ layers. Intrapericardial teratomas are far more common than intracardiac tumors.[6,112] Intracardiac teratomas are generally right-sided. They are lobulated and vary in size between 5 mm and 9 cm, often containing many multilocular cysts of varying diameter.[112] Figure 36–30 is an example of a right ventricular teratoma in a 6-year-old girl with congestive heart failure. The tumor appeared as a large multicystic mass attached to the upper portion of the interventricular septum and protruding into the right ventricular cavity.

Blood cysts are generally found on valvular endocardium in infants and children.[6] Figure 36–31, an unusual intraventricular blood cyst detected during routine echocardiographic examination,[113] appeared as a bilobed, mobile, cystic mass attached to the tip of the anterolateral papillary muscle and adjacent chordae tendineae.

Cardiac involvement in echinococcosis occurs in fewer than 2% of patients with echinococcal disease. The common sites of localization are the left ventricular free wall (50%) and the interventricular septum (20%); the right ventricle and the atria are less frequently involved.[114] Although they are intramyocardial, cysts may project into a cardiac chamber or into the pericardial space.[114] Intracardiac rupture is the most frequent complication, resulting in anaphylactic shock or cardiac tam-

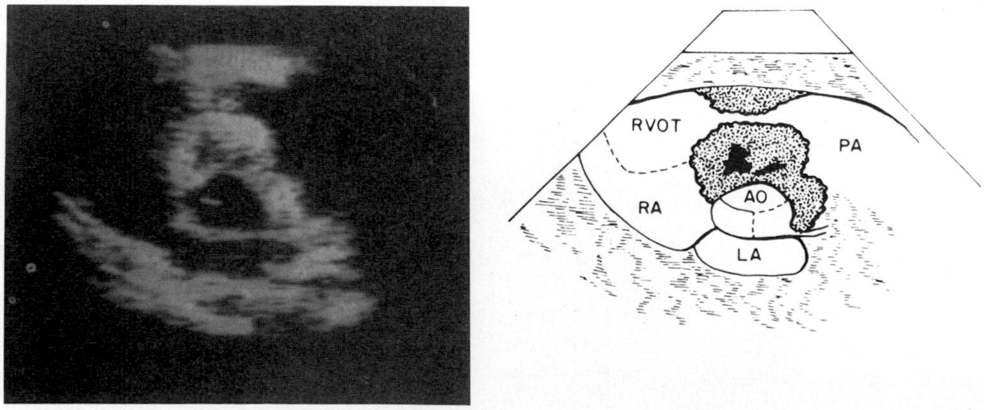

Fig. 36–28. Parasternal short axis recording from a patient with a large hemangioma involving the upper interventricular septum, the anterior margin of the aorta (AO), and encircling and partially obstructing the right ventricular outflow tract (RVOT). There are dilated feeding vessels within the tumor (echo-free spaces). PA = pulmonary artery; LA = left atrium; RA = right atrium.

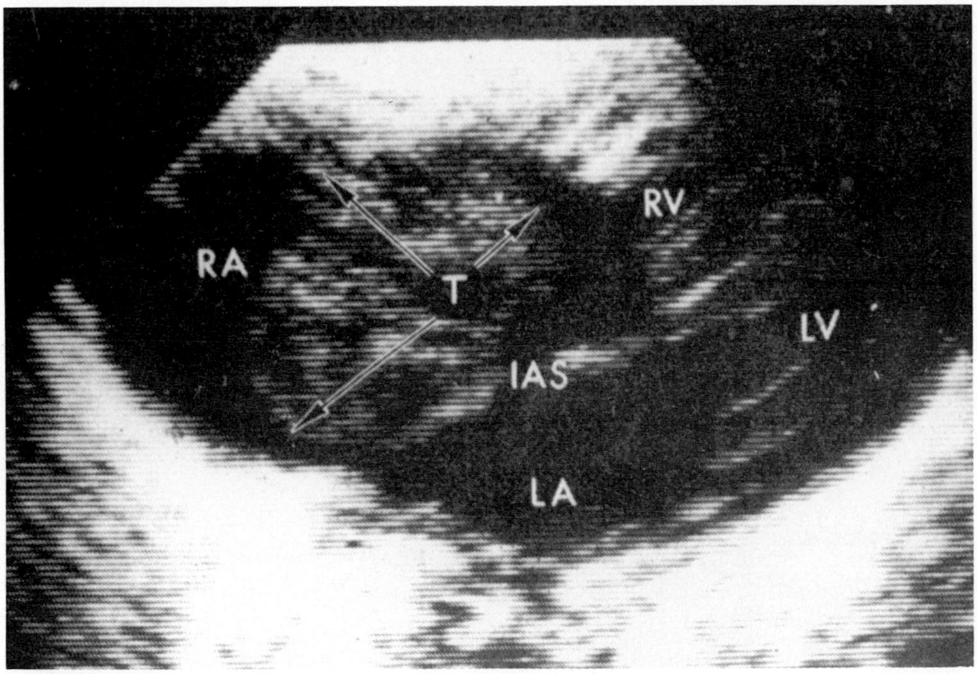

Fig. 36–29. Subcostal four-chamber recording from an infant with a right atrial hemangioendothelioma (T). RV = right ventricle; LV = left ventricle; LA = left atrium; RA = right atrium; IAS = interatrial septum. (From Riggs T, et al.: Two-dimensional echocardiography in evaluation of right atrial masses: five cases in pediatric patients. Am J Cardiol 48:961, 1981.)

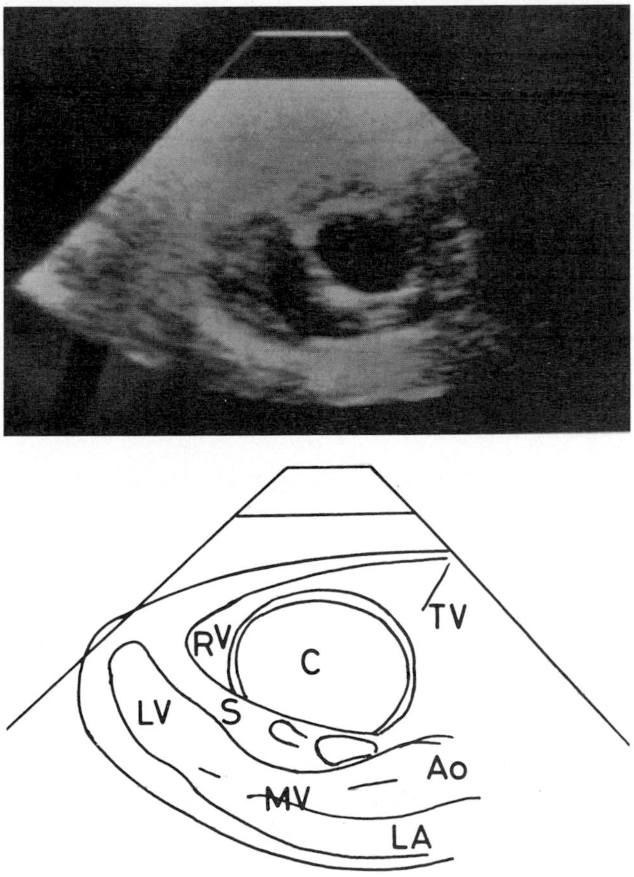

Fig. 36–30. Parasternal long axis recording demonstrating a cystic tumor (C) in the right ventricle (RV). LV = left ventricle; TV = tricuspid valve; MV = mitral valve; Ao = aorta; LA = left atrium. (From Cox, et al.: Teratoma of the heart: a case report and review of the literature. Virchows Arch [A] 402:163, 1983.)

ponade if a cyst ruptures into the pericardial space.[114] Echocardiography has been shown to be sensitive and specific in the detection of intracardiac echinococcal cysts.[115–118] The appearance of a large, cystic, thin-walled structure with multiple septa is diagnostic (Fig. 36–32), and it allows differentiation from other intracardiac masses.

Malignant Primary Tumors

Approximately 25% of all primary tumors of the heart are malignant.[6] Although reported in all age groups, these tumors are found predominantly in adults.[6] The majority of primary malignant tumors are sarcomas, which are second in overall frequency to myxomas.[6]

Sarcomas have many different histologic types including angiosarcoma, rhabdomyosarcoma, fibrosarcoma, lymphosarcoma, myxosarcoma, leiomyosarcoma, and undifferentiated sarcoma.[6] Primary extraskeletal osteosarcoma is a rare primary malignant tumor of the heart. Any of the cardiac chambers, and frequently the pericardium, may be involved, although right-sided tumors predominate.[6] Intramural tumors are more frequent than intracavitary lesions. Because of the rapid proliferation of these tumors, they commonly extend into the cardiac chambers, the pericardial space, or both.[6]

Clinical signs and symptoms are determined primarily by the location of the tumor. Common presentations include: congestive heart failure, particularly right-sided;[6,119,120] pericardial effusion, with pericarditis or tamponade;[119,121,122] precordial chest pain;[119,123] arrhythmias;[6,119] conduction disturbances;[6,119] obstruction of the venae cavae;[119,124] and sudden death.[6] Sarcomas tend to metastasize widely. Regardless of the histologic type, primary cardiac sarcomas are commonly associated with a brief clinical course and are almost uniformly fatal.[6,119,120]

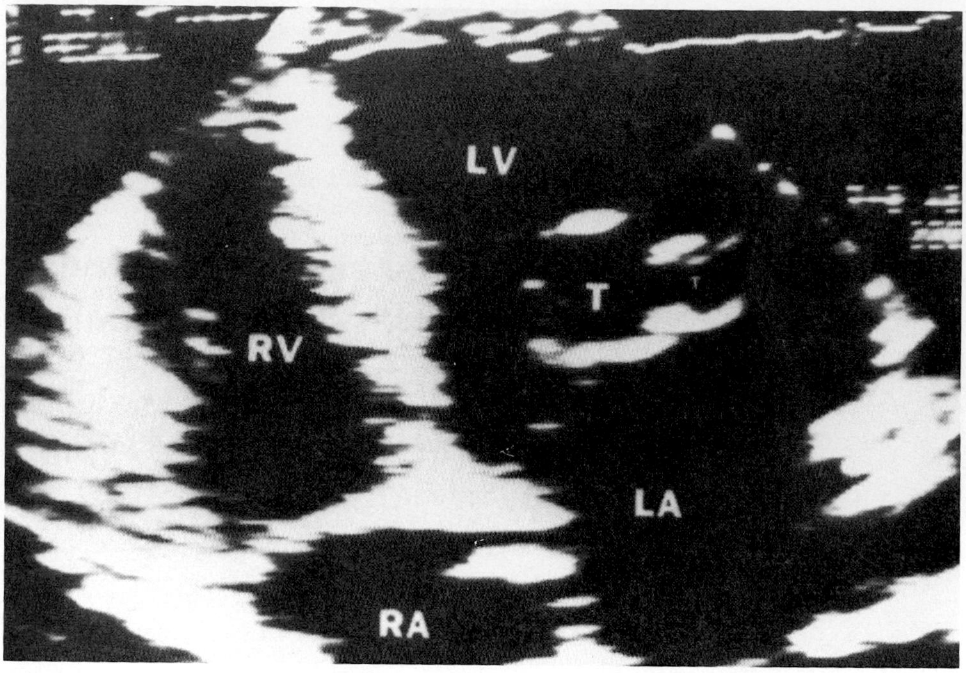

Fig. 36–31. Apical four-chamber recording of a blood cyst involving the papillary muscle. T = tumor; LV = left ventricle; LA = left atrium; RV = right ventricle; RA = right atrium. (From Hause AM, et al.: Blood cyst of the papillary muscle: clinical, echocardiographic and anatomic observations. Am J Cardiol 51:612, 1983.)

Two-dimensional echocardiography has enhanced the antemortem diagnosis of malignant cardiac tumors.[4,67,125,126] Intramural tumor infiltration of the myocardium appears as localized wall thickening, hypocontractility, or increased reflectivity on echocardiographic examination. Tumor infiltration through the myocardium into the pericardial space or into adjacent cardiac chambers may also be documented (Fig. 36–33). Serial echocardiographic studies may be useful in assessing tumor response to various treatment methods and may also be used to detect tumor recurrence.[4,67,94,126]

Angiosarcomas

Angiosarcoma is the most frequently occurring primary cardiac sarcoma (Table 36–1). These tumors occur predominantly in men.[6,119] Approximately 80% originate in the right atrium as large mural masses that frequently extend to the pericardium, venae cavae, or tricuspid valve, causing obstruction to filling of right-sided chambers.[6,119] Extensive involvement of the pericardium, generally in conjunction with a right atrial tumor, is seen in 30 to 40% of patients, resulting in hemopericardium with tamponade, or less commonly obliteration of the pericardial space with signs and symptoms of pericardial constriction.[119,127]

Figure 36–34A demonstrates a small mass in the superior aspect of the right atrium that was detected during a routine echocardiographic study. A repeat echocardiogram 1 year later (Fig. 36–34B) revealed a large echogenic mass filling the right atrium but not extending into the venae cavae. At thoracotomy, extensive tumor infiltration was found, encasing the right heart and lungs. Microscopic examination revealed an angiosarcoma.

Rhabdomyosarcomas

Rhabdomyosarcomas, the second most common primary sarcoma of the heart, originate in striated muscles. Approximately 25% of tumors occur in patients younger than 20 years of age.[6] Rhabdomyosarcomas can arise in any cardiac chamber and are typically multiple. Local pericardial extension is frequent. These tumors always develop intramurally, but they can grow into adjacent cardiac chambers and can cause partial obstruction of one or more valve orifices.[93,123] Unlike benign intracavitary cardiac tumors, however, rhabdomyosarcomas are locally invasive and often involve or partially replace the affected valve(s).[6,93]

Lymphosarcomas

Primary lymphoma of the heart or lymphosarcoma, defined as lymphoma involving only the heart and pericardium, is extremely rare.[6,128] Pericardial effusion, congestive heart failure, and heart block may be the initial presentation.[129–131] Myocardial infiltration by lymphoma may be nodular or diffuse. Right- and left-sided involvement occurs with equal frequency. The tumors may appear as multiple intracavitary polypoid nodules obliterating the heart chambers or valves. Figure 36–35 is an example of a B-cell lymphoma involving the cardiac apex, whereas Figure 36–36 illustrates a lymphosarcoma involving the right atrium and tricuspid valve. Primary cardiac lymphoma may mimic hypertrophic cardiomyopathy with thickening of the interventricular septum and left ventricular free wall and anterior motion of the mitral leaflets during ventricular systole.[130] Lymphosarcomas have no specific echocardiographic features that permit their differentiation from other car-

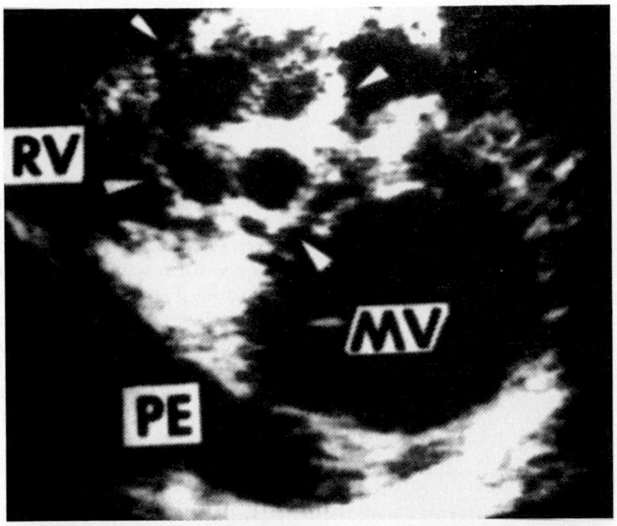

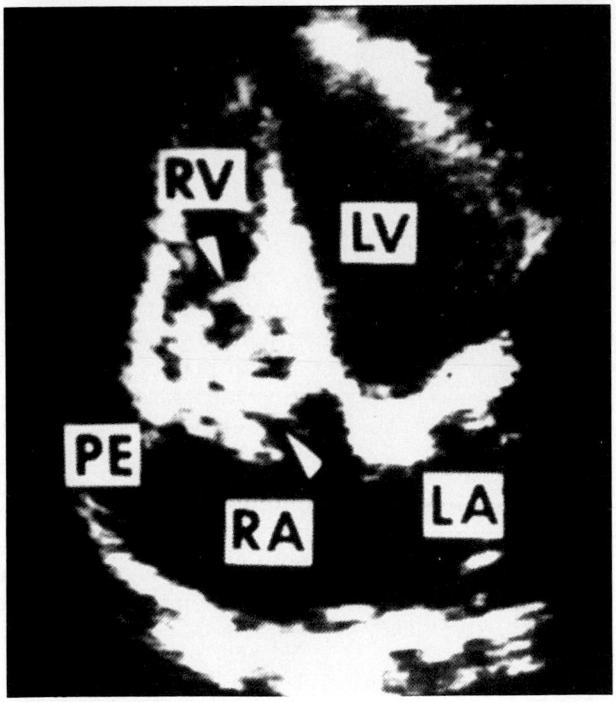

Fig. 36–32. Top. Parasternal short axis recording of the base of the right ventricle (RV) showing the typical appearance of an echinococchal cyst. Bottom. Apical four-chamber recording illustrating the extent of right ventricular involvement by the multicystic mass. MV = mitral valve; PE = pericardial effusion; RA = right atrium; LA = left atrium; LV = left ventricle. (From Erol C, et al.: Cardiac hydatid cyst simulating tricuspid stenosis. Am J Cardiol 56:833, 1985.)

diac tumors. Once diagnosed, however, initial reduction in tumor size in response to therapy may be dramatic.

Primary Extraskeletal Osteosarcomas

Primary extraskeletal osteosarcomas most commonly arise from the posterior wall of the left atrium near the entrance of the pulmonary veins.[6] Figure 36–37A illustrates a large, mobile osteosarcoma that prolapses through the mitral valve orifice during diastole, simulating a myxoma. Two features, however, namely, its site of origin from nonseptal atrial walls and tumor extension into the pulmonary veins (Fig. 36–37B), are useful in distinguishing osteosarcomas from myxomas and other left atrial tumors.[132]

Metastatic osteogenic sarcoma (Fig. 18–17) is more common than primary tumor. The echocardiographic appearance is similar, except metastatic tumor often involves multiple sites within the heart; the tumors are larger and more often intracavitary.[132–134] Calcifications are frequent in metastatic osteogenic sarcoma because metastases are composed, at least in part, of malignant osteoblasts.[133]

Other Primary Sarcomas

Rare primary sarcomas of the heart include fibrosarcomas,[39,135] malignant fibrous histiocytomas,[136,137] myxosarcomas,[138] liposarcomas,[139] leiomyosarcomas,[140] and sarcomas of other cell types.[141,142] Although individual cases have been reported, differential echocardiographic features have not been recognized.

Pericardial Tumors

Primary pericardial tumors are rare.[6] They include benign cysts and solid tumors. Primary tumors that may involve the pericardium include fibromas,[143] lipomas,[143] leiomyomas,[6] teratomas,[6,112] and heterotopic thymic or thyroid tissue.[144] Malignant pericardial tumors predominate, most frequently mesotheliomas, followed by sarcomas[6,127] (see also Chapter 35).

Pericardial Cysts

Pericardial cysts, the most common type of benign intrapericardial tumor, represent persistent blind-ended recesses of the parietal pericardium.[6] The cysts are usually detected on a routine chest radiograph or as an incidental finding at autopsy. One third of patients are symptomatic, however, with chest pain or dyspnea as the chief presenting complaints.[143,145] Seventy percent of cysts are located at the right cardiophrenic junction, and 22% occur at the left cardiophrenic junction, and they may occasionally be seen along the anterosuperior or posterior mediastinum, hilus, or left cardiac border.[145] Pericardial cysts range in size from 2 cm to more than 16 cm in diameter. The majority are filled with fluid and are unilocular. Foci of calcification may be present in the cyst wall.[6]

The clinical significance of pericardial cysts lies in their differentiation from solid tumors, left ventricular aneurysms and pseudoaneurysms, prominent left atrial appendage (see Chapter 18), and diaphragmatic and hiatal hernias (see Chapter 35). Two-dimensional echocardiography is a simple, noninvasive means of diagnosing pericardial cysts, as well as providing information on the size, shape, consistency, and spatial relationship of pericardial and extrapericardial masses.[146,147] Figure 36–38 is an example of a large pericardial cyst seen as a round, echo-free structure above the right hemidi-

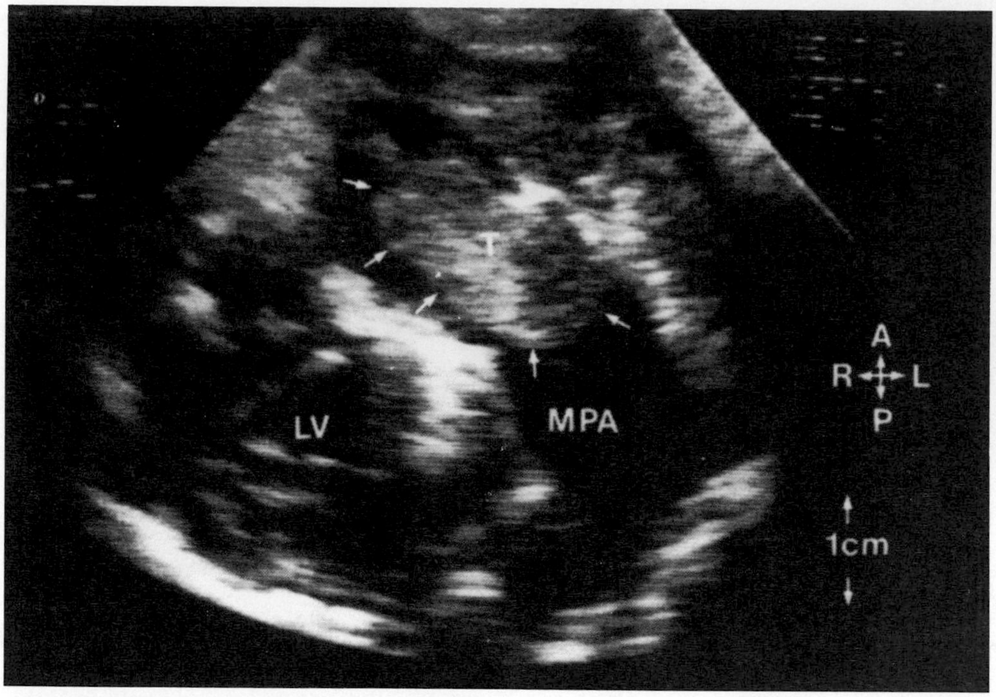

Fig. 36–33. Parasternal recording of the right ventricular outflow tract and pulmonary artery showing a large tumor mass (T) identified as an undifferentiated sarcoma. The tumor partially obstructed the outflow tract with an increase in outflow velocity to 3.6 m/sec. MPA = main pulmonary artery; LV = left ventricle. (From Ludomirsky A, et al.: Intracardiac undifferentiated sarcoma in infancy. Journal of the American College of Cardiology, 6:1362, 1985. Reprinted with permission from the American College of Cardiology.)

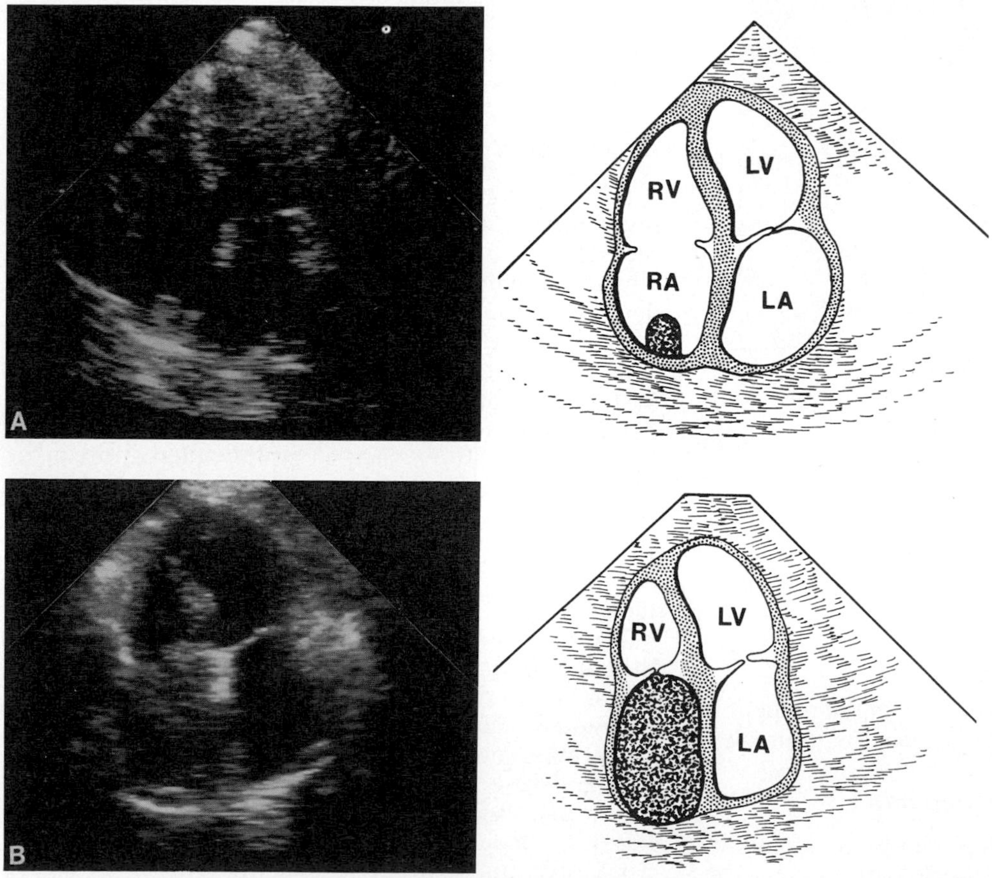

Fig. 36–34. A. Apical four-chamber recording showing a small (roughly 1 cm in diameter) mass arising from the superior border of the right atrium (RA). **B.** Similar recording obtained 1 year later. The mass has now grown to fill the RA. At surgery, the mass proved to be an angiosarcoma. RV = right ventricle; LV = left ventricle; LA = left atrium.

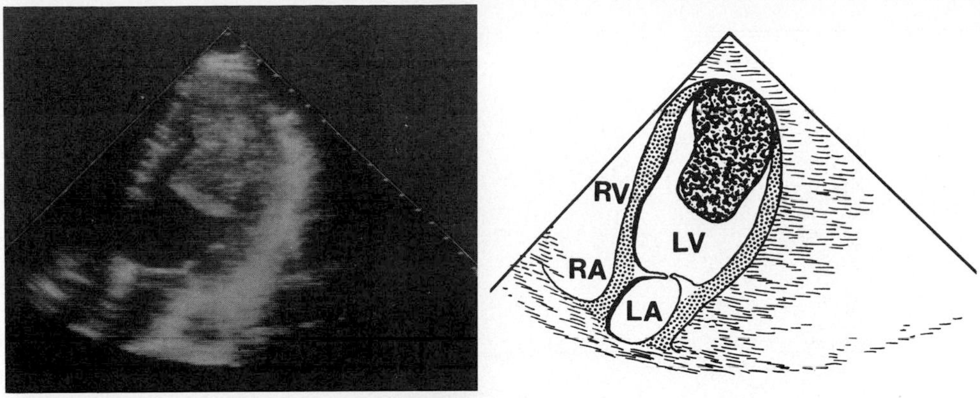

Fig. 36–35. Apical four-chamber recording of a B-cell lymphoma arising from the left ventricular apex. LV = left ventricle; RV = right ventricle; LA = left atrium; RA = right atrium.

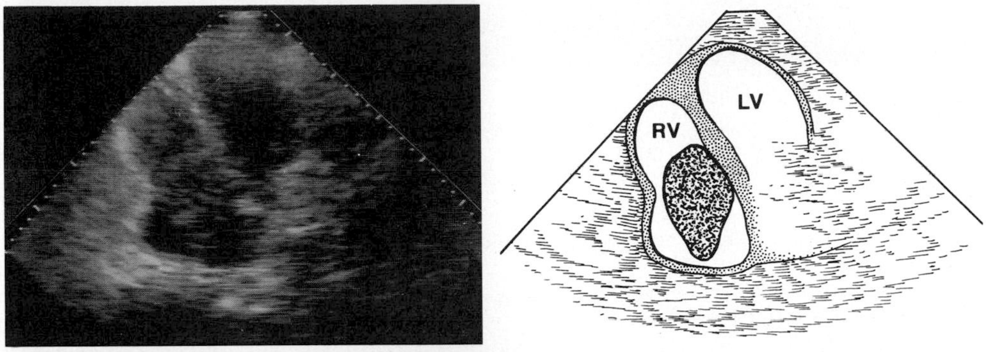

Fig. 36–36. Apical four-chamber recording illustrating a histiocytic lymphoma of the right atrium. RV = right ventricle; LV = left ventricle.

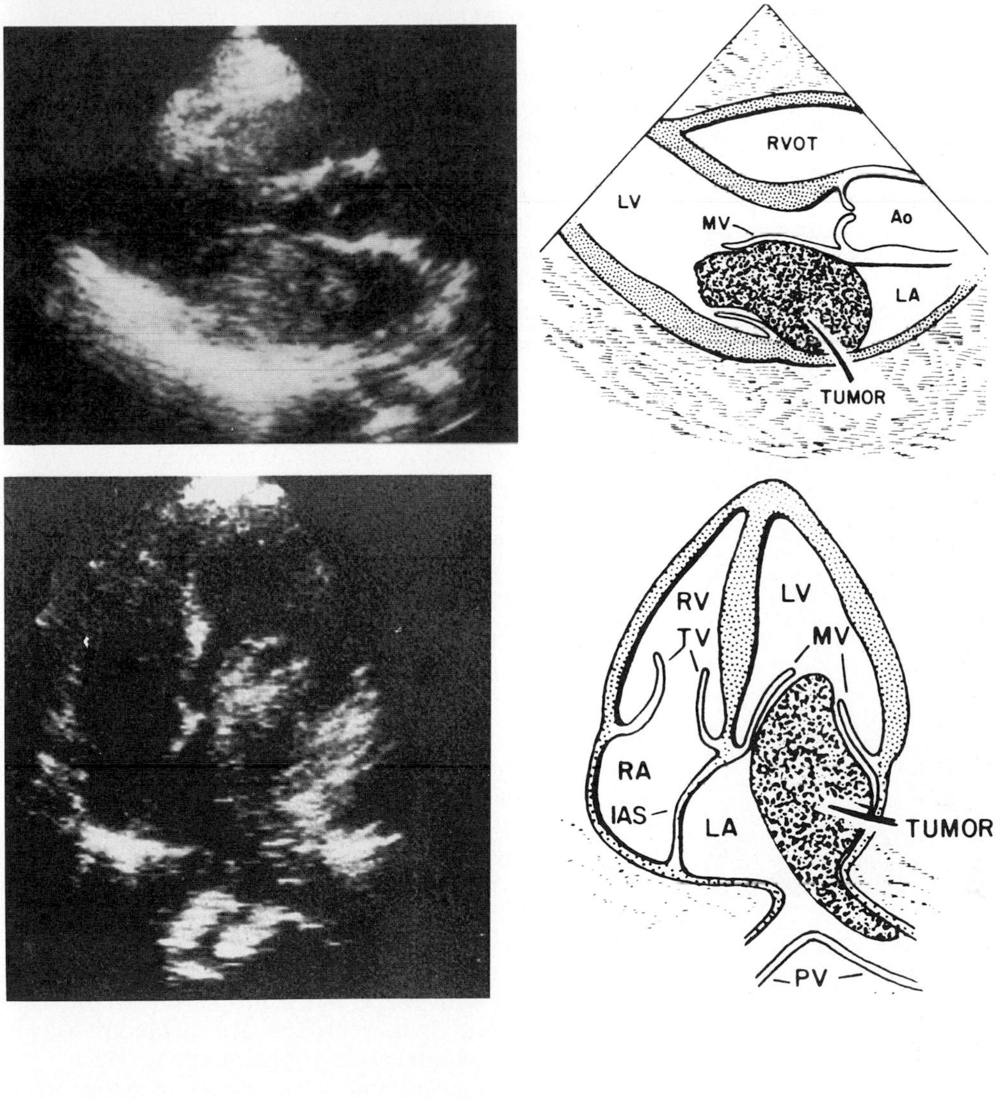

Fig. 36–37. A. Parasternal long axis recording of an osteogenic sarcoma of the left atrium (LA). Image is recording during diastole, and the tumor prolapses through the mitral valve (MV) into the left ventricle (LV), much like a typical myxoma. **B.** Apical four-chamber recording illustrating the origin of the tumor from the pulmonary veins (PV). The point of tumor origin helps to differentiate this osteogenic sarcoma from a typical myxoma. RVOT = right ventricular outflow tract; Ao = aorta; IAS = interatrial septum; RA = right atrium; TV = tricuspid valve; RV = right ventricle.

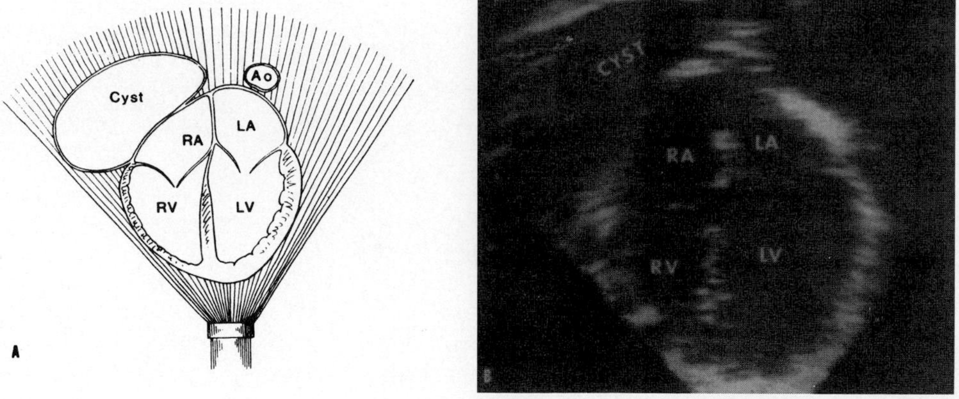

Fig. 36–38. Inverted apical four-chamber view illustrating a pericardial cyst lying superolateral to the right atrium (RA). Ao = aorta; LA = left atrium; LV = left ventricle; RV = right ventricle. (From Hynes JK, et al.: Two-dimensional echocardiographic diagnosis of pericardial cyst. Mayo Clin Proc 58:60, 1983.)

aphragm adjacent to, but clearly demarcated from, the right atrial cavity.

Pericardial Teratomas

Most teratomas of the heart and pericardium are extracardiac but intrapericardial, usually arising from the root of the pulmonary artery and aorta.[6,148] They are found predominantly in the pediatric age group and occur more often in females.[6] One case has been diagnosed in utero using echocardiography.[149] The tumors may be as large as 15 cm in diameter and often interfere with cardiac filling. Both solid and cystic areas may be present. The differentiation of pericardial tumors is aided by two-dimensional echocardiography, which typically demonstrates a rounded, well-circumscribed mass with echo-free areas of variable dimensions.[150,151]

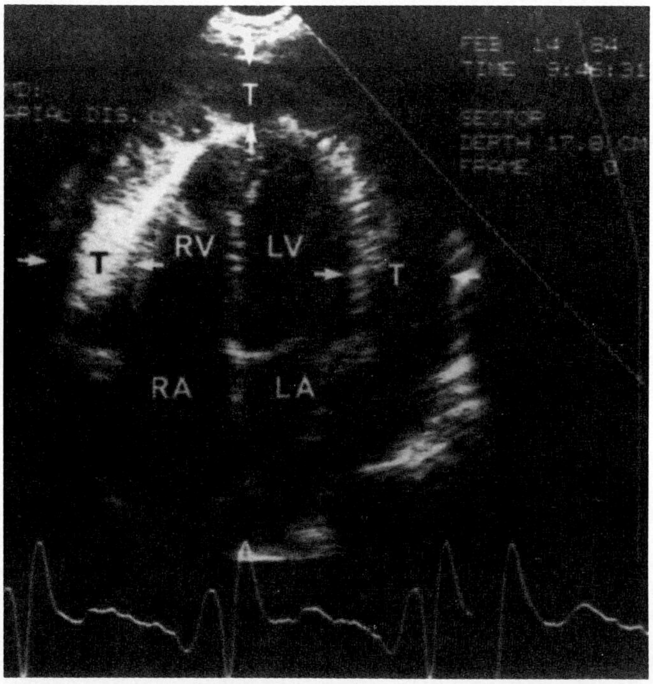

Fig. 36–39. Apical four-chamber recording of a pericardial mesothelioma. The tumor (T) fills the pericardial space, encasing the heart. RA = right atrium; RV = right ventricle; LA = left atrium; LV = left ventricle. (From Coplan NL, et al.: Pericardial mesothelioma masquerading as a benign pericardial effusion. J Am Coll Cardiol 4:1307, 1984. Reprinted with permission from the American College of Cardiology.)

Pericardial Mesotheliomas

Pericardial mesothelioma is the most common primary malignant tumor of the pericardium,[6,152–155] and it is the third most common primary malignant neoplasm of the heart and pericardium.[6] Most series indicate a male/female incidence ratio of nearly 2:1.[6,152] Most mesotheliomas diffusely involve both the visceral and parietal pericardium, encasing the heart. The tumor spreads by direct extension into contiguous structures including the epicardial layers of the myocardium, but, unlike primary cardiac sarcomas, it does not extend into the cardiac chambers. Primary pericardial mesothelioma may first appear as pericarditis with fever and chest pain, as constrictive pericarditis, or as cardiac tamponade.[152,155] Two-dimensional echocardiography may demonstrate thick, intense echoes arising from the pericardium, often with asymmetric echo-free spaces suggesting loculated effusion.[154,155] Figure 36–39 demonstrates an echodense mass encasing the heart in a patient with pericardial mesothelioma.

SECONDARY TUMORS OF THE HEART AND PERICARDIUM

Metastatic tumors to the heart and pericardium are 20 to 40 times more common than primary tumors.[6,8,10,39] Nearly every type of malignant tumor from every organ and tissue has been reported to metastasize to the heart and pericardium, with the exception of primary tumor of the central nervous system.[6] In autopsy series that included only patients with metastatic malignant tumors, the incidence of cardiac metastases ranged from 1.5 to 20%.[6,10,156] Carcinomas of the lung and breast, because of their prevalence, are the most common malignant tumors that metastasize to the heart.[6,10,156] Those tumors with the greatest propensity to metastasize to the heart or pericardium are melanoma (up to 64%),[157] and leukemia and lymphoma (up to 46%).[128,158]

Cardiac metastases generally appear late in the course

of the primary disease. Isolated cardiac involvement is rarely seen without dissemination to other organs or as the presenting symptom of a remote primary tumor.[159-161] Metastatic tumor typically involves the pericardium and myocardium and only rarely the endocardium, valves, or coronary arteries.[6] Pericardial metastases are more common than myocardial metastases.[6,10,156] Metastatic tumors to the myocardium are more often intramural than intracavitary.[6,157]

Metastatic spread may occur by direct extension from contiguous structures or through lymphatic or hematogenous spread. Most carcinomas metastasize to the heart and pericardium by lymphatic spread,[6] whereas hematogenous spread is the main route of metastases for melanoma, lymphoma, leukemia, and various soft tissue and skeletal sarcomas.[128,157,158,162] Tumor may reach the heart by direct venous extension along the venae cavae or pulmonary veins.[6,64,132]

The most common clinical findings associated with metastatic cardiac involvement include unexplained rapid cardiac enlargement with signs and symptoms of tamponade, congestive heart failure, and cardiac arrhythmias.[6,39] The clinical presentation may vary and is often nonspecific, however. Because metastatic cardiac involvement may be an important cause of morbidity and mortality in patients with malignant diseases, early detection has important therapeutic and prognostic implications. Two-dimensional echocardiography has proved to be useful not only in the detection of the presence of cardiac metastases, but also in the definition of their location and size, in the determination of the most appropriate therapy, and in evaluation of the results.[67,94,95,163-166] The most common echocardiographic finding suggesting metastasis is pericardial effusion. Wall thickening or protrusion of a tumor mass into a cardiac chamber, often producing obstruction, may also be seen.

Pericardial Involvement

Neoplastic involvement of the pericardium has been reported at autopsy in 5 to 15% of patients with malignant diseases.[6,10,156] Lung and breast carcinoma, leukemia, and lymphoma comprise over 80% of these tumors.[6] Other causes of malignant pericardial involvement include esophageal carcinoma, pancreatic carcinoma, thyroid carcinoma, ovarian and prostatic carcinoma, and sarcomas.[6] Malignant pericardial involvement may appear as pericardial effusion with or without cardiac tamponade, nodular epicardial tumor implants, effusive-constrictive pericarditis, or frank constrictive pericarditis.[6,167] Pericardial effusion is the most common manifestation.

Two-dimensional echocardiography is ideally suited for the detection of pericardial effusion and the assessment of related hemodynamic sequelae.[168-171] Discrete metastatic tumor nodules may be visualized as irregular echo-dense masses that protrude into the pericardial space (Fig. 36–40).[172] The motion of visceral pericardial metastases characteristically parallels the cyclic motion of the heart, whereas metastases to the parietal pericardium are fixed.[168]

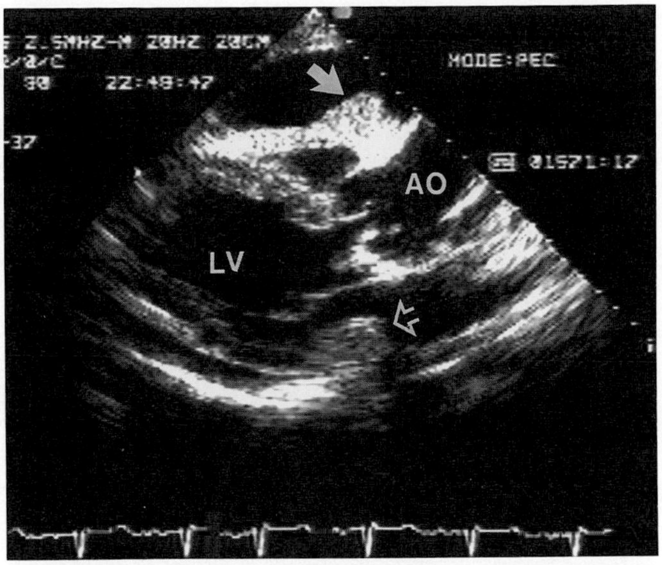

Fig. 36–40. Parasternal long axis recording from a patient with a metastatic gastric carcinoma. Tumor implants are evident anteriorly in the pericardial space (closed arrow) and posteriorly in the atrioventricular groove (open arrow). There is an associated large pericardial effusion. LV = left ventricle; AO = aorta.

Pericardial metastases may also appear as tumor encasement of the heart with abnormal thickening of the pericardium or obliteration of all or part of the pericardial space (see Fig. 35–19).[169] The presence of a large pericardial effusion without a recognized cause should always suggest the possibility of an underlying malignant disease. Isolated anterior echo-free spaces are caused by epicardial fat far more frequently than by tumor, however.[173-175]

The differential diagnosis of echogenic masses in the pericardial space includes intrapericardial adhesions, fibrin strands, and bridging bands that form dense linear echoes crossing the pericardial space.[176] Fibrinous deposits are usually seen in patients with chronic effusions secondary to chronic renal failure, radiation, trauma, or infection.[176] These deposits are generally easily distinguished from tumor masses, although fibrinous deposits and tumor masses may coexist.

Myocardial Involvement

Intramyocardial involvement by metastatic tumor may result in congestive heart failure, arrhythmias, outflow tract obstruction, or peripheral emboli.[6,8,156] On two-dimensional echocardiography, metastatic tumors involving the myocardium are most often evident as a focal area of wall thickening, often with increased reflectivity, and localized asynergy at the level of infiltration.[4,165,177,178] Metastatic tumor may also appear as more diffuse involvement, as in Figure 36–41, which is from a patient with malignant lymphoma with echocardiographic evidence of marked thickening of the left ventricular walls from extensive tumor invasion. Both carcinoma of the breast and bronchogenic carcinoma may directly invade adjacent cardiac structures and may dif-

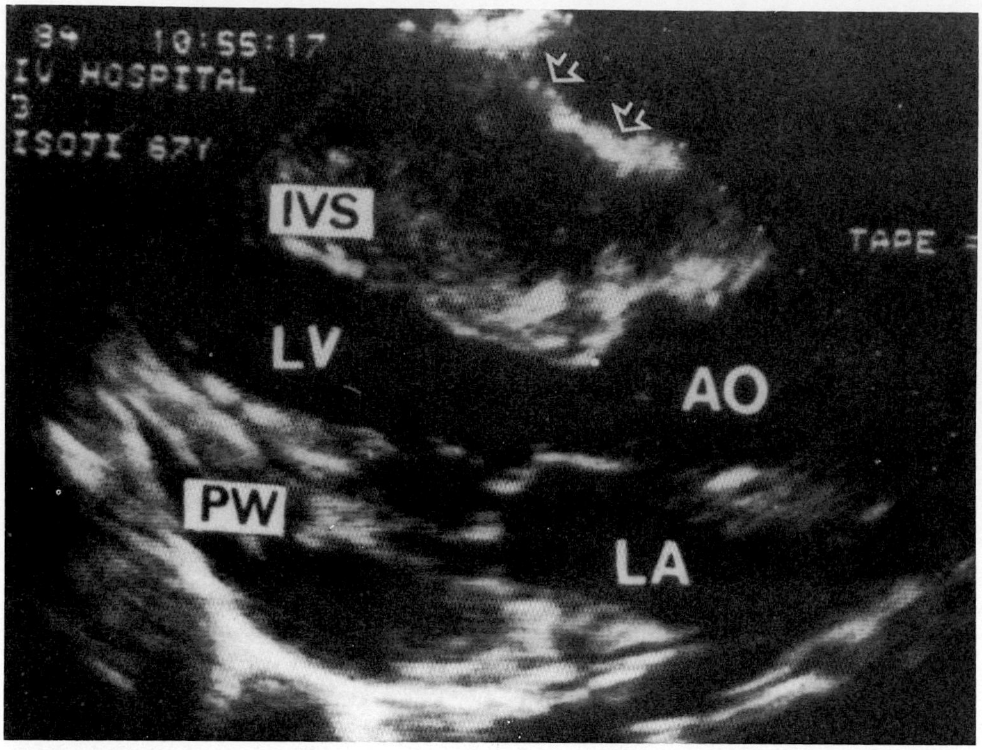

Fig. 36–41. Parasternal long axis recording from a patient with a malignant lymphoma infiltrating the interventricular septum (IVS) and posterior wall (PW). LV = left ventricle; LA = left atrium; AO = aorta. (From Miyazaki T, et al.: Intractable heart failure, conduction disturbances, and myocardial infarction by massive myocardial invasion of malignant lymphoma. J Am Coll Cardiol 6:937, 1985. Reprinted with permission from the American College of Cardiology.)

fusely infiltrate the myocardium or pericardium (see Figs. 35–18 and 35–19).

Intramural tumors may also project into a cardiac chamber.[164–166,179–181] Mural tumors may also involve the atria,[132,182] thereby thickening or distorting the normally smooth margins of the right atrial wall.[183]

Intracavitary Involvement

Intracavitary cardiac metastases are the least common type observed pathologically but the most obvious echocardiographically. Intracavitary metastases generally appear as fixed intracavitary masses of varying size or as mobile masses arising from the endocardium, valvular tissue, or systemic or pulmonary veins. Metastatic masses may be incidental findings, or they may grow to cause cavity obliteration, valve or vessel obstruction, often with associated congestive heart failure, or peripheral embolization.[6,8,10,160,161,179,184]

Tumor extension along the inferior vena cava and into the right atrium is the mechanism of intracardiac tumor spread most frequently described in renal cell carcinoma,[185–187] Wilms' tumor,[64,188] hepatoma,[179,189] and uterine leiomyomatosis.[190,191] Echocardiographically, such tumors may appear as large, immobile masses extending from the inferior vena caval-right atrial junction and filling the right atrial cavity (Fig. 36–42), or they may appear as mobile masses prolapsing across the tricuspid valve during diastole, often partially occluding the tricuspid valve orifice (Fig. 36–43). Right-to-left interatrial shunting resulting from partial tricuspid obstruction by

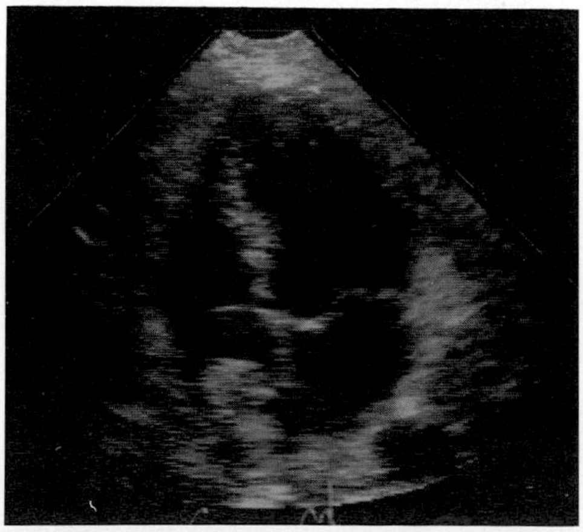

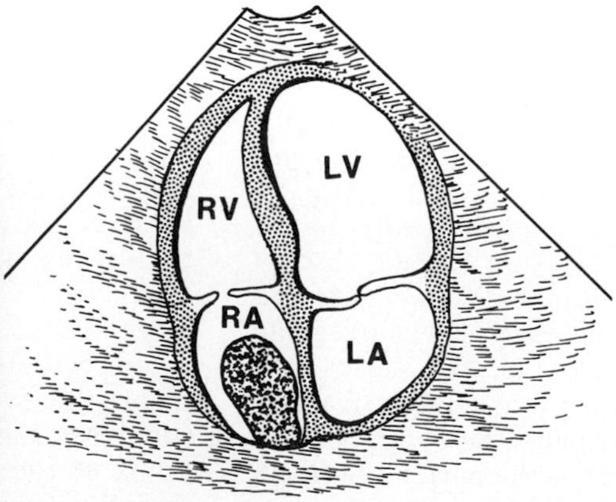

Fig. 36–42. Apical four-chamber recording from a patient with a metastatic hepatocellular carcinoma extending from the inferior vena cava into the right atrial cavity. RV = right ventricle; RA = right atrium; LV = left ventricle; LA = left atrium.

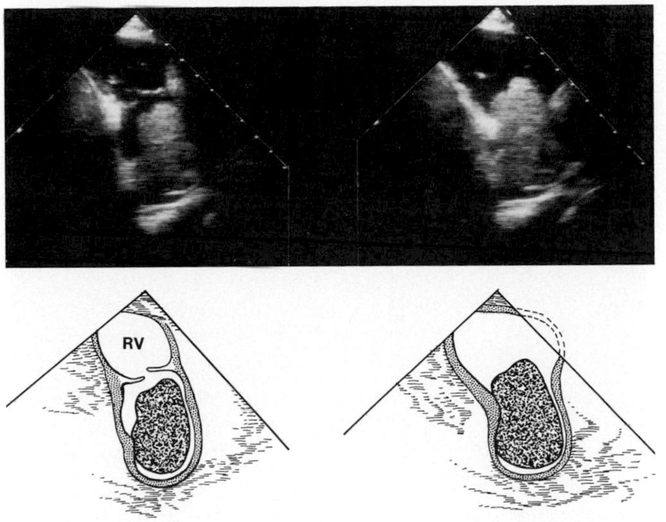

Fig. 36–43. Parasternal long axis right ventricular inflow recording from a second patient with a metastatic hepatocellular carcinoma. In this case, the tumor is larger, filling almost the entire right atrium during systole (right) and prolapsing through the mitral valve during diastole (left). RV = right ventricle.

metastatic carcinoma (Fig. 36–44) has also been noted.[199]

Intracavitary metastases to the right heart have also been reported in patients with testicular carcinoma,[192] ovarian carcinoma,[193] lymphoma,[183] adenocarcinoma of the colon,[194] and Ewing's sarcoma.[195] Secondary tumors involving the right atrium usually arise from the right atrial free wall or extend into the right atrium from the inferior vena cava, whereas primary tumors commonly originate from the interatrial septum.

The spread of pulmonary neoplasms, especially bronchogenic carcinomas and sarcomas, into the left atrium through the pulmonary veins has been documented by two-dimensional echocardiography and is illustrated in Figures 36–45 to 36–48.[132,196,197] Despite the widely differing cell types in these examples, there is little to distinguish one tumor from another. Although as a rule sarcomas appear soft, mobile, and pliable, whereas carcinomas appear solid and fixed and may deform surrounding structures, specific diagnosis is based on a known primary tumor or biopsy. Metastatic tumors to the left atrium, particularly sarcomas, may closely mimic an atrial myxoma, except for two helpful distinguishing features: (1) nonseptal attachment of the tumor mass; and (2) extension of the tumor into the pulmonary veins.

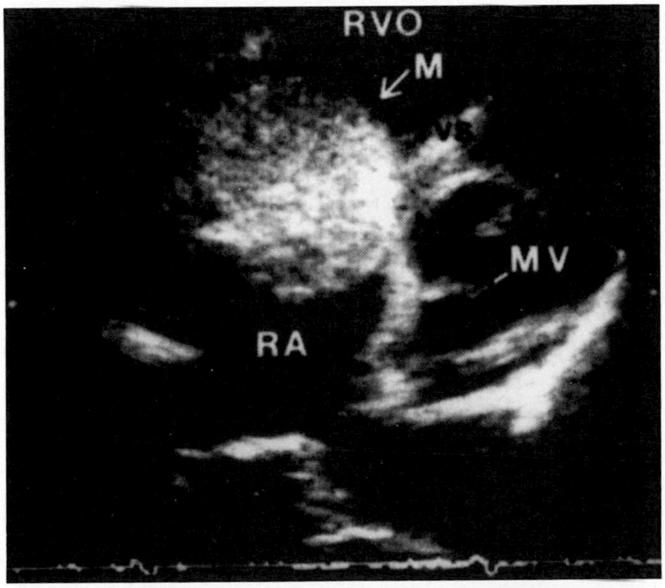

Fig. 36–44. Modified parasternal short axis recording from a patient with a metastatic nasopharyngeal carcinoma (M). RVO = right ventricular outflow tract; VS = interventricular septum; MV = mitral valve; RA = right atrium. (From Gallerstein PE, et al.: Right-to-left intracardiac shunt: a unique presentation of metastatic cardiac disease. J Am Coll Cardiol 3:865, 1984. Reprinted with permission from the American College of Cardiology. Journal of the American College of Cardiology 1984, 3, 865.)

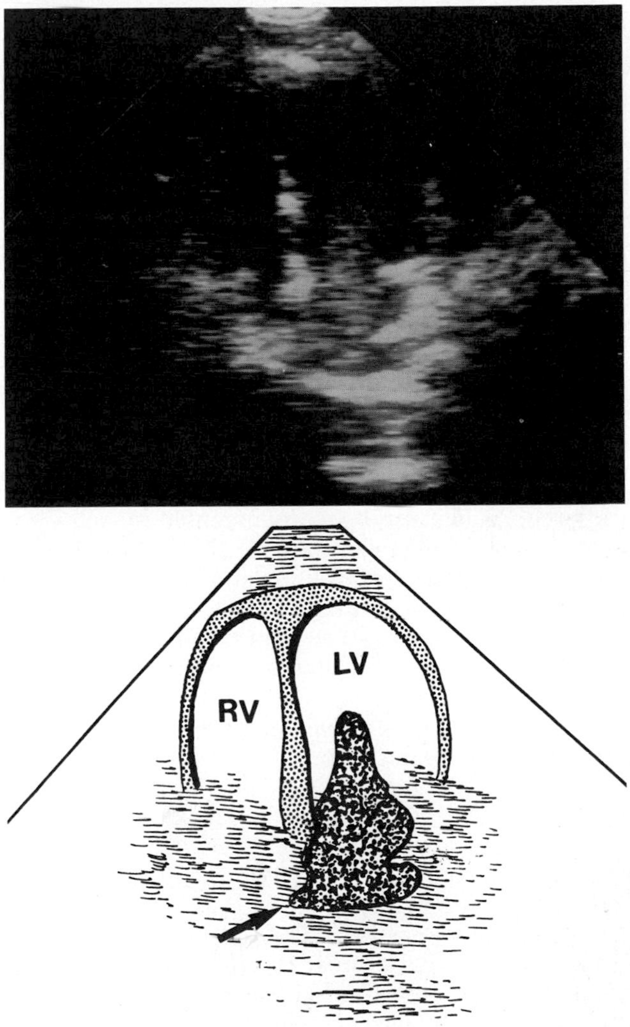

Fig. 36–45. Modified apical four-chamber recording showing a large cell undifferentated carcinoma of the lung extending into the left atrium from the pulmonary veins. LV = left ventricle; RV = right ventricle.

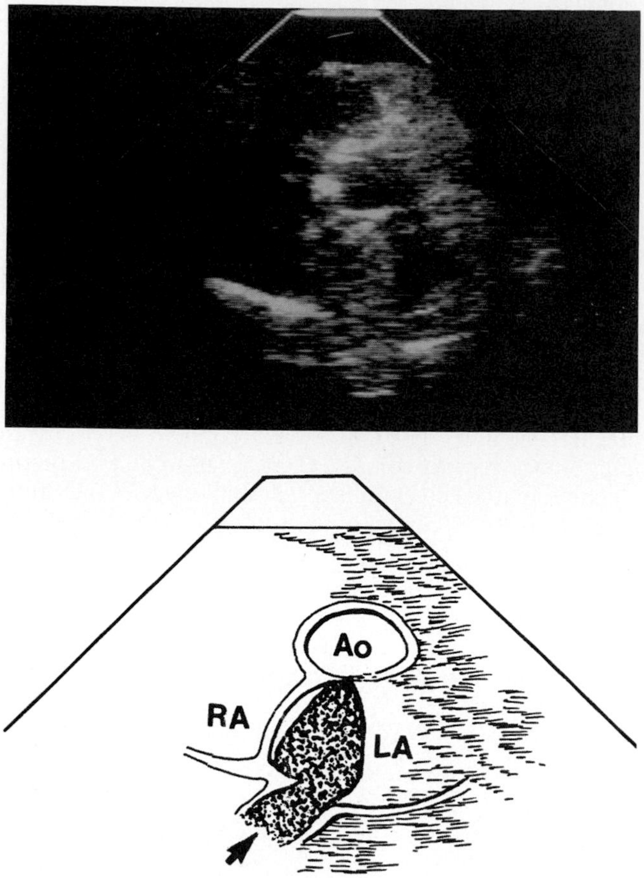

Fig. 36–46. Modified parasternal short axis view showing a primary bronchogenic carcinoma of the lung extending into the left atrium (LA) from one of the right pulmonary veins. RA = right atrium; Ao = aorta.

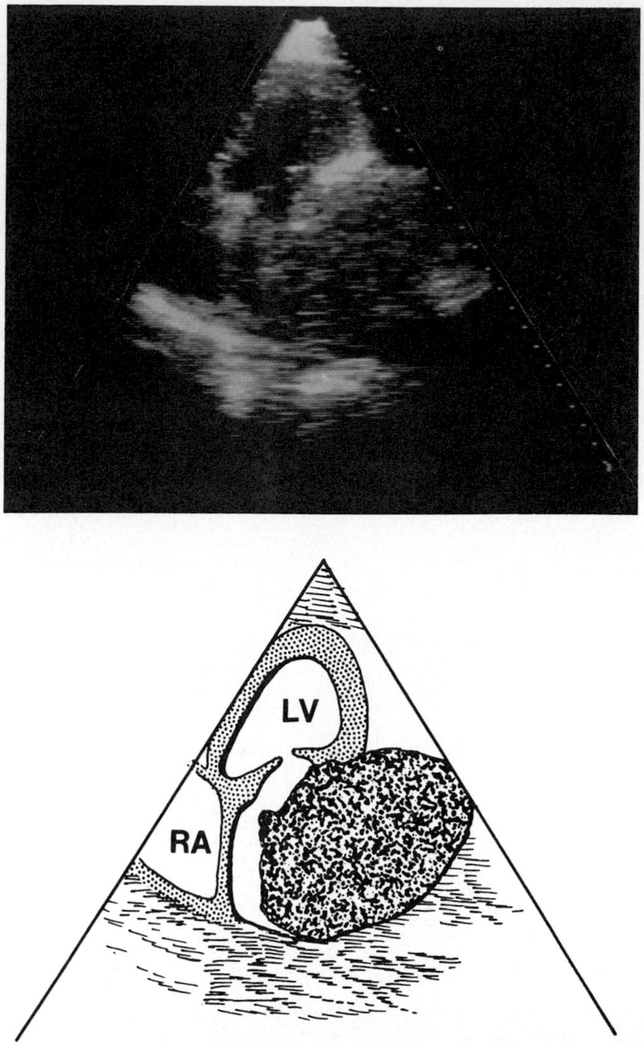

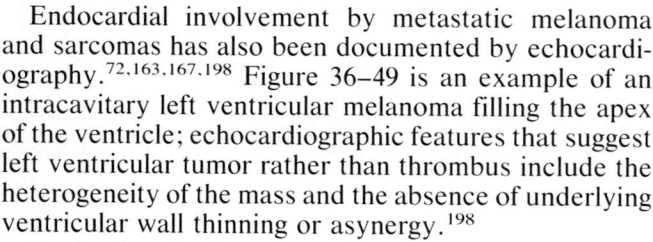

Fig. 36–47. Modified apical four chamber view showing a massive squamous cell carcinoma of the lung, which has metastasized to the left atrium, filling the chamber and distending the lateral wall. LV = left ventricle; RA = right atrium.

Endocardial involvement by metastatic melanoma and sarcomas has also been documented by echocardiography.[72,163,167,198] Figure 36–49 is an example of an intracavitary left ventricular melanoma filling the apex of the ventricle; echocardiographic features that suggest left ventricular tumor rather than thrombus include the heterogeneity of the mass and the absence of underlying ventricular wall thinning or asynergy.[198]

Lastly, breast, bronchogenic, and esophageal carcinoma may produce intracavitary masses by direct extension through the cardiac wall. Figure 36–50 demonstrates a large tumor mass obstructing the right ventricular outflow tract in a 67-year-old woman with breast carcinoma whose presenting sign was congestive heart failure. A pericardial effusion is also present.

Lesions that may be mistaken for intracavitary tumor masses include vegetations, thrombi, primary cardiac tumors, and prominent muscle bands. The clinical presentation and associated cardiac abnormalities are useful for distinguishing intracavitary tumors from thrombi or vegetations. Primary cardiac tumors are not always easily distinguished from metastatic tumors.

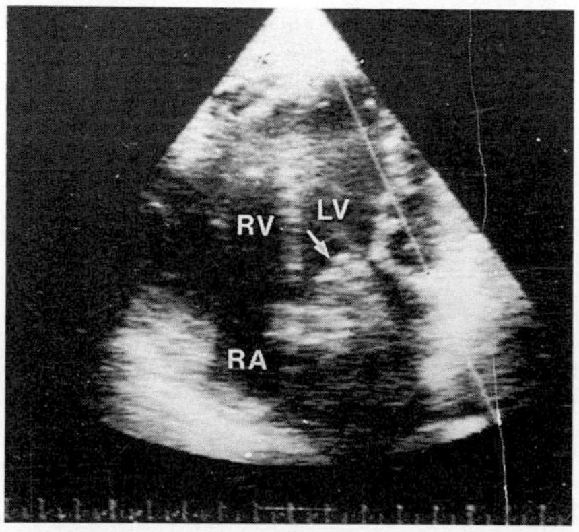

Fig. 36–48. Apical four-chamber view showing a large malignant mesenchymoma (arrow), which extends into the left atrium. LV = left ventricle; RV = right ventricle; RA = right atrium. (Courtesy of Dr. Zeng Shin Wang.)

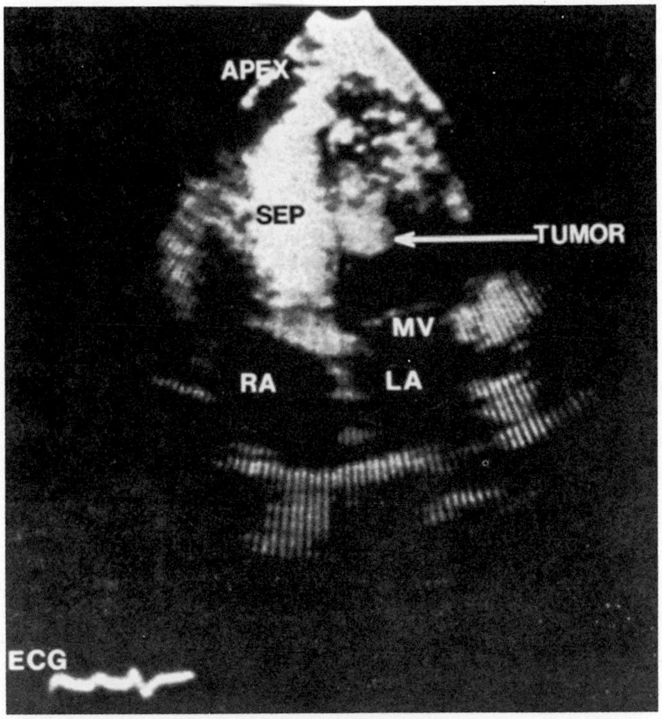

Fig. 36–49. Metastatic malignant melanoma within the left ventricular cavity. MV = mitral valve; SEP = interventricular septum; RA = right atrium; LA = left atrium. (From Ports TA, et al.: Echocardiography of left ventricular masses. Circulation 58:528, 1978.)

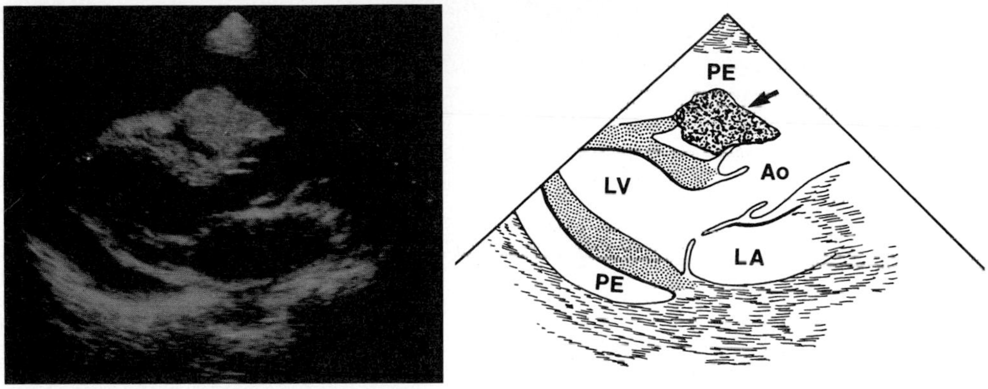

Fig. 36–50. Parasternal long axis recording showing a large solid mass of echoes (arrow) within and almost completely obstructing the right ventricular outflow tract. The echo-producing mass proved to be a metastatic carcinoma of the breast. There is also a large pericardial effusion (PE). LV = left ventricle; LA = left atrium; Ao = aorta.

EXTRACARDIAC TUMORS

Visualization of various types of extracardiac tumors (i.e., mediastinal and pleural) has been feasible with two-dimensional echocardiography.[147,200–206]

Anterior mediastinal masses including mediastinal cysts, hematoma, thymoma, teratoma, and other tumors may appear as displacement of the heart and/or compression of cardiac chambers, either causing or mimicking superior vena cava obstruction, cardiac tamponade, constrictive pericarditis, pulmonic stenosis, and tricuspid stenosis.[200,203,206–209] Mediastinal tumors may be nonhomogeneous, often because of hemorrhage and necrosis.[205] Some anterior mediastinal masses such as cysts,[206] as well as malignant tumors,[203,206,207] may appear as anterior echo-free spaces between the chest wall and right ventricle without a posterior echo-free space. The differential diagnosis includes blood or exudate, particularly in the immediate postoperative period,[208] or epicardial fat pads.[173,174]

Figure 36–51A is an example of right ventricular outflow tract compression by a superior mediastinal tumor. Biopsy revealed immunoblastic sarcoma. A repeat study (Fig. 36–51B), done after a course of chemotherapy, documented disappearance of the mediastinal tumor and the presence of a normal right ventricular outflow tract and pulmonary valve.

Posterior mediastinal masses may appear as posterior echo-free spaces and/or compression of the left atrium and left ventricle. Extension of a pancreatic pseudocyst into the posterior mediastinum may appear as a large echo-free space posterior to the left ventricle[210] (see Fig. 35–49). Several cases of extracardiac tumor compressing the left atrium have been described (see Fig. 18–9).[200] Figure 36–52 is an example of a large posterior mediastinal sarcoma that pushes against the posterior

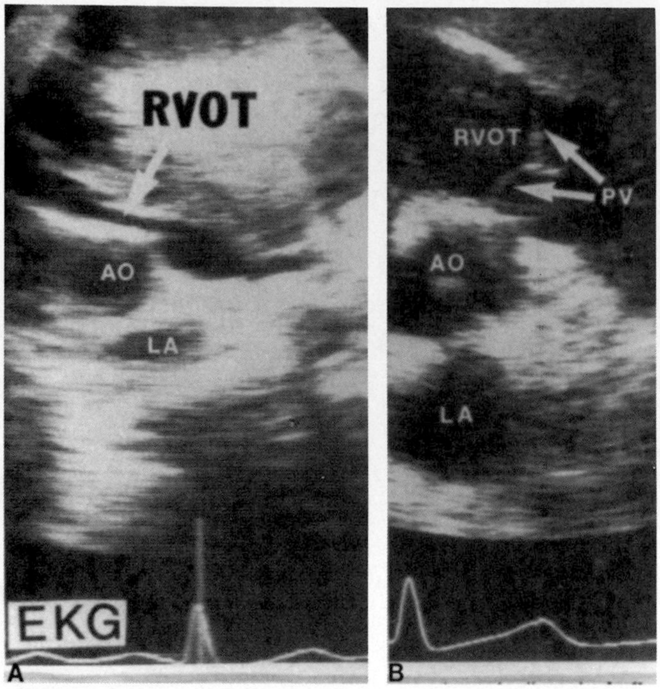

Fig. 36–51. **A.** Parasternal short axis recording of large anterior mediastinal tumor (immunoblastic sarcoma) compressing the right ventricular outflow tract (RVOT) from above. **B.** Similar recording from the same patient following chemotherapy. The tumor mass has decreased significantly, and the RVOT has returned to normal size. Ao = aorta; LA = left atrium; PV = pulmonary valve. (From Come PC, et al.: Reversible right ventricular outflow tract compression by immunoblastic sarcoma. Am J Cardiol 55:239, 1985.)

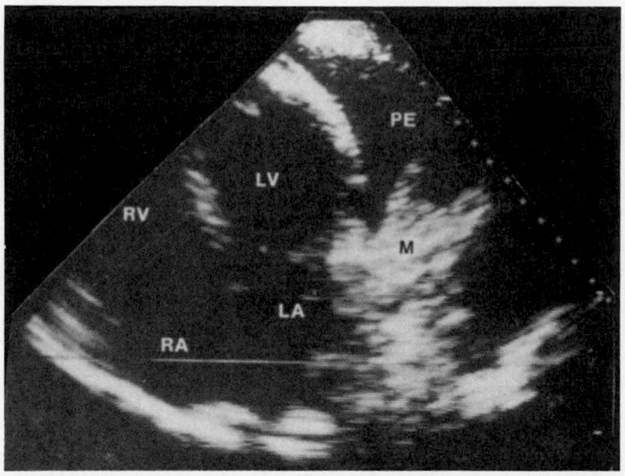

Fig. 36–53. Apical four-chamber recording from a patient with a large intrapleural mass (M) in the region of the atrioventricular groove and left atrium (LA) with finger-like projections into the pleural fluid (PE). The tumor proved to be an adenocarcinoma. The heart is shifted to the right. LV = left ventricle; RV = right ventricle; RA = right atrium. (From Cohen IS, et al.: Two-dimensional echocardiography in the detection of noneffusive cardiac involvement by intrathoracic neoplasms. Am Heart J 107:532, 1984.)

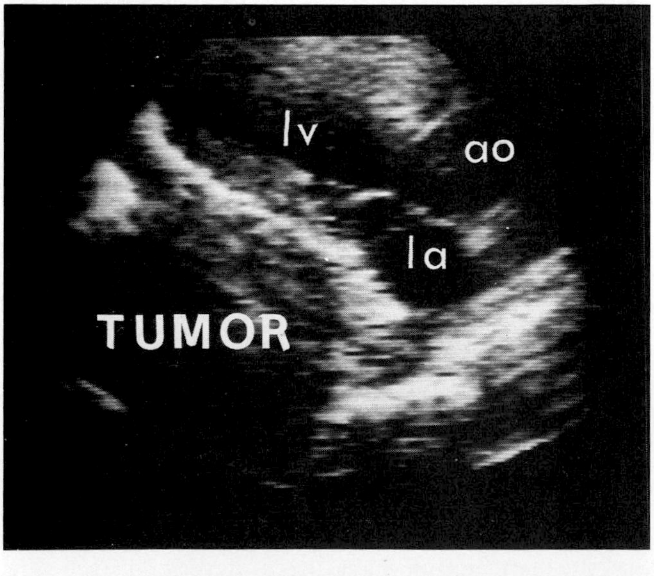

Fig. 36–52. Parasternal long axis recording of a posterior mediastinal sarcoma that compresses the left ventricle (lv) from behind, creating a posterior concavity in the ventricular wall. ao = aorta; la = left atrium; lv = left ventricle.

border of the left ventricle and produces a concavity in the left ventricular wall.

Pleural tumors may also compress the heart and invade the pericardium.[204,210,211] These masses are usually large and fixed to the parietal pleura and are frequently associated with pleural effusions. Figure 36–53 demonstrates displacement of the heart by an echo-free mass compressing the right ventricle in a patient with adenocarcinoma metastatic to the pleura. Structures in the pleural space, such as fibrin and collapsed left lung, may be confused with pleural tumors.[176]

INTRACARDIAC THROMBI

Intracardiac thrombi occur in the setting of underlying heart disease, including myocardial infarction, ventricular aneurysm, cardiomyopathy, valvular heart disease, prosthetic heart valves, and atrial arrhythmias. Before the development of two-dimensional echocardiography, these thrombi were recognized only after an embolic event or at the time of surgery or autopsy. Not only is two-dimensional echocardiography useful in the identification of intracardiac thrombi, but also it provides a noninvasive method of evaluating therapy through serial observations.[212–214]

Left Ventricular Thrombi

Left ventricular thrombi occur in conditions associated with stasis of blood flow and/or regional wall motion abnormalities including acute myocardial infarction,[212–215] left ventricular aneurysm,[216] and dilated cardiomyopathy.[217] Left ventricular mural thrombi are a common complication of acute infarction, noted in approximately 20 to 60% of cases in postmortem series.[218–220] The incidence of left ventricular thrombi is related to the size and location of the infarct, as well as the presence of akinesis, hypokinesis, or dyskinesis.[212–215,221] These thrombi are detected in approximately 30 to 40% of patients with acute anterior wall infarction and are especially common in patients with infarcts involving the cardiac apex. Left ventricular thrombi develop in fewer than 5% of patients with inferior infarctions.[212,214] They are generally visible echocardiographically 1 to 11 days after an infarct.[212,222]

Two-dimensional echocardiography has been used accurately to detect or to exclude the presence of left ventricular thrombi.[212,214,223,224] Several studies have documented 75 to 80% sensitivity and 90 to 95% specificity for two-dimensional echocardiographic detection of left ventricular thrombi, when compared to autopsy or surgical data.[225–227] Neither radionuclide ventriculography[227] nor angiography[216] is as sensitive in identifying left ventricular thrombi.

Echocardiographically, left ventricular thrombi appear as a mass of echoes superimposed on and interrupting the normal endocardial contour of the ventricle in regions of depressed wall motion. These thrombi are most commonly located in the apex.[212,214–216,224,227] Rarely, cases have been reported of left ventricular thrombi in patients with normal left ventricular contraction.[228]

Thrombi may be laminar and parallel to the endocardial surface (Fig. 36–54), spherical (Fig. 36–55), or pedunculated and freely mobile, or they may have a fixed base with mobile filaments extending from the base (Fig. 36–56). Thrombi characteristically have a speckled appearance, although some may be laminated and more homogeneous.[223] The echo density of thrombus is typically greater than that of adjacent myocardium, although the thrombus-blood interface is often variable in appearance.[223] When organized, thrombi may contain areas that are brighter than surrounding myocardium. When layered in appearance, the most echo-dense portion of the thrombus is along the intracavitary margin.[223] Protruding thrombi tend to be relatively more echo dense than mural thrombi, which may be more difficult to distinguish from myocardium.

Some studies have suggested that recent thrombi may be more shaggy and irregular in configuration, whereas organized thrombi may be more circumscribed and immobile.[215] Left ventricular thrombi usually move in concert with the underlying ventricular wall.

The clinical incidence of systemic embolization associated with myocardial infarction is 5 to 10%,[228–230] and it may be slightly higher in patients with left ventricular aneurysm[216,231] and idiopathic dilated cardiomyopathy.[217,232] Certain echocardiographic features are associated with a greater likelihood of embolization. Thrombi that protrude into the left ventricular cavity or those that are freely mobile are more likely to embolize, as well as thrombi with shaggy, irregular borders.[214,215,223–225,227,233] Two-dimensional echocardiography has helped investigators to define the natural history of left ventricular thrombi and the response to anticoagulation therapy.[212,215,219,223,233]

The differential diagnosis of left ventricular thrombus includes a variety of normal cardiac structures, benign and malignant cardiac tumors, and transducer-related

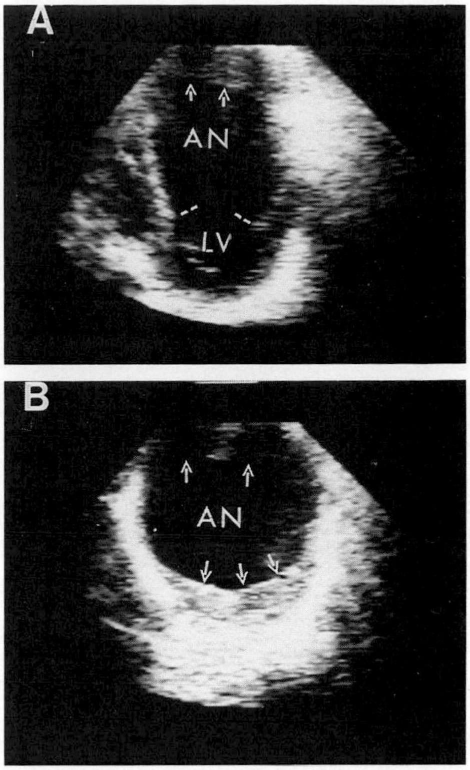

Fig. 36–54. **A.** Modified apical four-chamber recording from a patient with an anteroapical aneurysm (AN) containing a large laminar thrombus (vertical arrowheads). The origin of the aneurysm from the left ventricle (LV) is indicated by the interrupted lines. **B.** Short axis recording through the aneurysm. Anteriorly, the faint laminar thrombus is apparent, whereas posteriorly an equally large area of thrombus is more highly reflective, suggesting that it is better organized. (From Hsu TL, et al.: Two-dimensional echocardiographic features of floating left atrial thrombus. Am J Cardiol 57:701, 1986.)

artifacts. Normal cardiac structures that may be mistaken for thrombi include papillary muscles, prominent muscle trabeculations, chordal structures including false tendons, and technical artifacts.[223,226] A high index of clinical suspicion is crucial to the diagnosis. Because the majority of left ventricular thrombi are located at the

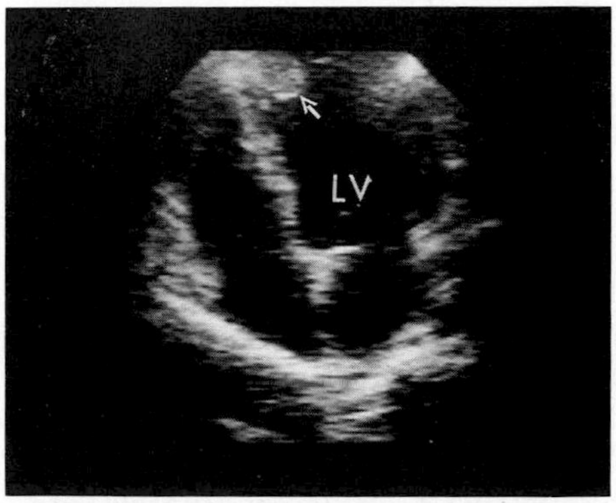

Fig. 36–55. Apical four-chamber recording illustrating a circumscribed spherical thrombus within the apex of the left ventricle (LV). The thrombus is clearly demarcated and has a speckled internal pattern.

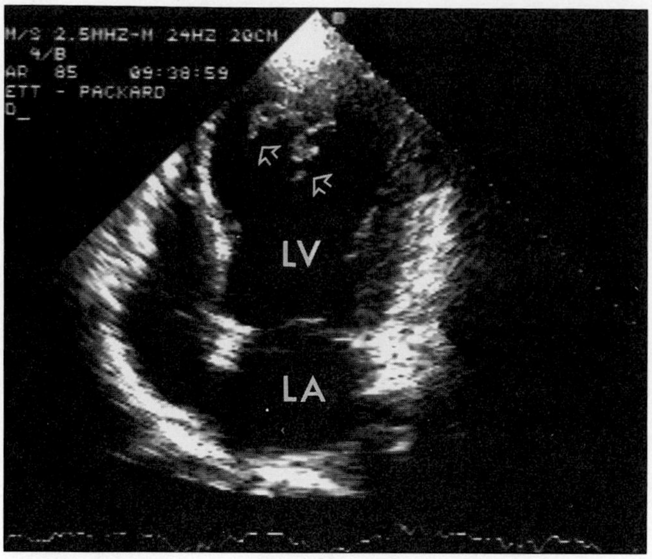

Fig. 36–56. Apical four-chamber view illustrating a large thrombus within an apical aneurysm. The thrombus has multiple mobile, serpentine fronds hanging from the large base into the left ventricular cavity. LV = left ventricle; LA = left atrium.

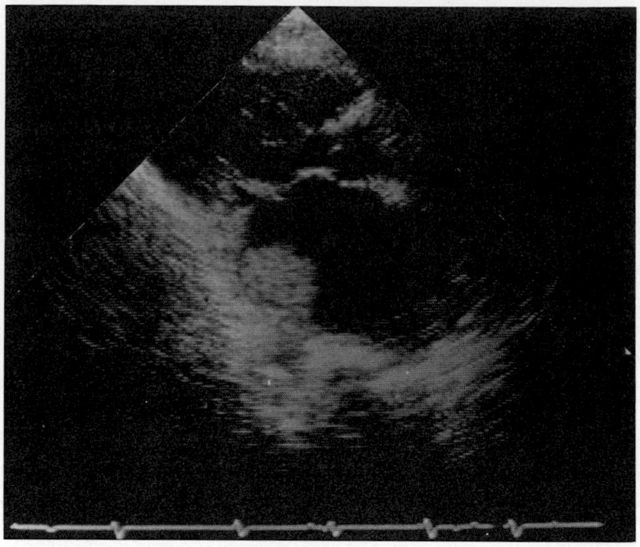

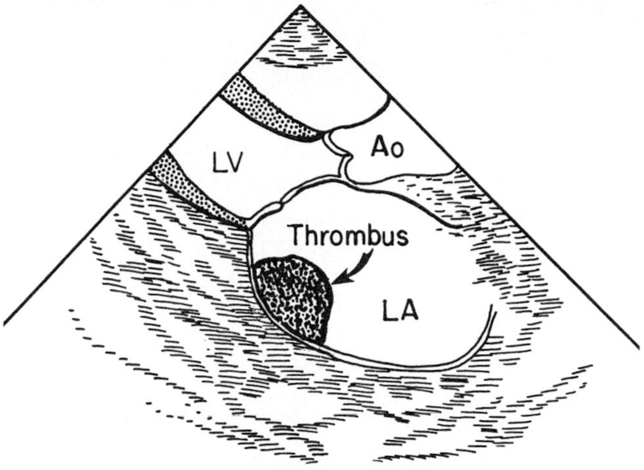

Fig. 36–57. Parasternal long axis recording from a patient with mitral stenosis and a large round thrombus attached to the left atrial posterior wall. The thrombus was strongly echogenic, immobile, and fixed by a broad base. LV = left ventricle; LA = left atrium; Ao = aorta.

cardiac apex, multiple views are required for their detection, including apical four- and two-chamber views, apical long axis views, parasternal short axis view at the apical level, and subcostal views. When thrombus is suspected, confirmation requires its visualization in at least two projections.[216,223] Several useful echocardiographic features can be reliably used to diagnose left ventricular thrombi: the presence of associated wall motion abnormalities, its apical location, differing acoustic properties of the thrombus and endocardial surface, and confirmation of thrombus in at least two views.[223] All true intracavitary masses have a constant, reproducible position within the left ventricular cavity and, unlike artifact, can generally be imaged in multiple planes.

Left Atrial Thrombi

Left atrial thrombi are associated with stasis of blood in the left atrium.[234–236] Predisposing factors in the formation of left atrial thrombi include atrial fibrillation, mitral valve disease, especially rheumatic mitral stenosis, left atrial enlargement, specifically of the atrial appendage, prosthetic mitral valves, and low cardiac output states. Because of their attendant embolic complications, left atrial thrombi are a clinically significant problem. Decisions concerning therapeutic anticoagulation, or possibly the approach to the left atrium for mitral valve replacement or mitral valvuloplasty, may be determined by the echocardiographic detection of left atrial clot.

Several studies have evaluated the efficacy of two-dimensional echocardiography in the detection of left atrial thrombus.[2,237–240] When thrombi are detected echocardiographically, they appear as well-demarcated round or oval masses of echoes usually within the left atrial cavity with broad-based attachment to the posterior and lateral walls (Figs. 36–57 and 36–58). The following characteristics are most useful in identifying left atrial thrombi: an acoustic density that differs from that of the left atrial blood pool and often from adjacent cardiac structures; a relatively well-circumscribed, defined border; synchronous motion with the underlying heart wall throughout the cardiac cycle; demonstration of the mass in two or more echocardiographic views; and a broad-based attachment to the left atrial wall in at least one echocardiographic plane.[239] Rarely, a left atrial thrombus may be free floating and larger than the mitral valve orifice, causing intermittent obstruction and sometimes sudden cardiac death (Fig. 36–59).[217,241–246] Doppler echocardiography may be used to characterize the mitral flow pattern.[245]

Differential diagnosis of left atrial thrombus includes myxoma, other tumors, and artifacts.[2,48] Often, the clinical setting aids in the diagnosis. Reverberations from a mitral prosthesis may simulate thrombus.[237]

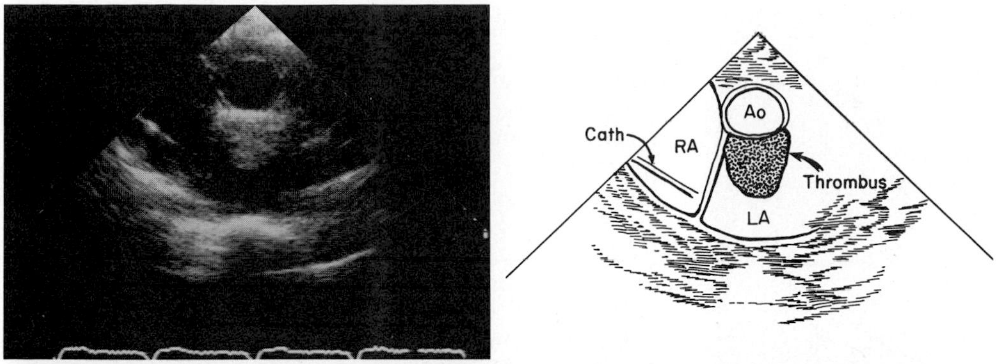

Fig. 36–58. Parasternal short axis recording from a patient with an unusual thrombus arising from the anterior wall of the left atrium (LA) beneath the aortic root. A catheter (Cath) is present in the right atrium (RA). Ao = aorta.

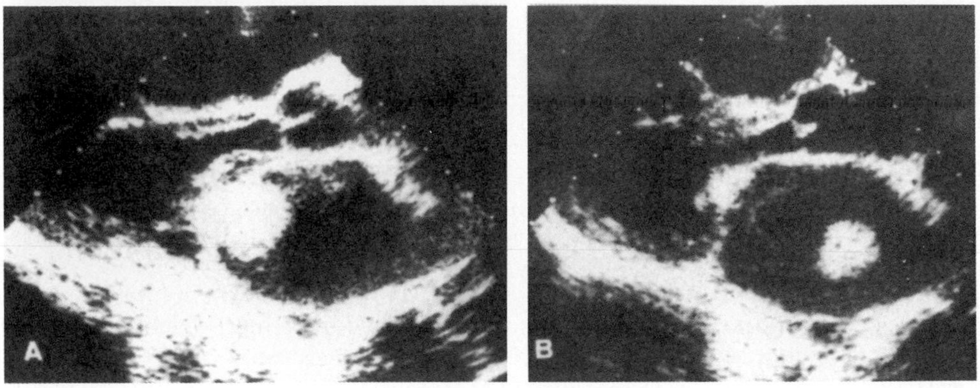

Fig. 36–59. Parasternal long axis recording from a patient with mitral stenosis and a freely mobile ball thrombus in the left atrium. **A.** The thrombus is within the mitral orifice during diastole and appears to occlude the valve. **B.** Also recorded during diastole, the thrombus is in the superior portion of the atrium. (From Hsu TL: Two-dimensional echocardiographic features of floating left atrial thrombus. Am J Cardiol 57:701, 1986.)

The sensitivity of transthoracic two-dimensional echocardiography in the detection of left atrial thrombi approaches 30 to 50% in surgical or autopsy series.[238,239,247] Several factors are responsible for the relative insensitivity of the technique. From 30 to 50% of left atrial thrombi are located in the atrial appendage,[238,239] and imaging of the left atrial appendage is often inadequate. In the largest series, 293 patients with rheumatic heart disease were examined before mitral valve replacement, and 54 were identified as having left atrial thrombi at surgery.[239] Thirty-three (61%) of the left atrial thrombi were identified by two-dimensional echocardiographic study, and 30 of 33 had thrombi confirmed at surgery. Twenty-one patients had left atrial thrombi that were not detected by echocardiography, 11 (52%) of which were located in the left atrial appendage. A modified parasternal short axis view may permit recognition of some appendage thrombi (Fig. 36–60).[240]

Occasionally, two-dimensional echocardiography may fail to show even large thrombi within the body of the left atrium if the acoustic properties of the thrombus do not differ sufficiently from those of surrounding blood or endocardium.[2,48] It may also be difficult to distinguish thin laminar thrombi from atrial wall,[2,239] particularly when there is a general increase in intra-atrial echoes because of blood stasis or redundant echoes along the posterior atrial wall because of beam width artifacts.[48] With the advent of transesophageal echocardiography, it has become possible to examine the entire left atrium including the appendage, and the result has been a marked increase in sensitivity and specificity (Fig. 36–61).

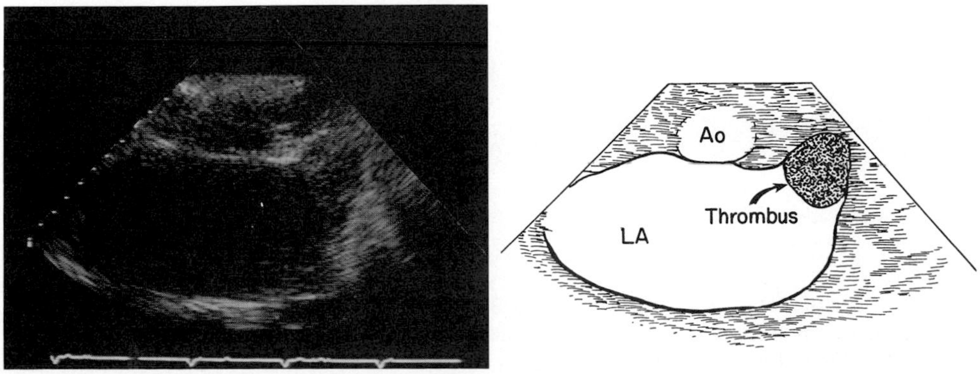

Fig. 36–60. Parasternal short axis recording of the left atrium (LA) illustrating a faint mass of echoes in the atrial appendage characteristic of an appendage thrombus. Ao = aorta.

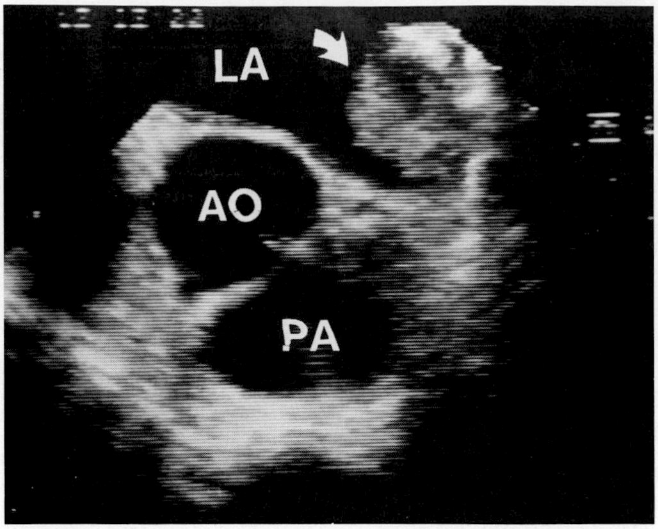

Fig. 36–61. Atrial appendage thrombus recorded by transesophageal echocardiography. LA = left atrium; AO = aorta; PA = pulmonary artery.

Right Atrial Thrombi

Before the development of two-dimensional echocardiography, the antemortem diagnosis of right atrial thrombus was rare.[248] The ability of two-dimensional echocardiography to show most of the right atrium, interatrial septum, superior and inferior venae cavae, and the tricuspid valve from multiple tomographic planes makes it a highly useful technique for detecting the presence of right atrial thrombus and assessing its hemodynamic effects.[63]

Right atrial thrombi tend to occur in two different settings. Most originate from venous thromboemboli that become trapped in the right heart.[249–259] Many of these patients develop pulmonary embolus, often with massive obstruction of the pulmonary artery resulting in acute pulmonary hypertension, cor pulmonale, and right heart failure.[249,254,255] The exact prevalence of echocardiographically identified right atrial thrombi in patients with suspected or impending pulmonary embolus is not well defined, particularly because the majority of the thromboemboli originating in systemic veins pass rapidly through the right atrium and may be missed.[249,254]

In situ thrombus formation in the right atrium is found in conditions associated with blood stasis and/or endocardial damage, as may occur in patients with right atrial dilation,[260,261] atrial arrhythmias, and/or cardiomyopathies.[249,260,262,263] In situ thrombi may form on foreign bodies in the right atrium including central venous catheters for parenteral nutrition,[64,253,264,265] ventriculoatrial shunts for hydrocephalus,[266] transvenous pacing electrodes,[267–269] and Swan-Ganz catheters,[270] or they may develop after right heart manipulation.[271–273]

The echocardiographic appearance of right atrial thrombi varies, depending on the underlying pathophysiology. Thromboemboli originating from peripheral veins appear echocardiographically as mobile, irregular, serpentine masses floating freely in the right atrium and often prolapsing across the tricuspid valve (Fig. 36–62). These thrombi do not have an obvious point of attachment to the right atrial wall. Highly mobile thrombi can become trapped in the tricuspid valve, chordae tendineae, or papillary muscles and can cause tricuspid regurgitation.[249,254,255] Fixation of the thrombus in the foramen ovale may be visualized by two-dimensional echocardiography as a pedunculated or bilobed mass asymmetrically attached to the mid portion of the in-

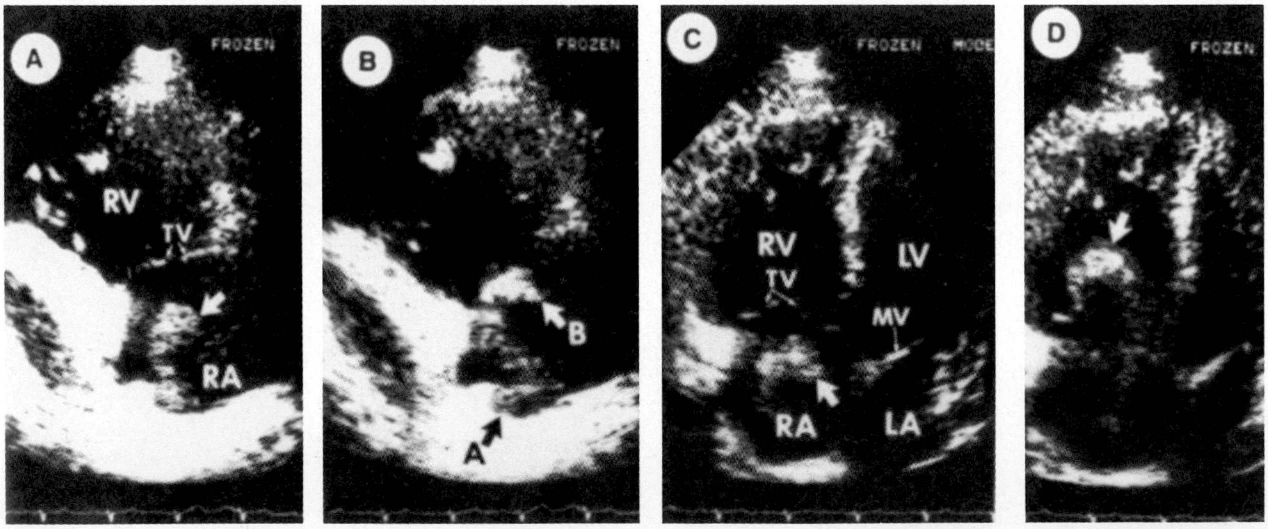

Fig. 36–62. Parasternal right ventricular inflow **(A, B)** and apical four-chamber views showing a mobile serpentine thromboembolism in the right atrium (RA). **A.** The thromboembolus is coiled in the RA. **B.** The mobile thromboembolus has uncoiled, and its proximal end is located at the level of the lateral right atrial wall (arrow A), whereas its distal end is at the level of the tricuspid valve (TV) (arrow B). **C.** The thromboembolism (large arrow) is completely contained within the RA. **D.** The thromboembolus (arrow) has prolapsed across the valve with the distal end curled in the right ventricle (RV). TV = tricuspid valve; LV = left ventricle; MV = mitral valve; LA = left atrium. (From Felner JM, et al.: Right atrial thromboemboli: clinical, echocardiographic and pathologic manifestations. J Am Coll Cardiol 4:1041, 1984. Reprinted with permission from the American College of Cardiology.)

teratrial septum. Displacement of part or all of the thrombus may be a cause of paradoxic embolism.[254,255]

Right atrial thrombi that develop in situ are typically nonhomogeneous, immobile, laminated masses adherent to the right atrial wall with distinct intracavitary margins (Fig. 36–63). Although in situ thrombi generally have a broad base of attachment to the atrial wall, they may also appear as fingerlike projections with a narrow stalk (Fig. 36–64). A less typical appearance is of a curvilinear band of echoes spanning the right atrium with a distinct echo-free area representing the interface between blood and thrombus.

Thrombi that form in situ around a foreign body (Fig. 36–65) typically have a gross motion pattern similar to that of the catheter or electrode to which they are attached. If the thrombus becomes large, it may develop secondary mobile portions at its free edges. Figure 36–66 is an example of a complex, infected thrombus with cystic and solid areas that arose from the tip of a venous catheter in the superior vena cava and extended into the right atrium.

Right atrial thrombi must be distinguished from other causes of right atrial masses including myxoma, sarcoma, and other primary and secondary tumors. Visualization of the site of attachment is often a useful differentiating feature. Right atrial myxomas are usually large, ovoid masses attached to the interatrial septum in a right atrium of normal size. Extension of secondary tumors from the inferior vena cava can usually be visualized using subcostal views. Tricuspid vegetations may simulate a right atrial mass, but vegetations are typically attached to the valve and move in concert with the valve in leaflets.[63] Right heart catheters and pacing wires are generally easily distinguished echocardiographically from right atrial thrombi.

Normal right atrial structures including the eustachian

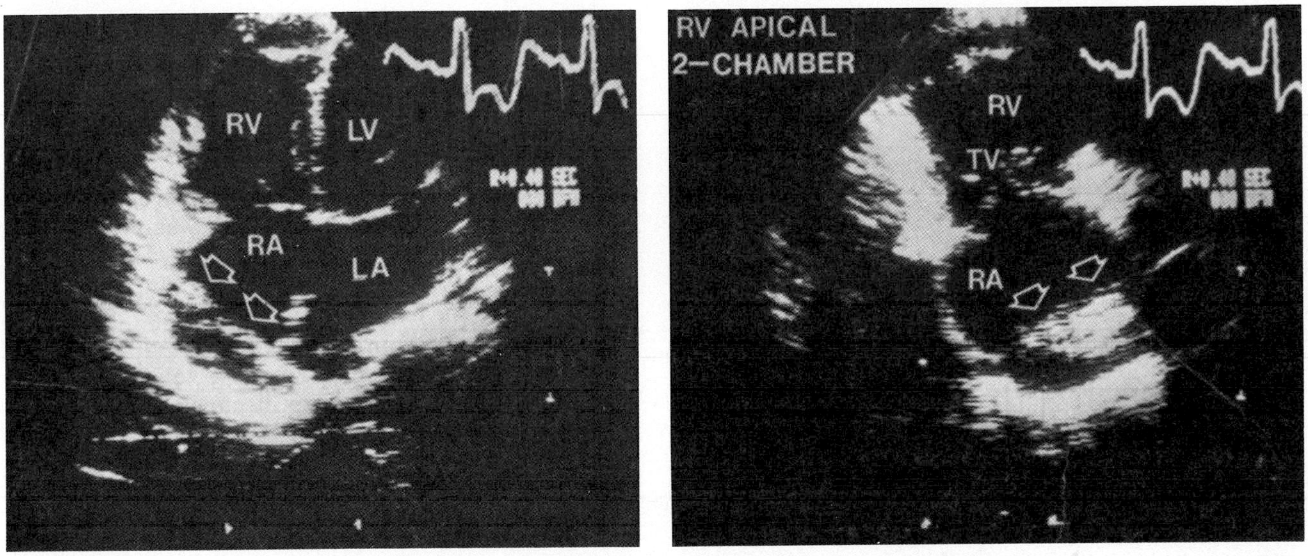

Fig. 36–63. Left. Apical four-chamber recording demonstrating thrombus (arrows) in the posterolateral right atrium (RA). Right. Right ventricular apical two-chamber view again demonstrating thrombus (arrows) in the RA. LA = left atrium; LV = left ventricle; RV = right ventricle; TV = tricuspid valve. (From Manno BV, et al.: Two-dimensional echocardiographic detection of right atrial thrombi. Am J Cardiol 51:615, 1983.)

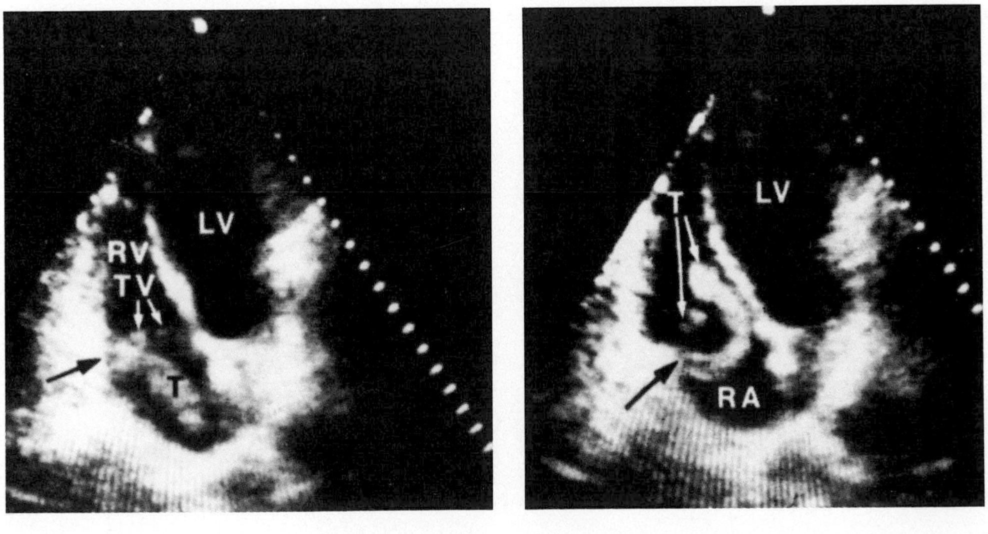

Fig. 36–64. Apical four-chamber recordings in systole (left) and diastole (right), demonstrate a large thrombus (T) attached to the lower lateral wall of the right atrium (RA). LV = left ventricle; RV = right ventricle; TV = tricuspid valve. (From Come, PC: Transient right atrial thrombus during acute myocardial infarction: diagnosis by echocardiography. Am J Cardiol 51:1228, 1983.)

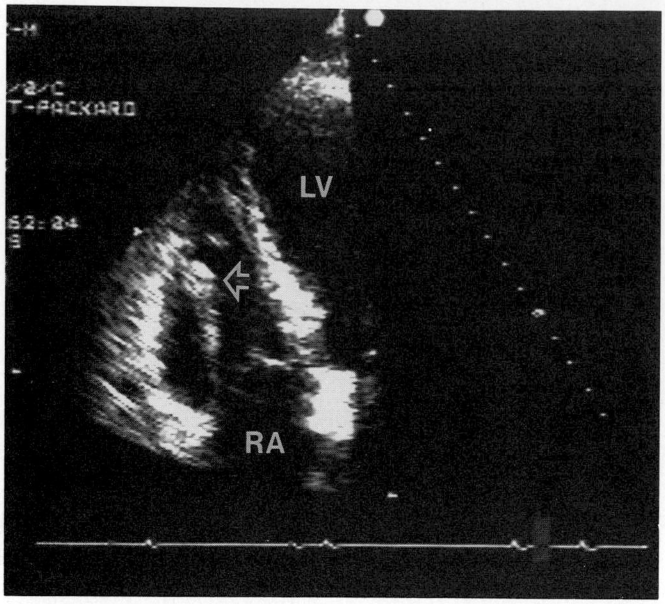

Fig. 36–65. Apical four-chamber recording illustrating a thrombus around catheter (open arrow) in the right ventricle. LV = left ventricle; RA = right atrium.

valve, Chiari network, and the tricuspid valve and its supporting structures may be mistaken for right atrial thrombi; however, their location and mobility are useful distinguishing features. In difficult cases, transesophageal echocardiography may clarify the diagnosis.

Right Ventricular Thrombi

Right ventricular thrombi are rarely diagnosed clinically. Two-dimensional echocardiography has been particularly helpful in their antemortem detection.[274–276] Right ventricular thrombi may be found in low output states including cor pulmonale,[274,277] right ventricular infarction,[275] or cardiomyopathy.[278] Right ventricular thrombi have been reported in patients with endomyocardial fibroelastosis,[279] Loeffler's endocarditis,[280] blunt chest trauma,[281] and ventriculoatrial shunts for hydrocephalus.[266] Patients with right ventricular thrombi may clinically have outflow obstruction or pulmonary emboli.[282] Right ventricular thrombi have also been reported to appear as calcified masses within the right ventricle.[174] Large right ventricular thrombi may obliterate the right ventricular cavity.[277] Right ventricular thrombi must be differentiated echocardiographically from tumors and vegetations, which are far more common. Although not always easily distinguished, the clinical setting often suggests the correct diagnosis.

VEGETATIONS

Echocardiography plays an important role in the assessment of patients with infective endocarditis. Historically, M-mode echocardiography identified valvular vegetations with a sensitivity approaching 50%.[63,283–287] With the advent of two-dimensional echocardiography, however, the reported sensitivity has increased to more than 80%. In addition, the information it provides about the size and shape, the site of attachment, and the hemodynamic sequelae of vegetations makes two-dimensional echocardiography the preferred technique.[284–288] The sensitivity of two-dimensional echocardiography is limited primarily by the size of vegetations, most of which are 1 to 3 mm in diameter, which is at or below the resolving capability of the technique.[286–289] Sensitivity is further limited in the presence of pre-existing val-

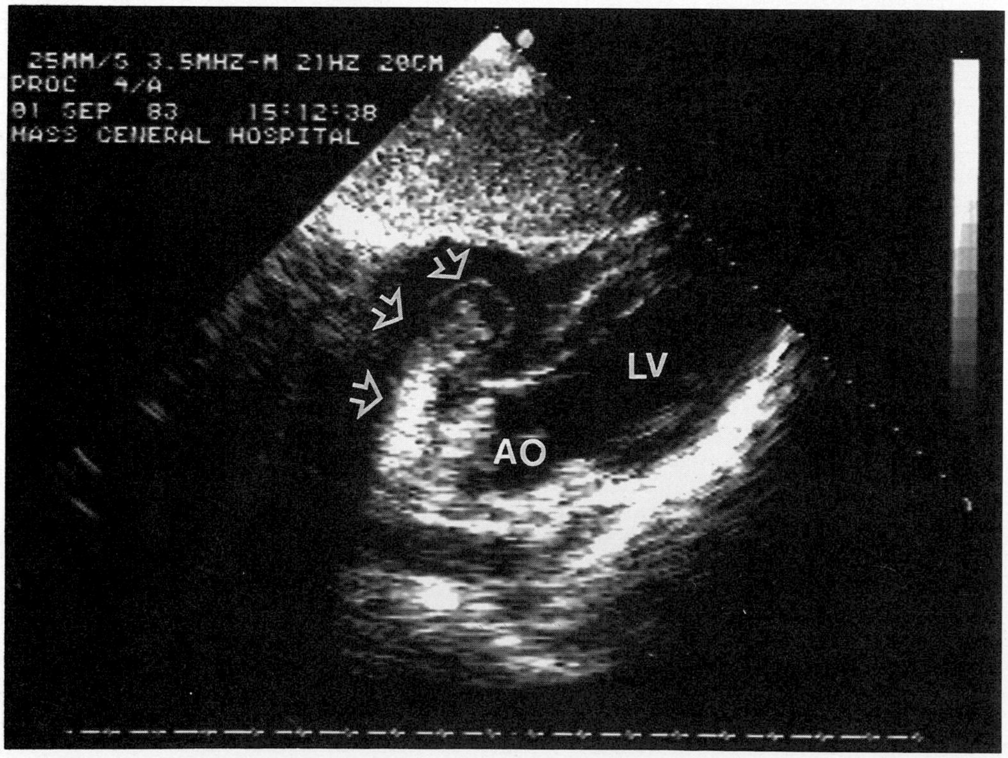

Fig. 36–66. Modified subcostal four-chamber view showing a hyperalimentation catheter in the right atrium. The catheter is covered with thrombus (arrows) and is secondarily infected. The infected thrombus at the tip of the catheter has formed a large complex cystic mass. LV = left ventricle; AO = aorta.

vular abnormalities or prosthetic valves. Transesophageal echocardiography is particularly useful in these settings.

In spite of these limitations, the echocardiographic detection of a vegetation defines a subset of patients at higher risk of complications including congestive heart failure, emboli, and death.[284,285,290] In addition, serial echocardiographic examinations may be used to follow the clinical course of patients with infective endocarditis. The technique enables one to identify flail leaflets, ring abscesses, sinus of Valsalva aneurysms, and paravalvular sinus tract formation that may complicate the course of infective endocarditis. The role of echocardiography in infective endocarditis is discussed in more detail in Chapter 37.

Valvular vegetations may simulate intracardiac tumors and thrombi. Their attachment to the valve leaflets and their movement in concert with valve opening and closure helps one to differentiate them from tumors and thrombi. In the case of valvular tumors (see Fig. 36–19), echocardiographic differentiation may be difficult, and the diagnosis is aided by the clinical setting.

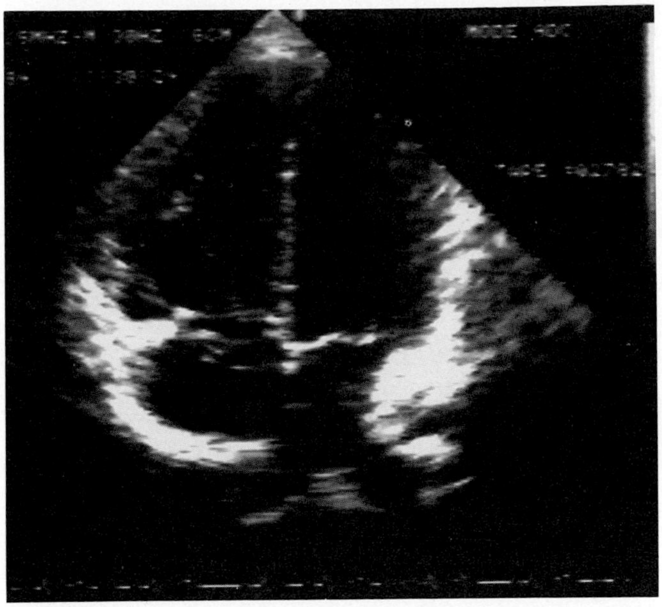

Fig. 36–67. Apical four-chamber view illustrating a mass of echoes behind the tricuspid valve consistent with the complex appearance of a Chiari network.

NORMAL VARIANTS SIMULATING INTRACARDIAC MASSES

Several congenital structures and normal variants may simulate pathologic intracardiac masses. These include the Chiari network, eustachian and thebesian valves, atrial septal aneurysms, moderator bands, false tendons and aberrant muscle bands, and calcification or prominence of the tricuspid and mitral annulus.

Chiari Network

The Chiari network, which is a remnant of the embryonic sinus venosus, is an anatomic variant found in 2 to 3% of normal hearts at autopsy.[291] This normal variant is a thin, weblike membrane with multiple fenestrations that usually extends from the inlet of the inferior vena cava to the interatrial septum. Echocardiographically, the Chiari network appears as a mobile, highly reflective structure in the right atrium, arising from the orifice of the inferior vena cava and extending to the interatrial septum or tricuspid valve with a characteristic flapping, chaotic motion (Fig. 36–67). The Chiari network is seldom clinically important, although it may rarely be a site of thrombus formation either de novo or after right heart catheterization with secondary pulmonary embolism.[291] Recognition of the Chiari network is important because this mobile structure is often confused with tricuspid valve vegetations, flail tricuspid leaflets, pedunculated tumors, and thrombi.[67,291] Unlike vegetations, however, the Chiari network is not attached to the tricuspid valve and has a random motion that is not synchronous with that of the tricuspid valve.

Eustachian Valve

Eustachian and thebesian valves are remnants of the embryonic right sinus venosus valve. A persistent eustachian valve is not uncommon in adults and is identified echocardiographically in nearly all children under 1 month of age and in approximately two thirds of older children.[67,292–294] The eustachian valve, also known as the valve of the inferior vena cava, is a ridge of tissue that extends from the orifice of the inferior vena cava across the posterior wall of the right atrium and attaches to the interatrial septum just beneath the fossa ovalis. In the fetus, the valve tends to be more prominent and directs blood returning from the inferior vena cava across the fossa ovalis. Figure 36–68 demonstrates the typical appearance of the eustachian valve as a horizontal linear echo rising along the inferior border of the right atrium just below the lower margin of the tricuspid annulus in the parasternal long axis right ventricular inflow view. Rarely, the eustachian valve may be large enough to cause nearly complete septation of the right atrium.[295] When large and mobile, a persistent eustachian valve in adults may simulate a Chiari network, vegetations, thrombi, or tumor.[292,294] The use of multiple imaging planes, however, including the parasternal long axis view of the right ventricular inflow tract, is valuable in differentiating the eustachian valve from truly pathologic masses in the right atrium.

Atrial Septal Aneurysm

Atrial septal aneurysm is an incidental finding at autopsy in approximately 1% of adults.[296] Although this lesion is frequently associated with longstanding elevation of atrial pressures, whether atrial septal aneurysms are congenital or acquired is uncertain.[69,296,297] Atrial septal aneurysms have been associated with systolic clicks, atrial arrhythmias, systemic and pulmonary emboli, atrioventricular valve prolapse, and atrial septal defects.[69,297] Echocardiographically, atrial septal aneurysms appear as a prominent linear bulge arising from the interatrial septum and protruding at least 1.5 cm beyond the plane of the atrial septum, generally exhibiting

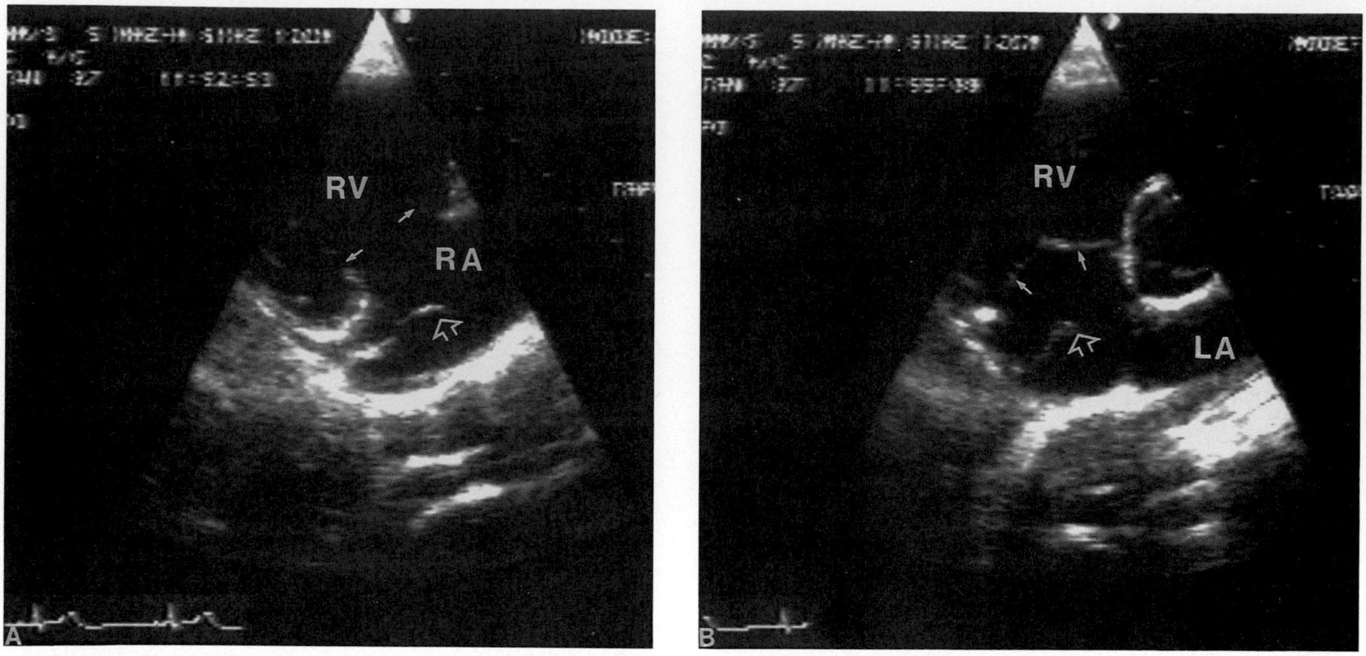

Fig. 36–68. A. Parasternal long axis right ventricular (RV) inflow view illustrating a prominent eustachian valve (open arrow) arising from the anterior margin of the orifice of the inferior vena cava behind the tricuspid valve leaflets (small closed arrows). **B.** Parasternal short axis recording of the same structure. LA = left atrium; RA = right atrium.

phasic excursion with respiration (see also Chapter 29).[69,297,298] Atrial septal aneurysms may involve only the region of the fossa ovalis, or the entire atrial septum may be involved.[69] In long axis views, atrial septal aneurysms may give the appearance of either right or left atrial masses, depending on the direction in which the aneurysm bulges (Fig. 36–69); however, the diagnosis of atrial septal aneurysm is usually obvious in short axis or apical views.

Moderator Band

The moderator band is a prominent muscular trabeculation or ridge found only in the right ventricle. Anatomi-

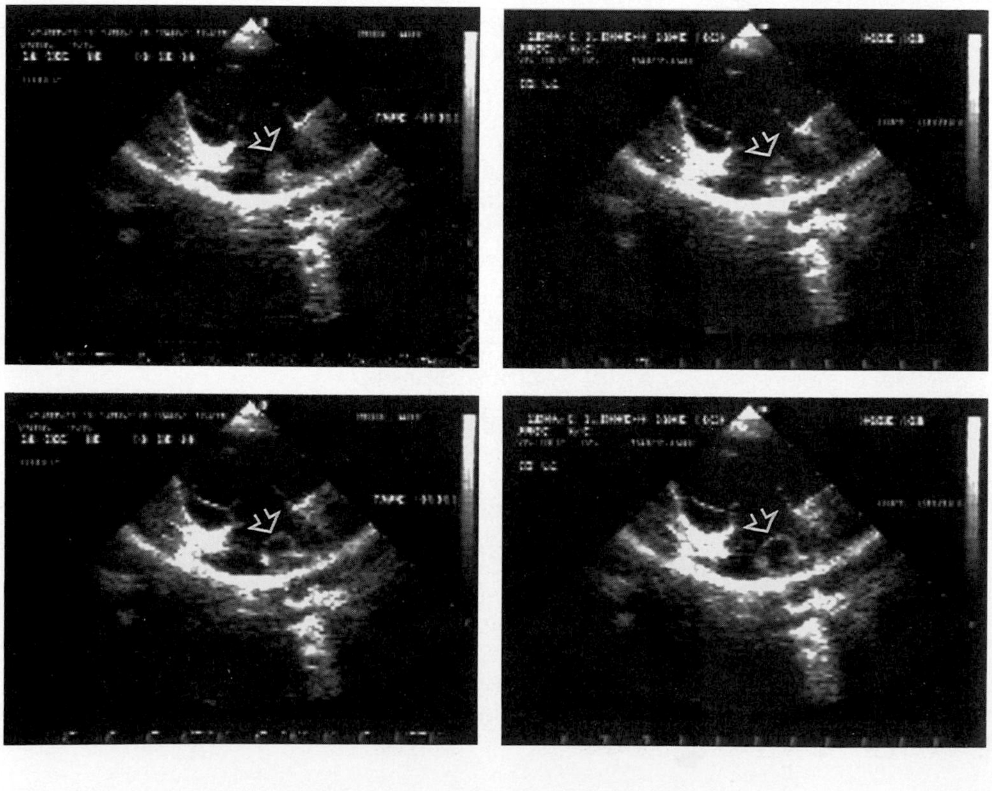

Fig. 36–69. Parasternal long axis recordings of the right atrium, tricuspid valve, and right ventricle illustrating the changing appearance of a transversely sectioned atrial septal aneurysm (open arrows) and its similarity to an intra-atrial mass in this tomographic plane.

cally, the moderator band is present in the majority of normal individuals and contains fibers of the right bundle branch, but it is often mistaken for a pathologic structure. Echocardiographically, the moderator band is best imaged in the apical four-chamber plane in which it appears as a thick, echo-dense band extending from the lower interventricular septum across the right ventricular cavity to the base of the anterior papillary muscle (Fig. 36–70). In addition to the moderator band, other muscular bands and prominent trabeculations may often be recorded in the distal third of the right ventricle.[299]

False Tendons

Left ventricular false tendons or aberrant bands are fibrous structures that traverse the left ventricular cavity in adults and children with and without coexisting heart disease.[299–303] Unlike true chordae tendineae, which originate from papillary muscles and insert onto valve leaflets, false tendons pass between papillary muscles, from papillary muscle to the ventricular septum, from free wall to free wall, or from free wall to interventricular septum.[302] They may be single or multiple. Echocardiographically, false tendons appear as linear, echo-dense structures that course through the left ventricular cavity in either an anteroposterior, a medial lateral, or a superior-inferior direction (Fig. 36–71). The echogenicity of these structures may vary considerably. Left ventricular false tendons are generally considered anatomic variants of no significance, although they may be associated with innocent murmurs in children.[300,302,304] Their major importance lies in their proper identification and differentiation from pedunculated tumors, thrombi, discrete subaortic membranes, flail aortic leaflets, vegetations, asymmetric septal hypertrophy, or other abnormalities of the mitral valve or septum.[302,303] Certain echocardiographic features aid in their differentiation, including the presence of an echo-free space on each side of the structure, constant motion of the structure during the cardiac cycle, and normal wall motion adjacent to the mass.[299]

Left ventricular false tendons must also be distinguished from prominent and/or abnormally arising papillary muscles. Figure 36–71 is an example of a large mobile structure oriented longitudinally in the left ventricular cavity that was initially thought to be a ventricular tumor. Off-axis imaging demonstrated normal attachment of a large anterolateral papillary muscle to the mitral valve by shortened chordal structures.

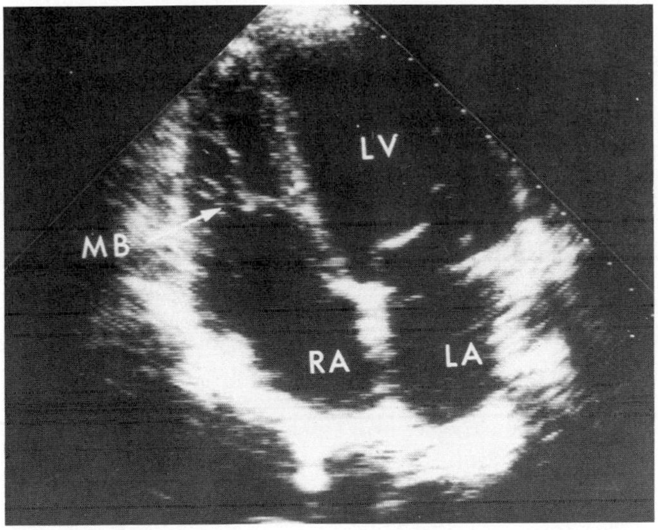

Fig. 36–70. Apical four-chamber recording illustrating a prominent moderator band (MB) in the right ventricle. LV = left ventricle; LA = left atrium; RA = right atrium.

Annular Calcification

Abnormal calcification in the region of the mitral or tricuspid annulus may simulate an intracardiac mass. On echocardiographic examination, mitral annular calcification appears as a circumscribed, echo-dense mass of variable size within the ventricular myocardium at the base of the posterior mitral valve leaflet. Annular calcium is immobile, and this immobility, together with the characteristic location, is useful in the differentiation of this lesion from pathologic masses.[305,306] Even in the absence of calcification, the right and left atrioventricular junctional regions may be prominent and may give the appearance of a soft tissue mass, particularly when sectioned obliquely (Fig. 36–72).

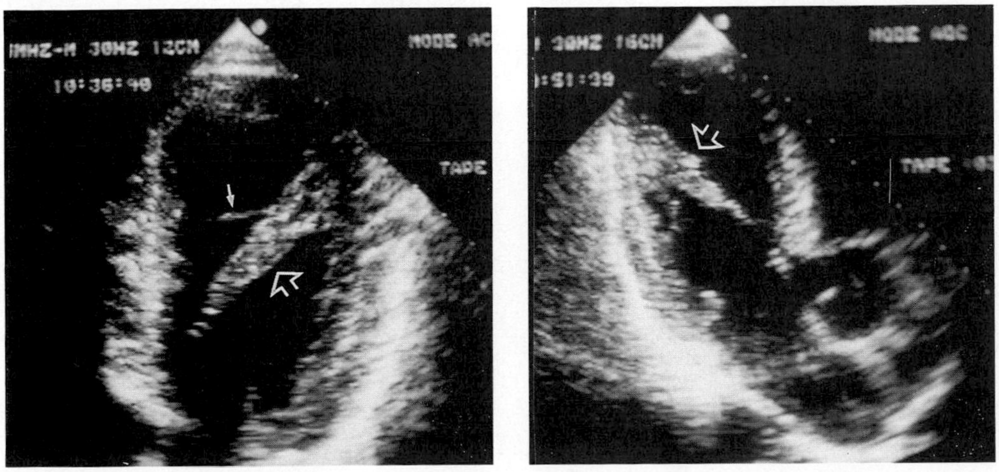

Fig. 36–71. Apical four-chamber (left) and long axis (right) recordings illustrating both an enlarged papillary muscle (open arrows) and false tendon (closed arrows). False tendons may vary in size from the small strand illustrated here to muscular bridges approximating the size of the papillary muscle in this example.

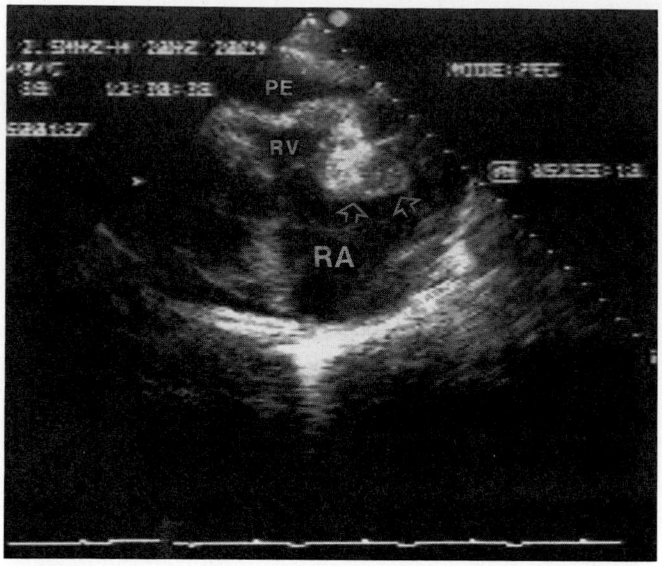

Fig. 36–72. Parasternal long axis right ventricular inflow view showing a prominent tricuspid annulus, which at this angle of section, simulated a right atrial mass (arrows). RV = right ventricle; RA = right atrium; PE = pericardial effusion.

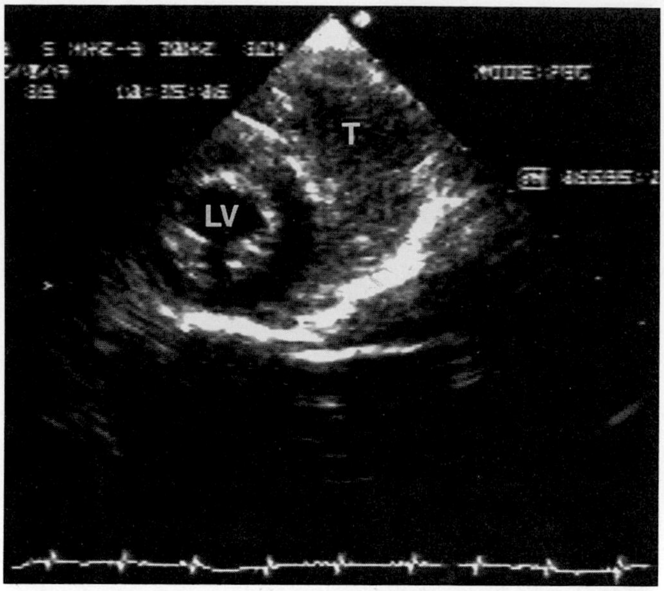

Fig. 36–73. Parasternal short axis recording at the midventricular level showing a large soft tissue mass lateral to the left ventricle in an infant. This mass (T) is produced by an enlarged thymus, which is often seen as a normal variant in this age group. LV = left ventricle.

Thymus

In the infant, the thymus is frequently large and may extend anterior and lateral to the heart. Thymus has the texture of soft tissue and can be misinterpreted as a pathologic extracardiac tumor. Figure 36–73 illustrates an enlarged thymus laying lateral to the left ventricle in a normal infant. The enlarged thymus can normally be recognized by its location in the anterior mediastinum, by its extension toward the neck, and by the age group in which it is found.

MAN-MADE OBJECTS IN THE HEART

Man-made objects in the heart may simulate intracardiac masses. Transvenous catheters including Swan-Ganz catheter and pacing catheters are the most common objects that may be visualized echocardiographically.[66,74,307,308] These catheters appear as elongated, thin, linear echoes that course through the right ventricular inflow tract and may be detected in the right ventricle, right atrium, or right ventricular outflow tract (Fig. 36–74). The catheter echoes may be single or associated with multiple linear reverberations that can be visualized posterior to the catheter. Occasionally, reverberations from a catheter may be detected within the left side of the heart even when the right heart catheter is not well seen. Recognition of this potential artifact, as well as knowledge of the clinical setting in which the study was recorded, reduces error in diagnosis. The subcostal transducer position is useful for evaluating the course of the catheter and can be used to detect dislodgment, perforation, thrombi, and vegetations.[309–312] Figure 36–75 is an example of a right ventricular pacing wire that has perforated the interventricular septum.

Two-dimensional echocardiography has also been used to locate bullets, nails, and needles in various cardiac structures.[313–316] More recently, two-dimensional echocardiography has been used to monitor biotome positioning during myocardial biopsy (Fig. 36–76),[317,318] to guide the positioning of the needle during pericardiocentesis, and to aid in pacemaker wire placement.

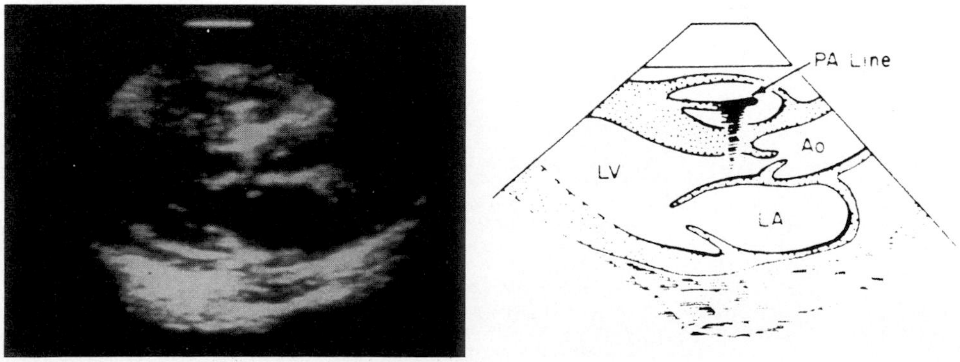

Fig. 36–74. Parasternal long axis recording of a pulmonary artery catheter as it passes through the right ventricular outflow tract. The catheter (PA line) produces multiple reverberations that extend through the septum into the left ventricular outflow tract, cross the mitral valve, and terminate in the anterior left atrium. LA = left atrium; LV = left ventricle; Ao = aorta.

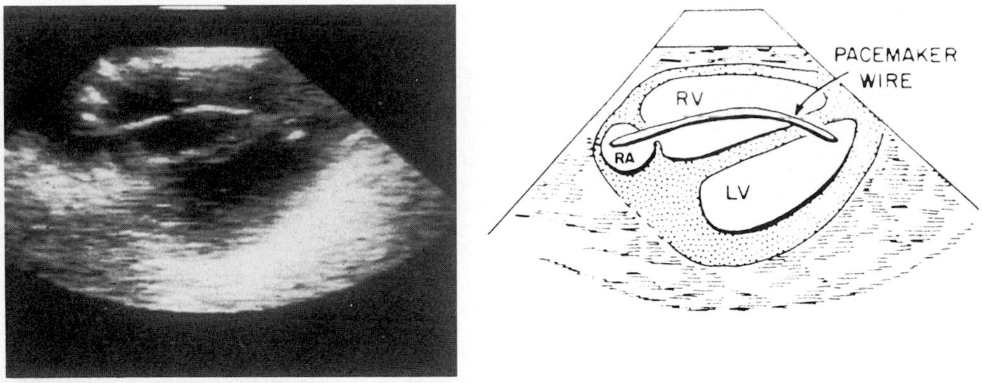

Fig. 36–75. Modified subcostal four-chamber recording of a pacemaker wire in the right ventricle that has perforated the interventricular septum and the tip of which is in the left ventricular cavity. LV = left ventricle; RV = right ventricle; RA = right atrium.

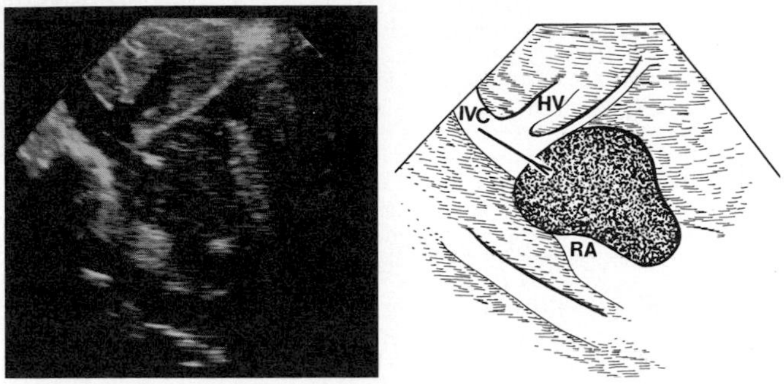

Fig. 36–76. Long axis recording of the inferior vena cava (IVC) and right atrium (RA) showing a biopsy forceps positioned to remove a sample from a large tumor mass in the RA. HV = hepatic vein.

REFERENCES

1. Lappe DL, Bulkley BH, Weiss JL: Two-dimensional echocardiographic diagnosis of left atrial myxoma. Chest 74:55, 1978.
2. DePace NL, Soulen RL, Kotler MN, Mintz GS: Two-dimensional echocardiographic detection of intra-atrial masses. Am J Cardiol 48:954, 1981.
3. St. John Sutton MG, Mercier LA, Giuliani ER, Lie JT: Atrial myxomas: a review of clinical experience in 40 patients. Mayo Clin Proc 55:371, 1980.
4. Duncan WJ, Rowe RD, Freedom RM: Space-occupying lesions of the myocardium: role of two-dimensional echocardiography in detection of cardiac tumors in children. Am Heart J 104:780, 1982.
5. Fyke FE III, et al.: Primary cardiac tumors: experience with 30 consecutive patients since the introduction of two-dimensional echocardiography. J Am Coll Cardiol 5:1465, 1985.
6. McAllister HA, Fenoglio JJ: Tumors of the cardiovascular system. *In* Atlas of Tumor Pathology. Washington, D.C., Armed Forces Institute of Pathology, Fascicle 15, Series 2, p. 1, 1978.
7. Nadas AS, Ellison RC: Cardiac tumors in infancy. Am J Cardiol 21:363, 1968.
8. Goodwin JF: The spectrum of cardiac tumors. Am J Cardiol 21:307, 1968.
9. Selzer A, Sakai FJ, Popper RW: Protean clinical manifestations of primary tumors of the heart. Am J Med 52:9, 1972.
10. Heath D: Pathology of cardiac tumors. Am J Cardiol 21:315, 1968.
11. Griffiths GD: A review of primary tumors of the heart. Prog Cardiovasc Dis 7:465, 1965.
12. Prichard RW: Tumors of the heart: review of the subject and report of 150 cases. Arch Pathol 51:98, 1951.
13. Wold LE, Lie JT: Atrial myxomas: a clinicopathologic profile. Am J Pathol 101:219, 1980.
14. Peters MN, et al.: The clinical syndrome of atrial myxomas. JAMA 230: 695, 1974.
15. Bulkley BH, Hutchins GM: Atrial myxomas: a fifty-year review. Am Heart J 97:639, 1979.
16. Farah MG: Familial atrial myxoma. Ann Intern Med 83:358, 1975.
17. Kleid JJ, Klugman J, Haas J, Battock D: Familial atrial myxoma. Am J Cardiol 32:361, 1973.
18. Siltanen P, et al.: Atrial myxoma in a family. Am J Cardiol 38:252, 1976.
19. Barold SS, et al.: Mitral valve myxoma diagnosed by two-dimensional echocardiography. Am J Cardiol 59:132, 1987.
20. Sandrasarga FA, Oliver WA, English TAH: Myxoma of the mitral valve. Br Heart J 42:221, 1979.
21. Suri RK, et al.: Myxoma of the tricuspid valve. Aust NZ J Surg 48:429, 1978.
22. Gosse P, et al.: Myxoma of the mitral valve diagnosed by echocardiography. Am Heart J 111:803, 1986.
23. Devig PM, Clark TA, Aaron BL: Cardiac myxoma arising from the inferior vena cava. Chest 78:784, 1980.
24. Meller J, et al.: Left ventricular myxoma: echocardiographic diagnosis and review of the literature. Am J Med 63:816, 1977.
25. Snyder SN, Smith DC, Lau FY, Turner AF: Diagnostic feature of right ventricular myxoma. Am Heart J 91:240, 1976.
26. Bjork VO, Bjork L: Left ventricular myxoma. Thorax 20:534, 1965.
27. Tway KP, Shah AA, Rahimtoola SH: Multiple biatrial myxomas demonstrated by two-dimensional echocardiography. Am J Med 71:896, 1981.
28. Imperio J, Summers D, Krasnow N, Piccone VA Jr: The distribution patterns of biatrial myxomas. Ann Thorac Surg 29:469, 1980.
29. Dashkoff N, et al.: Bilateral atrial myxomas: echocardiographic considerations. Am J Med 65:361, 1978.
30. Dang CR, Hurley EJ: Contralateral recurrent myxoma of the heart. Ann Thorac Surg 21:59, 1976.
31. Markel ML, Armstrong WF, Waller BF, Mohamed Y: Left atrial myxoma with multicentric recurrence and evidence of metastasis: a case report. Am Heart J 111:409, 1986.
32. Read RC, et al.: Malignant potentiality of left atrial myxoma. J Thorac Cardiovasc Surg 68:857, 1974.
33. DeSousa AL, et al.: Atrial myxoma: a review of neurological complications, metastasis, and recurrences. J Neurol Neurosurg Psychiatry 41:1119, 1978.
34. Hada Y, et al.: Recurrent multiple myxomas. Am Heart J 107:1280, 1984.
35. Cleveland DC, Westaby S, Karp RB: Treatment of intra-atrial cardiac tumors. JAMA 249:2799, 1983.
36. Ferrans VJ, Roberts WC: Structural features of cardiac myxomas: histology, histochemistry, and electron microscopy. Hum Pathol 4:111, 1973.
37. Graham HV, von Harititzsch B, Medina JR: Infected atrial myxoma. Am J Cardiol 38:658, 1976.
38. Rogers EW, Weyman AE, Noble RJ, Briuns SG: Left atrial myxoma infected with Histoplasma capsulatum. Am J Med 64:683, 1978.
39. Harvey WP: Clinical aspects of cardiac tumors. Am J Cardiol 21:328, 1968.
40. Greenwood WF: Profile of atrial myxoma. Am J Cardiol 21:367, 1968.
41. Nasser WK, et al.: Atrial Myxoma. II. Phonocardiographic, echocardiographic, hemodynamic, and angiographic features in nine cases. Am Heart J 83:810, 1972.
42. Sakakibara S, et al.: Myxoma of the right ventricle of the heart: report of a case with successful removal and review of the literature. Am Heart J 69:382, 1965.
43. Sasse L, Lorentzem D, Alvarez H: Paradoxical septal motion secondary to right ventricular tumor. JAMA 234:955, 1975.
44. Levisman JA, et al.: Echocardiographic diagnosis of a mobile pedunculated tumor in the left ventricular cavity. Am J Cardiol 36:957, 1975.
45. Heath D, Mackinnon J: Pulmonary hypertension due to myxoma of the right atrium with special reference to the behavior of emboli of myxoma in the lung. Am Heart J 68:227, 1964.
46. Gonzalez A, et al.: Massive pulmonary embolism associated with a right ventricular myxoma. Am J Med 69:795, 1980.
47. Effert S, Domanig E: The diagnosis of intra-atrial tumors and thrombi by the ultrasonic echo method. Ger Med Mth 4:1, 1959.
48. Come PC, Riley MF, Markis JE, Malagold M: Limitations of echocardiographic techniques in evaluation of left atrial masses. Am J Cardiol 48:947, 1981.
49. Giuliani ER, Lemire F, Schattenberg TT: Unusual echocardiographic findings in a patient with left atrial myxoma. Mayo Clin Proc 53:469, 1978.
50. DeMaria AN, et al.: Unusual echocardiographic manifestations of right and left heart myxomas. Am J Med 59:713, 1975.

51. Ciraulo DA: Mitral valve fluttering: an echocardiographic feature of left atrial myxoma. Chest 76:95, 1979.
52. Salcedo EE, et al.: Echocardiographic findings in 25 patients with left atrial myxoma. J Am Coll Cardiol 1:1163, 1983.
53. Popp RL, Harrison DC: Ultrasound for the diagnosis of atrial tumors. Ann Intern Med 71:785, 1969.
54. Wolfe SB, Popp RL, Feigenbaum H: Diagnosis of atrial tumors by ultrasound. Circulation 39:615, 1969.
55. Finegan RE, Harrison DC: Diagnosis of left atrial myxoma by echocardiography. N Engl J Med 282:1022, 1970.
56. Charuzi Y, Bolger A, Beeder C, Lew AS: A new echocardiographic classification of left atrial myxoma. Am J Cardiol 55:614, 1985.
57. Rahilly GT, Nanda NC: Two-dimensional echocardiographic identification of tumor hemorrhages in atrial myxomas. Am Heart J 101:237, 1981.
58. Thier [Aschenberg] W, et al.: Cysts in left atrial myxomas identified by transesophageal cross-sectional echocardiography. Am J Cardiol 51:1793, 1983.
59. Boughner DR, Persaud JA: Transcutaneous continuous wave Doppler ultrasound in the diagnosis of left atrial myxoma. Chest 79:322, 1981.
60. Vargas-Barron J, et al.: Pulsed Doppler echocardiographic analysis of atrioventricular flow changes in patients with atrial myxomas. Am Heart J 112:850, 1986.
61. Panidis IP, Mintz GS, McAllister M: Hemodynamic consequences of left atrial myxomas as assessed by Doppler ultrasound. Am Heart J 111:927, 1986.
62. Goli VD, et al.: Doppler echocardiographic profiles in obstructive right and left atrial myxomas. J Am Coll Cardiol 9:701, 1987.
63. Come PC, Kurland GS, Vine HS: Two-dimensional echocardiography in differentiating right atrial and tricuspid valve mass lesions. Am J Cardiol 44:1207, 1979.
64. Riggs T, Paul MH, DeLeon S, Ilbawi M: Two-dimensional echocardiography in evaluation of right atrial masses: five cases in pediatric patients. Am J Cardiol 48:961, 1981.
65. Panidis IP, Kotler MN, Mintz GS, Ross J: Clinical and echocardiographic features of right atrial masses. Am Heart J 107:745, 1984.
66. Kendrick MH, et al.: Ventricular pacemaker wire simulating a right atrial mass. Chest 72:649, 1977.
67. Marx GR, Bierman FZ, Matthews E, Williams R: Two-dimensional echocardiographic diagnosis of intracardiac masses in infancy. J Am Coll Cardiol 3:827, 1984.
68. Werner JA, et al.: Echocardiographic appearance of the Chiari network: differentiation from right-heart pathology. Circulation 63:1104, 1981.
69. Hanley PC, et al.: Diagnosis and classification of atrial septal aneurysm by two-dimensional echocardiography: report of 80 consecutive cases. J Am Coll Cardiol 6:1370, 1985.
70. Hada Y, Wolfe C, Murray GF, Craige E: Right ventricular myxoma: case report and review of phonocardiographic and auscultatory manifestations. Am Heart J 100:871, 1980.
71. Viswanathan B, Luber JM Jr, Bell-Thomson J: Right ventricular myxoma. Ann Thorac Surg 39:280, 1985.
72. Ports TA, Schiller NB, Strunk BL: Echocardiography of right ventricular tumors. Circulation 56:439, 1977.
73. Chandraratna PAN, Pedro SS, Elkins RC, Grantham N: Echocardiographic, angiographic, and surgical correlations in right ventricular myxoma simulating valvar pulmonic stenosis. Circulation 55:613, 1977.
74. Charuzi Y, Kraus R, Swan HJC: Echocardiographic interpretation in the presence of Swan-Ganz intracardiac catheters. Am J Cardiol 40:989, 1977.
75. Judson PL, Moore TB, Swank M, Ashworth HE: Two-dimensional echocardiograms of a transvenous left ventricular pacing catheter. Chest 80: 228, 1981.
76. Lo HM, et al.: Intracardiac goiter: a cause of right ventricular outflow obstruction and successful operative therapy. Am J Cardiol 53:976, 1984.
77. Mazer M, Harrigan P: Left ventricular myxoma: M-mode and two-dimensional echocardiographic features. Am Heart J 104:875, 1982.
78. Reyes LH, Rubio PA, Korompai FL, Guinn GA: Lipoma of the heart. Int Surg 61:179, 1976.
79. Olsen RE, Tangchai P: Large lipoma of the left ventricle. Arch Pathol 72: 58, 1961.
80. Esteves JM, Thompson DS, Levinson JP: Lipoma of the heart: a review of the literature and report of two autopsied cases. Arch Pathol 77:638, 1964.
81. Barberger-Gateau P, Paquet M, Desaulniers D, Chenard J: Fibrolipoma of the mitral valve in a child: clinical and echocardiographic features. Circulation 58:955, 1978.
82. Behnham R, et al.: Lipoma of the mitral valve and papillary muscle. Am J Cardiol 51:1459, 1983.
83. Fyke FE III, Tajik AJ, Edwards WD, Seward JB: Diagnosis of lipomatous hypertrophy of the atrial septum by two-dimensional echocardiography. J Am Coll Cardiol 1:1352, 1983.
84. Shub C, et al.: Cardiac papillary fibroelastomas: two-dimensional echocardiographic recognition. Mayo Clin Proc 56:629, 1981.
85. Almagro UA, Perry LS, Choi H, Pantar K: Papillary fibroelastoma of the heart: report of six cases. Arch Pathol Lab Med 106:318, 1982.
86. Ong LS, Nanda NC, Barold SS: Two-dimensional echocardiographic detection and diagnostic features of left ventricular papillary fibroelastoma. Am Heart J 103:917, 1982.
87. Frumin H, et al.: Two-dimensional echocardiographic detection and diagnostic features of tricuspid papillary fibroelastoma. J Am Coll Cardiol 2: 1016, 1983.
88. Flotte T, Dinar H, Fiener H: Papillary fibroelastoma of the left ventricular septum. Am J Surg Pathol 4:585, 1980.
89. Fenoglio JJ, McAllister HA, Ferrnas VJ: Cardiac rhabdomyoma: a clinicopathologic and electron microscopic study. Am J Cardiol 38:241, 1976.
90. Bass JL, Breningstall GN, Swaiman KF: Echocardiographic incidence of cardiac rhabdomyoma in tuberous sclerosis. Am J Cardiol 55:1379, 1985.
91. Golding R, Reed R: Rhabdomyoma of the heart: two unusual clinical presentations. N Engl J Med 276:957, 1967.
92. Mair DD, Titus JL, Davis GD, Riter DG: Cardiac rhabdomyoma simulating mitral atresia. Chest 71:102, 1977.
93. Shaher RM, et al.: Presentation of rhabdomyoma of the heart in infancy and childhood. Am J Cardiol 30:95, 1972.
94. Biancaniello TM, Meyer RA, Gaum WE, Kaplan S: Primary benign intramural ventricular tumors in children: pre- and postoperative electrocardiographic, echocardiographic, and angiocardiographic evaluation. Am Heart J 103:852, 1982.
95. Bini RM, et al.: Investigation and management of primary cardiac tumors in infants and children. J Am Coll Cardiol 2:351, 1983.
96. Birnbaum SE, McGahan JP, Janos GG, Meyers M: Fetal tachycardia and intramyocardial tumors. J Am Coll Cardiol 6:1358, 1985.
97. Geha AS, Weidman WH, Soule EH, McGoon DC: Intramural ventricular cardiac fibroma: successful removal in two cases and review of the literature. Circulation 36:420, 1967.
98. Rutkowski M, et al.: Successful excision of an atrial fibroma in a four-month-old male infant. Pediatr Cardiol 2:323, 1982.
99. Oliva PB, et al.: Left ventricular outflow obstruction produced by a pedunculated fibroma in a newborn: clinical, angiographic, echocardiographic and surgical observations. Chest 74:590, 1978.
100. Reul GJ, Howell JF, Rubio PA, Peterson PK: Successful partial excision of an intramural fibroma of the left ventricle. Am J Cardiol 36:262, 1975.
101. Aryanpur I, et al.: Calcified right ventricular fibroma causing outflow tract obstruction: report of a case with successful excision. Am J Dis Child 130: 1265, 1976.
102. Marin-Garcia J, Fitch CW, Shenefelt RE: Primary right ventricular tumor (fibroma) simulating cyanotic congenital heart disease in a newborn. J Am Coll Cardiol 3:868, 1984.
103. Reece IJ, Houston AB, Pollack JCS: Interventricular fibroma: echocardiographic diagnosis and successful surgical removal in infancy. Br Heart J 50:590, 1983.
104. Takahashi K, et al.: Echocardiographic demonstration of an asymptomatic patient with left ventricular fibroma. Am J Cardiol 53:981, 1984.
105. Taby IF, et al.: Cavernous hemangioma of the heart: case report and review of the literature. J Thorac Cardiovasc Surg 69:415, 1975.
106. Case records of the Massachusetts General Hospital: Case 4—1983. N Engl J Med 308:206, 1983.
107. Novitzky D, Rose AG, Morgan JA, Barnard CN: Primary cardiac hemangiomas. S Afr Med J 66:267, 1984.
108. Boden WE, et al.: Left ventricular hemangioma masquerading as mycoplasma pericarditis. Am Heart J 106:771, 1983.
109. Palmer TE, Tresch DD, Bonchek LI: Spontaneous resolution of a large, cavernous hemangioma of the heart. Am J Cardiol 58:184, 1986.
110. Case records of the Massachusetts General Hospital: Case 1—1982. N Engl J Med 306:32, 1982.
111. James TN, Galakov I: De subitaneis mortibus. XXVI. Fatal electrical instability of the heart associated with benign congenital polycystic tumor of the atrioventricular node. Circulation 56:667, 1977.
112. Cox JN, et al.: Teratoma of the heart: a case report and review of the literature. Virchows Arch (A) 402:163, 1983.
113. Hause AM, et al.: Blood cyst of the papillary muscle: clinical, echocardiographic, and anatomic observations. Am J Cardiol 51:812, 1983.
114. Perez-Gomez F, et al.: Cardiac echinococcosis: clinical picture and complications. Br Heart J 35:1326, 1973.
115. Erol C, et al.: Cardiac hydatid cyst simulating tricuspid stenosis. Am J Cardiol 56:833, 1985.
116. Farooki ZQ, Adelman S, Green EW: Echocardiographic differentiation of a cystic and solid tumor of the heart. Am J Cardiol 39:107, 1977.
117. Limacher MC, et al.: Cardiac echinococcal cyst: diagnosis by two-dimensional echocardiography. J Am Coll Cardiol 2:574, 1983.
118. Oliver JM, et al.: Cardiac hydatid cyst diagnosed by two-dimensional echocardiography. Am Heart J 104:164, 1982.
119. Glancy DL, Morales JB, Roberts WC: Angiosarcoma of the heart. Am J Cardiol 21:413, 1968.
120. Janigan DT, Husain A, Robinson NA: Cardiac angiosarcomas: a review and a case report. Cancer 57:852, 1986.
121. Lin TK, et al.: Pericardial angiosarcoma simulating pericardial effusion by echocardiography. Chest 73:881, 1978.
122. Panella JS, et al.: Angiosarcoma of the heart. Chest 76:221, 1979.
123. Orsmond GS, et al.: Alveolar rhabdomyosarcoma involving the heart: an echocardiographic, angiographic and pathologic study. Circulation 54:837, 1976.

124. McNalley MC, Kelble D, Pryor R, Blount SG Jr: Angiosarcoma of the heart: report of a case and review of the literature. Am Heart J 65:244, 1963.
125. Lutas EM, Stelzer P: Echocardiographic demonstration of right atrial rupture in a patient with right-sided cardiac tumor. Chest 83:921, 1983.
126. Ludomirsky A, et al.: Intracardiac undifferentiated sarcoma in infancy. J Am Coll Cardiol 6:1362, 1985.
127. Rossi NP, Kioschos JM, Aschenbrenner RA, Ehrenhaft JL: Primary angiosarcoma of the heart. Cancer 37:891, 1976.
128. Roberts WC, Glancy DL, DeVita VT: Heart in malignant lymphoma (Hodgkin's disease, lymphosarcoma, reticulum cell sarcoma and mycosis fungoides): a study of 196 autopsy cases. Am J Cardiol 22:85, 1968.
129. Cabin HS, et al.: Cardiac lymphoma mimicking hypertrophic cardiomyopathy. Am Heart J 102:466, 1981.
130. Chou S-T, et al.: Primary lymphoma of the heart: a case report. Cancer 52:744, 1983.
131. Gelman KM, et al.: Lymphoma with primary cardiac manifestations. Am Heart J 111:808, 1986.
132. Mich RJ, Gillam LD, Weyman AE: Osteogenic sarcomas mimicking left atrial myxomas: clinical and two-dimensional echocardiographic features. J Am Coll Cardiol 6:1422, 1985.
133. Seibert KA, et al.: Osteogenic sarcoma metastatic to the heart. Am J Med 73:136, 1982.
134. Dash H, et al.: Metastatic periosteal osteosarcoma causing cardiac and renal failure. Am J Med 75:145, 1983.
135. Herhusky MJ, et al.: Cardiac sarcomas presenting as metastatic disease. Arch Pathol Lab Med 109:943, 1985.
136. Shah AA, et al.: Malignant fibrous histiocytoma of the heart presenting as an atrial myxoma. Cancer 42:2466, 1978.
137. Hamada N, et al.: Malignant fibrous histiocytoma of the heart. Jpn Circ J 44:361, 1980.
138. Mahar LJ, et al.: Primary cardiac myxosarcoma in a child. Mayo Clin Proc 54:261, 1979.
139. Theodossi A, et al.: Budd-Chiari syndrome from myxosarcoma of the right atrium. J Pathol 128:159, 1979.
140. Elake S, Kealy WJ, Cloughlin S: Liposarcoma of the right atrium. J Ir Med Assoc 65:106, 1972.
141. Bearman RM: Primary leiomyosarcoma of the heart. Arch Pathol 98:62, 1974.
142. Bjerregard P, Baandrup U: Haemangioendotheliosarcoma of the heart: Diagnosis and treatment. Br Heart J 42:734, 1979.
143. Wychulis AR, Connolly DC, McGoon DC: Pericardial cysts, tumors, and fat necrosis. J Thorac Cardiovasc Surg 62:294, 1971.
144. Zanca P, Chuang TH, DeAvila R: True congenital mediastinal thymic cyst. Pediatrics 36:615, 1965.
145. Feigin DS, Fenoglio JJ, McAllister HA, Madewell JE: Pericardial cysts: a radiologic-pathologic correlation and review. Radiology 125:15, 1977.
146. Pezzano A, et al.: Value of two-dimensional echocardiography in the diagnosis of pericardial cysts. Eur Heart J 4:238, 1983.
147. Hynes JK, et al.: Two-dimensional echocardiographic diagnosis of pericardial cyst. Mayo Clin Proc 58:60, 1983.
148. Farooki ZQ, et al.: Real-time echocardiographic features of intrapericardial teratoma. J Clin Ultrasound 10:125, 1982.
149. DeGeeter B, et al.: Intrapericardial teratoma in a newborn infant: use of fetal echocardiography. Ann Thorac Surg 35:664, 1983.
150. Arciniegas E, Hakimi M, Farooki ZQ, Green EW: Intrapericardial teratoma in infancy. J Thorac Cardiovasc Surg 79:306, 1980.
151. Maeta H, et al.: Successful excision of intracardiac teratoma. J Thorac Cardiovasc Surg 83:909, 1982.
152. Sytman AL, MacAlpin RN: Primary pericardial mesothelioma: report of two cases and review of the literature. Am Heart J 81:760, 1971.
153. Yilling FP, Schlant RC, Hertzler GL, Krzyaniak R: Pericardial mesothelioma. Chest 81:520, 1982.
154. Coplan NL, et al.: Pericardial mesothelioma masquerading as a benign pericardial effusion. J Am Coll Cardiol 4:1307, 1984.
155. Agatston AS, et al.: Echocardiographic findings in primary pericardial mesothelioma. Am Heart J 111:986, 1986.
156. Hanfling SM: Metastatic cancer to the heart. Circulation 22:474, 1960.
157. Glancy DL, Roberts WC: The heart in malignant melanoma: a study of 70 autopsy cases. Am J Cardiol 21:555, 1968.
158. Roberts WC, Bouley GP, Wertlake PT: The heart in acute leukemia: a study of 420 autopsy cases. Am J Cardiol 21:388, 1968.
159. Birmingham CL, Peretz DI: Metastatic carcinoma, presenting as obstruction to the right ventricular outflow tract. Am Heart J 97:229, 1979.
160. Itoh K, et al.: Right ventricular metastasis of cervical squamous cell carcinoma. Am Heart J 108:1369, 1984.
161. Lagrange J-L, et al.: Cardiac metastasis: case report on an isolated cardiac metastasis of a myxoid liposarcoma. Cancer 58:2333, 1986.
162. Hallahan DE, et al.: Cardiac metastases from soft-tissue sarcomas. J Clin Oncol 4:1662, 1986.
163. Kutalik SP, et al.: Metastatic tumors of the heart detected by two-dimensional echocardiography. Am Heart J 109:343, 1985.
164. Grenadier E, et al.: Two-dimensional echocardiography for evaluation of metastatic cardiac tumors in pediatric patients. Am Heart J 107:122, 1984.
165. Lestuzzi C, et al.: Secondary neoplastic infiltration of the myocardium diagnosed by two-dimensional echocardiography in seven cases with anatomic confirmation. J Am Coll Cardiol 9:439, 1987.
166. Wiske PS, Gillam LD, Blyden G, Weyman AE: Intracardiac tumor regression documented by two-dimensional echocardiography. Am J Cardiol 58: 186, 1986.
167. Kralstein J, Frishman W: Malignant pericardial diseases: diagnosis and treatment. Am Heart J 113:785, 1987.
168. Chandraratna PAN, Aronow WS, Imaizumi T: Detection of pericardial metastases by cross-sectional echocardiography. Circulation 63:197, 1981.
169. Armstrong WF, et al.: Diastolic collapse of the right ventricle with cardiac tamponade: an echocardiographic study. Circulation 65:1491, 1982.
170. Gillam LD, et al.: Hydrodynamic compression of the right atrium: a new echocardiographic sign of cardiac tamponade. Circulation 68:294, 1983.
171. Tominaga K, et al.: The value of two-dimensional echocardiography in detecting malignant tumors in the heart. Cancer 58:1641, 1986.
172. Pizzarello RA, et al.: Tumor of the heart diagnosed by magnetic resonance imaging. J Am Coll Cardiol 5:989, 1985.
173. Come PC, Riley MF, Fortuin NJ: Echocardiographic mimicry of pericardial effusion. Am J Cardiol 47:365, 1981.
174. Isner JM, Carter BL, Roberts WC, Bankoff MS: Subepicardial adipose tissue producing echocardiographic appearance of pericardial effusion. Am J Cardiol 51:565, 1983.
175. Rifkin RD, Isner JM, Carter BL, Bankoff MS: Combined posteroanterior subepicardial fat simulating the echocardiographic diagnosis of pericardial effusion. J Am Coll Cardiol 3:1323, 1984.
176. Martin RP, Bowden R, Filly K, Popp RL: Intrapericardial abnormalities in patients with pericardial effusion. Circulation 61:568, 1980.
177. Koiwaya Y, et al.: Echocardiographic detection of metastatic cardiac mural tumor. J Clin Ultrasound 8:443, 1980.
178. Miyazaki T, et al.: Intractable heart failure, conduction disturbances, and myocardial infarction by massive myocardial invasion of malignant lymphoma. J Am Coll Cardiol 6:937, 1985.
179. Steffens TG, Mayer HS, Das SK: Echocardiographic diagnosis of a right ventricular metastatic tumor. Arch Intern Med 40:122, 1980.
180. Krivokapich J, et al.: M-mode and cross-sectional echocardiographic diagnosis of right ventricular cavity masses. J Clin Ultrasound 9:5, 1981.
181. Martin JL, Boak JG: Cardiac metastasis from uterine leiomyosarcoma. J Am Coll Cardiol 2:383, 1983.
182. Zelinger AB, Pouquet JM, Fishman PM: Two-dimensional echocardiographic demonstration of right atrial obstruction secondary to metastatic lung carcinoma. J Cardiovasc Ultrasonogr 1:347, 1982.
183. Garfein OB: Lymphosarcoma of the right atrium: angiographic and hemodynamic documentation of response to chemotherapy. Arch Intern Med 135:325, 1975.
184. Bryant J, Vuckovic G: Metastatic tumors of the endocardium: report of three cases. Arch Pathol Lab Med 102:206, 1978.
185. Ankless R: Renal carcinoma: how it metastasizes. Radiology 84:496, 1965.
186. Svane S: Tumor thrombus of the inferior vena cava resulting from renal carcinoma: a report of 12 autopsied cases. Scand J Urol 3:245, 1969.
187. Goldman A, et al.: Renal cell carcinoma and right atrial tumor diagnosed by echocardiography. Am Heart J 110:183, 1985.
188. Farooki ZQ, Henry JG, Green EW: Echocardiographic diagnosis of right atrial extension of Wilms' tumor. Am J Cardiol 36:363, 1975.
189. Kato Y, et al.: Growth of hepatocellular carcinoma into the right atrium: report of five cases. Ann Intern Med 99:472, 1983.
190. Maurer G, Nanda NC: Two-dimensional echocardiographic identification of intracardiac leiomyomatosis. Am Heart J 103:915, 1982.
191. Gonzalez-Lavin L, et al.: Tricuspid valve obstruction due to intravenous leiomyomatosis. Am Heart J 108:1544, 1984.
192. Pillai R, et al.: Intracardiac metastases from malignant teratoma of the testis. J Thorac Cardiovasc Surg 92:118, 1986.
193. Griffith DN, Myers A: Obstruction of right ventricular outflow tract by solitary ovarian metastases. Br Heart J 40:700, 1978.
194. Henuzet C, Franken P, Polis O, Fievez M: Cardiac metastasis of rectal adenocarcinoma diagnosed by two-dimensional echocardiography. Am Heart J 104:637, 1982.
195. Flinn RM, Foyce A, Montague TJ: Extraskeletal Ewing's sarcoma with fatal cardiac metastasis. Can Med Assoc J 133:1017, 1985.
196. Shuman RL: Primary pulmonary sarcoma with left atrial extension via left superior pulmonary vein. J Thorac Cardiovasc Surg 88:189, 1984.
197. D'Cruz IA, Roth RB: Left atrial extension of pulmonary adenocarcinoma mimicking left atrial myxoma. Echocardiography 4:59, 1987.
198. Hanley PC, Shub C, Seward JB, Wold LE: Intracavitary cardiac melanoma diagnosed by endomyocardial left ventricular biopsy. Chest 84:195, 1982.
199. Gallerstein PE, et al.: Right-to-left intracardiac shunt: a unique presentation of metastatic cardiac disease. J Am Coll Cardiol 3:865, 1984.
200. Canedo MI, Otken L, Stefadouros MA: Echocardiographic features of cardiac compression by a thymoma simulating cardiac tamponade and obstruction of the superior vena cava. Br Heart J 39:1038, 1977.
201. Chandraratna PAN, et al.: Echocardiographic evaluation of extracardiac masses. Br Heart J 40:741, 1978.
202. Cohen IS, Raible SJ, Anslnelli RA: Two-dimensional echocardiography in the detection of noneffusive cardiac involvement by intrathoracic neoplasms. Am Heart J 107:532, 1984.

203. Nishimura T, et al.: Two-dimensional echocardiographic findings of cardiovascular involvement by invasive thymoma. Chest 81:752, 1982.
204. Yoshikawa J, Sabah I, Yanagihara K: Cross-sectional echocardiographic diagnosis of a large left atrial tumor and extracardiac tumor compressing the left atrium. Am J Cardiol 42:853, 1978.
205. Kinney EL, et al.: Detection of posterior mediastinal lymphoma by pulsed Doppler echocardiography. Am Heart J 108:1365, 1984.
206. Baduini G, Paolillo V, DiSumma M: Echocardiographic findings in a case of acquired pulmonic stenosis from extrinsic compression by a mediastinal cyst. Chest 80:507, 1981.
207. Come PC, et al.: Reversible right ventricular outflow tract compression by immunoblastic sarcoma. Am J Cardiol 55:239, 1985.
208. Gondi B, Nanda NC: Two-dimensional echocardiographic diagnosis of mediastinal hematoma causing cardiac tamponade. Am J Cardiol 53:974, 1984.
209. Hsiung MC, et al.: Two-dimensional echocardiographic diagnosis of acquired right ventricular outflow obstruction due to external cardiac compression. Am J Cardiol 53:973, 1984.
210. Shah A, Schwartz H: Echocardiographic features of cardiac compression by mediastinal pancreatic pseudocyst. Chest 77:440, 1980.
211. Walters LL, Taxy JB: Malignant mesothelioma of the pleura with extensive cardiac invasion and tricuspid orifice occlusion. Cancer 52:1736, 1983.
212. Asinger RW, Mikell FL, Elsperger J, Hodges M: Incidence of left ventricular thrombosis after acute transmural myocardial infarction: serial evaluation by two-dimensional echocardiography. N Engl J Med 305:297, 1981.
213. Keating EC, et al.: Mural thrombi in myocardial infarctions: prospective evaluations by two-dimensional echocardiography. Am J Med 74:989, 1983.
214. Visser CA, et al.: Two-dimensional echocardiography in the diagnosis of left ventricular thrombus: a prospective study of 67 patients with anatomic validation. Chest 83:228, 1983.
215. DeMaria AN, et al.: Left ventricular thrombi identified by cross-sectional echocardiography. Ann Intern Med 90:14, 1979.
216. Reeder GS, et al.: Mural thrombus in left ventricular aneurysm: incidence, role of angiography, and relation between anticoagulation and embolization. Mayo Clin Proc 56:77, 1981.
217. Gottdeiner JS, et al.: Frequency and embolic potential of left ventricular thrombus in dilated cardiomyopathy: assessment by 2-dimensional echocardiography. Am J Cardiol 52:1281, 1983.
218. Abrams DL, Edelist A, Luria MH, Miller AJ: Ventricular aneurysm: a reappraisal based on a study of sixty-five consecutive autopsied cases. Circulation 27:164, 1965.
219. Dubnow MH, Burchell HB, Titus JL: Post-infarction ventricular aneurysm: a clinicopathologic and electrocardiographic study of 80 cases. Am Heart J 70:753, 1965.
220. Schlichter J, Hellerstein HK, Katz LN: Aneurysms of the heart: a correlative study of one hundred and two proven cases. Medicine 33:43, 1954.
221. Weinreich DJ, Burke JF, Pauletto FJ: Left ventricular mural thrombi complicating acute myocardial infarction: long-term follow-up with serial echocardiography. Ann Intern Med 100:789, 1984.
222. Spirito P, et al.: Prognostic significance and natural history of left ventricular thrombi in patients with acute anterior myocardial infarction: a two-dimensional echocardiographic study. Circulation 72:774, 1985.
223. Asinger RW, Midell FL, Sharma B, Hodges M: Observations on detecting left ventricular thrombus with two-dimensional echocardiography: emphasis on avoidance of false-positive diagnosis. Am J Cardiol 47:145, 1981.
224. Meltzer RS, Visser CA, Kan G, Roelandt J: Two-dimensional echocardiographic appearance of left ventricular thrombi with systemic emboli after myocardial infarction. Am J Cardiol 53:1511, 1984.
225. Ezekowitz MD, et al.: Comparison of indium-111 platelet scintigraphy and two-dimensional echocardiography in the diagnosis of left ventricular thrombi. N Engl J Med 306:1509, 1982.
226. Visser CA, et al.: Embolic potential of left ventricular thrombus after myocardial infarction: a two-dimensional echocardiographic study of 119 patients. J Am Coll Cardiol 5:1276, 1985.
227. Stratton JR, Lighty GW, Pearlman AS, Ritchie JL: Detection of left ventricular thrombi by two-dimensional echocardiography: sensitivity, specificity, and causes of uncertainty. Circulation 66:156, 1982.
228. DeGroat TS, Parameswaran R, Popper RM, Kotler MN: Left ventricular thrombi in association with normal left ventricular wall motion in patients with malignancy. Am J Cardiol 56:827, 1985.
229. Hilden T, Raaschou F, Iversen K, Schwartz M: Anticoagulants in acute myocardial infarction. Lancet 2:327, 1961.
230. Veterans Administration Cooperative Study Group: Anticoagulants in acute myocardial infarction: results of a cooperative clinical trial. JAMA 225:724, 1973.
231. Cooley DA, Hallman GL: Surgical treatment of left ventricular aneurysm: experience with excision of postinfarction lesions in 80 patients. Prog Cardiovasc Dis 11:222, 1968.
232. Fuster V, et al.: The natural history of idiopathic dilated cardiomyopathy. Am J Cardiol 47:525, 1981.
233. Haugland JM, et al.: Embolic potential of left ventricular thrombi detected by two-dimensional echocardiography. Circulation 70:588, 1984.
234. Jordan NA, Scheifly CH, Edwards JE: Mural thrombus and arterial embolism in mitral stenosis. Circulation 3:363, 1951.
235. Wallach JB, Lukash L, Angrist AA: An interpretation of the incidence of mural thrombi in the left auricle and appendage with particular reference to mitral commissurotomy. Am Heart J 45:252, 1953.
236. Nichols HT, et al.: Mitral commissurotomy: experience with 200 consecutive cases. JAMA 182:268, 1962.
237. Mikell FL, et al.: Two-dimensional echocardiographic demonstration of left atrial thrombi in patients with prosthetic mitral valves. Circulation 60: 1183, 1979.
238. Schweizer P, et al.: Detection of left atrial thrombi by echocardiography. Br Heart J 45:148, 1981.
239. Shrestha NK, et al.: Two-dimensional echocardiographic diagnosis of left atrial thrombus in rheumatic heart disease: a clinicopathologic study. Circulation 67:341, 1983.
240. Herzog CA, Bass K, Kane M, Asinger R: Two-dimensional echocardiographic imaging of left atrial appendage thrombi. J Am Coll Cardiol 3:1340, 1984.
241. Tabak SW, Maurer G: Echocardiographic detection of free-floating left atrial thrombus. Am J Cardiol 53:374, 1984.
242. Furukawa K, Katsume H, Matsukubo H, Inoue D: Echocardiographic findings of floating thrombus in the left atrium. Br Heart J 44:599, 1980.
243. Warda M, et al.: Auscultatory and echocardiographic features of mobile left atrial thrombus. J Am Coll Cardiol 5:379, 1985.
244. Hamada M, et al.: Left atrial mobile thrombus in hypertrophic cardiomyopathy. Am J Cardiol 56:812, 1985.
245. Hsu TL, et al.: Two-dimensional echocardiographic features of floating left atrial thrombus. Am J Cardiol 57:701, 1986.
246. Gottdeiner JS, Temeck BK, Patterson RH, Fletcher RD: Transient ("hole-in-one") occlusion of the mitral valve orifice by a free-floating left atrial ball thrombus: identification by two-dimensional echocardiography. Am J Cardiol 53:1730, 1984.
247. French P, Fletcher PJ, Bailey BP: Left atrial thrombus in severe mitral valve disease: prospective evaluation by two-dimensional echocardiography (abstr.). Circulation 68(Suppl. III):III-363, 1983.
248. Wartman WB, Hellerstein HL: The incidence of heart disease in 2000 consecutive autopsies. Ann Intern Med 28:41, 1948.
249. Felner JM, Churchwell AL, Murphy DA: Right atrial thromboemboli: clinical, echocardiographic, and pathophysiologic manifestations. J Am Coll Cardiol 4:1041, 1984.
250. Rosenzweig MS, Nanda NC: Two-dimensional echocardiographic detection of circulating right atrial thrombi. Am Heart J 103:435, 1982.
251. Spirito P, et al.: Right atrial thrombus detected by two-dimensional echocardiography after acute pulmonary embolism. Am J Cardiol 54:467, 1984.
252. Saner HE, Asinger RW, Daniel JA, Elsperger KJ: Two-dimensional echocardiographic detection of right-sided cardiac intracavitary thromboembolus with pulmonary embolism. J Am Coll Cardiol 4:1294, 1984.
253. Cameron J, et al.: Right heart thrombus: recognition, diagnosis, and management. J Am Coll Cardiol 5:1239, 1985.
254. Farfel Z, et al.: Review of echocardiographically diagnosed right heart entrapment of pulmonary emboli-in-transit with emphasis on management. Am Heart J 113:171, 1987.
255. Starkey IR, DeBano DP: Echocardiographic identification of right-sided intracavitary thromboembolus in massive pulmonary thromboembolism. Circulation 66:1322, 1982.
256. Ouyang P, et al.: Intracavitary thrombus in the right heart associated with multiple pulmonary emboli. Chest 84:296, 1983.
257. Nestico PF, et al.: Surgical removal of right atrial thromboembolus detected by two-dimensional echocardiography in pulmonary embolism. Am Heart J 107:1278, 1984.
258. Mancuso L, et al.: Echocardiographic detection of right-sided cardiac thrombi in pulmonary embolism. Chest 92:23, 1987.
259. Goldberg SM, Pizzarello RA, Goldman MA, Padmanabhan VT: Echocardiographic diagnosis of right atrial thromboembolism resulting in massive pulmonary embolization. Am Heart J 108:1371, 1984.
260. Manno BV, et al.: Two-dimensional echocardiographic detection of right atrial thrombi. Am J Cardiol 51:615, 1983.
261. Sheldon WC, Johnson CD, Favolaro RG: Idiopathic enlargement of the right atrium. Am J Cardiol 23:278, 1970.
262. Redish GA, Anderson AL: Echocardiographic diagnosis of right atrial thromboembolism. J Am Coll Cardiol 1:1167, 1983.
263. Lim SP, Hakim SZ, Van der Bel-Kahn JM: Two-dimensional echocardiography for detection of primary right atrial thrombus in pulmonary embolism. Am Heart J 108:1546, 1984.
264. Pliam MB, McGough EC, Nixon W, Ruttenberg H: Right atrial ball-valve thrombus: a complication of central venous alimentation in an infant. J Thorac Cardiovasc Surg 78:579, 1979.
265. Mahoney LJ, Silverman NH: Echocardiographic diagnosis of intracardiac thrombi complicating total parenteral nutrition. J Pediatr 98:469, 1981.
266. Schmaltz AA, Huenges R, Heil RP: Thrombosis and embolism complicating ventriculo-atrial shunt for hydrocephalus: echocardiographic findings. Br Heart J 43:241, 1980.
267. Chan W, Ikram H: Echocardiographic demonstration of tricuspid valvulitis and right atrial thrombus complicating an infected artificial pacemaker. Angiology 27:559, 1978.
268. Kinney EL, et al.: Recurrent pulmonary emboli secondary to right atrial thrombus around a permanent catheter: a case report. PACE 2:196, 1979.

269. Nicolosi GL, Charmet PA, Zanuttini D: Large right atrial thrombosis: rare complication during permanent transvenous endocardial pacing. Br Heart J 43:199, 1980.
270. Lange HW, Galliani CA, Edwards JE: Local complications associated with indwelling Swan-Ganz catheters: autopsy study of 36 cases. Am J Cardiol 52:1108, 1983.
271. Come PC: Transient right atrial thrombus during acute myocardial infarction: diagnosis by echocardiography. Am J Cardiol 51:1228, 1983.
272. Percy RF, Conetta DA, Perryman RA, Miller AB: Antemortem echocardiographic identification of right atrial thromboembolus. Am Heart J 109: 370, 1985.
273. Kunze K-P, et al.: Right atrial thrombus formation after transvenous catheter ablation of the atrioventricular node. J Am Coll Cardiol 6:1428, 1985.
274. Patel AK, et al.: Multiple calcified thrombi (rocks) in the right ventricle. J Am Coll Cardiol 2:1224, 1983.
275. Stowers SA, et al.: Right ventricular thrombus formation in association with acute myocardial infarction: diagnosis by two-dimensional echocardiography. Am J Cardiol 52:912, 1983.
276. Kessler KM, Mallon SM, Bolooki H, Myerburg RJ: Pedunculated right ventricular thrombus due to repeated blunt chest trauma. Am Heart J 102: 1064, 1981.
277. Shiu MF, Abrams LD: Echocardiographic features of free floating thrombus mimicking right ventricular myxoma. Br Heart J 49:612, 1983.
278. Kawamura Y, Nakamura Y, Handa S: Right ventricular thrombosis. Chest 73:435, 1978.
279. Isner JM, Roberts WC: Right ventricular infarction complicating left ventricular infarction secondary to coronary heart disease. Am J Cardiol 42: 885, 1978.
280. Guimaraes AC, Esteves JP, Filho AS, Macedo V: Clinical aspects of endomyocardial fibrosis in Bahia, Brazil. Am Heart J 81:7, 1971.
281. Bell J, Jankins B, Webb-Peploe M: Clinical, hemodynamic, and angiographic findings in Loeffler's eosinophilic endocarditis. Br Heart J 38:541, 1976.
282. Woolridge JD, Healey J: Echocardiographic diagnosis of right ventricular thromboembolism. Am Heart J 106:590, 1983.
283. O'Brien JT, Geiser EA: Infective endocarditis and echocardiography. Am Heart J 108:386, 1984.
284. Wann LS, Dillon JC, Weyman AE, Feigenbaum H: Echocardiography in bacterial endocarditis. N Engl J Med 295:135, 1976.
285. Stewart JA, et al.: Echocardiographic documentation of vegetative lesions in infective endocarditis: clinical implications. Circulation 61:374, 1980.
286. Dillon JC, et al.: Echocardiographic manifestations of valvular vegetations. Am Heart J 86:698, 1973.
287. Mintz GS, Kotler MN, Segal BL, Parry WR: Comparison of two dimension and M-mode echocardiography in the evaluation of patients with infective endocarditis. Am J Cardiol 43:738, 1979.
288. Wann LS, et al.: Comparison of M-mode and cross-sectional echocardiography in infective endocarditis. Circulation 60:728, 1979.
289. Gilbert BW, et al.: Two-dimensional echocardiographic assessment of vegetative endocarditis. Circulation 55:346, 1977.
290. Davis RS, et al.: Demonstration of vegetations by echocardiography in bacterial endocarditis: an indication for early surgical intervention. Am J Med 69:57, 1980.
291. Goldschlager A, Goldschlager N, Brewster H, Kaplan J: Catheter entrapment in a Chiari network involving an atrial septal defect. Chest 62:345, 1972.
292. Limacher MC, et al.: Echocardiographic anatomy of the eustachian valve. Am J Cardiol 57:363, 1986.
293. Battle-Diaz J, et al.: Manifestations of persistence of the right sinus venosus valve. Am J Cardiol 43:850, 1979.
294. Orita Y, et al.: Echocardiographic features of persistent right sinus venosus valve in adults. J Clin Ultrasound 10:461, 1982.
295. Hansing LE, Young WP, Rowe GG: Cor triatriatum dexter: persistent right sinus venosus valve. Am J Cardiol 30:559, 1972.
296. Silver MD, Dorsey JS: Aneurysms of the septum primum in adults. Arch Pathol Lab Med 102:62, 1978.
297. Wysham DG, McPherson DD, Kerber RE: Asymptomatic aneurysm of the interatrial septum. J Am Coll Cardiol 4:1311, 1984.
298. Vanderbossche JL, Englert M: Effects of respiration on atrial septal aneurysm of the fossa ovale shown by echocardiography study. Am Heart J 103:922, 1982.
299. Keren A, Billingham ME, Popp RL: Echocardiographic recognition and implications of ventricular hypertrophic trabeculations and aberrant bands. Circulation 70:836, 1984.
300. Perry LW, et al.: Left ventricular false tendons in children: prevalence as detected by two-dimensional echocardiography and clinical significance. Am J Cardiol 52:1264, 1983.
301. Vered Z, et al.: Prevalence and significance of false tendons in the left ventricle as determined by echocardiography. Am J Cardiol 53:330, 1984.
302. Nishimura T, Kondo M, Umadome H, Shimoto Y: Echocardiographic features of false tendons in the left ventricle. Am J Cardiol 48:177, 1981.
303. Brenner JI, Baker K, Ringel RE, Berman MA: Echocardiographic evidence of left ventricular bands in infants and children. J Am Coll Cardiol 3:1515, 1984.
304. Malouf J, Gharzuddine W, Kutayli F: A reappraisal of the prevalence and clinical importance of left ventricular false tendons in children and adults. Br Heart J 55:587, 1986.
305. D'Cruz IA, Devaraj N, Hirsch LJ, Glick G: Unusual echocardiographic appearance attributable to submitral calcification simulating left ventricular "masses." Clin Cardiol 3:260, 1980.
306. Dashkoff N, Karacuschansky M, Come PC, Fortuin NJ: Echocardiographic appearance of mitral annular calcification. Am Heart J 94:585, 1977.
307. Meier B, Felner JM: Two-dimensional echocardiographic evaluation of intracardiac transvenous pacemaker leads. J Clin Ultrasound 10:421, 1982.
308. Drinkovic N: Subcostal echocardiography to determine right ventricular pacing catheter position and control advancement of electrode catheters in intracardiac electrophysiologic studies: M-mode and two-dimensional studies. Am J Cardiol 47:1260, 1981.
309. Gondi B, Nanda NC: Real-time, two-dimensional echocardiographic features of pacemaker perforation. Circulation 64:97, 1981.
310. Cole WJ, et al.: Candida albicans-infected transvenous pacemaker wire: detection by two-dimensional echocardiography. Am Heart J 111:417, 1986.
311. Iliceto S, et al.: Two-dimensional echocardiographic recognition of complications of cardiac invasive procedures. Am J Cardiol 53:846, 1984.
312. Sakai K, Hoshino S, Osawa M: Needle in the heart: two-dimensional echocardiographic findings. Am J Cardiol 53:1482, 1984.
313. Portek IJ, Wright JS: Needle in the heart. Br Heart J 45:325, 1981.
314. Hsiung MC, et al.: Two-dimensional echocardiographic demonstration of multiple needles in the heart. Am J Cardiol 55:1245, 1985.
315. Hermoni Y, Engel PJ, Gallant TE: Sequelae of injury to the heart caused by multiple needles. J Am Coll Cardiol 8:1226, 1986.
316. Pierard L, et al.: Two-dimensional echocardiographic guiding of endomyocardial biopsy. Chest 85:759, 1984.
317. French JW, Popp RL, Pitlick PT: Cardiac localization of transvascular biotome using two-dimensional echocardiography. Am J Cardiol 51:219, 1983.
318. Chandraratna PAN, et al.: Application of two-dimensional contrast studies during pericardiocentesis. Am J Cardiol 52:1120, 1983.

CHAPTER

37

ECHOCARDIOGRAPHIC FINDINGS IN INFECTIVE ENDOCARDITIS

JAYASHRI R. ARAGAM and ARTHUR E. WEYMAN

The diagnosis and treatment of bacterial endocarditis remains one of the major challenges facing the clinical cardiologist. Although the classic clinical triad of persistent fever, changing heart murmurs, and positive blood cultures continues to be the foundation of diagnosis and may independently prompt treatment, direct visualization of valvular vegetations and the associated complications of intracardiac infection can alter management and can help to guide the timing of surgical intervention. Direct assessment of the infectious process has become particularly important because of the following: (1) the increased options for surgical management of complicated infections of native valves; (2) the growing number of postoperative patients with prosthetic valves that can potentially become a site of infection; and (3) the expanding population of patients with congenital heart disease who are undergoing complex surgical repairs that prolong life but that also place the patient at risk of infection for decades.

In the 20 years since the first descriptions of valvular vegetations by M-mode echocardiography were made,[1–3] the technique has assumed an increasingly important role in the assessment and management of the patient with known or suspected infective endocarditis. The development of cross-sectional, and later transesophageal, echocardiography has significantly improved the noninvasive detection, localization, and characterization of valvular vegetations.[4,5] Although vegetations are the hallmark of infective endocarditis, the complications of the infectious process are often the cause of major morbidity and mortality. Echo-Doppler studies provide clinically important information on the presence and degree of valvular destruction and its hemodynamic sequelae, as well as on the existence of perivalvular infection.

The potential of echocardiography to show valvular vegetations and to define other complications of endocarditis is particularly useful in the diagnosis of culture-negative endocarditis and in the management of patients whose clinical signs and symptoms are inconsistent with the severity of their infection. In this chapter, we summarize the echocardiographic findings in infective endocarditis, illustrate the complications of this disease, and discuss the significance of these findings.

CLINICAL CHARACTERISTICS OF VALVULAR VEGETATIONS

Vegetations are composed of clumps of microorganisms, platelet thrombi, fibrin, and erythrocytes attached to the surface of a valve leaflet, the chordae tendineae, or ventricular endocardium. Their morphologic features can vary, depending on the nature of the offending organism, the valve, and the activity of the disease. Some vegetations are discrete sessile masses closely adherent to the valve, others are pedunculated, friable clumps that prolapse freely, and still others appear as elongated fibrous strands.[4–6] Fungal vegetations are commonly larger than their bacterial counterparts, with bulky growth that may nearly occlude the valve orifice. In addition, fungal vegetations tend to embolize more readily and create less leaflet destruction than bacterial vegetations.[7] Tricuspid valve vegetations are generally larger than those located on left heart valves.[8] As vegetations heal, infiltration by fibroblasts occurs with hyalinization or calcification of the mass. Eventually, the healing vegetation is covered with endothelium.[6]

ECHOCARDIOGRAPHIC CHARACTERISTICS OF VALVULAR VEGETATIONS

The echocardiographic characteristics of valvular vegetations have been described in detail.[1,3,6,9] In M-mode studies, vegetations appeared as shaggy, irregular masses of echoes attached to valve leaflets that did not significantly impair the motion of the valve. Because vegetations generally move with the affected leaflet, the M-mode echocardiogram demonstrated them only during the portion of the cardiac cycle in which they were within the area encompassed by the ultrasonic beam (Fig. 37–1). The expanded field of vision and spatial orientation of two-dimensional imaging permitted the size, shape, location, reflective characteristics, and motion of vegetations to be more clearly defined. Analysis of these characteristics has facilitated the distinction between the vegetative mass and valve leaflets or other infected structures and has enabled one to define more clearly the spatial location and extent of the infectious process.[4]

Classic vegetations appear on two-dimensional echocardiographic images as circumscribed, echo-producing masses that arise from leaflet tips, either as an irregular area of highly reflective leaflet thickening (Fig. 37–2) or as one or more discrete, pedunculated, or fixed masses (Fig. 37–3). In acute endocarditis, the vegetations typically appear soft and friable, with varying degrees of independent motion, whereas chronic or healed vegetations become more echo dense and fixed. Vegetations may vary in size from a millimeter or less to several centimeters and can change appearance dramatically between studies because of embolization of part of the mass, growth of the vegetation, or intercurrent valvular disruption. Some vegetations, particularly those superimposed on foreign bodies, can develop a complex appearance with cystic components incorporated into or superimposed on the mass (Fig. 37–4). Because vegetations typically form on already diseased valves, their appearance is modified by the underlying valvular disor-

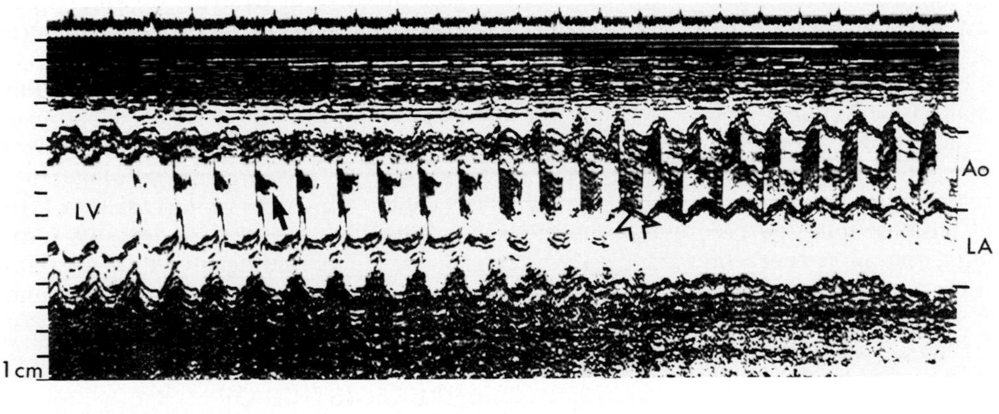

Fig. 37–1. M-mode scan from the left ventricular apex (left) to the aortic root (right), illustrating a large aortic valve vegetation prolapsing into the left ventricular outflow tract. The vegetation (small horizontal arrows) is evident in the aortic root during systole and is attached to the right coronary aortic cusp. During diastole it appears in the left ventricle anterior to the mitral valve (solid arrow). In the outflow tract immediately beneath the valve, the vegetation (open arrow) appears in both systole and diastole as it prolapses from the aorta to left ventricle. There is high frequency diastolic flutter of the vegetative mass, indicating leaflet destruction and aortic insufficiency. Ao = aorta; LA = left atrium; LV = left ventricle. (From King ME, Weyman AE: Echocardiographic findings in infective endocarditis. Cardiovasc Clin 13:3, 1983.)

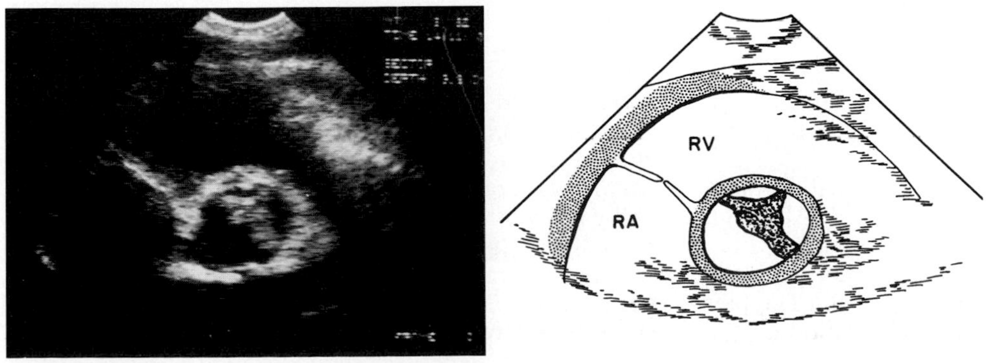

Fig. 37–2. Short axis recording of the aortic valve showing a large sessile vegetation superimposed on a bicuspid aortic valve. Both the valve leaflet tips and the raphe are involved in the vegetative process. RV = right ventricle; RA = right atrium.

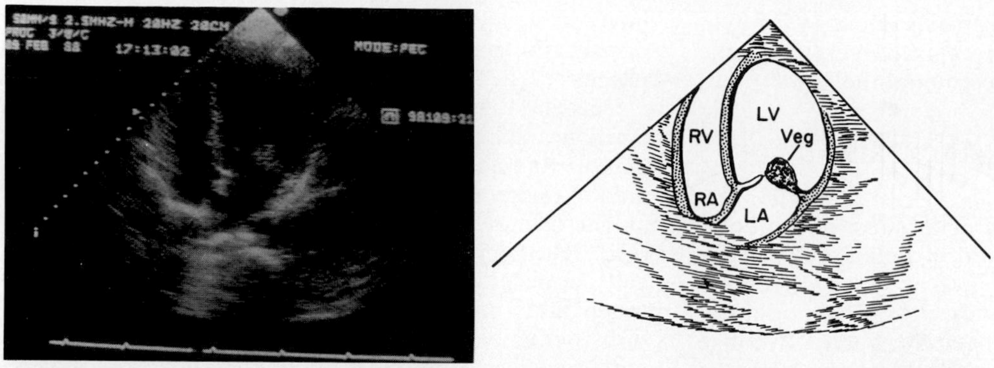

Fig. 37–3. Apical four-chamber recording of a mitral vegetation involving the posterior mitral leaflet. The vegetation appears as a roughly 1-cm, sessile mass that moves in concert with the valve leaflet. RV = right ventricle; RA = right atrium; LA = left atrium; LV = left ventricle; Veg = vegetation.

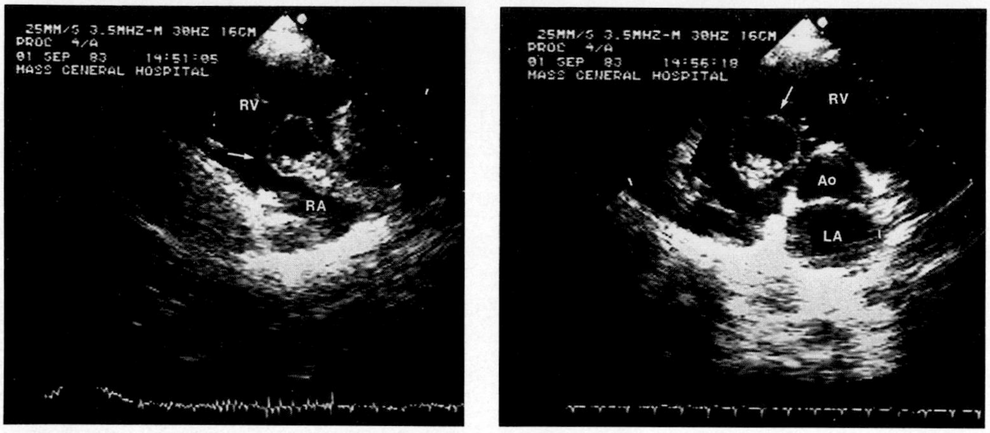

Fig. 37–4. Left. Right ventricular inflow view illustrating a vegetation superimposed on a catheter in the right ventricle (RV). Note the echolucency within the complex mass consistent with cystic degeneration of the vegetation. Right. The same cystic vegetation in a modified, short axis view at the level of the aortic valve. RA = right atrium; Ao = aorta; LA = left atrium.

der. Thus, a vegetation on a densely calcified, stenotic aortic valve in an elderly patient appears different from one involving an otherwise normally functioning bicuspid valve in a child. As a rule, the greater the degree of valvular deformity that existed before the infection began, the more difficult the superimposed vegetation is to define. Further, because valve disruption is part of the natural history of endocarditis, the appearance of the vegetation is often distorted by associated components of the infected valve, such as torn chordae tendineae or pieces of leaflet.

When vegetations are difficult to record on transthoracic studies or when vision is obscured by the intense reflections from prosthetic material, the esophagus provides an alternative window from which resolution is enhanced and diagnostic sensitivity and accuracy improved.

Aortic Valve Vegetations

The aortic valve is a common site of involvement in bacterial endocarditis. Although mitral valve endocarditis has been noted more frequently in postmortem studies,[10] the predominance of aortic valve involvement in surgical series suggests that operative intervention is more common when the aortic valve is affected.[10–14] Combined infections of both the aortic and mitral valves are also frequently observed.[10,11]

Predisposing factors in aortic valve endocarditis include rheumatic deformity of the valve leaflets,[15,16] bicuspid aortic valve,[17] and, in the elderly, atheromatous deposits, degeneration, and calcification of the aortic cusps.[18] Echocardiographically, aortic vegetations appear as masses or clumps of echoes attached to the ventricular surface of the leaflets. These echo-producing masses may be small or large, fixed or mobile, and have been described as fuzzy or shaggy in appearance (Fig. 37–5). When mobile and large, the vegetations may prolapse into the left ventricular outflow tract during dias-

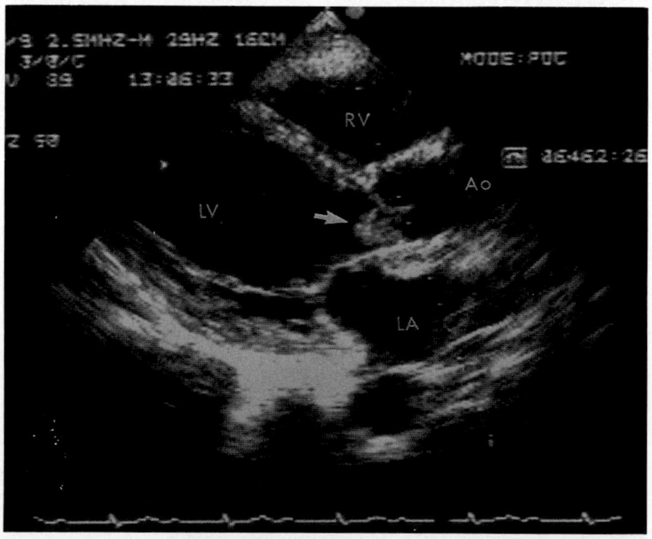

Fig. 37–5. Parasternal long axis recording illustrating a fixed, medium-sized vegetation on the ventricular surface of the aortic valve (arrow). LV = left ventricle; LA = left atrium; Ao = aortic valve; RV = right ventricle.

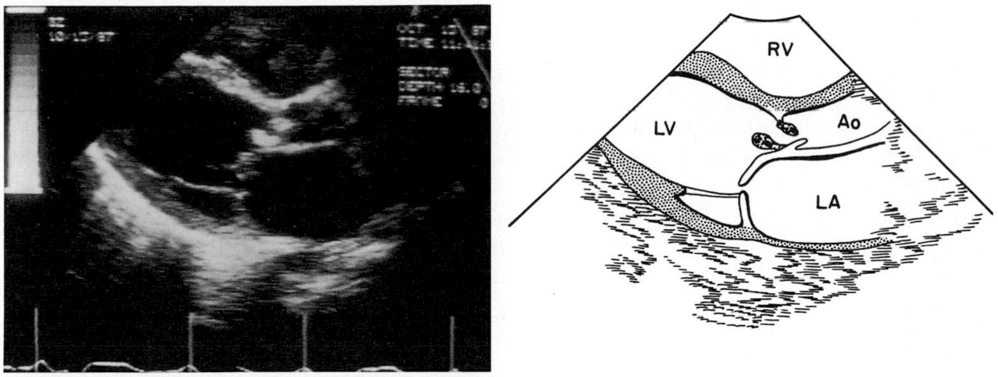

Fig. 37–6. Parasternal long axis view depicting an aortic valve vegetation that is prolapsing into the aortic outflow tract in diastole. Also note the pedunculated nature of the vegetation. LA = left atrium; LV = left ventricle; AO = aorta; RV = right ventricle.

tole and may swing forward with the stream of blood into the aorta during systolic ejection[1,5,6,19,20] (Fig. 37–6).

The identification of aortic vegetations depends on their location, size, relation to underlying valvular deformities, and association with valvular destruction. Aortic vegetations characteristically involve the bodies or free edges of the valve cusps. They are commonly focal, involving only one or two adjacent leaflets. Although visualization of vegetations as small as 2 mm has been reported,[1] larger lesions are obviously more easily detected. Prominent, underlying valvular deformities complicate the identification of vegetations, and when a vegetation is superimposed on a severely deformed, calcified valve, recognition of the vegetation as a distinct lesion may be difficult. Although vegetations generally move in unison with the leaflets to which they are attached, exaggerated motion of a pedunculated vegetation or of a friable portion of a fixed vegetation may aid in their recognition.

Vegetations may also arise in the left ventricular outflow tract immediately beneath the aortic valve. These vegetations usually originate from the base of the muscular septum and tend to be pedunculated. Figure 37–7 is an example of a pedunculated vegetation that is immediately beneath the aortic valve in this diastolic frame but prolapsed into the aortic valve orifice during systole.

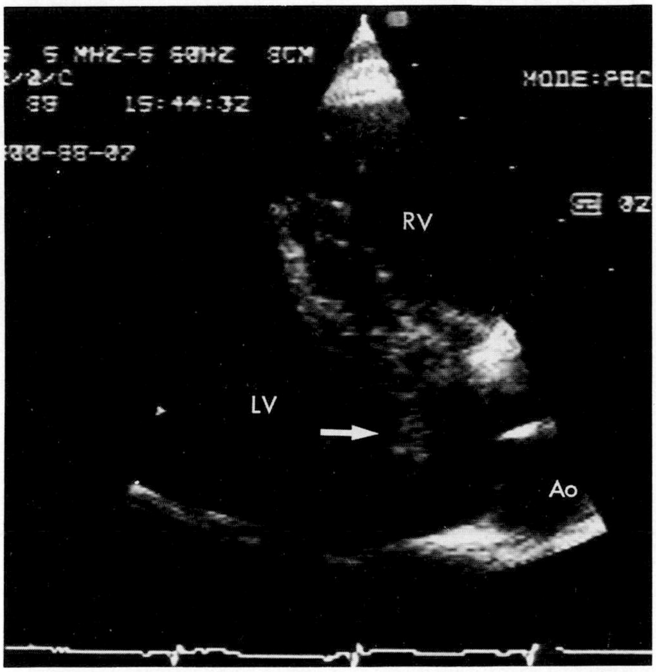

Fig. 37–7. Parasternal long axis recording of the left ventricular outflow tract illustrating a pedunculated vegetation (arrow) arising from the base of the interventricular septum immediately beneath the aortic valve. RV = right ventricle; LV = left ventricle; Ao = aorta.

Mitral Valve Vegetations

The mitral valve is more frequently involved in infective endocarditis than any other valve.[10] Mitral vegetations may involve the anterior or posterior leaflet but occur most often on the atrial surface. Infection of both mitral leaflets is not uncommon (Fig. 37–8).

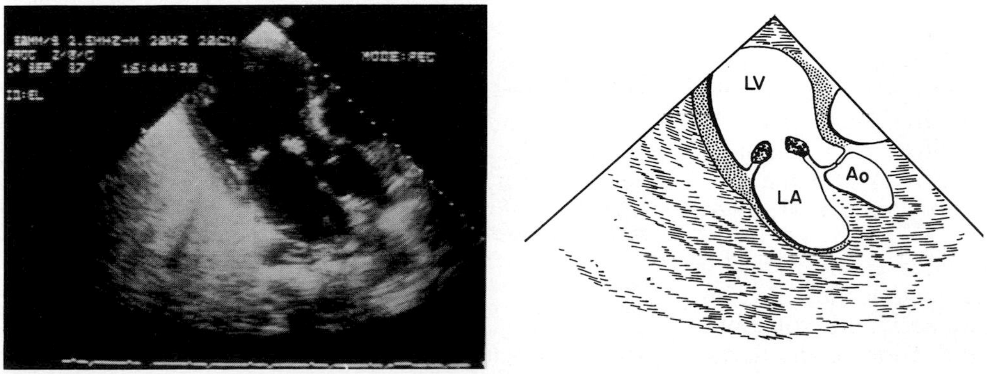

Fig. 37–8. Apical long axis recording illustrating bacterial vegetations involving the tips of both the anterior and posterior mitral leaflets. LV = left ventricle; LA = left atrium; Ao = aorta.

In addition to direct involvement of the mitral valve, seeding of the chordae tendineae or anterior mitral leaflet may occur because of extension of infection from an involved aortic valve. When mitral vegetations are large or pedunculated, they may prolapse into the left atrium during systole and may swing into the left ventricle in diastole (Fig. 37–9). Mitral valve vegetations can, on occasion, become large enough to cause severe mitral obstruction and can mimic the characteristic echocardiographic features of mitral stenosis.[21,22]

Mitral vegetations must be differentiated from a variety of other disorders that affect the valve, including myxomatous degeneration, rheumatic valvulopathy, and atrial and valvular tumors. Myxomatous degeneration of the valve may cause both leaflet thickening and increased echo production, simulating endocarditis. When myxomatous degeneration leads to systolic prolapse or to chordal rupture, the similarity may be even more striking.[23] The primary differential point lies in the degree of leaflet involvement. Myxomatous degeneration typically involves the leaflets diffusely and is associated with leaflet redundancy, whereas most vegetations are localized in their circumferential extent and have a predilection for the leaflet tips. In addition, myxomatous degeneration often involves the tricuspid valve, whereas involvement of both left- and right-sided valves by endocarditis is rare.

A thickened but mobile rheumatic mitral valve may also resemble an infected valve. The rheumatic valve can usually be identified by more restricted leaflet motion and fixation of the posterior leaflet. A prolapsing left atrial tumor may resemble a large vegetation; however, the point of origin of the prolapsing mass should aid in this distinction. When infection is superimposed on an underlying disease, the diagnosis depends on one's ability to distinguish the characteristics of the vegetation from those of the primary disease. Primary leaflet tumors such as myxomas and fibroelastomas may be impossible to differentiate from vegetations in the absence of clear clinical signs and symptoms, and it may be necessary to follow the natural history of the mass to determine whether intervention is necessary.

Tricuspid Valve Vegetations

Endocarditis involving the tricuspid valve was thought to be relatively infrequent, and earlier series reported an incidence as low as 2%.[24] The prevalence of right-sided endocarditis has increased significantly in recent years, however, especially among intravenous drug abusers.

Tricuspid endocarditis is typically an acute rather than a subacute process.[24] Staphylococcus aureus is the most common infecting organism.[24–26] Predisposing factors include intravenous drug abuse, alcohol abuse, virulent skin infections, and infected venous catheters. Among intravenous drug abusers, the valve is usually normal before the onset of infective endocarditis; however, patients with tricuspid valve endocarditis who are not drug addicts usually have an underlying cardiac disease. Congenital cardiac lesions associated with left-to-right shunts are more common in these patients.

The clinical diagnosis of tricuspid endocarditis is suggested by the triad of fever, narcotic addiction, and multiple lung lesions (septic emboli).[27] A pathologic murmur, which generally alerts the clinician to the possibility of endocarditis in lesions involving the left side of the heart, is frequently absent in patients with isolated tricuspid valve endocarditis.[24] Although significant tricuspid leaflet destruction and ruptured chordae tendineae are fairly common, the low pressure gradient between the right ventricle and the right atrium may be responsible for the absence of a murmur.[25] This frequent lack of clinical signs directing attention to the tricuspid valve makes the routine echocardiographic examination of this valve imperative in patients with suspected endocarditis.

Tricuspid vegetations generally appear as large, echo-producing masses that disrupt the normally smooth, thin contour of the tricuspid leaflets.[27,28] Vegetative growth may be on the atrial surface, the leaflet margins, or the ventricular surface, and it tends to be greater and more exophytic than in left-sided lesions. The echoes from these vegetations have been described as thick and shaggy (Fig. 37–10).

Large tricuspid vegetations may be difficult to differentiate from atrial tumors; however, their uniform association with the affected leaflet and their movement in unison with leaflet motion aid in their identification.[28] When vegetations arise on a stalk, their motion may be more erratic, but in these situations, identifying their point of origin should aid in diagnosis.

Pulmonic Valve Endocarditis

The pulmonic valve is the least commonly involved valve in infective endocarditis, and before the advent of echocardiography, the diagnosis of pulmonic valve

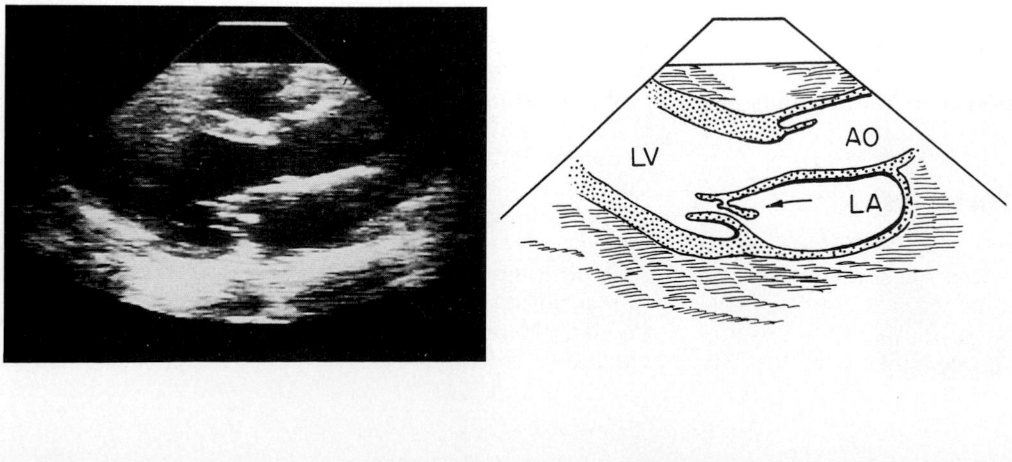

Fig. 37–9. Parasternal long axis recording depicting a pedunculated vegetation on the anterior mitral leaflet prolapsing into the left atrium in systole (arrow). LA = left atrium; AO = aorta; LV = left ventricle.

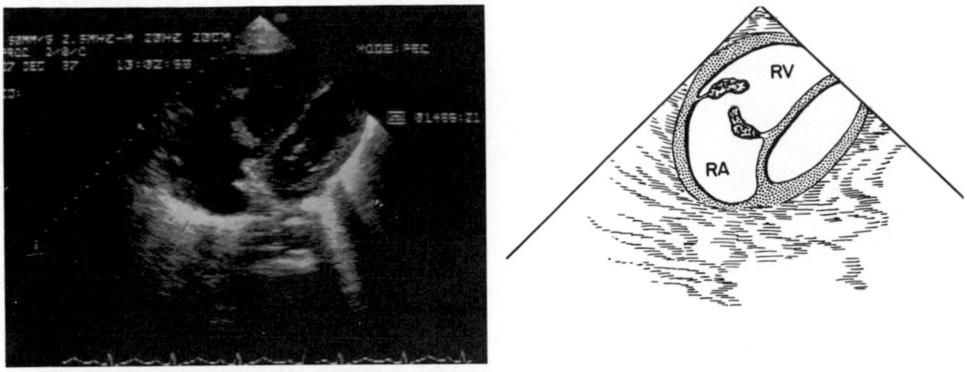

Fig. 37–10. Modified apical four-chamber view depicting large tricuspid valve vegetations involving both the septal and the anterior leaflets. Also note the enlarged right ventricle (RV) and right atrium (RA) that results from the hemodynamic burden of severe tricuspid regurgitation.

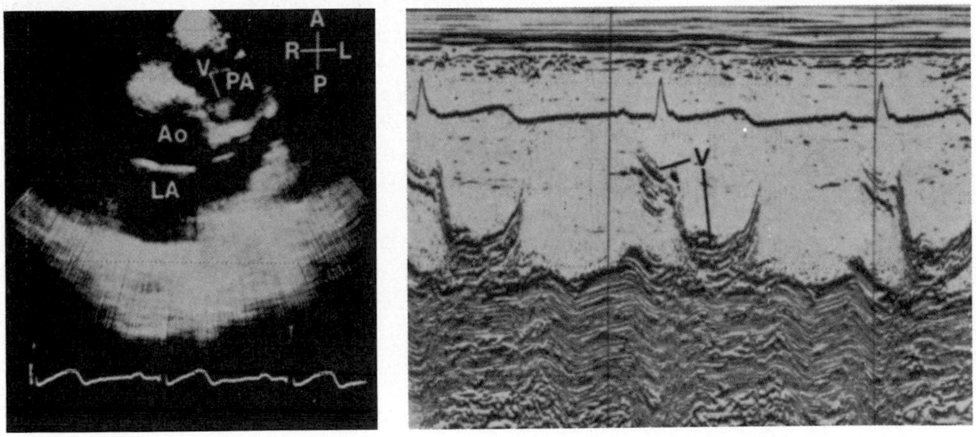

Fig. 37–11. Cross-sectional and M-mode echocardiograms demonstrating a pulmonic valve vegetation. Left. Parasternal short axis view of the aorta and pulmonary artery showing an echo-dense mass on the pulmonic valve (V). Right. M-mode tracing of the pulmonic valve with multiple dense echoes in systole and diastole from the pulmonic valve vegetation (V). Ao = aorta; LA = left atrium; PA = pulmonary artery. (From Berger M, et al.: Two-dimensional echocardiographic findings in right-sided infective endocarditis. Circulation 61:858, 1980. Reproduced by permission of the American Heart Association, Inc.)

endocarditis was usually made only at autopsy.[25,26] Unlike tricuspid endocarditis, pulmonic valve endocarditis usually occurs in patients with congenital heart disease, most commonly pulmonic stenosis, patent ductus arteriosus, tetralogy of Fallot, and ventricular septal defect.[29] In one report, seven of eight patients with pulmonic valve endocarditis had underlying congenital heart disease.[29] Involvement of the pulmonic valve in drug addicts is about ten times less common than tricuspid valve involvement in echocardiographic[30,31] and autopsy studies.[25,26]

Pulmonary valve vegetations resemble vegetations involving the other cardiac valves and are described as globular or shaggy, mobile masses of echoes that adhere to the valve leaflets (Fig. 37–11).[32]

Patients with ventricular septal defects may develop endocarditis at the site of the jet lesion on the endocardium of the right ventricular outflow tract, and detection of such a subpulmonic vegetation echocardiographically has been reported.[33]

PROSTHETIC VALVE VEGETATIONS

Vegetations on prosthetic valves are more difficult to detect than those involving native valves. The sewing ring and support structures of mechanical and bioprosthetic valves are strongly echogenic and tend to obscure vegetations within the valve apparatus or its shadow. By observation from multiple approaches and with careful attention to instrument gain settings, however, vegetations and associated leaflet/occluder malfunction can frequently be diagnosed. Transesophageal echocardiography has been especially useful in the diagnosis of prosthetic valve endocarditis.

Infection involving mechanical prosthetic valves usually begins in the perivalvular area at the annular insertion site.[34] Exuberant growth may extend down along the stents and may interfere with the motion of the ball or disc(s). This type of vegetative growth appears echocardiographically as thickening and irregularity of the normally smooth contour of the cage and sewing ring. Both thrombus and heavy pannus in this area have a similar appearance and cannot be distinguished from vegetative material. Necrosis of the supporting annular tissue with loosening of the sutures may lead to dehiscence of the sewing ring. Dehiscence appears during real-time study as excessive rocking of the prosthesis (Fig. 37–12).[35,36]

Bioprosthetic valves may demonstrate similar involvement of the sewing ring, with necrosis of the supporting annular tissue and loosening of the sutures leading to valve dehiscence. Investigators have reported that, although all dehiscent valves show some evidence of regurgitation, only valves with ring dehiscence affecting more than 40% of the annular circumference reveal excessive rocking.[36] Bioprosthetic valve leaflets may

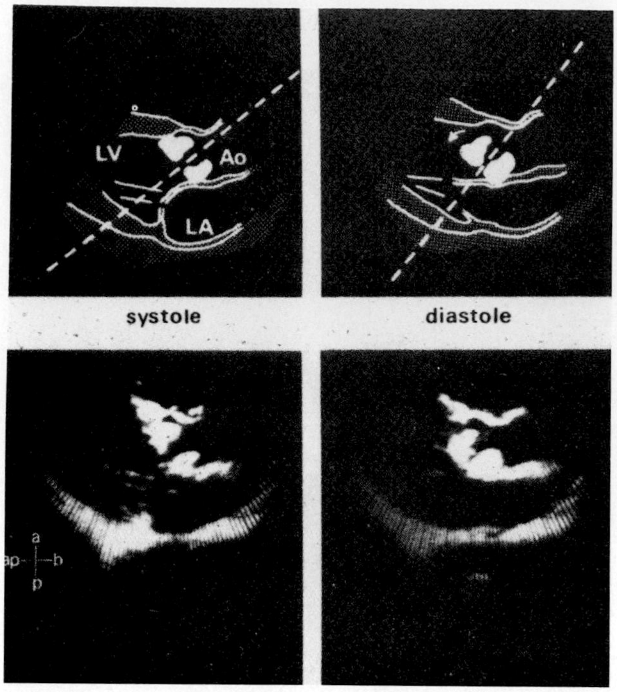

A B

Fig. 37–12. Cross-sectional echocardiogram of a patient with dehiscence of an aortic valve bioprosthesis. **A.** Parasternal long axis view of the left ventricle in systole, with the dashed line parallel to the long axis of the prosthetic valve stents. **B.** Parasternal long axis view in diastole showing excessive rocking motion of the prosthesis in the direction indicated by the small arrow. Ao = aorta; LA = left atrium; LV = left ventricle; a = anterior; p = posterior; ap = apex; b = base. (From Schapira JN, et al.: Two-dimensional echocardiographic assessment of patients with bioprosthetic valves. Am J Cardiol 43:510, 1979.)

also become infected, and this frequently leads to secondary destruction of leaflet tissue. The distinction between wear-and-tear degeneration of tissue valves and endocarditis is often difficult. Antegrade extension of echoes attached to a valve leaflet beyond the normal extent of the fully opened valve cusps can be a useful echocardiographic sign that distinguishes leaflet infection from leaflet degeneration (Fig. 37–13).[36] Although this sign appears highly specific, it is relatively insensitive, noted in only 25% of patients with documented vegetations in one clinicopathologic study.

Thus, although certain echocardiographic findings are characteristic of prosthetic valve endocarditis, definitive diagnosis may not be possible in all cases by echocardiography alone. In these patients, the clinician must rely on traditional clinical and laboratory methods to determine appropriate diagnosis and treatment (see also Chapter 38).

SENSITIVITY AND SPECIFICITY OF ECHOCARDIOGRAPHIC FINDINGS IN THE DIAGNOSIS OF VEGETATIVE ENDOCARDITIS

Multiple studies have examined the sensitivity of echocardiography in detecting vegetations in patients with clinical evidence of infective endocarditis. These studies are summarized in Table 37–1. Sensitivity varies with the population studied and the imaging technique used. In general, larger series evaluating all patients with suspected endocarditis report the lowest sensitivities, i.e., around 35 to 55%. When the clinical spectrum is narrowed to patients who require valve replacement, i.e., those with more serious disease, sensitivity improves to 80 to 100%.

The M-mode and cross-sectional techniques have nearly equal reported sensitivities in detecting left-sided vegetations; however, the accuracy in diagnosis of right-sided vegetations and of the complications of endocarditis is significantly better in studies using the two-dimensional technique.[30,37,38] The advent of transesophageal echocardiography has further increased sensitivity by its superior image quality and enhanced resolution. In one series that compared the transthoracic and transesophageal approaches for the identification of vegetations in hospitalized patients with clinically suspected endocarditis, the relative sensitivities were 63 and 100%, respectively, with equal specificities.[39] In another study of 105 patients with active infective endocarditis, transthoracic echocardiography enabled clinicians to visualize a definite vegetation in 58% of infected valves, whereas transesophageal echocardiography enabled them to visualize a definite vegetation in 90% of valves.[40] This difference in sensitivity between the two approaches was most striking in prosthetic valves.

The difference in sensitivity between transthoracic and transesophageal imaging can be directly attributed to vegetation size and, by inference, to relative image

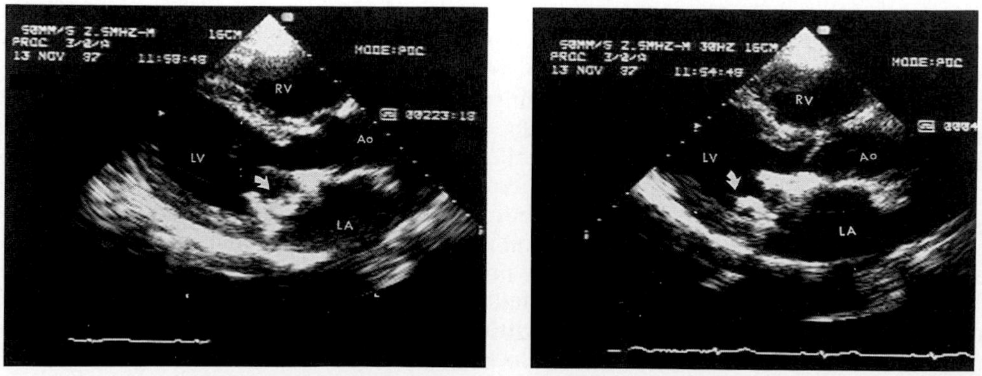

Fig. 37–13. Echocardiographic appearance of a large vegetation (arrow) attached to a leaflet of a mitral bioprosthesis in a patient with infective endocarditis. Note that the leaflet echoes remain within the prosthetic stents in systole (left) but extend beyond the stents in diastole (right). LA = left atrium; LV = left ventricle; AO = aorta; RV = right ventricle.

Table 37–1. Sensitivity of Echocardiographic Detection of Vegetations

Study (year)	No. of Patients	Disorder or Condition	Sensitivity M-mode (%)	Sensitivity 2-D (%)	Sensitivity Transesophageal (%)
Roy et al.[9] (1976)	32	Clinical endocarditis	69	—	—
Wann et al.[19] (1976)	65	Clinical endocarditis	34	—	—
Andy et al.[8] (1977)	25	Drug abuse in patients with active endocarditis and valvular regurgitation	80	—	—
Thomson et al.[41] (1977)	17	Clinical endocarditis	55	—	—
Gura et al.[105] (1978)	78	Clinical endocarditis	46	—	—
Young et al.[95] (1978)	59	Clinical endocarditis	39	—	—
Sheikh et al.[31] (1979)	10	Drug abuse in patients with right-sided endocarditis	70	—	—
Strom et al.[106] (1979)	30	Clinical endocarditis	57	—	—
Schapira et al.[35] (1979)	18	Bioprosthesis and suspected endocarditis	—	67	—
Gilbert et al.[5] (1977)	7	Clinical endocarditis (surgical or autopsy confirmation)	85	100	—
Mintz et al.[37] (1979)	21	Clinical endocarditis	48	—	—
Wann et al.[4] (1979)	23	Clinical endocarditis	78	83	—
Berger et al.[30] (1980)	12	Drug abuse in patients with clinical endocarditis	50	83	—
Martin et al.[107] (1980)	43	Clinical endocarditis	14	81	—
Stewart et al.[97] (1980)	87	Clinical endocarditis (surgical or autopsy confirmation)	—	54	—
Strom et al.[38] (1980)	24	Valve replacement for endocarditis	84	100	—
Rubenson et al.[94] (1981)	11	Abacteremic endocarditis (surgical confirmation)	45	100	—
Stafford et al.[101] (1985)	62	Clinical endocarditis	—	93	—
Lutas et al.[104] (1986)	77	Clinical endocarditis	45	56	—
Buda et al.[88] (1986)	50	Clinical endocarditis	—	42	—
Mügge et al.[40] (1989)	80	Clinical endocarditis (surgical or autopsy confirmation)	NV* PV†	68 27	94 77.7
Erbel et al.[39] (1988)	124	Clinical endocarditis	—	63	100

* NV = native valves.
† PV = prosthetic valves.

resolution. In the former study,[39] transthoracic recordings identified only 25% of vegetations smaller than 5 mm on transesophageal imaging, 69% between 6 and 10 mm, and all of those larger than 11 mm.

Several factors may contribute to the failure of echocardiography to show vegetations in patients thought to have endocarditis. In some cases, it is simply not possible to obtain an adequate study using the standard transthoracic approach; one hopes that these false-negative studies will be eliminated as the use of transesophageal imaging becomes more widespread. In others, no vegetations are detected because none are present. Many of the larger series included in Table 37–1 required only clinical evidence of endocarditis for inclusion, with no surgical or autopsy confirmation. Certainly, some of those patients may have had other undetected sources for bacteremia and fever; moreover, patients who have infective endocarditis but do not require surgical intervention probably represent a group with less virulent infection and hence might have small vegetations that fall below the limits of resolution of current ultrasound equipment. Finally, the presence of pre-existing valvular thickening and calcification or prosthetic heart valves may obscure the associated vegetations.

The specificity of echocardiographic findings consistent with valvular vegetations has not been clearly established. The reported false-positive rate is low in patients with proved endocarditis;[5,41] however, a study of patients with mitral valve prolapse reported 40% to have findings that might be interpreted as vegetations.[23] Other conditions predisposing patients to false-positive results have been discussed previously.

DIFFERENTIATION OF ACTIVE FROM HEALED VEGETATIONS

Some reports have suggested that valvular vegetations become smaller and more echo dense as they heal.[6,9] These observations are consistent with the fibrosis, collagen deposition, and calcification seen pathologically. Although these qualitative signs are used by many echocardiographers to differentiate active from healed vegetations, this distinction remains part of the "art" of echocardiographic diagnosis.

The observation that the echo amplitudes from vegetations increase as they heal has been confirmed quantitatively by measuring changes in mean gray level from serially digitized, two-dimensional images.[42] Unfortunately, routine clinical use of such techniques requires that serial studies be available or that some form of standardization between instruments and patients be achieved. Despite these limitations in quantitation, recognition of the characteristics of healed vegetations can be important in patients with prior endocarditis because evidence of the earlier infections may not completely disappear, and each new febrile episode must not be misinterpreted as a recurrence of endocarditis. This can be a particular problem in patients with right-sided vegetations and those of fungal origin, which may persist as large masses for years after the original infection.

VALVULAR AND EXTRAVALVULAR COMPLICATIONS OF ENDOCARDITIS

Valvular Complications

Primary valvular complications include valve disruption and mitral valve aneurysms.

Valvular Disruption

Among the more critical complications of infective endocarditis that lead to major morbidity and mortality is disruption of valvular tissue. This complication usually results in significant valvular regurgitation and may require urgent valve replacement.[43] Echocardiography provides important evidence of valvular destruction and its hemodynamic sequelae.

Aortic Valve. Some degree of valvular destruction is commonly seen in patients with aortic vegetations and may vary from a small fenestration in a cusp to a completely torn flail leaflet. Lesser degrees of cusp disruption (fenestration or torn leaflet margins) are characterized by valvular regurgitation with high frequency, diastolic fluttering within or at the margins of the echo-producing, vegetative mass.[37,44] This high frequency fluttering is caused by the regurgitant stream of blood flowing past the freely mobile piece of leaflet tissue and is readily appreciated on M-mode recordings (Fig. 37–14). To date, diastolic fluttering of the aortic valve has been noted only in cases of fenestrated or partially flail leaflets and may be considered pathognomonic for this type of disorder. Flail leaflets exhibit a more dramatic motion pattern, swinging freely into the left ventricular outflow tract during diastole, so their normal convex orientation toward the left ventricle is reversed and they become concave inferiorly.[37] During systole, the partially detached leaflet reverses its orientation, swinging in a 180° arc through the aortic annulus into the ascending aorta. When a flail leaflet is present, lack of diastolic coaptation with the remaining, normally attached leaflets is usually evident (Fig. 37–15).

When valvular destruction leads to severe aortic insufficiency, echo-Doppler studies are of particular importance in documenting the severity of the regurgitation and in assessing the effect of the increased hemodynamic burden on left ventricular volume and function. In addition, the timing of mitral leaflet closure may provide important hemodynamic information.[45–47] As discussed in Chapter 17, mitral valve closure is normally initiated by atrial relaxation and is completed by

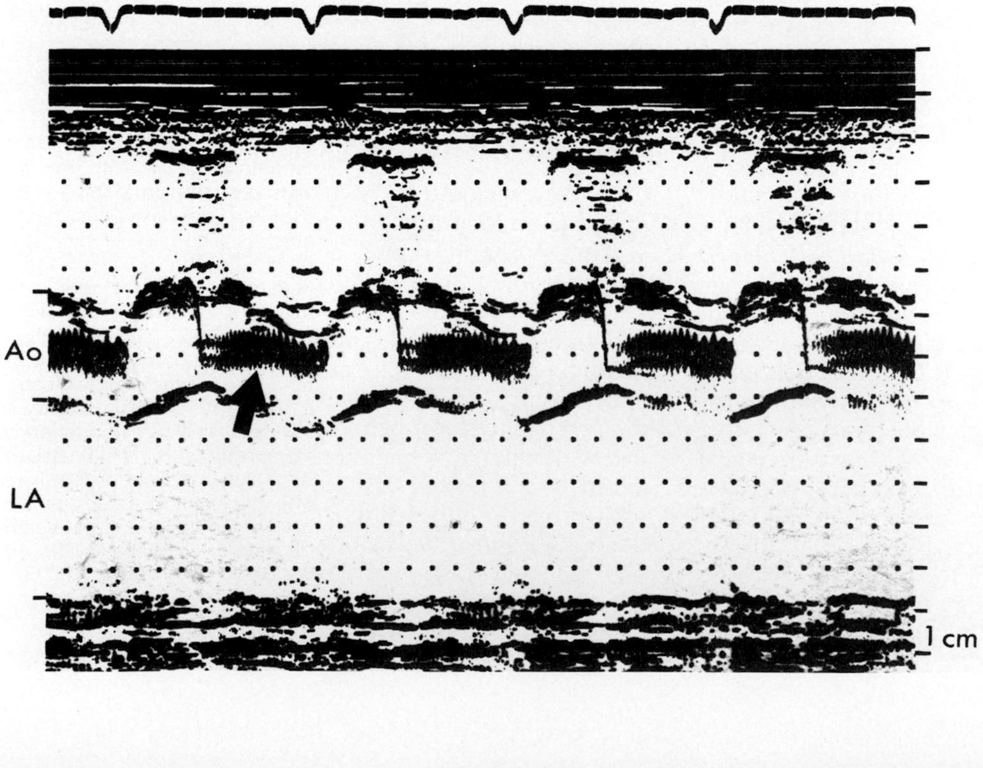

Fig. 37–14. M-mode recording illustrating diastolic fluttering (arrow) of the aortic valve leaflets caused by disruption of the cusp tissue and the resulting aortic regurgitation. Ao = aorta; LA = left atrium. (From King ME, Weyman AE: Echocardiographic findings in infective endocarditis. Cardiovasc Clin 13: 3, 1983.)

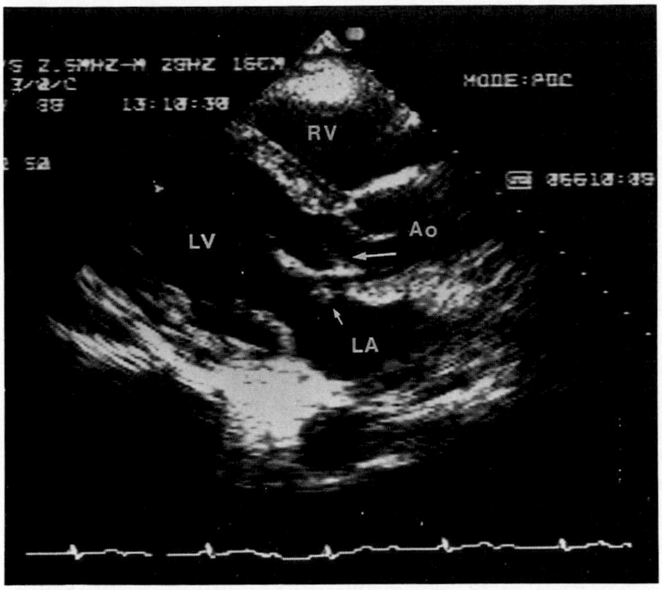

Fig. 37–15. Parasternal long axis view recording in a patient with aortic valve endocarditis depicting thickened aortic valve leaflets caused by superimposed vegetations and lack of diastolic coaptation caused by flail leaflet (large arrow). Also note the echo density on the atrial surface of the mitral leaflet consistent with a mitral valve vegetation (small arrow). RV = right ventricle; Ao = aorta; LA = left atrium; LV = left ventricle.

ventricular systole. In severe aortic insufficiency, diastolic pressure in the left ventricle may rise rapidly enough to exceed left atrial pressure before atrial contraction, causing the mitral valve to close prematurely (i.e., before the onset of atrial relaxation). Premature mitral valve closure is readily observed on M-mode recordings (Fig. 37–16), and in the setting of infective endocarditis, it has been associated with severe left ventricular failure, suggesting the need for urgent surgical intervention.[46–48] One caution must be observed: patients with extensive bacterial destruction of the aortic valve often develop septal abscesses with resulting conduction delay and prolongation of the PR interval. When first-degree heart block is present, the mitral valve normally closes completely in response to atrial relaxation, and as a result, closure before ventricular systole is neither unexpected nor abnormal. Therefore, truly premature mitral valve closure must occur earlier than would be expected as a result of atrial relaxation or ventricular systole.

Mitral Valve. Progressive destruction of the mitral valve results in ruptured chordae tendineae and ultimately in a flail leaflet. When there is limited loss of chordal support, the only evidence may be systolic prolapse. Often the ruptured chordae tendineae may be seen moving freely within the left ventricle. As additional chordal support is lost, the degree of systolic prolapse may increase, and/or a portion of the leaflet tip may evert during systole. Continued disruption of the leaflet results in a flail valve. A flail valve is characterized by a whipping motion of the tip of the affected leaflet through a 180° arc or greater about its point of annular attachment.[49,50] During diastole, the leaflet tip points into the left ventricular cavity, and the leaflet body is concave toward the left ventricle. With onset of systole, the leaflet is thrust upward into the left atrium. The leaflet tip completely reverses its direction and points toward the left atrium. Thus, the body of the leaflet is concave toward the left atrium or superiorly. This pattern is in contrast to the prolapsing leaflet, in which the leaflet body always remains concave toward the left ventricle. Normal systolic coaptation of the anterior and posterior leaflets is lost, and a clearly defined separation between these leaflets, in both parasternal long axis and apical four-chamber views, can usually be observed.

The range of motion of the anterior leaflet is normally greater than that of the posterior leaflet. This range is exaggerated when the leaflets become flail, and the anterior leaflet may actually arc upward into the left ventricular outflow tract during diastole. When such movement occurs, the leaflet swings through more than 270° from

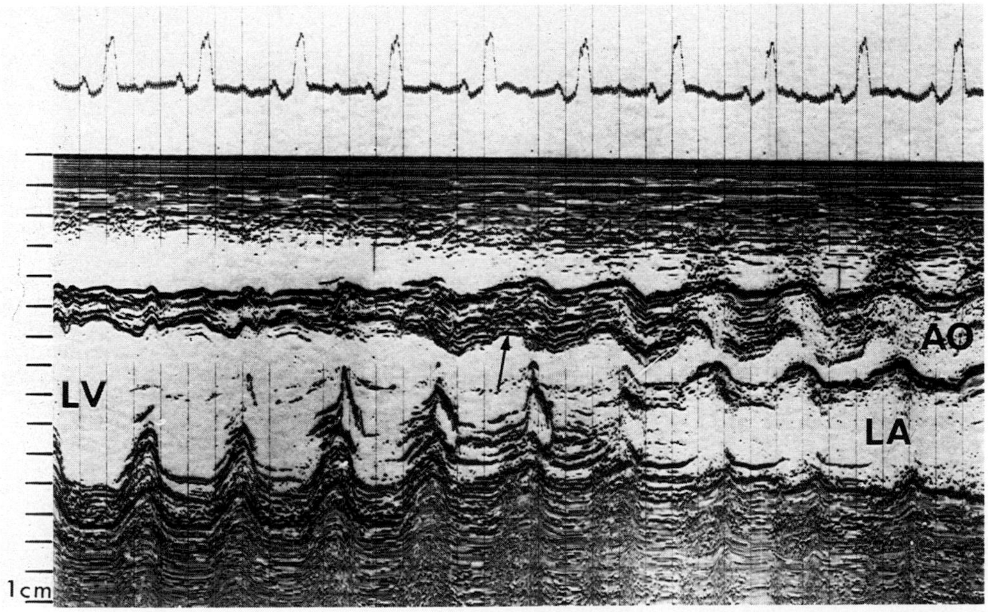

Fig. 37–16. M-mode echocardiographic scan from the left ventricle to the aorta in a patient with an interventricular septal abscess. The base of the interventricular septum (arrow) adjacent to the aortic annulus is unusually thick and echo dense compared with the myocardium of the lower portion of the septum. Also of note is early closure of the mitral valve secondary to severe aortic insufficiency. AO = aorta; LA = left atrium; LV = left ventricle. (From King ME, Weyman AE: Echocardiographic findings in infective endocarditis. Cardiovasc Clin 13: 3, 1983.)

full diastolic to full systolic excursion (Fig. 37–17). In contrast, the posterior leaflet is limited in its motion by the posterior wall of the left ventricle and normally cannot arc more than 180°.

Valvular disruption typically leads to mitral regurgitation, which can be detected by Doppler studies, as well as left atrial enlargement, left ventricular enlargement, increased excursion of the interventricular septum and left ventricular posterior wall, and, on occasion, early systolic closure of the aortic valve.

Tricuspid Valve. Right-sided infective endocarditis may also lead to valvular disruption. The echocardiographic features of ruptured chordae tendineae and flail tricuspid valve are similar to those for the mitral valve. The progression of valvular destruction is easily detected by serial studies and may signal the need for surgical intervention.[5] When tricuspid regurgitation occurs, the echocardiographic features of right ventricular volume overload appear, including right ventricular enlargement and paradoxic septal motion. The common association of tricuspid vegetations, tricuspid regurgitation, and right heart dilation facilitates echocardiographic recording of the tricuspid valve and appropriate diagnosis.

Pulmonic Valve. The pulmonic valve is rarely involved in infective endocarditis, and, as a result, echocardiographic reports of pulmonary valve disruption are not numerous. In general, pulmonary cusp disruption resembles that seen in aortic endocarditis. Coarse diastolic valve fluttering and visualization of a mass or everted leaflet in the right ventricular outflow tract suggest a flail pulmonic valve. Pulmonic regurgitation can be detected by Doppler studies, and its volume varies with the degree of valvular disruption and the pulmonary artery pressure.[29,31]

Mitral Valve Aneurysms

Aneurysm of the mitral valve, although uncommon, may be seen in association with aortic valve endocarditis.[51–54] Aneurysm formation appears to follow disruption of the aortic valve and to result from the regurgitant jet of aortic insufficiency striking the anterior mitral leaflet and creating a secondary site of infection. This localized mitral infection then destroys the endothelium and fibrosa of the valve, leading to the development of the aneurysm. Because of the higher left ventricular pressure, these aneurysms always bulge into the left atrium and are most prominent during systole. The aneurysms may remain intact, leak to varying degrees during systole, or rupture completely. The presence of the aneurysm is generally obscured by the dominant hemodynamic abnormalities produced by the more severe aortic disease; however, early and preoperative recognition of a mitral aneurysm is important because (1) the aneurysm may rupture and produce catastrophic mitral regurgitation in an already seriously ill patient or (2) it may be overlooked at the time of aortic valve replacement (mitral valve is usually examined through the aortotomy) and may remain as a site of continued infection or may later rupture spontaneously.[55]

A mitral valve aneurysm appears on the two-dimensional echocardiogram as a persistent bulge at the base of the anterior leaflet that protrudes toward the left atrium throughout systole and diastole (Fig. 37–18). This abnormal bulge is best visualized in the parasternal long

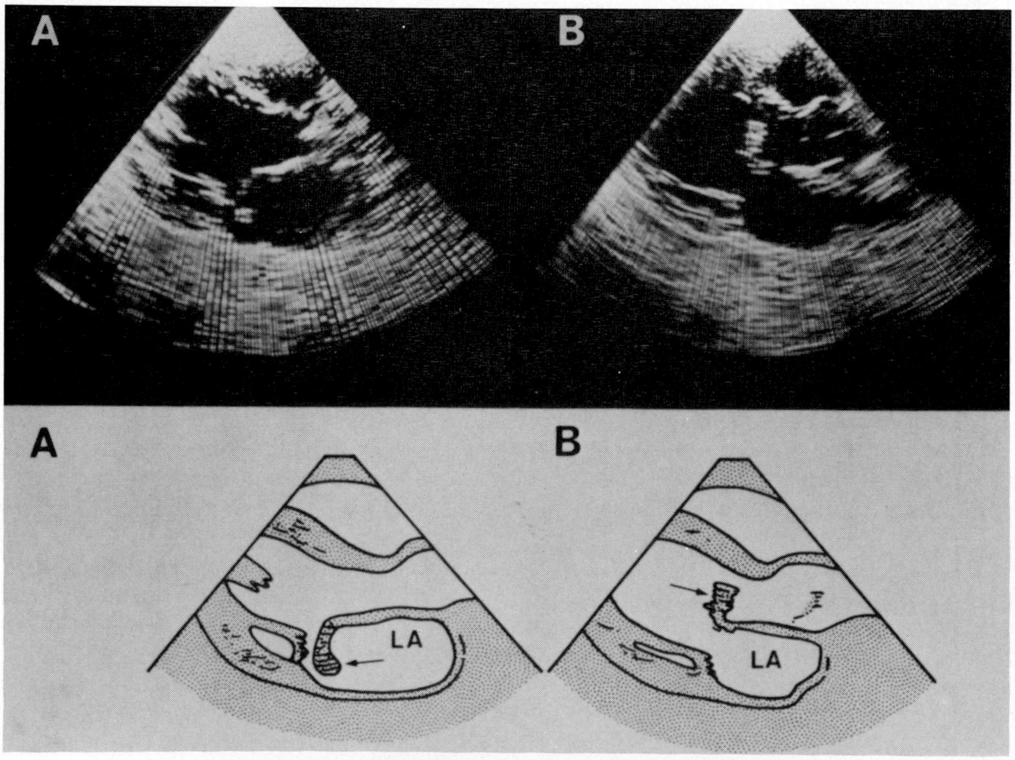

Fig. 37–17. Parasternal long axis recording of a flail, anterior, mitral leaflet in a patient with bacterial endocarditis. **A.** Recorded during systole, the leaflet arcs backward into the left atrium (LA). The body of the leaflet is concave toward the atrial chamber or superiorly. **B.** During diastole, the freely mobile leaflet is thrust upward into the left ventricular outflow tract and swings wildly in an arc about its point of attachment. The mass of echoes at the tip of the flail leaflet represents vegetative material (horizontal arrows in the diagram.) (From King ME, Weyman AE: Echocardiographic findings in infective endocarditis. Cardiovasc Clin 13:3, 1983.)

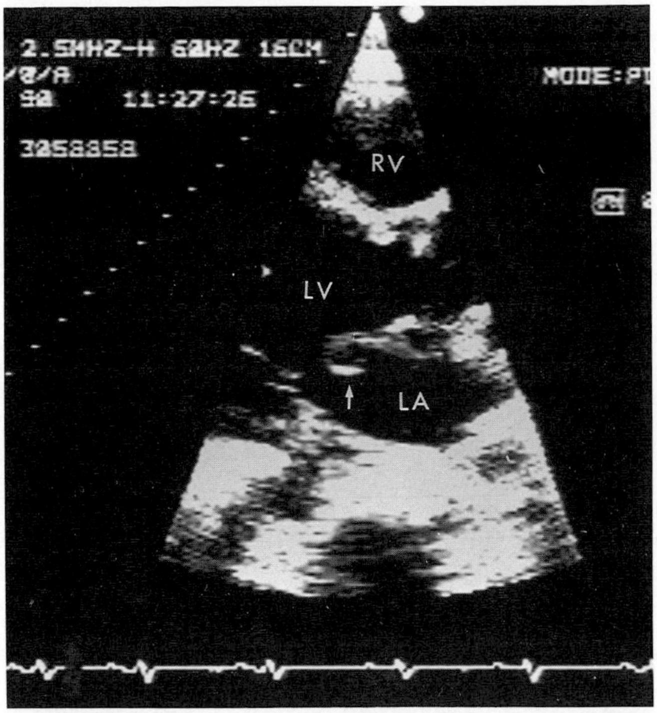

Fig. 37–18. Parasternal long axis recording of a mitral valve aneurysm in a patient with bacterial endocarditis. Arrow, LA = left atrium; LV = left ventricle; RV = right ventricle.

axis view, and a systolic jet of mitral regurgitation can often be seen on color flow recording to originate from the apex of the aneurysm. These aneurysms may be small and are easily overlooked;[55] therefore, the mitral valve should be carefully examined in all patients with aortic valve endocarditis.

Extravalvular Complications

Extension of the infectious process from the valve leaflets to surrounding tissue is an ominous step in the natural history of infective endocarditis.[56] Extravalvular extension may lead to endothelial erosion, perivalvular abscess, mycotic aneurysm, intracardiac fistulas, purulent pericarditis, and a variety of other complications. The nature and severity of these complications depend to a large extent on the valve and on the direction and degree of extravalvular extension.

Perivalvular Abscess

Perivalvular abscess is more common in acute bacterial endocarditis, particularly when staphylococci or enterococci are the offending agents.[57] Perivalvular abscesses often cause a new regurgitant murmur,[56] pericarditis,[58] or high grade atrioventricular block.[59–61] These features increase the index of suspicion for the presence of an abscess but are not definitive in themselves. Two-dimensional echocardiography has been found helpful in the identification and localization of perivalvular abscesses.

Aortic Root Abscess. An aortic root abscess is defined as purulent material contained within the fibrous capsule of the aortic root without intraluminal communication. Aortic root abscess is found in up to 52% of patients undergoing aortic valve replacement for endocarditis.[62–74] In a clinicopathologic, postmortem study, single or multiple abscesses of the valve ring were demonstrated by careful dissection in 86% of patients with treated bacterial endocarditis.[68]

Aortic root abscesses appear echocardiographically either as an echo-free space within the normally continuous echoes from the internal and external margins of the aortic wall[37,75,76] or contiguous myocardial tissue or as an area of increased echo production and thickening of the aortic wall or adjacent septum.[77] Figure 37–19 shows a series of recordings from a patient with a large aortic valve vegetation and evolving aortic root abscess illustrating progression from root thickening to the development of a discrete, echo-free abscess cavity.

Knowledge of the anatomic relation between the aortic valve cusps and adjacent structures is necessary for the successful use of two-dimensional echocardiography in the detection of aortic root abscess or mycotic aneurysm. If endocarditis of a specific cusp is suspected, careful inspection of the adjacent supporting tissues is essential.

Extension of native aortic valve endocarditis occurs in three different directions, depending on the respective aortic sinus involved:

1. From the left coronary sinus and the adjacent portion of the noncoronary cusp, infection usually extends to the base of the anterior mitral leaflet through the fibrous tissue between the aortic and mitral valves (Fig. 37–20).[69] Infection may also spread directly to the relatively avascular tissue bed between the aorta and the left atrium.[70,71] Further extension of the septic process from this region to the interatrial septum has also been noted.[72]
2. Infection involving the right coronary sinus typically extends through the aortic root into the membranous and muscular portions of the interventricular septum, with further extension to the right ventricle or right ventricular outflow tract.[73] Occasionally, a ventricular septal defect may result from rupture of the interventricular septum (Fig. 37–21).[74]
3. From the noncoronary sinus, infection extends toward the posterior portion of the interventricular septum, the right atrium, and occasionally the base of the right ventricle (see also Fig. 37–20).

In prosthetic valve endocarditis, extension of the septic process into adjacent tissue is also possible, and the pattern of spread is similar to that already described for native valves. Infection of the prosthesis usually begins at the sewing ring and extends to involve the adjacent annular connective tissue, however, resulting in loosening of the sutures and dehiscence of the prosthesis. Extensive necrosis of the annular connective tissue results in abscess formation. Both valvular dehiscence and aortic root abscess result in paravalvular regurgitation, a frequent manifestation of prosthetic valve endocarditis

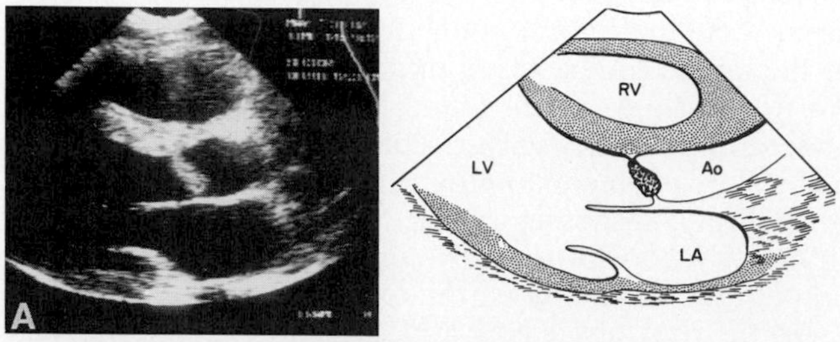

Fig. 37–19. Series of parasternal long axis recordings from a patient with Staphylococcus aureus endocarditis, illustrating the evolution of an aortic root abscess. **A.** Initial recording illustrating the valvular vegetation, with associated thickening of the aortic root extending from the superior portion of the interventricular septum to the sinotubular junction. **B.** Repeat study showing a linear echo-free band within the abscess just beneath the endocardium. **C.** Study recorded several days later showing a discrete echo-free cavity within the root abscess. Progression of the disease occurs despite presumably appropriate antibiotic therapy and clinical improvement. This area underwent postoperative aneurysm formation and rupture (see Fig. 37–22). RV = right ventricle; Ao = aorta; LA = left atrium; LV = left ventricle.

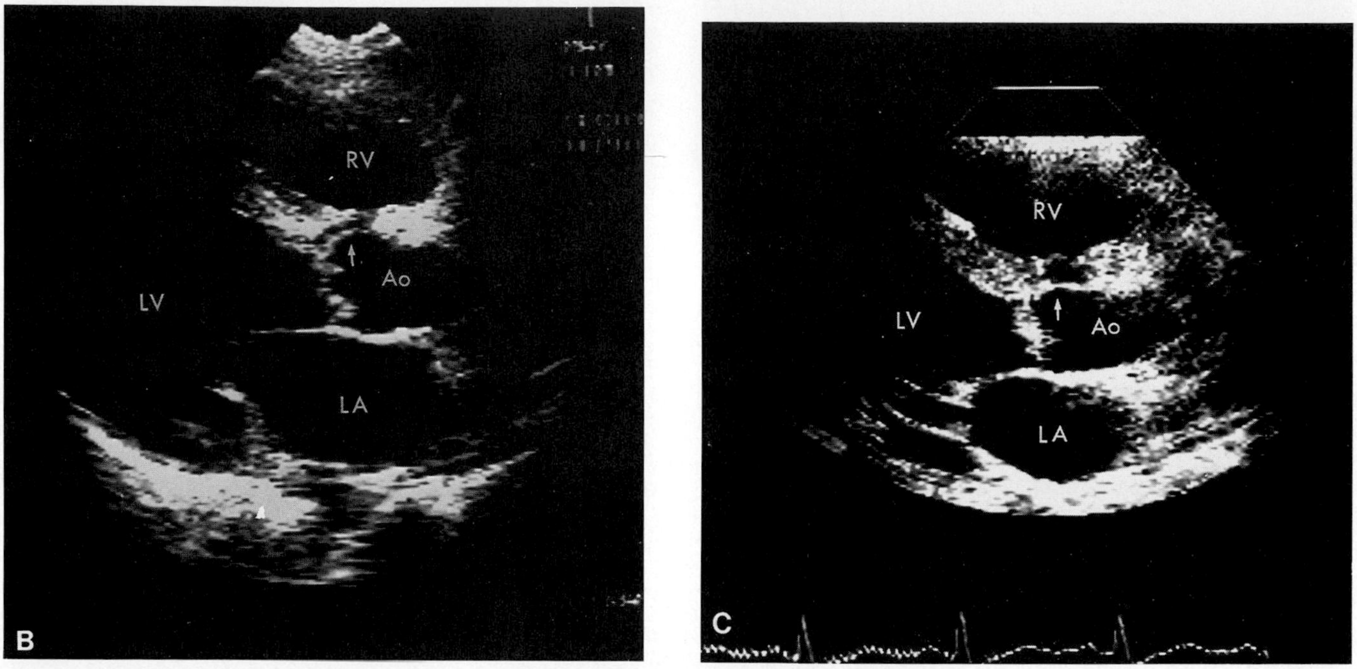

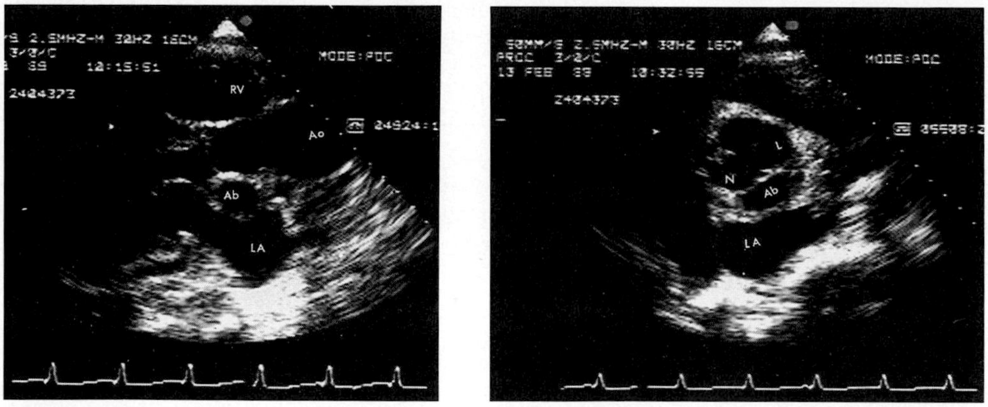

Fig. 37–20. Complicated posterior aortic root abscess in a patient with aortic valve endocarditis. Left. Parasternal long axis view of the aorta in diastole, indicating complicated aortic root abscess (Ab). Right. Parasternal short axis view of the abscess indicating the involvement of both the left (L) and the noncoronary (N) cusps. LA = left atrium; Ao = aorta; RV = right ventricle.

that can be readily diagnosed by color Doppler flow mapping. Localization of abscess or mycotic aneurysm in this setting should be suspected in the area of prosthetic valve dehiscence.[78]

Mitral Ring Abscess. This abscess is less common than aortic root abscess. Mitral ring abscesses appear as round, echo-free, circular spaces in the left ventricular wall behind the posterior mitral leaflet. They are best demonstrated in long and short axis views of the left ventricle.[79] If a valve ring abscess is not diagnosed before surgery, the infection may persist behind the site of attachment of the prosthesis, and significant paravalvular leakage may follow valve replacement.[80]

Septal Abscess. Progression of aortic annular infection into the adjacent interventricular septum results in septal abscess formation, which may be suspected clinically by the new onset of electrocardiographic conduction disturbances.[81] When inflammation and purulent

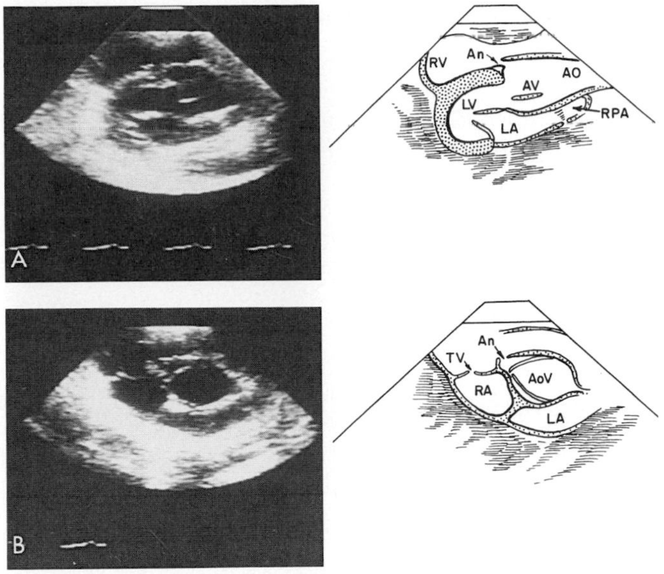

Fig. 37–21. Ruptured sinus of Valsalva aneurysm following Streptococcus viridans endocarditis. **A.** Parasternal long axis view of the aorta (AO) in diastole, indicating the dilated right coronary sinus of Valsalva (An) and a defect in its midportion, creating an aorta-to-right-ventricular shunt. **B.** Short axis parasternal view of the aorta in systole at the level of the aortic valve, again showing the distorted right coronary sinus (An) and the communication from Ao to right ventricle. AoV = aortic valve; AV = aortic valve; LA = left atrium; LV = left ventricle; RV = right ventricle; RA = right atrium; RPA = right pulmonary artery; TV = tricuspid valve. (From King ME, Weyman AE: Echocardiographic findings in infective endocarditis. Cardiovasc Clin 13:3, 1983.)

material extend into the myocardium, the septum appears thicker and more echo dense in the affected area. Echo-free cavities within the thickened myocardium have been described.[82]

Septic material from the mitral leaflets and valve apparatus may seed the mural endocardium by direct extension at other sites along the septum and may lead to abscess formation. Subsequent myocardial necrosis may result in a ventricular septal defect.[83] Spread of infection into the interventricular septum can also be seen in patients with tricuspid endocarditis, particularly when there is extensive leaflet involvement with aggressive organisms.

Mycotic Aneurysm

Most mycotic aneurysms of the heart involve the aortic root, although the mitral valve aneurysms described earlier might also be considered mycotic aneurysms. A mycotic aneurysm of the aortic root is defined as an aneurysm with its origin in the aortic annulus, sinuses, or wall that is caused by an infectious break in the intima, forming a blind sac connected with the aortic lumen. A mycotic aneurysm involving the sinuses of Valsalva is a rare complication of bacterial endocarditis (Fig. 37–22). Mycotic aneurysms are produced by the growth of microorganisms within the aortic wall that results in focal destruction of the media. The microorganisms may reach the aortic wall by embolization from bacterial vegetations or by direct extension from infected aortic valves. Internal rupture of the aneurysm and subsequent development of an intracardiac shunt, resulting in hemodynamic deterioration and requiring surgical intervention, are considered the natural history

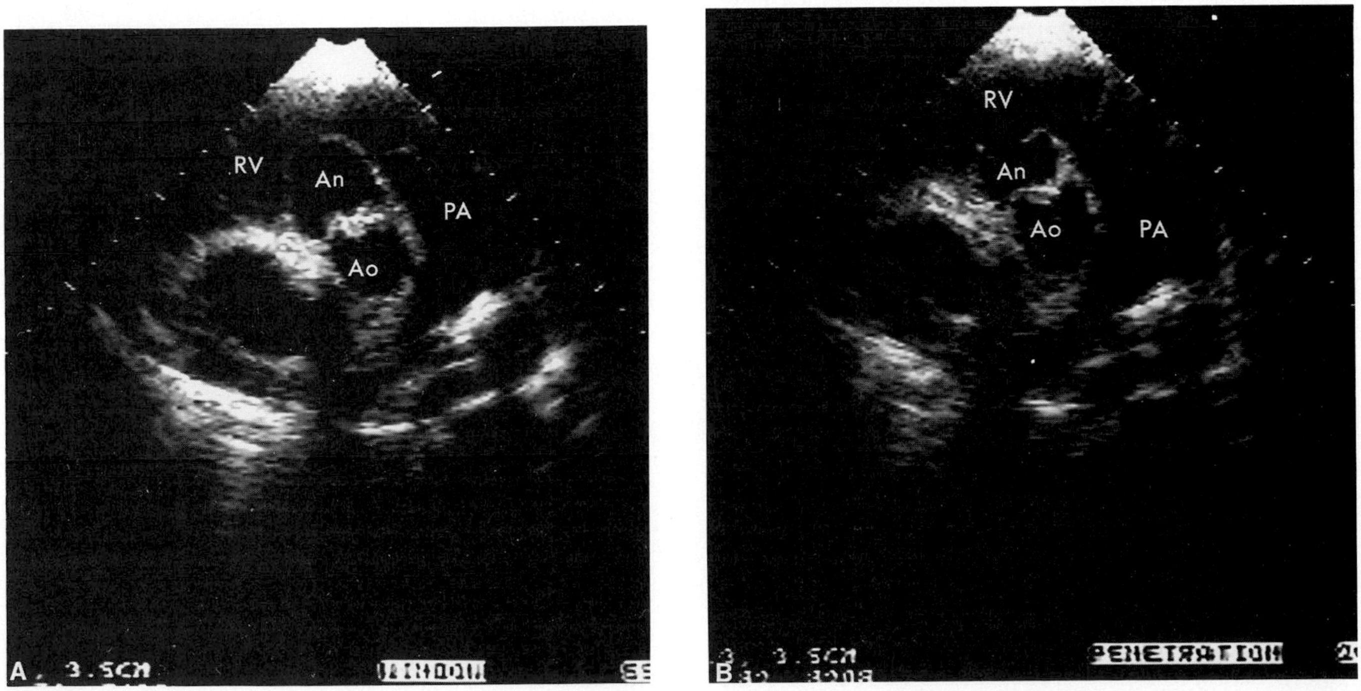

Fig. 37–22. **A.** Parasternal short axis view of the aortic root illustrating a mycotic aneurysm (An) of the right coronary sinus of Valsalva. The aneurysm expands and collapses from diastole to systole. **B.** As the aneurysm collapses, there is a perforation evident at its tip. Ao = aorta; PA = pulmonary artery, RV = right ventricle.

of this disorder. In some cases, however, this rare complication has been diagnosed and clinically followed by serial echocardiographic studies,[84] and thus its presence alone does not always necessitate surgical intervention. Color flow mapping has been helpful in diagnosing aneurysm rupture and the resulting fistulas that become manifest as continuous turbulent flow in systole and diastole.[85]

Intracardiac Fistula

Both aortic root abscesses and mycotic aneurysms may rupture into adjacent chambers and may thereby create intracardiac fistulous tracts. These fistulas may be single or multiple and generally extend from the aorta to the right ventricle, or the right or left atrium. Figure 37–23A illustrates a fistula from the aorta to the left atrium in a patient with aortic valve endocarditis and a flail noncoronary leaflet. Figure 37–23B is a color Doppler recording from the same patient demonstrating the turbulent jet traversing the fistula. In this case, multiple fistulas between the aorta and the right ventricle were also noted. The diastolic aortic-left atrial shunt in this example had the hemodynamic consequences of aortic insufficiency, with the shunt flow passing through the mitral valve rather than directly into the left ventricle. The systolic component had the effect of associated mitral regurgitation. The hemodynamic consequences of fistulas producing left-to-right shunts vary with the site of rupture and the size of the shunt. When rupture is into the right atrium and the shunt is large, all right-sided structures dilate, and the left ventricle is hyperdynamic. When rupture is into the right ventricle or right ventricular outflow tract, the right atrium may be spared unless tricuspid regurgitation is present. Small fistulas may have little effect on right or left ventricular hemodynamics.

Coronary Artery Obstruction

The proximity of the coronary ostia to an infected aortic valve places the coronary circulation in jeopardy, particularly when the right and left cusps are involved. If vegetative fragments embolize to the coronary arterial bed, myocardial infarction can result, which may be electrically inapparent, particularly in patients with heart block and/or bundle-branch block.[57] The new appearance of segmental wall motion abnormalities in such cases may be diagnostic.[86] Obstruction of coronary artery flow in diastole has been reported as a result of occlusion of the ostium by a large vegetation.[5]

Purulent Pericarditis

In acute infective endocarditis, a purulent pericardial effusion can be produced by hematogenous seeding, rupture of a myocardial abscess, or perforation of a mycotic aneurysm.[57] Subacute infections occasionally produce a serous reactive effusion. In either instance, the echocardiogram enables one to identify the effusion, to define its distribution within the pericardial space, and to indicate potential hemodynamic embarrassment.[87] Although an increase in echo density has been reported in patients with purulent effusion, this has not proved to be a reliable clinical sign (see Chapter 35).

INFECTED PROSTHETIC MATERIALS

Because of the characteristic increase in the reflections from prosthetic patch materials, detection of vegetations forming on septal patches or vascular conduits is difficult. If the patient has a discrete vegetative mass with motion distinct from that of the underlying prosthesis, detection is enhanced. Occasionally, infection may disrupt sutures or supporting tissues and may

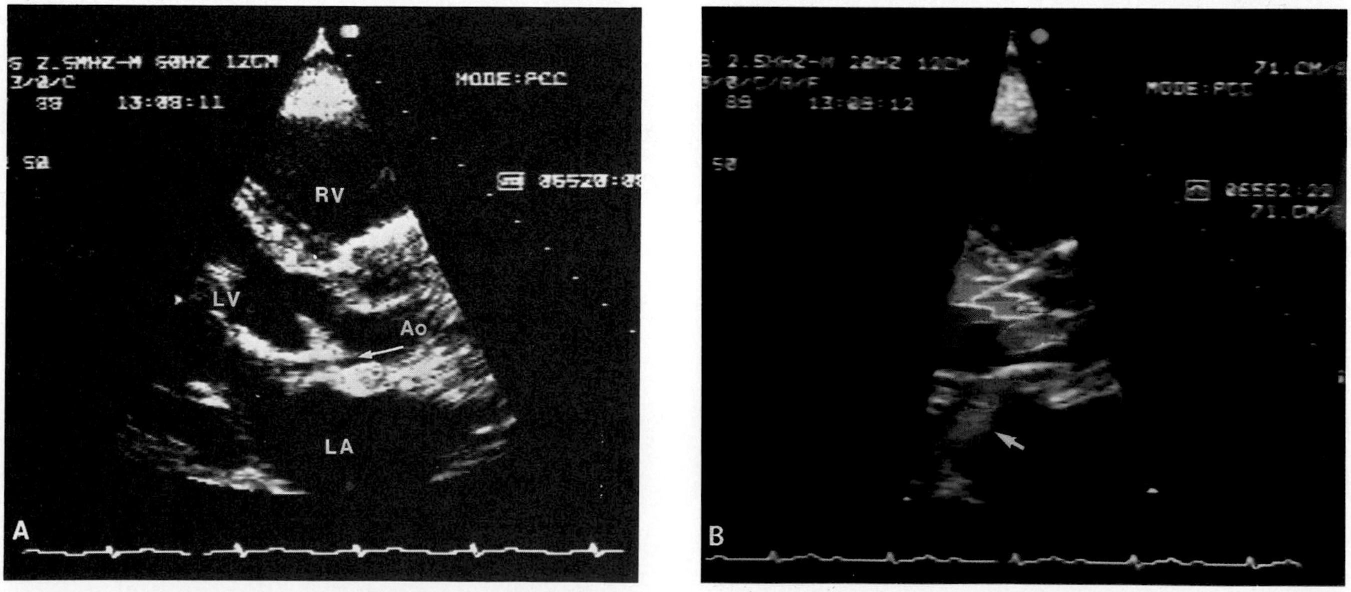

Fig. 37–23. A. Aorta to left atrial fistula in a patient with aortic valve endocarditis: parasternal long axis view depicting the fistulous communication between the aorta (Ao) and the left atrium (LA) (arrow). **B.** Superimposition of color Doppler flow. Again note the fistulous communication between the Ao and the LA (arrow). LV = left ventricle; RV = right ventricle.

thereby allow the patch material to move freely. Abnormal mobility can easily be detected during imaging studies, and patch dehiscence is usually associated with abnormal shunt or regurgitant flow, which can be recorded by Doppler techniques.

CLINICAL IMPLICATIONS OF VEGETATIONS DETECTED BY ECHOCARDIOGRAPHY

Although two-dimensional echocardiography is considered the most sensitive method for detecting vegetations in infective endocarditis, the independent clinical significance of these findings continues to be controversial.

Most available data suggest that patients with clinical endocarditis and echocardiographically detectable vegetations are at increased risk of complications such as systemic emboli, congestive heart failure, requirement for surgical intervention, and death (Table 37–2). Several reports, however, have questioned these findings. Even in studies that clearly indicate that patients with echocardiographically detected vegetations are at increased risk, the incidence of specific complications varies widely (Table 37–2). Much of this confusion appears to relate to the following factors: (1) the relatively small numbers of patients studied in most series; (2) the wide variation in populations of patients (this is suggested by the markedly different overall complication rates among different studies); (3) the nonuniform criteria used to diagnose endocarditis, to define vegetations and to diagnose complications; and (4) the failure to control for comorbid disease that may alter outcome independent of the cardiac infection.

Despite the wide variation in results from individual studies, if the data are pooled and analyzed, patients with clinical evidence of endocarditis and echocardiographically detected vegetations are at least twice as likely to have complications as patients without vegetations (Tables 37–2 and 37–3).

Similarly, although analysis of the morphologic char-

Table 37–2. Echocardiographic Reports on Complications in Infective Endocarditis with Vegetations

		Patients with Complications			
Reference and Type of Study	No. of Patients	Death (%)	CHF (%)	Embolus (%)	Surgery (%)
Roy et al.[9] (1976) M-mode	22	NA	NA	64	63
Wann et al.[19] (1976) M-mode	22	9	100	18	82
Young et al.[95] (1978) M-mode	23	26	78	67	65
Pratt et al.[96] (1978) M-mode	13	NA	100	0	92
Wann et al.[4] (1979) M-mode and 2-D	19	5	55	21	55
Stewart et al.[97] (1980) M-mode and 2-D	47	11	30	30	25
Davis et al.[98] (1980) M-mode and 2-D	17	35	82	47	100
Hickey et al.[99] (1981) M-mode	22	36	81	50	64
Come et al.[100] (1982) M-mode	19	26	53	16	32
Markiewicz et al.[102] (1983) M-mode	7	70	86	29	NA
Stafford et al.[101] (1985) 2-D	45	27	58	47	53
O'Brien and Geiser[103] (1984) M-mode and 2-D	23	23	83	37	65
Buda et al.[88] (1986) M-mode and 2-D	21	24	38	48	43
Lutas et al.[104] (1986) 2-D	43	7	53	26	12
Sanfilippo et al.[89] (1991) 2-D	98	11	21	41	24
Total	343	20	62	36	50

CHF = congestive heart failure; NA = not available.

Table 37–3. Echocardiographic Reports on Complications in Infective Endocarditis without Vegetations

Study	No. of Patients	Patients with Complications: Death (%)	CHF (%)	Embolus (%)	Surgery (%)
Roy et al.[9] (1976)	10	NA	NA	0	20
Wann et al.[19] (1976)	43	0	28	0	0
Young et al.[95] (1978)	36	3	36	13	17
Pratt et al.[96] (1978)	19	NA	11	0	11
Wann et al.[4] (1979)	5	0	0	0	0
Stewart et al.[97] (1980)	40	5	2	10	5
Davis et al.[98] (1980)	13	23	46	15	15
Hickey et al.[99] (1981)	14	14	28	35	21
Come et al.[100] (1982)	27	4	19	7	4
Markiewicz et al.[102] (1983)	18	33	28	17	NA
O'Brien and Geiser[103] (1984)	8	25	50	0	25
Stafford et al.[101] (1985)	17	0	53	12	53
Buda et al.[88] (1986)	29	7	21	14	24
Lutas et al.[104] (1986)	34	12	35	18	21
Sanfilippo et al.[89] (1991)	50	14	16	28	8
Total	363	9	24	12	12

CHF = congestive heart failure; NA = not available.

acteristics of vegetations has not been uniformly helpful in predicting complications, several studies have suggested that characteristics such as size, consistency, mobility, and extent of involvement can be useful in identifying a subset of patients with vegetative endocarditis who are likely to be at increased risk of complications.[40,88–90] For example, patients with vegetations larger than 10 mm in diameter have an increased risk of congestive heart failure, embolic events, need for surgical intervention, and death.[88] Table 37–4 lists reports that relate vegetation size to the occurrence of systemic emboli. Although all studies do not show a significant relationship, the majority of individual reports and the pooled data suggest that risk of systemic embolization is related to vegetation size. One explanation for the lack of statistical significance in some studies is that vegetation size is treated as a discrete variable, that is, the vegetation is either less than or greater than a set value. This approach will not fully address whether the complication rate is directly related to vegetation size. Figure 37–24 illustrates that a linear relationship does exist between vegetation size and complication rate, and supports prior analyses by demonstrating that the majority of complications occur in patients with vegetations over 10 mm.

Although patients with clinical endocarditis and echocardiographically detectable vegetations are at increased risk of complications and require careful moni-

Table 37–4. Size of Vegetation by Two-Dimensional Echocardiography Versus Risk of Embolism

Study	No.	Embolism: Total No. of Emboli	No Vegetation or ≤10 mm	Vegetation >10 mm	p Value
Lutas et al.[104]	76	17	16%(8/50)	45%(9/26)	0.06§
Buda et al.[88]*	42	14	26%(8/31)	55%(6/11)	0.08§
Wann et al.[4]†	21	7	21%(3/14)	57%(4/7)	0.16‖
Wong et al.[109]	31	6	20%(3/15)	19%(3/16)	0.64‖
Jaffe et al.[90]‡	50	10	11%(2/18)	26%(8/32)	0.19‖
Total	251	56	19%(24/128)	33%(30/92)	0.018§

* Excludes patients with right-sided endocarditis.
† Vegetation size graded qualitatively on a 1+ to 3+ scale; 3+ was considered >10 mm.
‡ Excludes patients with an embolism before echocardiography.
§ Chi-square analysis.
‖ Fisher's exact test.
(From Jaffe WM, Morgan DE, Pearlman AS, Otto CM: J Am Coll Cardiol 15:1232, 1990. Reproduced with permission from the American College of Cardiology.)

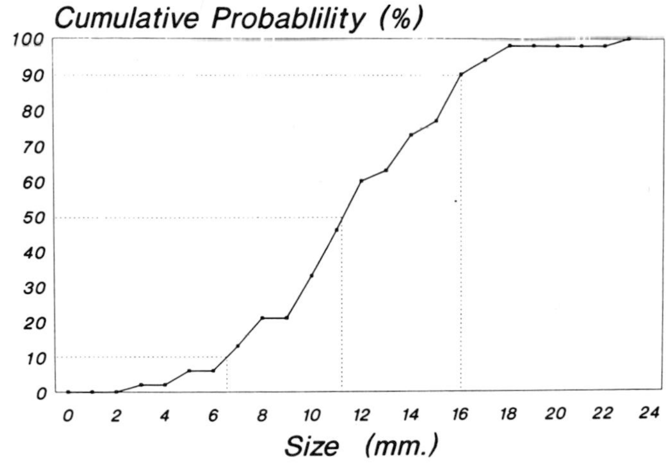

Fig. 37–24. Graph displaying the cumulative occurrence of complications relative to maximal vegetation diameter on transthoracic echocardiogram. It is seen that 75% of the complications in this population occurred with vegetations greater than 10 mm. (From Sanfilippo AJ, et al.: Echocardiographic assessment of patients with infectious endocarditis: Prediction of risk for complications. J Am Coll Cardiol 1991;18:1191. Reprinted with permission of the American College of Cardiology.)

toring, the mere presence of a vegetation, irrespective of its size, does not appear to be an indication for surgery.* Factors other than the presence and size of a vegetation clearly provide important information and may prompt early intervention, however. These include continued growth of the vegetation despite presumably adequate therapy, extension of the infectious process beyond the valve leaflets leading to perivalvular abscess or mycotic aneurysm, progressive valvular destruction and regurgitation, and more rarely, severe valvular or coronary obstruction by a large, critically placed, infected mass. Although the decision to intervene surgically is generally based on the clinical picture, clinical signs and symptoms may be misleading, particularly in well-trained athletes whose vital signs may remain near normal despite profound valvular destruction and in patients in whom endocarditis is superimposed on other disease processes that modify its presentation. Echocardiography, because of its ability to actually show the various complications of endocarditis as well as to permit evaluation of the total hemodynamic burden on the ventricle, can be helpful in timing surgical intervention in these patients.

ROLE OF ECHOCARDIOGRAPHY IN CULTURE-NEGATIVE ENDOCARDITIS

A subset of patients (10 to 25%) with infective endocarditis has persistently negative blood cultures in spite of active infection.[91–93] Excessive mortality has been reported in these patients with abacteremic endocarditis because of delay in establishing the diagnosis and in instituting therapy.[91] Echocardiography, by virtue of its ability to show valvular vegetations and to enable one to define other complications of endocarditis, appears to be useful in the evaluation of culture-negative endocarditis.[94] In one study of patients with abacteremic endocarditis, a correct diagnosis was established using either M-mode or two-dimensional studies in 9 of 11 cases.[94]

Although the sensitivity of echocardiography in the diagnosis of abacteremic endocarditis is not clear, in the appropriate clinical setting, identification of complications such as valve dehiscence, perivalvular abscess, and leaflet destruction can be critical in management of the patient. If the complications are not recognized in time, the needed surgical intervention may be delayed, resulting in increased mortality. In patients with suspected endocarditis without positive blood cultures, one must remember that the absence of an echocardiographically detected vegetation does not absolutely rule out the diagnosis of endocarditis, although it does reduce the likelihood of major cardiac complications.

In conclusion, echocardiography is currently the only noninvasive test that can enable one to detect the presence of vegetations in patients with infective endocarditis. It is reasonably sensitive and specific, and in difficult cases, reliability can be improved by performing transesophageal studies. The application of echocardiography in patients with active endocarditis has provided a better understanding of the natural history of the disease and has enabled the physician to identify complications accurately. Echocardiography can also permit one to identify a subset of patients with infective endocarditis who are at increased risk of complications, including death. In this subgroup of patients, the echocardiographic information, when integrated with the clinical data, can be helpful in timing surgical intervention. In patients cured of endocarditis but with chronic valvular incompetence, serial echocardiographic examinations can provide information about valvular integrity and ventricular function that may prove useful in timing valve replacement.

* An exception may be a vegetation large enough to occlude a major artery (i.e., the pulmonary artery) if it were to break loose intact. This is particularly true of chronic vegetations, which tend to be more rigid and probably should be treated as any other intracardiac mass.

REFERENCES

1. Dillon JC, et al.: Echocardiographic manifestations of valvular vegetations. Am Heart J 86:698, 1973.
2. Schelbert HR, Muller OF: Detection of fungal vegetations involving a Starr-Edwards mitral prosthesis by means of ultrasound. Vasc Surg 6:20, 1972.
3. Spangler RD, et al.: Echocardiographic demonstration of bacterial vegetations in active infective endocarditis. J Clin Ultrasound 1:126, 1973.
4. Wann LS, et al.: Comparison of M-mode and cross-sectional echocardiography in infective endocarditis. Circulation 60:728, 1979.
5. Gilbert BW, et al.: Two-dimensional echocardiographic assessment of vegetative endocarditis. Circulation 55:346, 1977.
6. Stafford A, et al.: Serial echocardiographic appearance of healing bacterial vegetations. Am J Cardiol 44:754, 1979.
7. Gura GM, Tajik AJ: Clinical usefulness of echocardiography in infective endocarditis. *In* Yu PN, Goodwin JF (eds.): Progress in Cardiology. Vol. 7. Philadelphia, Lea & Febiger, 1979.
8. Andy JJ, et al.: Echocardiographic observations in opiate addicts with active infective endocarditis. Am J Cardiol 40:17, 1977.
9. Roy P, et al.: Spectrum of echocardiographic findings in bacterial endocarditis. Circulation 53:474, 1976.
10. Lepeschkin E: On the relation between the site of valvular involvement in endocarditis and the blood pressure resting on the valve. Am J Med Sci 224:318, 1952.
11. Watanakunakorn C: Changing epidemiology and newer aspects of infective endocarditis. Adv Intern Med 22:21, 1977.

12. Pelletier LL Jr, Petersdorf RG: Infective endocarditis: a review of 125 cases from the University of Washington Hospitals, 1963–72. Medicine 56: 287, 1977.
13. Richardson JV, Karp RB, Kirklin JW, Dismukes WE: Treatment of infective endocarditis: a 10 year comparative analysis. Circulation 58:589, 1978.
14. Boyd AD, et al.: Infective endocarditis, an analysis of 54 surgically treated patients. J Thorac Cardiovasc Surg 73:23, 1977.
15. Lerner PI, Weinstein L: Infective endocarditis in the antibiotic era. N Engl J Med 274:199, 388, 1966.
16. Kelson SR, White PD: Notes on 250 cases of subacute bacterial (streptococcal) endocarditis studied and treated between 1927 and 1939. Ann Intern Med 22:40, 1945.
17. Roberts WC: The congenitally bicuspid aortic valve: a study of 85 autopsy cases. Am J Cardiol 26:72, 1970.
18. Braunwald E: Heart disease: A Text Book of Cardiovascular Medicine. Philadelphia, W.B. Saunders, 1980.
19. Wann LS, et al.: Echocardiography in bacterial endocarditis. N Engl J Med 295:135, 1976.
20. Gregoratos G, Karliner JS: Infective endocarditis: diagnosis and management. Med Clin North Am 63:173, 1979.
21. Pridie RB, Oakley CM: Echocardiographic evaluation of the mitral valve. Prog Cardivasc Dis 21:92, 1978.
22. Alam M, Lewis JW, Pickard SD, Goldstein S: Echocardiographic features of mitral obstruction due to bacterial endocarditis. Chest 76:331, 1979.
23. Chandraratna PAN, Langevin E: Limitations of the echocardiogram in diagnosing valvular vegetations in patients with mitral valve prolapse. Circulation 56:436, 1977.
24. Bain RC, et al.: Right-sided bacterial endocarditis and endoarteritis. Am J Med 24:98, 1958.
25. Roberts WC, Buchbinder NA: Right-sided valvular infective endocarditis: a clinicopathologic study of twelve patients. Am J Med 53:7, 1972.
26. Banks T, Fletcher R, Ali N: Infective endocarditis in heroin addicts. Am J Med 55:444, 1973.
27. Wright JS, Glennie JS: Excision of tricuspid valve with later replacement in endocarditis of drug addiction. Thorax 33:518, 1978.
28. Come PC, Kurland GS, Vine HS: Two-dimensional echocardiography in differentiating right atrial and tricuspid valve mass lesions. Am J Cardiol 44:1207, 1979.
29. Nakamura K, et al.: Clinical and echocardiographic features of pulmonary valve endocarditis. Circulation 67:198, 1983.
30. Berger M, et al.: Two-dimensional echocardiographic findings in right-sided infective endocarditis. Circulation 61:855, 1980.
31. Sheikh MU, et al.: Right-sided infective endocarditis: an echocardiographic study. Am J Med 66:283, 1979.
32. Berger M, et al.: M-mode and two-dimensional echocardiographic findings in pulmonic valve endocarditis. Am Heart J 107:391, 1984.
33. Aziz KN, Newfeld EA, Paul MH: Echocardiographic detection of bacterial vegetations in a child with ventricular septal defect. Chest 70:780, 1976.
34. Arnett EN, Roberts WC: Prosthetic valve endocarditis: clinicopathological analysis of 22 necropsy patients with comparison of observations in 74 necropsy patients with active infective endocarditis involving natural left-sided cardiac valves. Am J Cardiol 38:281, 1976.
35. Schapira JN, et al.: Two-dimensional echocardiographic assessment of patients with bioprosthetic valves. Am J Cardiol 43:510, 1979.
36. Effron MK, Popp RR: Two-dimensional echocardiographic assessment of bioprosthetic valve dysfunction and infective endocarditis. J Am Coll Cardiol 2:597, 1983.
37. Mintz GS, et al.: Comparison of two-dimensional and M-mode echocardiography in the evaluation of patients with infective endocarditis. Am J Cardiol 43:738, 1979.
38. Strom J, et al.: Echocardiographic and surgical correlations in bacterial endocarditis. Circulation 62(Suppl. I):164, 1981.
39. Erbel R, et al.: Improved diagnostic value of echocardiography in patients with infective endocarditis by trans-esophageal approach: a prospective study. Eur Heart J 9:43, 1988.
40. Mügge A, Daniel WG, Frank G, Lichtlen PR: Echocardiography in infective endocarditis: reassessment of prognostic complications of vegetation size determined by the transthoracic and transesophageal approach. J Am Coll Cardiol 14:631, 1989.
41. Thomson KR, Nanda N, Gramiak R: The reliability of echocardiography in the diagnosis of infective endocarditis. Radiology 125:473, 1977.
42. Tak T, et al.: Value of digital image processing of two dimensional echocardiograms in differentiating active from chronic vegetations of infective endocarditis. Circulation 78:116, 1988.
43. Mills J, Utley J, Abbott J: Heart failure in infective endocarditis: predisposing factors, course, and treatment. Chest 66:151, 1974.
44. Wray TM: Echocardiographic manifestations of flail aortic valve leaflets in bacterial endocarditis. Circulation 51:832, 1975.
45. Winsberg F: Aortic valve. *In* Cardiac Ultrasound. St. Louis, C.V. Mosby, 1975.
46. Pridie RB, Beham R, Oakley CM: Echocardiography of the mitral valve in aortic valve disease. Br Heart J 33:296, 1971.
47. Botvinick EH, et al.: Echocardiographic demonstration of early mitral valve closure in severe aortic insufficiency: its clinical implications. Circulation 51:836, 1975.
48. Mann T, McLaurin L, Grossman W, Craige E: Assessing the hemodynamic severity of acute aortic regurgitation due to infective endocarditis. N Engl J Med 293:108, 1975.
49. Child JS, et al.: M-mode and cross-sectional echocardiographic features of flail posterior mitral leaflets. Am J Cardiol 44:1383, 1979.
50. Mintz GS, et al.: Two-dimensional echocardiographic recognition of ruptured chordae tendineae. Circulation 57:244, 1978.
51. Saphir O, Leroy EP: True aneurysms of mitral valve in subacute bacterial endocarditis. Am J Pathol 24:83, 1948.
52. Morgan WL, Bland EF: Bacterial endocarditis in the antibiotic era. Circulation 19:753, 1959.
53. Maclean N, Macdonald MK: Aneurysm of the mitral valve in subacute bacterial endocarditis. Br Heart J 19:550, 1957.
54. Hoffman FG, Robinson JJ: Aneurysm of the mitral valve associated with bacterial endocarditis. Am Heart J 63:826, 1962.
55. Reid CL, Chandraratna AN, Harrison E: Mitral valve aneurysm: clinical features, echocardiographic-pathologic correlations. J Am Coll Cardiol 2: 460, 1983.
56. Arnett NE, Roberts WC: Valve ring abscess in active infective endocarditis. Circulation 54:140, 1976.
57. Weinstein L: Infective endocarditis. *In* Braunwald E (ed.): Heart Disease: A Textbook of Cardiovascular Medicine. Philadelphia, W.B. Saunders, 1980.
58. Utley JR, Mills J: Annular erosion and pericarditis: complications of endocarditis of the aortic root. J Thorac Cardiovasc Surg 64:76, 1972.
59. Meshel JC, Wachtel HL, Graham J: Bacterial endocarditis presenting as heart block. Am J Med 48:254, 1970.
60. Kleid JJ, et al.: Heart block complicating bacterial endocarditis. Chest 46: 939, 1972.
61. Wang K, Goberl F, Gleason DF, Edwards JE: Complete heart complicating bacterial endocarditis. Circulation 46:939, 1972.
62. Hudson REB: Infective endocarditis: aneurysm. *In* Cardiovascular Pathology. Vol. 2. London, Edward Arnold, p. 1191, 1965.
63. Nelson RJ, Harley DP, French WJ, Bayer AS: Favorable ten-year experience with valve procedures for active infective endocarditis. J Thorac Cardiovasc Surg 87:493, 1984.
64. Stinson EB, Copeland JG, Shaumway NE: Operative treatment of active endocarditis. J Thorac Cardiovasc Surg 71:659, 1976.
65. Syonbas PN, et al.: Immediate and long-term outlook for valve replacement in acute bacterial endocarditis. Ann Surg 195:721, 1982.
66. Mammana RB, et al.: Valve replacement for left-sided endocarditis in drug addicts. Ann Thorac Surg 35:431, 1983.
67. Arnett EN, Roberts WC: Valve ring abscess in active infective endocarditis: frequency, location, and clues to clinical diagnosis from the study of 95 necropsy patients. Circulation 54:140, 1976.
68. Sheldon WH, Golden A: Abscesses of the valve rings of the heart, frequent but not well recognized complication of acute bacterial endocarditis. Circulation 4:1, 1951.
69. Gonzales-Lavin L, Scappatura E, Lise M, Ross DN: Mycotic aneurysms of the aortic root: a complication of aortic valve endocarditis. Ann Thorac Surg 9:551, 1970.
70. Chesler E, et al.: False aneurysm of the left ventricle secondary to bacterial endocarditis with perforation of the mitral-aortic intervalvular fibrosa. Circulation 37:518, 1968.
71. Pirani CL: Erosive (mycotic) aneurysm of the heart with rupture. Arch Pathol 36:579, 1943.
72. Holt S, Martinez AA, Coulshed N: Interatrial abscess. Postgrad Med J 55: 207, 1979.
73. Fox S, Kotler MN, Segal BL, Parry W: Echocardiographic diagnosis of acute aortic valve endocarditis and its complications. Arch Intern Med 137:85, 1977.
74. Mansur AJ, et al.: Acquired ventricular septal defect and tricuspid valve disruption as a complication of infective endocarditis of the aortic valve. J Cardiovasc Surg 24:669, 1983.
75. Mardelli TJ, et al.: Cross-sectional echocardiographic detection of aortic ring abscess in bacterial endocarditis. Chest 74:576, 1978.
76. Scanlan JG, Seward JB, Tajik AJ: Valve ring abscess in infective endocarditis: visualization with wide angle two-dimensional echocardiography. Am J Cardiol 49:1794, 1982.
77. Come PC, Riley FM: Echocardiographic recognition of perivalvular infection complicating aortic bacterial endocarditis. Am Heart J 108:166, 1984.
78. Ellis SG, Goldstein J, Popp RL: Detection of endocarditis associated perivalvular abscesses by two dimensional echocardiography. J Am Coll Cardiol 5:647, 1985.
79. Nakamura K, et al.: Detection of mitral ring abscess by two-dimensional echocardiography. Circulation 65:816, 1982.
80. Crosby JK, Carrell R, Reed WA: Operative management of valvular complications of bacterial endocarditis. J Thorac Cardiovasc Surg 64:235, 1972.
81. Roberts NK, Somerville J: Pathological significance of electrocardiographic changes in aortic valve endocarditis. Br Heart J 31:395, 1969.
82. Scanlan JG, Seward JB, Tajik AJ: Myocardial abscess: direct visualization with wide-angle two-dimensional sector echocardiography. Circulation 59,60(Suppl.II):37, 1979.
83. Bierman FZ, Fellows K, Williams RG: Prospective identification of ven-

tricular septal defects in infancy using subxyphoid two-dimensional echocardiography. Circulation 62:807, 1980.
84. Burger AJ, Messineo FC, Schulman P, Geller D: Mycotic aneurysm of the sinus of valsalva due to eikenella corrodens bacterial endocarditis. Cardiology 71:220, 1984.
85. Aragam JR, Kerovac MA, Kemper AJ: Doppler echocardiographic diagnosis of aorto-pulmonary fistula following aortic valve replacement for endocarditis. Am Heart J 117:1392, 1989.
85a. Omoto R: Congenital heart disease. *In* Color Atlas of Real-Time Two-Dimensional Doppler Echocardiography. Tokyo, Shindan-to-chiryo, Lea & Febiger, 1984.
85b. Chia BL, Ee BK, Choo MH, Yan PC: Ruptured aneurysm of sinus of valsalva: recognition by doppler color flow mapping.
86. Heger JJ, et al.: Cross-sectional echocardiographic analysis of the extent of left ventricular asynergy in acute myocardial infarction. Circulation 61: 1113, 1980.
87. Feigenbaum H: Echocardiographic diagnosis of pericardial effusion. Am J Cardiol 26:475, 1970.
88. Buda AJ, Zotz RJ, Lemire MS, Bach DS: Prognostic significance of vegetations detected by two-dimensional echocardiography in infective endocarditis. Am Heart J 112:1291, 1986.
89. Sanfilippo AJ, et al.: Prediction of risk for complications in patients with left sided infectious endocarditis. J Am Coll Cardiol 13:72-A, 1989.
90. Jaffe WM, Morgan DE, Pearlman AS, Otto CM: Infective endocarditis, 1983–88: echocardiographic findings and factors influencing morbidity and mortality. J Am Coll Cardiol 15:1227, 1990.
91. Pesanti EL, Smith IM: Infective endocarditis with negative blood cultures: an analysis of 52 cases. Am J Med 66:43, 1979.
92. Cannady PB Jr, Sanford JP: Infective endocarditis with negative blood cultures: a review. South Med J 69:1420, 1976.
93. Gregoratos G, Karliner JS: Infective endocarditis: diagnosis and management. Med Clin North Am 63:173, 1979.
94. Rubenson DS, et al.: The use of echocardiography in diagnosing culture-negative endocarditis. Circulation 64:641, 1981.
95. Young JS, et al.: Prognostic significance of valvular vegetations identified by M-mode echocardiography in infective endocarditis. Circulation 58(Suppl. II):41, 1978.
96. Pratt C, et al.: Relationship of vegetations on echogram to the clinical course and systemic emboli in bacterial endocarditis. Am J Cardiol 41:384, 1978.
97. Stewart JA, et al.: Echocardiographic documentation of vegetative lesions in infective endocarditis: clinical implications. Circulation 61:374, 1980.
98. Davis RS, et al.: The demonstration of vegetations by echocardiography in bacterial endocarditis: an indication for early surgical intervention. Am J Med 69:57, 1980.
99. Hickey AJ, Wolfers J, Wilcken DE: Reliability and clinical relevance of detection of vegetations by echocardiography in bacterial endocarditis. Br Heart J 46:624, 1981.
100. Come PC, Isaacs RE, Riley MF: Diagnostic accuracy of M-mode echocardiography in active infective endocarditis and prognostic implications of ultrasound detectable vegetations. Am Heart J 103:839, 1982.
101. Stafford WJ, Petch J, Radford DJ: Vegetations in infective endocarditis: clinical relevance and diagnosis by cross-sectional echocardiography. Br Heart J 53:310, 1985.
102. Markiewicz W, et al.: Prognostic implication of detecting vegetations by M-mode echocardiography. Cardiology 70:194, 1983.
103. O'Brien JT, Geiser EA: Infective endocarditis and echocardiography. Am Heart J 108:386, 1984.
104. Lutas EM, Roberts RB, Devereux RB, Prieto LM: Relation between the presence of echocardiographic vegetation and the complication rate in infective endocarditis. Am Heart J 112:107, 1986.
105. Gura GM, Tajik AJ, Seward JB: Correlation of the initial echocardiographic findings with outcome in patients with bacterial endocarditis. Circulation 58(Suppl. II):232, 1978.
106. Strom J, et al.: The demonstration of vegetations by echocardiography in bacterial endocarditis: an indication for early surgical intervention. Circulation 60(Suppl. II):37, 1979.
107. Martin RP, et al.: Clinical utility of two-dimensional echocardiography in infective endocarditis. Am J Cardiol 46:379, 1980.
108. Sewatman T, et al.: Echocardiographic diagnosis of mitral regurgitation due to ruptured chordae tendineae. Circulation 46:580, 1972.
109. Wong D, et al.: Clinical implications of large vegetations in infective endocarditis. Arch Intern Med 143:1874, 1983.

CHAPTER

38

ECHO-DOPPLER ASSESSMENT OF PROSTHETIC HEART VALVES

GERARD THOMAS WILKINS, FRANK A. FLACHSKAMPF, and ARTHUR E. WEYMAN

In 1960, Starr and Harken implanted the first intracardiac prosthetic valves and in so doing began a new era in cardiology.[1,2] During the ensuing three decades, artificial heart valves have proved to be of enormous benefit, improving both survival times and quality of life. Unfortunately, no prosthetic valve currently exists that can be considered a faithful duplicate of the native valve in terms of hemodynamic performance, durability, or freedom from complications.[3] Indeed, prosthetic heart valve implantation can be viewed as the exchange of one disease (e.g., aortic stenosis) for another (i.e., the complications associated with the implanted prosthetic device), and until a "perfect" valve becomes available, all prosthetic valves should be considered palliative in that some type of malfunction can be expected if the implantation time is sufficiently long.

Regular, careful assessment of prosthetic valve function is therefore indicated. Prosthetic valves, however, present several unique diagnostic problems. Standard approaches such as the physical examination, chest radiograph, and electrocardiogram often lack the sensitivity required to assess prosthetic valve performance adequately. As a result, until recently cardiac catheterization was the basis of diagnosis in patients with suspected prosthetic valve malfunction.[4,5] Apart from its invasive nature, this form of investigation is complicated by the risks inherent in passing a catheter across a prosthetic valve,[6] and detailed study may require direct cardiac chamber puncture (transthoracic or transseptal).[7] In the presence of multiple prosthetic valves, the problem is compounded. As a result, invasive assessment of prosthetic valve function has been considered justifiable only when there is a significant clinical deterioration and routine assessment of the adequacy of the hemodynamic result immediately after implantation has been precluded.

Fortunately, echo-Doppler methods now provide the ability to: (1) determine baseline function immediately after valve implantation; (2) monitor valve performance serially over time; and (3) detect dysfunction when present. In this chapter, we present a *systematic* approach to the echo-Doppler examination of patients with implanted prosthetic heart valves, with particular emphasis on those aspects that differ from the routine examination of native valves.

SUMMARY OF VALVE TYPES

The echo-Doppler assessment of prosthetic valves is complicated by the variety and complexity of the prostheses in current use. All prosthetic valves have a sewing ring that forms the foundation of the valve and through which sutures are passed to attach the valve to surrounding tissues during implantation; however, the occluding portion of the valve can vary widely and may be composed of: (1) tissue leaflets; (2) single or multiple discs; or (3) a urethane ball in a cage. The occluding mechanism determines the echocardiographic appearance of the valve and the pattern in which blood flows through it. Therefore, to assess performance, the type of valve implanted must be known or recognized, and the normal appearance, movement, and pattern of flow

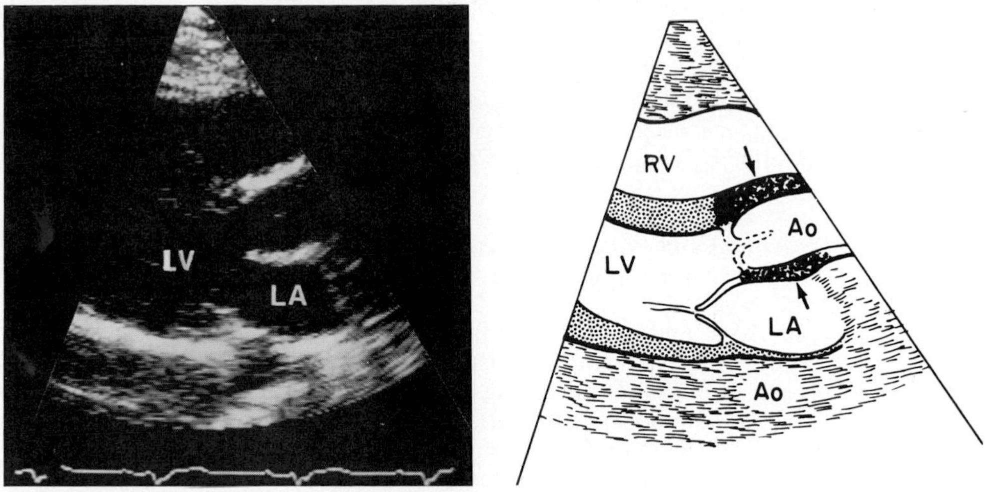

Fig. 38–1. Parasternal long axis view of a homograft valve in the aortic position. There is a slight increase in reflectivity from the anterior and posterior aortic root; however, the valve leaflets appear normal. LV = left ventricle; LA = left atrium; RV = right ventricle; Ao = aorta.

through that specific valve type must be understood. In this section, we describe the most common types of prosthetic valves, the characteristic flow patterns they produce, and the complications with which they are associated.

Biologic Prostheses

Homograft Valves

Human aortic and pulmonary valves have a proved role in prosthetic valve replacement.[8–10] These valves are harvested from cadaveric human hearts soon after death, when the valvular endothelium is still viable. In the past, the excised valve was generally prepared for implantation by storage in an antibiotic solution.[10] More recently, cryopreservation has become more common.[11] Implantation can be performed in two ways: stented or free sewn (unstented). When implantation is into the aortic site, the valve can be sewn into the existing aortic annulus without any additional support. This type of implantation is therefore valve transplantation. If implantation into sites such as the mitral orifice or a conduit is contemplated, the human homograft can be fitted to a stent similar to that used to support a porcine xenograft.

Unstented homografts in the aortic position have an appearance and flow characteristics that are difficult to distinguish from those of a native aortic valve.[12,13] The only evidence of homograft implantation is often an increase in the echo intensity and thickness of the aortic annulus as a result of the retaining sutures (Fig. 38–1). Stenosis of these valves is uncommon, and in the aortic site, eventual leaflet thickening is usually not a feature. Patients with isolated aortic valve homograft implants do not usually receive anticoagulants. In addition, a low incidence of homograft endocarditis is reported.[10] Valve failure is usually from gradually increasing aortic incompetence.[10]

Stented homografts in other sites, particularly the mitral orifice, have not proved as successful; they have a high incidence of failure reported within 5 years because of leaflet thickening, calcification, and the development of regurgitation. Stented homografts have an echocardiographic appearance and central flow characteristics similar to those of porcine xenograft prostheses (see later).

Porcine Bioprostheses

Two types of porcine bioprosthetic valve have been used extensively: the Hancock bioprosthesis and the Carpentier-Edwards bioprosthesis. Although they differ in manufacturing details and design, their echocardiographic appearance is similar, and thus they are considered together. These valves are constructed using a preserved porcine aortic valve fixed to a polypropylene mount and Dacron sewing ring (Fig. 38–2). The valve leaflets are treated with glutaraldehyde, which acts as a tanning agent and significantly reduces their antigenicity.[14] The "treated" valve leaflets are nonviable and become stiffer than their living human counterparts. This type of prosthesis has been used in a variety of intracardiac sites: aortic, mitral, tricuspid, and in valved conduits. Its major advantage is its low thrombogenicity, with the result that patients with this type of valve do not require anticoagulation. Flow occurs through a central, often triangular, orifice,[15] formed by the relatively stiff porcine leaflets opening to accommodate blood flow. This "incomplete opening" becomes more prominent at low flow rates and, when combined with a relatively unfavorable ratio of effective orifice to sewing ring size, can produce significant obstruction. This situation can be a particular problem when use is restricted to smaller valve sizes.[13]

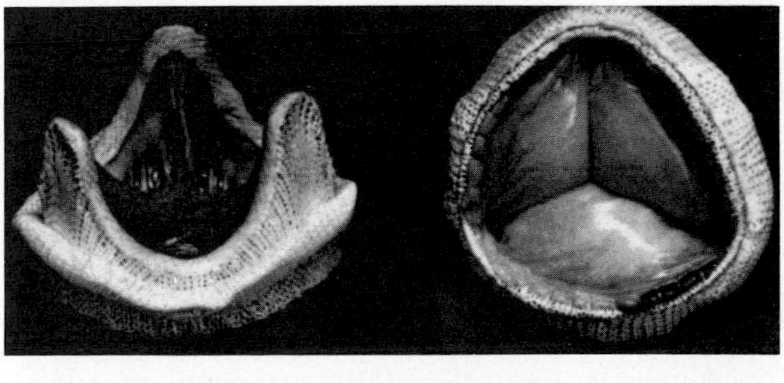

Fig. 38–2. Carpentier-Edwards bioprosthetic aortic valve.

Porcine prostheses cause little or no regurgitation in vitro.[16] In vivo, however, some leakage is reported in roughly 10% of apparently normal bioprosthetic valves.[17,18]

When these valves first became widely available,[19] the apparent advantages of low thrombogenicity and central flow profile led to widespread use. Time, however, has demonstrated some significant disadvantages inherent in this type of prosthesis. The major limitations have been durability and longevity, which are adversely influenced by implantation in young people, site (mitral worse than aortic), and ethnic group.[20–22] Few valves survive beyond 10 years, and replacement in the mitral site is common after 5 years. Dysfunction is usually associated with progressive leaflet thickening and calcification. As this process advances, the leaflets become more rigid and eventually develop fractures and tears or progressive stenosis. The degenerative process appears accelerated in valves in the mitral position because of the greater "backpressure" between the left ventricle and left atrium in systole, compared to that between the aorta and the left ventricle in diastole. It is postulated that the accelerated rate of failure in young patients is a reflection of their more active immune response to foreign (porcine) tissue.[23] The risk of bioprosthetic endocarditis involving either the leaflets or the sewing ring continues throughout the implanted life of the valve.[24]

Newer, "second generation," porcine prostheses are now available (e.g., Hancock II). These valves undergo preservation at lower pressures and with agents that should reduce the rate of calcification and primary tissue failure.[25] Additionally, a modification allowing the porcine leaflets to be mounted above the sewing ring (suprastent) allows a larger effective orifice in the smaller prostheses and thus better hemodynamic performance (mainly applicable to the aortic site).

Bovine Pericardial and Other Bioprosthetic Valves

Valves of this type are similar to porcine bioprostheses, except the leaflets are fashioned from some other biologic material such as bovine pericardium. The most commonly used valve of this type is the Ionescu-Shiley valve.[26] This prosthesis has three vertical stents rising from a circular base and sewing ring. Three "aortic leaflets" of bovine pericardium are then shaped and attached. The final appearance is not unlike a normal human aortic valve (Fig. 38–3). These prostheses offer several technical advantages over porcine prostheses. Because the entire prosthesis is constructed, progressive modifications can be made to improve its performance. In addition, the range of sizes available is unlimited, unlike in porcine valves, where the *aortic valve* size of the largest pig is the practical limit. The valve was first introduced in commercial form in 1976. Two common modes of failure appear to occur: abrasion of the pericardial elements at the point of contact with the Dacron-covered support frame and calcification of the pericardial leaflets. Both conditions lead to valvular regurgitation with sudden perforation occurring in the case of abrasions. Calcification also leads to gradual and progressive stiffening of the leaflets and an increasing transvalvular gradient.[27] Structural deterioration of pericardial prostheses leading to at least moderate regurgitation or stenosis appear to occur earlier than in porcine bioprostheses.[22]

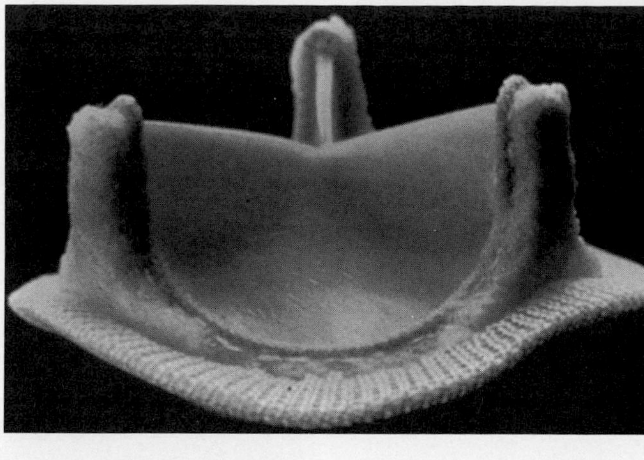

Fig. 38–3. Ionescu-Shiley low profile pericardial xenograft.

Several other bioprostheses have been used experimentally, including aortic valve xenografts from such donor animals as the kangaroo.[28] Valves have also been fashioned from a variety of other biologic membranes including human dura mater and fascia lata,[29] but these have not seen widespread use.

Mechanical Heart Prostheses

Ball-and-Cage Valves

The mechanical ball-and-cage prosthesis was the first type of artificial heart valve to be successfully implanted in man.[2] In the intervening three decades since Starr implanted the first such valve, the Starr-Edwards prosthesis has undergone several modifications, but in concept remains unchanged (Fig. 38–4). The Model 6120

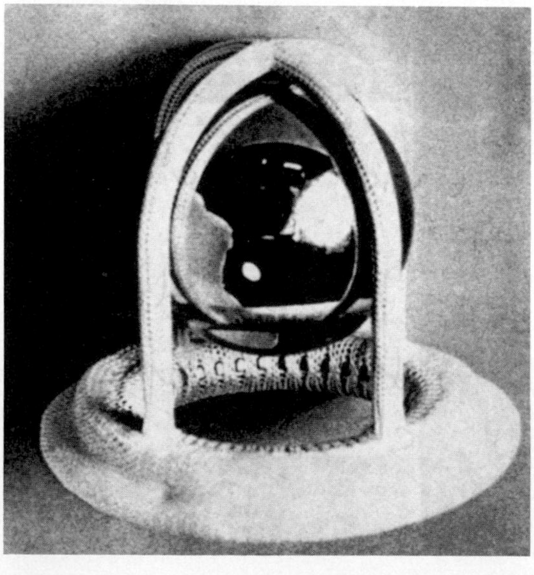

Fig. 38–4. Starr-Edwards ball-and-cage prosthesis.

valve has a circular sewing ring with a double cage formed by two U-shaped arches, crossing perpendicularly. The cage holds a Silastic ball, which is free to move up and down, opening and closing the primary orifice through the sewing ring. Flow through the valve is axisymmetric around the ball (Fig. 38–5). The streamlines of flow converge again downstream from the prosthesis and create an area of stagnant or vortical flow in the "shadow" of the ball. Doppler assessment of flow velocity (Fig. 38–6) must therefore be directed to the margins of the ball where the highest velocities are expected, rather than to the area of stagnant flow immediately behind or in front of the ball.

This valve offers proved durability; many prostheses are still functioning normally more than 20 years after implantation.[30] In the mitral position, the hemodynamic performance is satisfactory when the largest sizes (5M [34 mm] or 4M [32 mm]) are used. The smaller (3M [28 mm] and 2M [27 mm]) sizes are generally avoided for mitral replacement in the adult population. In the aortic site, small prostheses are required but can be associated with significant gradients.[31] The valve is also more likely

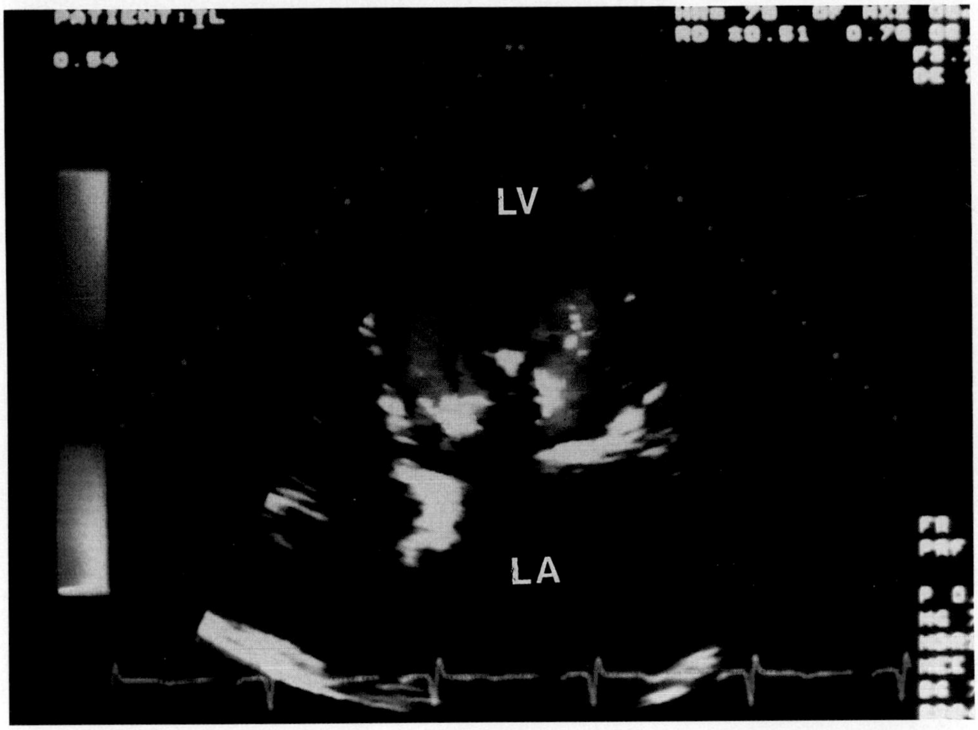

Fig. 38–5. Apical four-chamber, color flow recording of a Starr-Edwards prosthetic valve in the mitral position. Mitral inflow (red) is axisymmetric around the ball occluder. LV = left ventricle; LA = left atrium.

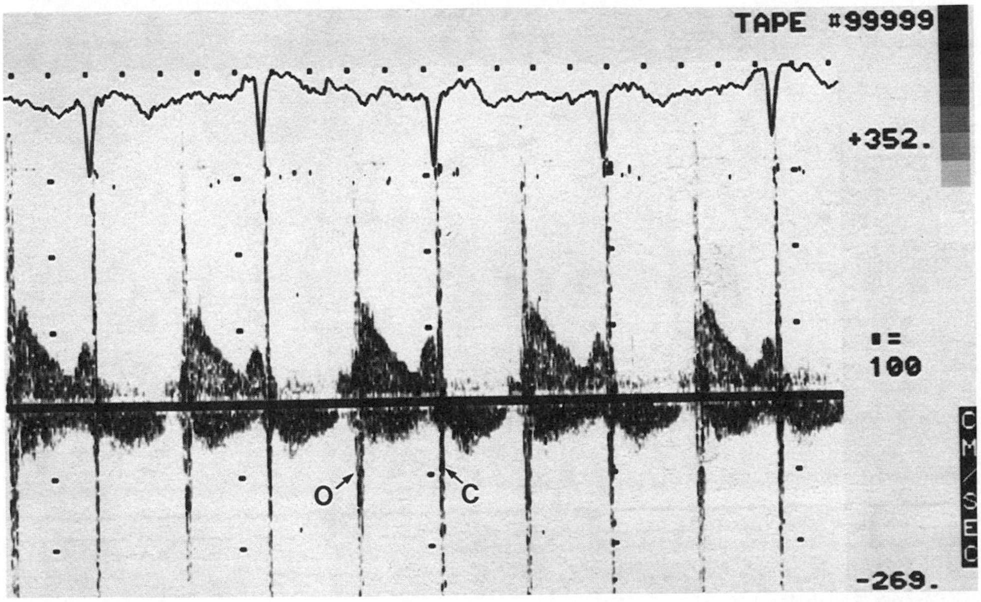

Fig. 38–6. Continuous wave recording of mitral valve inflow. Valve opening (O) and closing (C) clicks are recorded at the onset and completion of each diastolic inflow period.

to cause clinically significant hemolysis in the aortic position.

The Starr-Edwards prosthesis, like all mechanical valves, requires that the patient receive anticoagulants, and there is a continuing risk, even in adequately controlled patients, of thromboembolic events.[30] The valve carries a low incidence of late thrombotic occlusion or mechanical sticking and encasement compared to other mechanical prostheses, however. Implantation can at times be limited by the high profile of the device (the height from the base to the top of the struts). In the mitral site, the valve can affect the interventricular septum, and in the aortic site it can reach well up into the sinuses of Valsalva.

Because the ball fits snugly in the cage, regurgitation is generally restricted to closure backflow (see later).[17,31–33]

Tilting Disc Prostheses

Numerous valves are available in this category. They are best considered as single or double disc prostheses.

Single Disc Devices. Several different valves of this type exist, including the Bjork-Shiley spherical disc, Bjork-Shiley convex-concave disc, Bjork-Shiley monostrut (not available in the United States), Hall-Medtronics monostrut, Lillehei-Kaster, and several others (Fig. 38–7).

Significant manufacturing differences exist among these valves, but we consider them in general terms for simplicity. In principle, these valves are all similar in that they consist of a circular ring of prosthetic material (usually metallic) and a single hinged and mobile disc. The ring acts as both a sewing ring and the orifice of the prosthesis. The disc is attached eccentrically to the ring by the hinge mechanism, so closure occurs by backpressure on the largest portion of the disc. For this to occur reliably, the opening arc of the disc is restricted to less than 90° relative to the plane of the sewing ring (typically 55 to 70°). The flow orifice is therefore complex, consisting of a major and minor orifice,[13,16] with streamlines of flow passing through the sewing ring and then laterally out and around the prosthetic disc (Fig. 38–8).

Because the disc does not lie at a 90° angle to the sewing ring when the valve is fully open, there is, of necessity, a zone of stagnation behind the disc. This area

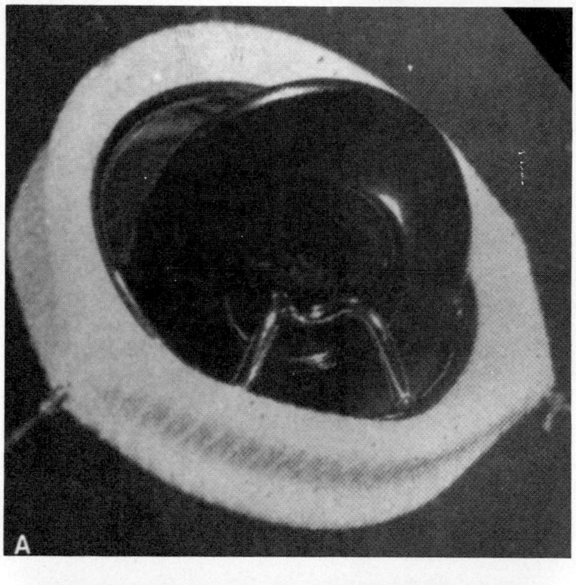

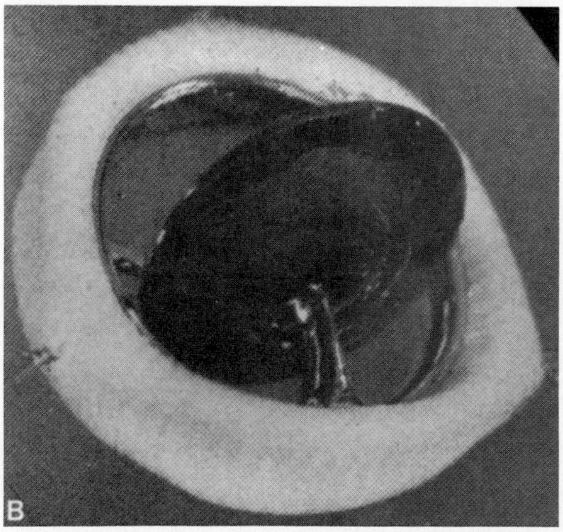

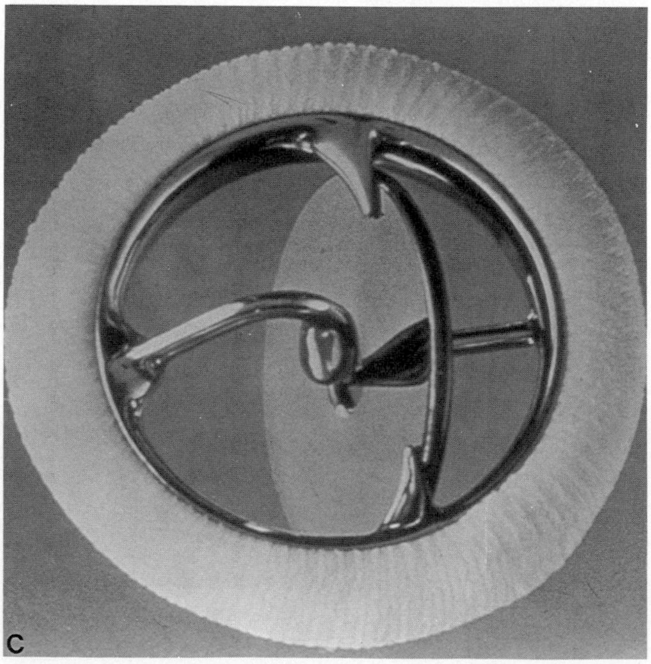

Fig. 38–7. Single disc mechanical prostheses. **A.** Bjork-Shiley convex-concave disc valve. **B.** Bjork-Shiley integral monostrut. **C.** Medtronics Hall.

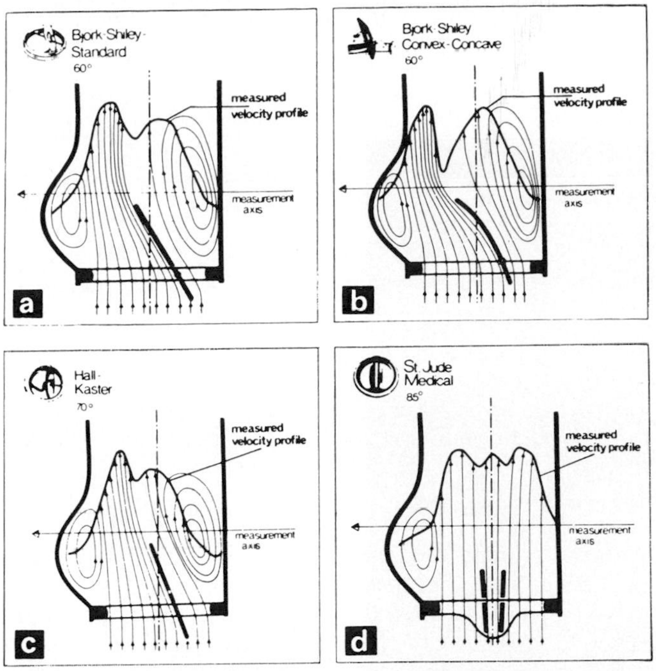

Fig. 38–8. Schematic representation of the velocity fields at t = 180 msec after start of systole, based on the measured velocity profiles. (From Bruss KH, et al.: Pressure drop and velocity fields at four mechanical heart valve prostheses: Bjork-Shiley standard, BS concave-convex, Hall-Kaster, and St. Jude Medical. Life Support Sys 1:3, 1983.)

of stagnation can become the site of thrombus formation leading to the common complications associated with this valve type: acute thrombotic occlusion and thromboembolism.[34,35] Improvements in design have resulted in an increase in the opening arc of the disc and thus in a decrease in the size of the stagnation zone. This should reduce the incidence of valvular thrombosis. Dysfunction can also occur from gradual ingrowth of fibrous tissue (pannus), which can obstruct the inlet orifice or interfere with the hinge mechanism. At times this can lead to intermittent sticking and clinical episodes of flash pulmonary edema. Moreover, the internal diameter of the sewing ring (primary orifice) is not the limiting orifice area through which flow must occur. The effective orifice is a result of the resistance to blood flow produced by the complex dual pathway through and around the disc that the streamlines of flow must follow. In spite of this complexity, the hemodynamic performance of single disc valves is generally satisfactory, especially when larger prostheses are implanted.[31]

Tilting disc valves characteristically leak around the central strut and between the occluding disc and sewing ring. The central regurgitation is predominant, creating a jet perpendicular to the ring plane (Fig. 38–9). If a tilting disc prosthesis is examined from a location (i.e., the esophagus) providing sufficient sensitivity, a large central and two smaller symmetric peripheral jets can be discerned using color flow mapping[35,36] (Fig. 38–10). The amount of leakage relative to the duration of closure has been evaluated in vitro[16,32,36] and in vivo.[17,18,33,37] Regurgitant volumes measured in vitro range, depending

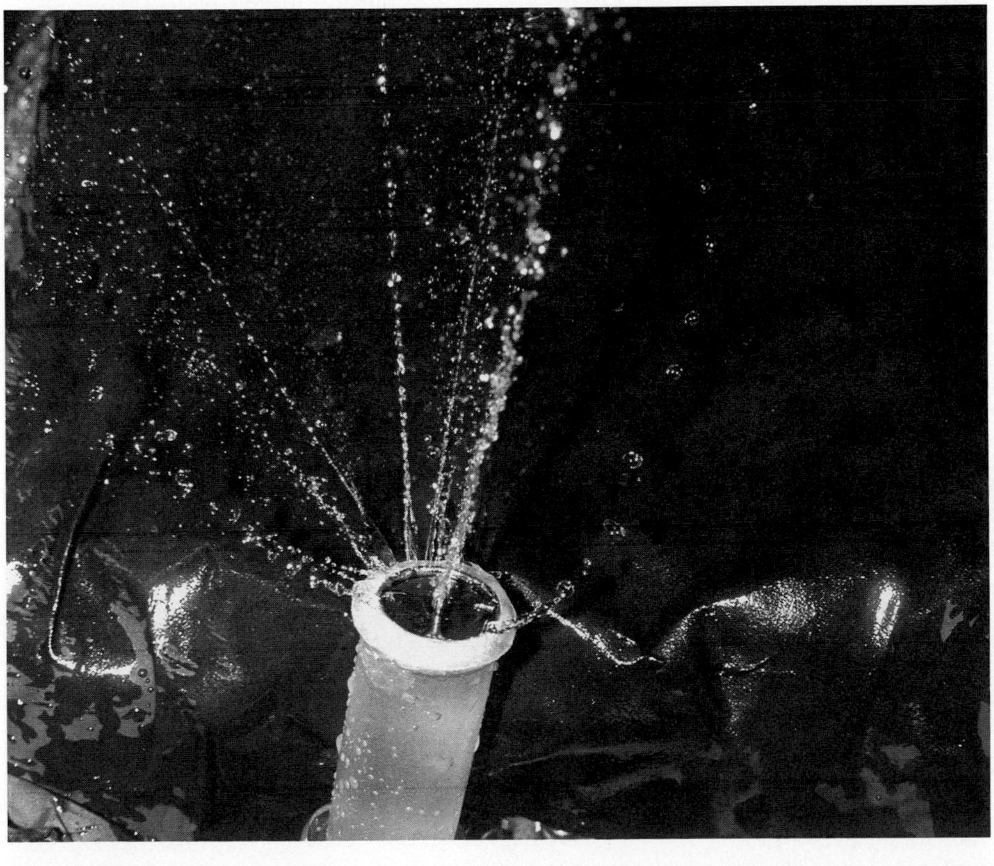

Fig. 38–9. Medtronics Hall valve mounted on a syringe and perfused retrogradely with water. There is one large central leakage jet along with multiple smaller jets around the periphery of the closed disc.

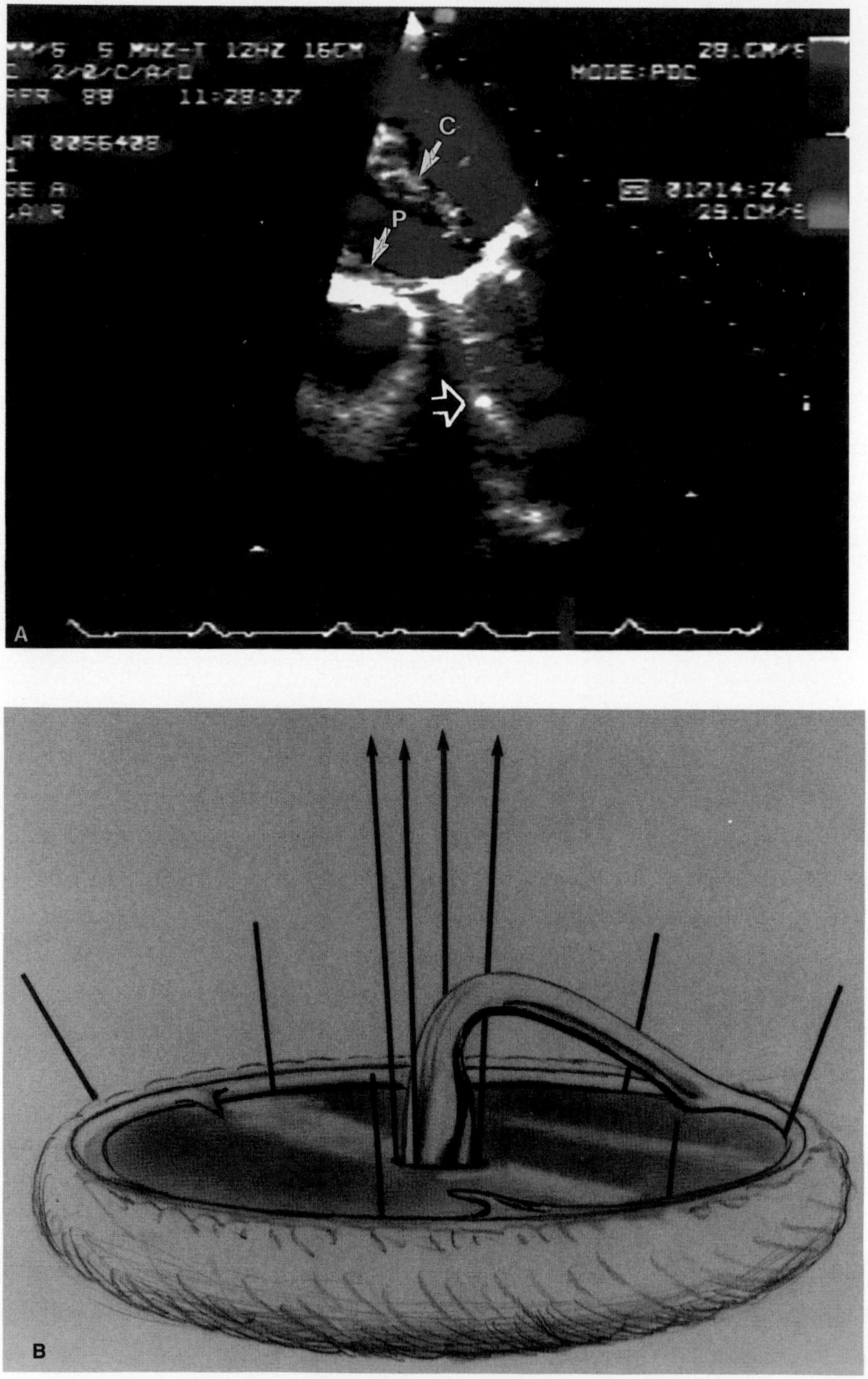

Fig. 38–10. A. Transesophageal color flow recording of a Medtronics Hall valve in the mitral position during systole. Note the large central regurgitant jet along with a smaller peripheral jet directed medially. The lateral margin of the valve is not visualized. There is an extensive area of reverberations in the left ventricular cavity distal to the closed valve (open arrow). **B.** The regurgitant flow pattern within a normal Medtronics Hall valve. P = peripheral; C = central.

on heart rate and cardiac output, between 6 and 16 ml per beat.[16,32] The combination of high heart rate and low cardiac output can result in in vitro regurgitant fractions of up to 37%, although under normal hemodynamic conditions the regurgitant fraction averages only about 12%.[32]

Bileaflet Mechanical Prostheses. The St. Jude medical prosthesis is the most commonly used device of this type. Unlike single disc valves, double disc devices consist of equal-sized, semicircular leaflets attached by a midline hinge (Fig. 38–11). This central hinge configuration results in two large, equally sized, lateral openings and a narrow rectangular slit between the discs in the open position. The hinge mechanism allows the discs to tilt in excess of 80°; thus, the effective orifice of the prosthesis is large relative to the sewing ring. Flow occurs equally through the two large lateral orifices and diverges little (less than 5°) (see Fig. 38–8D). Thus, unlike single disc devices where the streamlines of flow deviate to one side, flow through St. Jude valves is symmetric and along the axis of the valve inlet.[13,16] The large, unobstructed flow orifices, combined with an advantageous sewing ring/flow orifice ratio, result in excellent hemodynamic performance[30,38] (Fig. 38–12).

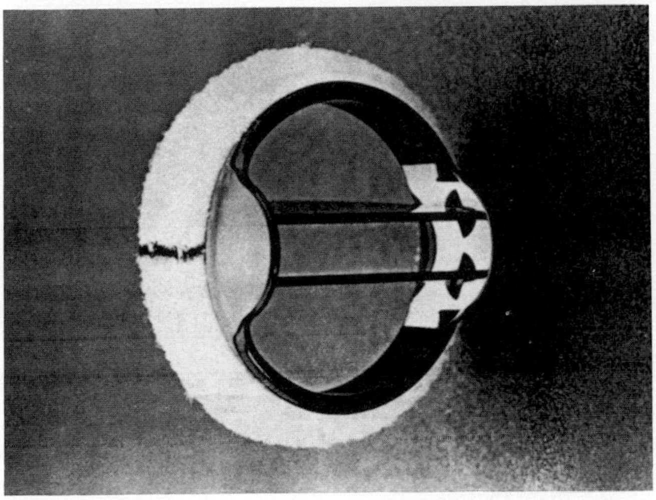

Fig. 38–11. St. Jude Medical bileaflet prosthesis.

The wide opening excursion, however, results in significant regurgitant backflow as backpressure swings the leaflets through their long closing arc. In addition, the St. Jude valve, like all tilting disc valves, normally leaks slightly when fully closed. This leakage occurs between the discs and sewing ring at the periphery and at the margins of the closure line centrally (Fig. 38–13). When viewed by color flow Doppler, the regurgitant flow jets at the disc margins converge toward the center of the valve (Fig. 38–14), whereas those arising at the margin of the closure line converge in planes parallel and diverge in planes perpendicular to the leaflets.[33,36] Anticoagulation is recommended,[39] although the valve probably has a lesser tendency to cause thromboembolic events than other mechanical devices. Valve dysfunction can occur from either microthrombi within the hinge mechanism or excessive tissue ingrowth into the hinge. Generally, this causes the leaflet(s) to stick in a semi-open position and the sudden onset of severe regurgitation.[40] More acute dysfunction around the time of implantation has been reported when loose suture ends or pledgets are not kept free of the valve mechanism, a problem made more difficult by the narrow sewing ring and proximity of the semicircular discs to the margin of the device. Despite these recognized complications, the St. Jude valve has performed well hemodynamically, with low thrombogenicity, has proven durable, and is now one of the most commonly implanted mechanical prostheses.[39,110]

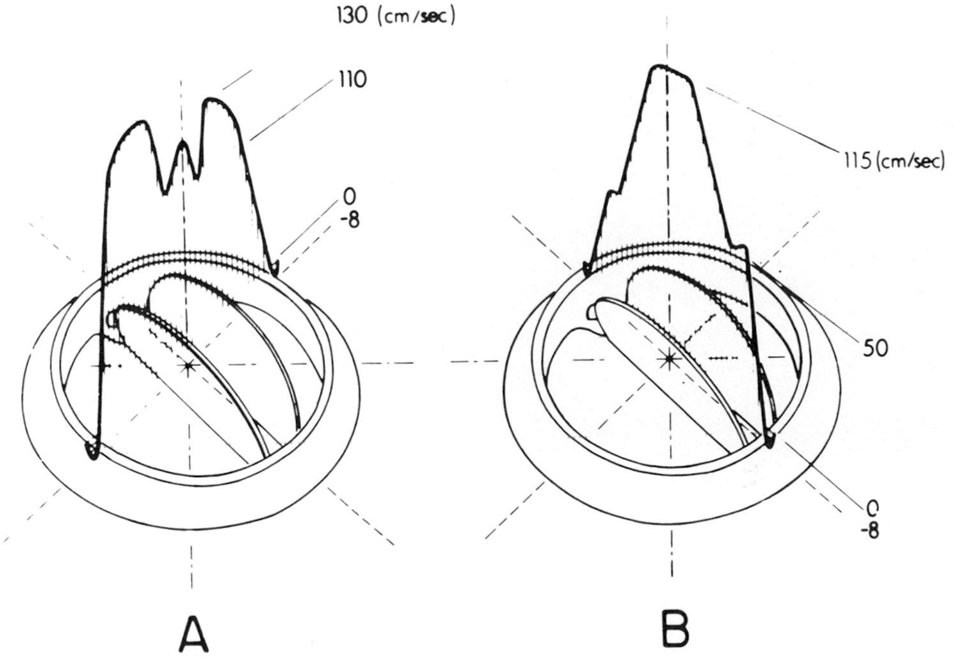

Fig. 38–12. Flow velocity measurements of the size 27 St. Jude Medical prosthesis. **A.** Measurements obtained in a plane perpendicular to the plane of the open leaflets. **B.** Measurement recorded in a plane parallel to the plane of the open leaflets. (From Yoganathan AP, et al.: Bileaflet, tilting disc and porcine aortic valve substitutes: in vitro hydrodynamic characteristics. J Am Coll Cardiol 3:313, 1984. Reprinted with permission of the American College of Cardiology.)

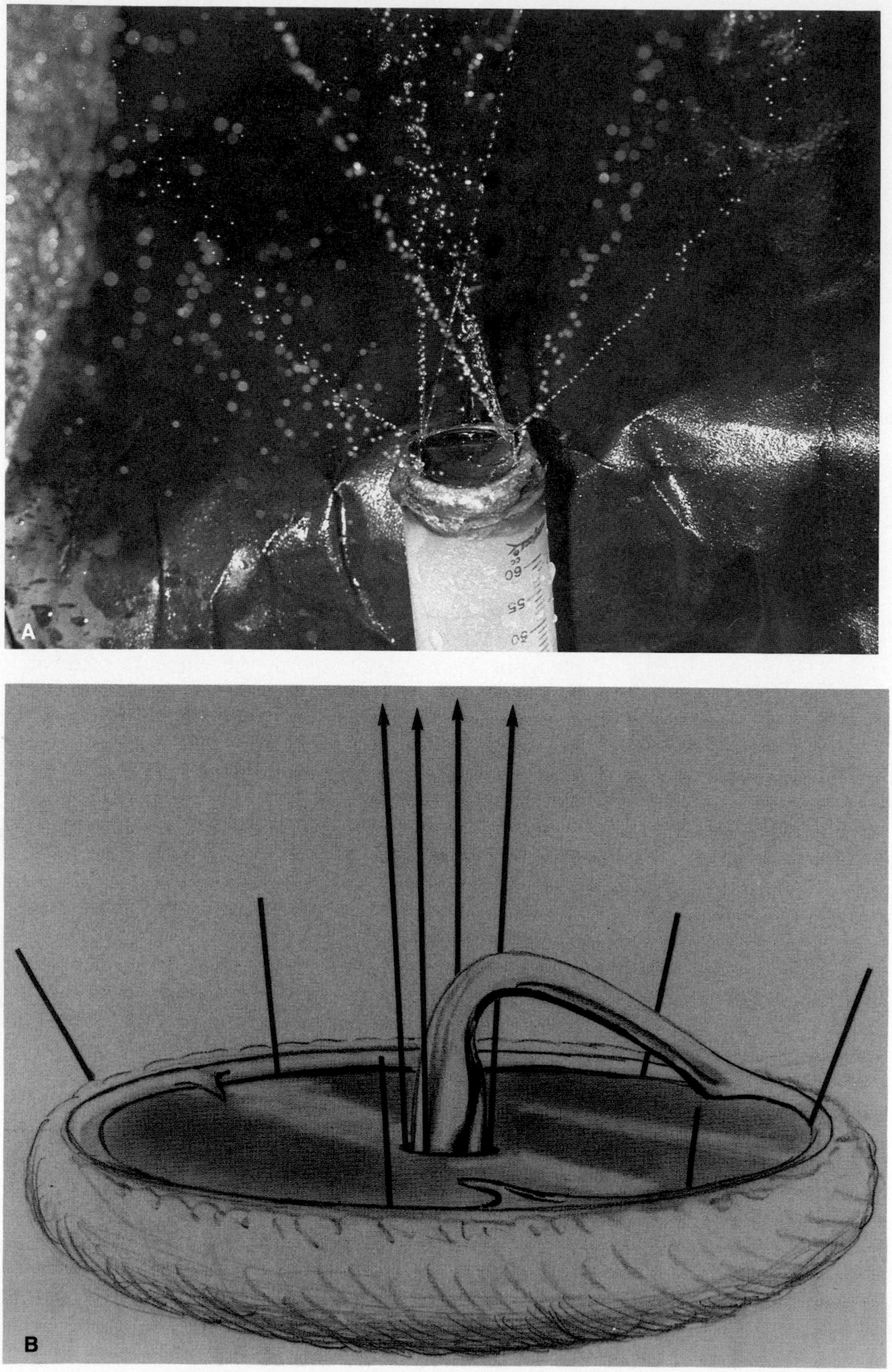

Fig. 38–13. St. Jude Medical valve mounted on a syringe and perfused retrogradely with water. Note the orientation of the leakage jets. (See text for details.)

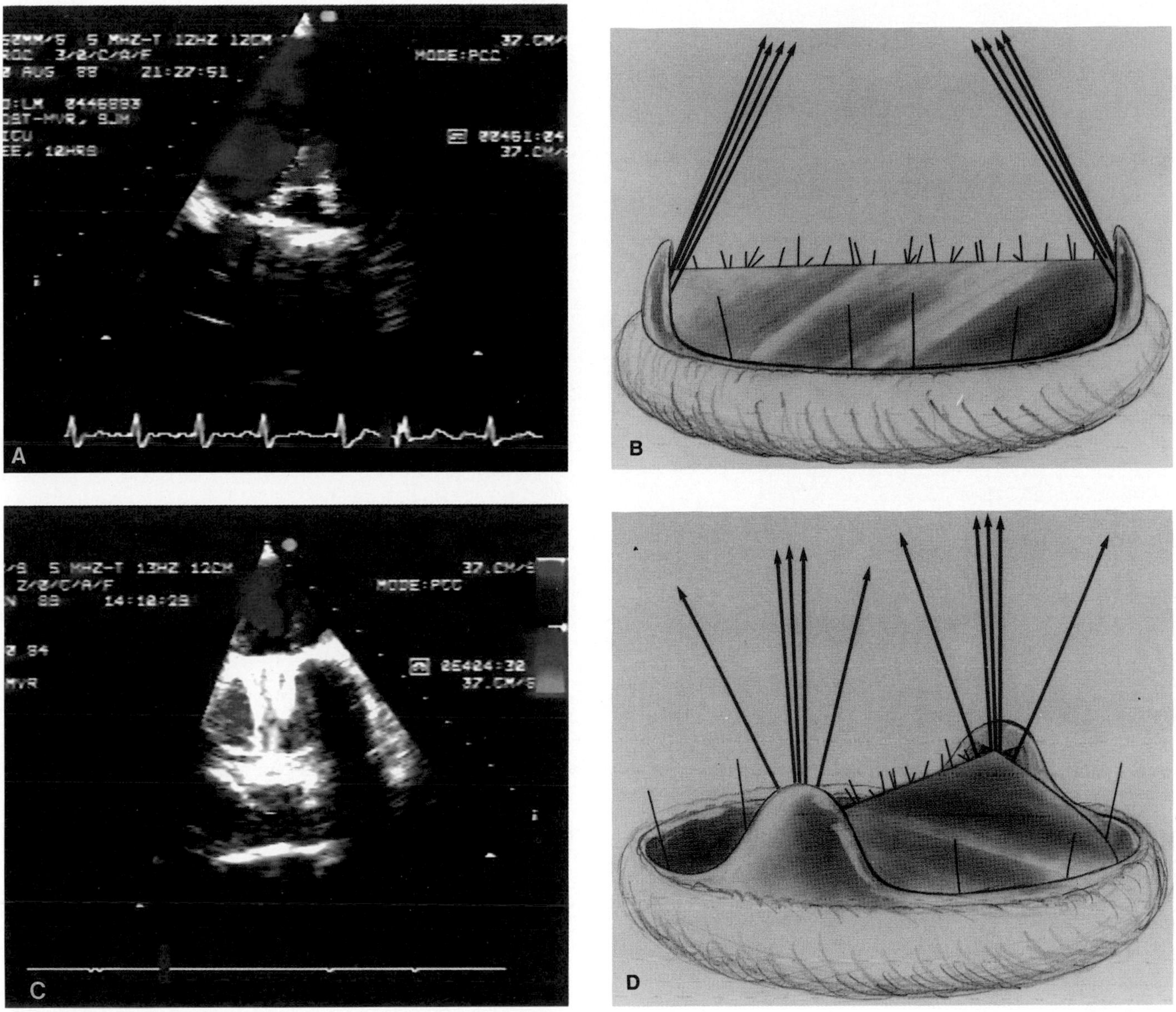

Fig. 38–14. Transesophageal color flow recording of a normal St. Jude valve in the mitral position with accompanying diagrams illustrating the normal pattern of regurgitant flow in planes parallel (**A** and **B**) and perpendicular (**C** and **D**) to the discs. During systole, regurgitation normally occurs at both the disc margins and at the extremes of the closure line. **A** and **B**. At the disc margins in parallel planes, the regurgitant jets converge toward the center of the valve. **C** and **D.** At the closure lIne, jet divergence is noted in planes perpendicular to the discs.

ECHOCARDIOGRAPHIC EXAMINATION OF PROSTHETIC VALVES—GENERAL PRINCIPLES

Imaging

Although the imaging principles described in Chapters 4, 5, and 13 apply to prosthetic as well as to native valves, artificial valves create special problems because the prosthetic materials used in their construction have far different acoustic properties than the surrounding cardiac tissue. For example, the speed of sound in prosthetic materials differs from that in tissue. Because all echocardiographs are calibrated to measure distance based on the speed of sound in tissue, this feature can alter the displayed size and location of the prosthesis and can distort the appearance of its component parts. Prosthetic materials also tend to be more dense than cardiac tissue, increasing their relative reflective and absorptive properties. Increased reflectivity tends to decrease the echocardiograph's ability to resolve the internal components of the prosthesis because of excessive point spreading in the lateral dimension and increased reverberations axially. The intense reverberations behind the prosthesis can obscure structures of interest or may create artifacts that mimic real intracardiac structures (e.g., atrial thrombus). Finally, the marked attenuation of the sound wave as it passes through the valve causes acoustic shadowing distal to the prosthesis, which may obscure structural echoes and Doppler signals from behind the valve (Fig. 38–15).

Several specific measures can be taken to reduce or

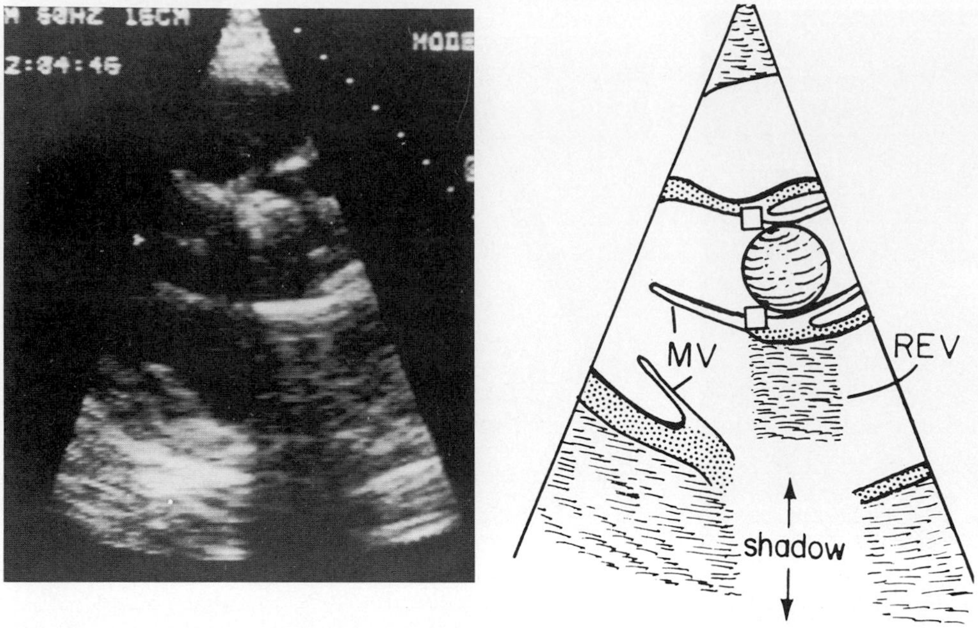

Fig. 38–15. Reverberations and acoustic shadowing distal to a Starr-Edwards prosthesis in the aortic position. The reverberations (REV) appear as a dense band of echoes beneath the valve in the left atrium, whereas the increased attenuation produced by the valve suppresses all reflections from the posterior atrial wall, creating an acoustic shadow. MV = mitral valve.

overcome these problems. First, gain and reject controls generally need to be specifically optimized to image the prosthesis. Often, considerably less overall gain leads to less reflection and reverberation from the nonbiologic components of the prosthesis and a better appreciation of its margins and internal components. When gain is reduced, the normal cardiac structures may be poorly defined, so it is appropriate to image at normal settings first and then to reduce the gain, to concentrate on the prosthetic device.

As with all cardiac imaging, multiple views of each structure should be recorded from the standard imaging planes. The use of multiple views often reveals one plane that allows better imaging of the valve components than others. By sweeping the scan plane gradually across the device, a detailed impression of the sewing ring integrity and the leaflet or disc structures can usually be obtained. No one view can be considered ideal for a specific intracardiac site. For example, the orifice of a disc valve in the mitral position may be best appreciated from a parasternal short axis view, whereas the movement of the disc may be best assessed from a plane originating at the apex.

The problem of acoustic shadowing (failure of sound to penetrate a prosthesis) hampers diagnosis when abnormalities are hidden in the shadow of a valve (Fig. 38–15). If a structure within the acoustic shadow requires careful examination, the best imaging information will usually come from a plane that does not require the sound to traverse the prosthetic valve. For example, examination of the left atrium from the standard apical imaging planes may be difficult in the presence of a highly reflective mitral prosthesis. This examination may easily be accomplished, however, from a high parasternal or, if warranted, esophageal window from which the path of the transmitted ultrasound is unobstructed by the mitral prosthesis. This problem can become more vexing when multiple prostheses are present, and although satisfactory data can usually be obtained from one of the transthoracic windows, in special cases a transesophageal study may be mandatory.

Doppler Examination

Doppler assessment of the pattern and velocity of flow through a prosthetic valve can provide valuable insights into valve function. In assessing Doppler data, however, one must remember that all prosthetic valves are inherently obstructive (Figs. 38–16 and 38–17), and many have some degree of normal regurgitation, so the definition of prosthetic obstruction or incompetence must take into account the complex interrelations among valve size and design, heart rate, and cardiac output.[32] Prosthetic stenosis and regurgitation therefore are more a matter of degree than presence.[31]

The recording of forward and regurgitant flow velocities across prosthetic valves follows the same general principles discussed in Chapter 13 for native valves; however, several characteristics of prosthetic valves must be considered if the same sensitivity and specificity are to be achieved. First, it is critical to remember that the increased reflection and attenuation of the ultrasonic signal caused by any prosthesis has a far greater impact on Doppler velocity recordings than image generation because the inherent Doppler signal/noise ratio is lower. Therefore, care should be taken, particularly when studying mechanical valves, to obtain Doppler data from transducer locations that do not require that the beam first pass through the prosthesis to record the signal of interest. For example, the diastolic flow profile of a prosthetic valve in the mitral position can be recorded from an apical transducer location without the need for the sound beam to pass through the prosthesis first. Regurgitant flow behind a prosthetic *aortic* valve could also be recorded from the same location. To record regurgitant flow behind a *mitral* prosthesis from the apex, however, would require that the beam pass through the valve, resulting in a significant loss of sensitivity. As a

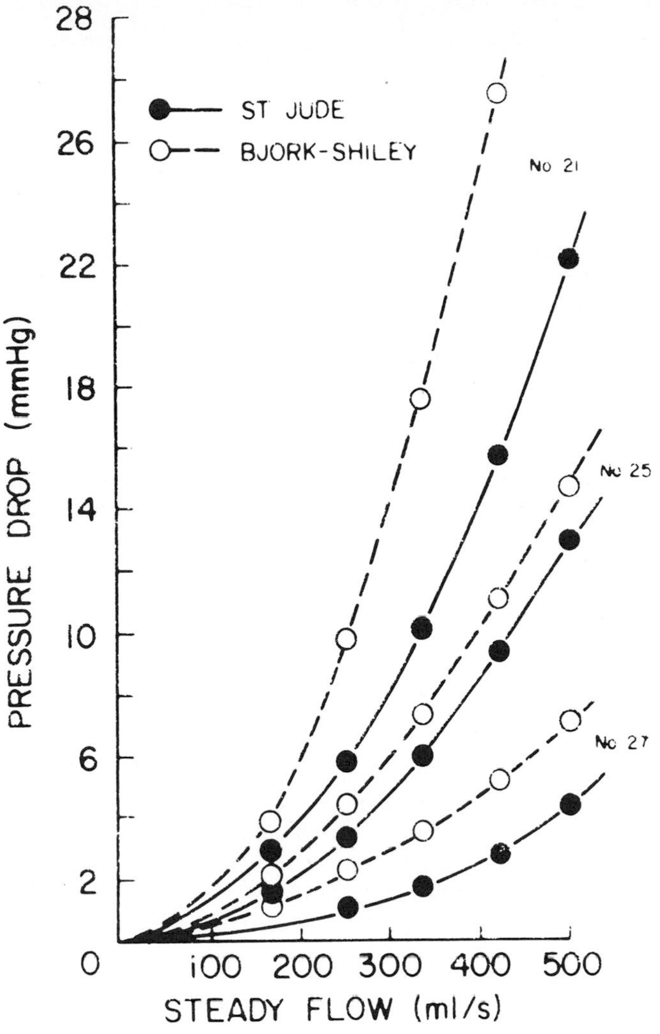

Fig. 38–16. Pressure drop (transvalvular gradient) across normal St. Jude and Bjork-Shiley valves of varying sizes at increasing steady flow rates from 0 to 500 ml/sec. (From Yoganathan AP, et al.: Bileaflet, tilting disc and porcine aortic valve substitutes: in vitro hydrodynamic characteristics. J Am Coll Cardiol; 3:313, 1984. Reprinted with permission of the American College of Cardiology.

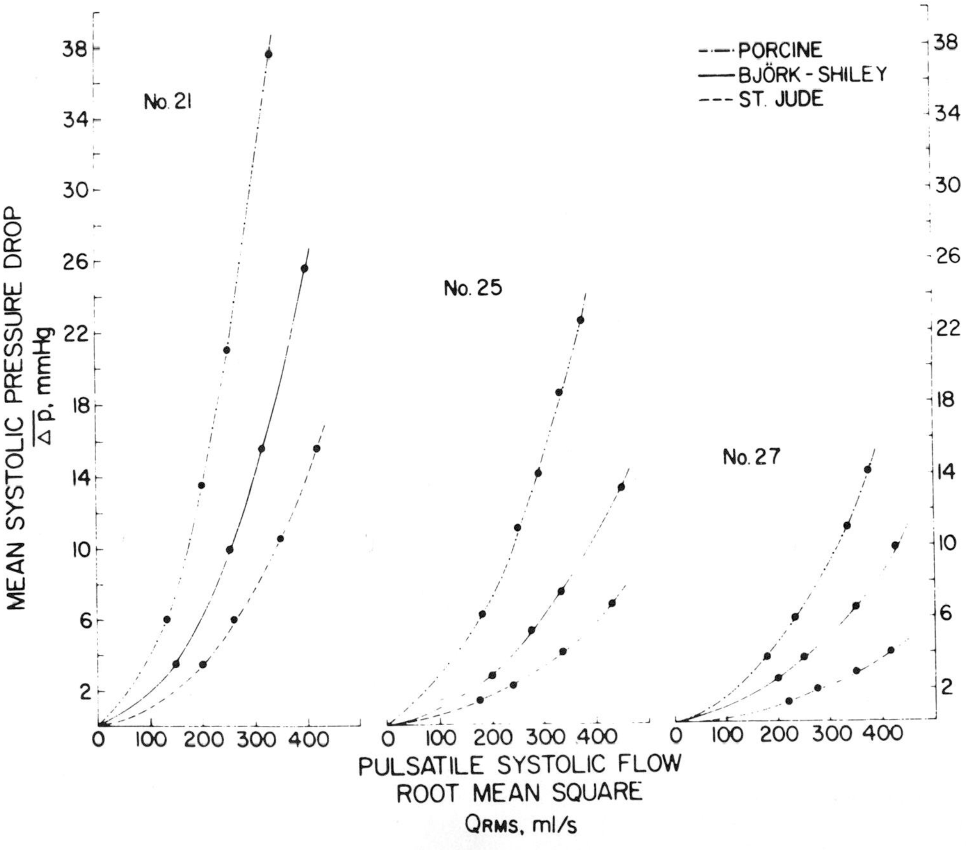

Fig. 38–17. Pressure drop (transvalvular gradient) measurements obtained during pulsatile flow for normally functioning valves of differing type (St. Jude, Bjork-Shiley, and porcine) and size. For each valve size and flow, the porcine valves produce the highest gradients and the St. Jude valves produce the lowest gradients. (From Yoganathan AP, et al.: Bileaflet, tilting disc and porcine aortic valve substitutes: in vitro hydrodynamic characteristics. J Am Coll Cardiol; 3:313, 1984. Reprinted with permission of the American College of Cardiology.

result, it is often better to sample for mitral regurgitant flow from a parasternal, subcostal, or esophageal transducer location. Second, the direction of flow through a prosthesis may differ greatly from that through a native valve in the same location, and flow through prostheses of the same type and size may vary depending on the orientation in which the valve is implanted and the surrounding cardiac morphology. Thus, to record peak velocities accurately across a potentially stenotic valve, it is necessary to understand the flow patterns characteristic of that valve and to either sample flow from several locations or map the spatial orientation of the peak velocities using color flow imaging. Once the direction of the streamlines of flow through the valve is known, the peak velocity can be determined by selecting the appropriate Doppler device (pulsed or continuous wave, depending on peak velocity),[41–45] and by aligning the beam appropriately or angle correcting if necessary.[37,46]

Assessment of Pressure Gradients Across Prosthetic Valves—Prosthetic Valve Stenosis

Pressure gradients across prosthetic valves are determined from the peak instantaneous transvalvular flow velocities using the modified Bernoulli equation (delta $p = 4 v^2$.) In a manner similar to that for native valves. This permits determination of a variety of parameters including the peak gradient, mean gradient, and gradient at the time of valve closing. Several reports of the range of transvalvular velocities and the derived gradients recorded in apparently normal prostheses of known type and size are available,[41–45,47–49,111,112] and they are summarized in Table 38–1.

Initially, the validity of applying the modified Bernoulli equation to prosthetic valves was questioned because the use of this equation requires certain assumptions that may not have been satisfied in the hydrodynamic states created by different prostheses. Specifically, the modified Bernoulli equation is valid only if: (1) the density of blood remains constant; (2) flow velocity is measured along streamlines of flow, which are lines tangential to the direction of flow (i.e., lines not crossed by fluid particles); (3) proximal velocity can be neglected; (4) viscous loss of kinetic energy is negligible; and (5) energy loss from acceleration of the inertial mass in the valve at the beginning of transvalvular flow can be ignored. The first of these assumptions, incompressibility of blood, may be considered valid for all cardiac applications. Measuring velocities along streamlines may be more difficult than in native valves because of the complex geometry of some prostheses. This is a technical problem, however, rather than a physical limitation that would invalidate the equation. Similarly, recognition of the importance of proximal velocities is fundamental in any analysis of stenotic lesions and is not unique to prosthetic valves.

Table 38–1. Normal Values of Doppler Parameters in Apparently Normal Prosthetic Valves

Parameter	Velocity (m/sec) V_{max}	Gradient (mm Hg) delta P_{max}	delta P_{mean}
Mitral Position			
Starr-Edwards (ball-in-cage)	1.9 ± 0.4	14.6 ± 5.5	4.6 ± 2.4
St. Jude Medical (bileaflet)	1.6 ± 0.3	10.0 ± 3.6	3.5 ± 1.3
Bjork-Shiley (tilting disc)	1.6 ± 0.3	10.7 ± 2.7	2.9 ± 1.6
Carpentier-Edwards (porcine bioprosthesis)	1.8 ± 0.2	12.5 ± 3.6?	6.5 ± 2.1?
Hancock (porcine bioprosthesis)	1.5 ± 0.3	9.7 ± 3.2	4.3 ± 2.1
Aortic Position			
Starr-Edwards (ball-in-cage)	3.2 ± 0.6	38.6 ± 11.7	23.0 ± 8.8
St. Jude Medical (bileaflet)	2.4 ± 0.3	25.5 ± 5.1	12.5 ± 6.4
Bjork-Shiley (tilting disc)	2.5 ± 0.6	23.8 ± 8.8	14.3 ± 5.3
Carpentier-Edwards (porcine bioprosthesis)	2.5 ± 0.5	23.2 ± 8.7	14.4 ± 5.7
Hancock (porcine bioprosthesis)	2.4 ± 0.4	23.0 ± 6.7	11.0 ± 2.3
Tricuspid Position (Case Reports)			
Bjork-Shiley (tilting disc)	1.6	10.2	5
Porcine bioprosthesis	1.3 ± 0.3	7 ± 2	3 ± 2

(Data summarized from refs. 18, 55, 111, and 112.)

That significantly increased viscous losses do not occur during passage of blood through the complex mechanism of a prosthesis or that additional energy is not lost by acceleration of the inertial mass in the valve at the beginning of flow, however, could only be determined by experimental and clinical studies. In vitro studies using models with a single circular orifice,[50] and irregular, multiple, and tunnel-like obstructions,[51] suggest that the condition of frictionless flow may be effectively fulfilled in prosthetic devices and should be independent of the position of the valve within the heart. In vitro tests of prosthetic valves in a pulsatile flow chamber have confirmed these observations and have indicated that the energy consumed accelerating blood or mobile valve parts during pulsatile flow is negligible for clinical purposes.[52,53]

In clinical studies, a similar excellent correlation has been demonstrated between simultaneously recorded Doppler and manometrically measured mean gradients across a variety of mitral valve types in patients with normally functioning valves,[41,42,54] and across mitral and tricuspid prostheses in patients with clinical evidence of prosthetic valve dysfunction (Figs. 38–18 and 38–19). These and further comparative studies in mitral and aortic prostheses[37,55–57] suggest that Doppler-derived pressure gradients are highly reliable and essentially interchangeable with those derived during cardiac catheterization (assuming the latter are accurately measured).

Surprisingly high velocities have been recorded in some patients with apparently normally functioning aortic prostheses.[58] Approximately 10% of patients with

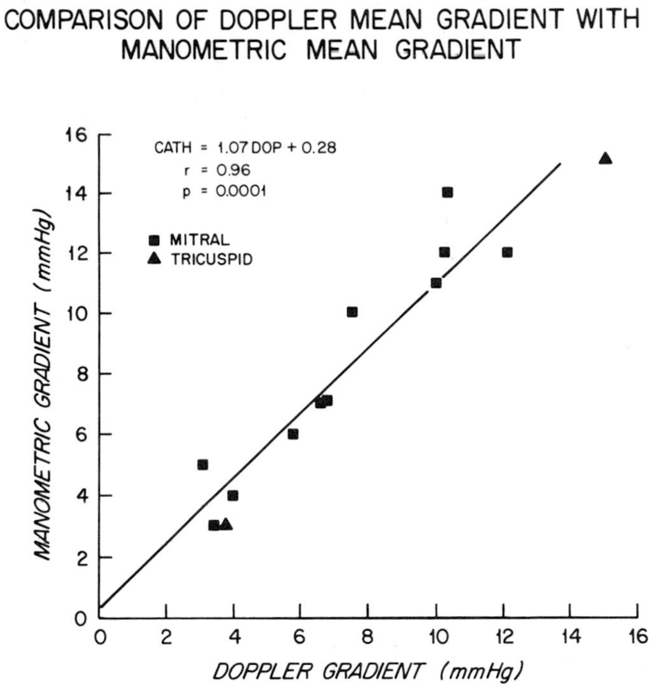

Fig. 38–19. Correlation of simultaneously measured Doppler and manometric mean gradients for both bioprosthetic and mechanical valves in the mitral and tricuspid positions. (From Wilkins GT, et al.: Validation of continuous-wave Doppler echocardiographic measurements of mitral and tricuspid prosthetic valve gradients: a simultaneous Doppler-catheter study. Circulation 74:786, 1986. Reproduced by permission of the American Heart Association, Inc.)

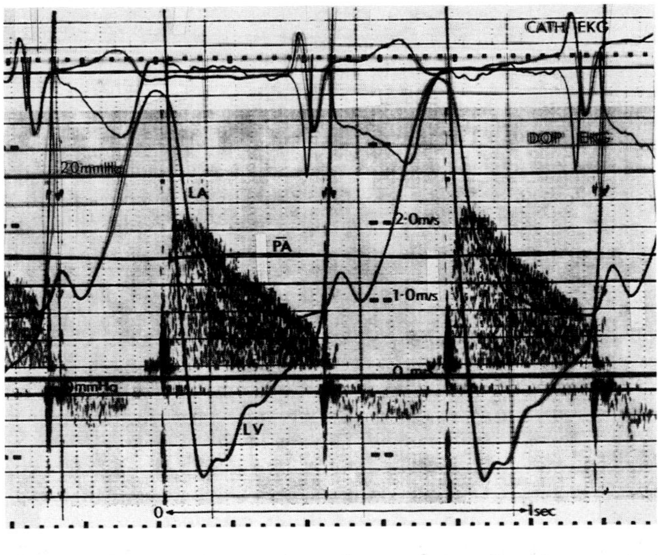

Fig. 38–18. Superimposed continuous wave Doppler spectral and manometric tracings obtained simultaneously during catheterization. Time on the horizontal scale is calibrated at 40-msec intervals. Pressure and velocity calibrations on the vertical scale are indicated. LA = left atrial pressure; LV = left ventricular pressure; PA = mean pulmonary artery pressure. (From Wilkins GT, et al.: Validation of continuous-wave Doppler echocardiographic measurements of mitral and tricuspid prosthetic valve gradients: a simultaneous Doppler-catheter study. Circulation 74:786, 1986. Reproduced by permission of the American Heart Association, Inc.)

aortic prostheses (St. Jude, Bjork-Shiley, or porcine) have been found to have maximal transvalvular velocities in excess of 3.5 m/sec or gradients of over 50 mm Hg. These high velocities are generally only present transiently at the instant the valve opens, and it is therefore routine practice also to report the mean transvalvular gradient, which is a better measure of the resistance to left ventricular emptying. As with native valves, comparison of the Doppler peak instantaneous gradient with the invasively derived peak to peak gradient can lead to confusion (see Chapter 19). This is a particular problem when studying prosthetic aortic valves where the initial Doppler gradient is often high and the peak to peak catheter-determined gradient is usually lower than the mean.[59] In these cases, the maximal instantaneous gradient derived by Doppler and the peak to peak gradient determined by cardiac catheterization may diverge even more than in native aortic valves. Nonetheless, mean gradients derived by either technique should be directly comparable.

Another potential source of transvalvular gradient "overestimation" is the effect of pressure recovery.[60] Pressure recovery occurs when part of the kinetic energy present at the valve level is converted back into pressure distal to the valve. Since kinetic energy is irretrievably dissipated in turbulent eddies, the amount of pressure energy that can be recovered depends on the smoothness of the transition from the valve to the postvalvular flow cross-section, which is determined by the geometry of the valve relative to surrounding cardiac structures. Thus, a clinically relevant amount of pressure recovery is more likely to occur at the aortic than at the mitral site, because the aortic valvular and postvalvular flow cross-sections are more similar than are the mitral valve and left ventricle. It should be noted, however, that even in the presence of pressure recovery distal to the prosthesis, the gradient calculated from the maximal flow velocity is real; but it is "localized" and, as pressure increases distal to the stenosis, the net gradient (which is the physiologically relevant gradient) between the left ventricle and aorta decreases. It is unclear how large this "overestimation" is in vivo, although it has been reported in vitro to range as high as 16 mmHg for peak and 10 mmHg for mean gradients across the central orifice of small St. Jude Medical prostheses under physiologic flow rates.[61]

Although transvalvular gradients are a useful measure of the impedance to blood flow across the valve, they depend on cardiac output. Nonetheless, an extremely high gradient or a rising gradient on successive studies with no apparent change in pump function is strong evidence of prosthetic valve stenosis.

Calculation of Valve Area

Because any transvalvular gradient is a function of flow rate (or cardiac output), the area through which flow must pass (i.e., the valve orifice area) is generally considered a better measure of "obstruction." The orifice area should be constant, particularly with mechanical devices, although some flow related increase in the physical opening of the valve leaflets has been demonstrated with porcine heterografts.[15] Fortunately, the Doppler approach provides an excellent method for estimating valve area and may indeed be superior to other techniques in this regard.

The primary Doppler method for calculating prosthetic valve areas is based on the continuity principle (discussed in Chapter 9), which states that in the absence of regurgitation or shunts, flow through the prosthetic valve must equal flow through other areas of the heart. Because flow is equal to mean velocity times area,

$$Q_{pr} = v_{pr} * A_{pr} \quad \text{or}$$

$$A_{pr} = Q_{pr}/v_{pr}$$

where Q is volume flow rate, v is the temporal and spatial mean flow velocity, and A is the area through which flow is occurring. As noted earlier, this equation measures the effective orifice area rather than the physical boundaries of an orifice. The effective orifice area corresponds to the vena contracta of the jet, which is its minimal cross section and is always smaller than the anatomic orifice area. Because the effective area accounts for differing orifice and inlet geometries, areas calculated from this equation are directly comparable regardless of the valve or prosthesis type.[62]

Applying this approach to a prosthetic valve requires that a cardiac output be calculated at some other site (for example, the aortic root for a mitral prosthesis or the left ventricular outflow tract for aortic prostheses) and that the time velocity integral across the valve be measured from Doppler spectra.[63] For aortic prostheses, only the instantaneous flow rate need be calculated using the peak velocity across the outflow tract and the peak transvalvular velocity (assuming these occur simultaneously).[64,65] Note that for the continuity equation to be applicable, flow through the prosthesis must be the same as flow at the reference site. For example, in the absence of mitral or aortic regurgitation, aortic flow can be used as the reference for calculating mitral valve area. If either mitral or aortic regurgitation is present, however, flow across the mitral prosthesis and the aortic outflow tract cannot be presumed to be the same, and the continuity equation would not be applicable. For an aortic prosthesis, use of the subvalvular outflow velocity and area would yield a valid reference flow in the presence of either a competent or a regurgitant valve. Mitral flow, in contrast, would only be valid if there were no aortic or mitral incompetence. Clinical usefulness of continuity-derived areas has been demonstrated in biological and mechanical prostheses in vivo.[66,67]

Another potentially useful but less well validated technique for measuring the area of mitral and tricuspid prostheses is the Doppler pressure half-time.[68] The half-time has been used to determine the area of a variety of mitral and tricuspid prostheses, with fair correlations to invasively derived valve areas.[37,45,47,49] Not surprisingly, however, considerable overestimation,[37,55] as well as underestimation,[49] by the pressure half-time method has been reported. The method was originally derived for native rheumatic mitral stenosis[69] (see Chapter 17), and the empiric constant 220 in the half-time equation implicitly reflects, among other factors, the geometry and discharge coefficient of this type of stenosis.[70] Application of this general equation and the cited constant to the wide range of available prostheses therefore cannot be expected to yield accurate results. In theory, however, the half-time method should be usable in longitudinal follow-up studies in the same patient.

Doppler Assessment of Prosthetic Regurgitation

Regurgitation in prosthetic heart valves can be divided into two primary types: transvalvular and paravalvular. Transvalvular regurgitation can be subdivided into normal or physiologic and pathologic regurgitation.

Normal Regurgitation

Normal or physiologic regurgitation or backflow is the result of the design characteristics of the prosthesis and includes closure backflow, which is caused by the reversal of flow required to move the occluding mechanism to the closed position, and leakage backflow, which takes place once the valve is in the fully closed position (Fig. 38–20).[32] Some closure backflow may be seen with all types of mechanical prostheses, as well as in roughly 10% of bioprosthetic valves; however, whether true closure backflow occurs in normally functioning bioprosthetic valves or whether the observed backflow is due to backward movement of the closed cusps is controversial.[71] Leakage backflow is most common with disc

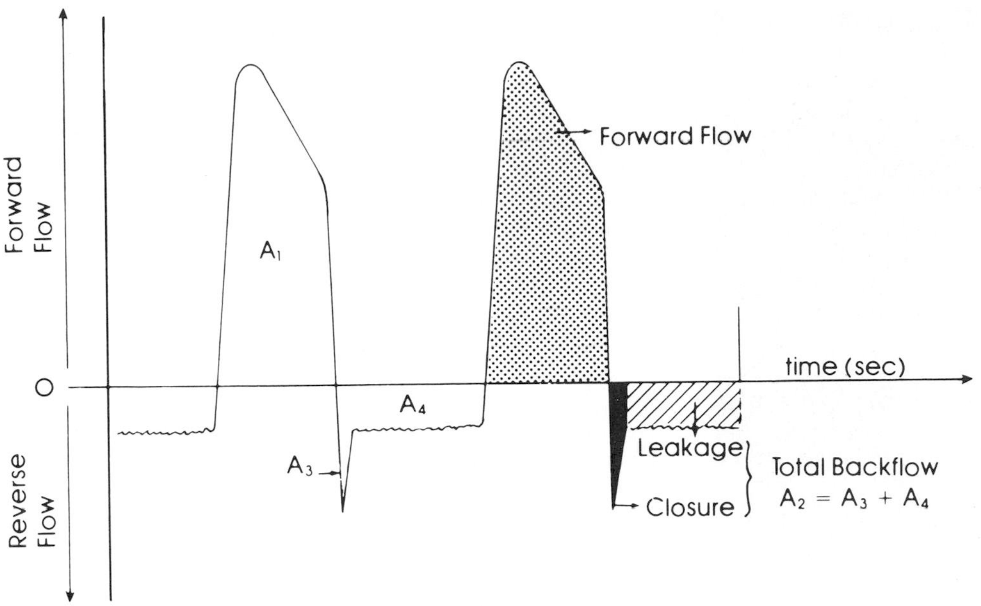

Fig. 38–20. In vitro recording of pulsatile aortic flow vs. time, indicating forward flow, closure backflow, and leakage backflow. Total backflow is the sum of closure backflow and leakage backflow. (From Dellsperger KC: Regurgitation of prosthetic heart valves: dependence on heart rate and cardiac output. Am J Cardiol 51:321, 1983.)

valves and varies in amount, depending on valve design and local hemodynamic state. Normal leakage backflow was not well recognized clinically until the use of transesophageal echocardiography became widespread, but it is routinely observed using this technique. This phenomenon is discussed earlier under the specific valve types.

Transvalvular Regurgitation

Transvalvular regurgitation is caused by valve malfunction, e.g., torn or flail leaflet, occluder immobilization, and improper seating. This condition can easily be differentiated from closure backflow by its volume and duration and from leakage backflow by its location and degree. Figure 38–21 is an example of regurgitation through the torn cusp of a bioprosthetic valve. Although in this case, the regurgitant jet is centrally directed, regurgitant jets emanating from prosthetic valves are often eccentric, they may impinge on adjacent walls, and their spatial extent and volume may be difficult to map.

Paravalvular Regurgitation

Paravalvular regurgitation results from failure of complete fixation of the valve along the suture line and may range from a pinhole leak to partial or complete valve dehiscence. Paravalvular leaks by definition occur between the sewing ring and the surrounding valve annulus, and their detection requires that the Doppler beam be directed to search the entire 360° margin of the valve. Searching the entire periphery of the valve without the beam's actually passing through the prosthetic material of the sewing ring may be difficult, particularly for valves in the mitral position. Detection is further complicated because the paravalvular leak frequently is not a free jet, but rather adheres to the receiving chamber wall (Coanda effect), limiting its spatial distribution. Figure 38–22 illustrates a paravalvular leak arising along the posterior margin of the sewing ring of a Hancock valve in the mitral position, whereas Figure 38–23 demonstrates a similar lesion medial to a bioprosthetic tricuspid valve. Differentiation of paravalvular regurgitation from transvalvular regurgitation occurring at the margins of an occluder may be difficult, and the following criteria have been suggested to help define paravalvular leaks using color flow mapping:[17,37] (1) regurgitation originating outside the sewing ring (i.e., flow occurring around, rather than through, the valve); (2) regurgitation originating from a point not clearly outside the sewing ring, but separate from the confines of the forward flow stream; and (3) presence of a proximal acceleration zone in the upstream chamber outside the confines of the prosthesis.

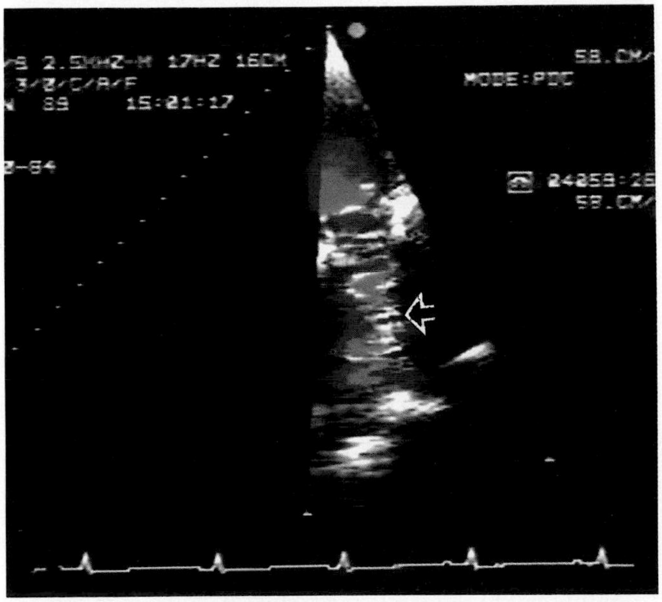

Fig. 38–21. Apical four-chamber color flow recording of a regurgitant jet (arrow) arising from a bioprosthetic valve with a partially flail leaflet.

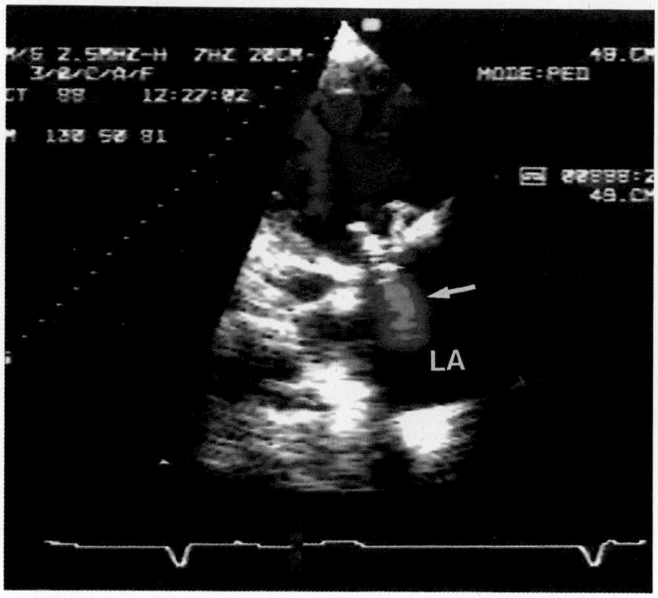

Fig. 38–22. Modified apical recording illustrating a paravalvular leak (arrow) at the posterior margin of a Hancock valve in the mitral position. LA = left atrium.

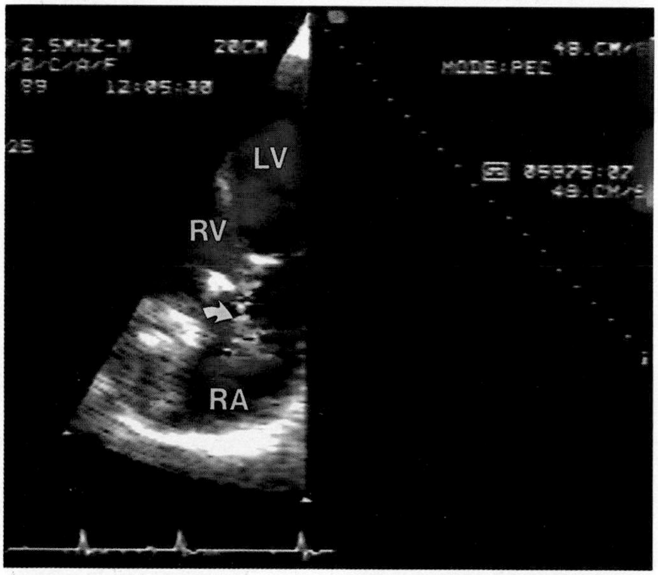

Fig. 38–23. Modified apical four-chamber recording illustrating a paravalvular leak (curved arrow) at the medial margin of a bioprosthetic valve in the tricuspid position. RA = right atrium; RV = right ventricle; LV = left ventricle.

Obviously, such assessment requires excellent image quality and Doppler sensitivity. Achievement of this degree of precision may require use of the transesophageal window, and on occasion, a paravalvular leak cannot be differentiated from a transvalvular leak at the margins of the occluder with absolute certainty.

Although in the past paravalvular leakage was always considered pathologic, increasing experience indicates that some paravalvular leakage is a common phenomenon immediately after valve replacement,[17] and its clinical significance depends more on extent than on mere presence.

PROSTHETIC VALVE EXAMINATION—ASSESSMENT BY LOCATION

The evaluation of prosthetic valves should be integrated into the routine echo-Doppler examination. The mere presence of a prosthesis often interferes with data acquisition through attenuation or artifact, however, and both forward and regurgitant prosthetic valve flow may differ in direction, location, and velocity from those expected for a native valve. Therefore, the specific views that provide the most meaningful information for each valve location and type may also differ. The following section therefore discusses the appropriate views to be used to record specific information about prostheses at each intracardiac site.

Mitral Prostheses

All prosthetic valves in the mitral position are normally imaged first in the parasternal long axis view. Figure 38–24 illustrates the parasternal long axis appearance of a ball-in-cage valve in the mitral position during diastole and systole. Figure 38–25 compares the diastolic images of bioprosthetic, single, and double disc valves in the same location. It is generally possible to determine valve type in this view, to record leaflet or occluder motion, to assess valve stability, and on occasion to identify masses attached to the sewing ring or other valve components. In patients with bioprosthetic valves, it is often possible to record leaflet motion, to measure leaflet thickness, and to detect thrombi or vegetations attached to the valve apparatus. In contrast, the dense reverberations arising from mechanical valves (Fig. 38–25C) often prevent any detailed assessment of

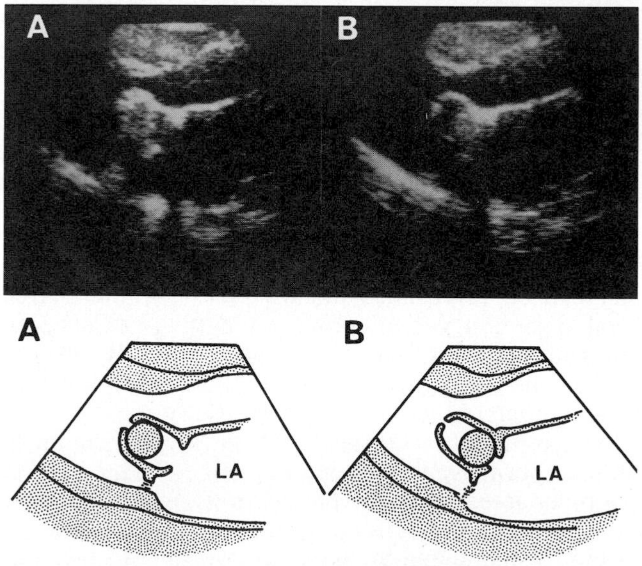

Fig. 38–24. Parasternal long axis recording of a Starr-Edwards prosthesis in the mitral position. **A.** Recorded during diastole. The ball moves forward or apically into the cage. **B.** Recorded during systole. The ball is seated within the sewing ring. LA = left atrium.

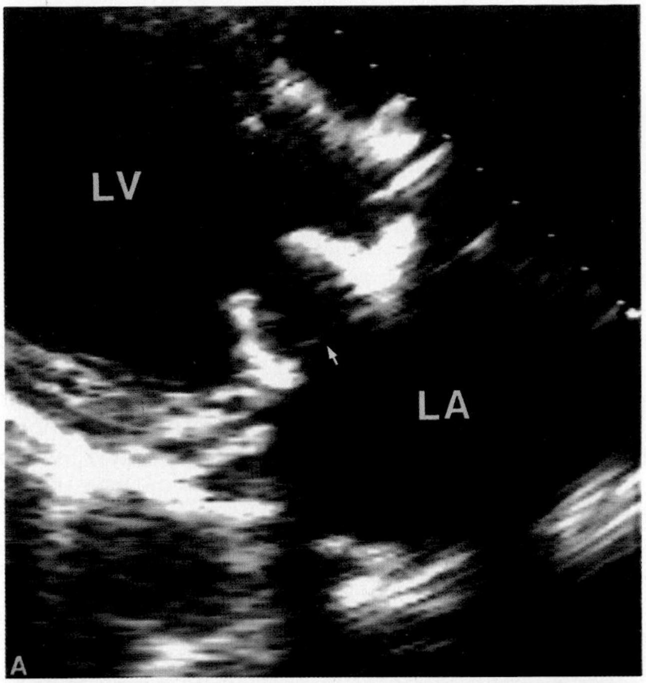

Fig. 38–25. Comparison of the parasternal long axis diastolic appearance in the mitral position. **A.** Bioprosthetic disc. **B.** Tilting disc. **C.** Double disc valve. An area of dense reverberations (REV) can be appreciated behind the double disc valve illustrated. LA = left atrium; LV = left ventricle; arrows point to valve leaflets/occluder(s).

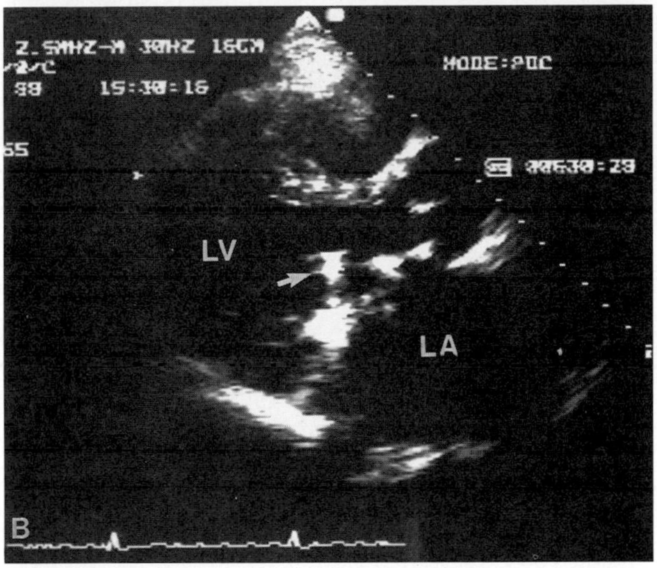

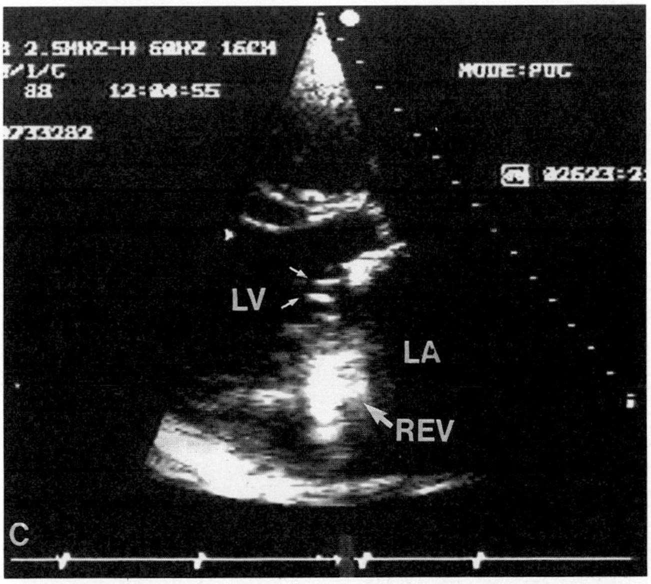

occluder motion and generally make it difficult to visualize the region immediately behind the valve. Valve stability can be determined in this view, but the degree of valve motion varies with the technique of surgical implantation. When the valve is sewn directly into the annulus, the sewing ring shows no motion independent of the annulus; however, when the valve is sutured to the base of the posterior leaflet, some independent motion may normally be detected.

Doppler assessment of forward flow varies with valve type and orientation relative to the ventricular long axis. For bioprosthetic and St. Jude valves, flow is centrivalvular and is normally directed toward and best recorded from the cardiac apex (Fig. 38–26). For ball-and-cage valves, flow normally curves around the ball, and the anterior component may be directed toward the left ventricular outflow tract or anterior septum depending on the orientation of the valve. Thus, it is necessary to define the direction of the dominant flow vector by color flow mapping or to record flow velocity from numerous locations along the anterior wall and at the apex, to establish the maximal transvalvular gradient. The same variation in forward flow patterns occurs in patients with tilting disc valves.

A high parasternal window generally permits access to the posterior surface of the valve and is particularly useful for detecting mitral regurgitation.

Parasternal short axis images often allow the leaflets of bioprosthetic valves to be examined in greater detail and the location of asymmetric leaflet thickening or vegetations to be defined. They also permit better visualization of the valve struts and, with the scan plane posi-

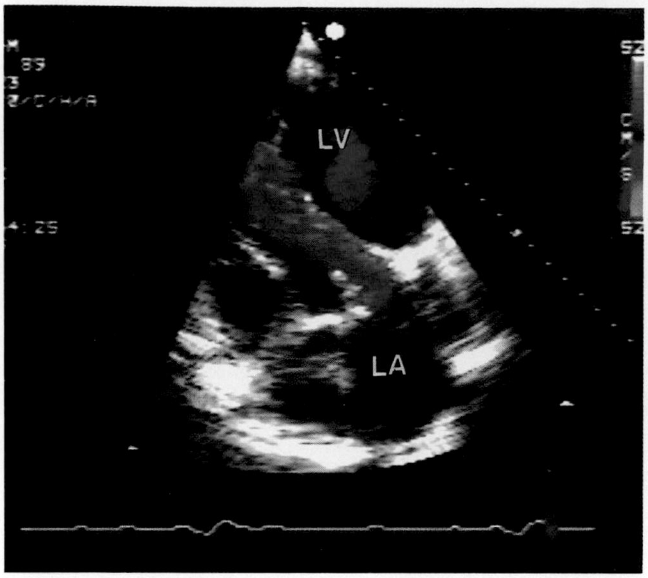

Fig. 38–26. Apical five-chamber color flow recording of diastolic inflow (red) through a bioprosthetic valve in the mitral position. LA = left atrium; LV = left ventricle.

tioned on the atrial side of the valve, can enable one to detect the spatial location of regurgitant jets, particularly those due to paravalvular leaks. Figure 38–27 is a parasternal short axis recording of a bioprosthetic valve illustrating the three valve struts and closed leaflets. Although placed in the mitral location, the valve is fabricated from a porcine aortic valve, and thus its short axis appearance is similar to that of a normal human aortic valve.

When ball valves are positioned so the direction of ball motion is on a more anteroposterior line, the full excursion of the ball may be best recorded from a low parasternal short axis location.

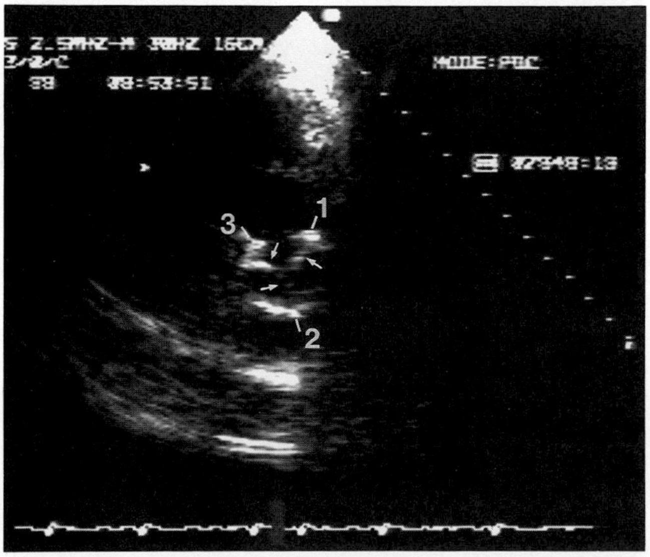

Fig. 38–27. Parasternal short axis recording of a bioprosthetic valve illustrating the three valve leaflets (small arrows) and struts (numbers). Recording is obtained during systole when the valve leaflets are closed.

Valve ring abscesses are also typically best visualized in a parasternal short axis view.

From the apex, a mitral prosthesis can be examined using any of the standard apical views (i.e., the four-chamber, two-chamber and long axis views). Figure 38–28 illustrates a ball-and-cage valve recorded in the apical four-chamber view during diastole (open) and systole (closed). In most instances, maximal opening excursion is toward the apex, and thus occluder motion can be best assessed from this location Figure 38–29. The apex is also the standard window for the Doppler assessment of mitral inflow because the flow vector is most commonly directed toward the transducer in this position. As a result, peak, mean and end-diastolic gradients and the Doppler half-time are most commonly determined from apical recordings (Fig. 38–30). The long axis of most mitral regurgitant jets is also typically closest to the beam path when the transducer is positioned at the apex. Unfortunately, from the apical transducer location the beam must also generally pass through the prosthesis to record regurgitant flow, so examination from alternative sites is critical. Timing of mitral inflow and regurgitation can be determined from Doppler spectral recordings. If the beam is angled superiorly to record both mitral inflow and ventricular outflow, the temporal relationship between the onset and termination of aortic outflow and the beginning and end of mitral inflow can be determined and isovolumic contraction and relaxation times measured (Fig. 38–31).

Subcostal images in long (Fig. 38–32) and short axis planes should also be included and often provide useful additional information, particularly in patients with suboptimal intercostal windows. If the information derived from the standard views is inadequate, a transesophageal examination may be performed to improve sensitivity and resolution (Fig. 38–33). Transesophageal studies may be of particular value when one is searching for prosthetic endocarditis and may reveal regurgitation that is inapparent during routine transthoracic study.[113]

Aortic Prostheses

The parasternal long axis view is also the first standard plane in which an aortic prosthesis is recorded; however, aortic prostheses in general are more difficult to recognize than mitral prostheses. This occurs because aortic prostheses are typically smaller than those in the mitral position, they are positioned horizontally in the scan plane, and thus the moving parts are most often recorded using the lateral resolution of the system, and they have an appearance not dissimilar to that of a calcified stenotic native valve (see Fig. 38–15). As a result, prosthetic valves in the aortic position are frequently misinterpreted as stenotic native valves by the inexperienced observer.

Once a prosthesis is identified in the aortic root, slowly reducing the gain while continuously imaging generally decreases reflections to a level that allows visualization of the sewing ring and valve components (Fig. 38–34). Once an appropriate gain level is achieved, the

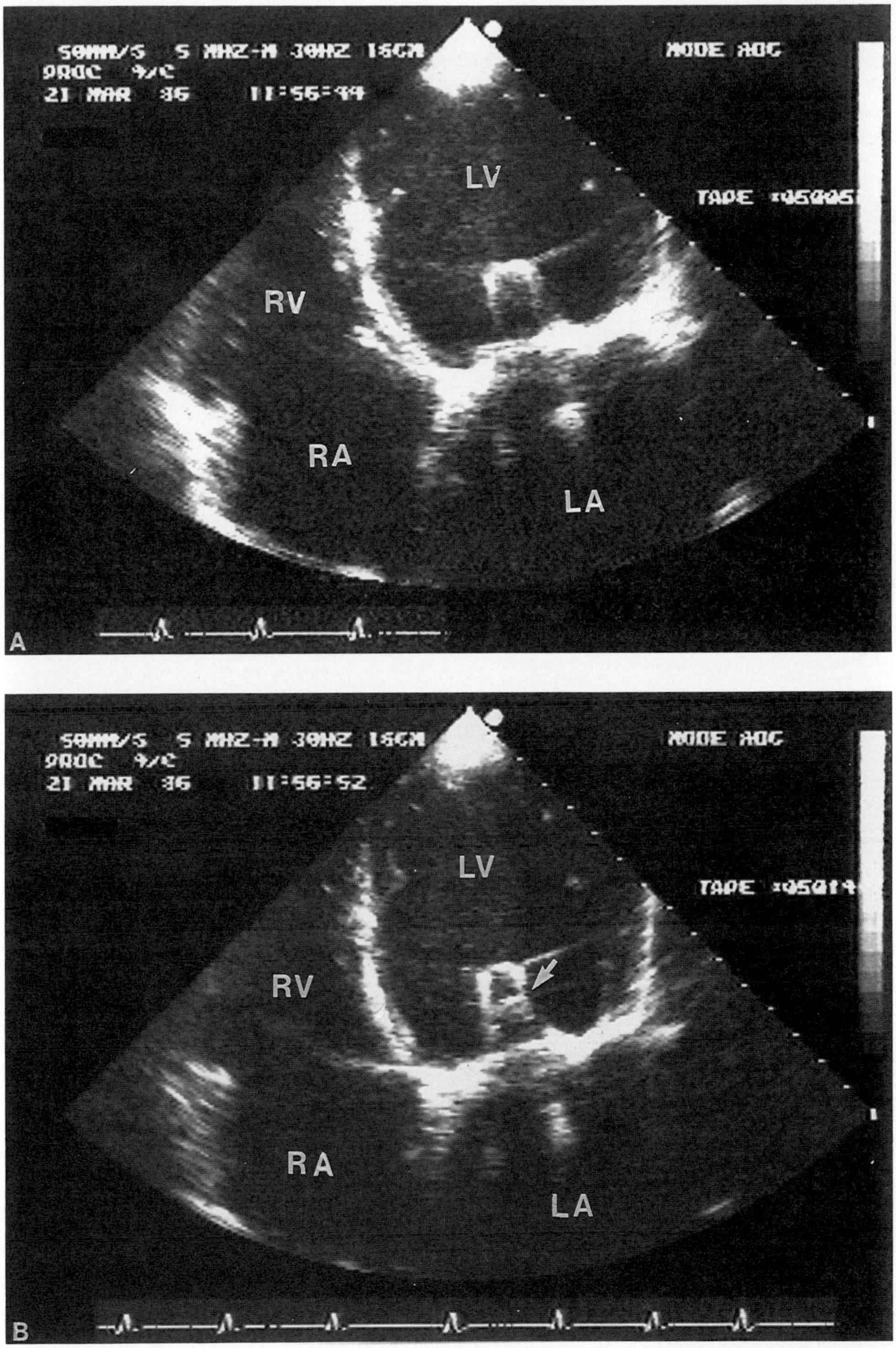

Fig. 38–28. A. Apical four-chamber recording of a Starr-Edwards valve in the mitral position during diastole. **B.** Same recording during systole. Arrow points to the front surface of the ball occluder. LV = left ventricle; LA = left atrium; RA = right atrium; RV = right ventricle.

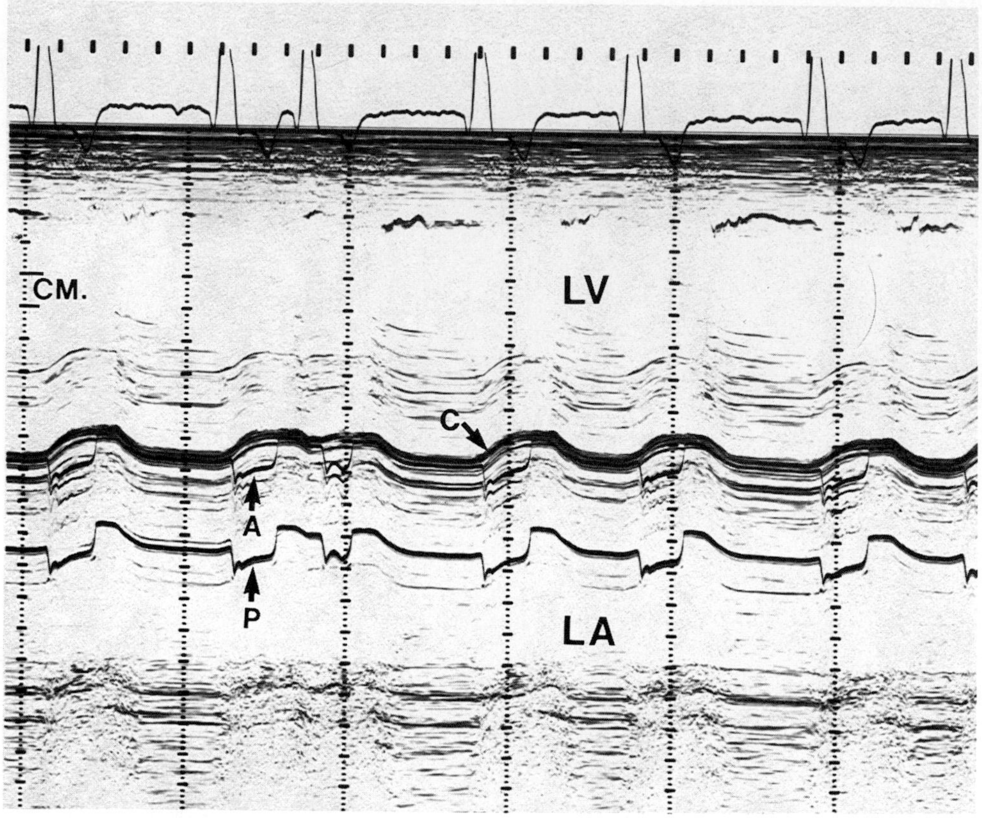

Fig. 38–29. M-mode recording of a Starr-Edwards valve from the apex illustrating the amplitude and timing of ball motion. LV = left ventricle; LA = left atrium; C = cage; A = anterior margin ball; P = posterior margin of ball. cm = centimeter.

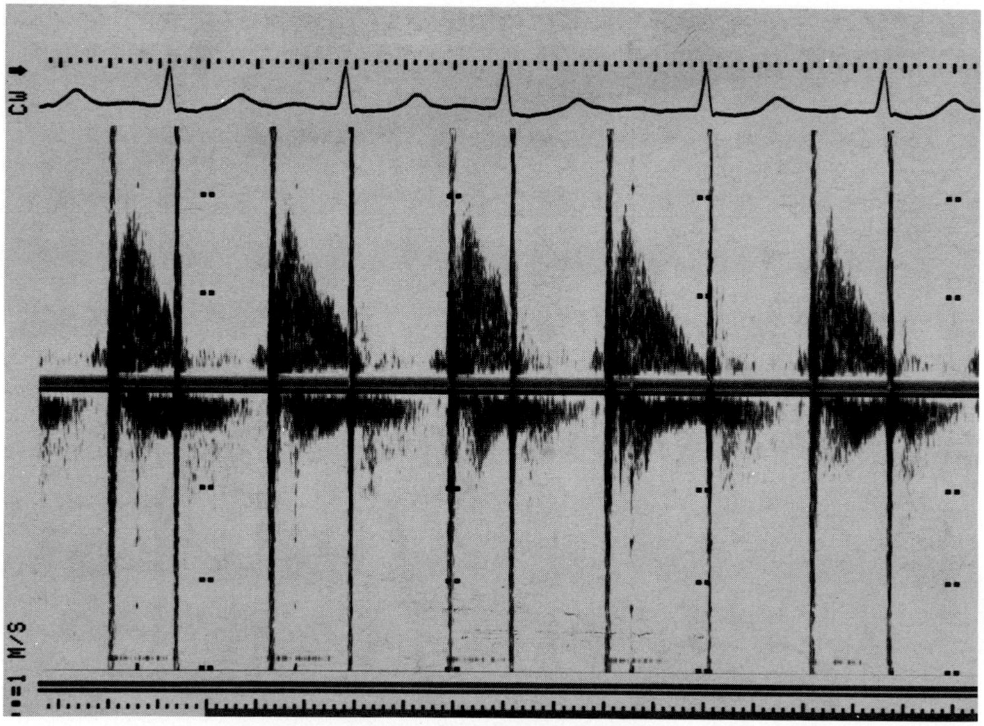

Fig. 38–30. Continuous wave Doppler recording of diastolic inflow across a Bjork-Shiley mitral prosthesis. Atrial fibrillation is present, and the velocity profile varies with cycle length. The peak gradient averages 14 mm Hg, the mean 6 mm Hg, and the end diastolic gradient falls to zero with longer cycles.

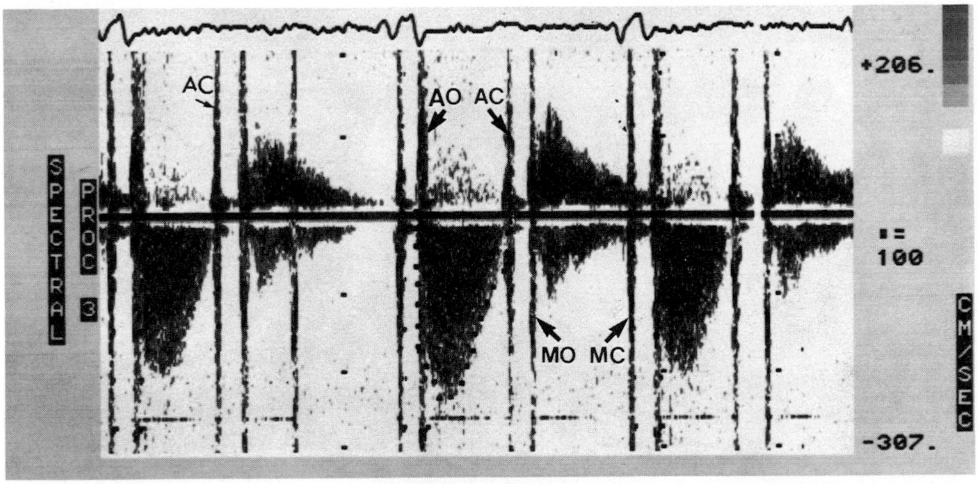

Fig. 38–31. Continuous wave Doppler recording of mitral inflow and aortic outflow in a patient with both mitral and aortic prostheses. Note the opening and closing clicks of both the mitral and aortic prostheses, which define the duration of both isovolumic contraction and relaxation. AO = aortic opening; AC = aortic closure; MO = mitral opening; MC = mitral closure.

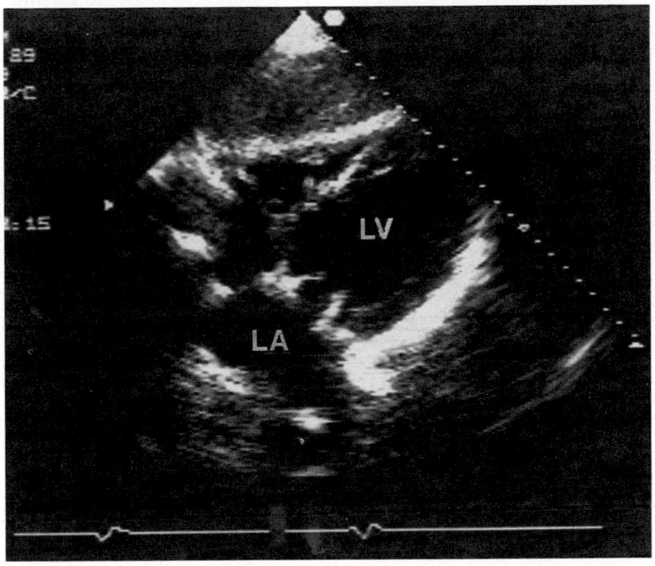

Fig. 38–32. Subcostal long axis recording of a bioprosthetic valve in the mitral position. LV = left ventricle: LA = left atrium.

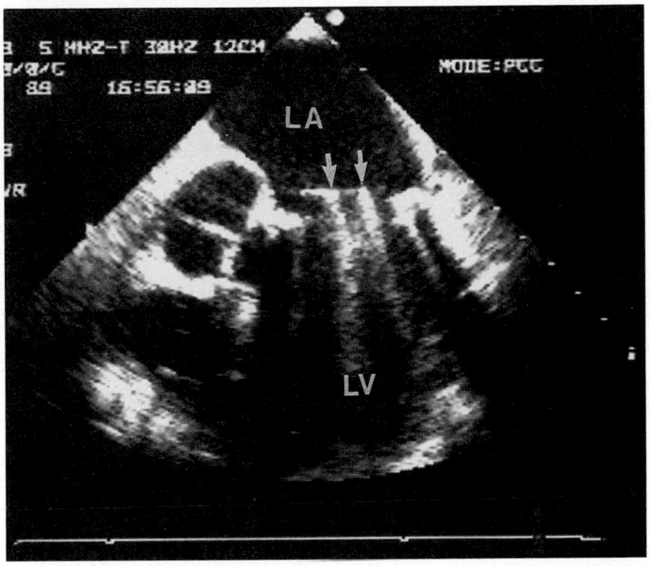

Fig. 38–33. Transesophageal recording of a St. Jude valve in the mitral position. From this transducer position, both discs of the open value can be clearly visualized (arrows). LA = left atrium; LV = left ventricle.

movement of valve components (i.e., leaflets, disc(s), or ball) can be clearly recorded. Angling the scan plane medially and laterally permits assessment of the sewing ring and its relationship with the aortic annulus. Regurgitant jets can also be recorded behind the valve and the jet diameter at the orifice measured. In patients with ball or disc valves in the mitral position, the transmitral flow is often directed anteriorly into the outflow tract and can be difficult to differentiate from aortic regurgitation using pulsed Doppler. Color flow mapping generally permits even complex local flows to be separated, and the differential velocities and timing on continuous wave recording can also facilitate differentiation.

In the parasternal short axis view, it is possible to examine the orifice of the aortic prosthesis directly. In patients with bioprosthetic valves, the leaflets and their opening can generally be clearly recorded if gain is optimized and the scan plane is precisely positioned. The short axis appearance of a bioprosthetic valve is illustrated in Figure 38–27. The movement and thickness of each leaflet should be assessed for uniformity. In this plane, ball movement in a Starr-Edwards valve or disc movement in other mechanical devices can be assessed, but the range requires a long axis plane. Remember that some prostheses have a considerable vertical height (e.g., Starr-Edwards), and thus several slow sweeps of the scan plane from the aortic annulus to the superior margin of the prosthesis are required to examine the valve apparatus completely. Using the short axis plane, it is also possible to record the sewing ring and perivalvular tissues. Color flow mapping should also be included in the short axis examination, to search for regurgitation, to identify its origin, and to determine the area of the jet at its base. Because of the large angle between

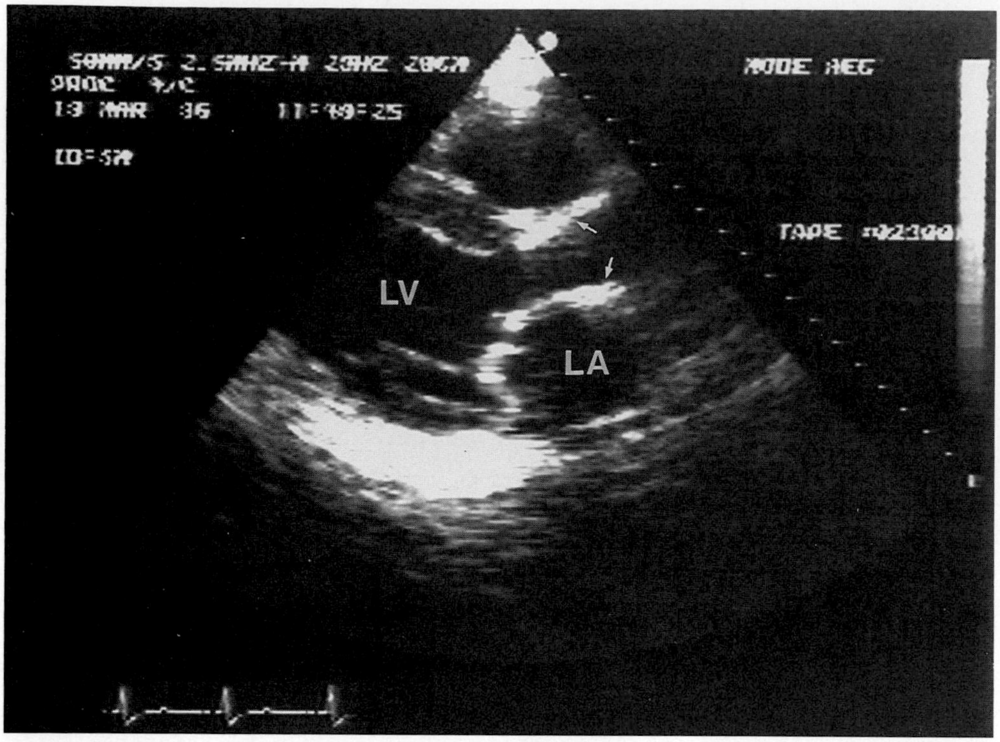

Fig. 38–34. Parasternal long axis recording of a bioprosthetic valve in the aortic position. In this systolic recording, the valve leaflets (arrows) are open and lie parallel to the valve stents. LA = left atrium; LV = left ventricle.

the direction of aortic outflow and the path of the ultrasonic beam, Doppler velocity measurements are unreliable.

From the apex, aortic prostheses can be imaged well in both long axis and anteriorly angulated four-chamber views (five-chamber view). In the apical views, the movements of the leaflets, disc, or ball are interrogated using the axial resolution of the instrument. These views are therefore most suitable for assessing the adequacy of opening. By carefully rotating the imaging plane while maintaining the valve in the center of the image, one can identify the maximal opening in those devices that open asymmetrically such as single disc valves. From this position two-dimensional guided M-mode studies can also be obtained, and the amplitude, velocity, and timing of valve opening and closure determined. The left ventricular outflow tract should also be interrogated using pulsed Doppler, to exclude a subvalvular gradient. Measurement of the outflow velocity immediately below the valve is also necessary for valve area calculations using the continuity equation (as discussed previously). If the outflow velocity is increased ($>$1.5 M/sec), the proximal velocity should be included in the calculation of transvalvular gradients using the Bernoulli equation. Because transvalvular velocities are typically above the Nyquist limits of a pulsed Doppler instrument, continuous wave Doppler is often necessary to record the highest transvalvular velocities. If stenosis is a concern, peak transprosthetic velocities should also be recorded from the right parasternal and suprasternal transducer locations. Color flow mapping should routinely be performed from the apex because the direction of regurgitant jets parallels the interrogating beam from this location. As a result, both the presence and the extent of regurgitation are most easily defined from the apical views (see later).

Subcostal imaging planes frequently provide additional high quality images of the aortic root and prosthetic valve. High resolution (long axis and short axis) views of aortic prostheses may also be obtained by transesophageal echocardiography if the transthoracic examination cannot satisfy the clinical needs.

Tricuspid Prostheses

Prosthetic valves in the tricuspid position are first recorded in the parasternal long axis view of the right ventricular inflow tract. The images obtained in this view should permit differentiation of valve type, stability, and leaflet/occluder motion. Tilting the imaging plane medially and laterally allows visualization of the valve margins. If the view is obtained from a high parasternal position, the right atrium is usually free of acoustic artifact, and abnormal structures (thrombi or vegetations) can be visualized. Because of the normal anterior tilt of the tricuspid annular plane, diastolic inflow is roughly parallel to the ultrasonic beam when the Doppler examination is performed from a low parasternal window. Tricuspid regurgitant flow can be recorded from either a high left or right parasternal window. Right parasternal recording is usually easier in patients with tricuspid prostheses than in normal subjects, because the conditions for which a prosthesis is inserted in the tricuspid position are generally associated with important right atrial dilation.

In the standard parasternal short axis view at the base of the heart, the orifice of the tricuspid prosthesis along with the circumference of the sewing ring can be visualized. As with valves in the mitral and aortic locations, this permits the bioprosthetic valve leaflets to be recorded and an assessment of their thickness and mobility to be made. The great anterior tilt of the tricuspid annulus also allows the excursion of the occluder in patients with mechanical valves to be better recorded than is the case for left-sided valves. Placement of the short axis plane superior to the sewing ring permits the spatial location of regurgitant jets to be defined and is particularly valuable for localizing paraprosthetic leaks.

From the apical transducer location, the standard four-chamber plane usually provides an excellent view of a tricuspid prosthesis (Fig. 38–35). As with a mitral prosthesis imaged from the apical window, the plane can be rotated to assess the full range of poppet or leaflet movement, and a two-dimensional guided M-mode image can be recorded. Diastolic flow is typically directed toward the transducer when it is positioned in the apical window, and as a result, this (or a low parasternal) view is most suitable for recording the timing and maximal velocity of tricuspid inflow and thus for the calculation of peak, mean, and end-diastolic gradients by Doppler. The pressure half-time can also be calculated, but as with mitral prosthesis, the appropriate constant is yet to be defined. In tricuspid bioprosthetic stenosis, inspiratory cessation of tricuspid regurgitation and persistent systolic antegrade flow due to excessive right atrial pressure have been reported.[72] When recording from the apex in patients with both pulmonary regurgitation and suspected tricuspid stenosis, it is possible to confuse the regurgitant jet with flow across the prosthesis and hence to misdiagnose stenosis. This can be a particular problem when one samples flow across the prosthesis using blind continuous wave Doppler recordings because the path of the pulmonary regurgitant jet may cross in front of the prosthesis and the velocities may not be inappropriate for those expected from a stenotic tricuspid valve. Placement of the pulsed Doppler sample volume at the orifice of the valve and careful measurement of the relative timing of the two flow streams should permit one to make the distinction.

The subcostal window frequently gives good two-dimensional and color Doppler views of a tricuspid prosthesis because the device is relatively close to the transducer from this position. This view also provides unobstructed visualization of the right atrium, so the presence of subtle abnormalities such as thrombus or spontaneous echo contrast resulting from stasis can be seen. Figure 38–36 illustrates the right atrium and interatrial septum recorded from the subcostal location. Note the swirling, smokelike echoes in the right atrium indicating stasis, in this case because of a severely stenotic tricuspid bioprosthesis. Against the margin of the

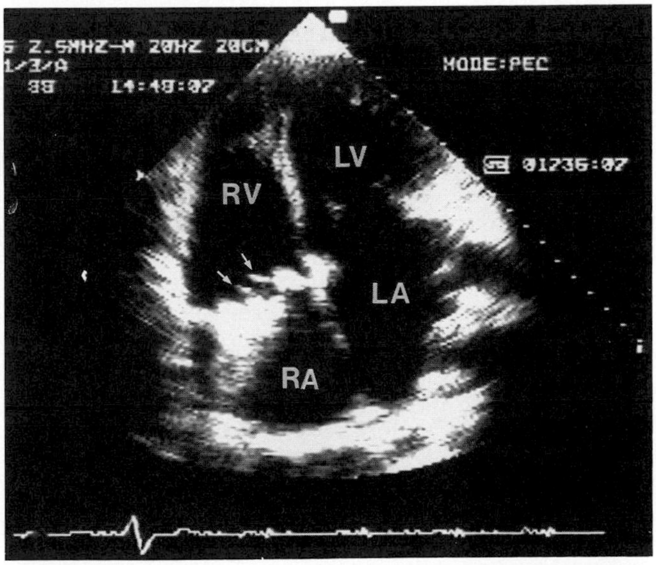

Fig. 38–35. Apical four-chamber recording of a St. Jude valve in the tricuspid position. In this diastolic image, the two discs of the valve (arrows) can be clearly seen in their open position, along with the typical area of dense reverberations behind the valve. RV = right ventricle; RA = right atrium; LA = left atrium; LV = left ventricle.

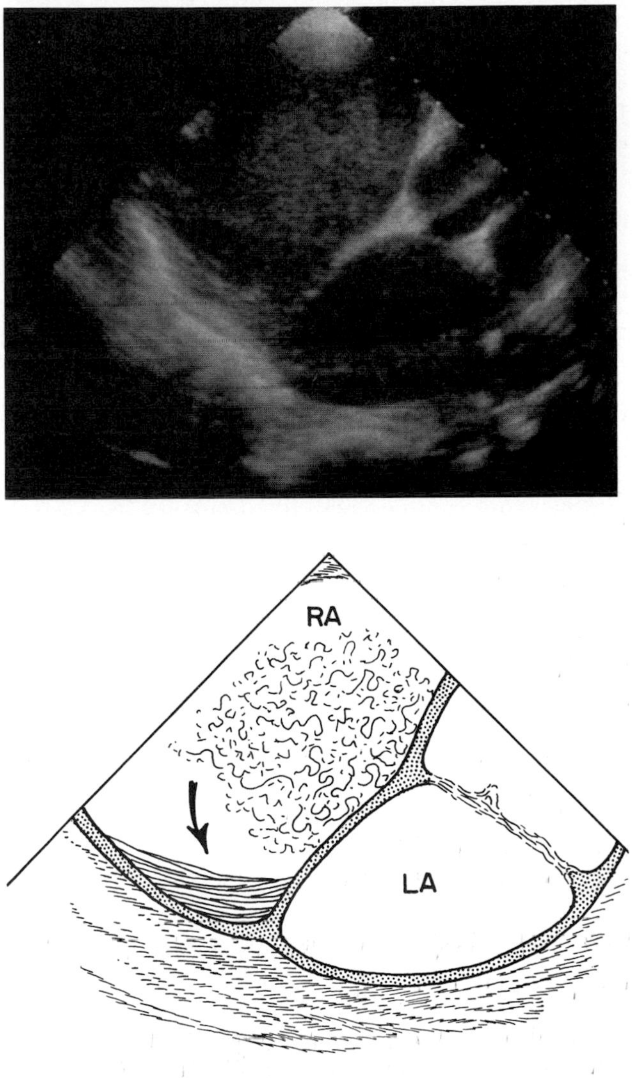

Fig. 38–36. Subcostal long axis recording of the right atrium (RA) and interatrial septum from a patient with stenosis of a bioprosthetic tricuspid valve. There is a diffuse granular echo pattern in the RA, which showed a swirling pattern in real-time, consistent with blood stasis. Along the superior border of the RA is a linear collection of echoes (downward pointing arrow) indicative of laminar thrombus. LA = left atrium.

right atrium is a linear collection of echoes indicative of thrombus.

When poorly recorded from all the standard transthoracic locations, the transesophageal window may yield additional information about the structure and function of a tricuspid prosthesis.

Pulmonary Prostheses and Valved Conduits

Several forms of severe congenital heart disease can be surgically managed using a valved conduit to establish more normal flow from the right heart to the pulmonary artery. These conditions include forms of pulmonary atresia, truncus arteriosus, D-transposition of the great vessels, and tricuspid atresia. These extracardiac communications can take the form of either a direct communication between the right ventricle and the pulmonary artery (Rastelli-type repair) or valved connections between the right atrium and the pulmonary artery (Fontan-type repair). Many such conduits are constructed using bioprosthetic valves or homografts.

Because the anatomic features on which these types of repairs are superimposed may vary greatly, only general guidelines can be given for evaluation of the conduit and valve.[73] First, the anatomic position and communications of the conduit must be defined relative to the three-dimensional anatomy of the heart. Second, the velocity of flow through the conduit including its distal and proximal anastomoses must be assessed. A complete examination of the conduit is important because stenosis can involve the prosthesis or can occur at any other site in the conduit or at its anastomoses. This examination is best conducted from an imaging plane in which conduit blood flow is directed either toward or away from the transducer. Identification of an appropriate plane may be difficult because of the atypical and varying orientation of these conduits, and it requires both an understanding of the surgical procedure and careful attention to imaging principles. Stenosis, as in native structures, is denoted by a sudden step up in velocity at any point along the conduit. Color flow mapping is also most helpful in defining flow direction, the presence of regurgitation, and the site of stenosis. Continuous wave Doppler can be used to define the maximal velocity and to provide the necessary data to calculate maximal and mean gradients. It is often difficult to obtain a transducer window where flow is parallel to the examining continuous wave ultrasound beam. Subcostal, left and right subclavicular, right parasternal, and transesophageal windows may all assist in recording the maximal velocity.

SPECIFIC PROSTHETIC VALVE ABNORMALITIES

Mismatch Dysfunction

Probably the most common type of prosthetic valve "dysfunction" is mismatch dysfunction in which the prosthetic device is functioning as designed, but its hemodynamic performance is inadequate for the specific intracardiac site or individual in whom it is implanted. The explanted valve in these cases appears normal. This form of dysfunction is usually associated with an inappropriately high pressure gradient and can result in persistence of the hemodynamic lesion for which valve replacement was originally undertaken.[31,74] Although mismatch dysfunction should be evident during a baseline postoperative study, it may become apparent only when cardiac output is increased during exercise.

Mismatch dysfunction must be differentiated from primary prosthetic valvular dysfunction in which the prosthesis itself functions abnormally and leads to stenosis or regurgitation or develops a superimposed process related to its presence (e.g., thrombosis or endocarditis). Because differences in surgical technique and in the morphologic features of individual patients may alter the appearance or function of valves of the same type and size, it may be difficult to differentiate mismatch from primary prosthetic valvular dysfunction from a single study.[75] Comparison of function and morphology on serial studies (particularly baseline and follow-up), however, usually permits mismatch and acquired dysfunction to be separated and facilitates clinical decision making.

Prosthetic Valve Endocarditis

A prosthetic valve is a foreign body at the center of the circulation that is always a potential site for infection. Infection involving prosthetic valves is particularly ominous because prosthetic endocarditis is difficult to eradicate and often leads to secondary complications requiring valve removal and replacement. The characteristic lesion of prosthetic endocarditis, like that of native valves, is vegetation. Prosthetic valve vegetations appear echocardiographically as irregular masses of echoes attached to the valve components (Figs. 38–37 and 38–38). When vegetations are small, they typically

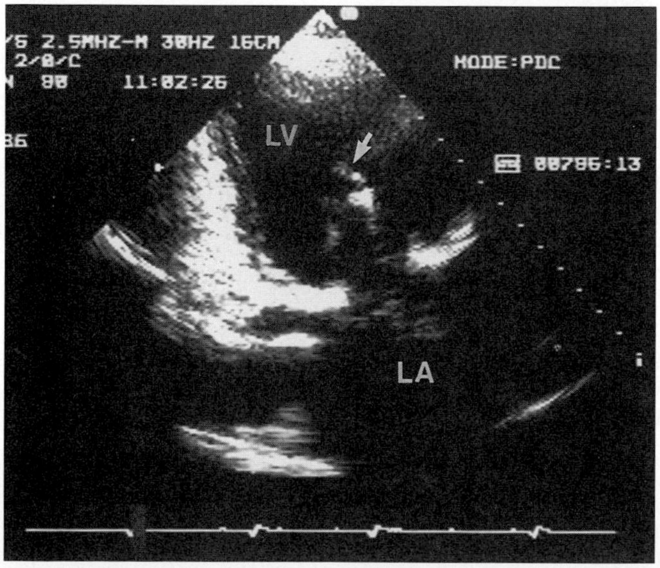

Fig. 38–37. Bacterial vegetation attached to the cage of a Starr-Edwards valve in the mitral position. In this still frame, the linear echoes from the vegetation (arrow) can be clearly separated from the prosthetic material. In real-time analysis, the vegetation moves in parallel with the path of blood flow into and out of the left ventricular outflow tract, further highlighting its presence. LA = left atrium; LV = left ventricle.

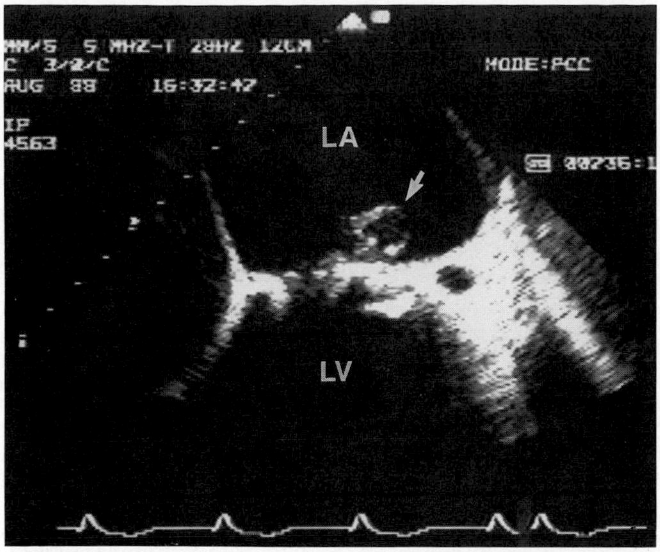

Fig. 38–38. Transesophageal recording of a large vegetation (arrow) attached to the inlet side of a mitral prosthesis. LV = left ventricle; LA = left atrium.

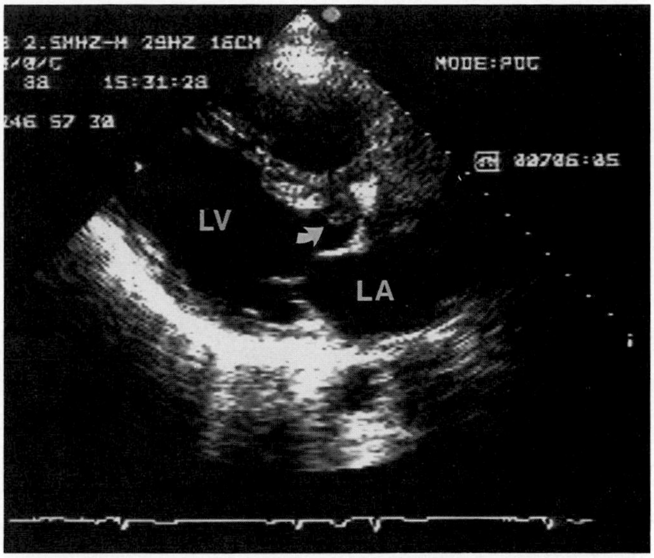

Fig. 38–39. Parasternal long axis recording from a patient with a bioprosthetic valve and aortic endocarditis. There is a large, mobile, spherical bacterial vegetation (arrow) on the inlet side of the valve, which moved into and obstructed the valve orifice during systole. LA = left atrium; LV = left ventricle.

appear as discrete, irregular, stationary echogenic masses superimposed on or attached to the margins of the valve. Small vegetations are extremely difficult to separate from the intensely reflective prosthetic materials of the artificial valve. As vegetations enlarge, they frequently become mobile (see Fig. 38–37) and can be observed to move parallel to the path of blood flow through the valve. Because of their size and independent motion, large vegetation are more easily detected (Fig. 38–38). Occasionally, the vegetations can spread to involve adjacent structures (e.g., superiorly from a mitral prosthesis along the surface of the left atrium or adjacent to the sewing ring of aortic prostheses).

The ability of transthoracic cross-section echocardiography to detect vegetations on prosthetic valves is poor compared to the diagnostic sensitivity for native valves.[76,77] This decrease in sensitivity is due both to the intense reflectivity of the prosthesis, which obscures small superimposed vegetations, and to the increased attenuation, which limits the access of the sound waves to the deeper portions of the valve apparatus. These limitations are most apparent when one tries to study the inlet side of a mechanical prosthesis in the mitral position. Fortunately, transesophageal echocardiography provides ready access to the areas that are most difficult to approach transthoracically and has significantly improved diagnostic accuracy (Fig. 38–38) (see also Chapter 16). This is especially true in the detection of small vegetations, owing to the higher spatial resolution that can be achieved using transesophageal echocardiography.[78]

Large vegetations can, at times, cause obstruction to flow through the valve orifice[79] (Fig. 38–39). When obstruction occurs, Doppler evidence of stenosis should be present (Fig. 38–40). It has also been suggested that the finding of large vegetations, greater than 0.5 cm, is associated with a poor clinical outcome,[80] and vegetation size may be useful information when deciding on more urgent surgical management. Endocarditis involving the leaflets of a bioprosthesis may lead to progressive destruction and increasing regurgitation. If a vegetation interferes with the mechanism of a mechanical valve, it can result in either regurgitation or stenosis.

Prosthetic valve endocarditis, at all intracardiac sites, may lead to paravalvular abscess formation and a higher complication rate.[81] In the mitral site, a paravalvular abscess generally appears as an echo-free space adjacent to the sewing ring, but it may simply be manifest as increased valvular mobility resulting from suture dehiscence and lack of local support. Unfortunately, ring or myocardial abscesses are frequently first detected at operation, suggesting that echocardiographic evaluation has been incomplete.[81,82] In the aortic site, abnormal thickening of the aortic root, with or without a central echo-free space confirmed in two views, suggests the presence of a ring abscess[83,84] (Fig. 38–41). Fistulous communications with the right atrium, left atrium, or right ventricle can be seen in these cases (Fig. 38–42). The resulting shunt(s) can be easily detected by a careful Doppler examination and may alert the examiner to the presence of endocarditis. Intraoperative epicardial echocardiography has been used to define complicated endocarditic lesions, e.g., abscesses.[82] Direct epicardial studies can be performed both before valve revision and immediately after valve implantation to assess the adequacy of the repair and to search for residual infected tissue.

Thus, although the demonstration of prosthetic valve vegetations often provides valuable clinical information, failure to demonstrate vegetations is common in prosthetic endocarditis. A negative transthoracic examination therefore does not exclude the diagnosis, and when

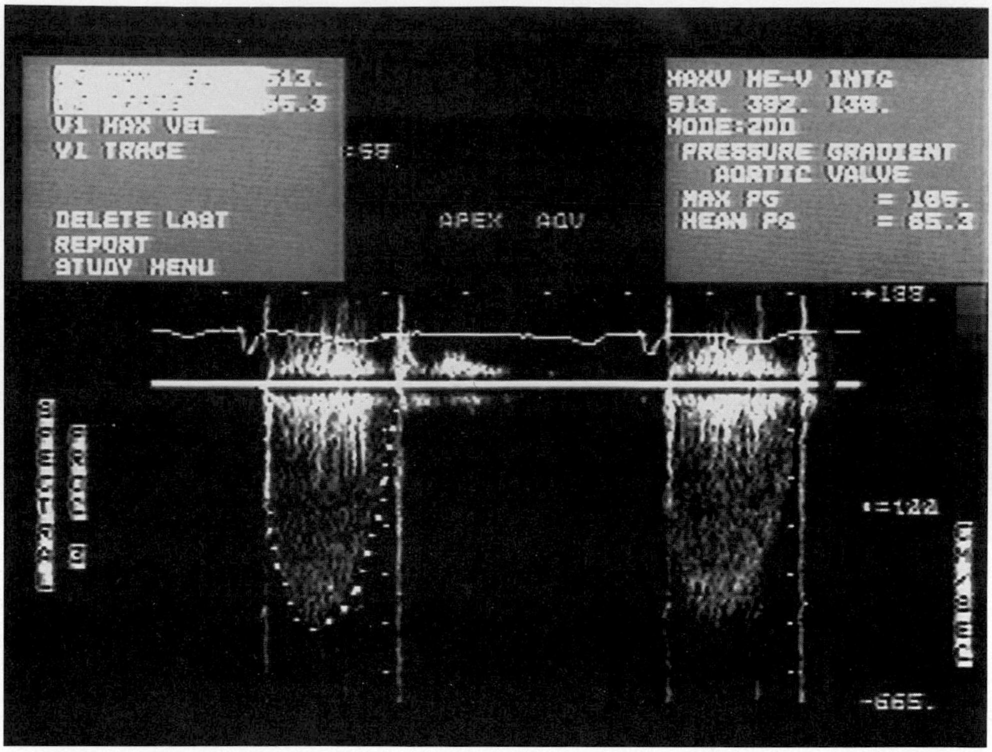

Fig. 38–40. Continuous wave Doppler recording of aortic outflow recorded from the cardiac apex in the same patient whose two-dimensional echo is illustrated in Figure 38–39. The valvular stenosis caused by the vegetation resulted in a 105-mm Hg transvalvular gradient and a 65-mm Hg mean gradient.

clinically warranted, transesophageal examination should be considered in such cases.

Thrombotic Occlusion of Prosthetic Valves

Acute thrombotic obstruction is seen almost exclusively in patients with mechanical prostheses who are receiving inadequate anticoagulation. Thrombotic occlusion of a prosthetic valve may be due to direct obstruction of the valve orifice by the thrombus, interference with the movement of the disc or poppet, or commonly some combination of both. Total thrombotic occlusion is incompatible with life. Patients with subtotal thrombotic obstruction often initially are seen in a moribund state, and the echocardiographic diagnosis can be critical in the institution of appropriate lifesaving therapy.[85] Thrombotic occlusion is recognized by an increase in echo density within the valve mechanism and decreased or absent occluder motion. On occasion, mobile echo densities representing thrombus or vegetation may also be present.

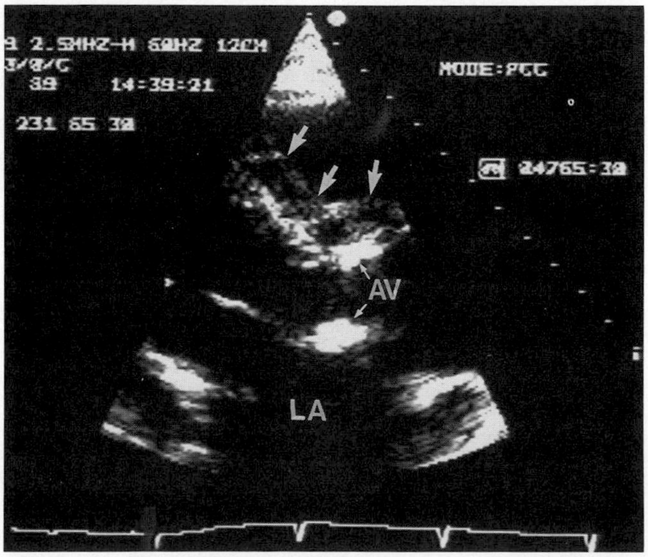

Fig. 38–41. Parasternal long axis recording of a patient with bacterial endocarditis involving a bioprosthetic valve in the aortic position (AV) complicated by an aortic root abscess. The abscess appears as a clear space (large vertical arrows) anterior to the valve that involves the sinus of Valsalva and extends downward into the interventricular septum. LA = left atrium.

Interference with normal occluder motion may be complete, partial, or intermittent (Figs. 38–43 and 38–44).[86] When hemodynamic dysfunction is due to restricted occluder motion, the predominant abnormality depends on the position in which the occluder is fixed. If the occluder is stuck in a fully open position, regurgitation will predominate, whereas fixation in a more closed position will result in predominant stenosis. To assess the range of occluder motion accurately, an extremely careful examination is necessary. With valves in the mitral, tricuspid, or aortic position, disc or poppet motion is generally best assessed from the cardiac apex because maximal excursion is directed toward (mitral and tricuspid) or away from (aortic) an apical window. Because disc motion may be eccentric, to record maximal excursion, the apically positioned transducer should be gradually rotated through a full 180° arc (with the valve as the center of rotation). Once the plane of maximal excursion is determined, M-mode recordings should be obtained to assess the rate and timing of occluder movement. The examination is less difficult in patients with ball valves

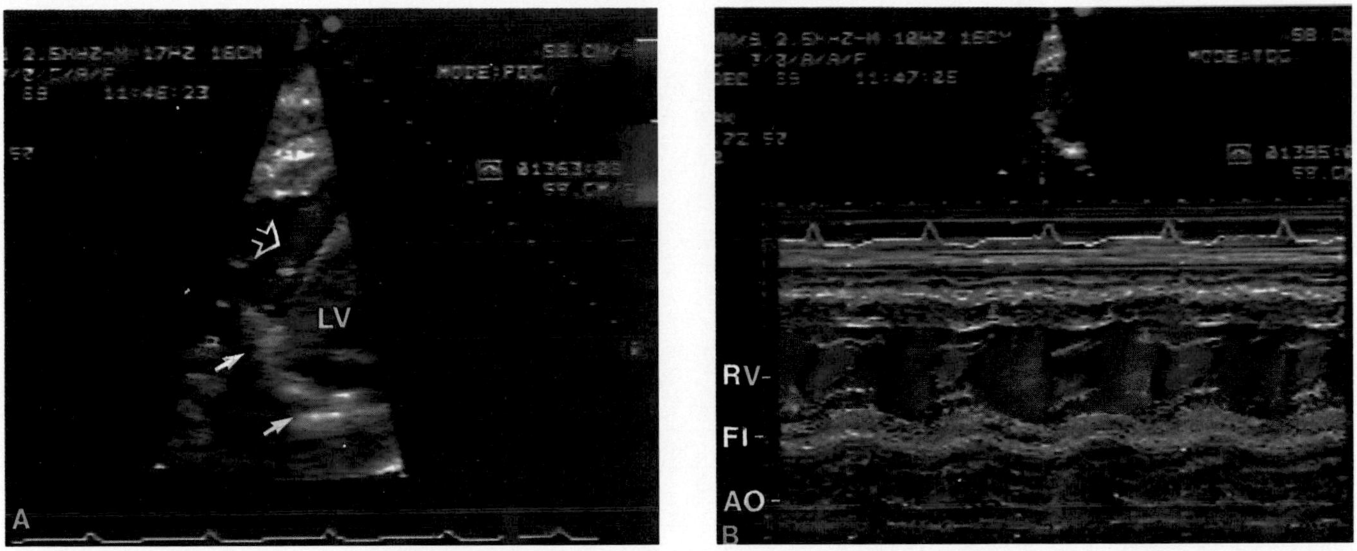

Fig. 38–42. **A.** Modified apical five-chamber color flow recording illustrating an aorto-right ventricular fistula (open arrow) caused by a paravalvular abscess surrounding a bioprosthetic aortic valve. The prosthesis lies between the two oblique arrows. LV = left ventricle. **B.** Color M-mode recording of the same fistula. The right ventricle (RV) is at the top of the scan, the abscess cavity and fistula (FI) in the center, and the prosthetic aortic valve at the bottom (AO). Turbulent flow through the fistula is displayed as turquoise, which changes to red, apically directed flow, as it passes from the outlet of the fistula into the RV. The majority of flow occurs during diastole.

because valve opening is axisymmetric, and the plane of maximal excursion is more easily defined. Double disc valves present a unique problem. Thrombotic obstruction frequently affects only one disc of the valve, and a superficial examination may inappropriately identify full opening of the unaffected disc as normal valve

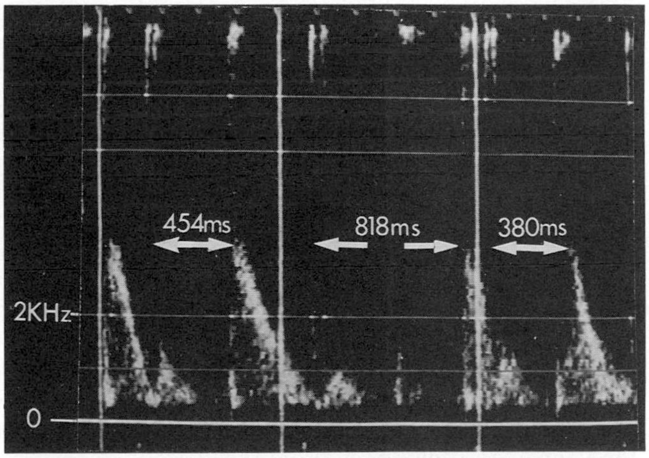

Fig. 38–43. Abnormal timing of prosthetic valve opening as illustrated by the onset of mitral valve inflow recorded during Doppler interrogation of the mitral valve. The patient is in normal sinus rhythm. The numbers depicted above the arrows refer to the time in milliseconds from prosthetic valve closing to valve opening. Note that the time to opening is very irregular, with the onset of opening in the third beat being significantly delayed relative to those preceding and following. This pattern is consistent with intermittent sticking of the valve disc. (From Mann DL, et al.: Doppler and two-dimensional echocardiographic diagnosis of Bjork-Shiley prosthetic valve malfunction: importance of interventricular septal motion and the timing of onset of valve flow. J Am Coll Cardiol; 8:971, 1986. Reprinted with permission of the American College of Cardiology.

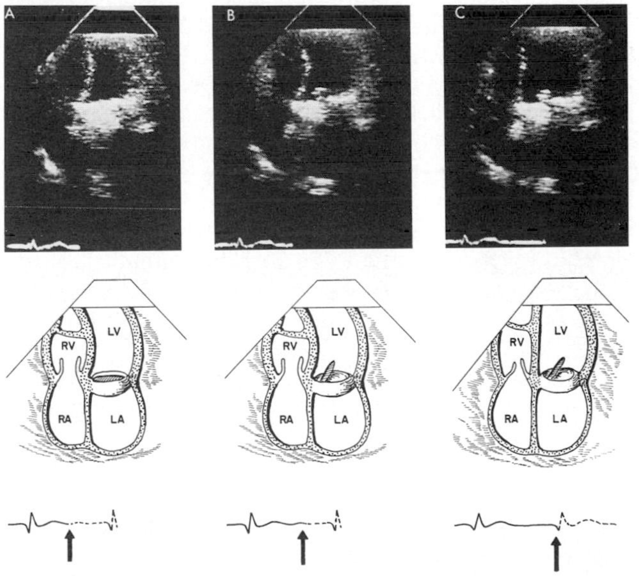

Fig. 38–44. Apical four-chamber recording showing early diastolic paradoxic septal motion. **A.** Early diastole (arrow) following tricuspid valve opening: the dysfunctioning tilting disc has remained closed. Note that the interventricular septum is displaced to the left and is convex toward the left ventricle (LV). **B.** As diastole progresses, the septum continues to shift toward the LV until the mitral valve opens. **C.** By end-diastole, the septum has returned to the midline position and its configuration has normalized. LA = left atrium; RA = right atrium; RV = right ventricle. (From Mann DL, et al.: Doppler and two-dimensional echocardiographic diagnosis of Bjork-Shiley prosthetic valve malfunction: importance of interventricular septal motion and the timing of onset of valve flow. J Am Coll Cardiol; 8:971, 1986. Reprinted with permission of the American College of Cardiology.

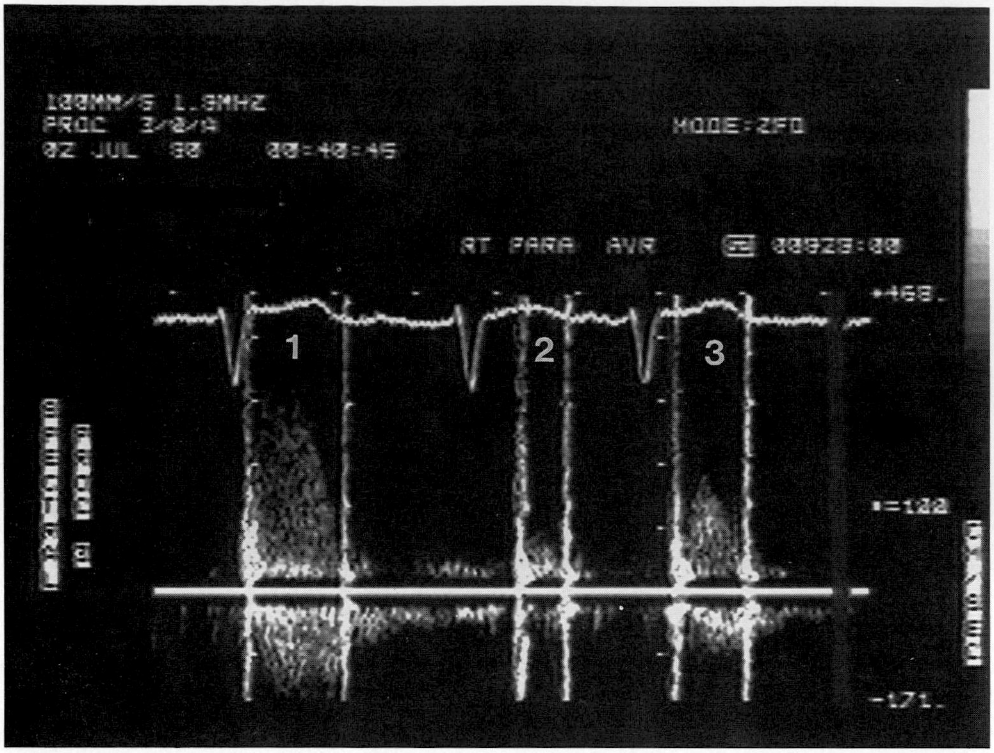

Fig. 38–45. Right parasternal continuous wave Doppler recording from a patient with a mechanical prosthesis in the aortic position. In the second complex valve, opening occurs late relative to the first beat and there is decreased outflow velocity. The third complex is intermediate with valve opening slightly delayed and the outflow velocity intermediate between complexes 1 and 2. This pattern is consistent with delayed valve opening because of ventricular failure, as opposed to a primary abnormality of the prosthetic valve. Relative timing of valve opening can be appreciated by comparing the delay between the S wave of the electrocardiogram and the valve opening clicks.

function. In cases of suspected thrombotic occlusion, therefore, it is critical to know that a double disc valve is present and to record the movement of both discs carefully, to avoid a false-negative examination.

When thrombotic occlusion fixes the valve in a partially closed position, the Doppler examination usually demonstrates markedly elevated transvalvular velocities, reflecting the pressure gradient produced by the obstruction.[87–89] Doppler imaging has also been used to demonstrate a progressive decrease in a transvalvular gradient after thrombolytic therapy. Significant gradients may be present even in predominant regurgitation, because the fixed valve mechanism and sewing ring cannot expand to accommodate the increased transvalvular flow.

When regurgitation is present, it should be clearly demonstrable by Doppler studies. One should use caution in grading the severity of the regurgitation by simply mapping the extent of the jet by pulsed or color flow Doppler, however. Thrombotic valve obstruction can result in an extremely large regurgitant orifice, profound degrees of regurgitation, and virtual abolition of the usual gradient between the chambers that drive and receive the regurgitant jet. In this situation, regurgitant velocities may be low and their spatial distribution limited, suggesting insignificant regurgitation when the opposite is really the case.

Valve obstruction may be intermittent and prolonged sampling may be required to identify a cycle in which the occluder fails to open properly. Moreover, when malfunction is intermittent, it may be difficult to separate transient loss of signal from true dysfunction. In such cases, all available confirmatory data should be sought to help establish the appropriate diagnosis. In one case, intermittent sticking of a mitral disc prosthesis resulted in abnormal timing of Doppler flow and abnormal septal movement.[90] Figure 38–43 illustrates the irregular timing of transmitral flow in relation to the regular electrocardiogram, whereas Figure 38–44 illustrates the marked shift in septal position that occurred during cycles when the mitral valve failed to open at the proper time and the septum was displaced by the resulting right-to-left pressure gradient. Although the Doppler signal was striking when properly recorded, the septal displacement first suggested the correct diagnosis.

Intermittent delay or failure of prosthetic valve opening may also occur because of severe ventricular failure. In these cases, differentiation from intermittent valve sticking is based on the Doppler velocity recorded during the shortened ejection. If the transvalvular gradient is normal or increased, as occurs with a sticking valve, the velocity during the abbreviated beat should be equal to or should exceed that of the beat during which the valve opens normally. In contrast, when the valve opens late because of poor ventricular function (Fig. 38–45), the velocity during the shorter beat will be low because the ventricle is unable to generate sufficient pressure to open in normally.

Mechanical Failure of Prosthetic Valves

The constant opening and closing of prosthetic valves leads to progressive wear on component parts, and ultimately, mechanical failure can occur. The mode of failure varies with valve type. Bioprosthetic valve leaflets are especially prone to failure and commonly show evidence of gradual thickening with increasing implantation time. Although thickening itself is not always associated with dysfunction, it does indicate morphologic change (i.e., infiltration and fibrosis,[91] and such changes eventually lead to functional abnormalities.[92–94] Figure 38–46 illustrates marked thickening of the leaflets of a porcine bioprosthesis in the tricuspid location. The leaflets in this example are intensely echogenic and have a roughened, irregular surface, in contrast to the smooth, thin leaflets of a normal bioprosthetic valve. Leaflet motion in this case was also reduced, and a continuous wave Doppler study demonstrated high transvalvular velocities consistent with severe tricuspid stenosis (Fig. 38–47).

Bioprosthetic valve deterioration more commonly leads to regurgitation than to stenosis. Repeated opening and closing of the nonviable leaflets causes fractures in the collagen fibers and, ultimately, rupture of the leaflets.[95–97] This is often associated with a dramatic clinical event.[98] Porcine valve rupture often results in a flail portion of the valve leaflet,[99,100] which can be visualized during the imaging study, confirming valve failure[12,76] (Fig. 38–48). Frequently, M-mode recordings reveals exaggerated fluttering of the flail or fenestrated portion of the valve leaflet produced by the turbulent regurgitant flow passing over the free leaflet surface. On occasion, the leaflet can become almost completely detached, so movement is exaggerated during both systole and diastole.

Pulsed Doppler or color flow mapping often demonstrates a distinct jet of regurgitation, variably directed into the left atrium. When regurgitation is significant, the jet is usually broad and penetrates deeply into the receiving chamber (see Fig. 38–21). As noted previously, a false-negative Doppler examination for the presence of mitral regurgitation can result if insufficient care is taken to adequately examine the region of the left atrium immediately adjacent to the mitral valve (see the section of this chapter on technique).[101,102] In some cases, an unusual high amplitude "banding" is present on the Doppler spectral recording that is the result of high velocity fluttering of the flail portion of the valve[103] (Fig. 38–49). The patterns of regurgitation for valves in other positions vary with location and severity.

Like porcine prostheses, bovine pericardial valves

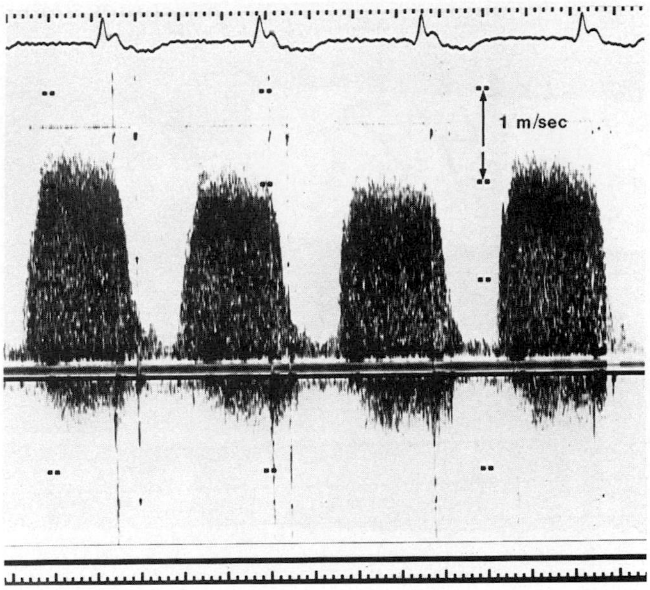

Fig. 38–47. Continuous wave Doppler recording from the cardiac apex of flow velocities across the tricuspid bioprosthesis shown in Figure 38–46. A peak diastolic velocity of 2.2 m/sec was recorded (peak gradient of 19 mm Hg) and a mean gradient of 15 mm Hg. (From Harrigan P, Wilkins GT: Stenosis of a Hancock bioprosthesis in the tricuspid position. J Diagn Med Sonography 2:287, 1986.)

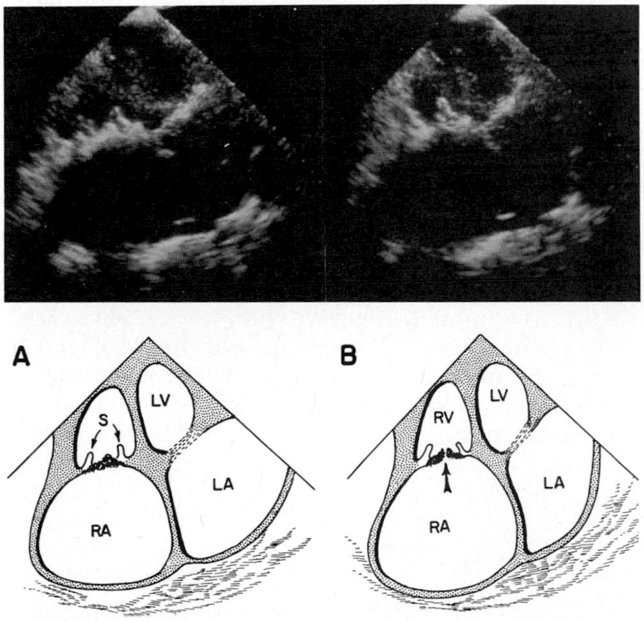

Fig. 38–46. **A.** Apical four-chamber view of a thickened stenotic tricuspid bioprosthesis. Right atrial (RA) and left atrial (LA) dilation are present. **B.** Diastolic recording illustrating significant restriction in leaflet motion and cusp separation. RV = right ventricle; LV = left ventricle; S = valve struts. (From Harrigan P, Wilkins GT: Stenosis of a Hancock Bioprosthesis in the tricuspid position. J Diagn Med Sonography 2:287, 1986.)

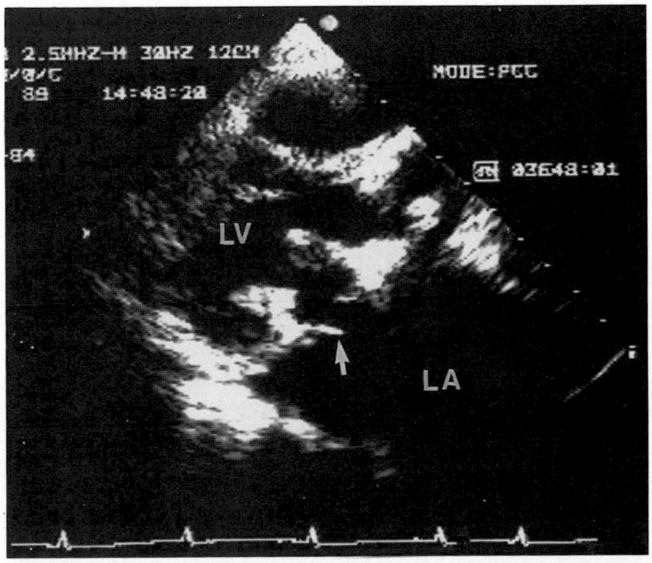

Fig. 38–48. Flail leaflet (arrow) of a degenerated porcine valve in the mitral position. LA = left atrium; LV = left ventricle.

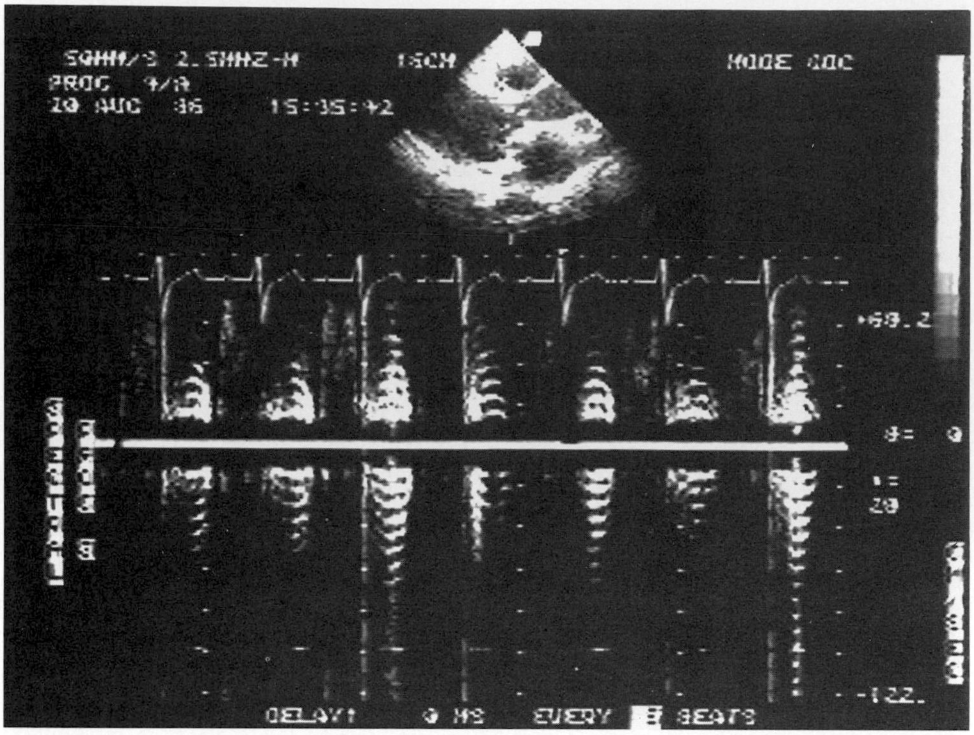

Fig. 38–49. High amplitude spectral peaks arising from the vibrations of a flail leaflet. Output at the base frequency and its harmonics produce a tiger-stripe-like appearance on the spectral output.

also deteriorate in time, and their failure is usually associated with increasing regurgitation.[71,104–107]

Paraprosthetic Leakage and Valve Dehiscence

Paraprosthetic regurgitation can occur as a result of either an incomplete seal between the sewing ring and the annulus at the time of insertion or suture failure after successful implantation. Small paravalvular leaks caused by an imperfect seal between the sewing ring and the annulus are not uncommon,[17] and their clinical significance depends on the size of the leak. They are typically present from the time of insertion and may decrease over time. When paraprosthetic regurgitation occurs de novo in the first days to weeks after valve insertion, it is usually because one or more sutures have pulled free from their annular insertion. Late (weeks to months) suture separation often heralds the insidious presence of prosthetic valve endocarditis and ring abscess formation.

Valve dehiscence results in loss of stability of the prosthesis and is characterized echocardiographically by abnormal rocking of the valve and sewing ring relative to the annulus.[91,108] The abnormal movement is usually more pronounced in the region of suture separation. Because the sewing ring is more easily defined in atrioventricular valve prostheses, this diagnosis is usually easier when mitral or tricuspid devices are affected. As previously noted, surgical technique can greatly influence the "normal" amount of prosthetic valve motion. In those centers where prosthetic mitral valves are sutured to the base of the mitral leaflets rather than to the annulus, some sewing ring motion is routinely noted, and differentiation of normal motion from dehiscence may be difficult without a baseline study.

The detection of aortic dehiscence may be hampered by the similarity in appearance of the sewing ring of an aortic prosthesis and the surrounding tubular aorta. Nonetheless, by using all available imaging windows, the full circumference of the prosthesis can usually be recorded and any independent motion relative to the annulus detected. Rocking of an aortic prosthesis is virtually always a pathologic finding and is frequently associated with severe regurgitation (Fig. 38–50).[109]

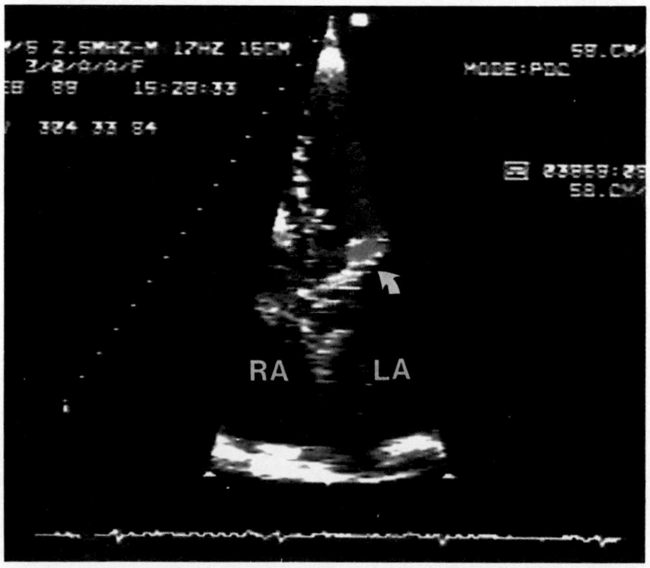

Fig. 38–50. Apical five-chamber view of a Bjork-Shiley valve in the aortic position. Color flow Doppler recording reveals a large paravalvular leak (arrow) caused by partial dehiscence of the prosthesis. LA = left atrium; RA = right atrium.

REFERENCES

1. Starr A, Edwards ML: MItral replacement: clinical experience with a ball valve prosthesis. Ann Surg 154:726, 1961.
2. Harken DE, et al.: Partial and complete prostheses in aortic insufficiency. J Thorac Cardiovasc Surg 40:744, 1960.
3. Roberts WC: Complications of cardiac valve replacement: characteristic abnormalities of prostheses pertaining to any or specific site. Am J Cardiol 103:11, 1982.
4. Wood EH, Leusen IR, Warner HR, Wright JL: Measurement of pressures in man by cardiac catheters. Circ Res 2:294, 1954.
5. Cournand A: Cardiac catheterization: development of the technique, its contributions to experimental medicine and its initial application in man. Acta Med Scand 579(Suppl.): 1, 1975.
6. Karsh DL, et al.: Retrograde left ventricular catheterization in patients with an aortic valve prosthesis. Am J Cardiol 41:893, 1978.
7. Schoenfeld MH, et al.: Underestimation of mitral valve area: role of transseptal catheterization in avoiding unnecessary repeat mitral valve surgery. J Am Coll Cardiol 5:1387, 1985.
8. Ross DN: Homograft replacement of the aortic valve. Lancet 2:487, 1962.
9. Barrett-Boyes BG: Homograft aortic valve replacement in aortic incompetence and stenosis. Thorax 19:131, 1964.
10. Barrett-Boyes BG, et al.: Long-term follow-up of patients with the antibiotic sterilized aortic homograft valve inserted free-hand in the aortic position. Circulation 75:768, 1987.
11. Angell WW, et al.: Long-term follow-up of viable frozen aortic homografts: a viable homograft valve bank. J Thorac Cardiovasc Surg 93:815, 1987.
12. Grenadier E, et al.: Detection of deterioration or infection of homograft and porcine xenograft bioprosthetic valves in mitral and aortic positions by two-dimensional echocardiographic examination. J Am Coll Cardiol 2: 452, 1983.
13. Schramm D, Baldauf W, Meisner H: Flow pattern and velocity field distal to human aortic and artificial heart valves as measured simultaneously by ultramicroscope anemometry in cylindrical glass tubes. Thorac Cardiovasc Surg 28:133, 1980.
14. Horowitz MS, Goodman DJ, Fogarty TJ, Harrison DC: Mitral valve replacement with the glutaraldehyde-preserved porcine heterograft. J Thorac Cardiovasc Surg 67:885, 1974.
15. Thomson FJ, Barrett-Boyes BG: The glutaraldehyde treated heterograft valve. Some engineering observations. J Thorac Cardiovasc Surg 74:317, 1977.
16. Yoganathan AP, et al.: Bileaflet, tilting disc and porcine aortic valve substitutes: in vitro hydrodynamic characteristics. J Am Coll Cardiol 3:313, 1984.
17. Chambers J, Monaghan M, Jackson G: Colour flow Doppler mapping in the assessment of prosthetic valve regurgitation. Br Heart J 62:1, 1989.
18. Reisner SA, Meltzer RS: Normal values of prosthetic valve Doppler echocardiographic parameters: a review. J Am Soc Echocardiogr 1:207, 1988.
19. Carpentier A, et al.: Biological factors affecting long-term results of valvular heterografts. J Thorac Cardiovasc Surg 58:467, 1969.
20. Oyer PE, et al.: Long-term evaluation of the porcine xenograft bioprosthesis. J Thorac Cardiovasc Surg 78:343, 1979.
21. Cohn LH, Mudge GH, Pratter F, Collins JJ Jr: Five to eight-year follow-up of patients undergoing porcine heart valve replacement. N Engl J Med 304:258, 1981.
22. Teoh KH, et al.: Clinical and Doppler echocardiographic evaluation of bioprosthetic valve failure after 10 years. Circulation 82(Suppl. IV):IV-110, 1990.
23. Kutsche LM, Oyer PE, Shumway NE, Baum D: An important complication of Hancock mitral valve replacement in children. Circulation 60:98, 1979.
24. Calderwood SB, et al.: Prosthetic valve endocarditis: analysis of factors affecting outcome of therapy. J Thorac Cardiovasc Surg 92:776, 1986.
25. Wright JTM, Eberhardt CE, Gibbs TS, Gilpin CB: Hancock II—an improved bioprosthesis. *In* Cohn LH, Gallucci V (eds.): Cardiac Bioprostheses: Proceedings of the Second International Symposium. New York, Yorke Medical Books, p. 425, 1982.
26. Ionescu MI, Tandon AP: The Ionescu-Shiley xenograft heart valve. *In* Ionescu MI (ed): Tissue Heart Valves. London, Butterworths, p. 201, 1979.
27. Ionescu MI: The pericardial xenograft valve: mode of failure and possible remedial developments. *In:* Bodnar E, Yacoub M (eds.): Biologic Bioprosthetic Valves: Proceedings of the Third International Symposium. New York, Yorke Medical Books, p. 245, 1986.
28. Weinhold C, et al.: In vivo investigation of kangaroo aortic valve xenobioprostheses: an experimental animal model. *In:* Bodnar E, Yacoub M (eds.): Biologic Bioprosthetic Valves: Proceedings of the Third International Symposium. New York, Yorke Medical Books, p. 668, 1986.
29. Ongcharit C, et al.: Findings in explanted homologous dura mater cardiac valves. *In:* Bodnar E, Yacoub M (eds.): Biologic Bioprosthetic Valves: Proceedings of the Third International Symposium. New York, Yorke Medical Books, p. 383, 1986.
30. Millar DC, et al.: Ten-to-fifteen year reassessment of the performance characteristics of the Starr-Edwards Model 6120 mitral valve prosthesis. J Thorac Cardiovasc Surg 85:1, 1983.
31. Rashtian MY, et al.: Flow characteristics of four commonly used mechanical heart valves. Am J Cardiol 58:743, 1986.
32. Dellsperger KC, et al.: Regurgitation of prosthetic heart valves: dependence on heart rate and cardiac output. Am J Cardiol 51:321, 1983.
33. van den Brink R, et al.: Comparison of transthoracic and transesophageal color Doppler flow imaging in patients with mechanical prostheses in the mitral valve position. Am J Cardiol 63:1471, 1989.
34. Bjork VO, Book K, Holgren A: The Bjork-Shiley mitral valve prosthesis. Ann Thorac Surg 18:379, 1974.
35. Ben-Zvi J, Hildner FJ, Chandraratna PA, Samet P: Thrombosis on Bjork-Shiley aortic valve prosthesis: clinical, arteriographic echocardiographic and therapeutic observations in seven cases. Am J Cardiol 34:538, 1974.
36. Flachskampf FA, et al.: Patterns of normal transvalvular regurgitation in mechanical valve prostheses. J Am Coll Cardiol 18:1493, 1991.
37. Kapur KK, et al.: Doppler color flow mapping in the evaluation of prosthetic mitral and aortic valve function. J Am Coll Cardiol 13:1561, 1989.
38. Gray RJ, et al.: Bileaflet, tilting disc and porcine aortic valve substitutes: in vitro hydrodynamic characteristics. J Am Coll Cardiol 3:321, 1984.
39. Myers ML, et al.: The St. Jude valve prosthesis: analysis of the clinical results in 815 implants and the need for systemic anticoagulation. J Am Coll Cardiol 13:57, 1989.
40. Zeimer G, Luhmer I, Oelert H, Borst H: Malfunction of a St. Jude valve in mitral position. Ann Thorac Surg 33:391, 1982.
41. Holen J, Simonsen S, Froysaker T: An ultrasound Doppler technique for the noninvasive determination of the pressure gradient in the Bjork-Shiley mitral valve. Circulation 59:436, 1979.
42. Holen J, Simonsen S, Froysaker T: Determination of pressure gradient in the Hancock mitral valve from noninvasive ultrasound Doppler data. Scand J Clin Lab Invest 41:177, 1981.
43. Holen J, Nitter-Hauge S: Evaluation of obstructive characteristics of mitral disc valve implants with ultrasound Doppler techniques. Acta Med Scand 201:429, 1977.
44. Holen J, Lhie J, Semb B: Obstructive characteristics of Bjork-Shiley, Hancock and Lillehei-Kaster prosthetic mitral valves in the immediate postoperative period. Acta Med Scand 204:5, 1978.
45. Ryan T, Armstrong WF, Dillon JC, Feigenbaum H: Doppler echocardiographic evaluation of patients with porcine mitral valves. Am Heart J 111: 237, 1986.
46. Omoto R, et al.: Doppler ultrasound examination of prosthetic function and ventricular blood flow after mitral valve replacement. Herz 11:346, 1986.
47. Williams GA, Labovitz AJ: Doppler hemodynamic evaluation of prosthetic (Starr-Edwards and Bjork-Shiley) and bioprosthetic (Hancock and Carpentier-Edwards) cardiac valves. Am J Cardiol 56:325, 1985.
48. Curtis JM, et al.: Dopplerechokardiographische Normwerte fur verschiedene mitral Prosthesentypen. Z Kardiol 76:25, 1987.
49. Fawzy ME, et al.: Hemodynamic evaluation of porcine bioprostheses in the mitral position by Doppler echocardiography. Am J Cardiol 59:643, 1987.
50. Holen J, et al.: Determination of effective orifice area in mitral stenosis from noninvasive ultrasound Doppler data and mitral flow rate. Acta Med Scand 201:83, 1977.
51. Teirstein P, Yock PG, Popp RL: The accuracy of Doppler ultrasound measurement of pressure gradients across irregular dual, and tunnel-like obstructions to blood flow. Circulation 72:577, 1985.
52. Arabia FA, Talbot TL, Jones M, Clark RE: Simultaneous in vitro maximum measured and Doppler derived pressure differences across prosthetic heart valves (abstr.). Circulation 76(Suppl. IV):IV-389, 1987.
53. Simpson IA, et al.: Comparison of Doppler ultrasound velocity measurements with pressure differences across bioprosthetic valves in a pulsatile flow model. Cardiovasc Res 20:317, 1986.
54. Wilkins GT, et al.: Validation of continuous-wave Doppler echocardiographic measurements of mitral and tricuspid prosthetic valve gradients: a simultaneous Doppler-catheter study. Circulation 74:786, 1986.
55. Alam M, et al.: Doppler and echocardiographic features of normal and dysfunctioning bioprosthetic valves. J Am Coll Cardiol 10:851, 1987.
56. Burstow DJ, et al.: Continuous wave Doppler echocardiographic measurement of prosthetic valve gradients. Circulation 80:504, 1989.
57. Nellessen U, et al.: Mitral prosthesis malfunction. Circulation 79:330, 1989.
58. Bhatia S, et al.: Frequency of unusually high transvalvular Doppler velocities in patients with normal prosthetic valves (abstr.). J Am Coll Cardiol 9(Suppl.A):238A, 1987.
59. Levang OW, et al.: Aortic valve replacement: A randomized study comparing the Bjork-Shiley and Lillehei-Kaster disc valves: late hemodynamics related to clinical results. Scand J Thorac Cardiovasc Surg 13:199, 1979.
60. Levine RA, et al.: Pressure recovery distal to a stenosis: potential cause of gradient "overestimation" by Doppler echocardiography. J Am Coll Cardiol 13:706, 1989.
61. Baumgartner H, et al.: Discrepancies between Doppler and catheter gradients in aortic prosthetic valves in vitro. Circulation 82:1467, 1990.
62. Flachskampf FA, Weyman AE, Guerrero JL, Thomas JD. Influence of orifice shape, size, and flow rate on effective valve area: an in vitro study. J Am Coll Cardiol 15:1173, 1990.
63. Warth DC, Stewart WJ, Block PC, Weyman AE: A new method to calculate aortic valve area without left heart catheterization. Circulation 70:978, 1984.
64. Skjaerpe T, Hegrenaes L, Hatle L: Noninvasive estimation of valve area

in patients with aortic stenosis by Doppler ultrasound and two-dimensional echocardiography. Circulation 72:810, 1985.

65. Dennig K, Rudolph W: Nichtinvasive Bestimmung der offnungsflache von Aortenklappenprothesen mit Hilfe der Doppler-Echokardiographie. Herz 11:341, 1986.
66. Rothbart RM, et al.: Determination of aortic valve area by two-dimensional and Doppler echocardiography in patients with normal and stenotic bioprosthetic valves. J Am Coll Cardiol 15:817, 1990.
67. Chafizadeh ER, Zoghbi WA. Doppler echocardiographic assessment of the St. Jude Medical prosthetic valve in the aortic position using the continuity equation. Circulation 83:213, 1991.
68. Hatle L, Angelson B, Tromsdal A: Noninvasive assessment of atrioventricular pressure half-time by Doppler ultrasound. Circulation 60:1096, 1979.
69. Hatle L, Anglesen B. Doppler Ultrasound in Cardiology: Physical Principles and Clinical Applications. Philadelphia, Lea & Febiger, 1982.
70. Thomas JD, Weyman AE: Doppler mitral pressure half-time: a clinical tool in search of theoretical justification. J Am Coll Cardiol 10:923, 1987.
71. Gabbay S, et al.: Long-term follow-up of the Ionescu-Shiley mitral pericardial xenograft. J Thorac Cardiovasc Surg 5:758, 1984.
72. Rosenzweig BP, et al.: Systolic antegrade tricuspid blood flow: a sign of severe prosthetic valve stenosis. Am Heart J 115:693, 1988.
73. Canale JM, et al.: Two-dimensional Doppler echocardiographic/M-mode echocardiographic and phonocardiographic method for study of extracardiac heterograft valved conduits in the right ventricular outflow tract position. Am J Cardiol 49:100, 1982.
74. Rahimtoola SH: The problem of valve prosthesis-patient mismatch. Circulation 58:20, 1978.
75. Rahimtoola SH. Valvular heart disease: a perspective. J Am Coll Cardiol 1:199, 1983.
76. Effron MK, Popp RL: Two-dimensional echocardiographic assessment of bioprosthetic valve dysfunction and infective endocarditis. J Am Coll Cardiol 2:597, 1983.
77. Alam M, et al.: Echocardiography evaluation of porcine bioprosthetic valves: experience with 309 normal and 59 dysfunctional valves. Am J Cardiol 52:309, 1983.
78. Erbel R, et al.: Improved diagnostic value of echocardiography in patients with infective endocarditis by transesophageal approach: a prospective study. Eur Heart J 9:43, 1988.
79. Lewis JF, et al.: Tricuspid stenosis in prosthetic valve endocarditis: diagnosis by Doppler echocardiography. Chest 91:276, 1987.
80. Come PC, Isaacs RE, Riley MF: Diagnostic accuracy of M-mode echocardiography in active infective endocarditis and prognostic implications of ultrasound-detectable vegetations. Am Heart J 103:839, 1982.
81. Ellis SG, Goldstein J, Popp RL: Detection of endocarditis associated perivalvular abscess by two-dimensional echocardiography. J Am Coll Cardiol 5:647, 1985.
82. Van Herwerden LA, et al.: Intraoperative two-dimensional echocardiography in complicated infective endocarditis of the aortic valve. J Thorac Cardiovasc Surg 93:587, 1987.
83. Pollak SJ, Felner JM: Echocardiographic identification of an aortic valve ring abscess. J Am Coll Cardiol 7:1167, 1986.
84. Come PC, Riley MF: Echocardiographic recognition of perivalvular infection complicating aortic bacterial endocarditis. Am Heart J 108:166, 1984.
85. Boskovic D, Pechacek LW, Krajcer Z: Thrombosis of a Bjork-Shiley aortic valve prosthesis diagnosed by two-dimensional echocardiography. J Clin Ultrasound 11:165, 1983.
86. Ledain LD, et al.: Acute thrombotic obstruction with disc valve prostheses: diagnostic considerations and fibrinolytic treatment. J Am Coll Cardiol 7:743, 1986.
87. Barzilai B, et al.: Detection of thrombotic obstruction of a Bjork-Shiley prosthesis by Doppler echocardiography. Am Heart J 112:1088, 1986.
88. Koblic M, Carey C, Webb-Peploe MM, Braimbridge MV: Streptokinase treatment of thrombosed mitral valve prosthesis monitored by Doppler ultrasound. Thorac Cardiovasc Surg 34:333, 1986.
89. Gonzalez-Santos JM, et al.: Thrombosis of a mechanical valve prosthesis late in pregnancy. Case report and review of the literature. Thorac Cardiovasc Surg 34:335, 1986.
90. Mann DL, et al.: Doppler and two-dimensional echocardiographic diagnosis of Bjork-Shiley prosthetic valve malfunction: importance of interventricular septal motion and the timing of onset of valve flow. J Am Coll Cardiol 8:971, 1986.
91. Schapira JN, et al.: Two-dimensional echocardiographic assessment of patients with bioprosthetic valves. Am J Cardiol 43:510, 1979.
92. Alam M, et al.: M-mode and two-dimensional echocardiographic features of porcine valve dysfunction. Am J Cardiol 43:502, 1979.
93. Alam M, Goldstein S: Echocardiographic features of a stenotic porcine valve. Am Heart J 100:517, 1980.
94. Harrigan P, Wilkins GT: Stenosis of a Hancock bioprosthesis in the tricuspid position. J Diagnostic Med Sonography 2:287, 1986.
95. Forman MB, Phelan BK, Robertson RM, Virmani R: Correlations of two-dimensional echocardiography and pathological findings in porcine valve dysfunction. J Am Coll Cardiol 5:224, 1985.
96. Ferrans VJ, Spray TL, Billingham ME, Roberts WC: Structural changes in glutaraldehyde treated porcine heterografts used as substitute cardiac valves: transmission and scanning electron microscopic observations in 12 patients. Am J Cardiol 41:1159, 1978.
97. Angell WW, Angell JD: Porcine valves. Prog Cardiovasc Dis 23:141, 1980.
98. Crupi G, Gibson D, Heard B, Lincoln C: Severe late failure of a porcine xenograft mitral valve: clinical, echocardiographic and pathological findings. Thorax 35:210, 1980.
99. Nicholson WJ, Gracey JG, Martin CE: Echocardiographic identification of prolapsing leaflet of a malfunctioning aortic porcine xenograft. Clin Cardiol 6:97, 1983.
100. Bansai RC, Morrison DL, Jacobson JG: Echocardiography of porcine aortic prosthesis with flail leaflets due to degeneration and calcification. Am Heart J 107:591, 1984.
101. Sprecher DL, et al.: In vitro color flow, pulsed and continuous wave Doppler ultrasound masking of flow by prosthetic valves. J Am Coll Cardiol 9:1306, 1987.
102. Come PC: Pitfalls in the diagnosis of peri-prosthetic valvular regurgitation by pulsed Doppler echocardiography. J Am Coll Cardiol 9:1176, 1987.
103. Kinney EL, Machado H, Cortado X: Cooing intracardiac sound in a perforated porcine mitral valve detected by pulsed Doppler echocardiography. Am Heart J 112:237, 1986.
104. Solana LG, et al.: Two-dimensional echocardiographic assessment of complications involving the Ionescu-Shiley pericardial valve in the mitral position. J Am Coll Cardiol 3:328, 1984.
105. Szkopiec RL, et al.: M-mode and 2-dimensional echocardiographic characteristics of the Ionescu-Shiley valve in the mitral and aortic positions. Am J Cardiol 51:973, 1983.
106. Ionescu MI, et al.: Clinical durability of the pericardial xenograft valve: 11 years experience in cardiac bioprostheses. *In* Cohn LH, Gallucci V (eds.): Cardiac Bioprostheses: Proceedings of the Second International Symposium. New York, Yorke Medical Books, 1982.
107. Robertson J, Burggraf G: Non-invasive assessment of the Ionescu-Shiley pericardial xenograft heart valve. Can J Cardiol 1:241, 1985.
108. Kotler MN, et al.: Noninvasive evaluation of normal and abnormal prosthetic valve function. J Am Coll Cardiol 2:151, 1983.
109. Mehta A, et al.: Two-dimensional echocardiographic observations in major detachment of a prosthetic aortic valve. Am Heart J 101:231, 1981.
110. Baudet EM, et al.: A 5-½ year experience with the St. Jude Medical cardiac valve prosthesis. J Thorac Cardiovasc Surg 90:137, 1985.
111. Miller FA, et al.: Normal aortic valve prosthesis hemodynamics: 609 prospective Doppler examinations (abstr.). Circulation 80(Suppl. II):II–169, 1989.
112. Panidis IS, Ross J, Mintz GS: Normal and abnormal prosthetic valve function as assessed by Doppler echocardiography. J Am Coll Cardiol 8:317, 1986.
113. Nellessen U, et al.: Transesophageal two-dimensional echocardiography and color Doppler flow velocity mapping in the evaluation of cardiac valve prostheses. Circulation 78:848, 1988.

CHAPTER

39

ECHOCARDIOGRAPHY IN CARDIAC TRANSPLANTATION

MICHAEL H. PICARD

Since the first human orthotopic cardiac transplant was performed in 1967,[1] the long-term survival of cardiac transplant patients has improved because of advances in donor and recipient selection, organ procurement, the treatment of transplant rejection, and the recognition and treatment of the side effects of immunosuppression. Although the echocardiogram has not met the initial hope of being an ideal noninvasive test by which to recognize acute cardiac transplant rejection, it plays an expanded role in the selection of potential donors and potential recipients and in the care of the cardiac transplant recipient.

EVALUATION OF POTENTIAL DONORS

The criteria for the potential heart donor include formal declaration of brain death, age less than 45 years, previous good general health, and no evidence of active or chronic infection. Additional goals are to exclude those hearts with left ventricular dysfunction, valve disease, or significant coronary artery disease. In an attempt to exclude those with left ventricular dysfunction, it has been the practice to exclude any potential donor with chest trauma, prolonged hypotension or hypoxemia, or cardiac arrest, or donors receiving high doses of catecholamines.[2,3] These clinical criteria lack a strong association with significant left ventricular dysfunction, however, and therefore echocardiographic assessment of left ventricular function has become an effective tool for screening of potential cardiac transplant donors.[3]

Many of the donors die as a result of motor vehicle accidents. In these potential donors, identifying patients with cardiac contusions due to blunt trauma becomes important. Electrocardiographic abnormalities are common in patients recovering from blunt trauma, but these abnormalities do not correlate strongly with structural cardiac damage.[4] The two-dimensional echocardiogram is a more sensitive detector of significant cardiac contusion, and functional cardiac abnormalities are observed by echocardiography in 10 to 30% of patients after blunt chest trauma.[4–6] The most common echocardiographic findings include pericardial effusion, wall motion abnormalities of the left and/or right ventricle, ventricular thrombi, and heterogeneous echo densities of the myocardium.[7] Because the main factor limiting cardiac transplantation today is the limited number of donor hearts available, two-dimensional echocardiography serves as an accurate screen by which to exclude those with significant cardiac contusions, while increasing the number of eligible donors who might have initially been excluded by clinical criteria. Pilot studies suggest that the number of hearts eligible for transplantation might increase by as much as 29% if echocardiograms were used as a screening tool.[3]

As discussed in previous chapters, echocardiography and Doppler together are sensitive and specific tools in the evaluation of valvular diseases such as significant valvular regurgitation, stenosis, and vegetation when these exclusion criteria are suggested during physical examination of the potential donor. The echocardiographic examination can also enable one to assess the size of the donor heart accurately when an initial screening test such as chest radiograph or electrocardiogram raises the question of cardiomegaly or left ventricular hypertrophy.

In potential donors who are comatose because of a primary central neurologic injury, an additional concern is an associated alteration in myocardial function. Electrocardiographic abnormalities are common after neurologic injury and can mimic patterns associated with myocardial infarction.[8] Unfortunately, in this setting, the electrocardiogram lacks the sensitivity and specificity required to discriminate between those with myocardial damage and those with normal myocardial function.[9–11] As in the case of cardiac contusions, the echocardiogram can permit one to identify those patients with significant myocardial abnormalities who must be excluded from the donor pool. Focal myocardial necrosis observed in the setting of neural injury has been hypothesized to be due to increased release of norepinephrine resulting from alterations in autonomic tone caused by ischemia of the hypothalamus.[10–13] Clouding this explanation, however, is the finding that patients with neurologic injury who have echocardiographic wall motion abnormalities tend to be older than comatose patients without wall motion abnormalities and have significant coronary artery disease on postmortem examination.[11] In our hospital, the echocardiogram is used as a screening test for comatose patients who are potential cardiac donors, to exclude significant left ventricular dysfunction, whether segmental or diffuse.

EVALUATION OF THE POTENTIAL RECIPIENT

Patients considered for cardiac transplantation are those with end-stage cardiomyopathy. The use of echocardiography to establish the cause of the cardiomyopathy serves several purposes. For example, the echocardiogram can enable the physician to identify cases of heart failure in which other means of treatment might first be attempted, such as severe aortic stenosis or ischemic cardiomyopathy amenable to revascularization. In addition, cases of heart failure that might require heart-lung transplantation rather than cardiac transplantation alone, such as in patients with complex congenital lesions and Eisenmenger's physiology, can be identified by the initial echo-Doppler examination.

Table 39–1 is a list of the indications for and relative contraindications to cardiac transplantation. Although the list may vary as techniques improve, certain contraindications such as irreversible pulmonary hypertension remain key variables in predicting a poor outcome after orthotopic cardiac transplantation. Elevation of the pulmonary vascular resistance above 8 Wood units was initially recognized as one of the major variables associated with a poor postoperative outcome.[14] When the donor right ventricle contracts against an increased pulmonary vascular resistance, it is unable to increase its work load acutely, and acute right ventricular dilatation and failure are commonly observed.[14,15] In some subsets of patients, the elevated pulmonary vascular resistance can be sufficiently reduced with pharmacologic therapy, so these recipients have successful outcomes after cardiac transplantation.[16] Those candidates with pulmonary hypertension defined by pulmonary artery systolic pressure higher than 50 mm Hg and/or a pulmonary vascular resistance of 4 to 8 Wood units should undergo further testing with vasodilatory drugs to assess the degree of reversibility of the process. Because patients with cardiomyopathy have a high prevalence of Doppler-detectable tricuspid regurgitation resulting from annular dilatation and incomplete tricuspid valve closure, the right ventricular and pulmonary artery systolic pressure can be accurately estimated noninvasively, as discussed in Chapter 26. Although this measurement only indirectly reflects the pulmonary artery resistance, it can be used as a primary screen to identify those patients with normal pulmonary artery pressures. When measured in conjunction with vasodilator therapy, the Doppler-estimated pulmonary artery systolic pressure can enable one to identify patients with cardiomyopathy who have reversible pulmonary hypertension.

The noninvasive assessment of left ventricular systolic dysfunction is of value in predicting the urgency for cardiac transplantation. In patients with idiopathic dilated cardiomyopathy who are awaiting cardiac transplantation, the ejection fraction is an accurate predictor of short-term mortality.[17] An ejection fraction of less than 10% predicts a 6-month survival of less than 20% and identifies a subgroup of patients who must be recognized promptly if they are to be given proper consideration for cardiac transplantation.

Right ventricular endomyocardial biopsy is commonly performed before one considers cardiac transplantation when the cause of heart failure is unclear. This is essential, to identify patients with diseases that may respond to medical therapy, such as acute myocarditis or sarcoidosis, and to exclude patients with diseases associated with multiorgan involvement such as hemochromatosis, carcinoid, and glycogen storage disease. By helping to identify patients with regional wall motion abnormalities and ischemic cardiomyopathy, the echocardiogram assists in the selection of patients who do not require a biopsy as part of the pretransplantation workup.

Table 39–1. Orthotopic Cardiac Transplantation

Indications
Functional class IV not remediable by conventional medical or surgical therapy: poor 6-month survival
Age: neonate to 60 years
Medically compliant, emotionally stable patient
Contraindications
Systemic diseases that would limit survival
Active infection
Pulmonary infiltrate including unresolved pulmonary infarction
Irreversible pulmonary hypertension
Moderate-to-severe renal or hepatic dysfunction

ASSESSMENT OF THE CARDIAC TRANSPLANT RECIPIENT

The unusual findings observed during echocardiography of the transplanted heart include visualization of anastomosis sites, variations in right ventricular size, transient myocardial edema, pericardial effusions, valvular regurgitation, and temporal variations in left ventricular filling. The echocardiographic appearance of the heart after transplantation is most easily appreciated if one understands the surgical procedure (Fig. 39–1). The original failing heart is excised from the recipient's chest by incisions through the pulmonary artery, the aorta, and the posterior walls of the right and left atria. As seen in Figure 39–1, by leaving the posterior portions of the right and left atria in situ, the inflow portions of the superior vena cava, inferior vena cava, and pulmonary veins are not disturbed. The donor heart is placed into the recipient's chest by suturing the heart to remnant recipient atria, proximal pulmonary artery, and proximal ascending aorta. Because the new donor heart is normal in size, it is typically smaller than the original dilated failing heart, and therefore it is positioned more medially in the chest and tends to be rotated clockwise. The remnant recipient atrial tissue includes the sinus node, and it is not uncommon for both the donor and remnant native atria to generate independent electrical and mechanical activity. Identifying these independent atrial events on the accompanying electrocardiographic lead is important when one interprets the Doppler flow signals in the vena cava and across the atrioventricular valves (discussed later).

Because of the rotation and medial displacement of the heart, the "standard" images of the heart may need to be obtained from nonstandard transducer locations, which vary from patient to patient. The long axis of the left atrium appears large because it is composed of both donor and recipient atrial tissue. In both parasternal and apical transducer positions, the suture lines within the left atrium and right atrium appear prominently as an echo-dense ridge (Figs. 39–2 and 39–3). The pulmonary artery anastomosis site is also represented as a ridge in the main pulmonary artery (Fig. 39–4). The anastomosis of the donor heart to the aorta is the least consistent finding, because of the variations in its position within the aorta.

In the early phase after cardiac transplantation, the right ventricle enlarges as a response to the increased pulmonary vascular resistance. Although the pulmonary artery hemodynamics normalize within weeks after cardiac transplantation, right ventricular size remains enlarged.[18–20] The persistence of the right ventricular enlargement in a subset of patients has been explained by the relative volume overload resulting from significant tricuspid regurgitation.[20] Commonly, because of the prominent suture line in the proximal pulmonary artery, the pulmonic outflow tract may appear narrowed; however, Doppler assessment of flow across this region confirms the lack of a hemodynamically significant gradient.

In the immediate postoperative state, an increase in left ventricular wall thickness and mass is observed. This initial increase in wall thickness is independent of rejection and has been hypothesized to represent myocardial edema resulting from manipulation and transport of the heart.[16,21]

In the normal transplanted heart, one sees no appreciable changes in the Doppler flow velocities across the pulmonic or aortic valve. Variability of the velocity profiles from the atrioventricular valves may be observed when the remnant recipient atria retain mechanical activity. These variations in transmitral or tricuspid diastolic velocities assessed by pulsed wave Doppler relate to the timing of contraction of the recipient atria.[22] The changes in the mitral inflow velocities assessed by pulsed Doppler are presented in Table 39–2.

Contraction of the recipient atrium in late diastole leads to an increased Doppler peak A-wave velocity be-

A

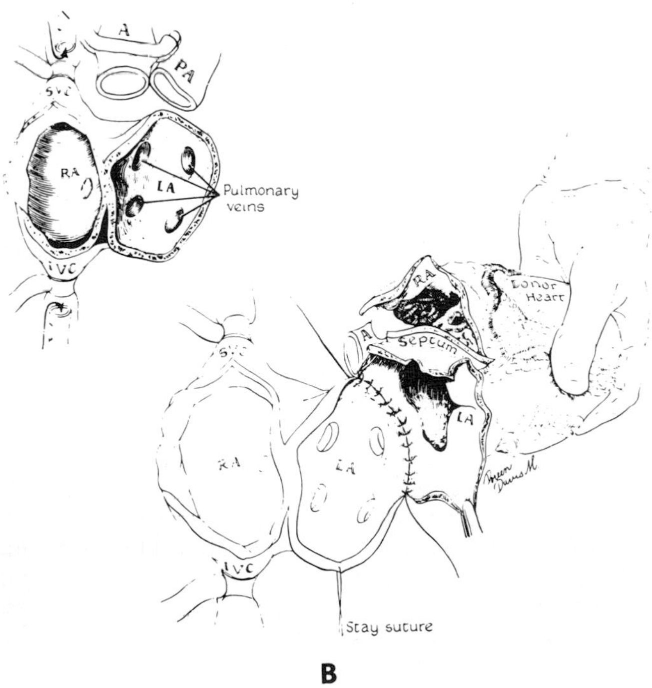

B

Fig. 39–1. The surgical technique of orthotopic cardiac transplantation. **A.** Preparation of recipient bed. **B.** Atrial anastomosis. A = aorta; PA = pulmonary artery; SVC = superior vena cava; RA = right atrium; LA = left atrium; IVC = inferior vena cava. (From Stinson EB, et al.: Initial clinical experience with heart transplantation. Am J Cardiol 22:799, 1968.)

Table 39–2. Alterations in Mitral Inflow Doppler Velocities: Relation to Timing of Recipient Atrial Contraction

Recipient Atrial Contraction	E	A	Isovolumic Relaxation Time	Deceleration Time
Early diastole	N	D	N	N
Late diastole	N	I	N	N
Early systole	D	N	N	I
Late systole	I	N	D	D

N = no change; I = increase; D = decrease.

(Data from Valantine HA, et al.: Influence of recipient atrial contraction on left ventricular filling dynamics of the transplanted heart assessed by Doppler echocardiography. Am J Cardiol 59:1159, 1987.)

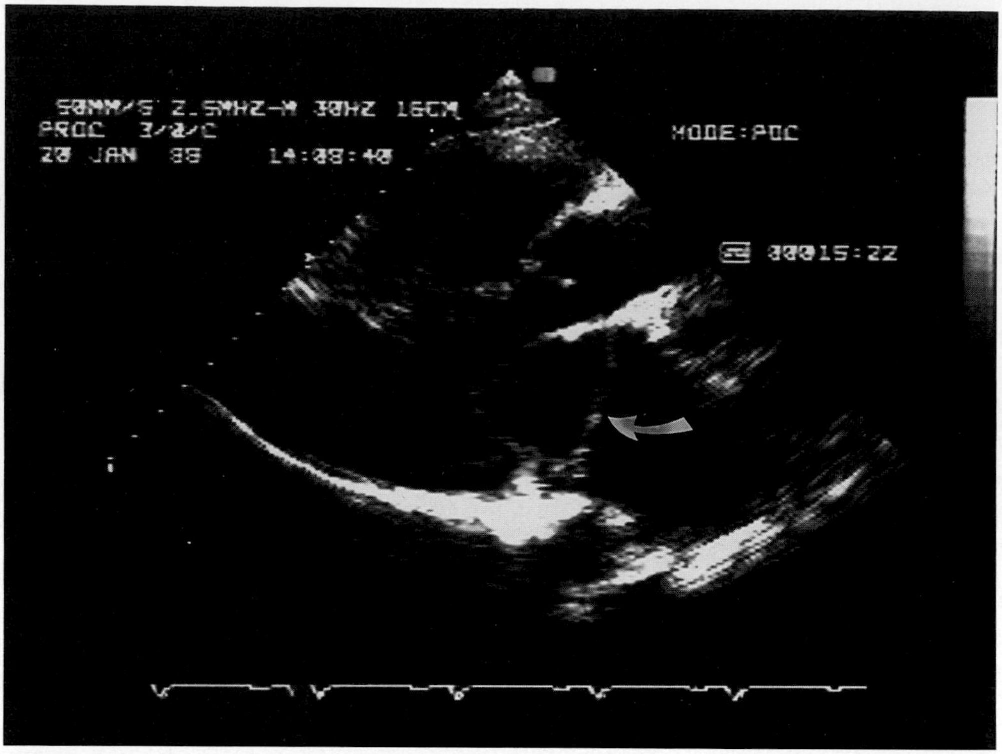

Fig. 39–2. Parasternal long axis view demonstrating the left atrial suture ridge (arrow).

cause of its synchrony with the donor atrial contraction (Fig. 39–5).

Contraction of the recipient atrium in early diastole is associated with a lower peak A-wave velocity from donor atrium, presumably reflecting a decrease in the peak left atrial pressure during donor atrial contraction resulting from relaxation of the recipient portion of the left atrium during the donor atrial contraction.

When the recipient atrium contracts during early systole, it leads to a decrease in the next Doppler peak E velocity along with an increase in the deceleration time. These findings are thought to be due to a lower left atrial pressure in early diastole resulting from coincident relaxation of the remnant recipient atria and a decrease in pulmonary venous filling of the left atrium during the prior systole associated with recipient atrial contraction.

Contraction of the recipient atrium in late systole leads to increases in the left atrial pressure and is associated with an increased peak E velocity. A shorter deceleration time occurs, suggesting a rapid decrease in

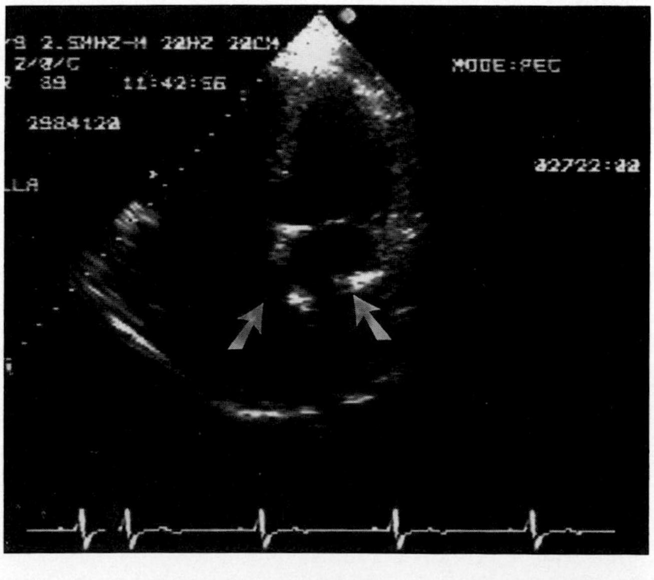

Fig. 39–3. Modified apical four-chamber view demonstrating left and right atrial suture ridges (arrows).

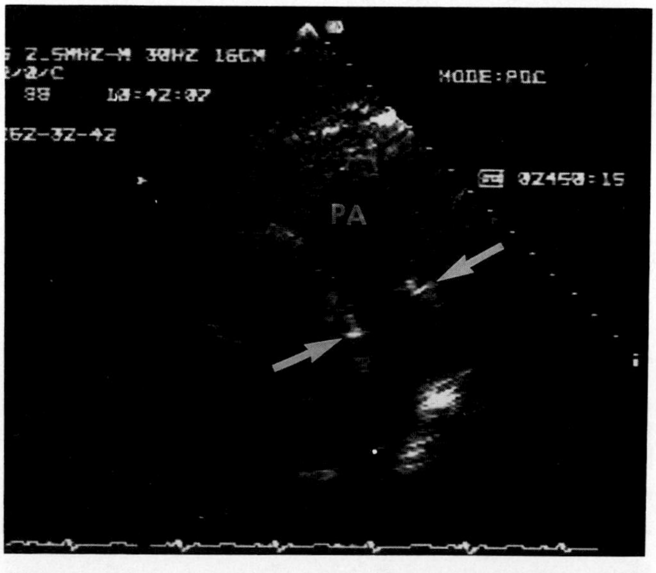

Fig. 39–4. Long axis view of the main pulmonary artery (PA) and its bifurcation. The suture ridge is noted by the arrows.

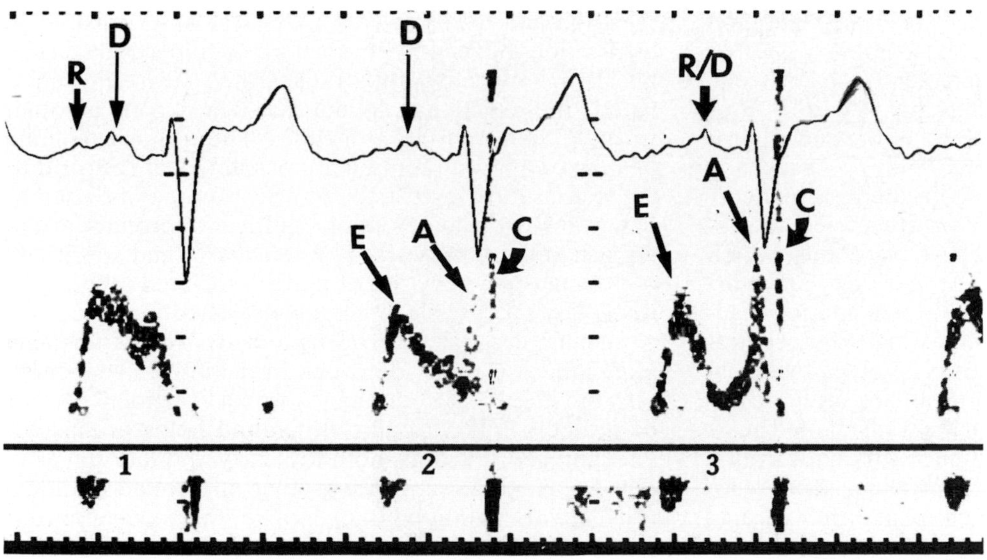

Fig. 39–5. Increase in peak A-wave velocity caused by recipient atrial contraction in late diastole. The baseline A-wave velocity in the second transmitral filling pattern (2) is contrasted with the increased A-wave velocity in the third diastolic cycle (3) caused by coordinated contraction of the recipient and donor portions of the atria in the third diastolic cycle. R = recipient P wave; D = donor P wave; R/D = combined donor and recipient P wave; E = E wave; A = A wave; C = valve closure.

the left atrial-left ventricular diastolic pressure gradient because of relaxation of the recipient atrium in early diastole. In addition, a decrease in the isovolumic relaxation time (IVRT) is observed with the earlier opening of the mitral valve because of the increased left atrial pressure (Fig. 39–6).

Moderate degrees of mitral, pulmonic, and tricuspid regurgitation are commonly found on Doppler examination in the early weeks after cardiac transplantation.[21,23] The natural history of these regurgitant lesions varies and is not related to episodes of rejection or alterations of myocardial function. Although some authors have reported a resolution in the severity of these lesions over time,[21] in some subsets of patients, multivalvular regurgitation is detected up to 4 years after cardiac transplantation.[24,25] Significant factors predicting a delay in resolution of tricuspid regurgitation include an elevated post-transplant pulmonary vascular resistance and structural abnormalities of the valvular and subvalvular apparatus.[24,25]

Posterior pericardial effusions of varying size are commonly observed early after the transplant operation and are thought to be due to hemorrhage, and cyclosporine effects; another cause is that the donor heart is often smaller than the cavity left by the former failing heart.[26–28] Over time, these effusions are resorbed. Late recurrences or increases in the size of effusion have been observed on two-dimensional echocardiography, and the significance of these findings is unclear. In the past, these late effusions were thought to be benign;[26] however, in a more recent, uncontrolled study, changes in effusion size were associated with inflammatory reactions of the pericardium resulting from acute rejection.[29] Unfortunately, this finding is a weak predictor of acute rejection, with a sensitivity of only 66%.

When relative hypotension or a persistent requirement for vasopressors occurs in the early postoperative period, the echocardiogram is used to exclude right ventricular failure, persistent pulmonary hypertension, left ventricular failure, or pericardial tamponade.

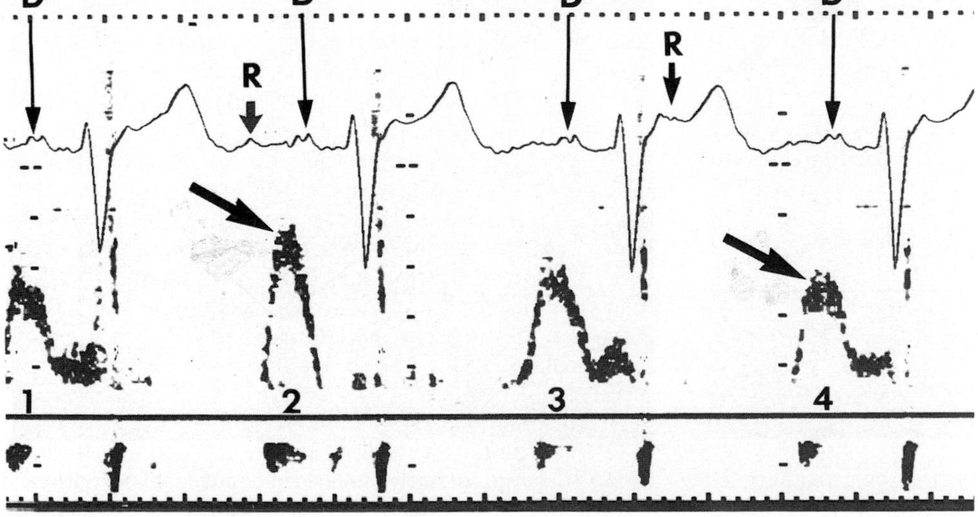

Fig. 39–6. Increased peak E-wave velocity (arrow, cycle 2) and shortened deceleration time is demonstrated because of recipient atrial contraction in late systole. A decrease in peak E-wave velocity is observed following a recipient atrial contraction earlier in systole (arrow, cycle 4). D = donor P wave; R = recipient P wave.

The major complications of cardiac transplantation are listed in Table 39–3. The echocardiogram is often used postoperatively to follow left ventricular systolic function and as an adjunct in the diagnoses of infections involving the heart and of transplant-associated atherosclerosis.

As a result of immunosuppressive therapy, patients who undergo cardiac transplantation are subject to systemic opportunistic infections. These infections, which account for a large proportion of the morbidity and mortality in the first year after cardiac transplantation, usually involve pulmonary, gastrointestinal, and central nervous systems. Rarely, the heart is involved by fungal endocarditis. Although the organisms are often different, the findings of endocarditis in the transplanted heart are the same as in the typical patient with endocarditis.

Frequent biopsies of the right ventricular septum are performed in the early convalescent phase after cardiac transplantation to detect rejection. In experienced hands, the frequency of perforation of the right ventricle as a complication of biopsy is less than 0.4%.[30] Because the pericardium is left open at the end of the operation, it is rare to observe tamponade of the right heart as a sequela of right ventricular perforation, and it occurs only when the residual anterior pericardium becomes fused. The biopsy is generally performed under fluoroscopic guidance. The disadvantages of this approach are the cumulative radiation exposure to the operator and patient, the limited portability of the equipment, and the limited appreciation by fluoroscopy of the three-dimensional relationships among the intracardiac structures. With a combination of modified apical and subcostal views, the echocardiogram can be used to guide the position and placement of the bioptome through the tricuspid valve and against the interventricular septum.[31] Because the complication rate is already low, echocardiographically guided biopsies do not necessarily lower it. Echocardiographic imaging is particularly helpful in children and adults with small right ventricles, however.[32] An additional advantage of the echocardiographically guided technique is the ability to sample specific sites of the heart selectively and to map the sampling site of each biopsy specimen accurately.

Although short-term survival is related to infectious complications and cardiac rejection, the major problem observed during the long-term management of the patient who has undergone cardiac transplantation is accelerated atherosclerosis.[33–35] At present, it is not known why this accelerated coronary disease occurs, although the suspected mechanism may relate to chronic rejection and localized vasculitis, HLA A2 mismatch, medication-induced hypertension, or hypertriglyceridemia.[33,35,36] Because the transplanted heart is denervated, these patients do not feel chest pain or other warning signs during ischemia. The echocardiogram demonstrating wall motion abnormalities at rest or during exercise in the absence of rejection may be used as one of the first indicators of significant coronary artery disease in these patients. The sensitivity and specificity of noninvasive detection of graft-associated atherosclerosis, however, has not been established.

Because coronary narrowing due to cardiac transplant graft atherosclerosis develops in a diffuse, concentric fashion, its early detection by coronary angiography can be difficult. Intravascular ultrasound holds promise as a technique to identify both the early and late stages of this disease process. Intravascular ultrasound has identified abnormal intimal thickening of the coronary arteries in up to 24% of transplant recipients with normal coronary angiograms.[37]

Intravascular ultrasound has also been combined with acetylcholine administration to assess endothelial function as a marker of early changes in the coronary arteries of transplant patients.[38] When allograft vasculopathy and endothelial dysfunction are present, acetylcholine provokes vasoconstriction instead of the expected normal dilatory response. Detection of intimal thickening by intravascular ultrasound may not be a sensitive marker for vasculopathy, because endothelial dysfunction has been demonstrated in transplant recipients without significant intimal thickening.[39] It remains to be determined whether the functional changes noted by acetylcholine testing are more important markers for clinically important accelerated atherosclerosis than the abnormal intimal thickening noted by intravascular ultrasound.

Table 39–3. Major Complications After Cardiac Transplantation

Allograft rejection
Opportunistic infection
Malignant disease (particularly lymphoma)
Allograft atherosclerosis
Medication-related disorders
Steroid-induced osteoporosis, glucose intolerance
Cyclosporine-induced nephrotoxicity, hypertension

NONINVASIVE INDICATORS OF TRANSPLANT REJECTION

Serial decreases in electrocardiographic voltage were originally used as a marker of cellular rejection; however, in patients treated with cyclosporine the accuracy of this measurement has diminished. It was hoped that the echocardiogram would replace the electrocardiogram as an indicator of the presence and evolution of tissue rejection. This task has not been simple. The clinical signs of rejection are multiple and nonspecific. These symptoms and signs include decreased cardiac output, weakness, and fatigue. Before the use of cyclosporine, the classic echocardiographic findings associated with rejection included an increase in left ventricular mass, which represented increases in wall thickening from diffuse cellular infiltration and interstitial edema.[40,41] Cellular rejection in the presence of cyclosporine is associated with less myocardial edema, and measurements of myocardial thickness have become less reliable markers of rejection.

Because echocardiographically detectable alterations in left ventricular systolic function are variable findings and often appear only late in the course of rejection,[42] the focus has shifted to echocardiographic assessment of diastolic function. Initial studies with M-mode echocardiography revealed prolongations of the early filling phase of diastole in patients with acute rejection,[42] suggesting changes in left ventricular relaxation and compliance caused by infiltration of the myocardium with mononuclear cells during acute rejection. In addition, a 10% reduction of the IVRT predicted myocardial necrosis with a sensitivity of 87% and a specificity of 90%.[43,44] This shortening of the IVRT is due to an earlier opening of the mitral valve, rather than to a change in the timing of aortic valve closure.

With the addition of Doppler techniques, interest has shifted to measurements of ventricular filling as a noninvasive means of recognizing transplant rejection. A correlation exists between the presence of acute transplant rejection and a shortened left ventricular IVRT, an increased peak E velocity, and a shortened early mitral flow deceleration time[45,46] (Fig. 39–7). The changes in

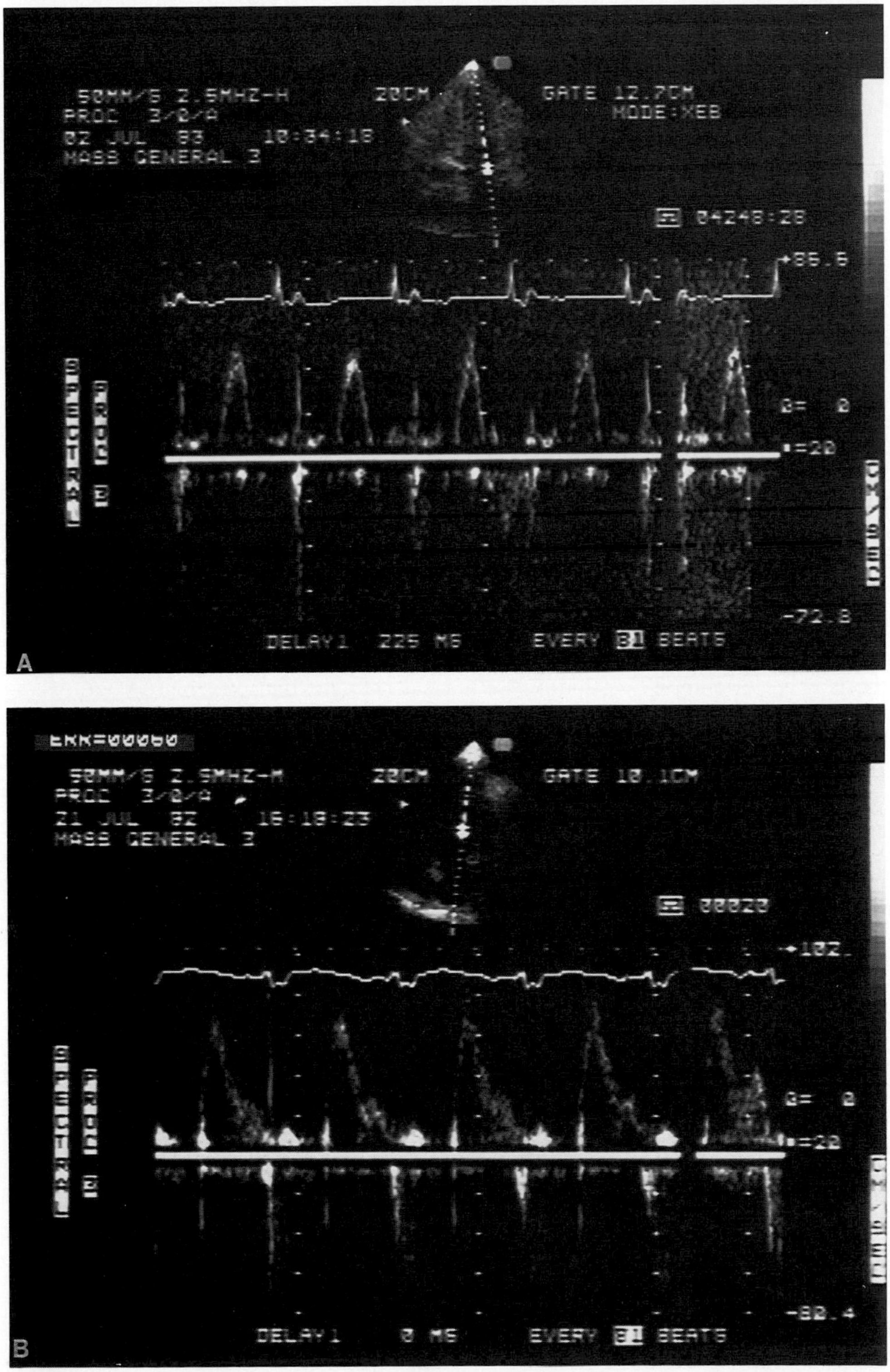

Fig. 39–7. Example of serial changes in left ventricle (LV) filling following cardiac transplant. **A.** Mitral inflow during clinical episode of rejection (peak E velocity = 49 cm/sec; deceleration time = 92.5 msec). **B.** Mitral inflow after improvement (peak E velocity = 75 cm/sec; deceleration time = 204 msec).

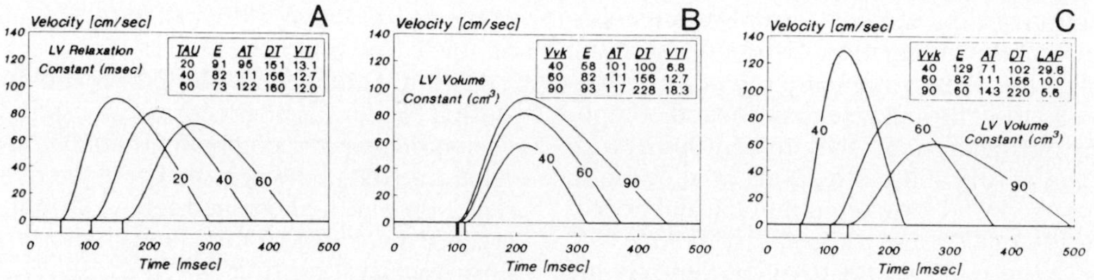

Fig. 39–8. Computer simulation illustrating the effect of changes in left ventricle (LV) relaxation, LV compliance, and left atrium (LA) pressure on the Doppler pattern of mitral inflow. **A.** Change in passive ventricular filling as a result of alterations in time constant of isovolumic relaxation (τ). As relaxation is prolonged and the LV relaxation constant increases from 20 to 60 msec—whereas other variables such as LV compliance and LA pressure are held constant—an increase in isovolumic relaxation time (IVRT), and a decrease in peak E-wave velocity are predicted on the transmitral Doppler filling pattern. **B.** Change in passive ventricular filling as a result of alterations in LV volume constant. The volume constant (V_{vk}, cm^3) is directly related to chamber compliance. As compliance decreases (represented by a decrease in LV volume constant from 90 to 40), an associated decrease in peak E velocity and increase in deceleration is predicted. **C.** Effect of atrial pressure **B.** As shown in the upper right corner of graph 8C, LV volume constant (V_{vk}) is inversely related to LA pressure (LAP). As LAP increases (represented by a decrease in LV volume constant), increases in the peak E-wave velocity and deceleration time are predicted along with a decrease in IVRT. These are the alterations in transmitral filling pattern that are noted during cardiac transplant rejection. AT = acceleration time; DT = deceleration time; VTI = velocity time integral.

transmitral flow that occur with alterations of left ventricular relaxation, compliance, and left atrial pressure have been described in both experimental and computer models.[47,48] The changes in the Doppler pattern of left ventricular filling observed during cardiac transplant rejection can be reproduced in a computer simulation by a decrease in left ventricular compliance with a compensatory increase in left atrial pressure to preserve stroke volume. As shown in Figure 39–8A, an isolated increase in the time constant of isovolumic relaxation (τ) would lead to changes in the early transmitral velocity that are opposite to those observed during rejection (i.e., increased IVRT, decreased peak E velocity, increased deceleration time). Figure 39–8B displays the effect of altered left ventricular compliance (represented by the left ventricular volume constant) on the E wave. If compliance decreases (represented by a decrease in left ventricular volume constant) and other variables such as filling pressure and relaxation rate are held constant, decreases in the peak E velocity and deceleration time are predicted. A compensatory increase in left atrial pressure (Fig. 39–8C) to preserve left ventricular stroke volume would predict a shortened IVRT, an increased peak E velocity, and a decreased deceleration time, identical to the findings observed during transplant rejection. To further delineate the relative contributions of preload, compliance, and relaxation rate to alterations in left ventricular filling during cardiac transplant rejection, variables that affect the Doppler profile such as heart rate, ventricular contractility, preload, and afterload must be examined in a controlled fashion. Although further work is required to understand completely the changes in myocardial function and noninvasive markers of left ventricular filling that occur during rejection, at present, serial recordings of the transmitral flow velocities are performed to identify patients who may be at higher risk of rejection and who may benefit from stricter surveillance for rejection of the donor heart.

Cyclosporine-associated interstitial myocardial fibrosis or multiple episodes of rejection may alter myocardial compliance on a long-term basis in subsets of patients who undergo cardiac transplantation.[49–51] Preliminary observations suggest that Doppler echocardiographic indices of left ventricular filling and systolic ejection can identify this subset of patients with restrictive physiology.[50] If these observations are confirmed, Doppler echocardiography may alter the manner in which acute and chronic rejection is treated.

In summary, the echocardiogram is valuable in the management of heart failure and potential cardiac transplantation. In particular, assessment of the potential cardiac donor by two-dimensional echocardiography can increase the number of donor hearts available to meet increasing demands for the procedure by improving the detection of regional myocardial dysfunction. Recognition of the normal changes that occur in structure and function of the heart after transplantation are important to differentiate them from abnormal. Although the original goal of echocardiography as a noninvasive indicator of transplant rejection has not yet been achieved, the addition of Doppler assessment of diastolic filling has improved our understanding of this complex process.

REFERENCES

1. Barnard CN: The operation: a human heart transplantation. An interim report of the successful operation performed at Groote Schuur Hospital, Cape Town, South Africa. S Afr Med J 41:1271, 1967.
2. Griepp RB, et al.: The cardiac donor. Surg Gynecol Obstet 133:792, 1971.
3. Gilbert EM, et al.: Echocardiographic evaluation of potential cardiac transplant donors. J Thorac Cardiovasc Surg 95:1003, 1988.
4. Hiatt JR, Yeatman LA Jr, Child JS: The value of echocardiography in blunt chest trauma. J Trauma 28:914, 1988.
5. Reid CL, Kawanishi DT, Rahimtoola SH, Chandraratna PAN: Chest trauma: evaluation by two dimensional echocardiography. Am Heart J 113:971, 1987.
6. Hersack KF, Moreno CA, Vanwar CW, Burdick DC: Frequency of cardiac contusion in nonpenetrating chest injury. Am J Cardiol 61:391, 1988.
7. Pandian NG, Skorton DJ, Doty DB, Kerber RE: Immediate diagnosis of acute myocardial contusion by two-dimensional echocardiography: studies in a canine model of blunt chest trauma. J Am Coll Cardiol 2:488, 1983.
8. Melin J, Fogelholm R: Electrocardiographic findings in subarachnoid hemorrhage. Acta Med Scand 213:5, 1983.
9. Koskelo P, Punsar S, Sipila W: Subendocardial haemorrhage and ECG changes in intracranial bleeding. Br Med J 1:1479, 1964.
10. Doshi R, Neil-Dwyer G: A clinicopathological study of patients following a subarachnoid hemorrhage. J Neurosurg 52:295, 1980.

11. Pollick C, Cujec B, Parker S, Tator C: Left ventricular wall motion abnormalities in subarachnoid hemorrhage: an echocardiographic study. J Am Coll Cardiol 12:600, 1988.
12. Benedict CR, Loach AB: Clinical significance of plasma adrenaline and noradrenaline concentrations in patients with subarachnoid hemorrhage. J Neurol Neurosurg Psychiatry 41:113, 1978.
13. Novitsky D, et al.: Prevention of myocardial injury during brain death by total cardiac sympathectomy in the Chacma baboon. Ann Thorac Surg 41: 520, 1986.
14. Griepp RB, et al.: Determinants of operative risk in human heart transplantation. Am J Surg 122:192, 1971.
15. Thompson ME, Kormos RL, Zerbe A, Hardesty RL: Patient selection and results of cardiac transplantation in patients with cardiomyopathy. Cardiovasc Clin 19:263, 1988.
16. Reemtsma K, et al.: Cardiac transplantation: changing patterns in evaluation and treatment. Ann Surg 202:418, 1985.
17. Keogh AM, Freund J, Baron DW, Hickie JB: Timing of cardiac transplantation in idiopathic dilated cardiomyopathy. Am J Cardiol 61:418, 1988.
18. Gavazzi A, et al.: Hemodynamic changes after orthotopic heart transplantation: 12 month follow-up of 28 patients. Circulation 76(Suppl. IV):IV-206, 1987.
19. Corcos T, et al.: Early and late hemodynamic evaluation after cardiac transplantation: a study of 28 cases. J Am Coll Cardiol 11:264, 1988.
20. Bhatia SJS, et al.: Time course of resolution of pulmonary hypertension and right ventricular remodeling after orthotopic cardiac transplantation. Circulation 76:819, 1987.
21. Cladellas M, et al.: Early transient multivalvular regurgitation detected by pulsed Doppler in cardiac transplantation. Am J Cardiol 58:1122, 1986.
22. Valantine HA, et al.: Influence of recipient atrial contraction on left ventricular filling dynamics of the transplanted heart assessed by Doppler echocardiography. Am J Cardiol 59:1159, 1987.
23. Hsiung MC, et al.: Value of color Doppler assessment of pulmonary artery pressure in cardiac transplant patients. J Am Coll Cardiol 7:140A, 1986.
24. Lewen MK, et al.: Tricuspid regurgitation after orthotopic cardiac transplant. Am J Cardiol 59:1371, 1987.
25. Tucker PA, et al.: Flail tricuspid leaflet after multiple biopsies following orthotopic cardiac transplantation: echocardiographic and hemodynamic correlation. J Am Coll Cardiol 21:142A, 1993.
26. Hastillo A, et al.: Cyclosporine induced pericardial effusion after cardiac transplantation. Am J Cardiol 59:1220, 1987.
27. Stevenson LW, Child JS, Laks H, Kern L: Incidence and significance of early pericardial effusions after cardiac surgery. Am J Cardiol 54:848, 1984.
28. Weitzman LB, et al.: The incidence and natural history of pericardial effusion after cardiac surgery: an echocardiographic study. Circulation 69:506, 1984.
29. Valantine HA, et al.: Increasing pericardial effusion in cardiac transplant recipients. Circulation 79:603, 1989.
30. Fowles RE, Mason JW: Endomyocardial biopsy. Ann Intern Med 97:885, 1982.
31. Williams GA, et al.: Clinical experience with two dimensional echocardiography to guide endomyocardial biopsy. Clin Cardiol 8:137, 1985.
32. French JW, Popp RL, Pitlick PT: Cardiac localization of transvascular bioptome using 2 dimensional echocardiography. Am J Cardiol 51:219, 1983.
33. Bieber CP, Hunt SA, Schwinn DA, et al.: Complications in long term survivors of cardiac transplantation. Transplant Proc 13:207, 1981.
34. Pennock JL, et al.: Cardiac transplantation in perspective for the future: survival, complications, rehabilitation and cost. J Thorac Cardiovasc Surg 83:168, 1982.
35. Uretsky BF, et al.: Development of coronary artery disease in cardiac transplant patients receiving immunosuppressive therapy with cyclosporine and prednisone. Circulation 76:827, 1987.
36. Gao SZ, Schroeder JS, Hunt SA, Stinson EB: Retransplantation for severe accelerated coronary artery disease in heart transplant recipients. Am J Cardiol 62:876, 1988.
37. St. Goar FG, et al.: Detection of coronary atherosclerosis in young adult hearts using intravascular ultrasound. Circulation 86:756, 1992.
38. Mills RM Jr, Billett JM, Nichols WW: Endothelial dysfunction early after heart transplantation. Assessment with intravascular ultrasound and Doppler. Circulation 86:1171, 1992.
39. Pinto FJ, et al.: Coronary endothelial function and vascular structure in cardiac transplant recipients. J Am Coll Cardiol 21:119A, 1993.
40. Griepp RB, et al.: Acute rejection of the allografted human heart. Ann Thorac Surg 12:113, 1971.
41. Sagar KB, et al.: Left ventricular mass by M-mode echocardiography in cardiac transplant patients with acute rejection. Circulation 64(Suppl. II): II-220, 1981.
42. Paulsen W, et al.: Left ventricular function of heart allografts during acute rejection: an echocardiographic assessment. Heart Transplantation 5:525, 1985.
43. Dawkins KD, et al.: Changes in diastolic function as a noninvasive marker of cardiac allograft rejection. Heart Transplantation 4:286, 1984.
44. Dawkins KD, et al.: Noninvasive assessment of cardiac allograft rejection. Transplantation Proc 17:215, 1985.
45. Valantine HA, et al.: Changes in Doppler echocardiographic indexes of left ventricular function as potential markers of acute cardiac rejection. Circulation 76(Suppl V):V-92, 1987.
46. Desruennes M, et al.: Doppler echocardiography for the diagnosis of acute cardiac allograft rejection. J Am Coll Cardiol 13:63, 1988.
47. Choong CY, et al.: Combined influence of ventricular loading and relaxation on the transmitral flow velocity profile in dogs measured by Doppler echocardiography. Circulation 78:672, 1988.
48. Levine RA, Thomas JD: Insights into the physiologic significance of the mitral inflow velocity pattern. J Am Coll Cardiol 14:1718, 1989.
49. Humen DP, McKenzie FN, Kostuk WJ: Restricted myocardial compliance one year following cardiac transplantation. Heart Transplantation 3:341, 1984.
50. Valantine HA, et al.: A hemodynamic and Doppler echocardiographic study of ventricular function in long-term cardiac allograft recipients: etiology and prognosis of restrictive-constrictive physiology. Circulation 79:66, 1989.
51. Wilensky RL, et al.: Restrictive hemodynamic patterns after cardiac transplantation: relationship to histologic signs of rejection. Am Heart J 122: 1079, 1991.

CHAPTER

40

THE ECHOCARDIOGRAM IN DISORDERS OF CARDIAC RHYTHM AND CONDUCTION

WENDY A. THOREAU, PAMELA HARRIGAN, and ARTHUR E. WEYMAN

The timing and sequence of cardiac events are determined by the rate and pattern of electrical activation of the heart. Disturbances of rate, rhythm, and conduction can alter the pattern, frequency, and amplitude of muscular contraction, valve motion, and intracardiac flow. Therefore, an understanding of the relationship between electrical and mechanical events is important lest secondary effects of altered electrical activity be misinterpreted as primary abnormalities of cardiac structure or function. In addition, because of the association between electrical depolarization and myocardial contraction, analysis of the pattern of wall and valve motion can provide important insight into the nature of an underlying rhythm disturbance as well as its functional effect.

The first section of this chapter describes the changes in valve motion and atrial and ventricular contraction that occur as a result of arrhythmias and conduction disturbances. The second section discusses how echo-Doppler parameters can be used to assess the structural and functional effects of arrhythmias, to predict natural history, and to evaluate response to therapy.

EFFECT OF DISORDERS OF RATE, RHYTHM AND CONDUCTION ON THE ECHOCARDIOGRAM

Echocardiography is an ideal noninvasive tool for defining alterations in the movement and function of intracardiac structures that result from disturbances in electrical activation. M-mode echocardiography, because of its superior temporal resolution, is the technique of choice for the analysis of arrhythmia-related changes in the motion of intracardiac structures. Doppler flow sampling is becoming increasingly important in identifying the hemodynamic effects of alterations in cardiac rhythm and conduction. Two-dimensional echocardiography is the most appropriate method of investigation in cases in which global ventricular function needs to be assessed or the spatial sequence of contraction needs to be defined (e.g., in Wolff-Parkinson-White [WPW] syndrome).

Supraventricular Rhythms

Supraventricular rhythms originate in the sinus node, the atrial myocardium, or the junctional tissue, or they arise through intranodal or other re-entrant pathways. Electrical activation originating at these sites has its primary mechanical expression in atrial contraction. Although atrial contraction can be recorded directly, it is more easily appreciated by its effects on the diastolic motion of the atrioventricular (AV) valves.

Atrial impulses are normally conducted to the ventricles by the AV node and the His-Purkinje system, where they initiate ventricular contraction after an interval of between 0.12 and 0.21 seconds.

Normal Sinus Rhythm

The pattern of motion of the AV valves in normal sinus rhythm depends on the length of the diastolic filling period, the AV (PR) interval, and the cardiac output. Figure 40–1 illustrates the effect of heart rate on the M-mode pattern of mitral valve motion. When the sinus rate is slow (sinus bradycardia), the early filling component (E wave) and atrial contraction component (A wave) are widely separated (Fig. 40–1, left), with a clearly defined period of diastasis between the two primary filling periods. As the heart rate increases, the separation between the E and A waves decreases and the period of diastasis shortens until the acceleration phase of the A wave arises directly from the deceleration slope of the E wave (Fig. 40–1, left center). During sinus tachycardia, the atrial component may be superimposed on the downslope of the rapid filling wave (Fig. 40–1, right center) or only one diastolic wave (representing fusion of the E and A waves) may be apparent (Fig. 40–1, right). Figure 40–2, an M-mode recording from a patient with sinus arrhythmia, illustrates the changes in mitral valve motion that occur as the sinus rate and duration of the diastolic filling period vary.

Doppler studies of mitral valve flow during sinus rhythm show similar variation with heart rate, as illustrated in Figure 40–3. During sinus bradycardia (Fig. 40–3, far left), the E and A waves of mitral inflow are clearly separated and a period of reduced flow during diastasis is present. As the heart rate increases, the E and A wave separation decreases and the period of diastasis shortens and eventually disappears (Fig. 40–3, right center). During sinus tachycardia (Fig. 40–3, far right), the A wave typically begins before passive filling is complete, and at extremely rapid heart rates, the E and A waves may be superimposed, leaving only a single diastolic filling wave representing fusion of the E and A components.

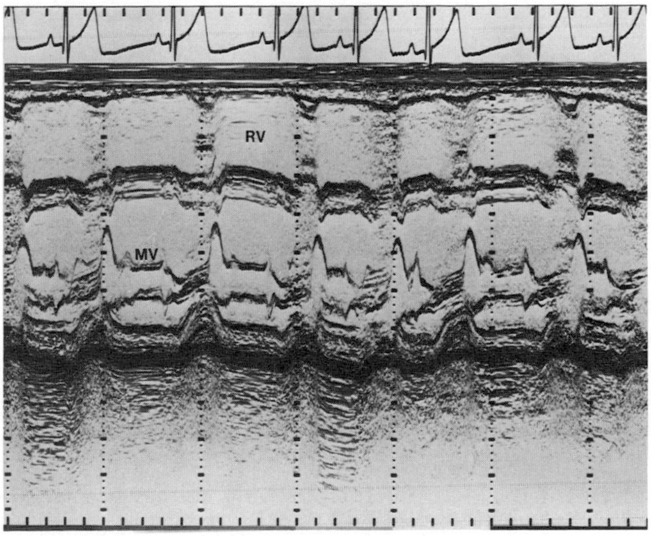

Fig. 40–2. M-mode recording of mitral valve (MV) motion illustrating the variation that occurs during sinus arrhythmia. RV = right ventricle.

Atrial Premature Beats

The effect of atrial premature beats on mitral valve motion and transmitral flow depends on the timing of the premature beat.[1] Figure 40–4 is a pulsed Doppler recording that illustrates the effect of coupling interval on the pattern of transmitral flow. Although there is some variability in cycle length, the first three diastolic filling periods are normal. The fourth beat is a supraventricular premature beat with a short coupling interval that interrupts the early filling wave and closes the mitral valve. The fifth beat occurs after a slightly longer RR interval, and atrial systole is superimposed on the initial passive filling wave (E-A fusion), producing a high ve-

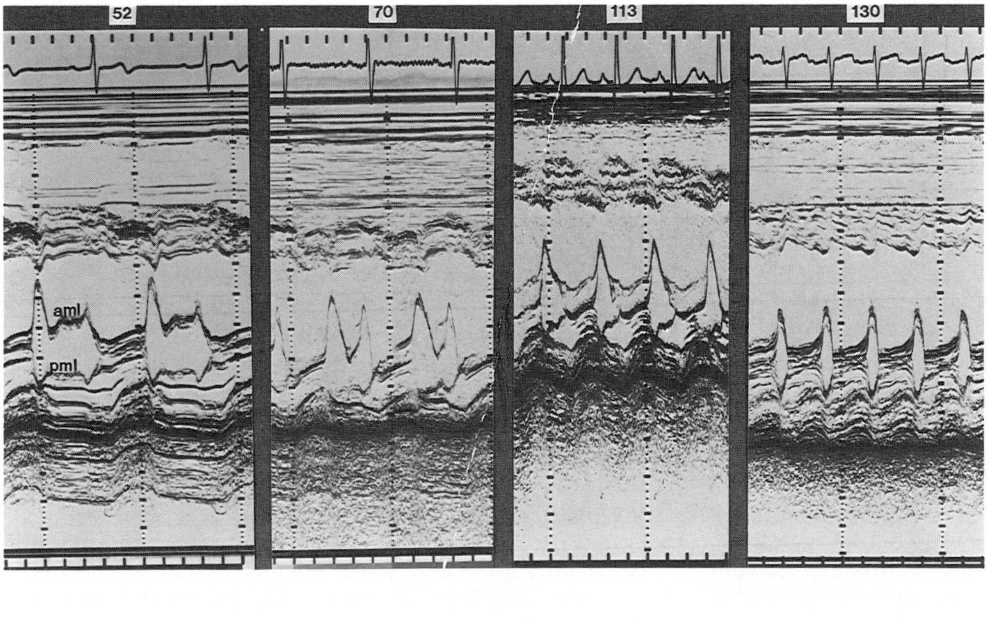

Fig. 40–1. M-mode recordings of normal mitral valve motion at different rates of sinus rhythm, from sinus bradycardia (far left), to sinus tachycardia (far right). Heart rates (beats/per minute) are indicated above each panel. aml = anterior mitral leaflet; pml = posterior mitral leaflet. (See text for details.)

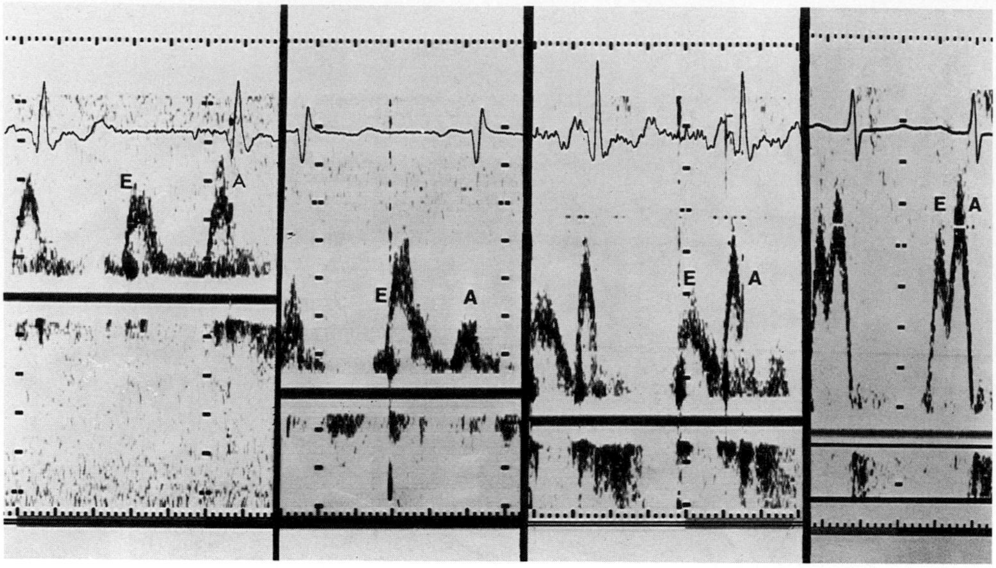

Fig. 40–3. Doppler spectral display of transmitral flow at different rates of sinus rhythm. E and A waves are indicated in each panel. (See text for description.)

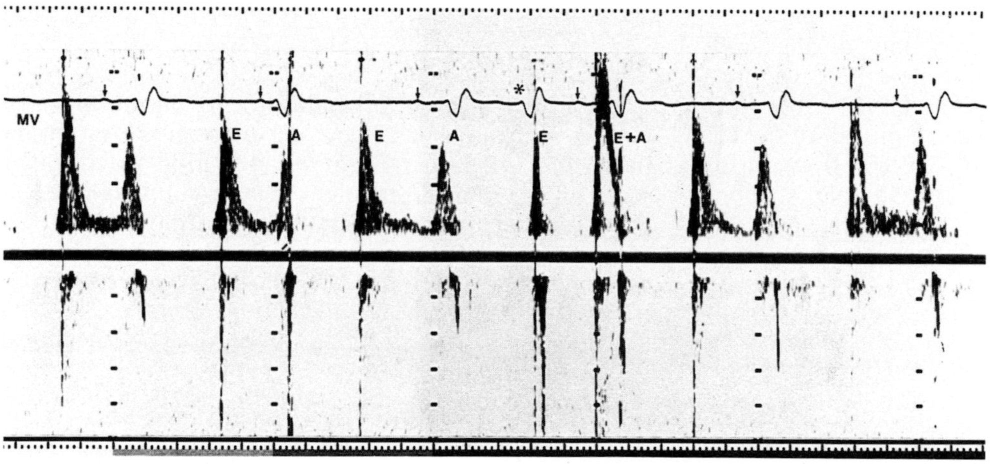

Fig. 40–4. Pulsed wave Doppler recording showing the changes in transmitral flow that result from a supraventricular ectopic beat. P waves on the electrocardiogram are arrowed; * = first supraventricular ectopic; E and A waves of mitral flow velocity are indicated. (See text for details.)

locity wave that is again interrupted by ventricular systole. Transmitral flow returns to normal after the premature beats.

Alterations in flow patterns across the aortic and pulmonary valves reflect the hemodynamic effects of atrial premature contractions (i.e., the interruption of diastolic filling caused by the premature contraction). The peak transaortic or transpulmonary flow velocity produced by an ectopic beat with a short coupling interval is reduced because of the decreased time available for ventricular filling, whereas the peak velocity and stroke velocity integral of the following sinus beat are increased slightly to compensate for the reduced ventricular filling during the short diastolic period (Fig. 40–5).

Junctional Rhythms

The effect of a junctional rhythm on the pattern of AV valve motion depends on the junctional rate and site of origin of the impulse. Accelerated junctional rhythms shorten the diastolic filling period, whereas junctional escape beats follow a prolonged diastolic period. High junctional rhythms result in retrograde atrial activation with a P wave that precedes the QRS complex, whereas impulses originating lower in the AV node usually result in atrial activation during or after the QRS complex.

When junctional rhythm with retrograde activation of the atria occurs before ventricular systole, there is usually an inverted P wave with a short PR interval on the electrocardiogram (ECG) and evidence of atrial contraction (A wave) on the M-mode and Doppler recordings. The A wave is frequently truncated because mitral closure, which begins with atrial relaxation, is accelerated by the closely coupled ventricular systole. A similar pattern of mitral valve motion and transmitral flow is sometimes seen during junctional escape rhythms when the slowed sinus rate results in atrial activation just before the escape focus stimulates ventricular contraction. Figure 40–6 is a recording from a patient whose rhythm varied from sinus at a rate of roughly 100 beats per minute to junctional at a rate of roughly 60 beats per minute. The two complexes on the far left and far right of Figure

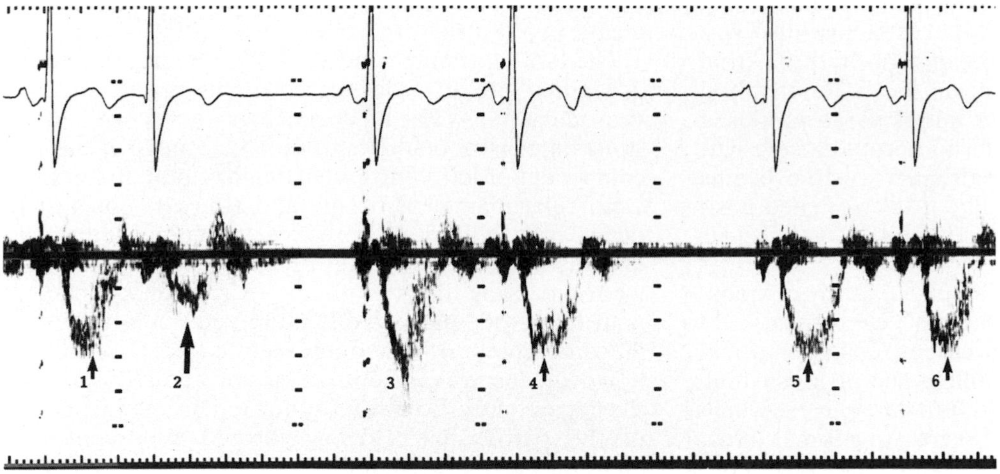

Fig. 40–5. Pulsed wave Doppler recording of transpulmonary flow illustrating the effect of a supraventricular ectopic beat (velocity profile 2). (See text for description.)

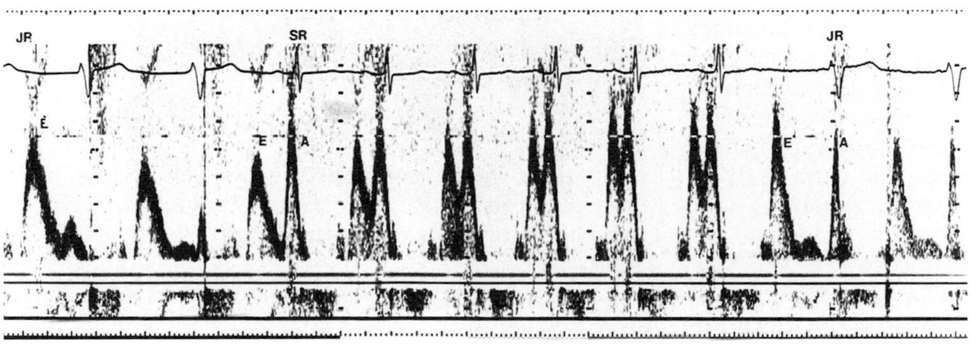

Fig. 40–6. Transmitral flow recorded by pulsed wave Doppler during intermittent junctional rhythm. JR = junctional rhythm; SR = sinus rhythm; E and A waves are indicated. (See text for details.)

40–6 are junctional beats and illustrate the effects of the PR interval on the morphology of the mitral Doppler flow pattern. In the first complex on the left of Figure 40–6, the P wave is buried in the QRS complex, and there is no evidence of atrial contraction related transmitral flow. In the second complex from the left of Figure 40–6, the P wave occurs slightly before the QRS complex, and flow secondary to atrial contraction begins but is terminated abruptly by ventricular systole, which closes the mitral valve. These two beats are followed by a run of six normal sinus beats at a more rapid rate that show the normal biphasic left ventricular filling pattern. The last two beats of the tracing are again of junctional origin, but now the PR interval is slightly longer and the atrial filling wave is able to reach a higher velocity before being terminated by ventricular systole. In each case the presence, duration, and form of the atrial filling wave is determined by the relationship between atrial and ventricular contraction.

During rhythms of junctional origin in which atrial activation occurs during ventricular systole, there is no P wave on the ECG, an absence of the atrial component of mitral valve opening on the M-mode recording, and the absence of an atrial filling wave on the Doppler spectral tracing. Figure 40–7 is an M-mode recording from a patient with an intermittent junctional rhythm. The left panel of Figure 40–7 was recorded during normal sinus

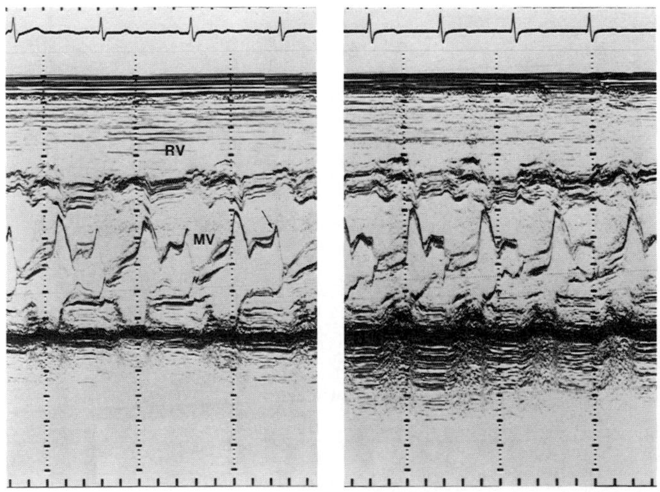

Fig. 40–7. M-mode recording of the mitral valve (MV) showing the difference in the pattern of motion between sinus rhythm (left) and junctional rhythm (right) in the same patient. RV = right ventricle; arrow indicates normal A-wave morphology.

rhythm and illustrates a normal PR interval and normal A wave morphology. The right panel of Figure 40–7 was recorded during an accelerated junctional rhythm. Atrial contraction is no longer evident on the ECG or mitral valve echocardiogram, and the mitral valve is closed abruptly by ventricular systole. This abrupt closure pattern typically occurs when ventricular systole begins with the mitral valve in a partially or fully opened position (i.e., when closure is not initiated by ventricular systole).

Figure 40–8 illustrates the Doppler pattern of transmitral flow in a patient with junctional escape beats. On the left of Figure 40–8 are three consecutive normal sinus beats, with typical rapid filling and atrial systolic velocity peaks. In the fourth and fifth complexes, which are junctional escape rhythms, there are normal initial diastolic filling waves but no ECG evidence of atrial contraction or late diastolic filling wave (A wave).

Supraventricular Tachycardia

Supraventricular tachycardias decrease the diastolic filling period, which shortens the time during which the AV valves are open. If the tachycardia has an atrial origin, the atrial component of mitral valve opening can usually be identified, although at extremely rapid rates it may be superimposed on the rapid filling wave (E-A fusion). Supraventricular tachycardias of a junctional or re-entrant origin usually show no atrial component of mitral valve opening on the M-mode recording, and no atrial filling wave is detectable by Doppler recording of transmitral flow. In these cases, the atrial rate must be determined by direct recording of atrial wall motion (see later). Figure 40–9 is an M-mode recording of mitral valve motion from a patient with intermittent supraventricular tachycardia. During sinus rhythm, the diastolic motion of the mitral valve is normal. With the onset of the tachycardia, diastole is abbreviated and the mitral valve opening time reflects the shortened diastolic filling period. Immediately after the onset of the tachycardia, the mitral valve fails to open (small arrow); however, opening amplitude and duration tend to increase as the

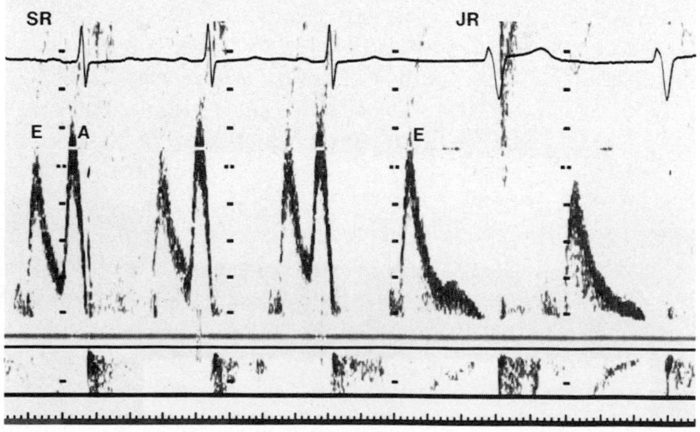

Fig. 40–8. Doppler spectral display of transmitral flow during sinus and junctional escape beats. SR = sinus rhythm; JR = junctional rhythm; E and W waves are indicated. (See text for description.)

tachycardia continues, presumably because of an increase in left atrial pressure.

The left ventricular end-diastolic dimension and cardiac output are often decreased during periods of supraventricular tachycardia because of the shortened diastolic filling period and the frequent absence of the atrial component of left ventricular filling. Comparison of the ventricular diameters before and after the onset of the tachycardia in Figure 40–9 (large double-headed arrows) demonstrates the decrease in left ventricular internal dimension during the arrhythmia. In one report,[2] patients with refractory paroxysmal supraventricular tachycardia were noted to have depressed left ventricular function even during transient periods of sinus rhythm, with the degree of dysfunction proportional to the frequency of the paroxysms. During chronic supraventricular tachycardia, left ventricular function was noted to be depressed but to return toward normal after successful surgical correction of the arrhythmia. Whether the changes observed in patients with intermittent arrhythmias are due to drug effects, are caused by primary myocardial abnormalities, or occur as a result of the arrhythmia remains to be determined.

Atrial Flutter

Atrial flutter is characterized by regular atrial contractions at a rate of 250 to 350 per minute that give rise to a characteristic saw-tooth contour on the ECG. The ventricular rate is determined by AV conduction and can range from 150 per minute (2:1 block) to extremely slow rates with greater degrees of AV block, and it is usually regular.

Atrial flutter is manifest on the M-mode echocardiogram by rapid, regular undulations of the AV valves that correspond to the rate of atrial contraction. Figure 40–10 is an M-mode recording from a patient with atrial flutter with variable AV conduction. The mitral valve opens normally during the rapid filling phase and then reopens slightly with each atrial contraction. Also of note is the concurrent undulation of the posterior wall, interventricular septum, and left atrial wall.[3,4] Atrial contraction can also be recorded directly using M-mode echocardiography. Figure 40–11 is a suprasternal M-mode recording of the left atrial superior wall that compares the timing of the flutter waves on the ECG with the contractions of the atrial wall. The subcostal approach can also be used to demonstrate the abnormal motion of the interatrial septum and the right atrial wall in patients with atrial flutter.[5]

Doppler studies of flow across the mitral valve during atrial flutter show an initial normal rapid filling wave (E wave) followed by regular atrial filling waves of varying amplitude that correspond to the flutter waves on the ECG and reflect organized atrial contraction (Fig. 40–12). With rapid ventricular response rates, the left ventricular end-diastolic dimension and output may be reduced, as occurs in other types of supraventricular tachycardia.

Atrial Fibrillation

Atrial fibrillation is characterized by disorganized atrial depolarization which is typically without effective

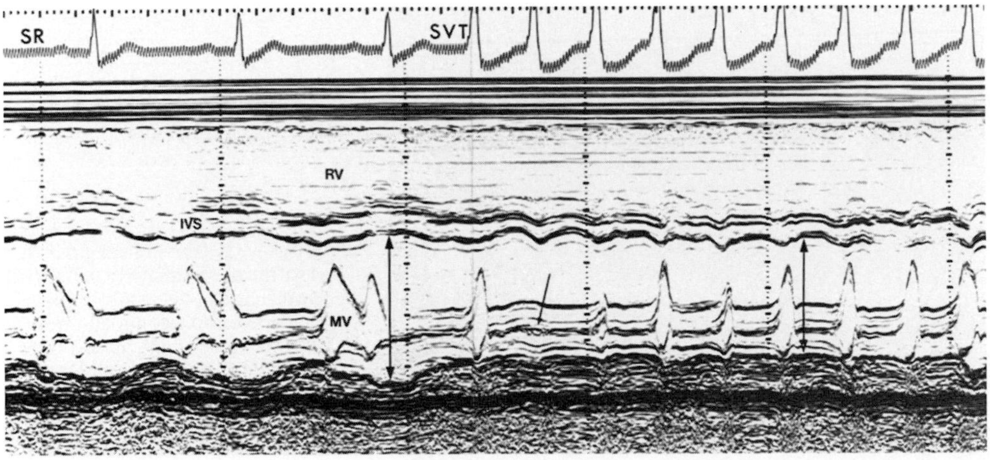

Fig. 40–9. M-mode recording illustrating the changes in the pattern of motion of the mitral valve, and the decrease in left ventricle dimensions (double-headed arrows), during an episode of supraventricular tachycardia. Single arrow indicates failure of mitral valve (MV) opening. SR = sinus rhythm; SVT = supraventricular tachycardia; RV = right ventricle; IVS = interventricular septum. (See text for details.) (From Harrigan P, Lee R: Principles of Interpretation in Echocardiography. New York; John Wiley & Sons, p. 332, 1985.)

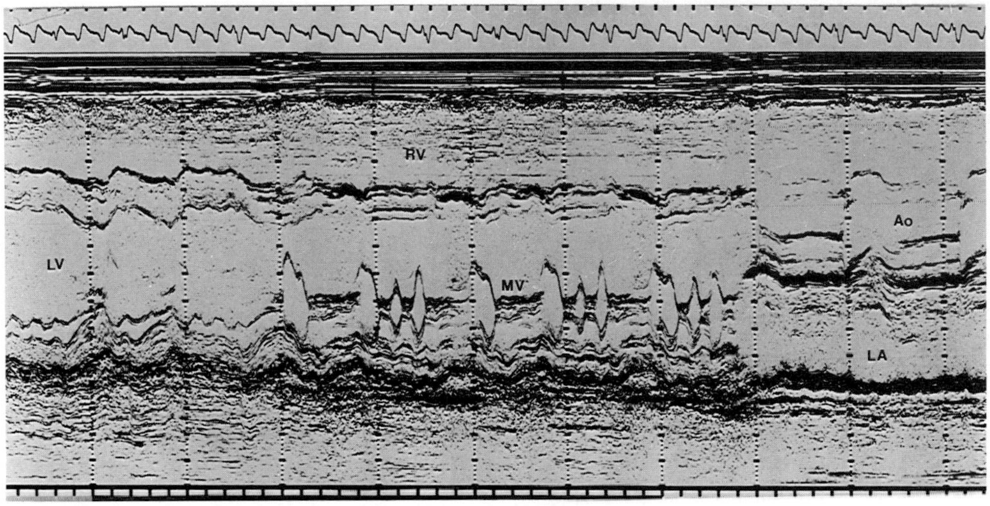

Fig. 40–10. M-mode recording illustrating the motion of the mitral valve (MV) and ventricular and left atrial walls during atrial flutter with variable atrioventricular (AV) conduction. RV = right ventricle; LV = left ventricle; Ao = aorta; LA = left atrium.

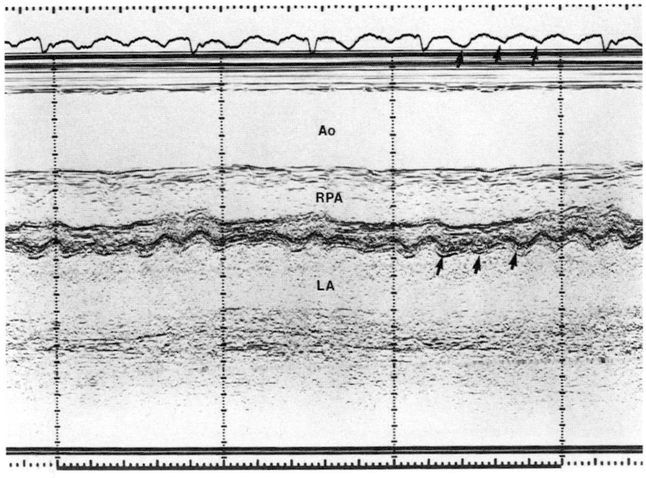

Fig. 40–11. M-mode recording of the left atrial wall from the suprasternal window during atrial flutter. Arrows indicate flutter waves on electrocardiogram and atrial wall. Ao = aorta; RPA = right pulmonary artery; LA = left atrium.

atrial contraction. The ventricular response is usually irregularly irregular.

Atrial fibrillation produces a variety of patterns on the echocardiogram that depend on the mechanical effectiveness of atrial contraction and on the rate and regularity of the ventricular response. Most commonly, the M-mode echocardiogram reveals diastolic filling periods of irregular length, undulation of the AV valves, and the absence of organized A waves. Occasionally, the left atrial wall near the AV junction also demonstrates the fibrillatory motion. Left ventricular dimensions and output vary depending on the length of the preceding diastolic filling period, with longer periods resulting in increased filling and therefore a greater stroke volume. Figure 40–13 is an example of the characteristic irregular motion of the mitral valve leaflets in a patient with atrial fibrillation. As illustrated in Figure 40–14, similar undulations can also be found on M-mode recordings of the aortic root. Figure 40–15 is an M-mode recording of the left ventricle from another patient with atrial fibrillation that illustrates variation in the rate and amplitude of ventricular contraction. During periods of rapid ventricular response, the left ventricular internal dimension becomes smaller because of decreased diastolic filling, and

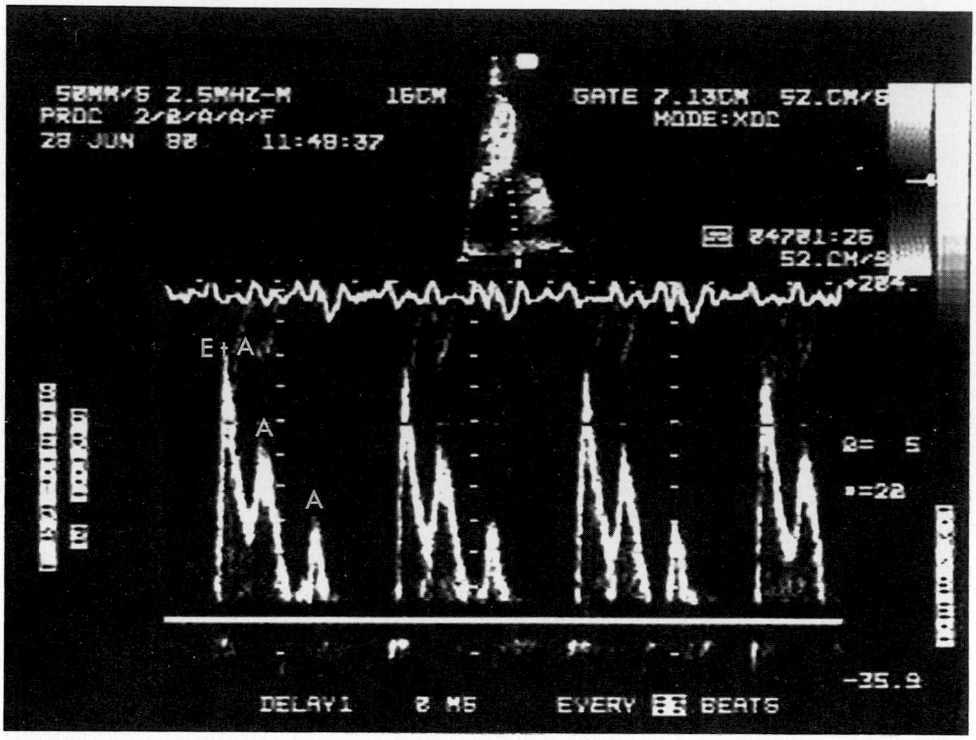

Fig. 40–12. Doppler spectral display of transmitral flow during atrial flutter with 4:1 atrioventricular (AV) block. The initial wave represents summation of the early ventricular filling wave and an atrial contraction. The following two waves also result from atrial contractions. The fourth atrial contraction occurs during ventricular systole, thus no transmitral flow results.

left ventricular contraction produces a smaller stroke volume.

Doppler echocardiography has provided important insight into the hemodynamic effects of atrial fibrillation on left ventricular function. In patients with normally functioning left ventricles and idiopathic atrial fibrillation, variations in cycle length and filling volume appear to regulate stroke volume, as predicted by Starling's law. Thus, when there is wide variation in RR interval, stroke volume varies inversely with preceding cycle length. Ventricular filling and stroke volume become constant and independent of cycle length when the RR intervals become longer than the time necessary for the completion of ventricular diastolic filling. In patients with impaired ventricular function, the relationship between cycle length and stroke volume is less apparent. Thus, in a study of patients with dilated cardiomyopathy and atrial fibrillation, no significant correlation was observed between the RR interval and either the filling or stroke volumes of the left ventricle.[6]

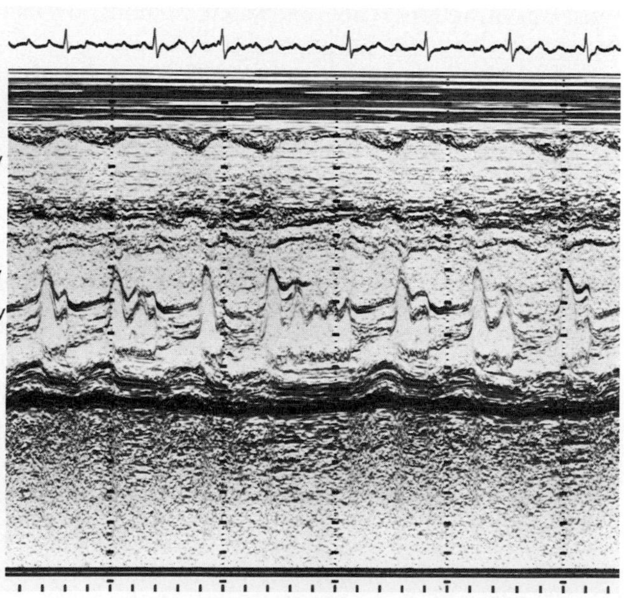

Fig. 40–13. M-mode recording of mitral valve (MV) motion during atrial fibrillation. RV = right ventricle; LV = left ventricle.

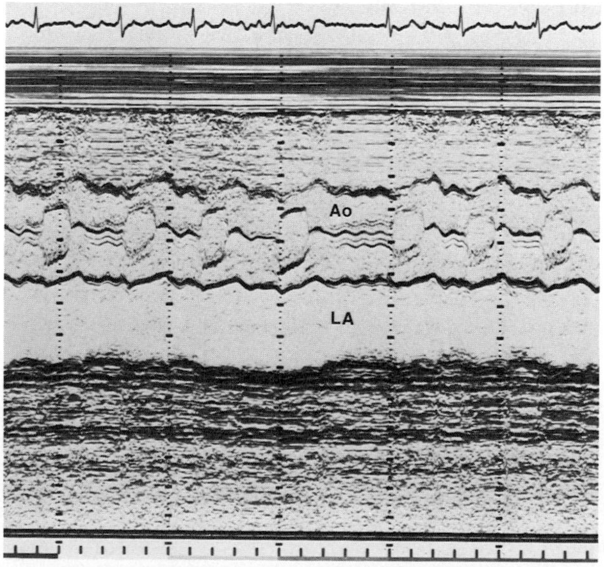

Fig. 40–14. M-mode recording of the aortic root illustrating the undulations sometimes seen during atrial fibrillation. Ao = aorta; LA = left atrium.

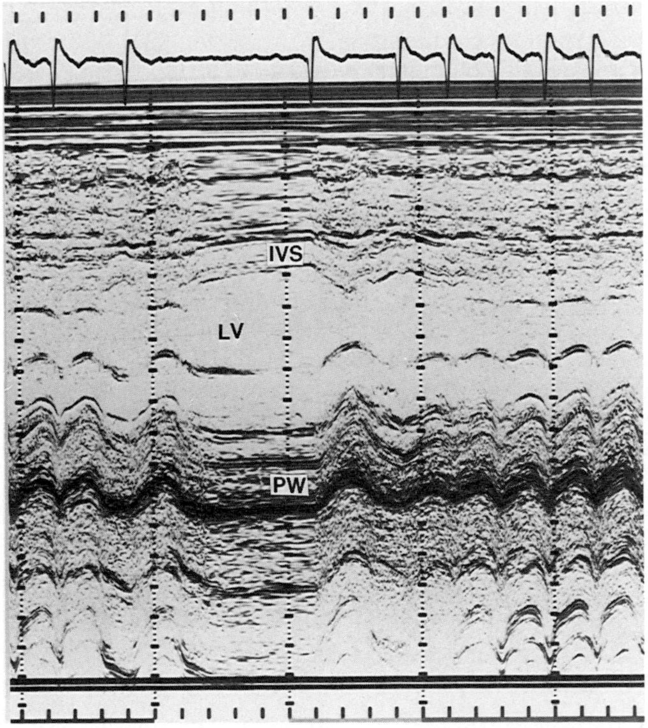

Fig. 40–15. M-mode of the left ventricle (LV) showing the fluctuations in dimensions that occur during atrial fibrillation with widely varying RR intervals. IVS = interventricular septum; PW = posterior wall.

The Doppler pattern of flow across the AV valves in patients with atrial fibrillation is characterized by variation in peak E-wave velocities and absence of A waves (Fig. 40–16). The peak pulmonary and aortic flow velocities are related to the RR interval of the preceding cycle, as detailed previously, and these patterns are illustrated in Figure 40–17.

Left atrial enlargement is commonly observed on M-mode and two-dimensional recordings in patients with atrial fibrillation and can be both a cause and an effect of the arrhythmia. Recent data demonstrate progressive left atrial enlargement in patients with initially normal left atrial dimensions and lone atrial fibrillation.[7] In patients with structural heart disease, such as mitral stenosis and regurgitation, however, the onset of atrial fibrillation usually follows considerable left atrial enlargement.

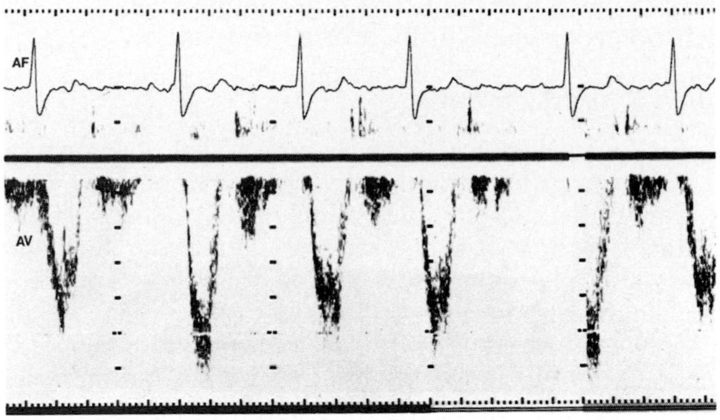

Fig. 40–17. Doppler spectral display illustrating the variation in transaortic flow during atrial fibrillation (AF). AV = aortic valve.

Simultaneous M-mode studies of the tricuspid and mitral valves (dual M-mode echocardiography) have been used to determine the sequence of atrial contraction in a variety of supraventricular rhythms. In normal patients, right atrial contraction precedes left atrial contraction, resulting in the occurrence of tricuspid valve A waves before that of mitral valve A waves. In atrial flutter, this sequence is reported to be reversed, and the interatrial conduction time, as determined by the delay between mitral and tricuspid valve A waves, is significantly prolonged. During coarse atrial fibrillation, the relative timing of contraction of the two atria varies, and coincident fibrillatory waves on both the mitral and tricuspid valves occur frequently. In patients with atrial tachycardia,

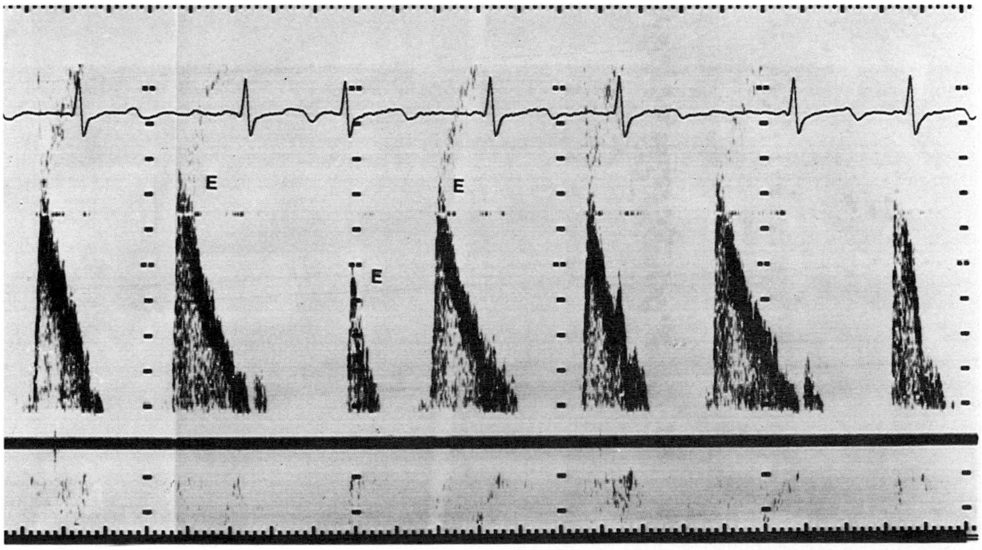

Fig. 40–16. A typical Doppler recording of transmitral flow during atrial fibrillation. E waves are indicated; A waves are absent.

atrial contractions either occur simultaneously, or the left precedes the right by a brief interval.[8]

Sick Sinus Syndrome

Sick sinus syndrome is a diagnosis that encompasses a range of supraventricular rhythm disturbances, including sinus node arrest, sinus bradycardia, sinoatrial block with or without AV block, supraventricular tachycardias, and alternating slow and fast rhythms known as the tachycardia-bradycardia syndrome. Surface and esophageal M-mode echocardiographic studies have been used to examine the left atrial contribution to left ventricle filling (atrial filling fraction) in patients with these disorders. Patients with sinoatrial block or sinus arrest, and those with transient atrial fibrillation, have atrial filling fractions during normally conducted sinus beats that are similar to those in patients with normal sinus rhythm. In contrast, patients with bradycardia-tachycardia syndrome have a significantly lower atrial filling fraction. These results suggest that within the group of sick sinus syndromes, patients with bradycardia-tachycardia syndrome have significantly impaired left atrial contraction in addition to the electrophysiologic abnormality.[9]

Dissimilar Atrial Rhythms

The coexistence of different rhythms in the two atria is a recognized electrophysiologic phenomenon. This condition, termed dissimilar atrial rhythms, is poorly diagnosed from the surface ECG, although it probably accounts for some cases of so-called impure flutter or flutter-fibrillation. The diagnosis requires the demonstration of different rhythms in the two atria, usually with the aid of either esophageal or direct intracardiac electrical recordings. The usual finding is a faster fibrillation-type rhythm in one atrium and a slower, more regular rhythm in the other. In these cases, the atria are probably not dissociated but exhibit a high degree of intra-atrial block or entrance and exit blocks of part of the atrial myocardium.[10,11] A more unusual condition of apparently completely dissociated atrial rhythms also exists.

Echocardiographic studies, including dual M-mode echocardiographic recordings, have been used to demonstrate dissimilar atrial rhythms.[8,12] The right atrial rate is reflected in the A-wave rate on the tricuspid valve M-mode echocardiogram, and the left atrial rate is similarly recorded from the mitral valve. Figure 40–18 is an interesting example of this condition in which the P waves on the surface ECG are related neither to the A waves on the mitral valve M-mode recording nor to the ventricular rate. The A waves recorded from the mitral valve, however, show a constant relation to the mitral valve E waves and the QRS complexes on the surface ECG. In this case, therefore, the left atrium appears to be controlled by a rhythm that is electrically silent on the surface ECG, but is conducted to the ventricles. In contrast, the right atrial electrical activity is dissociated from the left side of the heart, but results in the P waves recorded on the surface ECG.[13]

Ventricular Rhythms

Ventricular rhythms arise from foci within the ventricular myocardium or specialized conducting tissues and are characterized by broad QRS complexes on the ECG (duration longer than 0.12 seconds). The resultant ventricular contraction pattern is altered and the force of contraction is usually diminished. These rhythms range from benign single ventricular premature beats to fatal ventricular fibrillation.

Ventricular Premature Beats

Ventricular premature beats can produce changes in left and right ventricular free wall and interventricular septal motion, global ventricular function, and both AV and semilunar valve motion. Although many of these

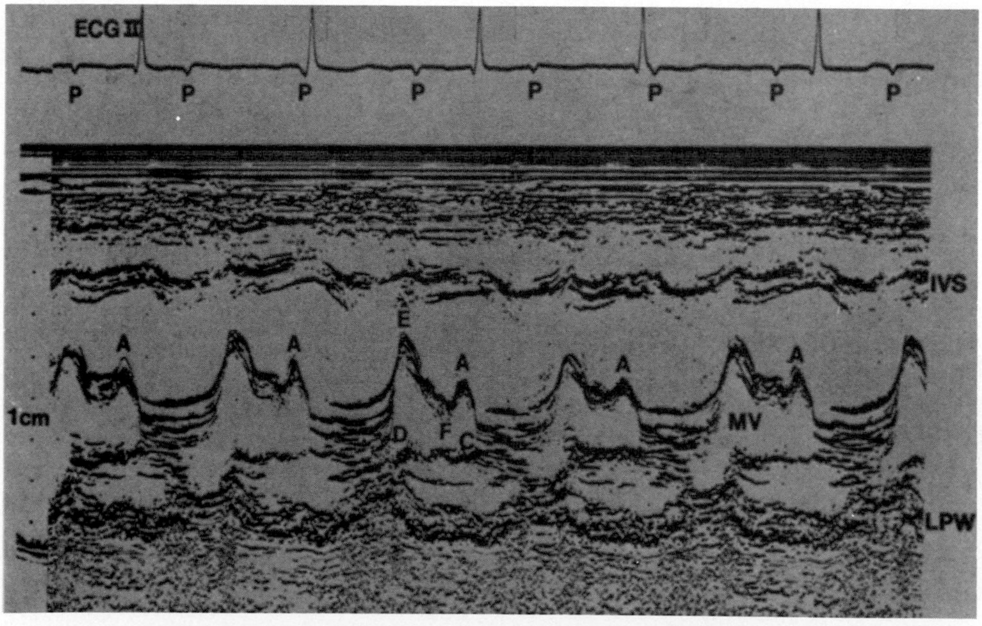

Fig. 40–18. In this example of dissimilar atrial rhythms, the atrial rate recorded on the surface electrocardiogram (P waves) is not related to the atrial rate demonstrated by M-mode echocardiography of the mitral valve (MV) (A waves). IVS = interventricular septum; LPW = left ventricular posterior wall. (See text for details.) (From Procacci PM, Levites R, Kotler MN, Anderson GJ: Dissimilar atrial rhythms diagnosed by echocardiography. Chest 73:429, 1978.)

changes are obvious, some are more subtle and require careful analysis of the M-mode tracing for correct interpretation. When appropriately analyzed, however, Echo-Doppler studies should permit the origin and functional significance of ventricular rhythms to be defined. Figure 40–19 is an M-mode recording of the left ventricle from a patient with ventricular bigeminy. Septal and posterior left ventricular wall motion are normal during each of the sinus beats. During the premature ventricular beats, however, septal motion is paradoxic (large arrow) and the septum fails to thicken normally. This pattern of motion is usually seen with ectopic beats originating in the right ventricle and results in "left bundle branch block" morphology on the ECG and a pattern of motion of the interventricular septum similar to that described for left bundle branch block (see later and also Chapter 29). Figure 40–20 is an M-mode of the left ventricle in a patient with intermittent ventricular bigeminy. Figure 40–20A was recorded during a period of sinus rhythm, and the excursions of the septum and posterior wall are normal. Figure 40–20B illustrates the effect of the ventricular premature beats. In this case, septal and

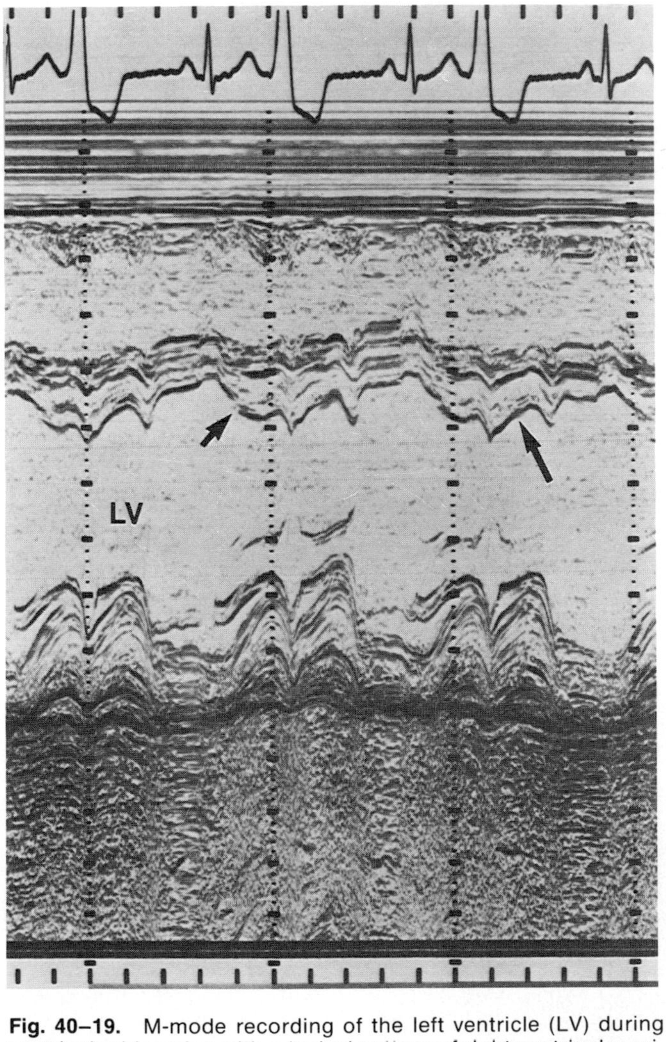

Fig. 40–19. M-mode recording of the left ventricle (LV) during ventricular bigeminy with a typical pattern of right ventricular origin. The small arrow indicates normal septal motion, and the large arrow indicates paradoxic septal motion. (See text for details.)

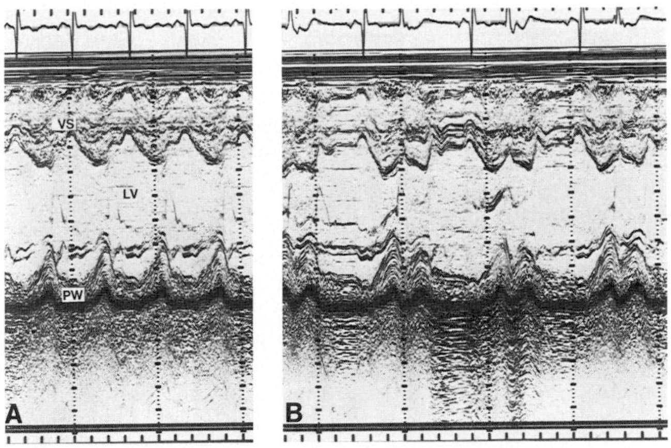

Fig. 40–20. M-mode recording comparing left ventricular wall motion. A. Motion during sinus rhythm. B. Motion during ventricular bigeminy typical of left ventricular origin. VS = ventricular septum; LV = left ventricle; PW = posterior wall.

posterior wall contraction remain normally directed and wall thickening is preserved. This suggests a left ventricular origin of the ventricular premature beats because septal depolarization appears normally directed from left to right. After the compensatory pause, the subsequent ventricular contraction is augmented compared to the normal beats in Figure 40–20A.

The effects of ventricular premature beats on valve motion can also be demonstrated by M-mode echocardiography. Figure 40–21 illustrates aortic valve motion in a patient with frequent ventricular premature beats. In this example, the normally conducted sinus beats (beats one and three) produce normal aortic valve opening. The second beat in this example is a ventricular premature beat that barely generates sufficient pressure to open the aortic valve. The fourth beat, also a ventricular premature beat, does not result in any opening of the aortic valve, a finding indicating that the left ventricle failed

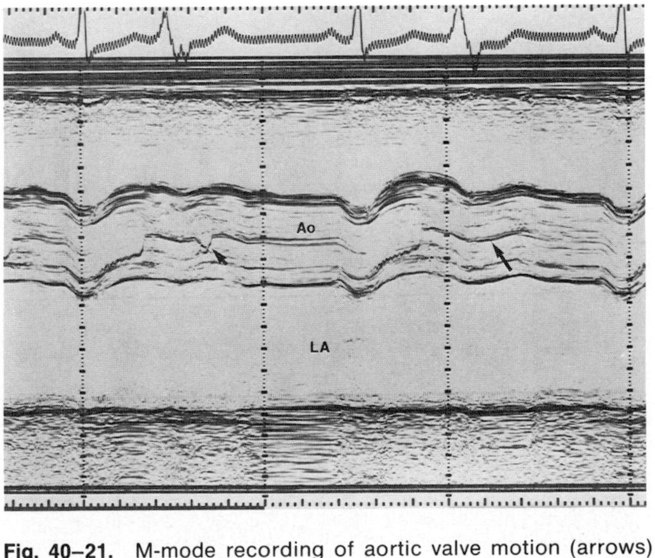

Fig. 40–21. M-mode recording of aortic valve motion (arrows) during ventricular premature beats. Ao = aorta; LA = left atrium. (See text for details.)

to generate enough pressure to propel blood into the aorta. Figures 40–22 and 40–23 illustrate the effects of ventricular premature beats on mitral and aortic valve motion. In the example in Figure 40–22, the premature beats occur soon after the preceding T wave, and the mitral valve does not open before the premature contraction (arrows). Because there is no ventricular filling, the stroke output after the premature contraction is reduced, as indicated by the limited duration of aortic valve opening in the right of Figure 40–22 panel. Figure 40–23 illustrates a slightly different pattern in which mitral valve opening begins normally but is abruptly terminated by the closely coupled premature ventricular contractions (arrows). The right panel of Figure 40–23 illustrates failure of aortic valve opening after the first of two ventricular premature beats, with opening similar to that of normally conducted beats after the second beat of the pair. These patterns have many variations which depend on the coupling interval between the premature and the preceding beat and on the underlying ventricular function.

Doppler recordings of flow across the AV valves show the effect of ventricular premature beats on ventricular filling. As with atrial premature beats, these effects primarily relate to the coupling interval between the premature and the preceding ventricular contraction. If the coupling interval is sufficiently short, the premature beat may prevent mitral opening and no ventricular filling will occur. If the coupling interval is slightly longer (Figure 40–24, VPB 1), the E wave may be truncated and further diastolic filling may be prevented by the rise in ventricular pressure. If the premature beat has a still longer coupling interval (Figure 40–24, VPB 2), passive filling may be completed and the premature beat will interrupt the atrial filling wave. When the premature beat interrupts ventricular filling, left atrial pressure rises, and there is often augmentation of the E wave in the diastolic period after the premature beat. Doppler recordings of flow through the aortic and pulmonary valves provide a direct measurement of the hemodynamic effect of ventricular premature beats. The timing of these ectopic beats within the cardiac cycle determines the hemodynamic consequence. Ventricular ectopic beats with short coupling intervals result in little or no flow across the semilunar valves, whereas those with longer coupling intervals result in stroke outputs proportional to the preceding

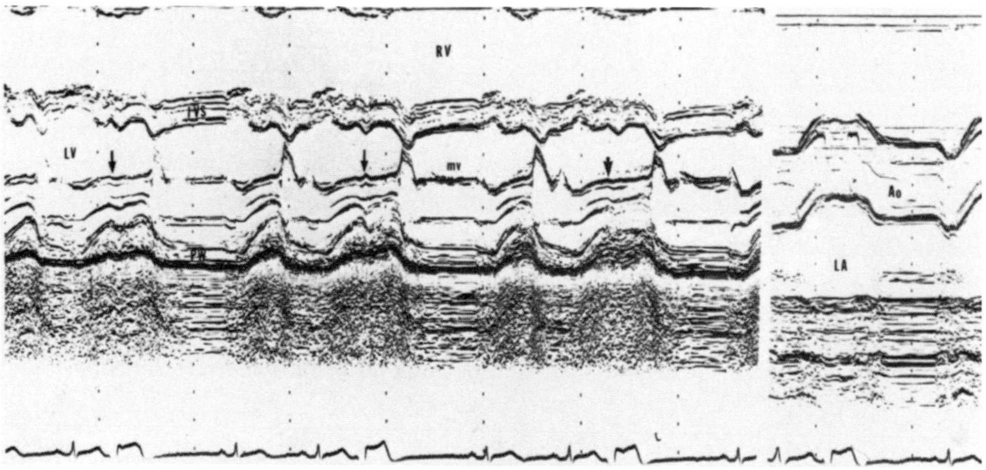

Fig. 40–22. M-mode pattern of mitral and aortic valve motion resulting from ventricular premature beats. Arrows indicate failure of mitral valve opening. RV = right ventricle; IVS = interventricular septum; LV = left ventricle; PW = posterior wall; Ao = aorta; LA = left atrium. (From Harrigan P, Lee R: Principles of Interpretation in Echocardiography. New York, John Wiley & Sons, p. 334, 1985.)

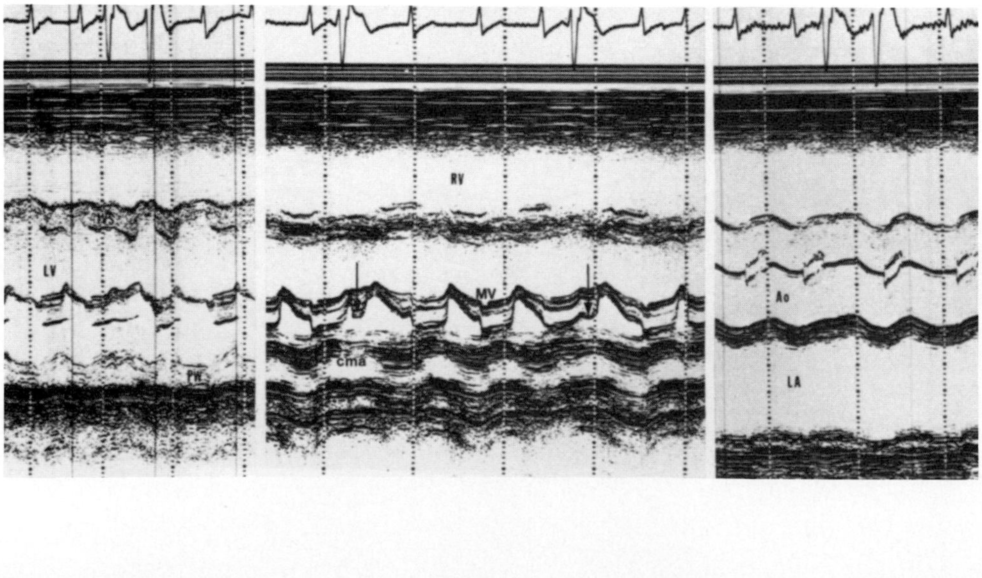

Fig. 40–23. M-mode recording of mitral valve (MV) (left) and aortic valve (right) motion during ventricular premature beats. Arrows indicate premature mitral valve closure. RV = right ventricle; LV = left ventricle; IVS = interventricular septum; PW = posterior wall; cma = calcified mitral annulus; Ao = aorta; LA = left atrium. (From Harrigan P, Lee R: Principles of Interpretation in Echocardiography. New York, John Wiley & Sons, p. 335, 1985.)

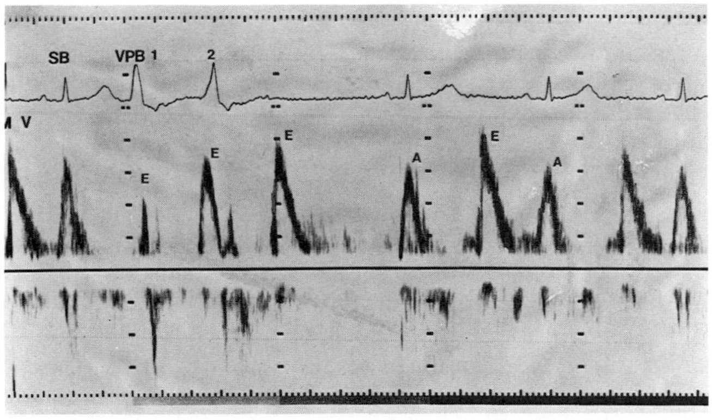

Fig. 40–24. Doppler spectral display of transmitral flow illustrating the effect of ventricular premature beats (VPB) of different coupling intervals. SB = sinus beat; MV = mitral valve.

RR interval (Figure 40–25). When a compensatory pause occurs, the first beat after the ventricular premature beat typically shows an increased flow velocity and volume as a result of the increased left ventricular filling period (VPB 1). These changes are also seen in Figure 40–26.

Ventricular Tachycardia

Ventricular tachycardia may originate anywhere within the ventricular chambers distal to the AV node and is characterized by a tachycardia of three or more broad, usually bizarre, QRS complexes on the surface ECG. Several features of a ventricular tachycardia aid in its differentiation from a supraventricular tachycardia with aberrant AV conduction. The first is AV dissociation, and this may be demonstrated by M-mode echocardiography, as shown in Figure 40–27. The second is the

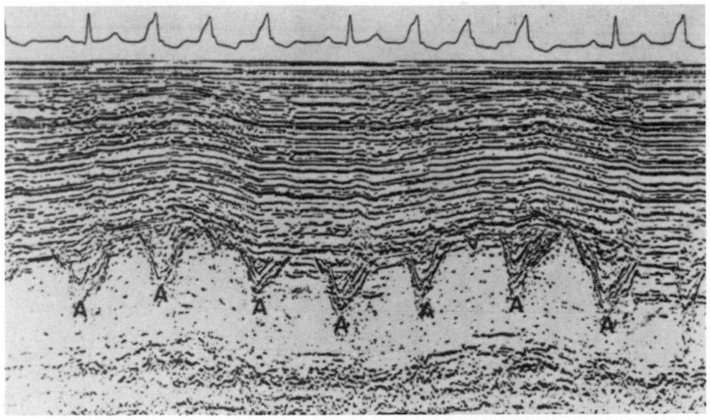

Fig. 40–27. Subcostal right atrial wall M-mode in a patient with runs of ventricular tachycardia. Atrioventricular dissociation is not easily seen on the electrocardiogram but may be identified on the echocardiogram. A = atrial contraction. (From Drinkovic N: Subcostal M-mode echocardiography of the right atrial wall for differentiation of supraventricular tachyarrhythmias with aberration from ventricular tachycardia. Am Heart J 107:326, 1984.)

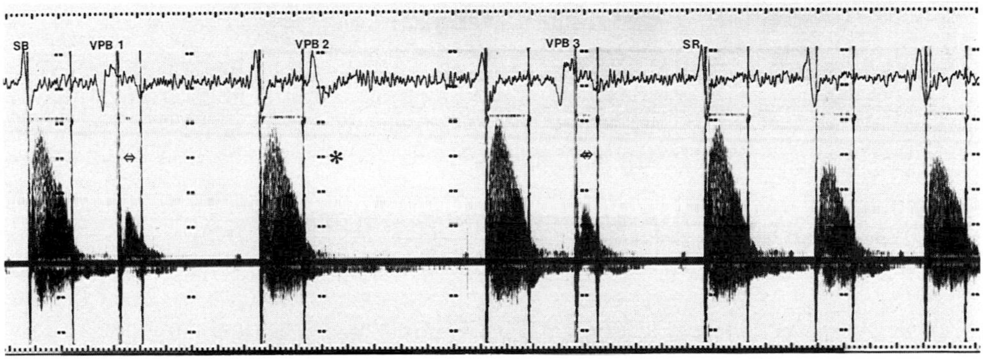

Fig. 40–25. Doppler spectral display of transaortic flow during ventricular premature beats (VPB) of varying coupling intervals. Double-headed arrows indicate shortened aortic valve opening times; * = absence of aortic valve opening; SB = sinus beat; SR = sinus rhythm.

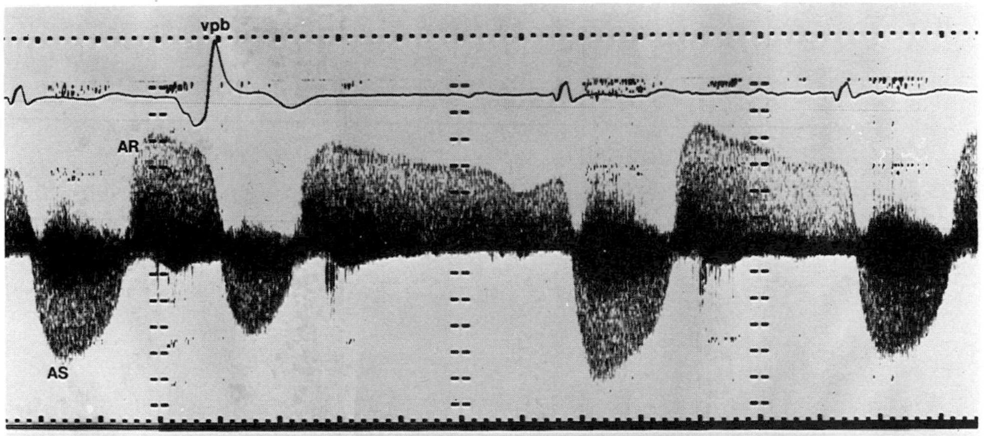

Fig. 40–26. Continuous wave Doppler recording of transaortic flow in a patient with aortic stenosis (AS) and regurgitation (AR). The ventricular premature beat (vpb) results in a shortened aortic ejection time and decreased peak flow velocity. The peak velocity generated by the next sinus beat is increased as a result of both the inefficient previous contraction and the increased diastolic filling period during the compensatory pause.

presence of fusion beats. These typically occur at the onset of the tachycardia when the ventricle is activated by the normal conducting system and the ectopic ventricular focus at the same time, and they represent this combined electrical activity. On the ECG, one usually sees a progressive change over several beats from the normal QRS complex to the broad QRS of the ventricular rhythm. Figure 40–28 is an M-mode recording (at 100 mm/sec) of mitral valve motion during the onset of ventricular tachycardia. Sinus rhythm (Fig. 40–28, left) is interrupted by a ventricular premature beat, which slightly shortens the mitral valve A-wave duration. A sinus beat follows, and the ventricular tachycardia begins with two fusion beats leading into the broad complex rhythm. After the onset of the arrhythmia, the heart rate increases, and evidence of atrial activity is lost on both the ECG and the mitral valve echocardiogram. In addition, the mitral valve E waves are shortened in duration and are irregular in amplitude, suggesting reduced ventricular filling.

The hemodynamic consequences of ventricular tachycardia can be illustrated by both M-mode and Doppler echocardiographic studies. The circulatory effects are typically adverse and result from both the reduced left ventricular filling and the inefficient pattern of ventricular contraction. In some patients, this rhythm is well tolerated and the left ventricular output, as assessed by Doppler recording of peak aortic velocity and systolic velocity interval, are reduced but still sufficient to maintain adequate resting circulation. In many patients, however, the rhythm results in hemodynamic collapse, either because of a rapid rate or an underlying cardiac disorder, and markedly diminished flow velocities are recorded across the aortic valve with each systole.

Ventricular Fibrillation and Asystole

Ventricular fibrillation is disorganized ventricular activity that results in no effective ventricular contraction. It is characterized on the surface ECG by irregular undulations of the baseline with no recognizable complexes. Untreated, it degenerates into asystole, which is the complete absence of all cardiac activity.

Experimental echocardiographic studies have shown that, after the onset of ventricular fibrillation, there is an initial progressive reduction in the left ventricular internal diameter with a concomitant increase in the right ventricular diameter. These changes are thought to reflect the different compliance characteristics of the two chambers and stabilize when the ventricular pressures equilibrate (usually 1 to 2 minutes). The ventricular walls initially show fibrillatory movements, which disappear when asystole supervenes. In addition, the majority of cases show continued atrial contraction, with A waves on the mitral valve echocardiogram, during ventricular fibrillation.[14]

Echocardiographic techniques have been used to assess the effectiveness of cardiopulmonary resuscitation. With low compressive forces on the chest, the mitral valve fails to close, and forward blood flow is mainly due to the chest pump mechanism. With higher compressive forces, however, direct heart compression and mitral valve closure occur. This cardiac pump action results in significantly higher cerebral and myocardial perfusion and should be the aim of all resuscitative techniques.[15]

Forceful, abrupt coughing is known to sustain circulation and consciousness in some patients with ventricular fibrillation and asystole. An echocardiographic study of this maneuver has shown that, although arterial pressures are maintained, there is little evidence of antegrade cardiac flow. The mitral valve remains open with minimal forward flow from the pulmonic veins. The aortic valve, however, remains closed with no Doppler evidence of forward flow, and there is an increase in the left ventricular dimensions. Arterial pressure maintenance has been postulated to result from a transmission of intrathoracic pressure, to a to-and-fro motion, rather than from antegrade blood flow.[16]

Conduction Disturbances

Disorders of intracardiac conduction result in a variety of echocardiographic abnormalities from both the altered electrical activation patterns and their resultant hemodynamic effects.

First-Degree Atrioventricular Block

First-degree AV block is characterized by prolongation of the interval between atrial and ventricular systole (i.e., the ECG PR interval). In normal subjects, relaxation of the atria causes atrial pressure to fall below ventricular pressure, thereby initiating valve closure, which is completed by ventricular systole. Prolongation of the PR interval gives the mitral valve leaflets time to reach full apposition before the onset of ventricular systole.

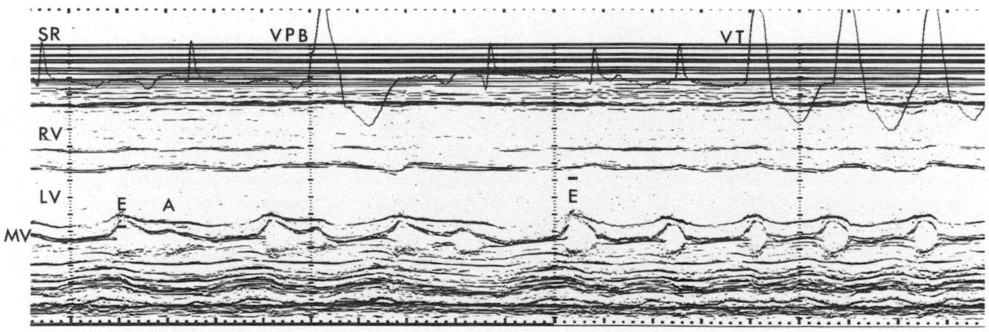

Fig. 40–28. M-mode echocardiogram of the mitral valve (MV) at the onset of an episode of ventricular tachycardia (VT). SR = sinus rhythm; VPB = ventricular premature beat; RV = right ventricle; LV = left ventricle. (See text for details.)

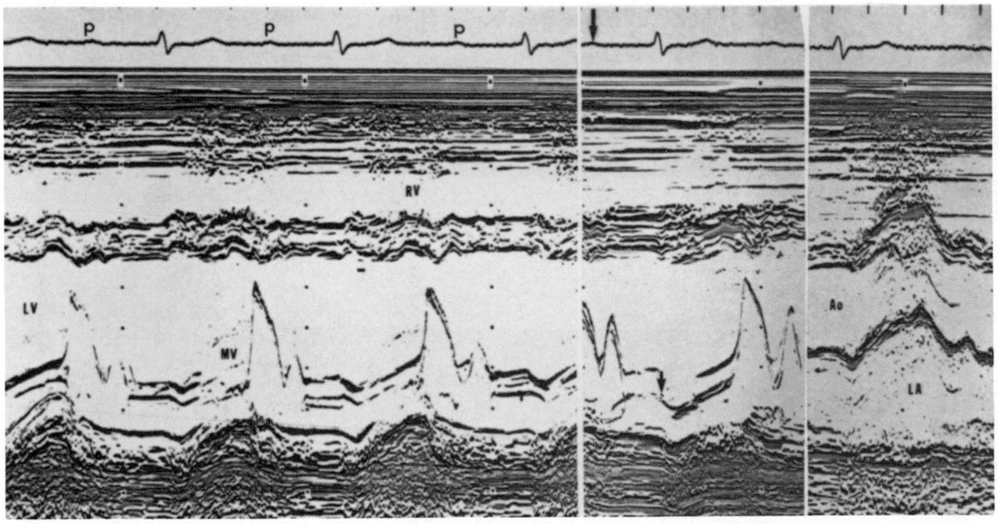

Fig. 40–29. M-mode recording of the mitral valve (MV) during first-degree heart block. Small arrow indicates MV position at the onset of ventricular systole. p = ECG P wave; RV = right ventricle; LV = left ventricle; Ao = aorta; LA = left atrium. (From Harrigan P, Lee R: Principles of Interpretation in Echocardiography. New York, John Wiley & Sons, p. 337, 1985.)

This early "closure" is easily detected on the M-mode echocardiogram (Figure 40–29) and is the expected pattern with first-degree heart block. Once the mitral leaflets are apposed, they tend to remain in this position until the ventricles are activated (Fig. 40–29, small arrow, middle panel) if the PR interval is not too long (less than 0.50 seconds). When the PR interval is longer than 0.50 seconds*, atrial pressure gradually rises and mitral reopening typically occurs. A direct relationship has been shown between the position of the mitral leaflets at the onset of systole and the intensity of the first heart sound. When the mitral leaflets are closely apposed, the first sound is soft because of minimal leaflet travel to full closure. As leaflet separation increases, the magnitude of the first heart sound also increases.[17]

Mitral valve closure before the QRS complex in patients with first-degree heart block should not be considered premature because it occurs as an appropriate response to atrial relaxation. This type of early closure must be differentiated from the *premature closure* of the mitral valve caused by acute severe aortic insufficiency. In the latter case, the valve is closed by the rapidly rising left ventricular pressure resulting from the massive regurgitant volume and typically precedes the end of the P wave of the ECG. Thus, by definition, mitral closure must precede atrial systole to be considered truly premature. This distinction is important because patients with aortic endocarditis often have septal involvement and first-degree heart block as well as truly premature closure due to aortic regurgitation, which has far different prognostic implications from normal closure due to atrial relaxation.

Second-Degree Atrioventricular Block

Second-degree heart block is characterized by intermittent block of atrial impulses before they can cause ventricular activation. Two primary types have been described and are termed Mobitz type I and type II. *Mobitz type I or Wenckebach block* is characterized by an incremental increase in the PR interval until a P wave is blocked and ventricular contraction fails to occur. In contrast, in *Mobitz type II block,* the PR interval remains constant and atrial contraction is intermittently blocked in a variable but typically ordered sequence (i.e., 2:1 block, 3:2 block, etc.). In patients with second-degree AV block of either type, the atrial rate is reflected both in excursion of the atrial walls and in the atrial components of AV valve motion on the M-mode echocardiogram. The degree of block determines the ventricular rate and thus the ventricular contraction pattern and aortic valve opening times. Figure 40–30, an M-mode recording of mitral valve motion during 2:1 Mobitz type II block, shows the characteristic pattern of alternating normal E and A waves during the conducted beats and lone A waves from the nonconducted atrial contractions.

The left ventricular stroke volumes and aortic valve opening times show typical patterns according to the type of block. During Wenckebach block, the left ventricular stroke volume is directly proportional to the preceding end-diastolic volume, which in turn is determined by the RR interval of the preceding diastole. During fixed second-degree AV block, such as 2:1 block, the left ventricular stroke volume is constant.[18]

Third-Degree Atrioventricular Block

Third-degree, or complete, AV block is characterized by independent action of the atria and ventricles. This results in a significantly altered pattern of AV valve motion, as illustrated in Figure 40–31. Typically, the A waves of the mitral valve follow the P waves on the ECG as they move through diastole. After atrial contraction, the left atrium relaxes, left atrial pressure falls, and mitral valve closure is initiated (Fig. 40–31, arrows). In the absence of ventricular activation, the mitral valve generally reopens gradually.

In the past, it was assumed that atrial relaxation closed the AV valves, and reopening of the mitral and tricuspid valves after atrial contraction in patients with

* These intervals were derived for complete heart block, but they apply equally to first-degree heart block.

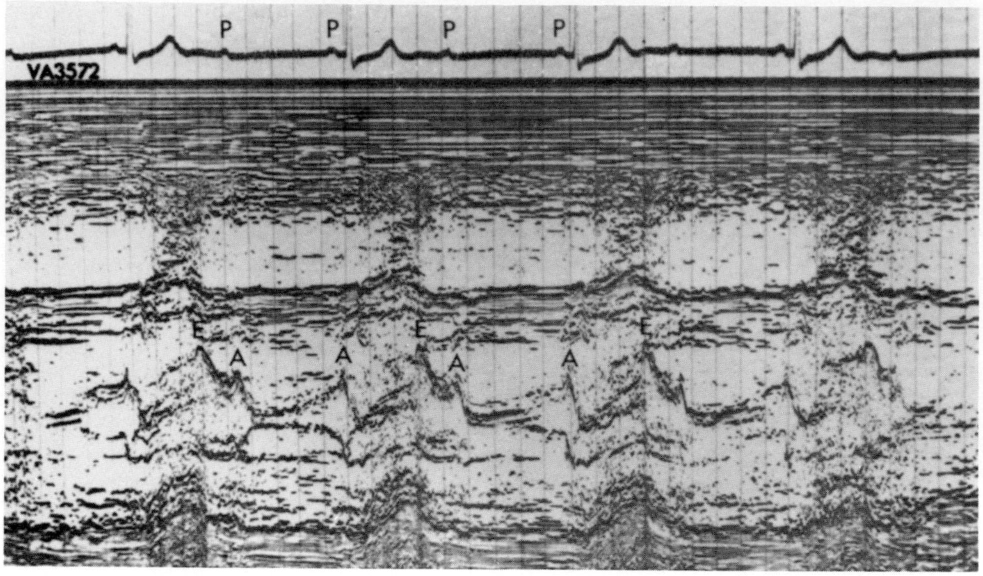

Fig. 40–30. M-mode recording of the left ventricle and mitral valve during second-degree atrioventricular block with 2:1 conduction. The mitral A waves follow each P wave on the electrocardiogram. (From Feigenbaum H: Echocardiography. 3rd Ed. Philadelphia, Lea & Febiger, p. 236, 1981.)

a prolonged PR interval was due to restoration of a positive AV gradient resulting from gradual atrial filling and a corresponding rise in atrial pressure. More recent Doppler studies have shown, however, that the apparent valve closure is generally associated with diastolic flow from the ventricle to atrium, or diastolic mitral regurgitation, as illustrated in Figure 40–32.[19–21] That the diastolic regurgitant flow begins immediately after atrial contraction suggests that, although the leaflets appear to close as a result of atrial relaxation, they are merely apposed and fail to seal the orifice. Because flow proceeds from ventricle to atrium, the initial pressure gradient must also be from ventricle to atrium, and the mitral valve must be held open against, rather than be closed by, the pressure acting on the leaflet surfaces. The force required to overcome this pressure can only come from the papillary muscles and chordae tendineae and must be secondary to tension in the ventricular wall created by atrial contraction. The diastolic regurgitant

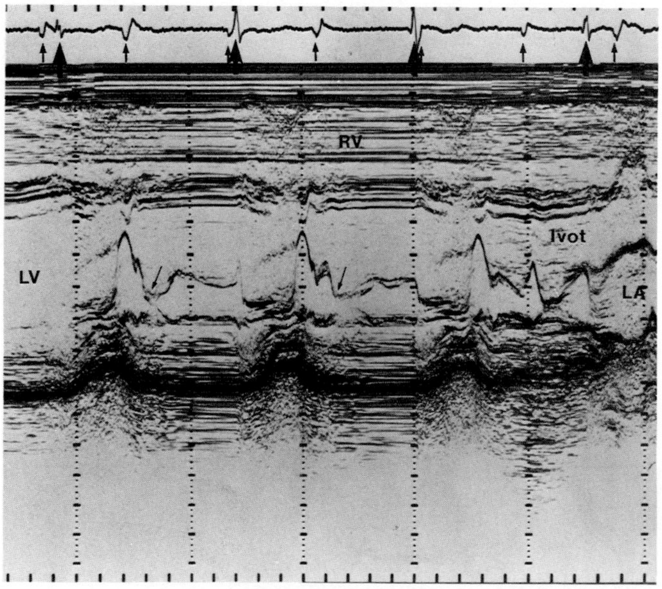

Fig. 40–31. M-mode pattern of motion of the mitral valve during third-degree (complete) atrioventricular block (thin arrows indicate mitral valve closure). Small arrows on electrocardiogram (ECG) = atrial rate; large arrows on ECG = ventricular rate; RV = right ventricle; LV = left ventricle; lvot = left ventricular outflow tract; LA = left atrium.

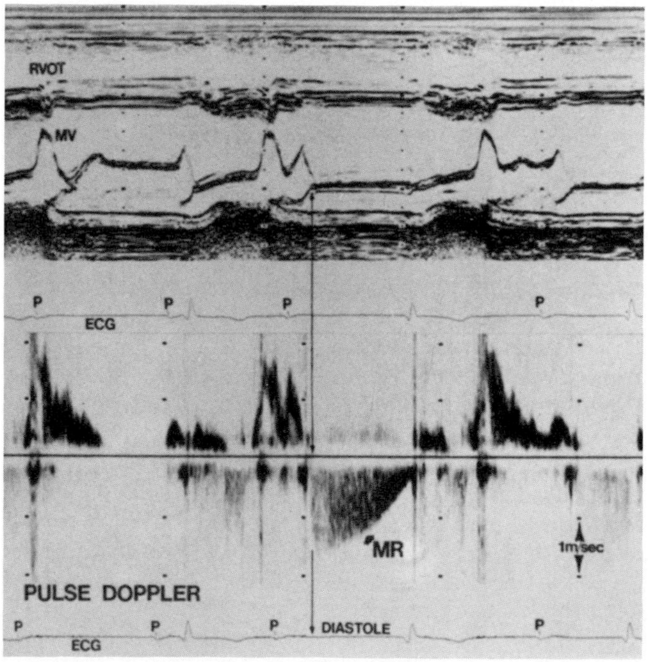

Fig. 40–32. Pulsed wave Doppler recording of transmitral flow during complete heart block illustrating diastolic mitral regurgitation. RVOT = right ventricular outflow tract; MV = mitral valve; MR = mitral regurgitation. (See text for full description.) (From Panidis IP, et al.: Diastolic mitral regurgitation in patients with atrioventricular conduction abnormalities: a common finding by Doppler echocardiography. Reprinted with permission from the American College of Cardiology. Journal of the American College of Cardiology 1986, 7, 768.)

flow velocity generally accelerates to a peak immediately after the cessation of forward flow and then decelerates as the ventriculoatrial pressure gradient decreases because of the post-A-wave fall in ventricular pressure and the rise in atrial pressure resulting from pulmonary and central venous inflow into the two atria. Once the atrial pressure exceeds that in the ventricle, obvious leaflet opening is recorded.

Left ventricular contraction and stroke output, although regular in rate, vary in magnitude in direct relation to the number of atrial contractions that occurred during the previous diastolic filling period.

Bundle Branch Block

Conduction abnormalities within the His-Purkinje system may give rise to right or left bundle branch block.

Right Bundle Branch Block. In patients with right bundle branch block, septal depolarization proceeds normally from left to right, and the pattern of left ventricular contraction is also normal. Although right bundle branch block is usually not associated with any significant cardiac disease, right ventricular activation is delayed, and this results in slightly delayed opening and closure of the pulmonary valve.[22] The right bundle branch comprises a single group of fibers that branch only at the periphery. A proximal interruption causes delay in right ventricular activation, which otherwise proceeds normally; however, a more diffuse condition causing delay in the progression of impulses to the whole ventricle results in a disorganized contraction sequence. Two subtypes of right bundle branch block have been identified based on the relationship of tricuspid and mitral closure with pulmonary opening. The first and most common subtype is a proximal block, and in these patients, the delay is mainly between mitral valve closure and tricuspid valve closure, with no prolongation of the interval between tricuspid and pulmonary valve closure. In the second subtype, with a distal block, the delay is mainly between tricuspid valve closure and pulmonary valve opening. Most patients in the first group are asymptomatic and presumably have the usual benign, nonprogressive form of right bundle branch block. Almost all the patients in the second group have myocardial disease, myocardial infarction, or diffuse idiopathic fibrosis of the conducting system, with a high incidence of syncope. In this study echocardiography is claimed to offer a noninvasive method of assessing prognosis in right bundle branch block.[22]

Left Bundle Branch Block. This disorder results in abnormal depolarization (from right to left) of the interventricular septum and delayed activation of the left ventricle. As a result, right ventricular depolarization occurs before that of the left ventricle, and the early unopposed rise in right ventricular pressure deflects the septum transiently to the left. Leftward movement of the septum continues until left ventricular contraction supervenes and left ventricular pressure rises. Once left ventricular pressure begins to rise, the normal left-to-right pressure gradient is rapidly restored and the initial leftward movement of the septum is reversed. The movement of the septum during the remainder of systole can be anterior (i.e., paradoxic), flat, or essentially normal (posterior).[23] Figure 40–33 illustrates the early systolic deflection of the septum that characterizes left bundle branch block. On this M-mode recording of the left ventricle, one notes an abrupt downward displacement of the septum in early systole (small arrow) and a posterior motion during ejection, followed by an early diastolic dip (large arrow). Note that the early diastolic dip was caused by dissociation of ventricular filling (right before left) and is a variable but not diagnostic feature of left bundle branch block. Figure 40–34 is another example of left bundle branch block in which both the presystolic and early diastolic dips were present; however, in this case, the septum remained flat during the ejection phase.

There is a higher incidence of anterior (paradoxic) septal motion in patients with left bundle branch block when this is associated with left axis deviation.[24] A normal axis is associated with a higher frequency of poste-

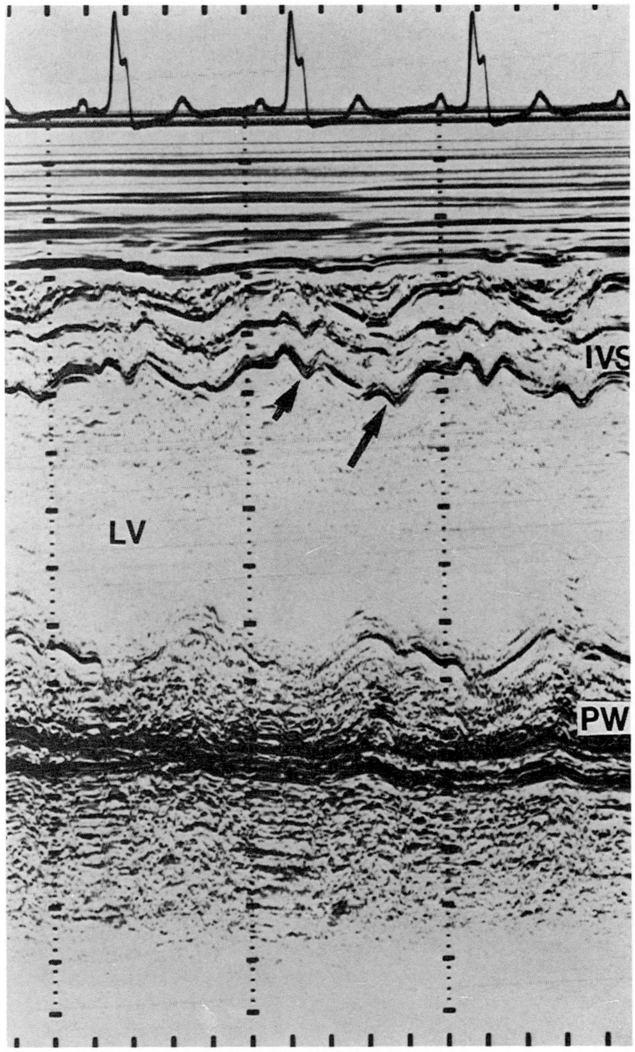

Fig. 40–33. M-mode recording of the left ventricle (LV) illustrating the typical early systolic downward movement (small arrow) of the interventricular septum (IVS) that occurs with left bundle branch block. PW = posterior wall; large arrow indicates early diastolic septal dip.

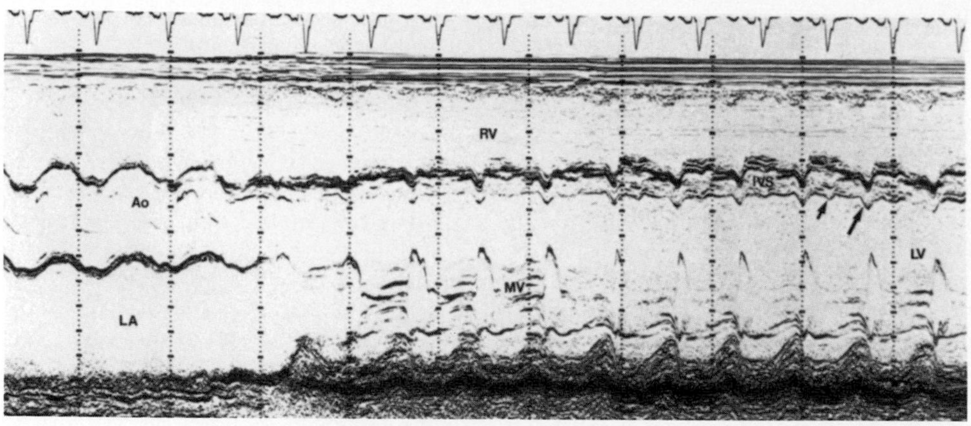

Fig. 40–34. M-mode recording of interventricular septal motion with left bundle branch block. In this case, the early systolic downward displacement (small arrow), is followed by flat septal motion. Ao = aorta; LA = left atrium; MV = mitral valve; RV = right ventricle; IVS = interventricular septum; LV = left ventricle; large arrow indicates early diastolic septal dip. (From Harrigan P, Lee R: Principles of Interpretation in Echocardiography. New York, John Wiley & Sons, p. 335, 1985.)

rior (normal) septal motion. Patients with ischemic heart disease and septal infarction are more likely to have flat septal motion. The correlation between axis and septal motion in combination with left bundle branch block may be explained by the pattern of activation or by the septal disease process producing both abnormalities.

Short axis two-dimensional imaging in patients with left bundle branch block reveals the same "presystolic" deflection of the interventricular septum, which may be followed by paradoxic, absent, or normal systolic septal motion.

Left bundle branch block can be subclassified based on the presence or absence of the presystolic dip and the type of systolic septal motion. In general, patients with a dip and paradoxic septal motion have enlarged left ventricles, severe dysfunction, and a poor prognosis.[25] In contrast, those with ECG evidence of left bundle branch block but no presystolic dip and normal septal motion have an interventricular conduction delay as demonstrated by vectorcardiography. Other combinations have no consistently reported pathologic association, although normal septal motion with left bundle branch block would appear to exclude associated infarction.[25]

Pre-excitation and Accessory Pathway Conduction

Pre-excitation of the left ventricle by an accessory conduction pathway from the atrium to the ventricle produces abnormal early local activation of the base of the ventricle at the point of entry of the bypass tract. The muscular contraction produced by this early activation can often be visualized by echocardiography. Accessory pathways allowing conduction between the atria and ventricles have been described in a variety of locations. The most common types are grouped together in the Wolff-Parkinson-White (WPW) syndrome. Type A WPW syndrome is characterized by an accessory pathway leading to pre-excitation of the left ventricular posterior wall. In type B WPW syndrome, the accessory pathway causes pre-excitation of the anterior right ventricular wall. M-mode echocardiography reveals contraction of the ventricular wall in the area of pre-excitation when antegrade conduction is occurring through the accessory pathway. In patients with type A WPW syndrome, initial contraction is noted in the posterobasal segment of the left ventricle and precedes the first heart sound and the onset of mechanical systole.[26] These patients usually have normal motion of the interventricular septum. Figure 40–35 is a recording from a patient with type A WPW syndrome that illustrates the characteristic early systolic contraction of the posterior wall (arrow).

M-mode studies in patients with type B WPW syndrome often reveal abnormal interventricular septal motion. A typical finding is an early systolic posterior septal deflection similar to the pattern seen in patients with left bundle branch block. An additional finding in patients with type B WPW syndrome is early posterior move-

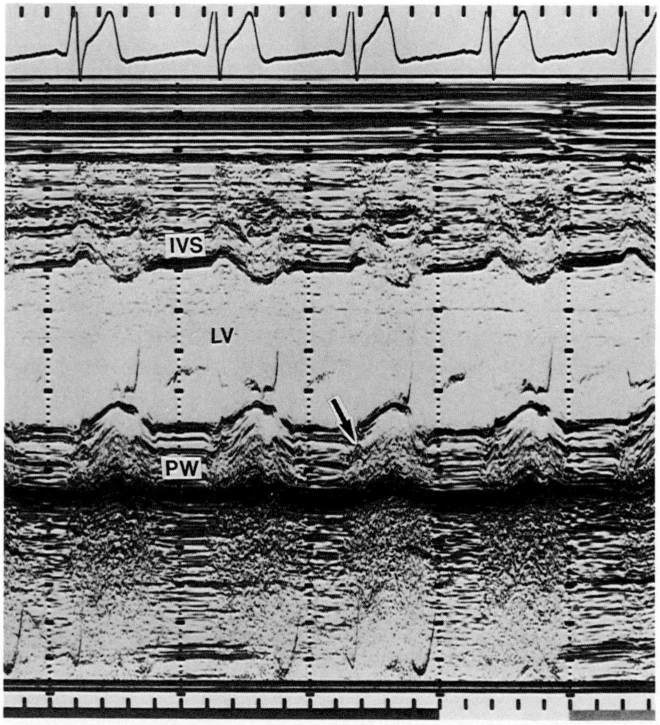

Fig. 40–35. M-mode recording of the left ventricle (LV) showing the typical movement of the posterior ventricular wall (PW) (arrow) in Wolff-Parkinson-White syndrome type A. IVS = interventricular septum. (See text for details.)

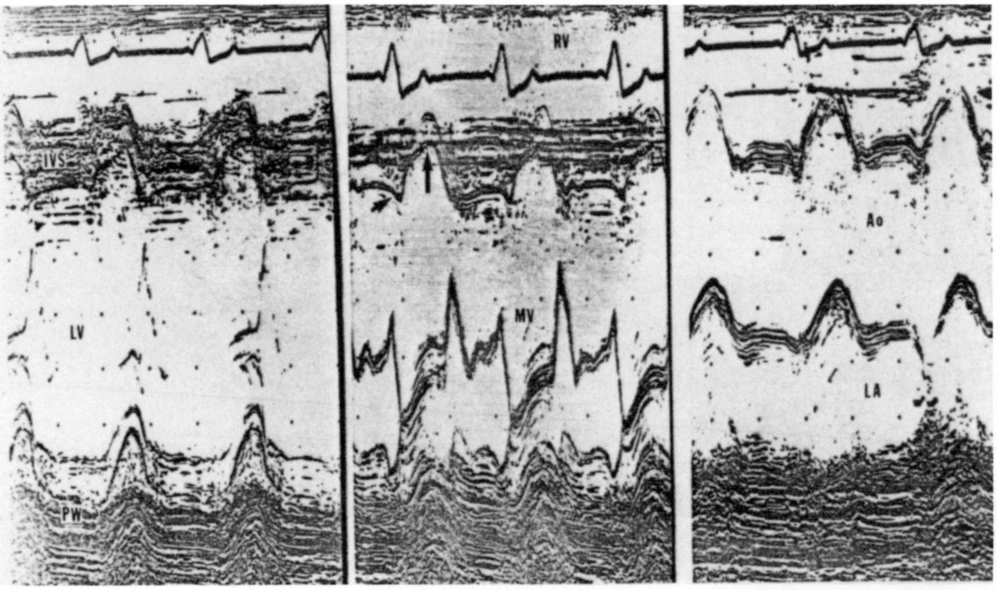

Fig. 40–36. M-mode recording of the left ventricle (LV) showing the typical movement of the interventricular septum (IVS) in Wolff-Parkinson-White syndrome type B. Small arrow indicates early systolic posterior septal motion; large arrow indicates anterior systolic septal motion. PW = posterior wall; RV = right ventricle; MV = mitral valve; Ao = aorta; LA = left atrium. (See text for details.) (From Harrigan P, Lee R: Principles of Interpretation in Echocardiography. New York, John Wiley & Sons, p. 336, 1985.)

ment of the right ventricular anterior wall at the onset of systole, in keeping with pre-excitation of this area.[27–33] Figure 40–36 was recorded in a patient with type B WPW syndrome. The typical early systolic posterior septal movement (small arrow) followed by anterior systolic motion (large arrow) is shown.

Type C WPW syndrome has also been described and is characterized by a negative delta wave in the left lateral leads on the ECG, with pre-excitation of the posterior right ventricle. Patients with this disorder have been reported to show a mixture of the echocardiographic changes seen in both other types of WPW syndrome, with no distinguishing features.[34]

Pacemaker Rhythms

Patients with pacemaker activation of the heart have a variety of echocardiographic findings that depend on the type and placement of the pacing electrode as well as the underlying condition leading to pacemaker insertion.

M-mode echocardiography is optimal for recording the motion of the ventricular walls and septum in patients with ventricular pacemakers. The most commonly noted finding in patients with right ventricular pacemakers is early posterior interventricular septal motion, immediately after the pacemaker artifact (Fig. 40–37), similar to that seen in left bundle branch block. In the example illustrated in Figure 40–37, there was also a simultaneous, brief anterior motion of the posterior wall, denoted by the small arrow. The motion of the interventricular septum throughout the remainder of the cardiac cycle is essentially normal.[35]

Doppler patterns of flow through the cardiac valves in patients with pacemakers are determined by the type of pacemaker, as well as the underlying cardiac disorder. In patients with complete AV dissociation and ventricular pacing, the findings are similar to those seen in patients with complete heart block, except the ventricular rate is usually faster. Diastolic regurgitation through the AV valves has been documented in such patients.[1]

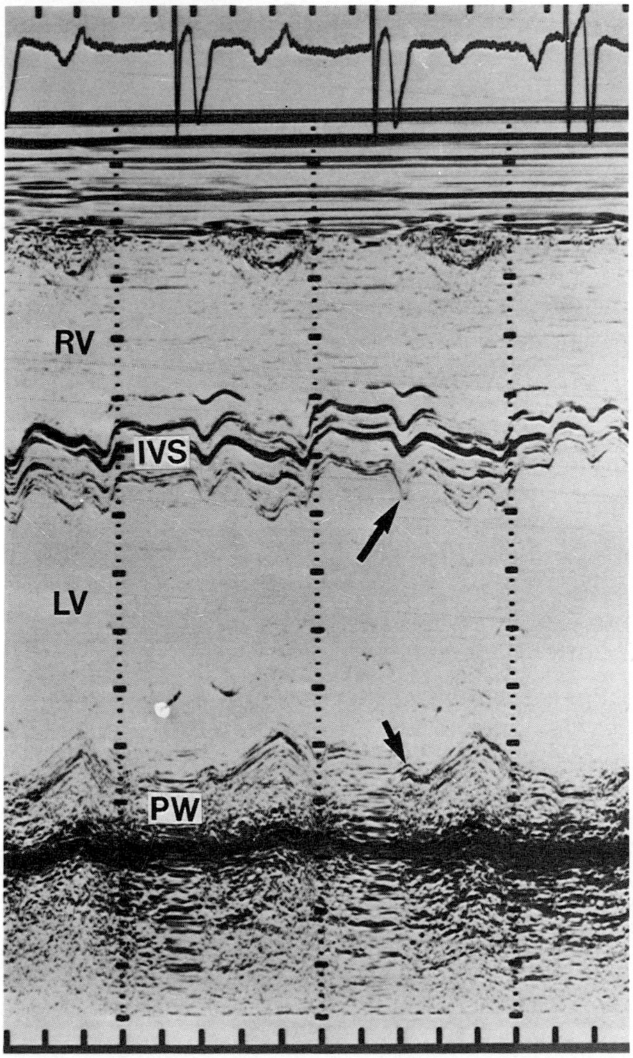

Fig. 40–37. M-mode recording of the left ventricle (LV) during a ventricular paced rhythm. Arrows indicate early systolic motion of the interventricular septum (IVS) and posterior wall (PW). RV = right ventricle. (See text for description.)

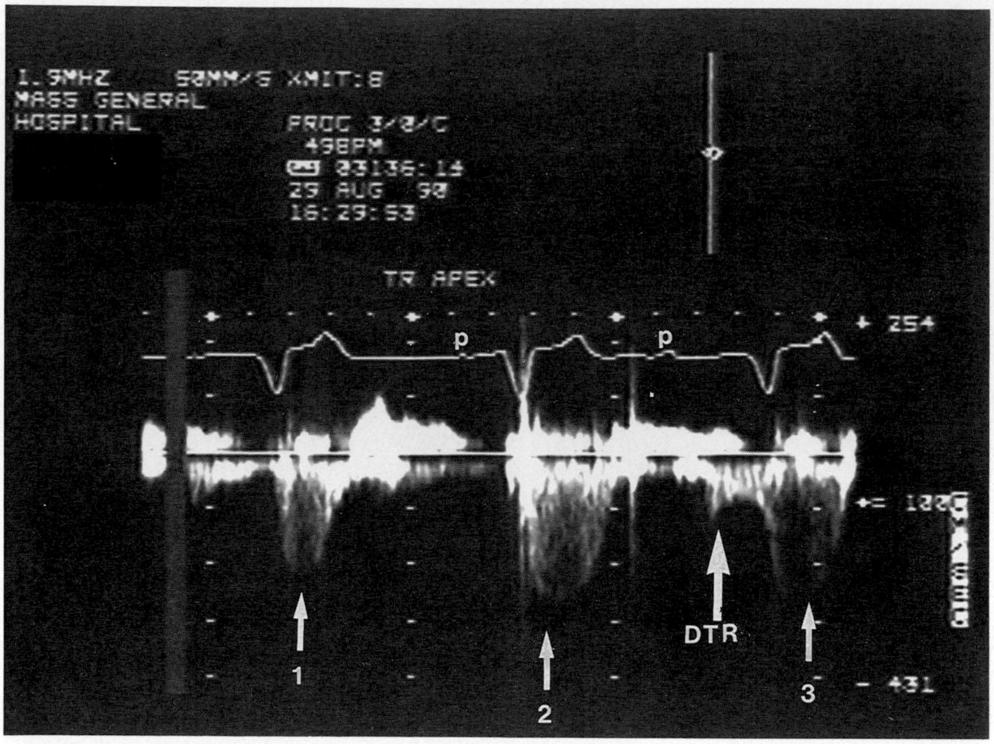

Fig. 40–38. Doppler spectral display of flow across the tricuspid valve during a paced rhythm showing variation in degree of systolic regurgitation and evidence of diastolic regurgitation according to the relationship between atrial and ventricular activation. P waves = atrial rate; TR = tricuspid regurgitation; DTR = diastolic tricuspid regurgitation. (See text for details.)

Figure 40–38 is a continuous wave Doppler recording from the apex in a patient with complete heart block, a right ventricular pacemaker, and systolic tricuspid regurgitation. After the first pacemaker complex, the tricuspid regurgitant jet reaches a maximum velocity of approximately 2.2 m/sec. Because of the timing of atrial contraction, there is presumably better filling of the right ventricle before the second complex, which results in a maximum velocity of the tricuspid regurgitant jet of 2.6 m/sec and a longer duration of regurgitation. The P wave that precedes the third pacemaker complex occurs early in diastole, and typical diastolic tricuspid regurgitation is recorded before the onset of systole and the higher velocity systolic tricuspid regurgitation. Figure 40–39 is

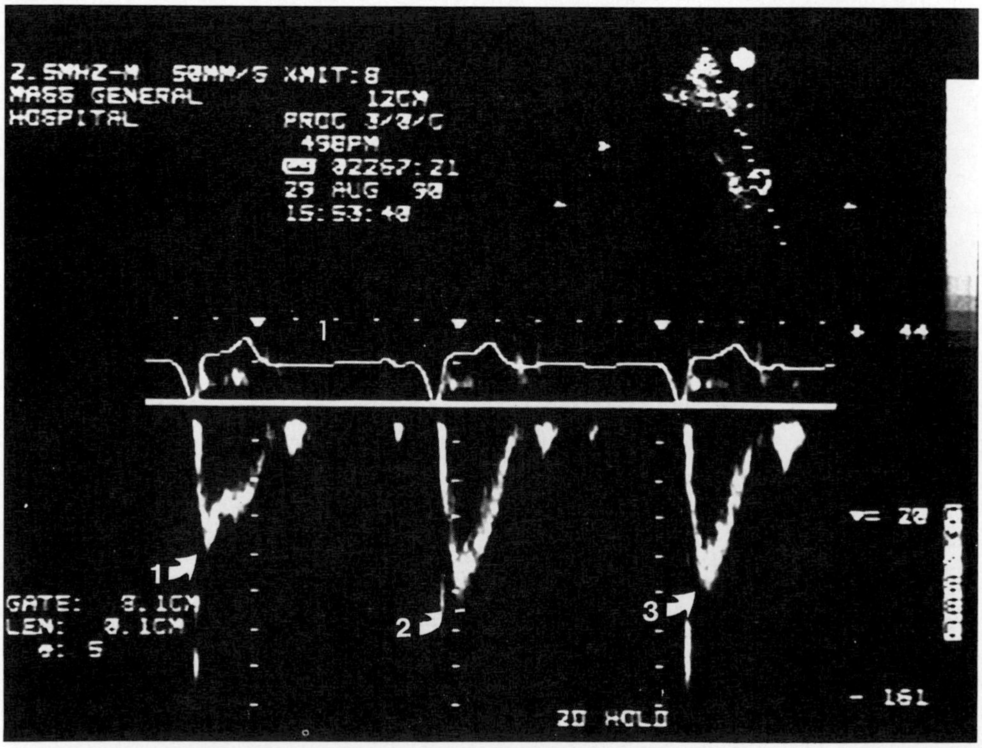

Fig. 40–39. Pulsed wave Doppler display of transpulmonary flow during a paced rhythm. (See text for description.)

a pulsed wave Doppler recording of flow in the proximal pulmonary artery from the same patient. Again, the diastolic filling of the right ventricle between the first and second complexes is greater, resulting in a greater peak velocity with this ejection.

CLINICAL APPLICATIONS OF ECHOCARDIOGRAPHY IN PATIENTS WITH DISTURBANCES OF RHYTHM AND CONDUCTION

In addition to describing the mechanical effects of arrhythmias on valvular motion and myocardial contraction and movement, echo-Doppler studies can provide useful clinical diagnostic and prognostic information on patients with abnormalities of rhythm and conduction. The areas of primary application include: (1) determining the nature of an arrhythmia when the surface ECG is nondiagnostic; (2) diagnosing an underlying cardiac disorder in a patient with an arrhythmia or conduction disorder; (3) defining primary structural or functional effects of arrhythmias and; (4) guiding therapy and management in patients with disturbances of cardiac rhythm and conduction.

Diagnosing an Arrhythmia

In some patients, it is not possible to identify the nature of an arrhythmia from the surface ECG along. Although additional maneuvers such as direct esophageal recording of atrial activity, or intracardiac electrophysiologic studies, can be used to obtain further information, the echocardiogram is often an ideal noninvasive tool by which to obtain the data necessary for diagnosis.

Both M-mode and two-dimensional echocardiogram recordings and analysis of the atrial walls and interatrial septal contraction patterns have been used extensively to diagnose arrhythmias. Atrial systole can be recorded in the majority of patients and can allow one to distinguish among supraventricular tachycardia, atrial flutter, and fibrillation (Fig. 40–40) and to differentiate ventricular arrhythmias from supraventricular arrhythmias with aberration based on the presence or absence of AV dissociation.[5,12,36–39]

This technique has also proved useful in the diagnosis of rhythm disturbances arising from physiologic pacemaker dysfunction. In these patients, atrial capture and sensing malfunctions can be reliably detected, and programming of the atrial output and sensitivity can be facilitated.[40]

Examination of the M-mode pattern of mitral valve motion and/or the Doppler spectral display of transmitral flow also permits identification of atrial and ventricular events. By comparing the timing of these events with the complexes on the surface ECG, further diagnostic information can be obtained in many patients with disordered cardiac rhythm and conduction, for example, in ventricular tachycardia or heart block, as discussed previously.

As discussed earlier in this chapter, the echocardiograph can be used to localize the site of a bypass tract in patients with anomalous AV connections, such as WPW syndrome. When combined with digital continuous loop two-dimensional echocardiographic analysis, the technique has been reported, in a small group of patients, to allow accurate localization of the site of the bypass tract in patients with WPW syndrome.[41] Theoretically, a similar application would enable one to identify the site of origin of ventricular arrhythmias.

Diagnosing an Underlying Cardiac Disorder

Echocardiography is a simple, noninvasive investigation frequently performed to diagnose or to exclude sig-

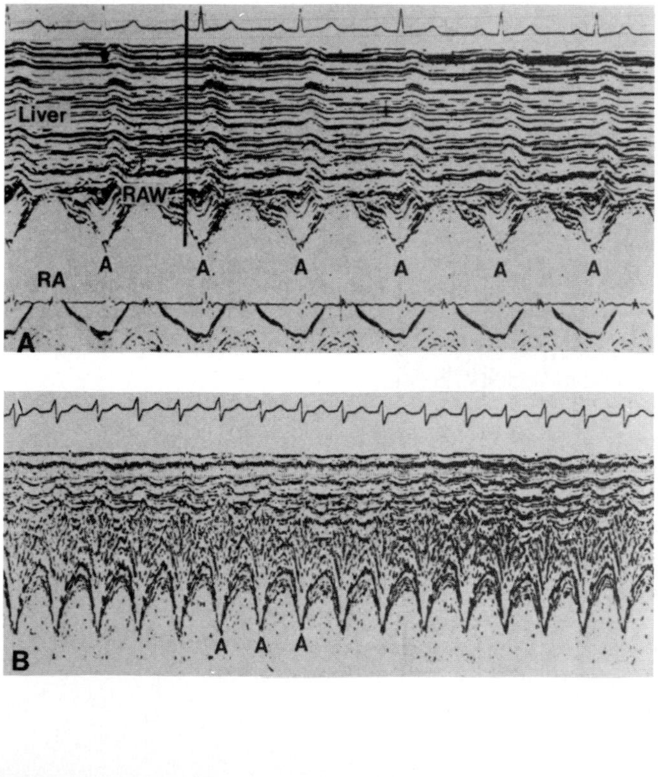

Fig. 40–40. **A.** M-mode of the right atrial wall (RAW) in sinus rhythm. A = atrial contraction; RA = right atrium. **B.** M-mode of the RAW during a supraventricular tachycardia with 1:1 atrioventricular conduction. A = atrial contraction. **C.** M-mode of the RAW during atrial flutter that was not apparent on the surface electrocardiogram. F = flutter waves. (From Drinkovic N: Subcostal M-mode echocardiography of the right atrial wall for differentiation of supraventricular tachyarrhythmias with aberration from ventricular tachycardia. Am Heart J 107:326, 1984.)

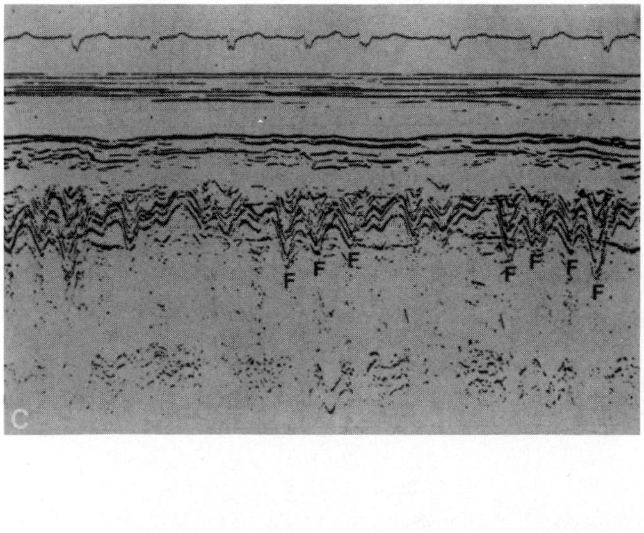

nificant cardiac abnormalities in patients who primarily have alterations in cardiac rhythm or conduction.

In patients with atrial fibrillation, without clinical evidence of any other cardiac abnormality, echocardiography shows an underlying cardiac disorder in approximately 10% of cases.[42,43] In patients with atrial fibrillation and minor or ambiguous symptoms, however, an underlying abnormality may be diagnosed in up to 60% of patients, emphasizing the value of the test.[42] Data concerning the relationship of atrial size and stroke in patients with atrial fibrillation without valvular disease are contradictory; some investigators report an increased risk of stroke in patients with enlarged left atria,[44] and others note no relationship.[45]

Patients with arrhythmias of ventricular origin are likely to have significant underlying cardiac disorders. In one study of over 3000 patients with complex or frequent ventricular premature beats (Lown grade 2 or greater) who were free of apparent heart disease, the left ventricular systolic diameter (which reflects both structure and function) was independently predictive of arrhythmia.[46] A similar relationship between cardiac abnormalities and rhythm disturbance is generally not detected in patients with isolated ventricular ectopic beats.[47] Frequent ventricular extrasystoles of presumed right ventricular origin (left bundle branch block morphology) may be associated with right ventricular dysplasia in children and careful echocardiographic study should be performed to locate an abnormal area in these patients.[48]

Ventricular tachycardias of left ventricular origin are frequently associated with poor left ventricular function, whose presence and origin can usually be well defined by echocardiography. Patients with ventricular tachycardia of a left bundle branch block morphology (suggesting right ventricular origin) and no clinical evidence of right ventricular dysfunction have been found to have right ventricular abnormalities in 30 to 50% of cases. These changes consisted of a quantifiable increase in interstitial fibrosis on biopsy and echocardiographic evidence of increased right ventricular dimensions with or without wall motion abnormalities.[49,50]

Assessing Primary and Secondary Functional Effects of an Arrhythmia

The role of cardiac arrhythmias as a cause, rather than an effect, of structural and functional abnormalities of the heart is beginning to gain recognition. The finding of progressive left atrial dilation in patients with lone atrial fibrillation and initially normal atrial size[7] is a good example of this concept. As more longitudinal echocardiographic studies are performed, the long-term effect of various disorders of rhythm and conduction may be elucidated. In particular, Doppler data may provide important insight into chronic functional changes resulting from these disorders.

Guiding Therapy

The information obtained from echocardiography, used in conjunction with clinical data and the results of other investigations, can guide the management of many patients with disorders of cardiac rhythm and conduction. The two areas of major focus have been the selection of patients with atrial fibrillation in whom cardioversion is most likely to be successful and the determination of pacemaker type and settings that result in optimal hemodynamic performance.

Atrial fibrillation is a common arrhythmia, and cardioversion is often required for patients with a persistence of this rhythm. Unfortunately, the maintenance of sinus rhythm after this procedure is not guaranteed, and atrial fibrillation has been reported to recur in anywhere from 30 to 86% of cases. The most important clinical predictor of response to cardioversion is the duration of atrial fibrillation; patients with the most recent onset are the most likely to remain in sinus rhythm after successful cardioversion.[51,52]

Echocardiography has been suggested as an ideal noninvasive method for determining the relationship of atrial size with maintenance of sinus rhythm after cardioversion. Several studies have suggested that patients with markedly enlarged left atria are less likely to maintain sinus rhythm than are those with normal or modestly enlarged chambers. In these reports, the chamber relevant size has varied widely, ranging from 45 to 60 mm.[53–55] Unfortunately, others have found no relationship between left atrial size and maintenance of sinus rhythm after cardioversion.[51,52] These conflicting results undoubtedly reflect differences in groups of patients and in the duration and causes of the arrhythmia, and they may be affected by the finding that patients with extremely large atria fail to convert to sinus rhythm initially, and hence their ability to maintain sinus rhythm cannot be assessed. It is clear, however, that no absolute value for atrial size uniformly identifies all patients who will revert to fibrillation or remain in sinus rhythm.

Atrial mechanical function is frequently depressed in patients with atrial fibrillation and may not immediately return to normal after successful cardioversion. It has been postulated that the return of normal atrial function after cardioversion can predict the long-term maintenance of sinus rhythm. Initially, A wave size from M-mode recordings of the mitral valve after cardioversion was examined as a marker of sustained sinus rhythm (Figure 40–41), but was found to have no predictive value.[56] Doppler-derived A-wave velocities are a more sensitive measure of the strength of atrial contraction and analysis of mitral A-wave velocity has provided important information on atrial function after cardioversion to sinus rhythm. Doppler studies have shown that, although successful cardioversion results in a return of normal atrial electrical activity, in many cases atrial mechanical activity, as assessed by A-wave velocities, is initially diminished or even absent. The degree and duration of atrial dysfunction after cardioversion has been shown to correlate with the duration of atrial fibrillation before the procedure. Patients with fibrillation of less than a week's duration generally show normal Doppler A-wave velocities, and by inference atrial function, immediately after successful cardioversion. Patients in whom atrial fibrillation is present for more than a week, however, have A waves that are significantly smaller and occasionally completely absent. In the second

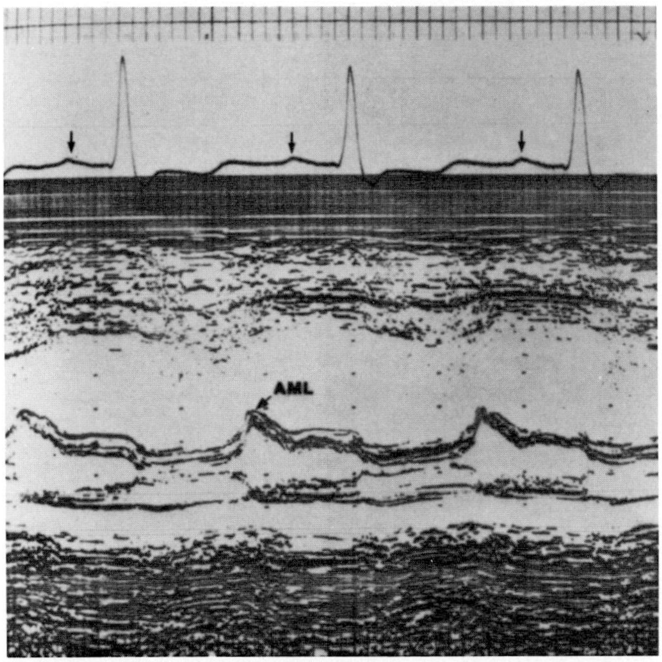

Fig. 40–41. M-mode recording of the mitral valve showing absence of atrial activity (no A wave) following cardioversion for atrial fibrillation. Arrows indicate electrocardiographic evidence of atrial contraction. AML = anterior mitral leaflet. (From Orlando JR, van Herick R, Aronow WS, Olson HG: Haemodynamics and echocardiograms before and after cardioversion of atrial fibrillation to normal sinus rhythm. Chest 76:521, 1979.)

group, the magnitude of the Doppler A wave increases over 24 hours after successful cardioversion and can continue to increase in function for several months while the patient remains in sinus rhythm.[57] The percentage of increase in peak A-wave velocity from 4 to 24 hours after cardioversion has been found to be the best prognostic indicator of maintenance of sinus rhythm 6 months after successful cardioversion.[51]

The second major area in which echo-Doppler studies can be of value in guiding therapy is in the assessment of the pacemaker type and settings required to attain optimal hemodynamic performance for each patient. This application has become increasingly important as the availability, complexity, and cost of newer types of pacemakers have increased. The two pacing techniques that improve hemodynamic performance over and above that seen with ventricular demand pacing are dual-chamber pacing and variable rate pacing.

Dual-chamber pacemakers provide rate responsiveness and AV synchrony. To obtain the optimal hemodynamic improvement from these pacemakers requires appropriate programming of the pacemaker, particularly the AV interval. As previously discussed, patients with AV dissociation or a prolonged AV interval may have a reduced left atrial contribution to ventricular filling. As assessed by Doppler echocardiography, the left ventricular inflow volume has been shown to be greater in AV sequential pacing at an optimal AV interval than in ventricular demand pacing. This is especially true in patients with an increased atrial contribution to left ventricular filling because of left ventricular dysfunction. The optimal AV interval can be determined for each patient by Doppler echocardiography because instantaneous changes in flow velocity are recorded as pacemaker settings are altered.[58]

In patients with sinus node disease or chronic atrial fibrillation, dual-chamber pacing is often an inappropriate mode. In these patients, especially those with reduced ventricular function, variable rate ventricular pacing may be superior to fixed rate demand pacing. Using two-dimensional and Doppler echocardiography to assess ejection fraction and cardiac output before and during exercise, the effect of variable rate pacing of the ventricle, using a movement-sensing pacemaker, has been assessed. Variable rate pacing resulted in a significant increase in duration of exercise and cardiac output compared with fixed rate pacing. Moreover, the benefit was unrelated to the baseline left ventricular function and included those patients with a left ventricular ejection fraction less than 40%.[59]

Two-dimensional echocardiography also provides accurate anatomic images of pacemaker electrode position. Cases have been described of incorrect electrode placement being diagnosed by this method and electrodes can be repositioned prior to firm attachment of the electrode tip.[60,61] In addition, permanent pacemaker positioning may be guided by two-dimensional echocardiography in patients such as women in early pregnancy, in whom standard x-ray screening is contraindicated.[62]

Other applications of echo-Doppler studies in patients with arrhythmias include the assessment of left ventricular function to aid in the choice of antiarrhythmic drugs, detailed analysis of regional left ventricular wall motion to enable identification of the site of pre-excitation in patients with WPW syndrome, which can reduce the time spent in electrophysiologic studies to locate the bypass before performing corrective surgery;[63] and the identification of early contraction sites at the margins of morphologic abnormalities, such as aneurysms and areas of dysplasia, which may predict the location of ectopic sites of activation.

In summary, arrhythmias and conduction disorders may interfere with the standard measurements used to assess valvular and ventricular function by echocardiography. It is important to understand the influence of rhythm on ventricular and valvular action, so abnormal results may be appropriately attributed either to the rhythm disturbance or to dysfunction of the structure in question. As discussed previously, a rapid ventricular rate from supraventricular tachycardia frequently reduces measured left ventricular function. In the majority of such patients, however, left ventricular function itself is normal as measured during a normal rate and rhythm. In such cases, it may be impossible to assess ventricular function during the arrhythmia, and the study should be repeated when the patient's heart rate is controlled.

The Doppler analysis of flow velocity across the cardiac valves is also affected by the heart rate and rhythm, as outlined earlier in this chapter. Therefore, during Doppler assessment of valvular function, it is imperative that these factors be taken into account. As outlined in relevant chapters on valvular function, the measurements of flow velocities and pressure half-times must be averaged over significantly more beats in patients with disorders of rhythm and conduction than in those with normal sinus rhythm. In particular, this situation applies to patients with atrial fibrillation with wide variation in the RR interval. The effect of varying rate and rhythm must also be considered in the evaluation of valvular regurgitation by color flow jets,[64] because a rapid heart rate can result in underestimation in color flow jet areas compared with area seen during a normal heart rate and rhythm (see Chapter 17), whereas irregular rhythms can result in variably sized or intermittent jets.

REFERENCES

1. Oki T, et al.: Pulsed Doppler echocardiographic observation of right and left ventricular inflow velocity patterns in various types of arrhythmia, with special reference to the mechanism of atrioventricular regurgitation. J Cardiography 13:617, 1983.
2. Bredikis Y, Vashkialite IV: Tachycardial disorders of cardiac rhythm as a cause of left ventricular dysfunction. Cor Vasa 31:110, 1989.
3. Fujii J, et al.: Cardiovascular echocardiograms of the left atrial wall, mitral valve, and tricuspid valve in atrial flutter. Sound Bull 5:751, 1975.
4. Sasse L, Frolich CR: Suprasternal notch echocardiography and atrial arrhythmias. Cardiovasc Dis 6:61, 1979.
5. Drinkovic N: Subcostal M-mode echocardiography of the right atrial wall in the diagnosis of cardiac arrhythmias. Am J Cardiol 50:1104, 1982.
6. Iwase M, et al.: Relationship between beat to beat interval and left ventricular function in patients with atrial fibrillation. Int J Card Imaging 3:217, 1988–1989.
7. Sanfilippo AJ, et al.: Atrial enlargement as a consequence of atrial fibrillation: a prospective echocardiographic study. Circulation 82:792, 1990.
8. Fujii J, et al.: Dual echocardiographic determination of atrial contraction sequence in atrial flutter and other related atrial arrhythmias. Circulation 58:314, 1978
9. Nawata T, et al.: Study of atrial contraction in sick sinus syndrome using conventional and esophageal echocardiography. J Cardiogr 13:981, 1983.
10. Zipes DP, DeJoseph RL: Dissimilar atrial rhythms in man and dog. Am J Cardiol 32:618, 1973.
11. Wu D, et al.: Limitation of the surface electrocardiogram in diagnosis of atrial arrhythmias: further observations on dissimilar atrial rhythms. Am J Cardiol 36:91, 1975.
12. Ichiyasu H, et al.: New echocardiographic observations in a patient with dissimilar atrial rhythms. Arch Intern Med 142:2215, 1982.
13. Procacci PM, Levites R, Kotler MN, Anderson GJ: Dissimilar atrial rhythms diagnosed by echocardiography. Chest 73:429, 1978.
14. Mashiro I, et al.: Left and right ventricular dimensions during ventricular fibrillation in the dog. Am J Physiol 235:H231, 1978.
15. Hackl W, Simon P, Mauritz W, Steinbereithner K: Echocardiographic assessment of mitral valve function during mechanical cardiopulmonary resuscitation in pigs. Anesth Analg 70:350, 1990.
16. Cohen A, Gottdeiner J, Wish M, Fletcher R: Limitations of cough in maintaining blood flow during asystole: assessment by two-dimensional and Doppler echocardiography. Am Heart J 118:474, 1989.
17. Burggraf GW, Craige E: The first heart sound in complete heart block. Circulation 50:17, 1974.
18. D'Cruz IA, Prabhu R, Cohen HC, Glick G: Echocardiographic features of second degree atrioventricular block. Chest 72:459, 1977.
19. Panidis IP, et al.: Diastolic mitral regurgitation in patients with atrioventricular conduction abnormalities: a common finding by Doppler echocardiography. J Am Coll Cardiol 7:768, 1986.
20. Schnittger I, Appleton CP, Hatle LK, Popp R: Diastolic mitral and tricuspid regurgitation by Doppler echocardiography in patients with atrioventricular block: new insights into the mechanism of atrioventricular valve closure. J Am Coll Cardiol 11:83, 1988.
21. Rokey R, et al.: Detection of diastolic atrioventricular valvular regurgitation by pulsed Doppler echocardiography and its association with complete heart block. Am J Cardiol 57:692, 1986.
22. Dancy M, Leech G, Leatham A: Significance of complete right bundle-branch block when an isolated finding: an echocardiographic study. Br Heart J 48:217, 1982.
23. Dillon JC, Chang S, Feigenbaum H: Echocardiographic manifestations of left bundle branch block. Circulation 49:876, 1974.
24. Strasberg B, et al.: M-mode echocardiography in left bundle branch block: significance of frontal plane QRS axis. Am Heart J 104:775, 1982.
25. Fujino M, Arakawa K: Echocardiographic assessment of left ventricular function in patients with complete left bundle branch block. Jpn Circ J 48: 119, 1984.
26. Hishida H, et al.: Echocardiographic patterns of ventricular contraction in the Wolff-Parkinson-White Syndrome. Circulation 54:567, 1976.
27. DeMaria AN, Mason DT: Echocardiographic evaluation of disturbances of cardiac rhythm and conduction. Chest 71:439, 1977.
28. Ticzon AR, et al.: Interventricular septal motion during pre-excitation and normal conduction in Wolff-Parkinson-White syndrome: echocardiographic and electrophysiological correlation. Am J Cardiol 37:840, 1976.
29. Francis GS, et al.: An echocardiographic study of interventricular septal motion in the Wolff-Parkinson-White syndrome. Circulation 54:174, 1976.
30. DeMaria AN, Vera Z, Neumann A, Mason DT: Alterations in ventricular activation pattern in the Wolff-Parkinson-White syndrome: detection by echocardiography. Circulation 53:249, 1976.
31. Lebovitz JA, et al.: Relationship between the electrical (electrocardiographic) and mechanical (echocardiographic) events in Wolff-Parkinson-White syndrome. Chest 71:463, 1977.
32. Chandra MS, Kerber RE, Brown DD, Funk DC: Echocardiography in Wolff-Parkinson-White syndrome. Circulation 53:943, 1976.
33. Okomura M, et al.: Echocardiographic evaluation of right ventricular anterior wall motion in the Wolff-Parkinson-White syndrome. Jpn Heart J 20: 577, 1979.
34. Okomura M, Okajima S, Sotobata I: Non-invasive localization of the pre-excitation site in patients with the Wolff-Parkinson-White syndrome: vectorocardiographic and echocardiographic correlations. Jpn Heart J 21:157, 1980.
35. Zoneraich S, Zoneraich O, Rhee JJ: Echocardiographic evaluation of septal motion in patients with artificial pacemakers: vectorocardiographic correlations. Am Heart J 93:596, 1977.
36. Egelblad H, Rasmussen V: Analysis of arrhythmias based on atrial wall motion: usefulness and feasibility of recording left and right atrial systole by echocardiography. Acta Med Scand 219:283, 1986.
37. Drinkovic N: Subcostal M-mode echocardiography of the right atrial wall for differentiation of supraventricular tachyarrhythmias with aberration from ventricular tachycardia. Am Heart J 107:326, 1984.
38. Goldbaum TS, Goldstein SA, Lindsay J Jr: Subcostal M-mode echocardiography of the atrial septum for diagnosis of atrial flutter. Am J Cardiol 54: 1143, 1984.
39. Zoneraich S, Zoneraich O, Rhee JJ: Echocardiographic findings in atrial flutter. Circulation 52:455, 1975.
40. Drinkovic N, Ferek B, Jursic M: Subcostal M-mode echocardiography of the right atrial wall in evaluation of cardiac arrhythmias and pacing. PACE 8:110, 1985.
41. Windle JR, et al.: Determination of the earliest site of ventricular activation in Wolff-Parkinson-White syndrome: application of digital continuous loop two-dimensional echocardiography. J Am Coll Cardiol 7:1286, 1986.
42. Godfredsen J, Egeblad H, Berning J: Echocardiography in lone atrial fibrillation. Acta Med Scand 213:111, 1983.
43. Kupari M, Leinonen H, Koskinen P: Value of routine echocardiography in new-onset atrial fibrillation. Int J Cardiol 16:106, 1987.
44. Caplan LR, et al.: Atrial size, atrial fibrillation, and stroke. Ann Neurol 19: 158, 1986.
45. BATAAF Study Investigators (Boston Area Anticoagulation Trial for Atrial Fibrillation): the effect of low dose warfarin on the risk of strokes in non-rheumatic atrial fibrillation. N Engl J Med 323:1505, 1990.
46. Levy D, et al.: Arrhythmias and conduction disturbances: echocardiographic determined left ventricular structural and functional correlates of complex and frequent ventricular arrhythmias on one-hour ambulatory electrocardiographic monitoring. Am J Cardiol 59:836, 1987.
47. Brodsky M, et al.: Arrhythmias documented by 24 hour continuous electrocardiographic monitoring in 50 male medical students without apparent heart disease. Am J Cardiol 39:390, 1977.
48. Patterson MW, De Souza E: Two-dimensional echocardiographic diagnosis of arrhythmogenic right ventricular dysplasia presenting as frequent ventricular extrasystoles in a child. Pediatr Cardiol 9:41, 1988.
49. Mehta D, et al.: Echocardiographic and histological evaluation of the right ventricle in ventricular tachycardias of left bundle branch block morphology without overt cardiac abnormality. Am J Cardiol 63:939, 1989.
50. Morgera T, et al.: Morphological findings in apparently idiopathic ventricular tachycardia: an echocardiographic, hemodynamic and histologic study. Eur Heart J 6:323, 1985.
51. Dethy M, Chassat C, Roy D, Mercier LA: Doppler echocardiographic predictors of recurrence of atrial fibrillation after cardioversion. Am J Cardiol 62:723, 1988.
52. Dittrich HC, et al.: Echocardiographic and clinical predictors for outcome of elective cardioversion for atrial fibrillation. Am J Cardiol 63:193, 1989.
53. Hoglund C, Rosenhamer G: Echocardiographic left atrial dimension as a predictor of maintaining sinus rhythm after conversion of atrial fibrillation. Acta Med Scand 217:411, 1985.
54. Henry WL, et al.: Relation between echocardiographically determined left atrial size and atrial fibrillation. Circulation 53:273, 1976.
55. Ieri A, et al.: Improvement of the cardiac function after electrical cardioversion of atrial fibrillation: echocardiographic study in patients with and without mitral stenosis. G Ital Cardiol 12:91, 1982.
56. Orlando JR, van Herick R, Aronow WS, Olson HG: Hemodynamics and

echocardiograms before and after cardioversion of atrial fibrillation to normal sinus rhythm. Chest 76:521, 1979.
57. Shapiro EP, et al.: Transient atrial dysfunction after conversion of chronic atrial fibrillation to sinus rhythm. Am J Cardiol 62:1202, 1988.
58. Iwase M, et al.: Evaluation by pulsed Doppler echocardiography of the atrial contribution to left ventricular filling in patients with DDD pacemakers. Am J Cardiol 58:104, 1986.
59. Buckingham TA, et al.: Effect of ventricular function on the exercise hemodynamics of variable rate pacing. J Am Coll Cardiol 11:1269, 1988.
60. Schwartz C, Nicolosi R, Lapinsky R, Grodman R: Use of two-dimensional echocardiography in the detection of an aberrantly placed transvenous pacing catheter. Am J Med 80:133, 1986.
61. Shettigar UR, Lougani RR, Smith CA: Inadvertent permanent ventricular pacing from the coronary vein: an electrocardiographic, roentgenographic, and echocardiographic assessment. Clin Cardiol 12:267, 1989.
62. Gudal M, et al.: Permanent pacemaker implantation in a pregnant woman with the guidance of ECG and two-dimensional echocardiography. PACE 10:543, 1987.
63. Okumura M, Okajima S, Sotobata I: Non-invasive localization of the pre-excitation site in patients with the Wolff-Parkinson-White syndrome: vectorocardiographic and echocardiographic correlations. Jpn Heart J 21: 157, 1980.
64. Wong M, Matsumara M, Suzuki K, Omoto R: Technical and biological sources of variability in the mapping of aortic, mitral and tricuspid color flow jets. Am J Cardiol 60:847, 1987.

CHAPTER

41

TISSUE CHARACTERIZATION

JUSTIN D. PEARLMAN and ARTHUR E. WEYMAN

When you can measure what you are speaking about and express it in numbers, you know something about it: but when you cannot measure it . . . your knowledge is of a meagre and unsatisfactory kind.

Lord Kelvin, lecture to the Institute of Civil Engineers, 1883

Previous chapters have demonstrated the wealth of information echocardiographic imaging and flow determination provide about cardiovascular structure and function. Although the assessment of macroscopic structure and function are enormously valuable, the diagnostic utility of ultrasound would be enhanced if it also included information about the ultrastructural basis of cardiac disease. This area of investigation, conventionally termed *tissue characterization,* seeks to define the nature of a tissue based on the changes that occur in a sound wave during their physical interaction. In the heart, most of the effort toward tissue characterization has centered around the identification and differentiation of normal from ischemic or infarcted myocardium. Whereas ischemia has been the primary area of interest, other cardiac structural abnormalities such as the infiltrative, hypertrophic, and toxic cardiomyopathies, the various forms of myocarditis, and cardiac tumors and thrombi offer fertile ground for similar types of studies.

Detection of changes in the sonographic properties of tissue resulting from changes in ultrastructure could be useful at many levels. Potential applications include: (1) identifying and localizing early changes within a tissue (e.g., ischemia or toxic myopathy) before gross changes in anatomic structure and function occur; (2) discerning the mechanism of an injury (e.g., differentiating among myocarditis, ischemia, and trauma as causes of abnormal segmental wall motion); (3) quantifying the extent of change or involvement (e.g., determining the transmural extent of infarction); and (4) differentiating tissue that is structurally intact but nonfunctioning from necrotic tissue (e.g., separating "stunned" from infarcted myocardium).

Interest in tissue characterization in cardiology has been stimulated by the general clinical experience that acoustically abnormal structures can often be recognized by simple inspection.[1] The intense reflections from calcified valvular tissue and the bright echoes returning from scarred myocardium are two familiar examples.[2,3] This interest has been reinforced by the experience in other areas of ultrasonic investigation where assessment of the intensity and pattern of ultrasonic reflections from organ parenchyma contributes significantly to clinical diagnosis. Unfortunately, the true diagnostic value of such clinical impressions is difficult to assess unless specific acoustic features can be measured and related to some underlying property of tissue. Although many approaches to this problem have been proposed and tested, none has reached the level of routine clinical application. This chapter is included, however, to familiarize the reader with the status of work in this area and to indicate the difficulties and future potential of this line of investigation.

GENERAL METHODS OF WAVEFORM ANALYSIS

Qualitative Assessment of Reflected Signal Amplitude and Distribution

The simplest approach to tissue characterization is based on the *qualitative* visual assessment of reflected signal amplitude and distribution.[4,5] Unfortunately, this method is subject to wide observer variability, and results are poor when data generated from selected groups are applied to more general populations. In addition, qualitative changes in echo amplitude and texture are rarely of clinical significance by themselves, but rely on their association with other findings to suggest the appropriate diagnosis (e.g., increased "speckle" is not typically related to hypertrophic myopathy unless there is associated focal myocardial hypertrophy, and intense echo production is attributed to scar only when the myocardium is also thinned and akinetic). Although inclusion of such findings in the diagnostic algorithm might be considered part of the "art" of echocardiography, it is our opinion that when viewed in isolation, these findings create confusion through inappropriate attribution far more frequently than they provide unique diagnostic information. Further, if such patterns are consistent, they should be quantifiable and show a clear relationship with some tissue property. As a result, only quantitative methods of tissue characterization are presented in the remainder of this chapter, and where appropriate, quantitative data are related to qualitative clinical impression.

Quantitative Analysis of Ultrasonic Waveforms

There are two general approaches to the *quantitative* ultrasonic waveform analysis on which tissue characterization is based. The first approach is *parameter estimation,* in which a specific characteristic of the sound wave such as its velocity, phase, attenuation, or the magnitude to which it is scattered is measured and is related directly to some fundamental tissue property such as fluid content or scatterer spacing. This approach treats tissue characterization as a problem of signal analysis, and relevant literature may be found in physics libraries under the topic of biomechanics.

The second approach is *classification,* which relies on pattern recognition and signal processing techniques similar to those used in voice or fingerprint analysis to define the major spatial and statistical features of individual waveforms and, based on these features, enables one to identify the tissue from which the signals arise.[6–9] This form of analysis treats tissue characterization as a mathematic and statistical problem, so relevant literature is found in mathematics libraries under the topic of classification.

Parametric analysis has the potential advantage of quantifying the extent of a change in tissue ultrastructure; however, definition of these relationships requires careful consideration of the signal paths and tissue/ultrasound interactions discussed later in this chapter. Tissue classification, on the other hand, is more flexible and may take advantage of multiple complex responses without requiring a model to explain them. Thus, tissue classification may be addressed without reference to the physical principles determining the signal responses.

Experimental Models

Two primary experimental models have been used to acquire the data for quantitative analysis: (1) the transmission model, which examines the changes in a sound wave during its passage through a sample of tissue (e.g., myocardium); and (2) the reflection model, in which the total energy content or spectral distribution of energy within the echoes reflected from a tissue sample is analyzed. Figure 41–1 compares the models used in transmission and reflection experiments. In the experimental transmission model (Fig. 41–1A), a matched pair of transmitting and receiving transducers is immersed in a water bath, and a broad-band ultrasonic pulse is initially transmitted between the two to define the free field system response. A sample of unknown tissue is then placed between the two transducers at the focal zone (B), and its effects on the ultrasonic waveform are measured.

In the reflection model (Fig. 41–1C), the same transducer is used as both a transmitter and a receiver. Typically, a pulse is first reflected off a glass or metal plate acting as a "perfect reflector," and the system response of the transceiver is measured. A piece of myocardium

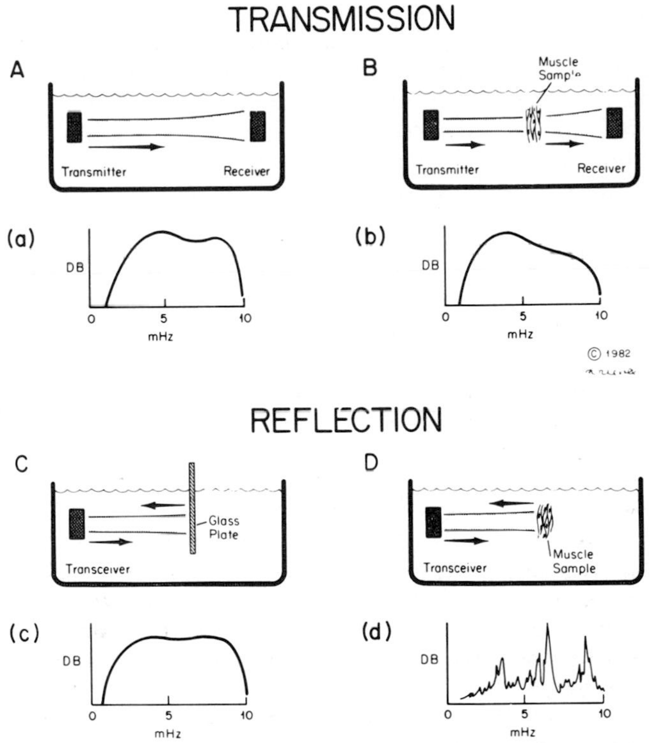

Fig. 41–1. The experimental models used in tissue characterization. **A.** In the transmission model, a transmitting transducer and a receiving transducer are initially immersed in a water bath. A pulse is then transmitted from one to the other to define the system response. **B.** An unknown sample of tissue is than placed between the two transducers. The effects of this tissue sample on the sound wave compared to the free field and system response. **C.** In the reflection model, a single transducer is used as both the transmitter and receiver. The system response (c) in this format is typically defined using a glass plate or some other "perfect reflector." An unknown tissue sample is then insonated using the pulsed echo format, and the reflected or backscattered signal from this sample is plotted as a function of frequency (d) and compared to that of the perfect reflector. (From Franklin TD, et al.: Tissue parameter characterization by ultrasound: state of the art in cardiology. *In* Hanrath P, Bleifeld W, Souquet J (eds.): Cardiovascular Diagnosis by Ultrasound. The Hague, Martinus Nijhoff, 1982.)

is then inserted in place of the plate, and an interrogating pulse is transmitted into the heart muscle. The energy content of the reflected echoes can then be measured absolutely, either as a function of frequency or relative to the signal from the perfect reflector.

TISSUE CHARACTERIZATION BY PARAMETER ESTIMATION

Because the identification of ischemia is of great clinical interest, and its time course and pathophysiologic concomitants have been so well characterized, most cardiac investigators have sought to examine changes in specific properties of the ultrasonic waveform that result from its interaction with ischemic/infarcted myocardium. The major acoustic parameters studied include: (1) acoustic impedance, which is the product of tissue density (ρ) and sound velocity (v); (2) attenuation, which is the loss of energy within the sound wave as it passes through tissue and is the result of absorption, reflection, dispersion, and scattering; and (3) backscatter, which is the amount of energy reflected back along the path of the sound wave and measurable by the transceiver. Scattering, in general, tends to be an omnidirectional phenomenon, with the result that the backscatter measured at the transducer reflects only a small but presumably representative portion of the total scattered energy. Both scatter and attenuation vary with frequency, and their appropriate analysis requires a broad-band transmitted pulse and the analysis of the reflected or transmitted energy as a function of frequency.

Acoustic Impedance and Ultrasonic Reflectance

Acoustic impedance is the product of mass density and sound speed.[10,11] Sound speed is related to tissue elasticity, so impedance is a reflection of tissue density and elasticity. Acoustic impedance is the basis of all clinical ultrasonic studies using the pulsed echo technique, because echo production results from the reflection of sound energy at points of impedance discontinuity.[10,11] When the impedance mismatch is large and the interface at which it occurs is extensive, such as the endocardial/blood interface in vivo or the epicardial/saline solution interface in vitro, large, specular (mirror-like) reflections occur, as discussed in Chapter 1. The proportion of the incident energy reflected is called the reflective index (R), and when the angle of incidence is 90°, this index can be calculated from the densities (ρ) of the two tissues by:

$$R = [(\rho_1 v_1 - \rho_2 v_2)/(\rho_1 v_1 + \rho_2 v_2)]^2 \qquad [41.1]$$

where v is the velocity of sound in each tissue. At smaller points of impedance discontinuity (relative to wavelength), which are present throughout tissue, scattering occurs which is lower in amplitude and more diffusely directed.

The first attempts to characterize myocardial tissue were based on expected difference in acoustic impedance between normal and infarcted myocardium. In these in vitro studies, the acoustic reflectance (i.e., specular reflections from the muscle/saline solution interface) of infarcted myocardium was consistently lower than that of normal heart muscle.[12] Although these findings were presumed to be due to a reduction in tissue density secondary to ischemia, more recent transmission studies suggest that the speed of sound is also significantly reduced in ischemic myocardium when compared to normal.[13]

The marked angular dependence of specular reflections (the amplitude of a specular reflection diminishes rapidly at angles <90° decreasing to $\frac{1}{10}$ at 84° and $\frac{1}{100}$ at 78°[14]) made it apparent at the outset that these reflections would be of limited utility as measures of impedance in the intact beating heart, and there has been little further work in this area. Note, however, that specular reflections cannot be excluded altogether from consideration in tissue analysis. In the simple transmission model described previously, specular reflections occur at both of the saline solution/muscle interfaces, whereas in the reflection model, the sound wave is subjected to specular losses as it enters and exits the surface of the muscle. Clinically, many tissues such as arterial wall contain both scatterers and specular reflectors and hence yield a complex response that contains both angle-dependent and angle-independent components (see later).

Attenuation

The next parameter to be studied was attenuation. Attenuation in homogeneous tissues is caused by absorption and scattering. Absorption is the result of viscous resistance to the high frequency oscillations of the sound wave that causes some of the sound energy to be converted to heat. Scattering results from the impedance discontinuities present in even the most homogeneous tissues. Beam characteristics also can cause attenuation in the far field where the sound beam spreads out conically and the sound intensity (per unit area of the beam cross section) drops proportionately. In nonhomogeneous tissues, specular reflections from tissue interfaces also diminish the amount of emitted sound energy that continues through the tissue along the beam axis.

The relative attenuation of normal and infarcted myocardium in vitro was first compared using the pulsed echo method with a standard reflector placed behind the interrogated tissue. Infarcted myocardium demonstrated greater frequency-dependent attenuation when compared to normal.[15,16] This frequency-dependent attenuation has subsequently been confirmed using a transmission model, and a good correlation ($r = .80$) demonstrated between myocardial necrosis, assessed by creatine kinase depletion, and the slope of attenuation in the chronically infarcted animal model.[17] Figure 41–2 illustrates this frequency-dependent attenuation. In this figure, amplitude is plotted against frequency for a range of 0 to 10 MHz. The upper curve in this plot illustrates the system response, which, for this transducer/receiver pair, is relatively flat over the frequency range of 3 to 9 MHz. The middle curve illustrates the attenuation produced when a sample of normal myocardium is placed in the path of the ultrasonic waveform. Normal muscle produces attenuation of the signal at all

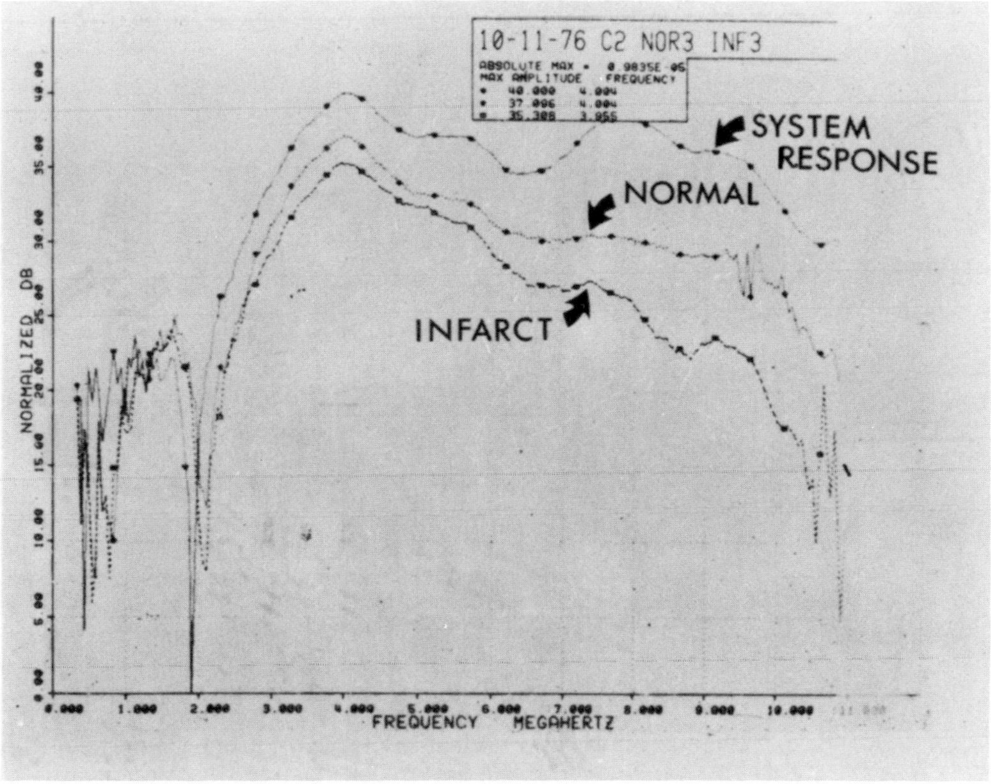

Fig. 41–2. Transmission experiment in which the frequency-dependent attenuation of normal and infarcted myocardium is compared to the free field system response. In the upper plot, the normalized amplitude of the broad band transducer/receiver pair is plotted against frequency. The response from 3 to 9 MHz is relatively flat. The middle curve illustrates the frequency-dependent decrease in signal amplitude (attenuation) that occurs when a sample of normal myocardium is placed between the transducer and receiver. The lower curve illustrates the additional increase in attenuation that occurs when infarcted myocardium is substituted for normal tissue. (From Franklin TD, et al.: Tissue parameter characterization by ultrasound: state of the art in cardiology. *In* Hanrath P, Bleifeld W, Souquet J (eds.): Cardiovascular Diagnosis by Ultrasound. The Hague, Martinus Nijhoff, 1982.)

frequencies, but this is more marked in the higher frequency range. The lower curve is produced by transmission of sound through a sample of infarcted myocardium: overall attenuation is increased relative to normal, but the difference is further exaggerated in the higher frequency ranges. The differences between these pairs of recordings and the measured thickness of the specimen are used to calculate the individual tissue attenuation coefficients (dB/cm) as a function of frequency:

$$A_t(f) = \frac{\ln[V_a(f)] - \ln[V_b(f)]}{T} \qquad [41.2]$$

where V_a is the control voltage and V_b is the attenuated signal, f is frequency, T is the tissue thickness, and ln is the natural logarithm (i.e., to the base: 2.71828 . . .). Absolute attenuation is also affected by energy losses resulting from specular reflections that increase attenuation at all frequencies, as a result absolute values are rarely reported. The slope of a least squares line fit to the attenuation coefficient as a function of frequency is, however, relatively independent of specular losses and has proved to be a useful measure of attenuation* (Fig. 41–3).[18,19]

Studies of the basic interactions of ultrasound with tissue suggest that protein content, particularly collagen, is an important determinant of ultrasonic attenuation in soft tissue.[20,21] Although in normal myocardium, collagen is responsible for no more than 15% of observed attenuation, it appears to be the major determinant of the increased attenuation noted in regions of healed myocardial infarction.[22] A direct relationship between attenuation and increasing collagen accumulation in the period 2 to 6 weeks after acute myocardial infarction has been demonstrated.[22] This relationship persists despite fragmentation of collagen with collagenase,[23] and it suggests that total collagen content (intact plus fragmented), not the structure of the protein, determines attenuation.

In studies of attenuation from the onset of ischemia (i.e., immediately after coronary ligation) to the phase of established infarction and scar formation, two distinct patterns have been observed.[24] In the early phase of evolution from ischemia to infarction (15 minutes to 24 hours), a slight decrease in attenuation is noted, whereas in myocardium subjected to ischemic injury for 3 days or more, attenuation progressively increases[25] (Fig. 41–4). In the early stages of infarction, edema and cellular dissolution appear to decrease tissue density by dilution of protein constituents and therefore reduce attenuation and impedance. During the evolution from necrotic tissue to scar, however, attenuation gradually increases as the tissue collagen content increases, and this is progressive over time up to 11 weeks after infarction.

Effects of Phase Cancellation

In addition to attenuation, early studies have also pointed out the importance of phase cancellation as a

* In in vitro studies, the slope of attenuation shows an inverse, approximately linear, relationship with temperature over the range 20.5 to 37°C, with the value at 37°C being about 20% less than at 20.5°. This slope has been shown to be relatively independent of time for up to 4 hours following excision at 19.5°, but increased by about 20% over the same 4-hour interval at 35°C.[29]

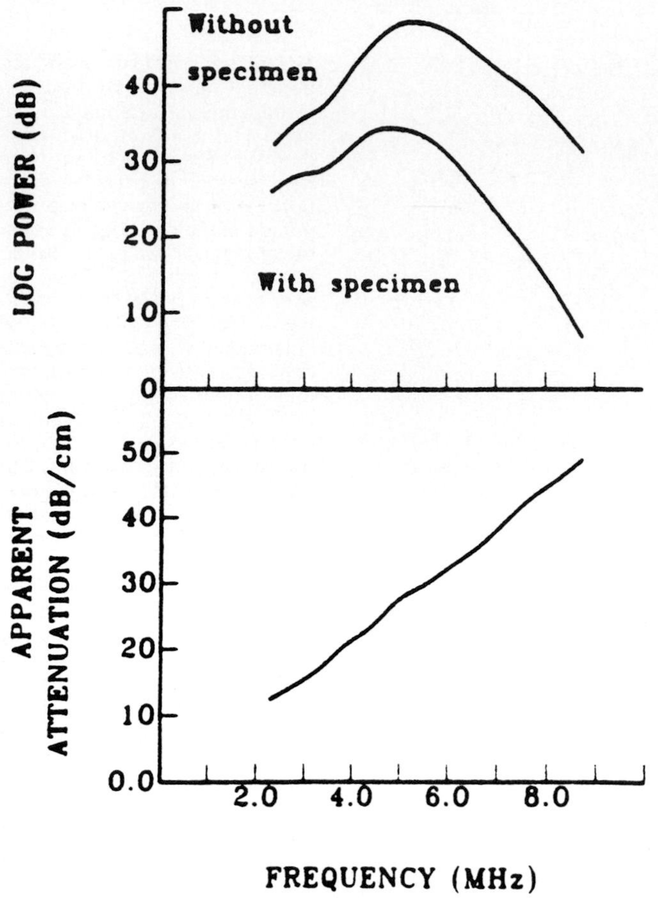

Fig. 41–3. Top. Attenuation vs. frequency with and without a specimen in the sample chamber. Bottom. Attenuation coefficient vs. frequency, calculated from the difference between the two curves at top ($S_n - S_s$) and the specimen thickness, T, by:

$$a = (S_n - S_s)/T \log_{10}:$$

Note from the bottom graph the linear relation between the attenuation coefficient (a) and frequency. (From O'Donnell M, et al.: Ultrasonic Tissue Characterization. National Bureau of Standards Special Publication No. 525, 1979, U.S. Government Printing Office, Washington, D.C.

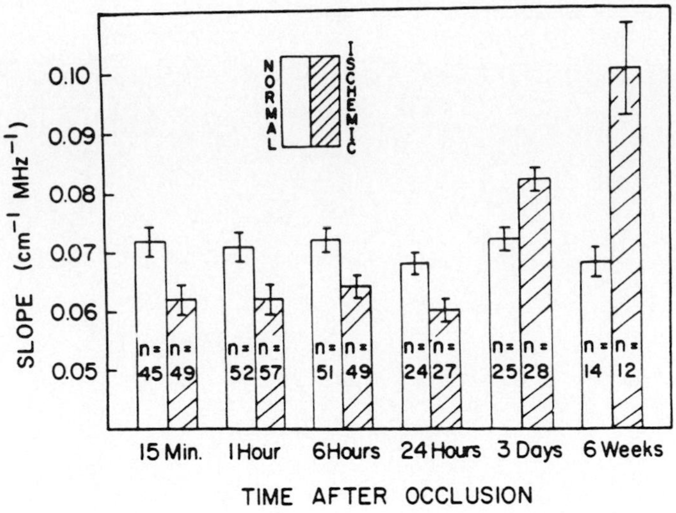

Fig. 41–4. Ultrasonic attenuation relative to time after coronary occlusion for normal and ischemic zones from the same canine hearts for four groups of animals studied in vitro at the intervals indicated. (From Mimbs JW, O'Donnell M, Miller JG, Soble BE: Changes in ultrasonic attenuation indicative of early myocardial ischemia injury. Am J Physiol 236:340, 1979.)

potential cause of signal loss, which must be considered in all tissue characterization studies.[26–28] Phase cancellation (see Chapter 2) occurs when inhomogeneities in tissue distort the ultrasonic wavefront presented to a spatially extended piezoelectric receiving transducer. These wavefront distortions may result from transmission of ultrasound through tissue with variations in surface characteristics, internal structural characteristics, or both. When the wavefronts incident on a piezoelectric receiver are distorted, the generated electrical signal is degraded because of the receiver's phase-sensitive nature. Phase cancellation effects can be reduced or eliminated by using (1) a small receiving transducer,[18] (2) identically focused transmitting and receiving transducers aligned to sample at the common focal point,[22] or (3) an acoustoelectric receiver.[30] Acoustoelectric receivers (i.e., cadmium sulfide) are sensitive to energy rather than pressure and thus are not affected by distortions in phase. Figure 41–5 compares attenuation with frequency plots for four adjacent portions of canine left ventricle in vitro using three different 1.3-cm diameter receivers.[31] Figure 40–5A illustrates the nonlinearity of attenuation with respect to frequency recorded using a planar piezoelectric receiver. The variation in response is due to distortions in the wavefront that cause phase cancellation at the transducer surface and variation in received intensities. Figure 41–5B illustrates the response obtained using a focused piezoelectric receiver. In this case, the response is more uniform, and the linearity and slope of attenuation are more consistent than observed with the nonfocused transducer. Figure 41–5C shows the response from a single crystal cadmium sulfide acoustoelectric receiver. Because this receiver is phase insensitive, it is not disturbed by phase cancellation, and the slopes of attenuation from each site are virtually superimposable. Unfortunately, phase-insensitive (acoustoelectric) transducers, while alleviating the problem of phase cancellation, lack sensitivity in comparison with conventional phase-sensitive (piezoelectric) transducers.[32]

Backscatter

Because transmission techniques are not readily adaptable to in vivo studies of the heart, quantitative approaches for characterizing the echoes arising from within the myocardium have been developed. These can be divided into techniques that analyze backscattered intensity as a function of frequency *(frequency domain analysis)* and those that analyze backscattered echo amplitude directly from the radiofrequency (RF) or video signal and hence operate in the time domain *(time domain analysis)*. Frequency domain analyses include integrated backscatter and frequency-dependent backscatter, whereas time domain analyses report mean and other statistical measures of backscatter amplitude within a region of interest.

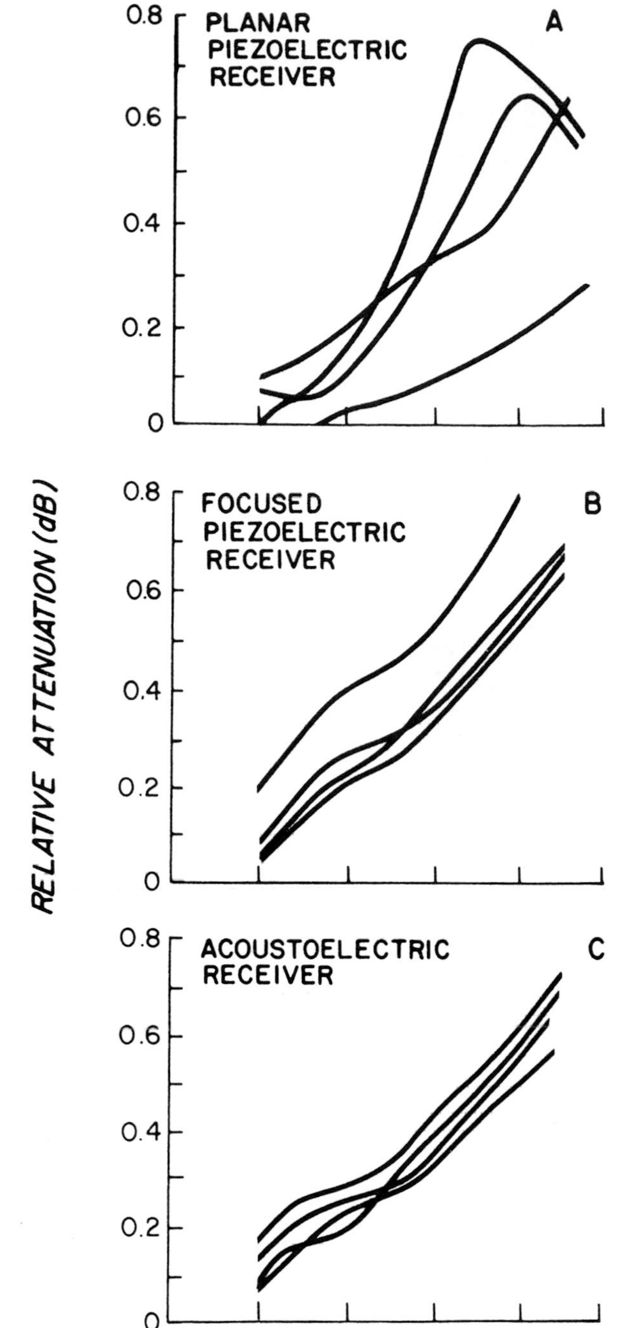

Fig. 41–5. Comparison with the relative phase sensitivity of a nonfocused piezoelectric and focused piezoelectric and acoustoelectric transducer. **A.** A standard planar piezoelectric receiver fails to exhibit the expected linear relation between attenuation and frequency of insonation. The nonlinearities are explained by interference of phase cancellation, which depends on the insonating frequency and its relation to the path length. **C.** A cadmium sulfide crystal, which is phase-insensitive, maintains the expected linear response to change of frequency. **B.** A focused piezoelectric receiver avoids phase cancellations, so the linearity of response vs. frequency is close to that of the phase-insensitive receiver. (From O'Donnell M, et al.: Ultrasonic Tissue Characterization. National Bureau of Standards Special Publication No. 525, 1979, U.S. Government Printing Office, Washington, DC.

Frequency Domain Analysis

Backscatter is generally measured as the reflected ultrasound power at each frequency over the bandwidth of the transducer. Backscatter, like attenuation, characteristically increases with frequency. A function that describes the efficiency with which ultrasound is backscattered at each frequency is called the *backscatter transfer function*.[33,34] The backscatter transfer function is typically determined by comparing the backscattered spectrum from a tissue volume to a reference spectrum from a "perfect" reflector, usually a metal or glass plate recorded at successive 5-dB decrements in input power (Fig. 41–6). The scattering volume from which the backscatter data are derived is typically selected by time or range gating the reflected signal to localize sampling to the myocardium and specifically excludes the specular reflections from the epicardial and endocardial interfaces. Consistency in the size of the scattering volume is sought by locating the volume of myocardium to be interrogated within the focal zone of the transducer. In experimental studies, the beam is aligned to maintain the highest amplitude specular reflection from the anterior surface of the myocardium and thereby "normalizes"

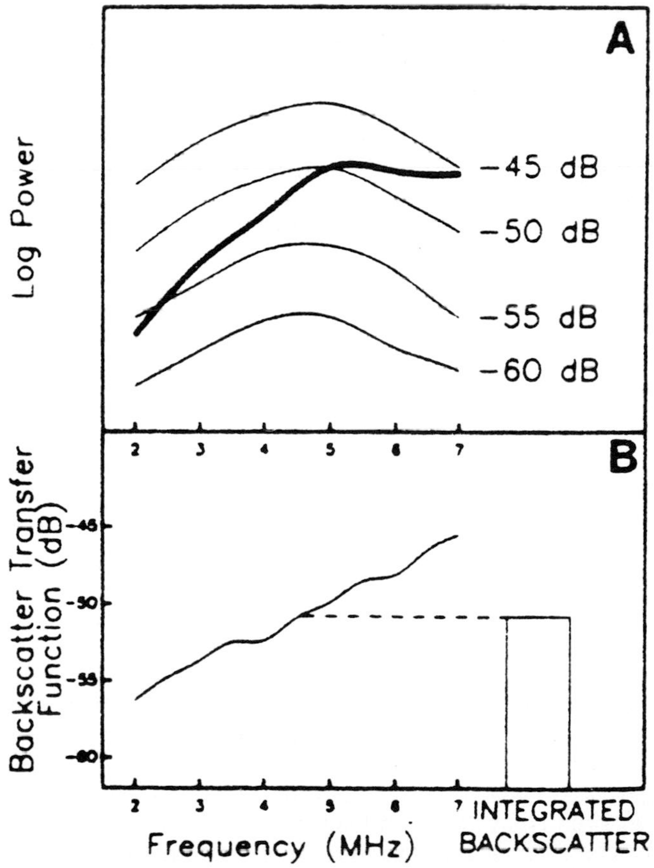

Fig. 41–6. Backscatter transfer function and integrated backscatter obtained by interpolating the received power spectrum (bold curve) backscattered from myocardium with respect to reference spectra from a stainless steel plate measured at 5-dB intervals. (From Miller JG, et al.: Myocardial tissue characterization: An approach based on quantitative backscatter and attenuation. Proc. IEEE Ultrasonics Symp. New York, Institute of Electrical and Electronic Engineers, 83:782, 1983.)

for reflective losses that attenuate the backscatter signal amplitude.

The spectrum reflected by any tissue volume is also affected by the attenuation of the pulse as it passes to and from the volume of interest and by frequency-related differences in the size of the sample volume for the same aperture size and degree of focusing. Thus, the higher frequency components of the pulse (1) are relatively weaker when they arrive at the volume of interest because of frequency-dependent attenuation and (2) encompass a smaller volume for the same aperture and degree of focusing because higher frequencies tend to remain better columnated, have a longer near field, show less dispersion in the far field, and can be brought to a sharper focus at a greater depth. To correct for these effects, the *backscatter coefficient,* which provides an absolute measure of the scattering properties of a volume of tissue, may be calculated by multiplying the backscatter transfer function by an attenuation factor and a measure of the inverse solid angle subtended by the scattering volume as a function of frequency[35–37] (Fig. 41–7).

Integrated Backscatter. Integrated backscatter, or the frequency average of the backscatter transfer function, can be calculated from the same data, as

$$\text{Integrated Backscatter} = \frac{B(f)df}{f\,df} \qquad [41.3]$$

where B is equal to the backscatter amplitude at each frequency (f). When integrated backscatter is averaged over one or more cardiac cycles, it is referred to as the *time averaged integrated backscatter.*[38]

Cyclic Variation. Cardiac contraction has long been known to change the volume and orientation of the muscle fibers within the sampled volume and hence to alter the characteristics of the reflected signal. As a result, most early in vivo studies either gated the samples,[39] so they were obtained at a consistent point in the cardiac cycle, or averaged the backscatter over one or more cycles (time averaged integrated backscatter). More recently, the variation in backscatter during the cardiac cycle has been directly examined to characterize its pattern and relationship with cardiac function.[40] Frequency domain measurement of cycle-related changes in integrated backscatter requires that the raw echo data be sampled at points in the cardiac cycle defined by a series of time gates, and data from similar windows can be subjected to Fourier analysis (Fig. 41–8). Importantly, measurement of cyclic variation in integrated backscatter does not require absolute calibration of the analysis system, and hence this parameter may be ideally suited for assessing tissue changes with conventional or adapted commercial instruments.

Phase Analysis of Time Variation. The phase or timing of variation in integrated back scatter can also be determined relative to a reference period usually taken to be the cardiac cycle. The cyclic variation in backscatter can then be phase weighted to express both the change in amplitude at the nadir and the shift of this point within the cardiac cycle. Another, simpler method for expressing the cycle-related time of minimum integrated backscatter is to relate the nadir of the integrated backscatter curve to the duration of systole as defined by the electrocardiographic QT interval*.[40]

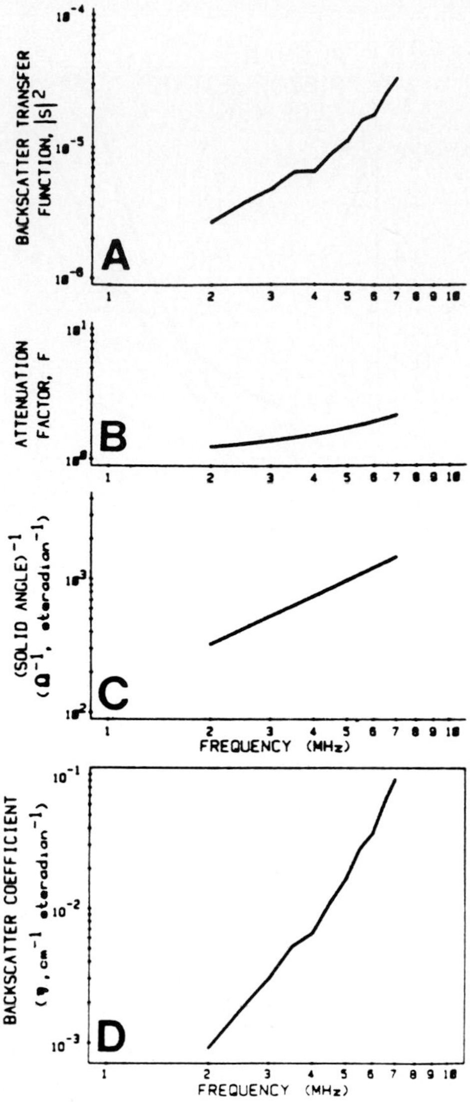

Fig. 41–7. **A.** The backscatter transfer function. **B.** The attenuation factor. **C.** The scattering volume. **D.** Backscatter coefficient from normal dog myocardium in vivo derived from the product of **A, B,** and **C.** (From Miller JG, et al.: Myocardial tissue characterization: An approach based on quantitative backscatter and attenuation. Proc. IEEE Ultrasonics Symp. New York, Institute of Electrical and Electronic Engineers, 83:782, 1983.)

Backscatter as a Function of Frequency. Integration of backscatter over the bandwidth of the transducer reduces fluctuations in resultant amplitude that arise from phase cancellations at the transducer or within tissue. Unfortunately, it also removes frequency-related maxima in the backscattered signal that might contain useful information about coherent internal scattering within the tissue of interest. An alternative approach to the analysis of backscatter seeks to capitalize on organizational patterns of normal and pathologic tissue at the micro-

* The delay ratio (Q-nadir of the backscatter curve/QT interval) for normal myocardium approximates unity). (From Miller JG, et al.: Myocardial tissue characterization: An approach based on quantitative backscatter and attenuation. Proc. IEEE Ultrasonics Symp. New York, Institute of Electrical and Electronic Engineers, 83:782, 1983.[31]

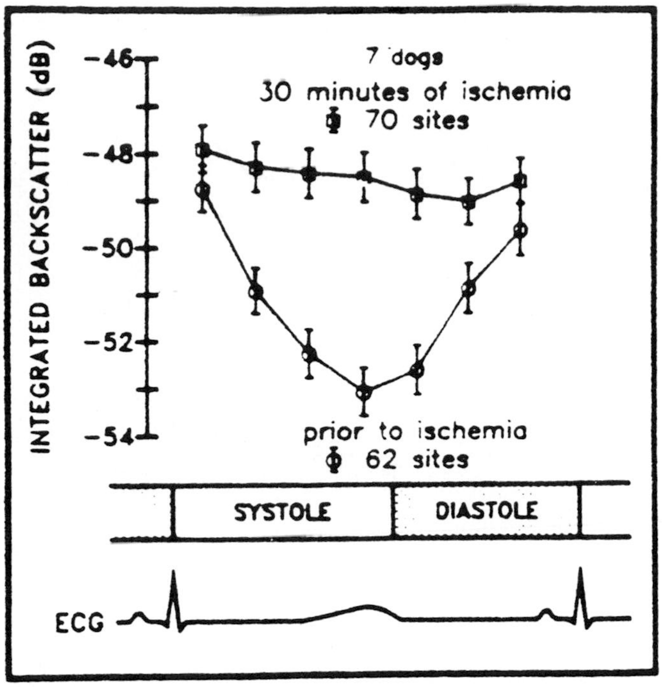

Fig. 41–8. Comparison of the normal cyclic variation in integrated backscatter to the increase in mean backscatter level and blunting of cyclic variation that occurs following 30 minutes of ischemia in a canine model. (From Miller JG, et al.: Myocardial tissue characterization: An approach based on quantitative backscatter and attenuation. Proc. IEEE Ultrasonics Symp. New York, Institute of Electrical and Electronic Engineers, 83:782, 1983.)

scopic level. These organizational patterns are assumed to result in a characteristic and relatively consistent spacing of acoustically different targets within the tissue, which, when struck by an acoustic wave, behave as a series of diffuse scatterers because of their small size relative to the ultrasonic wavelengths. The small, regularly spaced scatterers can then be predicted to produce interference patterns that depend specifically on the physical parameters (such as the spacings) of the array. These interference patterns use wavelengths within the frequency spectrum of the beam that are similar to the scatterer spacing to be selectively reinforced, whereas others are subject to phase cancellation. Ultrasound then may be used to determine the acoustical structure of tissue based on the selective reinforcement of certain frequencies when the Bragg scattering condition is satisfied:

$$n\lambda = 2d \sin \theta \qquad [41.4]$$

where λ is ultrasonic wavelength, n is number of wavelengths, d is distance between scatters, and θ is angle from the horizontal to the scattered signal. Integer multiples of the wavelength are required for constructive interference to occur.

Thus, either fixing the frequency (λ) and varying the angle or fixing the angle and sweeping the frequency will result in a succession of signal amplitude peaks whose spacing is indicative of the target's internal structure. For a perfect lattice, the scattered signal exhibits a periodic series of maxima as either the incident angle or the frequency is changed, with each maxima corresponding to a path length difference of an integer number of wavelengths.[15] The Fourier transform of this signal yields a single peak whose location is a measure of reflector spacing and whose amplitude is a measure of the scatter number n.

Instead of sweeping the frequency, a broad band ultrasonic pulse may be used to derive the frequency information over the bandwidth of the transducer. Expressing the Bragg equation in terms of frequency yields the relationship

$$f_n = nc/(2d \sin \theta) \qquad [41.5]$$

where c is the velocity of sound.

For a fixed angle and internal scatterer spacing (fixed d), "f_n" denotes the frequencies at which the signal achieves peaks resulting from constructive interference.

Figure 41–9 is an example that illustrates the variability of the frequency peaks arising from the subendocar-

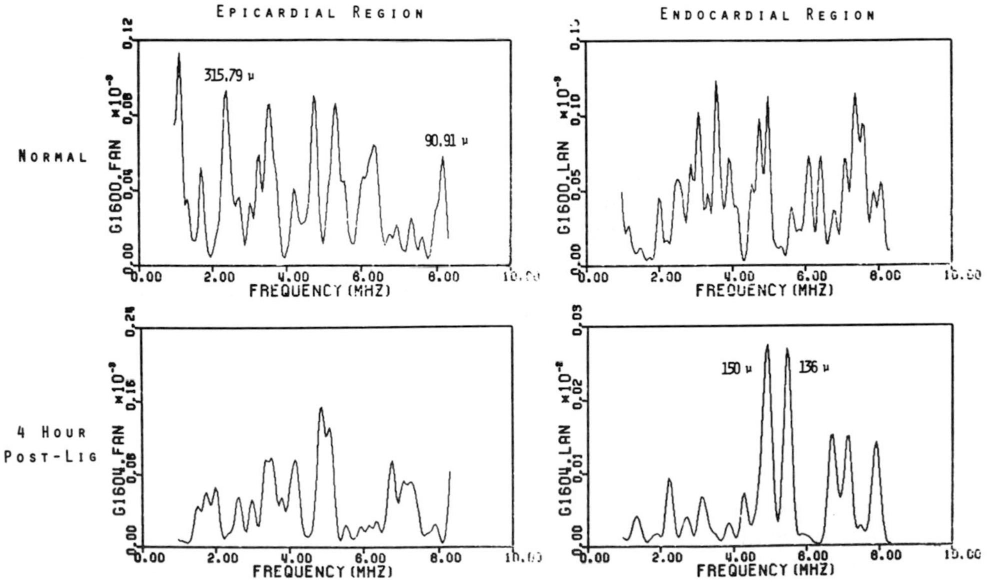

Fig. 41–9. Backscatter signal amplitude from myocardium vs. insonation frequency from the epicardial (left) and endocardial (right) regions of the myocardium before (upper panels) and 4 hours after coronary ligation (lower panels). Modeling this behavior as a function of wavelength suggests that the ischemic myocardium has a scatterer spacing of 150 to 180 μ. (From Franklin TD, et al.: Tissue parameter characterization by ultrasound: state of the art in cardiology. *In* Hanrath P, Bleifield W, Souquet J (eds.): Cardiovascular Diagnosis by Ultrasound. The Hague, Martinus Nijhoff, 1982.)

dium and subepicardium before and 4 hours after coronary artery ligation. These plots demonstrate how peaks occurring at specific frequencies can be related to internal organ structure. In this example, the frequency peaks recorded at 4 hours after coronary ligation from the subendocardium correspond to wavelengths in the range of 150 to 180 (μ). At the microscopic level, these distances correspond to the repetitive internal spacings between muscle bundles within ischemic tissue.[39]

In biologic tissues, change in acoustic impedance are expected to occur randomly. In any particular tissue, however, substructural spacings may vary widely but still fall within limits that can be statistically specified by the scattering profile shape. For instance, cardiac muscle fiber bundles tend to be regular in diameter despite the lack of one predominant orientation or direction. In disease processes where the structure is altered, the statistical values of d obtained from the scattering profile should be altered correspondingly. Thus, even an imperfect lattice may still yield distinct peaks (albeit broader and diminished in amplitude relative to those from a perfect lattice) at frequencies corresponding to the general structural pattern, whereas the amplitude at other frequencies will be increased by the wavelets reflected by random scatterers that do not cancel completely. This is the type of scattering expected from structures such as highly organized tissues and organs where the structural order is marked by small perturbations and where statistical fluctuation of interscatterer distance occurs around a certain mean value.

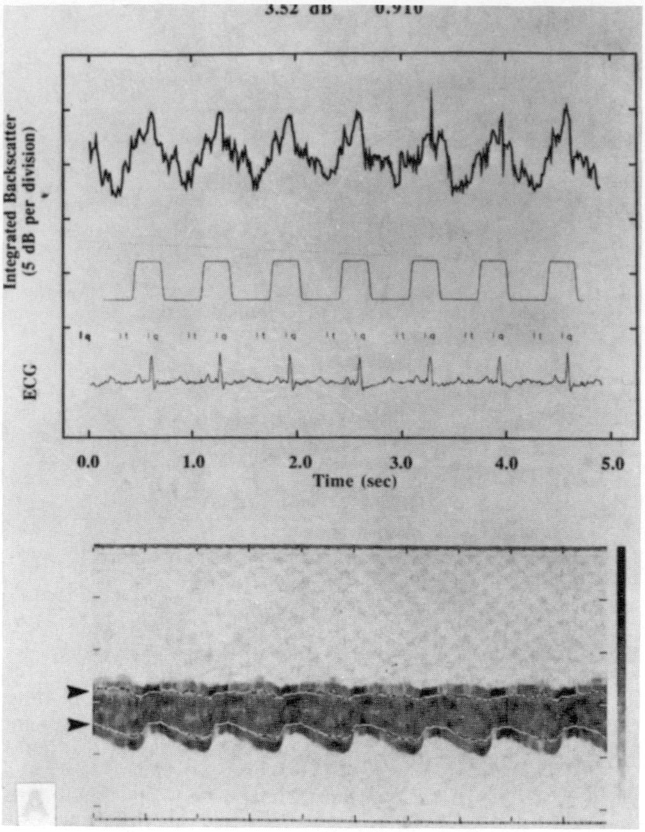

Fig. 41–10. Gray scale integrated backscatter M-mode image of normal cyclic variation of integrated backscatter. Top. The raw curve of cyclic variation of integrated backscatter. Bottom. The curve produced by a model function and the electrocardiogram (ECG). The boundaries of the region of analysis in the M-mode image are indicated by the dotted lines within the myocardial walls (arrows). (From Milunski MR, et al.: Early identification with ultrasonic integrated backscatter of viable but stunned myocardium in dogs. 1989. Journal of the American College of Cardiology 14: 462, 1989. Reprinted with permission from the American College of Cardiology.)

Time Domain Analysis

Radio Frequency (RF) Signals. Time domain analysis of reflected ultrasonic data is based on echo amplitude rather than frequency content and therefore does not require Fourier transformation of the received signals. Time domain amplitude analysis can be applied to the output of commercial echographs and is potentially available in real time. Such analyses can be approached in several ways. For off-line measurement, the gated and amplified RF signal from a piezoelectric transducer is digitized, squared, and integrated to determine the mean backscattered energy over the bandwidth of the transducer. This mean value is the same as the mean power computed from the power spectrum in the frequency domain. For real-time analysis, the RF data can be directly fed to an acoustoelectric energy detector that produces a peak output voltage proportional to the average energy contained in the signal over the bandwidth of the transducer. In the latter case, the resulting data can be output continuously to determine the cyclic variation in "integrated backscatter" or integrated over time to produce a time-averaged integrated backscatter (Fig. 41-10). In such analyses, the output values are compared to the backscatter from a "standard reflector" to correct for variation in the performance of the pulser, transducer, or receiver. Note that although the "backscatter" may be integrated over time, the frequency information is limited to the mean power over the bandwidth of the transducer.[41,42]

Analysis from Video Images. Backscatter has also been reported as the average intensity over an area of interest from digitized two-dimensional echo video images. Such analyses are based on the video envelope of the time domain RF signal. The output values are typically expressed as the mean gray level of the digitized area of the video image. For example, if the image is digitized at a resolution of 8 bits, there will be 256 shades of gray ranging from black (typically assigned a value of zero) to white (typically assigned the maximum value of 255) for each pixel, with the mean gray level equal to the sum of the values for each pixel divided by the total number of pixels in the sample. The gray values are typically preprocessed for visual appeal and are not calibrated. Some autoscaling and quantitation of the distribution of echo amplitudes within a region of interest are also possible; however, this type of analysis relies on nonparametric or statistical methods and therefore is discussed in the next section of this chapter.[43,44]

Color Encoding RF or Video Data. The final approach to time domain divides the amplitude of the RF or video signal into levels and assigns each level a color hue. Amplitude gradients within each range can be represented by varying the saturation or value (intensity) of the color. Such methods of analysis appear to provide little information beyond that contained in the gray scale display and are primarily used to highlight local amplitude differences.[45–48]

Clinical and Experimental Data

Normal Myocardium. Normal myocardium shows no significant regional or transmural variation in time-averaged integrated backscatter.[49–51] Cyclic variation in backscatter is normally recorded at all levels of the heart, with backscatter highest at end-diastole and lowest at end-systole. The reported normal cyclic variation in integrated backscatter has ranged from roughly 4.0 to 7.0 dB.[52–56] The amplitude of change in cyclic integrated backscatter is greatest at the apex and decreases at the mid ventricle and base.[50,57] Amplitude modulation is also reported to be greatest for the subendocardium (4.3 $\pm$ 0.6 dB) and decreases at the midwall (2.8 $\pm$ 0.5 dB) and subepicardium (2.9 $\pm$ 0.8 dB), reflecting contraction differences across the wall. Normal cyclic variation correlates with myocardial segment shortening and muscle thickening. Investigators have postulated that cyclic amplitude variation in integrated backscatter power results from changing acoustic impedance caused by variation in tissue elastic modulus during sarcomere shortening. This hypothesis predicts a decrease in backscatter power during systole as sarcomere shortening and series elastic stretch occur and the elastic modulus increases.[52] The nadir of the cyclic backscatter curve normally occurs at about 87% of the duration of systole as measured relative to the QT interval or roughly 120° before the nadir of the left ventricular pressure curve. The transmural gradient in amplitude modulation is abolished during ischemia and in the early stages of reperfusion. Although backscatter power decreases during systole for physiologic contraction, it increases during passive distension (dyskinesis). Note that these studies generally use a fixed sample volume. Hence as the myocardium contracts, the amount of muscle within the sample volume becomes a smaller percentage of wall thickness, and this phenomenon may account for some of the cycle-related variation in backscatter.

Data concerning the relative magnitude of integrated backscatter from the right and left ventricles have varied. In one study, integrated backscatter from the right ventricle was reported to be higher (-60.4 ± 1.6 dB) than that from the left ventricle (-66.9 ± 1.0 dB), and right ventricular collagen content was also increased.[58] No direct correlation between backscatter and hydroxyproline content was noted, however. This finding is consistent with other data suggesting that, in normal myocardium, tissue properties other than collagen content are the major determinants of ultrasonic backscatter[59] and attenuation.[22] In another study, where right and left ventricular integrated backscatter were rigorously measured, backscatter from both ventricles was similar. Amplitude modulation in the mid right ventricular anterior wall was also similar to that in the mid wall of the left ventricle, and both demonstrated significant transmural variation, with amplitude modulation in the subendocardium exceeding that in the mid wall and subepicardium.[49]

Ischemia/Infarction

Acute Ischemia. Numerous authors using a variety of approaches have reported an increase in backscatter amplitude or echo "brightness" from the zone of ischemia/infarction after coronary occlusion.[2,13,22,31,43,48,49,54,60,61] The reported increase in integrated backscatter has ranged from roughly 5 to 8 dB. This increase has been noted as early as 10 minutes[64] after coronary ligation and continues to increase over the first several hours after occlusion (Fig. 41–11).

When specific regions of the ischemic myocardium are analyzed, a small but consistent and significant increase in time-averaged integrated backscatter is observed in all layers.[49,62] This effect is independent of the simple diminution in blood flow, but instead appears to be related to structural concomitants of the ischemic injury. Increased myocardial water content has also been shown to increase backscatter.[60] Measurements of wet/dry weight ratios of myocardium suggest that the increased integrated backscatter seen in acute ischemia is secondary to myocardial edema,[60] and altered myocardial ultrastructure also plays a role.

Chronic Infarction. As the infarct matures, integrated backscatter increases[25] and is linearly related to myocardial collagen content estimated by hydroxyproline assay (r = .78).[35,59] However, quantitative histologic analysis reveals a variable relationship between the transmural distribution of collagen and the corresponding transmural pattern of the backscatter signal.[59]

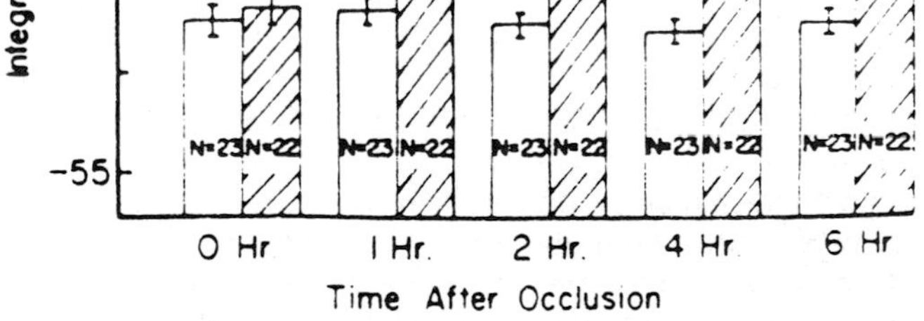

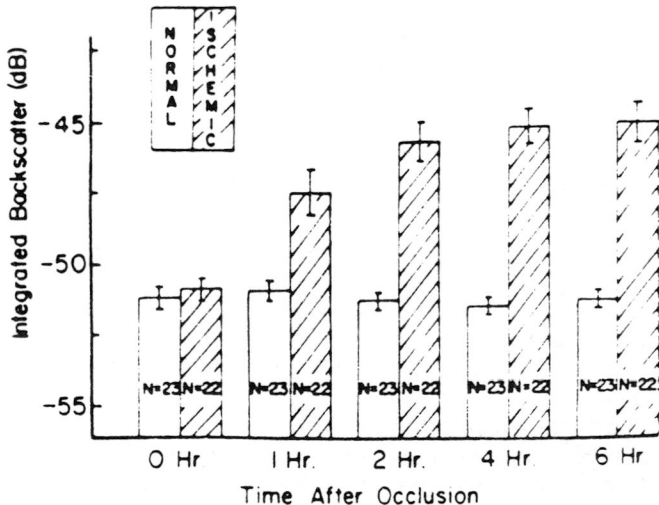

Fig. 41–11. Average integrated backscatter in 22 regions of ischemic canine myocardium (cross-hatched bars) and 23 normal regions (open bars) from seven hearts at several intervals of the occlusion. (From O'Donnell M, Bruwens D, Mimbs JW, Miller JG: Broadband integrated backscatter: an approach to spatially localized tissue characterization in vivo. Proc IEEE Ultrasound Symposium 79:175, 1979.)

Hydrolysis of intact collagen in regions of infarction and fibrosis by perfusion with clostridial collagenase type III decreased backscatter by a factor of 2. As previously noted, attenuation and hydroxyproline content are unaffected by hydrolysis of collagen. These data suggest that, although attenuation is sensitive to both intact and partially digested collagen, backscatter measurements report only the intact protein.[23]

Because scattering is one of the causes of attenuation, the increase in backscattered energy in chronic infarction is consistent with the increased attenuation noted in transmission studies. The reported increase in backscatter in the initial phases of ischemia when attenuation is decreasing is more difficult to reconcile. It may indicate that the edema thought to reduce the magnitude of attenuation by dilution of protein constituents may do so in a way that leaves tissue ultrastructure, and hence scattering, intact.

Blunting of cycle-dependent amplitude modulation occurs immediately after occlusion in all layers of myocardium.[49,63] Although the absolute changes in cycle-dependent amplitude modulation for the subendocardium, mid wall, and subepicardium were different, the percentage of decrease during ischemia was comparable. Values for phase delay relative to the QT interval in remote infarction increase to roughly 1.5.[42] When dyskinesis is present, backscatter power decreases as ischemic myocardium thins (i.e., sarcomeres are passively stretched).[56]

Reperfusion. Data concerning the effects of reperfusion on integrated backscatter and associated cyclic variation are less consistent and appear to vary with the duration of occlusion, the density of ischemia (i.e., the percentage of total wall thickness involved), and the sensitivity of the measurement technique. After a 15-minute occlusion, the backscatter ratio (the ratio of the amplitude of the myocardial signal to that from the posterior epicardial interface) returned to normal within 30 minutes in one study.[64] For the same occlusion period, time-averaged integrated backscatter began to decrease toward preischemic levels by 15 minutes and returned to normal after 2 hours of reperfusion.[49] When varying occlusion periods were studied, time-averaged backscatter increased by 5 dB during occlusion, and the early recovery after 5, 20, or 60 minutes of occlusion was 44%, 61%, or 89%, respectively, with late recovery approaching 100% in all cases.

Experimental studies have shown that the magnitude of cyclic variation of integrated backscatter bears a complex, nonlinear relation to wall thickening, and the recovery of endocardial motion lags behind the recovery of cyclic variation. After occlusion maintained for only 5 minutes followed by reperfusion, recovery of cyclic variation was rapid and complete.[41,54] However, a 15-minute occlusion caused a significant decrease in amplitude modulation that returned to control values only after 120 minutes of reperfusion. Occlusion for 20 minutes followed by reperfusion results in delayed but nearly complete recovery of cyclic variation, whereas occlusion for 60 minutes results in delayed and incomplete recovery (about 50% of baseline) at 3 hours.

Although early studies suggested that changes in cyclic variation parallel changes in recovery of function, more recent data suggest possible discordance in cyclic integrated backscatter and transmural wall function.[41,65] Because cycle-related variations should bear some relation to contraction, it has been hypothesized that this discordance is related to recovery of epicardial contraction before recovery of endocardial contraction, which is reflected by changes in integrated backscatter but not by recovery of wall thickening.

Cardiac Transplantation. Noninvasive diagnosis of early cardiac transplant rejection is an important clinical goal and one of the more promising potential applications of ultrasonic tissue characterization. Immediately after cardiac transplantation, control values for all backscatter parameters can be obtained, and the changes in these parameters associated with rejection can be anticipated because the alterations in tissue ultrastructure associated with transplant rejection are well recognized. In studies of early rejection after heterotopic cardiac transplantation, mean spatial gray levels measured from serial digitized two-dimensional images increased significantly during the first 3 days after cardiac transplantation, consistent with increased backscatter during early rejection. Histologically, the increased backscatter intensity was associated with myocardial edema, vascular engorgement, and cellular infiltration. Gray levels decreased from day 3 to 7 days in association with extensive cellular infiltration and myocytolysis, but without substantial edema.[66]

Cardiomyopathy. Primary disorders of cardiac muscle may be caused by inflammation or toxins, may occur as a familial disorder, or may arise spontaneously without recognized cause. Doxorubicin (Adriamycin), one of the most effective antineoplastic agents, is associated with a dose-related cardiomyopathy that limits its use. Doxorubicin-induced cardiomyopathy is noninflammatory and is characterized by cell death and replacement with fibrous tissue. Significant increases in backscatter from rabbit hearts subjected to cardiotoxic doses of doxorubicin have been reported in association with an increase in tissue collagen content.[67] Similarly, longitudinal studies in the cardiomyopathic Syrian hampster model in which calcium accumulation and fibrosis were compared to tissue acoustic properties revealed elevated values of both integrated backscatter and slope of attenuation when compared to age-matched control subjects.[68]

Atherosclerosis. Ultrasonic characterization of alterations in vascular tissue resulting from the accumulation of calcium, lipids, or fibrous connective tissue might make it possible to monitor the development of atherosclerotic lesions longitudinally in specific vessels. The 10-MHz backscatter from excised human arterial wall shows differences between normal and fibrofatty lesions compared to fibrous and calcified lesions.[69] Differences between normal vs. fatty and fibrous vs. fibrofatty lesions were not significant, however. In contrast to backscatter from myocardium, which is relatively independent of angle, that from arterial walls appears to be more specular. Thus, integrated backscatter fell off sharply as a function of angle for normal, fibrofatty, fibrous, and calcific lesions, but was relatively constant for fatty lesions. When data were pooled, a change of as little as a few degrees in the angle of incidence could completely blunt differences recorded at normal incidence. When data were corrected for the rate of fall off with angle, differentiation between fatty and normal and between fibrofatty and fibrous walls was also possible.[69]

Considerations in Assessing Data Based on Quantitative Analysis of Backscattered Signals

Quantitative measurements of backscatter are influenced by a variety of physical variables: (1) transducer power output; (2) transducer frequency and bandwidth; (3) attenuation between the transducer and target of interest; (4) signal threshold; (5) preprocessing digital signal level; (6) phase cancellation within the sample volume and at the transducer; and (7) tissue anisotropy, sample volume size, and the effects of fixation.

Transducer Power Output. Transducer power output has a direct effect on the amplitude of any reflected signal. In experimental studies, the system is calibrated at different transmit power levels and the backscatter transfer function is determined by comparing the received power spectrum to the power spectrum returned from a perfect reflector at known decrements in output power. In clinical studies, control of output power can be attempted by holding instrument settings constant or by scaling the strength of the reflections to those from a tissue phantom. The former approach is only valid if all of the components of the system remain unchanged. Different transducers, for example, may yield different output powers for the same input voltage. In one study, simply changing transducers of similar center frequency (12-MHz) resulted in up to a 300% difference in mean gray level.[63] Phantoms provide a reasonable method of calibration for relatively simple parameters such as mean gray level. The more complex the signal analysis, however, the more difficult it is to calibrate the backscatter from a tissue phantom. Differences in clinical instruments also can have a major effect on image data.

Transducer Frequency and Bandwidth. Transducer frequency and bandwidth both affect the amplitude of a backscattered signal. Because backscatter is frequency dependent, transducers with low center frequencies (i.e., 2.25 MHz) and narrow bandwidths (such as those used with clinical instruments) do not return the same scattered energy as higher frequency, broad-band transducers for the same input power. Although the term *integrated backscatter* is used in both cases, it obviously has a different meaning depending on the center frequency and bandwidth of the transducer. Reports of "integrated backscatter" calculated in the time domain correctly identify mean power over the transducer bandwidth, but may be misleading when compared to broad-band frequency analysis. Furthermore, the equivalence of mean power calculation for "integrated backscatter" computed from time domain vs. frequency domain analysis is restricted to a squared modeling formulation.

Attenuation. All absolute backscatter measurements must be corrected for any attenuation between the transducer and the sample volume of interest. User-adjusted depth compensation for attenuation (TGC) improves clinical image appearance but presents a nonstandard compensation. As a consequence, the image intensities for a given tissue type may vary significantly from image to image, case to case, user to user, and machine to machine. Maintenance of a constant TGC slope does not overcome this problem because attenuation varies from subject to subject, and hence a constant correction is inappropriate. Attempts to correct objectively for attenuation have included correction based on attenuation measurements of excised chest wall specimens,[70] correction for the amplitude of the backscattered signal along each line of sight,[71] correction based on the shift in mean frequency as a measure of cumulative frequency-dependent attenuation with distance, and minimizing the relationship of echo envelope peaks to associated variance. Unfortunately, none of these approaches have found widespread application.

Attenuation resulting from specular losses must also be considered. In experimental studies, the beam is directed such that the reflection from the anterior myocardial surface is optimized, and this orientation is held constant throughout the experiment. In clinical studies, such optimization is difficult because many interfaces encountered along the beam path lie at different angles relative to the direction of propagation of the beam. When two-dimensional images are recorded, the situation is even more complicated because each of the beam paths lateral to the central ray will intersect the endocardium at a different angle, so specular losses will vary within the same field of view. Thus, when studies of tissue properties are taken from the laboratory to the clinical environment, the problems increase many fold.

Although mathematic models to account for factors such as attenuation, diffraction, and reflection might be developed for individual cases, the degree of intersubject variability makes a general solution that would report precise absolute measures for backscatter probably intractable.

Another, potentially more clinically useful approach is to use relative values (i.e., cyclic variation in backscatter or changes in backscatter relative to control values). Thus, many investigators have used dominant specular reflectors such as the posterior wall endocardium or vascular walls as references to which backscatter from adjacent tissue can be related. Unfortunately, differences in the reflective properties of the specular and scattered echoes limits the success of such normalization.

Signal Threshold. The signal threshold in all echocardiographic instruments is controlled by a built-in reject function designed to eliminate electronic noise. In Doppler studies, variation in signal threshold can influence both the mean and peak frequency and hence the velocity estimate. In tissue characterization studies, a high signal threshold can alter the mean signal amplitude and the spatial distribution of low amplitude echoes (i.e., tissue texture).

Preprocessing Digital Signal Levels. Preprocessing of signals in commercial instruments also alters the amplitude assignment of individual signals and may cause the video output of the scan converter to differ markedly from the echo amplitudes contained in the raw RF signal. As a result, analysis of processed data without some correction for changes in the signal introduced in the processing path may yield spurious results. Measurements from video images also suffer from significant degradation because the video signal typically has a bandwidth of roughly 30 dB, whereas the RF signal has a bandwidth of 80 dB or more. In addition, the signals are generally interpolated in the digital scan converter before output in the video format. Thus, although analyses based on video data have the major advantage of being readily available, their significant theoretic limitations must not be ignored.

Phase Cancellation Within the Tissue Sample Volume and at the Transducer Backscatter is a phase-sensitive phenomenon and is affected both by phase cancellation at the transducer and random impedance discontinuities in tissue. Random regions of signal maxima and nulling in tissue vary depending on transducer bandwidth, and hence the same tissue may yield different amplitude responses to different interrogation frequencies. In most situations (i.e., electrical noise), the random signals cancel over time. In tissue this does not occur, however, and the same tissue yields the same response to comparable interrogating pulses, although it is possible to remove the random effects of phase cancellation within tissue by spatial averaging. Spatial averaging can be achieved either by increasing the sample volume length or by sampling from adjacent laterally displaced sites. Such averaging should emphasize amplitude peaks in the power spectrum resulting from coherent scatterer spacings and should suppress spurious peaks resulting from random associations. This occurs, however, at a loss of spatial resolution.[35] Correction for phase cancellation at the transducer has been previously discussed.

Tissue Anisotropy, Sample Volume Size, and the Effects of Fixation. Certain tissues exhibit structural anisotropy that affects their characteristic absorptive and scattering properties. Skeletal muscle, for example, displays frequency-dependent behavior when the ultrasonic beam impinges on the sample parallel to the orientation of the fibers different from that recorded when the beam is directed perpendicular to the fiber orientation. Structural anisotropy and dependence of scattering characteristics on fiber orientation have not been reported for cardiac muscle[16]

Integrated backscatter amplitude is a function of sample volume size or gate length as in Doppler flow sensing. Therefore, some correction for gate length (sample volume size) is often introduced.[58] In the analysis of the mean backscatter or gray levels from an extended spatial region of interest, the term integrated backscatter takes on yet another meaning because these data are spatially integrated rather than frequency integrated.

Because many of the studies cited in this chapter are based on fixed tissue specimens, the effects of fixation must also be considered. The velocity of sound in myocardium fixed with 10% formalin is faster than that recorded in freshly excised myocardium; however, myocardial integrated backscatter (2.25 MHz) was not significantly changed by formalin fixation.[58]

Ultrasonic Computed Tomography

Applying the same principles used in x-ray computed tomography (CT), it is possible to construct ultrasonic tomographic transmission or reflection images of velocity, attenuation, or backscatter. In experimental in vitro studies, these images are assembled by rotating a transmitting and receiving transducer pair around a sample and recording sequential angular views or by rotating a sample between two fixed transducers. Quantitative images have been obtained using acoustoelectric receivers that eliminate phase-cancellation errors, with reconstruction based on the frequency derivative (slope) of the attenuation coefficient to minimize reflective losses and to reduce refraction errors.[72] Reconstructive tomography is also affected by the anisotropy in the attenuation exhibited by many soft tissues.[35] Mathematic models have been developed that describe propagation of ultrasound through tissue in terms of refraction, deflection, and phase interference or diffraction*.[75] Once the relationship between external observations and internal properties of a tissue can be expressed mathematically, then computation of the inverse problem can produce CT images based on ultrasound instead of x-ray.[14]

Examples of backscatter, attenuation, and sound speed images of the ex vivo heart are shown in Figure 41–12.[13] Extension of this work to reflection studies of the beating heart is difficult, but it is theoretically possible. The increasingly widespread use of transesophageal echocardiography and the demonstration that transmission images can be reconstructed from a limited number of samples suggests a potential clinical application for this type of study.

Summary of Parametric Data

Investigators have convincingly demonstrated that alterations in the ultrastructure of cardiac tissue such as edema formation and collagen accumulation produce consistent and reproducible changes in tissue acoustic properties such as attenuation and backscatter. Unfortunately, these alterations in acoustic properties cannot be reported in absolute terms, nor have they been uniquely related to any specific abnormality. Integrated backscatter, for example, increases as a result of both edema and collagen accumulation, and similar changes are seen in transplant rejection, cardiomyopathy, and ischemia. The most clinically promising studies are based on serial changes in the same subject after some recognized insult or changes in the cyclic variation in backscatter amplitude. The former application, however, requires a priori

* These models offer a means of approaching the inverse problem of producing a three-dimensional map of intrinsic tissue properties based on observed refraction and diffraction patterns. An exact model yields viscoelastic wave equations that are too complicated for current methods of inverse solution. After some simplification (shear, mode conversion, and flow are ignored, yielding a Helmholtz inhomogeneous equation with constant coefficients), an exact solution of the inverse problem has been derived.[73,74] The validity of using simplified wave equations is supported by simulation and experimental studies.[76] An alternate approach to the inverse problem of forming an image of intrinsic tissue properties from external observations relates refractive index to scattered waves by Fourier analysis, providing a graphic description of scattering.[14]

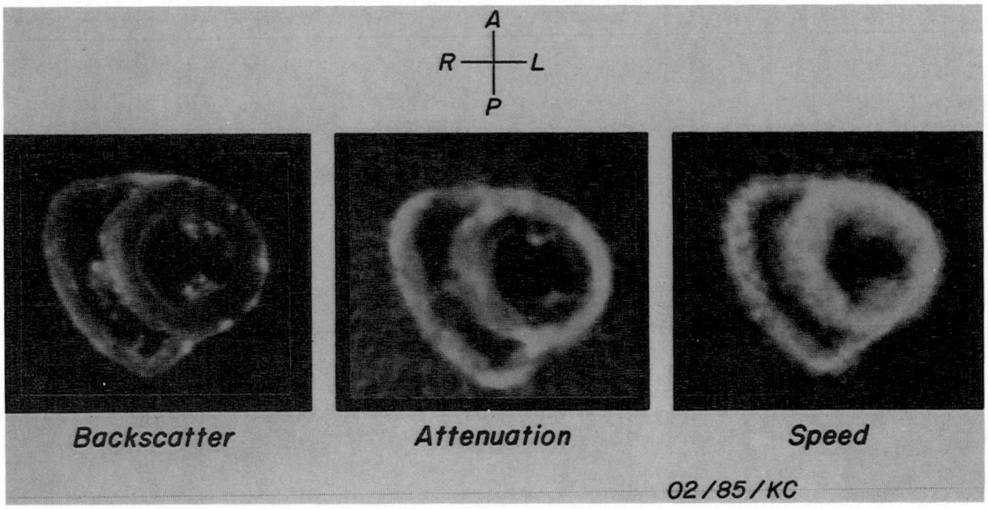

Fig. 41–12. Parametric images of the heart based on transmitted ultrasound. The images shown were obtained from ex vivo ultrasound transmission studies by computing an intrinsic tissue parameter vs. tomographic location. Left. Gray scale representation of localized backscatter. Middle. Map of attenuation to form an image of the heart. Right. Sound speed as a function of tissue location in the image plane represented as image brightness. (From Chandrasekaran MK, et al.: Echocardiographic visualization of acute myocardial ischemia: in vitro study. Ultrasound in Med. and Biol. 12:785, 1986.)

knowledge of the type of injury and the expected ultrastructural changes that occur over time for appropriate interpretation. Cyclic variation in backscatter amplitude provides little information not present in more basic measures such as endocardial excursion and wall thickening, although dissociation of backscatter variation from transmural function may provide unique insight into intramyocardial contraction. Thus, although much basic work has been done, clinical applicability remains to be demonstrated.

TISSUE CLASSIFICATION

The general topic of classification refers to a mathematic approach to organizing data into classes or types. Pattern recognition and cluster analysis are two methods of classification. Pattern recognition seeks, through examination of a set of observations, to determine the class to which each observation belongs. Studies relevant to pattern recognition include information theory, mathematic statistics, and biometrics. Closely related is cluster analysis, which examines a population of data to determine how it may be organized or subdivided into separate classes or subtypes. Thus, pattern recognition begins with prior knowledge of the possible types or classes and seeks to match each new case to one of the known types, whereas cluster analysis seeks to define types or classes based on examination of many observations.

Pattern Recognition

Pattern recognition requires objective rules for deciding which of several predefined groups (tissue types, disease states) best fits a new set of observations. The appropriate rules (known collectively as the *decision function*) are selected by examining how well they perform on training data. The rules are adjusted to achieve best performance (accurate classification). Typically, a new training set of observations is used to assess the performance of the proposed rules for classification. Depending on performance, the decision function may be validated and subsequently applied, or the process may be repeated iteratively, exploring different approaches until optimal classification is achieved.

Tissue characterization based on pattern recognition can proceed as follows: (1) selection of measurement parameters (observation); (2) acquisition of test data (preliminary acquisition); (3) simplification of the observations (data condensation and reduction); (4) examination of data and application of decision functions (training); (5) repetition of steps 1 to 4 until classification is optimal (reiteration); and (6) confirmation that classification remains good with new data (validation).

Observations

Echocardiographic observation parameters are the different types of information that may be acquired using ultrasound. The primary data for echocardiographic tissue classification are the spatial distribution of echo amplitudes, along individual lines of sight (RF data) or within regions in two-dimensional echo images (video data). The use of RF data appears preferable because it provides the widest dynamic range and is not altered by the internal processing and interpolation algorithms present in clinical instruments. Unfortunately, most echocardiographic instruments do not allow direct access to the ultrasound signal in its RF form, and when available, the analysis of RF signals requires that a large amount of digital data be acquired, stored, and processed. Therefore, despite the recognized limitations, many investigators have sought to correlate the patterns in ultrasonic video images with ultrastructural changes in myocardial tissue.

From these primary data, one selects observation parameters presumed to be useful in distinguishing different tissue types. The value for each observation parameter forms a coordinate of an observation vector. For example, mean signal intensity in a defined region could serve as an observed parameter, a second coordinate could report the variance in the intensity of internal reflections within a region of tissue, and attenuation, backscatter, and sound speed might contribute to three separate coordinates of an observation vector serving to characterize ischemic myocardium. Many choices for the component observations are possible. The number of component observations determines the dimensionality of the observation space. Once variables are selected and observations are collected, the results may be used to generate a multidimensional graph, a scatterplot in observation space. This may be visualized like stars in the sky. All points that relate to one tissue type may be displayed connected by line segments, and the points that belong to different groups then form separate constellations. As the number of dimensions increases, this becomes difficult to present, but for illustration, it suffices to visualize the three-dimensional case (Fig. 41–13). Each point represents a different result of observation, and the coordinates of that point represent the components of the vector that comprises the observation. If the different constellations form distinct patterns, then pattern recognition may be used to classify the points correctly.

In general, the choice of observation parameters is crucial to the success of pattern recognition—the observation parameters selected must be sensitive to the differences to be recognized. General classes of observations on echocardiographic data include: (1) classic statistics; (2) texture and tone; (3) histogram analysis, and (4) contiguity.

Statistical Observations. Although the spatial distribution of echoes in B-mode scans has been a major subject for tissue characterization, the random nature of these echoes is well recognized to result from coherent interference of the many wavelets reflected by scatterers located within the resolution cell. Because coherent interference diminishes the independence of echoes from individual scatterers, statistical analysis not only is necessary to associate tissue parameters with certain experimental data, but also is helpful in increasing computational efficiency by using only those components of the signal that are independent.[77] For example, the distinguishing factor between normal and contused myocardium may not be the intensity of echoes, but rather the local variation of intensity.[44]

Both mean and variance represent *statistical moments*. The mean reports the central value, whereas variance reports spread about that value. There are higher statistical moments as well, assessing the deviation about the prior central moment (Fig. 41–14). *Skewness* (third moment) measures deviation of variance, *kurtosis* (fourth moment) measures deviation of skewness, and so on.[78] The series of moments may be used to form an observation vector for pattern recognition.[79] In one study using a clinical instrument (2.25-MHz nominal center frequency), the first three statistical moments of the digitized RF signal were analyzed in an attempt to separate patients with hypertrophic myopathy, remote myocardial infarction, and cardiac amyloidosis from control subjects. Over the modest bandwidth of this instrument, it was not possible to differentiate normal from diseased myocardium.[80] Other investigators,[78] however, have reported that kurtosis alone may distinguish normal from ischemic myocardium.

Texture and Tone. Two observation variables commonly used to construct an observation vector are texture and tone. *Tone* represents the mean intensity from a region, whereas *texture* represents the patterns of variation within the region.[81] To exemplify the importance of texture vs. tone, consider a chessboard with alternating intensities of 0 (black) and 1 (white) compared to a gray slab the same size (8 × 8) with uniform intensity of ½ (Fig. 41–15).Over the 64 squares of the board, the average intensity is ½ in both cases; that number represents the tone for the regions, which is the dominant observation at low resolution. Thus, the gray slab and the chessboard are indistinguishable on the basis of

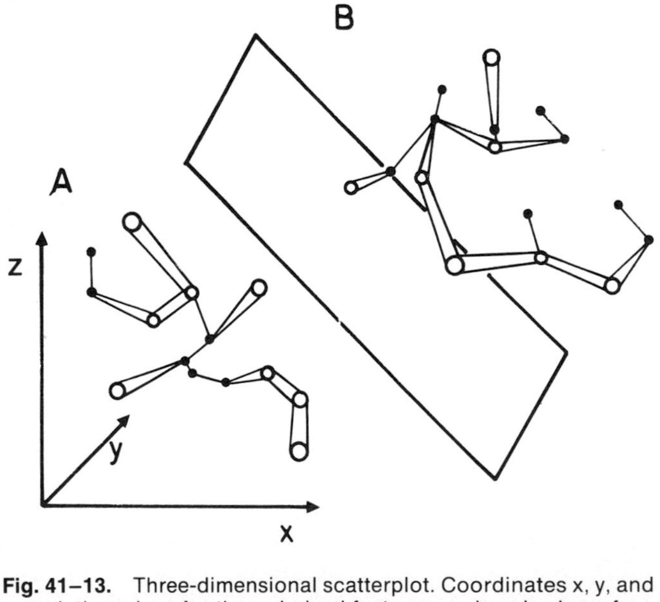

Fig. 41–13. Three-dimensional scatterplot. Coordinates x, y, and z mark the values for three derived features such as body surface area, integrated backscatter, and attenuation coefficient. Individual observations are plotted in this three-dimensional space and those from a particular class, such as ischemic myocardium are connected. **A.** The connected observations form a constellation disjoint from observations on another class, e.g., normal myocardium. **B.** Discriminant analysis seeks to identify a plane that separates these clusters.

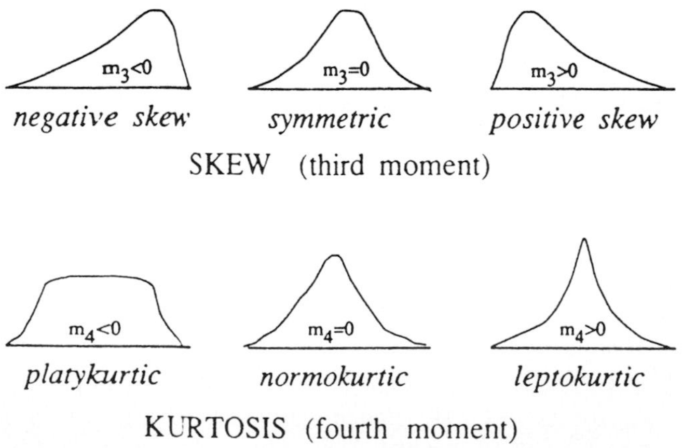

Fig. 41–14. Distributional moments describe the shape of a distribution or other curve f(x) in terms of a series of values computed by integrating or summing $x^n f(x)/n$. For n = 1, this yields the mean value, and for n = 2 with x centered at zero (subtracting the mean), this yields the variance of x. Higher moments include skew (top), which measures the degree of asymmetry or, in this example, leftward dominance, and kurtosis (bottom) measures peakedness.

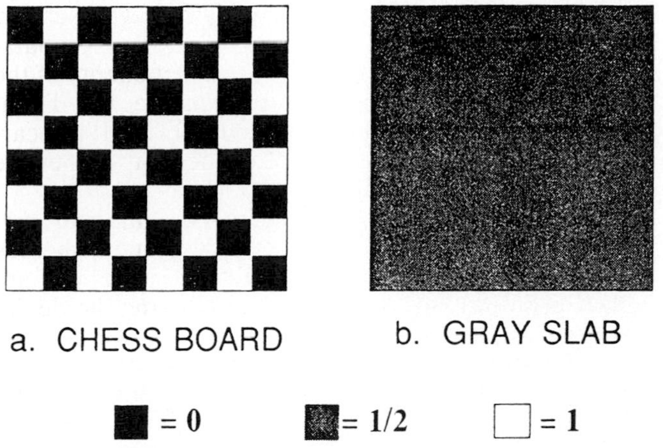

Fig. 41–15. The difference between texture and tone. **a.** white (1) and black (0) alternating squares. **b.** Uniform gray (½). At low resolution, only the overall tone or mean intensity is observed, which is the same for both (½). The distinction between **a** and **b** is in the texture or pattern of distribution of values within the respective regions.

tone (mean intensity). To distinguish between these two image patterns, it is necessary to make use of other information reflecting the difference in intensity distribution within the regions. The local distribution pattern defines the texture. One measure of the local intensity distribution is local variance, which reports the mean squared difference of neighboring points from their mean. Calculation of mean local variance (using 2 × 2 neighborhoods with edge wraparound to provide upper and left neighbors for each of 64 squares) produces a single number for each image that distinguishes all 3 example image patterns:

$$\text{gray slab: } 64\,[4(\tfrac{1}{2}-\tfrac{1}{2})^2/4]/64 = 0 \qquad [41.6]$$

$$\text{chessboard: } 64\,[4(\pm\tfrac{1}{2})^2/4]/64 = \tfrac{1}{4} \qquad [41.7]$$

$$\text{half-black image*: } (8[4(\pm\tfrac{1}{2})^2/4] + 24\,[4(0-0)^2/4] + 8[4(\pm\tfrac{1}{2})^2/4] + 24[4(1-1)^2/4])/64 = \tfrac{1}{16} \qquad [41.8]$$

Note that it was necessary to calculate the mean of 64 local (2 × 2) variance measurements to distinguish the foregoing on the basis of texture. The variance over the whole region in the latter 2 cases is $64(\pm\frac{1}{2})^2/64 = \frac{1}{4}$, which does not reflect their textural difference.

Texture measurement from echocardiographic images has been reported successful in identifying experimental myocardial contusion,[44] as well as acute ischemia.[63,82]

Histogram Analysis. A graph of a number of pixels of a given intensity or brightness is called an intensity histogram. An intensity histogram is basically a bar graph where the range of intensities is displayed on the abscissa and the ordinate values list the numbers of occurrences. The histogram of the gray slab has 64 entries at intensity ½ and 0 elsewhere, whereas the histogram of the chessboard is bimodal with 32 at 0, 32 at 1, and 0 elsewhere (Fig. 41–16). The chessboard may be identified by the computer as distinct from the gray slab by examining histograms of their images.[83] Based on histogram alone, however, it is not possible to distinguish a half-black image from the image of a chessboard because both have 32 values of 0 and 32 values of 1. Thus, although histograms tally intensities, they ignore their spatial relations.

Contiguity. Other commonly used observation variables measure the heterogeneity vs. contiguity of values. For example, gray level run lengths could be used to distinguish the gray slab from the chessboard of identical tone.[84] A gray level run consists of a count of consecutive picture elements (pixels) that agree within a chosen range (bin size) in intensity. Thus, if 0, ½, and 1 are selected as midpoints of separate bins, then the gray slab has a horizontal (and vertical) run length of 8 for the upper left pixel, whereas the corresponding pixel on the chessboard has a run length of only 1 before one encounters a pixel that maps to a different intensity bin. Run lengths may be computed for each pixel in a region, and various summary measures such as statistical moments for the run lengths may be reported as observations on texture.

Preliminary Acquisition

After selecting appropriate observation parameters, data should be collected on a training set of samples, preferably of known character. If the tissue types of the training sample are known before examination of the observations, the process of developing the pattern recognition decision function may be described as *supervised learning*. As evident from reading the section on cluster analysis, it is possible (although generally less desirable) too proceed with training even without the desired a priori information about tissue types *(unsupervised learning)*.[85–89] If a study of amyloid vs. normal

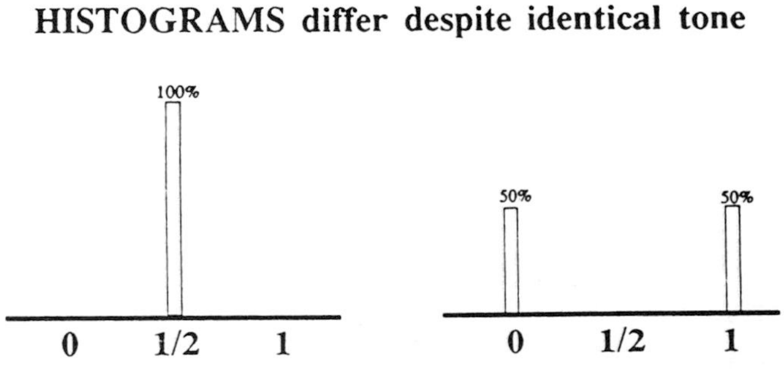

Fig. 41–16. A histogram is a graph of the distribution of intensity values in a region. Left. The uniform gray slab (Fig. 40–15b) has all squares (100%) at intensity ½. Right. The chessboard (Fig. 40–15a) has 32 white (1) squares and 32 black (0) squares, so the corresponding histogram is bimodal with an equal number (50%) of entries at 0 and 1.

* To calculate mean (2 × 2) variance on the half-black image, note by wraparound that the first column (8 squares of 0) has for each 0 a 0 above, a 1 to the left, and a 1 on the diagonal at the upper left by wraparound, so each 4-square region about these 8 has a mean of $(1 + 1 + 0 + 0)/4 = \frac{1}{2}$ and a deviation of either $0 - \frac{1}{2} = -\frac{1}{2}$ or $1 - \frac{1}{2} = +\frac{1}{2}$, netting a mean square deviation of $(\pm\frac{1}{2})^2/4$. The next 3 columns (24 regions) are all 0 deviation from the mean of 0. Columns 5 and 6 to 8 columns are a mirror of columns 1 and 2 to 4. The division by 64 completes the mean of the local variances.

myocardium is performed where all subjects have numerous myocardial biopsies, then the results of biopsy offer an independent standard that can be used to *supervise* the development of a pattern recognition decision function. If, on the other hand, the diagnosis is based on only the ultrasound data fed to the decision function so the performance of the decision function is judged on the basis of how distinctly it generates the expected classes, then it is *unsupervised*. Obviously, it is desirable to have a large and supervised training set that encompasses the variants of tissue type expected in real applications. If the training set is defined too narrowly, it will not represent borderline cases, which may be the most important classification problems.

Data Condensation and Reduction

Raw observations are typically voluminous. It is possible and often desirable to condense raw observations to a smaller set of numbers in categories called *feature variables*. The feature variables are typically represented in a list as a new, shorter vector called a feature vector or pattern vector. One manner of condensing the volume of raw observation data is to derive a tissue parameter, as discussed in the first half of this chapter. Thus, a large volume of backscattered intensity values may be replaced by the derived value for *integrated* backscatter. Another method of data condensation is to use summary statistics (mean amplitude and variance), rather than a multitude of measurements. The histogram of an image is much less data than the image itself, but also contains less information. Other summary parameters may be derived by ad hoc rules for convenience. A crucial consideration in data condensation is the balance between efficiency gained and information lost. If some of the data collected prove superfluous, then they should not simply be condensed. They should be eliminated from subsequent acquisitions. Methods by which to identify this situation are discussed later in reference to data reduction.

The choice of observed variables determines the structure of the *observation space* and modulates the distribution of points in the space to be partitioned. Through the process of data condensation, the observation space may be restructured by mapping it to *feature space* (Fig. 41–17), by applying a function that combines components of a given observation vector to derive another vector that is easier to interpret or has fewer components or (preferably) both. For example, observations on height and weight of subjects are often combined to the single derived parameter called body surface area, and subsequent data analysis relates to the derived feature (e.g., body surface area) rather than the original observation variables (e.g., height and weight).

Training

Training involves the examination of data to assess its separability into classes and the selection of the appropriate rules for separation. Data may be examined by plotting graphs and other graphic and computational methods, as discussed later in the section of this chapter on cluster analysis. Then, if the data appear to be separable into classes (Fig. 41–18), a decision function is applied to the training data to achieve classification. The decision function determines which class to assign to each new observation or pattern vector. Interpreted geometrically, a decision function divides the space spanned by all possible pattern vectors into regions representing distinct pattern types or states. Such a division of space is called a *partition*. Division of a space to construct partitions is accomplished by specifying boundaries that have one less dimension than that of the space to be partitioned. For example, a point (dimension =

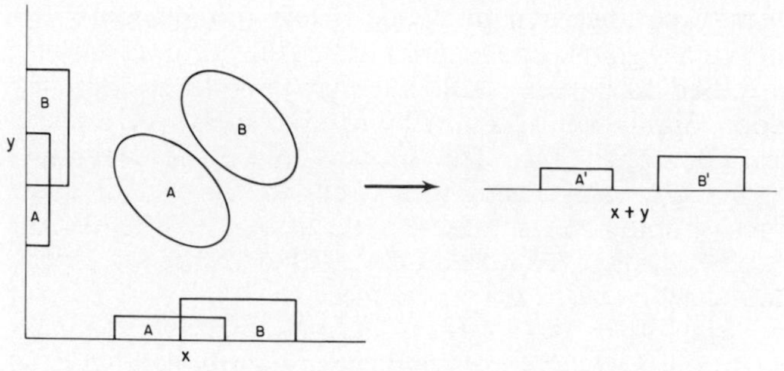

Fig. 41–17. The concept of feature space. A two-dimensional observation consists of a pair of observations (x, y) such as weight and height. The collection of all possible observations of this type forms "observation space." A cluster or group of observations occupying a region in observation space may have a priori significance such as women (A) vs. men (B). Regions A and B (ovals, left) are completely separable as viewed in two dimensions, but their projections onto the x axis are only partially separable, as are their projections on the y axis. However, if the observations are combined into a feature, for example combining (x, y) to yield x + y, then the groups A and B are completely separable using the single derived observation parameter or feature x + y. The space spanned by all possible features is called *feature space*.

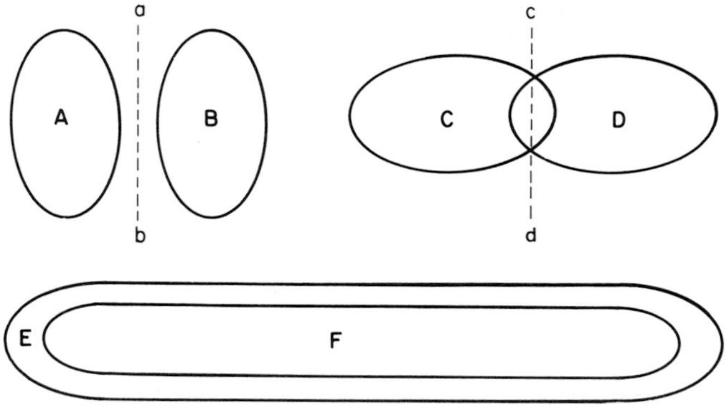

Fig. 41–18. The concept of separability. Two regions representing observations may be completely separable, partially separable, or inseparable depending on the degree of overlap and the manner of distinguishing them. Regions A and B are completely separable, distinguished by the side of the line a-b on which observations lie. Regions C and D are only partially separable as illustrated because these regions overlap. Classification of observations lying left of the line c-d as region C will misclassify the portion of D that also lies to the left of c-d, and similarly, classification of observations to the right of c-d as D will misclassify a portion of C. The line c-d is placed to minimize the total area of misclassification. Regions E and F are completely separable using a circle around F to distinguish observations inside the circle from those outside it, but E and F are only partially separable by a line.

0) may be specified to divide a line (dimension = 1) into two regions, and additional "cutoff" points may be specified to partition the line further into disjoint regions. Similarly, lines may be used to subdivide a plane into distinct regions. The dividing boundaries need not be linear, but imposing that boundary class restriction does simplify the mathematics. In higher dimensions (larger number of coordinates), the analogous linear boundary is called a hyperplane.

Although partitions that determine tissue type may be established arbitrarily and subsequently validated, in general, rules are applied, based either on a priori knowledge or on statistics. Figure 41–19 illustrates how probability may be used in specifying a decision function. In this example, it is known in advance that there are two tissue types of interest, labeled A and B. In examining a particular ultrasound parameter on training samples of A, a distribution of results is observed, with a mean of m_A. Similarly, examining training samples of B yields a distribution of values with a mean of m_B. With only a single observation parameter, two tissue types of interest, and the distributions as in Figure 41–19, left, the best choice of decision function is easily determined. The cutoff point c divides the observation space into a partition (P_A, P_B) as shown. If an unlabeled observation lies in the region of P_A, then it most likely came from A, and so it will be classified type A. Similarly, if an unlabeled observation lies in the region of P_B, then it most likely came from B, and so it will be classified type B. This decision function is not always successful because some observations on members of A lie in the region P_B and some observations on members of B lie in P_A. Varying the placement of the cutoff point c yields a family of decision functions. The preferred choice of decision function is selected by picking the point c, to minimize the probability or expected cost of classification error, computed by adding up the areas of error, each weighted by a fraction representing the relative clinical significance of the particular error. Figure

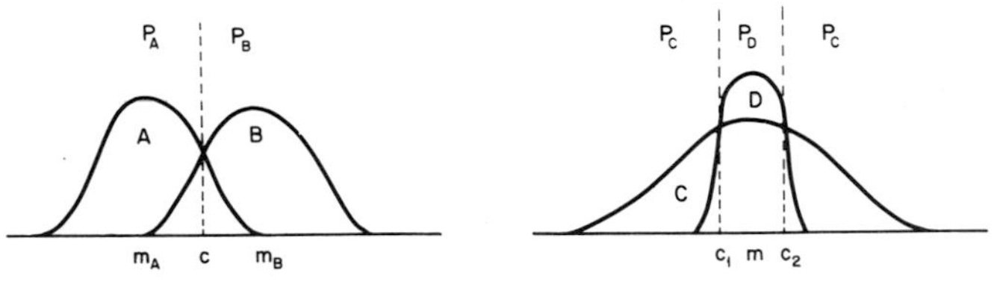

Fig. 41–19. A Bayesian decision function. Left. The distributions for two groups of observations, for example, weights of women (A) and men (B). The height of a distribution curve over a particular value on the horizontal axis represents the relative number of occurrences of that observed value. The values m_A and m_B represent the means or centers of the distributions for A and B, respectively. The point c on the horizontal axis partitions the observations into two regions: P_A (left) and P_B (right), which are used to classify observations as "A" or "B," respectively. Shifting the cutoff point c to the left changes P_A and P_B such that the portion of the B misclassified as "A" decreases, but the portion of A in P_B is smaller. Right panel illustrates the same concept for overlapping observation centered about the same mean. Expanding the separation between partitioning points C_1 and C_2 will increase the number of patients correctly classified as D. This will also increase the portion of C which is misclassified.

41–19, right, shows a slightly more complicated example in which the means are equal (m). The observations on C and D appear entirely inseparable, but using the partition (P_C, P_D) shown, partial separation is achieved—an unlabeled observation in region P_cs more likely to come from c than from D and an unlabeled observation in region P_D is more likely to come from D. As in the previous example, this is really a family of decision functions, this time depending on the selection of cutoff points c_1 and c_2, and the member of the family that performs best as a decision function is determined by setting these two parameters to minimize the probability or expected cost of error.

The foregoing classification methods apply to multivariate as well as univariate observations. Parameters are adjusted to minimize the expected cost of error, which in the multivariate normal case depends on the distribution for each component observation and also on the cross correlations. In general, one cannot assume that observations have the (multivariate) normal or Gaussian distribution; the distributions should be examined before choosing candidate decision function.[90–92] Transformation of variables to near normality, when possible, may simplify the analysis.

Statistical Methods. There are a number of statistical methods which are used for data separation or classification. These include: (1) discriminant analysis; (2) principal component analysis; (3) canonical variable analysis; (4) mixture modeling; and (5) nonparametric statistics.

Discriminant Analysis. Linear discriminant analysis divides the observation or pattern space by computing a linear combination of the observation variables (a set of coefficients that describes a hyperplane) such that all points above it are assigned to one class and all points below are assigned to another class. The predictive accuracy of the assignment is computed as a function of the coefficients, and this is solved to determine the set of coefficients that achieved the highest predictive accuracy. Higher order polynomial and other nonlinear discriminant methods may be implemented in a similar manner but are less commonly used. Logistic regression may be used similarly

Principal Component Analysis. Principal component analysis is a standard approach to condensation of a pooled data set. It creates serially uncorrelated artificial variables generated from the original observation variables. The method was originally described as a way of representing multivariate data with a series of linear models by finding the best linear fit to the observed data and then fitting a linear model in turn to the lower dimensional space spanned by the residual errors not addressed by the previous model.[93] Later, it was shown that this is equivalent to finding the transform of the data that are orthonormal and serially have maximal variance in each component.[94] The *first principal component* is a linear combination of the observation variables accounting for direction and amount of the maximum variance in the observations. The *second principal component* is selected from the subspace perpendicular to the first principal component, so it accounts for the direction and amount of maximum residual variance. Third, fourth, and higher components up to the number of observations are defined in succession by the maximal residual variance. The derived variables are uncorrelated; their covariance matrix is zero off the diagonal. Computer statistics analysis packages report the results from principal component analysis in terms of eigenvectors and eigenvalues (given a matrix C, a vector v and a scalar λ, λ is an eigenvalue and v is the corresponding eigenvector of C if v and λ satisfy the relation $Cv = \lambda v$; if a matrix C is zero off the diagonal then the values of the matrix elements on the diagonal are eigenvalues). If the eigenvectors of the covariance matrix are scaled to unit length, they represent the directions of the principal components of the variance, each eigenvalue of the covariance matrix can be interpreted as the variance of the corresponding eigenvector (principal component), and the sum of these variances is the same as the sum of variances from the original observations. Thus, each successive principal component may be interpreted as accounting for a portion of the original variance. Typically, a few components account for most of the variance, so if the variance reflects the information value, then principal component analysis followed by reporting only the first few principal components provides an effective means of data condensation.

Canonical Variable Analysis. Canonical variable analysis yields a serially orthogonal transform that maximizes the variance between two known tissue types. It requires a priori information (pathology), but in exchange its components reflect tissue differences rather than just variance (which need not align with the direction of maximal separability—see Fig. 41–8). Selection of any of these classic statistics techniques presupposes that one is dealing with a multivariate normal data distribution.

Mixture Modeling. Yet another way to analyze training data is to fit it to an equation describing a mixture of statistical distributions. The primary difficulty here is choosing the appropriate mixture model. Progress in that direction has been achieved by application of information theory to produce a model selection criterion.

Nonparametric Statistical Methods. Two commonly occurring circumstances favor the use of nonparametric statistic methods. One circumstance is when the assumptions of a classic statistics approach are violated. Note, for example, that intensities from adjacent points in an image are not independent samples. The other common obstacle is not knowing the values of all the parameters in a model, i.e., not knowing the variance for the alternate hypothesis "not X" when observations characterizing tissue type are presumed to have normal distributions. Mathematically, these circumstances indicate that the functional representation of one or more of the distributions of possible observations is incorrect or incomplete, and so a nonparametric approach may be more appropriate. The simplest nonparametric approach is a nearest-neighbor assignment.[95,96] Distances between a new, unlabeled observation and standard observations representing the tissue types of interest are compared, and the new observation is classified in accordance with its nearest neighbor among the standards. For an example such as that in Figure 41–9, left, m_A and m_B can serve as the standards for A and B, respectively, with fairly good results. For the example in Figure 41–19, right, the means of C and D are equal (m) and are thus useless for nearest-neighbor assignment. In that case, it is better to use multiple samples from C and from D as standards, distributed as C and D, respectively, so central observations tend to be closest to a member of D and peripheral observations tend to be closest to a member of C. Alternatively, one central sample can serve as standard for D and two peripheral samples can serve as standard for C. That corresponds to choosing the partition (P_C, P_D) illustrated. The choice of partition should be adjusted to minimize the expected cost of misclassification based on the training data.

Data Reduction. If the foregoing classification methods are repeated alternately with stepwise elimination or extension of the number of observation variables, then the performance with and without specific variables may be compared to determine the relative importance of each observation variable in the ability to classify. This can be used in data reduction because it indicates which variables are useful and which are redundant or useless.

For example, discriminant analysis may be applied repeatedly in a stepwise fashion. This test examines different combinations of the observation or pattern variables continually reassessing the ability to distinguish data from different tissue types, to find the best combination of predictors, and to determine the order of importance of the different components of observation in helping to identify the differences of interest. Its purpose is to separate "wheat from chaff," so only useful observations need be recorded and analyzed subsequently.

Similarly, the coordinates of the major principal components may be examined to estimate the relative importance of the observation or pattern variables. In accordance with the assumptions of principal component analysis, those variables that have the least weight in identifying the major components of variance may be eliminated from further examination. Similarly, canonical variable analysis can identify component observations that fail to contribute to the ability of distinguishing among the different known groups examined in training data.

Separability Assessment. Implicit in the comparison of different decision functions and in the ability to draw conclusions for data reduction is the ability to compare quality of classification results. Ultimately, the ability to classify the data correctly is limited by the data. It is possible to make an assessment of the intrinsic limit set by the data regarding its possible classification.

An example of a classic method that is widely used but limited in scope is generalized linear modeling. For data that are normally distributed with common variance, that method leads to the ANOVA (analysis of variance) or MANOVA (multivariate analysis of variance). ANOVA evaluates whether or not two or more groups of samples with common variance have the same mean value (thus deciding whether or not they represent the same distribution class). The decision is based on the F-statistic, a ratio of between-group variance to within-group variance. Information theory has allowed extension of that approach to methods for analysis of subgroups variable in number without assuming homoscedasticity (homogeneity of variance) and also to nonparametric separability evaluation without specification of the number of subgroups.[93]

Consider, for example, the task of distinguishing amyloid cardiomyopathy from normal myocardium based solely on observation of the mean intensity of their ultrasonic reflections. Amyloid myocardium might be brighter on average, but that is not sufficient for diagnostic purposes; there could be substantial overlap between values from normal and abnormal tissue. Measuring the separability of observations assesses that overlap. If knowing the mean signal intensity does not affect the likelihood of correct assignment of tissue type at all, then amyloid and normal myocardium are inseparable by mean intensity. If the knowledge is useful and improves the likelihood of correct classification, they are partially separable. If there were some cutoff value for observed mean intensity above which all hearts are amyloid and below which all are normal, then the mean intensity observations would be completely separable.*

In the examination of 13 features from A-mode signals (Fig. 41–20) of waveforms that were collected before, 1, 2, and 4 hours after ligation of the left anterior descending coronary artery in dogs, classification of individual waveforms as ischemic or normal based on a training set of 50 cases achieved 94% accuracy for data acquired 1 hour or 2 hours after occlusion, vs. preocclusion, and 96% classification accuracy for waveforms acquired 4 hours after occlusion.[39] It is important in studies of this sort that the training samples include stable control subjects, identical in all aspects except for the difference of interest, i.e., ischemic vs. normal. This problem is not simple because normal patterns from the same subject may differ over time, with vascular territory or in relation to the transducer position. As a result, large numbers of observations are needed to help randomize and diffuse effects not of interest. When applied more generally, the classification method also has to account for differences among subjects, machines, and acquisition techniques.

Reiteration

Failure to classify data adequately may relate to an inappropriate choice of observation data, feature vectors, or decision function. In practice, the foregoing steps often must be repeated iteratively, to select new observation variables, to combine observation variables into different feature variables, and to explore different decision functions until optimal classification is achieved (i.e., the best separation, using the least number of variables, and at the greatest computational efficiency).

* For data with a multivariate normal distribution, separability has been assessed by calculating the multivariate equivalent of z-scores, called *Mahalanobis distance*.[101] If the data include directional information or for other reasons are not multivariate normal, then a nonparametric measure of separability is needed.[93]

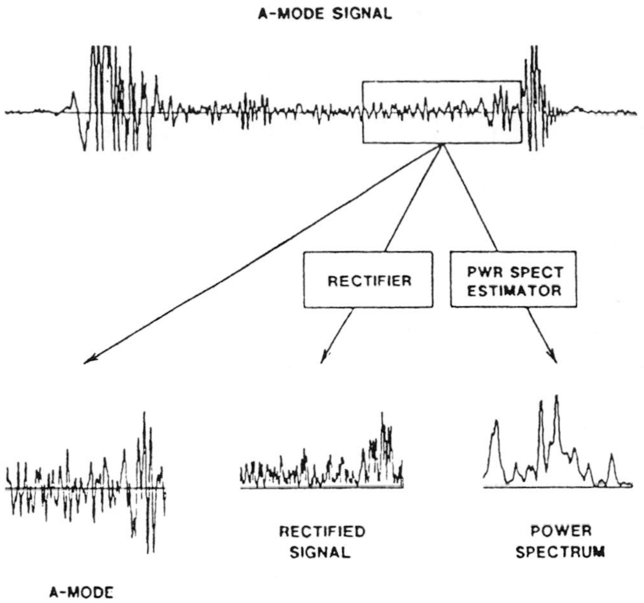

Fig. 41–20. A-mode waveforms obtained with a broad-band metaniobate transceiver through a saline bag on live intact beating canine hearts, synchronized by the R wave of the electrocardiogram to an isovolumic phase. Signals from the endocardial region were digitized at a sampling interval of 20 nsec and analyzed in a window of 256 data points (top). These data were normalized (bottom, left), rectified (bottom, middle), and also converted to a power spectrum (bottom, right). Feature extraction included computation of the first four central moments, periodicity, and randomness measures (determinant of the covariance and ratio of eigenvalues from the joint density function of successive data pairs) for each of the data sets. Multivariate discriminant analysis yielded a classifier whose performance on new waveforms achieved a positive predictive accuracy for identification of ischemia of 96%. (From Franklin TD, et al.: Tissue parameter characterization by ultrasound: state of the art in cardiology. *In* Hanrath P, Bleifeld W, Souquet J (eds.): Cardiovascular Diagnosis by Ultrasound. The Hague, Martinus Nijhoff, 1982.)

Validation

Subsequent validation of classification determines its success. There are techniques for accomplishing the validation from a single large data base (e.g., jackknifing, holdout[97]), or else separate data sets must be used for training vs. validation. It is unwise to use numerous parameters for a "hunting expedition" based on a small data set without testing the final decision function prospectively on a new data set. Small samples and numerous observation variables can lead to false conclusions because it is always possible to achieve perfect classification of the data set with a single derived observation variable just by numbering the samples and passing on that numbering as a case identifier (such a scheme would clearly fail to perform well on prospective classification of distinct data sets). An equivalent failing occurs inadvertently if numerous parameters are applied to a small data set with "validation" based on the same data because spurious differences can serve as case labels.

Cluster Analysis

Because it can be difficult to visualize the data that results from multiple simultaneous measurements taken to characterize tissue type or state, computer-based tools for multivariate data exploration play a valued role. This is addressed in a form of data analysis called cluster analysis. Cluster analysis refers to a broad range of tools used to examine data for the identification of subgroups, an important analysis that addresses the basic question: what distinguishable subgroups exist based on the chosen observations? If more than one subgroup is present, analysis of pathologic data corresponding to each subgroup may attach biologic significance and diagnostic value to the characterization. If the data do not cluster into distinct subgroups, however, then it is probably necessary to make different observations before proceeding further with tissue characterization.

The number of ways that observations may be sorted into various nonempty subgroups is typically large, so algorithms that explore data for subgroups do not generally explore every possible partition. Instead, rules are assumed for lumping and splitting, rules that simplify analysis but also affect the outcome. As a result, there are many different techniques for cluster analysis, but common themes allow an overview in the space allocated here.

Although some approaches to cluster analysis start with a fixed concept of how many subgroups or clusters suit the data and seek the best-fitting partition, the most general approaches aim to determine the number as well as the composition of subgroups. This may be approached graphically (Chernoff) or nongraphically (k-means). The main elements of a cluster analysis algorithm, which examines data to identify subgroups, are: *data type, similarity measure,* and *procedural order*. A change in any of these elements can alter the results of the cluster analysis. Data exploration by cluster analysis is therefore not definitive. Its importance lies in its ability to reveal unexpected data relations.

Data Type

The data type fed into a cluster algorithm may be taken as binary (yes/no, present/absent), discrete (3, 5, 7), or continuous (0.0 to 1.0). Different scales may be used including nominal, ordinal, interval, or ratio. Data may be converted from interval or ratio to binary by application of a threshold. The data type used in cluster analysis frequently is not the same as that used for the original measurements.

Similarity Measure

The similarity measure used for assignment of data points to clusters is any one of several distance functions that measure the closeness of data points. To assess the "naturalness" of a partition or subgroup selection, it is necessary to extend the concept of two-point distance to a measure of association of groups of points. Such a measure may be generated by comparing the dissimilarity of the groups (i.e., mean of intergroup pairwise distances) to the similarity within each group (i.e., mean of intragroup pairwise distances), so one may decide to merge groups into a single cluster if that ratio is below a chosen threshold. Alternative methods for measuring association include calculating correlation coefficients, or in the case of supervised learning, basing the measure of association on the confusion matrix (e.g., positive predictive value based on numbers of true-positives or false-positives results). Table 41–1 provides examples of distance measurement functions.

Euclidean distance is used commonly and represents the length of a vector from point a to point b, "as the crow flies." Mahalanobis distance includes Euclidean distance as a special case. It uses a matrix to scale or weight Euclidean distance in a prescribed fashion such as inverse to the pooled variance (in which case the distance measure is a multivariate equivalent to "z-scores" or number of standard deviations of separation). Minkowski's m-th distance measures city blocks (no diagonals) for m 1, Euclidean distance for m 2, and gives greater weight to the largest component difference for $m > 2$. Subjective scales use a variety of criteria, gaining flexibility at the expense of reproducibility.

Procedural Order

The *nearest-neighbor method* of cluster analysis exemplifies the role of similarity or distance measurement in cluster analysis. The method starts with values called "seeds" selected to represent the tissue types of interest. Biologic considerations may suggest the appropriate number of clusters (tissue types) in the data set, and training data may provide seed values representing the distinct tissue types. A new observation is associated with the closest seed (i.e., seed value at shortest distance) to form a cluster. Subsequent observations are assigned to the closest of the growing clusters defined as the cluster or group that has the smallest distance between the current observation and the center or mean observed value for that group. The mean changes as points are added, so a stepwise approach is sometimes adopted whereby following each addition, the point farthest from the mean in the selected group may be released from the group if it meets some prescribed threshold condition. A different choice of seed values can result in a different partition, as can a different application of distance measurement.

Table 41–1. Distance Measures

1. Euclidean distance:
   $d(a,b) = [(a - b)'(a - b)]^{1/2} = [\sum_i (a_i - b_i)^2]^{1/2}$

   Where a and b are column vectors and a′ is the transpose (to a row vector) of vector a, a_i is the ith compontent of vector a.
2. Mahalanobis distance:
   $d(a,b) = [(a - b)'M(a - b)]^{1/2}$
   Where M is a positive definite matrix which estimates the inverse of the variance-covariance matrix for vectors a and b.
3. Minkowski's m-th distance:
   $d_m(a,b) = [\sum_i (a_i - b_i)^{m}]^{1/m}$
4. Subjective distance:
   $0 \leq d(a,b) < 1$, where 0 signifies judged identical and 1 signifies judged maximally different.

Distance between a point and a group is called *linkage*. Linkage may be short (distance to the closest member of the group), long (distance to the farthest member of the group), or pairwise average or median. If one starts with some predefined groups, then individual points may be assigned one at a time to the current group with the shortest linkage (Fig. 41–21). On a second pass, each point in turn may be removed from its current group and reassigned by shortest linkage (which changes as the groups are redefined). Such a method is called *hierarchical clustering*.[98] Cluster analysis can proceed in many different ways. A procedure, as well as the resulting partitions or clusters, is considered robust if the results vary little despite reasonable changes in the approach. In techniques that require seed values, this means that the procedure should be repeated using different starting values.

Limitations to Classification Methods

Although the mathematic approaches to signal and image analysis described previously are well established, there are certain limitations inherent in their application to the images generated using currently available ultrasound instruments. First, all the factors discussed under tissue parameter determination analysis such as transducer power output, transducer bandwidth and frequency, attenuation by tissue interposed between the transducer and region of interest, signal threshold, and preprocessing of the signal as it is converted from RF to video format may affect echo amplitudes and distribution and hence the result of any numeric analysis. Physical and instrument-related factors have been shown to produce regional alterations in apparent image texture, even when one is imaging a uniformly scattering target,[44,83] and it has been demonstrated convincingly that the speckle pattern noted in ultrasonic images largely depends on the imaging system rather than on the microstructure of the scanned object.[83]

Classification schemes typically presume that the parameters to be characterized remain constant. For example, if tissue attenuation changes with time at room temperature, training data acquired at baseline would not be valid for a 4-hour sample. Similarly, if attenuation varies between two subjects, then training data used to define normal in one subject would not be applicable to the second. Fingerprint analysis only permits identification because fingerprints do not change. Thus, results for pattern recognition must be interpreted with caution. Although they do not require determination of physical parameters, they, in essence, assume that such parameters exist, albeit obscured by other aspects of the data provided by the imaging system.

In conclusion, experimental work demonstrates convincingly that changes in ultrasound signals contain information about tissue character, information highly desirable for clinical decision making. Unfortunately, the interactions between ultrasonic waves and a moving three-dimensional structurally variable target are sufficiently complex that accurate parameter measurement for tissue characterization is not yet available clinically. Methods for accomplishing these goals in vivo have been presented. Alternative methods for tissue classification without requiring precise parameter measurement have also been presented. Pattern recognition based on serial changes in the same subject, cycle-related variation, and multivariate analysis of reflected ultrasound intensities are most promising and can be expected to make rapid advances as newer ultrasonic imaging systems expand capabilities for digital processing.

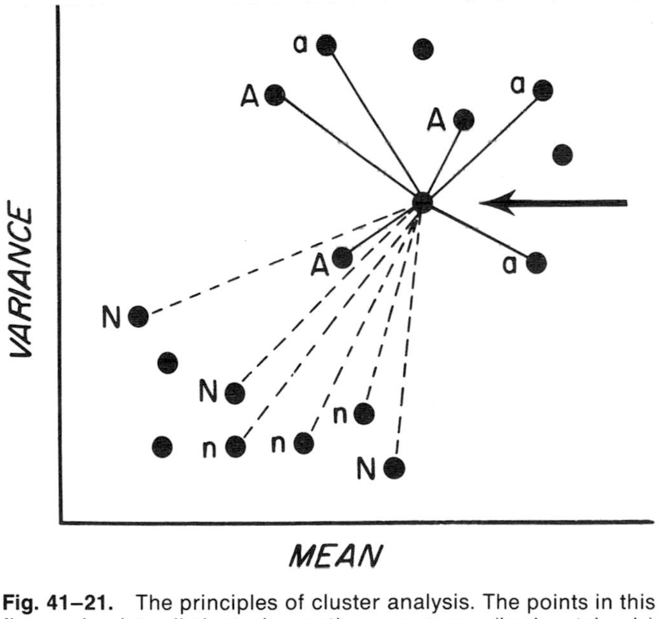

Fig. 41–21. The principles of cluster analysis. The points in this figure simulate distinct observations on mean (horizontal axis) and variance (vertical axis) of myocardial echo intensities from normal and amyloid hearts. The points labeled "A" represent biopsy-proven cases of amyloid heart, whereas those labeled "N" represent controls normal by biopsy. These serve as "seed" values to initialize assignment of the other observations. The points labeled "a" are presumed to be amyloid cases by proximity to all prior points labeled "A" and "a"; the points labeled "n" are similarly assigned as normal. The next point to be assigned (arrow) will be labeled "a" because the linkage from it to the growing amyloid cluster (solid lines) is less than the linkage from it to the growing normal cluster (broken lines).

REFERENCES

1. Siguerira-Filho SG, Cunha CLP, Tajik AJ: M-Mode and two-dimensional echocardiographic features in cardiac amyloidosis. Circulation 63:188, 1981.
2. Rasmussen S, Corya BC, Feigenbaum H, Knoebel SB: Detection of myocardial scar tissue by M-mode echocardiography. Circulation 57:230, 1978.
3. Wilkins GT, et al.: Percutaneous balloon dilatation of the mitral valve: an analysis of echocardiographic variables related to outcome and the mechanism of dilatation. Br Heart J 60:299, 1988.
4. Bhandari AK, Nanda NC: Myocardial texture characterization by two-dimensional echocardiography. Am J Cardiol 51:817, 1983.
5. Martin PR, Rakowski H, French, J Popp RL: Idiopathic hypertrophic subaortic stenosis viewed by wide-angle phased-array echocardiography. Circulation 59:1206, 1979.
6. Lerski RA, et al.: Discriminant analysis of ultrasonic texture data in diffuse alcoholic liver disease. Ultrason Imaging 3:164, 1981.
7. Franklin TDF, et al.: Tissue parameter characterization by ultrasound: state-of-the-art in cardiology. *In* Hanrath P, Bleifeld W, Souquet J, (eds.): Cardiovascular Diagnosis by Ultrasound. The Hague, Martinus Nijhoff, 1982.
8. Preston K, Czerwinski MJ, Skolnik JL, Leb DE: Recent developments in obtaining histopathological information from ultrasound tissue signatures. *In* Linzer M (ed.): National Bureau of Standards Special Publication No. 525. Washington, D.C., U.S. Government Printing Office, p. 303, 1979.
9. Preston K: Use of pattern recognition for signal processing in ultrasonic histopathology. *In* Linzer M (ed.): National Bureau of Standards Special

Publication No. 453. Washington, D.C., U.S. Government Printing Office, p. 51, 1976.
10. Edler I: The use of ultrasound as a diagnostic aid, and its effects on biological tissues. Acta Med Scand Suppl. 370, 1, 1961.
11. Wells PNT: Biomedical Ultrasonics. New York, Academic Press, 1977.
12. Lele PP, Namery J: Detection of myocardial infarction by ultrasound. *In* Proceedings of the 25th Annual Conference on Engineering in Medicine and Biology. Vol. 14, Arlington, VA, Alliance for Engineering in Medicine and Biology. p. 135, 1972.
13. Chandrasekaran K, et al.: Echocardiograhpic visualization of acute myocardial ischemia: in vitro study. Ultrasound Med Biol 12:785, 1986.
14. Greenleaf JF: Tissue characterization by computed tomography. *In* Thijssen JM, Berger G (eds): Ultrasound Tissue Characterization, and Echographic Imaging. Proceedings of the 6th European Communities Workshop. Luxembourg, Commission of the European Communities. Eur 10931, p. 3, 1986.
15. Lele PP, et al.: Tissue characterization by ultrasonic frequency-dependent attenuation and scattering. *In* Linzer M (ed.): Ultrasonic Tissue Characterization National Bureau of Standards Special Publication No. 435. Washington, D.C., U.S. Government Printing Office, p. 153, 1976.
16. Lele PP, Senapati N: The frequency spectra of energy backscattered and attenuated by normal and abnormal tissue. *In* White DN (ed.): Recent Advances in Ultrasound in Biomedicine. Vol. 1. Forest Grove, OR, Research Studies Press, p. 55, 1977.
17. Mimbs JW, et al.: Detection of myocardial infarction in vitro based on altered attenuation of ultrasound. Circ Res 41:192, 1977.
18. Miller JG, et al.: Ultrasonic tissue characterization: correlation between biochemical and ultrasonic indices of myocardial injury. *In* de Klerk J, McAvoy BR (eds): Proc IEEE Ultrason Symp. New York, Institute of Electrical and Electronic Engineers, 79:33, 1976.
19. Namery J, Lele PP: Ultrasonic detection of myocardial infarction in the dog. de Klerk J, McAvoy BR (eds): Proc IEEE Ultrason Symp New York, Institute of Electrical and Electronic Engineers, 72:491, 1972.
20. Field S, Dunn F: Correlation of echographic visualizability of tissue with biologic composition and physiologic state. J Acoust Soc Am 54:809, 1973.
21. O'Brien WD: Role of collagen in determining ultrasonic propagation properties in tissue. Acoust Hologr 7:37, 1977
22. O'Donnell M, Mimbs JW, Miller JG: The relationship between collagen and ultrasonic attenuation in myocardial tissue. J Acoust Soc Am 65:512, 1979.
23. Mimbs JW, et al.: The dependence of ultrasonic attenuation and backscatter on collagen content in dog and rabbit hearts. Circ Res 47:49, 1980.
24. O'Donnell M, Mimbs JW, Sobel BE, Miller JG: Ultrasonic attenuation in normal and ischemic myocardium. *In* Linzer M (ed.): Ultrasonic Tissue Characterization National Bureau of Standards Special Publication No. 525. Washington, D.C., U.S. Government Printing Office, p. 63, 1979.
25. Mimbs JW, et al.: Characterization of the evolution of myocardial infarction by ultrasonic backscatter. Circulation 60(Suppl. II):II-17, 1979.
26. Busse LJ, et al.: Phase cancellation effects: a source of attenuation artifact eliminated by a CdS acoustoelectric receiver. *In* White D, Brown AE (eds): Ultrasound in Medicine. Vol 3, 1977 New York, Plenum Press, p. 1519.
27. Busse LJ, Miller JG: Detection of spatially nonuniform ultrasonic radiation with phase-sensitive (piezoelectric) and phase insensitive (acoustoelectric) receivers. J Acoust Soc Am 70:1377, 1981.
28. Busse LJ, Miller JG: A comparison of finite-aperture phase-sensitive and phase-insensitive detection in the near field of inhomogenous material. Proc Ultrason Symp New York, Institute of Electrical and Electronic Engineers, 81:617, 1981.
29. O'Donnell M, Mimbs JW, Sobel BE, Miller JG: Ultrasonic attenuation of myocardial tissue: dependence of time after excixion and on temperature. J Acoust Soc Am 62:1054, 1977.
30. Busse LJ, Miller JG: Response characteristics of a finite-aperture, phase-insensitive ultrasonic receiver based upon the acoustoelectric effect. J Acoust Soc Am 70:1370, 1981.
31. Vered Z, et al.: Ultrasound integrated backscatter tissue characterization of remote myocardial infarction in human subjects. J Am Coll Cardiol 13: 84, 1989.
32. Greenleaf JF: A graphical description of scattering. Ultrasound Med Biol 12:603, 1986.
33. O'Donnell M, Mimbs JW, Miller JG: The relationship between collagen and ultrasonic attenuation in myocardial tissue. J Acoust Soc Am 65:512, 1979.
34. Miller JG, Perez JE, Sobel BE: Ultrasonic characterization of myocardium. Prog Cardiovasc Dis 28:85, 1985.
35. O'Donnell M, Mimbs JW, Miller JG: The relationship between collagen and ultrasonic backscatter in myocardial tissue. J Acoust Soc Am 69:580, 1981.
36. O'Donnell M, Miller JG: Quantitative broadband ultrasonic backscatter: an approach to nondestructive evaluation in acoustically inhomogeneous materials. J Appl Physiol 52:1056, 1981.
37. Perez JE, Madaras EI, Sobel BE, Miller JG: Quantitative myocardial characterization with ultrasound. Automedica 5:201, 1984.
38. O'Donnell M, Bauwens D, Mimbs JW, Miller JG: Broadband integrated backscatter: an approach to spatially localized tissue characterization in vivo. Proc IEEE Ultrason Symp. New York, Institute of Electrical and Electronic Engineers, 79:175, 1979.
39. Franklin TD, et al.: Multivariate discrimination and feature analysis of gated A-mode ultrasonic echoes from *in vivo* normal and ischemic myocardium. Circulation 66(Suppl. II):II-30, 1982.
40. Madaras EI, et al.: Changes in myocardial backscatter throughout the cardiac cycle. Ultrason Imaging 5:229, 1983.
41. Fitzgerald PJ, et al.: Two-dimensional ultrasonic tissue characterization: backscatter power, endocardial wall motion and their phase relationship for normal, ischemic and infarcted myocardium. Circulation 76:850, 1987.
42. Milunski MR, et al.: Ultrasonic tissue characterization with integrated backscatter: acute myocardial ischemia, reperfusion, and stunned myocardium in patients. J Am Coll Cardiol 80:491, 1989.
43. Skorton DJ, et al.: Detection of acute myocardial infarction in closed chest dogs by analysis of regional two-dimensional echocardiographic gray-level distributions. Circ Res 52:36, 1983.
44. Skorton DJ, et al.: Quantitative texture analysis in two-dimensional echocardiography: application to the diagnosis of experimental myocardial contusion. Circulation 68:217, 1983.
45. Logan-Sinclair RB, Wong CM, Gibson DG: Clinical applications of amplitude processing of echocardiographic images. Br Heart J 45:621, 1981.
46. Davies J, et al.: Echocardiographic features of eosinophilic endomyocardial disease. Am J Cardiol 48:434, 1982.
47. Shaw TRD, et al.: Relation between regional echo intensity and myocardial connective tissue in chronic left ventricular disease. Br Heart J 51:46, 1984.
48. Parisi AF, et al.: Enhanced detection of the evolution of tissue changes after acute myocardial infarction using color-encoded two-dimensional echocardiography. Circulation 66:764, 1982.
49. Sagar K, et al.: Intramyocardial variability in integrated backscatter: effects of coronary occlusion and reperfusion. Circulation 75:436, 1987.
50. Mottley JB, et al.: Regional differences in the cyclic variation of myocardial backscatter that parallel regional differences in contractile performance. J Acoust Soc Am 76:1617, 1984.
51. Barzilai B, et al.: Effects of myocardial contraction on ultrasonic backscatter before and after ischemia. Am J Physiol 247:H478, 1984.
52. Wickline SA, et al.: The dependence of myocardial ultrasonic integrated backscatter on contractile performance. Circulation 72:183, 1985.
53. Thomas LJ, et al.: A real-time integrated backscatter measurement system for quantitative tissue characterization. IEEE Trans Ultrason Ferroelect Freq Control 33:27, 1986.
54. Wickline SA, et al.: Sensitive detection of the effects of reperfusion on myocardium by ultrasonic tissue characterization with integrated backscatter. Circulation 74:389, 1986.
55. Milunski MR, et al.: Early identification with ultrasonic integrated backscatter of viable but stunned myocardium in dogs. J Am Coll Cardiol 14:462, 1989.
56. Wickline SA, et al.: A relationship between ultrasonic integrated backscatter and myocardial contractile function. J Clin Invest 76:2151, 1985.
57. Glueck RM, et al.: Effect of coronary artery occlusion and reperfusion on cardiac cycle-dependent variation of myocardial ultrasonic backscatter. Circ Res 56:683, 1985.
58. Hoyt RM, Skorton DJ, Collins SM, Melton HE: Ultrasonic backscatter and collagen in normal ventricular myocardium. Circulation 69:775, 1984.
59. Hoyt RH, et al.: Assessment of fibrosis in infarcted human hearts by analysis of ultrasonic backscatter. Circulation 71:740, 1985.
60. Mimbs JW, et al.: Effects of myocardial ischemia on quantitative ultrasonic backscatter and identification of responsible determinants. Circ Res 49:89, 1981.
61. Gramiak R, et al.: Ultrasonic detection of myocardial infarction by amplitude analysis. Radiolongy 130:713, 1979.
62. O'Donnell M, Bauwens D, Mimbs JW, Miller JG: *In vivo* detection of acute myocardial ischemia in the dog by quantitative ultrasonic backscatter. *In* Proceedings of the 4th International Symposium on Ultrasonic Imaging and Tissues Characterization. Gaithersburg, MD, National Bureau of Standards, p. 9, 1979.
63. Chandrasekaran K, et al.: Epicardial echocardiography in tissue characterization of ischemia myocardium in a canine model. Am J Cardiac Imaging 1:152, 1987.
64. Rassmussen S, et al.: Echocardiographic detection of ischemic and infarcted myocardium. J Am Coll Cardiol 3:733, 1984.
65. Milunski MR, et al.: Cardiac cycle-dependent variation of integrated backscatter is not distorted by abnormal myocardial wall motion in human subjects with paradoxical septal motion. Ultrasound Med Biol 15:311, 1989.
66. Chandrasekaran K, et al.: Early recognition of heart transplant rejection by backscatter analysis from serial 2D echoes in a heterotopic transplant model. J Heart Transplant 6:1, 1987.
67. Mimbs JW, O'Donnell M, MIller JG, Sobel BE: Detection of cardiomyopathic changes induced by doxorubicin based on quantitative analysis of ultrasonic backscatter. Am J Cardiol 47:1056, 1981.
68. Perez JE, et al.: Applicability of ultrasonic tissue characterization for longitudinal assessment and differentiation of calcification and fibrosis in cardiomyopathy. J Am Coll Cardiol 4:88, 1984.
69. Picano E, et al.: Angle dependence of ultrasonic backscatter in arterial tissues: a study in vitro. Circulation 72:572, 1985.
70. Cohen RD, et al.: Detection of ischemic myocardium in vivo through the chest wall by quantitative ultrasonic tissue characterization. Am J Cardiol 50:838, 1982.
71. Melton HE, Skorton DJ: Rational gain compensation for attenuation in cardiac ultrasonography. Ultrason Imaging 5:214, 1983.

72. Klepper JR, Brandenburger GH, Busse LJ, Miller JG: Phase cancellation, reflection and refraction effects of quantitative ultrasonic attenuation tomography. *In* deKlerk J, McAvoy BR, (eds), Proc IEEE Ultrason Symp New York, Institute of Electrical and Electronic Engineers. 77:182, 1977.
73. Johnson SA, et al.: Wave equations and inverse solutions for soft tissue. *In* Acoustic Imaging. vol. 11. New York, Plenum Press, p. 409, 1982.
74. Johnson SA, et al.: Inverse scattering solutions by a sinc basis, multiple source moment method. Part III: fast algorithms. Ultrason Imaging 6:103, 1984.
75. Mueller RK: Diffraction tomography I: The wave equation. Ultrason Imaging 2:213, 1980.
76. Robinson BS, Greenleaf JF: The scattering of ultrasound by cylinders: implications for diffraction tomography. J Acoust Soc Am 80:40, 1986.
77. He P, Greenleaf JF: Application of stochastic analysis to ultrasonic echo: estimation of attenuation and tissue heterogeneity from peaks of echo envelope. J Acoust Soc Am 79:526, 1986.
78. Kuc R: Ultrasonic tissue characterization using kurtosis. IEEE Trans Ultrason Ferroelect Freq Control (UFFC) 33:273, 1986.
79. Hu MK: Visual pattern recognition by moment invariants. IRE Trans Infor Theory 8:179, 1962.
80. Joynt L, et al.: Identification of tissue parameters by digital processing of real-time ultrasonic clinical cardiac data. Linzer M (ed.): Ultrasonic Tissue Characterization II. National Bureau of Standards Special Publication No. 525. Washington, D.C., U.S. Government Printing Office, p. 267, 1979.
81. Haralick RM: Statistical and structural approaches to texture. Proc IEEE 67:786, 1979.
82. McPherson DD, et al.: Ultrasound characterization of acute myocardial ischemia by quantitative texture analysis. Ultrason Imaging 8:227, 1986.
83. Kawamura K: Two-dimensional echocardiographic intensity distribution by histographic analysis. J Cardiogr 17:149, 1987.
84. Galloway MW: Texture analysis using gray level run lengths. Comput Graph Image Processing 4:172, 1975.
85. Cooper DB, Cooper PW: Nonsupervised adaptive signal detection and pattern recognition. Infor Control 7:416, 1964.
86. Fralick SC: Learning to recognize patterns without a teacher. IEEE Trans Info Theory 13:57, 1967.
87. Patrick EA: On a class of unsupervised estimation systems. IEEE Trans Info Theory 14:407, 1968.
88. Hilborn CG Jr, Laintiotis DG: Optimal unsupervised learning multicategory dependent hypotheses pattern recognition. IEEE Trans Info Theory 14:357, 1968.
89. Stanat DF: Unsupervised learning of mixtures of probability functions. *In* Kanal L (ed.): Pattern Recognition. Washington D.C., Thompson, p. 357, 1968.
90. Johnson RA, Wichern DW: Applied Multivariate Statistical Analysis. Englewood Cliffs, NJ, Prentice-Hall, p. 151, 1982.
91. Parzen E: On estimation of a probability density function and mode. Ann Math Stat 33:1065, 1962.
92. Murthy VK: Estimation of proability density. Ann Math Stat 36:1027, 1965
93. Pearson K: On lines and planes of closest fit to systems of points in space. Phil Mag 2:559, 1901.
94. Hotelling H: Analysis of a complex of statistical variables into principal components. Educ Psychol 24:417, 498, 1933.
95. Fix E, Hodges JL Jr: Discriminatory analysis, nonparametric discrimination. Project 21–49–004. Randolph Field, TX, United States Air Force, 1951.
96. Hellman ME: The nearest neighbor classification rule with a reject option. IEEE Trans Sys Sci Cyber 6:179, 1970.
97. Lachenbruch PA: Discriminant Analysis. New York, Hafner Press, 1975.
98. Fu KS: Sequential Methods in Pattern Recognition and Machine Learning. New York, Academic Press, 1968.

APPENDIX

A

NORMAL CROSS-SECTIONAL ECHOCARDIOGRAPHIC MEASUREMENTS

In Memoriam

This section is dedicated to the memory of Dr. Marco O. Triulzi, who spent more than a year of his much too brief life deriving these measurements, which have served for years as normative values for our laboratory and the many others who rely on this body of data.

Despite the large volume of published cross-sectional echocardiographic data, few normal cross-sectional echocardiographic values are available in the literature. Undoubtedly, development of these values has been delayed by the lack of accepted standards for making these measurements, which makes the selection of particular structures or areas for measurement difficult, and the acceptability of normal M-mode values for most of the major dimensions required in routine study analysis problematic. Despite these difficulties, it is obvious that normal cross-sectional values in both the adult and the child must be developed and made generally available.

In the following pages, we provide a series of normal cross-sectional values for most of the cardiac structures recorded in the primary echocardiographic views. These values were obtained from a group of 72 adult patients (38 males and 34 females) ranging in age from 15 to 76 years (mean 38 years). Subject height and weight were 155 to 180 cm (mean 169 cm) and 40 to 80 kg (mean 70 kg) respectively. Body surface area calculated in the standard fashion was 1.38 to 2.10 m^2 (mean 1.75 m^2). In several cases, the same structure is measured in several views. When this occurs, the preferable view is indicated and alternative measurements are included to provide some baseline values in those patients in whom the primary view is unobtainable. In addition, since there are no accepted standards for the point at which measurements should be taken, in many cases we have provided several alternatives (e.g., the left atrial anteroposterior dimension at the aortic valve level, which is comparable to the M-mode point of measurement and the largest dimension in the anteroposterior plane). All linear dimensions and area measurements are made using the inner-edge method, which is consistent with that discussed throughout the text. All these measurements were made in the Cardiac Ultrasound Laboratory at the Massachusetts General Hospital, and in some cases may differ slightly from values given in the text, which were taken from the literature.

NORMAL CROSS-SECTIONAL VALUES*

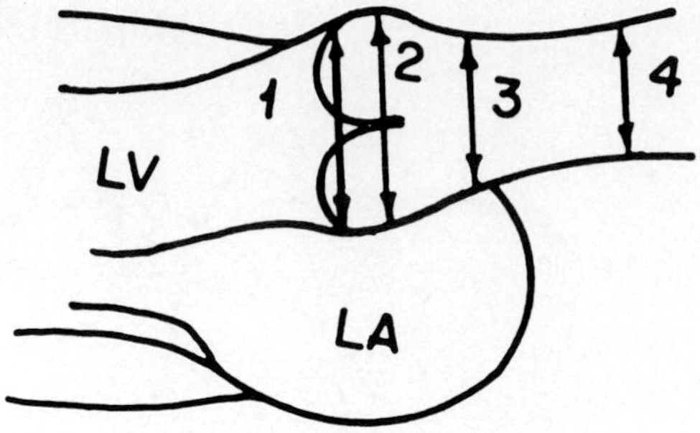

Parasternal Long Axis View	N	Mean ± SD*	Range
Aorta (end-diastole):			
1. Aortic annulus	68	1.9 ± 0.2	1.4–2.6
2. Sinus of Valsalva	68	2.8 ± 0.3	2.1–3.5
3. Sinotubular junction	64	2.4 ± 0.4	1.7–3.4
4. Ascending aorta	44	2.6 ± 0.3	2.1–3.4

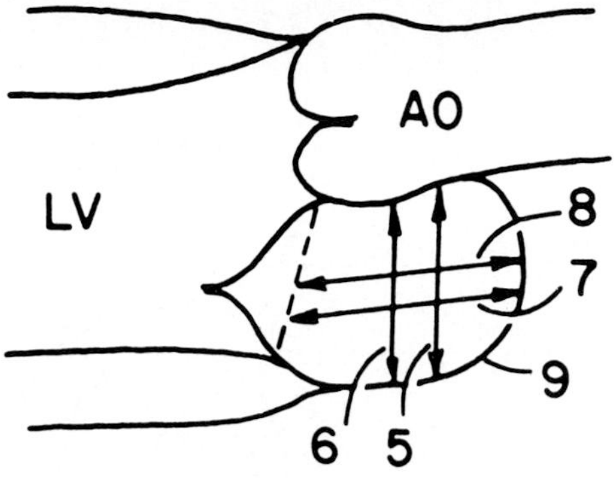

Left Atrium (end-systole):			
Antero-posterior dimension†			
5. Maximal	62	3.0 ± 0.3	2.3–3.8
6. Mid-cavity	62	3.0 ± 0.3	2.3–3.8
Supero-inferior dimension			
7. Maximal	59	4.8 ± 0.8	3.1–6.8
8. Mid-cavity	59	4.8 ± 0.8	3.1–6.8
9. Area	59	13.7 ± 3 cm^2	9.3–20.2 cm^2

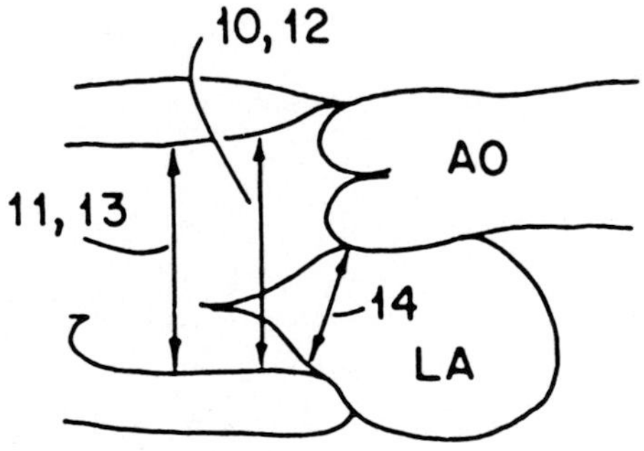

Left Ventricle			
Antero-posterior dimension:			
End-diastole			
10. Maximal	67	4.7 ± 0.4	3.6–5.4
11. "Mid-cavity" (chordal)	67	4.4 ± 0.4	3.4–5.2
End-systole			
12. Maximal	67	3.3 ± 0.5	2.3–4.0
13. "Mid-cavity" (chordal)	67	3.1 ± 0.4	2.3–3.8
14. Mitral annulus	61	2.5 ± 0.3	1.9–3.4

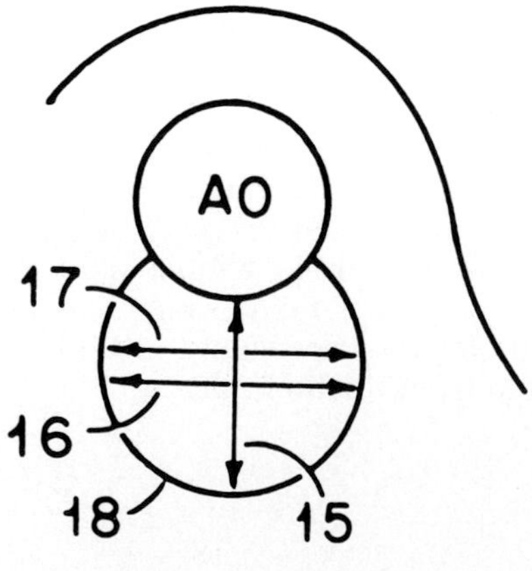

Parasternal Short Axis View at the Level of the Great Vessels	N	Mean ± SD*	Range
Left Atrium (end-systole):			
Antero-posterior dimension			
15. Maximal and mid-cavity	63	2.9 ± 0.4	2.2–4.1
Medio-lateral dimension†			
16. Maximal	64	4.2 ± 0.6	3.1–6.0
17. Mid-cavity	64	4.2 ± 0.6	3.0–6.0
18. Area	63	11.1 ± 2.1 cm^2	7–17.3 cm^2

* All linear dimensions are in cm, and areas are in cm^2.
† Indicates the preferable view for obtaining a particular measurement.

Parasternal Short Axis View at the Level of the Great Vessels	N	Mean ± SD*	Range
Pulmonary Artery (end-diastole):†			
19. Right ventricular outflow tract (subvalvular)	53	2.5 ± 0.4	1.8–3.4
20. Pulmonary valve	51	1.5 ± 0.3	1.0–2.2
21. Supravalvular	48	1.8 ± 0.3	0.9–2.9
22. Right pulmonary artery	39	1.2 ± 0.2	0.7–1.7
23. Left pulmonary artery	11	1.1 ± 0.2	0.6–1.4

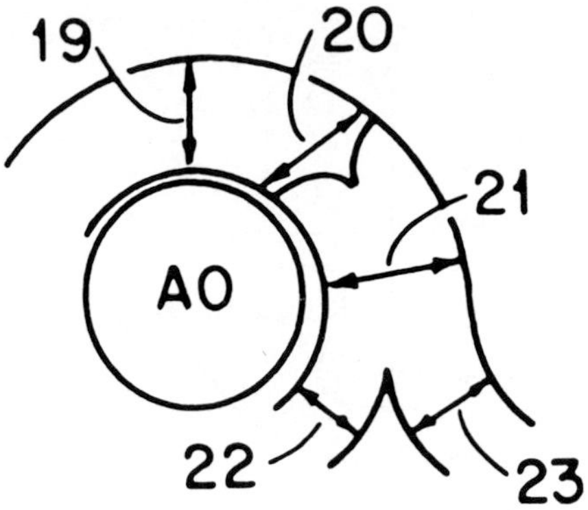

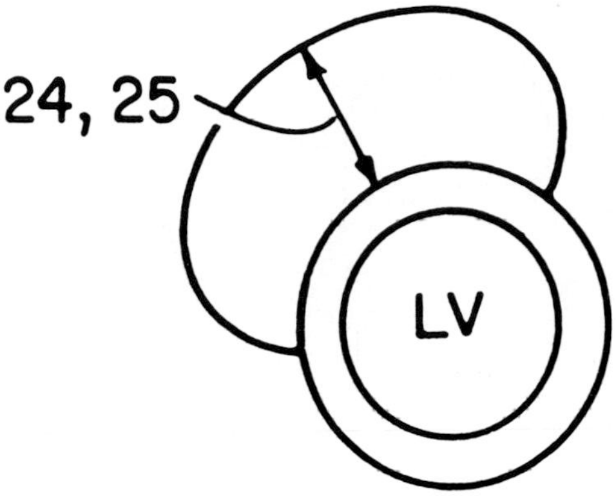

Parasternal Short Axis View at the Ventricular Level	N	Mean ± SD*	Range
Right Ventricle (tricuspid valve level):			
Septal-free wall maximal dimension			
24. Diastole	36	3.0 ± 0.4	2.5–3.8
25. Systole	36	2.6 ± 0.3	2.0–3.4
Left Ventricle (mitral valve level):			
Antero-posterior diameter			
26. Diastole	57	5.1 ± 0.5	3.4–5.8
27. Systole	57	3.6 ± 0.3	2.8–4.3
Medio-lateral diameter			
28. Diastole	57	5.0 ± 0.5	3.6–5.8
29. Systole	57	3.8 ± 0.5	2.6–4.8
Area			
30. Diastole	57	24.7 ± 5.1 cm^2	16.3–38.4 cm^2
31. Systole	57	12.3 ± 2.8 cm^2	6–20.2 cm^2
32. Fractional change	57	50.5 ± 6.8%	33.8–69.9%

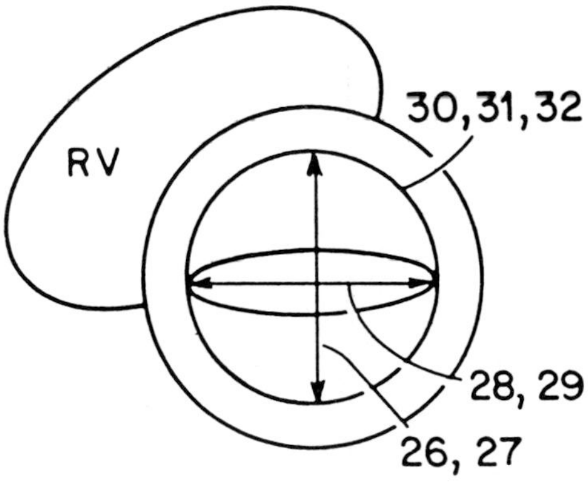

* All linear dimensions are in cm, and areas are in cm^2.
† Indicates the preferable view for obtaining a particular measurement.

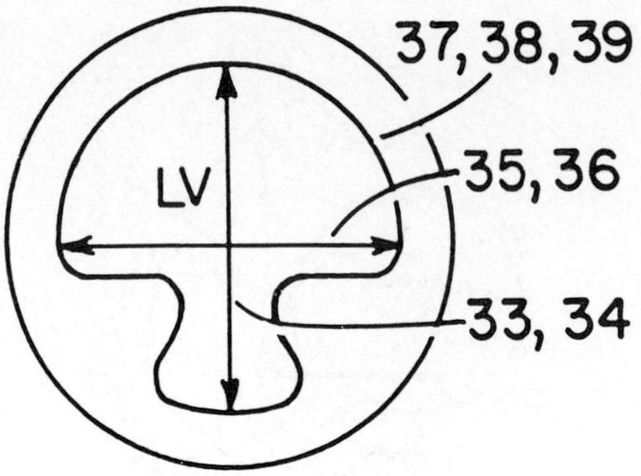

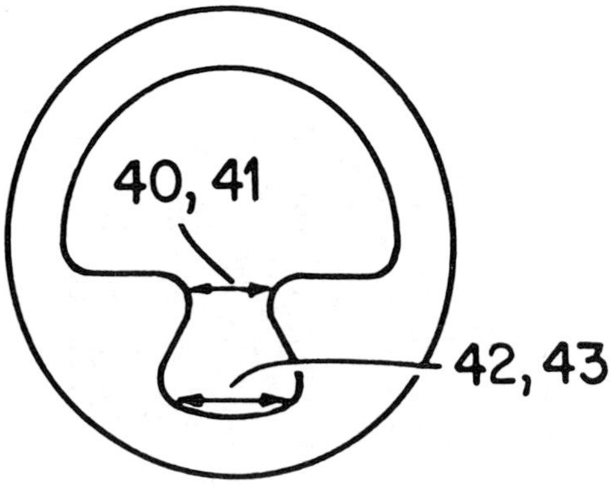

Parasternal Short Axis View at the Ventricular Level	N	Mean ± SD*	Range
Left Ventricle (papillary muscle level):			
Antero-posterior diameter			
33. Diastole	54	5.0 ± 0.5	3.5–5.7
34. Systole	54	3.5 ± 0.4	2.5–4.3
Medio-lateral diameter			
35. Diastole	54	4.9 ± 0.5	3.7–5.6
36. Systole	54	3.5 ± 0.6	2.5–4.8
Area			
37. Diastole	54	23.1 ± 4.1 cm^2	15.2–33.8 cm^2
38. Systole	54	9.8 ± 2.6 cm^2	5.2–16.8 cm^2
39. Fractional change	54	57.0 ± 8.3%	37.0–75.8%
Interpapillary muscle measurements:			
Tip			
40. Diastole	39	1.8 ± 0.4	1.1–3.0
41. Systole	39	1.1 ± 0.3	0.5–1.6
Base			
42. Diastole	39	2.8 ± 0.5	1.8–3.7
43. Systole	39	2.0 ± 0.5	1.3–3.3

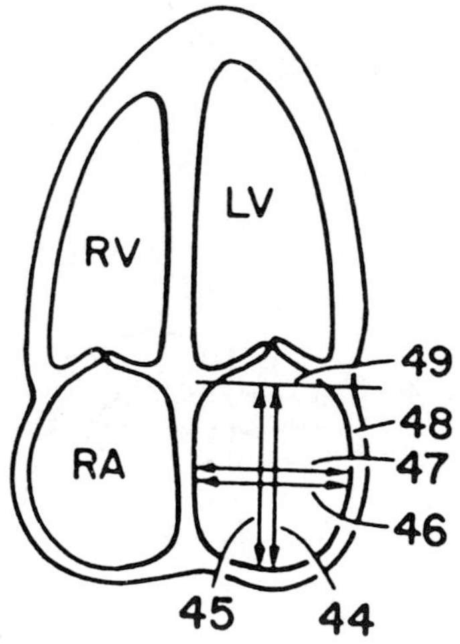

Apical Four Chamber View	N	Mean ± SD*	Range
Left Atrium (end-systole):			
Supero-inferior dimension†			
44. Maximal	68	4.1 ± 0.6	2.9–5.3
45. Mid-cavity	68	4.0 ± 0.6	2.9–5.3
Medio-lateral dimension			
46. Maximal	68	3.8 ± 0.4	2.9–4.9
47. Mid-cavity	68	3.7 ± 0.4	2.5–4.5
48. Area	68	14.2 ± 3.0 cm^2	8.8–23.4 cm^2
49. Mitral annulus	68	2.3 ± 0.5%	1.8–3.1%

* All linear dimensions are in cm, and areas are in cm^2.
† Indicates the preferable view for obtaining a particular measurement.

Apical Four Chamber View	N	Mean ± SD*	Range
Right Atrium (end-systole):			
Supero-inferior dimension			
50. Maximal	67	4.2 ± 0.4	3.4–4.9
51. Mid-cavity	67	4.2 ± 0.4	3.4–4.9
Medio-lateral dimension			
52. Maximal	67	3.7 ± 0.4	3.0–4.6
53. Mid-cavity	67	3.7 ± 0.4	2.9–4.6
54. Area	67	13.5 ± 2 cm^2	8.3–19.5 cm^2
55. Tricuspid annulus	53	2.2 ± 0.3	1.3–2.8
Left Ventricle			
Length (diastole)			
56. Maximal	67	7.8 ± 0.7	6.3–9.5
57. Mid-cavity	67	7.8 ± 0.7	6.2–9.5
Length (systole)			
58. Maximal	67	6.1 ± 0.8	4.6–8.5
59. Mid-cavity	67	6.1 ± 0.8	4.6–8.4
Medio-lateral dimension			
Diastole			
60. Maximal	67	4.7 ± 0.4	3.7–5.8
61. Mid-cavity	67	4.2 ± 0.5	3.3–5.2
Systole			
62. Maximal	67	3.7 ± 0.4	2.8–4.7
63. Mid-cavity	67	3.1 ± 0.4	2.4–4.2
Papillary muscle to mitral annulus			
64. Diastole	9	3.0 ± 0.4	2.2–3.6
65. Systole	9	2.2 ± 0.3	1.6–2.6
Area			
66. Diastole	62	33.2 ± 7.7 cm^2	17.7–47.3 cm^2
67. Systole	62	17.6 ± 5.2 cm^2	7.9–31.5 cm^2
68. Fractional change	63	47.2 ± 8.8%	31–67.9%
Right Ventricle:			
Length (diastole)			
69. Maximal	61	7.1 ± 0.8	5.5–9.1
70. Mid-cavity	61	7.1 ± 0.9	5.5–9.1
Length (systole)			
71. Maximal	61	5.5 ± 0.8	4.2–8.1
72. Mid-cavity	61	5.5 ± 0.8	4.2–8.1
Medio-lateral dimensions			
Diastole			
73. Maximal	61	3.5 ± 0.4	2.6–4.3
74. Mid-cavity	61	3.0 ± 0.5	2.1–4.2
Systole			
75. Maximal	61	2.9 ± 0.4	2.2–3.6
76. Mid-cavity	61	2.4 ± 0.3	1.9–3.1
Area			
77. Systole	41	20.1 ± 4.0 cm^2	10.7–35.5 cm^2
78. Diastole	41	10.9 ± 2.9 cm^2	4.5–20 cm^2
79. Fractional change	41	45.9 ± 7.3%	30–59.5%

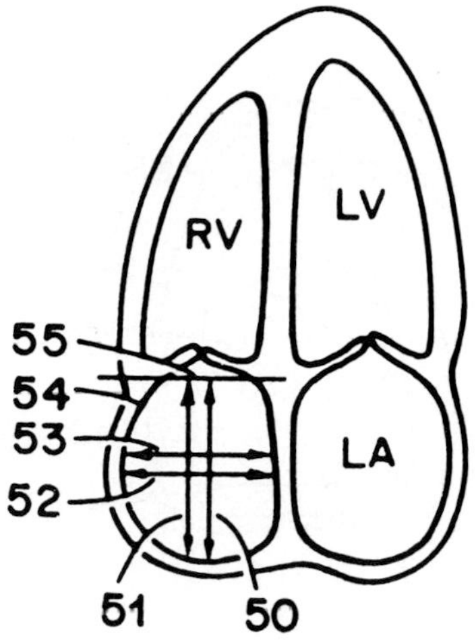

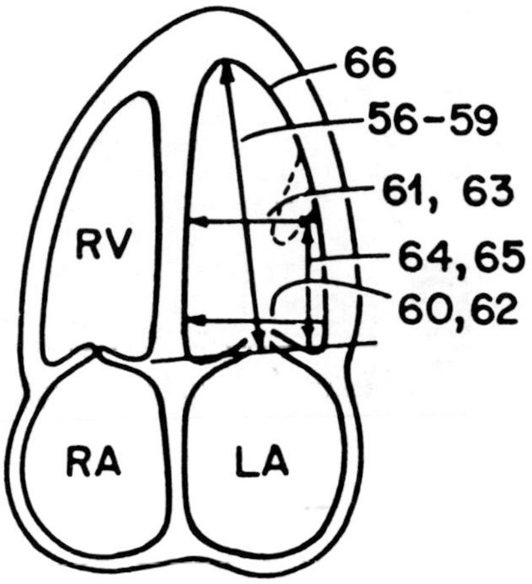

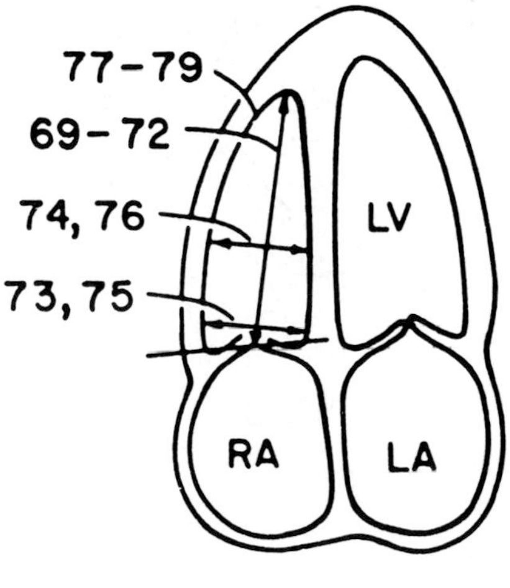

* All linear dimensions are in cm, and areas are in cm^2.

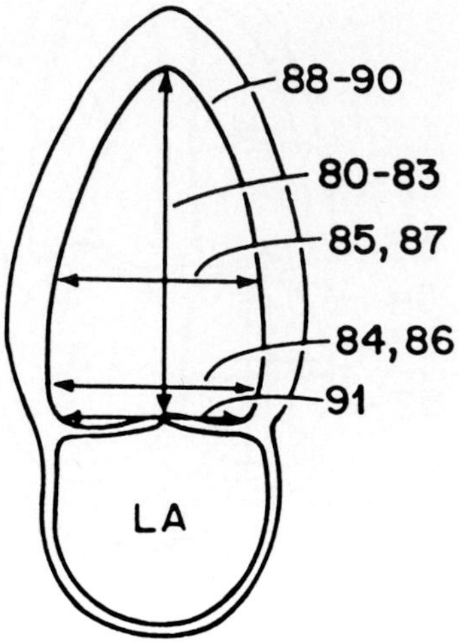

Apical Two Chamber View	N	Mean ± SD*	Range
Left Ventricle:			
Length (diastole)			
80. Maximal	54	8.0 ± 0.7	6.8–9.5
81. Mid-cavity	54	8.0 ± 0.7	6.8–9.5
Length (systole)			
82. Maximal	54	6.3 ± 0.9	4.4–7.8
83. Mid-cavity	54	6.2 ± 0.9	4.4–7.8
Transverse dimension			
Diastole			
84. Maximal	52	4.7 ± 0.6	3.8–5.8
85. Mid-cavity	52	4.2 ± 0.6	2.6–5.5
Systole			
86. Maximal	52	3.6 ± 0.6	2.6–4.8
87. Mid-cavity	52	3.2 ± 0.6	2.1–4.5
Area			
88. Diastole	42	34.2 ± 7.4 cm^2	19.3–48.8 cm^2
89. Systole	42	17.3 ± 5.2 cm^2	8.9–28.1 cm^2
90. Fractional change	42	49.8 ± 8.2%	33.7–69.0%
91. Mitral annulus	46	2.3 ± 0.3	1.8–2.8

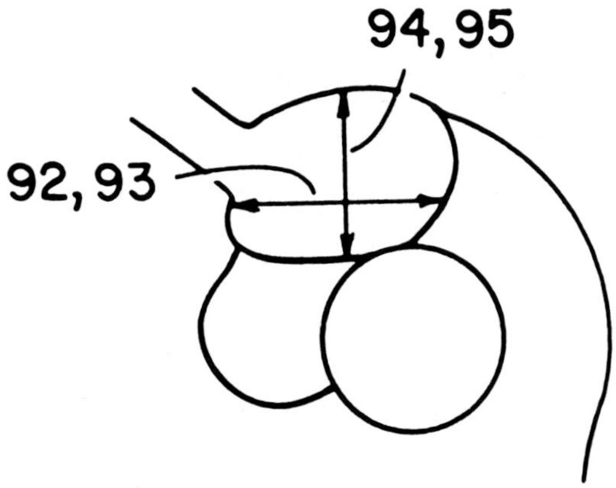

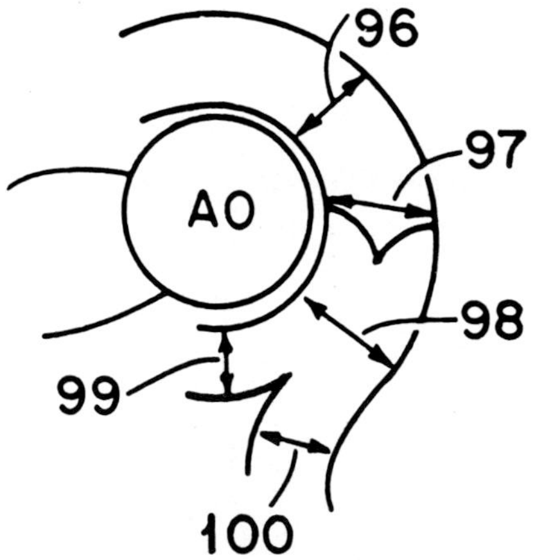

Subcostal View	N	Mean ± SD*	Range
Right Atrium (end-systole):			
Antero-posterior diameter			
92. Maximal	22	4.5 ± 0.5	3.7–5.7
93. Mid-cavity	22	4.5 ± 0.5	3.7–5.7
Medio-lateral diameter			
94. Maximal	31	4.0 ± 0.5	3.3–5.7
95. Mid-cavity	31	4.0 ± 0.4	3.3–4.9
Pulmonary Artery (end-diastole)§			
96. Right ventricular outflow tract (subvalvular)	18	2.0 ± 0.4	1.4–2.9
97. Pulmonary valve	19	1.4 ± 0.2	1.1–1.7
98. Supravalvular	19	1.6 ± 0.3	1.2–2.3
99. Right pulmonary artery	7	1.2 ± 0.2	0.9–1.3
100. Left pulmonary artery	5	1.1 ± 0.4	0.8–1.6

* All linear dimensions are in cm, and areas are in cm^2.

§ These values are consistently smaller than those obtained from the parasternal transducer location. The reason is that in the adult the pulmonary artery lies in the far field of the scan plane when viewed from the subcostal window and there is significant point-spreading of targets along the vessel walls caused by poor lateral resolution at this level. Therefore these measurements are more appropriately made from images recorded from the parasternal location, and the subcostal values are included only as a reference for patients in whom the parasternal window is unavailable.

Subcostal View	N	Mean ± SD*	Range
Inferior Vena Cava			
101. Proximal	52	1.6 ± 0.2	1.2–2.3
102. Distal	49	1.6 ± 0.3	1.1–2.5
103. Hepatic vein	12	0.8 ± 0.2	0.5–1.1

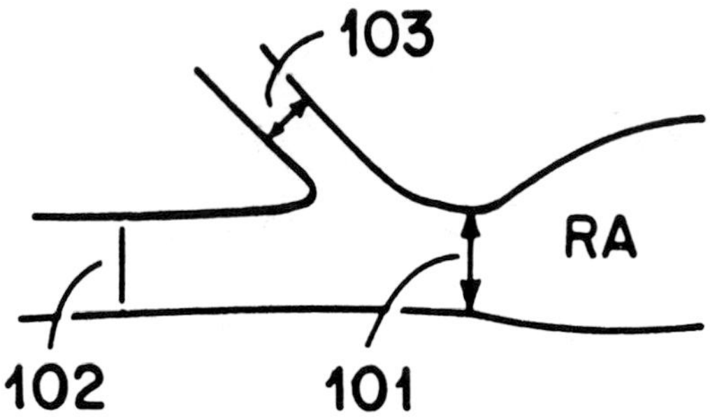

Suprasternal Notch View	N	Mean ± SD*	Range
End-diastole			
104. Aortic arch	42	2.7 ± 0.3	2.0–3.6
105. Right pulmonary artery	37	1.8 ± 0.3	1.4–2.7

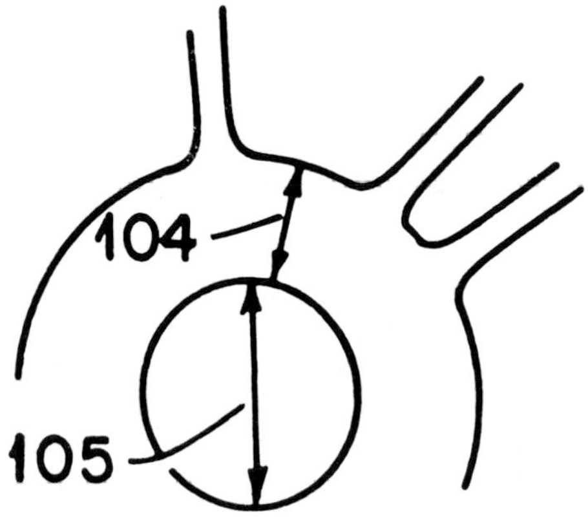

Data from Triulzi M et al.: Normal adult cross-sectional echocardiographic values: Linear dimensions and chamber areas. Echocardiography 1:403, 1984.
* All linear dimensions are in cm, and areas are in cm^2.

NORMALIZATION OF LINEAR CARDIAC DIMENSIONS

Although body surface area has been widely used as an index of body size for assessing the normality of cardiac dimensions, its use has been challenged on both theoretic[1] and mathematical grounds[2]. In addition, the body surface area index has certain clinical limitations. Specifically, it is difficult to estimate without reference to specialized tables, it is subject to variability in an individual due to changes in body weight, and it fails to present insight into the major determinant (height vs. weight) of cardiac dimensions during development. Finally, because the relationships between body surface area and cardiac dimensions are non-linear[3–5], the common clinical practice of dividing dimensions by body surface is mathematically incorrect and may lead to erroneous results in some clinical circumstances.

In view of these potential limitations, the relationship between cardiac dimensions and other indices of body size and growth including age, height, weight, and body surface area were reassessed in 72 adults (as described previously) and 196 children. This latter group included 99 males and 97 females selected from a healthy population of children without clinical, electrocardiographic or echocardiographic evidence of structural heart disease. The ages in this group ranged between 6 days and 18 years (mean 4.5 years), weight from 2.3 to 86 kg (mean 19 kg), and height ranged from 37 to 188 cm (mean 98 cm).

THE RELATIONSHIP BETWEEN AGE AND CARDIAC DIMENSION

Figures A–1A–A–1D demonstrate the relationships between age and the dimensions of the aortic annulus, the left atrium and the left ventricle in individuals <19 years of age. Although absolute values for each dimension differ, the rate of growth of each of these structures, expressed by the slope of each of these curves, is not significantly different. Further, regression analyses demonstrate that the rate of growth is independent of sex.

These data demonstrate that by birth the linear dimensions of the aorta, left atrium and left ventricle have reached almost 50% of their adult value, and by 12 to 18 months they have reached almost 65% of their adult size. The rate of growth slows subsequently, so that by 5 years these structures have attained 75%, and by puberty (12 to 15 years of age) they have reached almost 90% of their expected adult size. After this, the rate of cardiac growth slows even further, and significant increases in cardiac dimensions are not expected after 15 years of age.

While age offers a simple means of assessing cardiac

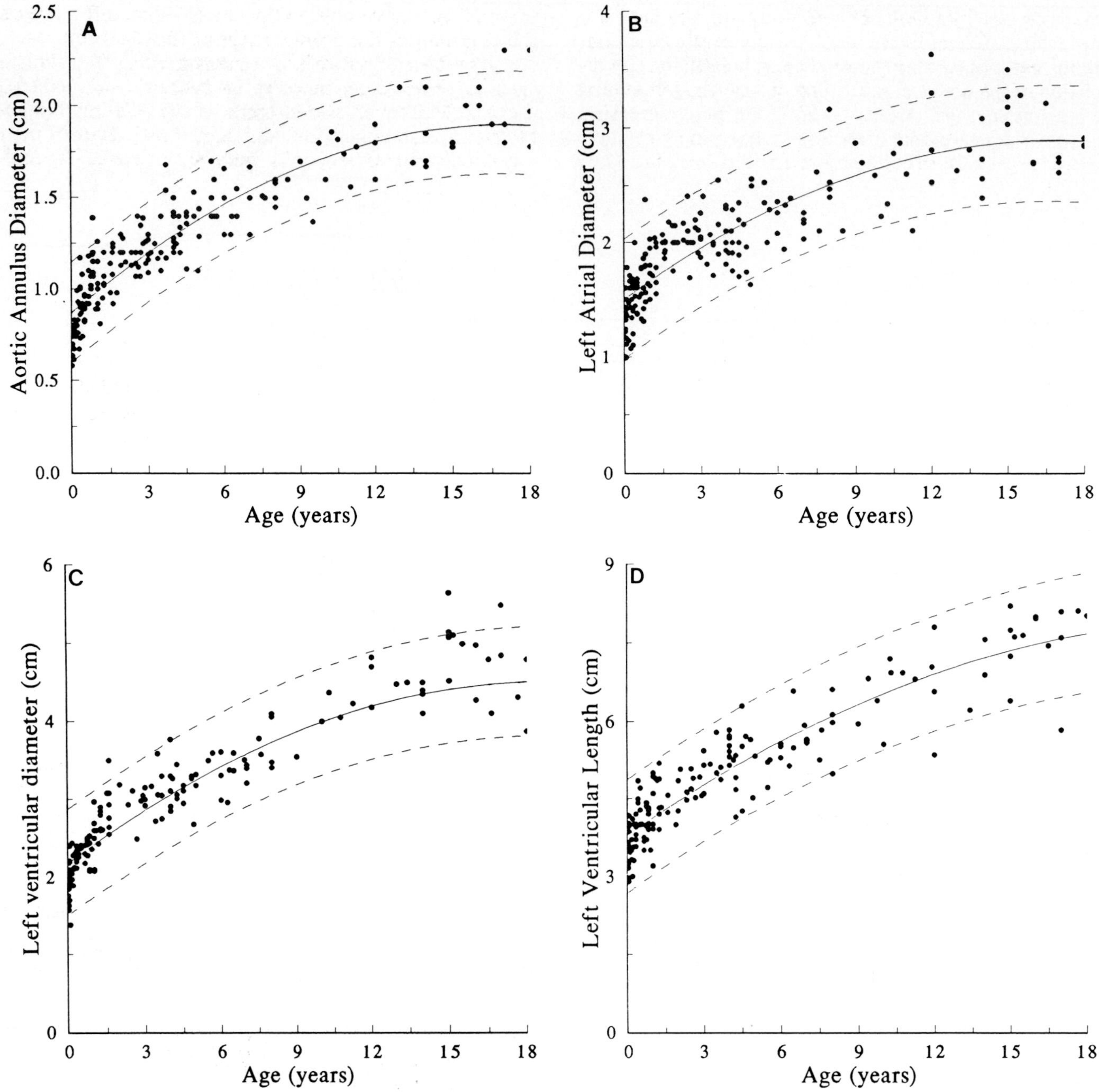

Fig. A–1. Relation between age and (A) aortic annulus diameter, (B) left atrial diameter, (C) left ventricular diameter, and (D) left ventricular length in 196 children—99 boys and 97 girls—less than 19 years of age, assessed as part of an echocardiographic study of well children. The mean and 95% confidence limits of the data are represented by the solid and dotted lines, respectively. (From Nidorf SM et al.: New perspectives in the assessment of cardiac chamber dimensions during development and adulthood. J Am Coll Cardiol *19*:983, 1992. Reproduced with permission of the American College of Cardiology.)

dimensions in a young healthy population, the relationship may be of less value in the assessment of cardiac dimensions in a population of chronically ill children in whom there might be disturbance of the normal age related growth curve. In these circumstances, indexing cardiac dimensions to an index of body size may be more appropriate.

THE RELATIONSHIP BETWEEN CARDIAC DIMENSIONS AND INDEXES OF BODY SIZE

Although a strong relationship could be demonstrated between linear cardiac dimensions and height (0.96), weight (0.90), and body surface area (0.93), it should be appreciated that the relationships between each cardiac dimension and both weight and body surface area are non-linear and best expressed by a quadratic equation. In contrast, the relationship between height and the dimension of the aortic annulus, left atrium and left ventricle are linear (Figs. A–2A–A–2D). Further, regression analysis confirmed that after adjusting for height, other univariate predictors of linear dimensions (weight, BSA, sex and age) have no significant additional influence on the estimate of the normal range of these structures.

These data therefore indicate that during development cardiac dimensions increase in concert with skeletal growth. Moreover, the strength of the relationship between cardiac dimensions and height may explain their non-linear relationship with body surface area. Specifi-

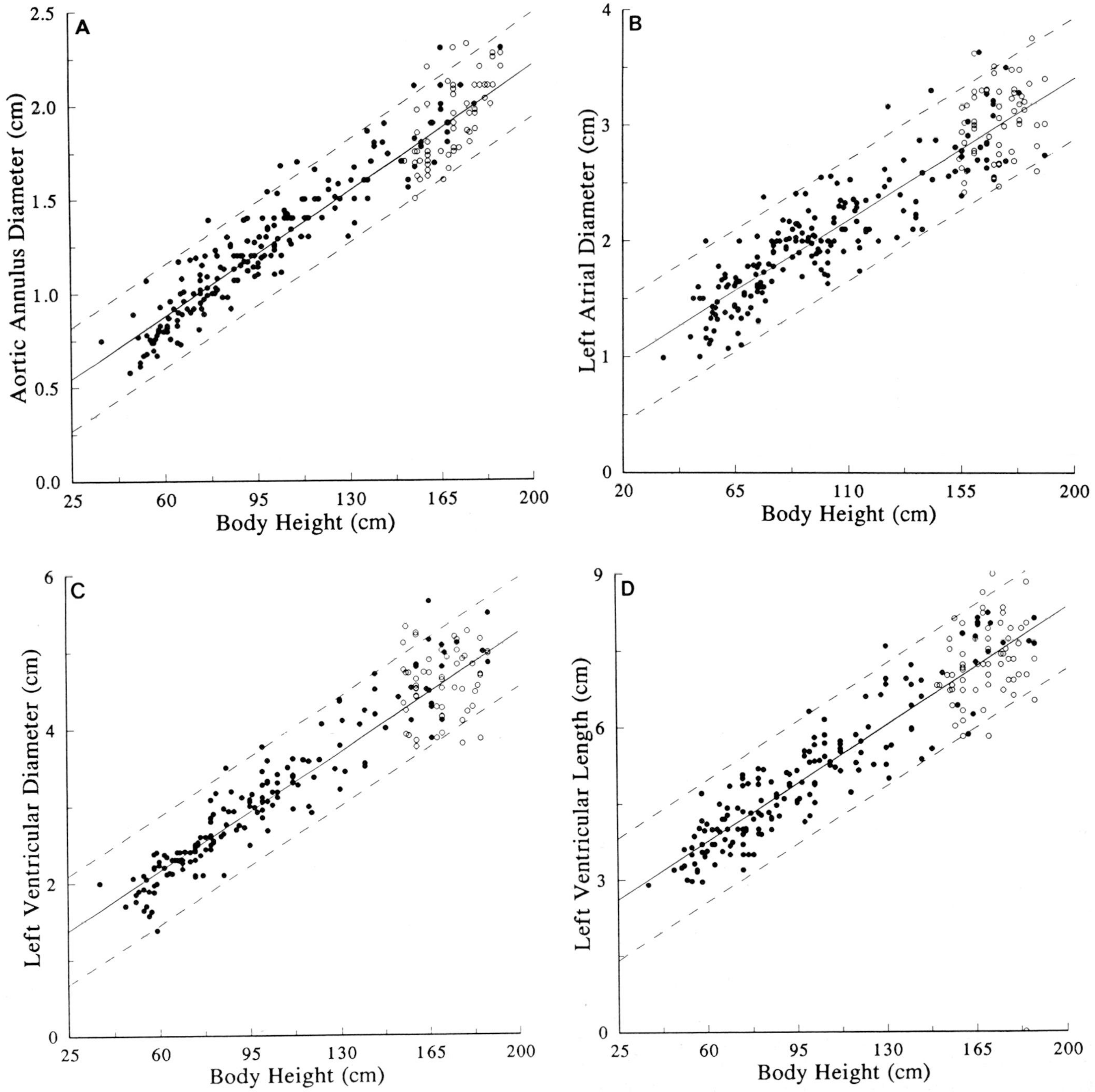

Fig. A–2. Relation between height and (A) aortic annulus diameter, (B) left atrial diameter, (C) left ventricular diameter, and (D) left ventricular length. • = Group I (196 children—99 boys and 97 girls—less than 19 years of age, assessed as part of an echocardiographic study of well children), ○ = Group II (38 male and 34 female adult volunteers with no cardiovascular or systemic disease, ranging in age from 18 to 76 years). (From Nidorf SM et al.: New perspectives in the assessment of cardiac chamber dimensions during development and adulthood. J Am Coll Cardiol *19*:983, 1992. Reproduced with permission of the American College of Cardiology.)

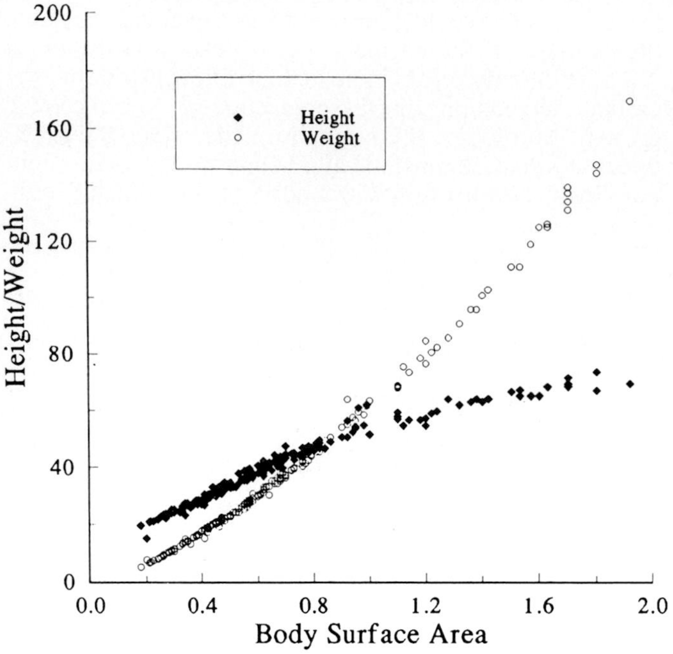

Fig. A–3. Relation between body surface area and height and weight in normals. As body surface area increases beyond 1, the major determinant of body surface area is weight rather than height. (From Nidorf SM et al.: New perspectives in the assessment of cardiac chamber dimensions during development and adulthood. J Am Coll Cardiol *19*:983, 1992. Reproduced with permission of the American College of Cardiology.)

cally, since height is no longer a major determinant of body surface area beyond values of 1.2[6] (Fig. A–3), it would be predicted that increases in body surface area due to increases in weight would not be associated with further increases in cardiac dimension. Hence, short obese individuals should have smaller cardiac dimensions than tall asthenic individuals even though their body surface areas may be the same.

For clinical purposes, then, body height appears to be an ideal means of indexing cardiac dimensions, as it is a simple, reliably obtained, non-derived variable that relates linearly to cardiac dimensions and is not subject to change during illness.

REFERENCES

1. Tanner JM. Fallacy of per weight and per surface area standards, and their relation to spurious correlation. J Applied Physiol. *2*:1, 1949.
2. Gutgesell HP, Remold CM. Growth of the human heart relative to body surface area. Am J Cardiol *65*:662, 1990.
3. Pearlman JD, Triulzi MO, King ME, Newell J, Weyman AE. Limits of normal left ventricular dimensions in growth and development: analysis of dimensions and variance in the two dimensional echocardiogram of 268 normal healthy subjects. J Am Coll Cardiol *12*:1432, 1988.
4. Epstein ML, Goldberg SJ, Allen HD, Konecke L, Wood J. Great vessel, cardiac chamber and wall growth pattern in normal children. Circulation *51*: 1124, 1975.
5. Henry WL, Ware J, Gardin JM, Hepner SI, McKay J, Weiner M. Echocardiographic measurements in normal subjects: growth related changes that occur between infancy and early adulthood. Circulation *57*:278, 1978.
6. Nidorf SM, Picard MH, Triulzi MO, et al. New perspectives in the assessment of cardiac chamber dimensions during development and adulthood. J Am Coll Cardiol *19*:983, 1992.

APPENDIX

B

APPLICATION OF FOURIER ANALYSIS IN ECHOCARDIOGRAPHY

JAMES D. THOMAS

In this appendix, I present a more technical description of Fourier analysis to supplement the earlier material. Although a full understanding of Fourier analysis requires a working knowledge of complex variable calculus, even a qualitative knowledge of this technique provides powerful insight into its applications. Furthermore, there are several important limitations to the way in which Fourier analysis is used in echocardiography, and one should be aware of these limitations to make intelligent use of the technique. Therefore, this discussion emphasizes a graphic, intuitive approach to the subject. For the mathematic details, interested readers are referred to several excellent texts.[1–3] It is hoped that even those less mathematically inclined will gain insight from this section into the fundamental principles and theoretic trade-offs inherent in the Fourier transform.

After introducing the notation for the discussion, I present the Fourier transform of a continuous, infinitely long signal, showing several Fourier transform pairs to give a sense of what the transform does. Then I introduce the concept of convolution (a more complicated type of multiplication). This notion is extremely important and turns up frequently as we explore signal smoothing, sampling theory, and the effects of imperfect measuring tools. Again, the full mathematic description is involved, but a graphic, intuitive understanding is accessible and provides insight into the physical origins of aliasing, signal broadening, and velocity resolution. With these two concepts introduced, I examine specific applications in cardiac imaging.

Fourier analysis is a technique by which to extract the frequency components from a function or signal. It is an extremely powerful mathematic tool and is used in many fields of science, from music synthesis to quantum mechanics to thermodynamics (the technique was originally devised by Joseph Fourier in the early nineteenth century to describe the distribution of temperature across a metal plate). In the past 10 years, Fourier analysis has achieved a prominent place in noninvasive cardiology. Perhaps its most familiar use is in Doppler echocardiography where the Fourier transform is used to convert the Doppler shifted ultrasound waveform into blood velocity. Beyond this, however, Fourier analysis is integral to image formation in magnetic resonance imaging (MRI) and computed tomography (CT) and is gaining utility in wall motion analysis in nuclear cardiology and echocardiography.[4]

NOTATIONAL CONVENTIONS

Throughout the discussion, functions of time and/or space (such as the Doppler-shifted signal) have lower case names and variables, $y(t)$, $f(x)$, $s(\theta)$, etc., whereas the corresponding functions of frequency are capitalized, $Y(T)$, $F(X)$, $S(\Theta)$, etc. Pairs of functions or variables that are related by the Fourier transform are indicated by $\Leftrightarrow$, as in $y(t) \Leftrightarrow Y(T)$. Note that the variables $t \Leftrightarrow T$ are reciprocal to each other. If t is time in seconds, then T is temporal frequency in sec^{-1} or Hertz. The functions of time and space are said to exist in the "time domain" or in "real space," whereas the frequency functions are said to exist in the "frequency domain" or in "Fourier space."

One must realize that $y(t)$ and $Y(T)$ are simply different representations of the *same thing,* much as a set of data can be displayed on a linear or logarithmic growth but are still the same data. A fluid relationship exists between y(t) and Y(T). Sometimes, it is more convenient to consider the real physical values of a signal, and for this one should use y(t). At other times, it is more informative to consider the component frequencies of the signal; here one should use Y(T).

FOURIER TRANSFORM PROPERTIES

Definition

Consider a signal that is a function of time, f(t), defined for all time from $-\infty$ to $+\infty$. The Fourier transform theorem states that it is possible to duplicate this signal by adding together sine and cosine waves of different frequencies. These sine and cosine waves are weighted by an amplitude coefficient that is a function of frequency (given as T in cycles per second or Hertz). This amplitude function exists for all frequencies from $-\infty$ to $+\infty$ and is by definition the Fourier transform of f(t), written F(T)*. I later consider the mathematics for converting f(t) to F(T) and vice versa, but first let us look graphically at a few transform pairs, to gain some insight into the meaning of the Fourier transform.

Linearity

The pair of graphs in Figure B–1A shows f(t), a signal composed of a single cosine wave of amplitude 1 and frequency 10 Hz, and F(T), its Fourier transform, which is zero everywhere except at ± 10 Hz, showing that these are the only frequencies that make up f(t). The presence of negative frequencies may be confusing. Note that, as drawn, f(t) is a function of time, but there is no way of telling whether it is running from left to right (positive frequency) or from right to left (negative frequency). Thus, F(T) consists of ± 10-Hz components in equal amounts.

In Figure B–1B, the frequency of the cosine wave is reduced to 6 Hz (g[t]), and the corresponding nonzero Fourier components (G[T]) are displaced inward to ± 6 Hz. This demonstrates the general observation that events close together in the time domain are far apart in the frequency domain.

Figure B–1C shows the sum of f(t) + g(t) and its corresponding Fourier transform with frequency components at ± 6 and ± 10. This demonstrates the important point that the Fourier transform is a *linear* process. We can either add two signals together and take the transform of the result or take the transform of the two signals separately and add these together. The result is the same.

Note that if we continue reducing the frequency below that in g(t), the two Fourier components get closer and closer together. Eventually, when the frequency is zero, the temporal function is a straight line displaced off the x axis, whereas the Fourier transform pairs have coalesced into a single positive value at T = 0 Hz.

Fourier Transform of a Square Wave

As stated previously, the Fourier transform enables one to extract the frequency spectrum from any signal, not just obvious sinusoidal combinations such as in Figure B–1. Consider the square wave in Figure B–2A, which is nonzero only between $\pm t_0$. The corresponding transformation is a damped sine wave (the sinc function, (sin x)/x) with most of the spectrum contained between $T = \pm 1/(2t_0)$ Hz. In the Figure B–2B, the square wave has had its duration cut in half but its amplitude doubled, so the area under the wave remains the same. Its transform has been spread out by a factor of 2, indicative of the higher frequencies necessary to generate the shorter duration pulse, but the maximum value remains the same as previously, at T = 0. In the extreme case (Fig. B–2C), the square wave has become a high narrow spike, though still with the same area, and the transformation now is a straight line with the same value as the previous maximal values. This indicates that to produce an infinitely brief pulse requires infinitely high frequency sinusoids all added together with just the right phase to produce the pulse at the proper place in time.

Delta Function

In Figures B–1 and B–2, we encountered tall, narrow spikes in either real-space or the Fourier domain. It will greatly simplify the following discussion if we give these spikes some formal mathematic characteristics. Such functions are termed delta functions and, in the temporal domain, are designated by $\delta(t)$; $\delta(t)$ is zero for all t except at t = 0; $\delta(0) = \infty$, so we see that the delta function is an infinitely high, infinitesimally narrow spike. We now consider what the area of the delta function is. This may seem counterintuitive; its height is ∞ and its width is 0, so how can $0 \cdot \infty$ be defined? In fact, it is defined analogously to Figure B–2. We start with a rectangle with finite height and width and an area = 1. As the width narrows, the spike becomes proportionally higher, so the area remains 1, *even in the limit of width = 0 and height = ∞*. To summarize, $\delta(t) = \infty$ at t = 0 and 0 everywhere else; and

$$\int_{-\infty}^{+\infty} \delta(t)\, dt = 1.$$

Similarly, $\delta(t - t_0)$ consists of a spike at $t = t_0$ (i.e., where $t - t_0 = 0$). We may now state mathematically the results from Figure B–1. For f(t), which is an infinitely long cosine wave of amplitude A and frequency f_0, its Fourier transform is a pair of delta functions, $Y(T) = \frac{1}{2}A\delta(T \pm f_0)$. Reduce f_0 as in g(t) (Fig. B–1) and the delta waves come closer together. Decrease f_0 to 0 and the two delta waves coalesce into one (with twice the area) as T = 0. In Figure B–2, when the square wave

* One source of confusion with the Fourier transform is that Y(T) is almost always a *complex* function; that is, it has one component made up of real numbers (the type of numbers we are most familiar with) and another component of *imaginary* numbers (an unfortunate term because they are neither more nor less "made up" than real numbers). Imaginary numbers are multiples of the imaginary constant, $i, \sqrt{-1}$. For our graphic presentations I show the *magnitude* of Y(T), the root summed square of the real and imaginary parts. Not shown is the *phase* of Y(T), essentially the ratio of the real and imaginary parts.

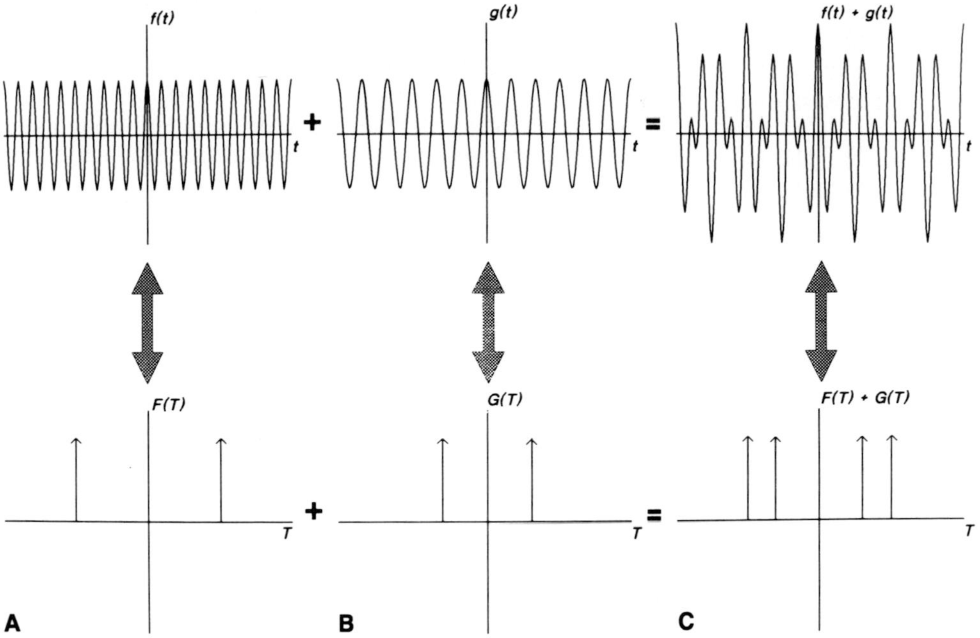

Fig. B–1. Fourier transformation is a linear process. **A.** f(t) Is a cosine wave with a frequency of 10 Hz, while its transform F(T) is nonzero only at 10 Hz. **B.** Similarly, g(t) is a lower frequency wave with G(T) positive at 6 Hz. **C.** The Fourier transform of the sum f(t) + g(t) is simply the sum of the two component transforms F(T) + G(T). (From Thomas JD: Principles of Imaging, in Fozzard HA, Haber E, Jennings RB, Katz AM, Morgan HE: The Heart and Cardiovascular System: Scientific Foundations. New York, Raven Press, 1991, p. 642.)

was squeezed into $2At_0\delta(t)$, the Fourier transform was a constant, $Y(T) = 2At_0$. Here are some transform pairs we have encountered so far, plus one new one:

Real		Fourier	
$A \cos 2\pi f_0 t$	$\Leftrightarrow$	$\frac{1}{2}A\delta(T \pm f_0)$	
$A\ \delta(t)$	$\Leftrightarrow$	A	
A	$\Leftrightarrow$	$A\ \delta(t)$	
$A\ \delta(t - nt_0)$	$\Leftrightarrow$	$(A/t_0)\ \delta(T - n/t_0)$	for $n = -\infty$ to ∞.

The last pair shows the transform for a *series* of delta functions, an infinite number of spikes spaced t_0 seconds apart. The transform is simply another infinite series of delta functions, now spaced $1/t_0$-Hz apart in the frequency domain. As before, notice the inverse relationship between real space and Fourier space. As shown in Figure B–3, as t_0 becomes smaller, and the temporal delta waves come closer together; at the same time, $1/t_0$ becomes larger, so the frequency delta waves get farther apart. This simple relationship between repeating delta waves proves extremely helpful in analyzing the effect of sampling interval on frequency resolution. Before we can discuss this, we must introduce the notion of *convolution*.

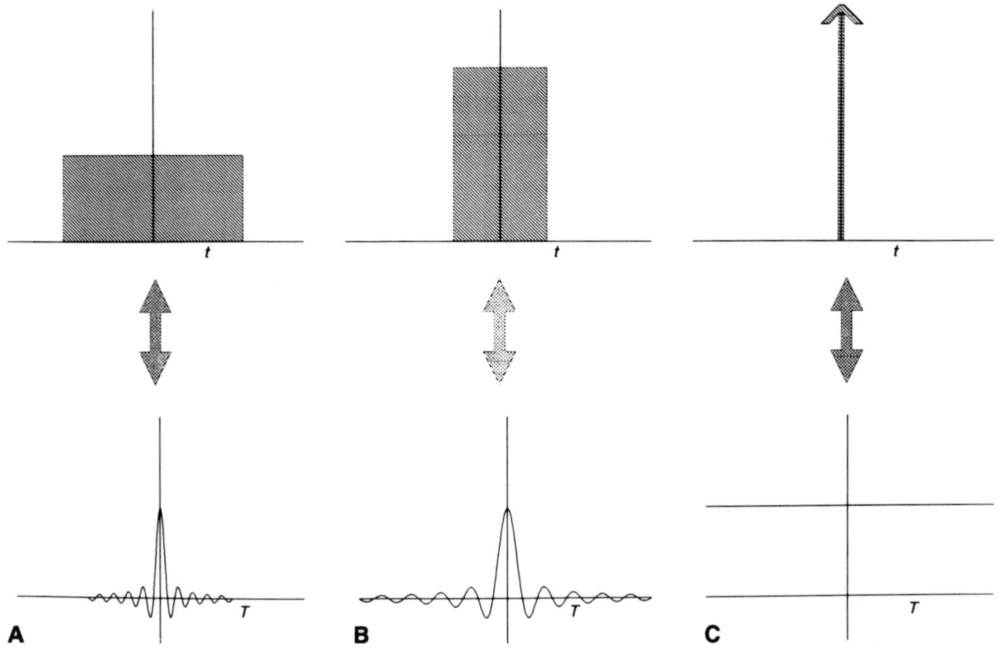

Fig. B–2. Fourier transforms of square waves. The transform of a square wave with positive values between $\pm t_0$ is a damped sine wave centered on 0 Hz with most of its significant components between $T = \pm 1/2t_0$ (though with nonzero values out to ∞, demonstrating that infinitely high frequency components are needed to produce sharp features such as the verticle lines at $\pm t_0$). **B.** The square wave is narrower and taller, and the transform has correspondingly broadened. **C.** In the extreme, the square wave shrinks to an infinitely tall, infinitesimally narrow impulse (a *delta wave,* $\delta(t)$). The corresponding Fourier transform is simply a constant, indicating that all frequencies are included with equal magnitude to produce a delta wave. (From Thomas JD: Principles of Imaging, in Fozzard HA, Haber E, Jennings RB, Katz AM, Morgan HE: The Heart and Cardiovascular System: Scientific Foundations. New York, Raven Press, 1991, p. 643.)

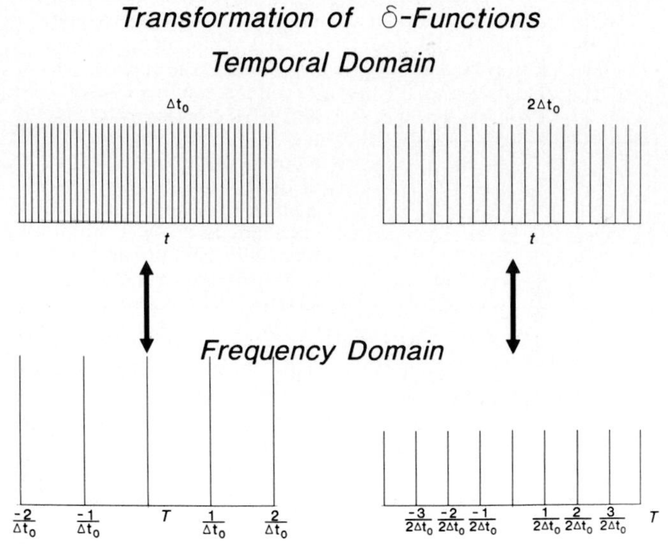

Fig. B–3. The delta function and its Fourier transform. In the temporal domain, there are a series of evenly spaced, infinitely high, infinitesimally narrow spikes (delta waves), which might correspond to a periodic sampling function. In Fourier space, these correspond to a series of delta waves whose spacing is inversely proportional to their spacing in real space ($\Delta T = 1/\Delta t$). (From Thomas JD: Principles of Imaging, in Fozzard HA, Haber E, Jennings RB, Katz AM, Morgan HE: The Heart and Cardiovascular System: Scientific Foundations. New York, Raven Press, 1991, p. 644.)

CONVOLUTION

Although its mathematic details are abstruse, convolution of two signals is extremely common in measuring physical values. Convolution is analogous to the simpler notion of multplying two signals, and I discuss this issue first.

Multiplication can occur in either the real domain or the Fourier domain and is done simply by multiplying the two curves point by point at each corresponding time (or frequency) value. For example, multiplying an infinite cosine wave in Figure B–4A by the square wave in Figure B–4B will produce a cosine wave of frequency f_0 between $\pm t_0$ and zero elsewhere (Fig. B–4C). Convolution, denoted by * rather than the × of multiplication is a more extensive procedure, much like smearing signal 2 by signal 1. Whereas in multiplication, each point in signal 1 is affected by just one point in signal 2, in convolution, each point in signal 1 is affected by every point in signal 2. A common example of convolution is in the smoothing of a noisy signal. Figure B–5A shows signal 1, a plot of ventricular diameter vs. time that has a significant amount of noise, and signal 2, a Gaussian curve (bell-shaped curve):

$$e^{-t^2/\tau^2}$$

When these curves are convolved, signal 2 is flipped about the y axis (which makes no difference in this case because it is symmetric) and then is superimposed on signal 1, shifted along the t axis point by point so it is centered in turn over each point in signal 1. At each of these points, the curves are multiplied by each other and this product is integrated so the output signal is similar to signal 1, but with each point replaced by a moving average weighted by the Gaussian smoothing operator as shown in Figure B–5C. The mathematic definition of the convolution for two signals, g(t) and h(t) is

$$g(t)*h(t) = \int_{-\infty}^{+\infty} g(\tau)h(t - \tau)\, d\tau$$

where τ is a dummy integration variable and emphasizes that each point t in the convolution output results from an integration of the two curves along their entire extent. The order of the curves, g(t) and h(t), does not matter: $g * h = h * g$. A particularly simple and important convolution results when either g(t) or h(t) is a delta function,

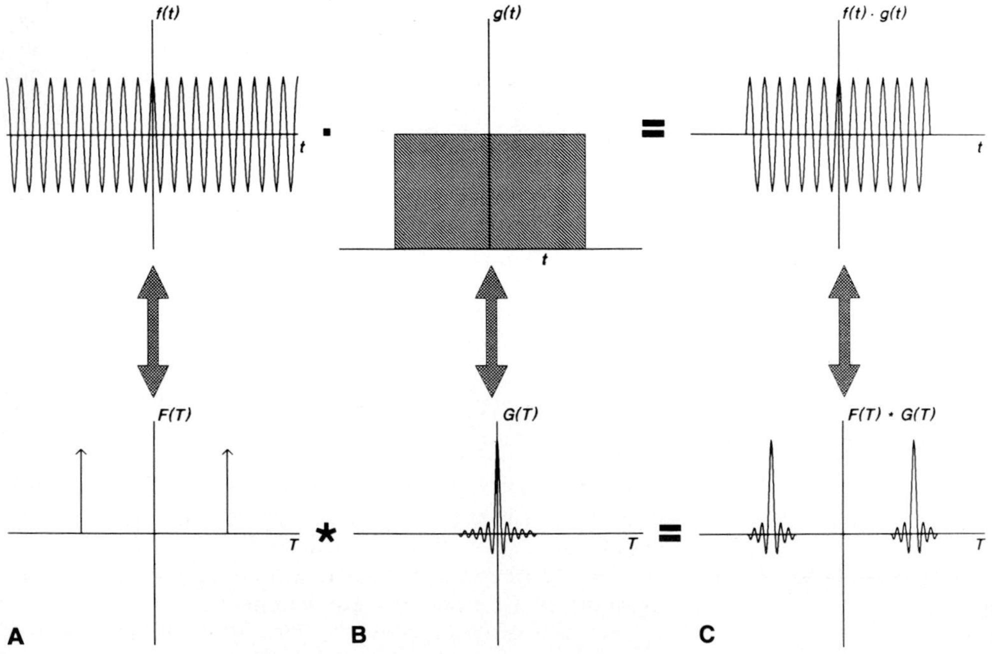

Fig. B–4. Multiplication in real space is equivalent to convolution in Fourier space. f(t) **A.** Is multiplied by a square wave **B.** to yield a truncated cosine wave **C.** The corresponding operations in Fourier space show the delta waves at f_0 being *convolved* with the damped sine wave, which has the effect of replicating the damped sine wave twice, centered on f_0. (From Thomas JD: Principles of Imaging, in Fozzard HA, Haber E, Jennings RB, Katz AM, Morgan HE: The Heart and Cardiovascular System: Scientific Foundations. New York, Raven Press, 1991, p. 645.)

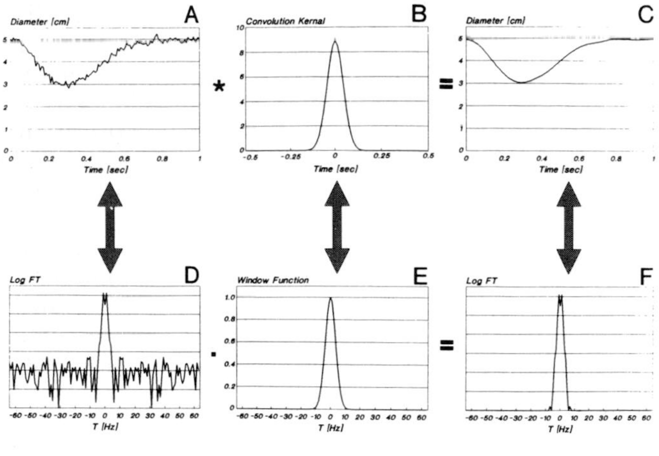

Fig. B–5. Convolution in real space is equivalent to multiplication in Fourier space. **A** to **C.** The noisy signal of ventricular volume is convolved with the Gaussian function in **B** to yield the smoothed curve in **C. D** to **F.** In Fourier space, the Fourier transform of the signal has most of its useful information in the low frequency components. These may be selected by multiplying the Fourier transform by the windowing function in **E** (the transform of a Gaussian function, itself a Gaussian function with width inversely proportional to the width of the real-space function). The result is the Fourier transform in **F** with the high frequency components set to zero. Because multiplication is numerically much simpler than convolution, it is often more efficient to perform the operations A → D, D·E = F, and F → C than the convolution A∗B = C. (From Thomas JD: Principles of Imaging, in Fozzard HA, Haber E, Jennings RB, Katz AM, Morgan HE: The Heart and Cardiovascular System: Scientific Foundations. New York, Raven Press, 1991, p. 646.)

the infinitely narrow, infinitely high function mentioned before. For instance, $\delta(t - t_0)$ is zero everywhere, except for an infinitely high spike at $t = t_0$. The area of this spike,

$$\int_{-\infty}^{+\infty} \delta(t - t_0)\, dt$$

is, by definition, 1. If we multiply $\delta(t - t_0)$ by any function $h(t)$ and integrate this product, we are left with simply $h(t_0)$, the only nonzero point from the delta function. Now we can evaluate the convolution of the delta function with any other function $h(t)$. If $g(t) = \delta(t - t_0)$, then

$$g(t) * h(t) = \int_{-\infty}^{+\infty} \delta(\tau - t_0)h(t - \tau)\, d\tau$$

which is nonzero only for $\tau = t_0$ and leaves us with $h(t - t_0)$. Thus, convolving any function with $\delta(t - t_0)$ simply replicates that function but shifts it by t_0 along the t axis (or T axis because these operations are equally well defined in Fourier space as real space). If, for example, $G(T)$ were two delta functions at T_0 and $-T_0$, $G(T)*H(T)$ would produce two copies of $H(T)$, one centered on $-T_0$ and the other centered on T_0.

Convolution Theorem

We are now in a position to state the convolution theorem, an extremely powerful theorem that ties together convolution, multiplication, and the Fourier transform:

> If $g(t)$ and $h(t)$ are functions of time and $G(T)$ and $H(T)$ their respective Fourier transforms (functions of frequency), then the Fourier transform of the product $g(t)\cdot h(t)$ is the convolution $G(T)*H(T)$. Conversely, the Fourier transform of the convolution $g(t)*h(t)$ is the product $G(T)\cdot H(T)$. This relationship also works with the inverse Fourier transform. If we start with $G(T)$ and $H(T)$, then the inverse transform of $G(T)\cdot H(T)$ is just $g(t)*h(t)$ and the inverse transform of $G(T)*H(T)$ is $g(t)\cdot h(t)$. Thus, multiplication in the time domain is the equivalent of convolution in the frequency domain and vice versa.

We can see how this works in Figures B–4 and B–5. In Figure B–4, multiplication is performed in the temporal domain, with $f(t)$ multiplied point by point with the square wave $g(t)$ to yield the truncated cosine wave. In the Fourier domain, the transform of the cosine wave is two delta waves at $\pm f_0$, whereas the transform of the square wave is the damped sine function, centered on $T = 0$. The Fourier transform of $f(t)\cdot g(t)$ is given by the *convolution* of the two component transforms, $F(T)*G(T)$. As discussed previously, the convolution of one function with a delta wave simply replicates that function centered on the delta wave. In the case of $F(T)$, there are two delta waves, and so the convolution simply replicates $G(T)$ twice, centered on $\pm f_0$. In essence, this means that the Fourier transform of a brief cosine wave no longer contains only frequency components at $\pm f_0$, but rather a spectrum of frequencies centered around $\pm f_0$. The longer the duration of the cosine wave, the narrower this spectrum becomes, until it converges on the two delta waves for an infinitely long cosine wave.

Data Smoothing

Figure B–5 illustrates another important kind of convolution: data smoothing in the temporal domain. We have already seen how Figure B–5A, a noisy signal of ventricular diameter, can be smoothed by convolving it with the Gaussian (bell-shaped) curve in Figure B–5B to yield the smoother curve in Figure B–5C. Figure B–5D to F show the equivalent operations in the Fourier domain. The Fourier transform of the original signal (Fig. B–5D) has a central peak in the low frequency components that represents most of the physiologic information. Beyond about ±6 Hz, the Fourier spectrum is flat, characteristic of random noise. Thus, the noise is represented predominantly in the high frequencies. Because convolution in the real domain is equivalent to multiplication in the Fourier domain, we multiply the Fourier signal in Figure B–5D by the Fourier transform of the Gaussian function in Figure B–5E (another Gaussian function with width inversely proportional to that in Fig. B–5B) to yield the transform in Figure B–5F, in which all the high frequency components are now zero. Performing the inverse Fourier transform on Figure B–5F yields the smoothed signal in Figure B–5C. Because convolution is a computationally intensive operation, it is frequently easier to perform a Fourier transform on the data, multiply the spectrum by a *windowing function* (such as the Gaussian function) to suppress the high frequencies, then perform the inverse transform to yield the smoothed data set. Mathematically, the two procedures are precisely equivalent.

This procedure, termed *Fourier filtration,* is not lim-

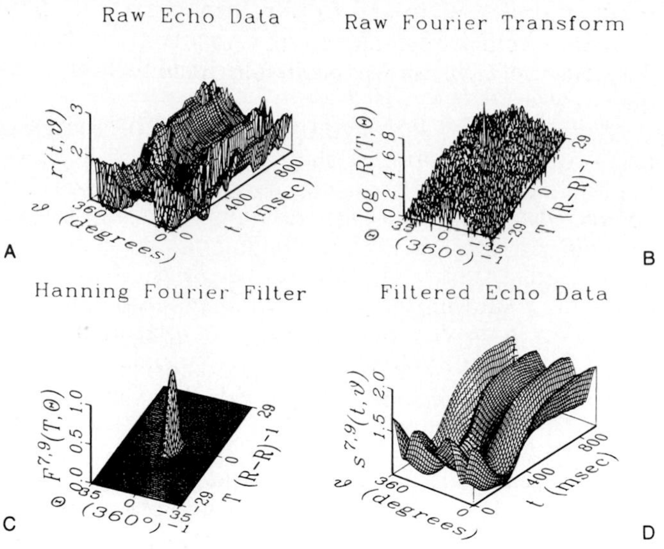

Fig. B–6. Spatiotemporal Fourier filtration. The noisy data in **A** (traced endocardial borders) are Fourier transformed in **B,** which are multiplied by the filter function in **C,** and then inverse transformed to yield the smoothed data set in **D.** (See text for discussion.) (From Thomas JD, Hagege AA, Choong CY, Wilkins GT, Newell JB, Weyman AE: Improved Accuracy of Echocardiographic Endocardial Borders by Spatiotemporal Filtered Fourier Reconstruction: Description of the Method with Optimization of the Cutoffs. Circulation, 1988; 77:415–428.)

ited to one-dimensional data sets such as Figure B–5A. For example, Figure B–6A displays the traced endocardial borders from a short axis echocardiogram throughout a complete cardiac cycle.[5] Thus, these data have both temporal (the t axis) and spatial dimensions (the θ axis, representing the angular distance around the border). The radial distance of the endocardium from the ventricular centroid is $r(t,\theta)$. Although one can discern gross systolic contraction (between 0 and 300 msec) and the location of the papillary muscles (at about 45 and 300°), much is lost in the random noise of the traced contours. The two-dimensional Fourier transform of these data (Fig. B–6B) shows physiologic information at low frequencies (center of the graph) with a noise spectrum in the high frequencies. These noisy frequencies are eliminated by multiplying Figure B–6B by the filter function in Figure B–6C. Performing the inverse Fourier transform on these filtered data yields the smoothed profile in Figure B–6D in which cardiac structure and function are much more evident.

Data Sampling and Windowing

An important consideration is the effect of discrete sampling in the real domain on the calculated Fourier transform. Recall that sampling a function $f(t)$ at intervals of t_0 simply multiplies $f(t)$ by $\delta(t - nt_0)$ (n is an integer ranging from $-\infty$ to $+\infty$), replacing $f(t)$ with its values at t_0 intervals, $f(nt_0)$. The Fourier transform of this sampled function is the "true" transform $F(T)$ convolved with the transform of the sampling function, itself another series of delta functions, $\delta(T - n/t_0)$. This convolution simply replicates $F(T)$ throughout Fourier space at intervals of $1/t_0$. In particular, copies of $F(T)$ are replicated at $T = 0$ (the "correct" location) and at $T = \ldots, -2/t_0, -1/t_0, 1/t_0, 2/t_0, \ldots$. Note that any components of $F(T)$ above $T = 1/(2t_0)$ will begin to be corrupted by components of $F(T)$ with $T < -1/(2t_0)$ which have been shifted to $T = 1/t_0$. This is the source of aliasing in signal processing: for signals sampled at an interval Δt, only frequencies between $\pm 1/(2\Delta t)$ can be fully resolved.

We are now in a position to describe fully (at least qualitatively) the sampling and resolution trade-offs in pulsed Doppler processing. There are two effects to consider: (1) the Doppler signal can only be sampled at an interval t_0 fixed by the range r of the sample of interest and the velocity of sound c: $t_0 = 2r/c$; and (2) because we wish to reproduce blood velocity dynamically throughout the cardiac cycle, we divide the Doppler signal into separate regimes, typically with a period p_0 of about 10 msec in duration, which are analyzed individually. The effect of this windowing is to multiply the Doppler signal by a square wave of duration p_0; equivalently, this 10-msec window of data is analyzed *as if it were periodic,* repeated every 10 msec. In other words, the data are convolved with a repeated delta function with interval p_0: $\delta(t - np_0)$. Thus, the effect of sampling and windowing the Doppler data is to multiply $f(t)$ by $\delta(t - nt_0)$ and convolve this with $\delta(t - np_0)$. Figure B–7 shows these two effects in the temporal domain along with the equivalent changes in Fourier space. The continuous Doppler signal (Fig. B–7A) has the frequency (velocity) spectrum in Figure B–7C. *Sampling* the data (Fig. B–7B) means that only data represented by the closed circles (at interval t_0) are available for analysis,

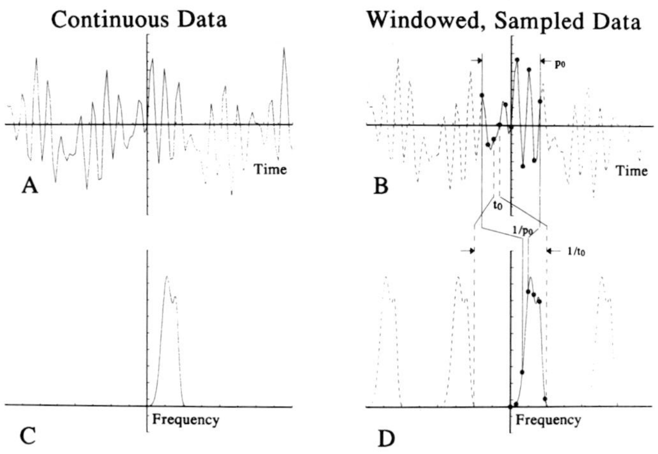

Fig. B–7. Effect of sampling and windowing of the Doppler waveform on its frequency representation. Left. The "true" Doppler signal in time **(A)** and frequency (Fourier) domains **(C)** are shown. The continuous temporal data are sampled at intervals of t_0 for a period of p_0 (a total of p_0/t_0 readings); in effect, the data are multiplied by $\delta(t - nt_0)$ and convolved with $\delta(t - np_0)$. In the frequency (velocity) domain, these effects are reversed and inverted: the data sampling leads to repetition of the velocity waveform at frequencies $1/t_0$ (i.e., convolving it with $\delta(T - n/t_0)$), while convolving the window leads to multiplication of the velocity profile by the repeating delta function, $\delta(T - n/p_0)$. Thus, unambiguous frequency data are available only for p_0/t_0 frequencies between $\pm\frac{1}{2}t_0$ at intervals of $1/p_0$. (From Thomas JD: Principles of Imaging, in Fozzard HA, Haber E, Jennings RB, Katz AM, Morgan HE: The Heart and Cardiovascular System: Scientific Foundations. New York, Raven Press, 1991, p. 648.)

whereas *windowing* means that only the data between $\pm 1/2p_0$ are analyzed at a given time, and these data are treated as if they were repeated over and over (i.e., convolved with $\delta(t - np_0)$). In the frequency domain (Fig. B–7D), the isolated effect of the windowing is that the frequency spectrum is sampled only for $T = n/p_0$, where n is integer ranging from $-\infty$ to $+\infty$ (i.e., the continuous spectrum is multiplied by $\delta(T - n/p_0)$; the isolated effect of the data sampling is to convolve the continuous frequency spectrum with $\delta(T - n/t_0)$, leading to periodic replication of the spectrum (dashed outlines). The net effect of these two operations is to take p_0/t_0 samples in

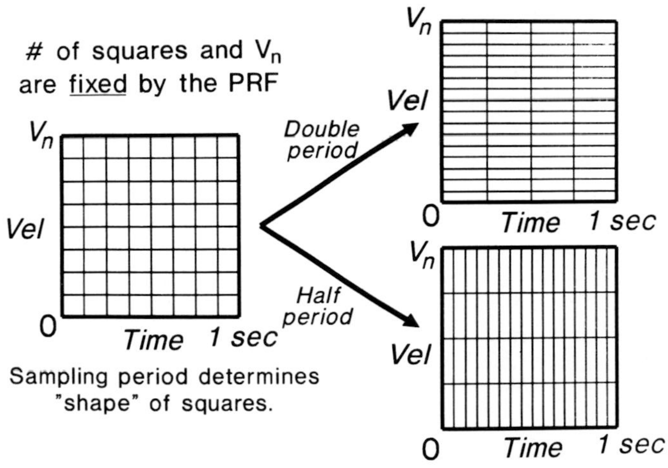

Fig. B–8. Trade-off between velocity and temporal resolution in pulsed Doppler. **A.** The pulse repetition frequency (PRF) fixes not only the maximal unambiguous velocity (v_n) but also the number of bins available for display in each second, where the (number of temporal windows per second) $\times$ (number of velocity bins displayed) equals the PRF. **B.** Increasing the velocity resolution is possible but only at the expense of decreasing the update rate of the Doppler output. **C.** Temporal resolution can be improved but only at the expense of coarser velocity resolution.

the temporal domain and to transform them into p_0/t_0 frequency velocity estimates with a minimum resolvable frequency of $1/p_0$ and a maximum unambiguous frequency of $\pm 1/(2t_0)$.

Another way of looking at the trade-off of temporal and velocity resolution is shown in Figure B–8. Here the pulse repetition frequency fixes both the *maximal velocity detectable* and the *total number of data points available in 1 second*. These data points can be divided up into any number of temporal windows. If the windows are made shorter (as in Fig. B–8C), the temporal resolution improves, but (because the total number of "boxes" is fixed) velocity resolution becomes coarser. Conversely, the velocity elimination can be made as fine as wanted (Fig. B–8B), but only by sacrificing temporal resolution.

We now see the trade-offs in Doppler velocity estimation (and analogous ones exist in CT and MRI processing). To increase the maximal unambiguous velocity, one must decrease t_0; however, t_0 is fixed by the depth of the sample volume, unless one is willing to accept range ambiguity in localizing the sample. To resolve the velocity into finer bins (i.e., to a lower minimum velocity), one can sample the Doppler waveform for a longer window p_0, but this leads to proportionally poorer temporal resolution in tracking dynamic cardiac events.

REFERENCES

1. Bracewell RN: The Fourier Transform and Its Applications. New York, McGraw-Hill, 1978.
2. Brigham EO: The Fast Fourier Transform. Englewood Cliffs, NJ, Prentice-Hall, 1974.
3. Arfken G: Mathematical Methods for Physicists. New York, Academic Press, 1985.
4. Thomas JD: Principles of imaging. *In* Fozzard HA, et al. (eds.): The Heart and Cardiovascular System. New York, Raven Press, p. 625, 1992.
5. Thomas JD, et al.: Improved accuracy of echocardiographic endocardial borders by spatiotemporal filtered Fourier reconstruction: description of the method and optimization of the cutoffs. Circulation 77:415, 1988.

Index

Page numbers in *italics* indicate illustrations; numbers followed by "t" indicate tables.